Stedman's

MEDICAL TERMS AND PHRASES:

A Complete Guide to Medical Language

Stedman's

MEDICAL TERMS AND PHRASES:

A Complete Guide to Medical Language

LIPPINCOTT
WILLIAMS
& WILKINS

Publisher: Julie K. Stegman
Series Managing Editor: Trista A. DiPaula
Associate Managing Editor: Steve Lichtenstein
Production Coordinator: Jason Delaney
Typesetter: Peirce Graphic Services, LLC.
Printer & Binder: Quebecor World Inc.

351 West Camden Street
Baltimore, Maryland 21201-2436

Printed in the United States of America

2005

Library of Congress Cataloging-in-Publication Data
Stedman's medical terms and phrases: a complete guide to medical language.
p. ; cm.
Includes bibliographical references.
ISBN 0–7817-4543–8
1. Medicine—Terminology. I. Title: Medical terms and phrases. II. Lippincott Williams & Wilkins.
[DNLM: 1. Medicine—Phrases—English. 2.
Medicine—Terminology—English. WB 15 S8127 2004]
R123.S715 2004
610′.1′4—dc22

2003024517
01
1 2 3 4 5 6 7 8 9 10

Contents

Acknowledgments

An important part of our editorial process is the involvement of medical transcriptionists—as advisors, reviewers, and/or editors. We extend special thanks to the following people who served as editors for this book:

Jeanne Bock, CSR, MT

Jeanne Bock has over 11 years' experience as a medical transcriptionist. She works for Medical Dictation Services, Inc. as a recruiter, supervisor of the QA department, and medical transcriptionist. She also actively serves as a researcher and editor for Stedman's.

R. Jo-Ann Clarke

Jo-Ann Clarke has over 25 years' experience as a medical transcriptionist, supervisor, editor, and educator in the medical transcription field. She currently owns a medical transcription business in Canada and is a researcher for Stedman's.

Carrie Donathan, CMT, FAAMT

Carrie Donathan is currently a CMT and Fellow of the American Association for Medical Transcription, and is employed as an Account Manager and Mentor for Healthscribe, Inc. She has been transcribing since 1964 in multiple settings, has owned her own transcription business, and managed several branch offices for national services over the past 15 years.

Nicole G. Peck, CMT

Nicole Peck has more than 10 years of experience in medical transcription, training on the job while attending the University of Utah and then later taking the transcription course at a local business college. She has worked in a variety of specialties over the years, from podiatry to a pain clinic. She has been a CMT for 2 years, as well as president of her local AAMT chapter.

Kathy Rockel, CMT, FAAMT

Kathy Rockel has been a medical transcriptionist for over 25 years, working in a variety of settings. She is currently the Transcription Manager for

Transcription Relief Services, LLC, in Greensboro, North Carolina and is a Fellow of the American Association for Medical Transcription.

Harriet R. Stewart, CMT, FAAMT

Harriet R. Stewart is a medical transcriptionist with over 25 years of experience. She has been a medical transcription instructor for over 10 years, currently with M-TEC. She resides in Sterling, Virginia and is a Fellow of the American Association for Medical Transcription.

Pat Vargo, RHIT

Pat Vargo is a graduate of Sinclair Community College with an AAS degree in Health Information Management. Pat has 13 years of experience in health care which includes coding at Good Samaritan Hospital, Baltimore MD; Health Information Management at Harford Memorial Hospital, Havre de Grace MD; and Quality Assurance for MedQuist. She is currently an Allied Health Instructor at Harford Community College in Bel Air, MD.

Special thanks goes to Holly Lukens for her editing assistance with the manuscript, as well as Jeanne Bock, Helen Littrell, and Terri Unkelhaeuser for their final prepublication review. We also thank Kathryn J. Cadle for her assistance with the content files. And, as always, Barb Ferretti played an integral role in the process by reviewing the content files for format, updating the content, and providing a final quality check.

As with all our *Stedman's* word references, this resource incorporates the suggestions and expertise of our many contacts in the medical transcriptionist community. Thanks to all of our advisory board participants, reviewers, and editors; AAMT meeting attendees; and others who have written us with requests and comments—keep talking, and we'll keep listening.

Publisher's Preface

Stedman's Medical Terms and Phrases offers an authoritative assurance of quality and exactness to the wordsmiths of the healthcare professions—medical transcriptionists, medical editors and copyeditors, health information management personnel, court reporters, and the many other users and producers of medical documentation.

Previously lacking in the Stedman's Word Book Series, this reference represents the most comprehensive listing of medical terms and phrases. This reference is particularly helpful for students and those new to the medical transcription profession, and we would be remiss in not thanking the Stedman's Editorial Advisory Board Members of 2002 and 2003 for their inspiration, and direction in helping *Stedman's* produce such a helpful compilation of medical terms and phrases.

Not only does this reference feature over 240,000 medical terms and phrases, we have also introduced new keyword referencing so that a medical term and phrase can not only be found by its first and last word, but all other significant words of the term and phrase. Now, no matter what portion of the term or phrase you hear, you can find it! In addition, we have included the following helpful appendices: Common Medical Abbreviations and Acronyms, as well as Medical Prefixes, Suffixes, and Combining Forms: The Building Blocks of Medical Language.

We at Lippincott Williams & Wilkins strive to provide you with the most up-to-date and accurate word references available. Your use of this reference will prompt new editions, which we will publish as often as updates and revisions justify. We welcome your suggestions for improvements, changes, corrections, and additions—whatever will make this *Stedman's* product more useful to you. Please complete the postage-paid card in this book for future suggestions and recommendations, or visit us online at *www.stedmans.com*.

Explanatory Notes

Medical transcription is an art as well as a science. Both approaches are needed to correctly interpret the dictation of a physician, whose language is a product of education, training, and experience. This variety in medical language means that there are several acceptable ways to express certain terms, including jargon. *Stedman's Medical Terms and Phrases* provides variant spellings and phrasings for many terms. These elements, in addition to complete cross-indexing, make *Stedman's Medical Terms and Phrases,* a valuable resource for determining the validity of terms as they are encountered.

Alphabetical Organization

Alphabetization of main entries is letter by letter as spelled, ignoring punctuation, spaces, prefixed numbers, or other characters. For example:

VSG 2/3F graphic card
V-slit lamp
VSR

Terms beginning or ending with Greek letters show the Greek letters spelled out and listed alphabetically. For example:

alpha, α
a. angle
a. crystallin

In subentry alphabetization, the abbreviated singular form or the spelled-out plural form of the noun main entry word is ignored.

Format and Style

All main entries are in **boldface** to expedite locating a sought-after term, to enhance distinction between main entries and subentries, and to relieve the textual density of the pages.

Irregular plurals and variant spellings are shown on the same line as the singular or preferred form of the word. For example:

ampulla, pl. ampullae
disc, disk

Hyphenation

As a rule of style, multiple eponyms (e.g., Smith-Fisher knife) are hyphenated. Also, hyphens have been added between a manufacturer and one or more eponyms (e.g., Storz-Duredge steel cataract knife). Please note that in many cases, hyphenation is a question of style, not of accuracy, and thus is a matter of choice.

Possessives

Possessive forms have been dropped in this reference for the sake of consistency and conformance with the guidelines of the American Association for Medical Transcription (AAMT) and other groups. Please note, however, that in many cases, retaining the possessive, like hyphenating, is a question of style, not of accuracy, and thus is a matter of choice. To form the possessive of a word, simply add the apostrophe or apostrophe "s" to the end of the word.

Cross-indexing

The word list is in an index-like main entry/subentry format. All phrases are cross-referenced by their first, last, as well as other key words in the phrase. This format of cross-referencing provides the user with several ways to find a multiple-word phrase. This format also allows the user to see together all terms that contain a particular descriptor, as well as all types, kinds, or variations of a noun entity.

relaxed	**pelvic**	**floor**
r. pelvic floor	relaxed pelvic floor	relaxed pelvic f.
sudden	**unexpected**	**death**
s. unexpected death	sudden unexpected death	sudden unexpected d.

References

In addition to the manufacturers' literature we gather at various medical meetings, scientific reports from hospitals, and the lists of our MT Editorial Advisory Board members (from their daily transcription work), we used the following sources for new terms in *Stedman's Medical Terms and Phrases.*

Books

The AAMT Book of Style, 2nd Edition. Modesto, CA: AAMT, 2002.

Lorenzini JA, Ley LL. Medical Phrase Index, 4th Edition. Los Angeles: PMIC, 2001.

Stedman's References.

A2
A. segment of anterior cerebral artery

A4
lipoxin A4, B4

A103
monoclonal antibody A103 fine-needle aspiration biopsy

A_{1c}
hemoglobin A.

1a
interferon-beta 1a

a-2
a. antiplasmin
a. antiplasmin coagulation inhibitor
a. antitrypsin inhibitor
a. macroglobulin
a. macroglobulin coagulation inhibitor

A1-A5 segments of anterior cerebral artery

A2 segment of anterior cerebral artery

A-a
alveolar-arterial gradient
aortic artery

AAA
abdominal aortic aneurysm
acquired aplastic anemia
acute anxiety attack

AAA
abdominal aortic aneurysm
acquired aplastic anemia
acute anxiety attack

AABR
automated auditory brainstem response

AAC
acute acalculous cholecystitis
antibiotic-associated colitis
antimicrobial agent-induced colitis
antimicrobial agents and chemotherapy
augmentative and alternative communication

AACD
abdominal aortic counterpulsation device
age-associated cognitive decline

AACG
acute angle-closure glaucoma

Aachen aphasia test

AACI
arachidonic acid cascade inhibitor

AAD
acid-ash diet
acute agitated delirium
antibiotic-associated diarrhea
atlantoaxial dislocation

Aagenaes syndrome

AAMD
atrophic age-related macular degeneration

AAO
amino acid oxidase
awake, alert, oriented

AARF
atlantoaxial rotatory fixation

AAROM
active-assisted range of motion

Aarskog-Scott syndrome

AAS
acute abdominal series

Ab
anti-HSV IgM Ab titer

abandoning
caregiver abandoning patient

abandonment
child a.
fear of a.
feeling of a.
intense abandonment fear
mode a.
perceived emotional a.
personal a.
separation or loss a.

abasia
atactic a.
ataxic a.
paralytic a.

abatement
sound a.

Abbe
A. flap
midline cross-lip Abbe flap
A. operation

Abbott operation

abbreviated
a. blood count
A. Conners Teacher Rating Scale
A. Injury Scale
A. Injury Score
A. Injury Score/Injury Severity Score
A. Parent Symptom Questionnaire
a. rapid processing

abbreviation
medical a.

ABC
absolute basophil count
airway, breathing, circulation
apnea, bradycardia, and cyanosis
applesauce, bananas, and cereal diet

ABCD
airway, breathing, circulation, differential

ABCDE
airway, breathing, circulation, disability, exposure

abdomen
acute surgical a.
anterior cutaneous nerve of a.
apertures of a.
ascitic fluid in a.
autopsy limited to a.
board-like rigidity of a.
cecum returned to a.
chest tube present in a.
circulation, respiration, abdomen, motor, and speech
a. closed in layers
a. contracted
a. distended
a. distended, tender, tympanitic
a. entered and explored
external oblique muscle of a.
a. flat
flat plate of a.
fluid aspirated from a.
fluid filled a.
fluid spilling into upper a.
free air in a.
fullness in a.
guarding of the a.
gunshot wound to a.
heart, lungs, and a.
horizontal incision across lower a.
hypogastric region of a.
internal oblique muscle of a.
left a.
left iliac of a.
left lower quadrant of a.
left upper quadrant of a.
manual exploration of a.
massively dilated a.

abdomen *(continued)*
membranous layer of subcutaneous tissue of a.
milk lines of a.
muscle of a.
oblique muscle of a.
pain in abdomen with constipation
pain in abdomen with diarrhea
pain in abdomen with vomiting
penetrating wound of the a.
percussion of a.
peristalsis of a.
plain film of a.
portable film of a.
preliminary film of a.
a. prepped and draped
right lower quadrant of a.
right upper quadrant of a.
rumbling in a.
a. scrubbed, prepped, and draped
a. showed evidence of weight loss
swelling of a.
taut and distended a.
tenderness of a.
tenderness in abdomen due to hepatitis
tenderness in abdomen from appendicitis
tenderness in abdomen from gastritis
a. tender to palpation
transverse muscle of a.
upright film of a.

abdominal
a. abscess
acute abdominal aortic occlusion
acute abdominal obstruction
acute abdominal series
acute abdominal tympany
a. adhesions
a. aneurysm
anterior abdominal cutaneous branch of intercostal nerve
anterior abdominal injury
anterior abdominal wall
anterior abdominal wall syndrome
anterior-posterior abdominal diameter
anterolateral abdominal wall
a. aorta
a. aortic aneurysm
a. aortic aneurysmectomy
a. aortic counterpulsation device
aplastic abdominal muscle syndrome
aponeurosis of abdominal oblique muscle
aponeurosis of transverse a.
a. approach
a. ascites
associated with abdominal pain
atrophied abdominal muscles
atrophy of abdominal muscle
a. auscultation
a. binder
a. bleeding
a. bloating
a. breathing
a. bruit
a. bulge
burning abdominal pain
a. cavity
a. cavity free of fluid
chronic abdominal tympany
a. circumference
classic abdominal Semm hysterectomy
a. compartment syndrome
a. compression
computed abdominal tomography
constant abdominal pain
a. content
continuous abdominal peritoneal dialysis
a. cramping
cramping abdominal pain
a. cramping pain
crampy abdominal pain
a. CT scan
a. curl exercise
a. decompression
deep abdominal complication
deep abdominal reflex
deep abdominal tenderness
a. delivery
a. diameter
diarrhea with abdominal pain and swelling
diffuse abdominal calcification
diffuse abdominal tenderness
a. discomfort
dissecting abdominal aneurysm
a. distention
a. distention and tenderness
a. distress
a. drainage
a. dressing
dull abdominal pain
ectasia of abdominal aorta
a. edema
a. effusion
a. epilepsy
a. examination
a. exploration
extended abdominal radiation therapy
external abdominal region
a. fat
a. fat deposit
fetal abdominal circumference
fetal abdominal diameter
a. flap
flap of abdominal tissue
a. fluid collection
a. foci of infection
focused abdominal sonography
focused abdominal sonography for trauma
free abdominal air
free abdominal fluid
a. fullness
a. gas
generalized abdominal pain
a. girth
a. guarding
a. heart
a. hemorrhage
a. hernia
high abdominal plain film
a. hysterectomy
ileus following abdominal surgery
a. incision
increased abdominal girth
increasing abdominal discomfort
a. infection
infrarenal abdominal aortic aneurysm
a. injury
intermittent abdominal pain
intermittent episode of acute abdominal pain
internal abdominal ring
interposed abdominal compression
interposed abdominal compressions-cardiopulmonary resuscitation
a. jugular test
a. kidney
laparoscopic-assisted abdominal hysterectomy
a. laparotomy
lateral abdominal region
a. leak-point pressure
left abdominal pain
a. left ventricular assist device
a. line
lining of abdominal cavity
localized abdominal sign
lower abdominal flap

lower abdominal pain
lower abdominal periosteal reflex
lower abdominal surgery
lower abdominal tenderness
lower abdominal transverse incision
lower transverse abdominal incision
a. lymph node
a. lymph node biopsy
major abdominal surgery
a. mass
maternal abdominal pressure
Mayo abdominal clamp
Mediterranean abdominal lymphoma
midline abdominal crease
a. muscle
a. muscle guarding
a. muscle strength
a. muscle tone
negative abdominal pressure
neonatal abdominal mass
a. nephrectomy
nonspecific abdominal pain
nonvascular abdominal surgery
a. obesity
oblique abdominal muscle
a. obstruction
a. opening
a. orifice
a. pain
a. pain associated with blood loss
a. pain with colitis
a. pain with Crohn disease
palpable abdominal mass
a. panniculus
a. paracentesis
paradoxical abdominal movement
paraumbilical anterior abdominal wall
parietal abdominal fascia
pectoral and abdominal anterior cutaneous branch of intercostal nerve
penetrating abdominal trauma
penetrating abdominal trauma index
penetrating abdominal wound
a. percussion
a. and perineal
peripancreatic abdominal drainage
a. peristalsis
a. peritoneum
plain abdominal radiograph
a. pocket
a. port
postoperative abdominal distention
a. pull-through procedure
a. pulse
a. radiation
radical abdominal hysterectomy
recurrent abdominal pain syndrome
a. reflex
a. region
a. respiration
right abdominal pain
a. rigidity
ruptured abdominal aortic aneurysm
a. scars
a. series
a. soft tissue density
staged abdominal repair
a. stimulus
a. stoma
a. stria
a. structure
subcutaneous a.
a. surgery
a. swelling and pain
a. tenderness
a. tenderness from appendicitis
a. testis
total abdominal colectomy
total abdominal evisceration
total abdominal fat
total abdominal hysterectomy
total abdominal hysterectomy and bilateral salpingo-oophorectomy
transverse abdominal diameter
a. trauma
a. trauma index
a. tumor
a. tympany
a. ultrasound
upper abdominal area
upper abdominal flap
upper abdominal pain
upper abdominal surgery
vague abdominal complaints
vague abdominal pain
a. viscera
visceral abdominal fat
visceral abdominal fat to total abdominal fat ratio
a. wall
a. x-ray

abdominalgia
periodic a.

abdominopelvic
whole abdominopelvic irradiation

abdominoperineal
Miles abdominoperineal resection
a. resection

abdominoplasty
Mladick a.
Monfort a.

abducens
alternating a.
mental retardation, skeletal dysplasia, abducens palsy syndrome
a. nerve sign
nervus a.
nucleus of abducens nerve

abducent
a. nerve
nucleus of abducent nerve

abducted and externally rotated

abduction
Atlanta-Scottish Rite abduction orthosis
congenital abduction deficiency
a. contracture of hip
a. exercise
fabere abduction test
flexion, abduction, external rotation
flexion, abduction, external rotation contracture
flexion, abduction, external rotation, extension
a. position

abduction/adduction
horizontal a./a.

abduction-external rotation

abductor
bilateral abductor vocal cord paralysis
a. digiti minimi muscle
a. digiti quinti
a. digiti quinti muscle
a. digiti quinti tendon
a. hallucis brevis muscle
a. hallucis tendon
Littler-Cooley abductor digiti quinti transfer
long abductor muscle of thumb
long abductor tendon
a. muscle
musculus a.
musculus abductor digiti minimi manus
musculus abductor digiti minimi pedis
musculus abductor digiti quinti

abductor *(continued)*
musculus abductor hallucis
musculus abductor pollicis brevis
musculus abductor pollicis longus
a. pollicis
pollicis brevis abductor muscle
a. pollicis brevis muscle
a. pollicis brevis tendon
a. pollicis longus
pollicis longus abductor muscle
a. spasmodic dysphonia

abductory
closing abductory wedge osteotomy
opening abductory wedge osteotomy

abductovalgus
adolescent hallux a.
hallux a.
McBride hallux abductovalgus reduction

abductus
hallux a.

Abelson
A. leukemia virus
A. murine leukemia virus

aberrans
vas a.

aberrant
a. artery
a. behavior
a. bundle
a. cell
a. crypt focus
a. cycle
a. right subclavian artery
a. sexual behavior
a. thyroid
a. ventricular conduction
a. vessel

aberration
angle of a.
autosomal a.
behavioral a.
chromatic-type a.
intraventricular a.
a. of judgment
longitudinal a.
mental a.
meridional a.
metabolic a.
monochromatic a.
newtonian a.
oblique a.
optic a.
optical a.
sexual a.
spherical a.
zona a.

ABG
arterial blood gas

ABI
ankle-brachial index

ability
attentional a.
attention shift a.
auditory a.
body's natural healing a.
body's tumor-killing a.
British A. Scale
Canadian Cognitive Abilities Test
cell refract a.
circulation, motor ability, sensation, and swelling
cognitive a.
College A. Test
Communication Abilities Diagnostic Test
Communicative Abilities in Daily Living
Comprehensive A. Battery
a. continuum
a. to cope with stress
coping a.
decline in ability to perform routine tasks
declining mathematical a.
decreased ability to concentrate
decreased ability to function
difficulty functioning at normal ability level
diminished ability to think or concentration
expressive a.
a. to function independently
heart rate condition a.
a. to hold head up
human a.
impaired ability to swallow
impaired pumping a.
independent functional a.
intellectual a.
kinesthetic ability trainer
knowledge, skills, and a.'s
language a.
learning a.
loss of ability to hold head up
mathematical a.
memory a.
mental a.
motor a.
muscle a.
nonverbal abstractive a.
Nonverbal A. Test
occupational a.
occupational ability pattern
olfactorial a.
Otis-Lennon Mental A. Test
Otis Quick Scoring Mental Abilities Test
parenting a.
patient's ability to perform
patient's functional a.
Perception of A. Scale for Students
perceptual-motor ability impairment
a. to perform
physical a.
physical abilities analysis
Physical A. Test
Porch Index of Communicative Abilities in Children
Predictive A. Test
primary mental a.
Primary Mental Abilities Test
problem-solving a.
psychic a.
pumping ability of failing heart
pumping ability of weakened heart
range of a.
red blood cell filter a.
Scales of Cognitive A. for Traumatic Brain Injury
School and College A. Test
social a.
a. to think or concentrate
thinking a.
word-finding a.

abiotrophy
retinal a.

ablation
accessory conduction a.
androgen ablation therapy
arrhythmogenic myocardial tissue a.
atrioventricular junctional a.
AV node a.
balloon endometrial a.
cold forceps a.
contact laser ablation of prostate
continuous wave a.
continuous wave laser a.
cryosurgical ablation of the prostate
electrical catheter a.
electrode catheter a.
endometrial resection and a.
endoscopic mucosal a.

excimer laser a.
His bundle a.
interstitial laser ablation of the prostate
laser uterosacral nerve a.
microwave cardiac ablation system
microwave endometrial a.
mucosal intact laser tonsillar a.
Nd:YAG laser a.
ovarian a.
percutaneous ethanol a.
percutaneous ethanol ablation of tumor
percutaneous transluminal coronary rotational a.
percutaneous transluminal septal myocardial a.
percutaneous tumor a.
peripheral retinal a.
pulsed laser a.
radiofrequency a.
radiofrequency catheter a.
radiofrequency thermal a.
supraventricular tachycardia a.
a. therapy
a. threshold
thyroid nodule a.
tissue ablation, incision and excision
transcoronary ablation of septal hypertrophy
transcoronary alcohol a.
transurethral needle a.
vaporization laser ablation of prostate
ventricular arrhythmia a.
visual laser ablation of prostate

ablation/resection
physiologic endometrial ablation/resection loop

ablatio placentae

ablative
androgen ablative monotherapy
a. device
a. hormonal therapy
peripheral ablative surgery
a. surgery
a. technique
a. therapy

ablepharon macrostomia syndrome

AB negative blood type

abnormal
a. activity
a. alignment
a. alpha activity
a. anatomic lesion
area of abnormal density
a. behavior
a. bladder contraction
a. bleeding
a. blood clotting
a. bone growth
a. brainstem
a. brain wave discharge
a. brain wave function
a. cardiac rhythm
a. cluster
conotruncal cardiac defect, abnormal face, thymic hypoplasia, cleft palate
a. coronary artery
a. curve
a. cytology
definitely abnormal tracing
a. development
a. development of scar tissue
a. diurnal weight gain
a. electrical activity
a. electrical events in heart
a. electrical impulse
a. electrical stimulus
a. endochondral ossification
a. eye movements
a. facies
a. fetal development
a. forms percent
a. frequency
a. functioning of heart
a. fusion
a. gait
a. gait and station
a. glucose tolerance
a. glucose tolerance test
a. growth
a. growth process
a. hair growth
a. heart activity
a. heartbeat
a. heart contraction
a. heart rhythm
a. increase in compliance
a. intolerance to light
a. intraluminal pressure
a. involuntary movement disorder
A. Involuntary Movement Scale
a. jugular reflex
a. karyotype
a. left axis deviation
life-threatening abnormal heartbeat
a. lipoprotein
a. liver function test
a. location of immature myeloid precursor
a. mammogram
a. mass
a. mass of tissue growth
mature abnormal chorionic villus
mature abnormal placenta
microcephalus, imperforate anus, syndactyly, hamartoblastoma, abnormal lung lobulation, polydactyly
microphallus, imperforate anus, syndactyly, hamartoblastoma, abnormal lung
a. motility
a. muscle movement
a. muscle response
a. muscle tone
no abnormal discovery
nothing abnormal detected
nothing abnormal discovered
a. oxygen affinity
a. Pap smear
a. pattern
a. peristaltic action of colon
a. position of infant
a. primary function
a. protrusion
a. pulmonary function
a. record
a. residual tissue
a. retinal correspondence
a. right axis deviation
a. sac containing gas
a. segment
a. spinal posture
a. sputum
a. tissue
a. tissue mass
transient abnormal myelopoiesis
transient abnormal Q wave
triple vessel disease with abnormal left ventricle
a. tubular myelin
a. uterine bleeding
a. vaginal bleeding
a. wave
a. wave form

abnormality
akinetic segmental wall motion a.
angle of a.
arch of aorta a.
arterial blood gas a.
asymmetry, range of motion abnormality, tissue texture a.

abnormality *(continued)*
calcinosis cutis, osteoma cutis, poikiloderma, and skeletal abnormalities syndrome
cardiac abnormality, abnormal facies, thymic hypoplasia, cleft palate, hypocalcemia
cardiac abnormality, T-cell deficit, clefting, hypocalcemia
cataract, motor system disorder, short stature, learning difficulty, skeletal abnormalities syndrome
characteristic of seizure a.
chemical abnormality in brain
coloboma, heart anomaly, ichthyosis, mental retardation, and ear abnormality syndrome
constitutional chromosome a.
electrographic background a.
electrophysiologic a.
enzymatic abnormality of adrenal gland
Gait A. Rating Scale Modified
a. in gas exchange
growth retardation, ocular abnormalities, microcephaly, brachydactyly, oligophrenia
heart muscle a.
a. in heart rate
heart rhythm a.
heart valve a.
immune function a.
inherited abnormality in brain
intracranial vascular a.
intraretinal microvascular a.
left atrial a.
left ventricular wall motion a.
lentigines, electrocardiographic abnormalities, ocular hypertelorism, pulmonary stenosis, abnormalities of genitalia, retardation of growth, deafness syndrome
limb abnormality syndrome
liver tissue a.
macrocephaly, facial abnormalities, disproportionate tall stature mental retardation syndrome
macrosomia, obesity, macrocephaly, ocular abnormality syndrome
major karyotypic a.
mental retardation, blepharonasofacial abnormalities, hand malformations syndrome
mental retardation, coarse face, microcephaly, epilepsy, skeletal abnormalities syndrome
minor karyotype a.
modified Gait A. Rating Scale
müllerian, renal, cervicothoracic, somite abnormalities syndrome
multiple congenital a.'s
multiple endocrine a.'s
nail fold capillarioscopy a.
nail fold capillary loop a.
neuritic cytoskeletal a.
no a.
no abnormality demonstrable
no abnormality of fetus
no apparent a.'s
no congenital a.'s
no essential a.'s
no evidence of a.
no histologic a.'s
no histopathologic a.
nondermatomal sensory a.
nonspecific abnormality of ST segment and T wave
nonspecific hepatocellular a.
nonspecific ST-T wave a.
no serious a.
no significant a.
nuclear membrane a.
oral cavity a.
palpable bony a.
potential abnormality of glucose tolerance
previous abnormality of glucose tolerance
protein binding a.
regional wall motion a.
right atrial a.
schizophrenic brain a.
segmental bronchus perfusion a.
segmental wall motion a.
skeletal abnormalities, cutis laxa, craniostenosis, psychomotor retardation, facial a.'s
sleep hygiene a.
sperm a.
spinal cord injury without radiographic a.
S-T and T-wave a.
tissue texture a.
ventricular wall motion a.
vertebral abnormality, anal imperforation, tracheoesophageal fistula, and radial, ray, or renal anomalies
wall motion a.
white matter signal a.

abnormally
a. contracting regions
a. fast activity
a. high concentration of urine
a. high content
a. low content
nonblanchable, abnormally colored lesion
a. rapid heart rate
a. slow heart rate
a. slow rhythm

ABO
A. antibody
A. antigen
A. blood group
A. blood type
blood type in ABO blood group
A. hemolytic disease
A. incompatibility
A. typing

aborted
a. human fetus
spontaneously aborted human fetus

abortion
ectopic pregnancy and a.
elective a.
equine abortion virus
full-term deliveries, premature deliveries, abortions, living children
gravida, para, multiple births, abortions, live birth
incomplete a.
induced a.
instillation abortion time
late a.
live birth a.
menstrual extraction a.
nonsurgical therapeutic a.
partial birth a.
recurrent spontaneous a.
repeated spontaneous a.
second trimester a.
spontaneous a.
suction aspiration a.
therapeutic a.
therapeutic abortion, dilation, aspiration, and curettage
total abortion rate

abortive
migraine abortive therapy

abortus
gravida, para, a.

abortus-Bang-ring test

about
confusion about time and place
drainage about shunt site
oozing about shunt site

above
amputated above ankle
amputated above knee
a. diaphragm
a. elbow
elevate feet above heart
fingers above umbilicus
fundus firm 1, 2 cm above umbilicus
a. knee
a. level of heart
one fingerbreadth above umbilicus
a. selected threshold
time above minimum inhibitory concentration
a. waist

above-elbow
short above-elbow cast
standard above-elbow cast

above-knee
femoral above-knee popliteal bypass

abraded skin

Abraham-Pankovich tendo calcaneus repair

Abrami disease

Abrams
A. disease
A. heart reflex

abrasion
air abrasion system
arthroscopic abrasion chondroplasty
a. of bowel
a. and contusion
a. of cornea
a. and laceration
multiple a.'s
perioperative corneal a.

abrasive
aluminum oxide a.
degree of fineness of abrasive particles

Abras virus

abreaction
motor a.

abridged ocular chart

abrupt
a. cessation
a. change in vision
a. closure
a. loss of consciousness
a. mood change
a. onset
a. recurrence
a. withdrawal

abruption
placental a.

abruptio placentae

abscess
anchovy paste a.
aortic annulus a.
aortic anulus a.
apical periodontal a.
Aspergillus brain a.
Aspergillus cerebral a.
breast abscess from breast-feeding
a. cavity
a. drainage
focal abscess formation
a. formation
Gram stain of facial a.
Gram stain of pelvic a.
a. of heel
iliac fossa a.
a. incised
incision and drainage of a.
incision and drainage of ischiorectal a.
intracranial a.
lumbar epidural a.
metastatic tuberculous a.
mixed aerobic and anaerobic a.
multiple a.'s
Mycobacterium chelonae a.
Nocardia brain a.
Paget abscess syndrome
parasitic brain a.
parotid gland a.
percutaneous abscess and fluid drainage
percutaneous drainage of epididymal a.
perianal fistula a.
perinephric abscess drainage
periodontal a.
periprosthetic breast a.
peritoneal cavity a.
peritonsillar a.
pyogenic abscess of liver
soft tissue a.
spinal cord a.
spinal epidural a.
subperiosteal a.
subperiosteal orbital a.
tuboovarian a.
tuboovarian abscess after previous tubal occlusion

abscessed
pseudocyst a.

abscessus
Mycobacterium abscessus infection

abscissic acid

absence
ApoB-100 a.
ApoB-48 a.
atonic a.
atonic absence seizure
atypical a.
atypical absence seizure
automatic a.
bilateral congenital absence of vas deferens
a. of branch pulmonary artery
a. of breathing
congenital absence of ureter
congenital absence of vagina
congenital absence of vas deferens
congenital bilateral absence of the vas deferens
congenital localized absence of skin
a. of consciousness
a. of electrical activity
epilepsy with myoclonic a.
epileptic a.
a. of facial and pubic hair
a. of feeling
a. of heartbeat
heat, absence of use, redness, pain, pus, swelling
a. of heat in a reaction
a. of immunoglobulin A, G, M
a. of infection
juvenile absence epilepsy
leave of a.
limb a.
a. of menstrual periods
microscopic a.
muscle a.
myoclonic a.
prothrombin induced by vitamin K absence or antagonist-II
a. of respiration
a. seizure
a. of sex chromosome
simple a.
surgical absence of breast
syndrome of absence of septum pellucidum with poerencephaly
temporary leave of a.

absence *(continued)*
timed therapeutic a.
unauthorized a.
unilateral absence of excretion
a. of voluntary muscle movement

absent
a. ankle jerk
a. bed occupancy
a. bowel function
a. bowel sounds
a. breath sounds
craniofacial dysmorphism, absent corpus callosum, iris colobomas, connective tissue dysplasia syndrome
a. heartbeat
a. kidney
a. menses
a. menstrual period from diabetes
a. pulse
a. reflex
septum pellucidum absent with porencephalia syndrome
thrombocytopenia and absent radius
a. without leave

absolute
a. amenorrhea
atmosphere a.
a. band count
a. basophil count
a. bedrest
a. blood eosinophil count
a. bone conduction
a. cardiac dullness
a. catabolic rate
a. cell count
a. dehydration
a. diet
a. dose intensity
a. free thyroxine
a. free triiodothyronine
a. glaucoma
a. granulocyte count
a. hemianopia
a. hypermetropia
hyperopia, a.
a. intensity
a. iodine uptake
a. latency
low absolute glomerular filtration rate
a. lymphocyte count
a. neutrophil count
a. nucleated red blood cell
a. phagocyte count
a. plasma concentration
a. proximal reabsorption
a. reaction of degeneration
a. refractory period
a. retention time
a. risk reduction
a. scotoma
a. temperature
a. temperature on the Rankine scale
a. viscosity
a. volume of trabecular bone

absorbable
a. catgut
a. collagen paste
fibrillar absorbable hemostat material
a. gelatin sponge
a. mesh
Mitek absorbable anchor
a. surgical suture
a. suture
synthetic absorbable suture

absorbance
light-induced absorbance change
time of-flight and a.
a. units, full scale

absorbancy
molar absorbancy index

absorbed
average target absorbed dose
a. dose
internal absorbed dose
maximum target absorbed dose
minimum target absorbed dose
a. normal pooled plasma
a. poison
a. radiation
roentgen absorbed dose
a. test plasma
to be a.

absorbent
antibody a.
a. gauze
a. gelling material
radar absorbent material
a. sterile towel
tumescent absorbent bandage

absorptiometer
single-energy x-ray a.

absorptiometry
dual-energy x-ray absorptiometry scan
dual-photon a.
dual-photon x-ray a.
peripheral dual-energy x-ray a.
radial photon a.
radiographic a.
single-photon a.

absorption
atomic a.
atomic absorption spectrometer
atomic absorption spectrophotometer
atomic absorption spectroscopy
a. coefficient
coefficient of a.
conglutinating complement absorption test
cytotoxicity negative, absorption positive
a., distribution, metabolism, and excretion
egg yolk-cobalamin absorption test
electrothermal atomic absorption spectrophotometry
a. enhancer
extended x-ray absorption fine structure spectroscopy
fat absorption study
fluorescence treponemal antibody a.
glucose absorption test
guinea pig kidney absorption test
linear absorption coefficient
mass absorption coefficient
mean absorption time
mean fraction a.
molar absorption coefficient
net calcium a.
neutron absorption process
a. of nutrients
paracetamol absorption test
peak absorption spike
photon absorption densitometry
a. process
radiation-equivalent-manikin a.
small intestine a.
specific absorption coefficient
specific absorption rate
spheroidal oral drug absorption system
a. study
surface extended x-ray absorption fine structure
total solute a.

absorption-equivalent thickness

absorptive
a. cell
a. endocytosis
a. hypercalciuria

absorptivity
molar a.
specific a.

abstinence
alcohol abstinence syndrome
alcoholic abstinence syndrome
conditioned a.
a. goal
Neonatal Abstinence Scoring System
neonatal abstinence sign
neonatal narcotic abstinence syndrome
opiate abstinence syndrome
period of a.
post treatment a.

abstinent
newly abstinent alcoholic

abstract
decreased capacity for abstract thought
a. form
a. functioning
a. idea
impaired abstract thinking
multiple abstract variance analysis
Personal Values A.
a. reasoning
a. thinking

abstractive
nonverbal abstractive ability

abundant
brief, small, abundant, polyphasic potential
brief, small, abundant motor-unit action potential

abuse
adolescent alcohol a.
adolescent chemical a.
adolescent drug a.
adolescent drug abuse unit
aerosol spray a.
alcohol a.
alcohol abuse among women
alcohol abuse scale
alcohol or drug a.
alcoholism and drug a.
alcohol and other drug a.
amyl nitrate a.
anabolic steroid a.
antibiotic use and a.
cardiovascular complications of drug a.
cardiovascular problems related to drug a.
a. case
cause of drug a.
Checklist for Child A. Evaluation
child a.
child abuse and neglect
childhood sexual a.
chronic alcohol a.
chronic child a.
chronic substance a.
comorbid alcohol a.
comorbid cocaine a.
comorbidity of schizophrenia and substance a.
complication of drug a.
continuous and confirmed memories of a.
a. counseling
cutaneous signs of drug a.
death due to drug a.
dissociation and sexual a.
drug abuse reporting program
drug abuse urine
drug and alcohol abuse death
Drug A. Screening Test
Drug A. Warning Network
early intervention in drug a.
economic costs of drug a.
fatal child a.
hepatic complications of drug a.
hepatic problems related to drug a.
history of a.
illicit drug a.
incidence of drug a.
a. intervention
intravenous drug a.
laxative abuse syndrome
long-term course of a.
maternal drug a.
maternal substance a.
medical history as screening device for drug a.
Michigan A. Screening Test
National Center for Child A. and Neglect
National Center on Elder A.
National Institute on Alcohol A. and Alcoholism
neonatal complications of drug a.
neuromuscular complication of drug a.
nonprescription drug a.
over-the-counter drug a.
patient education on drug a.
pattern of hallucinogen a.
PCP drug a.
perinatal substance a.
physical effect of hallucinogen a.
physical effects of drug a.
physician drug a.
polysubstance a.
polysubstance use and a.
potential of hallucinogen a.
prenatal abuse of illicit drug
prescription drug a.
prevalence of hallucinogen a.
psychoactive drug a.
psychoactive substance abuse and dependence
a. related depression
sexual abuse of child
sexual abuse group
sexual abuse history
sexual complications of drug a.
social history as screening device for drug a.
substance abuse counselor
substance abuse disorder
substance abuse evaluation screen unit
substance abuse treatment
substance abuse treatment clinic
substance abuse treatment program
substance abuse treatment unit
Substance A. Questionnaire
Substance A. Subtle Screening Inventory
surgical complication of drug a.
survivor of a.
suspected child abuse or neglect
symptom of drug a.
variety of abuse patterns
warning sign of drug a.

abuser
anxious substance a.
assessing needs of hallucinogen a.
child of substance a.
hard core drug a.
mentally ill chemical a.
parenteral drug a.

abusing
infant of drug abusing mother

abusive
a. family system
a. and hostile patient
a. invasive person
patient abusive and hostile
a. pattern
a. relationship

abutment
anterior a.
auxiliary a.

abutment *(continued)*
multiple a.
multiple abutment support
multirooted a.

academic
A. Alertness
a. aptitude test
assessment of academic achievement
a. health care
Kaufman Survey of Early A. and Language Skills
marked decline in academic functioning
Milwaukee A. Interest Inventory
a. orientation
poor academic achievement
A. Readiness Scale
Short Form Test of A. Aptitude

Acado virus

acalculia
aphasic a.

acalculous
acute acalculous cholecystitis
a. biliary colic
a. cholecystitis

Acanthamoeba
Acanthamoeba endophthalmitis
non-*Acanthamoeba* amebic keratitis

***Acanthocheilonema viteae* excretory-secretory antigen**

acantholytic
transient acantholytic dermatosis

acanthoma
pale cell a.

acanthosis
hirsutism, androgen excess, insulin resistance, acanthosis nigricans syndrome
hyperandrogenism, insulin resistance, and acanthosis nigricans syndrome
insulin-resistant diabetes, acanthosis nigricans, hypogonadism pigmentary retinopathy, deafness, mental retardation syndrome
malignant acanthosis nigricans
mental retardation, pre-and postnatal overgrowth, remarkable face, acanthosis nigricans syndrome
a. nigricans

accelerated
a. breathing
chronic myelocytic/myelogenous/myeloid leukemia accelerated phase
continuous hyperfractionated accelerated radiotherapy
a. destruction of red blood cells
a. freeze-drying
a. graft atherosclerosis
a. growth area
hyperfractionated accelerated radiation therapy
a. hyperfractionation
a. hypertension
a. idioventricular rhythm
a. idioventricular tachycardia
immediate good function followed by accelerated rejection
a. intraventricular rhythm
a. junctional rhythm
a. mental processes
a. painless labor
a. phase
premature accelerated lung maturation
a. reaction
a. respiration
a. ventricular rhythm

accelerating
a. heart rate
a. rate calorimetry

acceleration
angular a.
a. of blood flow
body acceleration synchronous with heart rate
early systolic a.
fetal activity acceleration determination
fetal growth a.
fetal heart rate a.
fetal movement acceleration test
a. force
a. index
movement-associated fetal heart rate a.'s
operant acceleration of heart rate
percentage of acceleration time
precordial acceleration tracing
resultant physiologic a.
a. time
unit of force of a.

accelerator
a. globulin
high-energy bent beam linear a.
linear accelerator isocenter motion
linear accelerator radiosurgery
low-energy linear a.
a. mass spectrometry
Mobetron mobile, self-shielded electron a.
plasma prothrombin conversion a.
proserum prothrombin conversion a.
serum accelerator factor
serum prothrombin conversion a.
serum thrombotic a.

accelerator-based
linear accelerator-based radiosurgery
linear accelerator-based SRS

accelerator-produced radiopharmaceuticals

accentuated heartbeat

accentuation
paramagnetic enhancement accentuation by chemical shift imaging
perifollicular a.

acceptable
a. daily intake
a. dental remedies
socially acceptable monitoring instrument

accepting illness

acceptor
methyl acceptor protein

access
central venous a.
central venous access device
controlled access to fluid
controlled fluid a.
dynamic random access memory
echo record a.
endoscopic access port
expandable access catheter
extracorporeal pneumoperititoneal access bubble
femoral access stabilization
implantable vascular access device
implantable venous access device
indwelling transcutaneous vascular access device
indwelling vascular access catheter
intravenous retrograde access port
A. Management Survey
minimal access general surgery
minimal access spinal technology
orbital exenteration gastroscopic access technique

patient-centered access to secure systems online
percutaneous access kit
Peripheral A. System
Peripheral A. System Port catheter system
piriform aperture a.
portal venous a.
prolonged venous access devices
public access defibrillation
public access defibrillator
radiology telephone access system
remote access perfusion
roaming optical access multiscope
side-entry a.
stable access cannula
static random access memory
Survey of Employee A.
transcervical tubal access catheter
ultrasound-guided vascular a.
uterine cornual access catheter
uterine ostial access catheter
vascular access device
vascular access dressing
vascular access in hemodialysis
venous access device
venous access port

accessibility

handicapped a.

accessorium

pancreas a.

accessory

a. clinical finding
a. bone
a. cholera enterotoxin
a. chromosome
a. clinical findings
a. collateral ligament
a. communicating tendon
a. conduction ablation
a. conduction pathway
a. cramp
a. cusp
a. ganglion
Gantzer accessory bundle
a. gland
a. lobe
lumbar accessory movement technique
male accessory gland fluid
medial accessory olivary nucleus
multiple accessory spleens
a. muscle
a. muscles of respiration
nasal accessory artery
a. nerve
a. nipple
nuclear accessory hormone
nucleus of accessory nerve
a. nucleus Monakow nucleus
a. olfactory bulb
a. optic tract
passive accessory intervertebral movements
passive accessory motion test
a. processes
a. pulmonary blood flow
spinal accessory nerve
spinal accessory nerve palsy
a. spleen
vagal accessory nerve

accident

acute cerebrovascular a.
alcohol-related risk for a.
automobile a.
cardiovascular a.
cerebrovascular a.
cerebrovascular accident dementia
date of a.
a. dispensary
health and accident insurance
a. insurance
motorcycle a.
motor vehicle a.
neonatal cerebrovascular a.
personal injury a.
personal watercraft a.
a. prone
property damage a.
right cerebrovascular a.
road traffic a.
thromboembolic cerebral vascular a.
traffic a.
a. victim

accidental

a. amputation
childhood accidental spiral tibial fracture
a. death
delayed closure of accidental wound
a. hypothermia
a. inhalation
a. injury
a. pregnancy

accidentally

incurred a.
a. incurred

acclimation to heat and work

accommodation

amplitude of a.
a. and compensation
far point of a.
light and a.
a. light
ocular vergance and accommodation sensor
paralysis of a.
pupils equal and reactive to light and a.
pupils equal, round, reactive to light and a.
pupils equal, round, reactive to light and accommodation directly and consensually
pupils react to light and a.
range of a.
a. reflex

accommodative

a. convergence
a. convergence/accommodation ratio
a. esophoria
nonrefractive accommodative esotropia

accompanying

convulsion accompanying fever
a. fever
orders accompanying patient on admission
a. vein
a. vein of hypoglossal nerve

accomplished

hemostasis a.

accomplishment

inflated judgment of a.'s
a. quotient

accordion

a. graft
a. sign

account

medical materials a.
narrative a.
on account of

accreditation

a. program/home health care
a. program/hospice care
a. program/long-term care

accredited

a. psychiatric hospital
a. rehabilitation worker

accreta

placenta a.

accretion

mass a.

accumulated alveolar ventilatory volume

accumulating
rapidly accumulating ascites

accumulation
a. of bile pigment
a. of blood within joint
excessive accumulation of glycogen
fluid accumulation and inflammation
niacin accumulation test
onset of blood lactate a.
platelet accumulation index

accuracy
assay a.
predictive a.
relative standard a.
standard a.
Test of Learning A. in Children
Test of Listening A. in Children
wavelength a.

accurate
intravenous accurate control device
limb accurate measurement

Ace bandage

acellular
antipertussis acellular vaccine
diphtheria, tetanus toxoid, and acellular pertussis vaccine
hyaline acellular area
pertussis, acellular antigens, vaccine
a. pertussis vaccine with diphtheria and tetanus toxoid

acetabular
anatomic porous replacement hemispheric acetabular component
a. anteversion
Aufranc-Turner acetabular cup
axial acetabular index
bipolar acetabular cup
chamfered cylinder acetabular component
custom-made acetabular cup
a. depth to femoral head diameter
a. fracture
a. head index
a. line
malignant acetabular osteolysis
metal-backed acetabular component
metal-backed acetabular cup
migration of acetabular cup
mild acetabular dysplasia
Modular A. Revision System
mold acetabular arthroplasty
a. notch
Osteolock acetabular component
porous-coated acetabular cup
a. rim
a. rim fracture
a. shell
threaded titanium acetabular prosthesis

acetabuloplasty
Albee a.
Pemberton a.

acetabulum
anterior lip of the a.
a. head index
lip of a.
lunate surface of a.
margin of a.
notch of a.
posterior lip of a.

acetaminophen
a. and codeine
hepatitis and a.
a. overdose
oxycodone and a.
a. poisoning
a. toxicity

acetate
betamethasone a.
cellular acetate propionate
cellulose a.
cellulose acetate butyrate
cellulose acetate dialysis device
cellulose acetate electrophoresis
cortisone a.
cresyl violet a.
deoxycorticosterone a.
depot medroxyprogesterone a.
desoxycorticosterone a.
a. dialysis
ethylene vinyl a.
ethylene-vinyl acetate copolymer
hydrocortisone a.
hypertonic acetate dextran
mafenide a.
mafenide acetate for burn
medroxyprogesterone a.
megestrol a.
methylazoxymethanol a.
methylprednisolone a.
norethindrone a.
phenylmercuric a.
polymyxin, lysozyme, EDTA, and thallous acetate in heart infusion agar
polyvinyl a.
tertiary butyl a.
tetradecadiene a.
triamcinolone acetomide *tert*-butyl a.

acetic
a. acid
a. acid reaction
a. acid test
flavone acetic acid
formaldehyde, acetic acid, and alcohol solution
formalin, acetic, and alcohol solution
naphthalene acetic acid
pyridine acetic acid

acetoacetic acid

acetomide
triamcinolone acetomide *tert*-butyl acetate

acetone
alcohol, ether, and acetone solution
buffered a.
hexone-extracted a.
a. powder extract
sugar and acetone determination
sugar, acetone, diacetic acid test
a. in water

acetone-extracted serum

acetone-killed
typhoid vaccine, acetone-killed and dried

acetonide
triamcinolone acetonide cream

acetophenetidin

acetowhite
a. epithelium
a. lesion
a. reaction
a. test

acetylase
choline a.

acetylcholine
antimuscarinic acetylcholine receptor
a. esterase
nicotinic acetylcholine receptor
a. receptor
a. receptor antibody
a. receptor-inducing activity

acetylcholinesterase inhibitor

acetylene reduction activity

acetylhydrolase
platelet-activating factor a.

acetyltransferase
choline a.
histone a.

achalasia
a. of esophagus
cricopharyngeal achalasia syndrome
megaesophagus of a.

achalasia-addisonism-alacrimia

ache
chronic a.'s and pains
generalized muscle aches
joint a.'s
a.'s and pains
psychosomatic a.'s and pains

achievable
as low as reasonably achievable radiation exposure

achieve
a. high dose
help patient achieve independence

achievement
a. age
assessment of academic a.
California A. Test
A. Checklist
creative a.
Diagnostic A. Battery, Second Edition
a. drive
Iowa A. Test
Kaufman Test of Educational A.
level of a.
manifest a.
Metropolitan A. Test, Seventh Edition
motive a.
Music A. Test 1-4
Norris Educational A. Test
a. orientation
Peabody Individual A. Test
poor academic a.
Progressive A. Tests of Listening Comprehension
a. quotient
a. ratio
Scaled Curriculum A. Levels Test
school a.
Stanford A. Test
a. test
a. through counseling and treatment
Wide Range A. Test-Revised

Achilles
A. bursa
A. heel
A. jerk
Lynn Achilles lengthening procedure
Lynn Achilles tendon repair technique
mop-end Achilles tendon tear
Murphy Achilles tendon advancement
percutaneous Achilles tendon repair
ruptured Achilles tendon
surgical Achilles tendon lengthening
A. tendinitis
A. tendinopathy
A. tendon
A. tendon advancement
A. tendon bursa
A. tendon bursitis
A. tendon enthesis
A. tendon enthesis calcification
A. tendon insertion
A. tendon lengthening
A. tendon pain
A. tendon reflex
A. tendon reflex test
A. tendon reflex time
A. tendon repair
A. tendon resurfacing
A. tendon rupture
A. tendon shortening
A. tendon taping technique
A. tendon test
A. tendon xanthoma
A. tendon Z-lengthening

Achillis
tendo A.
tendo Achillis lengthening and toe flexor release
tendo Achillis reflex

aching
diffuse dull, aching pressure discomfort
dull aching pain
fidgeting, aching, pulling, or itching feeling
generalized a.
a. joint
joint a.
a. and numbness
a. pain

achlorhydria
watery diarrhea, hypokalemia, and achlorhydria syndrome

acholic stool

acholuric hemolytic icterus

achondroplasia
hyperplastic a.

achromasia
neuronal a.

achromatopsia
atypical a.

achylic
macrocytic achylic anemia

acid
abscissic a.
acetic a.
acetic acid reaction
acetic acid test
acetoacetic a.
activated fatty a.
adenylic a.
adenylosuccinic a.
adult acid maltase deficiency
alanyl-transfer ribonucleic acid synthetase
all-trans-retinoic a.
alpha-allokainic a.
alpha amino a.
alpha-hydroxy a.
alpha-hydroxy acid gel
alpha-ketoisocaproic a.
alpha-linolenic a.
alpha-lipoic a.
amino a.
amino acid activating enzyme
amino acid decarboxylase
amino acid metabolic disorder
amino acid metabolism
amino acid mixture
amino acid nitrogen
amino acid oxidase
L-amino acid oxidase
amino acid sequence
amino acid that gives aspartic acid after hydrolysis
aminocaproic a.
aminocephalosporanic a.
p-aminohippuric a.
aminolevulinic acid dehydrase
5-aminolevulinic acid photodynamic therapy
aminolevulinic acid synthetase
5-aminosalicylic acid enema
antideoxyribonucleic acid antibody
anti-double-stranded deoxyribonucleic a.
anti-double-stranded deoxyribonucleic acid antibody

acid *(continued)*
antiglutamic acid decarboxylase autoantibody
arachidonic a.
arachidonic acid cascade
arachidonic acid cascade inhibitor
arachidonic acid level
arachidonic acid metabolism
arachidonic acid metabolite
arachidonic acid oxidation
arachidonic acid pathway
argininosuccinic acid lyase
argininosuccinic acid synthase deficiency
argininosuccinic acid synthetase deficiency
aromatic acid decarboxylase
aromatic amino a.
aromatic amino acid decarboxylase
aromatic D-amino acid decarboxylase
aromatic L-amino acid decarboxylase
ascorbic acid assay
ascorbic acid deficiency
ascorbic acid factor
ascorbic acid test
aspartic a.
a. aspiration syndrome
aurintricarboxylic acid stain
azelaic a.
a. balance control
basal acid output
bile a.
bile acid independent flow
a. bismuth yeast medium
blood uric a.
bone marrow acid phosphatase
boric a.
boric acid solution
branched-chain amino a.
branched-chain deoxyribonucleic a.
branched-chain fatty a.
branched deoxyribonucleic a.
a. challenge test
a. cholesterol ester hydrolase
chromosomal ribonucleic a.
chromotropic a.
cis-retinoic a.
13-*cis*-retinoic a.
9-*cis* retinoic acid receptor
citric a.
a. clearance test
clofibric a.
closed circle deoxyribonucleic a.
complementary deoxyribonucleic a.
conjugated linoleic a.
copolymer of polyinosinic and polycytidylic a.
crystalline amino a.
crystalline amino acid solution
cysteine sulfinic acid decarboxylase
deoxyribonucleic acid double stranded
deoxyribonucleic acid, histone
deoxyribonucleic acid phosphorus
deoxyribonucleic acid polymerase
deoxyribonucleic acid single stranded
1-dimethylamino-naphthalene-5-sulfonic a.
erythrocyte acid phosphatase
essential fatty acid deficiency
ethacrynic a.
excessive acid secretion
a. fast
fatty a.
fatty acid amide hydrolase
fatty acid free
fatty acid methyl ester
fatty acid oxidation
fatty acid poor
fatty acid translocase
fatty acid transport protein
fatty acids polyunsaturated
fecal bile a.
flavone acetic a.
folic a.
folic acid antagonist
formaldehyde, acetic acid, and alcohol solution
formiminoglutamic acid test
free a.
free fatty a.
free hydrochloric a.
free volatile fatty a.
fusaric a.
fusidic a.
gamma-aminobutyric acid transaminase
gastric acid inhibitor
gastric fluid, basal acid output
glucuronic acid lactone
glutamic acid decarboxylase
glutamic acid dehydrogenase
glycyrrhetinic acid like factor
a. heartburn
heart fatty acid binding protein
hepatoiminodiacetic a.
heterogeneous nuclear ribonucleic a.
heterogeneous ribonucleic a.
high acid level in blood
hippuric a.
homogentisic a.
homovanillic a.
hyaluronic a.
hydrobromic a.
hydrochloric a.
hydrocyanic a.
a. hydrolysis
12-hydroxyeicosatetraenoic a.
20-hydroxyeicosatetraenoic a.
21-hydroxyindoleacetic a.
hypoiodous a.
idiopathic bile acid malabsorption
iduronic a.
imidazoleacetic acid ribonucleotide
iminodiacetic a.
immune ribonucleic a.
a. indigestion
indoleacetic a.
infantile sialic acid storage disorder
infectious nucleic a.
informational ribonucleic a.
a. ingestion
inhibitory amino a.
insulin-induced peak acid output
a. intoxication
a. ionization dissociation constant
isobutyric a.
isonicotinic a.
isonicotinic acid hydrazide
kynurenic a.
lactic acid dehydrogenase
lactic acid mineral medium
large neutral amino a.
leukocyte ascorbic a.
linoleic acid depression
lipoteichoic a.
lithocolic a.
long-chain fatty a.
long-chain fatty acid oxidation
long-chain polyunsaturated fatty a.
long- and medium-chain fatty acid coenzyme-A dehydrogenase deficiency
low-branched-chain amino acid diet
low-saturated fatty acid diet
luminal acid clearance
Luna-Parker acid fuscin stain
lysergic acid amide
lysergic acid diethylamide

lysergic acid diethylamide assay
lysergic acid diethylamide and strychnine
lysophosphatidic a.
lysosomal acid lipase A, B
malic acid dehydrogenase
a. maltase deficiency
mandelic a.
maximal acid concentration
maximum acid output
Mayer acid alum hematoxylin stain
measure of acid strength
medium-chain fatty a.
2-mercaptoethanesulfonic a.
messenger ribonucleic a.
messenger ribonucleoprotein a.
methylbenzyl linoleic a.
2-methyl citric a.
methylmalonic a.
methyl tetrahydrofolic a.
mevalonic a.
mini-exon-derived ribonucleic acid gene
mitochondrial deoxyribonucleic acid analysis
mitochondrial deoxyribonucleic acid polymerase gamma
mitochondrial fatty acid beta-oxidation
mixed acid fermentation
modified amino a.
monosaturated fatty a.
monounsaturated fatty a.
morpholinoethanesulfonic a.
a. mucopolysaccharide
mucosal fatty a.
muramic a.
mycophenolic a.
nalidixic a.
nalidixic acid agar
nalidixic acid test
naphthalene acetic a.
naphthoxylactic a.
native deoxyribonucleic a.
negative logarithm of acid ionization constant
net acid flux
net acid input
neutral amino a.
a. neutralization capacity
neutralizing acid in stomach
nicotinic a.
nicotinic acid deficiency
nicotinic acid dehydrogenase
nicotinic acid maculopathy
nicotinic acid mononucleotide
nitric a.
nitric acid test
nitrilotriacetic a.
nitroblue tetrazolium-paraaminobenzoic a.
N-methyl D-aspartic a.
nocturnal acid reflux
nonessential amino a.
nonesterified fatty a.
nonpolar amino a.
noradrenaline acid tartrate
nordihydroguaiaretic a.
N-phosphonoacetyl-*l*-aspartic a.
nuclear ribonucleic a.
nucleic a.
nucleic acid amplification technique
nucleic acid amplification test
nucleic acid amplification testing
nucleic acid base
nucleic acid construct
nucleic acid detection
nucleic acid hybridization
nucleic acid hybridization analysis
nucleic acid hybridization test
nucleic acid immunization
nucleic acid phosphatase
nucleic acid probe
nucleic acid probe assay
nucleic acid sequence-band amplification
nucleic acid sequence-based amplification
nucleic acid sequence-based analysis
nucleic acid sequencing
nucleic acid vaccination
nucleic acid vector
oleic a.
oleic acid I 125
oleic acid uptake test
omega-3 fatty a.
omega-3, -6 fatty a.
omega-3 polyunsaturated fatty a.
oncogene ribonucleic a.
oral bile a.
organic acid metabolism
organic acid screen
orotic a.
orotidylic a.
orotidylic acid decarboxylase
orthoiodohippuric a.
orthophosphoric acid etch gel
osmic acid fixative
a. output
ovarian ascorbic acid depletion test
oxalic a.
oxalic acid assay
oxalic acid stain
oxaloacetic acid test
oxidation of fatty a.
oxolinic a.
Palmer acid test for peptic ulcer
p-aminobenzoic a.
p-aminosalicylic a.
pantothenic a.
pantothenic acid assay
pantothenic acid deficiency-induced colitis
pantothenic acid unit
paraaminobenzoic a.
paraaminomethylbenzoic a.
paraaminosalicylic a.
paraisopropyliminodiacetic acid scan
peak acid output after gastrin-releasing peptide
peak acid output after pentagastrin stimulation
peak acid output insulin-induced
pentose nucleic a.
peptide nucleic a.
perforated acid peptic ulcer
periodic a.
periodic acid staining
pharyngeal acid reflux
a. phosphatase
phosphatase acid serum
picric acid turbidity
pineapple test for butyric acid in stomach
placental acid phosphatase
plasma membrane fatty acid binding protein
polyunsaturated free fatty a.
polyunsaturated-to-saturated fatty acids ratio
primer-dependent deoxynucleic acid polymerase
primer-dependent deoxynucleic acid polymerase index
procaine and lactic a.
prostate-specific acid phosphatase
pure free a.
pyridine acetic a.
quisqualic a.
radioiodinated fatty a.
ratio of basal acid output to maximal acid output
recombinant deoxyribonucleic a.
a. reflux
a. reflux test
resorcylic acid lactone

acid *(continued)*
retinoic a.
retinoic acid metabolism blocking agent
retinoic acid receptor
ribonucleic a.
ribosomal deoxyribonucleic a.
ribosomal ribonucleic a.
ribosomal ribonucleic acid transcription unit
ribothymidylic a.
salicylic a.
salicylic and lactic acid paint
salicylsalicylic a.
saturated fatty a.
selenium-labeled homocholic acid conjugated with taurine
self-reinforcing polylevolactic a.
serum acid phosphatase
serum bile a.
serum folic a.
serum-free fatty a.
serum uric a.
short-chain fatty a.
short-chain polyunsaturated fatty a.
side chain in amino acid formula
silencing mediator of retinoic acid and thyroid hormone receptor
single-stranded deoxyribonucleic a.
small nuclear ribonucleic a.
soluble ribonucleic a.
a. stain
standard acid reflux test
sucrose-phosphate-glutamic a.
sugar, acetone, diacetic acid test
sulfated acid mucopolysaccharide
sulfosalicylic a.
synthetic amino a.
synthetic medium old tuberculin trichloroacetic acid precipitated
tannic acid, polyphosphomolybdic acid, and amido acid staining technique
tartrate-resistant acid phosphatase
taurodeoxycholic acid
tauroursodeoxycholic a.
technetium diisopropyliminodiacetic acid scan
technetium hepatoiminodiacetic acid scan
teichoic acid crude extract
a. test solution
thiobarbituric a.
titratable a.
toluene sulfonic a.
total a.
total bile a.
total cholic a.
total fatty a.
total serum bile a.
total serum prostatic acid phosphatase
trans fatty a.
transfer deoxyribonucleic a.
transfer ribonucleic a.
translational control ribonucleic a.
triiodothyronine, amino acids, glucagon, and heparin
unesterified free fatty a.
unknown amino a.
unsaturated fatty a.
unscheduled deoxynucleic acid synthesis
uric a.
uric acid calculus
uric acid infarct
uric acid nitrogen
uric acid urine spot test
uridine diphosphoglucuronic a.
uridylic a.
urine acid output
urocanic a.
ursodeoxycholic a.
valeric a.
valproic a.
vanillacetic a.
vanillylmandelic a.
very long chain fatty a.
viral ribonucleic a.
volatile fatty a.
xanthurenic a.

acidristocetin
arachidonic a.

acid-ash diet

acid-base ratio

acid-binding
cold-inducible ribonucleic acid-binding protein
fatty acid-binding protein
fatty acid-binding protein 2
folic acid-binding protein
intestinal fatty acid-binding protein
nucleic acid-binding protein
retinoic acid-binding protein
ribonucleic acid-binding motif

acid-creatinine

acid-dependent

acidemia
asymptomatic lactic a.
methylmalonic acidemia with homocystinemia
mixed umbilical arterial a.

acid-enriched
amino acid-enriched cardioplegic solution

acid-fast
a.-f. bacilli smear
a.-f. bacillus
a.-f. culture
modified Kinyoun acid-fast stain
modified acid-fast stain
a.-f. sputum smear
a.-f. stain
a.-f. staining method
a.-f. stain of sputum

acidic
antiglial fibrillary acidic protein
dimeric acidic glycoprotein
a. fibroblast growth factor
glial fibrillary acidic protein
immunosuppressive acidic protein
immunosuppressive acidic substance
monoclonal antiglial fibrillary acidic protein
a. proline-rich protein

acidified
a. complement
hereditary erythroblastic multinuclearity with positive acidified serum
not a.
a. serum, acidified complement

acidity
high titer, low a.
neutralize stomach a.
total a.
urinary titrable a.

acid-labile
organic acid-labile fluoride

acid-neutralizing capacity

acidophilus
Lactobacillus acidophilus vaccine

acidosis
anion gap a.
anion gap metabolic a.
chronic metabolic a.
diabetic a.
distal renal tubular a.
hyperchloremic metabolic a.
hyperchloremic renal a.
increasing respiratory a.
lactic acidosis threshold
metabolic a.

metabolic acidosis syndrome
mitochondrial myopathy, encephalopathy, lactic acidosis, strokelike episodes
myopathy, encephalopathy, lactic acidosis, strokelike episodes
nonanion gap a.
nonketotic hyperosmolar a.
nonketotic hypoglycemic a.
nonunion gap metabolic a.
renal tubular a.
terminal respiratory a.

acidotic
infant acidotic and hypoxic

acid-related
a.-r. disorder
retinoic acid-related orphan receptor

acid-Schiff
Alcian blue and periodic a.-S.
aldehyde-thionine-periodic acid-Schiff test
diastase-periodic a.-S.
peracetic acid-Schiff reaction
performic acid-Schiff reaction
periodic a.-S.
periodic acid-Schiff method
periodic acid-Schiff reaction
periodic acid-Schiff resistant
periodic acid-Schiff stain
periodic acid-Schiff test
a.-S. stain

acid-Schiff-positive
periodic a.-S.-p.
periodic acid-Schiff-positive material

acid-silver
periodic acid-silver methenamine
periodic acid-silver methenamine stain

acid-soluble
organic acid-soluble phosphorus

acidulated
Luride acidulated phosphate fluoride paste

aciduria
adult-onset combined methylmalonic aciduria and homocystinuria
organic a.
orotic a.
paradoxical a.
paroxysmal a.

acinar
atypical small acinar proliferation of prostate
a. cell carcinoma
central acinar emphysema
a. lumina
pancreatic acinar cell
pancreatic acinar cell carcinoma
pancreatic acinar mass
a. parenchyma
peripheral acinar vein
a. tissue

acini
malignant acini prostate gland

acinus
liver a.
lobular a.
pancreatic a.

Ackerman-Schoendorf Scales for Parent Evaluation of Custody

aclasis
metaphysial a.

acne
apocrine a.
atrophic facial acne scar
comedonal a.
common a.
a. cyst
Gram-negative a.
a. juvenilis
a. keloidalis
lupoid a.
mechanical a.
menstrual a.
miliary a.
neonatal a.
a. neonatorum
nodulocystic a.
occupational a.
oil a.
papular a.
pyogenic sterile arthritis, pyoderma gangrenosum, and a.
a. rosacea
a. scar
synovitis, acne, pustulosis, hyperostosis, osteomyelitis syndrome
tar a.
tropical a.
a. vulgaris

acneiform
a. dermatitis
a. eruption
a. lesion
a. rash

acneiformis
nevus acneiformis unilateralis

acontractility
detrusor a.

acorn-shaped implant

acoustic
a. agnosia
a. ambiguity
anterior acoustic stria
a. comfort index
contralateral acoustic stimulation
a. enhancement
a. evoked response
fetal acoustic stimulation testing
a. hair cell
a. imaging
a. impedance
internal acoustic meatus
internal acoustic orifice
longitudinal acoustic wave
maximum acoustic output
multicystic acoustic neuroma
a. muscle reflex
a. myography
a. nerve
a. nerve damage
nerve of external acoustic meatus
a. neuroma
a. noise test
notch in cartilage of acoustic meatus
nucleus of acoustic nerve
opening of external acoustic meatus
opening of internal acoustic meatus
oral-nasal acoustic ratio
orifice of external acoustic meatus
orifice of internal acoustic meatus
oronasal acoustic ratio
peak acoustic gain
a. pressure amplitude
a. quantification
a. reflex test
a. reflex threshold
a. resonance
a. respiratory motion sensor
a. response technology
a. rhinometry
scanning laser acoustic microscope
a. schwannoma

acoustic *(continued)*
sensitivity prediction by acoustic reflex
a. signal
slow-growing acoustic neuroma
spectral gradient acoustic reflectometry
a. stimulation test
a. tumor
vibratory acoustic stimulation
a. window

acquiescence
social a.

acquiescent response scale

acquired
a. abscess
adult acquired flatfoot
adult acquired micrognathia
alcohol acquired chronic hepatocerebral degeneration
a. angioedema
a. aplastic anemia
a. atelectasis
autoimmune acquired hemolytic anemia
blood product contaminated by acquired immune deficiency syndrome
a. brain injury
carrier of acquired immune deficiency syndrome
a. cellular immunodeficiency syndrome
chronic, acquired, pure red cell aplasia
a. cold urticaria
community a.
congenital versus acquired syndrome
congenital vs. acquired syndrome
a. cystic kidney disease
a. diabetes insipidus
distal acquired demyelinating symmetrical neuropathy
emotional effects of acquired immune deficiency syndrome
a. epilepsy
a. epileptic aphasia
Evaluating A. Skills in Communication
a. flatfoot
a. functional megacolon
a. gustolacrimal reflex
a. harelip
a. hemolytic anemia
a. hepatocerebral degeneration
a. hernia
hospital a.
a. hydrocephalus
a. hyperostosis syndrome
idiopathic acquired hemolytic disease
idiopathic acquired refractory sideroblastic anemia
idiopathic acquired sideroblastic anemia
a. idiopathic sideroblastic anemia
a. immune deficiency syndrome
a. immune deficiency syndrome antibody
a. immune deficiency syndrome antibody test
a. immune deficiency syndrome-associated transfusion
a. immune deficiency syndrome carrier
a. immune deficiency syndrome crisis
a. immune deficiency syndrome dementia complex
a. immune deficiency syndrome epidemic
a. immune deficiency syndrome infected child
a. immune deficiency syndrome mandatory testing
a. immune deficiency syndrome prevention
a. immune deficiency syndrome primary pathogen
a. immune deficiency syndrome-related complex
a. immune deficiency syndrome-related dementia
a. immune deficiency syndrome-related macular degeneration
a. immune deficiency syndrome residential treatment facility
a. immune deficiency syndrome tainted transfusion
a. immune deficiency syndrome transmission
a. immune deficiency syndrome treatment
a. immune deficiency syndrome virus infection
a. immune hemolytic disease
a. immunity
a. immunodeficiency syndrome
A. Immunodeficiency Syndrome Beliefs and Behavior Questionnaire
a. immunodeficiency syndrome health assessment questionnaire
a. immunodeficiency syndrome-related complex
a. immunodeficiency syndrome-related virus
a. immunodeficiency syndrome with Kaposi sarcoma
a. infection
juvenile acquired hypothyroidism
localized acquired cutaneous pseudoxanthoma elasticum
mandatory acquired immune deficiency syndrome testing
mechanical acquired ptosis
a. melanocytic nevus
a. monosaccharide intolerance
mother infected with acquired immune deficiency syndrome
multifocal acquired motor axonopathy
myogenic acquired ptosis
National Institute of A. Immune Deficiency
neurogenic acquired ptosis
neuropsychiatric acquired immunodeficiency syndrome rating scale
newly acquired disease
nosocomial acquired pneumonia
patient unknown acquired immune deficiency syndrome carrier
pediatric acquired immunodeficiency syndrome
a. perforating dermatosis
primary acquired melanosis
primary acquired nasolacrimal duct obstruction
primary acquired preleukemic syndrome
primary acquired sideroblastic anemia
a. progressive lymphangioma
a. prothrombin complex deficiency syndrome
a. red-cell aplasia
a. reflex
a. renal cystic disease
a. resistance to antibiotic
secretion and spill from acquired immune deficiency syndrome
a. severe aplastic anemia
sexually acquired reactive arthritis
Sheffield Screening Test for A. Language Disorders
simian acquired immunodeficiency syndrome
transfusion-associated acquired immune deficiency syndrome

transfusion-transmitted acquired immune deficiency syndrome
a. tufted angioma
a. valvular heart disease
a. ventricular septal defect
a. violence immune deficiency syndrome
a. von Willebrand disease
X-linked mental retardation, seizures, acquired microcephaly, agenesis of corpus callosum

acquisita
epidermolysis bullosa a.

acquisition
data acquisition processor
dual-isotope simultaneous acquisition single-photon emission computed tomography
fast acquisition multiple excitation
gradient-recalled acquisition in steady state
gradient-refocused acquisition in a steady state
half-Fourier acquisition single-shot turbo spin-echo
hybrid rapid acquisition with relaxation enhancement
language acquisition device
long axis a.
magnitude preparation-rapid acquisition gradient echo
multiple gated a.
multiple gated acquisition scan
multiple overlapping thin-slab a.
nuclear multiple gaited a.
parallel data acquisition coil
psychological information, acquisition, processing, and control system
rapid acquisition computed axial tomography
rapid acquisition with relaxation enhancement
rapid acquisition with resolution enhancement
stimulated echo acquisition mode
a. time
a. zoom

acral arteriovenous tumor

Acrel ganglion

acrid odor

acrocallosal syndrome

acrocephalosyndactyly syndrome

acrocyanosis
orthostatic a.
peripheral a.

acrodermatitis
papular a.
papular acrodermatitis of childhood
papulovesicular a.

acrofacial
Genée-Wiedemann acrofacial dysostosis
Nager acrofacial dysostosis
postaxial acrofacial dysostosis syndrome

acrokeratosis
paraneoplastic a.

acrolocated
papulovesicular acrolocated syndrome

acromandibular dysplasia

acromegalic
a. gigantism
a. heart disease

acromegaloid
a. facial appearance
a. facial syndrome

acromial
subcutaneous acromial bursa

acromiale
os a.

acromioclavicular
Allman acromioclavicular injury classification
articular disc of acromioclavicular joint
a. joint
a. joint injury
a. ligament
meniscus of acromioclavicular joint
Neviaser acromioclavicular technique

acromiodorsoanterior
left acromiodorsoanterior position of fetus
right acromiodorsoanterior fetal position

acromiodorsoposterior
left acromiodorsoposterior position of fetus
right acromiodorsoposterior fetal position

acromiohumeral interval

acromion
articular surface of a.
a. process

acromionectomy
Armstrong a.

acromioplasty
anterior a.
anterior acromioplasty approach
arthroscopic a.
McLaughlin a.
Neer a.
Neer acromioplasty for rotator cuff tear

acroparesthesia
Nothnagel-type a.

acropathy
mutilating a.

acrosomal
outer acrosomal membrane

acrospiroma
malignant clear cell a.

across
horizontal incision across lower abdomen

acrosyndactyly
Apert a.

acrylic
alveolar arch acrylic splint
antibiotic-loaded acrylic cement
autopolymerizing acrylic resin
a. bone cement
a. cement
a. implant
a. lens
lunate acrylic cement wrist prosthesis
multifunctional a.
a. plastic
prosthetic antibiotic-loaded acrylic cement
a. resin
a. splint
a. veneer crown

act
aggressive a.
Americans with Disabilities A.
assaultive a.
Baker A.
CARE A.
Clinical Laboratory Improvement A.
compulsive a.
Dangerous Drugs A.
Employee Retirement Income Security A.

act *(continued)*
Family and Medical Leave A. of 1993
Federal False Claims A.
Federal Food, Drug, and Cosmetic A.
Freedom of Information A.
a. of God
Good Samaritan A.
Hazardous Substances A.
Individuals with Disabilities Education A.
life-terminating acts without the explicit request
Medicare Bone Mass Measurement Standardization A.
mental a.
Mental Health Early Intervention, Treatment, and Prevention Act of 2000
Mental Health Parity Act of 1998
Nurse Training A.
Nutrition Labeling and Education A. of 1990
Prescription Drug User Fee A.
Safe Medical Device A.
Toxic Substance Control A.
a.'s of violence

acted
Baker a.

ACTH-independent bilateral macronodular hyperplasia

ACTH-producing adenoma

actin
alpha smooth muscle a.
antismooth muscle a.
filamentous a.
fluorescent actin staining
muscle a.
muscle-specific a.
neutrophil actin deficiency
neutrophil actin dysfunction
smooth muscle a.

acting
amphetamine or similarly acting sympathomimetic intoxication
asocial acting out
criminal acting out
impulsive acting out
locally acting paracrine effector
neurotic acting out
passive-aggressive acting out
patient acting inappropriately
peripherally acting anticholinergic medication

actinic
a. cheilitis
chronic actinic dermatitis
a. conjunctivitis
a. dermatitis
disseminated superficial actinic porokeratosis
a. granuloma
a. keratitis
a. keratosis
Miescher actinic granuloma
O'Brien actinic granuloma
precancerous actinic keratosis
a. ray
a. reticuloid dermatitis
a. reticuloid syndrome
a. retinitis

actinium emanation

actinomycosis
pelvic a.

actinotherapy
pulsed ultraviolet a.

action
abnormal peristaltic action of colon
addictive feeling and a.
a. against burns
agent, action, and object
brief, small, abundant motor-unit action potential
clot dissolving a.
clotting action of blood
compound motor action potential
compound muscle action potential
compound muscle-motor action potential
compound nerve action potential
consequences of a.
data, action, response
data, action, response, and evaluation
delayed a.
disordered action of heart
duration of a.
eighth nerve action potential
erythema a.
evoked muscle action potential
evoked sensory nerve action potential
Facial A. Coding System
faulty valve a.
fibrillating action potential
fixed action pattern
heart pumping a.
impulsive a.'s
increased action of reflex
individual motor unit action potential
ineffective heart a.
irregular heart a.
ligand-dependent action of thyroid hormone receptor
ligand-independent action of thyroid hormone receptor
lithium action on first messenger
lithium action on membranes
lithium action on second messenger
macro motor unit action potential
mass action law
mass action principle
mass action theory
mechanism of a.
membrane stabilizing a.
migrating action potential complex
mixed nerve action potential
mode of a.
monophasic action potential duration
motor unit action potential
multiple a.
multiple action cutter
muscle fiber action potential
National Arthritis A. Plan
nerve fiber action potential
no action indicated
no further action required
normal bowel a.
nursing a.
a. pattern
a. potential
a. potential duration
prolonged a.
rapid heart a.
repeat action tablet
repetitive bursts of action potential
Rincoe human action bionic
sensory nerve action potential
slowness of mental a.
specific action exercise
specific dynamic a.
sustained a.
test-estrin timed a.
triphasic action potential
virus-like a.
visual action time
voluntary muscle a.
wounded in a.

activated

autologous lymphokine activated killer cell
automated activated partial thromboplastin
carbonaceous activated water
a. charcoal
a. clotting factor
a. clotting time
a. coagulation time
electrically activated implant
a. endothelial cell
a. epilepsy
a. estrogen receptor
a. fatty acid
a. graft
a. hydrogen
magnetically activated cell sorter
mechanically activated implant
mitomycin adsorbed onto activated charcoal
multiple-dose activated charcoal
nuclear factor of activated T cell
a. partial thromboplastin time
peptide activated lymphocyte
pokeweed activated spleen conditioned medium
product of activated lymphocyte
a. protein C
a. protein C resistance
recalcified whole-blood activated clotting time
recombinant human activated protein C
repeated oral doses of activated charcoal
resistance activated protein C
semicontinuous activated sludge
a. thymus cell
tumor-derived activated cell
whole-blood activated clotting time

activates

a. chemical impulse of brain
a. facial expression
a. graft

activating

a. adjusting instrument
amino acid activating enzyme
apoptosis activating factor
endothelial-monocyte activating polypeptide II
a. enzyme
a. factor
human macrophage-monocyte chemotactic and activating factor
liver-enriched activating protein
monocyte chemotactic and activating factor
pituitary adenylate cyclase activating polypeptide
reticular activating system
smooth muscle activating factor
a. transcription factor
upstream activating sequence

activating/aggregating

platelet activating/aggregating factor

activation

anterior hippocampal a.
ascending reticular a.
atrial activation mapping
atrial activation time
cytotoxic lymphocyte activation antigen 4 immunoglobulin
endocardial activation mapping
a. energy
immunoreceptor tyrosine-based activation motif
instrumental neutron activation analysis
left ventricular activation time
light activation by stimulated emission of radiation
linker for activation of T cell
lyl-1 oncogene a.
lymphocyte activation factor
lyt-10 oncogene a.
a. map-guided surgical resection
mitogen a.
natural killer cell a.
NK cell a.
partial body neutron a.
phytohemagglutinin a.
platelet activation defect
protein kinase activation ratio
radiochemical neutron activation analysis
region of a.
regulated upon activation, normal T-cell expressed and secreted
right ventricular a.
signaling lymphocytic activation molecule
synaptic electronic a.
thrombin activation device
thromboplastin activation test
total body neutron a.
total body neutron activation analysis
trypsin activation peptide
ventricular activation time
ventricular premature a.
very late a.

activation-induced

a.-i. cell death
tumor necrosis factor-related activation-induced cytokine

activator

anisoylated plasminogen streptokinase activator complex
catabolite activator protein
catabolite gene a.
catabolite gene activator protein
2-chain urokinase plasminogen a.
extrinsic plasminogen a.
galactose enzyme a.
Janus kinase/signal transducer and activator of transcription
lung Hageman factor a.
plasminogen a.
plasminogen activator inhibitor type 1, 2
prekallikrein a.
a. protein
receptor activator of NF-κB
receptor activator of nuclear factor-kappa B
receptor activator of nuclear factor kappa B ligand
recombinant plasminogen a.
recombinant, single-chain, urokinase-type plasminogen a.
recombinant tissue-type plasminogen a.
signal transducer and activator of transcription-4
signal transducer and activator of transcription-5
sphingolipid activator protein-1
tissue plasminogen a.
urokinase plasminogen a.
urokinase plasminogen activator receptor
urokinase-type plasminogen a.
vascular plasminogen a.

activator-releasing

plasminogen activator-releasing hormone

active

a. alcoholic
a. alignment
a. ankle joint complex range of motion
anterior active mask rhinomanometry
arrest of active phase dystocia
artificial active immunity
a. assisted exercise
a. assistive exercise
attitude of active friendliness

active *(continued)*
autoimmune chronic active hepatitis
autoimmune-type chronic active hepatitis
a. avoidance
a. avoidance reaction
awake and active state
a. bending exercise
a. bilaterally
biologically active luteinizing hormone
a. bleeding
a. bowel sounds
bowel sounds normal and a.
bowel sounds present and a.
a. brain tissue
brisk and a.
centrally active phenethylamine derivative related to amphetamine and methamphetamine
chronic active cirrhosis
chronic active gastritis
chronic active hepatitis B
chronic active hepatitis with cirrhosis
chronic active liver disease
chronic active lupoid hepatitis
chronic active viral hepatitis
chronic active viral hepatitis, non-A, non-B
chronic active viral hepatitis, type B
a. chronic hepatitis
a. chronic inflammation
clinically active stage
a. compression-decompression
condemnation of active euthanasia
a. contractions
a. culture
deep tendon reflexes active and equal bilaterally
a. disease
a. disease process
a. electrode
enzymatic a.
a. epileptic process
a. euthanasia
a. exercise
fetus a.
a. flexion
a. hallucinations
a. hepatitis
highly active antiretroviral therapy
highly active antiretroviral treatment
a. hip movement
a. hostility index
a. hyperemia
a. hyperemia of retina
immediate active cutaneous anaphylaxis
a. immune system
a. immunity
a. immunization
a. incontinence
a. infection
a. infiltrate
a. inflammation
a. insufficiency
a. integral range of motion
a. intervention
a. invasive infectious process
a. involvement
a. knee extension
a. labor
a. life expectancy
a. lifestyle
a. listening
a. liver disease
lower fossa active, lateral knee pain, and long leg on the side ipsilateral to the weak fossa
a. medication
methylene blue active substance
minimal active muscle tendon tension
minimally active infant
a. motion
a. motion testing
a. movement
no active pulmonary disease
no evidence of active disease
normal and a.
not in active labor
a. oozing from site
a. oozing from wound
osmotically active substance
a. panic attack
a. and passive range of motion
patient admitted with active infection
patient physically a.
patient regained active status
a. pepsin
a. peristalsis
a. phase
a. phase of labor
photosynthetically active radiation
a. and present
present, active, equal
present and active reflexes
a. psychosis
a. pulmonary disease
a. quad strengthening exercise
a. range-of-motion exercise
released from active duty
a. renin concentration
a. resistance
a. resistive range of motion
rheumatoid biologically active factor
a. rosette-forming T cell
salvage highly active antiretroviral therapy
a. seizure
sexually active homosexual men
a. sleep
a. sleep state
slightly a.
a. specific immunotherapy
a. syphilis
systemic active immunotherapy
a. systemic anaphylaxis
total active motion
a. trabecular calcification surface
a. treatment
a. treatment period
a. tuberculosis
a. ulcer
upper fossa active, medial knee pain, and short leg on the side ipsilateral to the weak fossa
a. wrist rotation unit

active-assisted range of motion

actively
doctor actively caused death
a. suicidal

active-release technique

active-resistive exercises

activin
a. receptor
a. receptor IB, II, IIB

Activities-Specific Balance Confidence Scale

activity
abnormal alpha a.
abnormal electrical a.
abnormal heart a.
abnormally fast a.
absence of electrical a.
acetylcholine receptor-inducing a.
acetylene reduction a.
adenosine deaminase a.
adenosine triphosphatase a.
adolescent sexual a.
aimless motor a.
alkaline phosphatase activity of granular leukocyte

alpha frequency a.
alternative leisure a.
amylase inhibitor a.
antibacterial a.
anticomplement a.
antimuscarine cholinergic a.
antithymic a.
area of increased a.
arylsulfatase activity test
a. as tolerated
asymmetrical generalized epileptiform a.
background of slow a.
a. and behavior
Behavior A. Profile
biologic a.
Birmingham Vasculitis A. Score
blood granulocyte-specific a.
blood pool a.
bone-resorbing a.
bone scan reveals increased a.
bone scan showed increased a.
a. of both hemispheres
brain electrical a.
brain electrical activity map
brain electrical activity mapping
brain wave a.
burst of alpha a.
burst-promoting a.
bursts of beta a.
cancer cell-derived blood coagulating activity 1
cerebral activity of brain
cessation of a.
change in a.
chaotic activity of ventricular fibrillation
chaotic elcctrical a.
chemotactic a.
cholesterol-esterifying a.
chymotrypsin inhibitor a.
ciliary dyskinesia a.
Clinical Colitis A. Index
a. coefficient
colony-inhibiting a.
colony-stimulating a.
concentrated mental a.
continuous motor unit a.
continuous seizure a.
controlling alpha a.
Crohn Disease A. Index
cumulated a.
cystic fibrosis factor a.
cytotoxic T lymphocyte a.
a.'s of daily living
a.'s of daily living scale
day activity center
decreased brain a.
decreased brain wave a.
delta a.
delta activity of low amplitude
delusional type of a.
Developmental Activities Screening Inventory
diminished brain a.
diminution of background a.
diversional a.
diversional activity deficit
Duke A. Status Index
dynamic physical a.
efferent renal sympathetic nerve a.
efferent sympathetic a.
eighth nerve a.
electrical activity between electrodes
electrical activity of brain
electrical activity of heart
electrical response a.
electric control a.
electrodermal a.
electrographic seizure a.
Emotionality A. Sociability Scale
endogenous avidin-binding a.
endometrial cycling a.
endotoxin-like a.
energy expended with a.
esterase a.
evaluation of resting a.
excessive brain a.
excessive diffuse low and medium wave beta a.
excessive fast brain wave a.
excessive motor a.
extended activities of daily living
face, legs, activity, cry, consolability
factor VIII inhibitor bypassing a.
fetal activity acceleration determination
Fetal A. Test
fibrinolytic a.
filter paper a.
fine motor a.
fluids, aeration, nutrition, communication, activity, and pain
fluids, aeration, nutrition, communication, activity, and stimulation
focus of slow a.
frequent individual bursts of alpha a.
frontal intermittent rhythmic delta a.
frontal irregular rhythmic delta a.
functional a.
general gonadotropic a.
generalized fast a.
generalized slow a.
granulocyte-macrophage colony-stimulating a.
gross motor a.
a. group therapy
headache activity and desensitization
Health and A. Limitation Survey
heavy exertional a.
hemagglutinating a.
heparin-neutralizing a.
hepatitis activity index
highest level of a.
highly activity epileptic process
high-risk sexual a.
high-voltage fast a.
high-voltage slow a.
high-voltage slow-wave a.
His bundle a.
histamine-releasing a.
histologic activity index
history activity index
home uterine activity monitor
home uterine activity monitoring
hospital activity analysis
household a.
immunobiologic a.
impaired brain a.
impaired normal a.
impairment of activities of daily living
inactive renin a.
increase in amplitude of electrical a.
increased brain a.
increased physical a.
increased psychomotor a.
increased reflex a.
increased thyroid a.
independent in activities of daily living
insulin-degrading a.
insulin-like a.
a. interest and aptitude
intermittent rhythmic delta a.
a. intolerance
intrinsic a.
intrinsic stimulating a.
intrinsic sympathomimetic a.
involvement in reckless a.

activity *(continued)*
irregular spiking activity in electroencephalography
jaw muscle a.
large amplitude, slow wave a.
Leisure Activities Blank
leukemia-associated inhibitory a.
leukocyte alkaline phosphatase a.
leukocyte-specific a.
leukotactic factor a.
a. level
lipoprotein lipase a.
localized brain a.
A. Loss Assessment
loss of interest in peer social a.
loss of interest in usual a.
low-voltage electrocortical a.
low-voltage fast a.
lupus anticoagulant a.
lymphocyte chemoattractant a.
lymphocyte-transforming a.
lymphotoxin antitumor a.
lysosomal enzymatic a.
macrophage phagocytic a.
macrophage tumoricidal a.
Manning score of fetal a.
marrow repopulation a.
mast cell-enhancing a.
mean dose per unit cumulated a.
medium voltage a.
melanoma growth-stimulating a.
membrane-stabilizing a.
metabolic activity factor
a. metabolic rate
MHC class I-restricted cytolytic a.
mobility activities of daily living
monocyte chemoattractant and activity factor
monophasic endplate a.
monorhythmic frontal delta a.
motor activity log
multiple unit a.
multiplication-stimulating a.
muscle a.
muscle sympathetic nerve a.
mutagenic a.
myoclonic twitch a.
National Association of A. Professionals
natural killer a.
nerve growth stimulating a.
neutrophil aggregation a.
neutrophil chemotactic a.
neutrophil-inducing a.
neutrophil respiratory burst a.
no detectable a.
nonexercise activity thermogenesis
nonrhythmic electroencephalogram a.
nonsuppressible insulinlike a.
nonsuppressible insulinlike activity factor
normal electroencephalogram a.
normal heart a.
normal lactase a.
normal waking a.
no voluntary a.
occipital dominant intermittent rhythmic delta a.
opsonic a.
organically impaired brain a.
outside activity avoidance
paroxysmal alpha a.
partial agonist a.
pathologic spontaneous a.
patient global assessment of disease a.
patient independent in activities of daily living
patient with severe systemic disease limiting activity but not incapacitating
pattern of brain electrical a.
pattern of electrical a.
A. Pattern Indicator
Peabody Developmental Motor A. Cards
peak phrenic nerve a.
Pediatric Crohn Disease A. Index
Perianal Crohn Disease A. Index
peripheral androgen a.
peripheral androgen activity marker
peripheral cholinergic a.
peripheral electromyographic a.
peripheral vein renin a.
peroxidatic a.
personal self-maintenance a.
Physical A. Readiness Questionnaire
plasma insulin a.
plasma-recognition-factor a.
plasma renin substrate a.
plasmin renin a.
polyclonal B-cell a.
polymorphic delta a.
postheparin lipolytic a.
procoagulant a.
progression of a.
protection, restricted activity, ice, compression, elevation
proteolytic a.
prothrombin a.
pulseless electrical a.
radioreceptor a.
reckless and impulsive a.
recorded electrical brain a.
recording of electrical a.
reduced tolerance for physical a.
reflex vasculopathic a.
regular spiking a.
relative chemotactic a.
relative specific a.
renal vein plasma renin a.
renal vein/renal activity ratio
renal vein renin a.
renewed tumor a.
renin a.
resting muscle a.
a. restriction
retained alpha a.
retained cortical a.
retard bone a.
rheumatoid factorlike a.
runs of slow a.
scheduled nursing activities program
serum bactericidal a.
serum inhibitory a.
serum prothrombin a.
shift in direction and pattern of brain electrical a.
simulated activities of daily living
single potential analysis cavernous electrical a.
single unit a.
skin sympathetic a.
SLE Disease A. Index
slow waking a.
slow wave a.
snooze-induced excitation of sympathetic triggered a.
spastic muscle a.
specific a.
Specific A. Scale
spermatogenic activity test
spiking a.
spleen repopulating a.
spontaneous activity test
spontaneous electrical a.
spontaneous motor a.
spontaneous suppressor cell a.
steroid protein activity index
stimulated fibrinolytic a.
stromal osteoclast-forming a.
succinic dehydrogenase a.
suppressor cell a.
surfactant-like a.
sympathetic a.

sympathetic efferent nerve a.
Systemic Lupus Erythematosus Disease A. Index
Systemic Lupus A. Measure
thermic effect of physical a.
thermodynamic a.
a. threshold
thromblastic activity of amniotic fluid
thyrotropin-displacing a.
thyroxine-specific a.
tissue lactase a.
total antitryptic a.
total renin a.
a. training
transketolase a.
trypsin-binding a.
tumor activity test
tyrosine kinase a.
upright peripheral plasma renin a.
urinary muramidase a.
uterine a.
uterine activity integral
uterine activity unit
variations in electrical a.
ventricular ectopic a.
visual a.
vitiligo disease a.
vocal cord a.
wave lengths of rhythmic a.
whole-body a.
zone of polarizing a.

activity-interview group psychotherapy

activity-reactivity
autonomic a.-r.

activity-related heart problem

actual
a. body weight
a. immunity
a. mechanical advantage
a. suicide attempt
a. volume of lung

actuarial
multidimensional actuarial classification

actuation
direct mechanical ventricular a.

actuator
linear a.

acuity
best-corrected visual a.
Binocular Visual A. Test
Brightness A. Test
central visual a.
distance visual a.
distance visual acuity with correction
distance visual acuity without correction
dynamic visual a.
Functional A. Contrast Test
hearing acuity screening
laser interference a.
level of a.
Lighthouse Distance Visual A. Test
linear visual acuity test
loss of a.
loss of visual a.
minimum perceptible a.
minimum separable a.
motor discriminative a.
near acuity testing
near visual a.
normal visual a.
numerical visual a.
potential acuity meter
potential visual acuity meter
pure tone a.
Simultaneous Technique for A. and Readiness Testing
true visual a.
uncorrected visual a.
visual a.
visual acuity, left eye
visual acuity, left eye, left perception with projection
visual acuity loss
visual acuity, right eye
visual acuity screening
visual acuity test
visual discriminatory a.

acuminata
condylomata a.

acuminatum
condyloma a.
perianal condyloma a.

acuminatus
lichen ruber a.

acupoint
transcutaneous acupoint electrical stimulation

acupressure
self-massage acupressure for self-healing

acupuncture
a. analgesia
auricular a.
a. clinic
a. and transcutaneous electrical nerve stimulation

acustica
area a.

acusticae
maculae a.

acusticus
meatus acusticus externus
nervus a.
nucleus a.

acuta
parapsoriasis acuta et varioliformis

acute
a. abdomen
a. abdominal aortic occlusion
a. abdominal obstruction
a. abdominal series
a. abdominal tympany
a. abscess
a. acalculous cholecystitis
a. acidosis
a. adrenal insufficiency
a. adverse psychological reaction
a. agitated delirium
a. alcoholic hepatitis
a. alcohol intoxication
a. alcoholism
a. allergic encephalitis
a. allergic interstitial nephritis
a. allergic urticaria
a. allograft rejection
a. alveolar injury
a. amnesia
a. angle-closure glaucoma
anterior acute flexion elbow splint
anterior acute poliomyelitis
a. anterior uveitis
a. anxiety attack
a. anxiety reaction
a. aortic dissection
a. aortic insufficiency
a. appendicitis
a. articular rheumatism
a. aseptic meningitis
a. aseptic meningitis syndrome
a. asthma
a. asthma attack
a. atrophic spinal paralysis
a. attack of asthma
a. avulsion fracture
a. bacterial endocarditis
a. bacterial exacerbation of chronic bronchitis

acute *(continued)*
a. bacterial meningitis
a. bacterial myocarditis
a. bacterial rhinosinusitis
a. basophilic leukemia
B-cell acute lymphoblastic leukemia
bilateral acute retinal necrosis
bilateral otitis media, a.
a. blood loss
a. bovine pulmonary edema
a. brain disturbance
a. brain syndrome
a. bronchitis/bronchiolitis
a. bronchopulmonary asthma
Canadian A. Respiratory Illness and Flu Scale
a. canine idiopathic polyneuropathy
a. cardiac event
a. cardiac insufficiency
a. cardiogenic pulmonary edema
a. cardiorespiratory arrest
a. cardiovascular disease
a. care center
a. care for the elderly
a. care facility
a. care hospital
a. care unit
a. catarrhal inflammation
categories of acute nonlymphoblastic leukemia
a. cellular rejection
a. central cervical spinal cord injury
a. cerebellar ataxia
a. cerebral encephalopathy
a. cerebrospinal meningitis
a. cerebrovascular accident
a. cervical traumatic sprain or syndrome
a. change clinical score
a. change in mental status
a. chest syndrome
a. cholecystitis
a. and chronic alcohol ingestion
a. chronic glaucoma
a. and chronic inflammation
a. clinical illness
clinical manifestation of acute drug intoxication
a. cocaine intoxication
common acute lymphoblastic leukemia antigen
common acute lymphocytic leukemia antigen
a. compartment syndrome
compliance related acute complication
a. conditioned neurosis
conduction defect in acute myocardial infarction
a. confusional migraine
a. confusional state
a. congestive heart failure
contact lens-induced acute red eye
a. coronary event
a. coronary insufficiency
a. coronary occlusion
a. coronary syndrome
a. cutaneous lupus erythematosus
a. death syndrome
a. decubitus ulcer
a. delirium
a. dermatomyositis
a. diarrhea
a. diarrheal syndrome
differential diagnosis in acute drug intoxication
a. diffuse peritonitis
direct acute myocardial infarction angioplasty
a. disorder of cerebral circulation
a. disseminated encephalomyelitis
a. distress
a. diverticulitis
drug-associated primary acute pancreatitis
a. duodenal ulcer
a. dystonic reaction
a. edematous pancreatitis
a. enteritis
epidemic acute nonbacterial gastroenteritis
a. epidemic infectious adenitis
a. erosive gastritis
a. erythroleukemia
a. esophageal food impaction
a. event
a. exacerbation
a. exacerbation of chronic bronchitis
a. exertional compartment syndrome
a. exertional rhabdomyolysis
a. fatty liver
a. fatty liver of pregnancy
a. febrile illness
a. febrile neutrophilic dermatosis
a. febrile respiratory disease
a. febrile respiratory illness
a. fibropurulent pneumonia
a. flaccid paralysis
a. flank pain
a. focal bacterial nephritis
a. focal cerebral ischemia
a. food allergy
a. gallstone pancreatitis
a. gangrenous appendicitis
a. gastric dilatation
a. gastric mucosal lesion
a. gastritis
a. gastrointestinal hemorrhage
a. generalized exanthematous pustulosis
a. generalized tuberculosis
a. glaucoma
a. gonococcal arthritis
a. gout
a. gouty arthritis
a. graft-versus-host disease
a. granulocytic leukemia
a. hallucinatory mania
a. hallucinatory paranoia
a. hallucinosis
a. head trauma
a. heart attack
a. heart disease
a. heart failure
a. heart muscle degeneration
a. hematogenous osteomyelitis
a. hemiplegia
a. hemolytic anemia
a. hemolytic uremic syndrome
a. hemorrhagic bronchopneumonia
a. hemorrhagic conjunctivitis
a. hemorrhagic cystitis
a. hemorrhagic edema
a. hemorrhagic edema of infancy
a. hemorrhagic encephalomyelitis
a. hemorrhagic leukoencephalitis
a. hemorrhagic pancreatitis
a. hepatic coma
a. hepatic failure
a. hepatic rupture
a. hepatocellular necrosis
a. herpetic gingival stomatitis
a. HIV-1 infection
a. homosexual panic
a. humoral rejection
a. hydrocephalus
a. hypertensive episode
hypoplastic acute leukemia
a. hypoxemic respiratory failure
idiopathic acute eosinophilic pneumonia
a. idiopathic demyelinating polyradiculoneuritis
a. idiopathic inflammatory bowel disease

a. idiopathic pericarditis
a. idiopathic peripheral facial nerve palsy
a. idiopathic polyneuritis
a. idiopathic thrombocytopenic purpura
a. illness
a. incontinence
infant in acute respiratory distress
a. infarct
a. infection
a. infectious colitis
a. infectious diarrhea
a. infectious disease
a. infectious disease series
a. infectious gastroenteritis
a. infectious lymphocytosis
a. infectious mononucleosis
a. infectious nonbacterial gastroenteritis
a. infectious polyneuritis
a. infective endocarditis
a. inflammation
a. inflammatory cell
a. inflammatory demyelinating polyneuropathy
a. inflammatory demyelinating polyradiculoneuropathy
a. inflammatory demyelinating polyradiculopathy
a. injury
a. injury to brain
a. insulin response
a. intensive treatment
intermittent acute porphyria
intermittent episode of acute abdominal pain
a. intermittent porphyria
a. intermittent primary angle-closure glaucoma
interstitial acute inflammatory cell
a. interstitial pneumonia
a. interstitial pneumonitis
a. interstitial tubular nephritis
a. intestinal infection
a. intestinal obstruction
a. intoxication
a. intoxication with hallucinogen
a. intrapartum fetal distress
a. intraventricular hemorrhage
a. ionization detector
a. ischemia
ischemic acute renal failure
a. ischemic brain infarct
a. ischemic coronary syndrome
a. ischemic heart disease
a. ischemic stroke
a. isolated myocarditis
a. joint syndrome
a. kidney inflammation
a. laryngotracheobronchitis
a. lateral sclerosis
a. lead poisoning
a. left ventricular heart failure
a. lethal catatonia
a. leukemia protocol
lichenoid acute pityriasis
a. life-threatening event
a. liver failure
long-term acute care
A. Low Back Pain Screening Questionnaire
a. low back syndrome
a. lumbar trauma syndrome
a. lung injury
a. lung rejection
a. lupus pericarditis
a. lupus pneumonitis
a. lymphoblastic leukemia in children
a. lymphoblastic leukemia secondary to Burkitt lymphoma
a. lymphoblastic lymphoma
a. lymphoblastic myelogenous leukemia
a. lymphocytic leukemia
a. lymphocytic leukemia antigen
a. manic episode
a. maxillary sinusitis
a. medical illness
a. medical management intervention
a. megakaryoblastic leukemia
membranous acute inflammation
a. mesenteric vascular insufficiency
Miami A. Care
microgranular acute promyelocytic leukemia
a. miliary tuberculosis
minor acute illness
a. mitral regurgitation
a. monoblastic leukemia
a. monocytic leukemia
a. monophasic experimental autoimmune encephalomyelitis
a. motor-axonal neuropathy
a. motor-sensory axonal neuropathy
a. mountain sickness
a. multifocal posterior placoid pigment epitheliopathy
multiple acute rejection episode
a. multiple brain infarct
a. myeloblastic leukemia
a. myelocytic leukemia
a. myelofibrosis
a. myeloid leukemia
a. myelomonoblastic leukemia
a. myelomonocytic leukemia
a. myocardial ischemia
myoglobinuric rhabdomyolytic acute renal failure
a. narrow angle glaucoma
a. necrotizing myelitis
a. necrotizing pancreatitis
a. necrotizing ulcerative gingivitis
a. nephritis
nephrotoxic acute renal failure
a. nerve irritation
neuroleptic-induced acute dystonia
neuroleptic-induced acute movement disorder
NIH Classification Category I acute bacterial prostatitis
no acute change
no acute disease
no acute distress
no acute inflammation
no acute trauma
a. nonhemorrhagic infarct
a. nonlymphoblastic leukemia
a. nonlymphocytic leukemia
a. nonlymphoid leukemia
a. normovolemic hemodilution
no signs of acute disease
null cell acute lymphocytic leukemia
a. obstructive suppurative cholangitis
a. on chronic liver disease
a. on chronic renal failure
a. onset
a. organic brain syndrome
a. organ rejection
a. osteomyelitis
a. otitis media
otitis media, acute, catarrhal
otitis media, acute, suppurating
otitis media, catarrhal, a.
otitis media, purulent, a.
a. pain
a. paranoid schizophrenic reaction
a. parathyroidectomy
parenchymatous acute renal failure
a. pathology
Pediatric A. Admission Severity classification
a. pelvic inflammatory disease

acute *(continued)*
a. pelvic pain
a. pericarditis
a. peritonitis
a. pharyngitis
a. pharyngoconjunctival fever
a. phase
a. phase reactant
a. phase reaction
a. phase response
a. phase response element
a. physiology and chronic health evaluation score
a. polioencephalitis
a. polycystic disease
a. portal inflammation
a. posterior multifocal placoid pigment epitheliopathy
a. postinfectious glomerulonephritis
postischemic acute renal failure
postischemic acute tubular necrosis
a. postoperative renal failure
poststreptococcal acute glomerulonephritis
a. poststreptococcal glomerulonephritis
posttransplant acute renal failure
posttraumatic acute renal failure
a. posttraumatic stress syndrome
prerenal acute renal failure
a. primary angle-closure glaucoma
a. primary keratotic gingivostomatitis
a. progranulocytic leukemia
a. proliferative
a. proliferative glomerulonephritis
prolonged acute hepatitis
prolonged acute tissue expansion
a. promyelocytic leukemia
a. psychotic episode
a. pulmonary edema
a. pulmonary hemorrhage
a. pyelonephritis
a. radiation disease
a. radiation pneumonitis
a. rectal hemorrhage
a. recurrent pancreatitis
a. renal failure and chronic renal failure
a. renal insufficiency
a. renal necrosis
a. repetitive seizure
respiratory battery, a.
a. respiratory distress syndrome
a. respiratory insufficiency
a. respiratory tract illness
a. response
a. retinal necrosis syndrome
a. retroviral syndrome
a. rheumatic arthritis
a. rheumatic fever
a. rhinitis
a. right heart syndrome
right otitis media, suppurative, a.
a. right ventricular heart failure
a. salivary adenitis
schizophrenic reaction, acute, paranoid
schizophrenic reaction, acute undifferentiated
a. sclerosing hyaline necrosis
Score for Neonatal Acute Physiology-Perinatal Extension
screening and acute care
a. seizure
a. self-limited colitis
a. septicemia
a. serum sickness
severe acute pancreatitis
a. severe hypotension
a. shortness of breath
a. sickle chest syndrome
Simplified A. Physiology Score
Simplified A. Physiology Score version II
a. sinusitis
a. soft tissue injury
a. spinal cord injury
a. spinal stenosis
a. splenic sequestration crisis
spontaneous acute bacterial peritonitis
steroid acute regulatory protein
steroid acute respiratory protein
steroidogenic acute regulatory protein
a. stress disorder
a. stress erosion
a. stress reaction
a. stroke unit
subacute treatment of acute drug intoxication
a. subarachnoid hemorrhage
a. subdural hematoma
a. subendocardial myocardial infarction
superimposed acute inflammatory episode
a. suppurative appendicitis
a. suppurative cholangitis
a. suppurative parotitis
a. surgical abdomen
a. symmetric polyarthritis
a. symptom
symptoms of acute drug intoxication
a. systemic lupus erythematosus
a. tamponade
T-cell acute lymphoblastic leukemia
therapy-related acute myelogenous leukemia
therapy-related acute myeloid leukemia
a. throat infection
a. throat irritation
a. thrombosis
a. thyroiditis
a. thyroparathyroidectomy
a. toxic encephalopathy
a. toxic hepatitis
a. tracheobronchitis
transfusion-related acute lung injury
a. transverse myelitis
a. transverse myelopathy
a. traumatic aortic injury
a. treatment for acute drug intoxication
treatment of acute drug reaction to hallucinogen
treatment of acute intoxication
a. tubular necrosis
a. tumor lysis
a. tumor lysis syndrome
a. ulcerative colitis
a. ulcerative gingivitis
a. undifferentiated leukemia
a. undifferentiated schizophrenic reaction
a. upper gastrointestinal bleeding
a. upper gastrointestinal hemorrhage
a. urethral syndrome
a. urethritis
a. urinary retention
a. vascular compromise
a. vascular xenograft rejection
a. vasomotor nephropathy
a. ventricular assist device
a. viral hepatitis
a. viral infection
a. viral respiratory infection
a. viral syndrome
a. whiplash
a. wound
a. yellow atrophy
a. zonal occult outer retinopathy

acutely
a. decompensated congestive heart failure
a. ill
a. inflamed appendix
patient acutely ill

acute-phase
a.-p. protein
a.-p. reactant protein

acyanotic heart disease

acyl carrier protein

acylcoenzyme
a. A
a. A oxidase

ad
guardian ad litem
a. hoc
a. lib
a. lib feeding
patient up ad lib

adactyly
partial a.

adamantinum
odontoma a.

Adamkiewicz
arteria radicularis magna of A.
artery of A.

Adam's apple

Adam sign

Adams-Stokes
A.-S. attack
A.-S. disease
A.-S. syndrome

adaptability
Cross-Cultural A. Inventory
Family A. and Cohesion Evaluation Scale
poor a.

adaptation
air pollution a.
Arthur A. of the Leiter International Performance Scale
dark adaptation test
Employment and A. Index
general adaptation syndrome
a. level
light a.
local adaptation syndrome
maternal ocular a.
prism adaptation test
Profile of A. to Life
Social A. Self-Evaluation Scale
Social A. Status
Student A. to College Questionnaire
Suprathreshold A. Test

adapted
A. Sequenced Inventory of Communication Development

adapter
band a.
catheter a.
friction-fit a.
Mayfield a.
Olympus a.
peripheral interface a.

adaptive
Assessment of A. Areas
Balthazar Scales of A. Behavior
basic adaptive process
A. Behavior Evaluation Scale
A. Behavior Inventory for Children
Checklist of A. Living Skills
Clinical A. Test
Clinical A. Test/Clinical Linguistic and Auditory Milestone Scale
a. control of thought
a. equipment
a. hand skills
a. hypertrophy
modal adaptive task
Neurologic and A. Capacity Score
pacemaker adaptive rate
a. response
a. support ventilation
a. thermogenesis

adaptometer
Feldman a.

adaptor
female-female a.

add
estrogen add back therapy

added
salt a.

ADD-H: Comprehensive Teacher's Rating Scale, Second Edition

addict
drug a.
halfway house for drug a.'s

addicted
Rehabilitative A. Family Treatment

addiction
computer addiction disorder
cultural definition of a.
diagnostic, social and addiction history form
a. disorder
drug/alcohol a.
dual drug a.
MacAndrew A. Scale
medically managed intensive addiction treatment unit
neonatal drug addiction seizure
nonprescription drug a.
over-the-counter drug a.
prescription drug a.
sex and love a.'s
a. specialist
Teen A. Severity Index
a. treatment program
a. withdrawal

addictionologist
certified a.

addiction-prone personality

addictive
a. behavior group
comorbid addictive behavior
a. disease unit
a. feeling and action
highly addictive and isolated
a. illicit drug
a. illness
a. personality

Addison
A. disease
hypoparathyroidism, Addison disease, and mucocutaneous candidiasis syndrome
multiple endocrine deficiency, Addison disease, and candidiasis syndrome
A. syndrome
thyroiditis, Addison disease, Sjögren syndrome, sarcoidosis syndrome

addisonian crisis

addition
Paced Auditory Serial A. Test

additional
a. cost of false negatives
a. cost of false positives
a. diagnosis
a. films
a. personal injury protection
a. procedure
a. qualifying symptoms
School Health A. Referral Program

additional *(continued)*
a. surgery
a. testing

additive
a. hormonal therapy
a. solution

addresin
mucosal addresin cell adhesion molecule-1

addressed
regional lymph nodes cannot be a.

adductable
distillable nonurea a.

adducted
a. great toe

adduction
a. contracture
a. contracture of hip
a. fracture
a. weakness

adduction-internal rotation deformity

adductocavus
metatarsus a.
metatarsus adductocavus deformity

adductor
anterior adductor of the coxa
a. aponeurosis
a. brevis
a. brevis muscle
a. compartment of thigh
a. digiti quinti
great adductor muscle
a. hallucis
a. hallucis longus
a. hallucis muscle
a. hallucis tendon
hip adductor stretch exercise
laryngeal adductor reflex
long adductor muscle
a. longus
a. longus muscle
musculus adductor brevis
musculus adductor hallucis
musculus adductor longus
musculus adductor magnus
musculus adductor minimus
musculus adductor pollicis
percutaneous adductor tenotomy
a. pollicis
pollicis adductor muscle
a. pollicis brevis tendon
a. pollicis muscle
a. pollicis obliquus muscle
a. spasmodic dysphonia
a. spasticity of hip
a. sweep of thumb
a. tenotomy
a. tenotomy and obturator neurectomy
a. tuberosity

adductovarus
forefoot a.
metatarsus a.
metatarsus adductovarus deformity

adductus
a. clubfoot
forefoot a.
Ganley and Ganley metatarsus adductus procedure
metatarsus a.
metatarsus adductus angle
metatarsus adductus deformity
metatarsus primus a.
midfoot a.
pes a.
pes equinovarus a.
true metatarsus a.

Adelaide River virus

adenine
a. arabinoside
a. arabinoside monophosphate
a. deaminase
a. deoxyribonucleotide
flavin adenine dinucleotide
nicotinamide adenine dinucleotidase
nicotinamide adenine dinucleotide glycohydrolase
nicotinamide adenine dinucleotide phosphate positive
a. nucleotide
oxidized form of nicotinamide adenine dinucleotide
oxidized form of nicotinamide adenine dinucleotide phosphate
pyruvate, inosine, glucose phosphate, and a.
sodium chloride, adenine, glucose, mannitol
thymine, adenine, and guanine
total adenine deoxyribonucleotide
total adenine nucleotide
total adenine ribonucleotide
yeast, peptone, and adenine sulfate

adenitis
acute epidemic infectious a.
acute salivary a.
mesenteric a.
periodic fever, aphthous stomatitis, pharyngitis, cervical a.
phlegmonous a.
regional a.

adenoacanthoma
lymph node endometriotic a.

adenoadipose flap

adenoassociated
a. virus
a. virus 1–5
a. virus for cystic fibrosis

adenocarcinoma
aggressive digital papillary a.
Barrett a.
basal cell a.
cell kinetics of a.
clear cell a.
colorectal a.
distal gastric a.
distal rectal a.
endometrial secretory a.
esophageal a.
a. of the esophagus
ethmoid sinus a.
goblet cell-type a.
a. in head of pancreas
lung adenocarcinoma cell
lymphangitic spread of prostatic a.
metastatic a.
metastatic adenocarcinoma serosal surfaces
minimal deviation a.
moderately differentiated a.
a. of Moll
mucinous adenocarcinoma of ovary
mucinous adenocarcinoma tumor
mucinous cell a.
ovarian clear cell a.
ovarian papillary serous a.
oxyphilic endometrioid a.
pancreatic ductal a.
polymorphous low-grade a.
polypoid adenocarcinoma of colon
poorly differentiated a.
primary adenocarcinoma of the gallbladder
a. of prostate gland
prostatic a.
serous a.
sinonasal a.
a. in situ
slow-growing invasive a.
slowly growing invasive a.
small bowel a.

synchronous colonic a.
urinary bladder a.
a. of the uterus with sarcomatous overgrowth
villoglandular a.
vulvar adenocystic a.
well-differentiated fetal a.
a. with myometrial invasion
a. with squamous differentiation

adenocystic
a. carcinoma
vulvar adenocystic adenocarcinoma

adenocystoma
papillary adenocystoma lymphomatosum

adenofibroma
metanephric a.

adenohypophysial
a. corticotroph cell
a. gangliocytoma
neoplastic adenohypophysial cell
a. neuronal choristoma

adenohypophysial-thyroid axis

adenohypophysitis
lymphocytic a.

adenoid
a.'s appeared enlarged
a. cystic carcinoma
a. cystic carcinoma of head and neck
a. degeneration agent
a.'s did not appear enlarged
disorder of a.'s
a. facies
hypertrophied a.
a. hypertrophy
hypertrophy of a.'s
hypertrophy of tonsils and a.'s
a. pad
pseudovascular adenoid squamous cell carcinoma
a. tonsil
tonsils and a.'s

adenoidal
a. facies
nonmalignant adenoidal hypertrophy

adenoidal:nasopharyngeal ratio

adenoidal-pharyngeal-conjunctival virus

adenoidectomy
tonsillectomy and a.
a. and tonsillectomy
a. with radium

adenolike

adenoma
aggressive digital papillary a.
aldosterone-producing a.
autonomous thyroid a.
bile duct a.
a. of the breast
calcified thyroid a.
clinically nonfunctioning pituitary a.
ectopic parathyroid a.
a. familial polyposis
a. fibrosum
gonadotropin-producing pituitary a.
growth hormone cell a.
growth hormone-producing a.
hepatic a.
hepatocellular a.
hereditary flat adenoma syndrome
high-grade dysplastic a.
Hürthle cell a.
Leydig cell a.
liver cell a.
mammosomatotroph cell a.
mediastinal parathyroid a.
mixed GH-PRL cell a.
mixed GH- and prolactin-secreting a.
mixed growth hormone-prolactin cell a.
mixed growth hormone- and prolactin-secreting a.
moderately differentiated a.
monomorphic a.
mucous gland adenoma of bronchus
multicentric islet cell a.
multifocal autonomic a.
nephrogenic bladder a.
nonfamilial parathyroid a.
nonfunctional pituitary a.
nonfunctioning pituitary a.
nonsecreting pituitary a.
nonsecretory adrenal a.
nontoxic thyroid a.
null cell a.
papillary adenoma of large intestine
papillary cystic a.
papillary eccrine a.
parathyroid a.
periampullary a.
Pick tubular a.
pleomorphic a.
prolactin-producing pituitary a.
recurrent pleomorphic a.
salivary gland pleomorphic a.
sarcoma, breast and brain tumors, leukemia, laryngeal and lung cancer a.
a. sebaceum
small bowel a.
testicular tubular a.
toxic a.
TSH-secreting pituitary a.
undifferentiated cell a.

adenoma-associated
a.-a. antigen
a.-a. calcification

adenoma-carcinoma sequence

adenoma-gangliocytoma
mixed pituitary a.-g.

adenomatoid
ameloblastic adenomatoid tumor
congenital cystic adenomatoid malformation
a. hyperplasia
a. nodule
odontogenic adenomatoid tumor
a. odontogenic tumor
a. tumor

adenomatosis
a. of colon and rectum
hereditary adenomatosis of colon and rectum
multiple endocrine a.
multiple endocrine adenomatosis type I, II
a. oris
pancreatic islet a.
porcine intestinal a.
sheep pulmonary a.

adenomatous
attenuated adenomatous polyposis coli
attenuated familial adenomatous polyposis
atypical adenomatous hyperplasia
benign adenomatous polyp
carcinoma with adenomatous areas
a. crypt
cystic adenomatous malformation
a. focus
a. goiter
a. hyperparathyroidism
a. hyperplasia
a. hyperplastic nodule
multiple adenomatous polyps
papillary adenomatous polyp
pedunculated adenomatous polyp
a. polyp
a. polyp-cancer sequence

adenomatous *(continued)*
a. polyposis
a. polyposis coli
segmental colonic adenomatous polyposis syndrome
small pedunculated adenomatous polyps
sporadic adenomatous polyps

adenomectomy
medical a.

adenomyofibroma
atypical polypoid a.
atypical polypoid adenomyofibroma of low malignant potential

adenomyoma
atypical polypoid a.
a. of gallbladder

adenomyosis uteri

adenopapillary
a. carcinoma
mucus-producing adenopapillary carcinoma
a. tumor

adenopathy
anterior cervical chain a.
bilateral hilar a.
hemophiliac with a.
internal iliac a.
multiple endocrine a.
necrotizing inguinal a.
scalene a.
secondary axillary a.
tuberculous mediastinal a.

adenopolyposis coli gene

adenosarcoma
müllerian a.

adenosatellite virus

adenosine
concentration of adenosine monophosphate
cyclic adenosine monophosphate
a. 3′,5′-cyclic monophosphate
a. deaminase
a. deaminase activity
a. deaminase assay
a. deaminase deficiency
a. diphosphatase
a. diphosphate
a. 5′-diphosphate
a. diphosphate ribose
a. echocardiography imaging
F_1 adenosine triphosphatase
hydrogen adenosine triphosphatase
a. kinase
a. monophosphate
a. 5′-monophosphate
a. 5′ monophosphate
a. monophosphate deaminase deficiency
muscle adenosine monophosphate deaminase deficiency
nephrogenous cyclic adenosine monophosphate
nonselective adenosine receptor antagonist
a. nucleotide translocator
oxidized a.
polyethylene glycol-modified adenosine deaminase
a. radionuclide perfusion imaging
a. receptor
red blood cell adenosine deaminase
sodium- and potassium-activated adenosine triphosphatase
a. tetraphosphate
a. thallium scan
a. thallium test
a. triphosphatase
a. triphosphatase activity
a. triphosphate
a. 5′-triphosphate
a. triphosphate disodium
a. triphosphate single-photon emission computed tomography

adenosine-coupled spleen cell

adenosine-regulating agent

adenosis
apocrine a.
microglandular a.
nodular a.
sclerosing a.

adenosquamous
a. carcinoma
a. cell carcinoma

adenoviral
a. gene transfection
a. pneumonia
a. transfer
a. vector

adenovirus
a. 3
a. 7
a. 8
a. 19
Bos adenovirus 1–10
canine adenovirus 1
a. E1A protein
a. fiber knob
Galius adenovirus 1–2
human adenovirus 1–47
a. immunization
a. immunofluorescence
a. infection
Meleagris adenovirus 1–3
Mus adenovirus 1–2
ovine adenovirus 1–6
simian a.

adenovirus-mediated gene transfer

adenovirus-reactive T cell

adenoxyltransferase
ATP cobalamin a.

adenylate
a. cyclase
a. cyclase inhibitor
a. cyclase toxin
a. kinase
lymphocyte adenylate cyclase response
modulator of adenylate cyclase
muscle adenylate deaminase
pituitary adenylate cyclase activating polypeptide

adenylcyclase
human thyroid adenylcyclase stimulator

adenylic acid

adenylosuccinate lyase deficiency

adenylosuccinic acid

adequacy
a. of intravascular volume
nutritional a.
Social A. Index
a. of treatment

adequate
a. blood flow
a. blood supply
a. calorie intake
a. calories intake
a. cardiac output
a. coronary perfusion
estimated safe and adequate daily dietary intake
a. flow of blood
a. fluid replacement
a. gait and station
a. hemostasis
a. hemostasis maintained
a. hydration
a. patient care
perceptually adequate sound
stimulate adequate spontaneous breathing

a. stroke volume
a. urine output
zinc adequate pair-fed

adequately
bowel adequately evacuated
chest expands adequately bilaterally

adhalin gene

adherence
granulocyte a.
immune a.
immune adherence hemagglutination assay
immune adherence immunosorbent assay
leukocyte adherence inhibition factor
mitogenic adherence lectin
pollen adherence factor
a. ratio
red blood cell a.
red blood cell immune a.
specific red cell a.
Treponema pallidum immobilization immune a.

adherens
macula a.

adherent
bacterial adherent colony
barium adherent to esophageal walls
bowel adherent to omentum
a. cell
diffusely adherent *Escherichia coli*
a. macrophage-like cell
splenic adherent cell
surface adherent monocyte

adhesed
jejunum and ileum a.

adhesin-receptor interaction

adhesion
adnexal adhesion classification system
AFS adhesion scoring system
AFS classification of adnexal a.'s
amniotic adhesions of fetus
anomalous mesenteric a.
antiplatelet endothelial cell adhesion molecule
cell adhesion factor
cell adhesion molecule
cell-cell adhesion molecule
cellular adhesion molecule
circulating adhesion molecule
dense fibrous a.
disk-condyle a.
endothelial-leukocyte adhesion molecule
endothelial-leukocyte adhesion molecule-1
flexor tendon a.
focal adhesion kinase
freeing up of a.
intercellular adhesion molecule-1, -2, -3
intraperitoneal adhesion formation
intrauterine a.
leukocyte adhesion deficiency
leukocyte adhesion inhibitor
leukocyte adhesion molecule-1
leukocyte cell adhesion molecule
leukocyte adhesion deficiency type 1–4
lip adhesion operation
a. lysis
lysis of a.
lysis bladder neck a.'s
melanoma cell adhesion molecule
a. molecule
a. molecule cascade
a. molecule-like from the X-chromosome
monocyte adhesion molecule
mucosal addresin cell adhesion molecule-1
nerve cell adhesion molecule
neural cell adhesion molecule
pericardial diaphragmatic a.
a.'s of pericardium around heart
a. phenomenon
platelet endothelial cell adhesion molecule-1
A. Scoring Group
soluble intracellular adhesion molecule
takedown of a.
taking down of a.
vascular cell adhesion molecule
vascular cell adhesion molecule-1

adhesional and glide friction

adhesion/cohesion mechanism

adhesive
a. band
broad adhesive band
a. capsulitis
chronic adhesive otitis media
a. chronic pachymeningitis
a. disease
fibrin tissue a.
Marlen double-faced adhesive disc
Nexacryl tissue a.
omental adhesive band
plastic adhesive dressing
a. silicone implant
synthetic, adhesive, moisture vapor permeable
a. tissue
in vivo adhesive platelet

adhesiveness
platelet a.
platelet adhesiveness plasma factor

adiabatic
a. fast passage
fast adiabatic trajectory in steady state

Adie
A. pupil
A. syndrome
A. tonic pupil

Adie-Holmes pupil

adipocyte determination and differentiation factor-1

adipofascial
a. axial pattern cross-finger flap
a. flap
a. sural flap
a. turnover flap

adiposa
macrosomatia adiposa congenita
macrosomia adiposa congenita

adipose
brown adipose tissue
a. capsule of kidney
a. fold of the pleura
hernia a.
multilocular adipose tissue
orbital adipose tissue
palpebral adipose bag
a. renal capsule
subcutaneous adipose tissue
a. tissue
a. tissue extract
total adipose tissue
visceral adipose tissue
white adipose tissue

adiposis hepatica

adiposity
a. index
localized a.
painful a.
pituitary a.

adiposogenital
a. degeneration
a. dystrophy
a. syndrome

adiposus
ascites a.
panniculus a.

adipsic disorder

adjacent
brain adjacent tumor
necrotizing scleritis with adjacent inflammation
necrotizing scleritis without adjacent inflammation

adjective
A. Check List
Depression A. Check List
Depressive A. Checklist
Multiple Affect A. Check List
Personality A. Check List
A. Rating Form

adjudicating
independent adjudicating panel

adjunct
a. therapy
a. treatment

adjunctive
a. balloon angioplasty
a. glucocorticoid therapy
a. individual session
a. medication
a. procedure
a. screw fixation
a. technique
a. therapy

adjustable
A. Advanced Reciprocating Gait Orthosis
a. aiming apparatus
a. aiming device
a. articulator
a. axis facebow
a. brace
a. breast implant
a. cane
a. cane board
a. dynamic joint
a. external suture
laser adjustable silicone gastric banding
a. leg and ankle repositioning mechanism
a. nail
open adjustable silicone gastric banding
a. postoperative protective prosthetic socket
a. pressure shunt
a. ring gastroplasty
a. saline breast implant
a. screw
a. silicone gastric banding
a. splint
a. suture
a. thigh antiembolism stockings
wedge adjustable cushioned heel

adjustable-length
a.-l. gauge
a.-l. gauge needle

adjusted
a. age
a. body mass
corrected adjusted sinus node recovery time
a. gestational age
a. occlusion
per adjusted discharge
a. rate

adjusting
activating adjusting instrument
a. table

adjustive treatment

adjustment
anxiety adjustment disorder
anxious mood adjustment reaction
assessment adjustment pass
Bristol Social A. Guides
Children's Attention and A. Survey
conduct disturbance adjustment disorder
conduct disturbance adjustment reaction
control adjustment strap
a. depression
a. disorder
a. disorder, chronic
a. disorder with angry mood
a. disorder with anxiety
a. disorder with anxious mood
a. disorder with disturbance of conduct
a. disorder with mixed anxiety and depressed mood
a. disorder with mixed disturbance of emotions
early postoperative suture a.
emotional disturbance adjustment disorder
emotional disturbance adjustment reaction
family assessment adjustment pass
a. following migration
geographic adjustment factor
group adjustment therapy
improved psychological a.
a. interface disorder
intraoperative suture a.
a. inventory
late postoperative suture a.
Locke-Wallace Marital Adjustment test
Mandel Social A. Scale
Marriage A. Inventory
a. measure
a. mechanism
Mental A. to Cancer scale
a. method
occlusal adjustment armamentarium
occlusal adjustment instrument
Personal A. and Role Skills Scale
policy target adjustment factor
a. process
Psychosocial A. to Illness Scale
a. reaction of adolescence
a. reaction of childhood
a. reaction conduct disorder
a. reaction disturbance
a. reaction of infancy
a. reaction of later life
a. reaction of menopause
a. reaction of middle age
a. reaction physical symptom
Sexual A. Questionnaire
a. situational reaction
Social A. Self-Report Scale
Student A. Inventory
a. therapy
Veteran's A. Scale
Vocational Evaluation and Work A.
Weinberger A. Inventory

adjust repetitive behavior

adjuvant
a. alpha blockade
a. analgesic drug
a. arthritis
a. chemoradiation
a. chemoradiation therapy
a. chemotherapy
complete Freund a.
a. diagnostic modality
a. disease
a. drug therapy
Freund a.
Freund complete a.
Freund incomplete a.
a. hepatic arterial infusion chemotherapy
a. hormonal or chemotherapy treatment

human adjuvant disease
a. hyperthermia
incomplete Freund a.
a. irradiation
a. medical therapy
a. microwave thermotherapy
multimodal adjuvant therapy
neonatal adjuvant life support
a. polychemotherapy
a. post-radiation therapy
a. study
surgical adjuvant therapy
a. therapy for breast cancer
a. treatment
a. treatment option
a. whole-brain radiation therapy

adjuvant-induced arthritis

Adkins
A. spinal fusion
A. technique spinal arthrodesis

Adler
A. test
A. theory

adlerian
a. psychoanalysis
a. psychology
a. psychotherapy
a. theory

ADLs
patient independent in A.

administered
anesthesia a.
catheter administered treatment
oral administered drug
roentgen administered dose
to be a.
total administered dose

administration
avenues of a.
contract administration fees
drug administration device
electromotive drug a.
hospital a.
intracerebroventricular administration of morphine
intraperitoneal drug a.
intravenous administration of medication
intravesical electromotive drug a.
medical care a.
medication administration record
medication administration team
medication administration guideline
method of a.
mode of administration with hallucinogen
monitored administration of medication
ophthalmic administration of insulin
oral administration of insulin
parenteral drug a.
Pension and Welfare Benefits A.
percutaneous bacille Calmette-Guérin a.
peripheral intravenous a.
self-medication administration record
standard dose a.
subcutaneous peritoneal administration device
system for anesthetic and respiratory a.
treatment administration record

administrative
a. control center
a. medicine
other administrative reasons
Professional and A. Career Examination
a. psychiatry
a. segregation
a. therapy

administratively necessary days

administrator
health facility a.
third-party a.

admiration
demand for constant a.
need for a.

admissible
a. admission
a. evidence

admission
attending's admission notes
bedwetter a.
a. blood work
Certified Hospital A. Program
a. chest x-ray
condition on a.
conditions of a.
a. criteria
date of a.
day of a.
a. diagnosis
direct a.
a. and discharge
a., discharge, transfer
drug-related a.
a., entrance, and evaluation unit
expense-per-equivalent a.
a. hemoglobin
a. history
hospital a.
Hospital A. Risk Profile
intact on a.
intern admission note
laboratory admission baseline studies
morning a.
multiple a.
new a.
no previous a.
on a.
orders accompanying patient on a.
PAR Admissions Testing program
patient requesting a.
Pediatric Acute A. Severity classification
potential inpatient a.
prior to a.
resident's admission notes
routine admission laboratory test
same day a.
total infections versus total a.
voluntary a.

admittance
peak a.

admitted
not a.
patient admitted for evaluation and workup
patient admitted for observation
patient admitted for observation and treatment
patient admitted and transfused with whole blood
patient admitted with active infection
to be a.
treated but not a.

admitting
a. blood sugar
a. diagnosis
a. doctor
a. physician

admixture
a. lesion
a. lesion of heart
total nutrient a.
venous a.

adnexa
lids, lashes, and a.
lymphoma of ocular a.

adnexal
a. adhesion classification system
AFS classification of adnexal adhesions
a. embryo
female adnexal tumor of probable wolffian origin
a. mass
ocular adnexal inflammatory pseudotumor
ocular adnexal lesion
ocular adnexal lymphoid proliferation
ocular adnexal lymphoma
ocular adnexal tumor
a. skin tumor
a. torsion

adolescence
adjustment reaction of a.
anxiety disorder of a.
avoidant disorder of a.
complex disorder of a.
constitutional delay in growth and a.
a. developmental stage
disturbance of emotions specific to a.
emancipation disorder of a.
emotional disturbance of a.
gender identity disorder of a.
gender identity disorder of adolescence or adulthood, nontranssexual type
myoclonic epilepsy of a.
oppositional disorder of a.
overanxious disorder of a.
reaction of a.

adolescent
a. abuse
a. alcohol abuse
A. Alienation Index
a. anger management
a. anxiety
a. at risk
a. chemical abuse
child and adolescent burden assessment
child and adolescent psychoanalysis
Child and A. Functional Assessment Scale
Child Health and Illness Profile, A. Edition
Child and A. Psychiatric Assessment
Computerized Diagnostic Interview for Children and A.'s
controlled adolescent behavior
a. counseling
a. criminal
a. crisis
a. culture
a. day treatment program
a. depression
a. depression symptom
A. Diagnostic Interview
a. diversion project
A. Drinking Index
a. drug abuse
a. drug abuse unit
A. Drug and Alcohol Diagnostic Assessment
a. drug use
a. eczema
a. environment
a. experimentation with adult behavior
Fullerton Language Test for A.'s
Functional Impairment Scale for Children and A.'s
a. gambler
a. gang member
a. group therapy
a. guardedness
a. hallux abductovalgus
a. hallux valgus
high-risk adolescent population
a. hypertension
a. idiopathic scoliosis
a. inpatient unit
a. insanity
Interview Schedule for Children and A.'s
a. inventory
a. language quotient
A. Language Screening Test
A. Life Change Event Questionnaire
a. mania
a. medicine
Methodology for Epidemiology in Children and A.'s
Methods for the Epidemiology of Child and A. Disorders T score
Methods for Epidemiology of Child and A. Mental Disorders
Millon A. Clinical Inventory
Millon A. Personality Inventory
a. negativism
a. neurotic delinquency
Offer Self-Image Questionnaire for A.'s
a. onset
Opinions toward A.'s
Oregon Adolescent Depression Project-Conduct Disorder Screener
pediatric and adolescent epilepsy
A. and Pediatric Pain Tool Scale
a. pedophilia
a. personal identity
Personal Problems Checklist for A.'s
Pictorial Instrument for Children and A.'s
a. population
A. Problem Severity Index
a. psychiatry
a. psychologist
a. psychology
a. psychopharmacology
a. psychotherapy
a. rapist
a. rebellion
a. recovery
Responsibility and Independence Scale for A.'s
Reynolds A. Depression Scale
a.'s risk for violence
a. runaway
Service Assessment for Children and A.'s
a. sex offender
a. sexual activity
a. sexual change
a. sexual ideation
a. sexual identity
a. skepticism
a. spina bifida
a. stress hematuria
a. suicide
a. support group
a. support system
Test of A. Language
a. thinking
a. tibia vara
a. turmoil
a. turmoil reaction
a. violence
a. voice
a. voyeurism

Adolescent/Adult
Test of Adolescent/Adult Word Finding

adolescent-onset conduct disorder

adolescent-parent interview

adoptee
extrafamily a.
a. family method

adoption
baby for a.
baby up for a.
a. study

adoptive
a. care
a. caregiver
a. cellular therapy
a. family
a. father
a. immunity
a. immunotherapy
a. parent

adrenal
acute adrenal insufficiency
adult-onset congenital adrenal hyperplasia
a. androgen
a. androgen corticotropic stimulating hormone
a. androgenesis
a. androgen-stimulating hormone
autologous adrenal medullary tissue
autonomous adrenal hyperplasia
a. cell rest tumor
a. chromaffin cell
a. computerized tomography
congenital adrenal virilism
congenital hypoplasia of adrenal glands
congenital idiopathic adrenal hypoplasia
congenital lipoid adrenal hyperplasia
congenital virilizing adrenal hyperplasia
a. cortex
a. cortex cell
a. cortex estrogen-secreting tumor
a. cortex testosterone-secreting tumor
a. cortex zone
enzymatic abnormality of adrenal gland
a. epithelioid angiosarcoma
a. feminization syndrome
a. gland hormone
a. gland insufficiency
a. growth factor
hemorrhagic a.'s
hemorrhagic infarct of adrenal gland
a. hermaphroditism
a. hormone
hormone-secreting adrenal tumor
a. hyperandrogenism
a. hyperandrogenism marker
a. hyperplasia
a. hypertension
hypoparathyroidism, adrenal insufficiency, mucocutaneous candidiasis syndrome
a. hypoplasia
a. hypoplasia congenita
idiopathic adrenal hyperplasia
a. insufficiency
insufficiency
a. leukodystrophy
lipoid adrenal gland hypoplasia
lipoid adrenal hyperplasia
macronodular adrenal hyperplasia
malignant adrenal mass
Marchand a.'s
a. medulla
medulla of adrenal gland
a. medullary autograft
micronodular adrenal disease
miniature-type congenital adrenal hypoplasia
neonatal adrenal gland hemorrhage
neonatal adrenal ultrasound
nodular adrenal hyperplasia
nodular cortical adrenal hyperplasia
nonclassical adrenal hyperplasia
nonclassic congenital adrenal hyperplasia
nonfunctioning adrenal carcinoma
nonsalt-wasting congenital adrenal hyperplasia
nonsecretory adrenal adenoma
a. pheochromocytoma
a. primary aldosteronism
a. remodeling
a. rest tissue
salt-wasting congenital adrenal hyperplasia
simple virilizing congenital adrenal hyperplasia
a. steroid hormone
a. steroidogenesis
a. steroidogenic cascade
a. steroid precursor
a. vein aldosterone ratio
a. venous sampling
virilizing adrenal hyperplasia
a. virilizing syndrome
a. weight factor

adrenalectomy
laparoscopic a.
open a.
transperitoneal laparoscopic a.

Adrenalin
tetracaine, Adrenalin, and cocaine

adrenaline
lidocaine, adrenaline, tetracaine

adrenaline-Mecholyl test

adrenalitis
autoimmune a.
necrotizing a.

adrenal-sparing surgery

adrenal-to-spleen ratio

adrenergic
a. agent
alpha-1 adrenergic antagonist
alpha-1 adrenergic blocking agent
alpha-2 adrenergic receptor
a. beta-receptor
peripheral adrenergic agent
a. receptor
a. receptor binder
a. receptor kinase
a. receptor material
a. urticaria
a. vagal function

adrenergic-response state

adrenocortical
a. atrophy-cerebral sclerosis syndrome
a. autoantibody
a. carcinoma
a. coma
a. extract
a. hormone
a. hyperplasia
hypothalamic pituitary adrenocortical axis
idiopathic adrenocortical hyperplasia
a. insufficiency
lipid-laden homogeneous adrenocortical carcinoma
nodular adrenocortical hyperplasia
partial adrenocortical insufficiency
pigmented nodular adrenocortical disease
a. polypeptide
primary adrenocortical micronodular dysplasia
primary adrenocortical nodular dysplasia
primary pigmented nodular adrenocortical disease
a. steroid

adrenocorticotrophic
a. hormone-secreting pituitary tumor
little adrenocorticotrophic hormone

adrenocorticotrophin hormone

adrenocorticotropic
a. hormone
a. hormone-dependent Cushing syndrome
a. hormone-releasing factor
immunoreactive adrenocorticotropic hormone
a. peptide
a. polypeptide

adrenodoxin reductase

adrenogenital
adult adrenogenital syndrome
congenital adrenogenital hyperplasia
nonsalt-losing adrenogenital syndrome
salt-losing adrenogenital syndrome
a. syndrome

adrenoglomerulotropin hormone

adrenomedullin hormone

adrenoreceptor
alpha-1 a.

adrenotropic
pituitary adrenotropic hormone

Adriamycin-induced nephrosis

Adriamycin therapy toxicity

Adson
A. maneuver
A. sign
A. test

adsorbed
doxorubicin adsorbed to magnetic targeted carrier
mitomycin adsorbed onto activated charcoal
rabies vaccine a.

adsorbent
molecular adsorbent recirculating system

adsorption
agglutinin a.

adsorptive voltammetry

adult
a. abuse
a. acid maltase deficiency
a. acquired flatfoot
a. acquired micrognathia
adolescent experimentation with adult behavior
a. adrenogenital syndrome
Anxiety Scales for Children and A.'s
Apraxia Battery for A.'s
a. basic education
A. Basic Learning Examination
a. bone marrow
a. bovine serum
Brugia malayi adult antigen
a. bullous dermatosis
A. Career Concerns Inventory
Caucasian a.
a. celiac disease
a. child of alcoholic
a. child of dysfunctional family
children and adults with attention deficit disorder
children and adults with attention deficit disorder
a. congregate living facility
a. congruent living facility
a. cystic teratoma
a. cystinosis
a. day-care center
a. depressive disorder
a. depressive episode
a. development
a. diagnostic and treatment center
a. diarrhea rotavirus
disabled adult child
a. disease
a. dissociation
a. ego state
end-stage adult cardiac decompensation
a. environment
a. erythrocyte
a. familial hyaline membrane disease
a. female
a. foster care
a. foster home
gender identity disorder of adult life
a. granulosa cell tumor
a. group therapy
growth hormone deficiency syndrome in a.
growth hormone-deficient a.
a. hemoglobin
a. hypolactasia
individual adult children of alcoholics counseling
latent autoimmune diabetes of a.
a. life
a. lipofuscinosis
a. living facility
major component of adult hemoglobin
a. major depression
a. male
medically indigent a.
a. medulloepithelioma
minor fraction of adult hemoglobin
a.'s molested as children
a. monocyte
a. motivation
National A. Reading Test
Naylor-Harwood A. Intelligence Scale
A. Neuropsychological Questionnaire
a., normal
normal adult female
normal adult male
normal female adult genitalia
normal male adult genitalia
peak adult bone mass
A. Performance Level Survey
A. Personal Data Inventory
A. Personality Inventory
a. phimosis
a. polycystic kidney disease
a. polycystic liver disease
predicted adult height
a. psychiatric hospital
a. psychopathology
Rapid Estimation of A. Literacy in Medicine
a. recovery services
a. respiratory distress syndrome
a. Reye syndrome
a. schizophrenia
a. scoliosis
A. Self-Expression Scale
a. self-harm behavior
a. self-injury
a. situation stress reaction
a. social dysfunction
a. socialization
subclinical rhythmic epileptiform discharge of a.
A. Suicidal Ideation Questionnaire
a. survivor of neglect
a. T-cell leukemia
a. T-cell leukemia antigen
a. T-cell leukemia/lymphoma
a. T-cell leukemia virus
a. T-cell lymphoma
a. T-cell lymphoma-leukemia
tetanus-diphtheria toxoid, adult type
a. unit

Wechsler Intelligence for A.
young adult chronic patient
young adult psychiatric assessment

adult/adolescent spectrum of HIV disease

adult-child sex

adulterated rapeseed oil-associated toxic oil syndrome

adulthood

a. developmental stage
gender identity disorder of adolescence or adulthood, nontranssexual type
middle a.
a. psychiatry

adult-life psychosexual identity disorder

adult-onset

a.-o. asthma
a.-o. cataract
a.-o. combined methylmalonic aciduria and homocystinuria
a.-o. congenital adrenal hyperplasia
a.-o. diabetes
a.-o. diabetes mellitus
a.-o. dystonia
a.-o. enuresis
a.-o. epilepsy
a.-o. hypogammaglobulinemia
a.-o. myasthenia gravis
a.-o. obesity
a.-o. polycystic kidney disease
a.-o. polyglandular syndrome
a.-o. proband
a.-o. spinal muscular atrophy
a.-o. spinocerebellar ataxia
a.-o. systemic Still disease

adult-to-adult living related donor living transplant

adult-type

a.-t. polycystic kidney disease
a.-t. xanthogranuloma

advance

a. beneficiary notice
a. cochlear echo technique
a. directive
a. directive continuity
a. to regular diet

advanced

Adjustable A. Reciprocating Gait Orthosis
a. breast biopsy instrumentation
a. cardiac life support
a. cardiac mapping
a. care directive
A. Catheter System
a. combined encoder
a. communications function
a. coronary treatment
a. dementia
a. design LINAC radiosurgery
a. directive
early advanced hepatocellular carcinoma
familial advanced sleep-phase syndrome
far a.
a. first aid
a. glycation end-product
a. glycosylation end-product
a. gum disease
a. heart ailment
a. heart disease
a. hepatocellular carcinoma
a. injury
a. insulin infusion with a control loop
A. Interventional Systems
a. local invasion
locally advanced breast cancer
locally advanced cancer
locally advanced cervical carcinoma
locally advanced esophageal cancer
locally advanced and inflammatory breast carcinoma
locally advanced melanoma
locally advanced prostate cancer
locally advanced non-small-cell lung cancer
a. maternal age
medical ultrasound 3D portable, with advanced communication
mobile advanced real-time image
a. mobile-bearing prosthesis
moderately a.
a. multiple-beam equalization radiography
a. ovarian cancer
a. oxidation protein product
pediatric advanced life support
a. pediatric life support
A. Placement Examination
A. Placement Program
a. real-time motion analysis
a. resected head and neck cancer
scaphoid-lunate advanced collapse
scaphoid nonunion advanced collapse
scapholunate advanced collapse
a. sleep-phase pattern
a. sleep-phase syndrome
a. squamous cell cervical carcinoma
a. stage of congestive heart failure
a. stage group
a. trauma life support
a. ultrasonography
a. vessel analysis
Weber A. Spatial Perception test
a. x-ray facility

advancement

Achilles tendon a.
Antia-Buch chondrocutaneous advancement flap
Antia-Buch helical rim advancement flap
Atasoy-Kleinert volar V-Y advancement flap
Atasoy triangular advancement flap
Atasoy V-Y a.
Atasoy V-Y advancement flap
bilateral advancement transposition
calcaneonavicular ligament-tibialis posterior tendon a.
cumulative phase a.
en bloc a.
endorectal advancement flap
extended V-Y advancement flap
a. flap
a. flap graft
a. genioplasty
heel cord a.
lip border a.
local tissue advancement flap
mandibular advancement appliance
mandibular advancement device
maxillomandibular a.
maxillomandibular advancement procedure
meatal advancement and glanduloplasty procedure
meatal advancement glans-phalloplasty
meatal advancement and glansplasty
meatal advancement, glansplasty, penoscrotal junction meatotomy
meatal advancement, glanuloplasty, penoscrotal junction meatotomy

advancement *(continued)*
Millard advancement rotation flap reconstruction
Moberg advancement flap
Murphy Achilles tendon a.
Murphy heel cord a.
palmar advancement flap
patellar tendon a.
perialar crescentic advancement flap
a. procedure
a. of rectal flap
sagittal split a.
a. sleeve flap
triple advancement transposition
vastus medialis a.
V-Y advancement flap
V-Y advancement technique

advancing
a. wave-like epitheliopathy
mandibular advancing device

advantage
actual mechanical a.
a. by illness
right ear a.

adventitia
aortic tunica a.
a. of artery

adventitial
a. bed
a. cell
a. dermis
a. fibroplasia
a. forceps
a. neuritis
a. pulmonary sound
a. rupture
a. scissors
a. sheath
a. tissue

adventitious
a. albuminuria
a. breath sound
a. bursa
a. choreiform movement
a. cyst
a. deafness
a. dentin
a. membrane
a. motor flow
a. movement
a. reinforcement

adversarial relationship

adversary model

adverse
acute adverse psychological reaction
a. autonomic response
a. background factor
a. childhood experience
a. drug effect
a. drug-induced reaction
a. drug reaction
drug-related adverse patient event
a. effect
a. event
a. factor
herb-related adverse event
lowest observed adverse effect level
major adverse cardiac event
a. medication effect
a. negative immunosuppressive effect
neurologic adverse effect
a. neurologic complication
no adverse reaction
no observed adverse effect level
a. outcome
a. patient occurrences
peripheral neurologic adverse effect
a. psychological response
a. psychosocial environment
a. reaction
a. selection
serious adverse event
a. side-effects
suspected adverse drug reaction

advertising psychology

advice
discharged against medical a.
examination, opinion, and a.
home versus against a.
home with a.
Maastricht History and Advice Checklist-Revised
patient released against medical a.
remittance a.
signed out against medical a.

advise
discharge and a.
evaluate and a.

advised and released

advisory
pregnancy advisory service

advocacy
protection and a.

advocate
child a.
mental health a.
patient a.

adynamic
a. bone disease
a. ileus
a. intestinal obstruction

adynamic/paralytic ileus

aegyptius
Haemophilus influenzae biogroup *aegyptius*

aeration
fluids, aeration, nutrition, communication, activity, and pain
fluids, aeration, nutrition, communication, activity, and stimulation
lung a.

aeroallergen
mold a.

aerobe
facultative a.
Gram-negative a.
Gram-positive a.
negative a.
obligate a.

aerobic
a. and anaerobic blood culture
a. bacteria
a. bacterium
a. bone marrow culture
a. boxing
a. capacity
cardiovascular aerobic exercise
a. cellulitis
a. chair exercises
a. conditioning
a. conditioning functional assessment
condition muscles with aerobic exercise
a. culture
digital auditory a.'s
a. exercise
a. flora
functional aerobic capacity
functional aerobic impairment
a. glycolysis
Gram-negative aerobic organism
a. gram-negative rod
a. gram-positive coccus
high-impact aerobic dance
high-impact aerobic exercise
a. impairment

a. infection
low-impact a.'s
low-impact aerobic dance
low-impact aerobic exercise
maximal aerobic power
a. metabolism
a. microbial flora
mixed aerobic and anaerobic abscess
mixed aerobic and anaerobic flora
negative aerobic bacillus
nonhemolytic aerobic organism
personalized aerobics for cardiovascular enhancement
a. respiration
total aerobic bacteria count
a. walking

aerobiological property

***Aerococcus*-like organism**

aerodigestive
a. tract
upper a.
upper aerodigestive tract

aerodynamic
count median aerodynamic diameter
a. equivalent diameter
a. mass diameter
mass median aerodynamic diameter

aerogenic tuberculosis

aeromedical evacuation support team

aerosol
antigen a.
biologic aerosol detection
a. bolus dispersion
a. cloud enhancer
continuous heated a.
a. deposition
double aerosol face mask
drug a.
heated a.
a. inhalation monitor
manganese dioxide a.
a. mask
a. pentamidine
a. rebreathing method
a. sensitization
small-particle aerosol generator
a. spray
a. spray abuse
a. spray dependence
super-heated a.
a. tent
a. treatment chamber
a. ventilation scan
a. ventilation study

aerosol-derived airway morphometry

aerosolized
a. medication
a. plague weapon
a. pollutant exposure

aerospace medicine

aeruginosa
Pseudomonas a.
Pseudomonas aeruginosa bacteremia
Pseudomonas aeruginosa pneumonia

aesthetic
a. pleasure
a. value

afebrile
a. abortion
a., vital signs stable
vital signs stable, a.

affect
assessment of a.
a. attunement
A. Balance Scale
a., behavior, cognition
a. block
blunted or flat a.
Derogatis A.'s Balance Scale
diminution of a.
a. displacement
a. display
a. elicitation
a. energy
a. fantasy
a. fixation
full range of a.
a. hunger
a. intensity measure
a. intensity problem
a. inversion
a. memory
a. modulation
mood and/or a.
mood, orientation, judgment, affect, content
Multiple A. Adjective Check List
opposite affect state
patient has flat a.
profound change in a.
a. response
a. spasm
a. state
a. trauma model
a. within normal range

affected
to affected areas
apply to affected area
a. individual
inflammation within affected area
a. joint
part a.
a. parts
restore tissue to affected area
severely affected individual
shallow a.
a. site
a. by stress
swelling deformity of affected bone

affecting
extracorporeal membrane oxygenation affecting cognitive function

affection
a. and emotion
masked a.
patellar a.

affectional
a. attachment
a. bond

affectionate transference

affective
a. alcoholic psychosis
a. ambivalence
a. amnesia
a. arousal
a. arousal theory
atypical affective disorder
autonomic affective law
a. bipolar disorder
a. blunting
a. charge
Children's A. Rating Scale
a. constriction
daily affective rhythm
a. depressive reaction
a. determined disorder
a. discharge
a. disease
a. disharmony
a. disorder
a. disorders clinic
a. disorder syndrome
a. disturbance
a. dyscontrol
a. dysregulation
a. epilepsy
a. episode

affective *(continued)*
episodic affective disorder
a. experience
a. expression
a. expression disorder
a. feeble-mindedness
a. flattening
a. function
guided affective imagery
a. hallucination
a. illness
a. imagery
a. incontinence
a. insanity
a. instability
a. intensity
a. interaction
intermittent affective disorder
a. involvement
a. lability
major depressive affective psychosis
a. melancholia
melancholia affective psychosis
mixed bipolar affective psychosis
a. monomania
mutual affective responsiveness
a. need
a. neurotic personality disorder
normal affective processing
organic affective syndrome
a. paranoid organic psychosis
a. and paranoid state
a. personality
primary affective disorder
a. process
a. processing
a. prodrome of epilepsy
a. prodrome of migraine
a. property
a. ratio
a. reaction
a. reaction type
a. reactivity
a. responsiveness
a. rigidity
Schedule for A. Disorders and Schizophrenia-Change
Schedule for A. Disorders and Schizophrenia-Lifetime
Schedule for A. Disorders and Schizophrenia for School-Age Children
Schedule for A. Disorders and Schizophrenia for School-Age Children-Epidemiologic Version
Schedule for A. Disorders and Schizophrenia for School-Age Children-Present Episode
a. schematic mental model
a. schizophreniform psychosis
seasonal affective disorder syndrome
a. separation
a. significance
a. slumber
a. spectrum disorder
a. sphere
a. state
a. storm
a. stupor
A. Style Index
a. suggestion
a. symptom
a. symptom of seizure
a. tone
a. value

affective-arousal theory

affectivity
negative a.
a. ratio

affect-laden
a.-l. delusion
a.-l. paranoia

affectomotor pattern

affect-related
a.-r. information-processing biases
a.-r. meaning
a.-r. processing
a.-r. schematic mental model

afferent
a. artery
a. digital nerve
distended afferent loop
a. feedback
a. fiber
general somatic afferent nerve
general visceral afferent nerve
a. glomerular arteriole
a. ileal limb
a. impulse
a. innervation
a. loop
a. loop syndrome
a. lymphatic drainage
a. lymphatic vessel
Marcus Gunn relative afferent defect
a. motor aphasia
a. motor unit
a. nerve
a. neuron
a. pathway
primary afferent nociceptor neuron
a. pupillary defect
a. reflex
relative afferent pupillary defect
a. signal
special somatic a.
special visceral a.
a. stimulus interaction
Stoller afferent nerve stimulation
tactile a.
a. terminal
a. vessel
a. visual pathway

afferent-efferent pathway

affiliation
a. bonding
a. drive
lifelong a.
a. need
religious a.

affinity
abnormal oxygen a.
antibody affinity chromatography
anti-idiotypic affinity chromatography
a. attenuated total reflectance spectroscopy
a. constant
electric a.
eudismic affinity quotient
a. evanescent wave spectroscopy
a. fluorescence spectroscopy
high-pressure liquid affinity chromatography
immobilized metal affinity chromatography
low affinity antigen receptor
mutant hemoglobin with low affinity for oxygen
oxygen affinity anoxia
oxygen affinity hypoxia
relative binding a.
testosterone-binding a.

afflicted joint

affliction
age-related a.

aflatoxin
a. B1
a. B2
a. G
a. G1
a. G2
a. M

a. poisoning
a. Q

African
A. American
A. Burkitt lymphoma
A. cutaneous Kaposi sarcoma
A. endemic relapsing fever
A. furuncular myiasis
A. hemochromatosis
A. hemorrhagic fever
A. histoplasmosis
A. horse sickness
A. horse sickness virus 1–9
human African trypanosomiasis
A. iron overload
A. lymphadenopathic Kaposi sarcoma
A. meningitis
primary African green monkey kidney
A. sleeping sickness
South African tick-bite fever
South African tick fever
South African type porphyria
A. swine fever virus
A. swine pox
A. tick bite fever
A. tick typhus
A. tick virus
A. trypanosomiasis
West African fever
West African sleeping sickness

Africanized honeybee sting

africanum
Pygeum africanum extract

after
amino acid that gives aspartic acid after hydrolysis
amnesia after trance
back pain after childbirth
before and a.
biopsy after irradiation
bradycardia after arteriovenous fistula occlusion
breast reconstruction after mastectomy
a. bronchodilator
care of body after death
a. childbirth incontinence
days after birth
dead after arrival
delayed after polarization
designed after natural anatomy
a. diastase digestion
a. discharge
discharge patient after period of observation
a. feedings
fluorescence recovery after photobleaching
follow-through after barium meal
footdrop after stroke
fragment of immunoglobulin G after digestion with the enzyme pepsin
a. glide
growth after 48 hours incubation
headache after spinal tap
held after positioning
immediately after onset
Inventory of Functional Status A. Childbirth
junctional rhythm after cardiac surgery
Life A. Cancer Care
local recurrence after radiation therapy
male impotence after childbirth
a. meal
a. meals
a. meals and at bedtime
morning after pill
movement after effect
optokinetic after nystagmus
organism isolated after 48 hours
organism isolated after 72 hours
pancreas after kidney transplant
a. parturition
peak acid output after gastrin-releasing peptide
peak acid output after pentagastrin stimulation
salpingitis after previous tubal occlusion
sexual dysfunction after heart attack
tuboovarian abscess after previous tubal occlusion
urine specimen after prostate massage
vaginal birth after cesarean section
vaginal birth after cesarean—trial of labor
vaginal delivery after cesarean
wake after sleep onset
wake after sleep onset time
wakefulness after sleep onset

aftercare
a. agency
a. clinic
a. counseling
a. group
a. instruction
long-term aftercare treatment
methadone maintenance and aftercare treatment program
a. plan
a. planning
a. programs
a. treatment
a. worker

aftercoming
forceps to aftercoming head

afterdepolarization
delayed a.
early a.

afterdischarge
myotonic a.

aftereffect
contingent a.'s
a. of drinking

afterimage
memory a.
negative a.
a. test

afterload
LV a.
a. reduction
remote afterload brachytherapy

afterloading
a. brachytherapy
Fletcher afterloading colpostat
Fletcher-Suit afterloading ovoids
Fletcher-Suit afterloading tandem
Fletcher afterloading tandem
a. probe
a. radiation
a. screw
a. tandem and ovoids
a. technique

aftermath of trauma

afternoon
stitches out in a.

afternystagmus

afterpotential
depolarizing a.

aftershock
psychic a.

afterspike hyperpolarization

afunctional
a. neutrophil
a. occlusion
a. ulatrophy

again
had it before, got it a.

against
action against burns
astigmatism against the rule
autoantibodies against insulin
contract against self-harm
contract against suicide
crime against humanity
discharged against medical advice
monoclonal antibodies against gastric mucins
nonturning against self psychology
patient released against medical advice
signed out against medical advice
skin exposure reduction paste against chemical warfare agent
turning against object
turning against self

against-the-rule astigmatism

agalactia
mastitis, metritis, agalactia syndrome

agammaglobulinemia
late-onset a.
Swiss-type a.
X-linked a.

aganglionic
a. bowel
a. colon
a. megacolon
a. rectum
a. segment
a. segment of colon

aganglionosis
congenital intestinal a.
total aganglionosis coli
total colonic a.

agar
Bacteroides bile esculin a.
bismuth-sulfite a.
blood a.
blood agar base
blood agar plate
Bordet-Gengou a.
brain heart infusion a.
calcium nutrient a.
chocolate blood a.
cystine trypticase a.
Czapek-Dox a.
a. diffusion assay
a. diffusion for fungus
a. diffusion test
a. dilution test
a. disc elution
egg yolk a.
electrolyte-deficient a.
a. gel
a. gel diffusion
a. gel diffusion test
a. gel electrophoresis
a. gel precipitation test
heat infusion a.
Hektoen enteric a.
a. hydrocolloid
indulin a.
kanamycin-vancomycin blood a.
kanamycin-vancomycin laked blood a.
Lawrence Experimental Station a.
Lombard-Dowell a.
MacConkey II a.
mannitol salt a.
modified sea water yeast extract a.
Mueller-Hinton a.
nalidixic acid a.
neomycin egg yolk a.
NMN biphasic blood a.
nonnutrient agar plate
Novy and MacNeal blood a.
Novy-McNeal-Nicolle biphasic blood a.
nutrient gelatin a.
oatmeal-tomato paste a.
a. plate
a. plate count
polymyxin, lysozyme, EDTA, and thallous acetate in heart infusion a.
replicate organism direct agar contact
Salmonella-Shigella a.
sorbitol MacConkey a.
standard method a.
Thayer-Martin, modified a.
thermoacidurans agar modified
thiosulfate-citrate-bile salts-sucrose a.
triple sugar iron a.
trypticase-soy a.
tryptone glucose yeast a.
tryptophan deaminase a.
tryptose a.
Vogel-Johnson a.
well-developed a.
xylose-lysine-deoxycholate a.
yeast morphology a.

agar/agarose-gel diffusion method

agar-alginate impression

agarbase
purple agarbase medium

agarose electrophoresis

age
achievement a.
adjusted gestational a.
adjustment reaction of middle a.
advanced maternal a.
agonadism, mental retardation, short stature, retarded bone age syndrome
a. appropriate
appropriate for gestational a.
a. at first intercourse
a. at onset
a. at onset of use
average for gestational age
a. bias
birth weight for gestational a.
bone a.
bone age ratio
chronologic a.
chronological a.
conceptional a.
a. of consent
corrected gestational a.
a. correction
a. correction procedure
a. critique
debilitating effects of old a.
decrepitude with a.
a. dependent
developmental a.
diet for a.
a. discrimination
a., distant metastases, extent and size
educational a.
a. effect
a. equivalent
equivalent mean age at death
estimated gestational a.
fetal a.
full-term appropriate for gestational a.
full-term, large for gestational a.
full-term, small for gestational a.
Gesell Child Development A. Scale
gestational a.
glucose, age, LDH, AST, WBC
a. group
growth-adjusted sonographic a.
height a.
a. index
language a.
large for gestational a.
menstrual a.
mental a.

a., metastases, extent and size risk criteria
metastasis, age, completeness of resection, local invasion, and tumor size
middle age pedophilia
Moseley bone age graph
neurologic a.
new age suicide prevention
a. norm
old a.
old age benefits
old age pension
old age pensioner
Old A. Assistance
older maternal a.
a. peer
a. pigment
postconceptional a.
a. prejudice
premature appropriate for gestational a.
A. Projection Test
in proportion to a.
a. ratio
reading a.
a. of reasoning
a. regression
a. related
a. scale
a. score
skeletal a.
small for gestational a.
social a.
a. specific
A.'s and Stages Questionnaire
term birth appropriate for gestational a.
a. transition
years of potential life lost before age 65

age-adjusted prostate-specific antigen

age-appropriate
a.-a. behavior
a.-a. societal norm
a.-a. strategy

age-associated
a.-a. cognitive decline
a.-a. degenerative change
a.-a. memory impairment

aged
a., blind, and disabled
a. care assessment team
Medical Assistance for the A.
National Caucus and Center on Black A., Inc.
a. person
a. substrate plasma

age-dependent
a.-d. epilepsy syndrome
a.-d. epileptic encephalopathy
a.-d. slowing

Agee sign

age-grade scaling

age-group average

age-inappropriate knowledge of sexual behavior

age-indeterminate infarct

age-level behavior

age-matched individual

agency
health care a.
National Association of Area Agencies on Aging

agency-centered consultation

agenda
hidden a.
personal a.

agenesis
bilateral renal a.
congenital thrombocytopenia, Robin sequence, agenesis of corpus callosum, distinctive facies, developmental delay syndrome
a. of corpus callosum-mental retardation-osseous lesions syndrome
gonadal agenesis syndrome
Leydig cell a.
müllerian duct, unilateral renal agenesis, and anomalies of the cervicothoracic somites
partial agenesis of vermis
partial corpus callosum a.
patent renal a.
pure red blood cell a.
splenic agenesis syndrome
unilateral renal a.
X-linked mental retardation, seizures, acquired microcephaly, agenesis of corpus callosum

agenetic
a. fracture
a. porencephaly

agent
a., action, and object
adenoid degeneration a.
alkylating agent therapy
alpha-adrenergic blocking a.
alpha-1 adrenergic blocking a.
alpha blocking a.
alpha receptor blocking a.
androgenic anabolic a.
anesthetic induction a.
antiarrhythmic a.
antibacterial agent susceptibility testing
anticonvulsant agent hepatotoxicity
antidiabetic agent hepatotoxicity
antidiuretic hormone-like a.
antifibrin antibody imaging a.
antiinflammatory nonsteroidal a.
antimicrobial agents and chemotherapy
antineoplastic chemotherapeutic a.
atypical antipsychotic a.
augmentation agent overactivity in OCD
autologous growth factor binding a.
beta-adrenergic blocking a.
blood-borne infectious a.
blood thinning a.
A. Blue
cancer causing a.
cancer destroying a.
cell-cycle nonspecific a.
cell-cycle specific a.
a. of change
Change A. Questionnaire
chimpanzee coryza a.
chimpanzee coryza agent virus
chronic infectious neuropathic a.
cytotoxic chemotherapeutic a.
Eaton agent pneumonia
electron-transfer a.
extravasation of contrast a.
filterable a.
ganglionic blocking a.
glucose-lowering a.
gonadotropin-releasing a.
heat transfer a.
high-osmolar contrast a.
human reovirus-like a.
ingestion of toxic a.
intravenous anesthetic a.
life-threatening infectious a.
low molecular weight oxidizing a.
low-osmolality contrast a.
macrolide antimicrobial a.
mammary tumor a.
marrow agent bone scintigraphy
monkey intranuclear inclusion a.

agent *(continued)*
MS-1, -2 a.
multiple sclerosis-associated a.
natural anticancer a.
natural chemotherapy a.
negative contrast imaging a.
NeoTect imaging a.
neuromuscular blocking a.
noncorticosteroid antiinflammatory a.
nonglycoside inotropic a.
nonionic contrast a.
nonsteroidal antiinflammatory a.
Norwalk-like agent virus
oral antidiabetic a.
oral antifungal a.
oral antimotility a.
oral antiviral a.
oral contraceptive a.
oral contrast imaging a.
oral hypoglycemic a.
oral narcotic a.
A. Orange
osmotic driving a.
papilloma-polyoma-vacuolating agent virus
paramagnetic contrast a.
parenteral antihypertensive a.
parenteral antimicrobial a.
peripheral adrenergic a.
periurethral bulking a.
Pittsburgh pneumonia a.
prothrombin time fixing a.
a. provocateur
radiographic contrast a.
retinoic acid metabolism blocking a.
reverse transcriptase-producing a.
skin exposure reduction paste against chemical warfare a.
smooth muscle contracting a.
syphilis, toxoplasmosis, other agents, rubella, cytomegalovirus, herpes simplex virus
ultrasound contrast a.
vasodilator a.
virus-inactivating a.
virus-like infectious a.
viscoelastic a.

agent-induced
antimicrobial agent-induced colitis

age-related
a.-r. affliction
atrophic age-related macular degeneration
a.-r. brain change
a.-r. cataract
a.-r. change
a.-r. cognitive decline
a.-r. comorbidity
a.-r. dementia
a.-r. deterioration
a.-r. deterioration process
a.-r. developmental process
a.-r. diastolic dysfunction
a.-r. disease
a.-r. factor
a.-r. feature
a.-r. hearing loss
a.-r. macular degeneration
a.-r. maculopathy
maternal age-related risk
a.-r. memory impairment
a.-r. nocturia
nonneovascular age-related macular degeneration
a.-r. osteoporosis
a.-r. pharmacodynamic change
a.-r. pharmacodynamic response
a.-r. pharmacodynamics
a.-r. pharmacokinetic change
a.-r. ptosis
a.-r. risk
a.-r. trend
a.-r. visual impairment

age-specific
a.-s. cumulative incidence rate
a.-s. feature
a.-s. fertility rate
a.-s. rate
a.-s. risk factor

age-standardized mortality ratio

age-to-dose pattern

ageusia
peripheral a.

ageusic aphasia

agger nasi cell

agglutinating antibody

agglutination
Ashby differential agglutination method
a. assay
bacterial a.
capillary agglutination test
card agglutination trypanosomiasis test
chick-cell agglutination unit
differential agglutination test
differential agglutination titer
differential rheumatoid agglutination test
direct a.
direct agglutination test
direct latex agglutination pregnancy test
febrile antigen a.
gelatin agglutination test
granulocyte a.
head-to-head sperm a.
head-to-tail sperm a.
human erythrocyte agglutination test
a. immunoassay
immunosorbent agglutination assay
a. inhibition assay
latex a.
latex direct agglutination reaction
latex particle a.
latex particle agglutination inhibition
macroscopic agglutination test
microscopic a.
mixed agglutination test
mixed cell agglutination reaction
monoclonal antibody-based latex a.
particle agglutination test
pertussis agglutination test
polystyrene agglutination plate
red blood cell a.
reversed passive latex particle a.
ristocetin-induced platelet a.
sensitized sheep cell a.
sheep cell agglutination test
sheep cell agglutination titer
sheep erythrocyte agglutination test
slide agglutination test
slide latex a.
standard tube agglutination test
tanned red blood cell a.
a. technique
a. test
a. test for brucellosis
a. titer
tray agglutination test
Treponema pallidum a.
tube a.
tube slide agglutination test

agglutination-flocculation test

agglutination-inhibition
latex agglutination-inhibition test

agglutinative reactions

agglutinator
rheumatoid a.
serum normal a.

agglutinin
a. adsorption

Bauhinia purpura a.
cold a.
cold agglutinin disease
cold agglutinin syndrome
cold agglutinin titer
Dolichos biflorus a.
Helix pomatia a.
peanut a.
rheumatoid arthritis a.
salt-dependent a.
soybean a.
sperm a.
Ulex europaeus agglutinin I
wax bean a.
wheat germ a.

aggravated
a. assault
a. battery
pain aggravated by motion
pain aggravated by movement

aggregate
a. anaphylaxis
circulating platelet a.
cytoplasmic tubular a.
heart cell a.
mineral trioxide a.
nuclear aggregate lipid
nuclear crystalline a.
platelet aggregate ratio

aggregated
a. albumin
a. human gamma globulin
human stromelysin aggregated proteoglycan

aggregation
arachidonate-induced platelet a.
a. half-time
a. index
intravascular erythrocyte a.
intravascular red cell a.
labile aggregation stimulating substance
maximal aggregation index
maximal aggregation ratio
microscopic aggregation index
neutrophil aggregation activity
platelet a.
platelet aggregation as a risk of diabetes
platelet aggregation factor
platelet aggregation test
a. problem
side platelet aggregation test
spontaneous platelet a.
tumor-cell-induced platelet a.

aggression
a. and deceit impulsivity
a. factor
inattention-overactivity with a.
a. level
moment of a.
Overt A. Scale
pattern of a.
a. to people and animals
a. replacement training
a. scale
shock-elicited a.
situational anger disorder with a.
situational anger disorder without a.
a. without provocation

aggressive
a. act
a. action
a. adenoma
alleviating violence in aggressive behavior
a. angiomyxoma
a. approach
a. behavior
a. behavioral disturbance
a. behavior theory
a. care
a. chemotherapy
chronic aggressive hepatitis
a. conduct disorder
diffuse aggressive lymphoma
a. digital papillary adenocarcinoma
a. digital papillary adenoma
a. drive
dysrhythmic aggressive behavior
explosive aggressive behavior
a. fantasy
a. feeling
a. fibromatosis
a. good prognosis non-Hodgkin lymphoma
a. hepatitis
a. histology lymphoma
a. hostility
a. ideation
a. impulse
a. instinct
a. invasion
a. laser treatment
a. lesion
a. malignancy
a. medical care
moody, irritable and a.
multifocal aggressive infiltrate
a. objectionable behavior
a. obsession
oral a.
a. outburst
a. papillary middle ear tumor
passive a.
a. personality
physically a.
a. predatory type
a. psychotic behavior
a. psychotic inpatient
a. response
a. scale
a. surgical approach
a. therapeutic trial
a. therapy
a. thought
a. thyroid carcinoma
a. treatment
a. tumor
a. type undersocialized conduct disorder
a. undersocialized reaction
unusually hostile or aggressive behavior
a. or violent behavior
a. xanthomatosis

aggressively boisterous

aggressiveness
irritability and a.

aggressivity
drinking-related a.

agility
coordination and a.
a. drill
mental a.

aging
amyloidosis of a.
a. brain syndrome
Children of A. Parents
a. deformity
delay aging of cell
dizziness in a.
a. gamete
graying hair from a.
hearing loss from a.
heat stroke in a.
hypothermia in a.
a. issue
Lighthouse National Center for Vision and A.
National Asian Pacific Center on A.
National Association of Area Agencies on A.
National Institute on A.
natural aging process

aging *(continued)*
neuroanatomy of a.
normative aging process
Nuremberg A. Inventory
physiologic aging rate
problems from aging gums
a. theory
transient ischemic attack and a.

agitans
paralysis a.
paralysis agitans juvenilis

agitated
acute agitated delirium
a. behavior
combative and a.
depressed and a.
a. depression
disjointed agitated movement
a., irritable and easily annoyed
a. melancholia
a. patient
patient combative and a.
a. reaction
a. state

agitation
a. catatonic schizophrenia
intense motor a.
a. and irritability
irritability, agitation and restlessness
a. level
manic a.
mental a.
nighttime a.
nocturnal a.
onset of a.
overt a.
Overt A. Severity Scale
physical a.
psychomotor a.
reduced a.
a. response
severe a.

agitative feature

agnathia holoprosencephaly

agnogenic myeloid metaplasia

agnosia
aphasia, agnosia, apraxia, agraphia, and alexia
apperceptive visual a.
associative visual a.
auditory verbal a.
verbal-auditory a.

agnostic
a. alexia
a. behavior

agonadism, mental retardation, short stature, retarded bone age syndrome

agonal
a. expiration
a. gasp
a. gasping
a. respiration
a. rhythm
a. spinal cord hemorrhage
a. thrombosis
a. thrombus

agonic intussusception

agonist
alpha-adrenergic receptor a.
alpha-adrenoreceptor a.
beta-adrenoreceptor a.
beta agonist inhaler
calcium channel a.
contract relax agonist contract
dopamine receptor agonist property
gonadotropin agonist stimulation test
gonadotropin-releasing hormone a.
LH-releasing hormone agonist therapy
long-acting beta a.
low-dose dopaminergic a.
luteinizing hormone-releasing factor a.
luteinizing hormone-releasing hormone a.
a. medication
motilin receptor a.
muscarinic agonist carbamylcholine
muscarinic cholinergic a.
narcotic agonist drug
opiate receptor a.
opioid receptor a.
partial agonist activity
purinergic a.
a. therapy

agonist-antagonist
mixed a.-a.
mixed opioid a.-a.

agony
personal a.

agoraphobia
panic disorder with a.
panic disorder without a.
a. without history of panic disorder
a. with panic attack

agrammatic speech

agranular endoplasmic reticulum

agranulocytica
mucositis necroticans a.

agranulocytic angina

agranulocytosis
drug-induced a.
infantile genetic a.

agraphia
alexia with a.
alexia without a.
aphasia, agnosia, apraxia, agraphia, and alexia
aphasic a.
apraxic a.
atactic a.
a. atactica
atactica a.
jargon a.
lexical a.
literal a.
mental a.
motor a.
musical a.
optic a.
paretic a.
pure a.
verbal a.

agreed-on
a.-o. pattern
a.-o. routine

agriothymia hydrophobica

Aguacate virus

agyria
hydrocephalus, agyria, retinal dysplasia with or without encephalocele syndrome

agyria-pachygyria syndrome

ahead
impulsivity to plan a.

Ahlfeld sign

Aicardi-Goutieres syndrome

Aicardi syndrome

aid
advanced first a.
a.'s to ambulation
a. and attendance
Basic A. Training

behind-the-ear hearing a.
binaural hearing a.
a. to the blind
body worn hearing a.
bone-anchored hearing a.
bone conduction hearing a.
canal hearing a.
completely in the canal hearing a.
A. to Dependent Children
digital hearing a.
downsizing of hearing a.
in the ear hearing a.
first a.
first aid instruction
hearing a.
hearing aid amplifier
hearing aid dispenser
hearing aid evaluation
hearing aid microphone
hearing aid orientation
hearing aid problem
information overload testing a.
linear hearing a.
low vision a.
monaural hearing a.
mutual aid group
A. to Permanently and Totally Disabled
psychological first a.
refusal of medical a.
visual a.
walk with aid of cane

aide
health care a.
home-care a.
home health a.
patient care a.
psychiatric a.

aided equalization response

AIDS-associated
AIDS-a. BCBL
AIDS-a. KS
AIDS-a. lymphoma
AIDS-a. nephropathy
AIDS-a. retrovirus
AIDS-a. vacuolar myelopathy

AIDS-defining illness

AIDS-dementia complex

AIDS/HIV Treatment Directory

AIDS-related
AIDS-r. comp
AIDS-r. complex
AIDS-r. cryptococcal meningitis
AIDS-r. cryptococcosis
AIDS-r. encephalitis
AIDS-r. esophagitis
AIDS-r. Kaposi sarcoma
AIDS-r. lymphoma
AIDS-r. lymphoma of the lung
AIDS-r. lymphomatous meningitis
AIDS-r. myelopathy
AIDS-r. non-Hodgkin lymphoma
AIDS-r. primary central nervous system lymphoma
AIDS-r. retinitis
AIDS-r. syndrome
AIDS-r. toxoplasmosis
AIDS-r. tumor
AIDS-r. virus

ailment
advanced heart a.
chronic aspecific respiratory a.
heart a.

aim
a. inhibition
partial a.
a. transference

aiming
adjustable aiming apparatus
adjustable aiming device
a. test

aimless
a. behavior
a. motor activity
a. wandering

air
a. abrasion system
alternate inspiration and expiration of a.
ambient hospital a.
anterior ethmoidal air cell
apical air space
a. arthrography
average volume of a.
barium enema with air contrast
bladder distended with a.
a. bleed
a. block glaucoma
a. and bone conduction
bone conduction greater than air conduction
bone conduction less than air conduction
a. bronchogram
a. bronchogram sign
a. bubble
a. bubble instilled in anterior chamber
a. caloric test
capillary blood gas at room a.
captive air bubble
a. cell
a. cell cast
a. chamber
a. changes per hour
cold air challenge
a. in colon
compressed a.
a. compression osteotome
conditioned a.
a. conduction
a. conduction and bone conduction
a. conduction deafness
a. conduction testing
contamination from ambient hospital a.
a. contrast
a. contrast study
a. contrast view of the stomach
critical care air transport
a. critical-care transport
a. cystitome
a. cystogram
dead air space
diffuse air space disease
disturbance in air exchange
diving air embolism
a. dose
a. drinking
a. embolism
a. embolus
a. encephalogram
a. encephalography
a. encephalopathy
a. enema fluoroscopic imaging
a. entrainment
a. entry
equalize air pressure
escape of a.
a. esophagram
ethmoid air cell
a. exchange
expiratory trapping of a.
expired a.
expired air collection
extraalveolar a.
fatal air embolus
filterable a.
filtered a.
filtered hot a.
a. filtration machine
a. filtration system
a. flow
a. fluid cavity
foreign body in air passage
free abdominal a.

air *(continued)*
free air in abdomen
free air in diaphragm
free air passage
free air under diaphragm
free intraperitoneal a.
free peritoneal a.
a. gap correction
gasping for a.
gastric air bubble
a. greater than bone conduction
heating, ventilating, and air conditioning
high air flow with oxygen entrainment
high-efficiency particulate air filter
higher air pressure
high-speed air drill
high-viscosity barium and a.
a. hunger
indoor air quality
injection of a.
a. insufflation
intravascular fetal air sign
isocapnic hyperventilation with cold a.
isocapnic hyperventilation with room a.
laminar air flow room
laminar air flow unit
a. leak
low air loss
low air loss therapy mattress
mastoid air cell
a. mattress
medical air evacuation
a. medical transportation
microscopic air bubble
middle ethmoidal air cell
millions of particles per cubic foot of a.
minute volume of air or blood
a. monitor
Mosher air cell
a. movement
a. myelography
nasal air emission
neonatal air leak syndrome
normal hospital a.
obstruction of air passage
Ohio pediatric tent with compressed a.
open to a.
open air factor
oxygen in a.
a. passage
a. passage become inflamed
a. pathway
perinephric air injection
peripheral air space disease
perirenal air study
a. plasma spray
a. plethysmography
a. pocket
a. pollution adaptation
a. pollution index
a. pollution syndrome
poor air exchange
powered air loss
a. pressure effect
a. pressure enema reduction
a. pressure splint
a. pump
reflux of a.
residual a.
retrococcygeal air study
a. rifle
room air blood gas
a. sac
a. saccule
sequential impaction cascade sieve volumetric air sampler
shortness of a.
a. sickness
a. space
a. space disease
a. study
a. supply
a. swallowing
a. tight
total air volume
trapped a.
trapped air volume
a. trapping
trapping of a.
tubal air cell
tympanic air cell
ultralow particulate a.
a. velocity index
a. ventriculography
a. vesicle
a. volume
a. wastage

airbag
automobile airbag impulse noise
a. injury

air-bearing turbine handpiece

air-blade sound

air-block glaucoma

air-bone gap

air-bone-tissue boundary

airborne
a. allergen
a. bacterium
a. contact dermatitis
a. contaminant
a. contamination
a. droplet
a. infection
a. pathogen
a. precaution
a. spore
a. transmission

air-brain interface

air-conditioner lung

air-contrast
a.-c. barium enema
a.-c. enema
a.-c. fluoroscopy
a.-c. imaging
a.-c. study
a.-c. view

aircraft
simulated aircraft fire and emergency

air-displacement pipette

air-dried smear

air-driven
a.-d. artificial heart
a.-d. bur
compressed air-driven nebulizer
a.-d. oscillating saw

air-filled
a.-f. balloon
a.-f. cavity
a.-f. cushion
a.-f. cyst
a.-f. heart
a.-f. loop
a.-f. lung

air-filtration system

airflow
chronic airflow limitation
chronic airflow obstruction
obstruction of a.
a. obstruction
obstructive airflow disease
oral airflow in liters per second
volume airflow per unit of time

air-fluid
a.-f. exchange
a.-f. level
multiple air-fluid levels
pericardial air-fluid level

air-fluidized
a.-f. bed
Clinitron air-fluidized therapy

air-kerma
integrated reference a.-k.
total reference a.-k.

airless lung

airline flight radiation

airplane
a. cast
a. glue
a. glue dependence
a. position
a. shears
a. splint orthosis
a. splint shoulder brace

airport malaria

air-powered
compressed air-powered dermatome
a.-p. cutting drill

air-puff
a.-p. contact tonometer
a.-p. noncontact tonometer

air-space

airspace
a. consolidation
effective airspace dimension
a. ground-glass infiltrate
peripheral a.
a. process

airstream
a. mechanism
nasal a.

airway
aerosol-derived airway morphometry
alertness, airway, breathing, circulation, and cervical spine
asthmatic inflammatory airway disease
automated airway tree segmentation method
auto-titrating continuous positive airway pressure
a. bacterial colonization
bilevel positive airway pressure
binasal pharyngeal a.
a., breathing, circulation
a., breathing, circulation, cervical spine, and consciousness level
a., breathing, circulation, differential
a., breathing, circulation, disability, exposure
a., breathing, circulation, intravenous crystalloid
central a.
chronic airway disease
chronic airway obstruction
chronically inflamed a.
chronic obstructive airway disease
clearing of a.
complete obstruction of a.
a. conductance
congenital high airway obstruction syndrome
constant positive airway pressure
continuous distending airway pressure
continuous negative airway pressure
continuous positive airway pressure
continuous positive airway pressure device
a. dilation reflex
diminished airway perfusion
a.'s disease
distending airway pressure
end-inspiratory airway occlusion
a. eosinophilia
esophageal gastric tube a.
esophageal obturator a.
esophageal-tracheal double lumen a.
esophagogastric tube a.
exertional reactive airway disease
expiratory positive airway pressure
extrinsic compression of a.
a. function test
gastric laryngeal mask a.
a. hyperreactivity
a. hyperresponsiveness
increasing airway resistance
ineffective airway clearance
inflamed airway tissue
inspiratory positive airway pressure
intubation of a.
laryngeal mask a.
lingual airway dysfunction
lower airway disease
malignant airway obstruction
a. management
mean airway resistance
mineral dust airway disease
nasal airway clear
nasal airway obstructed
nasal airway obstruction
nasal bilevel biphasic positive airway pressure
nasal continuous positive airway pressure
nasal prong continuous positive airway pressure
nasopharyngeal a.
nasopharyngeal airway obstruction
obliterative airway disease
a. obstruction
obstruction of a.
a. obstruction in conscious patient
a. obstruction in unconscious patient
obstructive airway defect
occupational airway disease
oral a.
oral pharyngeal a.
oropharyngeal airway space
peripheral a.
peripheral airway obstruction
a. peroxidase
positive airway pressure ventilation
positive end-expiratory pressure/continuous positive airway pressure
posterior airway space
a. pressure
pressure at airway opening
a. pressure disconnect
a. pressure excursion
a. pressure release ventilation
a. protection
reactive upper airways dysfunction syndrome
a. reactivity
a. reactivity index
resistance a.
a. resistance
a. responsiveness
reversible obstructive airways disease
Sheen airway reconstruction
sleep apnea-hypersomnolence syndrome associated with upper airway obstruction
small airway disease
small airway dysfunction
small airway obstruction
a. smooth muscle
specific airway conductance
specific airway resistance
subsegmental a.
a. suction
a. suctioning

airway *(continued)*
total airway resistance
transmural pressure a.
a. tuberculosis
upper a.
upper airway closing pressure
upper airway congestion
upper airway disorder
upper airway opening pressure
upper airway resistance
upper airway resistance syndrome
upper airway respiratory syndrome
upper airway sleep apnea
variable positive airway pressure

Aitken
A. classification of epiphysial fracture
A. epiphysial fracture classification
A. femoral deficiency

AJCC TNM tumor classification

Akabane virus

akathisia
Barnes A. Scale
neuroleptic dose-dependent a.
neuroleptic-induced a.

Akerlund deformity

Akin
A. bunionectomy
A. operation
A. procedure
A. proximal phalangeal osteotomy

akinesia
a. amnestica
fetal akinesia deformation sequence
Nadbath a.
neuroleptic-induced a.
O'Brien akinesia technique
orbital a.
supraorbital a.

akinesia/diminished emotional expression

akinetic
apathetic akinetic mutism
a. apraxia
a. autism
a. depression
a. drop attack
a. epilepsy
a. left ventricle
a. mania
a. mutism
a. patient
a. psychosis
a. segment
a. segmental wall motion abnormality
a. seizure
a. stupor

akinetic-abulic syndrome

Akron midtarsal osteotomy

ala
a. of ethmoid
flaring of ala nasi
a. of ilium
nasal a.
a. of nose
sacral a.
a. of sacrum
a. of vomer

alae
flaring of alae nasi

Alagille syndrome

Alagille-Watson syndrome

Alagoas
vesicular stomatitis Alagoas virus

Alajouanine syndrome

Alajuela virus

alanine
a. amino transaminase
a. aminotransferase
ratio of serum alanine aminotransferase to serum aspartate aminotransferase
a. transaminase

Alanson amputation

alanyl-transfer ribonucleic acid synthetase

alar
a. bone
a. cartilage
a. chest
a. contour graft
a. crease
a. dome and cartilage
a. dysgenesis
a. flaring
a. flutter
a. incision
a. ligament
major alar cartilage
medial crus of major alar cartilage of nose
minor alar cartilage
nasal alar cartilage cleft
nasal alar rim
nasal alar rim reconstruction
a. notching
a. osteotome
a. plate
a. process
a. reconstruction
a. rim
a. rim excision
a. spine
a. wedge excision

alar-columella implant

alarm
a. clock voiding
digital display a.
a. mattress apnea
patient distress a.
a. reaction
a. reaction stage

alaryngeal speech

Albee
A. acetabuloplasty
A. hip arthrodesis
A. lumbar spinal fusion
A. operation
A. spinal fusion

Albee-Delbert
A.-D. operation
A.-D. procedure

Albert
A. disease
A. Einstein Neonatal Developmental Scale
A. suture technique

Alberta Infant Motor Scale

Albert-Lembert
A.-L. gastroplasty
A.-L. suture

Albert-Linder bone sectioning

albicans
corpus a.
Murex *Candida albicans* test

albinism
autosomal dominant oculocutaneous a.
autosomal recessive ocular a.
a. I, II
minimal pigment oculocutaneous a.
minimal-pigment oculocutaneous a.
Nettleship-Falls-type ocular a.
Nettleship-Falls X-linked ocular a.
ocular a.
ocular albinism 1, 2, 3
ocular albinism with late-onset sensorineural deafness

oculocutaneous a.
oculocutaneous albinism type I
partial albinism with immunodeficiency
tyrosinase-negative oculocutaneous a.
X-linked ocular a.

albinism-deafness syndrome

albinoidism
oculocutaneous a.

Albrecht syndrome

Albright
A. dimpling sign
A. disease
A. dystrophy
A. hereditary osteodystrophy
A. sign
A. solution
A. syndrome
A. synovectomy

Albright-Chase arthroplasty

Albright-Hadorn syndrome

Albright-McCune-Sternberg syndrome

albuginea
a. oculi
a. penis
a. testis
tunica albuginea oculi

albumin
aggregated a.
amoxicilloyl-human serum a.
ampicillin-human serum a.
antibovine serum albumin antibody
a. autoagglutinating factor
beef serum a.
bilirubin to albumin ratio
bovine a.
bovine plasma a.
bovine serum a.
a. clearance
a. cobalt binding
crystalline egg a.
Dubois oleic albumin complex
egg a.
a. excretion rate
guinea pig a.
human albumin microsphere
human albumin minimicrosphere
human serum a.
immunoreactive bovine serum a.
iodinated bovine serum a.
iodinated human serum a.
iodinated macroaggregated a.
iodinated rat serum a.
low plasma a.
macroaggregated a.
macroaggregated albumin arterial perfusion
macroaggregated radioiodinated a.
maleated bovine serum a.
methylated bovine serum a.
microaggregated a.
microaggregated human serum a.
mini-microaggregated albumin colloid
5% albumin, 1000 mL
5% albumin, 250 mL
mouse serum a.
narrow albumin gradient ascites
normal serum a.
polymerized human a.
polynitroxyl a.
predialyzed human a.
rabbit serum a.
radioactive iodinated human serum a.
radioactive iodinated serum a.
radioiodinated serum a.
rat serum a.
a. reading
recombinant human a.
salt-poor a.
serum a.
technetium-99m galactosyl-human serum a.
technetium-99m macroaggregated a.
technetium-99m mini-microaggregated a.
technetium albumin study
thyroxine-binding a.
total circulating a.
a. transfusion
urinary albumin excretion

albumin-globulin ratio

albumin-to-globulin ratio

albuminuria
adventitious a.
enterogenic a.
fractional albuminuria rate
lordotic a.
march a.
nephrogenous a.
neuropathic a.
orthostatic a.
postrenal a.
regulatory a.
residual a.

albumose-free tuberculin

albus
nevus spongiosus albus mucosa

albuterol
continuous albuterol nebulization
a. nebulizer

Alcian
A. blue
A. blue and periodic acid-Schiff
A. blue stain

Alcock canal

alcohol
a. absorption
a. abstinence
a. abstinence syndrome
a. abuse
a. abuse among women
a. abuse scale
a. acid
a. acquired chronic hepatocerebral degeneration
acute alcohol intoxication
acute and chronic alcohol ingestion
a. addiction
adolescent alcohol abuse
Adolescent Drug and A. Diagnostic Assessment
a. amnestic disorder
a. amnestic syndrome
a. anxiety disorder
a. as cause of seizure
Asian alcohol flush reaction
a. binge
blood a.
blood alcohol concentration
blood alcohol content
blood alcohol level
a. in bloodstream
a. in breast milk
a. breath tester
caffeine, alcohol, pepper, spicy foods
cardiovascular effects of a.
cellular effects of a.
a. cerebellar degeneration
a., chloroform, and ether mixture
chronic alcohol abuse
comorbid alcohol abuse
completely denatured a.
a. consumption behavior
a. counseling
a. craving
a. dehydrogenase
a. dependence
A. Dependence Scale
a. dependence syndrome

alcohol *(continued)*
a. dependence treatment program
a. dependence with tolerance
a. dependent
a. derivative
a. detoxification
a. diuresis
a. drinking
a. or drug abuse
drug and alcohol abuse death
drug and alcohol dependence
a. and drug dependence unit
a. and drugs
a. effect on brain
embryofetal alcohol syndrome
a., epilepsy, insulin, overdose, uremia, trauma, infection, psychiatric, stroke
a., ether, and acetone solution
excessive alcohol intake
excessive intake of a.
fetal alcohol baby
fetal alcohol effect
fetal alcohol retardation
formaldehyde, acetic acid, and alcohol solution
formalin, acetic, and alcohol solution
gastric alcohol dehydrogenase
gastritis from a.
gout from a.
a. group
a. habit
hallucination from a.
headache from a.
heat intolerance from a.
heavy alcohol consumption
heavy alcohol usage
heavy alcohol user
heavy consumption of a.
high blood alcohol level
horse liver alcohol dehydrogenase
idiosyncratic alcohol intoxication
a. idiosyncratic intoxication
impaired employee alcohol and drug treatment issue
incapacitated by a.
infertility from a.
initial levels of alcohol intake
a. injection of tumor
insomnia from a.
a. intake
a. intake withdrawal
a. interaction
a. intervention
a. intolerance
a. intoxication
a. intoxication-related disorder
isopropyl a.
a. level
limiting alcohol intake
liver alcohol dehydrogenase
local alcohol instillation effect
maternal alcohol consumption
a. metabolism
methyl alcohol peripheral neuropathy
methyl alcohol poisoning
methyl alcohol toxicity
methyl alcohol toxin
methylbenzyl a.
a. misuse
a. mood disorder
National Institute on A. Abuse and Alcoholism
a. offense
a. on breath
a. and other drug abuse
a. overdose
pathologic alcohol intoxication
a. pathological intoxication
percutaneous alcohol injection
percutaneous alcohol serotherapy
a. persisting dementia
phenol a.
a. pledget
a. poisoning
polyvinyl alcohol foam
polyvinyl alcohol fixative
positional alcohol nystagmus
a. potentiation
prenatal alcohol exposure
a. problem
Quantitative Inventory of A. Disorders
a. rehabilitation center
a. rehabilitation program
a. related
a. rub
a. sclerosis
a. sensitivity
serum alcohol level
serum methyl alcohol level
a. sleep disorder
a. sniff test
symptomatic alcohol heart muscle disease
a., tobacco, and other drugs
a. toxicity
transcoronary alcohol ablation
a. treatment unit
A. Usage Questionnaire
a. use
a. use disorder
A. Use Disorders Identification Test
a. use inventory
a. withdrawal delirium
a. withdrawal hallucinosis
a. withdrawal seizure
a. withdrawal syndrome
a. withdrawal tremulousness
yeast alcohol dehydrogenase

alcohol-Antabuse reaction

alcohol-associated dementia

alcohol-dependent
a.-d. individual
a.-d. sleep disorder

alcoholic
a. abstinence syndrome
active a.
acute alcoholic hepatitis
a. adolescent
adult child of a.
affective alcoholic psychosis
a. amblyopia
a. amentia
a. amnesia
a. amnestic disorder
A.'s Anonymous
a. ataxia
a. beverage
a. blackout
a. brain syndrome
a. cardiomyopathy
child of a.
children of a.'s
children of alcoholic screen testing
Children of A.'s Screening Test
chronic alcoholic brain syndrome
chronic alcoholic cirrhosis
chronic alcoholic delirium
chronic alcoholic heart muscle disease
chronic alcoholic pancreatitis
a. cirrhosis
a. classification
clinical alcoholic hepatitis
a. coma
a. confusional state
congenital alcoholic syndrome
decompensated alcoholic cirrhosis
a. delirium
a. dementia
a. deterioration
a. drunkenness
a. embryopathy
a. encephalopathy
a. epilepsy

a. family
a. gastritis
halfway house for a.'s
a. hallucination
a. hallucinosis
hard alcoholic user
hard core a.'s
a. heart muscle disease
a. hemorrhagic gastritis
a. hepatitis
a. hyaline inclusion body
inactive a.
a. individual
individual adult children of alcoholics counseling
a. insanity
a. jealousy
a. ketoacidosis
a. Korsakoff psychosis
a. Korsakoff syndrome
a. liver cirrhosis
a. liver disease
a. liver disease-type organic psychosis
a. malabsorption syndrome
a. mania
a. myocardiopathy
a. myopathy
newly abstinent a.
a. organic mental disorder
a. pancreatitis
a. paralysis
a. paranoia
a. paranoid psychosis
a. paranoid state
paranoid-type alcoholic psychosis
a. paraplegia
a. parent
a. paresis
a. pellagra encephalopathy
a. peripheral neuropathy
a. poisoning
a. polyneuritic psychosis
a. possible pancreatic encephalopathy
progressive perivenular alcoholic fibrosis
a. pseudoparesis
a. rehabilitation
a. steatohepatitis
a. stupor
a. symptom
a. twilight state
a. varix
a. withdrawal tremor

alcohol-induced
a.-i. anxiety
a.-i. birth defect
a.-i. cardiomyopathy
a.-i. delirium
a.-i. depression
a.-i. extracellular volume contraction
a.-i. functional impairment
a.-i. gastric injury
a.-i. gastrointestinal symptom
a.-i. hallucination
a.-i. hypertension
a.-i. hypoglycemia
a.-i. nighttime sleep
a.-i. organic mental syndrome
a.-i. pancreatitis
a.-i. paranoid state
a.-i. peripheral neuropathy
a.-i. persisting dementia
a.-i. psychotic disorder
a.-i. psychotic disorder with delusions
a.-i. psychotic disorder with hallucinations
a.-i. sexual dysfunction

alcoholism
a., leukopenia, pneumococcal sepsis
a. associated with dementia
Canterbury A. Screening Test
cardinal sign of a.
cognitive impairment in a.
a. and drug abuse
hepatitis and a.
hypothermia and a.
a. in isolation
male alcoholism subtype
McAndrews A. Scale
mental disorder due to a.
Michigan A. Screening Test
National Institute on Alcohol Abuse and A.
a. organic psychosis
Self-Administered A. Screening test
Short Michigan A. Screening Test
a. therapy class

alcohol-metabolizing system

alcohol-methadone interaction

alcohol-positive history

alcohol-precipitated epilepsy

alcohol-related
a.-r. behavior
a.-r. birth defect
a.-r. chronic pancreatitis
a.-r. dementia
a.-r. diagnosis
a.-r. disorder
a.-r. harm
a.-r. headache
a.-r. health hazard
a.-r. heart disorders
a.-r. hepatitis
a.-r. illness
a.-r. injury
a.-r. insomnia
a.-r. liver disease
a.-r. neurodevelopmental disorder
a.-r. offense
a.-r. phenotype
a.-r. physical problem
a.-r. psychiatric problem
a.-r. risk for accident
a.-r. risk for suicide
a.-r. risk for violence
a.-r. seizure
a.-r. use disorder, not otherwise specified

aldehyde
angular a.
a. dehydrogenase
a. fuchsin
methyl a.

aldehyde-fuchsin stain

aldehyde-thionine-periodic acid-Schiff test

Alden loop gastric bypass

alder
A. anomaly
A. body
a. tree
a. tree pollen

aldolase
fructose diphosphate a.
serum a.

aldose
a. reductase
a. reductase inhibitor

aldosterone
adrenal vein aldosterone ratio
a. antagonist
a. deficiency
a. excretion rate
low renin, normal a.
plasma a.
plasma aldosterone concentration
a. receptor
a. secretion defect
a. secretion rate
a. secretory rate
urinary a.

aldosterone-induced protein

aldosterone-producing adenoma

aldosterone-stimulating hormone

aldosteronism
- adrenal primary a.
- glucocorticoid-remediable a.
- primary a.
- syndrome of primary a.

aldoxime
- pyridine aldoxime methiodide

Aldrich syndrome

Alenquer virus

alert
- awake, alert, oriented
- a. awake state
- a. behavior
- a. check
- conscious and a.
- a. and cooperative
- a., cooperative, and oriented
- a. inactivity
- lymphedema alert bracelet
- medical alert bracelet
- medical alert center
- medical alert necklace
- oriented
- a. and oriented
- oriented and a.
- a. and oriented to person, place, and time
- a. and oriented to person, place, time, and date
- a. patient
- patient alert and cooperative
- patient alert and oriented
- patient awake, alert, and cooperative
- patient mentally a.
- patient alert to space, time, and person
- a. state of consciousness
- suicide a.
- a., verbal stimulus response, painful stimulus response, unresponsive
- a., vocal stimulus, painful stimulus, unresponsive

alerting
- a. effect
- a. maneuver on electroencephalogram
- a. mechanism
- a. stimulus
- a. stimulus on electroencephalogram

alertness
- Academic A.
- a., airway, breathing, circulation, and cervical spine
- attention alertness test
- gradual loss of a.
- impaired a.
- increased a.
- a. level
- mental a.
- Observer Assessment of A. and Sedation
- a., response to voice, response to pain, unresponsive
- state of a.

aleukemic
- a. granulocytic leukemia
- a. leukemia
- a. lymphocytic leukemia
- a. monocytic leukemia
- a. myelosis
- a. presentation

aleukia
- alimentary toxic a.
- a. hemorrhagica

aleukocythemic leukemia

Aleutian
- A. mink disease
- A. mink disease virus

Alexander anomaly

alexandrite
- a. laser lithotripsy
- a. long-pulsed laser

alexia
- aphasia, agnosia, apraxia, agraphia, and a.
- a. with agraphia
- a. without agraphia

alexin unit

Alexithymia
- Toronto Alexithymia Scale

alexithymic
- a. behavior
- a. personality

Alezzandrini syndrome

alfa
- epoetin a.
- interferon a.

alfalfa
- a. grass
- a. weed pollen

algae
- blue-green a.

Algebra
- Iowa Algebra Aptitude Test

algebraic
- a. reconstruction technique
- a. unknown or space coordinate

Al-Ghorab procedure

algid stage

alginate
- a. dressing
- a. wound cover

algogenic psychosyndrome

algolagnia
- passive a.

algorithm
- artificial neural network a.
- asthma care a.
- correlation a.
- genetic a.
- phase-invariant signature a.
- standard infertility treatment a.
- Swedish interactive thresholding a.

algorithm-oriented language

Alibert-Bazin
- A.-B. syndrome

Alibert disease

Alice in Wonderland syndrome

alien
- a. hand sign
- a. hand syndrome
- a. limb phenomenon
- a. limb sign
- myoclonic alien hand syndrome
- a. obsession
- a. thought

alienation
- Adolescent A. Index
- a. coefficient

aligning
- beam aligning holder

alignment
- abnormal a.
- active a.
- anatomic a.
- anatomical position and a.
- anatomic position and a.
- angular a.
- a. and apposition
- apposition and a.
- arch a.
- atlantoaxial a.
- bony a.
- a. chart
- a. curve

eye a.
femoral alignment jig
fiducial alignment system
field a.
a. of fracture
a. of fracture fragment
improper foot a.
a. index
joint alignment and motion
knee joint alignment disorder
long alignment rod
a. mark
a. measurement
normal anatomic a.
normalized alignment score
ocular a.
orbicular a.
overall a.
patellar a.
patellofemoral a.
a. pin
poor a.
position and a.
a. and position
position and a.
proper alignment of fracture
restoration of normal anatomic a.
structural a.
a. of tangential beam
tibiofemoral a.
a. of vertebral bodies

A-like non-A non-B hepatitis

alimentary
a. abstinence
a. bolus
a. canal
a. diabetes
a. glycosuria
a. hyperinsulinism
a. hypoglycemia
a. lipemia
a. obesity
oral alimentary automatism
a. osteopathy
a. pentosuria
a. seizure
a. system
a. toxic aleukia
a. tract
a. tract calcification
a. tract duplication

alimentation
elemental enteral a.
enteral a.
oral a.
total parenteral a.

aliquot
urine a.

alive and well

alizarin red S dye

alkali
ammonia alkali burn
Apt-Downey alkali denaturation test
a. burn
a. caustic
a. ingestion
milk alkali syndrome
a. patch test

alkaline
antidigoxigenin alkaline phosphatase antibody-conjugate
bacterial alkaline phosphatase
bone alkaline phosphatase
bone-specific alkaline phosphatase
a. buffer
a. diuresis
heat-stable alkaline phosphatase
a. injury
leukocyte alkaline phosphatase
leukocyte alkaline phosphatase activity
leukocyte alkaline phosphatase stain
microbial alkaline protease inhibitor
a. phosphatase
a. phosphatase activity of granular leukocyte
a. phosphatase antialkaline phosphatase
a. phosphatase isoenzyme
a. phosphatase isoenzyme tumor marker
a. phosphatase and pyrophosphate
a. phosphatase test
placental alkaline phosphatase
polyclonal antiplacental alkaline phosphatase
a. protease inhibitor
a. reflux esophagitis
a. reflux gastritis
serum alkaline phosphatase
soluble in alkaline medium
total alkaline phosphatase
a. toxicity
a. tuberculin

alkaline-ash diet

alkaline-encrusted cystitis

alkali-soluble nitrogen

alkali-stable pepsin

alkaloid
miotic a.
opium a.
pyrrolizidine a.
total a.

alkaloid-associated
ergot alkaloid-associated heart disease

alkalosis
altitude a.
metabolic a.
primarily respiratory a.
respiratory a.
uncompensated a.
watery diarrhea with hypokalemic a.

Alken approach

alkyl
arylated a.
linear alkyl sulfonate

alkylated androgenic steroid

alkylating
a. action
a. agent
a. agent therapy
a. chemotherapy
a. therapy

alkylbenzene sulfonate

6-alkyl guanine alkyl transferase

all
a. culture broth
failure of all vital forces
general all purpose
a. known allergies
lethal dose in all exposed subjects
longitudinal expert evaluation using all available data
massive all layer liposuction
moves all extremities
moves all extremities equally well
moves all extremities slowly
a. night sleep recording
a. or none
oriented in all spheres
a. 4 quadrants
summation of all quantities following the symbol
weak and dizzy all over

allachesthesia
optical a.

all-alumina socket

allantoic stalk

allantoidoangiopagous twins

allantoin vaginal cream

all-cause mortality

all-donor chimerism

alleged
- a. father
- a. onset date

allele
- frequency of the more common allele of a pair
- frequency of rarer allele of a gene pair
- human leukocyte antigen a.
- multiple a.

allele-specific
- mutant allele-specific amplification
- a.-s. oligomer
- a.-s. oligonucleotide
- a.-s. polymerase chain reaction

allelic
- a. exclusion
- a. gene
- a. heterogeneity
- a. polymorphism

allelotyping
- molecular a.
- p53 a.

Allen
- A. maneuver
- A. sign
- A. test
- A. vision test

Allen-Herndon-Dudley syndrome

allercoat enzyme allergosorbent unit

allergen
- airborne a.
- atopic a.
- cerebral a.
- environmental a.
- exposure to a.
- food a.
- greatest single allergen present
- a. inhalation challenge test
- *Lolium perenne* a.
- occupational a.
- a. specific nasal challenge
- total allergen content

allergenic
- a. arthritis
- a. epitope
- a. extract

allergen-induced asthma

allergic
- acute allergic encephalitis
- acute allergic interstitial nephritis
- acute allergic urticaria
- a. alveolitis
- a. angiitis
- a. angiitis and granulomatosis
- a. angioedema
- a. asthma
- biological allergic unit
- a. blepharitis
- a. blepharoconjunctivitis
- a. bowel disease
- a. bronchopulmonary aspergillosis
- a. bronchopulmonary mycosis
- a. colitis
- congestive seasonal allergic rhinitis
- a. conjunctivitis
- a. contact dermatitis
- a. contact stomatitis
- a. coryza
- a. cystitis
- a. dermatitis
- a. diaper rash
- a. diathesis
- a. disease
- a. drug reaction
- a. eczema
- eczematous allergic contact dermatitis
- a. eczematous contact dermatitis
- a. eczematous contact-type dermatitis
- a. encephalitis
- a. encephalomyelitis
- a. enterocolitis
- a. enteropathy
- a. eosinophilic gastroenteritis
- a. eosinophilic gastroenterocolitis
- a. esophagitis
- experimental allergic encephalitis
- experimental allergic encephalomyelitis
- experimental allergic neuritis
- experimental allergic orchitis
- a. extract
- extrinsic allergic alveolitis
- a. extrinsic alveolitis
- a. eye disease
- a. facies
- a. fungal sinusitis
- a. gingivitis
- a. gingivostomatitis
- a. gold dermatitis
- a. granulomatosis and angiitis
- a. granulomatous angiitis
- a. granulomatous arteritis
- a. granulomatous prostatitis
- a. importance
- a. inflammation
- a. interstitial nephritis
- a. keratoconjunctivitis
- a. laryngeal edema
- a. lung disorder
- a. manifestation
- nasal allergic disorder
- a. neuritis
- nonatopic allergic conjunctivitis
- a. nonthrombocytopenic purpura
- occupational allergic alveolitis
- a. orchitis
- a. pannus
- perennial allergic conjunctivitis
- perennial allergic rhinoconjunctivitis
- a. phenomenon
- photocontact a.
- a. pneumonia
- a. polyp
- possible allergic reaction
- probable allergic rhinitis
- a. proctitis
- a. psychogenic disorder
- a. pulmonary edema
- a. purpura
- a. reaction
- a. respiratory disease
- a. response
- a. rhinitis
- a. rhinitis perennial
- a. rhinobronchitis
- a. rhinoconjunctivitis
- a. salute
- seasonal allergic rhinitis
- seasonal allergic rhinoconjunctivitis
- a. sensitivity
- a. shiner
- a. shock
- a. sialadenitis
- a. sinusitis
- a. stomatitis
- a. transfusion reaction
- a. urticaria
- a. vasculitis

allergosorbent
- allercoat enzyme allergosorbent unit
- enzyme allergosorbent test
- fluorescent allergosorbent test
- multithread allergosorbent test

allergy
- acute food a.

all known a.'s
colic and a.
color allergy screening test
coughing from a.
cow's milk a.
cow's milk protein a.
house dust a.
a. immune system
a. and immunology
a. index
a. to insulin
known drug a.'s
laboratory animal dander a.
milk lactose a.
milk protein a.
minimal a.'s
moderate allergies
moderate-severe a.'s
muscle pain, allergy, tachycardia and tiredness, headache syndrome
National Institute of A. and Infectious Disease
natural rubber latex a.
no known a.'s
no known drug a.'s
no known food a.'s
no known medication a.'s
patch test for a.
pediatric a.
penicillin allergy skin testing
percutaneous allergy testing
photo a.
preventive allergy treatment
a. relief medicine
severe a.'s
severe latex a.
specific immunotherapy a.
a. testing
total allergy syndrome
a. treatment
a. unit

alleviating
a. violence
a. violence in aggressive behavior

all-fours
a.-f. maneuver
a.-f. maneuver for shoulder dystocia

Alliance
National Alliance of Breast Cancer Organization
National Alliance for Hispanic Health
National Alliance for the Mentally Ill

allied
a. health professional
a. reflex

alligator
a. bone-reduction forceps
a. forceps
a. scissors
a. skin

alligator-type grasping forceps

all-inclusive care

all-inside repair

Allis
A. maneuver
A. sign
A. test

Allison hiatal hernia repair

Allman
A. acromioclavicular injury classification
A. modification of Evans ankle reconstruction

all-median nerve hand

alloactivated killer cell

alloantibody
anti-HLA a.

alloantigen-independent risk factor

alloantigen response

allocating cadaveric kidney

allocation
a. of treatment
organ allocation policy

allochrome
Lillie allochrome connective tissue stain
Lillie allochrome method

allocortical cortex

AlloDerm
micronized AlloDerm tissue

allodonor lymphocyte infusion

allogeneic
a. antigen
a. antigen candidate
antigen-extracted allogeneic bone
autologous and allogeneic marrow transplantation
a. blood transfusion
a. bone marrow cell
a. bone marrow transplant
a. bone marrow transplantation
a. cellular immune therapy
devitalized allogeneic bone
a. disease
a. donor
a. engraftment
a. lymphocyte cytotoxicity
a. marrow transplantation
a. mixed leukocyte culture
nonmyeloablative allogeneic stem cell transplant
a. peripheral cell transplant
a. stem cell
a. stem cell transplant
a. stem cell transplantation
a. tumor cell immunization
a. tumor cell vaccine

allogenic
a. antigen
antigen-extracted a.
antigen-extracted allogenic bone
a. blood
a. blood component
a. blood transfusion
a. BMT
a. bone
a. bone crib
a. bone graft
a. bone marrow
a. bone marrow cell infusion
a. bone marrow transplantation
a. dendritic cell
a. disease
a. effect
a. effect factor
engrafted allogenic tissue
a. fetal graft
a. graft
a. hematopoietic stem cell transplantation
a. implant
a. inhibition
a. keratinocyte graft
a. kidney transplant
a. liver perfusion
a. lyophilized bone graft implant material
nonmyeloablative allogenic transplant
a. transplant
a. transplantation

allogenically vascularized prefabricated flap

allogenous bone graft

allograft
acute allograft rejection
aortic allograft conduit
a. bone grafting
cancellous freeze-dried a.
cardiac allograft vascular disease

allograft *(continued)*
cardiac allograft vasculopathy
chronic allograft nephropathy
a. corneal rejection
a. coronary artery disease
cortical bone a.
cryopreserved heart valve a.
cryopreserved human aortic a.
decalcified freeze-dried bone a.
demineralized freeze-dried bone a.
a. dermal matrix graft
a. extraction
femoral diaphysial a.
freeze-dried bone a.
freeze-dried cancellous a.
fresh frozen a.
a. iliac bone
a. irradiation
a. joint replacement
a. ligament replacement
a. membrane
napkin ring calcar a.
neonatal skin a.
a. nephropathy
osteoarticular allograft transplantation
a. parenchyma
a. pathology
a. reaction
a. reconstruction of fibular collateral ligament
a. rejection
renal allograft recipient
renal allograft rejection
a. strut
a. survival
a. survival rate
a. tissue transplantation
total lymphoid irradiation for allograft survival
a. transplantation
a. vasculopathy

allograft-bound lymphocyte

allograft-host junction

allografting
nerve a.

allograft-mediated hypertension

allographic stem cell transplant

alloimmune
a. disease
a. factor
fetomaternal alloimmune thrombocytopenia
a. hemolytic anemia
a. hemolytic disease of newborn
a. mechanism
neonatal alloimmune thrombocytopenic purpura
a. neonatal neutropenia
a. neonatal thrombocytopenic purpura
passive alloimmune thrombocytopenia
a. thrombocytopenia

alloimmunization
platelet a.

allomeric function

allopathic medicine

alloplastic
a. AMA
Aquaplast alloplastic material
a. biomaterial
a. chin augmentation
a. cranioplasty
a. crib
a. donor material
a. facial implant
a. graft
a. interpositional implant
malar alloplastic augmentation
a. material
midface alloplastic augmentation
a. plate
a. prostatic bladder
a. reconstruction
a. sandwich augmentation
a. spermatocele
a. temporomandibular joint prosthesis
a. transplant

allopsychic delusion

allopurinol hypersensitivity syndrome

all-or-none
a.-o.-n. law
a.-o.-n. phenomenon
a.-o.-n. reaction

all-or-nothing phenomenon

allosteric
full allosteric modulators
a. manner
partial allosteric modulators

allotransplantation
liver a.
total small intestinal a.

allotransplant recipient

allotropic personality

allotype
nominal a.
a. suppression

allotypic
a. determinant
a. marker

allowable
a. daily intake
a. limits of error
maximal allowable concentration
maximal allowable cost
maximal allowable dose
maximum allowable cost

allowance
approved dietary a.
recommended daily dietary a.
schedule of maximal a.

allowed
product selection a.

alloxan
hypophysectomized alloxan diabetic

alloy
base metal crown and bridge a.
forged cobalt-chromium alloy prosthesis
low-fusing a.
a. of mercury
metal a.
Midas a.
nickel-titanium a.
noble gold a.
Optaloy amalgam a.
a. restoration
shape memory a.

all-polyethylene socket

all-porcelain restoration

Allport
A. group relations theory
A. personality trait theory

Allport-Vernon-Linzey Study of Values

all-progestin contraceptive

all-purpose capsule

allspice oil

all-trans-retinoic acid

all-ulnar nerve hand

allusion in wit

allusive thinking

Almeida disease

Almeirim virus

almond
a. oil
oil of bitter a.

Almpiwar virus

aloin, belladonna, strychnine laxative

alone
intolerance of being a.
pancreas transplantation a.
pancreatic transplantation a.

along
induration along skin incision
propagated sensation along the channel
propagated sensation along the meridian
redness along incision site

alopecia
androgenetic a.
a. areata
central centrifugal scarring a.
a., contracture, dwarfism
a., contracture, dwarfism, mental retardation syndrome
a., epilepsy, oligophrenia syndrome
female pattern androgenetic a.
fibrosing alopecia in a pattern distribution
frontal fibrosing a.
growth retardation, alopecia, pseudoanodontia, and optic atrophy syndrome
ichthyosis, follicularis, atrichia or alopecia, photophobia syndrome
male pattern androgenetic a.
a., mental retardation, epilepsy, microcephaly syndrome
Moynahan alopecia syndrome
a. mucinosa/follicular mucinosis
a., nail dystrophy, ophthalmic complication, thyroid dysfunction, hypohidrosis, ephelides and enteropathy, and respiratory tract infection
ophiasic alopecia areata

Alouette
A. amputation
A. operation

alpha
abnormal alpha activity
a. activity
adjuvant alpha blockade
a. agonist
a. alcoholism
alternate with alpha rhythm
a. amino acid
a. antagonist
a. antigen
anti-interleukin-2 receptor alpha monoclonal antibody
a. antitrypsin level
a. apparent
a. arc
Army Alpha test
a., beta, gamma hypotheses
a. beta value
a. biofeedback
a. block
a. blocking
a. blocking agent
a. bone substitute material
a. brain wave
branched-chain alpha ketoacid dehydrogenase
a. burst
burst of alpha activity
a. cell
a. cell alternate
a. chain
a. chain disease
a. coefficient
colitis and alpha biofeedback
concept of alpha biofeedback
a. conditioning session
constituent of alpha protein plasma fraction
controlling alpha activity
a., delta sleep anomaly
a. error
estrogen receptor a.
a. examination
a. factor
fast alpha variant rhythm
a. feedback
a. fetoprotein
a. fetoprotein test
first in alpha series or group
a. frequency
a. frequency activity
a. frequency band
a. frequency coma
a. frequency range
frequent individual bursts of alpha activity
a. gene
a. globulin
a. globulin antibody
a. hemolysin
a. hemolysis
a. hemolytic streptococcus
immunoregulatory alpha globulin
a. index
interferon alpha 2-alpha
a. interferon therapy
interleukin-1 alpha converting enzyme
a. islet cell neoplasm
a. lactalbumin
a. level
low alpha coefficient
maternal alpha fetoprotein
mean alpha frequency
a. methyldopa
minor alpha asymmetry
MIP-1 a.
a. motor neuron
a. movement
a. nerve fiber
normal alpha rhythm
obsessional compulsive inventory a.
paroxysmal alpha activity
a. particle
a. pattern
a. radiation
a. ray
a. receptor
a. receptor blocking agent
recombinant human MIP-1 a.
recombinant interferon a.
recombinant tumor necrosis factor a.
a. response
retained alpha activity
a. rhythm
rhythm of alpha frequency
a. rhythm frequency
a. scan
a. sigmoid loop
slow alpha variant rhythm
a. smooth muscle actin
a. state
steady alpha rhythm
a. sympathetic blockade
a. test
a. thalassemia
a. threshold
a. tocopherol beta carotene
transforming growth factor a.
tumor necrosis factor-a.
a. units
a. variant
a. verbal test
a. wave
a. wave intrusion
waves of alpha frequency
a. wave strain
a. wave training

alpha-1
a.-1 adrenergic antagonist
a.-1 adrenergic blocking agent

alpha-1 *(continued)*
a.-1 adrenoreceptor
a.-1 agonist
a.-1 antichymotrypsin
a.-1 antitrypsin
a.-1 antitrypsin deficiency
a.-1 antitrypsin disease
a.-1 blocker
a.-1 fetoprotein assay
macrophage inflammatory protein a.-1
a.-1 PI
prostate-specific antigen bound to alpha-1 antichymotrypsin
recombinant alpha-1 antitrypsin

2-alpha
interferon alpha 2-a.

alpha-2
a.-2 adrenergic receptor
a.-2 antagonist
a.-2 antiplasmin
a.-2 globulin
pregnancy alpha-2 glycoprotein

$alpha_1$
human $alpha_1$-proteinase inhibitor
interferon $a._1$
thymosin $a._1$

alpha-1-adrenoceptor antagonist

alpha1-antichymotrypsin-prostate-specific antigen

alpha1-antitrypsin disease

alpha-21 antiplasmin

alpha-2-adrenoreceptor agonist

$alpha_1$-acid glycoprotein

alpha-adrenergic
a.-a. agent
a.-a. agonist
a.-a. antagonist
a.-a. blockade
a.-a. blocker
a.-a. blocking agent
a.-a. blocking drug
a.-a. receptor
a.-a. receptor agonist
a.-a. receptor antagonist
a.-a. receptors
a.-a. stimulating drug
a.-a. stimulation
a.-a. stimulator

alpha-1-adrenergic
a.-a. agonist
a.-a. antagonist

alpha-2-adrenergic
a.-a. agonist
a.-a. receptor
a.-a. receptor antagonist

alpha-adrenoceptor
a.-a. antagonist
a.-a. blocker

alpha-adrenoreceptor agonist

alpha-allokainic acid

alpha-amino nitrogen

alpha-amylase
pancreatic a.-a.

alpha-antilysin deficiency

$alpha_2$antiplasmin

alpha-1-antitrypsin
a.-a. deficiency
a.-a. deficiency disease
a.-a. disease
a.-a. disease-related emphysema
a.-a. globulin
a.-a. level

$alpha_1$-antitrypsin
$a._1$-a. deficiency
$a._1$-a. phenotyping

alpha-antitrypsin deficiency

alpha-blocker therapy

alpha-cell
pancreatic alpha-cell tumor

alpha-chain
a.-c. disease

alpha-fetoprotein
a.-f. elevation
a.-f. enzyme immunoassay
human a.-f.
maternal serum a.-f.

alpha-galactoside leukocyte

alpha-gliadin fraction

alpha-heavy-chain disease

alpha-hemolytic ***Streptococcus***

alpha-human chorionic gonadotropin

alpha-hydroxy
a.-h. acid
a.-h. acid gel

alpha-ketoisocaproic acid

alpha-linolenic acid

alpha-lipoic acid

alpha-melanocyte-stimulating hormone

alpha-methyldopa-induced mood disorder

alpha-nonrapid
a.-n. eye movement
a.-n. eye movement sleep

$alpha_1$-protease inhibitor

$alpha_1$-proteinase inhibitor

alpha-receptor
a.-r. antagonist
a.-r. blockade therapy

5-alpha-reductase
5-a.-r. inhibition
5-a.-r. inhibitor
5-a.-r. type I, II

alpha-reductase deficiency

alpha-thalassemia
a.-t. mental retardation
a.-t. minor

alpha-thalassemia-1, -2 trait

alpha-theta wave

$alpha_1$-trypsin inhibitor

Alport
autosomal-recessive Alport syndrome
A. syndrome
X-linked Alport syndrome

Alsberg
A. angle
A. triangle

also known as

Alström
A. disease
A. syndrome

Alstrom-Edwards syndrome

Alstrom-Hallgren syndrome

alta
patella a.

Altamira virus

alter
a.native alter ego
a.'s brain chemistry
a. ego
a. ego transference
a. gastric functioning

alteration
architectural alterations of bone
a. of blood brain barrier
blood gas a.
a. in consciousness
a. in hydration intake
a. in identity
a. of memory structure
metabolic a.
mitochondrial cristae a.
molecular genetic a.

neurocognitive a.
a. in nutrition intake
periodontium a.
qualitative a.
a. in rate of speech
a. in respiratory function
structural a.
a. in time perception

altered
a. appetite
a. auditory feedback
a. by behavior
a. body temperature
a. bowel habit
a. bowel movement
a. brain function
catalyst altered water
a. cognition
a. consciousness
a. development
a. facial appearance
a. function
a. gastric motility
a. growth and development
a. health maintenance
a. level of consciousness
a. life circumstance
a. mental state
a. mental status
a. mind-body perception
a. mood and perception
a. perception
a. performance
a. personal behavior
a. pharmacodynamics
a. sensation
a. sensory perception
a. set point
a. sleep schedule
a. spatial perception
a. sperm motility
a. state
a. state of conscious awareness
a. state of consciousness
a. tau processing
a. thought process
a. time perception
a. vision
a. voice

altering brain function

alternans
auditory a.
auscultatory a.
a. of the heart
parvus a.
T-wave a.

alternate
alpha cell a.
binaural alternate loudness balance
a. binaural loudness balance
a. cover test
a. forms reliability coefficient
a. hemianesthesia
a. hemiplegia
high single dose alternate day
a. identity
a. inspiration and expiration of air
a. level of care
a. monaural loudness balance test
a. motion rate
prism and alternate cover test
purified alternate pathway
a. response test
a. uses test
a. with alpha rhythm

alternate-day therapy

alternating
a. abducens
arrhythmia-insensitive flow-sensitive alternating inversion recovery
arrhythmia-insensitive flow-sensitive alternating IR
a. behavior
a. bidirectional tachycardia
a. bipolar disorder
a. current
a. current or direct current
a. days [L. *alternis dies*]
a. exotropia
a. failure of response mechanical to electrical depolarization
a. hemiplegia of childhood
a. hypertropia
a. hypotropia
a. insanity
low frequency alternating current
a. motion rate
a. mydriasis
a. nystagmus
a. oculomotor hemiplegia
periodic alternating gaze
periodic alternating gaze deviation
periodic alternating windmill nystagmus
a. personality
a. perspective
a. pressure mattress
a. pressure pad
a. psychosis
a. pulse
a. range of motion
rapid alternating movements
Rapidly A. Speech Perception Test
rapid rhythmic alternating movements
a. role
Speech with A. Masking Index
a. suture
a. tremor
a. triple therapy

alternation
electrical alternation of heart
mechanical alternation of the heart
Mental A. Test

alternative
a. alter ego
a. approach
augmentative and alternative communication
a. behavior
a. birth center
a. cancer therapy
complementary and alternative approach
complementary and alternative medicine
consent form to delivery by alternative physician
cost-effective a.
a. criterion B for dysthymic disorder
a. delivery system
a. diagnosis
a. dimensional descriptors for schizophrenia
a. donor
a. drug
a. explanation
a. health care
a. hypothesis
a. intervention
a. leisure activity
a. lifestyle
A. Lifestyle Checklist
a. lifestyle community
a.'s of management
a. medication
medicine
a. medicine
a. method
a. method of treatment
no a.
a. occipital artery middle cerebral artery
Office of A. Medicine

alternative *(continued)*
a. pathway of complement cascade
a. patterns of complement
a. perspective
positive a.
a. practitioner
procedure a.
procedures, a.'s, indications and complications
a. psychosis
risks, benefits, and a.'s
a. school
a. strategy
a. temporal forced choice
therapeutic a.
a. therapy
a. treatment
viable a.
a. viewpoint
a. to violent behavior

alternis
alternating days [L. *alternis dies*]

altitude
a. alkalosis
a. anoxia
General High A. Questionnaire
a. hypoxia
a. illness
a. sickness
a. syndrome

altitudinal scotoma

Altmann pulse

altruistic
a. behavior
a. personality
a. role
a. suicide

alum
Mayer acid alum hematoxylin stain

alumina
a. bioceramic joint replacement
a. cemented total hip prosthesis
magnesia and alumina oral suspension

alumina-alumina total hip replacement prosthesis

alumina-on-alumina prosthesis

alumina-reinforced porcelain crown

aluminous porcelain

aluminum
a. accumulation
a. bismuth oxide
a. bone disease
a. chloride solution
a. contouring template set
a. crown
a. deposit
a. foam splint
folded aluminum ear splint
a. hand splint
a. intoxication
magnesium aluminum hydroxide
magnesium aluminum silicate
Maloney stain for a.
a. master rod
neodymium:yttrium aluminum garnet laser
a. oxide abrasive
a. oxide arthroplasty material
a. oxide ceramic coating
a. oxide ceramic core
penicillin aluminum monostearate
a. pneumoconiosis
purified diphtheria toxoid precipitated by aluminum phosphate
a. salt
structural aluminum malleable
a. toxicity
a. wafer
a. wire splint
yttrium, aluminum, garnet

aluminum-associated osteomalacia

aluminum-induced osteomalacia

alum-precipitated
a.-p. diphtheria toxoid
a.-p. pyridine
a.-p. vaccine

alveolar
a. abscess
accumulated alveolar ventilatory volume
acute alveolar injury
anterior alveolar branch of maxillary nerve
anterior alveolar nerve
anterior middle superior a.
anterior superior alveolar artery
anterior superior alveolar branch of infraorbital nerve
a. arch acrylic splint
a. arch derangement
a. arch of mandible
a. arch of maxilla
arterial to a.
arterial to alveolar oxygen tension ratio
arterial to alveolar gradient
a. basement membrane
bilateral alveolar pulmonary infiltrate
a. bone
a. capillary membrane
a. cell
a. cell carcinoma
a. cell hyperplasia
central alveolar hypoventilation
central alveolar hypoventilation syndrome
a. density
difference in nitrogen tension between mixed alveolar gas and mixed arterial blood
difference in partial pressures of oxygen in mixed alveolar gas and mixed arterial blood
diffuse alveolar damage
diffuse alveolar hemorrhage
diffuse pulmonary alveolar hemorrhage
diffusion per unit of alveolar volume
a. disease
a. duct
effective alveolar ventilation
fluffy alveolar infiltrate
fraction of alveolar carbon dioxide
a. gingiva
a. hemorrhage
human alveolar macrophage
hyaline membranes lining alveolar space
a. hydatid disease
hyperplastic alveolar nodule
a. hypertension
a. hyperventilation
a. hypoventilation syndrome
a. hypoxia
idiopathic alveolar fibrosis
inferior alveolar nerve
a. lavage
lingual alveolar bone
lingual alveolar plate
lingual alveolar ridge
a. living material
lobular alveolar pattern
lower alveolar point
lower alveolar ridge
a. macrophage
mandibular alveolar mucosa
a. margin
maxillary alveolar buttress
maxillary alveolar protrusion

maxillary alveolar ridge
median alveolar cyst
median alveolar notch
mental branch of inferior alveolar artery
middle alveolar artery
minimum alveolar anesthetic concentration
1-minimum alveolar concentration
minute alveolar volume
a. minute ventilation
a. mucosa
mylohyoid branch of inferior alveolar artery
nodule-like alveolar lesion
a. occlusal border
a. occlusal plane
overdistention of alveolar populations
a. oxygen partial pressure
palatal alveolar fracture
partial pressure alveolar oxygen
a. partial pressure of inhalational anesthetic
passive alveolar molding appliance
patchy alveolar opacity
perforating alveolar artery
peribronchial alveolar space
a. permeability
a. pressure
a. process
proximal alveolar region
pulmonary alveolar hemorrhage
pulmonary alveolar hypoxic vasoconstriction
pulmonary alveolar macrophage
pulmonary alveolar microlithiasis
pulmonary alveolar proteinosis
a. pulmonary edema
regional alveolar damage
a. rhabdomyosarcoma
a. ridge
a. rupture
a. sac
a. sarcoidosis
segmental alveolar osteotomy
segmental alveolar pattern
a. sinus
a. soft part sarcoma
a. tidal volume
a. ventilation
ventilation of alveolar dead space
a. ventilation per minute
volume of alveolar dead space
a. wall
a. wall basement membrane
a. wash

alveolar-arterial
a.-a. carbon dioxide difference
a.-a. difference in partial pressure of oxygen
a.-a. gradient
a.-a. oxygen
a.-a. oxygen gradient
a.-a. oxygen tension difference
a.-a. oxygen tension gradient
a.-a. PO_2 difference
a.-a. pressure difference

alveolar-capillary
a.-c. block
a.-c. membrane permeability

alveolar-interstitial lung disease

alveolar-to-arterial oxygen difference

alveolectomy
maxillary mandibular odentectomy a.

alveoli (*pl. of* alveolus)

alveolitis
allergic a.
allergic extrinsic a.
cryptogenic fibrosing a.
extrinsic allergic a.
fibrosing a.
hypersensitivity a.
idiopathic fibrosing a.
occupational allergic a.

alveolocapillary partial pressure gradient

alveolodental
a. osteoperiostitis
a. periostitis

alveoloplasty
odontectomy and a.

alveolus, pl. **alveoli**
cleft lip and a.
cluster of milk-secreting alveoli
maxillary first molar a.
pulmonary alveoli

Alvis operation

ALV-related virus

alymphoplasia
Nezelof type of thymic a.
thymic a.

Alzheimer
A. basket
A. cell
degenerative dementia of Alzheimer type
A. dementia
dementia of Alzheimer type
A. disease
A. Disease Assessment Scale
A. Disease Assessment Scale, cognitive subscale
A. Disease Center
A. Disease Education and Referral
A. Disease Rating Scale
A. disease-related dementia
A. Disease and Related Disorders Association
early-onset Alzheimer disease
early-onset form of familial Alzheimer disease
familial Alzheimer dementia
A. fibrillary degeneration
A. II cell
late-onset Alzheimer disease
nonpsychotic Alzheimer patient
nosotropic drug dementia of Alzheimer type
A. precursor protein
A. presenile dementia
primary degenerative dementia of Alzheimer type
A. psychosis
A. sclerosis
senile dementia of the Alzheimer type
A. stain
structured interview for diagnosis of Alzheimer dementia
A. survivor
A. syndrome
A. type I, II astrocyte

Alzheimer-like senile dementia

Alzheimer-type
A.-t. dementia

amacrine cell

Amadori-type rearrangement

amalgam
Mowrey 695 a.
Optaloy amalgam alloy
a. tattoo

amalgamator
mechanical a.

***Amanita* mushroom hepatotoxicity**

Amapari virus

Amat
Marin Amat syndrome

Amato body

amaurosis
a. congenita of Leber
a. fugax
Leber congenital a.

amaurotic
a. axonal idiocy
a. cat's eye
a. familial idiocy
infantile amaurotic familial idiocy
juvenile amaurotic idiocy
late infantile amaurotic familial idiocy
a. mydriasis
a. nystagmus
a. pupil

amber fluid

ambient
chilly ambient temperature
contamination from ambient hospital air
a. factor
a. fissure
a. hospital air
a. light
a. noise
a. pressure
a. temperature
a. temperature and pressure
a. temperature and pressure, dry

ambiguity
acoustic a.
genital a.
lexical a.
linguistic a.

ambiguous
aniridia, ambiguous genitalia, mental retardation
aniridia, ambiguous genitalia, mental retardation triad syndrome
a. external genitalia
a. external stimuli
a. figure
a. genitalia

ambiguus
nucleus a.
situs ambiguus with polysplenia

AmB-induced reduction GFR

ambisexual development

ambivalence
affective a.

ambivalent
a. affect
a. feeling
positive-negative ambivalent quotient

amblyogenic
neonatal amblyogenic stimulus

amblyopia
alcoholic a.
anisometric a.
anisometropic a.
arsenic a.
astigmatic a.
axial a.
hysteric a.
meridional a.
microstrabismic a.
nocturnal a.
nutritional a.
occlusion a.
organic a.
pattern distortion a.
refractive a.
suppression a.
toxic a.

amblyopic eye

amblyoscope
major a.
major amblyoscope test

Amboyna button

Ambras syndrome

Ambu
infant Ambu resuscitator

ambulance
a. chaser
a. design criteria
field a.

ambulates
a. on parallel bars
patient ambulates with assistance
patient ambulates with walker
a. with assistance
a. with a cane
a. with minimal assist
a. with minimal assistance
a. with a quad cane

ambulation
aids to a.
a. balance
cardiac ambulation routine
contact assistance for a.
contact assisted a.
Functional A. Categories
a. goal
nonweightbearing a.
patient independent in a.
a. skills
standby assistance in transfers and a.
standby assist with a.
standby transfer and a.
a. training orthosis
a. with walker

ambulator
community a.

ambulatory
a. anesthesia
a. antibiotic treatment
a. basis
a. blood pressure
a. blood pressure monitor
cardiac ambulatory monitoring unit
a. care
a. care center
a. care research facility
a. care unit
chronic ambulatory peritoneal dialysis
comprehensive ambulatory care
computer-stored ambulatory record
continued ambulatory care
continuous ambulatory infusion
continuous ambulatory peritoneal dialysis
continuous ambulatory gamma globulin infusion
a. controls
a. electrocardiogram
a. electrocardiographic monitoring
a. electrocardiography
a. electroencephalogram
a. electroencephalography
a. electrogram monitor
free-standing ambulatory surgical center
a. Holter monitor
a. Holter monitoring
a. ischemia monitoring
late ambulatory monitoring
a. manometry
a. monitoring
National A. Medical Care Survey
a. oximetry monitoring
a. patient
patient discharged a.
a. patient group
a. payment classification group
a. peritoneal dialysis patient
a. polysomnography
a. schizophrenia
speech-controlled respirometer for ambulatory measurement
a. status
supervised intermittent ambulatory treatment
a. surgery

a. surgery center
a. surgical unit
a. traction
transtelephonic ambulatory monitoring system
a. urodynamics
a. uterine contraction test
a. venous pressure
a. visit
a. visit groups
a. with crutches

ameba
Page ameba saline

amebiasis
hepatic a.

amebic
a. abscess
a. appendicitis
a. colitis
a. dysentery
granulomatous amebic encephalitis
a. hepatitis
a. infection
a. keratitis
necrotizing amebic enterocolitis
non-*Acanthamoeba* amebic keratitis
a. prevalence rate
primary amebic meningoencephalitis
a. ulcer
a. vaginitis

amegakaryocytic thrombocytopenia

amelanotic
a. melanoma
a. tumor

ameliorated
headache a.

ameloblastic
a. adenomatoid tumor
a. fibroma
granular cell ameloblastic fibroma
peripheral ameloblastic fibroma

ameloblastoma
ghost cell a.
granular cell a.
unicystic a.

amelogenesis imperfecta

amenorrhea
chemotherapy-related a.
drug-induced a.
functional hypothalamic a.
a., galactorrhea, hypothyroidism
a. and hirsutism
a. and hyperprolactinemia
hypothalmic a.
lactation amenorrhea method
postpartum a.
postpill a.
primary a.
secondary a.

amenorrhea-galactorrhea syndrome

amenorrheic
a. patient
a. woman

amentia
alcoholic a.
nevoid a.

America
Assisted Living Federation of A.
Meals on Wheels Association of A.
Opticians Association of A.

American
African A.
A. cockroach
A. Diabetes Association
A. Diabetes Association diet
A. Diabetes Association guidelines
A. eel virus
A. Heart Association
A. Heart Association classification
A. Heart Association Step One Diet
A. Heart Association Stroke Outcome Classification
Hispanic A.
A. hookworm
A. Hospital Association
A. Indian Sign Language
A. Institute of Physics
Latin American female
Latin American male
A. leech
A. leishmaniasis
A. Lung Association
A. Medical Association
Mexican A.
Mexican American female
Mexican American male
Native A.
North American antisnakebite serum
North American blastomycosis
North American Brain Tumor Consortium
North American Malignant Hyperthermia protocol
North American Nursing Diagnosis Association
A. Nurses Association
A. Optical
Organization of Chinese A.'s
Pan American Health Organization grade 0–2
A. Pediatric Gross Assessment Record
A. Psychiatric Association
A. Psychoanalytical Association
A. Psychological Association
South American blastomycosis
South American hemorrhagic fever
South American trypanosomiasis
Spanish A.
Spanish American black
Spanish American female
Spanish American male
A. trypanosomiasis
A. Type Culture Collection
white A.
A.'s with Disabilities Act

amidase
penicillin a.
trypsin-like a.

amide
fatty acid amide hydrolase
lysergic acid a.

amido
fuchsin, amido black, and naphthol yellow
tannic acid, polyphosphomolybdic acid, and amido acid staining technique

amikacin level

amimia
ataxic a.

amine
heterocyclic aromatic a.
plasma amine oxidase
a. precursor uptake and decarboxylation cell
technetium-99m hexamethylpropylene amine oxime single-photon emission computed tomography
tricyclic a.
a. uptake and decarboxylation cell

amino
a. acid
a. acid activating enzyme

amino *(continued)*
a. acid decarboxylase
a. acid-enriched cardioplegic solution
a. acid metabolic disorder
a. acid metabolism
a. acid mixture
a. acid nitrogen
a. acid oxidase
a. acid sequence
a. acid that gives aspartic acid after hydrolysis
alanine amino transaminase
alpha amino acid
aromatic amino acid
aromatic amino acid decarboxylase
branched-chain amino acid
crystalline amino acid solution
crystalline amino acid
inhibitory amino acid
large neutral amino acid
low-branched-chain amino acid diet
modified amino acid
neutral amino acid
nonessential amino acid
nonpolar amino acid
side chain in amino acid formula
a. sugar
synthetic amino acid
a. terminal
triiodothyronine, amino acids, glucagon, and heparin
unknown amino acid

aminoaciduria
arginase deficiency a.
argininosuccinic a.
Marchiafava-Bignami a.
methylmalonic a.
overflow a.

aminocaproic acid

aminocephalosporanic acid

aminoglycoside
a. antibiotic
a. nephrotoxicity
once-daily a.
a. ototoxicity
serum aminoglycoside concentration
a. toxicity

aminoglycoside-impregnated methyl methacrylate bead

aminoglycoside-resistant
oxacillin aminoglycoside-resistant *Staphylococcus aureus*

aminoimidazole
a. carboxamide
a. carboxamide ribonucleotide
a. carboxamide ribotide
succinyl aminoimidazole carboxamide ribotide

aminolevulinic
a. acid dehydrase
a. acid synthetase

5-aminolevulinic acid photodynamic therapy

aminonucleoside
puromycin aminonucleoside nephropathy

aminooxypentane regulated-on-activation normal T-expressed and secreted

aminopeptidase
a. A
a. B
cystine a.
leucine a.
leucine aminopeptidase test
serum leucine a.

aminopyrine breath test

5-aminosalicylic acid enema

aminoterminal
procollagen type III aminoterminal peptide

aminotransferase
alanine a.
aspartate a.
aspartate aminotransferase assay
aspartate aminotransferase level
asymptomatic elevated a.
cytoplasmic aspartate a.
a. level
mitochondrial aspartate a.
ornithine a.
ornithine-ketoacid aminotransferase deficiency
ratio of serum alanine aminotransferase to serum aspartate a.
tyrosine a.
tyrosine aminotransferase deficiency
tyrosine aminotransferase regulator

amiodarone
a. hydrochloride
a. liver
a. lung
a. pigmentation

amiodarone-associated thyrotoxicosis

amiodarone-induced
a.-i. destructive thyrotoxicosis
a.-i. hypothyroidism

Amish
A. albinism
A. brittle hair syndrome

amitriptyline-induced mood disorder

Ammon
A. fissure
A. horn

ammonia
a. alkali burn
anhydrous a.
aromatic ammonia spirit
a. blood level
a., copper, arsenic
a. detoxication
a. fixation
a. intoxication
^{13}N ammonia radioactive tracer
^{13}N ammonia uptake
total ammonia nitrogen

ammoniac
Masson-Fontana ammoniac silver stain

ammoniagenic coma

ammoniated mercury

ammonium
a. chloride
ferric ammonium citrate
formalin ammonium bromide
magnesium ammonium phosphate stone
magnesium ammonium phosphate urinary lithiasis
quaternary ammonium compound
quaternary ammonium compounds
urinary a.

amnesia
acute a.
affective a.
a. after trance
alcoholic a.
amnesic a.
antegrade a.
anterograde a.
asymmetrical a.
audioverbal a.
auditory a.
autohypnotic a.

axial a.
childbirth a.
Children's Orientation and A. Test
circumscribed a.
concussion a.
Galveston Orientation and A. Test
generalized a.
global a.
localized a.
a. loss of memory
neurological a.
nonpathological a.
olfactory a.
organic a.
partial a.
patch a.
postconcussion a.
posttraumatic a.
profound a.
psychogenic a.
retroactive a.
retrograde a.
selective a.
a. for sleep and dreaming
a. for sleep terror event
tactile a.
temporary global a.
total a.
transient global a.
a. for trauma
traumatic a.

amnesic
a. amnesia
a. aphasia
a. apraxia
a. color blindness
a. patient
a. shellfish poisoning
a. state
a. syndrome

amnestic
alcohol amnestic disorder
alcohol amnestic syndrome
alcoholic amnestic disorder
anxiolytic amnestic disorder
a. aphasia
a. apraxia
a. disorder
a. dysnomia
a. effect
a. episode
organic amnestic syndrome
a. state
a. syndrome

amnestica
akinesia a.

amnifocal lens

amniocentesis
early a.
a. indicative of infection

amnioembryonic junction

amniography in hydatidiform mole

amnioinfusion therapy

amniotic
a. adhesion
a. adhesions of fetus
a. band sequence
a. cavity
a. fluid
a. fluid alpha-fetoprotein
a. fluid analysis
a. fluid aspiration
a. fluid at term
a. fluid bilirubin
a. fluid cell culture
a. fluid culture
a. fluid drained and preserved
a. fluid embolism
a. fluid embolization
a. fluid glucose
a. fluid index
a. fluid infection
a. fluid infection syndrome
a. fluid quantitation
a. fluid scan
a. fluid volume
a. fold
a. hernia
a. membrane
mouse amniotic fluid
a. sac
thromblastic activity of amniotic fluid
transvaginal amniotic puncture

amobarbital
intracarotid amobarbital procedure

amoebic
ocular amoebic keratitis

among
alcohol abuse among women

amoral
a. personality
a. psychopathic personality
a. trend

amorous paranoia

amorphous
electron-dense amorphous material
a. fetus
a. hydrogenated silicon carbide
a. material

Amoss sign

amotivational syndrome

amount
catalytic a.
a. of insulin extractable from pancreas
large a.
rapid ingestion of large amounts of food
time and a.
a. of use

amoxicillin
bismuth subsalicylate, metronidazole, and a.
metronidazole, amoxicillin, clarithromycin, *H. pylori*, one-week therapy
metronidazole, omeprazole, a.
omeprazole, amoxicillin, clarithromycin
omeprazole, amoxicillin, metronidazole
ranitidine bismuth citrate, amoxicillin, clarithromycin

amoxicilloyl-human serum albumin

AMP-activated protein kinase

ampere
mega a.
a.'s per kilogram
a.'s per meter
a. per second
a. turn
weber per a.

ampere-hour

ampere-second

ampere-square meter

amperometric
high-pH anion exchange chromatography coupled with pulsed amperometric detection

amphetamine
a. abuse
centrally active phenethylamine derivative related to amphetamine and methamphetamine
chronic amphetamine effect
cocaine and amphetamine regulated transcript
a. delirium
a. dependence
A. Interview Rating Scale

amphetamine *(continued)*
a. intoxication
a. look-alike
a. overdose
a. poisoning
a. psychosis
a. or similarly acting sympathomimetic intoxication
a. toxicity
trimethylxanthine a.
a. withdrawal

amphetamine-induced
a.-i. anxiety
a.-i. psychotic disorder with delusions
a.-i. psychotic disorder with hallucinations
a.-i. sexual dysfunction

amphetamine/methamphetamine, opiates, and phencyclidine

amphoric
a. resonance
a. respiration
a. respiratory sound

amphotericin
a. B colloid dispersion
a. B deoxycholate
a. B-induced reduction glomerular filtration rate
a. B lipid complex
liposomal amphotericin B

amphotropic murine leukemia virus

ampicillin
a. rash
a. resistant

ampicillin-human serum albumin

ampicillin-resistant ***Escherichia coli***

amplification
direct amplification fingerprinting
direct amplification test
group-specific a.
image a.
light amplification by stimulated emission of radiation
microwave amplification by stimulated emission of radiation
multiple biotin-avidin a.
mutant allele-specific a.
nucleic acid a.
nucleic acid amplification technique
nucleic acid amplification test
nucleic acid amplification testing
nucleic acid sequence-band a.
nucleic acid sequence-based a.
PCR amplification test
rapid amplification of polymorphic DNA
a. refractory mutation system
a. refractory mutation system-polymerase chain reaction
sequence-independent single primer a.
strand displacement a.
telomere repeat amplification protocol
telomeric repeat amplification protocol
transcription-mediated a.
tyramide signal a.

amplified
a. *Mycobacterium tuberculosis* direct test
random amplified polymorphic DNA
tumor amplified protein expression therapy

amplifier
endocardiographic a.
hearing aid a.
lock-in a.

amplifying
transiently amplifying cell

amplitude
a. of accommodation
acoustic pressure a.
aortic a.
apical interventricular septal a.
attenuated in a.
best a.
a. of convergence
delta activity of low a.
diastolic amplitude time index
frequency and form of a.
half amplitude pulse duration
increase in amplitude of electrical activity
large amplitude, slow wave activity
light/dark amplitude ratio
maximum amplitude constant
mean amplitude of glycerine excursion
mean distal contraction a.
minimal amplitude nystagmus
a. mode
a. modulation
peak amplitude period
point of maximum amplitude of wave
pulse amplitude ratio
a. ratio
reduction in a.
a. of signal
a. of successive responses
a. threshold
waves of increasing a.

amplitude-integrated electroencephalogram

amplitude-summation interferential current therapy

ampulla, pl. **ampullae**
a. of duodenum
a. of gallbladder
Henle a.
a. of lacrimal canal
a. of lacrimal duct
a. of lactiferous duct
Lieberkühn a.
membranous a.
membranous ampullae of the semicircular duct
a. of milk duct
osseous a.
a. of oviduct
rectal a.
a. of rectum
sphincter of a.
Thoma a.
a. tumor
a. of uterine tube
a. of vas deferens
a. of Vater
a. of Vater anatomy
a. of Vater cyst

ampullar
a. abortion
a. pregnancy

ampullary
anterior ampullary nerve
a. carcinoma
a. crest
a. groove
a. hamartoma
a. lesion
a. nerve
neuroepithelium of ampullary crest
posterior ampullary nerve
a. stenosis
a. stone
a. sulcus
a. tumor

ampullopancreatic carcinoma

amputated
a. above ankle
a. above knee
appendix ligated and a.
partially a.
a. stump

amputation
below-elbow a.
below-knee a.
cone-shaped amputation stump
a. in contiguity
a. in continuity
great toe a.
guillotine midfoot a.
a. index score
a. of joint
lower extremity a.
metacarpal a.
middle finger a.
modified Boyd a.
modified Boyd amputation of ankle and distal tibial physis
modified Chopart a.
a. neuroma
partial hand a.
pedicle tip a.
a. rehabilitation
revision of amputation stump
a. stump
a. stump neuroma
suprapatellar a.
transmetatarsal a.

amputation-related bone pain

amputee
a. athlete
a. cushion
unilateral a.

Amsel criteria

Amsler grid test

Amspacher-Messenbaugh
A.-M. closing wedge osteotomy
A.-M. technique

Amsterdam
A. Depression List
A. dwarfism
A. Rotterdam
A. syndrome

Amstutz
A. classification
A. reattachment
A. resurfacing

Amstutz-Wilson osteotomy

amusia
motor a.

Amussat
A. incision
A. operation

amygdalae
nucleus a.
nucleus amygdalae centralis
nucleus amygdalae corticalis
nucleus amygdalae lateralis
nucleus amygdalae medialis

amygdala-fear circuitry

amygdalofugal fiber

amygdaloid
anterior amygdaloid area
corticomedial amygdaloid nucleus
medial amygdaloid nucleus

amyl
a. acetate
a. alcohol
a. chloride
a. hydrate
a. nitrate
a. nitrate abuse
a. nitrate inhalant
a. nitrite
a. salicylate
a. valerate

amylase
a. clearance
a. concentration
a. to creatinine ratio
human pancreatic a.
a. inhibitor activity
serum a.
urinary a.
a. urine spot test
wheat amylase inhibitor

amylase-creatinine
a.-c. clearance
a.-c. clearance ratio

amylase-resistant starch

amyloid
a. A-degrading protease
a. angiopathy cerebral
a. A protein
a. arthropathy
a. body
a. cellulitis
a. degeneration
a. disease
familial amyloid polyneuropathy
a. goiter
a. heart disease
immunoglobulin light chain-origin amyloid deposit
a. of immunoglobulin origin
islet amyloid polypeptide
a. kidney
a. light chain
a. liver
2-microglobulin-origin amyloid deposit
a. nephrosis
a. neuropathy
neutral amyloid probe
a. P component
a. polyneuropathy
a. precursor protein
serum amyloid P component
serum amyloid type A
sporadic cerebral amyloid angiopathy
a. stain
a. staining
a. tumor
a. of unknown origin

amyloid-enhancing factor

amyloid-like glomerulopathy

amyloidoma
nodular a.

amyloidosis
a. of aging
dialysis-related a.
a. of heart
hereditary cerebral hemorrhage with a.
light chain-related a.
localized cutaneous a.
nodular pulmonary a.
nonneuropathic systemic a.

amyloidotic
familial amyloidotic polyneuropathy

amylolytic enzyme

amylosulfate
sodium a.

amyoplasia
oculomelic a.

amyotonia
Oppenheim a.

amyotrophic
a. cerebellar hypoplasia
a. choreoacanthocytosis
familial amyotrophic lateral sclerosis
lateral amyotrophic sclerosis
a. lateral sclerosis
a. syphilitic myelitis
a. type of spongiform encephalopathy

amyotrophy
Aran-Duchenne a.
asthmatic a.
monomelic a.
neuralgic a.
a. parkinsonism
spinal progressive a.

Amytal
carotid Amytal procedure

AN25S-1 virus

anabolic
a. agent
a. androgenic
androgenic anabolic agent
a. steroid
a. steroid abuse

anabolism
net a.

anabolism-promoting factor

anaclitic
a. depression
a. psychotherapy

Anaconda
Operation A.

anaerobe
facultative a.
obligate a.

anaerobic
aerobic and anaerobic blood culture
a. bacteria
a. cellulitis
a. culture
a. exercise
a. gram-negative rod
Gram-positive anaerobic coccus
a. infection
mixed aerobic and anaerobic abscess
mixed aerobic and anaerobic flora
mobile anaerobic laboratory
nonclostridial anaerobic cellulitis
nonclostridial anaerobic myonecrosis
a. respiratory infection
a. threshold
ventilatory anaerobic threshold

anaerobically
prereduced anaerobically sterilized medium

anagen
loose anagen hair syndrome

anagogic
a. interpretation
a. symbolism

anal
a. abscess
a. administration
a. anastomosis
a. atresia
a. bulge
a. bulging
a. canal
a. canal length
a. cancer
a. character
circular anal dilator
a. cleft
a. column
a. condyloma
a. continence
continent anal cap
a. crypt
a. cushion
a. dilation
a. dimplc
a. discharge
a. duct
a. effluent
a. encirclement
a. endoscopy
a. endosonography
a. erotism
external anal sphincter
a. fascia
a. fibrosis
a. fissure
a. fistula
a. foreign body
a. function
Gas A. F&T
a. gland
a. gland carcinoma
a. herpes
homosexual anal intercourse
a. human papilloma virus infection
a. humor
ileal pouch anal anastomosis
a. ileostomy with preservation of sphincter
a. impotence
a. incontinence
a. index
inhibitory anal reflex
a. intercourse
a. intermuscular septum
internal anal sphincter
a. intersphincteric groove
a. intraepithelial neoplasia
a. irritation
a. itching
a. itching and antibiotic
long anal sphincter
a. manometry
a. mapping
a. margin
a. masturbation
maximal resting anal pressure
a. membrane
multiple anal sphincterotomies
muscle of anal triangle
oral anal fistula
a. orifice
a. papilla
a. Pap smear
paroxysmal anal hyperkinesis
pecten of anal canal
a. penetration
perineal flexure of anal canal
a. personality
a. phase
a. phase of infancy
a. pitting
a. plate
a. pouch
a. procidentia
a. prolapse
a. protrusion
a. pruritus
a. rape
a. rape fantasy
a. reflex
a. rimming
a. sadism
a. sepsis
a. sex
a. sinus
a. skin tag
a. sphincter
a. sphincter dysplasia
a. sphincter laceration
a. sphincter squeeze pressure
a. squamous intraepithelial lesion
a. stage
a. stage psychosexual development
a. stretch
a. stricture
a. thrombosis
a. tone
a. transitional zone
a. tuberculosis
a. ulceration
a. valve
a. vein

a. verge
vertebral abnormality, anal imperforation, tracheoesophageal fistula, and radial, ray, or renal anomalies
a. wart
a. wink
a. wound

anal-aggressive character

anales
nervi anales inferiores

anal-expulsive stage

analgesia
acupuncture a.
continuous epidural a.
continuous infusion epidural a.
a. dolorosa
electrical stimulation-produced a.
electroacupuncture a.
fixed-dose patient-controlled a.
foot shock-induced a.
interpleural a.
on-demand analgesia computer
opiate a.
parenteral-controlled a.
patient-controlled analgesia anesthetic technique
patient-controlled epidural a.
patient-controlled intranasal a.
preemptive a.
procedural sedation and a.
segmental epidural a.
spinal opioid a.
stimulation-induced a.
stimulation-produced a.
stress-induced a.

analgesic
adjuvant analgesic drug
a. agent
chronic opioid analgesic therapy
a. dose
minimum effective analgesic concentration
minimum local analgesic concentration
parenteral analgesic medication
patient-controlled a.

analgesic-associated nephropathy

analgesic-rebound headache

analog
antihuman S5 a.
controlled substance a.
a. data
a. to digital
a. filter
juvenile hormone a.
linear analog pain scale
linear analog pain score
linear analog self-assessment
linear visual analog scale
luteinizing hormone-releasing hormone a.
a. of meperidine
nucleoside analog reverse transcriptase inhibitor
nucleoside analog RT inhibitor
nucleoside analog monotherapy
oxytocin a.
parallel analog mapping
a. signal
simultaneous analog stimulation
viral analog scale
visual analog pain score

analogies
Miller A. Test
Minnesota Engineering A. Test

analog-to-digital converter

analogue
Colored Visual A. Scale
Visual A. Mood Scale
Visual A. Self Assessment Scales For Pain Intensity

anal-retentive personality

anal-sadistic love

analysis
advanced real-time motion a.
advanced vessel a.
amniotic fluid a.
applied behavior a.
arch perimeter a.
arch width a.
arterial blood gas a.
astigmatic vector a.
Auditory A. Test
automated cell image a.
automated hematology a.
automated multiple a.
automatic voice a.
autoregressive model for signal a.
biochemical analysis and culture
bioelectrical impedance a.
bioimpedance venous a.
blood gas a.
carotid audiofrequency a.
cell block a.
cell cycle kinetics a.
cholesteric analysis profile
cholesteric analysis profile test
Classification and Regression Tree a.
Clinical A. Questionnaire
computer-assisted semen a.
a. of coping style
cost-benefit a.
cost-effectiveness a.
a. of covariance
directed heteroduplex a.
direct immunofluorescence a.
Doppler waveform a.
dose intensity a.
dot blot a.
drug analysis laboratory
electroencephalogram interval spectrum a.
electron spectroscopy for chemical a.
electrophoretic mobility shift a.
energy-dispersed x-ray a.
euclidean distance matrix a.
Everyman Contingency Table A.
failure a.
finite element stress a.
fluorometric analysis of DNA unwinding
forced vital capacity a.
Gardner A. of Personality Survey
gastric a.
gastric analysis, free and total
gene-linkage a.
Grammatical A. of Elicited Language
group of units of a.
hair analysis test
Hazard A. Critical Control Points
heart rate power spectral a.
heteroduplex a.
hospital activity a.
image display and a.
Immediate Response Mobile A.
immunoelectrophoresis a.
immunoradiometric a.
induced sputum a.
instrumental neutron activation a.
intention-to-treat a.
job task a.
joint fluid a.
Language Sampling A.
latent class a.
Leader Behavior A. II
limiting dilution a.
linear discriminant a.
linear displacement a.
linear regression a.
Linguistic A. of Speech Samples

analysis *(continued)*
logical analysis of automatic thought
logistic discriminant a.
Marriage Skills A.
mass isotopomer distribution a.
mass spectrometric a.
microprobe analysis generalized intensity correction
mitochondrial deoxyribonucleic acid a.
mixed dentition a.
molecular genetic a.
motion analysis system
motivation analysis test
motivation analysis testing
multicolor data a.
multidimensional analysis beam modifier
Multidimensional Scalogram A.
multilocus enzyme electrophoresis a.
multiple abstract variance a.
multiple analysis of variance
multiple factor a.
multiple linear regression a.
multivariant discriminant a.
multivariate analysis of covariance
multivariate analysis of variance
multivariate logistic regression a.
Nance analysis of arch length
neutron activation a.
nonlinear least squares regression a.
nonmetric principal component a.
Northern blot a.
nucleic acid hybridization a.
nucleic acid sequence-based a.
nucleotide sequence a.
occlusal cephalometric a.
optic nerve head a.
optimized microvessel density analysis
osteotomy analysis simulation software
PCR fragment a.
peripheral blood lymphocyte a.
physical abilities a.
plasmid pattern a.
platelet function a.
polymerase chain reaction analysis of prostate-specific antigen
power spectral a.
Prescription Analyses and Cost
principal components a.
qualitative a.
quantitative buffy-coat a.
radiochemical neutron activation a.
rank-order stability a.
regression a.
representational difference a.
restriction endonuclease a.
restriction enzyme a.
reversed passive hemagglutination by miniature centrifugal fast a.
root cause a.
routine urine a.
School Motivation A. Test
semen a.
seminal fluid a.
sequential analysis of twelve chemistry constituents
sequential multiple a.
serial analysis of gene expression
serial multiple a.
serum thyroxine measured by displacement a.
Shapes A. Test
simulation kinetics a.
single potential analysis cavernous electrical activity
slot-blot hybridization a.
Southern blot a.
Southern transfer a.
spectrum a.
spinal analysis machine
statistical analysis and quality control
Taylor-Johnson Temperament A.
total body neutron activation a.
transactional a.
Transactional A. Life Position Survey
unit of a.
urine a.
a. of variance
video dimensional a.
Vocal Profiles A.
Western blot a.

analyst anchor test

analyte-specific reagent

analytic
a. cytology
discriminant analytic model
a. group psychotherapy
a. interpretation
a. object
a. patient
a. psychiatry
a. reconstruction
a. rule
a. stalemate
a. study
subjective, objective, management, and a.
a. therapy
a. transmission electron microscope

analytical
a. electron microscope
a. electron microscopy
a. grade
a. philosophy
a. play therapy
a. process
a. profile index
a. psychology
a. reagent

analyzed
Factor A. Short Form

analyzer
automated biochemical a.
automatic clinical a.
automatic fluorescent image a.
blood color a.
digital differential a.
laser microprobe mass a.
medical gas a.
miniature centrifugal fast a.
MiniOX 1A oxygen a.
multichannel a.
Nerve Fiber A.
Nerve Fiber A. laser ophthalmoscope
nerve fiber layer a.
nondispersive infrared a.
octave band a.
organics-in-water a.
pacing system a.
pulse-height a.
sequential multiple a.
simultaneous multiple a.
single-channel a.
thermal energy a.

anamnesis
associative a.

anamnestic response

Ananindeua virus

anaphylactic
a. desensitization
a. intoxication
late cutaneous anaphylactic reaction
passive cutaneous anaphylactic reaction
a. purpura
a. reaction

a. shock
a. shock prophylaxis
a. syndrome
a. transfusion reaction

anaphylactoid
a. crisis
dextran-induced anaphylactoid reaction
a. food sensitivity
a. phenomenon
a. purpura
a. reaction
a. shock

anaphylactoid-type reaction

anaphylatoxin
classified a.
a. inactivator

anaphylaxis
active systemic a.
basophil kallikrein of a.
eosinophil chemotactic factor of a.
exercise-induced a.
immediate active cutaneous a.
inflammatory factor of a.
passive cutaneous a.
passive cutaneous anaphylaxis test
platelet-activating factor of a.
reverse passive a.
slow-reacting factor of a.
slow-reacting substance of a.

anaphylaxis-angioedema-frequent
idiopathic a.-a.-f.

anaphylaxis-angioedema-infrequent
idiopathic a.-a.-i.

anaphylaxis-generalized-frequent
idiopathic a.-g.-f.

anaphylaxis-generalized-infrequent
idiopathic a.-g.-i.

anaphylaxis-questionable
idiopathic a.-q.

anaphylaxis-variant
idiopathic a.-v.

anaplastic
a. anemia
a. astrocytoma
a. infiltrating single cell
large cell anaplastic lymphoma
a. large cell lymphoma
malignant teratoma, a.
multifocal anaplastic astrocytoma
null cell anaplastic large cell lymphoma
poorly differentiated anaplastic carcinoma
a. thyroid carcinoma
a. tumor
a. Wilms tumor

anarchic behavior

anasarca
dyspnea and a.

anastigmatic lens

anastomosed
gallbladder anastomosed to duodenum
a. graft
a. to loop of bowel

anastomosis
aneurysm by a.
arterial brain a.
arteriovenous a.
bidirectional cavopulmonary a.
bidirectional superior cavopulmonary a.
choledochocaval a.
circular end-to-end a.
coloanal a.‘
colorectal a.
Cooley intrapericardial a.
Cooley modification of Waterson a.
curved end-to-end a.
dog-ear of a.
end-to-end a.
end-to-end venous a.
end-to-side a.
end-to-side venous a.
flexor tendon a.
gastrointestinal a.
Hoyer a.'s
ileal pouch anal a.
ileoanal a.
ileocolic a.
ileorectal anastomosis with end-to-end a.
ileosigmoid a.
a. intact
intracranial to intracranial a.
laser-assisted vasal a.
laser-assisted vascular a.
LeDuc ureteral a.
low anterior resection in combination with coloanal a.
low coloanal a.
Ma-Griffith end-to-end a.
microsurgical tubocornual a.
onlay patch a.
pancreaticogastrostomy a.
pancreaticojejunostomy a.
portacaval a.
pulmonary artery a.
renal a.
right internal mammary a.
small bowel a.
stapled intestinal a.
temporary portacaval a.
venous-to-venous a.

anastomotic
a. abscess
a. aneurysm
atrial anastomotic branch of circumflex branch of left coronary artery
a. branch
a. complication
a. dehiscence
a. disruption
a. failure
a. fiber
a. fistula
a. flow
a. foramen
a. hemorrhage
a. leak
a. leakage
a. pseudoaneurysm
a. recurrence
a. site
a. stenosis
a. stoma
a. stricture
a. stricture formation
a. stump leak
a. suture
a. ulceration
a. vein
a. vessel

anatomic
abnormal anatomic lesion
a. alignment
a. assessment
a. bile duct variant
a. brain classification
chest closed in anatomic layers
clinical manifestations, etiologic factors, anatomic involvement, pathophysiologic features
closed in anatomic layers
a. closure
a. conjugate
a. dead space
a. defect
a. diagnosis
a. event
a. evidence
a. factor

anatomic *(continued)*
a. fracture
functional and anatomic loading
a. genu valgus
a. gift
a. gift statement
a. graduated component
a. hook
a. imaging
a. impotence
a. impression
a. insertion
a. integrity
a. intermetatarsal angle
a. leg length inequality
a. location
a. measurement
a. medullary locking
a. medullary locking hip system
a. modular knee
a. neck
normal anatomic alignment
normal anatomic position
normal anatomic variation
a. origin and distribution
a. pathology
a. plane
porous-coated anatomic prosthesis
a. porous replacement
a. porous replacement hemispheric acetabular component
a. position
a. position and alignment
preliminary anatomic diagnosis
a. profile
a. reduction
restoration of normal anatomic alignment
a. rigidity
a. root
a. short leg
a. site
a. stress incontinence
a. structure
a. surface prosthesis
usual anatomic position
a. variation
ventilation of anatomic dead space
volume of anatomic dead space

anatomical
a. anomaly
a. appearance
a. classification system of Severin
a. closure
a. considerations in radiation therapy
continuous anatomical passive exerciser
a. imaging
a. internal os of uterus
a. landmark
Link anatomical hip
a. neck of humerus
no anatomical cause of death
a. position and alignment
a. position of duodenum
a. snuffbox

anatomically
a. dominant
incision closed a.
a. normal
a. patent foramen ovale

anatomicum
ostium a.

anatomy
ampulla of Vater a.
coronary vessel a.
designed after natural a.
intracranial a.
lobar breast a.
native coronary a.
a. and physiology
a. response

ANCA-associated
ANCA-a. systemic vasculitis
ANCA-a. vasculitis

ANCA-positive
ANCA-p. granulomatous giant-cell arteritis
ANCA-p. vasculitis

ancestral
a. spirit
a. worship

anchor
analyst anchor test
axial anchor screw
a. hole
Mitek absorbable a.
a. plate
a. signs of withdrawal
a. suture
a. tooth
a. washer
a. with suture ligature

anchorage
facial a.
major a.
maxillomandibular a.
minimal a.
multiple a.
occipital a.

anchored
a. catheter

anchoring
a. balloon
a. fibril
perceptual a.
a. screw
a. suture
a. tendon

anchovy
a. paste abscess
a. procedure

ancient
a. schwannoma
a. tuberculous arthritis

anconeus
musculus a.

Andasibe virus

Andermann syndrome

Andernach ossicle

Andersch
A. ganglion
A. nerve

Anders disease

Andersen
A. disease
A. triad

Anderson
A. amputation
A. ankle fusion
A. classification
A. disease
A. and Goldberger test
A. marker
M.D. Anderson Cancer Center
M.D. Anderson cancer staging
M.D. Anderson grading system
M.D. Anderson tumor score system
A. modification of Berndt-Harty classification
A. operation
A. phenomenon
A. procedure
A. sampler
A. tibial pseudarthrosis classification
A. traction

Anderson-Collip test

Anderson-Fowler calcaneal displacement osteotomy

Anderson-Hynes dismembered pyeloplasty

Andes virus

Andresen Six-Basic-Factors-Model

Andrews
A. anterior instability test
A. disease

androgen
a. ablation
a. ablation therapy
a. ablative monotherapy
adrenal a.
adrenal androgen corticotropic stimulating hormone
a. antagonist
a. binding
a. binding protein
a. blockade
combined androgen blockade
complete androgen insensitivity
complete androgen insensitivity syndrome
a. deficiency
a. deprivation therapy
a. dynamics
a. gonadotropin feedback control
hirsutism, androgen excess, insulin resistance, acanthosis nigricans syndrome
a. hormone
human androgen receptor assay
human androgen receptor gene
a. insensitivity syndrome
a. interaction
intermittent androgen blockade
intermittent androgen deprivation
intermittent androgen suppression
a. level
luteinizing hormone-dependent androgen excess
a. metabolism
neoadjuvant androgen deprivation
neoadjuvant androgen derivation therapy
ovarian androgen secretion
partial androgen insensitivity
partial androgen insensitivity syndrome
partial androgen sensitivity
partial androgen insensitivity
peripheral androgen activity
peripheral androgen activity marker
peripheral androgen blockade
a. receptor
a. receptor antagonist
a. receptor element
a. receptor gene
a. receptor gene mutation
a. replacement therapy
a. resistance
a. resistance syndrome
a. secretion
a. sensitivity
a. suppression
a. suppression therapy
a. unit
a. withdrawal endocrine therapy
X-linked human androgen receptor

androgen-binding protein

androgen-dependent
a.-d. carcinoma
a.-d. prostate cancer
a.-d. syndrome

androgen-deprivation therapy

androgenesis
adrenal a.

androgenetic
a. alopecia
female pattern androgenetic alopecia
male pattern androgenetic alopecia

androgenic
alkylated androgenic steroid
a. alopecia
anabolic a.
a. anabolic agent
a. follicle
a. hormone
ovarian androgenic hyperfunction
a. property
a. steroid
a. zone

androgenic-anabolic steroid

androgen-independent
a.-i. prostate cancer
a.-i. prostate carcinoma

androgenital syndrome

androgenized woman

androgen-lowering therapy

androgen-producing tumor

androgen-secreting neoplasm

androgen-stimulating
adrenal androgen-stimulating hormone
cortical androgen-stimulating hormone

androgen-type hirsutism

androgynous individual

android
a. fat distribution
a. obesity
a. pattern
a. pelvis

androstane derivative

androstenedione test

androstenedione-to-testosterone ratio

Andy
A. Gump deformity
A. Gump facies

anecdotal
a. data
a. evidence
a. method
a. procedure

anechoic
a. area
a. center
a. chamber
a. cyst
a. fluid
a. fluid collection
a. foci
a. lesion
a. mantle
a. mass
a. space
a. thrombus
a. tissue

Anel
A. method
A. operation
A. probe

anelectrotonic
a. state
a. zone

anembryonic
a. gestation
a. pregnancy

anemia
acquired aplastic a.
acquired hemolytic a.
acquired idiopathic sideroblastic a.
acquired severe aplastic a.
acute hemolytic a.
alloimmune hemolytic a.
angiopathic hemolytic a.
antipernicious anemia factor
aplastic a.
aplastic anemia syndrome

anemia *(continued)*
aplastic crisis in hemolytic a.
appetite loss from pernicious a.
a. associated with chronic renal failure
autoallergic hemolytic a.
autoimmune acquired hemolytic a.
autoimmune hemolytic a.
blood loss a.
blurred vision from a.
breathing difficulty from a.
a. of chronic disease
chronic hemolytic a.
a. of chronic renal failure
combined cold and warm antibody autoimmune hemolytic a.
congenital anemia of newborn
congenital dyserythropoietic anemia types I–III
congenital Heinz body hemolytic a.
congenital hypoplastic a.
congenital inclusion-body hemolytic a.
congenital nonspherocytic hemolytic a.
constitutional aplastic a.
cow's milk a.
dementia from pernicious a.
Diamond-Blackfan a.
drug-induced immune a.
a. of end-stage renal disease
fainting from a.
familial hypoplastic a.
Fanconi a.
feline infectious a.
filterable hemolytic a.
Friend virus a.
a. from hookworm
GI bleed from a.
a. gravis
ground itch a.
heavy menstrual periods from a.
Heinz body hemolytic a.
a. of hemodialysis
hemolytic a.
hemolytic anemia antigen
hemolytic anemia of newborn
hereditary hemolytic a.
hereditary hemolytic anemia test
hereditary nonspherocytic hemolytic a.
idiopathic acquired refractory sideroblastic a.
idiopathic acquired sideroblastic a.
idiopathic autoimmune hemolytic a.
idiopathic hypochromic a.
idiopathic refractory sideroblastic a.
immune hemolytic a.
a. infantum pseudoleukemica
infectious equine a.
iron deficiency a.
juvenile pernicious a.
limp hair from a.
lysolecithin hemolytic a.
macrocytic achylic a.
macrocytic anemia of pregnancy
macrocytic anemia tropical
macrocytic hyperchromic a.
macrocytic normochromic a.
megaloblastic a.
megaloblastic anemia of pregnancy
memory loss from a.
microangiopathic hemolytic a.
microcytic hypochromic anemia
microcytic/normochromic anemia
microelliptopoikilocytic anemia of Rietti, Greppi, and Micheli
myopathy-lactic acidosis-sideroblastic anemia syndrome
a. neonatorum
nonmegaloblastic macrocytic a.
normochromic, normocytic a.
normocytic hypochromic a.
normocytic normochromic a.
nutritional macrocytic a.
pallor from a.
pernicious a.
a. of prematurity
primary acquired sideroblastic a.
a. pseudoleukemica infantum
pulmonary disease a.
refractory a.
refractory anemia, erythroblastic
refractory anemia with excess blasts
refractory anemia with excess of blasts in transformation
refractory anemia with excess blasts in transition
refractory anemia with excess myeloblasts
refractory anemia with partial myeloblastosis
refractory anemia with ring sideroblasts
a. related to chemotherapy
secondary a.
a. secondary to blood loss
severe aplastic a.
sickle cell a.
sickle cell anemia test
a. syndrome
target cell a.
tongue inflammation from pernicious a.
warm autoimmune hemolytic a.
weight loss from pernicious a.
white or pale nails from a.
white patches from a.

anemia-inducing
a.-i. factor
a.-i. factor-1

anemic
a. anoxia
a. effect
a. halo
a. headache
a. hypoxia
a. infarct
iron-sufficient, not a.
a. murmur
a. nevus
a. polyneuritis
a. polyneuropathy
a. urine

anemicus
nevus a.

anemometry
laser Doppler a.

anemone cell tumor

anencephalic infant

anencephaly
partial a.
a. screening

anencephaly-spina bifida syndrome

anenzymia catalasia

anergastic
a. organic psychosis
a. reaction

anergic
a. depression
a. leishmaniasis
a. schizophrenic
a. stupor
a. T cell

anergy
antigen-specific a.
native a.
natural a.
negative a.
nonspecific a.
a. panel

peripheral a.
a. skin test battery
specific a.
a. test

aneroid
a. chest bellows
a. device
a. gauge
a. manometer
a. manometry
a. sphygmomanometer

anesthesia
a. absorption
a. action
a. adjunct
a. adjuvant
a. administered
ankle block a.
automated anesthesia record
axillary block a.
a. bag
Bier block a.
a. breathing circuit
a. cartridge
a. circuit
circular block a.
combined spinal-epidural a.
congenital trigeminal a.
contamination from anesthesia equipment
continuous epidural a.
continuous intravenous regional a.
continuous lumbar epidural a.
continuous spinal a.
contralateral local a.
controlled partial rebreathing anesthesia method
craniosynostosis, ataxia, trigeminal anesthesia, parietal anesthesia and pons, vermis fusion syndrome
crash induction of a.
depth of a.
digital block a.
a. dolorosa
epidural a.
examination under a.
fairly good risk for a.
field block a.
first stage of a.
following satisfactory general a.
gas, oxygen, and ether a.
general a.
general anesthesia with endotracheal intubation
general endotracheal a.
general inhalational a.
halothane a.
high spinal a.
induction of a.
intravenous regional a.
laryngeal tracheal a.
local a.
local infiltrative a.
local tracheal a.
low central venous pressure a.
lumbar epidural a.
a. machine
management of a.
manipulation under a.
mask inhalation a.
Mayo block a.
modified Van Lint a.
Modulus CD anesthesia system
monitored anesthesia care anesthesia
monitored anesthesia care anesthetic technique
nasotracheal intubation a.
nerve block a.
nerve blocking a.
nerve compression a.
office-based a.
office laparoscopy under local a.
off-site a.
open anesthesia system
open drop a.
outpatient a.
palatine block a.
paracervical block a.
patient-controlled epidural a.
pediatric anesthesia system
pelvic examination under a.
poor risk for a.
Post A. Discharge Scoring System
rapid opiate detoxification under a.
a. record
regional block a.
respiratory depression inhalation a.
risk of a.
sacral a.
saddle block a.
segmental epidural a.
smart anesthesia multigas
spinal a.
a. standby
start of a.
stellate block a.
stress-induced a.
sympathetic block a.
a. time
topical oropharyngeal a.
total intravenous a.
tracheostomy mask a.
under satisfactory general a.
variable-dose patient-controlled a.
Vinethine and ether a.

anesthesia-related problem

anesthesiology critical care medicine

anesthetic
a. agent
alveolar partial pressure of inhalational a.
a. approach
arterial cannulation anesthetic technique
axillary block anesthetic technique
a. block
a. blockade
a. circuit
a. consideration
a. conversion reaction
a. cutoff
a. depth
a. emergence
endobronchial intubation anesthetic technique
epidural blood patch anesthetic technique
a. ether
eutectic mixture of local a.'s
a. and fluid management
a. gas
a. gas exposure
a. gas mixture
a. hepatitis
a. hepatotoxicity
a. immediate recovery
a. index
a. induction
a. induction agent
a. leprosy
local anesthetic reaction
low-flow anesthetic technique
lumbar anesthetic technique
a. management
minimum alveolar anesthetic concentration
monitored anesthesia care anesthetic technique
a. monitoring
a. needle
neuroleptanalgesia anesthetic technique
nitrous oxide-oxygen-opioid anesthetic technique

anesthetic *(continued)*
no apparent anesthetic complication
a. ointment
oral anesthetic technique
patient-controlled analgesia anesthetic technique
percutaneous anesthetic loss
peribulbar anesthetic technique
postspinal anesthetic headache
a. potency
a. record
a. risk
a. shock
a. skin lesion
start of a.
sympathetic blockade anesthetic technique
sympathetic ganglion block anesthetic technique
a. system
system for anesthetic and respiratory administration
a. technique
a. time
a. tolerance
a. tube
a. vapor
a. variant of schizoid behavior

anesthetizing effect of ice and snow

anestrous
a. condition
a. ovulation

anetoderma
a. of Jadassohn
a. of prematurity
a. of Schweninger-Buzzi
a. scleroatrophy

aneuploid
a. abortion
a. cell
a. cell line
a. colorectal carcinoma
a. tumor

aneuploidy
atypical a.
a. infant
mosaic a.
mucosal a.
Pallister mosaic a.
partial a.

aneurysm
abdominal aortic a.
a. by anastomosis
angled aneurysm clip
anterior circulation a.
anterior circulation intracranial a.
anterior communicating a.
anterior communicating artery a.
anterior parietal artery a.
aortic a.
aortic aneurysm graft
aortic aneurysm rupture
aortic aneurysm tissue
aortic arch a.
aortic sinus a.
arteriosclerotic aortic a.
arteriosclerotic intracranial a.
arteriosclerotic thoracoabdominal aortic a.
arteriosclerotic thrombosed a.
arteriovenous pulmonary a.
a. of ascending aorta
ascending aortic a.
atherosclerotic aortic a.
atrial septal a.
a. of atrial septum
axillary artery a.
berry intracranial a.
a. clip applicator
a. clip ligation
clip ligation of a.
a. clipping
clipping of a.
coiled intracranial a.
coiling of a.
communicating artery a.
coronary artery a.
DeBakey-Creech aneurysm repair
dilatation of a.
dissecting abdominal a.
dissecting aneurysm of the coronary artery
dissecting aortic a.
dissecting basilar artery a.
dissecting intracranial a.
dissecting renal artery a.
dissection aortic a.
embolization of a.
false a.
familial intracranial a.
a. of Galen vein
hemorrhage of a.
hepatic artery a.
hypogastric artery a.
iliac artery a.
inflammatory aortic a.
infrarenal abdominal aortic a.
interatrial septal a.
a. of internal carotid artery
interventricular septum a.
intracranial aneurysm clipped
intracranial arterial a.
left ventricular a.
lower basilar a.
luetic aortic a.
malignant bone a.
a. management
Mayfield aneurysm clip
a. of membranous ventricular septum
mesenteric artery a.
middle cerebral a.
mitral valve a.
multiple intracranial a.
mycotic aortic a.
mycotic brain a.
neck of a.
a. occlusion
ophthalmic artery a.
a. of orbit
oval aneurysm with bleb
pancreatic artery a.
pancreaticoduodenal artery a.
pararenal aortic a.
a. of persistent trigeminal artery
popliteal artery a.
portal vein a.
posterior communicating a.
a. of posterior communicating artery
posterior communicating artery a.
pulmonary arteriovenous a.
pulmonary artery a.
recurrent chronic dissecting a.
recurrent hemorrhage from a.
a. remnant neck
renal artery a.
a. repair
a. of retinal arteriole
ruptured abdominal aortic a.
ruptured brain a.
ruptured iliac a.
ruptured sinus of Valsalva a.
sacral a.
splenic artery a.
supraclinoid carotid a.
a. surgery
thoracic aortic a.
thoracoabdominal aortic a.
a. tissue
a. trapping
traumatic intracranial a.
unruptured brain a.
a. of vein of Galen
wall of a.
a. with simple shape

aneurysmal
aortic aneurysmal disease

a. benign fibrous histiocytoma
a. bleeding
a. bone cyst
a. bruit
a. bulging
cerebrovascular aneurysmal clip
a. clipping operation
a. cough
a. dilatation
a. dilation
a. disease
a. dissection
a. dome
a. fundus
a. hematoma
a. hemorrhage
a. murmur
a. neck
a. ostium
a. outpouching
peripheral arterial aneurysmal disease
a. phthisis
a. proportion
a. rebleed
a. rest
a. rupture
a. sac
a. subarachnoid hemorrhage
a. tissue
a. varix
a. vein
vein of Galen aneurysmal dilatation
vein of Galen aneurysmal malformation
a. wall
a. wall calcification
a. wall gas
a. widening of aorta

aneurysmectomy
abdominal aortic a.
left ventricular a.
ventricular a.

aneusomy
a. analysis
a. syndrome

angel
a. kisses lesion
a. wing

Angeles
Los Angeles classification
Los Angeles classification of GERD
Los Angeles Classification grade A, B, C, D esophagitis
Los Angeles preservation solution 1
Los Angeles variant galactosemia

angelica root

Angelo
San Angelo virus

angel-of-death hallucination

angel's
a. kiss
a. kiss capillary malformation
a. trumpet

angel-shaped phalangoepiphyseal dysplasia

ANGEL tumor

Angelucci
A. operation
A. syndrome

angel-wing
a.-w. deformity
a.-w. sign

anger
adolescent anger management
a. arousal
a. at God
a. attack
bursts of irritation and a.
child quick to a.
coping with a.
diffusing hostility and a.
a. disorder
a. dysregulation
expressions of a.
A. Expression Scale
externalized a.
feeling of a.
a. and frustration
A. gamma camera
inappropriate a.
inappropriate intense a.
inappropriate overt a.
integrated anger management
intense inappropriate a.
Inventory of A. Communications
level of a.
low anger threshold
a. mallet
a. management
a. management skill
marked a.
a. outburst
outburst of a.
outward expression of anger with impulsive feature
passivity in anger expression
permitting safe expression of a.
a. reaction
situational anger disorder with aggression
situational anger disorder without aggression
a. stage
State-Trait A. Expression Inventory
State-Trait A. Scale
stress, anger and hopelessness
unprovoked a.
a. and violence psychiatric syndrome

Anghelescu sign

angiectatic
a. skin rash
pleomorphic hyalinizing angiectatic tumor

angiitic
a. granulomatosis
a. luminal compromise

angiitis
allergic angiitis and granulomatosis
allergic granulomatosis and a.
allergic granulomatous a.
granulomatous angiitis of the central nervous system
isolated angiitis of central nervous system
isolated angiitis of the CNS
leukocytoclastic a.
lymphocytic angiitis and granulomatosis
primary angiitis of the central nervous system
primary angiitis of CNS

angiitis-granulomatosis disorder

angina
a. abdominis
agranulocytic a.
a. bullosa haemorrhagica
chronic stable a.
a. cordis
a. cruris
decubitus a.
a. decubitus
a. diphtheritica
a. dyspeptica
a. equivalent
ergonovine maleate provocation a.
ischemic rest a.
Ludwig a.
a. lymphomatosa
a. nervosa
a. pectoris

angina *(continued)*
preinfarction a.
Prinzmetal variant a.
a. scarlatinosa
stable angina pectoris
a. threshold heart rate
unstable a.
unstable angina pectoris
variant a.
variant angina pectoris
vasospastic a.

angina-guided therapy

anginal
a. attack
prevention of anginal attack

angio-Behçet disease

angioblastic
a. cell
a. cyst
a. lymphadenopathy
a. meningioma

angiocardiography
first-pass nuclear a.

Angiocath catheter

angiocentric
eosinophilic angiocentric fibrosis
a. immunoproliferative disorder
a. immunoproliferative lesion
a. lymphoma
a. lymphoproliferative lesion
nasal angiocentric lymphoma
a. NK-cell lymphoma
a. pattern
a. T-cell lymphoma

angiocholitis proliferans

angiodestructive
a. lymphoma
a. pattern

angiodysgenetic myelomalacia

angiodysplasia
a. of colon
intestinal a.
metaphysial a.

angiodysplastic lesion

angioedema
acquired a.
hereditary a.
a. profile

angioedema-induced urticaria

angioedema-urticaria-eosinophilia syndrome

angioendothelioma
malignant endovascular papillary a.

angioendotheliomatosis
malignant a.
neoplastic a.
neoplastic proliferating a.
a. proliferans
reactive cutaneous a.

angiofibroblastic
a. hyperplasia
a. hyperplasia tendinosis
a. proliferation

angiofibroma
a. contagiosum tropicum
juvenile nasopharyngeal a.
nasopharyngeal a.
a. of penis

angiofollicular
a. hyperplasia
a. hyperplasia lymph node
localized angiofollicular lymph node hyperplasia
a. lymph node hyperplasia
a. lymphoid hyperplasia
a. mediastinal lymph node hyperplasia
multicentric angiofollicular lymph node
multicentric angiofollicular lymphoid hyperplasia
a. and plasmacytic polyadenopathy

angiogenesis
endothelial cell-stimulating angiogenesis factor
a. factor
a. gene delivery
a. inhibitor
lymphocyte-induced angiogenesis factor
a. membrane
microscopic angiogenesis grading system
platelet-derived angiogenesis factor
tissue angiogenesis factor
a. tumor
tumor-induced a.

angiogenic
a. cell
a. cytokine
a. factor
a. growth factor
a. inducer
a. inhibitor
a. response
tumor angiogenic factor

angioglomoid tumor

angiogram
aortic root a.
coronary a.
digital subtraction a.
first-pass radionuclide a.
fundus fluorescein a.
intraarterial digital subtraction a.
left ventricular a.
multigated a.
nuclear cerebral a.
radionuclide cerebral a.
small-angle double-incidence a.
venous digital a.

angiogram-negative SAH

angiographic
a. assessment
a. blush
a. catheter
a. corkscrew artery
a. demonstration
a. embolization
a. end hole catheter
a. evaluation
a. finding
hemodynamic angiographic study
a. intervention
Multistar angiographic unit
a. muscle mass index
a. occlusion
orthogonal angiographic projection
a. recanalization
a. reference system
a. result
a. road-mapping technique
a. study
a. success
a. target
a. targeting
a. targetry
a. Teflon dilator
a. variceal embolization
a. vasospasm
a. 2-wire snare

angiographically
a. confirmed
a. occult intracranial vascular malformation
a. occult vascular malformation
a. occult vessel
a. visualized vascular malformation

angiography
anterior segment a.
aortic arch a.
cerebral radionuclide a.
computed tomographic a.

computed tomography a.
computerized tomographic hepatic a.
contrast-enhanced magnetic resonance a.
coronary a.
digital intravenous a.
digital rotational a.
digital subtraction indocyanine green a.
digital venous subtraction a.
directional color a.
dobutamine thallium a.
electron-beam angiography of coronary artery
equilibrium-gated radionuclide a.
equilibrium radionuclide a.
femorocerebral catheter a.
fluorescein a.
fluorescent a.
functional magnetic resonance a.
gated blood pool a.
gated radionuclide a.
helical computed tomographic a.
a. imaging
indocyanine green a.
indocyanine-green fundus a.
intraarterial digital subtraction a.
intraoperative digital subtraction a.
intraoperative vascular a.
intravenous digital subtraction a.
intravenous fluorescein a.
left coronary a.
magnetic resonance a.
magnetic resonance coronary a.
magnetic resonance tomographic a.
minimum basis set magnetic resonance a.
noninvasive coronary a.
nonselective arterial digital a.
nuclear cerebral a.
photoelectronic intravenous a.
pulmonary a.
quantitative coronary a.
radionuclide a.
right coronary a.
selective visceral a.
spiral CT a.
three-dimensional computed tomographic a.
three-dimensional contrast-enhanced magnetic resonance a.

angiohistiocytoma
multinucleate cell a.

angioid retinal streak

angioimmunoblastic
a. lymphadenopathy
a. lymphadenopathy-like T-cell lymphoma
a. lymphadenopathy with dysproteinemia
a. lymphadenopathy with dysproteinemia-like T-cell lymphoma
a. lymphoma
a. T-cell lymphoma

angioinvasive
a. adenoma
a. lesion

angiokeratoma
a. circumscription
a. circumscriptum
a. of Fordyce
localized a.
Mibelli a.
a. of Mibelli
a. of scrotum

angiolipoma
a., posttraumatic neuroma, glomus tumor, eccrine spiradenoma, and leiomyoma cutis
mediastinal a.

angiolithic
a. degeneration
a. sarcoma

angiolymphatic invasion

angiolymphoid
a. hyperplasia
a. hyperplasia with eosinophilia

angioma
acquired tufted a.
arteriovenous interhemispheric a.
a. cutis
extracerebral cavernous a.
littoral cell a.
nerve head a.
a. serpiginosum
a. simplex

angiomatoid
a. fibrous histiocytoma
a. malignant fibrous histiocytoma
a. myosarcoma
a. Spitz nevus
a. tumor

angiomatosis
bacillary a.
hemorrhagic familial a.
meningeal capillary a.
a. of retina

angiomatous
a. disease
a. involuting nevus
a. lymphoid hamartoma
a. meningioma
a. nasal polyp
a. neoplastic tissue
a. nevus
a. syndrome

angiomyoid
a. lesion
a. proliferation

angiomyolipoma
atypical angiomyolipoma of kidney
atypical angiomyolipoma of the kidney
a. rupture

angiomyoma of oviduct

angiomyxoma
aggressive a.

angioneurotic
a. anuria
a. dermatosis
a. edema
a. hematuria
intermittent angioneurotic edema

angioosteohypertrophy syndrome

angioparalytic neurasthenia

angiopathic
a. hemolytic anemia
a. neurasthenia
a. retinopathy
a. vertigo

angiopathy
amyloid angiopathy cerebral
cerebral amyloid a.
microvascular a.
sporadic cerebral amyloid a.

angioplastic meningioma

angioplasty
adjunctive balloon a.
balloon catheter a.
balloon dilation a.
carotid angioplasty and stenting
carotid stent-supported a.
complementary balloon a.
coronary a.
culprit lesion a.
cutting balloon a.
direct acute myocardial infarction a.

angioplasty *(continued)*
directional coronary a.
excimer laser-assisted a.
excimer laser coronary a.
excimer laser, rotational atherectomy, and balloon a.
laser-assisted balloon a.
new device a.
patch graft a.
percutaneous balloon a.
percutaneous coronary a.
percutaneous coronary transluminal a.
percutaneous excimer laser coronary a.
percutaneous excimer laser coronary angioplasty system
percutaneous low-stress a.
percutaneous rotational transluminal coronary a.
percutaneous transluminal a.
percutaneous transluminal angioplasty with stent placement
percutaneous transluminal balloon a.
percutaneous transluminal coronary a.
percutaneous transluminal renal a.
percutaneous transluminal ultrasonic coronary a.
peripheral balloon a.
peripheral excimer laser a.
peripheral laser a.
physiologic low stress a.
post balloon angioplasty restenosis
primary percutaneous transluminal coronary a.
renal percutaneous transluminal a.
right common femoral a.
salvage a.
smooth excimer laser coronary a.
standby a.
superficial femoral a.
thermal/perfusion balloon a.
transluminal coronary a.
valvuloplasty and angioplasty of congenital anomalies

angioplasty-related vessel occlusion

angioproliferative lesion

angioreticuloendothelioma of heart

angiosarcoma
adrenal epithelioid a.
a. bone tumor
a. of heart

angiosclerotica
myasthenia a.

angiosclerotic gangrene

angioscopic guidance

angioscopy
percutaneous transluminal a.

angiosomal flap

angiospastic
a. anesthesia
central angiospastic retinitis
a. retinopathy

angiotensin
a. amide
a. generation rate
a. I-converting enzyme
a. II
a. II antidiuretic hormone
a. III
a. I and II assay
a. I, II, III
a. I, II infusion test
a. II receptor
a. II receptor blocker
a. inhibitor
potent hormone angiotensin II
a. precursor
pulmonary angiotensin I converting enzyme
a. receptor
renin angiotensin blocker
a. sensitivity test

angiotensin-converting
a.-c. enzyme
a.-c. enzyme dysfunction syndrome
a.-c. enzyme gene
a.-c. enzyme gene polymorphism
a.-c. enzyme II
a.-c. enzyme inhibitor
a.-c. enzyme inhibitor cough

angiotensin-dependent hypertension

angiotensin-like substance

angiotensinogen test

angiotherapy
vasoocclusive a.

angiotrophic lymphoma

angiotropic
a. large cell lymphoma
a. lymphoma

angitis-granulomatosis disorder

angle
a. of aberration
a. of abnormality
acute narrow angle glaucoma
anatomic intermetatarsal a.
a. of anomaly
anterior angle of rib
anterior angulation a.
a. of anterior chamber
anterior chamber a.
a. of anterior rib
anterior talocalcaneal a.
anteroposterior talocalcaneal a.
a. of antetorsion
a. of anteversion
a. of aperture
articular facet a.
articular set a.
augmentation of mandibular a.
axial line a.
A. band
A. basic E arch appliance
a. bisection technique
calcaneal pitch a.
capital epiphysis angle of Wiberg
cardiophrenic a.
CE angle of Wiberg
cerebellopontine a.
A. classification
A. classification of malocclusion, class I–IV
condylar plateau a.
a. of convergence
costophrenic a.
costophrenic angle blunting
costovertebral a.
costovertebral angle tenderness
costovertebral angle tenderness to percussion
a. of declination
a. of declination of metatarsal
a. of depression
depressor muscle of angle of mouth
a. of deviation
a. of direction
distal articular set a.
distal metatarsal articular a.
a. of divergence
dorsiflexion a.
a. of eccentricity
electrocardiographic angle between QRS and T vectors
a. electron
a. of emergence
exaggerated craniocaudal lateral a.
a. of femoral torsion

femorotibial a.
a. finder
foot-progression a.
foot progression a.
a. former
a. fracture
Frankfort mandibular incisor a.
Frankfort mandibular plane a.
a. of Fuchs
a. of gait
gastroesophageal angle of His
a. of Gissane
a. of greatest extension
a. of greatest flexion
hallux dorsiflexion a.
hallux valgus a.
a. head
hip joint a.
a. of His
impedance a.
a. of incidence
incisal mandibular plane a.
a. of incision
a. of inclination of urethra
a. of incongruity
inferior a.
inferior lateral a.
a. of inferior scapula
a. of insonation
intermetatarsal a.
a. of iridocorneal
a. of iris
a. isometric testing
a. of jaw
a. of lateral eye
lateral talocalcaneal a.
left a.
logarithmic Minimum A. of Resolution
a. of Louis
a. of Ludwig
magic angle effect artifact
magic angle phenomenon
magic angle spinning NMR
A. malocclusion classification
a. of mandible
a. of Mary
mastoid angle of parietal bone
medial angle of eye
a. of medial eye
a. meningioma
Merchant congruence a.
metatarsus adductus a.
meter a.
minimal angle resolution
minimum separable a.
minimum visible a.
minimum visual a.
moderately narrow anterior chamber a.
moderately wide open anterior chamber a.
modiolus of angle of mouth
a. of mouth
a. of Mulder
nail-to-nail bed a.
navicular to first metatarsal a.
neck-shaft a.
negative congruence a.
nutation angle measurement
objective a.
occipital angle of parietal bone
a. of orientation
parietal angle of sphenoid
partial flip angle imaging
pectinate ligament of iridocorneal a.
pedicle axis a.
a. of polarization
a. position potentiometer
a. of posterior rib
proximal articular set a.
Q a.
quadriceps a.
quadriceps neutral a.
a. recession
a. of reflection
refracting angle of prism
a. of refraction
a. of retroversion
right a.
right angle clamp
A. splint
a. of squint
a. structure
a. of superior scapula
a. suture
a. suture technique
a. of Sylvius
talar axis–first metatarsal base a.
talocalcaneal a.
thigh-foot a.
thigh-leg a.
a. of thoracic inclination
tibiofemoral a.
a. of torsion
a.'s of trigone
ureterovesical a.
a. variation resolution
very narrow anterior chamber a.
a. of Wiberg
wide open anterior chamber a.
a. width

angle-closure
acute angle-closure glaucoma
acute intermittent primary angle-closure glaucoma
acute primary angle-closure glaucoma
chronic primary angle-closure glaucoma
a.-c. glaucoma
intermittent angle-closure glaucoma
mydriatic test for angle-closure glaucoma
neovascular angle-closure glaucoma
primary angle-closure glaucoma

angled
a. aneurysm clip
a. arthroscope
a. awl
a. bearing insert
a. blade plate fixation
a. cannula
a. capsule forceps
a. cartilage scissors
a. craniocaudal view
a. delivery device
a. dissecting forceps
a. dissector
a. elevator
a. iris hook and IOL dialer
a. jaw rongeur
a. left/right cannula
a. lens loupe
a. Lowman-type bone clamp
a. manipulator
multipurpose angled clamp
a. needle
a. nucleus removal loupe
a. pituitary rongeur
a. pleural tube
a. rasp
a. slice
a. suction tube
a. telescope
a. view

angled-down forceps
angled-lens endoscope
angled-shaft endoscope
angled-tip catheter
angled-up forceps
angled-vision lens system
angle-fixated lens
angle-recession glaucoma
angle-supported lens

angling
pantoscopic a.

Anglo-Saxon
A.-S. nomenclature
white Anglo-Saxon Protestant

angry
adjustment disorder with angry mood
a. affect
a. backfiring C nociceptor
a. back phenomenon
a. back reaction
a. back syndrome
a. behavior
a. outburst
a. reaction
a. reaction to minor stimuli
a. woman syndrome
a. word exchange

Ångström
Å. law
Å. scale
Å. unit

angular
a. acceleration
a. activation
a. aldehyde
a. alignment
a. aperture
a. aqueous sinus plexus
a. artery
artery of angular gyrus
artery of angular nasal branch
atomic orbital with angular momentum quantum number zero
axial plane angular deformity biomechanics
a. blepharitis
a. blepharoconjunctivitis
a. bolster
a. bone rongeur
a. bundle
a. cheilitis
a. cheilosis
a. conjunctivitis
constant angular velocity
a. convolution
a. coordinate variable
a. curvature
a. deformity
a. deviation
a. displacement
a. distance
a. eye velocity
a. facial vein
a. frequency
a. gyrus
a. gyrus syndrome
a. head velocity
a. hinge clamp
a. incision
a. incisure
a. junction
a. junction of eyelid
a. line
a. methyl
a. momentum
a. motion
a. movement
a. nasal artery
a. notch
a. notch of stomach
nuclear angular momentum
a. osteotomy
a. phenolization
a. position
a. position of ramus
a. process of orbit
a. resolved photoelectron spectroscopy
a. sampling
a. sphincter
a. spine
a. stomatitis
a. tilt
a. tract of cervical fascia
a. vein
a. vestibular nucleus

angularis
arteria a.
a. body
a. sulcus

angulated
ASSI breast dissector a.
a. buccal tube
a. cell
a. fracture
fracture, complete, a.
a. lesion
a. lysosome
a. segment

angulation
anterior angulation angle
apex anterior a.
apex dorsal a.
apex posterior a.
a. at fracture site
a. deformity
a. fracture
left a.
Marquardt angulation osteotomy
a. motion
a. osteotomy
a. of spine

angulatory malunion

anguli
modiolus anguli oris

Angus-Cowell scale

Anhanga virus

anhaustral colonic gas pattern

anhedonia
orgasmic a.
pervasive a.

Anhembi virus

anhemolytic streptococcus

anhepatic
a. jaundice
a. stage of liver transplantation

anhepatogenous jaundice

anhidrosis
chronic idiopathic a.

anhidrotic
a. congenital ectodermal dysplasia
a. ectodermal dysplasia
a. heat exhaustion
a. sweating

anhydrase
carbonic a.
carbonic anhydrase II
carbonic anhydrase inhibitor
a. glycerol

anhydrous
a. alcohol
a. ammonia
a. chloral
a. ethanol
a. lanolin
a. magnesium sulfate
a. sodium sulfite

ani
atresia a.
levator ani muscle
pruritus a.
tendinous arch of levator a.

anicteric
a. bile duct
a. cholestasis
a. hepatitis
sclerae a.
a. sclerae
a. skin
a. viral hepatitis
a. virus hepatitis

aniline
a., sulfur, formaldehyde

a. blue
a. blue modified trichrome stain
a. carcinoma
a. dye
a. fuchsin
a. gentian violet
Mallory aniline blue stain
a. red

animal
a. abuse
aggression to people and a.'s
anthrax-contaminated animal product
a. antisera
a. beanbag exerciser
a. bite
a. black
a. botulism
a. cell culture
a. charcoal
cruelty to a.'s
a. dander
a. dander sensitivity
a. dextran
a. force
frozen animal procedure
a. graft
a. hair
a. hemisphere
hydrolyzed animal protein
investigational new animal drug
laboratory animal dander allergy
low animal fat
a. magnetism
marine animal sting
a. model
a. pituitary gonadotropin
a. placenta lactogen
a. pole
a. protein diet
a. protein factor
a. psychology
a. scabies
a. soap
a. starch
a. toxin
tumor-bearing a.
a. virus
a. viruses
a. wax

animal-assisted therapy

animal-naming test

animal-scratch disease

animistic thinking

animo-terminal portion of heavy chain of immunoglobulin

anion
canicular multispecific organic anion transporter
a. exchanger
a. exchange resin
a. gap
a. gap acidosis
a. gap metabolic acidosis
a. gap test
high-pH anion exchange chromatography coupled with pulsed amperometric detection
a. of the Hofmeister series
a. interference
low anion gap
organic anion transporter polypeptide
a. transport inhibitor
voltage-dependent anion channel

anion-exchange
a.-e. chromatography
a.-e. resin

anionic
a. detergent
a. dye
a. IgG 4 fraction
a. neutrophil-activating peptide
organic anionic dye
a. trypsinogen

aniridia
a., ambiguous genitalia, mental retardation
a., ambiguous genitalia, mental retardation triad syndrome
a., cerebellar ataxia-oligophrenia syndrome
a., Wilms tumor association
a., Wilms tumor, gonadoblastoma syndrome

aniridia-Wilms
a.-W. tumor

anisakiasis
gastrointestinal a.

anisakid nematode

anise
oil of a.
a. oil

aniseikonic lens

anisic acid

anisocoria
a. contraction
a. with ipsilateral mydriasis

anisometric amblyopia

anisometropic amblyopia

anisotropic
a. band
a. band in striated muscle
a. bone property
a. conduction
a. 3DFT
a. diffusion
a. 3D imaging
a. disc
a. lipid
a. resolution
a. rotation
a. tissue
a. volume study

anisotropically
a. rotational diffusion
a. rotational diffusion imaging

anisotropine methylbromide

anisotropy
a. factor
magnetic a.
a. map
a. of white matter

anisoylated plasminogen streptokinase activator complex

Anitschkow
A. cell
A. myocyte

Ankara
modified vaccine virus A.

ankle
absent ankle jerk
active ankle joint complex range of motion
adjustable leg and ankle repositioning mechanism
Allman modification of Evans ankle reconstruction
amputated above a.
Anderson ankle fusion
annular atrophic connective tissue panniculitis of the a.
anterior ankle impingement
anterior ankle shift operation
anterior medial ankle ligament
anterior tibiotalar part of medial ligament of ankle joint
AO ankle fracture classification
AO-Danis-Weber ankle fracture classification
Arizona ankle brace
arthritic ankle joint narrowing
a. arthrocentesis
a. arthrodesis
a. arthrogram

ankle *(continued)*
a. arthrography
a. arthroplasty
a. arthroscopy
Ashhurst-Bromer ankle fracture classification
autologous reverse graft to a.
ball-and-socket ankle mortise
a. block
a. block anesthesia
a. bone
a. clonus
a. clonus test
a. contracture orthosis
controlled ankle motion
Danis-Weber classification for ankle fracture
a. disarticulation
a. disc device
a. disc training
a. dislocation
a. dorsiflexion range of motion
a. dorsiflexion test
eclipse ankle brace
a. edema
a. effusion
a. equinus
a. eversion
a. exercise machine
a. exerciser
fibular collateral ligament of a.
foot and ankle severity scale
forced inversion film of a.
a. fusion
a. guard
a. immobilizer
a. impingement
a. infectious arthritis
a. inferior transverse ligament
a. injury
a. instability
instability of the a.
a. inversion-eversion range of motion
a. inversion injury
a. jerk
a. jerk reflex
a. joint
a. joint complex
a. joint leg-curl
lateral collateral ligament of a.
a. laxity
a. ligament protector
a. ligament protector brace
long leg brace with free a.
a. loose body
Louisiana ankle wrap technique
a. magnet
Malleoloc ankle orthosis
Marcus-Balourdas-Heiple ankle fusion technique
Mayo ankle arthroplasty
Mazur ankle elevation classification
Mazur ankle evaluation
Mazur ankle rating
medial joint of a.
medial ligament of ankle joint
medical ankle orthosis
Merchant and Dietz ankle score
modified Boyd amputation of ankle and distal tibial physis
modified Boyd ankle arthrodesis
modified Chrisman-Snook ankle reconstruction
a. mortise
a. mortise axis
a. mortise diastasis
a. mortise fracture
a. mortise widening
Multi Axis A.
Nélaton ankle dislocation
a. osteoarthritis
a. osteomyelitis
paradoxical ankle reflex
pitting edema of a.
Pott ankle fracture
a. pressure
a. prosthesis
puffy a.'s
a. reconstruction
a. reflex time
a. region
resting ankle index
a. rheumatoid arthritis
rotary ankle instability
Scandinavian total ankle replacement
a. scoring system of Baird and Jackson
severely swollen a.
soft ankle, cushioned heel orthopaedic appliance
solid ankle flexible endoskeletal
a. sprain
a. stability
a. stabilizer
a. stabilizing orthosis
a. stabilizing orthosis support
stationary ankle flexible endoskeleton
a. stirrup brace
a. stirrup splint
a. strategy
swelling of a.'s
a. swelling
a. systolic pressure
timed repetitive ankle jerk
total ankle arthroplasty
total ankle replacement
trace ankle edema
a. traction bandage

ankle-arm
a.-a. index
a.-a. pressure
a.-a. pressure index

ankle-brachial
a.-b. blood pressure
a.-b. blood pressure ratio
a.-b. index
mean ankle-brachial systolic pressure index
a.-b. pressure index
a.-b. pressure measurement

ankle-foot
a.-f. electrogoniometer
a.-f. orthosis
a.-f. orthosis brace sock
a.-f. plastic orthosis
tone-reducing ankle-foot orthosis

ankle-hindfoot scale

ankle-level arteriotomy

ankle-pump exercise

ankle-type fibrous histiocytoma

ankyloblepharon
a., ectodermal defect, and cleft lip and/or palate
a., ectodermal dysplasia, clefting syndrome

ankyloglossia
a. superior
a. superior syndrome

ankylosed tooth

ankylosing
ankylosis and ankylosing enthesopathy
a. enthesopathy
a. hyperostosis
idiopathic ankylosing spondylitis
juvenile ankylosing spondylitis
a. spinal hyperostosis
a. spinal stenosis
a. spondylitis
a. spondylitis, lung
a. spondyloarthropathy
vertebral ankylosing hyperostosis

ankylosis
a. and ankylosing enthesopathy
artificial a.

cricoarytenoid joint a.
ligamentous a.
lung ankylosis spondylitis
a. nonunions
operative a.
osseous a.
partial a.
shoulder a.
a. spondylosis
a. of tooth
true a.

ankyrin deficiency

anlage
inner optic a.
outer optic a.
a. of pancreas
pancreatic dorsal a.
salivary gland anlage tumor

anlagen of the auditory ossicle

Ann
A. Arbor cancer staging
A. Arbor classification
A. Arbor classification of Hodgkin disease staging
A. Arbor double towel clamp
A. Arbor Hodgkin lymphoma stage I, IE, II, IIE, IIIE, IIIS, IIISE, IV
A. Arbor staging classification
A. Arbor tumor classification

Annandale operation

Annapolis lymphoblast globulin

annealing
a. algorithm
a. furnace
a. lamp
a. temperature
a. tray

Annie
Orphan Annie eye

annihilation
a. anxiety
a. coincidence detection
oblique annihilation photon pair
a. photon
a. radiation
a. reaction

anniversary
a. date
a. excitement
a. hypothesis
a. reaction

annotated imaging

announced
to be a.

announcement
public service a.

annoyance level

annoyed
agitated, irritable and easily a.

annual
a. bluegrass
a. cycle
a. goal
a. health evaluation
a. review

annually
complete gynecologic examination a.

annular (*var. of* anular)

annulare
a. bulbi
granuloma a.
localized granuloma a.
perforating granuloma a.

annuloaortic (*var. of* anuloaortic)

annuloplasty (*var. of* anuloplasty)

annulospiral (*var. of* anulospiral)

ano
fissure in a.

anococcygeal
a. body
a. ligament
a. nerve
a. raphe

anococcygei
nervi a.

anococcygeus
nervus a.

anocutaneous
a. line
a. reflex
a. stimulation

anodal
a. block
a. closure
a. closure contraction
a. closure picture
a. closure sound
a. closure tetanus
a. current
a. duration
a. duration contraction
a. duration tetanus
a. excitation
a. opening
a. opening clonus
a. opening contraction
a. opening picture
a. opening sound
a. opening tetanus

anode
molybdenum rotating anode x-ray tube
a. ray
a. tube reloading
a. voltage

anode-cathode axis

anoderm-preserving hemorrhoidectomy

anodic
a. stripping voltametry
circulating anodic antigen

anodontia
partial a.
a. vera

anogenital
a. band
a. cancer
a. disorder
a. epidermal cyst
a. herpes
a. neoplasm
a. pilar cyst
a. raphe
a. sebaceous cyst
a. squamous intraepithelial neoplasia
a. vestibular cyst
a. vestibular papilla
a. wart

anomalies/mental
multiple congenital anomalies/mental retardation syndrome

anomaloscope
Nagel a.

anomalous
a. anatomy
a. antigen expression
a. arrangement of pancreaticobiliary ductal system
a. atrioventricular excitation
a. branching
a. bronchus
a. calix
a. cerebral artery
a. complex
a. conduction
a. coronary artery
a. craniovertebral junction
a. development
a. disk

anomalous *(continued)*
a. distribution
a. fibular nutrient artery
a. fixation
a. genitalia
a. innervation
a. innominate artery compression syndrome
a. insertion
a. junction
a. junction of pancreaticobiliary ducts
a. junction of the pancreatobiliary duct
a. left coronary artery
a. left coronary artery from pulmonary artery
a. left coronary artery from pulmonary artery syndrome
a. left main coronary artery
a. left pulmonary artery
a. mesenteric adhesion
a. mitral arcade
a. movement
a. muscle
a. muscle band
a. muscle bundle
a. nonrecurrent right inferior laryngeal nerve
a. origin
a. origin of left coronary artery from pulmonary artery
a. pancreaticobiliary communication
a. pancreaticobiliary ductal union
a. pancreatobiliary duct junction
a. parental vocal pattern
partial anomalous pulmonary veins
partial anomalous pulmonary venous connection
partial anomalous pulmonary venous drainage
partial anomalous pulmonary venous return
a. pathway
a. position
pulmonary anomalous superior venous return
a. pulmonary vein
a. pulmonary venous connection, total or partial
a. pulmonary venous drainage
a. pulmonary venous return
a. rectification
a. result
a. retinal correspondence
a. right pulmonary vein dextroposition
a. right subclavian artery
a. serum chemistry
a. sexual behavior
a. sexual urge
a. tongue position
total anomalous pulmonary circulation
total anomalous pulmonary venous connection
total anomalous pulmonary venous drainage
total anomalous pulmonary venous return
a. trichromatism
a. trichromatopsia
a. uterus
a. vascular distribution
a. vertebral artery
a. vessel
a. viscosity

anomaly
alpha, delta sleep a.
a. angle
angle of a.
anophthalmos-limb anomalies syndrome
aortic arch a.
arthrogryposis-like hand a.
atrioventricular connection a.
atrioventricular junction a.
autosomal chromosomal a.
azoospermia, renal anomaly, cervicothoracic spine dysplasia
bell-clapper a.
branchial cleft a.
coloboma, heart anomaly, ichthyosis, mental retardation, and ear abnormality syndrome
coloboma, heart disease, atresia choanae, retarded growth and retarded development and/or CNS anomalies, genital hypoplasia, and ear anomalies and/or deafness syndrome
congenital anomaly of mitral valve
congenital heart a.
conjoined nerve root a.
conotruncal anomaly face syndrome
developmental venous a.
DiGeorge a.
digital anomalies, short palpebral fissures, atresia of esophagus or duodenum syndrome
distal arthrogryposis, hypopituitarism, mental retardation, facial anomalies syndrome
a. of drainage of pulmonary vein
immunodeficiency, centromeric instability, facial anomalies syndrome
May-Hegglin a.
mental retardation, facial anomalies, hypopituitarism, distal arthrogryposis syndrome
mental retardation, hearing impairment, distinct facies, skeletal anomalies syndrome
Meurmann external ear anomaly grade
microcephaly-cervical spine fusion a.'s
microcephaly-digital anomalies syndrome
microcephaly, mild mental retardation, short stature, skeletal anomalies syndrome
microphthalmia or anophthalmos with associated a.'s
minor physical a.
mitral valve prolapse, aortic anomalies, skeletal changes, and skin changes syndrome
Moore classification for vascular anomalies of the gastrointestinal tract
morning glory disc a.
morning glory optic disk a.
müllerian duct a.
müllerian duct, unilateral renal agenesis, and anomalies of the cervicothoracic somites
multiple congenital a.'s
nerve root a.
no significant a.
oculocephalic vascular a.
odontogenic keratocytosis-skeletal anomalies syndrome
optical disc a.
optic disc a.
partial DiGeorge a.
Pelger-Huët nuclear a.
Pelger-Huët nuclear a.
polydactyly, imperforate anus, vertebral anomalies syndrome
prune belly a.
pulmonary valve a.
severe congenital a.
short stature, hyperextensibility of joints or hernia or both, ocular

depression, Rieger anomaly, teething, delayed
spondylar changes, nasal anomaly, striated metaphyses
tracheoesophageal fistula, esophageal atresia, multiple congenital anomaly syndrome
true a.
urinary tract a.
valvuloplasty and angioplasty of congenital a.'s
vertebral abnormality, anal imperforation, tracheoesophageal fistula, and radial, ray, or renal a.'s
X-linked mental retardation-blindness-deafness-multiple congenital anomalies syndrome
a. of Zahn

anomer of carbohydrate

anomeric carbon

anomic
a. aphasia
a. error
a. suicide

anonyma
arteria a.

anonymous
Alcoholics A.
a. artery
Cocaine A.
Codependents A.
a. donor sperm
Gamblers A.
Narcotics A.
Parents A.
a. vein

***Anopheles* A, B virus**

anopheline
a. mosquito
a. vector

anophthalmia, hand-foot defects-mental retardation syndrome

anophthalmia-Waardenburg syndrome

anophthalmic
a. orbit syndrome
a. socket

anophthalmos
microphthalmia or anophthalmos with associated anomalies

anophthalmos-limb anomalies syndrome

anophthalmos-syndactyly syndrome

anoplasty
Martin a.
a. treatment

anopouch angle

anorectal
a. abscess
a. agenesis
a. angle
a. anomaly
a. atresia
a. band
a. carcinoma
a. disease
a. disorder
a. dressing
a. dysgenesis
a. endosonography
a. examination
a. fistula
a. flexure
a. foreign body
a. function test
a. gonorrhea
a. herpes
a. imaging
a. impalement
a. incontinence
a. junction
a. line
a. lymph node
a. lymphoma
a. malformation
a. manometry
a. measurement
a. melanoma
a. mobilization
a. mucosal prolapse
a. myectomy
a. nomenclature
a. outlet obstruction
perianal anorectal space
a. physiological dysfunction
a. physiology
a. physiology testing
a. plug
polypoid anorectal lesion
a. ring
a. sensorimotor dysfunction
a. sepsis
a. septum
a. space
a. spasm
a. sphincter
a. stenosis
a. surgery
a. syndrome
a. syphilis
total anorectal reconstruction
a. tuberculosis
a. variceal bleeding
a. varix

anorectic
a. drug
Goldberg A. Attitude Scale
patient a.
a. reaction

anorectoperineal muscle

anorectoplasty
anterior sagittal a.
Pena midsagittal a.

anorexia
a. athletica
bingeing behavior of a.
cancer, anorexia, cachexia syndrome
mild anorexia nervosa
National Association of A. Nervosa and Associated Disorders
a. nervosa
a. nervosa and associated disorders
A. Nervosa Inventory for Self-Rating
paraneoplastic a.
a. support group
unique facies, anorexia, cachexia, and eye and skin syndrome

anorexia-cachexia syndrome

anorexic
a. behavior
a. fast
patient a.

anoscopic aspirate

anosmia
a. and hypogonadotropic hypogonadism syndrome
mechanical a.

anosmic aphasia

anosognosic
a. epilepsy
a. seizure

anospinal center

another
hypersomnia related to another mental disorder

ANOTHER syndrome

anovaginal fistula

anovular
a. menstruation
a. ovarian follicle

anovulation
chronic a.
chronic anovulation syndrome
hyperandrogenic a.

anovulational menstruation

anovulatory
a. bleeding
a. cycle
delayed anovulatory syndrome
a. infertility
oligomenorrhea with anovulatory menses
a. patient

anoxemia test

anoxia
altitude a.
anemic a.
anoxic a.
global a.
hypoxia and a.
metabolic a.
myocardial a.
a. neonatorum
oxygen affinity a.
perinatal a.
perioperative a.
a. reaction

anoxic
a. anoxia
a. brain damage
a. brain injury
a. change
a. changes in brain
a. damage
a. encephalopathy
a. hypoxia
a. ischemia
a. seizure
severe anoxic encephalopathy
widespread anoxic change

anoxic-ischemic encephalopathy

ansa
a. cervicalis
a. cervicalis nerve
a. cervicalis root
a. hypoglossal nerve
a. hypoglossus muscle
a. pancreatica
a. pancreaticus
peduncular a.
a. peduncularis
peduncularis ansa peduncular
Reil a.
a. sacralis
thyrohyoid branch of ansa cervicalis
a. of Vieussens

anserine
a. bursa
a. bursitis
pes anserine transfer

anserinus
pes a.
pes anserinus bursa
pes anserinus bursitis

ansiform lobule

Anson-McVay
A.-M. femoral herniorrhaphy
A.-M. hernia repair
A.-M. operation

ansoparamedian fissure

Anstie
A. rule
A. test

answers
a. questions appropriately
approximate answers syndrome
syndrome of approximate relevant a.

ant
a. bite
a. sting

antacid
a. of choice
liquid a.

antagonism
metabolic a.
microbial a.
synalbumin-insulin a.

antagonist
alpha-1 adrenergic a.
alpha-adrenergic receptor a.
alpha-2-adrenergic receptor a.
androgen receptor a.
calcium a.
calcium channel a.
a. drug
folic acid a.
histamine-2 receptor a.
interferon
interleukin-1 receptor antagonist protein
intravenous H2 receptor a.
leukotriene receptor a.
a. medication
a. muscle
narcotic antagonist drug
neurokinin-1 receptor a.
NMDA antagonist ketamine
nonselective adenosine receptor a.
opioid receptor a.
partial agonist-partial a.
reversal of a.
serotonin/dopamine a.
tissue antagonist of interferon

antagonistic
a. behavior
downstream regulatory element antagonistic modulator gene
a. drug
a. effect
a. muscle
a. muscle strength
a. pattern
a. reflex
a. thermoeffector

antagonist-II
prothrombin induced by vitamin K absence or a.-I.

antagonist-induced gonadotropin deprivation

antalgic
a. gait
a. lean
a. limp
a. medication

antazoline hydrochloride

anteater nose

antebrachial
anterior antebrachial nerve
a. cutaneous nerve
a. fascia
a. fascial graft
medial antebrachial cutaneous nerve
median antebrachial vein
a. region
ulnar branch of medial antebrachial cutaneous nerve
a. vein

antecedent
a. event
a. pancreatic injury
plasma thromboplastin a.
platelet thromboplastin a.
a. sign
a. streptococcal infection
a. variable
a.'s of violence

antecedent-consequence variable

antecolic
a. anastomosis

a. gastrectomy
a. long-loop isoperistaltic gastrojejunostomy
a. position

antecubital
a. approach
a. arteriovenous fistula
a. crease
a. fossa
left a.
primary antecubital jump bypass
right a.
a. space
a. vein

anteflexed
anteverted and a.
normal size, shape, and position, anteverted and anteflexed uterus
a. uterus

anteflexion of iris

antegonial
a. angle
a. notch
a. notching

antegrade
a. amnesia
a. aortography
a. approach
a. bile flow
a. block
a. blood flow
a. cardioplegia
a. catheterization
a. colonic enema
a. conduction
a. continence enema
a. continence enema procedure
a. contrast study
a. cystography
a. diastolic flow
a. double balloon-double wire technique
a. ejaculation
a. endopyelotomy
a. fast pathway
a. femoral artery catheterization
a. femoral nail
a. filling of vessel
a. flow
a. instrumentation
ipsilateral antegrade arteriography
a. island flap
Malone antegrade colonic enema stoma procedure
Malone antegrade continence enema procedure
Malone antegrade continent enema channel
a. method
a. nailing
a. nephroscopy
percutaneous antegrade biliary drainage
percutaneous antegrade pyelography
percutaneous antegrade urography
a. perfusion
a. perfusion pressure measurement
a. pressure study
a. puncture
a. pyelogram
a. pyelography
a. pyelography imaging
a. pyeloureterography
a. refractory period
a. scrotal sclerotherapy
a. transluminal balloon dilatation
a. transseptal technique
a. ureteral drainage
a. ureteral stenting
a. urography
a. venography

antegrade/retrograde cardioplegia technique

antemortem
a. clot
a. thrombus

antenatal
a. anti-D immunoglobulin
a. Bartter syndrome
a. corticosteroid
a. corticosteroid therapy
a. corticosteroid treatment
a. diagnosis
a. disease process
a. dislocation
a. fetofetal transfusion
a. morbidity
a. patient
a. phenobarbital treatment
routine antenatal diagnostic imaging with ultrasound
a. screening
a. steroid
a. thyrotropin releasing hormone
a. treatment
a. ultrasound

antenatal-hypercalciuric variant

antenna
microwave antenna design
a. procedure

antepartum
a. asphyxia
a. bleeding
a. care
a. constipation
a. fetal BPP
a. fetal NST
a. fetal surveillance
a. hemorrhage
a. pyelonephritis
a. Rh isoimmunization

anteprostatic gland

Antequera virus

anterior
A1-A5 segments of anterior cerebral artery
a. abdominal cutaneous branch of intercostal nerve
a. abdominal injury
a. abdominal wall
a. abdominal wall syndrome
a. abutment
a. acoustic stria
a. acromioplasty
a. acromioplasty approach
a. active mask rhinomanometry
acute anterior uveitis
a. acute flexion elbow splint
a. acute poliomyelitis
a. adductor of the coxa
air bubble instilled in anterior chamber
a. alexia
a. alveolar branch of maxillary nerve
a. alveolar nerve
a. ampullary nerve
a. amygdaloid area
Andrews anterior instability test
angle of anterior chamber
angle of anterior rib
a. angle of rib
a. angulation
a. angulation angle
a. ankle impingement
a. ankle shift operation
a. antebrachial nerve
a. anular ligament
a. aortic wall
apex anterior angulation
a. aphasia
a. apical
a. apical vault defect
a. apprehension test
a. approach
a. apraxia
a. arch of atlas

anterior *(continued)*
a. arch length
a. arch width
arteria cecalis a.
arteria cerebri a.
arteria choroidea a.
arteria communicans a.
arteria conjunctivalis a.
arteria ethmoidalis a.
arteria malleolaris anterior lateralis
arteria malleolaris anterior medialis
arteria meningea a.
arteria pancreaticoduodenalis superior a.
arteria parietalis a.
arteria radicularis anterior magna
arteria temporalis a.
arteria tibialis a.
arteria tympanica a.
arteria vestibularis a.
arteritic anterior ischemic optic neuropathy
artery of anterior inferior segment of kidney
artery of anterior superior segment of kidney
arthroscopically assisted anterior cruciate ligament reconstruction
arthroscopic anterior cruciate ligament reconstruction
a. articular surface of dens
ascending anterior branch
A1 segment of anterior cerebral artery
A2 segment of anterior cerebral artery
a. aspect
a. aspiration
a. asynclitism
a. atlantodental interval
atlantooccipital anterior membrane
a. atlantooccipital membrane
a. atlantoodontoid interval
a. atlas arch
a. atrial myocardial bundle
a. auricular artery
a. auricular branch of superficial temporal artery
a. auricular groove
auricularis anterior muscle
a. auricular muscle
a. auricular nerve
a. auricular vein
a. axial developmental cataract
a. axial embryonal cataract
axial left anterior oblique ventriculogram
a. axillary approach
a. axillary fold
a. axillary line
a. axillary lymph node
a. axonal embryonal cataract
a. band
a. band of colon
a. band remover
a. basal
a. basal branch
a. basal bronchopulmonary segment
a. basal bronchus
a. basal encephalocele
a. basal segment
a. basal segmental artery
a. basal vein
a. basement membrane dystrophy
a. belly of digastric muscle
a. bending moment
a. border
a. border of body of pancreas
a. border of eyelid
a. border of fibula
a. border of heart
a. border of lung
a. border of radius
a. border of testis
a. border of tibia
a. border of ulna
a. bowing of sternum
a. bowing tibia
a. branch
a. branch of axillary nerve
a. branch of the renal artery
a. branch of thoracic nerve
a. bridge
a. bronchopulmonary segment
a. bulb syndrome
a. calcaneal osteotomy
a. calcaneal process fracture
a. callosotomy
a. canaliculus of chorda tympani
a. capsular distance
a. capsular shift
a. capsule
a. capsulectomy
a. capsule shagreen
a. capsulolabral reconstruction
a. capsulotomy
a. capsulotomy for treatment of OCD
a. cardiac vein
a. cardinal vein
a. carotid artery
a. cavernous sinus space
a. cavernous sinus syndrome
a. cavus
a. C1-C2 screw fixation
a. cecal artery
a. central beaking
a. central convolution
a. central curve
a. central gyrus
a. central indentation
a. centriole
a. cerebellar notch
a. cerebral artery
a. cerebral artery crawling under the skull
a. cerebral artery plexus
a. cerebral artery pulsatility index
a. cerebral vein
a. cervical approach to cervicothoracic junction
a. cervical body fusion
a. cervical chain adenopathy
a. cervical cord syndrome
a. cervical discectomy and fusion
a. cervical diskectomy
a. cervical diskectomy and fusion
a. cervical fascia
a. cervical fusion
a. cervical intertransverse muscle
a. cervical lip
a. cervical plate
a. cervical plate fixation system
a. cervical surgery vocal cord damage
a. cervicothoracic junction surgery
a. chamber
a. chamber angle
a. chamber aspiration
a. chamber-associated immune deviation
a. chamber cannula
a. chamber cleavage syndrome
a. chamber diameter
a. chamber dysgenesis syndrome
a. chamber of eye
a. chamber of eyeball
a. chamber hyphema
a. chamber inflammation
a. chamber intraocular lens
a. chamber irrigated with saline
a. chamber lymphoma
a. chamber paracentesis
a. chamber reaction
a. chamber reformation
a. chamber shallowing
a. chamber sinus
a. chamber tap

a. chamber trabecula
a. chamber tube
a. chamber washout
a. cheek electrode
a. chest diameter
a. chest wall flap
a. chest wall syndrome
a. choroidal artery
a. choroiditis
chronic anterior exertional compartment syndrome
chronic anterior uveitis
a. ciliary artery
a. ciliary vein
a. cingulate
a. cingulate cortex
a. cingulate flow
a. cingulate gyrus
a. cingulate gyrus tumor
a. cingulate pathway
a. cingulate prefrontal syndrome
a. cingulotomy for treatment of OCD
a. circulation
a. circulation aneurysm
a. circulation intracranial aneurysm
a. circulation stroke
a. circumflex humeral artery
a. circumflex humeral vein
a. clear space
a. cleavage syndrome
a. clinoid
a. clinoid process
a. collateral ligament
a. colliculus
a. column
a. column disruption
a. column fracture
a. column of medulla oblongata
a. column osteosynthesis
a. column of spinal cord
a. column of spine
a. commissure
a. commissure of labia
a. commissure of larynx
a. commissure ligament
a. commissure-posterior commissure
a. commissure-posterior commissure line
a. commissure-posterior commissure reference point
a. communicating aneurysm
a. communicating artery
a. communicating artery aneurysm
a. communicating artery complex
a. communicating artery distribution infarct
a. communicating artery distribution infarction
a. compartment
a. compartment of arm
a. compartment of forearm
a. compartment of leg
a. compartment syndrome
a. compartment of thigh
a. complete dislocation
a. component
a. component of force
a. compressive optic neuropathy
concave anterior surface
a. condylar canal
a. condylar vein
a. condyloid canal of occipital bone
a. condyloid foramen
congenital anterior staphyloma
a. conjunctival artery
a. conjunctival vein
a. construct
contoured anterior spinal plate
a. cord
a. cord compression
a. cord impingement
a. cord syndrome
a. cornea
a. corneal curvature
a. corneal dystrophy
a. corneal staphyloma
a. cornual syndrome
a. coronary periarterial plexus
a. corpectomy
a. corpus
a. correction
a. cortex
a. cortex penetration
a. corticospinal tract
a. costotransverse ligament
a. cranial base
a. cranial fossa
a. cranial fossa surgery
a. craniectomy
a. craniofacial resection
a. crest of stapes
a. cricoid split
a. cricoid split procedure
a. crossbite
a. cruciate
a. cruciate deficit knee
a. cruciate deficit of knee
a. cruciate ligament
a. cruciate ligament injury
a. cruciate ligament reconstruction
a. cruciate ligament repair
a. cruciate ligament tear
a. cruciate sprain
cruciform anterior spinal hyperextension
a. crural nerve
a. crural septum
a. crus
a. crus integrity
a. crus of stapes
a. current generator
a. curvature
a. cusp
a. cusp of left atrioventricular valve
a. cusp of mitral valve
a. cusp of right atrioventricular valve
a. cusp of tricuspid valve
a. cutaneous branch
a. cutaneous branch of femoral nerve
a. cutaneous branch of iliohypogastric nerve
a. cutaneous branch of intercostal nerve
a. cutaneous nerve
a. cutaneous nerve of abdomen
a. cylinder
a. cyst
a. decompression
deep anterior tibiotalar
a. deep cervical lymph node
degenerative anterior spurring
a. descending artery
a. descent
a. determinant
a. determinants of cusp occlusion
a. disc displacement without reduction
a. discectomy
a. diskectomy
a. dislocation
a. displacement
a. displacement no reduction
a. displacement with reduction
a. distraction
a. divergence
a. division
a. division of brachial plexus
a. dorsal nucleus
a. drainage
a. drawer sign
a. drawer stress radiograph
a. duodenal ulcer
a. elastic layer
a. embryotoxon

anterior *(continued)*
a. enterocele
a. epidural fat
a. epineurotomy
a. epithelium of cornea
a. epithelium corneae
a. equinus
a. esophagus
a. ethmoid
a. ethmoidal air cell
a. ethmoidal artery
a. ethmoidal branch of ophthalmic artery
a. ethmoidal cell
a. ethmoidal foramen
a. ethmoidal nerve
a. ethmoidal ostium
a. ethmoid canal
a. ethmoidectomy
a. ethmoid sinus
a. exenteration
exertional anterior compartment syndrome
a. extensile approach
a. external arcuate fiber
a. extradural clinoidectomy
a. extremity
a. extremity of caudate nucleus
a. extremity of spleen
a. facial height
a. facial vein
a. fascicle of palatopharyngeus muscle
a. fascicular block
a. fasciculus proprius
a. faucial pillar
a. feature English phoneme
a. fecal incontinence
a. feet view
a. femoral cutaneous nerve
a. fiber-region
a. fibular ligament
a. fissure
a. fistula
a. flared tooth
a. focal point
a. fontanelle
a. forceps
a. forearm
a. fornix of vagina
a. fossa skull base glabellar
a. fovea
a. fracture
a. frontal
frontodextra anterior position
a. fundoplasty
fundus anterior, normal size and shape, and mobile
a. funiculus
a. gastric branch of anterior vagal trunk
a. gastropexy
a. gastrotomy
a. glandular branch of superior thyroid artery
a. glenoid labrum
a. glide
gliosis of anterior column
a. gluteal line
a. gray column
a. gray column of cord
a. gray commissure
a. great vessel
a. ground bundle
a. guide
a. hairline incision
a. head cap
a. heart
a. heel
a. helical rim free flap
a. hemiblock
a. hiatal sign
a. hip dislocation
a. hippocampal activation
a. hip release
a. horizontal jugular vein
a. horizontal mandibular osteotomy
a. horn
a. horn cell
a. horn cell degeneration
a. horn cell disease
a. horn cell isolation
a. horn cell motor impairment
a. horn index
a. horn meniscal tear
a. horn of spinal cord
a. humeral circumflex artery
a. humeral line
a. hyaloidal fibrovascular proliferation
a. hyaloid membrane
a. hydrophthalmia
a. hypospadias
a. hypothalamic area
a. hypothalamic nucleus
a. hypothalamic preoptic area
a. hypothalamus
a. iliac crest
a. iliofemoral technique
a. impingement spur
a. impingement syndrome
a. incision
a. incisural space
a. infarction
a. inguinal herniorrhaphy
a. innominate
a. innominate osteotomy
a. innominate rotation
a. interbody fusion
a. intercavernous sinus
a. intercondylar area
a. intercondylar area of tibia
a. intercostal artery
a. intercostal branch of internal thoracic artery
a. intercostal vein
a. interhemispheric approach
a. interhemispheric cistern
a. interhemispheric fissure
a. intermediate groove
a. intermediate sulcus
a. intermuscular septum
a. internal cerebellar artery
a. internal fixation
a. internal stabilization
a. internal vertebral vein
a. internodal pathway
a. internodal tract of Bachmann
a. interosseous artery
a. interosseous nerve entrapment
a. interosseous nerve of forearm
a. interosseous nerve syndrome
a. interosseous vein
a. interpositus nucleus
a. interventricular branch of left coronary artery
a. interventricular groove
a. interventricular sulcus
a. intervertebral disc
a. intestinal portal
intramural left anterior descending artery
a. intraoccipital joint
a. intraoccipital synchondrosis
a. ischemic optic neuritis
a. ischemic optic neuropathy
a. joint capsule thickening
a. joint impingement
a. jugular lymph node
a. junction line
a. keratoconus
a. kyphosis
a. labial artery
a. labial branch of deep external pudendal artery
a. labial commissure
a. labial nerve
a. labial vein
a. labral avulsion

a. labral disruption
a. labroligamentous periosteal sleeve
a. labroligamentous periosteal sleeve avulsion lesion
a. labrum periosteal sleeve avulsion
a. labrum periosteum shoulder arthroscopic lesion
a. lacrimal crest
a. lateral malleolar artery
a. lateral myocardial infarct
a. lateral myocardial infarction
a. lateral nasal branch of anterior ethmoidal artery
a. latissimus dorsi
a. layer of rectus abdominis sheath
a. layer of thoracolumbar fascia
a. leaflet of the mitral valve
a. leaflet prolapse
left anterior bundle-branch block
left anterior descending coronary artery
left anterior fascicular block
left anterior hemiblock
left anterior internal diameter
left anterior measurement
left anterior oblique projection
left anterior occipital
left anterior small thoracotomy
left anterior spinal artery
left anterior superior
left anterior thigh
a. lens capsule
a. lie
a. ligament of fibular head
a. ligament of head of fibula
a. ligament of Helmholtz
a. ligament of malleus
ligamentous anterior dislocation
ligamentous anterior dislocation composite graft
limb of anterior capsule
a. limbic association area
a. limb of internal capsule
a. limb of stapes
limited anterior small thoracotomy
a. limiting lamina
limiting lamina a.
a. limiting layer of cornea
a. limiting ring
a. lingual gland
a. lip
a. lip of the acetabulum
a. lip of the cervix
a. lip of external os of uterus
a. lip of uterine os
a. lobe
a. lobe hormone
a. lobe of hypophysis
a. lobe of pituitary
a. locking plate system
a. long fiber
a. longitudinal ligament
a. long toe flexor
a. loop traction
low anterior resection
low anterior resection in combination with coloanal anastomosis
lower anterior axillary line
lower anterior dental height
lower anterior forceps
a. lower cervical spine surgery
a. lumbar interbody fusion
a. lumbar spine interbody fusion
a. lumbar vertebral interbody fusion
a. lunate lobule
lyophilized anterior pituitary
lyophilized anterior pituitary tissue
a. mallear fold
a. mallear ligament
malleolaris anterior medialis
a. mandibular posturing
a. mandibulectomy
a. margin
maxillary anterior tooth
a. maxillary spine
a. medial ankle ligament
medial anterior malleolus artery
medial anterior thoracic nerve
a. medial malleolar artery
median anterior maxillary cyst
a. median fissure
a. median fissure of medulla oblongata
a. median fissure of spinal cord
a. median line
a. median nucleus
a. mediastinal artery
a. mediastinal compartment
a. mediastinal lymph node
a. mediastinal mass
a. mediastinum
a. medullary velum
membrana atlantooccipitalis a.
a. membrane dystrophy
a. meningeal artery
a. meningeal branch of anterior ethmoidal artery
a. meniscofemoral ligament
mentum anterior position
a. mesial temporal resection
mesodermal dysgenesis of anterior segment
a. metallic fixation
a. metatarsal arch
a. microphthalmia
a. midbody of corpus callosum
a. middle meatus
a. middle superior alveolar
a. midpapillary
a. midpapillary level
a. mitral leaflet
mitral valve anterior leaflet
a. mitral valve leaflet
moderately narrow anterior chamber angle
moderately wide open anterior chamber angle
modified anterior hairline forehead lift
modified anterior scoring technique
a. mosaic crocodile shagreen
most anterior point of anterior contour of the sella turcica
a. motion of posterior mitral valve leaflet
multiple anterior pituitary hormone deficiency
musculus auricularis a.
a. myocardial infarct
a. myocardial infarction
a. myocutaneous flap
a. naris
a. nasal discharge
a. nasal meatus
a. nasal packing
a. nasal septum
a. nasal spine
a. nasal spine of maxilla
a. nasal valve
a. nephrectomy
a. nerve root
nervus ethmoidalis a.
a. neural tube closure
a. neural tube defect
a. neutralization
nonarteritic anterior ischemic optic neuropathy
nongranulomatous anterior uveitis
a. notch of auricle
a. notch of cerebellum
a. notch of ear
a. nucleus
nucleus cochlearis a.
a. nucleus of thalamus

anterior *(continued)*
a. nucleus of trapezoid body
nucleus ventralis anterior of thalamus
Ober anterior transfer
a. oblique
a. oblique ligament
a. oblique line of radius
a. oblique meniscal tear
a. oblique position
a. oblique projection
a. occipital artery-middle cerebral artery bypass
a. occipitocervical arthrodesis
a. occipitocervical spine
occiput a.
occiput right a.
a. occlusion
a. ocular segment
a. oesophageal sensor
a. olfactory nucleus
a. optical zone
a. optic chiasmal syndrome
ossification of anterior longitudinal ligament
a. osteophyte
a. palatal bar
a. palatal major connector
a. palatine arch
a. palatine foramen
a. palatine groove
a. palatine nerve
a. palatine suture
palmar branch of anterior interosseous nerve
palpation of anterior superior iliac spine
a. palpebral margin
a. papillary muscle
a. paracentral gyrus
a. paracentral lobule
a. pararenal space
paraumbilical anterior abdominal wall
paries anterior vaginae
paries anterior ventriculi
a. parietal artery
a. parietal artery aneurysm
a. parietal lesion
parietooccipital branch of anterior cerebral artery
a. parolfactory sulcus
pars anterior lobuli quadrangularis anterioris
pars anterior pedunculi cerebri
pars anterior pontis
a. part
a. part of anterior commissure of brain
a. part of diaphragmatic surface of liver
partial anterior cerebral infarct
partial anterior circulation infarct
partial anterior circulation syndrome
a. partial laryngectomy
a. part of pons
a. part of tongue
patchy anterior stromal infiltrate
pectoral and abdominal anterior cutaneous branch of intercostal nerve
a. pectoral cutaneous branch of intercostal nerve
a. peduncle of thalamus
a. pelvic exenteration
a. pelvic tilt
percutaneous anterior gastropexy
a. perforated substance
a. perforating artery
perforating branch of anterior interosseous artery
a. perichondrium
a. perineum
peripheral anterior stent keratopathy
peripheral anterior synechia
a. peripheral curve
a. periventricular nucleus
a. peroneal artery
perpendicular anterior wall
a. pes cavus
a. pillar
a. pillar of fauces
a. pillar of fornix
a. pillar tumor
a. piriform gyrus
a. pituitary
a. pituitary extract
a. pituitary function
a. pituitary gland
a. pituitary gonadotropin
a. pituitary hormone
a. pituitary insufficiency
a. pituitary-like hormone
a. pituitary-like substance
a. pituitary lobe
a. pituitary resection
a. planar image
a. planar imaging
a. plate fixation
a. platysma-cutaneous ligament
a. polar-amygdalar epilepsy
a. polar cataract
a. pole
a. pole cataract
a. pole of eyeball
a. pole of lens
a. Pólya procedure
a. pontomesencephalic vein
a. portion of left medial segment IV of liver
a. port scalp excision
a. and posterior
a. and posterior fusion
a. and posterior medialization thyroplasty
a. and posterior opposing portals
a. and posterior radicular artery
a. and posterior repair
a. and posterior superior pancreaticoduodenal artery
a. and posterior vestibular veins
a. precordium
a. predominance
preoptic anterior hypothalamic area
a. primary division
a. process of malleus
a. projection
a. pronator teres
proximal left anterior descending artery
a. pulmonary branch of vagus nerve
a. pulmonary plexus
a. puncture
a. pyramid
a. pyramidal cataract
a. pyramidal fasciculus
a. pyramidal tract
a. quadriceps musculocutaneous flap technique
a. quadrigeminal body
a. radial collateral artery
a. radicular artery
a. ramus of cervical nerve
a. ramus of lateral sulcus of cerebrum
a. ramus of lumbar nerve
a. ramus of sacral nerve
a. ramus of spinal nerve
a. ramus of thoracic nerve
a. raphespinal tract
a. recess
a. recess of interpeduncular fossa
a. recess of ischiorectal fossa
a. recess of tympanic membrane
a. rectoperineal fistula
a. rectus capitis
a. rectus fascia

a. rectus muscle
a. rectus muscle of head
a. recurrent tibial artery
a. release posterior fusion
a. renal fascia
a. resection
a. resection rectopexy
a. retinal orbital canal
a. retraction archwire
a. retroperitoneal decompression
a. retroperitoneal flank approach
a. retrosternal hernia of Morgagni
a. rhinoscopy
a. rhizotomy
a. rib impingement syndrome
right a.
right anterior caudocranial oblique
right anterior descending
right anterior descending coronary artery
right anterior hemiblock
right anterior measurement
right anterior oblique position
right anterior oblique projection
right anterior oblique view
right anterior quadrant
right anterior thigh
right sacrum a.
right ventricle anterior wall
a. right ventricular wall
a. root
a. root of spinal nerve
a. rotary drawer test
a. sacral foramen
a. sacral meningocele
a. sacrococcygeal ligament
a. sacroiliac joint plate
a. sacroiliac ligament
a. sacrosciatic ligament
a. sagittal anorectoplasty
a. sagittal diameter
a. sagittal pelvic inlet
a. sandwich patch technique
a. scalene muscle
scalene muscle, anterior, posterior, middle
scalenus anterior muscle
a. scalenus muscle
a. scaler
a. scalloping
a. scalloping of vertebra
a. scleritis
a. sclerochoroiditis
a. sclerotomy
a. scoring technique
a. screw fixation
a. scrotal branch of deep external pudendal artery
a. scrotal nerve
a. scrotal vein
a. segment
a. segmental artery
a. segmental dentoalveolar osteotomy
a. segment angiography
a. segment examination
a. segment of eye
a. segment inflammation
a. segment necrosis
a. segment sleeve
a. semicircular canal
a. semicircular duct
a. semilunar valve
a. septal branch of anterior ethmoidal artery
a. seromyotomy
serratus a.
serratus anterior muscle flap
a. serratus muscle
a. shear
a. sheath
a. shin splint
a. short-segment stabilization
a. shoulder dislocation
a. shoulder instability
a. shoulder release
a. sinus
a. skin flap
a. skull base
a. skull base malignancy
a. sliding tibial graft
a. slot graft arthrodesis
a. soft tissue impingement
a. speech zone
a. spinal artery syndrome
a. spinal cord syndrome
a. spinal fixation
a. spinal fusion
a. spinal instrumentation
a. spinal line
a. spinal plating
a. spine fusion
a. spinocerebellar tract
a. spinothalamic tract
split anterior tibial tendon transfer
a. spur
a. spurring
a. stabilization procedure
a. staphyloma
a. sternoclavicular joint
a. sternoclavicular ligament
a. sternomastoid approach
a. stromal micropuncture
a. subcapsular
a. subcapsular cataract
a. subperiosteal implant
a. superficial cervical lymph node
a. superior alveolar artery
a. superior alveolar branch of infraorbital nerve
a. superior dental artery
superior labrum anterior and posterior
a. superior pancreaticoduodenal artery
a. superior renal segment
a. superior segmental artery of kidney
a. supraclavicular nerve
a. surface
a. surgical exposure
a. suspension of hyoid bone
a. suspensory ligament
a. symblepharon
a. synchondrosis intraoccipital
a. synechia
a. synechia formation
systemic anterior motion
systolic anterior motion of mitral valve
a. talar articular surface of calcaneus
a. talar dome
a. talar translation
a. talocalcaneal angle
a. talocalcaneal ligament
a. talofibular ligament rupture
a. talofibular sprain
a. talotibial ligament
a. talus shift
a. tarsal resection
a. tarsal tendinitis
a. tarsal tendinous sheath
a. tarsal tunnel syndrome
a. tegmental decussation
a. temporal atrophy
a. temporal branch
a. temporal branch of posterior cerebral artery
a. temporal diploic vein
a. temporal focal spike
a. temporal lobectomy
a. temporobasal vein
a. terminal vein
a. thalamic radiation
a. thalamic tubercle
a. thalamotomy
a. thoracic meningocele

anterior *(continued)*
a. thoracic nerve
a. thoracic wall
a. thoracotomy
a. tibia
a. tibial artery
a. tibial bowing
a. tibial bursa
a. tibial compartment
a. tibial compartment syndrome
a. tibial fasciocutaneous flap
a. tibialis
tibialis anterior muscle
a. tibialis sign
a. tibialis tendon
a. tibialis transfer
a. tibial lymph node
a. tibial margin
a. tibial muscle
a. tibial nerve
a. tibial nerve dermatome
a. tibial recurrent artery
a. tibial sign
a. tibial spine
a. tibial subluxation
a. tibial tendon
a. tibial tubercle
a. tibial vein
a. tibiofibular ligament
a. tibiotalar fascicle
a. tibiotalar part
a. tibiotalar part of deltoid ligament
a. tibiotalar part of medial ligament of ankle joint
a. tip of temporal lobe
a. tonsillar pillar
total anterior circulation infarct
total anterior circulation syndrome
a. tracheal displacement
a. tracking
a. transabdominal approach
a. transfer
a. transhepatic approach
a. translation
a. translation of knee
transperitoneal anterior subcostal incision
a. transthoracic approach
a. transverse temporal gyrus
a. triangle
a. triangle approach
a. triangle of neck
a. tricuspid leaflet
a. tricuspid valve leaflet
a. trigeminothalamic tract
a. tubercle of atlas
a. tubercle of cervi
a. tubercle of cervical vertebrae
a. tubercle of thalamus
a. tympanic artery
a. ulnar recurrent artery
a. upper spine
a. urethra
a. urethral injury
a. urethral valve
a. urethritis
a. uveitis
a. vagal trunk
a. vaginal fornix
a. vaginal trunk
a. vaginotomy
a. vein of the leg
a. vein of septum pellucidum
ventralis oralis a.
a. vermis
a. vermis syndrome
a. vertebral body margin
a. vertebral vein
a. vertical canal
very narrow anterior chamber angle
a. vestibular artery
a. view
a. visual pathway
a. visual pathway dysfunction
a. vitrectomy
a. wall antral ulcer
a. wall infarction
a. wall ischemia
a. wall of middle ear
a. wall motion
a. wall myocardial infarct
a. wall myocardial infarction
a. wall of stomach
a. wall of tympanic cavity
a. wall of vagina
a. wedging
a. white commissure
wide open anterior chamber angle
a. wound

anterior-inferior
a.-i. capsular ligament dysfunction
a.-i. cerebellar
a.-i. cerebellar artery
a.-i. cerebral artery
a.-i. communicating artery
a.-i. compression
a.-i. dislocation
a.-i. fusion
a.-i. glide
a.-i. movement
a.-i. tibiofibular ligament

anterioris
pars anterior lobuli quadrangularis a.

anteriorization of midface

anterior/lateral/posterior glandular branch of superior thyroid artery

anteriorly
a. directed jet
a. displaced anus
opened a.

anterior-posterior
a.-p. abdominal diameter
a.-p. compression
a.-p. discrepancy
a.-p. dual energy radiography
a.-p. flow direction
a.-p. fusion with segmental spinal instrumentation
a.-p. fusion with SSI
a.-p. glide
a.-p. listhesis
a.-p. movement
a.-p. otoplasty
a.-p., posterior-anterior view
a.-p. repair

anterior-superior spine

anterior-to-posterior sagittal canal diameter

anteroapical
a. defect
a. trabecular septum

anterobasal segment

anterocentral arthroscopic portal

anterochiasmatic lesion

anterocrural celiac plexus block

anterodistal border

anterodorsal
a. nucleus of thalamus
a. thalamic nucleus

anterofacial dysplasia

anterofundal placenta

anterograde
a. amnesia
a. axonal transport
a. block
a. conduction
a. degeneration
a. direction
a. fast component neuropathy
a. flow
a. loss of memory
a. memory

a. memory interference
a. peristalsis
a. transseptal technique

anteroinferior
a. aspect
a. cerebellar artery
a. corner fracture
a. dislocation
a. glenohumeral ligament
a. myocardial infarct
a. myocardial infarction
nucleus anteroinferior thalami
a. portal
a. quadrant
a. spondylolisthesis
a. triangular fragment

anterolateral
a. abdominal wall
a. approach
a. aspect
a. capsule
a. central artery
a. column
a. column of spinal cord
a. compression fracture
a. cordotomy
a. decompression
a. dislocation
a. drainage
a. femorotibial ligament tenodesis
a. fontanelle
a. fontanelle
a. fragment
a. groove
a. gutter
a. impingement
a. impingement syndrome
a. intercostal nerve
a. intercostal perforator
Mueller anterolateral femorotibial ligament tenodesis
a. myocardial infarct
a. myocardial infarction
a. neck
a. portal
a. raphe
a. release
a. rotary knee instability
a. rotational instability
a. sclerosis
a. segment
a. striate artery
a. sulcus
a. surface
a. system
a. thalamostriate artery
a. thigh free flap
a. thoracotomy
a. thoracotomy incision
a. tibial bowing
a. tract
a. tractotomy
a. white matter of cord

anterolateral-anteromedial rotary instability

anteromedial
a. arm
a. bundle
a. capsule
a. caudate nucleus
a. central artery
a. central branch
a. drainage
a. frontal branch of callosomarginal artery
a. glenohumeral ligament
a. humeral head defect
a. incision
a. intercostal nerve
a. intercostal perforator
a. intermuscular septum
a. joint line
Maquet anteromedial osteoplasty
a. nucleus
a. nucleus of thalamus
a. portal
a. retropharyngeal approach
a. rotatory instability
a. superior humeral head impaction
a. surface
a. temporal lobe resection
a. thalamic nucleus
a. thalamostriate artery
a. tubercle transfer

anteromedial-posteromedial rotary instability

anteromedian groove

anteromesial temporal lobectomy

anteroposterior
a. analysis
a. aspect
a. axis
a. axis of Fick
a. chest x-ray
a. compression
a. control orthosis
a. correction
a. curve
a. diameter
a. diameter of pelvic inlet
a. dimension
a. drawer test
a. dysplasia
a. facial dysplasia
a. film
a. iliac spine
a. and lateral
a. lateral sway
a. and lateral views
a. laxity
a. lordotic projection
mandibular anteroposterior ridge slope
maximum anteroposterior diameter
a. movement
a. nail
narrow anteroposterior diameter
normal anteroposterior view
a. position
a. projection
a. stress test
a. talocalcaneal
a. talocalcaneal angle
a. talocalcaneal divergence
a. tilt
a. translation
a. tube
a. view

anteroseptal
a. commissure
a. infarct
a. myocardial infarct
a. myocardial infarction

anterosuperior
a. external ilium movement
a. glenohumeral ligament
a. iliac spine graft
a. ilium major
a. internal ilium movement
left anterosuperior hemiblock
nucleus anterosuperior thalami
a. quadrant

anterotransverse diameter

anteroventral
a. nucleus of thalamus
a. 3rd ventricle
a. thalamic nucleus

anteroventralis
nucleus a.
nucleus anteroventralis thalami

antetorsion
angle of a.
a. angle

antetracheal node

anteversion
acetabular a.

anteversion *(continued)*
angle of a.
a. determination
femoral a.
a. syndrome
a. of uterus
anteverted
a. and anteflexed
a. naris
normal size, shape, and position, anteverted and anteflexed uterus
a. nostril
a. pinna
a. uterus
antevesical hernia
anthelminthic drug
anthelmintic agent
Anthony
Saint Anthony dance
Saint Anthony fire
St. Anthony fire
anthracene
a. blue
a. glycoside
anthracene-type laxative
anthracotic
a. hilar node
a. material
a. pigment
a. tuberculosis
anthracycline
a. antibiotic
a. cardiomyopathy
a. cardiotoxicity
liposomal encapsulated a.
morpholino a.
anthracycline-based
a.-b. induction chemotherapy
a.-b. therapy
anthracycline-nave metastatic breast cancer
anthracycline-refractory metastatic breast carcinoma
anthranilic acid
anthraquinone
a. dye
a. laxative
anthrax
a. antiserum
a. anxiety
a. as a biological weapon
a. bacillus
a. capsule
a. epizootic
a. exposure
industrial a.
inhalation a.
inhalational a.
intestinal a.
a. malignant pustule
meningeal a.
oropharyngeal a.
a. pneumonia
a. septicemia
a. spore
a. toxin
anthrax-contaminated animal product
anthrax-infected
a.-i. animal
a.-i. body fluid
anthrone
a. colorimetric technique
a. method
anthropoid pelvis
anthropological
a. linguistics
a. philosophy
anthropologic baseline
anthropology
applied a.
medical a.
pathologic a.
anthropometric
a. analysis
a. calculation
a. caliper
a. evaluation
a. identification
a. imaging
a. marker
a. measure
a. measurement
a. measuring tape
a. method
a. total hip
a. value
anthropomorphic
a. baseline
a. face
a. measurement
a. parameter
a. test dummy
anthroponotic
a. cutaneous leishmaniasis
a. genotype
anti-33-kDa antibody
anti-37K antibody
anti-40 kDa colonic antigen
anti-70K antibody
anti-A
a.-A agglutinin
a.-A antibody
a.-A isohemagglutinin
anti-ABO antibody
Antia-Buch
A.-B. chondrocutaneous advancement flap
A.-B. helical rim advancement flap
antiacetylcholine
a. receptor antibody
a. receptor antibody assay
anti-ACh
a.-ACh antibody
a.-ACh receptor antibody
anti-acquired immune deficiency syndrome vaccine
antiactin antibody
antiadhesion agent
antiadhesive agent
antiadrenal antibody
antiadrenergic
a. drug
a. effect
antiaggressive
a. action
a. effect
anti-aging
a.-a. gene
a.-a. therapy
a.-a. treatment
antialias filtering
antialiasing technique
antialkaline
alkaline phosphatase antialkaline phosphatase
a. phosphatase method
antialopecia
a. factor
mouse antialopecia factor
anti-alpha-fodrin antibody
antiandrogen
nonsteroidal a.
nonsteroidal antiandrogen monotherapy
a. receptor blocker
a. therapy
a. treatment
a. withdrawal syndrome

antiandrogenic
neoadjuvant antiandrogenic treatment
antianemia
a. factor
a. principle
antianemic
a. factor
a. principle
antiangiogenesis
a. agent
a. factor
a. gene therapy
antiangiogenic
a. agent
a. effect
a. therapy
antiannexin V antibody
antianthrax serum
antiantibody formation
antianxiety
a. agent
a. and antidepressant medication
a. drug
a. medication
antiapoptotic
a. effect
a. molecule
a. properties
a. protein
a. signaling pathway
antiarrhythmic
a. agent
a. drug
oral antiarrhythmic therapy
a. therapy
anti-arteriosclerosis polysaccharide factor
antiasialoglycoprotein receptor
anti-B
a.-B agglutinin
a.-B antibody
a.-B isohemagglutinin
a.-B serum
anti-B19 antibody test
anti-B4 blocked ricin
antibacterial
a. activity
a. agent
a. agent susceptibility testing
a. drug
a. immunity
a. mouthwash
a. pillow
a. protein
a. substantivity
a. therapy
antibasement
a. membrane
a. membrane antibody
a. membrane antibody-induced glomerulonephritis
a. membrane nephritis
a. membrane zone autoantibody
anti-B-cell antibody
antiberiberi
a. factor
a. vitamin
anti-beta-1-adrenoreceptor antibody
antibiotic
acquired resistance to a.
ambulatory antibiotic treatment
anal itching and a.
a. antitumor drug
a. bead pouch
broad-spectrum a.
chronic antibiotic inhalation
a. combination therapy
a. concentrate
a. concentration in serum and tissue
copious antibiotic irrigation
a. course
a. diarrhea
a. drug
effective antibiotic concentration
a. enterocolitis
fever unresponsive to antibiotic therapy
hearing loss from a.
heartburn from a.
Heyden a.
home intravenous antibiotic therapy
home parenteral antibiotic therapy
a. infusion therapy
inhibiting antibiotic dose
intensive topical antibiotic therapy
intrapartum antibiotic prophylaxis
intrinsic resistance to a.
a. irrigation
lactose intolerance from a.
a. level
a. management
minimal antibiotic concentration
a. neurotoxicity
nonresponsive to a.
a. ointment
operative area irrigated with antibiotic solution
operative site irrigated with antibiotic solution
oral antibiotic medication
outpatient parenteral antibiotic therapy
a. penetration
perioperative antibiotic prophylaxis
perioperative antibiotic therapy
a. powder
prolonged antibiotic therapy
prophylactic a.
prophylactic antibiotic treatment
a. prophylaxis
protected environment units and prophylactic a.
a. protein
a. removal device
a. resistance
a. resistance gene
a. resistant
a. and saline solution
a. selection
a. sensitivity
a. sensitivity test
a. sensitivity testing
temporary articulating methylmethacrylate antibiotic spacer
a. therapy
tissue concentrations of a.'s
a. tongue
a. treatment
triple a.
a. use and abuse
a. utilization review
water-soluble a.
antibiotic-associated
a.-a. colitis
a.-a. colitis toxin test
a.-a. diarrhea
a.-a. enterocolitis
a.-a. pseudomembranous colitis
antibiotic-destroying enzyme
antibiotic-impregnated bead
antibiotic-induced
a.-i. diarrhea
a.-i. enterocolitis
antibiotic-loaded
a.-l. acrylic cement
prosthetic antibiotic-loaded acrylic cement
antibiotic-related colitis
antibiotic-resistant
a.-r. bacteria

antibiotic-resistant *(continued)*
a.-r. bacterial infection
a.-r. gram-negative organism
a.-r. organism

antibiotic-soaked swab

antibiotic-sterilized aortic valve homograft

antiblack-tongue factor

antibladder
rabbit antibladder antibody
rabbit antibladder cancer

antiblastic
hyperthermic antiblastic perfusion
a. immunity

anti-blood group A antiglobulin test

anti-BMZ autoantibody

antibody
a. absorbent
acetylcholine receptor a.
acquired immune deficiency syndrome a.
acquired immune deficiency syndrome antibody test
a. affinity chromatography
alpha globulin a.
antiacetylcholine receptor a.
antiacetylcholine receptor antibody assay
anti-ACh receptor a.
antiannexin V a.
anti-B19 antibody test
antibasement membrane a.
anti-beta-1-adrenoreceptor a.
anti-*Bordetella pertussis* a.
antibovine serum albumin a.
antibrush border a.
anticanalicular a.
anticarcinoembryonic antigen monoclonal a.
anticardiolipin a.
anticardiolipin antibody syndrome
anticardiolipin immunoglobulin M a.
anti-CD11a humanized monoclonal antibody for psoriasis
anti-CD18 humanized a.
anti-CD31 monoclonal a.
anti-CEA antibody immunoscintigraphy
anti-CEA monoclonal a.
anticentromere a.
anti-*Chlamydia* antibody test
anticholera toxin a.
anticyclic citrullinated peptide a.
anticytokeratin monoclonal a.
anticytoplasmic a.
anticytoplasmic antibody test
anti-D anti-Rh a.
anti-DCP monoclonal a.
antidelta IgM a.
antideoxyribonucleic acid a.
antidesmin monoclonal a.
anti-DNA antibody assay
anti-DNase B a.
anti-DNA-topoisomerase I a.
anti-double-stranded deoxyribonucleic acid a.
anti-double-stranded DNA a.
anti-E-cadherin monoclonal a.
anti-EGF receptor antibody for cancer
antiendomysial a.
antiendomysial antibody test
antiendomysium a.
antiendothelial cell a.
antiepidermal growth factor receptor antibody for cancer
antiepidermal growth factor receptor monoclonal a.
antiepithelial membrane antigen a.
anti-Epstein-Barr nuclear antigen a.
anti-Epstein-Barr virus a.
anti-*Escherichia coli*-derived protein a.
antiextractable nuclear a.
antifibrin antibody imaging agent
antigenic antibody lattice formation
anti-GFP polyclonal a.
antigliadin a.
antiglomerular a.
antiglomerular basement membrane a.
antiglomerular basement membrane antibody disease
antiglomerular basement membrane antibody nephritis
anti-GM_1 antibody test
anti-HAV IgM a.
anti-HBc IgM a.
anti-HCV antibody 3rd generation
anti-HCV core a.
antiheart a.
anti-HER2 monoclonal a.
anti-HHV8 antibody titer
antihistone a.
anti-HLA class I a.
antihuman alpha-catenin a.
antihuman beta-catenin a.
antihuman E-cadherin a.
antihuman herpesvirus 8 antibody titer
antihuman leukocyte antigen a.
anti-IgE humanized monoclonal a.
antiimmunoglobulin a.
antiimmunoglobulin E humanized monoclonal a.
antiinsulin a.
antiinsulin receptor a.
anti-interleukin-2 a.
anti-interleukin-2 receptor alpha monoclonal a.
antiislet cell a.
antikeratin a.
antilens protein a.
antiliver microsomal antibody detection
antilymphocyte a.
antimalignant antibody test
anti-M2 antimitochondrial antibody level
antimelanoma-associated antigen a.
antimetallothionein a.
anti-Mi-2 nuclear a.
antimitochondrial a.
antimitochondrial antibody assay
antimyeloperoxidase a.
antimyolemmal a.
antimyosin a.
antimyosin antibody imaging
antineuronal enteric antibody test
antineuronal nuclear a.
antineutrophil cytoplasmic a.
antineutrophil cytoplasmic antibody titer
antineutrophil cytoplasmic IgG a.
antineutrophilic cytoplasmic a.
antinuclear a.
antinuclear antibody assay
antinuclear antibody fluid
antinuclear antibody immunodiffusion
antinuclear antibody immunofluorescence
antinuclear antibody immunological study
antinuclear antibody screening by enzyme immunoassay
antinuclear antibody screening test
antinuclear antibody titer
antinuclear matrix a.
antinucleolar a.
anti-*Paracoccidioides brasiliensis* a.
antiparietal a.
antiparietal cell a.
antiparietal cell antibody assay

antiparvovirus 19 a.
antiparvovirus B19 IgG a.
antiparvovirus B19 IgM a.
antiperipheral nerve myelin a.
antiphosphatidylserine-prothrombin complex antibody testing
antiphospholipid a.
antiphospholipid antibody assay
antiphospholipid antibody syndrome
antiphospholipid antibodies in stroke study
antiplatelet antibody assay
antiplatelet immunoglobulin G a.
antireticulin a.
antiribosomal P a.
anti-RNA polymerase a.
antiscleroderma-70 a.
antisignal recognition particle a.
anti-Sjögren syndrome A, B a.
antiskeletal a.
antismooth muscle a.
antismooth muscle antibody assay
antispermicidal monoclonal a.
anti-tau monoclonal a.
antithymidylate synthase polyclonal a.
antithyroglobulin a.
antithyroid a.
antithyroid antibody titer
antithyroid microsomal a.
antithyroid peroxidase a.
antithyroid plasma membrane a.
antithyroid-stimulating hormone a.
antitopoisomerase I a.
anti-*Toxoplasma* a.
anti-*Toxoplasma gondii* a.
anti-*Toxoplasma gondii* antibody secretion assay
antitreponemal antibody test
antitubular basement membrane a.
anti-U1 RNP a.
anti-U3 RNP a.
antivascular endothelial growth factor monoclonal a.
antiviral a.
anti-von Willebrand factor a.
anti-Yo serum a.
Aspergillus antibody test
assay neutrophil cytoplasmic a.
ATGAM polyclonal a.
atypical antibody titer
automated enzyme immunoassay for antinuclear a.
bispecific monoclonal a.
blocking a.
a. blocking assay
bound hepatitis a.
brain-reactive a.
a. to bromodeoxyuridine
a. capture immunoassay
a. capture ligand assay
cardiolipin fluorescence a.
a. catabolism
cell mediated a.
cervicovaginal a.
Chido a.
circulation antineuronal a.
combined cold and warm antibody autoimmune hemolytic anemia
a. combining site
complement-binding a.
complement-dependent a.
complement fixation antibody test
complement-fixing a.
complement-fixing antibody consumption
Cost-Stirling a.
a. to c100 protein
cryptococcal a.
cytoplasmic antineutrophil cytoplasmic a.
cytotoxic a.
a. deficiency
a. deficiency disease
a. deficiency syndrome
a. deficiency with near-normal immunoglobulins
a. deposition
a. detection
dextran-reactive a.
a. directed cytotoxic response
direct fluorescent a.
direct fluorescent antibody examination for *Treponema pallidum*
direct fluorescent antibody test
Donath-Landsteiner a.
double antibody solid phase
drug-induced antinuclear a.'s
a. dysfunction
embryonic a.
endomysial a.
a. epitope
a.'s to the Epstein-Barr virus transactivator protein
erythrocyte a.
erythrocyte, antibody, and complement
erythrocyte antibody inhibition
a. excess
a. excess antibody
a. excess zone
extractable nuclear a.
Ferritin-conjugated a.
fluorescein treponemal antibody test
fluorescence antimembrane a.
fluorescence treponemal antibody absorption
fluorescent a.
fluorescent antibody dark-field
fluorescent antibody staining technique
fluorescent antimembrane antibody test
fluorescent antinuclear antibody assay
fluorescent-labeled a.
fluorescent antibody to membrane antigen test
fluorescent rabies a.
fluorescent antibody stain
fluorescent titer a.
a. formation
a. forming
fragment of a.
gonococcal antibody reaction
a. half-life
h-caldesmon a.
hemagglutinating a.
hemagglutinating antipenicillin a.
hemagglutinating inhibition a.
hemagglutinating penicillin a.
hemagglutination inhibition a.
heparin-dependent platelet-associated a.
hepatitis A a.
a. to hepatitis A–E virus
a. to hepatitis-associated antigen
hepatitis A virus a.
hepatitis B a.
hepatitis B core a.
a. to hepatitis B core antigen
a. to hepatitis Be antigen
hepatitis B early a.
hepatitis B surface a.
a. to hepatitis B surface antigen
herpes simplex antibody titer
heterophil a.
heterophil antibody titer
histone-reactive antinuclear a.
a.'s to HIV
homologous leukocyte a.
a. to HTLV-I
human antichimeric a.'s
human antimouse a.
human immunodeficiency virus a.
humanized antihuman IL-2 receptor a.
human leukocyte a.

antibody *(continued)*
human thyroid-stimulating a.
humoral antibody production
a. identification
IgA immunofluorescent a.
IgM immunofluorescent a.
immune fluorescent a.
a. immune response
immunofluorescence a.
immunofluorescent antibody assay
immunoglobulin A transglutaminase a.
immunoglobulin G antigliadin a.
immunoglobulin M antibody capture
indirect fluorescent a.
indirect fluorescent rabies antibody test
indirect hemagglutination antibody test
indirect immunofluorescent a.
a. induction therapy
insulin a.
interaction
intrathecal *Treponema pallidum* a.
islet cell surface a.
a. to keratin
a. Ki
a. labeling
leukocyte-specific antinuclear a.
a. level
Lewis a a.
Lewis b a.
a. linkage method
liposomally entrapped second a.
liver/kidney microsomal a.
liver-kidney-microsomal type 1 antibody target assay
liver membrane a.
lupus anticoagulant a.
Lutheran blood antibody type
Lyme disease antibody test
lymphocyte a.
lymphocyte antibody lymphocytolytic interaction
lymphocyte-dependent a.
lymphocytotoxic a.
MAb 12C3 monoclonal a.
MAb-170 monoclonal a.
maternal antiplatelet a.
maternal antithyroid a.
maternal-fetal transmission of a.
maternal IgG a.
maternal sperm a.
McCoy a.
microhemagglutination assay for antibodies to *Treponema pallidum*
microsomal antibody titer
microsome a.
MicroTrak direct fluorescent antibody staining
mirror-image complementary a.
mitochondrial a.
MoAb 425 a.
monoclonal a.
monoclonal antibodies against gastric mucins
monoclonal antibody ABX-CBL
monoclonal antibody A103 fine-needle aspiration biopsy
monoclonal antibody anticancer vaccine
monoclonal antibody B291
monoclonal antibody coagglutination test
monoclonal antibody ED1
monoclonal antibody imaging
monoclonal antibody M1G8
monoclonal antibody MIB-1
monoclonal antibody PC10
monoclonal antibody scintigraphic scan
monoclonal antibody staining
monoclonal antibody therapy
monoclonal antiendothelial cell a.
monoclonal antiendotoxin a.
monoclonal anti-IgE a.
monoclonal antimalignin a.
monoclonal anti-T-cell a.
monoclonal antibody BR96
mouse antibody production test
99mTc-labeled antigranulocyte a.
mumps antibody titer
a. to murine cardiac myosin
myelin-associated glycoprotein antibody detection
native type anti-DNA a.
nephrotoxic a.
nephrotoxic antiglomerular basement membrane antibody nephritis
neurofilament triplets a.
neuro-specific enolase a.
neutralizing a.
neutralizing antibody to vascular endothelial growth factor
neutralizing murine monoclonal antitumor necrosis factor a.
neutrophil a.
neutrophil antibody and transfusion reaction
a. nitrogen
no demonstrable a.'s
no detectable a.
nuclear a.
OKT3 anti-CD3 monoclonal a.
OKT3 anti-T-cell a.
OKT3 murine monoclonal a.
Oncolym radiolabeled monoclonal a.
organism-specific antibody index
osteosarcoma antigen-associated monoclonal a.
a. panel
panel of reactive a.'s
panel-reactive antibody testing
parainfluenza antibody test
parietal cell a.
parvovirus B19 IgG a.
parvovirus B19 IgM a.
parvovirus B19 neutralizing antibody assay
Paul-Bunnell antibody test
percent reactive a.
percent reactive antibody/panel reactive a.
perinuclear antineutrophil cytoplasmic a.
peroxidase antibody to peroxidase
peroxidase-labeled antibodies test
plasma antiendotoxin core a.
positive antinuclear a.
primary antiphospholipid antibody syndrome
a. production
a. production assay
proinsulin a.
protein a.
rabbit antibladder a.
rabbit antibody to human ovary
rabbit antibody to pig ovary
radiofluorescent a.
radioimmunoassay double antibody test
radioimmunologic assay antithyroid a.
radiolabeled antibody imaging
a. radionucleotide
a. radionucleotide conjugate
a. reaction site
a. replacement therapy
a. response
Rh antibody titer
rodent thyroid-stimulating a.
Rodgers a.
a. screen
a. screening
a. screening test
sectionally processed antibody coated

selective antipolysaccharide antibody deficiency
sensitizing a.
serum hepatitis-associated antigen a.
sheep erythrocyte a.
single antibody millipore filtration
skeletal a.
skin-sensitizing a.
smooth muscle a.
soluble antigen fluorescent antibody test
specific antibody deficiency
a. stain
staphylococcal hemagglutinating a.
steroidal-cell a.
a. test
tetanus toxoid a.
thyroglobulin a.
thyroid a.
thyroid-blocking a.
thyroid microsomal a.
thyroid-stimulating hormone-binding inhibitor a.
thyroid-stimulating hormone receptor a.
thyroid stimulation-blocking a.
thyroperoxidase a.
thyrotropin-receptor a.
thyrotropin receptor-stimulating a.
a. titer
a. to C22-3
a. transplacental transfer
treponemal antibody test
TSH-displacing a.
TSH receptor a.
TSH stimulation blocking a.
type-specific a.
virus-neutralizing a.
in vitro antibody production assay
whole-body antibody technique
xenoreactive natural a.
York a.

antibody-absorption
colony-stimulating factor
fluorescent treponemal antibody-absorption test

antibody-antigen complex

antibody-based detection system

antibody-coated
a.-c. bacteria
a.-c. suture

antibody-combining site

antibody-conjugate
antidigoxigenin alkaline phosphatase a.-c.

antibody-conjugated paramagnetic liposome

antibody-deficient syndrome

antibody-dependent
a.-d. cell cytotoxicity
a.-d. cell-mediated cytotoxicity
a.-d. cellular cytotoxicity
a.-d. cytotoxicity test
a.-d. enhancement
a.-d. enzyme-prodrug therapy
a.-d. lymphocyte-mediated cytotoxicity

antibody-directed
a.-d. catalysis
a.-d. cellular cytotoxicity
a.-d. enzyme prodrug therapy
a.-d., enzyme-producing therapy
a.-d. enzyme therapy

antibody-forming cell

antibody-labeled circulating granulocyte

antibody-mediated
a.-m. cell-dependent immunolympholysis
a.-m. cytotoxicity
a.-m. disorder
a.-m. immune suppression
a.-m. immunity

antibody/panel
percent reactive antibody/panel reactive antibody

antibody-phage display

antibody-positive
anticardiolipin a.-p.
a.-p. woman

antibody-producing cell

antibody-secreting cell

antibody-smooth muscle/ribonucleoprotein

anti-*Bordetella pertussis* antibody

antibotulinus serum

antibovine serum albumin antibody

anti-BrDU antibody

anti-bromodeoxyuridine antibody

antibrush border antibody

anti-C3 assay

anticachectic effect

anticanalicular antibody

anticancer
a. agent
a. cocktail
direct anticancer properties
a. drug
effective anticancer drug
monoclonal antibody anticancer vaccine
natural anticancer agent

anticapsular antibody

anticarcinoembryonic
a. antigen
a. antigen monoclonal antibody

anticardiac myosin

anticardiolipin
a. antibody
a. antibody-positive
a. antibody syndrome
a. autoantibody
a. immunoglobulin M antibody
a. lupus anticoagulant

anticatalyst
anticipatory a.

anticathepsin D autoantibody assay

anti-CD3
a.-CD3 antibody
a.-CD3 stimulated peripheral blood lymphocytes transduced with a gene encoding a chimeric

anti-CD11a humanized monoclonal antibody for psoriasis

anti-CD18 humanized antibody

anti-CD31 monoclonal antibody

anti-CD4 antibody

anti-CD54 antibody

anticentromere
a. antibody
a. autoantibody

anti-Centruroides antivenin

antichemokine antibody

antichimeric
human antichimeric antibodies

anti-*Chlamydia* antibody test

anticholera
a. serum
a. toxin antibody

anticholinergic
a. activity
a. agent
central anticholinergic syndrome

anticholinergic *(continued)*
a. delirium
a. dose
a. drug
a. effect
a. medication
a. medicine therapy
peripherally acting anticholinergic medication
a. property
a. side effect
a. syndrome
a. tricyclic

anticholinesterase
a. drug
a. medication
parasympathomimetic a.

antichromatin antibody

antichymotrypsin
alpha-1 a.
prostate-specific antigen bound to alpha-1 a.
serum a.
a. test

anticipated
a. blood loss
a. emotional suffering
a. lifespan

anticipate discharge tomorrow

anticipation
a. of role
a. of trigger

anticipatory
a. anticatalyst
a. anxiety
a. autocastration
a. avoidance
a. behavior
a. bogus heart rate feedback
a. coarticulation
a. control
a. emotion
a. error
a. goal response
a. grief
a. guidance
a. insanity
pictorial anticipatory guidance
a. reaction
a. response
a. and struggle behavior theories
a. vomiting

anticipatory-maturation principle

anti-class II MAb

anti-CMV
a.-CMV antibody
a.-CMV antiserum

anti-CNA antibody

anticoagulant
anticardiolipin lupus a.
a. bleed
circulating a.
a. effect
a. heparin solution
lupus anticoagulant activity
lupus anticoagulant antibody
lupus anticoagulant syndrome
lupus-like a.
Lupus A. Positive Control
a. monitoring
oral a.
oral anticoagulant therapy
a. therapy

anticoagulant-induced hematuria

anticoagulant-related bleed

anticoagulated blood

anticoagulation
a. monitoring
a. monitoring requirement
oral a.
a. regimen of aspirin
secondary anticoagulation system
a. therapy

anticoding strand

anticoincidence circuit

anticollagen autoantibody

anticolonic antibody

anticomplement
a. activity
a. immunofluorescence

anticomplementary
a. factor
a. serum

anticonstipation regimen

anticonvulsant
a. agent hepatotoxicity
a. drug
a. effect
a. hypersensitivity syndrome
a. intoxication
a. medication-induced postural tremor
parenteral a.
a. property
prophylactic a.
a. prophylaxis
a. therapy
a. treatment

anticonvulsant-induced dyskinesia

anticonvulsive activity

anticrotalus serum

anticurvature filing

anticus
a. reflex
scalenus anticus syndrome
a. sign

anticyclic citrullinated peptide antibody

anticytochrome P4502D6 assay

anticytokeratin
a. antibody
monoclonal a.
a. monoclonal antibody

anticytokine vaccination

anticytomegalovirus
a. antibody
a. immunoglobulin

anticytoplasmic
a. antibody
a. antibody test
a. autoantibody

anti-D
a.-D antibody
a.-D anti-Rh antibody
a.-D enzyme-linked immunosorbent assay
a.-D globulin treatment
a.-D immune globulin
a.-D immunoglobulin
a.-D therapy

anti-DCP monoclonal antibody

antidecubitus
a. mattress
a. pad

antidelta IgM antibody

antideoxyribonuclease B titer test

antidepressant
a. abuse
a. agent
antianxiety and antidepressant medication
bruising from a.
chronic antidepressant therapy
a. compound
constipation from a.
dizziness from a.
a. drug
a. drug hepatotoxicity
green urine from a.
hair loss from a.

heterocyclic a.
impotence from a.
a. inhibition
a. medication
nipple discharge from a.
noradrenergic and specific serotonergic a.
overdosed with a.
a. poisoning
a. response
tetracyclic a.
a. therapy
third-generation a.
a. toxicity
a. treatment

antidermatitis factor

antidesmin
a. antibody
a. monoclonal antibody

antidesmoplakin III

antidiabetic
a. agent
a. agent hepatotoxicity
a. medication
oral antidiabetic agent

antidiarrheal
a. agent
opioid a.

antidigoxigenin alkaline phosphatase antibody-conjugate

antidiphtheric serum

antidiphtheritic globulin

antidipsotropic agent

antidiuresis
syndrome of inappropriate a.

antidiuretic
a. action
a. activity
angiotensin II antidiuretic hormone
a. arginine vasopressin V2 receptor
a. hormone
a. hormone deficiency
a. hormone-like agent
inappropriate antidiuretic hormone
inappropriate antidiuretic hormone syndrome
inappropriate secretion of antidiuretic hormone
a. substance
syndrome of inappropriate antidiuretic hormone
syndrome of inappropriate antidiuretic hormone secretion
syndrome of inappropriate secretion of antidiuretic hormone

anti-DNase
a.-DNase B antibody
a.-DNase B assay
a.-DNase B titer

anti-DNA-topoisomerase I antibody

antidopaminergic
a. effect
a. potency

antidotally beneficial

antidote drug

anti-double-stranded
a.-d.-s. deoxyribonucleic acid
a.-d.-s. deoxyribonucleic acid antibody
a.-d.-s. DNA antibody

antidromic
a. conduction
a. potential
a. response
a. stimulation
a. tachycardia
a. volley

antidrug antibody

antiductal antibody

antidyskinetic agent

antidysrhythmic agent

anti-EA antibody

anti-EBNA antibody

anti-E-cadherin monoclonal antibody

anti-EGF receptor antibody for cancer

anti-ELAM-1

antiembolic
pneumatic antiembolic stocking
a. position
a. stockings
thigh-high antiembolic stocking

antiembolism
adjustable thigh antiembolism stockings
a. stocking

antiemetic
a. agent
a. drug
a. medication
a. therapy

antiendomysial
a. antibody
a. antibody test

antiendomysium antibody

antiendothelial
a. antibody
a. cell antibody
a. cell autoantibody
monoclonal antiendothelial cell antibody

antiendotoxin
a. measure
monoclonal antiendotoxin antibody
plasma antiendotoxin core antibody

antienterocyte antibody

antiepidermal
a. growth factor receptor
a. growth factor receptor antibody for cancer
a. growth factor receptor monoclonal antibody

antiepileptic
a. drug
a. drug hypersensitivity syndrome
a. drug-induced bone disease
a. medication

antiepiligrin cicatricial pemphigoid

antiepithelial
a. membrane antigen antibody
monoclonal antiepithelial membrane antigen
a. serum

anti-Epstein-Barr
a.-E.-B. nuclear antigen
a.-E.-B. nuclear antigen antibody
a.-E.-B. virus
a.-E.-B. virus antibody

anti-*Escherichia coli*-derived protein antibody

antiestrogen
a. drug
nonsteroidal a.
a. radiologic therapy
a. receptor
a. therapy

antiestrogenic
a. activity
a. effect
a. property

antiextractable nuclear antibody

antifactor
a. I–IX disorder
a. Xa
anti-Fas antibody
antifatty liver factor
antiferritin antibody
antifertility factor-1
antifibrin
a. antibody
a. antibody imaging agent
a. scintigraphy
antifibrinolytic
a. agent
a. therapy
antifibroblast serum
antifibronectin antibody
antifilaggrin antibody
antifoaming agent
antifolate
multitargeted a.
antifolic agent
antifungal
a. agent
a. azoles
a. drug
a. drug therapy
a. esophageal infection
oral antifungal agent
a. prophylaxis
a. regimen
a. therapy
a. treatment
antifungal-resistant opportunistic infection
antigas gangrene serum
antigen
Acanthocheilonema viteae excretory-secretory a.
a. activity
acute lymphocytic leukemia a.
adult T-cell leukemia a.
a. aerosol
age-adjusted prostate-specific a.
allogeneic antigen candidate
anomalous antigen expression
antibody to hepatitis-associated a.
antibody to hepatitis B core a.
antibody to hepatitis Be a.
antibody to hepatitis B surface a.
anticarcinoembryonic a.
anticarcinoembryonic antigen monoclonal antibody
antiepithelial membrane antigen antibody
anti-Epstein-Barr nuclear a.
anti-Epstein-Barr nuclear antigen antibody
antihepatitis a.
antihuman leukocyte antigen antibody
anti-40 kDa colonic a.
antimelanoma-associated antigen antibody
antineutrophil cytoplasmic a.
antiproliferating cell nuclear a.
antismooth muscle a.
antiviral capsid a.
Ascaris a.
Australia a.
Australia antigen protein
Australia antigen radioimmunoassay
Australia hepatitis-associated a.
Australian hepatitis a.
Australia serum hepatitis a.
autologous tumor rejection a.
bacterial antigen complex
B-cell antigen receptor
beef heart a.
beta-oncofetal a.
a. binding
a. binding protein
a. binding site
bladder tumor a.
blood group a.
bound/free antigen ratio
breast cancer a.
Brugia malayi adult a.
bullous pemphigoid a.
cancer a.
cancer antigen 125
cancer antigen 19-9
a. capture assay
a. capture ligand assay
carbohydrate a.
carcinoembryonic a.
carcinoembryonic antigen doubling time
cell surface a.
cephalin cholesterol a.
circulating anodic a.
circulating cathodic a.
colitis colon a.
collagen a.
colloid a.
colonization factor a.
colon-specific a.
colon-specific antigen protein
common a.
common acute lymphoblastic leukemia a.
common acute lymphocytic leukemia a.
a. 85 complex
complexed prostate-specific a.
cross-reactive antigen group
cryptococcal a.
cutaneous lymphocyte a.
cytotoxic lymphocyte activation antigen 4 immunoglobulin
a. deficiency
delta a.
a. detection
detection of early antigen fluorescent focus
a. detection test
a. determinant
Diego a.
differentiation a.
direct fluorescent a.
direct fluorescent antigen test
disease-resistant a.
disease-susceptible a.
Duffy antigen A, B positive phenotype
Duffy antigen A negative phenotype
Duffy antigen B negative phenotype
early a.
embryonic a.
enterobacterial common a.
envelope 2 a.
epidemic hepatitis-associated a.
epithelial membrane a.
Epstein-Barr viral capsid a.
Epstein-Barr virus early a.
Epstein-Barr virus nuclear a.
a. excess
a. excess antigen
a. expression
extractable nuclear a.
factor VII a.
factor VIII a.
factor X a.
febrile a.
febrile antigen agglutination
feline oncornavirus-associated cell membrane a.
fertilization a.
fetal sulfoglycoprotein a.
fibrinogen-related a.
fibrin-related a.
fluorescence overlay antigen mapping

fluorescent antibody to membrane antigen test
fragment antigen binding
fragment, antigen, and complement binding
fragment of immunoglobulin G involved in antigen binding
free to total prostate-specific a.
Friend-Moloney a.
Friend-Moloney-Rauscher a.
a. gain
gastrointestinal cancer a.
gastrointestinal cancer-associated a.
Gerbich red cell a.
gold-labeled antigen detection technique
Gross cell surface a.
Gross leukemia a.
Gross sarcoma virus a.
group-specific a.
H a.
Helicobacter pylori stool a.
hemagglutinating a.
hemolytic anemia a.
hepatitis A a.
hepatitis-associated a.
hepatitis B a.
hepatitis B_e a.
hepatitis B core a.
hepatitis B early a.
hepatitis B surface a.
hepatitis D a.
hepatitis surface antigen studies
Herpesvirus hominis membrane a.
heterophil transplantation a.
high molecular weight melanoma-associated a.
histocompatibility a.
histocompatibility leukocyte a.
histocompatibility locus a.
Histoplasma capsulatum a.
Histoplasma capsulatum polysaccharide a.
human B-lymphocyte a.
human erythrocyte a.
human leukocyte a.
human leukocyte antigen allele
human leukocyte antigen restriction element
human leukocyte antigen system
human lymphocyte a.
human platelet a.
human T-cell leukemia virus-associated membrane a.
human thymocyte a.
immediate early a.
immune complex-dissociated p24 a.
immune region-associated a.
induced complement-fixing a.
inhibitory a.
a. interferon
International Workshop and Conference on Human Leukocyte Differentiation A.'s
islet cell a.
killer inhibitor receptors-human leukocyte a.
late a.
latency-associated nuclear a.
latent nuclear a.
latex ELISA for antigen protein
lethal a.
leukemia a.
leukemia-associated a.
leukocyte antigen factor-3
leukocyte common a.
leukocyte function-associated a.
Lewis Y a.
LH 7:2 a.
a. load
low affinity antigen receptor
low-frequency blood group a.
low-temperature, heat-mediated antigen retrieval
lymphocyte detected membrane a.
lymphocyte function a.
lymphocyte function-associated a.
lymphocyte function-associated antigen 1
lymphocyte function-associated antigen 2
lymphocyte function-associated antigen 3
lymphogranuloma venereum a.
lytic-associated nuclear a.
macrophage lineage a.
major histocompatibility complex a.
major serologic a.
male specific a.
mammary serum a.
Marek associated tumor-specific a.
a. marker
MART-1 melanoma a.
melanoma antigen reacting to T cell
melanoma antigen recognized by T cell
melanoma-associated a.
melanoma-associated antigen GD2
melanoma-associated antigen GD3
melanoma-associated antigen GM2
melanoma specific a.
membrane a.
MHC antigen deficiency
MHC class I a.
MHC class I antigen deficiency
MHC class II a.
minor group antigen incompatibility
minor histocompatibility a.
mixed vespid a.
Moloney cell surface a.
monoclonal antibody-defined a.
monoclonal antiepithelial membrane a.
monocyte lineage a.
mouse-specific B-lymphocyte a.
mouse-specific bone marrow-derived lymphocyte a.
mucin-like carcinoma-associated a.
multiple antigen stimulation test
mumps skin test a.
myeloid associated a.
myeloid lineage a.
nasal antigen challenge test
natural killer cell a.
neoplasm embryonic a.
NK cell a.
nonhuman leukocyte antigen associated form
noninherited maternal a.
noninherited paternal a.
nonspecific cross-reacting a.
normal fecal a.
nuclear a.
oncofetal a.
ovarian carcinoma a.
pancreas antigen retrieval
pancreatic oncofetal a.
p24 antigen testing
parainfluenza virus a.
P blood group a.
a. peptide
perinuclear CD15 a.
pertussis, acellular antigens, vaccine
pertussis, whole-cell antigens, vaccine
phytohemagglutinin a.
platelet a.
polyclonal carcinoembryonic a.
polymerase chain reaction analysis of prostate-specific a.
polysaccharide egg a.
a. positive
a. presentation
a. processing

antigen *(continued)*
proliferating nuclear cell a.
prostate a.
prostate-specific antigen bound to alpha-1 antichymotrypsin
prostate-specific antigen density
prostate-specific antigen doubling time
prostate-specific antigen transition zone
prostate-specific antigen velocity
prostate-specific membrane a.
prostatic specific a.
protective a.
radioactive antigen microprecipitin
ragweed a.
ragweed antigen E
a. receptor
a. receptor gene
a. recognition
renal tubular a.
a. restriction
a. retrieval
rhesus antigen C
rhesus D a.
rhesus E a.
rheumatoid arthritis nuclear a.
rose bengal a.
a. screen
segmental antigen challenge
serum cryptococcal a.
serum hepatitis a.
serum hepatitis-associated antigen antibody
serum soluble a.
serum tissue polypeptide a.
sheep erythrocyte a.
Sjögren syndrome antigen A
soluble egg a.
soluble antigen fluorescent antibody test
soluble HLA a.
soluble human leukocyte a.
soluble liver a.
a. specific
sperm-coating a.
sperm-specific a.
squamous cell carcinoma a.
stage-specific embryonic a.
a. stimulation
a. stool detection test
surface a.
T-cell antigen receptor
T cell antigen receptor Vb
T-cell-restricted intracellular a.
testis-determining a.
thymic lymphocyte a.
thymus leukemia a.
tissue polypeptide a.
tissue-specific a.
a. titer
T-lymphocyte-associated a.
a. tolerance
toxic shock a.
toxoplasmin skin test a.
transplantation a.
trophoblast a.
tumor a.
tumor antigen 4
tumor-associated rejection a.
tumor-associated surface a.
tumor-associated transplantation a.
tumor polypeptide a.
tumor regression a.
tumor-resistant a.
tumor-specific cell surface a.
tumor-specific tissue a.
tumor-specific transplantation a.
tumor-susceptible a.
undenatured bacterial a.
a. unit
a. unmasking
variable antigen, surface
variable antigen type
variant-specific surface a.
varieties of human leukocyte a.
very-late a.
viral a.
viral capsid a.
viral capsid antigen, Epstein-Barr
viral cell surface a.
viral envelope a.
virus infection-associated a.
Wright a.

antigen-1
autoimmune thyroid-related a.-1
fertilization a.-1
leukocyte factor a.-1

antigen-3

antigen-4
cytotoxic T lymphocyte a.-4
very late a.-4

antigen-125
carcinoembryonic a.-125

antigen-A24
human leukocyte a.-A24

antigen-antibody
a.-a. complex
a.-a. crossed electrophoresis
a.-a. reaction
a.-a. system

antigen-antiglobulin
a.-a. reaction
red blood cell-linked antigen-antiglobulin reaction

antigen-associated
osteosarcoma antigen-associated monoclonal antibody

antigen-binding
a.-b. capacity
a.-b. diversity
a.-b. lymphocyte
a.-b. region
single-chain antigen-binding protein
a.-b. site

antigen-combining site

antigen-dependent pathway

antigenemia
a. assay
negative a.
p24 a.
a. test

antigenemically cross-reacting food

antigen-extracted
a.-e. allogeneic bone
a.-e. allogenic
a.-e. allogenic bone

antigenic
a. analysis
a. antibody lattice formation
a. assay
a. binding receptor
a. competition
a. complex
a. deletion
a. determinant
a. determinant of erythrocytes
a. drift
Heymann nephritis antigenic complex
microbial antigenic phase shift
a. mimicry
a. modulation
new antigenic determinant
a. paralysis
a. phenotype
a. property
a. shift
a. stimulation
a. stimulus
a. structural grouping
a. target
a. variation

antigenicity
lowered tumor a.
tumor a.

antigen-independent
a.-i. adhesion
a.-i. pathway
antigen-induced arthritis
antigen-inducing unit
antigen-modulated mini-stem cell transplant
antigen-nonspecific immune complex assay
antigen-positive
immune-associated a.-p.
antigen-presenting cell
antigen-pulsed autologous dendritic cell
antigen-reactive
a.-r. cell
a.-r. cell opsonization
a.-r. T cell
antigen-responsive cell
antigen-retrieval technique
antigen-sensitive cell
antigen-specific
a.-s. anergy
a.-s. antigen
a.-s. helper factor
a.-s. immune response
nucleocapsid a.-s.
a.-s. preventive therapy
a.-s. suppressor T cell
a.-s. T cell
a.-s. TCR
anti-GFAP staining
anti-GFP polyclonal antibody
anti-*Giardia* IgM
antiglare filter
antiglaucoma surgery
antigliadin
a. antibody
a. IgA ELISA autoimmune test
a. IgG ELISA autoimmune test
a. IgG, IgA test
immunoglobulin G antigliadin antibody
luminal a.
antiglial
a. fibrillary acidic protein
monoclonal antiglial fibrillary acidic protein
antiglide plate
antiglobulin
anti-blood group A antiglobulin test
direct antiglobulin rosette-forming
direct antiglobulin Coombs test
enzyme-linked antiglobulin test
indirect antiglobulin test
mixed antiglobulin reaction
mixed reverse passive antiglobulin hemagglutination
radioimmune antiglobulin test
antiglobulin-enhanced complement-dependent cytotoxicity
antiglomerular
a. antibody
a. basement membrane
a. basement membrane antibody
a. basement membrane antibody disease
a. basement membrane antibody nephritis
a. basement membrane disease
a. basement membrane glomerulonephritis
a. basement membrane-negative crescentic glomerular nephritis
nephrotoxic antiglomerular basement membrane antibody nephritis
antiglutamic acid decarboxylase autoantibody
anti-GM$_1$ antibody test
antigonadal action
antigonadotropic action
antigonadotropin
pineal a.
antigovernment feeling
antigranulocyte
a. antibody
99mTc-labeled antigranulocyte antibody
antigravity
a. activity
a. muscle
a. position
a. reflex
anti-HB antibody
anti-HBc
a.-H. IgM
a.-H. IgM antibody
anti-HBe antibody
anti-HBs
a.-H. antibody
a.-H. concentration
anti-HD antibody
antiheart
a. antibody
a. muscle autoantibody
antihelical fold
anti-*Helicobacter*
a.-*H.* pylori IgM
a.-*H.* pylori treatment
antihelix
a. area
a. unit
antihelminthic therapy
antihemophilic
cryoprecipitated antihemophilic factor
a. factor
factor VIII:C heat-treated antihemophilic factor
a. globulin
a. plasma
a. plasma human
prothrombin, proconvertin, Stuart factor, antihemophilic B factor
antihemorrhagic
a. factor
a. stent
a. vitamin
antiheparin factor
antihepatic serum
antihepatitis
a. A, E virus
a. A-IgM immunological study
a. antigen
a. C virus-positive cirrhosis
a. C virus seropositive
a. delta virus immunoglobulin
a. E virus immunoglobulin
anti-HER2 monoclonal antibody
antiherpetic agent
anti-HGF antibody
anti-HHV8 antibody titer
antihidrotic ectodermal dysplasia
antihidrotic ectodermal dysplasia
antihistamine
bruising from a.
confusion from a.
constipation from a.
drowsiness from a.
a. drug
dry mouth from a.
fatigue from a.
a. neurotoxicity
nonsedating a.

antihistamine *(continued)*
oral a.
voice change from a.

antihistaminergic effect

antihistocompatibility antibody

antihistone antibody

anti-*Histoplasma* antibody

anti-HIV
a.-HIV antibody
a.-HIV immune serum globulin
a.-HIV protease inhibitor

anti-HIV-1 antibody

anti-HLA
a.-HLA alloantibody
a.-HLA antibody
a.-HLA class I antibody

antihormonal therapy

anti-HSV IgM Ab titer

anti-HTLV-I antibody

anti-Hu
a.-Hu antibody
a.-Hu antineuronal autoantibody
a.-Hu test

antihuman
a. alpha-catenin antibody
a. beta-catenin antibody
a. E-cadherin antibody
equine antihuman lymphoblast globulin
equine antihuman lymphoblast serum
a. globulin
a. globulin crossmatch
a. globulin test
a. herpesvirus 8 antibody titer
horse antihuman thymocyte globulin
horse antihuman thymus globulin
humanized antihuman IL-2 receptor antibody
a. immunodeficiency virus immune serum globulin
a. immunodeficiency virus protease inhibitor
a. leukocyte antigen antibody
a. lymphocyte globulin
a. lymphocyte serum
a. S5 analog
a. thymocyte globulin
a. thymocyte plasma
a. thymus serum
a. transferrin

antihyaluronidase
a. antibody
a. assay
a. titer

antihyperlipidemic agent

antihypertensive
a. agent
a. drug
a. and lipid lowering
A. and Lipid-Lowering Treatment to Prevent Heart Attack Trial
a. medication
a. neural renomedullary lipids
parenteral antihypertensive agent
a. therapy

antihyperuricemic agent

anti-ICAM-1
monoclonal mouse a.-ICAM-1

antiidiotype
a. antibody
a. autoantibody
a. immune response
a. vaccine

antiidiotypic
a. antibody
a. immunoglobulin response

anti-IgA autoantibody

anti-IgE humanized monoclonal antibody

anti-IIb-IIIA mAB therapy

anti-I-kBa antibody

antiimmune body

antiimmunocytokeratin antibody

antiimmunoglobulin
a. antibody
a. E humanized monoclonal antibody
a. reagent

antiimpulse effect

antiincontinence procedure

antiinfective biomaterial

antiinflammatory
a. agent
compensatory antiinflammatory response syndrome
a. corticoid
a. cytokine
a. drug
a. effect
a. intervention
a. medication
noncorticosteroid antiinflammatory agent
a. nonsteroidal agent
nonsteroidal antiinflammatory compound
nonsteroidal antiinflammatory drug gastropathy
nonsteroidal antiinflammatory drug-induced intestinal stricture
nonsteroidal antiinflammatory medication
a. therapy
a. treatment

antiinflammatory-antibiotic combination

antiinhibitor coagulant complex

antiinstinctual force

antiinsulin
a. antibody
a. autoantibody
guinea pig antiinsulin serum
a. receptor antibody
a. serum

antiinterferon-alpha immunization

anti-interleukin-2
a.-i.-2 antibody
a.-i.-2 receptor alpha monoclonal antibody

antiinvasion factor

anti-IRF-1 antibody

anti-IRF-2 antibody

antiislet cell antibody

anti-itch medication

anti-Jo-1 antibody

anti-Jp-1 antibody

anti-Kaposi sarcoma

anti-Kell antibody

antikeratin
a. antibody
a. autoantibody

antikidney
a. antibody
a. serum nephritis

antiknock mix

anti-Ku antibody

anti-LA antibody

antilactoferrin antibody

anti-La/SSB antibody

anti-LA/SS-B test

antilens protein antibody

antileukemic therapy

antileukocyte antibody

anti-Lewis antibody

anti-Lewisite
British a.-L.
anti-LFLA test
antilipemic drug
antilipolytic effect
antiliver microsomal antibody detection
anti-LKM-1 antibody
antilymphocyte
a. antibody
a. globulin
a. heteroconjugate
a. induction
a. plasma
a. serum
a. therapy
antilymphocytic
a. antibody
a. globulin
a. serum
specified a.
antilymphoid therapy
anti-M
a.-M agglutinin
a.-M antibody
anti-M2 antimitochondrial antibody level
antimacrophage
a. globulin
a. serum
anti-MAG antibody
antimajor histocompatibility complex
antimalarial
a. agent
a. drug
antimalignant antibody test
antimalignin
monoclonal antimalignin antibody
antimanic treatment
antimegalin antiserum
antimelanocyte antibody
antimelanoma-associated antigen antibody
antimembrane
fluorescence antimembrane antibody
fluorescent antimembrane antibody test
antimeningococcus serum
antimesenteric
a. border
a. border of distal ileum
a. enterotomy
a. fat pad
a. side
a. surface
antimesocolic side of cecum
antimetabolite induction
antimetallothionein antibody
anti-Mi-2 nuclear antibody
antimicrobial
a. agent
a. agent-induced colitis
a. agents and chemotherapy
a. aminoglycoside
a. barrier
beta-lactamase-resistant a.
a. chemoprophylaxis
a. dosing regimen
intensive antimicrobial therapy
a. level
macrolide antimicrobial agent
oral antimicrobial prophylaxis
parenteral antimicrobial agent
a. prophylaxis
a. removal device
a. resistance
a. spectrum
a. substance
a. substantivity
a. susceptibility test
a. susceptibility testing
a. therapy
a. treatment
antimicrobial-resistant *Salmonella*
antimicrobiology susceptibility testing
antimicrosomal antibody
antimicrotubule agent
antimigraine therapy
antimigration system
antimitochondrial
a. antibody
a. antibody assay
anti-M2 antimitochondrial antibody level
antimitotic
a. drug
a. effect
antimongoloid
a. eyelid slant
a. eye slant
a. slanting
antimonial drug therapy for leishmaniasis
antimonous oxide
anti-Monson curve
antimony
a. assay
a. chloride
a. dimercaptosuccinate
a. hydride
a. monocrystalline electrode
a. poisoning
sodium antimony gluconate
a. spot
a. stain
a. trichloride
antimony-sulfur colloid
antimotility
a. agent
a. drug
oral antimotility agent
antimotivational syndrome
antimouse
a. lymphocyte serum
fowl antimouse lymphocyte globulin
goat antimouse immunoglobulin G
human antimouse antibody
antimouse-thymocyte
rabbit a.-t.
antimüllerian
a. derivative syndrome
a. hormone
antimuscarine cholinergic activity
antimuscarinic
a. acetylcholine receptor
a. agent
a. antagonist
a. drug
a. effect
peripheral antimuscarinic side effect
antimuscle factor
antimycobacterial
a. drug
a. prophylaxis
a. susceptibility testing
antimycoplasma titer
antimycotic
a. agent
a. resistance
antimyeloperoxidase antibody
antimyolemmal antibody

antimyosin
a. antibody
a. antibody imaging
anti-NADase
anti-N agglutinin
antinative DNA
antineoplastic
a. agent
a. chemotherapeutic agent
a. chemotherapy
a. drug
a. drug hepatotoxicity
selective apoptotic antineoplastic drugs
a. therapy
antineuritic
a. factor
a. vitamin
antineuronal
a. antibody
anti-Hu antineuronal autoantibody
circulation antineuronal antibody
a. cytoplasmic autoantibody
a. enteric antibody test
a. nuclear antibody
antineutrophil
a. antibody
a. cytoplasmic antibody
a. cytoplasmic antibody titer
a. cytoplasmic antigen
cytoplasmic antineutrophil cytoplasmic antibody
a. cytoplasmic autoantibody
a. cytoplasmic IgG antibody
pauciimmune antineutrophil cytoplasmic antibody-associated glomerulonephritis
perinuclear antineutrophil cytoplasmic antibody
perinuclear antineutrophil cytoplasmic autoantibody
antineutrophilic
a. cytoplasmic antibody
a. cytoplasmic autoantibody-small vessel vasculitis
a. serum
antinociceptive
a. action
a. agent
a. effect
a. procedure
antinodal behavior
antinuclear
a. antibody
a. antibody assay
a. antibody fluid
a. antibody immunodiffusion
a. antibody immunofluorescence
a. antibody immunological study
a. antibody screening by enzyme immunoassay
a. antibody screening test
a. antibody titer
a. autoantibody
automated enzyme immunoassay for antinuclear antibody
drug-induced antinuclear antibodies
a. factor
fluorescent antinuclear antibody assay
histone-reactive antinuclear antibody
leukocyte-specific antinuclear antibody
a. matrix antibody
positive antinuclear antibody
antinucleolar antibody
antinucleosomal autoantibody
antioncogene therapy
anti-O-specific polysaccharide
antiosteoclastic agent
antiovarian antibody
antioxidant
a. effect
a. enzyme
a. eye treatment
intravenous antioxidant therapy
lipid-soluble secondary a.
A. Polyp Prevention Trial
a. supplement
a. system
a. therapy
total peroxyl radical-trapping antioxidant potential
total radical-trapping antioxidant parameter
a. vitamin
anti-P
a.-P agglutinin
a.-P antibody
a.-P blood group specificity
antipanic agent
anti-*Paracoccidioides brasiliensis* antibody
antiparallel
a. B-sheet conformation
a. strand
antiparasitic
a. agent
a. drug therapy
antiparietal
a. antibody
a. cell antibody
a. cell antibody assay
antiparkinsonian response
antiparkinsonism agent
antiparvovirus
a. 19 antibody
a. B19 IgG antibody
a. B19 IgM antibody
a. B19-specific IgM
antipellagra factor
antipenicillin
hemagglutinating antipenicillin antibody
antipeptide antibody
antiperinuclear
a. autoantibody
a. factor
antiperipheral nerve myelin antibody
antiperistaltic
a. anastomosis
a. intestinal interposition
a. operation
a. reflux
a. technique
antipernicious anemia factor
antipertussis
a. acellular vaccine
a. serum
antiphagocytic
a. capsule
a. factor
antiphenyloxazolone antibody
antiphlogistic corticoid
antiphosphatidylserine-prothrombin complex antibody testing
antiphospholipid
a. antibodies in stroke study
a. antibody
a. antibody assay
a. antibody syndrome
paraneoplastic antiphospholipid syndrome
primary antiphospholipid antibody syndrome
antiphospholipid-anticardiolipin antibody

antipill finish
antipituitary antibody
antiplacental
polyclonal antiplacental alkaline phosphatase
antiplague serum
antiplasmin
a-2 antiplasmin coagulation inhibitor
a. deficiency
antiplatelet
a. agent
a. antibody
a. antibody assay
a. drug
a. endothelial cell adhesion molecule
a. immunoglobulin G antibody
maternal antiplatelet antibody
a. plasma
a. regimen
a. serum
a. therapy
a. trial
antipleiotrophin therapy
anti-PM-Scl antibody
antipneumococcal antibody
antipneumococcus serum
antipodal cone
antipode
optic a.
antipolysaccharide
selective antipolysaccharide antibody deficiency
anti-Pr cold autoagglutinin
antipredatory aggression
antiprogesterone receptor
antiproliferating cell nuclear antigen
antiproliferative
a. activity
a. agent
a. effect
a. property
antiprostaglandin agent
antiprotease therapy
antiproteinuric effect
antiprotozoal therapy
antiprotrusio cage
antipruritic
a. agent
a. therapy
anti-*Pseudomonas* human plasma
antipsoriatic action
antipsychotic
a. action
a. agent
atypical a.
atypical antipsychotic agent
atypical antipsychotic drug
atypical antipsychotic preparation
a. compound
a. drug
a. drug hepatotoxicity
a. drug therapy
a. drug treatment
a. effect
a. exposure
a. medication
neuroleptic antipsychotic drug
new-generation a.
new-generation antipsychotic drug
novel a.
novel antipsychotic drug
a. pharmacotherapy
a. preparation
a. response
second-generation a.
a. side effect
tricyclic a.
antipsychotic-associated sexual dysfunction
antipsychotic-induced
a.-i. tardive dyskinesia
a.-i. weight gain
antipyretic
a. agent
a. therapy
antipyretic/analgesic agent
antipyrine clearance
antipyrotic agent
antirabbit
goat antirabbit gamma globulin
antirabies serum
antirachitic
a. activity
a. effect
a. property
a. vitamin
antiradial
a. plane
a. technique
anti-RAP antibody
anti-RAP-GST antibody
antirat
mouse antirat serum
antireceptor antibody
antirecoverin antibody
antireflection coating
antireflux
a. double-J stent
a. flap-valve mechanism
laparoscopic antireflux surgery
a. nipple
Nissen antireflux operation
a. operation
a. procedure
a. prosthesis
a. regimen
a. surgery
a. therapy
a. ureteral implantation technique
a. valve
a. wrap
antirefluxing
a. colonic conduit
a. nipple
antiresorptive
a. agent
a. therapy
antirespiratory syncytial virus
antireticular cytotoxic serum
antireticulin antibody
antiretina antibody
antiretroviral
a. agent
a. chemotherapy
combined antiretroviral therapy
a. drug
genotypic antiretroviral resistance testing
highly active antiretroviral therapy
highly active antiretroviral treatment
a. medication
a. pregnancy registry
a. regimen
a. resistance
salvage highly active antiretroviral therapy
a. therapy
a. treatment
a. triple combination therapy
antiretroviral-exposed mother
antireward system
anti-Rh
a.-Rh agglutinin
a.-Rh antibody
a.-Rh gamma globulin
a.-Rh titer

anti-RhD immune globulin
antirheumatic
a. agent
disease-controlling antirheumatic therapy
disease-modifying antirheumatic drug
a. drug
immunomodulating antirheumatic drug
long-acting antirheumatic drug
slow-acting antirheumatic drug
anti-rhIL-3 antibody
anti-Rho-D titer test
anti-Ri
a.-Ri antibody
a.-Ri syndrome
antiribonucleoprotein antibody
antiribosomal
a. antibody
a. P antibody
antiribosomal-P antibody
antirlbosome antibody
anti-RNA polymerase antibody
anti-RNP antibody
anti-Ro antibody
anti-Ro/SSA antibody
anti-Ro/SS-A test
antirotation
a. cable
a. device
antirotavirus
a. antibody
a. IgA titer
anti-RT chemotherapy
antirubella antibody
anti-S
a.-S agglutinin
a.-S antibody
anti-S-100 protein
antisarcoma chemotherapy
antisarcomeric actin
antiscarlatinal serum
antiscatter grid
anti-Schiff stain
antiscleroderma-70 antibody
antiscorbutic vitamin
antisecretory
a. agent
a. drug
a. opioid
a. therapy
antiseizure
a. drug
a. effect
a. medication
antisense
antitelomerase antisense oligonucleotide
a. compound
a. DNA
a. DNA inhibition
a. drug
a. nucleotide
a. oligodeoxynucleotide
oligodeoxynucleotide antisense probe
a. oligonucleotide
a. oligonucleotide viral therapy
a. probe
a. riboprobe
a. RNA
a. rna
a. RNA probe
a. strand
a. strategy
a. therapy
antisepsis
disinfection and a.
antiseptic-impregnated central venous catheter
antiseptic solution
antisera
a. antibody
erythrocyte a.
antiserotonergic
a. agent
a. effect
antiserotoninergic effect
antiserum
a. anaphylaxis
anthrax a.
C-reactive protein a.
a., guinea pig
homologous canine distemper a.
a., horse
human thymus a.
a., monkey
nerve growth factor a.
a., rabbit
rat thymus a.
sperm-specific a.
staphylococcal enterotoxin B a.
antishock
a. garment
medical antishock trousers
military antishock trousers
pneumatic antishock garment
a. trousers
antisialosyl-Tn antigen
antisignal recognition particle antibody
antisiphon
a. device
a. valve
anti-Sjögren syndrome A, B antibody
antiskeletal antibody
anti-SLA test
anti-Sm
a.-Sm antibody
a.-Sm test
anti-Smith antibody
antismooth
a. muscle actin
a. muscle antibody
a. muscle antibody assay
a. muscle antigen
antisnakebite
North American antisnakebite serum
a. serum
antisnake venom
antisocial
a. activity
a. adolescent
a. aggression
a. alcoholism
a. behavior
childhood antisocial behavior
a. compulsion
a. feature
a. juvenile
a. lifestyle
a. neurotic personality
a. neurotic personality disorder
a. patient
pattern of antisocial behavior
a. personality trait
a. psychopathic Q factor
a. reaction
a. scale
a. teenager
a. tendency
a. trends psychopathic
a. trends psychopathic personality
antisomatostatin antibody
antispasmodic
a. agent

a. drug
opiate a.
antispastic drug
antispasticity index
antisperm antibody
antispermicidal monoclonal antibody
antispirochetal activity
antispleen globulin
anti-SRP antibody
anti-SSA
a.-SSA antibody
a.-SSA immunological study
anti-SS-A antibody
anti-SS-B antibody
anti-SSB immunological study
antistaphylococcal
a. agent
a. antibiotic
a. IgE
antistaphylococcus serum
antisterility
a. factor
a. vitamin
antistreptococcal
a. DNase-B titer
a. hyaluronidase
a. polysaccharide A test
antistreptococcus serum
antistreptolysin
a. O assay
a. O response
a. O titer
a. test
antistreptolysin-O test
antistreptozyme test
antistress effect
antistriational antibody
antisuppression exercise
antisynthetase
a. antibody
a. syndrome
antitachycardia
a. pacemaker
a. pacing
anti-Tamm-Horsfall protein
anti-tat
a.-t. antibody
a.-t. IgG
anti-tau monoclonal antibody
anti-TB cellular immunity
anti-TBM antibody
anti-T-cell
a.-T-c. antibody
a.-T-c. therapy
antitelomerase
a. agent
a. antisense oligonucleotide
antitension line
antitermination protein
antitetanic serum
antitetanus
a. booster
horse antitetanus toxoid globulin
a. serum
a. toxin
anti-Tg antibody
anti-Th antibody
antithoracic duct lymphocytic globulin
antithrombin
a. II
a. III
a. III coagulation inhibitor
a. III deficiency
a. III functional
a. III plasma level
a. III test
a. test
antithrombocyte antibody
antithromboembolic prophylaxis
antithrombogenic
antithrombotic
a. activity
a. therapy
antithrush treatment
antithrust seat
anti-Thy-1
a.-Thy-1 antibody
a.-Thy-1 nephritis
antithymic activity
antithymidylate synthase polyclonal antibody
antithymocyte
a. antibody
a. antibody-induced glomerulonephritis
a. gamma globulin
a. globulin
rabbit antithymocyte globulin
rabbit antithymocyte serum
a. serum
antithymocytic
specific a.
antithyroglobulin
a. antibody
a. autoantibody
antithyroid
a. antibody
a. antibody titer
a. autoantibody
a. drug
a. drug hepatotoxicity
a. drug therapy
maternal antithyroid antibody
a. medication
a. microsomal antibody
a. peroxidase
a. peroxidase antibody
a. plasma membrane antibody
radioimmunologic assay antithyroid antibody
antithyroid-stimulating
a.-s. hormone
a.-s. hormone antibody
antithyroperoxidase level
anti-TNF-alpha antibody
anti-TNF antibody
antitopoisomerase
a. I antibody
a. I autoantibody
antitorque suture
antitoxic
a. globulin
a. immunity
a. serum
tetanus antitoxic serum
antitoxin
botulism equine trivalent a.
diphtheria a.
gas a.
human tetanus a.
pentavalent gas gangrene a.
a. rash
scarlet fever a.
tetanus a.
tetanus antitoxin skin test
a. unit
antitoxoplasma
a. antibody
a. therapy
anti-*Toxoplasma*
a.-*T.* antibody
anti-*Toxoplasma gondii* antibody
anti-*Toxoplasma gondii* antibody secretion assay
a.-*T.* prophylaxis

antitoxoplasmosis
a. agent
a. therapy
anti-toxo therapy
anti-TPO antibody
antitragicus
a. muscle
musculus a.
antitragohelicine fissure
antitragus
muscle of a.
a. muscle
antitreponemal
a. antibody test
a. test
antitrichomonal therapy
antitrypsin
alpha-1 antitrypsin deficiency
alpha-1 antitrypsin disease
alpha antitrypsin level
a-2 antitrypsin inhibitor
a. deficiency
recombinant alpha-1 a.
serum a.
a. test
antitryptic
total antitryptic activity
antitryptic index
anti-tTG antibody
antitubercular therapy
antituberculosis
a. chemotherapy
a. drug
a. therapy
antituberculous
a. agent
a. chemoprophylaxis
a. drug
a. therapy
antitubular
a. basement membrane
a. basement membrane antibody
antitumor
a. activity
a. antibiotic
antibiotic antitumor drug
a. cytotoxic lymphocyte
a. drug
a. effect
a. enzyme
a. hormone
lymphotoxin antitumor activity
a. necrosis factor-based therapy
neutralizing murine monoclonal antitumor necrosis factor antibody
a. protein
rabbit ovarian antitumor serum
a. response
antitussive medication
antityphoid serum
antityrosinase antibody
anti-U1 RNP antibody
anti-U3 RNP antibody
anti-V3 antibody
antivariola
hyperimmune antivariola gamma globulin
antivascular endothelial growth factor monoclonal antibody
anti-VCA antibody
anti-VCAM-1
monoclonal mouse a.-V.
anti-VEGF antibody
antivenene unit
antivenin
anti-Centruroides a.
antivenomous serum
antivibration glove
antivimentin antibody
antiviral
a. activity
a. agent
a. antibody
a. capsid antigen
cell antiviral factor
a. chemotherapy
a. drug
a. factor
hepatitis C antiviral long-term treatment to prevent cirrhosis
a. immunity
a. lymphocyte serum
a. medication
oral antiviral agent
pokeweed antiviral protein
a. prophylactic
a. protein
a. regulator
a. therapy
Antivirogram test procedure
anti-von
a.-v. Willebrand factor
a.-v. Willebrand factor antibody
antiyeast factor
anti-Yo
a.-Yo antibody
a.-Yo serum antibody
Antley-Bixler syndrome
Anton
A. symptom
A. syndrome
A. test
Anton-Babinski syndrome
Antoni
A. A, B area
A. A, B tissue
A. A cell
A. A neurinoma classification
A. B cell
A. classification of schwannoma morphology
A. neurilemoma
A. pattern
A. type A, B neurilemoma
antonomic
parasympathetic division of antonomic nervous system
Antopol disease
Antopol-Goldman lesion
antra (*pl. of* antrum)
antral
anterior wall antral ulcer
a. atrophic gastritis
a. beaking
a. biopsy
a. cancer
a. carcinoma
a. cell
a. choanal polyp
diffuse antral gastritis
a. diverticulum of the colon
a. diverticulum of the ileum
a. edema
a. ethmoidal sphenoidectomy
a. exclusion
a. floor
a. fold
a. follicle
gastric antral erosion
gastric antral sessile polyp
gastric antral vascular ectasia
a. gastric cell
a. gastrin
a. gastrin cell hyperfunction
a. gastritis
a. G-cell hyperplasia
innervated antral pouch
a. irrigation
a. lavage

a. manometry
a. membrane
middle meatus nasal antral window
modified innervated antral pouch
a. mucosa
a. mucosal cyst
a. mucosal diaphragm
a. mucosal thickening
a. mycosis
a. nipple sign
a. nodularity
a. padding
a. peptide
a. peristalsis
a. polyp
a. pouch
a. pressure transducer
a. resection
a. sarcoma
a. scintigraphy
a. somatostatin
a. sphincter
a. stasis
a. stenosis
a. stenting
a. stomach narrowing
a. stricture
a. transplantation
a. tumor
a. ulcer
a. vascular ectasia
a. washout
a. web

antral-predominant gastritis

antral-type mucosa

antrectomy
selective vagotomy with a.
truncal vagotomy plus a.
vagotomy and a.

antrochoanal polyp

antrocolic transposition

antroduodenal
a. manometry
a. motility
a. ulcer

antroduodenojejunal manometry

antrofundal mucosa

antropyloric
a. canal
a. muscle thickness

antropyloroduodenal
a. common chamber
a. region

antrostomy
maxillary a.
nasal a.

antrum, pl. **antra**
aperture of mastoid a.
a. auris
a. cardiacum
a. cardiacum of Highmore
antra ethmoidale
a. ethmoidale
gastric a.
a. gastritis
a. of Highmore
a. mastoideum
maxillary antrum closure
polyp of antrum of stomach
a. punch forceps
a. pyloricum
retained gastric a.
retained gastric antrum syndrome
sphincter of gastric a.
a. of stomach
terminal a.
terminal antrum contraction
a. of Willis

antrum-predominant gastritis

antrum-sparing modified Whipple procedure

Antyllus method

anuclear cell

anucleate fragment

anular, annular
a. abscess
a. adenocarcinoma
anterior anular ligament
a. appearance
a. array
a. array transducer
a. atrophic connective tissue panniculitis of the ankle
a. band
a. bifocal contact lens
a. calcification
a. cartilage
a. cataract
a. constricting band syndrome
a. constricting lesion
a. corneal graft
a. corneal graft operation
a. detector
a. dilatation
a. disc bulge
a. disruption
a. distribution of lesion
a. elastolytic giant cell granuloma
a. epiphysis
a. erythema
a. erythema antigen
a. erythematous plaque
a. esophageal stricture
a. fiber
a. fibrosis
a. foreshortening
a. fracture
a. groove
a. hymen
a. hypoplasia
a. infiltrate
a. injury
a. keratitis
a. lamella
a. lesion
a. lichen planus
a. ligament
a. ligament entrapment
a. ligament of radius
a. ligament of stapes
a. ligament of trachea
a. lipid
a. lipoatrophy
a. macular dystrophy
mitral annular calcification
mitral annular calcium
napkin ring annular lesion
napkin ring anular stenosis
napkin ring anular tumor
nuclear anular differentiation
occult annular ciliary body
a. pancreas
a. part of fibrous digital sheath of digits of hand and foot
a. periradial recess
a. phased-array hyperthermia
a. placement
a. placenta
a. plexus
a. pulley
a. radial rupture
a. rim of cartilage
a. ring
a. scleritis
a. scotoma
sex cord tumors with annular tubules
a. sphincter
a. staphyloma
a. stenosis
a. stricture
a. synechia
a. syphilid
a. tear
a. tear classification

anular *(continued)*
a. tear extent
a. tear pattern
a. testis
tricuspid annular motion
a. tubule
a. ulcer

anularis
lichen planus a.
livedo a.
plexus a.

anular/posterior
outer anular/posterior longitudinal ligament complex

anuloaortic, annuloaortic
a. ectasia

anuloplasty, annuloplasty
mitral a.
prosthetic ring a.
a. ring
St. Jude annuloplasty ring
tricuspid a.

anulospiral, annulospiral
a. ending
a. ending of muscle spindle
a. fiber
a. organ

anum
per anum bleeding
per anum intersphincteric rectal dissection

anuria
angioneurotic a.
calculous a.
obstructive a.
postrenal a.
prerenal a.
renal a.

anus
anteriorly displaced a.
artificial a.
a. cerebri
imperforate a.
internal sphincter muscle of a.
itching in a.
low imperforate a.
a. malformation
manual dilatation of a.
microcephalus, imperforate anus, syndactyly, hamartoblastoma, abnormal lung lobulation, polydactyly
microphallus, imperforate anus, syndactyly, hamartoblastoma, abnormal lung
ocular coloboma-imperforate anus syndrome
Paget disease of a.
patent a.
patulous a.
polydactyly, imperforate anus, vertebral anomalies syndrome
a. vesicalis
a. vestibularis
vulvovaginal a.

anus-hand-ear syndrome

anvil
a. bone
a. sign
a. sound
a. test

anxiety
acute anxiety attack
acute anxiety reaction
a. adjustment disorder
adjustment disorder with a.
adjustment disorder with mixed anxiety and depressed mood
alcohol anxiety disorder
a. and apprehension
a. associated with depression
a. attack
attention span shortened from a.
atypical anxiety disorder
atypical neurotic anxiety state
behavioral, anxiety, mood, and other types of disorders
canker sore from a.
cheek biting from a.
childhood anxiety disorder
Children's Manifest A. Scale
chronic anxiety state
chronic tension and a.
circular interaction between anxiety and pain
Clinician Rated A. Scale
cognitive anxiety subscale
comorbid generalized a.
a. comorbidity
Concept-Specific A. Scale
confront source of a.
a. control technique
a. control training
coping with a.
crushing anxiety and depression
death anxiety scale
decreased signs and symptoms of a.
a. depression
a. and depression
depression and anxiety in elderly
a. diagnosis
a. discharge
a. disorder
a. disorder of adolescence
a. disorder of childhood
a. disorder clinic
A. Disorder Interview for Children
a. disturbance
a. dream
dream anxiety disorder
a. due to physical disorder
a. due to a substance
a. during pregnancy
Endler Multidimensional A. Scale
factors influencing a.
a. fixation
forgetfulness from a.
Free-Floating A. Test
Freeman A. Neurosis and Psychosomatic Test
a. from heat exhaustion
generalized anxiety disorder
generalized anxiety neurosis
Hamilton A. Rating Scale
a. hierarchy
high a.
high impulsiveness, high a.
high impulsiveness, low a.
high level of a.
Hospital A. and Depression
Hospital A. and Depression Scale
hyperactivity from a.
hyperactivity and irritability a.
hyperventilation from a.
a. hysteria
image patterns of a.
a. index
insomnia associated with a.
insomnia from a.
a. inventory
a. and irritability
irritability and/or a.
juvenile anxiety disorder
a. level
lifetime anxiety disorder
low a.
low impulsiveness, high a.
low impulsiveness, low a.
a. management
a. management training
Manifest A. Scale
Maternal Trait A. Score
means for a.
mild anxiety reaction
mixed anxiety depression disorder
morbid anxiety inventory
multiple anxiety comorbidity

a. neurosis
neurotic anxiety state
a. object
Objective-Analytic A. Battery
organic anxiety disorder
organic anxiety syndrome
pain determined by level of a.
Pain A. Symptoms Scale
pain-type anxiety neurosis
palpitations from a.
panic and anxiety disorder
panic attack neurotic anxiety state
a. and panic disorder clinic
a. panic reaction
parent anxiety rating scale
Patient Rated A. Scale
penalty, frustration, anxiety, guilt, hostility
phobic a.
a. preparedness
pretreatment a.
a. prevention
a. profile
a. psychogenic disorder
a. psychoneurosis
a. psychoneurotic reaction
a. rating for children
a. rating scale
a. reaction, intense
a. reduction
reduction of examination a.
relaxation-induced a.
a. relief response
a. resolution
Revised Children's Manifest A. Scale
Scale of A. and Depression
a. scale questionnaire
A. Scales for Children and Adults
a. sensitivity
a. sensitivity index
a. sensitivity theory
Sheehan Patient Rated A. Scale
Shipman A. Depression Scale
shortened attention span from a.
short-term anxiety intense
social anxiety disorder
a. source
Spielberger State-Trait A. Inventory
a. state
a. state neurotic disorder
State Trait A. Index-I
State-Trait A. Inventory
A. Status Index
A. Status Inventory
Suinn Test A. Behavior Scale
a. symptom
a. syndrome
Taylor Manifest A. Scale
a., tension, and headache
a. tension state
Test A. Inventory
throat clearing from a.
a. tolerance
total phobic a.
trench mouth from a.
a. typology
weight loss from a.

anxiety-avoiding personality disorder

anxiety-blissfulness psychosis

anxiety-depression

anxiety-induced impaired social functioning

anxiety-mood comorbidity

anxiety-provoking

a.-p. cue
short-term anxiety-provoking psychotherapy
a.-p. situation

anxiety-related

a.-r. diarrhea
a.-r. mental disorder
a.-r. psychiatric syndrome
a.-r. sensation

anxiety-withdrawal scale

anxiogenic stimulus

anxiolytic

a. abuse
a. activity
a. agent
a. amnestic disorder
a. delirium
a. dependence
a. drug
a. effect
a. intoxication
a. medication
a. property
a. response
a. sedative
a. stimuli
a. stimulus
a. substance
a. substance-use disorder
a. use disorder
a. withdrawal

anxiolytic-induced

a.-i. anxiety
a.-i. persisting dementia
a.-i. psychotic disorder with delusions
a.-i. psychotic disorder with hallucinations
a.-i. sexual dysfunction

anxious

adjustment disorder with anxious mood
a. arousal
a. delirium
depressed and a.
a. expectation
hostile and a.
a. look
a. mania
a. mood
a. mood adjustment reaction
a. rumination
a. somatic depression
a. substance abuser
a. thought

anxious-fearful cluster

anxious-neurotic personality trait

any quantity

any-angle splint

AO-ASIF

A.-A. compression technique
A.-A. orthopaedic implant
A.-A. screw

AO-Danis-Weber ankle fracture classification

AOFAS score

AOPE chemotherapy protocol

aorta

abdominal a.
aneurysmal widening of a.
aneurysm of ascending a.
anulus fibrosus of a.
arch of a.
arch of aorta abnormality
a. ascendens
ascending a.
ascending aorta dilatation
ascending aorta hypoplasia
ascending aorta synchronized pulsation
ascending hypoplasia of a.
ascending part of a.
coarctation of a.
cross clamping of a.

aorta *(continued)*
cystic medial necrosis of ascending a.
descending a.
descending thoracic a.
dextroposition of a.
a. dilation
ectasia of abdominal a.
ectasia of thoracic a.
embolectomy of a.
hardening of a.
hypoplastic a.
left ventricle to aorta pressure gradient
mediastinal branch of thoracic a.
medionecrosis of the a.
mitral valve, aorta, skeleton, skin
necrosis of ascending a.
pericardial branch of thoracic a.
root of a.
severe atheromatous change of a.
small aorta syndrome
symptomatic coarctation of a.
thoracic a.
a. thoracica
transposition of a.
traumatic rupture of thoracic a.

aorta-left ventricular fistula

aorta-right ventricular fistula

aortic
abdominal aortic aneurysm
abdominal aortic aneurysmectomy
abdominal aortic counterpulsation device
acute abdominal aortic occlusion
acute aortic dissection
acute aortic insufficiency
acute traumatic aortic injury
a. allograft
a. allograft conduit
a. amplitude
a. anastomosis
a. aneurysm
a. aneurysmal disease
a. aneurysmectomy
a. aneurysm graft
a. aneurysm rupture
a. aneurysm tissue
a. annulus abscess
a. anomaly
anterior aortic wall
antibiotic-sterilized aortic valve homograft
a. anulus abscess
a. aperture
a. arch
a. arch aneurysm
a. arch angiography
a. arch anomaly
a. arch anomaly-peculiar facies mental retardation syndrome
a. arch atresia
a. arch calcification
a. arch coarctation
a. arch disease
a. arch interruption
a. arch lesion
a. arch malformation
a. arch obstruction
a. arch rupture
a. area
a. area of auscultation
arteriosclerotic aortic aneurysm
arteriosclerotic thoracoabdominal aortic aneurysm
a. artery
ascending aortic aneurysm
a. atheromatous disease
a. atherosclerosis
atherosclerotic aortic aneurysm
atherosclerotic aortic ulcer
a. atresia
atretic aortic segment
a. attenuation
atypical aortic valve stenosis
bicommissural aortic valve
bicuspid aortic valve
a. bifurcation
a. bifurcation prosthesis
a. blood flow velocity waveform
a. blood pressure
a. body
a. body tumor
bovine aortic endothelium
brachydactyly, mesomelia, mental retardation, aortic dilation, mitral valve prolapse, characteristic facies syndrome
a. bruit
a. bud
a. bulb
a. button
calcific aortic valve stenosis
a. calcification
a. calcification sign
calcific nodular aortic stenosis
calcified aortic valve
calf aortic microsome
a. cannulation
carotid aortic dissection
a. cartilage
a. clamping
a. closure
a. coarctation
a. commissure
a. conduit
a. crossclamp
a. cross-clamping
a. cross clamp off
a. cross clamp on
cryopreserved aortic homograft
cryopreserved human aortic allograft
a. cuff
a. curtain
a. cusp
a. cusp prolapse
DeBakey-type aortic dissection
a. depressor nerve
a. deviation
a. diameter
a. dicrotic notch pressure
dilatation of aortic root
a. dilation
dissecting aortic aneurysm
dissecting aortic hematoma
a. dissection
dissection aortic aneurysm
a. distensibility
double aortic arch
a. dwarfism
dynamic aortic patch
ectatic aortic valve
a. ejection click
a. ejection sound
a. elongation
endovascular aortic graft
extended aortic root replacement
a. facies
a. first sound
floppy aortic valve
a. flow
a. flow volume
a. foramen
a. gland
a. glomus
a. graft
a. graft infection
a. graft placement
a. hiatus
a. homograft
human aortic endothelial cell
human aortic smooth muscle cell
a. hypoplasia
idiopathic hypertrophic aortic stenosis
a. idiopathic necrosis
a. impedance
a. impression of left lung
a. incisura
a. incompetence

incompetent aortic murmur
a. inflammation
inflammatory aortic aneurysm
a. inflow
infrarenal abdominal aortic aneurysm
infrarenal aortic thrombosis
a. injury
a. insufficiency
a. insult
intermittent aortic occlusion
interrupted aortic arch
interruption of aortic arch
a. intimal dehiscence
a. intramural hematoma
a. isthmus
a. jugular test
a. kinking
a. knob
a. knuckle
a. laceration
a. leaflet
a. and left ventricular tunnel
luetic aortic aneurysm
a. lumen
a. lymphatic plexus
a. lymph node
Martorell aortic arch syndrome
massive aortic regurgitation
mean aortic flow velocity
a. mean pressure
mental retardation, typical facies, aortic stenosis syndrome
middle aortic syndrome
mitral and aortic valve replacement
mitral valve prolapse, aortic anomalies, skeletal changes, and skin changes syndrome
mixed aortic valve disease
a. motion artifact
a. murmur
mycotic aortic aneurysm
narrowing of aortic valve
native aortic valve
native aortic valve closure
a. neck
a. nerve
a. nipple
a. nipple sign
a. node
a. node metastasis
nodular calcific aortic stenosis
nonrheumatic aortic insufficiency
a. notch
notched aortic knob
a. occlusion
a. occlusive disease
a. opening
opening of aortic valve
a. opening click
a. opening of heart
a. orifice
a. ostial stenosis
a. ostium
a. outflow gradient
a. outflow obstruction
a. override
a. oxygen content
a. oxygen saturation
palpable aortic ejection sound
a. paraganglion
pararenal aortic aneurysm
pararenal aortic atherosclerosis
a. paravalvular leak
a. patch
peak aortic flow velocity
peak systolic aortic pressure
a. penetrating ulcer
percutaneous balloon aortic valvuloplasty
perforated aortic cusp
a. perfusion
pig aortic endothelial cell
a. plexus
porcine aortic valve prosthesis
a. posterior wall
a. pressure gradient
prolapse of aortic valve
a. prominence
prosthetic aortic valve
a. pseudoaneurysm
a. pullback
a. pullback pressure
a. pulmonary
pulmonic heart sound less than aortic second heart sound
pulmonic second heart sound equal to aortic second heart sound
pulmonic second heart sound greater than aortic second heart sound
rat aortic tissue
a. reconstruction
a. reconstructive surgery
a. reflex
a. regurgitation
a. regurgitation murmur
rheumatic aortic valve disease
a. ring
a. root
a. root angiogram
a. root cineangiography
a. root diameter
a. root dilatation
a. root dimension
a. root echocardiography
a. root homograft
a. root pressure
a. root ratio
a. root reconstruction
a. root replacement
a. root velocity waveform
a. runoff
a. rupture
ruptured abdominal aortic aneurysm
a. sac
a. sclerosis
second aortic sound equals second pulmonic sound
second aortic sound greater than second pulmonic sound
second aortic sound less than second pulmonic sound
a. second sound, pulmonary second sound
a. segment
a. septal defect
a. septum
a. shag
a. sinotubular junction
a. sinus
a. sinus aneurysm
a. sinus fistula
a. sinus to right ventricle fistula
a. spindle
Stanford-type aortic dissection
a. stenosis and aortic insufficiency murmurs
a. stenosis, corneal clouding, growth and mental retardation syndrome
a. stiffness
a. stump blowout
a. sulcus
supravalvular aortic hypercalcemia syndrome
supravalvular hypertrophic aortic stenosis
a. systolic ejection murmur
a. systolic pressure
thickened aortic valve
thoracic aortic coarctation
thoracic aortic cross-clamping
thoracic aortic disease
thoracic aortic dissection
thoracoabdominal aortic aneurysm
a. thrill
a. thromboembolism

aortic *(continued)*
a. thrombosis
tortuous aortic arch
a. tract complex hypoplasia
a. transection
a. transsection
transvalvular aortic gradient
transverse aortic arch
tricuspid aortic valve
trileaflet aortic prosthesis
a. tube graft
tubular hypoplasia aortic arch
tubular hypoplasia left aortic arch
a. tunica adventitia
a. tunica intima
a. tunica media
a. valve anulus
a. valve area
a. valve atresia
a. valve calcification
a. valve cusp separation
a. valve deformity
a. valve disease
a. valve echocardiogram
a. valve echocardiography
a. valve endocarditis
a. valve insufficiency
a. valve leaflet
a. valve leaflet prolapse
a. valve lesion
a. valve nodule
a. valve obstruction
a. valve opening
a. valve opening to aortic valve closing ratio
a. valve peak instantaneous gradient
a. valve pressure gradient
a. valve prosthesis
a. valve regurgitation
a. valve repair
a. valve replacement
a. valve resistance
a. valve restenosis
a. valve sinus
a. valve stenosis
a. valve stroke volume
a. valve thickening
a. valve vegetation
a. valve velocity profile
a. valvotomy
valvular aortic disease
valvular aortic insufficiency
valvular aortic stenosis
a. valvular disease
a. valvular incompetence
a. valvular insufficiency
a. valvular stenosis
a. valvuloplasty
a. vasa vasorum
a. ventricle of heart
a. vent suction line
a. vestibule
a. vestibule of ventricle
a. wall
a. wall deterioration
a. wall necrosis
a. wall thickening
a. window
a. window node
a. wrap

aortic-brachiocephalic injury

aortic-enteric fistula

aortic-left ventricular tunnel

aorticopulmonary
major aorticopulmonary collateral arteries
a. paraganglioma
a. septal defect
a. septation
a. window
a. window defect
a. window shunt

aorticorenal
a. ganglion
a. graft

aorticosympathetic paraganglia

aortic/pulmonary

aortic-pulmonic window

aortic-superior mesenteric artery bypass

aortic-to-pulmonary shunt

aortitis
luetic a.
noninfectious a.
a. syndrome
syphilitic a.

aortoannular ectasia

aortoarteritis
transient emboligenic a.

aortobifemoral
a. bypass
a. bypass graft
a. reconstruction

aortobi-iliac bypass

aortobiprofunda femoral bypass

aortocaval fistula

aortocoronary
a. bypass
a. bypass graft
a. graft
a. valve
a. venous bypass

aortocoronary-saphenous vein bypass graft

aortocranial disease

aortoduodenal fistula

aortoenteric
a. fistula
a. fistula formation
a. graft

aortoesophageal fistula

aortofemoral
a. arteriography
a. bypass
a. bypass graft
a. bypass grafting
a. runoff

aortofemoral-femoral
descending thoracic aortofemoral-femoral bypass

aortogastric fistula

aortograft duodenal fistula

aortogram
arch a.
transbrachial arch a.
translumbar a.
a. with distal runoff

aortography
antegrade a.
arch a.
ascending a.
countercurrent a.
a. imaging
lumbar a.
postangioplasty a.
thoracic arch a.
translumbar a.

aortohepatic arterial graft

aortoiliac
a. anatomy
a. aneurysm
a. angioplasty
a. bypass
a. bypass graft
a. disease
a. inflow assessment
a. obstruction
a. occlusive disease
a. stenosis
a. thrombosis

aortoiliofemoral artery

aortojejunal fistula

aortoplasty
patch a.
subclavian flap a.
a. with patch graft

aortopulmonary
a. collateral coil embolization
a. fenestration
a. fistula
major aortopulmonary collateral artery
a. mediastinal stripe
multiple aortopulmonary collateral artery
a. septal defect
a. septum
a. transposition
a. trunk
a. window
a. window mass

aortorenal
a. bypass
a. bypass graft
a. reconstruction
a. reimplantation

aortoseptal continuity

aortosigmoid fistula

aorto-uni-iliac graft

aortovelography
transcutaneous a.
transvenous a.

aortovisceral bypass

AP-1 element

AP50 virus

APACHE-II
A.-I. point
A.-I. score
A.-I. system

Apak syndrome

apallic
a. state
a. syndrome

apathetic
a. affect
a. akinetic mutism
a. hyperthyroidism
a. thyrotoxicosis
a. withdrawal

apathetic-type personality disorder

apathy
A. gum syrup medium
a. and lack of interest in personal goals
a. syndrome

apatite
calcium apatite stone
a. calculus
carbonate apatite calculus
carbonate apatite stone
a. crystal
a. deposition disease

A-pattern
A-p. esotropia
A-p. exotropia
A-p. strabismus

APC-3 collimator

APC-4 collimator

A-P-C virus

ape
a. fissure
gibbon ape leukemia virus
gibbon ape lymphosarcoma virus
a. hand
a. hand of syringomyelia

apelike hand

aperiodic
a. biopolymer
a. complex
a. fibril
a. functional MR imaging
a. reinforcement
a. wave

aperiosteal amputation

aperistaltic
a. distal ureteral segment
a. esophagus

Apert
A. acrosyndactyly
A. disease
A. hirsutism
A. syndrome

aperta
spina bifida a.

Apert-Crouzon
A.-C. disease
A.-C. syndrome

apertognathia repair

apertural hypothesis

aperture
a.'s of abdomen
angle of a.
angular a.
aortic a.
congenital nasal pyriform aperture stenosis
a. current
a. current setting
a. diaphragm
a. disk
margin of piriform a.
a. of mastoid antrum
median a.
median aperture of fourth ventricle
nasal a.
nasal pyriform aperture stenosis
numeric a.
numerical a.
a. of orbit
orbital a.
a. pad
palpebral a.
pharyngeal a.
piriform a.
piriform aperture access
piriform aperture stenosis
a. ratio
a. of sphenoid sinus

Apeu virus

apex
a. anterior angulation
a. of arytenoid cartilage
a. of auricle
a. beat
a. of bladder
a. of brow
a. cardiogram
a. cordis
a. cornea
a. of cusp of tooth
a. of dens
a. dentis
derived value on apex cardiogram
a. dorsal angulation
a. of dorsal horn of spinal cord
a. of duodenal bulb
electronic apex locator
a. of external ring
a. of femur
a. of fibula
a. fracture
a. of head of fibula
a. of head of patella
a. of heart
a. impulse
a. of incision
a. of intussusception
a. of Koch triangle
a. of left ventricle
a. locator
a. of lung
a. nasi
a. of nose
notch of apex of heart

apex *(continued)*
notch of cardiac a.
a. of orbit
a. patellae
petrous apex mass
petrous apex tumor
a. of petrous part of temporal bone
a. of petrous portion of temporal bone
a. pin
a. plantar deformity
a. pneumonia
a. posterior angulation
a. of posterior horn
a. of posterior horn of spinal cord
a. of prism
a. prostatae
a. of prostate
a. pulmonis
a. radicis dentis
right ventricular a.
a. of sacrum
a. satyri
a. of tongue
upstroke pattern on apex cardiogram
a. of urinary bladder
a. of vagina
a. vertebra
a. vesicae

apexcardiogram
left apexcardiogram, calibrated displacement

apexcardiographic
handgrip apexcardiographic test
total apexcardiographic relaxation time index

Apfelbaum mirror

Apgar
initial Apgar score
newborn Apgar score
A. rating
A. scale
A. score

aphakia
monocular a.
pediatric a.

aphakic
a. bullous keratopathy
a. contact lens
a. correction
a. cystoid macular edema
a. detachment
a. eye
a. glaucoma
a. lens
a. pupillary block
a. retinal detachment
a. spectacles

aphalangia
partial a.

aphasia
Aachen aphasia test
acquired epileptic a.
afferent motor a.
a., agnosia, apraxia, agraphia, and alexia
Assessment of A. and Related Disorders, Second Edition
Boston Assessment of Severe A.
Boston Diagnostic A. Examination
Boston Test for Examining A.
Brief A. Screening Examination
A. Diagnostic Profiles
a. disorder
efferent motor a.
Frenchay A. Screening Test
Halstead A. Test
Language Modalities Test for A.
A. Language Performance Scale
migraine with a.
Minnesota Differential Diagnosis of A.
Minnesota Test for Differential Diagnosis of A.
motor aphasia transcortical
multilanguage a.
Multilingual A. Battery
Multilingual A. Examination
National A. Association
a. quotient
A. Screening Test
Sklar A. Scale
standard language test for a.
transcortical motor a.
Western A. Battery
Western A. Battery Test

aphasic
a. acalculia
a. agraphia
a. disturbance
a. error
fluent aphasic seizure
fluent aphasic speech
a. migraine
a. migraine headache
nonfluent aphasic seizure
nonfluent aphasic speech
a. patient
a. phonological impairment
promoting aphasics communicative effectiveness
Reitan-Indiana aphasic screening test
a. seizure

apheresis
a. catheter
low-density lipoprotein a.
a. platelet
single-donor apheresis platelet
stem cell a.

aphid lethal paralysis virus

aphonia
hysteric a.
a. paralytica
paralytica a.
a. paranoica
psychogenic a.
spastic a.

aphonic
a. episode
a. pectoriloquy

aphrasia paranoica

aphrodisiac drug

aphrodisia phrenitica

aphthae
major a.
Mikulicz a.
a. minor
oropharyngeal a.
periadenitis a.

aphthobullous stomatitis

aphthoid
a. proctocolitis
a. ulcer
a. ulceration

aphthosis
perianal a.

aphthous
a. erosion
a. fever
a. gastropathy
a. genital ulcer
a. ileal ulcer
oral aphthous ulcer
a. oral ulcer
periodic fever, aphthous stomatitis, pharyngitis, cervical adenitis
recurrent aphthous stomatitis
recurrent aphthous ulcer
a. stomach ulcer
a. stomatitis
a. ulcer

a. ulceration
a. ulitis

aphthous-type lesion

Aphthovirus
Aphthovirus A virus
Aphthovirus A virus
Aphthovirus SAT1
Aphthovirus SAT2
Aphthovirus SAT3

aphysiologic sway

apical
a. abscess
a. access
a. air space
a. angle
anterior a.
anterior apical vault defect
a. area
a. aspect
a. atelectasis
a. axillary lymph node
a. base
a. biopsy status
a. bleb
a. branch of inferior lobar branch of right pulmonary artery
a. branch of right superior pulmonary vein
a. bronchopulmonary segment
a. bronchus
a. canaliculus
a. cap
a. capping
a. cap sign
a. cardiac nodal enlargement
a. cell
a. cementum
central apical portion
a. 2-chamber
a. 2-chamber view
a. 4-chamber view
a. 2-chamber view echocardiogram
a. 4-chamber view echocardiogram
a. 5-chamber view echocardiogram
a. 2-chamber view echocardiography
a. 5-chamber view echocardiography
a. clearance
a. cochlea
a. complex
a. cone
a. corn
a. crest
a. curettage
a. curve
a. defect
a. delta
a. dendrite
a. dental foramen
a. dental ligament
a. dentin
a. distraction
double apical impulse
downward displacement of apical impulse
a. duodenal ulcer
a. ectodermal ridge
a. elevator
external apical root resorption
a. fenestration
a. fiber
first definite apical clearance lens
a. foramen
a. foramen of tooth
a. fragment ejector
a. fragment forceps
a. gland
a. granuloma
a. heave
a. hypertrophy
a. hypokinesis
a. hypoperfusion
a. impulse
a. infarction
a. infection
inferior a.
a. infiltrate
a. interventricular septal amplitude
a. iodide channel
lateral a.
a. left ventricular puncture
a. lesion
a. ligament
a. ligament of dens
a. lobe fibrosis
a. long axis
a. lordotic projection
a. lordotic view
a. lymph node
a. membrane
a. membrane of proximal convoluted tubule cell
a. middiastolic
a. mid-diastolic heart murmur
a. murmur
a. myocardial infarct
a. myocardial infarction
a. notch
a. pathosis
a. pericementitis
a. periodontal abscess
a. periodontal cyst
a. periodontitis
a. petrositis
a. pick
a. pleural stripping
a. pleural thickening
a. pneumonia
a. polar nephrectomy
a. portion of root
posterior apical radius
a. posterior artery
a. presystolic murmur
a. process
a. pulse
pulse a.
a. puncture
a. radicular cyst
a. radiolucency
a. radius
a. ramification
right ventricular a.
a. root perforation
a. root resorption
a. scarring
a. seal
a. segmental artery
a. segmental artery of superior lobar artery of right lung
a. segment of lung
septal a.
a. short-axis slice
a. sound
a. space
a. stitch
a. and subcostal four-chambered view
a. surface of heart
sustained apical impulse
a. suture
a. systolic
systolic apical impulse
a. systolic heart murmur
temporary master apical file
a. thickening
a. thickening of left ventricle
a. thinning
a. tissue
a. transportation
a. transverse
a. tumor
a. turn of the cochlea
a. vagina
a. vein
a. vertebra
a. view

apical *(continued)*
a. wall
a. wall motion
a. width
a. window
a. zip
a. zone
a. zone of cornea
apical-aortic conduit
apicalis
apical-lateral wall myocardial infarct
apically
a. directed chest tube
a. repositioned flap in mucogingival surgery
apical-radial pulse
apicomplexan parasite
apicoposterior
a. artery
a. branch of left superior pulmonary vein
a. bronchopulmonary segment
a. bronchus
a. segment
a. vein
apiculate waveform
apin-echo train
***Apis mellifera* sting**
aplanatic
a. focus
a. lens
a. objective
aplasia
acquired red-cell a.
chronic, acquired, pure red cell a.
a. cutis
a. cutis congenita
a. of deep vein
a. of dentition
germinal cell a.
idiopathic megakaryocytic a.
Leydig cell a.
membranous aplasia cutis
microphthalmia, dermal aplasia, sclerocornea syndrome
a. of optic nerve
optic nerve a.
parvovirus B19 red cell a.
pure red blood cell a.
pure red cell a.
vas deferens a.
aplastic
a. abdominal muscle syndrome
acquired aplastic anemia
acquired severe aplastic anemia
a. anemia
a. anemia syndrome
a. bone disease
a. bone disorder
a. bone lesion
a. bone marrow
constitutional aplastic anemia
a. crisis
a. crisis in hemolytic anemia
idiopathic aplastic bone marrow
a. leukemia
a. lymph
marrow
a. myelosis
a. pancytopenia
a. patella
severe aplastic anemia
transient aplastic crisis
a. uremic osteodystrophy
a. uterus
Apley
A. compression maneuver
A. compression test
A. distraction test
A. examination
A. grinding test
A. knee test
A. maneuver
A. scratch test
A. sign
A. traction
Apligraf tissue-engineered skin
apnea
alarm mattress a.
a. attack
a. and bradycardia
a., bradycardia, and cyanosis
central a.
central sleep a.
central sleep apnea syndrome
combined central and obstructive sleep a.
drowsiness from sleep a.
duration of voluntary apnea test
a. index
a. of infancy
infant apnea syndrome
infantile a.
infantile sleep a.
mixed a.
mixed sleep a.
a. monitored baby
monitored baby a.
a. neonatorum
obstructive a.
obstructive sleep a.
obstructive sleep apnea syndrome
a. of prematurity
prolonged cerebral a.
prolonged sleep a.
sleep a.
sleep apnea monitor
sleep apnea-hypersomnolence syndrome associated with upper airway obstruction
Sleep A. Quality of Life Index
symptom of a.
a. test
upper airway sleep a.
apnea/bradycardia
a. mild stimulation
a. ratio
a. self-stimulation
apnea:bradycardia ratio
apnea-hypopnea
a.-h. combination
a.-h. index
mixed obstructive apnea-hypopnea index
obstructive sleep apnea-hypopnea syndrome
apneahypoventilation
apnea-hypoventilation
obstructive sleep apnea-hypoventilation
apnea-like spell
apneic
a. event
a. infant with decreased heart rate
a. method
a. oxygenation
a. pause
a. period
a. seizure
silence of apneic episode
a. spell
a. spell associated with loud snoring
a. threshold
apneustic
a. breathing
a. center
a. period
a. respiration
ApoB-100 absence
ApoB-48 absence
ApoB gene

APOC2 region

apochromatic
a. lens
a. objective

apocrine
a. acne
a. adenocarcinoma
a. adenoma
a. adenosis
a. body odor
a. bromhidrosis
a. carcinoma
a. chromhidrosis
a. cyst
a. cystadenoma
a. duct
a. ductal carcinoma in situ
a. epithelioma
a. gland
a. gland of Moll
a. hidrocystoma
a. hyperplasia
a. malaria
a. metaplasia
a. miliaria
a. nevus
papillary apocrine change
a. poroma
a. region
a. retention cyst
a. secretion
a. sweat gland

ApoE4 gene

Apo E genotype

apoenzyme deficiency

apogeotropic nystagmus

Apoi virus

apolar
a. bond
a. cell
a. interaction

apolipoprotein
a. A-I
a. A-II
a. deficiency B
a. deficiency E
a. E epsilon 4
a. E epsilon 4 gene on chromosome 19
a. epsilon 4
a. type 3
a. B
a. B-100
a. B-48
a. B-containing lipoprotein
a. B gene
a. C-I, C-II, C-III
a. C-II
a. CII-CIII ratio
a. C-II deficiency
a. D
a. deficiency A-I
a. E
a. E epsilon 4 gene
a. epsilon
a. gene cluster
a. synthesis

Apollo
A. conjunctivitis
A. disease

apomorphine hydrochloride

aponeurogenic ptosis

aponeurosis
a. of abdominal oblique muscle
a. of biceps brachii
a. bicipitalis
a. epicranialis
external oblique a.
a. of external oblique
a. of external oblique muscle
a. of iliocostalis
a. of insertion
a. of internal oblique muscle
a. of investment
a. of musculus transversus abdominis
a. of origin
a. palatina
a. palmaris
a. pharyngea
a. plantaris
a. of plantar transverse fasciculi
a. of posterior superior serratus
a. reinsertion
a. of superior levator palpebra
a. of tendon
a. of transverse abdominal
a. of vastus muscle
a. of velum
a. of Zinn

aponeurotic
a. abscess
a. arch
a. band
a. blepharoptosis
a. closure
deep muscular aponeurotic system
a. defect
a. falx
a. fascia
a. fibroma
a. flap
a. galea
a. laxity
a. layer
a. lengthening
midline aponeurotic closure
a. musculature
a. portion of diaphragm
a. ptosis
a. reflex
submucosal aponeurotic system flap
a. tendon
a. triangle
a. troika

aponeurotica
galea a.

apoon-like protrusion of leaflet

apopathetic behavior

apophysary point

apophysial
a. complex
a. fracture
a. fracture
fused apophyseal joint
greater trochanteric apophysial arrest
a. injury
a. joint
a. joint
a. joint osteophyte
a. lesion
natural apophysial glide
obliteration of apophyseal space
open apophyseal joint
a. point
a. point
a. pouch
a. space
sustained natural apophysial glide

apophysis
a. cerebri
a. conchae
medial epicondylar a.
a. of Rau

apophysitis
olecranon a.
a. tibialis

apoplectic
a. coma
a. cyst
a. dementia
a. glaucoma
a. habit
a. hemorrhage

apoplectic *(continued)*
a. retinitis
a. type
a. vertigo

apoplectiform
a. convulsion
a. seizure

apoplexy
mesenteric a.
neonatal a.
occipital a.
parturient a.
a. of pituitary
Raymond a.
spinal a.

apoprotein A-1

apoptic
a. body
a. nuclear fragment

apoptosis
a. activating factor
a. assay
cellular inhibitors of a.
neuronal apoptosis inhibitory protein
neuronal cell a.
a. pathway
post heart attack a.
a. suppression
TNF-related apoptosis inducing ligand

apoptosis-associated molecule

apoptosis-inducing factor

apoptotic
a. bleb
a. body
a. cell
a. cell death
a. index
a. keratinocyte
neuronal apoptotic process
a. pathway
a. response
selective apoptotic antineoplastic drugs

aporic gland

apostematous cheilitis

apoT3R-mediated repression

apothecary's
a. ounce
a. weight

apotreptic therapy

AP-PA
A.-P. portal
A.-P. skull block
A.-P. skull immobilizer

apparatus
adjustable aiming a.
AO compression a.
AO contouring a.
Axer compression a.
4-bar external fixation a.
breathing a.
driver tunnel locator a.
a. extensor
eye movement measuring a.
Golgi a.
a. hyoideus
juxtaglomerular a.
a. lacrimalis
a. for maintaining pH of solution
mechanical joint a.
mitotic a.
mitotic spindle a.
mobile electroconvulsive therapy a.
Mueller compression a.
normal pilosebaceous a.
nuclear mitotic a.
optic apparatus glioma
a. of Perroncito
portable insulin dosage-regulating a.
quantitative inhalation challenge a.
rescue breathing a.
a. respiratorius
self-contained underwater breathing a.
a. urogenitalis

apparent
a. competence
a. death
a. diffuse coefficient
a. diffusion coefficient
a. digestible energy
a. digestive energy
a. distribution mass
a. exophthalmos
a. free testosterone concentration
a. half-life
a. leukonychia
a. life-threatening event
a. mineral corticoid excess syndrome
a. mineralocorticoid excess
a. mineralocorticoid excess syndrome
minimal apparent viscosity
a. net transfer rate
no apparent abnormalities
no apparent anesthetic complication
no apparent disease
no apparent disease seen in chest
in no apparent distress
no apparent distress
a. norepinephrine secretion rate
a. origin
a. oxygen utilization
a. paramagnetism
a. paresis
a. power
unexplained apparent life-threatening event
a. viscosity
a. volume of distribution

appear
adenoids did not appear enlarged
heart does appear enlarged
heart does not appear enlarged
lump in breast does appear enlarged

appearance
acromegaloid facial a.
altered facial a.
apple-peel appearance of the GI tract
apple sauce a.
asymmetric appearance time
asymmetric target a.
axon torpedo a.
bag of worms a.
candle wax appearance of bone
cockscomb appearance of cervix
coffee bean a.
congenital cataracts, sensorineural deafness, Down syndrome facial appearance, short stature, mental retardation syndrome
cord normal in a.
delusion concerning a.
a. deterioration
dirty lung a.
function, appearance, time
general a.
grape cluster a.
hemorrhagic appearance, mottled
jelly belly a.
light bulb a.
meconium ileus a.
a., mood, sensorium, intelligence, and thought process
myocardial contrast appearance time
normal in a.

normalized protein nitrogen a.
orange peel a.
owl's eye a.
Paget disease-like mosaic a.
pale facial a.
peau d'orange a.
peau d'orange appearance of the breast
peau d'orange appearance in breast carcinoma
plasma appearance rate
pruned tree a.
railroad track a.
scalloped appearance of white matter
urinary nitrogen a.

appeared
adenoids appeared enlarged
mucosa appeared inflamed

appearing
healthy appearing organ

Appelt-Gerkin-Lenz syndrome

appendage
atrial appendage juxtaposition
caudal appendage, short terminal phalanges, deafness, cryptorchidism, mental retardation syndrome
a. of eye
juxtaposition
left atrial a.
left auricular a.
right atrial a.
a. of skin
a. torsion

appendectomy
incidental a.
a. incision
laparoscopic a.
McBurney appendectomy incision
open a.
a. performed in routine fashion
a. scar
a. tape

appendiceal
a. abscess
a. adenocarcinoma
a. base
a. cancer
a. carcinoid
a. carcinoma
a. colic
a. cord
a. CT
a. fecalith
a. gangrene
a. intussusception
a. inversion
a. Kaposi sarcoma
a. lumen
a. mass
a. mesentery
a. mucocele
a. opening
a. orifice
a. perforation
a. stump
a. tissue

appendicitis
abdominal tenderness from a.
acute a.
acute gangrenous a.
acute suppurative a.
a. by contiguity
a. granulosa
indigestion from a.
a. obliterans
rule out a.
tenderness in abdomen from a.
vomiting from a.

appendicitis-like syndrome

appendicocystostomy
orthotopic a.

appendicostomy
Malone continent a.

appendicoumbilical stoma

appendicovesicostomy
Mitrofanoff a.

appendicular
a. aorta
a. artery
a. ataxia
a. bone mass measurement
a. colic
a. disease
a. dyspepsia
a. lymph node
a. muscle
a. sign
a. skeletal muscle
a. skeleton
a. tuberculosis
a. vein

appendiculares
lymphonodus a.
nodi lymphoidei a.

appendix
acutely inflamed a.
base of a.
a. brought into surgical incision
bury stump of a.
a. ceci
a. cerebri
a. dyspepsia
a. epididymidis
a. of epididymis
a. epiploica
a. fibrosa
focused appendix computed tomography
a. freed up
a. of laryngeal ventricle
a. ligated and amputated
ligation of a.
lumen of a.
mesentery of a.
a. of Morgagni
a. mucocele
obstruction of a.
perforated gangrenous a.
perforated retrocecal a.
removal of vermiform a.
a. rupture
a. testis
a. testis torsion
a. of ventricle of larynx
a. vermiform
a. vermiformis
a. vesiculosa

apperception
auditory apperception test
Children's A. Test-Human
Children's A. Test, Supplemental
Education A. Test
Family A. Test
Pain A. Test
Robert A. Test for Children
Senior A. Technique
Senior A. Test
a. test
thematic apperception test
visual apperception test
Vocational A. Test

apperceptive
a. agnosia
Children's A. Story-Telling Test
a. disorder
a. distortion
a. mass
a. prosopagnosia
a. visual agnosia

appetite
altered a.
change in a.
a. control
decrease in a.
decreased appetite and loss of energy

appetite *(continued)*
diminished a.
a. disorder
a. disturbance
fatigue and loss of a.
good a.
inability to control a.
increased a.
increased energy, decreased a.
increased sexual a.
insomnia, hyperactivity and decreased a.
a. juice
a. for life
a. loss
loss of appetite from gastritis
loss of appetite from heart failure
loss of appetite from hepatitis
loss of appetite with indigestion
loss of appetite with joint swelling
a. loss from pernicious anemia
loss of interest, appetite and concentration
patient's appetite is good
patient's appetite is poor
poor a.
a. psychogenic disorder
a. stimulant
a. suppressant
a. suppression
voracious a.

appetitive
a. behavior
a. center
a. disturbance
a. drive
a. phase
a. state

applanation
carotid applanation tonometry
a. pressure
a. tension
tension by a.
tonometry by a.
a. tonometry

apple
Adam's a.
a. jelly nodule
a. jelly papule of lupus vulgaris
May a.
May apple root
a. oil
a. pattern
a. sauce appearance

apple-core
a.-c. appearance
a.-c. carcinoma
a.-c. lesion
a.-c. tumor

apple-green birefringence

apple-peel
a.-p. appearance
a.-p. appearance of the GI tract
a.-p. atresia
a.-p. bowel
a.-p. bowel syndrome

applesauce
a. appearance
a., bananas, and cereal diet
bananas, rice cereal, applesauce, toast diet
bananas, rice, applesauce, tea, toast diet
bananas, rice, applesauce, toast diet

apple-shape body

appliance
Angle basic E arch a.
external cooling a.
lip habit a.
mandibular advancement a.
mandibular orthopedic repositioning a.
microstomia prevention a.
a. modification
occlusal appliance therapy
oral a.
oral appliance therapy
palatal expansion a.
passive alveolar molding a.
soft ankle, cushioned heel orthopaedic a.

application
arch bar a.
autologous serum a.
nonionizing nonthermal a.
open application test
point of a.
premarket approval a.
topical fluoride a.
a. of traction device

application-specific integrated circuit

applicator
aneurysm clip a.
Ernst radium a.
global force a.
intracavitary gynecologic a.
laryngotracheal a.
Multifire clip a.
multiple-site perineal applicator technique
Plummer-Vinson radium a.

applied
a. anatomy
a. anthropology
a. behavior analysis
a. chemistry
dressing and stockinette a.
dry sterile dressing a.
electrodes applied over cerebral cortex
a. extrasensory projection
eye pad and shield a.
gentle pressure bandage a.
heavy clamp a.
a. kinesiology
a. linguistics
a. load
a. phonetics
pressure dressing a.
a. psychoanalysis
a. psychology
a. relaxation
a. research
sterile drapes a.
sterile dressing a.
a. tourniquet
traction applied to extremity

applier
bulldog clamp a.
cotton-tipped a.

appliqué form

apply
a. to affected area
does not a.

Appolito
A. operation
A. suture
A. suture technique

apposing articular surface

apposition
a. and alignment
alignment and a.
central choroidal a.
a. of leaflet
margin of a.
margins of wound brought into a.
a. of skull suture
a. suture
a. suture technique

appositional
a. crystal proliferation
a. growth

appraisal
clinical appraisal of psychosocial problem
conflict management a.
health appraisal examination
health risk a.
a. of language disturbances
Management A. Survey

appreciable
no appreciable change
some appreciable change

apprehension
anterior apprehension test
anxiety and a.
a. expectation
patellar apprehension sign
patellar apprehension test
a. shoulder
a. sign
a. span
a. state
a. test

apprehensive
nervous and a.

apprentice
hospital a.
a. kyphosis

approach
aggressive surgical a.
anterior acromioplasty a.
anterior axillary a.
anterior cervical approach to cervicothoracic junction
anterior extensile a.
anterior interhemispheric a.
anterior retroperitoneal flank a.
anterior sternomastoid a.
anterior transabdominal a.
anterior transhepatic a.
anterior transthoracic a.
anterior triangle a.
anteromedial retropharyngeal a.
assertive-community treatment a.
Aufranc lateral a.
a. avoidance
axillary subpectoral a.
basal interhemispheric a.
cognitive behavioral a.
cognitive skills training a.
complementary and alternative a.
far lateral inferior suboccipital a.
a. gradient
gradient of a.
integrative neurobehavioral a.
language experience a.
long deltopectoral a.
low cervical a.
McConnell extensile a.
medial extradural a.
middle cranial fossa a.
middle fossa a.
middle fossa craniotomy a.
middle fossa transtentorial translabyrinthine a.
moisture fear-molar a.
multidisciplinary team a.
new approaches to brain tumor therapy
new approaches to coronary intervention
Ollier arthrodesis a.
pars plana a.
percutaneous femoral a.
posterior fossa a.
practical approach design

approach-approach conflict

approach-avoidance
a.-a. conflict
a.-a. stance
a.-a. theory

appropriate
a. affect
age a.
a. behavior
a. blood pressure cuff size
a. culture
a. disability
a. facial expression
full-term appropriate for gestational age
a. in gender
a. for gestational age
a. goal
a. learning experience
a. level of care
a. medical attention
multiples of the appropriate gestational median
a. nutritional supplementation
premature appropriate for gestational age
a. reduction
a. relationship
a. resection
a. response
term birth appropriate for gestational age
a. treatment

appropriately
answers questions a.

appropriateness
a. of emotional response
a. evaluation protocol
Managed Care A. Protocol

approval
Continuing Education A. and Recognition Program
emergency department approval for pediatrics
a. loss
premarket approval application

approved
British approved name
a. dietary allowance
a. drug product

approximal surface of tooth

approximate
a. answers syndrome
a. entropy
a. lethal concentration
a. skin edges
syndrome of approximate relevant answers
a. wound edges

approximated
breast tissue approximated with ties
internal oblique a.
subcutaneous tissues a.
wound loosely a.

approximating closure

approximation
a. conditioning
a. of cutaneous edges
glans approximation procedure
healing with a.
a. method
method of a.
a. suture
a. suture technique

approximator
clamp a.
a. clamp
nerve a.

apraxia
aphasia, agnosia, apraxia, agraphia, and alexia
a. battery
A. Battery for Adults
congenital ocular motor a.
developmental apraxia of speech
a. of eyelid opening
a. of gaze

apraxia *(continued)*
ideational a.
muscle atrophy-contracture-oculomuscle apraxia syndrome
ocular motor a.
A. Profile: A Descriptive Assessment Tool for Children

apraxia-ataxia-mental deficiency syndrome

apraxia-oculomotor contracture-muscle atrophy syndrome

apraxic
a. agraphia
a. behavior
a. disorder
a. dysarthria
a. gait
a. impairment

aprismatic enamel

apron
a. band
a. flap
a. flap procedure
lead apron shield
lingual a.
omental a.
a. pattern
a. shield
a. skin incision
a. U-shaped incision

apropulsive gait

aprosencephaly-atelencephaly syndrome

aprosencephaly syndrome

aprosody of speech

aprotic solvent

APRT deficiency

Apt-Downey
A.-D. alkali denaturation test
A.-D. test

aptitude
academic aptitude test
activity interest and a.
a. battery
Blind Learning Aptitude Test
Computer Operator A. Battery
Computer Programmer A. Battery
dental aptitude test
Detroit Tests of Learning A. - Primary, Second Edition
Detroit Tests of Learning A., Third Edition
Differential A. Test
Flanagan A. Classification Test
flight aptitude rating
General A. Test Battery
Guilford-Zimmerman A. Survey
Hiskey-Nebraska Test of Learning A.
a. inventory
Iowa Algebra A. Test
knowledge, a.'s, and practices
Manipulative A. Test
mechanical a.
Minnesota Clerical A. Test
Minnesota Scholastic A. Test
Musical A. Profile
Non-Reading A. Test Battery
Scholastic A. Test
Short Form Test of Academic A.
spatial a.
Special A. Test Battery
a. test
thematic aptitude test

apurinic acid

apyretic
a. tetanus
a. typhoid

apyrimidinic acid

aqua
a. oculi
a. PT dry physiotherapy
a. PT water massage

aquagenic
a. pruritus
a. urticaria

Aquaplast
A. alloplastic material
A. dressing

aquaporin-2 water channel

aquarium granuloma

aquatic
a. cardiac evaluation and testing
a. exercise
a. exercise program
a. rehabilitation
a. stabilization program
a. therapy
a. therapy pool
vertical float progression aquatic therapy
vertical float aquatic therapy

aqueduct
cerebral a.
a. of cerebrum
a. compression
enlarged vestibular aqueduct syndrome
gliosis of cerebral a.
hydrocephalus due to congenital stenosis of aqueduct of Sylvius
a. of midbrain
nonsyndromic familial enlarged vestibular a.
opening of aqueduct of midbrain
opening of cerebral a.
a. stenosis
a. of Sylvius
a. veil
vestibular aqueduct syndrome
a. of vestibule

aqueductal
a. CSF stroke volume
a. forking
a. gliosis
a. intubation
a. jet
a. obstruction
a. occlusion
a. plasty
a. stenosis
X-linked aqueductal stenosis

aqueductus
a. cerebri
a. cochlea
a. mesencephali
a. sylvii
a. vestibuli

aqueous
a. analysis
angular aqueous sinus plexus
a. procaine penicillin G
Ascher aqueous influx phenomenon
a. beclomethasone
budesonide aqueous nasal spray
a. chamber
a. cocaine
a. electron
a. extract
a. flare
a. flare response
a. flow
flow of aqueous humor
a. formaldehyde
fortified aqueous solution
a. humor
a. humor deficiency
a. humor drainage
a. humor eye
a. humor of the eye
a. inflow
a. influx phenomenon
a. layer of tear film
a. methyl cellulose

a. misdirected glaucoma
a. misdirection
a. mounting medium
a. outflow
a. paracentesis
penicillin G, parenteral, a.
a. phase
a. phenol
a. procaine penicillin
a. solution
sterile aqueous solution
sterile aqueous suspension
a. synthetic dual phenolic disinfectant
a. tear deficiency
a. tear layer
a. vaccine
a. vasopressin
a. vein

aqueous-influx phenomenon

arabic
a. acid
A. eye test

arabinose
a. fermentation test
a. operon

arabinoside
adenine a.
adenine arabinoside monophosphate

arabitol test

ara-C
a.-C + ADR
a.-C and Adriamycin
a.-C, daunorubicin, etoposide
a.-C, daunorubicin, prednisolone, mercaptopurine
a.-C + DNR + PRED + MP
a.-C + HU
a.-C and Platinol
a.-C plus 6-thioguanine
a.-C, VP-16, leucovorin

arachic acid

arachidic
a. acid
a. bronchitis

arachidonate-induced platelet aggregation

arachidonate metabolism

arachidonic
a. acid
a. acidristocetin
a. acid cascade
a. acid cascade inhibitor
a. acid level
a. acid metabolism
a. acid metabolite
a. acid oxidation
a. acid pathway
a. bronchitis

arachis oil

arachnid envenomation

arachnidism
necrotic a.

arachnodactyly
a. CHD
congenital contractural a.

arachnoid
a. adhesion
a. of brain
a. brain cyst
a. canal
a. cell
a. cyst
a. cyst of the middle fossa
a. diverticulum
a. fibrosis
a. foramen
a. granulation
a. granulation calcification
a. granulation villi
a. hemorrhage
a. layer
leptomeningeal arachnoid cyst
a. loculation of the spine
lumbar arachnoid peritoneal shunt
a. mater
a. mater cranialis
a. mater and pia mater
a. membrane
meningothelial arachnoid cell
a. nerve root sheath dilation
perineural arachnoid cyst
pia a.
a. plane
posterior fossa extra-axial arachnoid cyst
a. retrocerebellar pouch
a. sheath
a. sleeve
a. space
a. of spinal cord
a. spine cyst
a. tissue
a. trabecula
a. trabeculation
a. of uncus
a. villi
a. villi obstruction
a. villus

arachnoidal
a. cyst
a. foramen
a. gliomatosis
a. hyperplasia
a. root sleeve
a. sheet

arachnoidea
a. mater
a. mater cranialis
a. mater et pia mater

arachnoideus
nevus a.

arachnoiditis
neoplastic a.
obliterative a.
opticochiasmatic a.
a. of opticochiasmatic cistern
optochiasmatic a.
ossifying a.

arachnophlebectomy
a. needle
a. surgical device

Araki-Sako technique

araldehyde-tanned bovine carotid artery graft

Arana-Iniquez intracranial cyst removal technique

Arandel cell harvester

Aran-Duchenne
A.-D. amyotrophy
A.-D. disease
A.-D. muscular atrophy
A.-D. muscular dystrophy

araneus
nevus a.

Aransas Bay virus

Arantius
A. body
A. canal
canal of A.
A. duct
A. ligament

Arbaud
Grand Arbaud virus

Arbia virus

arbitrarily primer

arbitrarily-primed polymerase chain reaction

arbitrary
a. blockout

arbitrary *(continued)*
multiple arbitrary amplicon profiling
PCR with arbitrary primer
a. primed PCR
a. unit
a. valve unit

arbitrary-primed
a.-p. PCR
a.-p. polymerase chain reaction

Arboledas virus

Arbor
Ann Arbor cancer staging
Ann Arbor classification
Ann Arbor classification of Hodgkin disease staging
Ann Arbor double towel clamp
Ann Arbor Hodgkin lymphoma stage I, IE, II, IIE, IIIE, IIIS, IIISE, IV
Ann Arbor staging classification
Ann Arbor tumor classification

arbor
a. vitae
a. vitae cerebelli
a. vitae tree
a. vitae uterus

arborescens
lipoma a.

arborescent
a. cataract
a. keratitis
a. white substance of cerebellum

arborization
axonal a.
a. block
a. of duct
a. of ducts
a. pattern

arborizing pattern

arboviral
a. encephalitis
a. infection
a. meningoencephalitis
a. virus disease

arbovirus
a. group unclassified
a. infection
a. meningoencephalitis

arbovirus-associated arthritis

Arbuthnot Lane disease

arc
alpha a.
auricular a.
a. and bowl perimeter
a. burn
carbon arc lamp
a. of contact
coronal arc technique
a. de cercle
longitudinal arc of skull
mercury a.
mercury arc lamp
mobile a.
a. of motion
neural a.
noncoplanar arc technique
nuclear a.
painful arc sign
painful arc syndrome
a. perimetry
a. radiotherapy
a. radius system
a. ring
Riolan a.
a. of rotation
a. of rotation of fasciocutaneous flap
a. scotoma
a. staining
a. therapy
a. therapy technique
a. welder's lung
a. welding
xenon arc laser
xenon arc light

arcade
anomalous mitral a.
arterial a.
a. of Frohse
limbal a.
lower dental a.
lumbar a.
major a.
mandibular dental a.
marginal a.
maxillary dental a.
mesenteric a.
mitral a.
pancreaticoduodenal arcade vessel
pancreaticoduodenal arterial a.
peripheral arterial a.
Riolan a.
a. of Struthers
temporal a.
vascular a.

arcading effect

arcanobacterial pharyngitis

arc-beam pattern

arc-centered guidance system

Arcelin view

arc-flash conjunctivitis

arch
a. alignment
alveolar arch acrylic splint
alveolar arch derangement
alveolar arch of mandible
alveolar arch of maxilla
a. angle
Angle basic E arch appliance
anterior arch of atlas
anterior arch length
anterior arch width
anterior atlas a.
anterior metatarsal a.
anterior palatine a.
a. of aorta
a. of aorta abnormality
aortic a.
aortic arch aneurysm
aortic arch angiography
aortic arch anomaly
aortic arch anomaly-peculiar facies mental retardation syndrome
aortic arch atresia
aortic arch calcification
aortic arch coarctation
aortic arch disease
aortic arch interruption
aortic arch lesion
aortic arch malformation
aortic arch obstruction
aortic arch rupture
a. aortogram
a. aortography
arterial arch of colon
arterial arch of ileum
arterial arch of jejunum
arterial arch of lower eyelid
arterial arch of upper eyelid
a. of atlas
available arch length
axillary arch muscle
a. bar application
a. bar fixation
a. bar frame
a. binder
a. of bone
a. cookie
cortical arch of kidney
cricoid a.
a. of cricoid cartilage
a. of Cupid
a. cushion
a. discrepancy
double aortic a.

a. of fauces
a. of foot
a. form
a. fracture
a. of Frohse
high arch deformity
ideal arch wire
a. index
a. insole pad
interrupted aortic a.
interruption of aortic a.
jugular venous a.
a. length
a. length deficiency
a. length index
a. loading
longitudinal arch of foot
longitudinal arch support
mandibular arch bar
mandibular branchial a.
Martorell aortic arch syndrome
maxilla
medial longitudinal a.
medial lumbocostal a.
mental retardation, congenital contracture, low fingertip arches syndrome
Nance analysis of arch length
narrow pubic a.
neural arch cleft
neural arch defect
neural arch fracture
neural arch joint
neural arch resection technique
neural arch of vertebra
node of azygos a.
noncoplanar arch technique
orbital arch of frontal bone
a. of palate
palmar arterial a.
partially edentulous dental a.
a. peak area
pedicle of arch of vertebra
perforating branch of deep palmar a.
a. perimeter
a. perimeter analysis
plantar arch support orthosis
posterior arch vein
right aortic a.
a. of Riolan
a. rupture
a. and slouch position
superior dental a.
tendinous arch of levator ani
tendinous arch of pelvic fascia
tendinous arch of soleus muscle
thoracic arch aortography
a. of thoracic duct
tortuous aortic a.
transbrachial arch aortogram
transverse aortic a.
tubular hypoplasia aortic a.
tubular hypoplasia left aortic a.
a. of vertebra
vertebral arch defect
a. width
a. width analysis
Winter arch bar
a. wire
xenon arch photocoagulator

archaic
a. brain
a. inheritance
a. residue
a. thought

archaic-paralogical thinking

arch-and-slouch position

arched
a. crest
a. lower back

archenteric canal

archeological excavation

Archer lesion

archer's shoulder

arch-height
a.-h. index
a.-h. ratio

Archimedes spiral

arching of mitral valve leaflet

architectural
a. alterations of bone
a. barrier
a. disorder
a. distortion
a. disturbance
a. effacement
a. pattern
a. sheeting
a. symmetry

architecture
bony a.
a. of the brain
a. of brain
histologic a.
lobular a.
lobular architecture of liver
loculated a.
loss of normal a.
lung a.
mural a.
nasal a.
neural a.
pelvic a.
sleep a.
systems network a.

archival
picture archival communication system
a. system
a. tissue

arch-loop-whorl system

arch-up test

archwire
anterior retraction a.

arciform
a. artery
a. density
a. distribution of lesion
a. fiber
a. lesion
a. vein
a. vein of kidney
a. wave

arcing spring

Arco classification

arcon
a. articulator
a. semiadjustable articulator

arctic anemia

arcuate
anterior external arcuate fiber
a. aorta
a. artery
a. artery of foot
a. artery of kidney
a. Bjerrum scotoma
a. commissure
a. complex
a. course
a. crest
a. crest of arytenoid cartilage
a. eminence
a. fasciculus
a. fiber
a. fiber of cerebrum
a. fiber involvement
a. fibers
a. field defect
a. foramen
a. hypothalamus
a. incision
a. ligament
a. ligament of Clifford
a. ligament of diaphragm

arcuate *(continued)*
a. ligament of pubis
a. line
a. line of Douglas
a. line of ilium
a. line of rectus sheath
medial arcuate ligament
median arcuate ligament
median arcuate ligament of diaphragm
monocular temporal arcuate defect
a. movement
myometrial arcuate artery
a. nerve fiber bundle
a. nucleus
a. nucleus of brain
a. nucleus of the hypothalamus
a. nucleus of thalamus
a. osteotomy
a. popliteal ligament
a. pubic ligament
a. retinal fold
a. staining
a. suture technique
a. transverse keratotomy
a. uterus
a. vein
a. vein of kidney
a. vessel
a. visual field defect
a. zone

arcuatus
nucleus a.
nucleus arcuatus of intermediate hypothalamic area
nucleus arcuatus medullae oblongatae
nucleus arcuatus of medulla oblongata
nucleus arcuatus thalami
pes a.
pes arcuatus clawfoot deformity
a. uterus

arc-welder's disease

Arden grating

ardent
a. fever
a. spirit

area
a. of abnormal density
accelerated growth a.
a. acustica
to affected a.'s
anterior amygdaloid a.
anterior hypothalamic a.
anterior hypothalamic preoptic area
anterior intercondylar a.
anterior intercondylar area of tibia
anterior limbic association a.
Antoni A, B a.
aortic area of auscultation
aortic area of auscultation
aortic valve a.
apply to affected a.
arch peak a.
aspheric lenticular a.
Assessment of Adaptive A.'s
Atopic Dermatitis A. and Severity Index
atrophy in shoulder a.
auditory association a.
auditory cortical a.
auditory projection a.
average orifice a.
bearing area hair
biopsy of area taken
body surface a.
a. of bony destruction
brightness area product
calculated opening a.
carcinoma with adenomatous a.'s
a. of cardiac dullness
central chemosensitive a.
a. centralis
circumoral area of columnar epithelium
a. cochlea
concentrated care a.
a. of concern
a. of conscious regard
a. correction factor
cortical motor a.
a. cribrosa
a. cribrosa papillae renalis
critical care a.
a. of critical definition
cross-sectional a.
dead area of heart muscle
a. of denudation
a. diastolic pressure
discrete area of consolidation
discrete area of effusion
dose area product
Eczema A. and Severity Index
effective balloon-dilated a.
effective orifice a.
eloquent areas of brain
eloquent versus noneloquent a.
emergency a.
end-diastolic a.
epidemiologic catchment a.
a. for esophagus
a. of facial nerve
fibrin plate lysis a.
first auditory a.
focal area of hemorrhage
focal area of hyperemia
focal areas of intrapulmonary hemorrhage
focal areas of lymphoid infiltrate
follicular a.
a. of Forel
fractional area change
fractional area concentration
gastric cancerous a.
gastric noncancerous a.
gastrointestinal diagnostic a.
hand washing in critical care a.
a. health authority
a. health education center
health in underserved rural a.'s
hemorrhagic area, mottled
holding a.
hyaline acellular a.
hypoechoic area of ultrasound
a. of increased activity
a. of increased density
a. of increased pigmentation
a. of increased radiolabeling
a. of increased uptake
infected a.
inflammation within affected a.
a. of innervation
a. of interest magnification
intermediate care a.
internal surface a.
a. of intertrigo
intrastent minimal lumen cross-sectional a.
irrigated
jet a.
labyrinth area hammer
a. of Laimer
lateral hypothalamic a.
lateral preoptic a.
a. lavaged with sterile saline
left ventricular end-diastolic a.
left ventricular end-systolic a.
limbic midbrain a.
local area communications network
lytic area bone flap
a. Martegiani
mass transfer area coefficient
maximal noise a.
medial canthus a.
medial preoptic a.

medial superior temporal visual a.
medial temporal visual a.
mesial contact a.
metropolitan statistical a.
midarm fat a.
midarm muscle a.
middle temporal visual a.
minimal cross-sectional a.
mitral valve a.
mitral valve orifice a.
MST visual a.
MT visual a.
multifocal area of hyperintensity
nasal cross-sectional a.
National Association of A. Agencies on Aging
neocortical association a.
a. nervi facialis
neutral or gray a.
node bearing area of lymph nodes
noncontractile a.
normalized area under the curve
nucleus arcuatus of intermediate hypothalamic a.
nucleus of pretectal a.
occipital association cortical a.
open care a.
operative area irrigated with antibiotic solution
operative area irrigated with normal saline
osteoid a.
oval area of Flechsig
Paget disease of perianal a.
painful, inflamed a.
Panum fusion a.
paracentral gray a.
parietal association a.
a. parolfactoria
patchy area of bronchopneumonia
patchy area of consolidation
patchy area of density
patchy area of fibrosis
patchy area of pneumonia
patchy area of pneumonic consolidation
percussion of suprapubic a.
periaqueductal gray a.
permeability a.
popliteal node a.
postanesthesia recovery a.
posterior hypothalamic a.
postoperative holding a.
a. postrema
precoronary care a.
preoperative holding a.
a. preoptica
preoptic anterior hypothalamic a.
presumed circle area ratio
a. pretectalis
proximal isovelocity surface a.
proximal subcontact a.
psoriasis area sensitivity index
psoriasis area and severity index
pulmonary valve a.
punctate area of increased signal
radiation emergency a.
radiographic lung a.
raw area under curve
real-time dose area product
a. of recent hemorrhage
regurgitant jet a.
regurgitant orifice a.
relative area of cardiac dullness
relative medullary area of kidney
restore tissue to affected a.
a. retrochiasmatica
a. sampling
a. scar
second auditory a.
seizure-producing areas of brain
sewing ring a.
shade response to light gray a.
shading response to black a.'s
shading response to gray a.'s
standard metropolitan statistical a.
stimulation of trigger a.
a. of strength and weakness
a. of stricture
a. subcallosa
supplemental motor a.
supplementary motor a.
surface a.
surface area to volume ratio
a. systolic pressure
target area under the curve
total body surface a.
total burn surface a.
total graft area rejected
transverse fascicular a.
a. under the curve
a. under curve
a. under pH4
upper abdominal a.
a. ventralis of Tsai
ventral tegmental a.
a. vestibularis
a. vestibularis superior
xenograph surface a.

area/hemidiameter variation

areal
a. bone mineral density
a. density
a. stimulation

area-length
a.-l. method
a.-l. method for ejection fraction

areata
alopecia a.
ophiasic alopecia a.

areca nut

areflexia
detrusor a.

areflexic
a. bladder
a. paraparesis

aregenerative anemia

Arelin method

arena
association a.

Arenaviridae virus

arenavirus infection

Arenberg-Denver implant

areola
a. of bone
a. of breast
a. mammae
nevoid hyperkeratosis of nipple and a.
a. of nipple
a. papillaris
a. reduction
Wise areola mastopexy breast augmentation

areolar
a. central choroiditis
a. choroiditis
a. choroidopathy
a. complex
a. connective tissue
a. demarcation
a. enlargement
a. gingiva
a. gland
a. grafting
a. incision
loose areolar plane
a. mastopexy
a. plane
a. reconstruction
simultaneous areolar mastopexy and breast augmentation
a. thickening
a. tissue

areolar *(continued)*
a. tubercles
a. venous plexus
areolomammary complex
Arey rule
argentaffin
a. carcinoid tumor
a. cell
a. granule
Masson argentaffin stain
a. reaction
a. reaction test
a. stain
a. staining
Argentinian hemorrhagic fever
argentophilic plaque
arginase
a. deficiency
a. deficiency aminoaciduria
arginine
a. analog
antidiuretic arginine vasopressin V2 receptor
a., hypoxanthine, and uracil
a. codon
cyclic arginine monophosphate
a. deiminase
a. glutamate
a. hydrochloride
a., hypoxanthine, and uracil
a. infusion test
a. monohydrochloride
neonatal arginine vasopressin
a. oxytocin
a. stimulation test
a. test
a. vasopressin
a. vasopressin regulation
a. vasopressor precursor
a. vasotocin
arginine-insulin
a.-i. stimulation test
a.-i. tolerance test
argininosuccinate
a. lyase
a. lyase assay
a. lysate
a. synthetase
a. synthetase deficiency
argininosuccinic
a. acidemia
a. acid lyase
a. acid synthase deficiency
a. acid synthetase deficiency
a. aminoaciduria
arginosuccinate lyase deficiency
arginosuccinic acid
Argo corn starch test
argon
a. beam coagulation
a. beam coagulator
a. beam plasma coagulation
a. destruction
a. diode
a. fluoride
a. gas
a. ion
a. ionization detector
a. ion plasma coagulation
a. laser
a. laser coagulator
a. laser endophotocoagulation
a. laser-induced scar
a. laser iridectomy
a. laser iridotomy
a. laser peripheral iridoplasty
a. laser photocoagulation
a. laser therapy
a. laser trabeculectomy
a. laser trabeculopexy
a. laser trabeculoplasty
light argon laser burn
Ophthalas argon laser
panretinal argon laser photocoagulation
a. plasma coagulator
a. tuneable dye laser
yttrium, argon, garnet
argon-fluoride excimer laser
argon-krypton laser
argon-pumped
a.-p. dye laser
a.-p. tunable-dye laser
Argonz-Del Castillo syndrome
argument
semantic a.
Argyle
A. anti-reflux valve
A. arterial catheter
A. catheter
A. chest tube
Argyle-Salem sump tube
Argyll-Robertson
A.-R. instrument
A.-R. operation
A.-R. pupil
A.-R. pupil sign
A.-R. suture technique
argyophobic
argyrophilic and argyophobic neuron
argyria
local a.
argyrophil
a. cell
a. organizer region protein
a. plaque
a. stain
argyrophilic
a. and argyophobic neuron
a. cell
a. collagen fiber
a. ductal carcinoma in situ
a. fiber
a. fibril
a. granule
a. nucleolar organizer region
a. nucleolar organizer region staining
a. stain
Aria coronary bypass
Arias-Stella
A.-S. cell
A.-S. effect
A.-S. phenomenon
A.-S. reaction
Arias syndrome
Aries-Pitanguy
A.-P. breast reduction
A.-P. mammaplasty
A.-P. operation
A.-P. procedure
A-ring
aromatic A-r.
Arion
A. operation
A. sling
aristolochic acid
aristotelian method
Aristotle anomaly
arithmetic
A., Coding, Information, and Digit Span
completion, arithmetic problems, vocabulary, following directions
a. disorder
functioning, reasoning, orientation, memory, arithmetic, judgment, and emotion
a. grade equivalent
a. and logic unit
a. mean

mental arithmetic test
a. method
a. problem
a. progression
a. sign
a. subtest

arithmetical
a. developmental delay disorder
a. reasoning
a. skills learning retardation

Arizona
A. ankle brace
A. Articulation Proficiency Scale
A. ash
A. ash tree
A. Battery for Communication Disorders of Dementia
A. Cancer Center multiple myeloma staging system
A. coral snake
A. cypress
A. cypress tree
Arizona organism

Arizona/Fremont
A. cottonwood
A. cottonwood tree

Arkansas stone

Arkless-Graham syndrome

Arkonam virus

Arlt
A. disease
A. epicanthus repair
A. eyelid repair
A. lens
A. line
A. operation
A. pterygium
A. pterygium excision
A. recess
A. scoop
A. sinus
A. suture technique
A. trachoma
A. triangle

Arlt-Jaesche
A.-J. excision
A.-J. operation
A.-J. recess
A.-J. sinus
A.-J. trachoma

arm
anterior compartment of a.
augmented voltage unipolar left arm lead
augmented voltage unipolar right arm lead
a. band
blood pressure, right a.
a. bone
chest and left a.
chest and right a.
a. of chromosome
a. circumference
a. clasp
crook of the a.
a. cuff
a. cylinder cast
deletion of long arm of chromosome X
deletion of short arm of chromosome X
disabilities of the arm, shoulder, and hand
a. drift
a. duration maneuver
a. dysfunction
a. dystonia
end of short arm of chromosome
extended lateral arm free flap
extensor compartment of a.
a. flap
a. fossa test
functional arm brace
Gait, a.'s, Legs, and Spine
a. girth, chest depth, and hip width
grenade thrower's a.
a. hair
head, arms, and trunk
a. heel-strike synchrony
high-dose a.
a. holder
immobilization of injured a.
left arm electrode for electrocardiogram
left arm hemiparesis
left arm, reclining
left arm, recumbent
left arm, sitting
left upper a.
long arm brace
long arm cast
long arm of chromosome
long arm of chromosome X
long arm finger cast
long arm navicular cast
long arm posterior-molded splint
long arm of Y chromosome
low-dose a.
lower lateral cutaneous nerve of a.
mean arm muscle circumference
medial cutaneous nerve of a.
middle upper arm circumference
mobile arm support
movement arm vector
a. muscle circumference
nonsupported arm exercise
numbness in a.
numbness of a.
numbness, weakness and paralysis of a.
overhead movement of a.
pain down left a.
pain down right a.
pain spreading to a.
a. phenomenon
a. position
a. positioner
posterior compartment of a.
posterior cutaneous nerve of a.
a. presentation
a. raises maneuver
a. recoil
red patch or blister on a.
right a.
right arm electrode for electrocardiogram
right arm hemiparesis
right arm reclining
right arm recumbent
right arm, sitting
right lower a.
short arm brace
short arm of chromosome X
short arm cylinder cast
short arm fiberglass cast
short arm navicular cast
short arm plaster splint
short arm posterior-molded splint
short arm sugar-tong splint
short arm thumb spica cast
a. and shoulder
shoulder arm system
a. skate
a. span
spasticity of a.
a. straighten maneuver
supported arm exercise
a. swathe
total arm length
unsupported arm exercise
upper a.
upper arm flap
upper arm tourniquet
vaccination scar upper left a.
a. weakness

Armaly-Drance technique

armamentarium
occlusal adjustment a.
periodontal a.
Armand-Frappier strain
arm-ankle index
Armanni-Ebstein
A.-E. cell
A.-E. change
A.-E. disease
A.-E. kidney
A.-E. lesion
Armanni-Ehrlich degeneration
armchair splint
arm-down image
armed
a. combat
a. macrophage
a. rostellum
arm-extension position
arm-implanted subcutaneous reservoir-catheter system
Armistead
A. technique
A. ulnar lengthening operation
Armitage-Cochran test
armitage-doll model
arm-leg gradient
arm-lung time
armored heart
Armstrong
A. acromionectomy
A. disease
A. plate
A. prosthesis
A. tube
A. tube line
arms-up positioning
arm-tongue time test
arm-up image
Army
A. Alpha test
A. Beta test
A. General Classification Test
Arndorfer capillary perfusion system
Arndt-Gottron
A.-G. disease
A.-G. syndrome
Arndt law
Arneth
A. classification
A. count
A. formula
A. index
A. stage
Arning tincture
Arnold
auricular nerve of A.
A. body
A. bundle
A. canal
A. convolution
foramen of A.
A. ganglion
A. nerve
A. nerve reflex cough syndrome
A. tract
Arnold-Chiari
A.-C. anomaly
A.-C. deformity
A.-C. malformation
A.-C. syndrome
Arnold-Healy-Gordon syndrome
Aroa virus
aromatase
a. deficiency
a. enzyme complex
a. gene
a. inhibition
a. inhibitor
a. inhibitor testolactone
nonsteroidal aromatase inhibitor
P450 aromatase placental deficiency
aromatic
a. acid decarboxylase
a. amine
a. amino acid
a. amino acid decarboxylase
a. D-amino acid decarboxylase
a. ammonia spirit
a. A-ring
a. bitters
a. castor oil
a. compound
heterocyclic aromatic amine
a. hydrocarbon
a. L-amino acid decarboxylase
polycyclic aromatic hydrocarbon
polynuclear aromatic hydrocarbon
a. ring
a. series
a. solvent-induced shift
a. water
aromatization
peripheral a.
Aronson-Prager technique
around
adhesions of pericardium around heart
a. the clock
cord around infant neck
every hour around the clock
every 2 hours around the clock
glare around lights
halo around lights
light around wire technique
nuchal cord around infant's neck
numbness and tingling around mouth
pericardium around heart
pyorrhea around lower and upper teeth
tight nuchal cord around infant's neck
around-the-clock
a.-t.-c. dosing
a.-t.-c. observation
a.-t.-c. oral maintenance bronchodilator therapy
arousability factor
arousal
affective a.
affective arousal theory
anger a.
anxious a.
ascending reticular arousal system
autonomic a.
autonomic arousal disorder
a. boost
a. boost mechanism
a. category
a. component of consciousness
cortical arousal index
a. defect
a. detection
a. disorder
a. dysfunction
female sexual arousal disorder
a. from sleep
a. function
a. heart rate
high a.
high level of a.
increased a.
increased emotional a.
internal arousal insomnia
internal emotional a.
a. jag
a. level

mental a.
movement arousal index
nonspecific a.
NREM arousal parasomnia
object of a.
penile a.
physiological a.
a. reaction
a. reduction mechanism
a. reduction technique
sex arousal mechanism
sexual a.
sleep a.
a. state
a. symptom
a. theory
a. threshold

arouse
patient difficult to a.

aroused
a. motive
a. state of disturbed behavior

Arracacha
Arracacha A virus
Arracacha B virus
A. latent virus
A. virus A, B, Y

arrange
inability to arrange words
inability to arrange words properly

arranged
a. marriage
to be a.

arrangement
anomalous arrangement of pancreaticobiliary ductal system
community living a.'s
Kahn Test of Symbol A.
living a.
multiinstitutional a.
Picture A. psychology

array
annular phased array system
anular array transducer
a. coil
compressed spectral a.
density-modulated spectral a.
density spectral a.
diode array detector
linear array B-mode ultrasound transducer
linear array echoendoscope
linear array transrectal ultrasound probe
9- to 5-MHz convex a.
microchip DNA a.
MRCP using HASTE with a phased array coil
multicoil array technique
multiple coil a.
parallel a.'s
percutaneous electrode a.
subdural electrode a.
superficial linear a.
a. of symptoms
undedicated logic a.

arrayed library

arrector
a. muscle of hair
musculus arrector pili
a. pili
a. pili muscle
a. pilus

arrest
a. of active phase dystocia
acute cardiorespiratory a.
arrhythmia associated with cardiopulmonary a.
bone marrow a.
cardiac a.
cardiac arrest code
cardiac arrest following trauma
cardiopulmonary a.
complete maturation a.
coronary a.
deep hypothermic circulatory a.
a. of descent dystocia
a. of development
a. disorder
filed procedure in cardiac a.
full cardiac a.
greater trochanteric apophysial a.
a. of heartbeat
heart shocked during cardiac a.
hypothermic cardiac arrest surgery
hypothermic circulatory a.
hypothermic fibrillating a.
hypothermic hypokalemic cardioplegic a.
infant cardiac arrest tray
a. of labor
nontraumatic cardiac a.
patient in cardiac a.
patient suffered respiratory a.
postcardiac a.
profound hypothermic circulatory a.
profoundly hypothermic circulatory a.
a. reaction
a. of schizophrenia
secondary a.
a. signal
sinus a.
a. of speech
sudden cardiac a.
sudden cardiopulmonary a.
sustained cardiac a.
total circulatory a.
transient cardiac a.
traumatic cardiopulmonary a.

arrest/akinetic fit

arrest-and-reversal treatment

arrested
a. circulation
a. dental caries
a. development
a. follicular cyst
a. growth and development
a. hydrocephalus
a. tuberculosis

arrested-heart
a.-h. revascularization
a.-h. revascularization technique

arresting
a. consonant
high-efficiency particulate a.

Arrhenius
A. doctrine
A. equation
A. formula
A. theory

Arrhenius-Madsen theory

arrhinia
a., choanal atresia, microphthalmia syndrome
a., choanal atresia, microphthalmia syndrome
a. malformation

arrhythmia
a. associated with cardiopulmonary arrest
cardiac a.
cardiac arrhythmia evaluation center
cardiac arrhythmia suppression trial
a. circuit
clinically significant a.
a. control device
coronary arrhythmia monitoring unit
fatal heart a.
a. following defibrillation
intraoperative a.
life-threatening heart a.
malignant ventricular a.

arrhythmia *(continued)*
management of cardiac a.
a. mapping system catheter
nonspecific a.
paroxysmal supraventricular a.
potentially lethal a.
a. in pregnancy
primary atrial a.
reentrant ventricular a.
a. research technology
respiratory sinus a.
sinus a.
transtelephonic arrhythmia monitoring
ventricular a.
ventricular arrhythmia ablation
ventricular arrhythmia monitor
ventricular ectopic a.

arrhythmia-insensitive
a.-i. flow-sensitive alternating inversion recovery
a.-i. flow-sensitive alternating IR

arrhythmic
a. activity
high-voltage arrhythmic slow wave
a. myocardial infarct
pro arrhythmic effect
a. twitching

arrhythmogenesis
nocturnal a.

arrhythmogenic
a. area
a. border zone
a. myocardial tissue ablation
a. right ventricular cardiomyopathy
a. right ventricular dysplasia

arrival
born before a.
born on a.
date of a.
dead after a.
dead on a.
dead on arrival despite resuscitative attempts
estimated time of a.
hospital arrival time
on a.
prior to a.
time of a.
upon arrival patient found wearing patch on a.

arrogant
a. behavior
a. style

arrow
a. blade
A. catheter
a. clasp
meniscal a.
a. poison
A. Raulerson syringe

arrowhead
a. clasp
A. operation
a. sign

arrow-point
a.-p. tracer
a.-p. tracing

arrow-shaped graft

Arrow-Trerotola
A.-T. device
A.-T. percutaneous thrombectomy device

Arroyo
A. cataract extraction
A. dacryostomy
A. encircling suture
A. keratoplasty
A. operation
A. sign
A. tenotomy

Arruga
A. cataract extraction
A. dacryostomy
A. encircling suture
A. expressor
A. implant
A. keratoplasty
A. operation
A. tenotomy

Arruga-Berens operation

Arruga-Moura-Brazil implant

ARSB syndrome

arsenic
a. acid
a. amblyopia
ammonia, copper, a.
a. assay
a. keratosis
a. nickel silicon
a. peripheral neuropathy
a. pigmentation
a. poisoning
a. polyneuropathy
a. stain
a. tremor
a. trioxide
trioxide arsenic triosephosphate

arsenical
a. contact dermatitis
a. keratosis
organic a.
a. paralysis
a. polyneuropathy
a. tremor

arsenite
orthotoluidine a.

arsenous
a. acid
a. hydride
a. oxide

arsine gas

arsonic acid

arsphenamine dermatitis

art
Barron-Welsh A. Scale
Children's A. Project
a. test
a. therapy

artefactual density

arterial
a. access
a. adaptation
adjuvant hepatic arterial infusion chemotherapy
a. to alveolar
a. to alveolar gradient
a. to alveolar oxygen tension ratio
a. ammonia
a. anastomosis
a. anatomy
a. aneurysm
a. angioma
a. anomaly
aortohepatic arterial graft
a. arcade
a. arch
a. arch of colon
a. arch of ileum
a. arch of jejunum
a. arch of lower eyelid
a. arch of upper eyelid
Argyle arterial catheter
a. arteriolar resistance
a. avulsion
a. banding
a. baroreceptor
a. biopsy
a. bleeding
a. bleeding site
a. blockage
a. blood collection

a. blood gas
a. blood gas abnormality
a. blood gas analysis
a. blood gas point-of-care test
a. blood hydrogen tension
a. blood oximetry
a. blood pressure
a. blood sample
a. blood supply
a. border zone
brachial arterial pressure
brachiocephalic arterial trunk
a. brachiocephalic trunk
a. brain anastomosis
a. brain displacement
a. branch
a. branch to dura mater
a. bruit
a. bulb
a. bypass graft
a. calcification
a. canal
a. cannulation
a. cannulation anesthetic technique
a. cannulation support
a. capillary
a. carbon dioxide
a. carbon dioxide pressure
carotid arterial disease
a. catheter
a. catheterization
a. cerebral circle
a. chemoembolization
chronic peripheral arterial disease
a. circle
a. circle of cerebrum
a. circle of greater iris
a. circle of lesser iris
a. circle of Willis
a. circulation
a. collateral
collateral arterial flow to brain
computed tomography arterial portography
a. cone
continuous arterial spin-labeled perfusion magnetic resonance imaging
continuous regional arterial infusion
a. cutoff
a. decortication
a. deficiency pattern
a. degenerative disease
a. demand pacing
diastolic arterial pressure
a. dicrotic notch pressure
difference in nitrogen tension between mixed alveolar gas and mixed arterial blood
difference in partial pressures of oxygen in mixed alveolar gas and mixed arterial blood
a. dilatation
a. dilatation and rupture
a. dimension
a. disease
a. disorder
a. dissection
a. duct
a. ectasia
effective arterial blood volume
effective arterial elastance
a. embolectomy
a. embolism
a. embolization
a. embolus
a. endothelium
a. entry site
epi arterial bronchus
extracranial arterial disease
extracranial carotid arterial disease
extracranial-intracranial arterial bypass
feeding mean arterial pressure
femoral arterial cannulation
femoral arterial line
a. fenestration
fetal arterial oxygen saturation
a. fibrosing sclerosis
finger arterial blood pressure
a. flap
a. flow-phase image
Fogarty arterial embolectomy
a. gas embolism
a. gas sampling
a. gas volume
a. gland
a. graft
a. groove
a. hemangioma
a. hemorrhage
heparin arterial filter
hepatic arterial flow
hepatic arterial infusion
hepatic arterial infusional chemotherapy
hepatic arterial perfusion scintigraphy
hepatic arterial phase
hepatic arterial pulsatility index
a. hyperemia
a. hypertension
a. hypotension
a. hypoxemia
indwelling arterial catheter
a. inflammation
a. inflow
infundibular arterial inversion
a. infusion
inherent weakness in arterial wall
a. injury
a. insufficiency
a. intima
intracranial arterial aneurysm
a. invasion
isolated hepatic portal and arterial perfusion
a. kinking
lactate a.
a. lactate
a. lactate level
laser-induced arterial fluorescence
a. ligament
a. line
a. linear density
a. line culture
a. line flush solution
a. line insertion
a. loop
lower extremity a.
lower extremity arterial disease
a. lumen
macroaggregated albumin arterial perfusion
major arterial circle of iris
a. malformation
a. mean
mean a.
mean arterial blood pressure
a. mean line
mean systemic arterial pressure
mediastinal arterial variant
mesenteric arterial embolism
mesenteric arterial system
mesenteric arterial thrombosis
minor arterial circle
minor arterial circle of iris
mixed umbilical arterial acidemia
multilevel atherosclerotic arterial occlusive disease
a. murmur
a. narrowing
a. nephrosclerosis
a. network
a. NIVA
a. noninvasive vascular assessment

arterial *(continued)*
nonselective arterial digital angiography
a. obstruction
a. occlusion
a. occlusion sign
occlusive arterial disease
occlusive arterial thrombus
a. occlusive change
a. occlusive disease
a. opacification
a. oxygenation
a. oxygen concentration
a. oxygen desaturation
a. oxygen partial pressure
a. oxygen saturation
a. oxygen tension
a. oxyhemoglobin saturation
palmar arterial arch
pancreaticoduodenal arterial arcade
partial arterial gas tension of carbon dioxide
a. partial pressure
partial pressure of arterial carbon dioxide
partial pressure arterial oxygen
partial pressure of carbon dioxide in arterial gas
a. partial pressure of CO_2
particulate arterial embolization
a. patency
a. peak systolic pressure
pelvic arterial embolization
percutaneous arterial cannulation
percutaneous arterial closure device
peripapillary choroidal arterial system
peripheral arterial aneurysmal disease
peripheral arterial arcade
peripheral arterial catheter
peripheral arterial line
peripheral arterial occlusion
peripheral arterial occlusive disease
peripheral arterial tone
peripheral arterial vasodilation theory
peripheral occlusive arterial disease
a. pH
a. phase
a. photothrombosis
a. plaque
a. plasma input
a. plexus
a. port catheter system
a. pressure index
a. priapism
a. pseudoaneurysm
PTFE arterial graft
pulmonary arterial diastolic pressure
pulmonary arterial pressure-pulmonary venous pressure
pulmonary arterial stenosis
a. pulsatility
a. pulsation artifact
a. puncture site closure device
a. pyemia
radial arterial line
a. reconstructive procedure
a. reconstructive surgery
a. renal plasma flow
retinal arterial narrowing and straightening
a. return
a. revascularization
a. revascularization therapy study
a. ring
a. runoff
a. rupture
a. saturation
saturation of oxygen in arterial blood
a. sclerosis
a. scrotum supply
a. segment
segmental arterial disorganization
a. segment of kidney
a. sheath
a. smooth muscle cell
a. spasm
a. spider
a. steal
stenosing peripheral arterial disease
a. stenosis
a. stick
a. stiffening
subsegmental transcatheter arterial embolization
a. sump effect
a. supply
a. switch operation
a. switch procedure
a. system
systemic arterial hypertension
systemic mean arterial pressure
a. tension
tension, a.
a. thoracic outlet syndrome
a. thrombosis
a. tonus
a. topography
total systemic arterial resistance
transcatheter arterial chemoembolization
transcatheter arterial embolization
transcatheter arterial infusion
transcatheter splenic arterial embolization
a. transfusion
a. trauma
a. tree
twin reversed arterial perfusion
a. ulcer
umbilical a.
umbilical arterial line
a. underfilling
upper extremity a.
a. varix
a. vascular bed
a. vascular disease
a. vasospasm
a. vein
a. wall
a. wall dissection
a. wall integrity
a. wall thickness
a. wave
a. waveform
a. wedge

arterial-alveolar gradient

arterial-arterial fistula

arterial-ascitic fluid pH gradient

arterial/deep
a. venous
a. venous difference

arterial-ecchymotic type Ehlers-Danlos syndrome

arterial-enteric fistula

arterialization
a. of portal vein
a. of venous blood

arterialized
a. blood
a. capillary blood
a. flap
a. leptomeningeal vein

arterial-occlusive retinopathy

arterial-portal fistula

arterial-selective intravenous vasodilator

arteriobiliary fistula

arteriocapillary sclerosis

arteriococcygeal gland

arteriogenic impotence

arteriogram
bifemoral a.
percutaneous carotid a.
ultrasonic a.

arteriograph bath

arteriographic
a. embolization
a. presence

arteriography
carotid cerebral a.
coronary a.
digital subtraction a.
infusion hepatic a.
ipsilateral antegrade a.
magnetic resonance a.
percutaneous transluminal coronary a.
quantitative coronary a.
spiral computed tomography a.
x-ray a.

arteriohepatic dysplasia

arteriolar
arterial arteriolar resistance
a. atherosclerosis
a. attenuation
efferent arteriolar resistance
a. hyalinosis
hyperplastic arteriolar nephrosclerosis
a. infarction
a. ischemic ulcer
a. narrowing
a. necrosis
a. nephrosclerosis
a. network
a. nicking
a. occlusion
a. occlusive disease
pulmonary arteriolar resistance
a. resistance
a. sclerosis
a. sheathing
a. thrombonecrosis

arteriole
afferent glomerular a.
aneurysm of retinal a.
a. communication
copper-wire a.
efferent a.
efferent glomerular a.
glomerular a.
a. of kidney
macular a.
macular arteriole occlusion
main a.
medial arteriole of retina
middle macular a.
narrowed a.
narrowing of retinal a.
nasal arteriole of retina
occlusion of retinal a.
pancreatic a.
perifoveal a.
renal a.
terminal a.

arteriole-capillary-venous bed

arteriolitis
necrotizing a.

arteriolosclerotic kidney

arteriolovenous crossing

arteriolovenular
a. anastomosis
a. bridge

arteriomesenteric duodenal compression syndrome

arterionecrosis
hyaline a.

arteriopathy
autosomal dominant a.
autosomal-dominant a.
cerebral autosomal recessive arteriopathy with subcortical infarcts and leukoencephalopathy
hypertensive a.
Takayasu a.

arterioportal
a. fistula
a. vein shunting
a. venous shunt
a. venous shunting

arterioportobiliary fistula

arterioportographical examination

arteriosclerosis
calf pain from a.
cerebral a.
a. and diabetes
a. of eye vessel
generalized a.
idiopathic pulmonary a.
a. obliterans
a. of retina
severe coronary a.

arteriosclerotic
a. aneurysm
a. aortic aneurysm
a. brain disease
a. brain disease-type organic psychosis
a. brain disorder
a. brain syndrome
a. cardiovascular disease
a. cardiovascular renal disease
coronary arteriosclerotic heart disease
a. coronary artery disease
a. dementia
a. dementia confusional state
a. dementia with delirium
a. dementia with delusional feature
a. dementia with depressive feature
a. deposit
a. depression
a. encephalopathy
a. gangrene
a. heart disease
hypertensive a.
hypertensive arteriosclerotic cardiovascular disease
hypertensive arteriosclerotic heart disease
a. hypertensive heart disease
a. intracranial aneurysm
a. ischemic optic neuropathy
a. kidney
a. mesenteric vascular occlusive disease
a. nephritis
a. paranoid state
paranoid-type arteriosclerotic dementia
paranoid-type arteriosclerotic psychosis
peripheral arteriosclerotic occlusive disease
a. peripheral vascular disease
a. plaque
a. psychosis confusional state
a. renal artery disease
a. retinopathy
subcortical arteriosclerotic encephalopathy
a. thoracoabdominal aortic aneurysm
a. thrombosed aneurysm
uncomplicated arteriosclerotic dementia
a. vertigo

arteriosinusoidal
a. fistula
a. penile fistula

arteriosuperficial venous difference

arteriosus
artery of circulus a.
calcified ductus a.
ductus a.
fetal ductus arteriosus constriction
major circulus arteriosus of iris
minor circulus a.
minor circulus arteriosus of iris
patent ductus a.
persistent ductus a.
persistent truncus a.
premature ductus arteriosus closure
reversed ductus a.
right ductus a.
truncus a.

arteriotomy
ankle-level a.
end-to-side a.

arteriovascular calcification

arteriovenous
acral arteriovenous tumor
a. anastomosis
a. aneurysm
antecubital arteriovenous fistula
auditory arteriovenous malformation
a. block
bradycardia after arteriovenous fistula occlusion
a. brain malformation
a. canal defect
a. carbon dioxide
a. carbon dioxide difference
cerebral arteriovenous malformation
a. colon malformation
a. communication
a. conduction disturbance
continuous arteriovenous hemodiafiltration
continuous arteriovenous hemodialysis
continuous arteriovenous hemofiltration
continuous arteriovenous hemofiltration with dialysis
continuous arteriovenous ultrafiltration
a. cord malformation
a. crossing changes
a. crossing defect
a. dialysis
a. difference
dural arteriovenous fistula
dural arteriovenous malformation
extramedullary arteriovenous malformation
first-degree arteriovenous block
a. fist
a. fistula
a. fistula malformation
a. fistula transplant
a. fistula with good bruits
a. fistulous malformation
gastric arteriovenous malformation
a. glomus complex
a. hemangioma
a. hemofiltration
a. interhemispheric angioma
a. internal mammary fistula
intramedullary arteriovenous malformation
a. junctional rhythm
a. junctional tachycardia
a. kidney malformation
a. leaking
a. loop
a. malformation of brain
a. malformation nidus
a. malformation nidus definition
a. malformation radiosurgery
medial hemispheric arteriovenous malformation
mesenteric arteriovenous fistula
a. nicking
obliterated arteriovenous malformation
orbital arteriovenous malformation
osseous craniofacial arteriovenous malformation
a. oxygen content difference
a. oxygen difference
a. passage time
a. pattern
pelvic arteriovenous malformation
peripheral arteriovenous fistula
a. pressure gradient
a. pulmonary aneurysm
pulmonary arteriovenous aneurysm
a. ratio
Scribner arteriovenous shunt
a. shunt
a. shunt imaging
a. shunt infection
a. shunting
spinal dural arteriovenous fistula
a. strabismus syndrome
a. subclavian fistula
a. varix

arteritic anterior ischemic optic neuropathy

arteritis
allergic granulomatous a.
ANCA-positive granulomatous giant-cell a.
cranial granulomatous a.
giant cell a.
granulomatous temporal a.
Horton a.
necrotizing granulomatous systemic a.
a. nodosa
a. obliterans
occlusive retinal a.
occult temporal arteritis of Simmons
Takayasu a.
temporal a.
a. umbilicalis

artery
A1-A5 segments of anterior cerebral a.
aberrant right subclavian a.
abnormal coronary a.
absence of branch pulmonary a.
a. of Adamkiewicz
adventitia of a.
allograft coronary artery disease
alternative occipital artery middle cerebral a.
a. and/or nerve
aneurysm of internal carotid a.
aneurysm of persistent trigeminal a.
aneurysm of posterior communicating a.
angiographic corkscrew a.
a. of angular gyrus
angular nasal a.
a. of angular nasal branch
anomalous cerebral a.
anomalous coronary a.
anomalous fibular nutrient a.
anomalous innominate artery compression syndrome
anomalous left coronary a.
anomalous left coronary artery from pulmonary a.
anomalous left coronary artery from pulmonary artery syndrome
anomalous left main coronary a.
anomalous left pulmonary a.
anomalous origin of left coronary artery from pulmonary a.
anomalous right subclavian a.
anomalous vertebral a.
antegrade femoral artery catheterization

anterior auricular a.
anterior auricular branch of superficial temporal a.
anterior basal segmental a.
anterior branch of the renal a.
anterior carotid a.
anterior cecal a.
anterior cerebral a.
anterior cerebral artery crawling under the skull
anterior cerebral artery plexus
anterior cerebral artery pulsatility index
anterior choroidal a.
anterior ciliary a.
anterior circumflex humeral a.
anterior communicating a.
anterior communicating artery aneurysm
anterior communicating artery complex
anterior communicating artery distribution infarct
anterior communicating artery distribution infarction
anterior conjunctival a.
anterior descending a.
anterior ethmoidal a.
anterior ethmoidal branch of ophthalmic a.
anterior glandular branch of superior thyroid a.
anterior humeral circumflex a.
anterior-inferior cerebellar a.
anterior-inferior cerebral a.
anterior-inferior communicating a.
a. of anterior inferior segment of kidney
anterior intercostal a.
anterior intercostal branch of internal thoracic a.
anterior internal cerebellar a.
anterior interosseous a.
anterior interventricular branch of left coronary a.
anterior labial a.
anterior labial branch of deep external pudendal a.
anterior lateral malleolar a.
anterior lateral nasal branch of anterior ethmoidal a.
anterior/lateral/posterior glandular branch of superior thyroid a.
anterior medial malleolar a.
anterior mediastinal a.
anterior meningeal a.
anterior meningeal branch of anterior ethmoidal a.
anterior parietal a.
anterior parietal artery aneurysm
anterior perforating a.
anterior peroneal a.
anterior and posterior radicular a.
anterior and posterior superior pancreaticoduodenal a.
anterior radial collateral a.
anterior radicular a.
anterior recurrent tibial a.
anterior scrotal branch of deep external pudendal a.
anterior segmental a.
anterior septal branch of anterior ethmoidal a.
anterior spinal artery syndrome
anterior superior alveolar a.
anterior superior dental a.
anterior superior pancreaticoduodenal a.
anterior superior segmental artery of kidney
a. of anterior superior segment of kidney
anterior temporal branch of posterior cerebral a.
anterior tibial a.
anterior tibial recurrent a.
anterior tympanic a.
anterior ulnar recurrent a.
anterior vestibular a.
anteroinferior cerebellar a.
anterolateral central a.
anterolateral striate a.
anterolateral thalamostriate a.
anteromedial central a.
anteromedial frontal branch of callosomarginal a.
anteromedial thalamostriate a.
aortic a.
aortic-superior mesenteric artery bypass
apical branch of inferior lobar branch of right pulmonary a.
apical posterior a.
apical segmental a.
apical segmental artery of superior lobar artery of right lung
araldehyde-tanned bovine carotid artery graft
arcuate artery of foot
arcuate artery of kidney
arteriosclerotic coronary artery disease
arteriosclerotic renal artery disease
ascending branch of the inferior mesenteric a.
ascending branch of superficial cervical a.
ascending cervical a.
ascending frontoparietal a.
ascending ileocolic a.
ascending palatine a.
ascending pharyngeal a.
A1 segment of anterior cerebral a.
A2 segment of anterior cerebral a.
asymptomatic carotid artery stenosis
asymptomatic coronary artery disease
atherosclerotic carotid a.
atherosclerotic carotid artery disease
atherosclerotic carotid artery lesion
atherosclerotic coronary artery disease
atherosclerotic renal a.
atherosclerotic renal artery stenosis
atlantic part of vertebral a.
atrial anastomotic branch of circumflex branch of left coronary a.
atrial circumflex a.
atrioventricular node a.
a. to atrioventricular node
auricular branch of occipital a.
auricular branch of posterior auricular a.
axillary artery aneurysm
ballooning-out of artery wall
basilar a.
basilar artery insufficiency
bilateral inferior epigastric artery flap
bilateral internal carotid artery occlusion
bilateral internal mammary a.'s
blocked heart a.
blood flow from a.
brachial artery output
brachial artery mean pressure
brachiocephalic a.
a. of brain
branch retinal artery occlusion
bronchial artery embolization
bronchopulmonary segmental a.

artery *(continued)*
a. bronchus ratio
a. of bulb of penis
a. of bulb of vestibule
a. of calf
carotid a.
carotid artery canal
carotid artery stenosis
carotid artery system
carotid artery ultrasound
Carotid A. Stenosis with Asymptomatic Narrowing: Operation Versus Aspirin Study
a. of caudate lobe
celiac a.
celiac artery compression syndrome
central retinal a.
central retinal artery occlusion
a. of central sulcus
cerebral artery thrombosis
a. of cerebral hemorrhage
a. of chiasmal region
a. of circulus arteriosus
circumflex a.
circumflex coronary a.
coarctation of pulmonary a.'s
comitant artery of median nerve
common carotid a.
common carotid artery bifurcation
common carotid artery intima-media thickness
common femoral a.
common femoral artery-superficial femoral a.
common hepatic a.
common internal iliac a.
communicating artery aneurysm
complete transposition of great a.'s
compression of carotid a.
congenitally corrected transposition of the great a.'s
continuous hepatic artery infusion
a. of the conus medullaris
coronary a.
coronary artery aneurysm
coronary artery bypass graft
coronary artery bypass grafting
coronary artery bypass grafting surgery
coronary artery bypass graft patency
coronary artery bypass graft surgery
coronary artery calcification
coronary artery disease
coronary artery embolism
coronary artery embolization
coronary artery fistula
coronary artery lesion
coronary artery obstruction
coronary artery occlusive disease
coronary artery revascularization procedure
coronary artery scan
coronary artery spasm
coronary artery steal
deep circumflex iliac a.
deep circumflex iliac artery flap
deep inferior epigastric artery perforator
deep superior epigastric a.
degeneration of wall of a.
descending palatine a.
diagonal branch of a.
a. diameter
diastolic pulmonary artery pressure
a. disease
dissecting aneurysm of the coronary a.
dissecting basilar artery aneurysm
dissecting renal artery aneurysm
distal right coronary a.
dorsal digital a.
dorsal uterine a.
double coronary artery graft
a. of Drummond
D-transposition of great a.'s
a. to ductus deferens
a. ectasia
ectatic carotid a.
electron-beam angiography of coronary a.
endarterectomy and coronary artery bypass grafting
endoscopic coronary artery bypass grafting
a. entrapment
epibronchial right pulmonary artery syndrome
external carotid a.
external iliac a.
facial artery musculomucosal
facial artery myomucosal
facial artery pressure point
femoral a.
femoral artery blood flow
femoral artery catheter
femoral artery pressure
femoral artery thrombosis
femoral-popliteal artery bypass
femoropopliteal artery occlusion
first dorsal metatarsal a.
first obtuse marginal a.
first plantar metatarsal a.
a. forceps
frontopolar a.
gastroduodenal a.
gastroepiploic a.
greater palatine a.
greater superficial temporal artery biopsy
hardening of a.
hardening of coronary a.
hardening of walls of a.
hemorrhoidal artery ligation
hepatic a.
hepatic artery aneurysm
hepatic artery blood flow
hepatic artery chemoembolization
hepatic artery embolization
hepatic artery ligation
hepatic artery thrombosis
a. of Heubner
hyperdense middle cerebral artery sign
hypogastric artery aneurysm
iliac artery aneurysm
iliac artery occlusion
impaired coronary a.
increased pulmonary artery pressure
infarct-related a.
a. of inferior cavernous sinus
inferior epigastric a.
inferior mesenteric a.
inferior nasal a.
inferior temporal a.
infragenicular popliteal a.
innominate artery stenting
interlobar artery of kidney
interlobular artery of kidney
interlobular artery of liver
intermediate circumflex a.
intermediate coronary artery syndrome
internal carotid artery flow
internal carotid artery occlusion
internal iliac a.
internal mammary artery bypass
internal mammary artery catheterization
internal mammary artery graft
internal mammary artery implant
internal maxillary a.
internal thoracic artery graft
intramural left anterior descending a.

intramuscular artery of lower extremity
intramuscular artery of upper extremity
intrapulmonary a.
a. involvement
a. island flap
a. isolated
a. of labyrinth
lateral thoracic a.'s
left anterior descending coronary a.
left anterior spinal a.
left basal a.
left carotid a.
left circumflex a.
left circumflex coronary a.
left common carotid a.
left common femoral a.
left coronary a.
left femoral a.
left gastric a.
left hepatic a.
left iliac a.
left internal carotid a.
left internal mammary artery graft
left internal thoracic a.
left main coronary artery disease
left main stem coronary artery disease
left middle cerebral a.
left middle cerebral artery thrombosis
left posterior descending a.
left posterior internal carotid a.
left pulmonary artery oxygen saturation
left radial a.
left renal a.
left subclavian a.
left transposition of great a.
left vertebral a.
lesser palatine a.
a. ligation
long central a.
long ciliary a.
long posterior ciliary a.
long thoracic a.
a. of lower limb
lowest lumbar a.
lowest thyroid a.
lumbar branch of iliolumbar a.
lumen of bronchial a.
main pulmonary a.
main renal a.
main renal artery stenosis
major aortopulmonary collateral a.
major coronary a.
malignant middle cerebral artery infarction
malposition of the branch pulmonary a.
malposition of branch pulmonary a.
malposition of great a.'s
mammary artery graft
marginal artery of colon
marginal artery of Drummond
marginal atrial branch of right coronary a.
marginal branch of left circumflex coronary a.
marginal branch of right coronary a.
marginal circumflex a.
marginal tentorial branch of internal carotid a.
M2 artery segment
mastoid branch of occipital a.
mastoid branch of posterior auricular a.
mastoid branch of posterior tympanic a.
mean brachial artery pressure
mean pulmonary artery wedge pressure
medial anterior malleolus a.
medial basal branch of pulmonary a.
medial basal segmental a.
medial branch of artery of tuber cinereum
medial branch of pontine a.
medial circumflex artery of thigh
medial circumflex femoral a.
medial collateral a.
medial commissural a.
medial cutaneous branch of dorsal branch of posterior intercostal a.
medial femoral circumflex a.
medial frontobasal a.
medial geniculate a.
medial inferior genicular a.
medial malleolar branch of posterior tibial a.
median callosal a.
median commissural a.
mediastinal branch of internal thoracic a.
medullary artery of brain
medullary arteries of brain
meningeal artery groove
meningeal branch of cavernous part of internal carotid a.
meningeal branch of cerebral part of internal carotid a.
meningeal branch of intracranial part of vertebral a.
meningeal branch of occipital a.
mental branch of inferior alveolar a.
mesenteric artery aneurysm
mesenteric artery constriction
mesenteric artery occlusion
mesenteric artery syndrome
middle alveolar a.
middle cerebral a.
middle cerebral artery bifurcation
middle cerebral artery fenestration
middle cerebral artery infarct
middle cerebral artery occlusion
middle cerebral artery pressure
middle cerebral artery syndrome
middle cerebral artery thrombosis
middle colic a.
middle collateral a.
middle genicular a.
middle hemorrhoidal a.
middle hepatic a.
middle lobar a.
middle lobar artery of right lung
middle sacral a.
middle uterine a.
midmarginal branch of a.
minimally invasive direct coronary artery bypass graft
mobile artery and vein imaging system
M2 segment of middle cerebral a.
multiple aortopulmonary collateral a.
muscular artery of ophthalmic artery
mylohyoid branch of inferior alveolar a.
myometrial arcuate a.
narrowed coronary a.
narrowing of a.
narrowing of carotid a.
narrowing of coronary a.
narrowing of ostia of coronary a.
nasal accessory a.
native coronary a.
a. needle
nerve, artery, vein, empty space, lymphatics
normal coronary a.'s

artery *(continued)*
a. of nose
nutrient artery of femur
nutrient artery of fibula
nutrient artery growth
nutrient artery of humerus
nutrient artery of radius
nutrient artery of the tibia
nutrient artery of tibia
nutrient artery of ulna
obliterative coronary artery disease
obstruction of renal a.
obtuse marginal a.
occipital a.
a. occlusion
occlusion of a.
occlusion of internal carotid a.
occlusion of intramuscular a.
occlusion of left carotid a.
occlusion of right carotid a.
occlusive artery disease
occlusive carotid artery disease
occlusive coronary artery disease
off-pump coronary artery bypass
opening for dorsal artery of penis
ophthalmic a.
ophthalmic artery aneurysm
ophthalmic artery pressure
orbital branch of middle meningeal a.
origin of a.
ostial artery atherosclerosis
a. ostium
ovarian branch of uterine a.
palmar carpal branch of radial a.
palmar carpal branch of ulnar a.
palmar digital a.
palmar interosseous a.
pancreatic artery aneurysm
pancreaticoduodenal artery aneurysm
a. of the pancreatic tail
paracentral branch of callosomarginal a.
paracentral branch of pericallosal a.
parent artery occlusion
parietal branch of medial occipital a.
parietal branch of middle meningeal a.
parietal branch of superficial temporal a.
parietooccipital branch of anterior cerebral a.
parietooccipital branch of posterior cerebellar a.
parietooccipital branch of posterior cerebral a.
patency of a.
pectoral branch of thoracoacromial a.
pedal artery opacification
a. of Percheron
perforating alveolar a.
perforating artery of deep femoral artery
perforating artery of foot
perforating artery of hand
perforating artery infarct
perforating artery of internal mammary
perforating artery of internal thoracic artery
perforating artery of penis
perforating branch of anterior interosseous a.
perforating branch of fibular a.
perforating branch of internal thoracic a.
perforating branch of palmar metacarpal a.
perforating branch of peroneal a.
perforating branch of plantar metatarsal a.
perforating arteries of peronea
perfusion-assisted direct coronary artery bypass
pericallosal azygos a.
peridural a.
perineal artery axial flap
peripheral artery disease
peripheral pulmonary artery stenosis
persistent trigeminal a.
petrosal branch of middle meningeal a.
pharyngeal branch of artery of pterygoid canal
pharyngeal branch of ascending pharyngeal a.
pharyngeal branch of descending palatine a.
pharyngeal branch of inferior thyroid a.
plantar digital a.
plaque in a.
a.'s of pons
popliteal artery aneurysm
popliteal artery occlusive disease
popliteal artery pressure point
popliteal-tibial artery bypass
a. of postcentral sulcus
postciliary a.
post coronary artery bypass graft
posterior branch of obturator a.
posterior branch of recurrent ulnar a.
posterior branch of renal a.
posterior cerebral a.
posterior circumflex a.
posterior communicating a.
posterior communicating artery aneurysm
posterior descending a.
posterior descending coronary a.
posterior inferior cerebellar a.
posterior inferior communicating a.
posterior interosseous a.
a. of posterior segment of kidney
posterior tibial a.
posteroinferior cerebellar a.
posterolateral coronary a.
posterolateral spinal a.
posteromedial central a.
a. of precentral sulcus
primitive hypoglossal a.
primitive trigeminal a.
profunda brachii a.
profunda femoris a.
proximal circumflex a.
proximal left anterior descending a.
pseudo-renal artery syndrome
pterygoid branch of maxillary a.
pterygoid branch of posterior deep temporal a.
a. of pterygoid canal
pulmonary a.
pulmonary artery anastomosis
pulmonary artery aneurysm
pulmonary artery atresia
pulmonary artery balloon pump
pulmonary artery banding
pulmonary artery bifurcation
pulmonary artery blockage
pulmonary artery catheterization
pulmonary artery counterpulsation
pulmonary artery diastolic
pulmonary artery diastolic and wedge pressure
pulmonary artery embolization
pulmonary artery end-diastolic pressure
pulmonary artery filling defect
pulmonary artery hemorrhage
pulmonary artery hypotension

pulmonary artery line
pulmonary artery obstruction
pulmonary artery occlusion pressure
pulmonary artery pressure monitoring
pulmonary artery rupture
pulmonary artery steal
pulmonary artery stenting
pulmonary artery systolic
pulmonary artery systolic pressure
pulmonary artery thromboembolism
pulmonary artery thromboendarterectomy
pulmonary artery trunk
a. of pulp
radial artery bypass surgery
radial artery catheter
radial artery graft
radial artery pseudoaneurysm
radial artery systolic pressure
a. reconstitution
a. reconstruction
renal a.
renal artery aneurysm
renal artery bypass graft
renal artery pressure
renal artery response
renal artery stenosis
renal artery thrombosis
reoperative coronary artery bypass graft
reversed digital artery flap
reversed ophthalmic artery flow
right anterior descending coronary a.
right basilar a.
right brachial a.
right carotid a.
right colic a.
right common carotid a.
right common femoral a.
right coronary a.
right descending pulmonary a.
right external carotid a.
right femoral a.
right hepatic a.
right iliac a.
right innominate a.
right internal mammary a.
right internal thoracic a.
right main coronary a.
right middle cerebral artery thrombosis
right posterior internal carotid a.
right pulmonary artery withdrawal
right radial a.
right renal a.
right subclavian a.
right vertebral a.
rostral basilar artery syndrome
a. of round ligament of uterus
a. to sciatic nerve
second obtuse marginal a.
segmental artery of kidney
segmental artery of liver
segmental branch of a.
segmental bronchus renal artery waveform
segmented renal a.
single coronary artery bypass graft
single coronary artery graft
single internal mammary a.
single umbilical a.
a. to the sinoatrial node
sinoatrial node a.
a. spectrum
sphenopalatine a.
splanchnic artery occlusion
splenic a.
splenic artery aneurysm
spontaneous cervical artery dissection
spontaneous coronary artery dissection
a. stenosis
stented coronary a.
stenting in small a.'s
subclavian a.
superficial branch of medial circumflex femoral a.
superficial branch of medial plantar a.
superficial branch of superior gluteal a.
superficial branch of transverse cervical a.
superficial circumflex iliac a.
superficial external pudendal a.
superficial femoral a.
superficial inferior epigastric a.
superficial occipital artery to middle cerebral a.
superficial temporal artery-middle cerebral a.
superficial temporal artery-posterior cerebral a.
superficial temporal artery-superior cerebellar a.
superior carotid a.
superior cerebellar a.
superior epigastric a.
superior gluteal a.
superior gluteal artery perforator
superior hypophysial a.
superior mesenteric a.
superior mesenteric artery blood flow
superior mesenteric artery blood velocity
superior mesenteric artery embolus
superior mesenteric artery occlusion
superior mesenteric artery syndrome
superior nasal a.
superior temporal a.
supragenicular popliteal a.
supraorbital a.
systemic a.
systolic coronary artery narrowing
a. to tail of pancreas
takeoff of a.
temporal external a.
temporopolar a.
terminal internal carotid a.
thrombotic pulmonary a.
totally endoscopic coronary artery bypass
total occlusion of basilar a.
transplant coronary artery disease
transplant renal artery stenosis
transposition of the great a.'s
triple coronary artery bypass graft
a. of tuber cinereum
ulnar artery injury
umbilical a.
umbilical artery catheter
umbilical artery catheterization
umbilical artery line
unilateral renal artery stenosis
unstable coronary artery disease
a. of upper limb
ureteric branch of inferior suprarenal a.
ureteric branch of ovarian a.
ureteric branch of renal a.
uterine artery embolization
a. to vas deferens
vein, artery, nerve
velocity, common carotid a.
velocity internal carotid a.
vertebral a.
vertebral artery bypass graft
vertebral artery dissection
vertebral artery injury
vertebral artery occlusion

artery *(continued)*
vertebral artery test
vertebral arteries of intracerebral vessels
vertebrobasilar artery insufficiency
vertebrobasilar artery system
volar interosseous a.
a. weld strength
a. of Willis

artery:aortic velocity ratio

artery-clogging plaque in atherosclerosis patient

artery-like pattern of enhancement

artery-nerve conflict

artery-to-artery
a.-t.-a. anastomosis
a.-t.-a. embolism

artery-to-vein
a.-t.-v. anastomosis
a.-t.-v. ratio
a.-t.-v. shunt

artery-vein-nerve bundle

arthralgia
asymmetrical a.
migratory a.
nonspecific a.
periodic a.
psychogenic a.
recurrent a.
rheumatic a.
a. saturnina
a. saturnine
temporomandibular a.

arthrifluent abscess

arthritic
a. ankle joint narrowing
a. atrophy
a. calculus
degenerative arthritic change
a. deterioration
a. dose
a. general pseudoparalysis
a. joint
a. lipping
moderate arthritic condition
a. overgrowth
pantalocrural arthritic destruction
scapholunate arthritic collapse
a. shoe
a. talonavicular change
a. tuberculosis

arthritides
chronic idiopathic arthritides of childhood

arthritidis
Mycoplasma a.
Mycoplasma arthritidis mitogen

arthritis
acute gonococcal a.
acute gouty a.
acute rheumatic a.
adjuvant a.
adjuvant-induced a.
ancient tuberculous a.
ankle infectious a.
ankle rheumatoid a.
antigen-induced a.
a. arthrogram
arthropod-borne viral arthritis and rash
assignment criteria for rheumatoid a.
atypical mycobacterial a.
avian viral arthritis virus
axial psoriatic a.
caprine arthritis encephalitis virus
carcinomatous arthritis in hand
carcinomatous arthritis in wrist
chronic inflammatory a.
chronic, painful a.
chronic rheumatoid a.
chronic villous a.
collagen-induced a.
debilitating rheumatoid a.
degenerative a.
elderly-onset rheumatoid a.
facial pain from a.
fact joint a.
Gram-negative bacilli a.
A. Helplessness Index
a. hiemalis
idiopathic destructive a.
A. Impact Measurement Scale
joint problems from a.
joint rheumatoid a.
juvenile a.
juvenile chronic a.
Juvenile A. Functional Assessment Report
juvenile idiopathic a.
juvenile-onset rheumatoid a.
juvenile rheumatoid arthritis rash
juvenile rheumatoid arthritis type I, II
Lyme arthritis serology
Lyme disease a.
McMaster-Toronto A. Patient Reference
migratory peripheral a.
mixed rheumatoid and degenerative a.
monoarticular a.
monoarticular antigen-induced a.
monoarticular arthritis of unknown etiology
a. mutilans
National A. Action Plan
National A. Data Workgroup
National Institute of A. and Metabolic Diseases
a. nodosa
nonbacterial infectious a.
nongonococcal bacterial a.
nongonococcal septic a.
oligoarticular seronegative rheumatoid a.
Outerbridge degenerative arthritis staging
pain from a.
patellofemoral degenerative a.
pauciarticular juvenile chronic a.
pauciarticular juvenile rheumatoid a.
polyarticular gonococcal a.
polyarticular juvenile chronic a.
polyarticular juvenile rheumatoid a.
poststreptococcal reactive a.
primary gouty a.
psoriatic a.
pyogenic sterile arthritis, pyoderma gangrenosum, and acne
A. Quality of Life Scale
reactive a.
a. and rheumatic diseases
a. of rheumatic fever
rheumatoid a.
rheumatoid arthritis agglutinin
rheumatoid arthritis, diffuse idiopathic skeletal hyperostosis
rheumatoid arthritis nuclear antigen
rheumatoid arthritis precipitin
rheumatoid arthritis and Sjögren syndrome
rheumatoid arthritis factor test
rheumatoid arthritis serum factor
a. robustus
sexually acquired reactive a.
a. sock
spondylitis, enthesitis, a.
subacute infectious a.
systemic juvenile rheumatoid a.
a. of unknown diagnosis
a. urethritica
a. without deformity

Yersinia a.
younger-onset rheumatoid a.

arthritis-associated psoriasis

arthritisdermatitis
gonococcal arthritis/dermatitis syndrome

arthritis-dermatitis syndrome

arthritis-hives-angioedema syndrome

arthritogenic peptide

arthrocentesis
ankle a.
joint a.
knee a.

arthrochalasis
a. multiplex congenita
a. multiplex congenita Ehlers-Danlos syndrome

arthrodesed digit

arthrodesis
Adkins technique spinal a.
Albee hip a.
anterior occipitocervical a.
anterior slot graft a.
AO group shoulder a.
arthroscopic subtalar a.
calcaneocuboid distraction a.
flexion injury posterior atlantoaxial a.
Gant hip a.
hallux rigidus a.
a. of hip
Hoke triple a.
McKeever arthrodesis for hallux limitus
modified Boyd ankle a.
Ollier arthrodesis approach
scaphocapitolunate a.
a. screw

arthrodial
a. articulation
a. attachment
a. cartilage
a. joint
a. protractor

arthroereisis
axis-altering arthroereisis device
Maxwell-Brancheau a.
peg-in-hole a.
Smith subtalar joint arthroereisis peg

arthrogenic gait

arthrogram
ankle a.
arthritis a.
nuclear a.

arthrographic capsular distension and rupture technique

arthrography
coronal computed tomographic a.
double-contrast shoulder a.
a. imaging
magnetic resonance a.
osteochondral fracture a.
single shoulder contrast a.

arthrogryposis
a., ectodermal dysplasia, cleft lip/palate developmental delay syndrome
cataract, microcephaly, arthrogryposis, kyphosis
a. congenita, distal, type I, II syndrome
a. congenita multiplex
distal arthrogryposis, hypopituitarism, mental retardation, facial anomalies syndrome
a., ectodermal dysplasia, cleft lip/palate developmental delay syndrome
mental retardation-distal arthrogryposis syndrome
mental retardation, facial anomalies, hypopituitarism, distal arthrogryposis syndrome
mental retardation, overgrowth, craniosynostosis, distal arthrogryposis, sacral dimple, joint laxity
a. multiplex congenita
myopathic a.
myopathic arthrogryposis multiplex congenita
neurogenic a.
neuropathic arthrogryposis multiplex congenita

arthrogryposis-like hand anomaly

arthrogrypotic clubfoot

arthrokinetic nystagmus

arthrometer
a. measurement
a. test
a. testing

arthrometric knee laxity measurement

arthroonychodysplasia syndrome

arthropathia psoriatica

arthropathy
chronic pyrophosphate a.
cuff tear a.
cystic fibrosis a.
facet joint a.
neuropathic a.
pyrophosphate a.
secondary hypertrophic a.
seronegativity, enthesopathy, a.

arthroplastic implant

arthroplasty
aluminum oxide arthroplasty material
Ashworth hand a.
Aufranc cup a.
Austin Moore a.
autogenous interpositional shoulder a.
bipolar hip a.
a. bur
a. cement
cementless surface replacement a.
cementless total hip a.
convex condylar-implant a.
Crawford-Adams hip a.
cuff tear a.
cup-on-cup arthroplasty of the hip
double cup a.
extensor brevis a.
Ganley modification of Keller a.
a. gouge
great toe arthroplasty implant technique
laser image custom a.
low-friction a.
low friction a.
Matchett-Brown hip a.
Mayo ankle a.
Mayo modified total elbow a.
mold acetabular a.
Mueller hip a.
revision hip a.
Schlein-type elbow a.
total ankle a.
total articular replacement a.
total articular resurfacing a.
total elbow a.
total hip a.
total joint a.
total knee a.
total shoulder a.
total toe a.
total wrist a.
unicompartmental knee a.

arthropod
a. bite
a. dermatosis
extended-duration topical arthropod repellent
a. identification
a. sting
a. vector

arthropod-borne
a.-b. viral arthritis and rash
a.-b. viral disease
a.-b. viral encephalitis
a.-b. viral hemorrhagic fever
a.-b. virus
a.-b. virus encephalitis

arthropod-induced blister

arthroscope
angled a.
Panoview a.

arthroscopic
a. abrasion chondroplasty
a. acromioplasty
a. anterior cruciate ligament reconstruction
anterior labrum periosteum shoulder arthroscopic lesion
anterocentral arthroscopic portal
a. augmentation
a. Bankart repair
blunt arthroscopic cannula
a. cannula
a. cheilectomy
a. debridement
a. decompression
a. drilling
egress of arthroscopic fluid
a. entry portal
a. examination
a. grabber
a. knee surgery
a. knife
a. knot
a. laser instrument
a. laser surgery
a. legholder
a. lumbar laser diskectomy
a. lysis and lavage
a. meniscectomy
a. microdiskectomy
a. monopolar thermal stabilization
forefoot compression sleeve
a. mosaicplasty
a. osteotome
Panoview arthroscopic system
a. probe
a. pump
a. punch
same-day microsurgical arthroscopic lateral-approach laser-assisted
a. scissors
a. screw fixation
a. screw installation
a. shaver
a. shaving
a. sheath
a. shield
a. subtalar arthrodesis
a. synovectomy
a. tourniquet
a. transglenoid suture stabilization procedure
a. transhumeral reconstruction

arthroscopically
a. assisted anterior cruciate ligament reconstruction
a. assisted synovectomy

arthroscopy
a. and arthrotomy
a. basket forceps
calcaneonavicular joint a.
diagnostic a.
diagnostic arthroscopy, operative arthroscopy, and possible operative arthrotomy
diagnostic and operative a.
a. grasping forceps
total knee a.

arthroscopy-assisted patellar tendon substitution

arthrosis
a. deformity
subtalar a.

arthrotomographic image

arthrotomography of shoulder

arthrotomy
arthroscopy and a.
diagnostic arthroscopy, operative arthroscopy, and possible operative a.

Arthur Adaptation of the Leiter International Performance Scale

Arthus
A. hypersensitivity
passive Arthus reaction
A. phenomenon
A. reaction
A. response

Arthus-type reaction

articular
acute articular rheumatism
a. amyloid
anterior articular surface of dens
anterior talar articular surface of calcaneus
apposing articular surface
a. arch
arytenoidal articular surface
arytenoidal articular surface of cricoid
attenuated intercarpal articular cartilage
a. block
a. blockage
a. bone lamella
a. bone loss
a. bone tubercle
a. branch
a. branch of deep fibular nerve
a. calculus
a. capsule
capsule cartilage articular preservation
a. cartilage
a. cartilage attenuation
a. cartilage autograft
a. cartilage autografting
a. cartilage degeneration
a. cartilage lesion
a. cartilage violation
a. cartilage volume
a. cavity
a. chondrocalcinosis
a. chondrocyte
chronic articular rheumatism
chronic infantile neurological, cutaneous, and a.
a. circumference of head of radius
a. circumference of head of ulna
a. corpuscle
a. cortex
a. crepitus
a. crescent
a. crest
a. defect
a. derangement
a. disc of acromioclavicular joint
a. disc of distal radioulnar joint
a. disc of sternoclavicular joint
a. disc of temporomandibular joint
a. disease
a. disorder
distal articular set angle
distal metatarsal articular angle

a. eminence
a. eminence of temporal bone
a. erosion
erosion of articular surface
a. facet
a. facet angle
a. facet of head of fibula
a. facet of head of rib
a. facet of lateral malleolus
a. facet of medial malleolus
a. facet of radial head
a. facet of tubercle of rib
fibular articular facet of tibia
fibular articular surface of tibia
a. fluid
a. fossa
a. fossa of mandible
a. fossa of temporal bone
a. fracture
a. fragment
a. gout
a. of hand
a. hand disorder
a. instability
a. joint tissue catabolism
a. labrum
a. lamella of bone
a. leprosy
a. lip
Lisfranc articular interline
malleolar articular surface of fibula
malleolar articular surface of tibia
a. manifestation
a. margin
a. mass
a. mass separation
a. mass separation fracture
medial articular nerve
medial hemijoint articular space
a. meniscus
a. metaplasia
a. motion device
multiple articular contracture
multiple articular rigidity
a. muscle
a. muscle of elbow
a. muscle of knee
navicular articular surface of talus
a. nerve
a. network
opposing articular surfaces
a. overgrowth
painful articular syndrome
parallelism of articular surface
patellofemoral articular cartilage
phalangeal articular orientation
a. pillar
a. pillar fracture
a. pit
a. pit of head of radius
a. process
a. process of vertebra
proximal articular set angle
a. recurrent nerve
a. rheumatism
a. sensibility
a. set angle
a. strain
a. structure
superior articular process
a. surface
a. surface of acromion
a. surface of arytenoid cartilage
a. surface of head of fibula
a. surface of head of rib
a. surface of knee
a. surface of mandibular fossa
a. surface of mandibular fossa of temporal bone
a. surface on calcaneus for cuboid bone
a. surface of patella
a. surface of talus
a. surface of temporal bone
a. surface of tubercle of rib
a. syndrome
total articular replacement arthroplasty
total articular resurfacing arthroplasty
total hip articular replacement by internal eccentric shells
a. tubercle of temporal bone
a. tuberculosis
a. vascular circle
a. vascular network
a. vascular network of elbow
a. vascular network of knee
a. vascular plexus
a. wrist disorder

articular-ligamentous system

articular/nonarticular test

articulated

a. AFO
a. drainage catheter
a. partial denture
a. skeleton
a. tension device

articulate minifixator

articulating

a. arm
a. bone end
a. disc prosthesis
a. paper
a. surface
temporary articulating methylmethacrylate antibiotic spacer

articulation

a. area
Arizona A. Proficiency Scale
Austin Spanish A. Test
Children's A. Test
Clinical Probes of A. Consistency
a. curve
Denver A. Screening Exam
developmental articulation disorder
a. developmental delay disorder
Developmental A. Test
a. disorder
a. disturbance
Edinburgh A. Test
a. error
Fein A. Screening Test
Fein A. Screening Test
a. of fingers
Fisher-Logemann Test of A. Competence
Goldman-Fristoe Test of A.
a.'s of hand
a. index
Iowa Pressure A. Test
a. manipulation
manipulation of a.
McDonald Deep Test of A.
metatarsophalangeal a.'s
Ohio Tests of A. and Perception of Sounds
organic articulation disorder
Photo A. Test psychology
Picture A. and Language Screening Test
a. of pisiform bone
point of a.
a. programming
Riley A. and Language Test
Slosson Articulation Language Test with Phonology
a. of speech
a. test
Test of A. Performance-Diagnostic
Test of A. Performance-Screen
a. treatment

articulation-gain function

articulation-resonance
phonation, respiration, a.-r.

articulator
adjustable a.
arcon a.
arcon semiadjustable a.
a. articulation

articulatory
atypical articulatory contact
a. basis
a. loop component
a. phonetics
a. procedure
a. skill
a. specified neutral reference
a. tic

artifact
aortic motion a.
arterial pulsation a.
beam hardening a.
bone hardening a.
bowel gas a.
calibration failure a.
cardiac pacemaker a.
center line a.
chemical shift misregistration a.
data spike detection error a.
a. effect
flow artifact killer
foreign material a.
glass cye a.
a. image
magic angle effect a.
motion artifact rejection system
motion artifact suppression technique
noise spike a.
nuclear bubbling a.
a. on x-ray
overlying attenuation a.
phase shift a.
a. pronunciation
simulated echo a.
split image a.
stimulated echo a.
stimulus a.
temporal instability a.

artifactual
a. gap
a. hypoglycemia

artificial
a. abortion
a. active immunity
air-driven artificial heart
a. airway
a. anatomy
a. ankylosis
a. anus
a. assist
bacterial artificial chromosome
a. beta cell
a. bezoar
a. blood substrate
a. cardiac valve
CardioWest total artificial heart
a. chromosome
a. circus-movement tachycardia
a. classification cavity
a. cornea
a. crown
defective artificial heart valve
a. dentition
a. diabetes
a. disorder
a. divergence procedure
a. divergency surgery
a. diverticulum of the ileum
a. dream
a. ear
electromechanical artificial heart
electronic artificial larynx
a. endocrine pancreas
a. erection
a. erection test
a. fat pad
a. fecundation
a. fever
a. fistulation
a. fracture
a. genitourinary sphincter implantation
a. growth hormone
a. gut
a. heart
a. heart energy system
a. heart implant
a. heart recipient
a. heart valve
a. hepatic support
a. hip joint
homologous artificial insemination
human artificial chromosome
a. immunity
a. implant
implantable artificial heart
a. insemination
a. insemination by donor
a. insemination donor, husband
a. insemination, homologous
a. insemination with donor sperm
a. insulin
a. intelligence
a. intelligence in medicine
a. internal bladder
intrathoracic artificial lung
a. intravaginal insemination
a. joint implant material
a. kidney
a. knee joint
a. language
a. leech
a. left heart pump
a. left ventricular assist device
a. lens
a. lens implant
a. lens implantation
a. ligament
a. limb
a. lumen narrowing
a. lung-expanding compound
a. mastoid
a. melanin
a. membrane rupture
a. method
Myobock artificial hand
a. neural network
a. neural network algorithm
a. neurosis
nonpreserved artificial tears
a. nose
a. nutrition and hydration
a. organ
orthoptic biventricular artificial heart
orthotopic univentricular artificial heart
a. pacemaker-induced ventricular rhythm
a. passive immunity
a. penis
a. pleural effusion procedure
a. pneumothorax
a. pupil
a. radioactivity
a. respiration
a. root
a. rupture of bag of waters
a. rupture of membranes
a. saliva
Schafer method of artificial respiration
a. seawater
a. selection
silicone-based artificial joint
a. silk keratitis
a. skin
a. sound generator
a. spermatocele
a. spinal disk
a. stone

a. tears
a. temperature
a. tooth
total implantation of artificial heart
a. urethral sphincter
a. urinary sphincter
a. urinary sphincter implantation
a. UV radiation
a. vagina
a. vaginal epithelium
a. valve endocarditis
a. velum
a. ventilation
a. vertebral body
a. vichy salt
a. vision
yeast artificial chromosome

artificially
a. fed
a. ruptured

artiodactylous fold of Collier

Artisan
A. cement system
A. lens

artistic
a. anatomy
a. bias

arts
manual arts therapist
A. syndrome

art/trs gene

Aruac virus

arum
a. fixation pin
a. plant

Arumowot virus

Arvidsson dimension-length method for ventricular volume

arycorniculate synchondrosis

aryepiglottic
a. cyst
a. fascia
a. fold
a. fold carcinoma
a. fold neurofibroma
a. fold width
a. muscle
a. part of oblique arytenoid muscle

aryl
a. group
a. hydrocarbon receptor
a. hydrocarbon receptor nuclear translocator

arylalkanoic acid

arylamidase

arylarsonic acid

arylated alkyl

arylcarboxylic acid

aryl-ester hydrolase

arylhydrocarbon
a. hydroxylase
a. receptor

arylpropionic acid

arylsulfatase
a. A
a. activity test
a. A deficiency
a. B
a. B deficiency
a. b deficiency
a. B syndrome
a. C
a. a deficiency
a. test

arylsulfatase-activator deficiency

arytenoepiglottidean fold

arytenoid
a. adduction
apex of arytenoid cartilage
arcuate crest of arytenoid cartilage
articular surface of arytenoid cartilage
aryepiglottic part of oblique arytenoid muscle
a. cartilage
a. dislocation
a. gland
a. muscle
oblique a.
oblique arytenoid muscle
oblong fovea of arytenoid cartilage
a. perichondritis
a. process
a. sparing
a. subluxation
a. swelling
transverse arytenoid muscle

arytenoidal
a. articular surface
a. articular surface of cricoid

arytenoideus
musculus arytenoideus obliquus
musculus arytenoideus transversus

aryvocalis
musculus a.

AS-1 virus

ASA-induced gastric ulceration

Asbee-Hansen disease

asbestos
atelectatic asbestos pseudotumor
a. body
a. corn
a. exposure
a. fiber
a. liner
a. pleural plaque
a. transformation
a. wart

asbestos-induced pleural fibrosis

asbestosis
a. pneumoconiosis
pulmonary a.

asbestos-related
a.-r. illness
a.-r. lung carcinoma
a.-r. mesothelioma
a.-r. pleural disease
a.-r. pleural effusion
a.-r. pleural thickening

Asboe-Hansen
A.-H. disease
A.-H. sign

A-scan
A-s. imaging
A-s. ultrasonography
A-s. ultrasound

ascariasis
a. disorder
pancreatic a.
a. serological test

Ascaris
Ascaris antigen
Ascaris infestation
Ascaris pneumonitis

ascendant follicle

ascended healing

ascendens
aorta a.
arteria a.
arteria cervicalis a.
arteria palatina a.
arteria pharyngea a.
lumbalis a.
mesocolon a.
musculus cervicalis a.
palatina a.

ascendens *(continued)*
pars ascendens aortae
pars ascendens musculi trapezii

ascending
aneurysm of ascending aorta
a. anterior branch
a. aorta
a. aorta dilatation
a. aorta hypoplasia
a. aorta synchronized pulsation
a. aortic aneurysm
a. aortic pressure
a. aortography
a. bladder septum
a. branch
a. branch of the inferior mesenteric artery
a. branch of superficial cervical artery
a. cervical artery
a. cholangiopathy
a. cholangitis
a. chromatography
a. colon
a. contrast MR phlebogram
a. contrast phlebography
a. contrast phlebography imaging
a. contrast venography
cortical thick ascending limb
a. current
cystic medial necrosis of ascending aorta
a. degeneration
a. and descending
a. flaccid paralysis
a. frontal convolution
a. frontal gyrus
a. frontal parietal
a. frontoparietal
a. frontoparietal artery
a. gonococcal infection
a. hemiplegia
a. hypoplasia of aorta
a. ileocolic artery
a. intrauterine infection
a. limb
a. loop of Henle
a. lumbar vein
a. lymphangitis
medullary thick ascending limb
medullary thick ascending limb of Henle
a. medullary vein thrombosis
a. mesocolon
a. myelitis
necrosis of ascending aorta
a. neuritis
a. neurotransmitter system
nonsuppurative ascending cholangitis
a. palatine artery
a. paralysis
a. parietal convolution
a. parietal gyrus
a. part of aorta
a. part of duodenum
a. part of trapezius muscle
a. pathway
a. pathway of pain projection
a. pharyngeal artery
pharyngeal branch of ascending pharyngeal artery
a. pharyngeal plexus
a. pitch break
a. poliomyelitis
a. polyneuritis
a. polyradiculitis
a. posterior branch
a. process
a. pyelography
a. pyelonephritis
a. radiculomyelitis
a. ramus
a. ramus of ischium
a. ramus of lateral sulcus of cerebrum
a. ramus of mandible
a. reticular-activating system
a. reticular activation
a. reticular arousal system
Rosenthal ascending vein
a. technique
a. technique audiometry
thick ascending limb
thick ascending limb of Henle loop
a. tract
a. urethrogram
a. urography
a. venography

ascension
a. phase
A. PIP total joint replacement

ascertainment
a. bias
method of a.

Asch
A. operation
A. situation
A. splint

Ascher
A. aqueous influx phenomenon
A. glass-rod phenomenon
A. syndrome
A. vein

Aschheim-Zondek
A.-Z. hormone
A.-Z. test

Aschner
A. phenomenon
A. reflex

Aschner-Dagnini reflex

Aschoff
A. body
A. cell
A. node
node of Aschoff and Tawara
A. nodule

Aschoff-Rokitansky sinus

Aschoff-Tawara node

ascites
a. adiposus
a. chylosus
culture-negative neutrocytic a.
a. drainage tube
a. due to bile leak
Ehrlich ascites carcinoma
Ehrlich ascites tumor
Ehrlich ascites tumor cell
a. euglobulin lysis time
a. fluid tap
a. hepatoma
malignant ascites fluid
narrow albumin gradient a.
nephrogenous dialysis a.
obstruction with a.
ovarian carcinoma with a.
portal hypertension with a.
rapidly accumulating a.
refractory a.
a. tumor fluid
yellow-brown serous a.

ascites-albumin
serum ascites-albumin gradient

ascitic
a. agar
a. amylase
a. fluid
a. fluid in abdomen
a. fluid cytology
a. fluid tapped daily
a. fluid test
a. fluid total protein
a. tumor fluid

Ascoli
A. reaction
A. test
A. treatment

ascorbate-cyanide test

ascorbic
a. acid assay
a. acid deficiency
a. acid factor
a. acid test
a. free radical
leukocyte ascorbic acid
ovarian ascorbic acid depletion test

ascorbyl palmitate

ascospore-forming fungus

ascriptive responsibility

A1 segment of anterior cerebral artery

Aselli pancreas

asepsis
born out of a.
isolation and a.

aseptic
acute aseptic meningitis
acute aseptic meningitis syndrome
a. anastomosis
a. catheterization technique
a. condition
a. epiphysial necrosis
a. fashion
a. felon
a. fever
idiopathic aseptic necrosis
Lichtman aseptic necrosis classification
a. loosening
a. meningeal reaction
a. meningitis
a. meningitis syndrome
a. meningoencephalitis
a. necrosis of bone
a. peritonitis
a. surgery
a. technique
a. temperature
a. uremic meningitis
a. wound

asexual
a. dwarfism
a. generation
a. reproduction

ash
Arizona a.
Arizona ash tree
a. leaf patch
a. leaf spot
Oregon a.
a. tree
a. tree pollen
volcanic a.

ashamed
guilty, ashamed and intimidated

Ashby differential agglutination method

ashen
a. gray color
a. tuber
a. tubercle
a. wing

Asherman syndrome

Asher physical build assessment technique

Asherson syndrome

Ashford retracted nipple operation

ashgray
a. blister beetle
a. blister beetle sting

Ashhurst
A. fracture classification system
A. sign

Ashhurst-Bromer
A.-B. ankle fracture classification
A.-B. classification

Ashkenazi
A. Jew
A. Jewish community
A. Jewish heritage

ash-leaf
a.-l. macule
a.-l. patch
a.-l. spot
a.-l. spot in tuberous sclerosis

Ashley phenomenon

Ashman
A. index
A. phenomenon

Ashworth
A. hand arthroplasty
A. scale
A. score
A. score of muscle spasticity

ashy
a. dermatitis
a. dermatosis
a. dermatosis of Ramirez

Asia
Southeast Asia mosquito-borne hemorrhagic fever

ASIA impairment scale for classification of spinal cord injury

asialoglycoprotein receptor

Asian
A. alcohol flush reaction
A. influenza
National Asian Pacific Center on Aging
North Asian tick typhus
Southeast Asian ovalocytosis
A. taeniasis

Asiatic
A. cholera
A. schistosomiasis

asiatica
titrated extract of *Centella asiatica*

asiderotic anemia

ASIF
A. broad dynamic compression
A. chisel
A. system
A. T-plate

as-if
a.-i. hypothesis
a.-i. performance
a.-i. personality

Askanazy
A. cell
pathognomonic Askanazy cell

asked
frequently asked questions

Askin
A. biopsy
A. thoracopulmonary neuroepithelial tumor
A. tumor

Ask-Upmark renal segment

asleep
difficulty falling a.

ASLO titer

as-needed basis

Asnis
A. pinning
A. technique

asocial
a. acting out
a. trends psychopathic personality

Asopa
A. hypospadias repair
A. procedure

asparagine-linked
a.-l. glycosylation moiety
a.-l. oligosaccharide

asparaginic acid

asparic acid

aspartame-restricted diet

aspartate
a. aminotransferase
a. aminotransferase assay
a. aminotransferase level
a. carbamoyltransferase
cytoplasmic aspartate aminotransferase
a. 1-decarboxylase
a. 4-decarboxylase
a. kinase
mitochondrial aspartate aminotransferase
N-phosphoacetate-L a.
ratio of serum alanine aminotransferase to serum aspartate aminotransferase
a. target
a. transaminase
a. transferase

aspartic
a. acid
amino acid that gives aspartic acid after hydrolysis
a. proteinase

aspartoacylase deficiency

aspartyl
a. protease class
a. protease-mediated cleavage

aspecific
chronic aspecific respiratory ailment

aspect
anterior a.
anteroinferior a.
anterolateral a.
anteroposterior a.
apical a.
associative a.
axial a.
cognitive aspect of well-being
cultural aspect of chemical dependency
functional aspects of heart
health aspects of pesticides
ipsilateral a.
linguistic a.
lordotic a.
medial a.
mediolateral a.
mesial a.
mesial aspect of temporal lobe
normative a.
occipital a.
orbital aspect of frontal lobe
outer a.
paraspinous a.
perceptual a.
physiologic a.
plantar a.
plantar aspect of foot
posterior a.
posterior aspect of pharyngeal wall
posteroinferior a.
posterolateral a.
posteromedial a.
proximal a.
radial a.
superior a.
superolateral a.

Aspen sonography unit

Asperger
A. disorder
A. syndrome

aspergillic acid

aspergilloma formation

aspergillosis
allergic bronchopulmonary a.
bronchopulmonary a.
a. esophagitis
a. infection
invasive a.
invasive pulmonary a.
miliary pulmonary a.
obstructing bronchial a.
rhinocerebral a.
systemic a.
a. uveitis

aspergillotic
a. aneurysm
a. granuloma

Aspergillus
Aspergillus antibody test
Aspergillus arteritis
Aspergillus antibody test
Aspergillus brain abscess
Aspergillus cerebral abscess
Aspergillus fungus ball
Aspergillus IgG titer
Aspergillus bezoar
Aspergillus brain abscess
Aspergillus cerebral abscess
Aspergillus fungus ball
Aspergillus IgG titer

***Aspergillus*-specific IgE**

aspermatogenic sterility

aspermia
psychogenic a.

aspheric
a. contact lens
a. cornea
a. lens
a. lenticular area
a. spectacle lens

aspheric-viewing lens

asphyctic
a. infant
a. syndrome

asphyxia
antepartum a.
autoerotic a.
a. and death
a. livida
local a.
neonatal a.
a. neonatorum
perinatal a.
repeated partial a.

asphyxial
a. birth injury
a. brain injury
a. event
a. renal trauma

asphyxiant
thoracic asphyxiant dystrophy

asphyxia-related renal necrosis

asphyxiating
a. thoracic chondrodystrophy
a. thoracic dysplasia
a. thoracic dysplasia syndrome
a. thoracic dystrophy

aspidium oleoresin

aspiny
a. interneuron
a. neuron

aspirate
bone marrow a.
direct lung a.
endotracheal a.
nasopharyngeal a.
nipple aspirate fluid
orogastric gonococcal a.
protected catheter a.
protected transbronchial needle a.
tracheal a.
tracheobronchial aspirate fluid

aspirated
a. abdomen

catheter aspirated and flushed
catheter aspirated and flushed with saline
a. fat
fluid aspirated from abdomen
fluid aspirated from chest
fluid aspirated from joint
fluid aspirated from knee
a. and flushed
a. foreign body
a. foreign material
a. sample

aspirating
irrigating and a.
O'Gawa two-way aspirating cannula
specialized tissue aspirating resectoscope
uterine vacuum aspirating curette

aspirating/irrigating vectis

aspiration
acid aspiration syndrome
amniotic fluid a.
anterior chamber a.
a. biopsy
a. biopsy cytology
a. of blood material
a. of bloody material
a. of bone
bronchoscopic needle a.
a. cannula
a. catheter
cold knife cone a.
continuous aspiration of subglottic secretions
a. of cortex
a. cytology
dilatation and a.
dilation and a.
a. and dissection tube
elbow a.
endoluminal ultrasonography-guided fine-needle aspiration biopsy
a. of endometrium
endoscopic aspiration lumpectomy
endoscopic aspiration mucosectomy
endoscopic ultrasound-guided fine-needle a.
endotracheal a.
epididymal sperm a.
fine-needle a.
fine-needle aspiration biopsy
fine-needle aspiration cytology
follicle aspiration, sperm injection, and assisted rupture
a. of food of fluid
a. of food particle
a. of foreign body
a. of gastric contents
image-guided fine-needle aspiration biopsy
a. and injection of bursa
a. and injection of joint
a. and injection of tendons
intracoronary aspiration thrombectomy
intraoperative fine-needle a.
irrigation and a.
joint a.
large-needle aspiration biopsy
a. of lens
a. level
mammary aspiration specimen cytology test
manual vacuum a.
a. of mature oocyte
maxillary sinus a.
microepididymal sperm a.
microscopic epididymal sperm a.
microsurgical epididymal sperm a.
microsurgical epididymal sperm aspiration procedure
monoclonal antibody A103 fine-needle aspiration biopsy
a. mucosectomy
myringotomy with a.
a. needle
needle aspiration cytology
needle aspiration lung biopsy
a. needle biopsy
a. of newborn
nipple aspiration cytology
organizing aspiration pneumonia
a. of ova
pelvic aspiration biopsy
peptic aspiration pneumonia
peptic aspiration pneumonitis
percutaneous aspiration, instillation of hypertonic saline, respiration
percutaneous aspiration thromboembolectomy
percutaneous balloon a.
percutaneous bladder a.
percutaneous CT-guided a.
percutaneous cyst a.
percutaneous epididymal sperm a.
percutaneous fine-needle a.
percutaneous fine-needle aspiration biopsy
percutaneous needle a.
percutaneous needle aspiration biopsy
percutaneous needle lung a.
a. of pleural cavity
pleural fluid a.
a. pneumonia
a. pneumonitis
a. portal
preoperative gastric a.
a. prophylaxis
puncture, aspiration, injection, reaspiration
real-time fine-needle a.
rete testis a.
rotating aspiration thromboembolectomy
skinny needle a.
suction aspiration abortion
suprapubic a.
a. syndrome
a. syringe
terminal aspiration of gastric contents
testicular sperm a.
therapeutic abortion, dilation, aspiration, and curettage
transbronchial needle a.
translaryngeal a.
transthoracic needle a.
transthoracic needle aspiration biopsy
transtracheal a.
a. tube
ultrasound-guided fine-needle a.
ultrasound-guided fine-needle aspiration biopsy
uterine a.
vacuum a.

aspirational
a. biopsy
a. group

aspirative lipoplasty

aspirin
anticoagulation regimen of a.
bleeding from a.
burning mouth from a.
Carotid Artery Stenosis with Asymptomatic Narrowing: Operation Versus A. Study
a. and codeine
a. combination
a. effect
enteric coated a.
a. exposure
a. gastritis
gastritis from a.
hearing loss from a.
a. and heart attack
heart attack from a.

aspirin *(continued)*
high-dose aspirin therapy
hypersensitivity to a.
a. ingestion
a. interaction
liberal doses of a.
long-term aspirin therapy
low-dose aspirin therapy
oxycodone and a.
patient hypersensitive to a.
patient intolerant to aspirin therapy
phenacetin, aspirin, and caffeine
a. poisoning
preventive aspirin therapy
preventive aspirin therapy
a. sensitivity
ticlopidine plus a.
a. tolerance
a. tolerance test
a. tolerance therapy
a. tolerance time
a. toxicity
a. triad

aspiring
heart attack from a.

aspirin-induced
a.-i. asthma
a.-i. gastritis
a.-i. papillary necrosis

aspirin-intolerant asthma

aspirin-like disorder

aspirin-sensitive
a.-s. asthma
a.-s. asthma syndrome
a.-s. respiratory disease

aspiryl chloride

asplenia
congenital asplenia syndrome
a. syndrome

Assam fever

assassin
a. bug
a. bug bite

assault
aggravated a.
a. and battery
a. gun
personal a.
physical a.
radiation assault on tumor
a. rifle
sexual assault forensic evidence
sexual assault nurse examiner
Sexual A. Response Team
a. weapon
a. with deadly weapon
a. with a deadly weapon

assaultive
a. act
a. behavior
a. episode
management of assaultive behavior

assay
a. accuracy
adenosine deaminase a.
agar diffusion a.
agglutination inhibition a.
alpha-1 fetoprotein a.
angiotensin I and II a.
antiacetylcholine receptor antibody a.
antibody blocking a.
antibody capture ligand a.
antibody production a.
anticathepsin D autoantibody a.
anticytochrome P4502D6 a.
anti-D enzyme-linked immunosorbent a.
anti-DNA antibody a.
anti-DNase B a.
antigen capture a.
antigen capture ligand a.
antigen-nonspecific immune complex a.
antimitochondrial antibody a.
antinuclear antibody a.
antiparietal cell antibody a.
antiphospholipid antibody a.
antiplatelet antibody a.
antismooth muscle antibody a.
antistreptolysin O a.
anti-*Toxoplasma gondii* antibody secretion a.
APC gene mutation a.
argininosuccinate lyase a.
ascorbic acid a.
aspartate aminotransferase a.
autoantibody assay testing
automated LCx factor V Leiden a.
avidin-biotin complex a.
BCR-ABL multiplex reverse transcriptase polymerase chain reaction a.
a. buffer
clotting a.
cocaine metabolite a.
colony-forming a.
competitive-binding a.
competitive protein-binding a.
compressed spectral a.
cytotoxic a.
direct fluorescence a.
direct fluorescent a.
dot immunobinding a.
electrophoretic mobility shift a.
enzyme immunosorbent a.
enzyme-linked immunoabsorbent a.
enzyme-linked immunoelectrodiffusion a.
enzyme-linked immunofiltration a.
enzyme-linked immunosorbent a.
enzyme-linked immunospot a.
estradiol receptor a.
estrogen receptor a.
estrogen receptor immunocytochemistry a.
ethylene glycol a.
fluorescent a.
fluorescent antinuclear antibody a.
Folin-Denis assay
food immune complex a.
free radical assay technique
frozen section a.
glycoprotein-based enzyme-linked immunosorbent a.
gonadotropic hormone a.
Guthrie bacterial inhibition a.
hamster egg penetration a.
hemagglutination inhibition a.
hemagglutinin enzyme-linked immunosorbent a.
hemizona assay index
hemolytic complement a.
hemolytic plaque a.
heparin assay rapid easy method
heteroduplex mobility a.
histoculture drug response a.
human androgen receptor a.
human tumor colony a.
human tumor stem cell a.
hybrid capture a.
immune adherence hemagglutination a.
immune adherence immunosorbent a.
immunochemiluminescence a.
immunochemiluminescent a.
immunochemiluminometric a.
immunocytochemical a.
immunofluorescence a.
immunofluorescent antibody a.
immunometric a.
immunoperoxidase infectivity a.
immunoradiometric a.
immunosorbent agglutination a.

indirect fluorescent a.
indirect hemagglutination a.
indirect hemagglutinin a.
kinetic fibrinogen a.
leukocyte migration inhibition a.
ligase-chain reaction a.
limiting dilution a.
line probe a.
LiPA strip a.
liquid chromatographic a.
liver-kidney-microsomal type 1 antibody target a.
local lymph-node a.
Lyme enzyme-linked immunosorbent a.
lymphocyte function a.
lymphocyte proliferation a.
lysergic acid diethylamide a.
lysosomal hydrolase enzyme a.
a. marker
matrix metalloproteinase-2 a.
maximal static response a.
measles virus enzyme-linked immunosorbent a.
medical laboratory a.
mersalyl exchange a.
a. methodology
microbiologic a.
microculture tetrazolium dye a.
microcytotoxicity a.
microhemagglutination assay for antibodies to *Treponema pallidum*
micrometastases clonogenic a.
micrometastases detection a.
microplate plasma methotrexate a.
microplate plasma MTX a.
Minnesota-Hartford Personality A.
mobility shift a.
monocyte monolayer a.
multiple-allele-specific diagnostic a.
multiple marker reverse transcriptase-polymerase chain reaction a.
mutation-enriched restriction fragment length polymorphism a.
myelin basic protein a.
nephelometric inhibition a.
neuropilin 1 a.
neuropilin 2 a.
a. neutrophil cytoplasmic antibody
nonisotopic RNase cleavage a.
a. normalization
nuclear runoff a.
nucleic acid probe a.
ornithine carbamoyltransferase a.
Osteomark NTx a.
oxalic acid a.
oxidized lipoproteina a.
pantothenic acid a.
paper enzyme-linked immunosorbent a.
parathyroid hormone a.
parvovirus B19 neutralizing antibody a.
progesterone receptor a.
prolactin-binding a.
protein A hemolytic plaque a.
radioallergosorbent assay test
radioantigen-binding a.
radioenzymatic a.
radioimmunoblot a.
radioimmunologic assay antithyroid antibody
radioimmunoprecipitation a.
radioimmunosorbent a.
radioreceptor a.
radioreceptor assay pregnancy blood
Raji cell a.
rapid assay delivery systems
recombinant immunoblot a.
recombinant immunosorbent a.
recombinant virus a.
a. reference plasma
renal vein renin a.
replication-competent retrovirus a.
reverse hemolytic plaque a.
ribonuclease protection a.
seminal fluid a.
a. sensitivity
serum tobramycin a.
single-cell liquid cytotoxic a.
solid-phase immunoabsorbent a.
a. specificity
sperm penetration a.
spleen colony a.
stem cell indicated by transplantation a.
syncytia induction a.
a. target
a. technique
therapeutic drug a.
thyroxine radioisotope a.
tissue culture a.
tumor chemosensitivity a.
tumor clonogenic a.
tumor glycoprotein a.
Ultegra rapid platelet function a.
vasoconstrictor a.
in vitro antibody production a.

assembly

automated tray a.
blood pressure a.
emergency oxygen mask a.
fecal collection receptacle a.
infant nasal cannula a.
Minnesota Mechanical A. Test
multiple hook a.
multiple hook assembly C-D instrumentation
object assembly test

Asserachrom

A. APA
A. APA immunoassay
A. ATM
A. beta-TG
A. FPA
A. PF4
A. thrombospondin
A. VII:Ag10000
A. vWF
A. X:Ag

assertion structured therapy

assertive

a. behavior
a. conditioning
a. outreach
systematized assertive therapy
systemic assertive therapy
a. training

assertive-community treatment approach

assertiveness

a. skill
a. training

assess

a. functioning of heart
Structured and Scaled Interview to A. Maladjustment

assessed

to be a.

assessing

a. needs of hallucinogen abuser
a. severity: age of patient, systems involved, stage of disease, complications, response to therapy

assessment

a. of academic achievement
acquired immunodeficiency syndrome health assessment questionnaire
Activity Loss A.
A. of Adaptive Areas
a. adjustment pass
Adolescent Drug and Alcohol Diagnostic A.
aerobic conditioning functional a.

assessment *(continued)*

a. of affect
aged care assessment team
Alzheimer Disease A. Scale
Alzheimer Disease Assessment Scale, cognitive subscale
American Pediatric Gross A. Record
aortoiliac inflow a.
A. of Aphasia and Related Disorders, Second Edition
Apraxia Profile: A Descriptive A. Tool for Children
arterial noninvasive vascular a.
Asher physical build assessment technique
audiologic a.
awake neurological a.
Ballard A. Score
Barclay Learning Needs Assessment Inventory
a. of basic competency
a. battery
Behavioral A. of Pain Questionnaire
Behavioral A. Scale for Children
biological terrain a.
Boston A. of Severe Aphasia
Brazelton Neonatal Behavioral A. Scale
British Isles Lupus Assessment Group index
A. of Career Decision Making
A. of Career Development
Career A. Inventory
child and adolescent burden a.
Child and Adolescent Functional A. Scale
Child and Adolescent Psychiatric A.
Child Health A. Program
Childhood Health A. Questionnaire
Childhood Myositis A. Scale
Children's Global A. Scale
A. of Children's Language Comprehension
chronotropic exercise assessment protocol
cine densitometric assessment of transit time
Clifton A. Procedures for the Elderly
Clinical Health A. Questionnaire
clinical risk a.
Coarticulation A. in Meaningful Language
cognitive function a.
Cognitive Skills A.
communication skills a.
a. of competence
complete and ongoing a.
comprehensive assessment of symptoms and history
Comprehensive Career A. Scale
comprehensive geriatric a.
computer-assisted a.
computerized risk a.
A. of Conceptual Organization
Confusion A. Method
A. of Core Goals
A. of Dementia
Dementia Mood A. Scale
Developmental Indicators for A. of Learning
Developmental A. of Life Experiences
a. and diagnosis
Diagnostic A. Questionnaire
Diagnostic a.'s of Reading
Dimensional A. of Personality Pathology-Basic Questionnaire
Distress Risk A. Method
Early School A.
Edmonton Symptom A. Scale
Einstein Neonatal Neurobehavioral A. Scale
ergonomic assessment of risk and liability
Erhardt Developmental Prehension A.
Erhardt Developmental Vision A.
extensive hearing a.
external quality a.
fall risk a.
family assessment adjustment pass
Family A. Device
family risk assessment program
Final Comprehensive Consensus A.
focused assessment by sonography for trauma
Frenchay Dysarthria A.
functional assessment of human immunodeficiency
functional assessment inventory
functional assessment measure
Functional A. of Cancer Therapy
Functional A. of Cancer Therapy-Breast
Functional A. of Cancer Therapy-Fatigue
Functional A. of Cancer Therapy-General
Functional A. of Cancer Therapy–Head and Neck
Functional A. of Cancer Therapy-Lung
Functional A. of Cancer Therapy-Prostate
Functional Needs A.
Functional A. Staging
functional work capacity a.
General Audit Inpatient Psychiatric A. Scale
geriatric assessment team
geriatric assessment unit
Glasgow A. Schedule
global assessment of function
global assessment index
global assessment of functioning
Global A. of Relational Functioning
Headache A. Questionnaire
Health A. Questionnaire Disability Index
health-related quality-of-life a.
health risk a.
a. of health status
heart risk a.
individualized functional status a.
individual treatment a.
A. in Infancy Ordinal Scales of Psychological Development
initial assessment phase
initial case a.
initial head a.
a. instrument
intake assessment staff
Integrated A. System
A. of Intelligibility of Dysarthric Speech
Interpersonal Language Skills and A.
a. inventory
Juvenile Arthritis Functional A. Report
Kaufman A. Battery for Children
a. for limiting condition
Manchester and Oxford Universities Scale for the Psychopathological A. of Dementia
a. in mathematics
McGill Pain A. Questionnaire
McMaster Family A. Device
a. measure
A. Measure for Atopic Dermatitis
Memorial Delirium A. Scale
Memorial Pain A. Card

Memorial Symptom Assessment Scale-Physical
Memorial Symptom Assessment Scale-Psychological
Memory A. Scale
a. method
Meyer-Kendall A. Survey
Migraine Disability A. Scale
Miller A. for Preschoolers
Minnesota Clerical A. Battery
Modified Health A. Questionnaire
Morrow A. of Nausea and Emesis
Mother's A. of the Behavior of Her Infant
motor function a.
Motor A. Scale
movement assessment of infant
Multiaxial A. of Pain
multidimensional assessment of outcome
Multidimensional A. of Philosophy of Education
Multiphasic Environmental A. Procedure
Muma A. Program
Musculoskeletal Function A.
narrative, assessment, and plan
Neonatal Behavioral A. Scale
Neonatal Behavioral A. Scale with Kansas Supplements
neuromuscular maturity a.
Newborn Behavior A. Scale
noninvasive assessment of urinary flow
noninvasive vascular a.
nutritional status a.
OARS Multidimensional Functional A. Questionnaire
observation and a.
Observer A. of Alertness and Sedation
ocular hemodynamic a.
online assessment method
Outcomes and A. Information Set
overall a.
patient global assessment of disease activity
Patient A. Program
Performance-Oriented Mobility A.
Performance A. of Syntax Elicited and Spontaneous
peritoneal cytological a.
Personal A. for Continuing Education
Personal A. of Intimacy in Relationships
Personality A. Inventory
A. for Persons Profoundly or Severely Impaired
A. of Phonological Processes
Physical A. Center
a. and plan
a., plan, implementation, and evaluation
Postural A. Scale for Stroke Patients
preadmission screening and assessment team
premenstrual assessment form
preschool-age psychiatric a.
Preschool Evaluation and A. for Children with Handicaps
Preschool Evaluation and A. for Children with Handicaps
Preschool Language A. Instrument
pressure sore risk a.
A. of Preterm Infants Behavior
Prevocational A. and Curriculum Guide
a. procedure
Proficiency A. Report
A. Program of Early Learning Levels
Progress A. Chart of Social and Personal Development
psychosocial a.
Psychosocial A. of Childhood Experiences
Psychotherapy Competence A. Schedule
quality a.
a. questionnaire
resident assessment protocol
Rivermead motor a.
Rivermead Perceptual A. Battery
a. scale
Scale for the A. of Negative Symptoms
Scale for the A. of Positive Symptoms
Scale for the A. of Unawareness of Mental Disorder
Schedule for A. of Insight
Schema Assessment instrument
School A. Survey
Screening A. for Gifted Elementary Students, Primary
Seasonal Pattern A. Questionnaire
selective tubal assessment to refine reproductive therapy
Self Care A. Schedule
sepsis-related organ failure a.
sequential organ failure a.
Service A. for Children and Adolescents
Short Musculoskeletal Function A.
sideline assessment of concussion
Social Behavior A. Inventory
Social and Occupational Functioning A.
Standardized A. of Depressive Disorders
Stanford Health A. Questionnaire
subjective global a.
Support Team A. Schedule
Systematic A. for Treatment of Emergent Events
System of Multicultural A.
System of Multicultural Pluralistic A.
Tanner-Whitehouse Mark 2 bone-age a.
Teacher A. of Social Behavior
Toglia Category A. Test
Total Severity A.
Trainer's Assessment of Proficiency
Treatment Rating A. Matrix
Treatment Response A. Method
trial assessment procedure scale
Visual Analogue Self A. Scales For Pain Intensity
Vocational Interest, Experience, and Skill A.
Vocational Interest and Sophistication A.
vocational skills assessment and development program
Wide Range A. of Memory and Learning
work capacity a.
young adult psychiatric a.

assets-liabilities technique

Assézat triangle

ASSI

A. breast dissector angulated
A. breast dissector spatulated
A. cannula
A. coagulator

assident

a. sign
a. symptom

assign blame

assigned
a. responsibility
a. sex

assignment
a. criteria for rheumatoid arthritis
nursing a.
a. statement
a. therapy
treatment a.

assimilating
a. information
a. information disturbance

assimilation
atlantooccipital a.
atlas a.
a. effect
glucose a.
a. law
a. limit
nasal a.
a. pelvis
a. phonological process
a. regulatory protein
a. rule
a. sacrum

assimilative factor

assist
abdominal left ventricular assist device
acute ventricular assist device
ambulates with minimal a.
artificial left ventricular assist device
bilateral ventricular assist device
biventricular assist device
Bourns a.
a. control
dorsiflexion a.
extracorporeal liver assist device
extracorporeal lung a.
implantable left ventricular assist system
left ventricular assist device
light contact a.
permanently implanted ventricular assist device
proportional assist ventilation
proportional assist ventilator
right ventricular assist device
standby assist with ambulation
ventricular assist device
a. with bedpan
a. with urinal

assistance
AIDS Drug A. Program
ambulates with a.
ambulates with minimal a.
contact assistance for ambulation
continuous mechanical ventilatory a.
disability a.
disaster assistance center
disaster medical assistance team
emergency a.
emergency assistance to families
external pressure circulatory a.
general nursing a.
handheld a.
home care a.
intraaortic balloon a.
intraaortic balloon pumping a.
long-term mechanical a.
maximum assistance for lower body dressing
maximum assistance for upper body dressing
mechanical ventricular a.
medical a.
Medical A. for the Aged
minimal assistance for lower body dressing
minimal assistance for transfers
minimal assistance for upper body dressing
a. and mobility
National Organization of Victim A.
Old Age A.
passive assistance exercise
passive assistance range of motion
patient ambulates with a.
patient needs minimal assistance for wheelchair mobility
patient receiving respiratory a.
patient transfers with standby a.
physical a.
radiologic emergency assistance team
standby assistance in transfers and ambulation
total ventilatory a.
with a.
a. with walking

assistant
emergency a.
expanded function dental a.
family planning health a.
medical office a.
nonphysician surgical a.
patient care a.
physical therapy a.

assist-control
a.-c. mode ventilation
a.-c. ventilation

assist-controlled mechanical ventilation

assisted
active assisted exercise
a. ambulation
arthroscopically assisted anterior cruciate ligament reconstruction
arthroscopically assisted synovectomy
a. breech
a. breech delivery
a. cephalic delivery
a. circulation
contact assisted ambulation
a. control
electrothermally assisted capsulorrhaphy
endoscopically assisted duodenal intubation
ethical validity of assisted suicide
a. fertilization
follicle aspiration, sperm injection, and assisted rupture
a. health insurance plan
intermittent assisted ventilation
laparoscopically assisted distal partial gastrectomy
laparoscopically assisted surgery
a. living facility
A. Living Federation of America
a. living setting
maximum assisted transfer
mechanically a.
a. mechanical ventilation
a. medical procreation
memory impaired assisted living
micro assisted fertilization
minimal assisted transfer
a. reduction and internal fixation
a. reproduction
a. reproductive technique
a. respiration
right to be assisted to die
spontaneous assisted vaginal delivery
a. suicide
surgically assisted rapid maxillary expansion
surgically assisted rapid palatal expansion
a. zonal hatching

assisted-reproduction technology

assister
percutaneous breathing a.
pressure breathing a.

assistive
active assistive exercise
a. device
a. listening device
a. movement
progressive assistive exercise
a. technology device
unlicensed assistive personnel

Assmann
A. disease
A. focus
A. tuberculous infiltrate

associate
a. learning
National Association of Pediatric Nurse A.'s and Practitioners
paired associate learning
Paired A. Learning Subtest
Paired A. Learning Task
Remote A.'s Test
therapeutic recreation a.

associated
abdominal pain associated with blood loss
alcoholism associated with dementia
anemia associated with chronic renal failure
a. anomaly
anorexia nervosa and associated disorders
a. antagonist
anxiety associated with depression
apneic spell associated with loud snoring
arrhythmia associated with cardiopulmonary arrest
commissural a.
a. descriptive feature
a. disability
a. disorder
environmentally associated rheumatic disorder
eosinophilic, polymorphic, and pruritic eruption associated with radiotherapy
hepatitis B surface a.
human immunodeficiency virus associated dementia
human immunodeficiency virus associated motor cognitive disorder
human T-cell lymphotropic virus type I associated myelopathy
human T-lymphotrophic virus/lymphadenopathy associated virus
a. idea
a. imaging characteristic
a. infectious disease
a. injury
insomnia associated with anxiety
insomnia associated with depression
a. intervention
jaundice associated with sepsis
a. laboratory finding
a. macrophage
malignancy associated cellular marker
malignancy associated neutropenia
Marek associated tumor-specific antigen
microphthalmia or anophthalmos with associated anomalies
a. movement
multidrug resistance associated protein
myeloid associated antigen
a. myofascial trigger point
National Association of Anorexia Nervosa and A. Disorders
neurophysin associated with vasopressin
nonhuman leukocyte antigen associated form
pediatric autoimmune neuropsychiatric diseases associated with streptococcal infection
pediatric autoimmune neuropsychiatric disorders associated with streptococcal infection
a. physical examination finding
platelet a.
a. sequestrum
sleep apnea-hypersomnolence syndrome associated with upper airway obstruction
tropical spastic paraparesis/HTLV-I associated myelopathy
tumor a.
a. with abdominal pain

association
Alzheimer Disease and Related Disorders A.
American Diabetes Association
American Diabetes Association diet
American Diabetes A. guidelines
American Heart A.
American Heart Association classification
American Heart A. Step One Diet
American Heart A. Stroke Outcome Classification
American Hospital A.
American Lung A.
American Medical A.
American Nurses A.
American Psychiatric A.
American Psychoanalytical A.
American Psychological A.
aniridia, Wilms tumor a.
anterior limbic association area
a. areas
a. arena
auditory association area
auditory association cortex
a. center
a. characteristic
A. of Clinical Scientists
a. coefficient
a. constant
Controlled Oral Word A. Test
a. cortex
a. cortex of parietal lobe
a. deficit pathology
a. disease
equilibrium association constant
a. fibers
a. fluency
independent practice a.
a. learning
long association fiber
loosening of a.'s
Meals on Wheels A. of America
a. mechanism
Mental Health A.
multimodal association cortex
National A. of Activity Professionals
National A. of Anorexia Nervosa and Associated Disorders
National Aphasia A.
National A. of Area Agencies on Aging
National Bar A.
National Collegiate Athletic A. drug testing policy
National Collegiate Athletic A. prohibited drug
National A. of the Deaf

association *(continued)*
National Depressive and Manic-Depressive A.
National Family Caregivers A.
National A. for Health & Fitness
National A. for Hispanic Elderly
National A. for Home Care
National Lung Transplant Patient A.
National Mental Health A.
National A. of Pediatric Nurse Associates and Practitioners
National A. of Progressional Geriatric Care Managers
National A. of Psychiatric Health Systems
neocortical association area
a. neurosis
New York Heart A. classification of heart disease
North American Nursing Diagnosis A.
occipital association cortical area
Opticians Association of America
parietal association area
a. period
professional a.
a. reaction
a. reaction time
schizophrenia with premorbid a.
a. sensation ratio
a. of sounds and symbols
a. system
a. test
a. time
a. tract
visual, association, kinesthetic, tactile reading
a. with hydrocephalus syndrome
Word A. Test
World Medical A.

associative
a. anamnesis
a. aphasia
a. aspect
a. detail response to white space
a. facilitation
a. fluency
a. inhibition
a. learning
a. linkage
long-term associative memory
a. memory
a. play
a. prosopagnosia
a. reaction
a. response to a white space on a card
a. shifting
a. strength
a. thinking
a. visual agnosia
a. visual cortex

assortative
a. mating
negative assortative mating

assortive
assortive mating

assumed
a. mean
a. similarity

assumption of new identity

Assura
A. closed mini pouch
A. convex drainable pouch
A. convex urostomy pouch
A. pediatric pouch
A. stoma cap

assurance
basic assurance test
concurrent quality a.
nursing quality a.
quality a.
quality assurance monitor
quality assurance program
quality assurance reagent
quality assurance standards
quality assurance and utilization review
sterility assurance level

assurance/risk
quality assurance/risk management

assured
hemostasis a.

astacoid rash

AST/ALT ratio

astasia-abasia gait

astatic
myoclonic astatic epilepsy
a. seizure

asteatosis cutis

asteatotic
a. dermatitis
a. eczema

asteric seizure

asteroid
a. body
a. hyalitis
a. hyalosis

asthenia
mental a.
muscle a.
myalgic a.
neurocirculatory a.

asthenic
a. appearance
a. constitutional type
a. delirium
a. diathesis
grade, rough, breathy, asthenic, strained
a. habit
a. neurosis
a. orthophoria
a. personality
a. personality disorder
a. reaction
a. type

asthma
acute a.
acute asthma attack
acute attack of a.
acute bronchopulmonary a.
allergen-induced a.
aspirin-induced a.
aspirin-intolerant a.
aspirin-sensitive a.
aspirin-sensitive asthma syndrome
breathing difficulty from a.
bronchial a.
bronchiectasis, eosinophilia, asthma, pneumonia
a. care algorithm
a. care training
Childhood A. Management Program
Childhood A. Questionnaire
Chinese restaurant a.
chronic bronchitis with a.
cigarette smoke a.
conventional asthma therapy
corticosteroid sensitive a.
cotton dust a.
coughing from a.
a. crystal
daytime a.
eczema, asthma, and hay fever complex
effect of asthma on lung
a. exacerbation
exercise-induced a.
Free Running A. Test
Global Institute for A.
hyperventilation-induced a.
life-threatening asthma attack
Living with A. Questionnaire

malignant potentially fatal a.
mild intermittent a.
mild persistent a.
moderate persistent a.
a. morbidity
National A. Education Program
occupational a.
occupationally induced a.
occupational non-IgE-dependent a.
osmotically induced a.
Pediatric A. Quality of Life Questionnaire
a. of physical effort
poorly reversible a.
a. and pregnancy
premenstrual a.
premenstrual exacerbation of a.
A. Quality of Life Questionnaire
A. Severity Score
steroid resistant a.
a. symptom checklist
trigger of a.
a. with vasculitis

asthma-like
a.-l. symptom
a.-l. symptoms

asthma-related death

asthmatic
a. airway
a. amyotrophy
a. bronchitis
delayed asthmatic reaction
dual asthmatic reaction
early asthmatic response
immediate asthmatic reaction
a. inflammatory airway disease
late asthmatic response
nonsteroid-dependent a.
a. pneumonia
a. response
steroid-dependent a.

asthmatoid wheeze

astigmatic
a. amblyopia
a. axis
a. clock
a. dial
a. dial chart
a. hypermetropia
a. image
a. keratotomy
a. keratotomy enhancement
a. lens
radial and astigmatic keratotomy
a. refractive error
a. vector analysis

astigmatism
a. against the rule
compound hypermetropic a.
compound hyperopic a.
compound myopic a.
corneal irregular a.
a. correction
hypermetropic a.
hyperopic a.
mixed astigmatism with myopia predominating
myopic a.
a. of oblique pencils
penetrating keratoplasty a.
a. with the rule
with-the-rule a.

Astler-Coller
A.-C. A, B1, B2, C1, C2 classification
A.-C. modification of Dukes classification

Aston patterning

ASTRA
A. profile
A. profile test

astragalar bone

astragalocalcaneal bone

astragalocrural bone

astragaloid bone

astragalonavicular joint

astragaloscaphoid
a. bone
a. joint

astragalotibial bone

astragalus
aviator's a.
a. bone

astral
a. body
a. fiber
a. fibers
a. projection

Astrand 30-beat stopwatch method

astringent
a. mouthwash
a. soak

astrocyte
Alzheimer type I, II a.
atypical a.
a. footplate
protoplasmic a.
a. stain
a. staining

astrocytic
a. change
a. end foot
a. glioma
a. gliosis
a. hamartoma
a. neoplasm
a. proliferation
a. reaction
a. signal
a. tumor

astrocytoma
anaplastic a.
a. cell
a. cord
desmoplastic cerebral astrocytoma of infancy
a. gene
a. grade I–IV
high-grade a.
juvenile pilocytic a.
low-grade a.
low-grade diffuse a.
low-grade fibrillary a.
malignant pilocytic a.
multifocal anaplastic a.
pilocystic cerebellar a.
a. protoplasmaticum
subependymal giant cell a.

astrocytosis cerebri

astroglia cell

astroglial tumor

astrology chart

Astroturf toe

Astroviridae virus

astrovirus
a. gastroenteritis
human astrovirus serotype 1–7

Astrup
A. blood gas value
A. method

Astwood-Coller staging system for carcinoma

Astwood test

asymbolia
pain a.
a. to pain

asymmetric
a. appearance time
a. artifact
a. astigmatism
bilateral a.
a. bilateral cleft
a. bile duct

asymmetric *(continued)*
a. breast density
a. carbon atom
a. chin
a. chondrodystrophy
a. closure of cusp
a. crying facies
a. data sampling
a. dimethylarginine
a. distribution
a. disulfide
a. echo
fast asymmetric spin echo
a. fetal growth restriction
a. folds of eye
a. hyperopia
a. hyperplasia
a. hyperreflexia
a. incurvatum reflex
a. intrauterine growth retardation
isolated asymmetric septal hypertrophy
a. IUGR
a. jaws
a. limb uptake
a. lung opacity
a. maxillomandibular growth
a. motor neuropathy
a. nasopharyngeal lymphoid hyperplasia
a. negative T-wave
a. nystagmus
a. oligoarthritis
a. oligoarthropathy
a. palatal paresis
a. papilledema
a. parathyroid enlargement
a. periflexural exanthem of childhood
a. polyarthritis
a. pulmonary congestion
a. pupil
a. reflex
a. refractive error
a. short stature syndrome
a. skin fold
a. small foramen magnum
a. subtalar joint development
a. surgery
a. target appearance
a. thorax
a. tonic neck reflex
a. unit membrane
a. uterus
a. wear
a. Z-plasty

asymmetrical
a. amnesia
a. arthralgia
a. conjoined twins
a. generalized epileptiform activity
a. growth
reciprocal a.
a. signal change

asymmetry
a. amplitude
a., range of motion abnormality, tissue texture abnormality
a., border, color, and diameter of melanoma
a. of face
minor alpha a.
nasolabial fold a.
a. and order effect
surface asymmetry index
tenderness, asymmetry, restricted motion, and tissue texture changes
tissue texture changes, asymmetry, restriction of motion, tenderness

asymptomatic
a. angiomyolipoma
a. bacteriuria
a. cardiac ischemia
A. Cardiac Ischemia Pilot
a. carotid artery stenosis
Carotid Artery Stenosis with A. Narrowing: Operation Versus Aspirin Study
A. Carotid Atherosclerosis Study
a. carotid atherosclerosis study
a. carotid bruit
a. carotid surgery trial
a. cholecystitis
a. cholelithiasis
a. coarctation
a. coccidioidomycosis
a. coronary artery disease
a. cricoarytenoid synovitis
a. dehiscence
a. elevated aminotransferase
a. gallstone
a. heart attack
a. heart disease
a. hemodialysis patient
highest asymptomatic dose
a. hydrocephalus
a. hyperamylasemia
a. hyperlactemia
a. hypertrophy
a. hyperuricemia
a. hypocalcemia
a. hyponatremia
a. hypotonicity
a. infection
a. infertility
a. inflammatory prostatitis
a. ischemia
a. lactic acidemia
a. mass
Mayo Asymptomatic Carotid Endarterectomy Study
a. metastatic hormone-refractory prostate cancer
a. mild endometriosis
a. myoma
a. neck bruit
a. neoplasm
a. neurosyphilis
NIH Classification Category IV asymptomatic inflammatory prostatitis
a. optic neuritis
a. patient
a. pheochromocytoma
a. proteinuria
a. pyelonephritis
a. seizure
significant asymptomatic bacteriuria
a. synechia
a. urinary lithiasis
a. urinary tract infection
a. urolithiasis
a. viral shedding
a. viremia
a. visual field defect

asymptotic wish fulfillment

asynchronous
a. birth
a. breathing
continuous ventricular asynchronous pacing
a. data transmission
a. pulse generator
a. transfer mode
ventricular asynchronous pacemaker

asynchrony
marked a.

asynclitic
a. position
a. position of fetus

asynclitism
anterior a.

asyndetic
a. communication
a. thinking

asynergic myocardium

asystole
transient a.
ventricular a.

asystolic pause

A-T
A.-T. mutation
A.-T. mutation gene

at
a. autopsy tumor, nodes, and metastases
a. bedside
a. bedtime
a. large

AT1 receptor

AT2 receptor

AT3 deficiency type II

atactic
a. abasia
a. agraphia
a. ataxia

atactica
a. agraphia
agraphia a.

ataractic drug

Atasoy
A. palmar flap
A. triangular advancement flap
A. volar V-Y flap
A. V-Y advancement
A. V-Y advancement flap
A. V-Y technique

Atasoy-Kleinert
A.-K. flap
A.-K. volar V-Y advancement flap

Atasoy-type
A.-t. flap
A.-t. flap for nail injury repair

atavicus
metatarsus a.
metatarsus atavicus deformity

atavistic
a. cuneiform
a. epiphysial
a. epiphysis
a. foot
a. phenomenon
a. regression

ataxia
acute cerebellar a.
adult-onset spinocerebellar a.
a., myoclonic encephalopathy, macular degeneration, recurrent infections syndrome
autism, dementia, ataxia, loss of purposeful hand use syndrome
autosomal dominant cerebellar a.
autosomal recessive spastic ataxia of Charlevoix-Saguenay
canine inherited a.
cerebellar vermis hypoplasia, oligophrenia, congenital ataxia, coloboma, hepatic fibrosis
a. cordis
craniosynostosis, ataxia, trigeminal anesthesia, parietal anesthesia and pons, vermis fusion syndrome
episodic a.
feline ataxia virus
Friedreich a.
hereditary cerebellar a.
hereditary progressive a.
a. and intention tremor
mental retardation, ataxia, hypotonia, hypogonadism, retinal dystrophy syndrome
mental retardation, dystonic movements, ataxia, seizures syndrome
neurogenic muscle weakness, ataxia, and retinitis pigmentosa
progressive spinal a.
spinocerebellar a.
sporadic olivopontocerebellar a.
a. telangiectasia
a. with isolated vitamin E deficiency
X-linked cerebral a.
X-linked cerebral a.
X-linked olivopontocerebellar a.
X-linked olivopontocerebellar a.

ataxia-deafness-retardation
a.-d.-r. syndrome
a.-d.-r. with ketoaciduria

ataxia-deafness syndrome

ataxia-hemiparesis syndrome

ataxia-microcephaly-cataract syndrome

ataxia-telangiectasia syndrome

ataxic
a. abasia
a. amimia
a. aphasia
a. breathing
a. cerebral palsy
a. diplegia
a. dysarthria
a. feeling
a. gait
a. hemiparesis
a. nystagmus
a. paramyotonia
a. paraplegia
a. respiration
sensory ataxic neuropathy with dysarthria and ophthalmoplegia
a. and spastic dysarthria
a. speech
tropical ataxic neuropathy
a. writing

ataxin-1 gene

ataxin-2 gene

atelectasis
acquired a.
apical a.
dependent a.
linear a.
lobar a.
lobular a.
lobular patch of a.
massive a.
a. of middle ear
a. neonatorum
nonobstructive a.
obstructive a.
passive a.
patch of a.
patchy a.
periaortic a.
postoperative a.
primary a.
pulmonary a.
pulmonary immaturity and a.
segmental a.
slowly developing a.
subsegmental a.

atelectatic
a. asbestos pseudotumor
a. and edematous lung
firm and a.
a. lung
a. otitis
a. rale

atelencephalic syndrome

ateliotic dwarfism

AT/GC ratio

Athabascan type of severe combined immunodeficiency disease

atherectomized vessel

atherectomy
coronary rotational a.
directional coronary a.
excimer laser, rotational atherectomy, and balloon angioplasty
high-speed rotational a.
a. index
kissing atherectomy technique
percutaneous coronary rotational a.
percutaneous transluminal coronary rotational a.
peripheral directional a.
rotational atherectomy system
rotational coronary a.
transluminal extraction a.

atheroembolic
a. disease
a. renal disease

atherogenic
a. index
a. low-density lipoprotein pattern B phenotype

atherolytic reperfusion wire device

atheroma
calcified a.
a. embolism
a. molding

atheromata
calcified a.

atheromatosis cutis

atheromatous
a. abscess
aortic atheromatous disease
a. change
core of atheromatous material
a. debris
a. degeneration
a. disease
a. embolism
a. embolus
a. lesion
a. material
a. plaque
severe atheromatous change of aorta
a. stenosis
a. ulcer

atherosclerosis
accelerated graft a.
artery-clogging plaque in atherosclerosis patient
asymptomatic carotid atherosclerosis study
Asymptomatic Carotid A. Study
a. and blood flow
burning feet from a.
calcific mural a.
cardiac allograft a.
cerebral a.
diffuse calcific a.
gangrene from a.
a. graft
a. of intracerebral vessels
Mevacor Atherosclerosis Regression Study
mild systemic a.
moderate atherosclerosis with calcification
a. obliterans
ostial artery a.
pararenal aortic a.
progression of a.
trembling from a.

atherosclerosis-induced cavernosal ischemia

atherosclerotic
a. abnormality
a. aneurysm
a. aortic aneurysm
a. aortic ulcer
a. calcification
a. cardiovascular disease
a. carotid artery
a. carotid artery disease
a. carotid artery lesion
a. change
a. coronary artery disease
coronary atherosclerotic heart disease
a. debris
a. disease
a. encephalopathy
a. fatty streak
a. heart disease
a. hypertensive cardiovascular disease
a. infarction
intracranial atherosclerotic disease
a. ischemic neuritis
a. lesion
multilevel atherosclerotic arterial occlusive disease
a. narrowing
a. occlusive syndrome
ostial atherosclerotic plaque
peripheral atherosclerotic disease
a. plaque
a. plaque rupture
a. plaquing
a. pulmonary vascular disease
a. renal artery
a. renal artery stenosis
a. renovascular disease
a. stenosis
a. stroke
subcortical atherosclerotic encephalopathy
a. ulcer

atherothrombotic
a. brain infarct
a. brain infarction
a. stroke

athetoid
a. cerebral palsy
choreic athetoid movements
a. dysarthria
a. movement
a. spasm

athetosic
a. dysarthria
a. dystonia
a. idiocy

athetotic
a. movement disorder
a. posturing

athlete
amputee a.
female athlete triad
nail breaking from athlete's foot

athlete's
a. ankle
a. foot
a. heart
a. nodule
a. pseudoanemia
a. pseudonephritis

athletic
a. amenorrhea
a. brace
a. constitutional type
a. heart
a. heart syndrome
a. injury
a. nail
National Collegiate A. Association drug testing policy
National Collegiate A. Association prohibited drug
a. shoe carbon fiber plate

Standard Nomenclature of A. Injuries
a. trainer

athletica
anorexia a.

at-home recovery period

athyreotic
a. cretin
a. thyroglobulin

athyrotic
a. cretinism
a. hypothyroidism
a. neonate

AT-II-induced intraarterial chemotherapy

Atkin
A. epiphysial fracture
A. lid block

Atkin-Flaitz-Patil syndrome

Atkin-Flaitz syndrome

Atkins diet

Atkinson
A. block
A. lid block
A. Life Happiness
A. Life Happiness Rating
A. scoring system for dysphagia
A. technique
A. tube

Atlanta
A. brace orthosis
A. hip brace
Metropolitan Atlanta Congenital Defects Program

atlantal
a. fracture
a. ligament
a. transverse ligament

Atlanta-Scottish
A.-S. Rite abduction orthosis
A.-S. Rite brace

atlantic part of vertebral artery

atlantis
arcus posterior a.
massa lateralis a.

atlantoaxial
a. alignment
a. arthrodesis
a. articulation
a. dislocation
a. fixation
flexion injury posterior atlantoaxial arthrodesis
a. fracture-dislocation
a. fusion
a. impaction
a. instability
a. interval
a. joint
a. lesion
a. ligament
a. luxation
median atlantoaxial joint
a. relationship
a. rotary displacement
a. rotary fixation
a. rotatory fixation
a. rotatory subluxation
a. separation
a. stabilization

atlantodens interval

atlantodental
anterior atlantodental interval
a. dislocation
posterior atlantodental interval

atlantoepistrophic
a. ligament
middle atlantoepistrophic joint

atlantooccipital
anterior atlantooccipital membrane
a. anterior membrane
a. articulation
a. assimilation
a. disability
a. dislocation
a. extension
a. fusion
a. joint
a. joint dislocation
a. junction
a. ligament
a. membrane
a. separation
a. stabilization
a. subluxation
a. transection

atlantooccipitalis
articulatio a.
membrana atlantooccipitalis anterior
membrana atlantooccipitalis posterior

atlantoodontoid
anterior atlantoodontoid interval
a. interspace
a. joint

atlas
a. adjustment
a. anomaly
anterior arch of a.
anterior atlas arch
anterior tubercle of a.
a. arch
arch of a.
a. assimilation
a. burst fracture
a. facet
a. fracture
a. laterality
longitudinal bands of cruciform ligament of a.
a. matching
a. occipitalization
occipitalization of a.
a. odontoid distance
a. of Talairach and Tournoux
a. vertebral subluxation complex

atlas-axis
a.-a. combination fracture
a.-a. complex
a.-a. movement

atlas-dens interval

Atlas-Elite laser

atmosphere
a. absolute
a. effect
normal a.
a.'s of pressure
School A. Questionnaire
a. of trust
Ward A. Scale

atmospheric
a. condition
low atmospheric pressure
a. monitoring
oxygen at atmospheric pressure
a. perspective
a. pressure
transversely excited atmospheric pressure

A-T mutation gene

atom
asymmetric carbon a.
carbon atom farthest from principal functioning group
carbon separated from the carboxyl group by 2 other carbon a.'s
fast atom bombardment
fast atom bombardment mass spectrometry
mass of a.
number of a.'s

atomic
a. absorption

atomic *(continued)*
a. absorption spectrometer
a. absorption spectrophotometer
a. absorption spectroscopy
a., biological, chemical
a., biological, chemical warfare
a. core
electrothermal atomic absorption spectrophotometry
a. energy
a. force microscopy
a. heat
linear combination of atomic orbital-molecular orbital
linear combination of atomic orbitals
a. mass
a. mass unit
a. milk
a. number
number of neutrons in an atomic nucleus
a. orbital
a. orbital with angular momentum quantum number zero
a. resolution microscopy
a. spectrum
a. theory
unified atomic mass unit
a. volume
a. weight
a. weight unit

atomistic psychology

atomized
gas atomized dispersion strengthened

atonia
muscle a.

atonic
a. absence
a. absence seizure
a. bladder
a. cerebral palsy
congenital atonic pseudoparalysis
congenital atonic sclerotic muscular dystrophy
a. constipation
a. drop attack
a. dyspepsia
a. ectropion
a. entropion
a. epilepsy
a. epiphora
a. esophagus
a. impotence
a. sclerotic muscle dystrophy
a. seizure
a. ulcer
a. ureter
a. urinary bladder

atonic-astatic diplegia

atony
gastric a.
intestinal a.
postpartum a.
urinary bladder a.
uterine a.

atopic
a. allergen
a. allergy
Assessment Measure for A. Dermatitis
a. asthma
a. cataract
a. conjunctivitis
a. dermatitis
A. Dermatitis Area and Severity Index
a. dermatitis rash
a. dermatitis with keratoconjunctivitis
a. diaper rash
a. diathesis
a. disease
a. eczema
a. eczema keratoconjunctivitis
a. erythroderma
a. hypersensitivity
intractable atopic dermatitis
a. keratoconjunctivitis
a. line
mask of atopic dermatitis
moderate atopic dermatitis
ocular atopic dermatitis
a. reagin
a. respiratory disease
a. rhinitis
a. sensitivity
Severity Scoring of A. Dermatitis
six-area, six-sign atopic dermatitis

atopy patch test

ATP-binding cassette transporter

atrabiliary capsule

atractosylidic acid

atractylic acid

atracurium besylate

atraumatic
a., multidirectional, bilateral radial instability
a. bowel clamp
a. forceps
a. grasper
a. locking/grasping forceps
a. multidirectional instability
a. necrosis
normocephalic and a.
a. normocephalic
a. osteolysis of distal clavicle
a. suture
a. suture technique

atresia
a. ani
aortic arch a.
aortic valve a.
arrhinia, choanal atresia, microphthalmia syndrome
biliary a.
a. choanae
coloboma, heart disease, atresia choanae, retarded growth and retarded development and/or CNS anomalies, genital hypoplasia, and ear anomalies and/or deafness syndrome
congenital atresia of esophagus
congenital biliary a.
congenital bronchial a.
congenital duodenal a.
congenital intestinal a.
digital anomalies, short palpebral fissures, atresia of esophagus or duodenum syndrome
esophageal a.
extrahepatic bile duct a.
extrahepatic biliary a.
a. folliculi
a. of the foramen of Luschka and Magendie
intrahepatic a.
a. of larynx
mitral valve a.
a. plate
pulmonary artery a.
pulmonary atresia with intact ventricular septum
pulmonary atresia with ventricular septal defect
pure pulmonary a.
small bowel a.
small intestinal a.
tracheoesophageal fistula, esophageal atresia, multiple congenital anomaly syndrome
tricuspid a.

atresia/pulmonary
pulmonary atresia/pulmonary stenosis

atresic teratosis

atretic

a. aortic segment
a. cervix
a. corpus luteum
a. extrahepatic bile duct resection
a. follicle
a. follicular cyst
a. gallbladder
a. meningocele
a. outflow tract
a. ovarian follicle
a. segment
a. tube
a. ureter
a. vagina

atrial

a. activation mapping
a. activation time
a. anastomotic branch of circumflex branch of left coronary artery
aneurysm of atrial septum
anterior atrial myocardial bundle
a. appendage
a. appendage juxtaposition
a. arrhythmia
a. artery
a. auricle
automatic atrial tachycardia
a. baffle operation
balloon atrial septostomy
a. balloon septostomy
a. bigeminal rhythm
a. bigeminy
a. bolus dynamic computed tomography
a. branch
burst of rapid atrial pacing
a. canal
a. cannulation
a. capture
a. capture beat
cardiac atrial shunt
chaotic atrial tachycardia
a. chaotic tachycardia
chronic nonvalvular atrial fibrillation
a. circumflex artery
clamshell closure of atrial septal defect
combined atrial hypertrophy
a. complex
a. conduction disturbance
a. contraction
controlled atrial fibrillation/flutter
coupled atrial pacing
C-type atrial natriuretic peptide
a. cuff
a. defibrillation threshold
a. demand-inhibited pacemaker
a. diastole
diastolic atrial volume
a. diastolic gallop
a. disk
a. dissociation
a. diverticulum of brain
a. dome
a. echo
echo-guided balloon atrial septostomy
a. ectopic automatic tachycardia
a. ectopic beat
a. effective refractory period
electrical conversion of atrial fibrillation
a. electrogram
a. emptying index
a. emptying volume
end of atrial systole
a. extrastimulus method
a. extrasystole
extrasystolic atrial tachycardia
a. fetal flutter
a. fibrillation
a. fibrillation and/or flutter
a. fibrillation cycle length
a. fibrillation-flutter
a. filling fraction
a. filling pressure
filtered atrial rate interval
a. flutter
a. flutter response
a. focus
a. fusion
a. fusion beat
a. gallop
human atrial natriuretic peptide
a. hypertrophy
iatrogenic atrial septal defect
implantable atrial defibrillator
a. infarct
a. infarction
a. inhibited pacemaker
a. insufficiency
intraoperative atrial ischemia
a. inversion procedure
a. irritability
a. isomerism
a. kick
lateral atrial tunnel
left atrial abnormality
left atrial appendage
left atrial ball-valve thrombus
left atrial contraction
left atrial diameter
left atrial dimension
left atrial emptying index
left atrial end-diastolic pressure
left atrial end-diastolic volume
left atrial end-systolic volume
left atrial enlargement
left atrial function
left atrial hypertension
left atrial hypertrophy
left atrial involvement
left atrial isolation procedure
left atrial isomerism
left atrial myxoma
left atrial neovascularization
left atrial overloading
left atrial posterior wall
left atrial spontaneous echo contrast
left atrial transesophageal pacing test
left atrial transmural pressure
lentigines, atrial myxomas, cutaneous papular myxomas, blue nevi
a. liver pulse
lone atrial fibrillation
marginal atrial branch of right coronary artery
maximal left atrial dimension
mean atrial pressure
mean atrial rate
mean left atrial pressure
mean right atrial pressure
medial atrial vein
a. milliampere
Mustard atrial baffle repair
Mustard atrial switch procedure
a. myxoma
narrowed atrial ventricular valve
a. natriuretic factor
a. natriuretic factor receptor
a. natriuretic hormone
a. natriuretic peptide
a. natriuretic polypeptide
nevi, atrial myxoma, myxoid neurofibroma, and ephelides syndrome
nevi, atrial myxoma, myxoid neurofibroma, and ephelides syndrome
nonconducted premature atrial contraction
nonparoxysmal atrial tachycardia
nonrheumatic atrial fibrillation
nonvalvular atrial fibrillation

atrial *(continued)*
N-terminal atrial natriuretic peptide
onset of atrial fibrillation
a. ostium primum defect
a. overdrive stimulation rate
a. paroxysmal tachycardia
part of the electrocardio-graphic cycle representing atrial depolarization
a. partition
persistent atrial standstill
pharmacologic atrial defibrillator
postoperative atrial fibrillation
postventricular atrial blanking
postventricular atrial refractory period
premature atrial complex
premature atrial stimulus
a. premature beat
a. premature complex
a. premature contraction
a. premature depolarization
a. pressure
primary atrial arrhythmia
pulmonary vein atrial reversal
rapid atrial fibrillation
reentrant atrial tachycardia
a. regurgitation
right atrial abnormality
right atrial contraction
right atrial diameter
right atrial function
right atrial hypertrophy
right atrial involvement
right atrial mean pressure
right atrial pressure elevation
a. ring
secundum atrial septal defect
a. septal aneurysm
a. septal defect
a. septal defect occlusion
a. septal defect occlusion system
a. septal heart disease
a. septal resection
a. septectomy
a. septoplasty procedure
a. septostomy
a. septostomy procedure
a. septostomy via balloon
a. septum
a. septum excision
a. shunt
a. situs
a. situs solitus
slow paroxysmal atrial tachycardia
a. sound
a. standstill
a. stasis index
a. subendocardial hemorrhage
a. switch operation
a. switch procedure
a. synchronous pulse generator
a. synchronous ventricular inhibited pacing
a. systole
a. tachyarrhythmia
a. tachycardia detection rate
a. tachycardia with block
a. tachy response
a. thrombosis
a. thrombus
total atrial blanking
total atrial refractory period
a. tracking pacemaker
transesophageal atrial pacing
transesophageal atrial stimulation
a. transport function
a. transposition
a. triggered pulse generator
ventricular atrial distal coronary sinus
ventricular atrial height right atrium
ventricular atrial His bundle electrocardiogram
ventricular atrial proximal coronary sinus
a. ventricular canal defect
a. and ventricular implantable cardioverter-defibrillator
ventricular pacing, atrial sensing, triggered mode, pacemaker
wandering atrial pacemaker

atrialized ventricle

atrial-phase volumetric function

atrial-synchronous ventricular-inhibited pacemaker

atrial-well technique

atrichia
ichthyosis, follicularis, atrichia or alopecia, photophobia syndrome

atriocaval
a. junction
a. shunt

atriodextrofascicular tract

atriodigital dysplasia

atriofascicular tract

atriography
negative contrast left a.

atrio-His
a.-H. bypass tract
a.-H. fiber
a.-H. pathway
a.-H. tract

atrio-hisian bypass tract

atrionodal bypass tract

atriopressor reflex

atriopulmonary connection

atriosystolic murmur

atrioventricular
anomalous atrioventricular excitation
anterior cusp of left atrioventricular valve
anterior cusp of right atrioventricular valve
a. anulus
artery to atrioventricular node
atypical atrioventricular nodal reentrant tachycardia
a. band
a. block
a. block with first-degree conduction delay
a. bundle
a. canal
a. canal cushion
a. canal defect
a. canal septal defect
common atrioventricular canal
common atrioventricular orifice
complete atrioventricular block
complete atrioventricular dissociation
a. conduction
a. conduction delay
a. conduction system
a. conduction tissue
a. connection
a. connection anomaly
crisscross atrioventricular valve
deficient atrioventricular septation
a. delay
a. discordance
a. dissociation
enhanced atrioventricular conduction
enhanced atrioventricular nodal conduction
a. extrasystole
a. fistula
a. functional tachycardia
a. gradient
a. groove
a. groove branch

a. heart block
incompetent atrioventricular valve
incomplete atrioventricular block
incomplete atrioventricular dissociation
a. interval
a. junction
a. junctional ablation
a. junctional bigeminy
a. junctional escape beat
a. junctional heart block
a. junctional pacemaker
a. junctional reentrant
a. junctional rhythm
a. junctional tachycardia
a. junction anomaly
a. junction escape rhythm
a. malformation
Mobitz atrioventricular block
muscular atrioventricular septum
a. nodal branch
a. nodal bypass tract
a. nodal conduction
a. nodal function
a. nodal node mesothelioma
a. nodal orifice
a. nodal ostium
a. nodal reentrant tachycardia
a. nodal reentry
a. nodal rhythm
a. nodal septal defect
a. nodal septum
a. nodal valve
a. node
a. node artery
a. node dysfunction
a. node function
a. node of His
a. opening of His
a. orifice
paroxysmal atrioventricular nodal reciprocal tachycardia
partial atrioventricular canal
partial atrioventricular canal defect
a. pathway
persistent complete atrioventricular canal
premature atrioventricular junction complex
a. reciprocating tachycardia
a. reentrant paroxysmal tachycardia
a. reentry tachycardia
a. refractory period
a. ring
a. septal defect
a. septum
a. sequential pacing
sequential atrioventricular pacing
a. shunt
a. sulcus
third-degree atrioventricular block
a. time
a. trunk
univentricular atrioventricular connection
a. valve insufficiency
a. valve opening
Wenckebach atrioventricular block
a. Wenckebach block

at-risk

a.-r. adolescent
a.-r. infant
a.-r. patient
a.-r. period
a.-r. pregnancy

atrium

auricle of left a.
auricle of right a.
catheter stimulation of right a.
contraction of right a.
emptying of right a.
filling of right a.
giant left a.
a. glottidis
a. of glottis
a. of heart
high right a.
high right atrium electrocardiogram
hypoplastic left a.
a. of infection
a. of larynx
a. of lateral ventricle
left atrium of heart
low right a.
low septal right a.
a. of lungs
a. of middle nasal meatus
midright a.
a. pace
a. pulmonale
right a.
right atrium body
right atrium of heart
a. of ventricle
ventricular atrial height right a.
a. ventriculi lateralis

atrium-His bundle

atrophic

acute atrophic spinal paralysis
a. age-related macular degeneration
a. AMD
a. anemia
annular atrophic connective tissue panniculitis of the ankle
antral atrophic gastritis
a. appearance
a. arthritis
autoimmune metaplastic atrophic gastritis
a. brain lesion
a. breast
breast pendulous and a.
a. brown skin
a. candidiasis
a. change
chronic atrophic gastritis
a. chronic autoimmune thyroiditis
a. chronic gastritis
a. cirrhosis
a. degeneration
a. degenerative maculopathy
delirium, infection, atrophic urethritis and vaginitis, pharmaceuticals, psychological disorders, excessive urine output, restricted mobility, stool impaction
a. dementia
a. emphysema
a. endometrium
environmental metaplastic atrophic gastritis
a. excavation
a. facial acne scar
a. fenestration
a. fracture
fundic atrophic gastritis
a. gastric mucosa
a. gastritis
generalized atrophic benign epidermolysis bullosa
a. glossitis
a. Hashimoto thyroiditis
a. heterochromia
a. hole
a. hyperkeratotic lesion
a. inflammation
a. kidney
a. lesion
a. lesion of brain
a. lichen planus
a. macule
malignant atrophic papulosis
metaplastic atrophic gastritis
muscle of upper extremity a.

atrophic *(continued)*
a. muscular paralysis
a. neuroarthropathy
a. nonunion
a. pangastritis
a. papulosis
a. patch
peripheral chorioretinal atrophic spot
a. pharyngitis
a. plaque
a. polychondritis
a. pulp
a. pulposus
a. pyelonephritis
a. rhinitis
a. rhinitis of swine
a. senile gingivitis
a. skin
a. stria
a. testis
a. thrombosis
a. ulatrophy
a. urethritis
a. vagina
a. vaginal mucosa
a. vaginitis
a. villi
a. white scar

atrophica
macula a.
morphea a.
myotonia a.

atrophicans
epidermolysis bullosa a.
lichen sclerosus et a.
papulosis atrophicans maligna
poikiloderma atrophicans vasculare

atrophie
a. blanche
a. blanche lesion
a. noire

atrophied
a. abdominal muscles
a. ovary
a. papilla
shrunken atrophied neurons

atrophoderma
a. biotripticum
linear atrophoderma of Moulin
a. maculatum
neuritic a.
a. of Pasini and Pierini
Pasini-Pierini idiopathic a.
a. pigmentosum
a. scleroatrophy
senile a.
a. striatum
a. striatum et maculatum
a. ulerythematosa
a. vermicularis
a. vermiculatum

atrophy
a. of abdominal muscle
acute yellow a.
adult-onset spinal muscular a.
anterior temporal a.
apraxia-oculomotor contracture-muscle atrophy syndrome
Aran-Duchenne muscular a.
autosomal-dominant optic a.
autosomal-recessive optic a.
a. of bone
a. catarrh
cerebral a.
chronic spinal muscular a.
circumscribed atrophy of brain
cyanotic atrophy of liver
dentatorubral-pallidoluysian a.
diabetes insipidus, diabetes mellitus, progressive bilateral optic atrophy, and sensorineural deafness
diffuse muscle a.
disuse muscular a.
dominant juvenile optic a.
dominantly inherited juvenile optic a.
dominant optic a.
a. of dorsum sella
Duchenne-Aran muscular a.
Duchenne muscular a.
essential atrophy of iris
a. of fat
gastric mucosal a.
generalized white matter a.
a. of glandular tissue
glaucomatous optic nerve a.
granular atrophy of kidney
growth retardation, alopecia, pseudoanodontia, and optic atrophy syndrome
gyrate a.
healed yellow a.
hereditary atrophy optic nerve
hereditary optic a.
hyperornithinemia with gyrate a.
infantile spinal muscular a.
a. of iris
ischemic muscular a.
juvenile a.
juvenile muscular a.
late cortical cerebellar a.
Leber optic a.
Leydig cell a.
limb-girdle muscular weakness and a.
linear subcutaneous a.
lobar cerebral a.
Marie-Foix-Alajouanine cerebellar a.
mental retardation, dysmorphism, cerebral atrophy syndrome
mental retardation, optic atrophy, deafness, seizures syndrome
microvillus a.
morning glory optic a.
multiple system a.
muscular atrophy and cyanosis
myopic choroidal a.
neonatal olivopontocerebellar a.
neuritic muscular a.
neurogenic iris a.
neurogenic muscular a.
neuropathic muscular a.
olivopontocerebellar a.
optic a.
optical nerve a.
optic atrophy tremor
optic disc a.
a. of optic nerve
optic nerve a.
opticoacoustic nerve a.
osteogenesis imperfecta, optic atrophy, retinopathy, developmental delay syndrome
Parrot atrophy of newborn
partial villous a.
patchy atrophy of renal cortex
periorbital fat a.
peripapillary choroidal a.
peripheral chorioretinal a.
peroneal muscle a.
postpolio atrophy syndrome
postpoliomyelitis muscular a.
primary optic a.
progressive encephalopathy, edema, hypsarrhythmia, optic a.
progressive muscular a.
progressive postmyelitis muscular a.
progressive postpolio muscle a.
progressive spinal muscular a.
proximal spinal muscular a.
segmental iris a.
a. in shoulder area
small muscle a.
spinal muscular a.
spinal progressive muscular a.
subacute yellow a.

subcutaneous fat a.
subtotal villous a.
thenar muscle a.
toxic optic nerve a.
urogenital a.
vocal cord a.
weakness or a.
weakness, atrophy, and fasciculation
Werdnig-Hoffmann muscular a.

atropine
a. coma therapy
a. conjunctivitis
a. derivative
a. infusion
a. methylnitrate
a. psychosis
a. sulfate
a. suppression test
a. test

ATR-X syndrome

attachable cerumen loop

attached
a. cementicle
a. cranial section
a. craniotomy
a. denticle
a. gingiva
a. gingiva extension
a. gingival cuff
a. island
a. proton test
a. report

attaching
a. material implant superstructure
a. process

attachment
a. abuse
a. apparatus
ball-and-socket a.
bar-sleeve a.
a. behavior
a. bond
cell attachment protein
a. cuticle
a. disorder
a. disorder of infancy
a. dynamic
a. epithelium
a. fantasy
a. figure
a. to implant superstructure
a. in infancy
lateral disc a.
a. learning
a. level gain
liquidation of a.
major attachment figure
mesenteric attachments of colon
a. parenting
Pearson attachment to Thomas splint
a. plaque
a. plaques
a. relationship
stationary attachment flexible endoskeletal
a. style
tentorium cerebelli a.
a. theory
a. versatility
vesicle attachment site

attachment-retained construction

attachment-separation disorder

attack
active panic a.
acute anxiety a.
acute asthma a.
acute attack of asthma
acute heart a.
Adams-Stokes a.
agoraphobia with panic a.
akinetic drop a.
Antihypertensive and Lipid-Lowering Treatment to Prevent Heart A. Trial
aspirin and heart a.
asymptomatic heart a.
atonic drop a.
attitude of a.
atypical heart a.
cocaine heart a.
cocaine-related heart attack victim
crescendo transient ischemic a.
depressed heart attack patient
depressed heart attack survivor
dizziness from heart a.
exercise induced heart a.
fatal heart a.
full-blown panic a.
grand mal a.
heart a.
heart attack from aspirin
heart attack from aspiring
heart attack from blood clot
heart attack patient
heart attack rehabilitation
heart attack risk
heart attack risk factor
heart attack survivor
heart attack symptoms
heart attack trigger
heart attack victim
hypernatremia and fluid a.
initial attack of vertigo
initial heart a.
a. of intense fear
a. of intense terror
intermittent attacks of severe vertigo
life-threatening asthma a.
lightning attacks in infantile spasm
massive heart a.
Monday morning heart a.
nonepileptic attack disorder
nonfatal heart a.
pain of heart a.
panic a.
panic attack neurotic anxiety state
paroxysmal hypercyanotic a.
post heart attack apoptosis
pre-heart attack pain
prevention of anginal a.
a. rate
recurrent heart a.
repeat heart a.
reversible ischemic a.
risk of first heart a.
sexual dysfunction after heart a.
silent heart a.
Stokes-Adams a.
sudden fatal heart a.
sudden heart attack death
suspected heart a.
transient hemispheric a.
transient ischemic a.
transient ischemic attack and aging
transient ischemic attack, incomplete recovery
unprovoked rage a.
warning signs of heart a.

attacker role

attainment
Educational Goal A. Test
goal a.
goal attainment method
goal attainment scaling
Goal A. Scale

attar of rose

attempt
actual suicide a.
baby expired following resuscitation a.
dead despite resuscitation a.
dead on arrival despite resuscitative a.'s

attempt *(continued)*
despite resuscitation a.'s
expired following resuscitation a.
failed suicide a.
history of suicide a.
nonfatal attempt at suicide
suicide a.

attempted
a. cardiopulmonary resuscitation
hospitalized attempted suicide
not a.
a. passage of instrument
a. suicide

attend
did not a.

attendance
aid and a.

attendant
emergency medical a.
personal care a.
traditional birth a.

attending
a. behavior
a. to language stage
a. physician
a. physician's statement
a. skill
a. staff
a. surgeon

attending's admission notes

attention
a. alertness test
appropriate medical a.
attenuated by a.
auditory a.
children and adults with attention deficit disorder
Children's A. and Adjustment Survey
a. and concentration
a. concentration deficit
a. deficit
a. deficit disorder
A. Deficit Disorder Behavior Rating Scale
a. deficit disorder, residual type
a. deficit disorder with hyperactivity
a. deficit disorder without hyperactivity
a. deficit and disruptive behavior disorder
a. deficit hyperactivity disorder
a. deficit hyperactivity disorder, combined type
a. deficit hyperactivity disorder, predominantly hyperactive-impulsive type
a. deficit hyperactivity disorder-predominantly inattentive
deficits in attention, motor control, perception
a. deficit symptom
demand for constant a.
a. disorder
epileptic attention deficit disorder
evaluate orientation, attention, and recent recall
Flowers Auditory Test of Selective A.
a. fluctuation
focus of a.
a. focus
heightened a.
heightened attention state
impaired a.
a. impairment
inability to focus a.
inability to maintain a.
increased attention span
limited attention span
medical a.
National A. Test
need for constant a.
Numerical A. Test
a. overload
poor attention and memory
positive attention received
Positive A. Behavior
a. problem
a. reflex
a. reflex of pupil
shift in a.
a. shift ability
short attention span
shortened attention span from anxiety
a. to sound
a. span
a. span shortened from anxiety
spatial skills and a.
a. testing
Test of Variables of A.
a. time
Visual Search and A. Test

attentional
a. ability
a. abnormality
a. circuit
a. control
a. demand
a. difficulty
a. disturbance
a. dysfunction
a. dyslexia
a. failure
a. functioning
a. impairment
a. measure
a. mechanism
a. performance
a. problem
a. processing
a. skills

attention-distractibility problem

attention-focusing procedure

attention-getting behavior

attention-information processing

attention-seeking
a.-s. behavior
a.-s. manipulative behavior

attentive
responsive and a.
a. and responsive

attenuated
a. adenomatous polyposis coli
affinity attenuated total reflectance spectroscopy
a. in amplitude
a. androgen
a. by attention
a. bacterial vector
a. cortical surface
a. culture
a. dura
a. familial adenomatous polyposis
a. fever response
fluid attenuated inversion recovery
a. human rotavirus
a. image
influenza virus, attenuated live vaccine
a. intercarpal articular cartilage
a. ligament
live a.
a. lumen
a. media raphe
a. mumps virus
oral attenuated poliomyelitis virus vaccine
oral attenuated *Salmonella typhi* vaccine
oral attenuated poliovirus vaccine
a. poxvirus vector
a. pyloric canal
a. total reflection
a. tuberculosis

typhoid vaccine, attenuated live
a. vaccine
Venezuelan equine encephalitis vaccine, attenuated live
a. virus

attenuating
gonadotropin surge attenuating factor
minimally attenuating medical-grade foam
a. tissue

attenuation
a. activity
articular cartilage a.
a. artifact
blocking or a.
bone ultrasound a.
a. coefficient
a. coefficient on MRI scan
a. compensation
a. correction
diffuse low a.
diminished attenuation midbrain and pons
a. effect
a. factor
fluid attenuation inversion recovery
ground-glass a.
harmonic attenuation table
harmonic attenuation test
a. by hemidiaphragm
a. imaging
a. level
mass attenuation coefficient
a. measurement
mixed attenuation mass
mosaic attenuation pattern
a. number
overlying attenuation artifact
a. process
a. reflex
a. scan
a. of tendon
a. threshold
tissue attenuation and scattering
a. value
a. value on MRI scan
a. valve

attenuation-based on-line modulation of the tube current

attenuation-corrected image

attenuation-correction coefficient

attic
a. adhesion
a. cholesteatoma
a. fluid
a. mass
a. recess
a. temporal bone
tympanic a.

attical cholesteatoma

attitude
a. of active friendliness
a. adjustment
a. of attack
Cancer A. Survey
concrete a.
counterphobic a.
Creativity A. Survey
Cultural A. Inventory
Cultural A. Scale
a. to death
a. defense
Eating A.'s Test
Family A.'s Questionnaire
family attitudes test
Goldberg Anorectic A. Scale
Hereford Parental A. Survey
Heterosexual A.'s Toward Homosexuality scale
illness attitude scale
Insight and Treatment A.'s Questionnaire
a. inventory
Job A. Scale
knowledge, attitude, behavior
knowledge, attitude, behavior, and improvement in nutritional status
listening a.
Marital A.'s Evaluation
masculine a.
masculine attitude in female neurotic
maternal a.
Maternal A.'s Evaluation
a. to medication
Minnesota Teacher A. Inventory
negative a.
neutral a.
New Mexico A. Toward Work Test
object a.
oppositional a.
parental attitudes toward sex
Parent A. Scale
a. passionelle
paternal a.
Personal Experience and A. Questionnaire
pessimistic a.
phobic a.
positive a.
positive mental a.
a. reassessment
religious a.
a. restructuring
Risk-Taking, A., Values Inventory
Sales A. Check List
a. scale
A. to School Questionnaire
School A. Survey
School A. Test
Sex Knowledge and A. Test
sexual attitude reassessment
sexual attitude restructuring
Situational A. Scale
Study A.'s and Methods Survey
Survey of Pain A.'s
Survey of Study Habits and A.'s
Test of A. Toward School
a. theory
a. therapy
a. tic
A.'s Toward Disabled Persons
A.'s Toward Mainstreaming Scale
a. type
Work A.'s Questionnaire

attitudinal
a. group
a. hemianopia
a. pathosis
a. reflex
a. risk factor
a. type

Atton disease

attonita
melancholia a.

attorney
durable power of attorney for health care
power of a.

attracting
cutaneous T-cell attracting chemokine

attraction
magnetic a.
neurotropic a.
Pair A. Inventory
a. sphere

attractor field therapy

attributable
a. fraction
relative response attributable to the maneuver
a. risk

attribution
a. error
a. theory
Attributional Style Questionnaire
attrition
a. rate
a. rate scale
a. rupture of tendon
a. of tendon
attritional
a. occlusion
a. pattern change
a. perforation
a. tear
attunement
affect a.
spinal attunement technique
Attwood staining method
atubular glomerulus
ATX assay
A-type
A-t. nevus cell
A-t. reamer
atypia
basal cell a.
cellular a.
multinucleated atypia of the vulva
structural a.
atypical
a. absence
a. absence seizure
a. achromatopsia
a. adenomatous hyperplasia
a. affective disorder
a. aneuploidy
a. angina
a. angiomyolipoma
a. angiomyolipoma of the kidney
a. angiomyolipoma of kidney
a. antibody titer
a. antidepressant
a. antipsychotic
a. antipsychotic agent
a. antipsychotic drug
a. antipsychotic preparation
a. anxiety disorder
a. aortic valve stenosis
a. articulatory contact
a. astrocyte
a. atrioventricular nodal reentrant tachycardia
a. behavior
a. benign fibrous histiocytoma
a. bipolar disorder
a. brain teratoma
a. bronchial pneumonia
a. carcinoid
a. carcinoid tumor
a. cell
a. child
a. childhood psychosis
a. chondrocyte
a. chondrodystrophy
a. chronic myeloid leukemia
a. cleft
a. coloboma
complex atypical hyperplasia/metaplasia
a. conduct disorder
a. course
a. delusional experience
a. depression
a. development
a. diabetes
a. diabetes mellitus
a. dislocation
a. dissociative disorder
a. distribution of disease
a. ductal hyperplasia
a. ductular cell
a. eating disorder
a. endocervical cells of undetermined significance
a. endometrial hyperplasia
a. endosalpingiosis
a. epithelium
a. erythema multiforme
a. facial neuralgia
a. facial pain
a. factitious disorder with physical symptoms
familial atypical mole malignant melanoma
familial atypical multiple melanoma
familial atypical multiple-mole melanoma syndrome
a. favor reactive
a. feature
a. fibrous histiocytoma
a. fibroxanthoma
a. finding
a. gallbladder disease
a. gender identity disorder
a. giant cell tumor
a. gingivitis
a. gingivostomatitis
a. glandular cells of uncertain significance
a. glandular cells of unknown significance
a. glandular cell of undetermined significance
a. heart attack
a. hemolytic uremia syndrome
a. histiocytosis
a. hyperplasia
a. immune-mediated thrombocytopenia
a. impulse-control disorder
a. insulin
a. interest
a. interstitial pneumonia
a. junction
a. karyotype
a. Kawasaki disease
a. *Legionella*-like organism
a. leiomyoma
a. lichenoid stomatitis
a. lipoma
a. lobular breast hyperplasia
a. lobular hyperplasia
a. lymphocyte
a. lymphocytosis
a. lymphoepithelioid cell proliferation
a. lymphoproliferative disorder
a. mania
a. manifestation
a. measles
a. measles pneumonia
a. measles syndrome
a. medullary carcinoma
a. melanocytic hyperplasia
a. melanocytic nevus
a. meningioma
a. or mixed organic brain syndrome
a. mixed or other personality disorder
a. mole
a. mole syndrome
mood disorder with atypical features
a. mycobacteria
a. mycobacteria infection
a. mycobacterial arthritis
a. mycobacterial colonization
a. mycobacterial infection
a. mycobacteriosis
a. mycobacterium
a. neuralgia
a. neurotic anxiety state
a. nevus
a. pain
a. paranoid disorder
a. paraphilia

a. pervasive developmental disorder
a. petit mal seizure
a. pityriasis rosea
a. pneumonia
a. polypoid adenomyofibroma
a. polypoid adenomyofibroma of low malignant potential
a. polypoid adenomyoma
a. presentation
primary atypical pneumonia
a. primary pneumonia
a. pseudocholinesterase
a. psychosexual dysfunction
a. puberty
a. regeneration
a. regenerative hyperplasia
regressing atypical histiocytosis
a. renal cyst
a. schizophrenia
a. sensory modality
a. small acinar proliferation of prostate
a. somatoform disorder
a. specific developmental disorder
a. squamous cell of undetermined significance
a. stereotyped movement disorder
a. subisthmic coarctation
a. tamponade
a. teratoma
a. thymoma
a. tic disorder
a. transformation zone
a. trigeminal neuralgia
a. tuberculosis
a. vasculature
a. ventricular tachycardia
a. verrucous endocarditis
a. vessel colposcopic pattern

Atzpodien regimen for renal cell carcinoma

au
A. antigen
A. blood group
café au lait
café au lait spot

AUA
A. classification
A. Symptom Index

Aub-Dubois
A.-D. standard
A.-D. table

Auberger blood group

Aubert phenomenon

Auchincloss
A. modified radical mastectomy
A. operation

Auclair operation

audibility threshold

audible
a. blocking in speech
a. grunt
rales audible at bases
a. range
a. rub
a. speech blockade
a. stridor
a. thought

audience effect

audio
a. amplifier
central audio vestibular dysfunction
a. frequency

audiofrequency
a. eddy current
carotid audiofrequency analysis

audiogenic
a. epilepsy
a. seizure

audiogram configuration

audiokinetic nystagmus

audiologic
a. assessment
a. evaluation
a. habilitation
Medical A. Tinnitus Patient Protocol

audiological
a. evaluation
a. testing

audiology
masked a.
pediatric a.
speech pathology and a.

audiometer
automatic a.
evoked response a.
Filtered A. Speech Test

audiometric
a. brainstem response
a. evaluation
a. examination
a. test
a. testing
a. zero

audiometry
ascending technique a.
auditory brainstem response a.
average evoked response a.
behavioral observation a.
brainstem electrical response a.
brainstem electric response a.
brief tone a.
cardiac-evoked response a.
conditioned orientation reflex a.
condition orientation reflex a.
delayed feedback a.
electric response a.
electrodermal a.
electrodermal response a.
electroencephalic a.
electroencephalic response a.
electroencephalographic a.
evoked-response a.
evoked response a.
galvanic skin response a.
heart rate a.
operant conditioning a.
psychogalvanic skin response a.
pure tone a.
a. sweep test
tangible reinforcement of operant conditioned a.
visual reinforcement a.
visual response a.

audioverbal amnesia

audiovestibular
a. dysfunction
a. testing

audiovisual
a. electroencephalogram
a.'s on-line
a. stimulation
a. training

audio-visual-tactile stimulation

audit
General A. Inpatient Psychiatric Assessment Scale
human immunodeficiency virus quality audit marker
Management Transactions A.
medical a.
nursing a.

audition
mental a.
system universal verbotonol audition Guberina

auditory
a. ability
a. accommodation
a. acuity
a. adaptation
a. agnosia

auditory *(continued)*
a. alexia
altered auditory feedback
a. alternans
a. amnesia
a. analysis
A. Analysis Test
anlagen of the auditory ossicle
a. aphasia
a. apperception test
a. area
a. arteriovenous malformation
a. artery
a. association area
a. association cortex
a. attention
a. aura
automated auditory brainstem response
automated auditory brainstem response hearing screening
a. blending
blood in auditory canal
a. brain mapping
brainstem auditory evoked potential
brainstem auditory evoked response
a. brainstem-evoked potential
a. brainstem-evoked response
a. brainstem implant
a. brainstem response audiometry
a. brainstem response test
a. bulb
a. canal
a. capsule
Carrow Test for A. Comprehension
a. cartilage
central auditory nervous system
central auditory processing battery
central auditory processing disorder
Children's A. Verbal Learning Test-2
Clinical Adaptive Test/Clinical Linguistic and A. Milestone Scale
Clinical Linguistic and A. Milestone Scale
a. closure
command auditory hallucination
a. comprehension
a. comprehension impairment
a. comprehension of language
A. Comprehension Test for Sentences
a. continuous performance task
a. cortex
a. cortical area
cortical auditory evoked potential
cortical auditory evoked response
a. cue
Denver A. Phoneme Sequencing Test
a. differentiation
Differentiation of A. Perception Skill
digital auditory aerobics
a. discrimination
A. Discrimination Test
a. discrimination test
a. disorder
a. disorientation
a. distance cue
a. distortion
a. dysfunction
a. evoked potential
external a.
external auditory canal
a. fatigability
a. fatigue
a. feedback
a. field
a. figure-ground
a. figure-ground discrimination
first auditory area
Flowers A. Screening Test
Flowers A. Test of Selective Attention
a. flutter
a. flutter fusion
a. function
a. ganglion
Goldman-Fristoe-Woodcock A. Skills Test Battery
gradual loss of auditory discrimination
a. hair
a. hallucination
a. hyperalgesia
a. hyperesthesia
a. illusion
a. imagery
immediate auditory memory
immediate auditory recall
a. impairment
a. imperception
a. impulse
integrated visual and a.
a. integration thinking
a. integration training
internal auditory canal
internal auditory meatus
isthmus of auditory tube
Kindergarten A. Screening Test
a. and kinesthetic sensation
a. koniocortex
late auditory evoked response
a. learner
a. localization
a. meatus
medial lamina of cartilage of pharyngotympanic auditory tube
a. and medical evaluation
membranous lamina of cartilage of pharyngotympanic auditory plate
a. memory
a. memory span
a. method
a. middle latency response
Minimum A. Capabilities Test
a. modality
mucous gland of auditory tube
muscles of auditory ossicles
neonatal auditory response cradle
a. nerve
a. neuropathy
a. nucleus
occasional auditory hallucination
a. oculogyric reflex
a. oculogyric response
Oliphant A. Discrimination Memory Test
Oliphant A. Synthesizing Test
oral auditory method
a. organ
a. ossicle
a. ossicles
Paced A. Serial Addition Test
a. pathway
a. pattern
a. perception
a. perception of speech sounds
a. perceptual disability
a. perceptual disorder
peripheral auditory disorder
peripheral auditory function
a. phonetics
a. pit
a. placode
a. plate
A. Pointing Test
a. pore
a. process
a. processing
a. processing disorder
a. projection area
a. prosthesis
a. radiation

a. receptor cell
a. region
a. rehabilitation
a. response to bell
a. response cradle
Rey A. Verbal Learning Test
screening auditory brainstem response
Screening Test for A. Comprehension of Language
second auditory area
a. seizure
a. selective listening
a. sequencing
Short-Term A. Retrieval and Storage Test
simultaneous auditory feedback
a. skill
a. space perception
a. span
steady-state auditory evoked response
Stetson A. Discrimination Test
a. 3-stimuli oddball task
a. stimulus
a. striae
a. string
a. symptom
a. synesthesia
a. synthesis
a. system
a. teeth
Test of A. Discrimination
Testing-Teaching Module of A. Discrimination
Test of Nonverbal A. Discrimination
Tests for A. Comprehension of Language
Tests for A. Comprehension of Language-Revised
a. threshold
a. tooth
a. tract
a. training
a. training sessions
a. training units
a. transfer deficit
transient auditory evoked response
a. tube nerve
a. tubercle
a. vein
a. verbal agnosia
a. verbal memory
Verbal A. Screen for Children
a. vertigo
a. vesicle
visual auditory evoked response
visual auditory range
visual or auditory stimulation
a. visual evoked response
Visual A. Screen for Children
a. and visual signs
vivid visual, auditory and olfactory hallucinations
a. vocabulary
a. vocal sequencing
Weidel A. Processing Test
a. word center

auditory-evoked magnetic field

auditory-verbal dysgnosia

auditory-vocal

a.-v. association
a.-v. automaticity

Audouin microsporon

Auenbrugger sign

Auer

A. body
A. rod

Auerbach

A. ganglion
A. and Meissner plexus
A. mesenteric plexus
A. node
A. plexus
A. pseudohypoparathyroidism

Aufranc

A. awl
A. concentric hip mold
A. cup arthroplasty
A. lateral approach
A. osteotome
A. reamer

Aufranc-Turner

A.-T. acetabular cup
A.-T. arthroplasty
A.-T. femoral component
A.-T. operation
A.-T. stem

Aufrecht

A. disease
A. point
A. sign

Auger

A. effect
A. electron

augment

a. flow of blood
gastric augment and single pedicle tube
a. individual sense of self-worth

augmentation

a. agent overactivity in OCD
alloplastic chin a.
alloplastic sandwich a.
autologous human collagen a.
a. cystoplasty
demucosalized augmentation with gastric segment
diastolic a.
a. genioplasty
Gore-Tex augmentation material
Gore-Tex augmentation membrane
a. graft
ligament augmentation device
malar alloplastic a.
malar facial a.
a. mammaplasty
a. mammoplasty
a. of mandibular angle
midface alloplastic a.
Millard graft a.
orthotopic bladder a.
paraffin breast a.
periorbital volume a.
Pitocin augmentation of labor
a. plaque
pressure a.
simultaneous areolar mastopexy and breast a.
a. strategy
subcutaneous augmentation material
a. therapy
transumbilical breast a.
a. ureterocystoplasty
Wise areola mastopexy breast a.
a. with implant

augmentative

a. and alternative communication
a. communication
a. communication system
immune augmentative therapy

augmented

ASTM augmented soft tissue mobilization
a. biofeedback
a. bladder
a. breast
a. cardiac output
a. feedback
a. filling
a. filling of right ventricle
a. histamine test
a. reconstruction
a. repair
a. soft tissue mobilization
a. stroke volume

augmented *(continued)*
a. transition network
a. valved rectum
a. vector
a. voltage unipolar left arm lead
a. voltage unipolar left foot lead
a. voltage unipolar right arm lead

augmentor
a. fiber
a. nerve

Aujeszky
A. disease
A. disease virus

aunt
maternal a.
paternal a.

aura
auditory a.
classic headache preceded by a.
headache preceded by classic a.
a. hysterica
a. hysterics
a. intelligence
a. interpretation
migraine with a.
migraine without a.
migrainous a.
motor a.
olfactory a.
a. procursiva
a. sensation
sensory a.
somatosensory a.
A. virus
visual a.

aural
a. atresia
a. fistula
a. fullness
a. glomus
a. immittance measurement
a. keratosis
a. microtia
a. myiasis
a. nystagmus
a. pathology
a. polyp
a. pressure
a. rehabilitation
a. scotoma
a. temperature
a. vertigo
Visual A. Digit Span Test

aural-oral technique

auramine
a. fluorochrome stain
a. O fluorescent stain

auramine-phenol stain

auramine-rhodamine
a.-r. acid-fast stain
a.-r. stain

AuraTek rapid cancer test

aureus
borderline-resistant *Staphylococcus aureus*
epidemic methicillin-resistant *Staphylococcus aureus*
glycopeptide-insensitive *Staphylococcus aureus*
glycopeptide-intermediate *Staphylococcus aureus*
glycopeptide-resistant *Staphylococcus aureus*
hemolytic Staphylococcus a.
lichen a.
methicillin-aminoglycoside-resistant *Staphylococcus aureus*
mupirocin-resistant, methicillin-resistant *Staphylococcus aureus*
mupirocin-resistant *Staphylococcus aureus*
mutiresistant *Staphylococcus aureus*
oxacillin aminoglycoside-resistant *Staphylococcus aureus*
Staphylococcus aureus hyperimmunoglobulinemia E syndrome
Staphylococcus aureus pneumonia
Staphylococcus aureus protease
Staphylococcus aureus prosthetic joint infection
vancomycin-insensitive *Staphylococcus aureus*
vancomycin-intermediate-resistant *Staphylococcus aureus*
vancomycin-resistant *Staphylococcus aureus*

auricle
anterior notch of a.
apex of a.
concha of a.
left a.
a. of left atrium
ligament of a.
lobule of a.
right a.
a. of right atrium
a. scar
Tanzer auricle reconstruction
tip of a.

auricular
a. abscess
a. acupuncture
anterior auricular artery
anterior auricular branch of superficial temporal artery
anterior auricular groove
anterior auricular muscle
anterior auricular nerve
anterior auricular vein
a. appendage
a. appendectomy
a. appendix
a. arc
a. artery
a. branch
a. branch of occipital artery
a. branch of posterior auricular artery
a. branch of vagus nerve
a. canaliculus
a. cartilage
a. cartilage graft
cerebral, ocular, dental, auricular, skeletal syndrome
a. chondritis
communicating branch of glossopharyngeal nerve with auricular branch of vagus nerve
a. complex
a. composite graft
a. docimasia
a. endochondral pseudocyst
a. extrasystole
a. fibrillation
a. fissure
a. flutter
a. ganglion
a. glaucoma
a. helix
a. hematoma
a. index
Integrated A. Reconstruction Protocol
internal auricular vein
left auricular appendage
a. lesion
a. ligament
a. line
a. lymph node
mastoid branch of posterior auricular artery
a. muscle
a. nerve
a. nerve of Arnold
a. notch
oblique auricular muscle

oculogyric auricular reflex
paroxysmal auricular fibrillation
paroxysmal auricular tachycardia
a. perichondritis
a. point
posterior auricular flap
posterior auricular groove
posterior auricular muscle
posterior auricular nerve
posterior auricular vein
posterior branch of great auricular nerve
premature auricular beat
premature auricular systole
a. premature beat
a. reduction
a. reflex
a. repositioning
a. seroma
a. standstill
a. surface
a. surface of ilium
a. surface of sacrum
a. systole
a. tachycardia
a. tag
a. trauma
a. triangle
a. tubercle
a. tubercle of Darwin
a. vein

auricularis
a. anterior
a. anterior muscle
arteria anastomotica auricularis magna
arteria auricularis posterior
arteria auricularis profunda magna
a. magnus
musculus auricularis anterior
musculus auricularis posterior
musculus auricularis superior
nervus auricularis magnus
nervus auricularis posterior
a. posterior
a. posterior muscle
a. superior
a. superior muscle

auriculocephalic
a. angle
a. sulcus

auriculoinfraorbital plane

auriculomastoid
a. angle
a. area
a. crease
a. line

auriculopalpebral reflex

auriculopressor reflex

auriculotemporal
a. artery
a. branch
a. nerve
a. nerve syndrome
a. neuralgia
a. syndrome

auriculotemporalis
nervus a.

auriculoventricular
a. groove
a. interval
a. orifice
a. valve
a. valve opening

aurintricarboxylic
a. acid
a. acid stain

auris
a. dexter
a. hematoma
a. media
a. uterque

aurium
tinnitus a.

auropalpebral reflex

Aurora
A. diode soft-tissue laser
A. MR breast imaging

aurothiomalate
sodium a.

Aus antigen

ausculatory triangle

auscultation
aortic area of a.
a. of bowel sounds
chest clear to auscultation and percussion
chest clear to percussion and a.
chest percussion and a.
clear to a.
clear to auscultation and percussion
a. of heart
inspection, palpation, percussion, and a.
lungs clear to a.
lungs clear to auscultation and percussion
a. and palpation
palpation, percussion, and a.
percussion and a.
percussion and a.
a. and percussion
tympanicity auscultation of chest

auscultatory
a. alternans
a. finding
a. gap
a. percussion
a. sign
a. sound

Auspitz
A. dermatosis
A. sign

aussage test

Aussies-Isseis unstable scoliosis

austenitic stainless steel

Austin
A. bunionectomy
A. Flint murmur
A. Flint phenomenon
A. Flint respiration
A. Moore arthroplasty
A. Moore chisel
A. Moore hemiarthroplasty
A. Moore reamer
A. osteotomy
A. Spanish Articulation Test
A. syndrome

Austin-Akin bunionectomy

Austin-Kartush
A.-K. group A impairment
A.-K. group C patient related to ossiculoplasty

Australia
A. antigen
A. antigen protein
A. antigen radioimmunoassay
A. hepatitis-associated antigen
A. serum hepatitis antigen

Australian
A. antigen
A. hepatitis antigen
A. parrot feather
A. parrot protein
A. pine
A. pine tree
A. punch
A. Q fever
A. tick typhus
A. X disease
A. X disease virus

Australian *(continued)*
A. X encephalitis
A. X encephalitis virus

Austrian Breast Cancer Study Group

autacoid substance

Autenrieth and Funk method

Auth atherectomy

authentication
patient a.

authoritarian
a. aggression
a. character
a. conscience
a. leader
a. personality
a. rejecting-neglecting parent
a. submission

authoritative manner

authority
a. anxiety
area health a.
a. complex
a. confusion
district health a.
a. figure
a. figure fixation
Human Fertilization and Embryology A.

authorization
away without a.
cosmetic surgery authorization form
a. form for removal of tissue for grafting
medical a.
treatment authorization request
Treatment A. Number

authorized
duly authorized officer
a. leave
a. walk-in patient

autism
a., dementia, ataxia, loss of purposeful hand use syndrome
Childhood A. Rating Scale
a. diagnostic interview
A. Diagnostic Interview-Revised
A. Diagnostic Observation Schedule
high-functioning a.
infantile a.
prelinguistic autism diagnostic observation
a. spectrum screening questionnaire

autism-fragile X syndrome

autistic
a. behavior
a. child
a. disorder
a. fantasy
a. isolation
normal autistic phase
a. parasite
a. phase
a. proband
a. psychopathy
a. psychosis
a. spectrum disorder
a. syndrome
a. thinking
treatment and education of autistic and related communications handicapped children
Wing A. Disorder Interview Checklist

autistic-like behavior

autistic-presymbiotic adolescent

autistic-spectrum children

Autley-Bixler syndrome

autoagglutinating
albumin autoagglutinating factor

autoagglutinin
anti-Pr cold a.

autoaggressive behavior

autoallergic
a. disease
a. hemolytic anemia

autoamputation
a. of ovary
a. of penis

autoanalyzer
sequential multichannel a.
simultaneous multichannel a.

autoantibody
adrenocortical a.
a.'s against insulin
antibasement membrane zone a.
anticathepsin D autoantibody assay
anticentromere a.
anticollagen a.
antiendothelial cell a.
antiglutamic acid decarboxylase a.
antiheart muscle a.
anti-Hu antineuronal a.
anti-IgA a.
antineuronal cytoplasmic a.
antineutrophil cytoplasmic a.
antitopoisomerase I a.
a. assay testing
competitive insulin a.'s
gait disorder, autoantibody, late-age onset, polyneuropathy
a.'s to human thyroglobulin
insulin a.
liver cell membrane a.
microsomal a.'s
muscarinic receptor a.
myositis-specific a.
natural thymocytotoxic a.
perinuclear antineutrophil cytoplasmic a.
a. production
smooth muscle a.
a. to stratum corneum
thymocytotoxic a.
thyroid a.
thyroid hormone a.'s
thyroid-stimulating hormone receptor a.
thyrotropin receptor a.

autoantigen collagen

auto-antiidiotypic antibody

autoattenuation correction method

autoaugmentation cystoplasty

autobiographical
a. information
a. life chart
a. memory

autobiographic memory

autocastration
anticipatory a.

autocerebral cooling

autochthonous
a. delusion
a. gestalt
a. graft
a. idea
a. malaria
a. neoplasm
a. parasite
a. tumor
a. variable

autoclave
a. sterilization
a. sterilized

autoclaved India ink

autoclitic operant

autocoid substance

autocompression plate

autocorrelation

a. function
serial a.

autocrine

a. action
a. cell
a. communication
a. effect
a. growth factor
a. hormone
a. hypothesis
a. mechanism
a. motility factor
a. motility factor of the bladder
a. motility factor receptor
a. regulation
a. secretion
a. suppressor
a. system

autocrine-paracrine

a.-p. growth loop
a.-p. growth regulator

autocrine-paracrine-acting growth factor

autodermic graft

autodigestion of connective tissue

autoepidermic graft

autoerotic

a. asphyxia
a. rectal trauma

autoerythrocyte

a. sensitivity
a. sensitization
a. sensitization syndrome

autofluorescence

a. focal fluorescence
near-UV excited autofluorescence diagnosis system
a. test

autofluorescent endoscopic system

autogeneic graft

autogenic

a. drainage
a. graft
a. training
a. training for headache
a. training for hypertension
a. training for insomnia

autogenital stimulation

autogenous

a. bone
a. bone graft
a. bone grafting
a. bone slurry
a. cable graft interposition VII-VII neuroanastomosis
a. cancellous bone graft
a. cartilage graft
a. cartilage implantation
a. cartilage transplantation
a. composite tissue
a. control
a. corneal protector
a. corticocancellous graft
a. depression
a. dermis fat graft
a. donor material
a. fascia lata sling procedure
a. fascial heterograft
a. fat
a. fat graft
a. fibular graft
a. graft
a. grafting
a. iliac bone
a. interpositional shoulder arthroplasty
a. keratoplasty
a. meniscal cartilage replantation
a. nerve graft
a. osteocartilage transfer
a. patellar ligament graft
a. patellar tendon reconstruction
percutaneous autogenous dowel bone graft
a. semitendinosus-gracilis graft
a. spermatocele
split-thickness autogenous graft
a. strip
a. tooth transplantation
total autogenous latissimus
a. transplant
a. tunica vaginalis graft
a. union
a. vaccine
a. vein
a. vein bypass graft
a. vein graft conduit

autograft

adrenal medullary a.
articular cartilage a.
a. bone
a. bone grafting
a. bridge
a. extender
a. fusion
a. hair transplantation
a. harvesting
limbal autograft transplantation
meniscal autograft transplantation
osteochondral autograft transfer system
patellar bone-tendon-bone a.
patellar tendon a.
pulmonary a.

autografting

articular cartilage a.
limbal a.
peripheral blood stem cell a.

autohemolysis test

autohypnotic amnesia

autoimmune

a. acquired hemolytic anemia
acute monophasic experimental autoimmune encephalomyelitis
a. adrenalitis
a. antibody
antigliadin IgA ELISA autoimmune test
antigliadin IgG ELISA autoimmune test
atrophic chronic autoimmune thyroiditis
a. blistering mucocutaneous disease
a. cholangitis
a. chronic active hepatitis
a. chronic hepatitis
a. cirrhosis
collagen-induced autoimmune ear disease
a. collagen vascular disease
combined cold and warm antibody autoimmune hemolytic anemia
a. complement fixation
a. condition
a. connective tissue disorder
cryptogenic autoimmune cirrhosis
cryptogenic autoimmune hepatitis
a. deficiency
a. deficiency syndrome
a. demyelinating polyneuropathy
a. demyelination
a. diabetes
a. diabetes mellitus
a. disease
a. disorder
a. disorder immune disease
a. encephalomyelitis
a. endocrine disease
a. enteropathy

autoimmune *(continued)*
a. exocrinopathy
experimental autoimmune encephalitis
experimental autoimmune encephalomyelitis
experimental autoimmune gastritis
experimental autoimmune myasthenia gravis
experimental autoimmune thymitis
experimental autoimmune thyroiditis
experimental autoimmune uveitis
a. factor
a. glomerulonephritis
a. hearing loss
a. hemolysis
a. hemolytic anemia
a. hemolytic disease
a. hepatitis
a. hyperthyroidism
a. hypoparathyroidism
a. hypophysitis
idiopathic autoimmune hemolytic anemia
a. illness
a. immunoglobulin mediation
a. inflammatory demyelination
a. inner ear disease
a. interstitial nephritis
juvenile autoimmune myasthenia gravis
latent autoimmune diabetes of adult
a. leukopenia
a. lymphoproliferative syndrome
a. mechanism
a. metaplastic atrophic gastritis
a. myasthenia gravis
neonatal autoimmune neutropenia
neonatal autoimmune thrombocytopenia
a. neonatal thrombocytopenia
a. neuromuscular junction disorder
a. neutropenia
a. neutropenia of infancy
nonvasculitic autoimmune inflammatory meningoencephalitis
a. obsessive-compulsive tic disorder
a. oophoritis
a. orchitis
a. pancytopenia
a. panhypopituitarism
a. paraneoplastic syndrome
pediatric autoimmune neuropsychiatric diseases associated with streptococcal infection
pediatric autoimmune neuropsychiatric disorders associated with streptococcal infection
a. phenomenon
a. pituitary disease
a. polyendocrine-candidiasis syndrome
a. polyendocrine syndrome
a. polyendocrinopathy, candidiasis, ectodermal dysplasia
a. polyendocrinopathy, candidiasis, ectodermal dystrophy
a. polyglandular endocrinopathy
a. polyglandular failure
a. polyglandular hypofunction
a. polyglandular syndrome
polyglandular autoimmune syndrome type I, II
a. process
a. progenitor cell
a. progesterone dermatitis
a. purpura
a. reaction
a. regulator
a. regulator gene
a. regulatory
a. regulatory gene
a. response
a. sensorineural hearing loss
severe autoimmune disease
a. sialadenitis
a. signal
spontaneous autoimmune thyroiditis
symptomless autoimmune thyroiditis
a. thrombocytopenic purpura
a. thyroid disease
a. thyroid disorder
a. thyroid hyperfunction
a. thyroiditis
a. thyroid-related antigen-1
a. thyrotoxicosis
a. type of reaction
undifferentiated autoimmune syndrome
a. urticaria
warm autoimmune hemolytic anemia

autoimmune-associated congenital heart block

autoimmune-type chronic active hepatitis

autoimmunity
familial autoimmunity in diabetes

autokinetic
a. effect
a. visible light phenomenon

autologous
a. adrenal medullary tissue
a. and allogeneic marrow transplantation
a. antibody
a. antigen
antigen-pulsed autologous dendritic cell
a. blood
a. blood clot
a. blood collection
a. blood donation
a. blood and marrow transplantation
a. blood transfusion
a. blood unit
a. BMT
a. bone
a. bone marrow
a. bone marrow cell
a. bone marrow reinfusion
a. bone marrow rescue
a. bone marrow support
a. bone marrow transplant
a. cancellous bone graft
cartilaginous autologous thin septal graft
a. cellular therapy
a. chondrocyte
a. chondrocyte implantation
a. chondrocyte transplantation
a. clot
a. cord blood
a. cultured chondrocyte
a. cultured epithelium
a. cultured skin grafting
a. cultured skin transplantation
a. donor
a. fat
a. fat graft
a. fat injection
a. fat transfer
a. fibrin glue
a. fibrin sealant glue
a. graft
a. growth factor
a. growth factor binding agent
a. growth factor gel
a. HBcAg-specific CD4+
a. hemagglutinin

a. hematopoietic cell
a. hematopoietic progenitor cell transplantation
a. hematopoietic stem cell support
a. hematopoietic stem cell transplantation
a. human collagen
a. human collagen augmentation
a. iliac crest bone graft
a. implant
a. internal jugular vein
intraoperative autologous transfusion
a. labeled leukocyte
a. leukapheresis, processing, and storage
a. liver cell
a. lymphokine activated killer cell
a. melanoma
a. melanoma system
a. mixed leukocyte reaction
a. mixed lymphocyte culture
a. mixed lymphocyte reaction
a. ovarian transplantation
a. patch graft
a. patient donor
a. pearl fat graft
a. pericardial patch
a. pericardium
a. peripheral blood stem cell bone marrow transplantation
a. peripheral hematopoietic stem cell support
a. platelet gel
a. predeposit donation
preoperative autologous blood donation
preoperative autologous donation
a. protein
a. RBC unit
a. reactive T cell
a. rectus fascia sling
a. red blood cell
a. red cell salvage
a. reverse graft
a. reverse graft to ankle
a. rib
a. rib bone graft
a. serum application
a. skin transplant
a. stem
a. stem cell
a. stem cell rescue
a. stem cell transplantation
a. thrombin
a. tissue flap
a. T lymphocyte
a. T lymphocytes stimulated with the patient's tumor-specific mutated RAS peptides
a. traction
a. transfusion
a. transplantation
a. tumor
a. tumor cell immunization
a. tumor extract
a. tumor rejection antigen
a. tumor vaccine
a. vein graft
a. vein graft-coated stent
a. vein graft stent
a. white cell localization
zymosan-activated autologous serum

autolymphocyte-based

a.-b. treatment
a.-b. treatment for renal cell carcinoma

autolymphocyte therapy

autolytic

a. debridement
a. enzyme

autolyzed yeast protein

automated

a. activated partial thromboplastin
a. airway tree segmentation method
a. anesthesia record
a. assessment
a. auditory brainstem response
a. auditory brainstem response hearing screening
bacterial automated identification technique
a. bacteriology
a. biochemical analyzer
a. biopsy device
a. biopsy gun
a. blood pressure cuff
a. border detection
a. border detection by echocardiography
a. boundary protection
a. cardiac flow measurement
a. cardiac flow measurement ultrasound
a. cardiac output measurement
a. cell count
a. cell-counter technology
a. cell image analysis
a. cellular imaging system
a. chemistry profile
A. Child/Adolescent Social History
a. clinical record
a. computed axial tomography
a. computerized axial tomography
computerized automated psychophysiologic device
a. corneal shaper
a. cytochemical system
a. differential leukocyte counter
a. disposable keratome
a. dithionite test
a. edge detection
a. eligibility verification system
a. endoscopic system for optimal positioning
a. enzyme immunoassay for antinuclear antibody
a. external defibrillator
a. external defibrillator pacemaker
a. factor V Leiden mutation test
a. gamma counter
a. general experimental device
a. hematocrit
a. hematology analysis
a. hospital information system
a. Hough transform
hyperopic automated lamellar keratoplasty
a. immunoprecipitation
a. lamellar keratectomy
a. large-core breast biopsy
a. laser keratomileusis
a. LCx factor V Leiden assay
a. medical history
a. method
a. microkeratome
mini Vidas automated immunoassay system
a. mixture control
a. motility factor
motion automated perimetry
a. multiphasic health testing
a. multiphasic screening
a. multiple analysis
multiple automated sample harvester
a. multitest laboratory
Octopus automated perimetry
percutaneous automated diskectomy
a. percutaneous diskectomy
a. percutaneous lumbar discectomy
a. percutaneous lumbar diskectomy

automated *(continued)*
a. perimetry
a. peritoneal dialysis
a. physiologic profile
a. polyp detection
a. quantification
a. radioimmunoassay
a. radiometric technique
a. reagin
a. reagin test
a. reticulocyte counting
a. shaver
short wavelength automated perimetry
a. slide staining
a. static threshold perimetry
a. test target calibration
a. tray assembly
a. ventricular brain ratio
a. visual field
a. white blood cell differential

automatic
a. absence
a. action
atrial ectopic automatic tachycardia
a. atrial tachycardia
a. audiometer
a. audiometry
a. beat
a. behavior
a. bladder
cardiac automatic resuscitative device
chi-square automatic interaction detection
a. chorea
a. clinical analyzer
a. collimator
a. computed transverse axial scanning
a. computerized solvent litholysis
a. condenser
a. contraction
a. data processing
a. drawing
a. ectopic tachycardia
a. endoscopic reprocessor
a. endoscopic system for optimal positioning
a. epilepsy
a. exposure control
a. external cardioverter-defibrillator
a. external defibrillator
a. extraction
a. fluorescent image analyzer
a. gain control
a. hone
implantable automatic cardioverter-defibrillator
a. implantable cardioverter-defibrillator
a. implantable defibrillator
a. infrared optometer
a. internal cardioverter-defibrillator
a. intracardiac defibrillator
a. judgment
a. karyotype system database
a. language
leukocyte automatic recognition computer
logical analysis of automatic thought
a. lumen edge segmentation
a. memory
a. mode conversion
a. mode switching
a. motion correction
a. movement
a. movement reaction
a. neonatal walking reflex
a. obedience
a. peak tracking
a. phrase level
a. plugger
a. positioning system
a. processing
a. psychological process
a. reactivity
a. reflex
a. refractor
a. rotating tourniquet
a. seizure
a. signal processing
a. single-needle monitor
a. speech
a. spring-loaded biopsy device
a. staple
a. stop order
a. thought
time-resolved imaging by automatic data segmentation
a. tissue processing
a. titration system
a. tonometry
a. trephine
a. vibrator
a. voice analysis
a. volume control
a. walking
a. writing
a. zero set

automaticity
depolarization-induced a.
a. of performance
a. recovery phase
a. recovery time

automation
microbiology a.

automatism
command a.
motor a.
oral alimentary a.

automaton conformity

automobile
a. accident
a. airbag impulse noise
driver of a.
a. exhaust

automotility factor

automotor seizure

autonomic
a. activity
a. activity-reactivity
adverse autonomic response
a. affective law
a. apparatus
a. arousal
a. arousal disorder
a. ataxia
a. balance
a. blockade
a. column of spinal cord
a. conditioning
a. control
a. conversion reaction
a. cooling mechanism
a. crisis
a. denervation
diabetic autonomic neuropathy
a. disorganization
a. disruption
a. division of nervous system
a. dysfunction
a. dysnomia
a. dysreactivity
a. dysreflexia
a. dysregulation
a. epilepsy
a. epilepsy flush
familial autonomic dysfunction
a. function
a. function test
a. ganglion
a. ganglion block
a. ganglionic synapse
gastrointestinal autonomic nerve tumor

hereditary sensory and autonomic neuropathy types I-IV
a. hyperactivity
a. hyperactivity sign
a. hyperarousal
a. hyperreflexia
a. hyperventilation
a. imbalance
a. imbalance syndrome
a. impairment
incomplete development of autonomic nervous system
a. instability
a. insufficiency
Modified A. Perception Questionnaire
a. modulation
a. motor neuron
a. motor pool
multifocal autonomic adenoma
a. nerve
a. nerve block
a. nerve fiber
a. nerve preservation
a. nerve-preserving three-space dissection
a. nerve tumor
a. nervous system disorder
a. nervous system dysfunction
a. neurogenic bladder
a. neuropathy
a. nuclei
a. oculomotor nucleus
a. part
a. part of peripheral nervous system
a. pathway
pelvic autonomic nerve
pelvic autonomic nerve preservation
pelvic autonomic plexus
peripheral autonomic neuropathy
pharmacologic autonomic block
a. plexus
a. polyneuropathy
a. postganglionic nerve terminal
quantitative autonomic functioning testing
a. reactivity
a. response
a. seizure
severe autonomic insufficiency
a. side effect
sympathetic autonomic nervous system
a. sympathetic ganglion
a. sympathomimetic drug
a. urticaria
a. varicosity
a. visceral motor nucleus
a. walking reflex

autonomous
a. adenoma
a. adrenal hyperplasia
a. breathing
a. depression
a. ego function
a. function
a. functional component
a. hyperfunction
a. induction
a. nodular hyperplastic gland
a. nodule
a. parathyroid chief cell proliferation
a. psychotherapy
a. replication sequence
solitary autonomous nodule
a. stage
a. superego
a. thyroid adenoma
a. thyroid nodule
a. toxic nodule
a. zone

autonomously functioning thyroid nodule

autonomy
loss of a.
a. loss
masked thyroid a.
a. of motives
multifocal functional a.
nodular a.
patient a.
A. Preference Index
a. scale

autoparenchymatous
a. metaphysis
a. metaplasia

Autopath QC test

autophagic vacuole

autophagocytosed cellular material

autoplastic
a. adaptation
a. change
a. graft
a. suture
a. symptom

autoplasty
peritoneal a.

autopolymerizing
a. acrylic resin
a. resin

autopolymer resin

auto-positive end-expiratory pressure

autoprecipitin
thyroglobulin a.

autoprothrombin
a. I
a. IIa

autoprotolysis constant of water

autopsy
at autopsy tumor, nodes, and metastases
a. authorization
a. of brain
a. consent form
a. external description
a. external examination
a. internal examination
a. limited to abdomen
a. limited to brain
a. limited to heart and lungs
a. microscopic examination
permission for autopsy denied
permission for autopsy granted
a. permit signed
a. study
a. witness

autopsy-acquired hepatitis

autopsy-based neurochemical study

autopsychic
a. delusion
a. disorientation
a. orientation

autopsy-negative death

autoradiographic
a. image
a. localization
quantitative a.
a. study
a. technique

autoreactive B cell

autoregressive
a. model for signal analysis
a. moving average

autoregulation
a. of cerebral blood flow
a. filtration

auto-reinforced polyglycolide rod

autorotation
center of mandibular a.
vestibular autorotation test
autorotational
vestibular autorotational testing
autoscopic
a. phenomenon
a. psychosis
a. syndrome
autosensitization dermatitis
autoserum therapy
autosomal
a. aberration
a. abnormality
a. anomaly
cerebral autosomal recessive arteriopathy with subcortical infarcts and leukoencephalopathy
a. chromosomal anomaly
a. chromosome disorder
a. codominant
a. congenital tubular dysgenesis
deleted in azoospermia-like a.
a. deletion
a. dominant
a. dominant arteriopathy
a. dominant cardiomyopathy
a. dominant cerebellar ataxia
a. dominant compelling helioophthalmic outburst syndrome
a. dominant condition
a. dominant congenital cataract
a. dominant diabetes mellitus
a. dominant disorder
a. dominant febrile convulsion
a. dominant gene
a. dominant hemochromatosis
a. dominant hereditary optic neuropathy
a. dominant hypocalcemia
a. dominant hypoparathyroidism
a. dominant inheritance
a. dominant lamellar ichthyosis
a. dominant macrocephaly syndrome
a. dominant medullary cystic kidney disease
a. dominant migraine
a. dominant mild short limb dwarfism
a. dominant movement disorder
a. dominant nocturnal frontal lobe epilepsy
a. dominant nonsyndromic hearing loss
a. dominant oculocutaneous albinism
a. dominant Opitz syndrome
a. dominant osteosclerosis
a. dominant pattern
a. dominant temporal lobe epilepsy
a. dominant toxic thyroid hyperplasia
a. dominant trait
a. dominant transmission
a. gene
a. heredity
a. karyotypic disorder
a. monosomy
mosaic autosomal monosomy
nonsyndromic autosomal recessive disorder
a. recessive
a. recessive disorder
a. recessive hereditary optic neuropathy
a. recessive hypophosphatemic rickets
a. recessive ichthyosis
a. recessive inheritance
a. recessive juvenile parkinsonism
a. recessive kidney disease
a. recessive mode
a. recessive mutation
a. recessive nonsyndromic hearing loss
a. recessive ocular albinism
a. recessive ocular Ehlers-Danlos syndrome
a. recessive renal proximal tubulopathy and hypercalciuria
a. recessive severe combined immunodeficiency disorder
a. recessive spastic ataxia of Charlevoix-Saguenay
a. recessive syndrome of encephalopathy
a. recessive trait
severe childhood autosomal recessive muscular dystrophy
a. trisomy
type 1 autosomal recessive vitamin D dependency
autosomal-dominant
a.-d. arteriopathy
a.-d. benign form of osteopetrosis
a.-d. genetic defect
a.-d. ophthalmoplegia
a.-d. optic atrophy
a.-d. periodic fever syndrome
a.-d. polycystic kidney disease
a.-d. vitreoretinochoroidopathy
autosomally
a. inherited forms of nephrolithiasis
a. recessively inherited disease
autosomal-recessive
a.-r. Alport syndrome
a.-r. ophthalmoplegia
a.-r. optic atrophy
a.-r. polycystic kidney disease
a.-r. SCID
autosome translocation
autostapling device
autosuture technique
autosympathectomy secondary to neuropathy
autotaxin assay
auto-titrating continuous positive airway pressure
autotopagnosia agnosia
autotransformer formula
autotransfusion suction
autotransfusor
autotransplantation
jejunal a.
a. O
pancreatic a.
parathyroid a.
parathyroidectomy and a.
a. of splenic fragment
autotransplants
tandem a.
autotroph
obligate a.
autotrophic
a. bacterium
a. fixation
a. nutrition
autotrophy
nitrogen a.
autumn
a. fever
Russian autumn encephalitis
Russian autumn encephalitis virus
a. skullcap mushroom
autumnal fever
Auvray incision
auxanographic method
auxetic growth
auxiliary
a. abutment

a. canal
a. cone
dental auxiliary teacher education
Dental A. Utilization
a. ego
expanded duty dental a.
a. fiber
a. heterotopic liver transplantation
a. implant rest
a. liver transplantation
mechanical auxiliary ventricle
a. nurse midwife
a. occlusal rest
a. organ
a. orthotopic liver transplantation
partial auxiliary orthotopic liver transplantation
a. partial orthotopic living donor transplantation
a. rest implant substructure
a. solution
a. spring
a. therapist
a. transplant
a. ventricle
a. verb
a. wire

auxotrophic
a. mutant
a. mutation
a. strain

Auzduk disease virus

AV-1 virus

availability
a. of health care
oxygen a.
a. of weapons

available
a. arch length
chart not a.
free available chlorine
longitudinal expert evaluation using all available data
low available carbohydrate diet
no data a.
no information a.
not a.
not available at the present time
space available for the cord

avalanche
a. conduction
a. ionization
a. theory

Avalon virus

avascular
a. bone necrosis
a. brain mass
a. corneal stroma
a. cortical infarction necrosis
a. cuff technique
a. femoral head necrosis
a. fibrocartilage
foveal avascular zone
a. fragment
a. graft
a. keratitis
a. kidney mass
Marcus grading scale for avascular necrosis
a. necrosis of bone
a. necrosis of the femoral head
a. necrosis lunate
a. nonunion
a. peripheral retina
a. plaque
a. renal mass
a. scaphoid necrosis
a. sequestrum
a. tarsal scaphoid necrosis
a. tissue
a. vertebral body necrosis
a. zone

avascularity
periungual a.

Avellino dystrophy

Avellis
A. paralysis
A. syndrome

avenues of administration

average
autoregressive moving a.
baseline average peak velocity
a. body dose
calculated average life
computer of average transients
a. conditioning
a. cost of illness
a. daily census
a. daily dose
a. daily metabolic rate
a. daily patient load
a. day
a. deviation
a. diastolic pressure
a. diffusivity histogram
a. electroencephalic response
a. evoked potential
a. evoked response
a. evoked response audiometry
a. evoked response technique
a. extubation time
a. flow rate
a. for gestational age
a. gradient
a. gradient number
guessed a.
a. impairment rating
a. interocular difference
a. intravascular pressure
a. life
a. lymphocyte output
a. mean pressure
minimal average dose
multiple scan average dose
normalized average glandular dose
a. optical density
a. orifice area
a. path velocity
peak hyperemic average velocity
a. peak noise
a. peak velocity
a. perturbation quotient
a. pixel projection
a. positron energy
a. pulse magnitude
pure tone a.
a. radiation dose
rectified a.
relative average perturbation
a. remaining lifetime
a. response computer
spatial a.
spatial average-pulse a.
spatial average-temporal a.
spatial average temporal peak
spatial peak temporal a.
a. target absorbed dose
temporal a.
time-weighted a.
a. velocity
a. volume of air

averager
multichannel signed a.

averaging
computer averaging technique
evoked potential signal a.
Memorial dimension averaging method
volume a.

averse to risk

aversion
a. center
a. conditioning
a. depression
electrical aversion therapy

aversion *(continued)*
a. reaction
a. response
taste a.
a. therapy
aversion-covert conditioning
aversive
a. behavior
a. conditioning
a. control
a. drive
a. early environment
a. imagery
a. incentive
a. racism
a. stimulus
a. therapy
a. training
aVF
AVF-induced renal ischemia
aVF lead
avian
a. AAV
a. adenovirus
a. diphtheria
a. encephalomyelitis
a. encephalomyelitis virus
enterocytopathogenic avian orphan virus
a. erythroblastosis
a. erythroblastosis virus
a. herpesvirus
a. infectious bronchitis
a. infectious bronchitis virus
a. infectious encephalomyelitis
a. infectious laryngotracheitis
a. infectious laryngotracheitis virus
a. influenza
a. influenza virus
a. leukemia-sarcoma complex
a. leukosis
a. leukosis complex
a. leukosis-sarcoma complex
a. leukosis-sarcoma virus
a. leukosis virus
a. lymphomatosis
a. lymphomatosis virus
a. mite dermatitis
a. monocytosis
a. myeloblastosis
a. myeloblastosis leukemia virus reverse transcriptase
a. myeloblastosis virus reverse transcriptase
a. myelocytomatosis virus
a. neurolymphomatosis virus
a. orthoreovirus
a. pancreatic polypeptide
a. paramyxovirus virus 1–9
a. pneumoencephalitis
a. pneumoencephalitis virus
recovered avian sarcoma virus
a. reticuloendotheliosis
a. rotavirus
a. sarcoma
a. sarcoma and leukosis virus
a. tubercle bacillus
a. tumor virus
a. type C retrovirus group
a. viral arthritis virus
aviation
a. medicine
medicine
a. otitis
research aviation medicine
aviator's
a. astragalus
a. disease
a. ear
a. effort syndrome
a. neurasthenia
Avicine vaccine
avid
infarct avid hot spot scintigraphy
infarct avid imaging
infarct avid myocardial scintigraphy
avidin-biotin
a.-b. complex
a.-b. complex assay
a.-b. complex immunodetection system
a.-b. detection system
a.-b. immunoperoxidase technique
a.-b. peroxidase
a.-b. peroxidase complex
a.-b. stain technique
avidin-biotin-based detection system
avidin-biotin-horseradish peroxidase complex
avidin-biotin-peroxidase
a.-b.-p. complex
a.-b.-p. complex method
a.-b.-p. method
a.-b.-p. reagent
a.-b.-p. staining
avidity
a. antibody
low a.
a. testing
Avila
A. approach
A. operation
A. technique
avirulent
rough, noncapsulated, avirulent bacterial culture
A virus hepatitis
avis
nidus a.
avitaminosis B_{12} peripheral neuropathy
avium
Mycobacterium a.
Mycobacterium avium complex
Mycobacterium avium complex infection
Mycobacterium avium infection
avium-intracellulare
Mycobacterium a.-i.
aVL lead
avocational intervention
avoidance
active a.
active avoidance reaction
anticipatory a.
a. behavior
a. category
a. cluster
conditioned avoidance response
a. conditioning
escape and avoidance conditioning in human subjects
a. and escape learning
a. of exposure
Fear A. Beliefs Quest
a. gait
a. gradient
gradient of a.
a. maneuver
master of a.
a. measure
a. of others
outside activity a.
passive avoidance reaction
a. pattern
a. reflex
a. response
a. score
social avoidance and distress
a. speaking
a. of speech dysfluency
a. style
a. symptom

a. syndrome
a. therapy
a. training

avoidance-avoidance conflict

avoidant
a. attachment
a. disorder
a. disorder of adolescence
a. disorder of childhood
a. feature
a. neurotic personality disorder
a. personality
a. personality disorder
phobic avoidant behavior
a. scale
a. symptom

avoidant-attached behavior

aVR lead

avulsed
a. fracture fragment
a. fragment
a. laceration
a. ligament
a. tooth
a. wound

avulsion
acute avulsion fracture
a. amputation
anterior labral a.
anterior labroligamentous periosteal sleeve avulsion lesion
anterior labrum periosteal sleeve a.
a. of caruncula lacrimalis
a. chip fracture
epicondylar avulsion fracture
extension corner avulsion fracture
a. of eyelid
a. flap injury
a. fracture
a. fragment
humeral avulsion of the glenohumeral ligament
a. injury
midface avulsion flap
a. of nail plate
a. of nerve
obturator avulsion fracture
pelvic avulsion fracture
peroneus longus muscle a.
a. of portion of finger
root avulsion injury
a. stress fracture
a. technique
through-and-through avulsion injury
a. trauma

avulsive cortical irregularity

avuncular relationship

awake
a. and active state
alert awake state
a., alert, oriented
a. and aware
a. craniotomy
a. neurological assessment
oriented
patient awake, alert, and cooperative
a. recording
a. state
while a.
wide a.

awakening
early morning a.
epilepsy with grand mal seizures on a.
a. trauma

aware
awake and a.

awareness
altered state of conscious a.
cognitive awareness level
concept of a.
a. and consciousness
a. defect
a. deficit
delivery a.
Depression: A., Recognition, and Treatment
Diversity A. Profile
enhanced sensory a.
food awareness training
Galveston Orientation and A. Test
heart rate control learning and a.
heightened awareness state
heightened awareness of touch or taste
heightened sense of a.
length of awareness of illness
level of a.
momentary lapse of a.
Parent A. Skills Survey
sensory a.
speech awareness threshold
a. of spirituality
a. threshold
A. Through Movement
a. training model

A-wave pressure

away
tear a.
a. without authorization

awl
angled a.
Aufranc a.
Wangensteen a.

Axenfeld
A. anomaly
A. follicular conjunctivitis
A. suture technique
A. syndrome

Axenfeld-Fieger syndrome

Axenfeld-Krukenberg spindle

Axenfeld-Rieger
A.-R. anomaly
A.-R. syndrome

axenic medium

Axer
A. compression apparatus
A. compression device
A. lateral opening wedge osteotomy
A. operation
A. varus derotational osteotomy

Axer-Clark procedure

axial
a. acetabular index
adipofascial axial pattern cross-finger flap
a. amblyopia
a. ametropia
a. amnesia
a. anchor screw
a. aneurysm
a. angiography
a. angle
a. anisometropia
anterior axial developmental cataract
anterior axial embryonal cataract
a. aspect
automated computed axial tomography
automated computerized axial tomography
automatic computed transverse axial scanning
a. breath-hold gradient-echo cine magnetic resonance imaging
a. calcaneal projection
a. calcaneus view
a. carpal dislocation
a. cataract

axial *(continued)*
a. celloidin section
a. chamber
a. chordoma
a. cineangiography
a. closed-loop hydraulic mechanical testing
a. compression
a. compression fracture
a. compression injury
a. compression load
a. compression principle
a. compression screw
a. compression test
computer-assisted axial tomography
computerized axial tomography
computerized axial tomography scan
computer tomographic methods of axial skeleton
a. cornea
a. current
a. curvature map
a. curvature mapping
a. dimension
a. disease
a. dorsal flap
dynamic axial fixator
a. echo planar diffusion weighted imaging
a. embryonal cataract
emission computerized axial tomography
fasciocutaneous axial pattern flap
a. fat-suppressed T2-weighted image
a. filament
a. fixation
a. flag flap
a. flap
a. frontonasal flap
a. fusiform developmental cataract
a. grade echo imaging
a. gradient
a. gradient echo image
a. gripping strength
head computerized axial tomography
a. hernia
a. hiatal hernia
a. hyperkinesis
a. hyperopia
a. hypertonia
a. illumination
a. image
a. inclination
a. instability
a. joint dissection
a. left anterior oblique ventriculogram
a. length
a. length/corneal radius ratio
a. length of eye
a. lesion
a. line angle
a. load
a. loading
a. loading fracture
a. loading injury
a. loading of spine
a. load 3-part, 2-plane fracture
a. load teardrop fracture
a. load test
a. localizer
long axial oblique view
a. magnetic resonance image
a. manual traction test
a. melanoma
a. mesodermal dysplasia complex
multiecho axial image
a. multiplanar reformation technique
a. muscle
a. musculature
a. myopia
a. neuritis
oblique axial MR imaging
a. orientation
a. osteomalacia
a. partial childhood cataract
a. pattern scalp flap
a. pattern vascularized skin flap
perineal artery axial flap
a. pin technique
a. plane
a. plane angular deformity biomechanics
a. plane imaging
a. plate
a. point
a. posturing
a. projection
a. proptosis
proton-density axial image
a. proton-density-weighted image
a. psoriatic arthritis
a. QCT
a. quantified computed tomography
a. radiograph
rapid acquisition computed axial tomography
a. ray of light
a. resistance exerciser
a. resolution
a. rotation
a. rotation joint
a. scan
a. section
a. sesamoid projection
a. sesamoid view
a. single shot fast spin-echo
a. skeleton
a. slice
a. spillway
a. spinal system
a. spin density
a. spin-echo image
a. stiffness
a. stress
a. surface
a. surface cavity
a. temporoparietal fascial flap
thin-section axial image
a. tomography
total axial node irradiation
a. traction
a. transabdominal image
a. transabdominal imaging
transverse axial tomography
a. transverse tomography
a. T1-SE protocol
a. 0.2T T1-weighted spin-echo imaging
a. T2-weighed image
T1-weighted axial image
a. type
a. unenhanced CT scan
vertebral axial decompression
a. view
a. wall
a. wall of pulp chamber
a. weight loading

axial-based flap

axial-occipital ligament

axile corpuscle

axilla
a., shoulder, elbow bandage
suspensory ligament of a.
a. temperature
a. thermometer

axillary
a. abscess
a. adenopathy
a. anesthesia
a. aneurysm
anterior axillary approach
anterior axillary fold
anterior axillary line

anterior axillary lymph node
anterior branch of axillary nerve
apical axillary lymph node
a. approach
a. arch
a. arch muscle
a. arteriography
a. artery
a. artery aneurysm
a. bed
a. block
a. block anesthesia
a. block anesthetic technique
a. breast tissue
carotid axillary bypass
a. cataract
a. cavity
a. contracture
contralateral axillary metastasis
a. count rate
a. crutch
a. endoscopic reduction
a. envelope
a. fascia
a. fat pad
a. flap
a. fold
a. foramen
a. fossa
a. freckling
a. gland
a. hair
a. hematoma
a. hidradenitis
a. hidradenitis suppurativa
a. hyperhidrosis
a. incision
a. insertion
a. irradiation
a. irradiation therapy
left axillary line
a. line
lower anterior axillary line
a. lymphadenectomy
a. lymphadenopathy
a. lymph node
a. lymph node dissection
a. lymph node involvement
a. lymph node metastasis
a. lymphoscintigraphy
mean axillary count rate
metastatic axillary involvement
middle axillary line
a. muscle
a. nerve
a. nerve palsy
a. nodal metastasis in breast carcinoma
a. node
a. node dissection mastectomy
a. node negative
a. node positive
parallel development of axillary hair
pectoral axillary lymph node
a. perivascular technique
a. plexus
posterior axillary fold
a. pouch
a. projection
a. prolongation
quadrantectomy, axillary dissection, radiation therapy
quadrantectomy, axillary dissection and radiotherapy
a. region
secondary axillary adenopathy
a. sheath
a. space
a. subpectoral approach
superficial distal axillary node
a. tail of Spence
a. temperature
temperature, a.
a. thermometer
a. thoracotomy
a. triangle
tumorectomy, axillary dissection, radiotherapy
a. ultrasonography
a. vein
a. venom gland
a. vessel
a. view

axillary-axillary bypass graft

axillary-brachial bypass graft

axillary-femoral bypass graft

axillary-femorofemoral bypass graft

axis

abnormal left axis deviation
abnormal right axis deviation
adjustable axis facebow
ankle mortise a.
anteroposterior axis of Fick
apical long a.
borderline left axis deviation
cardinal axes X,Y,Z
celiac a.
central axis depth dose of electron beam therapy
central principal axis of inertia
coordinate axis in plane
cylinder a.
a. of cylindric lens
a. deviation
diagnosis or condition deferred on Axis I, II
distal reference a.
enteroinsular a.
femoral shaft a.
a. of Fick
helical axis of motion
horizontal axis of rectangular coordinate system
hypothalamic-pituitary a.
hypothalamic-pituitary-adrenal a.
hypothalamic pituitary adrenocortical a.
hypothalamo-hypophyseo-adrenal a.
hypothalamoneurohypophysial a.
a. I, II diagnosis
left axis deviation, minimal
left deviation of electrical a.
long a.
long axis acquisition
long axis of body
long axis of bone
long axis of kidney
long axis parasternal view
long axis ray
long axis of spleen
long axis technique
long axis traction chiropractic table
longitudinal axis of Fick
longitudinal midtarsal joint a.
long posterior ciliary a.
mean QRS a.
minor axis shortening of left ventricle
Multi A. Ankle
multiple axis knee joint
neural axis vascular malformation
neutral axis of straight beam
no deviation of electrical a.
normal a.
normal axis deviation
normal electrical a.
parasternal long a.
parasternal short a.
pedicle axis angle
proximal reference a.
right deviation of electrical a.
short a.
short axis image
short axis plane
subcostal long a.
subcostal short a.

axis *(continued)*
subtalar joint a.
superior axis deviation
superior QRS a.
a. of three-dimensional rectangular coordinate system
a. traction forceps
transcondylar a.
transmalleolar a.
vertical axis of rectangular coordinate system
visual a.

axis-altering arthroereisis device

axis-atlas combination fracture

axis–first
talar axis–first metatarsal base angle

axle lock and bumper

axon
giant axon formation
myelinated a.
myelination of a.
nerve fiber a.
nonmyelinated a.
Quantitative Sudomotor A. Reflex Test
a. torpedo appearance

axonal
acute motor-sensory axonal neuropathy
amaurotic axonal idiocy
anterior axonal embryonal cataract
anterograde axonal transport
a. arborization
diffuse axonal injury
focal axonal swelling
giant axonal neuropathy
motor-sensory axonal neuropathy
a. neuropathy
olfactory axonal growth
a. retraction ball
a. terminal

axonopathic neurogenic thoracic outlet syndrome

axonopathy
multifocal acquired motor a.

axoplasmic
fast axoplasmic transport

Ayerza syndrome

Ayurveda philosophy

azelaic acid

azide
buffered azide glucose glycerol
ethyl violet azide broth
iodine azide test

azidothymidine
glucuronide derivative of a.
a. monophosphate
a. triphosphate

azoles
antifungal a.

azoospermia
a., renal anomaly, cervicothoracic spine dysplasia
deleted in a.
a. factor

azoospermia-homologue
deleted in a.-h.

Azorean
Machado-Joseph Azorean disease

azotemia
extrarenal a.
nonrenal a.
postrenal a.
prerenal a.

azure
a. A
a. B
a. C
methylene a.

azurophilic granule

azygos
a. artery
lobe of azygos vein
lymphonodus arcus vena a.
musculus azygos uvulae
node of azygos arch
nodus lymphoideus arcus venae a.
pericallosal azygos artery

azygous ganglion

B1
aflatoxin B.
Astler-Coller A, B1, B2, C1, C2 classification
vitamin B_1 deficiency

B2
aflatoxin B.
Astler-Coller A, B1, B2, C1, C2 classification

B_6
vitamin B_6 deficiency

B-100
apolipoprotein B.

B_{12}
avitaminosis B_{12} peripheral neuropathy
total vitamin B_{12} binding capacity
unsaturated vitamin B_{12}-binding capacity
vitamin B_{12} deficiency
vitamin B_{12} level

B16
murine B16 cell

B19
antiparvovirus B19 IgG antibody
antiparvovirus B19 IgM antibody
parvovirus B19 DNA
parvovirus B19 IgG antibody
parvovirus B19 IgM antibody
parvovirus B19 infection
parvovirus B19 neutralizing antibody assay
parvovirus B19 red cell aplasia
parvovirus B19 serology

21B
cytochrome P450 enzyme 21B

B291
monoclonal antibody B.

B-48
apo B.
apolipoprotein B.

B_e
hepatitis B.

B_c
hepatitis B.

b_{558}
membrane-bound cytochrome b_{558}

Babahoya virus

babble
phonetic b.

Babinski
B. downgoing bilaterally
questionable Babinski sign
B. reflex
B. sign

Babinski-Vaquez syndrome

baboon
b. kidney
b. virus replication

baby
b. for adoption
apnea monitored b.
b. born dead
b. boy
Clinical Risk Index for B.'s
crack baby syndrome
b. expired following resuscitation attempt
father of b.
fetal alcohol b.
gray baby syndrome
b. hamster kidney cell
junior baby food
married, keeping b.
Michelin tire baby syndrome
monitored baby apnea
mother and baby endoscope
not keeping b.
not married, keeping b.
not married, not keeping b.
shaken baby syndrome
single parent keeping b.
single parent not keeping b.
b. soft diet
special baby Travesol
special care baby unit
b. up for adoption
well b.

Bachmann
anterior internodal tract of B.
B. bundle

bacillary
b. angiomatosis
b. emulsion
enteric Gram-negative b.
Gram-negative bacillary meningitis
parenchymal bacillary peliosis
b. peliosis
tuberculin bacillary emulsion
b. white diarrhea

bacille
b. bilié de Calmette-Guérin
b. Calmette-Guérin
b. Calmette-Guérin vaccine
heat-aggregated bacille Calmette-Guérin
percutaneous bacille Calmette-Guérin administration

bacillus, pl. **bacilli**
acid-fast b.
acid-fast bacillus smear
avian tubercle b.
b. Calmette-Guérin
b. emulsion
enteric Gram-negative b.
Gram-negative b.
Gram-negative bacilli
Gram-negative bacilli arthritis
Gram-negative bacilli infection
Gram-positive b.
Gram-positive bacilli
Legionnaire disease b.
methanol extraction residue of bacillus Calmette-Guérin vaccine
negative aerobic b.
nonfermentative gram-negative bacilli
nonmotile pleomorphic b.
nonpigment-producing acid-fast b.
Pasteur Institute bacillus Calmette-Guérin vaccine
b. species enzyme
tubercle b.

back
acute low back syndrome
Acute Low B. Pain Screening Questionnaire
angry back phenomenon
angry back reaction
angry back syndrome
arched lower b.
ball on b.
b. board
to call b.
b. care
chronic intermittent low back pain
chronic low back strain
chronic low intermittent back pain
debilitating back pain
elastic back strap
estrogen add back therapy
failed back surgery syndrome
failed back syndrome with documented pseudarthrosis
flat back syndrome
hump in upper b.
immobilization of back injury

back *(continued)*
inability to straighten b.
intense back pain
long back board
low back bend
low back disability
low back injury
low back neurosis
low back pain
low back pain psychogenic disorder
low back syndrome
low back tenderness
low back trouble
Low B. Pain Questionnaire
Low B. Pain Symptom Checklist
lumbar flat back syndrome
b. lying
mechanical low back pain
muscle of b.
muscle of back proper
nervousness from pain in b.
NordiCare Back Therapy System
numbness in b.
numbness in lower b.
b. optic zone radius
b. pain after childbirth
pain in b.
b. pain extends down legs
pain radiating to b.
pain radiating into b.
b. pain and weakness
pediatric back pain
postpartum low back pain
postural back problem
b. pressure
b. range of motion
b. range-of-motion instrument
region of b.
side to back to side
Taylor back brace
ureteral back pressure
b. vertex power
will call b.

backcutting osteotome

backfire fracture

backfiring
angry backfiring C nociceptor

backflow
b. bleeding
b. of blood
venous b.

backflush needle

background
b. activity
adverse background factor
computer-assisted blood background subtraction
b. corrected
b. counts
b. diabetic retinopathy
diminution of background activity
electrographic background abnormality
b. interval
b. of slow activity

backpack palsy

backscatter
ultrasound backscatter microscopy

back-scattered electron imaging

backscatter factor

backscattering
rutherford ion b.

backup ventilation

backward
b. bending
b. flow of blood
head b.
b. heart failure
held b.
b. internal rotation

backward-biting ostrum punch

backwardness
general reading b.

baclofen
continuous intrathecal baclofen infusion
intrathecal b.

bactercidal
minimal bactercidal level

bacteremia
coagulase-negative staphylococcus b.
Escherichia coli b.
Gram-negative b.
Gram-positive b.
Gram stain negative b.'s
Mycobacterium avium-intracellulare b.
Mycoplasma hominis b.
nontyphoid *Salmonella* b.
Pseudomonas aeruginosa b.
Pseudomonas cepacia b.

bacteremia-associated pneumococcal pneumonia

bacteria
antibody-coated b.
beta-lactamase-producing b.
black-pigmented b.
b. in blood smear
body's natural balance b.
cellulose breakdown b.
clinical isolates of b.
cluster of b.
colony of b.
b. in feces
harmful antibiotic-resistant b.
killed intracellular b.
lightly staining coiled b.
low bacteria diet
nonfermenting b.
nonmotile b.
phosphorus-dissolving b.
resistant strains of b.
smooth, capsulated, virulent b.
specific strain of b.
transmission of b.
b. in urine

bacteria-free environment

bacterial
acute bacterial endocarditis
acute bacterial exacerbation of chronic bronchitis
acute bacterial meningitis
acute bacterial myocarditis
acute bacterial rhinosinusitis
acute focal bacterial nephritis
b. adherent colony
b. adhesion
b. agglutination
airway bacterial colonization
b. alkaline phosphatase
b. allergy
antibiotic-resistant bacterial infection
b. antigen complex
b. artificial chromosome
attenuated bacterial vector
b. automated identification technique
b. cell lacking an F plasmid
b. cell with an F plasmid
b. chlorophyll
chronic bacterial prostatitis
coarse bacterial colonies
conjugative plasmid in F^+ bacterial cell
documented bacterial infection
b. endocarditis
b. food-borne illness
gastric bacterial overgrowth
gastrointestinal bacterial flora
Gram-positive bacterial infection
Gram-positive bacterial keratitis
b. growth
Guthrie bacterial inhibition assay

b. index
b. infection
b. infection of bloodstream
b. intravenous protein
b. levan
b. meningitis
mixed bacterial toxin
natural bacterial flora
neutropenia-related bacterial infection
NIH Classification Category I acute bacterial prostatitis
NIH Classification Category II chronic bacterial prostatitis
nongonococcal bacterial arthritis
nosocomial bacterial meningitis
b. overgrowth
pancreatic bacterial infection
b. phosphatidylethanolamine
rough bacterial colony
rough, noncapsulated, avirulent bacterial culture
small bowel bacterial overgrowth
small intestine bacterial overgrowth
smooth bacterial colony
smooth-rough bacterial colony
spontaneous acute bacterial peritonitis
systemic bacterial infection
b. toxin
undenatured bacterial antigen
b. vaginitis
b. vaginosis
b. vegetations

bactericidal
b. concentration
functional bactericidal concentration
b. index
maximal bactericidal dilution
microdilution serum bactericidal test
minimal bactericidal level
minimum bactericidal concentration test
neutrophil bactericidal index
serum bactericidal activity
serum bactericidal concentration
serum bactericidal level
serum bactericidal test
serum bactericidal titer

bactericidal/permeability-increasing protein

bacteriologic
chemical, bacteriologic, and radiologic warfare
serum bacteriologic titer
b. warfare

bacteriological index

bacteriolytic immunity

bacteriophage
mature b.

bacteriostatic water for injection

bacteriuria
asymptomatic b.
catheter-associated b.
screening b.
significant asymptomatic b.

***Bacteroides* bile esculin agar**

baculovirus
nonoccluded b.
occluded b.

bad
b. breath
b. breath from bronchitis
b. conduct discharge
b. dietary habit
prognostically bad signs during pregnancy

Baerveldt
pars plana Baerveldt tube insertion with vitrectomy

baffle
atrial baffle operation
Mustard atrial baffle repair
pericardial b.
posterior b.

bag
artificial rupture of bag of waters
b., valve, mask
bedside b.
bulging bag of waters
closed urinary drainage bag with drip chamber
gallbladder bag positioner
intact bag of waters
intact bag of waters
malar bag suctioning
manual ventilation b.
mask and bag ventilation
new bag hung
nuclear bag fiber
palpebral adipose b.
premature spontaneous rupture of bag of waters
purple urine bag syndrome
rupture of bag of waters
spontaneous rupture of bag of waters
straight bag drainage
b. ventilation
b. of waters
b. of waters ruptured
b. of worms appearance

bag-and-mask
b.-a.-m. resuscitation
b.-a.-m. ventilation

Bagaza virus

baggage
emotional b.

baggy heart

bag-valve-mask
b.-v.-m. device
b.-v.-m. ventilation

Bahig virus

Baillarger
outer band of B.

Bainbridge reflex

Baird
ankle scoring system of Baird and Jackson

baja
patella b.
b. patella

***Bakau* virus**

baked
b. brain phenomenon
b. tongue

Baker
B. Act
B. acted
ruptured Baker cyst

Baku virus

balance
acid balance control
Activities-Specific B. Confidence Scale
Affect B. Scale
alternate binaural loudness b.
alternate monaural loudness balance test
b., gait, and station
binaural alternate loudness b.
body's natural balance bacteria
chronic disordered water b.
Clinical Test of Sensory Interaction & B.
core body b.
Derogatis Affects B. Scale
deteriorating sense of b.
electrolyte balance and homeostasis
electrolyte balance restoration

balance *(continued)*
gait, balance and coordination
gait and balance disorder
gas-density b.
hearing and b.
hydrophilic-lipophilic b.
immune b.
loss of b.
mean daily nitrogen b.
measure of b.
metabolic balance of heart
mineral balance study
monaural bifrequency loudness b.
monaural loudness balance test
muscle b.
negative balance of body fluid
nitrogen b.
normal hormonal b.
sitting b.
sodium b.
standing b.
b. training
uniaxial balance evaluation

balanced
Earle balanced salt solution
b. electrolyte solution
b. forearm orthosis
Grey balanced saline solution
Hanks balanced salt solution
Hanks balanced salt solution plus glucose
b. ligamentous tension treatment
modified Hanks balanced salt solution
nutritionally balanced diet
performance versus intensity function for phonetically balanced words
phonetically b.
phonetically balanced rhyme test
phonetically balanced word
Phonetically B. Kindergarten
phonetically balanced percentage of word lists
pressure b.
b. saline solution
b. salt solution
b. skeletal traction

balanitis
gangrenous b.
b. xerotica obliterans

baldness
common b.
female-pattern b.
male pattern b.
moth-eaten b.
Norwood Classification of Male Pattern B.
partial b.
patchy b.

Balfour gastric resection

ball
Aspergillus fungus b.
axonal retraction b.
b. bearing
b. bur
b. dissector
b. forceps
hair b.
Marchi b.
massage b.
medicine b.
meshed ball implant
myelin b.
myelin ball formation
b. on back
prosthetic ball valve
b. reamer
sludge b.
b. tip electrode

ball-and-joint socket

ball-and-socket
b.-a.-s. ankle mortise
b.-a.-s. attachment
b.-a.-s. joint
b.-a.-s. prosthesis
b.-a.-s. trochanteric osteotomy

Ballard Assessment Score

ballasted contact lens

ballast prism

ball-bearing forearm orthosis

ball-catcher projection

Baller-Gerold syndrome

ball-in-cone valve

balloon
adjunctive balloon angioplasty
b. angioplasty
antegrade transluminal balloon dilatation
b. aortic valvotomy
b. aortic valvuloplasty
atrial balloon septostomy
b. atrial septostomy
atrial septostomy via b.
biliary balloon catheter
biliary balloon dilator
biliary balloon probe
b. buckle
cardiac balloon pump
cardiac catheter with balloon inserted
b. catheter
b. catheter angioplasty
catheter balloon valvuloplasty
b. catheter and basket-retrieval technique
complementary balloon angioplasty
b. coronary occlusion
cutting balloon angioplasty
detachable silicone b.
b. dilation
b. dilation angioplasty
b. dilation valvuloplasty
dual balloon perfusion catheter
echo-guided balloon atrial septostomy
endocardial balloon lead
b. endometrial ablation
endoscopic balloon dilation
endoscopic balloon sphincter dilation
endoscopic papillary balloon dilation
endoscopic retrograde balloon dilatation
endovascular balloon occlusion
esophageal balloon catheter
esophagogastric balloon tamponade
excimer laser, rotational atherectomy, and balloon angioplasty
b. expandable intravascular stent
flow-assisted short-term balloon catheter
fluoroscopy-guided balloon dilator
b. inflation
intraaortic balloon assistance
intraaortic balloon catheter
intraaortic balloon counterpulsation
intraaortic balloon pulsation
intraaortic balloon pump
intraaortic balloon pumping assistance
intraaortic counterpulsation b.
intracoronary thrombolysis balloon valvuloplasty
intraesophageal balloon distention
laser-assisted balloon angioplasty
mitral balloon commissurotomy
b. mitral commissurotomy
b. mitral valvotomy
b. mitral valvuloplasty
nondetachable balloon catheter
occlusion balloon catheter with silicone balloon
over-the-wire balloon catheter

percutaneous balloon angioplasty
percutaneous balloon aortic valvuloplasty
percutaneous balloon aspiration
percutaneous balloon commissurotomy
percutaneous balloon dilation
percutaneous balloon pericardiotomy
percutaneous balloon pulmonic valvuloplasty
percutaneous intraaortic balloon counterpulsation
percutaneous mitral balloon commissurotomy
percutaneous mitral balloon valvotomy
percutaneous mitral balloon valvuloplasty
percutaneous mitral balloon valvulotomy
percutaneous transluminal balloon angioplasty
percutaneous transluminal balloon dilatation
percutaneous transluminal balloon valvuloplasty
perfusion balloon catheter
peripheral balloon angioplasty
PET b.
positron emission tomography b.
post balloon angioplasty restenosis
preperitoneal distention b.
prostatic balloon dilatation
b. PTA catheter
pulmonary artery balloon pump
pulmonary balloon valvuloplasty
b. pulmonary valvuloplasty
b. reflex manometry
right ventricular copulsation b.
b. rupture
b. tamponade
b. test occlusion
thermal/perfusion balloon angioplasty
through-the-scope balloon dilation
transbronchoscopic balloon tipped
transcervical balloon tuboplasty
transluminal balloon valvuloplasty
b. tricuspid valvotomy
triple balloon valvuloplasty
uterine balloon therapy
b. uterine elevator cannula
b. valvuloplasty registry

balloon-assisted, endoscopic, retroperitoneal, gasless

balloon-expandable tantalum stent

ballooning-out
b.-o. of artery wall
b.-o. of blood vessel

balloon-occluded retrograde transvenous obliteration

balloon-shaped heart

balloon-tipped catheter

ballottable liver

ballottement
indirect b.
ocular b.
patella b.
b. tenderness

ball-tip
b.-t. microcatheter
b.-t. spike

ball-type
b.-t. disc prosthesis
b.-t. valve

ball-valve tumor

balm
butt b.
b. of Gilead
mountain b.

Balthazar Scales of Adaptive Behavior

bamboo hair

banana
applesauce, bananas, and cereal diet
b.'s, rice, applesauce, tea, toast diet
b.'s, rice, applesauce, toast diet
b.'s, rice cereal, applesauce, toast diet

band
A b.
absolute band count
b. adapter
alpha frequency b.
amniotic band sequence
anisotropic band in striated muscle
anomalous muscle b.
anterior band of colon
anterior band remover
anular constricting band syndrome
AO tension b.
b. and bar space maintainer
broad adhesive b.
b. of Broca
calciotraumatic b.
ciliary body b.
copper b.
creatine kinase-BB b.
creatine kinase myocardial b.
creatine phosphokinase-myocardial b.
b. and crib space maintainer
delta b.
diagonal b.
dysgenetic fibrous b.
elastic band ligation
endoscopic band ligation
endoscopic variceal band ligation
esophageal band ligation
b. form in sixth stage of myelocyte maturation
gamma band response
b. of Gennari
b. of Giacomini
high frequency b.
hypoechoic b.
I b.
iliotibial b.
iliotibial band friction syndrome
iliotibial band tendonitis
isotropic band striated muscle fiber
b. of Kaes-Bechterew
ligator
linear band of maximal radiolucency
lip furrow b.
longitudinal band of colon
longitudinal bands of cruciform ligament of atlas
longitudinal hyperpigmented b.
long leg brace with pelvic b.
low frequency b.
lupus band test
Mach band effect
medial epicanthal scar b.
metaphyseal lucent b.
modified band lid method
Muehrcke b.'s
multiple band ligator
myocardial b.
myocardial band enzymes of creatine phosphokinase
narrow band noise
narrow band spectrophotometer
narrow frequency b.
b. neutrophil
octave band analyzer
oligoclonal b.
omental adhesive b.

band *(continued)*
outer band of Baillarger
b. pliers
b. pusher
b. remover
rubber band hemorrhoidectomy
rubber band ligation of hemorrhoid
rubber band ligator
b. seater
b. and spur retainer
stabkernige band neutrophil
tension band fixation
wide band noise
b. wire

bandage
Ace b.
ankle traction b.
axilla, shoulder, elbow b.
cohesive b.
b. contact lens
cotton elastic b.
gentle pressure bandage applied
4-layer b.
Meditec bandage contact lens
Nu Gauze b.
rubber-reinforced b.
b. shears
T b.
thumb spica b.
tumescent absorbent b.

banded gastroplasty with a divided pouch

bandelette plate

Bandia virus

banding
adjustable silicone gastric b.
chromosome b.
b. cylinder
esophageal banding technique
Giemsa banding stain
laparoscopic tubal b.
laser adjustable silicone gastric b.
open adjustable silicone gastric b.
pulmonary artery b.
terminal banding of chromosome

band-pass filter

band-removing pliers

band-soldering pliers

bandwidth
critical bandwidth range of frequencies

banging
sleep-related head b.

Bangoran virus

Bangui virus

banjo
b. cast
b. traction

bank
blood b.
bone bank graft
hospital-based blood b.
hospital blood b.
human tumor b.
hybridoma b.
living b.
Pacific Coast Tissue B.
patient data b.
registry and tissue b.
Time-oriented Data B.
tumor immunology b.

Bankart
arthroscopic Bankart repair
B. dislocation
B. fracture
B. lesion
traumatic unidirectional Bankart lesion surgery

banked
b. breast milk
b. freeze-dried bone

banking
cryopreserved tissue b.

Bankson-Bernthal Test of Phonology

Bankson Language Screening Test

***Banna* virus**

Bannayan-Riley-Ruvalcaba syndrome

Bannayan-Zonna syndrome

bar
ambulates on parallel b.'s
anterior palatal b.
arch bar application
arch bar fixation
arch bar frame
band and bar space maintainer
cast bar splint
b. clasp
b. joint
lingual bar major connector
mandibular arch b.
median bar formation
median bar of Mercier
mesostructure conjunction b.
metatarsal bar shoe modification
metatarsal flatfoot b.
National B. Association
parallel b.'s
pterygoalar b.
T b.
tracheotomy b.
transpalatal b.
Winter arch b.

4-bar
4-b. external fixation
4-b. external fixation apparatus
4-b. external fixation device
4-b. linkage on knee prosthesis
4-b. linkage prosthetic knee mechanism
4-b. polycentric knee prosthesis

barbed
b. hypostome
b. staple
b. stinger

barber
b. chair position
b. pole sign

barbital
b. dependent
modified barbital buffer

barbiturate
b. dependence
nitrous oxide b.

Barbour-Stoenner-Kelly medium

Barclay
B. Classroom Climate Inventory
B. Learning Needs Assessment Inventory

Bardach
modified Bardach repair

bare lymphocyte syndrome

barely noticeable difference

barium
b. adherent to esophageal walls
air-contrast barium enema
b. bezoar
b. chloride
b. contrast radiology
b. contrast x-ray
double-contrast barium enema
double-contrast barium examination of the upper gastrointestinal tract
double tracking of b.
dual-contrast barium enema
dumping of barium meal
b. enema
b. enema with air contrast
b. filled esophagus

fleck of b.
follow-through after barium meal
b. granuloma
high-viscosity barium and air ingestion of b.
liquid barium suspension
b. meal
modified barium swallow with videofluoroscopy
normal evacuation of b.
oral barium suspension
b. passed through esophagus into stomach
b. peritonitis
pocketing of b.
reflux of b.
retrograde flow of b.
b. sediment in urine
single-contrast barium enema
b. sulfate
b. swallow
b. swallow study
transient time of b.
videofluoroscopic barium swallow

barium-based fecal tagging

bark
maple bark stripper disease

barking cough

Barkow
colliculus of B.

Barlow and Ortolani test

Barmah Forest virus

Barnes Akathisia Scale

baroceptor
noninvasive carotid baroceptor stimulation

barometric pressure

baroreceptor
arterial b.
low-pressure b.
low-pressure cardiopulmonary b.
b. reflex response
b. reflex sensitivity

baroreflex
b. dysfunction
b. sensitivity

barotrauma
otic b.

Barranqueras virus

Barr body

barrel
b. bur
b. chest
b. staved graft
b. stave osteotomy procedure

barreled sideplate

barrel-shaped thorax

Barrett
B. adenocarcinoma
B. carcinoma
B. disease
B. dysplasia
B. epithelium
B. esophagitis
B. esophagus
B. metaplasia
B. segment
short-segment Barrett esophagus
B. syndrome
B. ulcer

barrier
alteration of blood brain b.
blood-air b.
blood-brain b.
blood-brain-tumor b.
blood-cerebrospinal fluid b.
blood-nerve b.
blood-retinal b.
b. contraceptive
b. drape
fenestrated sterile field b.
b. filter
gastric component of reflex b.
gastric mucosal b.
b. isolation unit
b. method
mucosal barrier maturation
b. protection
b. sheet
small intestine as a defense b.

Barron-Welsh Art Scale

bar-sleeve attachment

Barthel
B. index
modified Barthel degree of disability index

Bartholin
B., urethral, and Skene glands, and external genitalia
B. cyst
B. duct
B. gland
B. gland duct cyst
B., Skene, and urethral glands

bartonellosis
ocular b.

Bartter
antenatal Bartter syndrome
B. syndrome

Barur virus

basal
b. acid output
anterior b.
anterior basal branch
anterior basal bronchopulmonary segment
anterior basal bronchus
anterior basal encephalocele
anterior basal segment
anterior basal segmental artery
anterior basal vein
b. body temperature
b. cell
b. cell adenocarcinoma
b. cell atypia
b. cell carcinoma
b. cell dysplasia
b. cell epithelioma
b. cell hyperplasia
b. cell liquefactive degeneration
b. cell nevus
b. cell nevus syndrome
cervical mucous basal body temperature
Eagle basal medium
b. energy expenditure
follicular basal lamina
b. ganglion
b. ganglion calcification
b. ganglion disease
b. ganglion disorder-mental retardation
gastric fluid, basal acid output
b. gastric secretion
glomerular basal lamina
b. heart rate
inferior b.
b. insulin level
b. interhemispheric approach
b. joint reflex
b. lamina
b. laminar deposit
lateral b.
left basal artery
magnocellular basal forebrain
medial basal branch of pulmonary artery
medial basal bronchopulmonary segment S VII
medial basal segment
medial basal segmental artery
medial basal segmental bronchus
b. medium

basal *(continued)*
b. membrane
b. metabolic rate
b. metabolism
metastatic basal cell carcinoma
mineral basal medium
morbilliform basal cell carcinoma
morpheaform basal cell
morpheaform basal cell carcinoma
morphea-type basal cell carcinoma
multicentric basal cell carcinoma
multiple basal cell carcinoma syndrome multiple basal cell nevus syndrome
multiple basal cell neuroma syndrome
multiple basal cell nevoid syndrome
multiple nevoid, basal cell epithelioma, jaw cysts, bifid rib syndrome
nevoid basal cell carcinoma syndrome
nevoid basal cell epithelioma, jaw cysts, bifid rib syndrome
nodular basal cell carcinoma
noduloulcerative basal cell carcinoma
obliterated basal cistern
b. optic root
oxidation-fermentation basal medium
b. pepsin output
pigmented basal cell carcinoma
point of basal convergence
b. promoter element
ratio of basal acid output to maximal acid output
b. secretory flow rate
septal b.
b. septal hypertrophy
b. skin resistance
b. skull fracture
symmetrical calcification of basal cerebral ganglion
b. temperature chart
b. vein of Rosenthal

basalis
nucleus b.
nucleus basalis of Ganser
nucleus basalis lesion
nucleus basalis of Meynert
pars b.
pars basalis arteriae pulmonalis

basaloid squamous cell carcinoma

base
anterior cranial b.
anterior fossa skull base glabellar
anterior skull b.
anterior skull base malignancy
b. of appendix
blood agar b.
blood buffer b.
Brown-Roberts-Wells phantom b.
buffer b.
closed base wedge osteotomy
compensated b.
curved base twin bracket
b. deficit
dissociation constant of a b.
b. excess
gonococcal b.
b. hospital
hydrophilic emollient b.
b. ionization constant
lung base infiltrate
meat base formula
meningitis of the b.
metal base denture
b. metal crown and bridge alloy
National Cancer Data B.
b. of natural logarithms
negative base excess
normal base deficit
nucleic acid b.
open base wedge osteotomy
open base wedge osteotomy/bunionectomy
b. out
b. pair
peg base plate
rales audible at bases
rubber base impression
saturated base excess
single base cane
b. of skull
skull base tumor
standard mineral b.
talar axis–first metatarsal base angle
tibial base plate
b. of tongue
b. of tongue carcinoma
total b.
Toxicology Data B.
tryptose/blood/agar b.
washable b.
wide base of support
yeast carbon b.
yeast nitrogen b.

baseball stitch

based
broad based scar
distally based fasciocutaneous flap
medial distally based fasciocutaneous flap
patient independent with small based quad cane

base-down prism

baseline
b. average peak velocity
delta over b.
B. Dyspnea Index
fetal heart rate b.
b. infection
initial baseline level
laboratory admission baseline studies
b. level of functioning
b. mammography
multiple baseline design
radiographic b.
b. rate
b. recovery
Reid b.
return to b.
b. variability of fetal heart rate

basement
alveolar basement membrane
alveolar wall basement membrane
anterior basement membrane dystrophy
antiglomerular basement membrane
antiglomerular basement membrane antibody
antiglomerular basement membrane antibody disease
antiglomerular basement membrane antibody nephritis
antiglomerular basement membrane disease
antiglomerular basement membrane glomerulonephritis
antiglomerular basement membrane-negative crescentic glomerular nephritis
antitubular basement membrane
antitubular basement membrane antibody
capillary basement membrane thickness
capillary basement membrane width
collagenase soluble glomerular basement membrane
epidermal basement zone
glomerular basement membrane

glomerular basement membrane disease
glomerular capillary b.
lung basement membrane
b. membrane
b. membrane thickness
b. membrane zone
muscle capillary basement membrane
muscle capillary basement membrane thickening
nephrotoxic antiglomerular basement membrane antibody nephritis
peripheral basement membrane
renal glomerular basement membrane thickness
subepithelial basement membrane
thin basement membrane disease
tubular basement membrane
urothelial basement membrane

base-up prism

bashful bladder syndrome

basic
b. adaptive process
adult basic education
Adult B. Learning Examination
B. Aid Training
Angle basic E arch appliance
assessment of basic competency
b. assurance test
Boehm Test of B. Concepts
Boston Diagnostic Inventory of B. Skills
b. calcium phosphate
California Test of B. Skills
Canadian Test of B. Skills
b. cycle length
Diabetes: B. Knowledge Test
b. drive cycle length
b. electrical rhythm
b. fibroblast growth factor
b. gastrin
Grassi B. Cognitive Evaluation
b. health profile
b. health unit
b. helix-loop-helix
b. human function
b. hygiene
b. immunization
b. incidence rate
Iowa Tests of B. Skills
b. metabolic panel
b. metabolic profile
M.O.M. basic kit
mouse-on-mouse basic kit
b. multicellular unit
myelin basic protein assay
myelin basic protein deficiency
myeloid basic protein
B. Occupational Literacy Test
B. Personality Inventory
b. plate
b. protein
B. Reading Inventory
b. rest-activity cycle
Riley Inventory of B. Learning Skills
B. School Skills Inventory
serum myelin basic protein
stratum corneum basic protein
b. structural unit
tests of basic experience
b. trauma life support
urinary basic fetoprotein

basilar
b. artery
b. artery insufficiency
cerebral basilar ischemia
b. crackle
dissecting basilar artery aneurysm
b. gliosis
b. hemiplegic migraine
b. impression
b. infiltrate
b. insufficiency
lower basilar aneurysm
b. membrane
b. pulmonary infiltrate
b. rales
right basilar artery
rostral basilar artery syndrome
total occlusion of basilar artery
vertebral basilar insufficiency

basilare
os b.

basilaris
arteria b.
membrana b.
norma b.
pars b.
pars basilaris ossis occipitalis
pars basilaris pontis

basilic
median basilic vein

basin
lymph node b.
nodal b.

basis
ambulatory b.
articulatory b.
as-needed b.
compassionate-use b.
empirical b.
minimum basis set magnetic resonance angiography
neurological b.
no known b.
nonimmunologic b.
outpatient b.
pathophysiological b.
patient followed on an outpatient b.
radiation therapy on prophylactic b.
treated on an outpatient b.

basket
Alzheimer b.
arthroscopy basket forceps
blind basket extraction
b. case
b. cell
b. crown
curved basket forceps
b. extraction
fibrillar b.
b. impaction
nitinol b.
b. rongeur
b. stockinette
Stokes b.

basketball heel

basketing
stone b.

basolateral membrane

basophil
absolute basophil count
b. chemotactic factor
fully granulated b.
b. granular leukocyte
b. granulation test
human basophil degranulation test
b. kallikrein of anaphylaxis
polymorphonuclear b.
systemic cutaneous basophil hypersensitivity

basophilia
paraneoplastic b.
peripheral b.

basophilic
acute basophilic leukemia
cutaneous basophilic hypersensitivity
b. degeneration
rat basophilic leukemia
b. stippling

basosquamous carcinoma

Bassini
B. inguinal hernia repair
modified Bassini herniorrhaphy
Bassini-type hernia repair
bastard suture technique
bat
Dakar bat virus
Entebbe bat virus
European bat lyssavirus 1
Mount Elgon bat virus
Phnom Penh bat virus
Batai virus
Batama virus
bath
b., laxative, enema, shampoo, and shower
bed b.
blanket b.
coal tar b.
contrast b.
demonstration b.
electric cabinet b.
healing power of warm b.'s
hot tub b.
own bed b.
paraffin b.
sedative cabinet b.
tub b.
whirlpool b.
bathing
inside bathing solution
patient independent in bathing with cueing
patient independent with b.
sink-side b.
bathmotropic
negatively b.
bathroom
out of bed with bathroom privileges
b. privileges
b. safety device
Battelle Developmental Inventory
battered
b. child syndrome
b. husband
b. husband syndrome
b. woman syndrome
battering
b. behavior
b. cycle
sexual b.
battery
anergy skin test b.
Apraxia B. for Adults
Arizona B. for Communication Disorders of Dementia
assault and b.
cardiac pacemaker battery change
central auditory processing b.
chemistry screening batteries I and II
Comprehensive Ability B.
Computer Operator Aptitude B.
Computer Programmer Aptitude B.
Coulter b.
Diagnostic Achievement B., Second Edition
Effective School B.
Environmental Pre-Language B.
Frostig Movement Skills Test B.
General Aptitude Test B.
Goldman-Fristoe-Woodcock Auditory Skills Test B.
Halstead-Reitan B.
Halstead-Reitan Neuropsychological B.
Halstead-Reitan Neuropsychological Test B.
B. of Health Improvement
Kaufman Assessment B. for Children
Luria-Nebraska Neuropsychological B.
MacArthur Story Stem B.
Mental Deterioration B.
mental deterioration b.
Minnesota Clerical Assessment B.
7-minute neurocognitive b.
Monas-Nitz Neuropsychological B.
Multilingual Aphasia B.
neurometric test b.
neuropsychological test b.
Non-Reading Aptitude Test B.
Objective-Analytic Anxiety B.
parietal lobe b.
Reitan-Indiana Neuropsychological B.
respiratory battery, acute
Right Hemisphere Language B.
Rivermead Perceptual Assessment B.
Social and Prevocational Information B.
Special Aptitude Test B.
b. of tests
Western Aphasia B.
Western Aphasia B. Test
Woodcock-Johnson Psychoeducational B.
battery-charging power supply
battery-powered electrocautery
battle
b. casualty
b. fatigue
b. neurosis
B. sign
batwing
perihilar batwing infiltrate
Baudelocque diameter
Bauhinia purpura **agglutinin**
Bauline virus
Baumé scale
bauxite
b. fibrosis of lung
b. pneumoconiosis
b. workers' disease
bay
Aransas Bay virus
Nelson Bay orthoreovirus
oil of b.
sick b.
bayesian image estimation
Bayley
B. Infant Neurodevelopmental Screener
B. Scales of Infant Development-II
Baylor bleeding score
bayonet
b. condenser
b. forceps
b. rongeur
b. saw
b. spacer
#11 bayonet-handled scalpel
bayonet-type
b.-t. forceps
b.-t. incision
Bayou **virus**
B-cell
B-c. acute lymphoblastic leukemia
B-c. antigen receptor
B-c. chronic lymphocytic leukemia
B-c. chronic lymphocytic leukemia/small lymphocytic lymphoma
B-c. chronic lymphoproliferative disorder
B-c. differentiation factor

B-c. enriched
B-c. growth factor
lymphocytosis
lymphoid precursor B-c.
B-c. lymphoma
B-c. lymphoproliferative disorder
monocytoid B-c.
B-c. non-Hodgkin lymphoma
B-c. precursor lymphoblastic leukemia
B-c. prolymphocytic leukemia
B-c. reactivity

B-cytomegalic inclusion disease of newborn

B_e

hepatitis B_e antigen

beach chair position

bead

aminoglycoside-impregnated methyl methacrylate b.
antibiotic bead pouch
glass b.
polyacrylamide b.
porous layer b.
b. pouch
b. sterilizer

bead-blasted prosthesis

beaded

b. hair
b. rod
b. transfixion wire

beaded-pin wrench

bead-loaded wire

beak

eagle beak bone-cutting forceps
medial metaphyseal b.
metacarpal b.
palmar beak ligament
parrot b.
parrot beak deformity

beaking

anterior central b.
antral b.

beam

b. aligning holder
alignment of tangential b.
argon beam coagulation
argon beam coagulator
argon beam plasma coagulation
beveled electron beam cone
cantilever b.
central axis depth dose of electron beam therapy
cold spots and hot spots with electron beam dosimetry
b. compensator
computer guided laser b.
cone b.
convergent beam irradiation
coplanar b.
electron beam boost
electron beam computerized tomography
electron beam dosimeter
electron beam scalp irradiation
external beam irradiation
external beam radiation therapy
external beam radiotherapy
external beam photon therapy
b. flattener
fractionated external beam irradiation
b. hardening artifact
helium ion b.
high beam intensity
high-dose beam of x-rays
high-energy bent beam linear accelerator
high-velocity electron b.
horizontal beam study
intensity-modulated photon b.
intraoperative electron beam therapy
intraoperative electron beam radiotherapy
intraoral cone for electron beam therapy
lateral-opposed b.
lens-sparing external beam radiation therapy
load b.
low LET external beam irradiation
lucite beam spoiler
measured beam data
b. monitor
multidimensional analysis beam modifier
multifield b.
narrow b.
narrow beam half-thickness
neutral axis of straight b.
neutron b.
neutron beam radiation
neutron beam therapy
nonaxial beam technique
noncoplanar b.
noncoplanar beam technique
open b.
orthovoltage b.
parallel b.
parallel-opposed b.
particle b.
particle beam radiation therapy
particle beam radiosurgery
photon beam radiosurgery
proton b.
proton beam radiation
proton beam radiosurgery
proton beam therapy
b. quality comparison
radiation b.
relative to rotation of a beam of polarized light
b. restrictor
b. shaper
tangential b.
total skin electron b.

beam-bending magnet

beam-modifying device

beam's eye view

bean

castor b.
coffee bean appearance
b. golden mosaic virus
lima bean trypsin inhibitor
northern bean extract
wax bean agglutinin

beanbag

animal beanbag exerciser

bearing

angled bearing insert
b. area hair
elbow b.
b. graft hair
hair bearing graft
ischial weight bearing leg brace
minimal weight b.
node bearing area of lymph nodes
patellar tendon b.
pretibial b.
quadriceps tendon b.
tumor b.

bearing-down

b.-d. pain
b.-d. sensation

beast fetishism

beat

apex b.
atrial capture b.
atrial ectopic b.
atrial fusion b.
atrial premature b.

beat *(continued)*
atrioventricular junctional escape b.
auricular premature b.
b.'s of clonus
coupled b.'s
ectopic junctional b.
ectopic ventricular b.
escape b.
frequency ectopic ventricular b.
funny-looking b.
fusion b.
b. generation
isolated premature b.
junctional escape b.
junctional premature b.
nodal premature b.
nonreassuring fetal heart beat pattern
paired b.'s
periodic dropped b.
b.'s per minute
premature atrial b.
premature auricular b.
premature junctional b.
premature nodal b.
premature ventricular b.
sinus breakthrough b.
standard deviation of normal-to-normal b.
supraventricular premature b.
tension-time index per b.
unifocal ventricular ectopic b.
ventricular capture b.
ventricular ectopic b.
ventricular extra b.
ventricular premature b.

beating
b. heart
b. heart brain-dead donor
b. heart muscle
rapid beating of heart

beating-heart bypass surgery

beat-to-beat
b.-t.-b. analysis
b.-t.-b. variability

Bebaru virus

Bechterew
line of B.

Beck
B. Depression Index Short Form
B. Depression Inventory
B. Hopelessness Scale

Becker
modified Becker repair
B. muscular dystrophy

beclomethasone
aqueous b.
b. dipropionate

become
air passage become inflamed

Becquerel ray

bed
absent bed occupancy
air-fluidized b.
arterial vascular b.
b. bath
b. board
b. to chair transfer
completion bed occupancy care
cyanosis of nail b.
dangle out of b.
draining lymphatic b.
edge of b.
elevate head of b.
elevation of head of b.
emergency observation b.
feet out of b.
feet over edge of b.
fell out of b.
foot of b.
gallbladder shelled out from the gallbladder b.
head of b.
head of bed up for shortness of breath
heated bed cradle
hospital b.
hot packs and bed rest
isolation b.
low air loss b.
b. mobility skill
mouse bed sign
nail b.
nail bed cyanosis
nail bed graft
nail bed hematoma evacuation
nail bed lesion
not out of b.
open bed warmer
out of bed with bathroom privileges
own bed bath
b. pan
patient at complete bed rest
place outpatient in inpatient b.
powder b.
raise head of b.
side of b.
simulated moving bed chromatography
strict bed confinement
strictly confined to b.
total bed capacity
total bed rest
up out of bed as tolerated
b. wetting

bed-mat
b.-m. activity
b.-m. mobility

bedpan
assist with b.
fracture b.

bedrest
absolute b.
complete b.
placed at b.
strict b.

bedridden
patient b.

bedside
at b.
b. bag
b. care
b. commode
b. drainage
may keep at b.
not at b.
b. scale
b. testing

bedtime
after meals and at b.
early b.
nothing by mouth at b.

bed-to-chair transfer

bedwetter admission

beef
b. heart antigen
b. heart infusion broth
b. insulin
b. liver catalase
proteose-peptone beef extract
b. serum albumin

beef-pork insulin

beekeeper serum

beer
b. heart
b. knife

Beery
B. Developmental Test of Visual-Motor Integration
B. Picture Vocabulary Screening

bee sting hypersensitivity

beeswax
penicillin in beeswax and oil
penicillin, oil, and b.

beetle
ashgray blister b.
ashgray blister beetle sting
black beetle virus

before
b. and after
born before arrival
detoxification before surgery
b. every meal
had it before, got it again
b. meals
mean time between or before failures
oxygenation before recirculation
b. present
b. sleep
b. time of operation
urine specimen before prostate massage
years of potential life lost before age 65

beggar
emotional b.

beginning
electrocardiographic interval from the beginning of QRS complex to end of the T wave
reference point following QRS complex, at beginning of ST segment
time between P wave and beginning of QRS complex in electrocardiography

behavior
aberrant sexual b.
Acquired Immunodeficiency Syndrome Beliefs and B. Questionnaire
activity and b.
B. Activity Profile
Adaptive B. Evaluation Scale
Adaptive B. Inventory for Children
addictive behavior group
adjust repetitive b.
adolescent experimentation with adult b.
adult self-harm b.
affect, behavior, cognition
age-inappropriate knowledge of sexual b.
aggressive behavior theory
aggressive objectionable b.
aggressive psychotic b.
aggressive or violent b.
alcohol consumption b.
alleviating violence in aggressive b.
altered by b.
altered personal b.
alternative to violent b.
anesthetic variant of schizoid b.
anomalous sexual b.
anticipatory and struggle behavior theories
applied behavior analysis
aroused state of disturbed b.
Assessment of Preterm Infants B.
Attention Deficit Disorder B. Rating Scale
attention deficit and disruptive behavior disorder
attention-seeking manipulative b.
Balthazar Scales of Adaptive B.
bingeing behavior of anorexia
bingeing behavior of bulimic
Burks B. Rating Scale
child behavior characteristic
child behavior rating form
Child B. Checklist
childhood antisocial b.
Child Sexual B. Inventory
classroom behavior of child
cognitive behavior therapy
cognitive behavior treatment
Cognitive B. Therapy Package
comorbid addictive b.
compulsive drug-taking b.
compulsive sexual b.
conditioned behavior response
consensual sexual b.
continued maladaptive b.
b. control
controlled adolescent b.
decondition pain b.
delusional b.
destructive sexual b.
Devereux Elementary School Behavior Rating Scale II
dialectical behavior therapy
differential reinforcement of other b.
direct self-destructive b.
b. disorder
B. Disorders Identification Scale
disruptive behavior disorder
drug-seeking b.
dynamics of human b.
dysfunctional staff b.
dysrhythmic aggressive b.
electrophysiologic behavior modification
Emotional and B. Problem Scale
ethnic relational b.
B. Evaluation Scale-2
explosive aggressive b.
Eyberg Child B. Inventory
full maternal b.
gender behavior disorder
global ward behavior scale
grossly disorganized b.
Health B. Scale
high-risk sexual b.
Hilton Drinking B. Questionnaire
human health and behavior questionnaire
Hutchins B. Inventory
hyperkinetic behavior syndrome
iatrogenic effects of behavior therapy
Illness B. Checklist
Illness B. Questionnaire
inability to sustain consistent work b.
inappropriate child b.
inappropriate dangerous b.
inappropriate sexual b.
inappropriate sexually provocative b.
inappropriate social b.
indirect self-destructive b.
infant exhibits hunger b.
Infant B. Record
Inpatient B. Rating Scale
Interpersonal B. Survey
Jesness B. Checklist
knowledge, attitude, b.
knowledge, attitude, behavior, and improvement in nutritional status
Leader B. Analysis II
Leader B. Description Questionnaire
life-threatening b.
localization of b.
management of assaultive b.
b. management plan
b. modification
b. modification technique
Mother's Assessment of the B. of Her Infant
multimodal behavior therapy
Newborn B. Assessment Scale
nonpharmacologic behavior management
b. objective
obsessive-compulsive b.
operant behavior theory
opiate-directed b.
Ottawa School B. Checklist

behavior *(continued)*
overt behavior consequences of divorce
b. pattern
pattern of antisocial b.
Pediatric B. Scale
phobic avoidant b.
Positive Attention B.
Preschool B. Questionnaire
preventive dental health b.
preventive health b.
B. Problem Checklist
profound change in b.
punishing behavior of bulimic
Pupil Record of Education B.
purging behavior of bulimic
radical behavior change
B. Rating Profile, Second Edition
B. Rating Scale
rational behavior therapy
REM behavior disorder
Revised Memory and B. Problems Checklist
Schedule-Controlled Operant B.
self-destructive b.
self-injurious b.
Smoking B. Questionnaire
Social B. Assessment Inventory
socially inappropriate b.
starving behavior of bulimic
B. Status Inventory
stereotyped b.
stimulation-bound b.
strong partial maternal b.
B. Style Questionnaire
Suinn Test Anxiety B. Scale
b. summarized evaluation
Supervisory B. Description
Teacher Assessment of Social B.
traditional behavior therapy
Transition B. Scale
type A b.
type B b.
unusually hostile or aggressive b.
Ward B. Rating Scale

behavioral
b. aberration
aggressive behavioral disturbance
B. Assessment of Pain Questionnaire
B. Assessment Scale for Children
b., anxiety, mood, and other types of disorders
Brazelton Neonatal B. Assessment Scale
Camelot B. Checklist
child behavioral study
childhood behavioral disorder
cognitive behavioral approach
cognitive behavioral intervention
cognitive behavioral technique
cognitive behavioral therapy
Cooper-Farran B. Rating Scale
b. disorder
B. Dyscontrol Scale
emotional and behavioral difficulties
B. and Emotional Rating Scale
b. family systems therapy
Family Therapist B. Scale
b. health
b. health treatment
b. hypnosis
b. inhibition system
b. intervention
maladaptive behavioral change
managed behavioral health plans
b. management technique
b. marital therapy
Miller B. Style Scale
Millon B. Health Inventory
multicomponent behavioral treatment
Neonatal B. Assessment Scale
Neonatal B. Assessment Scale with Kansas Supplements
b. observation audiometry
peak behavioral effect
Rivermead B. Memory Test
self-inhibiting behavioral injury device
Timed B. Rating Sheet
Time-Sample B. Checklist
youth risk behavioral survey

behaviorism
operant b.

Behçet syndrome

behind-the-ear hearing aid

Behnken unit of roentgen-ray exposure

Beighton
modified Beighton criteria

being
delusion of being controlled
intolerance of being alone
Quality of Well B. Index

Békésy
B. Ascending-Descending Gap Evaluation
B. comfortable loudness
B. Functionality Detection Test

belch
silent b.

belching
bloating or b.
b. and indigestion

Belem virus

belief
Acquired Immunodeficiency Syndrome B.'s and Behavior Questionnaire
Career B.'s Inventory
core b.
cultural belief and practice
delusional b.'s
endorsement of deviant thoughts and b.'s
Fear Avoidance B.'s Quest
Health B. Model
irrational b.'s
loss of b.
odd b.
paranoid belief system
paranoid delusional b.
personal b.
traditional b.

believe
This I Believe test

bell
auditory response to b.
long nerve of B.
B. palsy
b. sound

belladonna
aloin, belladonna, strychnine laxative
opium and b.
b. and opium
phenobarbital and b.

bell-clapper anomaly

Bellini
medullary ducts of B.
papillary duct of B.

bellows
aneroid chest b.
chest b.

belly
anterior belly of digastric muscle
b. button to medial malleolus
b. dancer dyskinesia
jelly belly appearance
muscle b.
occipital b.
occipital belly of occipitofrontalis muscle
prune belly anomaly

prune belly syndrome
swollen belly disease
swollen belly syndrome
wooden b.

Belmont virus

below
b. detectable levels
b. detectable limits
b. diaphragm
fingerbreadth below right costal margin
fingers below umbilicus
fundus firm 1, 2 cm below umbilicus
b. knee
left and b.
b. lower limit
one fingerbreadth below umbilicus
right and b.
b. right costal margin
b. the umbilicus
b. waist

below-elbow
b.-e. amputation
medium below-elbow cast
very short below-elbow cast

below-knee
b.-k. amputation
b.-k. orthosis
b.-k. walking cast
b.-k. walking plaster

below-knee-to-toe cast

Belsey
modified Belsey fundoplication
modified Belsey fundoplication procedure
modified Belsey fundoplication technique

belt
biomedical b.
body b.
crutch and belt femoral closed nailing
safety b.
waist b.

Belterra virus

Bem Sex Role Inventory

Bence
B. Jones
B. Jones protein
B. Jones proteinuria

bench
horizontal flow clean b.
horizontal laminar flow clean b.'s
park bench position
b. scale calorimeter
vertical flow clean b.

bend
cartilage-wearing knee b.'s
deep knee b.
low back b.
prone knee b.
side b.

bender
cast b.
B. Visual-Motor Gestalt Test

Bender-Gestalt test

bending
active bending exercise
anterior bending moment
backward b.
forward b.
lateral b.
left lateral b.
repetitive bending and stooping
right lateral b.
side b.
thoracolumbosacral orthosis—flexion, extension, lateral bending, and transverse rotation

benediction hand

beneficial
antidotally b.

beneficiary
advance beneficiary notice
qualified Medicare b.

benefit
coordination of b.'s
disability insurance b.'s
explanation of b.'s
Explanation of Medicare B.'s
health benefits of walking
maximal benefit from hospitalization
maximal hospital b.
maximum cytoreductive b.
maximum hospital b.
mental health b.
mental health insurance b.
nonspecific b.
objective b.
old age b.'s
patient reached maximum hospital b.
pedal disability b.
Pension and Welfare B.'s Administration
reached maximum hospital b.
risks, b.'s, and alternatives
therapeutic benefits of humor
Unemployment Insurance B.'s

benefit/cost ratio

Benevides virus

Benfica virus

bengal
radioiodinated rose bengal dye
rose bengal antigen
rose bengal dye
rose bengal scan
rose bengal staining

benign
b. adenomatous polyp
aneurysmal benign fibrous histiocytoma
b. anorectal disease
atypical benign fibrous histiocytoma
autosomal-dominant benign form of osteopetrosis
b. bile duct stricture
b. breast disease
b. breast syndrome
calcified benign granuloma
b. cellular change
central benign neoplasm
b. cephalic histiocytosis
b. childhood epilepsy
chronic benign hepatitis
chronic benign mucous membrane pemphigus
chronic benign neutropenia
chronic benign pain
chronic intractable benign pain
b. coital headache
complex benign disease
b. cystic endometrial hyperplasia
b. cystic teratoma
deep-seated benign tumor
b. early repolarization
b. epileptiform transients of sleep
b. epithelial tumor
b. essential blepharospasm
b. essential hypertension
b. essential tremor
familial benign chronic pemphigus
familial benign hypocalciuric hypercalcemia
b. familial hematuria
b. familial macrocephaly
b. familial neonatal convulsions

benign *(continued)*
b. febrile convulsion
b. focal epilepsy of childhood
b. gastric ulcer
generalized atrophic benign epidermolysis bullosa
b. glandular cell tumor
b. granuloma of thyroid
b. growth
b. gynecological disease
b. heart murmur
hereditary benign intraepithelial dyskeratosis
histologically b.
hospital course b.
b. hyperplastic gastropathy
b. hypertension
b. hypertrophy
b. hypertrophy of prostate
b. infantile familial convulsions
intracranial calcification benign glandular tissue
b. intracranial hypertension
b. intraductal papilloma
intraepithelial dyskeratosis syndrome, hereditary b.
b. lymphoepithelial disease
b. lymphoepithelial lesion
b. mesenchymal tumor
microscopic benign prostatic hyperplasia
b. monoclonal B-cell lymphocytosis
b. monoclonal gammopathy
b. mucous membrane pemphigoid
b. multinodular goiter
multiple benign circumferential skin creases on limb
multiple benign cystic epithelioma
b. necrotizing otitis externa
b. nephrosclerosis
b. ovarian mass
b. paroxysmal positional vertigo
b. paroxysmal positioning nystagmus
b. paroxysmal torticollis
b. partial epilepsy with centrotemporal spike
peripheral benign neoplasm
b. pheochromocytoma
b. pheochromocytoma with histological invasion
b. polyps of large intestine
b. proliferative lesion
prostate gland benign hyperplasia
b. prostatic enlargement
b. prostatic hyperplasia
b. prostatic hypertrophy
b. prostatic obstruction
recalcitrant benign paroxysmal positional vertigo
b. recurrent hematuria
b. recurrent intrahepatic cholestasis
b. rolandic epilepsy
Schaumann benign lymphogranuloma
b. symmetric lipomatosis
b. tertian malaria
b. ulcer
b. vascular neoplasm

Bennett
B. pressure ventilator
B. seal

Benoist scale

bent
high-energy bent beam linear accelerator

Benton
B. Visual Retention Test, Revised

bentonite flocculation test

benzathine
penicillin G b.
penicillin G benzathine and procaine combined

benzoate
caffeine sodium b.
estradiol b.
international benzoate unit

benzodiazepine
peripheral benzodiazepine receptor
b. receptor

benzoylarginine
b. ethyl ester
b. methyl ester

bereaved
b. husband
b. wife

bereavement
conjugal b.
b. disorder
home care b.
b. recovery group
unresolved b.

bereavement-related mood disorder

bergamot
oil of b.

Bergersen medium

Bergh
van den Bergh test

Bergmeister
papilla of B.

beriberi
b. heart
b. heart disease

Berlin
column of B.

Bernard-Soulier syndrome

Berne
B. pain questionnaire
B. virus

Bernie
method of Bernie Siegel

Bernoulli
modified Bernoulli equation

Bernse Coping Modes

Berrimah virus

berry
b. aneurysm
b. intracranial aneurysm
saw palmetto berry extract

beryllium
b. lung disease
chronic beryllium disease

Bessey-Lowry-Brock method or unit

Bessey-Lowry unit

best
b. amplitude
heard best at left lower sternal border
heard best at left upper sternal border
b. motor response

best-corrected visual acuity

besylate
atracurium b.
mesoridazine b.

beta
b. activity
b. agonist inhaler
alpha, beta, gamma hypotheses
alpha beta value
alpha tocopherol beta carotene
Army Beta test
artificial beta cell
b. blockade
b. blocker
b. blocker therapy
bursts of beta activity
b. carotene

estrogen receptor b.
excessive diffuse low and medium wave beta activity
frontocentral beta rhythm
b. globulin
group A beta hemolytic streptococcus
b. hemolytic
b. hemolytic strain
hydroxy beta methylbutyrate
immunoreactive beta endomorphin
interferon b.
interleukin-1 beta converting enzyme
b. lipoprotein
long-acting beta agonist
b. LP
luteinizing hormone beta core fragment
nicked free beta subunit of human chorionic gonadotropin
pancreatic islet beta cell
b. radiation
b. ray
sickle cell b.

beta-1
transforming growth factor beta-1, -2, -3

beta-adrenergic
b.-a. blocking agent
hyperdynamic beta-adrenergic circulatory
myocardial beta-adrenergic receptor
b.-a. receptor
b.-a. receptor kinase

beta-adrenoreceptor agonist

beta-agonist
b.-a. drug
b.-a. inhaler
long-acting inhaled b.-a.

beta-chain variable region

Betadine scrub solution

Betadine-soaked pledget

beta-endorphin immunoreactivity

beta-hemolytic streptococcus group A

beta-hexosaminidase A leukocyte

beta-human chorionic gonadotropin

3-beta-hydroxysteroid dehydrogenase

beta-lactam
double b.-l.

beta-lactamase
extended-spectrum b.-l.
b.-l. inhibiting protein
b.-l. inhibitor combination

beta-lactamase-producing
b.-l.-p. bacteria
b.-l.-p. organism

beta-lactamase-resistant antimicrobial

betamethasone acetate

beta-nerve growth factor

beta-oncofetal antigen

beta-oxidation
mitochondrial fatty acid b.-o.

beta-receptor
adrenergic b.-r.

beta-thyroid-stimulating hormone

Bethesda unit

betterment
potential for human b.

between
b. ischial tuberosities
circular interaction between anxiety and pain
difference in nitrogen tension between mixed alveolar gas and mixed arterial blood
distance between centers
distance between iliac spines
distance between nasal lines
electrical activity between electrodes
electrocardiographic angle between QRS and T vectors
electrocardiographic junction between QRS complex and ST segment
mean time between or before failures
pain between shoulders
time between P wave and beginning of QRS complex in electrocardiography
time interval between cessation of contraception and conception
time interval between doses
translocation between 2 X chromosome
transverse diameter between ischia

bevel
chamfer b.
marginal b.

beveled-edge lens

beveled electron beam cone

beveled-tip needle

beverage
carbonated b.
diet b.

beyond
patient burned beyond recognition

bezoar
artificial b.
Aspergillus b.
barium b.
medication b.

Bezold-type reflex

bias
affect-related information-processing b.'s
age b.
artistic b.
ascertainment b.
emotional b.
ethnic b.
b. flow down
memory b.
negativistic b.

biatrial hypertrophy

bibasilar
fluffy bibasilar infiltrate

bibeveled drill

bibliographic information and documentation

bicarbonate
b. dialysis
Krebs-Henseleit bicarbonate buffer
Krebs-Ringer bicarbonate solution
Krebs-Ringer bicarbonate buffer with glucose
plasma b.
sodium b.
sodium bicarbonate in invert sugar
standard b.

biceps
aponeurosis of biceps brachii
b. elevator
b. femoris muscle
b. femoris tendon
b. interval lesion
b. jerk
long head of b.
musculus biceps brachii

biceps *(continued)*
musculus biceps femoris
musculus biceps flexor cruris
b. semitendinosus
b. tendon reflex

bichloride
mercury b.

bicipital
medial bicipital groove
medial bicipital sulcus

bicipitalis
aponeurosis b.

bicolor
b. guaiac
b. guaiac test

bicommissural aortic valve

bicompartmental
b. implant
b. knee implant prosthesis

biconcave
b. disk
b. lens

bicornuate uterus

bicoronal
nonsyndromic bicoronal synostosis

Biculture
Toronto Biculture Test of Nonverbal Reasoning

bicuspid
b. aortic valve
mandibular cuspid-first bicuspid radiograph
maxillary bicuspid radiograph
b. valve
b. valvulotomy

bicycle
supine bicycle stress echocardiography

bidirectional
alternating bidirectional tachycardia
b. cardiac control
b. cavopulmonary anastomosis
b. Glenn procedure
b. ligation
periorbital bidirectional Doppler
b. shunt calculation
b. shunting
b. superior cavopulmonary anastomosis
b. telescopic distractor
b. traction

Bier
B. block
B. block anesthesia

bifascicular heart block

bifemoral arteriogram

bifenestratus
hymen b.

bifid
congenital bifid bladder
multiple nevoid, basal cell epithelioma, jaw cysts, bifid rib syndrome
nevoid basal cell epithelioma, jaw cysts, bifid rib syndrome
b. tongue

bifida
adolescent spina b.
anencephaly-spina bifida syndrome
spina b.
spina bifida aperta
spina bifida cystica
spina bifida occulta

biflorus
Dolichos biflorus agglutinin

bifocal glasses

biforis
hymen b.

bifrequency
monaural bifrequency loudness balance

bifrontal
b. headache
narrow bifrontal diameter

bifurcated

bifurcation
aortic b.
aortic bifurcation prosthesis
common carotid artery b.
b. graft
iliac b.
b. lesion
limb of bifurcation graft
middle cerebral artery b.
patent b.
pulmonary artery b.
b. of root
b. of trachea
tracheal b.
venous b.

big
B. Five Questionnaire
b. gastrin
b. heel

Bigelow
ligament of B.

bigeminal
atrial bigeminal rhythm

bigeminy
atrial b.
atrioventricular junctional b.
b. junctional
nodal b.
ventricular b.

bikini incision

bilateral
b. abductor vocal cord paralysis
b. ablation
ACTH-independent bilateral macronodular hyperplasia
b. acute retinal necrosis
b. advancement transposition
b. alveolar pulmonary infiltrate
b. asymmetric
asymmetric bilateral cleft
atraumatic, multidirectional, bilateral radial instability
atraumatic, multidirectional, bilateral rehabilitation inferior capsular shift
b., symmetrical, equal
b. breath sounds
b. bundle-branch block
b. carotid body resection
b. cleft lip and palate
b. congenital absence of vas deferens
congenital bilateral absence of the vas deferens
b. contralateral routing of signals
b. cortical necrosis
b. cryptorchidism
b. cystogram
diabetes insipidus, diabetes mellitus, progressive bilateral optic atrophy, and sensorineural deafness
b. diaphragm paralysis
en bloc bilateral lung transplant
equal bilateral breath sounds
equal bilateral expansion
b. equal breath sounds
b. firm hand grips
b. frame
b. fusion
b. gastrectomy
b. hemianopia
b. hemisphere damage
b. herniorrhaphy
b. hilar adenopathy

b. hilar infiltrates
b. hilar lymphadenopathy
b. hydrosalpinx
incomplete bilateral bundle-branch block
b. independent periodic lateralizing epileptiform discharge
infantile bilateral striatal necrosis syndrome
b. inferior epigastric artery flap
b. inguinal hernia
b. internal carotid artery occlusion
b. internal mammary arteries
laparoscopic bilateral partial salpingectomy
b. leg strength
b. lower lobes
b. lung transplant
b. mastectomy scar
Millard bilateral cleft lip repair
b. myringotomy and tubes
b. occipital lobe infarct
b. occipitoparietal
one-plane bilateral external fixator
one-plane bilateral frame
b. orbital decompression
b. otitis externa
b. otitis media, acute
b. otitis media with effusion
parietal lobe bilateral cerebral hemisphere lesion
b. partial oophorectomy
b. partial salpingectomy
b. pedal pulses present
b. pelvic lymph node
b. pelvic lymph node dissection
b. percutaneous cervical cordotomy
b. pleural rub
b. progressive hearing loss
radical hysterectomy and bilateral salpingo-oophorectomy
radioactive isotopic venogram, b.
rapidly progressing bilateral hearing loss
b. renal agenesis
b. renal tumor
b. renal vein thrombosis
b. sagittal split ramus osteotomies
b. salpingo-oophorectomy
b. serous otitis media
b. short leg cane
simultaneous bilateral percutaneous nephrolithotomy
simultaneous bilateral spontaneous pneumothorax
b. symmetric
b. tinnitus
total abdominal hysterectomy and bilateral salpingo-oophorectomy
b. tubal coagulation
b. tubal ligation
b. tubal occlusion
b. tympanic membranes
b. uncal herniation
b. upper dorsal sympathectomy
b. ureteral obstruction
b. ureterostomy takedown
b. vas ligation
b. ventilation tubes
b. ventricular assist device
b. vertical ramus osteotomy
b. vocal fold immobility
b. vocal fold paralysis
wall-eyed bilateral internuclear ophthalmoplegia
b. wheezes

bilaterally
active b.
Babinski downgoing b.
breath sounds equal b.
chest expands adequately b.
deep tendon reflexes active and equal b.
deep tendon reflexes b.
equal breath b.
equal breath sounds b.
fracture bilaterally in a horizontal plane
incision extended b.
b. independent
peripheral pulses full and equal b.

bilayer
human blood bilayer Tween
lipid b.
b. lipid membrane

bile
accumulation of bile pigment
b. acid
b. acid independent flow
anatomic bile duct variant
anicteric bile duct
antegrade bile flow
ascites due to bile leak
asymmetric bile duct
atretic extrahepatic bile duct resection
Bacteroides bile esculin agar
benign bile duct stricture
block passage of b.
chronic bile duct ligation
common bile duct
common bile duct diverticulum
common bile duct exploration
common bile duct microlithiasis
common bile duct obstruction
common bile duct stent
common bile duct stone
common bile duct stricture
concentrated b.
conjugated bile salts
dark green b.
dark green viscous b.
dilated bile duct
distal bile duct carcinoma
b. duct
b. duct adenoma
b. duct catheter
b. duct epithelia
b. duct-to-portal space ratio
b. esculin test
exploration of common bile duct
extrahepatic bile duct
extrahepatic bile duct atresia
extravasated b.
fecal bile acid
b. flow
high-density b.
idiopathic bile acid malabsorption
b. infarct
inspissated bile syndrome
intrahepatic bile duct
laparoscopic exploration of the common bile duct
laparoscopic transcystic common bile duct exploration
large bile duct
lithogenic b.
middle extrahepatic bile duct
muscle of common bile duct
nonsyndromic bile duct paucity
obstruction of bile flow
occluded common bile duct
occluded common bile duct stone
open common bile duct exploration
outflow of b.
papillary bile duct stenosis
partial bile outflow obstruction
passage of b.
patent opening for bile drainage
paucity of interlobular bile ducts
perforation of common bile duct
peripheral bile duct
b. phospholipid concentration
b. phospholipid output
proliferating bile ductules

bile *(continued)*
proximal bile duct
reflux of b.
reflux bile gastritis
regurgitation of b.
b. salt
b. salt concentrate
b. salt concentration
b. salt export pump
b. salt metabolism
b. salt output
b. salt-stimulated esterase
b. salt-stimulated lipase
segmental bile duct fibrosis
serum bile acid
sphincter of bile duct
sphincter of common bile duct
total bile acid
total serum bile acid

bilevel
b. positive airway pressure
nasal bilevel biphasic positive airway pressure

biliary
b. abscess
acalculous biliary colic
b. apparatus
b. ascites
b. atresia
b. balloon catheter
b. balloon dilator
b. balloon probe
b. cholesterol concentration
b. cholesterol output
chronic obstruction of biliary tract
b. coaxial dilator
b. colic
congenital biliary atresia
congenital biliary ectasia
controlled extrahepatic biliary drainage
b. cyst
b. cystadenoma
b. dilation
b. dilator catheter
b. diverticulum
b. drainage catheter
endoscopic biliary stent
endoscopic retrograde biliary drainage
endoscopic retrograde biliary stenting
b. epithelial cell
extrahepatic biliary atresia
extrinsic biliary compression
b. fistula
b. glycoprotein
b. imaging
b. immunoglobulin
internal biliary drainage
internal biliary stent
intrahepatic biliary calculus
b. leakage
malignant biliary obstruction
malignant biliary obstructive disease
b. manipulation catheter
Mayo Clinic system test for primary biliary cirrhosis
mechanical biliary obstruction
metallic biliary endoprosthesis
metallic biliary stent
metallic biliary stent migration
b. mud
neonatal biliary function
noncommunicating biliary cyst
obstructive biliary cirrhosis
occult biliary microlithiasis
operative biliary bypass
outflow biliary tract
partial external biliary diversion
percutaneous antegrade biliary drainage
percutaneous biliary bypass
percutaneous dilatation of biliary duct
percutaneous transhepatic biliary drainage
percutaneous transhepatic biliary drainage-enteric feeding
b. prosthesis
b. sclerosis
segmental biliary obstruction
b. sphincterotomy and stent placement
spontaneous biliary perforation
b. stent
b. tract
b. tract infection
b. tract obstruction
b. tract pain
b. tract stone
b. tract stricture
b. tree

Bili-Lite
infant placed under B.-L.

Bilingual Syntax Measure II Test

bilingualism
passive b.

biliointestinal bypass

biliopancreatic bypass

bilious
b. headache
hemoglobinuric bilious fever

bilirubin
b. to albumin ratio
amniotic fluid b.
b. clearance
conjugated b.
cord blood b.
b. diglucuronide
direct b.
fractionation of b.
b. icterus
indirect b.
indirect bilirubin test
b. infarct
minimal concentration of b.
minimum concentration of b.
neonatal b.
out of bilirubin light
overt bilirubin encephalopathy
plasma bilirubin concentration
b. production
serum b.
total serum b.
total-serum b.
transcutaneous b.
unconjugated b.
b. of undetermined origin
volume of distribution of b.

bilirubin-induced neurologic dysfunction

biliverdin reductase

bill
b. of health
patient's bill of rights

billion
b. electron volts
parts per b.

billowing mitral leaflet syndrome

Billroth
cord of B.
B. hypertrophy
vagotomy and Billroth gastroenterostomy

biloba
Ginkgo b.
Ginkgo biloba extract

bilobed
mesiolabial bilobed transposition flap
Zimany bilobed flap

Bimbo virus

Bimiti virus

Bimodality Lung Oncology Team

bimolecular liquid membrane

binangle chisel

binary
nearly ideal binary solvent

binary-coded decimal

binasal
b. cannula
b. hemianopia
b. pharyngeal airway
b. prongs

binaural
alternate binaural loudness balance
b. alternate loudness balance
b. hearing aid
simultaneous binaural bithermal
simultaneous binaural midplace localization
b. stethoscope

bindable
serum-platelet bindable immunoglobulin G

binder
adrenergic receptor b.

binding
albumin cobalt b.
androgen binding protein
antigen b.
antigen binding protein
antigen binding site
antigenic binding receptor
ATP binding site
autologous growth factor binding agent
buffer-soluble binding component
CCAAT/enhancer binding protein
competitive protein b.
estramustine binding protein
estrogen binding site
fragment antigen b.
fragment, antigen, and complement b.
fragment of immunoglobulin G involved in antigen b.
heart fatty acid binding protein
hepatic binding protein
hormone binding study
immobilized mismatch binding protein
intracellular binding protein
lipopolysaccharide binding protein
mammalian binding lectin deficiency
mannose binding molecule
maximal specific binding capacity
metenkephalin receptor b.
nonspecific b.
plasma membrane fatty acid binding protein
protein b.
protein binding abnormality
b. protein protease
relative binding affinity
rheumatoid factor b.
serum reserve cholesterol binding capacity
stereospecific b.
sterol regulatory element binding protein
surface binding protein
testis-specific binding protein
thyroid-specific enhancer binding protein-1
thyroxine binding globulin
total vitamin B_{12} binding capacity
unsaturated binding capacity

bind wire

Binet-Simon test

binge
alcohol b.
b. buyer
b. drinker
b. drinking
b. eater
b. eating
b. eating disorder
b. eating pattern
b. eating syndrome
episodic pattern of binge eating
b. gambler
b. and purge
b. and purge syndrome
b. spender

bingeing
b. behavior of anorexia
b. behavior of bulimic
b. and purging

binge-purge behavior

Bingham Button Test

biniodide
mercury b.

binocle dressing

binocular
AO binocular indirect ophthalmoscope
b. deprivation
b. dissecting microscope
b. eye patch
b. field
b. hemianopia
b. indirect ophthalmoscope
b. instrument
b. internuclear ophthalmoplegia
macular binocular vision
b. microscope
sensory binocular cooperation
single binocular vision
b. single vision
b. stereoscope
B. Visual Acuity Test
b. visual efficiency

Binswanger dementia

bioartificial
b. extracorporeal liver support system
b. liver

bioassay
cytochemical b.
b. of luteinizing hormone

bioavailabilty
oral b.

bioccipital headache

bioceramic
alumina bioceramic joint replacement

biochemical
b. analysis and culture
automated biochemical analyzer
b. change in brain
electrolyte biochemical oxygen demand
b. impairment
b. oxygen demand
physical and biochemical effect
b. profile

bioconcentration factor

biodegradable
b. calcium phosphate cement
b. fixation device
b. fixation instrumentation
b. implant

bioeffect dose

bioelectrical impedance analysis

bioenergy imbalance syndrome

bioerodible mucoadhesive

Bioethical Information On-Line

biofeedback
colitis and alpha b.
concept of alpha b.

biofeedback *(continued)*
concept of biofeedback control
electrodermal response b.
electroencephalogram biofeedback in control of hyperactivity
b. and headache
b. for hypertensives
nasopharyngoscopy biofeedback therapy
relaxation and b.
b. training

biofilm
microbial b.

biogenesis
mitochondrial b.

biographical
loss of biographical memory

biogroup
Haemophilus influenzae biogroup *aegyptius*

bioimpedance
multiple-frequency b.
single-frequency b.
thoracic electrical b.
b. venous analysis

biologic
b. activity
b. aerosol detection
b. and chemical warfare
b. detection system
direct biologic effect
b. effective dose
b. effects of ionizing radiation
b. factors in dose fractionation
b. false-positive
b. false-positive reactor
b. feedback
b. half-life
b. indicator
indirect biologic effect
nuclear, biologic, chemical
optimum biologic dose
relative biologic effectiveness
b. response
b. response modifier
roentgen-equivalent b.
b. value
b. weapon

biological
b. age
b. allergic unit
anthrax as a biological weapon
atomic, biological, chemical
atomic, biological, chemical warfare
chemical, biological, radiological or nuclear weapons
chemical and biological warfare
chemical, radiological, and b.
circadian biological rhythm
b. false-positive serologic test for syphilis
b. half-life
b. heart valve
high biological value protein
b. integration
low biological value
male biological status
opposite biological sex
b. oxygen demand
B. Response Modification Program
b. terrain assessment

biologically
b. active luteinizing hormone
b. designed hip
b. equivalent dose
b. inactive
rheumatoid biologically active factor

biology
engineering in medicine and b.
molecular cell b.

biomarker
surrogate end-point b.

biomaterial
alloplastic b.
antiinfective b.
b. interaction

biomechanical failure of implant

biomechanics
axial plane angular deformity b.
gait b.

biomedical
b. belt
b. monitoring system

biometal surface

biometry
ophthalmic biometry by ultrasound echography

biomicroscopy
ultrasound b.

biomolecule
psi-interactive b.

bionic
Rincoe human action b.

biophysical
fetal biophysical profile
placental grade biophysical profile
b. profile
b. profile score

biophysics
chiropractic b.

biopolymer
aperiodic b.
periodic b.

bioprosthesis
Carpentier-Edwards porcine b.
low-profile b.
porcine b.
porcine valve b.

bioprosthetic
b. heart valve
pericardial bioprosthetic tissue

biopsy
abdominal lymph node b.
advanced breast biopsy instrumentation
b. after irradiation
apical biopsy status
b. of area taken
aspiration biopsy cytology
aspiration needle b.
automated biopsy device
automated biopsy gun
automated large-core breast b.
automatic spring-loaded biopsy device
bone biopsy needle
bone marrow b.
breast b.
b. and brushings
cervical b.
cervical cone b.
chorionic villus b.
closed core needle b.
closed pleural b.
cold cone b.
cold cup b.
cold knife cone b.
cold knife conization b.
conventional core b.
core b.
core biopsy needle
core biopsy obturator
core breast b.
core needle b.
b. and curettage
curved needle b.
cutting needle b.
dilation, curettage, and b.
directional vacuum-assisted b.
endobronchial brush b.
endoluminal ultrasonography-guided fine-needle aspiration b.

endometrial b.
endomyocardial b.
excisional biopsy technique
excisional biopsy of tumor mass
excision and wedge b.
excision and wedge biopsy of breast
fasciotomy wound b.
fenestrated spiked open-span jumbo biopsy forceps
fine-needle aspiration b.
four quadrant b.
freehand CT-guided b.
greater superficial temporal artery b.
guided needle b.
guillotine needle b.
healing biopsy incision
hot biopsy technique
iliac crest b.
image-guided breast b.
image-guided fine-needle aspiration b.
imaging-guided open b.
inflammation of biopsy tissue
kidney ultrasound b.
large-core needle b.
large-needle aspiration b.
left breast b.
left breast biopsy examination
liver b.
lung b.
lung biopsy tissue
lymph node b.
median biopsy volume
Menghini biopsy technique
minimally invasive biopsy procedure
minimally invasive breast b.
mirror image breast b.
monoclonal antibody A103 fine-needle aspiration b.
Monopty core b.
MRI-based stereotactic b.
MRI-guided breast b.
multiple core b.'s
multiple biopsies taken
Multi-Pro biopsy needle
needle aspiration b.
needle aspiration lung b.
needle biopsy diagnosis
needle biopsy of liver
needle biopsy of prostate
needle biopsy specimen
needle core b.
needle liver b.
needle-localized open b.
negative breast b.
negative punch b.
nonoperative biopsy technique
open brain b.
open liver b.
open lung b.
open surgical b.
open-wedge biopsy specimen
Optical B. System
pelvic aspiration b.
percutaneous conchotome biopsy technique
percutaneous core bone b.
percutaneous excisional breast b.
percutaneous fine-needle aspiration b.
percutaneous fine-needle pancreatic b.
percutaneous liver b.
percutaneous needle aspiration b.
percutaneous peritoneal b.
percutaneous transhepatic liver biopsy with tract embolization
percutaneous transthoracic needle b.
pinch b.
prostate gland b.
prostate needle b.
prostate puncture b.
prostatic needle b.
punch b.
right breast b.
right breast biopsy examination
scalene fat pad b.
scalene lymph node b.
scalene node b.
selected mucosal b.
sentinel lymph node b.
shave excisional b.
Silverman needle b.
small bowel b.
specimen submitted for b.
Stanford biopsy method
stereotactically guided core needle b.
stereotactic brain b.
stereotactic breast b.
stereotactic core b.
stereotactic core-needle b.
stereotactic guided core-needle b.
stereotactic needle b.
submitted for b.
b. submitted for frozen section
suction biopsy instrument
supraclavicular node b.
surgical lung b.
temporal artery b.
tracheoscopy with b.
transbronchial brush b.
transbronchial lung b.
transcatheter b.
transrectal needle b.
transrectal needle biopsy of prostate
transrectal ultrasound-guided sextant b.
transthoracic needle aspiration b.
transurethral needle biopsy of the prostate
transvaginal fine-needle b.
Tru-Cut needle b.
ultrasonically guided needle b.
ultrasound-guided core breast b.
ultrasound-guided core-needle b.
ultrasound-guided fine-needle aspiration b.
b. under x-ray control
upper gastrointestinal b.
vacuum-assisted core b.
vaginal cone b.
video-assisted excisional b.
wedge excisional b.

biopsy-negative graft dysfunction

biopterin
neopterin to biopterin ratio

bioptic telescopic spectacle

bioreactor
MRI-compatible hollow-fiber b.

bioresorbable implant

biosafety level

biosynthetic
b. human growth hormone
b. human insulin
porphyrin biosynthetic pathway

biotherapy
cancer biotherapy study group

biothesiometry
penile b.

biotic potential

biotin
b. carboxylase
b. carboxyl carrier protein
labeled streptavidin b.
neonatal biotin deficiency

biotripticum
atrophoderma b.

biovar
Mycobacterium fortuitum third biovar complex

biparietal
b. diameter
fetal biparietal diameter
b. headache
b. hump
bipartite
placenta b.
bipedicle
mucosal bipedicle flap
bipennatus
musculus b.
biphasic
b. activity
helical biphasic contrast-enhanced CT
b. illness
nasal bilevel biphasic positive airway pressure
NMN biphasic blood agar
Novy-McNeal-Nicolle biphasic blood agar
overlapping biphasic impulse
b. synovial sarcoma
biplanar transducer
biplane
b. imaging
b. sector scanner
bipolar
b. acetabular cup
affective bipolar disorder
alternating bipolar disorder
atypical bipolar disorder
b. cauterization
b. cautery probe
b. cautery unit
b. cell
b. circumactive probe
circumferential bipolar montage
b. cutting loop
b. depression
b. disorder
b. disorder type 1, 2
b. electrocoagulation
b. electrocoagulation of hemorrhoid
b. electrosurgical scissors
b. femoral component
b. femoral head prosthesis
b. hip arthroplasty
b. hip replacement
b. hip replacement prosthesis
hyperpolarizing bipolar cell
b. illness
integrated bipolar sensing
manic bipolar disorder
mixed bipolar affective psychosis
mixed bipolar state
b. needle recording electrode
b. prosthetic cup
B. Psychological Inventory
b. psychosis
b. stimulating electrode
b. vertebral traction
Birao virus
bird fancier's lung
bird-headed dwarf
birefringence
apple-green b.
Birmingham Vasculitis Activity Score
birth
alcohol-related birth defect
alternative birth center
asphyxial birth injury
cesarean b.
Chlamydia from birth control pill
b. control
b. control clinic
b. control drug
b. control medication
b. control pill
b. control regimen
crude birth rate
date of b.
b. date
days after b.
b. defect
B. Defects Monitoring Program
extremely low birth weight
forceps birth trauma
full-term live b.
gravida, para, multiple births, abortions, live b.
hair loss from birth control pill
hepatitis from birth control pill
high birth weight
b. history
hospital birth certificate
b. injury
intrauterine pregnancy, term birth, cesarean section
intrauterine pregnancy, term birth, living infant
live b.
live birth abortion
low birth weight
low birth weight infant
mean birth weight
mechanical birth injury
moderately low birth weight
normal birth weight
normal spontaneous vaginal b.
oral birth control pill
partial birth abortion
b.'s per minute
place of b.
pregnancy and birth complication
premature birth live infant
prior to b.
severely low birth weight
spontaneous preterm b.
term birth appropriate for gestational age
term birth, living child
term birth, living female
term birth, living infant
term birth, living male
traditional birth attendant
trained participating father b.
trained participating husband b.
traumatic birth injury
twin birth weight discordance
ultralow birth weight
vaginal birth after cesarean section
vaginal birth after cesarean—trial of labor
very low birth rate
very low birth weight
very low birth weight infant
very low birth weight preterm neonate
viable b.
b. weight
b. weight for gestational age
woman who has given b.
year of b.
zero stool since b.
birthing
maternal birthing position
birthmark
port-wine stain b.
Birt-Hogg-Dubé syndrome
bisacetamide
hexamethylene b.
biscuit
low b.
low biscuit firing
medium b.
medium biscuit firing
bisection
angle bisection technique
AP malleolar b.
line bisection error
bisexual
gay, lesbian, b.

bismuth
acid bismuth yeast medium
aluminum bismuth oxide
b., metronidazole, tetracycline
butter of b.
colloidal bismuth subcitrate
emetine and bismuth iodide
b. germanate
b. hydroxide
iodide
b. iodoform paraffin
milk of b.
omeprazole, bismuth subcitrate, tetracycline, and metronidazole
ranitidine bismuth citrate
ranitidine bismuth citrate, amoxicillin, clarithromycin
ranitidine bismuth citrate, metronidazole, tetracycline
b. subgallate
b. subsalicylate
b. subsalicylate, metronidazole, and amoxicillin

bismuth-iodoform-paraffin paste

bismuth-sulfite agar

bispecific monoclonal antibody

bisphosphate
nucleoside b.

bispinous or interspinous diameter

bisque
low bisque firing
medium bisque firing

bit
check b.
diamond b.
b. drill
drill b.
drill bit fracture
femoral drill b.
most significant b.
parity b.

bitartrate
hydrocodone b.

bite
African tick bite fever
b. analysis
animal b.
ant b.
arthropod b.
assassin bug b.
deep bites of tissue
end-to-end b.
Gila monster b.
human b.
improper b.
insect b.
lizard b.
locked b.
mature b.
maxillary bite plate
maximum bite force
midge b.
mite b.
moccasin snake b.
molar bite position
mosquito b.
mosquito bite infection
normal b.
northern rat flea b.
occlusal bite force
open b.
posterior bite wing
vertical and centric b.
wax b.

bitemporal
b. headache
b. hemianopia

biter
nail b.

bite-wing radiograph

bithermal
simultaneous binaural b.

biting
cheek biting from anxiety
lip b.
nail b.
oral biting period

bitter
aromatic b.'s
oil of bitter almond
oil of bitter orange
styptic b.

bitterness
displays enduring b.

bitubal interruption

biundulant meningoencephalitis

bivalency
monogamous b.

bivalve overlap brace

bivalved
b. cylinder cast
b. pancake plaster hand cast
b. speculum

biventricular
b. assist device
b. dilatation and hypertrophy
b. enlargement
b. hypertrophy
mild biventricular dilatation hypertrophy
orthoptic biventricular artificial heart
b. support

bizarre
b. eating pattern
b. fixation
b. gait pattern
b. incoherent thinking
b. parosteal osteochondromatous proliferation
b. platelet
b. way of thinking

Bjerrum
arcuate Bjerrum scotoma

black
b. beetle virus
B. Creek Canal virus
b. death
fuchsin, amido black, and naphthol yellow
b. hairy tongue
b. induration
interrupted black silk suture
b. light
b. lipid membrane
b. male
matte black forceps
matte black instrument
National Caucus and Center on B. Aged, Inc.
nosologic black hole
pathognomonic black eschar
shading response to black areas
b. silk suture
Spanish American b.
Sudan Black B
tarry black bowel movement
tarry black stool
unknown black female
unknown black male
b. widow spider toxin
b. widow spider venom

blackmail
emotional b.

blackout
alcoholic b.
history of b.'s
recurring b.'s

black-pigmented bacteria

bladder
abnormal bladder contraction
b. agenesis
alloplastic prostatic b.

bladder *(continued)*
apex of b.
apex of urinary b.
artificial internal b.
ascending bladder septum
atonic urinary b.
autocrine motility factor of the b.
autonomic neurogenic b.
bashful bladder syndrome
bowel and b.
bowel and bladder dysfunction
bowel and bladder function
bowel and bladder incontinence
b. and bowel dysfunction
b. cancer
b. carcinoma in situ
b. carcinosarcoma
catheterized b.
change in bladder habit
change in bladder pattern
b. chimney procedure
b. choriocarcinoma
clean intermittent bladder catheterization
closed bladder drainage
community-acquired bladder infection
complete emptying of b.
congenital bifid b.
congestion of bladder mucosa
continence of bowel and b.
continuous bladder drainage
continuous bladder irrigation
b. cooling reflex
b. cuff
disruption of bladder function
distended urinary b.
b. distended with air
b. distended with water
b. emptied completely
b. emptied on voiding
b. empties normally
endoscopic bladder neck suspension
extraperitoneal laparoscopic bladder neck suspension
extrinsic bladder compression
filling of the b.
first voided bladder specimen
b. fistula
b. flap elevated
b. flap tube
b. habit
hemorrhage into wall of b.
b. hernia
hernia of b.
high bladder pressure
incomplete bladder emptying
incomplete emptying of b.
b. incontinence
indwelling bladder catheter
b. infection
infection or bladder involvement
inoperable bladder malignancy
intermittent bladder irrigation
intermittent catheterization of b.
invasive bladder cancer
b. involuntary contraction
b. irrigated
kidneys, ureters, bladder x-ray
kidneys and urinary b.
laparoscopic bladder neck suspension
liver, kidneys, spleen, and b.
loss of bladder control
loss of control of bladder function
low pressure b.
lysis bladder neck adhesions
malignant neoplasm of b.
mechanical bladder outlet resistance
modified Peyronie bladder neck suspension
b. mucosal hemorrhage
multifocal bladder tumor
muscular coat of urinary b.
muscular layer of urinary b.
b. neck
neck of b.
b. neck contracture
b. neck obstruction
b. neck resection
b. neck suspension
necrotic bladder mucosa
needle bladder neck suspension
neonatal exstrophic bladder repair
nephrogenic bladder adenoma
neuralgia of b.
neurogenic b.
neurogenic bladder disorder
neurogenic bladder dysfunction
neurologic bladder dysfunction
neurologic bladder lesion
normal bladder caliber
open bladder brachytherapy implant
orthotopic bladder augmentation
orthotopic bladder substitution
b. outflow obstruction
b. outlet obstruction
overactive b.
overdistension of b.
papilloma of b.
partial bladder denervation
partial obstruction of b.
b. patch
percutaneous bladder aspiration
percutaneous bladder neck stabilization
percutaneous bladder neck suspension
Pereyra bladder neck suspension
peripheral bladder denervation
poor bladder control
postoperative bladder dysfunction
b. pressure
prolapse of urethra and b.
b. regeneration
b. retraining drill
ruptured b.
second midstream bladder specimen
small cell cancer of b.
sound guided into b.
stammering of the b.
strangulation of b.
superficial bladder cancer
suprapubic bladder tap
thickened bladder wall
third midstream bladder specimen
total bladder capacity
total bladder resection
b. training
transitional bladder cell carcinoma
transitional cell carcinoma of b.
transurethral electrical bladder stimulation
transurethral incision of bladder neck
transurethral resection of b.
transvaginal bladder neck suspension
trigone of b.
b. tumor
b. tumor antigen
b. tumor check
b. tumor recheck
uninhibited neurogenic b.
uninhibited overactive b.
upper motor neurogenic b.
urinary b.
urinary bladder adenocarcinoma
urinary bladder atony
urinary bladder calculus
urinary bladder capacity
urinary bladder fistula
urinary bladder hernia
urinary bladder rupture
urinary bladder tumor

urinary bladder wall mass
urinary bladder wall thickening
voided b.
b. wall thickened
b. wall trabeculated
b. wall weakened
washed b.
b. washout
WHO classification for transitional cell carcinoma of the urinary bladder: stages Ta through T4
b. xanthoma

blade
angled blade plate fixation
arrow b.
cartilage shaver b.
b. catheter
diamond-dusted knife b.
b. gauge
Mullins blade technique
myringotomy b.
notchplasty b.
orbit b.
pediatric blade plate
b. plate
b. plate driver
prominent shoulder b.

blade-type holder

Blalock-Taussig
modified B.-T.
B.-T. operation
B.-T. procedure
B.-T. shunt

blame
assign b.
externalize b.
parental habits of b.
b. psychology

blanchable red lesion

blanche
atrophie b.
atrophie blanche lesion
tache b.

blanching of hand

bland diet

blank
Crowley Occupational Interests B.
Leisure Activities B.
order b.
Rotter Incomplete Sentences B.
Strong Vocational Interest B.
Vocational Interest B.

blanked ventricular sense

blanket
b. bath
cooling blanket for hyperthermia
hypothermia b.
hypothermic b.
mucus b.

blanking
postventricular atrial b.
total atrial b.

Blaschko
line of B.

blast
b. cell
chronic myelocytic/myelogenous/myeloid leukemia blast crisis
b. crisis
lung b.
refractory anemia with excess b.'s
refractory anemia with excess of blasts in transformation
refractory anemia with excess blasts in transition
resorbable blast media

blastema
metanephric b.
nephric b.
nodular b.

blastic
b. crisis
lytic blastic changes
megakaryocytic blastic phase

blastogenesis
spontaneous b.

blastogenic
b. factor
lymphocyte blastogenic factor

blastoid variant of mantel cell lymphoma

blastoma
b. mantel cell lymphoma
nodular renal b.
parenchymal b.
pineal b.
pleuropulmonary b.

blastomycosis
Lutz-Splendore-Almeida b.
nasopharyngeal b.
North American b.
peritoneal b.
South American b.
systemic b.

bleaching
melanin bleaching method
nonvital b.

bleb
apical b.
apoptotic b.
emphysematous b.
membrane bleb formation
nonleaking b.
oval aneurysm with b.
pulmonary b.
subpleural b.

bleed
air b.
GI bleed from anemia
massive intracerebral b.
subarachnoid b.

bleeder
b. cauterized
b. clamped
b. clamped and ligated
b. clamped and tied
b. electrocoagulated
episcleral b.
b. identified

bleeding
abnormal uterine b.
abnormal vaginal b.
acute upper gastrointestinal b.
anorectal variceal b.
arterial bleeding site
b. at site of injection
Baylor bleeding score
breakthrough b.
chronic gastrointestinal tract b.
b. controlled with clamp
b. controlled with hemostatic clamp
b. and cramping
cramping and b.
discrete bleeding source
dysfunctional b.
dysfunctional uterine b.
dysfunctional vaginal b.
electrodesiccated bleeding point
esophageal variceal b.
b. esophageal varix
esophagogastric variceal b.
estrogen breakthrough b.
estrogen-progesterone withdrawal b.
estrogen withdrawal b.
b. from aspirin
b. from multiple sites
functional uterine b.
gastric bleeding time

bleeding *(continued)*
b. gastric varix
gastrointestinal b.
gastrointestinal tract b.
gingival bleeding index
b. gums
hereditary bleeding disorder
b. and infection
b. inside skull
intermenstrual b.
b. into joint
intracranial b.
irregular uterine b.
irregular vaginal b.
lower gastrointestinal b.
lower GI b.
massive intestinal b.
midcycle b.
minute bleeding ulcer
nuclear bleeding scan
occult b.
occult gastrointestinal b.
b. on touch
b. and oozing
packing for b.
per anum b.
perforation and b.
placental bleeding site
pneumatic tourniquet-controlled b.
b. points secured
possible source of b.
postcoital b.
postmenopausal b.
pressure to control b.
prolonged bleeding time
rectal bleeding secondary to hemorrhoid
severe gastrointestinal b.
b. site cauterized
skin bleeding time
source of intraperitoneal b.
b. time
b. time template
b. ulcer
b. of undetermined origin
upper gastrointestinal b.
vitamin K deficiency b.
voluntary control of b.

blend
wheat soy b.

blenderized
b. diet
b. tube feeding

blending
auditory b.

blennorrhea
neonatal inclusion b.

blepharitis
chronic b.
mixed seborrheic-staphylococcal b.

blepharonasofacial
mental retardation, blepharonasofacial abnormalities, hand malformations syndrome

blepharophimosis, ptosis, epicanthus inversus syndrome

blepharoplasty
b. scissors
transconjunctival b.
transconjunctival blepharoplasty laser resurfacing

blepharoptosis
aponeurotic b.
mechanical b.
mental retardation, congenital heart disease, blepharophimosis, blepharoptosis, hypoplastic teeth
neurogenic b.

blepharospasm
benign essential b.
idiopathic b.

Blessed Dementia Rating Scale

Blessed-Roth Dementia Scale

blind
aged, blind, and disabled
aid to the b.
b. basket extraction
b. cautery
color b.
b. esophageal brushing
b. gut
b. headache
b. insertion
B. Learning Aptitude Test
b. lithotripsy
b. loop
Mariotte blind spot
b. matching
mental blind spot
physiologic blind spot
self-emptying blind loop
self-filling blind loop
single b.
b. thoracentesis

blinding head pain

blindness
amnesic color b.
congenital retinitis b.
congenital stationary night b.
night b.
total monocular b.
transient cortical b.
transient monocular b.

blink
corneal blink reflex
b. reflex

blinking
paroxysmal b.

blipped
modulus blipped echo-planar single-pulse technique

blister
arthropod-induced b.
ashgray blister beetle
ashgray blister beetle sting
burn b.
b. fluid
fracture b.
friction b.
healed b.
incision and drainage of b.
oral b.
painless, small intact b.
red patch or blister on arm
b. red, scaly, and itchy
sucking b.
water b.
b. without infection

blistering
autoimmune blistering mucocutaneous disease
b. distal dactylitis

bloated abdomen

bloater
blue b.

bloating
abdominal b.
b. and/or diarrhea, gas, cramps
b. or belching
b. and constipation
b. and cramping
b. or diarrhea
b. from lactose intolerance
b. and gas
b. and indigestion
b. and irritable bowel syndrome

bloc
en b.
en bloc advancement
en bloc bilateral lung transplant
en bloc dissection
en bloc esophagectomy
en bloc excision

en bloc no touch technique
en bloc removal
en bloc resection
en bloc running locking suture
en bloc vulvectomy
radical en bloc removal

Bloch method

block

air block glaucoma
alveolar-capillary b.
ankle block anesthesia
anterior fascicular b.
anterocrural celiac plexus b.
aphakic pupillary b.
AP-PA skull b.
Atkin lid b.
Atkinson lid b.
atrial tachycardia with b.
atrioventricular b.
atrioventricular block with first-degree conduction delay
atrioventricular heart b.
atrioventricular junctional heart b.
atrioventricular Wenckebach b.
autoimmune-associated congenital heart b.
autonomic ganglion b.
autonomic nerve b.
AV Wenckebach heart b.
axillary b.
axillary block anesthesia
axillary block anesthetic technique
Bier block anesthesia
bifascicular heart b.
bilateral bundle-branch b.
brachial plexus b.
bundle-branch b.
bundle branch heart b.
bundle-branch heart b.
cell block analysis
cervical, skull, and shoulder b.
circular block anesthesia
complete atrioventricular b.
complete AV b.
complete bundle-branch b.
complete heart b.
complete left bundle-branch b.
complete left bundle branch b.
complete right bundle branch b.
congenital complete heart b.
congenital heart b.
corticocancellous block graft
critical organ shielding b.'s
dedicated time b.
b. design test
digital block anesthesia
digital nerve b.
diversional heart b.
dorsal penile nerve b.
facet joint b.
facial nerve b.
fascicular heart b.
femoral nerve b.
field block anesthesia
first-degree arteriovenous b.
first-degree heart b.
four-in-one cutting b.
four-in-one positioning block system
graduated spinal b.
heart b.
3:1 heart b.
3:2 heart b.
heart-lung b.
His bundle branch b.
His bundle heart b.
humeral block in radiation therapy
iliohypogastric nerve b.
ilioinguinal-iliohypogastric nerve b.
incomplete atrioventricular b.
incomplete bilateral bundle-branch b.
incomplete heart b.
incomplete left bundle-branch b.
incomplete right bundle-branch b.
intercostal nerve b.
interventricular heart b.
intravenous regional sympathetic b.
intraventricular conduction b.
intraventricular heart b.
left anterior bundle-branch b.
left anterior fascicular b.
left anterior-superior fascicular b.
left bundle-branch system b.
left posterior fascicular b.
left posterior-inferior fascicular b.
left ventricular bundle-branch b.
local diagnostic b.
lower extremity nerve b.
lumbar epidural b.
lumbar spinal b.
lumbar sympathetic b.
Mayo block anesthesia
mental block injection
Mobitz atrioventricular b.
Mobitz I heart b.
Mobitz I, II b.
Mobitz type I, II b.
modified Van Lint b.
motor conduction b.
motor neuropathy with multifocal conduction b.
multiple b.'s
Nadbath facial b.
nerve block anesthesia
nerve block infusion
neurolytic celiac plexus b.
neurolytic nerve b.
neurosurgical nerve b.
O'Brien lid b.
b. pain impulse
palatine block anesthesia
paracervical b.
paracervical block anesthesia
paraffin block embedding
paravertebral b.
paroxysmal AV b.
partial heart b.
b. passage of bile
pentagonal block excision
percutaneous radiofrequency facet nerve b.
perichondrial double cartilage block technique
periinfarction b.
peripheral nerve b.
pharmacologic autonomic b.
plexus nerve b.
popliteal nerve b.
porous block hydroxyapatite
pudendal b.
rate-dependent left bundle-branch b.
regional block anesthesia
retrobulbar lid b.
right bundle-branch b.
right bundle-branch system b.
sacral b.
saddle block anesthesia
second-degree AV b.
second-degree heart b.
selective nerve root b.
short-acting b.
sinoatrial b.
sinoatrial entrance b.
sinoatrial heart b.
sinoauricular heart b.
stellate block anesthesia
stellate ganglion nerve b.
subarachnoid b.
subjunctional heart b.
submaximal neuromuscular b.
supraclavicular nerve b.
sympathetic block anesthesia
sympathetic ganglion block anesthetic technique
sympathetic nerve b.

block *(continued)*
third-degree atrioventricular b.
third-degree AV b.
third-degree heart b.
third degree heart b.
Three-Dimensional B. Construction Test
transient heart b.
trifascicular heart b.
upper extremity nerve b.
vocabulary, information, block design, and similarities
Wenckebach atrioventricular b.
Wenckebach heart b.

blockade
adjuvant alpha b.
alpha-adrenergic b.
alpha-receptor blockade therapy
alpha sympathetic b.
audible speech b.
beta b.
combined androgen b.
epidural neural b.
intercostal nerve b.
intermittent androgen b.
left stellate ganglionic b.
lumbar sympathetic b.
maximal androgen b.
muscarinic cholinergic b.
narcotic blockade drug
neuromuscular b.
neuromuscular blockade monitoring
neuromuscular transmission b.
nicotinic receptor blockade therapy
peripheral androgen b.
sympathetic blockade anesthetic technique

blockage
arterial b.
articular b.
intestinal b.
mechanical vessel b.
meconium blockage syndrome
nasal b.
neuromuscular b.
pulmonary artery b.

blocked
anti-B4 blocked ricin
b. blood flow
b. breathing passage
damaged or blocked fallopian tubes
b. heart artery
b. nasal passage

blocker
angiotensin II receptor b.
antiandrogen receptor b.
beta b.
beta blocker therapy
calcium b.
calcium channel b.
calcium entry b.
nondihydropyridine calcium channel b.
proton pump b.
renin angiotensin b.
slow channel b.

blocking
b. activity
alpha-adrenergic blocking agent
alpha-1 adrenergic blocking agent
alpha-adrenergic blocking drug
alpha blocking agent
alpha receptor blocking agent
b. antibody
antibody blocking assay
b. or attenuation
audible blocking in speech
beta-adrenergic blocking agent
b. factor
hemolysis b.
maternal thyrotropin receptor blocking antibody-induced congenital hypothyroidism
mixed lymphocyte reaction blocking factor
narcotic blocking drug
nerve blocking anesthesia
neuromuscular blocking drug
pain blocking illusion
progesterone-induced blocking factor
retinoic acid metabolism blocking agent
serum blocking factor
specific blocking factor
b. of thought process
TSH stimulation blocking antibody

blockout
arbitrary b.
parallel b.

Bloembergen, Purcell, and Pound theory

blood
abbreviated blood count
abdominal pain associated with blood loss
AB negative blood type
abnormal blood clotting
ABO blood group
ABO blood type
absolute blood eosinophil count
absolute nucleated red blood cell
accelerated destruction of red blood cells
acceleration of blood flow
accessory pulmonary blood flow
accumulation of blood within joint
acute blood loss
adequate blood flow
adequate blood supply
adequate flow of b.
admission blood work
admitting blood sugar
aerobic and anaerobic blood culture
b. agar
b. agar base
b. agar plate
AIDS blood culture
b. alcohol
b. alcohol concentration
b. alcohol content
b. alcohol level
allogeneic blood transfusion
allogenic blood component
allogenic blood transfusion
alteration of blood brain barrier
ambulatory blood pressure
ambulatory blood pressure monitor
ammonia blood level
anemia secondary to blood loss
ankle-brachial blood pressure
ankle-brachial blood pressure ratio
antegrade blood flow
anti-CD3 stimulated peripheral blood lymphocytes transduced with a gene encoding a chimeric
anticipated blood loss
anti-P blood group specificity
aortic blood flow velocity waveform
aortic blood pressure
appropriate blood pressure cuff size
arterial blood collection
arterial blood gas
arterial blood gas abnormality
arterial blood gas analysis
arterial blood gas point-of-care test
arterial blood hydrogen tension
arterial blood oximetry

arterial blood pressure
arterial blood sample
arterial blood supply
arterialization of venous b.
arterialized capillary b.
artificial blood substrate
aspiration of blood material
Astrup blood gas value
atherosclerosis and blood flow
Auberger blood group
Au blood group
b. in auditory canal
augment flow of b.
autologous blood clot
autologous blood collection
autologous blood donation
autologous blood and marrow transplantation
autologous blood transfusion
autologous blood unit
autologous cord b.
autologous peripheral blood stem cell bone marrow transplantation
autologous red blood cell
automated blood pressure cuff
automated white blood cell differential
autoregulation of cerebral blood flow
backflow of b.
backward flow of b.
bacteria in blood smear
ballooning-out of blood vessel
b. bank
blocked blood flow
blue skin from blood clot
B negative blood type
b. and body fluid precaution
borderline high blood pressure
bovine red blood cell
bright red blood per rectum
bronchial blood flow
b. buffer base
bulging eyes from blood clot
calf blood flow
cancer cell-derived blood coagulating activity 1
cancerous growth of blood cell
capillary b.
capillary blood flow
capillary blood gas
capillary blood gas at room air
capillary blood glucose
capillary blood flow velocity
capillary whole blood true sugar
cardiac blood pool imaging
b. cardioplegia
cardiopulmonary blood volume
carotid blood flow
b. cell profile
b. cell separator
b. center
central circulating blood volume
cerebral blood flow
cerebral blood flow studies
cerebral blood flow velocity
cerebral red blood cell volume
cerebral blood volume/cerebral blood flow ratio
charcoal blood medium culture
b. chemistry
b. chemistry profile
chicken red blood cell
chocolate blood agar
choroidal blood flow
choroidal blood volume
chronic blood loss
chronic high blood pressure
circulating blood lymphocyte
circulating blood volume
clotting action of b.
b. coagulation monitoring
b. coagulation time
cochlear blood flow
cold blood cardioplegia
collateral blood flow
collateral blood supply
b. color analyzer
compensatory blood supply
complete blood count
complete blood cell count
b. component therapy
computer-assisted blood background subtraction
concentrated red blood cell
constriction or spasm of blood vessel
contaminated blood culture
controlled high blood pressure
copious bright red b.
cord b.
cord blood bilirubin
cord blood cell therapy
cord blood erythropoietin level
cord blood gas
cord blood hemoglobin
cord blood mononuclear cell
cord blood registry
cord blood sample
cord blood transplantation
coronary blood flow
coronary blood flow velocity
coronary sinus blood flow
corrected blood volume
cortical blood flow
cortical blood volume
coughing up b.
coughing up blood with chest pain
b. count
crenated red blood cell
crying, requirement for oxygen supplementation, increases in heart rate and blood pressure
b. culture
dark blood stained fluid
decreasing blood count
denatured red blood cell
designated blood donation
designated donor b.
deteriorating blood gases
diastolic blood pressure
Diego blood group
difference in nitrogen tension between mixed alveolar gas and mixed arterial b.
difference in partial pressures of oxygen in mixed alveolar gas and mixed arterial b.
differential blood count
b. diffuses into heart muscle
digital blood perfusion
diminished blood flow
disseminated intravascular blood coagulation
diversion of flow of b.
dog red blood cell
donkey red blood cell
b. donor
donor-specific blood transfusion
drawing of blood sample
dried blood stain
drug-induced blood cytopenias
drug screen b.
dynamic cardiac blood flow
effective arterial blood volume
effective circulating blood volume
effective pulmonary blood flow
effective renal blood flow
electrolytes, blood urea nitrogen, and serum creatinine
electromagnetic blood flow imaging
elevation of blood lead level
b. eosinophilic nonallergic rhinitis
epidural blood patch
epidural blood patch anesthetic technique
equilibrium-gated blood pool study
erect diastolic blood pressure

blood *(continued)*
erratic blood glucose levels
erratic blood pressure
estimated blood loss
estimated hepatic blood flow
estimated liver blood flow
b. ethanol content
b. ethanol level
evening blood sugar
excessive blood loss
exchange blood transfusion
exercise hyperemia blood flow
exposure to blood or body fluid
b. extracellular fluid
extracorporeal irradiation of b.
extrahepatic blood flow clearance
b. factor in the MNS blood group system
fasting blood glucose
fasting blood sugar
fasting blood work
b. fasting sugar
fecal daily blood loss
fecal occult b.
fecal occult blood test
femoral artery blood flow
femoral blood pressure
fetal scalp b.
b. filtration rate
finger arterial blood pressure
fingerstick blood gas
fingerstick blood glucose
fingerstick blood sample
fingerstick blood sugar
finger systolic blood pressure
fingertip b.
flow of b.
b. flow
flow of blood and oxygen to heart
b. flow to brain
b. flow from artery
b. flow from capillary
b. flow in heart
b. flow rate
b. flow velocity
b. flow velocity waveform
forearm blood flow
b. forming tissues
frank blood in stool
b. from flow heart to lungs
frozen section red blood cell
full blood count
full blood examination
b. gas
b. gas alteration
b. gas analysis
b. gas at room temperature
b. gas measurement
b. gas stick
b. gas study
gastric mucosal blood flow
gated blood pool angiography
gated blood pool scanning
gated blood pool scintigraphy
gated blood pool ventriculogram
gated cardiac blood pool
gated cardiac blood pool imaging
gated blood pool study
gingival blood flow
b. glucose
b. glucose determination
b. glucose level
b. glucose levels
b. glucose monitor
b. glucose monitoring
b. glucose reagent strip
good blood return
b. granulocyte-specific activity
b. group
b. group antigen
b. group class
b. group degrading enzyme
b. group substance
guinea pig red blood cell
hand blood flow
heart attack from blood clot
heart circulates b.
heart rate-systolic blood pressure product
heel-stick blood gas
hemispheric blood flow
hemolytic blood transfusion disease
hemopoietic blood stem cell
hemorrhage and clotted b.
hepatic artery blood flow
hepatic blood flow
hepatotropic portal blood factor
high acid level in b.
high blood alcohol level
high blood cholesterol
high blood pressure
high-frequency blood group
b. histamine
hold breakfast for blood work
home blood glucose meter
home blood glucose monitor
home blood glucose monitoring
home blood pressure measurement
home blood pressure monitoring
home blood sugar monitoring
horse red blood cell
hospital-based blood bank
hospital blood bank
2-hour postprandial blood sugar
human blood bilayer Tween
human immunodeficiency virus infected b.
human peripheral blood leukocyte
human umbilical cord b.
hypothalamic blood flow
immature blood cell
immature red blood cell
immunological fecal occult blood test
impaired blood vessel elasticity
impairment of subendocardial blood flow
improved blood flow
inability to control blood pressure
inadequate blood flow
inadequate blood supply
b. incompatibility
incompatible blood transfusion
incompatible hemolytic blood transfusion
increased blood flow to ear
increased blood flow to heart muscle
increased blood pressure
increased cutaneous blood flow
increased level of blood sugar
increased pressure of b.
indirect blood pressure measuring system
inefficient pumping of b.
infected blood donor
infected red blood cell
inherited blood factor in MNS blood group
inner cortical blood flow
insufficient blood flow
insufficient blood flow to heart
insufficient blood supply
intermittent elevation of blood pressure
interruption of blood supply
interval blood count
intraarterial blood pressure
intracranial blood flow
intracranial blood pressure
intramyocardial coronary blood flow
intraoperative blood loss
intrapartum blood loss
intrathoracic blood volume
intravascular blood coagulation
intravitreal b.
invasive growth of blood cell

invasive growth of blood vessel
irradiated red blood cell
b. isotope clearance
kanamycin-vancomycin blood agar
kanamycin-vancomycin laked blood agar
Kell blood group
Kell blood system
b. lactate
b. lead level
lead level in b.
Lee-White blood clotting method
left heart blood volume
leukocyte-poor red blood cell
Lewis blood group
lidocaine blood concentration
life-threatening blood clot
limb blood flow
liver blood flow
local bone blood flow
local cerebral blood flow
Loeffler blood culture medium
longitudinal blood supply
b. loss
b. loss anemia
low blood gas partition
low blood pressure
low blood sugar
low-frequency blood group
low-frequency blood group antigen
Lu blood group
lung blood volume
Lutheran blood antibody type
Lutheran blood group system
b. and lymphatic system
lymphocytic blood cell
lysed horse b.
maintain blood glucose level
MAST blood test
maternal blood clot patch therapy
maternal blood type
maternal peripheral b.
maximal surgical blood order schedule
mean arterial blood pressure
mean blood glucose
mean cerebral blood flow
mean daily erect blood pressure
mean daily supine blood pressure
mean renal blood flow
mean resting diastolic blood pressure
mean sitting diastolic blood pressure
mediastinal shed b.
medullary blood flow
megakaryocytic blood cell
mesenteric blood flow
microtiter blood typing system
minimal blood loss
minimum blood pressure
a minor blood group
minute volume of air or b.
mixed venous b.
MN blood group
MNS blood group
MNSs blood group
monkey red blood cell
b. monocyte
monocytic blood cell
b. mononuclear cell
mouse red blood cell
mucosal blood flow
mucosal blood hemoglobin
mucosal blood vessel
MUGA cardiac blood pool imaging
multigated cardiac blood pool scanning
multigated blood pool image at rest
multigated blood pool image during exercise
muscle blood flow
myeloid blood element
nadir blood count
narrowed blood vessel
narrowing of blood vessel
National Heart, Lungs, and B. Institute Information Center
negative Rh b.
negligible blood loss
neonatal blood volume
NMN biphasic blood agar
no blood return
noninvasive blood pressure measurement
nonplacental blood flow
normal blood index
normal blood indices
normal blood loss
normal blood pressure
normal sheep red blood cell
Novy and MacNeal blood agar
Novy-McNeal-Nicolle biphasic blood agar
nucleated red blood cell mass
obstructed blood flow
occult b.
occult blood loss
occult blood in stool
occult blood test
occult blood testing
office blood pressure
onset of blood lactate accumulation
oozing of b.
oozing of blood from nose
oozing of blood from nostril
b. oozing from os
operative blood loss
orbital blood cyst
orbital blood flow
organ blood flow
Oriental blood fluke
orthostatic blood pressure
osmolarity of b.
osmolarity of blood and urine
outer cortical blood flow
ova, blood, and parasites
ox red blood cell
oxygenated blood supply
b. oxygenation level-dependent
b. oxygen capacity
oxygen capacity of b.
oxygen concentration in pulmonary capillary b.
oxygen content of b.
oxygen content of blood decreases
oxygen content of mixed venous b.
b. oxygen release rate
packed human blood cell
packed red blood cell
packed red blood cell transfusion
Pall-filtered whole b.
pancreatic blood flow
partial oxygen pressure in mixed venous b.
partial pressure of carbon dioxide in mixed venous b.
passage of b.
b. patch injection
patient admitted and transfused with whole b.
patient vomited large quantities of b.
patient vomiting b.
P blood group
P blood group antigen
P blood group system
peak blood level
peak blood pressure
peak reactive hyperemia blood flow
penile blood flow
penile blood flow study
penile blood pressure

blood *(continued)*
percutaneous umbilical blood sampling
b. perfusion monitor
periesophageal blood vessel
periodic blood transfusion
peripheral b.
peripheral blood $CD8^+$ lymphocytosis
peripheral blood cell
peripheral blood cell count
peripheral blood circulation
peripheral blood count
peripheral blood eosinophilia
peripheral blood eosinophils
peripheral blood labeling index
peripheral blood leukocyte
peripheral blood lymphocyte analysis
peripheral blood lymphocyte transformation
peripheral blood mononuclear cell
peripheral blood mononuclear cell hepatitis B virus measurement
peripheral blood preparation
peripheral blood preparation for microfilariae
peripheral blood pressure
peripheral blood progenitor cell
peripheral blood progenitor cell transplant
peripheral blood smear
peripheral blood stem cell
peripheral blood stem cell autografting
peripheral blood stem cell infusion
peripheral blood stem cell rescue
peripheral blood stem cell reserve
peripheral blood stem cell support
peripheral blood stem cell transplantation
peripheral blood studies
peripheral white blood cell
permission for blood transfusion
b. per rectum
placental residual blood volume
plaque in blood vessel
b. plasma measuring system
b. platelet disorder
platelet-poor b.
b. pool activity
b. pool imaging
poor blood circulation
portal vein blood flow velocity
postural blood pressure
potentially infectious blood specimen
predicted blood volume
preoperative autologous blood donation
b. pressure
b. pressure assembly
b. pressure decreased
b. pressure monitor
b. pressure and pulse
b. pressure, pulse, respiration, and temperature
b. pressure recorder
b. pressure, right arm
primary high blood pressure
b. product contaminated by acquired immune deficiency syndrome
b. production rate
production of red blood cells
pulmonary blood clot
pulmonary blood mixing volume
pulmonary blood volume index
pulmonary capillary blood volume
pulmonary capillary blood flow perfusion
pulsed ultrasonic blood velocity detector
pulse oximetry waveform systolic blood pressure
pure red blood cell agenesis
pure red blood cell aplasia
radioreceptor assay pregnancy b.
random blood glucose
random blood sugar
rapid whole blood test
Rasor blood pumping system
reactive hyperemia blood flow
recycled human blood substitute
red blood cell adenosine deaminase
red blood cell adherence
red blood cell count
red blood cell fallout
red blood cell fragility
red blood cell immune adherence
red blood cell mass
red blood cells per high-power field
red blood cell spun filtration
red blood cell transfusion
red blood cell volume
red blood corpuscle
red blood cell agglutination
red blood cell cast
red blood cell concentrate
red blood cell diameter width
red blood cell distribution width index
red blood cell filter ability
red blood cell folate
red blood cell iron turnover
red blood cell iron turnover rate
red blood cell-linked antigen-antiglobulin reaction
red blood cell to plasma ratio
red blood cell precursor production rate
red blood cell suspension
reduced blood flow to brain
reduced blood supply to heart
red venous b.
regional cerebral blood flow
regional cerebral blood volume
regional distribution of hepatic blood flow
regional myocardial blood flow
regional pulmonary blood flow
renal cortical blood flow
resting blood pressure
retrograde blood flow
revascularization of blood vessels of heart
reversed vertebral blood flow
Rh blood factor
Rh blood group
right heart blood volume
room air blood gas
ruptured blood vessels
saturation of oxygen in arterial b.
Sciana blood group
seated diastolic blood pressure
secondary high blood pressure
b. and secretion
b. sedimentation rate
self-monitored blood glucose
semen, hair and b.
serial blood sugar
b. serologic test
serum blood sugar
sheep red blood cell
sickle red blood cell
single-nephron glomerular blood flow
slow blood clotting
sluggish blood return
small blood pressure cuff
small vessel inadequate blood flow
spinal cord blood flow
splanchnic blood flow
splenic blood flow

sponge blood loss
standing diastolic blood pressure
stool positive for occult b.
b. sugar level
sulfation factor of blood serum
superior mesenteric artery blood flow
superior mesenteric artery blood velocity
supine diastolic blood pressure
b. supply of brain
b. supply to heart
surgical blood order equation
swallowed blood syndrome
systemic blood flow
systemic blood pressure
systolic, diastolic, mean blood pressure
tainted blood transfusion
tanned red blood cell agglutination
tanned red blood cell hemagglutination
tanned red blood cell hemagglutination inhibition
b. temperature chart
b. thinning agent
thin-walled blood vessel
toe blood pressure
tortuous blood vessel
total blood granulocyte pool
total cerebral blood flow
total pulmonary blood flow
total red blood cells
total renal blood flow
total blood volume predicted from body surface
total white blood cells
trace occult b.
tracheal blood flow
tracking blood flow to the brain
b. transfusion refusal form
b. transfusion therapy
trypsinized sheep red blood cell
b. type
b. type in ABO blood group
b. type A negative
b. type A, O positive
type and crossmatch b.
b. type O negative
b. typing
umbilical cord b.
umbilical cord blood culture
umbilical cord blood leukocyte
uncontrolled high blood pressure
unit of packed red blood cells
unit of whole b.
universal blood donor
b. urea
b. urea nitrogen
b. urea nitrogen/creatinine ratio
b. uric acid
velocity of sound of b.
venous b.
venous blood circulation
venous blood gas
venous blood pressure
venous blood sample
b. vessel
b. vessel endothelium
b. vessel graft
b. vessel inflammation
b. vessel invasion
b. vessel prosthesis
b. viscosity
b. volume
volume of blood flow
b. volume expander
b. volume expansion
volume of packed red blood cells
b. volume pulse
b. warmer
washed red blood cell
b. Wassermann
white blood cell count
white blood cell depletion
white blood cell scan
white blood cells per high-power field
white blood cell transfusion
white blood corpuscle
whole b.
whole blood transfusion
whole blood volume

blood-air barrier

blood-borne
b.-b. agent
b.-b. infection
b.-b. infectious agent
OSHA blood-borne pathogen standard

blood-brain barrier

blood-brain-tumor barrier

blood-cerebrospinal fluid barrier

blood-clot lysis time

blood-clotting mechanism effects

blood-forming organ

bloodletting
local b.

blood-negative
occult b.-n.

blood-nerve barrier

blood-positive
occult b.-p.

blood-retinal barrier

blood-starved heart muscle tissue

bloodstream
alcohol in b.
bacterial infection of b.
catheter-related bloodstream infection
hospital-acquired bloodstream infection
b. infection

blood-tinged
b.-t. fluid
b.-t. sputum
b.-t. stool
b.-t. urine

bloody
aspiration of bloody material
cough productive of bloody sputum
dark bloody material
dark bloody stool
b. discharge from breast
grossly b.
grossly bloody stool
b. tap
b. vaginal discharge
watery and bloody diarrhea

Bloom syndrome

blossom
orange b.

blot
dot blot analysis
enzyme-linked immunotransfer b.
ink blot test
Northern blot analysis
Northern blot technique
Northern blot test
Southern b.
Southern blot analysis
Western b.
Western blot analysis
Western blot test
Western ligand b.

blotch
palpebral b.

blotting
ligand b.
Western b.

blow
- b. bottle
- b. to head
- lethal b.

blow-in
- orbital blow-in fracture

blowing
- maximum duration of sustained b.
- b. systolic murmur

blow-out
- orbital floor b.-o.
- orbital blow-out fracture

blowout
- aortic stump b.
- b. pipette
- pure blowout fracture

blue
- Agent B.
- Alcian b.
- Alcian blue and periodic acid-Schiff
- Alcian blue stain
- aniline blue modified trichrome stain
- b. bloater
- brilliant cresyl blue stain
- bromothymol b.
- bromothymol blue lactose
- bromphenol b.
- carbolic methylene b.
- cellular blue nevus
- code b.
- Coomassie brilliant blue R-250 stain
- dextran b.
- b. diaper syndrome
- b. dome cyst
- Evans blue dye
- lentigines, atrial myxomas, cutaneous papular myxomas, blue nevi
- Loeffler methylene blue dye
- Loeffler methylene blue stain
- Luxol fast blue stain
- malignant blue nevus
- Mallory aniline blue stain
- Martius scarlet b.
- methylene b.
- methylene blue active substance
- methylene blue enema
- methylene blue instillation
- methylene blue line
- methylene blue, reduced
- methylene blue reduction time
- methylene blue stain
- methylene blue test
- methylthymol b.
- methylthymol blue complex
- Nair buffered methylene blue stain
- narrow-spectrum blue light
- new methylene blue N stain
- Nile blue A
- Nile blue fat stain
- no code b.
- out of the b.
- patent blue V
- patent blue V dye
- paternity b.'s
- periodic acid-Schiff-Alcian b.
- periodic acid-Schiff-Alcian blue combination stain
- polychrome methylene blue stain
- b. skin from blood clot
- b. tetrazolium
- b. toe syndrome
- toluidine b.
- toluidine blue stain
- b. tongue
- winter b.'s

blueberry
- nodular blueberry lips

bluegrass
- annual b.

blue-green algae

bluetongue virus 1–24

blunderbuss

blunt
- b. arthroscopic cannula
- b. caliper
- b. cardiac injury
- b. carotid injury
- b. dissection carried upward
- end-biting blunt nosed rongeur
- freed by blunt dissection
- b. hook
- b. injury
- b. injury to heart
- b. Metzenbaum scissors
- multiple blunt trauma
- b. nose hemostat
- b. probe
- sharp and blunt dissection
- b. and sharp dissection
- b. stylet
- b. tapered T-handled reamer
- b. trauma

blunted
- b. affect
- b. or flat affect

blunting
- affective b.
- caliceal b.
- costal border b.
- costophrenic b.
- costophrenic angle b.
- emotional b.
- Scale for Emotional B.

blunt-tip iris scissors

blunt-tipped epidural needle

blur
- b. artifact
- indistinct b.
- motion b.
- optical b.

blurred
- episode of blurred vision
- b. or fuzzy vision
- b. sensory perceptions
- b. vision from anemia
- b. vision from diabetes
- b. vision in one eye

blurring
- b. or dimming of vision
- gradual blurring of vision
- b. of vision
- visual b.

blurry
- distant objects b.

blush
- angiographic b.
- capillary b.
- erythematous b.
- marrow b.
- myocardial b.
- papillary b.
- terminal b.
- tumor b.

B-lymphocyte
- monocytoid B-l.
- B-l. stimulatory factor

board
- adjustable cane b.
- bed b.
- b. and care
- b. certified
- b. certified psychiatrist
- data monitoring b.
- b. eligible
- full spine b.
- b. of health
- health b.
- institutional review b.
- long back b.
- medical b.

Minnesota Paper Form B. Test
Permanent Disability Rating B.
powder b.
rating b.
research and development b.
slide b.

board-and-care
b.-a.-c. facility
b.-a.-c. home

boarding
b. home
personal care boarding home

board-like rigidity of abdomen

boat-shaped heart

Bobaya virus

bobbing
head b.
monocular bobbing movement
ocular b.
ocular bobbing nystagmus

Bobia virus

Bodansky unit

bodily
b. complaint
contaminated with bodily fluid
b. function
grievous bodily harm
b. injury
self-inflicted bodily injury

Bod unit

body
b. acceleration synchronous with heart rate
actual body weight
adjusted body mass
alcoholic hyaline inclusion b.
altered body temperature
altered mind-body perception
anal foreign b.
ankle loose b.
anorectal foreign b.
anterior border of body of pancreas
anterior cervical body fusion
anterior nucleus of trapezoid b.
anterior quadrigeminal b.
anterior vertebral body margin
anthrax-infected body fluid
aortic body tumor
apocrine body odor
artificial vertebral b.
asbestos b.
aspirated foreign b.
aspiration of foreign b.
avascular vertebral body necrosis
average body dose
basal body temperature
b. belt
bilateral carotid body resection
blood and body fluid precaution
bronchial foreign b.
Cabot ring b.
calcified free b.
care of body after death
carotid b.
carotid body denervation
carotid body tumor
carotid bodies resected
b. cavity-based lymphoma
b. cell mass
central fibrous b.
cervical mucous basal body temperature
ciliary body band
cognitive change of body image
computed body tomography
congenital Heinz body hemolytic anemia
conjunctival foreign b.
core body balance
core body temperature
cortical Lewy b.
curvilinear b.
cushingoid body habitus
cytomegalic inclusion b.
cytoplasmic inclusion b.
decalcified section of vertebral b.
decreased body hair
dementia with Lewy b.
dense b.
desirable body weight
diffuse Lewy body dementia
diffuse Lewy body disease
distorted body image
Döhle b.
Döhle body panmyelopathy
dry body weight
b. dysmorphic disorder
B. Dysmorphic Disorder Modification of Yale-Brown Obsessive-Compulsive Scale, McLean version
elementary b.
esophageal b.
esophageal foreign b.
esthetic body contouring
estimated fetal body weight
exchangeable body potassium
exposure to blood or body fluid
extracellular mass to body cell mass ratio
extracorporeal whole body hyperthermia
b. fat
field size in half body irradiation
flexion body cast
flexion body jacket
foreign b.
foreign body in air passage
foreign body in iris
foreign body removal
foreign body retained
foreign body soft tissue
foreign body of the cornea
foreign body-type granuloma
foreign body sensation
fractionated total body irradiation
full body immersion
generalized body irradiation
generalized body weakness
gluteal body fat
Gram stain of body fluid
granulomembranous b.
b. hair
b. hair distribution
head, limbs, and b.
b. heat
Heinz body hemolytic anemia
b. hematocrit-venous hematocrit ratio
hemolytic immune b.
Howell-Jolly b.
hyoid b.
ideal body mass
ideal body weight
b. identification
immune b.
impacted foreign b.
incidental Lewy b.
inclusion b.
inclusion body myositis
index of body build
infectious body fluid
inhalation of foreign b.
initial body mass index
internal body heat
internal body temperature
intraocular foreign b.
intrauterine foreign b.
intravascular foreign body retrieval
involuntary body function
involuntary body movement
involuntary trembling of b.
iodine-131 total body scan
iris ciliary b.
jerking of b.

body *(continued)*
ketone body ratio
lamellar b.
lamellar body count
lamellar body density
last body mass index
lateral geniculate b.
lean body mass
lean body muscle mass
lean body weight
Lewy body dementia
Lewy body disease
lipid b.
Lipschütz inclusion b.
long axis of b.
loose b.
loose body in joint
low body mass index
lower body negative pressure
lower GI tract foreign b.
lupus erythematosus b.
Luys body syndrome
lymphoid b.
lysosomal dense b.
Mallory b.
malpighian body of kidney
malpighian body of spleen
mamillary body volume
mammillary b.
mandible b.
mandibular body fracture
mandibular body length
marfanoid body habitus
b. mass
b. mass index
maximum assistance for lower body dressing
maximum assistance for upper body dressing
measles inclusion body encephalitis
medial geniculate b.
medial nucleus of trapezoid b.
medullary body of cerebellum
medullary body of vermis
membranous cytoplasmic b.
metallic foreign b.
minimal assistance for lower body dressing
minimal assistance for upper body dressing
Müller duct b.
multivesicular b.
navicular body fracture
negative balance of body fluid
negative body image
Negri b.
nerve cell b.
neuroendocrine b.
neuroepithelial body in lung
neuronal ceroid lipofuscinosis curvilinear b.
normal body temperature
nuclear inclusion b.
nucleus of mamillary b.
obstructed by foreign b.
occult annular ciliary b.
b. odor
opaque foreign b.
orbital fat b.
b. oscillation neuromuscular gain
osmiophilic lamellar inclusion b.
oval fat b.
owl's eye inclusion b.
oxytocinergic cell b.
Pappenheimer b.
b. part
partial body neutron activation
parts of human b.
patient independent in lower body dressing
patient independent in upper body dressing
peduncle of mamillary b.
perception of body image
perineal b.
pigmented layer of ciliary b.
pineal b.
plane of b.
b. plethysmography
polyp of body of stomach
poor body image
postmenopausal body mass
progressive weakness on one side of the b.
ramus, body, symphysis, palate
rapid body shaper
region of b.
regulation of body temperature
relative body weight
removal of foreign b.
Renaut b.
retained foreign b.
reticulate b.
right atrium b.
round b.
b. segment parameter
subacute inclusion body encephalitis
b. substance isolation
sudden body jerk
superior border of body of pancreas
b. surface area
b. surface burned
b. surface Laplacian mapping
b. surface potential mapping
surgical foreign b.
b. temperature
temperature, b.
b. temperature, pressure, dry
total b.
total blood volume predicted from body surface
total body bone mineral
total body bone mineral density
total body calcium
total body clearance
total body counting
total body density
total body electrical conductivity
total body fat
total body hematocrit
total body hyperthermia
total body irritation
total body mass
total body neutron activation
total body neutron activation analysis
total body nitrogen
total body phosphorus
total body photograph
total body potassium
total body protein
total body protein turnover
total body radiation
total body scan
total body scanning
total body sodium
total body solids
total body solute
total body surface
total body surface area
total body washout
total body water
tracheobronchial foreign b.
trapezoid b.
ultimobranchial b.
upper body ergometer
upper body segment to lower body segment ratio
usual body weight
vertebral body decompression
vertebral body endplate
vertebral body fracture
vertebral body shape
vertebral body size
vertebral body tenderness
b. water
b. weight
b. weight gain

whole b.
withdrawal body shakes
b. worn hearing aid
zebra b.

body's
b. natural defense mechanism
b. infection-fighting immune system
b. natural healing ability
b. tumor-killing ability

Boehm Test of Basic Concepts

Bogdanovac
Yug Bogdanovac virus

boggy uterus

bogus
anticipatory bogus heart rate feedback

Bohr
B. magneton
B. radius
ratio of magnetic moment of a particle to Bohr magneton

boil
b.'s at
Madura b.
Oriental b.

boiled
whole boiled milk

boiling
b. point
b. range

boisterous
aggressively b.

Boix-Ochoa score

bolete
pepper bolete mushroom

Boletus virus X

Bolivian hemorrhagic fever

bolster
angular b.
breast b.
cotton b.
b. dressing
muscular b.
padded b.
rubber b.
b. suture technique

bolt
b. cutter
b. fixation
Moreira b.
No-Lok b.

Bolton craniometric point

Bolton-Hunter reagent

Boltzmann constant

bolus
aerosol bolus dispersion
atrial bolus dynamic computed tomography
b. injection
magnetic bolus tracking
milk bolus obstruction
normal saline b.
obstructing bolus of food
peripheral bolus chase
b. thermodilution
b. tie-over graft

bombardment
end of saturated b.
fast atom b.
fast atom bombardment mass spectrometry
rhythmic sensory bombardment therapy

bomb calorimeter

bond
double b.
b. grafting
PDI-mediated disulfide bond reduction
Tc b.
technetium b.
type of molecular b.
valence b.

bondage
b. and discipline
physical b.

bonded
noncovalently bonded dimer of C-terminal immunoglobulin of Fc fragment
b. retainer
b. space maintainer

bonding
affiliation b.
direct bonding system
human b.
maternal-infant b.
mother-infant b.
parental bonding instrument

bone
abnormal bone growth
absolute bone conduction
absolute volume of trabecular b.
acrylic bone cement
adult bone marrow
adynamic bone disease
aerobic bone marrow culture
b. age
b. age ratio
agonadism, mental retardation, short stature, retarded bone age syndrome
air and bone conduction
air conduction and bone conduction
air greater than bone conduction
Albert-Linder bone sectioning
b. alkaline phosphatase
allogeneic bone marrow cell
allogeneic bone marrow transplant
allogeneic bone marrow transplantation
allogenic bone crib
allogenic bone graft
allogenic bone marrow
allogenic bone marrow cell infusion
allogenic bone marrow transplantation
allogenic lyophilized bone graft implant material
allogenous bone graft
allograft bone grafting
allograft iliac b.
alpha bone substitute material
alpha-BSM bone repair material
alpha-BSM bone substitute material
aluminum bone disease
amputation-related bone pain
aneurysmal bone cyst
angiosarcoma bone tumor
angled Lowman-type bone clamp
angular bone rongeur
anisotropic bone property
anterior condyloid canal of occipital b.
anterior suspension of hyoid b.
antiepileptic drug-induced bone disease
antigen-extracted allogeneic b.
antigen-extracted allogenic b.
apex of petrous part of temporal b.
apex of petrous portion of temporal b.
aplastic bone disease
aplastic bone disorder
aplastic bone lesion
aplastic bone marrow
appendicular bone mass measurement

bone *(continued)*
arch of b.
architectural alterations of b.
areal bone mineral density
areola of b.
articular bone lamella
articular bone loss
articular bone tubercle
articular eminence of temporal b.
articular fossa of temporal b.
articular lamella of b.
articular surface of mandibular fossa of temporal b.
articular surface on calcaneus for cuboid b.
articular surface of temporal b.
articular tubercle of temporal b.
articulating bone end
articulation of pisiform b.
aseptic necrosis of b.
aspiration of b.
atrophy of b.
attic temporal b.
autogenous bone graft
autogenous bone grafting
autogenous bone slurry
autogenous cancellous bone graft
autogenous iliac b.
autograft bone grafting
autologous bone marrow
autologous bone marrow cell
autologous bone marrow reinfusion
autologous bone marrow rescue
autologous bone marrow support
autologous bone marrow transplant
autologous cancellous bone graft
autologous iliac crest bone graft
autologous peripheral blood stem cell bone marrow transplantation
autologous rib bone graft
avascular bone necrosis
avascular necrosis of b.
banked freeze-dried b.
b. bank graft
b. biopsy needle
b. block
b. borer
both b.'s
both bones fracture
calcium bone index
cancellous cellular b.
cancellous cellular bone graft
cancellous chip bone graft
cancellous and cortical bone graft
cancellous morselized bone graft
cancellous versus cortical b.
candle wax appearance of b.
cantilevered bone graft
cantilevered split cranial bone graft
caries of b.
caries of petrous b.
carpal navicular b.
cavity of b.
b. cement implantation syndrome
central hyoid b.
cerebral yokes of bone of cranium
b. chip graft
chronic bone pain
coalition of b.
compact substance of b.
compensatory bone resorption
b. conduction
b. conduction greater than air conduction
b. conduction hearing aid
b. conduction less than air conduction
contour of nasal b.
b. core
cornu of hyoid b.
b. cortex
cortical bone allograft
cortical bone graft
cortical bone infarct
cortical bone lesion
cortical bone modeling
cortical bone plate
cortical bone remodeling
cortical bone resorption
cortical bone screw
cortical substance of b.
corticocancellous bone graft
creeping substitution of b.
crest of iliac b.
cryopreserved bone marrow
curved bone rongeur
cut end of b.
debilitating bone disease
débrided bone surfaces
decalcified freeze-dried bone allograft
decalcified freeze-dried cortical b.
decreased bone mineral density
degenerative bone change
degenerative bone marrow disease
demineralized b.
demineralized bone graft
demineralized bone matrix
demineralized bone powder
demineralized freeze-dried b.
demineralized freeze-dried bone allograft
density and strength of bone mass
depression of nasal b.
detection of bone spur
devitalized allogeneic b.
devitalized bone graft
devitalized portion of b.
diamond inlay bone graft
diastasis of cranial b.
direct-current bone growth stimulator
disordered bone growth
displacement bone marrow transplantation
donor bone marrow
donor bone marrow engraftment
donor site of bone graft
b. dowel
dowel bone graft
dowel-shaped bone graft
eburnated bone surface
eburnized bone end
ectopic bone growth
electrical bone stimulation
enchondral bone formation
end of bone covered with flap
endochondral bone deposits
eosinophilic fibrohistiocytic lesion of bone marrow
erosion surface per bone surface
ethmoidal crest of palatine b.
European compression technique bone screw and internal fixation
excessive bone loss
extensive new bone formation
b. extractor
b. felon
b. to femur graft
fetal bone marrow
first cuneiform b.
b. forceps
b. formation rate
fracture of both b.'s
fracture of both b.'s
fracture running length of b.
b. fragment
free-floating bone chip
freeze-dried bone allograft
freeze-dried bone pin
freeze-dried demineralized b.
b. Gla protein
gradual loss of bone tissue
b. graft
b. graft donor
b. graft punch

b. graft shoe horn
b. graft site
great toe b.
b. growth
b. growth and breakdown
guided bone regeneration
b. hardening artifact
harvest bone marrow
b. head
b. healing method
heel bone density scan
hereditary bone disease
hereditary bone dysplasia
b. holder
homogenous bone graft
human bone marrow
hypophosphatemic bone disease
idiopathic aplastic bone marrow
iliac cancellous b.
iliac crest bone graft
b. imaging
b. impactor
b. implant
implantable bone growth stimulator
b. implant material
incompatible bone marrow
incomplete fracture of b.
increased bone density
increased bone mass
b. infection
infection penetrated b.
inferior point of pubic b.
b. infusion
injecting bone cement
b. injury
inlay bone graft
insoluble bone gelatin
intact bone structure
interclavicular notch of occipital b.
interclavicular notch of temporal b.
interruption in continuity of b.
intractable bone pain
intramedullary bone graft
irradiated b.
irregularly shaped b.
ischemic bone necrosis
ischemic necrosis of b.
isotope bone scan
b. and joint examination
b. and joint infection
b. or joint pathology
joints and b.'s
b.'s, joints, and muscles
b.'s, joints, and muscles
jugular notch of temporal b.
lateral frontal bone window
limb bone length ratio
limbus of sphenoid b.
b. liner
lingual alveolar b.
liver, iron, red bone marrow
local bone blood flow
localized bone destruction
Locke bone clamp
long axis of b.
long bone deficiency
long bone fracture
long bone length
long bone osteomyelitis
long bone pseudoarthrosis
long bone survey
b. loss
loss of bone mass
low bone density
low bone mass
low bone turnover disease
lower frontal bone fracture
lower third of leg b.
low-turnover bone lesion
lumbar spine bone density
lumbar spine bone mineral density
lump growing in b.
lymphomatous bone marrow involvement
lyophilized bone graft
lytic area bone flap
lytic bone lesion
malar crest of great wing of sphenoid b.
malignant bone aneurysm
malignant fibrous histiocytoma of b.
malignant neoplasm of b.
marble bone disease
marble bone pattern
marble bone pin
marginal tubercle of zygomatic b.
b. marrow
b. marrow acid phosphatase
marrow agent bone scintigraphy
b. marrow arrest
b. marrow aspirate
b. marrow biopsy
b. marrow cell
b. marrow culture
b. marrow depression
b. marrow-derived cultured mast cell
b. marrow failure
b. marrow infection
b. marrow infusion
b. marrow lymphocyte
b. marrow lymphocytosis
b. marrow micrometastasis
b. marrow myeloid precursor
b. marrow necrosis
b. marrow neutrophil reserve
b. marrow pressure
b. marrow removed and stored
b. marrow stem cell
b. marrow suppression
b. marrow tap
b. marrow toxicity
b. marrow transplant
b. marrow transplant neutropenia
b. marrow transplant rejection
b. marrow transplant unit
mastoid angle of parietal b.
mastoid bone fracture
mastoid border of occipital b.
mastoid margin of occipital b.
matrix
Matti-Russe bone graft
McIndoe bone rongeur
McMaster bone graft
medial cuneiform b.
Medicare B. Mass Measurement Standardization Act
medullary bone graft
medullary bone infarct
medullary bone pain
membrane of b.
mesenchymal bone tumor
metabolic bone disorder
metabolic bone series
metabolic bone survey
metacarpal b.
metacarpophalangeal bone marrow development
b. metastasis
metastatic bone lesion
metastatic bone survey
metatarsophalangeal bone marrow development
methydiphosphonate bone scan
Michigan Bone Health Study
microvascular bone transfer
middle cuneiform b.
middle third of long b.
mildly hyperplastic bone marrow
b. mill
Miltner rotary bone rasp
b. mineral content
b. mineral densitometry
b. mineral density
b. mineralization

bone *(continued)*
mineralized bone histology
b. mineral mass
mixed bone lesion
mixed sclerosing bone dysplasia, small stature, seizures, mental retardation syndrome
mixed sclerosing bone dystrophy
morcellized bone graft
b. morphogenetic protein
b. morphogenetic protein type 2
b. mortise
mortise of b.
Moseley bone age graph
moth-eaten bone destruction
mouse-specific bone marrow-derived lymphocyte antigen
MPO bone marrow stain
multiple bone enchondromata
multiple bone myeloma
muscles of hyoid b.
b.'s, muscles, joints
b.'s, muscles, joints
myeloperoxidase bone marrow stain
nasal bone fragment
nasal border of frontal b.
nasal crest of horizontal plate of palatine b.
nasal margin of frontal b.
navicular bone of hand
necrotic bone pseudocyst
negative bone scan
new bone formation
Newcastle bone disease
new column of b.
Nicoll cancellous bone graft
no bone injury
no bone pathology
noncollagen bone matrix
noninvolved b.
nonvascularized bone graft
normal bone marrow
normal bone marrow extract
Northland bone density machine
nuclear bone imaging
nude bone graft transplantation
nutrient canal of b.
occipital angle of parietal b.
occipital bone jugular incisure
occipital border of parietal b.
occipital border of temporal b.
occipital margin of temporal b.
occult bone metastasis
onlay bone graft
onlay bone graft cast
onlay bone grafting
open bone graft epiphysiodesis
orbital arch of frontal b.
orbital bone hypoplasia
orbital border of sphenoid b.
orbital eminence of zygomatic b.
orbital lamina of ethmoid b.
orbital layer of ethmoid b.
orbital plane of frontal b.
orbital plate of ethmoid b.
orbital plate of frontal b.
orbital wing of sphenoid b.
orthopaedic bone file
os calcis b.
osseous bone contusion
ossifying bone fibroma
osteoblastic bone regeneration
osteoblast-mediated bone formation
osteoclast-activated bone resorption
osteoclast-driven bone resorption
osteoclastic bone resorption
osteoclast-mediated bone resorption
osteoconductive bone grafting material
osteogenic bone fibroma
Osteomin freeze-dried b.
osteonal bone union
osteopenic bone stock
osteoperiosteal bone graft
osteoperiosteal iliac bone graft
osteophytic bone lip
osteoplastic bone flap
osteoporosis of b.
osteosarcoma of b.
overlay cantilevered bone graft
Pacific Coast demineralized cortical bone powder
Paget disease of b.
pagetic bone lesion
palatal bone osteotomy
palatine bone fissure
palatine crest of horizontal process of palatine b.
palatomaxillary groove of palatine b.
Papineau bone graft
paraarticular bone remodeling
paramedian frontal bone window
parietal bone flap
parietal bone thickness
parietal bone thinning
parietal border of frontal b.
parietal border of sphenoid b.
parietal border of squamous part of temporal b.
parietal margin of frontal b.
parosteal bone lesion
particulate cancellous bone graft
particulate cancellous bone and marrow
b. paste
patellar bone-tendon-bone autograft
peak adult bone mass
peak bone mass
pediatric bone rongeur
pedicle bone graft
peg bone graft
b. pegging
percutaneous autogenous dowel bone graft
percutaneous bone marrow infection
percutaneous bone marrow injection
percutaneous core bone biopsy
periodic bone pain
periosteal bone collar
periprosthetic bone loss
periprosthetic bone resorption
b. phosphate of lime
photon-deficient bone lesion
b. plug cutter
b. plug extractor
b. plug setter
poor bone stock
porcine bone marrow transplantation
porous and spongy b.
postmenopausal bone loss
b. powder
predominant hyperparathyroid bone disease
primary bone cancer
primary bone lymphoma
primary bone sarcoma
primary lymphoma of b.
primary non-Hodgkin lymphoma of b.
proliferation of b.
prominence of b.
proximal third of b.
b. pulley
quantitative bone ultrasound
radiographic bone strength index
radionuclear bone scan
radionuclide bone scan
radiopaque bone cement
b. ramus
rapid bone loss
rapid loss of b.
b. rasp

Recklinghausen disease of b.
recombinant human bone morphogenetic protein
regenerating bone marrow extract
regional bone mass
replaced with new b.
retard bone activity
ring of b.
b. rongeur
Russe bone graft
b. scan reveals increased activity
b. scan showed increased activity
scaphoid fossa of sphenoid b.
b. seeker
segmental bone defect
segmental bone loss
severe bone loss
severed surface of b.
shaft of b.
shin bone fever
b. sialoprotein
sliding inlay bone graft
b. slurry
small bone structure
solid bone mass
solitary bone cyst
solitary bone lesion
solitary plasmacytoma of b.
b. spacer
sphenoid bone fracture
spongy part of b.
b. spreader
stimulate bone formation
stump of b.
b. suturing wire chisel-tip wire
swelling deformity of affected b.
syphilis of b.
tarsal bone fracture
temporal bone fracture
thinning process of b.
third cuneiform b.
three-phase bone scintigraphy
three-phase radionuclide bone scanning
total body bone mineral
total body bone mineral density
total trabecular bone volume
trabecular bone volume
trabeculated bone lesion
b. transfer
traumatic bone cyst
b. trough
tuberosity of carpal b.
tuberosity of cuboid b.
tuberosity of fifth metatarsal b.
b. tunnel
ulnar styloid b.
b. ultrasound attenuation
ultrasound bone imaging sonometer
Universal bone plate
upper third of long b.
vascularized bone graft
vascularized bone marrow transplantation
vertebral bone loss
volumetric bone mineral density
b. weapon
b. wedge
wedge-shaped cut into b.
whole-body bone scan
whole bone transplant graft
yellow bone marrow

bone-age
Tanner-Whitehouse Mark 2 bone-age assessment

bone-anchored
b.-a. hearing aid
b.-a. prosthesis

bone-biting
b.-b. punch
b.-b. trephine

bone-breaking forceps

bone-conduction
b.-c. oscillator
b.-c. receiver
b.-c. vibrator

bone-contacting surface ratio

bone-cutting forceps

bone-derived growth factor

bone-graft plug

bone-grasping forceps

bone-patellar
b.-p. ligament-bone
b.-p. tendon-bone

bone-reduction
alligator bone-reduction forceps

bone-resorbing activity

bone-specific alkaline phosphatase

bone-tendon-bone

Bonnet
Charles Bonnet syndrome

bonnet
gluteal b.

bony
b. abnormality
b. alignment
b. architecture
area of bony destruction
b. callus
coiled bony structure
demineralized bony structure
full bony impaction
b. growth
b. hard palate
b. healing
b. heart
b. hump
b. insertion
b. interorbital distance
b. landmark
lingual bony expansion
lingular mandibular bony defect
b. nonunion
palpable bony abnormality
partial bony impaction
periodontal bony defect
physeal bony bridging
plantar bony prominence
b. remodeling
b. thorax
b. union

book
doctor's order b.
open book fracture
oriented to time, place, person, and objects watch, pen, b.

booklet
Mentor b.

boost
arousal b.
arousal boost mechanism
electron beam b.
b. field
pelvic boost radiotherapy

booster
antitetanus b.
b. heart

boosting
patient independent in boosting and rolling

boot
cast boot brace
compression b.
intermittent pneumatic compression b.
Moon b.
oxygen disposable boot device
plaster b.
pneumatic compression b.
Unna b.
walking boot cast
Wilke boot brace

boot-shaped heart

Boraceia virus

border

alveolar occlusal b.
anterior border of body of pancreas
anterior border of eyelid
anterior border of fibula
anterior border of heart
anterior border of lung
anterior border of radius
anterior border of testis
anterior border of tibia
anterior border of ulna
antibrush border antibody
antimesenteric border of distal ileum
arrhythmogenic border zone
arterial border zone
asymmetry, border, color, and diameter of melanoma
automated border detection
automated border detection by echocardiography
brush b.
brush border membrane
cardiac border of dullness
costal border blunting
b. detection method
b. disease virus
Doctors Without B.'s
endocardial border delineation
heard best at left lower sternal b.
heard best at left upper sternal b.
indistinct cell b.
interosseous border of fibula
interosseous border of radius
interosseous border of tibia
interosseous border of ulna
intestinal brush b.
left border of cardiac dullness
left costal b.
left border dullness of heart to percussion
left lateral b.
left lower border of cardiac dullness
left lower scapular b.
left lower sternal b.
left sternal b.
left upper scapular b.
left upper sternal b.
lip border advancement
lower sternal b.
mastoid border of occipital bone
medial border of foot
medial border of forearm
medial border of humerus
medial border of kidney
medial border of scapula
medial border of suprarenal gland
medial border of tibia
mesovarian border of ovary
nasal border of frontal bone
nasal border of optic disc
occipital border of parietal bone
occipital border of temporal bone
occult border of nail
orbital border of sphenoid bone
outer border of iris
outer border of the uterus
parietal border of frontal bone
parietal border of sphenoid bone
parietal border of squamous part of temporal bone
peroneal border of foot
poorly differentiated defined b.
posterior border of eyelid
posterior border of fibula
posterior border of heart
right border cardiac dullness
right border of heart
right heart b.
right lower border of cardiac dullness
right lower scapular b.
right lower sternal b.
right middle sternal b.
right sternal b.
right upper sternal b.
rounded border of lung
shelving border of inguinal ligament
sternal b.
superior border of body of pancreas
tibial border of foot
ulnar border of forearm
upper left sternal b.
upper right sternal b.

bordering on insanity

borderline

b. of cardiac dullness
b. dull
endocervical mucinous borderline tumor
b. glucose tolerance test
b. high blood pressure
b. hypertensive
b. intellectual functioning
intestinal mucinous borderline tumor
b. left axis deviation
b. lepromatous
b. malignancy
mucinous borderline ovarian tumors
ovarian borderline tumor
ovarian serous borderline tumor
peritoneal borderline tumor
b. personality
b. personality disorder
b. schizophrenia
serous borderline tumor
symptom schedule for the diagnosis of borderline schizophrenia
b. syndrome index
b. systolic hypertension
b. tuberculoid

borderline-resistant *Staphylococcus aureus*

Bordetella

anti-*Bordetella pertussis* antibody

Bordet-Gengou agar

bore

magnetic b.

boredom

chronic emptiness and b.
inability to tolerate b.

borer

bone b.

boric

b. acid
b. acid solution

born

baby born dead
b. before arrival
full term, born dead
b. on arrival
b. out of asepsis

Borna disease virus

boron

b. neutron capture therapy
b. sulfhydryl

boronated porphyrin

Borrelia burgdorferi

borreliosis

Lyme borreliosis antibody

***Bos* adenovirus 1–10**

boss

carpal b.
parietal b.

bossing

frontal b.

occipital b.
tip b.

Boston
B. Assessment of Severe Aphasia
B. Diagnostic Aphasia Examination
B. Diagnostic Inventory of Basic Skills
B. Naming Test
B. Test for Examining Aphasia

Botallo
duct of B.
ligament of B.

Botambi virus

Boteke virus

both
activity of both hemispheres
b. bones
b. bones fracture
color and temperature normal, both lower extremities
b. end-expiratory pressures
b. eyes
b. eyes patched
finger count, both eyes
fracture of both bones
b. hands
Hering law-EOM innervation, both eyes
hydrosalpinx, both tubes
lateral rectus, both eyes
b. lower extremities
mast cell containing both tryptase and chymase
medial rectus, both eyes
peripheral pulses palpable both legs
short stature, hyperextensibility of joints or hernia or both, ocular depression, Rieger anomaly, teething, delayed
b. upper extremities

bottle
blow b.
child-resistant bottle top
hot water b.
left in b.
nursing bottle caries
water b.

bottle-fed infant

bottom
weaver b.

botulinum
b. toxin
b. toxin A

botulism
b. equine trivalent antitoxin
infantile b.
mean swell time botulism test
pentavalent botulism toxin
b. toxin

Bouboui virus

Bouchut respiration

bougie
following b.
Maloney b.
mercury b.
Savary b.

bougienage
mercury bougienage treatment

Boulogne
Duchenne de Boulogne muscular dystrophy
Duchenne de Boulogne muscular dystrophy/Becker muscular dystrophy

bouncing
ligamentous b.

bound
chemically bound residue
b. hepatitis antibody
nonprotein b.
nonsex hormone-binding globulin bound testosterone
out of b.'s
prostate-specific antigen bound to alpha-1 antichymotrypsin
protein b.
b. serum iron
total b.
total counts b.

boundary
air-bone-tissue b.
automated boundary protection
loss of ego b.
loss of boundaries of ego
moving boundary electrophoresis

bound/free antigen ratio

bouquet
Riolan b.

Bourns assist

bouton
synaptic b.
terminal b.

bout of rejection

Bovie
B. cautery
B. coagulation

Bovie-assisted uvulopalatoplasty

bovine
acute bovine pulmonary edema
adult bovine serum
b. albumin
b. aortic endothelium
araldehyde-tanned bovine carotid artery graft
b. chromogranin A
contagious bovine pleuropneumonia
despeciated bovine serum
embryonic bovine kidney
b. embryonic kidney cell
b. embryonic lung
b. embryonic spleen cell
b. embryo skeletal muscle
b. enteritis
enterocytopathogenic bovine orphan virus
b. ephemeral fever
fetal bovine endothelial cell
fetal bovine serum
b. gamma globulin
b. growth hormone
b. heart
b. heart valve
heat-inactivated fetal bovine serum
b. hemoglobin
b. heterograft
immunoreactive bovine serum albumin
infectious bovine keratoconjunctivitis
infectious bovine rhinotracheitis
infectious bovine rhinotracheitis virus
b. insulin
iodinated bovine serum albumin keratoconjunctivitis
b. kidney cell
b. lavage extract surfactant
b. leukemia virus
b. lumpy skin disease
Madin-Darby bovine kidney
Madin-Darby bovine kidney cell
maleated bovine serum albumin
methylated bovine serum albumin
microcrystalline bovine collagen
b. mucosal disease
oral bovine myelin
b. pancreatic polypeptide
b. pancreatic trypsin inhibitor
b. papillomavirus
b. papular stomatitis
b. parathyroid hormone
pegademase b.

bovine *(continued)*
b. plasma albumin
b. red blood cell
b. serum albumin
specified bovine offals
b. spinal cord protein
b. spongiform encephalopathy
b. thymus extract
b. thyroid-stimulating hormone
b. trypsin
b. trypsinogen
b. turbinate
Veronal-buffered saline-fetal bovine serum
b. viral diarrhea
b. viral diarrhea mucosal disease
b. viral diarrhea virus 1, 2

bovis
Mycobacterium bovis BCG

bow
Cupid bow configuration
Cupid's b.
Cupid's bow contour
Cupid's bow peak
Cupid's bow upper lip

bowed
dislocated elbow, bowed tibiae, scoliosis, deafness, cataract, microcephaly, mental retardation syndrome

bowel
abrasion of b.
absent bowel function
absent bowel sounds
active bowel sounds
acute idiopathic inflammatory bowel disease
b. adequately evacuated
b. adherent to omentum
allergic bowel disease
altered bowel habit
altered bowel movement
anastomosed to loop of b.
apple-peel bowel syndrome
atraumatic bowel clamp
auscultation of bowel sounds
b. and bladder
bladder and bowel dysfunction
b. and bladder dysfunction
b. and bladder function
b. and bladder incontinence
bloating and irritable bowel syndrome
brown bowel syndrome
bruising of b.
b. bypass
b. care of choice
change in bowel habit
change in bowel pattern
chronic inflammatory bowel disease
complete bowel obstruction
complete small bowel obstruction
contaminated small bowel syndrome
continence of bowel and bladder
b. continuity
debilitating bowel disease
decreased bowel function
dilated bowel loop
dilated bowel loop resection
dilated loops of b.
diminished bowel movement
diminished bowel sounds
diseased segment of b.
disturbed bowel function
b. emptying regimen
extensive inflammatory bowel disease
b. fills and evacuates satisfactorily
fixed segment of b.
fluid-filled loop of b.
fluid-filled small b.
frequent bowel movement
functional bowel disorder
functional bowel distress
functional bowel syndrome
Functional B. Disorder Severity Index
gangrene of b.
gangrenous small b.
b. gas artifact
b. gas pattern
granulomatous bowel disease
gurgling bowel sounds
b. habit
high-pitched bowel sound
hyperactive bowel sound
hyperactive bowel tones
hypoactive bowel sounds
hypoactive bowel tones
idiopathic inflammatory bowel disease
b. impaction
inadequate bowel preparation
incomplete bowel obstruction
b. incontinence
infectious bowel disease
inflammatory bowel disease
inflammatory bowel syndrome
Inflammatory B. Disease Questionnaire
intermittent functional bowel problem
intermittent small bowel obstruction
irregular bowel movements
irritable bowel syndrome with constipation
large bowel obstruction
last bowel movement
loop of b.
loose bowel movement
loss of bowel control
lumen of b.
malrotation of b.
malrotation of bowel loop
massive bowel resection
massive bowel resection syndrome
matted bowel loop
mechanical bowel obstruction
mid-small b.
b. movement
multiple bull's eye lesions bowel wall
multiple loops of small b.
narcotic bowel syndrome
necrosis of b.
necrotizing bowel vasculitis
Noble bowel plication
no bowel movement
nonrotation of bowel loop
nonspecific bowel gas pattern
normal bowel action
normal bowel function
normal bowel movement
normal bowel sounds
normoactive bowel tone
normoactive bowel sounds
b.'s not opened
b. obstruction
b.'s open
overlying bowel content
overlying bowel gas
overlying bowel shadows
partial bowel obstruction
partial small bowel obstruction
paucity of bowel gas
perforation of b.
peristalsis of b.
petechial hemorrhage of b.
positive bowel sounds
b. prep
b. preparation
proximal bowel distention
proximal small b.
radiation bowel reaction
b. rest

segmental bowel infarct
segment of b.
short bowel syndrome
Short Inflammatory B. Disease Questionnaire
short small b.
small b.
small bowel adenocarcinoma
small bowel adenoma
small bowel anastomosis
small bowel atresia
small bowel bacterial overgrowth
small bowel carcinoma
small bowel disease
small bowel dysmotility
small bowel enteroscopy
small bowel followthrough
small bowel ischemia
small bowel loop
small bowel motility
small bowel mucosa
small bowel peristalsis
small bowel phytobezoar
small bowel thickening
small bowel transit time
small bowel transplantation
small bowel tumor
small bowel volvulus
b. sounds
b. sounds normal
b. sounds normal and active
b. sounds present and active
b. sounds regular
spastic bowel syndrome
stimulation of lower b.
straining on bowel movement
strangulated bowel obstruction
strangulated small b.
superimposed bowel gas
superimposition of bowel shadow
tarry black bowel movement
thickened bowel loop
toxic dilatation of b.
b. training
b. training program
ulcerative bowel disease
upper gastrointestinal series with small bowel follow-through
b. wall hemorrhage
b. wall induration
water bowel movement

Bowen

extragenital Bowen disease

bowing

anterior bowing of sternum
anterior bowing tibia
anterior tibial b.
anterolateral tibial b.
b. of fracture
b. of mitral valve leaflet
tibial b.
b. tic

bowl

arc and bowl perimeter
mastoid b.

Bowman

capsule of B.
B. capsule

Bowman-Birk inhibitor

bow-tie

b.-t. knot
b.-t. stitch

box

b. chisel
ligamentous b.
negative-pressure b.
obstruction b.
orbital box osteotomy
b. osteotome
paired b.
paired box homeotic 3 gene
paired box homeotic 8 gene

box-end wrench

boxing

aerobic b.

box-type osteotomy

boy

baby b.
good old b.
sick b.

Boyd

modified Boyd amputation
modified Boyd amputation of ankle and distal tibial physis
modified Boyd ankle arthrodesis
Speed and Boyd reduction technique

BR96

monoclonal antibody B.

brace

airplane splint shoulder b.
ankle-foot orthosis brace sock
ankle ligament protector b.
ankle stirrup b.
Arizona ankle b.
Atlanta brace orthosis
Atlanta hip b.
Atlanta-Scottish Rite b.
bivalve overlap b.
cast boot b.
ceramic or plastic b.
chairback type b.
controlled position b.
donut support b.
b. drill
eclipse ankle b.
elastic knee sleeve b.
flexor-hinge hand-splint b.
four-poster cervical b.
functional arm b.
functional electronic peroneal b.
hinged knee b.
ischial weight bearing leg b.
knee b.
ligamentous control b.
long arm b.
long double upright b.
long leg brace with free ankle
long leg brace with pelvic band
Miami fracture b.
military brace maneuver
military brace position
Orthoplast fracture b.
patellar stabilizing b.
right short leg b.
R SL b.
short arm b.
short leg b.
sternooccipital-mandibular immobilization brace
Taylor back b.
tibial fracture brace proximal support
unilateral calcaneal b.
Wilke boot b.

bracelet

identification b.
lymphedema alert b.
medical alert b.
Nageotte b.
patient identification b.

brachial

anterior division of brachial plexus
b. arterial pressure
b. artery mean pressure
b. artery output
b., radial, femoral
b. cutaneous nerve
intercostal brachial nerve
interscalene brachial plexus
Klumpke brachial palsy
left brachial vein occlusion
lower brachial plexopathy
malignant brachial plexopathy
mean brachial artery pressure
medial brachial cutaneous nerve
medial brachial fascial compartment

brachial *(continued)*
medial brachial nerve
medial cord of brachial plexus
modified brachial technique
neoplastic brachial plexopathy
b. neuritis
obstetric brachial plexus injury
obstetric brachial plexus palsy
penile brachial index
b. plexus block
b. plexus injury
b. plexus neuropathy
b. plexus traction injury
b. radialis jerk
right brachial artery
right brachial vein
right brachial vein occlusion
trunks of brachial plexus

brachii
aponeurosis of biceps b.
arteria profunda b.
musculus biceps b.
profunda brachii artery

brachiocephalic
arterial brachiocephalic trunk
b. arterial trunk
b. artery
mirror-image brachiocephalic branching

brachiocephalicus
musculus b.

brachioradialis
musculus b.

brachioskeletogenital syndrome

Brachmann-Cornelia de Lange syndrome

brachycephaly
occipital b.

brachydactyly
b., mesomelia, mental retardation, aortic dilation, mitral valve prolapse, characteristic facies syndrome
growth retardation, ocular abnormalities, microcephaly, brachydactyly, oligophrenia

brachymicrocephaly
parietal foramina, brachymicrocephaly, mental retardation syndrome

brachymorphism, onychodysplasia, dysphalangism

brachy-tachy syndrome

brachytherapy
endolaryngeal brachytherapy mold
high dose rate b.
intracavitary b.
magnetic resonance spectroscopic imaging-guided b.
Manchester system for b.
open bladder brachytherapy implant
orbital plaque b.
palladium 103 ophthalmic plaque b.
remote afterload b.
transperineal interstitial permanent prostate b.
b. treatment

bracing
cast b.

bracket
curved base twin b.
longitudinal epiphysial b.
longitudinal epiphysial b.
metal frame reinforced plastic b.

bradycardia
b. after arteriovenous fistula occlusion
apnea and b.
apnea, bradycardia, and cyanosis
b. hypotensive
sinus b.

bradycardia-tachycardia syndrome

bradykinesia
end-of-dose b.

bradykinin
b. potentiating factor
b. potentiating peptide

Bragg
Fort Bragg evaluation project
sharp Bragg peak

braid
carbon fiber lamination b.

braided
b. occlusion device
silk braided suture

brain
abnormal brain wave discharge
abnormal brain wave function
acquired brain injury
activates chemical impulse of b.
active brain tissue
b. activity
acute brain disturbance
acute brain syndrome
acute injury to b.
acute ischemic brain infarct
acute multiple brain infarct
acute organic brain syndrome
b. adjacent tumor
age-related brain change
aging brain syndrome
alcohol effect on b.
alcoholic brain syndrome
alpha brain wave
alteration of blood brain barrier
altered brain function
altering brain function
alters brain chemistry
anatomic brain classification
anoxic brain damage
anoxic brain injury
anoxic changes in b.
anterior part of anterior commissure of b.
arachnoid of b.
arachnoid brain cyst
architecture of b.
architecture of the b.
arcuate nucleus of b.
arterial brain anastomosis
arterial brain displacement
arteriosclerotic brain disease
arteriosclerotic brain disease-type organic psychosis
arteriosclerotic brain disorder
arteriosclerotic brain syndrome
arteriovenous brain malformation
arteriovenous malformation of b.
artery of b.
Aspergillus brain abscess
asphyxial brain injury
atherothrombotic brain infarct
atherothrombotic brain infarction
atrial diverticulum of b.
atrophic brain lesion
atrophic lesion of b.
atypical brain teratoma
atypical or mixed organic brain syndrome
auditory brain mapping
automated ventricular brain ratio
autopsy of b.
autopsy limited to b.
avascular brain mass
baked brain phenomenon
biochemical change in b.
blood flow to b.
blood supply of b.
cancer of the prostate and brain gene
cerebral activity of b.
chemical abnormality in b.

chemical disruption in b.
chronic alcoholic brain syndrome
chronic organic brain syndrome
circumscribed atrophy of b.
collateral arterial flow to b.
compression of the b.
computed tomography brain scan
contrecoup injury of b.
contusion of the b.
b. cooling
cortical necrosis of b.
criteria for determination of brain death
damaged brain cell
b. damage from cerebral hemorrhage
b. dead
b. death
death of brain cell
decreased brain activity
decreased brain wave activity
definite brain damage
b. degeneration
degenerative brain disease
degenerative disease of b.
dementia due to traumatic brain injury
b. development
diffuse brain injury
diffuse brain swelling
diminished brain activity
diminished heart, kidney and brain function
direct brain stimulation
dorsal brain stem lipoma
b. dysfunction
b. edema
b. electrical activity
electrical activity of b.
b. electrical activity map
b. electrical activity mapping
electrical brain stimulation
electric stimulation of b.
eloquent areas of b.
endogenous brain mechanism
enhancing brain lesion
event-related brain potential
b. evoked potential
excessive brain activity
excessive fast brain wave activity
fixation and sectioning of the b.
focal brain lesion
full radiation of b.
glucose metabolism in b.
b. graft surgery
gray matter of b.
hallucination from b.
b. heart infusion agar
b. heart infusion broth
heart, kidney and brain function
b. hemisphere
hemisphere of b.
b. hemorrhage
hemorrhage in b.
b. herniation
herniation of the b.
higher brain center
high-resolution brain SPECT
high-voltage brain wave
b. hormone
human brain disease
human brain thromboplastin
b. hypersensitivity
hypoxia, intussusception, brain mass
hypoxic change in b.
b. imaging
b. imaging study
b. imaging technique
impaired brain activity
impairment of functions of brain stem
b. implant surgery
b. impulse
incipient degenerative brain disease
increased brain activity
infantile diffuse brain sclerosis
b. infarct
b. infection
inflammation of b.
inflammation and gliosis in b.
inherited abnormality in b.
b. injured
b. injury
b. injury center
inoperable brain tumor
invasive brain surgery
irregular brain function
irregularity in brain chemistry
irreversible brain death
irreversible catastrophic brain injury
irreversible damage to brain cell
ischemic brain infarction
labyrinth of b.
left brain damage
left hemisphere of b.
left hemisphere brain damage
life-threatening brain injury
lobe of b.
localized brain activity
low-voltage brain wave
malignant brain edema
malignant brain neoplasm
malignant brain tumor
massive infarct of brain stem
mediobasal brain structure
medullary arteries of b.
medullary artery of b.
membrane of b.
meninges of b.
metastatic brain disease
metastatic brain tumor
microscopically immature b.
midline of brain cyst
mild traumatic brain injury
miliary brain metastasis
Mini Inventory of Right B. Injury
minimal brain dysfunction
minimal brain dysfunction syndrome
minimally invasive brain surgery
multifocal brain tumor
multiple brain metastases
muscle, liver, brain, eye
muscle, liver, brain, eye disease
muscle, liver, brain, eye nanism
mycotic brain aneurysm
b. natriuretic peptide
navigated brain tumor surgery
necrosis of b.
negative brain scan
neonatal brain injury
neuron of b.
b. neurotransmitter
new approaches to brain tumor therapy
newborn mouse b.
no brain damage
Nocardia brain abscess
noninvasive brain imaging study
normal brain stem
normal immature brain tissue
North American Brain Tumor Consortium
occipital lobe of b.
olfactory lobe of b.
open brain biopsy
organically impaired brain activity
organically impaired brain function
organic brain changes
organic brain dysfunction
organic brain syndrome with hallucinogen
organic damage to b.
oxidative brain injury
parasellar brain mass
parasitic brain abscess

brain *(continued)*
parenchymal brain injury
parenchymal brain lesion
parenchymal brain metastasis
parenchymal brain neoplasm
parietal lobe of b.
partial brain irradiation
patient brain dead
pattern of brain electrical activity
pediatric brain stem glioma
penetrating brain injury
b. perfusion study
peritumoral brain edema
physical change in b.
pia mater of b.
plaque in b.
pressure on the b.
primary brain lymphoma
progressive brain disease
pronouncement of brain death
prophylactic brain irradiation
prophylactic whole brain radiation therapy
b. protein solvent
proximal brain shift
psychotic brain syndrome
recorded electrical brain activity
reduced blood flow to b.
reduce swelling in b.
right brain damage
right brain stroke
right hemisphere of b.
right hemisphere brain damage
ruptured brain aneurysm
Russell brain disease
sarcoma, breast and brain tumors, leukemia, laryngeal and lung cancer adenoma
Scales of Cognitive Ability for Traumatic B. Injury
schizophrenic brain abnormality
seizure-producing areas of b.
severely traumatized b.
shift in direction and pattern of brain electrical activity
silent brain infarction
silent ischemic brain damage
small brain hemorrhage
softening of the b.
SPECT brain perfusion scintigraphy
sponge-like holes in b.
b. spoon
b. stem glioma
b. stem hemorrhage
stereotactic brain biopsy
b. stimulation reinforcement
suckling mouse b.
suggested brain dysfunction
supporting tissue of b.
surgical treatment for brain tumor
thrombotic brain infarction
b. tickler
b. tissue implant
b. tissue partial pressure of oxygen
tracking blood flow to the b.
transient brain stem ischemia
transmitting electrochemical messages to the b.
traumatic brain death
unruptured brain aneurysm
b. uptake index
b. wave activity
b. wave cycle
b. wave frequency range
b. wave pattern
b. wave response
waxy deposit on b.
whole brain irradiation
whole brain radiation
whole brain versus local brain radiation therapy

brain-age quotient

brain-based pain control

brain-derived
b.-d. neurotrophic factor
b.-d. neurotropic factor

brain-heart infusion

brain/muscle ARNT-like protein 1

brain-reactive antibody

brainstem
abnormal b.
audiometric brainstem response
auditory brainstem implant
auditory brainstem response audiometry
auditory brainstem response test
b. auditory evoked potential
b. auditory evoked response
automated auditory brainstem response
automated auditory brainstem response hearing screening
b. compression
b. dysfunction
b. electrical response audiometry
b. electric response audiometry
b. evoked response
b. hemorrhage
b. infarction
b. injury
ischemic brainstem infarction
Navajo brainstem syndrome
pediatric brainstem glioma
b. reflex
screening auditory brainstem response
somatosensory brainstem evoked potential
b. tumor

brain-type glycogen phosphorylase

branch
absence of branch pulmonary artery
anterior abdominal cutaneous branch of intercostal nerve
anterior alveolar branch of maxillary nerve
anterior auricular branch of superficial temporal artery
anterior basal b.
anterior branch of axillary nerve
anterior branch of the renal artery
anterior branch of thoracic nerve
anterior cutaneous b.
anterior cutaneous branch of femoral nerve
anterior cutaneous branch of iliohypogastric nerve
anterior cutaneous branch of intercostal nerve
anterior ethmoidal branch of ophthalmic artery
anterior gastric branch of anterior vagal trunk
anterior glandular branch of superior thyroid artery
anterior intercostal branch of internal thoracic artery
anterior interventricular branch of left coronary artery
anterior labial branch of deep external pudendal artery
anterior lateral nasal branch of anterior ethmoidal artery
anterior/lateral/posterior glandular branch of superior thyroid artery
anterior meningeal branch of anterior ethmoidal artery
anterior pectoral cutaneous branch of intercostal nerve
anterior pulmonary branch of vagus nerve
anterior scrotal branch of deep external pudendal artery

anterior septal branch of anterior ethmoidal artery
anterior superior alveolar branch of infraorbital nerve
anterior temporal b.
anterior temporal branch of posterior cerebral artery
anteromedial central b.
anteromedial frontal branch of callosomarginal artery
apical branch of inferior lobar branch of right pulmonary artery
apical branch of right superior pulmonary vein
apicoposterior branch of left superior pulmonary vein
arterial branch to dura mater
artery of angular nasal b.
articular branch of deep fibular nerve
ascending anterior b.
ascending branch of the inferior mesenteric artery
ascending branch of superficial cervical artery
ascending posterior b.
atrial anastomotic branch of circumflex branch of left coronary artery
atrioventricular groove b.
atrioventricular nodal b.
auricular branch of occipital artery
auricular branch of posterior auricular artery
auricular branch of vagus nerve
bundle b.
bundle branch heart block
callosal marginal b.
circumflex b.
communicating branch of glossopharyngeal nerve with auricular branch of vagus nerve
complete left bundle branch block
complete right bundle branch block
diagonal branch of artery
distal communicating b.
external branch of superior laryngeal
first obtuse marginal b.
His bundle branch block
internal branch of superior laryngeal nerve
lateral cutaneous b.
lingual branch of facial nerve
lumbar branch of iliolumbar artery
macular branch retinal vein occlusion
malposition of branch pulmonary artery
malposition of the branch pulmonary artery
marginal atrial branch of right coronary artery
marginal branch of cingulate sulcus
marginal branch of left circumflex coronary artery
marginal branch of parietooccipital sulcus
marginal branch of right coronary artery
marginal mandibular branch of facial nerve
marginal tentorial branch of internal carotid artery
mastoid branch of occipital artery
mastoid branch of posterior auricular artery
mastoid branch of posterior tympanic artery
medial basal branch of pulmonary artery
medial branch of artery of tuber cinereum
medial branch C2
medial branch of pontine artery
medial branch of posterior branch of spinal nerve
medial branch of posterior rami of spinal nerve
medial calcaneal branch of tibial nerve
medial crural cutaneous branch of saphenous nerve
medial cutaneous b.
medial cutaneous branch of dorsal branch of posterior intercostal artery
medial malleolar branch of posterior tibial artery
medial mammary b.
mediastinal branch of internal thoracic artery
mediastinal branch of thoracic aorta
meningeal branch of cavernous part of internal carotid artery
meningeal branch of cerebral part of internal carotid artery
meningeal branch of intracranial part of vertebral artery
meningeal branch of mandibular nerve
meningeal branch of maxillary nerve
meningeal branch of occipital artery
meningeal branch of ophthalmic nerve
meningeal branch of spinal nerve
meningeal branch of vagus nerve
mental branch of inferior alveolar artery
mental branch of mental nerve
middle lobe branch of right superior pulmonary vein
midmarginal branch of artery
muscular branch of deep fibular nerve
mylohyoid branch of inferior alveolar artery
nasociliary branches of ophthalmic nerve
nonlingular branch of upper lobe bronchus
obturator branch of pubic branch of inferior epigastric vein
obtuse marginal b.
occlusion of branch vein
orbital branch of maxillary nerve
orbital branch of middle meningeal artery
orbital branch of pterygopalatine ganglion
ovarian branch of uterine artery
palmar branch of anterior interosseous nerve
palmar carpal branch of radial artery
palmar carpal branch of ulnar artery
palmar cutaneous branch of the median nerve
palmar cutaneous branch of the ulnar nerve
palpebral branch of infratrochlear nerve
pancreatic duct b.
paracentral branch of callosomarginal artery
paracentral branch of pericallosal artery
parietal branch of medial occipital artery
parietal branch of middle meningeal artery

branch *(continued)*
parietal branch of superficial temporal artery
parietooccipital branch of anterior cerebral artery
parietooccipital branch of posterior cerebellar artery
parietooccipital branch of posterior cerebral artery
pectoral and abdominal anterior cutaneous branch of intercostal nerve
pectoral branch of thoracoacromial artery
perforating branch of anterior interosseous artery
perforating branch of deep palmar arch
perforating branch of fibular artery
perforating branch of internal thoracic artery
perforating branch of palmar metacarpal artery
perforating branch of peroneal artery
perforating branch of plantar metatarsal artery
pericardial branch of phrenic nerve
pericardial branch of thoracic aorta
perineal branch of posterior cutaneous nerve of thigh
perineal branch of posterior femoral cutaneous nerve
peripheral branch retinal vein occlusion
peroneal communicating b.
petrosal branch of middle meningeal artery
pharyngeal branch of artery of pterygoid canal
pharyngeal branch of ascending pharyngeal artery
pharyngeal branch of descending palatine artery
pharyngeal branch of glossopharyngeal nerve
pharyngeal branch of inferior thyroid artery
pharyngeal branch of recurrent laryngeal nerve
pharyngeal branch of vagus nerve
posterior branch of great auricular nerve
posterior branch of medial cutaneous nerve of forearm
posterior branch of obturator artery
posterior branch of obturator nerve
posterior branch of recurrent ulnar artery
posterior branch of renal artery
posterior branch of spinal nerve
posterior descending b.
posterolateral b.
proximal communicating b.
pterygoid branch of maxillary artery
pterygoid branch of posterior deep temporal artery
pulmonary branch stenosis
b. retinal artery occlusion
b. retinal vein occlusion
second obtuse marginal b.
segmental branch of artery
sensory branch of radial nerve
superficial branch of lateral plantar nerve
superficial branch of medial circumflex femoral artery
superficial branch of medial plantar artery
superficial branch of superior gluteal artery
superficial branch of transverse cervical artery
superficial branch of ulnar nerve
sympathetic branch to submandibular ganglion
thyrohyoid branch of ansa cervicalis
ulnar branch of medial antebrachial cutaneous nerve
ureteric branch of inferior suprarenal artery
ureteric branch of ovarian artery
ureteric branch of renal artery
b. vein occlusion

branched-chain
b.-c. alpha ketoacid dehydrogenase
b.-c. amino acid
b.-c. deoxyribonucleic acid
b.-c. fatty acid

branched deoxyribonucleic acid

branchial
b. cleft anomaly
lip pseudocleft-hemangiomatous branchial cyst syndrome
mandibular branchial arch

branching
anomalous b.
linear branching microcalcification
linear branching pattern
mirror-image brachiocephalic b.
opaque branching structure
overlying branching pattern

branchiooculofacial syndrome

branchiootorenal syndrome

brash
water b.
weaning b.

brasiliensis
anti-*Paracoccidioides brasiliensis* antibody

Braun pinch graft technique

Bravo
Rio Bravo virus

brawny
b. induration
Stellwag brawny edema

Braxton-Hicks
B.-H. contraction
B.-H. sign

Brazelton
B. Neonatal Behavioral Assessment Scale

Brazilian purpuric fever

breach
naviculocuneiform b.

bread equivalent

breadth
length, breadth, height
maxilloalveolar b.
midfacial b.

breadwinner
loss of b.

break
ascending pitch b.
hangman's b.
major b.
material failure break point
mucosal b.
nonrejoining DNA strand b.
b. in the skin

breakage
low b.

breakdown
bone growth and b.

cellulose breakdown bacteria
fibrin breakdown product
fibrinogen breakdown product
germinal vesicle b.
gum tissue b.
potential for b.
social breakdown syndrome

breakfast
early dry b.
early light b.
hold b.
hold breakfast for blood work

breaking
impaired breaking and swallowing
nail breaking from athlete's foot
nail breaking from circulatory problem
b. strength

breakpoint
b. cluster region
b. cluster region negative
b. cluster region positive

breakthrough
b. bleeding
estrogen breakthrough bleeding
molybdenum-99 breakthrough test
normal perfusion pressure b.
sinus breakthrough beat

breakup
tear breakup time

breast
b. abscess from breast-feeding
adenoma of the b.
adjustable breast implant
adjustable saline breast implant
adjuvant therapy for breast cancer
advanced breast biopsy instrumentation
alcohol in breast milk
anthracycline-nave metastatic breast cancer
anthracycline-refractory metastatic breast carcinoma
areola of b.
Aries-Pitanguy breast reduction
ASSI breast dissector angulated
ASSI breast dissector spatulated
asymmetric breast density
atypical lobular breast hyperplasia
Aurora MR breast imaging
Austrian B. Cancer Study Group
automated large-core breast biopsy
axillary breast tissue
axillary nodal metastasis in breast carcinoma
banked breast milk
benign breast disease
benign breast syndrome
b. biopsy
bloody discharge from b.
b. bolster
b. caliper
b. cancer
b. cancer antigen
B. Cancer Detection Demonstration Project
b. cancer gene
b. cancer screening indicator
b. cancer-specific survival
carcinoma of b.
casting breast calcification
cellular breast cancer therapy
clinical breast examination
concentric circle pattern on breast self-examination
b. conservation therapy
core breast biopsy
b. cyst fluid
b. cyst fluid protein
cystic disease of b.
diarrhea and breast feeding
b. dimpling
dimpling of breast skin
direct injection of silicone into b.
double-lumen breast implant
dynamic optical breast imaging system
early detection of breast cancer
early stage breast cancer
electrical impedance breast scanning
b. enhancement surgery
b. examination
excessive breast firmness and discomfort
excision and wedge biopsy of b.
expandable breast implant
experimental breast cancer treatment
expressed breast milk
b. fed
fibrocystic breast disease
fibrocystic disease of b.
b. firm and lactating
fluid-filled cyst in b.
full-strength breast milk
gel-filled breast implant
growth monitoring, oral rehydration, breast feeding, and immunization
hardening of breast tissue
hereditary breast and ovarian cancer
high risk for breast cancer
high-risk breast cancer
high risk for breast cancer
high-risk primary breast cancer
hot vs. cold breast tumor
human breast milk
human breast tumor
hyperthermia in b.
b. hypertrophy
image-guided breast biopsy
b. imaging
immediate breast reconstruction
b. implant
b. implant valve
increased risk of breast cancer
infiltrating ductal carcinoma of the b.
inflammatory breast cancer
inflammatory carcinoma or b.
intraductal carcinoma of b.
intraductal papilloma of b.
invasive breast cancer
invasive carcinoma of b.
ipsilateral breast tumor recurrence
large operable breast cancer
leaking breast implant
left breast biopsy
left breast biopsy examination
lobar breast anatomy
lobular breast calcification
lobular breast microcalcification
b. localizer
locally advanced breast cancer
locally advanced and inflammatory breast carcinoma
locoregional breast cancer
locoregional breast carcinoma
low-pressure breast pump
lump in breast does appear enlarged
male breast carcinoma
malignant breast calcification
malignant breast tumor
mammaglobin breast cancer protein
manual breast pump
massive breast hypertrophy
maturation of breast cell
MCF-7 breast cancer cell
medullary breast carcinoma
medullary carcinoma of b.

breast *(continued)*
metastatic breast carcinoma
b. milk
minimally invasive breast biopsy
mirror image breast biopsy
b. mound reduction and nipple reconstruction with wraparound flap
MRI-guided breast biopsy
mucinous breast carcinoma
multifocal breast carcinoma
National Alliance of B. Cancer Organization
Nearly Me breast form
b. needle location
negative breast biopsy
neonatal breast hyperplasia
nipple discharge from breast injury
nodal involvement in breast carcinoma
nodal metastasis in breast carcinoma
nonhereditary breast cancer
noninvasive breast carcinoma
normal breast tissue
operable breast cancer
Page grade for breast tumor
Paget disease of b.
b. pain from breast-feeding
painful swelling of b.
papilla of b.
papillary breast carcinoma
papilloma of b.
papillomatosis of b.
paraffin breast augmentation
parenchymal breast pattern
b. parenchymal pattern
pathologic breast discharge
peau d'orange appearance of the b.
peau d'orange appearance in breast carcinoma
b. pendulous and atrophic
percutaneous excisional breast biopsy
periprosthetic breast abscess
phantom breast pain
pigeon breast deformity
b. plate
postmenopausal breast cancer
postpartum breast engorgement
primary operable breast cancer
proliferative breast disease
b. prosthesis rupture
b. pump
radiation therapy for intact b.
b. reconstruction after mastectomy
red spot on b.
red and warm b.
right b.
right breast biopsy
right breast biopsy examination
b.'s ropy or granular
saline filled breast implant
sarcoma, breast and brain tumors, leukemia, laryngeal and lung cancer adenoma
b. self-examination
self-sealing breast implant
shaping of b.
silicone-filled breast implant
silicone gel-filled breast implant
b. silicone implant
simultaneous areolar mastopexy and breast augmentation
b.'s soft and nontender
b. stimulation contraction test
b. strap
surgical absence of b.
survival relative to nodal involvement in breast carcinoma
suspensory ligament of b.
synchronous ipsilateral breast cancer
tail of b.
temporary breast implant
b. tissue approximated with ties
b. tissue expander
transumbilical breast augmentation
b. tumor
b. ultrasound
ultrasound-guided core breast biopsy
Wise areola mastopexy breast augmentation

breast-conserving therapy

breastfed
not b.

breastfeeding and seizure

breast-milk jaundice

breast-sparing mastectomy

breath
absent breath sounds
acute shortness of b.
adventitious breath sound
alcohol breath tester
alcohol on b.
aminopyrine breath test
bad b.
bad breath from bronchitis
bilateral breath sounds
bilateral equal breath sounds
carbon-13 urea breath test
carbon-14 urea breath test
coarse breath sounds
cough and deep b.
crowing breath sounds
C-urea breath test
deep b.
deep cleansing b.
diminished breath sounds
distant breath sound
equal bilateral breath sounds
equal breath bilaterally
equal breath sounds bilaterally
erythromycin breath test
Fowler single breath test
gasping for b.
good breath sound
head of bed up for shortness of b.
b. holding
b. hydrogen test
increased shortness of b.
lactose hydrogen breath testing
last living b.
nitrogen washout, multiple b.
nitrogen washout, single b.
palpitation and shortness of b.
b.'s per minute
phenacetin breath test
quiet breath sound
shortness of b.
shortness of breath on exertion
single b.
b. sounds
b. sounds equal bilaterally
sudden shortness of b.
tracheal breath sound
tubular breath sounds
turn, cough, deep b.
urea breath test
vesicular breath sounds
xylose breath test

breath-actuated inhaler

breathe
ceased to b.
encourage to cough and deep b.

breathed and cried

breath-holding
b.-h. index
pallid breath-holding spell
b.-h. spell

breathing
b. abnormality
absence of b.
airway, breathing, circulation

airway, breathing, circulation, cervical spine, and consciousness level
airway, breathing, circulation, differential
airway, breathing, circulation, disability, exposure
airway, breathing, circulation, intravenous crystalloid
alertness, airway, breathing, circulation, and cervical spine
anesthesia breathing circuit
b. apparatus
blocked breathing passage
ceased b.
chest pain on deep b.
Cheyne-Stokes b.
coarse and harsh b.
computerized diaphragmatic breathing retraining
constriction of breathing passages
continuous positive pressure b.
control of b.
decelerate breathing rhythm
deep breathing and coughing
depressed breathing and heartbeat
diaphragmatic b.
diaphragmatic and chest b.
b. difficulty from anemia
b. difficulty from asthma
b. difficulty from bronchitis
difficulty in nasal b.
disordered breathing rate
disordered breathing time
dizziness from rapid and deep b.
end positive pressure b.
enhancing normal b.
extrathoracic-assisted b.
fetal breathing movement
b. frequency
glossopharyngeal b.
grunting, flaring, and retracting b.
incentive spirometry b.
increased heart and breathing rate
increased and labored b.
indirect maximal breathing capacity
initial breathing difficulty
irregular breathing pattern
loaded breathing sensation
loaded breathing test
momentary lapse in normal b.
Ondine curse, periodic b.
pain on deep b.
pain with breathing difficulty
patient has labored b.
patient taught deep b.
pattern of b.
percutaneous breathing assister
periodic b.
periodic breathing in infants
periodic cessation of b.
positive-negative pressure b.
positive pressure b.
pressure b.
pressure breathing assister
prolonged and deep b.
rapid shallow b.
Rapid Shallow B. Index
b. rate
rating of perceived breathing difficulty
ratio of expiration time and total time of breathing cycle
ratio of inspiration time and total time of breathing cycle
b. and relaxation technique
rescue breathing apparatus
b. reserve
self-contained underwater breathing apparatus
sleep-disordered b.
spontaneously b.
stimulate adequate spontaneous b.
stretching and breathing exercise
b. supported by mechanical respirator
tidal breathing flow-volume
tidal breathing flow-volume loop
wheezing while b.
whistling in nose while b.
work of b.

breathing/inspiratory
intermittent positive pressure b./i.

breathlessness, insomnia and orthopnea

breathy
grade, rough, breathy, asthenic, strained

breech
assisted breech delivery
complete breech presentation
footling breech presentation
frank breech presentation
frank vaginal breech delivery
incomplete breech presentation
singleton breech presentation
spontaneous breech extraction
vaginal breech delivery

breeder
pigeon breeder disease
pigeon breeder lung

bregmocardiac reflex

Brent eyebrow reconstruction

bretylium tosylate

breve
os b.

brevis
abductor hallucis brevis muscle
abductor pollicis brevis muscle
abductor pollicis brevis tendon
adductor brevis muscle
adductor pollicis brevis tendon
arteria centralis b.
extensor brevis arthroplasty
extensor carpi radialis b.
extensor carpi radialis brevis muscle
extensor carpi radialis brevis tendon
extensor digitorum b.
extensor hallucis b.
extensor hallucis brevis muscle
extensor pollicis b.
extensor pollicis brevis tendon
flexor carpi radialis b.
flexor digiti quinti b.
flexor digitorum b.
flexor digitorum quinti b.
flexor hallucis b.
flexor hallucis brevis muscle
flexor pollicis b.
b. muscle
musculus abductor pollicis b.
musculus adductor b.
musculus extensor brevis pollicis
musculus extensor carpi radialis b.
musculus extensor hallucis b.
musculus extensor pollicis b.
musculus fibularis b.
musculus flexor brevis hallucis
musculus flexor digiti minimi brevis manus
musculus flexor digiti minimi brevis pedis
musculus flexor hallucis b.
musculus flexor pollicis b.
nervus ciliaris b.
palmaris brevis muscle
palmaris brevis tendon
peroneus b.
peroneus brevis elongation
peroneus brevis flap
peroneus brevis graft
peroneus brevis muscle
peroneus brevis tendon
peroneus brevis transfer

brevis *(continued)*
peroneus brevis transplant
pollicis brevis abductor muscle
pollicis brevis extensor muscle
pollicis brevis extensor tendon
pollicis brevis flexor muscle
pollicis longus b.
b. tendon

brewers' yeast

bridge
base metal crown and bridge alloy
broad nasal b.
crown and b.
found under b.
b. impression
intercellular b.'s
intracellular b.'s
Libra III bridge and crown
low nasal b.
narrow nasal b.
osseous bridge prevention
porcelain veneer b.

bridging
b. callus
internuclear b.
myocardial b.
b. osteophyte
physeal bony b.
subacute hepatitis with b.

bridle of clitoris

brief
B. Aphasia Screening Examination
b., small, abundant, polyphasic potential
B. Cognitive Rating Scale
detoxification and brief treatment
b. exposure to heat stress
Global Severity Index of B. Symptom Inventory
B. Index of Sexual Functioning for Women
B. Life History Inventory
b. maximal effort
B. Neuropsychological Mental Status Examination
B. Pain Inventory
B. Psychiatric Rating Scale for Children
b., small, abundant motor-unit action potential
B. Social Phobia Scale
b. stimulus therapy
B. Symptom Inventory
B. Test of Head Injury
b. tone audiometry
B. Vestibular Disorientation Test

Brigham prosthesis

bright
copious bright red blood
B. disease
morning bright light therapy
b. red blood per rectum
unidentified bright object

brightening
mood b.

brightness
B. Acuity Test
b. area product
b. modulation

Brill disease

brilliant
Coomassie brilliant blue R-250 stain
b. cresyl blue stain
b. green
b. green lactose broth
selenite brilliant green

brim
pelvic b.

Brinell hardness number

bring together

Brinster medium for ovum culture

brisk
b. and active
b. capillary refill
b. and equal
b. hemorrhage
b. reflex
b. wall motion

Brissaud
B. disease
B. syndrome

bristle
natural b.
nylon b.

Bristol
B. Language Development Scale
B. Social Adjustment Guides

British
B. Ability Scale
B. anti-Lewisite
B. anti-Lewisite therapy
B. approved name
familial British dementia
B. Isles Lupus Assessment Group index
B. Standard Unit
B. thermal unit

brittle
Amish brittle hair syndrome
ichthyosis, brittle hair, impaired intelligence, decreased fertility, short stature syndrome

brittle-bone disease

broach
cementless b.
drilling b.
femoral prosthesis b.
b. holder
Mittlemeir b.
orthopaedic b.

broad
b. adhesive band
b. affect
ASIF broad dynamic compression
b. based scar
leaf of broad ligament
b. nasal bridge

broadband
b. attenuation
b. noise
b. transducer

broad-based
b.-b. cane
b.-b. gait
b.-b. scar

broad-beam scattering

Broadbent registration point

broadcasting
thought b.

broadening
peak b.

broad-range effect

broad-spectrum
b.-s. antibiotic
b.-s. heater

Broca
band of B.
gyrus of B.
B. region

brochure
ASPS b.
professional information b.

Broden
Lund and Broden method

broken
b. injury
b. jaw
b. vs

bromcresol
b. green
b. purple

bromhidrosis
apocrine b.

bromide
cyanogen b.
ethidium b.
formalin ammonium b.
methyl b.
pancuronium b.
phenododecinium b.
potassium b.
tetraethylammonium b.
Walter bromide test

brominated vegetable oil

bromothymol
b. blue
b. blue lactose

brompheniramine maleate

bromphenol blue

bronchi (*pl. of* bronchus)

bronchial
b. artery embolization
b. asthma
atypical bronchial pneumonia
b. blood flow
b. carcinoma
ciliated bronchial epithelium
congenital bronchial atresia
double-sheath bronchial brushing
b. drainage
extensive bronchial mucosa hemorrhage
b. foreign body
b. glandular cell
human bronchial epithelial cell
hyperreactive bronchial tube
b. hyperreactivity
b. hyperresponsiveness
intraluminal typical bronchial carcinoid
b. irritation
b. lavage
lumen of bronchial artery
b. lymph node
b. mucous proteinase inhibitor
obstructing bronchial aspergillosis
plugging of bronchial tree
b. provocation challenge
b. rales
b. responsiveness
b. restriction
thick bronchial secretions
b. toilet
tracheal bronchial toilet
transtracheal selective bronchial brushing

bronchiectasis
b., eosinophilia, asthma, pneumonia
nodular b.
proximal b.

bronchioalveolar
b. carcinoma

bronchiolar
narrowing of bronchiolar passages

bronchiole
lobular b.
membranous b.
respiratory b.
terminal b.

bronchiolitis
b. obliterans
b. obliterans-organizing pneumonia
b. obliterans syndrome
obliterative fibroproliferative b.
pediatric b.
respiratory b.
respiratory syncytial virus b.
b. with interstitial pneumonitis

bronchioloalveolar
intravascular sclerosing bronchioloalveolar tumor

bronchitis
acute bacterial exacerbation of chronic b.
acute exacerbation of chronic b.
asthmatic b.
avian infectious b.
avian infectious bronchitis virus
bad breath from b.
breathing difficulty from b.
chronic b.
chronic bronchitis with asthma
chronic bronchitis with emphysema
chronic obstructive b.
infectious b.
infectious bronchitis vaccine
infectious bronchitis virus

bronchitis/bronchiolitis
acute b./b.

bronchoalveolar
b. cell
b. lavage
b. lavage fluid
protected bronchoalveolar lavage
b. washing

bronchocentric granulomatosis

bronchoconstriction
exercise-induced b.
hyperpnea-induced b.
reversal speed of bronchoconstriction in response to methacholine
speed of bronchoconstriction in response to methacholine

bronchocutaneous fistula

bronchodilation following deep inspiration

bronchodilator
after b.
around-the-clock oral maintenance bronchodilator therapy

bronchoesophageal fistula

bronchoesophageus
musculus b.

bronchogenic
b. carcinoma
mediastinal bronchogenic cyst
missed bronchogenic carcinoma
b. Pancoast-type tumor
small cell bronchogenic carcinoma

bronchogram
air b.
air bronchogram sign
mucinous b.
mucous b.
mucous bronchogram sign

bronchophony
whispered b.

bronchopleural fistula

bronchopleurocutaneous fistula

bronchopneumonia
acute hemorrhagic b.
hemorrhagic b.
necrotizing b.
patchy area of b.
tuberculous b.

bronchopneumonic infiltrate

bronchoprovocation
methacholine bronchoprovocation challenge

bronchopulmonale
lymphonodus b.

bronchopulmonary
acute bronchopulmonary asthma
allergic bronchopulmonary aspergillosis
allergic bronchopulmonary mycosis

bronchopulmonary *(continued)*
anterior basal bronchopulmonary segment
anterior bronchopulmonary segment
apical bronchopulmonary segment
apicoposterior bronchopulmonary segment
b. aspergillosis
b. dysplasia
b. histoplasmosis
medial basal bronchopulmonary segment S VII
b. segmental artery
b. segmental drainage
b. sequestration

bronchoscope
fiberoptic b.
flexible b.
b. inserted through vocal cords with ease

bronchoscopic needle aspiration

bronchoscopy
direct laryngoscopy and b.
fiberoptic b.
flexible fiberoptic b.
flexible fiberoptic bronchoscopy with protected brush
hypopharyngoscopy, bronchoscopy, and esophagoscopy
light-induced fluorescence endoscopic b.
virtual b.
b. with irrigation

bronchospasm
crying-induced b.
exercise-induced b.

bronchovascular markings

bronchus, pl. **bronchi**
anterior basal b.
artery bronchus ratio
epi arterial b.
left main stem b.
lower lobe b.
mainstem b.
malignant neoplasm of b.
medial basal segmental b.
middle lobe b.
mucoid impaction of b.
mucosa of bronchi
mucous gland adenoma of b.
muscular coat of bronchi
muscular layer of bronchi
nonlingular branch of upper lobe b.
occlusion of b.
occlusion of left b.
occlusion of mainstem b.
open bronchus sign
patent bronchus sign
right main b.
right main-stem b.
right middle lobe b.
segmental bronchus consolidation
segmental bronchus defect
segmental bronchus fracture
segmental bronchus ischemia
segmental bronchus lesion
segmental bronchus lower extremity Doppler pressure
segmental bronchus narrowing
segmental bronchus orifice
segmental bronchus perfusion abnormality
segmental bronchus plethysmography
segmental bronchus renal artery waveform
segmental bronchus sign
segmental bronchus symptom
small cell carcinoma of b.

bronchus-associated lymphoid tissue

bronzing
nuclear b.

brooding
obsessional b.

Broström-Evans
modified Broström-Evans procedure

broth
all culture b.
beef heart infusion b.
brain heart infusion b.
brilliant green lactose b.
Enterobacteriaceae enrichment b.
ethyl violet azide b.
fecal coli b.
Hajna-Damon b.
heart infusion b.
macroscopic broth dilution test
malt extract b.
membrane focal coli b.
microdilution broth dilution test
microdilution broth susceptibility test
nutrient b.
Penassay broth plus glucose
Penassay broth plus glucose plus menadione
peptone-yeast-glucose-maltose b.
selective broth medium
thioglycolate b.
trypticase soy b.
tryptone phosphate b.
tryptone soy b.
tryptophan peptone glucose b.

brought
appendix brought into surgical incision
b. in dead
drain brought out through stab wound
margins of wound brought into apposition
b. out near edge of incision

brow
apex of b.
b.s, lids, and lashes
hair of b.
ptotic b.

browlift
open coronal b.

brown
b. adipose tissue
atrophic brown skin
b. bowel syndrome
hereditary brown enamel
idiopathic brown induration
immature brown fat cell
b. induration
b. induration of lung
little brown mushroom
medium brown loose stool
passage of dark brown urine

Browne
Denis Browne splint

Brown-Roberts-Wells phantom base

Bruce
B. maximal stress test
B. treadmill protocol

Brucella
purified *Brucella* protein

brucellosis
agglutination test for b.

Brudzinski sign

***Brugia malayi* adult antigen**

bruisability
easy b.

bruising
b. of bowel
ecchymosis and b.
b. from antidepressant
b. from antihistamine

painful bruising syndrome
b. of undetermined origin

bruit
arteriovenous fistula with good b.'s
asymptomatic carotid b.
asymptomatic neck b.

Brunauer-Emmet-Teller method

Brunn
nest of von B.

Brunsting-Perry
localized pemphigoid of B.-P.

brush
b. biopsy
b. border
b. border membrane
b. catheter
b. cytology
endobronchial brush biopsy
flexible fiberoptic bronchoscopy with protected b.
intestinal brush border
protected brush catheter
transbronchial brush biopsy

brushing
biopsy and b.'s
blind esophageal b.
colposcopically directed b.
double-sheath bronchial b.
flossing, brushing, and irrigation
protected catheter brushing specimen
protected specimen b.
transtracheal selective bronchial b.
washing and b.

Bruton tyrosine kinase

bruxism
sleep b.

Bryan high titer

Bryant-Schwan Design Test

B-scan ultrasonogram

B-type natriuretic peptide

bubble
air bubble instilled in anterior chamber
captive air b.
b. chamber equipment
extracorporeal pneumoperititoneal access b.
gastric air b.
b. humidifier
microscopic air b.

bubble-like appearance

bubbling
middle chamber b.
nuclear bubbling artifact

bubo
malignant b.
nonvenereal b.
parotid b.

bubonic plague

buccal
angulated buccal tube
b. cartilage
b. developmental groove
b. ganglion
b. groove of central fossa
long buccal nerve
b. margin
b. mass
multiple buccal frenula
Nitrogard B.
parenzyme, b.
pedicled buccal fat pad flap
b. root
b. surface of tooth
b. triangular ridge
b. of upper and lingual of lower

buccinator
musculus b.

buccinator-orbicularis oris

buccolinguofacial dyskinesia

bucket-handle
b.-h. fracture
b.-h. meniscus tear
b.-h. plica
b.-h. tear
b.-h. tear of meniscus

buckle
balloon b.
encircling of scleral buckle operation
scleral b.
scleral buckle, left eye
scleral buckle, right eue

buckling
b. and/or locking of knee
midsystolic buckling of mitral valve
scleral b.

Bucky
tomogram with oscillating B.

bud
aortic b.
hair b.
limb b.
liver b.
lung b.
metanephric b.
periosteal b.
syncytial b.
taste b.
tooth b.

Budd-Chiari syndrome

budding
nonsynchronous b.

buddy taping

budesonide
b. aqueous nasal spray
b. inhalation suspension

Buenaventura virus

buffer
b. base
blood buffer base
b. capacity
gelatin, glucose, and Veronal b.
gelatin-veronal b.
glucose-gelatin Veronal b.
hypotonic lysis b.
kalium potassium phosphate b.
Krebs-Henseleit bicarbonate b.
Krebs-Ringer bicarbonate b.
Krebs-Ringer bicarbonate buffer with glucose
modified barbital b.
Neville upper reservoir b.
reticulocyte standard b.
tris-maleate b.
Veronal b.

buffered
b. acetone
b. analgesic
b. azide glucose glycerol
b. charcoal yeast extract
b. desoxycholate glucose
b. distilled water
gelatin Hanks buffered salt solution
hypertonic buffered medium
Nair buffered methylene blue stain
neutral buffered formalin fixative
b. Ringer solution
b. saline
b. saline solution
Seligmann buffered salt solution
b. single substrate

buffering
meal-related b.

buffer-soluble binding component

buffy
b. coat

buffy *(continued)*
quality buffy coat
quantitative buffy coat

bug
assassin b.
assassin bug bite

build
Asher physical build assessment technique
index of body b.
microcephaly, muscular build, rhizomelia-cataracts syndrome

builder
Fokes sentence b.

building
b. illness syndrome
medical office b.
power b.
power building exercise
sick building syndrome

buildup
composite b.
hyperventilation b.
b. time

build-up implant

built-up edge

bulb
accessory olfactory b.
anterior bulb syndrome
apex of duodenal b.
artery of bulb of penis
artery of bulb of vestibule
coarsening of duodenal b.
dry b.
dry bulb temperature
duodenal b.
duodenal bulb scarring
duodenal bulb and sweep
high jugular b.
irritable duodenal b.
Jackson-Pratt to bulb suction
light bulb appearance
molecular layers of olfactory b.
olfactory b.
onion bulb change
onion bulb formation
onion bulb neuropathy
penile bulb dosimetry
penile bulb imaging
polyp of duodenal b.
self-inflating b.
b. suction
wet b.
wet bulb temperature

bulbar
progressive bulbar palsy

bulbi
annulare b.
arteria bulbi penis
arteria bulbi urethrae
arteria bulbi vaginae
arteria bulbi vestibuli
atrophia b.
melanosis b.
musculi b.
musculus obliquus superior b.
musculus rectus lateralis b.
musculus rectus medialis b.
vagina b.
xanthomatosis b.

bulbocavernosus
Martius bulbocavernosus fat flap
musculus b.
b. reflex

bulbosa
myringitis b.

bulbous
b. nasal tip
b. tip reduction

bulbus chordae

bulgaricus
Lactobacillus bulgaricus factor

bulge
abdominal b.
anal b.
annular disc b.
anular disc b.
local bulge of kidney contour
local bulge renal contour
luminal b.
parasternal b.
parietal b.
periocular b.
precordial b.

bulging
anal b.
aneurysmal b.
b. bag of waters
b. disk
b. eyes from blood clot
b. infarct
b. tympanic membrane

bulimia
b. nervosa
b. test

bulimic
bingeing behavior of b.
punishing behavior of b.
b. purge
purging behavior of b.
starving behavior of b.

bulk
b. agent
high bulk diet
b. laxative
mediastinal b.
Modane B.
muscle b.
tumor b.

bulking
periurethral bulking agent

bulky compression dressing

bulla, pl. **bullae**
emphysematous b.
ethmoidal b.
b. ethmoidalis
friction b.
subpleural b.

bulldog
b. clamp applier
b. forceps
b. nasal scissors

bullet
full-jacketed bullet wound

bulletin

bullet-tip
b.-t. catheter
b.-t. dilator

bullosa
angina bullosa haemorrhagica
dominant epidermolysis bullosa simplex
dystrophic epidermolysis b.
epidermolysis b.
epidermolysis bullosa acquisita
epidermolysis bullosa atrophicans
epidermolysis bullosa, macular type
epidermolysis bullosa simplex
generalized atrophic benign epidermolysis b.
ichthyosis bullosa of Siemens
junctional epidermolysis b.
localized epidermolysis bullosa simplex
recessive dystrophic epidermolysis b.
recessive epidermolysis bullosa dystrophica–Hallopeau-Siemens syndrome

bullous
adult bullous dermatosis
aphakic bullous keratopathy

chronic bullous disease of childhood
chronic obstructive bullous emphysema
b. edema
b. emphysema
b. eruption
b. impetigo
b. keratopathy
linear IgA bullous dermatosis
linear IgA bullous disease
neonatal bullous dermatitis
b. pemphigoid
b. pemphigoid antigen
b. pemphigus
pseudophakic bullous keratopathy
b. systemic lupus erythematosus

bull's
liver bull's eye lesion
multiple bull's eye lesions bowel wall

bull's-eye lesion

bump
goose b.'s
hip b.
skin goose b.'s

bumper
axle lock and b.
gastrostomy b.
lip b.

bunching
Myers bunching technique

bundle
anomalous muscle b.
anterior atrial myocardial b.
anterior ground b.
arcuate nerve fiber b.
atrium-His b.
b. branch
b. branch heart block
complete left bundle branch block
complete right bundle branch block
deflection in His bundle in electrogram
desmosome with bundle of tonofilament
direct His bundle pacing
dorsal noradrenergic b.
fiber bundle volume
Gantzer accessory b.
glial b.
b. of His
His b.
His bundle ablation
His bundle activity
His bundle branch block
His bundle deflection
His bundle depolarization
His bundle electrocardiogram
His bundle electrode
His bundle electrogram deflection
His bundle electrogram, distal
His bundle electrogram, proximal
His bundle heart block
His bundle recording
left b.
light guide b.
longitudinal medial b.
longitudinal pontine b.
Mahaim bundle in heart
medial forebrain b.
medial longitudinal b.
myelinated fiber b.
nerve fiber b.
nerve fiber bundle defect
nerve fiber bundle layer
neurovascular b.
neurovascular bundle of Walsh
oblique bundle of pons
olivocochlear bundle of Rasmussen
papillomacular nerve fiber b.
paracentral nerve fiber b.
pigmented villonodular b.
b. of Rasmussen
right b.
right bundle ventricular
ventricular atrial His bundle electrocardiogram

bundle-branch
b.-b. block
b.-b. heart block
rate-dependent left bundle-branch block
b.-b. reentry
right b.-b.
right bundle-branch block

bunion
b. joint
McBride bunion hallux valgus operation

bunionectomy
Akin b.
Austin b.
Austin-Akin b.
chevron b.
Keller b.
Ludloff b.
Mann b.
Mayo b.
McBride b.
McKeever b.
Mitchell b.
modified Hohmann b.
osteotomy b.
Reverdin-Green b.
Silver b.

Bunsen solubility coefficient

Bunyamwera virus

Bunyip Creek virus

bur
dentate straight fissure b.
dentate tapered fissure b.
b. hole
b. holes drilled in skull
medium carbide cone b.
medium fine b.
narrow fissure b.
new happy b.
Oto-Flex carbide b.

Burch
laparoscopic Burch procedure
modified Burch colpourethropexy
transvaginal Burch procedure

burden
child and adolescent burden assessment
b. of disease
ischemic b.
stone b.
tumor b.
tumor burden index
tumor cell b.

bureau
Disease Detection Information B.

Buren
van Buren disease
van Buren sound
Van Buren catheter

burgdorferi
Borrelia b.

buried suture

Burke Stroke Time-Oriented profile

Burkitt
acute lymphoblastic leukemia secondary to Burkitt lymphoma
African Burkitt lymphoma
endemic Burkitt lymphoma
B. lymphoma
B. lymphoma cell line
B. tumor

Burkitt-like lymphoma

Burks Behavior Rating Scale

burn
action against b.'s
b. alopecia
ammonia alkali b.
b. blister
caloric requirements for burn patients
b. care unit
b. claw
b. contracture
b. depth indicator
b. dressing change
b. eschar
first-degree b.
b. healthy tissue
hypertrophic burn scar
b. index
b. injury
light argon laser b.
Lund-Browder burn diagram
Lund-Browder burn scale
Lund-Browder chart for burn estimation
mafenide acetate for b.
ocular chemical b.
Parkland burn resuscitation formula
Parkland fluid requirement formula for burn patients
Parkland formula for fluid resuscitation for burn trauma
b. scar contracture
second-degree b.
third-degree b.
total burn size
total burn surface area
traumatic burn injury

burned
body surface b.
patient burned beyond recognition

burnetii

burning
b. abdominal pain
b. chest discomfort
cold burning, pain and numbness
b. feet from atherosclerosis
b. feet syndrome
intense burning pain
itching or burning sensation
b. mouth from aspirin
b. mouth from cold sore
b. mouth from depression
b. mouth from diabetes
b. mouth syndrome
nasal b.
numbness, tingling, and b.
b. on urination
pain and b.
painful burning of feet
painful burning sensation in chest
prickly, burning, and tingling feeling
b. sensation in stomach
b. sensation in upper chest
substernal b.
tingling and burning sensation
urinary b.

burnout
caretaker b.
exhaustion, burnout and heart disease
mother b.
parent b.
staff burnout scale

burro
normal burro serum

burrowing hair

bursa, pl. **bursae**
Achilles b.
Achilles tendon b.
adventitious b.
anserine b.
anterior tibial b.
aspiration and injection of b.
calcaneal b.
b. cell
greater trochanteric b.
iliac b.
Luschka b.
MCL b.
medial malleolar subcutaneous b.
Monro b.
nasopharyngeal b.
olecranon b.
omental b.
ovarian b.
patellar b.
pes anserinus b.
pisiform b.
plantar b.
prepatellar b.
prepatellar bursa inflammation
retrocalcaneal b.
rider's b.
sacral b.
sartorius b.
semimembranous b.
subacromial b.
subcoracoid b.
subcutaneous acromial b.
subcutaneous bursa of lateral malleolus
subcutaneous bursa of medial malleolus
subcutaneous bursa of teres major
subdeltoid b.
sublingual b.
subscapular b.
suprapatellar b.
synovial b.
triceps b.
trochanteric b.

bursa-equivalent lymphocyte

bursal
infectious bursal disease
infectious bursal disease virus
partial bursal surface tear

bursata
exostosis b.

bursitis
Achilles tendon b.
anserine b.
gluteal b.
hip-associated b.
infrapatellar b.
ischial b.
medial gastrocnemius b.
olecranon b.
omental b.
patellar b.
pes anserinus b.
prepatellar b.
septic b.
subacromial b.
subcoracoid b.
subcutaneous b.
subdeltoid b.
traumatic hemorrhagic b.
trochanteric b.

burst
alpha b.
b. of alpha activity
atlas burst fracture
b.'s of beta activity
combined flexion-distraction injury and burst fracture
electroencephalogram burst suppression pattern
epileptiform b.
epileptiform burst discharge
epileptogenic b.
b. fracture
frequent individual bursts of alpha activity
high-voltage b.
b.'s of irritation and anger
isolated b.

long spike b.
macrophage oxidative b.
neutrophil respiratory burst activity
oxidative b.
pacemaker burst pacing
periodic bursts of high voltage
b. of rapid atrial pacing
repetitive bursts of action potential
respiratory b.
short spike b.
stable burst fracture
teardrop burst fracture
b. of ventricular pacing

burst-forming
b.-f. unit
b.-f. unit-erythroid

bursting
paroxysmal b.

burst-promoting
b.-p. activity
b.-p. factor

burst-suppression
electroencephalographic b.-s.

bury stump of appendix

Buschke
B. Memory Test
scleredema of B.

Bushbush virus

Bussuquara virus

buster
clot b.

busting
clot busting drug

butanol-extractable iodine

buthionine sulfoximine

butorphanol
transnasal b.

butt balm

butter
b. of bismuth
b. fat

butterfly
b. flap
malar butterfly rash
b. rash

buttock
heel to b.
left b.
left upper outer b.
perinatal gangrene of b.
right b.
symphysis, buttocks, and xiphoid

button
Amboyna b.
aortic b.
belly button to medial malleolus
Bingham B. Test
collar button tube
compression b.
b. drainage
b. infuser
lingual b.
nasal septal perforation b.
Oriental b.
padded b.
panic b.
penetrating keratoplasty b.
periosteal b.
Reuter b.
b. suture
tracheal b.
tracheostomy b.

buttonhole
b. incision
nasal buttonhole incision

Buttonwillow virus

buttress
maxillary alveolar b.
nasofrontal b.
nasomaxillary b.
b. pie plate
pretibial b.
pterygomaxillary b.
rotator cuff b.
b. thread screw

butyl
b. glycidyl ether
methyl tertiary butyl ether
tertiary butyl acetate

butylated
b. hydroxyanisole
b. hydroxytoluene

butyrate
cellulose acetate b.

buyer
binge b.

buying
compulsive b.

Bwamba virus

bypass
Alden loop gastric b.
anterior occipital artery-middle cerebral artery b.
aortic-superior mesenteric artery b.
aortobifemoral bypass graft
aortobiprofunda femoral b.
aortocoronary b.
aortocoronary bypass graft
aortocoronary-saphenous vein bypass graft
aortocoronary venous b.
aortofemoral b.
aortofemoral bypass graft
aortofemoral bypass grafting
aortoiliac bypass graft
aortorenal bypass graft
Aria coronary b.
arterial bypass graft
atrio-His bypass tract
atrio-hisian bypass tract
atrionodal bypass tract
atrioventricular nodal bypass tract
autogenous vein bypass graft
axillary-axillary bypass graft
axillary-brachial bypass graft
axillary-femoral bypass graft
axillary-femorofemoral bypass graft
beating-heart bypass surgery
biliointestinal b.
biliopancreatic b.
b. capacitor
cardiac b.
cardiac bypass graft
cardiopulmonary b.
cardiopulmonary bypass machine
cardiopulmonary bypass operation
cardiopulmonary bypass surgery
carotid axillary b.
carotid subclavian b.
b. circuit
clogged bypass graft
concealed bypass tract
b. conduit
coronary artery b.
coronary artery bypass graft
coronary artery bypass grafting
coronary artery bypass grafting surgery
coronary artery bypass graft patency
coronary artery bypass graft surgery
coronary bypass graft
cross femoral-femoral b.
descending thoracic aortofemoral-femoral b.
dilutional cardiopulmonary b.
endarterectomy and coronary artery bypass grafting

bypass *(continued)*
endoscopic coronary artery bypass grafting
extraanatomic b.
extracranial-intracranial arterial b.
femoral above-knee popliteal b.
femoral-femoral bypass graft
femoral-popliteal b.
femoral-popliteal artery b.
femoral-popliteal vein b.
femoral tibial b.
femoropopliteal bypass graft
gastric b.
gastric bypass operation
gastric bypass procedure
gastric bypass surgery
gastric ileal b.
gastric loop b.
b. graft
heart bypass surgery
ileal b.
infrapopliteal b.
internal mammary artery b.
intestinal bypass surgery
jejunoileal b.
left heart b.
left ventricle bypass pump
loop gastric bypass method
loop gastric bypass procedure
loop gastric bypass technique
lower extremity bypass graft
low-flow cardiopulmonary b.
mesenteric bypass graft
minimally invasive coronary bypass grafting
minimally invasive direct coronary artery bypass graft
nodoventricular bypass fiber
off-pump coronary artery b.
operative biliary b.
partial ileal b.
percutaneous biliary b.
percutaneous cardiopulmonary b.
percutaneous cardiopulmonary bypass support
percutaneous left heart b.
perfusion-assisted direct coronary artery b.
popliteal-tibial artery b.
popliteal tibial bypass vein graft
portacaval b.
post coronary artery bypass graft
primary antecubital jump b.
radial artery bypass surgery
renal artery bypass graft
reoperative coronary artery bypass graft
right heart b.
saphenofemoral b.
saphenous vein b.
saphenous vein bypass graft
Silastic ring vertical-banded gastric b.
single coronary artery bypass graft
substernal gastric b.
total b.
total cardiopulmonary b.
totally endoscopic coronary artery b.
triple bypass heart surgery
triple cardiac bypass surgery
triple coronary artery bypass graft
vein bypass graft
b. vein graft
venoarterial bypass pumping
venous bypass graft
venovenous b.
vertebral artery bypass graft
b. wire

bypassing
factor VIII inhibitor bypassing activity

Byrne and Euler formula

bystander dominates initial dominant

C1
Astler-Coller A, B1, B2, C1, C2 classification
C. esterase inhibitor
Niemann-Pick C1 disease

C2
Astler-Coller A, B1, B2, C1, C2 classification
C. deficiency
medial branch C.

C4
C. deficiency
leukotriene C.

C7
complement C.
C. deficiency

C8
complement C.

C9
complement C.

C22-3
antibody to C.

C_4
leukotriene C.

c100
antibody to c100 protein

cabin fever

cable
antirotation c.
c. artifact
autogenous cable graft interposition VII-VII neuroanastomosis
c. cerclage method
c. graft
c. pacing
c. suspension system
c. wire suture technique

cable-hook compression instrumentation

cable-twister brace

cabling
percutaneous c.

Cabot ring body

Cabral coronary reconstruction

cachectic
c. diarrhea
c. endocarditis
c. extremities
c. fever

cachecticorum
melanoderma c.
melanosis c.

Cache Valley virus

cachexia
cancer c.
cancer, anorexia, cachexia syndrome
c. and dehydration
malarial c.
malignant c.
muscle c.
neurogenic c.
neuropathic c.
c. and nutrition
c. ovaripriva
paraneoplastic c.
c. strumipriva
c. thyreopriva
unique facies, anorexia, cachexia, and eye and skin syndrome

cachexial fever

Cacipacore virus

cadaver
c. donor
homograft c.
c. homograft
procurement of cadaver organs for transplantation
c. renal transplant

cadaveric
allocating cadaveric kidney
c. donor
c. donor transplantation
c. dura
c. ecchymosis
freeze-dried cadaveric dura
c. graft
c. whole organ transplant

cadence of gait

cadmium fume

café
c. au lait macule
c. au lait spot

cafe coronary

caffeine
c., alcohol, pepper, spicy foods
c. and halothane contracture test
headache from c.
insomnia from c.
c. intake
c. intoxication
nervousness from c.
no caffeine or pepper
phenacetin, aspirin, and c.
salicylamide, phenacetin, c.
c. sodium benzoate

caffeine-induced
c.-i. anxiety
c.-i. sleep disorder
c.-i. vasoconstriction

caffeine-intolerant individual

caffeine-related sequela

Caffey disease

Caffey-Silverman syndrome

Caffey-Smyth-Roske syndrome

cage
disc cage valve
elastic knee cage orthosis
elastic knee cage with medial and lateral contoured knee joints
intact rib c.
lumbar intersomatic fusion expandable c.
manual splinting of thoracic c.
rib c.
thoracic c.
thoracic cage volume
threaded fusion c.
upper rib c.

caged-ball
c.-b. prosthesis
c.-b. prosthetic valve
c.-b. valve

Cagot ear

Caimito virus

Caisson disease

Cajal
interstitial cells of C.
interstitial nucleus of C.
nucleus of C.

cake
c. kidney
marble cake hyperpigmentation
omental c.

caked breast

Calabar swelling

calcaneal
Anderson-Fowler calcaneal displacement osteotomy
anterior calcaneal osteotomy
anterior calcaneal process fracture
axial calcaneal projection
c. bone
c. bursa
juvenile calcaneal fracture
medial calcaneal branch of tibial nerve
medial column calcaneal fracture

calcaneal *(continued)*
c. pitch angle
plantar calcaneal spur
c. region
resting calcaneal stance position
c. spur
unilateral calcaneal brace

calcaneocavus
pes c.

calcaneocuboid
c. articulation
c. bone
c. distraction arthrodesis
dorsal c.
c. joint
c. ligament
long calcaneocuboid ligament
short c.

calcaneofibular ligament

calcaneonavicular
inferior calcaneonavicular ligament
c. joint
c. joint arthroscopy
c. ligament
c. ligament-tibialis posterior tendon advancement

calcaneotibial
c. arthrodesis
c. fusion
c. ligament

calcaneovalgus
c. flatfoot
pes c.

calcaneus
Abraham-Pankovich tendo calcaneus repair
anterior talar articular surface of c.
articular surface on calcaneus for cuboid bone
axial calcaneus view
malunited calcaneus fracture
pes c.

calcar
napkin ring calcar allograft
c. pedis

calcarea
peritendinitis c.

calcareous
c. cataract
c. conjunctivitis
c. deposit
c. metastasis
c. nodules
pericardium calcareous deposit

calcarina
arteria c.

calcarine
c. fissure
c. sulcus

calcereous pancreatitis

Calchaqui virus

calcific
c. aortic valve stenosis
c. atherosclerosis
chronic calcific pancreatitis of the tropics
diffuse calcific atherosclerosis
medial calcific sclerosis
c. mitral stenosis
c. mural atherosclerosis
c. nodular aortic stenosis
nodular calcific aortic stenosis
perforating calcific elastosis
rotator cuff calcific tendinitis
tropical calcific pancreatitis

calcification
Achilles tendon enthesis c.
active trabecular calcification surface
alimentary tract c.
aneurysmal wall c.
aortic arch c.
aortic calcification sign
aortic valve c.
arachnoid granulation c.
basal ganglion c.
c., Raynaud phenomenon, scleroderma, telangiectasis syndrome
casting breast c.
coronary artery c.
diffuse abdominal c.
diffuse interstitial pulmonary c.
electrolyte steroid cardiopathy by c.
familial idiopathic nonarteriosclerotic cerebral c.
gyriform intracranial c.
c. intervertebral cartilage
intervertebral disc c.
intracranial calcification benign glandular tissue
juvenile intervertebral disc c.
lobular breast c.
malignant breast c.
mitral annular c.
mitral annulus c.
moderate atherosclerosis with c.
c. necrosis
optic disc drusen c.
partial subligamentous c.
radiographic coronary c.
c. rate
soft tissue c.
symmetrical calcification of basal cerebral ganglion
zone of preparatory c.

calcified
c. anulus
c. aorta
c. aortic valve
c. atheroma
c. atheromata
c. atherosclerosis
c. benign granuloma
c. ductus arteriosus
c. epithelioma
c. fecalith
c. fetus
c. free body
c. gallbladder
c. granuloma
c. hemangioma
c. hilar node
c. leiomyoma of uterus
c. metastasis
miliary calcified necrosis
c. myoma
c. plaque
c. thyroid adenoma
c. wall of gallbladder

calcifying
c. cell epithelioma
chronic calcifying pancreatitis
c. epithelial odontogenic tumor
c. epithelioma
large cell calcifying Sertoli cell tumor
Malherbe calcifying epithelioma
c. odotogenic cyst

calcinosis
c. cutis circumscripta
c. cutis, osteoma cutis, poikiloderma, and skeletal abnormalities syndrome
metastatic calcinosis cutis
striopallidodentate c.
c. universalis

calcinuric diabetes

calciobiotic root canal sealer

calciotraumatic band

calcis
os c.
os calcis bone
os calcis osteotomy
os calcis pin fixation

calcitonin
c. gene-related hormone
c. gene-related peptide
human c.
immunoreactive c.
porcine c.
salmon c.

calcitonin-forming cell

calcium
c. antagonist
c. apatite stone
basic calcium phosphate
biodegradable calcium phosphate cement
c. blocker
c. bone index
c. carbonate
c. channel
c. channel agonist
c. channel antagonist
c. channel blocker
c. chloride
cholesterol calcium content
citrated calcium carbimide
crystalline calcium pyrophosphate dihydrate
c. current
c. deposit
c. deposit on heart valves
dialysate calcium concentration
c. disodium edetate
endogenous fecal c.
c. entry blocker
c. excretion
c. gluconate
c. gout
c. heparin
c. homeostatic mechanism
c. hydroxide
c. hydroxyapatite
idiopathic calcium renal stone formation
c. intake
ionized c.
c. ionophore
c. leucovorin
L-type calcium channel
methotrexate, Platinol, 5-fluorouracil, leucovorin, c.
milk of calcium microcyst
milk of calcium urinary tract cyst
mitral annular c.
net calcium absorption
net calcium influx
nondihydropyridine calcium channel blocker
c. nutrient agar
c. oxalate
c. oxalate calculus
c. oxalate crystal
c. oxalate renal stone
c. oxalate stone former
paracellular calcium resorption
parathyroid hormone-mediated calcium efflux
c. phosphate crystal deposition disease
c. phosphate stone
c. phosphate urinary lithiasis
c. to phosphorus ratio
precipitated calcium carbonate
c. pyrophosphate crystal deposition disease
c. pyrophosphate dehydrate deposition disease
c. pyrophosphate deposition
c. pyrophosphate deposition disease
c. pyrophosphate dihydrate
c. pyrophosphate dihydrate crystal deposition
c. pyrophosphate dihydrate deposition disease
recurrent calcium urolithiasis
c. rigor
serum c.
c. sign
c. tolerance test
total c.
total body c.
urinary calcium volume excretion rate
c.-urine spot test
voltage-dependent calcium channel
voltage-gated calcium channel
voltage-sensitive calcium channel

calcium-activated neutral protease

calcium-binding protein

calcium-calmodulin kinase II

calcium-dependent regulator

calcium-magnesium free

calcium-sensing receptor

calcium-signal modulating cyclophilin B ligand

Calciviridae virus

calcofluor white stain

calculated
c. average life
c. date of confinement
c. mean organism
c. opening area
c. serum osmolality
Simple C. Osteoporosis Risk Estimation

calculation
bidirectional shunt c.
computer dose c.
Monte Carlo c.
multiplane dosage c.

calculosa
pericarditis c.

calculous
c. anuria
c. cholecystitis
chronic calculous cholecystitis
c. cirrhosis
c. gallbladder disease
c. pyelitis

calculus
calcium oxalate c.
caliceal diverticular c.
carbonate apatite c.
c. cholecystitis
c. cirrhosis
c. disease
c. formation
c. inhibitor
intrahepatic biliary c.
marginal line calculus index
Simplified C. Index
submandibular duct c.
C. Surface Index
uric acid c.
urinary bladder c.

Caldwell
C. position
C. x-ray view

Caldwell-Luc
C.-L. approach
C.-L. operation
C.-L. procedure

Caldwell-Moloy
C.-M. classification
C.-M. method

calf
c. aortic microsome
artery of c.
c. blood flow
c. embryonic heart cell
c. esophagus epithelial cell
external pneumatic calf compression
fetal calf serum
gamma globulin-free calf serum
heat-inactivated fetal calf serum

calf *(continued)*
inactivated fetal calf serum
c. kidney
lateral cutaneous nerve of c.
c. lung surfactant extract
Nebraska calf diarrhea virus
Nebraska calf scours virus
neonatal calf diarrhea virus
newborn calf serum
nighttime calf cramp
c. pain from arteriosclerosis
c. serum
stretching calf, thigh and hamstring
c. testis
c. thymus extract

calf-heel stretch exercise

caliber
normal bladder c.
normal caliber duct
small caliber vessel
c. of vessel

calibrated
c. electrical stimulation
international calibrated ratio
left apexcardiogram, calibrated displacement
c. loop
c. monofilament
c. triangle of septal cartilage

calibration
automated test target c.
c. of the cardia
c. curve
c. curve data
c. factor
c. failure artifact
radiation-equivalent-manikin c.
c. ruler

caliceal
c. blunting
c. diverticular calculus
c. fistula
c. fornix

calices (*pl. of* calix)

calicivirus
feline c.
human c.

caliculus ophthalmicus

caliectasis
localized c.

California
C. Achievement Test
C. Critical Thinking Dispositions Inventory
C. Critical Thinking Skills Test
C. disease
C. encephalitis
C. encephalitis virus
C. Infant Scale for Motor Development
C. Marriage Readiness Evaluation
C. mastitis test
C. Occupational Preference Inventory
C. Occupational Preference Survey
C. Personality Inventory
C. Preschool Social Competency Scale
C. Psychological Inventory
C. Relative Value Studies
C. soft spinal system
Southern California Figure Ground Test
Southern California Postrotary Nystagmus Test
Southern California Sensory Integration Tests
Southern California Space Visualization Test
C. Test of Basic Skills
C. Test of Mental Maturity-Short Form
C. Test of Personality
C. Verbal Learning Test

caliper
anthropometric c.
blunt c.
c. brace
breast c.
c. measurement
c. micrometer
Mitutoyo digital c.
c. orthosis
c. rib movement
skin c.
skin fold c.

calix, pl. **calices**
anomalous c.
effacement of c.
major c.
minor c.
multiple calices
pelvis and c.
pelvis, calix and ureter
pole of calices
renal c.

call
to call back
intern on c.
office c.
on c.
patient to c.
sick c.
will c.
will call back

Callahan operation

Callander amputation

Callaway test

Callison fluid

callosal
c. agenesis
c. gyrus
c. marginal branch
median callosal artery
c. sulcus
c. syndrome

callosity
metatarsal c.

callosomarginal
anteromedial frontal branch of callosomarginal artery
paracentral branch of callosomarginal artery

callosotomy
anterior c.

callosum
anterior midbody of corpus c.
congenital thrombocytopenia, Robin sequence, agenesis of corpus callosum, distinctive facies, developmental delay syndrome
craniofacial dysmorphism, absent corpus callosum, iris colobomas, connective tissue dysplasia syndrome
partial corpus callosum agenesis
peduncle of corpus c.
rostrum of corpus c.
trunk of corpus c.
X-linked mental retardation, seizures, acquired microcephaly, agenesis of corpus c.

callus
endogenous callus formation
c. formation
medium callus Podi-Burr
c. on hand
soft callus stage

Calmette-Guérin
bacille C.-G.
bacille bilié de C.-G.
bacille Calmette-Guérin vaccine
bacillus C.-G.
C.-G. bacillus

heat-aggregated bacille C.-G.
heat-aggregated bacille C.-G.
Pasteur Institute bacillus Calmette-Guérin vaccine
percutaneous bacille Calmette-Guérin administration

Calmette reaction

calmodulin-dependent protein kinase

calm-wakefulness state

calomel
saturated calomel electrode

caloric
air caloric test
cold caloric irrigation
daily caloric intake
Hallpike caloric stimulation test
high c.
high caloric density
c. intake
c. nystagmus
poor caloric intake
c. requirements for burn patients
c. stimulation
c. stimulation test for vestibular function
c. test
c. testing of vestibular function

calorie
adequate calorie intake
adequate calories intake
c. count
gram c.
high c.
high calorie and nitrogen
c. intake
International Table c.
kilogram c.
large c.
low c.
nonprotein carbohydrate c.
optimum calorie intake
c.'s per kilogram per day
c.'s per ounce
c. restricted
total dietary c.
very low calorie diet

calorimeter
bench scale c.

calorimetry
accelerating rate c.
indirect c.
infrared thermographic c.

Calot
C. node
C. triangle

calvarial hook

Calvé-Legg-Perthes syndrome

Calvé-Perthes disease

calyceal fistula

cambium
periosteal cambium layer

Cambridge
C. electrocardiograph
C. Mental Disorders in Elderly Examination

cameloid anemia

Camelot Behavioral Checklist

camera
Anger gamma c.
delayed gamma camera image
endoscopic c.
gamma scintillation c.
infrared c.
multicrystal gamma c.
retinal c.
single crystal gamma c.

camouflage
orthodontic c.

Campbell
C. Interest and Skill Survey
modified Crawford Campbell inlaid bone-grafting technique
C. operation

Camp-Coventry position

Camp fever

Camp-Gianturco method

camphor
monobromated c.
peppermint c.
tar c.

cAMP-response
cAMP-r. element
cAMP-r. element modulator

camptodactyly-arthropathy-pericarditis syndrome

camptomelic syndrome

***Campylobacter*-like organism**

Camurati-Engelmann syndrome

can
empty can test
high-voltage c.
c. opener capsulotomy

Canadian
C. Acute Respiratory Illness and Flu Scale
C. Cognitive Abilities Test
C. Heart Classification
C. Test of Basic Skills

canal
ampulla of lacrimal c.
anal canal length
anterior condylar c.
anterior condyloid canal of occipital bone
anterior ethmoid c.
anterior retinal orbital c.
anterior semicircular c.
anterior-to-posterior sagittal canal diameter
anterior vertical c.
c. of Arantius
arteriovenous canal defect
artery of pterygoid c.
atrial ventricular canal defect
atrioventricular c.
atrioventricular canal cushion
atrioventricular canal defect
atrioventricular canal septal defect
attenuated pyloric c.
Black Creek C. virus
blood in auditory c.
calciobiotic root canal sealer
carotid artery c.
cervical canal stenosis
common atrioventricular c.
completely in the canal hearing aid
c. of Corti
c. of Cuvier
c. and drum
external auditory c.
c. finder
floor of inguinal c.
greater palatine c.
c. of Guidi
c. of Guyon
c. hearing aid
c. of Hering
horizontal semicircular c.
incisive canal cyst
intact canal wall
internal auditory c.
c. of Kovalevsky
c. of Lambert
Lightspeed canal preparation technique
longitudinal canal of modiolus
lumbar canal stenosis
medial crus of facial c.

canal *(continued)*
medial crus of the horizontal part of the facial c.
middle ear c.
multiple cone root canal filling method
narrowing of spinal c.
neural foraminal c.
c. of Nuck
nutrient canal of bone
opening of carotid c.
outer ear c.
palmate fold of cervical c.
partial atrioventricular c.
partial atrioventricular canal defect
patent canal of Nuck
pecten of anal c.
perineal flexure of anal c.
persistent complete atrioventricular c.
petrous carotid c.
pharyngeal branch of artery of pterygoid c.
posterior semicircular c.
pulp c.
pulp canal sealer
pyloric c.
c. of Recklinghausen
c. resonance response
root canal therapy
root canal of tooth
root canal filling
c. of Scarpa
c. of Schlemm
c. of Schlemm
spinal canal tumor
spiral canal of cochlea
c. of Stilling
superior semicircular c.
superior semicircular canal deficiency
supplementary c.
vertebral c.
c. of Vesalius
c. wall down mastoidectomy
c. wall down tympanomastoidectomy
c. wall down tympanoplasty
c. wall up mastoidectomy
c. wall up tympanoplasty
c. of Wirsung

canalicular
dense canalicular system
c. duct
open canalicular system of platelets

canaliculum
papilloma c.

canaliculus
anterior canaliculus of chorda tympani
apical c.
auricular c.
c. chordae tympani
intracellular c.
c. lacrimalis
mastoid c.
polyp in c.

canaliform
medial canaliform dystrophy
median canaliform dystrophy

canalith
c. repositioning
c. repositioning maneuver
c. repositioning procedure

canalized thrombus

canal/wall-up technique

Cananeia virus

canarypox virus

cancellation
phase c.
Star C. Test

cancellous
autogenous cancellous bone graft
autologous cancellous bone graft
c. bone
c. cellular bone
c. cellular bone graft
c. chip bone graft
c. and cortical bone graft
cortical cancellous screw
c. freeze-dried allograft
freeze-dried cancellous allograft
c. graft
c. hematopoietic marrow
iliac cancellous bone
c. insert graft
marrow
morcellized cancellous graft
c. morselized bone graft
multiple cancellous chip graft
Nicoll cancellous bone graft
Nicoll cancellous insert graft
onlay cancellous iliac graft
Papineau cancellous graft
particulate cancellous bone graft
particulate cancellous bone and marrow
c. screw
c. tissue
c. versus cortical bone

cancer
adjuvant therapy for breast c.
advanced ovarian c.
advanced resected head and neck c.
alternative cancer therapy
androgen-dependent prostate c.
androgen-independent prostate c.
Ann Arbor cancer staging
anthracycline-nave metastatic breast c.
anti-EGF receptor antibody for c.
antiepidermal growth factor receptor antibody for c.
c. antigen
c. antigen 125
c. antigen 19-9
Arizona Cancer Center multiple myeloma staging system
asymptomatic metastatic hormone-refractory prostate c.
c. atrophicans
C. Attitude Survey
AuraTek rapid cancer test
Austrian Breast C. Study Group
c. biotherapy study group
bladder c.
breast c.
breast cancer antigen
breast cancer screening indicator
Breast C. Detection Demonstration Project
breast cancer gene
c. cachexia
c., anorexia, cachexia syndrome
c. care center
c. causing agent
c. cell-derived blood coagulating activity 1
cellular breast cancer therapy
centralized cancer patient data system
c. of cervix
clay pipe c.
clinical spectrum of c.
c. coagulation factor
colon c.
colorectal c.
comprehensive cancer center
c. destroying agent
detected in colon c.
c. detection center
early detection of breast c.
early gastric cancer of the upper stomach
early stage breast c.
epithelial ovarian c.

exenterative surgery for pelvic c.
experimental breast cancer treatment
familial colon c.
familial colonic c.
familial medullary thyroid c.
family history of c.
c. family syndrome
c. free
Functional Assessment of C. Therapy
Functional Assessment of C. Therapy-Breast
Functional Assessment of C. Therapy-Fatigue
Functional Assessment of C. Therapy-General
Functional Assessment of C. Therapy–Head and Neck
Functional Assessment of C. Therapy-Lung
Functional Assessment of C. Therapy-Prostate
gastric c.
gastric remnant c.
gastrointestinal cancer antigen
c. growth
head and neck c.
hepatitis-induced liver c.
hepatocellular c.
hereditary breast and ovarian c.
hereditary colon c.
hereditary nonpolyposis colon c.
hereditary nonpolyposis colorectal c.
hereditary papillary renal c.
hereditary prostate cancer 1 locus
hereditary site-specific colon c.
high-risk breast c.
high risk for breast c.
high risk for breast c.
high risk of developing cervical c.
high-risk primary breast c.
hormonal cancer treatment
hormone-dependent prostate c.
hormone-independent prostate c.
hormone-refractory metastatic prostate c.
hormone-refractory prostate c.
hormone-resistant prostate c.
human ovarian c.
immunocompromised cancer patient
increased risk of breast c.
infiltrating lobular c.
inflammatory breast c.
inoperable metastatic lung c.
inoperable ovarian c.
inoperable pancreatic c.
intradermal cancer test
invasive bladder c.
invasive breast c.
invasive cervical c.
invasive lobular c.
large operable breast c.
left-sided colon c.
c. and leukemia group B
Life After C. Care
limited-stage small cell lung c.
localization of prostate c.
locally advanced c.
locally advanced breast c.
locally advanced esophageal c.
locally advanced non-small-cell lung c.
locally advanced prostate c.
locoregional breast c.
lower urinary tract c.
lung c.
Lung C. Symptom Scale
Lung C. Symptom Score
Lynch cancer family syndrome I, II
male breast c.
c. malignant cell
mammaglobin breast cancer protein
mammary cancer virus of mice
MCF-7 breast cancer cell
M.D. Anderson cancer staging
M.D. Anderson C. Center
medullary thyroid c.
Memorial Sloan-Kettering C. Center
Mental Adjustment to C. scale
Merkel cell c.
metachronous colon c.
metastatic breast c.
metastatic cancer of spinal fluid
metastatic colon c.
metastatic colorectal c.
metastatic liver c.
metastatic lung c.
metastatic prostate c.
microinvasive cervical c.
Milan Cancer Institute
Muir-Torre syndrome of hereditary nonpolyposis colon c.
c. multistep therapy
mutated in colon c.
nasal cavity c.
nasal vestibule c.
nasopharyngeal c.
National Alliance of Breast C. Organization
National Comprehensive C. Network
National C. Data Base
National C. Institute
National C. Institute Cooperative Group
National C. Institute Protocol 89-C-41
National Prostatic C. Project criteria
neurologic complication of systemic c.
node-positive breast c.
nonhereditary breast c.
noninvasive cervical c.
nonmelanoma skin c.
nonpolyposis colorectal c.
non-small-cell lung c.
NSE lung cancer tumor marker
oat cell lung c.
obstructing colorectal c.
obstructive colorectal c.
obstructive esophagogastric c.
operable breast c.
oral cancer examination
oral cavity c.
ovarian c.
ovarian cancer metastasis
ovarian epithelial c.
pain from c.
pancreatic cancer marker
pancreatic cancer pain
pancreatic head c.
papillary thyroid c.
paranasal c.
pathological tumor, nodes, metastases staging of c.
pattern of cancer spread
performance status scale for head and neck c.
poorly differentiated lung c.
postmenopausal breast c.
C. Potential Index
preferred treatment in c.
preoperative staging of c.
primary bone c.
primary cancer site
primary colorectal c.
primary liver cell c.
primary operable breast c.
c. proneness phenotype
prostate c.
c. of prostate
c. of the prostate and brain gene

cancer *(continued)*
prostate cancer screening
prostate cancer treatment
rabbit antibladder c.
recurrent colorectal c.
c. registry
c. in remission
remnant gastric c.
renal cell c.
roentgenographically occult lung c.
sarcoma, breast and brain tumors, leukemia, laryngeal and lung cancer adenoma
c. serum index
c. in situ
slow down cancer growth
small cell cancer of bladder
small intestine c.
squamous cell c.
squamous cell head and neck c.
staging of c.
c. and steroid hormone
superficial bladder c.
C. Surveillance Program
C. Surveillance System
synchronous ipsilateral breast c.
terminal c.
testicular c.
c. therapy facility
transitional cell c.
c. of unknown primary
c. of unknown primary site

cancerous
gastric cancerous area
c. growth
c. growth of blood cell

Candida
Candida metabolic antigen
Ccandida granuloma
Murex *Candida albicans* test
Candida urinary tract infection

candidal
c. abscess
c. conjunctivitis
c. endocarditis
c. endophthalmitis
c. esophagitis
c. granuloma
c. granuloma infection
c. infection
c. intertrigo
c. leukoplakia
c. onychomycosis
c. osteomyelitis
c. overgrowth
c. pharyngitis
c. pneumonia
c. vaginitis
c. vulvovaginitis

candidate
allogeneic antigen c.
high-risk c.
organ donor c.
organ recipient c.

candidiasis
autoimmune polyendocrinopathy, candidiasis, ectodermal dysplasia
autoimmune polyendocrinopathy, candidiasis, ectodermal dystrophy
chronic mucocutaneous c.
esophageal c.
hypoparathyroidism, Addison disease, and mucocutaneous candidiasis syndrome
hypoparathyroidism, adrenal insufficiency, mucocutaneous candidiasis syndrome
localized mucocutaneous c.
mucocutaneous c.
multiple endocrine deficiency, Addison disease, and candidiasis syndrome
multiple endocrine deficiency-autoimmune c.
neonatal systemic c.
oropharyngeal c.
systemic c.
urinary tract c.
vulvovaginal c.

candidosis
mucocutaneous c.
oral c.
perianal c.

candle
mean horizontal candle power
mean spherical candle power
c. power
spherical candle power
c. wax appearance of bone

cane
adjustable cane board
ambulates with a c.
ambulates with a quad c.
bilateral short leg c.
large-base quad c.
narrow-base quad c.
patient independent with small based quad c.
quad c.
single base c.
small-based quad c.
walk with aid of c.
wide-base quad c.

canicularis
Fannia c.

canicular multispecific organic anion transporter

Caninde virus

canine
acute canine idiopathic polyneuropathy
c. adenovirus 1
c. distemper
c. distemper encephalitis
c. distemper virus
c. herpesvirus
homologous canine distemper antiserum
incisors, canines, premolars, and molars
infectious canine hepatitis
c. inherited ataxia
c. kala-azar
c. leishmaniasis
Madin-Darby canine kidney
mandibular c.
maxillary c.
maxillary canine cusp
maxillary canine eminence
minute virus of c.'s
c. pancreatic polypeptide
c. parvovirus
c. scabies
c. tooth

canker
oral c.
c. sore from anxiety
water c.

cannabinoid
cross-reacting c.
overdosed with c.
tetrahydrocannabinol cross-reacting c.

cannabis
c. abuse
c. delusional disorder
c. dependence
c. intoxication
c. intoxication-related disorder
c. intoxication, with perceptual disturbance
c. organic mental disorder
c. psychosis
c. sativa
c. use disorder

cannabis-induced
c.-i. mental changes
c.-i. psychotic disorder with delusions
c.-i. psychotic disorder with hallucinations

cannabis-related disorder, not otherwise specified

cannellata
manna c.

cannibalistic
c. fantasy
c. fixation

Cannon
C. ring
C. sound
C. theory

cannonball
c. lesion
c. metastasis
c. pattern
c. pulse

cannula
angled left/right c.
anterior chamber c.
balloon uterine elevator c.
binasal c.
blunt arthroscopic c.
curved cannula with locking dilator
four-pronged liposuction c.
high-flow nasal c.
infant nasal cannula assembly
c. insertion site
intragastric c.
liquid vitreous-aspirating c.
McIntyre nylon cannula connector
nasal c.
nasal cannula dermatitis
Nichamin hydrodissection c.
Oaks straight c.
O'Gawa two-way aspirating c.
O2 by nasal c.
O_2 by nasal c.
O2 saturation on three liters nasal c.
O2 saturation on two liters nasal c.
oxygen by nasal c.
oxygen saturation on 2 liters nasal c.
oxygen saturation on 3 liters nasal c.
Packo pars plana c.
Pautler infusion c.
Pearce coaxial irrigating/aspirating c.
Peczon I/A c.
stable access c.
c. tip
vacuum uterine c.

cannulated
c. drill point
c. expulsion piston
heart c.
c. hip screw
c. nail
c. percutaneously
c. reaming technique
c. screw
c. screwdriver
c. wrench

cannulation
arterial cannulation anesthetic technique
arterial cannulation support
ex vivo c.
femoral arterial c.
internal jugular vein c.
percutaneous arterial c.

canopy
surgical overhead c.

cant
occlusal c.

Canterbury Alcoholism Screening Test

canthal
inner canthal distance
internal canthal ligament
Lynch medial canthal incision
medial canthal fissure
medial canthal incision
medial canthal ligament
medial canthal repair
medial canthal tendon
outer canthal distance
c. raphe
c. recess

canthic
medial canthic fold

canthopexy
medial c.

canthoplasty
medial c.

canthus
inner c.
medial c.
medial canthus area
nasal c.
outer c.
outer canthus of eye
papilloma, inner c.

cantilever
c. beam
c. bridge
c. external fixator
c. fixed partial denture
c. space maintainer

cantilevered
c. bone graft
overlay cantilevered bone graft
c. split cranial bone graft

canting
occlusal c.

Cantor tube

Cantrell
pentalogy of C.
pentalogy of Cantrell syndrome

Cantwell
modified Cantwell technique

Canyon
Muerto Canyon virus
Sunday Canyon virus

cap
anterior head c.
apical cap sign
Assura stoma c.
continent anal c.
duodenal c.
endoscopic mucosal resection, cap method
heparin c.
radius cap prosthesis

capability
immune c.
inherent c.
metabolic c.
Minimum Auditory Capabilities Test
trypsin-inhibitory c.
wound healing c.

capable
c. of independent living
smallest unit of DNA capable of recombination

capacitance
c. factor
resistance and c.
segmental venous c.
segmented venous capacitance ratio
venous c.

capacitation
potassium-containing minimal capacitation medium

capacitive radiofrequency

capacitor

bypass c.
output c.
paper c.

capacity

acid neutralization c.
acid-neutralizing c.
aerobic c.
antigen-binding c.
blood oxygen c.
buffer c.
capillary diffusion c.
carbon dioxide diffusing capacity of the lung
cardiac functional c.
cardiovascular work c.
cerebrovascular reserve c.
colony-forming c.
corticosteroid-binding globulin-binding c.
decreased capacity for abstract thought
demand minimum functional c.
diffusing capacity for carbon dioxide
diffusing capacity for carbon monoxide
diffusing capacity of lung
diffusing capacity of lung for carbon monoxide
diffusing capacity of lungs for oxygen
dye-binding c.
elastase inhibition c.
electrostatic c.
forced expiratory c.
forced expiratory volume in one second to forced vital capacity ratio
forced expiratory volume timed to forced vital capacity ratio
forced inspiratory vital c.
forced vital capacity analysis
c. to function
functional c.
functional aerobic c.
functional capacity evaluation
functional residual c.
functional vital c.
functional work capacity assessment
galactose elimination c.
heart flow c.
heat c.
hemoglobin-binding c.
histamine-forming c.
c. for independent living
indirect maximal breathing c.
inspiratory c.
inspiratory reserve c.
inspiratory vital c.
inspired vital c.
job capacity evaluation
knot holding c.
latent iron-binding c.
maximal recycling c.
maximal specific binding c.
maximal sustainable ventilatory c.
maximal sustained ventilatory c.
maximum bladder c.
maximum breathing c.
maximum cystometric c.
maximum expiratory flow at 50% vital c.
membrane diffusing c.
mental capacity evaluation
midinspiratory flow at 50% of vital c.
molar heat c.
myeloid colony-forming c.
myocardial vascular c.
Neurologic and Adaptive C. Score
normal vital c.
oxygen c.
oxygen capacity of blood
peak work c.
physical dependence c.
physical work c.
predicted functional residual c.
predicted vital c.
proliferative c.
pulmonary diffusing c.
pulmonary diffusion c.
relative proliferative c.
relative storage c.
renal reserve filtration c.
residual functional c.
residual lung c.
residual volume/total lung capacity ratio
reticuloendothelial phagocytic c.
serum iron-binding c.
serum reserve cholesterol binding c.
serum trypsin inhibition c.
single-breath carbon monoxide diffusing capacity of lung
single-breath diffusing c.
slow vital c.
Smith physical capacities evaluation
specific heat c.
steady-state carbon monoxide diffusing capacity of lung
strong exchange capacity resin
submaximal working c.
timed ventilatory c.
timed vital c.
Toronto Functional C. Questionnaire
total c.
total bed c.
total bladder c.
total capacity of lung
total exchange c.
total iron-binding c.
total lung c.
total vital c.
total vitamin B_{12} binding c.
total volume c.
true total lung c.
trypsin-inhibitory c.
unbound iron-binding c.
uninhibited detrusor muscle c.
unsaturated binding c.
unsaturated iron-binding c.
unsaturated vitamin B_{12}-binding c.
urinary bladder c.
ventilatory c.
visual c.
vital c.
work c.
work capacity assessment
work capacity evaluation
work capacity specialist

Cape Wrath virus

CAP-free diet

Capgras

C. delusion
C. syndrome

capillarioscopy, capillaroscopy

nail fold c.
nail fold capillarioscopy abnormality

capillary

c. agglutination test
alveolar capillary membrane
angel's kiss capillary malformation
Arndorfer capillary perfusion system
arterial c.
arterialized capillary blood
c. basement membrane
c. basement membrane thickness
c. basement membrane width
c. blood
c. blood flow

blood flow from c.
c. blood flow velocity
c. blood gas
c. blood gas at room air
c. blood glucose
c. blood sugar
c. blush
brisk capillary refill
c. column gas chromatography
c. diffusion capacity
effective capillary flow
c. filling time
c. filtrate collector
c. filtration coefficient
c. fragility test
glomerular capillary basement
glomerular capillary wall
c. hemangioma
c. hemorrhage
c. hemostatic
hereditary capillary fragility
high-performance capillary electrophoresis
c. hydrostatic pressure
increasing capillary permeability
c. isotachophoresis
c. leak syndrome
liver capillary hemangioma
lobular capillary hemangioma
c. loop in dermal papilla
c. loop in hair papilla
c. lumen
lung capillary time
lymph c.
mean pulmonary capillary wedge pressure
meningeal capillary angiomatosis
micellar electrokinetic capillary chromatography
microhematocrit capillary tube
mixed capillary cavernous hemangioma
muscle capillary basement membrane
muscle capillary basement membrane thickening
nail fold capillary loop abnormality
orbital capillary hemangioma
c. osmotic pressure
oxygen concentration in pulmonary capillary blood
parafoveal capillary net
periocular capillary hemangioma
peripheral capillary filtration slit length
peritubular c.
prolonged capillary refill
pulmonary c.
pulmonary capillary blood flow perfusion
pulmonary capillary blood volume
pulmonary capillary gas volume
pulmonary capillary hemangiomatosis
pulmonary capillary protein leakage
pulmonary capillary wedge
pulmonary capillary wedge pressure
pulmonary venous c.
Quincke capillary pulse
c. refill
c. refill, sensation, motor function, temperature
c. refill time
retinal capillary microaneurysm
Rumpel-Leede capillary fragility
systemic capillary leak syndrome
terminal capillary network
venous c.
volume, c.
c. wedge pressure
c. whole blood true sugar
c. zone electrophoresis

capillary-free zone

capillary-leak phenomenon

capillary-lymphatic malformation

Capim virus

capita
per c.

capital
c. epiphysis
c. epiphysis angle of Wiberg
c. expenditure review
c. expenditure threshold
c. sin
slipped capital femoral epiphysis

capitate
c. bone
c. and hamate

capitated primary care network

capitate-hamate joint

capitate-lunate joint

capitatum
os c.

capitellum
osteochondritis of c.

capitis
anterior rectus c.
longissimus capitis muscle
longus c.
longus capitis muscle
musculus longissimus c.
musculus longus c.
oblique capitis muscle
obliquus capitis superior
obliquus capitis superior muscle
c. pediculosis
rectus and longus capitis muscle
semispinalis capitis muscle

capitular process

capitulum of stapes

Caplan syndrome

capnography
low-flow sidestream c.

capping
apical c.

caprine
c. arthritis encephalitis virus

caprylate
penicillin, bacitracin, streptomycin, c.

capsid
Epstein-Barr viral capsid antigen
major capsid protein gene
viral capsid antigen
viral capsid antigen, Epstein-Barr

capsular
anterior capsular distance
anterior capsular shift
anterior-inferior capsular ligament dysfunction
arthrographic capsular distension and rupture technique
atraumatic, multidirectional, bilateral rehabilitation inferior capsular shift
c. glaucoma
c. hemiplegia
inferior capsular shift
c. insufficiency
c. joint
ligamentous and capsular repair
L-shaped capsular incision
Macleod capsular rheumatism
medial capsular imbrication
medial capsular ligament
Neer capsular shift procedure
Neufeld capsular swelling
Neufeld capsular test
O'Brien capsular shift procedure
pelvis capsular dysplasia
pneumococcal capsular polysaccharide
posterior capsular cataract

capsular *(continued)*
posterior capsular opacification
posterior capsular polishing
specific capsular substance
c. surface smooth and glistening
c. synovial-like hyperplasia
c. thrombosis syndrome
c. tightness
typhoid vaccine, Vi capsular polysaccharide

capsulare
lipoma c.

capsularis
membrana c.
membrana capsularis lentis posterior

capsulated
smooth, capsulated, virulent bacteria

capsulatum
Histoplasma capsulatum antigen
Histoplasma capsulatum polysaccharide antigen

capsule
adipose capsule of kidney
adipose renal c.
all-purpose c.
angled capsule forceps
anterior capsule shagreen
anterior joint capsule thickening
anterior lens c.
anterior limb of internal c.
c. of Bowman
Bowman c.
c. cartilage articular preservation
contraceptive suppository c.
dry-filled c.
Ernst radium c.
c. fragment forceps
glomerular capsule of kidney
c. of glomerulus
hand-filled c.
hard gel c.
c. identified
internal c.
joint capsule defect
knee of internal c.
limb of anterior c.
medial carpal c.
olive-tip capsule polisher
periprosthetic fibrous c.
perirenal fat c.
placebo capsule or tablet
posterior c.
posterior capsule opacification
posterior limb of the internal c.
pseudoexfoliation of lens c.
right internal c.
soft elastic c.
soft elastic gelatin capsule
c. strip easily
c. of Tenon
vitamin c.
wireless endoscopy c.

capsulectomy
anterior c.

capsulitis
adhesive c.
c. joint

capsuloganglionic hemorrhage

capsulolabral
anterior capsulolabral reconstruction

capsulolenticular cataract

capsulopupillaris
membrana c.

capsulorrhaphy
electrothermally assisted c.

capsulorrhexis
continuous circular c.
continuous curvilinear c.
minicircular c.

capsulothalamic syndrome

capsulotomy
anterior capsulotomy for treatment of OCD
can opener c.
circular tear c.
YAG posterior c.

captioned media program

captive air bubble

captivus
penis c.

capture
antibody capture immunoassay
antibody capture ligand assay
antigen capture assay
antigen capture ligand assay
atrial capture beat
boron neutron capture therapy
electron c.
electron capture detector
c. gamma ray
hybrid capture assay
immunoglobulin M antibody c.
microparticle capture enzyme immunoassay
c. threshold
ventricular capture beat

caput stapedis

Carabello sign

Caraparu virus

carbachol inhalation challenge

carbamate
pyrindinol c.

carbamoyl
ornithine carbamoyl transferase deficiency

carbamoyltransferase
aspartate c.
ornithine c.
ornithine carbamoyltransferase assay
serum ornithine c.

carbazochrome sodium sulfonate

carbide
amorphous hydrogenated silicon c.
c. bur
medium carbide cone bur
Oto-Flex carbide bur
silicon c.
tungsten c.

carbimide
citrated calcium c.

carbohydrate
c. absorption
anomer of c.
c. antigen
critical carbohydrate level
fluorophore-assisted carbohydrate electrophoresis
gestational carbohydrate intolerance
hypocaloric carbohydrate feeding
c. intolerance
c. loading
low c.
low available carbohydrate diet
c. metabolism disorder
c. metabolism index
no concentrated c.'s
nonprotein carbohydrate calorie
Ross carbohydrate free

carbohydrate-active steroid

carbohydrate-binding protein

carbohydrate-deficient
c.-d. glycoprotein
c.-d. glycoprotein syndrome
c.-d. transferrin

carbohydrate-induced hyperglyceridemia

carbolic methylene blue

carbon
alveolar-arterial carbon dioxide difference
c. arc lamp
arterial carbon dioxide
arterial carbon dioxide pressure
arteriovenous carbon dioxide
arteriovenous carbon dioxide difference
asymmetric carbon atom
athletic shoe carbon fiber plate
c. atom farthest from principal functioning group
c., hydrogen, and nitrogen
concentration of total carbon dioxide
c. copy
diffusing capacity for carbon dioxide
diffusing capacity for carbon monoxide
diffusing capacity of lung for carbon monoxide
c. dioxide
c. dioxide combing power
c. dioxide diffusing capacity of the lung
c. dioxide electrode
c. dioxide elimination
c. dioxide gas
c. dioxide gas laser
c. dioxide insufflator
c. dioxide laser skin resurfacing
c. dioxide laser vaporization
c. dioxide output
c. dioxide pressure
c. dioxide therapy
c. dioxide with oxygen
end-tidal carbon dioxide monitoring
end-tidal carbon dioxide concentration
extracorporeal carbon dioxide removal
extrapolated end-tidal carbon dioxide tension
c. fiber fixator
c. fiber graft
c. fiber half ring
c. fiber lamination braid
c. fiber-reinforced plastic
c. fiber-reinforced plate
fractional concentration of carbon dioxide in expired gas
fraction of alveolar carbon dioxide
fraction of expired carbon dioxide
fraction of inspired carbon dioxide
functional uptake of carbon monoxide
inorganic c.
mixed expired carbon dioxide tension
c. monoxide
c. monoxide hemoglobin
c. monoxide myoglobin
c. monoxide oximetry
c. monoxide pressure or tension
c. monoxide transfer factor
nonpurgeable organic c.
organic c.
partial arterial gas tension of carbon dioxide
partial pressure of arterial carbon dioxide
partial pressure of carbon dioxide in arterial gas
partial pressure of carbon dioxide in mixed venous blood
partial pressure of intramuscular carbon dioxide
partial pressure of mesenteric venous carbon dioxide
partial pressure tension of carbon dioxide, vein
particulate organic c.
pressure of carbon dioxide
residual organic c.
c. separated from the carboxyl group by 2 other carbon atoms
single-breath carbon monoxide diffusing capacity of lung
steady-state carbon monoxide diffusing capacity of lung
c. steel drill point
subpleural reticulated carbon deposition
c. tetrachloride poisoning
total carbon dioxide content
total organic c.
transcutaneous carbon dioxide pressure
transcutaneous carbon dioxide tension
transcutaneous carbon dioxide monitor
ultrahigh c.
venous carbon dioxide production
yeast carbon base

carbon-14
c.-14 isotope
c.-14 urea breath test

carbonaceous
c. activated water
c. material
c. sputum

carbonate
c. apatite calculus
c. apatite stone
calcium c.
lithium c.
magnesium c.
precipitated calcium c.

carbonated beverage

carbon-hydrogen stretch

carbonic
c. anhydrase
c. anhydrase II
c. anhydrase inhibitor

carbonizing cellular debris

carbonless paper syndrome

carbon-to-nitrogen ratio

carbon-tungsten rasp

carbon-13 urea breath test

carborundum disc

carbovir monophosphate

carboxamide
aminoimidazole c.
aminoimidazole carboxamide ribonucleotide
aminoimidazole carboxamide ribotide
succinyl aminoimidazole carboxamide ribotide

carboxyl
biotin carboxyl carrier protein
carbon separated from the carboxyl group by 2 other carbon atoms
c. terminal
c. terminal peptide

carboxylase
biotin c.
3-methylcrotonyl-CoA carboxylase deficiency

carboxylic ester hydrolase

carboxymethylase
protein c.

carboxymethylcellulose
sodium c.

carboxypeptidase
c. A

carboxypeptidase *(continued)*
c. N
serum carboxypeptidase N

carboxyterminal
c. propeptide of type 1 procollagen

carbuncle
malignant c.

carbuncular fever

carcinoembryonic
c. antigen
c. antigen-125
c. antigen doubling time
polyclonal carcinoembryonic antigen

carcinogenesis
radiation-induced c.

carcinoid
argentaffin carcinoid tumor
atypical carcinoid tumor
goblet cell c.
c. heart disease
intestinal tract c.
intraluminal typical bronchial c.
metastatic carcinoid syndrome
multicentric carcinoid tumor
ovarian carcinoid tumor
rectal carcinoid tumor
c. syndrome
thymic carcinoid tumor
c. tumor of intestine
typical c.

carcinoma
acinar cell c.
adenoid cystic c.
adenoid cystic carcinoma of head and neck
adenosquamous cell c.
adrenocortical c.
advanced hepatocellular c.
advanced squamous cell cervical c.
aggressive thyroid c.
alveolar cell c.
anal gland c.
anaplastic thyroid c.
androgen-independent prostate c.
aneuploid colorectal c.
anthracycline-refractory metastatic breast c.
apocrine ductal carcinoma in situ
argyrophilic ductal carcinoma in situ
aryepiglottic fold c.
asbestos-related lung c.
Astwood-Coller staging system for c.
atypical medullary c.
Atzpodien regimen for renal cell c.
autolymphocyte-based treatment for renal cell c.
axillary nodal metastasis in breast c.
basal cell c.
basaloid squamous cell c.
base of tongue c.
basosquamous c.
c. to be ruled out
bladder carcinoma in situ
c. of breast
bronchial c.
bronchioalveolar c.
bronchogenic c.
c. cell line
cells consistent with invasive c.
central mucoepidermoid c.
cholangiocellular c.
choroid plexus c.
chromophobe renal cell c.
circumferential invasive c.
clear cell c.
clear cell hepatocellular c.
clear cell renal cell c.
collecting duct c.
colorectal c.
continuously cultured carcinoma cell line used for tissue cultures
conventional papillary c.
cribriform salivary carcinoma of excretory duct
cystic renal cell c.
differentiated c.
differentiated thyroid c.
distal bile duct c.
ductal carcinoma in situ
Duke classification of c.
early advanced hepatocellular c.
early gastric c.
early hepatocellular c.
Ehrlich ascites c.
embryonal c.
embryonal cell c.
endocrine ductal carcinoma in situ
endometrial c.
endometrial carcinoma in situ
endometrial intraepithelial c.
epithelial-myoepithelial carcinoma
Epstein-Barr nasopharyngeal c.
esophageal c.
esophageal squamous cell c.
extensive inoperable c.
extensive intraductal c.
extrapulmonary small cell c.
familial medullary thyroid c.
familial nonmedullary thyroid c.
fibrolamellar hepatocellular c.
follicular variant of papillary thyroid c.
c. of hard palate
head and neck squamous cell c.
c. head of pancreas
hepatic cell c.
hepatocellular c.
hepatoma carcinoma cell
hereditary clear cell renal c.
hereditary nonpolyposis colon c.
hereditary nonpolyposis colorectal c.
hereditary papillary renal cell c.
hormonal therapy in endometrial c.
human cervical carcinoma cell
human mammary carcinoma cell membrane proteinase
human oral epidermoid carcinoma cell
Hürthle cell c.
hyalinizing clear cell c.
infiltrating ductal c.
infiltrating ductal carcinoma of the breast
infiltrating ductal cell c.
infiltrating lobular c.
infiltrating squamous cell c.
inflammatory carcinoma or breast
inoperable esophageal c.
inoperable gastric c.
intraductal carcinoma of breast
intraductal papillary c.
intraepithelial carcinoma of cervix
invasive carcinoma of breast
invasive cervical c.
invasive ductal c.
invasive vulvar c.
islet cell c.
isolated gland carcinoma in situ
Kulchitsky cell c.
large cell lung c.
large cell neuroendocrine c.
laryngeal squamous cell c.
Lewis lung c.
lipid-laden homogeneous adrenocortical c.
liver cell c.
lobular carcinoma in situ
localized prostate c.
locally advanced cervical c.

locally advanced and inflammatory breast c.
locoregional breast c.
lymphoepithelioma-like c.
lymphoepithelioma-like carcinoma of skin
lymphoepithelioma-like thymic c.
macrofollicular thyroid papillary c.
male breast c.
maxillary sinus c.
medullary c.
medullary breast c.
medullary carcinoma of breast
medullary carcinoma flush
medullary carcinoma of the thyroid
medullary carcinoma of thyroid
medullary renal c.
medullary thyroid c.
meibomian gland c.
Merkel cell c.
Merkel cell carcinoma cell line
mesonephroid clear cell c.
metastatic basal cell c.
metastatic breast c.
metastatic carcinoma of unknown primary origin
metastatic colorectal c.
metastatic renal cell c.
metastatic squamous carcinoma of head and neck
microcystic adnexal c.
microcystic eccrine c.
microinvasive carcinoma classification
micropapillary serous c.
micropapillary serous ovarian c.
microtrabecular hepatocellular c.
minimally invasive follicular c.
missed bronchogenic c.
moderately differentiated neuroendocrine c.
morbilliform basal cell c.
morpheaform basal cell c.
morphea-type basal cell c.
mucinous breast c.
mucinous eccrine c.
mucoepidermoid c.
mucoepidermoid carcinoma of parotid
mucoepidermoid carcinoma of tongue
mucus-producing adenopapillary c.
multicentric basal cell c.
multicentric mammary c.
multifocal breast c.
multifocal infiltrated duct cell c.
multiple basal cell carcinoma syndrome multiple basal cell nevus syndrome
multiple nevoid-basal cell c.
multiple nevoid-basal cell carcinoma syndrome
multiple self-healing squamous c.
mutated colorectal c.
nasopharyngeal c.
nasopharyngeal carcinoma in situ
nasopharyngeal carcinoma with lymph node involvement
neuroendocrine ductal carcinoma in situ
neuroendocrine small cell c.
nevoid basal cell carcinoma syndrome
nodal involvement in breast c.
nodal metastasis in breast c.
nodular basal cell c.
noduloulcerative basal cell c.
nonfunctioning adrenal c.
noninfiltrating intraductal c.
noninvasive breast c.
nonkeratinizing epidermoid c.
nonpapillary thyrogenic c.
non-small-cell lung c.
oat cell c.
operable pancreatic c.
oral squamous cell c.
ovarian c.
ovarian carcinoma antigen
ovarian carcinoma debulking
ovarian carcinoma with ascites
ovarian clear cell c.
ovarian endometrioid c.
ovarian epithelial c.
pancreatic acinar cell c.
pancreatic duct cell c.
pancreatic ductectatic-type c.
papillary breast c.
papillary carcinoma of thyroid
papillary endometrial c.
papillary gastric c.
papillary renal cell c.
papillary serous carcinoma of the peritoneum
papillary thyroid c.
peau d'orange appearance in breast c.
perforating colorectal c.
perianal squamous cell c.
periurethral duct c.
pheochromocytoma, thyroid carcinoma syndrome
pigmented basal cell c.
pleomorphic lobular c.
polymorphous low-grade c.
poorly differentiated anaplastic c.
poorly differentiated ductal c.
poorly differentiated large-cell c.
poorly differentiated small-cell c.
poorly differentiated squamous cell c.
primary carcinoma unknown
primary fallopian tube c.
primary hepatic c.
primary hepatocellular c.
primary neuroendocrine carcinoma of skin
primary ovarian c.
primary ovarian carcinoma with metastasis
primary peritoneal c.
primary thymic c.
c. of prostate
prostatic c.
pseudovascular adenoid squamous cell c.
renal cell c.
reticulum cell c.
salivary duct c.
salivary gland c.
sarcomatoid renal cell c.
sarcomatoid thymic c.
sclerosing hepatic c.
sclerosing mucoepidermoid carcinoma with eosinophilia
secondary carcinoma of the upper mediastinum
secretory carcinoma of the endometrium
serous epithelial ovarian c.
sertoliform endometrioid c.
c. showing thymus-like differentiation
sigmoid colon c.
signet-ring cell c.
sinonasal undifferentiated c.
c. in situ
small bowel c.
small cell c.
small cell bronchogenic c.
small cell carcinoma of bronchus
small cell carcinoma of lung
small cell undifferentiated carcinoma of the prostate
small cell undifferentiated neuroendocrine c.
soft tissue c.
spindle cell c.
squamous carcinoma of cervix
squamous cell c.

carcinoma *(continued)*
squamous cell carcinoma antigen
squamous cell carcinoma dorsum of hand
squamous cell carcinoma of the esophagus
squamous cell carcinoma of head and neck
squamous cell carcinoma inhibitory factor
squamous cell carcinoma in situ
squamous cell carcinoma of the thyroid
squamous cell carcinoma of tongue
squamous cell carcinoma of vocal cord
squamous cell carcinoma of vulva
c. stage irresectable
superficial esophageal c.
superficial transitional cell c.
surface carcinoma in situ
survival relative to nodal involvement in breast c.
sweat gland c.
c. syndrome
terminal c.
thyroglossal duct c.
thyroid gland c.
tonsillar fossa c.
transitional bladder cell c.
transitional carcinoma in situ
transitional cell c.
transitional cell carcinoma of bladder
transplantable hepatocellular c.
c. of uncertain primary site
undifferentiated c.
undifferentiated large cell c.
c. of unknown primary
unknown primary c.
c. of unknown primary site
urothelial c.
usual type papillary c.
uterine endometrial c.
uterine papillary serous c.
vocal cord c.
well-differentiated hepatocellular c.
WHO classification for transitional cell carcinoma of the urinary bladder: stages Ta through T4
widely invasive follicular c.
c. with adenomatous areas
c. with metastasis
wolffian duct c.
yolk sac c.

carcinomatosa
lymphangitis c.
meningitis c.
peritonitis c.

carcinomatosis
extent of pleural carcinomatosis score
lymphangitic c.
meningeal c.

carcinomatous
c. arthritis in hand
c. arthritis in wrist

carcinosarcoma
bladder c.
embryonal c.
female genital tract c.

card
c. agglutination trypanosomiasis test
associative response to a white space on a c.
illuminated near c.
Macro-Vue RPR C. Test
c. made out
Memorial Pain Assessment C.
microendoscopic test c.
neonatal Guthrie c.
nursing care c.
organ donor c.
Peabody Developmental Motor Activity C.'s
rapid plasma reagin circle card test
Wisconsin C. Sorting Test

Cardarelli sign

cardia
calibration of the c.
gastric c.
c. incompetent
lymphatic ring of c.
patulous c.

cardiac
abnormal cardiac rhythm
c. abnormality, abnormal facies, thymic hypoplasia, cleft palate, hypocalcemia
c. abnormality, T-cell deficit, clefting, hypocalcemia
absolute cardiac dullness
c. accident
c. action
acute cardiac event
acute cardiac insufficiency
adequate cardiac output
c. adjustment scale
advanced cardiac life support
advanced cardiac mapping
c. allograft atherosclerosis
c. allograft vascular disease
c. allograft vasculopathy
c. ambulation routine
c. ambulatory monitoring unit
anterior cardiac vein
antibody to murine cardiac myosin
apical cardiac nodal enlargement
aquatic cardiac evaluation and testing
area of cardiac dullness
c. arrest
c. arrest code
c. arrest following trauma
c. arrhythmia
c. arrhythmia evaluation center
c. arrhythmia suppression trial
artificial cardiac valve
asymptomatic cardiac ischemia
Asymptomatic C. Ischemia Pilot
c. atrial shunt
augmented cardiac output
automated cardiac flow measurement
automated cardiac flow measurement ultrasound
automated cardiac output measurement
c. automatic resuscitative device
c. balloon pump
bidirectional cardiac control
c. blood pool imaging
blunt cardiac injury
c. border of dullness
borderline of cardiac dullness
c. bypass
c. bypass graft
c. catheter
c. catheterization
c. catheterization laboratory
c. catheterization recovery
c. catheterization technique
c. catheter microphone
c. catheter with balloon inserted
c. chest pain
closed chest cardiac massage
closed chest cardiac resuscitation
compensated cardiac status
comprehensive cardiac care unit
congestive cardiac failure

conotruncal cardiac defect, abnormal face, thymic hypoplasia, cleft palate
continuing cardiac care
continuous cardiac output
continuous cardiac output with SvO_2
c. contractility
c. cooling jacket
c. cripple
c. cushion
c. decompensation
c. defibrillation
c. depressor reflex
c. diagnostic center
c. diet
digital cardiac imaging system
direct cardiac compression
direct cardiac puncture
c. disease
disturbance in cardiac rhythm
c. Doppler examination
c. dropsy
c. dullness
dynamic cardiac blood flow
c. dysrrhythmia
c. edema
c. ejection fraction
c. electrophysiology
c. emergency
emergency cardiac care
end-diastolic cardiac wall thickness
endotracheal cardiac output monitor
end-stage adult cardiac decompensation
energetic dynamic cardiac insufficiency
enlarged cardiac silhouette
c. enlargement
c. event monitor
c. exercise laboratory
external cardiac compression
external cardiac massage
external cardiac pressure
c. failure
fatal cardiac event
fetal cardiac frequency
fetal cardiac motion
fetal cardiac reactivity test
c. fibrillation
filed procedure in cardiac arrest
c. fluoroscopy
full cardiac arrest
c. functional capacity
c. function index
c. ganglion
c. gap junction protein
gated cardiac blood pool
gated cardiac blood pool imaging
c. gated study
c. gating
c. gene expression
c. glycogenesis
great cardiac vein
great cardiac vein flow
heart shocked during cardiac arrest
c. hemodynamic monitoring
c. hemoptysis
c. herniation
heterotopic cardiac transplant
history and symptoms of emergency cardiac care
c. hypertrophy
hypothermic cardiac arrest surgery
c. imaging
c. imaging technique
impaired cardiac function
c. impairment
impedance cardiac output
implantable cardiac defibrillator
c. impression
c. impulse
inadequate cardiac output
c. incisura
incompetence of cardiac valve
infant cardiac arrest tray
c. infection
initial cardiac enzyme
c. injury
c. instability
instantaneous cardiac death
c. insufficiency
c. insult
internal cardiac massage
c. intervention
interventional cardiac catheterization
c. invasive procedure
c. irregularity
c. ischemia
isometric period of cardiac cycle
junctional rhythm after cardiac surgery
c. lacerations and hemopericardium
left border of cardiac dullness
left cardiac sympathetic ganglionectomy
left lower border of cardiac dullness
low cardiac output
low cardiac output syndrome
low-pressure cardiac tamponade
lymphatic ring of cardiac part of stomach
major adverse cardiac event
management of cardiac arrhythmia
mask-mode cardiac imaging
maximal cardiac width
mean cardiac index
mean cardiac vector
metastatic cardiac tumor
microwave cardiac ablation system
middle cardiac cervical nerve
middle cardiac vein
middle cervical cardiac nerve
minimally invasive cardiac surgery
c. minute output
mitral configuration of cardiac shadow
c. monitor
c. mucormycosis
MUGA cardiac blood pool imaging
multigated cardiac blood pool scanning
c. murmur
c. muscle
c. muscle wrap
c. myxoma
neonatal cardiac failure
c. neural chest
noninvasive cardiac evaluation
noninvasive cardiac testing
noninvasive cardiac output monitor
nontraumatic cardiac arrest
nontraumatic cardiac tamponade
normal cardiac sound
notch of cardiac apex
c. notch of left lung
c. notch of stomach
nuclear cardiac scan
c. nuclear probe scan
c. observation unit
c. obstruction in syncope
open-chest cardiac compression
open chest cardiac massage
open chest cardiac resuscitation
organic cardiac lesion
out-of-hospital sudden cardiac death
c. output index
c. output markedly reduced
c. output measurement

cardiac *(continued)*
c. output recorder
c. output by thermodilution
c. overload
c. pacemaker
c. pacemaker artifact
c. pacemaker battery change
c. pacing
c. pacing electrode
patient in cardiac arrest
patient in cardiac or respiratory distress
penetrating cardiac wound
c. performance
perioperative cardiac complication
peripartum cardiac failure
permanent cardiac pacemaker
c. pool
positive cardiac disease risk factors
positive risk factors for cardiac disease
postoperative low cardiac output
c. precautions
predicted cardiac output
progressive cardiac care
prosthetic cardiac valve
c. and pulmonary rehabilitation
c. puncture
c. refractory period
c. rehabilitation mental stress
c. rehabilitation program
c. rehabilitation team
c. rehabilitation unit
relative area of cardiac dullness
c. and respiratory
resting cardiac output
c. resuscitation team
c. revascularization procedure
c. rhythm
right border cardiac dullness
right lower border of cardiac dullness
c. risk factor
c. risk factor modification
C. Risk Index
c. risk reduction
c. roentgenography
c. rupture
c. sarcoidosis myocarditis
c. section of stomach
c. self-regulation
c. shock
c. shock wave therapy
c. shunt detection
c. silhouette enlargement
c. size and function
c. sounds normal
c. stepdown unit and telemetry
c. stress test
c. stump inverted
c. stun
sudden cardiac arrest
sudden cardiac death
c. surgery
c. surgery intensive care unit
c. surveillance unit
sustained cardiac arrest
c. sympathetic nerve
c. tamponade
thermodilution cardiac output
transient cardiac arrest
c. transplantation
transverse cardiac diameter
triple cardiac bypass surgery
c. troponin I
c. troponin T
c. ultrasonography
c. valve procedure
c. valve prosthesis
c. valvular regurgitation
c. vegetation
c. ventriculography
c. volume
c. wall hypokinesis
c. wall motion
c. wall thickening
c. work
c. work index
c. workup

cardiac-accelerator center

cardiac-evoked response audiometry

cardiac-imaging technique

cardiacum
antrum c.
antrum cardiacum of Highmore
ostium c.

cardia-intestinal metaplasia

cardinal
anterior cardinal vein
c. axes X,Y,Z
c. direction of gaze
c. ligament
c. sign of alcoholism

cardioaccelerating center

cardioauditory
Sanchez-Cascos cardioauditory syndrome

cardioauditory syndrome

cardiocentesis procedure

cardiocutaneous
c. myxoma
c. syndrome

CardioData MK-3 Holter scanner

cardioembolic
c. event
c. stroke

cardioesophageal
tear in mucosa at cardioesophageal junction

cardio-esophagus junction

cardiofacial syndrome

cardiofaciocutaneous syndrome

cardiogenic
acute cardiogenic pulmonary edema
patient in cardiogenic shock
c. pulmonary edema
c. shock

cardiogram
derived value on apex c.
diagnostic c.
impedance c.
ultrasonic c.
upstroke pattern on apex c.

cardiography
electrical impedance c.
ultrasonic c.
vector cardiography electrode right midaxillary line

cardioinhibitor center

cardioinhibitory syncope

cardiolipin
c. complement fixation
c. flocculation test
c. fluorescence antibody
c. micro flocculation
c. natural lecithin
c. synthetic lecithin
c. test
c. Wassermann test

Cardiolite
C. scan
C. stress test
technetium Cardiolite stress test

cardiology
c. intensive care unit
nuclear cardiology laboratory
pediatric c.

cardiomediastinal silhouette

cardiomegaly
glycogen c.

hypertrophy of c.
idiopathic c.

cardiometer center

cardiomyopathy
arrhythmogenic right ventricular c.
autosomal dominant c.
concentric hypertrophic c.
congestive c.
degenerative idiopathic c.
dilated c.
familial hypertrophic c.
familial hypertrophic obstructive c.
genetic hypertrophic c.
high-altitude hypertrophic cardiomyopathy syndrome
hypersensitive hypertrophic c.
hypertensive hypertrophic c.
hypertrophic c.
hypertrophic obstructive c.
idiopathic congestive c.
idiopathic dilated c.
idiopathic restrictive c.
inflammatory c.
latent c.
maternally inherited myopathy and c.
mental retardation, scapuloperoneal muscular dystrophy, lethal cardiomyopathy syndrome
mildly dilated congestive c.
postpartum c.
restrictive c.
right ventricular c.
c. transplant rejection
c. and woolly hair-coat syndrome
X-linked c.
X-linked dilated c.

cardiopathy
electrolyte steroid cardiopathy by calcification
electrolyte and steroid cardiopathy with necrosis
electrolyte steroid-produced cardiopathy characterized by hyalinization
nephropathic c.

cardiophrenic angle

cardioplegia
antegrade/retrograde cardioplegia technique
blood c.
cold blood c.
cold crystalloid c.
cold potassium c.
c. cooling
crystalloid c.
crystalloid potassium c.

cardioplegic
amino acid-enriched cardioplegic solution
c. perfusion solution
crystalloid cardioplegic solution
hypothermic hypokalemic cardioplegic arrest

cardiopneumographic recording

cardiopulmonary
c. abnormality
c. arrest
arrhythmia associated with cardiopulmonary arrest
attempted cardiopulmonary resuscitation
c. blood volume
c. bypass
c. bypass machine
c. bypass operation
c. bypass surgery
dilutional cardiopulmonary bypass
c. edema
c. exercise
c. exercise test
external cardiopulmonary resuscitation
hantavirus cardiopulmonary syndrome
c. insufficiency
low-flow cardiopulmonary bypass
low-pressure cardiopulmonary baroreceptor
no cardiopulmonary resuscitation
open-chest cardiopulmonary resuscitation
percutaneous cardiopulmonary bypass
percutaneous cardiopulmonary bypass support
c. resuscitation
c. sleep study
standard external cardiopulmonary resuscitation
c. stress test
sudden cardiopulmonary arrest
c. support
total cardiopulmonary bypass
traumatic cardiopulmonary arrest

cardiopulmonary-cerebral resuscitation

cardiorespiratory
acute cardiorespiratory arrest
c. endurance
home cardiorespiratory monitor
c. syndrome of obesity in child

cardiothoracic
c. intensive care unit
c. ratio
c. silhouette
c. surgery
c. trauma

cardiothymic silhouette

cardiotoxic
cumulative cardiotoxic dose
minimal cumulative cardiotoxic dose

cardiotoxicity
anthracycline c.
mitomycin c.

cardiovascular
c. accident
acute cardiovascular disease
c. aerobic exercise
arteriosclerotic cardiovascular disease
arteriosclerotic cardiovascular renal disease
atherosclerotic cardiovascular disease
atherosclerotic hypertensive cardiovascular disease
c. complications of drug abuse
c. computed tomography
congenital cardiovascular malformation
c. deconditioning
c. diagnostic study
c. disease
c. dysmetabolic syndrome
c. effects of alcohol
c. effects of methamphetamine
c. failure
hypertensive arteriosclerotic cardiovascular disease
hypertensive cardiovascular disease
c. incident
c. inpatient care unit
c. insufficiency
intensive thoracic cardiovascular unit
isolated cardiovascular malformation
c. malformation
C. Measurement system
c. monitor
c. morbidity and mortality
nuclear cardiovascular imaging
c. operating room

cardiovascular *(continued)*
c. patch graft
pediatric cardiovascular surgery
personalized aerobics for cardiovascular enhancement
c. problems related to drug abuse
c. recovery room
c. reflex conditioning
c. reflex conditioning system
c. renal disease
c. resistance
c. resistance index
c. review
c. risk factor
c. risk status
c. silhouette
c. specialty unit
c. steady state
c. surgery
c. surgery unit
c. work capacity

cardiovascular-thoracic
c.-t. intensive care unit
c.-t. surgery

cardioventricular pacing

cardioversion
congestive heart failure and c.
defibrillation and electrical c.
direct current c.
implantable defibrillator in c.
c. paddle

cardioverter
implantable c.
implantable cardioverter electrodes

cardioverter-defibrillator
atrial and ventricular implantable c.-d.
automatic external c.-d.
automatic implantable c.-d.
automatic internal c.-d.
external c.-d.
implantable c.-d.
implantable automatic c.-d.
implantable cardioverter-defibrillator catheter
internal c.-d.
pacer c.-d.
programmable c.-d.
subpectoral implantation of c.-d.
transvenous implantation of c.-d.
ventricular implantable c.-d.
wearable c.-d.

CardioWest total artificial heart

carditis
Lyme c.
rheumatic c.

care
academic health c.
accreditation program/home health c.
accreditation program/hospice c.
accreditation program/long-term c.
acute care center
acute care for the elderly
acute care facility
acute care hospital
acute care unit
adequate patient c.
adult foster c.
advanced care directive
aged care assessment team
aggressive medical c.
AIDS patient c.
alternate level of c.
alternative health c.
ambulatory c.
ambulatory care center
ambulatory care research facility
ambulatory care unit
anesthesiology critical care medicine
appropriate level of c.
asthma care algorithm
asthma care training
availability of health c.
back c.
bedside c.
board and c.
c. of body after death
bowel care of choice
burn care unit
cancer care center
capitated primary care network
cardiac surgery intensive care unit
cardiology intensive care unit
cardiothoracic intensive care unit
cardiovascular inpatient care unit
cardiovascular-thoracic intensive care unit
in care of
child care clinic
Children with Special Health C. Needs
community care unit
community-oriented primary c.
completion bed occupancy c.
comprehensive ambulatory c.
comprehensive cardiac care unit
comprehensive care clinic
comprehensive health care institution
comprehensive support care team
concentrated care area
continued ambulatory c.
continuing cardiac c.
continuing care center
continuing community c.
continuity of c.
continuous home c.
continuum of c.
coordinate home c.
coordination of c.
coronary care nursing
coronary care team
coronary intensive care unit
correctional health care program
critical care air transport
critical care area
critical care complex
critical care medicine
critical care medicine unit
critical care nursing
critical care recovery unit
day care center
day care surgical unit
dementia care mapping
dental health care provider
diabetes care clinic
diabetic eye c.
diabetic foot c.
direct care worker
direct patient c.
domiciliary c.
durable power of attorney for health c.
effective mental health c.
elected palliative c.
emergency cardiac c.
emergency care provider
emergency maternal and infant c.
emergency medical c.
emergency medical care and rescue
extended care facility
extended care hospital
extended care unit
extended health c.
eye c.
family-centered c.
family-centered care unit
family-centered maternity c.
fetal intensive care unit
foster c.
foster home c.
general care and treatment
general nursing c.

geriatric c.
geriatric care manager
geriatric skilled care unit
good prenatal c.
grossly pathogenic c.
habilitative day c.
hand washing in critical care
 area
health care agency
health care aide
health care cost reduction
health care coverage
health care decision-making
health care delivery
health care maintenance
health care management
health care review
health care worker
high level of c.
high-quality medical c.
history and symptoms of
 emergency cardiac c.
home c.
home-based hospital c.
home care assistance
home care bereavement
home care instruction
home health c.
home nursing c.
hospital care cost
immediate patient c.
improper foot c.
increased prenatal c.
industrial eye c.
infant intensive care unit
infant-toddler special care unit
informed health care decision
inpatient psychiatric c.
institutional c.
integrated c.
intensive care facility
intensive care medicine
intensive care nursery
intensive care, surgical
intensive care unit psychosis
intensive care ward
intensive coronary care unit
intensive nursing c.
intensive prenatal c.
intensive special care nursery
intensive special care unit
intensive supportive c.
intermediate care area
intermediate care facility
intermediate care nursery
intermediate coronary care unit
intermediate medical care unit
intermittent skilled nursing c.
intravenous needle site c.
juvenile residential c.
level of c.
Life After Cancer C.
long-term c.
long-term acute c.
long-term care insurance
lower level of c.
Managed C. Appropriateness
 Protocol
managed care environment
c. management continuity
c. management integration
maternal and child health c.
maternal and infant c.
maximal care unit
medical care administration
medical care organization
medical intensive care unit
medical progressive care unit
medical special care unit
mental health c.
mental health care professional
mental health care unit
Miami Acute C.
mobile coronary care unit
mobile intensive care nurse
mobile intensive care unit
monitored anesthesia c.
monitored anesthesia care
 anesthesia
monitored anesthesia care
 anesthetic technique
mouth c.
multilevel c.
nail infection and c.
National Ambulatory Medical C.
 Survey
National Association for
 Home C.
National Association of
 Progressional Geriatric C.
 Managers
need for c.
neighborhood family care center
neonatal intensive care unit
neurologic intensive care unit
neurosurgery intensive care unit
neurosurgical continuous care unit
neurosurgical intensive care unit
newborn convalescent care unit
newborn infant c.
newborn intensive c.
newborn intensive care unit
newborn special care unit
night care facility
nonbed c.
no prenatal c.
normal prenatal c.
not routine c.
nursing care card
nursing care continuity
nursing care integration
nursing care plan
nursing home c.
nursing home care unit
Nursing C. Intervention Tool
observation care unit
open care area
oral c.
oral health c.
organized care psychiatry
outpatient c.
palliative care service
palliative care unit
palliative home c.
Parental Stressor Scale: Neonatal
 Intensive C. Unit
patient care aide
patient care assistant
patient care coordinator
patient care plan
patient care report
patient care unit
patient discharged to home c.
patient-focused c.
Patient C. Information System
patient released in care of
 relative
patient treated with comfort care
 only
patient treated with supportive c.
pattern of c.
patterns of care study
pediatric critical care center
pediatric intensive care unit
pediatric special care unit
pediatric surgical intensive c.
perineum c.
periodontal gum c.
personal care attendant
personal care boarding home
personal care clinic
personal care home
personal care service
physician directed
 interdisciplinary c.
c. planning
plans of c.
point of c.
postanesthesia care unit
postcoronary care unit
posthospital c.

care *(continued)*
postoperative c.
prebed c.
precoronary c.
precoronary care area
prenatal c.
prenatal intensive care unit
primary care case management
primary care clinic
primary care intervention
primary care network
primary care nursing
primary care provider
primary care unit
Primary C. Evaluation of Mental Disorders
primary health c.
progressive cardiac c.
progressive care unit
progressive patient c.
prolonged hospital c.
protective care unit
psychiatric intensive care unit
pulmonary care team
pulmonary intensive care unit
quality of patient c.
referred c.
regional neonatal intensive care unit
regional perinatal intensive care center
residential care facility for the elderly
residential care home
respiratory c.
respiratory care plan
respiratory intensive care unit
Respiratory Special C. Unit
respiratory-surgical intensive care unit
respite and in-home c.
rising health care costs
routine health c.
routine home c.
routine medical c.
routine respiratory c.
screening and acute c.
c. seeker
Self C. Assessment Schedule
skilled nursing c.
skilled nursing extended care facility
special c.
special care baby unit
special care formula
special care nursery
special mouth c.
spinal intensive care unit
standard inpatient c.
standardized care plan
start of c.
subsequent hospital c.
supportive c.
surgical inpatient c.
surgical intermediate care unit
surgical pulmonary intensive care unit
surgical respiratory intensive care unit
tertiary care facility
thoracic intensive care unit
total patient c.
traditional home c.
transitional care unit
transplant intensive care unit
trauma intensive care unit
c. and treatment during pregnancy
under care of
urgent care center
urgent care clinic
urinary care unit
usual c.
weighted patient care unit
well-child c.

CARE Act

care-cure coordination

career
Adult C. Concerns Inventory
c. assessment
Assessment of C. Decision Making
Assessment of C. Development
C. Assessment Inventory
C. Beliefs Inventory
Comprehensive C. Assessment Scale
c. counseling
C. Decision-Making
Education and C. Exploration System
c. guidance
individual career exploration
C. Maturity Inventory
New Mexico C. Planning Test
c. planning program
Professional and Administrative C. Examination

careful
c. dissection
c. observation
c. watch

caregiver
c. abandoning patient
adoptive c.
designated c.
in-home c.
National Family C.'s Association
c. neglect
c. nutures patient
primary c.
C. Strain Index
c. withholding and uncaring

Caregiver's School Readiness Inventory

caretaker burnout

Carey-Coombs murmur

Carey Island virus

caries
arrested dental c.
c. of bone
early childhood c.
nursing bottle c.
c. of petrous bone
primary dental c.
c. resistant
c. susceptible

carina
c. freely movable
mainstem c.
c. midline sharp and mobile
c. of trachea

carinatum
pectus c.
pectus carinatum deformity

caring
c. environment
Partnership for C.
patient incapacitated of caring for self
quality of c.
C. Relationship Inventory
c. for self
totally incapacitated of caring for self

carinii
Pneumocystis c.
Pneumocystis carinii choroiditis

cariogenicity
intraoral cariogenicity test

carious teeth

Carlen tube

Carleton spot

Carlo
Markov chain Monte Carlo technique

Monte Carlo calculation
Monte Carlo modeling
Monte Carlo photon transport
Monte Carlo photon transport simulation
Monte Carlo technique

C-arm
fluoroscopic C-a.
C-a. fluoroscopy
C-a. fluoroscopy unit

Carmichael crown

carmine
contrast chromoscopy using indigo c.
indigo carmine dye
indigo carmine stain
indigo carmine test

carmustine
Adriamycin and c.
vincristine, carmustine, cyclophosphamide, melphalan, prednisone

Carnegie Interest Inventory

carnitine
muscle carnitine deficiency
muscle carnitine palmitoyltransferase deficiency
myopathic carnitine deficiency
palmitoyl c.
c. palmitoyltransferase
c. palmitoyltransferase I, II deficiency
systemic carnitine deficiency

carnosus
panniculus c.
panniculus carnosus muscle
pannus c.

Carolina
North Carolina macular dystrophy

carotene
alpha tocopherol beta c.
beta c.

carotenoid vesicle

caroticotympanicus
nervi c.

carotid
c. Amytal procedure
aneurysm of internal carotid artery
c. angioplasty and stenting
anterior carotid artery
c. aortic dissection
c. applanation tonometry
araldehyde-tanned bovine carotid artery graft
c. arterial disease
c. artery
c. artery canal
c. artery stenosis
C. Artery Stenosis with Asymptomatic Narrowing: Operation Versus Aspirin Study
c. artery system
c. artery ultrasound
Asymptomatic C. Atherosclerosis Study
asymptomatic carotid artery stenosis
asymptomatic carotid atherosclerosis study
asymptomatic carotid bruit
asymptomatic carotid surgery trial
atherosclerotic carotid artery
atherosclerotic carotid artery disease
atherosclerotic carotid artery lesion
c. audiofrequency analysis
c. axillary bypass
bilateral carotid body resection
bilateral internal carotid artery occlusion
c. blood flow
blunt carotid injury
c. bodies resected
c. body
c. body denervation
c. body tumor
c. cerebral arteriography
c. chemoreceptor stimulation
common carotid artery
common carotid artery bifurcation
common carotid artery intima-media thickness
common carotid compression
compression of carotid artery
c. compression tomography
c. compression tonography
c. Doppler
c. Doppler study
duplex carotid imaging
duplex carotid ultrasound
c. duplex imaging
c. duplex scan
c. duplex study
c. duplex ultrasonography
ectatic carotid artery
c. ejection time
c. endarterectomy
endovascular carotid sacrifice
external c.
external carotid artery
extracranial carotid arterial disease
extracranial carotid disease
c. foramen
c. ganglion
hyperactive carotid sinus reflex
hypersensitive carotid sinus syndrome
hypoglossal carotid entrapment
inferior carotid ganglion
c. insensitivity
internal carotid artery flow
internal carotid artery occlusion
internal carotid nerve
internal carotid stenosis
left carotid artery
left carotid endarterectomy
left common carotid artery
left internal carotid artery
left posterior internal carotid artery
marginal tentorial branch of internal carotid artery
massage of the carotid sinus
Mayo Asymptomatic Carotid Endarterectomy Study
mean carotid pressure
meningeal branch of cavernous part of internal carotid artery
meningeal branch of cerebral part of internal carotid artery
narrowing of carotid artery
nerve to carotid sinus
noninvasive carotid baroceptor stimulation
noninvasive carotid examination
noninvasive carotid study
occluded carotid vessel
occlusion of internal carotid artery
occlusion of left carotid artery
occlusion of right carotid artery
occlusive carotid artery disease
occlusive carotid disease
c. occlusive disease
c. occlusive disease retinopathy
opening of carotid canal
palpable carotid pulse
percutaneous carotid arteriogram
petrous carotid canal
c. phonoangiogram
c. phonoangiography
c. phonoangiography/oculoplethysmography
Pruitt-Inahara carotid shunt
c. pulse tracing

carotid *(continued)*
right carotid artery
right carotid endarterectomy
right common c.
right common carotid artery
right external c.
right external carotid artery
right posterior internal carotid artery
c. sheath
c. sinus
c. sinus compression
c. sinus denervation
c. sinus hypersensitivity
c. sinus massage
c. sinus nerve
c. sinus nerve stimulation
c. sinus pressure
c. sinus syncope
c. sinus syndrome
c. sinus test
c. siphon
c. steal syndrome
c. stent-supported angioplasty
c. subclavian bypass
superior carotid artery
superior carotid ganglion
supraclinoid carotid aneurysm
terminal internal carotid artery
c. ultrasound examination
c. upstroke
velocity, common carotid artery
velocity internal carotid artery

carotid-carotid bypass

carotid-cavernous sinus fistula

carpal
c. articulation
axial carpal dislocation
c. boss
endoscopic carpal tunnel release
idiopathic carpal tunnel syndrome
c. instability dissociation
c. instability nondissociative
c. ligament
c. lunate implant prosthesis
Mayo carpal instability classification
medial carpal capsule
middle carpal joint
c. navicular bone
open carpal tunnel release
Paine carpal tunnel retinaculotome
palmar carpal branch of radial artery
palmar carpal branch of ulnar artery
palmar carpal ligament
palmar carpal tendinous sheath
c. pedal spasm
perilunate carpal dislocation
radiate carpal ligament
Swanson carpal lunate implant
transverse carpal ligament
tuberosity of carpal bone
c. tunnel
c. tunnel decompression
c. tunnel endoscopy
c. tunnel release
c. tunnel release system
c. tunnel repair
c. tunnel syndrome

carpectomy
Omer-Capen c.

carpenter's
c. brace
c. knee

Carpentier-Edwards porcine bioprosthesis

carpet-layer's knee

carpet tack follicular keratotic plug

carpi
articulatio c.
extensor carpi radialis
extensor carpi radialis brevis
extensor carpi radialis brevis muscle
extensor carpi radialis brevis tendon
extensor carpi radialis longus
extensor carpi radialis longus flap
extensor carpi radialis longus muscle
extensor carpi radialis longus tendon
extensor carpi ulnaris
extensor carpi ulnaris muscle
extensor carpi ulnaris sheath
extensor carpi ulnaris tendon
flexor carpi radialis
flexor carpi radialis brevis
flexor carpi ulnaris
musculus extensor carpi radialis brevis
musculus extensor carpi radialis longus
musculus extensor carpi ulnaris
musculus flexor carpi radialis
musculus flexor carpi ulnaris
ossa c.

carpopedal
c. contraction
c. spasm

Carpue rhinoplasty

carpus
complex instability of c.

Carrel-Dakin fluid

Carrell operation

carriage
organism c.

carried
blunt dissection carried upward
incision carried down to the fracture site
regloving and regowning carried out

carrier
c. of acquired immune deficiency syndrome
acquired immune deficiency syndrome c.
acyl carrier protein
biotin carboxyl carrier protein
doxorubicin adsorbed to magnetic targeted c.
factor V Leiden c.
facultative yeast c.
c. free
hemoglobin-based oxygen c.
hepatitis B c.
c. of human immunodeficiency virus
human carriers of infection
linear in-line ligature c.
meningococcal carrier state
minus carrier contact lens
mutation carrier status
normal carrier hepatitis
patient unknown acquired immune deficiency syndrome c.
phosphate carrier compound
reduced folate c.
riboflavin carrier protein
sterol carrier protein-2
c. tube

Carrington pneumonia

Carrot
Therapy Carrot finger contracture orthosis

Carrow
C. Elicited Language Inventory
C. Test for Auditory Comprehension

Carr-Purcell-Meiboom-Gill
C.-P.-M.-G. sequence
C.-P.-M.-G. spin-echo technique

Carr-Purcell sequence

Carswell grapes

cartilage
alar dome and c.
angled cartilage scissors
anular rim of c.
apex of arytenoid c.
arch of cricoid c.
arcuate crest of arytenoid c.
articular cartilage attenuation
articular cartilage autograft
articular cartilage autografting
articular cartilage degeneration
articular cartilage lesion
articular cartilage violation
articular cartilage volume
articular surface of arytenoid c.
attenuated intercarpal articular c.
auricular cartilage graft
autogenous cartilage graft
autogenous cartilage implantation
autogenous cartilage transplantation
autogenous meniscal cartilage replantation
buccal c.
calcification intervertebral c.
calibrated triangle of septal c.
capsule cartilage articular preservation
chondritis intervertebral c.
convex cartilage graft
costal intraarticular c.
diced cartilage graft
displacement of cartilage padding
c. graft
c. implant
c. induction factor
c. intermediate layer protein
Luschka laryngeal c.
major alar c.
medial crus of major alar cartilage of nose
medial lamina of cartilage of pharyngotympanic auditory tube
membranous lamina of cartilage of pharyngotympanic auditory plate
minor alar c.
morselized cartilage onlay radix graft
nasal alar cartilage cleft
nasal dome c.
notch in cartilage of acoustic meatus
oblique line of thyroid c.
oblong fovea of arytenoid c.
c. oligomeric matrix protein
patellar cartilage thickness
patellar facet c.
patellofemoral articular c.
patellofemoral groove c.
pedicled cartilage graft
perichondrial double cartilage block technique
c. residue
rim of c.
c. of Santorini
c. shaver blade
softening of c.
c. strut
c. strut placement

cartilage-hair hypoplasia

cartilage-wearing knee bends

cartilaginous
c. autologous thin septal graft
congenital cartilaginous rest of neck
c. endplate
c. growth
low-grade malignant cartilaginous lesion
lumbosacral cartilaginous system
medial cartilaginous layer
medial cartilaginous plate
multiple cartilaginous exostoses
ossification of cartilaginous structure
c. ring incised
c. tissue

cartridge
inspiratory flow c.

caruncle
hymenal c.
Morgagni c.
myrtiform c.
Santorini major c.
sublingual c.
urethral c.

caruncula
avulsion of caruncula lacrimalis

Carvallo sign

Carvedilol
Multicenter Oral Carvedilol Heart Failure Assessment

CAS-200
morphology system C.

Casanellas operation

cascade
adhesion molecule c.
adrenal steroidogenic c.
alternative pathway of complement c.
arachidonic acid c.
arachidonic acid cascade inhibitor
c. filtration
MAPK c.
metastatic c.
mitogen-activated protein kinase c.
neurotoxic c.
pain c.
pathophysiological c.
c. phenomenon
sequential impaction cascade sieve volumetric air sampler
c. stomach

case
abuse c.
computer-based case tracing
consecutive case conference
data case report form
c. file
c. history
Individual C. Safety Reports
initial case assessment
intensive case management
c. management
multiple sib c.
neuro-ophthalmologic case history
primary care case management
c. report
c. report form
c. work
c. worker

caseating granuloma

case-fatality ratio

casein
c. hydrolysate
serum, casein, glucose, yeast extract medium
c. unit
c. yeast lactate medium

caseosa
nephritis c.

Casoni
C. intradermal test
C. reaction

Caspar ring opacity

Casser
C. fontanelle
C. muscle

cassette
ATP-binding cassette transporter
screen-containing c.
video cassette recorder

cast
air cell c.
arm cylinder c.
c. bar splint
below-knee-to-toe c.
below-knee walking c.
c. bender
bivalved cylinder c.
bivalved pancake plaster hand c.
c. boot brace
c. bracing
c. clasp
c. clinic
closed reduction and c.
c. cover
c. cushion
c. cutter
electric cast saw
extremity immobilized in c.
flexion body c.
full cast restoration
c. glass ceramics
c. gold inlay
granular c.
hip spica c.
hyaline c.
immobilized in plaster c.
c. immobilizer
long arm c.
long arm finger c.
long arm navicular c.
long below-elbow c.
long bent-knee leg c.
long leg c.
long leg cylinder c.
long leg fiberglass c.
long leg plaster c.
long leg walking c.
long leg weightbearing c.
maintainer cast space
medium below-elbow c.
modified Cotrel c.
myeloma cast nephropathy
c. off, to x-ray
onlay bone graft c.
out of c.
out of plaster c.
patellar dislocation c.
patellar tendon-bearing cast prosthesis
plaster of Paris c.
red blood cell c.
red cell c.
c. removed, take x-ray
c. resin lens
semirigid fiberglass c.
short above-elbow c.
short arm c.
short arm cylinder c.
short arm fiberglass c.
short arm navicular c.
short arm thumb spica c.
short below-elbow c.
short leg cylinder c.
short leg nonwalking c.
short leg nonweightbearing c.
short leg walking c.
c. sock
standard above-elbow c.
c. stroking maneuver during massage
sugar-tong c.
c. support
supportive halo c.
c. table
c. tape
very short below-elbow c.
c. walker
walking boot c.
walking heel c.
c. wedge
white cell c.
c. window
c. with dorsal toe plate extension
c. with volar toe plate extension

Castellino sign

Castelman disease

caster
sulfated hydrogenated caster oil

Castillo
Argonz-Del Castillo syndrome

casting
c. breast calcification
electric casting machine
fiberglass casting tape
foam c.
negative c.
postoperative c.
total contact c.

castione
proteose-yeast castione medium

Castleman
mesenterial Castleman lymphoma

cast-off x-ray

castor
aromatic castor oil
c. bean
c. oil

castration
c. anxiety
c. complex
c. fear
passive castration complex

casual
c. contact
c. drug user
c. sex

casualty
battle c.
c. clearing station
mass c.
no c.
nonbattle c.
c. staging unit

cat
c. cry
crying cat syndrome
enterocytopathogenic cat orphan virus
c. mite dermatitis

catabolic
absolute catabolic rate
fractional catabolic rate
normalized protein catabolic rate

catabolism
antibody c.
articular joint tissue c.
muscle c.
net c.

catabolite
c. activator protein
c. gene activator
c. gene activator protein
c. modular factor

catalase
beef liver c.
hepatic c.

catalasia
anenzymia c.

catalepsy schizophrenia

cataleptic somnambulism

catalysis
antibody-directed c.

catalyst
c. altered water
phase transfer c.

catalytic
c. activity
c. amount

apo B mRNA-editing catalytic polypeptide-1

catalyzed
- c. reporter deposition
- rate of reaction catalyzed by an enzyme

catalyzed reporter deposition

catamenial
- c. epilepsy
- c. migraine

cataphoria
- mature c.

cataplectic attack

cataplexy muscle weakness

cataract
- anterior axial developmental c.
- anterior axial embryonal c.
- anterior axonal embryonal c.
- anterior polar c.
- anterior pole c.
- anterior pyramidal c.
- anterior subcapsular c.
- Arroyo cataract extraction
- Arruga cataract extraction
- autosomal dominant congenital c.
- axial embryonal c.
- axial fusiform developmental c.
- axial partial childhood c.
- c., microcephaly, arthrogryposis, kyphosis
- c., microcephaly, failure to thrive, kyphoscoliosis
- c., motor system disorder, short stature, learning difficulty, skeletal abnormalities syndrome
- combined intracapsular cataract extraction
- congenital cataracts, sensorineural deafness, Down syndrome facial appearance, short stature, mental retardation syndrome
- cryo cataract extraction
- cryoextraction of c.
- dislocated elbow, bowed tibiae, scoliosis, deafness, cataract, microcephaly, mental retardation syndrome
- double needle operation on c.
- embryonal nuclear c.
- c. extraction
- c. flap operation
- c. glasses
- incipient cataract grade 11 to 41
- intracapsular cataract extraction with peripheral iridectomy
- c. lens implantation
- metabolic syndrome c.
- microcephaly, mental retardation, cataract, hypogonadism syndrome
- myotonic dystrophy c.
- nuclear developmental c.
- nutritional deficiency c.
- one-stitch cataract procedure
- open-sky cataract wound
- planned extracapsular cataract extraction
- posterior capsular c.
- posterior subcapsular c.
- round pupil intracapsular cataract extraction
- small incision cataract surgery
- c. surgery with implant
- sutureless cataract surgery
- c. with intraocular lens
- X-linked mental retardation, microphthalmia, microcornea, cataract, hypogenitalism-mental retardation-spasticity syndrome

cataractous
- posterior subcapsular cataractous plaque

catarrh
- atrophy c.
- hypertrophic c.
- nasal c.

catarrhal
- acute catarrhal inflammation
- c. disease
- c. gastritis
- malignant catarrhal fever
- malignant catarrhal fever disease
- malignant catarrhal fever virus
- marginal catarrhal ulcer
- otitis media, acute, c.
- otitis media, catarrhal, acute
- otitis media, catarrhal, chronic

catarrhalis
- herpes c.
- icterus c.
- *Moraxella* c.
- *Moraxella catarrhalis* vaccine

catastrophic
- c. event
- c. health insurance
- c. hemorrhaging
- c. illness
- irreversible catastrophic brain injury
- c. life-threatening illness
- c. migraine

catastrophizing
- pain catastrophizing scale

catatonia
- acute lethal c.
- c., coma and convulsions

catatonic
- agitation catatonic schizophrenia
- c. dementia
- c. excitation
- mood disorder with catatonic features
- patient in catatonic state
- c. rigidity
- c. schizophrenia
- schizophrenia, catatonic type, subchronic
- c. schizophrenic disorder
- c. state
- c. stupor
- c. syndrome

cat-bite fever

catch and clunk test

catching sensation

catchment
- epidemiologic catchment area

catecholamine
- peripheral catecholamine receptor
- plasma catecholamine concentration
- c. receptor
- total plasma c.'s

catechol methyltransferase

categorical
- newly emergent categorical change

category
- c.'s of acute nonlymphoblastic leukemia
- arousal c.
- avoidance c.
- Functional Ambulation C.
- grammatical c.
- high-risk c.
- lexical c.
- major diagnostic c.
- moderate c.
- NIH Classification Category I acute bacterial prostatitis
- NIH Classification Category II chronic bacterial prostatitis
- NIH Classification Category III inflammatory and noninflammatory chronic pelvic pain
- NIH Classification Category IV asymptomatic inflammatory prostatitis

category *(continued)*
NOS c.
Pediatric Overall Performance Category scale
c. ratio 0–10
C. Test
Toglia C. Assessment Test

catfish
channel catfish reovirus

catgut
absorbable c.
chromic catgut mattress suture
interrupted plain c.
c. ligature
plain c.
plain catgut suture
plain 2-0 catgut suture
plain 3-0 catgut suture
plain 4-0 catgut suture
c. plain tie
c. suture

catheter
c. ablation
c. adapter
c. administered treatment
Advanced C. System
anchored c.
angiographic end hole c.
antiseptic-impregnated central venous c.
Argyle arterial c.
Argyll trocar c.
arrhythmia mapping system c.
arterial port catheter system
articulated drainage c.
c. aspirated and flushed
c. aspirated and flushed with saline
balloon catheter angioplasty
balloon catheter and basket-retrieval technique
balloon PTA c.
c. balloon valvuloplasty
bile duct c.
biliary balloon c.
biliary dilator c.
biliary drainage c.
biliary manipulation c.
cardiac catheter microphone
cardiac catheter with balloon inserted
central venous c.
central venous catheter infection
c. cholangiogram
c. coiled upon itself
condom catheter collecting system
condom catheter endoscopic ultrasound
continuous catheter drainage
coronary seeking c.
dilation c.
double-lumen c.
double lumen subclavian c.
dual balloon perfusion c.
dual-lumen c.
electrical catheter ablation
electrode catheter ablation
c. embolus
esophageal balloon c.
c. exchange
expandable access c.
femoral artery c.
femoral cerebral c.
femorocerebral catheter angiography
fine-needle catheter jejunostomy
flow-assisted short-term balloon c.
Foley c.
c. guide
Hickman c.
implantable cardioverter-defibrillator c.
indwelling arterial c.
indwelling bladder c.
indwelling catheter drainage
indwelling Foley c.
indwelling subclavian c.
indwelling urethral c.
indwelling urinary c.
indwelling vascular access c.
indwelling venous c.
infant with umbilical c.
injection electrode c.
c. inserted
c. insertion site
inside-the-needle c.
c. instability
intermittent catheter routine
internal jugular c.
intraaortic balloon c.
intracardiac catheter recording
intracranial pressure c.
intramedullary c.
intrapleural c.
intratracheal oxygen c.
intrauterine c.
intrauterine insemination c.
intrauterine pressure c.
intravascular catheter culture
intravascular ultrasound c.
intravenous ultrasound c.
intraventricular c.
c. irrigation
jugular venous c.
long-term catheter use
long-term central venous access catheter placement
long-term venous c.
lumbar cerebrospinal fluid c.
membrane catheter technique
30-mHz transducer-tipped c.
microendoscopic optical c.
MR catheter imaging and spectroscopy system scanner
multiaccess c.
multilumen c.
nasobiliary drainage c.
nasocystic catheter lavage
nasovesicular catheter technique
needle catheter jejunostomy
nondetachable balloon c.
occlusion balloon catheter with silicone balloon
over-the-needle c.
over-the-wire balloon c.
passage of c.
c. passed with ease
c. patency
percutaneous catheter cecostomy
percutaneous catheter drainage
percutaneous catheter insertion
percutaneous central venous c.
percutaneous cholecystotomy c.
percutaneous femoral vein c.
percutaneous femoral venous c.
percutaneously inserted central line c.
percutaneous nephrostomy c.
perfusion balloon c.
Peripheral Access System Port catheter system
peripheral arterial c.
peripheral intravenous c.
peripherally inserted catheter line
peripherally inserted central venous c.
peritoneal dialysis c.
pigtail curl of c.
c. in place
c. probe-assisted endoluminal ultrasonography
prolonged indwelling c.
protected brush c.
protected catheter brushing specimen
pulled catheter out
pulmonary artery c.
quick c.
radial artery c.
radiofrequency catheter ablation

retention c.
retrograde femoral c.
return flow hemostatic c.
c. sepsis
Silastic mushroom c.
c. site
c. sonography
spiral tip c.
c. stimulation of right atrium
subclavian hemodialysis c.
suprapubic c.
surgically implanted hemodialysis c.
suspected catheter sepsis
Swan-Ganz c.
telescoping plugged c.
thermal dilution c.
transarterial catheter embolization
transcervical tubal access c.
transluminal endarterectomy c.
transluminal extraction c.
transluminal extraction-endarterectomy c.
transtracheal c.
transvenous catheter pacemaker
trial without c.
triple-lumen Arrow c.
triple lumen c.
Uldall c.
ultrasound catheter probe
umbilical artery c.
umbilical vein c.
umbilical venous c.
urethral catheter in
urethral catheter out
urinary c.
urinary catheter in
urinary catheter out
uterine cornual access c.
uterine ostial access c.
Van Buren c.

catheter-associated
c.-a. bacteriuria
c.-a. infection

catheter-based Maze procedure

catheter-guided
c.-g. biopsy
c.-g. endoscopic intubation

catheter-induced
c.-i. ablation
c.-i. spasm

catheterizable
Mitrofanoff catheterizable channel

catheterization
antegrade femoral artery c.
aseptic catheterization technique
cardiac catheterization laboratory
cardiac catheterization recovery
cardiac catheterization technique
clean intermittent bladder c.
combined heart c.
endoscopic transpapillary catheterization of gallbladder
c. of eustachian tube
heart c.
heart catheterization stylet
hepatic vein c.
intermittent c.
intermittent catheterization of bladder
intermittent catheterization protocol
intermittent clean c.
intermittent straight c.
internal mammary artery c.
interventional cardiac c.
c. lacrimonasal duct
left heart c.
long-term epidural c.
outpatient c.
percutaneous transhepatic c.
pulmonary artery c.
right heart c.
self-intermittent c.
subclavian vein c.
transseptal left heart c.
umbilical artery c.
umbilical vein c.
urethral c.

catheterized
c. bladder
c. urine specimen

catheter-related
c.-r. bacteremia
c.-r. bloodstream infection
c.-r. infection
c.-r. sepsis
c.-r. septicemia
c.-r. urinary tract infection

cathexis
object c.

cathodal
c. closing
c. closing contraction
c. closure clonus
c. closure contraction
c. closure tetanus
c. duration
monopolar cathodal stimulator
c. opening contraction

cathodal-duration tetanus

cathodal-opening
c.-o. contraction
c.-o. tetanus

cathode
Leonard cathode ray unit
c. ray
c. ray oscilloscope

cathode-duration tetanus

cathode-ray tube

cathodic
circulating cathodic antigen

cation
paramagnetic c.

cationic
c. colloidal gold
eosinophil cationic protein
eosinophilic cationic protein
lipophilic cationic complex
lipophilic cationic diphosphine
c. trypsinogen

cat's
amaurotic cat's eye
c. eye syndrome

cat-scratch
c.-s. disease
c.-s. fever

Cattell
C. Infant Intelligence Scale
C. Infant Scale Inventory

Catu virus

Caucasian
C. adult
C. female
C. male
young male C.

Caucus
National Caucus and Center on Black Aged, Inc.

cauda equina syndrome

caudal
c. appendage, short terminal phalanges, deafness, cryptorchidism, mental retardation syndrome
c. central nucleus
c. dysplasia syndrome
c. helix
left caudal quarter ganglion
c. mediastinal node
nuclei of caudal colliculus
c. regression syndrome
right caudal quarter ganglion
c. sac

caudal *(continued)*
spondylotic caudal myelopathy
spondylotic caudal radiculopathy

caudate
anterior extremity of caudate nucleus
anteromedial caudate nucleus
artery of caudate lobe
dorsal caudate putamen
left caudate nucleus
c. lobe of liver
native caudate lobe
c. nucleus
c. putamen
right caudate nucleus

caudocranial
c. hemiaxial view
right anterior caudocranial oblique
c. syndrome
c. view

cauliflower
c. ear
c. excrescence
c. mosaic virus

causal
probable causal relationship

causalgia
major c.
minor c.

causality assessment

causation
organismic c.

causative
c. agent
c. organism identified

cause
alcohol as cause of seizure
contributory cause of death
c. of death
death of other c.
c. of drug abuse
c. and effect
c.'s of heart disease
impaired memory of unknown c.
International Classification of Diseases and C.'s of Death
no anatomical cause of death
root cause analysis
c. undetermined
c. unknown

cause-and-effect relationship

caused
chronic ischemic colonic lesion caused by phlebosclerosis
constriction caused by light
doctor actively caused death
fever caused by infection
stress caused health problem

cause-specific survival

causing
cancer causing agent
minimal dose causing 100% death or malformation

caustic
alkali c.
c. ingestion
c. injury
Loeffler caustic stain
lunar c.
c. strictures of cervical esophagus
c. strictures of hypopharynx

cauterization
heater probe c.

cauterized
bleeder c.
bleeding site c.

cauterize lining of uterus

cautery
bipolar cautery probe
bipolar cautery unit
blind c.
Bovie c.
electric c.
endoscopic c.
galvanic c.
hook c.
c. incision
c. knife
laparoscopic tubal c.
Mira c.
Mueller c.
nasal tip c.
ophthalmic c.
ovarian c.
c. pencil
Rommel c.
snare c.
Wadsworth-Todd c.
Ziegler c.

cautery-assisted palatal stiffening operation

cava
Greenfield vena cava filter
inferior vena c.
inferior vena cava filter
inferior vena cava pressure
inferior vena cava reconstruction
inferior vena cava thrombosis
infrahepatic interruption of inferior vena c.
left inferior vena c.
left superior vena c.
ligament of left superior vena c.
ligament of left vena c.
membranous obstruction of the inferior vena c.
opening of inferior vena c.
orifice of inferior vena c.
radionuclide imaging of inferior vena c.
right inferior vena c.
right superior vena c.
superior vena c.
superior vena cava compression syndrome
superior vena cava obstruction
suprahepatic inferior vena c.
thoracic inferior vena c.
vena c.
vena cava inferior
vena cava superior

caval
vena caval filter

cavalryman's osteoma

cave
Meckel c.
Meckel cave lesion
C. operation
c. sickness
trigeminal c.

caved-in chest

cavernoma
familial cerebral c.

cavernosa
pars c.

cavernosal
atherosclerosis-induced cavernosal ischemia

cavernosography
dynamic infusion cavernosometry and c.

cavernosometry
dynamic infusion cavernosometry and cavernosography

cavernosum
lipoma c.
lymphangioma c.

cavernosus
nevus c.

cavernous
anterior cavernous sinus space
anterior cavernous sinus syndrome
artery of inferior cavernous sinus

extracerebral cavernous angioma
giant hepatic cavernous hemangioma
c. hemangioma
c. hemangioma of skin
meningeal branch of cavernous part of internal carotid artery
mixed capillary cavernous hemangioma
single potential analysis cavernous electrical activity
c. sinus
c. sinus infiltration
c. sinus sampling
c. sinus thrombosis
space of the cavernous sinus
c. transformation of the portal vein

Cave-Rowe operation

cavitary
c. infiltrate
c. tuberculosis

cavitating
c. neoplasm
c. pneumonia

cavitation
lobar c.
manual c.
pulmonary c.

cavitational
neuralgia-inducing cavitational osteonecrosis

cavity
abdominal cavity free of fluid
air fluid c.
anterior wall of tympanic c.
artificial classification c.
aspiration of pleural c.
axial surface c.
c. of bone
endometrial cavity sounded
incision through wall of c.
lining of abdominal c.
marrow cavity formation
medullary c.
nasal cavity cancer
nasal cavity wall
olfactory groove of nasal c.
opening of orbital c.
optic papilla c.
oral c.
oral cavity abnormality
oral cavity cytology
oral cavity proper
oral cavity tuberculosis
oral cavity tumors
oropharynx, oral c.
peripheral cavity wall
peritoneal cavity abscess
peritoneal cavity fluid
ventricles to peritoneal cavity shunt

cavography
radionuclide superior c.

cavopulmonary
bidirectional superior cavopulmonary anastomosis
total cavopulmonary connection
total cavopulmonary shunt

cavovalgus
pes c.

cavovarus
pes c.

cavus
anterior c.
anterior pes c.
c. foot deformity
forefoot c.
local c.
metatarsus c.
midfoot c.
pathological c.
pes c.
pes cavus clawfoot deformity
pes cavus deformity
talipes c.

Cayenne
mal de C.

C1–C9
serum complement C.

CCAAT/enhancer binding protein

C-clamp
pelvic C-c.

CD4
autologous HBcAg-specific C.
C. cell
C. count
C. helper-inducer cell
idiopathic CD4+ lymphocytopenia
idiopathic CD4 T-cell lymphocytopenia
normal clonal CD4+ T cell
recombinant soluble C.
soluble recombinant human C.
C. T-cell

CD4+
autologous HBcAg-specific C.

CD8
peripheral blood $CD8^+$ lymphocytosis

CD15
perinuclear CD15 antigen

CD20
low-grade CD20 positive lymphoma

cease
respiration c.

ceased
c. to breathe
c. breathing
c. to function
respiration has c.

cecal
anterior cecal artery
c. hernia
c. ligation and puncture
c. volvulus

cecalis
arteria cecalis anterior
arteria cecalis posterior

ceci
appendix c.

cecostomy
Malone c.
percutaneous c.
percutaneous catheter c.
percutaneous endoscopic c.

cecotomy
percutaneous c.

cecum
antimesocolic side of c.
c. grasped
hepatic c.
mesentery of c.
c. returned to abdomen

cedar
mountain c.
mountain cedar tree
salt c.

Cederschiöld massage

Cegka sign

celiac
adult celiac disease
anterocrural celiac plexus block
c. artery
c. artery compression syndrome
c. axis
childhood celiac disease
c. disease
c. flux
c. ganglion
c. lymph node metastasis
neurolytic celiac plexus block

celiac *(continued)*
c. plexus neurolysis
c. sprue
c. sprue disease

celiotomy
mandatory c.
negative c.

cell
aberrant c.
absolute cell count
absolute nucleated red blood c.
absorptive c.
accelerated destruction of red blood c.'s
accelerated destruction of red blood c.'s
acinar cell carcinoma
acoustic hair c.
activated endothelial c.
activated thymus c.
activation-induced cell death
active rosette-forming T c.
acute inflammatory c.
adenohypophysial corticotroph c.
adenosine-coupled spleen c.
adenosquamous cell carcinoma
adenovirus-reactive T c.
adherent c.
adherent macrophage-like c.
c. adhesion factor
c. adhesion molecule
adrenal cell rest tumor
adrenal chromaffin c.
adrenal cortex c.
adult granulosa cell tumor
advanced squamous cell cervical carcinoma
agger nasi c.
air cell cast
alloactivated killer c.
allogeneic bone marrow c.
allogeneic peripheral cell transplant
allogeneic stem c.
allogeneic stem cell transplant
allogeneic tumor cell immunization
allogeneic tumor cell vaccine
allogenic bone marrow cell infusion
allogenic dendritic c.
allogenic hematopoietic stem cell transplantation
allographic stem cell transplant
alpha cell alternate
alpha islet cell neoplasm
alveolar cell carcinoma
alveolar cell hyperplasia
Alzheimer II c.
amacrine c.
amine precursor uptake and decarboxylation c.
amine uptake and decarboxylation c.
amniotic fluid cell culture
anaplastic infiltrating single c.
anaplastic large cell lymphoma
anemone cell tumor
anergic T c.
aneuploid cell line
angioblastic c.
angiotropic large cell lymphoma
animal cell culture
annular elastolytic giant cell granuloma
anterior ethmoidal air c.
anterior ethmoidal c.
anterior horn c.
anterior horn cell degeneration
anterior horn cell disease
anterior horn cell isolation
anterior horn cell motor impairment
antibody-dependent cell cytotoxicity
antibody-forming c.
antibody-producing c.
antibody-secreting c.
antiendothelial cell antibody
antiendothelial cell autoantibody
antigen-modulated mini-stem cell transplant
antigen-presenting c.
antigen-pulsed autologous dendritic c.
antigen-reactive c.
antigen-reactive cell opsonization
antigen-reactive T c.
antigen-sensitive c.
antigen-specific suppressor T c.
antigen-specific T c.
antiislet cell antibody
antiparietal cell antibody
antiparietal cell antibody assay
antiplatelet endothelial cell adhesion molecule
antiproliferating cell nuclear antigen
c. antiviral factor
Antoni A c.
Antoni B c.
antral gastric c.
antral gastrin cell hyperfunction
apical membrane of proximal convoluted tubule c.
apoptotic cell death
Arandel cell harvester
argentaffin c.
argyrophilic c.
arterial smooth muscle c.
artificial beta c.
AS red c.
c. attachment protein
A-type nevus c.
atypical ductular c.
atypical endocervical cells of undetermined significance
atypical giant cell tumor
atypical glandular cell of undetermined significance
atypical glandular cells of uncertain significance
atypical glandular cells of unknown significance
atypical lymphoepithelioid cell proliferation
atypical squamous cell of undetermined significance
Atzpodien regimen for renal cell carcinoma
auditory receptor c.
autoimmune progenitor c.
autologous bone marrow c.
autologous hematopoietic c.
autologous hematopoietic progenitor cell transplantation
autologous hematopoietic stem cell transplantation
autologous liver c.
autologous lymphokine activated killer c.
autologous peripheral blood stem cell bone marrow transplantation
autologous peripheral hematopoietic stem cell support
autologous reactive T c.
autologous red blood c.
autologous red cell salvage
autologous stem c.
autologous stem cell rescue
autologous stem cell transplantation
autologous tumor cell immunization
autologous white cell localization
autolymphocyte-based treatment for renal cell carcinoma
automated cell count
automated cell image analysis

automated white blood cell differential
autonomous parathyroid chief cell proliferation
autoreactive B c.
baby hamster kidney c.
bacterial cell lacking an F plasmid
bacterial cell with an F plasmid
basal c.
basal cell adenocarcinoma
basal cell atypia
basal cell carcinoma
basal cell dysplasia
basal cell epithelioma
basal cell hyperplasia
basal cell liquefactive degeneration
basal cell nevus
basal cell nevus syndrome
basaloid squamous cell carcinoma
basket c.
benign glandular cell tumor
biliary epithelial c.
bipolar c.
blast c.
blast c.
blastoid variant of mantel cell lymphoma
blastoma mantel cell lymphoma
c. block analysis
blood cell profile
blood cell separator
blood mononuclear c.
body cell mass
bone marrow c.
bone marrow-derived cell or lymphocyte
bone marrow-derived cultured mast c.
bone marrow stem c.
bovine embryonic kidney c.
bovine embryonic spleen c.
bovine kidney c.
bovine red blood c.
bronchial glandular c.
bronchoalveolar c.
Burkitt lymphoma cell line
bursa c.
calcifying cell epithelioma
calcitonin-forming c.
calf embryonic heart c.
calf esophagus epithelial c.
cancer malignant c.
cancerous growth of blood c.
carcinoma cell line
CD4 helper-inducer c.
central giant cell granuloma
central giant cell lesion
central granular cell odontogenic tumor
centrocyte-like c.
cerebellar Purkinje c.
cerebral red blood cell volume
certified cell line
Chang conjunctiva c.
Chang liver c.
chicken red blood c.
chromophobe renal cell carcinoma
chronic, acquired, pure red cell aplasia
chronic inflammatory c.
chronic inflammatory cell infiltration
chronic lymphosarcoma cell leukemia
ciliated epithelial c.
c.'s of Claudius
clear cell adenocarcinoma
clear cell carcinoma
clear cell hepatocellular carcinoma
clear cell odontogenic tumor
clear cell renal cell carcinoma
clear cell sarcoma of the kidney
clear cell sarcoma of the liver
cluster of tumor c.'s
cluster of tumor c.'s
colony-forming c.
colony-forming unit-stem c.
columnar cell variant
combined germ cell tumor
committed progenitor c.
complete blood cell count
concentrated red blood c.
conductivity cell volume
conjugative plasmid in F^+ bacterial c.
c.'s consistent with invasive carcinoma
c.'s consistent with invasive carcinoma
contaminating tumor c.
continuously cultured carcinoma cell line used for tissue cultures
contractile function in cells of myocardium
cord blood cell therapy
cord blood mononuclear c.
crenated red blood c.
cryopreserved stem c.
crypt cell production rate
cultured T c.
c. cycle kinetics analysis
c. cycle redistribution
c. cycle redistribution and dose fractionation
cystic renal cell carcinoma
cytolytic T c.
cytotoxic T c.
damaged brain c.
Dameshek oval target c.
death of brain c.
degenerating c.
degenerative of dopamine-producing nerve c.
deglycerolized frozen red c.
delay aging of c.
denatured red blood c.
dendritic c.
dendritic reticulum c.
density-adjusted cell sorting
determined osteogenic precursor c.
differentiated c.
c. dissociation
c. division cycle
dog kidney c.
dog red blood c.
donkey red blood c.
donor c.
donor cell engraftment
donor dendritic c.
dorsal cell column
ectocervical cell yield
effector cell precursor
Ehrlich ascites tumor c.
embryonal cell carcinoma
embryonal cell tumor
embryonic stem c.
endothelial c.
endothelial cell growth factor
endothelial cell growth supplement
enterochromaffin c.
enterochromaffin cell hyperplasia
envelope of c.
enzymatic cell dispersion
enzyme-treated c.
epidermal c.
epidermal cell surface protein
epithelial c.
epithelioid-globoid c.
epitheloid c.
erythrocyte rosette-forming c.
erythropoietin-responsive c.
erythropoietin-sensitive stem c.
esophageal squamous cell carcinoma
ethmoid air c.

cell *(continued)*
extracellular mass to body cell mass ratio
c. extract
extrapulmonary small cell carcinoma
extruded c.
extrusion of cell cytoplasm
fatty liver c.
feline oncornavirus-associated cell membrane antigen
Ferrata c.
fetal bovine endothelial c.
fetal liver c.
fibroblast colony-forming c.
fixed cell immunofluorescence
c. and flare
flare and c.
fluorescence-activated cell sorter
fluorescence-activated cell sorter scan
fluorescence-activated cell sorting
fluorescent-activated cell sorting
follicle center lymphoma c.
follicular center c.
follicular center cell lymphoma
follicular dendritic c.
follicular large cell lymphoma
Friend erythroleukemia c.
Friend leukemia c.
frozen packed c.
frozen section red blood c.
ganglion c.
gap in cell cycle
gastric parietal c.
gastrointestinal pacemaker cell tumor
generation time of cell cycle
Gerbich red cell antigen
germ cell tumor
germinal cell aplasia
germ cell tumor with synchronous lesions in pineal and suprasellar region
ghost cell ameloblastoma
giant cell arteritis
giant cell collagenoma
giant cell fibroblastoma
giant cell hepatitis
giant cell thyroiditis
giant cell tumor
giant dopamine-containing c.
giant ganglion c.
giant cell interstitial pneumonia
giant cell interstitial pneumonitis
giant cell tumor of low malignant potential
giant cell tumor of tendon sheath
glandular neck c.
glial cell line-derived neurotropic factor
glomerular epithelial c.
goblet c.
goblet cell carcinoid
gonadal germ cell neoplasm
granular cell ameloblastic fibroma
granular cell ameloblastoma
granular cell layer
granular cell myeloblastoma
granular cell myoblastoma
granular cell schwannoma
granular cell tumor
granular chromophil c.
granular progenitor c.
granule c.
granulosa c.
granulosa-stromal cell tumor
granulosa-theca cell tumor
grivet monkey c.
Gross cell surface antigen
c. growth
growth hormone cell adenoma
growth hormone cell hyperplasia
growth hormone-expressing c.
guanosine-coupled spleen c.
guinea pig red blood c.
gut intestinal c.
hair c.
hair cell in ear
hairy c.
hairy cell leukemia variant
hamster embryo c.
hand-mirror c.
c.'s of Hansen
harvested stem c.
head and neck squamous cell carcinoma
healthy nerve c.
heart cell aggregate
heart cell death
heart disease c.
heart failure c.
heart lesion c.
heart muscle c.
helmet c.
helper T c.
hematopoietic progenitor c.
hematopoietic stem cell transplantation
hemopoietic blood stem c.
Henle c.
Henrietta Lacks c.
hepatic c.
hepatic cell carcinoma
hepatic reticuloendothelial c.
hepatic stellate c.
hepatoma c.
hepatoma carcinoma c.
hereditary clear cell renal carcinoma
hereditary papillary renal cell carcinoma
high cell passage
high-dose chemotherapy and stem cell rescue
high peroxide-containing c.
hippocampal pyramidal c.
Hodgkin-Reed-Sternberg c.
homozygous for sickle cell hemoglobin
homozygous typing c.
horizontally selective visual c.
horse red blood c.
human aortic endothelial c.
human aortic smooth muscle c.
human bronchial epithelial c.
human cervical carcinoma c.
human dermal microvascular endothelial c.
human diploid c.
human diploid cell strain
human diploid cell system
human diploid cell vaccine
human embryo kidney c.
human embryo lung cell culture
human embryonic intestine c.
human embryonic palatal mesenchymal c.
human endothelial c.
human epithelial c.
human fetal c.
human fetal diploid kidney c.
human fetal diploid lung c.
human foreskin epithelial c.
human genetic mutant cell repository
human immune c.'s
human kidney c.
human laryngeal tumor c.
human Lesch-Nyhan c.
human lymphoblastoid cell line
human mammary carcinoma cell membrane proteinase
human mesenchymal stem c.
human mesothelial cell membrane
human natural killer c.
human oral epidermoid carcinoma c.
human peripheral mononuclear c.
human skin nurse c.

human tumor stem cell assay
human umbilical vein
 endothelial c.
Hürthle cell adenoma
Hürthle cell carcinoma
Hürthle cell tumor
hyalinizing clear cell carcinoma
hyperdiploid c.
hypernephroma c.
hyperpolarizing bipolar c.
immature blood c.
immature brown fat c.
immature red blood c.
immune c.'s
c. immunity
immunocompetent c.
immunoglobulin-secreting c.
inclusion c.
inclusion cell disease
indirect cell division
indistinct cell border
individually viable c.
indolaminergic-accumulating c.
infected red blood c.
infection-fighting T c.
infection-fighting white c.
infectious cell protein
infiltrating ductal cell carcinoma
infiltrating squamous cell
 carcinoma
initial c.'s
inner cell mass
inner hair c.
c. integrity
c. interaction
c. interaction molecule
interdigitating c.
interdigitating dendritic cell
 sarcoma
intermediate cell column
interstitial c.
interstitial acute inflammatory c.
interstitial cells of Cajal
interstitial cell fluid
interstitial cell tumor
intestinal epithelial c.
intestinal mucosal mast c.
intratubular germ cell neoplasia,
 unclassified type
intravascular red cell aggregation
invasive growth of blood c.
irradiated red blood c.
irregular disfigured c.
irreversible damage to brain c.
irreversible sickle c.
islet cell antigen
islet cell carcinoma
islet cell surface antibody
islet cell transplant
islet cell of pancreas
c. isolation
juvenile granulosa cell tumor
juxtaglomerular c.
juxtaglomerular cell hyperplasia
juxtaglomerular cell tumor
killer c.
killer cell inhibitory receptor
c. kinetics of adenocarcinoma
c. kinetics of tumors
Kulchitsky cell carcinoma
Kupffer c.
Langerhans c.
Langerhans cell granule
Langerhans cell granulomatosis
Langerhans cell histiocytosis
large cell anaplastic lymphoma
large cell calcifying Sertoli cell
 tumor
large cell change
large cell lung carcinoma
large cell lymphoma
large cell neuroendocrine
 carcinoma
large cell non-Hodgkin lymphoma
large cleaved c.
large motile c.
large transformed c.
large unstained c.
laryngeal squamous cell
 carcinoma
laser cell and flare meter
left giant c.
lens epithelial c.
lesion on erythrocyte cell
 membrane at the site of
 complement fixation
leukocyte cell adhesion molecule
leukocyte-poor packed c.
leukocyte-poor red blood c.
Leydig cell adenoma
Leydig cell agenesis
Leydig cell aplasia
Leydig cell atrophy
Leydig cell embryology
Leydig cell hyperplasia
Leydig cell hypoplasia
Leydig cell insufficiency
Leydig cell secretion
Leydig cell secretory function
Leydig cell stimulation
Leydig cell tumor
Leydig cells of the testis
light cells of thyroid
limbal stem cell transplantation
limited-stage diffuse large cell
 lymphoma
limited-stage small cell lung
 cancer
limiting precursor c.
c. line
lineage
lining c.
lining cell layer hyperplasia
linker for activation of T c.
lipid cell neoplasm
lipid cell ovarian tumor
lipid-laden clear c.
lipoid cell tumor
littoral cell angioma
liver cell adenoma
liver cell carcinoma
liver cell dysplasia
liver cell plate
liver cell tumor
liver cell membrane autoantibody
live yeast cell derivative
log cell kill
long-lived memory T c.
long-term culture-initiating c.
low columnar c.
lung c.
lung adenocarcinoma c.
lupus erythematosus c.
lupus erythematosus cell test
luteinized theca c.
lymph node c.
lymph node mononuclear c.
lymphoblastoid cell line
lymphocytic blood c.
lymphoepithelioid cell lymphoma
lymphoid cell line
lymphoid dendritic c.
lymphoid stem c.
lymphokine-activated killer c.
lymphoplasmacytoid lymphoma c.
lymphosarcoma c.
lymphosarcoma-reticulum cell
 sarcoma
lysed tumor c.
macula densa c.
macular hair c.
Madin-Darby bovine kidney c.
magnetically activated cell sorter
magnocellular neuroendocrine c.
malfunctioning insulin
 receptor c.'s
malfunctioning insulin
 receptor c.'s
malignant clear cell acrospiroma
malignant giant cell tumor
malignant glandular cell tumor

cell *(continued)*
malignant granular cell myoblastoma
malignant islet cell tumor
malignant ovarian germ cell tumor
malignant small round cell tumor
mammalian cell culture
mammalian cell membrane
mammosomatotroph cell adenoma
mantle cell lymphocytic lymphoma
Marchand wandering c.
marginal zone c.
marginal zone cell lymphoma
marrow cell vacuolization
marrow hematopoietic stem c.
marrow mononuclear c.
Marschalko-type plasma c.
mast c.
mast cell containing both tryptase and chymase
mast cell containing tryptase but not chymase
mast cell degranulating peptide
mast cell degranulation
mast cell degranulation test
mast cell disease
mast cell growth factor
mast cell hyperplasia
mast cell inhibitor
mast cell leukemia
mast cell nevus
mast cell proteinase
mast cell reticulosis
mast cell sarcoma
mast cell stabilizer
mast cell staining
mast cell tryptase
mast cell tumor
mastoid air c.
matched unrelated donor stem cell transplant
maturation B c.
maturation of breast c.
mature B c.
mature cell leukemia
MCF-7 breast cancer c.
mean cell hemoglobin concentration
mean cell thickness
measles giant cell pneumonia
medial cell column
mediastinal germ cell tumor
c. mediated antibody
mediated cell death
c. mediated cytotoxicity
c. mediated immunity
megakaryocytic blood c.
melanoma c.
melanoma antigen reacting to T c.
melanoma antigen recognized by T c.
melanoma cell adhesion molecule
melanoma cell lysate
membrana granulosa c.
c. membrane
membrane lipid c.
memory B, T c.
memory T c.
meningeal cell tumor
meningothelial arachnoid c.
Merkel c.
Merkel cell cancer
Merkel cell carcinoma
Merkel cell carcinoma cell line
Merkel cell neoplasm
Merkel cell tumor
mesangial c.
mesangial cell proliferation
mesenchymal c.'s
mesenchymal intimal c.
mesenchymal progenitor c.
mesenchymal stem c.
mesenchymal stromal c.
mesonephroid clear cell carcinoma
mesothelial cell inclusion
mesothelial cell layer
metacerebral giant c.
metachronous testicular germ cell tumor
metaplastic epithelial c.
metaplastic mucus-secreting c.
metastatic basal cell carcinoma
metastatic renal cell carcinoma
Mexican hat c.
Meynert c.'s
MHC-restricted cytotoxic T c.
MIB-1 cell proliferation marker
microcytic red c.
microglial rod c.
microscopic granular cell tumor
middle ear c.
middle ethmoidal air c.
middle glial cell line-derived neurotrophic factor
Mikulicz c.'s
mild sickle cell disease
mitral c.'s
mitral cell layer
mixed cell agglutination reaction
mixed cell leukemia
mixed cell sarcoma
mixed germ cell tumor
mixed GH-PRL cell adenoma
mixed growth hormone-prolactin cell adenoma
mixed cell nodular lymphoma
mixed skin cell leukocyte reaction
mixed small cleaved and large cell lymphoma
molecular cell biology
Moloney cell surface antigen
MOLT-18, human T cell line
monkey c.
monkey kidney c.
monkey red blood c.
monoclonal antiendothelial cell antibody
monocyte-derived dendritic c.
monocytic blood c.
mononuclear cell infiltrate
mononuclear cell infiltration
mononuclear cell pleocytosis
mononuclear cell recruitment
mononuclear cell tissue factor
mononuclear Reed-variant c.
morbilliform basal cell carcinoma
morpheaform basal c.
morpheaform basal cell carcinoma
morphea-type basal cell carcinoma
Mosher air c.
mouse epithelial c.
mouse red blood c.
mouse rosette-forming c.
mouse stem cell-like c.
mucinous cell adenocarcinoma
mucosal addresin cell adhesion molecule-1
mucosal cell proliferation
mucosal mast c.
c.'s of Mueller
Müller cell footplate
multicentric basal cell carcinoma
multicentric islet cell adenoma
multifocal giant cell encephalitis
multifocal infiltrated duct cell carcinoma
multifocal Langerhans c.
multinucleate cell angiohistiocytoma
multinucleated cell encephalitis
multinucleated dentinoblastic c.
multinucleated giant epithelial c.
multinucleated osteoclastic giant c.

multiple basal cell carcinoma syndrome multiple basal cell nevus syndrome
multiple basal cell neuroma syndrome
multiple basal cell nevoid syndrome
multiple myeloma cell line
multiple nevoid-basal cell carcinoma
multiple nevoid-basal cell carcinoma syndrome
multiple nevoid, basal cell epithelioma, jaw cysts, bifid rib syndrome
multiple resistant cell lines
c. multiplication inhibition
multipotent hematopoietic c.
murine B16 c.
murine erythroleukemia c.
murine L c.
murine mesangial c.
murine myeloid leukemia cell line
murine tumor c.
mutant Ras peptide-pulsed dendritic cell therapy
Mycobacterium cell wall complex
myeloid cell infiltration
myeloid dendritic c.
myeloid precursor c.
myeloid stem c.
myenteric ganglion c.
myoepithelial c.
myoepithelial cell island
myoepithelial cell process
myoid visual c.
myxoid cell pattern
nave T c.
naive B c.
naive T c.
natural killer c.
natural killer cell activation
natural killer cell antigen
natural killer cell leukemia
natural killer T-c.
necrotic cell death
necrotic inflammatory c.
neonatal giant cell hepatitis
neoplastic adenohypophysial c.
neoplastic cell proliferation
nerve cell adhesion molecule
nerve cell body
nerve cell death
nerve cell degeneration
nerve cell disorder
nerve cell growth
nerve cell survival
nerve cell tumor
nests of nevus c.'s
nests of nevus c.'s
nests and strands of c.'s
Neumann c.'s
neural cell adhesion molecule
neural cell line
neural crest c.
neural crest-derived cell lineage
neural hamster c.
neuroendocrine c.
neuroendocrine small cell carcinoma
neuroepithelial c.'s
neuroepithelial cell migration
neuroepithelial cell proliferation
neuronal cell apoptosis
neuronal cell line
neuronal cell origin tumor
neurosecretory c.
nevoid basal cell carcinoma syndrome
nevoid basal cell epithelioma, jaw cysts, bifid rib syndrome
nevus cell, A-, B-, C-type
new host c.
NK cell activation
NK cell antigen
NK cell lymphoma
NK cell lysis
nodular basal cell carcinoma
nodular, mixed cell lymphoma
noduloulcerative basal cell carcinoma
no malignant c.
nonadherent c.
non-beta cell tumor
noncleaved follicular center c.
nonclonogenic proliferating c.
nondifferentiated c.
nongerminoma germ cell tumor
nongranular clear chromophobe c.
nonimmunogenic murine tumor c.
non-islet cell tumor hypoglycemia
nonmyeloablative allogeneic stem cell transplant
nonparenchymal liver c.
non–rosette-forming c.
nonseminomatous germ cell neoplasm
nonseminomatous germ cell testicular tumor
nonspecific effector c.
nonspecific suppressor c.
Noonan-like giant cell lesion
Noonan-like giant cell lesion syndrome
normal clonal CD4+ T c.
normal complement of c.'s
normal complement of c.'s
normal hematopoietic c.
normal sheep red blood c.
not enough c.'s
not enough c.'s
nuclear factor of activated T c.
nucleated cell count
nucleated endothelial c.
nucleated red blood cell mass
nucleated red c.
null cell acute lymphocytic leukemia
null cell adenoma
null cell anaplastic large cell lymphoma
null cell lymphoblastic leukemia
null cell lymphoma
null cell tumor
nurse cell environment
oat cell carcinoma
oat cell lung cancer
oat cell tumor
oculosensory cell reflex
oligodendroglialike c.
oncocytic epithelial c.
open cell foam
opioid cell membrane receptor
oral epithelial cell genetic fingerprinting
oral epithelial cell genotyping
oral squamous cell carcinoma
original host c.
Ortho-Kung T c.
osmotic cell injury
osteoclastic giant c.
osteoclast-like giant c.
outer hair c.
oval target c.
ovarian clear cell adenocarcinoma
ovarian clear cell carcinoma
ovarian germ cell tumor
ovarian granulosa c.
ovarian granulosa-stromal cell tumor
ovarian granulosa-theca cell tumor
ovarian hilar cell tumor
ovarian lipid cell neoplasm
ovarian malignant germ cell tumor
owl's eye c.
oxidative cell injury
ox red blood c.
oxytocinergic cell body

cell *(continued)*
packed c.'s
packed human blood c.
packed red blood c.
packed red blood cell transfusion
pale cell acanthoma
palisading epithelioid c.
Pall-filtered packed c.
pancreatic acinar c.
pancreatic acinar cell carcinoma
pancreatic duct cell carcinoma
pancreatic islet beta c.
pancreatic islet cell transplantation
pancreatic islet cell tumor
papillary renal cell carcinoma
parabasal cell layers
parafollicular calcitonin-producing c.
parathyroid cell membrane
parathyroid chief c.
parathyroid hormone-related protein-transfected RIN-141 c.
parenchymatous cell of corpus pineale
parent c.
parietal cell hyperplasia
parietal cell index
paroxysmal nocturnal hemoglobinuria c.
parvovirus B19 red cell aplasia
c. passaged
pathognomonic Askanazy c.
pathologic cell death
Pelger-Huët c.
peptic cell receptor
peptide-specific T c.
peptidoglycan rigid cell wall
percentage of goblet c.
percentage of multinucleated c.'s
perianal squamous cell carcinoma
perichondral cell seeding
peripheral blood c.
peripheral blood cell count
peripheral blood mononuclear c.
peripheral blood mononuclear cell hepatitis B virus measurement
peripheral blood progenitor c.
peripheral blood progenitor cell transplant
peripheral blood stem c.
peripheral blood stem cell autografting
peripheral blood stem cell infusion
peripheral blood stem cell rescue
peripheral blood stem cell reserve
peripheral blood stem cell support
peripheral blood stem cell transplantation
peripheral cytotrophoblast c.
peripheral giant cell reparative granuloma
peripheral giant cell tumor
peripheral lymphoid c.
peripheral nucleated c.
peripheral stem cell harvest
peripheral stem cell transplant
peripheral white blood c.
peritoneal c.
peritoneal exudate c.
peritubular contractile c.
peritubular endothelial c.
perivascular epithelioid c.
phase of mitosis in cell growth cycle
Pick c.'s
pig aortic endothelial c.
pig cell implant
pigmented basal cell carcinoma
pigmented retina epithelial c.
pigmented spindle c.
pineal cell tumor
plaque-forming c.
plasma c.
plasma cell count
plasma cell dyscrasia
plasma cell dyscrasia of unknown significance
plasma cell granuloma
plasma cell hepatitis
plasma cell interstitial pneumonitis
plasma cell labeling index
plasma cell leukemia
plasma-free red c.
platelet-derived endothelial cell growth factor
platelet endothelial cell adhesion molecule-1
pleural mesothelial c.
plexiform spindle cell nevus
pluripotent hemopoietic stem c.
pluripotent myeloid stem c.
poorly differentiated embryonal cell tumor
poorly differentiated squamous cell carcinoma
postmortem human kidney c.
potential erythropoietin-responsive c.
primary liver c.
primary liver cell cancer
primary mediastinal large cell lymphoma with sclerosis
primitive tumor c.
primordial germ c.
principal c.
producing c.
production of red blood c.'s
programmed cell death
proliferating nuclear cell antigen
proliferative helper c.
pseudovascular adenoid squamous cell carcinoma
pulmonary neuroendocrine c.
pure red cell aplasia
pure red blood cell agenesis
pure red blood cell aplasia
purified cell walls
purified chick embryo cell culture
Purkinje c.
pyramidal cell layer
quiescent phase of cells leaving the mitotic cycle
rabies vaccine, human diploid cell culture
rabies vaccine, purified chick embryo cell culture
radioactivity of vegetative c.'s
Raji cell-binding material
Raji cell-binding unit
Raji cell assay
rat mast cell protease
rat mast cell technique
reactive spindle cell nodule
receptor cells of hearing
red c.
red blood c.
red blood cell agglutination
red blood cell cast
red blood cell adenosine deaminase
red blood cell adherence
red blood cell count
red blood cell fallout
red blood cell fragility
red blood cell immune adherence
red blood cell mass
red blood cell spun filtration
red blood cell transfusion
red blood cell volume
red blood cell concentrate
red blood cell diameter width
red blood cell distribution width index
red blood cell filter ability
red blood cell folate
red blood cell iron turnover

red blood cell iron turnover rate
red blood cells per high-power field
red blood cell to plasma ratio
red blood cell precursor production rate
red blood cell suspension
red cell cast
red cell index
red cell morphology index
red cell peroxide hemolysis
red cell volume
c. redistribution and dose hyperfractionation
red cells too numerous to count
c. refract ability
regional lymph node c.
Reider cell leukemia
renal cell cancer
renal tubular c.
renomedullary interstitial c.
c. replication potential
c. repository line
c. resistance
resistant Friend leukemia c.
c. response to estrogen
reticulum c.
reticulum cell carcinoma
retinal ganglion c.
retinal pigment epithelial c.
reversible sickle c.
Rhesus diploid cell strain rabies vaccine
right giant c.
rosette-forming c.
c. salvage
sarcomatoid renal cell carcinoma
Schwann cell membrane
sedimented red c.
c. sensitivity to radiation
sensitization response c.
sensitized sheep cell agglutination
sensory hair c.'s
sensory hair c.'s
serous c.
Sertoli cell culture medium
Sertoli cell index
Sertoli cell mesenchyme tumor
sheep cell agglutination test
sheep cell agglutination titer
sheep red blood c.
sheep red cell rosette-forming c.
sickle c.
sickle cell anemia test
sickle cell beta
sickle cell chronic lung disease
sickle cell hemoglobin
sickle cell hemoglobin C disease
sickle cell hemoglobin D disease
sickle cell lung disease
sickle cell retinopathy
sickle cell screening
sickle cell thalassemia
sickle cell trait
sickle cell hemoglobin F
sickle red blood c.
sickle-shaped particle c.
signet-ring cell carcinoma
sinusoidal endothelial c.
small cell bronchogenic carcinoma
small cell cancer of bladder
small cell carcinoma of bronchus
small cell carcinoma of lung
small cell malignant lymphoma
small cell osteosarcoma
small cell sarcoma
small cell tumor
small cell undifferentiated carcinoma of the prostate
small cell undifferentiated neuroendocrine carcinoma
small cleaved c.
small noncleaved cell lymphoma
small noncleaved cell, non-Burkitt lymphoma
small pyramidal c.
smooth muscle c.
soft parts giant cell tumor
somatic cell human gene therapy
c. soupy cytoplasm
specific red cell adherence
spindle cell carcinoma
spindle cell lipoma
spindle cell nevus
spindle cell sarcoma
spindle cell epithelial tumor with thymus-like differentiation
spleen c.
spleen cell conditioned medium
splenic adherent c.
spontaneous killer c.
spontaneous suppressor cell activity
squamous cell carcinoma of vulva
squamous cell carcinoma
squamous cell carcinoma antigen
squamous cell carcinoma dorsum of hand
squamous cell carcinoma of the esophagus
squamous cell carcinoma of head and neck
squamous cell carcinoma inhibitory factor
squamous cell carcinoma in situ
squamous cell carcinoma of the thyroid
squamous cell carcinoma of tongue
squamous cell carcinoma of vocal cord
squamous cell head and neck cancer
squamous cell hyperplasia
squamous cell lung tumor
squamous cell papilloma
squamous epithelial c.
squamous epithelial c.
squamous intraepithelial c.
squamous intraepithelial lesion/atypical squamous cell of undetermined significance
stellate cell of cerebral cortex
stellate cell of liver
stem c.
stem cell apheresis
stem cell factor
stem cell indicated by transplantation assay
stem cell leukemia
stem cell proliferation factor
stem cell rescue
stem cell support
steroid cell tumor
streptococcal cell membrane
stromal cell tumor
subependymal giant cell astrocytoma
sunburn c.
superficial transitional cell carcinoma
suppressor c.
suppressor cell activity
c. surface antigen
c. surface protein
syncytiotrophoblastic giant c.
syngeneic spleen c.
synovial lining c.
systemic mast cell disease
T c.
tall cell variant
tanned red blood cell agglutination
tanned red blood cell hemagglutination
tanned red blood cell hemagglutination inhibition

cell *(continued)*
tanned red c.
tanycyte ependymal c.
target c.
target cell anemia
T cell antigen receptor Vb
T cell cytotoxic
theca cell tumor
T-helper suppressor c.
T-helper cell type 1, 2, 3
c. therapy
thromboplastic cell component
thymus c.
thymus cell growth factor
time required to complete G_1 phase of cell cycle
time required to complete G_2 phase of cell cycle
time required to complete M phase of cell cycle
time required to complete S phase of cell cycle
time required to double number of cells in given population
T/natural killer cell
total packed cell volume
total red blood c.'s
total red cell volume
total rosette-forming c.
total viable c.'s
total white blood c.'s
total white and differential cell count
totipotent hematopoietic stem c.
transferring immature muscle c.
transiently amplifying c.
transitional bladder cell carcinoma
transitional cell cancer-associated virus
transitional cell cancer
transitional cell carcinoma of bladder
transitional cell papilloma
transitional cell tumor
transitional cell zone
trypsinized sheep red blood c.
tubal air c.
tumor c.
tumor cell burden
tumor cell hypoxia
tumor-derived activated c.
tumor-draining lymph node c.
tumor cell migration-inhibition factor
tumor-specific cell surface antigen
tympanic air c.
ulcer-associated cell lineage
uncontrolled cell division growth
undifferentiated cell adenoma
undifferentiated large cell carcinoma
unidentified endosteal marrow c.
unit of packed red blood c.'s
untreated c.
vascular cell adhesion molecule
vascular cell adhesion molecule-1
vascular endothelial cell growth inhibitor
vascular smooth muscle c.
ventral cell column
vestibular hair c.
viral cell surface antigen
c. volume
volume-packed c.'s
volume of packed red blood c.'s
c. volume profile
c. wall
c. wall defective
c. wall skeleton
Walthard cell rest
washed packed c.'s
washed red blood c.
white c.
white blood c.
white blood cell count
white blood cell depletion
white blood cell scan
white blood cell transfusion
white blood cells per high-power field
white cell cast
white cell count
WHO classification for transitional cell carcinoma of the urinary bladder: stages Ta through T4
whorled c.'s
Wistar Institute Susan Hayflick c.
yeast c.

cell-bound
c.-b. antibody
c.-b. antigen

cell-cell adhesion molecule

cell-cycle
c.-c. nonspecific agent
c.-c. specific agent

cell-directed inhibitor

cell-linked
red blood cell-linked antigen-antiglobulin reaction

cell-mediated
c.-m. cytotoxicity
c.-m. immune
c.-m. immune response
c.-m. immunity
c.-m. lysis
c.-m. mutagenesis

celloidin
axial celloidin section

cells-spleen
colony-forming c.-s.

cell-to-slide transfer

cellular
c. abnormality
c. acetate propionate
acquired cellular immunodeficiency syndrome
c. activity
acute cellular rejection
c. adhesion molecule
adoptive cellular therapy
allogeneic cellular immune therapy
antibody-dependent cellular cytotoxicity
antibody-directed cellular cytotoxicity
anti-TB cellular immunity
c. atypia
autologous cellular therapy
automated cellular imaging system
autophagocytosed cellular material
benign cellular change
c. blue nevus
c. breast cancer therapy
cancellous cellular bone
cancellous cellular bone graft
carbonizing cellular debris
c. cutaneous fibrous histiocytoma
c. effects of alcohol
c. immunity
c. immunity deficiency syndrome
c. immunocompetence profile
c. immunologic reactivity
c. inhibitors of apoptosis
malignancy associated cellular marker
c. mediated immune response
Metchnikoff cellular immunity theory
mixed cellular Hodgkin disease
myocardial cellular degeneration
myocardial cellular hypertrophy
oxidative cellular injury
phosphorylation by the cellular double-stranded RNA-activated kinase

c. retinoic acid-binding protein
c. retinol-binding protein
total cellular receptor pool
total cellular score

cellularity
mixed cellularity Hodgkin disease

cellulite
c. of heel
indurated c.

cellulitis
aerobic c.
amyloid c.
anaerobic c.
cuff c.
gangrenous c.
monomicrobial necrotizing c.
necrotizing c.
nonclostridial anaerobic c.
orbital c.
pelvic c.
perianal streptococcal c.
periorbital c.
perirectal c.
peritonsillar c.
phlegmonous c.
Pseudomonas c.

celluloid implant material

cellulose
c. acetate
c. acetate butyrate
c. acetate dialysis device
c. acetate electrophoresis
aqueous methyl c.
c. breakdown bacteria
diethylaminoethyl c.
methyl cellulose paste
c. nitrate
o-diethylaminoethyl c.
oxidized c.
regenerated c.

Celsius
degree C.
temperature midpoint C.
C. temperature scale

cement
acrylic bone c.
antibiotic-loaded acrylic c.
Artisan cement system
biodegradable calcium phosphate c.
bone cement implantation syndrome
injecting bone c.
low-viscosity c.
lunate acrylic cement wrist prosthesis
c. mantle
c. mantle grade classification
methyl methacrylate c.
Morck cement bifocal
prosthetic antibiotic-loaded acrylic c.
radiopaque bone c.
removal of excess c.
segmental cement extraction system

cemental
periapical cemental dysplasia
peripheral cemental dysplasia
sclerotic cemental mass

cemented
alumina cemented total hip prosthesis

cementicle
attached c.

cementless
c. broach
c. femoral component
c. fixation
c. prosthesis
c. Sportono
c. surface replacement arthroplasty
c. total hip arthroplasty
c. total hip replacement

cementoenamel junction

cementoma

cementoosseous
c. dysphasia
c. dysplasia
florid local cementoosseous dysplasia
focal cementoosseous dysplasia
local cementoosseous dysphasia

cementoossifying fibroma

cementum
apical c.
c. hyperplasia
necrotic c.
periapical c.

censure
peer c.

census
average daily c.
daily c.

Centella
C. asiatica
titrated extract of *Centella asiatica*

center
acute care c.
administrative control c.
adult day-care c.
adult diagnostic and treatment c.
alcohol rehabilitation c.
alternative birth c.
Alzheimer Disease C.
ambulatory care c.
ambulatory surgery c.
area health education c.
Arizona Cancer Center multiple myeloma staging system
auditory word c.
blood c.
brain injury c.
cancer care c.
cancer detection c.
cardiac-accelerator c.
cardiac arrhythmia evaluation c.
cardiac diagnostic c.
cardioinhibitor c.
chest pain c.
clinical research c.
Communicable Disease C.
community health c.
community mental health c.
comprehensive cancer c.
conical protrusion of center of cornea
continuing care c.
crisis intervention c.
crisis resolution c.
day activity c.
day care c.
day treatment c.
Developmental Evaluation C.
diabetes management c.
diagnostic c.
diagnostic imaging c.
disaster assistance c.
distance between c.'s
drug information c.
c. edge
emergency center visits
Emergency Communications C.
emergency decontamination c.
emergency medical trauma c.
Emergency Operations C.
emergency and trauma c.
emetic c.
C.'s for Epidemiologic Studies Depression scale
excitatory c.
family health c.
family medicine c.
family practice c.
c. of field of vision
follicle center lymphoma cell

center *(continued)*
follicular center cell
follicular center cell lymphoma
Food and Nutrition Information C.
free-standing ambulatory surgical c.
free-standing emergency c.
germinal c.
c. of gravity
health evaluation c.
health screening c.
heat conservation c.
heat loss c.
c. hemodialysis
higher brain c.
hypothalamic feeding c.
incontinence treatment c.
c. for independent living
inpatient exercise c.
inspiratory c.
instrument recirculation c.
joint replacement c.
c. line artifact
lower limb ossification c.
malleolar ossification c.
c. of mandibular autorotation
c. of mass
M.D. Anderson Cancer C.
medical alert c.
medical training c.
Memorial Sloan-Kettering Cancer C.
mental health c.
microtubule organizing c.
mitotic organizing c.
motor cortical c.
multidisciplinary pain management c.
narcotics treatment c.
National Asian Pacific C. on Aging
National Caucus and C. on Black Aged, Inc.
National C. for Child Abuse and Neglect
National Health Information C.
National Heart, Lungs, and Blood Institute Information C.
National C. on Elder Abuse
National C. on Minority Health and Health Disparities
National C. on Poverty Law, Inc.
National Women's Health Information C.
neighborhood family care c.
neighborhood health c.
Neumann-Shepard oval optical center marker
neurotrauma c.
newborn c.
noncleaved follicular center cell
nurse-managed c.
occupational health c.
optical center of spectacle lens
organ transplant c.
outpatient diagnostic c.
outpatient rehabilitation c.
pain management c.
patient evaluation c.
pediatric critical care c.
Physical Assessment C.
pneumotaxic c.
pontine gaze c.
pontine micturition c.
Primary Children's Medical C.
progressive transformation of germinal c.
pseudofollicular growth c.
radiologic control c.
rape crisis c.
reaction c.
regional pediatric pulmonary c.
regional perinatal intensive care c.
rehabilitation center for physically handicapped
research and training c.
residential treatment c.
respiratory c.
c. of rotation
school-based health c.
sleep disorders c.
stroke treatment c.
Toxicology Information C.
transplant c.
trauma c.
trauma and emergency c.
urgent care c.
urgent visit c.
vasoconstrictor c.
vasodilator c.
vasoinhibitory c.
vasomotor c.
vomiting c.
X inactivation c.

centering
optical centering instrument

centesimal dilution

centigrade
c. temperature scale
c. thermal unit

centimeter
centimeters of water cuff pressure
cubic c.
cubic centimeter per hour
grams per cubic c.
liters per centimeter of water
nanogram per cubic c.
newton per square c.
reciprocal ohm c.
c.'s of water

central
c. acinar emphysema
acute central cervical spinal cord injury
AIDS-related primary central nervous system lymphoma
c. airway
c. alveolar hypoventilation
c. alveolar hypoventilation syndrome
c. angiospastic retinitis
anterior central beaking
anterior central convolution
anterior central curve
anterior central gyrus
anterior central indentation
anterolateral central artery
anteromedial central artery
anteromedial central branch
c. anticholinergic syndrome
antiseptic-impregnated central venous catheter
c. apical portion
c. apnea
areolar central choroiditis
artery of central sulcus
c. audio vestibular dysfunction
c. auditory nervous system
c. auditory processing battery
c. auditory processing disorder
c. axis depth dose of electron beam therapy
c. benign neoplasm
buccal groove of central fossa
caudal central nucleus
c., steady and maintained fixation
c. centrifugal scarring alopecia
c. cervical spinal cord syndrome
c. chemosensitive area
c. choroidal apposition
c. circulating blood volume
c. collodiaphysial
combined central and obstructive sleep apnea
congenital central hypoventilation syndrome

c. core disease
c. corneal thickness
c. counter-adaptive change
c. cyanosis
c. deafness
c. deposition
c. developmental groove
development and/or central nervous system anomalies, genital hypoplasia, ear anomalies
c. diabetes insipidus
c. disk-shaped retinopathy
c. emetic
c. episiotomy
c. episiotomy and repair
c. European encephalitis
c. European encephalitis virus
c. European tick-borne encephalitis
c. excitatory state
c. extensor mechanism
c. fibrous body
c. fossa
c. giant cell granuloma
c. giant cell lesion
c. granular cell odontogenic tumor
granulomatous angiitis of the central nervous system
c. gray
c. groove of central fossa
c. hemorrhagic necrosis
c. hyoid bone
idiopathic central nervous system hypersomnolence
idiopathic central serous chorioretinopathy
c. illumination
c. implantation
increased central venous pressure
information processing in central nervous system
c. inhibitory state
c. integrative deficit
isolated angiitis of central nervous system
c. language disorder
late central nervous system toxicity
left subclavian central venous pressure
c. line infection
long central artery
long-term central venous access catheter placement
low central venous pressure anesthesia
low-grade central osteogenic sarcoma
c. lung distance
lustrous central yellow point
mandibular central incisor
c. material section
c. material supply
maternal central hemodynamics
maxillary central incisor
measure of central tendency
medial central nucleus of thalamus
medial central tegmental field
mesencephalic central gray
midline central neuraxis
c. midline placement of electrodes in electroencephalography
c. motor conduction time
c. mucoepidermoid carcinoma
multilumen central venous pressure
c. nervous system
c. nervous system depression
c. nervous system leukemia
c. neurogenic hyperventilation
c. obesity
C. Obesity Index
organic central nervous system deterioration
partial central hypophysectomy
c. patient station
percutaneous central venous catheter
percutaneously inserted central line catheter
periaqueductal central gray
peripapillary central serous choroidopathy
peripherally inserted central venous catheter
c. pit
c. pontine myelinolysis
posterior central curve
c. posterior curve
posteromedial central artery
c. poststroke pain
c. precocious puberty
primary angiitis of the central nervous system
primary central nervous system
primary central nervous system lymphoma
c. primitive neuroectodermal tumor
c. principal axis of inertia
c. principal moments of inertia
c. processing unit
c. pulmonary vasculature
c. ray
c. reaction time
c. respiratory depression
c. retinal artery
c. retinal artery occlusion
c. retinal vein
c. retinal vein occlusion
right subclavian central venous
c. sacral line
c. scotoma
c. serous chorioretinopathy
c. serous choroidopathy
c. serous retinopathy
c. sharp wave transient
single central maxillary incisor
c. sleep apnea
c. sleep apnea syndrome
c. slow wave focus
c. somatosensory conduction time
c. spike focus
c. splanchnic venous thrombosis
c. sterile supply department
c. tegmental tract
c. terminal of Wilson
c. vein of hepatic lobule
c. venous
c. venous access
c. venous access device
c. venous catheter
c. venous catheter infection
c. venous line
c. venous nutrition
c. venous oxygen
c. venous pressure
c. venous temperature
c. vision loss
c. visual acuity
c. visual field
c. voluntary control
Wilson central terminal

centrale
os c.

centralis
area c.
arteria centralis brevis
c. lateralis
neurinomatosis c.
nucleus c.
nucleus amygdalae c.
nucleus caudalis c.
nucleus centralis lateralis
nucleus centralis lateralis thalami
nucleus centralis medialis thalami
nucleus centralis tegmenti superior

centralis *(continued)*
nucleus cuneatus, pars c.
nucleus centralis superior raphe
pars c.
pars centralis ventriculi lateralis
placenta previa c.

centralized cancer patient data system

centrally active phenethylamine derivative related to amphetamine and methamphetamine

centration
optical zone c.

centric
c. jaw relationship
long c.
mandibular centric relation
occluding centric relation record
c. position
c. relation
c. relation-centric occlusion
c. relation occlusion
vertical and centric bite

centrifugal
central centrifugal scarring alopecia
countercurrent centrifugal elutriation
c. counter-current chromatography
direct centrifugal flotation
c. force
indirect centrifugal flotation
miniature centrifugal fast analyzer
relative centrifugal field
relative centrifugal force
reversed passive hemagglutination by miniature centrifugal fast analysis

centrifugation
continuous-flow c.
continuous-flow centrifugation leukapheresis
continuous-flow zonal c.
c. extractable fluid
Ficoll-Hypaque c.
intermittent flow centrifugation leukapheresis
lysis centrifugation method
lysis centrifugation technique
sucrose density gradient c.

centrifuged
c. culture fluid
c. microaggregate filter

centrifuge microscope

centrilobar necrosis

centrilobular emphysema

centriole
anterior c.

centripetal
c. nystagmus
c. obesity
c. rub

centrocyte-like cell

centrocytic/mantle-cell lymphoma

centroid
c. frequency
myocardial c.

centromedullary nail

centromere
c. enumeration probe
c. protein

centromeric
immunodeficiency, centromeric instability, facial anomalies syndrome

centronuclear myopathy

centrotemporal
benign partial epilepsy with centrotemporal spike
c. epilepsy
c. sharp wave
c. spike

cepacia
Pseudomonas cepacia bacteremia

cephalad direction

cephalalgia
histamine c.
orgasmic c.

cephalic
assisted cephalic delivery
benign cephalic histiocytosis
c. delivery
external cephalic version
c. forceps
c. ganglion
c. index
median cephalic vein
c. presentation
c. vasomotor response

cephalin
c. cholesterol antigen
c. flocculation test

cephalin-cholesterol flocculation

cephalocaudad length

cephalocele
occipital c.
oral c.
orbital c.

cephalofacial deformity

cephalohematoma
parietal c.

cephalometric
c. laminagraphy
occlusal cephalometric analysis
c. radiograph

cephalometrics
sella to nasion c.

cephalometry
ultrasonic c.

cephalopelvic
c. disproportion
c. disproportion and fetal distress

cephalopharyngeus
musculus c.

cephalopolysyndactyly
Greig cephalopolysyndactyly syndrome

ceramic
aluminum oxide ceramic coating
aluminum oxide ceramic core
cast glass c.'s
esthetic c.'s
glass c.'s
orthoclase ceramic feldspar
c. or plastic brace
c. reconstruction
c. total hip

ceramide
c. dihexoside
c. trihexoside

ceratocricoideus
musculus c.

ceratoglossus
musculus c.

ceratopharyngeus
musculus c.

cerclage
cable cerclage method
cervical c.
Mann isthmic c.
McDonald cervical c.
c. operation
c. procedure
c. wire fixation
c. wire inserter
c. wire technique

cercle
arc de c.

cereal
applesauce, bananas, and cereal diet
bananas, rice cereal, applesauce, toast diet

cerebellar
acute cerebellar ataxia
alcohol cerebellar degeneration
amyotrophic cerebellar hypoplasia
aniridia, cerebellar ataxia-oligophrenia syndrome
anterior cerebellar notch
anterior-inferior c.
anterior-inferior cerebellar artery
anterior internal cerebellar artery
anteroinferior cerebellar artery
c. ataxia
autosomal dominant cerebellar ataxia
crossed cerebellar diaschisis
decussation of superior cerebellar peduncles
c. function
c. gait
c. gliosis
c. hemisphere
c. hemorrhage
hereditary cerebellar ataxia
c. impairment
c. infarct
late cortical cerebellar atrophy
Marie-Foix-Alajouanine cerebellar atrophy
middle cerebellar peduncle
molecular layer of cerebellar cortex
nonprogressive cerebellar disorder with mental retardation
paraneoplastic cerebellar degeneration
parenchymatous cerebellar degeneration
parietooccipital branch of posterior cerebellar artery
pilocystic cerebellar astrocytoma
posterior inferior cerebellar artery
posteroinferior cerebellar artery
precentral cerebellar vein
c. Purkinje cell
subacute cortical cerebellar degeneration
superficial temporal artery-superior cerebellar artery
superior cerebellar artery
superior cerebellar peduncle
c. vermis hypoplasia, oligophrenia, congenital ataxia, coloboma, hepatic fibrosis

cerebelli
arbor vitae c.
arteria cerebelli superior
arteria superior c.
lingula c.
mediastinum c.
monticulus c.
nodulus c.
nuclei c.
pedunculi c.
pons c.
tentorium cerebelli attachment

cerebelloparenchymal disorder IV

cerebellopontine angle

cerebellum
anterior notch of c.
arborescent white substance of c.
contralateral side of c.
lingula of c.
medullary body of c.
midline c.
pons and c.
tongue of c.
tonsil of c.

cerebral
A1-A5 segments of anterior cerebral artery
c. abscess
c. activity
c. activity of brain
acute cerebral encephalopathy
acute disorder of cerebral circulation
acute focal cerebral ischemia
c. allergen
alternative occipital artery middle cerebral artery
c. amyloid angiopathy
amyloid angiopathy c.
anomalous cerebral artery
anterior cerebral artery
anterior cerebral artery crawling under the skull
anterior cerebral artery plexus
anterior cerebral artery pulsatility index
anterior cerebral vein
anterior-inferior cerebral artery
anterior occipital artery-middle cerebral artery bypass
anterior temporal branch of posterior cerebral artery
c. aqueduct
arterial cerebral circle
c. arteriosclerosis
c. arteriovenous malformation
c. artery
artery of cerebral hemorrhage
c. artery thrombosis
A1 segment of anterior cerebral artery
A2 segment of anterior cerebral artery
Aspergillus cerebral abscess
c. ataxia
ataxic cerebral palsy
c. atherosclerosis
athetoid cerebral palsy
atonic cerebral palsy
c. atrophy
autoregulation of cerebral blood flow
c. autosomal recessive arteriopathy with subcortical infarcts and leukoencephalopathy
c. basilar ischemia
c. blood flow
c. blood flow studies
c. blood flow velocity
c. blood volume/cerebral blood flow ratio
brain damage from cerebral hemorrhage
carotid cerebral arteriography
closed cerebral trauma
c. contusion
c. cortex
c. cortex perfusion rate
delayed cerebral ischemia
delayed cerebral vasoconstriction
desmoplastic cerebral astrocytoma of infancy
drainage of cerebral epidural space
c. edema
electrodes applied over cerebral cortex
electrodes inserted in cerebral cortex
c. electrotherapy
embolic cerebral infarct
c. embolus
extension of cerebral infarct
extent of cerebral lesion
familial cerebral cavernoma
familial idiopathic nonarteriosclerotic cerebral calcification
femoral cerebral catheter

cerebral *(continued)*
c. fluid shunt
c. function monitor
c. gaze paresis
gliosis of cerebral aqueduct
c. glucose oxygen quotient
c. hemianesthesia
c. hemiplegia
hemiplegic form of cerebral palsy
c. hemisphere
c. hemorrhage
hemorrhage, c.
hereditary cerebral hemorrhage with amyloidosis
hereditary cerebral leukodystrophy
c. herniation
high-altitude cerebral edema
higher cerebral dysfunction
hyperdense middle cerebral artery sign
c. hypoxia
idiopathic paroxysmal cerebral dysrhythmia
infantile nuclear cerebral degeneration
c. infarct
c. infarction
c. infection
internal c.
internal cerebral vein
c. irritation
c. ischemia
c. ischemia steal
ischemic cerebral infarction
c. ischemic event
left cerebral hemisphere
left middle cerebral artery
left middle cerebral artery thrombosis
lobar cerebral atrophy
local cerebral blood flow
local cerebral glucose utilization
longitudinal cerebral fissure
c. malaria
malignant middle cerebral artery infarction
c. mantle
mapping of cerebral sulcus
massive cerebral edema
mean cerebral blood flow
medial cerebral surface
medial surface of cerebral hemisphere
meningeal branch of cerebral part of internal carotid artery
mental retardation, cerebral palsy
mental retardation, dysmorphism, cerebral atrophy syndrome
mesencephalic cerebral lymphoma
mesial cerebral structure
c. metabolic function
c. metabolic rate
c. metabolic rate of glucose
c. metabolic rate of lactate
c. metabolic rate of oxygen
c. microangiopathy
microcephaly-calcification of cerebral white matter syndrome
middle cerebral aneurysm
middle cerebral artery bifurcation
middle cerebral artery fenestration
middle cerebral artery infarct
middle cerebral artery occlusion
middle cerebral artery pressure
middle cerebral artery syndrome
middle cerebral artery thrombosis
mild spastic diplegic cerebral palsy
minor cerebral dysfunction
mixed cerebral dominance
mixed cerebral palsy
mixed form cerebral palsy
mixed-type cerebral palsy
molecular layer of cerebral cortex
M2 segment of middle cerebral artery
myelinoclastic diffuse cerebral sclerosis
neonatal cerebral hemorrhage
c. nerve ganglionectomy
nuclear cerebral angiogram
nuclear cerebral angiography
occipital cerebral vein
occipital lobe unilateral cerebral hemisphere lesion
occult cerebral vascular malformation
c., ocular, dental, auricular, skeletal syndrome
opening of cerebral aqueduct
other cerebral palsy
c. pacemaker
c. palsy
c. palsy clinic
paradoxical cerebral embolism
paradoxical cerebral embolus
paraneoplastic cerebral degeneration
parasagittal cerebral injury
parenchymal cerebral hemorrhage
parietal lobe bilateral cerebral hemisphere lesion
parietal lobe unilateral cerebral hemisphere lesion
parietooccipital branch of anterior cerebral artery
parietooccipital branch of posterior cerebral artery
partial anterior cerebral infarct
peduncle c.
perinatal cerebral hemorrhage
plexiform layer of cerebral cortex
primary cerebral non-Hodgkin lymphoma
primary degenerative cerebral disease
prolonged cerebral apnea
c. protective therapy
c. radiation necrosis
c. radionuclide angiography
radionuclide cerebral angiogram
c. rate of glucose metabolism
c. red blood cell volume
regional cerebral blood flow
regional cerebral blood volume
regional cerebral metabolic rate for oxygen
regional cerebral perfusion pressure
retrograde cerebral perfusion
right cerebral hemisphere
right middle cerebral artery thrombosis
c. salt wasting
c. seizure
c. shunt
c. sign
silent cerebral infarct
silent cerebral infarction
c. sinusography
sporadic cerebral amyloid angiopathy
stellate cell of cerebral cortex
stroke due to cerebral hemorrhage
c. subarachnoid venous pressure
superficial occipital artery to middle cerebral artery
superficial temporal artery-middle cerebral artery
superficial temporal artery-posterior cerebral artery
superior margin of cerebral hemisphere
symmetrical calcification of basal cerebral ganglion
c. tabes
c. tetany

thromboembolic cerebral vascular accident
c. tissue perfusion pressure
total cerebral blood flow
total cerebral ischemia
transient cerebral ischemic episode
c. transit time
c. trauma
c. tumor
two cerebral hemisphere vegetal hemisphere
c. vascular profile study
c. vasculitis
c. vasculopathy
c. vasospasm
c. vein thrombosis
c. venous malformation
c. venous sinus thrombosis
ventricle of cerebral hemisphere
c. ventriculography
white matter lesion c.
X-linked cerebral ataxia
c. yokes of bone of cranium

cerebri
anus c.
apophysis c.
appendix c.
aqueductus c.
arteria cerebri anterior
arteria cerebri media
arteria cerebri posterior
astrocytosis c.
falx c.
gyri c.
c. hernia
hypophysis c.
mediastinum c.
membrana c.
pars anterior pedunculi c.
pedunculus c.
pseudotumor c.
pseudotumor cerebri syndrome
tinnitus c.

cerebriform intradermal nevus

cerebritis
lupus c.
suppurative c.

cerebrobuccal connective

cerebrocostomandibular syndrome

cerebrofacioarticular syndrome

cerebrohepatorenal syndrome

cerebromacular degeneration

cerebroocular
c. dysgenesis
c. dysplasia-muscular dystrophy

cerebrooculofacial-skeletal syndrome

cerebrooculomuscular syndrome

cerebroosteonephrodysplasia

cerebrospinal
acute cerebrospinal meningitis
c. fluid
c. fluid glucose
c. fluid hypotension
c. fluid immunofixation electrophoresis
c. fluid leak
c. fluid pressure
c. fluid volume
c. fluid–Wassermann reaction
c. ganglion
lumbar cerebrospinal fluid catheter
c. meningitis
Orbis-Sigma cerebrospinal fluid shunt valve
palliative cerebrospinal shunt procedure
perioptic cerebrospinal fluid
c. pressure
radial immunodiffusion cerebrospinal fluid
subarachnoid cerebrospinal fluid
ventricular cerebrospinal fluid

cerebrospinalis
liquor c.

cerebrotendinous xanthomatosis

cerebrovascular
c. accident
c. accident dementia
acute cerebrovascular accident
c. aneurysmal clip
chronic cerebrovascular disease
c. disease
estimated cerebrovascular resistance
c. evaluation
c. event
c. incident
c. infarction
c. insufficiency
ischemic cerebrovascular headache
ischemic thrombotic cerebrovascular disease
neonatal cerebrovascular accident
c. obstructive disease
occlusive cerebrovascular disease
occlusive cerebrovascular insult
c. profile
c. reactivity
c. reserve capacity
c. resistance
right cerebrovascular accident
c. thrombosis

cerebroventricular hemorrhage

cerebrum
anterior ramus of lateral sulcus of c.
aqueduct of c.
arcuate fiber of c.
arterial circle of c.
ascending ramus of lateral sulcus of c.
cistern of lateral fossa of c.
convolution of c.
great transverse fissure of c.
lobe of c.
longitudinal fissure of c.
peduncle of c.

Cerenkov radiation

cerevisiae
anti-*Saccharomyces cerevisiae* antibody

ceroid
juvenile-onset neuronal ceroid lipofuscinosis
late infantile neural ceroid lipofuscinosis
lipofuscinosis
neural ceroid lipofuscinosis
neuronal ceroid lipofuscinosis
neuronal ceroid lipofuscinosis curvilinear body

certain
intolerance to certain foods

certificate
c. of disability for discharge
hospital birth c.
c. of incompetency
c. of need

certification
operator c.
preadmission c.
c. of terminal illness

certified
c. addictionologist
board c.
board certified psychiatrist
c. cell line
c. distinct part
C. Hospital Admission Program
c. for Medicare
c. nurse-midwife

certified *(continued)*
oncology certified nurse
c. raw milk
c. skilled nursing facility
c. sleep-disorder facility
c. social worker

CERULO

cerumen
attachable cerumen loop
c. curette
impacted c.
c. impaction
inspissated c.

ceruminal impaction

cervi
anterior tubercle of c.
c. coaxial

cervical
c. abortion
acute central cervical spinal cord injury
acute cervical traumatic sprain or syndrome
advanced squamous cell cervical carcinoma
airway, breathing, circulation, cervical spine, and consciousness level
alertness, airway, breathing, circulation, and cervical spine
angular tract of cervical fascia
anterior cervical approach to cervicothoracic junction
anterior cervical body fusion
anterior cervical chain adenopathy
anterior cervical cord syndrome
anterior cervical discectomy and fusion
anterior cervical diskectomy
anterior cervical diskectomy and fusion
anterior cervical fascia
anterior cervical fusion
anterior cervical intertransverse muscle
anterior cervical lip
anterior cervical plate
anterior cervical plate fixation system
anterior cervical surgery vocal cord damage
anterior deep cervical lymph node
anterior lower cervical spine surgery
anterior ramus of cervical nerve
anterior superficial cervical lymph node
anterior tubercle of cervical vertebrae
ascending branch of superficial cervical artery
ascending cervical artery
bilateral percutaneous cervical cordotomy
c. biopsy
c. canal stenosis
caustic strictures of cervical esophagus
central cervical spinal cord syndrome
c. cerclage
c., skull, and shoulder block
c., thoracic, and lumbar
c. cockscomb
c. collar
colposcopic grading of cervical dysplasia
c. cone biopsy
c. conization
c. cord injury
c. curettage
c. disc compression
c. disc decompression
c. disc disease
c. discectomy
c. disc herniation
c. disc syndrome
dorsal root, c.
c. dysplasia
c. dystonia
c. ectopic pregnancy
c. epidural steroid injection
c. epithelial neoplasia
flexion-extension control cervical orthosis
four-poster cervical brace
four-poster cervical orthosis
c. friability
full cervical spine
c. ganglion of uterus
c. goiter
headache secondary to cervical spinal disease
c. heart
herniated cervical disc
high risk of developing cervical cancer
home cervical traction unit
human cervical carcinoma cell
c. immobilization device
c. incision
c. incompetence
incompetent cervical os
c. infection
inferior cervical ganglion
c. insertion of radium
intermittent cervical traction
internal cervical device
internal cervical os
c. intraepithelial neoplasia, grade 1–3
invasive cervical cancer
invasive cervical carcinoma
c. invasive neoplasia
c. laminectomy
lateral cervical nucleus
c. line
locally advanced cervical carcinoma
loop diathermy cervical conization
c. lordotic curvature
low cervical approach
low cervical transverse
low cervical transverse cesarean section
lower cervical cesarean section
lower cervical spine fusion
lower cervical spine posterior stabilization
low cervical vertical incision
c. magnetic resonance phlebography
manual cervical traction
McDonald cervical cerclage
mechanical cervical dilator
c. mediastinal exploration
microglandular cervical hyperplasia
microinvasive cervical cancer
midcycle cervical mucus
middle cardiac cervical nerve
middle cervical cardiac nerve
middle cervical fascia
middle cervical ganglion
middle cervical peduncle
c. motion tenderness
c. mucous basal body temperature
c. mucous extract
c. mucous plug
c. mucous solution
c. mucus
c. mucus penetration test
c. myelography
c. nerves 1–8
Neurosurgical C. Spine Scale
noninvasive cervical cancer
odontogenic cervical necrotizing fasciitis

open double-decked hook cervical system
c. orthosis
c. os
osseous cervical spine injury
palmate fold of cervical canal
c. Pantopaque column
periodic fever, aphthous stomatitis, pharyngitis, cervical adenitis
portable cervical spine
c. portio
posterior c.
posterior cervical nodes
precancerous cervical growth
c. priming
c. probe
c. range of motion
c. range-of-motion instrument
rheumatoid cervical myelopathy
rigid cervical immobilization
c. ripening
c. scraper
c. skull pillow
c. somatosensory evoked potential
c. spine
c. spine injury
c. spine screw-plate fixation
c. spondylotic myelopathy
spontaneous cervical artery dissection
stable cervical spine injury
static cervical traction
c. stimulation
superficial branch of transverse cervical artery
c. tabes
c. tension myositis
c. and thoracic vertebrae
c. traction
urethral and cervical cultures
vaginal cervical endocervical smear
c. venous hum
c. vent-dependent quadriplegic
c. vertebra

cervicitis
granulomatous c.
mucopurulent c.
nongonococcal c.

cervicobrachial syndrome

cervicofacial face lift

cervicogenic headache

cervicoocular reflex

cervicooculoacusticus syndrome

cervicoprecordial maneuver

cervicothoracic
anterior cervical approach to cervicothoracic junction
anterior cervicothoracic junction surgery
azoospermia, renal anomaly, cervicothoracic spine dysplasia
c. ganglion
müllerian duct, unilateral renal agenesis, and anomalies of the cervicothoracic somites
müllerian, renal, cervicothoracic, somite abnormalities
müllerian, renal, cervicothoracic, somite abnormalities syndrome
c. orthosis

cervicouterine ganglion

cervicovaginal
c. antibody
c. fluid
c. hood

cervigram test

cervix
anterior lip of the c.
cancer of c.
cleft of c.
cockscomb appearance of c.
conglutination of c.
conization of c.
dilation of c.
effacement of c.
extirpation of uterus and c.
fishmouth c.
Gram stain of c.
c. granular
c. grasped
intraepithelial carcinoma of c.
lip of c.
long, closed, posterior c.
c. long, thick and closed
malignant tumor of c.
membrane of cervix uterus
neck of c.
polyp of c.
squamous carcinoma of c.
c. unripe

cesarean
c. birth
classic cesarean section
dehiscence of cesarean section scar
c. delivery
expected delivery, c.
c. hysterectomy
intrauterine pregnancy, term birth, cesarean section
low cervical transverse cesarean section
lower cervical cesarean section
lower segment c.
lower uterine segment transverse cesarean section
low flap cesarean section
low transverse c.
low vertical cesarean section
postmortem cesarean delivery
primary cesarean section
repeat low transverse cesarean section
c. section
vaginal birth after cesarean section
vaginal delivery after c.

cesium
c. implant
c. insertion
intracavitary cesium therapy
c. iodide
c. irradiation
radioactive c.

cessation
abrupt c.
c. of activity
habit c.
intermittent c.
c. of menstrual cycle
periodic cessation of breathing
smoking c.
time interval between cessation of contraception and conception

Cestan-Chenais syndrome

Chaco virus

Chaddock reflex

Chagres virus

chagrin
peau de c.

chain
allele-specific polymerase chain reaction
alpha chain disease
amplification refractory mutation system-polymerase chain reaction
amyloid light c.
animo-terminal portion of heavy chain of immunoglobulin
anterior cervical chain adenopathy
arbitrarily-primed polymerase chain reaction
arbitrary-primed polymerase chain reaction

chain *(continued)*
BCR-ABL multiplex reverse transcriptase polymerase chain reaction assay
closed kinetic c.
closed kinetic chain exercise
competitive polymerase chain reaction
competitive reverse transcription-polymerase chain reaction
constant domain of H c.
constant domain of L c.
c. of fetal hemoglobin
free monoclonal urinary light c.
gamma chain disease
gamma light c.
Gram-positive cocci in pairs and c.'s
heavy c.
heavy chain of immunoglobulin A
heavy chain of immunoglobulin D
heavy chain of immunoglobulin E
heavy chain of immunoglobulin G
heavy chain of immunoglobulin M
c. of hemoglobin
hemoglobin B c.
hemoglobin delta c.
hemoglobin gamma chain A
hemoglobin gamma chain G
c. initiating
kappa light c.
light chain deposition disease
light chain isotype suppression
light chain paraprotein
light chain of protein molecules
limiting dilution polymerase chain reaction
Markov chain Monte Carlo technique
mitochondrial respiratory chain defect
mitochondrial respiratory chain enzyme
mitochondrial respiratory chain enzyme complex
monoclonal free light c.
mu-heavy chain disease
multiple marker reverse transcriptase-polymerase chain reaction assay
multiplex polymerase chain reaction
myosin heavy c.
myosin light c.
nascent protein c.
nuclear chain fiber
open chain compound
open kinetic chain exercises
ossicular chain reconstruction
pairs and c.'s
paratracheal node c.
polymerase chain reaction analysis of prostate-specific antigen
polymerase chain reaction-restriction fragment length polymorphism
polymerase chain reaction–single-strand conformation polymorphism
polymerase chain reaction in situ hybridization
quantitative competitive polymerase chain reaction
repetitive extragenic palindromic polymerase chain reaction
reverse transcriptase polymerase chain reaction
ribonucleic acid-polymerase chain reaction
side chain in amino acid formula
in situ polymerase chain reaction
total ossicular chain replacement prosthesis
variable domain of heavy chain immunoglobulin
variable domain of light chain immunoglobulin
very long chain acyl-CoA dehydrogenase
very long chain fatty acid

2-chain urokinase plasminogen activator

chair
aerobic chair exercises
barber chair position
beach chair position
bed to chair transfer
computer-driven rotatory c.
dynamic integrated stabilization c.
geriatric c.
invalid c.
c. lift
patient up in c.
reclining c.
c. sit-up exercise

chairback
c. lumbosacral orthosis
c. type brace

chair-performance
Western Ontario and McMaster Universities Osteoarthritis Index Physical Functioning subscale and c.-p.

chalky
c. bones
c. gout

challenge
acid challenge test
allergen inhalation challenge test
allergen specific nasal c.
bronchial provocation c.
carbachol inhalation c.
clomiphene citrate challenge test
cold air c.
double-blind placebo-controlled food c.
histamine c.
histamine challenge test
methacholine bronchoprovocation c.
methacholine challenge test
methacholine inhalation c.
methacholine inhalation challenge response
methylphenidate challenge test
nasal allergen c.
nasal antigen challenge test
oral glucose challenge test
placebo-controlled oral challenge testing
progesterone challenge test
progestin challenge test
quantitative inhalation challenge apparatus
segmental antigen c.
c. virus strain

chamber
aerosol treatment c.
air c.
air bubble instilled in anterior c.
angle of anterior c.
anterior c.
anterior chamber angle
anterior chamber aspiration
anterior chamber cannula
anterior chamber cleavage syndrome
anterior chamber diameter
anterior chamber dysgenesis syndrome

anterior chamber of eye
anterior chamber of eyeball
anterior chamber hyphema
anterior chamber inflammation
anterior chamber intraocular lens
anterior chamber irrigated with saline
anterior chamber lymphoma
anterior chamber paracentesis
anterior chamber reaction
anterior chamber reformation
anterior chamber shallowing
anterior chamber sinus
anterior chamber tap
anterior chamber trabecula
anterior chamber tube
anterior chamber washout
antropyloroduodenal common c.
aqueous c.
axial wall of pulp c.
bubble chamber equipment
closed urinary drainage bag with drip c.
dual c.
dual chamber pacemaker implantation
end-diastolic chamber stiffness
heart pumping c.
hyperbaric oxygen c.
lower chamber of heart
middle chamber bubbling
moderately narrow anterior chamber angle
moderately wide open anterior chamber angle
multiwire proportional c.
parallel-plate flow c.
plasma clot diffusion c.
posterior c.
posterior chamber of eye
posterior chamber intraocular lens
posterior chamber lens implant
pulp c.
c. rupture
transsclerally sutured posterior chamber lens
upper chamber of heart
valved holding c.
very narrow anterior chamber angle
walk-in high-pressure c.
wide open anterior chamber angle
Wilson cloud c.

2-chamber
apical 2-c.

chamfer
c. bevel
c. cut
c. cut jig
c. preparation

chamfered cylinder acetabular component

Champion Trauma Score

chancre
mixed c.
monorecidive c.
mucous membrane c.
Nisbet c.

chancroid
mucous membrane c.
serpiginous c.

Chandipura virus

Chang
C. conjunctiva cell
C. liver cell

change
abrupt change in vision
abrupt mood c.
c. in activity
acute change clinical score
acute change in mental status
Adolescent Life C. Event Questionnaire
adolescent sexual c.
age-associated degenerative c.
agent of c.
C. Agent Questionnaire
age-related brain c.
age-related pharmacodynamic c.
age-related pharmacokinetic c.
air changes per hour
anoxic changes in brain
c. in appetite
arterial occlusive c.
arteriovenous crossing c.'s
arthritic talonavicular c.
asymmetrical signal c.
attritional pattern c.
benign cellular c.
biochemical change in brain
c. in bladder habit
c. in bladder pattern
c. in bowel habit
c. in bowel pattern
burn dressing c.
cannabis-induced mental c.'s
cardiac pacemaker battery c.
central counter-adaptive c.
Clinical Global Impression of C.
c. in cognition
cognitive change of body image
cognitive and motor c.'s
color change of skin
c. in color and consistency of stool
c. in color of pupil
complete change of drapes, gowns and instruments
degenerative arthritic c.
degenerative bone c.
c. description master
disorientation and personality c.
dressing c.
erosive prephloric c.
Family Inventory of Life Events and C.'s
focal inflammatory mucosal c.
fractional area c.
c. in gait
c. in gait and posture
c. in heart rate
c. in heart rhythm
hyaline fatty c.
hydrocephalus ex vacuo c.
hyperplastic-like mucosal c.
hypoxic change in brain
interstitial c.
interstitial fibrotic c.
irritability, depression and personality c.'s
c. in judgment
large cell c.
large magnitude voluntary heart rate c.'s
least significant c.
life change unit
life cycle c.
light-induced absorbance c.
lumbosacral skin pigment c.
lytic blastic c.'s
making change test
maladaptive behavioral c.
malignancy-associated c.
marked degenerative change of hip
mental status c.
minimal c.
minimal change idiopathic nephrotic syndrome
minimal change lesion
minimal change nephropathy
minimal change nephrotic syndrome
minimal glomerular c.

change *(continued)*
mitral valve prolapse, aortic anomalies, skeletal changes, and skin changes syndrome
myxoid degenerative c.
neuromuscular gait pattern c.
newly emergent categorical c.
no c.
no acute c.
no appreciable c.
no essential c.
nonspecific climatic c.
nonspecific ST c.
nonspecific ST-T wave c.
nonspecific ST wave segment changes on electroencephalogram
normal hypertrophic c.'s
no significant c.
no significant change from previous tracing
oil drop c.
onion bulb c.
organic brain c.'s
ovarian cycle c.
pancreatic ductal morphological c.
Paneth cell-like c.
papillary apocrine c.
Patterns of Individual C. Scale
personality change disorder
physical change in brain
c. of plaster
pleural inflammatory c.
polyneuropathy, organomegaly, endocrinopathy, monoclonal gammopathy, and skin changes syndrome
polyneuropathy, organomegaly, endocrinopathy, M protein, and skin changes syndrome
post ovulation hormone c.
profound change in affect
profound change in behavior
radical behavior c.
rate change induced
Readiness to C. questionnaire
schedule c.
severe atheromatous change of aorta
c. in sexual habit
c. of shift
sleep stage change frequency
some appreciable c.
c. in space and time
spondylar c.'s, nasal anomaly, striated metaphyses
structural change in heart
structural changes in joint
ST-T wave c.
tenderness, asymmetry, restricted motion, and tissue texture c.'s
therapeutic lifestyle c.
tissue texture changes, asymmetry, restriction of motion, tenderness
Totman C. Index
c. in urine flow from constipation
vascular c.
venous stasis c.'s
voice change from antihistamine
widespread anoxic c.

Changuinola virus

channel
apical iodide c.
aquaporin-2 water c.
calcium channel agonist
calcium channel antagonist
calcium channel blocker
c. catfish reovirus
diversion of drugs from illicit medical c.'s
c. down
epithelial sodium c.
c. 3 Holter monitor
L-type calcium c.
Malone antegrade continent enema c.
Mitrofanoff catheterizable c.
narrow spinal c.
nondihydropyridine calcium channel blocker
pancreatic duct-choledochus c.
pancreaticobiliary common c.
parallel channel sign
propagated sensation along the c.
pyloric channel ulcer
ren mai c.
slow channel blocker
voltage-dependent anion c.
voltage-dependent calcium c.
voltage-gated calcium c.
voltage-sensitive calcium c.

channel-forming integral protein

Chan wrist rest

chaos
mathematical c.
organizational c.
c. theory

chaotic
c. activity of ventricular fibrillation
atrial chaotic tachycardia
c. atrial tachycardia
c. electrical activity
c. eye movement
c. heart
c. heart rhythm
c. rhythm

chaperone
molecular c.

chapped
itchy or chapped skin

character
anal c.
anal-aggressive c.
authoritarian c.
c., onset, location, duration, exacerbation, remission
compound c.
c. disorder
c. education inquiry
emotionally unstable character disorder
masochistic c.
masochistic character defense
mendelian c.
narcissistic c.
narcissistic character structure
national c.
obsessional c.
optical character recognition
oral c.
out of c.
paranoiac c.
pathologic character formation

characteristic
associated imaging c.
brachydactyly, mesomelia, mental retardation, aortic dilation, mitral valve prolapse, characteristic facies syndrome
child behavior c.
codominant c.
electrooptical c.
c. frequency
c. inflammatory reaction
mental retardation, mitral valve prolapse, characteristic face syndrome
parental environment c.
receiver operating c.
receiver operating characteristic curve
relative operating c.
secondary sex c.
c. of seizure abnormality
specific c.
Summary of Product C.'s

characterized
electrolyte steroid-produced cardiopathy characterized by hyalinization

charcoal
activated c.
c. blood medium culture
buffered charcoal yeast extract
dextran c.
dextran-coated c.
c. hemoperfusion
mitomycin adsorbed onto activated c.
multidose activated c.
protein A immobilized in collodion c.
repeated oral doses of activated c.
c. viral transport medium
c. yeast extract medium

Charcot
C. arthritis
C. arthropathy
C. gait
C. joint
C. restraint orthotic walker
C. sign

Charcot-Leyden crystal

Charcot-Marie-Tooth
C.-M.-T. atrophy
C.-M.-T. disease/syndrome
C.-M.-T. syndrome, X-linked type II with deafness and mental retardation

charge
electric c.
electric charge density
elementary c.
ionic charge number
ligand-to-metal charge transfer
metal-to-ligand charge transfer
c. nurse
ratio of electron charge to mass
urine net c.
zero point of c.

charge-coupled device

charged
low-energy charged particle

Charles Bonnet syndrome

Charleville virus

Charlevoix-Saguenay
autosomal recessive spastic ataxia of C.-S.

charley horse

Charlson comorbidity index

chart
abridged ocular c.
A point c.
astigmatic dial c.
autobiographical life c.
basal temperature c.
blood temperature c.
computer screen c.
Lund-Browder chart for burn estimation
c. not available
Pelli-Robson contrast sensitivity c.
Pelli-Robson letter c.
Progress Assessment C. of Social and Personal Development
Reuss color c.
Snellen eye c.

charting
problem-oriented system of c.

char-zone depth

chase
peripheral bolus c.

chaser
ambulance c.

chat
cri du c.
cri du chat syndrome

chauffeur's fracture

check
Adjective C. List
c. bit
bladder tumor c.
Depression Adjective C. List
c. doctor's order
c. film
c. glaucoma
head c.
Health C. Test
medial check ligament of eyeball
Multiple Affect Adjective C. List
neurologic c.
neurovascular c.
Occupational Check List
c. out
Personality Adjective C. List
quantitative insulin sensitivity check index
Reality C. Survey
Rotterdam Symptom C. List
Sales Attitude C. List
symptom distress check list
c. valve

checkerboard analysis

Checklist-90

checklist
Achievement C.
C. of Adaptive Living Skills
Alternative Lifestyle C.
asthma symptom c.
Behavior Problem C.
Camelot Behavioral C.
C. for Child Abuse Evaluation
Child Behavior C.
Children's Coping Strategies C.
Depressive Adjective C.
Developing Skills C.
Everyday Problem C.
Fatigue Symptom C.
Illness Behavior C.
Jesness Behavior C.
life events c.
Life Experiences C.
Low Back Pain Symptom C.
Mooney Problem C.
Ottawa School Behavior C.
Pediatric Symptom C.
Personal Problems C. for Adolescents
Psychodevelopment C.
Revised Memory and Behavior Problems C.
Suicide-Depression Proneness C.
Symptoms C. 90 Revised
Time-Sample Behavioral C.
Trauma Symptom C. for Children
Wing Autistic Disorder Interview C.

Checklist-II
Gordon Occupational C.-II

Checklist-Revised
Maastricht History and Advice C.-R.

checkup
multiphasic health c.

check-up x-ray

check-valve sheath

Chédiak-Higashi syndrome

cheek
anterior cheek electrode
c. biting from anxiety
c. clamp
cracked mouth corners from sagging c.
facial implant of c.
c. implant
lower cheek flap
malar cheek pad
maxillectomy cheek flap

cheek *(continued)*
Mustardé rotational cheek flap
numb cheek syndrome
cheeking medication
cheese
Swiss cheese defect
Swiss cheese interventricular septum
cheesy pus
cheilectomy
arthroscopic c.
cheilitis
actinic c.
angular c.
apostematous c.
Miescher cheilitis granulomatosa
Miescher granulomatous c.
migrating c.
pseudomembranous c.
solar c.
Volkmann c.
cheilosis
angular c.
cheirooral syndrome
chelate
metal chelate complex
mixed ligand c.
chelated
gadolinium in chelated form
chelonae
Mycobacterium chelonae abscess
Mycobacterium chelonea infection
chemical
c. ablation
c. abnormality
c. abnormality in brain
c. abortion
activates chemical impulse of brain
adolescent chemical abuse
c. agent
atomic, biological, c.
atomic, biological, chemical warfare
c., bacteriologic, and radiologic warfare
c. and biological warfare
biologic and chemical warfare
c., biological, radiological or nuclear weapons
c., radiological, and biological
coughing from c.
cultural aspect of chemical dependency
c. dependence clinic
c. dependence disorder
c. dependency
c. dependency counselor
c. dependency and mental illness
c. dependency unit
c. detoxification
C. Dictionary On-Line
c. disruption in brain
c. dosimeter
electron spectroscopy for chemical analysis
emergency chemical restraint
c. energy
c. enzyme profile
c. exposure
external chemical messenger
c. face peeling
c. gastritis
c. history
c. hysterectomy
illegal c.
c. imbalance
c. impulse
c. incompatibility
c. indicator of ischemia
infertility from c.
c. injury
c. interaction
c. ionization
c. ionization mass spectrometry
c. knife
liquid chemical germicide
liquid chemical sterilization
mentally ill chemical abuser
multiple chemical sensitivity syndrome
narcotic chemical intoxication
new chemical entity
nuclear, biologic, c.
Obagi chemical peel
occupational exposure to c.'s
ocular chemical burn
optically inactive c.
c. oxygen demand
paramagnetic enhancement accentuation by chemical shift imaging
patient's chemical history
peripheral chemical sympathectomy
c. potential
c. sensitivity syndrome
c. shift imaging
c. shift misregistration artifact
c. shift selective
single c.
skin exposure reduction paste against chemical warfare agent
c. snap pack
c. straitjacket
c. sympathectomy
chemically
c. bound residue
c. defined medium
c. induced dynamic electron polarization
c. modified protein
c. pure
chemical-shift imaging
chemicoparasitic
Miller chemicoparasitic theory
chemiluminescence
electrogenerated c.
enhanced c.
chemiluminescent
c. immunoassay
chemistry
alters brain c.
anomalous serum c.
automated chemistry profile
blood c.
blood chemistry profile
executive 22 chemistry profile
fasting chemistry profile
hospital chemistry profile
irregularity in brain c.
c. panel
random chemistry profile
c. screening batteries I and II
c. screening profile
sequential analysis of twelve chemistry constituents
serum chemistry graft
serum chemistry graph
chemoattractant
lymphocyte chemoattractant activity
lymphocyte chemoattractant factor
monocyte chemoattractant and activity factor
chemoembolization
hepatic artery c.
transarterial c.
transcatheter arterial c.
transcatheter oily c.
chemogram
serum c.
chemokine
cutaneous T-cell attracting c.
growth factor-inducible c.
macrophage-derived c.

nonsyncytium-inducing c.
c. receptor 2, 3, 5
thymus and activation-regulated c.

chemokine-related receptor

chemoprevention
medical c.

chemoprophylaxis
antituberculous c.
course of c.
selective intrapartum c.

chemoradiation
adjuvant c.
adjuvant chemoradiation therapy
marrow-ablative c.
neoadjuvant c.
c. therapy

chemoradiotherapy
concurrent c.

chemoreceptor
carotid chemoreceptor stimulation
deficient transmission c.
macula densa c.
medullary c.
peripheral c.
c. trigger zone

chemoreflex
peripheral chemoreflex loop

chemosensitive
central chemosensitive area

chemosensitivity
tumor chemosensitivity assay

chemosis
orbital c.

chemosurgery
Mohs c.
Mohs fresh tissue chemosurgery technique

chemotactant
neutrophil chemotactant factor

chemotactic
c. activity
basophil chemotactic factor
crystal-induced chemotactic factor
c. difference
eosinophil chemotactic factor of anaphylaxis
eosinophilic chemotactic factor
eosinophilic chemotactic factor-complement
c. factor
c. factor for macrophage
fibroblast chemotactic factor
human macrophage-monocyte chemotactic and activating factor
c. index
c. migration
monocyte chemotactic and activating factor
monocyte chemotactic factor
monocyte-derived neutrophil chemotactic factor
neutrophil chemotactic activity
neutrophil chemotactic deficiency
neutrophil chemotactic peptide
neutrophil chemotactic response
neutrophilic chemotactic factor
polymorphonuclear neutrophil chemotactic factor
relative chemotactic activity

chemotactic-factor inactivator

chemotherapeutic
antineoplastic chemotherapeutic agent
cytotoxic chemotherapeutic agent
c. index

chemotherapy
adjuvant hepatic arterial infusion c.
adjuvant hormonal or chemotherapy treatment
anemia related to c.
anthracycline-based induction c.
antimicrobial agents and c.
AOPE chemotherapy protocol
APO chemotherapy protocol
AT-II-induced intraarterial c.
continuing maintenance c.
continuous infusion c.
course of c.
dose-intensive c.
Einhorn regimen of c.
heated intraoperative intraperitoneal c.
hepatic arterial infusional c.
high-dose c.
high-dose chemotherapy and stem cell rescue
home chemotherapy program
c. immunity
inhalation chemotherapy treatment
intense cycle of high-dose c.
intensive chemotherapy treatment
intensive combination c.
intraarterial c.
intraarterial hepatic c.
intraperitoneal hyperthermic c.
intravenous c.
irradiation and c.
metabolism in intraperitoneal c.
MOPP chemotherapy protocol
MVF chemotherapy protocol
MVT chemotherapy protocol
natural chemotherapy agent
neoadjuvant c.
neuropathy of c.
neurotoxicity of c.
novel form of consolidation c.
optimal dose of c.
PACE chemotherapy protocol
preoperative c.
primary c.
radiation and c.
c. and radiotherapy
sequential combination c.
sequential postremission c.
short course c.
single-agent c.

chemotherapy-induced
c.-i. emesis
c.-i. nausea and emesis
c.-i. neutropenia

chemotherapy-related amenorrhea

chemo wafers implanted

chenopodium
oil of c.

***Chenuda* virus**

cheoplastic teeth

Chernez incision

cherry
oil of cherry laurel
c. red spot

Cherry-Crandall unit

cherry-picking procedure

cherry-red
macular cherry-red spot
opacification cherry-red spot
c.-r. spot myoclonus

cherubic facies

cherubism
gingival fibromatosis, hypertrichosis, cherubism, mental retardation, epilepsy syndrome

Chesapeake
hemoglobin C.

chest
acute chest syndrome
acute sickle chest syndrome
admission chest x-ray
aneroid chest bellows
anterior chest diameter
anterior chest wall flap
anterior chest wall syndrome
anteroposterior chest x-ray
apically directed chest tube

chest *(continued)*
Argyle chest tube
arm girth, chest depth, and hip width
c. bellows
burning chest discomfort
burning sensation in upper c.
cardiac chest pain
cardiac neural c.
c. circumference
c. clear to auscultation and percussion
c. clear to percussion and auscultation
c. closed in anatomic layers
closed chest cardiac resuscitation
closed chest cardiac massage
closed chest commissurotomy
closed chest massage
closed chest pneumothorax
closed chest thoracostomy
coughing up blood with chest pain
crushed chest injury
crushing chest discomfort
crushing sensation in c.
deep chest therapy
diaphragmatic and chest breathing
diminished chest excursion
c. discomfort
double knee to c.
esophageal chest pain
exertional chest pain
c. expands adequately bilaterally
fluid aspirated from c.
good chest expansion
c. hair
c. heaviness
hematoma of chest wall
high-frequency chest wall compression
high-frequency chest wall oscillation
intact chest muscles
intercostal position for chest lead
knees to c.
c. and left arm
c. and left leg lead in electrocardiography
maximal chest width
modified chest lead
musculoskeletal chest wall pain
neonatal chest disease
no apparent disease seen in c.
nonischemic chest pain
normal chest film
notch chest sign
open chest cardiac massage
open chest cardiac resuscitation
PA chest film
c. pain
c. pain center
pain in chest, jaw, or extremity
c. pain from heart problem
painful burning sensation in c.
c. pain on deep breathing
c. pain on exertion
c. pain radiating to jaw and shoulder
c. pain and tightness
c. pain of unknown etiology
c. pain with hoarseness
paradoxical chest wall motion
passive chest drainage
passive chest expansion
c. percussion and auscultation
c. percussion and postural drainage
c. percussion and vibration
c. physical therapy
c. physician
c. physiotherapy
pleuritic chest pain
c. port
portable chest radiograph
portable chest x-ray
posterior chest tube
precordial chest leads
precordial chest pain
c. precordial lead in electrocardiography
pressure sensation in c.
prolonged chest pain intense
psychogenic chest pain
radiating chest pain
c. radiograph
region of c.
retrosternal chest pain
c. roentgenogram
c. roentgenography
single knee to c.
c. strap
c. stretch exercise
substernal chest pain
sucking chest wound
c. tube
c. tube drainage
c. tube output
c. tube placement
c. tube present in abdomen
tympanicity auscultation of c.
unipolar chest lead
upright chest film
c. wall
c. wall compliance
c. wall stimulation
water seal chest tube
c. x-ray film

chestnut
horse chestnut seed extract

chevron
c. bunionectomy
c. fracture
c. fusion
c. incision
c. marking technique
c. osteotomy
c. osteotomy with rigid screw fixation
c. procedure

chevron-shaped incision

chew
inability to chew or swallow

chewing
c., sucking, swallowing
pain on c.

Cheyne-Stokes
C.-S. breathing
C.-S. respiration

chiaie teeth

Chiari
Marchac and Chiari short scar technique

Chiari-Frommel syndrome

chiasm
cistern of c.
c. of digit of hand
glioma of optic c.
optic c.
optic chiasm compression
optic chiasm disease
optic chiasm tumor

chiasmal
anterior optic chiasmal syndrome
artery of chiasmal region
optic chiasmal lesion
optic and chiasmal neuropathy
optic chiasmal syndrome

chichiko dyspepsia

chick
c. embryo
c. embryo extract
c. embryo fibroblast
c. embryo kidney
embryonic chick muscle
c. embryo origin
C. Embryotoxicity Screening Test
c. infective dose

purified chick embryo cell culture
rabies vaccine, purified chick embryo cell culture
c. syncytial virus

chick-cell
c.-c. agglutination
c.-c. agglutination unit

chicken
c. ovalbumin
c. ovalbumin upstream promoter
c. red blood cell

chicken-embryo-lethal orphan

chickenpox
c. scar
varicella chickenpox vaccine

Chick-Martin coefficient

Chido antibody

chief
autonomous parathyroid chief cell proliferation
c. complaint
history of chief complaint
parathyroid chief cell

***Chikungunya* virus**

chilblain
necrotized c.

child
c. abandonment
c. abuse
c. abuse and neglect
c. abuser
acquired immune deficiency syndrome infected c.
c. and adolescent burden assessment
C. and Adolescent Functional Assessment Scale
C. and Adolescent Psychiatric Assessment
c. and adolescent psychoanalysis
adult child of alcoholic
adult child of dysfunctional family
c. advocate
c. of alcoholic
battered child syndrome
c. behavioral study
c. behavior characteristic
C. Behavior Checklist
c. behavior rating form
Brief Psychiatric Rating Scale for Children
cardiorespiratory syndrome of obesity in c.
c. care clinic
c. centered interaction
Checklist for C. Abuse Evaluation
chronic child abuse
classroom behavior of c.
Dennis Test of C. Development
c. development clinic
disabled adult c.
Down syndrome c.
c. endangerment
Eyberg C. Behavior Inventory
fatal child abuse
father of c.
female c.
full-term living female c.
full-term living male c.
Gesell C. Development Age Scale
growth hormone-deficient c.
C. Health Assessment Program
C. Health and Illness Profile, Adolescent Edition
c. health questionnaire
immature dead female c.
immature dead male c.
immature living female c.
immature living male c.
inappropriate child behavior
c. inattentive
inner child issue
Integrated C. Development Scheme
living female c.
living male c.
male c.
maternal and child health
maternal and child health care
maternal and child health service
Methods for the Epidemiology of C. and Adolescent Disorders T score
Methods for Epidemiology of C. and Adolescent Mental Disorders
Minnesota C. Development Inventory
modified Child technique
c. molester
mother of c.
National Center for C. Abuse and Neglect
c. neglect
neglect of c.
c. neurology
C. Neuropsychological Questionnaire
c. nutrition
only c.
out of wedlock and not keeping c.
parent to c.
Parent Perception of C. Profile
C. Personality Scale
premature dead female c.
premature dead male c.
premature living female c.
premature living male c.
c. prodigy
c. protection team
C. Protective Services
c. psychiatrist
c. psychiatry
c. psychology
c. quick to anger
c. restraint
Reynolds C. Depression Scale
Screen for C. Anxiety-Related Emotional Disorders
sexual abuse of c.
C. Sexual Behavior Inventory
c. speech impaired
c. of substance abuser
suspected child abuse or neglect
term birth, living c.
white c.
white female living c.
white male living c.
youngest living c.

child-adult mist

childbirth
after childbirth incontinence
c. amnesia
back pain after c.
hair loss from c.
c. injury
Inventory of Functional Status After C.
male impotence after c.
natural c.
c. organic psychosis
prepared c.
psychosis in c.
c. without pain

childcare worker

child-centered
c.-c. interaction
c.-c. literary orientation

childhood
c. accidental spiral tibial fracture
adjustment reaction of c.
adverse childhood experience
alternating hemiplegia of c.
c. antisocial behavior

childhood *(continued)*
- c. anxiety disorder
- anxiety disorder of c.
- C. Asthma Management Program
- C. Asthma Questionnaire
- asymmetric periflexural exanthem of c.
- atypical childhood psychosis
- C. Autism Rating Scale
- avoidant disorder of c.
- axial partial childhood cataract
- c. behavioral disorder
- benign childhood epilepsy
- benign focal epilepsy of c.
- c. celiac disease
- chronic bullous disease of c.
- chronic idiopathic arthritides of c.
- chronic nonspecific diarrhea of c.
- complex disorder of c.
- c. dermatomyositis
- c. disease
- c. disintegrative disorder
- disturbance of emotions specific to c.
- early childhood caries
- early childhood education
- emotional disturbance of c.
- gender identity disorder of c.
- granulomatous disease of c.
- C. Health Assessment Questionnaire
- c. history
- hyperkinetic reaction of c.
- hyperkinetic syndrome of c.
- c. immunization
- c. incest
- Indian childhood cirrhosis
- Integrated Management of C. Illness
- Inventory of C. Memories and Imaginings
- localized vulvar pemphigoid of c.
- Memorial Sloan-Kettering staging of childhood lymphoma
- c. migraine headache
- C. Myositis Assessment Scale
- neurobiology of early childhood development
- normal childhood development
- normal childhood diseases
- normal childhood disorders
- oppositional disorder of c.
- orbital childhood tumor
- ordinary disease of c.
- overanxious disorder of c.
- overwhelming childhood experience
- papular acrodermatitis of c.
- permanent childhood hearing impairment
- permanent childhood hearing loss
- c. polycystic kidney disease
- psychosis of c.
- Psychosocial Assessment of C. Experiences
- reaction of c.
- recurring digital fibroma of c.
- c. rheumatic disease
- severe childhood autosomal recessive muscular dystrophy
- c. severity of psychiatric illness
- c. sexual abuse
- c. shyness disorder
- transient erythroblastopenia of c.
- c. trauma questionnaire
- c. tuberculosis
- usual childhood diseases
- usual childhood illnesses
- usual diseases of c.
- c. visceral myopathy

childhood-onset schizophrenia

children
- acute lymphoblastic leukemia in c.
- Adaptive Behavior Inventory for C.
- adults molested as c.
- c. and adults with attention deficit disorder
- C. of Aging Parents
- Aid to Dependent C.
- c. of alcoholics
- c. of alcoholic screen testing
- C. of Alcoholics Screening Test
- Anxiety Disorder Interview for C.
- anxiety rating for c.
- Anxiety Scales for C. and Adults
- Apraxia Profile: A Descriptive Assessment Tool for C.
- Behavioral Assessment Scale for C.
- Brief Psychiatric Rating Scale for C.
- Computerized Diagnostic Interview for C. and Adolescents
- Coping Health Inventory for C.
- Creativity Tests for C.
- Diagnostic Interview for C. and Adolescents-Child Version
- Diagnostic Interview for C. and Adolescents-Parent Version
- Facial Impairment Scales for C.
- full-term deliveries, premature deliveries, abortions, living c.
- Functional Impairment Scale for C. and Adolescents
- Functional Independence Measure for C.
- group treatment for c.
- growth retardation in c.
- Hamburg-Wechsler Intelligence Test for C.
- hormone deficient c.
- c. of incarcerated parents
- individual adult children of alcoholics counseling
- Interview Schedule for C. and Adolescents
- It Scale for Children
- Kaufman Assessment Battery for C.
- living c.
- Methodology for Epidemiology in C. and Adolescents
- Murphy-Meisgeier Type Indicator for C.
- Neurological Examination for C.
- Pain Observation Scale for Young C.
- Pictorial Instrument for C. and Adolescents
- Porch Index of Communicative Abilities in C.
- Preschool Evaluation and Assessment for Children with Handicaps
- Preschool Evaluation and Assessment for C. with Handicaps
- Questionnaire for Identifying C. with Chronic Conditions
- Robert Apperception Test for C.
- Schedule for Affective Disorders and Schizophrenia for School-Age C.
- Screening C. for Related Early Educational Needs
- Service Assessment for C. and Adolescents
- Sheridan Tests for Young Children and Retardates
- Test of Learning Accuracy in C.
- Test of Listening Accuracy in C.
- Trauma Symptom Checklist for C.

treatment and education of autistic and related communications handicapped c.
Values Inventory for C.
Verbal Auditory Screen for C.
Visual Auditory Screen for C.
Wechsler Intelligence for C. Test
C. with Special Health Care Needs
Women, Infants, and Children Program

children's
C. Affective Rating Scale
C. Apperception Test-Human
C. Apperception Test, Supplemental
C. Apperceptive Story-Telling Test
C. Articulation Test
C. Art Project
Assessment of C. Language Comprehension
C. Attention and Adjustment Survey
C. Auditory Verbal Learning Test-2
C. Coma Score
C. Comprehensive Pain Questionnaire
C. Coping Strategies Checklist
crippled children's program
C. Depression Inventory
C. Depression Rating Scale-Revised
C. Depression Scale
C. Embedded Figures Test
C. Global Assessment Scale
C. Health Study
C. Interview for Psychiatric Disorders
C. Inventory of Self-Esteem
C. Manifest Anxiety Scale
c. mat
Missouri Children's Picture Series
Northwestern University C. Perception of Speech Test
C. Orientation and Amnesia Test
C. Perception of Support Inventory
C. Personality Questionnaire
Primary C. Medical Center
C. Psychiatric Rating Scale
Revised C. Depression Scale
Revised C. Manifest Anxiety Scale
C. Self-Concept Scale
c. service
C. Silapap
C. Vaccine Initiative
c. ward
C. Yale-Brown Obsessive Compulsive Scale

child-resistant
c.-r. bottle top
c.-r. container

child-restraint device

Child-Turcotte classification

***Chilibre* virus**

chill
fever and c.'s
c.'s and fever
fever, chills, and sweating
fever, chills, sweating, nausea, vomiting, and diarrhea
c.'s from myocardial infarction
c.'s from shingles
intermittent chills and fever
jaundice, chills and fever
nervous c.
onset of chills and fever
pain and c.'s
shaking c.'s and night sweats
c.'s with hypothermia

chilly
c. ambient temperature
c. sensation

chimeric
anti-CD3 stimulated peripheral blood lymphocytes transduced with a gene encoding a c.

chimerism
all-donor c.
mixed donor-host hematopoietic c.
mixed hematopoietic c.

chimney
bladder chimney procedure

chimpanzee
c. coryza agent
c. coryza agent virus

Chim virus

chin
alloplastic chin augmentation
asymmetric c.
facial implant of c.
head tilt and chin lift maneuver
head tilt with chin tilt
c. implant
c. lift maneuver
ptosis of c.
c. reflex
c. tuck
underdeveloped c.

Chinese
C. cucumber
C. hamster embryo fibroblast
C. hamster lung
C. hamster ovary
integral traditional Chinese medicine
medicine
Organization of Chinese Americans
C. restaurant asthma
C. restaurant syndrome
traditional Chinese herbal remedy
traditional Chinese herbal therapy
traditional Chinese medicine

chink
glottic c.

chip
avulsion chip fracture
bone chip graft
cancellous chip bone graft
corticocancellous chip graft
free-floating bone c.
ice c.
malleolar chip fracture
multiple cancellous chip graft
prostate c.'s
prostatic c.

chiropractic
c. biophysics
Doctor of C.
long axis traction chiropractic table
c. manipulation
c. manipulative reflex technique

chirospinal manipulation

chisel
ASIF c.
Austin Moore c.
binangle c.
box c.
c. fracture
Oratec c.
orthopaedic c.
Partsch c.
periodontal c.

chi-square automatic interaction detection

chi-squared test

Chlamydia
anti-*Chlamydia* antibody test
Chlamydia transport media
Chlamydia from birth control pill

Chlamydia (continued)
Chlamydia infection
LGV strain of *Chlamydia*
C. trachomatis
Chlamydia transport media

chloral
anhydrous c.
c. hydrate

chlorambucil, vinblastine, procarbazine, prednisone, etoposide, vincristine, Adriamycin

chlorhexidine
c. digluconate
c. gluconate

chloride
aluminum chloride solution
ammonium c.
aspiryl c.
barium c.
benzalkonium c.
c. current
cyanogen c.
10% invert sugar in 0.9% sodium chloride saline injection
liquid ethyl c.
manganese chloride contrast medium
mercuric chloride nephrotoxicity
mercury c.
methacholine chloride skin test
methylrosaniline c.
phenylmercuric c.
polyvinyl c.
potassium c.
potassium chloride sustained release tablet
potassium, sodium chloride, and sodium lactate solution
replacement normal saline
sodium chloride, adenine, glucose, mannitol
sodium-potassium-2 chloride cotransporter
succinylcholine c.
thallium c.
tolonium c.
vinyl c.
vinyl chloride monomer
xenon c.
zinc chloride poisoning

chlorine
free available c.
free from c.

chlormerodrin accumulation test

chloroacetate esterase

chloroethylene oxide

chlorohydrin
mustard c.

chloromethyl ketone

chlorophenyl
isopropyl c.
c. red

chlorophyll
bacterial c.

chloroquine
c., pyrimethamine, and sulfisoxazole
c. mustard
c. retinopathy

chlorpheniramine maleate

chlorpropamide-alcohol flushing

choana
primary c.
vomerine crest of c.

choanae
atresia c.
coloboma, heart disease, atresia choanae, retarded growth and retarded development and/or CNS anomalies, genital hypoplasia, and ear anomalies and/or deafness syndrome

choanal
antral choanal polyp
arrhinia, choanal atresia, microphthalmia syndrome
c. stenosis

Chobar Gorge virus

chocolate
c. blood agar
c. cyst
orbital chocolate cyst
pelvic chocolate cyst

chocolate-coated tablet

choice
alternative temporal forced c.
antacid of c.
bowel care of c.
diet of c.
drug of c.
enema of c.
fluid of c.
laxative of c.
multiple choice discrimination test
multiple choice question
Parent's Choice formula
c. reaction
c. reaction time

choking
c. from dentures
c. of optic nerve head

cholangiocarcinoma
intrahepatic c.
peripheral c.

cholangiocellular carcinoma

cholangio-drainage
percutaneous transhepatic c.-d.

cholangiogram
cholecystectomy and operative c.
drip-infusion c.
endoscopic retrograde c.
fine-needle percutaneous c.
fine-needle transhepatic c.
intraoperative c.
intravenous c.
magnetic resonance c.
percutaneous needle c.
percutaneous transhepatic c.
recurrent pyogenic c.
transhepatic c.
T-tube c.

cholangiography
direct percutaneous transhepatitic c.
drip-infusion c.
drip infusion c.
endoscopic retrograde c.
fine-needle transhepatic c.
intraoperative c.
intravenous c.
magnetic resonance c.
nasobiliary drain c.
operative c.
percutaneous hepatobiliary c.
percutaneous transhepatic c.
transhepatic c.

cholangiohepatitis
Oriental c.
recurrent pyogenic c.

cholangiolitic hepatitis

cholangiopancreatogram
endoscopic retrograde c.

cholangiopancreatography
endoscopic retrograde c.
magnetic resonance c.

cholangiopancreatoscopy
mother endoscopic retrograde cholangiopancreatoscopy system
peroral c.

cholangiopathy
AIDS c.
ascending c.

cholangioscopic
percutaneous cholangioscopic lithotomy
percutaneous transhepatic cholangioscopic lithotomy

cholangioscopy
percutaneous transhepatic c.
peroral c.

cholangitis
acute obstructive suppurative c.
acute suppurative c.
chronic nonsuppurative destructive c.
nonsuppurative ascending c.
nonsuppurative destructive c.
primary sclerosing c.

cholecystectomy
internal c.
laparoscopic c.
laparoscopic laser c.
laser laparoscopic c.
minilaparotomy c.
open c.
c. and operative cholangiogram
routine c.

cholecystitis
acalculous c.
acute c.
acute acalculous c.
chronic calculous c.

cholecystoendoprosthesis
endoscopic retrograde c.

cholecystogogic
oral c.

cholecystogram
cholecystokinin-gallbladder c.
double-dose gallbladder c.
oral c.
oral cholecystogram imaging

cholecystographic
oral cholecystographic dye

cholecystography
oral c.

cholecystokinin
c. A
c. B
c. octapeptide
secretin, cholecystokinin, pancreozymin
c. tetrapeptide

cholecystokinin-gallbladder cholecystogram

cholecystokinin-like immunoreactivity

cholecystolithotomy
percutaneous c.
percutaneous transhepatic c.

cholecystoscopy
percutaneous transhepatic c.

cholecystosis
hyperplastic c.

cholecystostomy
percutaneous c.

cholecystotomy
percutaneous cholecystotomy catheter
transpapillary endoscopic c.

choledochocaval anastomosis

choledochoscope
flexible fiberoptic c.
Machida c.

choledochoscopy
operative c.
percutaneous c.

choledochotomy
longitudinal c.

cholera
accessory cholera enterotoxin
Asiatic c.
c. exotoxin
pancreatic c.
pancreatic cholera syndrome
c. toxin
typhoid c.

choleriform
enteritis c.

cholescintigraphy
morphine c.
radionuclide c.

cholestasia
neonatal c.
pericentral c.
progressive familial intrahepatic c.

cholestasis
benign recurrent intrahepatic c.
extrahepatic c.
intrahepatic c.
intrahepatic cholestasis of pregnancy
neonatal c.
neonatal cholestasis workup

cholestatic
chronic cholestatic hepatitis
fibrosing cholestatic hepatitis
c. hepatitis
c. hepatosis of pregnancy
c. jaundice
neonatal cholestatic hepatitis
neonatal cholestatic jaundice
parenteral nutrition-associated c.
c. viral hepatitis

cholesteatoma
attic c.
attical c.
tympani c.

cholesteremic
normal cholesteremic xanthomatosis

cholesteric
c. analysis profile
c. analysis profile test

cholesterol
acid cholesterol ester hydrolase
biliary cholesterol concentration
biliary cholesterol output
c. calcium content
cephalin cholesterol antigen
c. crystal embolization
dietary cholesterol intake
c. ester
c. ester storage disease
free c.
c. granuloma
high blood c.
high cholesterol level
high cholesterol and tocopherol deficient
high cholesterol and tocopherol supplemented
inherited high c.
low c.
low-density lipoprotein c.
low fat and cholesterol diet
multiple cholesterol emboli syndrome
National C. Education guidelines
National C. Education Program
National C. Education Program criteria
National C. Evaluation Program
nonesterified c.
ovarian cholesterol depletion test
c. to phospholipid ratio
renal cholesterol embolization
c. saturated fat index
c. saturation index
serum reserve cholesterol binding capacity
c. stone
total c.
total-blood c.
total plasma c.
umbilical c.

cholesterol-esterifying activity

cholesterol-lecithin flocculation

cholesterol-lowering lipid

cholesteryl ester transfer protein

cholic
total cholic acid

choliformis
mycetism c.

choline
c. acetylase
c. acetyltransferase
c. dehydrogenase
c. glycerophosphatide
high-affinity choline transport
c. kinase
c. oxidase

cholinergic
antimuscarine cholinergic activity
c. innervation of lung
magnocellular cholinergic neuron
muscarinic cholinergic agonist
muscarinic cholinergic blockade
muscarinic cholinergic receptor
muscarinic cholinergic side effect
nicotinic cholinergic receptor
pedunculopontine cholinergic group
peripheral cholinergic activity
c. response

cholinesterase
serum c.
total c.

chondritis
auricular c.
c. intervertebral cartilage
nasal c.

chondrocalcinosis
articular c.

chondrocutaneous
Antia-Buch chondrocutaneous advancement flap

chondrocyte
articular c.
atypical c.
autologous c.
autologous chondrocyte implantation
autologous chondrocyte transplantation
autologous cultured c.

chondrodermatitis
nodular c.

chondrodynia
parasternal c.

chondrodysplasia
c. punctata
rhizomelic chondrodysplasia punctata

chondrodystrophia
c. fetalis
myotonia c.

chondrodystrophic

chondrodystrophy
asphyxiating thoracic c.
asymmetric c.
atypical c.
myotonic c.

chondroectodermal dysplasia

chondroglossus
musculus c.

chondroid
malignant chondroid syringoma

chondroitin
c. sulfate
c. sulfate A

chondroma
joint c.
malignant c.
nasal c.
periosteal c.

chondromalacia
c. fetalis
c. patellae

chondromatosis
Reichel c.
synovial c.

chondromyxoid
ectomesenchymal chondromyxoid tumor

chondromyxoid fibroma

chondropharyngeus
musculus c.

chondroplasty
arthroscopic abrasion c.

chondrosarcoma
extraskeletal myxoid c.
mesenchymal c.
skeletal myxoid c.
synovial c.

chop amputation

Chopart
modified Chopart amputation

chopped
c. meat-glucose-starch medium
c. meat medium

chopper
c. amplifier
Nichamin triple c.
Nichamin vertical c.
nonaspirating ultrasonic phaco chopper tip

chord
multiple c.'s

chorda
anterior canaliculus of chorda tympani
fold of chorda tympani

chordee
penile c.

chordoma
axial c.

chorea
chronic progressive hereditary c.
c. gravidarum
Huntington c.
involuntary movements of c.
oral contraceptive-induced c.

choreatic gait

choreic
c. ataxia
c. athetoid movements
c. insanity

choreiform
adventitious choreiform movement
c. disorder

choreoacanthocytosis
amyotrophic c.

choreoathetoid
peak-dose choreoathetoid dyskinetic movement

choreoathetosis
paroxysmal kinesigenic c.

chorioallantoic membrane

choriocapillaris
c. degeneration
membrana c.

choriocarcinoma

choriogenic gynecomastia

choriomeningitis
lymphatic c.
lymphocytic c.
lymphocytic choriomeningitis virus
lymphocytic choriomeningitis virus encephalitis
lymphocytic choriomeningitis virus group
murine lymphocytic choriomeningitis virus
pseudolymphocytic c.

chorionic
alpha-human chorionic gonadotropin
beta-human chorionic gonadotropin
c. gonadotropic hormone
c. gonadotropin
c. gonadotropin test
c. growth hormone-prolactin
human chorionic follicle-stimulating hormone
human chorionic gonadotropin
human chorionic gonadotropin level
human chorionic gonadotropin test
human chorionic somatotropin
human chorionic thyrotropin
human chorionic somatomammotropin
immunoradioassayable human chorionic somatomammotropin
immunoreactive human chorionic gonadotropin
immunoreactive human chorionic somatomammotropin
luteinizing hormone/human chorionic gonadotropin
mature abnormal chorionic villus
nicked free beta subunit of human chorionic gonadotropin
primate chorionic gonadotropin
c. somatomammotropin
urinary chorionic gonadotropin
c. villi
c. villus biopsy
c. villus infarction
c. villus ischemia
c. villus sampling

chorioretinal
c. degeneration
multifocal chorioretinal disease
peripheral chorioretinal atrophic spot
peripheral chorioretinal atrophy
senile macular chorioretinal degeneration

chorioretinitis
luetic c.
peripheral multifocal c.
toxoplasmosis c.

chorioretinopathy
central serous c.
idiopathic central serous c.
c. and pituitary dysfunction

choristoma
adenohypophysial neuronal c.
limbal c.
middle ear c.
neuromuscular c.
osseous c.
osseous choristoma of the tongue
pituitary adenoma-adenohypophysial neuronal c.

choroid
c. coat of eye
c. fissure
hemangioma of c.
malignant melanoma of c.
neonatal choroid plexus hemorrhage
peripapillary c.
c. plexus carcinoma
c. plexus cyst
c. plexus papilloma

choroidal
anterior choroidal artery
c. blood flow
c. blood volume
central choroidal apposition
circumscribed choroidal hemangioma
c. hemangioma
c. hypertensive disease
idiopathic polypoidal choroidal vasculopathy
lateral posterior c.
malignant choroidal melanoma
medial posterior c.
metastatic choroidal tumor
myopic choroidal atrophy
c. neovascular membrane
peripapillary choroidal arterial system
peripapillary choroidal atrophy
peripheral exudative choroidal hemorrhagic retinopathy
senile choroidal macular degeneration
c. or subretinal neovascularization
c. vasculature

choroidea
arteria c.
arteria choroidea anterior
arteria choroidea posterior

choroiditis
anterior c.
areolar c.
areolar central c.
macular c.
metastatic c.
multifocal c.
mycobacterial c.
nongranulomatous c.
Pneumocystis carinii c.
recurrent c.
tetanus toxoid toxoplasmic c.

choroidopathy
central serous c.
focal macular c.
multifocal and recurrent c.
peripapillary central serous c.
vitreoretinal choroidopathy syndrome

chosen
number of words c.

Christchurch chromosome

Christie-Atkins-Munch-Petersen test

Christmas factor

Christ-Siemens-Touraine syndrome

chromaffin
adrenal chromaffin cell

chromaffinoma
medullary c.

chromatic-type aberration

chromatic vision

chromatid
sister chromatid exchange
sister chromatid exchange rate

chromatin
c. clumps and nucleoli
marginated c.
nonhistone c.
oxyphil c.
sex c.

chromation
nuclear c.

chromatofocusing
high-performance c.

chromatographic
liquid chromatographic assay

chromatographic-fluorometric technique

chromatography
antibody affinity c.
anti-idiotypic affinity c.
capillary column gas c.
centrifugal counter-current c.
denaturing high-performance liquid c.
fibrinogen gel c.
gas c.

chromatography *(continued)*
gas-liquid c.
gas-liquid phase c.
gas-solid c.
gel c.
gel permeation c.
high-performance ion exchange c.
high-performance liquid c.
high-performance membrane c.
high-performance size-exclusion c.
high-pH anion exchange chromatography coupled with pulsed amperometric detection
high-power liquid c.
high-pressure liquid affinity c.
high-resolution c.
high-speed liquid c.
immobilized metal affinity c.
instant thin-layer c.
liquid c.
liquid chromatography coupled to tandem mass spectrometry
liquid chromatography with electrochemical detection
liquid-liquid c.
liquid-solid c.
low-pressure liquid c.
medium pressure liquid c.
micellar electrokinetic c.
micellar electrokinetic capillary c.
molecular exclusion c.
nitrogen-phosphorus detector in gas c.
optical c.
paper c.
precipitation thin-layer c.
radial flow c.
radio-gas c.
reversed phase high-performance liquid c.
reversed-phase liquid c.
serum thyroxine measured by column c.
simulated moving bed c.
size exclusion c.
steric exclusion c.
thin-layer c.
toroidal coil c.
vapor-phase c.

chromhidrosis
apocrine c.

chromic
c. catgut mattress suture
c. gut suture
interrupted chromic suture
c. ligature
mild chromic suture

chromium
c. isotope
c. release test

chromodynamics
quantum c.

chromoendoscopy
Lugol c.

chromogen
Porter-Silber c.
Porter-Silber chromogen test

chromoglycate
disodium c.

chromogranin
c. A
bovine chromogranin A

chromophil
granular chromophil cell

chromophobe
large c.
nongranular clear chromophobe cell
c. renal cell carcinoma

chromoscopy
contrast chromoscopy using indigo carmine
gastric c.

chromosomal
autosomal chromosomal anomaly
c. gonadal dysgenesis
c. instability
c. karyotype
c. marker
c. mediated resistance
nonhistone c.
nonhistone chromosomal protein
c. ribonucleic acid
c. satellite
c. segregation
c. trait

chromosomally
c. competent ovarian failure
c. incompetent ovarian failure
c. mediated resistant *Neisseria gonorrhoeae*

chromosome
absence of sex c.
apolipoprotein E epsilon 4 gene on chromosome 19
arm of c.
autosomal chromosome disorder
bacterial artificial c.
c. banding
Christchurch c.
constitutional chromosome abnormality
deletion of long arm of chromosome X
deletion of short arm of chromosome X
derivative c.
diploid chromosome number
double minute c.
end of short arm of c.
female sex c.
fragile chromosome site
fragile X chromosome
haploid chromosome number
homogeneous staining region of c.
human artificial c.
long arm of c.
long arm of chromosome X
long arm of Y c.
loss of heterozygosity chromosome 10
male sex c.
marker X c.
c. modification site
negatively staining region of c.
nonrandom X chromosome inactivation
normal female sex chromosome type
normal male sex chromosome type
Philadelphia c.
phosphatase and tensin homologue deleted on c.
premature chromosome condensation
presence of only one sex c.
recombinant c.
right X c.
ring chromosome 1–22
satellite c.
short arm of chromosome X
supernumerary marker c.
terminal banding of c.
translocation between 2 X c.
triploid chromosome number
whole chromosome paint
Y chromosome RNA recognition motif
yeast artificial c.

chromosome-mediated gene transfer

chromosome-negative
Philadelphia c.-n.

chromosome-positive
Philadelphia c.-p.

chromotropic acid

chronic

c. abdominal tympany
c. aches and pains
c. actinic dermatitis
active chronic hepatitis
active chronic inflammation
c. active cirrhosis
c. active gastritis
c. active hepatitis B
c. active hepatitis with cirrhosis
c. active liver disease
c. active lupoid hepatitis
c. active viral hepatitis
c. active viral hepatitis, non-A, non-B
c. active viral hepatitis, type B
acute bacterial exacerbation of chronic bronchitis
acute and chronic alcohol ingestion
acute chronic glaucoma
acute and chronic inflammation
acute exacerbation of chronic bronchitis
acute on chronic liver disease
acute on chronic renal failure
acute physiology and chronic health evaluation score
acute renal failure and chronic renal failure
adhesive chronic pachymeningitis
c. adhesive otitis media
adjustment disorder, c.
c. aggressive hepatitis
c. airflow limitation
c. airflow obstruction
c. airway disease
c. airway obstruction
c. alcohol abuse
alcohol acquired chronic hepatocerebral degeneration
c. alcoholic brain syndrome
c. alcoholic cirrhosis
c. alcoholic delirium
c. alcoholic heart muscle disease
c. alcoholic pancreatitis
alcohol-related chronic pancreatitis
c. allograft nephropathy
c. ambulatory peritoneal dialysis
c. amphetamine effect
anemia associated with chronic renal failure
anemia of chronic disease
anemia of chronic renal failure
c. anovulation
c. anovulation syndrome
c. anterior exertional compartment syndrome
c. anterior uveitis
c. antibiotic inhalation
c. antidepressant therapy
c. anxiety state
c. articular rheumatism
c. aspecific respiratory ailment
atrophic chronic autoimmune thyroiditis
atrophic chronic gastritis
c. atrophic gastritis
atypical chronic myeloid leukemia
autoimmune chronic active hepatitis
autoimmune chronic hepatitis
autoimmune-type chronic active hepatitis
c. bacterial prostatitis
B-cell chronic lymphocytic leukemia
B-cell chronic lymphocytic leukemia/small lymphocytic lymphoma
B-cell chronic lymphoproliferative disorder
c. benign hepatitis
c. benign mucous membrane pemphigus
c. benign neutropenia
c. benign pain
c. beryllium disease
c. bile duct ligation
c. blepharitis
c. blood loss
c. bone pain
c. bronchitis
c. bronchitis with asthma
c. bronchitis with emphysema
c. bullous disease of childhood
c. calcific pancreatitis of the tropics
c. calcifying pancreatitis
c. calculous cholecystitis
c. cerebrovascular disease
c. child abuse
c. cholestatic hepatitis
c., acquired, pure red cell aplasia
c., painful arthritis
c. compartment syndrome
c. congestive heart failure
c. constipation with hemorrhoid
c. coronary insufficiency
c. cutaneous lupus erythematosus
c. cystic gastritis
c. cystic infarct
c. daily headache
c. debilitating disease
c. degenerative disease
demyelinated inflammatory chronic polyneuropathy
c. depression
c. depressive personality disorder
c. destructive periodontitis
c. diabetes insipidus
c. diabetic neuropathic pain
c. diffuse interstitial lung disease
c. and dilute variant
c. disabling dermatosis
c. discoid lupus erythematosus
c. disease hospital
c. disordered water balance
c. electrophysiologic study
c. emotional suffering
c. emptiness and boredom
c. enthusiasm disorder
c. eosinophilic leukemia
c. eosinophilic pneumonia
c. Epstein-Barr virus
c. erosive gastritis
c. erythropoietic porphyria
c. esophageal dysphagia
c. factitious illness with physical symptoms
c. false-positive
familial benign chronic pemphigus
c. fatigue immune deficiency syndrome
c. fatigue and immune dysfunction syndrome
c. fecal shedding
c. feelings of deep emptiness
c. gastric ulcer
c. gastritis
c. gastrointestinal tract bleeding
c. glaucoma
c. glomerulonephritis
c. graft vascular disease
c. graft-versus-host disease
c. granulating wound
c. granulocytic leukemia
c. granulomatous disease
c. granulomatous inflammation
c. habit
c. haloperidol
c. headache
c. headache pain
c. health problem
c. heart disease
c. heart failure
c. heel pain syndrome
c. hemodialysis

chronic *(continued)*
c. hemolytic anemia
Hendler Test for C. Pain
c. hepatic encephalopathy
c. hepatitis B
c. hepatitis C
c. hepatitis C infection
hereditary chronic nephritis
c. high blood pressure
c. hydrocephalus
c. hyperplastic sinusitis with nasal polyposis
c. hypersomnia
c. hypertrophic emphysema
c. hypertrophic pachymeningitis
c. hyperventilation syndrome
c. hypoglycemia
c. hypoxia
c. hypoxic lung disease
c. idiopathic anhidrosis
c. idiopathic arthritides of childhood
c. idiopathic intestinal pseudo-obstruction syndrome
c. idiopathic myelofibrosis
c. idiopathic orthostatic hypotension
c. idiopathic urticaria
c. idiopathic xanthomatosis
c. illness
c. immune disorder
c. impotence
c. inactive cirrhosis
c. incontinence
c. or incurable disease
c. infantile hypotonic syndrome
c. infantile neurological, cutaneous, and articular
c. infarct
c. infection
c. infectious neuropathic agent
c. inflammation
c. inflammation of joint
c. inflammatory arthritis
c. inflammatory bowel disease
c. inflammatory cell
c. inflammatory cell infiltration
c. inflammatory demyelinating polyradiculoneuropathy
c. inflammatory demyelinating polyradiculopathy
c. inflammatory disease
c. inflammatory granulomatous process
c. inflammatory hyperplasia
c. inflammatory infiltrate
c. insomnia
c. insomniac
c. instability
c. intense envy
c. intermittent low back pain
c. intermittent peritoneal dialysis
c. interstitial hepatitis
c. interstitial inflammatory infiltrate
c. interstitial lung disease
c. interstitial nephritis
c. interstitial salpingitis
c. intestinal dysmotility
c. intractable benign pain
c. intractable shoulder pain
c. irritation
c. ischemia
c. ischemic colonic lesion caused by phlebosclerosis
c. ischemic heart disease
c. itch-and-scratch syndrome
c. itching syndromes
c. joint pain
juvenile chronic arthritis
juvenile chronic myelocytic leukemia
juvenile chronic myelogenous leukemia
lichenoid chronic dermatosis
c. liver disease
c. liver failure
c. lobular hepatitis
c. long term illness
c. low back strain
c. low intermittent back pain
c. low self-esteem
c. lung disease
c. lymphatic leukemia
c. lymphocytic leukemia
c. lymphocytic leukemia variant
c. lymphocytic thyroiditis
c. lymphoproliferative disorder
c. lymphosarcoma cell leukemia
c. medical illness
Meleney chronic undermining ulcer
c. membranoproliferative glomerulonephritis
c. membranous glomerulonephritis
c. mesenteric ischemia
c. metabolic acidosis
c. middle ear infection
c. migraine headache
mild chronic hepatitis
mild focal chronic inflammatory infiltrate
moderate chronic hepatitis
c. monoblastic leukemia
c. monocytic leukemia
c. motor tic
c. motor or vocal tic disorder
c. mucocutaneous candidiasis
c. mucus-producing cough
c. muscle pain syndrome
c. musculoskeletal pain syndrome
c. myelocytic/myelogenous/myeloid leukemia blast crisis
c. myelocytic/myelogenous/myeloid leukemia chronic phase
c. myelodysplastic syndrome
c. myeloid leukemia
c. myelomacrocytic leukemia
c. myelomonocytic leukemia
myelomonocytic leukemia, c.
c. myeloproliferative disorder
c. narrow-angle glaucoma
National Institutes of Health C. Prostatitis Symptom Index
neonatal chronic idiopathic neutropenia
neonatal chronic lung disease
c. nervous degenerative disease
c. nervous exhaustion
c. nervous exhaustion syndrome
c. neuromuscular disease
c. neutrophilic leukemia
NIH Classification Category II chronic bacterial prostatitis
NIH Classification Category III inflammatory and noninflammatory chronic pelvic pain
non-A–G chronic liver disease
c. nonbacterial prostatitis
non-B, non-C chronic liver disease
non-HIV chronic gingivitis
noninfectious chronic cystitis
nonspecific chronic lymphocytic thyroiditis
c. nonspecific diarrhea
c. nonspecific diarrhea of childhood
nonspecific chronic interstitial pneumonitis
c. nonspecific lung disease
c. nonsuppurative destructive cholangitis
c. nonvalvular atrial fibrillation
nonviral chronic hepatitis
c. obstruction of biliary tract
c. obstructive airway disease
c. obstructive bronchitis
c. obstructive bullous emphysema
c. obstructive lung disease

c. obstructive outflow disease
c. obstructive pulmonary disease
c. obstructive pulmonary emphysema
c. obstructive respiratory disease
c. open-angle glaucoma
c. opioid analgesic therapy
c. oral, facial, head pain
c. organic brain syndrome
c. organic mental syndrome
c. organ rejection
c. orthopedic impairment
c. orthostatic hypotension
otitis media, catarrhal, c.
otitis media, chronic, suppurating
c. otitis media with effusion
c. pain
pain disorder, c.
c. paranoid schizophrenic reaction
c. parathyroidectomy
c. paroxysmal hemicrania
c. passive congestion
patchy chronic inflammatory infiltrate
patient in chronic pain
pauciarticular juvenile chronic arthritis
c. pelvic inflammatory disease
c. pelvic pain
c. pelvic pain syndrome
c. perforating hyperplasia of pulp
c. peripheral arterial disease
persistent chronic hepatitis
c. persistent hepatitis
c. persisting hepatitis
c. phase chronic myelogenous leukemia
Philadelphia chromosome-negative chronic myelogenous leukemia
Philadelphia chromosome-positive chronic myelogenous leukemia
c. pigmental purpura
c. pneumonitis of infancy
c. polyarthritis
polyarticular juvenile chronic arthritis
c. postnasal drip
posttraumatic chronic osteomyelitis
c. posttraumatic headache
c. posttraumatic vertigo
c. primary angle-closure glaucoma
c. primary headache
c. progressive coccidioidal pneumonitis
c. progressive course
c. progressive external ophthalmoplegia
c. progressive headache
c. progressive hereditary chorea
c. and progressive illness
c. progressive multiple sclerosis
prolactin chronic growth hormone
c. proliferative glomerulonephritis
c. prostatitis/pelvic pain syndrome
c. pulmonary insufficiency of prematurity
c. pulmonary interstitial fibrosis
c. pyelonephritis
c. pyrophosphate arthropathy
Questionnaire for Identifying Children with C. Conditions
recurrent chronic depression
recurrent chronic dissecting aneurysm
c. recurrent multifocal osteomyelitis
c. recurring depression
c. relapsing demyelinating inflammatory polyneuropathy
c. relapsing disorder
c. relapsing pancreatitis
c. renal disease
c. renal failure
c. renal insufficiency
c. respiratory failure
c. respiratory insufficiency
C. Respiratory Questionnaire
c. restrictive pulmonary disease
c. rheumatoid arthritis
c. rheumatoid nodular fibrositis
right otitis media, suppurative, c.
scattered chronic inflammatory infiltrate
schizophrenia, chronic undifferentiated type
schizophrenic reaction, chronic, paranoid
schizophrenic reaction, chronic, undifferentiated
c. sensorimotor neuropathy
severe chronic neutropenia
sickle cell chronic lung disease
c. simple glaucoma
c. sleep schedule disturbance
c. slurred speech
c. spinal muscular atrophy
c. stable angina
c. stasis leg ulcer
c. subclinical scurvy
c. subdural hematoma
c. substance abuse
c. superficial gastritis
c. suppurative lung disease
c. suppurative otitis media
c. syphilitic infection
T-cell chronic lymphatic leukemia
c. T-cell leukemia
c. tension and anxiety
c. tension headache
c. thromboembolic pulmonary hypertension
c. thrombotic pulmonary vascular obstruction
c. tic disorder
c. total occlusion
c. transplant nephropathy
c. traumatic encephalopathy
c. ulcerative colitis
c. undifferentiated schizophrenia
c. untreatable condition
c. urinary retention
c. urinary tract infection
c. valvular heart disease
c. venous insufficiency
c. villous arthritis
c. widespread pain
young adult chronic patient

chronic,
c. acquired, pure red cell aplasia
c. painful arthritis

chronically
c. ill
c. infected
c. inflamed airway
c. inflamed gallbladder with stones
c. mentally ill
patient chronically ill

chronicus
lichen chronicus simplex
lichen simplex c.

chronologic
c. age
c. drinking record
postoperative chronologic year

chronological age

chronometry
mental c.

chronotropic
c. exercise assessment protocol
c. incompetence

chronotropism
negative c.

chyle
pericardial chyle with tamponade

chylocele
parasitic c.

chylosus
ascites c.

chylothorax
spontaneous neonatal c.
chylous
c. ascites
gynecological chylous reflux syndrome
c. hydrocele
chymase
mast cell containing both tryptase and c.
mast cell containing tryptase but not c.
chymotrypsin
c. inhibitor activity
c. unit
chymotrypsin-like protein
cicatricial
antiepiligrin cicatricial pemphigoid
c. contraction
drug-induced cicatricial conjunctivitis
c. ocular pemphigoid
cicatrix
cystoid cicatrix of limbus
hypertrophic c.
cicatrization
exuberant c.
cigarette
pack of c.'s
packs per year c.'s
c.'s per day
c. smoke
c. smoke asthma
c. smoke condensate
c. smoker
c. smoke solution
cilia (*pl. of* cilium)
ciliaris
musculus c.
nervus ciliaris brevis
nervus ciliaris longus
orbicularis c.
zonula c.
ciliary
c. action
anterior ciliary artery
anterior ciliary vein
c. beat frequency
c. body band
c. dyskinesia activity
c. ganglion
iris ciliary body
long ciliary artery
long ciliary nerve
longitudinal ciliary muscle
long posterior ciliary artery
long posterior ciliary axis
long root of ciliary ganglion
malignant ciliary epithelioma
meridional ciliary muscle fiber
meridional fibers of ciliary muscle
motor root of ciliary ganglion
c. neurotrophic factor
nonpigmented ciliary epithelium
occult annular ciliary body
oculomotor root of ciliary ganglion
c. particle transport
pigmented layer of ciliary body
primary ciliary dyskinesia
ciliary-derived neurotrophic factor receptor
ciliated
c. bronchial epithelium
c. epithelial cell
cilium, pl. **cilia**
dyskinetic cilia syndrome
immotile cilia syndrome
olfactory c.
cincture sensation
cine
axial breath-hold gradient-echo cine magnetic resonance imaging
c. computed tomography
c. densitometric assessment of transit time
high-spatial-resolution cine computed tomography
c. loop recording
c. magnetic resonance imaging
c. MRI
parallel c.
phase-contrast cine magnetic resonance imaging
c. phonation study
c. pulse system
velocity-encoded c.
cineangiography
aortic root c.
axial c.
radionuclide c.
c. and sensitometric ejection fraction
cinereum
artery of tuber c.
medial branch of artery of tuber c.
cingulate
anterior c.
anterior cingulate cortex
anterior cingulate flow
anterior cingulate gyrus
anterior cingulate gyrus tumor
anterior cingulate pathway
anterior cingulate prefrontal syndrome
c. gyrus
marginal branch of cingulate sulcus
c. sulcus
cingulotomy
anterior cingulotomy for treatment of OCD
cinnamon
oil of c.
cipher
numerical cipher method
circadian
c. biological rhythm
c. desynchronization
endogenous circadian pacemaker
endogenous circadian rhythm
endogenous circadian rhythm phase
c. event recorder
c. quotient
c. rhythm
c. rhythm-based sleep disorder
c. rhythm dyssomnia
c. testosterone pattern
circadian-modified floxuridine
circannual cycle
circinate retinopathy
circle
arterial c.
arterial cerebral c.
arterial circle of cerebrum
arterial circle of greater iris
arterial circle of lesser iris
arterial circle of Willis
articular vascular c.
closed circle deoxyribonucleic acid
concentric circle pattern on breast self-examination
c. of confusion
c. of Haller
major arterial circle of iris
minor arterial c.
minor arterial circle of iris
Minsky c.
Pagenstecher c.
Papez c.
presumed circle area ratio

rapid plasma reagin circle card test
T-cell receptor-rearrangement excision c.
c. of Vieussens
c. of Weber
c. of Willis
Zinn c.

circle-diamond
separation of c.-d.

circlet
Zinn c.

circling band

circuit
anesthesia c.
anesthesia breathing c.
application-specific integrated c.
error detection c.
feedback reduction c.
integrated c.
local circuit theory
open circuit method
printed c.
c. resistance training
short circuit current

circuitry
amygdala-fear c.
limbic c.
normal c.

circular
c. amputation
c. anal dilator
c. block anesthesia
c. cast
continuous circular capsulorrhexis
continuous circular inverting suture
c. dichroism
dispersion-induced circular dichroism
c. end-to-end anastomosis
c. hymen
c. incision
induced circular dichroism
c. insanity
c. interaction between anxiety and pain
lower esophageal sphincter circular muscle
magnetic circular dichroism
c. muscle
c. polarization
c. pressure maneuver during massage
c. Santorini muscles
c. stapler
c. stapler donut
c. sulcus of Reil
c. tape
c. tear capsulotomy
c. thinking
c. vesicomyotomy
vibrational circular dichroism
c. wire
c. wire fixator

circulates
heart circulates blood

circulating
c. adhesion molecule
c. anodic antigen
antibody-labeled circulating granulocyte
c. anticoagulant
c. blood lymphocyte
c. blood volume
c. cathodic antigen
central circulating blood volume
effective circulating blood volume
c. granulocyte pool
c. immune complex
lower circulating estrogen level
mean circulating filling pressure
mean circulating time
c. microemboli index
c. monocyte
c. pituitary hormone
c. platelet aggregate
total circulating albumin
total circulating protein

circulation
acute disorder of cerebral c.
airway, breathing, c.
airway, breathing, circulation, cervical spine, and consciousness level
airway, breathing, circulation, differential
airway, breathing, circulation, disability, exposure
airway, breathing, circulation, intravenous crystalloid
alertness, airway, breathing, circulation, and cervical spine
anterior c.
anterior circulation aneurysm
anterior circulation intracranial aneurysm
anterior circulation stroke
c. antineuronal antibody
c., respiration, abdomen, motor, and speech
c., sensation, mobility
decreased hand c.
enterohepatic c.
extracorporeal c.
general c.
general hepatic c.
good peripheral c.
hypothalamohypophysial portal c.
inadequacy of systemic c.
lacunar circulation infarct
lung-to-finger circulation time
c., motor ability, sensation, and swelling
nerves and c.
partial anterior circulation infarct
partial anterior circulation syndrome
peripheral blood c.
persistence of fetal c.
persistent fetal c.
persistent fetal circulation with pulmonary hypertension
poor blood c.
poor circulation in hand
posterior c.
posterior circulation infarct
posterior circulation syndrome
ratio of pulmonary to systemic c.
restoration of spontaneous c.
return of spontaneous c.
c. and sensation
sensation, circulation, motion
c. time
total anomalous pulmonary c.
total anterior circulation infarct
total anterior circulation syndrome
venous blood c.
venous collateral c.
well-developed collateral c.

circulatory
c. arrest
clamminess from circulatory problem
c. compromise
deep hypothermic circulatory arrest
c. embarrassment
external pressure circulatory assistance
hyperdynamic beta-adrenergic c.
hypothermic circulatory arrest
c. hypoxia
mean circulatory hematocrit
nail breaking from circulatory problem
c. overload
peripheral circulatory vasoconstriction

circulatory *(continued)*
postparacentesis circulatory dysfunction
c. problem from diabetes
c. problem with cold sensitivity
profound hypothermic circulatory arrest
profoundly hypothermic circulatory arrest
total circulatory arrest

circulus
artery of circulus arteriosus
major circulus arteriosus of iris
minor circulus arteriosus
minor circulus arteriosus of iris

circumactive
bipolar circumactive probe

circumareolar incision

circumcised
patient not c.

circumdental wire

circumduction
c. gait
McMurray circumduction maneuver

circumference
abdominal c.
arm c.
arm muscle c.
articular circumference of head of radius
articular circumference of head of ulna
chest c.
fetal abdominal c.
frontooccipital c.
head c.
head circumference measurement
left ventricular end-diastolic c.
mean arm muscle c.
midarm c.
midarm muscle c.
middle upper arm c.
occipitofrontal c.
ratio of waist to hip c.
right lung-to-head circumference ratio
thigh c.
thoracic c.
variable circumference suprapatellar socket

circumferential
c. bipolar montage
c. burn
c. clasp
end-diastolic circumferential stress
c. end-systolic stress
c. filing
c. grommet
c. implantation
c. incision
c. invasive carcinoma
loop circumferential wire
multiple benign circumferential skin creases on limb
c. pneumatic compression
c. pneumatic compression suit
sharply demarcated circumferential lesion
c. shortening fraction
c. suture tie
velocity of circumferential fiber shortening
c. wall stress
c. wire
c. wiring

circumflex
anterior circumflex humeral artery
anterior circumflex humeral vein
anterior humeral circumflex artery
c. artery
atrial anastomotic branch of circumflex branch of left coronary artery
atrial circumflex artery
c. branch
c. coronary artery
deep circumflex iliac artery
deep circumflex iliac vein
deep circumflex iliac artery flap
distal portion main c.
intermediate circumflex artery
left circumflex artery
left circumflex coronary artery
left circumflex marginal
marginal branch of left circumflex coronary artery
marginal circumflex artery
medial circumflex artery of thigh
medial circumflex femoral artery
medial circumflex femoral vein
medial femoral circumflex artery
osteomusculocutaneous deep circumflex iliac groin flap
posterior circumflex artery
proximal circumflex artery
superficial branch of medial circumflex femoral artery
superficial circumflex iliac artery
superficial circumflex iliac vein

circumoral
c. area of columnar epithelium
c. incision

circumoval precipitin

circumscribed
c. amnesia
c. atrophy of brain
c. choroidal hemangioma
c. gangrene
c. margin
c. nodule

circumscribing incision

circumscripta
calcinosis cutis c.
melanosis circumscripta precancerosa
myositis ossificans c.
osteoporosis c.
pachyderma c.

circumscription
angiokeratoma c.
monosymptomatic c.

circumscriptum
angiokeratoma c.
exophthalmos, myxedema circumscriptum praetibiale, and osteoarthropathia hypertrophicans syndrome
lymphangioma c.

circumstance
altered life c.
life circumstance problem

circumventricular organ

circumzygomatic
c. fixation
c. wire
c. wiring

cirrhosis
alcoholic c.
alcoholic liver c.
antihepatitis C virus-positive c.
chronic active c.
chronic active hepatitis with c.
chronic alcoholic c.
chronic inactive c.
cryptogenic autoimmune c.
decompensated alcoholic c.
decompensated liver c.
fatty nutritional c.
c. from hepatitis
functional renal failure of c.
hepatitis C antiviral long-term treatment to prevent c.
Indian childhood c.
indigestion from c.

Laënnec c.
liver c.
c. of liver
Mayo Clinic system test for primary biliary c.
micronodular liver c.
obstructive biliary c.
portal c.
postnecrotic c.
primary biliary c.

cirrhotic
c. ascites
c. gastritis
c. liver parenchyma

cis
9-*cis* retinoic acid
9-*cis* retinoic acid receptor

cisplatin
Adriamycin and c.
c., methotrexate, vinblastine
high-dose methotrexate and c.
methotrexate, cisplatin, vinblastine
methotrexate, vinblastine, Adriamycin, c.
mitomycin C, Oncovin, bleomycin, c.
c. nephropathy

cis-platinum

13-*cis*-retinoic acid

***cis*-retinoic acid**

cistern
anterior interhemispheric c.
arachnoiditis of opticochiasmatic c.
c. of chiasm
c. fossa of Sylvius
interpeduncular c.
c. of lateral fossa of cerebrum
mesencephalic cistern effacement
obliterated basal c.
quadrigeminal cistern lipoma
quadrigeminal plate c.

cisterna, pl. **cisternae**
cylindrical confronting c.
lymphatic c.
c. magna
mega cisterna magna

cisternogram
metrizamide CT c.

cisternography
computed tomographic c.
isotope c.
metrizamide computed tomographic c.
metrizamide computed tomography c.

citrate
ATP citrate lyase
clomiphene citrate challenge test
deoxycholate c.
ferric c.
ferric ammonium c.
gallium c.
gallium citrate contrast material
gallium-67 citrate contrast medium
gallium citrate scan
indole, methyl red, Voges-Proskauer, and citrate test
magnesium c.
oral transmucosal fentanyl c.
ranitidine bismuth c.
ranitidine bismuth citrate, amoxicillin, clarithromycin
ranitidine bismuth citrate, metronidazole, tetracycline
saline sodium c.
sodium c.
sodium chloride-sodium citrate solution
standard saline c.
c. synthase
triethyl c.

citrate-buffered saline

citrated
c. calcium carbimide
c. normal rabbit serum

citric
c. acid
2-methyl citric acid

citrine
Milian citrine skin

citronella
oil of c.

citrovorum
c. factor

citrovorum-factor rescue

citrullinated
anticyclic citrullinated peptide antibody

citrullinemia
neonatal c.

city
New York City medium
Sixgun City virus

civil defense

***c-Jun* N-terminal kinase**

c-kit
soluble c-k.

Clagett closure

claim
electronic claims processing
electronic claims submission
Federal False C.'s Act
c.'s inquiry form
original c.
unproven health c.

clairvoyant dream

clamminess
c. from circulatory problem
c. of skin

clammy
cold and c.
pale and clammy skin

clamp
angled Lowman-type bone c.
angular hinge c.
Ann Arbor double towel c.
aortic cross clamp off
aortic cross clamp on
approximator c.
c. approximator
atraumatic bowel c.
bleeding controlled with c.
bleeding controlled with hemostatic c.
bulldog clamp applier
cheek c.
columella c.
cross clamp time
endoscope holding c.
fine-toothed c.
c. fixator
heavy clamp applied
hook c.
c. lamp
Locke bone c.
Malis hinge c.
marking c.
Mayfield head c.
Mayo abdominal c.
metal c.
Mikulicz c.
Mixter c.
Mogen c.
Moria-France dacryocystorhinostomy c.
mosquito hemostatic c.
Moynihan c.
multipurpose angled c.
multipurpose curved c.
muscle c.
muscular c.

clamp *(continued)*
needle holder c.
nerve-approximating c.
nose c.
occlusive c.
Ochsner c.
osteoplastic flap c.
patch c.
patch clamp electrophysiology
patch clamp technique
Payr clamp method
right angle c.

clamp-and-sew technique

clamped
bleeder c.
bleeder clamped and ligated
bleeder clamped and tied
c., divided and tied
c. and cut
doubly c.
doubly clamped and divided
doubly clamped, transected and stump ligated
late clamped umbilical cord

clamping
aortic c.
cross clamping of aorta
c. habit
patch c.
selective vascular c.

clamshell
c. closure
c. closure of atrial septal defect
c. device

clandestine myocardial ischemia

clapping
c. hands
postural drainage and c.

Clarendon
Lake Clarendon virus

clarithromycin
metronidazole, amoxicillin, clarithromycin, *H. pylori*, one-week therapy
metronidazole, omeprazole, c.
omeprazole, amoxicillin, c.
omeprazole, metronidazole, c.
ranitidine bismuth citrate, amoxicillin, c.

clarity
optical c.

clash
paradigm c.

clasp
arm c.
arrow c.
arrowhead c.
bar c.
cast c.
circumferential c.
continuous clasp splint
embrasure c.
c. guideline
lingual c.
mesiodistal c.
multiple c.

clasp-knife
c.-k. reflex
c.-k. rigidity

class
alcoholism therapy c.
anti-HLA class I antibody
aspartyl protease c.
blood group c.
diabetes mellitus, pregnancy classification, class A–F
financial c.
functional c.
c. II invariant chain-derived peptide
latent class analysis
major histocompatibility complex class I
major histocompatibility complex class II
MHC class I antigen
MHC class I antigen deficiency
MHC class I deficiency
MHC class II
MHC class II antigen
MHC class II deficiency
MHC class I molecule
MHC class I-restricted cytolytic activity
middle class community
therapeutic class profile

classic
c. abdominal Semm hysterectomy
c. cesarean section
c. headache preceded by aura
headache preceded by classic aura
c. Hodgkin lymphoma
c. incision
c. interstitial pneumonitis with fibrosis
lymphocyte-rich classic Hodgkin
c. migraine
c. technique

classical
c. incision
c. pathway
c. signs of rejection

classifiable
not elsewhere c.

classification
adnexal adhesion classification system
AFS classification of adnexal adhesions
Aitken classification of epiphysial fracture
Aitken epiphysial fracture c.
AJCC TNM tumor c.
Allman acromioclavicular injury c.
ambulatory payment classification group
American Heart Association c.
American Heart Association Stroke Outcome C.
anatomical classification system of Severin
anatomic brain c.
Anderson modification of Berndt-Harty c.
Anderson tibial pseudarthrosis c.
Angle classification of malocclusion, class I–IV
Angle malocclusion c.
Ann Arbor c.
Ann Arbor classification of Hodgkin disease staging
Ann Arbor staging c.
Ann Arbor tumor c.
Antoni A neurinoma c.
Antoni classification of schwannoma morphology
anular tear c.
AO ankle fracture c.
AO-Danis-Weber ankle fracture c.
Army General C. Test
artificial classification cavity
Ashhurst-Bromer ankle fracture c.
Ashhurst fracture classification system
ASIA impairment scale for classification of spinal cord injury
Astler-Coller A, B1, B2, C1, C2 c.
Astler-Coller modification of Dukes c.
Canadian Heart C.
cement mantle grade c.
Child-Turcotte c.
contaminated operative wound c.
Crime Classification Manual

Danis-Weber classification for ankle fracture
diabetes mellitus, pregnancy classification, class A–F
dirty operative wound c.
Duke classification of carcinoma
elder malignant melanoma c.
Flanagan Aptitude C. Test
French-American-British leukemia classification system
c. of host
International C. of Diseases
International C. of Diseases and Related Health Problems, 10th Edition
International C. of Diseases and Causes of Death
International C. of Diseases–Clinical Modification
International C. of Diseases 9th Ed. Injury Severity Score
International Federation of Gynecology and Obstetrics classification of tumor staging
International C. of Impairments, Disabilities, and Handicaps
Le Fort c.
Lens Opacification C. System
Lens Opacities C. System II
Lichtman aseptic necrosis c.
Los Angeles c.
Los Angeles classification of GERD
Los Angeles Classification grade A, B, C, D esophagitis
Lugano classification for testicular tumor
Lukes-Collins classification of non-Hodgkin lymphoma
Lukes-Collins non-Hodgkin lymphoma c.
c. of malignant tumors
Marcus Gunn c.
Marx classification of microtia
Mason fracture classification system
Mayo carpal instability c.
Mayo classification of rheumatoid elbow
Mayo elbow fracture c.
Mazur ankle elevation c.
McLean classification of melanoma
microinvasive carcinoma c.
Milch classification of humeral fracture
Milch condylar fracture c.
Milch elbow fracture c.
Milch fracture classification syndrome
Minaar classification of coalition
Minaar classification system
Minaar coalition c.
Minnesota Occupational C. System
modified Dallas classification of disc morphology grades 0–7
modified Fischer c.
modified Frankel c.
Moore classification for vascular anomalies of the gastrointestinal tract
Mostofi classification of testicular tumor
Mueller femoral supracondylar fracture c.
Mueller humerus fracture c.
multiaxial classification system
multidimensional actuarial c.
Munro and Parker classification for laparoscopic hysterectomy
Neer classification of shoulder fracture
Neer femur fracture c.
Neer-Horowitz classification of humeral fracture
Neer humerus fracture c.
neonatal maturity classification of Dubowitz
Neviaser frozen shoulder c.
Newman classification of radial neck and head fracture
New York Heart Association classification of heart disease
NIH Classification Category I acute bacterial prostatitis
NIH Classification Category II chronic bacterial prostatitis
NIH Classification Category III inflammatory and noninflammatory chronic pelvic pain
NIH Classification Category IV asymptomatic inflammatory prostatitis
NIH C. System for Prostatitis
Norwood classification system
Norwood C. of Male Pattern Baldness
Nurick classification of spondylosis
Nursing Interventions C.
NYHA congestive heart failure c.
NYHA functional c.
O'Brien classification of radial fracture
Ogden epiphysial fracture c.
Ogden fracture classification system
osteoarthritis grading c.
Ovadia-Beals classification of tibial plafond fracture
Palmer classification of trapezial ridge fracture
Papavasiliou classification of olecranon fracture
Pauwels femoral neck fracture c.
Pediatric Acute Admission Severity c.
physical status patient c.'s
primary tumor, regional lymph node, remote metastases classification, staging
Rappaport classification of lymphoma
Reese Ellsworth c.
C. and Regression Tree analysis
Revised European-American Classification of Lymphoid Neoplasms
Salter-Harris classification of fracture
Standard Industrial C.
Structural C. of Proteins
suicide risk c.
WHO classification for transitional cell carcinoma of the urinary bladder: stages Ta through T4
World Health Organization classification of lupus nephritis I, IIA, IIB, III, IV, V

classified
c. anaphylatoxin
not c.
not elsewhere c.

classroom
Barclay C. Climate Inventory
c. behavior of child
C. Environmental Scale
Individual Learning Disabilities C. Screening Instrument

Claude
C. hyperkinesis sign
C. Mood Scale

claudication
intermittent c.
c. in the leg
c. limb pain

claudication *(continued)*
neurogenic c.
neurogenic peripheral intermittent c.
painful claudication of leg

Claudius
cells of C.

clavicle
atraumatic osteolysis of distal c.
penciling of the distal c.
perinatal clavicle fracture
shaft of c.

clavicular
c. fracture
c. notch of sternum

claw
burn c.
c. finger
c. foot
c. hand
lion's claw grasper
c. toe
c. toe position

clawfoot
pes arcuatus clawfoot deformity
pes cavus clawfoot deformity

clawhand
lobster c.
syringomyelic c.

clawing
toe c.

claw-like deformity

clay
c. pipe cancer
Symmers clay pipestem fibrosis

clay-colored stool

clay-like consistency

clay-shoveler's fracture

clean
horizontal flow clean bench
horizontal laminar flow clean benches
incision clean and dry
c. intermittent bladder catheterization
intermittent clean catheterization
c. intermittent self-catheterization
c., midstream urine
c. needle technique
operative wound clean and healed
vertical flow clean bench
c. wound
wound clean and healed

clean-catch
c.-c. midstream urinalysis
midstream clean-catch urine
c.-c. midstream urine
midstream clean-catch urine culture
c.-c. urine

clean-contaminated wound

cleaned, sutured, and dressed

cleaner
enzymatic c.

cleaning
ultrasonic c.

cleansing
deep cleansing breath
endoscope lens cleansing device

clean-voided specimen

clear
anterior clear space
c. to auscultation
c. to auscultation and percussion
c. cell adenocarcinoma
c. cell carcinoma
c. cell endothelioma
c. cell hepatocellular carcinoma
c. cell odontogenic tumor
c. cell renal cell carcinoma
c. cell sarcoma of the kidney
c. cell sarcoma of the liver
chest clear to auscultation and percussion
chest clear to percussion and auscultation
c. effluent
effluxed clear urine
hereditary clear cell renal carcinoma
hyalinizing clear cell carcinoma
lipid-laden clear cell
c. liquid
c. liquid diet
c. lung field
lungs clear to auscultation
lungs clear to auscultation and percussion
malignant clear cell acrospiroma
medial clear space
mesonephroid clear cell carcinoma
nasal airway c.
nongranular clear chromophobe cell
Orphan Annie-eyed clear nucleus
ovarian clear cell adenocarcinoma
ovarian clear cell carcinoma
regular rate, clear tones, no murmurs
c. sensorium
c. surgical diet
tap water enema til c.
c. thinking
c. urine

clearance
acid clearance test
albumin c.
p-aminohippurate c.
amylase c.
amylase-creatinine clearance ratio
ANP clearance receptor
bilirubin c.
blood isotope c.
creatinine c.
creatinine clearance test
enterohepatic c.
equivalent residual renal urea c.
estimated creatinine c.
extrahepatic blood flow c.
first definite apical clearance lens
fluorescein clearance test
fractional free-water c.
free water c.
gas clearance measurement
ineffective airway c.
insulin clearance test
lithium c.
low-hepatic clearance drug
luminal acid c.
lung clearance index
maximal c.
measure mucociliary c.
microciliary c.
mucociliary c.
mucociliary clearance rate
myoglobin clearance test
nasal c.
nitrogen clearance delay
nonrenal c.
osmolar c.
peritoneal dialysis creatinine clearance target
phosphate c.
pulmonary clearance delay
renal c.
steroid metabolic clearance rate
total body c.
urea c.
volume clearance rate
water c.

cleared
urinary tract infection c.

clearing
c. of airway

casualty clearing station
c. of infiltrate
interval c.
media c.
c. of mental symptoms
c. of sensorium
throat clearing from anxiety

Clearinghouse
National Diabetes Information C.
National Digestive Diseases Information C.
National Kidney and Urological Diseases Information C.
National Self-Help C.

Cleary
method of C.

cleavage
anterior chamber cleavage syndrome
anterior cleavage syndrome
aspartyl protease-mediated c.
c. fragment length polymorphism
lines of c.
manual c.
meridional c.
metal-catalyzed oxidative c.
mitochondrial glycine cleavage system
nonisotopic RNase cleavage assay
primary c.
pudendal c.
secondary c.
side-chain c.
tertiary c.
yolk c.

cleaved
large cleaved cell
mixed small cleaved and large cell lymphoma
c. polyprotein precursor molecule
c. polyprotein precursor molecule product

cleft
ankyloblepharon, ectodermal defect, and cleft lip and/or palate
arthrogryposis, ectodermal dysplasia, cleft lip/palate developmental delay syndrome
asymmetric bilateral c.
bilateral cleft lip and palate
branchial cleft anomaly
cardiac abnormality, abnormal facies, thymic hypoplasia, cleft palate, hypocalcemia
c. of cervix
congenital paucity of secondary synaptic clefts syndrome
conotruncal cardiac defect, abnormal face, thymic hypoplasia, cleft palate
ectodermal dysplasia, cleft lip and palate, mental retardation, syndactyly syndrome I, II
c. of Hahn
c. hand
c. lip
c. lip and alveolus
c. lip and cleft palate
c. lip, cleft palate, lobster-claw deformity syndrome
c. lip deformity
medial cleft of lip
medial cleft of palate
median cleft face
median cleft face syndrome
median cleft lip
median cleft of lower lip and mandible
median cleft upper lip, mental retardation, pugilistic facies syndrome
median facial c.
median facial cleft syndrome
middle ear c.
midline cleft palate
midline cleft syndrome
Millard bilateral cleft lip repair
nasal alar cartilage c.
neural arch c.
obesity, short stature, mental deficiency, hypogonadism, micropenis, finger contracture, cleft lip-palate syndrome
oblique facial c.
occult cleft palate
orbitofacial c.
c. palate knife
c. palate-lateral synechia syndrome
c. palate tenaculum
partial cleft palate
partial cricoid c.
Rathke cleft cyst
submucous cleft palate
c. tongue
unilateral cleft of lip and palate

clefting
ankyloblepharon, ectodermal dysplasia, clefting syndrome
cardiac abnormality, T-cell deficit, clefting, hypocalcemia
ectrodactyly, ectodermal dysplasia, clefting syndrome
midline cranioorbital c.
paramedian clefting syndrome

clenched
c. fist sign
hand c.
c. jaw
c. muscles in head and neck

clenching
extreme jaw c.
gnashing and clenching of teeth
jaw c.

Clerc-Levy-Cristeco syndrome

clergy intervention

clerical
General C. Test
Minnesota C. Aptitude Test
Minnesota C. Assessment Battery

clerk
unit c.

cleverness factor

click
aortic ejection c.
aortic opening c.
ejection c.
c. heard at hip joint
hip c.
late systolic c.
midsystolic c.
c. murmur
opening snap ejection systolic c.
pulmonary ejection c.
c. syndrome
systolic c.
systolic click murmur syndrome

clicking
c. of malfunctioning valve
palatal c.
c. rale
c. sensation

click-murmur syndrome

client
Rehabilitation C. Rating Scale

Clifford
arcuate ligament of C.

Clifton Assessment Procedures for the Elderly

climacteric
c. insanity
male c.
male climacteric syndrome
c. syndrome

climate
Barclay Classroom C. Inventory
occlusal c.
Social C. Scale

climatic
c. droplet keratopathy
nonspecific climatic change

climax
normal libido, coitus, and c.

climbing fiber

clindamycin
gentamicin, clindamycin, and polymyxin topical preparation

clinic
acupuncture c.
affective disorders c.
anxiety disorder c.
anxiety and panic disorder c.
birth control c.
cerebral palsy c.
chemical dependence c.
child care c.
child development c.
community hypertension evaluation c.
comprehensive care c.
diabetes care c.
diabetes disease management c.
family planning c.
flight medicine c.
free-standing c.
general medical c.
live c.
liver c.
low vision c.
Mayo Clinic forefoot score
Mayo Clinic hip scoring system
Mayo Clinic system test for primary biliary cirrhosis
Medical Walk-In Clinic
mental health c.
mental hygiene c.
outpatient c.
outpatient clinic substation
outpatient dialysis c.
pain clinic program
pediatric walk-in c.
personal care c.
preliminary diagnostic c.
primary care c.
private diagnostic c.
return to c.
substance abuse treatment c.
urgent care c.
well-baby c.

clinical
accessory clinical finding
accessory clinical findings
acute change clinical score
acute clinical illness
C. Adaptive Test
C. Adaptive Test/Clinical Linguistic and Auditory Milestone Scale
c. alcoholic hepatitis
C. Analysis Questionnaire
c. appraisal of psychosocial problem
c. assay
c. assessment
Association of C. Scientists
automated clinical record
automatic clinical analyzer
c. breast examination
C. Colitis Activity Index
complete clinical remission
composite clinical and laboratory index
controlled clinical trial
c. course
Cumulative Techniques and Procedures in C. Microbiology
C. Data Repository
c. decision-making
C. Dementia Rating
c. depression
c. diagnostic staging
double-blind placebo-controlled randomized clinical trial
early clinical drug evaluation unit
c. emphysema
c. estimation of survival
C. Evaluation of Language Function-Preschool
C. Evaluation of Language Functions
c. evidence of metastatic disease
expected value of clinical information
C. Global Impression of Change
C. Global Impression-Severity of Illness Scale
C. Global Improvement
C. Global Index
C. Health Assessment Questionnaire
c. heart disease
c. hepatitis
c. history
c. hyaline membrane disease
c. hypnosis
c. illness
c. impression
c. information
c. interaction and detoxification
c. interpretation
c. intervention
c. investigation
c. investigator
c. isolates of bacteria
c. judgment
C. Laboratory Improvement Act
C. Linguistic and Auditory Milestone Scale
Lovett clinical scale of strength
c. manifestation of acute drug intoxication
c. manifestation of drug reaction
c. manifestation of panic reaction
c. manifestations, etiologic factors, anatomic involvement, pathophysiologic features
c. manifestation of withdrawal
mean clinical value
c. medicine
Millon Adolescent C. Inventory
Millon Clinical Multiaxial Inventory test
Modified C. Technique test
Nephrolithiasis C. Guidelines Panel
c. nursing
objective structural clinical examination
c. obstetrics and gynecology
ongoing clinical trial
c. partial response
c. pathology
Pediatric AIDS C. Trial Group Protocol
c. performance score
c. pharmacokinetics consulting service
c. pharmacokinetics team
c. and pharmacological interaction
c. practice guidelines
c. practice issue
C. Practice Model
C. Probes of Articulation Consistency
c. procedure
c. pulmonary infection score
randomized controlled clinical trial
C. Rating Scale
c. record
c. remission
c. research
c. research center

c. research trial
c. research unit
results of clinical controlled trial
c. risk assessment
C. Risk Index for Babies
Short C. Rating Scale
c. significance
c. signs and symptoms
c. specialty unit
c. spectrum of cancer
c. stage
c. staging of tumors, nodes, and metastases as determined by noninvasive examination
c. status of node
structured clinical interview
Structured C. Interview for DSM
Structured C. Interview for DSM-IV Dissociative Disorders
Systematized Nomenclature of Medicine C. Terms
c. target volume
C. Test of Sensory Interaction & Balance
transient clinical hepatitis
c. transplant coordinator
c. trial
c. tumor volume
c. vascular laboratory
Working Formulation for C. Usage

clinically
c. active stage
c. isolated syndrome
minimum clinically important difference
c. nonfunctioning pituitary adenoma
c. observed seizure
c. significant arrhythmia

clinical-symptom/self-evaluation questionnaire

clinician
junior c.
C. Rated Anxiety Scale
C. Rated Anxiety Scale

Clinician's Global Rating Scale

clinicopathologic conference

Clinitron
C. air-fluidized therapy
C. bed

clinodactyly
facial dysplasia, hyperextensibility of joints, clinodactyly, growth retardation, mental retardation syndrome

clinoid
anterior c.
anterior clinoid process
middle clinoid process

clinoidal segment

clinoidectomy
anterior extradural c.

clip
aneurysm clip applicator
aneurysm clip ligation
angled aneurysm c.
cerebrovascular aneurysmal c.
c. gauge
c. ligation of aneurysm
Mayfield aneurysm c.
McKenzie hemostasis c.
Michel c.
mini-Sugita c.
Multifire clip applicator
nose c.
c. occlusion
Olivecrona c.
Omni clip gun
pelviscopic clip ligation technique

clipped
intracranial aneurysm c.
c. speech
c. word

clipping
aneurysm c.
c. of aneurysm
aneurysmal clipping operation
endoluminal c.
endoscopic c.
peak c.
proximal c.

clip-type electrode

clitoral therapy device

clitoris
bridle of c.
glans of c.
horn of c.
os c.
prepuce of c.
suspensory ligament of c.
c. tourniquet syndrome

clivus
lower c.
mucopyocele of the c.

cloaca
osteomyelitic cloaca formation

cloacogenic
inflammatory cloacogenic polyp

cloaking
periosteal c.
perivascular c.

clock
alarm clock voiding
around the c.
every hour around the c.
every 2 hours around the c.

clock-drawing test

clofibrate-induced muscular syndrome

clofibric acid

clogged bypass graft

clomiphene citrate challenge test

Clo Mor virus

clonal
normal clonal CD4+ T cell
occult clonal B-cell population

clone
molecular c.
neoplastic c.
overlapping c.'s

cloned enzyme donor immunoassay

clone-inhibiting factor

clonic
generalized tonic c.
c. jerk
c. movement
multifocal clonic convulsion
multifocal clonic movement
multifocal clonic seizure
c. perseveration
c. seizure
c. spasm

cloning
at c.
c. inhibitory factor
molecular c.
molecular cloning and sequencing

clonogenic
micrometastases clonogenic assay
tumor clonogenic assay

clonus
ankle clonus test
anodal opening c.
beats of c.
cathodal closure c.
c. index

Cloquet
C. ganglion
node of C.

close
inability to close eye
c. supervision

closed
abdomen closed in layers
c. amputation
c. in anatomic layers
Assura closed mini pouch
c. base wedge osteotomy
c. bladder drainage
c. cerebral trauma
cervix long, thick and c.
c. chest cardiac massage
c. chest cardiac resuscitation
chest closed in anatomic layers
c. chest commissurotomy
c. chest massage
c. chest pneumothorax
c. chest thoracostomy
c. circle deoxyribonucleic acid
continuous postoperative closed lavage
c. core needle biopsy
c. craniocerebral trauma
crutch and belt femoral closed nailing
c. drainage
eyes c.
c. head injury
c. head syndrome
c. head trauma
c. head unit
c. heart surgery
c. hospital
incision closed anatomically
incision closed in layers
incision closed musculofascially
incision closed in serial fashion
c. injury
c. iris forceps
c. kinetic chain
c. kinetic chain exercise
long, closed, posterior cervix
loosely closed incision
c. medullary nailing
c. mouth impression
nontubed closed distant flap graft
c. over wound
Parker-Kerr closed method of end-to-end enteroenterostomy
c. pleural biopsy
c. pleural drainage
c. reduction
c. reduction and cast
c. reduction of fracture
c. reduction and internal fixation
c. reduction and percutaneous pin fixation
c. reduction and percutaneous pin ring
skin closed with interrupted silk
skin incision c.
c. skull fracture
c. soft tissue injury
c. thoracotomy
c. unlocked nail
c. urinary drainage bag with drip chamber
c. vitrectomy
c. water seal drainage system
c. wedge osteotomy/bunionectomy

closed-angle glaucoma

closed-bite malocclusion

closed-end ostomy pouch

closed-eye surgery

closed-loop system passing electrode

close-fitting mask

closing
c. abductory wedge osteotomy
Amspacher-Messenbaugh closing wedge osteotomy
aortic valve opening to aortic valve closing ratio
cathodal c.
cathodal closing contraction
effect of closing of eyes in electroencephalography
medial closing wedge phalangeal osteotomy
oblique closing wedge osteotomy
upper airway closing pressure
c. volume
voluntary c.

clostridial
c. food poisoning
c. gas gangrene
c. myocarditis
c. nephritis
reinforced clostridial medium

Clostridium
C. difficile
Clostridium difficile-associated colitis
Clostridium difficile-associated diarrhea
Clostridium difficile-associated disease
Clostridium difficile colitis
Clostridium difficile culture filtrate
Clostridium perfringens enterotoxin

closure
anodal c.
anodal closure contraction
anodal closure picture
anodal closure sound
anodal closure tetanus
anterior neural tube c.
aortic c.
arterial puncture site closure device
asymmetric closure of cusp
cathodal closure clonus
cathodal closure contraction
cathodal closure tetanus
clamshell closure of atrial septal defect
c. of colostomy
delayed closure of accidental wound
delayed closure of operative wound
delayed primary c.
delayed secondary c.
double umbrella c.
early mitral valve c.
eyelid closure reflex
general c.
hemostatic puncture closure device
incomplete mitral leaflet c.
c. index
c. interatrial septal defect
interatrial septal defect c.
lid closure reaction
lid closure reflex
maxillary antrum c.
maximal closure pressure
maximum urethral closure pressure
membrane closure time
midline aponeurotic c.
mitral valve c.
native aortic valve c.
overlapping closure of peritoneum
palatal fistula c.
percutaneous arterial closure device
plastic c.
premature closure of valve
premature ductus arteriosus c.
premature mitral c.
premature tricuspid c.
primary c.
pulmonic c.
pulmonic closure sound
semilunar valve c.
c. of skin wound

c. of tracheal fistula
transcatheter c.
tricuspid valve c.
urethral closure pressure
urethral closure pressure profile
vacuum-assisted closure dressing

clot
antemortem c.
autologous c.
autologous blood c.
blue skin from blood c.
bulging eyes from blood c.
c. buster
c. busting drug
dilute blood clot lysis method
c. dissolving action
c. dissolving drug
c. dissolving thrombolytic drug
euglobulin clot lysis
euglobulin clot lysis time
euglobulin clot test
c. expressed from wound
heart c.
heart attack from blood c.
c. to hold
intramural c.
life-threatening blood c.
c. lysed
c. lysis
c. lysis time
marantic c.
maternal blood clot patch therapy
mucin clot prevention test
mucin clot test
mural c.
organized c.
passage of c.
passive c.
plasma clot diffusion chamber
poor c.
proximal c.
pulmonary blood c.
c. retraction
c. retraction test
c. retraction time
c. stabilization test

cloth binder

clothes
plucking at c.

clot-promoting factor

clottable protein

clotted
hemorrhage and clotted blood

clotting
abnormal blood c.
c. abnormality
c. action of blood
activated clotting factor
activated clotting time
c. assay
Dale-Laidlaw clotting time
disseminated intrauterine c.
c. factor
graft c.
ground-glass clotting time
high clotting risk
increased c.
Lee-White blood clotting method
Lee-White tritium clotting time
maximal extrapolated clotting time
plasma clotting time
recalcified whole-blood activated clotting time
slow blood c.
specific clotting factor and inhibitor
thrombin clotting time
c. time
venous clotting time
whole-blood activated clotting time

cloud
aerosol cloud enhancer
c. baby
Wilson cloud chamber

clouded
c. consciousness
c. cornea
c. lens
c. sensorium
c. vision

clouding
aortic stenosis, corneal clouding, growth and mental retardation syndrome
c. of consciousness
c. of cornea
hilar c.
mental c.
c. of sinuses
vitreous c.

cloudy
c. swelling
c. urine

cloudy-cornea syndrome

clove
oil of c.

clover
sweet clover disease

cloverleaf-type deformity

club
c. fungus
c. hair
c. hand
health c.
Lost Cord C.
mycotic club nail

clubbing
c., cyanosis, and edema
cyanosis, clubbing or edema
c. and cyanosis upper extremity
c. of distal phalanx
edema, clubbing, and cyanosis
c. of extremity
c. of finger
finger c.
no clubbing, cyanosis, or edema
c. of toe
c. or tremor

clucking
nervous c.
tongue c.

clue cell

clump
chromatin clumps and nucleoli
direct microscopic clump count
platelet c.

clumping
pigment c.
platelet c.
c. of platelet
staphylococcal clumping test

clumsy hand movement

cluneal
medial cluneal nerve
middle cluneal nerve

clunk
catch and clunk test
patellar clunk syndrome

cluster
abnormal c.
anxious-fearful c.
apolipoprotein gene c.
c. attack
avoidance c.
c. of bacteria
breakpoint cluster region
breakpoint cluster region negative
breakpoint cluster region positive
c. of differentiation
c. of differentiation 2–72
c. of differentiation 4 immunoglobulin G
emotional B c.
grape cluster appearance

cluster *(continued)*
c. headache
c. of infection
c. of isolates
macular c.
microcalcification c.
microglial c.
c. migraine
c. of milk-secreting alveoli
monophyletic c.
mood cluster score
c. of short gram-negative rods
sleep-related cluster headache
c. suicides
c. of symptom
c. of tubercles
c. of tumor cells

clustered
propagating clustered contraction
c. waves

cluster-of-grapes appearance

Clyde Mood Scale

C124M

coach in delivery

coach's finger

coactivator
NCoA-1 c.
NCoA-2 c.
receptor-associated coactivator 3

coagglutination
monoclonal antibody coagglutination test
c. test

coagulant
antiinhibitor coagulant complex

coagulase-negative
c.-n. staphylococcus
c.-n. staphylococcus bacteremia

coagulase-positive staphylococcus

coagulase-reacting factor

coagulated
Löffler coagulated serum medium

coagulating
cancer cell-derived blood coagulating activity 1

coagulation
activated coagulation time
a-2 antiplasmin coagulation inhibitor
antithrombin III coagulation inhibitor
APTT coagulation test
argon beam c.
argon beam plasma c.
argon ion plasma c.
AT-III coagulation inhibitor
bilateral tubal c.
blood coagulation monitoring
blood coagulation time
cancer coagulation factor
disseminated intravascular c.
disseminated intravascular blood c.
disseminated intravascular coagulation syndrome
factor VIII coagulation function
heater probe c.
c. and hemostatic resection of prostate
infrared coagulation of hemorrhoid
interstitial laser coagulation of the prostate
intradiscal electrothermal c.
intravascular blood c.
intravascular coagulation and fibrinolysis syndrome
laparoscopic tubal c.
laser coagulation vaporization procedure
light c.
lipoprotein-associated coagulation inhibitor
a-2 macroglobulin coagulation inhibitor
c. panel
percutaneous coagulation of gasserian ganglion
percutaneous microwave coagulation therapy
presurgical coagulation evaluation
c. profile–diagnosis
c. profile–presurgery
c. screen
c. study
c. time
c. of tissue

coagulative
maximum coagulative necrosis

coagulator
argon beam c.
argon laser c.
argon plasma c.
infrared c.

coagulin
thyroxine-binding c.

coagulopathic disorder

coagulopathy
diffuse intravascular c.
disseminated intravascular c.
intravascular consumption c.

coagulum
necrobiotic c.
necrotic c.
osseous coagulum trap

coal
crude coal tar
crude coal tar in petroleum
c. miner's lung
c. tar bath
c. tar pitch volatiles
c. worker's lung
c. worker's pneumoconiosis

coalition
c. of bone
Minaar classification of c.
Minaar coalition classification
naviculocuneiform c.
osseous c.

coaptation
nerve c.
c. site
c. suture

coarctation
c. of aorta
aortic arch c.
atypical subisthmic c.
c. of pulmonary arteries
symptomatic coarctation of aorta
thoracic aortic c.

coarse
c. bacterial colonies
c. breath sounds
c. crepitation
c. hand tremors
c. and harsh breathing
mental retardation, coarse face, microcephaly, epilepsy, skeletal abnormalities syndrome
mental retardation, coarse facies, epilepsy, joint contracture syndrome
c. murmur
numerous coarse rales
c. nystagmus
c. rales
c. rhonchi
c. scalp hair
c. thrill
c. trabeculation
c. tremor

coarsely
lungs coarsely granular

coarsening of duodenal bulb

coarticulation
anticipatory c.
C. Assessment in Meaningful Language

Coast
East Coast fever
Pacific Coast demineralized cortical bone powder
Pacific Coast Tissue Bank

coastal plains virus

coat
buffy c.
choroid coat of eye
longitudinal layer of muscle coat of small intestine
longitudinal layer of muscular c.
muscular coat of bronchi
muscular coat of colon
muscular coat of ductus deferens
muscular coat of esophagus
muscular coat of female urethra
muscular coat of gallbladder
muscular coat of intermediate part of male urethra
muscular coat of large intestine
muscular coat of pharynx
muscular coat of prostatic urethra
muscular coat of rectum
muscular coat of small intestine
muscular coat of spongy part of male urethra
muscular coat of stomach
muscular coat of trachea
muscular coat of ureter
muscular coat of urinary bladder
muscular coat of uterine tube
muscular coat of uterus
muscular coat of vagina
quality buffy c.
quantitative buffy c.
white coat effect
white coat syndrome

coated
c. compressed tablet
enteric coated aspirin
hydrophilic c.
sectionally processed antibody c.
silicone c.
c. tongue
wall coated open tubular

coating
aluminum oxide ceramic c.
antireflection c.
membrane coating granule
mirror c.
proteinaceous c.
pus coating stool

coat-sleeve amputation

coaxial
biliary coaxial dilator
cervi c.
Luxtec coaxial illumination
Pearce coaxial irrigating/aspirating cannula

coaxially
pass c.

cobalamin
ATP cobalamin adenoxyltransferase

cobalamin-binding protein

cobalt
albumin cobalt binding
external cobalt irradiation
c. isotope

cobbler's
c. chest
c. suture

cobblestone
c. appearance
c. tongue

cobblestoning
mucosal c.

coblation
tonsillar c.

cobra
c. toxin
c. venom factor

cocaine
acute cocaine intoxication
c. and amphetamine regulated transcript
c. anesthesia
C. Anonymous
comorbid cocaine abuse
c. and crack crisis
c. dependence
habitual cocaine smoker
c. heart attack
c. and heroin
heroin, morphine, and c.
c. high
c. injection
liquified powder c.
maternal cocaine use
c. metabolite assay
Minnesota C. Craving Scale
c. mood disorder
morphine and c.
c. and morphine
c. package ingestion
prenatal cocaine exposure
sudden death due to cocaine ingestion
tetracaine, Adrenalin, and c.

cocaine-induced
c.-i. anxiety
c.-i. death
c.-i. depression
c.-i. respiratory failure

cocaine-related
c.-r. heart attack victim
c.-r. vascular headache

cocci (*pl. of* coccus)

coccidioidal
chronic progressive coccidioidal pneumonitis
c. granuloma
c. meningitis

coccidioidomycosis
asymptomatic c.
disseminated c.
lung c.
c. meningitis

coccobacilli
small gram-negative c.

coccobacillus
Gram-negative c.

coccus, pl. **cocci**
aerobic gram-positive c.
Gram-negative cocci
Gram-negative rod and c.
Gram-positive cocci
Gram-positive anaerobic c.
Gram-positive cocci in pairs and chains
Gram-positive rod and c.
cocci granuloma
short-chain gram-positive cocci

coccygei
musculi c.

coccygeus
nervus c.
plexus c.

coccyx
muscle of c.

cochlea
apical c.
apical turn of the c.
aqueductus c.
area c.
membranous c.
outer spiral fibers of c.
radial fiber of c.
spiral canal of c.
spiral ganglion of c.

cochlear
advance cochlear echo technique
c. blood flow
c. implant
c. implantation
c. joint
little fossa of cochlear window
c. microphonic
c. nucleus
c. potential

cochlearis
arteria cochlearis communis
arteria cochlearis propria
nervus c.
nucleus cochlearis anterior
nucleus cochlearis posterior
pars c.

cochleitis
ossifying c.

cochleopalpebral reflex

cochleovestibular neurectomy

Cockayne syndrome

Cocklin
modified Cocklin toe operation

cockroach
American c.

cock-robin sign

cockscomb
c. appearance of cervix
cervical c.
c. cervix
c. ulcer

cocktail
anticancer c.
intramuscular c.
intravenous c.
lytic c.
MAK-6 c.
pain c.
c. party patter
pediatric c.
Rivers c.

cock-up
c.-u. deformity
c.-u. hand splint
c.-u. splint orthosis
c.-u. wrist splint

cocontraction
marked c.

code
c. blue
cardiac arrest c.
diagnostic c.
c. of ethics
evaluation and management c.'s
extended binary-coded decimal interchange c.
c. four
MMPI C. Type
Morse code pattern
no code blue
outpatient code editor
C. of Practice
pulse code modulation
c. red
c. of silence

coded
not elsewhere c.

coded-aperture imaging

codeine
acetaminophen and c.
aspirin and c.
elixir terpin hydrate with c.
c. neurotoxicity
Tylenol with c.

codependency disorder

codependent
C.'s Anonymous
individual codependent counseling
c. personality

coding
Arithmetic, C., Information, and Digit Span
Facial Action C. System
Medical Examination and Diagnostic C. System
Neonatal Facial Coding System

cod liver oil

codominant
autosomal c.
c. characteristic
c. circulation

codon
arginine c.
AUG c.
nonsense c.
ochre c.
opal c.
premature top c.

coefficient
absorption c.
c. of absorption
activity c.
alternate forms reliability c.
apparent diffuse c.
apparent diffusion c.
attenuation coefficient on MRI scan
Bunsen solubility c.
capillary filtration c.
Chick-Martin c.
correlation c.
c. of determination
c. of diffusion
distribution c.
c. of error
extinction c.
c. of fat retention
c. of heat transfer
inbreeding c.
c. of induction
c. of intelligence
internal conversion c.
linear absorption c.
linear attenuation c.
longitudinal random coefficient model
low alpha c.
mass absorption c.
mass attenuation c.
mass transfer c.
mass transfer area c.
molar absorption c.
molar extinction c.
noise reduction c.
obtained c.
osmotic c.
Ostwald solubility c.
partition c.
Pearson correlation c.
Pearson correlation coefficient pedantic
c. of performance
population correlation c.
prostatic pressure c.
rank correlation c.
reflection c.
regression c.
reliability c.
Rideal-Walker c.
sample correlation c.
c. of scleral rigidity
sedimentation c.
selection c.
sieving coefficient for sodium
specific absorption c.
temperature c.
transmission c.
c. of variation
water-retention c.
Yvon coefficient test

coenzyme
c. A-synthesizing protein complex
c. II
c. Q10

reduced coenzyme A
uncombined coenzyme A

coercive
c. behavior
c. communication
paraphiliac coercive disorder

coeur
cri de c.
c. en sabot

coexisting
c. medical condition
c. psychiatric disorders

cofactor
heparin cofactor II
ristocetin c.

coffee
c. bean appearance
c. ground emesis

coffee-ground
c.-g. drainage
c.-g. emesis
c.-g. hematemesis
c.-g. material
vomitus c.-g.

cognition
affect, behavior, c.
change in c.
c. disorder
c. and muscle control

cognitive
c. ability
c. activity
age-associated cognitive decline
age-related cognitive decline
Alzheimer Disease Assessment Scale, cognitive subscale
c. anxiety subscale
c. aspect of well-being
c. assessment
c. awareness level
c. behavior
c. behavioral approach
c. behavioral intervention
c. behavioral technique
c. behavioral therapy
c. behavior therapy
C. Behavior Therapy Package
c. behavior treatment
Brief C. Rating Scale
Canadian C. Abilities Test
c. capacity
c. change of body image
confrontational cognitive restructuring
c. coping skill
core cognitive disturbance
c. decline
deficient cognitive thinking
c. deterioration
c. disturbance
c. dysfunction
c. dysmetria
c. environmental stimulation
executive cognitive function
executive cognitive functioning
extracorporeal membrane oxygenation affecting cognitive function
C. Failures Questionnaire
c. function
c. function assessment
c. functioning
c. function tests
General C. Index
Grassi Basic C. Evaluation
higher cognitive function
HIV-associated cognitive disorder
human immunodeficiency virus associated motor cognitive disorder
impaired cognitive functioning
impaired cognitive performance
c. impairment
c. impairment in alcoholism
c. impairment of depression
c. improvement
c. information
Interpersonal C. Problem Solving
c. laterality quotient
measure of general cognitive functioning
c. and motor changes
multiple cognitive deficits
Neurobehavioral C. Status examination
C. Observation Guide
ongoing cognitive process
overall cognitive functioning
overall cognitive measure
perceptual cognitive mechanism
perceptual cognitive motor function
c. perceptual motor skills
c. performance
c. personality trait
postictal cognitive dysfunction
preexisting cognitive impairment
Primary Test of C. Skills
Rating Scale of Communication in C. Decline
c. remediation therapy
Scales of C. Ability for Traumatic Brain Injury
C. Skills Assessment
c. skills training approach
slow cognitive processing
c. slowing
c. status
c. symptom
c. testing
Test of C. Style in Mathematics
c. therapy group
c. training

cognitive-behavioral psychotherapy

cognitively
c. impaired
c. intact

cogwheel
c. phenomenon
c. respiration
c. rigidity
c. sign

coherence
ocular coherence tomography
optical coherence tomography in uveitis

coherent
optical coherent tomography

cohesion
Family Adaptability and C. Evaluation Scale
lexical c.

cohesive bandage

Cohn fraction II

cohort
Multicenter AIDS C. Study
Omega C.
relative risk c.

Coho salmon reovirus

coil
aortopulmonary collateral coil embolization
depth-resolved surface coil spectroscopy
electrically detachable c.
electrodetachable platinum c.
endoesophageal magnetic resonance imaging c.
endorectal surface coil MRI
Guglielmi detachable c.
magnetic field-search coil test
mechanically detachable platinum c.
MRCP using HASTE with a phased array c.

coil *(continued)*
multiple coil array
parallel data acquisition c.
pelvic phased-array c.
radiofrequency c.
secretory c.
surface coil MR
c. test
toroidal coil chromatography
torso phased-array c.

coiled
c. bony structure
catheter coiled upon itself
c. intracranial aneurysm
lightly staining coiled bacteria
c. spring sign

coiled-spring appearance

coiling
c. of aneurysm
endovascular c.
c. procedure
umbilical coiling index

coin
c. lesion
peripheral coin lesion

coincidence
annihilation coincidence detection
c. detection
loss c.

coital
c. age
benign coital headache
c. headache
c. orgasm
post coital headache

coitus
intestinal control in functional c.
normal libido, coitus, and climax
oral c.

coke-colored stool

cola tar soap

colchicine
quinine and c.

cold
acquired cold urticaria
c. agglutinin
c. agglutinin disease
c. agglutinin syndrome
c. agglutinin titer
c. air challenge
anti-Pr cold autoagglutinin
c. blood cardioplegia
burning mouth from cold sore
c. burning, pain and numbness
c. caloric irrigation
circulatory problem with cold sensitivity
c. and clammy
combined cold and warm antibody autoimmune hemolytic anemia
c. compressive dressing
c. cone biopsy
c. crystalloid cardioplegia
c. cup biopsy
c. food-related headache
c. forceps ablation
c. gangrene
c. gas sterilization
c. hand
c. hemagglutinin disease
hot and c.
hot or cold flash
hot and cold flushes
hot and cold sensation
hot vs. cold breast tumor
c. or ice whirlpool treatment
c. immersion
c. intolerance
intolerance to c.
c. ischemia time
c. ischemic time
isocapnic hyperventilation with cold air
c. knife
c. knife cone aspiration
c. knife cone biopsy
c. knife conization
c. knife conization biopsy
c. liquid diet
macromolecular insoluble cold globulin
c. mass
c. mist humidifier
c. mottled insensate leg
neonatal cold injury
c. nodule
c. to the opposite, warm to the same
paradoxical cold response
paroxysmal cold hemoglobinuria
c. potassium cardioplegia
c. pressor
c. pressor test
c. quartz mercury vapor lamp
right ear, cold stimulus
sinus headache from c.
c. spots and hot spots with electron beam dosimetry
c. storage
c. tolerance
c. water immersion foot
c. water soluble
c. water treatment

cold-adapted influenza virus vaccine, trivalent

cold-attenuated intranasal influenza vaccine

cold-induced
c.-i. angina
c.-i. vasoconstriction
c.-i. vasospasm

cold-inducible ribonucleic acid-binding protein

cold-insoluble globulin

cold-knife
c.-k. cone
c.-k. conization
c.-k. technique

cold-mist humidifier

coldness of extremity

cold-stimulation time test

colectomy
open c.
partial c.
subtotal c.
total c.
total abdominal c.

coli
adenomatous polyposis c.
adenopolyposis coli gene
ampicillin-resistant *Escherichia coli*
anti-*Escherichia coli*-derived protein antibody
arcus marginalis c.
arteria marginalis c.
attenuated adenomatous polyposis c.
diffusely adherent *Escherichia coli*
enteroadherent *Escherichia coli*
enteroaggregative *Escherichia coli*
enteroaggregative *Escherichia coli* heat-stable enterotoxin 1
enterohemorrhagic *Escherichia coli*
enteroinvasive *Escherichia coli*
enteropathogenic *Escherichia coli*
enterotoxigenic *Escherichia coli*
enterovirulent *Escherichia coli*
Escherichia c.
Escherichia coli bacteremia
Escherichia coli filtrate
Escherichia coli polypeptide
Escherichia coli enteropathic
Escherichia coli heat-labile toxin vaccine
Escherichia coli organism

Escherichia coli sepsis peritonitis
Escherichia coli septicemia
familial polyposis c.
fecal coli broth
membrane focal coli broth
polyposis c.
Shigella-like toxin-producing *Escherichia coli*
total aganglionosis c.
toxic *Escherichia coli*
verocytotoxin-producing *Escherichia coli*
verotoxin-producing *Escherichia coli*

colic
acalculous biliary c.
c. and allergy
biliary c.
middle colic lymph node
middle colic vein
Monday morning c.
right colic artery
right colic vein
c. tenia

colicin factor

colicky
c. infant
c. pain

coliform
lactose coliform count

colipase
pancreatic c.

colitis
abdominal pain with c.
acute infectious c.
acute self-limited c.
acute ulcerative c.
c. and alpha biofeedback
antibiotic-associated c.
antibiotic-associated colitis toxin test
antibiotic-associated pseudomembranous c.
antimicrobial agent-induced c.
chronic ulcerative c.
Clinical C. Activity Index
Clostridium difficile c.
Clostridium difficile-associated c.
c. colon antigen
Crohn and C. Knowledge
diarrhea from ulcerative c.
gangrenous ischemic c.
granulomatous c.
c. gravis
idiopathic ulcerative c.
indeterminate c.
lymphocytic c.
metachronous collagenous c.
microscopic colitis syndrome
mild ulcerative c.
moderate ulcerative c.
mucosal ulcerative c.
necrotic hemorrhagic c.
necrotizing pseudomembranous c.
pantothenic acid deficiency-induced c.
protein-induced eosinophilic c.
pseudomembranous c.
single-stripe c.
transmural c.
ulcerative c.
Yersinia enterocolitica c.

Collaborative
C. Home Infant Monitoring Evaluation
C. Perinatal Study
C. Transplant Study

collagen
absorbable collagen paste
c. antigen
argyrophilic collagen fiber
autoimmune collagen vascular disease
autologous human c.
autologous human collagen augmentation
C propeptide of type II c.
c. disease
fibroblast-populated collagen lattice
fibrous long-spacing c.
glutaraldehyde cross-linked c.
c. implant
c. injection
insoluble c.
interstitial and perivascular collagen network
localized collagen dystrophy
Mallory collagen stain
microcrystalline c.
microcrystalline bovine c.
microfibrillar collagen hemostat
nascent collagen molecule
N-terminal telopeptide of type I c.
periurethral collagen injection
pulmonary collagen vascular disease
purified fibrillar c.
segment long-spacing c.
c. skin treatment
c. sponge contraceptive
c. tape prosthesis
telopeptide-poor c.
c. vascular disease
c. vascular sealing

collagenase
human neutrophil c.
human skin c.
immunoreactive human skin c.
c. soluble glomerular basement membrane

collagenase-digestible protein

collagen-induced
c.-i. arthritis
c.-i. autoimmune ear disease

collagenoma
giant cell c.

collagenosis
mediastinal c.
reactive perforating c.

collagenous
dense collagenous tissue
metachronous collagenous colitis
onionskin configuration of collagenous fiber
posterior collagenous layer

collapse
extreme intervertebral disc c.
partial collapse of lung
scaphoid-lunate advanced c.
scaphoid nonunion advanced c.
scapholunate advanced c.
scapholunate arthritic c.

collapsed
c. jugular vein
c. tissue in throat
c. vertebra of spine

collapsing pulse

collar
c. button tube
cervical c.
c. and crown scissors
felt collar splint
heated tracheostomy c.
high-humidity tracheostomy c.
c. incision
periosteal bone c.
c. of Stokes
c. of tissue
tracheal c.

collar-and-cuff sling

collared cervix

collarless, polished, tapered

collateral
accessory collateral ligament

collateral *(continued)*
allograft reconstruction of fibular collateral ligament
anterior collateral ligament
anterior radial collateral artery
aortopulmonary collateral coil embolization
c. arterial flow to brain
c. artery
c. blood flow
c. blood supply
c. circulation
esophageal collateral vein
fibular collateral ligament
fibular collateral ligament of ankle
c. fibular ligament
c. hyperemia
c. immunization
lateral collateral ligament of ankle
lateral collateral ligament complex
lateral ulnar collateral ligament
c. ligament
c. ligament instability
c. ligament laxity
c. ligament rupture
c. ligament stability
major aorticopulmonary collateral arteries
major aortopulmonary collateral artery
medial collateral artery
medial collateral ligament degeneration
medial collateral ligament of elbow
medial collateral ligament of knee
medial collateral ligament tearing
medial collateral sprain
medial ulnar collateral ligament
mesenteric c.
middle collateral artery
moyamoya collateral enlargement
multiple aortopulmonary collateral artery
c. nerve sprouting
paraesophageal collateral vein
pelvic collateral vessel
peripelvic collateral vessel
proximal collateral ligament
c. radial ligament
systemic venous c.
c. tibial ligament
ulnar collateral ligament of elbow joint
ulnar collateral ligament of wrist joint
c. ulnar ligament
c. vein
venous collateral circulation
c. vessel
well-developed collateral circulation

collateralizing vessel

collected fluid

collecting
condom catheter collecting system
cortical collecting duct
c. duct
c. duct carcinoma
duplication of left collecting system
duplication of right collecting system
inner medullary collecting duct
lower collecting system
medullary collecting tubule
papillary collecting duct
c. tubule
c. vein

collection
abdominal fluid c.
American Type Culture C.
anechoic fluid c.
arterial blood c.
autologous blood c.
data collection form
expired air c.
fecal collection receptacle assembly
feces collection device
home c.
24-hour urine c.
National Type Culture C.
pancreatic fluid c.
Pasteur Culture C.
periarticular fluid c.
pericholecystic fluid c.
perinephric fluid c.
peripancreatic fluid c.
subarachnoid fluid c.
urine collection device
urine collection pads

collective volume

collector
capillary filtrate c.
pediatric urine c.

College
C. Ability Test
Community College Student Experiences Questionnaire
Medical College Admission Test
School and College Ability Test
Student Adaptation to College Questionnaire
C. Student Satisfaction Questionnaire
C. and University Environment Scales

Collegiate
National Collegiate Athletic Association drug testing policy
National Collegiate Athletic Association prohibited drug

Collet-Sicard syndrome

colli
longissimus c.
longus cervicis colli muscle
longus colli muscle
lordosis c.
musculus longus c.

colliculus
c. of Barkow
inferior c.
middle gray layer of superior c.
nuclei of caudal c.
superior c.

Collier
artiodactylous fold of C.

collimated
multiport collimated cobalt-60 therapy

collimation
narrow c.
parallel hole c.

collimator
APC-3 c.
APC-4 c.
automatic c.
micromultileaf c.
micromultileaf collimator system
multileaf c.
parallel-hole c.
segmental multileaf c.

Collin-Beard operation

Colling electrode

Collins solution

collision
mass collision stopping power
motor vehicle c.
personal injury c.
property damage c.
rearend c.

collodiaphysial
central c.

collodion
c. baby
protein A immobilized in collodion charcoal
c. solution

colloid
amphotericin B colloid dispersion
c. antigen
antimony-sulfur c.
c. bath
diffuse colloid goiter
c. droplet
c. goiter
c. hydrostatic pressure gradient
mild colloid depletion
mini-microaggregated albumin c.
nodular colloid goiter
c. nodule of thyroid
c. oncotic pressure
c. osmotic pressure
c. osmotic pressure in interstitial fluid
c. osmotic pressure in plasma
c. replacement solution
sulfur c.
technetium-99m sulfur c.
technetium sulfur c.

colloidal
c. bismuth subcitrate
cationic colloidal gold
c. gold
c. gold test
c. iron
red colloidal test

collutory
Miller c.

coloanal
c. anastomosis
low anterior resection in combination with coloanal anastomosis
low coloanal anastomosis

coloboma
atypical c.
cerebellar vermis hypoplasia, oligophrenia, congenital ataxia, coloboma, hepatic fibrosis
c., heart anomaly, choanal atresia, retardation, and genital and ear anomalies
c., heart anomaly, ichthyosis, mental retardation, and ear abnormality syndrome
macular c.
multiple ocular c.
ocular c.
optic c.
optic nerve c.
peripapillary c.
c. of vitreous

colocolic intussusception

colon
abnormal peristaltic action of c.
adenomatosis of colon and rectum
aganglionic segment of c.
air in c.
angiodysplasia of c.
anterior band of c.
antral diverticulum of the c.
arterial arch of c.
arteriovenous colon malformation
ascending c.
c. cancer
colitis colon antigen
Crohn disease of c.
descending c.
detected in colon cancer
distal c.
diverticular disease of c.
diverticulum of c.
duplication of c.
familial colon cancer
flexure of c.
Flint C. Injury Scale
foreshortening of the c.
hard, indurated colon mass
hepatic flexure of c.
hepatodiaphragmatic interposition of c.
hereditary adenomatosis of colon and rectum
hereditary colon cancer
hereditary nonpolyposis colon cancer
hereditary nonpolyposis colon carcinoma
hereditary site-specific colon cancer
iliac flexure of c.
inflammation of c.
irritable c.
irritable colon syndrome
large intestinal descending c.
left-sided colon cancer
longitudinal band of c.
longitudinal fasciculi of c.
marginal artery of c.
mesenteric attachments of c.
metachronous colon cancer
metastatic colon cancer
mucosa of c.
Muir-Torre syndrome of hereditary nonpolyposis colon cancer
multiple colon filling defect
muscular coat of c.
muscular layer of c.
mutated in colon cancer
neonatal small left colon syndrome
organic colon pathology
paradoxical colon dilatation
pedicled colon transfer
pelvic colon of Waldeyer
perforation of c.
peristalsis of c.
polyp of c.
polypoid adenocarcinoma of c.
proximal c.
c. resection
sacculation of c.
serosa of c.
sigmoid colon carcinoma
sigmoid flexure of c.
sphincter of hepatic flexure of c.
total colon examination
transverse c.

colonic
anhaustral colonic gas pattern
antegrade colonic enema
anti-40 kDa colonic antigen
antirefluxing colonic conduit
chronic ischemic colonic lesion caused by phlebosclerosis
c. diverticulum
familial colonic cancer
giant colonic diverticulum
c. hydrotherapy
inflammatory colonic polyp
c. irrigation
c. ischemia
Malone antegrade colonic enema stoma procedure
orthotopic colonic reservoir
paralytic colonic obstruction
patchy colonic ulcer
patchy colonic ulceration
pelvic colonic surgery
segmental colonic adenomatous polyposis syndrome
segmental colonic resection
segmental colonic tuberculosis
synchronous colonic adenocarcinoma
total colonic aganglionosis
c. transabdominal sonography

colonization
airway bacterial c.

colonization *(continued)*
atypical mycobacterial c.
c. factor
c. factor antigen
c. of host
perineal MRSA c.

colonizing organism

colonography
computed tomographic c.
magnetic resonance c.

colonoscope
fiberoptic c.
forward-viewing video c.
pediatric c.

colonoscopic
c. decompression
c. endoluminal ultrasound

colonoscopy
magnifying c.
pediatric c.
c. per rectum
c. per stoma
c. screening
surveillance c.
tandem c.
total c.
virtual c.

colon-specific
c.-s. antigen
c.-s. antigen protein

colony
c. of bacteria
bacterial adherent c.
coarse bacterial c.'s
c. count and culture
culture and sensitivity and colony count
endogenous erythroid c.
erythroid colony formation
human tumor colony assay
c. inhibition
mucoid c.
c. overlay test
c.'s per milliliter
rough bacterial c.
smooth bacterial c.
smooth-rough bacterial c.
spleen colony assay
surface c.

colony-forming
c.-f. assay
c.-f. capacity
c.-f. cell
c.-f. cells-spleen
c.-f. efficiency
c.-f. unit
c.-f. unit-culture
c.-f. unit-eosinophil
c.-f. unit-erythrocyte
c.-f. unit-erythroid
c.-f. unit-fibroblast
c.-f. unit-fibroblastoid
c.-f. unit-granulocyte, erythrocyte, megakaryocyte, macrophage
c.-f. unit-granulocyte-macrophage
c.-f. unit-lymphoid
c.-f. unit-megakaryocyte
c.-f. unit-neutrophil-monocyte
c.-f. units/mL
c.-f. unit-spleen
c.-f. unit-stem cell

colony-inhibiting activity

colony-stimulating
c.-s. activity
c.-s. factor
c.-s. factor-1
c.-s. factor developed by Venereal Disease Research Laboratory
c.-s. factor fluorescent treponemal antibody-absorption test
c.-s. factor microhemagglutination-*Treponema pallidum* test
granulocyte colony-stimulating factor
granulocyte-macrophage colony-stimulating activity
granulocyte-macrophage colony-stimulating factor

Colorado
C. tick fever
C. tick fever virus

ColorChecker
Macbeth C.

color-coded
c.-c. duplex sonography
c.-c. flow mapping

colorectal
c. adenocarcinoma
c. anastomosis
aneuploid colorectal carcinoma
c. cancer
c. carcinoma
c. dysmotility
hereditary nonpolyposis colorectal cancer
hereditary nonpolyposis colorectal carcinoma
metastatic colorectal carcinoma
mutated colorectal carcinoma
nonpolyposis colorectal cancer
obstructing colorectal cancer
obstructive colorectal cancer
perforating colorectal carcinoma
c. polyp
primary colorectal cancer
recurrent colorectal cancer
c. stricture
c. surgery

colored
nonblanchable, abnormally colored lesion
C. Progressive Matrices
Raven C. Progressive Matrices Test
c. vision
C. Visual Analogue Scale

color-flow
c.-f. Doppler
c.-f. Doppler sonography
c.-f. duplex imaging
c.-f. duplex scan
c.-f. imaging
c.-f. imaging Doppler echocardiography

colorimeter
differential scanning c.

colorimetric
anthrone colorimetric technique
c. assay
c. method
c. microtiter plate
c. test
c. titration

colorimetry, including spectrophotometry and photometry

colorless gas

colostomy
closure of c.
decompression c.
diverting c.
diverting colostomy with pull-through procedure
diverting loop c.
diverting proximal c.
double-barreled c.
end-to-side ileotransverse c.
ileotransverse c.
c. irrigation
longitudinal c.
loop c.
Mikulicz c.
nonirrigating descending c.
normal functioning ileal transverse c.
permanent c.

permanent end c.
resected end-to-end ileal c.
c. sac
sigmoid c.
sigmoid loop c.
c. takedown
takedown of c.
transverse c.
c. tube
Wangensteen c.

colovaginal fistula

colovesical fistula

colporrhaphy
posterior c.

colposcopic
atypical vessel colposcopic pattern
c. grading of cervical dysplasia

colposcopically directed brushing

colposcopy
intensive c.
normal transformation zone colposcopy

colpostat
Fletcher afterloading c.

colposuspension
Nottingham colposuspension needle

colpotomy
posterior c.

colpourethropexy
modified Burch c.

Columbia Mental Maturity Scale

columella
c. clamp
midline of c.

columellar strut

column
anterior c.
anterior column disruption
anterior column fracture
anterior column of medulla oblongata
anterior column osteosynthesis
anterior column of spinal cord
anterior column of spine
anterior gray c.
anterior gray column of cord
anterolateral column of spinal cord
autonomic column of spinal cord
c. of Berlin
capillary column gas chromatography
cervical Pantopaque c.
dorsal c.
dorsal cell c.
dorsal column nucleus
dorsal column stimulation
dorsal column stimulator
gliosis of anterior c.
gliosis of lateral c.
intermediate cell c.
lateral motor c.
medial cell c.
medial column calcaneal fracture
medial column instability
middle column injury
c. of Morgagni
Morgagni c.'s
new column of bone
ocular dominance c.
posterior c.
resin hemoperfusion c.
serum thyroxine measured by column chromatography
ventral c.
ventral cell c.
vertebral column defect

columnar
c. cell
c. cell variant
circumoral area of columnar epithelium
endocervical columnar mucosa
c. epithelium
low columnar cell
metaplastic columnar epithelium
mucinous columnar metaplasia
c. mucosa
papilla of columnar epithelium
specialized columnar epithelium

columnar-lined
c.-l. esophagus
c.-l. lower esophagus

coma
acute hepatic c.
alpha frequency c.
atropine coma therapy
catatonia, coma and convulsions
Children's C. Score
convulsion and c.
deep hepatic c.
Edinburgh 2 C. Scale
electrolyte imbalance c.
Glasgow Coma Scale
Glasgow C. Score
hyperosmolar hyperglycemic nonketotic c.
hyperosmolar nonketotic diabetic c.
hypotension and c.
induction of c.
insulin coma therapy
Maryland coma scale
nonketotic c.
nonketotic hyperglycmic-hyperosmolar c.
nonketotic hyperosmolar c.
paralysis and c.
c. secondary to head trauma

comatosa
malaria c.

comatose
patient deeply c.

combat
armed c.
c. casualty
c. crawl
c. fatigue
c. flashback
c. neurosis
c. reaction
c. rejection of transplanted organ
c. stress exposure
c. support hospital
c. trauma
c. veteran

combative
c. and agitated
c. and confused
confused and c.
patient combative and agitated

combination
antibiotic combination therapy
antiretroviral triple combination therapy
atlas-axis combination fracture
axis-atlas combination fracture
beta-lactamase inhibitor c.
c. chemotherapy
c. drug
esophagotracheal combination tube
fixed ratio combination drugs
c. high- and low-energy x-ray therapy
c. hormone therapy
intensive combination chemotherapy
c. of isotonics
light-induced fluorescence endoscopy in combination with pharmacoendoscopy
linear combination of atomic orbital-molecular orbital

combination *(continued)*
linear combination of atomic orbitals
linear combination of fragment configuration
linear combination model software
low anterior resection in combination with coloanal anastomosis
low-dose combination oral contraceptive
c. oral contraceptive
penicillin-inhibitor c.'s
periodic acid-Schiff-Alcian blue combination stain
c. product
c. retinoid and PUVA therapy
sequential combination chemotherapy

combined
adult-onset combined methylmalonic aciduria and homocystinuria
advanced combined encoder
c. androgen blockade
c. anesthesia
c. antiretroviral therapy
c. aphasia
Athabascan type of severe combined immunodeficiency disease
c. atrial hypertrophy
attention deficit hyperactivity disorder, combined type
autosomal recessive severe combined immunodeficiency disorder
c. central and obstructive sleep apnea
c. chemotherapy/radiation therapy
c. cold and warm antibody autoimmune hemolytic anemia
c. cortical thickness
c. diphtheria tetanus
c. drug and radiation modality
c. effects
epithelioid combined nevi
epithelioid combined nevi deep penetrating nevus
familial combined hyperlipidemia
c. fat- and carbohydrate-induced hyperlipidemia
c. flexion-distraction injury and burst fracture
c. fracture
c. germ cell tumor
c. heart catheterization
c. hemorrhoids
c. high-frequency ventilation
c. hormone therapy
c. hyperthermia and radiation treatment
c. immune deficiency disease
immune response and combined modality treatment
c. immunodeficiency
c. immunodeficiency disease
c. immunodeficiency syndrome
independent toxicity in combined modality therapy
c. intermittent therapy
c. intracapsular cataract extraction
c. kidney and pancreas transplant
low steroid content combined oral contraceptive
c. mechanical
c. mitral stenosis and regurgitation
c. modality therapy
multiple combined sclerosis
c. multisection diffuse-weighted and hemodynamically weighted echoplanar MR
c. nevi
c. oral contraceptive
partial combined immunodeficiency disorder
PCR combined with single-strand conformation polymorphism
penicillin G benzathine and procaine c.
c. pituitary hormone deficiency
severe combined immune deficiency
severe combined immune deficiency syndrome
severe combined immunodeficiency disease
severe combined immunodeficient mice
c. spinal-epidural anesthesia
subacute combined degeneration of spinal cord
c. system disease
c. testicular weight
c. ventricular hypertrophy
X-linked severe combined immunodeficiency

combing
carbon dioxide combing power

combining
antibody combining site
c. power
c. power test

comedo
c. carcinoma
c. nevus
open c.
solar c.

comedolytic agent

comedonal acne

comfort
acoustic comfort index
level of c.
maximal comfort level
c. measures only
patient treated with comfort care only
position of c.

comfortable
Békésy comfortable loudness
most comfortable frequency
most comfortable listening level
most comfortable loudness level
most comfortable loudness range
range of comfortable loudness
c. walking speed

comitant artery of median nerve

comma appearance

command
c. auditory hallucination
c. automatism
does not follow c.'s
follows c.'s
c. hallucination
negative c.
patient obeys c.'s
patient responsive to verbal c.
respond to verbal c.
time to following c.'s

commercial dialysis solution

commercially pure

comminuted
compound comminuted fracture
c. fracture
fracture complete, compound, and c.
fracture compound and c.
fracture simple complete and c.
c. intraarticular fracture
c. orbital fracture
c. skull fracture
c. tibial fracture

commissural
c. associated
median commissural artery

commissure
anterior c.
anterior commissure of labia
anterior commissure of larynx
anterior commissure ligament
anterior commissure-posterior c.
anterior gray c.
anterior labial c.
anterior part of anterior commissure of brain
anterior white c.
c. of fornix
Ganser c.
great transverse c.
c. of lips and mouth
medial commissure of eyelid
Meynert c.
nucleus of posterior c.
oral commissure movement
posterior c.

commissuroplasty
oral c.

commissurotomy
balloon mitral c.
closed chest c.
mitral c.
mitral balloon c.
open mitral c.
open mitral valve c.
percutaneous balloon c.
percutaneous mitral c.
percutaneous mitral balloon c.
percutaneous transatrial mitral c.
percutaneous transvenous mitral c.

commitment
legal c.
outpatient commitment order

committed
erythroid committed precursor
legally c.
c. progenitor cell

committee
hospital management c.
Human Investigation C.
human rights c.
National Joint C. on Learning Disabilities
peer review c.
radioactive drug research c.
residency review c.

commode
bedside c.

common
c. acne
c. acute lymphoblastic leukemia antigen
c. acute lymphocytic leukemia antigen
c. antigen
antropyloroduodenal common chamber
c. atrioventricular canal
c. atrioventricular orifice
c. baldness
c. bile duct
c. bile duct diverticulum
c. bile duct exploration
c. bile duct microlithiasis
c. bile duct obstruction
c. bile duct stent
c. bile duct stone
c. bile duct stricture
c. business-oriented language
c. carotid artery
c. carotid artery bifurcation
c. carotid artery intima-media thickness
c. carotid compression
c. duct
c. duct exploration
c. duct pigment stone
enterobacterial common antigen
exploration of common bile duct
c. femoral artery
c. femoral artery-superficial femoral artery
final common pathway
frequency of the more common allele of a pair
c. gateway interface
greatest common factor
c. hepatic artery
c. hepatic duct
highest common factor
c. iliac
c. iliac lymph nodes
c. iliac vein
c. immunodeficiency
c. internal iliac artery
laparoscopic common duct exploration
laparoscopic exploration of the common bile duct
laparoscopic transcystic common bile duct exploration
c. law marriage
least common factor
left common carotid artery
left common femoral artery
leukocyte common antigen
lowest common multiple
c. migraine
c. mode rejection
muscle of common bile duct
narrowing of common duct
occluded common bile duct
occluded common bile duct stone
open common bile duct exploration
c. palmar digital nerve
c. palmar digital nerve of lateral plantar nerves
c. palmar digital nerve of medial nerve
c. palmar digital nerve of ulnar nerve
pancreaticobiliary common channel
c. peak developed isovolumetric pressure
perforation of common bile duct
c. peroneal nerve
c. plantar digital nerve of medial plantar nerve
right common carotid
right common carotid artery
right common femoral angioplasty
right common femoral artery
c. sense judgment
c. source outbreak
sphincter of common bile duct
c. variable hypogammaglobulinemia
c. variable immunodeficiency
velocity, common carotid artery

communal traumatic experiences inventory

communicable
c. disease
C. Disease Center

communicans
arteria communicans anterior
arteria communicans posterior
macula c.
nervus communicans peroneus

communicate
inability to c.

communicated insanity

communicating
accessory communicating tendon
aneurysm of posterior communicating artery
anterior communicating aneurysm
anterior communicating artery

communicating *(continued)*
anterior communicating artery aneurysm
anterior communicating artery complex
anterior communicating artery distribution infarct
anterior communicating artery distribution infarction
anterior-inferior communicating artery
c. artery aneurysm
c. branch of glossopharyngeal nerve with auricular branch of vagus nerve
distal communicating branch
c. hydrocele
c. hydrocephalus
laser photocoagulation of the communicating vessel
peroneal communicating branch
posterior communicating aneurysm
posterior communicating artery aneurysm
posterior inferior communicating artery
proximal communicating branch
c. vein incompetence

communication
C. Abilities Diagnostic Test
Adapted Sequenced Inventory of C. Development
advanced communications function
anomalous pancreaticobiliary c.
Arizona Battery for C. Disorders of Dementia
augmentative and alternative c.
augmentative communication system
data c.
c. deviance
c. disorder
distorted communication in schizophrenia
Early Social C. Scale
Emergency C.'s Center
Evaluating Acquired Skills in C.
facilitated c.
fluids, aeration, nutrition, communication, activity, and pain
fluids, aeration, nutrition, communication, activity, and stimulation
gap junction intercellular c.
impaired verbal c.
c. impairment
interatrial c.
Interpersonal C. Inventory
Inventory of Anger C.'s
local area communications network
manipulation communication pattern
medical ultrasound 3D portable, with advanced c.
Mother/Infant C. Screening
nonconfrontational communication skills
nonverbal communication skill
order/results c.
parent-child communication schedule
picture archival communication system
Premarital C. Inventory
Rating Scale of C. in Cognitive Decline
c. in sign language
c. skills assessment
treatment and education of autistic and related communications handicapped children
visual communication therapy

communicative
C. Abilities in Daily Living
c. assessment
c. development inventory
c. disorder
c. function
c. gesture
Porch Index of C. Abilities in Children
promoting aphasics communicative effectiveness

communicatively impaired

communis
arteria cochlearis c.
arteria digitalis palmaris c.
arteria digitalis plantaris c.
arteria hepatica c.
extensor digiti c.
extensor digitorum c.
extensor digitorum communis muscle
extensor digitorum communis tendon
flexor digitorum c.

community
c. acquired
alternative lifestyle c.
c. ambulator
Ashkenazi Jewish c.
c. care unit
C. College Student Experiences Questionnaire
continuing community care
c. education
c. health center
c. health management information system
c. health network
hospital and community psychiatry
c. hypertension evaluation clinic
c. immunity
C. Integration Questionnaire
c. leave for reorientation
c. living arrangements
c. meeting
c. mental health center
mental health c.
middle class c.
c. nursing home
c. organization
c. periodontal index of treatment needs
c. resources
c. safety
sole community hospital
therapeutic c.

community-acquired
c.-a. bladder infection
c.-a. immunodeficiency syndrome
c.-a. infection
c.-a. meningitis
c.-a. organism
c.-a. pneumonia
c.-a. respiratory infection
c.-a. sepsis

community-based
c.-b. clinic
c.-b. distribution
c.-b. mental health treatment
c.-b. psychiatric program

community-oriented
c.-o. primary care
C.-o. Programs Environment Scale

comorbid
c. addictive behavior
c. alcohol abuse
c. cocaine abuse
c. condition
c. dementia
c. disease
c. generalized anxiety
c. illness

c. medical problem
c. mental disorder
c. psychopathology

comorbidity
age-related c.
anxiety c.
anxiety-mood c.
Charlson comorbidity index
medical c.
c. of mental disorder
multiple anxiety c.
National C. Study
psychiatric c.
c. of schizophrenia and substance abuse

compactor
McSpadden c.

compact substance of bone

company
neurologic c.

comparative
c. anatomy
c. genomic hybridization
C. Guidance and Placement Program
c. medicine
c. physiology

compared with previous study

compare with

comparison
beam quality c.
systematic c.

compartment
abdominal compartment syndrome
acute compartment syndrome
acute exertional compartment syndrome
adductor compartment of thigh
anterior compartment of arm
anterior compartment of forearm
anterior compartment of leg
anterior compartment syndrome
anterior compartment of thigh
anterior mediastinal c.
anterior tibial c.
anterior tibial compartment syndrome
chronic anterior exertional compartment syndrome
chronic compartment syndrome
deep c.
exertional anterior compartment syndrome
exertional deep posterior compartment syndrome
extensor compartment of arm
extensor compartment of forearm
extensor compartment of leg
extensor compartment of thigh
extracellular c.
extracellular fluid c.
c. fasciotomy
foot compartment syndrome
lateral compartment reconstruction
medial brachial fascial c.
medial compartment disruption
medial compartment injury
medial compartment of thigh
myeloblast-promyelocyte c.
orbital compartment syndrome
peroneal compartment syndrome
posterior compartment of arm
posterior compartment of forearm
posterior compartment of leg
posterior compartment of thigh
c. procedure
shallow c.
c. syndrome

compassionate
c. release
c. use

compassionate-use basis

compatibility
maternal-fetal HLA c.
MRI c.
Sexual C. Test

compatible
confirmed and c.
c. with
c. with grand mal

compelling
autosomal dominant compelling helioophthalmic outburst syndrome

compensable
designated compensable event
potentially compensable event

compensated
c. base
c. cardiac status
c. congestive heart failure
c. heart failure

compensation
accommodation and c.
c., pension, and education
flow c.
length contraction compensation element
mean frequency of c.
motion compensation gradient pulse
c. neurosis
c. and pension
c. reaction
reasonable compensation equivalent
special monthly c.
temperature c.
time compensation gain
time-gain c.
workers' c.

compensator
beam c.
Multivane Intensity Modulation C.
time-gain c.

compensatory
c. antiinflammatory response syndrome
c. blood supply
c. bone resorption
c. circulation
c. feedback
c. hypertrophy
c. hypertrophy of heart muscle
c. lordosis
c. scoliosis

competence
apparent c.
assessment of c.
Fisher-Logemann Test of Articulation C.
linguistic c.
measure of c.
mental c.
Psychotherapy C. Assessment Schedule
Test of Language C.
velopharyngeal c.
Vineland Measurement of Social C.

competency
c. assessment
assessment of basic c.
California Preschool Social C. Scale
c. standard
Test of Work C. and Stability

competent
chromosomally competent ovarian failure
conscious and mentally c.
mentally c.

competing
contralateral competing message

competing *(continued)*
ipsilateral competing message
c. message

competition
message competition ratio

competitive
c. insulin autoantibodies
c. polymerase chain reaction
c. protein binding
c. protein-binding assay
quantitative competitive PCR
quantitative competitive polymerase chain reaction
c. reverse transcription-polymerase chain reaction

competitive-binding assay

complainer
help-rejecting c.

complains
patient complains of

complaint
chief c.
entering c.
entrance c.
history of chief c.
history of present c.
Inventory of Psychic and Somatic C.'s in the Elderly
neck c.
no c.'s
no complaints offered
no previous c.
patient denies c.'s
present c.
vague abdominal c.'s

complement
c. 1–8
acidified c.
acidified serum, acidified c.
alternative pathway of complement cascade
alternative patterns of c.
autoimmune complement fixation
c. C7
c. C8
c. C9
cardiolipin complement fixation
conglutinating complement absorption test
c. control protein
erythrocyte, antibody, and c.
c. factor
first component of c.
c. fixation
c. fixation antibody test
c. fixation inhibition
c. fixing
fragment, antigen, and complement binding
guinea pig c.
hemolytic complement assay
immunodiffusion complement fixation
lesion on erythrocyte cell membrane at the site of complement fixation
c. level
lymphogranuloma venereum complement fixation test
normal complement of cells
platelet complement fixation test
progestin-binding c.
rapid plasma reagin complement fixation
c. receptor 1–4
c. receptor location
c. receptor lymphocyte
serum complement C1–C9
soluble complement receptor
c. test
total hemolytic c.
total serum hemolytic c.
Treponema pallidum complement fixation
Treponema pallidum cryolysis c.
whole c.

complement-activated plasma

complementarity-determining region

complementary
c. and alternative approach
c. and alternative medicine
c. balloon angioplasty
c. deoxyribonucleic acid
c. hypertrophy
c. induction
c. medical practice
c. metal-oxide semiconductor logic

complement-binding antibody

complement-dependent
c.-d. antibody
c.-d. cytotoxicity

complement-fixation
c.-f. reaction

complement-fixing
c.-f. antibody
c.-f. antibody consumption
immunodiffusion c.-f.

complement-mediated cytotoxicity

complete
c. abortion
c. abstinence
c. amputation
c. androgen insensitivity
c. androgen insensitivity syndrome
anterior complete dislocation
c. atrioventricular block
c. atrioventricular dissociation
c. AV block
c. A-V dissociation
c. bedrest
c. blood cell count
c. blood count
c. bowel obstruction
c. breech presentation
c. bundle-branch block
c. change of drapes, gowns and instruments
c. clinical remission
congenital complete heart block
continuous complete remission
c. continuous remission
c. denture impression
disease in complete remission
c. dislocation
c. emptying of bladder
fracture, complete, angulated
fracture complete and compound
fracture complete, compound, and comminuted
fracture complete and deviated
fracture complete and varus deformity
fracture simple and c.
fracture simple complete and comminuted
c. Freund adjuvant
Freund complete adjuvant
c. gynecologic examination annually
c. harelip
c. healing
c. heart block
c. hemianopia
c. hernia
c. hysterectomy
c. impairment of conduction
c. iridectomy
c. laparoscopic distal pancreatectomy
c. left bundle-branch block
c. left bundle branch block
longitudinal displaced complete tear
c. lower motor neuron lesion

c. lymph node dissection
c. maturation arrest
c. medium
c. myocardial infarction
nodular complete response
c. obstruction of airway
c. and ongoing assessment
c. and pain-free range of motion
pathologically confirmed complete remission
patient at complete bed rest
patient in complete restraint
patient c.'s independent transfers
persistent complete atrioventricular canal
c. physical
c. physical examination
c. placenta previa
c. psychosocial history
range of motion complete and pain-free
c. reaction of degeneration
c. responders
c. response
c. right bundle branch block
selective complete lymph node dissection
c. simple mastectomy
c. situs inversus
c. small bowel obstruction
c. subtalar release
c. surgical exploration
systematic, complete, objective, practical, empirical
time required to complete G_1 phase of cell cycle
time required to complete G_2 phase of cell cycle
time required to complete M phase of cell cycle
time required to complete S phase of cell cycle
c. transposition of great arteries
c. transposition of great vessels
unconfirmed/uncertain complete remission
c. upper and lower dentures
c. weightbearing

completed

not c.
c. stroke
c. suicide
treatment c.

completely

bladder emptied c.
c. in the canal hearing aid
c. denatured
c. denatured alcohol
c. follicular
lower completely edentulous
c. randomized design
upper completely edentulous

completeness

metastasis, age, completeness of resection, local invasion, and tumor size

completing

left without completing treatment
C. Sentence Test

completion

c., arithmetic problems, vocabulary, following directions
c. bed occupancy care
Forer Sentence C. Test
Franck Drawing C. Test
picture c.
Rotter Sentence C. Test
Sacks Sentence C. Test
Stein Sentence Completion Test

complex

acquired immune deficiency syndrome dementia c.
acquired immune deficiency syndrome-related c.
acquired immunodeficiency syndrome-related c.
active ankle joint complex range of motion
AIDS dementia c.
AIDS-related c.
amphotericin B lipid c.
anisoylated plasminogen streptokinase activator c.
ankle joint c.
anterior communicating artery c.
antigen 85 c.
antigen-nonspecific immune complex assay
antiinhibitor coagulant c.
antimajor histocompatibility c.
antiphosphatidylserine-prothrombin complex antibody testing
aortic tract complex hypoplasia
aromatase enzyme c.
arteriovenous glomus c.
atlas vertebral subluxation c.
atrial premature c.
c. atypical hyperplasia/metaplasia
avian leukemia-sarcoma c.
avian leukosis c.
avian leukosis-sarcoma c.
avidin-biotin c.
avidin-biotin complex assay
avidin-biotin-horseradish peroxidase c.
avidin-biotin peroxidase c.
avidin-biotin-peroxidase complex method
axial mesodermal dysplasia c.
bacterial antigen c.
c. benign disease
circulating immune c.
coenzyme A-synthesizing protein c.
contractile electrical c.
critical care c.
death-inducing signaling c.
c. disorder of adolescence
c. disorder of childhood
disseminated *Mycobacterium avium-intracellulare* c.
dissociation of enzyme-inhibitor c.
dorsal vein c.
Dubois oleic albumin c.
Dubois oleic serum c.
eczema, asthma, and hay fever c.
electrocardiographic interval from the beginning of QRS complex to end of the T wave
electrocardiographic junction between QRS complex and ST segment
electrocardiographic wave in QRS c.
enzyme inhibition c.
c. febrile seizure
C. Figure Test
c. fixation
food immune complex assay
Golgi c.
hemoglobin-haptoglobin c.
Heymann nephritis antigenic c.
hypothalamoneurohypophysial c.
immune c.
immune complex dissociation
immune complex glomerulonephritis
immune complex precipitation
immune complex reaction
immunostimulating c.
inferior glenohumeral ligament labral c.
c. instability of carpus
c. interaction
interdigestive migrating motor c.
interdigestive motility c.
interdigestive motor c.
interdigestive myoelectric c.

complex *(continued)*
intervertebral joint c.
ketoglutarate dehydrogenase c.
lateral collateral ligament c.
limb-body wall c.
lipophilic cationic c.
liver, iron, and B c.
c. loading
lymphomyeloid c.
major histocompatibility c.
major histocompatibility complex antigen
major histocompatibility complex class I
major histocompatibility complex class II
major histocompatibility complex haplotype
major histocompatibility complex restriction
major symptom c.
malar complex fracture
membrane attack c.
membranolytic attack c.
mesangial complex formation
mesenteric adenitis-ileitis c.
metal chelate c.
methylthymol blue c.
migrating action potential c.
migrating motor c.
migrating myoelectric c.
minor histocompatibility c.
mitochondrial respiratory chain enzyme c.
model immune c.
c. motor seizure
c. motor tic
c. motor unit
multiple complex developmental disorder
Mycobacterium avium c.
Mycobacterium avium complex infection
Mycobacterium avium-intracellulare c.
Mycobacterium fortuitum-chelonae c.
Mycobacterium fortuitum c.
Mycobacterium fortuitum third biovar c.
Mycobacterium terrae-triviale c.
narrow complex supraventricular tachycardia
narrow complex tachycardia
nephroblastomatosis c.
nipple-areola c.
nuclear pore c.
c. oncologic therapy protocol
optic complex tumor
organ inferiority c.
orthocresolphthalein c.
outer anular/posterior longitudinal ligament c.
Parkinson dementia c.
Parkinson disease and lateral sclerosis-dementia c.
parkinsonism-dementia c.
partial complex epilepsy
partial complex seizure
c. partial epilepsy
c. partial nocturnal seizure
c. partial status epilepticus
passive castration c.
peptide major histocompatibility c.
peptidomimetic inhibitor c.
periodic sharp wave c.
plasmin-inhibitor c.
polysaccharide-iron c.
polysaccharide iron c.
premature atrial c.
premature atrioventricular junction c.
premature junctional c.
premature ventricular c.
protein-lipid c.
prothrombin c.
c. psychophysiological process
pyruvate dehydrogenase complex deficiency
c. reaction time
receptor-chemoeffector c.
reference point following QRS complex, at beginning of ST segment
c. regional pain syndrome
c. repetitive discharge
c. retinal detachment
Rey-Estreich C. Figure Test
Rey-Osterrieth complex figure
rhodopsin-lipid c.
c. rotational movement
sign symptom c.
c. simple fracture
soluble c.
soluble fibrin-fibrinogen c.
soluble fibrin monomer c.
streptavidin-biotin peroxidase c.
synthesizing protein c.
temporal c.
time between P wave and beginning of QRS complex in electrocardiography
total symptom c.
transjugular fibrocartilage c.
triangular fibrocartilage c.
triangular fibrocartilage complex tear
triangular fibrocartilaginous c.
tuberous sclerosis c.
tuboovarian c.
tumor-inducing c.
c. unroofed coronary sinus
ventricular premature c.
vertebral subluxation c.
vitamin B c.
von Meyenburg c.
c. wave form
zygomatic malar c.
zygomatic maxillary c.
zygomaticomaxillary c.
zygomaxillary c.

complex-combined vascular malformation

complexed prostate-specific antigen

complexity
environmental c.
gradual increase in length and complexity of utterance
length complexity index
c. of mental processes

compliance
abnormal increase in c.
chest wall c.
c., rate, oxygenation, and pressure
c., rate, oxygenation, and pressure index
consistent medication c.
dynamic compliance of lung
effective dynamic c.
frequency dependence of c.
c. of heart
c. of lung
overt compliance masking covert resistance
quasistatic c.
c. rate
c. related acute complication
c. of the respiratory system
respiratory system compliance score
static lung c.
total lung c.
total static c.

compliant prestress system

complicated
c. delivery
c. grief disorder
c. postoperative course

postoperative course c.
pregnancy, term, complicated delivered, living female
pregnancy, term, complicated delivered, living male

complication

adverse neurologic c.
alopecia, nail dystrophy, ophthalmic complication, thyroid dysfunction, hypohidrosis, ephelides and enteropathy, and respiratory tract infection
assessing severity: age of patient, systems involved, stage of disease, complications, response to therapy
cardiovascular complications of drug abuse
compliance related acute c.
deep abdominal c.
c. of drug abuse
endocrine organ transplant c.
Epidemiology of Diabetes Interventions and C.'s
fatal complications of illicit drug use
hepatic complications of drug abuse
implant related c.'s
medical complications of obesity
metabolic organ transplant c.
neonatal complications of drug abuse
neurologic complication of systemic cancer
neuromuscular complication of drug abuse
no apparent anesthetic c.
no intraoperative c.'s
noninfectious disease c.
ocular complications of diabetes
operative site c.
perioperative cardiac c.
pregnancy and birth c.
procedures, alternatives, indications and c.'s
sexual complications of drug abuse
surgical complication of drug abuse
thromboembolic c.

component

allogenic blood c.
amyloid P c.
anatomic graduated c.
anatomic porous replacement hemispheric acetabular c.
anterior component of force
anterograde fast component neuropathy
arousal component of consciousness
articulatory loop c.
Aufranc-Turner femoral c.
autonomous functional c.
bipolar femoral c.
blood component therapy
buffer-soluble binding c.
cementless femoral c.
chamfered cylinder acetabular c.
expand internal c.'s of knee
extensive intraductal c.
fast component of neuron
femoral component pusher
first component of complement
free secretory c.
gastric component of reflex barrier
group-specific c.
high molecular weight c.
individual c.'s
late positive c.
major component of adult hemoglobin
membrane component of diffusion
Mental C. Summary
metal-backed acetabular c.
micropapillary c.
monoblock femoral c.
myeloma or macroglobulinemia c.
Neer II humeral c.
nonmetric principal component analysis
c. of occlusion
Osteolock acetabular c.
parallel elastic component of muscle
particulate c.
p55 component of the high-affinity interleukin-2
Physical C. Summary
plasma thromboplastin c.
Press-Fit c.
pressure at slow component intercept
principal c.'s analysis
proinsulin-like c.
risk reduction c.
secretory c.
series elastic component of muscles
serum amyloid P c.
slow c.
thromboplastic cell c.
thromboplastic plasma c.

composite

c. allograft
auricular composite graft
autogenous composite tissue
c. buildup
c. clinical and laboratory index
c. cultured skin
c. cyclic therapy
c. extrarenal rhabdoid tumor
c. filling
c. flap
c. fracture
c. free tissue transfer
c. ganglioneuroblastoma
c. graft
c. joint
C. Laryngeal Recurrence Staging System
ligamentous anterior dislocation composite graft
c. lymphoma
c. mandibular reconstruction
c. material
microfilled c.
microfilled composite resin
narcissistic c.
c. onlay
c. resin
C. Risk Index
c. treatment score
c. valve graft
void metal c.

compound

artificial lung-expanding c.
c. cathartic
c. character
c. comminuted fracture
debridement of compound skull fracture
evoked compound electromyography
fracture complete and c.
fracture complete, compound, and comminuted
fracture compound and comminuted
c. ganglion
c. hypermetropic astigmatism
c. hyperopic astigmatism
c. insanity
c. joint
liquid organic c.
macromolecular nonlipid c.
macromolecular polar c.
mechanical compound scan

compound *(continued)*
metallic compound inhalation
morphine-like c.
c. motor action potential
c. muscle action potential
c. muscle-motor action potential
c. myopic astigmatism
c. nerve action potential
N-nitroso c.
nonsteroidal antiinflammatory c.
open chain c.
organophosphorous compound poisoning
ouabain-like c.
pedicled compound rib-latissimus dorsi osteomusculocutaneous flap
phosphate carrier c.
Q c.
quaternary ammonium c.'s
spermicide-germicide c.
volatile organic c.'s
volatile organic c.
volatile sulfur c.

compound-Q treatment

comprehension
Assessment of Children's Language C.
auditory c.
auditory comprehension impairment
auditory comprehension of language
Auditory C. Test for Sentences
Carrow Test for Auditory C.
c. deficit
impaired c.
Listening C. Test
Miller-Yoder Test of Grammatical C.
passage c.
Progressive Achievement Tests of Listening C.
Screening Test for Auditory C. of Language
c. span
Test of Early Reading C.
Tests for Auditory C. of Language
Tests for Auditory C. of Language-Revised
verbal c.
verbal comprehension deviation quotient
verbal comprehension factor
Vocabulary C. Scale

comprehensive
C. Ability Battery
c. ambulatory care
c. assessment
c. assessment of symptoms and history
c. cancer center
c. cardiac care unit
c. care clinic
C. Career Assessment Scale
Children's C. Pain Questionnaire
Final C. Consensus Assessment
c. geriatric assessment
c. health care institution
c. health enhancement support system
c. health insurance plan
c. hospital infections project
c. identification process
c. inpatient treatment
C. Level of Consciousness Scale
c. medical history
c. medical plan
c. mental health
Minnesota C. Epilepsy Program
National C. Cancer Network
c. outpatient rehabilitation facility
c. outpatient treatment
C. Psychopathological Rating Scale
c. renal scintillation procedure
c. support care team
C. Test of Visual Functioning
c. treatment plan

compress
hot c.
hot moist c.'s
warm c.
warm compresses and lid scrubs
wet c.

compressed
c. air
c. air-driven nebulizer
c. air-powered dermatome
coated compressed tablet
c. electroencephalogram
c. fracture
multiple compressed tablet
Ohio pediatric tent with compressed air
c. spectral array
c. spectral assay
c. tablet triturate

compressed-air
c.-a. disease
c.-a. sickness

compression
abdominal c.
air compression osteotome
anomalous innominate artery compression syndrome
anterior cord c.
anterior-posterior c.
anterolateral compression fracture
AO-ASIF compression technique
AO compression apparatus
Apley compression maneuver
Apley compression test
arteriomesenteric duodenal compression syndrome
arthroscopic monopolar thermal stabilization forefoot compression sleeve
ASIF broad dynamic c.
Axer compression apparatus
Axer compression device
axial compression fracture
axial compression injury
axial compression load
axial compression principle
axial compression screw
axial compression test
c. bandage
c. boot
c. of the brain
bulky compression dressing
c. button
cable-hook compression instrumentation
c. of carotid artery
carotid compression tomography
carotid compression tonography
carotid sinus c.
celiac artery compression syndrome
cervical disc c.
circumferential pneumatic c.
circumferential pneumatic compression suit
common carotid c.
direct cardiac c.
dynamic c.
dynamic compression plate
dynamic compression plate fixation
eccentric dynamic compression plating
elastic compression stocking
epidural cord c.
epidural spinal cord c.
European compression technique bone screw and internal fixation
external cardiac c.
external pneumatic c.
external pneumatic calf c.

extrinsic biliary c.
extrinsic bladder c.
extrinsic compression of airway
extrinsic compression of trachea
c. flexion injury
c. fracture
c. fracture of spine
c. glove
graduated compression garment
graduated compression stockings
head c.
high-frequency chest wall c.
c. hip screw
ice, compression, and elevation
ice, compression, elevation, and support
c. injury
intermittent pneumatic compression boot
interposed abdominal c.
intervertebral disc c.
jugular compression test
c. lag screw
lateral c.
c. of liver cords
c. loading
local compression fracture
low-contact dynamic compression plate
lower sacral nerve root c.
metastatic cord c.
metastatic epidural spinal cord c.
microvascular compression syndrome
modulus of c.
Mueller compression apparatus
napkin ring c.
nerve compression anesthesia
nerve compression syndrome
nerve root c.
c. neuropathy
neurovascular compression syndrome
neurovascular cross c.
open-chest cardiac c.
optic chiasm c.
optic tract c.
osteoporotic compression fracture
c. paddle
c. paralysis
pathologic compression fracture
c. and percussion
peripheral root c.
c. plate fixation
c. plate and screw
c. plating
pneumatic compression boot
pneumatic compression sleeve
pneumatic compression stocking
pneumatic compression therapy
protection, rest, ice, compression, elevation, support
protection, restricted activity, ice, compression, elevation
rest, ice, compression, elevation
c. rod treatment
sciatic nerve c.
sequential compression device
c. sideplate
simultaneous compression ventilation-cardiopulmonary resuscitation
slow spinal cord compression syndrome
soft tissue compression injury
spinal compression fracture
spinal cord c.
c. of spinal nerve
c. stockings
subclavian vein c.
superior vena cava compression syndrome
suprascapular nerve c.
c. syndrome
c. therapy
c. to traction ratio
ulnar compression neuropathy
ulnar nerve c.
c. ultrasonography
c. ultrasound
ultrasound-guided compression repair
umbilical cord c.
uterine compression syndrome
c. and ventilation
wide dynamic range c.
c. wire
Wisconsin C. System
wrist hand extension compression support

compression-decompression
active c.-d.

compression-type deformity

compressive
anterior compressive optic neuropathy
cold compressive dressing

compressor
c. muscle of naris
orbital enucleation c.

compressor-generated nebulizer

compromise
acute vascular c.
angiitic luminal c.
circulatory c.
microcirculatory c.
neurovascular c.
organ c.
vascular c.

compromised
c. host
immune compromised host
c. ineffective family coping
c. renal function

Compton scatter tomography

compulsion
antisocial c.
hand washing c.
c. neurosis
c. psychoneurosis

compulsive
c. act
c. buying
Children's Yale-Brown Obsessive C. Scale
destructive compulsive disease
c. drug-taking behavior
c. eater
c. gambler
c. gambling
c. hair pulling
c. idea
c. impulse control disorder
c. insanity
c. mania
c. masturbation
Maudsley Obsessional C. Inventory
mixed compulsive states psychasthenia
National Institute of Mental Health-Global Obsessive C. Scale
c. neurosis
obsessional compulsive inventory alpha
patient highly c.
c. personality
c. personality disorder
c. self-mutilation
c. sexual behavior
c. spasms and tics
c. talking
c. tic

computed
c. abdominal tomography
adenosine triphosphate single-photon emission computed tomography

computed *(continued)*
atrial bolus dynamic computed tomography
automated computed axial tomography
automatic computed transverse axial scanning
axial quantified computed tomography
c. body tomography
cardiovascular computed tomography
cine computed tomography
contrast-enhanced computed tomography
coronal computed tomographic arthrography
cranial computed tomography
c. digital radiography
double-dose–delay computed tomography
dual-isotope simultaneous acquisition single-photon emission computed tomography
dynamic computed tomography
c. ejection fraction
c. electroencephalogram tomogram
electron-beam computed tomography
emission computed tomography
expiratory computed tomography
c. fluoroscopy
focused appendix computed tomography
gated single-photon emission computed tomography
gradient-echo single-photon emission computed tomography
head computed tomography
helical computed tomographic angiography
hepatic computed tomographic density
high-resolution computed tomography
high-resolution computed tomography scan
high-spatial-resolution cine computed tomography
intravenously enhanced computed tomography
megavoltage computed tomography
megavoltage computed tomography-assisted stereotactic radiosurgery
megavoltage computed tomography scanner
methoxyisobutyl isonitrile single-photon emission computed tomography
metrizamide-assisted computed tomography
metrizamide computed tomographic cisternography
metrizamide computed tomography cisternography
multidetector computed tomography
multiplanar computed tomography scan
multislice computed tomography
c. myelography
noncontrast helical computed tomography
parathyroid computed tomography
perfusion computed tomography
peripheral quantitative computed tomography
positron emission computed tomography
quantified computed tomography
c. radiology
rapid acquisition computed axial tomography
renal helical computed tomography
c. renal tomography
single-photon emission computed tomography
spinal computed tomography
spiral computed tomography arteriography
spiral x-ray computed tomography
technetium-99m hexamethylpropylene amine oxime single-photon emission computed tomography
thoracic computed tomography
three-dimensional computed tomographic angiography
three-dimensional computed tomography pancreatography
c. tomographic
c. tomographic angiography
c. tomographic cisternography
c. tomographic colonography
c. tomographic metrizamide myelography
c. tomographic myelography
c. tomographic pelvimetry
c. tomographic scan
c. tomographic scanner
c. tomography angiography
c. tomography arterial portography
c. tomography brain scan
c. tomography dose index
c. tomography-guided percutaneous radiofrequency denervation of the sacroiliac joint
c. tomography laser mammography
c. tomography number
c. tomography severity index
c. tomography under endoscopic retrograde pancreatography
c. tomography with multiplanar reconstructions
c. topographic scan
c. transaxial tomography
ultrasound computed tomography
unenhanced helical computed tomography
volumetric computed tomography
xenon-enhanced computed tomography
x-ray computed tomography

computer
c. addiction disorder
c. assisted menu planning
c. assisted stereotactic laser microsurgery
average response c.
c. of average transients
c. averaging technique
c. summation technique
delay computer tomographic myelography
c. dose calculation
electromechanical slope c.
c. enhanced image
c. graphic simulation
c. guided laser beam
c. imaging system
c. imaging system
leukocyte automatic recognition c.
c. liaison nurse
on-demand analgesia c.
C. Operator Aptitude Battery
c. output on microfilm
C. Programmer Aptitude Battery
c. screen chart
c. therapy program
c. tomographic methods of axial skeleton
c. tomographic methods of peripheral skeleton

triple-phase helical computer tomography
c. vision syndrome

computer-aided
c.-a. diagnosis
c.-a. fluency establishment trainer
c.-a. myelography
c.-a. surgery

computer-analyzed electroencephalography

computer-assisted
c.-a. assessment
c.-a. axial tomography
c.-a. blood background subtraction
c.-a. continuous infusion
c.-a. diagnosis
c.-a. instruction
c.-a. learning
c.-a. myelography
c.-a. myelography
c.-a. orthopedic surgery
C.-a. Psychiatric Evaluation and Review System
c.-a. real-time transcription
c.-a. reconstruction by tracing of serial sections
c.-a. research
c.-a. self-assessment
c.-a. semen analysis
c.-a. sensory examination
c.-a. stereotactic surgery
c.-a. ventilation

computer-automated measurement and control

computer-based
c.-b. case tracing
c.-b. continuing medical education
c.-b. examination
c.-b. patient record

computer-controlled radiotherapy

computer-driven rotatory chair

computer-generated artifact

computer-guided endoscopic sinus surgery

computerized
adrenal computerized tomography
c. assisted design prosthesis
automated computerized axial tomography
c. automated psycho-physiologic device
automatic computerized solvent litholysis
c. axial tomography
c. axial tomography scan
c. imaging technique
C. Diagnostic Interview for Children and Adolescents
c. diaphragmatic breathing retraining
c. digital mammography
c. display technique
c. dynamic platform posturography
c. edge detection
c. edge tracing
c. electroencephalographic map
electron-beam computerized tomography
electron beam computerized tomography
emergency room computerized tomography
emission computerized axial tomography
head computerized axial tomography
C. Healthcare And Record Transfer System
c. muscle-joint evaluation
c. notation system
c. nuclear morphometry
c. optical densitometry
c. patient record
c. pattern generator
c. pharmacokinetic model-driven drug infusion
c. risk assessment
c. scanning equipment
c. speech lab
c. tomographic hepatic angiography
c. tomographic holography
c. transaxial tomography
c. videokeratography
c. visual field machine

computerized dynamic platform posturography

computer-managed instruction

computer-patient management problem

computer-stored ambulatory record

Comrey Personality Scale

conative negative variation

concanavalin
c. A
c. A-horseradish peroxidase

concave
c. anterior surface
double c.
meniscus concave lens
periscopic c.
periscopic concave lens
c. posterior surface

concavity
c. and depression
c. of spine

concealed
c. bypass tract
c. hemorrhage
c. hernia
patient concealed illness

concentrate
ability to think or c.
antibiotic c.
bile salt c.
decreased ability to c.
fish protein c.
high oxygen c.
hog intrinsic factor c.
inability to c.
intrinsic factor c.
marine protein c.
platelet c.
pooled platelet c.
rat intrinsic factor c.
red blood cell c.
therapeutic c.
urine c.

concentrated
c. bile
c. care area
c. mental activity
no concentrated carbohydrates
no concentrated sweets
c. red blood cell
c. rust inhibitor
c. urine
c. volume

concentration
abnormally high concentration of urine
absolute plasma c.
active renin c.
c. of adenosine monophosphate
antibiotic concentration in serum and tissue
apo A-I c.
apparent free testosterone c.
approximate lethal c.
arterial oxygen c.
attention and c.
attention concentration deficit
bactericidal c.
bile phospholipid c.

concentration *(continued)*
bile salt c.
biliary cholesterol c.
blood alcohol c.
c. that inhibits 50%
constant initial c.
critical micellar c.
critical micelle c.
delayed concentration of dye
dialysate calcium c.
dialysate glucose c.
difficulty in c.
difficulty with c.
diminished ability to think or c.
dry gas fractional concentration
effective c.
effective antibiotic c.
c. effect relation
elastin fragment c.
end-tidal carbon dioxide c.
enhanced interest and c.
c. epidermal growth factor
extracellular c.
fractional area c.
fractional concentration of carbon dioxide in expired gas
fractional concentration of inspired oxygen
fractional concentration of oxygen in expired gas
fractional inhibitory c.
fractional inspired oxygen c.
functional bactericidal c.
functional inhibitory c.
geometric mean c.
hemoglobin c.
hepatic iron c.
hydrogen ion c.
hydroxyl c.
impaired thinking or c.
incipient lethal c.
information memory c.
inhibitory c.
c. of insulin in urine
integrated c.
intracellular hydrogen ion c.
lethal c.
lidocaine blood c.
lidocaine tissue c.
limiting isorrheic c.
loss of interest, appetite and c.
mass c.
maternal steroid c.
maximal c.
maximal acid c.
maximal allowable c.
maximal drug c.
maximal permissible c.
maximal permissible concentration of unidentified radionuclides
maximal tolerated c.
maximal urinary c.
maximum permissible c.
maximum urinary c.
mean cell hemoglobin c.
mean corpuscular hemoglobin c.
mean hemoglobin c.
mean plasma iron c.
median effective c.
median toxic c.
c. and memory
merthiolate, iodine, formaldehyde c.
methylene diphosphonate c.
microbubble concentration measurement
midnight plasma cortisol c.
minimal alveolar c.
minimal anesthetic c.
minimal antibiotic c.
minimal bacterial c.
minimal bactericidal c.
minimal complete-killing c.
minimal concentration of bilirubin
minimal detectable c.
minimal fungicidal c.
minimal inhibitory c.
minimal isorrheic c.
minimal medullary c.
minimal mycoplasmacidal c.
minimal protozoacidal c.
minimum alveolar c.
1-minimum alveolar c.
minimum alveolar anesthetic c.
minimum bactericidal c.
minimum bactericidal concentration test
minimum complete-killing c.
minimum concentration of bilirubin
minimum detectable c.
minimum effective c.
minimum effective analgesic c.
minimum inhibitory c.
minimum inhibitory concentration susceptibility test
minimum lethal c.
minimum local analgesic c.
minimum mycoplasmacidal c.
mixed leukocyte c.
mixed lymphocyte c.
molar c.
c. in moles per liter
c. multiplied by time
normal c.
number c.
oxygen concentration in pulmonary capillary blood
particle concentration fluorescence immunoassay
peak c.
peak maximum serum c.
peak plasma c.
plasma c.
plasma aldosterone c.
plasma bilirubin c.
plasma catecholamine c.
plasma digoxin c.
plasma renin c.
platelet c.
prothrombin-complex c.
pulmonary tissue c.
renal vein renin c.
serum aminoglycoside c.
serum bactericidal c.
serum digoxin c.
serum drug c.
serum gentamicin c.
serum inhibitory c.
serum insulin c.
serum phenylalanine c.
serum theophylline c.
target plasma c.
theophylline serum c.
time above minimum inhibitory c.
time-averaged urea c.
time of maximal c.
tissue c.'s of antibiotics
c. of total carbon dioxide
total L-chain c.
c. of total oxygen
total renin c.
transtubular potassium concentration gradient
trough minimum serum c.
urinary concentration of sodium
urinary concentration of urea
venous renin c.
xylose concentration test

concentration-camp syndrome

concentric
Aufranc concentric hip mold
c. circle pattern on breast self-examination
c. hypertrophic cardiomyopathy
c. hypertrophy
c. left ventricular hypertrophy
Mose concentric rings
multiple concentric GI rings
multiple concentric ring sign

c. needle electrode
c. needle electromyography

concept
c. of alpha biofeedback
c. of awareness
c. of biofeedback control
Boehm Test of Basic C.'s
concrete c.
C. Mastery Test
medicine c.
mental c.
Multidimensional Self C. Scale
no-threshold c.
object c.
Test of C. Utilization
three concept view

conception
cumulative conception rate
date of c.
estimated date of c.
estimated time of c.
evacuation of retained products of c.
prior to c.
products of c.
retained products of c.
time interval between cessation of contraception and c.

conceptional
c. age
c. vessel

Concept-Specific Anxiety Scale

conceptual
Assessment of C. Organization
molecular-based conceptual therapy
c. quotient
C. Systems Test

concern
Adult Career C.'s Inventory
area of c.
human spiritual c.'s
level of c.
Rating Form of IBD Patient C.'s

concerning
delusion concerning appearance

concha
c. of auricle
c. bullosa
ethmoidal process of inferior nasal c.
Morgagni c.
nasal c.
nasoturbinal c.
Santorini c.

conchae
apophysis c.

conchotome
percutaneous conchotome biopsy technique

concrete
c. attitude
c. concept
c. pelvis
c. thinking
c. thought process

concretion
fecal c.
tonsillar c.

concurrent
c. chemoradiotherapy
c. quality assurance
c. upper respiratory tract infection

concussion
c. amnesia
c. blindness
hydraulic c.
c. injury
sideline assessment of c.
spinal cord c.
c. syndrome

concussive
post concussive headache

condemnation of active euthanasia

condensate
cigarette smoke c.

condensation
c. of connective tissue
premature chromosome c.

condenser
automatic c.
bayonet c.
long-handled foil c.
mechanical c.

condition
c.'s of admission
assessment for limiting c.
autosomal dominant c.
chronic untreatable c.
coexisting medical c.
critical condition list
dementia due to hepatic c.
diagnosis or condition deferred on Axis I, II
general c.
general medical c.
good c.
heart rate condition ability
c. induced by medication
Living C.'s Rating Scale
local ovarian c.
mental disorder due to a general medical c.
moderate arthritic c.
mood disorder due to a general medical c.
c. muscles with aerobic exercise
obtained under test c.'s
c. on admission
c. on discharge
c. orientation reflex audiometry
c. of participation
patient discharged in good c.
patient dismissed in good c.
patient's condition deteriorated
patient's condition stabilized
patient in stable c.
persistent emotional c.
poor c.
Questionnaire for Identifying Children with Chronic C.'s
c. related to stress
satisfactory c.
School Handicap C. Scale
sexually transmitted c.
stress-related heart c.
teeth in good dental c.
unsatisfactory c.
ventriculoatrial c.

conditional
c. discharge
c. reflex

conditionally streptomycin dependent

conditioned
c. abstinence
acute conditioned neurosis
c. air
c. avoidance response
c. behavior response
c. cue
delayed conditioned necrosis
c. emotional response
c. fear response
c. insomnia
c. medium
c. orientation reflex audiometry
c. pitch level
c. place preference
pokeweed activated spleen conditioned medium
c. reflex
c. reflex skill
c. reflex therapy

conditioned *(continued)*
Roux conditioned medium
spleen cell conditioned medium
c. stimulus
stimulus, c.
tangible reinforcement of operant conditioned audiometry

conditioning
aerobic conditioning functional assessment
alpha conditioning session
cardiovascular reflex c.
cardiovascular reflex conditioning system
dynamic environmental conditioning cycle
escape and avoidance conditioning in human subjects
general conditioning exercise
heating, ventilating, and air c.
human operant heart rate c.
musculoskeletal evaluation, rehabilitation and c.
negative conditioning for sleep
nonmyeloablative conditioning regimen
operant conditioning audiometry
organic conditioning film
c. program
c. therapy

condom
c. catheter collecting system
c. catheter endoscopic ultrasound
foam and c.

conduct
adjustment disorder with disturbance of c.
adjustment reaction conduct disorder
adolescent-onset conduct disorder
aggressive conduct disorder
aggressive type undersocialized conduct disorder
atypical conduct disorder
bad conduct discharge
c. disorder
c. disorder type group
c. disturbance
disturbance of c.
c. disturbance adjustment disorder
c. disturbance adjustment reaction
hyperkinetic conduct disorder
moral c.
obsessive-compulsive conduct disorder
pattern of c.

conductance
airway c.
cystic fibrosis transmembrane conductance regulator
ion conductance modulator
skin conductance level
skin conductance orienting response
specific c.
specific airway c.
c. stroke volume
total respiratory c.

conducting vein

conduction
aberrant ventricular c.
c. abnormality
absolute bone c.
accessory conduction ablation
accessory conduction pathway
air c.
air and bone c.
air conduction and bone c.
air conduction deafness
air conduction testing
air greater than bone c.
anterograde c.
arteriovenous conduction disturbance
atrial conduction disturbance
atrioventricular c.
atrioventricular block with first-degree conduction delay
atrioventricular conduction delay
atrioventricular conduction system
atrioventricular conduction tissue
atrioventricular nodal c.
bone c.
bone conduction greater than air c.
bone conduction hearing aid
bone conduction less than air c.
central motor conduction time
central somatosensory conduction time
complete impairment of c.
c. defect
c. defect in acute myocardial infarction
c. delay
direct sinoatrial conduction time
effective conduction period
enhanced atrioventricular c.
enhanced atrioventricular nodal c.
functional conduction period
gap conduction phenomenon
interventricular conduction delay
intraatrial conduction defect
intraoperative conduction disturbance
intraventricular conduction block
intraventricular conduction delay
intraventricular conduction pattern
isolated conduction defect
maximum conduction velocity
motor conduction block
motor nerve conduction velocity
motor neuropathy with multifocal conduction block
muscle fiber conduction velocity
nerve c.
nerve conduction deafness
nerve conduction velocity study
nerve conduction velocity test
c. of nerve impulse
nonspecific intraventricular conduction defect
PA conduction time
partial impairment of c.
peripheral nerve c.
retrograde conduction time
sensory conduction velocity
sensory nerve conduction velocity
skin c.
c. system disease
ulnar nerve conduction velocity
c. velocity
c. velocity of slower fibers
ventricular conduction velocity
ventricular specialized conduction system
ventriculoatrial c.
zone of slow c.

conductive
coughing conductive of sputum
c. education
c. hearing loss
c. radiofrequency electric field

conductivity
c. cell volume
thermal c.
thermal conductivity detector
total body electrical c.

conductor
light c.

conduit
antirefluxing colonic c.
aortic allograft c.
autogenous vein graft c.
nonvalved c.

condylar
anterior condylar canal
anterior condylar vein
c. articulation

c. cartilage
cruciate condylar knee system
cruciate condylar unconstrained prosthesis
femoral condylar shaving
c. fracture
c. joint
lateral condylar fracture
mandibular condylar hypoplasia
Milch condylar fracture classification
mini condylar plate
osteotomy of condylar neck
c. plateau angle
progressive condylar resorption
c. screw fixation
total condylar prosthesis III

condyle
lateral condyle of femur
lateral condyle of humerus
lateral condyle of tibia
c. of mandible
mandibular condyle fracture
medial condyle of femur
medial condyle of humerus
medial condyle of tibia
medial femoral c.
medial humeral c.
medial/lateral femoral c.
neck of c.
occipital condyle fracture
occipital condyle hypoplasia
occipital condyle invasion
occipital condyle syndrome
odontoid condyle fracture

condylectomy
mandibular c.
phalangeal c.

condyloid
anterior condyloid canal of occipital bone
anterior condyloid foramen

condyloma
c. acuminatum
anal c.
oral condyloma planus
penile c.
perianal c.
perianal condyloma acuminatum
venereal c.

condylomata
c. acuminata
lata
perianal c.
perianal condylomata lata
vulvar c.

condylomatous carcinoma

cone
c. beam
beveled electron beam c.
cervical cone biopsy
cold cone biopsy
cold-knife c.
cold knife cone aspiration
cold knife cone biopsy
endocervical c.
intraoral cone for electron beam therapy
long cone technique
McIntyre truncated c.
M cone excitation
medium carbide cone bur
multiple cone root canal filling method
nose c.
outer cone fiber
paralleling cone position
peroral cone radiation therapy
rods and c.'s
surgical c.
transvaginal c.
vaginal cone biopsy

coned-down view

cone-down projection

cone-rod dystrophy

cone-shaped amputation stump

confabulans
paraphrenia c.

confabulated
c. detail response
c. whole response

confabulation
recent memory impairment and c.

conference
clinicopathologic c.
consecutive case c.
family c.
International Workshop and C. on Human Leukocyte Differentiation Antigens
treatment planning c.

confessor
mother c.

confidence
Activities-Specific Balance C. Scale
c. interval
c. level
lower confidence limit
upper confidence limit

confidential evaluation and treatment

confidentiality
c. of information
c. of record

configuration
Cupid bow c.
fishmouth configuration of mitral valve
linear combination of fragment c.
mitral configuration of cardiac shadow
mosaic detector c.
normal size and c.
onionskin configuration of collagenous fiber
c. and size
c. of uterus

confined
organ c.
c. placental mosaicism
strictly confined to bed

confinement
calculated date of c.
estimated date of c.
expected date of c.
strict bed c.
ward c.

confirmation
histologic c.

confirmatory incision

confirmed
angiographically c.
c. and compatible
continuous and confirmed memories of abuse
pathologically confirmed complete remission
c. transmission of viral hepatitis

conflict
c. avoidance
healthy conflict management
internal psychological c.
c. intervention
Korean c.
C. Management Appraisal
C. Management Survey
C. in Marriage Scale
c. mediation
parent-child conflict counseling
c. resolution

confluence
c. of nodules
superior mesenteric-portal vein c.

confluent, reticulate papillomatosis

confocal
laser-scanning confocal microscopy
c. laser scanning microscopy

conformal
c. radiation therapy
three-dimensional conformal radiation therapy

conformation
antiparallel B-sheet c.
PCR combined with single-strand conformation polymorphism
polymerase chain reaction–single-strand conformation polymorphism
c. of the skull

conformational
single-stranded conformational polymorphism

conformity
automaton c.
Group C. Rating
morality of conventional role c.
peer conformity inventory

conforms to social normal

confrontation
c. fields intact
full to c.
monocular confrontation visual field test
c. testing
c. of visual field
visual fields full to c.
c. visual field testing

confrontational
c. cognitive restructuring
c. tactic

confronting
cylindrical confronting cisterna

confront source of anxiety

confused
c. and combative
combative and c.
c. and disoriented
disoriented and c.
c. or impoverished thought and speech
c. language syndrome
patient c.

confusion
c. about time and place
C. Assessment Method
authority c.
circle of c.
c. and disorientation
disorientation and c.
episodic c.
c. from antihistamine
c. from heart failure
c. from insulin shock
c. from migraine headache
c. of ideas
increasing c.
intermittent c.
c. and lethargy
loss of recent memory, confusion and poor judgment
mental c.
nocturnal c.
Odorant Confusion Matrix scale
Odorant Confusion Matrix score
overstimulation and resulting c.
patient has forgetfulness, irritability, and c.
periodic c.
persistent vomiting or confusion headache
postictal c.
reactive c.
c. with head injury
c. with light sensitivity

confusional
acute confusional migraine
acute confusional state
alcoholic confusional state
arteriosclerotic dementia confusional state
arteriosclerotic psychosis confusional state
epileptic confusional state
c. episode
c. insanity
nocturnal confusional episode
pharmacogenic confusional syndrome
c. state
subacute confusional state

congenita
adrenal hypoplasia c.
amaurosis congenita of Leber
aplasia cutis c.
arthrochalasis multiplex c.
arthrochalasis multiplex congenita Ehlers-Danlos syndrome
arthrogryposis congenita, distal, type I, II syndrome
arthrogryposis congenita multiplex
arthrogryposis multiplex c.
dyskeratosis c.
ectopia pupillae c.
macrosomatia adiposa c.
macrosomia adiposa c.
myopathic arthrogryposis multiplex c.
neuropathic arthrogryposis multiplex c.
osteogenesis imperfecta c.
osteogenesis imperfecta congenita syndrome
pachyonychia congenita syndrome of nail

congenital
c. abducens-facial paralysis
c. abduction deficiency
c. abnormality
c. abscess
c. absence of ureter
c. absence of vagina
c. absence of vas deferens
c. adrenal virilism
c. adrenogenital hyperplasia
adult-onset congenital adrenal hyperplasia
c. alcoholic syndrome
c. anemia of newborn
anhidrotic congenital ectodermal dysplasia
c. anomaly of mitral valve
c. anterior staphyloma
c. asplenia syndrome
c. atonic pseudoparalysis
c. atonic sclerotic muscular dystrophy
c. atresia of esophagus
autoimmune-associated congenital heart block
autosomal congenital tubular dysgenesis
autosomal dominant congenital cataract
c. bifid bladder
c. bilateral absence of the vas deferens
bilateral congenital absence of vas deferens
c. biliary atresia
c. biliary ectasia
c. bronchial atresia
c. cardiovascular malformation
c. cartilaginous rest of neck
c. cataracts, sensorineural deafness, Down syndrome facial appearance, short stature, mental retardation syndrome
c. central hypoventilation syndrome

cerebellar vermis hypoplasia, oligophrenia, congenital ataxia, coloboma, hepatic fibrosis
c. complete heart block
c. contractural arachnodactyly
corrected congenital transposition of the great vessels
cyanotic congenital heart disease
c. cystic adenomatoid malformation
c. cytomegalovirus infection
c. defect interventricular septum of heart
c. diaphragmatic hernia
c. dislocation hip
c. dislocation of hip
c. disorder
c. displacement of heart
c. duodenal atresia
c. duodenal obstruction
c. dyserythropoietic anemia types I–III
c. dysplasia of hip
c. ectropion uveae
c. emphysema, cryptorchidism, penoscrotal web, deafness, mental retardation syndrome
c. endothelial corneal dystrophy
c. erythropoietic porphyria
c. eyelid tetrad
fetal congenital diaphragmatic hernia
c. fiber-type disproportion
c. fibrosarcoma
c. fibrous histiocytoma
Fukuyama congenital muscular dystrophy
giant congenital melanocytic nevus
c. glaucoma
c. goiter
c. heart anomaly
c. heart block
c. heart defect
c. heart disease
c. heart failure
c. Heinz body hemolytic anemia
c. hemidysplasia with ichthyosiform erythroderma and limb defects syndrome
hemihypertrophy, intestinal web, preauricular skin tag, and congenital corneal opacity syndrome
c. hemolytic icterus
c. hemolytic jaundice
c. hepatic fibrosis
c. hereditary retinoschisis
c. hernia
c. high airway obstruction syndrome
c. hip disease
c. hip dislocation
c. hip displacement
c. hip dysplasia
c. hip subluxation
c. HIV infection
c. hydrocephalus
hydrocephalus due to congenital stenosis of aqueduct of Sylvius
c. hyperphosphatasemic skeletal dysplasia
c. hypertrophy of retinal pigment epithelium
c. hypomyelinating neuropathy
c. hypoplasia of adrenal glands
c. hypoplastic anemia
c. hypothyroidism
c. ichthyosiform erythroderma
c. ichthyosis
c. idiopathic adrenal hypoplasia
c. immune deficiency
c. immunity
c. immunodeficiency
c. inclusion-body hemolytic anemia
c. infantile fibrosarcoma
c. infection
c. intestinal aganglionosis
c. intestinal atresia
isolated congenital folate malabsorption
Leber congenital amaurosis
c. limb deficiency
c. lipoid adrenal hyperplasia
c. lobar overinflation
c. localized absence of skin
long-segment congenital tracheal stenosis
c. malformation of heart
c. malrotation of the gut
maternal thyrotropin receptor blocking antibody-induced congenital hypothyroidism
c. melanocytic nevus
mental deficiency, spasticity, congenital ichthyosis syndrome
mental retardation, congenital contracture, low fingertip arches syndrome
mental retardation, congenital heart disease, blepharophimosis, blepharoptosis, hypoplastic teeth
c. mesoblastic nephroma
Metropolitan Atlanta Congenital Defects Program
miniature-type congenital adrenal hypoplasia
c. mitral regurgitation
c. multicystic kidney
multiple congenital anomalies/mental retardation syndrome
multiple congenital abnormalities
multiple congenital fibromatosis
c. muscle fiber-type disproportion
c. muscular dystrophy
c. myasthenia gravis
c. nasal pyriform aperture stenosis
c. nasolacrimal duct obstruction
neonatal cyanotic congenital heart disease
c. nephrogenic diabetes insipidus
c. nephrosis
c. nephrotic syndrome
c. nevocytic nevus
no congenital abnormalities
no congenital deformities
nonbullous congenital erythrodermic ichthyosis
nonbullous congenital ichthyosiform erythroderma
nonclassic congenital adrenal hyperplasia
nonsalt-wasting congenital adrenal hyperplasia
c. nonspherocytic hemolytic anemia
c. nonspherocytic hemolytic disease
nyctalopia with congenital myopia
c. nystagmus
c. ocular motor apraxia
c. onychodysplasia of the index finger
Oppenheim congenital hypotonia
c. palatopharyngeal incompetence
parenchymatous congenital syphilis
c. paucity of secondary synaptic clefts syndrome
c. penile deviation
c. polycystic disease
c. polyvalvular disease
pterygoarthromyodysplasia, c.
c. pulmonary cystic lymphangiectasia
c. pulmonary lymphangiectasia
c. radioulnar synostosis
c. retinitis blindness

congenital *(continued)*
c. rubella
c. rubella deafness
c. rubella infection
c. rubella syndrome
salt-wasting congenital adrenal hyperplasia
c. self-healing histiocytosis
severe congenital anomaly
severe congenital neutropenia
simple virilizing congenital adrenal hyperplasia
slow-channel congenital myasthenic syndrome
c. sodium diarrhea
c. stationary night blindness
c. syphilis
c. syphilitic conjunctivitis
c. syphilitic infection
c. syphilitic paralytic dementia
c. thrombocytopenia, Robin sequence, agenesis of corpus callosum, distinctive facies, developmental delay syndrome
c. thymic dysplasia
c. toxoplasmosis
tracheoesophageal fistula, esophageal atresia, multiple congenital anomaly syndrome
c. trigeminal anesthesia
c. urinary tract deformities
valvuloplasty and angioplasty of congenital anomalies
c. vascular-bone syndrome
c. vascular malformation
c. versus acquired syndrome
c. vertical talus
c. vertical talus foot deformity
c. virilizing adrenal hyperplasia
c. vs. acquired syndrome
X-linked mental retardation-blindness-deafness-multiple congenital anomalies syndrome
X-linked mental retardation/multiple congenital anomaly

congenitally
c. corrected transposition of the great arteries
patient delivered congenitally deformed infant

congenitum
megacolon c.

congested
parenchyma c.
parenchyma extremely c.
passively congested lung tissue
c. vascular structure

congestion
asymmetric pulmonary c.
c. of bladder mucosa
chronic passive c.
passive venous c.
pulmonary venous c.
upper airway c.
vascular congestion of interstitial vessel

congestive
acute congestive heart failure
acutely decompensated congestive heart failure
advanced stage of congestive heart failure
c. cardiac failure
c. cardiomyopathy
chronic congestive heart failure
c. cirrhosis
compensated congestive heart failure
decompensated congestive heart failure
c. edema
florid congestive heart failure
frank congestive failure
c. glaucoma
c. headache
c. heart disease
c. heart failure
c. heart failure and cardioversion
idiopathic congestive cardiomyopathy
mildly dilated congestive cardiomyopathy
c. myocardiopathy
natural history of congestive heart failure
NYHA congestive heart failure classification
passive congestive failure
portal vein congestive index
recurrent congestive heart failure
right-sided congestive heart failure
c. right ventricular failure
c. seasonal allergic rhinitis
sudden congestive heart failure

conglomerate
nonspecific c.

conglutinating complement absorption test

conglutination of cervix

conglutinogen-activating factor

congnita
spondyloepiphyseal dysplasia c.

Congo
intraoperative endoscopic Congo red test
C. red stain

congregate
adult congregate living facility

congruence
Merchant congruence angle
negative congruence angle
patellofemoral c.

congruent
adult congruent living facility
c. affect
Translating and Congruent Mobile-Bearing Knee test

congruous
c. cup-shaped reamer
c. hemianopia

conical
c. implant
c. obturator
c. protrusion of center of cornea
c. reamer
c. trocar

conidia
Aspergillus c.

conization
c. of cervix
cold-knife c.
cold knife c.
cold knife conization biopsy
laser vaporization and excisional c.
loop diathermy cervical c.
loop electrosurgical excision procedure c.

conjoined
asymmetrical conjoined twins
equal conjoined twins
c. heart
c. nerve root anomaly
c. tendon
c. twins
unequal conjoined twin

conjugacy
object/image c.

conjugal bereavement

conjugate
antibody radionucleotide c.
diagonal conjugate diameter

diphtheria, tetanus toxoids, whole-cell pertussis, and *Haemophilus influenzae* type b c.
external c.
extraocular movements full and c.
c. eye movement
c. fixed gaze
c. gaze
c. gaze palsy
Haemophilus b conjugate vaccine
Haemophilus influenzae type b conjugate vaccine
Haemophilus influenzae type b vaccine, PRP-D conjugate vaccine
Haemophilus influenzae type b vaccine, PRP-OMP conjugate vaccine
Haemophilus influenzae type b vaccine, PRP-T conjugate vaccine
Haemophilus influenzae type vaccine oligosaccharide-CRM197 vaccine c.
c. horizontal deviation
c. horizontal gaze
internal conjugate diameter
meningococcal c.
c. movement of eyes
nonvalent pneumococcal conjugate vaccine
obstetrical c.
obstetric conjugate diameter
obstetric conjugate of outlet
obstetric conjugate of pelvic outlet
c. ocular movement
paralysis of conjugate upward gaze
pneumococcal conjugate vaccine
pneumococcal 7-valent conjugate vaccine
polyribosylribitol phosphate-diphtheria toxoid c.
polysaccharide tetanus conjugate vaccine
sulfated lithocholic c.
true c.
c. upward gaze
7-valent pneumococcal c.

conjugated
c. bile salts
c. bilirubin
equine conjugated estrogen
c. equine estrogen
c. equine estrogen plus norgestrel
c. estrogen
c. linoleic acid
malondialdehyde conjugated low-density lipoprotein
neonatal conjugated hyperbilirubinemia
oral conjugated estrogen
rhodamine isothiocyanate c.
selenium-labeled homocholic acid conjugated with taurine

conjugated-immunoglobulin technique

conjugative plasmid in F^+ bacterial cell

conjunction
mesostructure conjunction bar

conjunctiva
annulus of c.
Chang conjunctiva cell
cornea, sclera, and c.
c. forceps
hemangioma of c.
sclera and c.
c. spreader

conjunctivae
anulus c.
corneas, conjunctivae, and sclerae
c. icteric
lithiasis c.
c. and sclerae
xerosis c.

conjunctival
anterior conjunctival artery
anterior conjunctival vein
c. cul-de-sac
c. edema
c. erythema
c. foreign body
c. fornix
c. hemorrhage
c. hyperemia
c. icterus
c. incision
c. infection
c. injection
c. intraepithelial neoplasia
c. limbus
Marquez-Gomez conjunctival graft
melanocytic conjunctival lesion
noncaseating conjunctival granuloma
papillary conjunctival hypertrophy
c. provocation test
c. reflex
c. ring
c. secretion
semilunar conjunctival fold
short duration, unilateral, neuralgic, conjunctival injection and tearing
c. telangiectasis
c. testing
total conjunctival flap
c. vascular injection

conjunctivalis
arteria conjunctivalis anterior
arteria conjunctivalis posterior
nodulus c.

conjunctivitis
acute hemorrhagic c.
Axenfeld follicular c.
congenital syphilitic c.
drug-induced cicatricial c.
feline c.
giant papillary c.
lymphogranuloma venereum c.
lymphogranuloma venereum-trachoma inclusion c.
necrotic infectious c.
neonatal inclusion c.
nonatopic allergic c.
nosocomial viral c.
ocular vaccinial c.
pain from c.
Parinaud oculoglandular c.
pediatric gonococcal c.
perennial allergic c.
pus from c.
seasonal allergic c.
Singapore epidemic c.
squirrel plague c.
trachoma and inclusion c.
virus inclusion c.
c. with eyelashes turning in

connected
service c.

Connecticut virus

connection
anomalous pulmonary venous connection, total or partial
atrioventricular connection anomaly
in connection with
internal c.
partial anomalous pulmonary venous c.
total anomalous pulmonary venous c.
total cavopulmonary c.
univentricular atrioventricular c.
ventriculoarterial c.

connective
annular atrophic connective tissue panniculitis of the ankle
areolar connective tissue
autodigestion of connective tissue
autoimmune connective tissue disorder
cerebrobuccal c.
condensation of connective tissue
craniofacial dysmorphism, absent corpus callosum, iris colobomas, connective tissue dysplasia syndrome
dense fibroelastic connective tissue
denuded connective tissue
diffuse connective tissue disease
elastic connective tissue
fibroelastic connective tissue
fibrous connective tissue
inflammation of connective tissue
Lillie allochrome connective tissue stain
loose fibroelastic connective tissue
mixed connective tissue disease
mixed connective tissue disorder
mucous connective tissue
myxomatous soft connective tissue
nodular connective tissue disease nevus
peribronchial connective tissue
pericanalicular connective tissue
perilobular connective tissue
c. tissue
c. tissue-activating peptide
c. tissue disease
c. tissue growth factor
c. tissue massage
c. tissue sheath
unclassifiable connective tissue disease
underlying connective tissue
undifferentiated connective tissue disease
undifferentiated connective tissue syndrome

connectivity
lung connectivity test

connector
anterior palatal major c.
lingual bar major c.
major c.
McIntyre nylon cannula c.
minor c.
palatal c.

Conners
Abbreviated Conners Teacher Rating Scale
C. Parent Questionnaire
C. Teacher Questionnaire
C. Teacher Rating Scale

connotation
lexical c.

conotruncal
c. anomaly face syndrome
c. cardiac defect, abnormal face, thymic hypoplasia, cleft palate

consanguineous donor

conscience
authoritarian c.
Ego-Ideal and C. Development Test

conscious
c. activity
airway obstruction in conscious patient
c. and alert
altered state of conscious awareness
c. anesthesia
area of conscious regard
c. avoidance
c. awareness
c. commitment
c. control of motor units
c. exploitation of others
c. memory
c. mental control
c. and mentally competent
meperidine conscious sedation
midazolam conscious sedation
parasomniac conscious state
c. recollection
c. sedation

consciousness
abrupt loss of c.
absence of c.
airway, breathing, circulation, cervical spine, and consciousness level
alert state of c.
alteration in c.
altered level of c.
altered state of c.
arousal component of c.
awareness and c.
clouding of c.
Comprehensive Level of C. Scale
decreased level of c.
fluctuating level of c.
gravity induced loss of c.
c. impaired
impairment of c.
level of c.
loss of c.
state of c.
stream of c.
transient loss of c.

conscious-subconscious relationships

consecutive
c. case conference
c. insanity
mean of consecutive differences

consensual
direct and c.
c. gaze
c. light reaction
c. light reflex
c. pupillary response
c. reflex
c. sexual behavior
c. validation consent

consensually
pupils equal, round, reactive to light and accommodation directly and c.
singly and c.

consensus
Final Comprehensive C. Assessment
c. interferon

consent
age of c.
ASPS informed consent form
autopsy consent form
consensual validation c.
cosmetic surgery consent form
c. form
c. form to delivery by alternative physician
c. form for removal of tissue for grafting
informed c.
informed waiver and c.
c. to intervention
leave without c.
medication release c.
operative informed c.
c. for organ donation
c. for surgery

consequence
c.'s of action
long-term c.

low probability, high consequence event
neurobehavioral c.
painful c.
psychiatric c.

conservation
breast conservation therapy
c. of energy
hearing conservation programs
heat c.
heat conservation center
c. surgery

conservative
failure of conservative management
c. management
c. subtraction-addition rhinoplasty
c. treatment

conservatively
patient treated c.

conservatorship
temporary c.

conserved helix-loop-helix ubiquitous kinase

conserver
high-flow oxygen c.

consideration
anatomical considerations in radiation therapy
anesthetic c.
oncologic c.

considered
not considered disabling
not considered disqualifying
not favorably c.

consistency
change in color and consistency of stool
clay-like c.
Clinical Probes of Articulation C.
moral c.
nectar-thick liquid diet c.
normal size, shape, and c.
object c.
perceptual c.
pudding-thick liquid diet c.
size/date c.

consistent
cells consistent with invasive carcinoma
inability to sustain consistent work behavior
c. medication compliance
c. with

consolability
face, legs, activity, cry, c.

console
direct display c.

Consolidated Standards Manual

consolidation
airspace c.
discrete area of c.
fracture line c.
c. and healing
hemorrhage c.
lobar c.
c. of lungs
memory c.
nonhomogeneous c.
novel form of consolidation chemotherapy
parenchymal c.
patchy area of c.
patchy area of pneumonic c.
peripheral c.
pneumonic c.
pulmonary c.
segmental bronchus c.
symmetric c.

consonant
arresting c.
deletion of final c.
final c.
final consonant deletion
final consonant position
initial consonant deletion
nasal c.
Percentage of C.'s Correct-Revised

Consortium
North American Brain Tumor C.

conspiracy
delusions with vague c.

constancy
location c.
object c.
perceptual c.

constant
c. abdominal pain
acid ionization dissociation c.
affinity c.
c. angular velocity
autoprotolysis constant of water
base ionization c.
Boltzmann c.
c., harsh pain
decay c.
demand for constant admiration
demand for constant attention
dielectric c.
dissociation c.
dissociation constant of a base
dissociation constant of water
c. domain of H chain
c. domain of L chain
Doppler-shifted constant frequency
c. dose rate
c. electric field
elimination rate c.
equilibrium c.
equilibrium association c.
equilibrium dissociation c.
c. error
c. estrus
c. exposure rate
flotation c.
c. frequency
gravitational c.
hemoglobin C. Spring
c. hypotropia
c. infusion excretory urogram
inhibition c.
c. initial concentration
kilovolt constant potential
c. linear velocity
low constant suction
c. magnetic field in nuclear magnetic resonance
maximum amplitude c.
method of constant stimuli
Michaelis c.
Michaelis-Menten dissociation c.
moderate constant suction
need for constant attention
negative logarithm of acid ionization c.
Newtonian constant of gravitation
newtonian constant of gravitation
c. passive-motion machine
permeability c.
Planck c.
c. positive airway pressure
radioactive c.
rate c.'s
rate of velocity c.
reaction rate c.
c. skin irritation and rubbing
specific gamma ray c.
specific heat at constant volume
c. spring
Stefan-Boltzmann c.
c. tension splint
velocity c.'s
c. verbal cueing

constipated
patient c.
small, yellow, constipated stool

constipation
antepartum c.
atonic c.
bloating and c.
change in urine flow from c.
chronic constipation with hemorrhoid
c. and fecal impaction
c. from antidepressant
c. from antihistamine
c. from intestinal obstruction
hiatal hernia and c.
incontinence and c.
indigestion from c.
intractable c.
irritable bowel syndrome with c.
nausea, vomiting, diarrhea, and c.
no nausea, vomiting, diarrhea or c.
pain in abdomen with c.
patient has c.
psychogenic c.
slow transit c.

constituent
c. of alpha protein plasma fraction
endocrine granule c.
c. of gamma protein plasma fraction
c. of plasma protein fraction
sequential analysis of twelve chemistry c.'s

constitutional
c. aplastic anemia
asthenic constitutional type
athletic constitutional type
c. chromosome abnormality
c. delayed growth
c. delay in growth and adolescence
c. delay in growth and development
c. hepatic dysfunction
melancholic constitutional type
c. psychopathic inferiority
c. psychopathic state
c. symptom

constitutive
endothelial constitutive nitric oxide synthase
endothelial constitutive nitric oxide synthetase
c. nitric oxide synthase
c. transcription unit

constraint
morality of c.
c. of thought

constraint-induced movement

constricted
c. affect
moderately constricted and equally reactive pupil
moderately constricted and slightly reactive pupil
c. pupil

constricting
annular constricting lesion
anular constricting band syndrome
anular constricting lesion
endothelium-derived constricting factor

constriction
affective c.
c. of breathing passages
c. caused by light
fetal ductus arteriosus c.
inferior esophageal c.
linguapalatal c.
mesenteric artery c.
middle esophageal c.
naris c.
pharyngoesophageal c.
pupillary c.
pyloric c.
ring c.
c. or spasm of blood vessel
upper esophageal c.
vacuum constriction device

constrictive
postoperative constrictive pericarditis

constrictor
middle constrictor muscle of pharynx
middle constrictor pharyngeal muscle
musculus constrictor urethrae
superior constrictor muscles of pharynx

construct
anterior c.
multidimensional c.
nucleic acid c.

construction
attachment-retained c.
McIndoe-Hayes c.
neovagina c.
phrase c.
Three-Dimensional Block C. Test

constructive
c. approach
c. support

consultant
lactation c.

consultation
c. and examination
inpatient geriatric consultation services
inpatient psychiatric c.
pathologic c.
c. psychiatry
c. service

consulting
clinical pharmacokinetics consulting service

consumed
oxygen c.

consumption
alcohol consumption behavior
complement-fixing antibody c.
decreasing consumption of oxygen
heavy alcohol c.
heavy consumption of alcohol
immunoglobulin consumption test
intravascular consumption coagulopathy
maternal alcohol c.
maximal oxygen c.
maximal venous oxygen c.
maximum oxygen c.
minimal venous oxygen c.
myocardial oxygen c.
O_2 consumption index
oxygen c.
oxygen consumption index
oxygen consumption per minute
peak exercise oxygen c.
poststress ethanol c.
prothrombin consumption index
prothrombin consumption time
relative consumption rate
volume oxygen c.
volume of oxygen consumption per unit of time

contact
airborne contact dermatitis
air-puff contact tonometer
allergic contact dermatitis
allergic contact stomatitis
allergic eczematous contact dermatitis
c. allergy

annular bifocal contact lens
aphakic contact lens
arc of c.
arsenical contact dermatitis
aspheric contact lens
c. assistance for ambulation
c. assisted ambulation
atypical articulatory c.
ballasted contact lens
bandage contact lens
c., control, test, evaluate, treatment
daily-wear contact lens
daily-wear soft contact lens
c. dermatitis
direct personal c.
eczematous allergic contact dermatitis
extended-wear contact lens
extended-wear soft contact lens
frequency of contact scale
gas permeable contact lens
c. glow discharge electrolysis
good contact with skin
c. guarding
hard contact lens
hospital-acquired penetration c.
c. hypersensitivity
c. illumination
immunological contact urticaria
implantable contact lens
indirect contact with contaminated instruments
indirect personal c.
c. infection
intraocular contact lens
irritant contact dermatitis
laparoscopic contact ultrasonography
c. laser ablation of prostate
c. laser vaporization of the prostate
last sexual c.
c. lens
c. lens-induced acute red eye
lichenoid contact dermatitis
light contact assist
linguapalatal contact pattern
liquid crystal contact thermography
loose contact lens
loss of contact point
macular contact lens
male homosexual c.
Meditec bandage contact lens
microthin contact lens
minus carrier contact lens
multicurve contact lens
nonimmunologic contact urticaria
nonpatient c.
opaque contact lens
optical contact lens
optical zone of contact lens
overall diameter of contact lens
patient contact record
peripheral curve on contact lens
photoallergic contact dermatitis
phototoxic contact dermatitis
c. potential difference
primary irritant contact dermatitis
Quality of C.
c. record
record of c.
replicate organism direct agar c.
retruded contact position
rigid contact lens
rigid gas-permeable contact lens
c. sensitivity
sperm-cervical mucus c.
squarely face person, open posture, lean toward person, eye contact, relaxed
T-cell-mediating contact sensitivity
tinted contact lens
toric contact lens
total contact casting
total contact orthosis
transmission by c.
c. transscleral laser cytophotocoagulation
c. urticaria
c. urticaria syndrome
c. with reality

contact-standby assist

contagiosum

angiofibroma contagiosum tropicum
molluscum c.
pemphigus c.

contagiosus

pemphigus c.

contagious

c. bovine pleuropneumonia
derivative of contagious tuberculin
c. disease
c. pustular dermatitis
c. pustular stomatitis
c. suicide syndrome
tuberculosis, c.

contained infection

container

child-resistant c.
cryogenic storage c.
instrument retrieval c.
intracavitary container placement
nonchild-resistant c.

containing

abnormal sac containing gas
mast cell containing both tryptase and chymase
mast cell containing tryptase but not chymase
region of sarcomere containing only myosin filaments
sulfur c.

containment

fecal containment device
fecal containment system
maximal containment laboratory

contaminant

airborne c.
measurable undesirable respiratory c.'s

contaminated

c. blood culture
blood product contaminated by acquired immune deficiency syndrome
indirect contact with contaminated instruments
c. needle
c. operative wound classification
c. sharps
c. small bowel syndrome
c. with bodily fluid

contaminating tumor cell

contamination

airborne c.
c. of exogenous sources
c. from ambient hospital air
c. from anesthesia equipment
c. from irrigating solutions
graft c.
gross fecal c.
hematogenous c.
c. index
indirect fetal c.
metastatic c.
source of c.

contemplative behavior

content

abnormally high c.
abnormally low c.
aortic oxygen c.

content *(continued)*
arteriovenous oxygen content difference
aspiration of gastric c.'s
blood alcohol c.
blood ethanol c.
bone mineral c.
cholesterol calcium c.
evacuation of uterine c.'s
exenteration of orbital contents operation
fasting intestinal c.'s
fasting intestinal c.'s
gastric c.'s
hemoglobin content index
hemoglobin content of reticulocyte
information c.
linguistic content of task
lipid content of storage fat
low steroid content combined oral contraceptive
mixed venous oxygen c.
mood, orientation, judgment, affect, c.
mucosal hexosamine c.
overlying bowel c.
oxygen c.
oxygen content of blood
oxygen content of blood decreases
oxygen content determination
oxygen content of mixed venous blood
poverty of c.
poverty of content of speech
poverty of content of thought
terminal aspiration of gastric c.'s
thematic content modification program
thoracic fluid c.
c. of thought
total allergen c.
total carbon dioxide c.

Contentment
Generalized Contentment Scale

context
performance c.
phonetic c.

contextual cue

contiguity
amputation in c.
appendicitis by c.

contiguum
per c.

continence
anal c.
antegrade continence enema
antegrade continence enema procedure
c. of bowel and bladder
c. line
Malone antegrade continence enema procedure
total c.

continent
c. anal cap
Malone antegrade continent enema channel
Malone continent appendicostomy
Mitrofanoff continent urinary stoma
orthotopic continent reservoir
patient c.

Contingency
Everyman Contingency Table Analysis

contingent
c. aftereffects
c. negative variation

continual skin peeling syndrome

continue
c.'s to do well
c. present management
c. same treatment

continued
c. ambulatory care
c. maladaptive behavior

continued-stay review

continuing
c. cardiac care
c. care
c. care center
c. community care
computer-based continuing medical education
c. disability review
c. education
C. Education Approval and Recognition Program
c. education unit
c. maintenance chemotherapy
c. medical education
c. smoker

continuity
advance directive c.
amputation in c.
c. of care
care management c.
interruption in continuity of bone
neuroma in c.
nursing care c.
segmental continuity defect
usual provider c.

continuous
c. abdominal peritoneal dialysis
c. albuterol nebulization
c. ambulatory gamma globulin infusion
c. ambulatory infusion
c. ambulatory peritoneal dialysis
c. anatomical passive exerciser
c. arterial spin-labeled perfusion magnetic resonance imaging
c. arteriovenous hemodiafiltration
c. arteriovenous hemodialysis
c. arteriovenous hemofiltration
c. arteriovenous hemofiltration with dialysis
c. arteriovenous ultrafiltration
c. aspiration of subglottic secretions
auditory continuous performance task
auto-titrating continuous positive airway pressure
c. bladder drainage
c. bladder irrigation
c. cardiac output
c. cardiac output with SvO_2
c. catheter drainage
c. circular capsulorrhexis
c. circular inverting suture
c. clasp splint
complete continuous remission
c. complete remission
computer-assisted continuous infusion
c. and confirmed memories of abuse
c. curvilinear capsulorrhexis
c. cycler-assisted peritoneal dialysis
c. cyclical peritoneal dialysis
c. cyclic peritoneal dialysis
c. cycling peritoneal dialysis
c. daytime drowsiness
c. distending airway pressure
c. distention-irrigation system
c. drainage
c. drip feeding
c. epidural analgesia
c. epidural anesthesia
epilepsy with continuous spikes and waves during sleep
c. extravascular infusion

c. flow ventilation
c. gastric drip
c. glucose monitoring system
c. heart murmur
c. heated aerosol
c. hemostatic suture
c. heparinization
c. hepatic artery infusion
c. high-amplitude electroencephalogram rhythmical synchronous slowing
c. home care
c. hormone replacement therapy
c. hyperfractionated accelerated radiotherapy
c. hyperthermic peritoneal perfusion
c. infusion
c. infusion chemotherapy
c. infusion epidural analgesia
c. insulin delivery system
c. insulin infusion
c. interleaved sampling
intermittent or continuous spasms
c. intrathecal baclofen infusion
c. intravenous insulin infusion
c. intravenous regional anesthesia
intubated continuous positive-pressure
c. invasive monitoring
c. inverting suture
c. irrigation
c. locking manner
c. long-term monitoring
c. loop exercise echocardiogram
c. loop wire
c. loop wiring
low continuous wall suction
low-dose continuous infusion
c. lumbar epidural anesthesia
c. mandatory ventilation
c. mattress suture
c. mechanical ventilation
c. mechanical ventilatory assistance
c. motor unit activity
c. narcosis
nasal continuous positive airway pressure
nasal prong continuous positive airway pressure
c. nebulization therapy
c. negative airway pressure
c. negative extrathoracic pressure
c. negative-pressure ventilation
neurosurgical continuous care unit
Neurotrend continuous multiparameter system
c. observation
c. over-and-over suture
c. oxygen therapy
c. passive motion
c. passive motion device
c. passive motion machine
c. performance task
c. performance test
c. pericardial lavage
c. positive airway pressure
c. positive airway pressure device
c. positive pressure breathing
c. positive-pressure ventilation
c. postoperative closed lavage
c. prophylaxis
c. pull-through technique
c. regional arterial infusion
c. reinforcement
c. renal replacement therapy
c. running lock suture
c. running monofilament suture
c. seizure activity
c. silk suture
c. sling suture
c. slow ultrafiltration
c. spinal anesthesia
c. stripping
subcutaneous continuous infusion
c. subcutaneous infusion
c. subcutaneous insulin infusion
c. subcutaneous insulin infusion pump
c. subcutaneous insulin injection
c. suction drainage
c. suture technique
therapeutic continuous penicillin
c. tone masking
c. tremor
c. tube feeding
c. venous infusion
c. venovenous hemodiafiltration
c. venovenous hemodialysis
c. venovenous hemofiltration
c. ventricular asynchronous pacing
C. Visual Memory Test
c. wave
c. wave ablation
c. wave laser ablation

continuous-combined hormone replacement therapy

continuous-flow
c.-f. centrifugation
c.-f. centrifugation leukapheresis
c.-f. tub
c.-f. zonal centrifugation

continuously cultured carcinoma cell line used for tissue cultures

continuous-wave
c.-w. Doppler
c.-w. Doppler echocardiogram
c.-w. Doppler echocardiography
c.-w. Doppler imaging
c.-w. Doppler ultrasound
c.-w. laser
c.-w. NMR
c.-w. technique

continuum
ability c.
c. of care
per c.

contortion
facial c.

contour
alar contour graft
Cupid's bow c.
distortion of c.
gum c.
c. of heart
lobulated c.
local bulge of kidney c.
local bulge renal c.
mandibular c.
c. mapping
most anterior point of anterior contour of the sella turcica
most posterior point on posterior contour of sella turcica
nasal c.
c. of nasal bone
normal contour of heart
patellar c.
proximal c.
smooth c.
tooth c.
uterus symmetrical in c.

contour-clamped homogeneous electric field

contoured
c. anterior spinal plate
elastic knee cage with medial and lateral contoured knee joints
c. femoral stem
c. T-plate plate

contour-facilitating instrument

contouring
aluminum contouring template set
AO contouring apparatus

contouring *(continued)*
esthetic body c.
occlusal c.
c. pliers
three-dimensional c.

contraception
long-acting c.
morning-after c.
oral c.
postcoital c.
time interval between cessation of contraception and conception
voluntary surgical c.

contraceptive
collagen sponge c.
combination oral c.
combined oral c.
c. device
c. diaphragm
c. effectiveness
emergency contraceptive pill
c. failure
c. failure rate
c. film
c. foam
c. implant
intrauterine contraceptive device
intrauterine progesterone contraceptive system
c. jelly
long-acting contraceptive steroid
low-dose combination oral c.
low-dose oral c.
low steroid content combined oral c.
c. method
monophasic oral c.
oral c.
oral contraceptive agent
oral contraceptive efficacy
oral contraceptive hormone
oral contraceptive medication
oral contraceptive steroid
oral contraceptive use
c. ring
sequential oral c.
c. sponge
c. suppository capsule
vaginal contraceptive film

contract
c. administration fees
c. against self-harm
c. against suicide
contract relax agonist c.
c. nursing home
c. for safety

contracted
abdomen c.
heart c.
c. heel
c. heel cord
shortened, held, resisted, c.

contractile
diminished contractile excursion
c. electrical complex
c. element
c. force
c. function in cells of myocardium
muscle contractile protein
myocardial contractile force
myocardial contractile function
myocardial contractile state
peritubular contractile cell
poorly contractile globular left ventricle
pre contractile heart
prolonged contractile duration
c. ring dysphagia
velocity of contractile element

contractility
detrusor hyperactivity with impaired c.
c. of heart muscle
impaired contractility of hypertrophied muscle
normal detrusor c.
ventricular contractility function

contracting
abnormally contracting regions
smooth muscle contracting agent

contraction
abnormal bladder c.
abnormal heart c.
active c.'s
alcohol-induced extracellular volume c.
ambulatory uterine contraction test
anodal closure c.
anodal duration c.
anodal opening c.
atrial premature c.
bladder involuntary c.
breast stimulation contraction test
cathodal closing c.
cathodal closure c.
cathodal opening c.
cathodal-opening c.
c. cycle of heart
c. during labor
escaped ventricular c.
external isovolumic contraction time
gastric interdigestive c.
giant migrating c.
c. of heart muscle
high-amplitude c.
hourglass contraction of stomach
improve muscular c.
inherent strength of myocardial c.
intensity of c.
intensity of labor c.'s
interdigestive migrating c.
intermittent tonic muscle c.'s
involuntary muscle c.
involuntary muscular c.
iris contraction reflex
isometric contraction period
isovolumic c.
isovolumic contraction time
junctional c.'s
junctional premature c.
left atrial c.
length contraction compensation element
low-amplitude c.
lower esophageal contraction ring
maximal voluntary c.
maximum voluntary c.
mean distal contraction amplitude
multifocal premature ventricular c.
nipple stimulation contraction stress test
nodal premature c.
nonconducted premature atrial c.
onset of c.'s
painful intestinal c.
painful muscle c.
c. peak force
physiology of heart c.
premature atrial c.
premature auricular c.
premature junctional c.
premature nodal c.
premature ventricular c.
premature ventricular contraction with coupling
propagating clustered c.
pulse-synchronized c.'s
c. of pupil
c. and relaxation of heart
repeated quick stretch superimposed upon an existing c.
rested state c.
right atrial c.

c. of right atrium
smooth muscle c.
spike-processed c.
c. stress test
suppress reflex c.
supraventricular premature c.
terminal antrum c.
thenar muscle c.
c. time
timed c.'s
c. tremor
unifocal premature ventricular c.'s
uterine c.
ventricular premature c.
ventricular premature contraction threshold
ventricular premature depolarization c.
c. wave

contraction-associated protein

contractual

c. behavior
c. psychiatry
c. psychotherapy

contractural

congenital contractural arachnodactyly

contracture

abduction contracture of hip
adduction contracture of hip
alopecia, contracture, dwarfism
alopecia, contracture, dwarfism, mental retardation syndrome
ankle contracture orthosis
bladder neck c.
burn scar c.
caffeine and halothane contracture test
c. deformity
Dupuytren c.
elbow flexion c.
c. exercise
fixed flexion c.
flexion c.
flexion, abduction, external rotation c.
flexion contracture of hip
infrapatellar contracture syndrome
intermittent facial c.
internal rotation contracture of hip
ischemic muscle c.
ischemic paralysis and c.
joint contracture and swelling
mental retardation, coarse facies, epilepsy, joint contracture syndrome
mental retardation, congenital contracture, low fingertip arches syndrome
multiple articular c.
obesity, short stature, mental deficiency, hypogonadism, micropenis, finger contracture, cleft lip-palate syndrome
pelvic flexion c.
permanent flexure c.
surgical relaxation of c.
Therapy Carrot finger contracture orthosis
vesical neck c.

contraindication

medical c.
medication c.
preoperative contraindication to surgery

contralateral

c. acoustic stimulation
c. axillary metastasis
bilateral contralateral routing of signals
c. competing message
decibel effective masking c.
focal contralateral routing of signals
c. head turning
c. hemiplegia
high-frequency contralateral routing of offside signals
c. knee
c. local anesthesia
metachronous contralateral hernias
c. optic tectum
c. remote masking
c. renal plasma flow
c. routing of signals
c. side
c. side of cerebellum
c. threshold shift

contrast

c. administration
c. agent
air contrast study
air contrast view of the stomach
c. angiography
antegrade contrast study
ascending contrast MR phlebogram
ascending contrast phlebography
ascending contrast phlebography imaging
ascending contrast venography
barium contrast radiology
barium contrast x-ray
barium enema with air c.
c. bath
c. chromoscopy using indigo carmine
corticomedullary c.
delayed contrast enhancement
dynamic susceptibility c.
c. echocardiology
c. enema
c. esophagography
Ethiodane contrast medium
Ethiodol contrast medium
extravasated iodinated contrast material
c. extravasation
extravasation of contrast agent
extravasation of contrast medium
c. filling
c. fluid
Functional Acuity C. Test
gallium citrate contrast material
gallium-67 citrate contrast medium
high-osmolar contrast agent
high-osmolar contrast medium
high-osmolarity contrast medium
injection of contrast media
intravenous contrast material
intravenous contrast medium
left atrial spontaneous echo c.
low-osmolality contrast agent
low-osmolality contrast material
low-osmolality contrast media
luminal contrast study
macromolecular contrast medium
magnesium contrast medium
manganese chloride contrast medium
c. material
maximum contrast method
c. media excretion
c. media-induced nephropathy
c. media leakage
c. media nephrotoxicity
c. medium
c. medium-enhanced magnetic resonance imaging
meglumine diatrizoate contrast medium
methylglucamine contrast medium
metrizamide contrast study
microbubble contrast enhancement
myocardial contrast appearance time

contrast *(continued)*
negative contrast echocardiography
negative contrast imaging agent
negative contrast left atriography
Nomarsky interference c.
nonionic contrast agent
nonionic contrast material
nonionic contrast medium
nonionic contrast radiography
nonionic dimer contrast medium
nonionic iodinated c.
oral contrast imaging agent
Pantopaque contrast medium
paramagnetic contrast agent
paramagnetic contrast enhancement
paramagnetic contrast injection
Pelli-Robson contrast sensitivity chart
prompt excretion of contrast material
pulse-inversion contrast harmonic imaging
c. radiograph
radiographic contrast agent
radiographic contrast medium
radiopaque contrast medium
retention of contrast material
Salpix contrast medium
c. sensitivity
single shoulder contrast arthrography
Sinografin contrast medium
spontaneous echo c.
c. study
c. subtraction mammography
c. threshold for motion perception
time to peak c.
time-resolved imaging contrast kinetics
ultrasound contrast agent
c. venography
c. ventriculography

contrast-enhanced
c.-e. computed tomography
dynamic contrast-enhanced magnetic resonance imaging
c.-e. endoscopic ultrasonography
c.-e. fast sequence
c.-e. Fourier-acquired steady state
c.-e. magnetic resonance angiography
c.-e. transcranial color-coded real-time sonography

contrast-induced
radiologic contrast-induced renal failure

contrast-to-noise ratio

contrecoup
c. fracture
c. injury of brain

contributing
paternally c.
c. role

contribution
maternal c.
primary c.

contributory
c. cause of death
c. element

control
acid balance c.
adaptive control of thought
c. adjustment strap
administrative control center
advanced insulin infusion with a control loop
ambulatory c.'s
androgen gonadotropin feedback c.
anteroposterior control orthosis
anxiety control technique
anxiety control training
arrhythmia control device
assist c.
assisted c.
automated mixture c.
automatic exposure c.
automatic gain c.
automatic volume c.
behavior c.
bidirectional cardiac c.
biopsy under x-ray c.
birth c.
birth control clinic
birth control drug
birth control medication
birth control pill
birth control regimen
brain-based pain c.
c. of breathing
central voluntary c.
Chlamydia from birth control pill
cognition and muscle c.
complement control protein
compulsive impulse control disorder
computer-automated measurement and c.
concept of biofeedback c.
conscious control of motor units
conscious mental c.
contact, control, test, evaluate, treatment
database input/output c.
deficits in attention, motor control, perception
diabetes mellitus out of c.
diabetic control with diet
c. diet
diffuse noxious inhibitory c.
disease control serum
disorder of impulse c.
dynamic range c.
effective infection c.
c. electrical rhythm
electric control activity
electroencephalogram biofeedback in control of hyperactivity
electronic pain c.
environmental control unit
evaluation, prediction, intervention, and c.
existing infection c.
experimental c.
external tachyarrhythmia control device
feedback mechanisms of hormonal c.
flexion-extension control cervical orthosis
foot pedal suction c.
forearm flexion control strap
gain control switch
c. gastric secretion
glucose level c.
c. group
hair loss from birth control pill
Hazard Analysis Critical C. Points
c. head movement
healthy c.
heart rate c.
heart rate control learning and awareness
c. of heart rate during oxygen deprivation
hepatitis from birth control pill
high-frequency filter c.
historic control trial
HIV prevention and c.
hospital infection c.
hospitalized c.'s
illusion of c.
impulse control difficulty
impulse control disorder
impulse control in eating

impulse control skills
impulse disorder c.
inability to control appetite
inability to control blood pressure
inability to control drinking
inability to control stool
inability to control urine
inability to control weight
inadequate impulse c.
individual voluntary c.
infant skin c.
infection c.
infection control policy
infection control professional
infection prevention and c.
infection surveillance and control program
Integrated Light C.
integrated vector c.
intent to c.
intestinal control in functional coitus
intravenous accurate control device
Isolette Servo c.
c. itching and sneezing
lack of c.
ligamentous control brace
c. of local and systemic disease
locus of c.
Locus of C. Scale
loss of bladder c.
loss of bowel c.
loss of control of bladder function
Lupus Anticoagulant Positive C.
magnetic control suturing
malaria control unit
maximum c.
measurement control handle
microbiologic quality c.
c. mode ventilation
monitored anesthesia c.
motion control limiter
motion control procedure
motor control of the ego
motor control test
c. motor skills
need to c.
negative control enzyme induction
negative control repression
negative control test
neuroendocrine control loop
neurohumoral control of motility
neurologic c.
neuromuscular c.
neuromuscular control exercise
normal c.
nutrition and weight c.
oral birth control pill
oral disease c.
out of c.
pain control infusion pump
pain control unit
parental control problem
partial thromboplastin time c.
pedal control venography
personal locus of c.
placebo control group
pneumatic tourniquet c.
poor bladder c.
poor impulse c.
pressure c.
pressure to control bleeding
pressure control ventilation
pressure-regulated volume c.
pronation spring c.
prothrombin time c.
psychological information, acquisition, processing, and control system
quality c.
quality control nurse
radiologic control center
respiratory control index
respiratory control ratio
c. serum
Sociopolitical Locus of C.
splatter control shield
statistical c.
statistical analysis and quality c.
Surveillance and C. of Pathogens of Epidemiologic Importance
c. test
thrombin c.
time-gain c.
time-varied gain c.
Total Environment C.
Toxic Substance C. Act
transairway laryngeal c.
translational c.
translational control ribonucleic acid
Trunk C. Test
c. unit
Universal C. Reference Plasma
volume c.
voluntary c.
voluntary control of bleeding
voluntary control of tension headache
voluntary heart rate c.
voluntary control of involuntary utterances
weight-matched c.

Control-Chance
Locus of C.-C.

control-dominated personality

Control-External
Locus of C.-E.

Control-Internal
Locus of C.-I.

controllable risk factor

controlled
c. access
c. access to fluid
c. activity
c. adolescent behavior
c. ankle motion
c. atrial fibrillation/flutter
bleeding controlled with clamp
bleeding controlled with hemostatic clamp
c. clinical trial
c. cord traction
delusion of being c.
c. depth osteotomy cutter
c. environment treatment
c. expansion
c. extrahepatic biliary drainage
c. fluid access
gestational diabetes mellitus, diet controlled, type 2
gestational diabetes mellitus, insulin controlled, type 1
c. heat-aided drug delivery
c. high blood pressure
illegal controlled substances
c. mechanical ventilation
microscopically controlled surgery
Obagi controlled variable-depth peel
C. Oral Word Association Test
pain well c.
c. partial rebreathing anesthesia method
c. position brace
power-oriented depth controlled osteotomy cutter
c. radial expansion
randomized controlled clinical trial
c. release
c. release infusion syndrome
c. respiration
results of clinical controlled trial
sterile spontaneous controlled vaginal delivery

controlled *(continued)*
c. substance analog
c. temperature
unsterile controlled vaginal delivery
c. ventricular response

controlled-release
morphine c.-r.

controller
venous flow c.
voice intensity c.

controlling
c. alpha activity
c. external entities
c. external spirit
c. fluid formation
c. identity
c. parent

contusion
abrasion and c.
c. of the brain
c. of heart
laceration and c.
osseous bone c.

conus
artery of the conus medullaris
low conus medullaris
low-placed conus medullaris
c. medullaris
medullaris
myopic c.

convalescence
c. and rehabilitation

convalescent
c. growing nursery
c. hospital
measles convalescent serum
newborn convalescent care unit
c. unit

convection-enhanced delivery

conventional
c. asthma therapy
c. core biopsy
c. cutaneous malignant melanoma
c. immunosuppressive therapy
c. insulin therapy
intensified conventional insulin therapy
intensive conventional therapy
c. magnetic resonance imaging
c. mechanical ventilation
morality of conventional role conformity
c. papillary carcinoma
c. planar imaging
c. reform eye implant
c. silicone elastomer
Snellen conventional reform implant
c. therapy group
c. transmission electron microscope
c. transmission electron microscopy
unchanged conventional treatment

convergence
accommodative c.
amplitude of c.
angle of c.
c. insufficiency
point of basal c.
range of c.
refractory convergence nystagmus
remote point of c.
unit of c.

convergent
c. beam irradiation
c. strabismus

conversation
hysterical conversation disorder
meaningful c.

conversational
ordinary conversational voice
Toxicology Information C. On-Line Network
c. voice

conversion
c. anesthesia
anesthetic conversion reaction
c. ataxia
automatic mode c.
autonomic conversion reaction
c. blindness
c. defect
c. disorder
c. disorder, mixed type
c. disorder, motor type
c. disorder, seizure type
dopachrome conversion factor
electrical conversion of atrial fibrillation
c. hysteria
hysterical conversion reaction
index of marrow c.
internal conversion coefficient
motor conversion symptom
c. paralysis
plasma prothrombin c.
plasma prothrombin conversion accelerator
plasma prothrombin conversion factor
proserum prothrombin conversion accelerator
prothrombin conversion factor
c. rate
c. reaction
c. seizure
serum prothrombin conversion accelerator
c. symptom

convertase
prohormone convertase 1, 2, 3
proprotein c.
proprotein c.

converter
analog-to-digital c.
digital-to-analog c.
multiplying digital-to-analog c.
time-to-pulse-height c.

converting
c. enzyme
c. enzyme inhibitor
interleukin-1 alpha converting enzyme
interleukin-1 beta converting enzyme
pulmonary angiotensin I converting enzyme

convex
Assura convex drainable pouch
Assura convex urostomy pouch
c. cartilage graft
c. condylar-implant arthroplasty
double c.
c. fusion
9- to 5-MHz convex array
c. nail
neuro convex transducer
periscopic c.
periscopic convex lens
c. rod

convexity
outer c.
paratracheal c.
parietal c.

convoluted
apical membrane of proximal convoluted tubule cell
distal convoluted tubule

convolution
angular c.
anterior central c.
Arnold c.
ascending frontal c.
ascending parietal c.

c. of cerebrum
c. of Gratiolet
middle frontal c.
nuclear c.
occipitotemporal c.
superior frontal c.
Zuckerkandl c.

convulsion
c. accompanying fever
autosomal dominant febrile c.
benign familial neonatal c.'s
benign febrile c.
benign infantile familial c.'s
catatonia, coma and c.'s
c. and coma
febrile c.
generalized tonic-clonic c.
grand mal c.
multifocal clonic c.
petit mal c.
postdecapitation c.
prolonged febrile c.'s

convulsive
c. disorder
c. dose
grand mal convulsive disorder
insulin convulsive therapy
c. seizure
c. shock therapy
c. status epilepticus
c. therapy
c. tic

co-occurring mood disorder

cooing murmur

cookie
arch c.
navicular cookie in shoe

cool
c. mist vaporizer
c. mist humidifier
c. mist vaporizer

Cooley
C. intrapericardial anastomosis
C. modification of Waterson anastomosis

cooling
autocerebral c.
autonomic cooling mechanism
bladder cooling reflex
c. blanket for hyperthermia
brain c.
cardiac cooling jacket
cardioplegia c.
external cooling appliance
immersion c.
nasopharyngeal c.
nerve c.
perfusion c.
rapid c.
c. rate

Coomassie brilliant blue R-250 stain

Coombs
direct antiglobulin Coombs test
indirect Coombs test
indirect Coombs titer
C. test

Cooper
C. fascia
C. ligament
suspensory ligament of C.

cooperation
morality of c.
sensory binocular c.

cooperative
alert and c.
alert, cooperative, and oriented
health maintenance c.
c. health statistics system
C. Human Tissue Network
c. institutional research program
National Cancer Institute C. Group
National C. Dialysis Study
National C. Growth Study
patient c.
patient alert and c.
patient awake, alert, and c.

cooperativity
negative c.

Cooper-Farran Behavioral Rating Scale

Coopernail sign

coordinate
algebraic unknown or space c.
angular coordinate variable
c. axis in plane
axis of three-dimensional rectangular coordinate system
c. home care
horizontal axis of rectangular coordinate system
object coordinate system
right-handed orthogonal coordinate system
vertical axis of rectangular coordinate system

coordination
c. and agility
c. of benefits
c. of care
care-cure c.
decrease in coordination or equilibrium
deterioration of coordination, gait, and speech
fine motor c.
finger-nose-finger coordination test
finger-to-nose coordination test
gait, balance and c.
hand-to-knee coordination
impaired motor c.
nursing c.
c. and posture

coordinator
clinical transplant c.
discharge planning c.
organ recovery c.
patient care c.

cope
ability to cope with stress
inability to c.
c. with daily stress

copied standing order

coping
c. ability
analysis of coping style
c. behavior
Bernse C. Modes
Children's C. Strategies Checklist
cognitive coping skill
compromised ineffective family c.
disabling ineffective family c.
C. Health Inventory for Children
C. Health Inventory for Parents
healthy coping strategy
inadequate c.
ineffective individual c.
maladaptive c.
maladaptive coping mechanism
maladaptive coping strategy
c. mechanism
C. Operations Preference Enquiry
C. Orientations to Problems Experienced
paralleling c.
C. Resources Inventory
c. skill
C. Strategies Questionnaire
c. strategy
c. strategy enhancement
c. style
c. technique
transfer c.
c. with anger
c. with anxiety

copious
c. antibiotic irrigation
c. bright red blood
c. discharge
c. irrigation
c. lavage of joint
c. lavage performed
c. mucoid material
c. peritoneal lavage
c. sputum

coplanar beam

copolymer
c. 1
ethylene-vinyl acetate c.
c. of polyinosinic and polycytidylic acid
polyolefin c.

copper
ammonia, copper, arsenic
c. band
c. half-value layer
nonceruloplasmin plasma c.
c. reduction test
serum copper level

copper-binding protein

copper-wire
c.-w. appearance
c.-w. arteriole
c.-w. artery
c.-w. effect
c.-w. reflex

coprolalia
mental c.

coproporphyria
erythropoietic c.
hereditary c.

coproporphyrin
erythrocyte c.
free erythrocyte c.
urinary c.
urinary coproporphyrin test

copulation
forced pair c.

copulatory mechanism

copulsation
right ventricular copulsation balloon

copy
carbon c.
c. intersecting pentagons test

copy-cat suicide

copying
digit c.
c. drawings
C. Drawings with Landmarks

coquetting
flirting and c.

coracoacromial ligament

coracobrachialis

coracoclavicular
c. arthrodesis
c. ligament
c. screw fixation
c. suture fixation

coracoid process

coral
Arizona coral snake

cord
acute central cervical spinal cord injury
acute spinal cord injury
agonal spinal cord hemorrhage
anterior cervical cord syndrome
anterior cervical surgery vocal cord damage
anterior column of spinal c.
anterior cord compression
anterior cord impingement
anterior cord syndrome
anterior gray column of c.
anterior horn of spinal c.
anterior median fissure of spinal c.
anterior spinal cord syndrome
anterolateral column of spinal c.
anterolateral white matter of c.
apex of dorsal horn of spinal c.
apex of posterior horn of spinal c.
arachnoid of spinal c.
c. around infant neck
arteriovenous cord malformation
ASIA impairment scale for classification of spinal cord injury
autologous cord blood
autonomic column of spinal c.
bilateral abductor vocal cord paralysis
c. of Billroth
c. blood
c. blood bilirubin
c. blood cell therapy
c. blood erythropoietin level
c. blood gas
c. blood hemoglobin
c. blood mononuclear cell
c. blood registry
c. blood sample
c. blood transplantation
bovine spinal cord protein
bronchoscope inserted through vocal cords with ease
central cervical spinal cord syndrome
cervical cord injury
c. compression
compression of liver c.'s
contracted heel c.
controlled cord traction
direct visualization of vocal c.'s
dorsal cord stimulation
dorsal horns of spinal c.
electrical spinal cord stimulation
c. embarrassment
epidural cord compression
epidural spinal cord compression
false vocal c.
gray matter of spinal c.
gray substance of spinal c.
head and spinal cord injury
heel c.
heel cord advancement
heel cord lengthening
hemisection of spinal c.
high thoracic cord lesion
human cord serum
human umbilical cord blood
c. insertion
intact spinal c.
intramedullary spinal cord metastasis
late clamped umbilical c.
lipoma of c.
Lost C. Club
lumbar enlargement of spinal c.
lumbosacral enlargement of spinal c.
medial cord of brachial plexus
medullary c.'s
mesenchymal sex cord stromal tumor
metastatic cord compression
metastatic epidural spinal cord compression
microsurgical denervation of the spermatic c.
milking of umbilical c.
mixed cord syndrome
mixed germ cell-sex cord stromal tumor
c. moves normally
mucoid degeneration of umbilical c.
Murphy heel cord advancement
needle cord length

neuron in spinal c.
c. normal in appearance
nuchal cord around infant's neck
oblique cord of interosseous membrane of forearm
occult cord prolapse
paradoxical vocal cord motion
c. paralysis
paralysis of vocal c.
paralyzed vocal c.
percutaneous cord cyst puncture
percutaneous heel cord lengthening
percutaneously inserted spinal cord electrical stimulation
pressure on spinal c.
prolapse of c.
sex cord tumors with annular tubules
slow spinal cord compression syndrome
space available for the c.
spermatic cord torsion
spinal c.
spinal cord abscess
spinal cord blood flow
spinal cord concussion
spinal cord decompression
spinal cord demyelinization
spinal cord disease
spinal cord disorder
spinal cord dysfunction
spinal cord infarction
spinal cord injury unit
spinal cord injury without radiographic abnormality
spinal cord laceration
spinal cord pain
spinal cord perfusion pressure
spinal cord stimulation
spinal cord tract
split spinal cord malformation
sport c.
squamous cell carcinoma of vocal c.
subacute combined degeneration of spinal c.
tethered cord release
tethered cord syndrome
tight nuchal cord around infant's neck
transected spinal c.
c. transection
true knot in c.
true vocal c.'s
umbilical c.
umbilical cord blood culture
umbilical cord blood leukocyte
umbilical cord compression
unilateral vocal cord paralysis
vocal c.
vocal cord activity
vocal cord atrophy
vocal cord carcinoma
vocal cord movement
vocal cord nodule
vocal cord palsy
vocal cord stripping

cordectomy
total c.

cordis
angina c.
anulus fibrosus dexter/sinister c.
apex c.
ataxia c.
ectasia c.
ectopia c.
foramen ovale c.
membrana c.
mucro c.
steatosis c.
theca c.

cordotomy
bilateral percutaneous cervical c.
percutaneous cervical c.

corduroy
c. artery
c. artifact

cordy pulse

core
aluminum oxide ceramic c.
antibody to hepatitis B core antigen
anti-HCV core antibody
Assessment of C. Goals
c. of atheromatous material
c. belief
c. biopsy
c. biopsy needle
c. biopsy obturator
c. body balance
c. body temperature
c. breast biopsy
central core disease
closed core needle biopsy
c. cognitive disturbance
conventional core biopsy
hard core alcoholics
hard core drug abuser
hepatitis B core antibody
hepatitis B core antigen
luteinizing hormone beta core fragment
magnetic core memory
Monopty core biopsy
mucin core protein
mucin core protein-1
multiple core biopsies
c. needle biopsy
percutaneous core bone biopsy
plasma antiendotoxin core antibody
stereotactically guided core needle biopsy
stereotactic core biopsy
ultrasound-guided core breast biopsy
vacuum-assisted core biopsy
c. values

corectopia
midbrain c.

corepraxy
mechanical c.

corepressor
nuclear receptor c.

Corfou virus

coriander
oil of c.

coring
myometrial c.

corium
papillae of c.

corkscrew
angiographic corkscrew artery
c. appearance
c. pattern
c. ureter
c. vessel

corn
apical c.
Argo corn starch test
asbestos c.
hard c.
Lister c.
neurovascular c.

cornea
abrasion of c.
anterior epithelium of c.
anterior limiting layer of c.
apex c.
apical zone of c.
clouding of c.
conical protrusion of center of c.
c.'s, conjunctivae, and sclerae
c., sclera, and conjunctiva
c. curvature
diabetic melanosis of c.

cornea *(continued)*
ectasia of c.
foreign body of the c.
herpes zoster of c.
limbus of c.
limiting layers of c.
marginal degeneration of c.
marginal ring ulcer of c.
meridian of c.
metaherpetic ulceration of the c.
periphery of c.
posterior polymorphic dystrophy of c.
sagittal depth of c.
tattoo of c.
ulceration of c.

corneae
anterior epithelium c.
herpes c.
limbus c.
liquor c.
macula c.

corneal
c. abrasion
allograft corneal rejection
anterior corneal curvature
anterior corneal dystrophy
anterior corneal staphyloma
anular corneal graft
anular corneal graft operation
aortic stenosis, corneal clouding, growth and mental retardation syndrome
autogenous corneal protector
automated corneal shaper
avascular corneal stroma
c. blink reflex
central corneal thickness
congenital endothelial corneal dystrophy
dendritic corneal ulcer
c. dystrophy
endothelial-epithelial corneal dystrophy
c. epithelial involvement
c. graft
granular corneal dystrophy
hemihypertrophy, intestinal web, preauricular skin tag, and congenital corneal opacity syndrome
c. implant
c. impression test
c. infiltrate
intrastromal corneal ring segments
c. irregular astigmatism
c. laceration
lattice corneal dystrophy
Londermann corneal trephine
macular corneal dystrophy
Manson-Aebli corneal section scissors
map-dot corneal dystrophy
map-dot-fingerprint corneal epithelial dystrophy
marginal corneal degeneration
marginal corneal ulcer
Mattis corneal scissors
Maurice corneal depot technique
mean corneal power
Meesman epithelial corneal dystrophy
microcystic corneal dystrophy
Mooren corneal ulcer
Moore-Troutman corneal scissors
mushroom corneal graft
mycotic corneal ulcer disease
Neumann-Shepard corneal marker
nodular corneal degeneration
noninvasive corneal redox fluorometry
c. opacification
c. opacity
organ-cultured corneal tissue
Osher-Neumann corneal marker
parenchymatous corneal dystrophy
partial-thickness corneal laceration
Paton corneal trephine
pattern-cut corneal graft
pattern-cut corneal graft operation
pellucid marginal corneal degeneration
penetrating corneal graft
penetrating corneal transplant
penetrating full-thickness corneal graft
perforated corneal ulcer
perimeter corneal reflex test
perioperative corneal abrasion
peripheral corneal opacity
peripheral corneal ulcer
polymorphous posterior corneal dystrophy
posterior corneal deposit
posterior polymorphous corneal dystrophy
pseudophakic corneal edema
recurrent corneal lesion
c. reflex
Reis-Bücklers superficial corneal dystrophy
Salzmann nodular corneal dystrophy
c. scar
c. scarring
Schnyder crystalline corneal dystrophy
serpiginous corneal ulcer
subepithelial corneal infiltrate
c. thickness
c. topography
c. transplant
c. transplantation
c. trauma
c. ulcer
c. ulceration
vitreal corneal touch syndrome

corneal-retinal potential

Cornelia de Lange syndrome

Cornell
C. exercise protocol
C. Learning and Study Skills Inventory
C. Medical Index
C. Scale for Depression, Dementia
C. Word Form

corneoscleral incision

corner
anteroinferior corner fracture
cracked mouth corners from sagging cheek
down-turned mouth c.'s
extension corner avulsion fracture
mesiolingual c.
c. stitch
c. suture

cornerstones of treatment

corneum
autoantibody to stratum c.
stratum c.
stratum corneum basic protein

cornification
disorder of c.
persistent vaginal c.

cornmeal, soybean, milk

cornpicker's pupil

corn-soy milk

cornu
hyoid c.
c. of hyoid bone
superior c.

cornual
anterior cornual syndrome
c. implantation

c. position of uterus
uterine cornual access catheter

cornuradicular zone

corollary incision

corona
human corona virus sensitivity
Zinn c.

coronal
c. adhesion
c. arc technique
c. computed tomographic arthrography
gradient-echo coronal image
c. incision
c. maximum-intensity projection
multiecho coronal image
nonsyndromic coronal craniosynostosis
oblique coronal plane
open coronal browlift
pearly coronal papule
c. section
c. suture synostosis
T1-weighted coronal image

corona-penetrating enzyme

coronary
abnormal coronary artery
acute coronary event
acute coronary insufficiency
acute coronary occlusion
acute coronary syndrome
acute ischemic coronary syndrome
adequate coronary perfusion
advanced coronary treatment
allograft coronary artery disease
c. angiogram
c. angiography
c. angioplasty
anomalous coronary artery
anomalous left coronary artery
anomalous left coronary artery from pulmonary artery
anomalous left coronary artery from pulmonary artery syndrome
anomalous left main coronary artery
anomalous origin of left coronary artery from pulmonary artery
anterior coronary periarterial plexus
anterior interventricular branch of left coronary artery
Aria coronary bypass
c. arrest
c. arrhythmia monitoring unit
c. arteriography
c. arteriosclerosis
arteriosclerotic coronary artery disease
c. arteriosclerotic heart disease
c. artery
c. artery aneurysm
c. artery bypass
c. artery bypass graft
c. artery bypass grafting
c. artery bypass grafting surgery
c. artery bypass graft patency
c. artery bypass graft surgery
c. artery calcification
c. artery disease
c. artery embolism
c. artery embolization
c. artery fistula
c. artery lesion
c. artery obstruction
c. artery occlusive disease
c. artery revascularization procedure
c. artery scan
c. artery spasm
c. artery steal
asymptomatic coronary artery disease
atherosclerotic coronary artery disease
c. atherosclerotic heart disease
atrial anastomotic branch of circumflex branch of left coronary artery
balloon coronary occlusion
c. blood flow
c. blood flow velocity
c. bypass graft
Cabral coronary reconstruction
c. care nursing
c. care team
chronic coronary insufficiency
circumflex coronary artery
complex unroofed coronary sinus
critical coronary stenosis
c. cusp
directional coronary angioplasty
directional coronary atherectomy
dissecting aneurysm of the coronary artery
distal coronary sinus
distal right coronary artery
double coronary artery graft
electron-beam angiography of coronary artery
endarterectomy and coronary artery bypass grafting
endoscopic coronary artery bypass grafting
excimer laser coronary angioplasty
c. flow
c. flow velocity reserve
hardening of coronary artery
c. heart disease
human coronary virus
c. imaging
impaired coronary artery
impaired coronary vascular reserve
c. insufficiency
c. insufficiency syndrome
c. intensive care unit
intensive coronary care unit
intermediate coronary artery syndrome
intermediate coronary care unit
intermittent coronary sinus occlusion
intervention
c. intervention
intramyocardial coronary blood flow
ischemic coronary heart disease
left anterior descending coronary artery
left circumflex coronary artery
left coronary angiography
left coronary artery
left coronary cusp
left coronary sinus
left coronary vein
left main coronary artery disease
left main stem coronary artery disease
magnetic resonance coronary angiography
mainstem coronary artery
major coronary artery
major coronary event
marginal atrial branch of right coronary artery
marginal branch of left circumflex coronary artery
marginal branch of right coronary artery
c. mastoid-to-mastoid incision
c. maximum-intensity projection
metabolic coronary dilation
minimal coronary vascular resistance index

coronary *(continued)*
minimally invasive coronary bypass grafting
minimally invasive direct coronary artery bypass graft
mobile coronary care unit
multivessel coronary disease
narrowed coronary artery
narrowing of coronary artery
narrowing of ostia of coronary artery
native coronary anatomy
native coronary artery
new approaches to coronary intervention
c. nodal rhythm
noncalcified coronary stenosis
noninvasive coronary angiography
normal coronary arteries
obliterative coronary artery disease
c. observation ratio
obstructive coronary disease
occluded coronary vessel
c. occlusion
occlusive coronary artery disease
occlusive coronary disease
off-pump coronary artery bypass
opening of coronary sinus
c. ostial dimple
percutaneous coronary angioplasty
percutaneous coronary rotational atherectomy
percutaneous coronary transluminal angioplasty
percutaneous excimer laser coronary angioplasty
percutaneous excimer laser coronary angioplasty system
percutaneous rotational transluminal coronary angioplasty
percutaneous transluminal coronary angioplasty
percutaneous transluminal coronary arteriography
percutaneous transluminal coronary recanalization
percutaneous transluminal coronary revascularization
percutaneous transluminal coronary rotational ablation
percutaneous transluminal coronary rotational atherectomy
percutaneous transluminal ultrasonic coronary angioplasty
perfusion-assisted direct coronary artery bypass
peripheral coronary pressure
post coronary artery bypass graft
posterior coronary plexus
posterior descending coronary artery
posterolateral coronary artery
preexisting coronary disease
premature coronary disease
pressure-controlled intermittent coronary sinus occlusion
primary percutaneous transluminal coronary angioplasty
c. prognostic index
proximal c.
proximal coronary sinus
qualitative coronary ultrasound
quantitative coronary arteriography
c. radiation therapy
radiographic coronary calcification
c. rehabilitation program
relative coronary flow reserve
c. remodeling
reoperative coronary artery bypass graft
c. reperfusion
c. reserve flow
right c.
right anterior descending coronary artery
right coronary angiography
right coronary sinus
right main coronary artery
c. risk factor
c. rotational atherectomy
rotational coronary atherectomy
c. sclerosis
c. seeking catheter
severe coronary arteriosclerosis
single coronary artery bypass graft
single coronary artery graft
c. sinus
c. sinus blood flow
c. sinus flow
c. sinus occlusion pressure
c. sinus stimulation
c. slow flow syndrome
smooth excimer laser coronary angioplasty
c. spasm induction
c. spasm and prolapse
spontaneous coronary artery dissection
c. steal
c. steal mechanism
c. steal phenomenon
c. steal syndrome
c. stenosis index
stented coronary artery
sudden coronary death
c. sulcus
systolic coronary artery narrowing
c. thrombosis
total coronary flow
total coronary score
totally endoscopic coronary artery bypass
transplant coronary artery disease
triple coronary artery bypass graft
unstable coronary artery disease
c. vascular resistance
c. vascular resistance index
c. vasculitis
c. vasospasm
ventricular atrial distal coronary sinus
ventricular atrial proximal coronary sinus
c. vessel anatomy
c. wedge pressure

coronary-pulmonary fistula

coronary-subclavian steal syndrome

coronavirus-like particle

coronoid
mandible c.
mandibular coronoid graft
c. process of ramus

corpectomy
anterior c.
median c.

corporal punishment

corporeal
Nesbit c.

corporis
pediculosis c.
tinea c.

corporoplasty
modified Essed-Schroeder c.

corpus
agenesis of corpus callosum-mental retardation-osseous lesions syndrome
c. albicans
anterior c.
anterior midbody of corpus callosum
atretic corpus luteum
congenital thrombocytopenia, Robin sequence, agenesis of corpus callosum, distinctive

facies, developmental delay syndrome
craniofacial dysmorphism, absent corpus callosum, iris colobomas, connective tissue dysplasia syndrome
hemorrhagic corpus luteum
c. luteum
c. luteum cyst
c. luteum deficiency syndrome
c. luteum dysfunction
c. luteum function
c. luteum hormone
c. luteum insufficiency
c. luteum of pregnancy
c. luteum stimulating hormone
parenchymatous cell of corpus pineale
partial corpus callosum agenesis
pediculosis c.
peduncle of corpus callosum
pedunculus corpus pinealis
persistent corpus luteum
prolapse of corpus luteum
rostrum of corpus callosum
c. striatum
trunk of corpus callosum
X-linked mental retardation, seizures, acquired microcephaly, agenesis of corpus callosum

corpuscle
articular c.
axile c.
Golgi c.
lingual c.
Lostorfer c.
lymph c.
lymphatic c.
lymphoid c.
malpighian c.
meconium c.
Meissner c.
Merkel c.
milk c.
molluscum c.
Negri c.
Nunn engorged c.'s
oval c.
pacchionian c.'s
pacinian c.
phantom c.
Purkinje c.
red c.
red blood c.
renal c.
reticulated c.
Ruffini c.
salivary c.
Schwalbe c.
shadow c.
splenic c.
tactile c.
taste c.
thymic c.
Traube c.
Vater c.
Vater-Pacini c.
Virchow c.
white blood c.
Zimmermann c.

corpuscular
mean corpuscular hemoglobin
mean corpuscular hemoglobin concentration
mean corpuscular hemoglobin count
medium corpuscular fragility
reticulocyte mean corpuscular volume
c. volume

correct
c. for inhomogeneity
needle and sponge count correct times three
needle and sponge count correct times two
needle, sponge, and instrument count correct times three
needle, sponge, and instrument count correct times two
c. response
sponge count c.
c. sponge and needle count

corrected
c. adjusted sinus node recovery time
background c.
c. blood volume
congenitally corrected transposition of the great arteries
c. congenital transposition of the great vessels
c. count increment
c. development quotient
c. ejection time
c. gestational age
c. perinatal mortality
c. preejection period
QT corrected for heart rate
relative corrected death rate
c. retention time
c. sedimentation rate
c. sinus nodal recovery time
c. survival rate
c. time of sinoatrial node function recovery
c. TIMI frame count
total corrected incremental score

correction
age correction procedure
air gap c.
area correction factor
autoattenuation correction method
automatic motion c.
distance visual acuity with c.
distance visual acuity without c.
laser vision c.
linear correction factor
loss of c.
mechanism of c.
microprobe analysis generalized intensity c.
navigator echo motion correction technique
one-stage esthetic c.
presurgical orthopedic c.
segmental correction using spine reconstruction
segmental correction using x-ray measurement
segmental spinal correction system
c. of strabismus
total c.
vision with c.
c. with glasses

correctional
c. health care program
C. Institutions Environment Scale
c. transfer

corrective
c. cast
c. orthodontics
c. orthosis
c. saccade
c. septorhinoplasty
c. shoe
c. therapy
c. therapy department

Correct-Revised
Percentage of Consonants C.-R.

correlated
negatively correlated region
spin-echo correlated spectroscopy

correlation
c. algorithm
c. coefficient
fluorescence correlation spectroscopy
mean intercriterion c.

correlation *(continued)*
Pearson correlation coefficient
Pearson correlation coefficient pedantic
population correlation coefficient
rank correlation coefficient
sample correlation coefficient

correlational
laser correlational spectroscopy

correlative
objective c.

correspondence
abnormal retinal c.
anomalous retinal c.
normal retinal c.

corresponding
critical corresponding frequency
electrocardiographic wave corresponding to repolarization of ventricles

Corriparta virus

corrosion
volatile corrosion inhibitor

cortex
adrenal c.
adrenal cortex cell
adrenal cortex estrogen-secreting tumor
adrenal cortex testosterone-secreting tumor
adrenal cortex zone
anterior cingulate c.
anterior cortex penetration
aspiration of c.
association cortex of parietal lobe
associative visual c.
auditory association c.
cerebral c.
cerebral cortex perfusion rate
dorsolateral prefrontal c.
electrodes applied over cerebral c.
electrodes inserted in cerebral c.
entorhinal c.
frontal c.
inferior temporal c.
lamina c.
medial frontal c.
mesial epileptogenic c.
molecular layer of cerebellar c.
molecular layer of cerebral c.
motor cortex unit
multimodal association c.
occipital cortex damage
occipital cortex tissue
parietal cortex damage
parietal cortex lesion
patchy atrophy of renal c.
pedicle cortex disruption
peristriate visual c.
piriform c.
plexiform layer of cerebral c.
posterior c.
premotor c.
prepiriform c.
primary sensorimotor c.
primary visual c.
provisional c.
receptive field of visual c.
sensorimotor c.
somatosensory c.
stellate cell of cerebral c.
visual c.

Corti
canal of C.
organ of C.
pillar of Corti organ

cortical
c. abrasion
c. androgen-stimulating hormone
c. arch of kidney
c. arousal index
attenuated cortical surface
auditory cortical area
c. auditory evoked potential
c. auditory evoked response
avascular cortical infarction necrosis
avulsive cortical irregularity
bilateral cortical necrosis
c. blood flow
c. blood volume
c. bone allograft
c. bone graft
c. bone infarct
c. bone lesion
c. bone modeling
c. bone plate
c. bone remodeling
c. bone resorption
c. bone screw
cancellous and cortical bone graft
c. cancellous screw
cancellous versus cortical bone
c. collecting duct
combined cortical thickness
decalcified freeze-dried cortical bone
diffuse c.
diffuse cortical sclerosis
direct cortical response
evoked cortical response
c. function testing
higher cortical dysfunction
higher cortical function
c. hyperplastic nodule
idiopathic cortical hyperostosis
infantile cortical hyperostosis
inner cortical blood flow
intraoperative electrical cortical stimulation
isolated cortical tubule
late cortical cerebellar atrophy
late cortical response
late distal cortical tubule
late proximal cortical tubule
c. Lewy body
c. lobules of kidney
c. magnification factor
malformation of cortical development
mapping of cortical function
c. mapping of memory function
maternal cortical vein
maternal cortical vein thrombosis
medial cortical overlap technique
c. medullary junction
metacarpal cortical density
metaphysial fibrous cortical defect
microscopic cortical dysplasia
mild focal cortical nodular hyperplasia
c. motor area
motor cortical center
c. motor output
movement-related cortical potential
multiple cortical infarction
multiple cortical infarcts
c. necrosis of brain
c. necrosis of kidney
nodular cortical adrenal hyperplasia
nodular cortical sclerosis
occipital association cortical area
occipital cortical dysplasia of Taylor
onlay cortical graft
outer cortical blood flow
Pacific Coast demineralized cortical bone powder
parasagittal cortical infarction
renal cortical blood flow
renal cortical vascular resistance
retained cortical activity
c. scarring of kidney
c. sensory loss
slow-growing cortical neoplasm
smooth cortical surface

somatosensory cortical evoked potential
c. somatosensory evoked potential
c. somatosensory evoked response
c. spoking
c. stromal hyperplasia
subacute cortical cerebellar degeneration
c. substance of bone
superficial cortical hemorrhage
superficial renal cortical perfusion
c. thick ascending limb
c. thickness
transcranial cortical magnetic stimulation
transient cortical blindness
visual-evoked cortical potential
c. visual impairment
visually evoked cortical potential

corticalis
nucleus amygdalae c.
pars c.

cortically spreading depression

corticectomy
occipital c.
parietal c.

corticobulbar tract

corticocancellous
autogenous corticocancellous graft
c. block graft
c. bone
c. bone graft
c. chip graft
c. strut

corticoid
antiinflammatory c.
antiphlogistic c.
apparent mineral corticoid excess syndrome
phlogistic c.
postinflammatory c.
c. sensitive

corticomedial amygdaloid nucleus

corticomedullary
c. contrast
c. differentiation

corticonuclear
mesencephalic corticonuclear fiber

corticospinal
anterior corticospinal tract
c. tract

corticosteroid
antenatal corticosteroid therapy
antenatal corticosteroid treatment
c. hormone
inhaled c.
c. receptor
c. sensitive asthma
c. therapy
c. treatment

corticosteroid-binding
c.-b. globulin
c.-b. globulin-binding capacity
c.-b. globulin variant

corticosterone methyl oxidase

corticotomy
maxillary c.
percutaneous c.

corticotroph
adenohypophysial corticotroph cell

corticotropic
adrenal androgen corticotropic stimulating hormone

corticotropin-releasing
c.-r. factor
c.-r. hormone
c.-r. hormone-binding protein
c.-r. hormone receptor type 1, 2

cortisol
diurnal cortisol test
midnight plasma cortisol concentration
plasma c.
c. production rate
c. secretion rate
urinary free c.
urine free c.

cortisol-binding globulin

cortisone
c. acetate
c. injection
c. resistant thymocyte

cortisone-glucose tolerance test

cortisone-primed oral glucose tolerance test

Corynebacterium
lipophilic *Corynebacterium*

coryneform bacteria

coryza
allergic c.
chimpanzee coryza agent
chimpanzee coryza agent virus
c. virus

cosmetic
c. defect
c. deformity
c. dentistry
elective cosmetic surgery
Federal Food, Drug, and C. Act
c. and functional purpose
good cosmetic result
c. implant
c. implant surgery
lip c.
MultiPulse cosmetic treatment laser
c. nasal surgery
c. orthodontics
c. reconstruction
c. result
c. skin resurfacing
c. surgery
c. surgery authorization form
c. surgery consent form

cost
additional cost of false negatives
additional cost of false positives
average cost of illness
economic costs of drug abuse
health care cost reduction
hospital care c.
c. of living
marginal cost per year of life saved
maximal allowable c.
maximum allowable c.
performance and cost efficiency
personal health c.
Prescription Analyses and C.
rising health care c.'s

costal
below right costal margin
c. border blunting
c. cartilage
c. facet
fingerbreadth below right costal margin
c. intraarticular cartilage
left costal border
left costal margin
lower costal margin
c. margin
c. notches of sternum
c. plaque
c. respiration
right costal margin

cost-benefit analysis

cost-effective
c.-e. alternative
c.-e. care

cost-effectiveness analysis

costimulatory
lymphocyte costimulatory molecule

costochondral
c. graft
c. junction
costochondritis syndrome
costoclavicular syndrome
costodiaphragmatic recess of pleura
costomediastinal recess of pleura
costophrenic
c. angle
c. angle blunting
c. blunting
costotransverse
anterior costotransverse ligament
middle costotransverse ligament
costovertebral
c. angle
c. angle tenderness
c. angle tenderness to percussion
c. joint
c. segmentation defect with mesomelia syndrome
Cost-Stirling antibody
cosyntropin stimulation test
Cotia virus
cotransmitter
peptide c.
cotransporter
monocarboxylate/proton c.
Na^+-phosphate c.
sodium glucose c.
sodium-potassium-2 chloride c.
taurine c.
Cotrel
modified Cotrel cast
cottage cheese-like discharge
cotton
c. bolster
c. dust asthma
c. elastic bandage
interrupted cotton suture
oxidized c.
c. pad
c. pledget
c. roll
c. sponge
c. swab
cotton-roll gingivitis
cotton-spot macular edema
cottontail rabbit herpesvirus
cotton-tipped
c.-t. applier
c.-t. swab
cottonwood
Arizona/Fremont c.
Arizona/Fremont cottonwood tree
cotton-wool
c.-w. appearance
c.-w. exudates
c.-w. spots
Cotunnius
nerve of C.
cotyledon
fetal c.
maternal c.
coudé catheter
cough
c. and/or hemoptysis
aneurysmal c.
angiotensin-converting enzyme inhibitor c.
Arnold nerve reflex cough syndrome
barking c.
chronic mucus-producing c.
c., dyspnea and headache
c. and deep breath
dry hacking c.
encourage to cough and deep breathe
c. and exercise
c. and expectoration
fever, cough, nausea, and vomiting
c. fracture
c. fracture of rib
c. frequency
hacking c.
c. headache
c. impulse
laryngeal cough reflex test
c. mechanism
nagging c.
nagging cough and hoarseness
nervous c.
nonproductive c.
paroxysmal c.
peak cough flow
persistent cough and phlegm
persistent cough with hemoptysis
persistent hacking c.
productive c.
c. productive of bloody sputum
productive cough and expectoration
reflex c.
c. reflex
c. resonance
seal-bark c.
c. and sputum
c. suppressant
c. syncope
c. threshold
turn and c.
turn, cough, deep breath
turn, cough, and hyperventilate
whooping c.
whooping cough vaccine
winter c.
c. with expectoration
coughing
c. and/or wheezing
c. conductive of sputum
deep breathing and c.
c. exercise
c. from allergy
c. from asthma
c. from chemical
impulse on c.
c. and straining
c. up blood
c. up blood with chest pain
c. with fever
c. with flatulence
c. with phlegm
coulomb
joule per c.
c.'s per kilogram
c. per volt
Coulter battery
Coumadin necrosis
counseling
achievement through counseling and treatment
identity and role c.
individual c.
individual adult children of alcoholics c.
individual codependent c.
individual counseling sessions
individual couple's c.
individual dependent c.
Inventory for C. and Development
leisure c.
long-term individual c.
mental health c.
multi-family group c.
parent-child conflict c.
perinatal mortality counseling program

perinatal mortality counseling team
Priority C. Survey
c. and testing
voluntary counseling and testing

counselor
chemical dependency c.
licensed professional c.
mental health c.
substance abuse c.
vocational rehabilitation c.

counselor-centered therapy

count
abbreviated blood c.
absolute band c.
absolute basophil c.
absolute blood eosinophil c.
absolute cell c.
absolute granulocyte c.
absolute lymphocyte c.
absolute neutrophil c.
absolute phagocyte c.
agar plate c.
automated cell c.
axillary count rate
background c.'s
blood c.
calorie c.
colony count and culture
complete blood cell c.
complete blood c.
corrected count increment
corrected TIMI frame c.
correct sponge and needle c.
culture and sensitivity and colony c.
daily fetal movement c.
decreasing blood c.
differential blood c.
differential leukocyte c.
direct microscopic clump c.
end-diastolic c.
end-systolic c.
eosinophil c.
ex vivo c.
fecal leukocyte count test
fetal movement c.
finger count, both eyes
c. fingers
full blood c.
full width of photopeak measured at half maximal c.
hemolysis, elevated liver enzymes, and low platelet c.
heterotopic plate c.
hundred c.
indirect platelet c.
c. information density
interval blood c.
interval platelet c.
lactose coliform c.
lamellar body c.
left to c.
leukocyte differential c.
lung count curve
lymphocyte c.
lymphocyte subset c.
mean axillary count rate
mean corpuscular hemoglobin c.
c. median aerodynamic diameter
c. median diameter of particles
c. median length
microvessel c.
nadir blood c.
needle and sponge count correct times two
needle and sponge c.
needle and sponge count correct times three
needle, sponge, and instrument count correct times three
needle, sponge, and instrument count correct times two
neutrophil leukocyte c.
neutrophil lobe c.
noise equivalent c.'s
nucleated cell c.
peak count density
percentage of lymphocytes in differential c.
peripheral blood cell c.
peripheral blood c.
peripheral eosinophil c.
peripheral lymphocyte c.
peripheral monocyte c.
c.'s per minute
plasma cell c.
platelet c.
platelet count decreased
platelet count increased
platelet count increment
platelet count posttransfusion
platelet count pretransfusion
polymorphonuclear leukocyte c.
posttetanic c.
red blood cell c.
red cells too numerous to c.
spinal fluid c.
sponge count correct
sponge and lap c.
sponge and needle c.
standard platelet c.
stroke c.
swollen joint c.
tender joint c.
too many to c.
too numerous to c.
total eosinophil c.
total lymphocyte c.
total ridge c.
total white and differential cell c.
white blood cell c.
white cell c.
white cell c.

counter
automated differential leukocyte c.
automated gamma c.
gamma well c.
Geiger-Müller counter
c. immunoelectrophoresis–colorimetric
c. immunoelectrophoresis–densitometric
c. incision
Michaelson counter pressure
over the c.
Pebax counter unit
pill c.
proportional counter spectrometry
c. rotating saw
c. stab wound incision

counteracting impulsivity

counteract spasticity

counter-adaptive
central counter-adaptive change

counterclockwise
c. direction
c. rotation

countercurrent
c. aortography
c. centrifugal elutriation
c. distribution
c. electrophoresis
c. exchange
c. exchanger
c. exchanger immunoelectrophoresis
c. extraction
c. flow-related enhancement
c. immunoelectrophoresis test
c. mechanism
c. multiplication
c. multiplier
c. multiplier principle

counterelectromotive force

counterelectrophoresis
sandwich c.
counterforce strap
counterimmunoelectrophoresis technique
counterintuitive relationship
counter/locator
digital c./l.
counterpart analysis
counterphobic
c. attitude
c. behavior
counterpressure
external counterpressure device
counterproductive training
counterpulsation
abdominal aortic counterpulsation device
enhanced external c.
external c.
intraaortic c.
intraaortic balloon c.
intraaortic counterpulsation balloon
percutaneous intraaortic balloon c.
pulmonary artery c.
counterregulation mechanism
counterregulatory
c. effect
glucose counterregulatory hormone
c. hormone
counterrolling
ocular c.
countershock
electrical c.
countersinking osteotomy
countersink screw head
countertorsion
ocular countertorsion reflex
countertraction splint
countertransference
c. behavior
c. experience
c. neurosis
c. reactions
countertransport
sodium-lithium c.
c. system
countertransporter
sodium-lithium c.
counter-wish dream
counting
automated reticulocyte c.
c. chamber
c. disruption
finger c.
c. fingers
liquid scintillation c.
c. money tremor
c. plate
replicate organism detection and c.
single photoelectron c.
single-photon counting system
single proton c.
time-resolved liquid scintillation c.
total body c.
couple
c. counseling
c.'s group therapy
integrative couple therapy
marital couples group therapy
coupled
c. atrial pacing
c. beats
G-protein c.
high-pH anion exchange chromatography coupled with pulsed amperometric detection
liquid chromatography coupled to tandem mass spectrometry
coupling
critical coupling interval
electromechanical c.
c. factor
intercellular c.
locomotor-respiratory c.
magnetic dipole-dipole c.
nasal c.
premature ventricular contraction with c.
variable c.
course
c. of chemoprophylaxis
c. of chemotherapy
chronic progressive c.
complicated postoperative c.
c. of dialysis
directly observed treatment, short c.
c. of disease
full course of radiation
full course radiation therapy
hospital c.
hospital course benign
c. of illness
longitudinal course specifier
long-term course of abuse
mutual self-help c.
onset and course of disease
patient's hospital course turbulent
patient tolerated full course of radiation
postoperative course complicated
postoperative course normal
postoperative course uncomplicated
postoperative course uneventful
postoperatively stormy c.
prenatal c.
progressive downhill c.
satisfactory postanesthesia c.
short course chemotherapy
short intense c.
split course technique
split course treatment
c. of treatment
uncomplicated postoperative c.
uneventful postoperative c.
coursing vessel
court
juvenile c.
c. referral for incest
court-appointed
c.-a. guardian
c.-a. psychiatrist
court-mandated
c.-m. evaluation
c.-m. treatment
court-ordered
c.-o. assessment
c.-o. examination
c.-o. involuntary outpatient treatment
c.-o. medical treatment
c.-o. obstetrical intervention
court-related problem
courtroom psychology
Courvoisier-Terrier syndrome
covariance
analysis of c.
multivariate analysis of c.
coven
member of a c.
cover
alginate wound c.
alternate cover test
cast c.
objective prism-neutralized cover test
pad c.
prism and alternate cover test

simultaneous prism and cover test
c. test

coverage
health care c.
mandated mental health c.
neocortical c.
skin c.

covered
end of bone covered with flap

covering
outermost c.

covert
c. behavior
c. dyskinesia
c. hostility
overt compliance masking covert resistance
c. resentment
c. resistance

cover-uncover
c.-u. eye test
c.-u. test

cow
c. kidney
c. lung lavage
mad cow disease

Cowbone Ridge virus

cowhorn forceps

Cowper
C. gland
C. ligament

cowpox virus

cow's
c. milk
c. milk allergy
c. milk anemia
c. milk protein
c. milk protein allergy
c. milk-sensitive enteropathy
whole cow's milk

COX-2
C. enzyme
C. inhibitor

coxa
anterior adductor of the c.
traumatic epiphysial coxa vara

COX-1 inhibitor

Coxsackie
C. viral infection
C. virus
C. virus myocarditis

coxsackievirus
group B c.

C-peptide
urinary C-p.

crab hand

crack
c. abuse
c. baby syndrome
cocaine and crack crisis
hairline c.

crack-addicted patient

cracked
c. heel
c. mouth corners from sagging cheek

cracked-pot
c.-p. resonance
c.-p. sound

cracking
knuckle c.

crackle
basilar c.
end-inspiratory c.
end-respiratory c.
fine inspiratory c.

crackling
dry crackling sound
parchment c.
c. rale
c. rales
c. sounds in lungs

cradle
auditory response c.
c. cap
heated bed c.
neonatal auditory response c.

cramp
accessory c.
bloating and/or diarrhea, gas, c.'s
c. and diarrhea
diarrhea with menstrual c.'s
intermittent c.'s
leg c.
menstrual c.
miner's c.'s
miner's c.
muscle c.
muscular c.
night c.
nighttime calf c.
nighttime leg c.
nocturnal leg c.
nocturnal leg muscle c.
occupational c.
painful leg c.
pelvic c.
potassium leg c.'s
recumbency c.
writer's c.

cramping
abdominal c.
abdominal cramping pain
c. abdominal pain
bleeding and c.
c. and bleeding
bloating and c.
intense c.
intermittent spotting and c.
spotting and c.
c. of toe
uterine c.

cramp-like
c.-l. pelvic pain
c.-l. sensation

crampy abdominal pain

cranial
anterior cranial base
anterior cranial fossa
anterior cranial fossa surgery
attached cranial section
c. autograft
BI cranial vascular headache
cantilevered split cranial bone graft
c. computed tomography
Cronqvist cranial index
diastasis of cranial bone
eighth cranial nerve
c. electrical stimulation
focal cranial radiation therapy
c. granulomatous arteritis
c. helmet
c. hemorrhage
middle cranial fossa
middle cranial fossa approach
middle cranial fossa cyst
middle cranial fossa line
migrainous cranial neuralgia
c. motor nuclei
c. nerve distribution
c. nerve impairment
c. nerve involvement
c. nerve palsy
c. nerves
c. nerves grossly intact
c. nerve sign
c. nerves I–XII
c. nerve transection
ninth cranial nerve
nuclei of cranial nerve
nucleus of cranial nerve
ocular motor cranial nerve
oculomotor cranial nerve palsy

cranial *(continued)*
olfactory cranial nerve
orbit, mandible, ear, cranial nerves, soft tissue syndrome
osteopathy in the cranial field
c. perfusion pressure
permanent cranial nerve deficit
posterior cranial fossa
prone cranial support device
prophylactic cranial irradiation
c. radiation therapy
c. rhythmic impulse
c. sector scan
seventh cranial nerve
c. sinus
tenth cranial nerve
third cranial nerve
c. tongs
transcutaneous cranial electrical stimulation
twelfth cranial nerve
c. vault

cranialis
arachnoidea mater c.
arachnoid mater c.

cranial-sacral respiratory mechanism

craniectomy
anterior c.
linear c.
metopic c.
partial-thickness c.
suboccipital c.

craniocardiac reflex

craniocaudal
angled craniocaudal view
exaggerated craniocaudal lateral angle
exaggerated craniocaudal lateral view
c. projection
c. view

craniocerebral
closed craniocerebral trauma injuries
penetrating craniocerebral injuries
perinatal craniocerebral trauma

craniocervical malformation

cranioectodermal dysplasia

craniofacial
anterior craniofacial resection
c. appliance
c. dysmorphism
c. dysmorphism, absent corpus callosum, iris colobomas, connective tissue dysplasia syndrome
c. dysostosis
c. microsomia
midline craniofacial tumor
osseocartilaginous craniofacial skeleton
osseous craniofacial arteriovenous malformation
c. stenosis

craniofrontonasal
c. dysostosis
c. dysplasia
c. syndrome

craniomandibular
c. dysfunction
c. orthopedic repositioning device

craniometric
Bolton craniometric point
glabellolambda line craniometric point
supramentale craniometric point

cranioorbital
midline cranioorbital clefting

cranioorbitozygomatic osteotomy

craniopathy
metabolic c.

craniopharyngioma
nasopharyngeal c.
papillary c.

cranioplastic
methylmethacrylate cranioplastic plug

cranioplasty
dynamic orthotic c.

craniosacral
c. therapy
c. vault
c. vault 4

craniospinal
c. defect
c. irradiation

craniostenosis
skeletal abnormalities, cutis laxa, craniostenosis, psychomotor retardation, facial abnormalities

craniosynostosis
c., ataxia, trigeminal anesthesia, parietal anesthesia and pons, vermis fusion syndrome
marfanoid craniosynostosis syndrome
mental retardation, overgrowth, craniosynostosis, distal arthrogryposis, sacral dimple, joint laxity
metopic c.
nonsyndromic coronal c.

craniotomy
left frontal c.
middle fossa craniotomy approach
right frontal c.

craniovertebral
anomalous craniovertebral junction

cranium
cerebral yokes of bone of c.
subarachnoid hemorrhage in c.
subdural hemorrhage in c.

crash
c. cart
c. induction of anesthesia

crate
egg crate foam mattress

crater
ulcer c.

craving
alcohol c.
increased craving for sweets
irritability, restlessness, and intense c.
Minnesota Cocaine C. Scale
nicotine c.
salt c.
c.'s and urges

Crawford
C. graft inclusion technique
modified Crawford Campbell inlaid bone-grafting technique

Crawford-Adams hip arthroplasty

crawl
combat c.

crawling
anterior cerebral artery crawling under the skull
skin crawling sensation
vehicle for initial c.

C-reactive
C.-r. protein
C.-r. protein antiserum

creaking
metatarsophalangeal c.
palmar c.

cream
allantoin vaginal c.
hydroquinone c.

ice cream headache
triamcinolone acetonide c.

creamy
turbid, no creamy layer

crease
distal palmar c.
earlobe c.
margin crease distance
midline abdominal c.
multiple benign circumferential skin c.'s on limb
nasolabial c.
proximal palmar c.
simian crease of palm
single palmar c.
thenar palmar c.

create physical need

creatine
c. kinase
c. kinase-BB band
c. kinase-BB isoenzyme
c. kinase fraction muscle
c. kinase isoenzyme electrophoresis
c. kinase MB
c. kinase MB fraction
c. kinase myocardial band
M and B isoenzyme of creatine kinase
muscle fraction enzyme of creatine phosphokinase
myocardial band enzymes of creatine phosphokinase
myocardial muscle creatine kinase isoenzyme
c. phosphokinase
c. phosphokinase isoenzyme
c. phosphokinase-myocardial band
rapid electrophoresis creatine kinase
serum creatine kinase
serum creatine phosphokinase

creatinine
amylase to creatinine ratio
BUN and c.
c. clearance
c. clearance test
electrolytes, blood urea nitrogen, and serum c.
estimated creatinine clearance
peritoneal dialysis creatinine clearance target
serum c.
serum creatinine test
urine c.
c. urine spot test

creatinine-height index

creation
diverting stoma c.
lordosis c.

creative
c. achievement
c. imagination
muscle-brain isoenzyme of creative kinase
c. outlet
Torrance Tests of Creative thinking

creative-associate thinking

creatively
thinking creatively with sounds and words

creativity
C. Attitude Survey
Scales of C. and Learning Environment
c. test
C. Tests for Children

Creek
Black Creek Canal virus
Bunyip Creek virus
Parry Creek virus

creep
mechanical creep of skin
periosteal c.

creeping
c. sensation in extremity
c. substitution of bone

creepy-crawly syndrome of legs

cremaster
musculus c.
c. ratio

cremasteric reflex

crenated red blood cell

creosote
naphthalene creosote and iodoform

crepitans
peritendinitis c.

crepitant
fine crepitant rales
c. rale

crepitation
coarse c.
patellofemoral c.

crepitus
articular c.
c. at fracture site
c. of eyeball

crescendo
c. angina
c. murmur
c. pain
c. sleep
c. transient ischemic attack

crescendo-decrescendo
c.-d. breathing
c.-d. murmur

crescent
articular c.
c. incision
malar c.
malarial c.
monocular temporal c.
myopic c.
radiolucent crescent sign
scleral c.
c. sign of hydronephrosis
sublingual c.

crescentic
antiglomerular basement membrane-negative crescentic glomerular nephritis
c. shelf osteotomy
necrotizing crescentic glomerulonephritis
pauciimmune crescentic glomerulonephritis
perialar crescentic advancement flap
perialar crescentic excision

crescenting
rapidly progressive crescenting glomerulonephritis

crescent-shaped
c.-s. flap of tissue
c.-s. incision

crest
anterior crest of stapes
anterior iliac c.
anterior lacrimal c.
arcuate crest of arytenoid cartilage
autologous iliac crest bone graft
ethmoidal crest of maxilla
ethmoidal crest of palatine bone
iliac c.
c. of iliac bone
iliac crest biopsy
iliac crest bone graft
left iliac c.
malar crest of great wing of sphenoid bone
marginal crest of tooth
maxilla

crest *(continued)*
medial crest of fibula
medial epicondylar c.
nasal crest of horizontal plate of palatine bone
nasal crest of maxilla
nasal crest of palatine process of maxilla
neural c.
neural crest cell
neural crest malformation
neural crest migration
neural crest origin
neural crest precursor
neural crest syndrome
neural crest tissue
neural crest tumor localization study
neuroepithelium of ampullary c.
outer lip of iliac c.
palatine crest of horizontal process of palatine bone
posterior iliac c.
right iliac c.
superior iliac c.
supraventricular c.
c. time
vomerine crest of choana

CREST syndrome

cresyl
brilliant cresyl blue stain
c. red
c. violet
c. violet acetate

cretin
athyreotic c.

cretinism
athyrotic c.
endemic c.
myxedematous endemic c.
neurologic endemic c.

Creutzfeldt-Jakob disease

Creveld
Ellis-van Creveld syndrome

crevice
gingival c.

crevicular
c. fluid flow rate
gingival crevicular fluid

cri
c. de coeur
c. du chat
c. du chat syndrome

crib
allogenic bone c.
alloplastic c.
band and crib space maintainer
c. death
lingual c.
open c.
sudden infant crib death

cribriform
c. fracture
c. growth pattern
c. hymen
meningioma of cribriform plate
c. plate
c. plate injury
c. salivary carcinoma of excretory duct
c. tissue

cribrosa
area c.
area cribrosa papillae renalis
macula c.
macula cribrosa inferior
macula cribrosa media
macula cribrosa quarta
macula cribrosa superior

cricoarytenoid
asymptomatic cricoarytenoid synovitis
c. joint ankylosis
lateral c.
posterior c.

cricoid
anterior cricoid split
anterior cricoid split procedure
c. arch
arch of cricoid cartilage
arytenoidal articular surface of c.
c. lamina
partial cricoid cleft

cricopharyngeal achalasia syndrome

cricothyroid
median cricothyroid ligament
c. muscle

cricothyroidotomy
needle c.
c. and tracheostomy

cricothyrotomy
needle c.

cricotracheal
partial cricotracheal resection

cricotracheal resection

cried
breathed and c.

Crieklair otoplasty

Crigler-Najjar syndrome

crime
c. against humanity
C. Classification Manual
c. a deux
nonviolent c.
c. of passion

Crimean-Congo
C.-C. hemorrhagic fever
C.-C. hemorrhagic fever virus

criminal
c. abortion
c. acting out
adolescent c.
habitual c.
c. sexual psychopath

crinkling
mucosal c.
patch c.

cripple
cardiac c.

crippled children's program

crisis
acquired immune deficiency syndrome c.
acute splenic sequestration c.
aplastic crisis in hemolytic anemia
blast c.
blastic c.
chronic myelocytic/myelogenous/myeloid leukemia blast c.
cocaine and crack c.
c. consultation
c. counseling
disaster crisis intervention
c. hotline
hypertensive c.
hypertensive vascular c.
c. intervention
c. intervention center
mobile crisis outreach team
oculogyric c.
periods of c.
potential fetal hypertensive c.
potential hypertensive c.
rape crisis center
rape crisis intervention program
c. resolution
c. resolution center
scleroderma renal c.
Screening and C. Intervention Program
sickle cell c.

transient aplastic c.
vasoocclusive c.

crisscross
c. atrioventricular valve
c. fashion
c. heart
c. heart malposition

cristae
mitochondrial cristae alteration

criteria
age, metastases, extent and size risk c.
ambulance design c.
assignment criteria for rheumatoid arthritis
damage risk c.
c. for determination of brain death
c. for discharge
extended criteria donor
family history research diagnostic c.
modified Beighton c.
National Cholesterol Education Program c.
National Prostatic Cancer Project c.
c. for organ donation
organ failure c.
patient inclusion c.
research diagnostic c.
response c.

criterion
alternative criterion B for dysthymic disorder
dose-intensity limiting c.
Individualized C. Reference Testing Mathematics
Individualized C. Reference Testing Reading
c. level
lifetime depression c.
method of defining c.
noise c.

critical
anesthesiology critical care medicine
area of critical definition
c. bandwidth range of frequencies
California C. Thinking Dispositions Inventory
California C. Thinking Skills Test
c. carbohydrate level
c. care air transport
c. care area
c. care complex
c. care medicine
c. care medicine unit
c. care nursing
c. care recovery unit
c. condition list
c. coronary stenosis
c. corresponding frequency
c. coupling interval
c. degree of deformation
c. experiment
c. flicker frequency
c. flicker fusion
c. flicker fusion test
c. frequency of photic driving
c. fusion frequency
hand washing in critical care area
Hazard Analysis C. Control Points
c. illness polyneuropathy
c. illumination
c. incident review
c. incident stress management
c. information
c. infrastructure protection
c. limb ischemia
c. micellar concentration
c. micelle concentration
c. off-time
c. organ shielding blocks
pediatric critical care center
c. point drying
c. problem-solving
c. ratio
C. Reasoning Test
c. stimulus duration
Sudeck critical point
c. value

critically ill

criticism
intolerance of c.
objective c.
overt c.
parental c.
peer c.

critique
age c.

crochet
main en c.

crocodile
anterior mosaic crocodile shagreen

crocodile tongue

Crohn
abdominal pain with Crohn disease
C. and Colitis Knowledge
diarrhea from Crohn disease
C. disease
C. Disease Activity Index
C. disease of colon
C. Disease Endoscopic Index of Severity
lower intestinal Crohn disease
luminal Crohn disease
obstructive gastroduodenal Crohn disease
oral Crohn disease
Pediatric Crohn Disease Activity Index
perianal Crohn disease
Perianal Crohn Disease Activity Index
perineal Crohn disease
refractory Crohn disease
steroid-dependent Crohn disease

Crombie ulcer

cromoglycate
disodium c.
sodium c.

Cronqvist cranial index

crook of the arm

cross
aortic cross clamp off
aortic cross clamp on
c. clamping of aorta
c. clamp time
c. femoral-femoral bypass
c. fiber friction
c. generational problem
c. immunity
Maltese c.
c. midline
monohybrid c.
motivation for cross dressing
nerve cross section
nosocomial and cross infection
oculocerebral syndrome of Cross and McKusick
optical c.
partial cross dressing
Ranvier c.

cross-addiction

crossarm flap

crossbar
outer c.

crossbite
anterior c.

crossbite *(continued)*
lingual c.
c. teeth
telescoping c.
cross-bite
crossbridge
myosin c.
cross-clamping
aortic c.-c.
thoracic aortic c.-c.
Cross-Cultural Adaptability Inventory
cross-cultural issue
crosscut
c. bur
c. saw
crossed
antigen-antibody crossed electrophoresis
c. cerebellar diaschisis
c. diagonal
c. electroimmunodiffusion
c. hemianesthesia
c. hemianopia
c. hemiplegia
c. immunoelectrophoresis
c. jerk
c. radioimmunoelectrophoresis
c. straight leg raising
c. with
cross-facial nerve grafting
cross-finger flap
cross-fire treatment
crossing
arteriovenous crossing changes
arteriovenous crossing defect
AV crossing defect
crossing-over
somatic c.-o.
cross-leg
c.-l. flap
c.-l. graft
cross-legged gait
cross-linkage theory
cross-linked
c.-l. fibrin degradation product
c.-l. protein
crossmatch
antihuman globulin c.
flow cytometry c.
T-cell c.
test and c.
c. to transfusion ratio
type and c.
type and crossmatch blood
crossmatched blood
crossmatch-positive recipient
cross-modal priming
crossover
medial crossover toe
c. value
cross-reacting
c.-r. cannabinoid
c.-r. material
cross-reactivation
cross-reactive
c.-r. antigen group
c.-r. idiotype
c.-r. protein
trophoblast-lymphocyte c.-r.
cross-reactivity
trophoblast-lymphocyte c.-r.
cross-section
normalized c.-s.
cross-sectional
c.-s. area
c.-s. echocardiography
c.-s. view
cross-shaped incision
cross-table
c.-t. lateral position
c.-t. lateral view
cross-talk pacemaker
cross-temporal processing
cross-tolerance
croup
membranous c.
crouposus
pemphigus c.
crowd
c. behavior
c. consciousness
c. control
c. fear
crowded dentition
crowding
molar c.
premolar c.
c. of teeth
crowing breath sounds
Crowley Occupational Interests Blank
crown
acrylic veneer c.
alumina-reinforced porcelain c.
aluminum c.
base metal crown and bridge alloy
c. and bridge
collar and crown scissors
full gold c.
full veneer c.
length of c.
Libra II crown and inlay
Libra III bridge and c.
mesiodistal diameter of c.
metal crown margin
partial veneer c.
porcelain jacket crown
porcelain veneer c.
c. rump
stainless steel c.
crown-crimping pliers
Crown-Crisp Experimental Index
crown-heel length
crowning
infant c.
c. of infant's head
crown-rump
c.-r. distance
c.-r. length
c.-r. measurement
crown-to-heel length
crucial incision
cruciate
anterior c.
anterior cruciate deficit of knee
anterior cruciate deficit knee
anterior cruciate ligament
anterior cruciate ligament injury
anterior cruciate ligament reconstruction
anterior cruciate ligament repair
anterior cruciate ligament tear
anterior cruciate sprain
arthroscopically assisted anterior cruciate ligament reconstruction
arthroscopic anterior cruciate ligament reconstruction
c. condylar knee system
c. condylar unconstrained prosthesis
c. hemianesthesia
c. incision
c. instability
c. ligament
c. ligament injury
c. ligament laxity
c. ligament of leg
c. ligament reconstruction

c. ligament rupture
c. ligament tear
median cruciate ligament
posterior cruciate ligament of knee
posterior cruciate ligament tear
posterior cruciate sprain

cruciform
c. anterior spinal hyperextension
longitudinal bands of cruciform ligament of atlas

crude
c. birth rate
c. coal tar
c. coal tar in petroleum
c. extract
c. marijuana extract
c. mortality ratio
c. protein
teichoic acid crude extract

cruel
c. impulse
c. punishment

cruelty to animals

cruenta
lochia c.

Crues
Lynch and Crues type 2 lesion

crunch
mediastinal c.

crunching
c. sound
xiphisternal crunching sound

crura
Oto-Flex crura saw

crural
anterior crural nerve
anterior crural septum
c. fold
c. hernia
lateral crural steal
medial crural cutaneous branch of saphenous nerve
medial crural cutaneous nerve
medial crural strut graft
medial crural suture
pectineal crural hernia

cruris
angina c.
musculus biceps flexor c.
tinea c.

crus
anterior c.
anterior crus integrity
anterior crus of stapes
c. of diaphragm
c. of helix
long crus of incus
medial c.
medial crus of facial canal
medial crus foot plate
medial crus of the horizontal part of the facial canal
medial crus of major alar cartilage of nose
medial crus of the superficial inguinal ring
muscular c.
muscular crus of diaphragm
penile c.
posterior c.
posterior crus of stapes
right c.
right crus of diaphragm
short crus of incus

crush
c. fracture
c. fracture syndrome
c. injury
c. injury renal problem
c. injury syndrome
nerve crush injury
c. syndrome

crushed
c. chest injury
c. eggshell fracture

crushing
c. anxiety and depression
c. chest discomfort
c. injury
c. of intervertebral disc
muscle crushing injury
c. procedure skull of fetus
c. sensation in chest

crust
milk c.

crusted excoriation

crustiness of ear

crusting
lid c.

crutch
c. ambulation
ambulatory with c.'s
axillary c.
c. and belt femoral closed nailing
c. glasses
lid crutch spectacles
nonweightbearing crutch walk
nonweightbearing crutch walking
c. palsy
c. paralysis
c. training
c. walking
weightbearing with c.'s

Crutchfield
C. reduction technique

Cruveilhier-Baumgarten
C.-B. cirrhosis
C.-B. murmur
C.-B. syndrome

crux of heart

cry
cat c.
color and cry good
face, legs, activity, cry, consolability
c. for help
high-pitched c.
hoarse c.
infant had weak c.
c. reflex
stimulate to c.
uterine c.

crying
asymmetric crying facies
c. cat syndrome
c., requirement for oxygen supplementation, increases in heart rate and blood pressure
head rolling, rocking and c.
inconsolable c.
c. jag
pathological c.
uncontrollable c.

crying-induced bronchospasm

cryo
c. cataract extraction
c. destruction procedure

cryoablation
encircling c.

cryoextraction
c. of cataract
open-sky c.
open-sky cryoextraction operation

cryogenic storage container

cryoglobulinemia
essential mixed c.
mixed c.
mixed cryoglobulinemia with glomerulonephritis
mixed essential c.

cryolysis
Treponema pallidum cryolysis complement

cryoprecipitated
c. antihemophilic factor
c. plasma
cryoprecipitate-depleted plasma
cryoprecipitate transfusion
cryopreservation
oocyte c.
cryopreserved
c. aortic homograft
c. bone marrow
c. cartilage
c. embryo
c. heart valve allograft
c. heart valve graft
c. homograft valve
c. human aortic allograft
c. stem cell
c. tissue
c. tissue banking
c. venous transplantation
cryostat
unfixed c.
cryosurgery and laser therapy
cryosurgical
c. ablation
c. ablation of the prostate
N_2O cryosurgical unit
cryothalamotomy procedure
crypt
aberrant crypt focus
adenomatous c.
anal c.
c. cell production rate
c. intraepithelial lymphocyte
Lieberkühn c.
lingual c.
Luschka c.
Morgagni c.
c. of Morgagni
mucous c.
mucous crypt of duodenum
multilocular c.
c.'s of pharyngeal tonsil
synovial c.
tonsillar c.
cryptic
c. tonsil
c. vascular malformation
cryptitis
neutrophilic c.
cryptococcal
AIDS-related cryptococcal meningitis
c. antibody
c. antigen
c. infection
c. meningitis
ocular cryptococcal infection
c. organism
pediatric cryptococcal epididymoorchitis
serum cryptococcal antigen
cryptococcosis
AIDS-related c.
cryptogenic
c. autoimmune cirrhosis
c. autoimmune hepatitis
c. fibrosing alveolitis
c. organizing pneumonia
cryptomeningitis
neurosyphilis c.
cryptorchidism
bilateral c.
caudal appendage, short terminal phalanges, deafness, cryptorchidism, mental retardation syndrome
congenital emphysema, cryptorchidism, penoscrotal web, deafness, mental retardation syndrome
crystal
appositional crystal proliferation
calcium oxalate c.
calcium phosphate crystal deposition disease
calcium pyrophosphate crystal deposition disease
calcium pyrophosphate dihydrate crystal deposition
Charcot-Leyden c.
cholesterol crystal embolization
c. examination screen
c. field stabilization energy
c. field theory
glycoprotein crystal growth inhibitor
c. healing
c. ligand field
lipid liquid c.
liquid crystal contact thermography
liquid crystal display projector
liquid crystal thermogram
liquid crystal thermography
monosodium urate monohydrate c.
oxalate c.'s
phosphate c.'s
single crystal gamma camera
sodium urate c.
thallium-activated sodium iodide c.
c. violet
crystal-induced chemotactic factor
crystalline
c. amino acid
c. amino acid solution
c. calcium pyrophosphate dihydrate
c. cataract
c. egg albumin
c. humor
infectious crystalline keratopathy
c. insulin
marginal crystalline dystrophy
nuclear crystalline aggregate
c. opacity
particulate crystalline material
particulate crystalline material deposition
Schnyder crystalline corneal dystrophy
Soemmerring crystalline swelling
c. zinc insulin
crystallography
optical c.
crystalloid
airway, breathing, circulation, intravenous c.
c. cardioplegia
c. cardioplegic solution
cold crystalloid cardioplegia
hepatic intramitochondrial c.
c. infusion
c. potassium cardioplegia
c. solution
CT
abdominal CT scan
axial unenhanced CT scan
enhanced CT scan
gated CT scanner
helical biphasic contrast-enhanced C.
high-resolution CT imaging
high-resolution CT mammography
high-resolution CT scan
LightSpeed CT scanner
low-dose CT scan
megavoltage CT scanner
metrizamide CT cisternogram
multidetector CT scanner
multiplanar CT scan
noncontrast CT scan
nonenhanced CT scan
orbital CT scan

panoramic CT scan
single enhancing CT lesion
spiral CT scan
two-phase CT imaging
ultrafast CT imaging

C-type
C-t. atrial natriuretic peptide
nevus cell, A-, B-, C-t.

Cuarto
mal de Rio Cuarto virus

cubic
c. centimeter
c. centimeter per hour
c. centimeters per kilogram per day
c. decimeter
c. feet per minute
c. foot
grams per cubic centimeter
c. inch
c. meter
c. micrometer
c. millimeter
millions of particles per cubic foot of air
mole per cubic meter
nanogram per cubic centimeter
pound per cubic foot
c. yard

cubital
median cubital vein
c. tunnel splint
c. tunnel syndrome

cuboid
articular surface on calcaneus for cuboid bone
tuberosity of cuboid bone

cucumber
Chinese c.
c. mosaic virus

cue
anxiety-provoking c.
auditory c.
auditory distance c.
conditioned c.
contextual c.
minimal c.
nonphotic c.
nonverbal c.
orientation c.
perceptual c.
peripheral cue test
Physiognomic Cue Test
verbal c.
visual c.

cued speech

cueing
constant verbal c.
patient independent in bathing with c.
semantic c.

cuff
c. abscess
aortic c.
appropriate blood pressure cuff size
arm c.
atrial c.
attached gingival c.
automated blood pressure c.
avascular cuff technique
bladder c.
c. cellulitis
centimeters of water cuff pressure
inflatable c.
Milch cuff resection of ulna technique
muscular c.
musculotendinous c.
Neer acromioplasty for rotator cuff tear
opacified c.
perivascular c.
pneumatic c.
pressure c.
rotator c.
rotator cuff buttress
rotator cuff calcific tendinitis
rotator cuff impingement syndrome
rotator cuff injury
rotator cuff of shoulder
rotator cuff tear
rotator cuff tendon
rotator cuff tendonitis
ruptured c.
small blood pressure c.
c. sphygmomanometer
suprapatellar c.
surrounding subretinal fluid c.
c. tear arthropathy
c. tear arthroplasty
tracheostomy c.
vaginal c.
Western Ontario Rotator C.

cuffed
c. endotracheal tube
c. tracheostomy tube

cuffing
lymphocytic c.
peribronchial c.
perivascular c.

cuirass
c. jacket
c. respiratory
c. ventilator

culdocentesis
nondiagnostic c.

culdoplasty
Marion-Moschcowitz c.
Mayo c.
McCall c.

culdotomy incision

culprit
c. lesion
c. lesion angioplasty
c. organism
c. vessel

cult
c. member
c. of personality

cultural
c. aspect of chemical dependency
C. Attitude Inventory
C. Attitude Scale
c. belief and practice
c. definition of addiction

cultural-ethnic background

cultural/ethnic diversity

culturally
microscopically positive, culturally negative

culture
acid-fast c.
aerobic and anaerobic blood c.
aerobic bone marrow c.
AIDS blood c.
all culture broth
allogeneic mixed leukocyte c.
American Type C. Collection
amniotic fluid cell c.
amniotic fluid c.
animal cell c.
arterial line c.
autologous mixed lymphocyte c.
biochemical analysis and c.
blood c.
bone marrow c.
Brinster medium for ovum c.
centrifuged culture fluid
charcoal blood medium c.
Clostridium difficile culture filtrate
colony count and c.
contaminated blood c.

culture *(continued)*
continuously cultured carcinoma cell line used for tissue c.'s
dog kidney tissue c.
endoscopic tissue c.
fetal thymus organ c.
fungus c.
fungus, smear, and c.
glass factor tissue c.
gonorrhea c.
gravity settling culture plate
hepatoma tissue c.
human embryo lung cell c.
infected tissue c.
intravascular catheter c.
Loeffler blood culture medium
lymph node c.
lymphocyte culture fluid
lymphoma c.
mammalian cell c.
McCoy culture medium
median tissue culture infective dose
c. medium
midstream clean-catch urine c.
c. midvoid specimen
mixed culture, leukocyte
mixed growth on c.
mixed leukocyte c.
mixed leukocyte-trophoblast c.
mixed lymphocyte c.
mixed lymphocyte culture reaction
mixed lymphocyte culture test
mixed lymphocyte culture, weak
monkey kidney tissue c.
mumps virus c.
Mycoplasma T-strain c.
nasal swab c.
c. of nasal washing
National Type C. Collection
c. negative for growth
c. negative for pathogens
Neisseria gonorrhoeae c.
Nicolle-Novy-MacNeal medium c.
NNN culture medium
organ c.
Organizational C. Inventory
in our c.
Oxgall media c.
parainfluenza virus c.
Pasteur C. Collection
pericardial fluid c.
c. of pleural effusion
purified chick embryo cell c.
pyogenic c.
quantitative tip c.
rabies vaccine, duck embryo c.
rabies vaccine, human diploid cell c.
rabies vaccine, purified chick embryo cell c.
rabies viral c.
rat embryo tissue c.
rat nephroma tissue c.
replacement culture medium
rough, noncapsulated, avirulent bacterial c.
semiquantitative c.
c. and sensitivity
c. and sensitivity and colony count
Sertoli cell culture medium
smear and c.
stained smear and c.
sterile urine c.
c. and susceptibility
throat c.
tissue c.
tissue culture assay
tissue culture infectious dose
tissue culture infective dose
tissue culture inoculated dose
umbilical cord blood c.
urethral and cervical cultures
urine c.
urine culture and sensitivity
urine sterile on c.

culture-bound syndrome

cultured
autologous cultured chondrocyte
autologous cultured epithelium
autologous cultured skin grafting
autologous cultured skin transplantation
bone marrow-derived cultured mast cell
composite cultured skin
continuously cultured carcinoma cell line used for tissue cultures
human cultured lymphoblast
c. macrophages
not c.
c. T cell
c. thymic epithelium

Culture-Free
C.-F. Intelligence Test
C.-F. Self-Esteem Inventories, Second Edition

culture-negative neutrocytic ascites

culture-positive
c.-p. toxin-negative
c.-p. toxin-positive

cumulated
c. activity
C. Index Medicus
mean dose per unit cumulated activity

cumulative
age-specific cumulative incidence rate
c. cardiotoxic dose
c. conception rate
c. dose unit
c. duration of the first remission
c. duration of survival
c. effects of trauma
c. effects of unprotected sun
minimal cumulative cardiotoxic dose
c. pain score
c. phase advancement
c. population doubling level
c. potency rate
c. probability of success
c. radiation effect
c. report
c. sleep deficit
c. survival rate
C. Tcchniques and Procedures in Clinical Microbiology
c. trauma disorder
c. urinary excretion

cuneate
main cuneate nucleus
nucleus of cuneate fasciculus

cuneiform
atavistic c.
first cuneiform bone
medial cuneiform bone
metatarsal cuneiform exostosis
middle cuneiform bone
navicular cuneiform ligament
third cuneiform bone

cuneonavicularis
articulatio c.

cup
c. arthroplasty
Aufranc cup arthroplasty
Aufranc-Turner acetabular c.
bipolar acetabular c.
bipolar prosthetic c.
cold cup biopsy
custom-made acetabular c.
double cup arthroplasty
c. feeding

c. forceps
c. holder
c. holder handle
metal-backed acetabular c.
MF heel c.
migration of acetabular c.
pencil and cup deformity
perilimbal suction c.
polyethylene vacuum c.
porous-coated acetabular c.
c. reamer

cup-and-ball osteotomy

cup-and-spill stomach

cup-cement interface

cup-disk ratio

Cupid
arch of C.
C. bow configuration

Cupid's
C. bow
C. bow contour
C. bow peak
C. bow upper lip

cup-on-cup arthroplasty of the hip

cupping
optic c.
optic disc c.
optic nerve c.
pathologic c.

cup-to-disc
c.-t.-d. ratio
c.-t.-d. ratio horizontal
c.-t.-d. ratio vertical

curable hypertension

curative
c. chemotherapy
c. dose
c. inoculation
c. irradiation
median curative dose
c. potential
c. result
c. treatment

curdy
c. discharge
c. pus

cure
five-year cure rate
high cure rate
no known c.
rest c.
test of c.

C-urea breath test

curettage
biopsy and c.
c. and desiccation
diagnostic dilatation and c.
dilatation and c.
dilation and c.
dilation, curettage, and biopsy
c. and electrodesication
electrodesiccation and c.
c. and electrodesiccation
endocervical c.
endometrial c.
excision and c.
excision, curettage and drilling
fractional dilatation and c.
fractional dilation and c.
c. and fulguration
gingival c.
c. and irrigation
irrigation and c.
root planing and c.
suction, dilation, and c.
therapeutic abortion, dilation, aspiration, and c.
vaginal interruption of pregnancy with dilatation and c.

curette
cerumen c.
curved c.
disposable c.
long c.
orthopaedic c.
oval curved-cup c.
uterine vacuum aspirating c.

curetting
uterine c.

curetting/curettage
endocervical c./c.

curies per milliliter

curl
abdominal curl exercise
hamstring c.
pigtail curl of catheter
pigtail curl of stent tube

curly
c. hair-ankyloblepharon-nail dysplasia syndrome
c. toe

currant jelly sputum

current
alternating c.
alternating current or direct c.
amplitude-summation interferential current therapy
anterior current generator
aperture c.
aperture current setting
attenuation-based on-line modulation of the tube c.
audiofrequency eddy c.
calcium c.
chloride c.
c. diagnosis
direct c.
direct current cardioversion
electric c.
electric current density
electrosurgical current intensity
equivalent current dipole
frequency-difference interferential current therapy
high-frequency c.
high-voltage pulsed c.
inhibitory postsynaptic c.
c. injury
integrated ion c.
interferential c.
c. liabilities
C. List of Medical Literature
low energy direct c.
low frequency alternating c.
low-frequency current field
low-intensity direct c.
c. medical evidence of record
c. medical information and terminology
miniature endplate c.
c. night terrors
pacemaker c.
C. and Past Psychopathology Scales
c. perception threshold
c. population survey
c. practice
C. Procedural Terminology
radiofrequency c.
resultant c.
short circuit c.
single-electrode current perception threshold
c. sleepwalker
sodium c.
c. strength
c. vital signs

curriculum
Prevocational Assessment and C. Guide
Scaled C. Achievement Levels Test
c. vitae

curse
Ondine c.

curse *(continued)*
Ondine curse, periodic breathing
Ondine curse syndrome

curtain
aortic c.
lip c.

curvature
anterior corneal c.
axial curvature map
axial curvature mapping
cervical lordotic c.
cornea c.
progressive curvature of radius

curve
abnormal c.
angulus on the lesser c.
anterior central c.
anterior peripheral c.
area under the c.
area under c.
calibration curve data
central posterior c.
dose-response c.
expiratory flow-volume c.
flattening of normal lordotic c.
frequency threshold c.
growth hormone dose-response c.
hemoglobin oxygen dissociation c.
Hunter and Driffield c.
increased lumbar c.
instantaneous resonance c.
intensity-duration curve
intermediate posterior c.
intracardiac pressure c.
kinetic hemolysis c.
length-tension c.
lumbar lordotic c.
lung count c.
maximal expiratory flow-static recoil curve
maximal expiratory flow volume c.
mechanical expiratory flow volume c.
milled-in c.'s
multiple event c.
nonlinear developmental c.
normal c.
normalized area under the c.
oxygen dissociation c.
partial expiratory flow-static recoil curve
passive length-tension c.
peripheral curve on contact lens
peripheral posterior c.
phase response c.
plasma disappearance c.
posterior central c.
posterior intermediate c.
posterior peripheral c.
pressure-volume curve
raw area under c.
receiver operating characteristic c.
scoliotic curve fixation
strength-duration c.
target area under the c.
time-activity c.
ventricular function c.

curved
c. base twin bracket
c. basket forceps
c. bone rongeur
c. cannula with locking dilator
c. curette
c., reformatted mandibular image
c. downward incision
c. end-to-end anastomosis
c. hemostat
c. incision
c. longitudinal incision
c. microneedle holder
multipurpose curved clamp
c. needle biopsy
c. osteotomy
c. passer
c. periosteal elevator
c. periscapular incision

curved-handle cane

curved-needle surgeon's knot

curvilinear
c. body
continuous curvilinear capsulorrhexis
c. incision
neuronal ceroid lipofuscinosis curvilinear body
c. skin incision
c. threshold shoulder
c. velocity

Cushing
C. adenoma
adrenocorticotropic hormone-dependent Cushing syndrome
ectopic Cushing syndrome
C. pressure response
C. reflex
C. virilizing syndrome

cushingoid
c. appearance
c. body habitus
c. facies
c. syndrome

cushion
air-filled c.
atrioventricular canal c.
endocardial cushion defect

cushioned
soft ankle, cushioned heel orthopaedic appliance
wedge adjustable cushioned heel

cusp
anterior cusp of left atrioventricular valve
anterior cusp of mitral valve
anterior cusp of right atrioventricular valve
anterior cusp of tricuspid valve
anterior determinants of cusp occlusion
aortic cusp prolapse
aortic valve cusp separation
apex of cusp of tooth
asymmetric closure of c.
distal c.
distal cusp ridge
distobuccal c.
distobuccal cusp ridge
distolingual c.
distolingual cusp ridge
fifth cusp groove
left coronary c.
lingual c.
maxillary canine c.
mesiobuccal c.
mesiolingual c.
noncoronary c.
perforated aortic c.
redundant cusp syndrome
right coronary c.

cusp-forming pliers

cuspid
mandibular cuspid radiograph
maxillary cuspid radiograph

custodial
c. care
c. parent

custody
Ackerman-Schoendorf Scales for Parent Evaluation of C.
parental c.

custom
c. fit in ear unit
laser image custom arthroplasty
c. prosthesis
c. rasp
c. tailoring

customary
c., prevailing, and reasonable
reasonable and c.
c. temperature
usual and c.
usual, customary, and reasonable fees

custom-fabricated graft

custom-fitted brace

customized joint repair

custom-made
c.-m. acetabular cup
c.-m. insert
c.-m. shoe

custom-molded shoe

custom-threaded prosthesis

cut
chamfer c.
chamfer cut jig
clamped and c.
electrosurgical c.
c. end of bone
field c.
freehand c.
intercostal nerve c.
notch c.
off-center c.
p c.
c. surface
tomographic c.
visual c.
visual field c.
wedge-shaped cut into bone

cutaneomandibular
multiple hereditary cutaneomandibular polyoncosis

cutaneous
c. abscess
acute cutaneous lupus erythematosus
African cutaneous Kaposi sarcoma
antebrachial cutaneous nerve
anterior abdominal cutaneous branch of intercostal nerve
anterior cutaneous branch
anterior cutaneous branch of femoral nerve
anterior cutaneous branch of iliohypogastric nerve
anterior cutaneous branch of intercostal nerve
anterior cutaneous nerve
anterior cutaneous nerve of abdomen
anterior femoral cutaneous nerve
anterior pectoral cutaneous branch of intercostal nerve
anthroponotic cutaneous leishmaniasis
approximation of cutaneous edges
c. basophilic hypersensitivity
c. B-cell lymphoma
brachial cutaneous nerve
cellular cutaneous fibrous histiocytoma
chronic cutaneous lupus erythematosus
chronic infantile neurological, cutaneous, and articular
conventional cutaneous malignant melanoma
delayed cutaneous hypersensitivity
delayed cutaneous reaction
diffuse cutaneous leishmaniasis
diffuse cutaneous scleroderma
disseminated cutaneous leishmaniasis
dorsal cutaneous nerve
femoral cutaneous nerve
florid cutaneous papillomatosis
c. graft-versus-host disease
c. graft-versus-host reaction
c. hepatic porphyria
hereditary cutaneous malignant melanoma
c. hyperesthesia
immediate active cutaneous anaphylaxis
increased cutaneous blood flow
c. infection
c. inoculation
intermediate dorsal cutaneous nerve
late cutaneous anaphylactic reaction
late-phase cutaneous reaction
lateral cutaneous branch
lateral cutaneous nerve of calf
lateral cutaneous nerve of forearm
lateral cutaneous nerve of thigh
lateral femoral c.
c. leishmaniasis
lentigines, atrial myxomas, cutaneous papular myxomas, blue nevi
localized acquired cutaneous pseudoxanthoma elasticum
localized cutaneous amyloidosis
localized cutaneous leishmaniasis
lower lateral cutaneous nerve of arm
c. lymphocyte antigen
c. lymphoid hyperplasia
c. malignant melanoma
c. malignant melanoma of head and neck
masseteric cutaneous ligament
medial antebrachial cutaneous nerve
medial brachial cutaneous nerve
medial crural cutaneous branch of saphenous nerve
medial crural cutaneous nerve
medial cutaneous branch
medial cutaneous branch of dorsal branch of posterior intercostal artery
medial cutaneous nerve
medial cutaneous nerve of arm
medial cutaneous nerve of forearm
medial cutaneous nerve of leg
medial cutaneous thigh flap
medial dorsal cutaneous nerve
necrotic cutaneous loxoscelism
c. necrotizing vasculitis
c. neural tumor
nondisseminated cutaneous leishmaniasis
palmar cutaneous branch of the median nerve
palmar cutaneous branch of the ulnar nerve
palmar cutaneous vein
pancreatic cutaneous fistula
passive cutaneous anaphylactic reaction
passive cutaneous anaphylaxis
passive cutaneous anaphylaxis test
pectoral and abdominal anterior cutaneous branch of intercostal nerve
perforating cutaneous nerve
perineal branch of posterior cutaneous nerve of thigh
perineal branch of posterior femoral cutaneous nerve
peripheral cutaneous vasoconstriction
posterior branch of medial cutaneous nerve of forearm
posterior cutaneous nerve of arm
posterior cutaneous nerve of forearm
posterior cutaneous nerve of thigh

cutaneous *(continued)*
primary cutaneous large B-cell lymphoma
primary cutaneous melanoma
reactive cutaneous angioendotheliomatosis
secondary cutaneous large B-cell lymphoma
septicemic cutaneous ulcerative disease
c. signs of drug abuse
subacute cutaneous lupus erythematosus
c. suture of palate
c. suture technique
systemic cutaneous basophil hypersensitivity
c. tag
c. T-cell attracting chemokine
c. T-cell leukemia
c. T-cell lymphoma
thick cutaneous melanoma
c. tuberculin test
ulnar branch of medial antebrachial cutaneous nerve
ulnar cutaneous vein
c. ureterostomy
c. water loss

cut-as-you-go technique

cutdown
c. access
greater saphenous vein c.
healed cutdown site
c. incision

cuticle
attachment c.
Nasmyth c.

cutis
angiolipoma, posttraumatic neuroma, glomus tumor, eccrine spiradenoma, and leiomyoma c.
aplasia cutis congenita
calcinosis cutis circumscripta
calcinosis cutis, osteoma cutis, poikiloderma, and skeletal abnormalities syndrome
membranous aplasia c.
metastatic calcinosis c.
skeletal abnormalities, cutis laxa, craniostenosis, psychomotor retardation, facial abnormalities

Cutler-Beard operation

Cutler implant

cutoff
c. frequency
liberal cutoff score

cutter
bone plug c.
controlled depth osteotomy c.
full radius c.
c. guide
multiple action c.
power-oriented depth controlled osteotomy c.
titanium linear c.
vitreous infusion suction c.

cutting
air-powered cutting drill
c. balloon angioplasty
bipolar cutting loop
c. block
c. cone
c. current
diamond cutting instrument
c. disk
c. electrode
electrosurgical cutting knife
c. endoscopic mucosal resection
four-in-one cutting block
c. instrument
c. needle biopsy
optimal cutting temperature
orthopaedic cutting instrument
c. shaver
c. wire

cuttlefish disc

Cuvier
canal of C.
duct of C.

cyanide
diphenylarsine c.
hydrogen c.
c. sulfonate
c. tablet

cyanogen
c. bromide
c. chloride

cyanosis
apnea, bradycardia, and c.
clubbing, cyanosis, and edema
clubbing and cyanosis upper extremity
c., clubbing or edema
edema, clubbing, and c.
c. of extremity
c. of fingernail
c. of fingertip
c. of lip
muscular atrophy and c.
c. of nail bed
nail bed c.
c. neonatorum
no clubbing, cyanosis, or edema
oral mucosa c.
pallor and c.
peripheral cyanosis of extremities
c. of retina

cyanotic
c. atrophy of liver
c. congenital heart disease
c. discoloration of skin
gasping and c.
c. heart disease
c. induration
c. infant
c. kidney
maternal cyanotic heart disease
neonatal cyanotic congenital heart disease
c. newborn
patient c.

cyclase
adenylate c.
adenylate cyclase inhibitor
adenylate cyclase toxin
lymphocyte adenylate cyclase response
modulator of adenylate c.
pituitary adenylate cyclase activating polypeptide

cycle
c. amplitude
atrial fibrillation cycle length
basic cycle length
basic drive cycle length
basic rest-activity c.
brain wave c.
cell cycle kinetics analysis
cell cycle redistribution
cell cycle redistribution and dose fractionation
cell division c.
cessation of menstrual c.
contraction cycle of heart
daily sleep-wake c.
disabled infectious single cycle virus
duty c.
dynamic environmental conditioning c.
gap in cell c.
generation time of cell c.
heart c.
intense cycle of high-dose chemotherapy
irregular menstrual c.
isometric period of cardiac c.
c. length
c. length, paced

life cycle change
life cycle of *Echinococcus*
life cycle theory
mean menstrual cycle hematocrit
menstrual cycle hemodynamic response
menstrual cycle induction
menstrual cycle regulation
menstrual cycle resumption
mitotic c.
nonrapid eye movement-rapid eye movement c.
ovarian cycle change
ovulatory menstrual c.
c. of pain and inactivity
part of the electrocardio-graphic cycle representing atrial depolarization
pentose phosphate c.
c.'s per degree
periodic breathing c.
c.'s per minute
phase of mitosis in cell growth c.
phosphate c.
purine nucleotide c.
quiescent phase of cells leaving the mitotic c.
ratio of expiration time and total time of breathing c.
ratio of inspiration time and total time of breathing c.
ratio of inspiratory time to total cycle time
c. redistribution and dose
sinus cycle length
sinus node cycle length
time required to complete G_2 phase of cell c.
time required to complete G_1 phase of cell c.
time required to complete M phase of cell c.
time required to complete S phase of cell c.
urea cycle enzymopathy
ventricular tachycardia cycle length

cyclic
c. adenosine monophosphate
c. AMP
c. AMP-binding protein
c. arginine monophosphate
composite cyclic therapy
continuous cyclic peritoneal dialysis
c. flow reduction
idiopathic cyclic edema
c. insanity
c. irregularity
nephrogenous cyclic adenosine monophosphate
oculomotor paresis with cyclic spasm
c. sedentary
c. total parenteral nutrition
c. uridine 3,′5′-monophosphate
c. vomiting syndrome

cyclin-dependent
c.-d. kinase
c.-d. kinase inhibitor

cycling
continuous cycling peritoneal dialysis
endometrial cycling activity
c. fibroblast
mood disorder with rapid c.
phase c.

cyclitis
Fuchs heterochromic c.

cyclodialysis

cyclophilin
calcium-signal modulating cyclophilin B ligand

cyclophotocoagulation
Nd:YAG c.
Nd:YAG laser c.

cycloplegic refraction

Cydia pomonella granulovirus

cylinder
arm cylinder cast
c. axis
bivalved cylinder cast
c. cast
chamfered cylinder acetabular component
long leg cylinder cast
osseointegrated cylinder implant
short arm cylinder cast
short leg cylinder cast

cylindric
axis of cylindric lens

cylindrical
c. confronting cisterna
c. lens

cylindroma
lung c.

cypress
Arizona c.
Arizona cypress tree
Monterey cypress tree

cyst
ampulla of Vater c.
aneurysmal bone c.
anogenital epidermal c.
anogenital pilar c.
anogenital sebaceous c.
anogenital vestibular c.
antral mucosal c.
apical periodontal c.
apical radicular c.
apocrine retention c.
arachnoid brain c.
arachnoid cyst of the middle fossa
arachnoid spine c.
Arana-Iniquez intracranial cyst removal technique
arrested follicular c.
atretic follicular c.
atypical renal c.
Bartholin gland duct c.
blue dome c.
breast cyst fluid
breast cyst fluid protein
calcifying odotogenic c.
choroid plexus c.
corpus luteum c.
endoscopic transpapillary cyst drainage
epidermal inclusion c.
excision of ganglionic c.
fluid-filled cyst in breast
Gartner duct c.
granular c.
hydatid cyst disease
implantation cyst of iris
incision and drainage of c.
incisive canal c.
infected pilonidal c.
c. of iris
leptomeningeal arachnoid c.
lip pseudocleft-hemangiomatous branchial cyst syndrome
liver cyst infection
luteal ovarian c.
massive ovarian c.
median alveolar c.
median anterior maxillary c.
median raphe cyst of the penis
mediastinal bronchogenic c.
mediastinal dorsal enteric c.
mediastinal duplication c.
middle cranial fossa c.
midline of brain c.
milk of calcium urinary tract c.
mucous retention c.
müllerian duct c.

cyst *(continued)*
multilocular hydatid c.
multilocular peritoneal inclusion c.
multilocular thymic c.
multiple luteinized theca c.
multiple nevoid, basal cell epithelioma, jaw cysts, bifid rib syndrome
nabothian c.
nasopalatine duct c.
nevoid basal cell epithelioma, jaw cysts, bifid rib syndrome
noncommunicating biliary c.
nonparasitic cyst of liver
omphalomesenteric duct c.
orbital blood c.
orbital chocolate c.
orbital dermoid c.
organizing hemorrhagic c.
osseous hydatid c.
ova, cysts, and parasites
ovarian cyst torsion
ovarian dermoid c.
ovarian endometriosis c.
ovarian inflammatory c.
paramesonephric duct c.
pars intermedia c.
pelvic chocolate c.
percutaneous cord cyst puncture
percutaneous cyst aspiration
pericardial duplication c.
perineural arachnoid c.
peritoneal mesothelial c.
popliteal c.
posterior fossa extra-axial arachnoid c.
Rathke cleft c.
ruptured Baker c.
salivary duct c.
solitary bone c.
tailgut c.
talar dome c.
third ventricle c.
thyroglossal duct c.
traumatic bone c.
vaginal inclusion c.

cystadenocarcinoma
mucinous c.
ovarian c.
pancreatic c.
papillary cystadenocarcinoma of ovary
papillary serous c.
parovarian c.

cystadenofibroma
ovarian c.

cystadenoma
apocrine c.
biliary c.
glycogen-rich c.
lymphomatosum
macrocystic c.
Moll gland c.
mucinous c.
mucinous cystadenoma of ovary
ovarian c.
pancreas c.
papillary cystadenoma lymphomatosum
papillary epididymal c.
serous c.

cystectomy
ovarian c.
palliative c.
partial c.
pilonidal c.
radical c.
salvage c.
total c.

cysteine
methyl cysteine hydrochloride
c. proteinase inhibitor
c. sulfinic acid decarboxylase

cystic
acquired cystic kidney disease
acquired renal cystic disease
adenoassociated virus for cystic fibrosis
adenoid cystic carcinoma
adenoid cystic carcinoma of head and neck
c. adenomatous malformation
adult cystic teratoma
autosomal dominant medullary cystic kidney disease
benign cystic endometrial hyperplasia
benign cystic teratoma
chronic cystic gastritis
chronic cystic infarct
congenital cystic adenomatoid malformation
congenital pulmonary cystic lymphangiectasia
c., partially differentiated nephroblastoma
c. disease of breast
c. duct
early cystic hyperplasia
familial juvenile nephrophthisis-medullary cystic disease
familial nephronophthisis-medullary cystic disease
c. fibrosis arthropathy
c. fibrosis factor
c. fibrosis factor activity
c. fibrosis protein
c. fibrosis-related diabetes
c. fibrosis transmembrane conductance regulator
c. fluid-filled mass
folliculosebaceous cystic hamartoma
c. goiter
gross cystic disease
gross cystic disease fluid protein
c. hernia
c. hygroma
c. hyperplasia
c. infarct
c. ischemia
Luschka cystic gland
c. mastitis
mature cystic ovarian teratoma
medial cystic necrosis
c. medial necrosis
c. medial necrosis of ascending aorta
c. mesothelioma
midline cystic structure
mucinous cystic neoplasm
multilocular cystic kidney
multilocular cystic lesion
multiple benign cystic epithelioma
neonatal cystic pulmonary emphysema
nephrophthisis-medullary cystic disease
nuchal cystic hygroma
old cystic infarct
ovarian cystic teratoma
pancreatic cystic fibrosis
pancreatic cystic lymphangioma
papillary cystic adenoma
papillary cystic neoplasm
parafoveal cystic space
pelvic cystic mass
c. periventricular leukomalacia
c. renal cell carcinoma
small cystic infarct
solid cystic tumor
solid and cystic tumor of the pancreas
c. suppurative necrosis
uremic medullary cystic disease

cystica
spina bifida c.

cystine
c. aminopeptidase

c. guanine
c. trypticase agar

cystine-tellurite medium

cystinosis
adult c.
nephropathic c.
neuropathic c.

cystitis
acute hemorrhagic c.
focal hemorrhagic c.
focal hemorrhagic necrotizing c.
interstitial c.
nonbacterial c.
noninfectious chronic c.

cystitome
air c.
McIntyre reverse c.

cystocele
paravaginal c.
paravaginal cystocele repair
protruding c.

cystocopy and retrograde

cystogram
bilateral c.
excretory c.
postvoiding c.
retrograde c.
triple voiding c.
voiding c.

cystography
excretory c.
indirect radionuclide c.

cystoid
aphakic cystoid macular edema
c. cicatrix of limbus
c. macular degeneration
c. macular edema
peripheral cystoid degeneration

cystoma
parvilocular c.

cystometric
maximum cystometric capacity

cystometrics
office c.

cystometry
filling c.
gas c.
multichannel c.
screening c.

cystoplasty
augmentation c.
autoaugmentation c.

cystosarcoma phyllodes

cystoscopy
c. and dilatation
c. and dilation
c. and fulguration
percutaneous fetal c.
c. and pyelography
c. and voiding urethrogram

cystoscopy-endoscopy dilation

cystosonography
echo-enhanced c.

cystostomy
percutaneous suprapubic c.

cystotomy
open c.
suprapubic c.

cystourethrogram
voiding c.

cystourethrograph
metallic bead-chain c.
voiding c.

cystourethrography
isotope voiding c.
metallic bead-chain c.
micturating c.
voiding c.

cystourethropexy
Marshall-Marchetti-Krantz c.
needle c.

cythemolytic icterus

cytoadhesion
reverse immune c.

cytoarchitecture
neural c.

cytochemical
automated cytochemical system
c. bioassay

cytochrome
c. c oxidase
membrane-bound cytochrome b_{558}
c. P450 11-beta-hydroxylase
c. P450 21-beta-hydroxylase
c. P450 enzyme 19, 27
c. P450 enzyme 1A1
c. P450 enzyme 11A
c. P450 enzyme 21B
c. pigment
c. protein
c. system

cytogenetic
M-FISH cytogenetic technique
multicolor FISH cytogenetic technique

cytogenetics

cytokine
angiogenic c.
antiinflammatory c.
osteoporotic c.
paracrine c.
suppressor of cytokine signaling 3
tumor necrosis factor-related activation-induced c.

cytokinin-regulated
c.-r. kinase
c.-r. kinase I, II, L

cytological
peritoneal cytological assessment

cytology
ascitic fluid c.
aspiration biopsy c.
fine-needle aspiration c.
histology and c.
mammary aspiration specimen cytology test
MAS cytology test
MASS cytology test
needle aspiration c.
negative peritoneal c.
nipple aspiration c.
nipple discharge c.
oral cavity c.
paracentesis fluid c.
pericardial fluid c.
peritoneal cytology sample
peritoneal fluid c.
positive peritoneal c.
voiding urine c.

cytolysis
lymphocyte-mediated c.

cytolytic
MHC class I-restricted cytolytic activity
c. T cell
c. T lymphocyte

cytoma
plasma c.

cytomegalic
c. disease
c. inclusion body
c. inclusion disease
c. inclusion disease virus

cytomegaloviral mononucleosis

cytomegalovirus
congenital cytomegalovirus infection
human cytomegalovirus infection
c. immune globulin
c. immunoglobulin

cytomegalovirus *(continued)*
macular c.
mouse c.
syphilis, toxoplasmosis, other agents, rubella, cytomegalovirus, herpes simplex virus
tissue-invasive c.
toxoplasmosis, other infections, rubella, cytomegalovirus infection, herpes simplex syndrome

cytomegalovirus-specific immune globulin

cytometric
flow cytometric platelet

cytometry
flow c.
flow cytometry crossmatch
multidimensional flow c.

cytopathic
c. effect
enteric cytopathic human orphan

cytopathogenic
c. effect
enteric cytopathogenic human orphan

cytopathy
mitochondrial c.

cytopenias
drug-induced blood c.

cytophagic
histiocytic cytophagic panniculitis

cytophotocoagulation
contact transscleral laser c.

cytophotometry
pulse c.

cytoplasm
cell soupy c.
extrusion of cell c.
granular eosinophilic c.
narrow rim of c.

cytoplasmic
antineuronal cytoplasmic autoantibody
c. antineutrophil cytoplasmic antibody
antineutrophil cytoplasmic antibody
antineutrophil cytoplasmic antibody titer
antineutrophil cytoplasmic antigen
antineutrophil cytoplasmic autoantibody
antineutrophil cytoplasmic IgG antibody
antineutrophilic cytoplasmic antibody
antineutrophilic cytoplasmic autoantibody-small vessel vasculitis
c. aspartate aminotransferase
assay neutrophil cytoplasmic antibody
c. immunoglobulin M
eosinophilic cytoplasmic inclusion
focal cytoplasmic degradation
hyaline cytoplasmic inclusion
c. inclusion body
c. lipid droplet
matrix
c. membrane
pauciimmune antineutrophil cytoplasmic antibody-associated glomerulonephritis
perinuclear antineutrophil cytoplasmic antibody
perinuclear antineutrophil cytoplasmic autoantibody
c. polyhedrosis virus
soluble cytoplasmic protein
structure of the cytoplasmic matrix
total cytoplasmic ribosome
c. tubular aggregate
c. vacuolization

cytoporphyrin
free cytoporphyrin in erythrocytes

cytoreduction
optimal c.

cytoreductive
maximum cytoreductive benefit
c. regimen
c. surgery
c. therapy

cytosine
c. arabinoside
guanine c.
hydroxymethyl c.
c. triphosphate

cytoskeletal
neuritic cytoskeletal abnormality
neuron-specific cytoskeletal protein

cytoskeleton-associated protein

cytosol
neuronal c.
c. protein

cytosolic
c. thymidine kinase
oxidase cytosolic factor

cytosome
lipid c.
multilamellar c.

cytotaxis
negative c.

cytotoxic
c. agent
c. antibody
antibody directed cytotoxic response
antireticular cytotoxic serum
antitumor cytotoxic lymphocyte
c. assay
c. chemotherapeutic agent
c. edema
c. factor
granulocyte c.
c. immunosuppressive therapy
c. index
c. lymphocyte
c. lymphocyte activation antigen 4 immunoglobulin
lymphocyte-mediated c.
MHC-restricted cytotoxic T cell
minimal cytotoxic epitope
c. necrosis
neuronal cytotoxic edema
c. reaction
single-cell liquid cytotoxic assay
soluble cytotoxic medium
sperm c.
T cell c.
c. T cell
c. T-cell lymphocyte response
c. T lymphocyte
c. T lymphocyte activity
c. T lymphocyte antigen-4
c. T lymphocyte-based immunotherapy
c. T lymphocyte line
c. T lymphocyte precursor

cytotoxicity
allogeneic lymphocyte c.
antibody-dependent cell c.
antibody-dependent cell-mediated c.
antibody-dependent cellular c.
antibody-dependent cytotoxicity test
antibody-dependent lymphocyte-mediated c.
antibody-directed cellular c.
antibody-mediated c.
antiglobulin-enhanced complement-dependent c.
c. assay
cell-mediated c.

cell mediated c.
complement-dependent c.
complement-mediated c.
immune c.
lymphocyte-mediated c.
macrophage cytotoxicity factor
natural c.
natural cell-mediated c.
natural cytotoxicity receptor
natural killer-mediated c.
c. negative, absorption positive
NK cell-mediated c.
spontaneous cell-mediated c.
spontaneous lymphocyte-mediated c.
tumor-induced marrow c.

cytotoxin-associated gene product A

cytotrophoblast
peripheral cytotrophoblast cell

cytourethropexy
retropubic c.

Czapek-Dox agar

d'accoucheur
main d.

dacryocystitis
trachomatous d.

dacryocystorhinostomy
endonasal laser d.
endoscopic intranasal d.
external d.
Moria-France dacryocystorhinostomy clamp

dacryolith
Nocardia d.

dacryostomy
Arroyo d.
Arruga d.

dactylitis
blistering distal d.

daily
acceptable daily intake
activities of daily living
activities of daily living scale
d. affective rhythm
allowable daily intake
ascitic fluid tapped d.
average daily census
average daily dose
average daily metabolic rate
average daily patient load
d. caloric intake
d. census
chronic daily headache
Communicative Abilities in D. Living
cope with daily stress
defined daily dose
d. dose
estimated safe and adequate daily dietary intake
extended activities of daily living
extended daily dialysis
fecal daily blood loss
d. fetal movement count
d. fetal movement record
d. fractionation rate of rad
d. group therapy
d. habits
d. high fiber supplement
impairment of activities of daily living
independent in activities of daily living
d. injection
d. intermittent peritoneal dialysis
d. irrigation
d. ischemia
d. living skills
maximal daily permissible intake
maximal tolerable daily intake
maximum recommended daily dose
mean daily dose
mean daily erect blood pressure
mean daily nitrogen balance
mean daily supine blood pressure
minimal daily requirement
mobility activities of daily living
multiple daily fraction
multiple daily injection
multiple daily insulin injection
d. observation for rejection
d. oral hygiene
patient independent in activities of daily living
d. permissible intake
physical daily living skills
postures of daily living
d. protein intake
recommended daily dietary allowance
recommended daily intake
d. replacement factor of lymphocytes
simulated activities of daily living
skills of daily living
d. sleep-wake cycle
three times daily with meal
times d.
tolerable daily intake
total daily dose
total daily energy expenditure
d. weight

daily-wear
d.-w. contact lens
d.-w. soft contact lens

Dakar bat virus

Dale-Laidlaw clotting time

Dalen-Fuchs nodule

Dallas
modified Dallas classification of disc morphology grades 0–7

dam
rubber d.

damage
acoustic nerve d.
anoxic brain d.
anterior cervical surgery vocal cord d.
bilateral hemisphere d.
brain damage from cerebral hemorrhage
definite brain d.
diffuse alveolar d.
drug-induced esophageal d.
end organ d.
glaucomatous optic nerve d.
d. to healthy tissue
heart and liver d.
heart muscle d.
heart valve d.
irreversible damage to brain cell
ischemic damage to heart
left brain d.
left hemisphere d.
left hemisphere brain d.
minimal brain d.
myocardial d.
no brain d.
noise-induced hearing d.
obturator nerve d.
occipital cortex d.
optic nerve d.
optic tract d.
organic damage to brain
parietal cortex d.
peripheral nerve d.
permanent joint d.
permanent kidney d.
potentially lethal d.
property damage collision
property damage accident
regional alveolar d.
repair of potentially lethal d.
repair of sublethal d.
residual thermal d.
retinal damage threshold
right brain d.
right hemisphere brain d.
d. risk criteria
seizure-brain d.
silent heart d.
silent ischemic brain d.
stress-related mucosal d.
tubal inflammatory d.
white matter d.

damaged
d. or blocked fallopian tubes
d. brain cell
d. disc syndrome
d. donor heart
external muscle layer d.
d. issue

damaging ultraviolet

Dameshek oval target cell

Damian graft procedure

D

dampening
Doppler waveform d.
Damus-Kaye-Stansel procedure
danazol
low-dose d.
dance
high-impact aerobic d.
low-impact aerobic d.
Saint Anthony d.
St. Vitus d.
dancer
belly dancer dyskinesia
dander
animal dander sensitivity
guinea pig d.
laboratory animal dander allergy
dandruff with itching
Dandy-Walker
D.-W. deformity
D.-W. syndrome
danger
fetal d.
fetal danger zone
d. list
d. to others
dangerous
d. behavior
d. delusion
d. drug
D. Drugs Act
inappropriate dangerous behavior
d. to one's self
d. to others
dangle out of bed
Danish Prostate Symptom Score
Danis-Weber classification for ankle fracture
Dantec
Le Dantec virus
D'Aoust Fineman virus
dapsone
motor dapsone neuropathy
D-arabitol fermentation test
Darier
D. disease
morbus D.
dark
d. adaptation test
d. blood stained fluid
d. bloody material
d. bloody stool
d. green bile
d. green viscous bile
d. ground
passage of dark brown urine
dark-adapted
d.-a. eye
d.-a. pupil size
darkening
immediate pigment d.
intermittent pigment d.
d. of nipple
d. vision
dark-field
fluorescent antibody d.-f.
d.-f. illumination
dark-ground illumination
darkly-staining gram-positive rods
darkness
paradoxical darkness reaction
dart and dome
dartos
d. fascia
d. muscle
d. muscle of scrotum
d. reflex
Darwin
auricular tubercle of D.
darwinism
neural d.
dashboard
d. dislocation
d. fracture
d. knee
d. knee injury
data
d. acquisition processor
Adult Personal D. Inventory
asymmetric data sampling
asynchronous data transmission
automatic data processing
calibration curve d.
d. case report form
centralized cancer patient data system
Clinical D. Repository
d. collection form
d. communication
d., action, response
d., action, response, and evaluation
derived hemodynamic d.
direct data entry
distributed data processing
electronic data processing
extended data stream
first set of followup d.
insufficient d.
investigational drug data form
investigational drug data sheet
laboratory d.
longitudinal expert evaluation using all available d.
long-term followup d.
material safety data sheet
measured beam d.
medical data screen
medical data system
minimum data set
d. monitoring board
multicolor data analysis
National Arthritis D. Workgroup
National Cancer D. Base
National Diabetes D. Group
no d.
parallel data acquisition coil
patient data bank
patient data system
Patient D. Management Systems
paucity of d.
Physician D. Query
d. processing
protocol data query
radiation experience d.
radiologic health d.
remote data entry
remote data entry system
second set of followup d.
d. spike detection error artifact
Time-oriented D. Bank
time-resolved imaging by automatic data segmentation
Toxicology D. Base
database
automatic karyotype system d.
incomplete d.
d. input/output control
date
d. of accident
d. of admission
alert and oriented to person, place, time, and d.
alleged onset d.
d. of arrival
d. of birth
birth d.
calculated date of confinement
d. of conception
d. of death
delivery d.
d. of discharge
due d.
estimated date of conception

estimated date of confinement
estimated date of delivery
estimated date of labor
estimated discharge d.
estimated due d.
d. of examination
expected date of confinement
expected date of delivery
d. of expected delivery
gestational sac and maternal d.
d. of injury
large for d.
d. of last drink
d. of last menstrual period
month, date, year
negative to d.
no d.
no expiration d.
d. of release
d. of transcription
d. of transfer
d. of treatment
up to d.
d. of visit
year to d.

dating
endometrial d.

d'Aubigné
Merle d'Aubigné hip score
Merle d'Aubigné and Postel hip rating scale

David
lyre of D.

David-O'Callaghan syndrome

Davidson protocol exercise test

Davies
Lloyd Davies Trendelenburg position

day
d. activity center
administratively necessary d.'s
d. of admission
adolescent day treatment program
d.'s after birth
average d.
calories per kilogram per d.
d. care center
d. care surgical unit
cigarettes per d.
cubic centimeters per kilogram per d.
d. of delivery
end of d.
episode free d.
every d.
every even d.
every other d.
expected day of delivery
female day equivalent
first day of last menstrual period
five times a d.
gestational d.
habilitative day care
habilitative day treatment
high single dose alternate d.
hospital d.
d. hospital
hospital day number
milligram per kilogram per d.
no-dialysis d.'s
one day at a time
packs per d.
patient d.
per d.
postburn d.
d.'s postburn
postentry d.
d.'s postinoculation
postlaser d.
postoperative d.
postoperative day one
postovulatory d.
postpartum d.
private day nurse
same day admission
d. surgery unit
d. treatment center
twice a d.

day-night cycle

daytime
d. asthma
continuous daytime drowsiness
excessive daytime sleepiness
excessive daytime somnolence
d. multiple sleep latency test
d. sleep episodes
d. somnolence
suppertime mixed insulin and daytime sulfonylureas

D-binding protein

dead
d. after arrival
d. air space
anatomic dead space
d. area of heart muscle
d. at scene
baby born d.
brought in d.
d. despite resuscitation attempt
discharged d.
d. fetus in utero
full term, born d.
d. hand
immature dead female child
immature dead male child
d. of intercurrent disease
mechanical dead space
d. on arrival
d. on arrival despite resuscitative attempts
patient brain d.
patient pronounced d.
physiologic dead space
premature dead female child
premature dead male child
d. space
ventilation of alveolar dead space
ventilation of anatomic dead space
ventilation per minute of dead space
volume of alveolar dead space
volume of anatomic dead space
volume of mechanical dead space

dead-in-bed syndrome

deadly
assault with a deadly weapon
assault with deadly weapon

dead-space
d.-s. gas volume to tidal gas volume ratio

deaf
National Association of the D.
telecommunication device for the d.

deafferentation
peripheral deafferentation pain

deafness
air conduction d.
caudal appendage, short terminal phalanges, deafness, cryptorchidism, mental retardation syndrome
Charcot-Marie-Tooth syndrome, X-linked type II with deafness and mental retardation
coloboma, heart disease, atresia choanae, retarded growth and retarded development and/or CNS anomalies, genital hypoplasia, and ear anomalies and/or deafness syndrome
congenital cataracts, sensorineural deafness, Down syndrome facial appearance, short stature, mental retardation syndrome
congenital emphysema, cryptorchidism, penoscrotal web,

deafness *(continued)*
deafness, mental retardation syndrome
congenital rubella d.
diabetes insipidus, diabetes mellitus, progressive bilateral optic atrophy, and sensorineural d.
dislocated elbow, bowed tibiae, scoliosis, deafness, cataract, microcephaly, mental retardation syndrome
d., femoral epiphysial dysplasia, short stature, developmental delay syndrome
insulin-resistant diabetes, acanthosis nigricans, hypogonadism pigmentary retinopathy, deafness, mental retardation syndrome
lentigines, electrocardiographic abnormalities, ocular hypertelorism, pulmonary stenosis, abnormalities of genitalia, retardation of growth, deafness syndrome
maternally inherited diabetes and d.
maturity onset d.
mental retardation, optic atrophy, deafness, seizures syndrome
motor-sensory neuropathy, X-linked Type II, with deafness and mental retardation
nerve conduction d.
ocular albinism with late-onset sensorineural d.
onychodystrophy-congenital deafness syndrome
d., onychoosteodystrophy, and mental retardation syndrome
ovarian dysgenesis-sensorineural deafness syndrome
progressive perceptive d.
total nerve d.
d. with tinnitus
X-linked progressive mixed deafness with perilymphatic gusher

deaminase
adenosine d.
adenosine deaminase activity
adenosine deaminase assay
adenosine deaminase deficiency
adenosine monophosphate deaminase deficiency
muscle adenosine monophosphate deaminase deficiency
muscle adenylate d.
myoadenylate d.
myoadenylate deaminase deficiency
polyethylene glycol-adenosine d.
polyethylene glycol-modified adenosine d.
porphobilinogen d.
red blood cell adenosine d.
tryptophan deaminase agar

deamination
oxidative d.

dearth
d. of evidence
d. of findings
d. of symptoms

death
activation-induced cell d.
acute death syndrome
d. anxiety scale
apoptotic cell d.
asphyxia and d.
attitude to d.
black d.
brain d.
d. of brain cell
care of body after d.
cause of d.
contributory cause of d.
criteria for determination of brain d.
date of d.
delirium and d.
died a natural d.
doctor actively caused d.
drug and alcohol abuse d.
d. due to drug abuse
early neonatal d.
embryonic d.
equivalent mean age at d.
exercise-induced sudden d.
expectation of d.
exposure-related hypothermia d.
Fas-associating protein with death domain
fast death factor
fear of imminent d.
fetal death in utero
heart cell d.
heart muscle d.
d. of heart muscle tissue
high death rate
indices of d.
infant d.
instantaneous cardiac d.
International Classification of Diseases and Causes of D.
intrauterine d.
intrauterine fetal d.
irreversible brain d.
ischemic sudden d.
late fetal d.
maternal death rate
mediated cell d.
minimal dose causing 100% death or malformation
mode of d.
moment of d.
National D. Index
natural d.
near death experience
near-miss sudden infant death syndrome
necrotic cell d.
neonatal d.
neonatal death rate
nerve cell d.
no anatomical cause of d.
nonrenal d.
notify of d.
oral radiation d.
Oriental nocturnal death syndrome
d. of other cause
out-of-hospital sudden cardiac d.
partially unexplained sudden infant death syndrome
pathologic cell d.
place of d.
postneonatal d.
programmed cell d.
pronouncement of brain d.
d. rattle
reaction to d.
relative corrected death rate
silencer of death domain
slow death factor
stillbirth, mummification, embryonic death, infertility syndrome
sudden cardiac d.
sudden coronary d.
sudden death due to cocaine ingestion
sudden death in infancy
sudden death ischemic heart disease
sudden heart attack d.
sudden inexplicable d.
sudden infant crib d.
sudden infant death syndrome
sudden sniffing d.
sudden unexpected infant d.

sudden unexpected, unexplained d.
sudden unexplained death syndrome
sudden unexplained infant d.
term delivery intrapartum d.
thermal death point
thermal death time
time of d.
totally unexplained sudden infant death syndrome
traumatic brain d.
treatment-related d.
d. in utero
very fast death factor
year of d.

death-inducing signaling complex

DeBakey-Creech aneurysm repair

DeBakey-type aortic dissection

debarquement
mal de d.

debilitating
d. back pain
d. bone disease
d. bowel disease
chronic debilitating disease
d. dementia
d. effects of old age
d. headache
d. illness
d. injury
painful and d.
d. rheumatoid arthritis
severe debilitating symptom

debilitative disease

debility
d. and/or pain
increasing debility and weakness
increasing weakness, debility, and dyspnea
nervous d.

debonded femoral stem prosthesis

debonding pliers

débrided
d. bone surfaces
d. necrotic tissue
d. wound edge

debridement
arthroscopic d.
autolytic d.
d. of bruised tissue
d. of compound skull fracture
d. and dressing
d. infected skin
irrigation and d.
maggot debridement therapy
Magnuson d.
minor mechanical d.
d. of necrotic tissue
open d.
d. and prosthesis retention
d. and revision
revision and d.
surgical d.
wound d.

debris
atheromatous d.
atherosclerotic d.
carbonizing cellular d.
desquamated epithelial d.
D. Index-Simplified
joint d.
loose d.
Malassez d.
metallic d.
necrotic d.
nuclear d.
oral d.
particulate d.
tissue d.
tonsillar d.

Debrix Index

debt
oxygen d.

debubbling procedure

debulking
ovarian carcinoma d.
percutaneous d.
d. surgery
surgical d.
d. therapy
tumor d.
d. of tumor

decaffeinated green tea

decalcified
d. freeze-dried bone allograft
d. freeze-dried cortical bone
d. section of vertebral body

decanoate
fluphenazine d.
haloperidol d.
nandrolone d.

decapacitation factor

decarboxylase
amino acid d.
antiglutamic acid decarboxylase autoantibody
aromatic acid d.
aromatic amino acid d.
aromatic D-amino acid d.
aromatic L-amino acid d.
cysteine sulfinic acid d.
glutamate d.
glutamic acid d.
histidine d.
lysine decarboxylase test
ornithine d.
orotidylate decarboxylase deficiency
orotidylic acid d.
uroporphyrinogen d.

1-decarboxylase
aspartate 1-d.

4-decarboxylase
aspartate 4-d.

decarboxylation
amine precursor uptake and decarboxylation cell
amine uptake and decarboxylation cell
Moeller decarboxylation test
oxidative d.

decay
d. constant
free induction d.
free-induction d.
modified tone decay test
rate of d.
reflex d.
tone d.
tone decay test

decay-accelerating factor

decayed
d., missing, and filled teeth
ratio of decayed and filled surfaces
ratio of decayed and filled teeth

deceit
aggression and deceit impulsivity

decelerate breathing rhythm

decelerating-flow
volume-cycled decelerating-flow ventilation

deceleration
fetal heart rate d.
d. injury
major deceleration injury
mitral deceleration slope
operant deceleration of heart rate
d. time

decelerator
graduated electronic d.

decerebrate
decorticate and d.
d. posture
d. posturing
d. rigidity
d. state

decibel
d. effective masking contralateral
d. hearing test
d.'s normal hearing level
d.'s sensation level
d.'s sound pressure level

decidual
d. cast
double decidual sac
d. prolactin
d. tissue

deciduitis
membranous d.

deciduoma
Loeb d.

deciliter
grams per d.
milligram per d.
milliliter per d.

decimal
binary-coded d.
extended binary-coded decimal interchange code
homeopathic symbol for decimal scale of potencies
d. reduction time
d. scale of potency or dilution

decimeter
cubic d.

decision
Assessment of Career D. Making
difficulty in decision making
end-of-life d.
evidence-based decision making
health d.'s
inability to make d.'s
incapacitated of making d.'s
informed d.
informed health care d.
Inquiry Mode Questionnaire: A Measure of How You Think and Make D.'s
interference with judgment and decision making
limiting d.
sensory decision theory

decision-maker
medical d.-m.

decision-making
Career D.-m.
clinical d.-m.
ethical d.-m.
health care d.-m.
d.-m. skills

declaration
dying d.

declarative
long-term declarative memory

declination
angle of d.
d. angle
angle of declination of metatarsal

decline
d. in ability to perform routine tasks
age-associated cognitive d.
age-related cognitive d.
d. in interest of opposite sex
d. in job performance
marked decline in academic functioning
d. in mental function
d. in personal grooming
progressive decline in function
Rating Scale of Communication in Cognitive D.
d. in sexual function
d. in social relationships

declined in function

declining
d. consciousness
d. mathematical ability
d. respiratory status

decoding
document image d.

decompensated
acutely decompensated congestive heart failure
d. alcoholic cirrhosis
d. congestive heart failure
d. heart failure
d. liver cirrhosis
d. liver disease

decompensation
cardiac d.
end-stage adult cardiac d.
vascular d.

decompensative neurosis

decomposition
singular value d.

decompression
anterior retroperitoneal d.
bilateral orbital d.
carpal tunnel d.
cervical disc d.
d. chamber
d. colostomy
d. disease
foramen magnum d.
d. of heart
d. injury
intramedullary metatarsal d.
laser disc d.
local decompression fracture
microvascular d.
Mubarak-Hargens decompression technique
optic nerve sheath d.
percutaneous laser disc d.
d. sickness
spinal cord d.
subacromial d.
d. surgery
tarsal tunnel d.
thoracic outlet d.
d. tube
vertebral axial d.
vertebral body d.

decompressive
d. laminectomy
d. lumbar laminectomy
d. osteotomy

deconditioning
cardiovascular d.

decondition pain behavior

decongestant
nasal d.
oral d.
topical d.

decongestion
local d.

decontamination
emergency decontamination center
d. factor
selective decontamination of the digestive tract
selective digestive d.
selective digestive tract d.
selective intestinal d.

decorticate
d. and decerebrate
d. posture
d. posturing
d. rigidity

decorticated flap

decortication
arterial d.

functional decortication from hypoglycemia
functional decortication from hypoxia
d. of heart
lung d.

decrease

d. in appetite
d. in coordination or equilibrium
d. in energy or fatigue
oxygen content of blood d.'s
relative volume d.
d. in respiratory effort

decreased

d. ability to concentrate
d. ability to function
d. activity
d. acuity
apneic infant with decreased heart rate
d. appetite and loss of energy
blood pressure d.
d. body hair
d. bone mineral density
d. bowel function
d. brain activity
d. brain wave activity
brittle hair, intellectual impairment, decreased fertility, short stature syndrome
d. capacity for abstract thought
d. energy, fatigue and weakness
d. estrogen receptor
d. fetal movement
d. hand circulation
d. hearing
d. heart rate
ichthyosis, brittle hair, impaired intelligence, decreased fertility, short stature syndrome
d. immune function
increased energy, decreased appetite
insomnia, hyperactivity and decreased appetite
d. intelligence
d. judgment
d. level of consciousness
markedly decreased reflex
d. need for sleep
platelet count d.
d. rebleeding risk
d. risk of heart disease
second stage of decreased intraocular tension
d. sensory perception
d. sexual interest
d. signs and symptoms of anxiety
d. signs and symptoms of depression
d. specific gravity
d. tension pressure
total decreased histamine
d. venous return to heart

decreasing

d. blood count
d. consumption of oxygen
d. hypertension
d. jaundice
d. peripheral vascular resistance

decrepitude with age

decubital

right lateral decubital position

decubitus

acute decubitus ulcer
d. angina
angina d.
dorsal decubitus position
d. heel
infected decubitus ulcer
lateral decubitus film
lateral decubitus position
lateral decubitus radiograph
left lateral decubitus muscle
left lateral decubitus position
d. position
sacral decubitus ulcer
d. ulcer
ventral d.

decussation

anterior tegmental d.
Meynert d.
Meynert fountain d.
motor d.
oculomotor d.
optic d.
d. of superior cerebellar peduncles
Wernekinck d.

dedicated time block

dedifferentiation

late d.

deep

d. abdominal complication
d. abdominal reflex
d. abdominal tenderness
anterior deep cervical lymph node
anterior labial branch of deep external pudendal artery
anterior scrotal branch of deep external pudendal artery
d. anterior tibiotalar
aplasia of deep vein
articular branch of deep fibular nerve
d. bites of tissue
d. brain stimulation
d. breath
d. breathing and coughing
d. breathing exercise
bronchodilation following deep inspiration
chest pain on deep breathing
d. chest therapy
chronic feelings of deep emptiness
d. circumflex iliac artery
d. circumflex iliac artery flap
d. circumflex iliac vein
d. cleansing breath
d. compartment
cough and deep breath
dizziness from rapid and deep breathing
d. dyspareunia
d. electroencephalogram
encourage to cough and deep breathe
epithelioid combined nevi deep penetrating nevus
exertional deep posterior compartment syndrome
extended deep inferior epigastric
d. fascia
d. friction massage
d. hepatic coma
hypoactive deep tendon reflex
d. hypothermic circulatory arrest
iliofemoral deep vein thrombosis
increased deep tendon reflex
d. inferior epigastric artery perforator
d. inguinal lymph node
d. inguinal ring
d. inspiration
d. knee bend
d. lamellar keratoplasty
d. lobe
McDonald D. Test of Articulation
migratory deep vein thrombophlebitis
d. muscular aponeurotic system
muscular branch of deep fibular nerve

deep *(continued)*
osteomusculocutaneous deep circumflex iliac groin flap
pain on deep breathing
d. palpation
parotid deep lobe
patient taught deep breathing
d. penetrating nevus
perforating artery of deep femoral artery
perforating branch of deep palmar arch
d. posterior tibiotalar
postoperative deep venous thrombosis
prolonged and deep breathing
prolonged deep inspiration
pterygoid branch of posterior deep temporal artery
d. pulse
d. quiet
recurrent deep vein thrombosis
regional deep heating
d. and regular respiration
d. shock insulin
d. sleep
d. sleep of short duration
small, deep, recent infarct
d. space neck infection
d. sternal wound infection
d. superior epigastric artery
d. temporal fascia
d. temporoparietal fascia
d. tendon reflex
d. tendon reflexes active and equal bilaterally
d. tendon reflexes bilaterally
d. tissue massage
d. transverse friction
turn, cough, deep breath
d. vastus lateralis
d. vein thrombosis
d. venous insufficiency
d. venous occlusion
d. venous thromboembolization
d. venous thromboscintigram
d. venous thrombosis
d. venous thrombosis prophylaxis
d. white matter hyperintensity
d. white matter infarct
d. white matter lesion
d. x-ray
d. x-ray therapy

deepened
incision d.

de-epithelialization
periareolar d.-e.

de-epithelialized
d.-e. flap
d.-e. rectus abdominis muscle graft

deeply
patient deeply comatose

deep-seated
d.-s. benign tumor
d.-s. cancer
d.-s. guilt
d.-s. psychopathology

deer
d. kidney virus
mule deer poxvirus

defatted
d. skin graft
skin graft d.

defecate
inability to d.

defecation
pain on d.
salivation, lacrimation, urination, defecation, gastrointestinal distress and emesis
d. syncope

defect
acquired ventricular septal d.
afferent pupillary d.
alcohol-induced birth d.
alcohol-related birth d.
aldosterone secretion d.
ankyloblepharon, ectodermal defect, and cleft lip and/or palate
anterior apical vault d.
anterior neural tube d.
anteromedial humeral head d.
aorticopulmonary septal d.
aorticopulmonary window d.
aortic septal d.
aortopulmonary septal d.
arcuate field d.
arcuate visual field d.
arteriovenous canal d.
arteriovenous crossing d.
asymptomatic visual field d.
atrial ostium primum d.
atrial septal d.
atrial septal defect occlusion
atrial septal defect occlusion system
atrial ventricular canal d.
atrioventricular canal d.
atrioventricular canal septal d.
atrioventricular nodal septal d.
atrioventricular septal d.
autosomal-dominant genetic d.
AV crossing d.
birth d.
Birth D.'s Monitoring Program
clamshell closure of atrial septal d.
closure interatrial septal d.
conduction d.
conduction defect in acute myocardial infarction
congenital defect interventricular septum of heart
congenital heart d.
congenital hemidysplasia with ichthyosiform erythroderma and limb defects syndrome
conotruncal cardiac defect, abnormal face, thymic hypoplasia, cleft palate
costovertebral segmentation defect with mesomelia syndrome
craniospinal d.
Eisenmenger ventricular septal d.
endocardial cushion d.
endocardial cushion-type ventricular septal d.
esophageal filling d.
heart valve d.
hereditary heart d.
humoral immune d.
hydrogen-detected ventricular septal d.
iatrogenic atrial septal d.
infundibular septal d.
interatrial septal d.
interatrial septal defect closure
interventricular septal d.
intolerance of d.
intraatrial conduction d.
intraluminal filling d.
intraventricular conduction d.
irradiated surgical d.'s
isolated conduction d.
joint capsule d.
labyrinthine d.
limb reduction d.'s
lingular mandibular bony d.
lobulated filling d.
luteal phase d.
mapping of d.
mapping the d.
Marcus Gunn relative afferent d.
membrane transport d.
mental retardation, spasticity, distal transverse limb defects syndrome
metaphysial fibrous cortical d.

metaphysial fibrous d.
Metropolitan Atlanta Congenital Defects Program
microphthalmia with linear skin d.'s
midline facial d.
midline fusion d.
mitochondrial respiratory chain d.
monocular field d.
monocular temporal arcuate d.
müllerian fusion d.
multiple colon filling d.
multiple sensory defect dizziness
muscular ventricular septal d.
napkin ring d.
nasal step d.
nerve fiber bundle d.
neural arch d.
neural tube d.
no d.'s
nonspecific intraventricular conduction d.
nonuniform rotational d.
no significant d.
obstructive airway d.
oval window d.
paravaginal defect repair
parietal lobe field d.
pars flaccida d.
partial atrioventricular canal d.
partial homonymous field d.
patchy window d.
periinfarction conduction d.
periodontal bony d.
persistent epithelial d.
plantar foot d.
plasma d.
platelet activation d.
pleiotrophic functional d.
pulmonary artery filling d.
pulmonary atresia with ventricular septal d.
relative afferent pupillary d.
right lower quadrant d.
secundum atrial septal d.
segmental bone d.
segmental bronchus d.
segmental continuity d.
septal d.
serum d.
structural heart d.
Swiss cheese d.
vascular septal d.
ventilation perfusion d.
ventral septal d.
ventral wall d.
ventricular septal heart d.
ventriculoseptal d.
vertebral arch d.
vertebral column d.
visual field d.
X-linked genetic d.
zero d.

defective
d. artificial heart valve
cell wall d.
d. immune response
d. implant
d. impression
d. interfering
d. leukemia virus

defense
body's natural defense mechanism
civil d.
immune defense mechanism
individual defense mechanism
maladaptive defense mechanism
masochistic character d.
d. mechanism inventory
Medical Education for National D.
natural defense mechanism
normal heat d.
small intestine as a defense barrier

defensive
D. Functioning Scale
host defensive factor

defensiveness
diminished denial and d.
emotional d.

deferens
ampulla of vas d.
artery to ductus d.
artery to vas d.
bilateral congenital absence of vas d.
congenital absence of vas d.
congenital bilateral absence of the vas d.
ductus deferens tumor
mouse vas d.
mucosa of ductus d.
muscular coat of ductus d.
muscular layer of ductus d.
vas d.
vas deferens aplasia
vas deferens obstruction

deferred
diagnosis or condition deferred on Axis I, II

defervesced
patient d.

defiance
oppositional d.
opposition defiance disorder

defibrillated
heart d.
heart defibrillated with single shock

defibrillation
arrhythmia following d.
atrial defibrillation threshold
d. and electrical cardioversion
paddle marks from d.
public access d.
d. response interval
d. threshold
transvenous defibrillation lead

defibrillator
automated external d.
automated external defibrillator pacemaker
automatic external d.
automatic implantable d.
automatic intracardiac d.
d. burn
d. implant
implantable atrial d.
implantable cardiac d.
implantable defibrillator in cardioversion
pacer-cardioverter d.
d. paddle
pharmacologic atrial d.
public access d.

defibrillator/atrial
implantable cardioverter-defibrillator/atrial tachycardia pacing

deficiency
acid maltase d.
acquired immune deficiency syndrome
acquired immune deficiency syndrome antibody
acquired immune deficiency syndrome antibody test
acquired immune deficiency syndrome carrier
acquired immune deficiency syndrome crisis
acquired immune deficiency syndrome dementia complex
acquired immune deficiency syndrome epidemic
acquired immune deficiency syndrome infected child

deficiency *(continued)*
acquired immune deficiency syndrome mandatory testing
acquired immune deficiency syndrome prevention
acquired immune deficiency syndrome primary pathogen
acquired immune deficiency syndrome residential treatment facility
acquired immune deficiency syndrome tainted transfusion
acquired immune deficiency syndrome transmission
acquired immune deficiency syndrome treatment
acquired immune deficiency syndrome virus infection
acquired immune deficiency syndrome-associated transfusion
acquired immune deficiency syndrome-related complex
acquired immune deficiency syndrome-related dementia
acquired immune deficiency syndrome-related macular degeneration
acquired violence immune deficiency syndrome
adenosine deaminase d.
adenosine monophosphate deaminase d.
adenylosuccinate lyase d.
adult acid maltase d.
Aitken femoral d.
alpha-1 antitrypsin d.
alpha-1-antitrypsin deficiency disease
anti-acquired immune deficiency syndrome vaccine
antibody deficiency disease
antibody deficiency syndrome
antibody deficiency with near-normal immunoglobulins
antidiuretic hormone d.
anti-müllerian hormone d.
antithrombin III d.
apolipoprotein C-II d.
apolipoprotein deficiency A-I
apolipoprotein deficiency B
apolipoprotein deficiency E
apraxia-ataxia-mental deficiency syndrome
aqueous humor d.
aqueous tear d.
arch length d.
arginase deficiency aminoaciduria
argininosuccinate synthetase d.
argininosuccinic acid synthase d.
argininosuccinic acid synthetase d.
arginosuccinate lyase d.
arterial deficiency pattern
arylsulfatase A d.
arylsulfatase B d.
arylsulfatase b d.
arylsulfatase a d.
ascorbic acid d.
ataxia with isolated vitamin E d.
AT3 deficiency type II
AT III d.
autoimmune d.
autoimmune deficiency syndrome
blood product contaminated by acquired immune deficiency syndrome
C2 d.
C4 d.
C7 d.
carnitine palmitoyltransferase I, II d.
carrier of acquired immune deficiency syndrome
cellular immunity deficiency syndrome
chronic fatigue immune deficiency syndrome
combined immune deficiency disease
combined pituitary hormone d.
congenital abduction d.
congenital immune d.
congenital limb d.
corpus luteum deficiency syndrome
dementia due to vitamin d.
dihydrotestosterone receptor d.
emotional effects of acquired immune deficiency syndrome
enzyme d.
essential fatty acid d.
d. factor
factor V deficiency Leiden mutation
factor VII d.
factor VIII d.
factor VIII, IX d.
factor X d.
factor XI d.
factor XII d.
factor XIII d.
familial glucocorticoid d.
familial high-density lipoprotein d.
familial idiopathic gonadotropin d.
familial multiple factor deficiency 1
fat-soluble vitamin d.
fetal iodine deficiency disorder
galactocerebrosidase d.
gamma A globulin d.
gamma A immunoglobulin d.
gamma globulin M d.
gay-related immune d.
glutathione synthetase d.
glycerol kinase d.
growth hormone d.
growth hormone receptor d.
human growth hormone d.
hypoglossia-limb deficiency phenotype
idiopathic growth hormone d.
idiopathic mental d.
iduronate sulfatase d.
immune d.
immunity deficiency state
immunoglobulin d.
intrinsic sphincter d.
iron deficiency anemia
isolated follicle-stimulating hormone deficiency syndrome
isolated gonadotropin d.
isolated growth hormone d.
isolated growth hormone deficiency type IB, II, III
isolated human growth d.
isolated lactase d.
isolated thyroid-stimulating hormone d.
late immunoglobulin d.
leukocyte adhesion d.
leukocyte adhesion deficiency type 1–4
limbal stem-cell d.
lipoprotein lipase d.
liver phosphorylase d.
long bone d.
long-chain acyl-CoA dehydrogenase d.
long-chain 3-hydroxyacyl-CoA dehydrogenase d.
long-chain very long-chain acyl-CoA dehydrogenase d.
long- and medium-chain fatty acid coenzyme-A dehydrogenase d.
low-density lipoprotein d.
luteal phase d.
luteinizing hormone-releasing hormone d.

macronutrient deficiency syndrome
magnesium d.
magnesium deficiency infantile tremor syndrome
mammalian binding lectin d.
mandatory acquired immune deficiency syndrome testing
mannan-binding lectin d.
medium-chain acyl-CoA dehydrogenase d.
mental d.
mental deficiency, spasticity, congenital ichthyosis syndrome
merosin deficiency dystrophy
methionine synthase d.
3-methylcrotonyl-CoA carboxylase d.
MHC antigen d.
MHC class I antigen d.
MHC class I d.
MHC class II d.
molybdenum cofactor d.
monoamine oxidase A d.
moral deficiency personality disorder
mother infected with acquired immune deficiency syndrome
multiple d.
multiple acyl-coenzyme A dehydrogenase d.
multiple anterior pituitary hormone d.
multiple carboxylase d.
multiple endocrine deficiency, Addison disease, and candidiasis syndrome
multiple glandular deficiency syndrome
multiple pituitary hormone d.'s
multiple sulfatase d.
multiple sulfatase deficiency syndrome
muscle adenosine monophosphate deaminase d.
muscle carnitine d.
muscle carnitine palmitoyltransferase d.
muscle phosphofructokinase d.
muscle phosphorylase d.
myelin basic protein d.
myoadenylate deaminase d.
myopathic carnitine d.
myophosphorylase deficiency glycogenosis
National Institute of Acquired Immune D.
neonatal biotin d.
neutrophil actin d.
neutrophil chemotactic d.
neutrophil-specific secondary granule d.
nicotinic acid d.
nonclassical hydroxylase d.
nonclassical 21-hydroxylase d.
no significant d.
nutritional deficiency cataract
nutritional deficiency dermatitis
nutritional deficiency disorder
nutritional deficiency eczema
obesity, short stature, mental deficiency, hypogonadism, micropenis, finger contracture, cleft lip-palate syndrome
ornithine carbamoyltransferase d.
ornithine carbamoyl transferase d.
ornithine-ketoacid aminotransferase d.
ornithine transcarbamylase d.
orotidylate decarboxylase deficiency
pancreatic exocrine d.
P450 aromatase placental d.
partial 21-hydroxylase d.
patient unknown acquired immune deficiency syndrome carrier
peripheral glucocorticoid d.
pernicious anemia-like syndrome and immunoglobulin d.
postnatal growth d.
pre-acquired immune deficiency syndrome
primary immune d.
protein C d.
protein S d.
proximal femoral focal d.
proximal femur focal d.
proximal focal femoral d.
pseudovitamin D deficiency rickets
pyruvate dehydrogenase complex d.
Qi and Yin d.
red-green color perception d.
secretion and spill from acquired immune deficiency syndrome
selective antipolysaccharide antibody d.
severe combined immune d.
severe combined immune deficiency syndrome
short-chain acyl-CoA dehydrogenase d.
somatropin deficiency syndrome
specific antibody d.
d. state immunity
sucrase-isomaltase d.
sulfoiduronate sulfatase d.
superior semicircular canal d.
systemic carnitine d.
thiamine deficiency encephalopathy
thymidine kinase d.
transfusion-associated acquired immune deficiency syndrome
transfusion-transmitted acquired immune deficiency syndrome
trifunctional protein d.
tyrosine aminotransferase d.
uridine diphosphate-galactose-4-epimerase d.
vertical maxillary d.
vitamin A d.
vitamin B_1 d.
vitamin B_6 d.
vitamin B_{12} d.
vitamin B d.
vitamin K deficiency bleeding

deficiens

orgasmic d.

deficient

d. atrioventricular septation
d. cognitive thinking
high cholesterol and tocopherol d.
hormone deficient children
mentally d.
nongrowth hormone deficient short stature
tocopherol d.
d. transmission chemoreceptor
zinc d.

deficit

anterior cruciate deficit of knee
anterior cruciate deficit knee
association deficit pathology
attention concentration d.
attention deficit disorder
attention deficit disorder, residual type
attention deficit disorder with hyperactivity
attention deficit disorder without hyperactivity
attention deficit and disruptive behavior disorder
attention deficit hyperactivity disorder
attention deficit hyperactivity disorder, combined type

deficit *(continued)*
attention deficit hyperactivity disorder, predominantly hyperactive-impulsive type
attention deficit hyperactivity disorder-predominantly inattentive
attention deficit symptom
Attention D. Disorder Behavior Rating Scale
d.'s in attention, motor control, perception
auditory transfer d.
base d.
cardiac abnormality, T-cell deficit, clefting, hypocalcemia
central integrative d.
children and adults with attention deficit disorder
cumulative sleep d.
delayed ischemic neurologic d.
dissolved oxygen d.
diversional activity d.
epileptic attention deficit disorder
executive function d.
focal neurologic d.
free water d.
gross motor d.
gross neurologic d.
gross sensory d.
hygiene self-care d.
juvenile memory d.
knowledge d.
left hemisphere d.
memory function d.
motor function d.
motor, pain, touch, reflex d.
multiple cognitive d.'s
multiple sensory d.
naming speed d.
neuropsychologic d.
neurosensory d.
normal base d.
pancreatic exocrine d.
peripheral vestibular d.
permanent cranial nerve d.
phonologic programming deficit syndrome
pituitary hormone d.
prolonged reversible ischemic neurologic d.
resolving ischemic neurologic d.
reversible ischemic neurologic d.
right hemisphere d.
sensory d.
severe d.
toileting self-care d.
visual field d.

definable illness index

defined
chemically defined medium
d. daily dose
d. exposure dose
d. formula diet
human lymphocyte antigen-lymphocyte d.
human lymphocyte antigen-serologically d.
lymphocyte d.
poorly differentiated d.
poorly differentiated defined border
serologically d.
d. substrate
within defined limits

defining
method of defining criterion

definite
d. brain damage
first definite apical clearance lens

definitely abnormal tracing

definition
area of critical d.
arteriovenous malformation nidus d.
AVM nidus d.
cultural definition of addiction
gender role d.
high definition power
loss of d.

definitive
d. diagnosis
d. irradiation
d. procedure
d. treatment

deflection
downward pen d.
full-scale d.
His bundle d.
d. in His bundle in electrogram
His bundle electrogram d.
indentation load d.
d. of nasal septum

deformation
critical degree of d.
fetal akinesia deformation sequence
minimal deformation target

deformed
d. gnarled joint
patient delivered congenitally deformed infant

deformity
adduction-internal rotation d.
Andy Gump d.
aortic valve d.
apex plantar d.
arthritis without d.
axial plane angular deformity biomechanics
cavus foot d.
cephalofacial d.
cleft lip, cleft palate, lobster-claw deformity syndrome
cleft lip d.
congenital urinary tract d.'s
congenital vertical talus foot d.
equinovarus hindfoot d.
equinovarus pes d.
fracture complete and varus d.
d. of gastric outlet
Haglund foot d.
hallux limitus d.
hallux valgus d.
high arch d.
limb reduction d.
lobster hand d.
main en griffe d.
mallet finger d.
metatarsal-phalangeal flexion d.
metatarsus adductocavus d.
metatarsus adductovarus d.
metatarsus adductus d.
metatarsus atavicus d.
nasal d.
neurogenic equinus d.
neuropathic foot d.
no congenital d.'s
pannus deformity of odontoid
parachute deformity of mitral valve
parrot beak d.
pectus carinatum d.
pectus excavatum d.
pencil and cup d.
pes arcuatus clawfoot d.
pes cavus clawfoot d.
pes cavus d.
pigeon breast d.
rigid flatfoot d.
rockerbottom flatfoot d.
rotational deformity of finger
saddle nose d.
skeletal d.
swan-neck finger d.
swelling deformity of affected bone
ulnar deviation d.
varus hindfoot d.

degenerated tissue disease

degenerating cell

degeneration

absolute reaction of d.
acquired hepatocerebral d.
acquired immune deficiency syndrome-related macular d.
acute heart muscle d.
adenoid degeneration agent
age-related macular d.
alcohol acquired chronic hepatocerebral d.
alcohol cerebellar d.
Alzheimer fibrillary d.
anterior horn cell d.
articular cartilage d.
ataxia, myoclonic encephalopathy, macular degeneration, recurrent infections syndrome
atrophic age-related macular d.
basal cell liquefactive d.
basophilic d.
cerebromacular d.
choriocapillaris d.
chorioretinal d.
complete reaction of d.
cystoid macular d.
diffuse hepatocellular d.
disciform macular degeneration with subretinal neovascular membrane
dry macular d.
fatty degeneration of heart
frontotemporal lobar d.
hepatolenticular d.
infantile nuclear cerebral d.
juvenile macular d.
d. of keratinocyte
lattice degeneration of retina
lipochondral d.
macular d.
macular disciform d.
marginal corneal d.
marginal degeneration of cornea
marginal furrow d.
medial collateral ligament d.
mucoid degeneration of umbilical cord
mucoid myoma d.
myocardial cellular d.
myocardial fiber d.
myopic retinal d.
d. of myxomatous heart valve
nerve cell d.
neurofibrillary d.
nodular corneal d.
nonexudative macular d.
nonneovascular age-related macular d.
olivopontocerebellar d.
paraneoplastic cerebellar d.
paraneoplastic cerebral d.
parenchymatous cerebellar d.
partial reaction of d.
pellucid marginal corneal d.
pellucid marginal retinal d.
peripheral cystoid d.
peripheral disciform d.
peripheral tapetochoroidal d.
rapid erythrocyte d.
reaction of d.
d. reaction
reticular degeneration of pigment epithelium
senile choroidal macular d.
senile macular d.
senile macular chorioretinal d.
Sorsby pseudoinflammatory macular d.
spinocerebellar d.
spongy degeneration of infancy
striatonigral d.
subacute combined degeneration of spinal cord
subacute cortical cerebellar d.
d. of vision
vitelliform macular d.
d. of wall of artery
wallerian d.

degenerative

age-associated degenerative change
d. anterior spurring
arterial degenerative disease
d. arthritic change
d. arthritis
atrophic degenerative maculopathy
d. bone change
d. bone marrow disease
d. brain disease
d. change
chronic degenerative disease
chronic nervous degenerative disease
d. dementia of Alzheimer type
d. dense microsphere
d. disc disease
d. disease
d. disease of brain
d. of dopamine-producing nerve cell
d. facet disease
generalized degenerative tic
d. heart disease
d. idiopathic cardiomyopathy
incipient degenerative brain disease
d. joint disease
linear degenerative signal intensity
marked degenerative change of hip
mixed rheumatoid and degenerative arthritis
d. myoclonus epilepsy
myxoid degenerative change
d. neurologic disease
Outerbridge degenerative arthritis staging
patellofemoral degenerative arthritis
primary degenerative cerebral disease
primary degenerative dementia
primary degenerative dementia of Alzheimer type
progressive degenerative disease process
d. spinal disease

degloved amputation

deglove injury

degloving

d. injury
midface d.
midface degloving incision
midface degloving procedure
midface degloving technique
midfacial d.
nasal d.
phalangeal d.
d. procedure

deglutition

muscle of d.

deglycerolized frozen red cell

Degos

Dowling Degos disease
malignant papillomatosis of D.

degradable starch microsphere

degradation

cross-linked fibrin degradation product
fibrin degradation product
fibrin/fibrinogen degradation product
fibrinogen degradation product
focal cytoplasmic d.
d. index
pollution and environmental d.
d. product
protein d.

degrading
blood group degrading enzyme
degranulating
mast cell degranulating peptide
degranulation
human basophil degranulation test
mast cell d.
mast cell degranulation test
piecemeal d.
degree
d. Celsius
critical degree of deformation
cycles per d.
d. of extension
d. Fahrenheit
d. of fineness of abrasive particles
d. of flexion
d. of freedom
d.'s of freedom
high degree of risk
level and degree of mental illness
modified Barthel degree of disability index
number of degrees of freedom
d. of physical functioning
d. of polymerization
third degree heart block
d. of voicelessness
dehiscence
anastomotic d.
aortic intimal d.
asymptomatic d.
d. of cesarean section scar
episiotomy d.
iris d.
perivalvular d.
scar d.
sternotomy d.
total d.
d. of uterus
dehydrase
aminolevulinic acid d.
serine d.
dehydrate
calcium pyrophosphate dehydrate deposition disease
dehydrated
emaciated and d.
d. and malnourished
dehydration
cachexia and d.
d., poisoning, trauma
diarrhea and d.
d. and exhaustion
osmolality dehydration test
d. of wound
dehydrogenase
alcohol d.
aldehyde d.
3-beta-hydroxysteroid d.
branched-chain alpha ketoacid d.
choline d.
dihydroorotate d.
dihydrouracil d.
electron transfer flavoprotein d.
gastric alcohol d.
glucose d.
glucose-6-phosphate d.
glutamate d.
glutamic acid d.
glyceraldehyde-3-phosphate d.
glycerophosphate d.
heat-stable lactic d.
horse liver alcohol d.
hydroxybutyrate d.
hydroxybutyric d.
hydroxysteroid d.
inosine monophosphate d.
isocitrate d.
ketoglutarate d.
ketoglutarate dehydrogenase complex
lactate dehydrogenase A
lactate dehydrogenase B
lactate dehydrogenase elevating virus
lactate dehydrogenase isoenzyme
lactate dehydrogenase, muscle
lactate dehydrogenase fraction 1–5
lactic acid d.
lactic dehydrogenase total
lactic dehydrogenase virus
lipoamide d.
liver alcohol d.
liver lactate d.
long-chain acyl-CoA d.
long-chain acyl-CoA dehydrogenase deficiency
long-chain acyl-coenzyme A d.
long-chain 3-hydroxyacyl-CoA dehydrogenase deficiency
long-chain hydroxyacyl-coenzyme A d.
long-chain very long-chain acyl-CoA dehydrogenase deficiency
long- and medium-chain fatty acid coenzyme-A dehydrogenase deficiency
long- and very-long-chain acyl-CoA d.
malate d.
malic d.
malic acid d.
medium-chain acyl-CoA d.
medium-chain acyl-CoA dehydrogenase deficiency
medium-chain acyl-coenzyme A d.
mitochondrial glutamate dehydrogenase pathway
multiple acyl-coenzyme A dehydrogenase deficiency
NADPH dehydrogenase quinone
nicotinic acid d.
plasma lactic d.
pyruvate d.
pyruvate dehydrogenase complex deficiency
serum hydroxybutyrate d.
serum hydroxybutyric d.
serum isocitrate d.
serum lactate d.
short-chain acyl-CoA dehydrogenase deficiency
short-chain hydroxyacyl-coenzyme A d.
sorbitol d.
succinate d.
succinate semialdehyde d.
succinic dehydrogenase activity
threonine d.
very long chain acyl-CoA d.
xanthine d.
yeast alcohol d.
dehydrogenated polymer
dehydrogenating
deiminase
arginine d.
deiodinase
type 1, 2, 3 d.
deionized water
Deiters nucleus
delay
d. aging of cell
arithmetical developmental delay disorder
arthrogryposis, ectodermal dysplasia, cleft lip/palate developmental delay syndrome
articulation developmental delay disorder
atrioventricular d.
atrioventricular block with first-degree conduction d.

atrioventricular conduction d.
d. computer tomographic myelography
congenital thrombocytopenia, Robin sequence, agenesis of corpus callosum, distinctive facies, developmental delay syndrome
constitutional delay in growth and adolescence
constitutional delay in growth and development
deafness, femoral epiphysial dysplasia, short stature, developmental delay syndrome
double-dose d.
echo delay time
gastric emptying d.
generalized d.'s
d. of gratification
interventricular conduction d.
intraventricular conduction d.
macrocephaly, hypertelorism, short limbs, hearing loss, developmental delay syndrome
microcephaly, mild developmental delay, short stature, distinctive face syndrome
minimize or delay urinary incontinence
mixed development developmental delay disorder
nitrogen clearance d.
osteogenesis imperfecta, optic atrophy, retinopathy, developmental delay syndrome
pulmonary clearance d.
tumor growth d.

delayed
d. action
d. afterdepolarization
d. after polarization
d. anovulatory syndrome
d. asthmatic reaction
d. auditory feedback
d. cerebral ischemia
d. cerebral vasoconstriction
d. closure
d. closure of accidental wound
d. closure of operative wound
d. concentration of dye
d. conditioned necrosis
constitutional delayed growth
d. contrast enhancement
d. cutaneous hypersensitivity
d. cutaneous reaction
d. delirium
d. development
developmentally d.
d. development of speech
d. diarrhea
d. double diffusion test
drug-induced delayed multiorgan hypersensitivity syndrome
d. erythema dose
d. feedback audiometry
fracture with delayed union
d. gamma camera image
d. gastric emptying
d. graft
d. graft function
d. healing
d. healing of fracture
d. hearing loss
d. hemolytic reaction
d. hypersensitivity test
immediate and delayed recall
immediate and delayed recognition
d. or impaired speech
d. intervention
d. ischemic neurologic deficit
d. light emission
d. microembolism syndrome
d. muscle soreness
d. neuropsychological sequela
d. pressure urticaria
d. primary closure
d. primary intention
d. primary intention healing
d. primary repair
d. puberty
d. pulmonary toxicity syndrome
d. recall
d. reflex
d. repair
d. response
d. secondary closure
d. sensitivity
d. sexual development
d. shock
short stature, hyperextensibility of joints or hernia or both, ocular depression, Rieger anomaly, teething, d.
d. skin hypersensitivity reaction
d. sleep phase
d. sleep phase syndrome
d. transfer flap
d. transit time
d. traumatic intracerebral hematoma
d. union
d. union of fracture
d. upstroke
d. work recall test
d. xenograft rejection

delayed-absorbable
Maxon delayed-absorbable suture

delayed-action tablet

delayed-blanch reaction

delayed-onset muscle soreness

delayed-type

DeLee suctioning

deleted
d. in azoospermia
d. in azoospermia-homologue
d. in azoospermia-like autosomal
phosphatase and tensin homologue deleted on chromosome

deletion
d. of long arm of chromosome X
d. of short arm of chromosome X
final consonant d.
d. of final consonant
initial consonant d.
4p deletion syndrome
weak syllable d.

deliberate
d. hyperventilation
d. hypotension
d. self-harm

deliberation
medical d.

delimiting keratotomy

delineation
endocardial border d.

delinquency
adolescent neurotic d.
neurotic d.
socialized d.

delinquent
juvenile d.

delipidized serum protein

delirium
acute agitated d.
alcohol withdrawal d.
arteriosclerotic dementia with d.
chronic alcoholic d.
d. and death
delayed d.
d., infection, atrophic urethritis and vaginitis, pharmaceuticals, psychological disorders, excessive

delirium *(continued)*
urine output, restricted mobility, stool impaction
Memorial D. Assessment Scale
multiinfarct dementia with d.
pathophysiology of d.
d. tremens
d. with high fever

delivered
infant d.
intrauterine pregnancy, d.
obstetrics-not d.
patient delivered congenitally deformed infant
patient delivered normal infant
placenta d.
placenta delivered intact
placenta delivered manually
pregnancy, not d.
pregnancy, term, complicated delivered, living male
pregnancy, term, uncomplicated delivered, living male
d. total dose

delivery
alternative delivery system
angiogenesis gene d.
angled delivery device
assisted breech d.
assisted cephalic d.
d. awareness
cesarean d.
coach in d.
complicated d.
consent form to delivery by alternative physician
continuous insulin delivery system
controlled heat-aided drug d.
convection-enhanced d.
d. date
date of expected d.
day of d.
demand oxygen delivery device
double footling d.
elective low forceps delivery
estimated date of d.
expected date of d.
expected day of d.
expected delivery, cesarean
failed forceps d.
father in d.
forceps d.
frank vaginal breech d.
full-term d.
full-term deliveries, premature deliveries, abortions, living children
full-term normal d.
full-term, normal, spontaneous d.
full-term uncomplicated pregnancy, labor, and d.
health care d.
high forceps d.
induction d.
instillation delivery time
instrumental delivery
integrated health delivery network
labor and d.
liposome drug d.
low forceps d.
low outlet forceps d.
method of d.
midforceps d.
midforceps vaginal d.
nonoral estradiol delivery system
normal d.
normal full-term d.
normal pregnancy and d.
normal spontaneous full-term d.
normal vaginal d.
open-loop insulin delivery system
operative delivery with forceps
operative vaginal d.
organized delivery system
outlet forceps d.
oxygen d.
oxygen delivery index
photon-activated drug delivery system
post delivery headache
postmortem cesarean d.
pregnancy, labor, and d.
prior to d.
rapid assay delivery systems
rotating delivery of excitation off resonance
single-unit delivery system
spontaneous d.
spontaneous assisted vaginal d.
spontaneous vertex vaginal d.
stent delivery system
sterile elective low forceps vaginal d.
sterile indicated low forceps vaginal d.
sterile low midforceps vaginal d.
sterile spontaneous controlled vaginal d.
sterile, spontaneous vaginal d.
term delivery intrapartum death
term normal d.
transdermal delivery system
traumatic vaginal d.
uncontrolled unsterile d.
unsterile controlled vaginal d.
unsterile uncontrolled vaginal d.
uterus d.
vacuum extraction d.
vacuum vaginal d.
vaginal breech d.
vaginal delivery after cesarean
vaginal vertex d.

Del Rio Language Screening Test

delta
d. activity
d. activity of low amplitude
alpha, delta sleep anomaly
d. antigen
antihepatitis delta virus immunoglobulin
d. band
enzyme-digested delta endotoxin
d. frame
d. frequencies
frontal intermittent rhythmic delta activity
frontal irregular rhythmic delta activity
d. gap
hemoglobin delta chain
hepatitis delta virus
intermittent rhythmic delta activity
monorhythmic frontal d.
monorhythmic frontal delta activity
negative delta sign
occipital dominant intermittent rhythmic delta activity
d. over baseline
polymorphic delta activity
d. ray
d. rhythm
d. rod
sheep factor d.
significant sharp spike or delta wave
d. sleep-inducing peptide
d. sleep stage
d. wave

delta-heavy-chain disease

deltoid
anterior tibiotalar part of deltoid ligament
left d.
d. ligament

Moberg deltoid muscle transfer
d. muscle
d. palsy
d. region
right d.
right deltoid muscle

delusion
alcohol-induced psychotic disorder with d.'s
amphetamine-induced psychotic disorder with d.'s
anxiolytic-induced psychotic disorder with d.'s
d. of being controlled
cannabis-induced psychotic disorder with d.'s
d. concerning appearance
d., hallucination, or illusion
d. and fantasy
d.'s of grandeur
d.'s of guilt
hallucinations and d.'s
d.'s and hallucinations
d. of jealousy and persecution
multiinfarct dementia with d.'s
multiple d.'s
object of a d.
paranoia and delusions psychiatric syndrome
paranoid grandiose d.
d. of power
d. of reference
schizophrenic hallucinations and d.'s
d.'s with vague conspiracy

delusional
arteriosclerotic dementia with delusional feature
atypical delusional experience
d. behavior
d. beliefs
cannabis delusional disorder
d. disorder
hallucinogen delusional disorder
d. or ideas of reference
litigious delusional state
marijuana delusional disorder
monosymptomatic delusional pseudocyesis
d. mood disorder
organic delusional disorder
organic delusional syndrome
paranoid delusional belief
d. paranoid disorder
persecutory delusional disorder
d. thinking
d. thought pattern
d. transient organic psychosis
d. type of activity

demand
arterial demand pacing
biochemical oxygen d.
biological oxygen d.
chemical oxygen d.
d. for constant admiration
d. for constant attention
dual demand pacemaker
electrolyte biochemical oxygen d.
d. feeding
increasing d.'s
intermittent demand ventilation
d. minimum functional capacity
d. oxygen delivery device
d. pacemaker
pacing on d.
permanent demand ventricular pacemaker
permanent transvenous demand pacemaker
ventricular demand pacing

demanding behavior

demarcated
sharply demarcated circumferential lesion

demarcation
areolar d.
d. line
line of d.
d. membrane system
nidus d.
no line of d.

demeanor
mild eccentricity in d.

dementia
acquired immune deficiency syndrome dementia complex
acquired immune deficiency syndrome-related d.
advanced d.
age-related d.
AIDS dementia complex
alcohol-induced persisting d.
alcoholism associated with d.
alcohol persisting d.
alcohol-related d.
Alzheimer d.
Alzheimer disease-related d.
Alzheimer-like senile d.
Alzheimer presenile d.
Alzheimer-type d.
d. of Alzheimer type
anxiolytic-induced persisting d.
Arizona Battery for Communication Disorders of D.
arteriosclerotic dementia confusional state
arteriosclerotic dementia with delirium
arteriosclerotic dementia with delusional feature
arteriosclerotic dementia with depressive feature
Assessment of D.
autism, dementia, ataxia, loss of purposeful hand use syndrome
Binswanger d.
Blessed D. Rating Scale
Blessed-Roth D. Scale
d. care mapping
cerebrovascular accident d.
Clinical D. Rating
congenital syphilitic paralytic d.
Cornell Scale for Depression, D.
debilitating d.
degenerative dementia of Alzheimer type
depression in d.
dialysis d.
diffuse Lewy body d.
drug-induced d.
d. due to Creutzfeldt-Jakob disease
d. due to head trauma
d. due to hepatic condition
d. due to multiple etiologies
d. due to traumatic brain injury
d. due to vitamin deficiency
epileptic d.
familial Alzheimer d.
familial British d.
d. from depression
d. from pernicious anemia
frontotemporal d.
full-blown d.
HIV human immunodeficiency virus-associated d.
HIV D. Scale
human immunodeficiency virus d.
human immunodeficiency virus associated d.
Lewy body d.
Manchester and Oxford Universities Scale for the Psychopathological Assessment of D.
Mattis D. Rating Scale
mnemonic d.
D. Mood Assessment Scale
multiinfarct d.

dementia *(continued)*
multiinfarct dementia, uncomplicated
multiinfarct dementia with delirium
multiinfarct dementia with delusions
multiinfarct dementia with depression
nosotropic drug dementia of Alzheimer type
d. paralytica juvenilis
paranoia dementia gravis
paranoid-type arteriosclerotic d.
Parkinson dementia complex
parkinsonian d.
primary degenerative d.
primary degenerative dementia of Alzheimer type
progressive d.
psychotic d.
senile d.
senile dementia of the Alzheimer type
socialized d.
structured interview for diagnosis of Alzheimer d.
d. syndrome of depression
transmissible virus d.
uncomplicated arteriosclerotic d.
vascular d.
d. with Lewy body

dementing illness

demineralized
d. bone
d. bone graft
d. bone matrix
d. bone powder
d. bony structure
d. freeze-dried bone
d. freeze-dried bone allograft
freeze-dried demineralized bone
Pacific Coast demineralized cortical bone powder

demise
fetal d.
intrauterine fetal d.

demographic information

demonstrable
no abnormality d.

demonstration
angiographic d.
d. bath
Breast Cancer Detection D. Project
patient d.

demosterol-to-cholesterol enzyme

demucosalized augmentation with gastric segment

demyelinated inflammatory chronic polyneuropathy

demyelinating
acute idiopathic demyelinating polyradiculoneuritis
acute inflammatory demyelinating polyneuropathy
acute inflammatory demyelinating polyradiculoneuropathy
acute inflammatory demyelinating polyradiculopathy
autoimmune demyelinating polyneuropathy
chronic inflammatory demyelinating polyradiculoneuropathy
chronic inflammatory demyelinating polyradiculopathy
chronic relapsing demyelinating inflammatory polyneuropathy
d. disease
d. disorder
distal acquired demyelinating symmetrical neuropathy
multifocal demyelinating motor neuropathy
neurologic demyelinating disease
optic demyelinating neuritis
segmental demyelinating polyneuropathy

demyelination
autoimmune d.
autoimmune inflammatory d.
nystagmus with d.
osmotic d.
osmotic demyelination syndrome

demyelinization
spinal cord d.

denaturation
Apt-Downey alkali denaturation test

denatured
completely d.
completely denatured alcohol
d. homograft
d. red blood cell

denaturing
d. density gradient electrophoresis
d. gradient gel electrophoresis
d. high-performance liquid chromatography

dendrite
apical d.
primary d.

dendritic
allogenic dendritic cell
antigen-pulsed autologous dendritic cell
d. cell
d. corneal ulcer
donor dendritic cell
d. expansion
follicular dendritic cell
interdigitating dendritic cell sarcoma
lymphoid dendritic cell
mutant Ras peptide-pulsed dendritic cell therapy
myeloid dendritic cell
d. reticulum cell
d. spine

denervated
evaluation of denervated heart at rest

denervation
carotid body d.
carotid sinus d.
computed tomography-guided percutaneous radiofrequency denervation of the sacroiliac joint
microsurgical denervation of the spermatic cord
partial bladder d.
percutaneous radiofrequency d.
peripheral bladder d.
reaction of d.
sinoaortic d.

dengue
d. fever
d. fever vaccine
d. hemorrhagic fever
d. hemorrhagic fever shock syndrome
d. virus 1–4

denial
color d.
diminished denial and defensiveness
d. and isolation
d. of lifesaving medical treatment

denied
permission for autopsy d.

denies
patient denies complaints

Denis Browne splint

Dennis Test of Child Development

Denonvilliers fascia

denotation
lexical d.

dens
anterior articular surface of d.
apex of d.
apical ligament of d.

densa
macula d.
macula densa cell
macula densa chemoreceptor
macula densa receptor

dense
d. adhesion
d. body
d. canalicular system
d. cataract
d. collagenous tissue
degenerative dense microsphere
d. deposit disease
d. fibroelastic connective tissue
d. fibrous adhesion
d. fibrous lamina
d. fibrous tissue
d. hemiplegia
d. intramembranous deposit disease
d. lobar infiltrate
longitudinal dense striation
lysosomal dense body
major dense line
d. microsphere
outer dense fibers of spermatozoon
d. parenchyma
d. plate
d. tubular system

densitometer
hair d.

densitometric
cine densitometric assessment of transit time

densitometry
bone mineral d.
computerized optical d.
dual-photon d.
photon absorption d.
video d.

density
abdominal soft tissue d.
alveolar d.
area of abnormal d.
area of increased d.
areal bone mineral d.
artefactual d.
arterial linear d.
asymmetric breast d.
average optical d.
axial spin d.
bone mineral d.
count information d.
decreased bone mineral d.
denaturing density gradient electrophoresis
electric charge d.
electric current d.
extravascular lung d.
d. of the fat-free mass
d. of the fat mass
femoral total d.
fluid d.
gradient d.
d. gradient
d. gradient electrophoresis
heel bone density scan
hepatic computed tomographic d.
high d.
high caloric d.
high-density humidity
hydrogen d.
increased d.
increased bone d.
increased linear d.
integrated optical d.
intermediate density lipoprotein
intramural microvessel d.
lamellar body d.
linear d.
low bone d.
lumbar spine bone d.
lumbar spine bone mineral d.
luminous flux d.
magnetic flux d.
mass d.
maximum d.
mean optical d.
metacarpal cortical d.
microvessel d.
mixed density mass
mixed fat-water density lesion
neutral d.
neutral density filter test
neutron number d.
nodular d.
Northland bone density machine
number of density of molecule
optical d.
optical density measurement
optical density method
optical density unit
d. optical standard
d. optical unknown
optimized microvessel density analysis
patchy area of d.
peak count d.
postsynaptic d.
power spectral d.
probability density function
prostate-specific antigen d.
PSA d.
relative vertebral d.
right vertebral d.
soft tissue d.
d. spectral array
spike occurrence d.
spin d.
strain energy d.
d. and strength of bone mass
sucrose density gradient
sucrose density gradient centrifugation
sucrose density gradient ultracentrifugation
total body d.
total body bone mineral d.
vapor d.
very high density lipoprotein
very low d.
very low density lipoprotein
very low density lipoprotein C
very low density lipoprotein-triglyceride
volumetric bone mineral d.

density-adjusted cell sorting

density-modulated spectral array

dental
acceptable dental remedies
accepted dental therapeutics
anterior superior dental artery
apical dental foramen
apical dental ligament
d. aptitude test
arrested dental caries
d. auxiliary teacher education
D. Auxiliary Utilization
cerebral, ocular, dental, auricular, skeletal syndrome
d. implant technique
d. distress syndrome
d. enamel dysplasia syndrome
expanded duty dental auxiliary
expanded function dental assistant
d. forceps

dental *(continued)*
d. granuloma
d. habits
d. health care provider
d. hygiene
d. impaction
d. implant
d. impression
d. inclusion
d. index
Index to D. Literature
d. injury
inner dental epithelium
intraoral dental molds
lower anterior dental height
lower dental arcade
mandibular dental arcade
maxillary dental arcade
osseointegrated dental implant
partially edentulous dental arch
past dental history
photostimulable phosphor dental radiography
poor dental hygiene
poor dental repair
D. Practitioners' Formulary
preventive dental health behavior
primary dental caries
d. prophylaxis
d. prosthesis
d. stain remover
superior dental arch
teeth in good dental condition
teeth in good dental repair

dental-alveolar abscess

dentale
osteoma d.

dentalis
arcus dentalis mandibularis
arcus dentalis maxillaris
arcus dentalis superior mandibularis
odontalgia d.
otalgia d.

dentate
d. gyrus
d. line
d. straight fissure bur
d. tapered fissure bur

dentatorubral-pallidoluysian atrophy

denticle
attached d.

denticular hymen

dentin
hereditary opalescent d.

dentinoblastic
multinucleated dentinoblastic cell
palisaded dentinoblastic layer

dentinoenamel junction

dentinogenesis imperfecta

dentistry
full-mouth restorative d.
operative d.

dentition
aplasia of d.
mandibular dentition odontectomy
mixed dentition analysis
d. in poor repair

dentoalveolar
anterior segmental dentoalveolar osteotomy

denture
articulated partial d.
cantilever fixed partial d.
choking from d.'s
complete denture impression
complete upper and lower d.'s
fixed partial d.
full d.
full lower d.
full mouth d.'s
full upper d.
full upper denture, partial lower d.
ill-fitting d.'s
improper fit of d.'s
metal base d.
model denture wax
mouth denture wax
partial d.'s
partial denture, distal extension
partial denture impression
partial denture prosthesis
partial denture prosthetics
partial denture retention
partial denture unit
partial lower d.
partial upper and lower d.'s
patient wears d.'s
poorly fitting d.'s
porcelain d.'s
red gums from d.'s
removable partial d.
slipping d.'s
standard d.'s

denudation
area of d.

denuded
d. bowel
d. connective tissue
d. jawbone
d. mucosa
d. surface
d. tissue

Denver
D. Articulation Screening Exam
D. Auditory Phoneme Sequencing Test
D. Developmental Screening Test
D. dialysis disease
D. Eye Screening Test
D. peritoneal venous shunt
D. pleuroperitoneal shunt
Revised Denver Prescreening Development Questionnaire

Denys-Drash syndrome

deodoratum
opium d.

deodorized
d. tincture of opium

deoxycholate
amphotericin B d.
d. citrate
sodium d.

deoxycorticosterone
d. acetate
d. glucoside
d. secretion rate
d. trimethylacetate

deoxycytidine
d. monophosphate
d. triphosphate

deoxyguanosine
d. monophosphate
d. triphosphate

deoxynucleic
primer-dependent deoxynucleic acid polymerase
primer-dependent deoxynucleic acid polymerase index
unscheduled deoxynucleic acid synthesis

deoxynucleotide
terminal deoxynucleotide transferase
d. triphosphate

deoxynucleotidyl
terminal deoxynucleotidyl transferase

deoxyribonucleic
d. acid double stranded
d. acid, histone

d. acid phosphorus
d. acid polymerase
d. acid single stranded
anti-double-stranded deoxyribonucleic acid
anti-double-stranded deoxyribonucleic acid antibody
branched deoxyribonucleic acid
closed circle deoxyribonucleic acid
complementary deoxyribonucleic acid
mitochondrial deoxyribonucleic acid analysis
mitochondrial deoxyribonucleic acid polymerase gamma
native deoxyribonucleic acid
recombinant deoxyribonucleic acid
ribonucleic acid-dependent deoxyribonucleic acid polymerase
ribosomal deoxyribonucleic acid
single-stranded deoxyribonucleic acid
transfer deoxyribonucleic acid

deoxyribonucleotide
total adenine d.

deoxyriboside
uracil d.

deoxythymidine
d. diphosphate
d. triphosphate

deoxyuridine
d. diphosphate
d. monophosphate
d. triphosphate

Depage-Janeway gastrostomy

department
central sterile supply d.
corrective therapy d.
died in emergency d.
district health d.
emergency d.
emergency department approval for pediatrics
emergency department physician
emergency department thoracotomy
hospital emergency d.
hospital outpatient d.
medical d.
mental health d.
nonsurgeon, emergency d.
outpatient d.
pediatric emergency d.
supply, processing, and distribution d.
walk-in emergency d.

departure
time of d.

dependence
aerosol spray d.
airplane glue d.
alcohol d.
alcohol dependence syndrome
alcohol dependence treatment program
alcohol dependence with tolerance
alcohol and drug dependence unit
Alcohol D. Scale
amphetamine d.
barbiturate d.
cannabis d.
chemical dependence clinic
chemical dependence disorder
cocaine d.
d. disorder
drug d.
drug and alcohol d.
drug dependence treatment program
emotional d.
Fagerstrom Test for Nicotine D.
frequency dependence of compliance
frequency dependence of resistance
increased emotional d.
narcotic drug d.
d. on hallucinogen
physical dependence capacity
physical dependence on nicotine gum
polysubstance d.
prescription drug d.
primary dependence study
primary physical d.
psychoactive substance abuse and d.
steroid d.
tobacco d.

dependency
chemical d.
chemical dependency counselor
chemical dependency and mental illness
chemical dependency unit
cultural aspect of chemical d.
Interpersonal D. Inventory
Nursing-Care Dependency scale
physical d.
psychological d.
Self-Administered D. Questionnaire
type 1 autosomal recessive vitamin D d.
unmet dependency need

dependent
Aid to D. Children
d. atelectasis
barbital d.
conditionally streptomycin d.
d. drainage
d. edema
head dependent position
hormone d.
individual dependent counseling
d. peripheral edema
d. personality disorder
d. pooling
d. rubor
T-cell d.
totally dependent individual
d. variable
ventilator dependent quadriplegia

depersonalization
d. or derealization
d. disorder
d. neurosis
d. psychoneurosis

depigmentation
periocular d.

depigmented
d. lesion
d. nevus

depleted
d. energy
Hodgkin disease of diffuse histiocytic lymphocyte depleted type
lymphocyte d.

depletion
extracellular fluid volume d.
glycogen d.
lipid d.
lymphocyte d.
mild colloid d.
neurotransmitter d.
ovarian ascorbic acid depletion test
ovarian cholesterol depletion test
potassium d.
salt depletion syndrome
thymic d.
volume d.
white blood cell d.
zinc depletion syndrome

deployment
stent d.

depolarization
alternating failure of response mechanical to electrical d.
atrial premature d.
ectopic d.
fluorescence d.
His bundle d.
long-lasting d.
onset of ventricular d.
part of the electrocardio-graphic cycle representing atrial d.
premature ventricular d.
rapid dyssynchronous d.
ventricular ectopic d.
ventricular premature d.
ventricular premature depolarization contraction

depolarization-induced automaticity

depolarizing
d. afterpotential
paroxysmal depolarizing shift
sustained depolarizing shift

deposit
abdominal fat d.
basal laminar d.
calcium deposit on heart valves
dense deposit disease
dense intramembranous deposit disease
endochondral bone d.'s
immunoglobulin light chain-origin amyloid d.
iron d.'s
lipofuscinosis granular osmiophilic d.
macrocephaly with feeblemindedness and encephalopathy with peculiar d.'s
2-microglobulin-origin amyloid d.
pericardium calcareous d.
plaque d.
posterior corneal d.
waxy deposit on brain

deposition
aerosol d.
apatite deposition disease
calcium phosphate crystal deposition disease
calcium pyrophosphate d.
calcium pyrophosphate crystal deposition disease
calcium pyrophosphate dehydrate deposition disease
calcium pyrophosphate deposition disease
calcium pyrophosphate dihydrate crystal d.
calcium pyrophosphate dihydrate deposition disease
catalyzed reporter d.
central d.
hydroxyapatite deposition disease
inhomogeneous d.
light chain deposition disease
malarial deposition pigment
marked hyaline d.
neonatal elastin d.
nonlinear IgA d.
normal d.
particulate crystalline material d.
perisinusoidal fibrin d.
subpleural reticulated carbon d.

depot
local depot injection
Maurice corneal depot technique
d. medroxyprogesterone acetate

depressant
motor d.
myocardial depressant substance

depressed
adjustment disorder with mixed anxiety and depressed mood
d. and agitated
d. and anxious
d. breathing and heartbeat
d. DNA synthesis
fracture simple and d.
d. fracture skull
d. heart attack patient
d. heart attack survivor
hostile and d.
immune depressed patient
d. individual
d. or irritable mood
resuscitation of depressed newborn
d. skull fracture
d. spectrum disease
d. ST segment

depressing
reticuloendothelial depressing substance

depression
abuse related d.
D. Adjective Check List
adolescent depression symptom
adult major d.
Amsterdam D. List
angle of d.
anxiety associated with d.
anxiety and d.
d. and anxiety in elderly
anxious somatic d.
D.: Awareness, Recognition, and Treatment
Beck D. Index Short Form
Beck D. Inventory
bone marrow d.
burning mouth from d.
Centers for Epidemiologic Studies D. scale
central nervous system d.
central respiratory d.
Children's D. Inventory
Children's D. Rating Scale-Revised
Children's D. Scale
chronic d.
chronic recurring d.
clinical d.
cognitive impairment of d.
concavity and d.
Cornell Scale for D., Dementia
cortically spreading d.
crushing anxiety and d.
decreased signs and symptoms of d.
d. in dementia
dementia from d.
dementia syndrome of d.
d., insomnia and fatigue
depression sine d.
downsloping ST-segment d.
drug-induced postanesthetic d.
drug-induced postanesthetic respiratory d.
Edinburgh Postnatal D. Scale
extreme d.
Family Drawing D. Scale
Geriatric D. Scale
Hamilton Rating Scale for D.
Hamilton D. Rating Scale
headache, insomnia, and depression syndrome
Hospital Anxiety and D.
Hospital Anxiety and D. Scale
hostility and d.
impact of d.
incapacitating d.
insomnia associated with d.
insomnia from d.
intermittent periods of d.
d. inventory
irritability and d.
irritability, depression and personality changes

lifetime depression criterion
linoleic acid d.
lunate fossa d.
major d.
manic d.
manifestation of d.
Martin Suicide D. Inventory
mental d.
mesial developmental d.
midlife d.
Minnesota Multiphasic Personality Inventory Depression Scale
mixed anxiety depression disorder
Montgomery-Asberg D. Rating Scale
multiinfarct dementia with d.
Multiscore D. Inventory
narcotic-induced respiratory d.
d. of nasal bone
nervousness from d.
neurotic d.
Oregon Adolescent Depression Project-Conduct Disorder Screener
orthogonal depression factor
pathological d.
Peer Nomination Inventory for D.
postanesthetic respiratory d.
postnatal d.
postpartum d.
poststroke d.
prevention and treatment of d.
profound d.
psychotic d.
d. pure disease
reactive neurotic d.
reciprocal ST d.
recurrent d.
recurrent chronic d.
respiratory depression inhalation anesthesia
Revised Children's D. Scale
Reynolds Adolescent D. Scale
Reynolds Child D. Scale
Scale of Anxiety and D.
Self-Assessment D. Scale
Self-Rating D. Scale
Shipman Anxiety D. Scale
short stature, hyperextensibility of joints or hernia or both, ocular depression, Rieger anomaly, teething, delayed
situational d.
sporadic d.
spreading d.
D. Status Inventory
ST segment d.
d. of transmission
treatment-resistant d.
d. triggered by physical illness
unipolar d.
Verdun D. Rating Scale
vital exhaustion and d.
Zung Self-Rating D. Scale

depressive
D. Adjective Checklist
adult depressive disorder
adult depressive episode
d. affect
affective depressive reaction
arteriosclerotic dementia with depressive feature
chronic depressive personality disorder
emotional stress depressive psychosis
D. Experiences Questionnaire
familial pure depressive disease
full-blown depressive episode
full-blown manic depressive illness
d. hallucination
d. illness
major depressive affective psychosis
manic d.
medication-induced depressive syndrome
minor depressive disorder
d. neurosis
neurotic depressive reaction
neurotic depressive state
overall depressive symptom
personal history of depressive disorders
d. psychosis
d. reaction
severe depressive illness
sporadic depressive disease
Standardized Assessment of D. Disorders

depressive-type psychosis

depressor
aortic depressor nerve
cardiac depressor reflex
muscle d.
d. muscle of angle of mouth
d. muscle of lower lip
d. muscle of septum of nose
O'Connor d.

deprivation
androgen deprivation therapy
antagonist-induced gonadotropin d.
binocular d.
control of heart rate during oxygen d.
intermittent androgen d.
long-term estrogen d.
maternal d.
monocular d.
neoadjuvant androgen d.
night sleep d.
nutritional deprivation syndrome
oxygen deprivation theory of narcosis
d. of sleep
d. syndrome

deprived
d. eye
nutritionally d.
protein d.

depth
acetabular depth to femoral head diameter
d. of anesthesia
arm girth, chest depth, and hip width
burn depth indicator
central axis depth dose of electron beam therapy
controlled depth osteotomy cutter
distorted depth perception
d. dose
d. electroencephalogram
d. electroencephalography
d. electrography
erosion d.
d. of focus
half-dose d.
high-dose d.
d. of insertion
invasion depth radiography
maximum d.
monocular depth perception
optical penetration d.
orthopaedic depth gauge
pocket d.
posterior mandibular d.
power-oriented depth controlled osteotomy cutter
probing d.
relative sagittal d.
sagittal depth of cornea
stereotactic depth electroencephalogram
temperature, depth, and salinity
volumetric lung d.

depth-resolved surface coil spectroscopy

Dera Ghazi Khan virus

deranged
mentally d.

derangement
alveolar arch d.
hemodynamic d.'s
internal derangement of knee joint
painful disc d.

derealization
depersonalization or d.

derivation
modeling d.
müllerian duct derivation syndrome
neoadjuvant androgen derivation therapy

derivative
antimüllerian derivative syndrome
centrally active phenethylamine derivative related to amphetamine and methamphetamine
d. chromosome
d. of contagious tuberculin
double radioisotope d.
fibrinogen d.
glucuronide derivative of azidothymidine
glycopeptide moiety modified d.
hematoporphyrin d.
hydroxyl derivative of GABA
live yeast cell d.
purified protein d.
purified protein derivative of tuberculin
purified protein derivative test
Siebert purified protein derivative of tuberculin

derivative–Battey
purified protein d.

derivative–standard
purified protein d.

derived
d. hemodynamic data
müllerian duct derived structure
originally d.
d. value on apex cardiogram

dermal
allograft dermal matrix graft
capillary loop in dermal papilla
d. fat free flap
d. fat free tissue transfer
d. fat graft
focal dermal hypoplasia
focal dermal hypoplasia syndrome
focal facial dermal dysplasia II
d. graft
d. grafting
human dermal microvascular endothelial cell
leishmaniasis
lumbosacral dermal sinus
d. lymphatic involvement
microphthalmia, dermal aplasia, sclerocornea syndrome
open dermal sinus
d. or oral herpes
d. overgrafting
papillary dermal peel
d. subcutaneous junction
d. ulcer

dermal-epidermal
d.-e. junction
d.-e. separation

dermatan sulfate

dermatis
papilla d.

dermatitis
actinic reticuloid d.
airborne contact d.
allergic contact d.
allergic eczematous contact d.
allergic eczematous contact-type d.
allergic gold d.
arsenical contact d.
Assessment Measure for Atopic D.
atopic d.
Atopic D. Area and Severity Index
atopic dermatitis rash
atopic dermatitis with keratoconjunctivitis
autoimmune progesterone d.
avian mite d.
cat mite d.
chronic actinic d.
contact d.
contagious pustular d.
diaper d.
distinctive exudative discoid and lichenoid d.
drug eruption d.
eczematous allergic contact d.
erythematous macular d.
exfoliative d.
herpes zoster d.
d. herpetiformis
hot tub d.
intractable atopic d.
irritant contact d.
juvenile plantar d.
lichenoid contact d.
machine worker d.
mask of atopic d.
medicamentosa d.
moderate atopic d.
monilial diaper d.
nasal cannula d.
nasal solar d.
neonatal bullous d.
nickel hand d.
nodules, eosinophilia, rheumatism, dermatitis, and swelling syndrome
nummular eczematous d.
nutritional deficiency d.
nylon stocking d.
occupational d.
occupational rubber d.
ocular atopic d.
onion mite d.
oozing from d.
papular dermatitis of pregnancy
photoallergic contact d.
phototoxic contact d.
primary irritant contact d.
seborrheic d.
Severity Scoring of Atopic D.
six-area, six-sign atopic d.
skin hardening from d.
stasis d.

dermatoarthritis
familial histiocytic d.

dermatofibrosarcoma
fibrosarcomatous variant of dermatofibrosarcoma protuberans
d. protuberans

dermatology
D. Index of Disease Severity
d. and syphilology

dermatomal somatosensory-evoked potential

dermatome
anterior tibial nerve d.
compressed air-powered d.
mechanical d.

dermatomyositis
acute d.
childhood d.
d. in hand
juvenile d.
polymyositis and d.

dermatomyositis/polymyositis
juvenile d./p.

dermatophyte
d. infection of hair
d. infection of nails
d. infection of scalp
d. infection of skin
d. test media

dermatosis
acquired perforating d.
acute febrile neutrophilic d.
adult bullous d.
ashy dermatosis of Ramirez
chronic disabling d.
febrile neutrophilic d.
juvenile plantar d.
lichenoid chronic d.
linear IgA bullous d.
linear IgA d.
neutrophilic intraepidermal IgA d.
d. papulosa nigra
papulosa nigra d.
subcorneal pustular d.
transient acantholytic d.
ulcerative d.

dermis
adventitial d.
autogenous dermis fat graft
new d.
papilla of d.
papillae d.
papillary d.

dermodistortive urticaria

dermoid
limbal d.
mediastinum d.
orbital d.
orbital dermoid cyst
ovarian d.
ovarian dermoid cyst
parasellar dermoid tumor

dermoids
mandibulofacial dysostosis with epibulbar dermoids syndrome

dermonecrotic toxin

Derogatis Affects Balance Scale

derogatory hallucination

derotating
ventral derotating spinal implant

derotation
elongation, derotation and lateral flexion
femoral derotation osteotomy
d. femoral osteotomy
d. osteotomy
ventral derotation spondylodesis

derotational
Axer varus derotational osteotomy
d. osteotomy
d. varus osteotomy

derotator splint

desaturation
arterial oxygen d.
oxygen desaturation index

Descemet
membrane of D.
D. membrane

descend
failure to d.

descending
anterior descending artery
d. aorta
ascending and d.
d. colon
intramural left anterior descending artery
large intestinal descending colon
left anterior descending coronary artery
left posterior descending artery
nonirrigating descending colostomy
d. palatine artery
pharyngeal branch of descending palatine artery
posterior descending artery
posterior descending branch
posterior descending coronary artery
proximal left anterior descending artery
d. rectal septum
right anterior d.
right anterior descending coronary artery
right descending pulmonary artery
d. thoracic aorta
d. thoracic aortofemoral-femoral bypass

descent
arrest of descent dystocia
diastolic descent rate
identical by d.
pelvic floor d.
spontaneous descent of testis

description
autopsy external d.
change description master
graphic d.
Job D. Index
Leader Behavior D. Questionnaire
narrative d.
Supervisory Behavior D.

descriptive
d. anatomy
Apraxia Profile: A D. Assessment Tool for Children
associated descriptive feature
Retirement D. Index
simple descriptive scale

descriptor
alternative dimensional descriptors for schizophrenia

desensitization
enzyme potentiated d.
eye movement desensitization reprocessing
headache activity and d.
palmar surface d.
d. and relaxation group
d. technique
d. test

desert fever

desertion
maternal d.
paternal d.

desiccated thyroid extract

desiccation
curettage and d.

design
advanced design LINAC radiosurgery
ambulance design criteria
block design test
Bryant-Schwan D. Test
completely randomized d.
computerized assisted design prosthesis
Graham-Kendall Memory for D.'s Test
Harris d.
longitudinal experimental study d.
memory for d.
Memory for D.'s test
microwave antenna d.
Morrison donor site d.
multiple baseline d.
Norwood donor site d.
practical approach d.
vocabulary, information, block design, and similarities

designated
d. blood donation
d. caregiver
d. compensable event
d. donor blood

designation
ordinal designation of the exanthemata
designed
biologically designed hip
d. after natural anatomy
designer
d. drug
d. hallucinogen
desirability
Marlowe-Crown Social D. Scale
social d.
desirable
d. body weight
mean percentage of desirable weight
desire
hypoactive sexual desire disorder
increased sexual d.
inhibited sexual d.
male hypoactive sexual desire disorder
personal desire for gain
desmoglein
recombinant d.
desmoid
periosteal d.
peritoneum desmoid tumor
desmoid-type fibromatosis
desmoplastic
d. cerebral astrocytoma of infancy
d. infantile ganglioglioma
neuraxial desmoplastic neuroepithelial tumor
d. neurotropic melanoma
d. small round-cell tumor
desmosome
modified d.
d. with bundle of tonofilament
desorption
electronic induction d.
electron-stimulated d.
field d.
d. ionization
matrix-assisted laser desorption and ionization mass spectrometry
matrix-assisted laser desorption ionization-time-of-flight mass spectrometry
photon-stimulated d.
desorption/ionization
laser desorption/ionization time-of-flight-mass spectrometer
surface enhanced laser d./i.
desoxycholate
buffered desoxycholate glucose
desoxycorticosterone
d. acetate
d. glucoside
d. triphenylacetate
despeciated bovine serum
despite
dead despite resuscitation attempt
dead on arrival despite resuscitative attempts
d. resuscitation attempts
desquamated
d. epithelial debris
d. epithelium
desquamating epithelium
desquamation
erosion d.
membranous d.
moist d.
peribronchial d.
perineal d.
periungual d.
plantar d.
desquamativa
otitis d.
desquamative
d. interstitial pneumonia
d. interstitial pneumonitis
destabilizing impact of trauma
destiny
manifest d.
destroyed
millicuries d.
destroy healthy tissue
destroying
cancer destroying agent
destruction
accelerated destruction of red blood cells
area of bony d.
cryo destruction procedure
laser destruction of intraepithelial neoplasia
localized bone d.
lung d.
moth-eaten bone d.
neoplastic destruction of spinal element
pantalocrural arthritic d.
pattern of d.
skin d.
thermal d.
tumor d.
weapons of mass d.
destructive
amiodarone-induced destructive thyrotoxicosis
chronic destructive periodontitis
chronic nonsuppurative destructive cholangitis
d. compulsive disease
idiopathic destructive arthritis
idiopathic midline destructive disease
d. illness
immune destructive process
d. injury
nonsuppurative destructive cholangitis
osseous destructive process
d. self-centeredness
d. sexual behavior
d. thought pattern
destructive-compulsive disease
Desus
Lee and Desus D test
desynchronization
event-related d.
desynchronized sleep
detachable
d. silicone balloon
electrically detachable coil
Guglielmi detachable coil
mechanically detachable platinum coil
detachment
aphakic retinal d.
complex retinal d.
macula-off rhegmatogenous retinal d.
medial meniscus d.
d. of medial meniscus
morning glory retinal d.
neurosensory retinal d.
nonrhegmatogenous retinal d.
pattern of d.
pigment epithelial d.
posterior vitreal d.
posterior vitreous d.
retinal d.
retinal detachment repair
retinal detachment, oculus dexter
retinal detachment, oculus sinister
retina pigment epithelium d.
rhegmatogenous retinal d.

sense of d.
total-retinal d.
tractional retinal d.
traction retinal d.

detail
associative detail response to white space
confabulated detail response
edge d.
inside d.
rare detail response
d. response
d. response elaborating the whole
d. response to small white space
unusual rare detail response
whole response to d.

detailed
d. evaluation of facial symmetry
d. medical history
d. rituals and routine

detained
fit to be d.

detectability
speech detectability threshold
threshold of d.

detectable
below detectable levels
below detectable limits
histologically detectable iron
immunologically detectable insulin
minimal detectable quantity
no detectable activity
no detectable antibody
none d.
serologically d.

detected
d. in colon cancer
lymphocyte detected membrane antigen
no gammopathy detected
none d.
not d.
nothing abnormal d.

detection
annihilation coincidence d.
antibody-based detection system
antigen detection test
antigen stool detection test
antiliver microsomal antibody d.
atrial tachycardia detection rate
automated border d.
automated border detection by echocardiography
automated edge d.
automated polyp d.
avidin-biotin-based detection system
avidin-biotin detection system
Békésy Functionality D. Test
biologic aerosol d.
biologic detection system
d. of bone spur
border detection method
Breast Cancer D. Demonstration Project
cancer detection center
cardiac shunt d.
chi-square automatic interaction d.
computerized edge d.
data spike detection error artifact
Disease D. Information Bureau
d. of early antigen fluorescent focus
early detection of breast cancer
electrochemical d.
error detection circuit
esophageal detection device
esophageal intubation d.
d. of gamma ray
gold-labeled antigen detection technique
heat detection test
hepatitis B DNA d.
high-pH anion exchange chromatography coupled with pulsed amperometric d.
Hypertension D. and Followup Program
infrared emission d.
limit of d.
liquid chromatography with electrochemical d.
lower limit of d.
Lyme disease DNA d.
micrometastases detection assay
molecular coincidence d.
motion detection threshold
multiple ion d.
Mycobacterium tuberculosis d.
myelin-associated glycoprotein antibody d.
Neisseria gonorrhoeae DNA detection test
noninvasive detection of trisomy 18
nonisotopic detection system
nucleic acid d.
pancreatic fungal d.
peripheral detection test
peripheral light d.
quantum detection efficiency
Rapid Rare Event D.
replicate organism detection and counting
resistive load d.
sensory detection method
sentinel lymph node d.
speech detection threshold
stone-tissue detection system
ultrasound gallstone d.
visual detection level

detective quantum efficiency

detector
acute ionization d.
argon ionization d.
diode array d.
Doppler flow d.
electrochemical d.
electron capture d.
emission spectrometric d.
evoked-response d.
flame ionization d.
flame photometric d.
mass spectrophotometric d.
mosaic detector configuration
multielectrode flame ionization d.
nitrogen-phosphorus d.
nitrogen-phosphorus detector in gas chromatography
nitrogen-specific d.
photoionization d.
pulsed ultrasonic blood velocity d.
quadrature phase d.
thermal conductivity d.
d. transfer function
ultrasonic flow d.

detention warrant

detergent
anionic d.
neutral detergent fiber
nonionic detergent soluble
synthetic d.

deteriorated
patient's condition d.

deteriorating
d. blood gases
d. effect of medication
d. function
d. neurological disorder
d. sense of balance

deterioration
age-related d.
age-related deterioration process
alcoholic d.
aortic wall d.
appearance d.
arthritic d.

deterioration *(continued)*
cognitive d.
d. of coordination, gait, and speech
end-of-dose d.
d. following improvement
Global D. Scale
gradual d.
d. of heart muscle
d. index
intellectual d.
manners d.
memory d.
mental d.
Mental D. Battery
mental deterioration battery
mood d.
motivation d.
neurologic d.
organic d.
organic central nervous system d.
organic CNS d.
personality d.
progressive d.
progressive intellectual and neurological d.
Progressive D. Scale
structural valve d.

determinant
anterior determinants of cusp occlusion
antigenic d.
antigenic determinant of erythrocytes
helper d.
ligand-binding d.
lymphocyte-activating d.
new antigenic d.
Oz isotypic d.
resistance d.
suppressor-activating d.

determination
adipocyte determination and differentiation factor-1
blood glucose d.
coefficient of d.
criteria for determination of brain death
disability determination service
d. of eligibility
environmental sex d.
fetal activity acceleration d.
gamma A immunoglobulin d.
gamma immunoglobulin D d.
gamma immunoglobulin E d.
gamma immunoglobulin G d.
gamma immunoglobulin M d.
hemoglobin d.
interim glucose d.
method of rapid d.
oxygen content d.
sugar and acetone d.

determine
unable to d.

determined
affective determined disorder
clinical staging of tumors, nodes, and metastases as determined by noninvasive examination
etiology to be d.
genetically determined immunodeficiency disease
lymphocytically d.
maximum determined heart rate
not d.
d. osteogenic precursor cell
pain determined by level of anxiety
serologically d.
to be d.

determinism
linguistic d.

detoxication
ammonia d.

detoxification
d. before surgery
d. and brief treatment
chemical d.
clinical interaction and d.
long-term detoxification program
major detoxification enzyme
medication-assisted d.
multidrug resistance d.
rapid d.
rapid opiate detoxification under anesthesia
rapid opioid d.
rehydration and d.
short-term d.

detrimental impact of fatigue

Detroit
D. Tests of Learning Aptitude - Primary, Second Edition
D. Tests of Learning Aptitude, Third Edition

detrusor
d. acontractility
d. areflexia
d. contraction
d. dyssynergia
d. external sphincter dyssynergia
d. hyperactivity
d. hyperactivity with impaired contractility
d. hypercontractility
d. hyperreflexia
d. hypocontractility
d. hyporeflexia
d. instability
instability
d. motor instability
d. muscle instability
d. muscle leak-point pressure
d. muscle pressure-flow micturition study
normal detrusor contractility
normal detrusor reflex
d. overactivity
perineobulbar detrusor facilitative reflex
perineobulbar detrusor inhibitory reflex
phasic detrusor instability
d. sphincter dyssynergia
spinal detrusor hyperreflexia
uninhibited detrusor muscle capacity

deuterium/hydrogen ratio

deutoiodide
mercury d.

deux
crime a d.

devascularization
esophagogastric devascularization and transection

devastating illness

developed
d. collateral
colony-stimulating factor developed by Venereal Disease Research Laboratory
common peak developed isovolumetric pressure
fairly well d.
maximal left ventricular developed pressure
normal well d.
patient well d.
patient well developed, well nourished
d. pressure

developing
high risk of developing cervical cancer
prone to developing pigment gallstones
D. Skills Checklist
slowly developing atelectasis

slowly developing lesion
d. stroke

develop isolation technique

development

abnormal development of scar tissue
abnormal fetal d.
Adapted Sequenced Inventory of Communication D.
altered growth and d.
anal stage psychosexual d.
arrest of d.
arrested growth and d.
Assessment of Career D.
Assessment in Infancy Ordinal Scales of Psychological D.
asymmetric subtalar joint d.
Bristol Language D. Scale
California Infant Scale for Motor D.
child development clinic
coloboma, heart disease, atresia choanae, retarded growth and retarded development and/or CNS anomalies, genital hypoplasia, and ear anomalies and/or deafness syndrome
communicative development inventory
constitutional delay in growth and d.
corrected development quotient
delayed d.
delayed development of speech
delayed sexual d.
Dennis Test of Child D.
d. of discharge plan
Ego-Ideal and Conscience D. Test
Ego D. Scale
embryonic growth and development factor
fetal growth and d.
fine motor d.
follow up intervention for normal d.
Frostig Program for the D. of Visual Perception
gel development time
Gesell Child D. Age Scale
grammar development stage
gross motor d.
growth and d.
d. of gut
heterosexual development of women
human development and family life
impaired sexual d.
incomplete development of autonomic nervous system
d. of inflammation
initial psychiatric d.
Integrated Child D. Scheme
Inventory for Counseling and D.
Inventory of Psychosocial D.
Kaufman D. Scale
Kent Infant D. Scale
lung growth and d.
male genital duct d.
malformation of cortical d.
Measures of Psychosocial D.
megakaryocyte growth and development factor
Mental Retardation and D. Disabilities
metacarpophalangeal bone marrow d.
metatarsophalangeal bone marrow d.
Minnesota Child D. Inventory
mixed development developmental delay disorder
motor development examination
neurobiology of early childhood d.
neurologic d.
neuromuscular development of speech
normal d.
normal childhood d.
normal fetal d.
normal growth and d.
normal human d.
normal muscle d.
organization d.
parallel development of axillary hair
parallel development of pubic hair
parental development questionnaire
perceptual motor d.
Prescreening D. Questionnaire
product development protocol
programmed multiple d.
Progress Assessment Chart of Social and Personal D.
Psychomotor D. Index
research and d.
research and development board
Revised Denver Prescreening D. Questionnaire
Screening Kit of Language D.
Sequenced Inventory of Language D.
slow expressive language d.
Tasks of Emotional D.
Test of Early Language D., Second Edition
Utah Test of Language D.
Verbal Language D. Scale
vocational skills assessment and development program

developmental

d. abnormality
D. Activities Screening Inventory
adolescence developmental stage
adulthood developmental stage
d. age
age-related developmental process
Albert Einstein Neonatal D. Scale
d. anatomy
anterior axial developmental cataract
d. aphasia
d. apraxia of speech
arithmetical developmental delay disorder
d. arrest
arthrogryposis, ectodermal dysplasia, cleft lip/palate developmental delay syndrome
articulation developmental delay disorder
d. articulation disorder
D. Articulation Test
D. Assessment of Life Experiences
atypical pervasive developmental disorder
atypical specific developmental disorder
axial fusiform developmental cataract
Battelle D. Inventory
Beery D. Test of Visual-Motor Integration
buccal developmental groove
central developmental groove
congenital thrombocytopenia, Robin sequence, agenesis of corpus callosum, distinctive facies, developmental delay syndrome
d. coordination disorder
deafness, femoral epiphysial dysplasia, short stature, developmental delay syndrome
Denver D. Screening Test

developmental *(continued)*
d. disability
d. disorders
distobuccal developmental groove
d. dysplasia of hip
Erhardt D. Prehension Assessment
Erhardt D. Vision Assessment
D. Evaluation Center
d. expressive language disorder
d. expressive writing disorder
D. Eye Movement
formal developmental history
Frostig D. Test of Visual Motor Perception
d. Gerstmann syndrome
Gesell D. Schedules
Griffiths Mental D. Scale
d. hand function test
d. history
D. Indicators for Assessment of Learning
d. language disorder
d. learning problem
d. level
lingual developmental groove
macrocephaly, hypertelorism, short limbs, hearing loss, developmental delay syndrome
mean developmental quotient
megalocornea, developmental retardation, dysmorphic syndrome
mesial marginal developmental groove
mesiolingual developmental groove
microcephaly, mild developmental delay, short stature, distinctive face syndrome
midline developmental lesion
mixed development developmental delay disorder
d. motor quotient
multiple complex developmental disorder
nonlinear developmental curve
nonverbal developmental index
nuclear developmental cataract
osteogenesis imperfecta, optic atrophy, retinopathy, developmental delay syndrome
Peabody D. Motor Activity Cards
Peabody D. Motor Scale
pediatric infectious disease developmental screening test
d. pediatrics
pervasive developmental disorder
pervasive developmental disorder not otherwise specified
D. Profile-II
d. quotient
d. receptive language disorder
Riley Preschool D. Screening Inventory
D. Sentence Scoring
d. sequence posture
sequential developmental exercises
specific developmental disorder
Tanner D. Scale
D. Test of Visual Perception
d. unit
d. venous anomaly

developmentally
d. delayed
d. disabled
mentally retarded and developmentally disabled

development-at-birth index

Development-II
Bayley Scales of Infant D.-II

Devereux Elementary School Behavior Rating Scale II

deviance
communication d.

deviant
color vision d.
endorsement of deviant thoughts and beliefs

deviate
involuntary deviate sexual intercourse
psychiatric deviate, subtle
psychopathic d.
standardized d.

deviated
fracture complete and d.
d. nasal septum
d. septum

deviation
abnormal left axis d.
abnormal right axis d.
angle of d.
anterior chamber-associated immune d.
average d.
axis d.
borderline left axis d.
congenital penile d.
conjugate horizontal d.
disconjugate eye d.
dissociated horizontal d.
dissociated vertical d.
Freedom from Distractibility D. Quotient
frequency d.
d. from norm
health deviation self-care requisite
d. to the left
left axis deviation, minimal
left deviation of electrical axis
mean d.
mean square d.
medial deviation of the second toe
memory deviation quotient
minimal deviation adenocarcinoma
minimal deviation melanoma
nasal septal d.
no deviation of electrical axis
normal axis d.
normal equivalent d.
no significant d.
out of specification deviation from standard
Perceptual Organization D. Quotient
periodic alternating gaze d.
population standard d.
qigong deviation syndrome
radial d.
relative standard d.
d. to the right
right axis d.
right deviation of electrical axis
root-mean-square d.
sample standard d.
standard deviation interval
standard deviation of mean
standard deviation of normal-to-normal beat
standard deviation score
standard normal d.
Standard D. Unit
sum of square d.'s
superior axis d.
d. of trachea
ulnar d.
ulnar deviation deformity
verbal comprehension deviation quotient
vertical d.

deviational nystagmus

device
abdominal aortic counterpulsation d.
abdominal left ventricular assist d.
acute ventricular assist d.
adjustable aiming d.

angled delivery d.
ankle disc d.
antibiotic removal d.
antimicrobial removal d.
antisiphon d.
application of traction d.
arachnophlebectomy surgical d.
arrhythmia control d.
Arrow-Trerotola percutaneous thrombectomy d.
arterial puncture site closure d.
articular motion d.
articulated tension d.
artificial left ventricular assist d.
assistive listening d.
assistive technology d.
atherolytic reperfusion wire d.
automated biopsy d.
automated general experimental d.
automatic spring-loaded biopsy d.
Axer compression d.
axis-altering arthroereisis d.
4-bar external fixation d.
bathroom safety d.
bilateral ventricular assist d.
biodegradable fixation d.
biventricular assist d.
braided occlusion d.
cardiac automatic resuscitative d.
cellulose acetate dialysis d.
central venous access d.
cervical immobilization d.
charge-coupled d.
child-restraint d.
clitoral therapy d.
computerized automated psycho-physiologic d.
continuous passive motion d.
continuous positive airway pressure d.
craniomandibular orthopedic repositioning d.
demand oxygen delivery d.
digital micromirror d.
Doppler sound d.
double umbrella d.
drowsiness monitoring d.
drug administration d.
electrode placement d.
electronic infusion d.
electronic portal imaging d.
electronic summation d.
emergency infusion d.
endoscope lens cleansing d.
esophageal detection d.
exoskeletal d.
expanded foam immobilization d.
external counterpressure d.
external tachyarrhythmia control d.
external urinary d.
extracorporeal liver assist d.
Family Assessment D.
fecal containment d.
feces collection d.
fluorescence capillary-fill d.
fog reduction elimination d.
frameless stereotactic d.
glaucoma drainage d.
hearing protection d.
hemostatic occlusive leverage d.
hemostatic puncture closure d.
home infusion d.
humanitarian device exemption
implantable middle ear hearing d.
implantable vascular access d.
implantable venous access d.
indwelling prosthetic medical d.
indwelling transcutaneous vascular access d.
insertion of fixation d.
intensified charge-coupled d.
internal cervical d.
intramedullary fixation d.
intrauterine contraceptive d.
intravascular device infection
intravenous accurate control d.
Investigational D. Exemption
language acquisition d.
lead locking d.
left uterine displacement d.
left ventricular assist d.
leg transfer d.
ligament augmentation d.
magnetic induction d.
mandibular advancement d.
mandibular advancing d.
McMaster Family Assessment D.
medical history as screening device for drug abuse
metered-dose inhaler-spacer device
Multitest CMI d.
negative pressure d.
new device angioplasty
oblique prism d.
oral temperature d.
oxygen disposable boot d.
percutaneous arterial closure d.
percutaneous thrombolytic d.
peripheral indwelling intermediate infusion d.
permanently implanted ventricular assist d.
personal heart d.
phonologic-acquisition d.
photoelectric registration d.
pneumatic compression d.
position indicating d.
positive pressure infusion d.
posterior reduction d.
pressure infusion d.
pressure monitoring d.
prolonged venous access d.'s
prolonged venous access d.'s
prone cranial support d.
psychological history as screening d.
pulsatile assist d.
Quantum inflation d.
radiant heat d.
right ventricular assist d.
right ventricular wall d.
Safe Medical D. Act
self-inhibiting behavioral injury d.
sequential compression d.
single needle d.
social history as screening device for drug abuse
specimen mass measurement d.
standardized d.
subcutaneous peritoneal administration d.
superconducting quantum interference device susceptometer
supportive device to restrain hernia
telecommunication device for the deaf
terminal d.
thrombin activation d.
tinnitus relief d.
tongue-retaining d.
transdermal fentanyl d.
d. for transverse traction
tubal occlusion d.
urine collection d.
urine specimen volume measuring d.
vacuum constriction d.
vacuum erection d.
vascular access d.
vascular hemostatic d.
venous access d.
ventricular assist d.

device-related urinary tract infection

devitalized

d. allogeneic bone
d. bone graft
d. epithelium
d. portion of bone

devitalized *(continued)*
d. pulp
d. soft tissue
d. tissue

dexter
auris d.
lower lid, oculus d.
retinal detachment, oculus d.

dexterity
fine hand d.
impaired d.
manual d.
O'Connor finger dexterity test

dextran
d. blue
d. charcoal
diethylaminoethyl d.
high molecular weight d.
hypertonic acetate d.
low molecular weight d.
low potassium d.
parenteral iron d.
d. sodium sulfate

dextran-coated charcoal

dextran-induced anaphylactoid reaction

dextran-reactive antibody

dextrans
limit d.

dextratransposition of great vessels

dextrin
limit d.

dextrinase
limit d.

dextrinosis
limit d.

dextrocardia with situs inversus

dextroduction
d. of left eye
d. of right eye

dextroposition
anomalous right pulmonary vein d.
d. of aorta
d. of heart

dextrorotation of uterus

dextrorotatory scoliosis

dextroscoliosis scoliosis

dextrotransposition of great arteries

dextroversion of heart

diabetes
absent menstrual period from d.
acquired diabetes insipidus
adult-onset diabetes mellitus
American Diabetes Association
American Diabetes Association diet
American D. Association guidelines
arteriosclerosis and d.
atypical diabetes mellitus
autoimmune diabetes mellitus
autosomal dominant diabetes mellitus
D.: Basic Knowledge Test
blurred vision from d.
burning mouth from d.
d. care clinic
central diabetes insipidus
chronic diabetes insipidus
circulatory problem from d.
congenital nephrogenic diabetes insipidus
cystic fibrosis-related d.
d. disease management clinic
Epidemiology of D. Interventions and Complications
familial autoimmunity in d.
family history of d.
fibrocalculous pancreatic d.
gangrene from d.
gestational d.
gestational diabetes mellitus
gestational diabetes mellitus, diet controlled, type 2
gestational diabetes mellitus, insulin controlled, type 1
immune-mediated d.
impotence from d.
incontinence from d.
infant of mother with gestational diabetes mellitus
infertility from d.
insipidus
d. insipidus
d. insipidus, diabetes mellitus, progressive bilateral optic atrophy, and sensorineural deafness
insulin-dependent diabetes mellitus
insulin-independent d.
insulin-independent diabetes mellitus
insulin-resistant diabetes, acanthosis nigricans, hypogonadism pigmentary retinopathy, deafness, mental retardation syndrome
insulin-resistant diabetes mellitus
intensive diabetes management
intensive diabetes treatment
juvenile diabetes mellitus
juvenile-onset d.
juvenile-onset diabetes mellitus
latent autoimmune diabetes of adult
lithium-induced nephrogenic diabetes insipidus
d. management center
maternally inherited diabetes and deafness
mature-onset diabetes of the young
mature-onset diabetes of youth
maturity-onset d.
maturity-onset diabetes of the young
maturity-onset diabetes of youth mellitus
d. mellitus
d. mellitus ketoacidosis
d. mellitus out of control
d. mellitus, pregnancy classification, class A–F
d. mellitus type 1
d. mellitus type 2
multiple epiphysial dysplasia-early onset diabetes mellitus syndrome
National D. Data Group
National D. Information Clearinghouse
neonatal diabetes mellitus
d. neonatorum
neurogenic diabetes insipidus
neurohypophysial diabetes insipidus
newly diagnosed d.
new-onset diabetes mellitus
non-insulin-dependent diabetes mellitus
non-insulin-dependent diabetes mellitus type 1, 2
d. nurse educator
obese type 2 noninsulin-dependent diabetes mellitus
obesity/type 2 diabetes syndrome
ocular complications of d.
oral diabetes drug
overt insulin-dependent diabetes mellitus
patients with d.
peripheral diabetes insipidus
permanent diabetes insipidus

platelet aggregation as a risk of d.
posttransplant diabetes mellitus
d. of pregnancy
D. Prevention Program
d. quality of life
supraoptical hypophysial diabetes insipidus
transient neonatal d.
transient neonatal diabetes mellitus
tropical pancreatic d.
type 1, 2 diabetes mellitus

diabetes-associated peptide

diabetes-related
d.-r. complication
d.-r. death

diabetic
d. acidosis
d. arthropathy
d. autonomic neuropathy
background diabetic retinopathy
d. cardiomyopathy
chronic diabetic neuropathic pain
d. coma
d. control with diet
d. dyslipidemia
early diabetic retinopathy
d. eye care
d. eye disease
familial diabetic history
d. father
d. fetopathy
fetus of diabetic mother
d. floor routine
d. foot care
d. foot syndrome
d. foot ulcer
full florid diabetic retinopathy
d. gangrene
d. gangrene of lung
d. gastropathy
d. glomerulosclerosis
hyperosmolar nonketotic diabetic coma
hyperosmolar nonketotic diabetic state
d. hypertension
hypophysectomized alloxan d.
infant of diabetic mother
d. iritis
d. ketoacidosis
d. macular edema
d. management
d. melanosis of cornea
Michigan D. Neuropathy Score
d. mother
d. muscle infarction
d. nephropathy
d. neuropathic osteoarthropathy
nonobese d.
offspring of diabetic parents
painful diabetic neuropathy
patient juvenile d.
peripheral diabetic neuropathy
peripheral diabetic retinopathy
d. peripheral neuropathy
d. polyneuropathy
preproliferative diabetic retinopathy
proliferative diabetic retinopathy
proliferative diabetic retinopathy with vitreous hemorrhage
d. retinitis
d. retinopathy
spontaneously diabetic rat
D. tabes
d. ulcer
d. urine
vascular disease in diabetic heart

diabetic-related disease

diabolical itch

diacetic
sugar, acetone, diacetic acid test

diaclastic amputation

diagnose
over d.

diagnosed
newly diagnosed diabetes
not d.
not yet d.
d. and treated

diagnosis
admitting d.
arthritis of unknown d.
assessment and d.
axis I, II d.
computer-aided d.
computer-assisted d.
d. or condition deferred on Axis I, II
current d.
differential d.
differential diagnosis in acute drug intoxication
discharge d.
dual diagnosis patient
dual diagnosis program
Early and Periodic Screening, Diagnosis, and Treatment program
entering d.
examination and d.
d. by exclusion
histologic d.
d. and implementation
incomplete diagnosis
initial d.
initial diagnosis and treatment
Minnesota Differential D. of Aphasia
Minnesota Test for Differential D. of Aphasia
near-UV excited autofluorescence diagnosis system
needle biopsy d.
nonorganic disorder d.
no pathologic d.
North American Nursing D. Association
nurse's d.
personality disorder d.
photodynamic d.
preimplantation genetic d.
preliminary anatomic d.
preoperative d.
principal d.
quick and early d.
referral, diagnosis, treatment, and discharge
d. responsible for length of stay
structured interview for diagnosis of Alzheimer dementia
suggested indication of d.
symptom schedule for the diagnosis of borderline schizophrenia
d. and treatment
d. undetermined

diagnosis-related group

diagnostant
pancreatic functioning d.

diagnostic
d. abnormality
D. Achievement Battery, Second Edition
adjuvant diagnostic modality
Adolescent Drug and Alcohol D. Assessment
Adolescent D. Interview
adult diagnostic and treatment center
Aphasia D. Profiles
d. arthroscopy
d. arthroscopy, operative arthroscopy, and possible operative arthrotomy
D. Assessment Questionnaire
D. Assessments of Reading
autism diagnostic interview

diagnostic *(continued)*
Autism D. Interview-Revised
Autism D. Observation Schedule
Boston D. Aphasia Examination
Boston D. Inventory of Basic Skills
d. bronchoscopy
cardiac diagnostic center
d. cardiogram
cardiovascular diagnostic study
d. center
clinical diagnostic staging
d. code
Communication Abilities D. Test
Computerized D. Interview for Children and Adolescents
d. criteria
Diagnostic Mathematics Inventory
d., social and addiction history form
d. dilatation and curettage
emergency diagnostic and treatment unit
d. error
family history research diagnostic criteria
gastrointestinal diagnostic area
general d.'s
Gordon diagnostic system
d. imaging
d. imaging center
D. Interview for Children and Adolescents-Child Version
D. Interview for Children and Adolescents-Parent Version
D. Interview for Genetic Study
D. Interview Schedule
invasive diagnostic evaluation
invasive diagnostic procedure
d. laparoscopy
local diagnostic block
major diagnostic category
Medical Examination and D. Coding System
d. medical sonography
Microsporidia diagnostic procedure
molecular diagnostic technique
multiple-allele-specific diagnostic assay
National Institute of Mental Health D. Interview Schedule
noninvasive diagnostic procedure
noninvasive diagnostic test
d. and operative arthroscopy
Oral Language Sentence Imitation D. Inventory
outpatient diagnostic center
d. peritoneal lavage
Personality D. Questionnaire-Revised
preliminary diagnostic clinic
prelinguistic autism diagnostic observation
private diagnostic clinic
d. procedure and treatment
process d.
d. and prognostic indicators
psychiatric diagnostic interview
d. radiology
research diagnostic criteria
d. roentgenology
routine antenatal diagnostic imaging with ultrasound
screening and diagnostic technique
d. spinal tap
Stanford D. Reading Test
d. and surgical
surgical diagnostic oncology
Szondi Experimental D.'s of Drives
d. test and procedure
d. and therapeutic team
d. therapy
d. thoracentesis
d. ultrasound
urinary diagnostic index
d. workup and staging

diagonal
d. band
d. branch of artery
d. conjugate diameter
crossed d.
d. 1, 2 lower extremity
d. 1, 2 upper extremity

diagram
Lund-Browder burn d.

dial
astigmatic d.
astigmatic dial chart
d. unit

dialectical behavior therapy

dialer
angled iris hook and IOL d.

dial-lock brace

dialogue
offensive chat-room d.

dialysance
insulin d.
urea d.

dialysate
d. calcium concentration
d. filtration rate
d. flow
d. glucose concentration
low-calcium d.
natriuretic plasma d.
peritoneal d.
d. protein loss
sodium d.
d. urea kinetic modeling
d. urea nitrogen

dialysis
acetate d.
ambulatory peritoneal dialysis patient
automated peritoneal d.
bicarbonate d.
cellulose acetate dialysis device
chronic ambulatory peritoneal d.
chronic intermittent peritoneal d.
commercial dialysis solution
continuous abdominal peritoneal d.
continuous ambulatory peritoneal d.
continuous arteriovenous hemofiltration with d.
continuous cycler-assisted peritoneal d.
continuous cyclical peritoneal d.
continuous cyclic peritoneal d.
continuous cycling peritoneal d.
course of d.
daily intermittent peritoneal d.
d. dementia
Denver dialysis disease
d. disequilibrium syndrome
d. encephalopathy
d. encephalopathy syndrome
equilibrium d.
equilibrium peritoneal d.
extended daily d.
home-automated peritoneal d.
home peritoneal d.
inpatient dialysis unit
intermittent peritoneal d.
LeVeen dialysis shunt
liver dialysis unit
long time d.
low-flux dialysis membrane
maintenance d.
maintenance dialysis unit
National Cooperative D. Study
nephrogenous dialysis ascites
nightly intermittent peritoneal d.
nocturnal tidal peritoneal d.
outpatient dialysis clinic
outpatient renal dialysis unit

peritoneal d.
peritoneal dialysis catheter
peritoneal dialysis creatinine clearance target
peritoneal dialysis effluent
peritoneal dialysis fluid
peritoneal dialysis system
peritoneal dialysis urea removal
portable dialysis unit
progressive dialysis encephalopathy
prolonged-dwell peritoneal d.
routine dialysis therapy
slow low-efficiency d.
subacute d.
sustained low-efficiency d.
title peritoneal d.
venous dialysis pressure

dialysis-related amyloidosis

dialytic ultrafiltration

dialyzable
d. free thyroxine
d. leukocyte extract
transfer factor, d.

dialyzed
patient d.

dialyzer
Dow hollow fiber d.
hollow fiber d.
hollow filter d.

diameter
abdominal d.
acetabular depth to femoral head d.
aerodynamic equivalent d.
aerodynamic mass d.
anterior chamber d.
anterior chest d.
anterior-posterior abdominal d.
anterior sagittal d.
anterior-to-posterior sagittal canal d.
anteroposterior d.
anteroposterior diameter of pelvic inlet
aortic d.
aortic root d.
asymmetry, border, color, and diameter of melanoma
Baudelocque d.
biparietal d.
bispinous or interspinous d.
count median aerodynamic d.
count median diameter of particles
diagonal conjugate d.
disc d.
disc d.
end-diastolic d.
end-systolic d.
external d.
fetal abdominal d.
fetal biparietal d.
follicular d.
frontooccipital d.
geometric mean d.
horizontal visible iris d.
increase in pupillary d.
D. Index Safety system
inlet
inner d.
inside d.
internal d.
internal conjugate d.
internal diameter to external diameter
left anterior internal d.
left atrial d.
left ventricular end-diastolic d.
left ventricular internal d.
left ventricular internal diastolic d.
left ventricular systolic d.
longitudinal diameter of heart
Mantoux d.
mass median aerodynamic d.
mass median diameter of particles
maximum anteroposterior d.
maximum diameter to minimum diameter ratio
mean cell d.
mean corpuscular d.
mean gestational sac d.
mean reference d.
mean tubular d.
median erythrocyte d.
mesiodistal diameter of crown
midsagittal d.
minimal effective d.
minimal port d.
minimum lumen d.
narrow anteroposterior d.
narrow bifrontal d.
obstetric conjugate d.
occipitofrontal d.
optical zone d.
outer d.
outside d.
overall d.
overall diameter of contact lens
papilla d.
particulate matter less than 10 micrometers d.
posterior sagittal d.
ratio of midsagittal d.
red blood cell diameter width
reference vessel d.
right atrial d.
right ventricular end-diastolic d.
sagittal d.
sternocleidomastoid d.
total end-diastolic d.
total end-systolic d.
tracheal d.
transcerebellar d.
transverse d.
transverse abdominal d.
transverse diameter between ischia
transverse cardiac d.
transverse diameter of heart
transverse heart d.
transverse thoracic d.
venous diameter ratio
visible iris d.

diamnionic
monochorionic diamnionic placenta

diamniotic
monochorionic diamniotic placenta
monochorionic diamniotic placenta twins
monochorionic diamniotic twin pregnancy

diamond
d. bit
d. bur
d. cutting instrument
d. disk
d. drill
d. ejection murmur
d. high-speed drill
d. inlay bone graft
d. knife
mounted diamond points
d. point needle
d. rotary instrument
d. stone
d. tip wire
d. wheel

Diamond-Blackfan
D.-B. anemia
D.-B. syndrome

diamond-dusted knife blade

diamond-point wire double-strand wire

diamond-shaped
d.-s. incision
d.-s. medullary nail
d.-s. murmur
d.-s. tracing

diaper
allergic diaper rash
atopic diaper rash
blue diaper syndrome
d. dermatitis
monilial diaper dermatitis
monilial diaper rash
psoriatic diaper rash
seborrheic diaper rash

diaphoretic
pale and d.
patient d.
skin pale and d.

diaphragm
above d.
antral mucosal d.
aponeurotic portion of d.
arcuate ligament of d.
below d.
bilateral diaphragm paralysis
crus of d.
eventration of the d.
excursion of d.
free air in d.
free air under d.
hernia of d.
involuntary spasm of d.
leaf of d.
lumbar part of d.
lumbocostal triangle of d.
median arcuate ligament of d.
muscular crus of d.
paradoxical diaphragm phenomenon
paralysis of d.
pillar of d.
right crus of d.
d. stimulation
tenting of d.
traumatic rupture of the d.
urogenital d.

diaphragmatic
anterior part of diaphragmatic surface of liver
d. breathing
d. and chest breathing
computerized diaphragmatic breathing retraining
congenital diaphragmatic hernia
d. excursion
fetal congenital diaphragmatic hernia
d. function
d. ganglion
d. hernia
d. injury
d. myocardial infarct
d. myocardial ischemia
d. nerve stimulation
occult diaphragmatic injury
paraesophageal diaphragmatic hernia
pericardial diaphragmatic adhesion
d. plaque
d. pulmonary infarct
d. respiration
d. surface of left lung
d. surface of right lung

diaphysial
femoral diaphysial fracture
femoral diaphysial allograft
metaphyseal diaphysial angle
metaphysial to diaphysial width ratio
phalangeal diaphysial fracture

diaphysis
humeral d.

diaphysitis
luetic d.

diarrhea
acute infectious d.
adult diarrhea rotavirus
antibiotic-associated d.
bacillary white d.
bloating and/or diarrhea, gas, cramps
bloating or d.
bovine viral d.
bovine viral diarrhea mucosal disease
bovine viral diarrhea virus 1, 2
d. and breast feeding
chronic nonspecific d.
chronic nonspecific diarrhea of childhood
Clostridium difficile-associated d.
congenital sodium d.
cramp and d.
d. and dehydration
delayed d.
d. and disorientation
epizootic diarrhea of infant mice
explosive watery d.
fever, chills, sweating, nausea, vomiting, and d.
d. from Crohn disease
d. from intestinal obstruction
d. from lactose intolerance
d. from toxic shock syndrome
d. from ulcerative colitis
idiopathic protracted d.
intractable diarrhea of infancy
nausea and d.
nausea, vomiting, and d.
nausea, vomiting, diarrhea, and constipation
Nebraska calf diarrhea virus
neonatal calf diarrhea virus
no nausea, vomiting, or d.
no nausea, vomiting, diarrhea or constipation
pain in abdomen with d.
pancreatogenous fatty d.
patient has d.
postvagotomy d.
precipitated withdrawal d.
protracted diarrhea of infancy
serous d.
traveler's d.
viral d.
vomiting and d.
watery and bloody d.
watery diarrhea with hypokalemic alkalosis
watery diarrhea, hypokalemia, and achlorhydria syndrome
d. with abdominal pain and swelling
d. with fever and vomiting
d. with menstrual cramps

diarrheal
acute diarrheal syndrome
noninfectious diarrheal disease
d. toxin

diarrheic shellfish poisoning

diary
Holter d.
voiding d.

diaschisis
crossed cerebellar d.

diaspirin
d. cross-linked hemoglobin

diaspirin cross-linked hemoglobin

diastase
after diastase digestion
pancreatic d.

diastase-periodic acid-Schiff

diastasis
ankle mortise d.
d. of cranial bone

fracture d.
frank d.
iris d.
d. of muscle
muscular d.
rectus d.

diastole
end d.
heart in d.
left ventricular end-d.
left ventricular internal dimension d.
right ventricle internal dimension d.

diastolic
age-related diastolic dysfunction
d. amplitude time index
antegrade diastolic flow
area diastolic pressure
d. arterial pressure
atrial diastolic gallop
d. atrial volume
d. augmentation
average diastolic pressure
d. blood pressure
d. descent rate
early diastolic relaxation
early diastolic wave
erect diastolic blood pressure
d. filling
d. filling period
d. gallop
d. gradient
d. grunt
d. heart disease
d. heart factor
d. heart failure
impairment of systolic and diastolic performance
instantaneous diastolic pressure
late diastolic potential
left ventricular diastolic dimension
left ventricular diastolic volume
d. left ventricular index
left ventricular initial diastolic pressure
left ventricular internal diastolic diameter
left ventricular internal diastolic dimension
mean d.
mean diastolic gradient
mean diastolic left ventricular pressure
mean resting diastolic blood pressure
mean sitting diastolic blood pressure
d. murmur
optimal diastolic pressure
peak diastolic filling rate
peak diastolic gradient
peak diastolic pressure
peak diastolic velocity
peak early diastolic filling velocity
d. pressure-flow relationship
d. pressure-time index
pulmonary arterial diastolic pressure
pulmonary artery d.
pulmonary artery diastolic and wedge pressure
d. pulmonary artery pressure
right ventricular diastolic overload
right ventricular diastolic pressure
right ventricular diastolic volume
right ventricular initial diastolic pressure
seated diastolic blood pressure
d. shock
standing diastolic blood pressure
supine diastolic blood pressure
syndrome of isolated diastolic dysfunction
systolic, diastolic, mean blood pressure
d. thrill
d. transmembrane voltage, maximum
unassisted diastolic pressure
ventricular diastolic fragmentation
ventricular diastolic gallop
ventricular diastolic pressure

diathermy
d., massage, and exercise
d., traction, and ultrasound
loop diathermy cervical conization
low-voltage diathermy loop
d. and massage
microwave d.
microwave diathermy treatment
Mira diathermy unit
needle diathermy excision of the transformation zone
d. short wave
shortwave d.
treated with ultrasound, diathermy, and traction

diathesis
allergic d.
asthenic d.
atopic d.
gouty d.
hemorrhagic d.
hemorrhagic diathesis secondary to hepatic failure
neuropathic d.
panic d.
seizure d.

diatrizoate
meglumine diatrizoate contrast medium
meglumine diatrizoate enema study

dibromide
ethylene d.

diced cartilage graft

dichloral urea

dichorionic
d. placenta
d. twins

dichorionic-diamniotic
d.-d. placenta
d.-d. twins

dichotic
d. environmental sounds test
d. pitch discrimination test
D. Word Test

dichroism
circular d.
dispersion-induced circular d.
induced circular d.
linear d.
magnetic circular d.
vibrational circular d.

Dickman
method of D.

dicrotic
aortic dicrotic notch pressure
arterial dicrotic notch pressure
d. notch

dictated
discharge summary d.
transfer summary d.
d. and typed

dictated/look
note has been dictated/look for report

Dictionary
Chemical Dictionary On-Line

did
adenoids did not appear enlarged
d. not attend
d. not exist prior to enlistment
d. not nurse
d. not pay

did *(continued)*
d. not respond
d. not test

didactic information

didelphys
uterus d.

die
right to be assisted to d.

died
d. of disease
d. of the disease
d. in emergency department
d. from wounds
d. in hospital
d. of injuries
d. a natural death
d. of
d. with disease

Diego
D. antigen
D. blood group

dielectric constant

diem
per d.

diencephalic syndrome

diet
acid-ash d.
advance to regular d.
d. for age
American Diabetes Association d.
American Heart Association Step One D.
animal protein d.
applesauce, bananas, and cereal d.
d. as tolerated
baby soft d.
bananas, rice, applesauce, tea, toast d.
bananas, rice, applesauce, toast d.
bananas, rice cereal, applesauce, toast d.
d. beverage
d. of choice
clear liquid d.
clear surgical d.
cold liquid d.
control d.
defined formula d.
diabetic control with d.
drugs, exercise, education, diet, and self-monitoring
elemental d.
d. and elimination
fat-free d.
full diet
full liquid d.
full and soft diet
gestational diabetes mellitus, diet controlled, type 2
gluten-free d.
high bulk d.
high-carbohydrate, high-fiber diet
high-carbohydrate, lowfiber d.
high-fat, high-cholesterol d.
high-fat, low-fiber d.
high-fiber d.
d. high in fiber
high-fruit/vegetable diet
high-protein d.
d. history
immune-enhancing d.
ketogenic d.
lactose-free d.
lactose reduced d.
Lorenzo oil d.
low available carbohydrate d.
low bacteria d.
low-branched-chain amino acid d.
low-calcium d.
low-calcium test d.
low-fat d.
low fat and cholesterol d.
low-fiber d.
low glycemic index d.
low-protein d.
low-salt d.
low-saturated fatty acid diet
low-sodium d.
low-sodium, high-potassium d.
low-sodium, low-fat d.
medically restricted d.
milk-free d.
mixed d.
nectar-thick liquid diet consistency
normal sodium d.
d. and nutrition
nutritionally balanced d.
d. order
phosphate restricted d.
phosphate supplemental d.
protein d.
prudent no-salt-added diet
pudding-thick liquid diet consistency
pureed, mechanical, soft d.
pyridoxine-deficient d.
residue-free d.
semielemental d.
six-meal bland d.
sodium-restricted d.
soy-free d.
staged ulcer d.
vegetable protein diet plus fiber
very low calorie d.

dietary
approved dietary allowance
bad dietary habit
d. cholesterol intake
estimated safe and adequate daily dietary intake
d. fat intake
d. fiber
d. guideline
d. habit
healthy dietary habit
d. insufficiency
d. intake
intensive dietary therapy
Pediatrician infant dietary supplement
poor dietary habit
poor dietary intake
d. protein intake
recommended daily dietary allowance
recommended dietary intake
d. thermogenesis
total dietary calorie

Dieterle
modified Dieterle stain

diethylamide
lysergic acid d.
lysergic acid diethylamide assay
lysergic acid diethylamide and strychnine

diethylaminoethyl
d. cellulose
d. dextran

diethylene glycol

diet-induced thermogenesis

dieting
hazard of yo-yo d.
obsessive d.

dietitian
therapeutic d.

Dietz
Merchant and Dietz ankle score

Dieulafoy lesion

difference
alveolar-arterial carbon dioxide d.
alveolar-arterial difference in partial pressure of oxygen
alveolar-arterial oxygen tension d.
alveolar-arterial PO_2 d.
alveolar-arterial pressure d.

alveolar-to-arterial oxygen d.
arterial/deep venous d.
arteriosuperficial venous d.
arteriovenous d.
arteriovenous carbon dioxide d.
arteriovenous oxygen d.
arteriovenous oxygen content d.
average interocular d.
barely noticeable d.
chemotactic d.
contact potential d.
honest significance d.
individual d.'s
intensity difference limen
just noticeable d.
least significant d.
light d.
d. limen threshold
masking level d.
mean consecutive d.
mean of consecutive d.'s
mean sorted d.
membrane potential d.
minimal perceptible d.
minimal perceptible color d.
minimum clinically important d.
d. in nitrogen tension between mixed alveolar gas and mixed arterial blood
noise tone d.
no significant d.
optical path d.
pain intensity difference score
d. in partial pressures of oxygen in mixed alveolar gas and mixed arterial blood
peak pain intensity difference score
potential difference in volts
rate d.
representational difference analysis
sex difference in life expectancy
d. spectroscopy
standard error of d.
summed pain intensity d.
temperature difference integrator
temporal difference limen
time interval d.
transmucosal potential d.

different

number of different words

differential

d. agglutination test
d. agglutination titer
airway, breathing, circulation, d.
D. Aptitude Test
Ashby differential agglutination method
automated differential leukocyte counter
automated white blood cell d.
d. blood count
d. diagnosis
d. diagnosis in acute drug intoxication
digital differential analyzer
electric differential therapy
d. leukocyte count
leukocyte differential count
light differential threshold
linear variable differential transformer
Minnesota D. Diagnosis of Aphasia
Minnesota Test for D. Diagnosis of Aphasia
percentage of lymphocytes in differential count
d. pulse polarography
d. reinforcement of low response rates
d. reinforcement of other behavior
d. rheumatoid agglutination test
d. scanning colorimeter
temperature d.
d. temperature sensor
d. thermoanalysis
d. time to positivity
total white and differential cell count
toxic granulation differential
zero differential overlap

differentiated

d. carcinoma
d. cell
cystic, partially differentiated nephroblastoma
diffuse lymphocytic poorly d.
diffuse lymphocytic, well d.
diffuse poorly differentiated lymphoma
further differentiated fibroblast
d. internal structure
malignant lymphoma, poorly differentiated lymphocytic
moderately d.
moderately differentiated adenocarcinoma
moderately differentiated adenoma
moderately differentiated neuroendocrine carcinoma
nodular-lymphocytic, poorly d.
nodular poorly differentiated lymphocytic lymphoma
poorly d.
poorly differentiated anaplastic carcinoma
poorly differentiated defined
poorly differentiated defined border
poorly differentiated ductal carcinoma
poorly differentiated embryonal cell tumor
poorly differentiated large-cell carcinoma
poorly differentiated lung cancer
poorly differentiated lymphocytes
poorly differentiated lymphocytic lymphoma
poorly differentiated lymphoma, diffuse
poorly differentiated small-cell carcinoma
poorly differentiated squamous cell carcinoma
poorly differentiated lymphocytic lymphoma-nodular
teratoma d.
d. thyroid carcinoma

differentiation

adenocarcinoma with squamous d.
adipocyte determination and differentiation factor-1
d. antigen
D. of Auditory Perception Skill
B-cell differentiation factor
carcinoma showing thymus-like d.
cluster of d.
cluster of differentiation 2–72
cluster of differentiation 4 immunoglobulin G
corticomedullary d.
early d.
erythroid differentiation factor
growth differentiation factor
growth differentiation factor-9
International Workshop and Conference on Human Leukocyte D. Antigens
light d.
male sex d.
NAP differentiation test
neu differentiation factor
new differentiation factor
nuclear anular d.
sexual differentiation scale
spindle cell epithelial tumor with thymus-like d.

differentiation-inducing factor

differently tested

difficile

Clostridium d.
Clostridium difficile colitis
Clostridium difficile culture filtrate

difficult

impaired difficult speech
patient difficult to arouse

difficult-denture patient

difficulty

attentional d.
breathing difficulty from anemia
breathing difficulty from asthma
breathing difficulty from bronchitis
cataract, motor system disorder, short stature, learning difficulty, skeletal abnormalities syndrome
d. in concentration
d. in decision making
emotional and behavioral d.'s
d. falling asleep
d. functioning at normal ability level
history of interpersonal d.
impulse control d.
d. or inability to speak
index of d.
initial breathing d.
d. initiating urinary stream
Interview Schedule for Events and D.'s
life d.
Life Events and D. Schedule Interview
memory d.
moderate d.
d. in nasal breathing
pain with breathing d.
passed without d.
patient has difficulty swallowing
rating of perceived breathing d.
d. in starting urinary stream
Surtees Difficulties Index
swallowing d.
voiding d.
d. with concentration
word-finding d.

diffraction

electron d.
low-energy electron d.
low-energy electron diffraction spectroscopy
neutrophil diffraction factor
photoelectron d.
reflection high-energy electron d.
x-ray d.

diffuse

d. abdominal calcification
d. abdominal tenderness
d. activity
acute diffuse peritonitis
d. aggressive lymphoma
d. air space disease
d. alveolar damage
d. alveolar hemorrhage
d. antral gastritis
apparent diffuse coefficient
d. axonal injury
blood d.'s into heart muscle
d. brain injury
d. brain swelling
d. calcific atherosclerosis
chronic diffuse interstitial lung disease
d. colloid goiter
d. connective tissue disease
d. cortical
d. cortical sclerosis
d. cutaneous leishmaniasis
d. cutaneous scleroderma
d. dull, aching pressure discomfort
d. esophageal spasm
excessive diffuse low and medium wave beta activity
d. fasciitis with eosinophilia
d. ganglion
d. gliosis
d. glomerulonephritis
d. hepatic softening
d. hepatocellular degeneration
hereditary diffuse leukoencephalopathy with spheroids
d. histiocytic lymphoma
d. histiocytic lymphoma of stomach
Hodgkin disease of diffuse histiocytic lymphocyte depleted type
d. idiopathic skeletal hyperostosis
infantile diffuse brain sclerosis
d. infiltrative lung disease
d. infiltrative lymphocytosis syndrome
d. interstitial fibrosing pneumonitis
d. interstitial fibrosis of the lung
d. interstitial hemorrhage
d. interstitial lung disease
d. interstitial pneumonia
d. interstitial pulmonary calcification
d. interstitial pulmonary disease
d. interstitial pulmonary fibrosis
d. intimal thickening
d. intravascular coagulopathy
isolated diffuse mesangial sclerosis
d. jaundice
d. large B-cell lymphoma
d. Lewy body dementia
d. Lewy body disease
limited-stage diffuse large cell lymphoma
d. liver disease
d. liver enlargement
d. low attenuation
low-grade diffuse astrocytoma
d. lung injury
d. and lymphoblastic
d. lymphocytic poorly differentiated
d. lymphocytic, well differentiated
d. lymphoma
d. malignant mesothelioma
d. malignant pleural mesothelioma
d. mesangial hypercellularity
d. mesangial proliferation
d. mesangial sclerosis
d. mixed lymphoma
d. muscle atrophy
myelinoclastic diffuse cerebral sclerosis
d. neuroendocrine system
nodular and diffuse fibrous proliferation
nodular and diffuse lymphoma
d. nodular hyperplasia
d. nodular lymphoma
nonautoimmune nontoxic diffuse goiter
d. non-Hodgkin lymphoma
d. noxious inhibitory control
d. obstructive pulmonary syndrome
d. panbronchiolitis
d. petechial hemorrhage
d. pigmented villonodular synovitis
d. poorly differentiated lymphoma
poorly differentiated lymphoma, d.
d. precipitation
primary symptomatic diffuse esophageal spasm
d. proliferative glomerulonephritis
d. pulmonary alveolar hemorrhage

d. pulmonary hemorrhage
d. pulmonary infiltrate
d. redness
d. reflectance spectroscopy
rheumatoid arthritis, diffuse idiopathic skeletal hyperostosis
d. sclerosing osteomyelitis
d. symmetrical uterine enlargement
symptomatic diffuse esophageal spasm
d. toxic non-nodular goiter
d. and undifferentiated
d. undifferentiated lymphoma
d. unilateral subacute neuroretinitis "wipe-out" syndrome
d. well-differentiated lymphocytic lymphoma

diffused
d. lung uptake
progressively diffused leukoencephalopathy

diffusely
d. adherent *Escherichia coli*
d. enlarged thyroid
d. infiltrated

diffusing
d. capacity
d. capacity for carbon dioxide
d. capacity for carbon monoxide
d. capacity of lung
d. capacity of lung for carbon monoxide
d. capacity of lungs for oxygen
carbon dioxide diffusing capacity of the lung
d. hostility and anger
membrane diffusing capacity
pulmonary diffusing capacity
pulmonary diffusing study
single-breath diffusing capacity
single-breath carbon monoxide diffusing capacity of lung
steady-state carbon monoxide diffusing capacity of lung

diffusion
agar/agarose-gel diffusion method
agar diffusion assay
agar diffusion for fungus
agar diffusion test
agar gel d.
agar gel diffusion test
anisotropically rotational d.
anisotropically rotational diffusion imaging
apparent diffusion coefficient
axial echo planar diffusion weighted imaging
capillary diffusion capacity
coefficient of d.
delayed double diffusion test
disc d.
double d.
gel diffusion precipitin
d. hypoxia
immune diffusion test
immunodouble diffusion test
impairment of d.
d. length
membrane component of d.
Ouchterlony double d.
Ouchterlony double diffusion technique
Ouchterlony gel diffusion technique
oxacillin disc diffusion test
oxygen d.
d. of oxygen and nutrients
d. per unit of alveolar volume
plasma clot diffusion chamber
d. pressure
pulmonary diffusion capacity
d. resistance
d. scan
single radial diffusion test
d. time

diffusion-tensor imaging

diffusion-weighted
d.-w. imaging
d.-w. imaging/magnetic resonance imaging
d.-w. imaging/perfusion imaging
d.-w. magnetic resonance imaging
d.-w. scanning

diffusive
volumetric diffusive respirator

diffusivity
average diffusivity histogram
mean d.

digastric
anterior belly of digastric muscle

DiGeorge
D. anomaly
partial DiGeorge anomaly
partial form of DiGeorge syndrome
D. syndrome

digest
soybean-casein digest medium

digestibility
in vitro protein d.

digestible
apparent digestible energy
d. protein
total digestible energy
total digestible nutrients

digestion
after diastase d.
fragment of immunoglobulin G after digestion with the enzyme pepsin
intracellular d.
pancreatic d.
peptic d.
proteinase K d.

digestive
apparent digestive energy
d. disease
d. energy
National D. Diseases Information Clearinghouse
pancreatic digestive zymogen
reroute digestive system
selective decontamination of the digestive tract
selective digestive decontamination
selective digestive tract decontamination
d. tract

digestive-respiratory fistula

digit
anular part of fibrous digital sheath of digits of hand and foot
Arithmetic, Coding, Information, and D. Span
arthrodesed d.
chiasm of digit of hand
d. copying
extensor digit minimi
first through fifth digits of hand
flail d.
d.'s of hand
most significant d.
multiple d.'s
sausage d.
d. span
d. substitution test
d. symbol
Symbol D. Modalities Test
d. symbol substitutional test
Visual Aural D. Span Test

digital
afferent digital nerve

digital *(continued)*
aggressive digital papillary adenocarcinoma
aggressive digital papillary adenoma
analog to d.
d. anomalies, short palpebral fissures, atresia of esophagus or duodenum syndrome
anular part of fibrous digital sheath of digits of hand and foot
d. auditory aerobics
d. block anesthesia
d. blood perfusion
d. cardiac imaging system
common palmar digital nerve
common palmar digital nerve of lateral plantar nerves
common palmar digital nerve of medial nerve
common palmar digital nerve of ulnar nerve
common plantar digital nerve of medial plantar nerve
computed digital radiography
computerized digital mammography
d. counter/locator
d. differential analyzer
direct digital radiography
d. display alarm
dorsal digital artery
d. echo quantification
endoscopic digital pancreatography
d. examination of prostate
extensor digital expansion
D. Finger Tapping Test
first digital interosseous muscle
d. fluoroscopy
d. gangrene
d. hearing aid
d. imaging
d. imaging processing
d. imaging spectrophotometer
intraarterial digital subtraction angiogram
intraarterial digital subtraction angiography
intraoperative digital subtraction angiography
d. intravenous angiography
intravenous digital subtraction angiography
d. ischemia
d. micromirror device
Mitutoyo digital caliper
d. nerve block
nonselective arterial digital angiography
pacing digital ventriculography
painless cold-sensitive digital vasospasm
palmar digital artery
palmar digital nerve
palmar digital vein
d. phase mapping
plantar digital artery
plantar digital nerve
quantitative digital radiography
d. radiography
d. rectal examination
d. rectal test
recurring digital fibroma of childhood
d. removal of stool
reversed digital artery flap
reversed dorsal digital flap
d. rotational angiography
d. runoff
scanning-beam digital x-ray
d. signal processing
d. sound processing
d. subtraction angiogram
d. subtraction arteriography
d. subtraction echocardiogram
d. subtraction echocardiography
d. subtraction imaging
d. subtraction indocyanine green angiography
d. subtraction phlebography
d. subtraction ventriculography
d. temperature recovery time test
tenderness to digital palpation
Trex digital mammography system
d. ultrasound
d. vascular imaging system
d. vascular reactivity
venous digital angiogram
d. venous subtraction angiography
d. voltmeter
whole-body digital scanner

digitalis
arteria digitalis palmaris communis
arteria digitalis palmaris propria
arteria digitalis plantaris communis
arteria digitalis plantaris propria
d. effect
d. intoxication
sensitize heart muscle to digitalis toxicity
d. toxicity

digitalis-like
d.-l. factor
d.-l. substances

digitalization of heart

digitalizing
total digitalizing dose

digitally reconstructed radiograph

digital-to-analog converter

digitate
multiple minute digitate hyperkeratosis

digiti
abductor digiti minimi muscle
abductor digiti quinti muscle
abductor digiti quinti tendon
adductor digiti quinti
extensor digiti communis
extensor digiti minimi
extensor digiti minimi muscle
extensor digiti minimi tendon
extensor digiti quinti
extensor digiti quinti muscle
extensor digiti quinti proprius
extensor digiti quinti tendon
flexor digiti minimi muscle
flexor digiti quinti brevis
flexor digiti quinti muscle
Littler-Cooley abductor digiti quinti transfer
musculus abductor digiti minimi manus
musculus abductor digiti minimi pedis
musculus abductor digiti quinti
musculus extensor digiti minimi
musculus extensor digiti quinti proprius
musculus extensor minimi d.
musculus flexor digiti minimi brevis manus
musculus flexor digiti minimi brevis pedis
opponens digiti minimi manus
opponens digiti minimi muscle
opponens digiti quinti
opponens digiti quinti muscle
panaritium d.

digitorenocerebral syndrome

digitorum
extensor d.
extensor digitorum brevis

extensor digitorum communis
extensor digitorum communis muscle
extensor digitorum communis tendon
extensor digitorum longus
flexor digitorum brevis
flexor digitorum communis
flexor digitorum longus
flexor digitorum quinti brevis
flexor digitorum profundus muscle
flexor digitorum profundus tendon
musculus extensor longus d.
profundus flexor digitorum muscle
profundus flexor digitorum tendon

digitus
d. minimus
d. primus

digluconate
chlorhexidine d.

diglucuronide
bilirubin d.

digoxin
d. investigators group
plasma digoxin concentration
d. reduction product
serum digoxin concentration
serum digoxin level
d. toxicity

digoxin-like
d.-l. immunoreactive factor
d.-l. immunoreactive substance

dihematoporphyrin ether

dihexoside
ceramide d.

dihydopteroate synthase

dihydrate
calcium pyrophosphate d.
calcium pyrophosphate dihydrate crystal deposition
calcium pyrophosphate dihydrate deposition disease
crystalline calcium pyrophosphate d.

dihydrobiopterin synthetase

dihydrochloride
histamine d.

dihydroepiandrosterone loading test

dihydrofolate reductase

dihydrogenarsenate
rubidium d.

dihydroorotate dehydrogenase

dihydropteridine reductase

dihydrostreptomycin sulfate

dihydrotestosterone
d. propionate
d. receptor deficiency

dihydrouracil dehydrogenase

diiodinated tyrosine

diisocyanate
methylene diphenyl d.
naphthalene d.
toluene d.

diisopropyl

dilatation
acute gastric d.
d. of aneurysm
aneurysmal d.
antegrade transluminal balloon d.
anular d.
d. of aortic root
aortic root d.
arterial d.
arterial dilatation and rupture
ascending aorta d.
d. and aspiration
biventricular dilatation and hypertrophy
d. and curettage
cystoscopy and d.
diagnostic dilatation and curettage
effacement and d.
endoscopic retrograde balloon d.
d. and evacuation
ex vacuo d.
fractional dilatation and curettage
gastric d.
gastric gaseous d.
d. and hypertrophy
idiopathic d.
manual dilatation of anus
megacolon d.
mild biventricular dilatation hypertrophy
mural d.
myocardial d.
pancreatic duct d.
paradoxical colon d.
pelvicaliceal d.
percutaneous dilatation of biliary duct
percutaneous stricture d.
percutaneous transluminal d.
percutaneous transluminal balloon d.
percutaneous ureteral d.
periodic d.
periodic dilatation of esophagus
posthemorrhagic ventricular d.
poststenotic d.
prostatic balloon d.
pupillary d.
d. thrombosis
toxic dilatation of bowel
d. of ureter
ureteral d.
urethral d.
vaginal interruption of pregnancy with dilatation and curettage
vein of Galen aneurysmal d.
d. of ventricle

dilatational
percutaneous dilatational tracheotomy

dilated
d. bile duct
d. bowel loop
d. bowel loop resection
d. cardiomyopathy
fixed and d.
fixed and dilated pupil
fully d.
d. fundus examination
heart hypertrophied and d.
d. loops of bowel
markedly dilated heart
massively dilated abdomen
mildly dilated congestive cardiomyopathy
moderately dilated and equally reactive pupil
moderately dilated and slightly reactive pupil
moderately dilated ureter
d. perivascular spaces
d. pupil
d. pupils and hypothermia
d. vein
d. ventricle
ventricles dilated and hypertrophied
X-linked dilated cardiomyopathy

dilation
airway dilation reflex
arachnoid nerve root sheath d.
d. and aspiration
balloon dilation angioplasty
balloon dilation valvuloplasty
brachydactyly, mesomelia, mental retardation, aortic dilation, mitral valve prolapse, characteristic facies syndrome
d. catheter

dilation *(continued)*
d. of cervix
d. and curettage
cystoscopy and d.
cystoscopy-endoscopy d.
d., curettage, and biopsy
endoscopic balloon d.
endoscopic balloon sphincter d.
endoscopic papillary balloon d.
d. and evacuation
d. and evaluation
flow-mediated d.
fractional dilation and curettage
d. of the heart
intrahepatic ductal d.
d. and irrigation
Lord dilation of hemorrhoid
metabolic coronary d.
percutaneous balloon d.
peroral esophageal d.
portal vein d.
posthemorrhagic ventricular d.
poststenotic d.
retinal venous dilation and tortuosity
d. and suction
suction, dilation, and curettage
therapeutic abortion, dilation, aspiration, and curettage
through-the-scope balloon d.
transient ischemic d.

dilational
percutaneous dilational tracheostomy
percutaneous dilational tracheotomy

dilator
angiographic Teflon d.
biliary balloon d.
biliary coaxial d.
biliary dilator catheter
circular anal d.
curved cannula with locking d.
dorsal root d.
fluoroscopy-guided balloon d.
mechanical cervical d.
musculus dilator naris
musculus dilator pupilla
musculus dilator pupillae
musculus dilator pylori gastroduodenalis
musculus dilator tubae
pyloric d.
sheath and dilator system
ventricular d.

dilaurate
fluorescein d.

dilemma
ethical d.
masking d.

diluent
lithium d.
Veronal-buffered d.
virus-adjusting d.

dilute
d. blood clot lysis method
chronic and dilute variant
d. intravenous Pitocin
d. strength
d. urine
d. volume of solution

diluting
Rees and Ecker diluting fluid

dilution
agar dilution test
centesimal d.
decimal scale of potency or d.
double-sampling dye dilution technique
d. end point
helium d.
limit dilution factor
limiting dilution analysis
limiting dilution assay
limiting dilution polymerase chain reaction
macroscopic broth dilution test
maximal bactericidal d.
maximum bactericidal d.
maximum inhibiting d.
microdilution broth dilution test
microtube d.
microtube dilution method
microtube dilution test
minimal hemolytic d.
minimal inhibitory d.
routine test d.
serial-agitated d.
standard peak d.
stream dilution factor
thermal d.
thermal dilution catheter
transpulmonary thermal-dye d.

dilutional
d. cardiopulmonary bypass

dilutional cardiopulmonary bypass

dimalonate
tartaric d.

dime
nickel and dime lesion

dimension
aortic root d.
effective airspace d.
end-diastolic d.
end-systolic d.
largest tumor d.
left atrial d.
left ventricular diastolic d.
left ventricular dimension in end-diastole
left ventricular end-diastolic d.
left ventricular end-systolic d.
left ventricular internal diastolic d.
left ventricular internal dimension at end systole
left ventricular internal dimension diastole
left ventricular internal dimension systole
left ventricular systolic d.
maximal left atrial d.
Memorial dimension averaging method
occlusal vertical d.
Organizational Value D.'s Questionnaire
postural vertical d.
right ventricle internal dimension diastole
right ventricular d.
right ventricular internal d.

dimensional
alternative dimensional descriptors for schizophrenia
D. Assessment of Personality Pathology-Basic Questionnaire
four d.
three d.
two d.
video dimensional analysis

3-dimensional
3-d. Fourier imaging
3-d. turbo-spin echo images

2-dimensional Fourier imaging

dimensioning
mathematical optimization and logical dimensioning for radiotherapy

dimer
noncovalently bonded dimer of C-terminal immunoglobulin of Fc fragment
nonionic d.
nonionic dimer contrast medium
type I, II regulatory d.

dimercaptosuccinate
pentavalent d.

dimeric acidic glycoprotein

dimethacrylate
ethylene glycol d.
tetraethylene glycol d.
urethane d.

dimethyl
d. disulfide
d. ether
d. sulfate
d. sulfide

dimethylamine sulfate

1-dimethylamino-naphthalene-5-sulfonic acid

dimethylarginine
asymmetric d.

diminished
d. ability to think or concentration
d. activity
d. airway perfusion
d. appetite
d. attenuation midbrain and pons
d. blood flow
d. bowel movement
d. bowel sounds
d. brain activity
d. breath sounds
d. capacity
d. chest excursion
d. contractile excursion
d. denial and defensiveness
d. fremitus
d. gag reflex
d. hearing
d. hearing and vision
d. heart, kidney and brain function
d. intensity of movement
d. libido
d. lung volume
d. recall
d. reflex
d. responsiveness
d. salt intake
d. sensation
d. sensation to pinprick

diminution
d. of affect
d. of background activity
d. of thought

diminutive polyp

dim light melatonin onset

dimming
blurring or dimming of vision

dimness or loss of vision

Dimon-Hughston intertrochanteric osteotomy technique

dimorphic
sexually dimorphic nucleus

dimple
anal d.
coronary ostial d.
lumbosacral d.
mental retardation, overgrowth, craniosynostosis, distal arthrogryposis, sacral dimple, joint laxity
palatal d.

dimpling
Albright dimpling sign
breast d.
d. of breast skin
d. of eyeball

dinitrate
glyceryl d.

dinucleotidase
nicotinamide adenine d.

dinucleotide
flavin adenine d.
nicotinamide adenine d.
nicotinamide adenine dinucleotide glycohydrolase
nicotinamide adenine dinucleotide phosphate positive
oxidized form of nicotinamide adenine d.
oxidized form of nicotinamide adenine dinucleotide phosphate

diode
d. array detector
Aurora diode soft-tissue laser
d. laser trabeculoplasty
light-emitting d.
OcuLight SL diode laser

diopter
prism d.
d. sphere

dioptric strength

diosmin
micronized d.

dioxalane guanine

dioxide
alveolar-arterial carbon dioxide difference
arterial carbon d.
arterial carbon dioxide pressure
arteriovenous carbon d.
arteriovenous carbon dioxide difference
carbon d.
carbon dioxide combing power
carbon dioxide diffusing capacity of the lung
carbon dioxide electrode
carbon dioxide elimination
carbon dioxide gas
carbon dioxide gas laser
carbon dioxide insufflator
carbon dioxide laser skin resurfacing
carbon dioxide laser vaporization
carbon dioxide output
carbon dioxide pressure
carbon dioxide with oxygen
concentration of total carbon d.
diffusing capacity for carbon d.
end-tidal carbon dioxide concentration
end-tidal carbon dioxide monitoring
extracorporeal carbon dioxide removal
extrapolated end-tidal carbon dioxide tension
fractional concentration of carbon dioxide in expired gas
fraction of alveolar carbon d.
fraction of expired carbon d.
fraction of inspired carbon d.
manganese dioxide aerosol
mixed expired carbon dioxide tension
nitrogen d.
nitrogen dioxide inhalation
partial arterial gas tension of carbon d.
partial pressure of arterial carbon d.
partial pressure of carbon dioxide in arterial gas
partial pressure of carbon dioxide in mixed venous blood
partial pressure of intramuscular carbon d.
partial pressure of mesenteric venous carbon d.
partial pressure tension of carbon dioxide, vein
pressure of carbon d.
sulfur d.
total carbon dioxide content

dioxide *(continued)*
transcutaneous carbon dioxide pressure
transcutaneous carbon dioxide tension
transcutaneous carbon dioxide monitor
venous carbon dioxide production
ventilation/carbon dioxide production

dipalmitoyl
linked to dipalmitoyl phosphatidylethanolamine

dipeptide
muramyl d.

diphasic
high-voltage diphasic slow wave
d. meningoencephalitis
d. milk fever
d. P-wave
d. T-wave

diphenyl
methylene diphenyl diisocyanate

diphenylarsine cyanide

diphenylhydantoin
sodium d.

diphosphatase
adenosine d.
fructose d.
inosine d.

diphosphate
adenosine d.
adenosine diphosphate ribose
deoxythymidine d.
deoxyuridine d.
fructose d.
fructose diphosphate aldolase
d. group
guanosine d.
hexose d.
inosine d.
manganese dipyridoxyl d.
menadiol sodium d.
methylene d.
nucleoside d.
nucleoside diphosphate sugar
thiamine d.
thymidine d.
uridine d.
uridine diphosphate glucuronosyltransferase
xanthine d.

5′-diphosphate
adenosine 5′-d.
guanosine 5′-d.
inosine 5′-d.
thymidine 5′-d.
uridine 5′-d.

diphosphine
lipophilic cationic d.

diphosphogalactose
uridine d.

diphosphoglucose
uridine d.

diphosphoglucuronic
uridine diphosphoglucuronic acid

diphosphoglucuronyl
uridine diphosphoglucuronyl transferase

diphosphoglycerate phosphatase

diphosphonate
hydroxymethylene d.
methylene d.
methylene diphosphonate concentration

diphosphopyridine
d. nucleotidase
d. nucleotide

diphtheria
acellular pertussis vaccine with diphtheria and tetanus toxoid
alum-precipitated diphtheria toxoid
d. antitoxin
combined diphtheria tetanus
d., pertussis, and tetanus
d., pertussis, and tetanus immunization
d., tetanus, pertussis, *Haemophilus influenzae* type b vaccine
d., tetanus toxoids, whole-cell pertussis, and *Haemophilus influenzae* type b conjugate
d., pertussis, tetanus, poliomyelitis, and measles vaccine
d., pertussis, and tetanus vaccine
purified diphtheria toxoid precipitated by aluminum phosphate
tetanus and d.
tetanus and diphtheria toxoid immunization
d., tetanus toxoid, and acellular pertussis vaccine
d., tetanus toxoids, whole-cell pertussis vaccine
d. toxin
d. toxin normal
d. toxin sensitivity
typhoid, paratyphoid A, B, tetanus toxoid, and diphtheria toxoid vaccine

diphtherial tonsillitis

diphtheria-pertussis immunization

diphtheria-tetanus
d.-t. immunization
d.-t. toxoid

diphtheric pseudotabes

diphtheritica
angina d.
otitis d.

diplegia
ataxic d.
atonic-astatic d.
masticatory d.
microcephaly-spastic diplegia syndrome

diplegic
mild spastic diplegic cerebral palsy

Diplocarpon rosae **virus**

diplococcus
Gram-negative d.

diploë thickness

diploic
anterior temporal diploic vein
occipital diploic vein

diploid
d. chromosome number
human diploid cell vaccine
human diploid cell
human diploid cell strain
human diploid cell system
human diploid fibroblast
human fetal diploid kidney cell
human fetal diploid lung cell
normal human diploid fibroblast
rabies vaccine, human diploid cell culture
Rhesus diploid cell strain rabies vaccine

dipole
equivalent current d.
magnetic dipole moment
d. tracing

dipole-dipole
proton-electron d.-d.

dipping
ocular d.

dipropionate
beclomethasone d.

dipstick
Micral urine dipstick test
screening d.
urine d.

dipyridamole
d. echocardiography imaging
d. echocardiography test
d. myocardial scintigraphy
d. thallium stress imaging

dipyridoxyl
manganese dipyridoxyl diphosphate

direct
d. ablation
d. access
d. acute myocardial infarction angioplasty
d. admission
d. agglutination
d. agglutination test
alternating current or direct current
d. amplification fingerprinting
d. amplification test
amplified *Mycobacterium tuberculosis* direct test
d. anticancer properties
d. antiglobulin Coombs test
d. antiglobulin rosette-forming
d. bilirubin
d. biologic effect
d. bonding system
d. brain stimulation
d. cardiac compression
d. cardiac puncture
d. care worker
d. centrifugal flotation
d. and consensual
d. cortical response
d. current
d. current cardioversion
d. data entry
d. digital radiography
d. display console
d. eighth nerve monitoring
d. electrical nerve stimulation
d. electronic urethrocystometry
d. fluorescence assay
d. fluorescent antibody
d. fluorescent antibody examination for *Treponema pallidum*
d. fluorescent antibody test
d. fluorescent antigen
d. fluorescent antigen test
d. fluorescent assay
d. forward gaze
group A streptococcus direct test
hepatic venous isolation by direct hemoperfusion
d. hernia
d. His bundle pacing
d. illumination
d. immunofluorescence analysis
d. immunofluorescence test
d. inguinal hernia
d. injection of silicone into breast
d. inoculation
d. insertion technique
d. intraperitoneal insemination
d. killing of incompetent individual
d. killing by lethal injection
d. laryngoscopy
d. laryngoscopy and bronchoscopy
d. latex agglutination pregnancy test
latex direct agglutination reaction
left direct inguinal hernia
d. linear plotting
low energy direct current
low-intensity direct current
d. lung aspirate
d. mechanical ventricular actuation
microfocal direct magnification in vitro x-ray tube
d. microscopic clump count
MicroTrak direct fluorescent antibody staining
MicroTrak direct fluorescent antibody test
d. migration inhibition
minimally invasive direct coronary artery bypass graft
Mycobacterium tuberculosis direct test
d. myocardial revascularization
d. observation evaluation
d. observation unit
on direct questioning
d. oocyte sperm transfer
d. patient care
d. percutaneous jejunostomy
d. percutaneous transhepatitic cholangiography
perfusion-assisted direct coronary artery bypass
d. personal contact
replicate organism direct agar contact
right direct inguinal hernia
d. self-destructive behavior
d. sinoatrial conduction time
d. suicide risk
thermostable direct hemolysin
d. transverse reaction
d. treatment
under direct vision
d. vesicoureteral scintigraphy
d. vision internal urethrotomy
d. vision times one
d. visualization of vocal cords

direct-current bone growth stimulator

directed
anteriorly directed jet
antibody directed cytotoxic response
apically directed chest tube
colposcopically directed brushing
dispense as d.
d. donor transfusion
d. heteroduplex analysis
d. listening
physician directed interdisciplinary care

direction
angle of d.
anterior-posterior flow d.
anterograde d.
cardinal direction of gaze
cephalad d.
completion, arithmetic problems, vocabulary, following d.'s
counterclockwise d.
Hostility and D. of Hostility Questionnaire
line of d.
neurotic direction profile
pelvic d.
Reach in Four D.'s Test
retrograde d.
rostral d.
shift in direction and pattern of brain electrical activity

directional
d. color angiography
d. coronary angioplasty
d. coronary atherectomy
d. Doppler sonography
periorbital directional Doppler ultrasonography
peripheral directional atherectomy
d. preponderance
d. vacuum-assisted biopsy

direction-changing positional nystagmus

directive
advanced d.
advanced care d.
advance directive continuity
d. group play therapy
d. play therapy group

directly
modified directly observed therapy
d. observed therapy
d. observed treatment, short course
pupils equal, round, reactive to light and accommodation directly and consensually

director
hospital field d.

directory
AIDS/HIV Treatment D.

dire straits

diribose
urine diribose phosphate

dirty
d. lung appearance
d. necrosis
d. needle
d. operative wound classification
d. surgery
d. urine

disability
airway, breathing, circulation, disability, exposure
Americans with Disabilities Act
appropriate d.
d.'s of the arm, shoulder, and hand
d. assistance
auditory perceptual d.
certificate of disability for discharge
continuing disability review
d. determination service
developmental d.
disease disability scale
Expanded Disability Status Scale
Facial D. Index
Facial D. Index Physical
Facial D. Index Social
Functional D. Index
glare d.
Health Assessment Questionnaire D. Index
d. impairment
inappropriate d.
Individual Learning Disabilities Classroom Screening Instrument
Individuals with Disabilities Education Act
individual with a d.
d. insurance
d. insurance benefits
International Classification of Impairments, Disabilities, and Handicaps
Kurtzke D. Status Scale
learning d.
Learning D. Evaluation Scale
long-term d.
low back d.
Mental Retardation and Development D.'s
Migraine D. Assessment Scale
Minimal Record of D.
moderate d.
modified Barthel degree of disability index
National Joint Committee on Learning D.'s
Neck D. Index
Nerve D. Score
Neurologic D. Score
non–service-connected d.
nonverbal learning d.
Oswestry D. Score
Owestry D. Questionnaire
Pain D. Index
pedal disability benefit
Pediatric Evaluation of D. Inventory
d. pension
Permanent Disability Rating Board
permanent partial d.
permanent total d.
person with a d.
physical d.
D. Rating Scale
reversible ischemic neurologic d.
service-connected d.
service-related d.
severe d.
specific reading d.
D. Status Scale
Student D. Survey
temporary d.
temporary partial d.
temporary total d.
total d.
total temporary d.
years of life with d.

disability-adjusted life years

disability-free life expectancy

disabled
d. adult child
aged, blind, and d.
Aid to Permanently and Totally D.
Attitudes Toward D. Persons
developmentally d.
emotionally disturbed and learning d.
gravely d.
d. infectious single cycle virus
learning d.
d. list
mentally retarded and developmentally d.
pre-aid to the d.
severely d.
totally d.

disabling
chronic disabling dermatosis
d. essential tremor
d. heartburn
d. illness
d. ineffective family coping
d. mental illness
not considered d.
d. positional vertigo
severe disabling handicap
d. shaking and trembling

disaccharide
nonabsorbable d.

disagreement
notice of d.

disappearance
dye disappearance test
fractional disappearance rate
plasma disappearance curve
plasma glucose disappearance rate
plasma iron d.
plasma iron disappearance time

disarray
lobular d.
myocardial d.
myofiber d.

disarticulation
elbow d.
hip d.
knee d.
shoulder d.
wrist d.

disaster
d. assistance center
d. crisis intervention
d. medical assistance team
natural d.
D. Warning System

disc

agar disc elution
anisotropic d.
ankle disc device
ankle disc training
annular disc bulge
anterior disc displacement without reduction
anterior intervertebral d.
anular disc bulge
anulus fibrosus of intervertebral d.
articular disc of acromioclavicular joint
articular disc of distal radioulnar joint
articular disc of sternoclavicular joint
articular disc of temporomandibular joint
articulating disc prosthesis
artificial spinal d.
ball-type disc prosthesis
d. cage valve
carborundum d.
carborundum d.
cervical disc compression
cervical disc decompression
cervical disc disease
cervical disc syndrome
cervical disc herniation
crushing of intervertebral d.
damaged disc syndrome
d. degeneration
degenerative disc disease
d. diameter
d. diameter
d. diffusion
d., macula, vessels, periphery
discs and vessels
elastic-type disc prosthesis
elastic-type disc replacement
elevated new vessels on the d.
extraforaminal lumbar disc herniation
extreme intervertebral disc collapse
extruded disc fragment
fibrovascular tissue on d.
frank disc herniation
free fragment d.
herniated d.
herniated cervical d.
herniated disc syndrome
herniated disc syndrome
herniated intervertebral d.
herniated lumbar d.
d. herniation
d. herniation
herniation of d.
I d.
d. impingement
intervertebral disc calcification
intervertebral disc disease
intervertebral disc protrusion
intervertebral disc space infection
intervertebral disc compression
intervertebral disc herniation
intervertebral disc rupture
isotropic disc striated muscle fiber
juvenile intervertebral disc calcification
laser disc decompression
lateral disc attachment
lumbar disc disease
lumbar disc herniation
lumbar disc rupture
lumbar disc syndrome
d. margin
Marlen double-faced adhesive d.
massive herniated d.
medial disc protrusion
microlumbar disc excision
midline disc herniation
modified Dallas classification of disc morphology grades 0–7
morning glory d.
morning glory disc anomaly
morning glory optic disc anomaly
narrowed disc space
narrowing of intervertebral disc space
nasal border of optic d.
neovascularization of d.
new vessel d.
nitrate disc test
noncontained disc herniation
open disc surgery
optical disc anomaly
optical disc swelling
optic disc anomaly
optic disc atrophy
optic disc cupping
optic disc dragging
optic disc drusen
optic disc drusen calcification
optic disc drusen retinopathy
optic disc dysplasia
optic disc edema
optic disc edema with a macular star
optic disc hyperemia
optic disc pallor
optic disc pit
optic disc swelling
optic disc topography
optic disc tubercle
oxacillin disc diffusion test
pain from herniated vertebral d.
pain from lumbar d.
painful disc derangement
pale optic d.
pallor of d.
pallor of optic d.
penicillin disc test
percutaneous laser disc decompression
posterior disc margin
prolapsed intervertebral d.
prosthetic disc nucleus
protruded intervertebral d.
protruding lumbosacral d.
d. protrusion
protrusion of d.
d. punch
pupils, tension, media, disc, and fundus
rod disc membrane
rudimentary disc space
d. rupture
ruptured d.
ruptured intervertebral d.
ruptured lumbar d.
rupture of intervertebral d.
d. space
d. space height
d. space narrowing
swelling of d.
vaporize water in herniated d.
video d.

discectomy

anterior d.
anterior cervical discectomy and fusion
automated percutaneous lumbar d.
cervical d.
lumbar d.
microendoscopic discectomy system
microsurgery d.
microsurgical d.

discernible

no discernible finding

discharge

abnormal brain wave d.
admission and d.
admission, discharge, transfer
d. and advise
after d.

discharge *(continued)*
anterior nasal d.
anticipate discharge tomorrow
bad conduct d.
bilateral independent periodic lateralizing epileptiform d.
bloody discharge from breast
bloody vaginal d.
certificate of disability for d.
complex repetitive d.
condition on d.
contact glow discharge electrolysis
cottage cheese-like d.
criteria for d.
date of d.
development of discharge plan
d. diagnosis
d. to duty
electrical organ d.
epileptiform d.
epileptiform burst d.
estimated discharge date
Gram stain of purulent d.
heavy vaginal d.
high-frequency d.'s
home evaluation prior to d.
hospital d.
hospital discharge survey
initiate discharge planning
involuntary discharge of feces
involuntary discharge of urine
itchy, whitish vaginal d.
nipple discharge cytology
nipple discharge from antidepressant
nipple discharge from breast injury
paroxysmal d.
paroxysmal epileptiform d.
paroxysmal high-voltage d.
partial epileptogenic d.
pathologic breast d.
d. patient after period of observation
per adjusted d.
perchlorate discharge test
period to d.
periodic lateralizing epileptiform d.
periodic synchronous d.
d. placement
d. planner
d. planning
d. planning coordinator
Post Anesthesia D. Scoring System
prior to d.
pseudoperiodic lateralized paroxysmal d.
D. Readiness Inventory
referral, diagnosis, treatment, and d.
rhythmical midtemporal d.
specific paroxysmal d.
subclinical rhythmic epileptiform discharge of adult
d. summary dictated
systolic d.
d. teaching
tentative discharge tomorrow
d. tomorrow
total urethral d.
undesirable d.
unilateral epileptiform d.'s
urethral d.
zero d.

discharged
d. against medical advice
d. dead
d. during referral
d. on visit
patient discharged ambulatory
patient discharged from hospital
patient discharged in good condition
patient discharged to home care
patient discharged improved
patient discharged to nursing home
patient discharged to office followup
patient discharged to skilled nursing facility
patient discharged to SNF

disciform
d. macular degeneration with subretinal neovascular membrane
macular disciform degeneration
peripheral disciform degeneration

discipline
bondage and d.

discission
Moncrieff d.

disclosure
d. of information
truth d.

discoid
chronic discoid lupus erythematosus
distinctive exudative discoid and lichenoid dermatitis
d. lupus
d. lupus erythematosus

discoides
lupus erythematosus d.

discoloration
cyanotic discoloration of skin
dusky d.
ecchymotic d.
d. of gums
heliotrope infraorbital d.
hemorrhagic d.
oil-spot d.
skin d.

discomfort
burning chest d.
crushing chest d.
diffuse dull, aching pressure d.
excessive breast firmness and d.
increasing abdominal d.
joint pain and d.
loudness discomfort level
pain and d.
d. relief quotient
threshold of d.

disconjugate
d. eye deviation
d. gaze
d. movement of eye
d. roving eye movement

disconnect
airway pressure d.

disconnected and racing thoughts

disconnection
internal d.

discontinuation
lithium d.

discontinued
therapy d.
treatment d.

discontinue previous medication

discontinuity
nerve d.
ossicular d.
pelvic d.

discord
marital d.

discordance
atrioventricular d.
twin birth weight d.

discordant behavior

discourse
Test of Word Finding in D.

discovered
nothing abnormal d.
not yet d.

discovery
no abnormal d.

discrepancy
leg length d.
limb-length d.

discrete
d. area of consolidation
d. area of effusion
d. bleeding source
d. Fourier transform
d. jerking musculature of face
d. lesion
d. mass
d. nodule
d. plaque
d. subaortic stenosis
d. symptom
d. time sample
d. tumor

discriminant
d. analytic model
d. function
linear discriminant analysis
logistic discriminant analysis
multivariant discriminant analysis

discriminating power

discrimination
auditory discrimination test
auditory figure-ground d.
Auditory D. Test
dichotic pitch discrimination test
dynamic two-point d.
gradual loss of auditory d.
D. by Identification of Pictures
impaired left d.
impaired right d.
index of d.
Kent State University Speech D. Test
light-dark d.
multiple choice discrimination test
ninety hue discrimination test
Oliphant Auditory D. Memory Test
pattern discrimination perimetry
d. score
speech d.
speech discrimination loss
speech discrimination score
speech discrimination test
speech discrimination testing
speech-sound d.
static two-point d.
Stetson Auditory D. Test
Test of Auditory D.
Testing-Teaching Module of Auditory D.
Test of Nonverbal Auditory D.
two-point d.
Visual Form D. Test
Visual Numerical D. Pretest
word discrimination score

discriminative
motor discriminative acuity
d. stimulus

discriminator
MR discriminator of osseous metastasis

discriminatory
impaired discriminatory, vibratory and position sensation
visual discriminatory acuity

discussion
heated d.
open d.

disease
abdominal pain with Crohn d.
ABO hemolytic d.
acquired cystic kidney d.
acquired immune hemolytic d.
acquired renal cystic d.
acquired valvular heart d.
acquired von Willebrand d.
acromegalic heart d.
active d.
active disease process
active liver d.
active pulmonary d.
acute cardiovascular d.
acute febrile respiratory d.
acute graft-versus-host d.
acute heart d.
acute idiopathic inflammatory bowel d.
acute infectious d.
acute infectious disease series
acute ischemic heart d.
acute on chronic liver d.
acute pelvic inflammatory d.
acute polycystic d.
acute radiation d.
acyanotic heart d.
addictive disease unit
adjuvant d.
adult d.
adult/adolescent spectrum of HIV d.
adult celiac d.
adult familial hyaline membrane d.
adult-onset polycystic kidney d.
adult-onset systemic Still d.
adult polycystic kidney d.
adult polycystic liver d.
adult-type polycystic kidney d.
advanced gum d.
advanced heart d.
adynamic bone d.
air space d.
alcoholic heart muscle d.
alcoholic liver d.
alcohol-related liver d.
Aleutian mink d.
Aleutian mink disease virus
allergic bowel d.
allergic eye d.
allergic respiratory d.
allograft coronary artery d.
alloimmune hemolytic disease of newborn
alpha1-antitrypsin d.
alpha-1-antitrypsin deficiency d.
alpha-1 antitrypsin d.
alpha-chain d.
alpha chain d.
alpha-heavy-chain d.
aluminum bone d.
alveolar hydatid d.
alveolar-interstitial lung d.
Alzheimer d.
Alzheimer D. Assessment Scale
Alzheimer Disease Assessment Scale, cognitive subscale
Alzheimer D. Center
Alzheimer D. Education and Referral
Alzheimer D. Rating Scale
Alzheimer D. and Related Disorders Association
amyloid heart d.
anemia of chronic d.
anemia of end-stage renal d.
Ann Arbor classification of Hodgkin disease staging
antenatal disease process
anterior horn cell d.
antibody deficiency d.
antiepileptic drug-induced bone d.
antiglomerular basement membrane antibody d.
antiglomerular basement membrane d.
aortic aneurysmal d.
aortic arch d.
aortic atheromatous d.

disease *(continued)*
aortic occlusive d.
aortic valve d.
aortic valvular d.
aortoiliac occlusive d.
APACHE II measure of disease severity
apatite deposition d.
aplastic bone d.
arboviral virus d.
Arbuthnot Lane d.
arterial degenerative d.
arterial occlusive d.
arterial vascular d.
arteriolar occlusive d.
arteriosclerotic brain d.
arteriosclerotic cardiovascular d.
arteriosclerotic cardiovascular renal d.
arteriosclerotic coronary artery d.
arteriosclerotic heart d.
arteriosclerotic hypertensive heart d.
arteriosclerotic mesenteric vascular occlusive d.
arteriosclerotic peripheral vascular d.
arteriosclerotic renal artery d.
arthritis and rheumatic d.'s
arthropod-borne viral d.
asbestos-related pleural d.
aspirin-sensitive respiratory d.
assessing severity: age of patient, systems involved, stage of disease, complications, response to therapy
associated infectious d.
asthmatic inflammatory airway d.
asymptomatic coronary artery d.
asymptomatic heart d.
Athabascan type of severe combined immunodeficiency d.
atheroembolic renal d.
atherosclerotic cardiovascular d.
atherosclerotic carotid artery d.
atherosclerotic coronary artery d.
atherosclerotic heart d.
atherosclerotic hypertensive cardiovascular d.
atherosclerotic pulmonary vascular d.
atherosclerotic renovascular d.
atopic respiratory d.
atrial septal heart d.
atypical distribution of d.
atypical gallbladder d.
atypical Kawasaki d.
Aujeszky disease virus
Australian X d.
Australian X disease virus
autoimmune d.
autoimmune blistering mucocutaneous d.
autoimmune collagen vascular d.
autoimmune disorder immune d.
autoimmune endocrine d.
autoimmune hemolytic d.
autoimmune inner ear d.
autoimmune pituitary d.
autoimmune thyroid d.
autosomal dominant medullary cystic kidney d.
autosomal-dominant polycystic kidney d.
autosomally recessively inherited d.
autosomal recessive kidney d.
autosomal-recessive polycystic kidney d.
Auzduk disease virus
basal ganglion d.
bauxite workers' d.
B-cytomegalic inclusion disease of newborn
benign anorectal d.
benign breast d.
benign gynecological d.
benign lymphoepithelial d.
beriberi heart d.
beryllium lung d.
border disease virus
Borna disease virus
bovine lumpy skin d.
bovine mucosal d.
bovine viral diarrhea mucosal d.
burden of d.
calcium phosphate crystal deposition d.
calcium pyrophosphate crystal deposition d.
calcium pyrophosphate dehydrate deposition d.
calcium pyrophosphate deposition d.
calcium pyrophosphate dihydrate deposition d.
calculous gallbladder d.
carcinoid heart d.
cardiac d.
cardiac allograft vascular d.
cardiovascular d.
cardiovascular renal d.
carotid arterial d.
carotid occlusive d.
carotid occlusive disease retinopathy
cat-scratch d.
causes of heart d.
celiac d.
celiac sprue d.
central core d.
cerebrovascular d.
cerebrovascular obstructive d.
cervical disc d.
childhood d.
childhood celiac d.
childhood polycystic kidney d.
childhood rheumatic d.
cholesterol ester storage d.
choroidal hypertensive d.
chronic active liver d.
chronic airway d.
chronic alcoholic heart muscle d.
chronic beryllium d.
chronic bullous disease of childhood
chronic cerebrovascular d.
chronic debilitating d.
chronic degenerative d.
chronic diffuse interstitial lung d.
chronic disease hospital
chronic graft vascular d.
chronic graft-versus-host d.
chronic granulomatous d.
chronic heart d.
chronic hypertensive d.
chronic hypoxic lung d.
chronic or incurable d.
chronic inflammatory bowel d.
chronic inflammatory d.
chronic interstitial lung d.
chronic ischemic heart d.
chronic liver d.
chronic lung d.
chronic nervous degenerative d.
chronic neuromuscular d.
chronic nonspecific lung d.
chronic obstructive airway d.
chronic obstructive lung d.
chronic obstructive outflow d.
chronic obstructive pulmonary d.
chronic obstructive respiratory d.
chronic pelvic inflammatory d.
chronic peripheral arterial d.
chronic renal d.
chronic restrictive pulmonary d.
chronic suppurative lung d.
chronic valvular heart d.
clinical evidence of metastatic d.
clinical heart d.
clinical hyaline membrane d.

Clostridium difficile-associated d.
cold agglutinin d.
cold hemagglutinin d.
collagen-induced autoimmune ear d.
collagen vascular d.
coloboma, heart disease, atresia choanae, retarded growth and retarded development and/or CNS anomalies, genital hypoplasia, and ear anomalies and/or deafness syndrome
colony-stimulating factor developed by Venereal D. Research Laboratory
combined immune deficiency d.
combined immunodeficiency d.
combined system d.
communicable d.
Communicable D. Center
d. in complete remission
complex benign d.
compressed-air d.
conduction system d.
congenital heart d.
congenital hip d.
congenital nonspherocytic hemolytic d.
congenital polycystic d.
congenital polyvalvular d.
congestive heart d.
connective tissue d.
contagious d.
control of local and systemic d.
d. control serum
coronary arteriosclerotic heart d.
coronary artery d.
coronary artery occlusive d.
coronary atherosclerotic heart d.
coronary heart d.
course of d.
Creutzfeldt-Jakob d.
Crohn D. Activity Index
Crohn disease of colon
Crohn D. Endoscopic Index of Severity
cutaneous graft-versus-host d.
cyanotic congenital heart d.
cyanotic heart d.
cystic disease of breast
cytomegalic d.
cytomegalic inclusion d.
cytomegalic inclusion disease virus
Darier d.
dead of intercurrent d.
debilitating bone d.
debilitating bowel d.
decompensated liver d.
decreased risk of heart d.
degenerated tissue d.
degenerative d.
degenerative bone marrow d.
degenerative brain d.
degenerative disc d.
degenerative disease of brain
degenerative facet d.
degenerative heart d.
degenerative joint d.
degenerative neurologic d.
degenerative spinal d.
delta-heavy-chain d.
dementia due to Creutzfeldt-Jakob d.
dense deposit d.
dense intramembranous deposit d.
Denver dialysis d.
depressed spectrum d.
depression pure d.
de Quervain d.
Dermatology Index of D. Severity
destructive compulsive d.
D. Detection Information Bureau
diabetes disease management clinic
diabetic eye d.
diarrhea from Crohn d.
diastolic heart d.
died of the d.
died of d.
died with d.
diffuse air space d.
diffuse connective tissue d.
diffuse infiltrative lung d.
diffuse interstitial lung d.
diffuse interstitial pulmonary d.
diffuse Lewy body d.
diffuse liver d.
digestive d.
d. disability scale
distant metastatic d.
diverticular disease of colon
double-vessel d.
Dowling Degos d.
drug-induced d.
drug-induced liver d.
drug-induced renal d.
Duchenne-Griesinger disease
duodenal peptic ulcer d.
dysgenetic polycystic d.
early-onset Alzheimer d.
early-onset form of familial Alzheimer d.
early-onset graft-versus-host d.
early-onset Parkinson d.
edema disease of swine
endocrine disease organic psychosis
end-stage heart and liver d.
end-stage kidney d.
end-stage liver d.
end-stage lung d.
end-stage organ d.
end-stage renal d.
enhancement Newcastle d.
epidemic disease of infant mice
epizootic hemorrhagic disease virus 1–8
Erdheim-Chester d.
ergot alkaloid-associated heart d.
evidence of d.
exertional reactive airway d.
exhaustion, burnout and heart d.
exophytic joint d.
extensive d.
extensive hyaline membrane d.
extensive inflammatory bowel d.
extent of d.
D. Extent Index
extracranial arterial d.
extracranial carotid d.
extracranial carotid arterial d.
extragenital Bowen d.
extramammary Paget d.
facet joint d.
familial Alzheimer d.
familial juvenile nephrophthisis-medullary cystic d.
familial nephronophthisis-medullary cystic d.
familial pure depressive d.
farmer's lung d.
fatal granulomatous d.
fatty liver d.
femoropopliteal occlusive d.
fetal heart d.
fibrocystic d.
fibrocystic breast d.
fibrocystic disease of breast
fibrocystic disease of the pancreas
fibrotic lung d.
Fiji disease virus
fish eye d.
flight into d.
focal d.
foot-and-mouth d.
foot-and-mouth disease virus
free of d.
Friend disease virus

disease *(continued)*
fulminant liver d.
functional bowel d.
gallbladder d.
gamma chain d.
gamma-heavy-chain d.
gastroesophageal reflux d.
Gaucher d.
Gee-Herter disease
genetically determined immunodeficiency d.
genital ulcer d.
Gerstmann-Straüssler-Scheinker d.
gestational trophoblastic d.
glassblower's d.
glomerular basement membrane d.
glomerular kidney d.
glomerulocystic kidney d.
glycogen storage disease, types 1–10
graft-versus-host disease reaction
graft-versus-host disease, grade 1–4
graft vessel d.
granulomatous bowel d.
granulomatous disease of childhood
Graves d.
gross cystic d.
gross cystic disease fluid protein
Guinea worm d.
gut-associated lymphoid d.
Hailey-Hailey d.
hand-foot-and-mouth d.
hantavirus d.
hard metal d.
headache secondary to cervical spinal d.
heart d.
heart disease cell
heart disease risk factor
heart disease screening
heart disease therapy
heart muscle d.
heart valve d.
heavy-chain disease protein
hemoglobin C-thalassemia d.
hemoglobin E-thalassemia d.
hemolytic d.
hemolytic blood transfusion d.
hemolytic disease of newborn
hemorrhagic disease of infant
hemorrhagic disease of newborn
hepatic venoocclusive d.
hepatobiliary tract d.
hepatocellular liver d.
hereditary bone d.
hereditary disease of nervous system
hereditary familial d.
hereditary respiratory d.
herpetic ocular d.
highest risk for d.
history of heart d.
Hodgkin disease of diffuse histiocytic lymphocyte depleted type
Hodgkin disease and HIV infection
Hodgkin disease, mixed nodular type
Hodgkin disease, nodular sclerosis
Hodgkin disease, recurrent
Hodgkin disease in relapse
Hodgkin disease staging
host-versus-graft d.
human adjuvant d.
human brain d.
human immunodeficiency virus-associated salivary gland d.
human retroviral d.
Hutchinson-Boeck disease
hyaline membrane d.
hydatid d.
hydatid cyst d.
hydroxyapatite deposition d.
hypersensitivity lung d.
hypertension secondary to renal d.
hypertensive arteriosclerotic cardiovascular d.
hypertensive arteriosclerotic heart d.
hypertensive cardiovascular d.
hypertensive heart d.
hypertensive ocular d.
hypertensive pulmonary vascular d.
hypoparathyroidism, Addison disease, and mucocutaneous candidiasis syndrome
hypophosphatemic bone d.
I-cell d.
ichthyosis and neutral lipid storage d.
idiopathic acquired hemolytic d.
idiopathic disease of myocardium
idiopathic inflammatory bowel d.
idiopathic midline destructive d.
idiopathic Parkinson d.
idiopathic Raynaud d.
immature lung d.
immune complex d.
immune kidney d.
immune renal d.
immunologically mediated d.
immunoproliferative small intestine d.
incipient degenerative brain d.
inclusion d.
inclusion cell d.
d. incurable, progressive
index of pulmonary vascular d.
infantile polycystic kidney d.
infectious bowel d.
infectious bursal d.
infectious bursal disease virus
infectious disease unit
infectious granulomatous d.
inflammatory bowel d.
Inflammatory Bowel D. Questionnaire
inflammatory joint d.
inflammatory lung d.
inflammatory pelvic d.
inhalational lung d.
International Classification of D.'s
International Classification of D.'s and Related Health Problems, 10th Edition
International Classification of D.'s and Causes of Death
International Classification of D.'s 9th Ed. Injury Severity Score
interstitial d.
interstitial lung d.
interstitial restrictive lung d.
intervertebral disc d.
intracranial atherosclerotic d.
intrastent recurrent d.
iron metabolism d.
iron storage d.
irreversible hereditary d.
ischemic coronary heart d.
ischemic disease of the growing hip
ischemic heart d.
ischemic leg d.
ischemic limb d.
ischemic myocardial d.
ischemic thrombotic cerebrovascular d.
ischemic vascular d.
Jakob-Creutzfeldt disease
juvenile-onset multisystem inflammatory d.
kinky hair d.
late-onset Alzheimer d.
left main coronary artery d.
left main stem coronary artery d.
Legg-Calvé-Perthes d.

Legionnaire d.
Legionnaire disease bacillus
lethal graft-versus-host d.
Lewy body d.
lichenoid graft-versus-host d.
life-threatening graft-versus-host d.
light chain deposition d.
limited d.
Lindau-von Hippel d.
linear IgA bullous d.
linear IgA d.
linear IgM disease of pregnancy
d. linkage disequilibrium
lipid storage d.
lipochrome histiocytosis d.
liver d.
liver disease organic psychosis
living with d.
localization of d.
long-term nonprogressive d.
low bone turnover d.
lower airway d.
lower extremity arterial d.
lower extremity occlusive d.
lower intestinal Crohn d.
lower motor neuron d.
lower risk of heart d.
low volume d.
lumbar disc d.
lumbar facet d.
lumbar root d.
luminal Crohn d.
lumpy skin d.
lung fluke d.
Lyme d.
Lyme disease antibody test
Lyme disease arthritis
Lyme disease DNA detection
Lyme disease immunoblot
Lyme disease keratitis
Lyme disease serology
Lyme disease stage 1–3
lymphocyte predominance Hodgkin d.
lymphocyte-predominant Hodgkin d.
lymphocytic infiltrative d.
lymphocytic nodular Hodgkin d.
lymphoproliferative d.
lysosomal storage d.
Machado-Joseph Azorean d.
macroscopic residual d.
mad cow d.
malignant biliary obstructive d.
malignant catarrhal fever d.
malignant lymphocytic proliferation d.
malignant metastatic d.
malignant neoplastic d.
malignant spinal d.
mammary Paget d.
maple bark stripper d.
maple syrup urine d.
marble bone d.
Marburg virus d.
Marek herpesvirus d.
market men d.
mast cell d.
maternal cyanotic heart d.
Mayaro virus d.
measurable d.
mediastinal d.
medullary cystic d.
medullary optic d.
Ménétrier d.
Menkes disease gene
mental retardation, congenital heart disease, blepharophimosis, blepharoptosis, hypoplastic teeth
mesenteric inflammatory venoocclusive d.
mesenteric vascular occlusive d.
metabolic bone d.
metabolic disease in newborn
metabolic disease organic psychosis
metabolic liver d.
metastatic brain d.
metastatic Crohn d.
metastatic trophoblastic d.
microcystic disease of renal medulla
micronodular adrenal d.
microvillus inclusion d.
middle ear d.
mild sickle cell d.
milk precipitin d.
Minamata d.
mineral dust airway d.
minimal change d.
minimal euthyroid Graves d.
minimal lesion d.
minimal renal d.
minimal residual d.
mitral d.
mitral valve d.
mitral valvular d.
mixed aortic valve d.
mixed cellular Hodgkin d.
mixed cellularity Hodgkin d.
mixed connective-tissue d.
mixed connective tissue d.
mixed mitral d.
Moschcowitz thrombotic thrombocytopenic purpura d.
motor neuron d.
mucopolysaccharide storage disease I–VIII
mucosal disease virus group
mu-heavy-chain d.
mu-heavy chain d.
multicentric Castleman d.
multicystic d.
multicystic kidney d.
multifocal chorioretinal d.
multilevel atherosclerotic arterial occlusive d.
multiple endocrine deficiency, Addison disease, and candidiasis syndrome
multivessel coronary d.
Münchausen disease by proxy
muscle-eye-brain disease of Santavuori
muscle, liver, brain, eye disease
mycotic corneal ulcer d.
myeloproliferative d.
myocardial d.
myocardial disease of unknown origin
myocardial ischemic d.
Nairobi sheep d.
Nairobi sheep disease virus
nasal sinus d.
National Digestive D.'s Information Clearinghouse
National Institute of Arthritis and Metabolic D.'s
National Kidney and Urological D.'s Information Clearinghouse
necrotizing bowel d.
neonatal chest d.
neonatal chronic lung d.
neonatal cyanotic congenital heart d.
neonatal gonococcal d.
neonatal hemorrhagic d.
neonatal hyaline membrane d.
neonatal iron-storage d.
neonatal staphylococcal d.
neoplastic trophoblastic d.
nephrophthisis-medullary cystic d.
neurogenic hip d.
neurological disease syndrome
neurologic demyelinating d.
neuronal intranuclear inclusion d.
neuropathic joint d.
neutral lipid storage d.
Newcastle bone d.

disease *(continued)*
Newcastle disease virus therapy
Newcastle virus d.
newly acquired d.
new variant Creutzfeldt-Jakob d.
New York Heart Association classification of heart d.
Niemann-Pick d.
Niemann-Pick C d.
Niemann-Pick C1 d.
Niemann-Pick disease, type A, B, C, D
Niemann-Pick disease type I, II
no d.
no active d.
no active pulmonary d.
no acute d.
no apparent d.
no apparent disease seen in chest
no appreciable d.
node-based malignant lymphoproliferative d.
no disease found
nodular connective tissue disease nevus
nodular sclerosing Hodgkin d.
no evidence of d.
no evidence of active d.
no evidence of disease-stationary d.
no evidence of pulmonary d.
no evidence of recurrent d.
no identifiable d.
no known d.'s
non-A–G chronic liver d.
nonalcoholic fatty liver d.
non-B, non-C chronic liver d.
noncaseating granulomatous d.
nonerosive gastroesophageal reflux d.
non-Graves disease hyperthyroidism
nonimmune renal d.
noninfectious diarrheal d.
noninfectious disease complication
nonmetastatic gestational trophoblastic d.
nonmetastatic trophoblastic d.
nonobstructive hepatic parenchymal d.
nonsexually transmitted d.
nonspecific granulomatous d.
nontreponemal genital ulcer d.
nontuberculin mycobacterial d.
nontuberculous mycobacterial d.
nonvalvular heart d.
normal childhood d.'s
no significant d.
no signs of acute d.
notifiable infectious d.
no venereal d.
oasthouse urine d.
obliterative airway d.
obliterative coronary artery d.
obliterative vascular d.
obstructive airflow d.
obstructive airway d.
obstructive coronary d.
obstructive gastroduodenal Crohn d.
obstructive intestinal d.
obstructive liver d.
obstructive lung d.
obstructive pulmonary d.
obstructive respiratory d.
occlusive arterial d.
occlusive artery d.
occlusive carotid artery d.
occlusive carotid d.
occlusive cerebrovascular d.
occlusive coronary artery d.
occlusive coronary d.
occlusive disease of liver
occlusive heart d.
occlusive vascular d.
occult extrahepatic d.
occult hepatic d.
occult metastatic d.
occupational airway d.
occupational immunologic lung d.
occupational lung d.
occupational parenchymal d.
ocular immune d.
ocular inflammatory d.
ocular surface d.
ocular syphilitic d.
oculocerebrorenal disease of Lowe
Ollier d.
onset and course of disease
ophthalmic Graves d.
optic chiasm d.
optic nerve d.
oral Crohn d.
oral disease control
orbital inflammatory d.
ordinary disease of childhood
organic brain d.
organic heart d.
Osgood-Schlatter d.
other neurologic d.
overt symptom of heart d.
Paget disease of anus
Paget disease of bone
Paget disease of breast
Paget disease of perianal area
Paget disease of vulva
Paget extramammary d.
paper mill worker's d.
parainfluenza viral d.
parenchymal lung d.
parenchymatous liver d.
Parkinson d.
Parkinson disease and lateral sclerosis-dementia complex
Parkinson D. Quality of Life Scale
Parkinson D. Questionnaire
pathologic parathyroid d.
patient global assessment of disease activity
patient with incapacitating systemic d.
patient with mild to moderate systemic d.
patient with severe systemic disease limiting activity but not incapacitating
pediatric autoimmune neuropsychiatric diseases associated with streptococcal infection
Pediatric Crohn D. Activity Index
pediatric infectious disease developmental screening test
pediatric spectrum of d.
Pelizaeus-Merzbacher d.
pelvic adhesive d.
pelvic inflammatory d.
peptic inflammatory d.
peptic ulcer d.
perforating disease of hemodialysis
Perianal Crohn D. Activity Index
perianal Crohn d.
perineal Crohn d.
periodontal disease rate
periodontal disease score
peripheral air space d.
peripheral arterial d.
peripheral arterial aneurysmal d.
peripheral arterial occlusive d.
peripheral arteriosclerotic occlusive d.
peripheral artery d.
peripheral atherosclerotic d.
peripheral occlusive arterial d.
peripheral vascular d.
peripheral vascular occlusive d.

peripheral venous d.
persistent trophoblastic d.
Pick d.
pigeon breeder d.
pigmented nodular
 adrenocortical d.
pilonidal sinus d.
polycystic disease of kidney
polycystic disease of liver
polycystic kidney d.
polycystic liver d.
polycystic ovarian d.
polycystic ovary d.
polycystic renal d.
polysaccharide storage d.
popliteal artery occlusive d.
popliteal occlusive d.
positive cardiac disease risk
 factors
positive risk factors for
 cardiac d.
postpartum thyroid d.
posttransplantation
 lymphoproliferative d.
posttransplant
 lymphoproliferative d.
potentially fatal d.
preclinical heart muscle d.
predominant hyperparathyroid
 bone d.
preexisting coronary d.
preexisting hepatic d.
premature coronary d.
premature heart d.
premature vascular d.
prevent heart d.
prevent transmission of d.
primary degenerative cerebral d.
primary hepatic d.
primary lung d.
primary myocardial d.
primary pigmented nodular
 adrenocortical d.
probability of having d.
probability of not having d.
d. progressed slowly
progression of d.
progressive brain d.
progressive degenerative disease
 process
progressive idiopathic
 neuromuscular d.
proliferative breast d.
proliferative kidney d.
protein loss in hepatic d.
pseudoheart d.
psychosomatic d.
pulmonary d.
pulmonary collagen vascular d.
pulmonary disease anemia
pulmonary heart d.
pulmonary hypoplasia
 membrane d.
pulmonary parenchymal d.
pulmonary thromboembolic d.
pulmonary valve d.
pulmonary vascular obstructive d.
pulmonary venoocclusive d.
radiation-induced heart d.
radiation-induced liver d.
radiation linked d.
Raynaud d.
Recklinghausen disease of bone
recurrent lower respiratory
 tract d.
refractory Crohn d.
rehabilitation of heart d.
Reiter d.
renal hypertensive d.
respiratory d.
respiratory bronchiolitis-associated
 interstitial lung d.
respiratory disease questionnaire
restrictive heart d.
reverse heart d.
reversible obstructive airways d.
Rhesus hemolytic d.
rheumatic aortic valve d.
rheumatic valvular heart d.
rheumatoid d.
rippling muscle d.
risk of heart d.
risk of infectious d.
Rosai-Dorfman d.
round heart d.
Rubarth disease virus
Russell brain d.
salivary gland d.
salivary gland virus d.
salmon-poisoning d.
Sandhoff d.
San Joaquin Valley d.
Schüller-Christian d.
sclerocystic disease of the ovary
septicemic cutaneous ulcerative d.
serious gum d.
serological marker of d.
severe autoimmune d.
severe combined
 immunodeficiency d.
sexually transmitted d.
Short Inflammatory Bowel D.
 Questionnaire
sickle cell d.
sickle cell chronic lung d.
sickle cell hemoglobin C d.
sickle cell hemoglobin D d.
sickle cell lung d.
sickle cell-thalassemia d.
silent ischemic heart d.
Sinding-Larsen-Johansson d.
single-vessel d.
sinovenous occlusive d.
site of d.
Skevas-Zerfus disease
SLE D. Activity Index
small airway d.
small bowel d.
small vessel d.
Spatz-Lindenberg d.
spinal cord d.
sporadic depressive d.
spouse's perception of d.
stable d.
Standard Nomenclature of D.'s
 and Operations
stenosing peripheral arterial d.
steroid-dependent Crohn d.
steroid resistant graft-versus-
 host d.
Still d.
stress of heart d.
structural heart d.
sudden death ischemic heart d.
sweet clover d.
swine vesicular d.
swine vesicular disease virus
swollen belly d.
symptomatic alcohol heart
 muscle d.
symptomatic gallbladder d.
symptomatic progression of d.
systemic inflammatory d.
Systemic Lupus Erythematosus D.
 Activity Index
systemic mast cell d.
target organ d.
Tay-Sachs d.
thin basement membrane d.
thoracic aortic d.
thromboembolic disease stocking
thyroid eye d.
thyroiditis, Addison disease,
 Sjögren syndrome, sarcoidosis
 syndrome
thyrotoxic heart d.
transfusion-associated graft-versus-
 host d.
transplant coronary artery d.
treatment of heart d.
triple vessel d.

disease *(continued)*
triple vessel disease with abnormal left ventricle
tuberculosis-respiratory d.
ulcerative bowel d.
unclassifiable connective tissue d.
undifferentiated connective tissue d.
undifferentiated respiratory d.
Unified Parkinson D. Rating Scale
unilateral renovascular d.
unstable coronary artery d.
unstable hemoglobin d.
upper airway d.
upper respiratory d.
uremic medullary cystic d.
usual diseases of childhood
usual childhood d.'s
valvular d.
valvular aortic d.
valvular disease of heart
valvular heart d.
van Buren d.
variant Creutzfeldt-Jakob d.
vascular d.
vascular disease in diabetic heart
vascular disease of heart
vascular heart d.
venereal d.
venereal disease, gonorrhea
venoocclusive d.
venous thromboembolic d.
ventricular heart d.
vertebrobasilar occlusive d.
viral hematodepressive d.
vitiligo disease activity
von Recklinghausen d.
von Willebrand d.
Warfarin-Aspirin Symptomatic Intracranial D.
Wesselsbron disease virus
wet tail d.
Wilson-Kimmelstiel d.
winter vomiting d.
with d.
X-linked lymphoproliferative d.
Yangtze River d.
yellow hyaline membrane d.

disease-controlling antirheumatic therapy

diseased
d. heart
d. human heart
d. joint with inflammation
d. kidney
d. region
d. segment of bowel

disease-free
d.-f. interval
d.-f. survival
d.-f. survival rate

disease-modifying
d.-m. antirheumatic drug
d.-m. drug

disease-oriented
d.-o. evidence
d.-o. physician education

disease-producing bacteria

disease-related
d.-r. symptom improvement
d.-r. symptoms

disease-resistant antigen

Diseases–Clinical
International Classification of Diseases–Clinical Modification

disease-specific survival

disease-susceptible antigen

disease/syndrome
Charcot-Marie-Tooth d./s.

disease-syphilis
venereal d.-s.

disembodied heart

disequilibrium
dialysis disequilibrium syndrome
disease linkage d.
single nucleotide polymorphisms - linkage d.
d. syndrome
transmission disequilibrium test

disfigured
irregular disfigured cell

disfluent speech

disharmonic
double disharmonic hearing

disharmony
affective d.
marital d.
maxillomandibular d.
midline d.
occlusal d.

disinfectant
aqueous synthetic dual phenolic d.

disinfection
d. and antisepsis
high-level d.

disinhibition
emotional d.
motor d.

disintegrating
orally disintegrating tablet

disintegration
endoscopic stone d.
increased personality d.
d. of judgment
mean disintegration time
d. of muscle
nuclear d.
d.'s per minute
d. of personality
personality d.
stone d.
timed d.

disintegrative
childhood disintegrative disorder

disjointed agitated movement

disk-condyle adhesion

diskectomy
anterior cervical d.
anterior cervical diskectomy and fusion
arthroscopic lumbar laser d.
automated percutaneous d.
automated percutaneous lumbar d.
endoscopic transformational d.
microlumbar d.
microsurgical d.
microsurgical lumbar d.
percutaneous automated d.
percutaneous endoscopic lumbar d.
percutaneous laser d.
percutaneous lumbar d.
percutaneous transpedicular d.

diskography
lumbar d.
microlumbar d.

dislocated
d. elbow, bowed tibiae, scoliosis, deafness, cataract, microcephaly, mental retardation syndrome
d. hip
manipulation of dislocated joint

dislocation
anterior complete d.
anterior hip d.
anterior shoulder d.
atlantoaxial d.
atlantooccipital joint d.
axial carpal d.

congenital dislocation hip
congenital dislocation of hip
congenital hip d.
gamekeeper's thumb d.
d. head of radius
ligamentous anterior d.
ligamentous anterior dislocation composite graft
luxatio erecta shoulder d.
milkmaid's elbow d.
multiple d.'s
Nélaton ankle d.
orbitonasal d.
Osborne-Cotterill elbow dislocation operation
d. of patella
patellar dislocation cast
perilunate carpal d.
posterior dislocation injury
posterior facet d.
radial head d.
shoulder d.
temporomandibular joint d.
unilateral interfacetal dislocation or subluxation

dislodgement
partial d.

disloyalty
guilt over d.

dismembered
Anderson-Hynes dismembered pyeloplasty

dismissed
patient dismissed in good condition

dismutase
human superoxide d.
manganese superoxide dismutase gene
polyethylene glycol-conjugated superoxide dismutase pegorgotein
recombinant human superoxide d.

disodium
adenosine triphosphate d.
calcium disodium edetate
d. chromoglycate
d. cromoglycate
d. monomethanearsonate

disomy
uniparental d.

disorder
abnormal involuntary movement d.
acid-related d.
acute disorder of cerebral circulation
acute stress d.
d. of adenoids
adjustment disorder, chronic
adjustment disorder with angry mood
adjustment disorder with anxiety
adjustment disorder with anxious mood
adjustment disorder with disturbance of conduct
adjustment disorder with mixed anxiety and depressed mood
adjustment disorder with mixed disturbance of emotions
adjustment interface d.
adjustment reaction conduct d.
adolescent-onset conduct d.
adult depressive d.
adult-life psychosexual identity d.
affective d.
affective bipolar d.
affective disorders clinic
affective determined d.
affective disorder syndrome
affective expression d.
affective neurotic personality d.
affective spectrum d.
aggressive conduct d.
aggressive type undersocialized conduct d.
agoraphobia without history of panic d.
alcohol amnestic d.
alcohol anxiety d.
alcohol-dependent sleep d.
alcoholic amnestic d.
alcoholic organic mental d.
alcohol-induced psychotic d.
alcohol-induced psychotic disorder with delusions
alcohol-induced psychotic disorder with hallucinations
alcohol intoxication-related d.
alcohol mood d.
alcohol-related heart d.'s
alcohol-related neurodevelopmental d.
alcohol-related use disorder, not otherwise specified
alcohol sleep d.
alcohol use d.
Alcohol Use D.'s Identification Test
allergic lung d.
allergic psychogenic d.
alpha-methyldopa-induced mood d.
alternating bipolar d.
alternative criterion B for dysthymic d.
Alzheimer Disease and Related D.'s Association
amino acid metabolic d.
amitriptyline-induced mood d.
amphetamine-induced psychotic disorder with delusions
amphetamine-induced psychotic disorder with hallucinations
angiocentric immunoproliferative d.
anorexia nervosa and associated d.'s
antifactor I–IX d.
antisocial neurotic personality d.
anxiety adjustment d.
anxiety-avoiding personality d.
anxiety disorder of adolescence
anxiety disorder of childhood
anxiety disorder clinic
anxiety due to physical d.
Anxiety D. Interview for Children
anxiety and panic disorder clinic
anxiety psychogenic d.
anxiety-related mental d.
anxiety state neurotic d.
anxiolytic amnestic d.
anxiolytic-induced psychotic disorder with delusions
anxiolytic-induced psychotic disorder with hallucinations
anxiolytic substance-use d.
anxiolytic use d.
apathetic-type personality d.
aplastic bone d.
appetite psychogenic d.
arithmetical developmental delay d.
Arizona Battery for Communication D. of Dementia
arteriosclerotic brain d.
articular hand d.
articular wrist d.
articulation developmental delay d.
Asperger d.
Assessment of Aphasia and Related D.'s, Second Edition
asthenic personality d.
athetotic movement d.
attachment disorder of infancy
attention deficit d.

disorder *(continued)*
Attention Deficit D. Behavior Rating Scale
attention deficit disorder, residual type
attention deficit disorder with hyperactivity
attention deficit disorder without hyperactivity
attention deficit and disruptive behavior d.
attention deficit hyperactivity d.
attention deficit hyperactivity disorder, combined type
attention deficit hyperactivity disorder, predominantly hyperactive-impulsive type
atypical affective d.
atypical anxiety d.
atypical bipolar d.
atypical conduct d.
atypical dissociative d.
atypical eating d.
atypical factitious disorder with physical symptoms
atypical gender identity d.
atypical impulse-control d.
atypical lymphoproliferative d.
atypical mixed or other personality d.
atypical paranoid d.
atypical pervasive developmental d.
atypical somatoform d.
atypical specific developmental d.
atypical stereotyped movement d.
atypical tic d.
auditory perceptual d.
auditory processing d.
autistic spectrum d.
autoimmune connective tissue d.
autoimmune disorder immune disease
autoimmune neuromuscular junction d.
autoimmune obsessive-compulsive tic d.
autoimmune thyroid d.
autonomic arousal d.
autonomic nervous system d.
autosomal chromosome d.
autosomal dominant d.
autosomal dominant movement d.
autosomal karyotypic d.
autosomal recessive d.
autosomal recessive severe combined immunodeficiency d.
avoidant disorder of adolescence
avoidant disorder of childhood
avoidant neurotic personality d.
avoidant personality d.
B-cell chronic lymphoproliferative d.
B-cell lymphoproliferative d.
behavioral d.
behavioral, anxiety, mood, and other types of d.'s
Behavior D.'s Identification Scale
bereavement-related mood d.
binge eating d.
bipolar disorder type 1, 2
blood platelet d.
body dysmorphic d.
Body Dysmorphic D. Modification of Yale-Brown Obsessive-Compulsive Scale, McLean version
borderline personality d.
caffeine-induced sleep d.
Cambridge Mental D.'s in Elderly Examination
cannabis delusional d.
cannabis-induced psychotic disorder with delusions
cannabis-induced psychotic disorder with hallucinations
cannabis intoxication-related d.
cannabis organic mental d.
cannabis-related disorder, not otherwise specified
cannabis use d.
carbohydrate metabolism d.
cataract, motor system disorder, short stature, learning difficulty, skeletal abnormalities syndrome
catatonic schizophrenic d.
central auditory processing d.
central language d.
cerebelloparenchymal disorder IV
character d.
chemical dependence d.
childhood anxiety d.
childhood behavioral d.
childhood disintegrative d.
childhood shyness d.
children and adults with attention deficit d.
Children's Interview for Psychiatric D.'s
chronic depressive personality d.
chronic enthusiasm d.
chronic immune d.
chronic lymphoproliferative d.
chronic motor or vocal tic d.
chronic myeloproliferative d.
chronic relapsing d.
chronic tic d.
circadian rhythm-based sleep d.
cocaine mood d.
coexisting psychiatric d.'s
communication d.
comorbidity of mental d.
comorbid mental d.
complex disorder of adolescence
complex disorder of childhood
complicated grief d.
compulsive impulse control d.
compulsive personality d.
computer addiction d.
conduct d.
conduct disorder type group
conduct disturbance adjustment d.
conversion disorder, mixed type
conversion disorder, motor type
conversion disorder, seizure type
convulsive d.
co-occurring mood d.
d. of cornification
cumulative trauma d.
delirium, infection, atrophic urethritis and vaginitis, pharmaceuticals, psychological disorders, excessive urine output, restricted mobility, stool impaction
delusional d.
delusional mood d.
delusional paranoid d.
dependent personality d.
deteriorating neurological d.
developmental d.'s
developmental articulation d.
developmental coordination d.
developmental expressive language d.
developmental expressive writing d.
developmental language d.
developmental receptive language d.
disorganized schizophrenic d.
disruptive behavior d.
dissociation in eating d.
dissociative disorder not otherwise specified
dissociative identity d.
distinct psychiatric d.
dream anxiety d.
drug-induced movement d.'s
dual d.
eating d.

eating disorder unit
eating disorders examination
Eating D. Inventory
electroconvulsive therapy-induced mood d.
emancipation disorder of adolescence
emotional d.
emotional disturbance adjustment d.
emotional dyscontrol d.
emotionally unstable character d.
environmentally associated rheumatic d.
epileptic attention deficit d.
episodic affective d.
esophageal motility d.
d.'s of excessive sleepiness
d.'s of excessive somnolence
explosive personality d.
factitious disorder by proxy
factitious disorder with physical symptoms
female sexual arousal d.
fetal iodine deficiency d.
functional bowel d.
Functional Bowel D. Severity Index
functional gastrointestinal d.
gait and balance d.
gait disorder, autoantibody, late-age onset, polyneuropathy
gastric tract d.
gender behavior d.
gender identity d.
gender identity disorder of adolescence
gender identity disorder of adolescence or adulthood, nontranssexual type
gender identity disorder of adult life
gender identity disorder of childhood
generalized anxiety d.
glycogen storage d.
gonadal endocrine d.
grand mal convulsive d.
granular lymphocyte-proliferative d.
Grid Test of Schizophrenic Thought D.
hallucinogen delusional d.
hallucinogen mood d.
hallucinogen persisting perception d.
Hamburg Rating Scale for Psychiatric D.'s
heart rate d.
heart rhythm d.
heart valve d.
heat-related d.'s
hereditary bleeding d.
high altitude-related d.
histrionic personality d.
HIV-associated cognitive d.
human genetic d.
human immunodeficiency virus associated motor cognitive d.
hyperkinetic conduct d.
hyperkinetic impulse d.
hypersomnia related to another mental d.
hypoactive sexual desire d.
hysterical conversation d.
idiopathic gait disorders of elderly
idiopathic seizure d.
impairment from d.
impulse control d.
d. of impulse control
impulse disorder control
impulse dyscontrol in eating d.
infantile sialic acid storage d.
inflammatory intestinal d.
inherited giant platelet d.
inherited metabolic d.
d.'s of initiating and maintaining sleep
insomnia related to mental d.
intermittent affective d.
intermittent explosive personality d.
involuntary movement d.
isolated explosive d.
juvenile anxiety d.
knee joint alignment d.
late luteal phase dysphoric d.
learning d.
lifetime anxiety d.
lipid metabolism d.
low back pain psychogenic d.
low-density lipoprotein receptor d.
lysosomal enzyme d.
lysosomal storage d.
major affective d.
major depressive d.
male dyspareunia male erectile d.
male erectile d.
male hypoactive sexual desire d.
malignant lymphoproliferative d.
manic bipolar d.
manic-depressive d.
marijuana delusional d.
mendelian genetic d.
mental disorder due to alcoholism
mental disorder due to a general medical condition
mental and physical retardation, speech disorders, peculiar facies syndrome
metabolic bone d.
metabolic disorder screening
metabolic disorder with hepatic dysfunction
metabolic disorder with neurologic dysfunction
metabolic and electrolyte disorder
metabolic, endocrine, and gastrointestinal d.'s
metabolic screening d.
metal metabolism d.
Methods for Epidemiology of Child and Adolescent Mental D.'s
Methods for Epidemiology of Child and Adolescent Mental D.'s
Methods for the Epidemiology of Child and Adolescent D.'s T score
mineral-related nutritional d.
minor depressive d.
mixed acid-base d.
mixed anxiety depression d.
mixed connective tissue d.
mixed development developmental delay d.
mixed receptive-expressive language d.
mood disorder due to a general medical condition
mood disorder patient
mood disorder with atypical features
mood disorder with catatonic features
mood disorder with melancholic features
mood disorder with postpartum onset
mood disorder with rapid cycling
mood disorder with seasonal pattern
moral deficiency personality d.
motion perception d.
movement d.
movement disorder effect
multihormonal system d.

disorder *(continued)*
multiple complex developmental d.
multiple personality d.
multiple tic d.
narcissistic personality d.
nasal allergic d.
National Association of Anorexia Nervosa and Associated D.'s
nerve cell d.
neurogenic bladder d.
neuroleptic-induced acute movement d.
neuromuscular d.
neuronal migration d.'s
neuronal migration d.
neurotic hysteric d.
neutrophil functional d.
nicotine-related disorder NOS
nicotine-related disorder, not otherwise specified
nonaffective psychotic d.
nonepileptic attack d.
nonorganic disorder diagnosis
nonprogressive cerebellar disorder with mental retardation
nonspecific esophageal motility d.
nonsyndromic autosomal recessive d.
normal childhood d.'s
nutritional deficiency d.
obsessive-compulsive conduct d.
obsessive-compulsive disorder with poor insight type
obsessive-compulsive personality d.
obstructive sleep d.
occupational lung d.
ocular inflammatory d.
ocular motility d.
oppositional defiant d.
oppositional disorder of adolescence
oppositional disorder of childhood
opposition defiance d.
optic nerve d.
Oregon Adolescent Depression Project-Conduct Disorder Screener
organic anxiety d.
organic articulation d.
organic brain d.
organic delusional d.
organic mental d.
organic mood d.
organic personality d.
other neurologic d.
overactive thyroid d.
overanxious d.
overanxious disorder of adolescence
overanxious disorder of childhood
over-the-counter drug-related d.
pain disorder, chronic
painful nerve d.
panic d.
panic and anxiety d.
panic disorder with agoraphobia
panic disorder without agoraphobia
paranoid personality d.
paraphiliac coercive d.
parkinsonian movement d.
Parkinson tremor d.
paroxysmal pain d.
partial combined immunodeficiency d.
passive-aggressive personality d.
pathological habit d.
pathologic gambling d.
pediatric autoimmune neuropsychiatric disorders associated with streptococcal infection
pelvic floor d.
perforating disorder of uremia
periodic limb movement d.
periodic movement d.
peripheral auditory d.
peripheral nervous system d.
persecutory delusional d.
personal history of depressive d.'s
personality d.
personality change d.
personality disorder diagnosis
personality disorder NOS
personality disorder profile
personality disorder score
personality trait d.
pervasive developmental d.
pervasive developmental disorder not otherwise specified
pituitary endocrine d.
posttransplant lymphoproliferative d.
posttraumatic stress d.
premenstrual dysphoric d.
previous seizure d.
primary affective d.
Primary Care Evaluation of Mental D.'s
primary sleep d.
psychoactive substance use d.
psychoaffective d.
d.'s of psychosexual identity
psychotic thought d.
pulmonary heart valve d.
pulmonary interstitial d.
pulmonary vascular d.
Quantitative Inventory of Alcohol D.'s
rapid movement d.
rectal evacuatory d.
REM behavior d.
repetitive motion d.
repetitive trauma d.
rheumatic pain modulation d.
rhythm of heartbeat d.
Scale for the Assessment of Unawareness of Mental D.
Schedule for Affective D.'s and Schizophrenia-Change
Schedule for Affective D.'s and Schizophrenia-Lifetime
Schedule for Affective D.'s and Schizophrenia for School-Age Children
Schedule for Affective D.'s and Schizophrenia for School-Age Children-Epidemiologic Version
Schedule for Affective D.'s and Schizophrenia for School-Age Children-Present Episode
schizoid personality d.
schizoid-schizotypal personality d.
schizophrenic spectrum d.
schizotypal personality d.
Screen for Child Anxiety-Related Emotional D.'s
seasonal affective d.
seasonal affective disorder syndrome
senile gait d.
d. of sensation
separation anxiety d.
Sheffield Screening Test for Acquired Language D.'s
single gene d.
situational anger disorder with aggression
situational anger disorder without aggression
sleep disorders center
sleep terror d.
slowly progressive hereditary d.
social anxiety d.
sociopathic personality d.
specific developmental d.
specific language d.
spinal cord d.

Standardized Assessment of Depressive D.'s
stereotype habits d.
stereotypic movement d.
Structured Clinical Interview for DSM-IV Dissociative D.'s
Structured Clinical Interview for DSM-IV Dissociative D.'s
Structured Clinical Interview for DSM-IV Psychotic D.'s
substance abuse d.
substance use d.
temporomandibular d.
temporomandibular joint d.
transient tic d.
upper airway d.
whiplash-associated d.
Wing Autistic D. Interview Checklist

disordered
d. action of heart
d. bone growth
d. breathing rate
d. breathing time
chronic disordered water balance
mentally disordered sex offender
d. thinking

disorganization
autonomic d.
linguistic d.
mental d.
segmental arterial d.

disorganized
d. globe
grossly disorganized behavior
d. schizophrenia
schizophrenia, disorganized type, subchronic
d. schizophrenic disorder
d. thinking
d. type schizophrenia

disorientation
auditory d.
autopsychic d.
Brief Vestibular D. Test
d. and confusion
confusion and d.
diarrhea and d.
d. and fever
graphic d.
d. and irritability
patient has disorientation and hallucinations
d. and personality change
right-left d.
senility and d.
d. to time and place

disoriented
d. and confused
confused and d.
d. and dysfunctional
d. or slow thought process

disparity
National Center on Minority Health and Health D.'s
phase d.

dispensary
accident d.
general d.
outpatient d.

dispense
d. as directed
d. as written

dispenser
hearing aid d.

dispensing
d. information
d. tablet

dispersed
molecular dispersed solution

dispersion
aerosol bolus d.
amphotericin B colloid d.
enzymatic cell d.
extra-low d.
gas atomized dispersion strengthened
magnetic optical rotatory d.
optical rotatory d.
pigment dispersion syndrome
QT d.

dispersion-induced circular dichroism

displaced
anteriorly displaced anus
longitudinal displaced complete tear
minimally displaced fracture
d. person

displacement
Anderson-Fowler calcaneal displacement osteotomy
anterior d.
anterior disc displacement without reduction
anterior displacement no reduction
anterior displacement with reduction
anterior tracheal d.
arterial brain d.
atlantoaxial rotary d.
d. bone marrow transplantation
d. of cartilage padding
congenital displacement of heart
congenital hip d.
downward displacement of apical impulse
lateral head d.
left apexcardiogram, calibrated d.
left uterine displacement device
linear displacement analysis
medial displacement osteotomy
motion and displacement perimetry
oblique displacement osteotomy
odontoid process d.
d. placentogram
posterior facet d.
serum thyroxine measured by displacement analysis
strand displacement amplification
subcoracoid type d.

display
computerized display technique
digital display alarm
direct display console
d.'s enduring bitterness
d.'s extreme sarcasm
head-mounted d.
high-definition video d.
d.'s hopelessness
image display and analysis
liquid crystal display projector
monocular heads-up display imaging system
multiplanar d.
shaded-surface d.
variable life-adjusted d.
video display terminal
video display terminal glare screen
video display terminal simulator
video display unit
visual display terminal
visual display unit
visual feedback d.

disposable
automated disposable keratome
d. curette
d. elbow protector
d. glove
d. heel protector
d. needle
one-piece disposable plug
d. one-piece osteotome
oxygen disposable boot device

disposable *(continued)*
Passport disposable injection system
d. pudendal nerve electrode
d. trocar

disposal
glucose disposal rate
maximal glucose d.

disposition
California Critical Thinking D.'s Inventory

disproportion
cephalopelvic d.
cephalopelvic disproportion and fetal distress
congenital fiber-type d.
congenital muscle fiber-type d.
fetopelvic d.
muscle fiber type d.

disproportionate
d. growth
macrocephaly, facial abnormalities, disproportionate tall stature mental retardation syndrome
d. micromelia
d. septal thickening

disqualifying
not considered d.

disquietude
patient d.

disregard
d. for others
d. rights of others

disruption
anastomotic d.
anterior column d.
anterior labral d.
anular d.
autonomic d.
d. of bladder function
chemical disruption in brain
counting d.
ligamentous d.
marital d.
medial compartment d.
myofascial d.
ossicular d.
pancreatic duct d.
pattern disruption point
pedicle cortex d.
perivalvular d.
skeletal d.
sleep d.

disruptive
attention deficit and disruptive behavior disorder
d. behavior disorder

dissatisfaction
marital d.

dissecans
endometritis d.
osteochondritis d.
osteochondrosis d.

dissecta
lingua d.

dissecting
d. abdominal aneurysm
d. aneurysm
d. aneurysm of the coronary artery
angled dissecting forceps
d. aortic aneurysm
d. aortic hematoma
d. basilar artery aneurysm
binocular dissecting microscope
d. hemorrhage of midbrain
d. intracranial aneurysm
recurrent chronic dissecting aneurysm
d. renal artery aneurysm

dissection
acute aortic d.
aortic d.
d. aortic aneurysm
arterial wall d.
aspiration and dissection tube
autonomic nerve-preserving three-space d.
axial joint d.
axillary lymph node d.
axillary node dissection mastectomy
bilateral pelvic lymph node d.
blunt dissection carried upward
blunt and sharp d.
carotid aortic d.
complete lymph node d.
DeBakey-type aortic d.
elective lymph node d.
elective neck d.
elective regional lymph node d.
en bloc d.
epiphenomena of d.
extraperitoneal endoscopic pelvic lymph node d.
field of d.
freed by blunt d.
functional neck d.
d. of heart
laparoscopic pelvic lymph node d.
left radical neck d.
lymph node d.
middle fossa floor/petrous d.
modified neck d.
neck d.
partial neck d.
partial zona d.
partial zonal d.
pelvic lymph node d.
pelvic node d.
per anum intersphincteric rectal d.
plane of d.
quadrantectomy, axillary dissection, radiation therapy
quadrantectomy, axillary dissection and radiotherapy
radical neck d.
regional lymph node d.
retroperitoneal pelvic lymph node d.
right radical neck d.
selective complete lymph node d.
selective neck d.
sharp and blunt d.
sharp dissection technique
d. and snare
d. and snare tonsillectomy
spontaneous cervical artery d.
spontaneous coronary artery d.
Stanford-type aortic d.
d. and stripping
therapeutic lymph node d.
thoracic aortic d.
tongue, jaw, neck d.
tumorectomy, axillary dissection, radiotherapy
vertebral artery d.

dissector
angled d.
ASSI breast dissector angulated
ASSI breast dissector spatulated
ball d.
dura d.
hockey-stick d.

disseminated
acute disseminated encephalomyelitis
d. aspergillosis
d. candidiasis
d. carcinomatosis
d. coccidioidomycosis
d. cutaneous leishmaniasis
fatal disseminated infection
d. fat necrosis

d. foci
d. gonococcal infection
d. herpes zoster infection
d. histoplasmosis
d. infection
d. intrauterine clotting
d. intravascular blood coagulation
d. intravascular coagulation
d. intravascular coagulation syndrome
d. intravascular coagulopathy
d. lupus erythematosus
d. *Mycobacterium avium-intracellulare* complex
d. necrotizing leukoencephalopathy
d. nontuberculous mycobacterial infection
progressive disseminated histoplasmosis
d. sclerosis
d. superficial actinic porokeratosis
d. tuberculosis

disseminating fungal infection

dissemination

lymphatic dissemination theory of endometriosis

disseminatum

xanthoma d.

dissimilar

number of dissimilar matches

dissociated

d. double hypertropia
d. horizontal deviation
d. sensation
d. state
d. vertical deviation

dissociation

acid ionization dissociation constant
carpal instability d.
cell d.
complete atrioventricular d.
complete A-V d.
d. constant
d. constant of a base
d. constant of water
d. in eating disorder
electromechanical d.
d. of enzyme-inhibitor complex
equilibrium dissociation constant
hemoglobin oxygen dissociation curve
immune complex d.
incomplete atrioventricular d.
intracavitary pressure electrogram d.
light-near d.
Michaelis-Menten dissociation constant
molecular dissociation theory
d. and repression
d. and sexual abuse

dissociative

atypical dissociative disorder
d. disorder
d. disorder not otherwise specified
d. identity disorder
severe dissociative symptom
Structured Clinical Interview for DSM-IV D. Disorders

dissolution

mean dissolution time
percutaneous dissolution of thrombus
rapid dissolution formula

dissolved

d. organic matter
d. oxygen
d. oxygen deficit
partially dissolved gutta-percha
d. solids

dissolving

clot dissolving action
clot dissolving drug
clot dissolving thrombolytic drug

distal

d. acquired demyelinating symmetrical neuropathy
antimesenteric border of distal ileum
aortogram with distal runoff
aperistaltic distal ureteral segment
arthrogryposis congenita, distal, type I, II syndrome
d. arthrogryposis, hypopituitarism, mental retardation, facial anomalies syndrome
articular disc of distal radioulnar joint
d. articular set angle
atraumatic osteolysis of distal clavicle
d. bile duct carcinoma
blistering distal dactylitis
clubbing of distal phalanx
d. colon
d. communicating branch
complete laparoscopic distal pancreatectomy
d. convoluted tubule
d. coronary sinus
d. cusp
d. cusp ridge
early distal proximal tubule
d. effective potassium secretion
d. femoral epiphysis
d. forearm
d. fossa
d. gastric adenocarcinoma
His bundle electrogram, d.
d. ileal obstruction syndrome
d. ileitis
d. ileum
d. interphalangeal joint
d. intestinal obstruction syndrome
junction of distal third
laparoscopically assisted distal partial gastrectomy
late distal cortical tubule
d. marginal ridge
mean distal contraction amplitude
d. mean wave pressure
mental retardation, facial anomalies, hypopituitarism, distal arthrogryposis syndrome
mental retardation, overgrowth, craniosynostosis, distal arthrogryposis, sacral dimple, joint laxity
mental retardation, spasticity, distal transverse limb defects syndrome
mesial, occlusal, d.
metallic distal end of tube
metaphyseal lesion of distal femur
d. metatarsal articular angle
Mitchell distal osteotomy
modified Boyd amputation of ankle and distal tibial physis
d. motor latency
nonarticular distal radial fracture
d. oblique groove
osteitis distal phalanx
d. over-shoulder strap
d. palmar crease
d. pancreatectomy
partial denture, distal extension
penciling of the distal clavicle
d. perfusion system
d. phalangeal width
d. phalanx
d. pit
poor distal runoff
d. portion main circumflex
d. portion of small intestine
d. and proximal

distal *(continued)*
proximal and distal portion of vessel
d. radioulnar joint
d. rectal adenocarcinoma
d. reference axis
d. renal tubular acidosis
d. right coronary artery
d. root
d. sensory latency
d. sensory polyneuropathy
d. soft tissue release
d. splenorenal
d. splenorenal shunt
d. subungual onychomycosis
superficial distal axillary node
superficial distal esophagus hemorrhage
d. symmetrical polyneuropathy
d. symmetric sensory neuropathy
d. symmetric sensory polyneuropathy
d. third
Tinel sign distal tingling on percussion
d. tingling on percussion
d. triangular fossa
d. tuft
d. urethral stenosis
ventricular atrial distal coronary sinus

distally
d. based fasciocutaneous flap
medial distally based fasciocutaneous flap

distance
anterior capsular d.
atlas odontoid d.
auditory distance cue
d. between centers
d. between iliac spines
d. between nasal lines
bony interorbital d.
central lung d.
crown-rump d.
E-point to septal d.
esophoria for d.
esotropia at d.
euclidean distance matrix analysis
exophoria d.
focal d.
focal film d.
focus film d.
focus object d.
focus-skin d.
d. glasses
hearing d.
hearing distance with watch
inner canthal d.
intercanthal d.
internodal d.
interpupillary d.
intramammary d.
judgment of d.
light and d.
Lighthouse D. Visual Acuity Test
marginal reflex d.
margin crease d.
margin reflex d.
maximum interincisal d.
maximum walking d.
medial osseous interorbital d.
MPH distance measurement
d. and near vision
neck-capsule d.
noncycloplegic distance static retinoscopy
one-leg hop for distance test
outer canthal d.
pupillary d.
shallow d.
short distance group
skin-film d.
skin-to-tumor d.
source film d.
source image d.
source-skin d.
source to skin d.
source-surface d.
source-to-axis d.
source-to-image receptor d.
source-to-skin d.
source-tray d.
symptom-free walking d.
target-film d.
target-skin d.
d. visual acuity
d. visual acuity with correction
d. visual acuity without correction
working d.

distant
age, distant metastases, extent and size
d. breath sound
freedom from distant metastases
free from distant metastases
d. gaze
d. heart sounds
lateral distant view
d. metastases
d. metastasis
d. metastatic disease
no evidence of distant metastases
nontubed closed distant flap graft
d. objects blurry
d. objects fuzzy
d. recurrence-free survival
d. spread
time to distant failure

distant-disease-free survival

distemper
canine d.
canine distemper encephalitis
canine distemper virus
homologous canine distemper antiserum
d. virus

distended
abdomen d.
d. abdomen
abdomen distended, tender, tympanitic
d. afferent loop
d. bladder
bladder distended with air
bladder distended with water
d. colon
d. gallbladder
neck vein d.
taut and distended abdomen
d. urinary bladder

distending
continuous distending airway pressure
d. airway pressure
positive distending pressure

distensibility
aortic d.
venous distensibility index

distension
arthrographic capsular distension and rupture technique

distention
abdominal distention and tenderness
intraesophageal balloon d.
jugular neck vein d.
jugular venous d.
neck vein d.
no venous d.
postoperative abdominal d.
preperitoneal distention balloon
proximal bowel d.
uterine d.
venous distention or mass

distillable nonurea adductable

distillate
primary flash d.

distilled
buffered distilled water
double distilled water
d. water

distinct
certified distinct part
d. psychiatric disorder
mental retardation, hearing impairment, distinct facies, skeletal anomalies syndrome
multiple distinct identities

distinction
loss of distinction at gray/white matter interface

distinctive
congenital thrombocytopenia, Robin sequence, agenesis of corpus callosum, distinctive facies, developmental delay syndrome
d. exudative discoid and lichenoid dermatitis
microcephaly, mild developmental delay, short stature, distinctive face syndrome

distobuccal
d. cusp
d. cusp ridge
d. developmental groove
d. root

distolingual
d. cusp
d. cusp ridge
d. fossa
d. groove

distomiasis
hepatic d.

distorted
d. anatomy
d. body image
d. communication in schizophrenia
d. depth perception
d. grief
d. ideas of reference
d. negative thinking
d. perception
d. sense of time and perception
d. thinking
d. visual images and hallucinations

distortion
apperceptive d.
architectural d.
auditory d.
d. of contour
d. of dots
gradual distortion of sound
illusion or perceptual d.'s
local field d.
memory d.
memory, and distortion hypnosis
nonlinear d.
parataxic d.
pattern distortion amblyopia
perceptual d.
pituitary stalk d.
d. or retraction of nipple
d. of sensory perception
d. of time and space
visual d.
visual distortion test
waveform d.

distortion-product otoacoustic emission

distractability
freedom from d.

distractibility
easy d.
Freedom from D. Deviation Quotient

distractible speech

distraction
anterior d.
apical d.
Apley distraction test
calcaneocuboid distraction arthrodesis
flexion d.
head distraction test
hearing distraction test
d. injury
joint d.
d. lengthening
longitudinal d.
lumbar distraction manipulation
MacroPore distraction mesh
mandibular d.
mandibular distraction osteogenesis
maxillary distraction osteogenesis
Monticelli-Spinelli d.
Monticelli-Spinelli distraction technique
multiplanar d.
muscle d.
d. osteogenesis
palatal d.
relaxation, distraction and imagery
skeletal d.
d. technique

distractor
bidirectional telescopic d.
intramedullary skeletal kinetic d.

distress
acute intrapartum fetal d.
acute respiratory distress syndrome
adult respiratory distress syndrome
cephalopelvic disproportion and fetal d.
dental distress syndrome
epigastric distress syndrome
exercise-induced respiratory distress syndrome
fetal d.
functional bowel d.
gastrointestinal d.
idiopathic respiratory distress of newborn
idiopathic respiratory distress syndrome
infant in acute respiratory d.
infant respiratory distress syndrome
intrapartum fetal d.
intrauterine fetal d.
Menstrual D. Management Questionnaire
neonatal respiratory distress syndrome
newborn respiratory distress syndrome
no acute d.
no apparent d.
in no apparent d.
not in d.
pain and distress score
patient in cardiac or respiratory d.
patient distress alarm
perinatal distress prediction
Positive Symptom D. Index
Premenstrual D. Questionnaire
respiratory d.
respiratory distress index
respiratory distress syndrome
D. Risk Assessment Method
salivation, lacrimation, urination, defecation, gastrointestinal distress and emesis
D. Scale for Ventilated Newborn Infants

distress *(continued)*
silent heart muscle d.
social avoidance and d.
Subjective Units of D. Scale
symptom distress check list
Symptom D. Scale
transient respiratory distress of the newborn
transient respiratory distress syndrome
Urogenital D. Inventory

distressing
d. psychedelic experience
d. recollection of incident

distributed data processing

distribution
absorption, distribution, metabolism, and excretion
anatomic origin and d.
android fat d.
annular distribution of lesion
anomalous vascular d.
anterior communicating artery distribution infarct
anterior communicating artery distribution infarction
apparent distribution mass
apparent volume of d.
arciform distribution of lesion
atypical distribution of disease
body hair d.
d. coefficient
community-based d.
countercurrent d.
cranial nerve d.
ed blood cell distribution width index
extracellular volume of d.
extrahepatic d.
d. factor
fibrosing alopecia in a pattern d.
hepatic distribution volume
linear distribution of lesion
liquid-liquid d.
mass isotopomer distribution analysis
d. of median nerve
molecular weight d.
multistate drug distribution ring
normal distribution of hair
normal hair d.
organ and tissue d.
particle size d.
patchy distribution of tracer
pattern of d.
platelet distribution width
Quimby dose distribution system
d. ratio
regional distribution of hepatic blood flow
reticulocyte hemoglobin distribution width
spectral frequency d.
spectral power d.
stocking glove d.
stress distribution factor
supply, processing, and distribution department
ulnar nerve d.
vascular volume of d.
velocity distribution function
d. of ventilation
volume of d.
volume of distribution of bilirubin

district
d. health authority
d. health department

distrust
malevolent d.

disturbance
acute brain d.
adjustment disorder with disturbance of conduct
adjustment disorder with mixed disturbance of emotions
adjustment reaction d.
aggressive behavioral d.
d. in air exchange
appraisal of language d.'s
arteriovenous conduction d.
assimilating information d.
atrial conduction d.
attentional d.
cannabis intoxication, with perceptual d.
d. in cardiac rhythm
chronic sleep schedule d.
color and space perceptual d.
d. of conduct
conduct disturbance adjustment disorder
conduct disturbance adjustment reaction
core cognitive d.
Draw-A-Person Screening Procedure for Emotional D.
emotional d.
emotional disturbance adjustment disorder
emotional disturbance adjustment reaction
emotional disturbance of adolescence
emotional disturbance of childhood
emotional disturbance stress reaction
d. of emotions specific to adolescence
d. of emotions specific to childhood
executive functioning d.
fatal heart rhythm d.
fluctuating mood d.
focal neurologic d.
d. of function occlusion syndrome
d.'s in gait
d. of gait and stance
heart rhythm d.
increased rhythm d.'s
initial sleep d.
intraoperative conduction d.
d. of mental equilibrium
midsleep d.
mixed disturbance stress reaction
persistent identity d.
personal identity d.
respiratory disturbance index
d. in self-concept
d. in self-image
d. of sensation
serious emotional d.
Thinking D. Factor
visual field d.
d. of visual function

disturbed
aroused state of disturbed behavior
d. bowel function
emotionally d.
emotionally disturbed individual
emotionally disturbed and learning disabled
d. interpersonal relationships
patient very d.
d. sense of time
d. sleep pattern
socially and emotionally d.

disulfide
dimethyl d.
PDI-mediated disulfide bond reduction
protein disulfide isomerase

disuse
d. atrophy
d. muscular atrophy
d. syndrome

dithionite
automated dithionite test

diuretic
d. agent
hearing loss from d.'s
heat intolerance from d.'s
indirect d.
intermittent diuretic therapy
intravenous d.
loop d.
mechanical d.
mercurial d.
osmotic d.
parenteral d.

diurnal
abnormal diurnal weight gain
d. cortisol test
d. and matutinal variation
d. rhythm
d. weight fluctuation

divalent ion metabolism

divergence
angle of d.
anteroposterior talocalcaneal d.
artificial divergence procedure
d. excess
d. insufficiency
negative vertical d.
positive vertical d.

divergency
artificial divergency surgery

diver's
pearl diver's keratopathy

diversion
adolescent diversion project
d. of drugs from illicit medical channels
d. of flow of blood
loop d.
orthotopic d.
partial external biliary d.

diversional
d. activity
d. activity deficit
d. heart block
d. therapy

diversionary tactic

diversity
D. Awareness Profile
cultural/ethnic d.
generation of d.
variable diversity joining

diverticula (*pl. of* diverticulum)

diverticular
d. bleeding
caliceal diverticular calculus
d. disease
d. disease of colon
d. hernia

diverticulectomy
Meckel d.
open d.

diverticulitis
jejunal d.

diverticulosis
jejunal d.

diverticulum, pl. **diverticula**
antral diverticulum of the colon
antral diverticulum of the ileum
artificial diverticulum of the ileum
atrial diverticulum of brain
d. of colon
colonic d.
common bile duct d.
giant colonic d.
intraluminal duodenal d.
jejunal d.
Meckel d.
meningeal d.
periampullary duodenal d.
pharyngoesophageal d.

diverting
d. colostomy
d. colostomy with pull-through procedure
d. enterostomy
d. loop colostomy
d. loop ileostomy
d. proximal colostomy
d. stoma creation

divide-and-conquer
d.-a.-c. method
d.-a.-c. technique

divided
banded gastroplasty with a divided pouch
clamped, divided and tied
doubly clamped and d.

diving
d. air embolism
d. injury
mammalian diving response

division
anterior d.
anterior division of brachial plexus
anterior primary d.
autonomic division of nervous system
cell division cycle
indirect cell d.
lingular division of the left lung
parasympathetic division of antonomic nervous system
posterior d.
trigeminal nerve, mandibular d.
trigeminal nerve, maxillary d.
trigeminal nerve, ophthalmic d.
uncontrolled cell division growth

divisum
incomplete pancreas d.
pancreas d.

divorce
overt behavior consequences of d.
parental d.
d. support group

divorced
single, divorced, married
white divorced female

divot
liposuction d.

Dix-Hallpike maneuver

dizygotic twins

dizziness
d. in aging
d. and faintness
d. from antidepressant
d. from heart attack
d. from heat stroke
d. from infection of ear
d. from insect sting
d. from rapid and deep breathing
d. from tic douloureux
D. Handicap Inventory
d. or lightheadedness
multiple sensory defect d.
d. and nausea
weakness, dizziness and joint pain

DNA
anti-double-stranded DNA antibody
antisense DNA inhibition
depressed DNA synthesis
DNA image cytometry
D. topoisomerase I
fluorometric analysis of DNA unwinding
hepatitis B DNA detection
immunostimulatory DNA sequence
D. index
inhibitor of DNA synthesis
Lyme disease DNA detection

DNA *(continued)*
microchip DNA array
mitochondrial DNA mutation
mitochondrial DNA polymerase gamma
mitochondrial DNA syndrome
naked DNA encoding
naked DNA vector vaccine
naked plasmid D.
Neisseria gonorrhoeae DNA detection test
nonrejoining DNA strand break
parvovirus B19 D.
PCR for HIV D.
random amplified polymorphic D.
rapid amplification of polymorphic D.
recombinant D.
ribosomal D.
sequence-specific DNA primer
single-stranded D.
smallest unit of DNA capable of recombination

DNA-binding domain

dobutamine
d. echocardiogram
d. echocardiography
d. holiday
low-dose dobutamine stress radionuclide ventriculography
d. stress echocardiography
d. stress test
d. thallium angiography
transesophageal dobutamine stress echocardiograph

dobutamine-atropine stress echocardiography

docimasia
auricular d.

doctor
d. actively caused death
admitting d.
D. of Chiropractic
family d.
family medical d.
local medical d.
naturopathic d.
no family d.
outside d.
private medical d.
referring d.
D.'s Without Borders

doctor-patient relationship

doctor/population ratio

doctor's
check doctor's order
d. order
d. order book

doctrine
Arrhenius d.
Monro d.
neuron d.

document
d. image decoding
D.'s On-Line
Portable D. Format
resubmission turnaround d.

documentation
bibliographic information and d.
emergency room triage d.

documented
d. bacterial infection
failed back syndrome with documented pseudarthrosis
d. silent ischemia
d. viral infection

docusate sodium

dodecyl
sodium dodecyl sulfate
sodium dodecyl sulfate-polyacrylamide gel electrophoresis

Doerfler-Stewart test

does
heart does appear enlarged
heart does not appear enlarged
lump in breast does appear enlarged
d. not apply
d. not follow commands
patient does ADL with supervision

doffing
donning and d.
d. prosthesis

dog
d. ear
enterocytopathogenic dog orphan virus
guide d.
d. kidney cell
d. kidney tissue culture
medial dog ear
nonshedding d.
normal dog serum
d. red blood cell
d. unit
wet dog shakes syndrome

dog-ear
d.-e. of anastomosis
d.-e. deformity
d.-e. repair

Doheny

Döhle
D. body
D. body panmyelopathy

doing well

Dolichos biflorus **agglutinin**

doll's
d. eyes
d. eye sign

dolorimetric unit of pain intensity

dolorosa
analgesia d.
anesthesia d.
atrophia d.
hallux d.
nephritis d.
neurolipomatosis d.
paraplegia d.

domain
constant domain of H chain
constant domain of L chain
DNA-binding d.
extracellular d.
Fas-associating protein with death d.
frequency domain imaging
hormone-binding d.
ligand-binding d.
membrane-spanning d.
multiple domains of self
nucleotide-binding d.
phosphotyrosine-binding d.
silencer of death d.
time domain signal processor
time domain ultrasound
variable domain of heavy chain immunoglobulin
variable domain of light chain immunoglobulin

dome
alar dome and cartilage
aneurysmal d.
anterior talar d.
atrial d.
blue dome cyst
dart and d.
d. fragment
gallbladder d.
injection d.
liver d.

Maquet dome osteotomy
midtarsal dome osteotomy
nasal d.
nasal dome cartilage
osteochondral fracture of the dome of the talus
patellar d.
talar d.
talar dome cyst
talar dome fracture

domestic violence

domiciliary
d. care
d. visit

dominance
Lateral D. Examination
mixed cerebral d.
ocular dominance column

dominant
autosomal d.
autosomal dominant compelling helioophthalmic outburst syndrome
autosomal dominant arteriopathy
autosomal dominant cardiomyopathy
autosomal dominant cerebellar ataxia
autosomal dominant condition
autosomal dominant congenital cataract
autosomal dominant diabetes mellitus
autosomal dominant disorder
autosomal dominant febrile convulsion
autosomal dominant gene
autosomal dominant hemochromatosis
autosomal dominant hereditary optic neuropathy
autosomal dominant hypocalcemia
autosomal dominant hypoparathyroidism
autosomal dominant inheritance
autosomal dominant lamellar ichthyosis
autosomal dominant macrocephaly syndrome
autosomal dominant medullary cystic kidney disease
autosomal dominant migraine
autosomal dominant mild short limb dwarfism
autosomal dominant movement disorder
autosomal dominant nocturnal frontal lobe epilepsy
autosomal dominant nonsyndromic hearing loss
autosomal dominant oculocutaneous albinism
autosomal dominant Opitz syndrome
autosomal dominant osteosclerosis
autosomal dominant pattern
autosomal dominant temporal lobe epilepsy
autosomal dominant toxic thyroid hyperplasia
autosomal dominant trait
autosomal dominant transmission
bystander dominates initial d.
d. epidermolysis bullosa simplex
d. exudative vitreoretinopathy
d. hand
d. hemisphere
inheritance
d. juvenile optic atrophy
left-hand d.
mixed foot d.
occipital dominant intermittent rhythmic delta activity
d. optic atrophy
right-hand d.
X-linked d.

dominantly inherited juvenile optic atrophy

dominates
bystander dominates initial dominant

domino heart transplantation

donated
heart d.
d. human organs

Donath-Landsteiner antibody

donation
autologous blood d.
autologous predeposit d.
consent for organ d.
criteria for organ d.
designated blood d.
d. of heart
oocyte d.
preoperative autologous d.
preoperative autologous blood d.
segmental pancreas d.

Donders
space of D.

done
not d.
nothing d.
routine laboratory work d.
skin test d.

donkey red blood cell

donner
long-handled sock d.

donning
d. and doffing
d. prosthesis

donning-doffing skill

donor
adult-to-adult living related donor living transplant
alloplastic donor material
anonymous donor sperm
artificial insemination by d.
artificial insemination donor, husband
artificial insemination with donor sperm
autogenous donor material
autologous patient d.
auxiliary partial orthotopic living donor transplantation
beating heart brain-dead d.
d. biopsy
blood d.
bone graft d.
d. bone marrow
d. bone marrow engraftment
cadaver d.
cadaveric donor transplantation
d. cell
d. cell engraftment
cloned enzyme donor immunoassay
consanguineous d.
damaged donor heart
d. dendritic cell
designated donor blood
directed donor transfusion
extended criteria d.
d. graft
d. heart
heart-beating d.
d. heart retrieved
d. hepatic duct
d. hospital
hydrotropic electron d.
infected blood d.
infected organ d.
d. insemination
kidney d.
laparoscopic donor nephrectomy
d. leukocyte infusion
live donor nephrectomy

donor *(continued)*
living d.
living donor bilobar transplant
living-related donor transplantation
living relative transplant d.
living renal d.
living segmental donor pancreas transplantation
living unrelated d.
d. lymphocyte infusion
matched related d.
matched unrelated d.
matched unrelated donor stem cell transplant
d. material
mismatched related d.
Morrison donor site design
National Marrow D. Program
non-heart-beating d.
non-heart-beating donor liver transplantation
nonmatching donor relative
Norwood donor site design
organ donor candidate
organ donor card
d. organ ischemic time
patellar tendon graft donor site
pedicled enteric donor site
d. procurement
procurement of donor organs and tissue
random single donor platelet
replica of donor tissue
d. site
d. site of bone graft
d. site dressing
d. site of skin graft
skin graft d.
d. team
therapeutic donor insemination
d. tissue
d. transfusion, specific
universal blood d.
unrelated d.
unrelated donor transplant

donor-related warm ischemia

donor-specific
d.-s. blood transfusion
d.-s. transfusion

donor's plasma

do-not-resuscitate
d.-n.-r. order
d.-n.-r. status

donovanosis
oral d.

donut
circular stapler d.
d. support brace

Doo
Humpty Doo virus

doom
fear of impending d.

door
locked door seclusion
open door laminoplasty
out the d.
rotary door flap

dopachrome conversion factor

dopamine
d. agonist
endorphin, dopamine, and prostaglandin theory
d. hydroxylase
irregular dopamine transmission
limbic dopamine receptor
mesocortical dopamine pathway
mesolimbic dopamine pathway
mesolimbic dopamine system
mesolimbic dopamine tract
nigrostriatal dopamine system
d. receptor agonist property
renal dose d.
d. reuptake inhibitor
saline and dopamine infusion
tuberoinfundibular dopamine system

dopamine-beta hydroxylase

dopamine-boosting drug

dopamine-releasing drug

dopaminergic
low-dose dopaminergic agonist
mesocortical dopaminergic system
nigrostriatal dopaminergic system
tuberohypophyseal dopaminergic neuron
tuberoinfundibular d.
tuberoinfundibular dopaminergic neuron

dopa-responsive dystonia

Doppler
cardiac Doppler examination
D. cardiography
carotid Doppler study
color Doppler echocardiography
color Doppler energy
color Doppler flow
color Doppler flow imaging
color Doppler scan
color Doppler signal
color Doppler sonography
color Doppler ultrasonography
color-flow D.
color flow D.
color flow Doppler imaging
color-flow Doppler sonography
color flow Doppler ultrasound
D. color-flow imaging
color-flow imaging Doppler echocardiography
D. color-flow mapping
D. color jet
continuous-wave D.
continuous-wave Doppler echocardiogram
continuous-wave Doppler echocardiography
continuous-wave Doppler imaging
continuous-wave Doppler ultrasound
directional Doppler sonography
duplex B-mode D.
duplex Doppler imaging
duplex Doppler scan
duplex Doppler ultrasound
D. echocardiography
D. effect
epicardial Doppler echocardiography
esophageal Doppler monitor
D. evaluation
extracranial Doppler sonography
D. flow
D. flow detector
D. flowmetry
D. flow study
D. flow test
functional transcranial Doppler sonography
high-frequency D.
D. imaging
D. interrogation
laser Doppler anemometry
laser Doppler flowmetry
laser Doppler flux
laser Doppler velocimetry
microvascular Doppler ultrasonography
mitral pressure half-time Doppler
D. monitoring of fetus
myocardial Doppler velocity
ophthalmic Doppler sonogram
D. ophthalmic test
ovarian Doppler signal
D. perfusion index
periorbital bidirectional D.
periorbital directional Doppler ultrasonography

periorbital Doppler imaging
power Doppler imaging
D. pressure gradient
D. probe
D. pulse
pulsed Doppler cross-sectional echocardiography
pulsed Doppler echo
pulsed Doppler echocardiogram
pulsed Doppler flowmetry
pulsed Doppler ultrasonic flowmeter
pulsed-wave Doppler echocardiogram
pulsed-wave Doppler echocardiography
pulsed-wave Doppler mapping
pulsed-wave tissue D.
range-gated D.
D. recording
D. Resistive Index
D. scanning
segmental bronchus lower extremity Doppler pressure
D. shift
D. signal
D. sonography
D. sound device
D. study
D. systolic velocity index
D. tissue imaging
transcranial Doppler sonography
transcranial Doppler ultrasound
transesophageal Doppler color flow imaging
transthoracic color Doppler echocardiography
transvaginal color Doppler sonography
D. ultrasonic flowmeter
D. ultrasonography
D. ultrasound
D. ultrasound imaging
D. ultrasound stethoscope
D. velocity probe
venous Doppler study
D. venous examination
D. venous imaging
D. waveform
D. waveform analysis
D. waveform dampening

Doppler-shifted constant frequency

Dor

Heller myotomy with Dor fundoplication

d'orange

peau d'orange appearance
peau d'orange appearance
peau d'orange in breast carcinoma

dornase

pancreatic d.

dorsal

anterior dorsal nucleus
apex dorsal angulation
apex of dorsal horn of spinal cord
axial dorsal flap
bilateral upper dorsal sympathectomy
d. brain stem lipoma
d. calcaneocuboid
cast with dorsal toe plate extension
d. caudate putamen
d. cell column
d. column
d. column nucleus
d. column stimulation
d. column stimulator
d. cord stimulation
d. cutaneous nerve
d. decubitus position
d. digital artery
d. elevated position
first dorsal interosseous
first dorsal metatarsal artery
first through twelfth dorsal vertebrae
d. glide
d. hippocampus
d. horn
d. horns of spinal cord
d. hump
d. intercalated segment instability
intermediate dorsal cutaneous nerve
d. interosseous metacarpal vein
d. interosseous muscle of foot
d. interosseous muscle of hand
d. interosseous vein of foot
d. lateral geniculate
low-profile dorsal plate
Marchac dorsal nasal flap
medial cutaneous branch of dorsal branch of posterior intercostal artery
medial dorsal cutaneous nerve
medial dorsal nucleus of thalamus
mediastinal dorsal enteric cyst
medullary dorsal horn
d. medullary reticular formation
Mendel dorsal foot reflex
d. motor nucleus of vagus
navicular dorsal lip fracture
d. nerve root
d. noradrenergic bundle
nucleus of dorsal field
opening for dorsal artery of penis
opening for dorsal nerve of penis
palmar and dorsal aspects
pancreatic dorsal anlage
d. penile nerve block
d. radiocarpal ligament
d. raphe
d. raphe nucleus
d. recumbent position
d. respiratory group
reversed dorsal digital flap
d. root, cervical
d. root dilator
d. root entry zone
d. root ganglion
d. root, lumbar
d. root potential
d. root reflex
d. root, sacral
d. root, thoracic
selective dorsal rhizotomy
spinal dorsal horn
d. spine
d. spinocerebellar tract
subjacent dorsal horn
d. uterine artery
d. vagal nucleus
d. vein complex
d. wire-loop fixation
d. wrist splint
d. wrist syndrome

dorsalis

nucleus d.
nucleus dorsalis of Clarke
d. pedis
d. pedis pulse
d. tibialis

dorsi

anterior latissimus d.
latissimus dorsi fasciocutaneous flap
latissimus dorsi muscle
latissimus dorsi musculocutaneous flap
latissimus dorsi myocutaneous flap
pedicled compound rib-latissimus dorsi osteomusculocutaneous flap

dorsi *(continued)*
pedicled endoscopic latissimus dorsi harvest
posterior latissimus dorsi muscle

dorsiflexed intercalated segment instability

dorsiflexion
d. angle
ankle dorsiflexion range of motion
ankle dorsiflexion test
d. assist
hallux dorsiflexion angle
superimposed dorsiflexion of foot

dorsiflexory wedge osteotomy

dorsoanterior
left d.
right d.

dorsogluteal
right d.

dorsolateral
d. funiculus
d. prefrontal cortex
d. surface of knee
d. tract

dorsomedial
d. hypothalamic nucleus lesion
d. nucleus

dorsomedialis-ventromedialis
nucleus d.-v.

dorsoplantar projection

dorsoposterior
left d.
right d.

dorsoradial ligament

dorsotransverse
left dorsotransverse fetal position

dorsum
atrophy of dorsum sella
nasal d.
squamous cell carcinoma dorsum of hand

dosage
gradual dosage schedule
high d.
hypnotic d.
medium d.
minimal d.
minimal intermittent dosage of heparin
multiplane dosage calculation
multiple dosage insulin
new dosage form
d. regimen
safe and effective d.
unit of neutron d.

dosage-sensitive sex reversal

dose
absolute dose intensity
absorbed d.
achieve high d.
air d.
analgesic d.
d. area product
arthritic d.
average body d.
average daily d.
average radiation d.
average target absorbed d.
bioeffect d.
biologically equivalent d.
biologic effective d.
biologic factors in dose fractionation
cell cycle redistribution and dose fractionation
cell redistribution and dose hyperfractionation
central axis depth dose of electron beam therapy
chick infective d.
computed tomography dose index
computer dose calculation
constant dose rate
convulsive d.
cumulative cardiotoxic d.
cumulative dose unit
curative d.
cycle redistribution and d.
defined daily d.
defined exposure d.
delayed erythema d.
delivered total d.
depth d.
double d.
drug dose intensity
effective d.
effective pressor d.
egg-infectious d.
egg lethal d.
d. equivalent
equivalent d.
erythema d.
fatal d.
fractionated high dose rate
growth hormone d.
hemolysing d.
heparin dose response
high d.
high dose rate
high dose rate brachytherapy
highest asymptomatic d.
highest nontoxic d.
high heparin d.
high single dose alternate day
human infectious d.
human therapeutic d.
identical midplane D.'s
inactivating d.
increased dose size per fraction
d. increase factor
individual d.
infective d.
inhibiting antibiotic d.
inhibitory d.
initial d.
injected d.
d. intensity analysis
intermediate dose group
intermediate dose methotrexate
internal absorbed d.
intraoperative high dose rate
intravenous loading d.
intravenous push dose
last d.
least fatal d.
lethal d.
lethal dose in all exposed subjects
liberal doses of aspirin
loading d.
lowest effective d.
lowest effective toxic d.
maintenance d.
matched peripheral d.
maximal d.
maximal allowable d.
maximal human d.
maximal permissible d.
maximal recommended human d.
maximal tolerated d.
maximum accumulated d.
maximum dose permissible d.
maximum permissible d.
maximum recommended daily d.
maximum recommended human d.
maximum target absorbed d.
maximum tolerated d.
mean d.
mean central d.
mean daily d.
mean dose per unit cumulated activity
mean episcleral heat d.
mean hemolytic d.
mean marrow d.
mean total d.

median curative d.
median effective d.
median fatal d.
median lethal dose
median paralyzing d.
median tissue culture infective d.
median toxic d.
medical internal radiation d.
minimal average d.
minimal cumulative cardiotoxic d.
minimal dose causing 100% death or malformation
minimal dose possible
minimal effective d.
minimal erythema d.
minimal fatal d.
minimal hemolytic d.
minimal infecting d.
minimal inhibitory d.
minimal irradiation d.
minimal lethal d.
minimal morbidostatic d.
minimal necrosing d.
minimal peripheral d.
minimal phototoxic erythema d.
minimal popular d.
minimal reacting d.
minimal urticarial d.
minimum effective d.
minimum effective naproxen d.
minimum hemolytic d.
minimum infective d.
minimum lethal d.
minimum reacting d.
minimum target absorbed d.
minimum tolerance d.
minimum toxic d.
d. modification
multiple d.
multiple dose vial
multiple scan average d.
nominal single d.
nominal standard d.
d. nonuniformity ratio
no observed effect d.
normal d.
normalized average glandular d.
normal single d.
occlusion dose monitor
off-axis dose inhomogeneity
optimal d.
optimal dose of chemotherapy
optimal dose selection
optimal immunomodulating d.
optimal therapeutic d.
optimum biologic d.
organ tolerance d.
paralyzing d.
pediatric d.
percentage depth d.
pharmacy to d.
precision high d.
pressor d.
provocation d.
psychoactive doses of hallucinogen
Quimby dose distribution system
radiation absorbed d.
radiation-absorbed d.
radiation dose limit
rad surface d.
real-time dose area product
d. reduction effectiveness factor
renal dose dopamine
repeated oral doses of activated charcoal
roentgen absorbed d.
roentgen administered d.
single dose suppression
single saturating d.
skin d.
skin epidermis dose radiation
skin erythema d.
skin test d.
skin unit d.
standard dose administration
standard test d.
suberythemal d.
test d.
threshold d.
threshold erythema d.
time interval between d.'s
tissue culture infectious d.
tissue culture infective d.
tissue culture inoculated d.
tissue tolerance d.
titrated initial d.
tolerance d.
total d.
total administered d.
total daily d.
total digitalizing d.
total dose infusion
total tumor d.
toxic d.
toxic dose, low
tumor dose fractionation
tumor lethal d.
tumor-producing d.
ultralow dose rate
unit d.
d. unit
very high dose phenobarbital
virtually safe d.
warfarin dose index

dose-intensity limiting criterion

dose-intensive chemotherapy

dose-limiting toxicity

dose-response curve

dose-volume histogram

dosimeter
chemical d.
electron beam d.
pencil d.
thermoluminescent dosimeter rod
transluminescent d.

dosimetry
cold spots and hot spots with electron beam d.
Fricke d.
marrow d.
penile bulb d.
d. and technique
x-ray d.

dosing
antimicrobial dosing regimen
around-the-clock d.
ATC d.
heparin dosing nomogram
neuroleptic d.
once-daily d.
pediatric dosing information
pharmacologic d.
tapered steroid dosing package
weight-based heparin dosing

dot
d. blot analysis
distortion of d.'s
d. ELISA test
d. hemorrhage
hemorrhagic d.
d. immunobinding
d. immunobinding assay
line frequency noise d.
Marcus Gunn d.
Maurer d.
Mittendorf d.
Morgan d.
multiple evanescent white dot syndrome
nuclear dot pattern
Schüffner d.
Trieger D. Test
Ziemann d.

double
d. aerosol face mask
Ann Arbor double towel clamp

double *(continued)*
antegrade double balloon-double wire technique
d. antibody solid phase
d. aortic arch
d. apical impulse
d. autograft
d. beta-lactam
d. bond
d. concave
d. convex
d. coronary artery graft
d. cup arthroplasty
d. decidual sac
delayed double diffusion test
deoxyribonucleic acid double stranded
d. diffusion
d. disharmonic hearing
dissociated double hypertropia
d. distilled water
d. dose
electron nuclear double resonance
esophageal-tracheal double lumen airway
d. filtration plasmapheresis
d. footling delivery
d. gloving
d. harelip
d. helix
d. immunodiffusion technique
d. indemnity
d. induction
intermittent double vision
d. isomorphous replacement
d. knee to chest
d. label index
long double upright brace
d. lumen
d. lumen subclavian catheter
d. lung transplant
d. membrane
d. minute chromosome
d. minute sphere
d. needle operation on cataract
Ouchterlony double diffusion
Ouchterlony double diffusion technique
perichondrial double cartilage block technique
d. radial immunodiffusion
radioimmunoassay double antibody test
d. radioisotope derivative
d. seated straight leg raise
short double upright
simultaneous double kidney transplantation
d. simultaneous recording
d. simultaneous stimulation
d. stapling technique
d. strength
d. subordinance
d. tachycardia
time required to double number of cells in given population
d. tongue
d. tracking of barium
d. umbrella
d. umbrella closure
d. umbrella device
d. valve replacement
d. vein graft
d. ventricular response
d. vibration
d. vision
d. vision from myasthenia gravis
d. vision with headache
d. wrap

double-armed mattress suture

double-balloon
d.-b. valvotomy
d.-b. valvuloplasty

double-barrel aorta

double-barreled colostomy

double-blind
d.-b. experiment
d.-b. placebo-controlled food challenge
d.-b. placebo-controlled randomized clinical trial
d.-b. procedure
d.-b. study

double-blinded trial

double-bubble
d.-b. appearance
d.-b. flushing reservoir

double-button suture

double-charge exchange

double-contrast
d.-c. barium enema
d.-c. barium examination of the upper gastrointestinal tract
d.-c. shoulder arthrography

double-dose
d.-d. delay
d.-d. gallbladder cholecystogram

double-dose–delay computed tomography

double-dummy technique

double-end
d.-e. flap
d.-e. graft

double-fusion fluorescent in situ hybridization

double-inlet ventricle

double-J
d.-J. catheter
d.-J. stent

double-limb progression

double-looped semitendinous and gracilis hamstring graft knee reconstruction technique

double-lumen
d.-l. breast implant
d.-l. catheter
d.-l. endobronchial tube

double-normal solution

double-outlet
d.-o. left ventricle
d.-o. right ventricle

double-sampling dye dilution technique

double-sheath bronchial brushing

double-shock sound

double-stapled ileoanal reservoir

double-step gait

double-stranded

double-vessel disease

doubling
carcinoembryonic antigen doubling time
cumulative population doubling level
mass doubling time
mean population d.
mortality rate doubling time
population doubling level
population doubling time
prostate-specific antigen doubling time
d. time
d. time of tumor size

doubly
d. clamped
d. clamped and divided
d. clamped, transected and stump ligated
d. labeled water
d. ligated

d. ligated and sectioned
d. ligated with transfixion suture

doubt
fear, uncertainty, and d.

doubting insanity

douche
fan d.

doughnut
d. configuration
d. headrest

doughy mass

Douglas
arcuate line of D.
D. cul-de-sac
line of D.
pouch of D.
D. pouch
D. virus

douloureux
dizziness from tic d.
tic d.

dovetail
d. joint osteotomy
lingual d.
occlusal d.

Dow
D. hollow fiber dialyzer
D. Hollow Fiber kidney

dowager's hump

dowel
d. arthrodesis
bone d.
d. bone graft
graft d.
d. graft
percutaneous autogenous dowel bone graft
d. spinal fusion

dowel-shaped bone graft

Dowling Degos disease

down
back pain extends down legs
bias flow d.
canal wall down mastoidectomy
canal wall down tympanomastoidectomy
canal wall down tympanoplasty
channel d.
congenital cataracts, sensorineural deafness, D. syndrome facial appearance, short stature, mental retardation syndrome
d. drain
incision carried down to the fracture site
milk let d.
morbus D.
pain down left arm
pain down leg
pain down right arm
pain radiating down legs
slow down cancer growth
D. syndrome
D. syndrome child
taking down of adhesion

downgoing
Babinski downgoing bilaterally
plantar response d.
toes d.

downgrafting
maxillary d.

downhill
d. course
progressive downhill course

downsizing of hearing aid

downsloping
d. activity
d. palpebral fissure
d. ST-segment depression

downstream
d. regulatory element antagonistic modulator gene
d. venous pressure

down-turned mouth corners

downward
curved downward incision
d. deviation
d. displacement of apical impulse
d. drift
d. gaze
d. pen deflection

drafting
overlay d.

dragging
macular d.
optic disc d.

drag-to gait

drain
d. brought out through stab wound
down d.
fluted silicone d.
free d.
d. inserted
Mentor pre-cut d.
Mikulicz drain technique
nasobiliary d.
nasobiliary drain cholangiography
open fracture wound d.
percutaneous d.
d. placed into wound
surgical d.

drainable
Assura convex drainable pouch

drainage
d. about shunt site
afferent lymphatic d.
anomalous pulmonary venous d.
anomaly of drainage of pulmonary vein
antegrade ureteral d.
aqueous humor d.
articulated drainage catheter
ascites drainage tube
d. at incision site
autogenic d.
bedside d.
biliary drainage catheter
bronchial d.
bronchopulmonary segmental d.
d. of cerebral epidural space
chest percussion and postural d.
chest tube d.
closed bladder d.
closed pleural d.
closed urinary drainage bag with drip chamber
closed water seal drainage system
continuous d.
continuous bladder d.
continuous catheter d.
continuous suction d.
controlled extrahepatic biliary d.
dependent d.
drilling and d.
endoscopic nasobiliary d.
endoscopic retrograde biliary d.
endoscopic transpapillary cyst d.
external ventricular d.
glaucoma drainage device
d. of hematoma
incision and d.
incision and drainage of abscess
incision and drainage of blister
incision and drainage of cyst
incision and drainage of fistulous tract
incision and drainage of ischiorectal abscess
incision and drainage of paronychia
indwelling catheter d.
internal biliary d.
interrupted lymphatic d.

drainage *(continued)*
intrapleural sealed drainage unit
irrigation and d.
d., irrigation, fibrinolytic therapy
lymphatic drainage of genitalia
lymphatic drainage pattern
lymph node d.
manual lymph d.
mucociliary drainage pathway
nasobiliary drainage catheter
nasolacrimal drainage system
open flap d.
overside d.
partial anomalous pulmonary venous d.
passive chest d.
patent opening for bile d.
pattern of d.
percussion and postural d.
percutaneous abscess d.
percutaneous abscess and fluid d.
percutaneous antegrade biliary d.
percutaneous biliary d.
percutaneous catheter d.
percutaneous drainage of epididymal abscess
percutaneous external d.
percutaneous transhepatic d.
percutaneous transhepatic biliary d.
percutaneous transhepatic gallbladder d.
perinephric abscess d.
peripancreatic abdominal d.
portal venous and enteric drainage technique
postnasal d.
postnasal drainage syndrome
postural d.
postural drainage and clapping
postural drainage and percussion
postural drainage, percussion and vibration
primary peritoneal d.
d. of purulent material
purulent nasal d.
serosanguineous d.
straight d.
straight bag d.
straight gravity d.
d. subretinal fluid
suprapubic d.
tear drainage system
thoracic duct d.
total anomalous pulmonary venous d.
transmural d.
d. tube
water seal d.

drainage-enteric
percutaneous transhepatic biliary drainage-enteric feeding

drained
d. abscess
amniotic fluid drained and preserved

draining
d. abscess
d. fistula
gaping, draining sore
incisional site d.
d. infected nonunion
d. lymphatic bed
d. lymph node
d. otitis media
d. sinus

Draize
modified Draize test

dram
fluid d.
half a d.
liquid d.

drape
complete change of d.'s, gowns and instruments
foot d.
perineal prep and d.
short foot d.
sterile d.'s applied

draped
abdomen prepped and d.
abdomen scrubbed, prepped, and d.
operative field prepared and d.
operative field prepped and d.
patient is prepped and d.
patient is prepped and draped for surgery
patient is prepped and draped in usual sterile fashion
sterilely prepped and d.

Draw-A-Family test

Draw-A-Person
D.-A.-P. Screening Procedure for Emotional Disturbance
D.-A.-P. test

drawer
anterior drawer sign
anterior drawer stress radiograph
anterior rotary drawer test
anteroposterior drawer test
posterior drawer test
d. sign
d. test

drawing
automatic d.
d. of blood sample
copying d.'s
Copying D.'s with Landmarks
Family D. Depression Scale
Franck D. Completion Test
Goodenough Figure D.
Human Figure D.
Kinetic Family D.
line d.
mirror d.
pain d.

dread
sensation of intense d.

dream
anxiety d.
d. anxiety disorder
artificial d.
clairvoyant d.
counter-wish d.
d. elements
embarrassment d.
erotic d.
d. interpretation
manifest d.
parallel d.
pipe d.
recurring d.
terror d.
d. time

dreaming
amnesia for sleep and d.

dream-like image

drenching
hyperbaric oxygen d.
d. night sweats

dressed
cleaned, sutured, and d.

dressing
anorectal d.
bulky compression d.
burn dressing change
d. change
cold compressive d.
debridement and d.
donor site d.
dry d.
d. dry and intact
dry and occlusive d.
dry sterile d.
dry sterile dressing applied
fluff d.

fluffed gauze d.
highly permeable transparent d.
hydrocolloid d.
long-handled dressing reacher
maximum assistance for lower body d.
maximum assistance for upper body d.
minimal assistance for lower body d.
minimal assistance for upper body d.
moistened fine mesh gauze d.
motivation for cross d.
occlusive and dry d.
open wet d.
partial cross d.
patient independent in d.
patient independent in lower body d.
patient independent in upper body d.
plastic adhesive d.
polyurethane foam d.
pressure d.
pressure dressing applied
sterile d.
sterile dressing applied
sterile dry d.
d. and stockinette applied
tap water wet d.
thin film d.
vacuum-assisted closure dressing
vascular access d.
wet d.
wound dressing emulsion

DREZotomy
microsurgical D.

dribble
postmicturition d.
postvoid d.

dribbling
d. at end of urination
involuntary dribbling of urine
d. on urination
postvoid dribbling of urine
terminal d.

dried
d. blood stain
d. skim milk
typhoid vaccine, acetone-killed and d.
typhoid vaccine, heat and phenol inactivated, d.

Driffield
Hunter and Driffield curve

drift
antigenic d.
arm d.
downward d.
field d.
mesial d.
observer d.
osseous d.
physiologic d.
radial d.
ulnar d.

drill
air-powered cutting d.
d. bit
d. bit fracture
bladder retraining d.
cannulated drill point
carbon steel drill point
diamond high-speed d.
femoral drill bit
high-speed air d.
d. hole
microsurgical drill system
offset drill hole
d. pin
d. sleeve

drilled
bur holes drilled in skull

drilling
d. broach
d. and drainage
excision, curettage and d.
d. jig
partial zona d.
zona d.

drink
date of last d.

drinker
heavy social d.'s
incurable problem d.
patient heavy d.
problem d.
d. respirator

drinker's
milk drinker's syndrome

drinking
Adolescent D. Index
aftereffect of d.
chronologic drinking record
emergency drinking water germicidal tablet
d. habit
has been d.
hazard of d.
Hilton D. Behavior Questionnaire
d. history
inability to control d.
long-term heavy d.
nocturnal drinking syndrome
Obsessive-Compulsive D. Scale
prolonged heavy d.
shock-induced suppression of d.
voluntarily stopping eating and d.

drinking-related aggressivity

drip
chronic postnasal d.
closed urinary drainage bag with drip chamber
continuous drip feeding
continuous gastric d.
d. infusion
d. infusion cholangiography
d. infusion technique
d. infusion valve
intravenous d.
intravenous Pitocin d.
nasal drip pad
nasogastric drip feeding
Pitocin intravenous d.
postnasal d.
postnasal drip due to rhinitis
postnasal drip due to sinusitis
postnasal drip syndrome
d. rate of infusion
slow intravenous d.
sterile water gastric d.

drip-infusion
d.-i. cholangiogram
d.-i. cholangiography
d.-i. pyelogram

drive
achievement d.
basic drive cycle length
fundamental human d.
heightened sexual d.
hypoxic ventilatory d.
stimulus d.
Szondi Experimental Diagnostics of D.'s

driven equilibrium Fourier transform

drivenness
organic d.

driver
d. of automobile
blade plate d.
impaired d.'s
nail d.
remove intoxicated d.
D. Risk Inventory
d. tunnel locator apparatus

drivethrough sign

driving
- critical frequency of photic d.
- osmotic driving agent
- d. under the influence of drugs
- d. under the influence of intoxicants
- d. while impaired
- d. while intoxicated

dromotropic
- negatively d.

dromotropism
- negative d.

droop
- facial d.
- lid d.
- nasolabial d.
- neck d.

drop
- akinetic drop attack
- atonic drop attack
- dual drop pelvis
- egg drop syndrome
- d. hand
- hanging d.
- hanging drop examination
- head d.
- d. heart
- lubricating d.'s
- Luride D.'s
- Micro D. yeast identification system
- navicular drop test
- nose d.'s
- oil drop change
- oil drop lesion
- oil drop sign
- open drop anesthesia
- open drop technique
- Pearl D.'s
- d.'s per minute
- d. shoulder
- voltage d.
- wrist d.

drop-arm
- d.-a. sign
- d.-a. test

drop-foot
- d.-f. gait
- d.-f. procedure

droplet
- climatic droplet keratopathy
- colloid d.
- cytoplasmic lipid d.
- macrovesicular fat d.
- secretion d.

dropout
- myofibrillar d.
- nerve fiber layer d.
- D. Prediction and Prevention

dropped
- d. beat
- periodic dropped beat

dropsy
- cardiac d.
- nutritional d.
- peritoneal d.

Drosophila
- *Drosophila* A, C, P, X virus

drowned
- d. lung
- d. newborn syndrome

drowning
- near d.

drowsiness
- continuous daytime d.
- drug-induced morning d.
- d. from antihistamine
- d. from glomerulonephritis
- d. from sleep apnea
- d. monitoring device

Drucker
- Lucas and Drucker Motor Index

drug
- d. absorption
- d. abuse reporting program
- D. Abuse Screening Test
- d. abuse urine
- D. Abuse Warning Network
- acute treatment for acute drug intoxication
- d. addict
- addictive illicit d.
- adjuvant analgesic d.
- adjuvant drug therapy
- d. administration device
- Adolescent D. and Alcohol Diagnostic Assessment
- adolescent drug abuse
- adolescent drug abuse unit
- adolescent drug use
- adverse drug effect
- adverse drug reaction
- d. aerosol
- AIDS D. Assistance Program
- alcohol and d.'s
- alcohol and d.'s
- d. and alcohol abuse death
- d. and alcohol dependence
- alcohol or drug abuse
- alcohol and drug dependence unit
- alcoholism and drug abuse
- alcohol and other drug abuse
- alcohol, tobacco, and other d.'s
- allergic drug reaction
- d. allergy
- alpha-adrenergic blocking d.
- alpha-adrenergic stimulating d.
- d. analysis laboratory
- antiarrhythmic d.
- antibiotic antitumor d.
- anticonvulsant d.
- antidepressant drug hepatotoxicity
- antiepileptic drug hypersensitivity syndrome
- antifungal drug therapy
- antihypertensive d.
- antiinflammatory d.
- antimonial drug therapy for leishmaniasis
- antineoplastic drug hepatotoxicity
- antiparasitic drug therapy
- antipsychotic d.
- antipsychotic drug hepatotoxicity
- antipsychotic drug therapy
- antipsychotic drug treatment
- antithyroid d.
- antithyroid drug hepatotoxicity
- antithyroid drug therapy
- approved drug product
- atypical antipsychotic d.
- autonomic sympathomimetic d.
- birth control d.
- cardiovascular complications of drug abuse
- cardiovascular problems related to drug abuse
- casual drug user
- cause of drug abuse
- d. of choice
- clinical manifestation of acute drug intoxication
- clinical manifestation of drug reaction
- clot busting d.
- clot dissolving d.
- clot dissolving thrombolytic d.
- combination d.
- combined drug and radiation modality
- complication of drug abuse
- computerized pharmacokinetic model-driven drug infusion
- controlled heat-aided drug delivery
- curb intravenous use of d.'s

cutaneous signs of drug abuse
dangerous d.
Dangerous D.'s Act
death due to drug abuse
d. dependence
d. dependence treatment program
differential diagnosis in acute drug intoxication
d. discontinuation
disease-modifying d.
disease-modifying antirheumatic d.
d. dose intensity
driving under the influence of d.'s
dual drug addiction
early clinical drug evaluation unit
early intervention in drug abuse
economic costs of drug abuse
effective anticancer d.
effective drug duration
d. efficacy study implementation
electromotive drug administration
d. eruption dermatitis
d. evaluation
d. evaluation matrix
exanthematous drug rash
excessive drug use
d.'s, exercise, education, diet, and self-monitoring
extreme drug resistance
fatal complications of illicit drug use
Federal Food, D., and Cosmetic Act
d. fever
final drug evaluation
fixed drug eruption
fixed ratio combination d.'s
forensic urine drug testing
d. free
d. habit
halfway house for drug addicts
hallucinatory state induced by d.
hallucinogenic drug interaction
hallucinogenic drug intoxication
hard core drug abuser
hard drug usage
hazard of d.'s
hazard of d.'s
heart rhythm d.
hepatic complications of drug abuse
hepatic drug metabolism
hepatic problems related to drug abuse
herb drug interaction
histoculture drug response assay
d. hypersensitivity
idiosyncratic drug reaction
illegal drug traffic
illegal intravenous drug use
illicit drug abuse
illicit drug use
immunomodulating antirheumatic d.
immunosuppressive d.
immunosuppressive drug therapy
impaired employee alcohol and drug treatment issue
implantable drug infusion pump
inactive dummy d.
incidence of drug abuse
indirect drug effect
infant of drug abusing mother
infected intravenous drug needle
d. information
d. information center
d. information log
d. infusion
d. ingestion
ingestion of d.
ingestion of toxic d.
initial drug screening test
injecting drug user
injection drug user
inpatient drug treatment
intense psychoactive drug effect
d. intervention program
d. intolerance
intolerance to specific d.'s
intolerance to specific d.'s
d. intoxication
intranasal drug intake
intraperitoneal drug administration
intrathecal drug infusion
intrauterine drug exposure
intravenous drug abuse
intravenous drug use
intravesical electromotive drug administration
investigational drug data form
investigational drug data sheet
investigational new animal d.
kicking drug habit
known drug allergies
d. level
lichenoid drug eruption
life-threatening drug interaction
liposome drug delivery
long-acting drug
long-acting antirheumatic d.
low-hepatic clearance d.
maintenance drug therapy
marrow toxic d.
master drug list
D. Master File
maternal drug abuse
maximal drug concentration
maximum residue limits of veterinary d.'s
medical history as screening device for drug abuse
mind-altering d.
multistate drug distribution ring
narcotic agonist d.
narcotic antagonist d.
narcotic blockade d.
narcotic blocking d.
narcotic drug dependence
National Collegiate Athletic Association drug testing policy
National Collegiate Athletic Association prohibited d.
neonatal complications of drug abuse
neonatal drug addiction seizure
neuroleptic antipsychotic d.
neuromuscular blocking d.
neuromuscular complication of drug abuse
neuromuscular disorder-causing d.
new d.
newborn drug toxicity
newborn drug withdrawal
new drug therapy
new-generation antipsychotic d.
New and Nonofficial D.'s
nitrous oxide-donor d.
no known drug allergies
nonimmediate-type immunologic drug reaction
nonimmunologic drug reaction
nonprescription drug abuse
nonprescription drug addiction
nonsteroidal antiinflammatory d.
nonsteroidal antiinflammatory drug gastropathy
nosotropic drug dementia of Alzheimer type
novel antipsychotic d.
online prospective drug utilization review
d.'s only
oral administered d.
oral diabetes d.
oral drug therapy
oral steroid d.
outpatient drug treatment
d. overdose
overdosed with multiple d.'s
over-the-counter drug abuse

drug *(continued)*
over-the-counter drug addiction
over-the-counter nonprescription d.
overuse of d.'s
overuse of d.'s
parenteral drug abuser
parenteral drug administration
pathologic drug intoxication
pathologic drug intoxication drug psychosis
patient education on drug abuse
patient's drug history
PCP drug abuse
periocular drug sensitivity
photoallergic drug reaction
photon-activated drug delivery system
physical effects of drug abuse
physician drug abuse
placebo-controlled drug study
pleiotropic drug resistance
potentially harmful d.
prenatal abuse of illicit d.
prenatally exposed to d.'s
prescription d.
prescription drug abuse
prescription drug addiction
prescription drug dependence
pressure lowering d.
primary drug resistance
D. Product Information File
d. prophylaxis
prospective drug review
psychedelic drug ingestion
psychoactive drug abuse
psychotropic d.
radioactive drug research committee
radiopharmaceutical drug product
d. rash
d. reaction-monitoring system
d. receptor
d. regimen
d. regimen review
remission-inducing d.
d. resistance
d. screen blood
second-line d.
selective apoptotic antineoplastic d.'s
self-administration of psychoactive d.
self-administration of psychotropic d.
serum drug concentration
serum drug level
sexual complications of drug abuse
sharing infected intravenous drug needle
slow-acting antirheumatic d.
social history as screening device for drug abuse
spheroidal oral drug absorption system
subacute treatment of acute drug intoxication
sulfur-carbon d.
surgical complication of drug abuse
suspected adverse drug reaction
symptom of drug abuse
symptoms of acute drug intoxication
therapeutic drug assay
therapeutic drug monitoring
d. tolerance
d. toxicity
toxicity or drug interaction
treatment of acute drug reaction to hallucinogen
d. treatment group
tricyclic antidepressant d.
United States Pharmacopeia D. Information
urine drug panel
d. use evaluation
d. use monitoring
d. use review
in utero drug exposure
warning sign of drug abuse
d. withdrawal insomnia

drug-affected
d.-a. baby
d.-a. kid

drug/alcohol addiction

drug-associated
d.-a. fatality
d.-a. primary acute pancreatitis

drug-dependent illness

drug-drug interaction

drug-exposed baby

drug-food interaction

drug-impaired
d.-i. baby
d.-i. child

drug-induced
d.-i. abortion
d.-i. agranulocytosis
d.-i. amenorrhea
d.-i. antinuclear antibodies
d.-i. blood cytopenias
d.-i. cicatricial conjunctivitis
d.-i. delayed multiorgan hypersensitivity syndrome
d.-i. dementia
d.-i. disease
d.-i. esophageal damage
d.-i. esophagitis
d.-i. galactorrhea
d.-i. hallucination
d.-i. hallucinosis
d.-i. heartburn
d.-i. hepatic encephalopathy
d.-i. hepatic injury
d.-i. hyperplasia
d.-i. immune anemia
d.-i. liver disease
d.-i. lupus
d.-i. lupus erythematosus
d.-i. lupus syndrome
d.-i. lymphocyte stimulation test
d.-i. morning drowsiness
d.-i. movement disorders
d.-i. parkinsonism
d.-i. postanesthetic depression
d.-i. postanesthetic respiratory depression
d.-i. renal disease
d.-i. skin reactions
d.-i. thrombocytopenia

drug-metabolizing enzyme

drug-prescribing index

drug-related
d.-r. admission
d.-r. adverse patient event
d.-r. impairment
d.-r. infection
d.-r. involuntary movement
d.-r. lupus
d.-r. morbidity
d.-r. neutropenia
d.-r. problem
d.-r. thrombocytopenia

drug-resistant
multiple d.-r.
d.-r. plasmid
d.-r. *Streptococcus pneumoniae*

drug-seeking
d.-s. behavior
d.-s. index

drug-sensitive cancer

drug-taking behavior

drug-using peer group

drum
canal and d.

intact d.
optokinetic d.

Drummond
artery of D.
marginal artery of D.

drunk
highly probably d.

drunkenness
alcoholic d.
pathologic d.

drusen
macular d.
maculopathy
nerve head d.
optic disc d.
optic disc drusen calcification
optic disc drusen retinopathy
optic nerve d.
soft d.
soft drusen maculopathy

dry
ambient temperature and pressure, d.
aqua PT dry physiotherapy
body temperature, pressure, d.
d. body weight
d. bulb
d. bulb temperature
d. crackling sound
d. dressing
dressing dry and intact
early dry breakfast
estimated dry weight
d. eye symptom
fat-free dry weight
d. gangrene
d. gas fractional concentration
d. hacking cough
d. heaves
d. hernia
high dry field
incision clean and d.
d. itching skin
d. joint
d. macular degeneration
d. matter
d. mouth from antihistamine
mucus membranes d.
d. and occlusive dressing
occlusive and dry dressing
oral mucosa d.
oral mucous membrane d.
d. powder inhaler
d. rale
d. skin and hair
standard temperature and pressure, d.
d. sterile dressing
d. sterile dressing applied
sterile dry dressing
d. sterile fluff
d. sterile gauze
d. swallow
target dry weight
warm and d.
d. to wet

dry-filled capsule

drying
critical point d.
d. and wrinkling of skin

dryness
redness, dryness and itching

DSM
Structured Clinical Interview for D.

D-transposition of great arteries

du
cri du chat
cri du chat syndrome
mal perforant du pied

dual
anterior-posterior dual energy radiography
aqueous synthetic dual phenolic disinfectant
d. asthmatic reaction
d. balloon perfusion catheter
d. chamber
d. chamber pacemaker implantation
d. demand pacemaker
d. diagnosis
d. diagnosis patient
d. diagnosis program
d. disorder
d. drop pelvis
d. drug addiction
d. lock total hip replacement
d. pacing
d. pathology
d. percutaneous endoscopic gastrostomy
d. therapy
d. ventricle

dual-chambered
d.-c. implant
d.-c. prosthesis

dual-chamber rate-responsive

dual-coil imaging

dual-contrast
d.-c. barium enema
d.-c. study

dual-diagnosis patient

dual-energy
d.-e. radiograph
d.-e. x-ray absorptiometry scan

dualism
mind-body d.
molecular d.

dual-isotope simultaneous acquisition single-photon emission computed tomography

dual-lumen catheter

dually diagnosed

dual-mode, dual-pacing, dual-sensing pacemaker

dual-photon
d.-p. absorptiometry
d.-p. densitometry
d.-p. x-ray absorptiometry

Duane syndrome retraction

Dubois
D. oleic albumin complex
D. oleic serum complex

Dubowitz
neonatal maturity classification of D.
D. score

Duchenne
D. de Boulogne muscular dystrophy
D. de Boulogne muscular dystrophy/Becker muscular dystrophy
D. muscular atrophy
D. muscular dystrophy

Duchenne-Aran muscular atrophy

Duchenne-Griesinger disease

Duchenneís muscular dystrophy

duck
d. hepatitis B
d. embryo fibroblast
d. embryo origin vaccine
d. embryo virus
d. hepatitis B virus
rabies vaccine, duck embryo culture
d. virus enteritis

duckbill
d. forceps
d. voice prosthesis

duct
alveolar d.
ampulla of lacrimal d.
ampulla of lactiferous d.
ampulla of milk d.
anatomic bile duct variant
anicteric bile d.
anomalous junction of pancreaticobiliary d.'s
anomalous junction of the pancreatobiliary d.
anomalous pancreatobiliary duct junction
anterior semicircular d.
antithoracic duct lymphocytic globulin
arborization of d.'s
arborization of d.
arch of thoracic d.
asymmetric bile d.
atretic extrahepatic bile duct resection
Bartholin gland duct cyst
benign bile duct stricture
bile d.
bile duct adenoma
bile duct catheter
bile duct epithelia
d. of Botallo
catheterization lacrimonasal d.
chronic bile duct ligation
collecting d.
collecting duct carcinoma
common d.
common bile d.
common bile duct diverticulum
common bile duct exploration
common bile duct microlithiasis
common bile duct obstruction
common bile duct stent
common bile duct stone
common bile duct stricture
common duct exploration
common duct pigment stone
common hepatic d.
congenital nasolacrimal duct obstruction
cortical collecting d.
cribriform salivary carcinoma of excretory d.
d. of Cuvier
cystic d.
dilated bile d.
distal bile duct carcinoma
donor hepatic d.
exploration of common bile d.
extrahepatic bile d.
extrahepatic bile duct atresia
Gartner duct cyst
hepatic duct stone
hyperplasia of d.'s
inferior lacrimal d.
inner medullary collecting d.
intrahepatic bile d.
laparoscopic common duct exploration
laparoscopic exploration of the common bile d.
laparoscopic transcystic common bile duct exploration
large bile d.
left hepatic d.
longitudinal duct of epoöphoron
Luschka d.'s
Luschka duct leak
main d.
main duct of Wirsung
main pancreatic d.
main papillary d.
major sublingual d.
male genital d.
male genital duct development
mammary duct ectasia
mammary duct obstruction
mechanical duct obstruction
medullary ducts of Bellini
medullary collecting d.
medullary duct epithelium
membranous ampullae of the semicircular d.
membranous limb of semicircular d.
middle extrahepatic bile d.
mucinous duct ectasia
Müller duct body
müllerian duct anomaly
müllerian duct cyst
müllerian duct derivation syndrome
müllerian duct derived structure
müllerian duct fusion
müllerian duct inhibitory factor
müllerian duct syndrome
müllerian duct, unilateral renal agenesis, and anomalies of the cervicothoracic somites
multifocal infiltrated duct cell carcinoma
muscle of common bile d.
narrowing of common d.
nasolacrimal d.
nasolacrimal duct probe
nasopalatine duct cyst
nonsyndromic bile duct paucity
normal caliber d.
obstruction of d.
occluded common bile d.
occluded common bile duct stone
omphalomesenteric duct cyst
omphalomesenteric duct remnant
open d.
open common bile duct exploration
opening of left parotid d.
pancreatic d.
pancreatic duct branch
pancreatic duct cell carcinoma
pancreatic duct dilatation
pancreatic duct disruption
pancreatic duct encasement
pancreatic duct hyperplasia
pancreatic duct manipulation
pancreatic duct obstruction
pancreatic duct sphincterotomy
pancreatic duct stone
pancreatic duct stricture
papillary bile duct stenosis
papillary collecting d.
papillary duct of Bellini
paramesonephric duct cyst
parotid duct ligation
parotid duct transposition
patent pancreatic d.
patent vitelline d.
paucity of interlobular bile d.'s
percutaneous dilatation of biliary d.
perforation of common bile d.
peripheral bile d.
periurethral duct carcinoma
persistent müllerian duct syndrome
primary acquired nasolacrimal duct obstruction
probing of lacrimal d.
proximal bile d.
right hepatic d.
salivary duct cyst
salivary duct obstruction
segmental bile duct fibrosis
sphincter of bile d.
sphincter of common bile d.
Stensen d.
subareolar duct papillomatosis
submandibular duct calculus
superior lacrimal d.
thoracic d.
thoracic duct drainage

thoracic duct fistula
thoracic duct flow
thoracic duct lymphocyte
thoracic duct pressure
thoracic lymphatic d.
thyroglossal d.
thyroglossal duct carcinoma
transcystic d.
vitellointestinal d.
d. of Wirsung
wolffian duct carcinoma

ductal
d. abnormality
anomalous arrangement of pancreaticobiliary ductal system
anomalous pancreaticobiliary ductal union
apocrine ductal carcinoma in situ
argyrophilic ductal carcinoma in situ
atypical ductal hyperplasia
d. carcinoma in situ
endocrine ductal carcinoma in situ
d. glandular mastectomy
d. hyperplasia
infiltrating ductal carcinoma
infiltrating ductal carcinoma of the breast
infiltrating ductal cell carcinoma
intrahepatic ductal dilation
invasive ductal carcinoma
d. lavage fluid
microsurgical extraction of ductal sperm
mucinous ductal ectasia of the pancreas
neuroendocrine ductal carcinoma in situ
pancreatic ductal adenocarcinoma
pancreatic ductal hypertension
pancreatic ductal morphological change
pancreaticobiliary ductal junction
pancreaticobiliary ductal system
poorly differentiated ductal carcinoma
d. shunt
terminal ductal lobular unit

ductectatic
mucinous ductectatic tumor of pancreas

duction
ocular d.
passive d.
passive forced duction test
d.'s and versions

ductlike structure

ductogram
mammary d.
mammary ductogram imaging
pancreatic d.

ductography
pancreaticobiliary d.

duct-to-duct

ductular
atypical ductular cell

ductule
efferent d.
proliferating bile d.'s

ductus
d. arteriosus
artery to ductus deferens
calcified ductus arteriosus
d. deferens tumor
fetal ductus arteriosus constriction
mucosa of ductus deferens
muscular coat of ductus deferens
muscular layer of ductus deferens
papilla ductus parotidei
patent d.
patent ductus venosus
persistent ductus arteriosus
premature ductus arteriosus closure
reversed ductus arteriosus
right ductus arteriosus

due
anxiety due to physical disorder
anxiety due to a substance
ascites due to bile leak
d. date
death due to drug abuse
dementia due to Creutzfeldt-Jakob disease
dementia due to head trauma
dementia due to hepatic condition
dementia due to multiple etiologies
dementia due to traumatic brain injury
dementia due to vitamin deficiency
eclampsia due to uremia
estimated due date
hydrocephalus due to congenital stenosis of aqueduct of Sylvius
mental disorder due to alcoholism
mental disorder due to a general medical condition
mood disorder due to a general medical condition
postnasal drip due to rhinitis
postnasal drip due to sinusitis
stroke due to cerebral hemorrhage
sudden death due to cocaine ingestion
tenderness in abdomen due to hepatitis
d. to void

Duffy
D. antigen A, B positive phenotype
D. antigen A negative phenotype
D. antigen B negative phenotype

Dugbe virus

Duke
D. Activity Status Index
D. classification of carcinoma
D. treadmill prognostic score

Dukes
Astler-Coller modification of Dukes classification
D. classification
D. stage
D. staging

Dulbecco
D. modified Eagle medium
D. phosphate-buffered saline

dull
d. abdominal pain
d. aching pain
borderline d.
d. curettage
diffuse dull, aching pressure discomfort
d. epigastric pain
d. and lethargic
d. on questioning
d. psychopathy

dullness
absolute cardiac d.
area of cardiac d.
borderline of cardiac d.
cardiac d.
cardiac border of d.
left border of cardiac d.
left border dullness of heart to percussion
left lower border of cardiac d.
d. on percussion
d. over left lung
d. over right lung
d. to percussion
relative area of cardiac d.

dullness *(continued)*
relative hepatic d.
retromanubrial d.
right border cardiac d.
right lower border of cardiac d.
right manubrial d.
submanubrial d.

duly authorized officer

dummy
anthropomorphic test d.
inactive dummy drug

dumping
d. of barium meal
late dumping syndrome
d. provocation test
d. syndrome

duodenal
acute duodenal ulcer
anterior duodenal ulcer
aortograft duodenal fistula
apex of duodenal bulb
apical duodenal ulcer
arteriomesenteric duodenal compression syndrome
d. bulb
d. bulb scarring
d. bulb and sweep
d. cap
coarsening of duodenal bulb
congenital duodenal atresia
congenital duodenal obstruction
endoscopically assisted duodenal intubation
d. exclusion
extramucosal duodenal myotomy
healing duodenal ulcer
intraluminal duodenal diverticulum
intramural duodenal hematoma
d. irritability
irritable duodenal bulb
major duodenal papilla
malignant duodenal tumor
microcephaly, oculodigital, esophageal, duodenal syndrome
minor duodenal papilla
mosaic duodenal mucosal pattern
d. mucosa
narrow duodenal opening
d. opening narrow
d. peptic ulcer disease
d. peptone infusion
perforated duodenal ulcer
periampullary duodenal diverticulum
periampullary duodenal tumor
polyp of duodenal bulb
refractory duodenal ulcer
d. secretin test
d. string test
superior duodenal flexure
superior duodenal fold
superior duodenal fossa
superior duodenal recess
thickened duodenal fold
d. ulcer perforation

duodenal-gastric reflux gastropathy

duodenitis
nonspecific nonerosive d.

duodenogastric reflux

duodenogastroesophageal reflux

duodenogastroscopy
retrograde d.

duodenography
hypotonic d.

duodenojejunal
d. hernia
d. junction

duodenopancreatectomy
partial d.

duodenoscope
master d.

duodenostomy
nasal duodenostomy tube

duodenum
ampulla of d.
anatomical position of d.
ascending part of d.
digital anomalies, short palpebral fissures, atresia of esophagus or duodenum syndrome
esophagus, stomach, and d.
flexure of d.
gallbladder anastomosed to d.
longitudinal fold of d.
malrotation of d.
mucous crypt of d.
polyp of d.
prompt spill into d.
stomach and d.
stomach, duodenum, and pancreas
suspensory ligament of d.

duodenum-preserving pancreatic head resection

duplex
d. B-mode Doppler
d. B-mode ultrasound
carotid duplex imaging
carotid duplex scan
carotid duplex study
carotid duplex ultrasonography
d. carotid imaging
d. carotid ultrasound
color-coded duplex sonography
color duplex imaging
color duplex ultrasonography
color duplex ultrasound
color-flow duplex imaging
color-flow duplex scan
d. color ultrasonography
d. Doppler imaging
d. Doppler scan
d. Doppler ultrasound
d. echocardiography
Ferribacterium d.
d. imaging
penile duplex ultrasonography
renal duplex scan
d. scan
d. scanner
serial duplex scan
d. sonography
transcranial color-coded duplex sonography
d. ultrasonography
venous duplex scanning

duplicated
partially duplicated ureter

duplication
alimentary tract d.
d. of colon
d. of esophagus
d. of left collecting system
d. of left kidney
mediastinal duplication cyst
pericardial duplication cyst
d. of right collecting system
d. of right kidney

Dupuytren
D. contracture
D. hydrocele

dura
arterial branch to dura mater
attenuated d.
cadaveric d.
d. dissector
effacement of d.
freeze-dried cadaveric d.
d. hook
lyophilized d.
lyophilized dura graft
d. mater
d. mater prosthesis
meningeal layer of dura mater
Olivecrona dura scissors
periosteal layer of dura mater

durable
d. medical equipment
d. power of attorney for health care

dural
d. arteriovenous fistula
d. arteriovenous malformation
d. carotid-cavernous fistula
d. cul-de-sac
d. graft
d. grafting
d. graft matrix
long dural tail
lyophilized dural patch
d. microclip
partial dural resection
d. punch
d. sac
d. shunt
spinal dural arteriovenous fistula

duration
d. of action
action potential d.
anodal d.
anodal duration contraction
anodal duration tetanus
arm duration maneuver
cathodal d.
character, onset, location, duration, exacerbation, remission
critical stimulus d.
cumulative duration of the first remission
cumulative duration of survival
deep sleep of short d.
effective drug d.
d. of ejection
d. of epoch
d. of expiration
exposure duration threshold
half amplitude pulse d.
increased overall treatment of d.
d. of inspiration
insufficient severity of d.
intensity/time duration of contractions
maximum duration of phonation
maximum duration of sustained blowing
maximum inhibiting d.
median duration of response
monophasic action potential d.
d. of positive pressure
prolonged contractile d.
pulse d.
short duration, unilateral, neuralgic, conjunctival injection and tearing
signal-averaged P-wave d.
d. of sleep interruption
d. of systole
d. of tetany
d. of voluntary apnea test

during
anxiety during pregnancy
care and treatment during pregnancy
cast stroking maneuver during massage
circular pressure maneuver during massage
contraction during labor
control of heart rate during oxygen deprivation
discharged during referral
ejection fraction during exercise
epilepsy with continuous spikes and waves during sleep
fan stroking maneuver during massage
heart shocked during cardiac arrest
multigated blood pool image during exercise
pain during urination
periodic limb movements during sleep
prognostically bad signs during pregnancy
psychosis during pregnancy
rearranged during transfection

durotomy
paramedian d.

duroxide uptake

durum
fibroma d.
heloma d.
osteoma d.
palatine d.
palatum d.
papilloma d.

dusky discoloration

dust
cotton dust asthma
house dust allergy
house dust mite
mineral dust airway disease
organic dust toxic syndrome

duty
d. cycle
discharge to d.
entry on d.
expanded duty dental auxiliary
injured on d.
light d.
line of d.
neglect of d.
not fit for d.
omission of d.
on d.
overseas d.
private duty nurse
released from active d.

dwarfism
alopecia, contracture, d.
alopecia, contracture, dwarfism, mental retardation syndrome
autosomal dominant mild short limb d.
microcephalic primordial dwarfism 1
mulibrey nanism or d.
osteodysplastic primordial d.
short limb d.

dyad
mother-child d.
parent-child d.

Dyadic
Marital Dyadic Inventory

dye
alizarin red S d.
argon-pumped dye laser
argon tuneable dye laser
delayed concentration of d.
d. disappearance test
double-sampling dye dilution technique
endoscopic pulsed dye laser
endoscopic pulsed dye laser lithotripsy
Evans blue d.
flashlamp pulsed dye laser
flashlamp-pumped pulsed dye laser
d. fluorescence index
d. free
indigo carmine d.
indocyanine green d.
injection of d.
liquid organic dye laser
Loeffler methylene blue d.
Lugol dye esophagoscopy
lunate facet dye punch injury
materials primary d.
methylene blue d.
methyl green pyronin dye

dye *(continued)*
microculture tetrazolium dye assay
Molulsky dye reduction test
NBT dye test
nitroblue tetrazolium d.
nitroblue tetrazolium dye test
oral cholecystographic d.
orange dye laser
organic anionic d.
patent blue V d.
pooling of d.
prompt excretion of d.
radioiodinated rose bengal d.
rose bengal d.
Sabin dye test
Sabin-Feldman dye test
thermal green d.
tracking d.

dye-binding capacity

dying
d. declaration
d. trajectory

Dyke Davidoff-Masson syndrome

dynamic
adjustable dynamic joint
androgen d.'s
d. aortic patch
ASIF broad dynamic compression
atrial bolus dynamic computed tomography
attachment d.
d. axial fixator
d. cardiac blood flow
chemically induced dynamic electron polarization
d. compliance of lung
d. compression
d. compression plate
d. compression plate fixation
d. computed tomography
computerized dynamic platform posturography
d. contrast-enhanced magnetic resonance imaging
eccentric dynamic compression plating
effective dynamic compliance
d. electrocardiogram
energetic dynamic cardiac insufficiency
d. enhanced magnetic resonance imaging
d. environmental conditioning cycle
d. equilibrium
d. finger exerciser
d. flow study
group d.'s
d. hip screw
d.'s of human behavior
d. hyperinflation
d. infusion cavernosometry and cavernosography
d. infusion pharmacocavemosometry
d. integrated stabilization chair
d. light scattering
d. locking nail
low-contact dynamic compression plate
medial hemispheric d.'s
monocular-estimate-method dynamic retinoscopy
d. movement of inertia
narcissistic d.'s
Neufeld dynamic method
d. nuclear polarization
d. optical breast imaging system
d. orthotic cranioplasty
pathogenesis d.
d. pedobarography
personality d.'s
D. Personality Inventory
d. physical activity
d. planar reconstructor
d. pulmonary imaging
d. random access memory
d. range control
d. renal scintigraphy
d. spatial reconstructor
specific dynamic action
specific dynamic effect
d. stabilizing innersole system
d. subaortic stenosis
d. susceptibility contrast
d. tone-reducing orthosis
d. two-point discrimination
d. ultrasound of shoulder
d. urinary graciloplasty
d. viscosity
d. visual acuity
d. wall walk
wide dynamic range compression

dynamism
lust d.
mental d.

dynamite
d. headache
d. heart

dynamometer
hand-held d.
handheld d.
Hand D. Test

dysalbuminemic
familial dysalbuminemic hyperthyroxinemia

dysarthria
apraxic d.
ataxic d.
ataxic and spastic d.
athetoid d.
athetosic d.
Frenchay D. Assessment
neurogenic d.
parkinsonian d.
peripheral d.
progressive d.
pure d.
sensory ataxic neuropathy with dysarthria and ophthalmoplegia
spastic d.

dysarthria-clumsy hand syndrome

dysarthric
Assessment of Intelligibility of D. Speech
patient d.
d. speech

dysarthrosis
patellofemoral d.

dysautonomia
familial d.

dysautonomic
d. feature
d. illness

dyschondroplasia
Ollier d.

dysconjugate
d. gaze
d. movement

dyscontrol
affective d.
Behavioral D. Scale
emotional dyscontrol disorder
impulse d.
impulse dyscontrol in eating disorder
organic d.
serious impulsive d.

dyscrasia
lymphatic d.
plasma cell d.
plasma cell dyscrasia of unknown significance

dysembryoplastic neuroepithelial tumor

dysentery
amebic d.
institutional d.
malarial d.
malignant d.
protozoal d.
schistosomal d.
scorbutic d.
Shigella d.
swine d.
typhoid d.
viral d.
winder d.

dysequilibrium syndrome

dyserythropoietic
congenital dyserythropoietic anemia types I–III

dysesthesia
d. disorder
palmar d.

dysesthetic pain syndrome

dysfluency
avoidance of speech d.

dysfunction
adult social d.
age-related diastolic d.
alcohol-induced sexual d.
alopecia, nail dystrophy, ophthalmic complication, thyroid dysfunction, hypohidrosis, ephelides and enteropathy, and respiratory tract infection
amphetamine-induced sexual d.
angiotensin-converting enzyme dysfunction syndrome
anorectal physiological d.
anorectal sensorimotor d.
anterior-inferior capsular ligament d.
anterior visual pathway d.
antipsychotic-associated sexual d.
anxiolytic-induced sexual d.
atrioventricular node d.
atypical psychosexual d.
autonomic nervous system d.
AV node d.
baroreflex d.
bilirubin-induced neurologic d.
biopsy-negative graft d.
bladder and bowel d.
bowel and bladder d.
brain d.
central audio vestibular d.
chorioretinopathy and pituitary d.
chronic fatigue and immune dysfunction syndrome
constitutional hepatic d.
corpus luteum d.
craniomandibular d.
end organ d.
erectile d.
eustachian tube d.
extensor mechanism d.
eye-tracking d.
familial autonomic d.
female sexual d.
global neurologic d.
higher cerebral d.
higher cortical d.
hypertonic uterine d.
immune dysfunction problem
intrinsic sphincter d.
lacrimal gland d.
left ventricular d.
left ventricular systolic d.
lingual airway d.
Logistic Organ D. Score
lower urinary tract d.
male erectile d.
male sexual d.
mandibular pain dysfunction syndrome
maternal postpartum thyroid d.
meibomian gland d.
metabolic disorder with hepatic d.
metabolic disorder with neurologic d.
minimal brain d.
minimal brain dysfunction syndrome
minimal cerebral d.
minor cerebral d.
minor neurologic d.
motor perception d.
multiorgan d.
multiple organ d.
multiple organ dysfunction syndrome
multiple organ system d.
neonatal thyroid d.
neurogenic bladder d.
neurogenic erectile d.
neurologic bladder d.
neurovesicle d.
neutrophil actin d.
nonspecific esophageal motor d.
optic nerve d.
organic brain d.
orofacial dysfunction syndrome
ovarian d.
ovarian steroidogenic d.
pain dysfunction syndrome
painful minor intervertebral d.
pancreatic exocrine d.
papillary muscle d.
paradoxical vocal fold d.
parathyroid gland d.
patellofemoral d.
pelvic floor d.
phagocytic dysfunction immunodeficiency
posterior tibial tendon d.
postictal cognitive d.
postoperative bladder d.
postparacentesis circulatory d.
postpartum thyroid d.
prosthetic valve d.
psychogenic erectile d.
reactive upper airways dysfunction syndrome
sexual d.
sexual dysfunction after heart attack
sinus node d.
small airway d.
somatic d.
somatic dysfunction lower extremity
somatic dysfunction upper extremity
sphincter of Oddi d.
spinal cord d.
suggested brain d.
syndrome of isolated diastolic d.
temporomandibular joint d.
temporomandibular joint-pain dysfunction syndrome
thyroid gland d.
velopharyngeal d.
vocal cord d.
vocal fold d.

dysfunctional
adult child of dysfunctional family
d. bleeding
disoriented and d.
d. group
heart dysfunctional episode
d. immune system
d. labor
obstructive dysfunctional ileitis
d. parenting style
primary dysfunctional labor
d. staff behavior
d. uterine bleeding
d. vaginal bleeding
d. voiding scoring system

dysgenesis
anterior chamber dysgenesis syndrome
autosomal congenital tubular d.
cerebroocular d.
chromosomal gonadal d.
gonadal d.
gonadal dysgenesis syndrome
gonadal dysgenesis of Turner type
mesodermal dysgenesis of anterior segment
mixed gonadal d.
partial gonadal d.
pure gonadal d.
renal tubular d.
reticular d.
thyroid d.

dysgenetic
d. fibrous band
d. male pseudohermaphroditism
multicystic dysgenetic kidney
d. polycystic disease

dysgerminoma
mediastinum d.
ovarian d.
parasellar d.

dysgnosia
auditory-verbal d.
number d.

dysharmonic luteal phase

dysjunction
pterygomaxillary d.

dyskaryosis index

dyskeratosis
d. congenita
hereditary benign intraepithelial d.
intraepithelial dyskeratosis syndrome, hereditary benign

dyskinesia
antipsychotic-induced tardive d.
belly dancer d.
buccolinguofacial d.
ciliary dyskinesia activity
covert d.
initial d.
neuroleptic-induced tardive d.
paroxysmal exertional d.
paroxysmal exertion-induced d.
paroxysmal hypnogenic d.
paroxysmal kinesigenic d.
paroxysmal nonkinesigenic d.
poststatic d.
primary ciliary d.
D. Rating Scale
tardive d.
withdrawal d.
withdrawal-emergent d.
without d.

dyskinetic
d. cilia syndrome
peak-dose choreoathetoid dyskinetic movement

dyslalia
organic d.

dyslexia
attentional d.
neglect d.

dyslipidemia
diabetic d.

dysmaturity
placental d.

dysmenorrhea
essential d.
mechanical d.
membranous d.
obstructive d.
ovarian d.
primary d.
psychogenic d.
secondary d.
spasmodic d.
uterine d.

dysmetabolic
cardiovascular dysmetabolic syndrome

dysmetria
cognitive d.
ocular d.
ocular dysmetria nystagmus
ocular dysmetria test
ocular motor d.

dysmigration
nephrosis-neuronal dysmigration syndrome

dysmorphia
mandibulo-oculofacial d.
Simpson dysmorphia syndrome

dysmorphic
Body D. Disorder Modification of Yale-Brown Obsessive-Compulsive Scale, McLean version
body dysmorphic disorder
d. facies
megalocornea, developmental retardation, dysmorphic syndrome

dysmorphism
craniofacial d.
craniofacial dysmorphism, absent corpus callosum, iris colobomas, connective tissue dysplasia syndrome
lobar d.
major d.
mental retardation, dysmorphism, cerebral atrophy syndrome
minor d.

dysmorphogenesis
otomandibular facial d.

dysmorphology
orbital d.

dysmotility
chronic intestinal d.
small bowel d.
d. syndrome

dysmyelopoietic syndrome

dysnomia
amnestic d.
autonomic d.

dysostosis
craniofacial d.
craniofrontonasal d.
Genée-Wiedemann acrofacial d.
mandibular dysostosis and peromelia
mandibulofacial d.
mandibulofacial dysostosis with epibulbar dermoids syndrome
mandibulofacial dysostosis with limb malformations syndrome
Nager acrofacial d.
nasal hypoplasia, peripheral dysostosis, mental retardation syndrome
peripheral dysostosis, nail hypoplasia, mental retardation syndrome
postaxial acrofacial dysostosis syndrome

dysotosis
mandibulofacial dysotosis syndrome

dyspareunia
deep d.
female d.
lifelong-type d.
male d.
male dyspareunia male erectile disorder
psychogenic d.

dyspepsia
appendicular d.
appendix d.

atonic d.
chichiko d.
gastric d.
Glasgow D. Severity Score
intestinal d.
mononuclear d.
nervous d.
nonulcer d.
psychogenic d.
recurrent nonulcer d.
reflux d.
ulcer d.

dyspeptica
angina d.

dysperception
metabolic d.

dysphagia
Atkinson scoring system for d.
chronic esophageal d.
contractile ring d.
liquid food d.
malignant d.
motility-related d.
nervous d.
neurogenic d.
nonneurogenic d.
oropharyngeal d.
receptive d.
recurrent d.
sideropenic d.

dysphagic
patient d.

dysphalangism
brachymorphism, onychodysplasia, d.

dysphasia
cementoosseous d.
local cementoosseous d.

dysphonia
abductor spasmodic d.
adductor spasmodic d.
spasmodic d.
spastic d.

dysphoria
intense episodic d.
neuroleptic-induced d.

dysphoric
late luteal phase dysphoric disorder

dysplasia
acromandibular d.
anal sphincter d.
angel-shaped phalangoepiphyseal d.
anhidrotic congenital ectodermal d.
anhidrotic ectodermal d.
ankyloblepharon, ectodermal dysplasia, clefting syndrome
anteroposterior facial d.
antihidrotic ectodermal d.
arrhythmogenic right ventricular d.
arteriohepatic d.
arthrogryposis, ectodermal dysplasia, cleft lip/palate developmental delay syndrome
asphyxiating thoracic d.
asphyxiating thoracic dysplasia syndrome
autoimmune polyendocrinopathy, candidiasis, ectodermal d.
axial mesodermal dysplasia complex
azoospermia, renal anomaly, cervicothoracic spine d.
basal cell d.
bronchopulmonary d.
caudal dysplasia syndrome
cementoosseous d.
chondroectodermal d.
colposcopic grading of cervical d.
congenital dysplasia of hip
congenital hip d.
congenital hyperphosphatasemic skeletal d.
congenital thymic d.
cranioectodermal d.
craniofacial dysmorphism, absent corpus callosum, iris colobomas, connective tissue dysplasia syndrome
craniofrontonasal d.
curly hair-ankyloblepharon-nail dysplasia syndrome
deafness, femoral epiphysial dysplasia, short stature, developmental delay syndrome
dental enamel dysplasia syndrome
developmental dysplasia of hip
ectodermal d.
ectodermal dysplasia, cleft lip and palate, mental retardation, syndactyly syndrome I, II
ectodermal dysplasia, ectrodactyly, macular dystrophy syndrome
ectodermal and mesodermal dysplasia with osseous involvement ectodermal dysplasia-central
ectrodactyly, ectodermal dysplasia, clefting syndrome
endocervical glandular d.
facial dysplasia, hyperextensibility of joints, clinodactyly, growth retardation, mental retardation syndrome
fibrocystic d.
fibromuscular d.
fibrous d.
fibrous dysplasia of the mandible
florid local cementoosseous d.
focal cementoosseous d.
focal facial dermal dysplasia II
frontometaphyseal d.
frontonasal d.
hereditary bone d.
high-grade d.
hydrocephalus, agyria, retinal dysplasia with or without encephalocele syndrome
hypohidrotic ectodermal d.
hypohidrotic ectodermal dysplasia with hypothyroidism
inherited epidermal d.
intestinal neuronal d.
lateral facial d.
lichenoid d.
liver cell d.
low-grade d.
lymphopenic thymic d.
mammary d.
Margarita Island type ectodermal d.
mental retardation, epilepsy, short stature, skeletal dysplasia syndrome
mental retardation, skeletal dysplasia, abducens palsy syndrome
microscopic cortical d.
mild acetabular d.
mixed sclerosing bone dysplasia, small stature, seizures, mental retardation syndrome
monostotic fibrous d.
multicystic d.
multicystic renal d.
multiple epiphysial d.
multiple epiphysial dysplasia tarda syndrome
necrotic facial d.
neonatal osseous d.
neurogenic dysplasia of hip
neurogenic hip d.
occipital d.

dysplasia *(continued)*
occipital cortical dysplasia of Taylor
occipito-faciocervico-thoraco-abdomino-digital dysplasia
oculodentoosseous d.
optic disc d.
optic nerve d.
orbitozygomaticomaxillary fibrous d.
osteodental d.
otospondylometaphyseal d.
pelvis capsular d.
periapical cemental d.
peripheral cemental d.
polyostotic fibrous d.
postradiation d.
primary adrenocortical micronodular d.
primary adrenocortical nodular d.
pulmonary valve d.
skeletal dysplasia in fetus
split hand-cleft lip/palate and ectodermal d.
spondyloepimetaphyseal dysplasia with joint laxity
spondyloepiphyseal d.
spondyloepiphyseal dysplasia congnita
vaginal intraepithelial d.
valves, unilateral reflux, d.
ventricular radial d.

dysplasia-associated lesion or mass

dysplasia-central
ectodermal and mesodermal dysplasia with osseous involvement ectodermal d.-c.

dysplastic
epidermal dysplastic verruciformis
familial dysplastic nevus syndrome
high-grade dysplastic adenoma
d. nevus
d. nevus syndrome

dyspnea
d. and anasarca
Baseline D. Index
cough, dyspnea and headache
exertional d.
external d.
d. and flushing
increased dyspnea on exertion
increasing weakness, debility, and d.
d. index
d. on exercise
d. on exertion
onset of d.
paroxysmal dyspnea on exertion
paroxysmal nocturnal d.
postexertional d.
Pulmonary Functional Status and D. Questionnaire

dyspneic
patient d.

dyspraxia
limb-kinetic d.

dysproteinemia
angioimmunoblastic lymphadenopathy with d.

dysraphism
occult d.
spinal d.
tracheoesophageal d.

dysreactivity
autonomic d.

dysreflexia
autonomic d.

dysregulation
affective d.
anger d.
autonomic d.
limbic d.
neurologic d.

dysrhythmia
idiopathic paroxysmal cerebral d.
paroxysmal cerebral d.

dysrhythmic
d. aggressive behavior
d. movement

dysrrhythmia
cardiac d.

dyssomnia
circadian rhythm d.

dyssynchronous
rapid dyssynchronous depolarization

dyssynergia
detrusor d.
detrusor external sphincter d.
detrusor sphincter d.
pelvic floor d.
vesical external sphincter d.

dystaxia
heel-to-knee d.

dysthymic
alternative criterion B for dysthymic disorder
d. disorder

dystocia
all-fours maneuver for shoulder d.
arrest of active phase d.
arrest of descent d.
maternal d.
placental d.
shoulder d.

dystonia
cervical d.
dopa-responsive d.
golfer's focal d.
neurocirculatory d.
neuroleptic-induced acute d.
nocturnal paroxysmal d.
oromandibular d.
torsion d.

dystonia-improvement-dystonia

dystonic
acute dystonic reaction
mental retardation, dystonic movements, ataxia, seizures syndrome
d. phenomenon
d. reaction

dystopia
orbital d.
pituitary d.

dystrophic
d. epidermolysis bullosa
recessive dystrophic epidermolysis bullosa

dystrophy
alopecia, nail dystrophy, ophthalmic complication, thyroid dysfunction, hypohidrosis, ephelides and enteropathy, and respiratory tract infection
annular macular d.
anterior basement membrane d.
anterior corneal d.
anterior membrane d.
Aran-Duchenne muscular d.
asphyxiating thoracic d.
atonic sclerotic muscle d.
autoimmune polyendocrinopathy, candidiasis, ectodermal d.
Becker muscular d.
cerebroocular dysplasia-muscular d.
cone-rod d.
congenital atonic sclerotic muscular d.
congenital endothelial corneal d.
congenital muscular d.
corneal d.

Duchenne de Boulogne
 muscular d.
Duchenne de Boulogne muscular
 dystrophy/Becker muscular d.
Duchenne muscular d.
ectodermal dysplasia, ectrodactyly,
 macular dystrophy syndrome
Emery-Dreifuss muscular d.
endothelial-epithelial corneal d.
facioscapulohumeral muscular d.
Fukuyama congenital muscular d.
granular corneal d.
idiopathic muscular d.
infantile neuroaxonal d.
lattice corneal d.
Leyden-Möbius muscular d.
limb-girdle muscular d.
localized collagen d.
macular corneal d.
map-dot corneal d.
map-dot-fingerprint corneal
 epithelial d.
marginal crystalline d.
medial canaliform d.
median canaliform d.
median nail d.
Meesman epithelial corneal d.
Meesman juvenile epithelial d.
mental retardation, ataxia,
 hypotonia, hypogonadism, retinal
 dystrophy syndrome
mental retardation, scapuloperoneal
 muscular dystrophy, lethal
 cardiomyopathy syndrome
merosin deficiency d.
microcystic corneal d.
microcystic epithelial d.
micropolygyria with muscular d.
mild X-linked recessive
 muscular d.
mixed sclerosing bone d.
muscular d.
muscular dystrophy, progressive
myotonic d.
myotonic dystrophy cataract
myotonic dystrophy effect
myotonic dystrophy gene
myotonic muscular d.
myxedema-myotonic dystrophy
 syndrome
North Carolina macular d.
ocular muscle d.
ocular muscular d.
oculogastrointestinal muscular d.
oculopharyngeal muscular d.
ophthalmoplegic muscular d.
parenchymatous corneal d.
pericentral rod-cone d.
polymorphous posterior corneal d.
posterior polymorphic dystrophy
 of cornea
posterior polymorphous corneal d.
progressive muscular d.
reflex sympathetic d.
Reis-Bücklers superficial
 corneal d.
Salzmann nodular corneal d.
Schnyder crystalline corneal d.
severe childhood autosomal
 recessive muscular d.
tardive muscular d.
thoracic asphyxiant d.
thoracic-pelvic-phalangeal d.

dystrophy-dystocia syndrome

each bedtime, every night

eagle

E. basal medium
e. beak bone-cutting forceps
Dulbecco modified Eagle medium
E. minimal essential medium
supplemented Eagle minimal essential medium
E. syndrome

Eagle-Barrett syndrome

Eales disease

ear

aggressive papillary middle ear tumor
anterior notch of e.
anterior wall of middle e.
atelectasis of middle e.
autoimmune inner ear disease
chronic middle ear infection
collagen-induced autoimmune ear disease
coloboma, heart anomaly, ichthyosis, mental retardation, and ear abnormality syndrome
coloboma, heart disease, atresia choanae, retarded growth and retarded development and/or CNS anomalies, genital hypoplasia, and ear anomalies and/or deafness syndrome
crustiness of e.
custom fit in ear unit
development and/or central nervous system anomalies, genital hypoplasia, ear anomalies
dizziness from infection of e.
external e.
eyes and e.'s
eyes, e.'s, nose and throat
folded aluminum ear splint
e. glue
hair cell in e.
hairy e.'s
head, eyes, ears, nose, and throat
head, eyes, ears, nose, and throat unremarkable
in the ear hearing aid
hearing loss from infection of ear
hot weather e.
e. implant
implantable middle ear hearing device
increased blood flow to e.
e. infection
inner e.
inner ear electronic implantation
inner ear hearing loss
inner ear implant
inner ear infection
inner ear mass
internal e.
laser office ventilation of e.'s with insertion of tubes
left e.
left middle ear exploration
low-set e.'s
medial dog e.
Meurmann external ear anomaly grade
middle ear canal
middle ear cell
middle ear choristoma
middle ear cleft
middle ear disease
middle ear endoscopy
middle ear exploration
middle ear impedance
middle ear implantable
middle ear implantable system
middle ear infection
middle ear mass
middle ear muscle reflex
middle ear neoplasm
middle ear segment
middle ear space
middle ear surgery
Mladick ear reconstruction
e. mold
mouse ear erosion
nontest e.
nose to ear to xiphoid
e.'s, nose, and throat
opposite ear masked
orbital, mandibular, ear, neural, soft tissue
orbit, mandible, ear, cranial nerves, soft tissue syndrome
outer ear canal
e. ox
e. oximetry
paracentesis and tubing of ears
e., patella, short stature syndrome
e. pulling
pus in e.
repeated ear infection
right e.
right ear, cold stimulus
right ear advantage
right middle ear exploration
right ear, warm stimulus
simulated real ear measurement
skin, head, eyes, ears, nose, and throat
test e.
tip of e.

eardrum

perforated e.
ruptured e.

Earle

E. balanced salt solution
hydrolysate lactalbumin Earle glucose

earlobe crease

early

e. abortion
e. advanced hepatocellular carcinoma
e. afterdepolarization
e. ambulation
e. amniocentesis
e. antigen
Assessment Program of E. Learning Levels
e. asthmatic response
aversive early environment
e. bedtime
benign early repolarization
e. childhood caries
e. childhood education
e. clinical drug evaluation unit
e. cystic hyperplasia
e. deceleration
e. defibrillation
e. detection of breast cancer
detection of early antigen fluorescent focus
e. diabetic retinopathy
e. diastolic murmur
e. diastolic relaxation
e. diastolic wave
e. differentiation
e. distal proximal tubule
e. dry breakfast
Early and Periodic Screening, Diagnosis, and Treatment program
Epstein-Barr early region protein
Epstein-Barr virus early antigen
e. exercise testing
e. gastric cancer of the upper stomach
e. gastric carcinoma
e. gastric emptying
Hawaii E. Learning Profile
e. healed
hepatitis B early antibody
hepatitis B early antigen

E

early *(continued)*
e. hepatocellular carcinoma
e. identification of symptom
immediate early antigen
inducible cAMP early repressor
e. infantile epileptic encephalopathy
e. infection
e. interstitial fibrosis
e. intervention in drug abuse
e. intervention program
e. ischemic recurrence
Kaufman Survey of E. Academic and Language Skills
e. labeled peak
E. Language Milestone Scale
e. latent
e. light breakfast
e. memory
Mental Health Early Intervention, Treatment, and Prevention Act of 2000
e. mitral valve closure
e. morning awakening
e. morning specimen of urine
e. morning stiffness
Mullen Scales of E. Learning
e. neonatal death
E. Neonatal Neurobehavior Scale
neurobiology of early childhood development
onset of early menstruation
e. onset Parkinsonism-mental retardation syndrome
e. opening of valve
peak early diastolic filling velocity
Pediatric E. Elemental Examination
e. postoperative period
postoperative regimen for oral early feeding
e. postoperative suture adjustment
e. posttraumatic epilepsy
e. pregnancy factor
e. pregnancy loss
e. pregnancy test
e. pregnancy wastage
e. prenatal karyotype
prevention and early intervention
e. progressing stroke
e. progressive resistance
e. proliferative phase
quick and early diagnosis
quick early warning
e. receptor potential
e. receptor potential mottling
recurrent early pregnancy loss
e. repolarization
e. repolarization pattern
e. reticulocyte
E. School Assessment
E. School Personality Questionnaire
Screening Children for Related E. Educational Needs
E. Social Communication Scale
E. Speech Perception Test
e. stage breast cancer
e. stages of sleep
e. systolic acceleration
e. systolic paradox
Test of E. Language Development, Second Edition
Test of E. Reading Comprehension
too early to evaluate
e. traumatic epilepsy
e. ventricular repolarization syndrome
very early onset schizophrenia
Williams syndrome, early puberty
E. Years Easy Screen

early-onset
e.-o. Alzheimer disease
e.-o. form of familial Alzheimer disease
e.-o. graft-versus-host disease
e.-o. Parkinson disease
e.-o. schizophrenia

early-phase
e.-p. reaction
e.-p. termination

earmold
open e.
perimeter e.

earth
rare earth element

earthy tongue

ease
bronchoscope inserted through vocal cords with e.
catheter passed with e.
ill at e.
passed with e.
position of e.
scope inserted into trachea with e.

easily
agitated, irritable and easily annoyed
capsule strip e.

East
E. Coast fever
Near East equine encephalomyelitis

eastern
E. equine encephalitis
E. equine encephalitis virus
E. equine encephalomyelitis
E. equine encephalomyelitis virus
Far Eastern tick-borne encephalitis
E. subtype Russian spring-summer encephalitis
E. tick-borne rickettsiosis
E. and Western encephalomyelitis vaccine

easy
e. bruisability
e. distractibility
Early Years E. Screen
e. fatigability
heparin assay rapid easy method
e. normal
e. normal left
e. normal right

eat
refusal to e.

eater
binge e.
compulsive e.
liver e.

eating
E. Attitudes Test
atypical eating disorder
binge eating disorder
binge eating pattern
binge eating syndrome
bizarre eating pattern
e. disorder
E. Disorder Inventory
e. disorders examination
e. disorder unit
dissociation in eating disorder
episodic pattern of binge e.
erratic eating habits
freely e.
good eating habit
e. habit
impulse control in e.
impulse dyscontrol in eating disorder
night eating syndrome
nocturnal eating syndrome
stable eating habit
voluntarily stopping eating and drinking

Eaton agent pneumonia

Eaton-Lambert
myasthenic syndrome of E.-L.

Ebbinghaus test

Ebola
E. hemorrhagic fever
E. virus
E. virus outbreak

eboris
membrana e.
membrana eboris of Kölliker

Ebstein
E. anomaly
E. diet
E. disease
E. lesion
E. sign

eburnated bone surface

eburnation
trapezium-metacarpal e.

eburnized bone end

eccentric
e. arteriosclerosis
e. atrophy
e. behavior
e. dynamic compression plating
e. fixation
e. gaze
e. hypertrophy
e. narrowing
e. personality
e. stenosis
total hip articular replacement by internal eccentric shells
e. vessel

eccentricity
angle of e.
mild eccentricity in demeanor

ecchymosis
e. and bruising
endocervical e.
e. and swelling
Tardieu e.
widespread ecchymosis and hematoma

ecchymotic
e. discoloration
e. hemorrhage
e. purpura

eccrine
angiolipoma, posttraumatic neuroma, glomus tumor, eccrine spiradenoma, and leiomyoma cutis
malignant eccrine poroma
malignant eccrine spiradenoma
microcystic eccrine carcinoma
mucinous eccrine carcinoma
neutrophilic eccrine hidradenitis
palmoplantar eccrine hidradenitis
papillary eccrine adenoma

echinococcosis
liver e.
lung e.

Echinococcus
life cycle of *Echinococcus*

echo
advance cochlear echo technique
axial echo planar diffusion weighted imaging
axial grade echo imaging
axial gradient echo image
e. delay time
digital echo quantification
3-dimensional turbo-spin echo images
fast asymmetric spin e.
fast-field e.
gradient-recalled echo technique
gradient-refocused e.
e. guidance
e. guided pericardiocentesis
e. guided ultrasound
e. imaging
e. intensity
left atrial spontaneous echo contrast
magnitude preparation-rapid acquisition gradient e.
mitral valve e.
navigator echo motion correction technique
partial saturation spin e.
pulsed Doppler e.
pulsed-gradient spin e.
rapid-acquisition spin e.
e. record access
simulated echo artifact
single shot fast spin e.
spin echo imaging
spontaneous echo contrast
stimulated echo acquisition mode
stimulated echo artifact
turbo spin e.

echocardiogram
e. adenosine
aortic valve e.
apical 2-chamber view e.
apical 4-chamber view e.
apical 5-chamber view e.
continuous loop exercise e.
continuous-wave Doppler e.
digital subtraction e.
dobutamine e.
exercise e.
M-mode echocardiogram imaging
pulsed Doppler e.
pulsed-wave Doppler e.
transesophageal e.
transthoracic e.

echocardiograph
transesophageal dobutamine stress e.

echocardiographic
e. gating
e. transducer

echocardiography
adenosine echocardiography imaging
aortic root e.
aortic valve e.
apical 2-chamber view e.
apical 5-chamber view e.
automated border detection by e.
color Doppler e.
color-flow imaging Doppler e.
continuous-wave Doppler e.
cross-sectional e.
digital subtraction e.
dipyridamole echocardiography imaging
dipyridamole echocardiography test
dobutamine e.
dobutamine-atropine stress e.
dobutamine stress e.
epicardial Doppler e.
exercise stress e.
high-frequency epicardial e.
intracardiac e.
intraoperative e.
intraoperative transesophageal e.
M-mode e.
myocardial contrast e.
negative contrast e.
pulsed Doppler e.
pulsed Doppler cross-sectional e.
pulsed-wave Doppler e.
supine bicycle stress e.
three-dimensional e.
transesophageal echocardiography-dobutamine stress e.
transesophageal echocardiography with pacing
transthoracic color Doppler e.

echocardiography *(continued)*
two-dimensional transesophageal e.
two-dimensional transthoracic e.

echocardiography-radionuclide ventriculography

echocardiology
contrast e.

echodense
e. mass
e. pattern
e. structure

echoencephalograph
midline e.

echoendoscope
linear array e.

echo-enhanced cystosonography

echo-enhancing agent

echo-free area

echogenic
e. appearance
e. area
e. foci
e. interface
e. intraluminal thrombus
e. mass
mixed echogenic solid mass
e. plug
e. tissue
e. tumor

echogenicity
increased e.
normal e.
parenchymal e.
periventricular e.
e. of periventricular white matter

echogram
M-mode e.
prostatic e.

echography
ocular e.
ophthalmic biometry by ultrasound e.
orbital e.
ultrasonic e.

echo-guided balloon atrial septostomy

echoing words of others

echolucency
periventricular e.

echolucent
e. pattern
e. plaque

echophonocardiography
M-mode e.

echoplanar
combined multisection diffuse-weighted and hemodynamically weighted echoplanar MR

echo-poor
e.-p. area
e.-p. lesion

echo-train length

echoviral infection

echovirus
e. infection
e. meningitis
e. myocarditis

Ecker
E. fluid
Rees and Ecker diluting fluid

eclampsia
e. due to uremia
puerperal e.

eclamptic
e. convulsion
e. idiocy
e. seizure
e. toxemia

eclectic psychotherapy

eclipse
e. ankle brace
e. blindness
mental e.

ecology
microbial e.
mucosal e.
physiologic e.

economic
e. costs of drug abuse
medical economic index
Test of E. Literacy

Economo
E. encephalitis
von Economo encephalitis

economy
token economy unit

ecosystem
parasite-host e.

ecstasy
religious e.

ectasia
e. of abdominal aorta
antral vascular e.
anuloaortic e.
congenital biliary e.
e. cordis
e. of cornea
gastric antral vascular e.
gastric vascular e.
e. iridis
mammary duct e.
mucinous ductal e.
mucinous ductal ectasia of the pancreas
mucinous duct e.
e. of sclera
e. of thoracic aorta

ectatic
e. aneurysm
e. aortic valve
e. artery
e. carotid artery
e. emphysema
e. vessel

ectethmoid bones

ectocervical cell yield

ectocervix
vagina, ectocervix, and endocervix

ectocuneiform bone

ectoderm
extraembryonic e.
neural e.

ectodermal
anhidrotic congenital ectodermal dysplasia
anhidrotic ectodermal dysplasia
ankyloblepharon, ectodermal defect, and cleft lip and/or palate
ankyloblepharon, ectodermal dysplasia, clefting syndrome
e. anomaly
antihidrotic ectodermal dysplasia
apical ectodermal ridge
arthrogryposis, ectodermal dysplasia, cleft lip/palate developmental delay syndrome
autoimmune polyendocrinopathy, candidiasis, ectodermal dysplasia
autoimmune polyendocrinopathy, candidiasis, ectodermal dystrophy
e. defect
e. dysplasia
e. dysplasia, cleft lip and palate, mental retardation, syndactyly syndrome I, II
e. dysplasia, ectrodactyly, macular dystrophy syndrome

ectrodactyly, ectodermal dysplasia, clefting syndrome
hypohidrotic ectodermal dysplasia
hypohidrotic ectodermal dysplasia with hypothyroidism
Margarita Island type ectodermal dysplasia
e. and mesodermal dysplasia with osseous involvement
ectodermal dysplasia-central
split hand-cleft lip/palate and ectodermal dysplasia
e. tumor

ectodermogenic neurosyphilis

ectoenzyme
TRH-degrading e.

ectomesenchymal chondromyxoid tumor

ectophytic parasite

ectopia
e. cordis
gastric mucosal ectopia in rectum
e. of lens
e. lentis
macular e.
no e.
e. pupillae congenita
renal e.
e. testis
testis e.
ureteral e.
e. vesicae

ectopic
e. ACTH syndrome
e. activity
e. adenoma
atrial ectopic automatic tachycardia
atrial ectopic beat
e. atrial tachycardia
automatic ectopic tachycardia
e. bone growth
cervical ectopic pregnancy
e. Cushing syndrome
e. depolarization
fimbrial ectopic pregnancy
e. focus
frequency ectopic ventricular beat
e. gestation
e. hormone production
e. hyperparathyroidism
e. impulse
e. junctional beat
ligamentous ectopic pregnancy
multifocal ectopic gastric mucosa
paraneoplastic ectopic ACTH production
parasitic ectopic pregnancy
e. parathyroid adenoma
persistent ectopic pregnancy
e. pregnancy
e. pregnancy and abortion
e. rhythm
e. tachycardia
unifocal ventricular ectopic beat
unruptured ectopic pregnancy
e. ventricular beat
ventricular ectopic activity
ventricular ectopic arrhythmia
ventricular ectopic depolarization

ectopy
sinus rhythm, no e.
supraventricular e.
ventricular e.

ectrodactyly
e., ectodermal dysplasia, clefting syndrome
ectodermal dysplasia, ectrodactyly, macular dystrophy syndrome
microcephaly, microphthalmia, ectrodactyly, prognathism syndrome

ectrodactyly-cleft palate syndrome

ectropion
atonic e.
congenital ectropion uveae
e. of eyelid
lid e.
mechanical e.
medial e.
nasal e.
paralytic e.
e. uveae

eczema
E. Area and Severity Index
e., asthma, and hay fever complex
atopic eczema keratoconjunctivitis
e. herpeticum
e. intertrigo
nutritional deficiency e.
oozing from e.

eczematoid
e. blepharitis
e. dermatitis
e. seborrhea
e. skin rash

eczematous
e. allergic contact dermatitis
allergic eczematous contact dermatitis
allergic eczematous contact-type dermatitis
e. conjunctivitis
e. dermatitis
nummular eczematous dermatitis
e. pannus
e. patch
e. reaction
e. skin lesion

ED1
monoclonal antibody ED1

eddy
audiofrequency eddy current
e. current
E. hot plate test
e. sound

Edelmann anemia

edema
acute bovine pulmonary e.
acute cardiogenic pulmonary e.
acute hemorrhagic e.
acute hemorrhagic edema of infancy
acute pulmonary e.
allergic laryngeal e.
allergic pulmonary e.
alveolar pulmonary e.
aphakic cystoid macular e.
brain e.
cardiogenic pulmonary e.
e., clubbing, and cyanosis
clubbing, cyanosis, and e.
cotton-spot macular e.
cyanosis, clubbing or e.
cystoid macular e.
dependent peripheral e.
diabetic macular e.
e. disease of swine
e., erythema, and exudate
e. factor
four plus e.
fulminant pulmonary e.
e. of hand
hereditary angioneurotic e.
high-altitude cerebral e.
high-altitude pulmonary e.
high permeability e.
hydrostatic pulmonary e.
idiopathic cyclic e.
injury pulmonary e.
intermittent angioneurotic e.
interstitial pulmonary e.
e. of iris
lower extremity e.

edema *(continued)*
macular e.
malignant brain e.
massive cerebral e.
neurogenic pulmonary e.
neuronal cytotoxic e.
no clubbing, cyanosis, or e.
noncardiac pulmonary e.
noncardiogenic pulmonary e.
nonhydrostatic pulmonary e.
optic disc e.
optic disc edema with a macular star
pedal e.
pericyte edema generation
peripheral extremity e.
peritumoral brain e.
permeability pulmonary e.
pitting edema of ankle
pitting edema of lower extremity
pretibial e.
progressive encephalopathy, edema, hypsarrhythmia, optic atrophy
e., proteinuria, hypertension
pseudophakic corneal e.
pulmonary e.
pulmonary edema fluid
pulmonary interstitial e.
remitting seronegative symmetric synovitis with pitting e.
sacral e.
septic pulmonary e.
Stellwag brawny e.
trace ankle e.
upper lobe pulmonary e.
white matter e.

edematous
acute edematous pancreatitis
atelectatic and edematous lung
parenchyma e.

edentulous
jaw
lower completely e.
lower partially e.
partially edentulous dental arch
partially edentulous jaw
upper completely e.
upper partially e.

edetate
calcium disodium e.
trisodium e.

edge
approximate skin e.'s
approximate wound e.'s
approximation of cutaneous e.'s
automated edge detection
automatic lumen edge segmentation
e. of bed
brought out near edge of incision
built-up e.
center e.
computerized edge detection
computerized edge tracing
débrided wound e.
e. detail
feathered edge proximal finishing
feet over edge of bed
gaping wound e.'s
E. Hill virus
labioincisal e.
left sternal e.
ligament reflecting e.
ligament shelving e.
linguoincisal e.
microbevel edge lens
palpable liver e.
e. response function
right sternal e.
Short Transitional E. Protection
spectral edge frequency
e. thickness
e.'s undermined

edible portion

Edinburgh
E. Articulation Test
E. 2 Coma Scale
E. Handedness Inventory
E. Postnatal Depression Scale
E. Rehabilitation Status Scale

Edinger-Westphal nucleus

edition
ADD-H: Comprehensive Teacher's Rating Scale, Second E.
Assessment of Aphasia and Related Disorders, Second E.
Behavior Rating Profile, Second E.
Child Health and Illness Profile, Adolescent E.
Culture-Free Self-Esteem Inventories, Second E.
Detroit Tests of Learning Aptitude - Primary, Second E.
Detroit Tests of Learning Aptitude, Third E.
Diagnostic Achievement Battery, Second E.
Gray Oral Reading Test, Third E.
International Classification of Diseases and Related Health Problems, 10th E.
Metropolitan Achievement Test, Seventh E.
Minnesota Multiphasic Personality Inventory, Second E.
Stanford-Binet Fourth E.
Test of Early Language Development, Second E.

editor
outpatient code e.

Edmondson
E. grade
E. grading

Edmonston-Zagreb high-titer vaccine

Edmonton Symptom Assessment Scale

educable
e. mentally handicapped
e. mentally retarded

education
adult basic e.
Alzheimer Disease E. and Referral
E. Apperception Test
area health education center
E. and Career Exploration System
character education inquiry
community e.
compensation, pension, and e.
computer-based continuing medical e.
conductive e.
continuing e.
Continuing E. Approval and Recognition Program
continuing education unit
continuing medical e.
dental auxiliary teacher e.
disease-oriented physician e.
drugs, exercise, education, diet, and self-monitoring
early childhood e.
graduate medical e.
Health Media E.
health-oriented physical e.
indirect medical e.
individualized education program
Individuals with Disabilities E. Act
lifestyle e.
medical e.
Medical E. for National Defense

Multidimensional Assessment of Philosophy of E.
National Asthma E. Program
National Cholesterol E. guidelines
National Cholesterol E. Program
National Cholesterol E. Program criteria
Nutrition Labeling and E. Act of 1990
patient education on drug abuse
patient education program
Personal Assessment for Continuing E.
physical e.
psychodynamic and therapeutic e.
public health education program
e. quotient
regular e.
research and e.
special e.
Stroke E. Program
treatment and education of autistic and related communications handicapped children
vocational rehabilitation and e.

educational
e. age
E. Goal Attainment Test
Kaufman Test of E. Achievement
low educational level
National E. Longitudinal Survey
Norris E. Achievement Test
Pediatric Examination of E. Readiness
e. quotient
Rucker-Gable E. Programming Scale
Screening Children for Related Early E. Needs
Screening Instrument for Targeting E. Risk
Screening Test for E. Prerequisite Skills
Sequential Tests of E. Progress, Series III
e. therapy

educationally
e. mentally handicapped
e. subnormal
e. subnormal-moderate
e. subnormal-severe

educator
diabetes nurse e.

Edwards
E. Personal Preference Schedule
E. syndrome

eel
American eel virus

effaced cervix

effacement
architectural e.
e. of calix
e. of cervix
e. and dilatation
e. of dura
mesencephalic cistern e.
e. of mucosa

effect
adverse drug e.
adverse medication e.
adverse negative immunosuppressive e.
air pressure e.
alcohol effect on brain
allogenic effect factor
anesthetizing effect of ice and snow
anticholinergic side e.
antipsychotic side e.
arterial sump e.
e. of asthma on lung
asymmetry and order e.
autonomic side e.
biologic effects of ionizing radiation
blood-clotting mechanism e.'s
cardiovascular effects of alcohol
cardiovascular effects of methamphetamine
cause and e.
cellular effects of alcohol
chronic amphetamine e.
e. of closing of eyes in electroencephalography
combined E.
concentration effect relation
cumulative radiation e.
cumulative effects of trauma
cumulative effects of unprotected sun
cytopathic e.
cytopathogenic e.
debilitating effects of old age
deteriorating effect of medication
digitalis e.
direct biologic e.
emotional effects of acquired immune deficiency syndrome
estrogen-agonist uterine e.
extrapyramidal e.
extrapyramidal side e.
fetal alcohol e.
first-pass e.
graft-versus-leukemia effect
health effects of environmental pollutants
health effects of ionizing radiation
iatrogenic effects of behavior therapy
indirect biologic e.
indirect drug e.
insufficient therapeutic e.
insulated gate field effect transistor
intense psychoactive drug e.
late effects of normal tissue
local alcohol instillation e.
local side e.
long-term effects of trauma
loss of e.
lowest effect level of toxicity
lowest observed adverse effect level
Mach band e.
magic angle effect artifact
maternal toxic e.
50% maximal e.
maximal possible e.
metal oxide semiconductor field effect transistor
movement after e.
movement disorder e.
muscarinic cholinergic side e.
myotonic dystrophy e.
negative immunosuppressive e.
nervous system e.
neurologic adverse e.
no e.
nongenomic glucocorticoid e.
no observed adverse effect level
no observed effect dose
ocular motility e.
on-off effect of L-dopa
e. of opening eyes
partial-reinforcement e.
partial reinforcement extinction e.
peak behavioral e.
peripheral antimuscarinic side e.
peripheral neurologic adverse e.
photographic e.
physical and biochemical e.
physical effects of drug abuse
physical effect of hallucinogen abuse
pituitary gonadotropin e.

effect *(continued)*
postantibiotic e.
pro arrhythmic e.
psychological effects of hallucinogen
quinidine e.
radiation effect unit
rapid extinction e.
secondary effect of treatment
side e.
specific dynamic e.
thermal effect of exercise
thermal effect of food
thermic effect of exercise
thermic effect of feeding
thermic effect of food
thermic effect of physical activity
white coat e.

effective
e. airspace dimension
e. alveolar ventilation
e. antibiotic concentration
e. anticancer drug
e. arterial blood volume
e. arterial elastance
atrial effective refractory period
e. balloon-dilated area
biologic effective dose
e. capillary flow
e. circulating blood volume
e. concentration
e. conduction period
decibel effective masking contralateral
e. direct radiation
distal effective potassium secretion
e. dose
e. drug duration
e. dynamic compliance
equivalent effective photon
e. filtration pressure
e. filtration rate
e. focal length
Generally Recognized as Safe and E.
generally regarded as e.
e. half-life
e. half-life of radioactive substance
e. heartbeat
high-quality and effective treatment
e. infection control
e. intervention
e. isotropic radiated power
less than e.
lowest effective dose
lowest effective toxic dose
e. mandibular length
e. masking
mean effective life
mean effective pressure
median effective concentration
median effective dose
e. mental health care
minimum effective analgesic concentration
minimum effective naproxen dose
e. orifice area
e. oxygen transport
e. path length
e. patient life
e. perceived noise level
e. pressor dose
e. pulmonary blood flow
e. refractory length
e. refractory period
e. refractory period of the left ventricle
e. regurgitant orifice
e. renal blood flow
e. renal plasma flow
safe and effective dosage
E. School Battery
e. sensory projection
e. systolic pressure
e. temperature
e. thyroxine ratio
e. thyroxine test
ventricular effective refractory period

effectiveness
contraceptive e.
dose reduction effectiveness factor
interpersonal e.
long-term e.
promoting aphasics communicative e.
relative biologic e.
Team E. Survey
Youth E. Training

effector
e. cell
e. cell precursor
linkage e.
locally acting paracrine e.
e. molecule
nephritogenic e.
nonspecific effector cell
e. to target ratio

efferent
e. arteriolar resistance
e. arteriole
e. artery
e. duct
e. ductule
e. fiber
general somatic efferent nerve
general visceral efferent nerve
e. glomerular arteriole
e. limb
e. loop
e. loop syndrome
e. motor aphasia
e. nerve
e. nerve impulse
e. neuron
e. pathway
e. renal sympathetic nerve activity
special visceral e.
e. sympathetic activity
sympathetic efferent nerve activity
e. vessel

efferentes
neurofibrae e.

efficacy
drug efficacy study implementation
Falls E. Scale
Global Evaluation of E.
oral contraceptive e.
e. ratio

efficiency
binocular visual e.
colony-forming e.
detective quantum e.
enhanced intellectual e.
geometric e.
hair removal e.
improve efficiency of heart and lungs
luminous e.
oxygen uptake efficiency slope
performance and cost e.
physical efficiency index
plating e.
protein efficiency ratio
quantum detection e.
relative fluorescence e.
respiratory isolation implementation e.
safety and e.
secondary plating e.
visual e.

Effler hiatal hernia repair

effleurage technique

effluence
hepatic venous e.

effluent
anal e.
clear e.
peritoneal dialysis e.
efflux
net e.
parathyroid hormone-mediated calcium e.
effluxed clear urine
effort
asthma of physical e.
aviator's effort syndrome
brief maximal e.
decrease in respiratory e.
e. intolerance
maximal e.
poor respiratory e.
relative inspiratory e.
voluntary e.
effort-induced thrombosis
effortless regurgitation
effusion
artificial pleural effusion procedure
asbestos-related pleural e.
bilateral otitis media with e.
chronic otitis media with e.
culture of pleural e.
discrete area of e.
endotoxin-mediated otitis media with e.
loculated pleural e.
malignant pericardial e.
malignant pleural e.
middle ear e.
mucopurulent hemorrhagic e.
neoplastic pericardial e.
otitis media with e.
otitis media without e.
pericardial e.
pericarditis with e.
pleural e.
pleurisy with e.
primary effusion lymphoma
reactive subdural e.
subdural effusion with hydrocephalus
transudative pleural e.
effusive-constrictive pericarditis
egg
e. albumin
e. crate foam mattress
crystalline egg albumin
e. drop syndrome
hamster egg penetration assay
hen egg lysozyme
implantation of fertilized e.
e. lecithin
e. lethal dose
Locke egg serum medium
neomycin egg yolk agar
operculate e.
polysaccharide egg antigen
e. retrieval procedure
soluble egg antigen
e. transfer
e. yolk
e. yolk agar
e. yolk-cobalamin absorption test
Eggers
E. operation
E. procedure
egg-infectious dose
egg-laying
e.-l. hormone
e.-l. release hormone
egg-shaped heart
eggshell
crushed eggshell fracture
e. fracture
e. pattern
egg-white lysozyme
ego
adult ego state
alter e.
alter ego transference
alternative alter e.
autonomous ego function
auxiliary e.
E. Development Scale
executive ego function
e. ideal
loss of boundaries of e.
loss of ego boundary
mental e.
motor control of the e.
multiple ego state
narcissistic ego ideal
negation of the e.
oral e.
parent ego state
perception e.
E. State Inventory
E. Strength test
egocentric thought process
ego-defense
Ego-Ideal and Conscience Development Test
ego-oriented individual therapy
egress
e. of arthroscopic fluid
neutrophil e.
Egyptian
E. conjunctivitis
E. hematuria
E. ophthalmia
E. splenomegaly
Ehlers-Danlos
arterial-ecchymotic type Ehlers-Danlos syndrome
arthrochalasis multiplex congenita Ehlers-Danlos syndrome
autosomal recessive ocular Ehlers-Danlos syndrome
Mitis-type Ehlers-Danlos syndrome
ocular-scoliotic type Ehlers-Danlos syndrome
periodontitis Ehlers-Danlos syndrome
E.-D. syndrome
Ehrlich
E. ascites carcinoma
E. ascites tumor
E. ascites tumor cell
E. granule
E. reaction
E. test
E. unit
ehrlichiosis
human e.
human granulocytic e.
human monocytic e.
Eichhorst atrophy
eicosanoid excretion
eidetic
e. image
increase in eidetic imagery
E. Parents Test
eighth
e. cranial nerve
direct eighth nerve monitoring
e. nerve action potential
e. nerve activity
Einhorn regimen of chemotherapy
Einstein
Albert E. Neonatal Developmental Scale
E. Neonatal Neurobehavioral Assessment Scale
Einthoven triangle
Eisenmenger
E. complex

Eisenmenger *(continued)*
E. disease
E. reaction
E. syndrome
E. tetralogy
E. ventricular septal defect

ejaculation
antegrade e.
premature e.
retrograde e.

ejaculator
musculus ejaculator seminis

ejection
aortic ejection click
aortic ejection sound
aortic systolic ejection murmur
area-length method for ejection fraction
cardiac ejection fraction
carotid ejection time
cineangiography and sensitometric ejection fraction
e. click
computed ejection fraction
corrected ejection time
diamond ejection murmur
duration of e.
excess ejection fraction
e. fraction
e. fraction at rest
e. fraction during exercise
e. fraction of heart
e. fraction systolic
e. fraction/wall motion
gallbladder ejection fraction
gallbladder ejection rate
global left ventricular ejection fraction
left ventricular e.
left ventricular ejection fraction
left ventricular ejection time
left ventricular ejection time index
mean normalized systolic ejection rate
mean systolic ejection rate
milk ejection reflex
e. murmur
normal ejection fraction
opening snap ejection systolic click
palpable aortic ejection sound
peak ejection rate
peak ejection time
peak ejection velocity
preejection period/left ventricular ejection time
pulmonary ejection click
e. rate
regional ejection fraction image
resting radionuclide ejection fraction
right ventricular ejection fraction
right ventricular ejection time
e. sound
systolic ejection murmur
systolic ejection period
systolic ejection time
e. time
two-dimensional echo-derived ejection fraction
e. velocity
volume e.

ejective time index

ejector
apical fragment e.

Ekbom syndrome

elaborating
detail response elaborating the whole

elastance
effective arterial e.
maximum ventricular e.
respiratory system e.
static e.

elastase
human leukocyte e.
human neutrophil e.
e. inhibition capacity
neutrophil e.
plasma polymorphonuclear e.
porcine pancreatic e.

elastase-like protein

elastic
anterior elastic layer
e. artery
e. back strap
e. bandage
e. band ligation
e. cartilage
e. compression stocking
e. connective tissue
cotton elastic bandage
e. equilibrium volume
external elastic lamina
external elastic membrane
e. fiber
e. fibril
e. fixation
Henle elastic membrane
e. hook
intermaxillary e.
internal elastic lamina
intimal elastic lamina
e. knee cage orthosis
e. knee cage with medial and lateral contoured knee joints
e. knee sleeve brace
e. ligature
e. limit
lung elastic recoil pressure
maxillomandibular e.
maximum expiratory airflow-static lung elastic recoil pressure
parallel elastic component of muscle
parallel elastic element
e. pressure-volume
e. recoil pressure of lung
series elastic component of muscles
series elastic element
soft elastic capsule
soft elastic gelatin capsule
e. soft tissue
e. stable intramedullary nailing
e. stocking
e. suspensor
e. tissue
titanium elastic nailing
e. tubing
e. twister orthosis
e. wrap
e. wristlet

elastica
internal e.

elasticity
impaired blood vessel e.
modulus of e.
ventricular e.

elastic-type
e.-t. disc prosthesis
e.-t. disc replacement

elasticum
localized acquired cutaneous pseudoxanthoma e.
pseudoxanthoma e.

elastin
e. fragment concentration
neonatal elastin deposition

elastofibroma
e. dorsi
mediastinal e.

elastography
magnetic resonance e.

elastolysis
middermal e.

elastolytic
annular elastolytic giant cell granuloma

elastoma
Miescher e.

elastomer
e. catheter
conventional silicone e.
silicone elastomer ring vertical gastroplasty
thermoplastic e.

elastomeric balloon

elastosis
linear focal e.
nodular e.
perforating calcific e.
solar e.

elation
inappropriate e.

elbow
above e.
anterior acute flexion elbow splint
articular muscle of e.
articular vascular network of e.
e. aspiration
axilla, shoulder, elbow bandage
e. bearing
e. disarticulation
dislocated elbow, bowed tibiae, scoliosis, deafness, cataract, microcephaly, mental retardation syndrome
disposable elbow protector
e. flexion contracture
golfer's elbow test
e. jerk
e. joint
Little League e.
lymph node of e.
Mayo classification of rheumatoid e.
Mayo elbow fracture classification
Mayo elbow performance score
Mayo modified total elbow arthroplasty
McKeever-Buck elbow operation
McKeever-Buck elbow technique
medial collateral ligament of e.
Milch elbow fracture classification
Milch elbow operation
Milch elbow technique
milkmaid's elbow dislocation
Mital elbow release
Mital elbow release operation
Mital elbow release technique
oblique ligament of elbow joint
e. orthosis
Osborne-Cotterill elbow dislocation operation
Osborne-Cotterill elbow technique
prone on e.'s
e. prosthesis
Schlein-type elbow arthroplasty
e. sensory potential
shoulder, elbow, wrist, hand orthosis
tennis e.
tip of e.
total elbow arthroplasty
total elbow replacement
transverse ligament of e.
ulnar collateral ligament of elbow joint
under e.

elbow-wrist-hand orthosis

elder
e. abuse
e. malignant melanoma classification
marsh e.
National Center on E. Abuse

elderly
acute care for the e.
Cambridge Mental Disorders in E. Examination
Clifton Assessment Procedures for the E.
depression and anxiety in e.
e. fibromyalgia
Hearing Handicap Inventory for the E.
idiopathic gait disorders of e.
Inventory of Psychic and Somatic Complaints in the E.
e. and mentally infirm
National Association for Hispanic E.
Pacemaker Selection in the E.
e. primigravida
psychosis in the e.
residential care facility for the e.
Salamon-Conte Life Satisfaction in the E. Scale
systolic hypertension in the e.

elderly-onset rheumatoid arthritis

elected palliative care

elective
e. abortion
e. cosmetic surgery
e. induction
e. induction of labor
e. interruption of pregnancy
e. irradiation
e. low forceps delivery
e. lymph node dissection
e. midforceps
e. neck dissection
e. neck irradiation
e. regional lymph node dissection
e. replacement indicator
sterile elective low forceps vaginal delivery
e. termination of pregnancy

Electra complex

electric
e. affinity
e. anesthesia
brainstem electric response audiometry
e. cabinet bath
e. casting machine
e. cast saw
e. cautery
e. charge
e. charge density
e. coagulation
conductive radiofrequency electric field
constant electric field
contour-clamped homogeneous electric field
e. control activity
e. current
e. current density
e. differential therapy
e. field
e. field mediated transfer
e. field stimulation
e. field vector
fine-tooth electric saw
intensity of electric field
e. knife
regressive electric shock therapy
e. response audiometry
e. shock therapy
e. shock treatment
e. skin resistance
e. stimulation
e. stimulation of brain
e. susceptibility
transthoracic electric impedance respirogram

electrical
abnormal electrical activity
abnormal electrical events in heart

electrical *(continued)*
abnormal electrical impulse
abnormal electrical stimulus
absence of electrical activity
e. activity
e. activity between electrodes
e. activity of brain
e. activity of heart
acupuncture and transcutaneous electrical nerve stimulation
alternating failure of response mechanical to electrical depolarization
e. alternation of heart
e. aversion therapy
basic electrical rhythm
e. bone-growth stimulation
e. bone-growth stimulator
e. bone stimulation
brain electrical activity
brain electrical activity map
brain electrical activity mapping
brainstem electrical response audiometry
e. brain stimulation
calibrated electrical stimulation
e. cardioversion
e. catheter ablation
chaotic electrical activity
e. conductivity
contractile electrical complex
control electrical rhythm
e. conversion of atrial fibrillation
e. countershock
cranial electrical stimulation
defibrillation and electrical cardioversion
direct electrical nerve stimulation
e. evoked potential
e. fulguration
functional electrical stimulation
e. function of heart
heart electrical rhythm
e. heart position
e. impedance breast scanning
e. impedance cardiography
e. impedance tomography
e. implant
e. impulse
e. impulse to heart
e. inactivity
increase in amplitude of electrical activity
e. instability of heart
e. intervention
e. intracranial stimulation
intraoperative electrical cortical stimulation
lateral electrical spine stimulation
lateral electrical surface stimulation
left deviation of electrical axis
e. membrane property
microamperage electrical nerve stimulation
e. muscle stimulation
muscular response to electrical stimulation of motor nerve
e. nerve stimulation
neuromuscular electrical stimulation therapy
neuromuscular electrical stimulator
no deviation of electrical axis
normal electrical axis
e. organ discharge
paired electrical stimulation
pattern of brain electrical activity
pattern of electrical activity
pelvic floor electrical stimulation
percutaneous electrical nerve stimulation
percutaneously inserted spinal cord electrical stimulation
e. potential in volts
programmed electrical stimulation
pulseless electrical activity
recorded electrical brain activity
recording of electrical activity
e. resistivity
e. response activity
right deviation of electrical axis
sharp, jabbing or electrical pain
shift in direction and pattern of brain electrical activity
single potential analysis cavernous electrical activity
e. spinal cord stimulation
spontaneous electrical activity
e. stimulation of hand
e. stimulation of heart
e. stimulation mapping
e. stimulation-produced analgesia
therapeutic electrical stimulation
thoracic electrical bioimpedance
total body electrical conductivity
e. transcranial stimulation
transcutaneous acupoint electrical stimulation
transcutaneous cranial electrical stimulation
transcutaneous electrical nerve stimulation
transcutaneous electrical nerve stimulator
transmural electrical field stimulation
transurethral electrical bladder stimulation
variations in electrical activity
e. waveform

electrically
e. activated implant
e. detachable coil
heart electrically unstable
e. induced spinal reflex

electroacupuncture analgesia

electroaerosol therapy

electrocardiogram
ambulatory e.
dynamic e.
fetal e.
graded exercise e.
high right atrium e.
His bundle e.
intraarterial e.
intraatrial e.
left arm electrode for e.
left leg electrode for e.
maternal e.
poor R-wave progression electrocardiogram
right arm electrode for e.
scalp e.
signal-averaged e.
e. tracing
vector e.
ventricular atrial His bundle e.
wave on e.

electrocardiographic
ambulatory electrocardiographic monitoring
e. angle between QRS and T vectors
e. complex
e. gating
e. interval from the beginning of QRS complex to end of the T wave
e. junction between QRS complex and ST segment
e. lead
lentigines, electrocardiographic abnormalities, ocular hypertelorism, pulmonary stenosis, abnormalities of genitalia, retardation of growth, deafness syndrome
e. monitoring

precordial electrocardiographic mapping
e. response
e. time-wave interval
transtelephonic electrocardiographic monitoring
e. wave
e. wave corresponding to repolarization of ventricles
e. wave in QRS complex
e. wave segment

electrocardiography
ambulatory e.
chest and left leg lead in e.
chest precordial lead in e.
endocoronary e.
exercise stress e.
high-resolution e.
long-term e.
P wave in e.
R-wave threshold electrocardiography
signal-averaged e.
stress e.
time between P wave and beginning of QRS complex in e.

electrocautery
battery-powered e.
e. conization
hook e.
light e.
low-current e.
Mentor wet-field e.
multipolar e.
needle-knife e.
needlepoint e.
e. unit

electrocerebral
e. inactivity
record of electrocerebral inactivity
e. silence
tracings of electrocerebral inactivity

electrochemical
e. detection
e. detector
liquid chromatography with electrochemical detection
net electrochemical potential gradient
e. potential gradient
e. relaxation method
shortened electrochemical systole
transmitting electrochemical messages to the brain

electrocoagulated
bleeder e.

electrocoagulating
e. current
e. forceps

electrocoagulation
bipolar e.
bipolar electrocoagulation of hemorrhoid
e. diathermy
monopolar e.
multipolar e.

electrocochleography
round window e.

electroconvulsive
mobile electroconvulsive therapy apparatus
multimonitored electroconvulsive treatment
multiple monitored electroconvulsive therapy
e. seizure
e. shock therapy
e. shock treatment
e. therapy-induced mood disorder
e. treatment

electrocorticogram study

electrocorticography study

electrode
anterior cheek e.
antimony monocrystalline e.
e.'s applied over cerebral cortex
ball tip e.
bipolar needle recording e.
bipolar stimulating e.
carbon dioxide e.
cardiac pacing e.
e. catheter ablation
central midline placement of electrodes in electroencephalography
closed-loop system passing e.
concentric needle e.
disposable pudendal nerve e.
electrical activity between electrodes
fetal scalp e.
frontal midline placement of electrodes in electroencephalography
frontal polar electrode placement in electroencephalography
His bundle e.
hydrogen e.'s
e. impedance
implantable cardioverter e.'s
implantable unipolar endocardial e.
injection electrode catheter
e.'s inserted in cerebral cortex
internal fetal scalp e.
left arm electrode for electrocardiogram
left leg electrode for electrocardiogram
nasopharyngeal electrode placement
nasopharyngeal electrode placement in electroencephalography
needle electrode electromyography
needle electrode examination
optically transparent e.
pacing electrode wire
paired electrode recording
parietal midline zero electrode placement in electroencephalography
percutaneous electrode array
e.'s placed on the surface of head
e. placement device
e. potential
return electrode monitor
right arm electrode for electrocardiogram
saturated calomel e.
single reference e.
single-use e.
standard electrode potential
subcutaneous electrode implantation
subdural electrode array
vectorcardiography e.
vector cardiography electrode right midaxillary line

electrodermal
e. activity
e. audiometry
e. response
e. response audiometry
e. response biofeedback

electrodesication
curettage and e.

electrodesiccated bleeding point

electrodesiccation
curettage and e.
e. and curettage

electrodetachable
e. balloon
e. platinum coil

electrodiagnostic
e. medicine
e. study
electrodialysis with reversed polarity
electrodispersive skin potential
electrodynamics
quantum e.
electroencephalic
e. audiometry
average electroencephalic response
e. response audiometry
electroencephalogram
alerting maneuver on e.
alerting stimulus on e.
amplitude-integrated e.
audiovisual e.
e. biofeedback
e. biofeedback in control of hyperactivity
e. burst suppression pattern
computed electroencephalogram tomogram
continuous high-amplitude electroencephalogram rhythmical synchronous slowing
depth e.
fetal e.
e. interval spectrum analysis
nonrhythmic electroencephalogram activity
nonspecific ST wave segment changes on e.
normal e.
normal electroencephalogram activity
normal waking e.
normal waking electroencephalogram pattern
quantitative e.
resting e.
stereotactic e.
stereotactic depth e.
e. tracing
vigilance-controlled e.
electroencephalographic
e. audiometry
e. burst-suppression
computerized electroencephalographic map
e. dysrhythmia
localized electroencephalographic seizure pattern
e. response
e. sleep study
electroencephalography
central midline placement of electrodes in e.
computer-analyzed e.
depth e.
effect of closing of eyes in e.
frontal midline placement of electrodes in e.
frontal polar electrode placement in e.
intracranial e.
irregular spiking activity in e.
nasopharyngeal electrode placement in e.
parietal midline zero electrode placement in e.
quantitative e.
scalp-sphenoidal e.
vertex sharp transient electroencephalography
electrofulguration hemostasis
electrogalvanic
e. stimulation
e. stimulator
electrogenerated chemiluminescence
electrogram
ambulatory electrogram monitor
atrial e.
deflection in His bundle in e.
His bundle e.
His bundle electrogram deflection
His bundle electrogram, distal
His bundle electrogram, proximal
intracavitary pressure electrogram dissociation
sinus node e.
electrographic
e. background abnormality
e. seizure
e. seizure activity
electrography
depth e.
electrohydraulic
e. extracorporeal lithotripsy
e. fragmentation
intracorporeal electrohydraulic lithotripsy
e. lithotripsy
e. shock wave lithotripsy
electrohydrodynamic ionization mass spectrometry
electroimmunodiffusion
crossed e.
electrokinetic
micellar electrokinetic capillary chromatography
micellar electrokinetic chromatography
electrokymography study
electroluminescent sensitometer
electrolysis
contact glow discharge e.
electrolyte
balanced electrolyte solution
e. balance and homeostasis
e. balance restoration
e. biochemical oxygen demand
e. depletion
e. derangement
e. disturbance
fluid and electrolyte imbalance
e. imbalance
e. imbalance coma
maintenance electrolyte solution
metabolic and electrolyte disorder
nonstandard electrolyte solution
e. panel
polyethylene glycol electrolyte lavage solution
renal and e.
e. replacement
e. replacement with glucose
serum protein e.'s
standard electrolyte solution
e. steroid cardiopathy by calcification
e. and steroid cardiopathy with necrosis
e. steroid-produced cardiopathy characterized by hyalinization
urine e.'s
electrolyte-deficient agar
electrolytes
e., blood urea nitrogen, and serum creatinine
fluids, electrolytes, nutrition
serum protein e.
electromagnetic
e. blood flow imaging
e. fields
e. flowmeter
e. focusing field probe
e. force
e. induction
e. interference/radiofrequency interference
e. molecular electronic resonance
e. moment

nonionizing electromagnetic radiation
pulsating electromagnetic field
e. pulse
pulsed electromagnetic field
pulsed electromagnetic stimulator
e. radiation
transverse e.
transverse electromagnetic mode
e. unit
e. waves

electromechanical
e. artificial heart
e. coupling
e. dissociation
e. impactor
e. slope computer
total electromechanical systole

electromedical
Ortho DX electromedical stimulator

electromembrane
therapeutic e.

electromolecular propulsion

electromotive
e. drug administration
e. force
intravesical electromotive drug administration

electromyogram
evoked e.
integrated e.
e. sensors

electromyographic
peripheral electromyographic activity

electromyography
concentric needle e.
evoked e.
evoked compound e.
laryngeal e.
needle electrode e.
pelvic floor e.
single fiber e.
surface e.

electron
analytical electron microscope
analytical electron microscopy
analytic transmission electron microscope
aqueous e.
back-scattered electron imaging
e. beam boost
e. beam computerized tomography
e. beam dosimeter
e. beam scalp irradiation
beveled electron beam cone
billion electron volts
e. capture
e. capture detector
central axis depth dose of electron beam therapy
chemically induced dynamic electron polarization
cold spots and hot spots with electron beam dosimetry
conventional transmission electron microscope
conventional transmission electron microscopy
e. diffraction
e. donor-acceptor interaction
e. energy loss spectroscopy
field emission scanning electron microscopy
freeze fracture electron microscopy
high-resolution transmission electron microscopy
high-velocity electron beam
high-voltage electron microscope
high-voltage transmission electron microscopy
hydrotropic electron donor
e. impact
intraoperative electron beam radiotherapy
intraoperative electron beam therapy
intraoral cone for electron beam therapy
e. ionization
e. ionization mass spectrometry
light and electron immunoperoxidase observation
light electron microscope
low-energy electron diffraction
low-energy electron diffraction spectroscopy
low-voltage high-resolution scanning electron microscopy
medical free electron laser
e. micrograph
e. microscope
e. microscopic examination
e. microscopy
e. microscopy of stool
Mobetron mobile, self-shielded electron accelerator
negative e.
e. nuclear double resonance
e. paramagnetic resonance
e. paramagnetic response
peak electron volt
photoemission electron microscopy
e. and photon therapy
positron positive e.
e. probe x-ray microanalyzer
e. radiography
ratio of electron charge to mass
reflection high-energy electron diffraction
e. rest mass
scanning electron micrograph
scanning electron microscopy
scanning transmission electron microscope
e. spectroscopy for chemical analysis
e. spin resonance
e. time-of-flight
total skin electron beam
e. transfer flavoprotein
e. transfer flavoprotein dehydrogenase
transmission electron microscope
transmission electron microscopy
transmission scanning electron microscopy
e. transport particle
universal electron microscope
e. volt
Xonics electron mammography

electron-beam
e.-b. angiography of coronary artery
e.-b. computed tomography
e.-b. computerized tomography
e.-b. intraoperative radiation therapy
e.-b. intraoperative radiotherapy

electron-dense
e.-d. amorphous material
e.-d. iron-containing particle

electroneurodiagnostic technologist

electronic
e. apex locator
e. artificial larynx
e. claims processing
e. claims submission
e. data processing
direct electronic urethrocystometry
electromagnetic molecular electronic resonance
e. fetal monitoring

electronic *(continued)*
functional electronic peroneal brace
e. glucose monitor
graduated electronic decelerator
e. implant
e. induction desorption
e. infusion device
inner ear electronic implantation
e. microanalyzer
e. pacemaker
e. pain control
e. patient medical record
peroral electronic pancreatoscope
e. portal imaging device
e. prescription
e. pupillography
e. speckle pattern interferometry
e. summation device
synaptic electronic activation
e. transducer
e. voltmeter

electronically provoked response

electron-probe microanalysis

electron-stimulated desorption

electron-transfer agent

electro-oculogram
monocular e.-o.

electrooptical characteristic

electrophilic stress

electrophoresis
agar gel e.
agarose e.
antigen-antibody crossed e.
capillary zone e.
cellulose acetate e.
cerebrospinal fluid immunofixation e.
countercurrent e.
creatine kinase isoenzyme e.
denaturing density gradient e.
denaturing gradient gel e.
density gradient e.
fluorophore-assisted carbohydrate e.
free flow e.
gel e.
gradient gel e.
hemoglobin e.
high-performance capillary e.
high-resolution protein e.
high-voltage e.
high-voltage paper e.
immunofixation e.
isoelectric focusing electrophoresis
isoelectric focusing electrophoresis in polyacrylamide gel
lipoprotein electrophoresis test
moving boundary e.
multilocus enzyme e.
multilocus enzyme electrophoresis analysis
nonequilibrium pH gradient gel e.
paper e.
polyacrylamide gel e.
polyacrylamide gel electrophoresis with silver stain
protein e.
pulsed-field gradient gel e.
rapid e.
rapid electrophoresis creatine kinase
e. scanning
serum e.
serum immunofixation e.
serum protein e.
serum protein and immunofixation electrophoresis system
sodium dodecyl sulfate-polyacrylamide gel e.
temperature-gradient gel e.
temporal temperature gradient gel e.
thin-layer e.
timed-temperature gradient e.
urine immunofixation e.
urine protein e.

electrophoretic
e. analysis
e. immunoblotting
e. karyotyping
macrophage electrophoretic mobility
e. mobility
e. mobility shift analysis
e. mobility shift assay
e. pattern
tanned erythrocyte electrophoretic mobility

electrophoretogram
serum protein e.

electrophrenic respiration

electrophysiologic
e. abnormality
e. behavior modification
chronic electrophysiologic study
e. function
e. mapping
e. monitoring
e. study
e. testing

electrophysiological stimulation

electrophysiology
patch clamp e.

electroresection
transurethral e.

electroretinogram
focal e.
local e.
macular e.
pattern-evoked e.
peak latencies of pattern e.
e. study

electrosensitive point

electrosensitivity
mucosal e.

electroshock
maximal electroshock model
regressive electroshock treatment
e. seizure threshold
e. therapy
e. threshold
e. treatment

electroshock-induced
e.-i. psychosis
e.-i. psychotic syndrome

electrosleep therapy

electrospinal orthosis

electrospinogram
evoked e.

electrospray ionization mass spectrometry

electrostatic
e. capacity
e. imaging
e. unit

electrostimulation
e. therapy
transcranial electrostimulation therapy

electrosurgery pencil

electrosurgical
bipolar electrosurgical scissors
e. current intensity
e. cut
e. cutting knife
e. desiccation
e. dissection
e. excision
e. filter
e. fulguration
e. instrument

large loop excision of transformation zone/loop electrosurgical excision procedure
loop electrosurgical excisional procedure
loop electrosurgical excision procedure
loop electrosurgical excision procedure conization
e. loop excision
e. pencil
e. scaling
e. snare
e. snare polypectomy
e. unit
e. wire

electrotaxis
negative e.

electrotherapeutic
e. point stimulation
e. sleep

electrotherapy
cerebral e.
transcerebral e.

electrothermal
e. atomic absorption spectrophotometry
intradiscal electrothermal coagulation
intradiscal electrothermal therapy

electrothermally assisted capsulorrhaphy

electrovaporization
transurethral electrovaporization of prostate

electuary confection

Elejalde syndrome

element
acute phase response e.
androgen receptor e.
basal promoter e.
cAMP-response e.
cAMP-response element modulator
contractile e.
downstream regulatory element antagonistic modulator gene
dream e.'s
elements on urinalysis
estrogen-response e.
finite element method
finite element stress analysis
glucocorticoid response e.
glucocorticoid-responsive e.
hormone response e.
human leukocyte antigen restriction e.
inhibitory response e.
length contraction compensation e.
long interspersed e.'s
lysozyme F_2 e.
multiple trace e.'s
myeloid blood e.
negative T_3 response e.
negative triiodothyronine response e.
neoplastic destruction of spinal e.
neuroepithelial element of retina
neuronal element firing
parallel elastic e.
peroxisome proliferator response e.
picture e.
rare earth e.
series elastic e.
short interspersed e.'s
sterol regulatory element binding protein
thyroid hormone response e.
thyroid response e.
trace e.
trace metal elements injection
T_3 responsive e.
velocity of contractile e.
vitamin D-response e.
volume e.
xenobiotic-response e.

elemental
e. diet
e. enteral alimentation
Pediatric Early E. Examination

elementary
e. body
e. charge
Devereux Elementary School Behavior Rating Scale II
Screening Assessment for Gifted E. Students, Primary

element-binding
cAMP response e.-b.

elephantiasis
lymphangiectatic e.
neuromatosis e.
nevoid e.
nonfilarial e.
nostras e.
e. of vulva

elevate
e. feet above heart
e. head of bed

elevated
asymptomatic elevated aminotransferase
bladder flap e.
dorsal elevated position
e. heart rate
hemolysis, elevated liver enzymes, and low platelet count
legs elevated higher than heart
liver fraction e.
may be e.
e. new vessels elsewhere
e. new vessels on the disc
not e.
e. triglycerides

elevated-arm stress test

elevating
lactate dehydrogenase elevating virus

elevation
e. of blood lead level
finger-assisted malar e.
e. of head of bed
ice, compression, and e.
ice, compression, elevation, and support
intermittent elevation of blood pressure
liver enzyme e.
Mazur ankle elevation classification
protection, rest, ice, compression, elevation, support
protection, restricted activity, ice, compression, e.
rest, ice, compression, e.
right atrial pressure e.

elevator
balloon uterine elevator cannula
curved periosteal e.
fine periosteal e.
fracture reducing e.
lumbosacral fusion e.
modified Darrach-type e.

eleventh nerve

elfin
e. facies
e. facies hypercalcemia syndrome

Elgon
Mount Elgon bat virus

elicitation
affect e.
Patterned E. Syntax Screening Test
problem elicitation technique

elicited
e. behavior
Carrow E. Language Inventory
Grammatical Analysis of E. Language
Performance Assessment of Syntax E. and Spontaneous
e. response

eligibility
automated eligibility verification system
determination of e.
e. on-site
proof of e.

eligible
board e.

eliminate gravity

elimination
carbon dioxide e.
e. diet
diet and e.
fog reduction elimination device
galactose elimination capacity
e. half-life
multiple inert gas elimination technique
nonpulmonary route of e.
process of e.
e. rate constant
transepithelial e.

ELISA-I, -II, -III test

ELISPOT
E. assay
E. test

elixir
e. terpin hydrate
e. terpin hydrate with codeine

Ellestad
E. exercise stress test
E. protocol

Elliot operation

Elliott treatment

ellipsoid
e. joint
e. of spleen

ellipsoidal
e. articulation
e. cell

elliptical
e. amputation
e. anastomosis
e. biopsy
e. flap
e. incision
e. nystagmus
e. trephination

elliptocytosis
hereditary e.

elliptocytotic anemia

Ellis-Jones operation

Ellis sign

Ellis-van Creveld syndrome

Ellsworth
Reese Ellsworth classification

Elmslie-Cholmeley operation

Eloesser
E. flap
E. operation

elongated
muscle in elongated state

elongation
aortic e.
e., derotation and lateral flexion
e. factor
e. factor G
gradual elongation intramedullary nailing
ligament e.
peroneus brevis e.
repeated quick stretch from e.

elongation-derotation flexion

elopement
e. ideation
e. precaution
e. status

eloper
suicidal and e.
violence and e.

eloquent
e. areas of brain
e. versus noneloquent area

Elschnig
E. body
E. conjunctivitis
E. operation
E. pearl
E. spot
E. syndrome

elsewhere
elevated new vessels e.
fibrovascular tissue e.
neovascularization elsewhere on retina
neovascularization of new vessels e.
new vessels e.
not elsewhere classifiable
not elsewhere classified
not elsewhere coded
not elsewhere specified
vascularization elsewhere in the retina

Elsner asthma

eluted antibody

elution
agar disc e.

elutriation
countercurrent centrifugal e.

Ely
E. operation
E. test

emaciated and dehydrated

emanation
actinium e.
radium e.

emancipated adolescent

emancipation disorder of adolescence

emancipatory striving

embarrassed respiration

embarrassment
circulatory e.
cord e.
e. dream
e. psychosis

Embden-Meyerhof
E.-M. glycolytic pathway

embedded
Children's E. Figures Test
E. Figures Test
Group E. Figures Test
e. tooth

embedding
paraffin e.
paraffin block e.

embolectomy
e. of aorta
e. catheter
Fogarty arterial e.
shredding embolectomy thrombectomy

emboli (*pl. of* embolus)

embolic
e. aneurysm
e. cerebral infarct
e. disease
e. event
e. gangrene
e. infarct
e. infarction
e. occlusion

e. phenomenon
e. shower
e. source
e. stroke

emboligenic
transient emboligenic aortoarteritis

embolism
air e.
amniotic fluid e.
arterial gas e.
coronary artery e.
diving air e.
fat embolism syndrome
fibrocartilaginous e.
mesenteric arterial e.
paradoxical air e.
paradoxical cerebral e.
pulmonary e.
source of e.
submassive pulmonary e.
venous air e.

embolization
amniotic fluid e.
e. of aneurysm
angiographic variceal e.
aortopulmonary collateral coil e.
bronchial artery e.
cholesterol crystal e.
coronary artery e.
hepatic artery e.
partial splenic e.
particulate arterial e.
pelvic arterial e.
percutaneous embolization therapy
percutaneous transhepatic liver biopsy with tract e.
portal e.
pulmonary artery e.
renal cholesterol e.
subsegmental transcatheter arterial e.
e. therapy
transarterial catheter e.
transcatheter arterial e.
transcatheter splenic arterial e.
transhepatic e.
e. treatment
uterine artery e.

embolotherapy
transcatheter e.

embolus, pl. **emboli**
fatal air e.
massive pulmonary e.
e. migration
multiple cholesterol emboli syndrome
occult pulmonary e.
paradoxical cerebral e.
pulmonary e.
pulmonary embolus with small infarct
recurrent pulmonary emboli
superior mesenteric artery e.

embolus-to-blood ratio

embrace reflex

embrasure
e. clasp
e. hook
lingual e.
occlusal e.

embryo
bovine embryo skeletal muscle
chick e.
chick embryo extract
chick embryo fibroblast
chick embryo kidney
chick embryo origin
Chinese hamster embryo fibroblast
duck embryo fibroblast
duck embryo origin vaccine
duck embryo virus
e. extract
e. fetal
frozen embryo replacement
guinea pig e.
hamster embryo cell
hamster embryo fibroblast
human embryo fibroblast
human embryo lung cell culture
human embryo kidney cell
e. intrafallopian transfer
live e.
mouse e.
mouse embryo fibroblast
preimplantation e.
pronucleate stage embryo transfer
purified chick embryo cell culture
rabies vaccine, duck embryo culture
rabies vaccine, purified chick embryo cell culture
rat embryo tissue culture
Syrian hamster e.
tubal embryo stage transfer

embryofetal alcohol syndrome

embryofetoscopy
transabdominal thin-gauge e.

embryoic
human embryoic lung fibroblast

embryology
Human Fertilization and E. Authority
Leydig cell e.

embryonal
e. adenoma
anterior axial embryonal cataract
anterior axonal embryonal cataract
axial embryonal cataract
e. carcinoma
e. carcinosarcoma
e. cell carcinoma
e. cell tumor
e. cyst
e. leukemia
e. nephroma
e. nuclear cataract
ovarian embryonal teratoma
poorly differentiated embryonal cell tumor
e. rhabdomyosarcoma
e. sarcoma
e. tumor
undifferentiated embryonal sarcoma

embryonic
e. antibody
e. antigen
bovine embryonic lung
bovine embryonic spleen cell
e. bovine kidney
bovine embryonic kidney cell
calf embryonic heart cell
e. chick muscle
e. death
e. development
e. growth and development factor
e. heart
e. heart motion
human embryonic kidney
human embryonic lung fibroblast
human embryonic skin
human embryonic spleen
human embryonic intestine cell
human embryonic palatal mesenchymal cell
neoplasm embryonic antigen
stage-specific embryonic antigen
e. stem cell
stillbirth, mummification, embryonic death, infertility syndrome
thyrotroph embryonic factor

embryopathy
alcoholic e.

embryotoxicity
Chick E. Screening Test

embryotoxon
anterior e.

emergence
anesthetic e.
angle of e.

emergency
e. admission
e. area
e. assistance
e. assistance to families
e. assistant
cardiac e.
e. cardiac care
e. care provider
e. center visits
e. chemical restraint
E. Communications Center
e. contraceptive pill
e. decontamination center
e. department
e. department approval for pediatrics
e. department physician
e. department thoracotomy
e. diagnostic and treatment unit
died in emergency department
e. drinking water germicidal tablet
extreme medical e.
e. facility
free-standing emergency center
Heroin E. Life Project
history and symptoms of emergency cardiac care
e. hospital
hospital emergency department
hypertensive e.'s
e. hysterectomy
in-flight e.
e. infusion device
e. maternal and infant care
e. mechanical restraint
e. medical attendant
e. medical care
e. medical care and rescue
medical emergency treatment
e. medical information
e. medical team
e. medical trauma center
e. medical treatment
e. medicine
medicine
national e.
nonsurgeon, emergency department
e. observation bed
E. Operations Center
e. outpatient
e. oxygen mask assembly
personal emergency response system
e. physical restraint
e. procedure
psychiatric emergency service
psychiatric emergency team
radiation emergency area
radiologic emergency assistance team
e. reperfusion
e. room computerized tomography
e. room physician
e. room triage documentation
simulated aircraft fire and e.
e. thoracentesis
e. thoracotomy
e. tracheotomy
e. and trauma center
trauma and emergency center
e. and trauma unit
e. vehicle
walk-in emergency department
e. ward

emergent
newly emergent categorical change
Systematic Assessment for Treatment of E. Events
treatment of emergent symptom
Treatment E. Symptom Scale

emery disc

Emery-Dreifuss muscular dystrophy

emesis
chemotherapy-induced e.
chemotherapy-induced nausea and e.
coffee ground e.
fecal e.
e. gravidarum
induced e.
Morrow Assessment of Nausea and E.
nausea and e.
radiation induced e.
salivation, lacrimation, urination, defecation, gastrointestinal distress and e.

emetic
e. center
central e.
e. episodes
indirect e.

emetine and bismuth iodide

eminence
arcuate e.
articular e.
articular eminence of temporal bone
hypothenar e.
iliopubic e.
intercondylar e.
malar e.
maxillary e.
maxillary canine e.
medial e.
medial eminence resection
medial eminence of rhomboid
median e.
nasal e.
olivary e.
omental eminence of pancreas
orbital e.
orbital eminence of zygomatic bone
parietal e.
pyramidal e.
radial eminence of wrist
round e.
thenar e.
tibial e.

emissary
mastoid emissary vein
occipital emissary vein
parietal emissary vein

emission
adenosine triphosphate single-photon emission computed tomography
e. angiography
e. computed tomography
e. computer-assisted tomography
e. computerized axial tomography
delayed light e.
distortion-product otoacoustic e.
dual-isotope simultaneous acquisition single-photon emission computed tomography
evoked otoacoustic e.
field emission scanning electron microscopy
flame emission spectroscopy
fluoride ion positron emission tomography
gated single-photon emission computed tomography
gradient-echo single-photon emission computed tomography
inductively-coupled plasma-optical emission spectrometry

infrared emission detection
laser-induced fluorescence e.
light activation by stimulated emission of radiation
light amplification by stimulated emission of radiation
methoxyisobutyl isonitrile single-photon emission computed tomography
microwave amplification by stimulated emission of radiation
nasal air e.
optical emission spectroscopy
otoacoustic emission test
otoacoustic emission testing
particle-induced x-ray e.
positron emission computed tomography
positron emission tomography balloon
positron emission tomography scan
positron emission tomography technique
positron emission transaxial tomography
positron emission transverse tomography
proton-induced x-ray e.
single-photon emission computed tomography
single-photon emission imaging tomography
e. spectrometric detector
e. spectrometry
e. spectroscopy
spontaneous otoacoustic e.
technetium-99m hexamethylpropylene amine oxime single-photon emission computed tomography
e. tomography
transient evoked otoacoustic e.
true radiation e.

emitter-coupled logic

Emmet operation

emollient

hydrophilic emollient base

Emory Pain Estimate Model

emotion

adjustment disorder with mixed disturbance of e.'s
affection and e.
disturbance of emotions specific to adolescence
disturbance of emotions specific to childhood
expressed e.
functioning, reasoning, orientation, memory, arithmetic, judgment, and e.
handling e.'s
manifestation of e.
memory by e.
E.'s Profile Index

emotional

e. abuse
akinesia/diminished emotional expression
e. anesthesia
anticipated emotional suffering
appropriateness of emotional response
e. avoidance
e. baggage
e. B cluster
e. beggar
e. and behavioral difficulties
Behavioral and E. Rating Scale
E. and Behavior Problem Scale
e. bias
e. blackmail
e. blunting
chronic emotional suffering
conditioned emotional response
e. defensiveness
e. dependence
e. disinhibition
e. disorder
e. disturbance
e. disturbance adjustment disorder
e. disturbance adjustment reaction
e. disturbance of adolescence
e. disturbance of childhood
e. disturbance stress reaction
Draw-A-Person Screening Procedure for E. Disturbance
e. dyscontrol disorder
e. effects of acquired immune deficiency syndrome
e., spiritual, and social
episodic emotional instability
e. excitability
e. factor
e. flattening
e. gratification
hallucinatory emotional experience
e. handicap
e. health
e. illness
illness of emotional origin
increased emotional arousal
increased emotional dependence
e. insanity
e. instability
interference with intellectual and emotional growth
internal emotional arousal
e. irritability
paroxysmal emotional state
perceived emotional abandonment
persistent emotional condition
preexisting emotional problem
e. reactivity
Scale for E. Blunting
Screen for Child Anxiety-Related E. Disorders
serious emotional disturbance
severe emotional handicap
spatial emotional stimuli
e. stimulation
e. stress depressive psychosis
e. stress precipitating tremor
Tasks of E. Development
e. trajectory
underlying emotional issue
e. upheaval
e. well-being
e. withdrawal

emotionality

E. Activity Sociability Scale
negative e.
pathologic e.
pathological e.

emotionally

e. disturbed
e. disturbed individual
e. disturbed and learning disabled
e. handicapped
e. impaired
e. isolated
patient emotionally ill
socially and emotionally disturbed
e. unavailable
e. unstable
e. unstable character disorder

emotive

e. imagery
perceptual emotive stimulus

empathize

recognize, empathize, think, hear, integrate, notice, keep

empathy

accurate e.
support, empathy, and truth

emphysema

alpha-1-antitrypsin disease-related e.

emphysema *(continued)*
central acinar e.
centrilobular e.
chronic bronchitis with e.
chronic hypertrophic e.
chronic obstructive bullous e.
chronic obstructive pulmonary e.
clinical e.
congenital emphysema, cryptorchidism, penoscrotal web, deafness, mental retardation syndrome
glassblower's e.
idiopathic unilobar e.
infantile lobar e.
interstitial pulmonary e.
intrapulmonary interstitial e.
neonatal cystic pulmonary e.
obstructive pulmonary e.
panlobular e.
persistent interstitial pulmonary e.
pink puffer sign of e.
pleuritis and e.
pulmonary e.
pulmonary interstitial e.
e. secondary to heavy smoking
subcutaneous e.

emphysematous
e. alveolus
e. asthma
e. bleb
e. bulla
e. COPD
e. cystitis
e. gallbladder
e. gangrene
e. gastritis
e. pyelonephritis

empiric
e. antibiotic
e. therapy
e. treatment

empirical
e. approach
e. basis
e. data
e. finding
systematic, complete, objective, practical, e.
e. treatment

empirically
patient empirically treated
patient treated e.
treat e.

employee
E. Health Maintenance Examination
impaired employee alcohol and drug treatment issue
e. mental illness
E. Reliability Inventory
E. Retirement Income Security Act
Survey of E. Access

employing
sequential treatment employing pharmacologic support

employment
E. and Adaptation Index
Professional E. Test

emptied
bladder emptied completely
bladder emptied on voiding

emptiness
chronic emptiness and boredom
chronic feelings of deep e.

empty
bladder empties normally
e. can test
e., measure, and record
e. gestational sac
lowest empty molecular orbital
nerve, artery, vein, empty space, lymphatics
optically e.
primary empty sella syndrome
e. sella turcica syndrome
supine empty stress test

empty-chair technique

emptying
atrial emptying index
atrial emptying volume
bowel emptying regimen
complete emptying of bladder
delayed gastric e.
early gastric e.
gastric e.
gastric emptying delay
gastric emptying half-time
gastric emptying procedure
gastric emptying scan
gastric emptying of solids
incomplete bladder e.
incomplete emptying of bladder
left atrial emptying index
partial emptying of stomach
peak emptying rate
radionuclide gastric emptying study
e. of right atrium
time of peak emptying rate of mouth
time of peak emptying rate of pharynx
venous e.

empyema
e. of gallbladder
interlobar e.
loculated e.
mastoid e.
Müller e.
parapneumonic e.
e. of pericardium
pleural e.
pneumococcal e.
pulsating e.
recurrent e.
streptococcal e.
subdural e.

empyematic scoliosis

emulgent vein

emulsion
bacillary e.
bacillus e.
ethiodized oil e.
intravenous fat e.
magnesium hydroxide and mineral oil e.
nuclear track e.
oil in water e.
oxygenated fluorocarbon nutrient e.
radiodermatitis e.
tuberculin bacillary e.
wound dressing e.

en
e. bloc
e. bloc advancement
e. bloc bilateral lung transplant
e. bloc dissection
e. bloc esophagectomy
e. bloc excision
e. bloc no touch technique
e. bloc removal
e. bloc resection
e. bloc running locking suture
e. bloc vulvectomy
coeur en sabot
e. face
e. face irradiation field
main en crochet
main en griffe
main en griffe deformity
main en lorgnette
main en singe
meningioma en plaque

milia en plaque
parapsoriasis en plaque
parapsoriasis en plaques
radical en bloc removal
sclerose en plaques

enamel
dental enamel dysplasia syndrome
hereditary brown e.
hereditary enamel hypoplasia
e. hypoplasia
inner enamel epithelium
e. prism
e. surface index

enanthem
oral e.

enarthrodial joint

encapsulans
peritonitis e.

encapsulated
liposomal encapsulated anthracycline

encapsulating
sclerosing encapsulating peritonitis

encapsulation
peritoneal e.

encased heart

encasement
pancreatic duct e.

encasing cell

encephalic
e. angioma
e. infant
e. region
e. vertigo

encephalitis
acute allergic e.
AIDS-related e.
arthropod-borne viral e.
arthropod-borne virus e.
Australian X e.
Australian X encephalitis virus
California e.
canine distemper e.
caprine arthritis encephalitis virus
central European e.
central European encephalitis virus
central European tick-borne e.
Eastern equine e.
Eastern equine encephalitis virus
Eastern subtype Russian spring-summer e.
equine e.
experimental allergic e.
experimental autoimmune e.
Far Eastern tick-borne e.
focal tick-borne e.
granulomatous amebic e.
herpes simplex e.
herpes simplex virus e.
Japanese B e.
Japanese encephalitis virus vaccine
Japanese equine e.
Langat e.
lymphocytic choriomeningitis virus e.
measles inclusion body e.
meningeal tick-borne e.
meningitis or encephalitis, metabolic, Reye syndrome
multifocal giant cell e.
multinucleated cell e.
Murray Valley e.
Murray Valley encephalitis virus
neonatal HSV-1, -2 e.
Powassan encephalitis
progressive form of tick-borne e.
pyretic tick-borne e.
Russian autumn e.
Russian autumn encephalitis virus
Russian spring-summer e.
Russian spring-summer encephalitis virus
St. Louis encephalitis virus
subacute inclusion body e.
tick-borne e.
tick-borne encephalitis virus
Toxoplasma e.
Venezuelan equine encephalitis vaccine, attenuated live
Venezuelan equine encephalitis vaccine, inactivated
Venezuelan equine encephalitis virus
viral e.
von Economo e.
western equine e.
West Nile e.
West Nile encephalitis virus

encephalitogenic factor

encephalization quotient

encephalocele
anterior basal e.
hydrocephalus, agyria, retinal dysplasia with or without encephalocele syndrome
nasal e.
nasoethmoidal e.
occipital e.
orbital e.
parietal e.

encephalocraniocutaneous lipomatosis

encephalogram
air e.

encephalography
air e.
slow volume e.
slow-wave e.
ultrasonic e.

encephaloid
e. cancer
e. carcinoma

encephalomalacia
multicystic e.
periventricular e.

encephalomyelitis
acute disseminated e.
acute hemorrhagic e.
acute monophasic experimental autoimmune e.
avian e.
avian encephalomyelitis virus
avian infectious e.
Eastern equine e.
Eastern equine encephalomyelitis virus
Eastern and Western encephalomyelitis vaccine
experimental allergic e.
experimental autoimmune e.
hemagglutinating e.
hemagglutination encephalomyelitis virus
infectious porcine e.
mouse encephalomyelitis virus
myalgic e.
Near East equine e.
perivenous e.
postinfectious e.
progressive encephalomyelitis with rigidity and myoclonus
Theiler murine encephalomyelitis virus
Venezuelan equine encephalomyelitis virus
western equine e.
western equine encephalomyelitis virus

encephalomyeloneuropathy
nonspecific e.

encephalomyelopathy
infantile necrotizing e.
subacute necrotizing e.

encephalomyocarditis virus

encephalomyopathy
mitochondrial e.
mitochondrial encephalomyopathy with sensorimotor polyneuropathy
mitochondrial encephalomyopathy with sensorimotor polyneuropathy, ophthalmoplegia, and paralysis
mitochondrial neurogastrointestinal e.

encephalopathy
acute cerebral e.
acute toxic e.
age-dependent epileptic e.
alcoholic pellagra e.
alcoholic possible pancreatic e.
amyotrophic type of spongiform e.
anoxic e.
ataxia, myoclonic encephalopathy, macular degeneration, recurrent infections syndrome
atherosclerotic e.
autosomal recessive syndrome of e.
bovine spongiform e.
chronic hepatic e.
chronic traumatic e.
dialysis e.
dialysis encephalopathy syndrome
drug-induced hepatic e.
early infantile epileptic e.
epidemic fatal e.
hemorrhagic shock and e.
hepatic e.
human immunodeficiency virus e.
hypoxic-ischemic e.
hypoxic ischemic e.
macrocephaly with feeblemindedness and encephalopathy with peculiar deposits
mitochondrial myopathy, encephalopathy, lactic acidosis, strokelike episodes
multicystic e.
myoclonic encephalopathy syndrome
myoneuro-gastrointestinal e.
myopathy, encephalopathy, lactic acidosis, strokelike episodes
neonatal e.
neonatal hypoxic-ischemic e.
overt bilirubin e.
paraneoplastic limbic e.
portal-systemic e.
portosystemic e.
postanoxic e.
postshunt e.
progressive dialysis e.
progressive encephalopathy, edema, hypsarrhythmia, optic atrophy
progressive multifocal leuko-J e.
prolonged postictal e.
severe anoxic e.
spongiform e.
subclinical hepatic e.
subcortical arteriosclerotic e.
subcortical atherosclerotic e.
subcortical vascular e.
thiamine deficiency e.
toxic metabolic e.
transmissible mink e.
transmissible spongiform e.
Wernicke e.

encephalotrigeminal angiomatosis

enchondral bone formation

enchondroma
multiple e.

enchondromata
multiple bone e.

enchondromatosis
multiple e.

enchondromatosum
myxoma e.

encirclement
anal e.

encircling
Arroyo encircling suture
Arruga encircling suture
e. cryoablation
e. endocardial ventriculotomy
e. explant
e. implant
partial encircling endocardial ventriculotomy
e. of scleral buckle operation
e. wire

encoder
advanced combined e.
precision encoder and pattern recognizer

encoding
anti-CD3 stimulated peripheral blood lymphocytes transduced with a gene encoding a chimeric
memory e.
naked DNA e.
respiratory ordered phase e.
uniform food e.

encopresis
overflow e.

encounter
forced sexual e.
Group E. Scale
Group E. Survey
marriage e.
online e.
sexual e.
stressful e.

encourage to cough and deep breathe

encroachment
hypertrophic e.
osseous foraminal e.
scrotal e.

encrusted
e. pyelitis
e. tongue

encysted
e. calculus
e. hernia
e. hydrocele
e. pleurisy

end
angiographic end hole catheter
articulating bone e.
astrocytic end foot
e. of atrial systole
e. of bone covered with flap
cut end of bone
e. cutter
e. of day
e. diastole
dilution end point
dribbling at end of urination
eburnized bone e.
electrocardiographic interval from the beginning of QRS complex to end of the T wave
e. exhalation
e. expiration
e. expiratory
e. of field
e. of file
fimbriated end of fallopian tube
fimbriated end of oviduct
hemolysis end point
identified proximal ends of tendon
e. ileostomy
e. inhalation
e. inspiration
left ventricular end-diastole

left ventricular dimension in end-diastole
left ventricular internal dimension at end systole
e. of life
loop end ileostomy
e. of message
metallic distal end of tube
open end flow-through radiopaque tip
e. organ
e. organ damage
e. organ dysfunction
perineuronal end foot
perivascular end foot
permanent end colostomy
e. point
e. positive pressure breathing
e. product
proximal end of rib
proximal end of ulna
e. range of motion
rostral e.
e. of saturated bombardment
e. of short arm of chromosome
in situ end labeling
spontaneous positive end expiratory pressure
e. stoma
terminal or e.
e. tube

endangerment
child e.

endarterectomy
carotid e.
e. and coronary artery bypass grafting
e. knife
left carotid e.
Mayo Asymptomatic Carotid Endarterectomy Study
right carotid e.
transluminal endarterectomy catheter

endarteritis
obliterating e.
obliterative e.

endaural
e. mastoid incision
Shambaugh endaural incision

end-bearing amputation

end-biting blunt nosed rongeur

end-cutting
e.-c. reciprocating saw
tissue-protective, e.-c.

end-diastole
left ventricular dimension in e.-d.
posterior wall thickness at e.-d.

end-diastolic
e.-d. aortic-left ventricular pressure gradient
e.-d. area
e.-d. cardiac wall thickness
e.-d. chamber stiffness
e.-d. circumferential stress
e.-d. count
e.-d. diameter
e.-d. dimension
e.-d. flow
left atrial end-diastolic volume
left ventricular end-diastolic volume
e.-d. left ventricular pressure
e.-d. load
right ventricular end-diastolic volume
e.-d. segment length
e.-d. velocity
e.-d. velocity measurement
e.-d. volume
e.-d. volume index

endemic
African endemic relapsing fever
e. Burkitt lymphoma
e. cretinism
e. disease
e. fungal infection
e. goiter
e. hematuria
e. hemoptysis
e. influenza
malaria e.
myxedematous endemic cretinism
neurologic endemic cretinism

end-expiratory
e.-e. esophageal pressure
e.-e. lung volume
e.-e. phase
e.-e. wheeze

end-filling pressure

end-flow
right ventricular e.-f.

end-gaze
e.-g. nystagmus
e.-g. physiologic nystagmus

ending
anulospiral e.
anulospiral ending of muscle spindle
nerve e.
rat synaptic e.
synaptic e.
terminal nerve e.

end-inspiratory
e.-i. airway occlusion
e.-i. crackle
e.-i. crackles
e.-i. lung volume
e.-i. pause
e.-i. volume

Endler Multidimensional Anxiety Scale

endless
e. loop tachycardia
e. rumination

end-loop stoma

endoanal
e. probe
e. ultrasound

endobronchial
e. anesthesia
e. biopsy
e. brachytherapy
e. brush biopsy
double-lumen endobronchial tube
e. fistula
e. intubation anesthetic technique
e. stent
e. tree

endocardial
e. activation mapping
e. balloon lead
e. border delineation
e. cushion defect
e. cushion-type ventricular septal defect
encircling endocardial ventriculotomy
extended endocardial resection
extended endocardial resection procedure
e. fibroelastosis
e. fibrosis
e. flow
implantable unipolar endocardial electrode
e. mapping
e. murmur
nonbacterial thrombotic endocardial lesion
partial encircling endocardial ventriculotomy
e. potential
e. resection
e. resection procedure
right ventricular endocardial potential

endocardial *(continued)*
e. thickening
e. thrombus
e. vegetation
e. viability ratio

endocardiographic amplifier

endocarditis
acute bacterial e.
acute infective e.
aortic valve e.
artificial valve e.
atypical verrucous e.
bacterial e.
experimental enterococcal e.
infectious e.
infective e.
isolated parietal e.
mitral valve e.
native valve e.
Neisseria mucosa e.
nonbacterial thrombotic e.
nonbacterial verrucous e.
nosocomial infective e.
e. parietalis fibroplastica
prosthetic infectious e.
prosthetic valve e.
Streptococcus viridans e.
subacute bacterial e.

endocarditis parietalis fibroplastica

endocavitary
e. irradiation
e. pelvic lymphadenectomy
e. radiation

endocervical
atypical endocervical cells of undetermined significance
e. canal
e. columnar mucosa
e. cone
e. culture
e. curettage
e. curetting/curettage
e. ecchymosis
e. glandular dysplasia
e. mucinous borderline tumor
mucopurulent endocervical exudate
e. os
e. polypectomy
e. resection
vaginal cervical endocervical smear

endocervix
vagina, ectocervix, and e.

endochondral
abnormal endochondral ossification
auricular endochondral pseudocyst
e. bone deposits

endochondromatosis
multiple e.

endocoronary electrocardiography

endocrine
androgen withdrawal endocrine therapy
artificial endocrine pancreas
autoimmune endocrine disease
e. disease organic psychosis
e. ductal carcinoma in situ
familial multiple endocrine neoplasia
e. gland failure
gonadal endocrine disorder
e. granule constituent
e. hormone
e. hormone imbalance
e. imbalance
e. inactive pituitary tumor
e. and infertility
lymphoepithelial endocrine gland
e. and metabolic
metabolic, endocrine, and gastrointestinal
metabolic, endocrine, and gastrointestinal disorders
multiple endocrine adenomatosis type I, II
multiple endocrine deficiency, Addison disease, and candidiasis syndrome
multiple endocrine adenomatosis
multiple endocrine deficiency-autoimmune candidiasis
multiple endocrine neoplasm
multiple endocrine neoplasia syndrome, type 1, 2A, 2B, 3
multiple endocrine neoplasia type 1, 2, 2a, 2b, 3
e. organ transplant complication
pancreatic endocrine tumor
pathological endocrine tissue
pituitary endocrine disorder
pulmonary neuroepithelial e.

endocrinology
pediatric e.
reproductive e.

endocrinoma
multiple e.

endocrinopathy
autoimmune polyglandular e.
multiple e.
polyneuropathy, organomegaly, endocrinopathy, monoclonal gammopathy, and skin changes syndrome
polyneuropathy, organomegaly, endocrinopathy, M protein, and skin changes syndrome

endocrinoplasia
multiple e.

endocytosis
absorptive e.

endodermal
e. cyst
pulmonary endodermal tumor
e. sinus tumor

endodonic material

endodontic
e. implant
McSpadden endodontic technique
temporary endodontic restorative material
e. treatment

endoergic reaction

endoesophageal
e. magnetic resonance imaging
e. magnetic resonance imaging coil

end-of-dose
e.-o.-d. bradykinesia
e.-o.-d. deterioration

end-of-life
e.-o.-l. care
e.-o.-l. decision
e.-o.-l. issues
pacemaker e.-o.-l.

endofluoroscopy
percutaneous e.

endoforehead-biplanar face technique

endoforehead-endomidface lift

endoforehead fixation technique

endoforehead-periorbital-cheek lift

end-of-phase 1

end-of-phase 2

end-of-treatment response

endogenous
e. avidin-binding activity
e. brain mechanism
e. callus formation

e. circadian pacemaker
e. circadian rhythm
e. circadian rhythm phase
e. depression
e. digitalis-like factor
e. digitalis-like substance
e. erythroid colony
e. estrogen
e. fecal calcium
e. GAD inhibitor
e. glucose production
e. hormone
e. hyperlipidemia
e. hypothermia
e. infection
e. inhibitor of prostaglandin synthase
e. insulin
leukocyte endogenous mediator
e. limbic potential
e. obesity
e. opioid peptide
porcine endogenous retrovirus
e. pyrogen
e. steroid
e. toxin

endolaryngeal
e. brachytherapy mold
e. stent

endolaser
e. photocoagulation
e. probe tip

endolumenal gastroplication

endoluminal
e. brachytherapy
catheter probe-assisted endoluminal ultrasonography
e. clipping
colonoscopic endoluminal ultrasound
e. endoscopy
e. enlargement
e. graft
high-resolution endoluminal sonography
percutaneous endoluminal gastrostomy tube
e. prosthesis
e. radiation therapy
e. rectal ultrasonography
e. sonography
e. stenting
e. ultrasonography-guided fine-needle aspiration biopsy

endolymphatic
e. fluid
e. hydrops
e. sac
e. stromal myosis

endolymph filtration and excretion

endometrial
e. ablation
atypical endometrial hyperplasia
balloon endometrial ablation
benign cystic endometrial hyperplasia
e. biopsy
e. carcinoma
e. carcinoma in situ
e. cavity sounded
e. culture
e. curettage
e. cycling activity
e. cyst
e. dating
fragment of endometrial tissue
e. gland
hormonal therapy in endometrial carcinoma
e. hyperplasia
e. implant
e. intraepithelial carcinoma
e. intraepithelial neoplasia
e. laser intrauterine thermal therapy
microwave endometrial ablation
obesity in endometrial sarcoma
outpatient endometrial resection/ablation procedure
papillary endometrial carcinoma
physiologic endometrial ablation/resection loop
e. polyp
progestogen-dependent endometrial protein
e. resection and ablation
secretory e.
e. secretory adenocarcinoma
e. sloughing
e. stimulation
e. stripe
e. stroma
e. stromal sarcoma
e. thickness
e. tissue
uterine endometrial carcinoma

endometrioid
e. adenocarcinoma
ovarian endometrioid carcinoma
oxyphilic endometrioid adenocarcinoma
sertoliform endometrioid carcinoma

endometrioma
ovarian e.

endometriosis
asymptomatic mild e.
e. externa
ovarian endometriosis cyst
thoracic endometriosis syndrome

endometriosis-associated infertility

endometritis
e. dissecans
glandular e.
hyperplastic e.
nosocomial postpartum e.
postpartum e.
puerperal e.

endometrium
aspiration of e.
atrophic e.
hyperplastic e.
menstrual e.
nonpregnant e.
proliferative e.
prolonged phase e.
secretory carcinoma of the e.
transcervical resection of the e.

endomorphin
immunoreactive beta e.

endomyocardial
e. biopsy
e. disease
e. fibroelastosis
e. fibroplasia
e. fibrosis
e. lymphocytic infiltrates
percutaneous transluminal endomyocardial revascularization

endomyometrial resection

endomysial
e. antibody
e. staining

endomysium antibody

endonasal
e. dacryocystorhinostomy
e. fenestration
e. laser dacryocystorhinostomy
e. skull-base endoscopy

endoneural fluid pressure

endonuclease
restriction endonuclease analysis

endonucleases
restriction endonucleases from *Haemophilus influenzae*

endopeduncularis
nucleus e.

endopeptidase
neutral e.
neutral endopeptidase inhibition
pancreatic e.

endoperoxide steal

endophlebitis of retinal vein

endophotocoagulation
argon laser e.

endophthalmitis
Acanthamoeba e.
Aspergillus e.
candidal e.
granulomatous e.
metastatic e.
nocardial e.
parasitic e.
postoperative e.
posttraumatic e.

endophytic parasite

endophytum glioma

endoplasmic
agranular endoplasmic reticulum
Golgi endoplasmic reticulum lysosome
granular endoplasmic reticulum
rough endoplasmic reticulum
smooth endoplasmic reticulum
total endoplasmic reticulum

endoprosthesis
metallic biliary e.
Moore hip endoprosthesis system
peroral e.
total e.

endoprosthetic femoral head replacement

endopyelotomy
antegrade e.

endopyeloureterotomy
percutaneous e.

endorectal
e. advancement flap
e. flap
e. ileal pouch
e. ileal pull-through
e. ileoanal pull-through
e. ileoanal pull-through procedure
e. magnetic resonance imaging
e. probe
e. surface coil MRI
e. ultrasonography
e. ultrasound

end-organ
e.-o. damage
e.-o. degeneration
e.-o. failure
motor e.-o.
e.-o. resistance
e.-o. response

endorphin
e., dopamine, and prostaglandin theory
human e.

endorsement of deviant thoughts and beliefs

endosalpingiosis
atypical e.

endoscope
flexible fiberoptic e.
e. holder
e. holding clamp
e. lens cleansing device
lung imaging fluorescence e.
mother and baby e.
e. shaft

endoscope-assisted technique

endoscope-controlled microsurgery

endoscopic
e. access port
e. aspiration lumpectomy
e. aspiration mucosectomy
autofluorescent endoscopic system
automated endoscopic system for optimal positioning
automatic endoscopic reprocessor
automatic endoscopic system for optimal positioning
axillary endoscopic reduction
balloon-assisted, endoscopic, retroperitoneal, gasless
e. balloon dilation
e. balloon sphincter dilation
e. band ligation
e. biliary stent
e. bladder neck suspension
e. camera
e. carpal tunnel release
e. cautery
e. clipping
computed tomography under endoscopic retrograde pancreatography
computer-guided endoscopic sinus surgery
condom catheter endoscopic ultrasound
contrast-enhanced endoscopic ultrasonography
e. control
e. coronary artery bypass grafting
Crohn Disease E. Index of Severity
cutting endoscopic mucosal resection
e. decompression
e. digital pancreatography
e. dissection
dual percutaneous endoscopic gastrostomy
extraperitoneal endoscopic pelvic lymph node dissection
fetal e.
fiberoptic endoscopic evaluation of swallowing
fiberoptic endoscopic evaluation of swallowing with sensory testing
fiberoptic endoscopic examination of swallowing
flexible endoscopic evaluation of swallowing
flexible endoscopic evaluation of swallowing with sensory testing
flexible endoscopic swallowing examination
e. forceps
e. fulguration
functional endoscopic sinus
functional endoscopic sinus surgery
e. guidance
e. harvest
e. hemorrhoid ligation
image-guided functional endoscopic sinus surgery
e. India ink injection
e. injection sclerosis
e. injection sclerotherapy
e. injection therapy
e. in-line needle holder
e. intranasal dacryocystorhinostomy
intraoperative endoscopic Congo red test
e. intubation
jejunal tube through percutaneous endoscopic gastrostomy
e. knot pusher
e. laser
e. laser foraminotomy
e. laser recanalization

e. laser therapy
lift-and-cut endoscopic mucosal resection
light-induced fluorescence endoscopic bronchoscopy
e. light source
e. magnetic resonance
mechanical endoscopic management
mini-functional endoscopic sinus surgery
mother endoscopic retrograde cholangiopancreatoscopy system
e. mucosal ablation
e. mucosal resection
e. mucosal resection, cap method
e. mucosal resection, tube method
e. mucosal resection with ligation
multiplanar endoscopic facial rejuvenation technique
e. muscle plication
nasal endoscopic surgery
e. nasobiliary drainage
needle-knife endoscopic pancreatic sphincterotomy
e. pancreatic sphincterotomy
e. pancreatic stenting
e. pancreatocholangiography
e. papillary balloon dilation
e. papillotomy
pedicled endoscopic latissimus dorsi harvest
percutaneous e.
percutaneous endoscopic cecostomy
percutaneous endoscopic gastrostomy
percutaneous endoscopic gastrostomy insertion
percutaneous endoscopic gastrostomy and jejunal extension tube
percutaneous endoscopic gastrostomy tube
percutaneous endoscopic jejunostomy
percutaneous endoscopic lumbar diskectomy
percutaneous endoscopic placement of jejunal tube
percutaneous endoscopic recanalization
percutaneous endoscopic removal
e. photography
e. plantar fasciotomy
powered endoscopic sinus surgery
e. pulsed dye laser
e. pulsed dye laser lithotripsy
e. raking
rectal endoscopic ultrasonography
rectal-expander-assisted transanal endoscopic microsurgery
e. removal
e. retrograde balloon dilatation
e. retrograde biliary drainage
e. retrograde biliary stenting
e. retrograde cholangiogram
e. retrograde cholangiography
e. retrograde cholangiopancreatogram
e. retrograde cholangiopancreatography
e. retrograde cholecystoendoprosthesis
e. retrograde pancreatogram
e. retrograde pancreatography
e. retrograde parenchymography of pancreas
e. retrograde sphincterotomy
e. sinus surgery
e. snare
e. stone disintegration
e. stone manipulation
e. stone removal
subfascial endoscopic perforator surgery
subperiosteal minimally invasive laser endoscopic facelift
e. surveillance
e. technique
e. tissue culture
totally endoscopic coronary artery bypass
transanal endoscopic microsurgery
e. transformational diskectomy
transnasal endoscopic ethmoidectomy
e. transpapillary catheterization of gallbladder
e. transpapillary cyst drainage
transpapillary endoscopic cholecystotomy
e. transthoracic symphathectomy
e. ultrasound
e. ultrasound-guided fine-needle aspiration
e. unroofing
e. variceal band ligation
e. variceal sclerosis
e. variceal sclerotherapy
e. video-assisted surgery
e. visualization

endoscopically assisted duodenal intubation

endoscopy
carpal tunnel e.
endonasal skull-base e.
esophageal e.
gastrointestinal e.
intraoperative e.
laser-assisted spinal e.
light-induced fluorescence endoscopy in combination with pharmacoendoscopy
lumbar epidural e.
lung imaging fluorescent e.
microscopic endoscopy surgery
middle ear e.
Olympus endoscopy system
open access e.
perform e.
e. suite
upper gastrointestinal e.
virtual e.
wireless endoscopy capsule

endoscopy-related emphysema

endoskeletal
solid ankle flexible e.
stationary attachment flexible e.

endoskeleton
stationary ankle flexible e.

endosmotic equivalent

endosonography
anal e.

endosseous implant

endosteal
e. implant
unidentified endosteal marrow cell

endothelial
activated endothelial cell
antiplatelet endothelial cell adhesion molecule
antivascular endothelial growth factor monoclonal antibody
e. cell
e. cell growth factor
e. cell growth supplement
e. cell-stimulating angiogenesis factor
congenital endothelial corneal dystrophy
e. constitutive nitric oxide synthase
e. constitutive nitric oxide synthetase
fetal bovine endothelial cell
human aortic endothelial cell

endothelial *(continued)*
human dermal microvascular endothelial cell
human endothelial cell
human umbilical vein endothelial cell
intravascular papillary endothelial hyperplasia
iridocorneal endothelial syndrome
Masson intravascular endothelial proliferation
neutralizing antibody to vascular endothelial growth factor
e. nitric oxide synthase
nucleated endothelial cell
e. PAS-domain protein-1
peritubular endothelial cell
pig aortic endothelial cell
platelet-derived endothelial cell growth factor
platelet endothelial cell adhesion molecule-1
e. proliferating factor
pulmonary endothelial membrane
recombinant human vascular endothelial growth factor
sinusoidal endothelial cell
e. specular microscope
e. tissue
vascular endothelial cell growth inhibitor
vascular endothelial growth factor/vascular permeability factor
vascular endothelial growth factor 2, 3
vasoablative endothelial sarcoma

endothelial-epithelial corneal dystrophy

endothelial-leukocyte
e.-l. adhesion molecule
e.-l. adhesion molecule-1

endothelial-monocyte activating polypeptide II

endotheliitis
linear e.
peripheral e.

endothelin
e. A
e. B

endothelin-converting enzyme

endothelin-1–endothelin-3

endothelin-receptor-B

endotheliochorial placenta

endothelioid habit

endothelioma
clear cell e.

endothelium
blood vessel e.
bovine aortic e.

endothelium-derived
e.-d. constricting factor
e.-d. hyperpolarizing factor
e.-d. nitric oxide
e.-d. relaxing factor

endothoracic fascia

endotoxic
Gram-negative endotoxic shock
e. reaction
e. shock

endotoxin
e. antibody
enzyme-digested delta endotoxin
e. unit

endotoxin-like activity

endotoxin-mediated otitis media with effusion

endotracheal
e. anesthesia
e. aspirate
e. aspiration
e. cardiac output monitor
cuffed endotracheal tube
general anesthesia with endotracheal intubation
general endotracheal anesthesia
e. induction
e. insufflation
e. intubation and mechanical ventilation
nasal endotracheal intubation
nasal endotracheal tube
open endotracheal suction
open endotracheal suctioning
oral endotracheal intubation
oral endotracheal tube
e. stylet
e. suction
e. tube
e. tube placement

endovaginal ultrasound

endovascular
e. aneurysm
e. aortic graft
e. approach
e. balloon
e. balloon occlusion
e. brachytherapy
e. carotid sacrifice
e. coagulation
e. coiling
e. embolism
e. grafting
e. graft insertion
e. graft treatment
e. hemolytic-uremic syndrome
e. intervention
intracaval endovascular ultrasound
e. irradiation
malignant endovascular papillary angioendothelioma
percutaneous endovascular treatment
e. proliferation
e. repair
e. stent graft
e. stenting
e. surgery
e. technique
e. treatment

endovasculitis
hemorrhagic e.

endovasculopathy
hemorrhagic e.

endplate
cartilaginous e.
giant miniature endplate potential
miniature endplate current
miniature endplate potential
monophasic endplate activity
motor e.
muscle e.
e. ossification
posterior e.
e. potential
superior e.
e. of vertebrae
vertebral e.
vertebral body e.

endpoint
e. measurement
e. nystagmus
skin endpoint titration
therapeutic e.

endpoints
multiple e.

end-position nystagmus

end-pressure artifact

end-product
advanced glycation e.-p.
advanced glycosylation e.-p.

end-respiratory crackle

end-stage
e.-s. adult cardiac decompensation
e.-s. cardiomyopathy

e.-s. cirrhosis
e.-s. dementia
e.-s. heart factor
e.-s. heart failure
e.-s. heart and liver disease
e.-s. kidney disease
e.-s. liver disease
e.-s. liver failure
e.-s. lung disease
e.-s. organ disease
e.-s. renal disease
e.-s. renal failure

end-state functioning

end-systolic
e.-s. count
e.-s. diameter
e.-s. dimension
e.-s. force velocity index
left atrial end-systolic volume
left ventricular end-systolic volume
e.-s. left ventricular pressure
e.-s. pressure-length relationship
right ventricular end-systolic volume
e.-s. segment length
e.-s. ventricular volume
e.-s. volume index
e.-s. wall index
e.-s. wall stress
e.-s. wall thickness

end-tidal
e.-t. carbon dioxide concentration
e.-t. carbon dioxide monitoring
e.-t. CO2 monitoring

end-to-end
e.-t.-e. anastomosis
e.-t.-e. bite
e.-t.-e. invaginating
e.-t.-e. reconstruction
e.-t.-e. reconstruction technique
e.-t.-e. suture
e.-t.-e. tendon repair
e.-t.-e. venous anastomosis

end-to-side
e.-t.-s. anastomosis
e.-t.-s. arteriotomy
e.-t.-s. ileotransverse colostomy
e.-t.-s. portacaval shunt
e.-t.-s. splenorenal shunt
e.-t.-s. venous anastomosis

endurance
cardiorespiratory e.
e. factor
isometric endurance time
isotonic endurance test
e. level
e. limit
metal endurance limit
e. time
tolerance and e.
e. training

enduring
displays enduring bitterness

enema
air-contrast barium e.
air enema fluoroscopic imaging
air pressure enema reduction
5-aminosalicylic acid e.
antegrade colonic e.
antegrade continence e.
antegrade continence enema procedure
barium e.
barium enema with air contrast
bath, laxative, enema, shampoo, and shower
e. of choice
double-contrast barium e.
dual-contrast barium e.
Gastrografin e.
glycerin and water e.
high soapsuds e.
magnesium sulfate, glycerin, and water e.
Malone antegrade colonic enema stoma procedure
Malone antegrade continence enema procedure
Malone antegrade continent enema channel
meglumine diatrizoate enema study
methylene blue e.
normal saline e.
oil retention e.
return flow e.
saline e.
saline solution e.
single-contrast barium e.
tap water e.
tap water enema til clear
tepid water e.

energetic dynamic cardiac insufficiency

energy
activation e.
anterior-posterior dual energy radiography
apparent digestible e.
apparent digestive e.
artificial heart energy system
average positron e.
basal energy expenditure
chemical e.
color Doppler e.
e. conservation
conservation of e.
crystal field stabilization e.
decreased appetite and loss of e.
decreased energy, fatigue and weakness
decrease in energy or fatigue
depleted e.
depleted
digestive e.
electron energy loss spectroscopy
estimated energy needs
e. expended with activity
e. expenditure
fluorescence energy transfer immunoassay
fluorescence resonance energy transfer
free e.
Gibbs free e.
Helmholtz e.
Helmholtz free e.
high linear energy transfer radiation
increased energy, decreased appetite
internal e.
ion kinetic e.
kinetic energy of a particle
kinetic energy released in the medium
lack of e.
linear energy transfer
loss of energy metabolism
low energy direct current
low energy level
low energy transfer
low-linear energy transfer radiation
mass-analyzed ion kinetic e.
measured energy expenditure
metabolic e.
metabolizable e.
muscle e.
muscle energy technique
potential e.
e. quotient
radiant e.
rate of energy loss
reaction e.
resting e.
resting energy expenditure
standard free e.

energy *(continued)*
strain energy density
thermal energy analyzer
threshold e.
total daily energy expenditure
total digestible e.
total energy expended
total energy expenditure
total energy requirement
total metabolizable e.
e. unit
x-ray energy spectrometry

energy/alertness
increased e.

energy-dispersed x-ray analysis

energy-dispersive
e.-d. spectrometer
e.-d. x-ray fluorescence

energy-protein malnutrition

engaged
e. head
head not e.

engine
high-speed e.
Mity engine T-file

engineering
e. in medicine and biology
Minnesota E. Analogies Test
sanitary e.

English
anterior feature English phoneme
E. as a second language
manual E.
Pidgin Sign E.
Seeing Essential E.
Signed E.
Signing Exact E.

engorged
e. breast
Nunn engorged corpuscles

engorgement
liver e.
postpartum breast e.

engraft
failure to e.

engrafted allogenic tissue

engraftment
allogeneic e.
donor bone marrow e.
donor cell e.
myeloid e.
neutrophil e.
sustained e.

enhanced
e. atrioventricular conduction
e. atrioventricular nodal conduction
e. chemiluminescence
color enhanced view
computer enhanced image
e. CT scan
dynamic enhanced magnetic resonance imaging
e. external counterpulsation
e. green fluorescent protein
e. inactivated polio vaccine
e. intellectual efficiency
e. interest and concentration
intravenously enhanced computed tomography
pulsed irrigation for enhanced evacuation
e. reactivation
e. sensory awareness
surface enhanced laser desorption/ionization
visually enhanced vestibuloocular reflex
Weinstein enhanced sensory test

enhancement
antibody-dependent e.
artery-like pattern of e.
astigmatic keratotomy e.
breast enhancement surgery
comprehensive health enhancement support system
coping strategy e.
countercurrent flow-related e.
delayed contrast e.
flow-related e.
hybrid rapid acquisition with relaxation e.
leukocyte migration e.
e. of magnetic resonance imaging
microbubble contrast e.
migration enhancement factor
motivational enhancement therapy
e. Newcastle disease
paramagnetic contrast e.
paramagnetic enhancement accentuation by chemical shift imaging
penile girth e.
personalized aerobics for cardiovascular e.
proton relaxation e.
rapid acquisition with relaxation e.
rapid acquisition with resolution e.
e. ratio
ring e.
self-applied health enhancement method
signal enhancement ratio
thermal enhancement ratio

enhancer
aerosol cloud e.
pancreatic islet cell-specific enhancer sequence
thyroid-specific enhancer binding protein-1

enhancing
e. brain lesion
health enhancing trait
e. lesion
multifocal enhancing lesion
neurotrophic enhancing molecule
e. normal breathing
e. ring
e. ring lesion
single enhancing CT lesion

enkephalin
leucine e.
methionine e.

enlarged
adenoids appeared e.
adenoids did not appear e.
e. cardiac silhouette
diffusely enlarged thyroid
e. heart
heart does appear e.
heart does not appear e.
e. heart muscle
lump in breast does appear e.
nonsyndromic familial enlarged vestibular aqueduct
not e.
e. vestibular aqueduct syndrome

enlargement
apical cardiac nodal e.
asymmetric parathyroid e.
benign prostatic e.
biventricular e.
cardiac e.
cardiac silhouette e.
diffuse liver e.
diffuse symmetrical uterine e.
excessive enlargement of head
generalized glandular e.
e. of heart
hereditary hypertrophic e.
left atrial e.
left ventricular e.
lumbar enlargement of spinal cord

lumbosacral enlargement of spinal cord
lymph node e.
moyamoya collateral e.
no e.
noncancerous enlargement of prostate gland
no palpable e.
parathyroid gland e.
parotid gland e.
right atrial e.
right ventricular e.
salivary gland e.
significant glandular e.

enlistment
did not exist prior to e.
existed prior to e.

enolase
muscle-specific e.
neuron-specific e.
neuron-specific enolase stain
neuron-specific enolase tumor marker
neuro-specific enolase antibody
nonneuronal e.

enough
not enough cells

Enquiry
Coping Operations Preference E.
Life Interpersonal History E.

enriched
B-cell e.
T-cell e.

enrichment
Enterobacteriaceae enrichment broth
language enrichment therapy
osmotic erythrocyte e.
primary enrichment medium
secondary enrichment medium

Enseada virus

ensheathing callus

ensiform
e. appendix
e. cartilage

Entebbe bat virus

enteral
e. alimentation
elemental enteral alimentation
e. feeding
e. feeding tube
home enteral nutrition
home enteral tube feeding
e. hyperalimentation
e. nutrition
e. nutritional supplement
e. nutritional support
e. nutritional therapy
e. nutrition solution
parenteral and enteral nutrition
total enteral nutrition

entered
abdomen entered and explored

enteric
e. anastomosis
antineuronal enteric antibody test
e. coated aspirin
e. cytopathic human orphan
e. cytopathogenic human orphan
e. drainage
e. feeding
graft enteric erosion
graft enteric fistula
e. Gram-negative bacillary
e. Gram-negative bacillus
Hektoen enteric agar
human enteric virus
mediastinal dorsal enteric cyst
e. nervous system
e. organism
e. pathogen
pedicled enteric donor site
portal venous and enteric drainage technique
respiratory enteric orphan virus

enterically transmitted non-A, non-B hepatitis

enteric-coated aspirin

entericus
liquor e.

entering
e. complaint
e. diagnosis

enteritis
bovine e.
e. choleriform
duck virus e.
e. gravis
mink enteritis virus
necrotic e.
e. necroticans
regional e.
transmural e.

enteroadherent *Escherichia coli*

enteroaggregative
e. *Escherichia coli*
e. *Escherichia coli* heat-stable enterotoxin 1

Enterobacteriaceae
Enterobacteriaceae enrichment broth
extended-spectrum beta-lactamase-producing E.

enterobacterial common antigen

enterocele
anterior e.
partial e.

enterochromaffin
e. cell
e. cell hyperplasia

enterochromaffin-like type

enterocleisis
omental e.

enterocoated
e. microspheres of pancrelipase

enterococcal
e. bacteremia
e. endocarditis
experimental enterococcal endocarditis
e. infection
e. sepsis

Enterococcus
VanB *Enterococcus faecium*
vancomycin-resistant *Enterococcus*
vancomycin-resistant *Enterococcus faecium*

enterococcus
glycopeptide-resistant e.
group D e.
e. microorganism
multiple-drug-resistant e.'s

enterocolic fistula

enterocolitica
Yersinia enterocolitica colitis

enterocolitis
gangrenous ischemic e.
Hirschsprung-associated e.
necrotizing e.
necrotizing amebic e.
neonatal necrotizing e.
neutropenic e.
pseudomembranous necrotizing e.

enterocutaneous
e. fistula
e. intubation

enterocystoplasty
seromuscular enterocystoplasty lined with urothelium

enterocytopathogenic
e. avian orphan virus
e. bovine orphan virus

enterocytopathogenic *(continued)*
e. cat orphan virus
e. dog orphan virus
e. equine orphan virus
e. human orphan
e. human orphan-rhinocoryza virus
e. human orphan virus
e. monkey orphan virus
e. porcine orphan virus
e. rodent orphan virus
e. swine orphan virus

enteroenteric fistula

enteroenterostomy
Parker-Kerr closed method of end-to-end e.

enterogastric reflex

enterogenic
e. albuminuria
e. proteinuria

enterohemorrhagic *Escherichia coli*

enterohepatic
e. circulation
e. clearance
e. shunt
e. shunting

enteroinsular axis

enteroinvasive *Escherichia coli*

enteromesenteric occlusion

enteropathic
Escherichia coli e.

enteropathogenic
Escherichia e.
e. *Escherichia coli*

enteropathy
alopecia, nail dystrophy, ophthalmic complication, thyroid dysfunction, hypohidrosis, ephelides and enteropathy, and respiratory tract infection
autoimmune e.
cow's milk-sensitive e.
gluten-sensitive e.
proliferative hemorrhagic e.
protein-losing e.

enteropathy-associated T-cell lymphoma

enteroscope
magnifying e.

enteroscopy
intraoperative e.
small bowel e.
transgastrostomic e.

enterostomal
e. therapist
e. therapy

enterostomy
diverting e.
percutaneous e.
proximal e.

enterotomy
antimesenteric e.
longitudinal e.
occult e.

enterotoxigenic *Escherichia coli*

enterotoxin
accessory cholera e.
Clostridium perfringens e.
enteroaggregative *Escherichia coli* heat-stable enterotoxin 1
staphylococcal enterotoxin A, B, D, F
staphylococcal enterotoxin B antiserum

enterovirulent *Escherichia coli*

enterovirus
neonatal enterovirus infection
nonpolio e.

enthalpy
e. physics
specific e.

enthesis
Achilles tendon e.
Achilles tendon enthesis calcification

enthesitis
spondylitis, enthesitis, arthritis

enthesopathy
ankylosis and ankylosing e.
seronegativity, enthesopathy, arthropathy

enthusiasm
chronic enthusiasm disorder

entire treatment period

entity
controlling external e.'s
new chemical e.
new molecular e.
pathologic e.

Entner-Doudoroff metabolic pathway

entocuneiform bone

entomological inoculation rate

entopic pulse

entorbital fissure

entorhinal cortex

entozoic parasite

entrainment
high air flow with oxygen e.

entrance
admission, entrance, and evaluation unit
e. complaint
e. of fetal head into superior pelvic strait
pedicle entrance point
sinoatrial entrance block

entrapment
anterior interosseous nerve e.
anular ligament e.
hypoglossal carotid e.
long thoracic nerve e.
e. mononeuropathy
nerve entrapment neuralgia
nerve entrapment site
nerve entrapment syndrome
e. neuropathy
peroneal entrapment neuropathy
peroneal nerve e.
sciatic nerve e.
supracapsular nerve entrapment syndrome
ulnar nerve e.

entrapped
liposomally entrapped doxorubicin
liposomally entrapped second antibody
e. nerve

entropion
atonic e.
marginal e.
spastic e.

entropy
approximate e.
e. unit

entry
air e.
arterial entry site
arthroscopic entry portal
calcium entry blocker
direct data e.
dorsal root entry zone
internal ribosome entry site
nurse's late e.
e. on duty
point of e.
point of entry, traction and twist
port of e.
posterior root entry zone
provider order e.
remote data e.
remote data entry system

sperm entry point
virus entry mediator, a receptor expressed by T lymphocyte

entubulation
nerve e.

enucleation
e. of eyeball
e. of eyeball operation
orbital e.
orbital enucleation compressor
e. technique

enumeration
centromere enumeration probe

enuresis
adult-onset e.
monosymptomatic nocturnal e.
nocturnal e.
primary nocturnal e.
psychogenic e.
secondary e.
sleep e.

envelope
e. 2 antigen
e. of cell
glycosylated protein spanning viral e.
maximal flow-volume e.
skin-soft tissue e.
viral envelope antigen

envenomation
arachnid e.
marine e.

environment
adverse psychosocial e.
aversive early e.
e. characteristic
College and University E. Scales
Community-Oriented Programs E. Scale
controlled environment treatment
Correctional Institutions E. Scale
Family E. Scale
Group E. Scale
health and e.
heredity and e.
e. and heredity
Home Observation for Measurement of the E.
hostile work e.
Infant/Toddler E. Rating Scale
least restrictive e.
managed care e.
medical toxic e.
neutral thermal e.
nurse cell e.
parental environment characteristic
parental environment item
patient's home e.
perception of the e.
protected environment units and prophylactic antibiotic
Restricted E. Stimulation Therapy
Scales of Creativity and Learning E.
The Instructional E. Scale
Total E. Control
total protective e.
University Residence E. Scale

environmental
e. allergen
e. allergy
Classroom E. Scale
cognitive environmental stimulation
e. complexity
e. control unit
dichotic environmental sounds test
dynamic environmental conditioning cycle
e. exposure unit
e. hazard
e. health
health effects of environmental pollutants
E. Health Laboratory
e. heat injury
idiopathic environmental intolerance
e. illness
E. Impact Statement
e. irritation
E. Language Inventory
e. metaplastic atrophic gastritis
Multiphasic E. Assessment Procedure
occupational and environmental medicine
pollution and environmental degradation
potentially pathogenic environmental mycobacterial
E. Pre-Language Battery
e. protection
e. resistance
E. Response Inventory
restriction of environmental stimulation therapy
e. sex determination
social environmental therapy
e. stimulation
e. tobacco smoke
e. toxin
e. variance

environmentally associated rheumatic disorder

envy
chronic intense e.
penis e.
phallus e.

enzootic nasal tumor

enzygotic twins

enzymatic
e. abnormality of adrenal gland
e. active
e. activity
e. cell dispersion
e. cleaner
e. debridement
e. imbalance
e. immunoassay
lysosomal enzymatic activity
e. pancreatic secretion
self-contained enzymatic membrane immunoassay

enzyme
allercoat enzyme allergosorbent unit
e. allergosorbent test
alpha-fetoprotein enzyme immunoassay
amino acid activating e.
angiotensin-converting e.
angiotensin-converting enzyme dysfunction syndrome
angiotensin-converting enzyme gene
angiotensin-converting enzyme gene polymorphism
angiotensin-converting enzyme II
angiotensin-converting enzyme inhibitor
angiotensin-converting enzyme inhibitor cough
angiotensin I-converting e.
antibody-directed enzyme prodrug therapy
antibody-directed enzyme therapy
antinuclear antibody screening by enzyme immunoassay
AP marker e.
aromatase enzyme complex
automated enzyme immunoassay for antinuclear antibody
bacillus species e.
blood group degrading e.
chemical enzyme profile
cloned enzyme donor immunoassay
converting e.

enzyme *(continued)*
converting enzyme inhibitor
corona-penetrating e.
cytochrome P450 enzyme 19, 27
cytochrome P450 enzyme 1A1
cytochrome P450 enzyme 11A
cytochrome P450 enzyme 21B
e. deficiency
demosterol-to-cholesterol e.
drug-metabolizing e.
endothelin-converting e.
erythropoietin-producing e.
fluorescent enzyme immunoassay
fragment of mmunoglobulin G after digestion with the enzyme pepsin
galactose enzyme activator
e. glaucoma
hepatic enzyme study
hepatitis C virus enzyme immunoassay
hepatocellular e.'s
high-strength pancreatic e.'s
hollow e.
homogeneous enzyme immunoassay
hormone-receptor e.
human milk reverse transcriptase e.
imbalance of e.'s
e. immunoassay
immunoglobulin-complexed e.
e. immunosorbent assay
indirect enzyme immunoassay for anti-*Mycoplasma pneumoniae* IgM
e. inhibition complex
e. inhibitor
initial cardiac e.
insulin-degrading e.
interleukin-1 alpha converting e.
interleukin-1 beta converting e.
lipogenic enzyme propensity
liver enzyme elevation
liver enzyme serum level
liver enzyme test
lymphocyte enzyme stain
lysosomal enzyme disorder
lysosomal hydrolase enzyme assay
lysozymal enzyme release
major detoxification e.
malic e.
malic enzyme gene
microparticle capture enzyme immunoassay
microsomal enzyme system
mitochondrial hydroxylase e.
mitochondrial respiratory chain e.
mitochondrial respiratory chain enzyme complex
multilocus enzyme electrophoresis analysis
muscle enzyme serum level
muscle enzyme test
muscle fraction enzyme of creatine phosphokinase
myocardial band enzymes of creatine phosphokinase
negative control enzyme induction
old yellow e.
oligosaccharide transferase e.
pancreatic enzyme replacement therapy
pancreatic enzyme secretion
penicillin-sensitive e.
phosphorylase-rupturing e.
photoreacting e.
photoreactivating e.
e. potentiated desensitization
e. product
pulmonary angiotensin I converting e.
rapid rabies enzyme immunodiagnosis
rate of reaction catalyzed by an e.
receptor-destroying e.
reduced yellow e.
restriction enzyme analysis
second-generation enzyme immunoassay
serum angiotensin-converting e.
serum enzyme study
e. substrate
e. substrate inhibitor
e. unit
yellow e.

enzyme-digested delta endotoxin

enzyme-labeled immunoassay

enzyme-linked
e.-l. antiglobulin test
e.-l. fluorescent immunoassay
e.-l. immunoabsorbent assay
e.-l. immunocytochemical technique
e.-l. immunoelectrodiffusion assay
e.-l. immunofiltration assay
e.-l. immunosorbent as
e.-l. immunosorbent assay
e.-l. immunospot assay
e.-l. immunotransfer blot

enzyme-multiplied
e.-m. immunoassay technique
e.-m. immunoassay test

enzymes
hemolysis, elevated liver enzymes, and low platelet count
high-strength pancreatic e.
imbalance of e.
myocardial band enzymes of creatine phosphokinase

enzyme-treated cell

enzymopathy
urea cycle e.

eosin
hematoxylin and e.
hematoxylin and eosin stain

eosinophil
absolute blood eosinophil count
e. cationic protein
e. chemotactic factor of anaphylaxis
e. count
e. protein X
peripheral eosinophil count
polymorphonuclear e.
polynuclear e.
e. stimulation promoter
total eosinophil count

eosinophil-derived neurotoxin

eosinophilia
angiolymphoid hyperplasia with e.
bronchiectasis, eosinophilia, asthma, pneumonia
diffuse fasciitis with e.
nodules, eosinophilia, rheumatism, dermatitis, and swelling syndrome
nonallergic rhinitis with eosinophilia syndrome
peripheral blood e.
pulmonary infiltrate with e.
pulmonary infiltration with e.
radiation-related e.
sclerosing mucoepidermoid carcinoma with e.
tumor-associated tissue e.

eosinophilia-myalgia syndrome

eosinophilic
e. adenoma
allergic eosinophilic gastroenteritis
allergic eosinophilic gastroenterocolitis
e. angiocentric fibrosis
blood eosinophilic nonallergic rhinitis

e. cationic protein
e. chemotactic factor
e. chemotactic factor-complement
chronic eosinophilic leukemia
chronic eosinophilic pneumonia
e. cytoplasmic inclusion
e., polymorphic, and pruritic eruption associated with radiotherapy
e. fasciitis
e. fibrohistiocytic lesion of bone marrow
e. gastritis
e. gastroenteritis
granular eosinophilic cytoplasm
e. granuloma
e. granuloma of lung
idiopathic acute eosinophilic pneumonia
e. index
nodular eosinophilic panniculitis
e. nonallergic rhinitis
oil-associated pneumoparalytic eosinophilic syndrome
e. pneumonia
protein-induced eosinophilic colitis
e. pustular folliculitis
reactive eosinophilic pleuritis
unifocal eosinophilic granuloma

eosinophil protein X

eosinophils
peripheral blood e.

ependymal
e. cell
e. glioma
tanycyte ependymal cell

ependymitis granularis

ependymoma
malignant e.
myxopapillary e.
papillary e.

ephelides
alopecia, nail dystrophy, ophthalmic complication, thyroid dysfunction, hypohidrosis, ephelides and enteropathy, and respiratory tract infection
nevi, atrial myxoma, myxoid neurofibroma, and ephelides syndrome
nevi, atrial myxoma, myxoid neurofibroma, and ephelides syndrome

ephemeral
bovine ephemeral fever
e. fever
e. pneumonia

epi arterial bronchus

epibronchial right pulmonary artery syndrome

epibulbar
e. carcinoma
mandibulofacial dysostosis with epibulbar dermoids syndrome

epicanthal
medial epicanthal scar band

epicanthus
Arlt epicanthus repair
blepharophimosis, ptosis, epicanthus inversus syndrome

epicardial
e. Doppler echocardiography
e. fat pad
e. fat pad sign
e. fat tag
e. monitoring
e. pacing

epichlorohydrin and triethanolamine

epic microscope

epicondylar
e. avulsion fracture
medial epicondylar apophysis
medial epicondylar crest
medial epicondylar fracture
medial epicondylar ridge
e. ridge

epicondyle
medial epicondyle of femur
medial epicondyle humeral fracture
medial epicondyle of humerus

epicondylectomy
medial e.

epicondylitis
external humeral e.
medial e.

epicranialis
aponeurosis e.

epicritic sensibility

epidemic
acquired immune deficiency syndrome e.
acute epidemic infectious adenitis
e. acute nonbacterial gastroenteritis
e. disease of infant mice
e. fatal encephalopathy
e. gangrenous proctitis
e. hemorrhagic fever
e. hepatitis
e. hepatitis-associated antigen
hibernal epidemic viral infection
e. influenza
e. keratoconjunctivitis
e. methicillin-resistant *Staphylococcus aureus*
e. observation unit
Singapore epidemic conjunctivitis
toxic epidemic syndrome
toxic oil epidemic syndrome

epidemiologic
Centers for E. Studies Depression scale
e. catchment area
Surveillance and Control of Pathogens of E. Importance

epidemiology
E. of Diabetes Interventions and Complications
Human Genome E. Network
Methodology for E. in Children and Adolescents
Methods for the E. of Child and Adolescent Disorders T score
Methods for E. of Child and Adolescent Mental Disorders
Rochester E. Project
e. year

epidermal
anogenital epidermal cyst
e. basement zone
e. cell
e. cell surface protein
concentration epidermal growth factor
e. dysplastic verruciformis
erythema multiforme/toxic epidermal necrolysis
esophageal epidermal growth factor
e. growth factor
e. growth factor receptor
heparin-binding epidermal growth factorlike growth factor
human epidermal growth factor
human epidermal growth receptor 2
e. inclusion cyst
inflamed linear verrucous epidermal nevus
inflammatory linear verrucous epidermal nevus
inherited epidermal dysplasia
lichen striatus epidermal nevus

epidermal *(continued)*
linear epidermal nevus
linear inflammatory verrucous epidermal nevus
mouse epidermal growth factor
pagetoid epidermal involvement
platelet-derived epidermal growth factor
salivary epidermal growth factor
e. soluble protein
total epidermal necrolysis
toxic epidermal necrolysis
toxic epidermal necrosis

epidermidis
methicillin-resistant *Staphylococcus epidermidis*

epidermin

epidermis
interfollicular e.
skin epidermis dose radiation
uninvolved e.

epidermodysplasia verruciformis

epidermoid
human oral epidermoid carcinoma cell
nonkeratinizing epidermoid carcinoma

epidermolysis
e. bullosa
e. bullosa acquisita
e. bullosa atrophicans
e. bullosa, macular type
e. bullosa simplex
dominant epidermolysis bullosa simplex
dystrophic epidermolysis bullosa
generalized atrophic benign epidermolysis bullosa
junctional epidermolysis bullosa
localized epidermolysis bullosa simplex
recessive epidermolysis bullosa dystrophica–Hallopeau-Siemens syndrome
recessive dystrophic epidermolysis bullosa

epidermolytic hyperkeratosis

epidermotropic metastatic malignant melanoma

epididymal
microscopic epididymal sperm aspiration
microsurgical epididymal sperm aspiration
microsurgical epididymal sperm aspiration procedure
papillary epididymal cystadenoma
percutaneous drainage of epididymal abscess
percutaneous epididymal sperm aspiration
e. sperm aspiration

epididymidis
vas e.

epididymis
appendix of e.
ligament of epididymis inferior and superior
lobule of e.
lobule of e.
microsurgical extraction of sperm from e.
superior ligament of e.

epididymitis
mumps e.

epididymoorchitis
pediatric cryptococcal e.

epididymovasostomy
microsurgical e.

epidural
e. abscess
e. anesthesia
e. anesthetic
anterior epidural fat
e. block
e. blockade
e. blood
e. blood patch
e. blood patch anesthetic technique
blunt-tipped epidural needle
e. catheter
e. cavity
cervical epidural steroid injection
continuous epidural analgesia
continuous epidural anesthesia
continuous infusion epidural analgesia
continuous lumbar epidural anesthesia
e. cord compression
e. delivery
drainage of cerebral epidural space
e. fat
e. fibrosis
e. hematoma
e. hemorrhage
e. implant
e. injection
intracranial epidural pressure
intraspinal epidural pressure
long-term epidural catheterization
lumbar epidural abscess
lumbar epidural anesthesia
lumbar epidural block
lumbar epidural endoscopy
lumbar epidural steroid
lumbar epidural steroid injection
e. meningitis
metastatic epidural spinal cord compression
e. needle
e. neural blockade
patient-controlled epidural anesthesia
percutaneous epidural nerve stimulator
percutaneous epidural neurostimulator
e. pressure waveform
segmental epidural analgesia
segmental epidural anesthesia
e. space
e. space infection
e. spinal cord compression
spinal epidural abscess
spinal epidural hematoma
spinal epidural hemorrhage
spontaneous spinal epidural hematoma
e. steroid
e. steroid injection
surgical treatment for epidural hemorrhage
thoracic epidural steroid injection

epigastric
bilateral inferior epigastric artery flap
deep inferior epigastric artery perforator
deep superior epigastric artery
e. distress syndrome
dull epigastric pain
extended deep inferior e.
e. hernia
inferior epigastric artery
Marfan epigastric puncture
noncolicky epigastric pain
obturator branch of pubic branch of inferior epigastric vein
pulsatile epigastric mass
e. region
superficial inferior epigastric artery
superior epigastric artery
superior epigastric vein

epiglottic
e. fold
e. vallecula

epiglottis
hyperplasia of e.

epilepsy
affective prodrome of e.
age-dependent epilepsy syndrome
alcohol, epilepsy, insulin, overdose, uremia, trauma, infection, psychiatric, stroke
alopecia, epilepsy, oligophrenia syndrome
alopecia, mental retardation, epilepsy, microcephaly syndrome
anterior polar-amygdalar e.
autonomic epilepsy flush
autosomal dominant nocturnal frontal lobe e.
autosomal dominant temporal lobe e.
benign childhood e.
benign focal epilepsy of childhood
benign partial epilepsy with centrotemporal spike
benign rolandic e.
complex partial e.
degenerative myoclonus e.
early posttraumatic e.
early traumatic e.
extratemporal lobe e.
frontal lobe e.
generalized e.
generalized tonic-clonic e.
gingival fibromatosis, hypertrichosis, cherubism, mental retardation, epilepsy syndrome
grand mal e.
Grenoble-Paris-Rennes e.
juvenile absence e.
juvenile myoclonic e.
localization-related epilepsy seizure
malignant familial myoclonic e.
medial temporal-lobe e.
mental retardation, coarse face, microcephaly, epilepsy, skeletal abnormalities syndrome
mental retardation, coarse facies, epilepsy, joint contracture syndrome
mental retardation, epilepsy, short stature, skeletal dysplasia syndrome
Minnesota Comprehensive E. Program
e. monitoring unit
myoclonic astatic e.
myoclonic epilepsy of adolescence
neocortical temporal-lobe e.
nonconvulsive e.
Northern epilepsy with mental retardation
partial complex e.
pediatric and adolescent e.
people with e.
petit mal e.
posttraumatic e.
primary generalized e.
progressive myoclonus e.
quality of life in e.
secondary generalized e.
severe myoclonic e.
severe myoclonic epilepsy in infancy
support group for e.
temporal lobe e.
tonic postural e.
e. with continuous spikes and waves during sleep
e. with grand mal seizures on awakening
e. with multiple independent spike focus
e. with myoclonic absence

epileptic
e. absence
acquired epileptic aphasia
active epileptic process
age-dependent epileptic encephalopathy
e. attention deficit disorder
e. confusional state
e. convulsion
e. dementia
e. discharge
early infantile epileptic encephalopathy
e. encephalopathy
e. focus
e. fugue
highly activity epileptic process
e. migraine
e. myoclonus
e. nystagmus
partial epileptic seizure
e. postictal sleep
e. prodrome
e. seizure
sleep-related epileptic seizure
e. syndrome

epilepticus
complex partial status e.
convulsive status e.
febrile status e.
limbic status e.
nonconvulsive status e.
refractory status e.
status e.

epileptiform
e. abnormality
e. activity
asymmetrical generalized epileptiform activity
benign epileptiform transients of sleep
bilateral independent periodic lateralizing epileptiform discharge
e. burst
e. burst discharge
e. convulsion
e. discharge
e. neuralgia
paroxysmal epileptiform discharge
periodic lateralizing epileptiform discharge
e. seizure
subclinical rhythmic epileptiform discharge of adult
unilateral epileptiform discharges

epileptogenic
e. burst
e. center
e. cortex
e. focus
mesial epileptogenic cortex
partial epileptogenic discharge
e. stimulation
e. structural lesion
e. temporal lesion

epileptoid
orthostatic e.

epiluminescent microscopy

epimacular proliferation

epineurotomy
anterior e.
local e.

epinosic gain

epiotic center

epiphenomena of dissection

epiphora
atonic e.

epiphrenic diverticulum

epiphysealis

epiphysial, epiphyseal
Aitken classification of epiphysial fracture
Aitken epiphysial fracture classification
aseptic epiphysial necrosis
atavistic e.
Atkin epiphysial fracture
deafness, femoral epiphysial dysplasia, short stature, developmental delay syndrome
e. growth plate
longitudinal epiphysial bracket
longitudinal epiphysial bracket
multiple epiphysial dysplasia-early onset diabetes mellitus syndrome
multiple epiphysial dysplasia tarda syndrome
multiple epiphysial dysplasia
Ogden epiphysial fracture classification
traumatic epiphysial coxa vara

epiphysiodesis
open bone graft e.
percutaneous e.

epiphysis
capital e.
capital epiphysis angle of Wiberg
distal femoral e.
proximal tibial e.
radial head e.
slipped capital femoral e.
slipped upper femoral e.

epiploic
e. abscess
e. appendage
e. appendicitis
e. appendix
e. foramen
e. foramen of Winslow

epiploica
appendix e.

epiretinal
idiopathic epiretinal membrane
macular epiretinal membrane
e. membrane
e. membrane proliferation

episcleral
e. bleeder
e. lamina
mean episcleral heat dose
Molteno episcleral explant
e. venous pressure

episcleritis
gouty e.
nodular e.
nonrheumatoid e.

episiotomy
central e.
central episiotomy and repair
e. dehiscence
left mediolateral e.
mediolateral e.
midline e.
e. repair
right mediolateral e.
e. stitch

episode
acute hypertensive e.
acute manic e.
acute psychotic e.
adult depressive e.
e. of blurred vision
daytime sleep e.'s
emetic e.'s
e. free day
full-blown depressive e.
heart dysfunctional e.
hypoxemic e.
intermittent episode of acute abdominal pain
intermittent episode of pain
major depressive e.
manic e.
metabolic stress e.
mitochondrial myopathy, encephalopathy, lactic acidosis, strokelike e.'s
most recent e.
multiple acute rejection e.
myopathy, encephalopathy, lactic acidosis, strokelike e.'s
nocturnal confusional e.
nocturnal hypotensive e.
nonprimary first e.
Schedule for Affective Disorders and Schizophrenia for School-Age Children-Present E.
silence of apneic e.
superimposed acute inflammatory e.
total episode of illness
transient cerebral ischemic e.
transient ischemic e.
transient episodes of myocardial ischemia
vascular occlusive e.

episodic
e. affective disorder
e. angioedema
e. ataxia
e. confusion
e. emotional instability
e. hypertension
e. incontinence
intense episodic dysphoria
e. nocturnal wandering
e. paroxysmal hemicrania
e. pattern of binge eating
e. tension-type headache
e. treatment group
e. weight gain

epispadias
male e.
penile e.
penopubic e.

epistaxis
Merocel epistaxis packing

episternal impulse

epistropheus axis

epitestosterone
testosterone to epitestosterone ratio

epithelia
bile duct e.
oral mucosal e.

epithelial
benign epithelial tumor
biliary epithelial cell
calcifying epithelial odontogenic tumor
calf esophagus epithelial cell
e. cell
cervical epithelial neoplasia
ciliated epithelial cell
corneal epithelial involvement
desquamated epithelial debris
e. focus
e. focus-forming unit
glomerular epithelial cell
e. glycoprotein-2
human bronchial epithelial cell
human epithelial cell
human foreskin epithelial cell
e. hyperplasia
e. hyperplastic laryngeal lesion
intestinal epithelial cell
lens epithelial cell
e. lining fluid
lobular epithelial hyperplasia
low malignant potential epithelial ovarian tumor
Malassez epithelial rests
malignant epithelial tumor
map-dot-fingerprint corneal epithelial dystrophy
Meesman epithelial corneal dystrophy

Meesman juvenile epithelial dystrophy
e. membrane antigen
metaplastic epithelial cell
microcystic epithelial dystrophy
mouse epithelial cell
multinucleated giant epithelial cell
odontogenic gingival epithelial hamartoma
oncocytic epithelial cell
oral epithelial cell genetic fingerprinting
oral epithelial cell genotyping
oral epithelial nevus
e. ovarian cancer
ovarian epithelial carcinoma
ovarian epithelial metasepithelial
ovarian malignant epithelial neoplasm
persistent epithelial defect
pigmented retina epithelial cell
pigment epithelial detachment
polymorphic epithelial mucin
predominantly epithelial thymoma
punctate epithelial erosion
punctate epithelial keratopathy
renal tubular e.
retinal pigment epithelial cell
serous epithelial ovarian carcinoma
e. sodium channel
spindle cell epithelial tumor with thymus-like differentiation
thymic epithelial supernatant
e. tumor

epithelial-myoepithelial carcinoma

epitheliochorial placenta

epithelioid

adrenal epithelioid angiosarcoma
e. angiomatosis
e. combined nevi
e. combined nevi deep penetrating nevus
e. hemangioendothelioma
e. leiomyosarcoma
palisading epithelioid cell
perivascular epithelioid cell
renal epithelioid oxyphilic neoplasm
e. sarcoma
e. soft-tissue neoplasm

epithelioid-globoid cell

epithelioma

basal cell e.
calcifying cell e.
Malherbe calcifying e.
malignant ciliary e.
multiple benign cystic e.
multiple nevoid, basal cell epithelioma, jaw cysts, bifid rib syndrome
nevoid basal cell epithelioma, jaw cysts, bifid rib syndrome

epitheliomatocylindromatosus

nevus e.

epitheliopathy

acute multifocal posterior placoid pigment e.
acute posterior multifocal placoid pigment e.
advancing wave-like e.
multifocal posterior pigment e.

epithelium

anterior epithelium of cornea
anterior epithelium corneae
artificial vaginal e.
autologous cultured e.
ciliated bronchial e.
circumoral area of columnar e.
columnar e.
congenital hypertrophy of retinal pigment e.
cultured thymic e.
glandular e.
human intestinal e.
inner dental e.
inner enamel e.
iris pigment e.
maceration of e.
medullary duct e.
metaplastic columnar e.
mouse mammary e.
native squamous e.
nonpigmented ciliary e.
normal ovarian surface e.
outer enamel e.
ovarian germinal e.
ovarian surface e.
papilla of columnar e.
pigmented e.
reticular degeneration of pigment e.
retinal pigment e.
retina pigment epithelium detachment
specialized columnar e.
squamous e.
surface e.
thymus e.

epithelium-derived relaxation factor

epitheloid cell

epithet

national e.

epitope

allergenic e.
antibody e.
heat-induced epitope retrieval
linear e.
microwave epitope retrieval technique
minimal cytotoxic e.
myc e.
nephritogenic e.
neutralization e.
sonication-induced epitope retrieval

epitrochleoanconeus

e. muscle
musculus e.

epitympanic recess

epiurethral suprapubic vaginal suspension

epizootic

anthrax e.
e. diarrhea of infant mice
e. hemorrhagic disease virus 1–8

epizootica

lymphangitis e.

epoch

duration of e.

epoetin

e. alfa
e. beta

E-point

E.-p. to septal distance
E.-p. to septal separation

eponychial fold

epoophoron

e. cyst
longitudinal duct of e.

epoxide hydratase

epsilometer test

epsilon

apolipoprotein E epsilon 4
apolipoprotein E epsilon 4 gene
apolipoprotein E epsilon 4 gene on chromosome 19
apolipoprotein epsilon 4
e. granule
e. staphylolysin

Epstein-Barr

chronic Epstein-Barr virus
E.-B. early region protein
E.-B. mononucleosis

Epstein-Barr *(continued)*
E.-B. nasopharyngeal carcinoma
E.-B. viral capsid antigen
viral capsid antigen, E.-B.
E.-B. virus
E.-B. virus early antigen
E.-B. virus-encoded RNA in situ hybridization
E.-B. virus nuclear antigen

Epworth Sleepiness Scale

equal
e. bilateral breath sounds
bilateral equal breath sounds
e. bilateral expansion
bilateral, symmetrical, e.
e. breath bilaterally
e. breath sounds bilaterally
breath sounds equal bilaterally
brisk and e.
e. conjoined twins
deep tendon reflexes active and equal bilaterally
firm and e.
grips equal and good
grips strong and e.
handgrasp equal and strong
E. Listener Response scale
not e.
number equal to one; single patient trial
e. ocular movement
parallel line equal spacing
pedal pulses equal and strong
peripheral pulses full and equal bilaterally
present, active, e.
e. probability of selection method
pulmonic second heart sound equal to aortic second heart sound
pupils equal, reactive, and contracting
pupils equal and reactive to light and accommodation
pupils equal, round, reactive to light and accommodation
pupils equal, round, reactive to light and accommodation directly and consensually
pupils equal in size and reaction
e. and reactive
round and e.
round, regular, and e.
round, regular, and equal pupil
second aortic sound e.'s second pulmonic sound
e. to

equality
point of subjective e.

equalization
advanced multiple-beam equalization radiography
aided equalization response
pressure e.
pressure equalization tube
scanning equalization radiography
unaided equalization reference

equalization-cancellation

equalize air pressure

equalizing
pressure equalizing tube

equally
moderately constricted and equally reactive pupil
moderately dilated and equally reactive pupil
moves all extremities equally well

equal-pressure point

equation
Goldman-Hodgkin-Katz equation
modified Bernoulli e.
respiratory gas e.
simultaneous e.
surgical blood order e.

equational division

equatorial staphyloma

equilateral hemianopia

equilibrating
forced equilibrating expiration

equilibration
helium equilibration time
mandibular e.
occlusal e.

equilibrium
e. association constant
e. constant
decrease in coordination or e.
e. dialysis
e. dissociation constant
disturbance of mental e.
driven equilibrium Fourier transform
elastic equilibrium volume
multiple gated equilibrium scintigraphy
e. peritoneal dialysis
e. radionuclide angiography
sense of e.

equilibrium-gated
e.-g. blood pool study
e.-g. radionuclide angiography

equina
cauda equina syndrome

equine
e. abortion virus
e. antihuman lymphoblast globulin
e. antihuman lymphoblast serum
botulism equine trivalent antitoxin
conjugated equine estrogen plus norgestrel
conjugated equine estrogen
e. conjugated estrogen
Eastern equine encephalitis virus
Eastern equine encephalomyelitis
Eastern equine encephalomyelitis virus
e. encephalitis
e. encephalomyelitis
enterocytopathogenic equine orphan virus
e. estrogen
e. gait
e. growth hormone
e. herpesvirus
infectious equine anemia
e. influenza
Japanese equine encephalitis
e. morbilli virus
Near East equine encephalomyelitis
e. rhinopneumonia
e. rhinopneumonitis
e. rhinopneumonitis virus
e. serum hepatitis
Venezuelan equine encephalitis virus
Venezuelan equine encephalomyelitis virus
Venezuelan equine encephalitis vaccine, attenuated live
Venezuelan equine encephalitis vaccine, inactivated
western equine encephalitis
western equine encephalomyelitis
western equine encephalomyelitis virus

equinovalgus
e. deformity
e. foot
pes e.
talipes e.

equinovarus
e. deformity

e. foot
e. hindfoot deformity
pes e.
e. pes deformity
pes equinovarus adductus
e. posturing
talipes e.

equinus
ankle e.
anterior e.
e. clubfoot
e. contracture
e. deformity
e. foot
forefoot e.
e. gait
neurogenic equinus deformity
osseous e.
pes e.
e. position

equipment
bubble chamber e.
computerized scanning e.
contamination from anesthesia e.
durable medical e.
home medical e.
lower extremity equipment related
medical support e.
personal protective e.

equipotential
e. electrode
e. line

equivalency

equivalent
aerodynamic equivalent diameter
age e.
arithmetic grade e.
biologically equivalent dose
bread e.
e. current dipole
e. dose
dose e.
e. effective photon
female day e.
fibrinogen equivalent unit
e. focus
generic e.
genome e.
highest equivalent heart rate
histamine equivalent prick
human skin e.
joule e.
leukocyte equivalent unit
living skin e.
loudness e.
lymph node seeking e.
male e.
e. mean age at death
mean spherical e.
meconium ileus e.
metabolic e.
metabolic equivalent level
metabolic equivalent of task
milliroentgen equivalent man
milliroentgen equivalent physical
minimal pure radium e.
Monteggia equivalent lesion
noise equivalent counts
noise equivalent power
normal equivalent deviation
e. oxygen performance
oxygen ventilation e.
peak equivalent sound pressure level
Pharmacy E. Name
plasma equivalent unit
rad equivalent therapeutic
radiation equivalent in man
radiation equivalent therapy
radiobiologic e.
reasonable compensation e.
e. residual renal urea clearance
retinol e.
e. roentgen unit
spherical e.
starch e.
tissue e.
toxic e.
whiskey e.
whole time e.

equivalent-physical
roentgen e.-p.

equivocal
e. diagnosis
e. findings
e. response
e. symptom

era
Vietnam e.

eradicated
infection e.

eradication
Helicobacter pylori eradication therapy
e. rates

erasable programmable read-only memory

Erb
E. area
E. atrophy
E. disease
E. dystrophy
E. palsy
E. paralysis
E. point
E. sclerosis
E. sign
E. syndrome
E. wave

Erb-Charcot
E.-C. disease
E.-C. syndrome

Erb-Duchenne paralysis

Erben reflex

Erb-Goldflam
E.-G. disease
E.-G. syndrome

Erb-Landouzy disease

Erdheim-Chester disease

erect
e. diastolic blood pressure
mean daily erect blood pressure
e. posterior-anterior projection

erecta
luxatio e.
luxatio erecta shoulder dislocation

erectile
e. dysfunction
e. function
e. impairment
e. impotence
International Index of E. Function
male dyspareunia male erectile disorder
male erectile disorder
male erectile dysfunction
neurogenic erectile dysfunction
psychogenic erectile dysfunction
e. tissue

erection
artificial e.
artificial erection test
Japanese erection ring
medication-associated e.
nocturnal e.
nocturnal penile erection monitoring
nonsustained e.
penile e.
pharmacologic erection program
vacuum erection device

erector
musculus erector penis

erethismic
e. idiocy

erethismic *(continued)*
e. idiot
e. shock

ergometer
rowing e.
upper body e.

ergonomic
e. assessment of risk and liability
e. intervention

ergonovine
e. challenge
e. echocardiography
e. maleate
e. maleate provocation angina
e. provocation test

ergosterol
irradiated e.

ergot
e. alkaloid-associated heart disease
e. derivative

ergotamine derivative

Erhardt
E. Developmental Prehension Assessment
E. Developmental Vision Assessment

Erhard test

Erichsen
E. disease
E. ligature
E. sign

Eristalis tenax

Erlacher-Blount syndrome

Ernst
E. applicator
E. radium applicator
E. radium capsule
E. radium tandem

eroding gum tissue

erosion
acute stress e.
e. of articular surface
e. depth
e. desquamation
gastric antral e.
gastric mucosal e.
graft enteric e.
intramucosal hemorrhage and e.
mouse ear e.
punctate epithelial e.
recurrent erosion syndrome
superficial punctate e.
e. surface per bone surface

erosive
acute erosive gastritis
e. arthritis
chronic erosive gastritis
e. esophagitis
e. gastritis
e. gastritis with ulceration
e. gastropathy
hemorrhagic erosive gastritis
nonspecific erosive gastritis
e. osteoarthritis
e. prephloric change
e. tracheitis

erotic
e. delusion
e. dream
e. drive
e. epilepsy
e. paranoia
e. pyromania
e. seizure
e. transference
e. vomiting

erotism
anal e.
lip e.
muscle e.
olfactory e.
oral e.
organ e.
paranoid e.

erotized
e. anxiety
e. hanging

erotomanic
e. delusion
e. disorder

errant thought

erratic
e. behavior
e. blood glucose levels
e. blood pressure
e. eating habits
e. heart rhythm
mamma e.
e. mood
e. sleep
e. speech rhythm
e. thinking
e. weight gain

errector pilus

error
allowable limits of e.
astigmatic refractive e.
asymmetric refractive e.
coefficient of e.
constant e.
data spike detection error artifact
e. detection circuit
diagnostic e.
e. of the first kind
e. function
inborn error of metabolism
integrated square e.
line bisection e.
maximal possible e.
mean prediction e.
mean square e.
e. of measurement
payment error prevention program
probability of type I, II e.
probable e.
probable error of measurement
replication error negative
replication error positive
root-mean-square e.
Spondee E. Index
standard error of difference
standard error of estimate
standard error of the mean
therapeutic error signal
trial and e.
wrong test requested-floor e.

eructation
nervous e.

erupted wisdom teeth

eruption
drug eruption dermatitis
eosinophilic, polymorphic, and pruritic eruption associated with radiotherapy
fixed drug e.
Kaposi varicelliform e.
lichenoid drug e.
monomorphous papular e.
noneczematous persistent papular gold e.
polymorphous light e.
pruritic papular e.

eruptive
multiple eruptive milia

eruptivum
xanthoma e.

erysiphake
New York e.
Nugent-Green-Dimitry e.

erythema
e. action
atypical erythema multiforme

delayed erythema dose
e. dose
edema, erythema, and exudate
generalized erythema multiforme
herpes-associated erythema multiforme
e. infectiosum
linear extensor e.
linear gingival e.
e. migrans
migratory necrolytic e.
minimal phototoxic erythema dose
mouth erythema multiforme
e. multiforme major
e. multiforme/toxic epidermal necrolysis
necrolytic migratory e.
e. neonatorum
oral erythema multiforme
prolonged postpeel e.
skin erythema dose
threshold erythema dose

erythema-edema reaction

erythematosis
subcutaneous lupus e.

erythematosus
acute cutaneous lupus e.
acute systemic lupus e.
bullous systemic lupus e.
chronic cutaneous lupus e.
chronic discoid lupus e.
discoid lupus e.
disseminated lupus e.
drug-induced lupus e.
lupus e.
lupus erythematosus body
lupus erythematosus cell
lupus erythematosus cell test
lupus erythematosus discoides
lupus erythematosus factor
lupus erythematosus inhibitor
lupus erythematosus, neonatal
lupus erythematosus panniculitis
lupus erythematosus peripheral neuropathy
lupus erythematosus phenomenon
lupus erythematosus preparation
lupus erythematosus profundus
lupus erythematosus, systemic
lupus erythematosus tumidus
neonatal lupus e.
neuropsychiatric syndrome of systemic lupus e.
pseudolupus erythematosus syndrome
subacute cutaneous lupus e.
Systemic Lupus E. Disease Activity Index

erythematous
anular erythematous plaque
e. blush
e. confluent plaque
e. hyperpigmented papule
e. lesion
e. macular dermatitis
e. macule
e. maculopapular rash
Mediterranean erythematous fever
e. papule
e. plaque
e. rash
reticular erythematous mucinosis
e. satellite lesion
e. wheal

erythroblast
polychromatic e.

erythroblastic
hereditary erythroblastic multinuclearity with positive acidified serum
e. island
e. leukemia
refractory anemia, e.

erythroblastopenia
transient erythroblastopenia of childhood

erythroblastosis
avian e.
avian erythroblastosis virus
fetal e.
e. fetalis
murine erythroblastosis virus
e. neonatorum

erythrocyte
e. acid phosphatase
adult e.
e. antibody
e. antibody inhibition
antigenic determinant of e.'s
e. antisera
colony-forming unit-granulocyte, erythrocyte, megakaryocyte, macrophage
e. coproporphyrin
e., antibody, and complement
fixed erythrocyte turnover
fluorescing e.
formalin-treated pyruvaldehyde-stabilized human e.'s
e. fragility test
free cytoporphyrin in e.'s
free erythrocyte coproporphyrin
free erythrocyte porphyrin
free erythrocyte protoporphyrin
e. glutamic oxaloacetic transaminase
e. glutathione reductase
human erythrocyte agglutination test
human erythrocyte antigen
e. initiation factor
intravascular erythrocyte aggregation
lesion on erythrocyte cell membrane at the site of complement fixation
macrocytic e.
e. mass
e. maturation factor
median erythrocyte diameter
e. membrane protein
Mexican hat e.
microcytic e.
normochromic normocytic erythrocyte
osmotic erythrocyte enrichment
packed e.'s
polychromic e.'s
e. protoporphyrin
rabbit e.
rapid erythrocyte degeneration
e. receptor
e. rosette-forming cell
e. rosette inhibitor
e. sedimentation rate
sheep e.
sheep erythrocyte agglutination test
sheep erythrocyte antibody
sheep erythrocyte antigen
tanned erythrocyte electrophoretic mobility
e. transketolase
e. triiodothyronine
Westergren erythrocyte sedimentation rate
Wintrobe erythrocyte sedimentation rate
zeta erythrocyte sedimentation rate

erythrocytic fragmentation

erythrocytosis
paraneoplastic e.
pathologic secondary e.

erythroderma
congenital hemidysplasia with ichthyosiform erythroderma and limb defects syndrome
congenital ichthyosiform e.

erythroderma *(continued)*
nonbullous congenital ichthyosiform e.

erythrodermic
nonbullous congenital erythrodermic ichthyosis
e. psoriasis

erythrodysesthesia
palmar-plantar e.
palmar-plantar erythrodysesthesia syndrome
palmoplantar e.
palmoplantar erythrodysesthesia syndrome

erythrogenesis imperfecta

erythrohepatic protoporphyria

erythroid
e. colony formation
e. committed precursor
e. differentiation factor
endogenous erythroid colony
e. iron turnover
e. leukemia virus
mature burst-forming unit e.
myeloid to e.
myeloid to erythroid ratio
e. precursor

erythrokeratodermia
progressive symmetric e.
e. variabilis

erythroleukemia
acute e.
Friend erythroleukemia cell
Friend murine e.
human erythroleukemia line
mouse e.
murine e.
murine erythroleukemia cell

erythromycin
e. breath test
e. topical solution

erythronormoblastic anemia

erythrophagocytic
familial erythrophagocytic lymphohistiocytosis

erythroplasia
Queyrat e.
Zoon e.

erythropoiesis
idiopathic ineffective e.

erythropoietic
chronic erythropoietic porphyria
congenital erythropoietic porphyria
e. coproporphyria
e. porphyria
e. protoporphyria
renal erythropoietic factor

erythropoietic-stimulating factor

erythropoietin
e. assay
cord blood erythropoietin level
human e.
recombinant human e.

erythropoietin-producing enzyme

erythropoietin-responsive cell

erythropoietin-sensitive stem cell

escalation
opioid escalation index

escalator
mucous e.

escape
e. of air
atrioventricular junctional escape beat
atrioventricular junction escape rhythm
e. and avoidance conditioning in human subjects
avoidance and escape learning
e. beat
heat escape lessening posture
e. impulse
junctional escape beat
e. mechanism
mucus escape reaction
nodal escape rhythm
pacemaker escape interval
e. rhythm
transcapillary escape rate
ventricular e.
ventricular escape rhythm

escaped ventricular contraction

eschar
burn e.
neuropathic e.
pathognomonic black e.

Escherichia
ampicillin-resistant *Escherichia coli*
anti-*Escherichia coli*-derived protein antibody
E. coli
Escherichia coli bacteremia
Escherichia coli enteropathic
Escherichia coli filtrate
Escherichia coli heat-labile toxin vaccine
Escherichia coli K1
Escherichia coli organism
Escherichia coli polypeptide
Escherichia coli sepsis peritonitis
Escherichia coli septicemia
diffusely adherent *Escherichia coli*
enteroadherent *Escherichia coli*
enteroaggregative *Escherichia coli*
enteroaggregative *Escherichia coli* heat-stable enterotoxin 1
enterohemorrhagic *Escherichia coli*
enteroinvasive *Escherichia coli*
E. enteropathogenic
enteropathogenic *Escherichia coli*
enterotoxigenic *Escherichia coli*
enterovirulent *Escherichia coli*
Escherichia coli filtrate
Escherichia coli K1
Shigella-like toxin-producing *Escherichia coli*
toxic *Escherichia coli*
verocytotoxin-producing *Escherichia coli*
verotoxin-producing *Escherichia coli*

escort
staff e.

esculin
Bacteroides bile esculin agar
bile esculin test

escutcheon
male e.

esodeviation
nonaccommodative e.

esodic nerve

esophageal
acute esophageal food impaction
e. adenocarcinoma
antifungal esophageal infection
anular esophageal stricture
anular esophageal stricture
e. atresia
e. balloon catheter
e. banding
e. banding technique
e. band ligation
barium adherent to esophageal walls
bleeding esophageal varix
blind esophageal brushing
e. body
e. candidiasis
e. carcinoma
e. chest pain
chronic esophageal dysphagia
e. collateral vein
e. detection device

diffuse esophageal spasm
e. dilation
e. Doppler monitor
drug-induced esophageal damage
e. dysmotility
end-expiratory esophageal pressure
e. endoscopy
e. epidermal growth factor
expandable esophageal stent
e. filling defect
e. fistula
e. foreign body
e. gastric tube airway
e. hiatal hernia
e. hiatus
e. hiatus hernia
idiopathic esophageal ulcer
incompetent esophageal sphincter
ineffective esophageal motility
inferior esophageal constriction
inferior esophageal sphincter
inoperable esophageal carcinoma
e. introitus
e. intubation
e. intubation detection
lesser esophageal sphincter
locally advanced esophageal cancer
longitudinal esophageal stricture
lower esophageal B ring
lower esophageal contraction ring
lower esophageal high-pressure zone
lower esophageal mucosal ring
lower esophageal ring
lower esophageal segment
lower esophageal sphincter
lower esophageal sphincter circular muscle
lower esophageal sphincter locator
lower esophageal sphincter pressure
lower esophageal sphincter relaxation
lower esophageal sphincter tone
lower esophageal stricture
lower esophageal transection
e. manometric sequence
e. manometry
maximal esophageal pressure
maximal sniff-induced esophageal pressure
mechanical esophageal obstruction
medication-induced esophageal injury
microcephaly, oculodigital, esophageal, duodenal syndrome
middle esophageal constriction
e. motility
e. motility disorder
mucosal esophageal ring
e. mucosal ring
muscular esophageal ring
e. muscular ring
e. narrowing
nonspecific esophageal motility disorder
nonspecific esophageal motor dysfunction
e. obstruction
e. obturator airway
oral esophageal stethoscope
oral esophageal tube
pacing esophageal stethoscope
peptic esophageal stricture
peroral esophageal dilation
e. pH
e. polyp
e. pressure
primary symptomatic diffuse esophageal spasm
radionuclide esophageal scintigraphy
e. radionuclide transit
e. reflux
e. resection
e. rupture
e. scintigraphy
e. shunt
sliding esophageal hiatal hernia
e. sound
e. spasm
e. sphincter
e. squamous cell carcinoma
superficial esophageal carcinoma
symptomatic diffuse esophageal spasm
e. tamponade
tracheoesophageal fistula, esophageal atresia, multiple congenital anomaly syndrome
transient lower esophageal relaxation
e. transit scan
e. transit time
e. ultrasound
upper esophageal constriction
upper esophageal sphincter pressure
upper esophageal sphincter relaxation
e. valve
e. variceal bleeding
e. variceal hemorrhage
e. variceal sclerosis
e. variceal sclerotherapy
e. varices
e. varix
e. wall thickness
e. web
Wickwitz esophageal stricture

esophageal-directed pressure support

esophageal-tracheal double lumen airway

esophagectomy
en bloc e.
near-total e.
open e.
total e.
total thoracic e.
transhiatal e.

esophagitis
alkaline reflux e.
drug-induced e.
erosive e.
Los Angeles Classification grade A, B, C, D e.
reflux e.

esophagogastric
e. balloon tamponade
e. devascularization and transection
e. junction
ligation of esophagogastric junction
obstructive esophagogastric cancer
e. tube airway
e. variceal bleeding
e. varix

esophagography
contrast e.

esophagojejunostomy
loop e.
mechanical e.
mediastinal e.

esophagomyotomy
modified Heller e.
open e.

esophagoplasty
patch e.
pediatric e.

esophagorespiratory fistula

esophagoscopy
hypopharyngoscopy, bronchoscopy, and e.
Lugol dye e.
transnasal e.

esophagostomy
palliative e.

esophagotracheal combination tube

esophagram
air e.
oropharyngeal e.

esophagus
achalasia of e.
adenocarcinoma of the e.
area for e.
A ring of e.
barium filled e.
barium passed through esophagus into stomach
Barrett e.
calf esophagus epithelial cell
caustic strictures of cervical e.
columnar-lined e.
columnar-lined lower e.
congenital atresia of e.
digital anomalies, short palpebral fissures, atresia of esophagus or duodenum syndrome
duplication of e.
e., stomach, and duodenum
hernia of e.
long-segment Barrett e.
mucosa of e.
muscular coat of e.
muscular layer of e.
narrowing of e.
nutcracker e.
obstruction of e.
passed through esophagus into stomach
perforation of e.
periodic dilatation of e.
primary malignant melanoma of the e.
scarring and narrowing of e.
serosa of e.
short-segment Barrett e.
spontaneous intramural hematoma of the e.
squamous cell carcinoma of the e.
superficial distal esophagus hemorrhage
suspensory ligament of e.
time of peak filling rate of e.
upper e.

esophoria
e. for distance
e. for near

esotropia
e. at distance
e. at 6 meters
e. at near
intermittent e.
intermittent esotropia at near
left e.
near e.
e. for near
nonrefractive accommodative e.
right e.

essential
e. anemia
e. atrophy of iris
benign essential blepharospasm
benign essential hypertension
benign essential tremor
e. bradycardia
e. cryoglobulinemia
disabling essential tremor
e. dysmenorrhea
Eagle minimal essential medium
factor essential for resistance to methicillin
e. fatty acid deficiency
e. findings
e. hematuria
e. hemorrhage
hereditary essential tremor
high-renin essential hypertension
e. hypercholesterolemia
e. hyperlipidemia
e. hypernatremia
e. hypertension
e. hypertensive patient
improved minimal essential medium, hormone supplemented
low-renin essential hypertension
e. macroglobulinemia
e. metabolism ratio
Minimum E.'s Test
e. mixed cryoglobulinemia
e. monoclonal gammopathy
no essential abnormalities
no essential change
normal renin essential hypertension
e. phospholipid
e. pulmonary hemosiderosis
renin essential hypertension
Seeing Essential English
supplemented Eagle minimal essential medium
e. tachycardia
e. thrombocythemia
e. thrombocytopenia
e. thrombocytosis
e. thrombopenia
e. tremor
e. uterine hemorrhage

essentially negative

Esser graft

Essex-Lopresti
E.-L. fracture
E.-L. method
E.-L. reduction technique

established
e. extraprostatic extension
e. patient

establishment
computer-aided fluency establishment trainer

ester
acid cholesterol ester hydrolase
benzoylarginine ethyl e.
benzoylarginine methyl e.
carboxylic ester hydrolase
cholesterol e.
cholesterol ester storage disease
cholesteryl esters transfer protein
fatty e.
fatty acid methyl e.
long-acting testosterone e.
orthophosphoric ester monohydrolase
polyphosphoric e.
sterol e.
tosylarginine methyl e.
tyrosine ethyl e.
wax e.

esterase
e. activity
bile salt-stimulated e.
C1 esterase inhibitor
chloroacetate e.
e. D
human serum e.
leukocyte e.
leukocyte esterase test
lymphocyte serine e.
neurotoxic e.
nonspecific e.
nonspecific esterase stain
postheparin e.
toxoid-antitoxoid mixture e.
e. unit

esterification
fractional esterification rate
molar esterification rate

Estero Real virus

Estes operation

esthesiometer
monofilament pressure e.

esthetic
e. appearance
e. body contouring
e. ceramics
e. dentistry
one-stage esthetic correction
e. surgery

esthetically pleasing

estimate
Emory Pain E. Model
maximal risk e.
monocular estimate method
platelet e.
standard error of e.

estimated
e. blood loss
e. cerebrovascular resistance
e. creatinine clearance
e. date of conception
e. date of confinement
e. date of delivery
e. date of labor
e. discharge date
e. dry weight
e. due date
e. energy needs
e. fetal body weight
e. gestational age
e. hepatic blood flow
E. Learning Potential
e. length of program
e. liver blood flow
e. protein needs
e. protein requirement
e. safe and adequate daily dietary intake
e. thyroid ratio
thyroxine-binding globulin, e.
e. time of arrival
e. time of conception
e. time of ovulation
e. weight loss

estimation
bayesian image e.
clinical estimation of survival
holistic orthogonal parameter e.
Lund-Browder chart for burn e.
magnitude e.
maximal likelihood e.
point estimation by sequential testing
Rapid E. of Adult Literacy in Medicine
Simple Calculated Osteoporosis Risk E.
time e.

estimator
maximum likelihood e.

Estlander
E. flap
E. operation

estradiol
e. benzoate
maternal estradiol rhythm
micronized 17beta e.
nonoral estradiol delivery system
e. production rate
e. receptor
e. receptor assay
e. valerate

estradiol-binding
e.-b. index
e.-b. protein

estradiol-testosterone-binding globulin

estramustine binding protein

estriol
maternal estriol level
unconjugated e.

estrogen
activated estrogen receptor
e. add back therapy
e. binding site
e. breakthrough bleeding
cell response to e.
conjugated e.
conjugated equine e.
conjugated equine estrogen plus norgestrel
decreased estrogen receptor
e. deficiency
e. deprivation
equine conjugated e.
increased estrogen receptor
e. level
long-term estrogen deprivation
e. loss
low-dose estrogen replacement
low-dose vaginal e.
lower circulating estrogen level
membrane-associated estrogen receptor
menopausal estrogen replacement therapy
e. monotherapy
oestrogen estrogen-replacement therapy
oral conjugated e.
oral estrogen therapy
ovarian estrogen synthesis
persistent estrogen secretion
postmenopausal e.
postmenopausal estrogen replacement
postmenopausal estrogen therapy
e. and progesterone
e. receptor
e. receptor alpha
e. receptor assay
e. receptor beta
e. receptor immunocytochemistry assay
e. receptor-negative
e. receptor-positive
e. receptor-positive tumor
e. receptor/progesterone receptor
e. receptor protein
e. replacement
e. replacement therapy
selective estrogen receptor modulator
selective estrogen response modifier
e. surge
total estrogen excretion
total placental e.
unopposed e.
e. withdrawal
e. withdrawal bleeding

estrogen-agonist uterine effect

estrogen-only HRT

estrogen-producing tumor

estrogen-progesterone withdrawal bleeding

estrogen/progestin
postmenopausal estrogen/progestin intervention

estrogen-progestin contraceptive

estrogen-response element

estrogen-stimulated neurophysin

estropia
infantile e.

estrus
constant e.
e. cycle

etch
orthophosphoric acid etch gel

etched porcelain veneer

etching
tooth e.

ethacrynic acid

ethane
tetrachlorodiphenyl e.
ethanesulfate
ethyl e.
ethanol
e. abuse
blood ethanol content
blood ethanol level
formalin and e.
formalin, ethanol, xylol, and e.
e. gelation test
e. ingestion
e. metabolic rate
microsomal ethanol oxidizing system
mitochondrial ethanol oxidase system
percutaneous ethanol ablation
percutaneous ethanol ablation of tumor
percutaneous fine-needle ethanol injection
poststress ethanol consumption
sustained ethanol release tube
tetradecyl sulfate, ethanol, and saline
e. volume fraction
ethanol-induced tumor necrosis
ether
alcohol, ether, and acetone solution
alcohol, chloroform, and ether mixture
butyl glycidyl e.
dihematoporphyrin e.
dimethyl e.
gas, oxygen, and ether anesthesia
methyl-*tert*-butyl ether therapy
methyl tertiary butyl e.
oxygen and ether gas
Vinethine and ether anesthesia
ether-chloroform mixture
ethical
e. decision-making
e. dilemma
e., legal, and social implications
e. issue
e. judgment
e. validity of assisted suicide
ethics
code of e.
medical e.
normative e.
professional e.
situational e.
ethidium bromide
Ethiodane contrast medium
ethiodized oil emulsion
Ethiodol contrast medium
ethmoid
e. air cell
ala of e.
anterior ethmoid canal
anterior ethmoid sinus
orbital lamina of ethmoid bone
orbital layer of ethmoid bone
orbital plate of ethmoid bone
e. sinus
e. sinus adenocarcinoma
ethmoidal
anterior ethmoidal air cell
anterior ethmoidal artery
anterior ethmoidal branch of ophthalmic artery
anterior ethmoidal cell
anterior ethmoidal foramen
anterior ethmoidal nerve
anterior ethmoidal ostium
anterior lateral nasal branch of anterior ethmoidal artery
anterior meningeal branch of anterior ethmoidal artery
anterior septal branch of anterior ethmoidal artery
antral ethmoidal sphenoidectomy
e. bulla
e. crest of maxilla
e. crest of palatine bone
e. infundibular system
middle ethmoidal air cell
e. process of inferior nasal concha
e. rongeur
e. scissors
e. sinus
e. spine
ethmoidale
antra e.
antrum e.
os e.
ethmoidalis
arteria ethmoidalis anterior
arteria ethmoidalis posterior
bulla e.
nervus ethmoidalis anterior
nervus ethmoidalis posterior
ethmoidectomy
anterior e.
partial e.
total e.
transnasal endoscopic e.
ethnic
e. bias
e. hate
e. heritage
e. profiling
e. relational behavior
ethyl
e. alcohol
benzoylarginine ethyl ester
e. ethanesulfate
liquid ethyl chloride
e. methanesulfonate
tin e.
tyrosine ethyl ester
e. violet azide broth
ethylene
e. dibromide
ethylene tetrafluor e.
e. glycol assay
e. glycol dimethacrylate
e. glycol poisoning
e. glycol succinate
e. glycol toxicity
e. oxide
e. oxide gas
e. vinyl acetate
ethylene-vinyl acetate copolymer
etiocholanolone
e. fever
e. test
etiologic
e. agent
clinical manifestations, etiologic factors, anatomic involvement, pathophysiologic features
e. diagnosis
e. factor
etiology
e. to be determined
chest pain of unknown e.
dementia due to multiple e.'s
fever of unknown e.
monoarticular arthritis of unknown e.
ocular etiology of headache
pyrexia of unknown e.
toxic metabolic e.
uncertain e.
e. undetermined
undetermined e.
e. unknown
villitis of unknown e.

etiopathogenesis
MS e.

Eubenangee virus

euclidean distance matrix analysis

eudismic affinity quotient

eugenics
negative e.

euglobulin
ascites euglobulin lysis time
e. clot lysis
e. clot lysis time
e. clot test
e. lysis test

eukaryotic initiation factor

Euler
Byrne and Euler formula
E. number

eunuchism
pituitary e.

eunuchoid
e. gigantism
e. habitus
e. state
e. voice

eunuchoidism
hypogonadotropic e.

euphoria
increased e.
initial feeling of e.
intense e.

euphoric
e. affect
e. mood
e. presentation
e. speech

euphorigenic effect

eupraxic center

europaeus
Ulex europaeus agglutinin I

European
central European encephalitis
central European encephalitis virus
central European tick-borne encephalitis
E. Community
E. compression technique bone screw and internal fixation
E. bat lyssavirus 1
E. Stroke Scale

European-American
Revised European-American Classification of Lymphoid Neoplasms

eurytrophic parasite

Eustace Smith murmur

eustachian
catheterization of eustachian tube
e. tube
e. tube dysfunction
e. tube function
e. tube obstruction
e. tube pressure

eutectic mixture of local anesthetics

euthanasia
active e.
condemnation of active e.
passive e.

euthymic
e. mood
e. state

euthyroid
e. goiter
minimal euthyroid Graves disease
multinodular euthyroid goiter
e. sick syndrome
e. state

evacuated
bowel adequately e.
e. tissue

evacuates
bowel fills and evacuates satisfactorily

evacuation
aeromedical evacuation support team
dilatation and e.
dilation and e.
e. hospital
medical air e.
nail bed hematoma e.
normal evacuation of barium
pulsed irrigation for enhanced e.
e. of retained products of conception
e. of uterine contents

evacuator
high-volume e.

evacuatory
rectal evacuatory disorder

evagination
optic e.

evaluate
e. and advise
contact, control, test, evaluate, treatment
e. extent of injury or illness
e. implant
e. orientation, attention, and recent recall
e. safety and stability at home
too early to e.

evaluated
not e.
to be e.

Evaluating Acquired Skills in Communication

evaluation
Ackerman-Schoendorf Scales for Parent E. of Custody
acute physiology and chronic health evaluation score
Adaptive Behavior E. Scale
admission, entrance, and evaluation unit
annual health e.
appropriateness evaluation protocol
aquatic cardiac evaluation and testing
assessment, plan, implementation, and e.
auditory and medical e.
Behavior E. Scale-2
behavior summarized e.
Békésy Ascending-Descending Gap E.
California Marriage Readiness E.
cardiac arrhythmia evaluation center
cerebrovascular e.
Checklist for Child Abuse E.
Clinical E. of Language Function-Preschool
Clinical E. of Language Functions
Collaborative Home Infant Monitoring E.
community hypertension evaluation clinic
Computer-Assisted Psychiatric E. and Review System
computerized muscle-joint e.
confidential evaluation and treatment
data, action, response, and e.
e. of denervated heart at rest
detailed evaluation of facial symmetry
Developmental E. Center

evaluation *(continued)*
dilation and e.
direct observation e.
drug e.
drug evaluation matrix
drug use e.
early clinical drug evaluation unit
e., prediction, intervention, and control
Fairview Language E. Scale
Fairview Language E. Test
Family Adaptability and Cohesion E. Scale
Family E. Form
fiberoptic endoscopic evaluation of swallowing
fiberoptic endoscopic evaluation of swallowing with sensory testing
final drug e.
flexible endoscopic evaluation of swallowing
flexible endoscopic evaluation of swallowing with sensory testing
Fort Bragg evaluation project
foster home e.
functional capacity e.
geriatric evaluation and management unit
Gifted E. Scale
Global E. of Efficacy
Grassi Basic Cognitive E.
health evaluation center
health hazard e.
Health E. and Learning Program
hearing aid e.
Holter monitor e.
home evaluation prior to discharge
human immunodeficiency virus overview of problems evaluation system
initial evaluation and treatment
initial hypertension e.
intracranial vascular e.
invasive diagnostic e.
job capacity e.
Learning Disability E. Scale
longitudinal expert evaluation using all available data
longitudinal interval followup e.
e. and management codes
Marital Attitudes E.
Maternal Attitudes E.
Mazur ankle e.
McMaster Overall Treatment E.
medical care e.
medication use e.
mental capacity e.
mental status e.
monitored self-care e.
Mother-Child Relationship E.
multiple outcomes of raloxifene evaluation trial
musculoskeletal evaluation, rehabilitation and conditioning
National Cholesterol E. Program
noninvasive cardiac e.
noninvasive evaluation of radiation output
Nurses' Observation Scale for Inpatient E.
e. and observation
outpatient e.
overnight sleep e.
parent-child interaction e.
patient admitted for evaluation and workup
patient evaluation center
patient evaluation rating scale
Patient E. Grid
Pediatric E. of Disability Inventory
performance evaluation procedure
periodic evaluation record
peripheral nerve e.
physical e.
physical capacity e.
Prematurity Risk E. Measure
Preschool E. and Assessment for Children with Handicaps
Preschool Evaluation and Assessment for Children with Handicaps
presurgical coagulation e.
Primary Care E. of Mental Disorders
professional performance e.
program evaluation and review technique
prospective evaluation of radial keratotomy
prospective outcomes monitoring evaluation system
Psychiatric E. Form
Psychiatric E. Profile
e. of resting activity
safety, monitoring, intervention, length of stay, and e.
Smith physical capacities e.
substance abuse evaluation screen unit
Teacher E. Scale
testing and e.
testing, orientation, work, evaluation, rehabilitation
theoretical growth e.
toddler and infant motor e.
e. and treatment
tridimensional evaluation scale
uniaxial balance e.
Vane E. of Language Scale
verbal sample evaluation method
videofluorographic evaluation of swallowing
Vietnam Veterans E. and Treatment Program
vocational e.
Vocational E. and Work Adjustment
work capacity e.
work evaluation systems technology

evanescent
affinity evanescent wave spectroscopy
multiple evanescent white dot syndrome

Evans
Allman modification of Evans ankle reconstruction
E. blue dye

evaporated milk formula

evaporation
transurethral evaporation of prostate
e. water loss

evasion
macular e.

even
every even day

evening
e. blood sugar
e. interrupted suture
oil of evening primrose
e. primrose oil

event
abnormal electrical events in heart
acute cardiac e.
acute coronary e.
acute life-threatening e.
Adolescent Life Change E. Questionnaire
amnesia for sleep terror e.
apparent life-threatening e.
cardiac event monitor
cerebral ischemic e.
circadian event recorder

designated compensable e.
drug-related adverse patient e.
Family Index of Life E.'s
Family Inventory of Life E.'s and Changes
fatal cardiac e.
herb-related adverse e.
Impact of E.'s Scale
impaired memory for recent e.'s
important medical e.
inability to recall e.'s
Interview Schedule for E.'s and Difficulties
life events checklist
Life E.'s and Difficulty Schedule Interview
low probability, high consequence e.
main timing e.
major adverse cardiac e.
major coronary e.
medical e.'s
medication monitoring event system
e. monitor
multiple event curve
Pleasant E.'s Schedule
potentially compensable e.
prescription event monitoring
quality-related e.
Rapid Rare E. Detection
recent event memory
recent life e.
report of e.
sequence of e.'s
serious adverse e.
significant medial e.
skeletal related e.
Suretee E.'s Index
Systematic Assessment for Treatment of Emergent E.'s
thromboembolic e.
transient focal neurologic e.
transient ischemic e.
e. transmitter
unexplained apparent life-threatening e.
Unpleasant E.'s Schedule
ventricular tachycardia e.

event-free survival

eventration of the diaphragm

event-related

e.-r. brain potential
e.-r. desynchronization
e.-r. slow-brain potential

Everglades virus

Eversbusch operation

eversion

maximum eversion velocity
Potts eversion osteotomy

every

before every meal
e. day
e. even day
e. four weeks
e. hour
e. hour around the clock
e. 2 hours
e. 3 hours
e. 4 hours
e. 2 hours around the clock
e. night
e. other day
e. week
e. weekend

Everyday Problem Checklist

Everyman Contingency Table Analysis

evidence

abdomen showed evidence of weight loss
clinical evidence of metastatic disease
current medical evidence of record
dearth of e.
e. of disease
disease-oriented e.
e. of insurability
medical e.
no evidence of abnormality
no evidence of active disease
no evidence of disease
no evidence of disease-stationary disease
no evidence of distant metastases
no evidence of malignancy
no evidence of pathology
no evidence of primary tumor
no evidence of pulmonary disease
no evidence of recurrence
no evidence of recurrent disease
patient-oriented e.
rule of e.
sexual assault forensic e.
there is no evidence of malignancy

evidence-based

e.-b. decision making
e.-b. medicine
e.-b. outcomes
e.-b. recommendations

evidenced

as evidenced by

evisceration

pelvic e.
total abdominal e.

evoked

acoustic evoked response
auditory evoked potential
auditory visual evoked response
average evoked potential
average evoked response
average evoked response audiometry
average evoked response technique
brainstem auditory evoked potential
brainstem auditory evoked response
brainstem evoked response
cervical somatosensory evoked potential
e. compound electromyography
cortical auditory evoked potential
cortical auditory evoked response
e. cortical response
cortical somatosensory evoked potential
cortical somatosensory evoked response
electrical evoked potential
e. electromyogram
e. electromyography
e. electrospinogram
extreme somatosensory evoked potential
late auditory evoked response
left somatosensory evoked potential
localized evoked potential
lower extremity somatosensory evoked potential
median nerve somatosensory evoked potential
multimodality evoked response
e. muscle action potential
neurogenic motor evoked potential
neurological evoked response
neurologically evoked response
e. otoacoustic emission
paced ventricular evoked response
paroxysmal evoked pain
pattern evoked retinal response

evoked *(continued)*
pattern reversal visual evoked potential
e. potential response
e. potential signal averaging
e. potential study
pudendal evoked response
e. response audiometer
e. response audiometry
e. response test
right somatosensory evoked potential
sensory evoked response
e. sensory nerve action potential
somatically evoked field
somatosensory brainstem evoked potential
somatosensory cortical evoked potential
e. somatosensory response
spinal evoked potential
steady-state auditory evoked response
e. synaptic potential
transient auditory evoked response
transient evoked otoacoustic emission
trigeminal evoked potential
upper extremity somatosensory evoked potential
visual auditory evoked response
visually evoked cortical potential
visually evoked field
visually evoked flow response
e. visual potential
e. visual response

evoked-potential index

evoked-response
e.-r. audiometry
e.-r. detector

evolution
stroke in e.

evolving
e. dementia
e. hematoma
e. myocardial infarction

evulsion
nerve e.

Ewald
E. node
E. test meat

Ewart sign

Ewing
extraosseous Ewing sarcoma
E. sarcoma family of tumors
E. sarcoma/peripheral neuroectodermal tumor
E. sign

ex
hydrocephalus ex vacuo
hydrocephalus ex vacuo change
e. situ
e. utero intrapartum tracheloplasty
e. utero intrapartum treatment
e. vacuo dilatation
e. vivo
e. vivo cannulation
e. vivo count
e. vivo fertilization
e. vivo perfusion
e. vivo technique

exacerbated
headache e.
e. symptoms

exacerbating-remitting multiple sclerosis

exacerbation
acute e.
acute bacterial exacerbation of chronic bronchitis
acute exacerbation of chronic bronchitis
character, onset, location, duration, exacerbation, remission
e. and hemorrhage
e. of illness
e. of preexisting psychiatric illness
premenstrual exacerbation of asthma
e. and remission

exact
Fisher exact test
Signing Exact English

exaggerated
e. craniocaudal lateral angle
e. craniocaudal lateral view
e. response

exam
Denver Articulation Screening E.
Parkland Rapid E.

examination
Adult Basic Learning E.
Advanced Placement E.
anterior segment e.
ARM method of physical e.
associated physical examination finding
autopsy external e.
autopsy internal e.
autopsy microscopic e.
bone and joint e.
Boston Diagnostic Aphasia E.
breast e.
Brief Aphasia Screening E.
Brief Neuropsychological Mental Status E.
Cambridge Mental Disorders in Elderly E.
cardiac Doppler e.
carotid ultrasound e.
clinical breast e.
clinical staging of tumors, nodes, and metastases as determined by noninvasive e.
complete gynecologic examination annually
complete physical e.
computer-assisted sensory e.
computer-based e.
consultation and e.
court-ordered e.
crystal examination screen
date of e.
e. and diagnosis
digital examination of prostate
digital rectal e.
dilated fundus e.
direct fluorescent antibody examination for *Treponema pallidum*
Doppler venous e.
double-contrast barium examination of the upper gastrointestinal tract
eating disorders e.
electron microscopic e.
Employee Health Maintenance E.
e., opinion, and advice
external eye e.
fiberoptic endoscopic examination of swallowing
flexible endoscopic swallowing e.
full blood e.
e. glove
Graduate Record E.
gross examination of tissue
hanging drop e.
health appraisal e.
health and nutrition examination survey
history and physical e.
independent medical e.
initial physical e.
initial screening e.
Lateral Dominance E.
left breast biopsy e.
manual internal e.

Medical E. and Diagnostic Coding System
mental status e.
mental status examination report
Mental Status E. Record
Mini-Mental State Examination of Folstein
Modified Mini-Mental State E.
modified version of the mini mental status e.
motility e.
motor development e.
Multilingual Aphasia E.
muscle e.
National Health and Nutrition E. Follow-Up Study
National Health and Nutrition E. Survey
needle electrode e.
Neurobehavioral Cognitive Status e.
neurologic e.
Neurological E. for Children
neurological examination of extremities
neuropsychologic e.
neurosurgical e.
noninvasive carotid e.
nonrehydrated guaiac e.
normal pelvic e.
not found this e.
objective structural clinical e.
observation and e.
on e.
oral cancer e.
oral peripheral e.
orthopedic e.
orthopedic examination, special
ova and parasites e.
panoral x-ray e.
pathological tissue e.
Pediatric Early Elemental E.
Pediatric E. of Educational Readiness
Pediatric Extended E. at Three
pediatric orthopedic e.
pelvic examination under anesthesia
pelvic and rectal examination
pericardial fluid e.
periodic health e.
peritoneal fluid e.
personality disorder e.
physical e.
physical and neurologic examination for soft signs
preparticipation sports e.
present e.
Present State E.
Professional and Administrative Career E.
programmed physical e.
rectal e.
reduction of examination anxiety
e. and report
right breast biopsy e.
routine gynecological e.
Schizophrenic Subscale of Present State E.
self-breast e.
Sensory Perceptual E.
slit-lamp e.
sterile vaginal e.
total colon e.
total skin e.
tuning fork e.
e. under anesthesia
vaginal e.
visual e.
Wood light examination of eye

examined
e. hormone levels
not e.
wound examined for hemostasis

examiner
sexual assault nurse e.

examining
Boston Test for E. Aphasia
Nightingale examining lamp
Test for E. Expressive Morphology

exanthem
asymmetric periflexural exanthem of childhood
maculopapular e.
measles e.
papular e.
petechial e.
unilateral laterothoracic e.

exanthema
rheumatic e.
e. subitum
vesicular e.
vesicular exanthema of swine virus

exanthemata
ordinal designation of the e.

exanthematous
acute generalized exanthematous pustulosis
e. disease
e. drug rash
e. fever
Mediterranean exanthematous fever

excavation
archeological e.
atrophic e.
physiologic e.

excavatum
pectus e.
pectus excavatum deformity
pes e.

exceed
not to e.

excess
antibody excess antibody
antibody excess zone
antigen excess antigen
apparent mineral corticoid excess syndrome
apparent mineralocorticoid e.
apparent mineralocorticoid excess syndrome
base e.
divergence e.
e. ejection fraction
extracellular fluid volume e.
e. facial hair
e. hemorrhoidal tissue
hirsutism, androgen excess, insulin resistance, acanthosis nigricans syndrome
e. incidence
e. lactate
luteinizing hormone-dependent androgen e.
negative base e.
parathyroid hormone e.
refractory anemia with excess blasts
refractory anemia with excess of blasts in transformation
refractory anemia with excess blasts in transition
refractory anemia with excess myeloblasts
removal of excess cement
repetitive excess mixed anhydride method
saturated base e.
vertical maxillary e.
yin deficiency-yang excess syndrome

excessive
e. accommodation
e. accumulation of glycogen
e. acid secretion
e. activity

excessive *(continued)*
e. alcohol intake
e. blood loss
e. bone loss
e. brain activity
e. breast firmness and discomfort
e. daytime sleepiness
e. daytime somnolence
delirium, infection, atrophic urethritis and vaginitis, pharmaceuticals, psychological disorders, excessive urine output, restricted mobility, stool impaction
e. diffuse low and medium wave beta activity
disorders of excessive sleepiness
disorders of excessive somnolence
e. drug use
e. enlargement of head
e. facial hair growth
e. fast brain wave activity
e. fluid intake
e. food intake
e. gambling
e. gas formation
e. guilt
e. hair growth
e. hair shedding
e. heat production
e. or inappropriate guilt
e. ingestion
e. insulin secretion
e. intake of alcohol
e. intestinal gas
e. joint play
e. lateral pressure syndrome
e. motor activity
e. tearing
e. thirst
e. urination
e. ventilation
e. volubility
e. weight gain
e. weight loss

excessively rapid heart rate

exchange
abnormality in gas e.
angry word e.
anion exchange resin
e. blood transfusion
disturbance in air e.
double-charge e.
extracorporeal exchange hypothermia
extracorporeal gas e.
gas e.
guidewire e.
guidewire exchange technique
half-time of e.
high-performance ion exchange chromatography
high-pH anion exchange chromatography coupled with pulsed amperometric detection
hydrogen e.
impaired gas e.
mersalyl exchange assay
mersalyl exchange method
e. nailing
needle exchange program
neonatal exchange transfusion
partial exchange transfusion
partial plasma e.
perfluorocarbon-associated gas e.
plasma e.
plasma exchange number three
e. plasmapheresis
poor air e.
pulmocutaneous e.
pulmonary gas e.
rapid e.
regional gas e.
respiratory exchange ratio
respiratory heat e.
sister chromatid e.
sister chromatid exchange rate
strong exchange capacity resin
syringe exchange program
therapeutic plasma e.
total exchange capacity

exchangeable
e. body potassium
total exchangeable potassium
total exchangeable sodium
total exchangeable thyroxine

exchange/education-practice
role e.-p.

exchanger
countercurrent exchanger immunoelectrophoresis
heat e.
heat/moisture e.
sodium/hydrogen e.

exchanging
heat and moisture exchanging filter

excimer
argon-fluoride excimer laser
e. laser
e. laser ablation
e. laser-assisted angioplasty
e. laser coronary angioplasty
e. laser photorefractive keratectomy
e. laser phototherapeutic keratectomy
e. laser, rotational atherectomy, and balloon angioplasty
percutaneous excimer laser coronary angioplasty
percutaneous excimer laser coronary angioplasty system
peripheral excimer laser angioplasty
smooth excimer laser coronary angioplasty
e. vascular recanalization

excised
old incision e.

excision
alar rim e.
alar wedge e.
anterior port scalp e.
Arlt pterygium e.
e. arthroplasty
atrial septum e.
e. biopsy
e. and curettage
electrosurgical e.
electrosurgical loop e.
en bloc e.
e., curettage and drilling
full-thickness local e.
e. of ganglionic cyst
e. head of pancreas
heel spur e.
e. of joint
large loop excision of transformation zone/loop electrosurgical excision procedure
large loop excision of transition zone
local tumor e.
local tumor excision with irradiation
loop electrosurgical excision procedure
loop electrosurgical excision procedure conization
loop excision of the transformation zone
lymph node e.
Malawer excision technique
marginal e.
McKeever-Buck fragment e.
microlumbar disc e.
modified fishtail e.
needle diathermy excision of the transformation zone

nuclear excision repair instability
pentagonal block e.
perialar crescentic e.
probe e.
split-thickness skin e.
surgical e.
T-cell receptor-rearrangement excision circle
thymus gland e.
tissue ablation, incision and e.
total mesorectal e.
e. and wedge biopsy
e. and wedge biopsy of breast
wide local e.

excisional
e. biopsy technique
e. biopsy of tumor mass
laser vaporization and excisional conization
loop electrosurgical excisional procedure
percutaneous excisional breast biopsy
shave excisional biopsy
video-assisted excisional biopsy
wedge excisional biopsy
well-healed previous excisional scars

excitability
emotional e.
membrane e.
neuronal e.
supernormal e.

excitability-inducing material

excitable gap

excitation
anodal e.
anomalous atrioventricular e.
fast acquisition multiple e.
fluorescence excitation transfer immunoassay
generator of e.
magnetization-prepared rapid gradient echo-water e.
M cone e.
multiphoton e.
neural e.
neurohumoral excitation state
number of e.
paradoxic levator e.
rotating delivery of excitation off resonance
slice excitation wave
snooze-induced excitation of sympathetic triggered activity
tilted optimized nonsaturating e.
variable-angle uniform signal e.
e. wave

excitation-contraction

excitative-type psychosis

excitatory
e. center
e. junction potential
local excitatory state
low excitatory state
e. postsynaptic potential
e. transmitter

excited
e. skin syndrome
near-UV excited autofluorescence diagnosis system
transversely excited atmospheric pressure

excitement
inhibited sexual e.

excitoreflex nerve

excitor substance

exclusion
diagnosis by e.
duodenal e.
hepatic vascular e.
molecular exclusion chromatography
partial hepatic vascular e.
proximal gastric e.
size exclusion chromatography
steric exclusion chromatography

exclusive
e. operating room
e. provider organization

excoriation
crusted e.
necrotic e.
neurotic e.

excrement
secreta and e.

excrescence
cauliflower e.
papillary e.
polypoid e.

excreted mass

excretion
absorption, distribution, metabolism, and e.
albumin excretion rate
aldosterone excretion rate
calcium e.
contrast media e.
cumulative urinary e.
endolymph filtration and e.
fecal fat e.
fractional excretion of lithium
fractional excretion of potassium
fractional excretion of sodium
increased excretion of protein
increasing urinary e.
net acid e.
phosphate excretion index
prompt excretion of contrast material
prompt excretion of dye
protein e.
renal e.
renal excretion rate
sebum excretion rate
secretion and e.
titrated norepinephrine e.
total estrogen e.
unilateral absence of e.
urinary albumin e.
urinary calcium volume excretion rate
urinary excretion of protein
urinary potassium volume excretion rate
urinary sodium e.
urinary urea nitrogen e.

excretory
constant infusion excretory urogram
cribriform salivary carcinoma of excretory duct
e. cystogram
e. cystography
e. index
e. phase
total excretory nitrogen
e. urogram
e. urography

excruciating
recurrent excruciating headache

excursion
airway pressure e.
e. of diaphragm
diaphragmatic e.
diminished chest e.
diminished contractile e.
interventricular septal e.
mean amplitude of glycerine e.
mean indices of meal e.
mitral valve leaflet e.
posterior wall e.
total-head e.

executive
e. 22 chemistry profile
e. cognitive function

executive *(continued)*
e. cognitive functioning
e. ego function
e. function deficit
e. functioning disturbance
health and safety e.

exemption
humanitarian device e.
Investigational Device E.

exenterated orbit

exenteration
anterior e.
anterior pelvic e.
orbital e.
e. of orbital contents operation
orbital exenteration gastroscopic access technique
pelvic e.
radical e.
total pelvic e.

exenterative surgery for pelvic cancer

exercise
abdominal curl e.
active e.
active assisted e.
active assistive e.
active bending e.
active quad strengthening e.
active range-of-motion e.
active-resistive e.'s
e. addiction
aerobic e.
aerobic chair e.'s
ankle exercise machine
aquatic exercise program
calf-heel stretch e.
e. capacity
cardiac exercise laboratory
cardiopulmonary e.
cardiopulmonary exercise test
cardiovascular aerobic e.
chair sit-up e.
chest stretch e.
chronotropic exercise assessment protocol
closed kinetic chain e.
condition muscles with aerobic e.
continuous loop exercise echocardiogram
Cornell exercise protocol
cough and e.
Davidson protocol exercise test
deep breathing e.
diathermy, massage, and e.
drugs, exercise, education, diet, and self-monitoring
dyspnea on e.
early exercise testing
e. echocardiogram
e. echocardiography
ejection fraction during e.
e. electrocardiogram
e. electrocardiography
Ellestad exercise stress test
field training e.
functional exercise program
general conditioning e.
general therapeutic e.
graded exercise electrocardiogram
graded exercise program
graded exercise test
graded resistive e.
graded treadmill exercise test
gradual exercise progression
hamstring stretch e.
hand grip exercise
heart helping e.
e.'s for heart patient
e. heart rate
heat, massage, and e.
heel squat e.
high-impact aerobic e.
hip adductor stretch e.
home exercise program
e. hyperemia blood flow
e. imaging
inability to e.
independent progressive home exercise program
e. index
e. induced heart attack
inpatient exercise center
e. intolerance
e. ischemia
isometric quad strengthening e.
knee extension e.
knee sling e.'s
e. lability index
e. limit
low-impact aerobic e.
low-level graded exercise test
manual active-resistive e.
manual resistance e.
maximal exercise systolic pressure
maximal exercise tolerance test
maximal exercise ventilation
maximal restrictive e.
McKenzie extension e.
moderate intensity e.
modified treadmill exercise testing
e. MUGA
MUGA exercise stress test
multigated blood pool image during e.
multistage graded exercise test
e. myopathy
neuromuscular control e.
nonsupported arm e.
normal exercise study
nutrition and e.
open kinetic chain e.'s
overhead exercise test
passive e.
passive assistance e.
passive resistance e.
e.'s for patient in home
peak exercise oxygen consumption
peak exercise ventilation
pelvic floor e.
pelvic floor muscle e.
pelvic muscle e.
pelvic tilt e.
physical e.
physical reconditioning e.
poor exercise tolerance
postoperative e.
power building e.
predischarge graded exercise test
e. pressure index
progressive assistive e.
progressive exercise test
progressive home exercise program
progressive resistance e.
progressive-resistive e.
quadriceps extension e.
Regen flexion e.
regressive resistive e.
resistive e.
resistive exercise product
resistive e.'s to upper extremities
rest and e.
sequential developmental e.'s
shoulder shrug e.
single-stage exercise stress test
specific action e.
steady-state e.
strength training e.
e. stress echocardiography
e. stress electrocardiography
e. stress test
stretching and breathing e.
e. study
submaximal treadmill exercise test
supported arm e.
sustained maximal inspiratory lung e.

symptom-limited graded exercise test
e. thallium
thallium exercise heart scan
thallium-graded exercise test
e. thallium 201 scintigraphy
therapeutic e.
thermal effect of e.
thermic effect of e.
e. tidal flow-volume loop
toe touch e.
e. tolerance
e. tolerance test
transtelephonic exercise monitor
e. treadmill
treadmill e.
treadmill exercise stress test
e. treadmill test
e. treadmill test with thallium
unsupported arm e.
visual imagery e.
weight training e.
whirlpool, massage, e.
work hardening e.
written home exercise program

exercise-induced
e.-i. amenorrhea
e.-i. anaphylaxis
e.-i. arrhythmia
e.-i. asthma
e.-i. bronchoconstriction
e.-i. bronchospasm
e.-i. hives
e.-i. respiratory distress syndrome
e.-i. silent myocardial ischemia
e.-i. sudden death
e.-i. urticaria
e.-i. ventricular tachycardia

exerciser
animal beanbag e.
axial resistance e.
continuous anatomical passive e.
dynamic finger e.
microcomputer upper limb e.
Nelson finger e.

exercise-related
e.-r. amenorrhea
e.-r. headache

exeresis
palliative e.

exertion
chest pain on e.
dyspnea on e.
increased dyspnea on e.
pain on e.
pain related to e.
paroxysmal dyspnea on e.
rated perceived e.
rate of perceived e.
rating of perceived e.
shortness of breath on e.

exertional
e. activity
acute exertional compartment syndrome
acute exertional rhabdomyolysis
e. anterior compartment syndrome
e. asthma
e. chest pain
chronic anterior exertional compartment syndrome
e. deep posterior compartment syndrome
e. dyspnea
e. headache
e. heat illness
e. heat stroke
heavy exertional activity
e. hypotension
paroxysmal exertional dyskinesia
e. reactive airway disease

exfoliation
e. syndrome
e. syndrome glaucoma

exfoliative
e. dermatitis
e. gastritis

exhalation
end e.

exhaled
e. nitric oxide
e. tidal volume

exhaust
automobile e.
local exhaust ventilation

exhaustion
anhidrotic heat e.
anxiety from heat e.
chronic nervous e.
chronic nervous exhaustion syndrome
dehydration and e.
e., burnout and heart disease
obvious physical e.
ovarian follicle e.
e. syndrome
vital exhaustion and depression

exhibited
patient exhibited muscle guarding

exhibitionistic tendency

exhibits
e. irritable negativism
infant exhibits hunger behavior
patient exhibits overt hostility

exist
did not exist prior to enlistment

existed
e. prior to enlistment
e. prior to service

existing
e. infection control
repeated quick stretch superimposed upon an existing contraction

exit
open exit foramen
root exit zone
e. site
wound of e.
e. wound

exocardial murmur

exocrine
e. insufficiency
pancreatic e.
pancreatic exocrine deficiency
pancreatic exocrine deficit
pancreatic exocrine dysfunction
pancreatic exocrine function insufficiency
pancreatic exocrine function test
pancreatic exocrine insufficiency
e. pancreatic insufficiency
e. tissue

exocrinopathy
autoimmune e.

exocytosis
misplaced e.

exogenous
contamination of exogenous sources
e. disease
e. hormone
e. hyperthyroidism
e. lipoid pneumonia
e. natural surfactant
e. obesity

exomphalos, macroglossia, gigantism syndrome

exopeptidase
pancreatic e.

exophoria
e. distance
e., near viewing

exophthalmic
e. factor
e. goiter
exophthalmometer
Luedde e.
Marco prism e.
exophthalmos
e., myxedema circumscriptum praetibiale, and osteoarthropathia hypertrophicans syndrome
thyrotoxic e.
exophthalmos-hyperthyroid factor
exophthalmos-producing
e.-p. factor
e.-p. substance
exophytic
e. carcinoma
e. growth
e. joint disease
e. lesion
e. mass
e. nodule
e. skin lesion
exophytic-type growth
exophytum glioma
exopolysaccharide
mucoid e.
exoprotein
toxic shock syndrome e.
exoskeletal device
exostectomy
medial e.
exostosis
e. bursata
e. formation
hereditary multiple e.
metatarsal cuneiform e.
multiple e.'s
multiple cartilaginous e.'s
multiple exostoses of jaw
multiple exostoses mental retardation syndrome
multiple hereditary e.'s
multiple hereditary osteochondral e.'s
tricho-rhino-auriculo-phalangeal multiple e.'s
trichorhinophalangeal multiple e.'s
exotoxin
cholera e.
Pseudomonas e.
pyrogenic e.
pyrogenic exotoxin C
streptococcal pyrogenic e.
streptococcal pyrogenic exotoxin B, C
toxic shock syndrome e.
exotoxin-A
streptococcal e.-A.
exotropia
alternating e.
left e.
paralytic pontine e.
right e.
V-pattern e.
expand
chest expands adequately bilaterally
e. internal components of knee
expandable
e. access catheter
balloon expandable intravascular stent
e. breast implant
e. esophageal stent
lumbar intersomatic fusion expandable cage
e. olive
expanded
e. consciousness
e. duty dental auxiliary
Expanded Disability Status Scale
e. foam immobilization device
e. free scalp flap
e. function dental assistant
e. plasma
e. polytetrafluoroethylene
poorly expanded lungs
expander
blood volume e.
breast tissue e.
Miami STAR tissue e.
e. pocket
subperiosteal tissue e.
expansile
familial expansile osteolysis
expansion
blood volume e.
controlled e.
controlled radial e.
dendritic e.
equal bilateral e.
extensor digital e.
extracellular volume e.
good chest e.
intravascular volume e.
lingual bony e.
medial extensor e.
membrane expansion theory
palatal expansion appliance
paradoxical systolic e.
passive chest e.
prolonged acute tissue e.
rapid maxillary e.
relative gas e.
surgically assisted rapid maxillary e.
surgically assisted rapid palatal e.
expansive
e. delusion
e. idea
e. mood
expectancy
active life e.
disability-free life e.
Pre-Reading E. Screening Scale
quality-adjusted life e.
remission, relapse, and life e.
sex difference in life e.
total life e.
e. wave
expectant
e. management
e. treatment
expectation
e. of death
e. of life
mathematical e.
E. Score
expected
e. date of confinement
e. date of delivery
date of expected delivery
e. day of delivery
e. delivery, cesarean
e. intervention strategy
lost years of expected life
medical improvement e.
medical improvement not e.
moribund patient not expected to live
reasonably expected as safe
standard observed minus e.
e. upper limit
e. value
e. value of clinical information
e. weight gain
expectoration
cough and e.
cough with e.
productive cough and e.
expelled
infant e.
placenta e.

expended
energy expended with activity
total energy e.

expenditure
basal energy e.
capital expenditure review
capital expenditure threshold
energy e.
measured energy e.
resting energy e.
resting metabolic e.
total daily energy e.
total energy e.

expense
out-of-pocket e.

expense-per-equivalent admission

experience
adverse childhood e.
appropriate learning e.
atypical delusional e.
communal traumatic experiences inventory
Community College Student E.'s Questionnaire
Depressive E.'s Questionnaire
Developmental Assessment of Life E.'s
distressing psychedelic e.
Grief E. Inventory
hallucinatory emotional e.
human immunodeficiency virus-patient-reported status and e.
language experience approach
Learning Inventory of Kindergarten E.'s
Life E.'s Checklist
Life E. Survey
near-death e.
near death e.
overwhelming childhood e.
Personal E. and Attitude Questionnaire
Personal E. Screening Questionnaire
Profile of Out-of-Body E.'s
Psychosocial Assessment of Childhood E.'s
radiation experience data
Schedule of Recent E.'s
Stress From Life E.
subjective paranormal e.
tests of basic e.
training and e.
Vocational Interest, E., and Skill Assessment

Experienced
Coping Orientations to Problems E.

Experiential World Inventory

experiment
critical e.
labeled release experiment

experimental
acute monophasic experimental autoimmune encephalomyelitis
e. allergic encephalitis
e. allergic encephalomyelitis
e. allergic neuritis
e. allergic orchitis
e. autoimmune encephalitis
e. autoimmune encephalomyelitis
e. autoimmune gastritis
e. autoimmune myasthenia gravis
e. autoimmune thymitis
e. autoimmune thyroiditis
e. autoimmune uveitis
automated general experimental device
e. breast cancer treatment
e. control
Crown-Crisp E. Index
e. enterococcal endocarditis
e. glomerulonephritis
Lawrence Experimental Station agar
longitudinal experimental study design
Szondi E. Diagnostics of Drives

experimentally induced Köbner phenomenon

experimentation
adolescent experimentation with adult behavior

expert
longitudinal expert evaluation using all available data
mental health e.

expiration
alternate inspiration and expiration of air
duration of e.
forced equilibrating e.
inhalation and e.
inspiration and e.
no expiration date
pressure on e.
ratio of expiration time and total time of breathing cycle
e. time
time to peak expiratory flow and total expiration time

expiration-inspiration ratio

expiration-synchronized intermittent mandatory ventilation

expiratory
e. attenuation
e. computed tomography
e. dyspnea
e. excursion
e. flow volume
e. flow-volume curve
forced e.
forced expiratory capacity
forced expiratory flow
forced expiratory flow volume
forced expiratory spirogram
forced expiratory time in seconds
forced expiratory volume at one second
forced expiratory volume in one second as percent of FVC
forced expiratory volume in one second to forced vital capacity ratio
forced expiratory volume timed
forced expiratory volume timed to forced vital capacity ratio
forced volume, e.
e. grunting
inspiratory to expiratory ratio
inspiratory expiratory ratio
e. to inspiratory ratio
inspiratory resistance and positive expiratory pressure
maximal expiratory flow
maximal expiratory flow rate
maximal expiratory flow-static recoil curve
maximal expiratory flow volume
maximal expiratory flow volume curve
maximal expiratory mouth pressure
maximal forced expiratory flow
maximal forced expiratory maneuver
maximum expiratory airflow-static lung elastic recoil pressure
maximum expiratory flow
maximum expiratory flow at 50% vital capacity
maximum expiratory flow rate
maximum expiratory flow volume
mean maximal expiratory flow
mechanical expiratory flow volume curve
e. murmur

expiratory *(continued)*
negative expiratory force
negative expiratory pressure
partial expiratory flow-static recoil curve
partial expiratory flow volume
peak expiratory flow
peak expiratory flow rate
peak expiratory flow time
peak tidal expiratory flow
percent predicted peak expiratory flow
e. phase
e. positive airway pressure
positive expiratory pressure
positive expiratory pressure plateau
e. prolongation
e. reserve
e. reserve volume
resting expiratory level
e. rhonchi
e. sibilant
spontaneous positive end expiratory pressure
e. stridor
e. threshold load
tidal expiratory flow at 25% of tidal volume
tidal expiratory flow at 50% of tidal volume
tidal expiratory flow at 75% of tidal volume
tidal expiratory volume
e. time
timed forced expiratory volume
time to peak expiratory flow
time to peak expiratory flow and total expiration time
time to peak tidal expiratory flow
total expiratory time
e. trapping of air
volume to peak expiratory flow and total expiratory volume
e. wheeze
e. wheezing

expiratory time
forced expiratory time in seconds

expired
e. air
e. air collection
baby expired following resuscitation attempt
e. following resuscitation attempt
fractional concentration of carbon dioxide in expired gas
fractional concentration of oxygen in expired gas
fraction of expired carbon dioxide
mixed expired carbon dioxide tension
mixed expired gas
e. volume
volume of expired gas

explanation
alternative e.
e. of benefits
E. of Medicare Benefits

explant
encircling e.
Molteno episcleral e.

explanted heart

expleomorphic adenoma

explicit
e. behavior
life-terminating acts without the explicit request

exploitation
conscious exploitation of others

exploration
cervical mediastinal e.
e. of common bile duct
common bile duct e.
common duct e.
complete surgical e.
Education and Career E. System
individual career e.
laparoscopic common duct e.
laparoscopic exploration of the common bile duct
laparoscopic transcystic common bile duct e.
left middle ear e.
manual exploration of abdomen
middle ear e.
open common bile duct e.
Picture Interest E. Survey
e. and revision
right middle ear e.
thoracotomy with e.

exploratory
e. incision
e. insight-oriented psychotherapy
e. laparotomy
e. operation
e. surgery
e. thoracotomy

explored
abdomen entered and e.

Explorer
Occupational Interests E.

explosion fracture

explosive
e. aggressive behavior
e. decompression
e. diarrhea
e. follicular hyperplasia
intermittent explosive personality disorder
isolated explosive disorder
e. outburst
e. personality
e. personality disorder
e. psychotic state
e. speech
e. vomiting
e. watery diarrhea

exponential
e. function
time-delayed e.

export
bile salt export pump

exposed
hilar vessels e.
lethal dose in all exposed subjects
never e.
prenatally exposed to drugs
e. protruding form

exposure
aerosolized pollutant e.
airway, breathing, circulation, disability, e.
e. to allergen
anesthetic gas e.
anterior surgical e.
as low as reasonably achievable radiation e.
automatic exposure control
avoidance of e.
Behnken unit of roentgen-ray e.
e. to blood or body fluid
brief exposure to heat stress
combat stress e.
constant exposure rate
defined exposure dose
e. duration threshold
environmental exposure unit
e. factor
filtered smoke e.
good exposure obtained
hundred woman years of e.
e. to industrial substances
intrauterine drug e.
ionization exposure rate

Kienböck unit of x-ray e.
limitation of e.
maternal mercury e.
measurement of e.
middle fossa e.
mucous membrane e.
narrow band UVB therapeutic light e.
noise exposure meter
occupational exposure to chemicals
parotid gland exposure guideline
passive smoke e.
patient at high-risk of e.
patient exposure guideline
percutaneous exposure risk
permissible exposure limits
person-years of e.
prenatal alcohol e.
prenatal cocaine e.
prior to e.
radiation exposure guide
radiation exposure in pregnancy
recommended exposure level
risk of e.
short-term exposure limit
skin exposure reduction paste against chemical warfare agent
smoke e.
smoke exposure machine
targeted systemic e.
in utero drug e.
volumetric multiple exposure transmission holography
willful exposure to unwanted pregnancy

exposure-related hypothermia death

expressed
e. breast milk
clot expressed from wound
e. emotion
patient expressed guilt feeling
e. prostatic secretions
regulated upon activation, normal T-cell expressed and secreted
e. sequence tag
virus entry mediator, a receptor expressed by T lymphocyte

expression
activates facial e.
affective expression disorder
akinesia/diminished emotional e.
e.'s of anger
e.'s of anger
Anger E. Scale
anomalous antigen e.
appropriate facial e.
cardiac gene e.
Human Gene E.
involuntary facial e.
lines of e.
MHC receptor e.
muscles of facial e.
neurotrophic factor e.
outward expression of anger with impulsive feature
passivity in anger e.
pattern of e.
permitting safe expression of anger
Rb protein e.
e. sequence tagged
serial analysis of gene e.
State-Trait Anger E. Inventory
tumor amplified protein expression therapy
in vivo expression technology

expressive
e. ability
developmental expressive language disorder
developmental expressive writing disorder
E. One-Word Picture Vocabulary Test
paucity of expressive gestures
slow expressive language development
specific expressive language impairment
Structure Photographic E. Language Test-II
Test for Examining E. Morphology

expressor
Arruga e.
meibomian gland e.

expulsion
cannulated expulsion piston
graft e.

expulsive hemorrhage

exsanguinating
e. hemorrhage
e. intraperitoneal hemorrhage

exstrophic
neonatal exstrophic bladder repair

extended
e. abdominal radiation therapy
e. activities of daily living
e. aortic root replacement
e. binary-coded decimal interchange code
e. care facility
e. care hospital
e. care unit
e. criteria donor
e. daily dialysis
e. data stream
e. deep inferior epigastric
e. electron-loss line fine structure
e. endocardial resection
e. endocardial resection procedure
e., rotated, sidebent
e. external rotation
e. family therapy
e. field radiation
e. field radiation therapy
head e.
head and neck in extended position
e. health care
incision extended bilaterally
e. jaundice of newborn
e. lateral arm free flap
e. length of utterance
e. lymphadenopathy syndrome
e. mandatory minute ventilation
medial extended facial translocation
Pediatric E. Examination at Three
e. radical mastectomy
e. release tablet
e. resistance
skilled nursing extended care facility
e. supraplatysmal plane
surface extended x-ray absorption fine structure
e. V-Y advancement flap
e. x-ray absorption fine structure spectroscopy

extended-care nursery

extended-duration topical arthropod repellent

extended-spectrum
e.-s. beta-lactamase
e.-s. beta-lactamase-producing Enterobacteriaceae

extended-wear
e.-w. contact lens
e.-w. soft contact lens

extender
autograft e.
nail e.

extends
back pain extends down legs

extensibility
penile e.

extensible markup language

extensile
anterior extensile approach
McConnell extensile approach

extension
active knee e.
angle of greatest e.
attached gingiva e.
cast with dorsal toe plate e.
cast with volar toe plate e.
e. of cerebral infarct
e. contracture
e. corner avulsion fracture
e. deformity
degree of e.
established extraprostatic e.
external rotation in e.
extracapsular e.
extraprostatic e.
fabere extension test
finger extension test
flexion, abduction, external rotation, e.
flexion and e.
flexion, extension, and rotation
focal extraprostatic e.
full knee e.
gravity extension locking system
hand held in position of e.
e. instability
internal rotation in e.
jejunal extension tube
knee extension exercise
lumbar extension test
McKenzie extension exercise
McKenzie extension maneuver
medial hip rotation in e.
midline vertical uterine e.
e. nail
neck extension position
e. 50% of normal
e. osteotomy
paraplegia in e.
partial denture, distal e.
pear-shaped extension tube
percutaneous endoscopic gastrostomy and jejunal extension tube
quadriceps extension exercise
reverse transcriptase primer e.
Score for Neonatal Acute Physiology-Perinatal E.
e. teardrop fracture
terminal e.
terminal knee e.
thoracolumbosacral orthosis—flexion, extension, lateral bending, and transverse rotation
tonic hind limb e.
venous e.
wrist hand extension compression support

extensive
e. bronchial mucosa hemorrhage
e. disease
e. fecal impaction
e. hearing assessment
e. hyaline membrane disease
e. inflammatory bowel disease
e. inoperable carcinoma
e. interstitial fibrosis
e. intraductal carcinoma
e. intraductal component
e. manipulation of joint
e. metastatic involvement
e. new bone formation

extensor
apparatus e.
e. apparatus
e. brevis arthroplasty
e. carpi radialis
e. carpi radialis brevis
e. carpi radialis brevis muscle
e. carpi radialis brevis tendon
e. carpi radialis longus
e. carpi radialis longus flap
e. carpi radialis longus muscle
e. carpi radialis longus tendon
e. carpi ulnaris
e. carpi ulnaris muscle
e. carpi ulnaris sheath
e. carpi ulnaris tendon
central extensor mechanism
e. compartment of arm
e. compartment of forearm
e. compartment of leg
e. compartment of thigh
e. digital expansion
e. digiti communis
e. digiti minimi
e. digiti minimi muscle
e. digiti minimi tendon
e. digiti quinti
e. digiti quinti muscle
e. digiti quinti proprius
e. digiti quinti tendon
e. digit minimi
e. digitorum
e. digitorum brevis
e. digitorum communis
e. digitorum communis muscle
e. digitorum communis tendon
e. digitorum longus
e. hallucis
e. hallucis brevis
e. hallucis brevis muscle
e. hallucis longus
e. indicis
e. indicis proprius
e. lengthening
linear extensor erythema
long extensor muscle of great toe
long extensor muscle of thumb
long radial extensor muscle of wrist
lumbar extensor muscle
e. mechanism dysfunction
medial extensor expansion
musculus extensor brevis pollicis
musculus extensor carpi radialis brevis
musculus extensor carpi radialis longus
musculus extensor carpi ulnaris
musculus extensor digiti minimi
musculus extensor digiti quinti proprius
musculus extensor hallucis brevis
musculus extensor hallucis longus
musculus extensor indicis
musculus extensor indicis proprius
musculus extensor longus digitorum
musculus extensor longus pollicis
musculus extensor minimi digiti
musculus extensor ossis metacarpi pollicis
musculus extensor pollicis brevis
musculus extensor pollicis longus
paradoxical extensor reflex
e. pollicis brevis
pollicis brevis extensor muscle
pollicis brevis extensor tendon
e. pollicis brevis tendon
e. pollicis longus
pollicis longus extensor muscle
e. proprius hallucis
e. quinti proprius
radial extensor muscle
reactive extensor postural synergy
e. rigidity
e. tendon
e. tendon lengthening
e. tendon tenolysis
e. tendon transfer
e. tenodesis
e. tenosynovectomy

e. tenotomy
terminal extensor mechanism
toe extensor muscle
wrist extensor tendon

extent
age, distant metastases, extent and size
age, metastases, extent and size risk criteria
anular tear e.
e. of cerebral lesion
e. of disease
Disease E. Index
evaluate extent of injury or illness
e. of pleural carcinomatosis score
e. of skin involvement

exterior surface

externa
benign necrotizing otitis e.
bilateral otitis e.
left otitis e.
malignant necrotizing otitis e.
malignant otitis e.
membrana granulosa e.
otitis e.
right otitis e.

external
e. abdominal region
adjustable external suture
ambiguous external genitalia
ambiguous external stimuli
e. anal sphincter
anterior external arcuate fiber
anterior labial branch of deep external pudendal artery
anterior lip of external os of uterus
anterior scrotal branch of deep external pudendal artery
anterosuperior external ilium movement
AO external fixation
apex of external ring
e. apical root resorption
aponeurosis of external oblique
aponeurosis of external oblique muscle
e. auditory
e. auditory canal
e. auditory meatus
automated external defibrillator
automated external defibrillator pacemaker
automatic external cardioverter-defibrillator
automatic external defibrillator
autopsy external description
autopsy external examination
4-bar external fixation
4-bar external fixation apparatus
4-bar external fixation device
Bartholin, urethral, and Skene glands, and external genitalia
e. beam irradiation
e. beam photon therapy
e. beam radiation therapy
e. beam radiotherapy
e. branch of superior laryngeal
cantilever external fixator
e. cardiac compression
e. cardiac massage
e. cardiac pressure
e. cardiopulmonary resuscitation
e. cardioverter-defibrillator
e. carotid
e. carotid artery
e. cephalic version
e. chemical messenger
chronic progressive external ophthalmoplegia
e. cobalt irradiation
e. conjugate
controlling external entities
controlling external spirit
e. cooling appliance
e. counterpressure device
e. counterpulsation
e. dacryocystorhinostomy
detrusor external sphincter dyssynergia
e. diameter
e. dyspnea
e. ear
e. elastic lamina
e. elastic membrane
extended external rotation
for external use only
e. eye examination
fabere external rotation test
female external genitalia
e. fetal heart rate monitoring
e. fetal maternal monitor
e. fetal monitoring
flexion, abduction, external rotation
flexion, abduction, external rotation contracture
flexion, abduction, external rotation, extension
e. fluid loss
fractionated external beam irradiation
e. genitalia
half-pin external fixator
e. hemorrhage
e. hemorrhoid
e. hernia
high-dose external irradiation
e. humeral epicondylitis
e. iliac
e. iliac artery
e. iliac lymph nodes
e. iliac vein
e. ilium
e. impulsive form
e. inguinal ring
e. injury
e. insulin pump
e. intercostal muscle
internal and e.
internal diameter to external diameter
internal versus e.
e. intervention
e. irradiation
e. irradiation therapy
e. isovolumic contraction time
e. jugular
e. jugular vein
lens-sparing external beam radiation therapy
e. lids
e. limiting membrane
long external lateral ligament
long external rotator
low LET external beam irradiation
male external genitalia
malignant external otitis syndrome
megavoltage external radiotherapy
e. membrane protein
Meurmann external ear anomaly grade
molecular external layer
e. movement
e. muscle layer damaged
nerve of external acoustic meatus
normal external female genitalia
nuclear external layer
e. oblique aponeurosis
e. oblique fascia
e. oblique muscle
e. oblique muscle of abdomen
e. oculomotor ophthalmoplegia
one-plane bilateral external fixator
opening of external acoustic meatus
open reduction and external fixation

external *(continued)*
orifice of external acoustic meatus
e. os of uterus
e. otitis media
partial external biliary diversion
passive external rewarming
e. plexiform layer
e. pneumatic calf compression
e. pneumatic compression
popliteal external nerve
posteroinferior e.
e. pressure circulatory assistance
progressive external ophthalmoparesis
progressive external ophthalmoplegia
e. quality assessment
e. reduction
e. resistance
right external carotid
right external carotid artery
e. rotation-abduction stress test
e. rotation in extension
e. rotation in flexion
e. rotation/internal rotation
seborrheic external otitis
e. skeletal fixation
e. spinal skeletal fixator
standard external cardiopulmonary resuscitation
superficial external pudendal artery
supination external rotation
e. tachyarrhythmia control device
temporal external artery
therapeutic external radiation
e. ultrasound-assisted lipoplasty
e. urethral meatus
e. urethral orifice
e. urethral sphincter
e. urinary device
e. ventricular drainage
e. version
vesical external sphincter dyssynergia
volume treated in external irradiation

externalize blame

externalized anger

externalizing behavior

externally
abducted and externally rotated
e. supported

externus
malleolus e.
meatus acusticus e.
obliquus abdominis externus muscle
obliquus externus abdominis
obturator externus muscle

extinction
e. coefficient
molar extinction coefficient
order of e.
partial reinforcement extinction effect
perceptual e.
Quality E. Test
rapid extinction effect
tactile e.

extirpation
nodal e.
e. of uterus and cervix

extra
e. ABL signal fluorescent in situ hybridization
e. food
e. heart sound
e. high potency
e. large
e. point
e. strength
e. uterine life
ventricular extra beat

extraalveolar
e. air
e. vessel

extraamniotic saline infusion

extraanatomic bypass

extraarticular
MacIntosh extraarticular tenodesis

extracapillary
e. lesion
e. proliferative glomerulonephritis

extracapsular
e. cataract extraction
e. extension
planned extracapsular cataract extraction
e. spread

extracardiac murmur

extracellular
alcohol-induced extracellular volume contraction
blood extracellular fluid
e. compartment
e. concentration
e. domain
e. fluid
e. fluid compartment
e. fluid volume
e. fluid volume depletion
e. fluid volume excess
functional extracellular fluid volume
e. granular material
e. kalium
e. mass to body cell mass ratio
e. material
e. matrix
e. matrix metalloproteinase inducer
multifunctional extracellular glycoprotein
normal extracellular fluid volume
parathyroid extracellular calcium-sensing receptor
e. regulated kinase
e. space
e. tachyzoite
e. tissue
e. volume of distribution
e. volume expansion
e. water

extracellular-like, calcium-free solution

extracerebral cavernous angioma

extracolonic malignancy

extracorporal
neonatal extracorporal membrane oxygenation

extracorporeal
bioartificial extracorporeal liver support system
e. carbon dioxide removal
e. circulation
e. dialysis
electrohydraulic extracorporeal lithotripsy
e. exchange hypothermia
e. gas exchange
e. heart
heparin-induced extracorporeal low-density lipoprotein precipitation
e. irradiation of blood
e. irradiation of lymph
e. life support
e. liver assist device
e. liver perfusion
e. lung assist
e. membrane
e. membrane oxygenation
e. membrane oxygenation affecting cognitive function

e. membrane oxygenator
e. photochemotherapy
e. photopheresis
e. photophoresis
e. piezoelectric lithotripsy
e. pneumoperititoneal access bubble
e. rewarming
e. shockwave lithotripsy
e. shock wave therapy
e. ultrafiltration
e. volume
e. whole body hyperthermia

extracranial
e. arterial disease
e. carotid arterial disease
e. carotid disease
e. Doppler sonography

extracranial-intracranial
e.-i. arterial bypass
e.-i. bypass

extract
acetone powder e.
adipose tissue e.
adrenocortical e.
anterior pituitary e.
autologous tumor e.
bovine lavage extract surfactant
bovine thymus e.
buffered charcoal yeast e.
calf lung surfactant e.
calf thymus e.
cell e.
cervical mucous e.
charcoal yeast extract medium
chick embryo e.
crude e.
crude marijuana e.
desiccated thyroid e.
dialyzable leukocyte e.
embryo e.
fluid e.
Ginkgo biloba e.
green tea e.
horse chestnut seed e.
hot water e.
malt extract broth
malt soup e.
modified sea water yeast extract agar
nonferrous e.
normal bone marrow e.
northern bean e.
pancreatic e.
parathyroid e.
peptone, glucose, and yeast extract medium
peptone-yeast e.
platelet granule e.
powdered e.
proteose-peptone beef e.
purified spleen e.
Pygeum africanum e.
rabbit thymus e.
regenerating bone marrow e.
saw palmetto berry e.
serum, casein, glucose, yeast extract medium
smoke e.
solid e.
soluble viral e.
soy phytoestrogen e.
teichoic acid crude e.
titrated extract of *Centella asiatica*
total lipid e.
tryptone glucose e.
whole-body e.
whole ragweed e.
yeast e.

extractable
amount of insulin extractable from pancreas
centrifugation extractable fluid
e. nuclear antibody
e. nuclear antigen
e. nucleoprotein

extracted
placenta e.
tooth e.

extraction
Arroyo cataract e.
Arruga cataract e.
blind basket e.
cataract e.
combined intracapsular cataract e.
cryo cataract e.
extracapsular cataract e.
e. fraction
full-mouth e.
gallbladder e.
intracapsular cataract extraction with peripheral iridectomy
intracapsular lens e.
lactate e.
lens e.
Marshall-Taylor vacuum e.
Masimo SET signal extraction pulse oximetry
menstrual extraction abortion
micro liquid e.
microsurgical extraction of ductal sperm
microsurgical extraction of sperm from epididymis
oxygen extraction index
oxygen extraction ratio
partial breech e.
peripheral fractional oxygen e.
planned extracapsular cataract e.
e. ratio
round pupil intracapsular cataract e.
segmental cement extraction system
signal extraction technology
solid-phase e.
spontaneous breech e.
supercritical fluid e.
testicular sperm e.
transluminal extraction atherectomy
transluminal extraction catheter
transurethral e.
vacuum e.
vacuum extraction delivery

extractor
bone e.
bone plug e.
metatarsal head e.
M-type e.
mucus e.
vacuum e.

extracutaneous sporotrichosis

extradimensional shift

extradural
anterior extradural clinoidectomy
e. fluid
e. hematoma
e. hemorrhage
medial extradural approach

extraembryonic ectoderm

extrafamily adoptee

extrafascial hysterectomy

extraforaminal lumbar disc herniation

extrafusion defect

extragenic
repetitive extragenic palindromic polymerase chain reaction

extragenital
e. Bowen disease
e. teratoma

extraglandular manifestation

extragonadal seminoma

extrahepatic
atretic extrahepatic bile duct resection
e. bile duct
e. bile duct atresia
e. biliary atresia
e. blood flow clearance
e. cholestasis
controlled extrahepatic biliary drainage
e. distribution
mechanical extrahepatic obstruction
e. metastasis
middle extrahepatic bile duct
e. obstructive jaundice
occult extrahepatic disease
e. portal hypertension
e. portal vein obstruction

extraintestinal manifestation

extralobar sequestration

extra-low dispersion

extralymphatic organ site

extramammary
e. Paget disease
Paget extramammary disease

extramedullary
e. arteriovenous malformation
e. hematopoiesis
e. site
e. solitary plasmacytoma

extramembranous glomerulonephritis

extramucosal duodenal myotomy

extranodal
primary extranodal lymphoma

extranodular tissue

extraocular
e. eye movements normal
full extraocular motion
full extraocular movement
medial rectus extraocular muscle
e. motility
e. motion
e. movement
e. movements full and conjugate
e. movements intact
e. muscle
e. muscles intact
muscular fascia of extraocular muscle
normal extraocular movements
e. palsy
e. paralysis

extraoral
mental extraoral radiography
panoramic extraoral radiography

extraordinary meridian

extraosseous
e. Ewing sarcoma
e. plasmacytoma of the mediastinum

extraparenchymal resistance

extraperitoneal
e. endoscopic pelvic lymph node dissection
e. laparoscopic bladder neck suspension
total extraperitoneal laparoscopic hernia repair
totally e.

extrapleural
e. air
e. pneumonectomy
e. pneumothorax

extrapolated
e. end-tidal carbon dioxide tension
maximal extrapolated clotting time

extrapolation
half-scan with e.

extraprostatic
established extraprostatic extension
focal extraprostatic extension

extrapulmonary
e. pneumocystosis
e. small cell carcinoma

extrapyramidal
e. effect
e. involvement
e. side effect
e. sign
e. symptom
e. symptom rating scale
e. syndrome
e. system

extrarenal
e. azotemia
composite extrarenal rhabdoid tumor
malignant extrarenal rhabdoid tumor
e. rhabdoid tumor
e. uremia

extraretinal eye position information

extrasaccular hernia

extrasensory
applied extrasensory projection
e. perception

extraskeletal myxoid chondrosarcoma

extrastimulus
atrial extrastimulus method

extrasystole
atrioventricular e.
premature ventricular e.
ventricular e.

extrasystolic atrial tachycardia

extratemporal lobe epilepsy

extrathoracic
continuous negative extrathoracic pressure
noninvasive extrathoracic ventilator

extrathoracic-assisted breathing

extrathyroidal
e. neck radioactivity
e. thyroxine

extrauterine
e. gestation
e. pregnancy

extravasated
e. bile
e. blood
e. contrast
e. iodinated contrast material

extravasation
e. of contrast agent
e. of contrast medium
e. extrusion
e. feces
e. gas
e. injury
e. irrigation solution
e. phenomenon

extravascular
continuous extravascular infusion
e. lung density
e. lung mass
e. lung water
e. mass
pulmonary extravascular water volume
pulmonary extravascular fluid volume
e. thermal volume

extravesical
Lich extravesical technique

extreme
e. depression

displays extreme sarcasm
e. drug resistance
e. hostility
e. hunger
e. impairment
e. intervertebral disc collapse
e. jaw clenching
e. medical emergency
e. pressure
e. somatosensory evoked potential
e. ultraviolet
e. ultraviolet laser

extremely
e. high factor
e. high frequency
e. low birth weight
e. low frequency
parenchyma extremely congested
e. premature infant

extremity
anterior extremity of caudate nucleus
anterior extremity of spleen
both lower e.'s
both upper e.'s
cachectic e.'s
clubbing and cyanosis upper e.
clubbing of e.
coldness of e.
color and temperature normal, both lower e.'s
creeping sensation in e.
cyanosis of e.
diagonal 1, 2 lower e.
diagonal 1, 2 upper e.
gangrene in e.
e. immobilized in cast
intention tremor of e.
intramuscular artery of lower e.
intramuscular artery of upper e.
e. ischemia
jerking of e.
left lower e.
left upper e.
long thin e.
lower e.
lower extremity amputation
lower extremity arterial
lower extremity arterial disease
lower extremity bypass graft
lower extremity edema
lower extremity equipment related
lower extremity fracture
lower extremity nerve block
lower extremity noninvasive
lower extremity occlusive disease
lower extremity prosthesis
lower extremity reconstruction
lower extremity revascularization
lower extremity somatosensory evoked potential
lower extremity surgery
lower extremity venous
Lower E. Functional Scale
lower and upper extremities
mangled extremity syndrome index
Mangled E. Severity Score
movement of e.'s
moves all e.'s
moves all extremities equally well
moves all extremities slowly
e. MRI
muscle of upper extremity atrophic
neurological examination of e.'s
nondiabetic e.
numbness in e.
pain in chest, jaw, or e.
paresthesia of e.
peripheral cyanosis of e.'s
peripheral extremity edema
pitting edema of lower e.
e. preservation
progressive weakness of e.
Quality of Upper Extremities Test
resistive exercises to upper e.'s
right lower e.
right upper e.
segmental bronchus lower extremity Doppler pressure
somatic dysfunction lower e.
somatic dysfunction upper e.
traction applied to e.
upper e.
upper extremity arterial
upper extremity nerve block
upper extremity somatosensory evoked potential
upper and lower extremities within normal limits

extrinsic
e. allergic alveolitis
allergic extrinsic alveolitis
e. biliary compression
e. bladder compression
e. compression of airway
e. compression of trachea
e. factor
e. plasminogen activator

extrinsically supported

extruded
e. cell
e. disc fragment
e. disk
e. teeth

extruding mucus

extrusion
e. of cell cytoplasm
extravasation e.
implant e.
oocyte e.
pellet e.
placental e.

extubation
average extubation time

exuberant
e. callus
e. cicatrization
e. granulation tissue
e. infection

exudate
cotton-wool e.'s
edema, erythema, and e.
fluffy cotton-wool e.
hard e.
hemorrhage and e.
hemorrhage, papilledema, e.
hemorrhages, e.'s, and/or nicking
mucopurulent endocervical e.
peritoneal e.
peritoneal exudate lymphocyte
peritoneal exudate macrophage
soft e.
waxy exudate hard

exudative
distinctive exudative discoid and lichenoid dermatitis
dominant exudative vitreoretinopathy
peripheral exudative choroidal hemorrhagic retinopathy

exudative tonsillitis

Eyach virus

Eyberg Child Behavior Inventory

eye
abnormal eye movements
e. alignment
allergic eye disease
alpha-nonrapid eye movement
alpha-nonrapid eye movement sleep
amaurotic cat's e.
angle of lateral e.
angle of medial e.

eye *(continued)*
angular eye velocity
anterior chamber of e.
anterior segment of e.
antimongoloid eye slant
antioxidant eye treatment
appendage of e.
appendages of e.
aqueous humor of the e.
aqueous humor e.
Arabic eye test
arteriosclerosis of eye vessel
asymmetric folds of e.
axial length of e.
beam's eye view
binocular eye patch
blurred vision in one e.
both e.'s
both eyes patched
bulging eyes from blood clot
e. care
cat's eye syndrome
chaotic eye movement
choroid coat of e.
e.'s closed
conjugate eye movement
conjugate movement of e.'s
contact lens-induced acute red e.
conventional reform eye implant
cover-uncover eye test
Denver E. Screening Test
deprived e.
Developmental E. Movement
dextroduction of left e.
dextroduction of right e.
diabetic eye care
diabetic eye disease
disconjugate eye deviation
disconjugate movement of e.
disconjugate roving eye movement
dry eye symptom
e.'s and ears
e.'s ears, nose and throat
effect of closing of eyes in electroencephalography
effect of opening eyes
external eye examination
extraocular eye movements normal
extraretinal eye position information
finger count, both e.'s
fish eye disease
fixing left e.
fixing right e.
Fox eye shield
frontal eye field
glass eye artifact
globe of the e.
habitual eye rubbing
head, eyes, ears, nose, and throat
head, eyes, ears, nose, and throat unremarkable
e. hemorrhage
Hering law-EOM innervation, both e.'s
herpes eye infection
herpes virus of the e.
horizontal eye movement
e. implant
inability to close e.
increased eye tension
increased pressure inside the e.
increased rapid eye movement sleep
industrial eye care
inferior oblique eye muscle
internal eye pressure
involuntary eye movement
itchy, watery e.
jerking eye movements
lateral eye movement
lateral rectus, both e.'s
lateral rectus eye muscle
left e.
left eye patched
left lateral rectus eye muscle
left medial rectus eye muscle
lightning eye movement
Listing reduced e.
Listing schematic e.
liver bull's eye lesion
lower lid, left e.
Manson eye worm
medial angle of e.
medial rectus, both e.'s
micro eye movement
e.'s motor, verbal
e. movement desensitization reprocessing
e. movement gauge
e. movement measuring apparatus
e. movement recording
Mueller eye shield
multiple bull's eye lesions bowel wall
Murdoon eye speculum
muscle of e.
e. muscle imbalance
muscle, liver, brain, e.
muscle, liver, brain, eye disease
muscle, liver, brain, eye nanism
National E. Institute Visual Function Questionnaire
nonoptic reflex eye movement
nonrapid eye movement-rapid eye movement cycle
nonrapid eye movement sleep
nosocomial eye infection
occipital eye field
one-stage reconstruction of eye socket and eyelids
e.'s open
orbicular muscle of e.
Orphan Annie e.
outer canthus of e.
oval eye patch
owl's eye appearance
owl's eye cell
owl's eye inclusion body
owl's eye nucleus
owl's eyes view of hydrocele
e. pad and shield applied
part-time occlusion eye patch
periphery of e.
phacoemulsification of the left e.
phacoemulsification of the right e.
posterior chamber of e.
posterior pole of e.
protective eye pad
protective eye shield
protrusion of e.
pursuit eye movement
pyramidal eye implant
rapid eye movement
rapid eye movement sleep
e. research
restricted eye movement
reverse sutured e.
right e.
right eye patched
runny nose and eyes itchy
saccadic eye movement
scleral buckle, left e.
scleral buckle, right e.
Seeing E.
skin, eye, mucocutaneous
skin, head, eyes, ears, nose, and throat
sleep-onset rapid eye movement period
slow eye movement
slow lateral eye movement
smooth pursuit eye movement
Snellen eye chart
Snellen reform e.
sphincter of e.

squarely face person, open posture, lean toward person, eye contact, relaxed
subconjunctival hemorrhage of e.
sursumduction of e.
suspensory ligament of e.
thyroid eye disease
unique facies, anorexia, cachexia, and eye and skin syndrome
unpatched left e.
unpatched right e.
upper lid right e.
vergence eye movements
vision left e.
vision right e.
visual acuity, left e.
visual acuity, left eye, left perception with projection
visual acuity, right e.
Wood light examination of e.

eyeball
anterior chamber of e.
anterior pole of e.
crepitus of e.
dimpling of e.
enucleation of e.
enucleation of eyeball operation
luxation of e.
medial check ligament of e.
meridian of e.
muscle of e.
oblique muscle of e.
protruded e.
protrusion of e.
rhythmic horizontal oscillation of e.

eyeball-heart reflex

eyebrow
Brent eyebrow reconstruction
hair of e.
ptotic e.

eye-hand coordination

eyelashes
conjunctivitis with eyelashes turning in

eyelid
angular junction of e.
anterior border of e.
antimongoloid eyelid slant
apraxia of eyelid opening
Arlt eyelid repair
arterial arch of lower e.
arterial arch of upper e.
avulsion of e.
e. closure reflex
congenital eyelid tetrad
ectropion of e.
left upper eyelid
lower e.
margin of e.
medial commissure of e.
melanoma of e.
myopathic eyelid retraction
neuromuscular eyelid retraction
neuropathic eyelid retraction
one-stage reconstruction of eye socket and e.'s
orbital margin of e.
orbital portion of e.
paradoxical movement of e.'s
posterior border of e.
ptosis of e.
right upper eyelid
upper e.

eyepiece
wide-field e.

eyesight

eyes-open coma

eye-tracking dysfunction

eyewear
protective e.

Eysenck
Junior Eysenck Personality Inventory
E. Personality Inventory
E. Personality Questionnaire

Faber
F. disease
F. syndrome

fabere
f. abduction test
f. extension test
f. external rotation test
f. fixation test
f. sign

Fabian
method of F.

fabric
neoprene f.

fabricated illness

fabrication
illness f.

Fabry disease

face
asymmetry of f.
cervicofacial face lift
chemical face peeling
conotruncal anomaly face syndrome
conotruncal cardiac defect, abnormal face, thymic hypoplasia, cleft palate
discrete jerking musculature of f.
double aerosol face mask
endoforehead-biplanar face technique
en face irradiation field
face to f.
f., legs, activity, cry, consolability
high-humidity face mask
inner fracture f.
f. laser skin resurfacing
long face syndrome
f. lying position
f. mask
median cleft f.
median cleft face syndrome
median face syndrome
mental retardation, coarse face, microcephaly, epilepsy, skeletal abnormalities syndrome
mental retardation, mitral valve prolapse, characteristic face syndrome
mental retardation, polydactyly, phalangeal hypoplasia, syndactyly, unusual face, uncombable hair
mental retardation, pre-and postnatal overgrowth, remarkable face, acanthosis nigricans syndrome
microcephaly, mild developmental delay, short stature, distinctive face syndrome
middle one-third of face underdevelopment
nonrebreather face mask
numbness of f.
open face mask
pHisoHex face wash
f. presentation
puffiness of f.
region of f.
squarely face person, open posture, lean toward person, eye contact, relaxed
whistling face syndrome

facebow
adjustable axis f.

facelift
subperiosteal minimally invasive laser endoscopic f.

facet
f. arthropathy
articular facet angle
articular facet of head of fibula
articular facet of head of rib
articular facet of lateral malleolus
articular facet of medial malleolus
articular facet of radial head
articular facet of tubercle of rib
f. degeneration
degenerative facet disease
fibular articular facet of tibia
inferior f.
f. joint
f. joint arthropathy
f. joint block
f. joint disease
f. joint osteoarthritis
lateral facet syndrome
lumbar facet disease
lumbar facet injection
lunate facet dye punch injury
medial malleolar facet of talus
medial talocalcaneal f.
middle greater tubercle of facet of humerus
oblique facet wiring
patellar facet cartilage
percutaneous radiofrequency facet nerve block
posterior facet dislocation
posterior facet displacement
f. rhizotomy
f. subluxation
superior f.
f. surface
worn facet joint

facetectomy
O'Donoghue f.
partial f.

facial
absence of facial and pubic hair
acromegaloid facial appearance
acromegaloid facial syndrome
F. Action Coding System
activates facial expression
acute idiopathic peripheral facial nerve palsy
alloplastic facial implant
altered facial appearance
f. anchorage
angular facial vein
f. anomaly
anterior facial height
anterior facial vein
anteroposterior facial dysplasia
appropriate facial expression
area of facial nerve
f. artery musculomucosal
f. artery myomucosal
f. artery pressure point
f. asymmetry
atrophic facial acne scar
f. atrophy
atypical facial neuralgia
atypical facial pain
chronic oral, facial, head pain
congenital cataracts, sensorineural deafness, Down syndrome facial appearance, short stature, mental retardation syndrome
f. contortion
detailed evaluation of facial symmetry
F. Disability Index
F. Disability Index Physical
F. Disability Index Social
distal arthrogryposis, hypopituitarism, mental retardation, facial anomalies syndrome
f. droop
f. dysplasia
f. dysplasia, hyperextensibility of joints, clinodactyly, growth retardation, mental retardation syndrome
f. edema
excess facial hair
excessive facial hair growth

F

facial *(continued)*
f. flushing
focal facial dermal dysplasia II
F. Grading System
Gram stain of facial abscess
f. grimacing
growth phase of facial hair
f. hair
hard tissue replacement-malleable facial implant
f. hemihyperplasia
f. hemiparesis
f. hemiplegia
f. hemispasm
idiopathic facial paralysis
immunodeficiency, centromeric instability, facial anomalies syndrome
F. Impairment Scales for Children
f. implant of cheek
f. implant of chin
f. implant of jaw
incomplete facial paralysis
intermittent facial contracture
involuntary facial expression
involuntary facial pain
f. laceration
lateral facial dysplasia
ligamentous facial fence
lingual branch of facial nerve
Lyme-associated peripheral facial nerve palsy
macrocephaly, facial abnormalities, disproportionate tall stature mental retardation syndrome
malar facial augmentation
malleable facial implant
marginal mandibular branch of facial nerve
medial crus of facial canal
medial crus of the horizontal part of the facial canal
medial extended facial translocation
median facial cleft
median facial cleft syndrome
mental retardation, facial anomalies, hypopituitarism, distal arthrogryposis syndrome
mesial occlusal f.
midline facial defect
multiplanar endoscopic facial rejuvenation technique
mumps facial nerve palsy
muscles of facial expression
f. myoclonus
Nadbath facial block
necrotic facial dysplasia
Neonatal Facial Coding System
Neonatal F. Pain Inventory
f. nerve
f. nerve block
f. nerve injury
f. neuralgia
oblique facial cleft
odontogenic facial pain
onset of facial weakness
otomandibular facial dysmorphogenesis
f. pain from arthritis
pale facial appearance
f. palsy
f. paralysis
f. paresis
partial facial paralysis
peripheral facial nerve palsy
peripheral facial paralysis
persistent facial palsy
resting phase of facial hair
f. rhytidectomy
f. ridge
f. rosacea
severe, jabbing facial pain
skeletal abnormalities, cutis laxa, craniostenosis, psychomotor retardation, facial abnormalities
f. spasm
f. tic
unusual facial features
f. weakness

facialis
area nervi f.
arteria f.
herpes f.
nervus facialis [CN VII]
neuralgia facialis vera
norma f.
nucleus f.

facies
Andy Gump f.
aortic arch anomaly-peculiar facies mental retardation syndrome
asymmetric crying f.
brachydactyly, mesomelia, mental retardation, aortic dilation, mitral valve prolapse, characteristic facies syndrome
cardiac abnormality, abnormal facies, thymic hypoplasia, cleft palate, hypocalcemia
congenital thrombocytopenia, Robin sequence, agenesis of corpus callosum, distinctive facies, developmental delay syndrome
elfin facies hypercalcemia syndrome
femoral hypoplasia unusual facies syndrome
Marshall Hall f.
median cleft upper lip, mental retardation, pugilistic facies syndrome
mental and physical retardation, speech disorders, peculiar facies syndrome
mental retardation, coarse facies, epilepsy, joint contracture syndrome
mental retardation, hearing impairment, distinct facies, skeletal anomalies syndrome
mental retardation, typical facies, aortic stenosis syndrome
unique facies, anorexia, cachexia, and eye and skin syndrome

facilitate
f. interaction
f. transfer

facilitated
f. angioplasty
f. communication
f. positional release

facilitation
associative f.
neuromuscular f.
posttetanic f.
proprioceptive neuromuscular f.

facilitative
perineobulbar detrusor facilitative reflex

facility
acquired immune deficiency syndrome residential treatment f.
acute care f.
adult congregate living f.
adult congruent living f.
adult living f.
advanced x-ray f.
ambulatory care research f.
assisted living f.
cancer therapy f.
certified skilled nursing f.
certified sleep-disorder f.
comprehensive outpatient rehabilitation f.
emergency f.
extended care f.

health facility administrator
health-related f.
inpatient non-psychiatric medical f.'s
inpatient treatment f.
intensive care f.
intermediate care f.
long-term care f.
long-term healthcare f.
f.'s management
medical treatment f.
mental health treatment f.
narcotic treatment f.
National Biomedical Tracer F.
night care f.
nursing f.
other medical/surgical f.
patient discharged to skilled nursing f.
patient transferred to skilled nursing f.
personal hygiene f.
residential care facility for the elderly
skilled nursing f.
skilled nursing extended care f.
specialized treatment f.
state medical facilities plan
tertiary care f.

faciobrachial hemiplegia

faciolingual hemiplegia

facioscapulohumeral

f. artery
f. muscular dystrophy

fact

f. and fantasy
f. joint arthritis
well-known f.

factitial

f. dermatitis
f. lesion

factitious

atypical factitious disorder with physical symptoms
chronic factitious illness with physical symptoms
f. disorder by proxy
f. disorder with physical symptoms
f. illness with psychological symptoms

factor

acidic fibroblast growth f.
activated clotting f.
activating transcription f.
adrenal growth f.
adrenal weight f.
adrenocorticotropic hormone-releasing f.
adverse background f.
age-specific risk f.
albumin autoagglutinating f.
alloantigen-independent risk f.
allogenic effect f.
amyloid-enhancing f.
anabolism-promoting f.
F. Analyzed Short Form
androgen-induced growth f.
anemia-inducing f.
angiogenesis f.
angiogenic growth f.
animal protein f.
anti-arteriosclerosis polysaccharide f.
antiepidermal growth factor receptor
antiepidermal growth factor receptor antibody for cancer
antiepidermal growth factor receptor monoclonal antibody
antifatty liver f.
antigen-specific helper f.
antiinvasion f.
antimuscle f.
antineuritic f.
antinuclear f.
antiperinuclear f.
antipernicious anemia f.
antisocial psychopathic Q f.
antivascular endothelial growth factor monoclonal antibody
antiviral f.
anti-von Willebrand f.
anti-von Willebrand factor antibody
antiyeast f.
apoptosis activating f.
area correction f.
ascorbic acid f.
atrial natriuretic f.
atrial natriuretic factor receptor
attenuation f.
attitudinal risk f.
autocrine growth f.
autocrine motility f.
autocrine motility factor of the bladder
autocrine motility factor receptor
autocrine-paracrine-acting growth f.
autologous growth f.
autologous growth factor binding agent
autologous growth factor gel
automated factor V Leiden mutation test
automated LCx factor V Leiden assay
automated motility f.
azoospermia f.
backscatter f.
basic fibroblast growth f.
basophil chemotactic f.
B-cell differentiation f.
B-cell growth f.
beta-nerve growth f.
bioconcentration f.
biologic factors in dose fractionation
blastogenic f.
blocking f.
blood factor in the MNS blood group system
B-lymphocyte stimulatory f.
bone-derived growth f.
bradykinin potentiating f.
brain-derived neurotrophic f.
brain-derived neurotropic f.
burst-promoting f.
calibration f.
cancer coagulation f.
carbon monoxide transfer f.
cardiac risk f.
cardiac risk factor modification
cardiovascular risk f.
cartilage induction f.
catabolite modular f.
cell adhesion f.
cell antiviral f.
chemotactic f.
chemotactic factor for macrophage
Christmas f.
ciliary-derived neurotrophic factor receptor
ciliary neurotrophic f.
citrovorum f.
cleverness f.
clinical manifestations, etiologic f.'s, anatomic involvement, pathophysiologic features
clone-inhibiting f.
cloning inhibitory f.
clot-promoting f.
clotting f.
coagulase-reacting f.
cobra venom f.
colicin f.
colonization f.

factor *(continued)*
colonization factor antigen
colony-stimulating f.
colony-stimulating factor developed by Venereal Disease Research Laboratory
colony-stimulating factor microhemagglutination-*Treponema pallidum* test
colony-stimulating factor fluorescent treponemal antibody-absorption test
complement f.
concentration epidermal growth f.
conglutinogen-activating f.
connective tissue growth f.
controllable risk f.
coronary risk f.
cortical magnification f.
corticotropin-releasing f.
coupling f.
cryoprecipitated antihemophilic f.
crystal-induced chemotactic f.
cystic fibrosis f.
cystic fibrosis factor activity
cytotoxic f.
daily replacement factor of lymphocytes
decapacitation f.
decay-accelerating f.
decontamination f.
deficiency f.
diastolic heart f.
differentiation-inducing f.
digitalis-like f.
digoxin-like immunoreactive f.
distribution f.
dopachrome conversion f.
dose increase f.
dose reduction effectiveness f.
early pregnancy f.
edema f.
elongation f.
elongation factor G
embryonic growth and development f.
emotional f.
encephalitogenic f.
endogenous digitalis-like f.
endothelial cell growth f.
endothelial cell-stimulating angiogenesis f.
endothelial proliferating f.
endothelium-derived constricting f.
endothelium-derived hyperpolarizing f.
endothelium-derived relaxing f.
end-stage heart f.
endurance f.
eosinophil chemotactic factor of anaphylaxis
eosinophilic chemotactic f.
epidermal growth f.
epidermal growth factor receptor
epithelium-derived relaxation f.
erythrocyte initiation f.
erythrocyte maturation f.
erythroid differentiation f.
erythropoietic-stimulating f.
esophageal epidermal growth f.
f. essential for resistance to methicillin
eukaryotic initiation f.
exophthalmic f.
exophthalmos-hyperthyroid f.
exophthalmos-producing f.
exposure f.
extremely high f.
extrinsic f.
familial multiple factor deficiency 1
fast death f.
father f.
feedback inhibition f.
fertility f.
fibrin-stabilization f.
fibroblast-activating f.
fibroblast chemotactic f.
fibroblast-derived growth f.
fibroblast growth factor receptor
fibroblast growth factor receptor 2
fibroblastic growth f.
fibroblast pneumocyte f.
filtration f.
follicle-stimulating hormone-releasing f.
free thyroxine f.
geographic adjustment f.
GH-releasing f.
glass factor tissue culture
glia-activating f.
glial cell line-derived neurotropic f.
glial-derived neurotrophic f.
glia maturation f.
glucose tolerance f.
glycosylation-inhibiting f.
glycyrrhetinic acid like f.
gonadotropin-enhancing f.
gonadotropin-inhibitory factor
gonadotropin-releasing f.
gonadotropin surge attenuating f.
granulocyte colony-stimulating f.
granulocyte colony-stimulating factor receptor
granulocyte-macrophage colony-stimulating f.
granulocytosis-promoting f.
greatest common f.
growth differentiation f.
growth hormone-inhibiting f.
growth hormone release-inhibiting f.
growth hormone releasing f.
growth hormone-releasing factor test
growth hormone-releasing factor tumor
guanine nucleotide-releasing f.
Hageman f.
health risk f.
heart attack risk f.
heart disease risk f.
heat-labile f.
heat transfer f.
helper f.
hemorrhagic f.
heparin-binding epidermal growth factorlike growth f.
heparin-binding growth f.
heparin-binding neurotrophic f.
hepatocyte growth f.
hepatocyte nuclear f.
hepatotropic portal blood f.
heterothyrotropic f.
highest common f.
histamine-induced suppressor f.
histamine inhibitory releasing f.
histamine releasing f.
histamine-sensitizing f.
histoplasma tissue inhibitory f.
HIV-inducing f.
hog intrinsic factor concentrate
host defensive f.
human epidermal growth f.
human growth f.
human macrophage-monocyte chemotactic and activating f.
human serum thymus f.
human skeletal growth f.
humoral thymic f.
hyperglycemic-glycogenolytic f.
hypermobility as a risk f.
hypersomnia related to a known organic f.
hypothalamic-releasing f.
hypothalamic secretory f.
immunoglobin M-rheumatoid f.
immunoglobulin-binding f.
immunoglobulin G rheumatoid f.

immunoreactive corticotropin-releasing f.
infection-potentiating f.
inflammatory factor of anaphylaxis
f.'s influencing anxiety
inherited blood factor in MNS blood group
inhibiting f.
initiation f.
injury f.
insomnia related to a known organic f.
insulin growth f.
insulin-like growth f.
insulinlike growth factor-1, -2
intellectual power f.
intrinsic factor concentrate
f. I through XIII
f. IX nine
Kaposi sarcoma human growth f.
Kell f.
keratinocyte growth factor receptor
labile f.
lactating rat serum f.
Lactobacillus bulgaricus factor
least common f.
leg protection f.
lethal f.
leukemia-inhibiting f.
leukemia inhibitory f.
leukocyte-activating f.
leukocyte adherence inhibition f.
leukocyte factor antigen-1
leukocyte infiltration f.
leukocyte inhibitory f.
leukocyte migration inhibition f.
leukocyte mitogenic f.
leukocytosis-inducing f.
leukocytosis-promoting f.
leukokinesis-enhancing f.
leukopenia f.
leukotactic factor activity
f. level
limit dilution f.
linear correction f.
lipopolysaccharide f.
lipotropic f.
liver migration inhibitory f.
liver regenerating serum f.
liver residue f.
low-affinity platelet f.
luminal CCK-releasing f.
lung-derived neurotrophic f.
lung Hageman factor activator
lupus erythematosus f.
luteinizing hormone/follicle-stimulating hormone-releasing f.
luteinizing hormone-releasing factor agonist
lymph node permeability f.
lymphocyte-activating f.
lymphocyte activation f.
lymphocyte blastogenic f.
lymphocyte chemoattractant f.
lymphocyte-induced angiogenesis f.
lymphocyte mitogenic f.
lymphocyte-stimulating f.
lymphocyte-transforming f.
lytic nephritic f.
macrophage-activating f.
macrophage activation f.
macrophage-agglutinating f.
macrophage agglutination f.
macrophage chemotactic f.
macrophage colony-stimulating f.
macrophage cytotoxicity f.
macrophage-derived growth f.
macrophage-derived tumor necrosis f.
macrophage immunogenic antigen-recruiting f.
macrophage-inhibiting f.
macrophage migration-inhibiting f.
macrophage migration inhibitory f.
macrophage slowing f.
macrophage spreading f.
magnification f.
male factor infertility
Marsh-Bendall f.
mass transfer f.
mast cell growth f.
maternal health risk f.
maturation-promoting f.
Mayneord F f.
megakaryocyte colony-stimulating f.
megakaryocyte growth and development f.
melanocyte-inhibiting f.
melanocyte release-inhibiting f.
melanocyte-releasing f.
melanocyte-stimulating hormone-inhibiting f.
melanocyte-stimulating hormone-releasing f.
metabolic activity f.
microscopic f.
middle glial cell line-derived neurotrophic f.
migration enhancement f.
migration-inhibitory f.
mitogenic f.
mitosis-promoting f.
mixed lymphocyte reaction blocking f.
modulation transfer f.
monoclonal rheumatoid f.
monocyte chemoattractant and activity f.
monocyte chemotactic and activating f.
monocyte chemotactic f.
monocyte colony-stimulating f.
monocyte-derived neutrophil chemotactic f.
monocyte tissue f.
mononuclear cell tissue f.
morphine-like f.
mortality risk f.
mouse antialopecia f.
mouse epidermal growth f.
M protein f.
müllerian duct inhibitory f.
müllerian inhibiting f.
müllerian inhibiting f.
müllerian regression f.
multilineage colony-stimulating f.
multiple factor analysis
Multiple Risk F. Intervention Trial
multiplication f.
murine granulocyte-macrophage colony-stimulating growth f.
myeloid growth f.
myeloid leukemia inhibitory f.
myeloid progenitor factor 1
myeloid progenitor inhibitory f.
myeloma growth f.
myocardial depressant f.
natural killer cell-stimulating f.
negative f.
nephritic f.
nerve growth f.
nerve growth factor antiserum
nerve growth factor receptor
neu differentiation f.
neural growth f.
neural growth factor receptor
Neurotic Personality F. Test
neurotrophic factor expression
neutralizing antibody to vascular endothelial growth f.
neutralizing murine monoclonal antitumor necrosis factor antibody
neutrophil activating f.
neutrophil chemotactant f.

factor *(continued)*
neutrophil chemotactic f.
neutrophil diffraction f.
neutrophilic chemotactic f.
neutrophil-immobilizing f.
neutrophil migration-inhibition f.
new differentiation f.
NF-1 transcription f.
noise f.
nonhematopoietic growth f.
nonsuppressible insulinlike activity f.
no predisposing f.
nuclear factor of activated T cell
nuclear factor kappa B ligand
nuclear factor kappa B transcription factor protein
nuclear transcription f.
obstetric risk f.
octamer-binding transcription f.
off-axis f.
oocyte maturation-inhibiting f.
open air f.
opioid growth f.
oral transfer f.
orthogonal depression f.
osteoclast differentiation f.
osteoclastogenesis inhibitory f.
osteoprotegerin f.
ouabain-like f.
ovarian growth f.
Ovenstone f.
ovine corticotropin-releasing f.
oxidase cytosolic f.
oxygen gain f.
peak scatter f.
pellagra preventive f.
pelvic infertility f.
peptide growth f.
peptide growth factor receptor signal
peptide growth factor signaling mechanism
peptide regulatory f.
permeability f.
personality f.
personality factor questionnaire
16 Personality F. Questionnaire
phagocytosis promoting f.
phosphodiesterase-activating f.
pigment inspiratory f.
placental growth f.
plasma prothrombin conversion f.
plasma thromboplastin f.
platelet factor 1–4
platelet-activating f.
platelet activating/aggregating f.
platelet-activating factor acetylhydrolase
platelet-activating factor of anaphylaxis
platelet adhesiveness plasma f.
platelet-aggregating f.
platelet aggregation f.
platelet-derived angiogenesis f.
platelet-derived endothelial cell growth f.
platelet-derived epidermal growth f.
platelet-derived growth factor A, B
platelet-derived histamine-releasing f.
platelet-derived wound healing f.
policy target adjustment f.
pollen adherence f.
polyclonal rheumatoid f.
polymorphonuclear neutrophil chemotactic f.
polypeptide growth f.
positive cardiac disease risk f.'s
positive risk factors for cardiac disease
power f.
primary pulmonary hypertension risk f.
proatrial natriuretic f.
progesterone-induced blocking f.
prolactin-inhibiting f.
prolactin-releasing f.
proliferation-inhibiting f.
proliferation inhibitory f.
properdin factor B
prostacyclin-stimulating f.
prostacyclin synthesis-stimulating plasma f.
protection f.
prothrombin conversion f.
prothrombin, proconvertin, Stuart factor, antihemophilic B f.
psychological, social, and vocational
pulmonary f.
pyrogen-releasing f.
pyruvate oxidation f.
Rathke pouch homeobox transcription f.
rat intrinsic factor concentrate
receptor activator of nuclear factor kappa B ligand
recognition f.
recombinant factor VIIA
recombinant human granulocyte-macrophage colony-stimulating f.
recombinant human insulinlike growth f.
recombinant human platelet-derived growth f.
recombinant human tissue factor pathway inhibitor
recombinant human vascular endothelial growth f.
recombinant tumor necrosis factor alpha
releasing f.
renal erythropoietic f.
resistance-inducing f.
resistance transfer f.
retardation f.
Rh blood f.
rheumatoid arthritis serum f.
rheumatoid arthritis factor test
rheumatoid biologically active f.
rheumatoid factor binding
rheumatoid factor test
risk f.
risk factor for mortality
risk factor reduction
rosette inhibitory f.
salivary epidermal growth f.
sarcoma growth f.
screen-intensifying f.
serologic-blocking f.
serum f.
serum accelerator f.
serum blocking f.
serum inhibitory f.
serum thymus f.
sheep factor delta
Simon septic f.
Sixteen Personality F.'s Test
skeletal growth f.
skin protection f.
skin-reactive f.
slow death f.
slow-reacting f.
slow-reacting factor of anaphylaxis
smooth muscle activating f.
soluble suppressor f.
somatic cell-derived growth f.
somatotropin release f.
somatotropin release-inhibiting f.
specific blocking f.
specific clotting factor and inhibitor
specific immune-response-enhancing f.
specific macrophage-arming f.
squamous cell carcinoma inhibitory f.

stable f.
stem cell f.
stem cell proliferation f.
stimulating f.
stream dilution f.
streptococcal proliferative f.
stress distribution f.
Stuart-Prower f.
sulfation factor of blood serum
sun protection f.
suntan photoprotection f.
T-cell replacing f.
temperature f.
testis-determining f.
test for rheumatoid f.
therapeutic gain f.
Thinking Disturbance F.
thrombopoiesis-stimulating f.
thymic humoral f.
thymus cell growth f.
thymus permeability f.
thymus tolerance f.
thymus transfer f.
thyroid-stimulating hormone-releasing f.
thyroid transcription f.
thyroid transcription factor 2
thyrotroph embryonic f.
thyrotropic hormone-releasing f.
thyrotropin release f.
thyrotropin-releasing f.
time-dose fractionation f.
tissue angiogenesis f.
tissue-coding f.
tissue-damaging f.
tissue factor pathway inhibitor
tissue necrosis f.
transactivation f.
transcriptional intermediary factor 2
transfer f.
transfer factor, dialyzable
transfer factor test
transforming growth f.
transforming growth factor beta-1, -2, -3
transforming growth factor alpha
trefoil factor family
trypanosome growth f.
T-suppressor f.
tumor angiogenesis f.
tumor angiogenic f.
tumor cell migration-inhibition f.
tumor growth f.
tumor-inducing f.
tumor-inhibiting f.
tumor necrosis factor-alpha
tumor necrosis f.
tumor necrosis factor receptor
tumor necrosis factor receptor-associated f.
tumor necrosis factor receptor-associated periodic syndrome
tumor receptor-associated f.
undegraded insulin f.
unidentified growth f.
unknown f.
urethral resistance f.
uterine-relaxing f.
vascular endothelial growth factor 2, 3
vascular endothelial growth factor/vascular permeability f.
f. V deficiency Leiden mutation
verbal comprehension f.
very fast death f.
f. VII
f. VII antigen
f. VII deficiency
f. VIII
f. VIII antigen
f. VIII:C heat-treated antihemophilic factor
f. VIII:C inhibitor
f. VIII coagulation function
f. VIII deficiency
f. VIII gene
f. VIII hemophilia
f. VIII inhibitor
f. VIII inhibitor bypassing activity
f. VIII, IX deficiency
f. VII inhibitor
f. VII, VIII inhibitor
f. V Leiden
f. V Leiden carrier
f. V Leiden gene
f. V Leiden mutation test
f. V Leiden thrombophilia
von Willebrand f.
f. X antigen
f. X deficiency
F. XI
f. XI deficiency
f. XII deficiency
f. XIIIa
f. XIII deficiency
f. XII inhibitor
f. X inhibitor

factor-1
adipocyte determination and differentiation f.-1
anemia-inducing f.-1
antifertility f.-1
colony-stimulating f.-1
heparin-binding growth f.-1
human stomach cancer-transforming f.-1
insulin promoter f.-1
interferon regulatory f.-1
myeloid progenitor inhibitory f.-1
pituitary-specific transcription f.-1
preadipocyte f.-1
recombinant human insulin-like growth f.-1
steroidogenic f.-1
stromal cell-derived f.-1
thyroid transcription f.-1
transforming growth f.-1

factor-2
heparin-binding growth f.-2
human stomach cancer-transforming f.-2
interferon regulatory f.-2
keratinocyte growth f.-2

factor-3
hepatocyte nuclear f.-3
leukocyte antigen f.-3

factor-4
hepatocyte nuclear f.-5
recombinant platelet f.-5

factor-9
growth differentiation f.-9

factor-A

factor-4a
hepatocyte nuclear f.-4a

factor-alpha

factor-1-alpha
hypoxia-inducible f.-1-a.

factor-beta
tumor necrosis f.-b.

factor-complement
eosinophilic chemotactic f.-c.

factorlike
heparin-binding epidermal growth factorlike growth factor
rheumatoid factorlike activity
rheumatoid factorlike substance

factor-related
tumor necrosis factor-related activation-induced cytokine

factor/vascular
vascular endothelial growth factor/vascular permeability factor

facultative
f. aerobe
f. anaerobe
f. hyperopia

facultative *(continued)*
- f. parasite
- f. yeast carrier

faculty
- gradual loss of mental f.'s
- loss of intellectual f.'s
- mental f.

Faden procedure

faecium
- VanB *Enterococcus faecium*
- vancomycin-resistant *Enterococcus faecium*

Fagerstrom
- F. Test for Nicotine Dependence
- F. tolerance questionnaire

Fahey operation

Fahrenheit
- degree F.
- F. temperature scale

failed
- f. anesthesia
- f. back surgery syndrome
- f. back syndrome with documented pseudarthrosis
- f. forceps delivery
- f. graft
- f. intubation
- f. joint replacement
- patient failed to respond
- f. procedure
- f. reduction
- f. to report
- f. to respond
- f. suicide attempt
- f. transplant

failing
- f. lung sign
- f. ovary syndrome
- pumping ability of failing heart

fail-safe mechanism

failure
- acute congestive heart f.
- acute heart f.
- acute hepatic f.
- acute hypoxemic respiratory f.
- acute left ventricular heart f.
- acute liver f.
- acutely decompensated congestive heart f.
- acute on chronic renal f.
- acute postoperative renal f.
- acute renal failure and chronic renal f.
- acute right ventricular heart f.
- advanced stage of congestive heart f.
- f. of all vital forces
- alternating failure of response mechanical to electrical depolarization
- f. analysis
- anemia associated with chronic renal f.
- anemia of chronic renal f.
- autoimmune polyglandular f.
- backward heart f.
- biomechanical failure of implant
- bone marrow f.
- calibration failure artifact
- cardiac f.
- cardiovascular f.
- cataract, microcephaly, failure to thrive, kyphoscoliosis
- chromosomally competent ovarian f.
- chromosomally incompetent ovarian f.
- chronic congestive heart f.
- chronic heart f.
- chronic liver f.
- chronic renal f.
- chronic respiratory f.
- cocaine-induced respiratory f.
- Cognitive F.'s Questionnaire
- compensated congestive heart f.
- compensated heart f.
- confusion from heart f.
- congenital heart f.
- congestive cardiac f.
- congestive heart f.
- congestive heart failure and cardioversion
- congestive right ventricular f.
- f. of conservative management
- contraceptive failure rate
- decompensated congestive heart f.
- decompensated heart f.
- f. to descend
- diastolic heart f.
- endocrine gland f.
- end-stage heart f.
- end-stage liver f.
- end-stage renal f.
- f. to engraft
- fear of f.
- f. of fixation suppression
- florid congestive heart f.
- forward heart f.
- frank congestive f.
- fulminant hepatic f.
- functional renal failure of cirrhosis
- gonadal failure, short stature, mitral valve prolapse, mental retardation syndrome
- growth f.
- growth hormone f.
- heart failure cell
- heart failure treatment
- hemorrhagic diathesis secondary to hepatic f.
- high-output heart f.
- high-output renal f.
- hyperacute liver f.
- hypertensive renal f.
- f. of immediate recall
- impending renal f.
- incipient heart f.
- intractable heart f.
- ischemic acute renal f.
- ischemic heart f.
- lasting impression of impending f.
- late-onset hepatic f.
- late-stage heart f.
- left heart f.
- left-sided heart f.
- left ventricular f.
- left ventricular heart f.
- local-regional f.
- loss of appetite from heart f.
- low-output heart f.
- marginal heart f.
- marrow failure syndrome
- massive hepatic f.
- material failure break point
- mean time between or before f.'s
- mild thyroid f.
- mixed respiratory f.
- moderate renal f.
- Multicenter Oral Carvedilol Heart F. Assessment
- multiorgan system f.
- multiple organ f.
- multiple organ failure syndrome
- multiple organ system f.
- multisystem organ f.
- myoglobinuric rhabdomyolytic acute renal f.
- natural history of congestive heart f.
- neonatal cardiac f.
- nephrotoxic acute renal f.
- nonorganic failure to thrive
- NYHA congestive heart failure classification

onset of overt heart f.
organ failure criteria
organic failure to thrive
organ system failure index
overt heart f.
parenchymatous acute renal f.
parental failure to guide
passive congestive f.
pericardial constriction-growth failure syndrome
peripartum cardiac f.
peripheral circulatory f.
postischemic acute renal f.
postoperative heart f.
postoperative hepatic f.
postpartum renal f.
posttransplant acute renal f.
posttraumatic acute renal f.
premature gonadal f.
premature ovarian f.
prerenal acute renal f.
primary graft f.
primary ovarian f.
f. to progress in labor
progressive renal f.
radiologic contrast-induced renal f.
recurrent congestive heart f.
refractory heart f.
renal failure index
renal vascular f.
reverse heart f.
right heart f.
right-sided congestive heart f.
right-sided heart f.
right ventricular f.
right ventricular heart f.
sense of f.
sepsis-related organ failure assessment
sequential organ failure assessment
severe renal f.
subacute liver f.
sudden congestive heart f.
sudden heart f.
symptoms of heart f.
systolic heart f.
f. to thrive
time to distant f.
time to local f.
time-to-treatment f.
ventilator-dependent respiratory f.
f. to wean

failure-free survival

faint
fight, flee, freeze, or f.

fainting
f. from anemia
hysterical f.

faintness
dizziness and f.

fair
nursed f.

fairly
f. good risk for anesthesia
nursed fairly well
f. well developed

Fairview
F. Language Evaluation Scale
F. Language Evaluation Test

faith
good f.
f. healing
religious f.

Fajersztajn sign

faking
patient faking illness

falciform
f. body
f. cartilage
f. fold of fascia lata
f. hymen
f. ligament
f. lobule
f. process

falcine region

Falk operation

Falk-Shukuris operation

fall
F. Efficacy Scale
f.'s and fractures immobility
f. precautions
f. risk assessment

fallacy
pathologic f.

fallback theory

fallen arch

falling
difficulty falling asleep
f. hematocrit
f. risk
f. sickness
f. spells of Tumarkin
f. of the womb

fallopian
f. aqueduct
damaged or blocked fallopian tubes
fimbriated end of fallopian tube
obstruction of fallopian tube
patent fallopian tube
primary fallopian tube carcinoma
f. tube
f. tube sperm perfusion

Fallopio
foramen of F.

Fallot
pentalogy of F.
F. tetrad
tetralogy of F.
F. tetralogy
F. triad
trilogy of F.

fallout
red blood cell f.

false
additional cost of false negatives
additional cost of false positives
f. aneurysm
Federal F. Claims Act
f. ganglion
f. hematuria
f. high
f. hypercholesterolemia
f. hypertrophy
idiosyncratic false idea
idiosyncratic false ideas
f. joint
f. membrane
f. morel
f. negative
f. neurochemical transmitter
overvalued false ideas
f. positive
f. pregnancy
superstitious false ideas
f. transmitter
treponemal false positive
unpersuasive false ideas
f. vocal cord
f. vocal fold

false-negative
f.-n. fraction
f.-n. rate
f.-n. results

false-positive
biologic f.-p.
chronic f.-p.
f.-p. fraction
f.-p. reaction
f.-p. results

falsification
memory f.

Falta triad

falx
aponeurotic f.
f. cerebri
ligamentous f.
parasagittal f.

familial
adenoma familial polyposis
f. adenomatous polyposis
adult familial hyaline membrane disease
f. advanced sleep-phase syndrome
f. Alzheimer dementia
f. Alzheimer disease
amaurotic familial idiocy
f. amyloidotic polyneuropathy
f. amyloid polyneuropathy
f. amyotrophic lateral sclerosis
attenuated familial adenomatous polyposis
f. atypical mole malignant melanoma
f. atypical multiple melanoma
f. atypical multiple-mole melanoma syndrome
f. autoimmunity in diabetes
f. autonomic dysfunction
f. benign chronic pemphigus
benign familial hematuria
benign familial macrocephaly
benign familial neonatal convulsions
f. benign hypocalciuric hypercalcemia
benign infantile familial convulsions
f. British dementia
f. cerebral cavernoma
f. colon cancer
f. colonic cancer
f. combined hyperlipidemia
f. diabetic history
f. dysalbuminemic hyperthyroxinemia
f. dysautonomia
f. dysplastic nevus syndrome
early-onset form of familial Alzheimer disease
f. erythrophagocytic lymphohistiocytosis
f. expansile osteolysis
f. exudative vitreoretinopathy
f. multiple factor deficiency 1
f. glucocorticoid deficiency
f. hemiplegic migraine
f. hemophagocytic lymphohistiocytosis
hemorrhagic familial angiomatosis
f. hepatitis
hereditary familial disease
hereditary familial illness
heterozygous familial hypercholesterolemia
f. Hibernian fever
f. high-density lipoprotein deficiency
f. histiocytic dermatoarthritis
homozygous familial hypercholesterolemia
f. hypercalcemia with hypocalciuria
f. hypercholesterolemia
f. hypercholesterolemia, low-density lipoprotein
f. hypertriglyceridemia
f. hypertrophic cardiomyopathy
f. hypertrophic obstructive cardiomyopathy
f. hypertrophy
f. hypobetalipoproteinemia
f. hypophosphatemia
f. hypophosphatemic rickets
f. hypoplastic anemia
f. idiopathic gonadotropin deficiency
f. idiopathic nonarteriosclerotic cerebral calcification
f. immunity
infantile amaurotic familial idiocy
f. intracranial aneurysm
f. isolated hypoparathyroidism
f. isolated primary hyperparathyroidism
f. juvenile nephrophthisis
f. juvenile nephrophthisis-medullary cystic disease
f. juvenile polyposis
late infantile amaurotic familial idiocy
Li-Fraumeni familial cancer syndrome
male-limited familial precocious puberty
malignant familial myoclonic epilepsy
f. Mediterranean fever
f. medullary thyroid cancer
f. medullary thyroid carcinoma
mixed hyperlipoproteinemia familial type 5 hyperlipidemia
f. multiple endocrine neoplasia
multiple familial polyposis
f. nephronophthisis-medullary cystic disease
nonautoimmune familial hyperthyroidism
f. nonmedullary thyroid carcinoma
nonsyndromic familial enlarged vestibular aqueduct
f. paroxysmal polyserositis
f. periodic paralysis
f. polyposis coli
f. porencephaly
f. primary pulmonary hypertension
progressive familial intrahepatic cholestasia
f. progressive hyperpigmentation
f. pure depressive disease
f. spastic paraplegia
f. tremor
f. visceral myopathy
f. visceral neuropathy

familiar
matching familiar figures
Matching F. Figures Test
F. Sensory Stimulation

family
abusive family system
F. Adaptability and Cohesion Evaluation Scale
adoptee family method
adult child of dysfunctional f.
F. Apperception Test
f. assessment adjustment pass
F. Assessment Device
F. Attitudes Questionnaire
f. attitudes test
behavioral family systems therapy
compromised ineffective family coping
f. conference
disabling ineffective family coping
f. doctor
F. Drawing Depression Scale
emergency assistance to f.'s
F. Environment Scale
F. Evaluation Form
Ewing sarcoma family of tumors
extended family therapy
f. goal
f. group therapy
f. health center
f. health insurance plan
herpes family of viruses
f. history
f. history of cancer
f. history of diabetes
f. history of hirsutism

f. history of mental illness
f. history negative
f. history noncontributory
f. history not remarkable
f. history of obesity
f. history positive
f. history research diagnostic criteria
human development and family life
F. Index of Life Events
Individualized F. Service Plan
intake interview of f.
f. interaction
f. intervention
f. intervention program
F. Inventory of Life Events and Changes
F. Inventory of Resources for Management
f. issue
Janus family tyrosine kinase
Kinetic F. Drawing
Lynch cancer family syndrome I, II
McMaster F. Assessment Device
f. medical doctor
f. medical history
F. and Medical Leave Act of 1993
f. medicine center
melanoma antigen-encoding gene f.
f. member presence
multidimensional family therapy
multiple family therapy
National F. Caregivers Association
natural family planning
neighborhood family care center
no family doctor
no family physician
noncontributory family history
notch gene f.
f. ocular history
f. participation unit
pathogenic family pattern
f. physician
f. planning
f. planning clinic
f. planning health assistant
f. practice
f. practice center
f. practitioner
psychiatric family history
f. psychiatric history
f. reaction to illness
Rehabilitative Addicted F. Treatment
F. Relations Test
f. risk assessment program
schizophrenia family history
F. Therapist Behavioral Scale
F. Tracking System
trefoil factor f.

family-centered
f.-c. care
f.-c. care unit
f.-c. maternity care
f.-c. maternity nursing

family-oriented issue

fan
f. douche
f. stroking maneuver during massage

Fanconi
F. anemia
F. pancytopenia
F. syndrome

Fannia canicularis

fanning of toes

fantasies
preoccupation with fantasies of grandeur

fantasizer
habitual f.

fantastica
paraphrenia f.

fantasy
affect f.
aggressive f.
anal rape f.
attachment f.
autistic f.
cannibalistic f.
delusion and f.
fact and f.
flight into f.
highly prone to f.
magic f.
masturbation f.
night f.
obsessive f.
paraphiliac f.
pathognomonic f.

far
f. advanced
f. infrared
f. lateral inferior suboccipital approach
f. point of accommodation

faradization
galvanic f.

Farallon virus

Farber test

farm
Royal Farm virus

farmer's lung disease

farnesyltransferase inhibitor

Farnsworth panel D-15 color vision test

Farre
line of F.
F. line

Farris test

farthest
carbon atom farthest from principal functioning group

Fas
F. ligand
ligation of F.

Fasanella-Servat operation

Fas-associating protein with death domain

fascia, pl. **fasciae**
angular tract of cervical f.
anterior cervical f.
anterior layer of thoracolumbar f.
anterior rectus f.
anterior renal f.
autogenous fascia lata sling procedure
autologous rectus fascia sling
deep temporal f.
deep temporoparietal f.
endothoracic f.
external oblique f.
falciform fold of fascia lata
f. graft
f. incised
f. incised transversely
internal spermatic f.
lata
f. lata graft
lumbodorsal f.
medial geniculate f.
membranous layer of superficial f.
membranous layer of superficial fascia of perineum
middle cervical f.
muscular fascia of extraocular muscle
orbital fasciae

fascia *(continued)*
parietal abdominal f.
pedicled fascia lata musculocutaneous flap
plantar fascia syndrome
quadratus lumborum f.
rim of f.
skin and fascia stapler
superficial temporal f.
temporalis fascia proper
tendinous arch of pelvic f.
tensor fasciae latae muscle

fascial
antebrachial fascial graft
autogenous fascial heterograft
axial temporoparietal fascial flap
f. closure
f. defect
f. dilator
f. flap
f. graft
f. hemiatrophy
f. herniation
f. layer
Martius flap and fascial sling
medial brachial fascial compartment
Mersilene fascial strip
f. necrosis
paravaginal fascial repair
f. plane
plantar fascial release
f. sheath
superficial fascial system
temporoparietal fascial flap
underlay fascial graft

fascicle
anterior fascicle of palatopharyngeus muscle
anterior tibiotalar f.
oculomotor nerve f.

fascicular
anterior fascicular block
f. graft
f. heart block
left anterior fascicular block
left anterior-superior fascicular block
left posterior fascicular block
left posterior-inferior fascicular block
transverse fascicular area

fasciculata
zona f.

fasciculated bladder

fasciculation
f. potential
proprioceptive neuromuscular fasciculation reaction
weakness, atrophy, and f.

fasciculus, pl. **fasciculi**
anterior fasciculus proprius
anterior pyramidal f.
aponeurosis of plantar transverse fasciculi
arcuate f.
f. cuneatus
f. gracilis
f. interfascicularis
longitudinal fasciculi of colon
f. longitudinalis medialis
medial longitudinal f.
nucleus of cuneate f.
f. retroflexus

fasciectomy
limited f.
partial f.

fasciitis
diffuse fasciitis with eosinophilia
eosinophilic f.
necrotizing fasciitis of the scrotum
necrotizing myositis f.
nodular pseudosarcomatous f.
odontogenic cervical necrotizing f.
palmar fasciitis and polyarthritis syndrome
plantar fasciitis orthosis
plantar fasciitis syndrome
pseudosarcomatous f.
Universal plantar fasciitis orthotic

fascination
obsessional f.

fasciocutaneous
anterior tibial fasciocutaneous flap
arc of rotation of fasciocutaneous flap
f. axial pattern flap
distally based fasciocutaneous flap
f. flap
latissimus dorsi fasciocutaneous flap
medial distally based fasciocutaneous flap
f. vessel

fasciogram study

Fasciola hepatica

fasciotome
Moseley f.

fasciotomy
endoscopic plantar f.
percutaneous plantar f.
f. wound biopsy

fashion
appendectomy performed in routine f.
aseptic f.
crisscross f.
incision closed in serial f.
interrupted f.
inverted-T f.
McLean f.
Moschowitz f.
multiaxial f.
nonaxial f.
patient is prepped and draped in usual sterile f.
perpendicular f.
retrograde f.
simple interrupted f.

fast
abnormally fast activity
acid f.
f. acquisition multiple excitation
f. activity
adiabatic fast passage
f. adiabatic trajectory in steady state
f. alpha variant rhythm
antegrade fast pathway
anterograde fast component neuropathy
f. asymmetric spin echo
f. atom bombardment
f. atom bombardment mass spectrometry
axial single shot fast spin-echo
f. axoplasmic transport
f. component of neuron
contrast-enhanced fast sequence
f. death factor
excessive fast brain wave activity
f. feedback
f. food intake
generalized fast activity
f. green
f. growth rate
f. heartbeat
f. heart rate
f. hemoglobin
high-voltage fast activity
14-hour fast required
f. imaging steady precession sequence three-dimensional magnetic resonance imaging
f. imaging with steady precession

f. imaging with steady-state free precession
left ventricular fast filling time
f. low-angle shot
Luxol fast blue stain
miniature centrifugal fast analyzer
f. multiplanar spoiled gradient-recalled imaging
nuclear fast red stain
f. oxidative
protein-sparing modified f.
f. red B salt
reversed passive hemagglutination by miniature centrifugal fast analysis
reverse fast imaging with steady-state free precession
single shot fast spin echo
f. track program
f. twitch
very fast death factor
f. wave

fast-acting insulin

fast-binding target-attaching globulin

fast-field echo

fast-frequency repetitive transcranial magnetic stimulation

fast-glycolytic muscle fiber

fastigial

f. nucleus
f. pressor response

fasting

blood fasting sugar
f. blood glucose
f. blood sugar
f. blood work
f. chemistry profile
f. gastrin level
f. glucose level
f. hyperbilirubinemia
impaired fasting glucose
f. insulin resistance index
f. intestinal contents
f. intestinal flow rate
f. laboratory work
f. lipid profile
f. metabolic panel
partial f.
f. plasma glucose
f. plasma lipid
preoperative f.
f. serum glucose
f. serum level
f. test

fast-repeating high sequence

fat

abdominal fat deposit
f. absorption
f. absorption study
android fat distribution
anterior epidural f.
antimesenteric fat pad
artificial fat pad
atrophy of f.
autogenous dermis fat graft
autogenous fat graft
autologous fat graft
autologous fat injection
autologous fat transfer
autologous pearl fat graft
axillary fat pad
body f.
butter f.
cholesterol saturated fat index
coefficient of fat retention
density of the fat mass
dermal fat free flap
dermal fat free tissue transfer
dermal fat graft
dietary fat intake
disseminated fat necrosis
f. embolism
f. embolism syndrome
f. embolization
f. embolus
epicardial fat pad
epicardial fat pad sign
epicardial fat tag
f. and fat-free mass
fecal fat excretion
f. flap
f. free
free fat graft
f. globule
gluteal body f.
f. graft
f. grafting
f. heart
f. hernia
herniated fat pad
Hoffa fat pad
human milk fat globule
immature brown fat cell
infrapatellar fat pad
f. injection
f. intake
intravenous fat emulsion
lipid content of storage f.
liposuction fat fillant implant
low animal f.
low fat and cholesterol diet
low saturated f.
macrovesicular fat droplet
f. malabsorption
malar fat pad
f. maldigestion/malabsorption
Martius bulbocavernosus fat flap
Martius fat pad
f. mass
masticatory fat pad
metastatic fat necrosis
midarm fat area
milk fat globule membrane
milk fat globule protein
mouse milk fat globule
mutton f.
f. necrosis
Nile blue fat stain
orbital fat body
orbital fat pad
orbital fat suppression
parapharyngeal fat pad
patellar fat pad
pedicled buccal fat pad flap
pedicle fat graft
percent body f.
pericapsular fat infiltration
pericardial fat pad
periorbital fat atrophy
peripancreatic fat plane
peripheral fat wasting
perirectal fat infiltration
perirenal fat capsule
pre-Achilles fat pad
retroorbicularis oculi f.
retropatellar fat pad
saturated f.
saturated fat intake
scalene fat pad biopsy
scrotal fat necrosis
subcutaneous fat atrophy
subcutaneous fat necrosis
submental fat pad
suborbicularis oculi f.
supraclavicular fat pad
f. tolerance test
total abdominal f.
total body f.
total fat intake
total fat mass
traumatic fat necrosis
ultrasonic fat suctioning
visceral abdominal f.
visceral abdominal fat to total abdominal fat ratio

fatal

f. accident
f. air embolus

fatal *(continued)*
f. arrhythmia
f. cardiac event
f. child abuse
f. complications of illicit drug use
f. disseminated infection
f. dose
epidemic fatal encephalopathy
f. familial insomnia
f. genetic illness
f. granulomatous disease
f. heart arrhythmia
f. heart attack
f. heart rhythm disturbance
f. hemorrhage
f. hepatitis
f. hypersensitivity reaction
f. hypothermia
f. illness
f. infection
least fatal dose
malignant potentially fatal asthma
median fatal dose
minimal fatal dose
f. nosocomial infection
potentially fatal disease
f. pulmonary hemorrhage
sudden fatal heart attack

fatality
drug-associated f.

fat-blood interface

fat-free
f.-f. diet
f.-f. dry weight
f.-f. solid
f.-f. supper
f.-f. wet weight

father
alleged f.
f. of baby
f. of child
f. in delivery
diabetic f.
f. factor
foster f.
mother and f.
trained participating father birth

father's
f. grandfather
f. grandmother

fatigability
auditory f.
easy f.
nervous f.

fatigue
auditory f.
battle f.
chronic fatigue immune deficiency syndrome
chronic fatigue and immune dysfunction syndrome
combat f.
decreased energy, fatigue and weakness
decrease in energy or f.
depression, insomnia and f.
detrimental impact of f.
f. from antihistamine
inactivity, lethargy and f.
inappropriate f.
increased f.
increasing f.
f. and insomnia
f. and loss of appetite
mental f.
metal f.
Multidimensional F. Symptom Inventory
nervous f.
neurotic f.
olfactory f.
operational f.
overwhelming f.
pain and f.
pain, fatigue, and insomnia
postviral fatigue syndrome
progressive fatigue and weakness
quadriceps f.
severe joint pain and f.
F. Symptom Checklist
weakness and f.

fat-induced hyperglycemia

fat-mobilizing
f.-m. hormone
f.-m. substance

fatness
intense fear of f.

fat-pad

fat-soluble vitamin deficiency

fat-suppressed spin-echo

fatty
f. acid
f. acid amide hydrolase
f. acid-binding protein
f. acid free
f. acid methyl ester
f. acid oxidation
f. acid poor
f. acids polyunsaturated
f. acid translocase
f. acid transport protein
activated fatty acid
acute fatty liver
acute fatty liver of pregnancy
atherosclerotic fatty streak
branched-chain fatty acid
f. degeneration of heart
essential fatty acid deficiency
f. ester
f. acid-binding protein 2
f. food intolerance
free fatty acid
free volatile fatty acid
f. heart
heart fatty acid binding protein
hyaline fatty change
intestinal fatty acid-binding protein
f. liver
f. liver cell
f. liver disease
f. liver and kidney syndrome
long-chain fatty acid
long-chain fatty acid oxidation
long-chain polyunsaturated fatty acid
long- and medium-chain fatty acid coenzyme-A dehydrogenase deficiency
low-saturated fatty acid diet
macrovesicular fatty liver
f. meal sonogram
mitochondrial fatty acid beta-oxidation
monosaturated fatty acid
mucosal fatty acid
muscle layer in fatty layer of subcutaneous tissue
nonalcoholic fatty liver disease
f. nutritional cirrhosis
omega-3 fatty acid
omega-3, -6 fatty acid
omega-3 polyunsaturated fatty acid
oxidation of fatty acid
pancreatogenous fatty diarrhea
pediatric fatty marrow
plasma membrane fatty acid binding protein
polyunsaturated free fatty acid
polyunsaturated-to-saturated fatty acids ratio
Quain fatty heart
radioiodinated fatty acid
serum-free fatty acid
short-chain fatty acid

short-chain polyunsaturated fatty acid
total fatty acid
trans fatty acid
unesterified free fatty acid
unsaturated fatty acid
f. vacuolization
very long chain fatty acid
volatile fatty acid

fatty acid-binding protein 2

fauces
anterior pillar of f.
arch of f.

Fauchard disease

faucial
anterior faucial pillar

faucial arch

faulty valve action

favor
atypical favor reactive

favorable histology

favorably
not favorably considered

favosa
mycosis f.

Favre disease

Fazio-Londe atrophy

fear
f. of abandonment
attack of intense f.
F. Avoidance Beliefs Quest
castration f.
conditioned fear response
crowd f.
f. of failure
f., uncertainty, and doubt
f. of imminent death
f. of impending doom
incapacitating f.
intense abandonment f.
intense fear of fatness
life f.
marriage f.
masking f.
maturity f.
mirror f.
morbid f.
motion f.
mouse f.
night f.
obligations f.
obsessive f.
odor f.
paranoid f.
patient has fear of hospital
penis f.
performance f.
f. of personal harm
F. Survey Schedule
unreasonable f.
Wolpe F. Survey Schedule

feather
f. analysis
Australian parrot f.
mixed f.
parrot f.

feathered
f. edge
f. edge proximal finishing

feature
age-related f.
age-specific f.
agitative f.
anterior feature English phoneme
antisocial f.
arteriosclerotic dementia with delusional f.
arteriosclerotic dementia with depressive f.
associated descriptive f.
atypical f.
avoidant f.
clinical manifestations, etiologic factors, anatomic involvement, pathophysiologic f.'s
dysautonomic f.
manic f.
manometric f.
melancholic f.
mixed f.
mood-congruent psychotic f.
mood disorder with atypical f.'s
mood disorder with catatonic f.'s
mood disorder with melancholic f.'s
morphologic f.
myofibroblastic f.
narcissistic f.
neurobehavioral f.
neurologic f.
neuropsychiatric f.
neurotic f.
obsessional f.
obsessive-compulsive f.
outward expression of anger with impulsive f.
paranoid f.
passive-aggressive f.
pathologic f.
pathological f.
personality f.
predominant f.
unusual facial f.'s

febrile
acute febrile illness
acute febrile neutrophilic dermatosis
acute febrile respiratory disease
acute febrile respiratory illness
f. agglutinin
f. antigen
f. antigen agglutination
autosomal dominant febrile convulsion
f. baby
benign febrile convulsion
complex febrile seizure
f. convulsion
f. crisis
f. delirium
f. disease
f. epilepsy
f. illness
maternal febrile morbidity
f. morbidity
f. neutropenia
f. neutrophilic dermatosis
nonhemolytic febrile transfusion reaction
f. nonhemolytic transfusion react
other febrile illness
f. paroxysm
patient f.
prolonged febrile convulsions
f. psychosis
f. seizure
f. status epilepticus
f. urine
f. urticaria

febrilis
herpes f.
placenta f.

fecal
f. abscess
anterior fecal incontinence
barium-based fecal tagging
f. bile acid
chronic fecal shedding
f. coli broth
f. collection receptacle assembly
f. concretion
constipation and fecal impaction
f. containment device
f. containment system
f. daily blood loss
f. emesis

fecal *(continued)*
endogenous fecal calcium
extensive fecal impaction
f. fat excretion
f. fistula
f. frequency
gross fecal contamination
immunological fecal occult blood test
impacted fecal material
f. impaction
f. incontinence
f. leukocyte count test
f. occult blood
f. occult blood test
overflow fecal incontinence
passing fecal material
f. seepage
f. smear
f. soiling
f. spillage
f. tagging
total fecal nitrogen
f. tumor
unclassified fecal virus
f. urobilinogen
f. vomiting

fecalith
appendiceal f.
calcified f.

feces
bacteria in f.
f. collection device
f. and gas
gas and f.
hard f.
incontinence of f.
involuntary discharge of f.
patient incontinent of f.
soft f.

fecundation
artificial f.

fecundity
natural f.

fed
artificially f.
breast f.

federal
F. False Claims Act
F. Food, Drug, and Cosmetic Act
f. immunization program

Federation
Assisted Living Federation of America
International Federation of Gynecology and Obstetrics classification of tumor staging

fee
contract administration f.'s
medical fee schedule
sliding fee scale
usual, customary, and reasonable fees

feeble-mindedness
affective f.-m.

feeblemindedness
macrocephaly with feeblemindedness and encephalopathy with peculiar deposits

feedback
altered auditory f.
androgen gonadotropin feedback control
anticipatory bogus heart rate f.
biologic f.
delayed auditory f.
delayed feedback audiometry
fast f.
heart rate f.
f. inhibition factor
long-loop feedback signal
f. mechanism
f. mechanisms of hormonal control
negative feedback loop
negative feedback regulation
neuromuscular feedback training
neuronal feedback loop
positional feedback stimulation trainer
f. reduction circuit
f. regulation
respiratory f.
f. signal
simultaneous auditory f.
supplementary sensory f.
tubuloglomerular f.
visual feedback display

feeder
leukocyte feeder layer
universal f.
f. vessel

feeding
ad lib f.
after f.'s
blenderized tube f.
continuous drip f.
continuous tube f.
diarrhea and breast f.
enteral feeding tube
gastrostomy tube f.
f. gastrostomy tube
gavage f.
glucose water f.
growth monitoring, oral rehydration, breast feeding, and immunization
home enteral tube f.
house tube f.
hypocaloric carbohydrate f.
hypocaloric protein f.
hypothalamic feeding center
infant feeding tube
jejunal feeding tube
jejunostomy tube f.
f. mean arterial pressure
modified sham f.
by mouth f.
nasogastric f.'s
nasogastric drip f.
nasogastric feeding tube
nasogastric tube f.
nasojejunal feeding tube
NJ feeding tube
orogastric feeding
parental feeding practice
patient independent in f.
pediatric feeding tube
percutaneous transhepatic biliary drainage-enteric f.
postoperative regimen for oral early f.
sham f.
special tube f.
standard tube f.
thermic effect of f.
tube f.
f. tube placement
with f.'s

feel
f.'s hollow and empty
inability to feel pleasure
patient feels guilty
patient feels isolated

feeling
f. of abandonment
absence of f.
addictive feeling and action
aggressive f.
ambivalent f.
f. of anger
antigovernment f.
ataxic f.
chronic feelings of deep emptiness

fidgeting, aching, pulling, or itching f.
guilt f.
f. of guilt, worthlessness and helplessness
f.'s of hopelessness
f. of immobilization
inferiority f.
initial feeling of euphoria
f. of intellectual and physical power
intense f.
intensified f.
internal f.
f. of isolation
lack of f.
loving f.
maladaptive f.
negative f.
obsessive f.
obsessive feelings of responsibility
painful f.
patient expressed guilt f.
patient feeling hostile
positive f.
premonitory f.
premorbid inferiority f.
prickly, burning, and tingling f.
repressed f.
f.'s of social inadequacy
suicidal or homicidal f.
tight feeling in head

feet
anterior feet view
burning feet from atherosclerosis
burning feet syndrome
cubic feet per minute
elevate feet above heart
flat f.
hand motion at 3 feet vision test
neuropathy of f.
numbness in f.
f. out of bed
f. over edge of bed
painful burning of f.
paresthesia of f.
peeling of feet and hands
f. per minute
puffiness of f.
swelling of hands or f.
tingling and numbness in f.

Fehr dystrophy

Feigenbaum echocardiogram

feigned eruption

feigning symptoms

Fein Articulation Screening Test

Feingold diet

Feist-Mankin position

Feldman
F. adaptometer
McGlamry and Feldman modification

feldspar
orthoclase ceramic f.

feline
f. ataxia virus
f. calicivirus
f. conjunctivitis
f. fibrosarcoma virus
f. immunodeficiency virus
f. infectious anemia
f. infectious peritonitis
f. infectious peritonitis virus
f. kidney
f. leukemia
f. leukemia virus
McDonough feline sarcoma virus
f. oncornavirus-associated cell membrane antigen
f. panleukopenia virus
f. urologic syndrome
f. viral rhinotracheitis

Felix-Weil reaction

fell
f. on outstretched hand
f. out of bed

felon
aseptic f.
bone f.
f. drainage
f. infection
subcutaneous f.

felt
f. brace
f. collar splint
fetal movement f.
f. pad
f. padding
f. patch

Felty syndrome

female
f. adnexal tumor of probable wolffian origin
adult f.
f. athlete triad
Caucasian f.
f. child
f. day equivalent
f. dyspareunia
f. external genitalia
full-term living female child
f. genitalia
f. genital mutilation
f. genital tract
f. genital tract carcinosarcoma
f. genital tract mutilation
Hispanic f.
f. hormone
immature dead female child
immature living female child
f. infertility
Latin American f.
level of female gonadotropin
masculine attitude in female neurotic
Mexican American f.
mucosa of female urethra
muscular coat of female urethra
muscular layer of female urethra
newborn, term, normal, f.
nonwhite f.
normal adult f.
normal external female genitalia
normal female adult genitalia
normal female sex chromosome type
f. pattern androgenetic alopecia
f. pattern hair loss
pregnancy, term, complicated delivered, living f.
pregnancy, term, uncomplicated delivered, living f.
premature dead female child
premature living female child
f. pseudo-Turner syndrome
f. reproductive tract
f. sex chromosome
f. sex hormone
f. sexual arousal disorder
f. sexual dysfunction
Spanish American f.
spongy layer of female urethra
sterile f.
term birth, living f.
unknown black f.
unknown white f.
viable female infant
well-nourished f.
white divorced f.
white female living child

female-female adaptor

female-pattern baldness

feminization
adrenal feminization syndrome

feminization *(continued)*
incomplete testicular feminization syndrome
testicular f.
testicular feminization mutation
testicular feminization syndrome

feminizing testis syndrome

femoral
f. above-knee popliteal bypass
f. access stabilization
acetabular depth to femoral head diameter
Aitken femoral deficiency
f. alignment jig
angle of femoral torsion
Anson-McVay femoral herniorrhaphy
antegrade femoral artery catheterization
antegrade femoral nail
anterior cutaneous branch of femoral nerve
anterior femoral cutaneous nerve
f. anteversion
aortobiprofunda femoral bypass
f. arterial cannulation
f. arterial line
f. artery
f. artery blood flow
f. artery catheter
f. artery pressure
f. artery thrombosis
Aufranc-Turner femoral component
avascular femoral head necrosis
avascular necrosis of the femoral head
bipolar femoral component
bipolar femoral head prosthesis
f. blood pressure
brachial, radial, f.
cementless femoral component
f. cerebral catheter
common femoral artery
common femoral artery-superficial femoral artery
f. component pusher
f. condylar shaving
contoured femoral stem
crutch and belt femoral closed nailing
f. cutaneous nerve
deafness, femoral epiphysial dysplasia, short stature, developmental delay syndrome
debonded femoral stem prosthesis
derotation femoral osteotomy
f. derotation osteotomy
f. diaphysial allograft
f. diaphysial fracture
distal femoral epiphysis
f. drill bit
endoprosthetic femoral head replacement
f. graft
greater trochanteric femoral fracture
f. head
f. head line
f. hernia
f. herniorrhaphy
f. hypoplasia
f. hypoplasia unusual facies syndrome
intertrochanteric femoral fracture
f. intertrochanteric fracture
f. intratrochanteric fracture
ischemic necrosis of femoral head
lateral femoral cutaneous
lateral femoral torsion
left common femoral artery
left femoral artery
left femoral hernia
f. length
low-profile femoral prosthesis
medial circumflex femoral artery
medial circumflex femoral vein
medial femoral circumflex artery
medial femoral tuberosity
medial/lateral femoral condyle
monoblock femoral component
monoblock femoral stem prosthesis
Mueller femoral supracondylar fracture classification
f. neck
f. neck fracture
f. neck nail
f. neck prosthesis
f. neck version
f. nerve block
painful femoral head prosthesis
palpable femoral pulse
patellar femoral syndrome
Pauwels femoral neck fracture classification
percutaneous femoral approach
percutaneous femoral vein
percutaneous femoral vein catheter
percutaneous femoral venous catheter
perforating artery of deep femoral artery
perineal branch of posterior femoral cutaneous nerve
f. prosthesis broach
f. prosthesis fixation
prosthetic femoral head
proximal femoral focal deficiency
proximal femoral fracture
proximal focal femoral deficiency
f. pulsatility index
retrograde femoral catheter
right common femoral angioplasty
right common femoral artery
right femoral artery
right femoral vein
right lateral f.
self-articulating femoral hip replacement
f. shaft axis
f. shaft malunion
slipped capital femoral epiphysis
slipped upper femoral epiphysis
superficial branch of medial circumflex femoral artery
superficial femoral angioplasty
superficial femoral artery
superficial femoral vein
f. supracondylar fracture
f. tibial bypass
f. total density
transcervical femoral fracture
f. vein
f. vein ligation
Zimaloy femoral head prosthesis

femoral-femoral
f.-f. bypass
f.-f. bypass graft

femoral-popliteal
f.-p. artery bypass
f.-p. bypass
f.-p. vein bypass

femoral-tibial-peroneal bypass

femoris
biceps femoris muscle
biceps femoris tendon
left rectus f.
musculus biceps f.
os f.
profunda f.
profunda femoris vein
quadratus f.
quadratus femoris muscle
quadriceps femoris muscle
rectus f.
rectus femoris muscle

rectus femoris muscle flap
rectus femoris tendon
right rectus f.
trochlea f.

femoroaxillary bypass

femorocerebral catheter angiography

femoropopliteal
f. artery
f. artery occlusion
f. bypass
f. bypass graft
f. occlusive disease
f. vein

femorotibial
f. angle
anterolateral femorotibial ligament tenodesis
f. bypass
f. joint
Mueller anterolateral femorotibial ligament tenodesis

femtomoles per milligram

femur
apex of f.
bone to femur graft
head of f.
intercondylar notch of f.
lateral condyle of f.
ligament of head of f.
medial condyle of f.
medial epicondyle of f.
metaphyseal lesion of distal f.
nail inserted into neck and head of f.
neck of f.
neck and head of f.
Neer femur fracture classification
notch of f.
NSA of f.
nutrient artery of f.
osteonecrosis of f.
pectineal line of f.
proximal femur focal deficiency
shaft of f.
universal proximal femur prosthesis

femur-fibula-ulna syndrome

fence
ligamentous facial f.

fenestrated
f. compress
f. drape
f. forceps
Henle fenestrated membrane
f. hymen
f. reamer
f. spiked open-span jumbo biopsy forceps
f. splint
f. sterile field barrier
f. tracheostomy tube

fenestration
aortopulmonary f.
apical f.
arterial f.
atrophic f.
endonasal f.
middle cerebral artery f.
optic nerve sheath f.
f. of oval window
f. procedure
f. technique
tracheal f.

fentanyl
intraoperative f.
oral transmucosal fentanyl citrate
transdermal fentanyl device

fer-de-lance virus

Ferguson method

fermentation
adonitol fermentation test
arabinose fermentation test
D-arabitol fermentation test
maltose fermentation test
mannitol fermentation test
mannose fermentation test
D-mannose fermentation test
melezitose fermentation test
melibiose fermentation test
mixed acid f.
modified rapid fermentation test
mucate fermentation test
N-acetylglucosamine fermentation test
nonlactose f.

Ferment fever

fermenting
lactose fermenting Gram-negative rod
nonlactose fermenting gram-negative rod

fern
Nitrazine fern test
f. test

ferning
f. technique
vaginal fluid f.

fern-positive Nitrazine

Ferrata cell

ferredoxin-reducing substance

Ferree-Rand perimeter

Ferrein canal

Ferribacterium duplex

ferric
f. ammonium citrate
f. citrate

ferritin
serum f.

Ferritin-conjugated antibody

ferrokinetic data

ferromagnetic
f. artifact
f. metal plate
f. rod
f. tamponade

ferrous
f. citrate
f. fumarate
f. gluconate
f. iron
Lillie ferrous iron stain
macroaggregated ferrous hydroxide
f. sulfate

ferrugineus
locus f.

fertility
age-specific fertility rate
brittle hair, intellectual impairment, decreased fertility, short stature syndrome
f. factor
ichthyosis, brittle hair, impaired intelligence, decreased fertility, short stature syndrome
impairment of f.
total fertility rate

fertilization
f. antigen
f. antigen-1
ex vivo f.
Human F. and Embryology Authority
micro assisted f.
in vitro f.
in vivo f.

fertilized
implantation of fertilized egg
implantation of fertilized ovum

fescue
meadow f.
meadow fescue grass

festinating gait

festoon
McCall f.

festooning
periocular f.

fetal
f. abdominal circumference
f. abdominal diameter
abnormal fetal development
f. abnormality
f. acoustic stimulation testing
f. activity
f. activity acceleration determination
F. Activity Test
acute intrapartum fetal distress
f. adenocarcinoma
f. age
f. akinesia deformation sequence
f. alcohol baby
f. alcohol effect
f. alcohol retardation
f. alcohol syndrome
allogenic fetal graft
f. allograft
antepartum fetal BPP
antepartum fetal NST
antepartum fetal surveillance
f. arterial oxygen saturation
asymmetric fetal growth restriction
atrial fetal flutter
baseline variability of fetal heart rate
f. biophysical profile
f. biparietal diameter
f. bone marrow
f. bovine endothelial cell
f. bovine serum
f. breathing movement
f. calf serum
f. cardiac frequency
f. cardiac motion
f. cardiac reactivity test
f. catecholamine
cephalopelvic disproportion and fetal distress
chain of fetal hemoglobin
f. congenital diaphragmatic hernia
f. cotyledon
daily fetal movement count
daily fetal movement record
f. danger
f. danger zone
f. death in utero
decreased fetal movement
f. demise
f. distress
f. ductus arteriosus constriction
f. electrocardiogram
f. electroencephalogram
electronic fetal monitoring
embryo f.
f. endoscopic
entrance of fetal head into superior pelvic strait
f. erythroblastosis
estimated fetal body weight
f. estrogen-binding protein
external fetal heart rate monitoring
external fetal maternal monitor
external fetal monitoring
f. fibronectin
f. foot length
frontooccipital fetal position
f. gigantism-renal hamartoma-nephroblastomatosis syndrome
good fetal movement
f. growth
f. growth acceleration
f. growth and development
f. growth restriction
f. growth retardation
f. head
f. heart
f. heartbeat
f. heart disease
f. heart frequency
f. heart heard
f. heart monitor
f. heart monitor tracing
f. heart motion
f. heart not heard
f. heart rate
f. heart rate acceleration
f. heart rate baseline
f. heart rate deceleration
f. heart rate monitoring
f. heart rate nonstress test
f. heart rate reactivity
f. heart rate reading
f. heart rate variability
f. heart rhythm
f. heart sound
f. heart tones
heat-inactivated fetal bovine serum
heat-inactivated fetal calf serum
f. hemoglobin
f. hemoglobin test
hereditary persistence of fetal hemoglobin
hourly fetal urine production rate
human fetal diploid kidney cell
human fetal diploid lung cell
human fetal cell
human fetal lung fibroblast
human fetal pancreas transplant
f. hydantoin syndrome
f. hydrops
f. hyperthyroidism
f. hypothyroidism
immature fetal lung
inactivated fetal calf serum
f. inclusion
indirect fetal contamination
f. intensive care unit
internal fetal heart rate monitoring
internal fetal monitoring
internal fetal scalp electrode
f. intervention
intrapartum fetal distress
intrauterine fetal death
intrauterine fetal demise
intrauterine fetal distress
intrauterine fetal growth retardation
intrauterine fetal monitoring
intrauterine fetal transfusion
intravascular fetal air sign
intravenous fetal transfusion
f. iodine deficiency disorder
f. karyotyping
late fetal death
left dorsotransverse fetal position
left frontoanterior fetal position
left frontoposterior position fetal
left frontotransverse fetal position
left mentoanterior fetal position
left mentoposterior fetal position
left mentotransverse fetal position
left occipitoanterior fetal position
left occipitolateral fetal position
left occipitotransverse fetal position
left occiput posterior fetal position
left sacroposterior fetal position
f. length
f. liver cell
f. lung maturity
f. macrosomia
Manning score of fetal activity
maternal fetal hemorrhage
maternal fetal medicine
maternal hyperglycemia-induced fetal hyperinsulinemia
membranes
mentum posterior fetal position
f. mesencephalic tissue

monomer in fetal hemoglobin
f. movement acceleration test
movement-associated fetal heart rate accelerations
f. movement count
f. movement felt
f. movement record
nonimmune fetal hydrops
nonreassuring fetal heart beat pattern
nonreassuring fetal status
nonreassuring fetal testing
nonstress test fetal monitoring
normal fetal development
normal fetal growth
occipitosacral fetal position
percutaneous fetal cystoscopy
percutaneous fetal tissue sampling
percutaneous fetal transfusion
persistence of fetal circulation
persistent fetal circulation with pulmonary hypertension
persistent mentoposterior fetal position
persistent occipitoposterior fetal position
poor intrauterine fetal growth
potential fetal hypertensive crisis
premature rupture of fetal membranes
primary human fetal glia
primitive fetal hemoglobin
prolonged rupture of fetal membranes
protrusion of fetal part
f. quickening
recurrent fetal loss
f. respiration
retained fetal lung fluid
retard fetal growth
f. rhabdomyomatous nephroblastoma
right acromiodorsoanterior fetal position
right acromiodorsoposterior fetal position
right frontoanterior fetal position
right frontolateral fetal position
right frontoposterior fetal position
right frontotransverse fetal position
right mentoanterior fetal position
right mentolateral fetal position
right mentoposterior fetal position
right occipitolateral fetal position
right occipitotransverse fetal position
right sacroanterior fetal position
right sacrolateral fetal position
right sacroposterior fetal position
rotate fetal head
f. scalp blood
f. scalp electrode
f. scalp sampling
slow fetal growth
f. souffle
stable fetal heart tones
f. sulfoglycoprotein antigen
f. thrombotic vasculopathy
f. thymus organ culture
f. tissue transplant
f. tobacco syndrome
f. tonsil
transplanting human fetal tissue
f. valproate syndrome
f. varicella syndrome
f. viability
f. warfarin syndrome
f. wastage
wedged fetal head
f. weight
well-differentiated fetal adenocarcinoma

Fetaldex test

fetalis
chondrodystrophia f.
erythroblastosis f.
maternal hydrops f.
maternal parvovirus f.
nonimmune hydrops f.

fetal-maternal
f.-m. communication
f.-m. hemoglobin
f.-m. hemorrhage

fetal-renal hamartoma

fetid odor

fetishism
beast f.
transvestic f.

fetofetal
antenatal fetofetal transfusion

fetomaternal
f. alloimmune thrombocytopenia
f. hemorrhage
f. incompatibility

fetopathy
diabetic f.

fetopelvic disproportion

fetoplacental unit

fetoprotein
alpha-1 fetoprotein assay
alpha fetoprotein test
maternal alpha f.
urinary basic f.

fetus, pl. **fetuses**
aborted human f.
f. active
amniotic adhesions of f.
appendages of f.
asynclitic position of f.
crushing procedure skull of f.
dead fetus in utero
f. of diabetic mother
Doppler monitoring of f.
head of f.
impact on f.
left acromiodorsoanterior position of f.
left acromiodorsoposterior position of f.
no abnormality of f.
nuchal translucency in a f.
f. papyraceus
position of f.
presentation of f.
presenting part of f.
size/date inconsistency
skeletal dysplasia in f.
small third-trimester f.
spontaneously aborted human f.
f. with hydrocephalus

Feuerstein
nevus sebaceous of Feuerstein and Mims

fever
acute pharyngoconjunctival f.
acute rheumatic f.
African endemic relapsing f.
African hemorrhagic f.
African swine fever virus
African tick bite f.
Argentine hemorrhagic f.
Argentine hemorrhagic fever virus
Argentinian hemorrhagic f.
arthritis of rheumatic f.
arthropod-borne viral hemorrhagic f.
attenuated fever response
Australian Q f.
autosomal-dominant periodic fever syndrome
Bolivian hemorrhagic f.
bovine ephemeral f.
Brazilian purpuric f.
f. caused by infection
f. and chills
chills and f.
chills, fever, and night sweats
Colorado tick f.

fever *(continued)*
Colorado tick fever virus
convulsion accompanying f.
coughing with f.
Crimean-Congo hemorrhagic f.
Crimean-Congo hemorrhagic fever virus
delirium with high f.
dengue f.
dengue fever vaccine
dengue hemorrhagic f.
dengue hemorrhagic fever shock syndrome
diarrhea with fever and vomiting
diphasic milk f.
disorientation and f.
East Coast f.
Ebola hemorrhagic f.
eczema, asthma, and hay fever complex
epidemic hemorrhagic f.
familial Hibernian f.
familial Mediterranean f.
f., chills, and sweating
f., chills, sweating, nausea, vomiting, and diarrhea
f., cough, nausea, and vomiting
hay f.
hay fever symptoms
hemoglobinuric bilious f.
hemorrhagic f.
hemorrhagic fever with renal symptoms
hemorrhagic fever with renal syndrome
intermittent chills and f.
intermittent hepatic f.
Japanese spotted f.
jaundice, chills and f.
jaundice, lethargy and f.
jungle yellow f.
Korean hemorrhagic f.
Lassa fever virus
Lone Star f.
louse-borne relapsing f.
malignant catarrhal f.
malignant catarrhal fever disease
malignant catarrhal fever virus
malignant tertian f.
Manchurian hemorrhagic f.
Marburg hemorrhagic f.
Mediterranean erythematous f.
Mediterranean exanthematous f.
Mediterranean spotted f.
metal fume f.
Mexican spotted f.
miniature scarlet f.
New World hemorrhagic f.
f. and night sweats
nonseasonal hay f.
North Queensland tick f.
Omsk hemorrhagic f.
Omsk hemorrhagic fever virus
onset of chills and f.
onset of f.
Pahvant Valley f.
pain and f.
pappataci fever virus
paratyphoid fever, types A, B, C
patient spiked a f.
perennial hay f.
periodic fever, aphthous stomatitis, pharyngitis, cervical adenitis
periodic fever syndrome
pharyngoconjunctival f.
pharyngoconjunctival fever virus
polymer fume f.
prison fever typhus
prolonged fever of unknown origin
pulmonary infiltrate f.
Queensland f.
recrudescent typhus f.
remittent malarial f.
rheumatic f.
rheumatic fever vaccine
Rift Valley fever virus
Rocky Mountain spotted fever vaccine
Ross River f.
routine fever therapy
sandfly fever Naples virus
sandfly fever Sicilian virus
São Paulo f.
scarlet f.
scarlet fever antitoxin
shin bone f.
simian hemorrhagic f.
South African tick-bite f.
South African tick f.
South American hemorrhagic f.
Southeast Asia mosquito-borne hemorrhagic f.
spotted fever group
f. of undetermined origin
f. of unknown etiology
f. of unknown origin
f. unresponsive to antibiotic therapy
viral hemorrhagic f.
West African f.
West Nile f.
West Nile-like f.
yellow f.
yellow fever vaccine
yellow fever virus

few fine rales

fiber
adenovirus fiber knob
alpha nerve f.
anterior external arcuate f.
anterior long f.
arcuate fiber of cerebrum
arcuate fiber involvement
arcuate nerve fiber bundle
argyrophilic collagen f.
athletic shoe carbon fiber plate
autonomic nerve f.
f. bundle volume
carbon fiber fixator
carbon fiber graft
carbon fiber half ring
carbon fiber lamination braid
climbing f.
conduction velocity of slower f.'s
cross fiber friction
daily high fiber supplement
dietary f.
diet high in f.
Dow hollow fiber dialyzer
Dow Hollow Fiber kidney
elastic f.
fast-glycolytic muscle fiber
fine f.
f. glass graft
heart muscle f.
f. and hemorrhoid
hollow fiber dialyzer
hyperplastic muscle f.
ischemic muscle f.
isotropic band striated muscle f.
isotropic disc striated muscle fiber
F.'s of Kent
lateral giant f.
long association f.
f.'s of Luschka
man-made mineral f.
man-made vitreous f.
medullated nerve f.
meridional fibers of ciliary muscle
meridional ciliary muscle f.
mesencephalic corticonuclear f.
mossy fiber sprouting
muscle fiber action potential
muscle fiber conduction velocity
muscle fiber type disproportion
myelinated fiber bundle
myelinated retinal nerve f.

myocardial fiber degeneration
Nerve F. Analyzer
Nerve F. Analyzer laser ophthalmoscope
nerve fiber action potential
nerve fiber axon
nerve fiber bundle
nerve fiber bundle defect
nerve fiber bundle layer
nerve fiber layer analyzer
nerve fiber layer dropout
nerve fiber layer hemorrhage
nerve fiber layer infarct
nerve fiber myelination
neurogenic fiber type group
neutral detergent f.
nodoventricular bypass f.
nuclear bag f.
nuclear chain f.
nylon f.
oblique gastric f.
oblique fibers of muscular layer of stomach
onionskin configuration of collagenous f.
optic nerve f.
outer cone f.
outer dense fibers of spermatozoon
outer spiral fibers of cochlea
oxytalan fiber stain
papillomacular nerve fiber bundle
paracentral nerve fiber bundle
parallel f.
perforating fibers of Sharpey
periodontal ligament f.
peripapillary nerve fiber layer
peripapillary retinal nerve f.
plasma-resistant fiber oxygenator
Purkinje f.
radial fiber of cochlea
ragged red f.
f. of Remak
retinal nerve fiber layer
f. shortening velocity
single fiber electromyography
slow twitch f.
T f.
total-dietary f.
ultrafine f.
vegetable protein diet plus f.
velocity of circumferential fiber shortening

fiberglass
f. cast
f. casting tape
flexible glass f.
f. jacket
long leg fiberglass cast
semirigid fiberglass cast
short arm fiberglass cast
f. splint

fiberoptic
f. bronchoscope
f. bronchoscopy
f. cable
f. catheter
f. colonoscope
f. endoscopic evaluation of swallowing
f. endoscopic evaluation of swallowing with sensory testing
f. endoscopic examination of swallowing
f. examination
flexible fiberoptic bronchoscopy
flexible fiberoptic bronchoscopy with protected brush
flexible fiberoptic choledochoscope
flexible fiberoptic endoscope
flexible fiberoptic sigmoidoscopy
f. headband
f. headlight
f. injection sclerotherapy laryngoplasty
f. laryngoscope
f. laryngoscopy
f. light
f. phototherapy
f. proctosigmoidoscopy
f. rhinoscopy
f. sigmoidoscope
f. sigmoidoscopy
transnasal fiberoptic laryngoplasty

fiber-region
anterior f.-r.

fiberscope
gastrointestinal f.
nasopharyngeal f.
pediatric f.
tracheal intubation f.

fibril
anchoring f.
elastic f.
globule f.

fibrillar
f. absorbable hemostat material
f. basket
f. collagen
f. contraction
f. material
purified fibrillar collagen

fibrillary
Alzheimer fibrillary degeneration
antiglial fibrillary acidic protein
glial fibrillary acidic protein
low-grade fibrillary astrocytoma
monoclonal antiglial fibrillary acidic protein

fibrillating
f. action potential
hypothermic fibrillating arrest

fibrillation
atrial f.
atrial fibrillation and/or flutter
atrial fibrillation cycle length
auricular f.
chaotic activity of ventricular f.
chronic nonvalvular atrial f.
electrical conversion of atrial f.
idiopathic ventricular f.
lone atrial f.
nonrheumatic atrial f.
nonvalvular atrial f.
onset of atrial f.
paroxysmal atrial f.
paroxysmal auricular f.
positive sharp wave f.'s
postoperative atrial f.
f. potential
primary ventricular f.
rapid atrial f.
repetitive fibrillation potential
f. rhythm
spontaneous f.
f. threshold
ventricular fibrillation threshold

fibrillation-flutter
atrial f.-f.

fibrillationflutter
controlled atrial fibrillation/flutter

fibrillation/flutter
controlled atrial f.

fibrin
autologous fibrin glue
autologous fibrin sealant glue
f. breakdown product
cross-linked fibrin degradation product
f. degradation product
f. glue
f. matrix gel
f. monomer
perisinusoidal fibrin deposition
f. plate lysis area
soluble fibrin monomer
soluble fibrin monomer complex
f. split product

fibrin *(continued)*
split products of f.
f. tissue adhesive
fibrin/fibrinogen degradation product
fibrinogen
f. breakdown product
f. deficiency
f. degradation product
f. derivative
f. equivalent unit
f. gel chromatography
kinetic fibrinogen assay
f. qualitative test
radioactive fibrinogen uptake
f. related
serum f.
f. split product
f. uptake test
fibrinogen-related antigen
fibrinolysis
intravascular coagulation and fibrinolysis syndrome
local intraarterial f.
fibrinolytic
f. activity
drainage, irrigation, fibrinolytic therapy
intraoperative intraarterial fibrinolytic therapy
f. potential
f. split product
stimulated fibrinolytic activity
fibrinopeptide
f. A
f. B
thrombin-increasing fibrinopeptide B
fibrinous
f. exudate
f. tissue
fibrin-related antigen
fibrin-stabilization factor
fibroadenomatosis hyperplasia of prostate gland
fibroblast
acidic fibroblast growth factor
basic fibroblast growth factor
f. chemotactic factor
chick embryo f.
Chinese hamster embryo f.
f. colony-forming cell
cycling f.
duck embryo f.
f. growth factor receptor 2
further differentiated f.
galactosemic f.
genital skin f.
f. growth factor receptor
hamster embryo f.
human diploid f.
human embryo f.
human embryoic lung f.
human embryonic lung f.
human fetal lung fibroblast
human fibroblast interferon
human foreskin f.
human lung f.
interferon
monkey kidney fibroblast monolayer
mouse embryo f.
murine fibroblast transformation
neonatal lung f.
nongenital skin f.
nonintestinal f.
normal human diploid f.
normal sheep lung f.
f. pneumocyte factor
skin f.
transformed mink f.
fibroblast-activating factor
fibroblast-conditioned medium
fibroblast-derived growth factor
fibroblast growth factor receptor 2
fibroblastic growth factor
fibroblast-like synoviocyte
fibroblastoma
giant cell f.
fibroblast-populated collagen lattice
fibrocalculous pancreatic diabetes
fibrocartilage
avascular f.
intervertebral f.
meniscal f.
transjugular fibrocartilage complex
triangular f.
triangular fibrocartilage complex tear
fibrocartilaginous
f. embolism
f. joint
f. material
nuchal fibrocartilaginous pseudotumor
f. plate
f. ring
f. ring of tympanic membrane
f. tissue
triangular fibrocartilaginous complex
fibrocystic
f. breast
f. breast disease
f. change
f. disease
f. disease of breast
f. disease of the pancreas
f. dysplasia
f. mastitis
fibrodysplasia ossificans progressiva
fibroelastic
f. cartilage
f. connective tissue
dense fibroelastic connective tissue
loose fibroelastic connective tissue
f. membrane
f. tissue
fibroelastoma
papillary f.
fibroelastosis
endocardial f.
fibrofatty
f. plaque
f. tissue
fibrofibrinous adhesion
fibrohistiocytic
eosinophilic fibrohistiocytic lesion of bone marrow
hemosiderotic fibrohistiocytic lipomatous lesion
marrow
fibrohistiocytoma
malignant f.
fibroid
f. adenoma
f. degeneration
f. embolization
f. heart
f. induration
inflammatory fibroid polyp
intramural f.
pedunculated f.
f. polyp
subserosal f.
subserous f.
symptomatic f.
uterine f.
fibrointimal hyperplasia

fibrolamellar
f. hepatocellular carcinoma

fibrolamellar hepatocellular carcinoma

fibrolipoma
massive f.
myxoid f.

fibrolipomatosis
macrodactylia f.

fibroma
ameloblastic f.
cementoossifying f.
chondromyxoid f.
f. durum
granular cell ameloblastic f.
malignant rabbit fibroma virus
f. molle
nasopharyngeal f.
nonossifying f.
ossifying bone f.
osteogenic bone f.
perifollicular f.
peripheral ameloblastic f.
recurring digital fibroma of childhood

fibromatosis
desmoid-type f.
gingival fibromatosis, hypertrichosis, cherubism, mental retardation, epilepsy syndrome
multiple congenital f.
retroperitoneal f.

fibromuscular
f. dysplasia
f. hyperplasia
f. junction

fibromyalgia
elderly f.
F. Impact Questionnaire
posttraumatic fibromyalgia syndrome
primary f.
primary fibromyalgia syndrome
f. syndrome

fibromyoadenomatous hyperplasia

fibromyoma uteri

fibromyxoid
low-grade fibromyxoid sarcoma
pseudosarcomatous fibromyxoid tumor

fibronectin
fetal f.
immunoreactive f.
plasma f.

fibroosseous pseudotumor

fibroplasia
idiopathic f.
retrolental f.

fibroplastica
endocarditis parietalis f.
gastritis granulomatosa f.

fibroproliferative
obliterative fibroproliferative bronchiolitis

fibropurulent
acute fibropurulent pneumonia

fibrosa
appendix f.
meninx f.
myodysplasia fibrosa multiplex
myositis f.
osteitis f.
pericardium f.

fibrosarcoma
congenital f.
congenital infantile f.
feline fibrosarcoma virus
f. of soft tissue

fibrosarcomatous variant of dermatofibrosarcoma protuberans

fibrosclerosis
multifocal f.

fibrosing
f. alopecia in a pattern distribution
f. alveolitis
arterial fibrosing sclerosis
f. cholestatic hepatitis
cryptogenic fibrosing alveolitis
diffuse interstitial fibrosing pneumonitis
frontal fibrosing alopecia
idiopathic fibrosing alveolitis

fibrosis
adenoassociated virus for cystic f.
apical lobe f.
asbestos-induced pleural f.
bauxite fibrosis of lung
cerebellar vermis hypoplasia, oligophrenia, congenital ataxia, coloboma, hepatic f.
chronic pulmonary interstitial f.
classic interstitial pneumonitis with f.
congenital hepatic f.
cystic fibrosis arthropathy
cystic fibrosis factor
cystic fibrosis factor activity
cystic fibrosis protein
cystic fibrosis transmembrane conductance regulator
diffuse interstitial fibrosis of the lung
diffuse interstitial pulmonary f.
early interstitial f.
endomyocardial f.
eosinophilic angiocentric f.
extensive interstitial f.
focal interstitial f.
focal subpleural interstitial f.
idiopathic alveolar f.
idiopathic interstitial pulmonary f.
idiopathic retroperitoneal f.
interstitial left ventricular myocardial f.
lymph node f.
myocardial f.
nodular subepidermal f.
noncirrhotic portal f.
obliterative granulomatous f.
oral submucous f.
pancreatic cystic f.
papillary muscle f.
patchy area of f.
patchy interstitial f.
progressive interstitial pulmonary f.
progressive massive f.
progressive perivenular alcoholic f.
pulmonary interstitial f.
radiation-induced f.
segmental bile duct f.
Symmers clay pipestem f.

fibrositis
chronic rheumatoid nodular f.

fibrosum
adenoma f.
lipoma f.
molluscum f.
molluscum fibrosum gravidarum
molluscum fibrosum pendulum
myxoma f.
pericardium f.

fibrosus
anulus f.
anulus fibrosus of aorta
anulus fibrosus dexter/sinister cordis
anulus fibrosus tear
anulus fibrosus of intervertebral disc
nucleus fibrosus lingua

fibrotic
f. change
f. focus
interstitial fibrotic change
f. lung disease

fibrous
f. adhesion
aneurysmal benign fibrous histiocytoma
angiomatoid malignant fibrous histiocytoma
ankle-type fibrous histiocytoma
anular part of fibrous digital sheath of digits of hand and foot
anulus of fibrous sheath
atypical benign fibrous histiocytoma
atypical fibrous histiocytoma
cellular cutaneous fibrous histiocytoma
central fibrous body
congenital fibrous histiocytoma
f. connective tissue
dense fibrous adhesion
dense fibrous lamina
dense fibrous tissue
dysgenetic fibrous band
f. dysplasia
f. dysplasia of the mandible
f. goiter
hyalinized fibrous tissue
indistinct semi-circumferential fibrous thickening
f. insulin
f. intimal thickening
f. joint
localized fibrous mesothelioma
localized fibrous tumor
f. long-spacing collagen
malignant fibrous histiocytoma
malignant fibrous histiocytoma of bone
malignant fibrous histiocytoma of soft tissue
malignant fibrous xanthoma
metaphysial fibrous cortical defect
metaphysial fibrous defect
monostotic fibrous dysplasia
nodular and diffuse fibrous proliferation
orbitozygomaticomaxillary fibrous dysplasia
outer fibrous layer
periprosthetic fibrous capsule
f. plaque
polyostotic fibrous dysplasia
f. proliferation
f. protein
right fibrous trigone
f. sheath
solitary fibrous tumor
f. synovium
f. tumor
f. union

fibrovascular
anterior hyaloidal fibrovascular proliferation
f. tissue elsewhere
f. tissue on disc

fibroxanthoma
atypical f.

fibula
anterior border of f.
anterior ligament of head of f.
apex of f.
apex of head of f.
articular facet of head of f.
articular surface of head of f.
f. free flap
head of f.
interosseous border of f.
ligaments of head of f.
malleolar articular surface of f.
medial crest of f.
neck of f.
nutrient artery of f.
posterior border of f.
shaft of f.
f. shortening
tibia and f.

fibular
f. allograft
allograft reconstruction of fibular collateral ligament
anomalous fibular nutrient artery
anterior fibular ligament
anterior ligament of fibular head
articular branch of deep fibular nerve
f. articular facet of tibia
f. articular surface of tibia
autogenous fibular graft
collateral fibular ligament
f. collateral ligament
f. collateral ligament of ankle
f. hemimelia
long fibular muscle
Maisonneuve fibular fracture
f. metaphysis
muscular branch of deep fibular nerve
nonvascularized fibular strut graft
f. notch
paraxial fibular hemimelia
pedicled fibular transfer
perforating branch of fibular artery
f. sesamoid
f. sesamoidectomy
f. transfer
f. transplant

fibularis
musculus fibularis brevis
musculus fibularis longus

fibulectomy
partial f.

fibulotalar arthrodesis

fibulotalocalcaneal ligament

Fick
anteroposterior axis of F.
axis of F.
F. bacillus
longitudinal axis of F.
F. method
F. principle
F. technique

Ficoll-Hypaque
F.-H. centrifugation
F.-H. technique

fidelity
lineage f.

fidgeting, aching, pulling, or itching feeling

fidgety leg syndrome

fiducial
f. alignment system

field
f. alignment
f. ambulance
arcuate field defect
arcuate visual field defect
asymptomatic visual field defect
attractor field therapy
auditory-evoked magnetic f.
automated visual f.
f. block
f. block anesthesia
center of field of vision
central visual f.
clear lung f.
computerized visual field machine
conductive radiofrequency electric f.
confrontation fields intact
confrontation of visual f.
confrontation visual field testing
constant electric f.

constant magnetic field in nuclear magnetic resonance
contour-clamped homogeneous electric f.
crystal field stabilization energy
crystal field theory
crystal ligand f.
f. cut
f. defect
f. desorption
f. of dissection
f. drift
electric f.
electric field mediated transfer
electric field stimulation
electric field vector
electromagnetic f.'s
electromagnetic focusing field probe
f. emission scanning electron microscopy
end of f.
en face irradiation f.
extended field radiation
extended field radiation therapy
fenestrated sterile field barrier
f. focused nuclear magnetic resonance
f.'s of Forel
four field technique
frontal eye f.
f. gain
glaucomatous visual field loss
good visual f.'s
gradient field transform
gradient magnetic f.
high dry f.
high-power f.
high-power field microscope
f. hospital
hospital field director
human lung f.
Humphrey visual f.
insulated gate field effect transistor
intensity of electric f.
involved f.
f. ion microscopy
large field of view
left visual f.
local field distortion
locoregional field radiotherapy
low-frequency current f.
low-power f.
magnetic f.
magnetic field strength
magnetic field vector
main field magnet
medial central tegmental f.
metal oxide semiconductor field effect transistor
minimal audible f.
minimum acceptable f.
minimum audible f.
monocular confrontation visual field test
monocular field defect
narrowing of visual f.
nasal field loss
near field scanning optical microscope
nonphysiologic visual field loss
nucleus of dorsal f.
occipital eye f.
oil immersion field microscopy
operative field anesthetized
operative field anesthetized with 1% lidocaine
operative field prepared and draped
operative field prepped and draped
optic fundi and peripheral f.'s
organisms per high power f.
osteopathy in the cranial f.
paracentral visual f.
parietal lobe field defect
partial homonymous field defect
peripheral field image
peripheral visual f.
peripheral visual field loss
polymorphonuclear per low-power f.
pulsating electromagnetic f.
pulsed electromagnetic f.
f. of radiation
radiofrequency magnetic field in nuclear magnetic resonance
receptive field of visual cortex
red blood cells per high-power f.
relative centrifugal f.
right visual f.
sedimentation field flow fractionation
f. shift
shrinking field technique
f. size in half body irradiation
somatically evoked f.
sound f.
f. stimulation
temporal field of vision
Thought F. Therapy
f. training exercise
transmural electrical field stimulation
useful field of view
f. of view
f. of vision
f. of vision intact
visual f.
visual field cut
visual field defect
visual field deficit
visual field disturbance
visual field floater
visual field intact
visual field loss
visual field test
visual field testing
visual fields full to confrontation
visual fields by Goldmann-type perimeter
visually evoked f.
white blood cells per high-power f.
wide f.

field-echo sequence with even-echo rephasing

field-electrical neural stimulation

field-flow fractionation

fifth

f. cusp groove
first to fifth sacral nerves
first to fifth sacral vertebrae
first through fifth digits of hand
first through fifth lumbar vertebrae or lumbar nerve
f. intercostal space
lumbar fifth vertebra to sacral first vertebra
point of maximum impulse fifth intercostal space
tuberosity of fifth metatarsal
tuberosity of fifth metatarsal bone

fight

f., flee, freeze, or faint
f. or flight reaction

fight-and-flight response

fighting

f., injuries, sex, threats, self-defense

fight-or-flight

f.-o.-f. reaction
f.-o.-f. stress

Figurative

F. Language Interpretation Test

figure
authority figure fixation
Children's Embedded F.'s Test
Complex F. Test
Embedded F.'s Test
Goodenough F. Drawing
Group Embedded F.'s Test
Human F. Drawing
human figure parts response
matching familiar f.'s
Matching Familiar F.'s Test
f. of merit
mitotic f.
myelin f.
Rey-Estreich Complex F. Test
Rey-Estreich Complex F. Test
Rey-Osterrieth complex f.
Sorting of F.'s Test
Southern California F. Ground Test

figure-four position

figure-ground
auditory f.-g.

figure-of-eight
f.-o.-e. apparatus
f.-o.-e. cast
f.-o.-e. harness
f.-o.-e. splint
f.-o.-e. stitch
f.-o.-e. strapping
f.-o.-e. suture
f.-o.-e. suture technique
f.-o.-e. taping
f.-o.-e. wire
f.-o.-e. wire loop

figure-of-four test

Fiji disease virus

filament
intermediate f.
intermediate filament protein
f. keratitis
paired helical f.'s
region of sarcomere containing only myosin f.'s

filamentous
f. actin
f. hemagglutinin

filariasis
lymphatic f.
lymphatic filariasis granuloma
Malayan f.
occult f.
f. of orbit
periodic f.

file
case f.
Drug Master F.
Drug Product Information F.
end of f.
master apical f.
orthopaedic bone f.
patient treatment f.
temporary master apical f.

filed procedure in cardiac arrest

filial
first filial generation
f. generation
f. piety
second filial generation

filiform
f. and follower
f. lesion

filing
anticurvature f.
circumferential f.

fillant
liposuction fat fillant implant

filled
barium filled esophagus
decayed, missing, and filled teeth
f. voiding flow rate
fluid filled abdomen
fluid filled ganglion
ratio of decayed and filled surfaces
ratio of decayed and filled teeth
saline filled breast implant

filler
Multidex f.
omental f.

fillet
medial f.
osteocutaneous fillet flap

filling
antegrade filling of vessel
atrial filling fraction
atrial filling pressure
augmented filling of right ventricle
f. of the bladder
capillary filling time
f. cystometrogram
f. cystometry
f. defect
diastolic f.
diastolic filling period
esophageal filling defect
f. gallop
intraluminal filling defect
left ventricular fast filling time
left ventricular filling pressure
left ventricular peak filling rate
left ventricular slow filling time
lobulated filling defect
mean circulating filling pressure
multiple colon filling defect
multiple cone root canal filling method
PA filling pressure
peak diastolic filling rate
peak early diastolic filling velocity
f. pressure
pulmonary artery filling defect
rapid f.
rapid filling period
rapid filling rate
rapid filling wave
reverse filling procedure
f. of right atrium
right ventricular filling pressure
right ventricular peak filling rate
root canal f.
slow filling wave
f. time
time to peak filling rate
time of peak filling rate of esophagus
venous filling time

fills
bowel fills and evacuates satisfactorily

film
additional f.
anteroposterior f.
aqueous layer of tear f.
check f.
chest x-ray f.
contraceptive f.
focal film distance
focus film distance
forced inversion film of ankle
gallbladder f.
high abdominal plain f.
lateral decubitus f.
malaria film test
measurement f.
noninvasive tear film break-up time
normal chest f.
occlusal f.
occlusal film radiography
organic conditioning f.
PA chest f.
periapical f.

plain film of abdomen
polyurethane f.
portable f.
portable film of abdomen
posteroanterior f.
postreduction f.
postvoiding f.
preliminary film of abdomen
preocular tear f.
review of outside f.
scoliosis f.
scout f.
f. screen radiography
semipermeable f.
semiupright f.
source film distance
spine spot f.
thin film dressing
upright chest f.
upright film of abdomen
vaginal contraceptive f.
wet f.
x-ray f.

filmy adhesion

Filoviridae virus

filter
antiglare f.
ARI Group I–IV f.
centrifuged microaggregate f.
electrosurgical f.
Greenfield vena cava f.
heat and moisture exchanging f.
heparin arterial f.
high-efficiency particulate air f.
high-frequency filter control
high-pass f.
high pass f.
hollow filter dialyzer
inferior vena cava f.
Kimray-Greenfield filter
leukoreduction f.
membrane filter technique
millipore filter method
neutral density filter test
f. paper
f. paper activity
f. paper microscopic test
polysulfone f.
red blood cell filter ability
vena caval f.

filterable
f. agent
f. air
f. hemolytic anemia

filtered
f. air
f. atrial rate interval
F. Audiometer Speech Test
f. hot air
f. load
f. mass
not f.
f. phosphate
silica gel f.
f. smoke exposure
f. sodium

filtering
antialias f.
glaucoma filtering surgery
perceptual f.
f. scotoma

filtrate
capillary filtrate collector
Clostridium difficile culture f.
Escherichia coli f.
glomerular f.
tuberculin f.

filtration
air filtration machine
air filtration system
amphotericin B-induced reduction glomerular filtration rate
blood filtration rate
cascade f.
dialysate filtration rate
double filtration plasmapheresis
effective filtration pressure
effective filtration rate
endolymph filtration and excretion
f. factor
f. fraction
glomerular f.
low absolute glomerular filtration rate
membrane filtration method
peripheral capillary filtration slit length
f. rate
rate of fluid f.
red blood cell spun f.
renal reserve filtration capacity
f. replacement fluid
screen filtration pressure
single antibody millipore f.
single-nephron glomerular filtration rate
tangential flow f.
urine filtration rate

filtrum
Merkel filtrum ventriculi

filum
olfactory f.
tight filum terminale

fimbria, pl. **fimbriae**
mushrooming of f.
ovarian f.
fimbriae of ovarian tube
fimbriae of uterine tube

fimbrial
f. adhesion
f. ectopic pregnancy
f. hemagglutinin

fimbriated
f. end of fallopian tube
f. end of oviduct

final
f. common pathway
F. Comprehensive Consensus Assessment
f. consonant
f. consonant deletion
f. consonant position
deletion of final consonant
f. diagnosis
f. drug evaluation
f. impression
f. nitrogen
f. outcome
f. printed labeling

financial class

finder
angle f.
canal f.

finding
accessory clinical f.
angiographic f.
associated laboratory f.
associated physical examination f.
atypical f.
auscultatory f.
dearth of f.'s
empirical f.
essential f.
incidental f.
mammographic f.
manometric f.
motor f.
negative f.
neurophysiological f.
neuropsychologic f.
no discernible f.
f. of no significant impact
object f.
objective f.
operative f.
pathologic f.

finding *(continued)*
pathological f.
paucity of f.'s
pelvic f.
pertinent physical f.'s
physical f.
prognostic f.
sensory f.
subjective f.
tentative f.
Test of Adolescent/Adult Word F.
Test of Word F.
Test of Word F. in Discourse
x-ray f.

fine
f. crepitant rales
extended electron-loss line fine structure
extended x-ray absorption fine structure spectroscopy
few fine rales
f. fiber
f. fraction
f. hair
f. hair movement
f. hand dexterity
f. inspiratory crackle
interrupted fine silk suture
f. intestinal needle
medium fine bur
f. mesh gauze
moistened fine mesh gauze dressing
f. motor
f. motor activity
f. motor coordination
f. motor development
f. motor function
f. motor movement
f. motor skill
f. periosteal elevator
f. postural tremor
f. rapid nystagmus
f. structure
surface extended x-ray absorption fine structure
f. suspended particulate
f. tactile sensation

finely granular

Fineman
D'Aoust Fineman virus

fine-needle
f.-n. aspirate
f.-n. aspiration
f.-n. aspiration biopsy
f.-n. aspiration cytology
f.-n. biopsy
f.-n. catheter jejunostomy
f.-n. percutaneous cholangiogram
f.-n. transhepatic cholangiogram
f.-n. transhepatic cholangiography

fineness
degree of fineness of abrasive particles

fine-tooth
f.-t. electric saw

fine-toothed
f.-t. clamp
f.-t. forceps

finger
f.'s above umbilicus
f. arterial blood pressure
articulation of f.'s
avulsion of portion of f.
f.'s below
f. clubbing
clubbing of f.
congenital onychodysplasia of the index f.
count f.'s
f. count, both eyes
counting f.'s
f. counting
Digital F. Tapping Test
dynamic finger exerciser
f. extension test
f. flexion
f. jerk
f. joint size
left index f.
left middle f.
left ring f.
long arm finger cast
mallet finger deformity
mallet finger orthotic
MCP finger joint prosthesis
middle finger amputation
Nelson finger exerciser
numbness of f.
numbness and tingling in f.
obesity, short stature, mental deficiency, hypogonadism, micropenis, finger contracture, cleft lip-palate syndrome
O'Connor finger dexterity test
opposing muscle of little f.
F. Oscillation Test
f. oximeter
promyelocytic leukemia zinc f.
f. pulp
f. ray
replantation of f.
right index f.
right middle f.
rotational deformity of f.
septic finger joint
swan-neck finger deformity
f. systolic blood pressure
Tactile F. Recognition Test
f. tension
Therapy Carrot finger contracture orthosis
f. trap traction
trigger finger release
f. tuft
vibration-induced white f.
web of f.
zinc finger protein

finger-assisted malar elevation

fingerbreadth
f. below right costal margin
one fingerbreadth above umbilicus
one fingerbreadth below umbilicus

finger-counting vision test

finger-in-glove appearance

fingernail
cyanosis of f.
gnarled f.

finger-nose-finger
f.-n.-f. coordination test
f.-n.-f. test

finger-nose test

fingerprint
high-resolution f.

fingerprinting
direct amplification f.
oral epithelial cell genetic f.

fingerstick
f. blood gas
f. blood glucose
f. blood sample
f. blood sugar
f. device
f. test

fingertip
f. blood
cyanosis of f.
mental retardation, congenital contracture, low fingertip arches syndrome
outstretched f.
f. unit

fingertips-to-floor test

finger-to-finger-to-nose test

finger-to-nose
f.-t.-n. coordination test
f.-t.-n. testing

fingertrap
f. suspension
f. traction

finish
antipill f.

finished
until f.

finishing
feathered edge proximal f.

finite
f. element method
f. element stress analysis

Finkelstein test

Finney pyloroplasty

Finochietto stirrup

Finsen
F. lamp
F. unit

fire
nosocomial f.
Saint Anthony f.
f. setter
simulated aircraft fire and emergency
St. Anthony f.

fire-related injury

firing
high-voltage f.
low biscuit f.
low bisque f.
medium biscuit f.
medium bisque f.
neuromuscular f.
neuromuscular firing in normal subject
neuromuscular firing in spastic subject
neuronal element f.

firm
f. and atelectatic
bilateral firm hand grips
breast firm and lactating
f. and equal
fundus f.
fundus firm 1, 2 cm above umbilicus
fundus firm 1, 2 cm below umbilicus
fundus firm at umbilicus
f. and midline uterus

firmness
excessive breast firmness and discomfort

first
advanced first aid
age at first intercourse
f. aid
f. aid instruction
f. in alpha series or group
aortic first sound
f. auditory area
f. component of complement
cumulative duration of the first remission
f. cuneiform bone
f. day of last menstrual period
f. definite apical clearance lens
f. digital interosseous muscle
f. dorsal interosseous
f. dorsal metatarsal artery
error of the first kind
f. to fifth sacral nerves
f. to fifth sacral vertebrae
f. filial generation
f. to fourth heart sounds
f. full-term pregnancy
healing by first, second, or third intention
f. heart sound
f. impression
intention
f. jejunal vein
lithium action on first messenger
lumbar fifth vertebra to sacral first vertebra
f. lumbar ventral nerve root
f. malignant neoplasm
maxillary first molar alveolus
Mendel first law
f. menstrual period
f. metatarsal head
f. morning urine
navicular to first metatarsal angle
nonprimary first episode
f. obtuse marginal artery
f. obtuse marginal branch
f. parental generation
f. pass
f. plantar metatarsal artery
psychological first aid
f. rank symptom
f. responder
risk of first heart attack
f. set of followup data
f. stage of anesthesia
f. stage of labor
f. through fifth digits of hand
f. through fifth lumbar vertebrae or lumbar nerve
f. through fourth heart sounds
f. through twelfth dorsal vertebrae
tricuspid first heart sound
f. to twelfth thoracic nerves
f. to twelfth thoracic vertebrae
f. twitch height
f. voided bladder specimen
wound healed by first, second or third intention
X-linked first site of fragility

first-degree
f.-d. arteriovenous block
f.-d. burn
f.-d. heart block

first-dose reaction

first-pass
f.-p. effect
f.-p. metabolism
f.-p. nuclear angiocardiography
f.-p. radionuclide angiogram

first-phase insulin response

first-stage repair

first-trimester
f.-t. abortion
f.-t. bleeding
f.-t. maternal seizure

first-use syndrome

first-void urine

fiscal
f. intermediary
f. year

Fischer
modified Fischer classification
F. sign

fish
f. eye disease
f. mouth incision
f. protein concentrate

Fisher
F. exact test
Miller Fisher syndrome

Fisher-John melting point method

Fisher-Race notation

fishhook lead

fishmouth
f. amputation
f. anastomosis
f. cervix
f. configuration of mitral valve
f. incision

fishmouth *(continued)*
f. meatus
Pulvertaft fishmouth incision

fishnet pattern

fishtail
modified fishtail excision

fissurata
lingua f.

fissure
f. in ano
anterior interhemispheric f.
anterior median f.
anterior median fissure of medulla oblongata
anterior median fissure of spinal cord
choroid f.
dentate straight fissure bur
dentate tapered fissure bur
digital anomalies, short palpebral fissures, atresia of esophagus or duodenum syndrome
downsloping palpebral f.
great horizontal f.
great transverse fissure of cerebrum
Henle f.'s
interhemispheric f.
longitudinal cerebral f.
longitudinal fissure of cerebrum
medial canthal f.
mild down-slant to palpebral f.
narrow fissure bur
oblique fissure of lung
orbital fissure width
orbital superior f.
palatine bone f.
palpebral fissure height
palpebral fissure inclination
palpebral fissure length
palpebral fissure widening
f. of Rolando
f. of Santorini
superior orbital f.
superior orbital fissure syndrome
f. of Sylvius

fissured
f. tongue
f. tongue syndrome

fist
arteriovenous f.
clenched fist sign

fistula
antecubital arteriovenous f.
anterior rectoperineal f.
aorta-left ventricular f.
aorta-right ventricular f.
aortic sinus f.
aortic sinus to right ventricle f.
aortoduodenal f.
aortoenteric fistula formation
aortograft duodenal f.
arteriosinusoidal penile f.
arteriovenous f.
arteriovenous fistula malformation
arteriovenous fistula transplant
arteriovenous fistula with good bruits
arteriovenous internal mammary f.
arteriovenous subclavian f.
bradycardia after arteriovenous fistula occlusion
bronchoesophageal f.
bronchopleural f.
bronchopleurocutaneous f.
carotid-cavernous sinus f.
closure of tracheal f.
coronary artery f.
coronary-pulmonary f.
digestive-respiratory f.
dural arteriovenous f.
dural carotid-cavernous f.
esophagorespiratory f.
gastric f.
graft enteric f.
mesenteric arteriovenous f.
microcephaly, mesobrachyphalangy, tracheoesophageal fistula syndrome
oozing of f.
oral anal f.
palatal fistula closure
pancreatic cutaneous f.
perianal fistula abscess
perilymphatic f.
perilymphatic fistula syndrome
peripheral arteriovenous f.
persistent bronchopleural f.
pulmonary arteriovenous f.
spinal dural arteriovenous f.
Thiry-Vella f.
thoracic duct f.
tracheoesophageal f.
tracheoesophageal fistula, esophageal atresia, multiple congenital anomaly syndrome
f. tract
urinary bladder f.
vertebral abnormality, anal imperforation, tracheoesophageal fistula, and radial, ray, or renal anomalies
vesicovaginal f.
vesicovaginal fistula repair

fistulation
artificial f.

fistulotomy
needle-knife f.

fistulous
arteriovenous fistulous malformation
incision and drainage of fistulous tract
f. tract

fit
arrest/akinetic f.
f. to be detained
custom fit in ear unit
improper fit of dentures
mixed flexor/extensor f.
not fit for duty
parental f.

fitness
health and f.
maternal f.
National Association for Health & F.
physical f.

fittest
survival of the f.

fitting
immediate postoperative prosthetic f.
immediate postsurgical fitting of prosthesis
poorly fitting dentures

Fitz-Hugh-Curtis syndrome

five
Big F. Questionnaire
f. times a day
f. times a week

five-chamber transverse

five-factor score

five-finger movement

five-minute format

five-year
f.-y. cure rate
f.-y. survival rate

fixate and follow

fixation
adjunctive screw f.
angled blade plate f.
anterior C1-C2 screw f.

anterior cervical plate fixation system
anterior internal f.
anterior metallic f.
anterior plate f.
anterior screw f.
anterior spinal f.
AO external f.
AO spinal internal f.
arch bar f.
arthroscopic screw f.
arum fixation pin
assisted reduction and internal f.
atlantoaxial rotary f.
atlantoaxial rotatory f.
authority figure f.
autoimmune complement f.
4-bar external f.
4-bar external fixation apparatus
4-bar external fixation device
biodegradable fixation device
biodegradable fixation instrumentation
cardiolipin complement f.
central, steady and maintained f.
cerclage wire f.
cervical spine screw-plate f.
chevron osteotomy with rigid screw f.
closed reduction and internal f.
closed reduction and percutaneous pin f.
complement f.
complement fixation antibody test
complement fixation inhibition
complex f.
compression plate f.
condylar screw f.
coracoclavicular screw f.
coracoclavicular suture f.
dorsal wire-loop f.
dynamic compression plate f.
eccentric f.
endoforehead fixation technique
European compression technique bone screw and internal f.
external skeletal f.
fabere fixation test
failure of fixation suppression
femoral prosthesis f.
flexible intramedullary f.
f. fluid
f. graft
immunodiffusion complement f.
insertion of fixation device
intermaxillary f.
internal fixation of fracture
intramedullary fixation device
intramedullary rod f.
iris fixation lens
latex f.
latex fixation test
lesion on erythrocyte cell membrane at the site of complement f.
line of f.
locus of f.
lymphogranuloma venereum complement fixation test
mandibulomaxillary f.
maxillomandibular f.
microcomplement f.
myoma fixation instrument
near fixation position of gaze
odontoid fracture internal f.
open reduction and external f.
open reduction and internal f.
open reduction metallic f.
os calcis pin f.
Peak F. System
phalangeal fracture f.
platelet complement fixation test
plate and screw fixation of fracture
point of f.
f. protein
rapid plasma reagin complement f.
rigid internal f.
scoliotic curve f.
f. and sectioning of the brain
spinopelvic transiliac f.
standard fixation preference test
tantalum wire f.
tension band f.
Treponema pallidum complement f.
uterine positioning via ligament investment fixation truncation

fixative
mercuric f.
methanol f.
neutral buffered formalin f.
osmic acid f.
polyvinyl alcohol f.

fixator
AO internal f.
cantilever external f.
carbon fiber f.
circular wire f.
dynamic axial f.
external spinal skeletal f.
Ganz anti-shock pelvic f.
half-pin external f.
one-plane bilateral external f.
Vermont spinal f.

fixator-augmented nailing

fixed
f. action pattern
cantilever fixed partial denture
f. cell immunofluorescence
conjugate fixed gaze
f. and dilated
f. and dilated pupil
f. drug eruption
f. erythrocyte turnover
f. flexion contracture
f. frequency response
f. ideas
f. interval
f. mandibular implant
f. parenchymal turnover
f. partial denture
f. P-R interval
f. pupil
pupils mid-position, f.
f. rate pacemaker
f. ratio
f. ratio combination drugs
f. segment of bowel
f. slit lamp

fixed-dose
f.-d. patient-controlled analgesia
f.-d. procedure

fixes and follows

fixing
complement f.
f. fluid
f. left eye
prothrombin time fixing agent
f. right eye

fixture
osseointegrated f.

FK-binding
FK-b. protein 12
FK-b. protein rapamycin-associated protein

flaccid
acute flaccid paralysis
ascending flaccid paralysis
f. gait
f. hemiplegia
f. leg
f. paralysis
f. tone

flaccida
membrana f.
pars f.
pars flaccida defect

flag
axial flag flap

flail
f. chest
f. digit
f. foot
f. joint
f. mitral leaflet
f. segment
f. shoulder

flair valve

Flajani operation

flaking
periungual f.

flame
f. emission spectroscopy
f. ionization
f. ionization detector
multielectrode flame ionization detector
osteolytic f.
f. photometric detector

flame-shaped hemorrhage

Flanagan
F. Aptitude Classification Test
F. Industrial Test

Flanders virus

flange
lingual f.

flank
acute flank pain
anterior retroperitoneal flank approach
f. incision
lateral flank incision
subcostal flank incision

flap
f. of abdominal tissue
adipofascial axial pattern cross-finger f.
adipofascial sural f.
adipofascial turnover f.
advancement flap graft
advancement of rectal f.
advancement sleeve f.
allogenically vascularized prefabricated f.
antegrade island f.
anterior chest wall f.
anterior helical rim free f.
anterior myocutaneous f.
anterior quadriceps musculocutaneous flap technique
anterior skin f.
anterior tibial fasciocutaneous f.
anterolateral thigh free f.
Antia-Buch chondrocutaneous advancement f.
Antia-Buch helical rim advancement f.
apically repositioned flap in mucogingival surgery
apron flap procedure
arc of rotation of fasciocutaneous f.
artery island f.
Atasoy-Kleinert volar V-Y advancement f.
Atasoy palmar f.
Atasoy triangular advancement f.
Atasoy-type flap for nail injury repair
Atasoy volar V-Y f.
Atasoy V-Y advancement f.
autologous tissue f.
avulsion flap injury
axial dorsal f.
axial flag f.
axial frontonasal f.
axial pattern scalp f.
axial pattern vascularized skin f.
axial temporoparietal fascial f.
bilateral inferior epigastric artery f.
bladder flap elevated
bladder flap tube
breast mound reduction and nipple reconstruction with wraparound f.
cataract flap operation
crescent-shaped flap of tissue
deep circumflex iliac artery f.
delayed transfer f.
dermal fat free f.
distally based fasciocutaneous f.
end of bone covered with f.
endorectal advancement f.
expanded free scalp f.
extended lateral arm free f.
extended V-Y advancement f.
extensor carpi radialis longus f.
fasciocutaneous axial pattern f.
fibula free f.
free forearm f.
free transverse rectus abdominis musculocutaneous f.
free transverse rectus abdominis myocutaneous f.
galeal frontalis f.
galeal myofascial f.
galeal occipital f.
galeal periosteal f.
glabellar rotation f.
gluteal free f.
gluteus maximus musculocutaneous f.
great toe wraparound f.
horseshoe-shaped skin f.
immediate transfer f.
inverted horseshoe f.
jejunal free f.
latissimus dorsi fasciocutaneous f.
latissimus dorsi musculocutaneous f.
latissimus dorsi myocutaneous f.
lingual tongue f.
liver flap sign
local tissue advancement f.
lower abdominal f.
lower cheek f.
low flap cesarean section
low flap transverse
lytic area bone f.
maple leaf f.
Marchac dorsal nasal f.
Marchac glabella f.
Martius bulbocavernosus fat f.
Martius flap and fascial sling
maxillectomy cheek f.
McCraw gracilis myocutaneous f.
McFarlane skin f.
McGregor forehead f.
medial cutaneous thigh f.
medial distally based fasciocutaneous f.
mesiolabial bilobed transposition f.
microsurgical free f.
microsurgical free pulp f.
microvascular free f.
microvascular free flap transfer
microvascular free muscle f.
microvascular free posterior interosseous f.
midface avulsion f.
midline cross-lip Abbe f.
midline forehead f.
Millard advancement rotation flap reconstruction
Millard forked flap technique
Moberg advancement f.
modified double-opposing tab flap nipple reconstruction
modified flap operation
mucoperiosteal flap technique
mucoperiosteal flap trimming
mucosal bipedicle f.
musculocutaneous flap harvest
musculocutaneous free f.

Mustardé rotational cheek f.
neurosensorial free medial plantar f.
neurovascular free f.
nontubed closed distant flap graft
open flap drainage
open flap technique
osteocutaneous fillet f.
osteomusculocutaneous deep circumflex iliac groin f.
osteomyocutaneous free f.
osteoplastic bone f.
osteoplastic flap clamp
palmar advancement f.
palmar cross-finger f.
paramedian forehead f.
parietal bone f.
partial conjunctival f.
pectoralis major myocutaneous f.
pedicled buccal fat pad f.
pedicled compound rib-latissimus dorsi osteomusculocutaneous f.
pedicled fascia lata musculocutaneous f.
pedicled galeal frontalis f.
pedicled groin f.
pedicle flap operation
pedicle flap urethroplasty
perialar crescentic advancement f.
perineal artery axial f.
peroneus brevis f.
posterior auricular f.
radial forearm free f.
rectus abdominis free f.
rectus abdominis muscle f.
rectus abdominis musculocutaneous f.
rectus abdominis myocutaneous f.
rectus femoris muscle f.
reversed digital artery f.
reversed dorsal digital f.
reverse flow island f.
reverse forearm island f.
rotary door f.
sequential free f.
serratus anterior muscle f.
skin-muscle free f.
subclavian flap aortoplasty
submucosal aponeurotic system f.
tailoring of f.
temporoparietal fascial f.
total conjunctival f.
f. transplant technique
transverse rectus abdominis musculocutaneous f.
transverse rectus abdominis musculoperitoneal f.
trapezoidal paddle pectoralis major myocutaneous f.
tubed pedicle f.
upper abdominal f.
upper arm f.
vascularized double-sided preputial island flap and W flap glanuloplasty hypospadias repair
V-Y advancement f.
Waldhausen subclavian flap technique
Wookey neck f.
Zimany bilobed f.

flapping
hand f.

flare
aqueous flare response
cell and f.
f. cell
f. and cell
laser cell and flare meter
laser flare meter
f. response
wheal and f.

flared
anterior flared tooth
f. spinal rod

flaring
f. of alae nasi
f. of ala nasi
alar f.
f. and grunting
grunting and f.
grunting, flaring, and retracting breathing
metaphyseal f.
nasal f.

flash
hot f.
hot or cold f.
hot flash trigger
intermittent flash of light
isolated flash of light
menopausal hot f.
onset of flashes and floaters
primary flash distillate

flashback
combat f.
marijuana f.
f. reaction with hallucinogen

flashing lights and/or scotoma

flashlamp pulsed dye laser

flashlamp-pumped pulsed dye laser

flask
f. culture
volumetric f.

flask-shaped heart

flat
abdomen f.
f. affect
f. back syndrome
blunted or flat affect
f. feet
f. hand
hereditary flat adenoma syndrome
f. hook
f. jugular vein
lumbar flat back syndrome
metatarsal flat head
patient has flat affect
f. plate
f. plate of abdomen
f. plate radiography
soft and f.
f. splint

flat-bladed nasal speculum

flatfoot
adult acquired f.
metatarsal flatfoot bar
Miller flatfoot operation
modified Hoke-Miller flatfoot procedure
rigid flatfoot deformity
rockerbottom flatfoot deformity

flatness
malar f.

flattener
beam f.

flattening
affective f.
emotional f.
f. of normal lordotic curve
occipital f.
T-wave f.

flatulence
coughing with f.

flatus
passage of f.
passage of flatus per vagina
passing f.

flatworm
parasitic f.

flava
macula f.

flavin
f. adenine dinucleotide
f. mononucleotide
f. phosphate, reduced

flavin *(continued)*
reduced form of flavin mononucleotide

flavin-containing mono-oxygenase metabolic system

flavone acetic acid

flavonidic
micronized flavonidic fraction

flavonoid
micronized purified flavonoid fracture

flavoprotein
electron transfer f.
electron transfer flavoprotein dehydrogenase

flaw
perioral f.

flea
northern rat f.
northern rat flea bite

flea-bitten kidney

Flechsig
oval area of F.

fleck of barium

flecked retinopathy

flee
fight, flee, freeze, or faint

fleeting illusion

Fleischer dystrophy

Fleischmann hygroma

flesh
goose f.
goosebump f.

fleshy
soft fleshy lesion
soft fleshy nodule

fleshy growth

Fletcher
F. afterloading colpostat
F. afterloading tandem

Fletcher-Suit
F.-S. afterloading ovoids
F.-S. afterloading tandem

Flexal virus

flexed
f., rotated, sidebent
hand flexed at wrist
neck passively f.
volar flexed intercalated segment instability
well f.

flexibility
improved f.
increased f.
joint f.
mental f.
f. training
trunk and hip f.

flexible
f. bronchoscope
f. endoscope
f. endoscopic evaluation of swallowing
f. endoscopic evaluation of swallowing with sensory testing
f. endoscopic swallowing examination
f. fiberoptic
f. fiberoptic bronchoscopy
f. fiberoptic bronchoscopy with protected brush
f. fiberoptic choledochoscope
f. fiberoptic endoscope
f. fiberoptic sigmoidoscopy
f. fluoropolymer
f. forceps
f. forward-viewing panendoscope
f. gastroscope
f. glass fiberglass
f. hinge implant
f. intramedullary fixation
f. intramedullary nail
f. medullary nail
f. medullary reamer
multiple flexible medullary nail
f. nephroscope
f. orthosis
f. sigmoidoscope
f. silicone implant
solid ankle flexible endoskeletal
f. sound
f. spiral wire retainer
stationary ankle flexible endoskeleton
stationary attachment flexible endoskeletal
f. ureteroscope
f. video laparoscope

flexion
angle of greatest f.
anterior acute flexion elbow splint
f. body cast
f. body jacket
compression flexion injury
f. contracture
f. contracture of hip
f. crease
degree of f.
f. distraction
elbow flexion contracture
elongation, derotation and lateral f.
f. and extension
external rotation in f.
finger f.
fixed flexion contracture
f., abduction, external rotation
f., abduction, external rotation contracture
f., abduction, external rotation, extension
f., extension, and rotation
forced flexion injury
forced passive full forward f.
forced plantar f.
forearm flexion control strap
forward f.
forward flexion posture
further f.
hand splinted in f.
f. injury posterior atlantoaxial arthrodesis
internal rotation in f.
left lateral f.
metatarsal-phalangeal flexion deformity
normal flexion of great toe
paraplegia in f.
passive flexion of leg
plantar f.
plantar flexion of foot
f. reflex testing
Regen flexion exercise
shoulder horizontal f.
variable flexion overhinge
wrist flexion reflex
wrist flexion test

flexion-burst fracture

flexion-compression
f.-c. fracture
f.-c. spine injury stabilization

flexion-extension
f.-e. axis
f.-e. control cervical orthosis
f.-e. exercise
hip f.-e.
f.-e. injury
knee f.-e.

flexion-rotation-compression maneuver

flexion-rotation-drawer knee instability test

flexor
anterior long toe f.
f. carpi radialis
f. carpi radialis brevis
f. carpi ulnaris
f. digiti minimi muscle
f. digiti quinti brevis
f. digiti quinti muscle
f. digitorum brevis
f. digitorum communis
f. digitorum longus
f. digitorum profundus muscle
f. digitorum profundus tendon
f. digitorum quinti brevis
f. hallucis brevis
f. hallucis brevis muscle
f. hallucis longus
f. hinge orthosis
f. hinge splint
increased flexor tone
long flexor muscle of great toe
long flexor muscle of thumb
medial flexor muscle of forearm
musculus biceps flexor cruris
musculus flexor brevis hallucis
musculus flexor carpi radialis
musculus flexor carpi ulnaris
musculus flexor digiti minimi brevis manus
musculus flexor digiti minimi brevis pedis
musculus flexor hallucis brevis
musculus flexor hallucis longus
musculus flexor pollicis brevis
musculus flexor pollicis longus
neck flexor tendon
paradoxical flexor reflex
plantar flexor reflex
f. plantar response
f. pollicis
f. pollicis brevis
pollicis brevis flexor muscle
f. pollicis longus
pollicis longus flexor muscle
postoperative flexor tendon
f. profundus
profundus flexor digitorum muscle
profundus flexor digitorum tendon
f. profundus tendon
tendo Achillis lengthening and toe flexor release
f. tendon
f. tendon adhesion
f. tendon anastomosis
f. tendon graft
f. tendon grafting
f. tendon laceration
f. tendon repair
f. tendon rupture
f. tendon sheath
f. tenosynovectomy
f. tenosynovitis
f. tenotomy

flexorextensor
mixed flexor/extensor fit

flexor-hinge hand-splint brace

flexure
anorectal f.
f. of colon
f. of duodenum
hepatic f.
hepatic flexure of colon
iliac flexure of colon
lumbar f.
mesencephalic f.
perineal f.
perineal flexure of anal canal
perineal flexure of rectum
permanent flexure contracture
pontine f.
f. of rectum
sacral f.
sigmoid f.
sigmoid flexure of colon
sphincter of hepatic flexure of colon
splenic f.
splenic flexure syndrome
superior duodenal f.

flicker
critical flicker fusion
f. fusion frequency test
f. fusion threshold

flight
airline flight radiation
f. aptitude rating
fight or flight reaction
f. from reality
f. of ideas
f. into disease
f. into fantasy
f. into health
f. into illness
f. medicine clinic
f. nurse

flint
Austin Flint murmur
Austin Flint phenomenon
Austin Flint respiration
F. Colon Injury Scale
F. Infant Security Scale

flip
partial flip angle imaging

flipped
f. T wave
f. T-wave

flipper hand

flirtatious behavior

flirting and coquetting

float
vertical float aquatic therapy
vertical float progression aquatic therapy

floater
meniscus f.
onset of flashes and f.'s
pigment f.
visual f.
visual field f.
vitreous f.

floating
f. harbor syndrome
f. hospital
f. mass transducer
f. rib
f. spherical gaussian orbital

flocculation
bentonite flocculation test
cardiolipin flocculation test
cardiolipin micro f.
cephalin-cholesterol f.
cephalin flocculation test
cholesterol-lecithin f.
Hinton flocculation test for syphilis
latex flocculation test
limit of f.
limit flocculation unit
liver flocculation test
nontreponemal flocculation test
f. rate in antigen-antibody reaction
thymol f.
zinc flocculation test

floccule
toxoid-antitoxin f.
toxoid-antitoxoid f.

flocculus
peduncle of f.

floor
diabetic floor routine
general medical f.
f. of inguinal canal
leave on f.
f. manager
maternal floor infarction

floor *(continued)*
f. of mouth
orbital floor blow-out
orbital floor fracture
orbital floor implant
orbital floor plate
orbital floor prosthesis
orbital floor syndrome
pelvic floor descent
pelvic floor disorder
pelvic floor dysfunction
pelvic floor dyssynergia
pelvic floor electrical stimulation
pelvic floor electromyography
pelvic floor movement
pelvic floor muscle
pelvic floor muscle exercise
pelvic floor nerve
pelvic floor pressure
pelvic floor relaxation
pelvic floor syndrome
pelvic floor weakness
regular nursing f.
relaxed pelvic f.

flopping tremor

floppy
f. aortic valve
f. infant
infant f.
f. infant syndrome
f. larynx
f. mitral valve

flora
aerobic microbial f.
gastrointestinal bacterial f.
mixed aerobic and anaerobic f.
natural bacterial f.
normal gut f.
normal throat f.
usual throat f.

floral
f. variant of follicular lymphoma
nectary of floral unit

florid
f. congestive heart failure
f. cutaneous papillomatosis
full florid diabetic retinopathy
f. local cementoosseous dysplasia
oral florid papillomatosis

flossing, brushing, and irrigation

flotation
f. constant
direct centrifugal f.
indirect centrifugal f.
Svedberg flotation unit

flounce
meniscal f.

flow
acceleration of blood f.
accessory pulmonary blood f.
adequate blood f.
adequate flow of blood
adventitious motor f.
antegrade bile f.
antegrade blood f.
antegrade diastolic f.
anterior cingulate f.
anterior-posterior flow direction
aortic f.
aortic blood flow velocity waveform
aortic flow volume
f. of aqueous humor
arterial renal plasma f.
f. artifact killer
atherosclerosis and blood f.
augment flow of blood
automated cardiac flow measurement
automated cardiac flow measurement ultrasound
autoregulation of cerebral blood f.
average flow rate
backward flow of blood
basal secretory flow rate
bias flow down
bile f.
bile acid independent f.
blocked blood f.
blood f.
f. of blood
blood flow to brain
blood flow from artery
blood flow from capillary
blood flow in heart
blood flow rate
blood flow velocity
blood flow velocity waveform
blood from flow heart to lungs
f. of blood and oxygen to heart
bronchial blood f.
calf blood f.
capillary blood f.
capillary blood flow velocity
carotid blood f.
cerebral blood f.
cerebral blood flow studies
cerebral blood flow velocity
cerebral blood volume/cerebral blood flow ratio
change in urine flow from constipation
choroidal blood f.
cochlear blood f.
collateral arterial flow to brain
collateral blood f.
color-coded flow mapping
color Doppler f.
color Doppler flow imaging
color flow Doppler
color flow Doppler imaging
color flow Doppler ultrasound
color flow imaging
color flow mapping
f. compensation
continuous flow ventilation
contralateral renal plasma f.
coronary f.
coronary blood f.
coronary blood flow velocity
coronary flow velocity reserve
coronary reserve f.
coronary sinus f.
coronary sinus blood f.
coronary slow flow syndrome
cortical blood f.
crevicular fluid flow rate
cyclic flow reduction
f. cytometric platelet
f. cytometry
f. cytometry crossmatch
dialysate f.
diminished blood f.
diversion of flow of blood
Doppler flow detector
Doppler flow study
Doppler flow test
dynamic cardiac blood f.
dynamic flow study
effective capillary f.
effective pulmonary blood f.
effective renal blood f.
effective renal plasma f.
electromagnetic blood flow imaging
end-diastolic f.
estimated hepatic blood f.
estimated liver blood f.
exercise hyperemia blood f.
expiratory flow volume
extrahepatic blood flow clearance
fasting intestinal flow rate
femoral artery blood f.
filled voiding flow rate
forced expiratory f.
forced expiratory flow volume
forced inspiratory f.

forced midexpiratory f.
forearm f.
forearm blood f.
fractional flow reserve
free flow electrophoresis
fresh gas f.
gastric mucosal blood f.
gingival blood f.
glomerular plasma f.
great cardiac vein f.
hand blood f.
Harris return f.
heart flow capacity
heavy menstrual f.
hemispheric blood f.
hepatic arterial f.
hepatic artery blood f.
hepatic blood f.
hepatic plasma f.
high f.
high air flow with oxygen entrainment
horizontal flow clean bench
horizontal laminar flow clean benches
hypothalamic blood f.
impairment of subendocardial blood f.
improved blood f.
inadequate blood f.
increased blood flow to ear
increased blood flow to heart muscle
increased cutaneous blood f.
increased flow rate
increased urinary f.
inner cortical blood f.
inspiratory flow cartridge
inspiratory flow rate
insufficient blood f.
insufficient blood flow to heart
intermittent flow centrifugation leukapheresis
internal carotid artery f.
interrupted urine f.
interruption of flow of urination
intracranial blood f.
intramyocardial coronary blood f.
intrinsic flow resistance
laminar air flow room
laminar air flow unit
left ventricular minute f.
limb blood f.
f. limitation
liver blood f.
liver plasma f.
local bone blood f.
local cerebral blood f.
low flow principle
low flow rate
maximal expiratory f.
maximal expiratory flow rate
maximal expiratory flow volume
maximal expiratory flow volume curve
maximal flow per unit of time
maximal forced expiratory f.
maximal inspiratory f.
maximal inspiratory flow rate
maximal midexpiratory f.
maximal midexpiratory flow rate
maximal midexpiratory flow volume
maximal terminal f.
maximal urinary flow rate
maximum expiratory f.
maximum expiratory flow at 50% vital capacity
maximum expiratory flow rate
maximum expiratory flow volume
maximum free flow rate
maximum midexpiratory flow rate
mean aortic flow velocity
mean cerebral blood f.
mean inspiratory f.
mean maximal expiratory f.
mean midexpiratory flow rate
mean renal blood f.
measurement
mechanical expiratory flow volume curve
medullary blood f.
mesenteric blood f.
f. meter
meter
f. microfluorometry
midexpiratory f.
midinspiratory f.
midinspiratory flow at 50% of vital capacity
midinspiratory flow rate
minimum flow rate
mitral regurgitant f.
mucosal blood f.
mucus flow rate
multidimensional flow cytometry
muscle blood f.
myocardial blood f.
myocardial fractional flow reserve
nipple flow rate
noninvasive assessment of urinary f.
noninvasive flow study
nonplacental blood f.
normal f.
normal urine f.
oblique flow misregistration
obstructed blood f.
obstruction of bile f.
orbital blood f.
organ blood f.
outer cortical blood f.
pancreatic blood f.
pancreatic secretory flow rate
parallel-plate flow chamber
parotid flow rate
partial expiratory flow volume
peak f.
peak aortic flow velocity
peak cough f.
peak expiratory f.
peak expiratory flow rate
peak expiratory flow time
peak flow measurement
peak flow meter monitor
peak flow sensitivity
peak flow whistle
peak inspiratory f.
peak inspiratory flow rate
peak jet flow rate
peak nasal inspiratory f.
peak reactive hyperemia blood f.
peak secretory flow rate
peak tidal expiratory f.
peak tidal inspiratory f.
penile blood f.
penile blood flow study
percent predicted peak expiratory f.
perfusion flow rate
peripheral blood f.
physiologic shunt f.
placental blood f.
point of identical f.
portal vein blood flow velocity
portal venous f.
postperfusion low f.
pressure flow gradient
pulmonary blood f.
pulmonary capillary blood flow perfusion
pulmonary-to-systemic flow ratio
pulmonary venous f.
radial flow chromatography
f. rate
rate of f.
f. ratio
reactive hyperemia blood f.
reduced blood flow to brain
regional cerebral blood f.

flow *(continued)*
regional distribution of hepatic blood f.
regional myocardial blood f.
regional pulmonary blood f.
relative f.
relative coronary flow reserve
relative shunt f.
renal blood f.
renal cortical blood f.
renal plasma f.
retrograde blood f.
retrograde flow of barium
return to f.
return flow enema
return flow hemostatic catheter
reversed ophthalmic artery f.
reversed vertebral blood f.
reverse flow island flap
scanty menstrual f.
sedimentation field flow fractionation
selected ion flow tube
shunt f.
single-nephron glomerular blood f.
single-nephron glomerular plasma f.
small vessel inadequate blood f.
spinal cord blood f.
splanchnic blood f.
splenic blood f.
stenotic flow reserve
stopped flow pressure
superior mesenteric artery blood f.
systemic blood f.
tangential flow filtration
thoracic duct f.
tidal expiratory flow at 25% of tidal volume
tidal expiratory flow at 50% of tidal volume
tidal expiratory flow at 75% of tidal volume
tidal inspiratory f.
tidal inspiratory flow at 50% of tidal volume
time to peak expiratory f.
time to peak expiratory flow and total expiration time
time to peak inspiratory f.
time to peak tidal expiratory f.
total f.
total cerebral blood f.
total coronary f.
total flow resistance
total pulmonary blood f.
total renal blood f.
total systemic f.
tracheal blood f.
tracking blood flow to the brain
transesophageal Doppler color flow imaging
ultrasonic flow detector
urodynamic flow study
uterine blood f.
vascular flow headache
f. velocity
venous flow controller
venous renal plasma f.
venous stop flow pressure
vertical flow clean bench
visually evoked flow response
f. volume
volume of blood f.
volume to peak expiratory flow and total expiratory volume

flow-assisted
f.-a. short-term
f.-a. short-term balloon catheter

flower
heated soybean f.

Flowers
F. Auditory Screening Test
F. Auditory Test of Selective Attention

flow-limiting segment

flow-mediated
f.-m. dilation
f.-m. vasodilation

flowmeter
Doppler ultrasonic f.
electromagnetic f.
O_2 flowmeter nipple
peak f.
pulsed Doppler ultrasonic f.
Wright peak f.

flowmetry
laser Doppler f.
magnetic resonance f.
pulsed Doppler f.

flow-related enhancement

flow-relieving
pressure-retaining f.-r.

flow-velocity waveforms

flow-volume
f.-v. loop
tidal breathing f.-v.

floxuridine
circadian-modified f.

fluctuant
f. abscess
f. drainage
f. mass
soft fluctuant nodular lesion

fluctuated
hemoglobin f.

fluctuating
f. affect
f. course
f. hearing loss
f. hormone levels
f. level of consciousness
f. mental status
f. mood disturbance
periodically fluctuating protein kinase
f. periods of remission and relapse
f. sensorineural hearing loss

fluctuation
attention f.
diurnal weight f.
hormonal f.
Luria-Delbruck fluctuation test
motor f.
orthostatic f.
spontaneous f.
temperature f.

fluency
association f.
associative f.
computer-aided fluency establishment trainer
Verbal F. Test
word f.

fluent
f. aphasia
f. aphasic seizure
f. aphasic speech
f. paraphasic speech
f. speech

fluff
f. dressing
dry sterile f.
f. gauze

fluffed gauze dressing

fluffy
f. alveolar infiltrate
f. bibasilar infiltrate
f. cotton-wool exudate
f. infiltrate
f. pulmonary infiltrate

Fluharty Preschool Speech and Language Screening Test

fluid

abdominal cavity free of f.
abdominal fluid collection
f. accumulation
f. accumulation and inflammation
adequate fluid replacement
f.'s aeration, nutrition, communication, activity, and pain
f.'s aeration, nutrition, communication, activity, and stimulation
air fluid cavity
amniotic f.
amniotic fluid alpha-fetoprotein
amniotic fluid analysis
amniotic fluid aspiration
amniotic fluid at term
amniotic fluid bilirubin
amniotic fluid cell culture
amniotic fluid culture
amniotic fluid drained and preserved
amniotic fluid embolism
amniotic fluid embolization
amniotic fluid glucose
amniotic fluid index
amniotic fluid infection
amniotic fluid infection syndrome
amniotic fluid quantitation
amniotic fluid scan
amniotic fluid volume
anechoic fluid collection
anesthetic and fluid management
anthrax-infected body f.
antinuclear antibody f.
arterial-ascitic fluid pH gradient
ascites fluid tap
ascites tumor f.
ascitic f.
ascitic fluid in abdomen
ascitic fluid cytology
ascitic fluid tapped daily
ascitic fluid test
ascitic fluid total protein
ascitic tumor f.
f. aspirated from abdomen
f. aspirated from chest
f. aspirated from joint
f. aspirated from knee
aspiration of food of f.
f. attenuated inversion recovery
f. attenuation inversion recovery
blister f.
blood and body fluid precaution
blood-cerebrospinal fluid barrier
blood extracellular f.
breast cyst f.
breast cyst fluid protein
bronchoalveolar lavage f.
Carrel-Dakin f.
centrifugation extractable f.
centrifuged culture f.
cerebral fluid shunt
cerebrospinal f.
cerebrospinal fluid glucose
cerebrospinal fluid hypotension
cerebrospinal fluid immunofixation electrophoresis
cerebrospinal fluid leak
cerebrospinal fluid pressure
cerebrospinal fluid volume
cervicovaginal f.
f. of choice
collected f.
colloid osmotic pressure in interstitial f.
contaminated with bodily f.
controlled access to f.
controlled fluid access
controlling fluid formation
crevicular fluid flow rate
dark blood stained f.
f. density
drainage subretinal f.
f. dram
ductal lavage f.
egress of arthroscopic f.
f. and electrolyte imbalance
f.'s electrolytes, nutrition
endoneural fluid pressure
epithelial lining f.
excessive fluid intake
exposure to blood or body f.
external fluid loss
extracellular f.
extracellular fluid compartment
extracellular fluid volume
extracellular fluid volume depletion
extracellular fluid volume excess
f. extract
extradural f.
f. filled abdomen
f. filled ganglion
filtration replacement f.
fixation f.
fixing f.
follicular f.
force f.'s
free abdominal f.
free peritoneal f.
functional extracellular fluid volume
gastric f.
gastric fluid, basal acid output
gingival crevicular f.
f. gradient
gradient of fluid inflow
Gram stain of body f.
Gram stain of peritoneal f.
gross cystic disease fluid protein
harvest f.
hazardous spills of f.
f. in heart sac
human lung f.
human oviduct f.
hyperalimentation f.
hypernatremia and fluid attack
f. imbalance
inadequate intake of f.'s
infectious body f.
insufficient fluid intake
f. intake
interstitial f.
interstitial cell f.
interstitial fluid space
interstitial fluid volume
f. intoxication
intracellular fluid volume
intraocular f.
intravascular f.
intravenous f.
intravenous nutritional f.
joint fluid analysis
lavage f.
leaking of f.
loculated pleural f.
loculation of f.
lumbar cerebrospinal fluid catheter
lymphocyte culture f.
male accessory gland f.
malignant ascites f.
meconium-stained amniotic f.
metal working f.
metastatic cancer of spinal f.
middle ear f.
monitor fluid intake and output
mouse amniotic f.
f. movement
mucosal f.
negative balance of body f.
net gradient of fluid outflow
nipple aspirate f.
normal extracellular fluid volume
normal spinal f.
f.'s and nutrition
oozing of f.
Orbis-Sigma cerebrospinal fluid shunt valve

fluid *(continued)*
f. ounce
f. output
pancreatitis-associated ascites f.
paracentesis fluid cytology
parenteral f.'s
Parkland fluid requirement formula for burn patients
Parkland formula for fluid resuscitation for burn trauma
parotid f.
patient treated initially with intravenous f.'s
percutaneous abscess and fluid drainage
periarticular fluid collection
pericardial f.
pericardial fluid culture
pericardial fluid cytology
pericardial fluid examination
pericholecystic fluid collection
perinephric fluid collection
perioptic cerebrospinal f.
peripancreatic fluid collection
peritoneal cavity f.
peritoneal dialysis f.
peritoneal fluid cytology
peritoneal fluid examination
piggyback intravenous fluids
pleural f.
pleural fluid aspiration
precursor f.
f. pressure
prostatic interstitial f.
pseudoamniotic f.
pulmonary edema f.
pulmonary extravascular fluid volume
push f.'s
radial immunodiffusion cerebrospinal f.
rate of fluid filtration
red hemorrhagic f.
Rees and Ecker diluting f.
respiratory tract f.
respiratory tract lining f.
restricted f.'s
f. restriction
retained fetal lung f.
retained lung f.
f. retention
f. retention syndrome
seminal f.
seminal fluid analysis
seminal fluid assay
serosal f.
serous f.
simulated gastric f.
simulated intestinal f.
f. spilling into upper abdomen
spinal f.
spinal fluid count
spinal fluid Gram stain
spinal fluid leak
spinal fluid pressure
standard perfusion f.
subarachnoid cerebrospinal f.
subarachnoid fluid collection
subretinal f.
supercritical f.
supercritical fluid extraction
surrounding subretinal fluid cuff
synovial f.
synovial fluid lymphocyte
temporomandibular joint synovial f.
testicular interstitial f.
f. thioglycolate medium
thoracentesis f.
thoracic fluid content
thromblastic activity of amniotic f.
total fluid movement
tracheobronchial aspirate f.
tubular f.
vaginal fluid ferning
ventricular f.
ventricular cerebrospinal f.
ventricular fluid pressure
f. volume
f. volume overload
f. wave

fluid-electrolyte malnutrition

fluid-filled
f.-f. balloon
f.-f. catheter
f.-f. cyst
f.-f. cyst in breast
f.-f. diverticulum
f.-f. loop of bowel
f.-f. sac
f.-f. small bowel

fluid-gas exchange

fluidity
lipid fluidity unit

fluid–Wassermann
cerebrospinal fluid–Wassermann reaction

fluke
liver f.
lung fluke disease
Oriental blood f.

flu-like syndrome

fluoracetate
methyl f.

fluorescein
f. angiography
f. clearance test
f. dilaurate
f. dye
fundus fluorescein angiogram
intravenous fluorescein angiography
f. isothiocyanate
M.O.M. fluorescein kit
mouse-on-mouse fluorescein kit
f. to protein ratio
sodium f.
f. treponemal antibody test
f. uptake

fluorescein-labeled serum protein

fluorescence
affinity fluorescence spectroscopy
f. antimembrane antibody
autofluorescence focal fluorescence
f. capillary-fill device
cardiolipin fluorescence antibody
f. correlation spectroscopy
f. depolarization
direct fluorescence assay
dye fluorescence index
energy-dispersive x-ray f.
f. energy transfer immunoassay
f. excitation transfer immunoassay
formaldehyde-induced f.
indirect f.
intercellular f.
laser-induced f.
laser-induced arterial f.
laser-induced fluorescence emission
laser-induced fluorescence spectroscopy
light-induced fluorescence endoscopic bronchoscopy
light-induced fluorescence endoscopy in combination with pharmacoendoscopy
lung imaging fluorescence endoscope
f. overlay antigen mapping
particle concentration fluorescence immunoassay
f. photobleaching recovery
f. plus Giemsa stain
f. polarization
f. polarization immunoassay
quantitative light induced f.

f. recovery after photobleaching
relative f.
relative fluorescence efficiency
f. resonance energy transfer
simulated fluorescence process
skin f.
solid phase fluorescence immunoassay
solid-phase immunoassay f.
f. thiourea
f. treponemal antibody absorption
ultrasensitive fluorescence in situ hybridization
wavelength-dispersive x-ray f.
x-ray f.

fluorescence-activated
f.-a. cell sorter
f.-a. cell sorter scan
f.-a. cell sorting

fluorescence-lactose-denitrification medium

fluorescence-polarization immunoassay

fluorescent
f. actin staining
f. allergosorbent test
f. angiography
f. antibody
f. antibody dark-field
f. antibody to membrane antigen test
f. antibody stain
f. antibody staining technique
f. antimembrane antibody test
f. antinuclear antibody assay
f. assay
auramine O fluorescent stain
automatic fluorescent image analyzer
colony-stimulating factor
fluorescent treponemal antibody-absorption test
detection of early antigen fluorescent focus
direct fluorescent antigen test
direct fluorescent antibody
direct fluorescent antibody examination for *Treponema pallidum*
direct fluorescent antibody test
direct fluorescent antigen
direct fluorescent assay
double-fusion fluorescent in situ hybridization
enhanced green fluorescent protein
f. enzyme immunoassay
enzyme-linked fluorescent immunoassay
extra ABL signal fluorescent in situ hybridization
f. focus
f. focus inhibition test
f. gonorrhea test
green fluorescent protein
immune fluorescent antibody
f. immunoassay
indirect fluorescent antibody
indirect fluorescent assay
indirect fluorescent rabies antibody test
f. lamp
f. light intensity
lung imaging fluorescent endoscopy
mean fluorescent intensity
f. microscopy
MicroTrak direct fluorescent antibody staining
multispectral fluorescent in situ hybridization
f. polarization immunoassay
f. rabies antibody
rapid fluorescent focus inhibition test
f. shift
f. in situ hybridization
small, intensely fluorescent ganglion
soluble antigen fluorescent antibody test
f. staining
substrate-labeled fluorescent immunoassay
substrate-linked fluorescent immunoassay
f. thyroid imaging
f. titer antibody

fluorescent-activated cell sorting

fluorescent-labeled antibody

fluorescing erythrocyte

fluoride
argon f.
f. ion positron emission tomography
lithium f.
Luride acidulated phosphate fluoride paste
neodymium:yttrium lithium fluoride laser
f. number
organic acid-labile f.
prenatal f.
stannous f.
sustained-release sodium f.
topical fluoride application
yttrium lithium f.

fluoroallergosorbent test

fluorocarbon
oxygenated fluorocarbon nutrient emulsion

fluorochrome
auramine fluorochrome stain

fluorometholone and neomycin sulfate

fluorometric
f. analysis of DNA unwinding
f. study

fluorometry
noninvasive corneal redox f.

fluorophore-assisted carbohydrate electrophoresis

fluorophotometry
vitreous f.

fluoropolymer
flexible f.

fluoroscopic
air enema fluoroscopic imaging
f. assistance
f. C-arm
f. control
f. examination
f. guidance
f. image guidance
f. imaging
f. insertion
f. monitoring
f. placement
radiographic and f.
f. table
f. visualization

fluoroscopic-assisted lumbar puncture

fluoroscopy
C-arm fluoroscopy unit
computed f.
digital f.
orthogonal C-arm f.

fluoroscopy-guided balloon dilator

fluorouridine
f. monophosphate
f. triphosphate

fluorourodynamic study

fluphenazine decanoate

flush
arterial line flush solution
Asian alcohol flush reaction
autonomic epilepsy f.
heparin f.
f. heparin lock
hot f.
hot and cold f.'s
mahogany f.
malar f.
medullary carcinoma f.
orgasmic f.
peroxide f.
saline f.

flushed
aspirated and f.
catheter aspirated and f.
catheter aspirated and flushed with saline

flushing
chlorpropamide-alcohol f.
double-bubble flushing reservoir
dyspnea and f.
f. and heat
idiopathic f.
on-off flushing reservoir
f. sensation of heaviness
vasomotor f.

fluted
f. drain
f. medullary rod
f. reamer
f. silicone drain
f. titanium nail

flute needle

flutter
atrial f.
atrial fetal f.
atrial fibrillation and/or f.
atrial flutter response
auditory flutter fusion
ocular flutter nystagmus
ventricular f.
f. wave

flutter-fibrillation

flux
laser Doppler f.
leucine f.
luminous f.
luminous flux density
magnetic f.
magnetic flux density
net acid f.
radiant f.

fly
louse f.
mangrove f.
may f.
screwworm f.

foam
aluminum foam splint
f. casting
f. and condom
contraceptive f.
f. cushion
egg crate foam mattress
expanded foam immobilization device
intravaginal f.
minimally attenuating medical-grade f.
open cell f.
polyurethane f.
polyurethane foam dressing
polyvinyl alcohol f.
f. stability index
f. tape
urea formaldehyde foam insulation

foamy
f. interstitial plaque
intimal foamy plaques
simian foamy viruses

focal
f. abnormality
f. abscess formation
f. accumulation
acute focal bacterial nephritis
acute focal cerebral ischemia
f. adhesion kinase
anterior focal point
anterior temporal focal spike
f. area of hemorrhage
f. area of hyperemia
f. areas of intrapulmonary hemorrhage
f. areas of lymphoid infiltrate
autofluorescence focal fluorescence
f. axonal swelling
benign focal epilepsy of childhood
f. brain lesion
f. cementoosseous dysplasia
f. contralateral routing of signals
f. cranial radiation therapy
f. cytoplasmic degradation
f. dermal hypoplasia
f. dermal hypoplasia syndrome
f. disease
f. distance
f. edema
effective focal length
f. electroretinogram
f. epithelial hyperplasia
f. extraprostatic extension
f. facial dermal dysplasia II
f. film distance
global focal sclerosis
f. global glomerulosclerosis
f. hemorrhage
f. hemorrhagic cystitis
f. hemorrhagic infarct
f. hemorrhagic necrotizing cystitis
f. hepatic hemorrhage
f. herpes of vulva
f. hypertrophy
f. hypoechoic lesion
f. illumination
f. immunoassay
f. infarct
f. infarct of liver
f. infection
f. inflammatory mucosal change
f. interstitial fibrosis
f. interstitial hemorrhage
f. interstitial scarring
f. intrapulmonary hemorrhage
f. involvement
f. length
linear focal elastosis
f. lymphoid hyperplasia
f. macular choroidopathy
membrane focal coli broth
mild focal chronic inflammatory infiltrate
mild focal cortical nodular hyperplasia
mild focal interstitial scarring
multiple focal lesion
f. necrosis
f. neurological impairment
f. neurologic deficit
f. neurologic disturbance
f. nodular hyperplasia
f. nonfatty infiltration of liver
oral focal mucinosis
f. petechial hemorrhage
f. proliferative glomerulonephritis
proximal femoral focal deficiency
proximal femur focal deficiency
proximal focal femoral deficiency
f. sclerosing glomerulonephritis
secondary focal point of lens
f. segmental glomerular hyalinosis and sclerosis
f. segmental glomerulosclerosis
f. and segmental hyalinosis

f. seizure
f. shallow subpleural hemorrhage
f. spot
f. spot size
f. subendocardial hemorrhage
f. subpleural interstitial fibrosis
superficial subendocardial focal hemorrhage
f. tenderness
f. tick-borne encephalitis
transient focal neurologic event
f. vascular headache
f. zone

focus, pl. **foci**
abdominal foci of infection
aberrant crypt f.
f. of attention
central slow wave f.
central spike f.
depth of f.
detection of early antigen fluorescent f.
disseminated foci
ectopic f.
epilepsy with multiple independent spike f.
epithelial f.
equivalent f.
fibrotic f.
f. film distance
fluorescent f.
fluorescent focus inhibition test
Friend spleen focus virus
inability to f.
inability to focus attention
foci of infarct
f. of infection
line focus principle
low-voltage foci
multicentric foci
natural focus of infection
nodular hyperintense f.
f. object distance
occult frontal f.
f. out
rapid fluorescent focus inhibition test
serial focus seizures
f. of slow activity
small focus hemorrhage
small focus of hepatic necrosis

focused
f. abdominal sonography
f. abdominal sonography for trauma
f. appendix computed tomography
f. assessment by sonography for trauma
field focused nuclear magnetic resonance
high-intensity focused ultrasonography
high-intensity focused ultrasound
f. medical review
f. segmented ultrasound machine
solution focused group therapy

focus-forming unit

focusing
electromagnetic focusing field probe
isoelectric focusing electrophoresis
isoelectric focusing electrophoresis in polyacrylamide gel
isoelectric focusing in polyacrylamide
polyacrylamide gel isoelectric f.

focus-reduction neutralization test

focus-skin distance

fog
mental f.
f. reduction elimination device

Fogarty arterial embolectomy

foil
long-handled foil condenser
noncohesive gold f.

Fokes sentence builder

folate
isolated congenital folate malabsorption
red blood cell f.
reduced folate carrier
whole-blood f.

fold
adipose fold of the pleura
anterior axillary f.
anterior mallear f.
arcuate retinal f.
artiodactylous fold of Collier
aryepiglottic f.
aryepiglottic fold carcinoma
aryepiglottic fold neurofibroma
aryepiglottic fold width
asymmetric folds of eye
asymmetric skin f.
bilateral vocal fold immobility
bilateral vocal fold paralysis
f. of chorda tympani
falciform fold of fascia lata
false vocal f.
f. forceps
glossoepiglottic f.
horizontal fold of rectum
f. increase in resistance
inframammary f.
inframammary fold incision
f. of iris
junctional f.
f.'s of Kerckring
f.'s of large intestine
lateral nail f.
lateral nasal f.
longitudinal fold of duodenum
Marshall vestigial f.
medial canthic f.
median glossoepiglottic f.
middle glossoepiglottic f.
mucosal fold of gallbladder
nail fold capillarioscopy abnormality
nail fold capillarioscopy
nail fold capillary loop abnormality
nail fold removal
nasolabial f.
nasolabial fold asymmetry
palmate fold of cervical canal
paradoxical vocal fold dysfunction
patellar synovial f.
pharyngoepiglottic f.
posterior axillary f.
semilunar conjunctival f.
skin fold incision
skin fold measurement
skin fold thickness test
f. of stapes
superior duodenal f.
synovial fold of hip
thickened duodenal f.
thickness of skin f.
transverse fold of rectum
true vocal f.
vocal fold dysfunction
vocal fold injection

foldable intraocular lens

folded aluminum ear splint

folded-lung syndrome

Foley
F. catheter
indwelling Foley catheter

folic
f. acid
f. acid antagonist
f. acid-binding protein
serum folic acid

Folin-Denis assay

Folin-Wu
F.-W. method
F.-W. reaction

folium
lingual f.

follicle
androgenic f.
anovular ovarian f.
antral f.
ascendant f.
f. aspiration, sperm injection, and assisted rupture
atretic f.
atretic ovarian f.
f. center lymphoma cell
hair f.
hair follicle nevus
hair follicle tumor
Lieberkühn f.
limbal f.
lingual f.
lollipop f.
luteinized unruptured f.
luteinized unruptured follicle syndrome
lymph f.
lymphatic f.
lymphatic follicle of larynx
lymphatic follicle of tongue
lymphoid f.
f. lysis
mature f.
Montgomery f.
Naboth f.
nabothian f.
neck of hair f.
necrotic f.
neoplastic f.
ovarian f.
ovarian follicle exhaustion
ovulatory f.
f. puncture for oocyte retrieval
f. regulatory protein
rupture f.
solitary f.

follicle-stimulating
f.-s. hormone
f.-s. hormone and luteinizing hormone-releasing hormone
f.-s. hormone-releasing factor
f.-s. hormone-releasing hormone
human follicle-stimulating hormone

follicular
f. adenocarcinoma
f. adenoma
f. area
arrested follicular cyst
atretic follicular cyst
Axenfeld follicular conjunctivitis
f. basal lamina
carpet tack follicular keratotic plug
f. center cell
f. center cell lymphoma
completely f.
f. dendritic cell
f. diameter
explosive follicular hyperplasia
floral variant of follicular lymphoma
f. fluid
f. gait
f. gastritis
giant follicular hyperplasia
giant follicular lymphoma
f. goiter
f. hyperplasia
indolent follicular lymphoma
f. iritis
f. large cell lymphoma
lymphoid follicular reticulosis
f. lymphoma
f. lymphosarcoma
minimally invasive follicular carcinoma
mixed follicular hyperplasia
multiclonal follicular lymphoma
f. nodular hyperplasia
noncleaved follicular center cell
f. non-Hodgkin lymphoma
partially f.
tumor of the follicular infundibulum
f. variant of papillary thyroid carcinoma
widely invasive follicular carcinoma

follicularis
hydrosalpinx f.
ichthyosis, follicularis, atrichia or alopecia, photophobia syndrome
lichen planus f.
nevus follicularis keratosis

folliculi (*pl. of* folliculus)

folliculitis
eosinophilic pustular f.
Malassezia f.

folliculorum
pityriasis f.

folliculosebaceous cystic hamartoma

folliculus, pl. **folliculi**
atresia folliculi
hydrops folliculi
liquor folliculi

follow
does not follow commands
fixate and f.
incomplete resolution, scan to f.
results to f.
to f.
f. up
f. up intervention for normal development
will follow in office

followed
f. by
immediate good function followed by accelerated rejection
patient to be followed as an outpatient
patient followed on an outpatient basis
f. with

follower
filiform and f.

following
adjustment following migration
arrhythmia following defibrillation
baby expired following resuscitation attempt
f. bougie
bronchodilation following deep inspiration
cardiac arrest following trauma
completion, arithmetic problems, vocabulary, following directions
deterioration following improvement
expired following resuscitation attempt
ileus following abdominal surgery
f. ingestion
reference point following QRS complex, at beginning of ST segment
f. satisfactory general anesthesia
summation of all quantities following the symbol
time to following commands

follows
f. commands
fixes and f.

follow-through
f.-t. after barium meal

small bowel f.-t.
upper gastrointestinal series with small bowel f.-t.

followup
first set of followup data
Hypertension Detection and F. Program
longitudinal interval followup evaluation
long-term f.
long-term followup data
lost to f.
lost to f.
medical f.
naturalistic followup study
f. note
patient discharged to office f.
second set of followup data
surgical f.

follow-up office visit

Folstein
Mini-Mental State Examination of F.

Fomede virus

fomentation
hot f.

Fontan
modified Fontan operation
modified Fontan procedure

fontanelle
anterior f.
anterolateral f.
mastoid f.
open posterior f.
f. reflex

food
acute esophageal food impaction
acute food allergy
f. allergen
f. allergy
anaphylactoid food sensitivity
antigenemically cross-reacting f.
aspiration of food of fluid
aspiration of food particle
f. awareness training
caffeine, alcohol, pepper, spicy foods
clostridial food poisoning
double-blind placebo-controlled food challenge
excessive food intake
extra f.
fast food intake
fatty food intolerance
Federal F., Drug, and Cosmetic Act
hard food orientation
idiosyncratic food preference
f. immune complex assay
intake of f.
f. intolerance
intolerance to certain f.'s
intolerance to specific f.'s
junior baby f.
liquid food dysphagia
microatomized protein f.
F.'s and Moods Inventory
neurotrophic food ulcer
no known food allergies
F. and Nutrition Information Center
obstructing bolus of f.
f. poisoning
rapid ingestion of large amounts of f.
restricting food intake
thermal effect of f.
thermic effect of f.
tube-fed f.
uniform food encoding

food-borne
bacterial food-borne illness
f.-b. illness
f.-b. illness outbreak
f.-b. transmission of viral hepatitis

food-chemical intolerance

food-drug interaction

foot
f. and ankle severity scale
anular part of fibrous digital sheath of digits of hand and f.
arch of f.
arcuate artery of f.
articulations of f.
astrocytic end f.
augmented voltage unipolar left foot lead
f. of bed
cavus foot deformity
cold water immersion f.
f. compartment syndrome
congenital vertical talus foot deformity
cubic f.
diabetic foot care
diabetic foot syndrome
diabetic foot ulcer
dorsal interosseous muscle of f.
dorsal interosseous vein of f.
f. drape
fetal foot length
F. Function Index
Haglund foot deformity
immersion f.
improper foot alignment
improper foot care
improper functioning of f.
incomplete foot presentation
indirect foot hazard
interphalangeal joint of f.
intrinsic muscle of f.
joint of f.
left f.
left foot switch
ligament of f.
longitudinal arch of f.
lumbrical of f.
lumbrical muscle of f.
lumen per square f.
Maryland F. Score
Maryland Foot Score Profile
McElvenny foot procedure
medial border of f.
medial crus foot plate
Mendel dorsal foot reflex
metal foot plate
Miller foot procedure
millions of particles per cubic foot of air
mixed foot dominant
nail breaking from athlete's f.
neuropathic foot deformity
numbness in f.
one hand-two foot syndrome
f. orthosis
Osmond-Clarke foot procedure
f. pedal suction control
perforating artery of f.
perineuronal end f.
perivascular end f.
peroneal border of f.
phantom foot pain
plantar aspect of f.
plantar flexion of f.
plantar foot defect
f. poundal
f. pound-force
pound-force f.
pound per cubic f.
f. process
f. progression angle
pronation of f.
puncture wound of f.
regular foot hygiene
right f.
right foot switch

foot *(continued)*
f. shock-induced analgesia
short foot drape
f. slap
superimposed dorsiflexion of f.
supination of f.
tibial border of f.
tropic immersion f.
warm water immersion f.
f. yaw

foot-and-mouth
f.-a.-m. disease
f.-a.-m. disease virus

footballer migraine

footdrop
f. after stroke
neurological f.

footling
double footling delivery
f. breech presentation

footpad swelling

footplate
astrocyte f.
Müller cell f.
f. of the stapes

footprint
f. identification
Musgrave footprint pedobarograph
Musgrave Footprint System

foot-progression angle

for
f. external use only
f. internal use only
not otherwise provided f.

foramen, pl. **foramina**
anatomically patent foramen ovale
anterior condyloid f.
anterior ethmoidal f.
anterior palatine f.
anterior sacral f.
apical f.
apical dental f.
apical foramen of tooth
f. of Arnold
asymmetric small foramen magnum
atresia of the foramen of Luschka and Magendie
carotid f.
epiploic foramen of Winslow
f. of Fallopio
greater palatine f.
greater sciatic f.
interventricular f.
intravertebral f.
f. of Key and Retzius
Luschka and Magendie f.
f. magnum decompression
median foramen of Magendie
f. of Monro
f. of Morgagni
f. of Morgagni hernia
multiple foramina
neural foramina
neural foramen remodeling
open exit f.
outlet foramina
f. ovale
f. ovale cordis
f. ovale of heart
oval foramen of heart
papillary foramina of kidney
parietal foramina, brachymicrocephaly, mental retardation syndrome
patent neural foramina
f. of Vesalius
f. of Winslow

foraminal
f. hernia
neural foraminal canal
osseous foraminal encroachment

foraminotomy
endoscopic laser f.
f. operation

force
acceleration f.
anterior component of f.
atomic force microscopy
centrifugal f.
contractile f.
contraction peak f.
counterelectromotive f.
electromagnetic f.
electromotive f.
end-systolic force velocity index
failure of all vital f.'s
f. fluids
global force applicator
inspiratory f.
lateral force microscopy
magnetomotive f.
maximal force at rest length
maximal inspiratory f.
maximum bite f.
moment of f.
myocardial contractile f.
negative expiratory f.
negative inspiratory f.
occlusal bite f.
proton motive f.
relative centrifugal f.
scanning force microscopy
spontaneous peak inspiratory f.
f. translation
unit of f.
unit of force of acceleration
van der Waals f.
f., velocity, length

forced
alternative temporal forced choice
f. end-expiratory wheeze
f. equilibrating expiration
f. expiratory
f. expiratory capacity
f. expiratory flow
f. expiratory flow volume
f. expiratory spirogram
f. expiratory time
f. expiratory time in seconds
f. expiratory volume at one second
f. expiratory volume in one second as percent of FVC
f. expiratory volume in one second to forced vital capacity ratio
f. expiratory volume timed
f. expiratory volume timed to forced vital capacity ratio
f. flexion injury
f. inspiration
f. inspiratory flow
f. inspiratory oxygen
f. inspiratory spirogram
f. inspiratory vital capacity
f. inspiratory volume
f. inspiratory volume in one second
f. inversion
f. inversion film of ankle
f. mandatory intermittent ventilation
maximal forced expiratory flow
maximal forced expiratory maneuver
f. midexpiratory flow
f. oscillation
f. oscillation technique
f. pair copulation
passive forced duction test
f. passive full forward flexion
f. passive internal rotation
f. plantar flexion
f. respiration
f. sexual encounter
timed forced expiratory volume
f. vital capacity analysis

f. volume, expiratory
f. whisper

forced-duction test

forceps

adventitial f.
f. to aftercoming head
alligator f.
alligator bone-reduction f.
alligator-type grasping f.
angled capsule f.
angled dissecting f.
angled-down f.
angled-up f.
anterior f.
antrum punch f.
apical fragment f.
artery f.
arthroscopy basket f.
arthroscopy grasping f.
atraumatic f.
atraumatic locking/grasping f.
axis traction f.
ball f.
bayonet f.
bayonet-type f.
f. birth trauma
bone f.
bone-breaking f.
bone-cutting f.
bone-grasping f.
bulldog f.
capsule fragment f.
cephalic f.
closed iris f.
cold forceps ablation
conjunctiva f.
cowhorn f.
cup f.
curved basket f.
f. delivery
dental f.
duckbill f.
eagle beak bone-cutting f.
elective low forceps delivery
electrocoagulating f.
endoscopic f.
f. extraction
failed forceps delivery
fenestrated f.
fenestrated spiked open-span jumbo biopsy f.
fine-toothed f.
flexible f.
fold f.
f. fracture
galea f.
gallstone f.
hook f.
lid f.
lower anterior f.
low forceps delivery
low outlet f.
low outlet forceps delivery
major f.
mandibular f.
f. maneuver
matte black f.
meniscus f.
microsurgery f.
microvascular f.
midcavity f.
miniature f.
minor f.
mosquito f.
mosquito hemostatic f.
muscle f.
nonfenestrated f.
obstetric f.
occipital f.
operative delivery with f.
orthopaedic f.
outlet forceps delivery
oval f.
ovum f.
packing f.
papilloma f.
f. passed up through incision
pediatric f.
pelvic f.
perforating f.
f. removal
right-angle f.
f. rotation
sterile elective low forceps vaginal delivery
sterile indicated low forceps vaginal delivery

force-time integral

force-velocity curve

force-velocity-length relation

Fordyce

angiokeratoma of F.

forearm

anterior compartment of f.
anterior interosseous nerve of f.
balanced forearm orthosis
ball-bearing forearm orthosis
f. blood flow
distal f.
extensor compartment of f.
f. flexion control strap
f. flow
free forearm flap
lateral cutaneous nerve of f.
left f.
loop forearm graft
malunited forearm fracture
medial border of f.
medial cutaneous nerve of f.
medial flexor muscle of f.
minimal forearm vascular resistance
Monteggia forearm fracture
oblique cord of interosseous membrane of f.
posterior branch of medial cutaneous nerve of f.
posterior compartment of f.
posterior cutaneous nerve of f.
posterior interosseous nerve of f.
f. pronated
radial forearm free flap
reverse forearm island flap
right f.
f. supination
supination of f.
ulnar border of f.
f. vascular resistance

forebrain

limbic f.
limbic forebrain structure
magnocellular basal f.

Forecariah virus

forefoot

f. abduction
f. abductus
f. adduction
f. adductovarus
f. adductus
f. angulation
f. arthroplasty
arthroscopic monopolar thermal stabilization forefoot compression sleeve
f. cavus
f. equinus
Mayo Clinic forefoot score
narrowing of f.
neuropathic forefoot ulceration
f. valgus
f. varus

forefoot-to-rearfoot striker

forehead

McGregor forehead flap
midline forehead flap
modified anterior hairline forehead lift
olympian f.

forehead *(continued)*
paramedian forehead flap
prominent f.

foreheadplasty
male f.
open f.

foreign
anal foreign body
anorectal foreign body
aspirated foreign body
aspirated foreign material
aspiration of foreign body
f. body
f. body in air passage
f. body of the cornea
f. body in iris
f. body, metallic
f. body removal
f. body retained
f. body sensation
f. body soft tissue
f. body-type granuloma
bronchial foreign body
conjunctival foreign body
esophageal foreign body
impacted foreign body
inhalation of foreign body
inhalation of foreign substance
intraocular foreign body
intrauterine foreign body
intravascular foreign body retrieval
lower GI tract foreign body
f. material artifact
metallic foreign body
f. military
f. object
f. object/body
obstructed by foreign body
opaque foreign body
removal of foreign body
retained foreign body
surgical foreign body
tracheobronchial foreign body
unidentified foreign object

Forel
area of F.
fields of F.

forelock
occipital f.

forensic
maximum-security forensic psychiatric hospital
f. medicine
military forensic psychiatry
f. pathology
sexual assault forensic evidence
f. urine drug testing

foreperiod
preceding f.

Forer Sentence Completion Test

foreshortening
anular f.
f. of the colon

foreskin
human foreskin epithelial cell
human foreskin fibroblast

Forest
Barmah Forest virus
Gabek Forest virus
Semliki Forest virus
Telok Forest virus

forged cobalt-chromium alloy prosthesis

forgetfulness
f. from anxiety
patient has forgetfulness, irritability, and confusion

forgetting
motivated f.

fork
f. implant
knife and fork
tuning f.
tuning fork examination
tuning fork test

forked
Millard forked flap technique

forking
aqueductal f.

form
abnormal forms percent
abnormal wave f.
Adjective Rating F.
alternate forms reliability coefficient
ASPS informed consent form
authorization form for removal of tissue for grafting
autopsy consent f.
autosomal-dominant benign form of osteopetrosis
autosomally inherited forms of nephrolithiasis
band form in sixth stage of myelocyte maturation
Beck Depression Index Short F.
blood transfusion refusal f.
California Test of Mental Maturity-Short F.
case report f.
child behavior rating f.
claims inquiry f.
color and f.
complex wave f.
consent form to delivery by alternative physician
consent form for removal of tissue for grafting
Cornell Word F.
cosmetic surgery authorization f.
cosmetic surgery consent f.
data case report f.
data collection f.
diagnostic, social and addiction history f.
early-onset form of familial Alzheimer disease
exposed protruding f.
external impulsive f.
Factor Analyzed Short F.
Family Evaluation F.
frequency and form of amplitude
Fuzzy Functional F.
gadolinium in chelated f.
good form response
Harvard Group Scale of Hypnotic Susceptibility, Form A
hemiplegic form of cerebral palsy
Historical Information F.
intramural protruding f.
investigational drug data f.
36-item short form health survey
Minnesota Paper F. Board Test
mixed form cerebral palsy
Nearly Me breast f.
new dosage f.
nonhistocompatibility locus antigen-associated f.
nonhuman leukocyte antigen associated f.
novel form of consolidation chemotherapy
oral form recognition
oxidized form of nicotinamide adenine dinucleotide
oxidized form of nicotinamide adenine dinucleotide phosphate
partial form of DiGeorge syndrome
patient release f.
patient report f.
patient transfer f.
Personality Research F.
physician's order f.
poor form response

premenstrual assessment f.
progressive form of tick-borne encephalitis
Psychiatric Evaluation F.
Rating F. of IBD Patient Concerns
reduced form of flavin mononucleotide
replicative f.
f. response
Self-Analysis F.
Short F. Test of Academic Aptitude
Teacher Rating F.
Teacher Report F.
f. of thought
ulcerating f.
variable-width forms tractor
Visual F. Discrimination Test

forma

formal
f. developmental history

formaldehyde
f., acetic acid, and alcohol solution
aniline, sulfur, f.
gelatin, resorcinol, f.
latex and resorcinol f.
merthiolate formaldehyde solution
merthiolate, iodine, formaldehyde concentration
merthiolate, iodine, formaldehyde method
resorcinol f.
urea f.
urea formaldehyde foam insulation
f. vapors

formaldehyde-induced fluorescence

formaldehyde-releasing preservative

formal developmental history

formalin
f., acetic, and alcohol solution
f. ammonium bromide
f. and ethanol
f., ethanol, xylol, and ethanol
f. fixation
merthiolate, iodine, formalin solution
neutral buffered formalin fixative
phosphate-buffered f.
f. solution

formalin-fixed paraffin-embedded

formalin-treated pyruvaldehyde-stabilized human erythrocytes

format
five-minute f.
Portable Document F.

formation
anastomotic stricture f.
anterior synechia f.
antigenic antibody lattice f.
aortoenteric fistula f.
bone formation rate
controlling fluid f.
dorsal medullary reticular f.
enchondral bone f.
endogenous callus f.
erythroid colony f.
excessive gas f.
extensive new bone f.
focal abscess f.
giant axon f.
grammar formation stage
idiopathic calcium renal stone f.
intraperitoneal adhesion f.
localized plaque f.
macular star f.
marrow cavity f.
median bar f.
membrane bleb f.
mesangial complex f.
mesencephalic reticular f.
midbrain reticular f.
myelin ball f.
new bone f.
new lesion f.
onion bulb f.
osteoarthritic hypertrophic spur f.
osteoblast-mediated bone f.
osteomyelitic cloaca f.
paramedian pontine reticular f.
pathologic character f.
pontine paramedian reticular f.
pontine parareticular f.
pontine reticular f.
f. and release of hormones
reticular f.
rosette f.
f. scar
sinus node f.
stimulate bone f.
syncytial knot f.
thrombus formation time
total matrix formation rate

former
angle f.
calcium oxalate stone f.

forming
antibody f.
blood forming tissues

formocresol pulpotomy

formol toxoid

formula
Byrne and Euler f.
defined formula diet
evaporated milk f.
house f.
MCT oil f.
meat base f.
Parent's Choice f.
Parkland burn resuscitation f.
Parkland fluid requirement formula for burn patients
Parkland formula for fluid resuscitation for burn trauma
f. protein intolerance
rapid dissolution f.
Sanders-Retzlaff-Kraff f.
side chain in amino acid f.
special care f.
stress f.
f. translation

formulary
Dental Practitioners' F.
National F.

formulated

formulation
new working f.
Working F. for Clinical Usage

fornix
anterior fornix of vagina
anterior pillar of f.
anterior vaginal f.
commissure of f.

Förster uveitis

Fort
F. Bragg evaluation project
Le Fort classification
Le Fort fracture
Le Fort osteotomy
F. Morgan virus
F. Sherman virus

fortified
f. aqueous solution
f. hexachlorocyclohexane

fortifier
human milk f.

fortuitum
Mycobacterium fortuitum complex
Mycobacterium fortuitum infection
Mycobacterium fortuitum third biovar complex

forum
physicians f.

forward
f. bending
f. conduction
direct forward gaze
f. flexion
f. flexion posture
forced passive full forward flexion
head f.
f. head posture
f. heart failure
f. protrusion
f. stroke volume
f. tandem gait

forward-cutting knife

forward-viewing
f.-v. endoscope
f.-v. telescope
f.-v. video colonoscope

fossa
anterior cranial f.
anterior cranial fossa surgery
anterior fossa skull base glabellar
anterior recess of interpeduncular f.
anterior recess of ischiorectal f.
arachnoid cyst of the middle f.
arm fossa test
articular fossa of mandible
articular fossa of temporal bone
articular surface of mandibular f.
articular surface of mandibular fossa of temporal bone
buccal groove of central f.
central f.
central groove of central f.
cistern fossa of Sylvius
cistern of lateral fossa of cerebrum
distal f.
distal triangular f.
distolingual f.
glenoid fossa mandibularis
greater supraclavicular f.
iliac fossa abscess
left iliac f.
limiting sulcus of rhomboid f.
lingual f.
little fossa of cochlear window
little fossa of oval vestibular window
lower fossa active, lateral knee pain, and long leg on the side ipsilateral to the weak f.
lunate fossa depression
mandibularis
margin of fossa ovalis
medial inguinal f.
mesial triangular f.
mesiolingual f.
middle cranial f.
middle cranial fossa approach
middle cranial fossa cyst
middle cranial fossa line
middle fossa approach
middle fossa craniotomy approach
middle fossa exposure
middle fossa floor/petrous dissection
middle fossa plate
middle fossa syndrome
middle fossa transtentorial translabyrinthine approach
middle fossa vestibular nerve section
middle fossa vestibular neurectomy
navicular fossa of male urethra
patellar fossa of vitreous
popliteal fossa tumor
posterior cranial f.
posterior fossa approach
posterior fossa extra-axial arachnoid cyst
posterior fossa tumor
pterygoid f.
pterygomaxillary f.
pterygopalatine fossa syndrome
right iliac f.
scaphoid fossa of sphenoid bone
superior duodenal f.
suprasternal f.
tonsillar fossa carcinoma
upper fossa active, medial knee pain, and short leg on the side ipsilateral to the weak fossa

foster
adult foster care
adult foster home
f. care
f. father
f. home
f. home care
f. home evaluation
f. home placement
f. mother

foul
purulent and foul smelling

foul-smelling urine

found
no disease f.
none f.
not f.
not found this examination
f. under bridge
upon arrival patient f.

fountain
Meynert fountain decussation

four
f. dimensional
every four weeks
f. field technique
f. plus edema
f. quadrant biopsy
Reach in F. Directions Test

four-chambered human heart

four-chamber transverse

fourchette
posterior f.

four-compartment fasciotomy

four-flanged nail

four-flap procedure

Fourier
2-dimensional Fourier imaging
3-dimensional Fourier imaging
discrete Fourier transform
driven equilibrium Fourier transform
inverse Fourier transform
multidimensional Fourier transform
partial Fourier imaging
F. series
three-dimensional Fourier transform
F. transform infrared spectroscopy
two-dimensional Fourier transform

Fourier-acquired steady-state technique

four-in-one
f.-i.-o. arthroplasty
f.-i.-o. cutting block
f.-i.-o. positioning block system

Fournier gangrene

four-point
f.-p. gait
f.-p. restraint
f.-p. walker

four-poster
f.-p. cervical brace
f.-p. cervical orthosis
f.-p. frame

four-pronged liposuction cannula

four-quadrant biopsy

fourth
- f. circulation
- first to fourth heart sounds
- first through fourth heart sounds
- f. heart sound
- median aperture of fourth ventricle
- myelocyte at fourth stage of maturation
- f. in a series or group
- Stanford-Binet F. Edition

fovea
- anterior f.
- Morgagni f.
- oblong fovea of arytenoid cartilage
- obscured f.
- trochlear f.

foveal
- f. avascular zone
- simultaneous foveal perception
- f. vision

fowl
- f. antimouse lymphocyte globulin
- f. gamma globulin
- northern fowl mite
- f. plague virus

Fowler
- F. position
- F. single breath test

Fox eye shield

foxtail
- meadow foxtail grass

fraction
- f. of alveolar carbon dioxide
- anionic IgG 4 f.
- area-length method for ejection f.
- atrial filling f.
- attributable f.
- cardiac ejection f.
- cineangiography and sensitometric ejection f.
- circumferential shortening f.
- Cohn fraction II
- computed ejection f.
- constituent of alpha protein plasma f.
- constituent of gamma protein plasma f.
- constituent of plasma protein f.
- creatine kinase MB f.
- creatine kinase fraction muscle
- ejection f.
- ejection fraction at rest
- ejection fraction during exercise
- ejection fraction of heart
- ejection fraction systolic
- ethanol volume f.
- excess ejection f.
- f. of expired carbon dioxide
- extraction f.
- false-negative f.
- false-positive f.
- filtration f.
- fine f.
- free f.
- free thyroxine f.
- gallbladder ejection f.
- global left ventricular ejection f.
- growth f.
- heparin-precipitable f.
- hepatocycle volume f.
- increased dose size per f.
- f. of inspired carbon dioxide
- f. of inspired oxygen
- intrapulmonary shunt f.
- lactate dehydrogenase fraction 1–5
- left ventricular ejection f.
- lipoprotein-deficient f.
- liver fraction elevated
- mean fraction absorption
- Melcher acid-soluble f.
- micronized flavonidic f.
- minor fraction of adult hemoglobin
- mole f.
- multiple daily f.
- muscle fraction enzyme of creatine phosphokinase
- neutral f.
- nonmigrating fraction of spermatozoa
- normal ejection f.
- oxygen extraction f.
- plasma protein f.
- precipitable fraction heparin
- quick f.
- regional ejection fraction image
- regurgitant f.
- resting radionuclide ejection f.
- right ventricular ejection f.
- shortening fraction percentage
- survival f.
- thymosin fraction 5
- true negative f.
- true positive f.
- two-dimensional echo-derived ejection f.
- ultrafine f.
- f. unbound
- ventricular ejection f.
- whole lymphocyte f.

fractional
- f. albuminuria rate
- f. area change
- f. area concentration
- f. catabolic rate
- f. clearance
- f. concentration of carbon dioxide in expired gas
- f. concentration of inspired oxygen
- f. concentration of oxygen in expired gas
- f. dilatation and curettage
- f. dilation and curettage
- f. disappearance rate
- f. dose
- dry gas fractional concentration
- f. esterification rate
- f. excretion
- f. excretion of lithium
- f. excretion of potassium
- f. excretion of sodium
- f. flow reserve
- f. free-water clearance
- high-dose fractional radiation therapy
- f. inhibitory concentration
- f. inspired oxygen concentration
- long-axis fractional shortening
- myocardial fractional flow reserve
- f. osteoid surface
- f. percentage of inspired oxygen
- percent fractional shortening
- peripheral fractional oxygen extraction
- f. proximal resorption
- f. reabsorption
- f. shortening
- f. test meal
- f. turnover rate
- f. urinalysis
- f. urines
- f. velocity reserve

fractionated
- f. external beam irradiation
- f. high dose rate
- f. radiotherapy
- f. stereotactic radiosurgery
- f. stereotactic radiotherapy
- f. total body irradiation

fractionation
f. of bilirubin
biologic factors in dose f.
cell cycle redistribution and dose f.
daily fractionation rate of rad
field-flow f.
gravitational field-flow f.
high-dose fractionation radiation therapy
sedimentation field flow f.
time-dose fractionation factor
tumor dose f.

fracture
acetabular rim f.
acute avulsion f.
Aitken classification of epiphysial f.
Aitken epiphysial fracture classification
alignment of f.
alignment of fracture fragment
angulation at fracture site
ankle mortise f.
anterior calcaneal process f.
anterior column f.
anteroinferior corner f.
anterolateral compression f.
AO ankle fracture classification
AO-Danis-Weber ankle fracture classification
AO fracture pattern
articular mass separation f.
articular pillar f.
Ashhurst-Bromer ankle fracture classification
Ashhurst fracture classification system
Atkin epiphysial f.
atlas-axis combination f.
atlas burst f.
avulsed fracture fragment
avulsion chip f.
avulsion stress f.
axial compression f.
axial loading f.
axial load 3-part, 2-plane f.
axial load teardrop f.
axis-atlas combination f.
basal skull f.
f. bedpan
f. bilaterally in a horizontal plane
f. blister
both bones f.
f. of both bones
bowing of f.
f. callus
childhood accidental spiral tibial f.
f. classification
clavicular f.
clay-shoveler's f.
closed reduction of f.
closed skull f.
combined flexion-distraction injury and burst f.
comminuted intraarticular f.
comminuted orbital f.
comminuted skull f.
comminuted tibial f.
f., complete, angulated
f. complete and compound
f. complete, compound, and comminuted
f. complete and deviated
f. complete and varus deformity
complex simple f.
f. compound and comminuted
compound comminuted f.
compression fracture of spine
cough fracture of rib
crepitus at fracture site
crushed eggshell f.
crush fracture syndrome
Danis-Weber classification for ankle f.
debridement of compound skull f.
f. decompression
f. deformity
delayed healing of f.
delayed union of f.
depressed fracture skull
depressed skull f.
de Quervain f.
f. deviation
f. diastasis
f. dislocation
drill bit f.
epicondylar avulsion f.
extension corner avulsion f.
extension teardrop f.
falls and f.'s immobility
femoral diaphysial f.
femoral intertrochanteric f.
femoral intratrochanteric f.
femoral neck f.
femoral supracondylar f.
f. fixation
f. fragment
f. frame
freeze fracture electron microscopy
Galeazzi fracture of radius
greater trochanteric femoral f.
greater tuberosity f.
grenade thrower's f.
growth plate f.
hamate hook f.
head fracture frame
high fracture risk
humeral shaft f.
immobilization mandibular f.
incision carried down to the fracture site
incomplete fracture of bone
incomplete vertical root f.
inner fracture face
intercondylar fracture of hip
internal fixation of f.
intertrochanteric femoral f.
intertrochanteric region f.
F. Intervention Trial
intracapsular f.
juvenile calcaneal f.
lateral condylar f.
Le Fort f.
linear f.
linear skull f.
f. line consolidation
Lloyd-Roberts fracture technique
local compression f.
local decompression f.
long bone f.
lower extremity f.
lower frontal bone f.
Maisonneuve fibular f.
major fracture fragment
malar complex f.
malleolar chip f.
malunited calcaneus f.
malunited forearm f.
mandibular body f.
mandibular condyle f.
manual fracture reduction
Mason fracture classification system
mastoid bone f.
Mayo elbow fracture classification
medial column calcaneal f.
medial epicondylar f.
medial epicondyle humeral f.
metacarpal head f.
metatarsal stress f.
Miami fracture brace
micronized purified flavonoid f.
Milch classification of humeral f.
Milch condylar fracture classification

Milch elbow fracture classification
Milch fracture classification syndrome
minimally displaced f.
Monteggia forearm f.
Mueller femoral supracondylar fracture classification
Mueller humerus fracture classification
navicular body f.
navicular dorsal lip f.
naviculocapitate fracture syndrome
Neer classification of shoulder f.
Neer femur fracture classification
Neer-Horowitz classification of humeral f.
Neer humerus fracture classification
neural arch f.
Newman classification of radial neck and head f.
Nicoll fracture operation
Nicoll fracture repair procedure
nonarticular distal radial f.
nonunion of f.
nonunion of fracture site
nonunion fracture trauma
nonunion horse-hoof f.
O'Brien classification of radial f.
obturator avulsion f.
occipital condyle f.
odontoid condyle f.
odontoid fracture internal fixation
odontoid fracture stabilization
Ogden epiphysial fracture classification
Ogden fracture classification system
old healed f.
open book f.
open fracture wound drain
open reduction of skull f.
f. of orbit
orbital blow-in f.
orbital blow-out f.
orbital floor f.
orbital rim f.
orbital wall f.
ORIF of f.
Orthoplast fracture brace
osteochondral fracture arthrography
osteochondral fracture of the dome of the talus
osteoporotic compression f.
outlet strut f.
Ovadia-Beals classification of tibial plafond f.
pacemaker lead f.
palatal alveolar f.
Palmer classification of trapezial ridge f.
Papavasiliou classification of olecranon f.
pathologic compression f.
Pauwels femoral neck fracture classification
pelvic avulsion f.
pelvic fracture frame
perinatal clavicle f.
perinatal humerus f.
phalangeal diaphysial f.
phalangeal fracture fixation
plate and screw fixation of f.
Pott ankle f.
pronation-lateral rotation fracture
proper alignment of f.
proximal femoral f.
proximal humeral f.
pure blowout f.
radial head f.
reduced nasal f.
f. reducing elevator
f. reduction
f. remodeling
remottling fracture site
f. repair
rotation and reduction of f.
f. running length of bone
sacral insufficiency f.
Salter-Harris classification of f.
segmental bronchus f.
f. simple and complete
f. simple complete and comminuted
f. simple and depressed
f. site
skull f.
sphenoid bone f.
spinal compression f.
f. splint
spontaneous f.
spontaneous osteoporotic fracture of sacrum
f. stabilization
stable burst f.
f. table
talar dome f.
tarsal bone f.
teardrop burst f.
temporal bone f.
tibial fracture brace proximal support
tibial plateau f.
transcervical femoral f.
tripartite fracture of patella
vertebral body f.
wagon wheel f.
f. with delayed union
f. with malunion
f. with nonunion

fracture-dislocation
Monteggia fracture-dislocation of ulna
perilunate f.-d.

fractured jaw

fracturing wall

fragile
f. chromosome site
f. gene
f. histidine triad
f. site mental retardation 1, 2
f. X chromosome
f. X-E
f. X gene
f. X mental retardation protein
f. X syndrome
f. X type A

fragility
capillary fragility test
erythrocyte fragility test
hereditary capillary f.
medium corpuscular f.
osmotic fragility test
red blood cell f.
Rumpel-Leede capillary f.
vascular fragility syndrome
X-linked first site of f.
X-linked second site of f.

fragment
alignment of fracture f.
anteroinferior triangular f.
f. of antibody
f. antigen binding
f., antigen, and complement binding
apical fragment ejector
apical fragment forceps
apoptic nuclear f.
autotransplantation of splenic f.
avulsed fracture f.
bone f.
capsule fragment forceps
cleavage fragment length polymorphism
dome f.
elastin fragment concentration
f. of endometrial tissue
extruded disc f.

fragment *(continued)*
free fragment disc
free fragment herniation
f. of immunoglobulin G after digestion with the enzyme pepsin
f. of immunoglobulin G involved in antigen binding
limited fragment proteolysis
linear combination of fragment configuration
luteinizing hormone beta core f.
major fracture f.
major proglucagon f.
McKeever-Buck fragment excision
multiple fragment wounds
mutation-enriched restriction fragment length polymorphism assay
nasal bone f.
noncovalently bonded dimer of C-terminal immunoglobulin of Fc f.
PCR fragment analysis
polymerase chain reaction-restriction fragment length polymorphism
prothrombin fragment 1.2
restriction fragment length polymorphism
shell f.
shell fragment wound
shrapnel fragment wound
single-chain variable f.
urinary beta-core f.
urinary gonadotropin f.
f. wound

fragmentation
electrohydraulic f.
erythrocytic f.
Ocutome II fragmentation system
ventricular diastolic f.

fragmented sarcoplasmic reticulum

fragmentography
mass f.

fragmentor
Lieberman f.

fragrance mix

frame
arch bar f.
corrected TIMI frame count
head fracture f.
metal frame reinforced plastic bracket
mouth gag f.
nonferromagnetic MR-compatible f.
one-plane bilateral f.
open reading f.
overhead f.
overhead frame trapeze
pelvic fracture f.
peripheral frame implant substructure
unidentified reading f.
universal frame outer socket

frameless
f. stereotactic device
f. stereotactic guidance
f. stereotactic microsurgery
f. stereotaxy
f. stereotaxy system

framework
multidimensional f.
osteocartilaginous f.
third framework region

Franchesseti
oculodigital sign of F.

Franck Drawing Completion Test

Franconi anemia

frank
f. blood
f. blood in stool
f. breech
f. breech presentation
f. congestive failure
f. delirium
f. diastasis
f. disc herniation
f. dislocation
f. hemorrhage
f. pus
f. rale
f. rigors
f. vaginal breech delivery
f. vertigo

Frankel
modified Frankel classification

Frankfort
F. horizontal plane of skull
F. mandibular incisor angle
F. mandibular plane angle

Franz-O'Rahilly classification

Fraser
nasal Fraser suction technique

fraternal twins

fraud
health f.

frayed
f. disk
f. meniscus

fraying of meniscus

freckle
melanotic f.
melanotic freckle of Hutchinson

freckling
axillary f.
periorbital f.

free
f. abdominal air
abdominal cavity free of fluid
f. abdominal fluid
absolute free thyroxine
absolute free triiodothyronine
f. acid
f. air
f. air in abdomen
f. air in diaphragm
f. air passage
f. air under diaphragm
anterior helical rim free flap
anterolateral thigh free flap
apparent free testosterone concentration
ascorbic free radical
f. available chlorine
calcified free body
calcium-magnesium f.
cancer f.
carrier f.
f. cholesterol
composite free tissue transfer
f. cytoporphyrin in erythrocytes
dermal fat free flap
dermal fat free tissue transfer
f. dermal-fat graft
dialyzable free thyroxine
f. of disease
f. drain
drug f.
dye f.
f. energy
episode free day
f. erythrocyte coproporphyrin
f. erythrocyte porphyrin
f. erythrocyte protoporphyrin
expanded free scalp flap
extended lateral arm free flap
fast imaging with steady-state free precession
fat f.
f. fat graft
f. fatty acid
fatty acid f.

f. fatty-acid phase
fibula free flap
f. flow electrophoresis
f. forearm flap
f. fraction
f. fragment disc
f. fragment herniation
f. from chlorine
f. from distant metastases
f. from infection
f. from progression
full, free range of motion
gastric analysis, free and total
Gibbs free energy
f. gingival groove
gluteal free flap
f. graft
Helmholtz free energy
hepatic vein free pressure
f. hepatic venous pressure
f. hydrochloric acid
f. induction decay
f. intraperitoneal air
iris scraped f.
jejunal free flap
left ventricular free wall
long leg brace with free ankle
maximum free flow rate
mean free path
meat f.
medical free electron laser
metatarsal free vascularized graft
microsurgical free flap
microsurgical free pulp flap
microvascular free flap
microvascular free flap transfer
microvascular free muscle flap
microvascular free posterior interosseous flap
microvascular free tissue transfer
microvascular free toe transfer
mitochondrial free radical generation
Moberg free tendon graft
monoclonal free light chain
f. monoclonal urinary light chain
musculocutaneous free flap
neurosensorial free medial plantar flap
neurovascular free flap
nicked free beta subunit of human chorionic gonadotropin
osteomyocutaneous free flap
oxygen free radical
f. peritoneal air
f. peritoneal fluid
polyunsaturated free fatty acid
f. portal pressure
f. position gravity
preservative f.
proportion free thyroxine
pure free acid
f. pyrophosphate
radial forearm free flap
f. radical
f. radical assay technique
rectus abdominis free flap
reverse fast imaging with steady-state free precession
Ross carbohydrate f.
F. Running Asthma Test
salt f.
f. secretory component
f. secretory piece
sequential free flap
skin-muscle free flap
specific pathogen f.
standard free energy
steady-state free precession
steady-state free progression
symptom f.
f. testosterone
f. testosterone level
f. thyroxine factor
f. thyroxine fraction
f. thyroxine index
f. T_4 index
f. tissue transfer
f. to total prostate-specific antigen
f. transverse rectus abdominis musculocutaneous flap
f. transverse rectus abdominis myocutaneous flap
f. triiodothyronine
f. triiodothyronine index
f. unbound thyroxine
unesterified free fatty acid
urinary free cortisol
urine free cortisol
f. volatile fatty acid
f. water
f. water clearance
f. water deficit

freed
appendix freed up
f. by blunt dissection

freedom
degree of f.
degrees of f.
f. from distant metastases
f. from distractability
F. from Distractibility Deviation Quotient
f. from metastases
f. from progression
f. from relapse
F. of Information Act
loss of f.
number of degrees of f.

free-floating
f.-f. anxiety
F.-f. Anxiety Test
f.-f. bone chip
f.-f. thrombus

free-flow oxygen

freehand
f. biopsy
f. cannulation
f. CT-guided biopsy
f. cut
f. method
f. suturing technique
f. technique

free-hand
f.-h. injection
f.-h. knife

free-induction decay

freeing up of adhesion

freely
carina freely movable
f. eating
f. movable joint

Freeman Anxiety Neurosis and Psychosomatic Test

free-standing
f.-s. ambulatory surgical center
f.-s. clinic
f.-s. emergency center

freeze
fight, flee, freeze, or faint
f. fracture electron microscopy
quick f.

freeze-dried
f.-d. allograft
f.-d. bone allograft
f.-d. bone pin
f.-d. cadaveric dura
f.-d. cancellous allograft
f.-d. demineralized bone
f.-d. graft

freeze-drying
accelerated f.-d.

freeze-thaw cryotherapy

freeze-thawed graft

freezing
gastric f.
methanol freezing method

freezing *(continued)*
f. point
f. point osmometer
sudden transient f.
temperature, f.

Fregoli delusion

Freiberg disease

Freiburger Personality Inventory

Freiburg method

fremitus
diminished f.
hydatid f.
pleural f.
subjective f.
tactile f.
tactile vocal f.
vocal f.

French
F. catheter
F. scale
F. steel sound

French-American-British leukemia classification system

Frenchay
F. Aphasia Screening Test
F. Dysarthria Assessment

frenulum, pl. **frenula**
lingual f.
f. of M'Dowel
multiple buccal frenula
multiple oral frenula

frenum
lingual f.
Morgagni f.

frequency
abnormal f.
alpha frequency activity
alpha frequency band
alpha frequency coma
alpha frequency range
alpha rhythm f.
angular f.
audio f.
brain wave frequency range
breathing f.
centroid f.
characteristic f.
ciliary beat f.
constant f.
f. of contact scale
cough f.
critical bandwidth range of f.'s
critical corresponding f.
critical flicker f.
critical frequency of photic driving
critical fusion f.
cutoff f.
delta f.'s
f. dependence of compliance
f. dependence of resistance
f. deviation
f. domain imaging
Doppler-shifted constant f.
f. ectopic ventricular beat
extremely high f.
extremely low f.
fecal f.
fetal cardiac f.
fetal heart f.
fixed frequency response
flicker fusion frequency test
f. and form of amplitude
fundamental f.
fundamental frequency indicator
haplotype f.
hearing f.
heart f.
Hertz f.
high f.
high-filter f.
high frequency band
high frequency of recording
increased frequency of urination
f. of infection
intermediate f.
line frequency noise dot
low-filter f.
low frequency alternating current
low frequency band
maximum frequency range
mean alpha f.
mean dominant f.
mean frequency of compensation
mean power f.
medium f.
f. modulation
f. of the more common allele of a pair
most comfortable f.
mutation f.
narrow frequency band
night frequency of voiding
nocturnal urinary f.
observed intrinsic f.
peak repetition f.
preferred frequency speech interference level
pulse repetition f.
range of f.
f. of rarer allele of a gene pair
reduced hearing at high f.
reduce tension headache f.
f. of respiration
respiratory f.
rhythm of alpha f.
rotational f.
running frequency and intensity
seizure f.
sleep stage change f.
speaking fundamental f.
spectral edge f.
spectral frequency distribution
square waves of high f.
super high f.
Thorndike-Lorge written f.
f. threshold curve
f. to tidal volume
transformation f.
ultrahigh f.
ultrasonic f.
f. and urgency of urination
urinary urgency and f.
variant f.
very high f.
very low f.
video f.
waves of alpha f.
weight transferral f.
zero f.

frequency-difference interferential current therapy

frequency-duration index

frequency-following response

frequency-selective saturation

frequent
f. bowel movement
f. heartburn
f. individual bursts of alpha activity
f. intoxication
f. urinary incontinence

frequently
f. asked questions
f. relapsing nephrotic syndrome

fresh
f. frozen
f. frozen allograft
f. frozen plasma
f. frozen plasma transfusion
f. gas flow
f. hemorrhage
Mohs fresh tissue chemosurgery technique
f. water

Freund
F. adjuvant
F. complete adjuvant
complete Freund adjuvant
F. incomplete adjuvant
incomplete Freund adjuvant

friability
cervical f.

friable necrotic tissue

Fricke
F. dosimetry
F. operation

friction
adhesional and glide f.
f. artifact
f. blister
f. bulla
cross fiber f.
deep friction massage
deep transverse f.
iliotibial band friction syndrome
iliotibial tract friction syndrome
internal f.
f. lock pin
low friction arthroplasty
f. murmur
pericardial friction rub
pericardial friction sound
peritoneal friction rub
pleural friction rub
f. rub
single-axis friction knee prosthesis
f. sound
transverse friction massage

friction-fit adapter

friction-retained pin

Friedman test for pregnancy

Friedreich
F. ataxia
F. tabes

Friend
F. disease virus
F. erythroleukemia cell
F. leukemia cell
F. leukemia virus
F. murine erythroleukemia
resistant Friend leukemia cell
F. spleen focus virus
F. virus anemia
F. virus polycythemia

friendliness
attitude of active f.

Friend-Moloney antigen

Friend-Moloney-Rauscher antigen

Friesinger score

Frijoles virus

Frimberger-Karpiel 12 o'clock papillotome

fringe
synovial f.

Fritz-Lang operation

frog
male frog test

frogleg
f. position
f. view

frog-legged position

Frohse
arcade of F.
arch of F.

frond
intravitreal neovascular f.
f. of vessel

frond-like appearance

front
mineralization f.
f. optic zone radius
f. routing of signal
f. support strap
f. wheel walker

frontal
anterior f.
anteromedial frontal branch of callosomarginal artery
ascending frontal convolution
ascending frontal gyrus
ascending frontal parietal
autosomal dominant nocturnal frontal lobe epilepsy
f. bossing
f. cortex
f. eye field
f. fibrosing alopecia
f. headache
f. horn index
inferior frontal gyrus
inferior frontal lobe
f. intermittent rhythmic delta activity
ipsilateral frontal routing of signals
f. irregular rhythmic delta activity
lateral frontal bone window
left frontal craniotomy
left frontal hematoma
f. lobe
f. lobe epilepsy
f. lobe seizure
lower frontal bone fracture
medial frontal cortex
medial frontal gyrus
medial frontal lobe syndrome
median frontal sulcus
metallic frontal needle
middle frontal convolution
middle frontal gyrus
middle frontal sulcus
f. midline placement of electrodes in electroencephalography
monorhythmic frontal delta
monorhythmic frontal delta activity
nasal border of frontal bone
nasal margin of frontal bone
occult frontal focus
opening of frontal sinus
orbital arch of frontal bone
orbital aspect of frontal lobe
orbital plane of frontal bone
orbital plate of frontal bone
osteoplastic frontal sinus procedure
f. outflow tract
paramedian frontal bone window
parietal border of frontal bone
parietal margin of frontal bone
persistent frontal suture
f. polar electrode placement in electroencephalography
right frontal craniotomy
right frontal hematoma
right frontal lobe
right frontal sinus
sagittal, frontal, transverse, rotation
superior frontal convolution
superior frontal gyrus
superior frontal sulcus
synostotic frontal plagiocephaly
transseptal frontal sinusotomy

frontale
operculum f.
os f.

fronting
palatal f.

front-loading ultrasound probe

frontoanterior
left frontoanterior fetal position
right frontoanterior fetal position

frontobasal
medial frontobasal artery

frontocentral beta rhythm

frontodextra
f. anterior position
f. posterior position

frontoethmoidal suture

frontoethmoidectomy
Lynch frontoethmoidectomy procedure

frontolateral
left f.
right frontolateral fetal position

frontomaxillonasal suture

frontometaphyseal dysplasia

frontonasal
axial frontonasal flap

frontonasal dysplasia

frontooccipital
f. circumference
f. diameter
f. fetal position

frontoparietal
f. area
ascending f.
ascending frontoparietal artery

frontopolar artery

frontoposterior
left frontoposterior position fetal
right frontoposterior fetal position

frontosphenoid suture

frontotemporal
f. dementia
f. lobar degeneration

frontotransverse
left frontotransverse fetal position
f. position
right frontotransverse fetal position

frontozygomatic suture

frostbite
f. hand
f. injury
superficial f.
third-degree f.

frosted heart

Frostig
F. Developmental Test of Visual Motor Perception
F. Movement Skills Test Battery
F. Program for the Development of Visual Perception

frosting heart

frothy
f. discharge
f. sputum

frowning
oral f.

frozen
f. animal procedure
biopsy submitted for frozen section
deglycerolized frozen red cell
f. embryo replacement
fresh f.
fresh frozen allograft
fresh frozen plasma
fresh frozen plasma transfusion
f. hand
Neviaser frozen shoulder classification
f. packed cell
f. plasma
rapid frozen section
f. section assay
f. section red blood cell
single-donor frozen plasma

fructose
f. diphosphatase
f. diphosphate
f. diphosphate aldolase
f. intolerance
f. tolerance test

fructose-terminated oligosaccharide

Frühsommer meningoencephalitis

frustration
anger and f.
low frustration tolerance
penalty, frustration, anxiety, guilt, hostility
picture frustration study

Fuchs
angle of F.
F. atrophy
F. heterochromic cyclitis
F. heterochromic iridocyclitis
F. iritis

fuchsin
aldehyde f.
f., amido black, and naphthol yellow

fugax
amaurosis f.

fugue
epileptic f.
psychogenic f.
f. state

fugu poisoning

Fukuyama congenital muscular dystrophy

fulcrum fracture

fulfillment
asymptotic wish f.

fulguration
curettage and f.
cystoscopy and f.

full
absorbance units, full scale
f. allosteric modulators
f. blood count
f. blood examination
f. body immersion
f. bony impaction
f. cardiac arrest
f. cast restoration
f. cervical spine
f. to confrontation
f. course of radiation
f. course radiation therapy
f. denture
f. diet
f. extraocular motion
f. extraocular movement
extraocular movements full and conjugate
f. florid diabetic retinopathy
forced passive full forward flexion
f., free range of motion
f. gold crown
f. head of hair
f. inspiration
f. joint range of motion
f. joint range of movement
f. knee extension
f. liquid diet
f. lower denture
f. maternal behavior
f. mouth dentures
neck full range of motion
f. outpatient rate
f. passive movements
patient tolerated full course of radiation
f. period
peripheral pulses full and equal bilaterally
physiologic full value
f. radiation of brain
f. radius cutter
f. range
f. range of affect
f. recovery time
f. ROM

f. scan with interpolation projection
f. and soft diet
f. spine board
f. strength
stroke with full recovery
f. term, born dead
f. upper denture
f. upper denture, partial lower denture
f. veneer crown
visual fields full to confrontation
f. weightbearing
f. width at half maximum
f. width of photopeak measured at half maximal count
within full limits
f. year

full-blown
f.-b. AIDS
f.-b. delirium
f.-b. dementia
f.-b. depressive episode
f.-b. infection
f.-b. manic depressive illness
f.-b. panic attack
f.-b. psychosis

full-breech presentation

Fullerton Language Test for Adolescents

full-jacketed
f.-j. bullet wound
f.-j. military round

full-mouth
f.-m. extraction
f.-m. periapicals
f.-m. restorative dentistry
f.-m. series
f.-m. x-ray

fullness
f. in abdomen
abdominal f.
aural f.
hilar f.
periorbital f.
postprandial f.

full-on gain

full-radius
f.-r. resector
f.-r. resector knife

full-scale
f.-s. deflection
F.-s. Intelligence Quotient
f.-s. IQ
f.-s. score
F.-s. Score Total

full-strength breast milk

full-term
f.-t. appropriate for gestational age
f.-t. deliveries, premature deliveries, abortions, living children
f.-t. delivery
f.-t., small for gestational age
f.-t. infant
f.-t. intrauterine pregnancy
f.-t., large for gestational age
f.-t. live birth
f.-t. living female child
f.-t. living male child
f.-t. newborn
f.-t. normal delivery
f.-t., normal, spontaneous delivery
f.-t. nursery
f.-t., small for gestational age
f.-t. uncomplicated pregnancy, labor, and delivery

full-thickness
f.-t. local excision
f.-t. skin graft

fully
f. dilated
f. granulated basophil
f. resonant nucleus

fulminans
purpura f.

fulminant
f. abscess
f. disease
f. glaucoma
f. hepatic failure
f. hepatitis
f. hyperthermia
f. liver disease
non-A–G fulminant hepatitis
f. pulmonary edema
f. sepsis
f. viral hepatitis

fumarate
f. hydratase, mitochondrial
f. hydratase, soluble

fume
cadmium f.
polymer fume fever

function
ability to function independently
abnormal brain wave f.
abnormal liver function test
abnormal primary f.
abnormal pulmonary f.
absent bowel f.
adrenergic vagal f.
advanced communications f.
airway function test
alteration in respiratory f.
altered brain f.
altering brain f.
anorectal function test
anterior pituitary f.
f., appearance, time
atrial-phase volumetric f.
atrial transport f.
atrioventricular nodal f.
atrioventricular node f.
autonomic function test
autonomous ego f.
basic human f.
bowel and bladder f.
caloric stimulation test for vestibular f.
caloric testing of vestibular f.
capacity to f.
capillary refill, sensation, motor function, temperature
cardiac function index
cardiac size and f.
ceased to f.
cerebral metabolic f.
Clinical Evaluation of Language F.'s
cognitive function assessment
cognitive function tests
compromised renal f.
contractile function in cells of myocardium
corpus luteum f.
corrected time of sinoatrial node function recovery
cortical function testing
cortical mapping of memory f.
declined in f.
decline in mental f.
decline in sexual f.
decreased ability to f.
decreased bowel f.
decreased immune f.
delayed graft f.
detector transfer f.
developmental hand function test
diaphragmatic f.
diminished heart, kidney and brain f.
discriminant f.
disruption of bladder f.

function *(continued)*
disturbance of function occlusion syndrome
disturbance of visual f.
disturbed bowel f.
edge response f.
electrical function of heart
error f.
eustachian tube f.
executive cognitive f.
executive ego f.
executive function deficit
expanded function dental assistant
exponential function
extracorporeal membrane oxygenation affecting cognitive f.
factor VIII coagulation f.
fine motor f.
Foot F. Index
gallbladder function test
global assessment of f.
Gross Motor F. Measure
heart, kidney and brain f.
heart and lung f.
heart valve f.
hepatocyte f.
higher cognitive f.
higher cortical f.
higher integrative f.
higher intellectual f.
higher mental f.
high level of f.
Hipputope renal f.
host leukotactic f.
immediate good function followed by accelerated rejection
immune function abnormality
impaired cardiac f.
impaired hepatic f.
impaired kidney f.
impaired left ventricular f.
impaired liver f.
impaired motor f.
impaired neurological f.
impaired renal f.
impaired systolic f.
impairment of functions of brain stem
impairment in liver f.
impairment of liver f.
impairment of social f.
improved immune f.
inability to f.
inadequate sexual f.
increased kidney f.
intellectual function or memory
International Index of Erectile F.
involuntary body f.
irregular brain f.
kidney f.
left atrial f.
left ventricular f.
level of independent f.
Leydig cell secretory f.
line-spread f.
line spread f.
liver function profile
liver function series
liver function tests
localization of f.
loss of control of bladder f.
loss of f.
low thyroid f.
lung function testing
lymphocyte function antigen
lymphocyte function assay
mapping of cortical f.
mathetic function of language
measuring heart f.
medial rectus f.
memory function deficit
mixed function oxidase
mixed function oxidase system
modulation transfer f.
monocyte function test
motor function assessment
motor function deficit
mucosa-associated lymphoid tissue f.
muscle function test
myocardial contractile f.
National Eye Institute Visual F. Questionnaire
neonatal biliary f.
nerve function impairment
normal bowel f.
normal heart f.
normal immune system f.
normal jaw f.
normal pulmonary f.
normal renal f.
normal urinary f.
nuclear ventricular function study
organically impaired brain f.
pancreatic exocrine function insufficiency
pancreatic exocrine function test
parietal lobe f.
perceptual cognitive motor f.
performance-intensity function test
performance versus intensity function for phonetically balanced words
peripheral auditory f.
peripheral rod f.
phagocytosis and killing f.
pituitary function test
pituitary gland f.
pituitary hormone f.
placental function test
platelet function analysis
platelet function study
platelet function test
point-spread f.
position of f.
postoperative pulmonary f.
prior level of f.
probability density f.
progressive decline in f.
pulmonary f.
pulmonary function score
pulmonary function study
pumping function of heart
renal function panel
renal function study
renal function test
residual renal f.
right atrial f.
right ventricular f.
sciatic function index
Self-Evaluation of Life Function scale
sensation and motor f.
severely impaired renal f.
sexual function score
sexual function of women
Sexual F. Inventory Questionnaire
Short Musculoskeletal F. Assessment
slowed intellectual f.
slow initial f.
Social F. Index
split function study
split renal f.
stabilize heart f.
f. study
subtalar joint f.
f. test
thymus gland f.
thyroid function profile
thyroid function study
Ultegra rapid platelet function assay
unimpaired motor f.
velocity distribution f.
ventricular contractility f.
ventricular function curve
wave f.
Wolf Motor F. Test

functional
acquired functional megacolon

f. activity
F. Acuity Contrast Test
f. aerobic capacity
aerobic conditioning functional assessment
f. aerobic impairment
alcohol-induced functional impairment
F. Ambulation Categories
f. and anatomic loading
antithrombin III f.
aperiodic functional MR imaging
f. arm brace
f. aspects of heart
F. Assessment of Cancer Therapy
F. Assessment of Cancer Therapy-Breast
F. Assessment of Cancer Therapy-Fatigue
F. Assessment of Cancer Therapy-General
F. Assessment of Cancer Therapy–Head and Neck
F. Assessment of Cancer Therapy-Lung
F. Assessment of Cancer Therapy-Prostate
f. assessment of human immunodeficiency
f. assessment inventory
f. assessment measure
F. Assessment Staging
atrioventricular functional tachycardia
autonomous functional component
f. bactericidal concentration
f. bowel disease
f. bowel disorder
F. Bowel Disorder Severity Index
f. bowel distress
f. bowel syndrome
f. capacity
f. capacity evaluation
cardiac functional capacity
Child and Adolescent F. Assessment Scale
f. class
f. communication
f. conduction period
cosmetic and functional purpose
f. decortication from hypoglycemia
f. decortication from hypoxia
demand minimum functional capacity
F. Disability Index
f. electrical stimulation
f. electronic peroneal brace
f. endoscopic sinus
f. endoscopic sinus surgery
f. exercise program
f. extracellular fluid volume
Fuzzy F. Form
f. gastrointestinal disorder
Hand F. Index
f. headache
f. hearing loss
f. hearing test
f. heart
f. heart murmur
hepatic functional panel
highest functional level
f. hypertrophy
f. hypothalamic amenorrhea
f. illness
image-guided functional endoscopic sinus surgery
f. imaging
f. impairment
F. Impairment Scale for Children and Adolescents
f. incontinence
F. Independence Measure for Children
independent functional ability
f. indigestion
individualized functional status assessment
f. inhibitory concentration
f. inquiry
F. Integration test
intermittent functional bowel problem
intestinal control in functional coitus
Inventory of F. Status After Childbirth
Juvenile Arthritis F. Assessment Report
left ventricular functional shortening
f. length
F. Life Scale
F. Limitation Profile
F. Living Index-Cancer
F. Living Index-Emesis
Lower Extremity F. Scale
f. magnetic resonance angiography
f. magnetic resonance imaging
f. maintenance program
major functional impairment
mandibular functional reconstruction
mechanical functional loss
f. movement
f. MRI
multifocal functional autonomy
f. muscle test
f. neck dissection
F. Needs Assessment
f. neuromuscular stimulation
neutrophil functional disorder
NYHA functional classification
OARS Multidimensional F. Assessment Questionnaire
F. Outcomes of Sleep Questionnaire
partially functional neutrophil
patient's functional ability
F. Performance Record
pleiotrophic functional defect
predicted functional residual capacity
Pulmonary F. Status and Dyspnea Questionnaire
radionuclide functional lymphoscintigraphy
f. reach
f. refractory period
F. Related Groups
f. renal failure of cirrhosis
f. reserve capacity of lungs
f. residual capacity
f. residual capacity of lungs
residual functional capacity
f. residual volume
f. resting position splint
restrictive functional impairment
severe functional insufficiency
f. shortening
f. spinal unit
f. status
F. Status Index
f. status measures
F. Status Questionnaire
f. subunit
f. terminal innervation ratio
Toronto F. Capacity Questionnaire
totally functional neutrophil
f. transcranial Doppler sonography
f. transcutaneous nerve stimulation
f. trial visit
f. uptake of carbon monoxide
f. urethral length
f. uterine bleeding

functional *(continued)*
f. vital capacity
f. well-being
within functional limits
f. work capacity assessment

functionality
Békésy F. Detection Test
social stress and functionality inventory

functionally
f. illiterate
f. independent

functioning
abnormal functioning of heart
alter gastric f.
anxiety-induced impaired social f.
assess functioning of heart
autonomously functioning thyroid nodule
baseline level of f.
borderline intellectual f.
Brief Index of Sexual F. for Women
carbon atom farthest from principal functioning group
Comprehensive Test of Visual F.
Defensive F. Scale
degree of physical f.
difficulty functioning at normal ability level
executive cognitive f.
executive functioning disturbance
global assessment of f.
Global Assessment of Relational F.
global level of f.
grossly impaired f.
impaired cognitive f.
impaired mental f.
impairment in occupational f.
improper functioning of foot
improved overall f.
Institutional Functioning Inventory
level of f.
major impairment of f.
marked decline in academic f.
measure of general cognitive f.
neurovegetative functioning or symptom
normal functioning ileal transverse colostomy
normally functioning kidney
optimal level of f.
overall cognitive f.
pancreatic functioning diagnostant
previous level of f.
quantitative autonomic functioning testing
f., reasoning, orientation, memory, arithmetic, judgment, and emotion
Sexual F. Index
Social and Occupational F. Assessment
Visual F. index
Western Ontario and McMaster Universities Osteoarthritis Index Physical F. subscale and chair-performance
Western Ontario and McMaster Universities Osteoarthritis Index Physical F. subscale and chair-stand performance

Function-Preschool
Clinical Evaluation of Language F.-P.

fund
f. of information
f. of intelligence
f. of knowledge

fundal
f. height
f. plication
f. portion of uterus
f. pressure

fundamental
f. frequency
f. frequency indicator
f. human drive
f. imaging
F. Interpersonal Relations Orientation-Behavior
F. Interpersonal Relations Orientation-Feelings
f. predisposition
speaking fundamental frequency

fundi (*pl. of* fundus)

fundic
f. atrophic gastritis
f. gland polyp
metaplastic gastric fundic gland

fundoplasty
anterior f.
Nissen f.

fundoplication
gastroesophageal f.
Heller myotomy with Dor f.
laparoscopic f.
laparoscopic Nissen f.
modified Belsey f.
modified Belsey fundoplication procedure
modified Belsey fundoplication technique
Nissen 360-degree wrap f.
Nissen fundoplication method
Nissen fundoplication operation
Nissen fundoplication procedure
Nissen fundoplication technique
Nissen fundoplication wrap
Nissen-Rosseti fundoplication method
Nissen-Rosseti fundoplication procedure
Nissen-Rosseti fundoplication technique
open Nissen f.
Rossetti modification of Nissen f.
Thal fundoplication procedure
total fundoplication procedure
Toupet hemifundoplication fundoplication

fundus, pl. **fundi**
f. anterior, normal size and shape, and mobile
dilated fundus examination
f. firm
f. firm at umbilicus
f. firm 1, 2 cm above umbilicus
f. firm 1, 2 cm below umbilicus
f. fluorescein angiogram
f. of the gallbladder
height of f.
indocyanine-green fundus angiography
mottling of f.
optic f.
optic fundi and peripheral fields
f. photo
polyp of fundus of stomach
pupils, tension, media, disc, and f.
retinal fundus photography
xerophthalmic f.

funduscopic examination

funeral
f. home arrangements
f. home notification

fungal
f. abscess
allergic fungal sinusitis
f. arthritis
disseminating fungal infection
endemic fungal infection
f. growth
f. immunodiffusion

f. infection
f. intracellular pathogen
mixed fungal organism
nondermatophyte fungal infection
nosocomial fungal infection
opportunistic systemic fungal infection
f. overgrowth
pancreatic fungal detection
peritoneal fungal infection

fungal/bacterial
mixed fungal/bacterial infection

fungating
f. growth
f. lesion
f. mass
f. sore
f. tumor
f. wound

fungicidal
minimal fungicidal concentration
serum f.

fungistatic
serum f.

fungoides
microabscess of mycosis f.
mycosis fungoides palmaris et plantaris

fungus
agar diffusion for f.
Aspergillus fungus ball
f. culture
generalized infection involving f.
f. infected nail
f. infection
mycelial phase of fungus
f. smear
f., smear, and culture

funicular hernia

funiculus
dorsolateral f.

funisitis
necrotizing f.

Funk
Autenrieth and Funk method

funnel
Martegiani f.
muscular f.

funny-looking
f.-l. beat
f.-l. kid
f.-l. rash

furnace
annealing f.

furred tongue

furrow
Liebermeister f.
lip furrow band
marginal f.
marginal furrow degeneration
median furrow of prostate
mentolabial f.
nasolabial f.
orbitopalpebral f.
palpebral f.

furrowed tongue

furrowing
scarring and f.

further
f. differentiated fibroblast
f. flexion
no further action required
no further information
no further treatment
prevent further outbreak
until further notice

furuncular
African furuncular myiasis

fusaric acid

fuscin
Luna-Parker acid fuscin stain

fused apophyseal joint

fusidic acid

fusiform
f. aneurysm
axial fusiform developmental cataract
f. skin revision

fusion
Adkins spinal f.
Albee lumbar spinal f.
Albee spinal f.
Anderson ankle f.
anterior cervical f.
anterior cervical body f.
anterior cervical discectomy and f.
anterior cervical diskectomy and f.
anterior interbody f.
anterior lumbar interbody f.
anterior lumbar spine interbody f.
anterior lumbar vertebral interbody f.
anterior and posterior f.
anterior-posterior fusion with segmental spinal instrumentation
anterior-posterior fusion with SSI
anterior release posterior f.
anterior spinal f.
anterior spine f.
atrial f.
atrial fusion beat
auditory flutter f.
f. beat
craniosynostosis, ataxia, trigeminal anesthesia, parietal anesthesia and pons, vermis fusion syndrome
critical flicker f.
critical flicker fusion test
critical fusion frequency
dowel spinal f.
flicker fusion frequency test
flicker fusion threshold
f. inhibitor
laminectomy and f.
lower cervical spine f.
lumbar intersomatic fusion expandable cage
lumbosacral fusion elevator
Marcus-Balourdas-Heiple ankle fusion technique
microcephaly-cervical spine fusion anomalies
midline fusion defect
müllerian duct f.
müllerian fusion defect
Panum fusion area
partial labioscrotal f.
f. point
posterior lumbar interbody f.
posterior spinal f.
posterolateral interbody f.
purified fusion protein
spinal fusion surgery
threaded fusion cage
unilateral posterior lumbar interbody f.
ventricular f.
Worth four-dot test for f.

fusion-inferred threshold test

fusobacteria microorganisms

futility
medical f.

future order screen

fuzzy
blurred or fuzzy vision
distant objects f.
F. Functional Form

G
G. inhibiting protein
G. protein-coupled receptor

G_1
immunoglobin G.
time required to complete G_1 phase of cell cycle

G_2
time required to complete G_2 phase of cell cycle

Gabek Forest virus

Gadget's Gully virus

gadolinium in chelated form

gadolinium-enhanced magnetic resonance imaging

gadolinium-enhancing tumor volume

Gaenslen sign

Gaffky scale

gag
diminished gag reflex
hair-trigger gag reflex
g. junction
mouth g.
mouth gag frame
g. reflex
g. response

gage gene

gain
abnormal diurnal weight g.
antipsychotic-induced weight g.
attachment level g.
automatic gain control
body oscillation neuromuscular g.
body weight g.
g. control
g. control switch
episodic weight g.
erratic weight g.
excessive weight g.
expected weight g.
field g.
full-on g.
gradual weight g.
infant weight g.
manipulates to gain power
manipulates to gain profit
maternal weight g.
modified gain ratio
oxygen gain factor
peak acoustic g.
personal desire for g.
g. perspective
postmenopausal weight g.
rapid weight g.
significant gain in weight
significant weight g.
subsequent weight g.
sudden weight g.
therapeutic gain factor
time compensation g.
time-varied g.
time-varied gain control
total weight g.
g. weight

gait
abnormal gait and station
g. abnormality
G. Abnormality Rating Scale Modified
adequate gait and station
Adjustable Advanced Reciprocating G. Orthosis
g. analysis
angle of g.
g. apraxia
G., Arms, Legs, and Spine
g. assessment
g. ataxia
g., balance and coordination
g. and balance disorder
balance, gait, and station
g. biomechanics
bizarre gait pattern
cadence of g.
change in g.
change in gait and posture
deterioration of coordination, gait, and speech
g. deviation
g. disorder, autoantibody, late-age onset, polyneuropathy
g. disturbance
disturbance of gait and stance
disturbances in g.
g. dysfunction
forward tandem g.
idiopathic gait disorders of elderly
g. imbalance
g. imbalance and oscillopsia
intermittent double-step g.
g. lock splint
g. and mobility
modified G. Abnormality Rating Scale
neuromuscular gait pattern change
patient unsteady in g.
g. pattern
Peak gait module
progressive gait imbalance
reciprocating gait orthosis
g. reeling, staggering
senile gait disorder
g. and stance
g. and station
tandem gait test
g. training
g. trait

gaited
nuclear multiple gaited acquisition

gaiter cast

galactocerebrosidase deficiency

galactokinase deficiency

galactorrhea
amenorrhea, galactorrhea, hypothyroidism
drug-induced g.

galactorrhea-amenorrhea hyperprolactinemia syndrome

galactose
g. elimination capacity
g. enzyme activator
neuraminidase and galactose oxidase
g. tolerance test

galactose-binding protein

galactosemia
g. diet
lactose intolerance and g.
Los Angeles variant g.

galactosemic fibroblast

galactosidase deficiency

galactosyl transferase

galanthamine hydrobromide

galea
aponeurotic g.
g. aponeurotica
g. forceps
tendinous g.

galea-frontalis advancement

galea-frontalis-occipitalis release

galeal
g. flap
g. frontalis flap
g. myofascial flap
g. occipital flap
pedicled galeal frontalis flap
g. periosteal flap

Galeazzi fracture of radius

Galen
aneurysm of Galen vein
aneurysm of vein of G.
great vein of G.
vein of G.

Galen *(continued)*
vein of Galen aneurysmal dilatation
vein of Galen aneurysmal malformation

Galius adenovirus 1–2

gallate

gallbladder
adenomyoma of g.
ampulla of g.
g. anastomosed to duodenum
atypical gallbladder disease
g. bag positioner
g. bed
calcified wall of g.
calculous gallbladder disease
g. calculus
g. cancer
chronically inflamed gallbladder with stones
g. contraction
g. disease
g. dome
double-dose gallbladder cholecystogram
g. dysmotility
g. ejection fraction
g. ejection rate
empyema of g.
endoscopic transpapillary catheterization of g.
g. extraction
g. films
g. fossa
g. function
g. functioning
g. function test
g. fundus
fundus of the g.
g. hydrops
hydrops of the g.
hydrops of g.
inflammation of the g.
laparoscopic gallbladder surgery
g. and liver scan
g. meridian
mucocele of g.
mucosa of g.
mucosal fold of g.
muscular coat of g.
muscular layer of g.
neck of g.
Niemeier gallbladder perforation
nonvisualization of g.
notch of g.
pelvis of g.
percutaneous transhepatic gallbladder drainage
perforation of g.
g. pigment stones
poorly visualized g.
poorly visualizing g.
primary adenocarcinoma of the g.
g. series
serosa of g.
g. shadow
g. shelled out from the gallbladder bed
g. sludge
g. stasis
symptomatic gallbladder disease
thickened gallbladder wall
g. trocar
g. visualized
g. wall

gallium
g. citrate
g. citrate contrast material
g. citrate scan
g. imaging
limited gallium scan
radioactive g.
g. scanning
g. scintography

gallium-67
g.-67 citrate contrast medium
g.-67 imaging
g.-67 scan
g.-67 scintigraphy

gallons per minute

gallop
atrial g.
atrial diastolic g.
diastolic g.
murmurs, rubs, and g.'s
murmurs, g.'s, or rubs
presystolic g.
g. rhythm
g. sound
summation g.
systolic gallop rhythm
ventricular diastolic g.

galloping
g. consumption
g. paresis

Galloway-Mowat syndrome

gallows humor

gallstone
acute gallstone pancreatitis
g. colic
g. detection
g. disease
g. forceps
g. formation
g. ileus
g. imaging
Moore gallstone scoop
Moynihan gallstone scoop
multiple g.'s
g. pancreatitis
pancreatitis secondary to g.'s
g. probe
prone to developing pigment g.'s
g. removal
g. surgery
ultrasound gallstone detection

galvanic
g. bath
g. cautery
g. contractility
g. current
g. faradization
high-voltage pulsed galvanic stimulation
g. muscle stimulation
g. nystagmus
g. resistance
g. response
g. skin potential
g. skin reflex
g. skin resistance
g. skin response audiometry
g. stimulation
g. tetanus ratio
g. threshold
g. vertigo
g. vestibular stimulation

galvanocaustic amputation

galvanotonic contraction

Galveston
G. Orientation and Amnesia Test
G. Orientation and Awareness Test

gambler
adolescent g.
G.'s Anonymous
binge g.
compulsive g.
occasional g.
pathologic g.
problem g.
professional g.

gambling
g. addiction
compulsive g.
excessive g.
pathologic g.
pathological g.
pathologic gambling disorder
video g.

Gamboa virus

game
middle g.
model g.

gamekeeper's
g. injury
g. thumb
g. thumb dislocation

gamete
aging g.
g. intrafallopian tube transfer
g. manipulation
g. micromanipulation

gamete-shedding substance

gametic
g. nucleus
g. selection

gametocyte
person gametocyte week

gametogenesis
ovarian g.

gamma
aggregated human gamma globulin
g. A globulin deficiency
g. A immunoglobulin deficiency
g. A immunoglobulin determination
alpha, beta, gamma hypotheses
Anger gamma camera
anti-Rh gamma globulin
antithymocyte gamma globulin
automated gamma counter
g. band response
bovine gamma globulin
capture gamma ray
g. chain disease
constituent of gamma protein plasma fraction
continuous ambulatory gamma globulin infusion
g. decay
delayed gamma camera image
detection of gamma ray
g. fibers
fowl gamma globulin
g. fungus
gamma immunoglobulin G.
g. globule
g. globulin
g. globulin-free calf serum
g. globulin injection
g. globulin M deficiency
g. globulin replacement
g. globulin therapy
goat antirabbit gamma globulin
guinea pig gamma globulin
hemoglobin gamma chain A
hemoglobin gamma chain G
human gamma globulin
g. hydroxybutyrate
hyperimmune antivariola gamma globulin
g. immunoglobulin A, D, G, M
g. immunoglobulin D determination
g. immunoglobulin E determination
g. immunoglobulin G determination
g. immunoglobulin M determination
g. interferon
intramuscular gamma globulin
intravenous gamma globulin
g. knife
g. knife stereotactic radiosurgery
g. light chain
g. locking nail
mitochondrial deoxyribonucleic acid polymerase g.
mitochondrial DNA polymerase g.
g. motoneuron
mouse gamma globulin
multicrystal gamma camera
neurosurgical gamma knife
peroxisome proliferator-activated receptor g.
photon gamma ray
polyclonal gamma globulin
g. probe guided lymphoscintigraphy
g. probe radiolocalization
prophylactic gamma globulin
g. radiation
g. ray
g. ray spectrometer
g. ray surgery
g. ray therapy
recombinant interferon g.
retroplacental gamma globulin
g. rhythm
g. roentgen
g. scintillation camera
single crystal gamma camera
single-photon gamma scintigraphy
specific gamma ray constant
g. staphylolysin
g. streptococcus
synthesize gamma globulin
turkey gamma globulin
g. wave
g. well counter

gamma-aminobutyric acid transaminase

gamma-chain disorder

gamma-glutamyl
g.-g. transferase
g.-g. transpeptidase

gamma-glutamyltransferase
serum g.-g.

gamma-glycoprotein
glycine-rich g.-g.

gamma-heavy-chain disease

gamma-melanocyte-stimulating hormone

gammopathy
benign monoclonal g.
essential monoclonal g.
IgA monoclonal g.
monoclonal g.
monoclonal gammopathy of undetermined significance
monoclonal gammopathy of unknown significance
no gammopathy detected
polyclonal gammopathy identified
polyneuropathy, organomegaly, endocrinopathy, monoclonal gammopathy, and skin changes syndrome

Gamna disease

Gamna-Gandy
G.-G. body
G.-G. nodule
G.-G. spleen

gang
adolescent gang member

Gan Gan virus

ganglia (*pl. of* ganglion)

gangliocytoma
adenohypophysial g.

ganglioglioma
desmoplastic infantile g.

ganglion, pl. **ganglia**
aorticorenal g.
Auerbach g.
autonomic g.

ganglion *(continued)*
autonomic ganglion block
autonomic sympathetic g.
basal ganglion calcification
basal ganglion disease
basal ganglion disorder-mental retardation
buccal g.
g. cell
cervical ganglion of uterus
cervicothoracic g.
dorsal root g.
fluid filled g.
giant ganglion cell
histologic section of g.
inferior carotid g.
inferior cervical g.
inferior ganglion of vagus nerve
inferior jugular g.
inferior mesenteric g.
inferior vagal g.
jugular ganglion of vagus nerve
left caudal quarter g.
left rostral quarter g.
long root of ciliary g.
lower ganglion of glossopharyngeal nerve
lower ganglion of vagus nerve
lumbar g.
middle cervical g.
motor root of ciliary g.
myenteric ganglion cell
nodose g.
oculomotor root of ciliary g.
optic g.
orbital branch of pterygopalatine g.
paracervical g.
parasympathetic g.
paravertebral g.
pelvic g.
percutaneous coagulation of gasserian g.
posterior intervertebral ganglion of head
retinal ganglion cell
right caudal quarter g.
right rostral quarter g.
right stellate g.
right visceral g.
sacral ganglia
small, intensely fluorescent g.
sphenopalatine g.
spiral ganglion of cochlea
stellate ganglion nerve block
superior carotid g.
superior cervical g.
superior ganglion of vagus nerve
superior mesenteric g.
superior vagal g.
symmetrical calcification of basal cerebral g.
sympathetic branch to submandibular g.
sympathetic ganglion block anesthetic technique
g. of sympathetic plexus
g. of sympathetic trunk
Wrisberg g.

ganglionectomy
cerebral nerve g.
left cardiac sympathetic g.

ganglioneuroblastoma
composite g.

ganglionic
autonomic ganglionic synapse
g. blocking agent
g. center
g. cyst
excision of ganglionic cyst
g. glioma
left stellate ganglionic blockade
g. saliva

ganglionitis
herpetic geniculate g.

gangliosidosis
neuronal GM1 g.

gangrene
angiosclerotic g.
antigas gangrene serum
appendiceal g.
arteriosclerotic g.
g. of bowel
circumscribed g.
clostridial gas g.
cold g.
diabetic g.
diabetic gangrene of lung
digital g.
dry g.
embolic g.
emphysematous g.
g. in extremity
Fournier g.
g. from atherosclerosis
g. from diabetes
gas g.
gas gangrene wound
hot g.
incipient g.
ischemic g.
g. of lung
major g.
mammary g.
Meleney synergistic g.
moist g.
necrotic gangrene tissue
nosocomial g.
oral g.
penile g.
pentavalent gas gangrene antitoxin
perinatal gangrene of buttock
peripheral g.
Pott g.
primary g.
Raynaud g.
senile g.
static g.
g. stomatitis
symmetrical peripheral g.
thrombotic g.
trophic g.
wet g.

gangrene-like infection

gangrenosum
pyoderma g.
pyogenic sterile arthritis, pyoderma gangrenosum, and acne

gangrenosus
pemphigus g.

gangrenous
g. abscess
acute gangrenous appendicitis
g. appendicitis
g. appendix
g. balanitis
g. bowel
g. cellulitis
g. cholecystitis
g. colon
g. cystitis
g. emphysema
epidemic gangrenous proctitis
g. ischemic colitis
g. ischemic enterocolitis
g. necrosis
necrotic gangrenous tissue
perforated gangrenous appendix
g. pharyngitis
g. pneumonia
g. pulp necrosis
g. rhinitis
g. skin
g. small bowel
g. stomatitis

Ganley
G. and Ganley metatarsus adductus procedure

G. modification of Keller arthroplasty
G. technique
G. tendon transfer

Ganser
G. commissure
G. diverticulum
G. ganglion
nucleus basalis of G.
G. syndrome

Gant
G. hip arthrodesis
G. operation
G. osteotomy

gantry
g. angulation
g. rotation
g. tilt

Gantzer
G. accessory bundle
G. muscle

Ganz
G. anti-shock pelvic fixator
G. cup
G. fixation
G. osteotomy

Ganzfeld stimulation

gap
air-bone g.
air gap correction
anion g.
anion gap acidosis
anion gap metabolic acidosis
anion gap test
g. arthroplasty
Békésy Ascending-Descending G. Evaluation
g. calculation
cardiac gap junction protein
g. in cell cycle
g. conduction phenomenon
delta g.
g. detection
g. function
g. healing
g. junction
g. junction intercellular communication
g. junction protein
low anion g.
mean residual g.
nonanion gap acidosis
g. nonunion
nonunion gap metabolic acidosis
g. paradigm
g. 0, 1, 2 period
g. 0 phase
velopharyngeal g.

gaping
g., draining sore
g. wound
g. wound edges

garbled speech

Gardner Analysis of Personality Survey

garment
antishock g.
graduated compression g.
pneumatic g.
pneumatic antishock g.

garnet
holmium yttrium-aluminum garnet laser
neodymium:yttrium aluminum garnet laser
yttrium, aluminum, g.
yttrium, argon, g.

Gartner
G. duct
G. duct cyst

gas
abnormality in gas exchange
abnormal sac containing g.
G. Anal F&T
g. analyzer
g. anesthetic
anesthetic gas exposure
anesthetic gas mixture
aneurysmal wall g.
anhaustral colonic gas pattern
g. antitoxin
arterial blood g.
arterial blood gas abnormality
arterial blood gas analysis
arterial blood gas point-of-care test
arterial gas embolism
arterial gas sampling
arterial gas volume
Astrup blood gas value
g. atomized dispersion strengthened
bloating and/or diarrhea, gas, cramps
bloating and g.
blood gas alteration
blood gas analysis
blood gas at room temperature
blood gas measurement
blood gas stick
blood gas study
bowel gas artifact
bowel gas pattern
g. bubble
capillary blood g.
capillary blood gas at room air
capillary column gas chromatography
carbon dioxide g.
carbon dioxide gas laser
g. chromatographic-mass spectrometry
g. chromatography
g. clearance
g. clearance measurement
clostridial gas gangrene
cold gas sterilization
cord blood g.
g. cystometry
dead-space gas volume to tidal gas volume ratio
deteriorating blood g.'s
difference in nitrogen tension between mixed alveolar gas and mixed arterial blood
difference in partial pressures of oxygen in mixed alveolar gas and mixed arterial blood
g. distribution
dry gas fractional concentration
g. embolism
g. embolus
ethylene oxide g.
excessive gas formation
excessive intestinal g.
g. exchange
extracorporeal gas exchange
g. and feces
feces and g.
fingerstick blood g.
fractional concentration of carbon dioxide in expired g.
fractional concentration of oxygen in expired g.
fresh gas flow
g. gangrene
g. gangrene wound
heel-stick blood g.
hepatic portal venous g.
impaired gas exchange
inspiratory phase g.
intestinal gas pattern
intestinal tract g.
intrathoracic gas volume
intrauterine g.
g. isotope ratio mass spectrometry
g. level
liquified natural g.

gas *(continued)*
liquified petroleum g.
low blood gas partition
medical gas analyzer
mixed expired g.
multiple gas rebreathing
multiple inert gas elimination technique
mustard g.
nerve gas poisoning
nitrate to g.
nitrogen-phosphorus detector in gas chromatography
nonspecific bowel gas pattern
overlying bowel g.
overlying gas shadow
overlying intestinal g.
g. and oxygen
g., oxygen, and ether anesthesia
oxygen and ether g.
g. pack
partial arterial gas tension of carbon dioxide
g. partial pressure
partial pressure of carbon dioxide in arterial g.
partial venous gas tension of oxygen
g. pattern
paucity of bowel g.
paucity of g.
pentavalent gas gangrene antitoxin
perfluorocarbon-associated gas exchange
perfluoropropane g.
g. permeable contact lens
pulmonary capillary gas volume
pulmonary gas exchange
regional gas exchange
relative gas expansion
respiratory gas equation
retroperitoneal gas insufflation
room air blood g.
g. sterilization
g. sterilized instrument
g. in stomach
superimposed bowel g.
g. tamponade
thoracic gas volume
tracheal gas insufflation
g. transfer
trapped gas volume
g. tube
venous blood g.
g. volume
volume of expired g.
volume of inspired gas per minute
volume thoracic g.

gas-density balance

gaseous
g. cholecystitis
g. distention
gastric gaseous dilatation
g. microembolus
g. pulse

gas-fluid exchange

gas-forming food

gasless
g. abdomen
balloon-assisted, endoscopic, retroperitoneal, g.

gas-liquid
g.-l. chromatography
g.-l. chromatography/mass spectrometry
g.-l. phase chromatography

gasp
agonal g.
g. reflex

gasping
agonal g.
g. for air
g. for breath
g. and cyanotic
g. respiration

gasserian
g. fissure
g. ganglion
g. ganglionectomy
percutaneous coagulation of gasserian ganglion

gas-solid chromatography

gastrectomy
laparoscopically assisted distal partial g.
partial g.
pylorus-preserving g.
total g.

gastric
g. acid inhibitor
g. acidity
g. acid secretion
acute gastric dilatation
acute gastric mucosal lesion
adjustable silicone gastric banding
g. air bubble
g. alcohol dehydrogenase
alcohol-induced gastric injury
Alden loop gastric bypass
altered gastric motility
alter gastric functioning
g. analysis
g. analysis, free and total
anterior gastric branch of anterior vagal trunk
g. antral erosion
antral gastric cell
g. antral sessile polyp
g. antral vascular ectasia
g. antrum
g. arteriovenous malformation
g. artery
ASA-induced gastric ulceration
g. aspirate
g. aspiration
aspiration of gastric contents
g. atony
atrophic gastric mucosa
g. atrophy
g. augment and single pedicle tube
g. bacterial overgrowth
Balfour gastric resection
g. banding
basal gastric secretion
benign gastric ulcer
g. bleeding
bleeding gastric varix
g. bleeding time
g. bubble
g. bypass
g. bypass operation
g. bypass procedure
g. bypass surgery
g. cancer
g. cancerous area
g. carcinoma
g. cardia
g. chromoscopy
chronic gastric ulcer
g. component of reflex barrier
g. contents
continuous gastric drip
control gastric secretion
g. culture
g. cycle
g. cytology
g. decompression
deformity of gastric outlet
delayed gastric emptying
demucosalized augmentation with gastric segment
g. dilatation
g. disorder
distal gastric adenocarcinoma
g. distention
g. distress

g. diverticulum
g. dyspepsia
early gastric cancer of the upper stomach
early gastric carcinoma
early gastric emptying
g. emptying
g. emptying delay
g. emptying half-time
g. emptying procedure
g. emptying scan
g. emptying of solids
g. emptying time
g. erosion
esophageal gastric tube airway
g. first-pass metabolism
g. fistula
g. fluid
g. fluid, basal acid output
g. fold
g. freezing
g. fundus
g. gaseous dilatation
giant gastric ulcer
g. gland
hog gastric mucin
g. hypersecretion
g. ileal bypass
g. indigestion
g. inhibitory peptide
g. inhibitory polypeptide
inoperable gastric carcinoma
g. insufficiency
g. interdigestive contraction
g. irritation
isolated gastric varices type 1, 2
g. juice
g. laryngeal mask airway
laser adjustable silicone gastric banding
g. lavage
g. lavage tube
left gastric artery
left gastric lymph node
left gastric vein
g. loop bypass
loop gastric bypass method
loop gastric bypass procedure
loop gastric bypass technique
g. lung
g. lymphoma
maximal sniff-induced gastric pressure
metaplastic gastric fundic gland
monoclonal antibodies against gastric mucins
g. mucosa
g. mucosal atrophy
g. mucosal barrier
g. mucosal blood flow
g. mucosal ectopia in rectum
g. mucosal erosion
mucosal gastric ulcer
g. mucosal hemorrhage
multifocal ectopic gastric mucosa
narrowing of gastric outlet
g. nerve
g. neurectomy
nocturnal gastric reflux
g. noncancerous area
nonerosive gastric mucosal lesion
normal human gastric juice
g. notch
NSAID-induced gastric injury
oblique gastric fiber
open adjustable silicone gastric banding
oral g.
oral gastric tube
g. outlet
g. outlet irritability
g. outlet obstruction
g. pacemaker
papillary gastric carcinoma
g. parietal cell
g. pars media
partial gastric resection
pentagastrin gastric secretory test
perforated gastric ulcer
g. pits
preoperative gastric aspiration
g. pressure
primary gastric lymphoma
primary gastric non-Hodgkin lymphoma
proximal gastric exclusion
proximal gastric resection
proximal gastric vagotomy
psychogenic gastric ulcer
g. pull-through procedure
g. pull-up procedure
g. pylorus
radionuclide gastric emptying study
g. reduction surgery
g. remnant
g. remnant cancer
remnant gastric cancer
g. resection
g. residence time
g. residual volume
retained gastric antrum
retained gastric antrum syndrome
reversed gastric tube
right gastric lymph node
right gastric vein
g. sclerosis
secretes gastric juice
g. secretory testing
selective gastric vagotomy
g. shield
short gastric vein
Silastic ring vertical-banded gastric bypass
simulated gastric fluid
sphincter of gastric antrum
g. stapling procedure
sterile water gastric drip
g. stoma
substernal gastric bypass
g. suction
superficial gastric ulcer
terminal aspiration of gastric contents
g. tract disorder
g. tumor
g. varix
g. vascular ectasia
g. vertical stapling
g. volvulus
g. washing
g. wrap

gastric-inhibitory hormone

gastric-intrapleural pressure

gastrin

antral gastrin cell hyperfunction
basic g.
big g.
fasting gastrin level
immunoreactive g.
immunoreactive human g.
integrated gastrin response
plasma g.
synthetic human g.

gastrin-releasing peptide

gastritis

acute erosive g.
alcoholic hemorrhagic g.
alkaline reflux g.
antral atrophic g.
atrophic chronic g.
autoimmune metaplastic atrophic g.
chronic active g.
chronic atrophic g.
chronic cystic g.
chronic erosive g.
chronic superficial g.
diffuse antral g.

gastritis *(continued)*
environmental metaplastic atrophic g.
erosive gastritis with ulceration
experimental autoimmune g.
g. from alcohol
g. from aspirin
fundic atrophic g.
giant hypertrophic g.
g. granulomatosa fibroplastica
hemorrhagic erosive g.
hypertrophic lymphocytic g.
loss of appetite from g.
lymphocytic g.
metaplastic atrophic g.
multifocal atrophic g.
nonspecific erosive g.
nonspecific nonerosive g.
reflux bile g.
tenderness in abdomen from g.

gastrocnemius
g. aponeurosis
g. flap
g. lengthening
medial gastrocnemius bursitis
medial gastrocnemius muscle
medial head of the gastrocnemius rupture
g. muscle
musculus g.
g. recession
g. soleus
g. and soleus muscles
g. tendon

gastrocnemius-soleus
g.-s. complex
g.-s. muscle
g.-s. recession
g.-s. tendon

gastrocolonic response

gastroduodenal
g. artery
obstructive gastroduodenal Crohn disease
g. pylorus

gastroduodenalis
arteria g.
musculus dilator pylori g.

gastroduodenitis
neutrophilic g.

gastroenteritides
parasitic g.

gastroenteritis
acute infectious g.
acute infectious nonbacterial g.
allergic eosinophilic g.
eosinophilic g.
epidemic acute nonbacterial g.
nonbacterial gastroenteritis virus
nonbacterial infantile g.
transmissible g.
transmissible gastroenteritis virus
viral g.

gastroenterocolitis
allergic eosinophilic g.

gastroenterostomy
percutaneous g.
posterior g.
vagotomy and Billroth g.

gastroenterotomy
vagotomy and g.

gastroepiploic
g. artery
g. vein
g. vessel

gastroesophageal
g. angle of His
g. fundoplication
g. hernia
g. incompetence
g. junction
nonerosive gastroesophageal reflux disease
normal gastroesophageal reflux of infancy
patulous gastroesophageal junction
g. pressure gradient
g. reflux
g. reflux disease
g. sphincter

Gastrografin enema

gastrointestinal
acute gastrointestinal hemorrhage
acute upper gastrointestinal bleeding
acute upper gastrointestinal hemorrhage
alcohol-induced gastrointestinal symptom
g. anastomosis
g. anisakiasis
g. autonomic nerve tumor
g. bacterial flora
g. bleeding
g. cancer antigen
g. cancer-associated antigen
chronic gastrointestinal tract bleeding
g. diagnostic area
g. distress
double-contrast barium examination of the upper gastrointestinal tract
g. endoscopy
g. fiberscope
functional gastrointestinal disorder
g. hemorrhage
g. hormone
g. hypermotility
g. infection
g. intubation
g. irritation
g. irritation and ulceration
g. lavage
lower g.
lower gastrointestinal bleeding
lower gastrointestinal hemorrhage
massive gastrointestinal hemorrhage
metabolic, endocrine, and g.
metabolic, endocrine, and gastrointestinal disorders
Moore classification for vascular anomalies of the gastrointestinal tract
g. motility
g. mucormycosis
multiple gastrointestinal polyps
neonatal gastrointestinal hemorrhage
nonfamilial gastrointestinal polyposis
nosocomial gastrointestinal infection
occult gastrointestinal bleeding
g. pacemaker cell tumor
g. polyposis
postoperative gastrointestinal motility
g. procedure unit
psychophysiologic gastrointestinal reaction
G. Quality of Life Index
salivation, lacrimation, urination, defecation, gastrointestinal distress and emesis
g. series
severe gastrointestinal bleeding
g. smooth muscle tumor
g. stromal tumor
g. symptom
G. Symptom Rating Scale
g. therapeutic system
g. tract
g. tract bleeding
g. tract lymphoma
g. transit time

upper gastrointestinal biopsy
upper gastrointestinal bleeding
upper gastrointestinal endoscopy
upper gastrointestinal series with small bowel follow-through
upper gastrointestinal tract hemorrhage
g. virus
g. workup

gastrointestinal-associated lymphoid tissue

gastrojejunostomy
antecolic long-loop isoperistaltic g.
percutaneous endoscopic g.
g. tube

gastroparesis
nondiabetic g.
postsurgical gastroparesis syndrome
transient g.

gastropathy
benign hyperplastic g.
duodenal-gastric reflux g.
hypertrophic hypersecretory g.
nonsteroidal antiinflammatory drug g.
portal hypertensive g.
prolapse gastropathy syndrome

gastropexy
anterior g.
percutaneous anterior g.

gastroplasty
adjustable ring g.
banded gastroplasty with a divided pouch
silicone elastomer ring vertical g.
vertical banded g.
vertical ring g.

gastroplication
endolumenal g.

gastroprotective
g. agent
g. drug

gastrosalivary reflex

gastroscope
flexible g.
pediatric g.

gastroscopic
orbital exenteration gastroscopic access technique

gastrostomy
g. bumper
dual percutaneous endoscopic g.
feeding gastrostomy tube
jejunal tube through percutaneous endoscopic g.
open gastrostomy tube placement
percutaneous endoluminal g.
percutaneous endoluminal gastrostomy tube
percutaneous endoscopic g.
percutaneous endoscopic gastrostomy insertion
percutaneous endoscopic gastrostomy and jejunal extension tube
percutaneous endoscopic gastrostomy tube
retrograde percutaneous g.
g. tube feeding
g. tube migration
venting percutaneous g.

gastrotomy
anterior g.
g. tube

gate
insulated gate field effect transistor
locking g.
OR g.

gated
g. blood pool angiography
g. blood pool scanning
g. blood pool scintigraphy
g. blood pool study
g. blood pool ventriculogram
g. cardiac blood pool
g. cardiac blood pool imaging
cardiac gated study
g. CT scanner
g. 3D reconstruction
multiple gated acquisition scan
quantitative gated SPECT
g. radionuclide angiography
g. single-photon emission computed tomography
g. sweet magnetic imaging

gateway
common gateway interface
g. drug

gating
cardiac g.
echocardiographic g.
electrocardiographic g.
navigator echo-based real-time respiratory gating and triggering

Gaucher disease

gauge
adjustable-length gauge needle
eye movement g.
g. of needle
orthopaedic depth g.
peak-flow g.
standard wire g.
water g.

gauntlet
g. anesthesia
g. atrophy
g. bandage
g. cast
g. flap

gaussian
floating spherical gaussian orbital

gauze
g. dissection
g. dressing
dry sterile g.
fine mesh g.
fluffed gauze dressing
iodoform gauze packing
moistened fine mesh gauze dressing
narrow gauze roll
Nu Gauze bandage
Nu Gauze packing
g. pack
packed with g.
g. packing
g. pad
g. sponge
g. wick
g. wrap

gavage
g. feeding
nasal g.

gay-related
g.-r. immune deficiency

gaze
apraxia of g.
cardinal direction of g.
cerebral gaze paresis
conjugate fixed g.
conjugate gaze palsy
conjugate horizontal g.
conjugate upward g.
g. deficit
direct forward g.
downward g.
g. fixation
g. following
horizontal gaze nystagmus
horizontal gaze palsy
g. impairment
left lateral g.
midline position of g.
near fixation position of g.

gaze *(continued)*
near gaze reflex
nuclear horizontal gaze paralysis
g. nystagmus
nystagmus on upward g.
g. palsy
parallelism of g.
g. paralysis
paralysis of conjugate upward g.
g. paresis
periodic alternating g.
periodic alternating gaze deviation
pontine gaze center
g. preference
right lateral g.
g. saccade
supranuclear gaze palsy
upward gaze weakness
vertical gaze palsy

gaze-evoked
g.-e. amaurosis
g.-e. blindness
g.-e. nystagmus
g.-e. visual loss

Gee-Herter disease

Geiger-Müller counter

gel
agar gel diffusion
agar gel electrophoresis
alpha-hydroxy acid g.
autologous growth factor g.
autologous platelet g.
g. chromatography
denaturing gradient gel electrophoresis
g. development time
g. diffusion precipitin
g. electrophoresis
fibrin matrix g.
fibrinogen gel chromatography
hard gel capsule
instant thin-layer chromatography-silica g.
isoelectric focusing electrophoresis in polyacrylamide g.
localized hemolysis in g.
malleolar gel sleeve
mucous gel thickness
nonequilibrium pH gradient gel electrophoresis
orthophosphoric acid etch g.
Ouchterlony gel diffusion technique
g. permeation chromatography
polyacrylamide g.
polyacrylamide gel electrophoresis with silver stain
polyacrylamide gel isoelectric focusing
pulsed-field gradient gel electrophoresis
radial hemolysis in g.
silica gel filtered
silicone gel sheeting
sodium dodecyl sulfate-polyacrylamide gel electrophoresis
temperature-gradient gel electrophoresis
temporal temperature gradient gel electrophoresis

gelatin
absorbable gelatin sponge
g. agglutination test
g., glucose, and Veronal buffer
g. Hanks buffered salt solution
g. infusion medium
insoluble bone g.
modified heat-degraded g.
nutrient gelatin agar
g., resorcinol, formaldehyde
soft elastic gelatin capsule
soluble g.

gelatinous
g. substance of gray substance
Rolando gelatinous substance

gelatin-veronal buffer

gelation
ethanol gelation test

gel-filled
g.-f. breast implant
g.-f. implant

gel-filtered platelet

gelling
absorbent gelling material

gender
appropriate in g.
atypical gender identity disorder
g. behavior disorder
g. gap
g. identity disorder
g. identity disorder of adolescence
g. identity disorder of adolescence or adulthood, nontranssexual type
g. identity disorder of adult life
g. identity disorder of childhood
male gender identity
personality and g.
g. role definition

gene
adenopolyposis coli g.
adenoviral gene transfection
adenovirus-mediated gene transfer
androgen receptor g.
androgen receptor gene mutation
angiogenesis gene delivery
angiotensin-converting enzyme g.
angiotensin-converting enzyme gene polymorphism
antiangiogenesis gene therapy
antibiotic resistance g.
anti-CD3 stimulated peripheral blood lymphocytes transduced with a gene encoding a chimeric
antigen receptor g.
APC gene mutation assay
APC tumor suppressor g.
apolipoprotein B g.
apolipoprotein E epsilon 4 g.
apolipoprotein E epsilon 4 gene on chromosome 19
apolipoprotein gene cluster
A-T mutation g.
autoimmune regulator g.
autoimmune regulatory g.
autosomal dominant g.
breast cancer g.
cancer of the prostate and brain g.
CAPB g.
cardiac gene expression
catabolite gene activator protein
catabolite gene activator
chromosome-mediated gene transfer
cytotoxin-associated gene product A
downstream regulatory element antagonistic modulator g.
factor VIII g.
factor V Leiden g.
fragile g.
fragile X g.
frequency of rarer allele of a gene pair
growth g.
growth hormone-1 g.
growth hormone-2 g.
homeobox gene
human androgen receptor g.
human ether-a-go-go-related g.
Human G. Expression
human gene therapy

human jagged-1 g.
human kidney glandular kallikrein-1 g.
identical g.'s
identification of g.
lipoprotein lipase g.
listeriolysin O g.
luciferase reporter g.
lymphocyte gene rearrangement
malic enzyme g.
manganese superoxide dismutase g.
master regulator g.
melanoma antigen-encoding gene family
melanoma-associated g.
Menkes disease g.
methylenetetrahydrofolate reductase g.
mini-exon-derived ribonucleic acid g.
mini-exon-derived RNA g.
multidrug resistance g.
multiple-drug resistance g.
multiple sclerosis susceptibility g.
myotonic dystrophy g.
neurofibromatosis 2 g.
nitric oxide synthase g.
notch gene family
paired box homeotic 3 g.
paired box homeotic 8 g.
parathyroid hormone gene transcription
Pendred syndrome g.
peripheral myelin protein 22 g.
pituitary tumor transforming g.
PMP22 g.
g. product
protein gene product
retinitis pigmentosa GTPase regulator g.
retinoblastoma g.
rhesus gene CE, D
serial analysis of gene expression
serine threonine kinase gene 11
short stature homeobox gene
single gene disorder
SMN telomeric g.
somatic cell human gene therapy
survival motor neuron telomeric g.
g. therapy
g. therapy for heart
tumor-suppressor g.
type II procollagen g.
vacuolating toxin gene A

gene-activating sequence

Genée-Wiedemann acrofacial dysostosis

gene-linkage analysis

general

g. adaptation syndrome
g. all purpose
g. anatomy
g. anesthesia
g. anesthesia with endotracheal intubation
g. appearance
G. Aptitude Test Battery
Army G. Classification Test
arthritic general pseudoparalysis
G. Audit Inpatient Psychiatric Assessment Scale
automated general experimental device
g. care and treatment
g. circulation
G. Clerical Test
g. closure
G. Cognitive Index
g. condition
g. conditioning exercise
g. diagnostics
g. dispensary
g. duties
g. endotracheal anesthesia
following satisfactory general anesthesia
g. gonadotropic activity
G. Health Perception Questionnaire
g. health problem
g. hepatic circulation
G. High Altitude Questionnaire
g. immunocompetence
g. inhalational anesthesia
involuntary general paroxysm
g. joint pain
juvenile general paralysis
g. linear model
Massachusetts G. Hospital Utility Multi-Programming System
measure of general cognitive functioning
g. medical clinic
g. medical condition
g. medical floor
g. medical panel
g. medicine and surgery
mental disorder due to a general medical condition
g. mental health
minimal access general surgery
molecular and general genetics
mood disorder due to a general medical condition
National Institute of G. Medical Sciences
g. nursing assistance
g. nursing care
g. paralysis
g. paralysis of the insane
g. paresis
g. paresis of insane
g. practice
g. practitioner
g. preventive medicine
g. procedure
g. proprioception
Psychological G. Well-Being Scale
G. Purpose Psychiatric Questionnaire
g. reading backwardness
g. relief
g. research
rural general practitioner
g. somatic afferent nerve
g. somatic efferent nerve
g. therapeutic exercise
under satisfactory general anesthesia
g. visceral afferent nerve
g. visceral efferent nerve
g. ward
G. Well-Being Index

generalization

stimulus g.

generalized

g. abdominal pain
g. aching
acute generalized exanthematous pustulosis
acute generalized tuberculosis
g. amnesia
g. anxiety disorder
g. anxiety neurosis
g. arteriosclerosis
asymmetrical generalized epileptiform activity
g. atrophic benign epidermolysis bullosa
g. body irradiation
g. body weakness
comorbid generalized anxiety
G. Contentment Scale
g. degenerative tic
g. delays
g. dystonia
g. epilepsy
g. erythema multiforme

generalized *(continued)*
g. fast activity
g. glandular enlargement
g. headache
immediate generalized reaction
g. infection involving fungus
itching g.
late generalized tuberculosis
g. linear interactive model
g. lymphadenopathy syndrome
microprobe analysis generalized intensity correction
g. muscle aches
g. nephrographic
g. osteoarthritis
partial seizures with or without generalized tonic-clonic seizures
persistent generalized lymphadenopathy
primary generalized epilepsy
g. rash
g. resistance to thyroid hormone
g. Sanarelli-Shwartzman reaction
secondarily generalized tonic-clonic seizure
secondary generalized epilepsy
Shwartzman generalized reaction
g. Shwartzman reaction
g. slow activity
g. social phobia
syndrome of generalized thyroid hormone resistance
g. thyroid hormone resistance
g. time reflex
g. tonic clonic
g. tonic-clonic convulsion
g. tonic-clonic epilepsy
g. tonic-clonic seizure
uncontrolled generalized grand mal seizure
g. visceral hypersensitivity
g. weakness
g. white matter atrophy

generally regarded as effective

generated
pulse generated runoff

generation
angiotensin generation rate
anti-HCV antibody 3rd g.
g. of diversity
filial g.
first filial g.
first parental g.
mean generation time
mitochondrial free radical g.
parental g.
pericyte edema g.
second filial g.
second generation sulfonylurea
thromboplastin generation test
thromboplastin generation time
g. time
g. time of cell cycle

generational
cross generational problem

generator
anterior current g.
artificial sound g.
asynchronous pulse g.
atrial synchronous pulse g.
atrial triggered pulse g.
computerized pattern g.
g. of excitation
pacemaker pulse g.
small-particle aerosol g.

generic equivalent

genetic
g. abnormality
g. algorithm
autosomal-dominant genetic defect
Diagnostic Interview for G. Study
g. disorder
fatal genetic illness
g. hemochromatosis
g. heterogeneity
high genetic risk
human genetic disorder
human genetic material
human genetic mutant cell repository
human molecular g.'s
g. hypertension
g. hypertrophic cardiomyopathy
g. immunity
g. impairment
g. induction
infantile genetic agranulocytosis
g. information
g. intervention
g. manipulation
mendelian genetic disorder
molecular and general g.'s
molecular genetic alteration
molecular genetic analysis
molecular genetic study
molecular genetic technique
M-type genetic group
ochre suppressor genetic mutation
oral epithelial cell genetic fingerprinting
p-ANC genetic marker
polymorphic genetic marker
g. prediabetes
g. predisposition
g. predisposition to psychiatric illness
preimplantation genetic diagnosis
g. susceptibility
g. therapy
g. variance
X-linked genetic defect

genetically
g. determined immunodeficiency disease
G. Handicapped Persons Program
g. heterogeneous
g. modified
g. modified organisms

geneticist
medical g.

genicular
medial genicular vein
medial inferior genicular artery
middle genicular artery
middle genicular vein

geniculate
g. artery
g. body
g. branch
dorsal lateral g.
g. ganglion
herpetic geniculate ganglionitis
lateral geniculate body
lateral geniculate nucleus
medial g.
medial geniculate artery
medial geniculate body
medial geniculate fascia

geniculohypothalamic tract

genioplasty
advancement g.
augmentation g.
osseous g.
osteoplastic g.

genital
g. ambiguity
aphthous genital ulcer
coloboma, heart disease, atresia choanae, retarded growth and retarded development and/or CNS anomalies, genital hypoplasia, and ear anomalies and/or deafness syndrome
development and/or central nervous system anomalies, genital hypoplasia, ear anomalies
female genital mutilation
female genital tract

female genital tract carcinosarcoma
female genital tract mutilation
g. herpes
g. herpes infection
g. herpes virus
g. lichen sclerosus
lower genital tract infection
male genital duct
male genital duct development
massive genital prolapse
multicentric lower genital tract neoplasia
multisite lower genital tract involvement
g. neoplasm-papilloma syndrome
nontreponemal genital ulcer disease
recurrent genital herpes
g. self-examination
g. skin fibroblast
Tanner genital stage
g. ulcer disease

genitalia
ambiguous external g.
aniridia, ambiguous genitalia, mental retardation
aniridia, ambiguous genitalia, mental retardation triad syndrome
Bartholin, urethral, and Skene glands, and external g.
external g.
female external g.
lentigines, electrocardiographic abnormalities, ocular hypertelorism, pulmonary stenosis, abnormalities of genitalia, retardation of growth, deafness syndrome
lymphatic drainage of g.
male external g.
male genitalia melanoma
male internal g.
mesomelic dwarfism-small genitalia syndrome
normal external female g.
normal female adult g.
normal male adult g.

genitalis
herpes g.
herpes simplex g.

genitoanorectal syndrome

genitofemoralis
nervus g.

genitourinary
artificial genitourinary sphincter implantation
g. infection
g. sphincter

Gennari
band of G.
line of G.

genodermatosis
neurologic g.

genome
g. equivalent
Human G.
Human G. Epidemiology Network
Human G. Initiative
Human G. Project
G. Initiative
G. Institute
minus sense-RNA g.
mosaic g.
mosaic genome structure
negative-sense g.

genomic
comparative genomic hybridization
restriction landmark genomic scanning

genotype
anthroponotic g.
Apo E g.

genotypic antiretroviral resistance testing

genotyping
oral epithelial cell g.

gentamicin
g. bead
g., clindamycin, and polymyxin topical preparation
high-level gentamicin resistance
g. implant
g. ototoxicity
g. peak level
serum gentamicin concentration
g. trough level
g., vancomycin, and nystatin

gentian
aniline gentian violet
g. violet

gentle pressure bandage applied

genu
anatomic genu valgus
idiopathic genu valgum
g. recurvatum
g. valgum
g. valgus
g. varum
g. varus

genuine stress urinary incontinence

geographic
g. adjustment factor
g. tongue

geometric
g. efficiency
g. mean
g. mean concentration
g. mean diameter
g. mean titer
g. progression
reciprocal geometric mean titer

Georges
St. Georges Respiratory Questionnaire

Gerbich red cell antigen

geriatric
g. assessment team
g. assessment unit
g. care
g. care manager
g. chair
G. Depression Scale
g. evaluation and management unit
inpatient geriatric consultation services
National Association of Progressional G. Care Managers
neurologic g.'s
Philadelphia G. Center Morale Scale
g. skilled care unit

germ
g. cell tumor
g. cell tumor with synchronous lesions in pineal and suprasellar region
combined germ cell tumor
gonadal germ cell neoplasm
hair g.
intratubular germ cell neoplasia, unclassified type
male germ line tumor
malignant ovarian germ cell tumor
mediastinal germ cell tumor
metachronous testicular germ cell tumor
mixed germ cell-sex cord stromal tumor

germ *(continued)*
mixed germ cell tumor
nongerminoma germ cell tumor
nonseminomatous germ cell neoplasm
nonseminomatous germ cell testicular tumor
ovarian germ cell tumor
ovarian malignant germ cell tumor
tooth g.
g. warfare
wheat germ agglutinin

germanate
bismuth g.

germanium
high-purity g.

germ-free isolation unit

germicidal
emergency drinking water germicidal tablet
ultraviolet germicidal irradiation

germicide
liquid chemical g.

germinal
g. cell aplasia
g. center
g. layer hemorrhage
g. matrix
g. matrix hemorrhage
ovarian germinal epithelium
progressive transformation of germinal center
g. vesicle
g. vesicle breakdown

Germiston virus

germ-laden air

Gerstmann
developmental Gerstmann syndrome

Gerstmann-Straüssler-Scheinker
G.-S.-S. disease
G.-S.-S. syndrome

Gesell
G. Child Development Age Scale
G. Developmental Schedules

gestalt
autochthonous g.
Bender Visual-Motor G. Test
Visual-Motor G. Test

gestation
extrauterine g.
intrauterine g.

gestational
adjusted gestational age
g. age
appropriate for gestational age
average for gestational age
birth weight for gestational age
g. carbohydrate intolerance
corrected gestational age
g. day
g. diabetes
g. diabetes mellitus
g. diabetes mellitus, diet controlled, type 2
g. diabetes mellitus, insulin controlled, type 1
empty gestational sac
estimated gestational age
full-term appropriate for gestational age
full-term, large for gestational age
full-term, small for gestational age
infant of mother with gestational diabetes mellitus
intrauterine gestational sac
large for gestational age
mean gestational sac diameter mellitus
multiples of the appropriate gestational median
nonmetastatic gestational trophoblastic disease
premature appropriate for gestational age
g. sac
g. sac and maternal date
g. sac size
small for gestational age
term birth appropriate for gestational age
g. transient thyrotoxicosis
g. trophoblastic disease
g. trophoblastic neoplasm
g. trophoblastic tumor

gesture
communicative g.
obscene g.
overt g.
paucity of expressive g.'s
suicidal g.

Getah virus

Ghazi
Dera Ghazi Khan virus

ghost
g. cell ameloblastoma
separation of g.'s

ghoul hand

GH-releasing
GH-r. factor
GH-r. peptide

GI
apple-peel appearance of the GI tract
G. bleed from anemia
lower GI bleeding
lower GI tract foreign body
major GI surgery
multiple concentric GI rings
upper GI lesion
upper GI series

Giacomini
band of G.

Giannetti Online Psychosocial History

giant
annular elastolytic giant cell granuloma
atypical giant cell tumor
g. axonal neuropathy
g. axon formation
g. cell arteritis
g. cell collagenoma
g. cell fibroblastoma
g. cell hepatitis
g. cell interstitial pneumonia
g. cell interstitial pneumonitis
g. cell thyroiditis
g. cell transformation
g. cell tumor
g. cell tumor of low malignant potential
g. cell tumor of tendon sheath
central giant cell granuloma
central giant cell lesion
g. colonic diverticulum
g. congenital melanocytic nevus
g. dopamine-containing cell
g. follicular hyperplasia
g. follicular lymphoma
g. ganglion cell
g. gastric ulcer
g. hepatic cavernous hemangioma
g. hive
g. hypertrophic gastritis
inherited giant platelet disorder
lateral giant fiber
g. left atrium
left giant cell
g. lymph node hyperplasia

malignant giant cell tumor
measles giant cell pneumonia
g. melanosome
metacerebral giant cell
g. migrating contraction
g. miniature endplate potential
multifocal giant cell encephalitis
multinucleated giant epithelial cell
multinucleated osteoclastic giant cell
neonatal giant cell hepatitis
Noonan-like giant cell lesion
Noonan-like giant cell lesion syndrome
osteoclastic giant cell
osteoclast-like giant cell
g. papillary conjunctivitis
g. papillary hypertrophy
peripheral giant cell reparative granuloma
peripheral giant cell tumor
g. pigmented hairy nevus
g. pigment melanosome
g. platelet
g. prosthetic reinforcement of the visceral sac
g. ragweed test
g. retinal tear
right giant cell
g. serotonin-containing neuron
soft parts giant cell tumor
subependymal giant cell astrocytoma
syncytiotrophoblastic giant cell

giantism
hyperpituitary g.

gibbon
g. ape leukemia virus
g. ape lymphosarcoma virus
G. hydrocele

Gibbs free energy

gibbus
lumbar g.

Gibson
modified Gibson incision
G. rule

Gibson-Cooke sweat test

Giemsa
G. banding stain
fluorescence plus Giemsa stain
overnight Giemsa stain

Gieson
hematoxylin and van Gieson stain

gift
anatomic g.
anatomic gift statement

Gifted
G. Evaluation Scale
Screening Assessment for Gifted Elementary Students, Primary

gigaelectron volt

giganteum
molluscum g.

gigantism
acromegalic g.
eunuchoid g.
exomphalos, macroglossia, gigantism syndrome
hyperpituitary g.
lipodystrophy-acromegaloid gigantism syndrome
pituitary g.
primordial g.

gigantocellularis
nucleus gigantocellularis medullae oblongatae

giggling
nervous g.

Gila monster bite

Gilbert-Behçet syndrome

Gilchrist disease

Gilead
balm of G.

Gilles de la Tourette syndrome

Gillquist procedure

Gilmore Oral Reading Test

Gilsbach
modified Gilsbach technique

gingiva
attached g.
attached gingiva extension
g. treatment

gingival
acute herpetic gingival stomatitis
attached gingival cuff
g. bleeding
g. bleeding index
g. blood flow
g. crevice
g. crevicular fluid
g. curettage
g. fibromatosis, hypertrichosis, cherubism, mental retardation, epilepsy syndrome
g. flap
free gingival groove
g. hemorrhage
g. hyperplasia
G. Index
g. line
linear gingival erythema
lingual gingival papilla
g. margin
g. margin trimmer
g. mucosa
odontogenic gingival epithelial hamartoma
g. onlay graft
g. sulcus
g. surface
g. tissue

gingival-buccal sulcus

gingivalis
papilla g.

gingival-labial sulcus

Gingival-Periodontal Index

gingivitis
acute necrotizing ulcerative g.
acute ulcerative g.
atrophic senile g.
human immunodeficiency virus g.
necrotizing ulcerative g.
non-HIV chronic g.

gingivostomatitis
acute primary keratotic g.
herpes simplex g.

Ginkgo
G. biloba
Ginkgo biloba extract

Giraldes
organ of G.

girdle
hip g.
Hitzig g.
limbal girdle of Vogt
limbus g.
pectoral g.
pelvic g.
shoulder g.
thoracic g.

Girdlestone-Taylor procedure

girth
abdominal g.
arm girth, chest depth, and hip width
increased abdominal g.
midthigh g.
penile girth enhancement

Gissane
angle of G.

given
time required to double number of cells in given population
woman who has given birth

gives
amino acid that gives aspartic acid after hydrolysis

Gla
bone Gla protein

glabella
Marchac glabella flap

glabellar
anterior fossa skull base g.
g. region
g. rotation flap

glabellolambda line craniometric point

glabellomeatal line

glabelloopisthion line

glancing wound

gland
adenocarcinoma of prostate g.
adrenal gland hormone
adrenal gland insufficiency
anal gland carcinoma
anterior lingual g.
anterior pituitary g.
apocrine gland of Moll
apocrine sweat g.
autonomous nodular hyperplastic g.
axillary venom g.
Bartholin gland duct cyst
Bartholin, Skene, and urethral g.'s
congenital hypoplasia of adrenal g.'s
endocrine gland failure
enzymatic abnormality of adrenal g.
fibroadenomatosis hyperplasia of prostate g.
fundic gland polyp
g.'s, goiter, or stiffness of neck
greater vestibular g.
great vestibular g.
hemorrhagic infarct of adrenal g.
high-lying thyroid g.
human immunodeficiency virus-associated salivary gland disease
infected lymph g.
inferior thyroid g.
isolated gland carcinoma in situ
isthmus of thyroid g.
labial salivary g.
lacrimal gland dysfunction
lingual thyroid g.
lipoid adrenal gland hypoplasia
lobe of mammary g.
lobe of pituitary g.
lobe of thyroid g.
lobule of mammary g.
lobule of thyroid g.
Luschka cystic g.
lymph g.
lymphoepithelial endocrine g.
major salivary g.
male accessory gland fluid
malignant acini prostate g.
mammary gland mass
medial border of suprarenal g.
medulla of adrenal g.
meibomian gland carcinoma
meibomian gland expressor
meibomian gland obstruction
meibomian gland orifice metaplasia
metaplastic gastric fundic g.
metaplastic pyloric g.
minor gland obstruction
mixed tumor of salivary g.
Moll gland cystadenoma
mouse salivary gland virus
mucous gland adenoma of bronchus
mucous gland of auditory tube
multinodular thyroid g.
multiple gland hyperplasia
muscular layer of seminal g.
neonatal adrenal gland hemorrhage
nodular hyperplasia of prostate g.
noncancerous enlargement of prostate g.
overactive thyroid g.
painful swollen g.
parathyroid g.
parathyroid gland dysfunction
parathyroid gland enlargement
parathyroid gland hyperplasia
parathyroid gland immaturity
parotid g.
parotid gland abscess
parotid gland enlargement
parotid gland exposure guideline
parotid gland tuberculosis
pineal gland tumor
pituitary gland function
pituitary gland tumor
pretragal parotid g.
prostate gland benign hyperplasia
prostate gland biopsy
prostate gland innervation
prostate gland lymphoma
prostate gland sarcoma
prostate gland secretion
pyramidal lobe of thyroid g.
g. removal
salivary g.
salivary gland anlage tumor
salivary gland carcinoma
salivary gland disease
salivary gland enlargement
salivary gland lymphocyte
salivary gland pleomorphic adenoma
salivary gland swelling
salivary gland virus
salivary gland virus disease
sebaceous g.
sebaceous gland hyperplasia
sublabial salivary g.
submandibular g.
submandibular gland renin
submucosal gland hypertrophy
suspensory ligament of thyroid g.
sweat gland carcinoma
thymus gland excision
thymus gland function
thyroid gland carcinoma
thyroid gland dysfunction
ultimobranchial g.
underactive thyroid g.

glandular
g. abnormality
anterior glandular branch of superior thyroid artery
anterior/lateral/posterior glandular branch of superior thyroid artery
g. atrophy
atrophy of glandular tissue
atypical glandular cells of uncertain significance
atypical glandular cells of unknown significance
atypical glandular cell of undetermined significance
benign glandular cell tumor
bronchial glandular cell
g. cancer
g. carcinoma
g. cell
g. disease
ductal glandular mastectomy
g. element
endocervical glandular dysplasia
g. endometritis
g. enlargement
g. epithelioma

g. epithelium
g. fever
g. fluid
generalized glandular enlargement
human kidney glandular kallikrein-1 gene
g. hyperplasia
intracranial calcification benign glandular tissue
g. involvement
malignant glandular cell tumor
malignant glandular schwannoma
g. mastitis
multiple glandular deficiency syndrome
g. neck cell
normalized average glandular dose
pancreatic glandular necrosis
g. pharyngitis
radiation treatment of glandular tissue
g. replacement therapy
g. secretion
significant glandular enlargement
g. structure
g. swelling
g. therapy
g. tissue
g. vaginitis

glandularity
normal g.

glans
g. approximation procedure
g. of clitoris
neck of g.
neck of glans penis
g. penis
septum of glans penis

glans-phalloplasty
meatal advancement g.-p.

glansplasty
meatal advancement and g.
meatal advancement, glansplasty, penoscrotal junction meatotomy
g. in situ tubularization of urethral plate

glanuloplasty
meatal advancement, glanuloplasty, penoscrotal junction meatotomy
meatoplasty and g.
g. in situ tubularization of urethral plate
vascularized double-sided preputial island flap and W flap glanuloplasty hypospadias repair

Glanzmann thrombasthenia

glare
g. around lights
g. disability
peripheral g.
scatter and veiling g.
sensitivity to light and g.
specular g.
video display terminal glare screen

Glasgow
G. Assessment Schedule
G. Coma Scale
G. Coma Score
G. Dyspepsia Severity Score
G. Meningococcal Septicemia Prognostic Score
G. Outcome Scale
G. Outcome Score

glass, pl. **glasses**
g. bead
cast glass ceramics
g. ceramics
correction with glasses
g. eye artifact
g. factor tissue culture
fiber glass graft
flexible glass fiberglass
has not worn glasses
has worn prescription glasses
nonreflective glass screen
optical g.
g. pipe
g. ray
red glass test
single vision glasses
g. thermometer
g. transition temperature
g. vial
wearing glasses
without correction/without glasses

glassblower's
g. cataract
g. disease
g. emphysema

glass-distilled water

glasses (*pl. of* glass)

glassy
g. degeneration
g. swelling

glaucoma
acute angle-closure g.
acute chronic g.
acute intermittent primary angle-closure g.
acute narrow angle g.
acute primary angle-closure g.
air block g.
angle-closure g.
aqueous misdirected g.
chronic narrow-angle g.
chronic open-angle g.
chronic primary angle-closure g.
chronic simple g.
g. drainage device
exfoliation syndrome g.
g. filtering surgery
high-tension g.
g. imminens
intermittent angle-closure g.
juvenile open-angle g.
laser glaucoma surgery
low-tension g.
mydriatic test for angle-closure g.
narrow-angle g.
neovascular g.
neovascular angle-closure g.
normal-tension g.
ocular hypertension g.
ocular hypertensive g.
open-angle g.
painful hemorrhagic g.
penetrating keratoplasty and g.
primary angle-closure g.
primary glaucoma triple procedure
primary open-angle g.
pseudoexfoliative g.
g. screening
g. simplex
g. surgery
g. therapy
g. treatment

glaucomatosus
halo g.

glaucomatous
g. cataract
g. cup
g. habit
g. halo
g. optic nerve atrophy
g. optic nerve damage
g. visual field loss

glaze
low g.

glazed
g. eyes
g. look

Gleason
G. score
surgical Gleason score

Glees
method of G.

Glenn
bidirectional Glenn procedure

glenohumeral
anteroinferior glenohumeral ligament
anteromedial glenohumeral ligament
anterosuperior glenohumeral ligament
g. articulation
humeral avulsion of the glenohumeral ligament
inferior glenohumeral ligament
inferior glenohumeral ligament labral complex
g. joint
g. ligament

glenoid
anterior glenoid labrum
g. cavity
g. fossa
g. fossa mandibularis
g. labrum
labrum
g. ligament
lip of g.
g. process

glia
g. maturation factor
primary human fetal g.

glia-activating factor

Gliadel wafer treatment protocol

glial
g. bundle
g. cell line-derived neurotropic factor
g. fibrillary acidic protein
middle glial cell line-derived neurotrophic factor
peritumor glial reaction
g. tumor

glial-derived neurotrophic factor

glicentin-related pancreatic polypeptide

glide
adhesional and glide friction
after g.
anterior g.
anterior-inferior g.
anterior-posterior g.
dorsal g.
mandibular g.
natural apophysial g.
occlusal g.
off g.
patellar g.
patellar glide test
posterior g.
side g.
sustained natural apophysial g.

gliding
g. joint
mandibular gliding movement
passive gliding technique

glioblastoma
g. multiforme
recurrent glioblastoma multiforme

glioma
brain stem g.
low-grade g.
multicentric malignant g.
g. multiforme
optic apparatus g.
g. of optic chiasm
g. of optic nerve
optic nerve g.
pediatric brain stem g.
pediatric brainstem g.
g. sarcomatosum

gliomatosis
arachnoidal g.
meningeal g.

gliosis
g. of anterior column
aqueductal g.
astrocytic g.
basilar g.
cerebellar g.
g. of cerebral aqueduct
diffuse g.
hemispheric g.
hypertrophic nodular g.
inflammation and gliosis in brain
g. of lateral column
lobar g.
neonatal g.
perivascular g.
spinal g.
unilateral g.

glistening
capsular surface smooth and g.
peritoneum smooth and g.

global
g. amnesia
g. anoxia
g. aphasia
g. assessment of function
g. assessment of functioning
g. assessment index
G. Assessment of Relational Functioning
Children's G. Assessment Scale
Clinical G. Impression of Change
Clinical G. Impression-Severity of Illness Scale
Clinical G. Improvement
Clinical G. Index
Clinician's G. Rating Scale
Current, G., Psychiatric-Social Status
G. Deterioration Scale
g. distribution
g. evaluation
G. Evaluation of Efficacy
focal global glomerulosclerosis
g. focal sclerosis
g. force applicator
g. hypokinesis
G. Improvement Rating
G. Institute for Asthma
g. left ventricular ejection fraction
g. level of functioning
g. neurologic dysfunction
NIMH global scale
Nurse's G. Impressions
G. Obsessive-Compulsive Scale
patient global assessment of disease activity
G. Severity Index of Brief Symptom Inventory
G. Sexual Satisfaction Index
subjective global assessment
temporary global amnesia
transient global amnesia
g. ward behavior scale
g. well-being
Yale G. Tic Severity Scale

globe
disorganized g.
g. of the eye
luxation of g.
ocular g.
ulceration of the g.

globe-cell anemia

globoid leukodystrophy

globular
g. abdomen
g. heart

poorly contractile globular left ventricle
g. protein

globular-fibrous protein

globule
fat g.
g. fibril
human milk fat g.
milk fat g.
milk fat globule membrane
milk fat globule protein
mouse milk fat g.

globulin
accelerator g.
aggregated human gamma g.
alpha globulin antibody
Annapolis lymphoblast g.
anti-D globulin treatment
anti-D immune g.
antihemophilic g.
anti-HIV immune serum g.
antihuman g.
antihuman globulin crossmatch
antihuman globulin test
antihuman immunodeficiency virus immune serum g.
antihuman lymphocyte g.
antihuman thymocyte g.
antilymphocyte g.
antimacrophage g.
anti-RhD immune g.
anti-Rh gamma g.
antispleen g.
antithoracic duct lymphocytic g.
antithymocyte g.
antithymocyte gamma g.
bovine gamma g.
cold-insoluble g.
continuous ambulatory gamma globulin infusion
corticosteroid-binding g.
corticosteroid-binding globulin variant
cortisol-binding g.
cytomegalovirus immune g.
cytomegalovirus-specific immune g.
equine antihuman lymphoblast g.
estradiol-testosterone-binding g.
fast-binding target-attaching g.
fowl antimouse lymphocyte g.
fowl gamma g.
gamma g.
gamma A globulin deficiency
gamma globulin injection
gamma globulin M deficiency
gamma globulin replacement
gamma globulin therapy
goat antirabbit gamma g.
gonadal steroid-binding g.
guinea pig gamma g.
heat-aggregated g.
homologous tetanus immune g.
horse antihuman thymocyte g.
horse antihuman thymus g.
horse anti-Rhesus lymphocyte g.
horse antitetanus toxoid g.
human gamma g.
human immune serum g.
human rabies immune g.
human tetanus immune g.
hyperimmune antivariola gamma g.
hyperimmune serum g.
immune globulin to an Rh-negative woman
immune serum g.
immunoregulatory alpha g.
intramuscular gamma g.
intravenous gamma g.
intravenous immune serum g.
lymphocyte immune g.
macromolecular insoluble cold g.
measles immune globulin
Minnesota antilymphoblast g.
Minnesota antilymphocyte g.
modified immune serum g.
mouse gamma g.
Nonne globulin test
nonsex hormone-binding globulin bound testosterone
normal human g.
nuclear globulin inclusion
pertussis immune g.
plasma protein globulin
polyclonal gamma g.
pregnancy-associated g.
prophylactic gamma g.
rabbit antithymocyte g.
respiratory syncytial virus immune g.
retinol-binding g.
retroplacental gamma g.
Rhesus immune g.
Rh immune g.
RhO D immune g.
serum g.
sex hormone-binding g.
sex steroid-binding g.
slow-binding target-attaching g.
steroid hormone-binding g.
synthesize gamma g.
target-attaching g.
target-attaching globulin precursor
testosterone-binding g.
testosterone-estradiol-binding g.
tetanus immune g.
thyroid-binding g.
thyroid-binding globulin index
thyroxine-binding g.
thyroxine binding g.
thyroxine-binding globulin, estimated
thyroxine-binding globulin index
turkey gamma g.
unbound thyroxine-binding g.
vaccinia-immune g.
varicella-zoster immune g.
zoster immune g.

globulin-bound insulin

globus
g. hystericus
g. pallidus

glomerular
afferent glomerular arteriole
amphotericin B-induced reduction glomerular filtration rate
antiglomerular basement membrane-negative crescentic glomerular nephritis
g. arteriole
g. basal lamina
g. basement membrane
g. basement membrane disease
g. capillary basement
g. capillary wall
g. capsule
g. capsule of kidney
collagenase soluble glomerular basement membrane
g. cyst
g. disease
g. disorder
efferent glomerular arteriole
g. epithelial cell
g. filtrate
g. filtration
g. filtration rate
focal segmental glomerular hyalinosis and sclerosis
focal segmental glomerular sclerosis and hyalinosis
hemoglobinuria and glomerular thrombosis
g. hyalinization
ICR strain-derived glomerular nephritis
g. index
g. insufficiency
g. kidney disease
g. layer

glomerular *(continued)*
local glomerular lesion
low absolute glomerular filtration rate
g. membrane antibodies
minimal glomerular change
minor glomerular lesion
g. nephritis
pauciimmune glomerular nephritis
g. plasma flow
renal glomerular basement membrane thickness
g. sclerosis
single-nephron glomerular blood flow
single-nephron glomerular filtration rate
single-nephron glomerular plasma flow
g. tip lesion

glomerular-stimulating hormone

glomerulocapsular nephritis

glomerulocystic
g. kidney
g. kidney disease

glomerulonephritis
acute postinfectious g.
acute poststreptococcal g.
acute proliferative g.
antibasement membrane antibody-induced g.
antiglomerular basement membrane g.
antithymocyte antibody-induced g.
chronic g.
chronic membranoproliferative g.
chronic membranous g.
chronic proliferative g.
diffuse g.
diffuse proliferative g.
drowsiness from g.
experimental g.
extracapillary proliferative g.
extramembranous g.
focal proliferative g.
focal sclerosing g.
hypocomplementemic g.
idiopathic rapidly progressive g.
immune complex g.
lobular g.
membranoproliferative glomerulonephritis type I, II
membranous g.
mesangial g.
mesangial proliferative g.
mesangiocapillary glomerulonephritis type I, II
mesangioproliferative g.
minimal-change g.
minimal lesion g.
mixed cryoglobulinemia with g.
necrotizing crescentic g.
pauciimmune antineutrophil cytoplasmic antibody-associated g.
pauciimmune crescentic g.
postinfectious g.
poststreptococcal g.
poststreptococcal acute g.
proliferative g.
rapidly progressive crescenting g.
rapidly progressive necrotizing g.

glomerulonephropathy
membranous g.

glomerulopathy
immunotactoid g.
membranous g.

glomerulosa
zona g.
zona glomerulosa protein

glomerulosclerosis
diabetic g.
focal global g.
focal segmental g.

glomerulus
atubular g.
capsule of g.
immature g.
malpighian g.
olfactory g.

glomerulus-stimulating hormone

glomus
angiolipoma, posttraumatic neuroma, glomus tumor, eccrine spiradenoma, and leiomyoma cutis
aortic g.
arteriovenous glomus complex
aural g.
neuromyoarterial g.
g. tumor

glory
morning glory disc anomaly
morning glory disc
morning glory optic atrophy
morning glory optic disk anomaly
morning glory retinal detachment
morning glory syndrome

gloss
loss of g.

glossectomy
partial g.
total g.

glossitis
atrophic g.
Hunter g.
median rhomboid g.
migratory g.
Moeller g.
parenchymatous g.

glossoepiglottic
g. fold
median glossoepiglottic fold
middle glossoepiglottic fold

glossopalatal junction

glossopalatine arch

glossopharyngeal
g. breathing
communicating branch of glossopharyngeal nerve with auricular branch of vagus nerve
lower ganglion of glossopharyngeal nerve
g. muscle
g. nerve
g. nerve sign
g. neuralgia
g. neurotomy
pharyngeal branch of glossopharyngeal nerve

glossy skin

glottic
g. atresia
g. carcinoma
g. chink
g. extension
posterior glottic stenosis
g. spasm
total glottic transverse laryngectomy

glottidis
atrium g.

glottis
atrium of g.

glove
antivibration g.
compression g.
disposable g.
examination g.
papular-purpuric gloves and socks syndrome
protective g.
g.'s and socks syndrome

stocking glove distribution
stocking and glove type hypesthesia
g. wearing

glove-and-stocking anesthesia

gloving
double g.

glow
contact glow discharge electrolysis

glucagon
immunoreactive g.
large glucagon immunoreactivity
g. receptor
g. secretion
g. test
triiodothyronine, amino acids, glucagon, and heparin

glucagon-free insulin

glucagon-like
g.-l. immunoreactivity
g.-l. peptide
g.-l. peptide-1

glucagonoma
nonsecretory g.

glucanotransferase

glucocorticoid
adjunctive glucocorticoid therapy
familial glucocorticoid deficiency
nongenomic glucocorticoid effect
peripheral glucocorticoid deficiency
g. receptor
g. response element
g. steroid-induced osteoporosis
trabecular meshwork-inducible glucocorticoid response

glucocorticoid-remediable
g.-r. aldosteronism
g.-r. hyperaldosteronism

glucocorticoid-responsive element

glucogen
mitochondria lipid g.

glucometer
One Touch g.

gluconate
calcium g.
chlorhexidine g.
sodium antimony g.
zinc gluconate glycine

glucosamine sulfate

glucose
abnormal glucose tolerance
abnormal glucose tolerance test
g. absorption test
g., age, LDH, AST, WBC
amniotic fluid g.
g. assimilation
blood g.
blood glucose determination
blood glucose levels
blood glucose monitor
blood glucose reagent strip
buffered azide glucose glycerol
buffered desoxycholate g.
capillary blood g.
cerebral glucose oxygen quotient
cerebral metabolic rate of g.
cerebral rate of glucose metabolism
cerebrospinal fluid g.
g. concentration
continuous glucose monitoring system
g. control
cortisone-primed oral glucose tolerance test
g. counterregulatory hormone
g. dehydrogenase
dialysate glucose concentration
g. disposal rate
electrolyte replacement with g.
electronic glucose monitor
endogenous glucose production
erratic blood glucose levels
fasting blood g.
fasting glucose level
fasting plasma g.
fasting serum g.
g. feeding
fingerstick blood g.
gelatin, glucose, and Veronal buffer
Hanks balanced salt solution plus g.
hepatic glucose output
hepatic glucose production
high g.
home blood glucose meter
home blood glucose monitor
home blood glucose monitoring
5-hour glucose tolerance test
human glucose monitoring
human glucose output
hydrolysate lactalbumin Earle g.
immunoreactive g.
immunoreactive insulin to serum or plasma glucose ratio
impaired fasting g.
impaired glucose tolerance
implantable glucose sensor
insulin-mediated glucose uptake
g. insulinotropic peptide
g., insulin, and potassium
interim glucose determination
g. intolerance
intraperitoneal glucose tolerance test
intravenous glucose tolerance test
Krebs-Ringer bicarbonate buffer with g.
g., lactalbumin, serum, and hemoglobin
g. level
g. level control
local cerebral glucose utilization
low g.
maintain blood glucose level
maximal glucose disposal
maximal tubular reabsorption rate for g.
mean blood g.
mean maternal g.
g. metabolism
g. metabolism in brain
g. monitor
g. monitoring
negative arterial-portal glucose gradient
net hepatic glucose uptake
noninvasive glucose monitor
normal glucose tolerance
g. in normal saline
one-hour glucose tolerance test
oral glucose challenge test
oral glucose tolerance test
oral glucose tolerance testing
g. oxidase
g. oxidase-perioxidase method
g. oxidase test
g. oxidation quotient
Penassay broth plus g.
Penassay broth plus glucose plus menadione
peptone, glucose, and yeast extract medium
peripheral glucose uptake
phosphate, saline, g.
plasma g.
plasma glucose disappearance rate
plasma glucose tolerance rate
g. polymer
g., postprandial
postprandial plasma g.
potassium, glucose, and insulin
g. potassium insulin

glucose *(continued)*
potential abnormality of glucose tolerance
prednisolone glucose tolerance test
pregnancy-induced glucose intolerance
previous abnormality of glucose tolerance
g. production
g. production rate
pyruvate, inosine, glucose phosphate, and adenine
random blood g.
g. response
g. and saline
self-monitored blood g.
serum g.
serum, casein, glucose, yeast extract medium
serum glucose monitoring
sodium chloride, adenine, glucose, mannitol
sodium glucose cotransporter
standard glucose tolerance test
steady-state plasma g.
g. strip
g. tolerance
g. tolerance factor
g. tolerance test
g. toxicity
g. transport
g. transporter
g. transport system
tryptone glucose extract
tryptone glucose yeast agar
tryptophan peptone glucose broth
g. uptake
urinary g.
urine glucose ketone
urine glucose spot test
g. in water
g. water feeding

glucose-controlled insulin infusion

glucose-dependent insulin-releasing peptide

glucose-electrolyte solution

glucose-free Hanks solution

glucose-galactose malabsorption

glucose-gelatin Veronal buffer

glucose-insulin-potassium solution

glucose-insulin tolerance test

glucose-lactate tolerance test

glucose-lowering agent

glucose/nitrogen
glucose/nitrogen ratio in urine
glucose/nitrogen ratio in water

glucose-6-phosphate
g.-p. dehydrogenase

glucose-Ringer-phosphate solution

glucose-stimulated insulin secretion

glucoside
deoxycorticosterone g.
desoxycorticosterone g.

glucuronic acid lactone

glucuronide
g. derivative of azidothymidine
pregnanediol g.
sodium pregnanediol g.
testosterone g.

glucuronosyltransferase
uridine diphosphate g.

glucuronyl transferase

glue
airplane glue dependence
autologous fibrin g.
autologous fibrin sealant g.
fibrin g.
methyl methacrylate g.
g. sniffer's rash

glutamate
arginine g.
g. decarboxylase
g. dehydrogenase
metabotropic g.
metabotropic glutamate receptor
mitochondrial glutamate dehydrogenase pathway
monosodium g.
monosodium glutamate poisoning

glutamic
g. acid decarboxylase
g. acid dehydrogenase
erythrocyte glutamic oxaloacetic transaminase

glutamic-oxaloacetic
g.-o. transaminase, mitochondrial
g.-o. transaminase, soluble

glutamic-pyruvic transaminase

glutamide receptor subunit

glutaminase
phosphate-dependent g.
phosphate-independent g.

glutamine synthetase

glutamyl
g. transferase
g. transpeptidase

glutamylcysteine synthetase

glutaraldehyde cross-linked collagen

glutathione
erythrocyte glutathione reductase
g. peroxidase
reduced g.
reduced glutathione peroxidase
g. reductase
g. synthetase deficiency

glutathione-insulin transhydrogenase

gluteal
anterior gluteal line
g. artery
g. body fat
g. bonnet
g. bursitis
g. erythema
g. fold
g. free flap
g. gait
greatest gluteal muscle
g. hernia
inferior gluteal nerve
inferior gluteal vein
left g.
g. limp
g. line
middle gluteal muscle
middle gluteal nerve
g. muscle
g. nerve
g. reflex
g. region
right g.
right ventrolateral g.
g. sets
superficial branch of superior gluteal artery
superior gluteal artery
superior gluteal artery perforator
superior gluteal nerve
superior gluteal vein

gluten
g. allergy
g. intolerance

gluten-free diet

gluten-restricted diet

gluten-rich diet

gluten-sensitive enteropathy

gluteus
left g.
g. maximus
g. maximus muscle
g. maximus musculocutaneous flap
g. minimus
g. minimus muscle
musculus gluteus maximus
musculus gluteus quartus
nervus gluteus superior
right gluteus maximus

gluthathione
oxidized g.
g. reductase

glycated hemoglobin

glycation
advanced glycation end-product
nonenzymatic g.
nonenzymatic protein g.

glycemic
g. control
low glycemic index diet

glyceraldehyde-3-phosphate dehydrogenase

glyceral methacrylate

glycerin
magnesium sulfate, glycerin, and water enema
g. suppository
g. and water
g. in water
g. and water enema

glycerine
mean amplitude of glycerine excursion

glycerine-buffered saline

glycerol
buffered azide glucose g.
g. kinase
g. kinase deficiency
percutaneous glycerol rhizolysis
percutaneous retrogasserian glycerol injection
g. test

glycerophosphate dehydrogenase

glycerophosphatide
choline g.
serine g.

glyceryl
g. dinitrate
g. monostearate
transdermal glyceryl trinitrate
g. trinitrate

glycidyl
butyl glycidyl ether

glycinate
zinc glycinate marker

glycine
mitochondrial glycine cleavage system
zinc gluconate g.

glycine-rich
g.-r. gamma-glycoprotein
g.-r. glycoprotein
g.-r. RNA-binding protein

glycoalkaloids
total g.

glycoconjugate
respiratory g.

glycogen
brain-type glycogen phosphorylase
g. cardiomegaly
g. depletion
excessive accumulation of g.
g. loading
g. nephrosis
g. storage disease, types 1–10
g. storage disorder
g. storage test
g. synthase kinase-3
g. synthetase kinase
g. synthetase phosphatase

glycogenesis
cardiac g.

glycogen- and fat-free solid

glycogenic unit

glycogenosis
myophosphorylase deficiency g.

glycogen-rich cystadenoma

glycohydrolase
nicotinamide adenine dinucleotide g.

glycol
diethylene g.
ethylene glycol assay
ethylene glycol dimethacrylate
ethylene glycol poisoning
ethylene glycol succinate
ethylene glycol toxicity
g. methacrylate
neopentyl glycol succinate
polyethylene glycol electrolyte lavage solution
polypropylene g.
recombinant polyethylene g.
tetraethylene glycol dimethacrylate

Glycolic

glycolysis
aerobic g.

glycolytic
Embden-Meyerhof glycolytic pathway

glycopeptide
g. moiety modified derivative

glycopeptide-insensitive
Staphylococcus aureus

glycopeptide-intermediate
Staphylococcus aureus

glycopeptide-resistant
g.-r. enterococcus
g.-r. *Staphylococcus aureus*

glycoprotein
$alpha_1$-acid g.
biliary g.
carbohydrate-deficient g.
carbohydrate-deficient glycoprotein syndrome
g. crystal growth inhibitor
dimeric acidic g.
glycine-rich g.
high molecular weight g.
g. hormone
g. IIa, IIb-IIIa
intestinal g.
membrane glycoprotein IB/IX
microfil-associated g.
mucous g.
multifunctional extracellular g.
myelin-associated g.
myelin-associated glycoprotein antibody detection
myelin-oligodendrocyte g.
novel glycoprotein tapasin
pregnancy alpha-2 g.
soluble g.
thrombomodulin g.
tobacco g.
tumor-associated g.
tumor glycoprotein assay
tumor-specific g.
variant surface g.
viral g.

glycoprotein-1
lysosomal membrane g.-1

glycoprotein-2
epithelial g.-2
lysosomal membrane g.-2
sulfated g.-2

glycoprotein-72
tumor-associated g.-72
glycoprotein-based enzyme-linked immunosorbent assay
glycoprotein-producing
g.-p. adenoma
g.-p. tumor
glycoprotein-secreting
g.-s. adenoma
g.-s. pituitary tumor
glycoside
anthracene g.
glycosuria
alimentary g.
nondiabetic g.
nonhyperglycemic g.
normoglycemic g.
orthoglycemic g.
overt g.
pathologic g.
renal g.
glycosylated
g. hemoglobin
g. hemoglobin level
g. hemoglobin test
N-linked glycosylated site
g. protein
g. protein spanning viral envelope
g. serum protein
glycosylation
advanced glycosylation end-product
asparagine-linked glycosylation moiety
N-linked g.
glycosylation-inhibiting factor
glycyrrhetinic acid like factor
G-myeloma protein
gnarled
deformed gnarled joint
g. enamel
g. fingernail
gnashing and clenching of teeth
gnawing
g. pain
g. sensation
go
timed up and g.
goal
abstinence g.
ambulation g.
annual g.
anticipatory goal response
apathy and lack of interest in personal g.'s
apathy and lack of interest in personal g.'s
appropriate g.
Assessment of Core G.'s
g. attainment
g. attainment method
G. Attainment Scale
g. attainment scaling
g. behavior
Educational G. Attainment Test
family g.
Institutional G.'s Inventory
life g.
long-term g.
manifest g.
negotiating g.'s skills
nursing g.
g. orientation
g. oriented task
outcome g.
overall therapeutic g.
patient g.
performance g.
personal g.
primary g.
pursuit g.
rehabilitation team g.
safety technique g.
g. setting
shifting g.
short-term g.
g.'s of treatment
treatment g.
ultimate g.
g. weight
goal-directed behavior
goal-oriented
g.-o. behavior
g.-o. psychotherapy
goat
g. antimouse immunoglobulin G
g. antirabbit gamma globulin
normal goat serum
g. serum
goblet
g. cell
g. cell carcinoid
g. cell-type adenocarcinoma
percentage of goblet cell
God
act of G.
anger at G.
G. complex
goiter
adenomatous g.
amyloid g.
benign multinodular g.
cervical g.
colloid g.
congenital g.
cystic g.
g. development
diffuse colloid g.
diffuse toxic non-nodular g.
endemic g.
euthyroid g.
g. excision
exophthalmic g.
fibrous g.
follicular g.
glands, goiter, or stiffness of neck
hypothyroid g.
intrathoracic g.
lobulated g.
multiheteronodular toxic g.
multinodular euthyroid g.
myxedematous g.
neonatal g.
nodular colloid g.
nonautoimmune nontoxic diffuse g.
nontoxic multinodular g.
nontoxic nodular g.
nontoxic sporadic g.
ovarian g.
papillomatous g.
parenchymatous g.
plunging g.
g. recurrence
g. reduction
g. regrowth
simple g.
g. or stiffness of glands
substernal g.
suffocative g.
thoracic g.
thyrotoxic g.
toxic multinodular g.
toxic nodular g.
vascular g.
wandering g.
Golabi-Rosen syndrome
gold
allergic gold dermatitis
cast gold inlay
cationic colloidal g.
colloidal g.
colloidal gold test

g. equivalent
full gold crown
g. grain implant
g. implant material
g. injection
injection gold probe
g. inlay
g. marker
noble gold alloy
noncohesive gold foil
noneczematous persistent papular gold eruption
radioactive g.
g. salt
g. salt therapy
g. sodium thioglucose
g. sodium thiomalate
g. standard
g. thioglucose
g. treatment
triethylphosphine g.

Goldberg Anorectic Attitude Scale

Goldberger
Anderson and Goldberger test

Goldberg-Maxwell-Morris syndrome

golden
bean golden mosaic virus
g. shiner virus

gold-labeled
g.-l. antigen detection technique
g.-l. optical rapid immunoassay

Goldman elevator

Goldman-Fristoe Test of Articulation

Goldman-Fristoe-Woodcock Auditory Skills Test Battery

Goldman-Hodgkin-Katz equation

Goldmann-Favre
G.-F. disease
G.-F. dystrophy
G.-F. syndrome

golfer's
g. elbow
g. elbow test
g. focal dystonia
g. wrist

Golgi
G. apparatus
G. body
G. cell
G. complex
G. corpuscle
G. endoplasmic reticulum lysosome
mechanoreceptor Golgi tendon organ
G. reflex
G. stain
G. staining
G. tendon
G. tendon organ

Goll
nucleus of G.
tract of G.

Golombok-Rust Inventory of Marital State

Gomco
low Gomco suction

Gomoka virus

Gomori
G. methenamine silver
modified Gomori trichrome reaction

gonad
male g.
maternal g.
palpable g.
streak g.
suspensory ligament of g.

gonadal
g. agenesis
g. agenesis syndrome
g. aplasia
g. artery
g. branch
chromosomal gonadal dysgenesis
g. complication
g. cord
g. cycle
g. differentiation
g. disease
g. dose
g. dysfunction
g. dysgenesis
g. dysgenesis syndrome
g. dysgenesis of Turner type
g. dysplasia
g. endocrine disorder
g. failure
g. failure, short stature, mitral valve prolapse, mental retardation syndrome
g. germ cell neoplasm
g. hormone
g. irradiation
g. mosaicism
normal gonadal steroid level
partial gonadal dysgenesis
g. peptide
pineal gonadal syndrome
premature gonadal failure
pure gonadal dysgenesis
g. shield
g. steroid
g. steroid-binding globulin
g. steroidogenesis
g. steroid suppression
g. streak
g. stroma
g. suppression
g. suppression treatment
g. vein
g. vessel

gonadoblastoma
aniridia, Wilms tumor, gonadoblastoma syndrome
ovarian g.

gonadotrophic hormone

gonadotrophin-resistant ovary syndrome

gonadotropic
g. adenoma
chorionic gonadotropic hormone
g. deficiency
general gonadotropic activity
g. hormone
g. hormone assay
pituitary gonadotropic hormone

gonadotropin
g. agonist stimulation test
alpha-human chorionic g.
androgen gonadotropin feedback control
animal pituitary g.
antagonist-induced gonadotropin deprivation
anterior pituitary g.
beta-human chorionic g.
chorionic g.
chorionic gonadotropin test
g. deficiency
familial idiopathic gonadotropin deficiency
human g.
human chorionic g.
human chorionic gonadotropin level
human chorionic gonadotropin test
human menopausal g.
human pituitary g.
immunoreactive human chorionic g.

gonadotropin *(continued)*
inappropriate gonadotropin secretion
isolated gonadotropin deficiency
level of female g.
luteinizing hormone-chorionic gonadotropin hormone
luteinizing hormone/human chorionic g.
menopausal g.
menopausal urinary g.
nicked free beta subunit of human chorionic g.
pituitary g.
pituitary gonadotropin effect
pituitary gonadotropin inhibition
pituitary gonadotropin secretion
pituitary gonadotropin suppression
pregnant mare serum g.
primate chorionic g.
g. surge attenuating factor
g. titer
total urinary g.
urinary chorionic g.
urinary gonadotropin fragment
urinary gonadotropin peptide

gonadotropin-enhancing factor

gonadotropin-inhibiting material

gonadotropin-inhibitory
g.-i. factor
g.-i. material

gonadotropin-producing pituitary adenoma

gonadotropin-releasing
g.-r. agent
g.-r. factor
g.-r. hormone
g.-r. hormone agonist
g.-r. hormone-associated peptide
g.-r. hormone receptor

gonadotropin-secreting
g.-s. adenoma
g.-s. tumor

gondii
anti-*Toxoplasma gondii* antibody
anti-*Toxoplasma gondii* antibody secretion assay
Toxoplasma g.

gone
until g.

goniodysgenesis, mental retardation, short stature

goniometer
O'Brien g.
orthopaedic g.

goniometric
parallel goniometric measure

genioposterior

goniopuncture knife

gonioscopic
g. implant
g. lens
g. prism

goniotomy knife

gonococcal
acute gonococcal arthritis
g. antibody reaction
g. arthritis
g. arthritis/dermatitis syndrome
g. arthropathy
ascending gonococcal infection
g. base
g. complement-fixation test
g. conjunctivitis
g. dermatitis
disseminated gonococcal infection
g. endocarditis
g. gingivitis
g. infection
g. meningitis
neonatal gonococcal disease
g. ophthalmia
g. ophthalmia neonatorum
orogastric gonococcal aspirate
pediatric gonococcal conjunctivitis
pediatric gonococcal infection
polyarticular gonococcal arthritis
g. stomatitis
g. urethritis

gonorrhea
g. complement-fixation test
g. culture
fluorescent gonorrhea test
insomnia from g.
venereal disease, g.

gonorrheal
g. invasive peritonitis
g. proctitis
g. urethritis

gonorrhoeae
chromosomally mediated resistant *Neisseria gonorrhoeae*
Neisseria gonorrhoeae culture
Neisseria gonorrhoeae DNA detection test
Neisseria gonorrhoeae susceptibility testing
Neisseria gonorrhoeae urethritis
non–penicillinase-producing *Neisseria gonorrhoeae*
quinolone-resistant *Neisseria gonorrhoeae*
tetracycline-resistant *Neisseria gonorrhoeae*

good
aggressive good prognosis non-Hodgkin lymphoma
g. appetite
arteriovenous fistula with good bruits
g. blood return
g. breath sound
g. chest expansion
color and cry g.
g. concentration
g. condition
g. contact with skin
g. cosmetic result
g. eating habit
g. exposure obtained
fairly good risk for anesthesia
g. faith
g. fetal movement
g. form response
g. functioning
grips equal and g.
g. hemostasis
immediate good function followed by accelerated rejection
g. impression
introitus with good support
g. laboratory practice
no g.
g. nutrition
g. old boy
g. partial response
patient discharged in good condition
patient dismissed in good condition
patient has good rapport with others
patient's appetite is g.
g. pelvic support
g. peripheral circulation
g. prenatal care
prognosis is g.
g. recovery
g. response
G. Samaritan Act
g. self-image
suggestive of g.
teeth in good dental condition
teeth in good dental repair
g. tissue turgor
uterus has good support
very g.

very good health
g. visual fields

Goodenough Figure Drawing

Goodenough-Harris Drawing Test

Goodpasture
G. disease
G. syndrome

goose
g. bumps
g. flesh
g. hepatitis virus
g. honk murmur
skin goose bumps

goosebump flesh

goose-honk murmur

gooseneck deformity

Gordil virus

Gordon
G. diagnostic system
G. Occupational Checklist-II
G. Personal Inventory
G. Personal Profile
G. Personal Profile Inventory

Gore-Tex
G.-T. augmentation material
G.-T. augmentation membrane

Gorge
Chobar Gorge virus

Gorlin-Goltz syndrome

goserelin

Gossas virus

got
had it before, got it again

gouge
arthroplasty g.
orthopaedic g.
oscillating g.
g. spud

Gougerot-Carteaud
papillomatosis of G.-C.

Goulian
G. mammaplasty
G. mastopexy
G. technique

gourd-shaped sella

gout
acute g.
articular g.
calcium g.
chalky g.
g. from alcohol
latent g.
lead g.
masked g.
misplaced g.
oxalic g.
polyarticular g.
retrocedent g.
rheumatic g.
saturnine g.
tophaceous g.

gouty
acute gouty arthritis
g. arthritis
g. arthropathy
g. diabetes
g. diathesis
g. diet
g. episcleritis
g. iritis
g. nephropathy
g. node
g. phlebitis
primary gouty arthritis
g. proteinuria
g. tophus
g. urethritis
g. urine

governing vessel

government
g. mandated guideline
insufficient government reimbursements

Gower
panatrophy of G.

gown
complete change of drapes, g.'s and instruments
sterilized gown and mask
g.'s and towels

G-protein coupled

grab bar

grabber
arthroscopic g.

gracilis
double-looped semitendinous and gracilis hamstring graft knee reconstruction technique
fasciculus g.
g. flap
McCraw gracilis myocutaneous flap
g. muscle
g. myocutaneous unit
nucleus fasciculi g.
nucleus gracilis tubercle
g. tendon

graciloplasty
dynamic urinary g.

grade
analytical g.
arithmetic grade equivalent
astrocytoma grade I–IV
axial grade echo imaging
cement mantle grade classification
cervical intraepithelial neoplasia, grade 1–3
Edmondson g.
graft-versus-host disease, grade 1–4
g. 1–6 heart murmur
high g.
incipient cataract grade 11 to 41
intraventricular hemorrhage grade 1–4
ligamentous injury grade I–III
Los Angeles Classification grade A, B, C, D esophagitis
lymphedema grade II, III
g. of marijuana
Meurmann external ear anomaly g.
modified Dallas classification of disc morphology grades 0–7
modified Dallas classification of disc morphology grades 0–7
Page grade for breast tumor
PAHO grade 0, 1, 2
Pan American Health Organization grade 0–2
placental grade biophysical profile
g., rough, breathy, asthenic, strained
tumor regression g.
vesicoureteral reflux grade I–V

graded
g. exercise electrocardiogram
g. exercise program
g. exercise test
low-level graded exercise test
multistage graded exercise test
predischarge graded exercise test
g. resistive exercise
symptom-limited graded exercise test
g. treadmill exercise test

gradient
g. acquisition
alveolar-arterial g.
alveolar-arterial oxygen g.
alveolar-arterial oxygen tension g.
alveolocapillary partial pressure g.
g. amplitude
aortic outflow g.

gradient *(continued)*
aortic pressure g.
aortic valve peak instantaneous g.
aortic valve pressure g.
g. of approach
arterial to alveolar g.
arterial-ascitic fluid pH g.
arteriovenous pressure g.
average gradient number
g. of avoidance
axial g.
axial gradient echo image
g. bandwidth
g. coil
colloid hydrostatic pressure g.
denaturing density gradient electrophoresis
denaturing gradient gel electrophoresis
g. density
density gradient electrophoresis
Doppler pressure g.
g. echo
electrochemical potential g.
end-diastolic aortic-left ventricular pressure g.
g. field transform
g. of fluid inflow
gastroesophageal pressure g.
g. gel electrophoresis
hepatic venous pressure g.
interatrial pressure g.
intracavitary pressure g.
left ventricle to aorta pressure g.
magnetic field g.
g. magnetic field
magnetization-prepared rapid gradient echo-water excitation
magnitude preparation-rapid acquisition gradient echo
mean diastolic g.
mitral valve g.
g. moment nulling
g. moment reduction
g. moment rephasing
motion compensation gradient pulse
g. motion rephasing
multiplanar gradient recall
multiplanar gradient refocused
narrow albumin gradient ascites
negative arterial-portal glucose g.
net electrochemical potential g.
net gradient of fluid outflow
nonequilibrium pH gradient gel electrophoresis
peak diastolic g.
peak instantaneous g.
peak systolic gradient pressure
peak transaortic valve g.
pleural pressure g.
portosystemic g.
pressure flow g.
pulmonary valve g.
pulsed-field gradient gel electrophoresis
g. reduction
serum ascites-albumin g.
spectral gradient acoustic reflectometry
spoiled gradient recalled
sucrose density g.
sucrose density gradient centrifugation
sucrose density gradient ultracentrifugation
temporal temperature gradient gel electrophoresis
thyroid uptake g.
timed-temperature gradient electrophoresis
transaortic valve g.
transmembrane potential g.
transplacental g.
transtubular potassium concentration g.
transvalvular aortic g.
transvalvular pressure g.
tricuspid valve g.
venous pressure gradient support stockings
ventricular pleural pressure g.

gradient-echo
g.-e. coronal image
g.-e. method
g.-e. sequence
g.-e. single-photon emission computed tomography

gradient-recalled
g.-r. acquisition in steady state
g.-r. echo technique
multiple planar g.-r.

gradient-refocused
g.-r. acquisition in a steady state
g.-r. echo

grading
colposcopic grading of cervical dysplasia
Edmondson g.
Facial G. System
House-Brackmann G. Scale
Marcus grading scale for avascular necrosis
McAllister grading system
M.D. Anderson grading system
mean rejection g.
microscopic angiogenesis grading system
Nelson grading system
Nottingham modification of Scarff-Bloom-Richardson g.
osteoarthritis grading classification
g. parameter
von Herrick grading system

gradual
g. ambulation
g. blurring of vision
g. curve
g. desensitization
g. deterioration
g. distortion of sound
g. dosage schedule
g. effect
g. elongation intramedullary nailing
g. exercise progression
g. increase
g. increase in length and complexity of utterance
g. lifestyle modification
g. loss of alertness
g. loss of auditory discrimination
g. loss of bone tissue
g. loss of mental faculties
g. memory loss
g. onset
g. relaxation
g. weightbearing
g. weight gain
g. withdrawal

graduate
g. medical education
G. Record Examination

graduated
anatomic graduated component
g. compress
g. compression garment
g. compression stockings
g. electronic decelerator
g. spinal block
g. tenotomy

Graefe
G. sign
von Graefe sign

Grafenberg spot

graft
accelerated graft atherosclerosis

advancement flap g.
alar contour g.
allogenic bone g.
allogenic fetal g.
allogenic keratinocyte g.
allogenic lyophilized bone graft implant material
allogenous bone g.
allograft dermal matrix graft
g. anastomosis
antebrachial fascial g.
anterior sliding tibial g.
anterior slot graft arthrodesis
anterosuperior iliac spine g.
anular corneal g.
anular corneal graft operation
aortic aneurysm g.
aortic graft infection
aortic graft placement
aortic tube g.
aortobifemoral bypass g.
aortocoronary g.
aortocoronary bypass g.
aortocoronary-saphenous vein bypass g.
aortofemoral bypass g.
aortohepatic arterial g.
aortoiliac bypass g.
aortoplasty with patch g.
aortorenal bypass g.
araldehyde-tanned bovine carotid artery g.
arterial bypass g.
g. atherosclerosis
g. atrophy
auricular cartilage g.
auricular composite g.
autogenous bone g.
autogenous cable graft interposition VII-VII neuroanastomosis
autogenous cancellous bone g.
autogenous cartilage g.
autogenous corticocancellous g.
autogenous dermis fat g.
autogenous fat g.
autogenous fibular g.
autogenous nerve g.
autogenous patellar ligament g.
autogenous semitendinosus-gracilis g.
autogenous tunica vaginalis g.
autogenous vein bypass g.
autogenous vein graft conduit
autologous cancellous bone g.
autologous fat g.
autologous iliac crest bone g.
autologous patch g.
autologous pearl fat g.
autologous reverse g.
autologous reverse graft to ankle
autologous rib bone g.
autologous vein g.
autologous vein graft stent
axillary-axillary bypass g.
axillary-brachial bypass g.
axillary-femoral bypass g.
axillary-femorofemoral bypass g.
barrel staved g.
bearing graft hair
g. bed
biopsy-negative graft dysfunction
blood vessel g.
bolus tie-over g.
bone g.
bone bank g.
bone chip g.
bone to femur g.
bone graft donor
bone graft punch
bone graft shoe horn
bone graft site
brain graft surgery
Braun pinch graft technique
bypass vein g.
cancellous cellular bone g.
cancellous chip bone g.
cancellous and cortical bone g.
cancellous insert g.
cancellous morselized bone g.
cantilevered bone g.
cantilevered split cranial bone g.
carbon fiber g.
cardiac bypass g.
cardiovascular patch g.
cartilaginous autologous thin septal g.
chronic graft vascular disease
clogged bypass g.
g. clotting
composite valve g.
g. contamination
convex cartilage g.
coronary artery bypass g.
coronary artery bypass graft patency
coronary artery bypass graft surgery
coronary bypass g.
cortical bone g.
corticocancellous block g.
corticocancellous bone g.
corticocancellous chip g.
costochondral g.
Crawford graft inclusion technique
cryopreserved heart valve g.
Damian graft procedure
de-epithelialized rectus abdominis muscle g.
defatted skin g.
delayed graft function
demineralized bone g.
dermal fat g.
devitalized bone g.
diamond inlay bone g.
diced cartilage g.
donor site of bone g.
donor site of skin g.
double coronary artery g.
double-looped semitendinous and gracilis hamstring graft knee reconstruction technique
double vein g.
g. dowel
dowel bone g.
dowel-shaped bone g.
dural graft matrix
g. edema
endoluminal g.
endovascular aortic g.
endovascular graft insertion
endovascular graft treatment
endovascular stent g.
g. enteric erosion
g. enteric fistula
g. epithelium
g. expulsion
g. failure
fascia lata g.
femoral-femoral bypass g.
femoropopliteal bypass g.
fiber glass g.
g. fixation
flexor tendon g.
g. fracture
g. fragmentation
free dermal-fat g.
free fat g.
full-thickness skin g.
g. function
gingival onlay g.
hair bearing g.
g. harvest
g. harvesting
homogenous bone g.
iliac crest bone g.
immediate graft rejection
g. impingement
g. implantation
g. infection

graft *(continued)*
g. injury
inlay bone g.
intermediate split-thickness skin g.
internal mammary artery g.
internal thoracic artery g.
g. interstice
intramedullary bone g.
intramedullary and spongiosa g.
late graft rejection
left internal mammary artery g.
ligamentous anterior dislocation composite g.
limb of bifurcation g.
liver g.
loop forearm g.
g. loss
lower extremity bypass g.
lyophilized bone g.
lyophilized dura g.
mammary artery g.
mandibular coronoid g.
Marquez-Gomez conjunctival g.
marrow graft rejection
massive sliding g.
Matti-Russe bone g.
McMaster bone g.
medial crural strut g.
medial graft technique
medullary bone g.
mesenteric bypass g.
mesh graft urethroplasty
metatarsal free vascularized g.
g. migration
Millard graft augmentation
minimally invasive direct coronary artery bypass g.
Moberg free tendon g.
morcellized bone g.
morcellized cancellous g.
morselized cartilage onlay radix g.
mucosal membrane g.
mucous membrane g.
multiple cancellous chip g.
mushroom corneal g.
nail bed g.
Nicoll cancellous bone g.
Nicoll cancellous insert g.
nontubed closed distant flap g.
nonvascularized bone g.
nonvascularized fibular strut g.
nude bone graft transplantation
g. occlusion
onlay bone g.
onlay bone graft cast
onlay cancellous iliac g.
onlay cortical g.
open bone graft epiphysiodesis
oral mucous membrane g.
osteoperiosteal bone g.
osteoperiosteal iliac bone g.
overlay cantilevered bone g.
Papineau bone g.
Papineau cancellous g.
particulate cancellous bone g.
patch Gore-Tex g.
patch graft angioplasty
patch graft urethroplasty
patellar tendon graft donor site
g. patency
pattern-cut corneal g.
pattern-cut corneal graft operation
pedicle bone g.
pedicled cartilage g.
pedicle fat g.
peg bone g.
penetrating corneal g.
penetrating full-thickness corneal g.
percutaneous autogenous dowel bone g.
peroneus brevis g.
g. placement
popliteal tibial bypass vein g.
portacaval H g.
post coronary artery bypass g.
g. preparation
primary graft failure
PTFE arterial g.
PTFE Gore-Tex g.
PTFE graft material
radial artery g.
g. reinfection
g. rejection
renal artery bypass g.
reoperative coronary artery bypass g.
g. replacement
g. resorption
g. restenosis
reversed saphenous vein g.
Russe bone g.
saphenous vein g.
saphenous vein bypass g.
saphenous vein graft de novo
saphenous vein graft stenosis
Seddon nerve g.
g. sensation
g. septoplasty
serum chemistry g.
single coronary artery g.
single coronary artery bypass g.
g. site
skin g.
skin graft defatted
skin graft donor
skin graft slough
sliding inlay bone g.
g. spatulation
split-thickness autogenous g.
split-thickness skin g.
stent g.
g. strength
g. structure
g. surveillance
g. survival
g. survival rate
synthetic graft material
tantalum mesh g.
tendon g.
g. tension
g. thrombosis
total graft area rejected
g. treatment
triple coronary artery bypass g.
underlay fascial g.
valise handle g.
vascular access g.
vascular graft infection
vascularized bone g.
g. vasculopathy
vein g.
vein bypass g.
venous bypass g.
vertebral artery bypass g.
g. vessel disease
g. weight
whole bone transplant g.

graft-coated
autologous vein graft-coated stent

graft-host interface

grafting
allograft bone g.
g. anastomosis
aortofemoral bypass g.
authorization form for removal of tissue for g.
autogenous bone g.
autograft bone g.
autologous cultured skin g.
consent form for removal of tissue for g.
coronary artery bypass g.
coronary artery bypass grafting surgery
cross-facial nerve g.
endarterectomy and coronary artery bypass g.

endoscopic coronary artery bypass g.
endovascular g.
flexor tendon g.
minimally invasive coronary bypass g.
onlay bone g.
osteoconductive bone grafting material
repeated skin g.
g. vein

graft-to-recipient weight ratio

graft-versus-host
g.-v.-h. disease, grade 1–4
g.-v.-h. disease reaction
g.-v.-h. response

graft-versus-leukemia effect

Graham-Kendall
G.-K. Memory for Designs Test

grain
g. alcohol
gold grain implant

gram
g. calorie
G. iodine
g. negative
g.'s of nitrogen to nonprotein kilocalories
g. percent
g.'s per cubic centimeter
g.'s per deciliter
g.'s per liter
g.'s per milliliter
g. positive
spinal fluid Gram stain
sputum Gram stain
G. stain of body fluid
G. stain of cervix
G. stain of exudates
G. stain of facial abscess
G. staining technique
G. stain of pelvic abscess
G. stain of peritoneal fluid
G. stain procedure
G. stain of purulent discharge
G. stain of skin lesion
G. stain of stool test
G. stain of throat
G. stain of UN spun urine
G. stain of urethra

grammar
g. development stage
g. formation stage

grammatic
g. closure
g. method

grammatical
g. analysis
G. Analysis of Elicited Language
g. category
g. component
g. equivalent
g. meaning
Miller-Yoder Test of G. Comprehension
g. structure

gram-molecular
g.-m. volume
g.-m. weight

Gram-negative
G.-n. acne
G.-n. aerobe
G.-n. aerobic organism
aerobic Gram-negative rod
anaerobic Gram-negative rod
antibiotic-resistant Gram-negative organism
G.-n. bacillary meningitis
G.-n. bacilli
G.-n. bacilli arthritis
G.-n. bacilli infection
G.-n. bacillus
G.-n. bacteremia
G.-n. bacteria
cluster of short Gram-negative rods
G.-n. cocci
G.-n. coccobacillus
G.-n. diplococcus
G.-n. endocarditis
G.-n. endotoxic shock
G.-n. endotoxin
G.-n. endotoxin-induced shock
enteric Gram-negative bacillary
enteric Gram-negative bacillus
G.-n. enterococcus
G.-n. infection
lactose fermenting Gram-negative rods
G.-n. medium
G.-n. microorganism
nonfermentative Gram-negative bacilli
nonlactose fermenting Gram-negative rod
nosocomial Gram-negative infection
nosocomial Gram-negative organism
G.-n. rod
G.-n. rod and coccus
G.-n. sepsis
G.-n. septicemia
small Gram-negative coccobacilli
G.-n. species

Gram-positive
G.-p. aerobe
aerobic Gram-positive coccus
G.-p. anaerobic coccus
G.-p. bacilli
G.-p. bacillus
G.-p. bacteremia
G.-p. bacterial infection
G.-p. bacterial keratitis
G.-p. cocci
G.-p. cocci in pairs and chains
darkly-staining Gram-positive rods
G.-p. identification
G.-p. microorganism
G.-p. nosocomial infection
G.-p. rod
G.-p. rod and coccus
short-chain Gram-positive cocci
G.-p. surgical pathogen

Gram-stain morphology

Gram-variable bacteria

Gram-Weigert stain

grand
G. Arbaud virus
compatible with grand mal
epilepsy with grand mal seizures on awakening
isolated grand mal seizure
g. lamella
g. mal
g. mal attack
g. mal convulsion
g. mal convulsive disorder
g. mal epilepsy
g. mal seizure
g. mal status
g. multiparity
g. rounds
g. total
uncontrolled generalized grand mal seizure

granddad syndrome

granddaughter cyst

Grande
Rio Grande virus

grandeur
g. delusion
delusions of g.
ideas of g.

grandeur *(continued)*
preoccupation with fantasies of g.
grandfather
g. complex
father's g.
maternal g.
paternal g.
grandiose
g. delusion
g. idea
g. ideas
g. ideation
g. mania
g. notion
paranoid grandiose delusion
g. sense of self-importance
g. thought
grandiosity
sustained periods of g.
grandmother
father's g.
paternal g.
granny knot
granted
permission for autopsy g.
granular
alkaline phosphatase activity of granular leukocyte
g. appearance
g. atrophy of kidney
basophil granular leukocyte
breasts ropy or g.
g. cast
g. cell
g. cell ameloblastic fibroma
g. cell ameloblastoma
g. cell layer
g. cell myeloblastoma
g. cell myoblastoma
g. cell schwannoma
g. cell tumor
central granular cell odontogenic tumor
cervix g.
g. chromophil cell
g. component
g. conjunctivitis
g. corneal dystrophy
g. cyst
g. endoplasmic reticulum
g. eosinophilic cytoplasm
extracellular granular material
finely g.
g. formation
g. induration
g. inflammation
g. inflammatory nodule
g. kidney
large granular leukocyte
large granular lymphocyte
large granular vesicle
g. layer
g. lesion
lipofuscinosis granular osmiophilic deposit
lungs coarsely g.
g. lymphocyte-proliferative disorder
malignant granular cell myoblastoma
g. material
microscopic granular cell tumor
g. osmiophilic material
g. pharyngitis
g. precipitate
g. progenitor cell
g. protoplasm
g. respiration
small granular vesicle
g. stricture of urethra
g. surface
g. urethritis
g. vaginitis
granularis
ependymitis g.
granulated
g. cell
fully granulated basophil
granulating
chronic granulating wound
g. in and healing
g. in
incision granulating in
wound granulating in
granulation
arachnoid g.
arachnoid granulation calcification
arachnoid granulation villi
basophil granulation test
exuberant granulation tissue
healing by g.
juxtaglomerular granulation index
pacchionian g.
g. phase
g. stenosis
g. time
g. tissue
toxic granulation differential
granulatum
opium g.
granule
azurophilic g.
g. cell
g. deficiency
endocrine granule constituent
immature g.
lamellar g.
Langerhans cell g.
membrane coating g.
mucigen g.
mucous g.
neurosecretory g.
neutrophil-specific secondary granule deficiency
pigment g.
platelet granule extract
secretory g.
serous g.
granulocyte
absolute granulocyte count
g. adherence
g. agglutination
antibody-labeled circulating g.
circulating granulocyte pool
g. colony-stimulating factor
g. colony-stimulating factor receptor
g. count
g. cytotoxic
g. immunofluorescence test
macrophage and granulocyte inducer
marginal granulocyte pool
marginated granulocyte pool
polymorphonuclear g.
polymorphonuclear neutrophilic granulocyte
g. substance
total blood granulocyte pool
g. transfusion
g. turnover rate
granulocyte-macrophage
g.-m. colony-forming unit
g.-m. colony-stimulating activity
g.-m. colony-stimulating factor
granulocytic
acute granulocytic leukemia
aleukemic granulocytic leukemia
chronic granulocytic leukemia
human granulocytic ehrlichiosis
myeloid granulocytic leukemia
orbital granulocytic sarcoma
granulocytosis
paraneoplastic g.
granulocytosis-promoting factor

granuloma
g. annulare
annular elastolytic giant cell g.
benign granuloma of thyroid
calcified benign g.
Candida g.
candidal granuloma infection
caseating g.
central giant cell g.
eosinophilic g.
eosinophilic granuloma of lung
foreign body-type g.
lethal midline g.
localized granuloma annulare
g. of lung
lymphatic filariasis g.
massive granuloma of sclera
midline lethal g.
Miescher actinic g.
mixed inflammatory g.
multifocal eosinophilic g.
noncaseating conjunctival g.
O'Brien actinic g.
g. of orbit
palisading orbital g.
perforating granuloma annulare
peripheral giant cell reparative g.
plasma cell g.
pulmonary hyalinizing g.
g. sarcoid
g. of sinus
swimming pool g.
unifocal eosinophilic g.

granulomatosa
gastritis granulomatosa fibroplastica
Miescher cheilitis g.

granulomatosis
allergic angiitis and g.
allergic granulomatosis and angiitis
bronchocentric g.
Langerhans cell g.
limited Wegener g.
lymphocytic angiitis and g.
lymphomatoid g.
malignant g.
necrotizing respiratory g.
necrotizing sarcoid g.
pulmonary g.
g. siderotica
Wegener pulmonary g.

granulomatous
g. abscess
allergic granulomatous angiitis
allergic granulomatous arteritis
allergic granulomatous prostatitis
g. amebic encephalitis
ANCA-positive granulomatous giant-cell arteritis
g. angiitis of the central nervous system
g. arteritis
g. bowel disease
g. calcification
g. cervicitis
g. change
g. cholangitis
chronic granulomatous inflammation
chronic inflammatory granulomatous process
g. colitis
g. conjunctivitis
cranial granulomatous arteritis
g. cystitis
g. disease
g. disease of childhood
g. disorder
g. encephalitis
g. endophthalmitis
g. enteritis
g. enterocolitis
g. gastritis
g. hypersensitivity reaction
g. ileitis
g. ileojejunitis
g. infection
infectious granulomatous disease
g. inflammation
g. iridocyclitis
g. lesion
g. lesions of unknown significance
g. lining
g. lymphadenitis
g. lymphoma
massive granulomatous orchitis
g. mastitis
g. meningitis
Miescher granulomatous cheilitis
miliary granulomatous inflammation
g. myositis
necrotizing granulomatous inflammation
necrotizing granulomatous lymphadenitis
necrotizing granulomatous systemic arteritis
necrotizing granulomatous vasculitis
nodular granulomatous vasculitis
g. nodule
noncaseating granulomatous disease
nonspecific granulomatous disease
nonspecific granulomatous orchitis
obliterative granulomatous fibrosis
g. panuveitis
g. peritonitis
g. perivasculitis
g. pneumonitis
g. process
g. prostatitis
g. reaction
g. salpingitis
g. sialadenitis
g. synovitis
g. temporal arteritis
g. tenosynovitis
g. thyroiditis
g. tissue
g. uveitis
g. vasculitis
g. zone

granulomembranous body

granulopoiesis
neutrophil g.

granulosa
adult granulosa cell tumor
appendicitis g.
g. cell
g. cell tumor
juvenile granulosa cell tumor
membrana g.
membrana granulosa cell
membrana granulosa externa
membrane g.
ovarian granulosa cell
pars g.
pyelitis g.

granulosa-stromal cell tumor

granulosa-theca cell tumor

granulosis virus

granulosum
stratum g.

granulovirus
Cydia pomonella g.

grape
Carswell g.'s
g. cluster appearance

grapefruit juice

graph
Moseley bone age g.
serum chemistry g.

graphic
g. analysis
g. aphasia

graphic *(continued)*
computer graphic simulation
g. description
g. disorientation
g. impairment
g. level recorder
G. Rating Scale
selective imaging and graphics for stereotactic surgery
g. stress telethermometry
g. stress thermography
video graphic tool technology
g. violence

graphite
g., benzalkonium, heparin
polyurethane-polyvinyl g.
g. treatment

grasp
hand grasp reflex
ipsilateral instinctive grasp reaction
palmar grasp reflex
palmar reflex g.
pen g.
pinch g.
reflex g.
g. reflex
response g.
strength g.
toe g.

grasped
cecum g.
cervix g.
tonsil g.

grasper
atraumatic g.
lion's claw g.
nonsuction g.
pituitary g.
4-pronged polyp g.

grasping
alligator-type grasping forceps
arthroscopy grasping forceps

grass
individually polymerized g.
meadow fescue g.
meadow foxtail g.
orchard grass pollen

Grassi
G. Basic Cognitive Evaluation
nerve of G.

gratification
delay of g.
emotional g.
material g.
oral g.

grating
Arden g.
g. pain
g. sensation
g. sensation under kneecap
g. sound

Gratiolet
convolution of G.

gravely disabled

grave prognosis

Graves
G. disease
G. hyperthyroidism
minimal euthyroid Graves disease
neonatal Graves hyperthyroidism
ophthalmic Graves disease
G. ophthalmopathy
G. scapula

gravida
g., para, abortus
g., para, multiple births, abortions, live birth

gravidarum
chorea g.
emesis g.
hyperemesis g.
melasma g.
molluscum fibrosum g.
nausea g.
nephritis g.
pyelitis g.
retinitis g.

gravid uterus

gravis
adult-onset myasthenia g.
autoimmune myasthenia g.
congenital myasthenia g.
double vision from myasthenia g.
experimental autoimmune myasthenia g.
icterus gravis neonatorum
juvenile autoimmune myasthenia g.
muscle weakening myasthenia g.
myasthenia g.
myasthenia gravis and mediastinal tumors
myasthenia gravis pseudoparalytica
myasthenia gravis syndrome
neonatal myasthenia g.
ocular myasthenia g.
paranoia dementia g.
persistent neonatal myasthenia g.

gravitating hemorrhage

gravitation
Newtonian constant of g.
newtonian constant of g.

gravitational
g. constant
g. field-flow fractionation
lumbar gravitational line
g. ulcer
g. unit

gravity
center of g.
g. concentration
decreased specific g.
g. drainage
g. extension locking system
free position g.
g. induced loss of consciousness
line of g.
g. lumbar reduction
Parvin gravity technique
g. settling culture plate
specific g.
specific gravity test
straight gravity drainage
g. stress test
g. unit
g. urinary incontinence

gravity-induced loss of consciousness

gravity-setting culture

gray
anterior gray column
anterior gray column of cord
anterior gray commissure
ashen gray color
g. atrophy
g. baby syndrome
g. cataract
central g.
gelatinous substance of gray substance
g. induration
g. line
G. Lodge virus
g. matter
g. matter of brain
g. matter of spinal cord
mesencephalic central g.
middle gray layer of superior colliculus
neutral or gray area
occipital gray matter
G. Oral Reading Test-Revised
G. Oral Reading Test, Third Edition

paracentral gray area
g. patches
periaqueductal central g.
periaqueductal gray area
periaqueductal gray matter
periaqueductal gray nucleus
periaqueductal gray substance
periventricular gray matter
periventricular gray substance
g. platelet syndrome
pontine gray matter
shade response to light gray area
shading response to gray areas
g. softening
g. substance
g. substance of spinal cord
tympanic membrane g.

graying
g. hair from aging
macular g.

gray-scale
g.-s. imaging
g.-s. median
g.-s. ultrasonography
g.-s. ultrasound

gray/white
loss of distinction at gray/white matter interface

greasy stool

great
adducted great toe
g. adductor muscle
anterior great vessel
g. cardiac vein
g. cardiac vein flow
g. cistern
complete transposition of great arteries
complete transposition of great vessels
congenitally corrected transposition of the great arteries
corrected congenital transposition of the great vessels
dextratransposition of great vessels
dextrotransposition of great arteries
D-transposition of great arteries
heart and great vessels
g. horizontal fissure
G. Island virus
left transposition of great artery
long extensor muscle of great toe
long flexor muscle of great toe
malar crest of great wing of sphenoid bone
malposition of great arteries
medial great muscle
normal flexion of great toe
palliation of great vessels
posterior branch of great auricular nerve
G. Smoky Mountains Study of Youth
g. toe
g. toe amputation
g. toe arthroplasty implant technique
g. toe bone
g. toe implant
g. toe implant prosthesis
g. toe reflex
g. toe transplant
g. toe wraparound flap
transposition of the great arteries
transposition of great vessel
g. transverse commissure
g. transverse fissure of cerebrum
g. vein of Galen
g. vessel
g. vestibular gland

greater
air greater than bone conduction
arterial circle of greater iris
bone conduction greater than air conduction
g. cul-de-sac
g. curvature
middle greater tubercle of facet of humerus
g. occipital neuritis
g. omentum
g. palatine artery
g. palatine canal
g. palatine foramen
g. palatine groove
g. palatine nerve
parietal margin of greater wing of sphenoid
g. psoas muscle
pulmonic second heart sound greater than aortic second heart sound
g. rhomboid muscle
g. ring of iris
g. sacrosciatic notch
g. saphenous phlebectomy
g. saphenous vein
g. saphenous vein cutdown
g. sciatic foramen
g. sciatic notch
second aortic sound greater than second pulmonic sound
g. splanchnic nerve
g. superficial petrosal neurectomy
g. superficial temporal artery biopsy
g. supraclavicular fossa
g. trochanter
g. trochanteric apophysial arrest
g. trochanteric bursa
g. trochanteric femoral fracture
g. trochanter muscle
g. tubercle
g. tuberosity
g. tuberosity fracture
g. tuberosity osteotomy
g. tympanic spine
g. vestibular gland
g. zygomatic muscle

greatest
angle of greatest extension
angle of greatest flexion
g. common factor
g. gluteal muscle
g. single allergen present

great-grandfather
paternal g.-g.

great-grandmother
paternal g.-g.

green
brilliant g.
brilliant green lactose broth
bromcresol g.
dark green bile
dark green viscous bile
decaffeinated green tea
digital subtraction indocyanine green angiography
enhanced green fluorescent protein
fast g.
g. fluorescent protein
indocyanine green angiography
indocyanine green dye
large green soft stool
methyl green pyronin dye
orange green stain
primary African green monkey kidney
selenite brilliant g.
g. tea extract
g. tea polyphenol
thermal green dye
tincture of green soap
g. urine from antidepressant

Greenfield vena cava filter

greenstick
g. fracture
g. injury

Greig cephalopolysyndactyly syndrome

grenade
g. thrower's arm
g. thrower's fracture

Grenoble-Paris-Rennes epilepsy

grenz ray

Greppi
microelliptopoikilocytic anemia of Rietti, Greppi, and Micheli

Grey
G. balanced saline solution
tris-buffered Grey solution
G. Turner sign

grid
g. 1
g. 2
Amsler grid test
antiscatter g.
g. laser photocoagulation
g. method
Patient Evaluation G.
G. Test of Schizophrenic Thought Disorder
Wetzel g.

grief
anticipatory g.
complicated grief disorder
g. counselor
distorted g.
G. Experience Inventory
impacted g.
mutual g.
pathologic grief reaction
prolonged g.
g. support group
g. therapy
unresolved g.

Griesinger
G. disease
G. sign

grieving
pathologic g.
g. process

grievous bodily harm

griffe
main en g.
main en griffe deformity

Griffiths Mental Developmental Scale

grimacing
facial g.

grinding
Apley grinding test
habitual g.
jaw g.
night grinding of teeth
nonfunctional g.
selective g.
tooth g.

grind test

grip
bilateral firm hand g.'s
g.'s equal and good
hand grip exercise
hand grip strength
isometric hand grip test
left-hand g.
right hand g.
g. strength
g.'s strong and equal

gripping
axial gripping strength

Griscelli syndrome

griseofulvin peripheral neuropathy

gritty tumor

grivet monkey cell

groaning
nocturnal g.

Grocott-Gomori methenamine silver nitrate

Grocott methenamine silver stain

groin
g. dissection
g. exploration
g. flap
g. hernia
g. incision
g. mass
osteomusculocutaneous deep circumflex iliac groin flap
g. pain
pedicled groin flap

grommet
circumferential g.
myringotomy and grommet insertion
g. tube

groomed
poorly g.
well g.

grooming
decline in personal g.
g. and hygiene
loss of interest in personal g.

groove
anal intersphincteric g.
anterior auricular g.
anterior intermediate g.
anterior interventricular g.
anterior palatine g.
atrioventricular groove branch
buccal developmental g.
buccal groove of central fossa
central developmental g.
central groove of central fossa
distal oblique g.
distobuccal developmental g.
distolingual g.
fifth cusp g.
free gingival g.
greater palatine g.
interdental g.
lingual developmental g.
maxilla
medial bicipital g.
median groove of tongue
meningeal artery g.
mesial marginal developmental g.
mesiobuccal developmental g.
mesiolingual developmental g.
olfactory groove meningioma
olfactory groove of nasal cavity
olfactory groove tumor
palatine groove of maxilla
palatomaxillary groove of palatine bone
patellofemoral groove cartilage
posterior auricular g.
g. sign
supplemental g.
supraorbital g.
transverse groove of oblique ridge

grooved
g. incision
g. tongue

gross
American Pediatric G. Assessment Record
g. anatomy
G. cell surface antigen
g. cystic disease
g. cystic disease fluid protein
g. deformity
g. examination of tissue
g. fecal contamination
g. fracture

g. hematuria
g. hemorrhage
g. impairment
g. insensitivity
g. lesion
G. leukemia antigen
G. leukemia virus
g. manipulation
g. and microscopic
g. motor
g. motor activity
g. motor deficit
g. motor development
G. Motor Function Measure
g. motor skill
g. neurologic deficit
persistent gross splenomegaly
recurrent gross hematuria
G. sarcoma virus antigen
g. sensory deficit
g. specimen
g. total resection
g. tumor volume
g. weight

grossly

g. bloody
g. bloody stool
cranial nerves grossly intact
g. disorganized behavior
g. impaired functioning
g. pathogenic care

grotesque features

ground

anterior ground bundle
coffee ground emesis
dark g.
interstitial fluids and ground substance
g. itch anemia
g. lamella
lateral g.
Southern California Figure G. Test

ground-fault interrupter

ground-glass

airspace ground-glass infiltrate
g.-g. appearance
g.-g. attenuation
g.-g. clotting time
g.-g. opacification
g.-g. opacity
g.-g. pathway
g.-g. pattern

group

g. A beta hemolytic streptococcus
ABO blood g.
g. activity
activity group therapy
activity-interview group psychotherapy
addictive behavior g.
g. adjustment therapy
adolescent group therapy
adolescent support g.
adult group therapy
advanced stage g.
AIDS group home
Allport group relations theory
ambulatory patient g.
ambulatory payment classification g.
ambulatory visit groups
g. analysis
analytic group psychotherapy
anorexia support g.
anti-blood group A antiglobulin test
anti-P blood group specificity
AO group shoulder arthrodesis
arbovirus group unclassified
ARI Group I–IV filter
g. A streptococcus
g. A streptococcus direct test
g. A streptococcus infection
Auberger blood g.
Au blood g.
Austin-Kartush group A impairment
Austin-Kartush group C patient related to ossiculoplasty
Austrian Breast Cancer Study G.
avian type C retrovirus g.
g. B coxsackievirus
g. behavior
bereavement recovery g.
beta-hemolytic streptococcus group A
blood group degrading enzyme
blood factor in the MNS blood group system
blood group class
blood group substance
blood group system
blood type in ABO blood g.
British Isles Lupus Assessment Group index
g. B streptococcal infection
g. B streptococcal meningitis
g. B streptococcal pneumonia
g. B streptococcal sepsis
g. B streptococcus
cancer biotherapy study g.
cancer and leukemia group B
carbon atom farthest from principal functioning g.
carbon separated from the carboxyl group by 2 other carbon atoms
g. care
cognitive therapy g.
conduct disorder type g.
G. Conformity Rating
control g.
conventional therapy g.
g. counseling
couples group therapy
cross-reactive antigen g.
g. C streptococcus
daily group therapy
g. D enterococcus
desensitization and relaxation g.
diagnosis-related g.
Diego blood g.
digoxin investigators g.
diphosphate g.
directive group play therapy
directive play therapy g.
divorce support g.
dorsal respiratory g.
drug treatment g.
drug-using peer g.
g. D streptococcus
g. dynamics
G. Embedded Figures Test
G. Encounter Scale
G. Encounter Survey
G. Environment Scale
episodic treatment g.
family group therapy
g. feedback
first in alpha series or g.
fourth in a series or g.
Functional Related G.'s
grief support g.
g. G streptococcus
Harvard Group Scale of Hypnotic Susceptibility, Form A
high-dose g.
high-frequency blood g.
high mobility g.
g. home
hydroxyl g.
inherited blood factor in MNS blood g.
intensive group therapy
g. interaction
interdisciplinary g.
intermediate dose g.
interpersonal group therapy

group *(continued)*
Kell blood g.
Lewis blood g.
g. living
long-distance g.
long-term support g.
low-dose g.
low-frequency blood g.
low-frequency blood group antigen
low mobility g.
Lu blood g.
Lutheran blood group system
lymphocytic choriomeningitis virus g.
lymphoproliferative virus g.
mammalian type B, C, D oncovirus g.
marathon group psychotherapy
Marburg virus g.
marital couples group therapy
measles-rinderpest-distemper virus g.
medical group practice
g. method
middle group of mesenteric lymph node
a minor blood g.
minor group antigen incompatibility
minority group psychiatry
MN blood g.
MNS blood g.
MNSs blood g.
Morphine-Benzedrine G. Scale
M-type genetic g.
mucosal disease virus g.
multidisciplinary group psychiatry
multi-family group counseling
muscle g.
mutual aid g.
National Cancer Institute Cooperative G.
National Diabetes Data G.
neurogenic fiber type g.
nonocular muscle g.
nontreatment g.
nonventilated g.
optimal group size
pain support g.
parent-child group therapy
g. participation
P blood g.
P blood group antigen
P blood group system
Pediatric AIDS Clinical Trial G. Protocol
pedunculopontine cholinergic g.
placebo control g.
play group therapy
psychoeducational group therapy
radiation therapy oncology g.
g. reaction
G. Reading Test
resource utilization g.
Rh blood g.
risk group for infection
Sciana blood g.
self-help support g.
g. setting
sexual abuse g.
short distance g.
small group therapy
solution focused group therapy
special interest g.
g. specific
spotted fever g.
g. striction
G. Styles Inventory
g. support
support group for epilepsy
g. support session
g. tension
therapeutic play g.
g. therapist
g. therapy session
topic-oriented process g.
training g.
treated g.
g. treatment for children
g. treatment for insomnia
g. of units of analysis
ventilated g.
g. work
xeroderma pigmentosum group A, C
youth/parent support g.

grouping
antigenic structural g.
symptom g.

group-living program

group-specific
g.-s. amplification
g.-s. antigen
g.-s. component

grow
plug the lung until it g.'s

growing
convalescent growing nursery
g. fracture
ischemic disease of the growing hip
g. lesion
lump growing in bone
g. pain
rapidly growing lesion
rapidly growing tumor
slowly growing invasive adenocarcinoma
slowly growing tumor
g. tumor

growth
abnormal bone g.
abnormal growth process
abnormal hair g.
g. abnormality
abnormal mass of tissue g.
accelerated growth area
acidic fibroblast growth factor
adrenal growth factor
g. after 48 hours incubation
altered growth and development
androgen-induced growth factor
angiogenic growth factor
antiepidermal growth factor receptor
antiepidermal growth factor receptor antibody for cancer
antiepidermal growth factor receptor monoclonal antibody
antivascular endothelial growth factor monoclonal antibody
aortic stenosis, corneal clouding, growth and mental retardation syndrome
g. arrest
arrested growth and development
artificial growth hormone
asymmetric fetal growth restriction
asymmetric intrauterine growth retardation
asymmetric maxillomandibular g.
autocrine growth factor
autocrine-paracrine-acting growth factor
autocrine-paracrine growth loop
autocrine-paracrine growth regulator
autologous growth factor
autologous growth factor binding agent
autologous growth factor gel
basic fibroblast growth factor
B-cell growth factor
beta-nerve growth factor
biosynthetic human growth hormone
bone-derived growth factor
bone growth and breakdown

bovine growth hormone
cancerous growth of blood cell
chorionic growth hormone-prolactin
coloboma, heart disease, atresia choanae, retarded growth and retarded development and/or CNS anomalies, genital hypoplasia, and ear anomalies and/or deafness syndrome
concentration epidermal growth factor
connective tissue growth factor
constitutional delayed g.
constitutional delay in growth and adolescence
constitutional delay in growth and development
cribriform growth pattern
culture negative for g.
g. curve
g. cycle
g. deficiency
g. and development
g. differentiation factor
g. differentiation factor-9
direct-current bone growth stimulator
disordered bone g.
ectopic bone g.
embryonic growth and development factor
endothelial cell growth factor
endothelial cell growth supplement
epidermal growth factor
epidermal growth factor receptor
epiphysial growth plate
equine growth hormone
esophageal epidermal growth factor
excessive facial hair g.
excessive hair g.
facial dysplasia, hyperextensibility of joints, clinodactyly, growth retardation, mental retardation syndrome
g. factor-inducible chemokine
g. failure
fast growth rate
fetal growth acceleration
fetal growth and development
fetal growth restriction
fetal growth retardation
fibroblast-derived growth factor
fibroblast growth factor receptor
fibroblast growth factor receptor 2
fibroblastic growth factor
g. fraction
g. gene
glycoprotein crystal growth inhibitor
heparin-binding epidermal growth factorlike growth factor
heparin-binding growth factor-1
heparin-binding growth factor-2
heparin-binding growth factor
hepatocyte growth factor
g. hormone
g. hormone-binding protein
g. hormone cell adenoma
g. hormone cell hyperplasia
g. hormone deficiency
g. hormone deficiency syndrome in adult
g. hormone-deficient adult
g. hormone-deficient child
g. hormone dose
g. hormone dose-response curve
g. hormone-expressing cell
g. hormone failure
g. hormone-1 gene
g. hormone-2 gene
g. hormone hypersecretion
g. hormone immunoassay
g. hormone-inhibiting factor
g. hormone-inhibiting hormone
g. hormone inhibitory hormone
g. hormone insensitivity
g. hormone insufficiency
g. hormone insulin
g. hormone-producing adenoma
g. hormone receptor deficiency
g. hormone release
g. hormone release-inhibiting factor
g. hormone release-inhibiting hormone
g. hormone releasing factor
g. hormone-releasing factor test
g. hormone-releasing factor tumor
g. hormone-releasing hormone
g. hormone-releasing hormone receptor
g. hormone-releasing peptide
g. hormone replacement
g. hormone response
g. hormone secretagogue
g. hormone secretagogue receptor
g. hormone secretion
g. hormone stimulation test
g. hormone therapy
g. hormone variant
human epidermal growth factor
human epidermal growth receptor 2
human growth factor
human growth hormone
human growth hormone deficiency
human pituitary growth hormone
human skeletal growth factor
idiopathic growth hormone
idiopathic growth hormone deficiency
immunoreactive human growth hormone
implantable bone growth stimulator
g. inhibiting
g. inhibition
insulin growth factor
insulin growth factor-binding protein
insulinlike growth factor-1, -2
insulinlike growth factor-binding protein-1–6
insulinlike growth factor-II receptor
interference with intellectual and emotional g.
intrauterine fetal growth retardation
intrauterine growth rate
intrauterine growth restriction
invasive growth of blood cell
invasive growth of blood vessel
isolated growth hormone deficiency
isolated growth hormone deficiency type IB, II, III
isolated human growth deficiency
Kaposi sarcoma human growth factor
keratinocyte growth factor
keratinocyte growth factor-2
keratinocyte growth factor receptor
lentigines, electrocardiographic abnormalities, ocular hypertelorism, pulmonary stenosis, abnormalities of genitalia, retardation of growth, deafness syndrome
linear growth retardation
linear growth velocity
little growth hormone
loudness growth perception
lung growth and development

growth *(continued)*
macrophage-derived growth factor
mast cell growth factor
g. and maturation of new skin
maximal increment in growth and weight
g. medium
megakaryocyte growth and development factor
mental and growth retardation-amblyopia syndrome
mixed growth hormone-prolactin cell adenoma
mixed growth hormone- and prolactin-secreting adenoma
mixed growth on culture
g. monitoring, oral rehydration, breast feeding, and immunization
mouse epidermal growth factor
murine granulocyte-macrophage colony-stimulating growth factor
mycobacteria growth indicator tube
mycobacteria growth indicator tube system
Mycobacteria Growth Indicator tube
myeloid growth factor
myeloma growth factor
National Cooperative G. Study
natural growth hormone
nerve cell g.
nerve growth factor antiserum
nerve growth factor receptor
nerve growth inhibitor
nerve growth stimulating activity
neural growth factor
neural growth factor receptor
neutralizing antibody to vascular endothelial growth factor
new skin g.
nodular growth of tissue
noncancerous skin g.
nonhematopoietic growth factor
normal fetal g.
normal growth and development
normotensive intrauterine growth restriction
nutrient artery g.
olfactory axonal g.
ovine growth hormone
g. parameter
paraneoplastic growth hormone
g. pattern
peak growth velocity
peptide growth factor
peptide growth factor receptor signal
peptide growth factor signaling mechanism
g. period
g. phase of facial hair
phase of mitosis in cell growth cycle
pituitary growth hormone
plasma growth hormone
g. plate fracture
g. plate injury
platelet-derived endothelial cell growth factor
platelet-derived epidermal growth factor
platelet-derived growth factor A, B
pleiotrophin/midkine growth enhancer
polypeptide growth factor
poor intrauterine fetal g.
porcine growth hormone
postnatal growth deficiency
precancerous cervical g.
prolactin chronic growth hormone
pseudofollicular growth center
rapid muscle g.
g. rate
rat growth hormone
recombinant human growth hormone
recombinant human insulinlike growth factor
recombinant human insulin-like growth factor-1
recombinant human platelet-derived growth factor
recombinant human vascular endothelial growth factor
relative growth rate
g. retardation
g. retardation, alopecia, pseudoanodontia, and optic atrophy syndrome
g. retardation in children
g. retardation, ocular abnormalities, microcephaly, brachydactyly, oligophrenia
retard fetal g.
revitalize hair g.
salivary epidermal growth factor
sarcoma growth factor
skeletal growth factor
slow down cancer g.
slow fetal g.
slow growth rate
somatic cell-derived growth factor
g. spurt
stimulate new vessel g.
g. stimulating hormone
g. stunting
supplemental growth hormone therapy
suppression for tumor g.
synthetic human growth hormone
T-cell growth factor-1
T-cell growth factor-2
theoretical growth evaluation
thymus cell growth factor
thyroid growth immunoglobulin
g. and transformation
transforming growth factor beta-1, -2, -3
transforming growth factor
transforming growth factor-1
transforming growth factor alpha
trypanosome growth factor
tumor g.
tumor growth delay
tumor growth factor
uncontrolled cell division g.
unidentified growth factor
vascular endothelial cell growth inhibitor
vascular endothelial growth factor 2, 3
vascular endothelial growth factor/vascular permeability factor
g. velocity
zero population g.

growth-adjusted sonographic age

growth-associated
g.-a. protein
g.-a. protein-43

growth-discordant twins

growth-inhibiting hormone

growth-related oncogene

growth-releasing hormone

growth-stimulating
g.-s. antibody
g.-s. hormone

Gruber syndrome

grunt
audible g.
diastolic g.

grunting
expiratory g.
g. and flaring
flaring and g.

g., flaring, and retracting breathing
infant retracting and g.
g. maneuver
g. respiration
g. and retraction
retraction or g.
g. or retraction

G-stimulating protein

guaiac
bicolor guaiac test
g. negative
nonrehydrated guaiac examination
g. positive
g. stool test
g. test
g. testing
test of stool g.

guaiac-negative stool

guaiac-positive stool

Guajara virus

Guama virus

guanethidine
parenteral g.

guanidinoacetate methyltransferase

guanine
6-alkyl guanine alkyl transferase
cystine g.
g. cytosine
dioxalane g.
g. nucleotide regulatory protein
g. nucleotide-releasing factor
penta-acetylglucopyranosyl g.
thymine, adenine, and g.

guanosine
g. diphosphate
g. 5′-diphosphate
g. triphosphatase
g. triphosphate
g. 5′ triphosphate
g. 5′-triphosphate

guanosine-coupled spleen cell

guaranteed yield strength

guard
ankle g.
mouth g.
occlusal g.
off g.
old g.
palm g.

guarded
g. manner
postoperative period g.
prognosis is g.

guardedness
adolescent g.

guardian ad litem

guarding
g. of the abdomen
abdominal muscle g.
g. and/or rebound
g. and/or rigidity
contact g.
patient exhibited muscle g.
rebound and/or g.
rebound guarding or rigidity
g. reflex
rigidity and/or g.
g. sign

guar gum

Guaroa virus

Guberina
system universal verbotonol audition G.

gubernacular
g. attachment
g. canal
g. vein

gubernaculum
Hunter g.

Gubler hemiplegia

Guérin
G. fold
G. fracture
G. gland
G. sinus
G. valve

Guérin-Stern syndrome

guessed average

Guglielmi detachable coil

guidance
arc-centered guidance system
Comparative G. and Placement Program
fluoroscopic image g.
frameless stereotactic g.
hip guidance orthosis
memory guidance saccade test
parent guidance work
pictorial anticipatory g.
stroke guidance system

guide
Bristol Social Adjustment G.'s
Cognitive Observation G.
g. dog
g. hole
image g.
light g.
light guide bundle
mandibular guide prosthesis
parental failure to g.
patient guide to medication
g. plane
Prevocational Assessment and Curriculum G.
radiation exposure g.
radiation protection g.
relative value g.

guided
g. affective imagery
g. biopsy
g. bone regeneration
computer guided laser beam
g. drainage
echo guided pericardiocentesis
echo guided ultrasound
g. eruption
gamma probe guided lymphoscintigraphy
g. imagery
g. imagery therapist
g. needle biopsy
sound guided into bladder
stereotactically guided core needle biopsy
stereotactic guided core-needle biopsy
g. tissue regeneration
ultrasonically guided needle biopsy

guideline
American Diabetes Association g.'s
clasp g.
clinical practice g.'s
dietary g.
government mandated g.
income poverty g.
Mallinckrodt Institute g.'s
medication administration g.
mucosal guideline pattern
National Cholesterol Education g.'s
Nephrolithiasis Clinical G.'s Panel
parotid gland exposure g.
patient exposure g.

guidewire
g. exchange
g. exchange technique
g. manipulation
g. passage
g. perforation

guidewire *(continued)*
g. reflection
g. sphincterotomy
Guidi
canal of G.
guiding
g. incline
g. plane
Guilford-Zimmerman
G.-Z. Aptitude Survey
G.-Z. Interest Inventory
G.-Z. Personality Test
G.-Z. Temperament Survey
Guillain-Barré-Landry syndrome
Guillain-Barré syndrome
guillotine
g. incision
g. midfoot amputation
g. needle biopsy
guillotine-type
g.-t. amputation
g.-t. cutter
guilt
g. complex
deep-seated g.
delusions of g.
excessive g.
excessive or inappropriate g.
g. feeling
feeling of guilt, worthlessness and helplessness
inappropriate g.
increased g.
low self-esteem or g.
neurotic g.
g. over disloyalty
pathologic g.
patient expressed guilt feeling
penalty, frustration, anxiety, guilt, hostility
g. reaction
sense of g.
g. and shame
shame and g.
surviving and survival g.
survivor g.
guilty
g., ashamed and intimidated
g. but mentally ill
not guilty by reason of insanity
patient feels g.
g. rumination
guinea
antiserum, guinea pig
g. pig
g. pig albumin
g. pig antiinsulin serum
g. pig complement
g. pig dander
g. pig embryo
g. pig gamma globulin
g. pig ileum
g. pig inoculation
g. pig keratocyte
g. pig kidney absorption test
g. pig lung strip
g. pig maximization test
g. pig myelin-basic protein
g. pig red blood cell
g. pig spleen
g. pig trachea
g. pig tracheal smooth muscle
g. pig unit
Guinea worm disease
Gulf War syndrome
gull
modified gull wing incision
gullwing
g. flap
g. incision
g. pattern
Gully
Gadget's Gully virus
gum
advanced gum disease
Apathy gum syrup medium
bleeding g.'s
g. bleeding
g. contour
discoloration of g.'s
g. disease
eroding gum tissue
guar g.
heat, steam, gum, yawn, and Valsalva maneuver
g. hyperplasia
g.'s infected
g. infection
inflamed g.'s
g. inflammation
g. lancet
g. line
periodontal gum care
physical dependence on nicotine g.
problems from aging g.'s
puffy g.'s
receded g.'s
g. recession
red g.'s from dentures
g.'s red and puffy
red, swollen, tender g.'s
g. resection
serious gum disease
g. shrinkage
g.'s shrinking
swelling of g.'s
swollen and tender g.'s
g. tissue
g. tissue breakdown
Gumbo Limbo virus
gumma, pl. **gummata, gummas**
multiple g.
gummatous
g. abscess
g. necrosis
g. syphilis
gummosa
periarteritis g.
Gump
Andy Gump deformity
Andy Gump facies
gun
assault g.
automated biopsy g.
g. control
Mentor g.
Omni clip g.
paint gun injury
pressure gun injury
Gunn
G. jaw-winking phenomenon
Marcus G.
Marcus Gunn classification
Marcus Gunn dot
Marcus Gunn jaw-winking phenomenon
Marcus Gunn jaw-winking ptosis
Marcus Gunn jaw-winking syndrome
Marcus Gunn pupillary sign
Marcus Gunn relative afferent defect
Marcus Gunn test
G. pupillary reflex
gunpowder lesion
gunshot
multiple gunshot wound
g. wound
g. wound to abdomen
g. wound to head
gurgling
g. bowel sounds
g. rale
Gurupi virus

gusher
X-linked progressive mixed deafness with perilymphatic g.

gustatory
g. anesthesia
g. hallucination
g. lacrimation
rhombencephalic gustatory nucleus
g. sweating
thalamic gustatory nucleus

gustolacrimal
acquired gustolacrimal reflex
paradoxic gustolacrimal reflex

gut
artificial g.
blind g.
chromic gut suture
congenital malrotation of the g.
development of g.
g. intestinal cell
lumen of the g.
lumen of g.
g. mucosal lymphocyte
nervous g.
normal gut flora
plain g.
plain gut suture
postanal g.
preoral g.
primitive g.
g. rest
ribbon g.
silkworm gut suture
g. suture
upper g.

gut-associated
g.-a. lymphoid disease
g.-a. lymphoid tissue

gut-derived infectious toxic shock

Guthrie
G. bacterial inhibition assay
neonatal Guthrie card

guttata
morphea g.
parapsoriasis g.
psoriasis g.

guttate
idiopathic guttate hypomelanosis

gutter
anterolateral g.
g. cast
g. fracture
packing of paracolic g.
paracolic g.
paravertebral g.
pelvic g.
posterior g.
right g.
g. splint
g. wound

guttering
limbal g.
limbus g.

guttural
g. pulse
g. rale
g. sound

Guyon
G. amputation
canal of G.
G. canal
G. operation
G. sign
G. sound

gymnastics
ocular g.

gynecologic
complete gynecologic examination annually
g. cryosurgery
g. disease
g. examination
g. infection
intracavitary gynecologic applicator
g. laparoscopy
g. lesion
g. malignancy
g. oncology
g. urology

gynecological
benign gynecological disease
g. care
g. chylous reflux syndrome
g. examination
g. history
g. malignancy
nosocomial gynecological infection
routine gynecological examination

gynecology
clinical obstetrics and g.
International Federation of G. and Obstetrics classification of tumor staging
obstetrics and g.
surgery, gynecology, and obstetrics

gynecomastia
choriogenic g.
mastectomy for g.
mental retardation, gynecomastia, obesity syndrome

gyrate
g. atrophy
hyperornithinemia with gyrate atrophy

gyratum
ovarium g.

gyri (*pl. of* gyrus)

gyriform intracranial calcification

gyrous area

gyrus, pl. **gyri**
angular g.
angular gyrus syndrome
anterior central g.
anterior cingulate g.
anterior cingulate gyrus tumor
anterior paracentral g.
anterior piriform g.
anterior transverse temporal g.
artery of angular g.
ascending frontal g.
ascending parietal g.
g. of Broca
gyri cerebri
cingulate g.
dentate g.
g. frontalis inferior
g. frontalis medialis
g. frontalis superior
g. herniation
Heschl g.
inferior frontal g.
medial frontal g.
middle frontal g.
occipital gyri
orbital gyri
superior frontal g.
superior temporal g.
supramarginal g.
g. temporalis inferior
g. temporalis superior

H
H. antigen
H. band
H. chain
H. space
H. spike

H-2
H-2 antigen
H-2 complex

H2
H2 antagonist
H2 blocker
intravenous H2 receptor antagonist

habenula, pl. **habenulae**
nucleus h.

habenular
medial h.
medial habenular nucleus

habenularis
nucleus habenularis lateralis
nucleus habenularis medialis

Habermann disease

habilitation
audiologic h.

habilitative
h. day care
h. day treatment

habit
alcohol h.
altered bowel h.
apoplectic h.
asthenic h.
bad dietary h.
bladder h.
bowel h.
h. cessation
change in bladder h.
change in bowel h.
change in sexual h.
chronic h.
clamping h.
daily h.'s
dental h.'s
dietary h.
drinking h.
drug h.
eating h.
endothelioid h.
erratic eating h.'s
h. forming
glaucomatous h.
good eating h.
health h.
healthy dietary h.
healthy lifestyle h.
kicking the h.
kicking drug h.
kicking smoking h.
lip habit appliance
mentalis h.
modify stressful living h.'s
motor h.
narcotic h.
nicotine h.
occlusal habit neurosis
opium h.
oral h.
parental habits of blame
parental habits of praise
pathological habit disorder
personal h.
physiologic h.
poor dietary h.
h. reversal
h. reversal training
revising sleep h.'s
sedentary h.
self-injurious h.
severe nail-biting h.
smoking h.
stable eating h.
stereotype habits disorder
Survey of Study H.'s and Attitudes
visual h.

habit-forming drug

habitual
h. abortion
h. behavior
h. cocaine smoker
h. criminal
h. dislocation
h. drinking
h. eye rubbing
h. fantasizer
h. grinding
h. labor
h. occlusion
h. offender
h. patterns
h. snoring

habitus
cushingoid body h.
eunuchoid h.
marfanoid body h.

hack
smoker's h.

hacking
h. cough
dry hacking cough
persistent hacking cough

had
h. it before, got it again
infant had weak cry

haemophilum
Mycobacterium haemophilum infection

Haemophilus
Haemophilus b conjugate vaccine
diphtheria, tetanus, pertussis, *Haemophilus influenzae* type b vaccine
diphtheria, tetanus toxoids, whole-cell pertussis, and *Haemophilus influenzae* type b conjugate
Haemophilus b conjugate vaccine
Haemophilus influenzae type b
Haemophilus test medium
H. influenzae
Haemophilus influenzae biogroup *aegyptius*
Haemophilus influenzae type b
Haemophilus influenzae type b conjugate vaccine
Haemophilus influenzae type b polysaccharide vaccine
Haemophilus influenzae type b vaccine, PRP-D conjugate vaccine
Haemophilus influenzae type b vaccine, PRP-OMP conjugate vaccine
Haemophilus influenzae type b vaccine, PRP-T conjugate vaccine
Haemophilus influenzae type vaccine oligosaccharide-CRM197 vaccine conjugate
H. parainfluenzae
Haemophilus pertussis vaccine
restriction endonucleases from *Haemophilus influenzae*
Haemophilus test medium

***Haemophilus-Neisseria* identification**

haemorrhagica
angina bullosa h.

Hagedorn
neutral protamine Hagedorn insulin

Hageman
H. factor
lung Hageman factor activator

Haglund
H. disorder

Haglund *(continued)*
H. exostosis
H. foot deformity
hag teeth
Hahn
cleft of H.
Hailey-Hailey disease
hair
abnormal hair growth
absence of facial and pubic h.
acoustic hair cell
Amish brittle hair syndrome
h. analysis test
arrector muscle of h.
autograft hair transplantation
axillary h.
h. ball
bearing area h.
h. bearing graft
bearing graft h.
body hair distribution
brittle hair, intellectual impairment, decreased fertility, short stature syndrome
h. of brow
h. bud
h. bulb
capillary loop in hair papilla
h. cell
h. cell in ear
coarse scalp h.
compulsive hair pulling
h. cycle
decreased body h.
h. densitometer
dermatophyte infection of h.
dry skin and h.
excess facial h.
excessive facial hair growth
excessive hair growth
excessive hair shedding
h. of eyebrow
female pattern hair loss
fine hair movement
h. follicle
h. follicle nevus
h. follicle tumor
full head of h.
h. germ
h. graft
graying hair from aging
h. growth
growth phase of facial h.
ichthyosis, brittle hair, impaired intelligence, decreased fertility, short stature syndrome
inner hair cell
kinky hair disease
kinky hair syndrome
limp hair from anemia
loose anagen hair syndrome
h. loss
h. loss from antidepressant
h. loss from birth control pill
h. loss from childbirth
h. loss and nausea
lumbosacral tuft of h.
macular hair cell
male pattern hair loss
mare's hair line
Marzola hair restoration surgery
masculine pubic h.
h. matrix
medulla of hair shaft
Menkes kinky h.
Menkes kinky hair syndrome
mental retardation, polydactyly, phalangeal hypoplasia, syndactyly, unusual face, uncombable h.
mental retardation-sparse hair syndrome
microcephaly, sparse hair, mental retardation, seizures syndrome
minoxidil and hair loss
nasal h.
neck of hair follicle
normal distribution of h.
normal hair distribution
h. normal texture
h. of nose
h. on head
h. papilla
parallel development of axillary h.
parallel development of pubic h.
pathological hair pulling
patient pulls h.
h. plucking
pubic h.
pubic hair line
h. of pubis
radioimmunoassay of h.
h. removal
h. removal efficiency
h. removal treatment
h. replacement
h. replacement surgery
resting phase of facial h.
h. restoration surgery
restore lost or thinning h.
revitalize hair growth
h. root
semen, hair and blood
sensory hair cells
h. shaft
h. teeth
temporary hair loss
h. testing
h. transplant
h. transplantation
h. transplanting
treatment for hair loss
tuft of h.
h. unit
vestibular hair cell
hair-bearing
h.-b. area
h.-b. graft
hair-like
h.-l. cell
h.-l. tumor
hairline
anterior hairline incision
h. crack
h. fracture
h. incision
low occipital h.
modified anterior hairline forehead lift
hair-matrix carcinoma
hair-trigger gag reflex
hairy
black hairy tongue
h. cell
h. cell leukemia
h. cell leukemia variant
h. ears
giant pigmented hairy nevus
h. heart
h. leukoplakia
h. nevus
oral hairy leukemia
h. tongue
Hajdu-Cheney syndrome
Hajna-Damon broth
half
h. amplitude pulse duration
carbon fiber half ring
h. crown
h. a dram
field size in half body irradiation
full width at half maximum
full width of photopeak measured at half maximal count
inner h.
lower h.

lower half headache of Sluder
h. relaxation time
h. strength
upper h.
h. vision

half-axial projection

half-cap crown

half-dose depth

half-field
visual h.-f.

half-Fourier
h.-F. acquisition single-shot turbo spin-echo
h.-F. imaging

half-hour interval

half-life
apparent h.-l.
biologic h.-l.
effective h.-l.
elimination h.-l.
h.-l. elimination
physical h.-l.
radiologic h.-l.

half-normal
h.-n. saline
h.-n. solution

half-pin
h.-p. external fixator
h.-p. fixation

half-power distance

half-scan with extrapolation

half-strength saline

half-thickness
narrow beam h.-t.

half-time
aggregation h.-t.
h.-t. of exchange
gastric emptying h.-t.
h.-t. method
pressure h.-t.
reaction h.-t.

half-value
h.-v. layer
h.-v. thickness

halfway
h. house
h. house for alcoholics
h. house for drug addicts
h. house for penal rehabilitation
h. house for physically handicapped
h. house placement
h. house for runaways

Hall
H. Occupational Orientation Inventory
Marshall Hall facies

Haller
H. cell
circle of H.

Hallermann syndrome

Hallpike
H. caloric stimulation test
H. maneuver
H. position

hallucination
alcohol-induced psychotic disorder with h.'s
amphetamine-induced psychotic disorder with h.'s
anxiolytic-induced psychotic disorder with h.'s
cannabis-induced psychotic disorder with h.'s
command auditory h.
delusion, hallucination, or illusion
delusions and h.'s
distorted visual images and h.'s
h. from alcohol
h. from brain
inhalant induced h.
h.'s and loss of reality
occasional auditory h.
occasional tactile h.
patient has disorientation and h.'s
schizophrenic h.'s and delusions
sexually oriented h.
visual h.'s
vivid visual, auditory and olfactory h.'s

hallucinatory
acute hallucinatory mania
acute hallucinatory paranoia
h. behavior
h. drug
h. emotional experience
h. experience
mania
h. neuralgia
h. odor
h. paranoia
h. state induced by drug
h. vision
h. voice

hallucinogen
h. abuse
acute intoxication with h.
assessing needs of hallucinogen abuser
h. delusional disorder
dependence on h.
designer h.
flashback reaction with h.
h. hallucinosis
mode of administration with h.
h. mood disorder
organic brain syndrome with h.
overdose with h.
panic reactions with h.
patient overdosed with h.
pattern of hallucinogen abuse
h. persisting perception disorder
physical effect of hallucinogen abuse
potential of hallucinogen abuse
potential tolerance to h.
prevalence of hallucinogen abuse
psychoactive doses of h.
psychoactive properties of h.
psychological effects of h.
short-acting h.
tolerance to h.
toxicity of h.
treatment of acute drug reaction to h.
withdrawal from h.

hallucinogenic
h. amphetamine
h. drug
h. drug interaction
h. drug intoxication
h. effect
h. mushroom

hallucinosis
acute h.
alcoholic h.
alcohol withdrawal h.
drug-induced h.
hallucinogen h.
organic h.
organic hallucinosis syndrome
peduncular h.

hallucis
abductor hallucis brevis muscle
abductor hallucis tendon
adductor hallucis longus
adductor hallucis muscle
adductor hallucis tendon
extensor hallucis brevis muscle
extensor hallucis longus
extensor proprius h.
flexor hallucis brevis
flexor hallucis brevis muscle
flexor hallucis longus
musculus abductor h.
musculus adductor h.

hallucis *(continued)*
musculus extensor hallucis brevis
musculus extensor hallucis longus
musculus flexor brevis h.
musculus flexor hallucis brevis
musculus flexor hallucis longus

hallux
h. abductovalgus
h. abductus
adolescent hallux abductovalgus
adolescent hallux valgus
h. dolorosa
h. dorsiflexion angle
h. limitus
h. limitus deformity
h. malleus
Mayo hallux valgus modified operation
McBride bunion hallux valgus operation
McBride hallux abductovalgus reduction
McBride hallux valgus reduction
McKeever arthrodesis for hallux limitus
mental retardation-absent nails of hallux and pollex syndrome
h. metatarsophalangeal interphalangeal scale
Mitchell hallux valgus procedure
h. rigidus
h. rigidus arthrodesis
h. valgus
h. valgus angle
h. valgus deformity
h. valgus orthosis
h. varus

halo
h. around lights
h. cast
h. glaucomatosus
low-profile halo traction
h. melanoma
h. nevus
object h.'s
h. phenomenon
h. sign
supportive halo cast
h. traction
h. vest
h. vision

halogen
h. lamp
h. ophthalmoscope
h. phosphorus

halo-pelvic traction

haloperidol
chronic h.
h. decanoate
reduced h.

halothane
h. anesthesia
caffeine and halothane contracture test
h. hepatitis

Halstead Aphasia Test

Halstead-Reitan
H.-R. Battery
H.-R. Neuropsychological Battery
H.-R. Neuropsychological Test Battery
H.-R. test

Halsted
H. maneuver
H. method
H. radical mastectomy

halter
head h.
head halter traction
h. traction

halting
h. gait
h. nystagmus
h. speech

hamartoblastoma
microcephalus, imperforate anus, syndactyly, hamartoblastoma, abnormal lung lobulation, polydactyly
microphallus, imperforate anus, syndactyly, hamartoblastoma, abnormal lung

hamartoma
angiomatous lymphoid h.
folliculosebaceous cystic h.
inverted polypoid hamartoma of rectum
iris h.
h. of lung
multiple hamartoma syndrome
odontogenic gingival epithelial h.

hamate
h. bone
capitate and h.
h. hook
hook of the h.
h. hook fracture
h. ligament

Hamburg Rating Scale for Psychiatric Disorders

Hamburg-Wechsler Intelligence Test for Children

Hamilton
H. Anxiety Rating Scale
H. Depression Rating Scale
H. Rating Scale for Depression

Hamman-Rich syndrome

hammer
h. bone
h. defect
h. finger
hypothenar hammer syndrome
labyrinth area h.
neurological h.
h. nose
orthopaedic h.
percussion h.

hammering head pain

hammertoe
h. correction
h. defect
h. deformity
h. repair
h. syndrome

hammock
omental h.

Hampshire
New Hampshire rule

hamster
baby hamster kidney cell
Chinese hamster embryo fibroblast
Chinese hamster lung
Chinese hamster ovary
h. egg penetration assay
h. embryo cell
h. embryo fibroblast
h. kidney
h. leukemia virus
neural hamster cell
h. oocyte penetration test
Syrian hamster embryo
h. tumor line
h. zona-free ovum test

hamstring
h. curl
double-looped semitendinous and gracilis hamstring graft knee reconstruction technique
h. lengthening
medial h.
h. muscle
outer h.
h. reflex
h. release

h. sets
h. stretch exercise
stretching calf, thigh and h.
h. tightness

hamulus
medial h.

hand
adaptive hand skills
alien hand sign
alien hand syndrome
all-median nerve h.
all-ulnar nerve h.
aluminum hand splint
anular part of fibrous digital sheath of digits of hand and foot
ape hand of syringomyelia
arthrogryposis-like hand anomaly
h. arthroplasty
articular of h.
articular hand disorder
articulations of h.
Ashworth hand arthroplasty
h. ataxia
autism, dementia, ataxia, loss of purposeful hand use syndrome
bilateral firm hand grips
bivalved pancake plaster hand cast
blanching of h.
h. blood flow
both h.'s
callus on h.
carcinomatous arthritis in h.
chiasm of digit of h.
clapping h.'s
h. clenched
clumsy hand movement
coarse hand tremors
cock-up hand splint
h. contracture
h. control
decreased hand circulation
h. deficit
dermatomyositis in h.
developmental hand function test
digits of h.
disabilities of the arm, shoulder, and h.
h. disorder
dominant h.
dorsal interosseous muscle of h.
H. Dynamometer Test
dysarthria-clumsy hand syndrome
edema of h.
electrical stimulation of h.
h. exercise
fell on outstretched h.
fine hand dexterity
first through fifth digits of h.
h. flapping
h. flexed at wrist
H. Functional Index
h. grasp reflex
h. grip exercise
h. grip strength
h. held in position of extension
infant passive h.
h. injury
intercostal vein of h.
interphalangeal joint of h.
inverted hand position
isometric hand grip test
joint of h.
left h.
lobster hand deformity
Luck hand procedure
lumbrica of h.
lumbrical muscle of h.
Marinesco succulent h.
McCash hand procedure
McCash hand surgery
mental retardation, blepharonasofacial abnormalities, hand malformations syndrome
Michigan H. Outcomes Questionnaire
h. motion
h. motion at 3 feet vision test
h. motion and light perception
h. movement
Myobock artificial h.
myoclonic alien hand syndrome
navicular bone of h.
nickel hand dermatitis
on h.
h. orthosis
outstretched hand or tongue
h. pain
palmar ligament of interphalangeal joint of h.
palm of h.
paroxysmal hand hematoma
partial hand amputation
peeling of feet and h.'s
perforating artery of h.
poor circulation in h.
puffiness of h.'s
pulling-boat h.'s
repetitive hand motion
right h.
right hand grip
shoulder, elbow, wrist, hand orthosis
h. splinted in flexion
squamous cell carcinoma dorsum of h.
h. strength test
h. surgery
surgical hand scrub
swelling of hands or feet
h. thrust test
tingling sensation in h.
h. transplant
trembling of h.
h. tremor
h. washing compulsion
h. washing in critical care area
h. washing in nursery
h. washing technique
weakness in h.
h. wringing
wrist hand extension compression support

hand-assisted
h.-a. laparoscopic radical nephrectomy
h.-a. laparoscopic surgery
h.-a. laparoscopy

hand-breath coordination

handedness
Edinburgh Handedness Inventory

hand-eye coordination

hand-filled capsule

hand-foot-and-mouth disease

hand-foot-genital syndrome

hand-foot-mouth
h.-f.-m. disease
h.-f.-m. syndrome

hand-foot syndrome

hand-foot-uterus syndrome

handgrasp equal and strong

handgrip apexcardiographic test

handgun
licensed h.

handheld
h. assistance
h. defibrillator
h. dynamometer
h. nebulizer
h. probe
h. weight

handicap
Dizziness H. Inventory
emotional h.
Hearing H. Inventory for the Elderly
Hearing H. Scale

handicap *(continued)*
International Classification of Impairments, Disabilities, and H.'s
learning h.
multiple h.
Preschool Evaluation and Assessment for Children with H.'s
School H. Condition Scale
severe disabling h.
severe emotional h.
violence-induced h.
voice handicap index

handicapped
h. accessibility
educable mentally h.
educationally mentally h.
emotionally h.
Genetically H. Persons Program
halfway house for physically h.
multiple h.
neurologically h.
parking for h.
h. patient
h. person
rehabilitation center for physically h.
severely and profoundly h.
trainable mentally h.
treatment and education of autistic and related communications handicapped children

handle
cup holder h.
love h.
malleus h.
measurement control h.
metal handle mixing spatula
only handle it once rule
h. traction
valise handle graft

handling emotions

hand-mirror cell

handpiece
air-bearing turbine h.
Lightning high-speed vitrectomy h.
oral surgery h.

hands-off violence

hands-on care

hand-to-hand transmission

hand-to-knee coordination

hand-to-mouth movement

hand-wringing movement

hand/wrist joint replacement

handwriting progressively shaky

hanging
h. cast
h. drop
h. drop examination
erotized h.
h. heart
liver hanging maneuver
Mensor-Scheck hanging hip operation
h. skin

hanging-block culture

hanging-drop
h.-d. culture
h.-d. test

hangman's
h. break
h. fracture
h. injury
h. surgery

hangover headache

Hanks
H. balanced salt solution
H. balanced salt solution plus glucose
gelatin Hanks buffered salt solution
glucose-free Hanks solution
modified Hanks balanced salt solution

Hanover Intensive Score

Hansen
cells of H.

Hansen-Street nail

Hantaan virus

hantavirus
h. cardiopulmonary syndrome
h. disease
h. pulmonary syndrome
Puumala h.

haploid chromosome number

haploscope
mirror h.

haplotype
h. frequency
major histocompatibility complex h.
maternal HLA h.
MHC h.
h. relative risk
shared h.'s

happiness
Atkinson Life H.
Memorial University of Newfoundland Scale of H.

happy
new happy bur

hapten
molecule h.

haptic
h. hallucination
H. Intelligence Scale
one-piece plate haptic silicone intraocular lens

harassment
sexual h.

harbor
floating harbor syndrome

hard
h. abdomen
h. adhesion
h. alcoholic user
bony hard palate
h. cancer
carcinoma of hard palate
h. cataract
h. contact lens
h. core alcoholics
h. core drug abuser
h. corn
h. cyst
h. drug
h. drug usage
h. exudate
h. feces
h. food orientation
h. gel capsule
h. of hearing
h., indurated colon mass
h. lens
h. metal disease
h. nevus
h. pulse
h. rays
rough hard sphere
h. and soft palates
h. stool
h. subcutaneous nodule
h. tick
h. tissue replacement
h. tissue replacement-malleable facial implant
h. tumor
waxy exudate h.
h. x-ray imaging spectrometer

hardening
h. of aorta
h. of artery
beam hardening artifact
bone hardening artifact
h. of breast tissue
h. of coronary artery
skin hardening from dermatitis
h. tissue
h. of walls of artery
work h.
work hardening exercise
work hardening program

Harding-Passey melanoma

hardness
Brinell hardness number
Knoop hardness number of solids
Mohs h.
Mohs hardness scale
Mohs hardness test
Rockwell hardness number
Vickers hardness number

hard-nose strategy

hardware
orthopaedic h.

Hardy-Rand-Ritter color vision test kit

hare
snowshoe hare virus

Harleco synthetic resin

harlequin
h. deformity
h. sign

harm
alcohol-related h.
h. avoidance
fear of personal h.
grievous bodily h.
physical h.
physical harm or violence
h. reduction
h. reduction psychotherapy
self h.

harmful
h. antibiotic-resistant bacteria
potentially harmful drug

harmonic
h. attenuation table
h. attenuation test
h. imaging
h. mean
native tissue harmonic imaging
h. phase
pulse-inversion contrast harmonic imaging
h. scalpel
second harmonic imaging
simple harmonic motion

harmony
occlusal h.

harness
figure-of-eight h.
head h.

Harrington
modified Harrington rod
H. rod

Harris
H. design
H. hip score
H. Infant Neuromotor Test
modified Harris hip score
H. return flow

harsh
coarse and harsh breathing
constant, harsh pain
h. murmur
h. respiration
h. systolic murmur

Hartmann
H. operation
H. pouch
pouch of H.
H. procedure
H. solution

Hartnup
H. disease
H. syndrome

Hart Park virus

Harvard
H. Group Scale of Hypnotic Susceptibility, Form A

harvest
h. bone marrow
endoscopic h.
h. fluid
graft h.
marrow h.
h. mites
musculocutaneous flap h.
h. organ
organ h.
pedicled endoscopic latissimus dorsi h.
peripheral stem cell h.
h. tissue

harvested stem cell

harvester
Arandel cell h.
h. lung
multiple automated sample h.

harvesting
autograft h.
graft h.
open harvesting technique
organ h.
Ostrup harvesting technique

Harvey-Bradshaw Index

Harvey murine sarcoma virus

Harwood

Hashimoto
atrophic Hashimoto thyroiditis
H. disease
H. thyroiditis

Hassan
modified Hassan open technique

Hasse rule

Hasson
open Hasson technique

hastening phenomenon

hat
measuring h.
Mexican hat cell
Mexican hat erythrocyte
Mexican hat sign

hatchet job

hatching
assisted zonal h.

hate
ethnic h.

Hatha yoga

Hatter
Mad Hatter syndrome

haustral
h. fold
h. marking
h. pouch

have
men who have sex with men

Haven
New Haven study

haversian
h. canal
h. lamella
h. space
h. system

having
probability of having disease
probability of not having disease

Hawaii Early Learning Profile

Haw River syndrome

hay
eczema, asthma, and hay fever complex
h. fever
h. fever symptoms
nonseasonal hay fever
perennial hay fever
Hayflick
Wistar Institute Susan Hayflick cell
Hazara virus
hazard
alcohol-related health h.
H. Analysis Critical Control Points
h.'s awareness
h. of drinking
h. of drugs
environmental h.
h.'s from microwave radiation
health h.
health hazard evaluation
indirect foot h.
infection h.
moral h.
occupational h.
public health h.
radiation h.
h. ratio
relapse h.
h. of smoking
h. of yo-yo dieting
hazardous
h. activity
h. blood
h. drug
job hazardous to health
H. Materials Response Unit
h. spills of fluid
h. stress
H. Substances Act
h. waste
haze
hilar h.
hazy
h. appearance
h. density
h. infiltrate
h. lung
urine h.
h. vision
HBe antibody
h-caldesmon antibody
head
ability to hold head up
acetabular depth to femoral head diameter
acetabular head index
acetabulum head index
acute head trauma
adenocarcinoma in head of pancreas
adenoid cystic carcinoma of head and neck
advanced resected head and neck cancer
angular head velocity
anterior head cap
anterior ligament of fibular h.
anterior ligament of head of fibula
anterior rectus muscle of h.
anteromedial humeral head defect
anteromedial superior humeral head impaction
apex of head of fibula
apex of head of patella
h., arms, and trunk
articular circumference of head of radius
articular circumference of head of ulna
articular facet of head of fibula
articular facet of head of rib
articular facet of radial h.
articular pit of head of radius
articular surface of head of fibula
articular surface of head of rib
avascular femoral head necrosis
avascular necrosis of the femoral h.
h. backward
h. of bed
h. of bed up for shortness of breath
bipolar femoral head prosthesis
h. birth
blinding head pain
blow to h.
h. bobbing
h. brace
Brief Test of H. Injury
h. cancer
h. cap
carcinoma head of pancreas
h. check
choking of optic nerve h.
chronic oral, facial, head pain
h. circumference
h. circumference measurement
clenched muscles in head and neck
closed head injury
closed head syndrome
closed head trauma
closed head unit
h. cold
coma secondary to head trauma
h. compression
h. computed tomography
h. computerized axial tomography
confusion with head injury
contralateral head turning
h. control
control head movement
countersink screw h.
crowning of infant's h.
cutaneous malignant melanoma of head and neck
dementia due to head trauma
h. dependent position
dislocation head of radius
h. distraction test
h. drop
duodenum-preserving pancreatic head resection
electrodes placed on the surface of h.
elevate head of bed
elevation of head of bed
endoprosthetic femoral head replacement
entrance of fetal head into superior pelvic strait
excessive enlargement of h.
excision head of pancreas
h. extended
h. extension
h., eyes, ears, nose, and throat
h., eyes, ears, nose, and throat unremarkable
femoral head line
h. of femur
fetal h.
h. of fetus
h. of fibula
first metatarsal h.
h. fold
forceps to aftercoming h.
h. forward
forward head posture
h. fracture frame
full head of hair
h. growth
gunshot wound to h.
hair on h.
h. halter

h. halter traction
hammering head pain
h. harness
h. higher than heart
h. hood
h. of humerus
initial head assessment
h. injury
h. injury routine
h. injury unit
innervation of head and neck
ipsilateral head turning
ischemic necrosis of femoral h.
h. jerking
lateral head displacement
lateral head of malleolus
h. lice
ligament of head of femur
ligaments of head of fibula
h., limbs, and body
little head of humerus
little head of mandible
long head of biceps
longissimus muscle of h.
long muscle of h.
loss of ability to hold head up
h. louse
lymph node of head and neck
malformed radial h.
h. of malleus
mandible h.
h. of mandible
h. maneuver
Mayfield head clamp
medial head of the gastrocnemius rupture
metacarpal head fracture
metaphysial head resection with prosthesis
metastatic squamous carcinoma of head and neck
metatarsal flat h.
metatarsal head extractor
metatarsal head osteochondritis
metatarsal head osteotomy
metatarsal head resection
minor head injury
molding of h.
h. movement
muscle of h.
nail inserted into neck and head of femur
h. and neck
h. and neck cancer
h. and neck in extended position
neck and head of femur
h. and neck motion
h. and neck normal
h., neck, and shaft
h. and neck squamous cell carcinoma
h. and neck tremor
nerve head angioma
nerve head drusen
Newman classification of radial neck and head fracture
nodding of h.
nonpenetrating head trauma
normal head and neck
h. not engaged
h. nurse
occipital regions of h.
occult head trauma
open head injury
ophthalmology, otorhinolaryngology, and head and neck surgery
optic nerve h.
optic nerve head analysis
h. pain
painful femoral head prosthesis
h. of pancreas
pancreatic head cancer
pancreatic head origin
pancreatic head resection
panmetatarsal head resection
past head injury
performance status scale for head and neck cancer
Philadelphia H. Injury Questionnaire
h. position
h. positioner
posterior intervertebral ganglion of h.
h. posture
primary head vein
prosthetic femoral h.
h. of pterygium
radial head epiphysis
radial head fracture
radiate ligament of head of rib
radiation-induced sarcoma of the head and neck
h. of radius
raise head of bed
rapid head movement
region of h.
resection head of pancreas
resection head of radius
resting head pressure
rhabdomyosarcoma of head and neck
rhythmic instability of head and trunk
rhythm instability of head and trunk
h. rolling
h. rolling, rocking and crying
rotate fetal h.
h. rotation to right
h. to rump length
Sayre head sling
segmenting dual-echo MR head scan
semispinal muscle of h.
severe head trauma
skin, head, eyes, ears, nose, and throat
sleep-related head banging
h. sling
h. and spinal cord injury
squamous cell carcinoma of head and neck
squamous cell head and neck cancer
h. of stapes
surface of h.
Swanson radial head implant
h. of talus
throbbing pain in h.
h. thrust test
tight feeling in h.
h. tilt
h. tilt and chin lift maneuver
h. tilting
h. tilt method
h. tilt test
h. tilt with chin tilt
h. tilt with neck lift
tomographic image of the h.
h. trauma
h. trauma syndrome
h. tremor
unilateral head pain
h. unremarkable
Veley head rest
h. weaving
wedged fetal h.
Yaquina Head virus
Zimaloy femoral head prosthesis

headache

h. activity
h. activity and desensitization
h. after spinal tap
h. ameliorated
anxiety, tension, and h.
aphasic migraine h.
H. Assessment Questionnaire
autogenic training for h.

headache *(continued)*
benign coital h.
BI cranial vascular h.
biofeedback and h.
cervicogenic h.
childhood migraine h.
chronic daily h.
chronic headache pain
chronic migraine h.
chronic posttraumatic h.
chronic primary h.
chronic progressive h.
chronic tension h.
classic headache preceded by aura
h. clinic
cluster h.
cocaine-related vascular h.
cold food-related h.
confusion from migraine h.
cough, dyspnea and h.
double vision with h.
episodic tension-type h.
h. exacerbated
focal vascular h.
h. frequency
h. from alcohol
h. from caffeine
h. Assessment Questionnaire
hemicranial vascular h.
high-altitude h.
ice cream h.
Idiopathic H. Score
h., insomnia, and depression syndrome
intense headache pain
intensity of h.
intracranial neoplasm h.
ischemic cerebrovascular h.
lower half headache of Sluder
lumbar puncture h.
h. medication
medication-induced h.
migraine with interparoxysmal h.
miner's h.
Monday morning h.
monosodium glutamate-induced h.
muscle contraction h.
muscle pain, allergy, tachycardia and tiredness, headache syndrome
muscle tension h.
nervous tension h.
occipitofrontal h.
ocular etiology of h.
h. pain
patient has h.
h. pattern
persistent vomiting or confusion h.
post coital h.
post concussive h.
post delivery h.
postdural puncture h.
postlumbar puncture h.
postspinal anesthetic h.
h. preceded by classic aura
recurrent excruciating h.
reduce tension headache frequency
relaxation response in headache therapy
h. secondary to cervical spinal disease
severe throbbing h.
sinus headache from cold
sleep-related cluster h.
sudden, severe h.
syncopal migraine h.
temporary relief of headache pain
h. and tension
h. therapy
h. triggers
unilateral throbbing h.
h. unit index
vascular flow h.
vascular headache syndrome
voluntary control of tension h.
vomiting and h.

headband
fiberoptic h.

head-down
h.-d. position
h.-d. presentation
h.-d. tilt
h.-d. tilt test

head-dropping test

head-drop unit

headholder
Mayfield-Kees h.

headlight
fiberoptic h.

head-mounted display

head-neck replacement

headrest
doughnut h.
Mayfield horseshoe h.
Mayfield-Kees h.
neurosurgical h.
pediatric h.
3-prong h.

head-tilt
h.-t. maneuver
h.-t. test

head-to-abdomen ratio

head-to-head sperm agglutination

head-to-tail sperm agglutination

head-up
h.-u. tilt
h.-u. tilt-table test

healed
h. blister
h. cutdown site
early h.
h. fracture
incision healed per primam
h. incision site
late h.
h. myocardial infarction
old healed myocardial infarction
operative wound clean and h.
h. perforation
h. rheumatic valvulitis
h. superficial laceration
h. ulcer
well h.
wound clean and h.
wound healed by first, second or third intention
wound healed per primam
wound healed by secondary intention
h. yellow atrophy

healing
h. biopsy incision
body's natural healing ability
bone healing method
complete h.
consolidation and h.
delayed healing of fracture
delayed primary intention h.
h. duodenal ulcer
h. by first, second, or third intention
h. fracture
granulating in and h.
h. by granulation
h. incision site
incomplete h.
h. injury
manual healing method
natural healing method
per primam h.
per secundum h.
platelet-derived wound healing factor

poor wound h.
h. power of warm baths
Pressure Ulcer Scale for H.
h. by primary intention
h. process
rate of h.
satisfactory wound h.
h. by secondary intention
stall the healing process
h. surgical incision
h. touch
h. well
h. with approximation
wound h.
h. wound
wound healing capability
wound healing well

health

academic health care
h. and accident insurance
accreditation program/home health care
acquired immunodeficiency syndrome health assessment questionnaire
H. and Activity Limitation Survey
acute physiology and chronic health evaluation score
alcohol-related health hazard
allied health professional
altered health maintenance
alternative health care
annual health evaluation
h. appraisal examination
area health authority
area health education center
h. aspects of pesticides
h. assessment
assessment of health status
H. Assessment Questionnaire Disability Index
assisted health insurance plan
automated multiphasic health testing
availability of health care
h. awareness
basic health profile
basic health unit
Battery of H. Improvement
behavioral health treatment
H. Behavior Scale
H. Belief Model
h. benefits of walking
bill of h.
board of h.
h. board
h. care
h. care agency
h. care aide
h. care cost reduction
h. care coverage
h. care decision-making
h. care delivery
h. care maintenance
h. care management
h. care review
h. care worker
catastrophic health insurance
h. center
H. Check Test
Child H. Assessment Program
child health questionnaire
Childhood H. Assessment Questionnaire
Child H. and Illness Profile, Adolescent Edition
Children's H. Study
Children with Special H. Care Needs
chronic health problem
Clinical H. Assessment Questionnaire
h. club
community-based mental health treatment
community health center
community health management information system
community health network
community mental health center
comprehensive health care institution
comprehensive health enhancement support system
comprehensive health insurance plan
comprehensive mental h.
h. conscious
cooperative health statistics system
Coping H. Inventory for Children
Coping H. Inventory for Parents
correctional health care program
h. decisions
dental health care provider
h. deviation self-care requisite
district health authority
district health department
durable power of attorney for health care
h. education
h. educator
effective mental health care
h. effects of environmental pollutants
h. effects of ionizing radiation
Employee H. Maintenance Examination
h. enhancing trait
h. and environment
Environmental H. Laboratory
h. evaluation
h. evaluation center
H. Evaluation and Learning Program
extended health care
h. facility administrator
family health center
family health insurance plan
family planning health assistant
h. and fitness
flight into h.
h. food
h. fraud
general health problem
general mental h.
General H. Perception Questionnaire
h. habit
h. hazard
h. hazard evaluation
h. history
holistic h.
holistic health spa
home h.
home health aide
home health care
home health nurse
home health visit
human health and behavior questionnaire
h. illness profile
improve health self-esteem
h. information management
informed health care decision
h. insurance
h. insuring organization
integrated health delivery network
H. Intention Scale
International Classification of Diseases and Related H. Problems, 10th Edition
36-item short form health survey
job hazardous to h.
Juvenile Wellness and H. Survey
h. level seven
Life H. Monitoring Program
h. maintenance cooperative
h. maintenance organization
h. maintenance plan

health *(continued)*
managed behavioral health plans
managed mental h.
mandated mental health coverage
maternal and child h.
maternal and child health care
maternal and child health service
maternal health program
maternal health risk factor
H. Media Education
mental h.
Mental H. Association
Mental Health Early Intervention, Treatment, and Prevention Act of 2000
mental health advocate
mental health benefit
mental health care professional
mental health care unit
mental health center
mental health community
mental health counseling
mental health department
mental health expert
mental health hold
mental health inpatient
mental health insurance benefit
mental health law
mental health legislation
mental health and mental retardation
mental health patient
mental health practitioner
mental health professional
mental health provider
mental health reform
mental health resource
mental health status
mental health system
mental health treatment
mental health treatment facility
Mental Health Parity Act of 1998
Michigan Bone Health Study
Millon Behavioral H. Inventory
Modified H. Assessment Questionnaire
multiphasic health checkup
multiphasic health screen test
multiphasic health testing
multiple health screening
National Alliance for Hispanic H.
National Association for H. & Fitness
National Association of Psychiatric H. Systems
National Center on Minority H. and H. Disparities
national health insurance
National H. Information Center
National Institute of Mental H.
National Institute of Mental H. Diagnostic Interview Schedule
National Institute for Occupational Safety and H.
National Institutes of H.
National Institutes of H. Chronic Prostatitis Symptom Index
National Mental H. Association
National H. and Nutrition Examination Follow-Up Study
National H. and Nutrition Examination Survey
National Women's H. Information Center
National Women's H. Network
neighborhood health center
no medical health history
h. and nutrition examination survey
occupational h.
occupational health center
occupational health risk
occupational health and safety
Office on Smoking and H.
oral health care
oral health status
Pan American Health Organization grade 0–2
h. perception
personal health cost
Physicians Health Study II
poor h.
prepaid health plan
preservation of h.
preventive dental health behavior
preventive health behavior
Preventive H. Model
primary health care
h. professional
public h.
public health education program
public health hazard
public health nurse
public health official
radiologic h.
radiologic health data
rising health care costs
h. risk
h. risk appraisal
h. risk assessment
h. risk factor
h. risks from smoking
routine health care
routine health management
h. and safety executive
School H. Additional Referral Program
school-based health center
h. screening
h. screening center
h. screening test
self-applied health enhancement method
H. Self-Determination Index
serious health risk
stable health status
Stanford H. Assessment Questionnaire
h. status
stress caused health problem
h. in underserved rural areas
unproven health claim
H. Utilities Index
very good h.
vital health information
weight-related health problem
h. wellness
Women's Health Initiative
World Health Organization classification of lupus nephritis I, IIA, IIB, III, IV, V
World Health Organization Quality of Life 100-Item

healthcare
Computerized H. And Record Transfer System
h. facility
home h.
h. industry
h. institution
long-term healthcare facility
medical h.
h. product
h. professional
h. provider
h. proxy
quality h.
h. questionnaire
h. rationing plan
h. service
h. specialist
h. system
h. team
h. technology
total h.
utilization h.
h. worker

health-impaired
physically or otherwise h.-i.

health-oriented physical education

health-related
h.-r. facility
h.-r. legislation
h.-r. quality of life
h.-r. quality-of-life assessment
h.-r. quality-of-life questionnaire

Health-Sickness Rating Scale

healthy
h. appearing organ
burn healthy tissue
h. conflict management
h. control
h. coping strategy
damage to healthy tissue
destroy healthy tissue
h. diet
h. dietary habit
heart healthy lifestyle
h. hemophiliac
h. lifestyle
h. lifestyle habit
h. mobile sperm
h. nerve cell
h. patient with localized pathological process
h. patient with localized pathologic process
h. pregnant women
h. reaction
h. self-assertion
h. tissue
h. tissue stained
years of healthy life
h. years of life
h. years of life lost

healthy-appearing organ

hear
recognize, empathize, think, hear, integrate, notice, keep

heard
h. best at left lower sternal border
h. best at left upper sternal border
click heard at hip joint
fetal heart h.
fetal heart not h.

hearing
h. acuity
h. acuity screening
age-related hearing loss
h. aid
h. aid amplifier
h. aid dispenser
h. aid evaluation
h. aid microphone
h. aid orientation
h. aid problem
autoimmune hearing loss
autoimmune sensorineural hearing loss
automated auditory brainstem response hearing screening
autosomal dominant nonsyndromic hearing loss
autosomal recessive nonsyndromic hearing loss
h. and balance
bilateral progressive hearing loss
binaural hearing aid
body worn hearing aid
bone-anchored hearing aid
bone conduction hearing aid
canal hearing aid
completely in the canal hearing aid
conductive hearing loss
h. conservation programs
h. damage
decibel hearing test
decibels normal hearing level
h. defect
delayed hearing loss
digital hearing aid
diminished hearing and vision
h. disorder
h. distance
h. distance with watch
h. distraction test
h. disturbance
double disharmonic h.
downsizing of hearing aid
in the ear hearing aid
extensive hearing assessment
fluctuating hearing loss
fluctuating sensorineural hearing loss
h. frequency
functional hearing loss
functional hearing test
H. Handicap Inventory for the Elderly
H. Handicap Scale
hard of h.
high-frequency sensorineural hearing loss
high-tone hearing loss
idiopathic sudden sensorineural hearing loss
idiopathic sudden sensory hearing loss
h. impaired
impaired hearing loss
h. impairment
implantable middle ear hearing device
inner ear hearing loss
in-the-canal hearing aid
h. level
linear hearing aid
h. loss
h. loss from aging
h. loss from antibiotic
h. loss from aspirin
h. loss from diuretics
h. loss from infection of ear
h. loss studies
low-frequency sensorineural hearing loss
macrocephaly, hypertelorism, short limbs, hearing loss, developmental delay syndrome
mental retardation, hearing impairment, distinct facies, skeletal anomalies syndrome
mild hearing impairment
mild hearing loss
minor hearing loss
mixed hearing impairment
mixed hearing loss
moderate hearing impairment
moderate hearing loss
modified rhyme hearing test
modify hearing patterns
monaural hearing aid
monaural hearing loss
Mondini hearing impairment
natural hearing loss
h. nerve
neural hearing loss
noise-induced hearing damage
noise-reduced hearing loss
nonsyndromic hereditary hearing impairment
normalized hearing level
occupational hearing loss
organ of h.
organic hearing impairment
partial hearing loss
perceptive hearing impairment
perceptive hearing loss
permanent childhood hearing impairment
permanent childhood hearing loss
permanent hearing loss
h. problem
profound hearing impairment
profound hearing loss

hearing *(continued)*
progressive hearing loss
progressive unilateral hearing loss
h. protection device
psychogenic hearing impairment
psychogenic hearing loss
rapidly progressing bilateral hearing loss
receptor cells of h.
receptor organ of h.
reduced hearing at high frequency
retrocochlear hearing loss
Rinne hearing test
Scheibe hearing impairment
h. screening
selective hearing loss
sensation level of h.
sense of h.
sensorineural hearing impairment
sensory neural hearing loss
severe hearing loss
severe impairment of h.
severe sensorineural hearing loss
slight hearing impairment
slight hearing loss
speech and h.
speech and hearing impairment
Stenger hearing test
STYCAR H. Test
symptomatic hearing loss
h. system
temporary hearing loss
h. threshold
h. threshold level
unilateral hearing loss
Universal Neonatal H. Screening
universal newborn hearing screening program
visual hearing loss
h. voices
warning signs of hearing loss

hearing-for-speech test

heart
abnormal electrical events in h.
abnormal functioning of h.
abnormal heart activity
abnormal heart contraction
abnormal heart rhythm
abnormality in heart rate
abnormally rapid heart rate
abnormally slow heart rate
above level of h.
accelerating heart rate
acquired valvular heart disease
acromegalic heart disease
h. action
h. activity
activity-related heart problem
acute congestive heart failure
acute heart attack
acute heart disease
acute heart failure
acute heart muscle degeneration
acute ischemic heart disease
acute left ventricular heart failure
acutely decompensated congestive heart failure
acute right heart syndrome
acute right ventricular heart failure
acyanotic heart disease
adhesions of pericardium around h.
admixture lesion of h.
advanced heart ailment
advanced heart disease
advanced stage of congestive heart failure
h. ailment
air-driven artificial h.
alcoholic heart muscle disease
alcohol-related heart disorders
alternans of the h.
American H. Association
American Heart Association classification
American H. Association Step One Diet
American H. Association Stroke Outcome Classification
amyloid heart disease
amyloidosis of h.
angina threshold heart rate
angioreticuloendothelioma of h.
angiosarcoma of h.
h. anomaly
anterior border of h.
anticipatory bogus heart rate feedback
Antihypertensive and Lipid-Lowering Treatment to Prevent H. Attack Trial
aortic opening of h.
aortic ventricle of h.
apex of h.
apical mid-diastolic heart murmur
apical surface of h.
apical systolic heart murmur
apneic infant with decreased heart rate
arousal heart rate
h. arrest
h. arrhythmia
arteriosclerotic heart disease
arteriosclerotic hypertensive heart disease
artificial h.
artificial heart energy system
artificial heart implant
artificial heart recipient
artificial heart valve
artificial left heart pump
aspirin and heart attack
assess functioning of h.
h. assessment
asymptomatic heart attack
asymptomatic heart disease
atherosclerotic heart disease
athletic heart syndrome
atrial septal heart disease
atrioventricular heart block
atrioventricular junctional heart block
atrium of h.
h. attack
h. attack from aspirin
h. attack from aspiring
h. attack from blood clot
h. attack patient
h. attack rehabilitation
h. attack risk
h. attack risk factor
h. attack survivor
h. attack symptoms
h. attack trigger
h. attack victim
atypical heart attack
auscultation of h.
autoimmune-associated congenital heart block
autopsy limited to heart and lungs
AV Wenckebach heart block
backward heart failure
basal heart rate
baseline variability of fetal heart rate
beating heart brain-dead donor
beating heart muscle
beef heart antigen
beef heart infusion broth
benign heart murmur
beriberi heart disease
bifascicular heart block
biological heart valve
bioprosthetic heart valve
h. biopsy
h. block
blocked heart artery
blood diffuses into heart muscle

blood flow in h.
blood from flow heart to lungs
blood-starved heart muscle tissue
blood supply to h.
blunt injury to h.
body acceleration synchronous with heart rate
h. border
bovine heart valve
brain heart infusion agar
brain heart infusion broth
bundle branch heart block
bundle-branch heart block
h. bypass surgery
calcium deposit on heart valves
calf embryonic heart cell
Canadian H. Classification
h. cannulated
carcinoid heart disease
CardioWest total artificial h.
h. catheterization
h. catheterization stylet
causes of heart disease
h. cell
h. cell aggregate
h. cell death
h. chamber
4-chambered human h.
change in heart rate
change in heart rhythm
chaotic heart rhythm
chest pain from heart problem
chronic alcoholic heart muscle disease
chronic congestive heart failure
chronic heart disease
chronic ischemic heart disease
chronic valvular heart disease
h. circulates blood
clinical heart disease
closed heart surgery
h. clot
cocaine heart attack
cocaine-related heart attack victim
coloboma, heart anomaly, ichthyosis, mental retardation, and ear abnormality syndrome
coloboma, heart disease, atresia choanae, retarded growth and retarded development and/or CNS anomalies, genital hypoplasia, and ear anomalies and/or deafness syndrome
combined heart catheterization
compensated congestive heart failure
compensated heart failure
compensatory hypertrophy of heart muscle
complete heart block
compliance of h.
h. condition
h. configuration
confusion from heart failure
congenital complete heart block
congenital defect interventricular septum of h.
congenital displacement of h.
congenital heart anomaly
congenital heart block
congenital heart defect
congenital heart disease
congenital heart failure
congenital malformation of h.
congestive heart disease
congestive heart failure
congestive heart failure and cardioversion
continuous heart murmur
contour of h.
h. contracted
contractility of heart muscle
h. contraction
contraction cycle of h.
contraction of heart muscle
contraction and relaxation of h.
control of heart rate during oxygen deprivation
contusion of h.
coronary arteriosclerotic heart disease
coronary atherosclerotic heart disease
coronary heart disease
crisscross heart malposition
crux of h.
crying, requirement for oxygen supplementation, increases in heart rate and blood pressure
cryopreserved heart valve allograft
cryopreserved heart valve graft
cyanotic congenital heart disease
cyanotic heart disease
h. cycle
h. damage
damaged donor h.
dead area of heart muscle
death of heart muscle tissue
decompensated congestive heart failure
decompensated heart failure
decompression of h.
decortication of h.
decreased heart rate
decreased risk of heart disease
decreased venous return to h.
h. defect
defective artificial heart valve
h. defibrillated
h. defibrillated with single shock
degeneration of myxomatous heart valve
degenerative heart disease
depressed heart attack patient
depressed heart attack survivor
deterioration of heart muscle
dextroposition of h.
dextroversion of h.
h. in diastole
diastolic heart disease
diastolic heart factor
diastolic heart failure
digitalization of h.
h. dilated
dilation of the h.
diminished heart, kidney and brain function
h. disease
h. disease cell
diseased human h.
h. disease history
h. disease, low risk
h. disease risk factor
h. disease screening
h. disease therapy
h. disorder
disordered action of h.
dissection of h.
distant heart sounds
h. disturbance
diversional heart block
dizziness from heart attack
h. does appear enlarged
h. does not appear enlarged
domino heart transplantation
h. donated
donation of h.
donor heart retrieved
h. dysfunction
h. dysfunctional episode
ejection fraction of h.
electrical activity of h.
electrical alternation of h.
electrical function of h.
electrical heart position
electrical impulse to h.
electrical instability of h.
h. electrically unstable
h. electrical rhythm
electrical stimulation of h.

heart *(continued)*
electromechanical artificial h.
elevated heart rate
elevate feet above h.
embryonic heart motion
end-stage heart factor
end-stage heart failure
end-stage heart and liver disease
enlarged h.
enlarged heart muscle
enlargement of h.
ergot alkaloid-associated heart disease
erratic heart rhythm
evaluation of denervated heart at rest
excessively rapid heart rate
exercise heart rate
exercise induced heart attack
exercises for heart patient
exhaustion, burnout and heart disease
external fetal heart rate monitoring
extra heart sound
h. failure cell
h. failure treatment
fascicular heart block
fast heart rate
fatal heart attack
fatal heart rhythm disturbance
h. fatty acid binding protein
fatty degeneration of h.
fetal h.
fetal heart disease
fetal heart frequency
fetal heart heard
fetal heart monitor
fetal heart monitor tracing
fetal heart motion
fetal heart not heard
fetal heart rate
fetal heart rate acceleration
fetal heart rate baseline
fetal heart rate deceleration
fetal heart rate monitoring
fetal heart rate nonstress test
fetal heart rate reactivity
fetal heart rate reading
fetal heart rate variability
fetal heart rhythm
fetal heart tones
first-degree heart block
first to fourth heart sounds
first heart sound
first through fourth heart sounds
florid congestive heart failure
flow of blood and oxygen to h.
h. flow capacity
fluid in heart sac
h. flutter
foramen ovale of h.
forward heart failure
four-chambered human h.
fourth heart sound
h. frequency
h. function
functional aspects of h.
functional heart murmur
gene therapy for h.
grade 1–6 heart murmur
h. and great vessels
head higher than h.
h. health
h. healthy lifestyle
3:1 heart block
3:2 heart block
height of h.
Heimlich heart valve
h. helping exercise
hereditary heart defect
heterotopic heart transplant
highest equivalent heart rate
high-output heart failure
His bundle heart block
history of heart disease
holiday heart syndrome
h. hormone
human operant heart rate conditioning
hypertensive arteriosclerotic heart disease
hypertensive heart disease
h. hypertrophied and dilated
hypertrophy of h.
hypoplasia of left h.
hypoplastic left heart syndrome
hypoplastic right heart syndrome
h. icing
idiopathic hyperkinetic heart syndrome
h. imaging
immune rejection of transplanted h.
implantable artificial h.
improve efficiency of heart and lungs
incipient heart failure
incomplete heart block
increased blood flow to heart muscle
increased heart and breathing rate
increased heart size
increase heart production
increasing heart rate
ineffective heart action
h. infection
inflammation of h.
inflammation of heart lining
inflammation of heart muscle
infundibulum of h.
h. infusion
h. infusion broth
initial heart attack
injured heart muscle
innocent heart murmur
instrumental heart rate responses
insufficient blood flow to h.
intermittent heart pain
internal fetal heart rate monitoring
interventricular heart block
interventricular sulcus of h.
h. intracorporeal
intractable heart failure
intraventricular heart block
h. irregular
irregular heart action
irregular heart rhythm
h. irritable
ischemic coronary heart disease
ischemic damage to h.
ischemic heart disease
ischemic heart failure
ischemic heart muscle
ischemic heart wall
h., kidney and brain function
laceration of h.
large magnitude voluntary heart rate changes
laser heart surgery
h. laser revascularization
late-stage heart failure
law of the h.
leaking heart valve
leaky heart valve
left atrium of h.
left border dullness of heart to percussion
left heart blood volume
left heart bypass
left heart failure
left heart strain
left-sided heart failure
left ventricle of h.
left ventricular heart failure
legs elevated higher than h.
h. lesion
h. lesion cell
life-threatening heart arrhythmia
life-threatening heart rhythm

h. lining
h. and liver damage
h., liver, and kidney
longitudinal diameter of h.
longitudinal sulcus of h.
long-term survivor of heart transplant
h. loop
loss of appetite from heart failure
lower chamber of h.
lower risk of heart disease
low-output heart failure
h. and lung
h. and lung function
h., lungs, and abdomen
h. and lungs normal
magnetic heart vector
h. malformation
malformed heart or heart valve
marginal heart failure
markedly dilated h.
h. massage
massive heart attack
maternal cyanotic heart disease
maximal predicted heart rate
maximum determined heart rate
maximum predicted heart rate
measuring heart function
mechanical alternation of the h.
mechanical heart pump
mechanical heart valve
mental retardation, congenital heart disease, blepharophimosis, blepharoptosis, hypoplastic teeth
h. meridian
metabolic balance of h.
metal heart valve
middle lobe of h.
h. minute output
Mobitz I heart block
Monday morning heart attack
h. monitor
movement-associated fetal heart rate accelerations
movement of h.
muffled heart sound
Multicenter Oral Carvedilol H. Failure Assessment
h. murmur
h. muscle
h. muscle abnormality
h. muscle cell
h. muscle damage
h. muscle death
h. muscle disease
h. muscle fiber
h. muscle tissue
h. muscle weakness
myocytolysis of h.
narrowing of heart valve
National H., Lungs, and Blood Institute Information Center
natural history of congestive heart failure
neonatal cyanotic congenital heart disease
New York H. Association classification of heart disease
nonfatal heart attack
nonreassuring fetal heart beat pattern
nonvalvular heart disease
normal contour of h.
normal heart activity
normal heart function
normal heart rhythm
normal heart size
normal rhythm of h.
normal sinus heart rhythm
normal size h.
notch of apex of h.
NYHA congestive heart failure classification
h. observed
occlusive heart disease
one ventricle h.
onset of overt heart failure
operant acceleration of heart rate
operant deceleration of heart rate
orthoptic biventricular artificial h.
orthotopic heart transplant
orthotopic univentricular artificial h.
oval foramen of h.
overt heart failure
overt symptom of heart disease
oxygen-starved heart muscle
pacemaker of h.
pain from heart problem
pain of heart attack
h. palpitations
partial heart block
h. patient
penetrating wound of h.
percutaneous left heart bypass
pericardium around h.
personal heart device
physiologic third heart sound
physiology of heart contraction
plastic heart valve
polymyxin, lysozyme, EDTA, and thallous acetate in heart infusion agar
porcine heart valve
h. position
posterior border of h.
posterior wall of h.
post heart attack apoptosis
postoperative heart failure
postoperative open heart surgery
pounding of h.
preclinical heart muscle disease
pre contractile h.
precordial heart rate
predicted maximal heart rate
premature heart disease
prevent heart disease
h. problem
prosthetic heart valve
prosthetic heart valve surgery
prudent living h.
pulmonary heart disease
pulmonary heart valve disorder
pulmonic heart sound less than aortic second heart sound
pulmonic second heart sound equal to aortic second heart sound
pulmonic second heart sound greater than aortic second heart sound
h. pump
h. pumping
pumping ability of failing h.
pumping ability of weakened h.
h. pumping action
h. pumping chamber
pumping function of h.
QT corrected for heart rate
Quain fatty h.
quiet heart sound
racing heart rhythm
radiation-induced heart disease
rapid beating of h.
rapid heart action
rapid heart rhythm
h. rate audiometry
h. rate condition ability
h. rate control
h. rate control learning and awareness
h. rate disorder
h. rate feedback
h. rate monitor
h. rate monitored
h. rate peak
h. rate perception
h. rate power spectral analysis
h. rate range
h. rate reserve

heart *(continued)*
h. rate responses
h. rate-systolic blood pressure product
h. rate variability
h. recipient
reconstruct heart muscle
recurrent congestive heart failure
recurrent heart attack
reduced blood supply to h.
reduced heart rate
h. reduced to normal size
h. reduction surgery
h. reflex
refractory heart failure
regular heart rate
regular heart rhythm
regular heart tones
rehabilitation of heart disease
h. rehabilitation program
h. rejected
relaxation of heart muscle
h. relaxed phase
h. remodeling
repeat heart attack
h. reshaping
h. response to stress
h. resting
restrictive heart disease
h. resuscitated
revascularization of blood vessels of h.
reverse heart disease
reverse heart failure
rheumatic valvular heart disease
rheumatism of h.
h. rhythm
h. rhythm abnormality
h. rhythm disorder
h. rhythm disturbance
h. rhythm drug
h. rhythm problem
right atrium of h.
right border of h.
right heart blood volume
right heart border
right heart mixing volume
right heart strain
right margin of h.
right-sided congestive heart failure
right-sided heart failure
right ventricle of h.
right ventricular heart failure
rising heart rate
h. risk
h. risk assessment
risk of first heart attack
risk of heart disease
round heart disease
rubbing heart sound
rupture of h.
h. sac
scarring of heart muscle
scarring of heart valve
h. screening
second-degree heart block
semihorizontal heart position
sensitize heart muscle to digitalis toxicity
septation of h.
septum of h.
severe heart valve narrowing
severely weakened h.
sexual dysfunction after heart attack
h. shadow
h. shock
h. shocked during cardiac arrest
shock heart into normal rhythm
silent heart attack
silent heart damage
silent heart muscle distress
silent ischemic heart disease
h. silhouette
silhouette of h.
sinoatrial heart block
sinoauricular heart block
sinusoidal heart rate
h. size and outline
h. size and shape
slow heart rate
slow heart rhythm
small vein of h.
Smeloff heart valve
smoker's h.
sonogram of h.
h. sounds
h. sounds normal
splitting of heart sound
stabilize heart function
stable fetal heart tones
standing heart rate
staphylococcal infection of heart valve
steady-state heart rate
h. stimulant
stimulate heart muscle
stress of heart disease
stress-related heart condition
h. stroke
stroke volume of h.
structural change in h.
structural heart defect
structural heart disease
h. study
subjunctional heart block
sudden congestive heart failure
sudden death ischemic heart disease
sudden fatal heart attack
sudden heart attack death
sudden heart failure
h. sugar
superior lobe of h.
h. surgery
suspected heart attack
symptomatic alcohol heart muscle disease
symptoms of heart failure
synthetic heart valve
systolic heart failure
systolic heart murmur
h. tamponade
target heart rate zone
temporary heart transplant
h. test
thallium exercise heart scan
thickened heart muscle
third degree heart block
third-degree heart block
third heart sound
thyrotoxic heart disease
h. tissue
h. tones
tonic heart level
total artificial h.
total implantation of artificial h.
transient heart block
h. transplant patient
h. transplant recipient
transseptal left heart catheterization
transverse diameter of h.
transverse heart diameter
transverse section of h.
transverse sulcus of h.
treatment of heart disease
tricuspid first heart sound
tricuspid heart valve
tricuspid second heart sound
trifascicular heart block
h. trimming procedure
triple bypass heart surgery
underlying heart rhythm
univentricular h.
upper chamber of h.
h. valve
h. valve abnormality
h. valve damage
h. valve defect

h. valve disease
h. valve disorder
h. valve function
h. valve infection
h. valve prosthesis
h. valve replacement
h. valve surgery
h. valve vegetation
valvular disease of h.
vascular disease of h.
vascular disease in diabetic h.
vascular heart disease
venous return to h.
ventricular heart disease
ventricular septal heart defect
h. volume
voluntary heart rate control
vortex of h.
h. wall thickening
warning signs of heart attack
weakened heart muscle
h. weight
Wenckebach heart block
h. with pericardium
h. worm

heart-assist pump

heartbeat

abnormal h.
absence of h.
absent h.
accentuated h.
arrest of h.
depressed breathing and h.
effective h.
fast h.
fetal h.
initiate h.
irregular heartbeat rhythm
h. irregularities
h. irregularity
life-threatening abnormal h.
monitoring h.
multifocal h.
nocturnal h.
normal h.
racing h.
rapid h.
rhythm of heartbeat disorder
slow h.
symptom of h.
synchronous with h.

heart-beating donor

3:1 heart block

3:2 heart block

heartburn

acid h.
disabling h.
drug-induced h.
frequent h.
h. from antibiotic
nighttime h.
nocturnal h.
patient has h.
h. of pregnancy
severe h.

heart-circulation training

heart-hand syndrome

heart-healthy lifestyle

heart-lung

h.-l. block
h.-l. bypass
h.-l. machine
h.-l. resuscitation
h.-l. resuscitator
h.-l. transplant
h.-l. transplantation

heartrate-corrected OT interval

heart-threatening hypertension

heart-to-lung ratio

heartworm disease

heat

absence of heat in a reaction
h., absence of use, redness, pain, pus, swelling
acclimation to heat and work
anhidrotic heat exhaustion
anxiety from heat exhaustion
brief exposure to heat stress
h. capacity
coefficient of heat transfer
h. conservation
h. conservation center
h. detection test
dizziness from heat stroke
environmental heat injury
h. escape lessening posture
h. exchanger
exertional heat illness
exertional heat stroke
h. exhaustion
flushing and h.
humidify and h.
h. illness syndrome
h. inactivated
increased local h.
h. infusion agar
h. injury
h. input
internal body h.
h. intolerance
h. intolerance from alcohol
h. intolerance from diuretics
isolated heat perfusion
h. killed
h. lesion
life-threatening heat stroke
h. loss
h. loss center
h. loss by radiation
h., massage, and exercise
h. and massage therapy
mean episcleral heat dose
metabolic heat load stimulator
metabolic heat production
moist h.
moist heat therapy
moist heat treatment
h. and moisture exchanging filter
molar heat capacity
normal heat defense
overexposure to h.
paraffin heat therapy
prickly heat rash
h. production
radiant h.
radiant heat device
radiant heat warmer
h. rash
h., reddening, swelling, or tenderness
respiratory heat exchange
h. sensitivity
h. shock protein
specific heat at constant volume
specific heat capacity
specific latent h.
h. stable
h., steam, gum, yawn, and Valsalva maneuver
h. sterilization
h. stress
h. stress index
h. stroke
h. stroke in aging
h. syncope
h. temperature vulcanized
h. therapy
h. tolerance
h. transfer agent
h. transfer factor
h. treatment
typhoid vaccine, heat and phenol inactivated, dried
h., ultrasound, and massage
unit of h.
h. urticaria
warm moist h.

heat-activated recoverable temporary stent

heat-aggregated
h.-a. bacille Calmette-Guérin
h.-a. globulin

heat-curing resin

heated
h. aerosol
h. bed cradle
continuous heated aerosol
h. discussion
h. intraoperative intraperitoneal chemotherapy
Puritan heated nebulizer
h. serum reagent
h. soybean flower
h. tracheostomy collar

heater
broad-spectrum h.
h. probe
h. probe cauterization
h. probe coagulation
h. probe therapy
h. probe unit

heat-inactivated
h.-i. fetal bovine serum
h.-i. fetal calf serum

heat-induced
h.-i. epitope retrieval
h.-i. illness

heating
regional deep h.
h., ventilating, and air conditioning

heat-killed ***Listeria monocytogenes***

heat-labile
h.-l. factor
h.-l. toxin

heat/moisture exchanger

heat-related
h.-r. disorders
h.-r. illness
h.-r. injury

heat-shock protein

heat-stable
h.-s. alkaline phosphatase
h.-s. lactic dehydrogenase

heave
apical h.
dry h.'s
parasternal h.
precordial h.
right ventricular h.
systolic h.
ventricular h.

heaviness
chest h.
flushing sensation of h.
h. in legs
h. of limbs
sensation of h.
stiffness or heaviness of limbs

heavy
h. alcohol consumption
h. alcohol usage
h. alcohol user
animo-terminal portion of heavy chain of immunoglobulin
h. chain
h. chain of immunoglobulin A
h. chain of immunoglobulin D
h. chain of immunoglobulin E
h. chain of immunoglobulin G
h. chain of immunoglobulin M
h. clamp applied
h. consumption of alcohol
emphysema secondary to heavy smoking
h. exertion
h. exertional activity
h. flow
h. infection
h. ion irradiation
h. lifting
long-term heavy drinking
long-term heavy use
h. menstrual flow
h. menstrual periods
h. menstrual periods from anemia
h. meromyosin of muscle
h. metal
h. metal poisoning
h. metal screen
h. metal stain
patient heavy drinker
h. period
prolonged heavy drinking
h. resistance strength training
h. retention suture
h. scaling of skin
h. sedation
h. social drinkers
h. vaginal discharge
variable domain of heavy chain immunoglobulin

heavy-chain disease protein

hebephrenia
manic h.

Heberden
H. disease
H. node
H. rheumatism
H. sign

Hebra
melanotic prurigo of H.

Hedstrom number

heel
abscess of h.
Achilles h.
anterior h.
basketball h.
big h.
h. bone
h. bone density scan
h. to buttock
cellulite of h.
chronic heel pain syndrome
contracted h.
contracted heel cord
h. cord
h. cord advancement
h. cord lengthening
cracked h.
decubitus h.
disposable heel protector
inner heel wedge
h. lance
left heel strike
h. lift
lift-off of heel in walk
medial heel skive technique
medial heel wedge orthosis
MF heel cup
Murphy heel cord advancement
network of h.
obligatory heel valgus
h. pad
h. pain
painful heel pad
painful heel spur
painful heel syndrome
percutaneous heel cord lengthening
prominent h.
h. protector
right heel strike
rump heel length
soft ankle, cushioned heel orthopaedic appliance
h. spur
h. spur excision
h. spur syndrome
h. squat exercise
h. stick pain
h. strike

Stryker walking h.
h. tap
h. tendon
h. and toe walking
toe walking and heel walking
walking h.
h. walking
walking heel cast
h. wedge
wedge h.
wedge adjustable cushioned h.

heel-and-toe
h.-a.-t. gait
h.-a.-t. walking

heel-cord stretches

heel-knee-shin test

heeloff
right h.

heel-stick blood gas

heel-tap reflex

heel-toe gait

heel-to-knee
h.-t.-k. dystaxia
h.-t.-k. test

heel-to-shin test

heel-to-toe
h.-t.-t. gait
h.-t.-t. walking

Hegar sign

Heidelberg retina tomograph

height
h. age
anterior facial h.
disc space h.
first twitch h.
fundal h.
h. of fundus
h. of heart
length, breadth, h.
h. loss
lower anterior dental h.
maximum laryngeal h.
midparental h.
minimal acceptable h.
minimal height velocity
minimum laryngeal h.
h. of occlusion
palatal height index
h. of palate
palpebral fissure h.
peripapillary retinal h.
predicted adult h.
Roche, Wainer, and Thissen method of height prediction
sitting h.
h. velocity
ventricular atrial height right atrium
h. vertigo

heightened
h. anxiety
h. attention
h. attention state
h. awareness
h. awareness state
h. awareness of touch or taste
lapse into heightened irritability
h. perception of colors
h. sense of awareness
h. sensitivity to odors
h. sensitivity to sounds
h. sexual drive
h. startle reactions
h. stress

Heimlich
H. heart valve
H. maneuver

Heineke-Mikulicz
H.-M. pyloroplasty
H.-M. strictureplasty

Heinz
H. body
H. body hemolytic anemia
congenital Heinz body hemolytic anemia

Hektoen enteric agar

HeLa cell

held
h. after positioning
h. backward
hand held in position of extension
shortened, held, resisted, contracted

helical
anterior helical rim free flap
Antia-Buch helical rim advancement flap
h. axis of motion
h. biphasic contrast-enhanced CT
h. computed tomographic angiography
h. fold
low-dose helical scanning technique
noncontrast helical computed tomography
paired helical filaments
renal helical computed tomography
h. rim
triple-phase helical computer tomography
unenhanced helical computed tomography

Helicobacter
anti-*Helicobacter pylori* IgM
anti-*Helicobacter pylori* treatment
H. pylori
Helicobacter pylori eradication therapy
Helicobacter pylori-like organism
Helicobacter pylori stool antigen
Helicobacter pylori vaccine

helicoidal
long pitch helicoidal layer

helioophthalmic
autosomal dominant compelling helioophthalmic outburst syndrome

heliotrope
h. infraorbital discoloration
h. rash
h. sign

helium
h. dilution
h. equilibration time
h. ion beam
h. and oxygen

helium-oxygen mixture

helix
auricular h.
caudal h.
crus of h.
double h.
limb of h.
root of h.
spine of h.
tail of h.
triple h.
Watson-Crick h.

helix-bundle peptide

helix-loop-helix
basic h.-l.-h.

***Helix pomatia* agglutinin**

Heller
modified Heller esophagomyotomy
H. myotomy
H. myotomy with Dor fundoplication
H. operation
H. plexus

Heller-Dor procedure

helmet
h. cell
cranial h.
h. headache
neurasthenic h.

Helmholtz
anterior ligament of H.
H. energy
H. free energy
H. line

helminth
multicellular h.

heloma
h. durum
h. molle

help
cry for h.
home h.
h. patient achieve independence

helper
antigen-specific helper factor
h. cell
h. determinant
h. factor
magic h.
proliferative helper cell
T h.
h. T cell

helpful
newborn helpful hints

helping
heart helping exercise

helplessness
Arthritis H. Index
feeling of guilt, worthlessness and h.
sense of h.
sense of increasing h.

help-rejecting complainer

help-seeking behavior

hemacytology index

hemadsorption
h. inhibition
mixed h.
h. test
h. virus

hemagglutinating
h. activity
h. antibody
h. antigen
h. antipenicillin antibody
h. encephalomyelitis
h. inhibition antibody
h. penicillin antibody
staphylococcal hemagglutinating antibody
h. unit
h. virus of Japan

hemagglutination
h. encephalomyelitis virus
immune adherence hemagglutination assay
indirect h.
indirect hemagglutination antibody test
indirect hemagglutination assay
h. inhibition antibody
h. inhibition assay
h. inhibition immunoassay
h. inhibition morphine test
h. inhibition titer
mannose-resistant h.
mannose-sensitive h.
Middlebrook-Dubos hemagglutination test
mixed reverse passive antiglobulin h.
passive h.
passive hemagglutination inhibition
passive hemagglutination test
reversed passive h.
reversed passive hemagglutination by miniature centrifugal fast analysis
reversed passive hemagglutination reaction
tanned red blood cell h.
tanned red blood cell hemagglutination inhibition
h. treponemal test for syphilis
Treponema pallidum hemagglutination assay
Treponema pallidum hemagglutination test

hemagglutinin
cold hemagglutinin disease
h. enzyme-linked immunosorbent assay
filamentous h.
fimbrial h.
indirect hemagglutinin assay
h. neuraminidase
h. unit

hemalum
Mayer h.

hemangioblastoma
inoperable h.
optic nerve h.

hemangioendothelioma
epithelioid h.

hemangioma, pl. **hemangiomata**
cavernous hemangioma of skin
h. of choroid
circumscribed choroidal h.
h. of conjunctiva
giant hepatic cavernous h.
h. of iris
h. of liver
liver capillary h.
lobular capillary h.
macrocephaly, multiple lipomas, hemangiomata syndrome
macrocephaly, pseudoepithelioma, multiple hemangiomas syndrome
h. of meningeal vessels
mixed capillary cavernous h.
h. of orbit
orbital capillary h.
periocular capillary h.
port wine h.
h. of retina
h. simplex
targetoid hemosiderotic h.

hemangioma-thrombocytopenia syndrome

hemangiomatosis
Osler h.
pulmonary capillary h.

hemangiopericytoma
lipomatous h.

hemapheresis
h. methodology
h. technology
therapeutic h.

hematemesis
h. and melena
melena, hematochezia or h.
h. neonatorum

Hematest stools

hematocele
pelvic h.

hematochezia
melena, hematochezia or hematemesis

hematocrit
h. concentration
hemoglobin and h.
large vessel h.
mean circulatory h.
mean menstrual cycle h.
platelet h.
total body h.

venous h.
whole-blood h.

hematocystic spot

hematodepressive
viral hematodepressive disease

hematogenous
h. contamination
h. dissemination
h. embolism
h. jaundice
h. metastases
h. pigmentation
h. proteinuria
h. pyelitis
h. siderosis
h. tuberculosis

hematologic
h. abnormality
h. disease
h. disorder
h. dysfunction
h. effect
h. malignancy
h. parameters
h. reaction
h. toxicity
h. workup

hematological
h. disease
h. disorder

hematology
automated hematology analysis

hematology-oncology
pediatric h.-o.

hematoma
acute subdural h.
aortic intramural h.
h. aspiration
h. of chest wall
chronic subdural h.
delayed traumatic intracerebral h.
dissecting aortic h.
h. dissection
h. drainage
drainage of h.
epidural h.
h. evacuation
extradural h.
interhemispheric subdural h.
intracerebral h.
intramural duodenal h.
left frontal h.
liquefaction of subdural h.
nail bed hematoma evacuation
h. of orbit
paraaortic h.
parenchymal h.
paroxysmal hand h.
pelvic viscera surrounded by h.
periaortic mediastinal h.
h. of placenta
rectus sheath h.
right frontal h.
h. of scalp
soft tissue h.
sonography of subfascial h.
spinal epidural h.
spontaneous intramural hematoma of the esophagus
spontaneous spinal epidural h.
subcapsular hematoma of liver
subdural h.
subgaleal h.
widespread ecchymosis and h.

hematopoiesis
extramedullary h.
Ogawa model for h.

hematopoietic
allogenic hematopoietic stem cell transplantation
autologous hematopoietic cell
autologous hematopoietic progenitor cell transplantation
autologous hematopoietic stem cell transplantation
autologous peripheral hematopoietic stem cell support
autologous hematopoietic stem cell support
cancellous hematopoietic marrow
infectious hematopoietic necrosis virus
marrow hematopoietic stem cell
mixed donor-host hematopoietic chimerism
mixed hematopoietic chimerism
multipotent hematopoietic cell
multipotent hematopoietic progenitor
mutation in hematopoietic tissue
normal hematopoietic cell
h. progenitor cell
h. stem cell transplantation
totipotent hematopoietic stem cell

hematoporphyrin derivative

hematoxylin
h. and eosin
h. and eosin stain
iron h.
Mayer acid alum hematoxylin stain
h. and van Gieson stain
Weigert hematoxylin stain

hematoxylin-eosin stain

hematoxylin-phloxine-saffron stain

hematuria
adolescent stress h.
benign familial h.
benign recurrent h.
loin pain hematuria syndrome
nonfamilial h.
painless intermittent h.
pyuria and h.
recurrent gross h.

hematuria-dysuria syndrome

heme
microsomal heme oxygenase
h. negative
h. oxygenase
h. positive
h. synthase
h. synthetase
total heme mass

heme-controlled repressor

heme-negative stool

heme-positive stool

hemianesthesia
alternate h.
cerebral h.
crossed h.
cruciate h.
mesocephalic h.
pontile h.
spinal h.

hemianopia
h. in intracranial neoplasm
left homonymous h.
right homonymous h.

hemianopsia
heteronymous h.
homonymous h.
lower h.
nasal h.

hemiarthroplasty
Austin Moore h.
McKeever and MacIntosh h.
Miller-Galante I h.
Neer h.
h. procedure

hemiatrophy
fascial h.
lingual h.
progressive lingual h.

hemiaxial
caudocranial hemiaxial view
hemiazygos
superior hemiazygos vein
Hemiballism/Hemichorea Outcome Rating Score
hemiblock
left anterior h.
left anterior-superior h.
left anterosuperior h.
left posterior h.
left posterior inferior h.
right anterior h.
hemibody
h. irradiation
sequential hemibody irradiation
upper hemibody irradiation
hemicentral, lateral
hemicolectomy
left h.
right h.
hemicondylar fracture
hemiconvulsion-hemiplegia-epilepsy syndrome
hemicrania
chronic paroxysmal h.
episodic paroxysmal h.
migraine sine h.
hemicranial vascular headache
hemideficit
motor h.
hemidiaphragm
attenuation by h.
h. rupture
hemidiaphragmatic
ipsilateral hemidiaphragmatic paresis
hemidysplasia
congenital hemidysplasia with ichthyosiform erythroderma and limb defects syndrome
hemifacial
h. hyperplasia
h. hypertrophy
h. microsomia
h. spasm
h. weakness
hemifield
h. loss
nasal h.
hemifundoplication
Toupet hemifundoplication fundoplication
hemigastrectomy and vagotomy
hemihyperplasia
facial h.
hemihypertrophy, intestinal web, preauricular skin tag, and congenital corneal opacity syndrome
hemijoint
medial hemijoint articular space
hemilaminectomy
lumbar h.
partial h.
hemilaryngopharyngectomy
supracricoid h.
hemilingual
periodic hemilingual numbness
hemimandibular hyperplasia
hemimelia
fibular h.
paraxial fibular h.
partial h.
hemiparesis
ataxic h.
left arm h.
pure motor h.
right arm h.
hemiparetic gait
hemiplegia
alternating hemiplegia of childhood
alternating oculomotor h.
left h.
right h.
hemiplegic
basilar hemiplegic migraine
familial hemiplegic migraine
h. foot
h. form of cerebral palsy
h. gait
h. hand
h. idiocy
h. migraine
patient h.
h. rigidity
hemisection
h. of kidneys
mandibular h.
h. of spinal cord
hemispasm
facial h.
hemisphere
activity of both h.'s
bilateral hemisphere damage
h. of brain
h. implant
left cerebral h.
left hemisphere of brain
left hemisphere brain damage
left hemisphere damage
left hemisphere deficit
left hemisphere lesion
left hemisphere stroke
medial surface of cerebral h.
nondominant hemisphere lesion
occipital lobe unilateral cerebral hemisphere lesion
parietal lobe bilateral cerebral hemisphere lesion
parietal lobe unilateral cerebral hemisphere lesion
right h.
right cerebral h.
right hemisphere of brain
right hemisphere brain damage
right hemisphere deficit
right hemisphere lesion
Right H. Language Battery
h. spikes
superior margin of cerebral h.
h. thrombotic infarction
two cerebral hemisphere vegetal hemisphere
ventricle of cerebral h.
h. width
hemispheric
h. activity
anatomic porous replacement hemispheric acetabular component
h. blood flow
h. gliosis
h. infarction
lateral ventricular width to hemispheric width
medial hemispheric arteriovenous malformation
medial hemispheric dynamics
transient hemispheric attack
hemisuccinate of hydrocortisone
hemitransfixion incision
hemizona assay index
hemoblast
lymphoid h.
lymphoid hemoblast of Pappenheim
hemoblastic leukemia
Hemoccult
H. negative stools
H. positive stools

H. screening
H. slide test

hemochromatosis
autosomal dominant h.
genetic h.
hereditary h.
idiopathic h.
neonatal h.

hemodiafiltration
continuous arteriovenous h.
continuous venovenous h.

hemodialysis
anemia of h.
h. arthropathy
asymptomatic hemodialysis patient
center h.
chronic h.
continuous arteriovenous h.
continuous venovenous h.
home h.
in-center h.
intermittent h.
joint swelling in h.
h. maintenance
maintenance h.
h. patient
perforating disease of h.
h. prognostic nutrition index
regular hemodialysis treatment
simplified nocturnal home h.
subclavian hemodialysis catheter
surgically implanted hemodialysis catheter
h. therapy
h. transmission of viral hepatitis
h. treatment
h. unit
vascular access in h.

hemodialyzer
ultrafiltration h.

hemodilution
acute normovolemic h.

hemodynamic
h. abnormality
h. angiographic study
h. assessment
h. calculation
cardiac hemodynamic monitoring
h. collapse
h. derangements
derived hemodynamic data
h. effect
h. gradient
h. instability
left ventricular hemodynamic abnormalities
h. maneuver
h. measurement
menstrual cycle hemodynamic response
h. monitoring
ocular hemodynamic assessment
ocular hemodynamic value
h. parameters
postanesthesia h.
h. pressure
h. principle
h. study
h. support
systemic hemodynamic parameters
h. tolerance
h. vise

hemodynamically
combined multisection diffuse-weighted and hemodynamically weighted echoplanar MR
h. significant stenosis
h. stable

hemodynamically-weighted MRI

hemodynamics
intraoperative h.
maternal central h.
systemic h.

hemofiltration
continuous arteriovenous h.
continuous arteriovenous hemofiltration with dialysis
continuous venovenous h.
h. therapy

hemoflagellate
mitochondrion of h.

hemoglobin
h. A
h. A_{1c}
adult h.
h. B chain
bovine h.
h. C
carbon monoxide h.
chain of h.
chain of fetal h.
h. Chesapeake
h. concentration
h. Constant Spring
h. content index
h. content of reticulocyte
cord blood h.
h. C-thalassemia disease
h. D
h. delta chain
h. determination
diaspirin cross-linked h.
h. E
h. electrophoresis
h. E-thalassemia disease
h. F
fetal h.
fetal hemoglobin test
h. fluctuated
h. gamma chain A
h. gamma chain G
glucose, lactalbumin, serum, and h.
glycosylated h.
glycosylated hemoglobin level
glycosylated hemoglobin test
h. H
h. and hematocrit
hereditary persistence of fetal h.
heterozygosity for hemoglobin A and hemoglobin S
high molecular weight h.
homozygosity for hemoglobin S
homozygous for sickle cell h.
h. I
h. Lepore
liposome-encapsulated h.
h. M
major component of adult h.
mean cell h.
mean cell hemoglobin concentration
mean corpuscular h.
mean corpuscular hemoglobin concentration
mean corpuscular hemoglobin count
mean hemoglobin concentration
minor fraction of adult h.
monomer in fetal h.
mucosal blood h.
mutant hemoglobin with low affinity for oxygen
nitric oxide h.
nonionized h.
oxygenated h.
h. oxygen dissociation curve
oxygen half-saturation pressure of h.
peripheral ring of h.
primitive fetal h.
h. production
pyridoxalated stroma-free h.
pyridoxylated h.
reduced h.
relative h.
reticulocyte hemoglobin distribution width
h. S

hemoglobin *(continued)*
saturation of h.
serum-free h.
sickle cell h.
sickle cell hemoglobin F
sickle cell hemoglobin C disease
sickle cell hemoglobin D disease
sickle hemoglobin screen
h. S-thalassemia
stroma-free h.
stroma-free hemoglobin pyridoxalated
total h.
total circulating h.
unstable hemoglobin disease
h. Z
h. zeta
h. Zürich

hemoglobinate
potassium h.

hemoglobin-based oxygen carrier

hemoglobin-binding capacity

hemoglobin-haptoglobin complex

hemoglobin-polyoxyethylene
pyridoxylated h.-p.

hemoglobinuria
h. and glomerular thrombosis
malarial h.
march h.
nocturnal h.
paroxysmal cold h.
paroxysmal nocturnal h.
paroxysmal nocturnal hemoglobinuria cell

hemoglobinuric
h. bilious fever
h. fever

hemolysate
membrane-free h.
sheep hemolysate supernatant

hemolysin
alpha h.
natural h.
thermostable direct h.

hemolysing dose

hemolysis
h. blocking
h., elevated liver enzymes, and low platelet count
h. end point
h. inhibition
kinetic hemolysis curve
localized hemolysis in gel
massive intravascular h.
peroxide hemolysis test
radial h.
radial hemolysis in gel
red cell peroxide h.
single radial h.

hemolytic
ABO hemolytic disease
acholuric hemolytic icterus
acquired immune hemolytic disease
acute hemolytic anemia
acute hemolytic uremic syndrome
alloimmune hemolytic anemia
alloimmune hemolytic disease of newborn
alpha hemolytic streptococcus
h. anemia
h. anemia antigen
h. anemia of newborn
angiopathic hemolytic anemia
aplastic crisis in hemolytic anemia
atypical hemolytic uremia syndrome
autoallergic hemolytic anemia
autoimmune acquired hemolytic anemia
autoimmune hemolytic anemia
autoimmune hemolytic disease
beta hemolytic strain
h. blood transfusion disease
combined cold and warm antibody autoimmune hemolytic anemia
h. complement assay
congenital Heinz body hemolytic anemia
congenital hemolytic icterus
congenital hemolytic jaundice
congenital inclusion-body hemolytic anemia
congenital nonspherocytic hemolytic anemia
congenital nonspherocytic hemolytic disease
delayed hemolytic reaction
h. disease
h. disease of newborn
filterable hemolytic anemia
group A beta hemolytic streptococcus
Heinz body hemolytic anemia
hereditary hemolytic anemia
hereditary hemolytic anemia test
hereditary hemolytic syndrome
hereditary nonspherocytic hemolytic anemia
h. icterus
idiopathic acquired hemolytic disease
idiopathic autoimmune hemolytic anemia
h. immune body
immune hemolytic anemia
incompatible hemolytic blood transfusion
h. index
h. jaundice
lysolecithin hemolytic anemia
microangiopathic hemolytic uremic syndrome
minimal hemolytic dilution
minimal hemolytic dose
h. plaque assay
h. process
protein A hemolytic plaque assay
h. resistance
reverse hemolytic plaque assay
Rhesus hemolytic disease
h. splenomegaly
h. Staphylococcus aureus
h. streptococcus
h. substance
thrombotic thrombocytopenic purpura and hemolytic uremic syndrome
total hemolytic complement
total serum hemolytic complement
h. transfusion react
h. unit
h. uremic syndrome
h. uremic syndrome/thrombotic thrombocytopenia purpura
warm autoimmune hemolytic anemia

hemolyticus
icterus h.
morbus hemolyticus neonatorum

hemopathy
maternal h.

hemoperfusion
charcoal h.
hepatic venous isolation by direct h.
resin hemoperfusion column

hemopericardium
cardiac lacerations and h.

hemopexin serum protein

hemophagocytic
familial hemophagocytic lymphohistiocytosis

infection-associated hemophagocytic syndrome
h. lymphohistiocytosis
h. syndrome
virus-associated hemophagocytic syndrome

hemophilia
factor VIII h.
Leyden hemophilia B

hemophiliac
healthy h.
h. with adenopathy

hemopoietic
h. blood stem cell
h. factor
h. histocompatibility
h. inductive microenvironment
pluripotent hemopoietic stem cell

hemoptysis
cardiac h.
cough and/or h.
endemic h.
intermittent h.
Manson h.
massive h.
oriental h.
parasitic h.
persistent cough with h.
vicarious h.

hemorrhage
acute gastrointestinal h.
acute intraventricular h.
acute pulmonary h.
acute rectal h.
acute subarachnoid h.
acute upper gastrointestinal h.
agonal spinal cord h.
h. of aneurysm
aneurysmal subarachnoid h.
antepartum h.
area of recent h.
areas of hemorrhage and necrosis
artery of cerebral h.
atrial subendocardial h.
bladder mucosal h.
bowel wall h.
h. in brain
brain damage from cerebral h.
brain stem h.
h., cerebral
cerebroventricular h.
h. and clotted blood
h. consolidation
h. control
diffuse alveolar h.
diffuse interstitial h.
diffuse petechial h.
diffuse pulmonary alveolar h.
diffuse pulmonary h.
dissecting hemorrhage of midbrain
esophageal variceal h.
essential uterine h.
exacerbation and h.
exsanguinating intraperitoneal h.
extensive bronchial mucosa h.
h. and exudate
h.'s, exudates, and/or nicking
fatal pulmonary h.
fetomaternal h.
focal area of h.
focal areas of intrapulmonary h.
focal hepatic h.
focal interstitial h.
focal intrapulmonary h.
focal petechial h.
focal shallow subpleural h.
focal subendocardial h.
gastric mucosal h.
gastrointestinal h.
germinal layer h.
germinal matrix h.
hereditary cerebral hemorrhage with amyloidosis
high-altitude retinal h.
hypertensive intracerebral h.
idiopathic pulmonary h.
infiltration by h.
interhemispheric subarachnoid h.
h. into submucosa
h. into wall of bladder
intracerebral h.
intracerebral and subarachnoid h.
intracranial h.
intractable postpartum h.
intramucosal hemorrhage and erosion
intramural h.
intraparenchymal h.
intraperitoneal h.
intraretinal h.
intraventricular hemorrhage grade 1–4
h. of iris
h. or laceration
laceration or h.
late postpartum h.
lower gastrointestinal h.
macular h.
massive gastrointestinal h.
massive intracerebral h.
massive midbrain h.
massive pulmonary h.
massive variceal h.
massive vitreous h.
maternal fetal h.
h. in medulla
h. and microaneurysm
multiple interstitial pulmonary h.
multiple lobar h.
multiple punctuate h.
necrotizing hemorrhage leukomyelitis
neonatal adrenal gland h.
neonatal cerebral h.
neonatal choroid plexus h.
neonatal gastrointestinal h.
nerve fiber layer h.
h. of newborn
h. in orbit
h., papilledema, exudate
parenchymal h.
parenchymal cerebral h.
patchy purpuric h.
periadrenal h.
periesophageal h.
perimesencephalic nonaneurysmal subarachnoid h.
perinatal cerebral h.
peripheral intraretinal h.
periventricular h.
periventricular-intraventricular h.
petechial hemorrhage of bowel
petechial hemorrhage of kidney
petechial hemorrhage of pericardium
petechial hemorrhage of peritoneum
petechial hemorrhage of skin
postoperative h.
postpartum h.
posttonsillectomy h.
preretinal h.
preventricular intraventricular h.
primary intracerebral h.
primary postpartum h.
proliferative diabetic retinopathy with vitreous h.
pulmonary alveolar h.
pulmonary artery h.
punctate h.
recent soft tissue h.
rectocolic h.
recurrent hemorrhage from aneurysm
recurrent lobar h.
recurrent variceal h.
renal pelvic h.
h. in retina
retinal h.

hemorrhage *(continued)*
retroperitoneal h.
h. and shock
signs of recent h.
small brain h.
small focus h.
soft tissue h.
soft tissue hemorrhage into mesentery
spinal epidural h.
spinal subdural h.
spontaneous intracerebral h.
stigmata of recent h.
h. and stroke
stroke due to cerebral h.
subarachnoid h.
subarachnoid hemorrhage in cranium
subconjunctival hemorrhage of eye
subdural hemorrhage in cranium
subendocardial petechial h.
subependymal h.
superficial cortical h.
superficial distal esophagus h.
superficial subendocardial focal h.
suprachoroidal h.
surface infiltration by h.
surgical procedure for subarachnoid h.
surgical treatment for epidural h.
symptomatic h.
thrombolysis-related intracranial h.
transplacental h.
traumatic multiple h.'s
traumatic subarachnoid h.
upper gastrointestinal tract h.
h. in vitreous
vitreous h.

hemorrhagic
acute hemorrhagic bronchopneumonia
acute hemorrhagic conjunctivitis
acute hemorrhagic cystitis
acute hemorrhagic edema
acute hemorrhagic edema of infancy
acute hemorrhagic encephalomyelitis
acute hemorrhagic pancreatitis
h. adrenals
African hemorrhagic fever
alcoholic hemorrhagic gastritis
h. anemia
h. appearance, mottled
h. area, mottled
Argentine hemorrhagic fever
Argentine hemorrhagic fever virus
Argentinian hemorrhagic fever
arthropod-borne viral hemorrhagic fever
h. ascites
h. bronchitis
h. bronchopneumonia
central hemorrhagic necrosis
h. colitis
h. corpus luteum
Crimean-Congo hemorrhagic fever
Crimean-Congo hemorrhagic fever virus
h. cyst
h. cystitis
dengue hemorrhagic fever shock syndrome
dengue hemorrhagic fever
h. diathesis
h. diathesis secondary to hepatic failure
h. discoloration
h. disease
h. disease of infant
h. disease of newborn
h. dot
Ebola hemorrhagic fever
h. edema
h. encephalitis
h. encephalopathy
h. endovasculitis
h. endovasculopathy
h. enterocolitis
epizootic hemorrhagic disease virus 1–8
h. erosive gastritis
h. esophagitis
h. extravasation
h. factor
h. familial angiomatosis
h. fever
h. fever with renal symptoms
h. fever with renal syndrome
h. fluid
focal hemorrhagic cystitis
focal hemorrhagic infarct
focal hemorrhagic necrotizing cystitis
h. gastritis
h. gingivitis
h. glaucoma
h. infarct
h. infarct of adrenal gland
h. infiltration
h. lesion
Manchurian hemorrhagic fever
h. manifestation
Marburg hemorrhagic fever
h. material
h. measles
h. metastasis
mucopurulent hemorrhagic effusion
h. mucosa
multifocal hemorrhagic sarcoma
multiple hereditary hemorrhagic telangiectasis
multiple idiopathic hemorrhagic sarcoma
necrotic hemorrhagic colitis
necrotizing hemorrhagic leukoencephalitis
neonatal hemorrhagic disease
h. nephritis
New World hemorrhagic fever
h. omental lymph nodes
Omsk hemorrhagic fever virus
organizing hemorrhagic cyst
h. pain
painful hemorrhagic glaucoma
h. pancreatitis
h. pericarditis
peripheral exudative choroidal hemorrhagic retinopathy
h. peritonitis
h. petechiae
h. pleurisy
h. pneumonitis
proliferative hemorrhagic enteropathy
pulmonary hemorrhagic necrosis
purplish hemorrhagic spot on skin
h. purpura
h. pyelitis
red hemorrhagic fluid
h. retinopathy
h. salpingitis
h. scurvy
severe hemorrhagic pancreatitis
h. shock
h. shock and encephalopathy
h. shock-encephalopathy syndrome
h. shock syndrome
simian hemorrhagic fever
h. softening
South American hemorrhagic fever
Southeast Asia mosquito-borne hemorrhagic fever
spontaneous hemorrhagic necrosis
h. sputum
h. stool
h. stroke

superior hemorrhagic polioencephalitis
h. telangiectasia
h. telangiectasis
h. transformation
traumatic hemorrhagic bursitis
h. tumor metastasis
uncontrolled hemorrhagic shock
viral hemorrhagic fever
viral hemorrhagic septicemia virus
h. virus

hemorrhagica
aleukia h.
metropathia h.
osteopathia hemorrhagica infantum
purpura h.
urticaria h.

hemorrhagic-septicemia group

hemorrhagicus
lichen h.
pemphigus h.

hemorrhaging
catastrophic h.
petechial h.
uncontrollable h.

hemorrhoid
bipolar electrocoagulation of h.
chronic constipation with h.
combined h.'s
endoscopic hemorrhoid ligation
fiber and h.
infrared coagulation of h.
internal hemorrhoid of rectum
laser therapy of h.
ligation of h.
ligator
Lord dilation of h.
mixed h.'s
nonsymptomatic h.
rectal bleeding secondary to h.
h. reduction
rosette of h.'s
rubber band ligation of h.
shrinkage of h.

hemorrhoidal
h. artery ligation
h. banding
h. cushion
h. disease
excess hemorrhoidal tissue
inferior hemorrhoidal nerves
inferior hemorrhoidal vein
middle hemorrhoidal artery
middle hemorrhoidal plexus
middle hemorrhoidal vein
h. plexus
h. prolapse
h. sclerotherapy
h. skin tag
superior hemorrhoidal plexus
superior hemorrhoidal vein
h. tag
vaporized hemorrhoidal tissue
h. vessels
h. zone

hemorrhoidectomy
anoderm-preserving h.
ligation h.
limited h.
Lord h.
Milligan-Morgan h.
open h.
Parks h.
radical h.
rubber band h.

hemosiderin-laden macrophages

hemosiderosis
essential pulmonary h.
idiopathic pulmonary h.
secondary pulmonary h.

hemosiderotic
h. fibrohistiocytic lipomatous lesion
targetoid hemosiderotic hemangioma

hemostasis
h. accomplished
adequate h.
adequate hemostasis maintained
h. assured
h. complete
electrofulguration h.
good h.
h. good
McKenzie hemostasis clip
metabolic h.
meticulous h.
h. obtained
osmotic h.
h. secured
h. secured with ties
h. valve
wound examined for h.

hemostat
blunt nose h.
curved h.
fibrillar absorbable hemostat material
microfibrillar collagen h.
mosquito h.
orthopaedic h.

hemostatic
bleeding controlled with hemostatic clamp
capillary h.
coagulation and hemostatic resection of prostate
continuous hemostatic suture
h. control
h. disorder
h. material
mosquito hemostatic clamp
mosquito hemostatic forceps
natural hemostatic process
h. occlusive leverage device
h. puncture closure device
return flow hemostatic catheter
rotating hemostatic valve
h. screening profile
h. suture
h. therapy
vascular hemostatic device

hemothorax
right h.
spontaneous left h.
spontaneous right h.
traumatic h.

hemotoxylin

Hemovac
H. drain
H. suction
H. tube
H. unit

hen
h. egg lysozyme
h. egg-white lysozyme

Hendler Test for Chronic Pain

Henle
H. ampulla
ascending loop of H.
H. canal
H. cell
H. elastic membrane
H. fenestrated membrane
H. fissures
H. gland
ligament of H.
H. loop
loop of H.
medullary thick ascending limb of H.
H. membrane
H. reaction
H. sphincter
H. spine
thick ascending limb of Henle loop

Henoch
H. chorea
H. disease
H. purpura
Henoch-Schönlein
H.-S. purpura
H.-S. purpura nephritis
H.-S. syndrome
Henrietta Lacks cell
Henry
H. knot
H. law
ligament of H.
heparin
anticoagulant heparin solution
h. arterial filter
h. assay rapid easy method
benzalkonium and h.
h. block
calcium h.
h. cap
h. cofactor II
h. dose response
h. dosing nomogram
h. drip
h. flush
flush heparin lock
graphite, benzalkonium, h.
high heparin dose
h. lock
low-dose h.
low-dose unfractionated h.
low molecular weight h.
minimal intermittent dosage of h.
h. neutralized thrombin time
precipitable fraction h.
h. protamine titration
h. response test
standard heparin infusion
h. sulfate
h. surface-modified intraocular lens
h. therapy
h. thrombocytopenia
triiodothyronine, amino acids, glucagon, and h.
unfractionated h.
weight-based heparin dosing
h. well
heparin-associated
h.-a. thrombocytopenia
h.-a. thrombocytopenia and thrombosis
heparin-binding
h.-b. epidermal growth factorlike growth factor
h.-b. growth factor
h.-b. growth factor-1
h.-b. growth factor-2
h.-b. neurotrophic factor
h.-b. protein
heparin-dependent platelet-associated antibody
heparin-induced
h.-i. extracorporeal low-density lipoprotein precipitation
h.-i. thrombocytopenia
h.-i. thrombocytopenia-thrombosis
h.-i. thrombosis-thrombocytopenia syndrome
heparinization
continuous h.
intermittent h.
regional h.
heparinized
h. blood
patient h.
h. saline
h. solution infusion
heparin-neutralizing activity
heparin-precipitable fraction
hepatectomy
laparoscopic-assisted h.
living donor partial h.
partial h.
hepatic
h. abnormality
h. abscess
acute hepatic coma
acute hepatic failure
acute hepatic rupture
h. adenoma
h. adhesion
adjuvant hepatic arterial infusion chemotherapy
h. amebiasis
h. angiography
h. angiosarcoma
h. angle
h. arterial-dominant phase
h. arterial flow
h. arterial infusion
h. arterial infusional chemotherapy
h. arterial perfusion scintigraphy
h. arterial phase
h. arterial pulsatility index
h. artery
h. artery aneurysm
h. artery blood flow
h. artery chemoembolization
h. artery embolization
h. artery ligation
h. artery thrombosis
artificial hepatic support
h. bed
h. binding protein
h. bleeding
h. blood flow
h. calculus
h. cancer
h. capsule
h. carcinoma
h. catalase
h. catheterization
h. cecum
h. cell
h. cell carcinoma
central vein of hepatic lobule
cerebellar vermis hypoplasia, oligophrenia, congenital ataxia, coloboma, hepatic fibrosis
chronic hepatic encephalopathy
h. cirrhosis
h. colic
h. coma
common hepatic duct
h. complications of drug abuse
h. computed tomographic density
computerized tomographic hepatic angiography
congenital hepatic fibrosis
h. congestion
constitutional hepatic dysfunction
continuous hepatic artery infusion
h. cord
cutaneous hepatic porphyria
h. cyst
deep hepatic coma
dementia due to hepatic condition
diffuse hepatic softening
h. disease
h. disorder
h. distention
h. distomiasis
h. distribution volume
h. diverticulum
donor hepatic duct
drug-induced hepatic encephalopathy
drug-induced hepatic injury
h. drug metabolism
h. duct
h. duct stone
h. dullness
h. dysfunction
h. effect

h. encephalopathy
h. enzyme
h. enzyme study
estimated hepatic blood flow
h. failure
h. fever
h. fistula
h. flexure
h. flexure of colon
h. flux
h. fossa
free hepatic venous pressure
fulminant hepatic failure
h. function
h. functional panel
h. ganglion
general hepatic circulation
giant hepatic cavernous hemangioma
h. glucose output
h. glucose production
h. hemorrhage
hemorrhagic diathesis secondary to hepatic failure
h. hemosiderosis
h. hydrothorax
impaired hepatic function
h. impairment
h. infarct
infusion hepatic arteriography
h. injury
h. insufficiency
intermittent hepatic fever
intraarterial hepatic chemotherapy
intraarterial hepatic infusion
h. intramitochondrial crystalloid
h. iron concentration
h. iron index
h. iron overload
h. ischemia and reperfusion
isolated hepatic portal and arterial perfusion
late-onset hepatic failure
left hepatic artery
left hepatic duct
left hepatic lobe
left hepatic vein
h. lipoperoxidation
h. lobe
h. lobule
h. lymph node
malignant hepatic neoplasm
massive hepatic failure
metabolic disorder with hepatic dysfunction
h. metabolism
h. metastases
microvesicular hepatic steatosis
middle hepatic artery
mixed hepatic porphyria
h. necrosis
h. neoplasm
net hepatic glucose uptake
h. non-Hodgkin lymphoma
nonobstructive hepatic parenchymal disease
h. obstruction
occult hepatic disease
orthotopic hepatic transplant
h. outflow
h. parenchyma
partial hepatic vascular exclusion
h. perfusion index
h. plasma flow
h. portal
h. portal vein
h. portal venous gas
h. portoenterostomy
postoperative hepatic failure
preexisting hepatic disease
primary hepatic carcinoma
primary hepatic disease
h. problems related to drug abuse
protein loss in hepatic disease
h. pulse
h. radical
regional distribution of hepatic blood flow
h. reticuloendothelial cell
right hepatic duct
h. scan
h. schistosomiasis
sclerosing hepatic carcinoma
h. segment
segment-oriented hepatic resection
h. siderosis
small focus of hepatic necrosis
sphincter of hepatic flexure of colon
h. stellate cell
h. stimulant
h. stimulatory substance
subacute hepatic necrosis
subclinical hepatic encephalopathy
terminal hepatic vein obliteration
h. triad
h. triglyceride lipase
h. tumor
h. tumor index
h. vascular exclusion
h. vascular isolation
h. vein catheterization
h. vein free pressure
h. vein injury
h. vein occlusion
h. venoocclusive disease
h. venous effluence
h. venous isolation by direct hemoperfusion
h. venous outflow obstruction
h. venous pressure gradient
wedge hepatic venous pressure
h. wedge pressure
woodchuck hepatic virus

hepatica
adiposis h.
arteria hepatica communis
arteria hepatica propria
Fasciola h.
ophthalmia h.
pars h.
porphyria h.
pseudohemophilia h.

hepatic-occluded portal pressure

hepatis
porta h.

hepatitis
h. A
h. A antibody
h. A antigen
h. A, B, C, E,G vaccine
h. and acetaminophen
active chronic h.
h. activity index
acute alcoholic h.
acute toxic h.
acute viral h.
h. A–G virus
alcoholic h.
h. and alcoholism
A-like non-A non-B h.
anicteric viral h.
anicteric virus h.
antibody to hepatitis A–E virus
antibody to hepatitis Be antigen
antibody to hepatitis B core antigen
antibody to hepatitis B surface antigen
Australian hepatitis antigen
Australia serum hepatitis antigen
autoimmune h.
autoimmune chronic active h.
autoimmune chronic h.
autoimmune-type chronic active h.
h. A virus antibody
A virus h.

hepatitis *(continued)*
h. B
h. B_c
h. B_e
h. B antibody
h. B antigen
h. B_e antigen
h. B carrier
h. B core antibody
h. B core antigen
h. B DNA detection
h. B early antibody
h. B early antigen
h. B infection
h. B oligosaccharide-CRM197 vaccine
bound hepatitis antibody
h. B surface
h. B surface antibody
h. B surface antigen
h. B surface associated
h. B virus immunoglobulin
h. C
h. C antiviral long-term treatment to prevent cirrhosis
cholestatic viral h.
chronic active hepatitis B
chronic active hepatitis with cirrhosis
chronic active lupoid h.
chronic active viral h.
chronic active viral hepatitis, non-A, non-B
chronic active viral hepatitis, type B
chronic aggressive h.
chronic hepatitis B
chronic benign h.
chronic hepatitis C
chronic cholestatic h.
chronic hepatitis C infection
chronic interstitial h.
chronic lobular h.
chronic persistent h.
chronic persisting h.
cirrhosis from h.
clinical alcoholic h.
confirmed transmission of viral h.
cryptogenic autoimmune h.
h. C serology
h. C virus enzyme immunoassay
h. C virus RNA
h. D
h. D antigen
h. delta virus
duck hepatitis B
duck hepatitis B virus
h. E
enterically transmitted non-A, non-B h.
equine serum h.
h. F
fibrosing cholestatic h.
food-borne transmission of viral h.
h. from birth control pill
fulminant viral h.
h. G
giant cell h.
goose hepatitis virus
h. G virus RNA
halothane h.
hemodialysis transmission of viral h.
hospital-acquired viral h.
human hepatitis A virus
icteric serum h.
h. infection
infectious h.
infectious canine h.
infectious human h.
h. inoculation
inoculation transmission of viral h.
long incubation h.
loss of appetite from h.
maternal-neonatal transmission of viral h.
mild chronic h.
moderate chronic h.
multiple hepatitis virus infection
murine h.
neonatal cholestatic h.
neonatal giant cell h.
neonatal hepatitis syndrome
non-A–G fulminant h.
non-A hepatitis virus
non-A, non-B h.
non-A non-B h.
non-A, non-B hepatitis virus
non-A, non-B, non-C h.
non-B hepatitis virus
nonviral chronic h.
normal carrier h.
oral transmission of viral h.
parenterally transmitted non-A non-B h.
patient has natural immunity to hepatitis B virus
patient immune to hepatitis B infection
peliosis h.
peripheral blood mononuclear cell hepatitis B virus measurement
persistent chronic h.
persistent viral h.
persistent viral hepatitis, non-A, non-B
persistent viral hepatitis, type B
plasma cell h.
posttransfusion h.
posttransfusion non-A, non-B hepatitis
h. profile
prolonged acute h.
relapsing hepatitis B
secretion spills from hepatitis patients
h. serodiagnosis
serum h.
serum hepatitis antigen
sexual transmission of viral h.
subacute hepatitis with bridging
h. surface antigen studies
tenderness in abdomen due to h.
transfusion transmission of viral h.
transient clinical h.
turkey virus h.
h. vaccine
viral h.
viral hepatitis panel
h. viremia
h. virus
h. virus A, B, IH
virus A h.
virus B h.
h. virus social history
waterborne transmission of viral h.

hepatitis-associated
h.-a. antigen
h.-a. virus

hepatitis-induced liver cancer

hepatitis-infectious mononucleosis

hepatitis-tainted blood

hepatobiliary
h. disease
h. imaging
nuclear hepatobiliary imaging
percutaneous hepatobiliary cholangiography
quantitative hepatobiliary scintigraphy
h. scan
h. tract disease

hepatocatalase peroxidase

hepatocellular
acute hepatocellular necrosis
h. adenoma
advanced hepatocellular carcinoma
h. cancer
h. carcinoma
clear cell hepatocellular carcinoma
h. damage
diffuse hepatocellular degeneration
h. disease
early advanced hepatocellular carcinoma
early hepatocellular carcinoma
h. enzymes
h. failure
fibrolamellar hepatocellular carcinoma
h. injury
h. liver disease
microtrabecular hepatocellular carcinoma
oncocytic hepatocellular tumor
primary hepatocellular carcinoma
transplantable hepatocellular carcinoma
h. tumor
well-differentiated hepatocellular carcinoma

hepatocerebral
acquired hepatocerebral degeneration
alcohol acquired chronic hepatocerebral degeneration

hepatocycle volume fraction

hepatocyte
h. function
h. growth factor
lipid-laden h.
h. nuclear factor
h. nuclear factor-3
h. nuclear factor-4
h. nuclear factor-4a
periportal h.
h. proliferation inhibitor

hepatodiaphragmatic interposition of colon

hepatoencephalomyelitis virus

hepatoerythrocytic porphyria

hepatoerythropoietic porphyria

hepatoiminodiacetic
h. acid
technetium hepatoiminodiacetic acid scan

hepatojejunostomy
palliative h.
pediatric h.
peripheral h.
side-to-side h.

hepatojugular
h. reflex
h. reflex test

hepatolenticular degeneration

hepatoma
ascites h.
h. carcinoma cell
h. cell
h. tissue culture

hepatopathy
paraneoplastic h.

hepatopulmonary syndrome

hepatorenal
h. angle
h. disease
h. failure
h. syndrome

hepatorenale

hepatosis
cholestatic hepatosis of pregnancy

hepatosplenic
primary hepatosplenic lymphoma

hepatosplenomegaly with liver metastases

hepatotoxicity
Amanita mushroom h.
anesthetic h.
anticonvulsant agent h.
antidepressant drug h.
antidiabetic agent h.
antineoplastic drug h.
antipsychotic drug h.
antithyroid drug h.
nutritional h.

hepatotropic portal blood factor

herald patch

herbal
h. medicine
h. remedy
h. supplement
h. therapy
traditional Chinese herbal remedy
traditional Chinese herbal therapy
h. treatment

herb drug interaction

herb-related adverse event

herd
h. immunity
h. instinct

hereditary
h. adenomatosis of colon and rectum
Albright hereditary osteodystrophy
h. angioedema
h. angioneurotic edema
h. ataxia
h. atrophy optic nerve
autosomal dominant hereditary optic neuropathy
autosomal recessive hereditary optic neuropathy
h. benign intraepithelial dyskeratosis
h. bleeding disorder
h. bone disease
h. bone dysplasia
h. breast and ovarian cancer
h. brown enamel
h. capillary fragility
h. cerebellar ataxia
h. cerebral hemorrhage with amyloidosis
h. cerebral leukodystrophy
h. chorea
h. chronic nephritis
chronic progressive hereditary chorea
h. clear cell renal carcinoma
h. colon cancer
congenital hereditary retinoschisis
h. coproporphyria
h. cutaneous malignant melanoma
h. deafness
h. defect
h. diffuse leukoencephalopathy with spheroids
h. disease of nervous system
h. elliptocytosis
h. enamel hypoplasia
h. erythroblastic multinuclearity with positive acidified serum
h. essential tremor
h. factors
h. familial disease
h. familial illness
h. flat adenoma syndrome
h. fructose intolerance
h. heart defect
h. hemochromatosis
h. hemolytic anemia
h. hemolytic anemia test
h. hemolytic syndrome
h. hypertrophic enlargement

hereditary *(continued)*
h. hypophosphatemic rickets with hypercalciuria syndrome
h. insanity
intraepithelial dyskeratosis syndrome, hereditary benign
irreversible hereditary disease
Leber hereditary optic neuropathy
h. motor sensory neuropathy II-deafness-mental retardation
h. motor-sensory neuropathy type IA, II, III–VII
Muir-Torre syndrome of hereditary nonpolyposis colon cancer
h. multifocal relapsing inflammation
h. multiple exostosis
multiple hereditary cutaneomandibular polyoncosis
multiple hereditary exostosis
multiple hereditary hemorrhagic telangiectasis
multiple hereditary osteochondral exostosis
h. nephritic protein
h. neuropathy with liability for pressure palsy
h. neuropathy with susceptibility to pressure palsy
h. nonpolyposis colon cancer
h. nonpolyposis colon carcinoma
h. nonpolyposis colorectal cancer
h. nonpolyposis colorectal carcinoma
h. nonspherocytic
h. nonspherocytic hemolytic anemia
nonsyndromic hereditary hearing impairment
h. onychoosteodysplasia syndrome
h. opalescent dentin
h. optic atrophy
h. osteoonychodysplasia
h. pancreatitis
h. papillary renal cancer
h. papillary renal cell carcinoma
h. persistence of fetal hemoglobin
h. predisposition
h. progressive ataxia
h. prostate cancer 1 locus
h. psychoses
h. pyropoikilocytosis
h. respiratory disease
h. sclerosing poikiloderma
h. sclerosis
h. sensory and autonomic neuropathy types I-IV
h. sensory motor neuropathy type I–III
h. sensory neuropathy
h. site-specific colon cancer
slowly progressive hereditary disorder
h. spastic paraparesis
h. spastic paraplegia
h. spherocytosis
h. tabes
h. tendency

heredity
environment and h.
h. and environment

heredodegeneration
macular h.

Hereford Parental Attitude Survey

Hering
canal of H.
H. law-EOM innervation, both eyes

Hering-Breuer inflation reflex

heritage
Ashkenazi Jewish h.
ethnic h.

hermaphroditism
adrenal h.
male h.
transverse h.

HER-2/neu
HER-2/neu gene
HER-2/neu oncogene
HER-2/neu oncoprotein
HER-2/neu protooncogene

hernia
h. adipose
Allison hiatal hernia repair
Anson-McVay hernia repair
anterior retrosternal hernia of Morgagni
axial hiatal h.
Bassini inguinal hernia repair
Bassini-type hernia repair
bilateral inguinal h.
h. of bladder
congenital diaphragmatic h.
h. of diaphragm
diaphragmatic h.
direct inguinal h.
Effler hiatal hernia repair
esophageal hiatal h.
esophageal hiatus h.
h. of esophagus
fetal congenital diaphragmatic h.
foramen of Morgagni h.
hiatal h.
hiatal hernia and constipation
hiatal hernia repair
high ligation of hernia sac
incarcerated inguinal h.
indirect inguinal h.
inguinal h.
inguinal hernia repair
intraperitoneal onlay mesh hernia repair
h. knife
laparoscopic paraesophageal hernia repair
laparoscopic repair of paraesophageal h.
large inguinal hernia sac
left direct inguinal h.
left femoral h.
left oblique inguinal h.
Lotheissen hernia repair
lower midline scar with h.
h. of lung
Macewen hernia operation
Marcy hernia repair
McVay repair of h.
metachronous contralateral h.'s
microcephaly, hiatus hernia, nephrotic syndrome
Moloney hernia repair
nephrosis, microcephaly, hiatus hernia syndrome
nontender incarcerated inguinal h.
open hernia operation
ovary in inguinal h.
pantaloon inguinal h.
paraesophageal diaphragmatic h.
paraesophageal hiatal h.
paraesophageal hiatus h.
paraesophageal hernia type I, II
pectineal crural h.
posterior labial h.
posterior vaginal h.
h. in recto
h. repair
right direct inguinal h.
right inguinal h.
right oblique inguinal h.
short stature, hyperextensibility of joints or hernia or both, ocular depression, Rieger anomaly, teething, delayed
sliding esophageal hiatal h.
supportive device to restrain h.

total extraperitoneal laparoscopic hernia repair
transabdominal preperitoneal laparoscopic hernia repair
umbilical h.
urinary bladder h.
videoscopic hernia surgery

hernial
h. aneurysm
h. defect
indirect hernial sac
Lichtenstein hernial repair
Marlex hernial repair
pants-over-vest hernial repair
h. protrusion
h. repair
h. sac

herniated
h. bowel
h. cervical disc
h. disc
h. disc syndrome
h. disc syndrome
h. fat pad
h. intervertebral disc
h. lumbar disk
massive herniated disc
h. nucleus pulposus
pain from herniated vertebral disc
vaporize water in herniated disc
h. viscus

herniation
bilateral uncal h.
h. of the brain
cervical disc h.
h. of disc
extraforaminal lumbar disc h.
frank disc h.
free fragment h.
intervertebral disc h.
lumbar disc h.
midline disc h.
h. of muscle
noncontained disc h.
nucleus pulposus h.
h. of nucleus pulposus
traumatic transtentorial h.

hernioplasty
tension-free h.

herniorrhaphy
Anson-McVay femoral h.
anterior inguinal h.
laparoscopic inguinal h.
modified Bassini h.

herniotomy
Petit h.

hero
negative h.

heroic
no heroic measures

heroin
h. addiction
cocaine and h.
H. Emergency Life Project
h., morphine, and cocaine
h. overdose
h. withdrawal

heroin-associated nephropathy

herpes
anal h.
anogenital h.
anorectal h.
h. catarrhalis
h. corneae
dermal or oral h.
disseminated herpes zoster infection
h. esophagitis
h. eye infection
h. facialis
h. family of viruses
h. febrilis
focal herpes of vulva
genital h.
genital herpes infection
genital herpes virus
h. genitalis
h. infection
h. keratitis
keratitis h.
McKrae herpes simplex virus
mucocutaneous herpes simplex
multidermatomal herpes zoster
nasal h.
neonatal h.
neonatal herpes simplex
neonatal herpes simplex virus
neonatal herpes simplex virus infection
ocular h.
ocular herpes infection
ocular herpes simplex
ophthalmic h.
h. ophthalmicus
oral h.
oral herpes lesion
orofacial herpes simplex
orolabial h.
h. oticus
h. pain
penile h.
perianal h.
perinatal h.
h. pneumonia
h. praeputialis
h. progenitalis
recurrent genital h.
recurrent herpes labialis
simian herpes virus
h. simplex
h. simplex antibody titer
h. simplex encephalitis
h. simplex genitalis
h. simplex gingivostomatitis
h. simplex infection
h. simplex keratitis
h. simplex labialis
h. simplex neonatorum
h. simplex pneumonitis
h. simplex retinitis
h. simplex type 1, 2
h. simplex viral shedding
h. simplex virus 1, 2
h. simplex virus encephalitis
h. simplex virus thymidine kinase
h. simplex virus type 1, 2, 6, 7
h. stomatitis
syphilis, toxoplasmosis, other agents, rubella, cytomegalovirus, herpes simplex virus
toxoplasmosis, other infections, rubella, cytomegalovirus infection, herpes simplex syndrome
h. virus of the eye
h. virus vesicles
visceral herpes simplex
h. vulvitis
h. zoster
h. zoster of cornea
h. zoster dermatitis
h. zoster of iris
h. zoster ophthalmicus
h. zoster pain
h. zoster virus
h. zoster virus infection

herpes-associated erythema multiforme

herpes-like
h.-l. lesions
h.-l. virus

herpes-type virus

herpesvirus
antihuman herpesvirus 8 antibody titer

herpesvirus *(continued)*
avian h.
canine h.
cottontail rabbit h.
h. encephalitis
equine h.
Herpesvirus hominis membrane antigen
h. hominis
human herpesvirus 1–8
human herpesvirus 6A
human herpesvirus 8/Kaposi sarcoma h.
h. infection
Kaposi sarcoma h.
h. saimiri
h. sensitivity
h. of turkeys

herpetic
acute herpetic gingival stomatitis
h. fever
h. geniculate ganglionitis
h. gingivitis
h. gingivostomatitis
h. keratitis
h. lesion
h. ocular disease
h. stomatitis
stromal herpetic keratitis
h. stromal keratitis
h. tonsillitis
h. ulcer
h. ulceration
h. vulvovaginitis
whitlow h.

herpetica
pharyngitis h.
stomatitis h.

herpeticum
eczema h.

herpetiform
h. lesion
h. pemphigus

herpetiformis
dermatitis h.

Herrick
von Herrick grading system

herring
red h.

Hertz frequency

Heschl gyrus

hesitancy
patient h.
urinary h.

hesitant speech

Hesselbach
H. fascia
H. hernia
H. ligament
H. triangle

Hess School Readiness Scale

Heston
H. Personality Index
H. Personality Inventory Test

heterochromia
atrophic h.
monocular h.
sympathetic h.

heterochromic
Fuchs heterochromic cyclitis
Fuchs heterochromic iridocyclitis
h. uveitis

heteroconjugate
antilymphocyte h.

heterocyclic
h. antidepressant
h. aromatic amine

heterodimeric luteinizing hormone

heterodisomy
maternal uniparental h.

heteroduplex
h. analysis
directed heteroduplex analysis
h. mobility assay

heterogeneity
allelic h.
genetic h.
lineage h.
locus h.
loss of h.
neurophysiological h.
optical h.

heterogeneous
h. appearance
h. attenuation
h. cation-exchange membrane
genetically h.
h. graft
h. noise
h. nuclear ribonucleic acid
h. nuclear ribonucleoprotein
h. resistance to vancomycin
h. ribonucleic acid

heterogenicity
locus h.
osteoblast h.

heterograft
autogenous fascial h.
bovine h.
porcine h.
stent-mounted heterograft valve

heteronymous
h. diplopia
h. hemianopia
h. hemianopsia
h. motoneurons
h. parallax

heterophil
h. antibody
h. antibody titer
h. transplantation antigen

heteroplasia
osseous h.

heterosexual
H. Attitudes Toward Homosexuality scale
h. behavior
h. development of women
h. intercourse
h. orientation
h. relationship
h. relations scale

heterothyrotropic factor

heterotopia
mesodermal h.
neuronal h.
nodular h.

heterotopic
auxiliary heterotopic liver transplantation
h. cardiac transplant
h. heart transplant
h. kidney transplant
h. ossification
h. pain
paraarticular heterotopic ossification
h. plate count
h. pregnancy
h. stimulus
h. tissue

heterotropia
noncomitant h.
paralytic h.

heterotropic ossification

heterozygosity
h. for hemoglobin A and hemoglobin S
loss of h.
loss of heterozygosity chromosome 10

heterozygous
h. familial hypercholesterolemia
h. ornithine transcarbamylase

Heubner
H. arteritis
artery of H.
H. artery

hex
h. implant
h. screw
h. wrench

hexachloride
gamma-benzene hexachloride

hexachlorocyclohexane
fortified h.

hexafluoride
sulfur h.

hexamethylenamine
h., Adriamycin, melphalan
h., Adriamycin, methotrexate

hexamethylene bisacetamide

hexamethylenetetramine
methenamine h.

hexamethylmelamine
h., Adriamycin, melphalan
h., Adriamycin, methotrexate

hexamethylphosphoric triamide

hexamethylpropylene
technetium-99m hexamethylpropylene amine oxime single-photon emission computed tomography

hexamethylpropyleneamine oxime

hexone-extracted acetone

hexosamine
mucosal hexosamine content

hexosaminidase
h. A
h. B

hexose
h. diphosphate
h. monophosphate
h. monophosphate pathway
h. monophosphate shunt

Heyden antibiotic

Heymann
H. nephritis antigenic complex
passive Heymann nephritis

6-HIAA tumor marker

hiatal
Allison hiatal hernia repair
anterior hiatal sign
axial hiatal hernia
Effler hiatal hernia repair
esophageal hiatal hernia
h. hernia
h. hernia and constipation
h. hernia repair
h. insufficiency
paraesophageal hiatal hernia
sliding esophageal hiatal hernia

hiatus
aortic h.
esophageal h.
esophageal hiatus hernia
h. hernia
maxillary h.
microcephaly, hiatus hernia, nephrotic syndrome
nephrosis, microcephaly, hiatus hernia syndrome
paraesophageal hiatus hernia
patulous h.
pleuropericardial h.
pleuroperitoneal h.
sacral h.
scalene h.
Scarpa h.
semilunar h.

hibernal epidemic viral infection

hibernation
myocardial h.

Hibernian
familial Hibernian fever

Hickman
H. catheter
H. line

hidden
h. agenda
h. meaning
h. rage
h. testis

hidradenitis
axillary h.
axillary hidradenitis suppurativa
neutrophilic eccrine h.
palmoplantar eccrine h.
h. suppurativa

hidradenoma
malignant nodular h.
nodular h.
papillary h.

hidrocystoma
apocrine h.

hiemalis
arthritis h.

hierarchy
anxiety h.
lifetime h.
motivational h.
occupational h.

high
h. abdominal plain film
abnormally high concentration of urine
abnormally high content
achieve high dose
h. acid level in blood
h. air flow with oxygen entrainment
h. altitude-related disorder
h. altitude-related sickness
h. amplitude
h. anxiety
h. arch deformity
h. arousal
h. beam intensity
h. biological value protein
h. birth weight
h. bladder pressure
h. blood alcohol level
h. blood cholesterol
h. blood pressure
borderline high blood pressure
Bryan high titer
h. bulk diet
h. caloric
h. caloric density
h. calorie
h. calorie and nitrogen
h. cell passage
h. cholesterol level
h. cholesterol and tocopherol deficient
h. cholesterol and tocopherol supplemented
chronic high blood pressure
h. clotting risk
h. concentration
congenital high airway obstruction syndrome
controlled high blood pressure
h. cure rate
daily high fiber supplement
h. death rate
h. definition power
h. degree of risk
delirium with high fever
h. density
diet high in fiber
h. dosage
h. dose
h. dose rate

high *(continued)*
h. dose rate brachytherapy
h. dry field
extra high potency
extremely high factor
extremely high frequency
fast-repeating high sequence
h. flow
h. forceps delivery
fractionated high dose rate
h. fracture risk
h. frequency
h. frequency band
h. frequency of recording
h. functioning
General H. Altitude Questionnaire
h. genetic risk
h. glucose
h. grade
h. heparin dose
h. impulsiveness
h. impulsiveness, high anxiety
h. impulsiveness, low anxiety
h. incision
h. index of suspicion
inherited high cholesterol
h. intermittent suction
h. intracranial pressure
intraoperative high dose rate
h. irradiance response
h. jugular bulb
h. lateral tension
h. level of anxiety
h. level of arousal
h. level of care
h. level of function
h. level of kidney protein rennin
h. ligation
h. ligation of hernia sac
h. ligation and stripping
h. linear energy transfer radiation
low impulsiveness, high anxiety
low probability, high consequence event
h. lung volume
h. medical-social risk
h. membranous interventricular septum
h. methacholine sensitivity
h. mobility group
h. molecular weight
h. molecular weight component
h. molecular weight dextran
h. molecular weight glycoprotein
h. molecular weight hemoglobin
h. molecular weight kininogen
h. molecular weight melanoma-associated antigen
h. molecular weight polyethylene
h. myopia
h. occlusion
organisms per high power field
h. oxygen
h. oxygen concentrate
h. oxygen percentage
h. oxygen percentage in retinopathy of prematurity
h. oxygen pressure
oxygen under high pressure
h. partial pressure of oxygen
h. pass filter
patient on a h.
periodic bursts of high voltage
h. permeability edema
h. peroxide-containing cell
h. potency
precision high dose
primary high blood pressure
h. probability of survival
h. profile
reduced hearing at high frequency
h. regional wall motion velocity
h. resolution
h. right atrium
h. right atrium electrocardiogram
h. right parasternal view
h. risk
h. risk for breast cancer
h. risk for breast cancer
h. risk of developing cervical cancer
h. risk of HIV
h. risk of HIV infection
h. risk of suicide
h. saphenous vein ligation
H. School Personality Questionnaire
secondary high blood pressure
h. self-expectation
h. serum-bound iron
h. single dose alternate day
h. soapsuds enema
h. spinal anesthesia
square waves of high frequency
super high frequency
super high speed
h. temperature-short time pasteurization
h. testis
h. thoracic cord lesion
h. tibial osteotomy
h. titer, low acidity
h. tone
h. toxicity
h. tracheotomy
h. transection
uncontrolled high blood pressure
h. vacuum
very high density lipoprotein
very high dose phenobarbital
very high frequency
h. vitamin

high-affinity
p55 component of the high-affinity interleukin-2

high-affinity choline transport

high-altitude
h.-a. cerebral edema
h.-a. headache
h.-a. hypertrophic cardiomyopathy syndrome
h.-a. illness
h.-a. pulmonary edema
h.-a. retinal hemorrhage
h.-a. retinopathy
h.-a. simulation test

high-amplitude
continuous high-amplitude electroencephalogram rhythmical synchronous slowing
h.-a. contraction
hyperventilation-induced high-amplitude rhythmic slowing
h.-a. peristalsis
h.-a. sucking technique

high-anxiety sensitivity

high-arched palate

high-beam intensity

high-calorie diet

high-carbohydrate
h.-c. diet
h.-c., high-fiber diet
h.-c., low-fiber diet

high-definition
h.-d. image
h.-d. imaging
h.-d. video display

high-density
h.-d. bile
h.-d. humidity
h.-d. lipoprotein C
h.-d. lipoprotein-cell surface receptor
h.-d. lipoprotein-cholesterol
h.-d. nebulizer
h.-d. polyethylene

high-dose
h.-d. arm
h.-d. aspirin therapy
h.-d. beam of x-rays
h.-d. chemotherapy
h.-d. chemotherapy and stem cell rescue
h.-d. depth
h.-d. external irradiation
h.-d. fractional radiation therapy
h.-d. fractionation radiation therapy
h.-d. group
h.-d. immunosuppressive therapy
h.-d. infusion
h.-d. intravenous methylprednisolone
h.-d. methotrexate
h.-d. methotrexate and cisplatin
h.-d. methotrexate and 5-fluorouracil
h.-d. methylprednisolone
h.-d. morphine
h.-d. radiation
h.-d. radiation therapy
h.-d. radiation to tumor mass
h.-d. thrombin time
h.-d. urea in invert sugar

high-efficiency
h.-e. particulate air filter
h.-e. particulate arresting

high-endothelial venule

high-energy
h.-e. accelerator
h.-e. behavior
h.-e. bent beam linear accelerator
h.-e. cardioversion
h.-e. electron
h.-e. intermediate
h.-e. ionizing radiation
h.-e. ion scattering
h.-e. phosphate
h.-e. pulsed ruby laser
h.-e. radiation
h.-e. transthoracic shock
h.-e. transurethral microwave thermotherapy

higher
h. air pressure
h. brain center
h. cerebral dysfunction
h. cognitive function
h. cortical dysfunction
h. cortical function
head higher than heart
h. integrative function
h. intellectual function
legs elevated higher than heart
h. level skill
h. mental function
h. rate
h. than

highest
h. asymptomatic dose
h. common factor
h. equivalent heart rate
h. functional level
h. intercostal vein
h. level of activity
h. nontoxic dose
h. occupied molecular orbital
h. risk for disease

high-fat
h.-f. food
h.-f., high-cholesterol diet
h.-f., low-fiber diet

high-fiber diet

high-filter frequency

high-flow
h.-f. nasal cannula
h.-f. oxygen conserver

high-frequency
h.-f. activity
h.-f. audiometry
h.-f. blood group
h.-f. chest wall compression
h.-f. chest wall oscillation
h.-f. contralateral routing of offside signals
h.-f. current
h.-f. deafness
h.-f. discharges
h.-f. Doppler
h.-f. epicardial echocardiography
h.-f. filter
h.-f. filter control
h.-f. jet ventilator
liquid-assisted high-frequency oscillatory ventilation
h.-f. murmur
h.-f. oscillation ventilation
h.-f. oscillation ventilator
h.-f. oscillatory
h.-f. oscillatory ventilation
h.-f. percussive ventilation
h.-f. positive pressure
h.-f. positive-pressure ventilation
h.-f. recombination
h.-f. response
h.-f. sensorineural hearing loss
h.-f. sound wave
h.-f. stimulation
h.-f. thrombolysis
h.-f. transduction
h.-f. transfer
h.-f. ultrasound probe sonography
h.-f. ventilation trial

high-fruit/vegetable diet

high-functioning
h.-f. autism
h.-f. patient

high-grade
h.-g. astrocytoma
h.-g. defect
h.-g. dysplasia
h.-g. dysplastic adenoma
h.-g. lesion
h.-g. obstruction
h.-g. squamous intraepithelial lesion
h.-g. stenosis
h.-g. tumor

high-humidity
h.-h. face mask
h.-h. tracheostomy collar
h.-h. tracheostomy mask
h.-h. tracheostomy shield

high-impact
h.-i. activity
h.-i. aerobic dance
h.-i. aerobic exercise
h.-i. exercise

high-input impedance

high-intensity
h.-i. exercise
h.-i. focused ultrasonography
h.-i. focused ultrasound
h.-i. lesion
h.-i. light source
h.-i. transient signal
h.-i. zone

high-jumper's strain

Highlands J virus

high-level
h.-l. disinfection
h.-l. gentamicin resistance

highly
h. active antiretroviral therapy
h. active antiretroviral treatment
h. activity epileptic process
h. addictive
h. addictive and isolated monocomponent highly purified pork insulin
h. motivated
patient highly compulsive
h. permeable transparent dressing

highly *(continued)*
h. probably drunk
h. prone to fantasy
h. purified
h. reactive oxygen molecules
salvage highly active antiretroviral therapy
h. selective vagotomy

high-lying thyroid gland

Highmore
antrum of H.
antrum cardiacum of H.

high-osmolar
h.-o. contrast agent
h.-o. contrast medium
h.-o. contrast agent

high-osmolarity contrast medium

high-output
h.-o. heart failure
h.-o. renal failure

high-pass filter

high-performance
h.-p. capillary electrophoresis
h.-p. chromatofocusing
h.-p. ion exchange chromatography
h.-p. liquid chromatography
h.-p. membrane chromatography
h.-p. size-exclusion chromatography

high-pH anion exchange chromatography coupled with pulsed amperometric detection

high-pitched
h.-p. bowel sound
h.-p. cry
h.-p. murmur
h.-p. voice
h.-p. wheezing

high-potency vitamin

high-potential iron protein

high-power
h.-p. field
h.-p. field microscope
h.-p. liquid chromatography

high-powered magnification

high-pressure
h.-p. chamber
h.-p. liquid affinity chromatography
h.-p. neurologic syndrome
h.-p. oxygen
h.-p. treatment
h.-p. zone

high-profile research

high-protein
h.-p. diet
h.-p. supplement

high-purity germanium

high-quality
h.-q. care
h.-q. and effective treatment
h.-q. medical care

high-renin essential hypertension

high-residue diet

high-resolution
h.-r. brain SPECT
h.-r. chromatography
h.-r. computed tomography
h.-r. computed tomography scan
h.-r. CT
h.-r. CT imaging
h.-r. CT mammography
h.-r. CT scan
h.-r. electrocardiography
h.-r. endoluminal sonography
h.-r. fingerprint
h.-r. infrared imaging
h.-r. light microscopy
h.-r. MRI
h.-r. multisweep
h.-r. protein electrophoresis
h.-r. transmission electron microscopy
h.-r. ultrasound

high-riding bladder

high-risk
h.-r. adolescent population
h.-r. angioplasty
h.-r. baby
h.-r. behavior
h.-r. breast cancer
h.-r. candidate
h.-r. category
h.-r. factor
h.-r. followup
h.-r. group
h.-r. of HIV infection
h.-r. infant
h.-r. lifestyle
h.-r. model of threat perception
h.-r. mother
h.-r. patient
h.-r. population
h.-r. potential victims
h.-r. pregnancy
h.-r. primary breast cancer
h.-r. procedure
h.-r. recipient
h.-r. register
h.-r. sexual activity
h.-r. sexual behavior
h.-r. transfer

high-salt diet

high-spatial-resolution cine computed tomography

high-speed
h.-s. air drill
h.-s. bur
h.-s. drill
h.-s. engine
h.-s. handpiece
h.-s. liquid chromatography
h.-s. rotational atherectomy
h.-s. supernatant
h.-s. volumetric imaging

high-strength pancreatic enzymes

high-stress
h.-s. job
h.-s. workout

high-strung
patient h.-s.

high-tension
h.-t. glaucoma
h.-t. pulse

high-throughput screening

high-tone hearing loss

high-velocity
h.-v. electron beam
h.-v. lead therapy
h.-v. low-amplitude

high-viscosity barium and air

high-voltage
h.-v. activity
h.-v. arrhythmic slow wave
h.-v. brain wave
h.-v. burst
h.-v. can
h.-v. diphasic slow wave
h.-v. electron microscope
h.-v. electrophoresis
h.-v. fast activity
h.-v. firing
h.-v. paper electrophoresis
paroxysmal high-voltage discharge
h.-v. pattern
h.-v. pulsed current
h.-v. pulsed galvanic stimulation
h.-v. slow activity
h.-v. slow-wave activity

h.-v. transformer
h.-v. transmission electron microscopy

high-volume
h.-v. evacuator
h.-v., low-pressure

hilar
h. adenopathy
anthracotic hilar node
bilateral hilar adenopathy
bilateral hilar infiltrates
bilateral hilar lymphadenopathy
calcified hilar node
h. cell
h. clouding
h. dance
h. fullness
h. haze
h. infiltrate
left hilar lymph node
h. lesion
h. lymphadenopathy
h. lymph node
h. mass
h. node metastasis
ovarian hilar cell tumor
h. prominence
h. region
right hilar lymph node
h. scarring
h. shadow
h. structure
h. substance of lung
h. vasculature
h. vessels exposed

Hill
Edge Hill virus
H. Interaction Matrix
Prospect Hill virus

hillock
seminal h.

Hill-Sachs lesion

Hilson Personnel Profile/Success Quotient

Hilton Drinking Behavior Questionnaire

hilum
h. of kidney
h. of lung
h. of ovary
prominence of right h.
pulmonary h.
renal h.
h. of spleen
splenic h.

hilus
kidney h.
liver h.
lung h.
neurovascular h.
renal h.

Himmelsbach Rating Scale

hind
h. leg paralysis
tonic hind limb extension

hindfoot
h. deformity
equinovarus hindfoot deformity
h. fracture
h. instability
h. motion
h. orthosis
h. pronation
h. supination
varus h.
varus hindfoot deformity

hinge
angular hinge clamp
h. articulation
h. axis
flexible hinge implant
flexor hinge orthosis
flexor hinge splint
h. joint
Malis hinge clamp

hinged knee brace

hint
newborn helpful h.'s

Hinton flocculation test for syphilis

hip
h. abduction
abduction contracture of h.
active hip movement
adduction contracture of h.
adductor spasticity of h.
h. adductor stretch exercise
Albee hip arthrodesis
alumina-alumina total hip replacement prosthesis
alumina cemented total hip prosthesis
anatomic medullary locking hip system
anterior hip dislocation
anterior hip release
anthropometric total h.
APR hip stem
arm girth, chest depth, and hip width
h. arthritis
arthrodesis of h.
h. arthroplasty
artificial hip joint
Atlanta hip brace
Aufranc concentric hip mold
biologically designed h.
bipolar hip arthroplasty
bipolar hip replacement
bipolar hip replacement prosthesis
h. bone
h. bump
cannulated hip screw
cementless total hip arthroplasty
cementless total hip replacement
ceramic total h.
h. click
click heard at hip joint
compression hip screw
congenital dislocation of h.
congenital dislocation h.
congenital dysplasia of h.
congenital hip disease
congenital hip dislocation
congenital hip displacement
congenital hip dysplasia
congenital hip subluxation
h. contracture
Crawford-Adams hip arthroplasty
cup-on-cup arthroplasty of the h.
h. deformity
developmental dysplasia of h.
h. disarticulation
h. dislocation
dual lock total hip replacement
dynamic hip screw
h. dysplasia
h. extension
h. fixation
h. flexed
h. flexion
flexion contracture of h.
h. flexion-extension
h. fracture
Gant hip arthrodesis
h. girdle
h. guidance orthosis
Harris hip score
intercondylar fracture of h.
internal rotation contracture of h.
ischemic disease of the growing h.
h. joint
h. joint angle
Link anatomical h.
h. lipectomy
Lorenz hip reduction

hip *(continued)*
marked degenerative change of h.
Matchett-Brown hip arthroplasty
Mayo Clinic hip scoring system
McKay hip procedure
medial hip rotation
medial hip rotation in extension
medial snapping hip syndrome
Mensor-Scheck hanging hip operation
Merle d'Aubigné hip score
Merle d'Aubigné and Postel hip rating scale
metal-on-metal hip replacement
metal-on-plastic hip replacement
h. mobility
modified Harris hip score
Moore hip endoprosthesis system
h. motion
Mueller hip arthroplasty
h. musculature
h. nailing
neurogenic dysplasia of h.
neurogenic hip disease
neurogenic hip dysplasia
neutral hip position
Newport hip system
orbicular zone of h.
h. orthosis
h. osteoarthritis
osteoarthritis of the h.
h. pain
P.C.A. E-Series hip replacement
h. and pelvis
pelvis and h.
h. pinning
h. pointer
h. prosthesis
reconstructive hip surgery
h. reduction
repeat hip replacement surgery
h. replacement
h. replacement surgery
revision hip arthroplasty
revision hip replacement surgery
h. roll
h. rotation
h. rotation test
self-articulating femoral hip replacement
h. snapping
h. spica
h. spica cast
h. stiffness
synovial fold of h.
total hip articular replacement by internal eccentric shells
total hip prosthesis
total hip replacement operation
total hip replacement procedure
transient osteoporosis of h.
trunk and hip flexibility

hip-associated bursitis

hip-knee-ankle-foot orthosis

hip-knee-ankle orthosis

hip-knee orthosis splint

Hippel
Lindau-von Hippel disease

hippocampal
anterior hippocampal activation
h. complex
h. gyrus
h. pyramidal cell
h. sclerosis
h. synaptic plasma membrane
h. volume loss

hippocampus
dorsal h.
h. major
h. minor

Hippocratic oath

Hippuran
radioactive Hippuran test

hippurate
methenamine h.

hippuric acid

Hipputope renal function

Hirschberg
H. method
H. reflex
H. test

Hirschfeld canal

Hirschsprung-associated enterocolitis

Hirschsprung disease

hirsutism
amenorrhea and h.
h., androgen excess, insulin resistance, acanthosis nigricans syndrome
family history of h.
idiopathic h.

hirudin
recombinant h.

His
angle of H.
atrioventricular node of H.
atrioventricular opening of H.
H. band
H. bundle
bundle of H.
H. bundle ablation
H. bundle activity
H. bundle branch block
H. bundle deflection
H. bundle depolarization
H. bundle electrocardiogram
H. bundle electrode
H. bundle electrogram
H. bundle electrogram deflection
H. bundle electrogram, distal
H. bundle electrogram, proximal
H. bundle heart block
H. bundle recording
H. canal
deflection in His bundle in electrogram
direct His bundle pacing
gastroesophageal angle of H.
isthmus of H.
H. perivascular space
H. rule
space of H.
H. spindle
ventricular atrial His bundle electrocardiogram

Hiskey-Nebraska Test of Learning Aptitude

Hispanic
H. American
H. female
H. male
National Alliance for Hispanic Health
National Association for Hispanic Elderly

His-Purkinje
H.-P. conduction
H.-P. fiber
H.-P. system
H.-P. tissue

histamine
h. antagonist
augmented histamine test
h. cephalalgia
h. challenge
h. challenge test
h. dihydrochloride
h. equivalent prick
h. headache
h. inhalation test
h. inhibitory releasing factor
intravenous histamine test
h. ion transfer

leukocyte histamine release test
h. methyltransferase
h. phosphate
h. provocation test
h. receptor type 1
h. releasing factor
h. shock
h. stimulation test
subcutaneous histamine test
h. test
total decreased h.

histamine-2
h.-2 blocker
h.-2 receptor
h.-2 receptor antagonist

histamine-containing neuron

histamine-forming capacity

histamine-induced suppressor factor

histamine-releasing activity

histamine-sensitizing factor

His-Tawara node

histidine
h. decarboxylase
fragile histidine triad
peptide histidine methionine

histidine-rich
h.-r. calcium-binding protein
h.-r. protein-II

histiocyte
palisading h.
sea-blue h.

histiocytic
h. cytophagic panniculitis
diffuse histiocytic lymphoma of stomach
familial histiocytic dermatoarthritis
h. fibroma
Hodgkin disease of diffuse histiocytic lymphocyte depleted type
h. hyperplasia of lymph node
h. leukemia
h. lymphoma
malignant histiocytic lymphoma
malignant lymphoma, h.
h. medullary reticulosis
mononuclear histiocytic portal infiltrate
h. necrotizing lymphadenitis
nodular and h.
true histiocytic lymphoma

histiocytoma
aneurysmal benign fibrous h.
angiomatoid fibrous h.
angiomatoid malignant fibrous h.
ankle-type fibrous h.
atypical benign fibrous h.
atypical fibrous h.
cellular cutaneous fibrous h.
congenital fibrous h.
malignant fibrous h.
malignant fibrous histiocytoma of bone
malignant fibrous histiocytoma of soft tissue
h. of soft tissue

histiocytosis
benign cephalic h.
congenital self-healing h.
Langerhans cell h.
lipochrome histiocytosis disease
malignant h.
malignant histiocytosis of intestine
nodular non-X h.
regressing atypical h.
sinus h.
sinus histiocytosis with massive lymphadenopathy

histochemistry
in situ hybridization h.

histocompatibility
h. antigen
antimajor histocompatibility complex
hemopoietic h.
h. leukocyte antigen
h. locus
h. locus antigen
major histocompatibility complex antigen
major histocompatibility complex class I
major histocompatibility complex class II
major histocompatibility complex haplotype
major histocompatibility complex restriction
major histocompatibility region
major histocompatibility system
major histocompatibility type
minor histocompatibility antigen
minor histocompatibility complex
net histocompatibility ratio
peptide major histocompatibility complex

histoculture drug response assay

histocytic hyperplasia of lymph nodes

histocytoid hemangioma-like lesion

histogram
average diffusivity h.
dose-volume h.
joint interval h.
poststimulus time h.
time interval h.

histograph
poststimulus time h.

histoincompatibility
maternal-fetal h.

histologic
h. activity index
h. analysis
h. anatomy
h. appearance
h. architecture
h. confirmation
h. diagnosis
h. evaluation
h. examination
h. factor
h. lesion
h. morphology
Mostofi histologic typing
no histologic abnormalities
nonspecific histologic pattern
h. section
h. section of ganglion
h. technologist

histological
benign pheochromocytoma with histological invasion
h. diagnosis

histologically
h. benign
h. detectable iron
h. malignant

histologic/histochemical
Mankin histologic/histochemical scale

histology
aggressive histology lymphoma
h. and cytology
favorable h.
lymph node h.
mineralized bone h.
mixed histology tumor
tumor h.

histone
h. acetyltransferase
deoxyribonucleic acid, h.

histone-reactive antinuclear antibody

histopathologic
myxoid histopathologic subtype
no histopathologic abnormality

histopathological study

histopathologic examination

histoplasma
Histoplasma capsulatum antigen
Histoplasma capsulatum polysaccharide antigen
h. tissue inhibitory factor
h. tissue inhibitory factor

histoplasmin skin test

histoplasmosis
disseminated h.
h. of lung
macular ocular histoplasmosis syndrome
presumed ocular histoplasmosis syndrome
progressive disseminated h.
pseudopresumed ocular histoplasmosis syndrome

historian
poor h.

Historical Information Form

historic control trial

history
h. of abuse
h. activity index
agoraphobia without history of panic disorder
alcohol-positive h.
Automated Child/Adolescent Social H.
Automated Child/Adolescent Social H.
automated medical h.
birth h.
h. of blackouts
Brief Life History Inventory
case h.
h. of chief complaint
complete psychosocial h.
comprehensive assessment of symptoms and h.
comprehensive medical h.
detailed medical h.
developmental h.
diagnostic, social and addiction history form
familial diabetic h.
family h.
family history of cancer
family history of diabetes
family history of hirsutism
family history of mental illness
family history negative
family history noncontributory
family history not remarkable
family history of obesity
family history positive
family history research diagnostic criteria
family medical h.
family ocular h.
family psychiatric h.
formal developmental h.
Giannetti Online Psychosocial H.
heart disease h.
h. of heart disease
hepatitis virus social h.
h., physical, impression, and plan
h. of interpersonal difficulty
interval h.
Life Interpersonal H. Enquiry
long smoking h.
Maastricht History and Advice Checklist-Revised
h. of maladjustment
marital h.
medical h.
medical history as screening device for drug abuse
medical history review
h. of medical illness
menstrual h.
natural history of congestive heart failure
h. of needle sharing
h. of neglect
neuro-ophthalmologic case h.
no medical health h.
no medical ocular h.
noncontributory family h.
noncontributory past h.
noncontributory past medical h.
no previous h.
occupational h.
ocular h.
h. of
h. of presenting problem
packs per year h.
past dental h.
past history noncontributory
past history not remarkable
past medical h.
past medical history noncontributory
past medical history unremarkable
past ocular h.
past pertinent h.
past relevant h.
past social h.
past surgical h.
h. of pathological use
pathophysiology and natural h.
patient's chemical h.
patient's drug h.
patient's medical h.
personal h.
personal history of depressive disorders
personal and social h.
h. and physical
h. and physical examination
h., physical, impression, and plan
positive family h.
post h.
h. of present complaint
h. of present illness
previous h.
previous psychiatric h.
programmed medical h.
psychiatric family h.
psychological history as screening device
Psychosocial H. Screening Questionnaire
Psychosocial H. Screening Test
h. of research
schizophrenia family h.
schizophrenia non-family h.
sexual abuse h.
social h.
social history as screening device for drug abuse
h. of stroke
h. of suicide attempt
surgical h.
h. and symptoms of emergency cardiac care
h. of tobacco use
unfavorable h.

histrionic
h. patient
h. personality
h. personality disorder
h. personality trait

hit
pedestrian hit by motor vehicle

hitchhiker's thumb

Hitzig girdle

HIV
adult/adolescent spectrum of HIV disease
antibodies to H.

H. antibody
carrier of H.
congenital HIV infection
H. Dementia Scale
H. encephalitis
H. encephalopathy
high risk of H.
high risk of HIV infection
high-risk of HIV infection
Hodgkin disease and HIV infection
H. human immunodeficiency virus-associated dementia
H. immunoglobulin
infected with H.
H. infection
macrophage-tropic HIV strain
morphine-potentiated HIV replication
H. nucleocapsid protein
PCR for HIV DNA
perinatal HIV transmission
H. positive
H. prevention and control
H. retinopathy
H. screening
H. seroconversion
H. serology
H. seropositivity
symptomatic HIV infection
H. test
H. therapy

HIV-associated
HIV-a. cognitive disorder
HIV-a. dementia

hive
exercise-induced h.'s
giant h.

HIV-inducing factor

HIV-infected blood

HIV-tainted blood

hoarse
h. cry
h. voice

hoarseness
chest pain with h.
nagging cough and h.
pain with h.
persistent h.
progressive h.

hobbling gait

Hoboken
H. nodule
H. valve

hoc
ad h.

hockey-stick
h.-s. deformity
h.-s. dissector
h.-s. fracture
h.-s. incision

Hodgkin
Ann Arbor classification of Hodgkin disease staging
Ann Arbor Hodgkin lymphoma stage I, IE, II, IIE, IIIE, IIIS, IIISE, IV
H. cell
classic Hodgkin lymphoma
H. cycle
H. disease
H. disease of diffuse histiocytic lymphocyte depleted type
H. disease and HIV infection
H. disease, mixed nodular type
H. disease, nodular sclerosis
H. disease, recurrent
H. disease in relapse
H. disease staging
H. granuloma
lymphocyte predominance Hodgkin disease
lymphocyte-rich classic H.
lymphocytic nodular Hodgkin disease
H. lymphoma
mixed cellular Hodgkin disease
mixed cellularity Hodgkin disease
nodular sclerosing Hodgkin disease
H. sarcoma

Hodgkin-like growth

Hodgkin-Reed-Sternberg cell

Hodkinson Mental Test

Hoechst Marion Roussel stain

Hoeve
Van der Hoeve syndrome

Hoffa
H. fat pad
H. operation

Hoffmann
H. phenomenon
H. reflex
H. sign

Hofmeister
anion of the Hofmeister series

hog
h. gastric mucin
h. intrinsic factor concentrate

Hohmann
modified Hohmann bunionectomy

Hoke
H. triple arthrodesis

hold
ability to hold head up
h. breakfast
h. breakfast for blood work
clot to h.
loss of ability to hold head up
mental health h.
sample and h.
type and h.

holder
arm h.
beam aligning h.
blade-type h.
bone h.
broach h.
cup h.
cup holder handle
curved microneedle h.
endoscope h.
endoscopic in-line needle h.
knee h.
limb h.
McPherson needle h.
needle h.
needle holder clamp
neurosurgery needle h.
pin h.
tube h.

holding
h. area
breath h.
h. chamber
endoscope holding clamp
knot holding capacity
liquid holding recovery
low-temperature holding pasteurization
postoperative holding area
preoperative holding area
valved holding chamber

hole
anchor h.
angiographic end hole catheter
atrophic h.
bur h.
bur holes drilled in skull
drill h.
guide h.
macular h.
macular hole surgery
Murphy h.
nosologic black h.

hole *(continued)*
offset drill h.
operculated h.
parallel hole collimation
retinal h.
sponge-like holes in brain

hole-in-one technique

holiday
h. anxiety
h. depression
dobutamine h.
h. heart
h. heart syndrome

holistic
h. approach
h. healing
h. health
h. health spa
h. medicine
natural holistic technique
h. orthogonal parameter estimation
h. perspective

hollow
Dow Hollow Fiber kidney
Dow hollow fiber dialyzer
h. enzyme
feels hollow and empty
h. fiber dialyzer
h. filter dialyzer
h. needle
h. organ
h. sphere prosthesis
h. viscus injury
h. viscus organ

hollow-sphere
h.-s. implant
h.-s. implant material

holmium
h. laser
h. laser resection of the prostate
h. YAG laser
h. yttrium-aluminum garnet laser

holmium:yttrium
noncontact holmium:yttrium-argon-garnet laser thermal keratoplasty

holmium:yttrium-aluminum-garnet

holocarboxylase synthetase

holography
computerized tomographic h.
volumetric multiple exposure transmission h.

holoprosencephaly
agnathia h.

holosystolic murmur

Holter
ambulatory Holter monitor
ambulatory Holter monitoring
CardioData MK-3 Holter scanner
channel 3 Holter monitor
3-channel Holter monitor
H. diary
H. monitor
H. monitor evaluation
H. shunt
H. technology
H. tube
H. valve

Holtzman Inkblot Technique

Holzknecht unit

homatropine methylbromide

home
adult foster h.
AIDS group h.
h. assessment
h. birth
h. blood glucose meter
h. blood glucose monitor
h. blood glucose monitoring
h. blood pressure measurement
h. blood pressure monitoring
h. blood sugar monitoring
h. cardiorespiratory monitor
h. care
h. care assistance
h. care bereavement
h. care instruction
h. cervical traction unit
h. chemotherapy program
Collaborative H. Infant Monitoring Evaluation
h. collection
community nursing h.
continuous home care
contract nursing h.
coordinate home care
h. dialysis
h. enteral nutrition
h. enteral tube feeding
h. environment
evaluate safety and stability at h.
h. evaluation
h. evaluation prior to discharge
h. exercise program
exercises for patient in h.
foster home care
foster home evaluation
foster home placement
funeral home arrangements
funeral home notification
h. health
h. health aide
h. healthcare
h. health care
h. health nurse
h. health visit
h. help
h. hemodialysis
impaired home maintenance management
H. Incapacity Scale
independent progressive home exercise program
h. infusion device
h. infusion therapy
h. intravenous antibiotic therapy
life-care at h.
h. management
Masimo SET home monitor
h. medical equipment
h. medical test kit
h. modification
h. monitoring
National Association for H. Care
h. nebulizer
h., no services needed
h. nursing
nursing h.
h. nursing care
nursing home care
nursing home care unit
nursing home placement
nursing home transfer
h. nutrition therapy
H. Observation for Measurement of the Environment
h. oxygen
h. oxygen therapy
palliative home care
h. parenteral antibiotic therapy
patient discharged to home care
patient discharged to nursing h.
patient's home environment
patient transferred to nursing h.
h. peritoneal dialysis
personal care h.
personal care boarding h.
h. pregnancy test
progressive home exercise program
h. prothrombin time monitoring
rebellion in h.
residential care h.
rest h.
routine home care
h. setting
simplified nocturnal home hemodialysis

take home pack
therapeutic home pass
therapeutic home trial visit
h. therapist
h. total parenteral nutrition
traditional home care
transfer to nursing h.
h. treatment
h. uterine activity monitor
h. uterine activity monitoring
h. uterine monitoring
h. versus against advice
h. with advice
written home exercise program

home-automated peritoneal dialysis

home-based
h.-b. hospital care
h.-b. telemetry

homebound
h. individual
h. needs
h. patient
h. person

home-care aide

home-delivered meal

homeless
h. child
h. children
h. family
h. person
h. population

homeobox
h. gene
Rathke pouch homeobox transcription factor
short stature homeobox gene

homeopathic
h. drug
magnetically influenced homeopathic remedy
h. medicine
h. remedy
h. symbol for decimal scale of potencies
h. therapy
h. treatment

homeostasis
electrolyte balance and h.
mineral h.
osmotic h.
osseous h.
physiologic h.

homeostatic
calcium homeostatic mechanism
h. thymus hormone

homeotic
paired box homeotic 3 gene
paired box homeotic 8 gene

home-related activity

Homes-Rahe Scale

homicidal
h. behavior
h. ideation
h. insanity
h. intent
h. plan
h. risk
h. state
suicidal or homicidal feeling
h. tendency
h. thought

homing
lymphocyte homing receptor

hominis
herpesvirus h.
Herpesvirus hominis membrane antigen
Mycoplasma hominis bacteremia
poliovirus h.

homocholic
selenium-labeled homocholic acid conjugated with taurine

homochronous insanity

homocysteine
total homocysteine level

homocysteine level

homocystinemia
methylmalonic acidemia with h.

homocystinuria
adult-onset combined methylmalonic aciduria and h.

homogenate
liver h.
lung h.
whole h.

homogeneous
contour-clamped homogeneous electric field
h. enzyme immunoassay
lipid-laden homogeneous adrenocortical carcinoma
h. staining region of chromosome

homogenous
h. bone graft
h. graft
h. immersion
h. transplant

homogentisic
h. acid

homograft
antibiotic-sterilized aortic valve h.
aortic root h.
h. cadaver
cryopreserved aortic h.
cryopreserved homograft valve
h. implant
h. implant material
h. incus prosthesis
h. reaction
h. rejection

homolog
meniscus h.
murine h.

homologous
h. antigen
h. antiserum
h. artificial insemination
artificial insemination, h.
h. canine distemper antiserum
h. graft
h. leukocyte antibody
mammalian achaete-scute homologous protein-2
h. serotype
h. serum
h. serum jaundice
h. tetanus immune globulin

homologue
phosphatase and tensin homologue deleted on chromosome
TNF-weak h.

homonymous
h. diplopia
h. hemianopia
h. hemianopsia
left homonymous hemianopia
h. motoneurons
h. parallax
partial homonymous field defect
right homonymous hemianopia

homophobia
pathological h.

homoplasmy
mutant h.

homosexual
h. activity
acute homosexual panic
h. anal intercourse
h. community

homosexual *(continued)*
h. male
male homosexual contact
h. neurosis
h. panic
h. patient
h. relationship
sexually active homosexual men
h. transmission

homosexuality
Heterosexual Attitudes Toward H. scale
latent h.
male h.
masked h.
overt h.

homotransplantation
renal h.

homovanillic acid

homozygosity for hemoglobin S

homozygous
h. familial hypercholesterolemia
h. for sickle cell hemoglobin
h. typing cell

Honan pressure reducer

hone
automatic h.

honest significance difference

honey
mad honey intoxication

honeybee
Africanized honeybee sting
h. venom

honeycomb
h. appearance
h. lesion
h. lung
h. pattern

honeycombed
h. appearance
h. bone

honeymoon cystitis

honk
goose honk murmur
precordial h.
systolic h.

honking murmur

hood
cervicovaginal h.
head h.

hoof-and-mouth disease

hook
anatomic h.
angled iris hook and IOL dialer
blunt h.
calvarial h.
h. cautery
h. clamp
dura h.
elastic h.
h. electrocautery
embrasure h.
h. fixation
flat h.
h. forceps
h. of the hamate
hamate h.
hamate hook fracture
iris h.
LIH hook pin
locking hook instrumentation
loop and hook strapping
lower hook trial
MegaDyne arthroscopic hook electrode
meniscus h.
multiple hook assembly
multiple hook assembly C-D instrumentation
muscle h.
nerve h.
neutral h.
oblique muscle h.
open double-decked hook cervical system
ophthalmic h.
scleral h.

hook-plate fixation

hookworm
American h.
h. anemia
anemia from h.
h. disease
h. larva

Hooper
H. Visual Organization Test

hop
one-leg hop for distance test

hope
misplaced h.

hopelessness
Beck H. Scale
displays h.
feelings of h.
level of h.
H. Scale
sense of h.
stress, anger and h.

Hopkins
H. Symptom Checklist-90 Total Score

horizon
open h.
Streeter h.

horizontal
h. abduction/adduction
anterior horizontal jugular vein
anterior horizontal mandibular osteotomy
h. axis
h. axis of rectangular coordinate system
h. beam study
h. canal
h. cell
conjugate horizontal deviation
conjugate horizontal gaze
cup-to-disc ratio h.
h. deviation
dissociated horizontal deviation
h. eye movement
h. fissure
h. flap
h. flow clean bench
h. fold of rectum
fracture bilaterally in a horizontal plane
Frankfort horizontal plane of skull
h. gaze
h. gaze nystagmus
h. gaze palsy
great horizontal fissure
h. heart
h. hemianopia
h. incision across lower abdomen
h. laminar flow clean benches
locking horizontal mattress suture
h. mattress stitch
h. mattress suture
mean horizontal candle power
medial crus of the horizontal part of the facial canal
h. meridian
nasal crest of horizontal plate of palatine bone
nuclear horizontal gaze paralysis
h. nystagmus
h. overlap
palatine crest of horizontal process of palatine bone
h. plane
h. position
rhythmic horizontal oscillation of eyeball

sacral horizontal plane line
h. semicircular canal
shoulder horizontal flexion
h. sternotomy
h. strabismus
supraglottic horizontal laryngectomy
sustained horizontal nystagmus
h. tube
h. uterine incision
h. vertigo
h. visible iris diameter

horizontally selective visual cell

hormonal

ablative hormonal therapy
h. abnormality
h. activity
additive hormonal therapy
adjuvant hormonal or chemotherapy treatment
h. agent
h. assay
h. balance
h. cancer treatment
h. change
h. component
h. control
h. deficiency
h. disorder
h. disturbance
h. factor
feedback mechanisms of hormonal control
h. fluctuation
h. gingivitis
h. imbalance
h. influence
h. level
h. manipulation
h. migraine
normal hormonal balance
postmenopausal hormonal status
postmenopausal hormonal therapy
h. reaction
h. receptor
h. replacement therapy
h. response
h. stimulation
h. therapy
h. therapy in endometrial carcinoma
h. treatment

hormone

adrenal androgen corticotropic stimulating h.
adrenal androgen-stimulating h.
adrenal gland h.
adrenal steroid h.
adrenocortical h.
adrenocorticotropic h.
adrenoglomerulotropin h.
aldosterone-stimulating h.
alpha-melanocyte-stimulating h.
h. analysis
angiotensin II antidiuretic h.
antenatal thyrotropin releasing h.
anterior lobe h.
anterior pituitary h.
anterior pituitary-like h.
antidiuretic h.
antidiuretic hormone deficiency
antimüllerian h.
anti-müllerian hormone deficiency
antithyroid-stimulating h.
antithyroid-stimulating hormone antibody
artificial growth h.
atrial natriuretic h.
beta-thyroid-stimulating h.
h. binding study
bioassay of luteinizing h.
biologically active luteinizing h.
biosynthetic human growth h.
bovine growth h.
bovine parathyroid h.
bovine thyroid-stimulating h.
brain h.
calcitonin gene-related h.
cancer and steroid h.
h. change
chorionic gonadotropic h.
circulating pituitary h.
combination hormone therapy
combined hormone therapy
combined pituitary hormone deficiency
continuous-combined hormone replacement therapy
continuous hormone replacement therapy
corpus luteum h.
corpus luteum stimulating h.
cortical androgen-stimulating h.
corticotropin-releasing h.
corticotropin-releasing hormone receptor type 1, 2
h. deficiency
h. deficient children
h. dependent
h. disorder
ectopic hormone production
egg-laying h.
egg-laying release h.
endocrine hormone imbalance
equine growth h.
examined hormone levels
fat-mobilizing h.
female sex h.
fluctuating hormone levels
follicle-stimulating h.
follicle-stimulating hormone and luteinizing hormone-releasing h.
follicle-stimulating hormone-releasing h.
formation and release of h.'s
gamma-melanocyte-stimulating h.
gastric-inhibitory h.
gastrointestinal h.
generalized resistance to thyroid h.
generalized thyroid hormone resistance
glomerulus-stimulating h.
glucose counterregulatory h.
gonadotropic h.
gonadotropic hormone assay
gonadotropin-releasing h.
gonadotropin-releasing hormone agonist
gonadotropin-releasing hormone receptor
growth h.
growth hormone cell adenoma
growth hormone cell hyperplasia
growth hormone deficiency
growth hormone dose
growth hormone dose-response curve
growth hormone failure
growth hormone hypersecretion
growth hormone immunoassay
growth hormone-inhibiting h.
growth hormone inhibitory h.
growth hormone insensitivity
growth hormone insufficiency
growth hormone insulin
growth hormone normal
growth hormone receptor deficiency
growth hormone release
growth hormone release-inhibiting h.
growth hormone release-inhibiting factor
growth hormone-releasing h.
growth hormone releasing factor
growth hormone replacement
growth hormone response
growth hormone secretagogue
growth hormone secretagogue receptor

hormone *(continued)*
growth hormone secretion
growth hormone stimulation test
growth hormone therapy
growth-inhibiting h.
growth-stimulating h.
growth stimulating h.
growth hormone variant
h. heart
heterodimeric luteinizing h.
homeostatic thymus h.
human chorionic follicle-stimulating h.
human corticotropin-releasing h.
human follicle-stimulating h.
human growth h.
human growth hormone deficiency
human luteinizing h.
human parathyroid h.
human pituitary follicle-stimulating h.
human pituitary growth h.
human placental uterotropic h.
human thyroid hormone receptor
human thyroid-stimulating h.
human urinary follicle-stimulating h.
h. hypercalcemia
hypothalamic hypophysiotropic-releasing h.
hypothalamic-releasing h.
idiopathic growth h.
idiopathic growth hormone deficiency
imbalance of h.'s
immunoreactive adrenocorticotropic h.
immunoreactive human growth h.
immunoreactive parathyroid h.
h. implant
improved minimal essential medium, hormone supplemented
inappropriate antidiuretic h.
inappropriate antidiuretic hormone syndrome
inappropriate secretion of antidiuretic h.
h. ingestion
inhibiting h.
h. insensitive
intact parathyroid h.
interstitial cell-stimulating h.
isolated follicle-stimulating hormone deficiency syndrome
isolated growth hormone deficiency type IB, II, III
isolated growth hormone deficiency
isolated thyroid-stimulating hormone deficiency
juvenile hormone analog
lactogenic h.
h. level
h. levels
LH-releasing hormone agonist therapy
ligand-dependent action of thyroid hormone receptor
ligand-independent action of thyroid hormone receptor
lipid-mobilizing h.
lipotropic h.
lipotropic pituitary hormone
little adrenocorticotrophic h.
little growth h.
long-acting thyroid-stimulating h.
luteinizing h.
luteinizing hormone beta core fragment
luteinizing hormone-chorionic gonadotropin h.
luteinizing hormone-follicle-stimulating h.
luteinizing hormone/follicle-stimulating hormone-releasing
luteinizing hormone/follicle-stimulating hormone-releasing factor
luteinizing hormone receptor
luteinizing hormone receptor-binding inhibitor
luteinizing hormone-releasing h.
luteinizing hormone secretion
lutein-stimulating h.
luteomammotrophic h.
luteotropic h.
lymphocyte-stimulating h.
male hormone production
male hormone testosterone
male sex h.
mammotropic h.
h. manipulation
melanin-concentrating h.
melanocyte release-inhibiting h.
melanocyte-releasing h.
melanocyte-stimulating h.
melanocyte-stimulating hormone-releasing hormone
melanocyte-stimulating hormone sequence
melanophore-stimulating h.
melanotropin release-inhibiting h.
melanotropin-releasing h.
methasone-suppressed corticotropin-releasing hormone test
mid-molecule parathyroid h.
morning corticotropin-releasing hormone test
müllerian-inhibiting h.
müllerian inhibiting h.
müllerian inhibitory h.
multiple anterior pituitary hormone deficiency
multiple pituitary hormone deficiencies
natriuretic h.
natural growth h.
natural or synthetic h.
neurohypophyseal h.
nocturnal thyroid-stimulating hormone surge
nongrowth hormone deficient short stature
Novel erythropoiesis-stimulating h.
nuclear accessory h.
nuclear hormone receptor
oral contraceptive h.
oral hormone replacement therapy
ovine corticotropin-releasing h.
ovine growth h.
ovine lactogenic h.
ovine leuteinizing h.
paraneoplastic growth h.
parathyroid h.
parathyroid hormone assay
parathyroid hormone excess
parathyroid hormone gene transcription
parathyroid hormone level
parathyroid hormone resistance syndrome
parathyroid hormone secretion rate
partial thyroid-stimulating hormone hyporesponsiveness
peak thyroid-stimulating hormone response
peripheral hormone level
peripheral thyroid hormone metabolism
peripheral tissue resistance to thyroid h.
pituitary adrenotropic h.
pituitary gonadotropic h.
pituitary growth h.
pituitary hormone deficit
pituitary hormone function
pituitary hormone hypofunction
pituitary hormone release

pituitary hormone trigger ovulation
pituitary reproductive h.
pituitary resistance to thyroid h.
pituitary thyroid hormone resistance
placental growth h.
placental lactogenic h.
plasma growth h.
plasma parathyroid h.
plasminogen activator-releasing h.
porcine growth h.
posterior pituitary h.
postmenopausal hormone therapy
post ovulation hormone change
potent hormone angiotensin II
pregnancy urine h.
premenopausal hormone receptor positive
production of sex h.
prolactin chronic growth h.
prolactin-inhibiting h.
prolactin inhibitory h.
prolactin release-inhibiting h.
prolactin-releasing h.
prostate hormone therapy
prothoracotropic h.
rat growth h.
h. receptor
h. receptor site
h. receptor test
recombinant follicle-stimulating h.
recombinant human growth h.
recombinant human thyroid-stimulating h.
regulatory h.
release of h.'s
releasing h.
h. replacement
h. replacement medication
h. replacement therapy
resistance to thyroid h.
h. response element
h. response unit
secretion of h.'s
selective pituitary resistance to thyroid h.
h. sensitive lipase
serum immunoreactive parathyroid h.
sex h.
silencing mediator of retinoic acid and thyroid hormone receptor
slow release of h.'s
somatotroph h.
somatotropic h.
somatotropin release-inhibiting h.
somatotropin-releasing h.
h. supplement
supplemental growth hormone therapy
supplemental thyroid h.
syndrome of generalized thyroid hormone resistance
syndrome of inappropriate antidiuretic h.
syndrome of inappropriate antidiuretic hormone secretion
syndrome of inappropriate secretion of antidiuretic h.
synthetic human growth h.
synthetic male h.
synthetic thyroid h.
h. therapy
thyroid h.
thyroid hormone autoantibodies
thyroid hormone production
thyroid hormone receptor
thyroid hormone receptor-retinoid X receptor
thyroid hormone replacement
thyroid hormone resistance
thyroid hormone treatment
thyroid-releasing h.
thyroid hormone response element
thyroid-stimulating hormone receptor
thyroid-stimulating hormone receptor antibody
thyroid-stimulating hormone receptor autoantibody
thyroid-stimulating hormone-releasing h.
thyrotropic h.
thyrotropin-releasing h.
thyrotropin-releasing hormone receptor
thyrotropin-releasing hormone stimulation test
thyrotropin-stimulating h.
h. titer
total parathyroid hormone secretion
h. treatment
urinary-derived human follicle-stimulating h.
urinary follicle-stimulating h.
urinary luteinizing h.

hormone-beta
luteinizing h.-b.

hormone-binding
h.-b. domain
growth hormone-binding protein
thyroid hormone-binding index
thyroid hormone-binding ratio

hormone-dependent prostate cancer

hormone/follicle
luteinizing hormone/follicle-stimulating hormone-releasing
luteinizing hormone/follicle-stimulating hormone-releasing factor

hormone/human
luteinizing hormone/human chorionic gonadotropin

hormone-independent prostate cancer

hormone-prolactin
chorionic growth h.-p.

hormone-receptor enzyme

hormone-refractory
h.-r. metastatic prostate cancer
h.-r. prostate cancer

hormone-releasing
follicle-stimulating hormone-releasing factor
follicle-stimulating hormone-releasing hormone
growth hormone-releasing factor tumor
growth hormone-releasing peptide
luteinizing hormone/follicle-stimulating h.-r.
thyroid-stimulating hormone-releasing hormone

hormone-resistant prostate cancer

hormone-secreting
h.-s. adrenal tumor
h.-s. pituitary tumor
h.-s. tumor

horn
anterior horn cell
anterior horn cell degeneration
anterior horn cell disease
anterior horn cell isolation
anterior horn cell motor impairment
anterior horn index
anterior horn meniscal tear
anterior horn of spinal cord
apex of dorsal horn of spinal cord
apex of posterior h.
apex of posterior horn of spinal cord
bone graft shoe h.

horn *(continued)*
h. of clitoris
dorsal h.
dorsal horns of spinal cord
frontal horn index
long-handled shoe h.
medullary dorsal h.
noncommunicating uterine h.
occipital h.
occipital horn syndrome
posterior horn of medial meniscus
pulp h.
spinal dorsal h.
subjacent dorsal h.
h. of uterus

Horner
H. muscle
H. pupil
H. syndrome

hornet
white-faced h.
yellow-faced h.

horse
African horse sickness
African horse sickness virus 1–9
h. antihuman thymocyte globulin
h. antihuman thymus globulin
h. anti-Rhesus lymphocyte globulin
antiserum, h.
h. antitetanus toxoid globulin
h. chestnut seed extract
h. immunoglobulin
inactivated horse serum
h. liver alcohol dehydrogenase
lysed horse blood
h. red blood cell
h. serum

horseradish
h. peroxidase

horseshoe
h. configuration
h. incision
inverted horseshoe flap
h. lung
Mayfield horseshoe headrest
h. placenta
h. tear

horseshoe-shaped skin flap

horseshoe-type kidney

Horton arteritis

hospice
h. approach
h. care
h. coordinator
inpatient hospice unit
h. inquiry
h. nurse
h. philosophy
h. program
h. support
h. team
h. volunteer

hospital
accredited psychiatric h.
h. acquired
h. activity analysis
acute care h.
h. administration
h. admission
H. Admission Risk Profile
adult psychiatric h.
ambient hospital air
American H. Association
H. Anxiety and Depression
H. Anxiety and Depression Scale
h. apprentice
h. arrival time
automated hospital information system
base h.
h. bed
h. birth certificate
h. blood bank
h. camp
h. care cost
Certified H. Admission Program
h. chemistry profile
chronic disease h.
combat support h.
h. and community psychiatry
comprehensive hospital infections project
contamination from ambient hospital air
convalescent h.
h. course
h. course benign
h. day
day h.
h. day number
died in h.
h. discharge
h. discharge survey
h. emergency department
h. environment
h. epidemiology
extended care h.
h. fever
h. field director
floating h.
h. flora
home-based hospital care
Hospital Indicator for Physicians Orders
h. induced
h. infection control
inpatient h.
h. inservice program
h. inservice training
h. insurance
h. insurance program
h. isolation
locked hospital unit
h. management
h. management committee
Massachusetts General H. Utility Multi-Programming System
maximal hospital benefit
maximum hospital benefit
maximum-security forensic psychiatric h.
Naval H.
normal hospital air
h. onset of infection
h. operation
orientation to h.
osteopathic h.
out of h.
outpatient h.
h. outpatient department
outside h.
Parkland Hospital technique
partial hospital patient population
partial hospital setting
partial hospital treatment program
h. participation
patient discharged from h.
patient has fear of h.
patient reached maximum hospital benefit
patient's hospital course turbulent
patient treated in h.
h. peer review
h. policy
prevention of hospital infection
private psychiatric h.
prolonged hospital care
h. protocol
reached maximum hospital benefit
h. report
h. residency program
h. resources
h. setting
h. ship
sole community h.
standard hospital treatment
state mental h.

h. study
subsequent hospital care
h. systems
h. team
h. transfer order
h. treatment
H. Utilization Project
Veteran's Administration h.
h. visit

hospital-acquired
h.-a. bloodstream infection
h.-a. infection
h.-a. lower respiratory infection
h.-a. organism
h.-a. organism infection
h.-a. penetration contact
h.-a. pneumonia
h.-a. urinary tract infection
h.-a. viral hepatitis

hospital-associated respiratory tract infection

hospital-based
h.-b. blood bank
h.-b. physician
h.-b. stress management

hospitalization
intensive structured h.
maximal benefit from h.
multiple h.'s
h. not indicated
prior to h.
psychological stress of h.
throughout h.
h. and treatment

hospitalize
do not h.

hospitalized
h. attempted suicide
h. controls
patient h.
patient hospitalized for workup
patient previously h.

hospital-related infection

hospital-wide practice

host
h. body
h. cell
h. chromosome
classification of h.
colonization of h.
h. defense
h. defensive factor
immune compromised h.
immunocompromised h.
h. leukotactic function
living host cell
new host cell
nonimmunocompromised h.
original host cell
h. resistance
h. susceptibility
transmission of microbe to h.

host-cell reactivation

hostile
abusive and hostile patient
h. and anxious
h. behavior
h. conflict
h. dependence
h. dependency
h. and depressed
h. patient
patient abusive and h.
patient feeling h.
h. personality
h. relationship
unusually hostile or aggressive behavior
h. work environment

hostility
active hostility index
aggressive h.
covert h.
h. and depression
diffusing hostility and anger
H. and Direction of Hostility Questionnaire
extreme h.
open h.
overcontrolled hostility scale
paranoid h.
patient exhibits overt h.
penalty, frustration, anxiety, guilt, h.
pent-up h.
thoughtless h.

host-versus-graft
h.-v.-g. disease
h.-v.-g. response

hot
h. abscess
h. appendix
h. biopsy
h. biopsy technique
h. and cold
h. or cold flash
h. and cold flushes
h. and cold sensation
cold spots and hot spots with electron beam dosimetry
h. compress
h. cone
Eddy hot plate test
h. environment
filtered hot air
h. flash
h. flash trigger
h. flush
h. fomentation
h. gangrene
heat, ultrasound, and massage
infarct avid hot spot scintigraphy
h. knife
h. lesion
menopausal hot flash
h. moist compresses
h. moist packs
h. moist poultice
h. node
h. packs and bed rest
h. pad
h. plate reaction time
h. plate test
h. reactor syndrome
h. spot
h. spot imaging
h. stage
h., swollen, and tender
h. tip laser probe
h. tub bath
h. tub dermatitis
h. vs. cold breast tumor
h. water
h. water bottle
h. water extract
h. water soluble
h. weather ear
h. wet pack

hot-cold
h.-c. lysis
h.-c. system

hotline
crisis h.
National STD and AIDS H.'s

Hough
automated Hough transform
H. transform

Hounsfield unit

hour
air changes per h.
cubic centimeter per h.
every h.
every 2 h.'s
every 3 h.'s
every 4 h.'s
every hour around the clock
lumen h.

hour *(continued)*
miles per h.
milliequivalents per 24 h.'s
milligram per h.
milligram per kilogram per h.
milliroentgens per hour at one meter
organism isolated after 48 h.'s
organism isolated after 72 h.'s
roentgen per h.
roentgen per hour at one meter
service h.'s
sighs per h.
urobilinogen—2 h.'s
Wagner-Nelson time 50 h.'s
watt h.

2-hour
-h. postprandial blood sugar
-h. pregnancy test

24-hour
-h. period of observation and hydration
-h. urine
-h. urine collection

hourglass
h. contraction of stomach
h. deformity
h. vertebra

hour-glass murmur

5-hour glucose tolerance test

hourly
h. fetal urine production rate
h. output

house
H. classification
h. dust allergy
h. dust mite
h. formula
halfway h.
halfway house for alcoholics
halfway house for drug addicts
halfway house for penal rehabilitation
halfway house for physically handicapped
halfway house placement
medical house officer
notify house officer
h. officer
h. staff
h. tube feeding

House-Brackmann Grading Scale

household activity

housemaid's knee

House-Tree-Person Projective Technique psychologic test

House-Tree Test

Houston
H. fold
H. muscle

How
Inquiry Mode Questionnaire: A Measure of How You Think and Make Decisions
H. I See Myself Scale

Howell-Jolly body

Hoyer
H. anastomoses
H. canal
H. lift
H. traction

Hoyeraal-Hreidarsson syndrome

Huacho virus

Hubbard tank

Huber
noncoring Huber needle

hue
ninety hue discrimination test
violaceous h.

Hughes
H. reflex
H. virus

Huhner test

hum
cervical venous h.

human
h. ability
aborted human fetus
h. adenovirus 1–47
h. adjuvant disease
h. African trypanosomiasis
aggregated human gamma globulin
h. albumin microsphere
h. albumin minimicrosphere
h. alpha-fetoprotein
h. alpha$_1$-proteinase inhibitor
h. alveolar macrophage
anal human papilloma virus infection
h. androgen receptor assay
h. androgen receptor gene
h. antichimeric antibodies
antihemophilic plasma h.
h. antimouse antibody
anti-*Pseudomonas* human plasma
h. aortic endothelial cell
h. aortic smooth muscle cell
h. artificial chromosome
h. astrovirus serotype 1–7
h. atrial natriuretic peptide
attenuated human rotavirus
autoantibodies to human thyroglobulin
autologous human collagen
autologous human collagen augmentation
basic human function
h. basophil degranulation test
h. behavior
biosynthetic human growth hormone
biosynthetic human insulin
h. bite
h. blood bilayer Tween
h. B-lymphocyte antigen
h. B lymphotropic virus
h. body
h. bonding
h. bone marrow
h. brain disease
h. brain thromboplastin
h. breast milk
h. breast tumor
h. bronchial epithelial cell
h. calcitonin
h. calicivirus
carrier of human immunodeficiency virus
h. carriers of infection
h. cervical carcinoma cell
4-chambered human heart
h. chorionic follicle-stimulating hormone
h. chorionic gonadotropin
h. chorionic gonadotropin level
h. chorionic gonadotropin test
h. chorionic somatomammotropin
h. chorionic somatotropin
h. chorionic thyrotropin
h. condition
Cooperative H. Tissue Network
h. cord serum
h. coronary virus
h. corona virus sensitivity
h. corticotropin-releasing hormone
cryopreserved human aortic allograft
h. cultured lymphoblast
h. cytomegalovirus infection
h. dermal microvascular endothelial cell
h. development
h. development and family life
h. diploid cell

h. diploid cell strain
h. diploid cell system
h. diploid cell vaccine
h. diploid fibroblast
diseased human heart
donated human organs
dynamics of human behavior
h. ehrlichiosis
h. embryo fibroblast
h. embryoic lung fibroblast
h. embryo kidney cell
h. embryo lung cell culture
h. embryonic intestine cell
h. embryonic kidney
h. embryonic lung fibroblast
h. embryonic palatal mesenchymal cell
h. embryonic skin
h. embryonic spleen
h. endorphin
h. endothelial cell
enteric cytopathic human orphan
enteric cytopathogenic human orphan
h. enteric virus
enterocytopathogenic human orphan
enterocytopathogenic human orphan-rhinocoryza virus
enterocytopathogenic human orphan virus
h. epidermal growth factor
h. epidermal growth receptor 2
h. epithelial cell
h. erythrocyte agglutination test
h. erythrocyte antigen
h. erythroleukemia line
h. erythropoietin
escape and avoidance conditioning in human subjects
h. ether-a-go-go-related gene
H. Fertilization and Embryology Authority
h. fetal cell
h. fetal diploid kidney cell
h. fetal diploid lung cell
h. fetal lung fibroblast
h. fetal pancreas transplant
h. fibroblast interferon
H. Figure Drawing
h. figure parts response
h. follicle-stimulating hormone
h. foreskin epithelial cell
h. foreskin fibroblast
formalin-treated pyruvaldehyde-stabilized human erythrocytes
four-chambered human heart
functional assessment of human immunodeficiency
fundamental human drive
h. gamma globulin
H. Gene Expression
h. gene therapy
h. genetic disorder
h. genetic material
h. genetic mutant cell repository
h. genetics
H. Genome
H. Genome Epidemiology Network
H. Genome Initiative
H. Genome Project
h. glucose monitoring
h. glucose output
h. gonadotropin
h. granulocytic ehrlichiosis
h. growth factor
h. growth hormone
h. growth hormone deficiency
h. health and behavior questionnaire
h. hepatitis A virus
h. hepatoma
h. herpesvirus
h. herpesvirus 1–8
h. herpesvirus 8/Kaposi sarcoma herpesvirus
HIV-associated dementia
h. host
human leukocyte interferon
h. hypopituitary serum
h. immune cells
h. immune serum globulin
h. immune status survey
h. immunodeficiency virus
h. immunodeficiency virus antibody
h. immunodeficiency virus associated dementia
h. immunodeficiency virus associated motor cognitive disorder
h. immunodeficiency virus-associated nephropathy
h. immunodeficiency virus-associated non-Hodgkin lymphoma
h. immunodeficiency virus-associated periodontitis
h. immunodeficiency virus-associated salivary gland disease
h. immunodeficiency virus dementia
h. immunodeficiency virus encephalopathy
h. immunodeficiency virus gingivitis
h. immunodeficiency virus immunoglobulin
h. immunodeficiency virus infected blood
h. immunodeficiency virus overview of problems evaluation system
h. immunodeficiency virus-patient-reported status and experience
h. immunodeficiency virus quality audit marker
h. immunodeficiency virus seroconversion
h. immunodeficiency virus-1 subtype C
h. immunodeficiency virus type 1, 2
immunoradioassayable human chorionic somatomammotropin
immunoreactive human chorionic gonadotropin
immunoreactive human chorionic somatomammotropin
immunoreactive human gastrin
immunoreactive human growth hormone
immunoreactive human placental lactogen
immunoreactive human skin collagenase
h. infection
h. infectious dose
infectious human hepatitis
h. insulin
h. insulin antibodies
h. insulin regular
h. intelligence
h. interaction
h. interferon
International Workshop and Conference on H. Leukocyte Differentiation Antigens
h. intestinal epithelium
h. intracisternal A-type particle
H. Investigation Committee
iodinated human serum albumin
isolated human growth deficiency
h. jagged-1 gene
Kaposi sarcoma human growth factor
h. kidney cell
h. kidney glandular kallikrein-1 gene

human *(continued)*
h. laryngeal tumor cell
h. Lesch-Nyhan cell
h. leukocyte
h. leukocyte antibody
h. leukocyte antigen
h. leukocyte antigen-A24
h. leukocyte antigen allele
h. leukocyte antigen restriction element
h. leukocyte antigen system
h. leukocyte elastase
h. lipotropin
liquid human serum
live-attenuated human immunodeficiency virus
h. lung fibroblast
h. lung field
h. lung fluid
h. lung surfactant
h. luteinizing hormone
h. lymphoblastoid cell line
h. lymphoblastoid interferon
h. lymphocyte
h. lymphocyte antigen
h. lymphocyte antigen-lymphocyte defined
h. lymphocyte antigen-serologically defined
h. lymphocyte interferon
h. lymphocyte transformation
lyophilized human AT-III
h. macrophage-monocyte chemotactic and activating factor
macrophage-tropic human immunodeficiency virus strain
h. mammaglobin RNA
h. mammary carcinoma cell membrane proteinase
h. mammary tumor virus
maximal human dose
maximal recommended human dose
maximum recommended human dose
h. menopausal gonadotropin
h. mesenchymal stem cell
h. mesothelial cell membrane
microaggregated human serum albumin
h. milk fat globule
h. milk fortifier
h. milk lysozyme
h. milk reverse transcriptase enzyme
h. molar thyrotropin
h. molecular genetics
MOLT-18, human T cell line
h. monocytic ehrlichiosis
morphine-potentiated human immunodeficiency virus replication
Multidimensional Quality of Life Questionnaire for Persons with H. Immunodeficiency Virus
h. myoglobulin radioimmunoassay
natural human interferon-beta
natural human interferon-gamma
h. natural killer cell
h. needs
h. neuroblastoma
h. neurophysin
h. neutrophil collagenase
h. neutrophil elastase
h. neutrophil peptide-4
nicked free beta subunit of human chorionic gonadotropin
nonsyncytia-forming human immunodeficiency virus
normal human development
normal human diploid fibroblast
normal human gastric juice
normal human globulin
normal human kidney
normal human pooled plasma
normal human serum
normal human white matter
h. nutrition
h. old tuberculin
h. oncology
h. operant heart rate conditioning
h. oral epidermoid carcinoma cell
h. osteogenic sarcoma
h. osteosarcoma
h. ovarian cancer
h. oviduct fluid
packed human blood cell
h. pancreas-specific protein
h. pancreatic amylase
h. pancreatic polypeptide
h. pancreatic trypsin inhibitor
h. papillomavirus
h. papilloma virus
h. papillomavirus type 16
h. parathyroid hormone
h. parotid lysozyme
partially pure human leukocyte interferon
parts of human body
h. parvovirus
h. peripheral blood leukocyte
h. peripheral lymphocyte
h. peripheral mononuclear cell
h. pituitary
h. pituitary follicle-stimulating hormone
h. pituitary gonadotropin
h. pituitary growth hormone
h. placental thyrotropin
h. placental uterotropic hormone
h. platelet antigen
h. platelet-rich plasma
h. platelet suspension
h. poliovirus
polymerized human albumin
pooled human plasma
pooled human serum
postmortem human kidney
postmortem human kidney cell
potential for human betterment
predialyzed human albumin
predialyzed human serum
primary human fetal glia
h. prolactin
h. proximal tubule
h. psychopathology
purified placental protein, h.
rabbit antibody to human ovary
h. rabies immune globulin
h. rabies immunoglobulin
rabies vaccine, human diploid cell culture
radioactive iodinated human serum albumin
recombinant human activated protein C
recombinant human albumin
recombinant human bone morphogenetic protein
recombinant human erythropoietin
recombinant human granulocyte-macrophage colony-stimulating factor
recombinant human growth hormone
recombinant human IL-10
recombinant human insulinlike growth factor
recombinant human insulin-like growth factor-1
recombinant human leukocyte interferon A
recombinant human MIP-1 alpha
recombinant human platelet-derived growth factor
recombinant human superoxide dismutase
recombinant human thyroid-stimulating hormone
recombinant human tissue factor pathway inhibitor

recombinant human TSH
recombinant human vascular endothelial growth factor
recombinant human interleukin-2, -3, -11
recycled human blood substitute
h. relations
h. reovirus-like
h. reovirus-like agent
h. respiratory syncytial virus
h. retroviral disease
h. retrovirus
h. rights committee
Rincoe human action bionic
h. rotavirus
h. seminal plasma inhibitor
h. semisynthetic insulin
h. serum albumin
h. serum esterase
h. serum prealbumin
h. serum protein
h. serum thymus factor
h. sialoglycoprotein
h. skeletal growth factor
h. skin collagenase
h. skin equivalent
h. skin nurse cell
soluble human leukocyte antigen
soluble recombinant human CD4
somatic cell human gene therapy
h. spiritual concerns
spontaneously aborted human fetus
h. stomach cancer-transforming factor-1
h. stomach cancer-transforming factor-2
h. stromelysin aggregated proteoglycan
h. subject
h. superoxide dismutase
synthetic human gastrin
synthetic human growth hormone
synthetic human relaxin
h. T-cell leukemia-lymphoma virus
h. T-cell leukemia virus
h. T-cell leukemia virus-associated membrane antigen
h. T-cell leukemia virus type 1, 2, 3
h. T-cell lymphoma virus
h. T-cell lymphotrophic virus type I–III
h. T-cell lymphotropic virus
h. T-cell lymphotropic virus II
h. T-cell lymphotropic virus III
h. T-cell lymphotropic virus type I associated myelopathy
h. telomerase reverse transcriptase
h. testing
h. tetanus antitoxin
h. tetanus immune globulin
h. tetanus immunoglobulin
h. therapeutic dose
h. therapy
h. thrombin
h. thymic leukemia
h. thymocyte antigen
h. thymus antiserum
h. thyroglobulin
h. thyroid adenylcyclase stimulator
h. thyroid hormone receptor
h. thyroid-stimulating antibody
h. thyroid-stimulating hormone
h. tissue
h. T-lymphotrophic virus/lymphadenopathy associated virus
h. T-lymphotropic virus 1, 2
h. transmission
transplanting human fetal tissue
h. tumor bank
h. tumor colony assay
h. tumor stem cell assay
h. umbilical cord blood
h. umbilical vein
h. umbilical vein endothelial cell
h. urinary
h. urinary CSF
urinary-derived human follicle-stimulating hormone
h. urinary follicle-stimulating hormone
h. urinary kallikrein
h. urine
varieties of human leukocyte antigen
h. violence
X-linked human androgen receptor

human-controlled repressor

humanitarian device exemption

humanity

crime against h.

humanized

anti-CD11a humanized monoclonal antibody for psoriasis
anti-CD18 humanized antibody
h. antihuman IL-2 receptor antibody
anti-IgE humanized monoclonal antibody
antiimmunoglobulin E humanized monoclonal antibody

human-specific thyroid stimulator

humeral

anterior circumflex humeral artery
anterior circumflex humeral vein
anterior humeral circumflex artery
anterior humeral line
anteromedial humeral head defect
anteromedial superior humeral head impaction
h. avulsion of the glenohumeral ligament
h. block in radiation therapy
h. bone
h. canal
h. condyle
h. diaphysis
h. epicondyle
external humeral epicondylitis
h. fracture
h. head
medial epicondyle humeral fracture
medial humeral condyle
Milch classification of humeral fracture
h. neck
Neer-Horowitz classification of humeral fracture
Neer II humeral component
proximal humeral fracture
h. reamer
h. shaft
h. shaft fracture

humeroradial

h. joint
h. synostosis

humerus

anatomical neck of h.
head of h.
lateral condyle of h.
h. length
little head of h.
medial border of h.
medial condyle of h.
medial epicondyle of h.
middle greater tubercle of facet of h.
Mueller humerus fracture classification
neck of h.

humerus *(continued)*
Neer humerus fracture classification
nutrient artery of h.
open reduction of h.
perinatal humerus fracture
shaft of h.
surgical neck of h.

humidified air

humidifier
bubble h.
cold mist h.
cold-mist h.
cool mist h.
jet h.
h. lung
Ohio h.
h. and oxygen
passover h.
ultrasonic h.
warm mist h.

humidify and heat

humidity
high-density h.
increased fluids and h.
h. mask
relative h.

humor
anal h.
aqueous h.
aqueous humor deficiency
aqueous humor drainage
aqueous humor of the eye
aqueous humor eye
crystalline h.
flow of aqueous h.
gallows h.
Morgagni h.
ocular h.
peccant h.
therapeutic h.
therapeutic benefits of h.
therapeutic humor movement
h. therapist
vitreous h.

humoral
acute humoral rejection
h. antibody production
h. host
h. hypercalcemia of malignancy
h. immune defect
h. immunity
h. immunocompetence profile
malignancy-associated humoral hypercalcemia
maternal humoral immune response
passive humoral immunotherapy
h. response
h. signal
h. thymic factor
thymic humoral factor

hump
biparietal h.
bony h.
dorsal h.
dowager's h.
parietal h.
h. in upper back
widow's h.

Humphrey visual field

Humpty Doo virus

hundred
h. count
parts per hundred million
H. Pictures Naming Test
h. woman years of exposure

hundredth molar solution

hung
new bag h.

hunger
affect h.
air h.
extreme h.
h. headache
infant exhibits hunger behavior
narcotic h.
h. pain
h. pang
h. respiration
stimulus h.
stimulus-action h.
h. strike
h. swelling

Hunner ulcer

Hunter
H. canal
H. and Driffield curve
H. glossitis
H. gubernaculum
H. ligament

Huntington
H. chorea
H. disease

Hurler
H. disease
mucopolysaccharidosis type I H.
H. syndrome

Hurler-Scheie
mucopolysaccharidosis type I H.-S.

Hürthle
H. cell
H. cell adenoma
H. cell carcinoma
H. cell tumor

husband
artificial insemination donor, h.
battered husband syndrome
trained participating husband birth

husband-insemination
therapeutic h.-i.

Huschke
H. cartilage
H. foramen
H. valve

Hutchins Behavior Inventory

Hutchinson
melanotic freckle of H.

Hutchinson-Boeck disease

hyaline
h. acellular area
acute sclerosing hyaline necrosis
adult familial hyaline membrane disease
alcoholic hyaline inclusion body
h. arterionecrosis
h. body
h. cartilage
h. cast
clinical hyaline membrane disease
h. cytoplasmic inclusion
extensive hyaline membrane disease
h. fatty change
intracytoplasmic hyaline inclusion
marked hyaline deposition
h. membrane
h. membrane disease
h. membranes lining alveolar space
neonatal hyaline membrane disease
pulmonary hyaline membrane
h. sclerosis
h. thrombus
yellow hyaline membrane disease

hyalinization
electrolyte steroid-produced cardiopathy characterized by h.
glomerular h.

hyalinized fibrous tissue

hyalinizing
h. clear cell carcinoma
pleomorphic hyalinizing angiectatic tumor
pulmonary hyalinizing granuloma
segmental hyalinizing vasculitis

hyalinosis
focal and segmental h.
focal segmental glomerular hyalinosis and sclerosis

hyalitis
asteroid h.

hyaloid
anterior hyaloid membrane
h. artery
h. body
h. canal
h. fossa
posterior hyaloid membrane

hyaloidal
anterior hyaloidal fibrovascular proliferation

hyaloplasm
nuclear h.

hyalosis
asteroid h.

hyaluronic acid

hyaluronidase
antistreptococcal h.
physiologic hyaluronidase inhibitor
h. unit for semen

hybrid
h. capture assay
h. F plasmid
mutant h.
h. neural network
h. rapid acquisition with relaxation enhancement

hybridization
comparative genomic h.
double-fusion fluorescent in situ h.
Epstein-Barr virus-encoded RNA in situ h.
extra ABL signal fluorescent in situ h.
fluorescent in situ h.
molecular hybridization study
molecular probe h.
multiple in situ h.
multispectral fluorescent in situ h.
nonisotopic in situ h.
nonradioactive in situ h.
nucleic acid h.
nucleic acid hybridization analysis
nucleic acid hybridization test
polymerase chain reaction in situ h.
sequence-specific oligonucleotide probe hybridization
sequencing by h.
in situ h.
in situ hybridization histochemistry
slot-blot hybridization analysis
ultrasensitive fluorescence in situ h.

hybridoma
h. bank
h. product

hydantoin
fetal hydantoin syndrome

hydatid
alveolar hydatid disease
h. cyst
h. cyst disease
h. disease
h. fremitus
h. mole
h. of Morgagni
Morgagni h.
multilocular hydatid cyst
osseous hydatid cyst
h. polyp
h. pregnancy
sessile h.
stalked h.

hydatidiform
amniography in hydatidiform mole
h. mole
partial hydatidiform mole

hydramnios
maternal h.

hydratase
epoxide h.
fumarate hydratase, mitochondrial
fumarate hydratase, soluble

hydrate
chloral h.
elixir terpin h.
elixir terpin hydrate with codeine

hydrated
h. to hydration
inadequately h.
patient well h.
h. pyelogram

hydration
alteration in hydration intake
artificial nutrition and h.
24-hour period of observation and h.
hydrated to h.
h. of mucous membranes
observation and h.
h. and turgor

hydraulic
axial closed-loop hydraulic mechanical testing
h. chamber
h. concussion

hydrazide
isonicotinic acid h.

hydrobromic acid

hydrobromide
galanthamine h.

hydrocarbon
aryl hydrocarbon receptor
aryl hydrocarbon receptor nuclear translocator
lipid hydrocarbon inclusion
polycyclic aromatic h.
polynuclear aromatic h.

hydrocele
h. coli
communicating h.
owl's eyes view of h.

hydrocephalus
h., agyria, retinal dysplasia with or without encephalocele syndrome
association with hydrocephalus syndrome
h. due to congenital stenosis of aqueduct of Sylvius
h. ex vacuo
h. ex vacuo change
fetus with h.
infantile h.
normal-pressure h.
posthemorrhagic h.
h. shunt
subdural effusion with h.

hydrochloric
h. acid
free hydrochloric acid

hydrochloride
methyl cysteine h.
neopyrithiamin h.
phencyclidine h.

hydrochlorothiazide
methyldopa and h.

hydrocodone bitartrate

hydrocolloid
h. dressing
h. impression
irreversible h.

hydrocortisone
h. acetate
hemisuccinate of h.
h. injection
h. test

hydrocyanic acid

hydrodissection
Nichamin hydrodissection cannula

hydrodissector
Pearce nucleus h.

hydrogen
h. adenosine triphosphatase
arterial blood hydrogen tension
breath hydrogen test
h. breath test
carbon, hydrogen, and nitrogen
h. cyanide
h. density
h. electrodes
h. exchange
h. fluoride
h. gas
intracellular hydrogen ion concentration
h. iodide
h. ion
h. ion concentration
lactose hydrogen breath testing
nonradioactive hydrogen isotope
h. peroxide ultrasound
radioactive hydrogen isotope
h. transport
vaporized hydrogen peroxide

hydrogenated
amorphous hydrogenated silicon carbide
sulfated hydrogenated caster oil

hydrogen-detected ventricular septal defect

hydrolaparoscopy
transvaginal h.

hydrolase
acid cholesterol ester h.
carboxylic ester h.
fatty acid amide h.
lysosomal hydrolase enzyme assay
maleylacetoacetate hydrolase, type Ib
monoglyceride h.

hydrolysate
casein h.
lactalbumin h.
h. lactalbumin Earle glucose
milk protein h.

hydrolysis
acid h.
amino acid that gives aspartic acid after h.
nucleus hydrolysis needle

hydrolyzed animal protein

hydromotive pressure

hydronephrosis
crescent sign of h.

hydroperoxide
total h.

hydrophilic
h. coated
h. emollient base
h. ointment
h. petrolatum
psyllium hydrophilic mucilloid

hydrophilic-lipophilic balance

hydrophobic
h. bond
h. gel
h. protein
short h.

hydrophobica
agriothymia h.

hydrophthalmia
anterior h.

hydrops
endolymphatic h.
h. fetalis
h. folliculi
h. of gallbladder
h. of the gallbladder
hypertensive meningeal h.
maternal hydrops fetalis
maternal hydrops syndrome
nonimmune fetal h.
h. pericardii
h. of pleura
h. spurious

hydroquinone cream

hydrosalpinx
bilateral h.
h., both tubes
h. follicularis
intermittent h.
h. simplex

hydrostatic
colloid hydrostatic pressure gradient
h. gradient
h. indifference point
intravascular hydrostatic pressure
h. pressure
h. pulmonary edema
tissue hydrostatic pressure
transmembrane hydrostatic pressure

hydrothorax
hepatic h.

hydrotropic electron donor

hydroxide
bismuth h.
calcium h.
macroaggregated ferrous h.
magnesium aluminum h.
magnesium hydroxide and mineral oil emulsion
magnesium hydroxide suspension
potassium hydroxide stain
tetramethylammonium h.

hydroxy
h. beta methylbutyrate

hydroxyacyl

hydroxyanisole
butylated h.

hydroxyapatite
calcium h.
h. cement
h. deposition disease
porous block h.
total h.

hydroxybutyrate
h. dehydrogenase
gamma h.
serum hydroxybutyrate dehydrogenase

hydroxybutyric
h. dehydrogenase
serum hydroxybutyric dehydrogenase

12-hydroxyeicosatetraenoic acid

20-hydroxyeicosatetraenoic acid

2-hydroxyethyl methacrylate

hydroxyethyl starch solution

21-hydroxyindoleacetic acid

hydroxyl
h. concentration
h. derivative of GABA
h. group
h. radical

hydroxylase
arylhydrocarbon h.
dopamine h.
dopamine-beta h.
mitochondrial hydroxylase enzyme
nonclassical hydroxylase deficiency
protocollagen proline h.
tryptophan h.
tyrosine h.

hydroxylation
microsomal h.

hydroxymethyl cytosine

hydroxymethylene diphosphonate

hydroxyphenylpyruvate oxidase

hydroxypropyl methylcellulose

hydroxysteroid dehydrogenase

hydroxytoluene
butylated h.

5-hydroxytryptamine
5-h. 2A
5-h. serotonin

hygiene
daily oral h.
grooming and h.
industrial h.
mental h.
mental hygiene clinic
oral h.
oral hygiene instruction
Oral H. Index-Simplified
personal hygiene facility
personal oral h.
poor dental h.
regular foot h.
h. self-care deficit
Simplified Oral H. Index
sleep hygiene abnormality

hygienic laboratory

hygroma
cystic h.
Fleischmann h.
nuchal cystic h.
perioptic h.
subdural h.

hymen
anular h.
h. bifenestratus
h. biforis
circular h.
cribriform h.
denticular h.
falciform h.
fenestrated h.
imperforate h.
infundibuliform h.
intact h.
lunar h.
microperforate h.
rigid h.
septate h.
stenotic h.
subseptus h.
vertical h.

hymenal
h. band
h. caruncle
h. cyst
h. membrane
h. orifice
h. ring
h. syndrome

hyoglossus
h. muscle
musculus h.

hyoid
anterior suspension of hyoid bone
h. arch
h. body
h. bone
central hyoid bone
h. cornu
cornu of hyoid bone
muscles of hyoid bone
h. region

hyoideum
os h.

hyoideus
apparatus h.

hyothyroideum

hypalgesia
stimulation-induced h.

hyperactive
h. asthma
h. behavior
h. bowel sound
h. bowel tones
h. carotid sinus reflex
h. child
h. children
h. immune system
h. malarial splenomegaly syndrome
patient h.
h. reflex
h. tendon reflex
h. thyroid
h. and violent

hyperactivity
attention deficit disorder with h.
attention deficit disorder without h.
attention deficit hyperactivity disorder
attention deficit hyperactivity disorder, combined type
attention deficit hyperactivity disorder, predominantly hyperactive-impulsive type
attention deficit hyperactivity disorder-predominantly inattentive
autonomic hyperactivity sign
detrusor hyperactivity with impaired contractility
h. disorder
electroencephalogram biofeedback in control of h.
h. from anxiety
insomnia, hyperactivity and decreased appetite
h. and irritability anxiety
pharmacotherapy for h.
progressive relaxation under h.
relaxation therapy for h.

hyperacute
h. liver failure
h. phase
h. xenograft rejection

hyperaldosteronism
glucocorticoid-remediable h.
idiopathic h.

hyperalgesia
auditory h.
muscular h.

hyperalimentation
h. catheter
enteral h.
h. feeding
h. fluid
infected hyperalimentation line
intravenous h.
h. kit
h. management
peripheral intravenous h.
h. solution
standard h.
h. therapy
h. tubing

hyperammonemia
transient hyperammonemia of newborn
transient neonatal h.

hyperamylasemia
asymptomatic h.

hyperandrogenic anovulation

hyperandrogenism
adrenal hyperandrogenism marker
h., insulin resistance, and acanthosis nigricans syndrome
ovarian h.

hyperarousal
autonomic h.
physiological h.

hyperbaric
h. bed
h. medicine
h. oxygen
h. oxygenation
h. oxygen chamber
h. oxygen drenching
h. oxygen therapy
h. oxygen treatment
h. pressure
systemic hyperbaric oxygen therapy
h. tank

hyperbilirubinemia
fasting h.
neonatal conjugated h.

hyperbolic glasses

hypercalcemia
elfin facies hypercalcemia syndrome
familial benign hypocalciuric h.
familial hypercalcemia with hypocalciuria
h. hormone
humoral hypercalcemia of malignancy
idiopathic infantile h.
immobilization h.
infantile hypercalcemia stenosis
h. of malignancy
malignancy
malignancy-associated humoral h.
supravalvular aortic hypercalcemia syndrome
tumor-inducing h.

hypercalcemia-osteolysis-T-cell syndrome

hypercalcemic
h. crisis
h. encephalopathy
h. nephropathy

hypercalcinuria
idiopathic h.

hypercalciuria
absorptive h.
autosomal recessive renal proximal tubulopathy and h.
hereditary hypophosphatemic rickets with hypercalciuria syndrome
idiopathic h.

hypercalciuric
X-linked hypercalciuric nephrolithiasis

hypercapnia
permissive h.

hypercapnic ventilatory response

hypercarbia pulmonary hypertension

hypercellularity
diffuse mesangial h.
segmental mesangial h.

hyperchloremic
h. metabolic acidosis
h. renal acidosis

hyperchlorhydria
hypergastrinemic h.
nontumorous hypergastrinemic h.

hypercholesterolemia
essential h.
familial h.
familial hypercholesterolemia, low-density lipoprotein
heterozygous familial h.
homozygous familial h.

hyperchromatic
oval hyperchromatic nucleus

hyperchromatism
macrocytic h.

hyperchromemia
idiopathic h.

hyperchromic
h. acidosis
macrocytic hyperchromic anemia

hypercoagulability
paraneoplastic h.

hypercoagulable state

hypercontractility
detrusor h.

hypercortisolemia
pathologic h.

hypercortisolism
metyrapone-induced h.

hypercyanotic
paroxysmal hypercyanotic attack

hyperdense middle cerebral artery sign

hyperdiploid cell

hyperdynamic
h. beta-adrenergic circulatory
h. ventricle

hyperemesis
h. gravidarum

hyperemia
active h.
active hyperemia of retina
arterial h.
h. of arytenoids
collateral h.
conjunctival h.
exercise hyperemia blood flow
focal area of h.
h. of iris
occlusive h.
passive h.
passive hyperemia of retina
peak reactive hyperemia blood flow
peristaltic h.
postocclusive reactive h.
postoperative reactive h.
pulp h.
reactive h.
reactive hyperemia blood flow
relative h.
h. unit
unit h.
venous h.

hyperemic
h. headache
h. laryngeal mucosa
h. membrane
h. mucosal pattern
h. nasal mucosa
peak hyperemic average velocity

hypereosinophilia
tropical h.

hypereosinophilic syndrome

hyperesthesia
auditory h.
cutaneous h.
muscular h.
olfactory h.
oneiric h.
optic h.
tactile h.

hyperexcitability
neuronal h.

hyperextensibility
facial dysplasia, hyperextensibility of joints, clinodactyly, growth retardation, mental retardation syndrome
short stature, hyperextensibility of joints or hernia or both, ocular depression, Rieger anomaly, teething, delayed

hyperextensible joint

hyperextension
h. brace
cruciform anterior spinal h.
h. deformity
h. dislocation
h. exercise
h. postures and maneuvers
h. of spine

hyperfine structure

hyperfractionated
h. accelerated radiation therapy
continuous hyperfractionated accelerated radiotherapy

hyperfractionation
accelerated h.
cell redistribution and dose h.

hyperfunction
antral gastrin cell h.
autoimmune thyroid h.
autonomous h.
ovarian androgenic h.
pituitary h.

hypergammaglobulinemia
M-component h.
polyclonal h.

hypergastrinemic
h. hyperchlorhydria
nontumorous hypergastrinemic hyperchlorhydria

hyperglobulinemia purpura

hyperglycemia
fat-induced h.
isolated postchallenge h.
nonketotic h.

hyperglycemia-induced
maternal hyperglycemia-induced fetal hyperinsulinemia

hyperglycemic
hyperosmolar hyperglycemic nonketotic coma
h. hyperosmolar nonketotic syndrome
hyperosmolar hyperglycemic nonketotic syndrome
h. index

hyperglycemic-glycogenolytic factor

hyperglyceridemia
carbohydrate-induced h.

hyperglycinemia
nonketotic h.

hypergonadotropic
microcephaly, hypergonadotropic hypogonadism, short stature syndrome

hyperhidrosis
paroxysmal localized h.

hyper-IgM syndrome

hyperimmune
h. antivariola gamma globulin
h. reaction
h. serum
h. serum globulin

hyperimmunized suppressed

hyperimmunoglobulinemia
h. D syndrome
Staphylococcus aureus hyperimmunoglobulinemia E syndrome
h. syndrome

hyperimmunoglobulin E syndrome

hyperinfection
strongyloidiasis with massive h.

hyperinflation
dynamic h.

hyperinsulinemia
maternal hyperglycemia-induced fetal h.

hyperinsulinemic
nonfamilial hyperinsulinemic hypoglycemia
persistent hyperinsulinemic hypoglycemia of infancy

hyperinsulinism
alimentary h.
nonfamilial hyperinsulinism of infancy
obesity of h.

hyperintense
nodular hyperintense focus
periventricular hyperintense lesion

hyperintensity
deep white matter h.
multifocal area of h.
periventricular h.
pontine h.
white matter h.

hyperirritability
posttraumatic hyperirritability syndrome

hyperkeratosis
epidermolytic h.
mental retardation, spastic paraplegia, palmoplantar hyperkeratosis syndrome
multiple minute digitate h.
nevoid hyperkeratosis of nipple and areola
h. of sole

hyperkeratotic
h. area
atrophic hyperkeratotic lesion
h. lesion
h. verrucoid surfaced lesion

hyperkinesis
axial h.
Claude hyperkinesis sign
paroxysmal anal h.
h. syndrome

hyperkinetic
h. behavior syndrome
h. conduct disorder
h. heart syndrome
idiopathic hyperkinetic heart syndrome
h. impulse disorder
organic hyperkinetic syndrome
h. pulse
h. reaction of childhood
h. state
h. syndrome
h. syndrome of childhood

hyperkyphoscoliosis
neuropathic h.

hyperlactemia
asymptomatic h.

hyperlinearity
palmar h.

hyperlipemia
mixed h.

hyperlipidemia
combined fat- and carbohydrate-induced h.
endogenous h.
essential h.
familial combined h.
mixed hyperlipoproteinemia familial type 5 h.

hyperlipoproteinemia
mixed hyperlipoproteinemia familial type 5 hyperlipidemia

hyperlucent
h. lung
h. lung syndrome
hypermature cataract
hypermelanosis
linear and whorled nevoid h.
nevoid h.
hypermetropia
absolute h.
astigmatic h.
h., right
h., total
hypermetropic astigmatism
hypermineralocorticoidism
licorice-induced h.
hypermobile
h. joint
h. kidney
hypermobility
h. as a risk factor
marfanoid hypermobility syndrome
marfanoid hypermobility syndrome
posterior occipitoatlantal h.
h. syndrome
hypermotility
gastrointestinal h.
intestinal h.
hypernatremia
essential h.
h. and fluid attack
hypernatremic
h. dehydration
h. encephalopathy
hypernephroma cell
hyperopia
h., absolute
manifest h.
h., total
total h.
hyperopic
h. astigmatism
h. automated lamellar keratoplasty
compound hyperopic astigmatism
hyperornithinemia with gyrate atrophy
hyperosmolality
iatrogenic h.
hyperosmolar
h. coma
hyperglycemic hyperosmolar nonketotic syndrome
h. hyperglycemic nonketotic coma
h. hyperglycemic nonketotic syndrome
nonketotic h.
h. nonketotic diabetic coma
h. nonketotic diabetic state
nonketotic hyperosmolar acidosis
nonketotic hyperosmolar state
h. syndrome
hyperosmotic
nonketotic h.
hyperostosis
acquired hyperostosis syndrome
ankylosing spinal h.
diffuse idiopathic skeletal h.
idiopathic cortical h.
idiopathic skeletal h.
infantile cortical h.
rheumatoid arthritis, diffuse idiopathic skeletal h.
sternocostoclavicular h.
synovitis, acne, pustulosis, hyperostosis, osteomyelitis syndrome
h. totalis
vertebral ankylosing h.
hyperoxic normocapnic
hyperparathyroid
predominant hyperparathyroid bone disease
hyperparathyroidism
familial isolated primary h.
neonatal severe h.
normocalcemic primary h.
nutritional secondary h.
primary h.
secondary h.
tertiary h.
hyperpeptic gastritis
hyperphagia
hypotonia, hyperphagia, hypogonadism, obesity
hyperphenylalaninemia
malignant h.
maternal h.
mild h.
persistent h.
hyperphoria
left h.
Maddox rod h.
right h.
hyperphosphatasemic
congenital hyperphosphatasemic skeletal dysplasia
hyperphosphatasia
osteoectasia with h.
hyperpigmentation
familial progressive h.
longitudinal nail h.
marble cake h.
oral postinflammatory h.
hyperpigmented
erythematous hyperpigmented papule
h. lesion
longitudinal hyperpigmented band
h. skin
hyperpituitary
h. giantism
h. gigantism
hyperplasia
ACTH-independent bilateral macronodular h.
adenomatous h.
adult-onset congenital adrenal h.
alveolar cell h.
angiofibroblastic hyperplasia tendinosis
angiofollicular h.
angiofollicular hyperplasia lymph node
angiofollicular lymph node h.
angiofollicular lymphoid h.
angiofollicular mediastinal lymph node h.
angiolymphoid h.
angiolymphoid hyperplasia with eosinophilia
antral G-cell h.
apocrine h.
asymmetric nasopharyngeal lymphoid h.
atypical h.
atypical adenomatous h.
atypical ductal h.
atypical endometrial h.
atypical lobular h.
atypical lobular breast h.
atypical melanocytic h.
atypical regenerative h.
autonomous adrenal h.
autosomal dominant toxic thyroid h.
basal cell h.
benign cystic endometrial h.
benign prostatic h.
capsular synovial-like h.
chronic inflammatory h.
chronic perforating hyperplasia of pulp
complex atypical hyperplasia/metaplasia
congenital adrenogenital h.
congenital lipoid adrenal h.
congenital virilizing adrenal h.

cortical stromal h.
cutaneous lymphoid h.
diffuse nodular h.
ductal h.
h. of ducts
early cystic h.
endometrial h.
enterochromaffin cell h.
h. of epiglottis
explosive follicular h.
fibroadenomatosis hyperplasia of prostate gland
fibromuscular h.
focal epithelial h.
focal lymphoid h.
focal nodular h.
follicular h.
follicular nodular h.
giant follicular h.
giant lymph node h.
gingival h.
growth hormone cell h.
hemifacial h.
histiocytic hyperplasia of lymph node
histocytic hyperplasia of lymph nodes
idiopathic adrenal h.
idiopathic adrenocortical h.
inflammatory papillary h.
inflammatory papillary hyperplasia of the palate
intimal h.
intravascular papillary endothelial h.
juxtaglomerular cell h.
Leydig cell h.
lining cell layer h.
lipoid adrenal h.
lobular epithelial h.
localized angiofollicular lymph node h.
lymph node h.
macronodular adrenal h.
mantle zone h.
massive macronodular h.
mast cell h.
mediastinal lymph node h.
mesothelial h.
microglandular h.
microglandular cervical h.
micronodular pneumocyte h.
microscopic benign prostatic h.
mild focal cortical nodular h.
mixed follicular h.
mucosal inflammatory h.
mucous cell h.
multicentric angiofollicular lymphoid h.
multiple gland h.
myointimal h.
neonatal breast h.
nodular adrenal h.
nodular adrenocortical h.
nodular cortical adrenal h.
nodular hyperplasia of ovary
nodular hyperplasia of prostate gland
nodular lymphoid h.
nodular regenerative h.
nodular regenerative hyperplasia of liver
nonclassical adrenal h.
nonclassic congenital adrenal h.
nonsalt-wasting congenital adrenal h.
ovarian stromal h.
pancreatic duct h.
parathyroid gland h.
parietal cell h.
persistent hyperplasia of primary vitreous
postatrophic h.
prostate gland benign h.
pseudoangiomatous stromal h.
pseudointimal h.
pulmonary lymphoid h.
pulmonary vascular h.
reactive lymphoid h.
salt-wasting congenital adrenal h.
sebaceous gland h.
simple virilizing congenital adrenal h.
squamous cell h.
Swiss cheese h.
virilizing adrenal h.

hyperplasia/metaplasia
complex atypical h./m.

hyperplastic
h. achondroplasia
adenomatous hyperplastic nodule
h. alveolar nodule
h. arteriolar nephrosclerosis
h. arteriosclerosis
autonomous nodular hyperplastic gland
benign hyperplastic gastropathy
h. bone
h. cholecystosis
chronic hyperplastic sinusitis with nasal polyposis
cortical hyperplastic nodule
h. cyst
h. endometritis
h. endometrium
epithelial hyperplastic laryngeal lesion
h. gingivitis
h. graft
h. liver nodule
h. membrane
mildly hyperplastic bone marrow
h. muscle fiber
h. nodule
persistent hyperplastic primary vitreous
persistent primary hyperplastic vitreous
h. persistent pupillary membrane
primary persistent hyperplastic vitreous
h. rectal polyp
h. sclerosis
h. synovium
h. tissue

hyperplastic-like mucosal change

hyperpnea-induced bronchoconstriction

hyperpolarization
afterspike h.

hyperpolarizing
endothelium-derived hyperpolarizing factor
h. bipolar cell
passive hyperpolarizing potential

hyperprolactinemia
amenorrhea and h.
galactorrhea-amenorrhea hyperprolactinemia syndrome

hyperpyrexia
malignant h.

hyperreactive
h. airway
h. bronchial tube

hyperreactivity
airway h.
bronchial h.
h. to stimuli
vestibular h.

hyperreflexia
autonomic h.
spinal detrusor h.

hyperreflexic bladder

hyperresonance
h. to percussion
lungs revealed hyperresonance to percussion

hyperresponsiveness
airway h.
bronchial h.

hypersecretion
ACTH h.
gastric h.
growth hormone h.
mucus h.
pituitary h.

hypersecretory
hypertrophic hypersecretory gastropathy

hypersegmented neutrophil

hypersensitive
h. carotid sinus syndrome
h. dentin
h. hearing
h. hypertrophic cardiomyopathy
patient h.
patient hypersensitive to aspirin
h. skin

hypersensitivity
allopurinol hypersensitivity syndrome
h. alveolitis
h. angiitis
anticonvulsant hypersensitivity syndrome
antiepileptic drug hypersensitivity syndrome
h. to aspirin
bee sting h.
carotid sinus h.
contact h.
cutaneous basophilic h.
delayed cutaneous h.
delayed hypersensitivity test
delayed skin hypersensitivity reaction
h. disorder
drug h.
drug-induced delayed multiorgan hypersensitivity syndrome
fatal hypersensitivity reaction
generalized visceral h.
granulomatous hypersensitivity reaction
immediate h.
immediate-type h.
immunologic hypersensitivity reaction
interstitial hypersensitivity pneumonitis
h. lung disease
h. myocarditis
h. pneumonia
h. pneumonitis
h. pneumonitis panel
h. reaction
skin test for delayed-type h.
summer-type hypersensitivity pneumonitis
systemic cutaneous basophil h.
tumor-direct cell-mediated h.
h. vasculitis

hypersexuality
paroxysmal h.

hypersomnia
chronic h.
menstrual-associated periodic h.
paroxysmal h.
periodic h.
persistent h.
primary h.
h. related to another mental disorder
h. related to a known organic factor

hypersomnolence
idiopathic central nervous system h.
sleep apnea-hypersomnolence syndrome associated with upper airway obstruction

hyperstimulation
ovarian h.
severe ovarian hyperstimulation syndrome
h. syndrome

hypertelorism
lentigines, electrocardiographic abnormalities, ocular hypertelorism, pulmonary stenosis, abnormalities of genitalia, retardation of growth, deafness syndrome
macrocephaly, hypertelorism, short limbs, hearing loss, developmental delay syndrome
mental retardation, short stature, hypertelorism syndrome
ocular h.
orbital h.

hypertelorism-microtia-clefting syndrome

hypertension
arterial h.
autogenic training for h.
benign essential h.
benign intracranial h.
borderline systolic h.
chronic thromboembolic pulmonary h.
community hypertension evaluation clinic
H. Detection and Followup Program
edema, proteinuria, h.
essential h.
extrahepatic portal h.
familial primary pulmonary h.
genetic h.
high-renin essential h.
hypercarbia pulmonary h.
hypoxia-induced pulmonary h.
idiopathic intracranial h.
idiopathic portal h.
initial hypertension evaluation
intracerebral h.
intracranial h.
intrahepatic portal h.
isolated systolic h.
left atrial h.
low-renin essential h.
malignant h.
normal renin essential h.
ocular h.
ocular hypertension glaucoma
ocular hypertension indicator
h. optical treatment study
h. optimal treatment
oral contraceptive-induced h.
pancreatic ductal h.
passive pulmonary h.
persistent fetal circulation with pulmonary h.
persistent pulmonary h.
persistent pulmonary hypertension of newborn
h. plus proteinuria
portal h.
portal hypertension of the liver
portal hypertension with ascites
portopulmonary h.
h. in pregnancy
pregnancy-induced h.
primary plexogenic h.
primary pulmonary h.
primary pulmonary hypertension murmur
primary pulmonary hypertension risk factor
pulmonary artery h.
pulmonary hypertension pressure
pulmonary vascular h.
renin essential h.
renovascular h.
h. screening program

secondary pulmonary h.
h. secondary to renal disease
superimposed pregnancy-induced h.
systemic arterial h.
systemic vascular h.
systemic venous h.
systolic-diastolic h.
systolic hypertension in the elderly
h. and tachycardia
thromboembolic pulmonary h.
white coat h.

hypertensive
acute hypertensive episode
h. agent
h. arteriopathy
h. arteriosclerosis
h. arteriosclerotic
h. arteriosclerotic cardiovascular disease
h. arteriosclerotic heart disease
arteriosclerotic hypertensive heart disease
atherosclerotic hypertensive cardiovascular disease
biofeedback for h.'s
borderline h.
h. cardiomyopathy
h. cardiovascular disease
choroidal hypertensive disease
h. choroidopathy
chronic hypertensive disease
h. crisis
h. emergencies
h. emergency
h. encephalopathy
h. episode
essential hypertensive patient
h. heart disease
h. hemorrhage
h. hypertrophic cardiomyopathy
h. hypervolemic therapy
h. intracerebral hemorrhage
h. meningeal hydrops
minor hypertensive infant
h. nephropathy
h. nephrosclerosis
h. neuroretinopathy
obese hypertensive patient
h. ocular disease
ocular hypertensive glaucoma
h. optic neuropathy
h. patient
patient is h.
h. personality
portal hypertensive gastropathy
portal hypertensive intestinal vasculopathy
potential fetal hypertensive crisis
potential hypertensive crisis
h. pulmonary vascular disease
rational hypertensive therapy
h. renal failure
renal hypertensive disease
h. retinitis
h. retinopathy
h. smoker
stress in hypertensive patient
stroke-prone spontaneous h.
h. therapy
h. urgency
h. vascular crisis
h. vasculopathy

hypertext markup language

hyperthecosis
ovarian h.

hyperthermia
anular phased-array h.
h. in breast
combined hyperthermia and radiation treatment
cooling blanket for h.
h. effect
extracorporeal whole body h.
local tumor h.
malignant h.
malignant hyperthermia resistance
malignant hyperthermia syndrome
microwave hyperthermia of the prostate
h. in newborn
North American Malignant Hyperthermia protocol
h. in pelvis
sensitivity to h.
stress-induced h.
systemic h.
thermometer monitoring in h.
total body h.
transrectal prostatic h.
whole-body h.

hyperthermic
h. antiblastic perfusion
continuous hyperthermic peritoneal perfusion
intraperitoneal hyperthermic chemotherapy
intraperitoneal hyperthermic perfusion
isolated hyperthermic limb perfusion
h. isolated limb perfusion
malignant hyperthermic rhabdomyolysis
h. rhabdomyolysis

hyperthyroid heart

hyperthyroidism
neonatal Graves h.
nonautoimmune familial h.
non-Graves disease h.
h. in pregnancy
primary h.
spontaneously responding h.

hyperthyroxinemia
familial dysalbuminemic h.
prealbumin-associated h.

hypertonia
axial h.
sympathetic h.

hypertonic
h. acetate dextran
h. bladder
h. buffered medium
percutaneous aspiration, instillation of hypertonic saline, respiration
h. saline
h. solution
h. sphincter
h. uterine dysfunction

hypertonica
polycythemia h.

hypertrichosis
cataract, hypertrichosis, mental retardation
gingival fibromatosis, hypertrichosis, cherubism, mental retardation, epilepsy syndrome
nevoid h.

hypertriglyceridemia
familial h.

hypertrophic
h. adenoids
h. arthritis
h. burn scar
h. cardiomyopathy
h. catarrh
h. change
chronic hypertrophic emphysema
chronic hypertrophic pachymeningitis
h. cicatrix
h. cirrhosis
h. dystrophy
h. emphysema
h. encroachment
h. enlargement
h. exostosis

hypertrophic *(continued)*
familial hypertrophic obstructive cardiomyopathy
h. gastritis
genetic hypertrophic cardiomyopathy
giant hypertrophic gastritis
hereditary hypertrophic enlargement
high-altitude hypertrophic cardiomyopathy syndrome
h. hypersecretory gastropathy
hypersensitive hypertrophic cardiomyopathy
hypertensive hypertrophic cardiomyopathy
idiopathic hypertrophic aortic stenosis
idiopathic hypertrophic osteoarthropathy
idiopathic hypertrophic subaortic stenosis
infantile hypertrophic pyloric stenosis
h. infiltrative tendinitis
h. lipping
h. lymphocytic gastritis
h. muscular subaortic stenosis
h. myopathy
h. neuropathy
h. nodular gliosis
normal hypertrophic changes
h. obstructive cardiomyopathy
h. ossification
osteoarthritic hypertrophic spur formation
persistent hypertrophic vitreous
h. pharyngitis
progressive hypertrophic interstitial neuropathy
pulmonary hypertrophic osteoarthropathy
h. pulmonary osteoarthritis
h. pulmonary osteoarthropathy
h. pyloric stenosis
h. rhinitis
h. salpingitis
secondary hypertrophic arthropathy
h. smooth muscle layer
h. spondylitis
h. spur
h. spurring
supravalvular hypertrophic aortic stenosis
h. synovitis
h. tonsil
h. zone

hypertrophicans
exophthalmos, myxedema circumscriptum praetibiale, and osteoarthropathia hypertrophicans syndrome

hypertrophied
h. adenoid
heart hypertrophied and dilated
impaired contractility of hypertrophied muscle
h. inferior turbinate
h. muscle
h. papilla
h. scar
h. tonsil
ventricles dilated and h.

hypertrophy
h. of adenoids
basal septal h.
benign hypertrophy of prostate
benign prostatic h.
biventricular h.
biventricular dilatation and h.
h. of cardiomegaly
combined atrial h.
combined ventricular h.
compensatory hypertrophy of heart muscle
concentric left ventricular h.
congenital hypertrophy of retinal pigment epithelium
dilatation and h.
eccentric h.
familial h.
giant papillary h.
h. of heart
idiopathic myocardial h.
isolated asymmetric septal h.
left atrial h.
left ventricular h.
marked left ventricular h.
massive breast h.
mild biventricular dilatation h.
muscular hypertrophy syndrome
myocardial cellular h.
myocardial idiopathic h.
nodular prostatic h.
nonmalignant adenoidal h.
papillary conjunctival h.
prostatic h.
right atrial h.
right ventricular h.
submucosal gland h.
h. of tonsils and adenoids
transcoronary ablation of septal h.
h. of trigone
ventricular h.
volume load h.

hypertropia
alternating h.
dissociated double h.
intermittent h.
left h.
right h.

hyperuricemia
asymptomatic h.

hypervariable segment II

hyperventilate
turn, cough, and h.

hyperventilating
patient h.
patient is h.
h., sweating and shaking

hyperventilation
h. buildup
central neurogenic h.
chronic hyperventilation syndrome
h. from anxiety
isocapnic hyperventilation with cold air
isocapnic hyperventilation with room air
h. maneuver
h. procedure
prolonged intensive h.
h. provocation test
h. syndrome
h. tetany

hyperventilation-induced
h.-i. asthma
h.-i. high-amplitude rhythmic slowing

hyperviscosity syndrome

hypervolemic
hypertensive hypervolemic therapy

hypesthesia
h. of left leg
median nerve h.
numbness and h.
h. and paralysis
h. of right leg
stocking and glove type h.

hyphema
anterior chamber h.
microscopic h.

hypnagogic
h. hallucination
h. imagery
h. phenomena
h. startle

h. starts
h. state

hypnic jerk

hypnogenic
paroxysmal hypnogenic dyskinesia

hypnopompic hallucination

hypnosis
memory, and distortion h.
h. study
h. technique

hypnotic
h. agent
h. delirium
h. dosage
Harvard Group Scale of Hypnotic Susceptibility, Form A
h. imagery
h. induction
H. Induction Profile
h. relaxation for insomnia
Stanford H. Susceptibility Scale
h. state

hypoactive
h. bowel sounds
h. bowel tones
h. deep tendon reflex
male hypoactive sexual desire disorder
h. movement
h. sexual desire disorder

hypoadrenalism
primary h.

hypoaldosteronism
hyporeninemic h.
syndrome of hyporeninemic h.

hypoandrogenism
ovarian h.

hypobaric hypoxia

hypobetalipoproteinemia
familial h.

hypocalcemia
autosomal dominant h.
cardiac abnormality, abnormal facies, thymic hypoplasia, cleft palate, h.
cardiac abnormality, T-cell deficit, clefting, h.
neonatal h.

hypocalcemic
simple hypocalcemic tetany

hypocalcification
linear h.

hypocalciuria
familial hypercalcemia with h.

hypocalciuric
familial benign hypocalciuric hypercalcemia

hypocaloric
h. carbohydrate feeding
h. protein feeding

hypochlorite
sodium h.

hypochondriacal
h. delusion
monosymptomatic h.
monosymptomatic hypochondriacal psychosis
h. neurosis
h. patient
h. personality
h. reflex

hypochondriac region

hypochondriasis
monosymptomatic h.
h. scale

hypochondrium
left h.
right h.

hypochromic
h. anemia
h. erythrocyte
idiopathic hypochromic anemia
microcytic hypochromic anemia
normocytic hypochromic anemia

hypocomplementemic
h. glomerulonephritis
h. urticarial vasculitis syndrome
h. vasculitis urticaria syndrome

hypocontractility
detrusor h.

hypodensity
nodal h.

hypodermic
h. implantation
h. microscope
h. morphine sulfate
h. needle
per h.
h. syringe
h. tablet

hypodermoclysis infusion

hypoechoic
h. area
h. area of ultrasound
h. band
focal hypoechoic lesion

hypofibrinogenic plasma

hypofractionated stereotactic radiotherapy

hypofunction
autoimmune polyglandular h.
pituitary hormone h.

hypogammaglobulinemia
common variable h.
transient hypogammaglobulinemia of infancy

hypogastric
h. artery
h. artery aneurysm
h. ganglion
inferior hypogastric plexus
h. ligation
h. nerve
h. occlusion
h. plexus
h. pressure
h. region
h. region of abdomen
h. vein

hypogeusia
postinfluenza-like hyposmia and h.

hypoglossal
accompanying vein of hypoglossal nerve
ansa hypoglossal nerve
h. carotid entrapment
h. ganglion
loop of hypoglossal nerve
h. muscle
h. nerve
h. nerve sign
nucleus of hypoglossal nerve
primitive hypoglossal artery
h. trigone

hypoglossal-facial neuroanastomosis

hypoglossalis
nucleus h.

hypoglossia-limb deficiency phenotype

hypoglossus
ansa hypoglossus muscle

hypoglycemia
functional decortication from h.
insulin hypoglycemia test
nonfamilial hyperinsulinemic h.
non-islet cell tumor h.
nonislet-cell tumor-induced h.
persistent hyperinsulinemic hypoglycemia of infancy
symptomatic h.

hypoglycemic
h. agent
h. coma
h. encephalopathy
h. episode
h. index
neonatal hypoglycemic seizure
nonketotic hypoglycemic acidosis
oral h.
patient h.
patient is h.
h. reaction
h. shock
h. syncope

hypogonadism
anosmia and hypogonadotropic hypogonadism syndrome
hypogonadotropic h.
hypotonia, hyperphagia, hypogonadism, obesity
hypotonia, hypomentia, hypogonadism, and obesity syndrome
idiopathic hypogonadotropic h.
idiopathic hypothalamic h.
insulin-resistant diabetes, acanthosis nigricans, hypogonadism pigmentary retinopathy, deafness, mental retardation syndrome
isolated hypogonadotropic h.
mental retardation, ataxia, hypotonia, hypogonadism, retinal dystrophy syndrome
mental retardation, short stature, obesity, hypogonadism syndrome
microcephaly, hypergonadotropic hypogonadism, short stature syndrome
microcephaly, mental retardation, cataract, hypogonadism syndrome
obesity, short stature, mental deficiency, hypogonadism, micropenis, finger contracture, cleft lip-palate syndrome

hypogonadotropic
anosmia and hypogonadotropic hypogonadism syndrome
h. eunuchoidism
h. hypogonadism
h. hypogonadism-anosmia syndrome
idiopathic hypogonadotropic hypogonadism
isolated hypogonadotropic hypogonadism

hypohidrosis
alopecia, nail dystrophy, ophthalmic complication, thyroid dysfunction, hypohidrosis, ephelides and enteropathy, and respiratory tract infection

hypohidrotic
h. ectodermal dysplasia
h. ectodermal dysplasia with hypothyroidism

hypoiodous acid

hypokalemia
renal tubule h.
watery diarrhea, hypokalemia, and achlorhydria syndrome

hypokalemia-induced arrhythmia

hypokalemic
hypothermic hypokalemic cardioplegic arrest
watery diarrhea with hypokalemic alkalosis

hypokinesis
apical h.
cardiac wall h.
global h.

hypolactasia
adult h.

hypomagnesemia
neonatal h.

hypomelanosis
idiopathic guttate h.
h. of Ito

hypomentia
hypotonia, hypomentia, hypogonadism, and obesity syndrome

hypomyelinating
congenital hypomyelinating neuropathy

hyponatremia
asymptomatic h.
psychosis, intermittent hyponatremia, polydipsia syndrome

hypoosmotic
h. shock treatment
h. swelling

hypoparathyroidism
h., Addison disease, and mucocutaneous candidiasis syndrome
h., adrenal insufficiency, mucocutaneous candidiasis syndrome
autosomal dominant h.
familial isolated h.
idiopathic h.
surgical h.

hypoperfusion
apical h.
ocular hypoperfusion syndrome
organ h.
parietooccipital h.
peripheral h.

hypoperistalsis
megacystis-microcolon-intestinal hypoperistalsis syndrome
megalocystis microcolon intestinal hypoperistalsis syndrome

hypopharyngeus
musculus h.

hypopharyngoscopy, bronchoscopy, and esophagoscopy

hypopharynx
caustic strictures of h.

hypophonic aphasia

hypophosphatemia
familial h.
X-linked h.

hypophosphatemic
autosomal recessive hypophosphatemic rickets
familial hypophosphatemic rickets
hereditary hypophosphatemic rickets with hypercalciuria syndrome
h. bone disease
sex-linked hypophosphatemic rickets
X-linked hypophosphatemic rickets

hypophysectomized alloxan diabetic

hypophysectomy
partial central h.

hypophysial
superior hypophysial artery
supraoptical hypophysial diabetes insipidus

hypophysiotropic

hypophysis
anterior lobe of h.
h. cerebri
peduncle of h.
h. sicca
tentorium of h.

hypophysitis
autoimmune h.

lymphocytic h.
lymphoid h.

hypopigmentation
oculocerebral hypopigmentation syndrome
oculocutaneous h.
perianal h.

hypopigmented
marbled hypopigmented streak

hypopituitarism
distal arthrogryposis, hypopituitarism, mental retardation, facial anomalies syndrome
idiopathic h.
mental retardation, facial anomalies, hypopituitarism, distal arthrogryposis syndrome

hypopituitary
human hypopituitary serum

hypoplasia
adrenal h.
adrenal hypoplasia congenita
amyotrophic cerebellar h.
aortic tract complex h.
ascending aorta h.
ascending hypoplasia of aorta
cardiac abnormality, abnormal facies, thymic hypoplasia, cleft palate, hypocalcemia
cartilage-hair h.
cerebellar vermis hypoplasia, oligophrenia, congenital ataxia, coloboma, hepatic fibrosis
coloboma, heart disease, atresia choanae, retarded growth and retarded development and/or CNS anomalies, genital hypoplasia, and ear anomalies and/or deafness syndrome
congenital hypoplasia of adrenal glands
congenital idiopathic adrenal h.
conotruncal cardiac defect, abnormal face, thymic hypoplasia, cleft palate
development and/or central nervous system anomalies, genital hypoplasia, ear anomalies
femoral h.
femoral hypoplasia unusual facies syndrome
focal dermal h.
focal dermal hypoplasia syndrome
hereditary enamel h.
h. of left heart
Leydig cell h.
lipoid adrenal gland h.
mandibular condylar h.
mental retardation, polydactyly, phalangeal hypoplasia, syndactyly, unusual face, uncombable hair
midface hypoplasia syndrome
miniature-type congenital adrenal h.
mitral valve h.
nasal hypoplasia, peripheral dysostosis, mental retardation syndrome
occipital condyle h.
optic nerve h.
orbital bone h.
peripheral dysostosis, nail hypoplasia, mental retardation syndrome
pulmonary hypoplasia membrane disease
right ventricular h.
secondary pulmonary h.
tubular hypoplasia aortic arch
tubular hypoplasia left aortic arch

hypoplastic
h. acute leukemia
h. anemia
h. aorta
h. emphysema
h. enamel
familial hypoplastic anemia
h. heart
h. kidney
h. left atrium
h. left heart syndrome
h. left ventricle
h. left ventricular syndrome
h. lung syndrome
mental retardation, congenital heart disease, blepharophimosis, blepharoptosis, hypoplastic teeth
nonprogressive hypoplastic syndrome
h. right heart syndrome

hypopnea
obstructive h.

hyporeflexia
detrusor h.

hyporeninemic hypoaldosteronism

hyporesponsiveness
partial thyroid-stimulating hormone h.
partial TSH h.

hyposensitization
oral h.

hyposmia
postinfluenza-like hyposmia and hypogeusia

hyposomatotropism
obesity-related h.

hypospadias
anterior h.
Asopa hypospadias repair
Magpi hypospadias repair
penoscrotal h.
perineal h.
perineoscrotal h.
pseudovaginal perineoscrotal h.
third-degree h.
vascularized double-sided preputial island flap and W flap glanuloplasty hypospadias repair

hypostome
barbed h.

hypotelorism
ocular h.
orbital h.

hypotension
acute severe h.
cerebrospinal fluid h.
chronic idiopathic orthostatic h.
chronic orthostatic h.
h. and coma
deliberate h.
idiopathic orthostatic h.
increased peripheral vasodilation and h.
instantaneous orthostatic h.
intradialytic h.
neurally mediated h.
neurogenic orthostatic h.
obliterative pulmonary h.
orthostatic h.
postexercise h.
pulmonary artery h.
spontaneous intracranial h.
sympathetic orthostatic h.
h. and tachycardia
vertigo, syncope and h.

hypotensive
h. agent
bradycardia h.
nocturnal hypotensive episode
patient h.
patient weak, hypotensive and unresponsive
h. period
supine hypotensive syndrome
h. and ventilatory support

hypothalamic
anterior hypothalamic area
anterior hypothalamic nucleus
anterior hypothalamic preoptic area
h. blood flow
dorsomedial hypothalamic nucleus lesion
h. epilepsy
h. feeding center
functional hypothalamic amenorrhea
h. hormone
h. hypophysiotropic-releasing hormone
idiopathic hypothalamic hypogonadism
lateral hypothalamic area
lateral hypothalamic nucleus
lateral hypothalamic syndrome
h. lesion
nucleus arcuatus of intermediate hypothalamic area
h. obesity
h. pituitary adrenocortical axis
h., pituitary, thyroid
posterior hypothalamic area
preoptic anterior hypothalamic area
h. pubertal syndrome
pulmonary hypothalamic stimulation
h. secretory factor
supraoptic hypothalamic nucleus
h. ventromedial nucleus

hypothalamic-hypophysial-adrenal system

hypothalamic-pituitary-adrenal axis

hypothalamic-pituitary-adrenocortical system

hypothalamic-pituitary axis

hypothalamic-releasing
h.-r. factor
h.-r. hormone

hypothalamo-hypophyseo-adrenal axis

hypothalamohypophysial
h. portal circulation
h. portal system

hypothalamoneurohypophysial
h. axis
h. complex
h. tract

hypothalamus
anterior h.
arcuate h.
arcuate nucleus of the h.
lateral h.
mamillary tubercle of h.
medial h.
medial basal h.
paraventricular nucleus of the h.
posterior h.
posteromedial h.
ventrolateral nucleus of h.
ventromedial nucleus of the h.

hypothalmic amenorrhea

hypothenar
h. eminence
h. fascia
h. hammer syndrome

hypothermia
accidental h.
h. in aging
h. and alcoholism
h. blanket
chills with h.
dilated pupils and h.
exposure-related hypothermia death
extracorporeal exchange h.
malignant hypothermia susceptibility
h. oxygen warmer
topical h.

hypothermic
h. blanket
h. cardiac arrest surgery
h. circulatory arrest
deep hypothermic circulatory arrest
h. fibrillating arrest
h. hypokalemic cardioplegic arrest
h. ischemia
h. mattress
h. procedure
profound hypothermic circulatory arrest
profoundly hypothermic circulatory arrest
h. surgery
h. technique

hypothesis, pl. **hypotheses**
alpha, beta, gamma hypotheses
alternative h.
large number h.
log-kill h.
missing self h.
Neyman-Pearson statistical h.
null h.
overworked B-cell h.
tension-reducing h.

hypothetical
h. mean organism
h. mean strain

hypothromboplastinemia

hypothyroid goiter

hypothyroidism
amenorrhea, galactorrhea, h.
congenital h.
hypohidrotic ectodermal dysplasia with h.
juvenile acquired h.
maternal thyrotropin receptor blocking antibody-induced congenital h.
minimally symptomatic h.
spontaneous primary h.

hypothyroxinemia
maternal h.
h. of prematurity

hypotonia
h., hyperphagia, hypogonadism, obesity
h., hypomentia, hypogonadism, and obesity syndrome
mental retardation, ataxia, hypotonia, hypogonadism, retinal dystrophy syndrome
muscle h.
muscular h.
neonatal h.
nonparalytic h.
Oppenheim congenital h.
paralytic h.
uterine h.

hypotonic
h. bladder
chronic infantile hypotonic syndrome
h. colon
h. duodenography
h. lysis buffer

hypotonicity
asymptomatic h.

hypotony
ocular h.
persistent postdrainage h.

hypotrichosis
Matie-Unna h.

hypotropia
alternating h.
constant h.

hypoventilation
alveolar hypoventilation syndrome
central alveolar h.
central alveolar hypoventilation syndrome
congenital central hypoventilation syndrome
h. failure

hypovitaminosis D osteopathy

hypovolemic shock

hypoxanthine
arginine, hypoxanthine, and uracil
h., azaserine, and thymidine
h. riboside

hypoxemia
arterial h.
nocturnal h.
perinatal h.

hypoxemic
acute hypoxemic respiratory failure
h. episode

hypoxia
altitude h.
alveolar h.
anemic h.
h. and anoxia
anoxic h.
cerebral h.
chronic h.
circulatory h.
diffusion h.
functional decortication from h.
hypobaric h.
hypoxic h.
h., intussusception, brain mass
ischemic h.
mixed venous h.
neonatal h.
orbital h.
oxygen affinity h.
perinatal h.
relative h.
sleep h.
stagnant h.
tumor cell h.

hypoxia-induced pulmonary hypertension

hypoxia-inducible factor-1-alpha

hypoxic
h. change in brain
chronic hypoxic lung disease
h. hypoxia
infant acidotic and h.
h. ischemic encephalopathy
paroxysmal hypoxic spell
pulmonary alveolar hypoxic vasoconstriction
h. pulmonary vasoconstriction
h. responder
h. ventilatory drive
h. ventilatory response

hypoxic-ischemic
h.-i. encephalopathy
h.-i. lesion
h.-i. neuronal injury

hypsarrhythmia
progressive encephalopathy, edema, hypsarrhythmia, optic atrophy

hysterectomy
abdominal h.
classic abdominal Semm h.
laparoscopic-assisted abdominal h.
laparoscopic-assisted vaginal h.
laparoscopic supracervical h.
modified radical h.
Munro and Parker classification for laparoscopic h.
h. and radiation
radical abdominal h.
radical hysterectomy and bilateral salpingo-oophorectomy
Schauta radical vaginal h.
h. and sterilization
subtotal h.
h. support
total h.
total abdominal h.
total abdominal hysterectomy and bilateral salpingo-oophorectomy
total vaginal h.
vaginal h.
Wertheim radical h.

hysteria psychosis

hysteric
h. amaurosis
h. amblyopia
h. angina
h. aphonia
h. ataxia
aura h.'s
h. insanity
h. joint
h. lethargy
megalopia h.'s
neurotic hysteric disorder
h. pregnancy
h. stigma

hysterica
aura h.
megalopia h.

hysterical
h. ataxia
h. blindness
h. chorea
h. conversation disorder
h. conversion reaction
h. convulsion
h. deafness
h. disorder
h. epilepsy
h. fainting
h. fever
h. laughter
h. mania
h. mutism
h. neurosis
h. paralysis
h. personality
h. reaction
h. state
h. stricture
h. syncope
h. tremor
h. vertigo
h. vomiting

hystericus
globus h.

hysterogram study

hysteroid conversion

hysterosalpingogram study

hysteroscopy
laparoscopic-assisted vaginal h.

hysterosonography
transvaginal h.

hysterotomy
low transverse h.
Pelosi h.

I band

Iaco virus

iatrogenic

i. anemia
i. atrial septal defect
i. bladder
i. disorder
i. effect
i. effects of behavior therapy
i. effusion
i. fracture
i. hyperosmolality
i. illness
i. injury
i. multiple pregnancy
i. pneumothorax
i. trauma
i. ureteral injury

Ibaraki virus

ice

anesthetizing effect of ice and snow
i. bag
i. chip
cold or ice whirlpool treatment
i., compression, and elevation
i., compression, elevation, and support
i. cream headache
i. mapping
i. massage
i. pack
protection, rest, ice, compression, elevation, support
protection, restricted activity, ice, compression, elevation
rest, ice, compression, elevation
slipped on i.
therapeutic qualities of i.
i. therapy
i. victim
i. water test

iced saline

ice-pick view

ichthyosiform

congenital hemidysplasia with ichthyosiform erythroderma and limb defects syndrome
congenital ichthyosiform erythroderma
nonbullous congenital ichthyosiform erythroderma

ichthyosis

autosomal dominant lamellar i.
autosomal recessive i.
i., brittle hair, impaired intelligence, decreased fertility, short stature syndrome
i. bullosa of Siemens
coloboma, heart anomaly, ichthyosis, mental retardation, and ear abnormality syndrome
i. congenita
i. fetalis
i. fetus
i., follicularis, atrichia or alopecia, photophobia syndrome
lamellar i.
mental deficiency, spasticity, congenital ichthyosis syndrome
i. and neutral lipid storage disease
nonbullous congenital erythrodermic i.
recessive X-linked i.
i. vulgaris
X-linked i.

ichthyosis-cheek-eyebrow syndrome

icing

i. compression
i. heart
heart i.

Icoaraci virus

icteric

conjunctivae i.
i. hepatitis
i. index
infant mildly i.
mildly icteric infant
i. necrosis
i. sclerae
sclerae markedly i.
i. serum hepatitis
i. sputum

icterus

acholuric hemolytic i.
i. catarrhalis
congenital hemolytic i.
i. gravis
i. gravis neonatorum
i. hemolyticus
i. index
i. index test
i. infectiosus
i. melas
i. praecox
i. simplex
i. viridans

idea

abstract i.
associated i.
autochthonous i.
compulsive i.
confusion of i.'s
delusional or ideas of reference
distorted ideas of reference
expansive i.
flight of i.'s
i.'s of grandeur
grandiose i.
idiosyncratic false i.
morbid i.
obsessional i.
overvalued false i.'s
overvalued obsessional i.'s
persistent inappropriate i.
poverty of i.'s
i.'s of reference
superstitious false i.'s
transient ideas of reference
unpersuasive false i.'s

ideal

i. arch wire
i. body mass
i. body weight
ego i.
narcissistic ego i.
nearly ideal binary solvent
i. occlusion

ideation

adolescent sexual i.
Adult Suicidal I. Questionnaire
homicidal i.
suicidal i.
suicidal/homicidal i.
transient paranoid i.

ideational apraxia

identical

i. by descent
i. genes
i. midplane doses
i. patterns
point of identical flow
i. stimulus
i. twin
i. twin transplants

identifiable

minimal identifiable odor
no identifiable disease

identification

Alcohol Use Disorders I. Test
antibody i.

identification *(continued)*
bacterial automated identification technique
Behavior Disorders I. Scale
i. bracelet
comprehensive identification process
Discrimination by I. of Pictures
early identification of symptom
i. of gene
Gram-positive i.
Haemophilus-Neisseria i.
isolation and i.
Micro Drop yeast identification system
number user i.
organism identification number
patient identification bracelet
personal identification number
Picture I. for Children-Standardized Index
Picture I. Test
rapid identification method
rapid identification method-*Neisseria*
Rhode Island Pupil I. Scale
standard mycological identification technique
synthetic sentence i.
University of Pennsylvania Smell I. Test
warning sign i.
Word Intelligibility by Picture I.

identified
bleeder i.
capsule i.
causative organism i.
i. criteria
i. high-risk mother
i. and ligated
not i.
patient's needs i.
polyclonal gammopathy i.
i. proximal ends of tendon
tumor i.

Identifying
Questionnaire for Identifying Children with Chronic Conditions

identity
adolescent personal i.
adolescent sexual i.
adult-life psychosexual identity disorder
alteration in i.
alternate i.
assumption of new i.
atypical gender identity disorder
controlling i.
i. disorder
disorders of psychosexual i.
i. disturbance
gender identity disorder
gender identity disorder of adolescence
gender identity disorder of adolescence or adulthood, nontranssexual type
gender identity disorder of adult life
gender identity disorder of childhood
loss of i.
male gender i.
masculine i.
multiple distinct i.'s
new i.
persistent identity disturbance
personal i.
personal identity disturbance
i. problem
psychosexual i.
reaction of i.
i. and role counseling
sense of i.
sexual i.

idiocy
amaurotic axonal i.
amaurotic familial i.
infantile amaurotic familial i.
juvenile amaurotic i.
late infantile amaurotic familial i.

idiojunctional
i. rhythm
i. tachycardia

idiopathic
i. acquired hemolytic disease
acquired idiopathic sideroblastic anemia
i. acquired refractory sideroblastic anemia
i. acquired sideroblastic anemia
acute canine idiopathic polyneuropathy
i. acute eosinophilic pneumonia
acute idiopathic demyelinating polyradiculoneuritis
acute idiopathic inflammatory bowel disease
acute idiopathic pericarditis
acute idiopathic peripheral facial nerve palsy
acute idiopathic polyneuritis
acute idiopathic thrombocytopenic purpura
adolescent idiopathic scoliosis
i. adrenal hyperplasia
i. adrenocortical hyperplasia
i. alveolar fibrosis
i. anaphylaxis-angioedema-frequent
i. anaphylaxis-angioedema-infrequent
i. anaphylaxis-generalized-frequent
i. anaphylaxis-generalized-infrequent
i. anaphylaxis-questionable
i. anaphylaxis-variant
i. anemia
i. ankylosing spondylitis
aortic idiopathic necrosis
i. aplastic bone marrow
i. aseptic necrosis
i. autoimmune hemolytic anemia
i. bile acid malabsorption
i. blepharospasm
i. bradycardia
i. brown induration
i. calcium renal stone formation
i. cardiomegaly
i. cardiomyopathy
i. carpal tunnel syndrome
i. CD4+ lymphocytopenia
i. CD4 T-cell lymphocytopenia
i. central nervous system hypersomnolence
i. central serous chorioretinopathy
chronic idiopathic anhidrosis
chronic idiopathic arthritides of childhood
chronic idiopathic myelofibrosis
chronic idiopathic orthostatic hypotension
chronic idiopathic urticaria
chronic idiopathic xanthomatosis
chronic idiopathic intestinal pseudo-obstruction syndrome
congenital idiopathic adrenal hypoplasia
i. congestive cardiomyopathy
i. cortical hyperostosis
i. cyclic edema
degenerative idiopathic cardiomyopathy
i. destructive arthritis
diffuse idiopathic skeletal hyperostosis
i. dilatation
i. dilated cardiomyopathy
i. disease of myocardium
i. disorder

i. environmental intolerance
i. epilepsy
i. epiretinal membrane
i. esophageal ulcer
i. facial paralysis
familial idiopathic gonadotropin deficiency
familial idiopathic nonarteriosclerotic cerebral calcification
i. fibroplasia
i. fibrosing alveolitis
i. fibrosis
i. flushing
i. gait disorders of elderly
i. genu valgum
i. growth hormone
i. growth hormone deficiency
i. guttate hypomelanosis
I. Headache Score
i. hemochromatosis
i. hirsutism
i. hyperaldosteronism
i. hypercalcemia
i. hypercalcinuria
i. hypercalciuria
i. hyperchromemia
i. hypereosinophilic syndrome
i. hyperkinetic heart syndrome
i. hypertension
i. hypertrophic aortic stenosis
i. hypertrophic osteoarthropathy
i. hypertrophic subaortic stenosis
i. hypochromic anemia
i. hypogonadotropic hypogonadism
i. hypoparathyroidism
i. hypopituitarism
i. hypothalamic hypogonadism
i. ineffective erythropoiesis
i. infantile hypercalcemia
i. inflammatory bowel disease
i. inflammatory myopathy
i. interstitial pneumonia
i. interstitial pulmonary fibrosis
i. intestinal pseudo-obstruction
i. intracranial hypertension
i. isosexual puberty
juvenile idiopathic arthritis
juvenile idiopathic scoliosis
i. juvenile osteoporosis
i. leucine sensitivity
i. long Q-T interval syndrome
i. lymphadenopathy syndrome
i. megacolon
i. megakaryocytic aplasia
i. mental deficiency
i. midline destructive disease
minimal change idiopathic nephrotic syndrome
i. minimal lesion nephrotic syndrome
i. mitral valve prolapse
multiple idiopathic hemorrhagic sarcoma
i. muscular dystrophy
i. myelofibrosis
i. myeloid proliferation
i. myocardial hypertrophy
myocardial idiopathic hypertrophy
i. myocardiopathy
i. myocarditis
i. myoglobinuria
neonatal chronic idiopathic neutropenia
i. nephritis
i. nephrotic syndrome
i. neutropenia
i. orbital inflammatory syndrome
i. orthostatic hypotension
i. Parkinson disease
i. paroxysmal cerebral dysrhythmia
Pasini-Pierini idiopathic atrophoderma
i. pericarditis
i. polypoidal choroidal vasculopathy
i. polyserositis
i. portal hypertension
i. postprandial syndrome
progressive idiopathic neuromuscular disease
i. protracted diarrhea
i. pulmonary arteriosclerosis
i. pulmonary hemorrhage
i. pulmonary hemosiderosis
i. purpura
i. rapidly progressive glomerulonephritis
i. Raynaud disease
i. recurrent pancreatitis
i. recurring stupor
i. refractory sideroblastic anemia
i. respiratory distress of newborn
i. respiratory distress syndrome
i. restrictive cardiomyopathy
i. retroperitoneal fibrosis
rheumatoid arthritis, diffuse idiopathic skeletal hyperostosis
i. seizure disorder
i. short stature
i. skeletal hyperostosis
i. steatorrhea
steroid-sensitive idiopathic nephrotic syndrome
i. sudden sensorineural hearing loss
i. sudden sensory hearing loss
i. thrombocytopenia
i. thrombocytopenia purpura
i. thrombocytopenic purpura
i. toe-walker
i. toe-walking
i. trigeminal neuralgia
i. ulcerative colitis
i. unilobar emphysema
i. ventricular fibrillation
i. ventricular tachycardia
i. vertigo
i. white matter lesion

idiophrenic insanity

idiosyncratic

alcohol idiosyncratic intoxication
i. alcohol intoxication
i. drug reaction
i. false idea
i. false ideas
i. food preference
i. intoxication
i. obsessions and rituals
i. reaction

idiot

erethismic i.
mongolian i.

idiotype

cross-reactive i.

idioventricular

accelerated idioventricular tachycardia
i. bradycardia
i. kick
pulsed idioventricular rhythm
pulseless idioventricular rhythm
i. rhythm
i. tachycardia

I disc

iduronate sulfatase deficiency

iduronic acid

Ieri virus

Ife virus

ifosfamide

L-asparaginase, ifosfamide, methotrexate
doxorubicin, cyclophosphamide, etoposide, ifosfamide, vincristine, methotrexate, bleomycin

ifosfamide *(continued)*
vincristine, doxorubicin, cyclophosphamide, dactinomycin plus ifosfamide with mesna

IGF-binding protein

IgG
immunoglobulin G, G2, G2a, G4
IgG AGA
anionic IgG 4 fraction
antigliadin IgG ELISA autoimmune test
antigliadin IgG, IgA test
antineutrophil cytoplasmic IgG antibody
antiparvovirus B19 IgG antibody
Aspergillus IgG titer
maternal IgG antibody
parvovirus B19 IgG antibody
IgG RF

Ignatius
Saint Ignatius itch

ileal
afferent ileal limb
aphthous ileal ulcer
i. artery
i. atresia
i. bladder
i. bypass
i. conduit
distal ileal obstruction syndrome
endorectal ileal pouch
endorectal ileal pull-through
gastric ileal bypass
i. loop
i. loop stoma
normal functioning ileal transverse colostomy
orifice of ileal papilla
i. pouch anal anastomosis
rabbit ileal loop test
resected end-to-end ileal colostomy
i. resection
i. segment
i. stasis
terminal ileal loop
i. vein

ileitis
distal i.
granulomatous i.
nonsclerosing i.
nonspecific i.
obstructive dysfunctional i.
regional i.
terminal i.

ileoanal
double-stapled ileoanal reservoir
endorectal ileoanal pull-through
endorectal ileoanal pull-through procedure

ileoanal anastomosis

ileocecal
i. bladder
i. fold
i. incompetence
i. insufficiency
i. intussusception
i. junction
i. opening
i. region
i. sphincter
i. valve

ileocecale
ostium i.

ileocolic
i. anastomosis
i. artery
ascending ileocolic artery
i. fold
i. intussusception
i. junction
i. lymph node
i. region
i. valve

ileocolitis
regional i.

ileogastric reflex

ileoileal intussusception

ileojejunitis
granulomatous i.
nongranulomatous i.

ileorectal anastomosis with end-to-end anastomosis

ileosigmoid anastomosis

ileostomy
anal ileostomy with preservation of sphincter
i. bag
diverting loop i.
loop i.
loop end i.
i. pouch
i. sac

ileotransverse
i. colostomy
end-to-side ileotransverse colostomy

Ilesha virus

ileum
antimesenteric border of distal i.
antral diverticulum of the i.
arterial arch of i.
artificial diverticulum of the i.
guinea pig i.
inflammation of i.
jejunum and ileum adhesed
reflux into terminal ileum normal
terminal i.
terminal ileum intubation

ileus
adynamic i.
adynamic/paralytic i.
i. following abdominal surgery
gallstone i.
mechanical i.
meconium i.
meconium ileus appearance
meconium ileus equivalent
myxedema i.
occlusive i.
paralytic i.
postoperative i.
reflex i.
reflexive i.
reflex-type i.
spastic i.
terminal i.

Ilheus virus

iliac
allograft iliac bone
anterior iliac crest
anteroposterior iliac spine
anterosuperior iliac spine graft
i. artery
i. artery aneurysm
i. artery occlusion
i. augmentation
autogenous iliac bone
i. autograft
autologous iliac crest bone graft
i. bifurcation
i. bone
i. bursa
i. cancellous bone
i. chain
i. colon
common i.
common iliac lymph nodes
common internal iliac artery
i. crest
i. crest biopsy
i. crest bone graft
crest of iliac bone
deep circumflex iliac artery flap
deep circumflex iliac artery

deep circumflex iliac vein
distance between iliac spines
i. endarterectomy
external i.
external iliac artery
external iliac lymph nodes
i. flexure of colon
i. fossa abscess
i. graft
i. horn
internal iliac adenopathy
internal iliac artery
internal iliac lymph node
internal iliac vein
left iliac of abdomen
left iliac artery
left iliac crest
left iliac fossa
i. lymph nodes
i. muscle
onlay cancellous iliac graft
osteomusculocutaneous deep circumflex iliac groin flap
osteoperiosteal iliac bone graft
outer lip of iliac crest
palpation of anterior superior iliac spine
posterior iliac crest
posterior inferior iliac spine
posterior superior iliac spine
i. pulse
i. region
right iliac artery
right iliac crest
ruptured iliac aneurysm
i. spine
i. steal
superficial circumflex iliac artery
superficial circumflex iliac vein
superior iliac crest
superior iliac spine
i. vein
i. vein thrombosis
i. vessel

iliacum
os i.

iliacus
musculus i.
musculus iliacus minor

ilial segment

iliocostal
lumbar iliocostal muscle

iliofemoral
anterior iliofemoral technique
i. artery
i. deep vein thrombosis
i. ligament

iliohypogastric
anterior cutaneous branch of iliohypogastric nerve
i. nerve block

ilioinguinal-iliohypogastric nerve block

iliolumbar
i. artery
i. ligament
lumbar branch of iliolumbar artery
i. vein

iliopectineal
i. fascia
i. fossa
i. ligament
i. line

iliopsoas muscle

iliopubic
i. eminence
i. tract

iliosacral articulation

iliotibial
i. band
i. band friction syndrome
i. band tendonitis
i. tract
i. tract friction syndrome

ilium
ala of i.
anterosuperior external ilium movement
anterosuperior ilium major
anterosuperior internal ilium movement
arcuate line of i.
arteria circumflexa ilium profunda
auricular surface of i.
external i.

Ilizarov procedure

ill
i. at ease
chronically mentally i.
i. defined
guilty but mentally i.
louping ill virus
mentally ill chemical abuser
National Alliance for the Mentally I.
patient acutely i.
patient chronically i.
patient emotionally i.
patient incurably i.
patient mentally i.
patient terminally i.
seriously ill list

ill-defined
i.-d. density
i.-d. mass

illegal
i. chemical
i. controlled substances
i. drug traffic
i. intravenous drug use

ill-fitting
i.-f. dentures
i.-f. shoes

illicit
addictive illicit drug
i. drug
i. drug abuse
i. drug use
fatal complications of illicit drug use
prenatal abuse of illicit drug
i. sex
i. substance use

illiterate
functionally i.

illness
acute clinical i.
acute febrile i.
acute febrile respiratory i.
acute medical i.
advantage by i.
i. attitude scale
average cost of i.
bacterial food-borne i.
I. Behavior Checklist
I. Behavior Questionnaire
bipolar i.
building illness syndrome
Canadian Acute Respiratory I. and Flu Scale
catastrophic life-threatening i.
certification of terminal i.
chemical dependency and mental i.
Child Health and I. Profile, Adolescent Edition
childhood severity of psychiatric i.
chronic factitious illness with physical symptoms
chronic long term i.
chronic medical i.
chronic and progressive i.
Clinical Global Impression-Severity of I. Scale

illness *(continued)*
course of i.
critical illness polyneuropathy
definable illness index
depression triggered by physical i.
disabling mental i.
i. of emotional origin
employee mental i.
environmental i.
evaluate extent of injury or i.
exacerbation of i.
exacerbation of preexisting psychiatric i.
exertional heat i.
i. fabrication
factitious illness with psychological symptoms
family history of mental i.
family reaction to i.
fatal genetic i.
flight into i.
food-borne i.
food-borne illness outbreak
full-blown manic depressive i.
genetic predisposition to psychiatric i.
health illness profile
heat illness syndrome
hereditary familial i.
history of medical i.
history of present i.
increased risk for i.
influenza-like i.
i. or injuries
insight into i.
Integrated Management of Childhood I.
length of awareness of i.
length of i.
level and degree of mental i.
lower respiratory tract i.
major mental i.
manic-depressive i.
mass psychogenic i.
mass sociogenic i.
mental i.
minor acute i.
model of i.
Multiple Severity of I. System
nature of i.
no mental i.
noncontributory to present i.
nonspecific building-related i.
nonthyroid i.
nonthyroidal illness syndrome
no present i.
no recent i.'s
opportunistic i.
other febrile i.
outcome of i.
past medical i.
patient concealed i.
patient faking i.
perceived illness threat
persistent mental i.
petition of mental i.
potentially life-threatening i.
predisposition towards i.
present medical i.
prevention of mental i.
previously unrecognized mental i.
previous medical i.
prolonged symptomatic i.
proof of i.
Psychosocial Adjustment to I. Scale
respiratory i.
self-awareness in i.
serious i.
severe depressive i.
severe mental i.
severe paralytic i.
severe and persistent mental i.
site of i.
terminal stage of i.
total episode of i.
treatment of mental i.
underlying physical i.
upper respiratory tract i.
usual childhood i.'s
warning signs of serious i.
waterborne illness outbreak

illogical thinking

illuminated near card

illumination
axial i.
central i.
contact i.
critical i.
dark-field i.
dark-ground i.
direct i.
focal i.
lateral i.
Luxtec coaxial i.
Macbeth i.
narrow-slit i.
oblique i.
red laser i.
through i.

illusion
auditory i.
i. of control
delusion, hallucination, or i.
fleeting i.
memory i.
movement i.
oculogravic i.
oculogyral i.
oculoparalytic i.
optic i.
optical i.
pain blocking i.
passive i.
perception i.
i. or perceptual distortions
i. of transparency
visual i.

illusional seizure

image
i. acquisition
i. amplification
anterior planar i.
arterial flow-phase i.
automated cell image analysis
automatic fluorescent image analyzer
axial fat-suppressed T2-weighted i.
axial gradient echo i.
axial magnetic resonance i.
axial proton-density-weighted i.
axial spin-echo i.
axial transabdominal i.
axial T2-weighed i.
bayesian image estimation
cognitive change of body i.
computer enhanced i.
curved, reformatted mandibular i.
delayed gamma camera i.
3-dimensional turbo-spin echo images
i. display and analysis
distorted body i.
DNA image cytometry
document image decoding
fluoroscopic image guidance
gradient-echo coronal i.
i. guide
high-definition i.
i. intensifier
laser image custom arthroplasty
mirror image breast biopsy
mirror image interpretation
mobile advanced real-time i.
model-based image processing
multiecho axial i.
multiecho coronal i.

multigated blood pool image at rest
multigated blood pool image during exercise
negative body i.
i. patterns of anxiety
perception of body i.
peripheral field i.
persistent inappropriate i.
poor body i.
proton-density axial i.
regional ejection fraction i.
short axis i.
source image distance
split image artifact
stress myocardial i.
thin-section axial i.
tomographic image of the head
T2-weighted i.
T1-weighted axial i.
T1-weighted coronal i.
T2 weighted i.

image-guided
i.-g. breast biopsy
i.-g. fine-needle aspiration biopsy
i.-g. functional endoscopic sinus surgery
i.-g. surgical technique

imagery
i. device
guided affective i.
guided imagery therapist
increase in eidetic i.
relaxation, distraction and i.
stress management and i.
visual imagery exercise
i. and visualization
vivid visual i.

imagination
creative i.

imagined
irrational obsession with imagined ugliness
I. Process Inventory

imaging
adenosine echocardiography i.
adenosine radionuclide perfusion i.
i. agent
air enema fluoroscopic i.
anisotropically rotational diffusion i.
anisotropic 3D i.
antegrade pyelography i.
anterior planar i.
antifibrin antibody imaging agent
antimyosin antibody i.
aperiodic functional MR i.
i. of arteries
arteriovenous shunt i.
Artoscan MRI i.
ascending contrast phlebography i.
associated imaging characteristic
ATL real-time Neurosector scan i.
Aurora MR breast i.
automated cellular imaging system
axial breath-hold gradient-echo cine magnetic resonance i.
axial echo planar diffusion weighted i.
axial grade echo i.
axial plane i.
axial transabdominal i.
axial 0.2T T1-weighted spin-echo i.
back-scattered electron i.
blood pool i.
brain imaging study
brain imaging technique
cardiac blood pool i.
cardiac imaging technique
carotid duplex i.
i. chain
chemical-shift i.
chemical shift i.
cine magnetic resonance i.
color Doppler flow i.
color duplex i.
color flow Doppler i.
color-flow duplex i.
color-flow imaging Doppler echocardiography
computer imaging system
computerized imaging technique
continuous arterial spin-labeled perfusion magnetic resonance i.
continuous-wave Doppler i.
contrast medium-enhanced magnetic resonance i.
conventional magnetic resonance i.
conventional planar i.
i. device
diagnostic i.
diagnostic imaging center
diffusion-tensor i.
diffusion-weighted imaging/magnetic resonance i.
diffusion-weighted imaging/perfusion i.
diffusion-weighted magnetic resonance i.
digital cardiac imaging system
digital imaging processing
digital imaging spectrophotometer
digital subtraction i.
digital vascular imaging system
2-dimensional Fourier i.
3-dimensional Fourier i.
dipyridamole echocardiography i.
dipyridamole thallium stress i.
Doppler color-flow i.
Doppler tissue i.
Doppler ultrasound i.
Doppler venous i.
duplex carotid i.
duplex Doppler i.
dynamic contrast-enhanced magnetic resonance i.
dynamic enhanced magnetic resonance i.
dynamic optical breast imaging system
dynamic pulmonary i.
electromagnetic blood flow i.
electronic portal imaging device
endoesophageal magnetic resonance i.
endoesophageal magnetic resonance imaging coil
endorectal magnetic resonance i.
enhancement of magnetic resonance i.
fast imaging steady precession sequence three-dimensional magnetic resonance i.
fast imaging with steady precession
fast imaging with steady-state free precession
fast multiplanar spoiled gradient-recalled i.
fluorescent thyroid i.
frequency domain imaging
functional magnetic resonance i.
fundamental i.
gadolinium-enhanced magnetic resonance i.
gated cardiac blood pool i.
gated sweet magnetic i.
half-Fourier i.
hard x-ray imaging spectrometer
harmonic i.
hepatobiliary i.
high-definition i.
high-resolution CT i.
high-resolution infrared imaging

imaging *(continued)*
high-speed volumetric i.
hot spot i.
infarct avid i.
intensified radiographic imaging system
live x-ray i.
low-field magnetic resonance i.
lung imaging fluorescence endoscope
lung imaging fluorescent endoscopy
macromolecular contrast-enhanced MR i.
magnetic resonance i.
magnetic resonance imaging thermometry
magnetic source i.
magnetization transfer i.
magnetization transfer magnetic resonance i.
mammary ductogram i.
mask-mode cardiac i.
mediastinal cross-sectional i.
medical optimal i.
M-mode echocardiogram i.
mobile artery and vein imaging system
monoclonal antibody i.
monocular heads-up display imaging system
MR catheter imaging and spectroscopy system scanner
MUGA cardiac blood pool i.
multiple line-scan i.
multisection diffuse-weighted magnetic resonance i.
myocardial perfusion i.
native tissue harmonic i.
negative contrast imaging agent
NeoTect imaging agent
neuroradiologic imaging procedure
Niamtu video imaging system
noninvasive brain imaging study
nuclear bone i.
nuclear cardiovascular i.
nuclear hepatobiliary i.
nuclear magnetic resonance i.
oblique axial MR i.
one-dimensional chemical-shift i.
optical intrinsic signal imaging
optical surface i.
oral cholecystogram i.
oral contrast imaging agent
paramagnetic enhancement accentuation by chemical shift i.
partial flip angle i.
partial Fourier i.
penile bulb i.
perfusion-weighted magnetic resonance i.
periorbital Doppler i.
phase-contrast cine magnetic resonance i.
phase-sensitive gradient-echo MR i.
phosphorus magnetic resonance i.
planar myocardial i.
power Doppler i.
i. procedures
pulse-inversion contrast harmonic i.
radiographic imaging system
radiolabeled antibody i.
radionuclide imaging of inferior vena cava
radionuclide joint i.
radionuclide thyroid i.
reverse fast imaging with steady-state free precession
routine antenatal diagnostic imaging with ultrasound
second harmonic i.
segmenting dual-echo MR i.
selective imaging and graphics for stereotactic surgery
short inversion imaging recovery
single-photon emission imaging tomography
single-photon planar i.
sonic imaging technique
spin echo i.
staging process and i.
stone imaging and localization
i. study
i. system
technetium-99m MIBI i.
i. technique
i. technology
thallium perfusion i.
time-resolved imaging by automatic data segmentation
time-resolved imaging contrast kinetics
tissue Doppler i.
transesophageal Doppler color flow i.
transient response i.
two-phase CT i.
ultrafast CT i.
ultrasound bone imaging sonometer
velocity-encoded cine-magnetic resonance i.
video imaging system
i. window
xenon lung ventilation i.

imaging-guided open biopsy

imaging/magnetic
diffusion-weighted imaging/magnetic resonance imaging

imaging/perfusion
diffusion-weighted imaging/perfusion imaging

Imaginings
Inventory of Childhood Memories and I.

imbalance
autonomic imbalance syndrome
bioenergy imbalance syndrome
electrolyte i.
electrolyte imbalance coma
endocrine hormone i.
i. of enzymes
eye muscle i.
fluid and electrolyte i.
gait imbalance and oscillopsia
hormonal i.
i. of hormones
i. in neurotransmitter level
i. of oxygen
progressive gait i.
salt and water i.
vertigo and i.

imbecile
moral i.

imbecility
old age i.

imbricating
i. layer
i. suture

imbrication
lid imbrication syndrome
medial capsular i.

imidazoleacetic acid ribonucleotide

imidazole-buffered saline

imidazoline receptor

iminodiacetic acid

imitation
morbid i.
Oral Language Sentence I. Diagnostic Inventory
Oral Language Sentence I. Screening Test

immature
abnormal location of immature myeloid precursor
i. blood cell
i. brown fat cell
i. cataract
i. cell
i. dead female child
i. dead male child
i. erythrocyte
i. fetal lung
i. glomerulus
i. granule
i. infant
kidneys i.
i. labor
i. living female child
i. living male child
i. lung
i. lung disease
microscopically immature brain
normal immature brain tissue
i. oocyte retrieval
ovarian immature teratoma
i. ovarian teratoma
oxygen toxicity in immature lung
patient i.
i. phage
i. phenomenon
i. prostate
i. red blood cell
i. teratoma
transferring immature muscle cell

immaturity
i. of lung
interstitial immaturity of lung
i. of lung
parathyroid gland i.
pulmonary immaturity and atelectasis
pulmonary immaturity of prematurity

immediate
i. active cutaneous anaphylaxis
i. allergy
i. amputation
anesthetic immediate recovery
i. asthmatic reaction
i. auditory memory
i. auditory recall
i. auscultation
i. breast reconstruction
i. cause
i. contact
i. contagion
i. and delayed recall
i. and delayed recognition
i. diagnosis
i. discharge
i. early antigen
i. effect
failure of immediate recall
i. generalized reaction
i. good function followed by accelerated rejection
i. graft rejection
i. hypersensitivity
intense need to void i.
i. intense need to void
i. interpretation
morphine sulfate immediate release
i. patient care
i. phase reaction
i. pigment darkening
i. postexercise
i. postoperative prosthesis
i. postoperative prosthetic fitting
i. postoperative stability
i. postsurgical fitting of prosthesis
i. response
I. Response Mobile Analysis
i. sensitivity
i. sensory trace recall
i. transfer flap
i. transfusion
i. transfusion reaction
i. transport
i. visual memory

immediately after onset

immediate-release tablet

immediate-type hypersensitivity

immersion
cold i.
cold water immersion foot
i. cooling
i. foot
full body i.
homogenous i.
i. injury
i. lens
i. objective
oil i.
oil immersion field microscopy
restraint and water immersion stress
silicone i.
tropic immersion foot
warm water immersion foot
water i.

imminens
glaucoma i.

imminent
i. abortion
i. death
fear of imminent death

immittance
aural immittance measurement

immobility
bilateral vocal fold i.
falls and fractures i.
postictal i.
stiffness, tremors and i.
tonic i.

immobilization
i. of back injury
cervical immobilization device
expanded foam immobilization device
feeling of i.
i. hypercalcemia
i. of injured arm
i. of injured leg
i. mandibular fracture
i. of neck injury
rigid cervical i.
Sperm I. Test-Fjabrant
Sperm I. Test-Isojima
i. of spinal injury
sternal occipital mandibular i.
sternooccipital-mandibular immobilization brace
sternooccipital-mandibular immobilization orthosis
surgical immobilization of joint
Treponema pallidum immobilization test
Treponema pallidum immobilization immune adherence

immobilized
extremity immobilized in cast
knee i.
i. knee
i. metal affinity chromatography
i. mismatch binding protein
patient i.
i. in plaster cast
protein A immobilized in collodion charcoal
i. and unconscious

immobilizer
AP-PA skull i.
knee i.
sternooccipital-mandibular i.

immotile cilia syndrome

immovable joint

immune

acquired immune deficiency syndrome-associated transfusion
acquired immune deficiency syndrome-related complex
acquired immune deficiency syndrome-related dementia
acquired immune deficiency syndrome-related macular degeneration
acquired immune deficiency syndrome
acquired immune deficiency syndrome antibody
acquired immune deficiency syndrome antibody test
acquired immune deficiency syndrome carrier
acquired immune deficiency syndrome crisis
acquired immune deficiency syndrome dementia complex
acquired immune deficiency syndrome epidemic
acquired immune deficiency syndrome infected child
acquired immune deficiency syndrome mandatory testing
acquired immune deficiency syndrome prevention
acquired immune deficiency syndrome primary pathogen
acquired immune deficiency syndrome residential treatment facility
acquired immune deficiency syndrome tainted transfusion
acquired immune deficiency syndrome transmission
acquired immune deficiency syndrome treatment
acquired immune deficiency syndrome virus infection
acquired immune hemolytic disease
acquired violence immune deficiency syndrome
active immune system
i. adherence
i. adherence hemagglutination assay
i. adherence immunosorbent assay
i. agglutinin
allergy immune system
allogeneic cellular immune therapy
anterior chamber-associated immune deviation
anti-acquired immune deficiency syndrome vaccine
antibody immune response
antibody-mediated immune suppression
anti-D immune globulin
antigen-nonspecific immune complex assay
antigen-specific immune response
anti-HIV immune serum globulin
antihuman immunodeficiency virus immune serum globulin
antiidiotype immune response
anti-RhD immune globulin
i. augmentative therapy
autoimmune disorder immune disease
i. balance
blood product contaminated by acquired immune deficiency syndrome
i. body
body's infection-fighting immune system
i. capability
carrier of acquired immune deficiency syndrome
cell-mediated immune response
i. cells
cellular mediated immune response
chronic fatigue immune deficiency syndrome
chronic fatigue and immune dysfunction syndrome
chronic immune disorder
circulating immune complex
combined immune deficiency disease
i. complex
i. complex disease
i. complex-dissociated p24 antigen
i. complex dissociation
i. complex glomerulonephritis
i. complex precipitation
i. complex reaction
i. compromised host
congenital immune deficiency
cytomegalovirus immune globulin
cytomegalovirus-specific immune globulin
i. cytotoxicity
decreased immune function
defective immune response
i. defense
i. defense mechanism
i. deficiency
i. depressed patient
i. destructive process
i. deviation
i. diffusion test
drug-induced immune anemia
i. dysfunction
dysfunctional immune system
i. dysfunction problem
i. electron microscopy
i. elimination
emotional effects of acquired immune deficiency syndrome
i. factor
i. fluorescent antibody
food immune complex assay
i. function
i. function abnormality
gay-related immune deficiency
i. globulin
i. globulin to an Rh-negative woman
i. hemolytic anemia
hemolytic immune body
homologous tetanus immune globulin
human immune cells
human immune serum globulin
human immune status survey
human rabies immune globulin
human tetanus immune globulin
humoral immune defect
hyperactive immune system
i. illness
improved immune function
inhibit immune system
initial immune response
i. interferon
interleukin regulation of immune system
intravenous immune serum globulin
i. kidney disease
localized immune reaction
lymphocyte immune globulin
i. lysis
malfunctioning immune system
mandatory acquired immune deficiency syndrome testing
maternal humoral immune response
measles immune globulin
mesangial immune injury
model immune complex
modified immune serum globulin

i. modulating nutrition
i. modulation procedure
mother infected with acquired immune deficiency syndrome
mucosal immune response
National Institute of Acquired I. Deficiency
nephropathic immune response
normal immune system function
ocular immune disease
overactive immune system
patient immune to hepatitis B infection
patient's immune response
patient unknown acquired immune deficiency syndrome carrier
i. potential
pre-acquired immune deficiency syndrome
i. precipitate
primary immune deficiency
primary immune response
i. reaction
red blood cell immune adherence
i. region-associated antigen
i. to rejection
i. rejection of transplanted heart
i. renal disease
respiratory syncytial virus immune globulin
i. response
i. response and combined modality treatment
reverse immune cytoadhesion
Rhesus immune globulin
Rh immune globulin
RhO D immune globulin
i. ribonucleic acid
secondary immune response
secretion and spill from acquired immune deficiency syndrome
i. serum
i. serum globulin
severe combined immune deficiency
severe combined immune deficiency syndrome
slow immune response
soluble immune response suppressor
specific immune release
i. state
stimulate the immune system
i. stromal keratitis
suppressed immune response
i. suppression
i. suppressor
i. system
tetanus immune globulin
i. therapy
i. thrombocytopenic purpura
tolerate immune state
transfusion-associated acquired immune deficiency syndrome
transfusion-transmitted acquired immune deficiency syndrome
Treponema pallidum immobilization immune adherence
underactive immune system
weakened immune system
zoster immune plasma
zoster immune platelet

immune-associated antigen-positive

immune-based therapy

immune-enhancing diet

immune-mediated
i.-m. diabetes
i.-m. disease

immune-suppressive medication

immunity
antibody-mediated i.
anti-TB cellular i.
artificial active i.
artificial passive i.
cell i.
cell-mediated i.
cell mediated i.
cellular immunity deficiency syndrome
i. deficiency state
deficiency state i.
humoral i.
Metchnikoff cellular immunity theory
patient has natural immunity to hepatitis B virus
i. response
i. test
tumor-specific transplantation i.

immunization
allogeneic tumor cell i.
autologous tumor cell i.
diphtheria-pertussis i.
diphtheria, pertussis, and tetanus i.
diphtheria-tetanus i.
federal immunization program
growth monitoring, oral rehydration, breast feeding, and i.
measles, mumps, rubella i.
National I. Program
nucleic acid i.
oral polio i.
passive immunization therapy
i. rate
Standards for Pediatric I.
tetanus and diphtheria toxoid i.
tetanus toxoid i.
i. therapy
i.'s up-to-date
yellow fever i.

immunizing unit

immunoabsorbent
enzyme-linked immunoabsorbent assay
solid-phase immunoabsorbent assay

immunoactivity
trypsin-like i.

immunoassay
alpha-fetoprotein enzyme i.
antibody capture i.
antinuclear antibody screening by enzyme i.
Asserachrom APA i.
automated enzyme immunoassay for antinuclear antibody
chemiluminescent i.
cloned enzyme donor i.
enzymatic i.
enzyme i.
enzyme-labeled i.
enzyme-linked fluorescent i.
enzyme-multiplied immunoassay technique
enzyme-multiplied immunoassay test
fluorescence energy transfer i.
fluorescence excitation transfer i.
fluorescence-polarization i.
fluorescence polarization i.
fluorescent i.
fluorescent enzyme i.
fluorescent polarization i.
focal i.
gold-labeled optical rapid i.
growth hormone i.
hemagglutination inhibition i.
hepatitis C virus enzyme i.
homogeneous enzyme i.
indirect enzyme immunoassay for anti-*Mycoplasma pneumoniae* IgM
microlatex particle-mediated i.
microparticle capture enzyme i.
microparticle enzyme i.
microparticulate enzyme i.

immunoassay *(continued)*
mini Vidas automated immunoassay system
optical i.
optimal i.
particle concentration fluorescence i.
particle-enhanced turbidimetric inhibition i.
potentiometric ionophore mediated i.
second-generation enzyme i.
self-contained enzymatic membrane i.
solid-phase i.
solid phase fluorescence i.
solid-phase immunoassay fluorescence
sperm-ubiquitin tag i.
substrate-labeled fluorescent i.
substrate-linked fluorescent i.

immunoaugmentative therapy

immunobead test

immunobinding
dot i.
dot immunobinding assay

immunobiologic activity

immunoblastic
i. lymphadenopathy
i. lymphoma
i. plasma

immunoblot
Lyme disease i.
recombinant immunoblot assay

immunoblotting
electrophoretic i.

immunochemiluminescence assay

immunochemiluminescent assay

immunochemiluminometric assay

immunocompetence
cellular immunocompetence profile
general i.
humoral immunocompetence profile

immunocompetent
i. cell
i. host

immunocompromised
i. cancer patient
i. host
i. individual
i. patient
i. person

immunocytochemical
i. assay
enzyme-linked immunocytochemical technique

immunocytochemistry
estrogen receptor immunocytochemistry assay

immunocytoma
lymphoplasmacytic i.
lymphoplasmacytoid i.

immunodeficiency
acquired cellular immunodeficiency syndrome
acquired immunodeficiency syndrome
acquired immunodeficiency syndrome health assessment questionnaire
acquired immunodeficiency syndrome-related complex
acquired immunodeficiency syndrome-related virus
acquired immunodeficiency syndrome with Kaposi sarcoma
Acquired I. Syndrome Beliefs and Behavior Questionnaire
antihuman immunodeficiency virus immune serum globulin
antihuman immunodeficiency virus protease inhibitor
Athabascan type of severe combined immunodeficiency disease
autosomal recessive severe combined immunodeficiency disorder
carrier of human immunodeficiency virus
i., centromeric instability, facial anomalies syndrome
combined immunodeficiency disease
combined immunodeficiency syndrome
common variable i.
community-acquired immunodeficiency syndrome
i. disease
i. disorder
feline immunodeficiency virus
functional assessment of human i.
genetically determined immunodeficiency disease
HIV-associated dementia
human immunodeficiency virus
human immunodeficiency virus antibody
human immunodeficiency virus associated dementia
human immunodeficiency virus associated motor cognitive disorder
human immunodeficiency virus-associated nephropathy
human immunodeficiency virus-associated non-Hodgkin lymphoma
human immunodeficiency virus-associated periodontitis
human immunodeficiency virus-associated salivary gland disease
human immunodeficiency virus dementia
human immunodeficiency virus encephalopathy
human immunodeficiency virus gingivitis
human immunodeficiency virus immunoglobulin
human immunodeficiency virus infected blood
human immunodeficiency virus overview of problems evaluation system
human immunodeficiency virus-patient-reported status and experience
human immunodeficiency virus quality audit marker
human immunodeficiency virus seroconversion
human immunodeficiency virus-1 subtype C
human immunodeficiency virus type 1, 2
live-attenuated human immunodeficiency virus
macrophage-tropic human immunodeficiency virus strain
morphine-potentiated human immunodeficiency virus replication
Multidimensional Quality of Life Questionnaire for Persons with Human I. Virus
neuropsychiatric acquired immunodeficiency syndrome rating scale
nonsyncytia-forming human immunodeficiency virus

partial albinism with i.
partial combined immunodeficiency disorder
pediatric acquired immunodeficiency syndrome
phagocytic dysfunction i.
primary i.
primary immunodeficiency syndrome
severe combined immunodeficiency disease
simian acquired immunodeficiency syndrome
X-linked severe combined i.

immunodeficiency-associated virus

immunodeficient
i. disorder
severe combined immunodeficient mice

immunodepressed
patient i.

immunodetection

immunodiagnosis
rapid rabies enzyme i.

immunodiffusion
antinuclear antibody i.
i. complement fixation
i. complement-fixing
double radial i.
double immunodiffusion technique
fungal i.
i. procedure
radial immunodiffusion cerebrospinal fluid
single radial i.
i. test
i. tube precipitin

immunodouble diffusion test

immunoelectrodiffusion
enzyme-linked immunoelectrodiffusion assay

immunoelectron microscopy

immunoelectrophoresis
i. analysis
countercurrent exchanger i.
countercurrent immunoelectrophoresis test
crossed i.
quantitative i.
rocket i.
serum i.
urine i.

immunoelectrophoresis-–colorimetric
counter i.

immunoelectrophoresis–densitometric
counter i.

immunofiltration
enzyme-linked immunofiltration assay

immunofixation
cerebrospinal fluid immunofixation electrophoresis
i. electrophoresis
serum immunofixation electrophoresis
serum protein and immunofixation electrophoresis system
urine immunofixation electrophoresis

immunofluorescence
i. antibody
anticomplement i.
antinuclear antibody i.
i. assay
direct immunofluorescence analysis
direct immunofluorescence test
fixed cell i.
granulocyte immunofluorescence test
indirect membrane i.
lymphocyte immunofluorescence test
i. method
i. microscopy
mixed i.
multicolor immunofluorescence measurement
platelet suspension immunofluorescence test
rapid immunofluorescence staining
i. technique
i. test

immunofluorescent
i. antibody
i. antibody assay
IgA immunofluorescent antibody
IgM immunofluorescent antibody
indirect i.
indirect immunofluorescent antibody
i. stain

immunogenic
macrophage immunogenic antigen-recruiting factor

immunoglobin
i. G1
i. M-rheumatoid factor

immunoglobulin
i. A
i. A1
absence of immunoglobulin A, G, M
amyloid of immunoglobulin origin
animo-terminal portion of heavy chain of i.
antenatal anti-D i.
anticardiolipin immunoglobulin M antibody
antihepatitis delta virus i.
antihepatitis E virus i.
antiidiotypic immunoglobulin response
antiplatelet immunoglobulin G antibody
i. A subclass 1, 2
i. A transglutaminase antibody
autoimmune immunoglobulin mediation
cluster of differentiation 4 immunoglobulin G
i. consumption test
cytomegalovirus i.
cytoplasmic immunoglobulin M
cytotoxic lymphocyte activation antigen 4 i.
i. D
i. deficiency
i. D subclass 1, 2
i. E
i. F
fragment of immunoglobulin G after digestion with the enzyme pepsin
fragment of immunoglobulin G involved in antigen binding
gamma immunoglobulin A, D, G, M
gamma A immunoglobulin deficiency
gamma A immunoglobulin determination
gamma immunoglobulin D determination
gamma immunoglobulin E determination
gamma immunoglobulin Gamma
gamma immunoglobulin G determination
gamma immunoglobulin M determination

immunoglobulin *(continued)*
i. G antigliadin antibody
i. G, G2, G2a, G4
goat antimouse immunoglobulin G
i. G rheumatoid factor
heavy chain of immunoglobulin A
heavy chain of immunoglobulin D
heavy chain of immunoglobulin E
heavy chain of immunoglobulin G
heavy chain of immunoglobulin M
hepatitis B virus i.
HIV i.
horse i.
human immunodeficiency virus i.
human rabies i.
human tetanus i.
insulin-reactive i.
intracytoplasmic i.
intramuscular i.
intravenous i.
late immunoglobulin deficiency
i. light chain-origin amyloid deposit
i. M
malaria i.
i. M antibody capture
measles i.
membrane i.
noncovalently bonded dimer of C-terminal immunoglobulin of Fc fragment
oligoclonal i.
pernicious anemia-like syndrome and immunoglobulin deficiency
platelet-associated immunoglobulin G
i. quantitation
quantitative i.
rabies i.
respiratory syncytial virus intravenous i.
Rous sarcoma virus immunoglobulin intravenous
serum i.
serum-platelet bindable immunoglobulin G
subclass of immunoglobulin E, M
subcutaneous i.
surface immunoglobulin A
surface membrane i.
tetanus i.
thyroid-binding inhibitory i.
thyroid growth i.
thyroid growth-blocking i.
thyroid-stimulating i.
thyrotropin-binding inhibitory i.
TSH-binding inhibitory i.
vaccinia i.
variable domain of heavy chain i.
variable domain of light chain i.
zoster serum i.

immunoglobulin-binding factor

immunoglobulin-complexed enzyme

immunoglobulin-secreting cell

immunogold-silver staining

immunologic
cellular immunologic reactivity
i. deficiency
i. disorder
i. disturbance
i. hypersensitivity reaction
nonimmediate-type immunologic drug reaction
occupational immunologic lung disease
i. response
i. test

immunological
anti-DNA immunological study
antihepatitis A-IgM immunological study
antinuclear antibody immunological study
anti-SSA immunological study
anti-SSB immunological study
i. contact urticaria
i. fecal occult blood test
i. host

immunologically
i. detectable insulin
i. measurable insulin
i. mediated disease

immunology
allergy and i.
tumor immunology bank

immunolympholysis
antibody-mediated cell-dependent i.

immunometric assay

immunomodulating
i. antirheumatic drug
optimal immunomodulating dose

immunoperoxidase
avidin-biotin immunoperoxidase technique
indirect i.
i. infectivity assay
light and electron immunoperoxidase observation
PAP i.
paraffin i.
silver nitrate i.
i. technique

immunopotentiating reconstituted influenza virosomes

immunoprecipitation
automated i.

immunoproliferative
angiocentric immunoproliferative disorder
angiocentric immunoproliferative lesion
i. disorder
i. small intestine disease

immunoprophylaxis
passive i.

immunoradioassayable human chorionic somatomammotropin

immunoradiometric
i. analysis
i. assay

immunoreactive
i. adrenocorticotropic hormone
i. beta endomorphin
i. bovine serum albumin
i. calcitonin
i. corticotropin-releasing factor
digoxin-like immunoreactive factor
digoxin-like immunoreactive substance
i. fibronectin
i. gastrin
i. glucagon
i. glucose
i. human chorionic gonadotropin
i. human chorionic somatomammotropin
i. human gastrin
i. human growth hormone
i. human placental lactogen
i. human skin collagenase
i. substance P
i. insulin
i. insulin to serum or plasma glucose ratio
i. methionine-enkephalin

i. parathyroid hormone
i. plasma
plasma immunoreactive insulin
plasma immunoreactive secretion
i. proinsulin
i. prostaglandin E
i. secretin
serum immunoreactive parathyroid hormone
total i.
total immunoreactive serum pepsinogen
i. trypsin
i. trypsinogen
i. trypsin output

immunoreactivity
beta-endorphin i.
cholecystokinin-like i.
glucagon-like i.
large glucagon i.
metenkephalin-like i.
motilin-like i.
neurotensin-like i.
secretin-like i.
somatostatin-like i.
tachykinin-like i.
vasoactive intestinal polypeptide i.

immunoreceptor tyrosine-based activation motif

immunoregulatory alpha globulin

immunoscintigraphy
anti-CEA antibody i.

immunosorbent
anti-D enzyme-linked immunosorbent assay
enzyme immunosorbent assay
enzyme-linked immunosorbent as
glycoprotein-based enzyme-linked immunosorbent assay
hemagglutinin enzyme-linked immunosorbent assay
immune adherence immunosorbent assay
i. agglutination assay
Lyme enzyme-linked immunosorbent assay
measles virus enzyme-linked immunosorbent assay
paper enzyme-linked immunosorbent assay
recombinant immunosorbent assay

immunospot
enzyme-linked immunospot assay
solid-phase enzyme-linked i.

immunostimulating complex

immunostimulatory
i. DNA sequence
i. oligodeoxynucleotide

immunosuppressant therapy

immunosuppressed
patient i.
i. protocol

immunosuppression method

immunosuppressive
i. acidic protein
i. acidic substance
adverse negative immunosuppressive effect
i. agent
conventional immunosuppressive therapy
cytotoxic immunosuppressive therapy
i. drug
i. drug therapy
i. effect
high-dose immunosuppressive therapy
i. medication
negative immunosuppressive effect
x-ray immunosuppressive measure

immunotactoid glomerulopathy

immunotherapy
active specific i.
adoptive i.
cytotoxic T lymphocyte-based i.
passive humoral i.
short-term i.
specific immunotherapy allergy
specific injection i.
sublingual i.
systemic active i.
venom i.

immunotoxin therapy

immunotransfer
enzyme-linked immunotransfer blot

impact
Arthritis I. Measurement Scale
BPH impact index
i. of depression
destabilizing impact of trauma
detrimental impact of fatigue
electron i.
Environmental I. Statement
Fibromyalgia I. Questionnaire
finding of no significant i.
Incontinence I. Questionnaire-Revised
i. on fetus
Sickness I. Profile
Stress I. Scale
Stroke I. Scale

impacted
i. bowel
i. calculus
i. cerumen
i. fecal material
i. feces
i. foreign body
i. fracture
i. grief
i. molar
partially impacted wisdom teeth
patient i.
i. stone
i. stool
i. teeth
i. tooth
i. twin
i. wisdom teeth

impaction
acute esophageal food i.
anteromedial superior humeral head i.
bowel i.
constipation and fecal i.
delirium, infection, atrophic urethritis and vaginitis, pharmaceuticals, psychological disorders, excessive urine output, restricted mobility, stool i.
extensive fecal i.
i. fracture
full bony i.
i. lesion
mucoid impaction of bronchus
partial bony i.
sequential impaction cascade sieve volumetric air sampler

impactor
electromechanical i.

impaired
i. ability to swallow
i. abstract thinking
i. adjustment
i. affect
i. alertness
anxiety-induced impaired social functioning
Assessment for Persons Profoundly or Severely I.

impaired *(continued)*
i. attention
i. balance
i. behavior
i. blood vessel elasticity
i. brain activity
i. breaking and swallowing
i. cardiac function
i. cartilage
child speech i.
i. circulation
i. cognition
i. cognitive functioning
i. cognitive performance
i. communication
i. comprehension
i. concentration
i. consciousness
i. contractility of hypertrophied muscle
i. coordination
i. coronary artery
i. coronary vascular reserve
delayed or impaired speech
detrusor hyperactivity with impaired contractility
i. development
i. dexterity
i. difficult speech
i. discriminatory, vibratory and position sensation
i. drivers
driving while i.
emotionally i.
i. employee alcohol and drug treatment issue
i. fasting glucose
i. function
i. gas exchange
i. glucose tolerance
grossly impaired functioning
i. growth
hearing i.
i. hearing
i. hearing loss
i. hepatic function
i. home maintenance management
i. host
ichthyosis, brittle hair, impaired intelligence, decreased fertility, short stature syndrome
i. immunity
i. intelligence
i. interpersonal relations
i. judgment
i. kidney function
learning i.
i. left discrimination
i. left ventricular function
i. liver function
i. memory
memory impaired assisted living
i. memory for recent events
i. memory of unknown cause
i. mental functioning
mentally i.
mild to moderately i.
i. mobility
i. motor coordination
i. motor function
i. neurological function
i. normal activity
organically impaired brain activity
organically impaired brain function
i. parent
patient physically i.
physically i.
i. physical mobility
i. pumping ability
i. reality testing
i. regeneration syndrome
i. renal function
renal impaired patient
i. right discrimination
i. sensation
sensory impaired support
severely impaired renal function
severely mentally i.
i. sexual development
i. short-term memory
i. side
i. skin integrity
i. social interaction
i. speech
speech impaired individual
speech and language i.
i. swallowing
i. systolic function
i. thinking or concentration
i. tissue integrity
i. ventilation
i. verbal communication
i. vision
visually i.

impair immunity

impairment
i. of activities of daily living
age-associated memory i.
age-related memory i.
age-related visual i.
alcohol-induced functional i.
anterior horn cell motor i.
aphasic phonological i.
ASIA impairment scale for classification of spinal cord injury
auditory comprehension i.
Austin-Kartush group A i.
average impairment rating
brittle hair, intellectual impairment, decreased fertility, short stature syndrome
chronic orthopedic i.
cognitive impairment in alcoholism
cognitive impairment of depression
complete impairment of conduction
i. of consciousness
cortical visual i.
cranial nerve i.
i. of diffusion
Facial I. Scales for Children
i. of fertility
focal neurological i.
i. from disorder
functional aerobic i.
Functional I. Scale for Children and Adolescents
i. of functions of brain stem
International Classification of I.'s, Disabilities, and Handicaps
i. of judgment
language i.
i. of liver function
i. in liver function
major functional i.
major impairment of functioning
McDowell I. Index
i. of memory
mental retardation, hearing impairment, distinct facies, skeletal anomalies syndrome
mild cognitive i.
mild hearing i.
mixed hearing i.
moderate hearing i.
Mondini hearing i.
musculoskeletal i.
nerve function i.
neurosensory i.
nonprogressive motor impairment syndrome
nonsyndromic hereditary hearing i.
i. in occupational functioning
occupational and social i.
organic hearing i.
orgasmic i.

partial impairment of conduction
partial permanent i.
perceptive hearing i.
perceptual-motor ability i.
permanent childhood hearing i.
permanent visual i.
i. of power of voluntary movement
preexisting cognitive i.
profound hearing i.
progressive impairment of vision
psychogenic hearing i.
pulmonary ventilation i.
recent memory impairment and confabulation
restrictive functional i.
Scheibe hearing i.
sensorineural hearing i.
severe impairment of hearing
severe impairment in interpretation of reality
severe impairment in thinking
severe impairment of ventricle
severe neurological i.
sexual/reproductive system i.
i. of skin integrity
slight hearing i.
i. of social function
specific expressive language i.
speech and hearing i.
i. of subendocardial blood flow
i. of systolic and diastolic performance
visual i.
Visual I. Service

impalement
anorectal i.

impedance
acoustic i.
i. angle
aortic i.
bioelectrical impedance analysis
i. cardiac output
i. cardiogram
electrical impedance breast scanning
electrical impedance cardiography
electrical impedance tomography
electrode i.
high-input i.
middle ear i.
output i.
pacemaker i.
i. phlebograph
i. plethysmography
skin i.
i. threshold valve
transthoracic electric impedance respirogram
venous impedance plethysmography

impediment
language i.

impending
i. doom
fear of impending doom
lasting impression of impending failure
i. myocardial infarction
i. renal failure

imperception
auditory i.

imperfecta
dentinogenesis i.
osteogenesis imperfecta congenita syndrome
osteogenesis imperfecta, optic atrophy, retinopathy, developmental delay syndrome
osteogenesis imperfecta tarda
osteogenesis imperfecta type I–IV
perinatal lethal osteogenesis i.

imperforate
i. anus
i. hymen
low imperforate anus
microcephalus, imperforate anus, syndactyly, hamartoblastoma, abnormal lung lobulation, polydactyly
microphallus, imperforate anus, syndactyly, hamartoblastoma, abnormal lung
polydactyly, imperforate anus, vertebral anomalies syndrome

imperforation
vertebral abnormality, anal imperforation, tracheoesophageal fistula, and radial, ray, or renal anomalies

impersistence
motor i.
Motor I. Test

impetigo
i. bullosa
bullous i.
i. contagiosa
i. herpetiformis
i. neonatorum
nonbullous i.
i. simplex
i. staphylogenes
i. streptogenes
i. vulgaris

impingement
ankle i.
anterior ankle i.
anterior cord i.
anterior impingement spur
anterior impingement syndrome
anterior joint i.
anterior rib impingement syndrome
anterior soft tissue i.
anterolateral i.
anterolateral impingement syndrome
disc i.
graft i.
nerve i.
i. on spinal nerve
rotator cuff impingement syndrome
i. syndrome

implant
adhesive silicone i.
adjustable breast i.
adjustable saline breast i.
allogenic lyophilized bone graft implant material
alloplastic facial i.
alloplastic interpositional i.
anterior subperiosteal i.
AO-ASIF orthopaedic i.
artificial heart i.
artificial joint implant material
artificial lens i.
attaching material implant superstructure
attachment to implant superstructure
auditory brainstem i.
augmentation with i.
auxiliary implant rest
auxiliary rest implant substructure
bicompartmental knee implant prosthesis
biomechanical failure of i.
bone implant material
brain implant surgery
brain tissue i.
breast implant valve
breast silicone i.
carpal lunate implant prosthesis
cataract surgery with i.
celluloid implant material
cesium i.
cochlear i.
conventional reform eye i.

implant *(continued)*
cosmetic implant surgery
dental implant technique
double-lumen breast i.
electrically activated i.
i. erosion
expandable breast i.
i. extrusion
facial implant of cheek
facial implant of chin
facial implant of jaw
fixed mandibular i.
flexible hinge i.
flexible silicone i.
gel-filled breast i.
gold grain i.
gold implant material
great toe arthroplasty implant technique
great toe i.
great toe implant prosthesis
hard tissue replacement-malleable facial i.
hollow-sphere implant material
homograft implant material
inner ear i.
insertion of polyethylene i.
insert radioactive i.
internal mammary artery i.
intraocular lens i.
jaw
leaking breast i.
leaky saline i.
levonorgestrel subdermal i.
liposuction fat fillant i.
lumbar anterior-root stimulator i.
malleable facial i.
mechanically activated i.
meshed ball i.
metal hemi-toe i.
metatarsophalangeal i.
methyl methacrylate i.
microstructured i.
mucoperiosteal implant placement
open bladder brachytherapy i.
orbital floor i.
orbital implant operation
orthopedic implant infection
osseointegrated cylinder i.
osseointegrated dental i.
paraffin implant material
peripheral frame implant substructure
peritoneal implant metastasis
permanent implant therapy
pig cell i.
i. placement
plastic implant material
plastic sphere i.
polyethylene implant material
polyvinyl sponge i.
posterior chamber lens i.
pump-operated penile i.
pyramidal eye i.
radioactive seed i.
radium i.
i. related complications
rupture of i.
saline-filled breast i.
saline filled breast i.
salt water i.
self-sealing breast i.
silicone-filled breast i.
silicone gel-filled breast i.
silicone gel-filled mammary i.
silicone implant material
silicone rod i.
silicone sponge i.
i. site
Snellen conventional reform i.
stainless steel i.
subdermal implant material
subdermal levonorgestrel i.
subperiosteal implant material
subthalamic nucleus i.
Swanson carpal lunate i.
Swanson radial head i.
Swanson wrist joint i.
tantalum mesh implant material
temporary breast i.
temporary pacemaker i.
transmandibular i.
ureteral implant material
ventral derotating spinal i.
wire mesh i.
wire mesh implant material

implantable
i. artificial heart
i. atrial defibrillator
atrial and ventricular implantable cardioverter-defibrillator
i. automatic cardioverter-defibrillator
automatic implantable cardioverter-defibrillator
automatic implantable defibrillator
i. bone growth stimulator
i. cardiac defibrillator
i. cardioverter
i. cardioverter-defibrillator
i. cardioverter-defibrillator/atrial tachycardia pacing
i. cardioverter-defibrillator catheter
i. cardioverter electrodes
i. contact lens
i. defibrillator
i. defibrillator in cardioversion
i. device
i. drug infusion pump
i. glucose sensor
i. insulin infusion pump
i. left ventricular assist system
i. lens
middle ear i.
i. middle ear hearing device
middle ear implantable system
i. pacemaker
programmable implantable medication system
i. pulse generator
i. rings in eyes
i. unipolar endocardial electrode
i. vascular access device
i. venous access device
ventricular implantable cardioverter-defibrillator

implantation
antireflux ureteral implantation technique
artificial genitourinary sphincter i.
artificial lens i.
artificial urinary sphincter i.
autogenous cartilage i.
autologous chondrocyte i.
i. bleeding
bone cement implantation syndrome
cataract lens i.
cochlear i.
i. cyst
i. cyst of iris
dual chamber pacemaker i.
i. of fertilized egg
i. of fertilized ovum
i. graft
inner ear electronic i.
interstitial implantation of radioactive isotope
intraocular lens i.
i. metastasis
i. of pacemaker
permanent pacemaker i.
i. of radium
radon seed i.
i. response
subcutaneous electrode i.
subpectoral implantation of cardioverter-defibrillator
surgical orthotopic i.
i. techniques
i. test

total implantation of artificial heart
transvenous implantation of cardioverter-defibrillator
i. of ureter into rectum

implanted
chemo wafers i.
pacemaker implanted under skin
permanently implanted ventricular assist device
surgically implanted hemodialysis catheter

implementation
assessment, plan, implementation, and evaluation
diagnosis and i.
drug efficacy study i.
respiratory isolation implementation efficiency
respiratory isolation implementation sensitivity

implication
ethical, legal, and social i.'s

importance
allergic i.
Minnesota I. Questionnaire
Surveillance and Control of Pathogens of Epidemiologic I.

important
i. medical event
minimum clinically important difference
very important patient

imposed abstinence

impotence
anal i.
anatomic i.
arteriogenic i.
atonic i.
chronic i.
erectile i.
i. from antidepressant
i. from diabetes
male impotence after childbirth
male impotence test
organic i.
orgastic i.
paretic i.
penile i.
psychic i.
psychogenic i.
rage i.
sexual i.
symptomatic i.
temporary i.
vasculogenic i.

impoverished
confused or impoverished thought and speech

impression
aortic impression of left lung
basilar i.
Clinical Global I. of Change
closed mouth i.
complete denture i.
corneal impression test
i. cup
history, physical, impression, and plan
hydrocolloid i.
lasting impression of impending failure
i. material
Nurse's Global I.'s
partial denture i.
rubber base i.
i. tonometer

imprinting
loss of i.

improper
i. bite
i. exercise
i. fit of dentures
i. foot alignment
i. foot care
i. functioning of foot
i. management
i. nail trimming
i. use of prescription

improve
i. circulation
i. efficiency of heart and lungs
i. health self-esteem
i. muscular contraction
i. quality of life
i. self-image

improved
i. blood flow
i. condition
i. energy
i. flexibility
i. immune function
i. minimal essential medium, hormone supplemented
i. muscle tone
i. overall functioning
patient discharged i.
patient partially i.
patient symptomatically i.
i. performance and tolerance
i. pregnancy outcome
i. psychological adjustment
i. self-concept
i. symptom relief
i. thought process

improvement
Battery of Health I.
Clinical Global I.
Clinical Laboratory I. Act
deterioration following i.
disease-related symptom i.
Global I. Rating
knowledge, attitude, behavior, and improvement in nutritional status
maximal medical i.
medical improvement expected
medical improvement not expected
medical improvement possible
neurologic i.
no i.
no improvement with pinhole
no manifest i.
objective i.
performance i.
pinhole no i.
quality i.

impulse
abnormal electrical i.
activates chemical impulse of brain
apical i.
automobile airbag impulse noise
block pain i.
compulsive impulse control disorder
conduction of nerve i.
i. control
i. control difficulty
i. control disorder
i. control in eating
i. control skills
cranial rhythmic i.
i. disorder control
disorder of impulse control
double apical i.
downward displacement of apical i.
i. dyscontrol
i. dyscontrol in eating disorder
efferent nerve i.
electrical impulse to heart
i. formation
hyperkinetic impulse disorder
inadequate impulse control
intensity of i.
irresistible impulse test
left parasternal i.
loss of nerve i.

impulse *(continued)*
maximal point of i.
milliampere i.
i. on coughing
overlapping biphasic i.
pacing i.
paradoxical rocking i.
i.'s per minute
persistent inappropriate i.
point of maximal i.
point of maximum i.
point of maximum impulse fifth intercostal space
poor impulse control
i. propagation
right parasternal i.
sinus node i.
stimulate nerve i.
i. stimulator
i. summation
sustained apical i.
systolic apical i.
i. transmission
i. transmitted pain
i. violence

impulse-conducting system

impulse-dominated personality

impulsive
i. acting out
i. actions
i. aggression
i. behavior
i. child
i. eating
external impulsive form
i. insanity
outward expression of anger with impulsive feature
i. patient
reckless and impulsive activity
serious impulsive dyscontrol

impulsiveness
high i.
high impulsiveness, high anxiety
high impulsiveness, low anxiety
i. and inattention
low i.
low impulsiveness, high anxiety
low impulsiveness, low anxiety

impulsivity
aggression and deceit i.
counteracting i.
i. and inattentiveness
lifetime i.
marked i.
pattern of i.
i. to plan ahead

impurities
limit of i.

inability
i. to arrange words
i. to arrange words properly
i. to chew or swallow
i. to close eye
i. to communicate
i. to concentrate
i. to control appetite
i. to control blood pressure
i. to control drinking
i. to control stool
i. to control urine
i. to control weight
i. to cope
i. to defecate
difficulty or inability to speak
i. to exercise
i. to feel pleasure
i. to focus
i. to focus attention
i. to function
i. to interpret written word
i. to maintain attention
i. to make decisions
i. to move a joint
i. to move tongue
painful inability to urinate
i. to pass urine
i. to perform purposeful movements
progressive inability to walk
i. to recall
i. to recall events
i. to recognize objects
i. to relate to people
i. to relax
i. to remember spoken words
i. to sleep
i. to speak
i. to straighten back
i. to suckle
i. to sustain consistent work behavior
i. to talk
i. to tolerate boredom
total inability to urinate
i. to walk

inaction
passivity and i.

inactivated
enhanced inactivated polio vaccine
i. fetal calf serum
heat i.
i. horse serum
influenza virus inactivated vaccine
influenza virus inactivated vaccine, split virion, types A, B, trivalent
normal inactivated rabbit serum
i. pepsin
poliomyelitis vaccine i.
i. polio vaccine
i. poliovirus vaccine
i. serum
typhoid vaccine, heat and phenol inactivated, dried
Venezuelan equine encephalitis vaccine, i.

inactivating
i. dose
kallikrein inactivating unit

inactivation
kallikrein inactivation unit
nonrandom X chromosome i.
thermal inactivation point
X inactivation center

inactivator
chemotactic-factor i.

inactive
i. alcoholic
chronic inactive cirrhosis
i. colon
i. dummy drug
i. electrode
endocrine inactive pituitary tumor
i. hormone
i. lifestyle
medically inactive placebo
i. medication
i. muscles
optically inactive chemical
physically inactive lifestyle
i. placebo
i. renin activity
i. tuberculosis
X inactive, specific transcript

inactivity
cycle of pain and i.
electrocerebral i.
i., lethargy and fatigue
obesity and i.
record of electrocerebral i.
tracings of electrocerebral i.

inadequacy
feelings of social i.
luteal phase i.

sexual i.
i. of systemic circulation

inadequate
i. blood flow
i. blood supply
i. bowel preparation
i. cardiac output
i. coping
i. impulse control
i. intake of fluids
i. literacy skills
i. luteal phase
i. pelvis
i. personality
i. sexual function
small vessel inadequate blood flow
i. tissue maintenance
i. tissue repair
i. ventilation

inadequately hydrated

inappropriate
i. action
i. admission
i. affect
i. anger
i. antidiuretic hormone
i. antidiuretic hormone syndrome
i. behavior
i. child behavior
i. dangerous behavior
i. disability
i. elation
excessive or inappropriate guilt
i. fatigue
i. gonadotropin secretion
i. guilt
inconsistent and inappropriate thinking
i. intense anger
intense inappropriate anger
i. irritability
i. laughing
i. overt anger
patient i.
persistent inappropriate idea
persistent inappropriate image
persistent inappropriate impulse
i. polycythemia
i. secretion of antidiuretic hormone
i. sexual behavior
i. sexually provocative behavior
i. social behavior
socially inappropriate behavior
i. suspicion
syndrome of inappropriate antidiuresis
syndrome of inappropriate antidiuretic hormone
syndrome of inappropriate antidiuretic hormone secretion
syndrome of inappropriate secretion of antidiuretic hormone
i. vasopressin secretion
i. verbalization

inappropriately
patient acting i.
patient laughs i.

inarticulate
patient i.

inattention
impulsiveness and i.

inattention-overactivity with aggression

inattentive
attention deficit hyperactivity disorder-predominantly i.

inattentiveness
impulsivity and i.

inborn
i. error of metabolism
i. immunity

inbred
recombinant inbred strain

inbreeding coefficient

incalculable
triglycerides i.

incapacitated
i. by alcohol
i. of making decisions
patient incapacitated of caring for self
totally incapacitated of caring for self

incapacitating
i. depression
i. fear
patient with incapacitating systemic disease
patient with severe systemic disease limiting activity but not i.

incapacity
Home Incapacity Scale
Ward Incapacity Scale

incarcerated
children of incarcerated parents
i. hernia
i. inguinal hernia
nontender incarcerated inguinal hernia
i. placenta

in-center hemodialysis

incentive
aversive i.
i. spirometer
i. spirometry
i. spirometry breathing
i. therapy

incessant
i. coughing
i. movements
i. tachycardia

incest
childhood i.
court referral for i.
memories of i.
unverifiable memories of i.

inch
cubic i.

incidence
age-specific cumulative incidence rate
angle of i.
basic incidence rate
i. of drug abuse
excess i.
permanent i.
plane of i.
relapse i.
standardized incidence ratio

incident
cardiovascular i.
cerebrovascular i.
critical incident review
critical incident stress management
distressing recollection of i.

incidental
i. appendectomy
i. exposure
i. finding
i. Lewy body
i. murmur
i. parasite

incipient
i. cataract
i. cataract grade 11 to 41
i. degenerative brain disease
i. gangrene
i. glaucoma
i. heart failure
i. lethal concentration
i. respiratory infection

incisal
i. edge
i. guide
i. mandibular plane angle
i. margin
mesial incisal lingual surface
i. opening
i. ridge

incised
abscess i.
cartilaginous ring i.
fascia i.
fascia incised transversely
mediastinal pleura i.
periosteum i.
periosteum incised and retracted
peritoneum i.
i. perpendicular
platysma i.
pleura i.
i. renal parenchyma
trachea i.
tubularized incised plate
visceral pleura i.
i. wound

incision
angle of i.
anterior hairline i.
anterolateral thoracotomy i.
apex of i.
appendix brought into surgical i.
apron skin i.
apron U-shaped i.
brought out near edge of i.
i. carried down to the fracture site
i. clean and dry
i. closed anatomically
i. closed in layers
i. closed musculofascially
i. closed in serial fashion
coronary mastoid-to-mastoid i.
counter stab wound i.
curved downward i.
curved longitudinal i.
curved periscapular i.
curvilinear skin i.
i. deepened
i. and drainage
i. and drainage of abscess
drainage at incision site
i. and drainage of blister
i. and drainage of cyst
i. and drainage of fistulous tract
i. and drainage of ischiorectal abscess
i. and drainage of paronychia
endaural mastoid i.
i. enlarged
i. extended bilaterally
fish mouth i.
forceps passed up through i.
i. granulating in
healed incision site
i. healed per primam
healing biopsy i.
healing incision site
healing surgical i.
hockey stick i.
horizontal incision across lower abdomen
horizontal uterine i.
induration along skin i.
infected incision site
inframammary fold i.
i. into intestine
i. into joint
inverted T i.
irritation of incision site
lateral flank i.
lateral to the i.
lateral rectus i.
i. line
loosely closed i.
low cervical vertical i.
lower abdominal transverse i.
lower pole of i.
lower transverse abdominal i.
low segment transverse i.
low transverse uterine i.
low vertical uterine i.
L-shaped capsular i.
Lynch medial canthal i.
McBurney appendectomy i.
medial canthal i.
median sternotomy i.
Mercedes-Benz i.
midface degloving i.
midline skin i.
minimum incision surgery
modified Gibson i.
modified gull wing i.
muscle splitting i.
nasal buttonhole i.
old incision excised
pain at incision site
para muscular i.
Pulvertaft fishmouth i.
pus at incision site
rectus muscle splitting i.
redness along incision site
redness at incision site
scleral tunnel i.
Shambaugh endaural i.
shape of surgical incisions W-plasty
shape of surgical incision Z-plasty
shape of incisions in V-Y plasty
i. site
skin fold i.
skin incision closed
skin line i.
smaller rib i.
small incision cataract surgery
stab wound i.
standard Y i.
sternal splitting i.
stocking seam i.
subcostal flank i.
swelling at incision site
tenderness at site of i.
i. through wall of cavity
tissue ablation, incision and excision
transperitoneal anterior subcostal i.
transurethral i.
transurethral incision of bladder neck
transurethral incision of prostate
transverse linear i.
upper pole of uterine i.
vertical uterine i.
warmth at incision site
i. widened
wide skin i.

incisional
i. biopsy
i. care
i. discomfort
i. edge
i. hernia
i. pain
i. site draining
i. surgical wound infection

incisive
i. bone
i. canal cyst
i. duct

incisor
Frankfort mandibular incisor angle
mandibular central i.
maxillary central i.
medial incisor tooth
single central maxillary i.
winged i.

incisura
aortic i.
cardiac i.

incisural
anterior incisural space

incisure
angular i.
occipital bone jugular i.
Rivinus i.
Santorini i.
Schmidt-Lanterman i.

inclination
angle of inclination of urethra
angle of thoracic i.
axial i.
palpebral fissure i.
pelvic i.

incline
guiding i.

including
colorimetry, including spectrophotometry and photometry

inclusion
alcoholic hyaline inclusion body
B-cytomegalic inclusion disease of newborn
i. body
i. body myositis
i. cell
i. cell disease
i. conjunctivitis
Crawford graft inclusion technique
i. cyst
cytomegalic inclusion disease
cytomegalic inclusion disease virus
cytomegalic inclusion virus
cytoplasmic inclusion body
i. disease
eosinophilic cytoplasmic i.
epidermal inclusion cyst
hyaline cytoplasmic i.
intracytoplasmic hyaline i.
intracytoplasmic tuboreticular i.
lipid hydrocarbon i.
Lipschütz inclusion body
lupus-type i.
lymphogranuloma venereum-trachoma inclusion conjunctivitis
mascara particle i.
measles inclusion body encephalitis
mesothelial cell i.
monkey intranuclear inclusion agent
multilocular peritoneal inclusion cyst
neonatal inclusion blennorrhea
neonatal inclusion conjunctivitis
neuronal intranuclear inclusion disease
nuclear globulin i.
nuclear inclusion body
osmiophilic lamellar inclusion body
owl's eye inclusion body
patient inclusion criteria
subacute inclusion body encephalitis
trachoma and inclusion conjunctivitis
tubuloreticular i.
vaginal inclusion cyst
virus inclusion conjunctivitis
Walthard i.

incoherent
bizarre incoherent thinking
i. ideation
patient i.
i. speech
i. thinking
i. thoughts

income
Employee Retirement I. Security Act
low i.
oxygen i.
i. poverty guideline

incompatibility
minor group antigen i.
i. number
parental Rh i.

incompatible
i. bone marrow
i. hemolytic
i. hemolytic blood transfusion

incompetence
aortic i.
aortic valvular i.
i. of cardiac valve
cervical i.
communicating vein i.
congenital palatopharyngeal i.
level of i.
mitral i.
pelvic venous i.
plea of mental i.
pulmonary i.
tricuspid i.
velopharyngeal i.

incompetency
certificate of i.

incompetent
i. aortic murmur
i. atrioventricular valve
cardia i.
i. cervical os
i. cervix
chromosomally incompetent ovarian failure
direct killing of incompetent individual
i. esophageal sphincter
legally incompetent patient
mentally i.
patient i.
i. perforating vein
i. perforator vein
socially i.
i. valve
i. vein

incomplete
i. abortion
i. angiography
i. atrioventricular block
i. atrioventricular dissociation
i. bilateral bundle-branch block
i. bladder emptying
i. bowel obstruction
i. breech presentation
i. closure
i. database
i. development of autonomic nervous system
i. diagnosis
i. dislocation
i. emptying of bladder
i. facial paralysis
i. filling
i. fistula
i. foot presentation
i. fracture
i. fracture of bone
i. Freund adjuvant
Freund incomplete adjuvant
i. harelip
i. healing
i. heart block
i. hemianopia
i. hernia
i. left bundle-branch block
i. male pseudohermaphroditism
i. mitral leaflet closure
i. Moro reflex
i. opening

incomplete *(continued)*
i. pancreas divisum
i. paralysis
i. pregnancy
i. resolution, scan to follow
i. right bundle-branch block
Rotter I. Sentences Blank
i. separation
i. situs inversus
i. testicular feminization syndrome
i. thrombosis
transient ischemic attack, incomplete recovery
i. vertical root fracture

incongruity
angle of i.

incongruous hemianopia

inconsistency
size/date inconsistency
Zinsser i.

inconsistent and inappropriate thinking

inconsolable crying

incontinence
after childbirth i.
anatomic stress i.
anterior fecal i.
bowel and bladder i.
i. and constipation
i. of feces
frequent urinary i.
i. from diabetes
genuine stress urinary i.
gravity urinary i.
I. Impact Questionnaire-Revised
increased stress i.
micturition urinary i.
minimize or delay urinary i.
mixed type of i.
Miyazaki-Bonney test for stress i.
nocturnal urinary i.
overflow fecal i.
i. product
i. of stool
stress i.
stress urinary i.
i. treatment center
urinary i.
urinary stress i.
i. of urine

incontinent
patient incontinent of feces
patient incontinent of stool
patient incontinent of urine

increase
abnormal increase in compliance
i. in amplitude of electrical activity
crying, requirement for oxygen supplementation, increases in heart rate and blood pressure
dose increase factor
i. in eidetic imagery
fold increase in resistance
gradual increase in length and complexity of utterance
i. heart production
i. in life span
i. in pupillary diameter

increased
i. abdominal girth
i. action of reflex
i. activity
i. alertness
i. amplitude
i. anxiety
i. appetite
area of increased activity
area of increased density
area of increased pigmentation
area of increased radiolabeling
area of increased uptake
i. arousal
i. attention span
i. attenuation
i. blood flow to ear
i. blood flow to heart muscle
i. blood pressure
i. bone density
i. bone mass
bone scan reveals increased activity
bone scan showed increased activity
i. brain activity
i. central venous pressure
i. clotting
i. correlation
i. craving for sweets
i. cutaneous blood flow
i. deep tendon reflex
i. density
i. depression
i. dosage
i. dose size per fraction
i. drowsiness
i. dyspnea on exertion
i. echogenicity
i. emotional arousal
i. emotional dependence
i. energy
i. energy/alertness
i. energy, decreased appetite
i. estrogen receptor
i. euphoria
i. excretion of protein
i. eye tension
i. fatigue
i. flexibility
i. flexor tone
i. flow
i. flow rate
i. fluids and humidity
i. frequency of urination
i. guilt
i. heart and breathing rate
i. heart size
i. intake
i. intracranial pressure
i. intraocular pressure
i. intraocular tension
i. kidney function
i. knee jerk
i. and labored breathing
i. lacrimation
i. level of blood sugar
i. libido
i. linear density
i. local heat
i. lumbar curve
i. lung permeability
i. medical risk
i. memory
i. mental tension
i. metabolism
i. muscle mass
i. muscle strength
i. muscle tone
i. obtundation
i. overall treatment of duration
i. pain threshold
i. pain tolerance
i. peripheral vasodilation and hypotension
i. personality disintegration
i. phlegm
i. physical activity
platelet count i.
i. prenatal care
i. pressure
i. pressure of blood
i. pressure inside the eye
i. psychomotor activity
i. pulmonary artery pressure
i. pulse
i. pulse rate
punctate area of increased signal
i. rapid eye movement sleep

i. recoil
i. reflex
i. reflex activity
i. respiratory rate
i. rhythm disturbances
i. rigidity
i. risk of breast cancer
i. risk for illness
i. sadness
i. sensitivity
i. sexual appetite
i. sexual desire
i. shortness of breath
i. skin temperature
i. stress
i. stress incontinence
i. susceptibility to infection
i. sweating
symptoms increased in severity
i. talking
i. tension line
i. thirst
i. thyroid activity
i. tolerance of pain
i. toxicity
tumor increased in size
i. uptake of isotope
i. urinary flow
i. urination
i. urine osmolality
i. venous pressure
i. wandering
i. weight

increasing
i. abdominal discomfort
i. airway resistance
i. capillary permeability
i. confusion
i. congestion
i. debility
i. debility and weakness
i. demands
i. fatigue
i. heart rate
i. insomnia
i. jaundice
i. oncotic pressure
pain increasing in severity
i. respiratory acidosis
sense of increasing helplessness
i. symptomatology
i. urinary excretion
waves of increasing amplitude
i. weakness, debility, and dyspnea

increasingly irritable

increment
corrected count i.
maximal increment in growth and weight
platelet count i.
pressure increment rate
short increment sensitivity index
small increment sensitivity index
suggested minimum i.

incremental
total corrected incremental score

increta
placenta i.

incubation
growth after 48 hours i.
long incubation hepatitis
i. period
placed in i.

incubator
infant placed in i.

incudostapedia
articulatio i.

incurable
chronic or incurable disease
disease incurable, progressive
i. illness
i. problem drinker

incurably
patient incurably ill

incurred
accidentally i.
i. accidentally
i. but not reported

incurvatum
asymmetric incurvatum reflex

incus
homograft incus prosthesis
ligament of i.
long crus of i.
long limb of i.
long process of i.
i. replacement prosthesis
short crus of i.
superior ligament of i.

indecent exposure

indecisiveness
parental i.

indemnity
double i.

indentation
anterior central i.
i. load deflection

independence
Functional I. Measure for Children
help patient achieve i.
loss of i.
moral i.
optimal level of i.
physical i.
Responsibility and I. Scale for Adolescents

independent
i. in activities of daily living
i. adjudicating panel
i. in ADL
i. ambulation
bilateral independent periodic lateralizing epileptiform discharge
bile acid independent flow
capable of independent living
capacity for independent living
center for independent living
epilepsy with multiple independent spike focus
i. evaluation
i. functional ability
i. functioning
i. laboratory
level of independent function
i. lifestyle
i. living
i. living needs
i. living skills
maximum level of independent mobility
i. medical examination
i. metabolism
patient completes independent transfers
patient independent in activities of daily living
patient independent in ADLs
patient independent in ambulation
patient independent in bathing with cueing
patient independent in boosting and rolling
patient independent in dressing
patient independent in feeding
patient independent in lower body dressing
patient independent in upper body dressing
patient independent with bathing
patient independent with small based quad cane
i. practice
i. practice association

indirect *(continued)*
i. fetal contamination
i. fluorescence
i. fluorescent antibody
i. fluorescent assay
i. fluorescent rabies antibody test
i. foot hazard
i. fraction
i. fracture
i. fulguration
i. hemagglutination
i. hemagglutination antibody test
i. hemagglutination assay
i. hemagglutinin assay
i. hernia
i. hernial sac
i. immunofluorescent
i. immunofluorescent antibody
i. immunoperoxidase
i. infection
i. inguinal hernia
i. lead
i. maximal breathing capacity
i. medical education
i. membrane immunofluorescence
i. method
i. microhemagglutination test
monocular indirect ophthalmoscope
monocular indirect ophthalmoscopy
i. murmur
i. ophthalmoscope
i. ophthalmoscopy
i. optic nerve injury syndrome
i. personal contact
i. platelet count
i. radioimmunoassay
i. radionuclide cystography
i. rays
i. reflex
i. self-destructive behavior
i. sequela
i. transfusion
i. treatment
i. vision

indiscriminate lesion

indistinct
i. blur
i. cell border
i. margin
i. semi-circumferential fibrous thickening
slurred indistinct speech

indium
i. pentate
I. scan

indium-labeled leukocyte scan

individual
adjunctive individual session
i. adult children of alcoholics counseling
augment individual sense of self-worth
i. career exploration
I. Case Safety Reports
i. cell
i. codependent counseling
i. complex
i. components
i. counseling
i. counseling sessions
i. couple's counseling
i. defense mechanism
i. dependent counseling
i. differences
direct killing of incompetent i.
i. dose
ego-oriented individual therapy
emotionally disturbed i.
frequent individual bursts of alpha activity
i. gene
ineffective individual coping
i. layer
I. Learning Disabilities Classroom Screening Instrument
long-term individual counseling
i. medical record
i. motor unit action potential
Patterns of I. Change Scale
Peabody I. Achievement Test
i. preference
i. psychodynamic psychotherapy
i. psychology
i. reaction
I. Self-Rating Scale
i. sensory modality
severely affected i.
i. solution-based therapy
speech impaired i.
i. stress
i. subject
totally dependent i.
i. treatment
i. treatment assessment
i. treatment plan
i. voluntary control
i. vulnerability
i. wave
i. well-being
I.'s with Disabilities Education Act
i. with a disability

individualized
I. Criterion Reference Testing Mathematics
I. Criterion Reference Testing Reading
i. education program
I. Family Service Plan
i. functional status assessment
i. plan

individually
i. polymerized grass
i. viable cell

indocyanine
digital subtraction indocyanine green angiography
i. green
i. green angiography
i. green dye

indocyanine-green fundus angiography

indolaminergic-accumulating cell

indole
methyl i.
i., methyl red, Voges-Proskauer, and citrate test
sulfide, indole, motility medium

indoleacetic acid

indolent
i. disease
i. follicular lymphoma
i. papule
i. ulcer

indoor air quality

induced
i. abortion
i. allergy
chemically induced dynamic electron polarization
i. circular dichroism
i. complement-fixing antigen
condition induced by medication
electrically induced spinal reflex
i. emesis
exercise induced heart attack
experimentally induced Köbner phenomenon
i. fever
gravity induced loss of consciousness
hallucinatory state induced by drug
hospital i.
inhalant induced hallucination
malaria
i. muscular tension

i. nitric oxide synthase
osmotically induced asthma
i. potential
prothrombin induced by vitamin K absence or antagonist-II
quantitative light induced fluorescence
radiation induced emesis
rate change i.
recurrent induced malaria
remission i.
i. sputum
i. sputum analysis

inducer
extracellular matrix metalloproteinase i.
macrophage and granulocyte i.

inducible
i. arrhythmia
i. cAMP early repressor
i. nitric oxide synthase
i. nitric oxide synthetase
prolactin inducible protein

inducing
TNF-related apoptosis inducing ligand
tumor i.

inductance
respiratory inductance plethysmography

induction
i. of anesthesia
i. anesthesia
anesthetic induction agent
anthracycline-based induction chemotherapy
antibody induction therapy
cartilage induction factor
i. chemotherapy
coefficient of i.
i. of coma
coronary spasm i.
crash induction of anesthesia
i. delivery
elective induction of labor
electronic induction desorption
free induction decay
Hypnotic I. Profile
i. of labor
magnetic i.
magnetic induction device
menstrual cycle i.
menstruation i.
negative control enzyme i.
i. period
rapid-sequence i.
rapid sequence induction orotracheal intubation
remission i.
i. of sleep
syncytia induction assay
tumor i.

induction-delivery interval

inductive
hemopoietic inductive microenvironment
respiratory inductive plethysmography
surface inductive plethysmography

inductively-coupled
i.-c. plasma-mass spectrometer
i.-c. plasma-optical emission spectrometry

indulin agar

indurated
i. border
i. cellulite
hard, indurated colon mass
i. mass
i. papule
i. plantar keratoma

induration
i. along skin incision
black i.
bowel wall i.
brawny i.
brown i.
brown induration of lung
cyanotic i.
fibroid i.
granular i.
gray i.
idiopathic brown i.
laminate i.
mass, induration, or tenderness
parchment i.
penile i.
plastic i.
red i.
i. and swelling
i. of tissue

industrial
i. accident
i. anthrax
i. chemistry
i. clinic
i. disease
exposure to industrial substances
i. eye care
Flanagan I. Test
i. hygiene
i. injury
i. medicine
i. methylated spirit
i. monitoring
i. physical therapist
i. population
i. psychiatry
i. psychology
i. rehabilitation unit
Standard I. Classification

industry
healthcare i.
Personnel Tests for I.

indwelling
i. arterial catheter
i. bladder catheter
i. catheter drainage
i. Foley catheter
i. line
peripheral indwelling intermediate infusion device
prolonged indwelling catheter
i. prosthetic joint
i. prosthetic medical device
i. subclavian catheter
i. transcutaneous vascular access device
i. urethral catheter
i. urinary catheter
i. vascular access catheter
i. venous catheter
i. venous line

ineffective
i. airway clearance
compromised ineffective family coping
disabling ineffective family coping
i. esophageal motility
i. heart action
idiopathic ineffective erythropoiesis
i. individual coping
i. intervention
i. iron turnover
i. treatment

ineffectively treated

inefficient pumping of blood

inequality
anatomic leg length i.
i. in leg length
leg length i.
limb length i.

inert
multiple inert gas elimination technique

inertia
central principal axis of i.
central principal moments of i.
dynamic movement of i.
moment of i.

inertial
segment inertial properties

inevitable abortion

inexplicable
sudden inexplicable death

infancy
acute hemorrhagic edema of i.
adjustment reaction of i.
anal phase of i.
apnea of i.
Assessment in I. Ordinal Scales of Psychological Development
attachment disorder of i.
attachment in i.
autoimmune neutropenia of i.
chronic pneumonitis of i.
desmoplastic cerebral astrocytoma of i.
intractable diarrhea of i.
melanotic neuroectodermal tumor of i.
minipuberty of i.
nonfamilial hyperinsulinism of i.
normal gastroesophageal reflux of i.
persistent hyperinsulinemic hypoglycemia of i.
protracted diarrhea of i.
severe myoclonic epilepsy in i.
spongy degeneration of i.
sudden death in i.
transient hypogammaglobulinemia of i.

infant
abnormal position of i.
i. acidotic and hypoxic
i. in acute respiratory distress
Alberta I. Motor Scale
i. Ambu resuscitator
i. apnea syndrome
apneic infant with decreased heart rate
Assessment of Preterm I.'s Behavior
Bayley Infant Neurodevelopmental Screener
Bayley Scales of Infant Development-II
I. Behavior Record
California I. Scale for Motor Development
i. cardiac arrest tray
Cattell I. Intelligence Scale
Cattell I. Scale Inventory
Collaborative Home I. Monitoring Evaluation
cord around infant neck
i. crowning
i. death
i. delivered
i. development
i. of diabetic mother
Distress Scale for Ventilated Newborn I.'s
i. of drug abusing mother
emergency maternal and infant care
epidemic disease of infant mice
epizootic diarrhea of infant mice
i. exhibits hunger behavior
i. expelled
extremely premature i.
i. feeding tube
Flint I. Security Scale
i. floppy
floppy infant syndrome
i. had weak cry
Harris I. Neuromotor Test
hemorrhagic disease of i.
i. of high-risk mother
i. of infected mother
i. intensive care unit
intrauterine pregnancy, term birth, living i.
i. intubated
i. jaundice
i. jaundiced
Kent I. Development Scale
limp infant syndrome
low birth weight i.
i. massage
maternal and infant care
i. mildly icteric
mildly icteric i.
minimally active i.
minor hypertensive i.
i. morbidity
i. morbidity and mortality
i. mortality
i. mortality rate
Mother's Assessment of the Behavior of Her I.
i. of mother with gestational diabetes mellitus
movement assessment of i.
i. nasal cannula assembly
near-miss sudden infant death syndrome
Neonatal I. Pain Scale
newborn infant care
i. of nondiabetic mother
nonthrombocytopenic preterm infant
normal male i.
i. nutrition
partially unexplained sudden infant death syndrome
i. passive hand
patient delivered congenitally deformed i.
patient delivered normal i.
Pediatrician infant dietary supplement
periodic breathing in i.'s
i. placed in incubator
i. placed under Bili-Lite
i. placed in warmer
position of i.
postperinatal infant mortality
postterm i.
premature i.
premature birth live i.
Premature I. Pain Profile
i. respiratory distress syndrome
i. retracting and grunting
i. rotated
i. skin control
i. stillborn
i. of substance-abusing mother
i. suck is poor
sudden infant crib death
sudden infant death syndrome
sudden unexpected infant death
sudden unexplained infant death
term birth, living i.
Test of I. Motor Performance
toddler and infant motor evaluation
totally unexplained sudden infant death syndrome
i. tracks movement
transmission of infected mother to i.
very low birth weight i.
viable female i.
viable male i.
i. vision
i. weight gain
i. weight loss
i. with oxygen
i. with seizures
i. with sepsis
i. with umbilical catheter
Women, Infants, and Children Program

infantile
i. amaurotic familial idiocy
i. aphasia
i. apnea
i. astrocytoma
i. autism
benign infantile familial convulsions
i. bilateral striatal necrosis syndrome
i. botulism
i. cataract
chronic infantile hypotonic syndrome
chronic infantile neurological, cutaneous, and articular
congenital infantile fibrosarcoma
i. cortical hyperostosis
desmoplastic infantile ganglioglioma
i. diarrhea
i. diffuse brain sclerosis
early infantile epileptic encephalopathy
i. eczema
i. estropia
i. gastroenteritis
i. genetic agranulocytosis
i. glaucoma
i. hemangioma
i. hemiplegia
i. hernia
i. hydrocephalus
i. hypercalcemia stenosis
i. hypertrophic pyloric stenosis
idiopathic infantile hypercalcemia
late infantile amaurotic familial idiocy
late infantile neural ceroid lipofuscinosis
lightning attacks in infantile spasm
i. lobar emphysema
magnesium deficiency infantile tremor syndrome
microcephaly, infantile spasm, psychomotor retardation, nephrotic syndrome
mixed infantile spasm
i. myoclonic jerk
i. myoclonic seizure
i. necrotizing encephalomyelopathy
i. nephrotic syndrome
i. neuroaxonal dystrophy
nonbacterial infantile gastroenteritis
i. nuclear cerebral degeneration
i. paralysis
paralytic infantile paralysis
i. periarteritis nodosa
periorbital infantile myofibromatosis
i. polyarteritis nodosa
i. polycystic kidney disease
i. Refsum syndrome
i. sialic acid storage disorder
i. sleep apnea
i. spasm
i. spinal muscular atrophy
i. tibia vara

infantilis
roseola i.

infantilism
Lorain i.
Lorain-Lévi i.
muscular i.
myxedematous i.
pancreatic i.
pituitary i.

infant's
crowning of infant's head
nuchal cord around infant's neck
tight nuchal cord around infant's neck

Infant/Toddler Environment Rating Scale

infant-toddler special care unit

infantum
anemia infantum pseudoleukemica
anemia pseudoleukemica i.
lichen i.
osteopathia hemorrhagica i.
roseola i.
tabes i.

infarct
acute ischemic brain i.
acute multiple brain i.
acute nonhemorrhagic i.
anterior communicating artery distribution i.
anterior lateral myocardial i.
anterior myocardial i.
anterior wall myocardial i.
anteroinferior myocardial i.
anterolateral myocardial i.
anteroseptal myocardial i.
apical-lateral wall myocardial i.
apical myocardial i.
arrhythmic myocardial i.
atherothrombotic brain i.
i. avid hot spot scintigraphy
i. avid imaging
i. avid myocardial scintigraphy
bilateral occipital lobe i.
brain i.
chronic cystic i.
cortical bone i.
deep white matter i.
diaphragmatic myocardial i.
diaphragmatic pulmonary i.
embolic cerebral i.
i. expansion
i. extension
extension of cerebral i.
focal hemorrhagic i.
focal infarct of liver
foci of i.
hemorrhagic infarct of adrenal gland
inferior myocardial i.
internal borderzone i.
lacunar circulation i.
left ventricular infarct volume
massive infarct of brain stem
medullary bone i.
middle cerebral artery i.
multiple pulmonary i.
myocardial i.
i. of myocardium
nerve fiber layer i.
old cystic i.
partial anterior cerebral i.
partial anterior circulation i.
perforating artery i.
pontine i.
posterior circulation i.
posterior wall i.
pulmonary embolus with small i.
rule out myocardial i.
i. scar
segmental bowel i.
silent cerebral i.
i. size index
size of i.
small cystic i.
small, deep, recent i.
subendocardial i.
total anterior circulation i.
uric acid i.

infarcted bowel

infarction
acute subendocardial myocardial i.
anterior communicating artery distribution i.
anterior lateral myocardial i.
anterior myocardial i.
anterior wall i.
anterior wall myocardial i.
anteroinferior myocardial i.

infarction *(continued)*
anterolateral myocardial i.
anteroseptal myocardial i.
apical myocardial i.
atherothrombotic brain i.
avascular cortical infarction necrosis
cerebral i.
cerebrovascular i.
chills from myocardial i.
chorionic villus i.
complete myocardial i.
conduction defect in acute myocardial i.
diabetic muscle i.
direct acute myocardial infarction angioplasty
evolving myocardial i.
healed myocardial i.
hemisphere thrombotic i.
hemorrhagic i.
impending myocardial i.
inferior wall myocardial i.
inferoposterior myocardial i.
ischemic brain i.
ischemic brainstem i.
ischemic cerebral i.
lacunar i.
large-vessel i.
lateral medullary i.
malignant middle cerebral artery i.
maternal floor i.
medial medullary i.
multiple cortical i.
multiple subcortical i.
myocardial i.
myocardial infarction recovery index
myocardial infarction rehabilitation program
myocardial infarction research unit
myocardial infarction triage and intervention
nonocclusive mesenteric i.
non–Q-wave myocardial i.
non-ST-elevation myocardial i.
nontransmural myocardial i.
old healed myocardial i.
old inferior wall myocardial i.
parasagittal cortical i.
perioperative myocardial i.
posterior myocardial i.
posterior wall myocardial i.
postmyocardial i.
postmyocardial infarction syndrome
previous posterior myocardial i.
primary i.
pulmonary i.
Q-wave myocardial i.
recurrent myocardial i.
right ventricle i.
rule out myocardial i.
silent brain i.
silent cerebral i.
silent myocardial i.
small-vessel i.
spinal cord i.
status post myocardial i.
subendocardial myocardial i.
threatened myocardial i.
thrombotic brain i.
transmural myocardial i.
unstable angina/non-Q-wave myocardial i.
i. zone

infarct-related
i.-r. artery
i.-r. vessel

infected
acquired immune deficiency syndrome infected child
i. aneurysm
i. area
i. blood donor
i. callus
chronically i.
debridement infected skin
i. decubitus ulcer
draining infected nonunion
i. eye
fungus infected nail
human immunodeficiency virus infected blood
i. hyperalimentation line
i. incision
i. incision site
infant of infected mother
i. intravenous drug needle
i. joint
i. joint lining
i. lymph gland
i. membrane
mother infected with acquired immune deficiency syndrome
i. organ donor
i. pancreatic necrosis
i. pilonidal cyst
i. red blood cell
sharing infected intravenous drug needle
i. tissue
i. tissue culture
i. tonsil
transmission of infected mother to infant
i. with HIV

infection
abdominal foci of i.
absence of i.
acquired immune deficiency syndrome virus i.
acute HIV-1 i.
acute intestinal i.
acute throat i.
acute viral i.
acute viral respiratory i.
alcohol, epilepsy, insulin, overdose, uremia, trauma, infection, psychiatric, stroke
alopecia, nail dystrophy, ophthalmic complication, thyroid dysfunction, hypohidrosis, ephelides and enteropathy, and respiratory tract i.
amniocentesis indicative of i.
amniotic fluid i.
amniotic fluid infection syndrome
anaerobic respiratory i.
anal human papilloma virus i.
antecedent streptococcal i.
antibiotic-resistant bacterial i.
antifungal esophageal i.
antifungal-resistant opportunistic i.
aortic graft i.
arteriovenous shunt i.
ascending gonococcal i.
ascending intrauterine i.
asymptomatic urinary tract i.
ataxia, myoclonic encephalopathy, macular degeneration, recurrent infections syndrome
atrium of i.
atypical mycobacteria i.
atypical mycobacterial i.
bacterial infection of bloodstream
biliary tract i.
i. or bladder involvement
bleeding and i.
blister without i.
bloodstream i.
bone and joint i.
bone marrow i.
candidal granuloma i.
Candida urinary tract i.
catheter-associated i.
catheter-related i.
catheter-related bloodstream i.

catheter-related urinary tract i.
central line i.
central venous catheter i.
Chlamydia i.
chronic hepatitis C i.
chronic middle ear i.
chronic syphilitic i.
chronic urinary tract i.
clinical pulmonary infection score
cluster of i.
community-acquired bladder i.
community-acquired respiratory i.
i. complication
comprehensive hospital infections project
concurrent upper respiratory tract i.
congenital cytomegalovirus i.
congenital HIV i.
congenital rubella i.
congenital syphilitic i.
i. control
i. control policy
i. control professional
Coxsackie viral i.
deep space neck i.
deep sternal wound i.
delirium, infection, atrophic urethritis and vaginitis, pharmaceuticals, psychological disorders, excessive urine output, restricted mobility, stool impaction
dermatophyte infection of hair
dermatophyte infection of nails
dermatophyte infection of scalp
dermatophyte infection of skin
device-related urinary tract i.
disseminated gonococcal i.
disseminated herpes zoster i.
disseminated nontuberculous mycobacterial infection
disseminating fungal i.
dizziness from infection of ear
documented bacterial i.
documented viral i.
effective infection control
endemic fungal i.
epidural space i.
i. eradicated
existing infection control
fatal disseminated i.
fatal nosocomial i.
fever caused by i.
focus of i.
free from i.
frequency of i.
fungal i.
generalized infection involving fungus
genital herpes i.
genitourinary i.
Gram-negative bacilli i.
Gram-positive bacterial i.
Gram-positive nosocomial i.
group A streptococcus i.
group B streptococcal i.
i. hazard
hearing loss from infection of ear
heart valve i.
hepatitis B i.
herpes eye i.
herpes simplex i.
herpes zoster virus i.
hibernal epidemic viral i.
high risk of HIV i.
high-risk of HIV i.
Hodgkin disease and HIV i.
hospital-acquired bloodstream i.
hospital-acquired lower respiratory i.
hospital-acquired organism i.
hospital-acquired urinary tract i.
hospital-associated respiratory tract i.
hospital infection control
hospital onset of i.
human carriers of i.
human cytomegalovirus infection
i. immunity
incipient respiratory i.
incisional surgical wound i.
increased susceptibility to i.
i. and inflammation
inner ear i.
insertion site i.
intervertebral disc space i.
intraabdominal i.
intraamniotic infection syndrome
intrauterine i.
intrauterine viral i.
intravascular device i.
intravenous infection site
intravenous line i.
intravenous site of i.
Kaposi sarcoma and opportunistic i.
laboratory-acquired i.
liver cyst i.
lowered resistance to i.
lower genital tract i.
lower respiratory tract i.
lower urinary tract i.
lymphogranuloma venereum i.
Mansonella ozzardi i.
Mansonella perstans i.
Mansonella streptocerca i.
i. medium
middle ear i.
mixed fungal/bacterial i.
mixed nail i.
mixed vaccine, respiratory i.
mixed virus respiratory i.
mosquito bite i.
multiple hepatitis virus i.
multiple opportunistic pathogen i.
multiplicity of i.
Mycobacterium abscessus i.
Mycobacterium avium complex i.
Mycobacterium avium i.
Mycobacterium avium-intracellulare i.
Mycobacterium chelonea i.
Mycobacterium fortuitum i.
Mycobacterium haemophilum i.
Mycobacterium kansasii i.
Mycobacterium marinum i.
Mycobacterium xenopi i.
nail infection and care
natural focus of i.
necrotizing soft-tissue i.
neonatal enterovirus i.
neonatal herpes simplex virus i.
neutropenia-related bacterial i.
no infection present
nondermatophyte fungal i.
nonrespiratory i.
nontuberculous mycobacterial i.
nontyphoidal salmonella i.
no sign of i.
nosocomial bacterial i.
nosocomial and cross i.
nosocomial eye i.
nosocomial fungal i.
nosocomial gastrointestinal i.
nosocomial Gram-negative i.
nosocomial Gram-positive i.
nosocomial gynecological i.
nosocomial respiratory tract i.
nosocomial rotavirus i.
nosocomial urinary tract i.
nosocomial wound i.
ocular cryptococcal i.
ocular herpes i.
operative site i.
opportunistic i.
opportunistic systemic fungal i.
oral yeast i.
organ transplant i.
orofacial odontogenic i.
orthopedic implant i.

infection *(continued)*
overwhelming postsplenectomy i.
pancreatic bacterial i.
paravaccinia virus i.
parvovirus B19 i.
patient admitted with active i.
patient immune to hepatitis B i.
pediatric autoimmune neuropsychiatric diseases associated with streptococcal i.
pediatric autoimmune neuropsychiatric disorders associated with streptococcal i.
pediatric gonococcal i.
i. penetrated bone
percutaneous bone marrow i.
peritoneal fungal i.
persistent tolerant i.
postnatal i.
postoperative wound i.
potential for i.
potential source of i.
i. prevention
i. prevention and control
prevention of hospital i.
prevention of i.
prevent spread of i.
primary i.
prosthetic joint i.
recurrent upper respiratory tract i.
reduce risk of hospital-associated i.
reemerging i.
repeated ear i.
resistance to i.
respiratory tract i.
i. risk
risk group for i.
risk of i.
route of i.
severe intestinal i.
sexually transmitted i.
soft tissue i.
source of i.
spread of i.
staphylococcal infection of heart valve
Staphylococcus aureus prosthetic joint i.
subclinical papillomavirus i.
surgical wound i.
i. surveillance and control program
symptomatic HIV i.
symptomatic urinary tract i.
systemic bacterial i.
total infections versus total admission
toxoplasmosis, other infections, rubella, cytomegalovirus infection, herpes simplex syndrome
toxoplasmosis, other infections, rubella, cytomegalovirus infection, herpes simplex syndrome
transmission of i.
upper respiratory tract i.
urinary tract i.
urinary tract infection cleared
vaginal yeast i.
varicella virus i.
vascular graft i.
viral respiratory i.
wheezing-associated respiratory i.

infection-associated hemophagocytic syndrome

infection-fighting
i.-f. T cell
i.-f. white cell

infection-potentiating factor

infection-related crisis

infectiosa
mononucleosis i.

infectiosum
erythema i.

infectiosus
icterus i.

infectious
i. abortion
active invasive infectious process
acute epidemic infectious adenitis
acute infectious colitis
acute infectious diarrhea
acute infectious disease
acute infectious disease series
acute infectious gastroenteritis
acute infectious lymphocytosis
acute infectious mononucleosis
acute infectious nonbacterial gastroenteritis
acute infectious polyneuritis
i. agent
ankle infectious arthritis
associated infectious disease
avian infectious bronchitis
avian infectious bronchitis virus
avian infectious encephalomyelitis
avian infectious laryngotracheitis
avian infectious laryngotracheitis virus
blood-borne infectious agent
i. body fluid
i. bovine keratoconjunctivitis
i. bovine rhinotracheitis
i. bovine rhinotracheitis virus
i. bowel disease
i. bronchitis
i. bronchitis vaccine
i. bronchitis virus
i. bursal disease
i. bursal disease virus
i. canine hepatitis
i. carcinoma
i. cardiomyopathy
i. cause
i. cell protein
chronic infectious neuropathic agent
i. colitis
i. conjunctivitis
i. crystalline keratopathy
i. diarrhea
disabled infectious single cycle virus
i. disease unit
i. disorder
i. endocarditis
i. equine anemia
i. esophagitis
i. etiology
feline infectious anemia
feline infectious peritonitis
feline infectious peritonitis virus
i. fluid
i. gastritis
i. granuloma
i. granulomatous disease
gut-derived infectious toxic shock
i. hematopoietic necrosis virus
i. hepatitis
i. human hepatitis
human infectious dose
i. illness
life-threatening infectious agent
log infectious virus titer
i. mononucleosis
i. mononucleosis receptor
i. morbidity
i. myocarditis
National Institute of Allergy and I. Disease
necrotic infectious conjunctivitis
nonbacterial infectious arthritis
notifiable infectious disease
i. nucleic acid
i. organism

other potentially infectious material
i. pancreatic necrosis virus
i. papilloma virus
patient i.
pediatric infectious disease developmental screening test
i. pericarditis
i. porcine encephalomyelitis
potentially i.
potentially infectious blood specimen
i. process
prosthetic infectious endocarditis
i. pustular vaginitis
i. rhinitis
risk of infectious disease
subacute infectious arthritis
tissue culture infectious dose
i. units per million
virus-like infectious agent

infective

acute infective endocarditis
chick infective dose
i. dose
i. endocarditis
i. granuloma
median tissue culture infective dose
minimum infective dose
nosocomial infective endocarditis
tissue culture infective dose

infectivity

immunoperoxidase infectivity assay
macrophage infectivity potentiator
macrophage infectivity potentiator protein

inference

logical i.
Test of Social I.'s

inferior

i. alveolar nerve
i. angle
angle of inferior scapula
angulus inferior scapulae
ankle inferior transverse ligament
anomalous nonrecurrent right inferior laryngeal nerve
apertura pelvis i.
apertura thoracis i.
i. apical
apical branch of inferior lobar branch of right pulmonary artery
artery of anterior inferior segment of kidney
artery of inferior cavernous sinus
ascending branch of the inferior mesenteric artery
atraumatic, multidirectional, bilateral rehabilitation inferior capsular shift
i. basal
bilateral inferior epigastric artery flap
i. border
i. calcaneonavicular ligament
i. capsular shift
i. carotid ganglion
i. cervical ganglion
i. colliculus
deep inferior epigastric artery perforator
i. dislocation
i. edge
i. epigastric artery
i. esophageal constriction
i. esophageal sphincter
ethmoidal process of inferior nasal concha
extended deep inferior epigastric
i. facet
far lateral inferior suboccipital approach
i. flap
i. frontal gyrus
i. frontal lobe
i. ganglion of vagus nerve
i. glenohumeral ligament
i. glenohumeral ligament labral complex
i. gluteal nerve
i. gluteal vein
gyrus frontalis i.
gyrus temporalis i.
i. hemorrhoidal nerves
i. hemorrhoidal vein
i. horn
hypertrophied inferior turbinate
i. hypogastric plexus
infrahepatic interruption of inferior vena cava
i. jugular ganglion
i. lacrimal duct
i. lateral angle
left inferior oblique muscle
left inferior pulmonary vein
left inferior rectus
left inferior vena cava
left posterior inferior hemiblock
ligament of epididymis inferior and superior
macula cribrosa i.
i. margin
i. margin of liver
medial inferior genicular artery
membranous obstruction of the inferior vena cava
mental branch of inferior alveolar artery
i. mesenteric artery
i. mesenteric ganglion
i. mesenteric vein
mylohyoid branch of inferior alveolar artery
i. myocardial infarct
i. nasal artery
i. nasal quadrant
i. nasal vein
i. oblique eye muscle
i. oblique overaction
i. oblique recession
obturator branch of pubic branch of inferior epigastric vein
old inferior wall myocardial infarction
i. olive
opening of inferior vena cava
orbital inferior rim
i. orbital rim
orifice of inferior vena cava
i. parietal and superior temporal lobe
i. part
i. petrosal sinus sampling
pharyngeal branch of inferior thyroid artery
i. point of pubic bone
i. pole
posterior inferior cerebellar artery
posterior inferior communicating artery
posterior inferior iliac spine
i. radicular vein
radionuclide imaging of inferior vena cava
i. rectus
i. rectus muscle
right inferior oblique muscle
right inferior rectus
right inferior vena cava
sacrococcygeal to inferior pubic point
i. sagittal sinus
segment i.
shunt index via the inferior mesenteric vein
i. spermatic plexus
superficial inferior epigastric artery

inferior *(continued)*
suprahepatic inferior vena cava
i. tarsal muscle
i. temporal
i. temporal artery
i. temporal cortex
i. temporal quadrant
i. temporal vein
thoracic inferior vena cava
i. thyroid gland
i. thyroid notch
i. turbinate
ureteric branch of inferior suprarenal artery
i. vagal ganglion
i. vena cava
i. vena cava filter
vena cava i.
i. vena cava pressure
i. vena cava reconstruction
i. vena cava thrombosis
i. venacavogram
i. venacavography
ventral posterior i.
i. wall ischemia
i. wall myocardial infarction

inferiority
i. complex
constitutional psychopathic i.
i. feeling
organ inferiority complex
premorbid inferiority feeling

inferoposterior myocardial infarction

infertile patient

infertility
endocrine and i.
endometriosis-associated i.
i. evaluation
i. from alcohol
i. from chemical
i. from diabetes
male factor i.
male infertility problem
pelvic infertility factor
i. perceptions inventory
standard infertility treatment algorithm
stillbirth, mummification, embryonic death, infertility syndrome
i. studies
i. tests
i. in women
i. workup

infestation
Ascaris i.
louse i.
mite i.
parasitic i.

infiltrate
active i.
airspace ground-glass i.
annular i.
apical i.
Assmann tuberculous i.
basilar i.
basilar pulmonary i.
bilateral alveolar pulmonary i.
bilateral hilar i.'s
bronchopneumonic i.
cavitary i.
chronic inflammatory i.
chronic interstitial inflammatory i.
clearing of i.
corneal i.
dense lobar i.
diffuse pulmonary i.
endomyocardial lymphocytic i.'s
fluffy i.
fluffy alveolar i.
fluffy bibasilar i.
fluffy pulmonary i.
focal areas of lymphoid i.
hazy i.
hilar i.
interstitial i.
left lower lobe i.
liver i.
localized i.
lung base i.
lymphocytic infiltrate of Jessner
lymphoid i.
lymphoplasmacytic i.
mild focal chronic inflammatory i.
miliary i.
moderate i.
mononuclear cell i.
mononuclear histiocytic portal i.
multifocal aggressive i.
multilobe i.
nodular i.
parapneumonic i.
parenchymal i.
patchy anterior stromal i.
patchy chronic inflammatory i.
patchy pneumonic i.
peribronchial inflammatory i.
perihilar batwing i.
peripheral ring i.
pneumonic i.
polymorphonuclear leukocyte i.
pulmonary i.
pulmonary infiltrate fever
pulmonary infiltrate with eosinophilia
punctate subepithelial i.
residual i.
right lower lobe i.
scattered chronic inflammatory i.
strandy i.
streaky i.
subepithelial corneal i.

infiltrated
diffusely i.
multifocal infiltrated duct cell carcinoma

infiltrating
i. adenocarcinoma
anaplastic infiltrating single cell
i. ductal carcinoma
i. ductal carcinoma of the breast
i. ductal cell carcinoma
i. glioma
i. irregular tumor mass
i. lesion
i. lobular cancer
i. lobular carcinoma
i. squamous cell carcinoma
i. tumor

infiltration
cavernous sinus i.
chronic inflammatory cell i.
focal nonfatty infiltration of liver
i. ganglion
i. by hemorrhage
leukocyte infiltration factor
lymphocytic infiltration of the skin
mononuclear cell i.
myeloid cell i.
pancreatic lymphocytic i.
patchy infiltration of medullary parenchyma
pericapsular fat i.
perirectal fat i.
pulmonary infiltration with eosinophilia
surface infiltration by hemorrhage

infiltrative
diffuse infiltrative lung disease
diffuse infiltrative lymphocytosis syndrome
hypertrophic infiltrative tendinitis
local infiltrative anesthesia
lymphocytic infiltrative disease

patchy infiltrative process
i. tendonitis

infirm
elderly and mentally i.

inflamed
acutely inflamed appendix
air passage become i.
i. airway tissue
i. appendix
i. area
chronically inflamed airway
chronically inflamed gallbladder with stones
i. diverticulum
i. gallbladder
i. gums
i. intestine
i. joint
joint swollen and i.
i. linear verrucous epidermal nevus
mucosa appeared i.
i. nasal passage
painful, inflamed area
i. swollen joint
swollen, stiff, inflamed joint
i. tissue
trachea markedly i.

inflammation
active chronic i.
acute i.
acute catarrhal i.
acute and chronic i.
acute kidney i.
acute portal i.
i. and/or swelling
anterior chamber i.
anterior segment i.
i. of biopsy tissue
blood vessel i.
i. of brain
chronic i.
chronic granulomatous i.
chronic inflammation of joint
i. of colon
i. of connective tissue
development of i.
diseased joint with i.
fluid accumulation and i.
i. of the gallbladder
i. and gliosis in brain
i. of heart
i. of heart lining
i. of heart muscle
hereditary multifocal relapsing i.
i. of ileum
infection and i.
i. of intestine
ischemic ocular i.
jaundice without i.
i. of joint
lower respiratory tract i.
membranous acute i.
miliary granulomatous i.
nasal passage i.
necrotizing granulomatous i.
necrotizing scleritis with adjacent i.
necrotizing scleritis without adjacent i.
neutrophil-mediated joint i.
no acute i.
no inflammation present
no sign of i.
painful inflammation of joint
parietal peritoneal i.
prepatellar bursa i.
redness and i.
respiratory tract i.
tongue inflammation from pernicious anemia
tympanic membrane i.
i. within affected area

inflammatory
i. activity
acute idiopathic inflammatory bowel disease
acute inflammatory cell
acute inflammatory demyelinating polyneuropathy
acute inflammatory demyelinating polyradiculoneuropathy
acute inflammatory demyelinating polyradiculopathy
acute pelvic inflammatory disease
i. adhesion
i. aneurysm
i. aortic aneurysm
i. arthritis
asthmatic inflammatory airway disease
asymptomatic inflammatory prostatitis
i. atrophy
autoimmune inflammatory demyelination
i. bowel disease
I. Bowel Disease Questionnaire
i. bowel syndrome
i. breast cancer
i. carcinoma
i. carcinoma or breast
i. cardiomyopathy
i. cell
i. change
characteristic inflammatory reaction
chronic inflammatory arthritis
chronic inflammatory bowel disease
chronic inflammatory cell
chronic inflammatory cell infiltration
chronic inflammatory demyelinating polyradiculoneuropathy
chronic inflammatory demyelinating polyradiculopathy
chronic inflammatory disease
chronic inflammatory granulomatous process
chronic inflammatory hyperplasia
chronic inflammatory infiltrate
chronic interstitial inflammatory infiltrate
chronic pelvic inflammatory disease
chronic relapsing demyelinating inflammatory polyneuropathy
i. cloacogenic polyp
i. colonic polyp
i. condition
i. cyst
demyelinated inflammatory chronic polyneuropathy
i. diarrhea
i. disease
i. disorder
extensive inflammatory bowel disease
i. factor of anaphylaxis
i. fibroid polyp
focal inflammatory mucosal change
i. fracture
i. glaucoma
i. glomerulopathy
granular inflammatory nodule
i. headache
i. hyperplasia
idiopathic inflammatory bowel disease
idiopathic inflammatory myopathy
idiopathic orbital inflammatory syndrome
interstitial acute inflammatory cell
i. intestinal disorder
i. joint disease

inflammatory *(continued)*
juvenile-onset multisystem inflammatory disease
i. lesion
linear inflammatory verrucous epidermal nevus
i. linear verrucous epidermal nevus
local inflammatory response
locally advanced and inflammatory breast carcinoma
i. lung disease
lymphoid inflammatory pseudotumor
macrophage inflammatory protein-1
macrophage inflammatory protein alpha-1
macrophage inflammatory protein-1-alpha
macrophage inflammatory protein-1-beta
macrophage inflammatory protein I, II
i. mass
maternal inflammatory response
mesenteric inflammatory venoocclusive disease
mild focal chronic inflammatory infiltrate
mixed inflammatory granuloma
mucosal inflammatory hyperplasia
multifocal white matter inflammatory lesion
i. myofibroblastic tumor
i. myopathy
necrotic inflammatory cell
NIH Classification Category III inflammatory and noninflammatory chronic pelvic pain
NIH Classification Category IV asymptomatic inflammatory prostatitis
no inflammatory signs
nonvasculitic autoimmune inflammatory meningoencephalitis
ocular adnexal inflammatory pseudotumor
ocular inflammatory disease
ocular inflammatory disorder
orbital inflammatory disease
ovarian inflammatory cyst
i. papillary hyperplasia
i. papillary hyperplasia of the palate
patchy chronic inflammatory infiltrate
i. pelvic disease
peptic inflammatory disease
peribronchial inflammatory infiltrate
pleural inflammatory change
i. process
i. pseudotumor
i. reaction
i. response
scattered chronic inflammatory infiltrate
Short I. Bowel Disease Questionnaire
superimposed acute inflammatory episode
i. suppression
systemic inflammatory disease
systemic inflammatory response syndrome
i. tissue
tubal inflammatory damage

inflatable
i. balloon
i. cuff
i. limb splint
i. penile prosthesis

inflated
i. judgment of accomplishments
i. self-esteem

inflation
balloon i.
Hering-Breuer inflation reflex
intermittent positive pressure inflation with oxygen
peak inflation pressure
Quantum inflation device

in-flight emergency

inflow
aortic i.
aortoiliac inflow assessment
aqueous i.
arterial i.
i. cannula
gradient of fluid i.
left ventricular inflow volume
right ventricular inflow tract
i. tract

influence
driving under the influence of drugs
driving under the influence of intoxicants
interpersonal i.'s

influenced
magnetically influenced homeopathic remedy

influencing
factors influencing anxiety

influenza
i. A, B, C
avian influenza virus
i. bacillus
cold-adapted influenza virus vaccine, trivalent
cold-attenuated intranasal influenza vaccine
i. immunization
immunopotentiating reconstituted influenza virosomes
i. nostras
swine influenza strain
swine influenza virus
i. vaccination
i. vaccine
i. virion vaccine, split virion
i. virion vaccine, whole virion
i. virus
i. virus, attenuated live vaccine
i. virus inactivated vaccine
i. virus inactivated vaccine, split virion, types A, B trivalent
i. virus pneumonia

influenzae
diphtheria, tetanus, pertussis, *Haemophilus influenzae* type b vaccine
diphtheria, tetanus toxoids, whole-cell pertussis, and *Haemophilus influenzae* type b conjugate
Haemophilus i.
Haemophilus influenzae biogroup *aegyptius*
Haemophilus influenzae type b
Haemophilus influenzae type b conjugate vaccine
Haemophilus influenzae type b polysaccharide vaccine
Haemophilus influenzae type b vaccine
Haemophilus influenzae type b vaccine, PRP-D conjugate vaccine
Haemophilus influenzae type b vaccine, PRP-OMP conjugate vaccine
Haemophilus influenzae type b vaccine, PRP-T conjugate vaccine

Haemophilus influenzae type
vaccine oligosaccharide-CRM197
vaccine conjugate
restriction endonucleases from *Haemophilus influenzae*

influenza-like illness

influenza-related illness

influx
aqueous influx phenomenon
Ascher aqueous influx phenomenon
net calcium i.

information
Arithmetic, Coding, I., and Digit Span
assimilating information disturbance
automated hospital information system
bibliographic information and documentation
Bioethical Information On-Line
community health management information system
confidentiality of i.
i. content
count information density
current medical information and terminology
disclosure of i.
Disease Detection I. Bureau
dispensing i.
drug i.
drug information center
drug information log
Drug Product I. File
emergency medical i.
expected value of clinical i.
extraretinal eye position i.
Food and Nutrition I. Center
Freedom of I. Act
fund of i.
health information management
Historical I. Form
HIV/AIDS Treatment Information Service
management information system
medication information leaflet for seniors
i. memory concentration
National Diabetes I. Clearinghouse
National Digestive Diseases I. Clearinghouse
National Health I. Center
National Heart, Lungs, and Blood Institute I. Center
National Kidney and Urological Diseases I. Clearinghouse
National Prevention I. Network
National Women's Health I. Center
no further i.
no information available
no more i.
nuclear medicine information system
optimum information size
Outcomes and Assessment I. Set
i. outflow rate
i. overload testing aid
Patient Care I. System
patient information leaflet
pediatric dosing i.
perception, thought and recognition of i.
permission, limited information, specific suggestions, and intensive therapy
preadmission i.
problem solving i.
i. processing
i. processing in central nervous system
professional information brochure
psychological information, acquisition, processing, and control system
quality information monitoring system
release of i.
retaining new i.
social information system
Social and Prevocational I. Battery
i. storage and retrieval
strict no information in paper
time i.
Toxicology I. Center
Toxicology I. Conversational On-Line Network
Tri-Service Medical I. System
United States Pharmacopeia Drug I.
Utilization I. Service
Vaccine I. Statement
visual information storage
vital health i.
vocabulary, information, block design, and similarities

informational ribonucleic acid

informed
ASPS informed consent form
i. consent
i. decision
i. health care decision
operative informed consent
i. waiver and consent

infraclavicular
i. block
i. region

infracostalis
musculus i.

infracostal margin

infracted bowel

infragenicular popliteal artery

infrahepatic interruption of inferior vena cava

infrahyoid strap

inframammary
i. fold
i. fold incision
i. region

infraorbital
anterior superior alveolar branch of infraorbital nerve
i. block
i. foramen
i. groove
heliotrope infraorbital discoloration
i. incision
i. line
i. margin
i. nerve
i. region
i. suture

infraorbitomeatal line

infrapatellar
i. bursitis
i. contracture syndrome
i. fat pad

infrapopliteal bypass

infrared
automatic infrared optometer
i. camera
i. coagulation of hemorrhoid
i. coagulator
i. emission detection
far i.
Fourier transform infrared spectroscopy
high-resolution infrared imaging
i. light
i. liver scanner
nondispersive infrared analyzer
nondispersive infrared spectrometer
i. photocoagulation

infrared *(continued)*
i. radiation
i. ray
reflection-absorption infrared spectroscopy
i. refractometry
i. spectrophotometry
i. thermographic calorimetry

infrarenal
i. abdominal aortic aneurysm
i. aortic thrombosis
i. node
periaortic infrarenal node

infraspinatus
musculus i.

infraspinous muscle

infrasternalis
angulus i.

infrasternal retraction

infrastructure
critical infrastructure protection

infratemporal approach

infratrochlear
palpebral branch of infratrochlear nerve

infratrochlear nerve

infraumbilical
i. area
i. fold
i. incision

infraumbilically
opened i.

infundibular
i. arterial inversion
ethmoidal infundibular system
myocardial infundibular stenosis
i. nucleus
i. obstruction
i. pouch
i. process
i. pulmonary stenosis
i. septal defect
i. stalk
i. stenosis
i. wedge resection

infundibularis
pars i.

infundibuliform hymen

infundibulopelvic ligament

infundibulum
i. of heart
i. of neurohypophysis
pars i.
tumor of the follicular i.

infused
volume to be i.

infuser
button i.

infusion
adjuvant hepatic arterial infusion chemotherapy
advanced insulin infusion with a control loop
allodonor lymphocyte i.
allogenic bone marrow cell i.
angiotensin I, II infusion test
antibiotic infusion therapy
arginine infusion test
beef heart infusion broth
bone marrow i.
brain heart infusion broth
brain heart infusion agar
computer-assisted continuous i.
computerized pharmacokinetic model-driven drug i.
constant infusion excretory urogram
continuous i.
continuous ambulatory gamma globulin i.
continuous ambulatory i.
continuous extravascular i.
continuous hepatic artery i.
continuous infusion chemotherapy
continuous infusion epidural analgesia
continuous insulin i.
continuous intrathecal baclofen i.
continuous intravenous insulin i.
continuous regional arterial i.
continuous subcutaneous i.
continuous subcutaneous insulin i.
continuous subcutaneous insulin infusion pump
continuous venous i.
controlled release infusion syndrome
donor leukocyte i.
donor lymphocyte i.
drip infusion cholangiography
drip infusion technique
drip infusion valve
drip rate of i.
duodenal peptone i.
dynamic infusion cavernosometry and cavernosography
dynamic infusion pharmacocavemosometry
electronic infusion device
emergency infusion device
extraamniotic saline i.
gelatin infusion medium
glucose-controlled insulin i.
heart i.
heart infusion broth
heat infusion agar
heparinized solution i.
hepatic arterial i.
i. hepatic arteriography
home infusion device
home infusion therapy
hypodermoclysis i.
implantable drug infusion pump
implantable insulin infusion pump
intermittent high-dose i.
intermittent infusion set
intraamniotic saline i.
intraarterial hepatic i.
intraosseous infusion needle
intrathecal drug i.
large-volume parenteral infusion
low-dose continuous i.
multivitamin i.
nerve block i.
neuraxial opioid i.
pain control infusion pump
Pautler infusion cannula
pediatric multivitamin i.
peripheral blood stem cell i.
peripheral indwelling intermediate infusion device
polymyxin, lysozyme, EDTA, and thallous acetate in heart infusion agar
portable insulin infusion pump
portal insulin infusion system
portal vein i.
positive pressure infusion device
postoperative narcotic i.
pressure infusion device
protracted venous i.
i. pump
i. pyelogram
i. pyelographic study
rapid infusion pump
i. rate
regular insulin i.
saline i.
saline and dopamine i.
saline infusion sonography
saline infusion sonohysterography
slow intravenous i.
small volume parenteral i.
standard heparin i.
subcutaneous continuous i.
target-controlled i.
total-dose i.
total dose i.

total infusion period
transcatheter arterial i.
transdermal infusion system
i. urogram
vitreous infusion suction cutter

infusional
hepatic arterial infusional chemotherapy

infusoria killing unit

ingested
orally i.

ingestion
acid i.
acute and chronic alcohol i.
alkali i.
aspirin i.
i. of barium
caustic i.
cocaine package i.
i. of drug
drug i.
ethanol i.
excessive i.
following i.
hormone i.
L-tryptophan i.
oral i.
organophosphate i.
paraquat i.
i. of poisonous substance
i. of potentially poisonous substance
psychedelic drug i.
rapid i.
rapid ingestion of large amounts of food
sudden death due to cocaine i.
i. of toxic agent
i. of toxic drug
water i.

ingress
neutrophil i.

ingressive-egressive sequence

ingrown
i. hair
i. nail
i. positive strain
i. toenail

inguinal
anterior inguinal herniorrhaphy
i. arch
i. area
Bassini inguinal hernia repair
bilateral inguinal hernia
i. canal
i. crease
deep inguinal lymph node
deep inguinal ring
direct inguinal hernia
external inguinal ring
floor of inguinal canal
i. fold
i. fossa
i. hernia
i. hernia repair
i. herniorrhaphy
i. impulse
incarcerated inguinal hernia
i. incision
indirect inguinal hernia
internal inguinal ring
laparoscopic inguinal herniorrhaphy
large inguinal hernia sac
left direct inguinal hernia
left inguinal hernia
left oblique inguinal hernia
i. ligament
i. lymph nodes
medial crus of the superficial inguinal ring
medial inguinal fossa
necrotizing inguinal adenopathy
i. nodes
nontender incarcerated inguinal hernia
i. orchiectomy
ovary in inguinal hernia
pantaloon inguinal hernia
i. reflex
i. region
right direct inguinal hernia
right inguinal hernia
right oblique inguinal hernia
i. ring
shelving border of inguinal ligament
i. sphincter
superficial inguinal lymph node

inguinocrural hernia

inguinofemoral hernia

inguinoproperitoneal hernia

inguinosuperficial hernia

Ingwavuma virus

inhalant
amyl nitrate i.
i. induced hallucination
i. intoxication
nitrite i.
overdosed with i.

inhalation
aerosol inhalation monitor
i. agent
allergen inhalation challenge test
i. analgesia
i. anesthesia
i. anesthetic
i. anthrax
budesonide inhalation suspension
carbachol inhalation challenge
i. challenge
i. chemotherapy treatment
chronic antibiotic i.
i. and expiration
i. fever
i. of foreign body
i. of foreign substance
histamine inhalation test
i. injury
mask inhalation anesthesia
metallic compound i.
methacholine inhalation challenge
methacholine inhalation challenge response
nitrogen dioxide i.
patient treated for smoke i.
i. pneumonia
quantitative inhalation challenge apparatus
respiratory depression inhalation anesthesia
i. solution
steam inhalation therapy
i. test
i. therapist
i. therapy
tobramycin solution for i.
i. tuberculosis

inhalational
alveolar partial pressure of inhalational anesthetic
i. anesthesia
i. anthrax
general inhalational anesthesia
i. lung disease

inhaled
i. bronchodilator
i. corticosteroid
long-acting inhaled beta-agonist
i. nitric oxide
i. nitrous oxide

inhaler
beta agonist i.
breath-actuated i.
dry powder i.
metaproterenol i.
metered-dose i.

inhaler *(continued)*
metered solution i.
pressurized metered-dose i.
steam spray i.

inherent
i. capability
i. density
i. filter
i. mechanism
i. risk
i. strength of myocardial contraction
i. weakness in arterial wall

inheritance
archaic i.
autosomal dominant i.
autosomal recessive i.
maternal i.
matroclinous i.
mendelian i.
Mendelian I. in Man
mitochondrial i.
mode of i.
monofactorial i.
multifactorial i.
oligogenic i.
pattern of i.
X-linked i.

inherited
i. abnormality in brain
autosomally inherited forms of nephrolithiasis
autosomally recessively inherited disease
i. blood factor in MNS blood group
canine inherited ataxia
i. disease
i. disorder
dominantly inherited juvenile optic atrophy
i. epidermal dysplasia
i. giant platelet disorder
i. high cholesterol
i. immunity
i. infertility
maternally inherited diabetes and deafness
maternally inherited myopathy and cardiomyopathy
i. metabolic disorder
i. releasing mechanism

inhibited
atrial inhibited pacemaker
atrial synchronous ventricular inhibited pacing
i. sexual desire
i. sexual excitement

inhibit immune system

inhibiting
i. antibiotic dose
beta-lactamase inhibiting protein
i. factor
G inhibiting protein
growth i.
i. hormone
kallikrein inhibiting unit
liver-enriched inhibiting protein
maximum inhibiting dilution
maximum inhibiting duration
müllerian inhibiting factor
müllerian inhibiting hormone
müllerian inhibiting factor
müllerian inhibiting hormone
müllerian inhibiting substance
self-injurious-behavior inhibiting system

inhibition
agglutination inhibition assay
antisense DNA i.
behavioral inhibition system
cell multiplication i.
colony i.
complement fixation i.
i. constant
direct migration i.
elastase inhibition capacity
enzyme inhibition complex
erythrocyte antibody i.
feedback inhibition factor
fluorescent focus inhibition test
growth i.
Guthrie bacterial inhibition assay
hemadsorption i.
hemagglutinating inhibition antibody
hemagglutination inhibition antibody
hemagglutination inhibition assay
hemagglutination inhibition immunoassay
hemagglutination inhibition morphine test
hemagglutination inhibition titer
hemolysis i.
latex particle agglutination i.
leukocyte adherence inhibition factor
leukocyte migration inhibition assay
leukocyte migration inhibition factor
leukocyte migration inhibition reaction
leukocyte migration inhibition test
macrophage migration i.
macrophage migration inhibition test
mental inhibition level
metabolism inhibition test
migration i.
nephelometric inhibition assay
neuraminidase i.
neutral endopeptidase i.
paradoxic levator i.
particle-enhanced turbidimetric inhibition immunoassay
passive hemagglutination i.
patellar inhibition test
phosphodiesterase III i.
pituitary gonadotropin i.
prepulse i.
proactive i.
rapid fluorescent focus inhibition test
release i.
retroactive i.
rosette i.
rosette inhibition titer
serum trypsin inhibition capacity
tanned red blood cell hemagglutination i.
tetrazolium reduction i.
tissue thromboplastin inhibition test
translational i.

inhibitor
acetylcholinesterase i.
adenylate cyclase i.
aldose reductase i.
alkaline protease i.
$alpha_1$-protease i.
$alpha_1$-proteinase i.
amylase inhibitor activity
angiogenesis i.
angiotensin i.
angiotensin-converting enzyme i.
angiotensin-converting enzyme inhibitor cough
anion transport i.
anti-HIV protease i.
antihuman immunodeficiency virus protease i.
a-2 antiplasmin coagulation i.
antithrombin III coagulation i.
a-2 antitrypsin i.
arachidonic acid cascade i.
aromatase inhibitor testolactone
AT-III coagulation i.

beta-lactamase inhibitor combination
bovine pancreatic trypsin i.
Bowman-Birk i.
bronchial mucous proteinase i.
carbonic anhydrase i.
cell-directed i.
cellular inhibitors of apoptosis
C1 esterase i.
chymotrypsin inhibitor activity
concentrated rust i.
converting enzyme i.
cyclin-dependent kinase i.
cysteine proteinase i.
i. of DNA synthesis
dopamine reuptake i.
endogenous GAD i.
endogenous inhibitor of prostaglandin synthase
enzyme i.
enzyme substrate i.
erythrocyte rosette i.
factor VIII:C i.
factor VIII i.
factor VIII inhibitor bypassing activity
factor VII i.
factor VII, VIII i.
factor XII i.
factor X i.
farnesyltransferase i.
fusion i.
gastric acid i.
glycoprotein crystal growth i.
hepatocyte proliferation i.
human alpha$_1$-proteinase i.
human pancreatic trypsin i.
human seminal plasma i.
killer inhibitor receptors-human leukocyte antigen
Kunitz pancreatic trypsin i.
leukocyte adhesion i.
leukotriene pathway i.
lima bean trypsin i.
lipophilic topoisomerase I i.
lipoprotein-associated coagulation i.
liposomal topoisomerase I i.
lupus erythematosus i.
luteinizing hormone receptor-binding i.
a-2 macroglobulin coagulation i.
mammary-derived growth i.
mast cell i.
matrix metalloproteinase i.
matrix metalloproteinase inhibitor, marimastat
microbial alkaline protease i.
mitotic spindle i.
monoamine oxidase i.
monoamine oxidase B i.
myosin ATPase i.
nerve growth i.
nitric oxide synthase i.
N-methyl-D-aspartate i.
non-ergot long-acting prolactin i.
nonnucleoside reverse transcriptase i.
nonnucleoside RT i.
nonsteroidal aromatase i.
noradrenaline reuptake i.
norepinephrine reuptake i.
nucleoside analog reverse transcriptase i.
nucleoside analog RT i.
nucleoside reverse transcriptase i.
nucleotide reverse transcriptase i.
oocyte maturation i.
oocyte meiotic i.
ovomucoid trypsin i.
pancreatic secretory trypsin i.
pancreatic trypsin i.
peptidomimetic inhibitor complex
periventricular i.
phosphodiesterase type 5 i.
physiologic hyaluronidase i.
plasminogen activator i.
plasminogen activator inhibitor type 1, 2
potato kallikrein i.
prolactin i.
prostaglandin synthetase i.
protease i.
proton pump i.
i. of radical processes
recombinant human tissue factor pathway i.
reverse transcriptase i.
reversible inhibitor of monoamine oxidase-type A
secretory leukocyte protease i.
secretory leukoprotease i.
secretory leukoproteinase i.
selective serotonin reuptake i.
serine protease i.
serotonin noradrenergic reuptake i.
serotonin-norepinephrine reuptake i.
serum inhibitor of streptolysin S
serum trypsin i.
shoulder subluxation i.
soybean trypsin i.
specific clotting factor and i.
specific COX-2 i.
i. substance
target of rapamycin i.
thyroid-stimulating hormone-binding inhibitor antibody
tissue factor pathway i.
tissue inhibitor of metalloproteinase
urinary trypsin i.
vascular endothelial cell growth i.
vasopeptidase i.
volatile corrosion i.
wheat amylase i.

inhibitor-containing minimal medium

inhibitory

i. amino acid
i. anal reflex
i. antigen
central inhibitory state
cloning inhibitory factor
i. concentration
diffuse noxious inhibitory control
i. dose
fractional inhibitory concentration
functional inhibitory concentration
i. ganglion
gastric inhibitory peptide
gastric inhibitory polypeptide
growth hormone inhibitory hormone
histamine inhibitory releasing factor
histoplasma tissue inhibitory factor
i. junction potential
killer cell inhibitory receptor
kinase inhibitory protein
leukemia-associated inhibitory activity
leukemia inhibitory factor
leukocyte inhibitory factor
liver migration inhibitory factor
macrophage migration inhibitory factor
minimal inhibitory dilution
minimal inhibitory dose
minimum inhibitory concentration susceptibility test
müllerian duct inhibitory factor
myeloid leukemia inhibitory factor
myeloid progenitor inhibitory factor
myeloid progenitor inhibitory factor-1

inhibitory *(continued)*
neuronal apoptosis inhibitory protein
nonadrenergic inhibitory response
perineobulbar detrusor inhibitory reflex
i. postsynaptic current
i. postsynaptic potential
proliferation inhibitory factor
i. receptor
rectoanal inhibitory reflex
i. response element
rhythmic inhibitory pattern
rosette inhibitory factor
serum inhibitory activity
serum inhibitory concentration
serum inhibitory factor
serum inhibitory titer
slow inhibitory potential
squamous cell carcinoma inhibitory factor
thyroid-binding inhibitory immunoglobulin
thyrotropin-binding inhibitory immunoglobulin
time above minimum inhibitory concentration
i. transmitter
TSH-binding inhibitory immunoglobulin

in-home
i.-h. caregiver
i.-h. chemotherapy

inhomogeneity
correct for i.
off-axis dose i.

inhomogeneous deposition

Inini virus

initial
i. Apgar score
i. apnea
i. assessment
i. assessment phase
i. attack
i. attack of vertigo
i. baseline level
i. bleed
i. body mass index
i. breathing difficulty
bystander dominates initial dominant
i. cardiac enzyme
i. case assessment
i. cells
i. complaint
i. consonant deletion
constant initial concentration
i. consultation
i. contact
i. crisis
i. cryotherapy
i. diagnosis
i. diagnosis and treatment
i. dosage
i. dose
i. dose period
i. drug screening test
i. dyskinesia
i. evaluation
i. evaluation and treatment
i. examination
i. feeling of euphoria
i. head assessment
i. heart attack
i. hypertension evaluation
i. immune response
i. implant
i. impression
i. infection
i. insomnia
i. interview
i. investigation
law of initial value
left ventricular initial diastolic pressure
i. levels of alcohol intake
i. management
i. manifestation
no middle i.
i. office visit
i. onset
i. opening pressure
i. physical examination
i. planning option
i. prognostic score
i. psychiatric development
i. psychiatric treatment plan
i. reaction
i. resuscitation
right ventricular initial diastolic pressure
i. screening
i. screening examination
i. segment
i. sleep disturbance
i. slope index
slow initial function
i. stage
i. stroke
i. study
i. symptom
i. syphilitic lesion
i. target volume
i. therapy
i. trauma
i. treatment
i. tumor
i. urinalysis
i. urine specimen
vehicle for initial crawling
i. venous shunt
i. visit

initially
patient treated i.
patient treated initially with intravenous fluids

initiate
i. discharge planning
i. heartbeat

initiating
chain i.
difficulty initiating urinary stream
disorders of initiating and maintaining sleep

initiation
erythrocyte initiation factor
eukaryotic initiation factor
i. factor
labor i.
rhythmic i.
Ward I. Scale

Initiative
Children's Vaccine I.
Human Genome I.
Women's Health I.

injectable
long-acting injectable medication
i. medication
sterile injectable solution
sterile injectable suspension

injected
i. dose
posterior pharynx not i.
i. radiation
throat i.
tympanic membrane i.

injecting
i. bone cement
i. drug user

injection
i. of air
alcohol injection of tumor
aspiration and injection of bursa
aspiration and injection of joint
aspiration and injection of tendons
autologous fat i.
bacteriostatic water for i.

bleeding at site of i.
blood patch i.
cervical epidural steroid i.
conjunctival vascular i.
continuous subcutaneous insulin i.
i. of contrast media
direct injection of silicone into breast
direct killing by lethal i.
i. dome
i. drug user
i. of dye
i. electrode catheter
endoscopic India ink i.
endoscopic injection sclerosis
endoscopic injection sclerotherapy
endoscopic injection therapy
epidural steroid i.
fiberoptic injection sclerotherapy
follicle aspiration, sperm injection, and assisted rupture
gamma globulin i.
i. gold probe
intracardiac i.
intracytoplasmic sperm head i.
intramuscular i.
intrathecal anesthesia injection
10% invert sugar in 0.9% sodium chloride saline i.
10% invert sugar injection in water
left ventricular i.
local depot i.
local methotrexate i.
long-term injection sclerotherapy
lumbar epidural steroid i.
lumbar facet i.
lump at site of i.
Medralone I.
mental block i.
Monistat IV I.
M-Prednisol I.
multiple daily i.
multiple daily insulin i.
multiple injection regimen
multiple injection therapy of insulin
multiple vitamin i.
Nebcin I.
needle-free injection system
Neosar I.
original injection site
pain relieving i.
paramagnetic contrast i.
Passport disposable injection system
percutaneous alcohol i.
percutaneous bone marrow i.
percutaneous ethanol i.
percutaneous fine-needle ethanol i.
percutaneous retrogasserian glycerol i.
perinephric air i.
peripheral glycerol i.
periurethral collagen i.
puncture, aspiration, injection, reaspiration
i. of radiopaque material
round spermatid nuclear i.
saline i.
i. scan interval
i. sclerotherapy
short duration, unilateral, neuralgic, conjunctival injection and tearing
single i.
i. site
i. site reaction
specific injection immunotherapy
sterile water for i.
subureteric Teflon i.
subzonal i.
i. therapy
thoracic epidural steroid i.
trace metal elements i.
i. treatment
trigger point i.
ultrasound-guided injection therapy
vocal fold i.
water for i.

injector's

morphine injector's septicemia

injunction

paradoxical i.

injured

brain i.
i. heart muscle
immobilization of injured arm
immobilization of injured leg
left i.
i. on duty

injury

Abbreviated I. Scale
Abbreviated I. Score
Abbreviated I. Score/Injury Severity Score
accidental i.
acquired brain i.
acromioclavicular joint i.
acute alveolar i.
acute central cervical spinal cord i.
acute injury to brain
acute lung i.
acute soft tissue i.
acute spinal cord i.
acute traumatic aortic i.
additional personal injury protection
alcohol-induced gastric i.
Allman acromioclavicular injury classification
ankle inversion i.
anoxic brain i.
antecedent pancreatic i.
anterior abdominal i.
anterior cruciate ligament i.
anterior urethral i.
ASIA impairment scale for classification of spinal cord i.
asphyxial birth i.
asphyxial brain i.
Atasoy-type flap for nail injury repair
avulsion flap i.
axial compression i.
axial loading i.
blunt cardiac i.
blunt carotid i.
blunt injury to heart
bodily i.
bone i.
brachial plexus i.
brachial plexus traction i.
brain i.
brain injury center
brainstem i.
Brief Test of Head I.
cervical cord i.
cervical spine i.
closed head i.
closed soft tissue i.
combined flexion-distraction injury and burst fracture
compression flexion i.
confusion with head i.
contrecoup injury of brain
cribriform plate i.
cruciate ligament i.
crushed chest i.
crush injury renal problem
crush injury syndrome
dashboard knee i.
date of i.
dementia due to traumatic brain i.
de Quervain i.
died of i.'s
diffuse axonal i.

injury *(continued)*
diffuse brain i.
diffuse lung i.
drug-induced hepatic i.
environmental heat i.
evaluate extent of injury or illness
facial nerve i.
i. factor
fighting, injuries, sex, threats, self-defense
flexion-compression spine injury stabilization
flexion injury posterior atlantoaxial arthrodesis
Flint Colon I. Scale
forced flexion i.
growth plate i.
head i.
head injury routine
head injury unit
head and spinal cord i.
hepatic vein i.
hollow viscus i.
hypoxic-ischemic neuronal i.
iatrogenic ureteral i.
illness or i.'s
immobilization of back i.
immobilization of neck i.
immobilization of spinal i.
indirect optic nerve injury syndrome
International Classification of Diseases 9th Ed. I. Severity Score
intraabdominal i.
intracranial i.
irreversible catastrophic brain i.
ischemic reperfusion i.
level of i.
life-threatening brain i.
ligamentous injury grade I–III
liver injury test
low back i.
lumbosacral plexus i.
lunate facet dye punch i.
lung injury score
major deceleration i.
major injury vector
mechanical birth i.
mechanism of i.
medial compartment i.
medication-induced esophageal i.
mesangial immune i.
microwave radiation i.
middle column i.
mild head i.
mild traumatic brain i.
Mini Inventory of Right Brain I.
Mini Inventory of Right Brain I.
minor head i.
Modified I. Severity Score
motor vehicle i.
multiple soft tissue i.'s
muscle crushing i.
needle stick i.
neonatal brain i.
neonatal cold i.
nerve crush i.
New I. Severity Score
nipple discharge from breast i.
no bone i.
nonaccidental i.
nonbattle i.
i. not known
NSAID-induced gastric i.
obstetric brachial plexus i.
obstetric traction i.
occult diaphragmatic i.
old nerve i.
open head i.
optic nerve i.
Organ I. Scaling
osmotic cell i.
osseous cervical spine i.
overuse strain i.
oxidative brain i.
oxidative cell i.
oxidative cellular i.
paint gun i.
parasagittal cerebral i.
parenchymal brain i.
past head i.
patient has whiplash i.
pelvic nerve i.
penetrating brain i.
penetrating craniocerebral i.'s
penetrating renal i.
percutaneous i.
perinatal i.
peripheral nerve i.
personal i.
personal injury collision
personal injury accident
personal injury protection
Philadelphia Head I. Questionnaire
postcardiac injury syndrome
posterior dislocation i.
posterior urethral i.
post-head injury syndrome
postischemic reperfusion i.
pressure gun i.
i. pulmonary edema
reality of i.
repetitive motion i.
repetitive strain i.
repetitive stress i.
root avulsion i.
rotator cuff i.
Scales of Cognitive Ability for Traumatic Brain I.
Scales of Cognitive Ability for Traumatic Brain I.
self-inflicted bodily i.
self-inhibiting behavioral injury device
i. severity index
severity of i.
I. Severity Scale
I. Severity Score
i. site
smoke-induced lung i.
soft tissue compression i.
spinal cord i.
spinal cord injury unit
spinal cord injury without radiographic abnormality
stable cervical spine i.
Standard Nomenclature of Athletic I.'s
steering wheel i.
stress injury stage
subendocardial myocardial i.
The I. Prevention Program
through-and-through avulsion i.
tracheobronchial i.
transfusion-associated lung i.
transfusion-related acute lung i.
Trauma and I. Severity Scores
traumatic birth i.
traumatic brain i.
traumatic burn i.
twisting injury to joint
ulnar artery i.
ventilator-associated lung i.
ventilator-induced lung i.
vertebral artery i.

ink
autoclaved India i.
i. blot test
endoscopic India ink injection
India ink stain

Inkblot
Holtzman Inkblot Technique
Rorschach Inkblot Test

Inkoo virus

inlaid
modified Crawford Campbell inlaid bone-grafting technique

inlay
i. bone graft
cast gold i.
diamond inlay bone graft
gold i.
Libra II crown and i.
Mowrey B i.
sliding inlay bone graft

inlet
anterior sagittal pelvic i.
anteroposterior diameter of pelvic i.
pelvic i.
i. pouch
thoracic i.
transverse i.

innate
i. behavior
i. immunity
i. releasing mechanism

inner
autoimmune inner ear disease
i. canthal distance
i. canthus
i. cell mass
i. child issue
i. cortical blood flow
i. dental epithelium
i. diameter
i. ear
i. ear electronic implantation
i. ear hearing loss
i. ear implant
i. ear infection
i. ear mass
i. enamel epithelium
i. fracture face
i. hair cell
i. half
i. hamstrings
i. heel wedge
low inner quadrant
i. medullary collecting duct
i. membrane
molecular inner layer
nuclear inner layer
i. optic anlage
papilloma, inner canthus
i. plexiform layer
i. table thickness
i. wall

innermost intercostal muscle

innersole
dynamic stabilizing innersole system

innervated
i. antral pouch
modified innervated antral pouch

innervation
area of i.
cholinergic innervation of lung
functional terminal innervation ratio
Hering law-EOM innervation, both eyes
i. of head and neck
prostate gland i.
terminal innervation ratio

innocent heart murmur

innominate
i. aneurysm
anomalous innominate artery compression syndrome
anterior i.
anterior innominate osteotomy
anterior innominate rotation
i. artery
i. artery stenting
i. bone
left innominate vein
i. osteotomy
right innominate artery
right innominate vein
i. vein

innovative psychiatric nursing intervention

inoculated
tissue culture inoculated dose

inoculation
curative i.
cutaneous i.
direct i.
entomological inoculation rate
guinea pig i.
hepatitis i.
intracerebral i.
parenteral i.
periodic i.
physical i.
protective i.
stress i.
i. transmission of viral hepatitis

inoperable
i. bladder malignancy
i. brain tumor
i. esophageal carcinoma
extensive inoperable carcinoma
i. gastric carcinoma
i. hemangioblastoma
i. malignancy
i. metastatic lung cancer
i. ovarian cancer
i. pancreatic cancer
patient totally i.
shrink inoperable tumor
tumor i.

inorganic
i. carbon
i. compound
inosine, pyruvate, and inorganic phosphate
i. orthophosphate
i. phosphate
i. phosphorus
plasma inorganic iodine
i. pyrophosphate

inosine
i. diphosphatase
i. diphosphate
i. 5′-diphosphate
i. 5′-monophosphate
i. monophosphate dehydrogenase
i., oxidized
i., pyruvate, and inorganic phosphate
pyruvate, inosine, glucose phosphate, and adenine
i. triphosphatase
i. triphosphate
i. 5′-triphosphate

inositol triphosphate

inotrope
pulsed inotrope therapy

inotropic
i. agent
i. arrhythmia
i. drug
i. effect
i. medication
negatively i.
nonglycoside inotropic agent
i. state
i. support

inpatient
adolescent inpatient unit
aggressive psychotic i.
I. Behavior Rating Scale
cardiovascular inpatient care unit
i. care
comprehensive inpatient treatment
i. counselor
i. day
i. detoxification
i. dialysis
i. dialysis unit
i. drug treatment
i. exercise center

inpatient *(continued)*
i. facility
General Audit I. Psychiatric Assessment Scale
i. geriatric consultation services
i. hospice unit
i. hospital
mental health i.
I. Multidimensional Psychiatric Scale
i. non-psychiatric medical facilities
Nurses' Observation Scale for I. Evaluation
i. to outpatient transfer
place outpatient in inpatient bed
potential inpatient admission
i. psychiatric care
i. psychiatric consultation
i. psychiatric treatment
Psychotic I. Profile
i. rehabilitation
i. setting
specialty inpatient service
standard inpatient care
i. status
i. surgery
surgical inpatient care
i. treatment
i. treatment facility
i. treatment protocol

input
arterial plasma i.
heat i.
mean input time
net acid i.
i. resistor
i. signal processor

input/output
database input/output control

inquest
mental inquest warrant

inquiry
character education i.
claims inquiry form
functional i.
I. Mode Questionnaire: A Measure of How You Think and Make Decisions
Systematic I.

insane
general paralysis of the i.
general paresis of i.

insanity
adolescent i.
affective i.
alcoholic i.
alternating i.
anticipatory i.
bordering on i.
choreic i.
circular i.
climacteric i.
communicated i.
compound i.
compulsive i.
confusional i.
consecutive i.
cyclic i.
doubting i.
emotional i.
hereditary i.
homicidal i.
homochronous i.
hysteric i.
idiophrenic i.
impulsive i.
manic-depressive i.
moral i.
not guilty by reason of i.
perceptional i.
periodic i.
polyneuritic i.
primary i.
puerperal i.
recurrent i.
senile i.
simultaneous i.
toxic i.

insect
i. bite
dizziness from insect sting
i. sting

insecticide
organochlorine i.
organophosphate i.

insemination
artificial i.
artificial insemination by donor
artificial insemination donor, husband
artificial insemination, homologous
artificial insemination with donor sperm
artificial intravaginal i.
direct intraperitoneal i.
donor i.
homologous artificial i.
intraperitoneal i.
intrauterine insemination catheter
intravaginal i.
sperm-washing insemination method
subzonal i.
therapeutic donor i.

insensate
cold mottled insensate leg

insensible water loss

insensitive
hormone i.
ouabain i.

insensitivity
androgen insensitivity syndrome
complete androgen i.
complete androgen insensitivity syndrome
growth hormone i.
partial androgen i.
partial androgen i.
partial androgen insensitivity syndrome

insert
angled bearing i.
cancellous insert graft
custom-made i.
intramucosal i.
Nicoll cancellous insert graft
package i.
patient package i.
i. radioactive implant

inserted
bronchoscope inserted through vocal cords with ease
cardiac catheter with balloon i.
catheter i.
drain i.
electrodes inserted in cerebral cortex
monitoring lines inserted and positioned
nail inserted into neck and head of femur
percutaneously inserted central line catheter
percutaneously inserted spinal cord electrical stimulation
peripherally inserted catheter line
peripherally inserted central venous catheter
pillow inserted under shoulder
rib spreader i.
scope inserted into trachea with ease
speculum i.
suction tubes i.
tracheostomy tube i.
tube i.

inserter
cerclage wire i.

insertion
Achilles tendon i.
i. activity
aponeurosis of i.
arterial line i.
cannula insertion site
catheter insertion site
cervical insertion of radium
cord i.
depth of i.
direct insertion technique
endovascular graft i.
i. of fixation device
i. of intraocular lens
inverted i.
laser office ventilation of ears with insertion of tubes
low insertion of placenta
medial transplantation of patellar tendon i.
muscle reflected from i.
myringotomy and grommet i.
pars plana Baerveldt tube insertion with vitrectomy
patellar tendon i.
percutaneous catheter i.
percutaneous endoscopic gastrostomy i.
permanent pacemaker i.
i. of polyethylene implant
i. of prosthesis
i. and removal
Rush rod i.
i. sequence
i. site
i. site infection
i. of stent
subzonal i.
Teflon tube i.
thought i.
tympanostomy tube i.
tympanotomy and tube i.

inservice
hospital inservice program

inside
i. bathing solution
bleeding inside skull
i. detail
i. diameter
increased pressure inside the eye
i. radius

inside-out
i.-o. technique
i.-o. vesicle

inside-the-needle catheter

insight
i. into illness
obsessive-compulsive disorder with poor insight type
Schedule for Assessment of I.
I. and Treatment Attitudes Questionnaire

insignificant allergies

insipidus
acquired diabetes i.
central diabetes i.
chronic diabetes i.
congenital nephrogenic diabetes i.
diabetes i.
diabetes insipidus, diabetes mellitus, progressive bilateral optic atrophy, and sensorineural deafness
lithium-induced nephrogenic diabetes i.
nephrogenic diabetes i.
neurogenic diabetes i.
neurohypophysial diabetes i.
peripheral diabetes i.
permanent diabetes i.
supraoptical hypophysial diabetes i.

insole
arch insole pad

insoluble
i. bone gelatin
i. collagen
macromolecular insoluble cold globulin
i. residue

insomnia
i. associated with anxiety
i. associated with depression
autogenic training for i.
breathlessness, insomnia and orthopnea
depression, insomnia and fatigue
drug withdrawal i.
fatal familial i.
fatigue and i.
i. from alcohol
i. from anxiety
i. from caffeine
i. from depression
i. from gonorrhea
group treatment for i.
headache, insomnia, and depression syndrome
i., hyperactivity and decreased appetite
hypnotic relaxation for i.
internal arousal i.
Livingston insomnia scale
management of i.
middle i.
i. and nightmares
pain, fatigue, and i.
i. and paranoia
patient has i.
progressive relaxation for i.
i. related to a known organic factor
i. related to mental disorder
sleep maintenance i.
sleep onset i.

insomniac
chronic i.
paranoid i.
patient i.
sleep patterns of i.

insonation
angle of i.

inspection
medical i.
i., palpation, percussion, and auscultation
visual i.

inspiration
alternate inspiration and expiration of air
bronchodilation following deep i.
duration of i.
i. and expiration
forced i.
pressure in i.
pressure on i.
prolonged deep i.
ratio of inspiration time and total time of breathing cycle
sustained maximal i.
i. time
wheezing on i.

inspiratory
i. capacity
i. center
i. dyspnea
expiratory to inspiratory ratio
i. to expiratory ratio
i. expiratory ratio
fine inspiratory crackle
i. flow cartridge
i. flow rate
i. force
forced inspiratory flow
forced inspiratory oxygen

inspiratory *(continued)*
forced inspiratory spirogram
forced inspiratory vital capacity
forced inspiratory volume
forced inspiratory volume in one second
i. loading
maximal inspiratory flow
maximal inspiratory flow rate
maximal inspiratory force
maximal inspiratory mouth pressure
mean inspiratory flow
medium i.
minimal inspiratory pressure
i. murmur
i. muscle
i. muscles
i. muscle training
negative inspiratory force
partial pressure of inspiratory oxygen
peak inspiratory flow
peak inspiratory flow rate
peak inspiratory ventilator pressure
peak nasal inspiratory flow
peak tidal inspiratory flow
i. phase
i. phase gas
pigment inspiratory factor
i. positive airway pressure
i. rale
ratio of inspiratory time to total cycle time
relative inspiratory effort
i. reserve capacity
i. reserve volume
i. resistance
i. resistance and positive expiratory pressure
i. respiration
i. rhonchi
i. sound
i. spasm
spontaneous peak inspiratory force
i. standstill
i. stridor
sustained maximal inspiratory lung exercise
i. threshold load
tidal inspiratory flow
tidal inspiratory flow at 50% of tidal volume
tidal inspiratory volume
i. time
time to peak inspiratory flow
i. vital capacity
i. wheeze
i. wheezing

inspired
fractional concentration of inspired oxygen
fractional inspired oxygen concentration
fractional percentage of inspired oxygen
fraction of inspired carbon dioxide
fraction of inspired oxygen
i. oxygen tension
i. ventilation
i. vital capacity
volume of inspired gas per minute

inspissated
i. bile syndrome
i. cerumen

inspissation
mucous i.

instability
Andrews anterior instability test
i. of the ankle
anterior shoulder i.
anterolateral-anteromedial rotary i.
anterolateral rotary knee i.
anterolateral rotational i.
anteromedial rotatory i.
atraumatic, multidirectional, bilateral radial i.
atraumatic multidirectional i.
carpal instability dissociation
carpal instability nondissociative
chromosomal i.
collateral ligament i.
complex instability of carpus
detrusor i.
detrusor motor i.
detrusor muscle i.
dorsal intercalated segment i.
dorsiflexed intercalated segment i.
electrical instability of heart
episodic emotional i.
flexion-rotation-drawer knee instability test
immunodeficiency, centromeric instability, facial anomalies syndrome
i. of knee
i. of lumbosacral joint
Mayo carpal instability classification
medial column i.
microsatellite i.
microsatellite instability screening
microsatellite instability testing
midcarpal i.
multidirectional i.
nuclear excision repair i.
pervasive pattern of i.
phasic detrusor i.
rhythmic instability of head and trunk
rhythm instability of head and trunk
rotary ankle i.
temporal instability artifact
volar flexed intercalated segment i.
Western Ontario I. Index

installation
arthroscopic screw i.

instant
i. thin-layer chromatography
i. thin-layer chromatography-silica gel

instantaneous
aortic valve peak instantaneous gradient
i. cardiac death
i. diastolic pressure
i. orthostatic hypotension
peak instantaneous gradient
i. pressure
i. resonance curve

in-stent restenosis

instillation
i. abortion time
i. delivery time
local alcohol instillation effect
methylene blue i.
percutaneous aspiration, instillation of hypertonic saline, respiration

instilled
air bubble instilled in anterior chamber

instinct
aggressive i.
herd i.

instinctive
ipsilateral instinctive grasp reaction

institution
comprehensive health care i.
Correctional I.'s Environment Scale

healthcare i.
mental i.

institutional
i. care
cooperative institutional research program
i. dysentery
I. Functioning Inventory
I. Goals Inventory
i. review board

instruction
aftercare i.
computer-assisted i.
computer-managed i.
first aid i.
home care i.
oral hygiene i.
patient medical i.
patient medication i.
postoperative i.
programmed i.
tooth-brushing i.

instrument
activating adjusting i.
arthroscopic laser i.
attempted passage of i.
back range-of-motion i.
cervical range-of-motion i.
complete change of drapes, gowns and i.'s
contour-facilitating i.
diamond cutting i.
diamond rotary i.
gas sterilized i.
indirect contact with contaminated i.'s
Individual Learning Disabilities Classroom Screening I.
matte black i.
myoma fixation i.
needle, sponge, and instrument count correct times three
needle, sponge, and instrument count correct times two
Newport medical i.
oblique forward-viewing i.
occlusal adjustment i.
optical centering i.
orthopaedic cutting i.
parental bonding i.
Pictorial I. for Children and Adolescents
Preschool Language Assessment I.
Problem-Oriented Screening I. for Teenagers
i. recirculation center
i. retrieval container
Schema Assessment i.
Screening I. for Targeting Educational Risk
socially acceptable monitoring i.
stuttering severity i.
suction biopsy i.
Yasargil neurological i.
Zeiss i.'s

instrumental
i. delivery
i. heart rate responses
i. neutron activation analysis

instrumentation
advanced breast biopsy i.
anterior-posterior fusion with segmental spinal i.
anterior spinal i.
biodegradable fixation i.
cable-hook compression i.
locking hook i.
multiple hook assembly C-D i.
segmental spinal i.

insufficiency
acute adrenal i.
acute aortic i.
acute cardiac i.
acute coronary i.
acute mesenteric vascular i.
acute renal i.
acute respiratory i.
adrenal gland i.
adrenocortical i.
anterior pituitary i.
aortic i.
aortic stenosis and aortic insufficiency murmurs
aortic valve i.
aortic valvular i.
atrial i.
atrioventricular valve i.
basilar artery i.
cardiac i.
cardiovascular i.
cerebrovascular i.
chronic coronary i.
chronic pulmonary insufficiency of prematurity
chronic renal i.
chronic respiratory i.
chronic venous i.
convergence i.
coronary i.
coronary insufficiency syndrome
corpus luteum i.
deep venous i.
energetic dynamic cardiac i.
exocrine pancreatic i.
growth hormone i.
hepatic i.
hypoparathyroidism, adrenal insufficiency, mucocutaneous candidiasis syndrome
left ventricular i.
Leydig cell i.
luteal phase i.
mitral i.
mitral valve i.
moderate renal i.
i. murmur
Neonatal Pulmonary I. Index
nonrheumatic aortic i.
pancreatic exocrine function i.
pancreatic exocrine i.
pancreatic insufficiency syndrome
partial adrenocortical i.
peripheral vascular i.
posttraumatic pulmonary i.
pulmonary insufficiency of the premature
pulmonary insufficiency of prematurity
pulmonic i.
renal i.
sacral insufficiency fracture
severe autonomic i.
severe functional i.
severe pancreatic i.
severe renal i.
severe respiratory i.
tricuspid i.
uteroplacental i.
valvular aortic i.
velopharyngeal i.
venous insufficiency syndrome
venous valvular i.
vertebral basilar i.
vertebrobasilar i.
vertebrobasilar artery i.

insufficient
i. blood flow
i. blood flow to heart
i. blood supply
i. data
i. fluid intake
i. government reimbursements
i. severity of duration
i. signal
i. therapeutic effect

insufflation
i. needle
retroperitoneal gas i.
tracheal gas i.
transtracheal i.

insufflator
carbon dioxide i.

insular
i. cistern
i. gyrus

insulated gate field effect transistor

insulation
urea formaldehyde foam i.

insulin
acute insulin response
advanced insulin infusion with a control loop
alcohol, epilepsy, insulin, overdose, uremia, trauma, infection, psychiatric, stroke
allergy to i.
amount of insulin extractable from pancreas
i. antibody
autoantibodies against i.
i. autoantibody
basal insulin level
beef-pork i.
biosynthetic human i.
i. clearance
i. clearance test
i. coma
i. coma therapy
competitive insulin autoantibodies
concentration of insulin in urine
confusion from insulin shock
continuous insulin delivery system
continuous insulin infusion
continuous intravenous insulin infusion
continuous subcutaneous insulin infusion
continuous subcutaneous insulin infusion pump
continuous subcutaneous insulin injection
conventional insulin therapy
i. convulsive therapy
crystalline i.
crystalline zinc i.
deep shock i.
i. deficiency
i. delivery
i. dialysance
i. dosage
excessive insulin secretion
external insulin pump
fasting insulin resistance index
fibrous i.
first-phase insulin response
gestational diabetes mellitus, insulin controlled, type 1
globulin-bound i.
glucagon-free i.
glucose-controlled insulin infusion
glucose, insulin, and potassium
glucose potassium i.
glucose-stimulated insulin secretion
i. growth factor
i. growth factor-binding protein
growth hormone i.
hirsutism, androgen excess, insulin resistance, acanthosis nigricans syndrome
human i.
human insulin antibodies
human insulin regular
human semisynthetic i.
hyperandrogenism, insulin resistance, and acanthosis nigricans syndrome
i. hypoglycemia test
immunologically detectable i.
immunologically measurable i.
immunoreactive i.
immunoreactive insulin to serum or plasma glucose ratio
implantable insulin infusion pump
i. inhaler
i. injection
intensified conventional insulin therapy
intensive insulin therapy
internal insulin pump
intranasal i.
i. level
low-dose intravenous insulin therapy
low insulin therapy
malfunctioning insulin receptor cells
mechanical insulin pump
monocomponent highly purified pork i.
multidose insulin treatment
multiple daily insulin injection
multiple dosage i.
multiple injection therapy of insulin
nasal spray i.
neutral protamine Hagedorn i.
neutral regular i.
NPH i.
open-loop insulin delivery system
ophthalmic administration of i.
oral administration of i.
partial insulin resistance
i. pen pump
peripheral insulin sensitivity
plasma immunoreactive i.
portable insulin dosage-regulating apparatus
portable insulin infusion pump
portal insulin infusion system
potassium, glucose, and i.
i. preparation
i. production rate
i. promoter factor-1
protamine zinc i.
i. pump
purified porcine i.
purified pork i.
quantitative insulin sensitivity check index
i. radioimmunoassay
rat insulin receptor
i. receptor binding test
i. receptor knockout
i. receptor-related receptor
i. receptor species
regular i.
regular insulin infusion
i. regulation
i. requirement
i. resistance index
i. secretion rate
i. secretory response
i. sensitivity test
serum i.
serum insulin concentration
i. shock therapy
i. shock treatment
sliding scale i.
sliding scale insulin therapy
soluble i.
i. standard
steady-state plasma i.
stimulating insulin resistance
i. stimulation
subcoma insulin treatment
subshock insulin treatment
sulfated i.
suppertime mixed insulin and daytime sulfonylureas
i. therapy
i. tolerance test
undegraded insulin factor
i. variable
i. zinc suspension

insulin-degrading
i.-d. activity
i.-d. enzyme

insulin-dependent
i.-d. diabetes
i.-d. diabetes mellitus
i.-d. diabetic
insulin-independent
i.-i. diabetes
i.-i. diabetes mellitus
insulin-induced
peak acid output i.-i.
i.-i. peak acid output
insulinlike
i. growth factor-1, -2
i. growth factor-binding protein-1–6
i. growth factor-II receptor
nonsuppressible insulinlike activity factor
recombinant human insulinlike growth factor
insulin-like
i.-l. activity
i.-l. growth factor
i.-l. material
insulin-mediated glucose uptake
insulinoma
malignant i.
rat i.
insulinotropic
glucose insulinotropic peptide
insulin-producing cell
insulin-protamine zinc
insulin-reactive immunoglobulin
insulin-releasing polypeptide
insulin-resistance syndrome
insulin-resistant
i.-r. diabetes
i.-r. diabetes, acanthosis nigricans, hypogonadism pigmentary retinopathy, deafness, mental retardation syndrome
i.-r. diabetes mellitus
insult
aortic i.
cardiac i.
occlusive cerebrovascular i.
pathologic i.
perinatal i.
vascular i.
insurability
evidence of i.
insurance
accident i.
assisted health insurance plan
catastrophic health i.
comprehensive health insurance plan
disability i.
disability insurance benefits
family health insurance plan
health i.
health and accident i.
hospital i.
hospital insurance program
i. index
long-term care i.
major medical insurance
mental health insurance benefit
national health i.
no-fault i.
primary private practice i.
supplementary medical i.
Unemployment I. Benefits
insuring
health insuring organization
intact
i. bag of waters
i. bone structure
i. canal wall
i. chest muscles
confrontation fields i.
cranial nerves grossly i.
dressing dry and i.
i. drum
extraocular movements i.
extraocular muscles i.
field of vision i.
i. hymen
i. implant
membrane i.
i. motor skills
i. motor tract
i. movement
mucosal intact laser tonsillar ablation
i. neuron
i. on admission
i. outer rim
painless, small intact blister
i. parathyroid hormone
i. pedicle
peripheral pulses i.
placenta delivered i.
pulmonary atresia with intact ventricular septum
radiation therapy for intact breast
i. rib cage
i. round window
sensory tract i.
skin suture i.
i. spinal cord
i. tissue
i. ventricular septum
i. vision
visual field i.
intake
acceptable daily i.
adequate calorie i.
adequate calories i.
alcohol intake withdrawal
allowable daily i.
alteration in hydration i.
alteration in nutrition i.
i. assessment staff
daily caloric i.
daily permissible i.
daily protein i.
i. data
dietary cholesterol i.
dietary fat i.
dietary protein i.
diminished salt i.
estimated safe and adequate daily dietary i.
excessive alcohol i.
excessive fluid i.
excessive food i.
excessive intake of alcohol
fast food i.
i. of food
inadequate intake of fluids
initial levels of alcohol i.
insufficient fluid i.
i. interview of family
intranasal drug i.
limiting alcohol i.
limit salt i.
i. of liquid
low sodium i.
maximal daily permissible i.
maximal oxygen i.
maximal permitted i.
maximal tolerable daily i.
monitor fluid intake and output
optimum calorie i.
i. and output
output and i.
oxygen i.
poor caloric i.
poor dietary i.
poor oral i.
poor p.o. i.
recommended daily i.
recommended dietary i.
recommended nutrient i.
reduce salt i.
reduce sodium i.
reduction of salt i.
restricting food i.

intake *(continued)*
saturated fat i.
saturated for i.
therapeutic nutritional i.
tolerable daily i.
total fat i.

integral
active integral range of motion
channel-forming integral protein
i. dose
force-time i.
pressure-time i.
systolic velocity integral
time velocity i.
i. traditional Chinese medicine
uterine activity i.

integrate
recognize, empathize, think, hear, integrate, notice, keep

integrated
i. anger management
application-specific integrated circuit
i. approach
I. Assessment System
I. Auricular Reconstruction Protocol
i. bipolar sensing
i. care
I. Child Development Scheme
i. circuit
i. concentration
dynamic integrated stabilization chair
i. electromyogram
i. gastrin response
i. health delivery network
i. ion current
i. isometric tension
I. Light Control
I. Management of Childhood Illness
i. medical services
i. medicine
i. optical density
i. pancreatic polypeptide response
i. psychotherapy
i. reference air-kerma
i. secretory response
i. square error
I. Summary of Safety
i. therapy
i. treatment
i. vector control
i. visual and auditory

integrating regulatory transcription unit

integration
auditory integration thinking
auditory integration training
Beery Developmental Test of Visual-Motor I.
care management i.
Community I. Questionnaire
Functional I. test
large-scale i.
medium-scale i.
nursing care i.
plan-do i.
sensory i.
sensory integration training
sensory motor i.
Sensory I. and Praxis Tests
small-scale i.
Southern California Sensory I. Tests
temporal i.
very large scale i.
visual-motor i.
visual-motor integration test

integrative
central integrative deficit
i. couple therapy
higher integrative function
key integrative social system
i. neurobehavioral approach

integrator
temperature difference i.

integrity
anatomic i.
anterior crus i.
arterial wall i.
cell i.
impaired skin i.
impaired tissue i.
impairment of skin i.
Nerve Integrity Monitor 2
Nicolet Nerve I. Monitor
Organic I. Test
skin i.

intellect
structure of i.

intellectual
i. ability
borderline intellectual functioning
brittle hair, intellectual impairment, decreased fertility, short stature syndrome
i. decline
i. deficiency
i. deficit
i. deterioration
i. development
i. dysfunction
enhanced intellectual efficiency
i. environment
i. evaluation
i. exertion
feeling of intellectual and physical power
i. functioning
i. function or memory
higher intellectual function
i. impairment
interference with intellectual and emotional growth
i. level
i. life
loss of intellectual faculties
i. and motor skills
i. power factor
progressive intellectual and neurological deterioration
slowed intellectual function
i. stimulation
i. stimulus

intellectually
i. conscious
i. stimulated

intelligence
appearance, mood, sensorium, intelligence, and thought process
artificial i.
artificial intelligence in medicine
Cattell Infant I. Scale
coefficient of i.
Culture-Free I. Test
Full-Scale I. Quotient
fund of i.
Hamburg-Wechsler I. Test for Children
Haptic I. Scale
ichthyosis, brittle hair, impaired intelligence, decreased fertility, short stature syndrome
Kahn intelligence test
Naylor-Harwood Adult I. Scale
Non-Reading Intelligence Test, Levels 1-3
Oral Verbal I. Test
Performance I. Quotient
Pictorial Test of I.
i. quotient test
i. ratio
Slosson I. Test
Stanford-Binet Intelligence Test-Form LM

Test of Nonverbal I.
Verbal I. Quotient
Wechsler I. for Adult
Wechsler Adult Intelligence Scale-Third Edition
Wechsler I. for Children Test
Wechsler Preschool and Primary Scale of I.
Wechsler I. Scale

intelligibility
Assessment of I. of Dysarthric Speech
Pediatric Speech I. Test
threshold of i.
Word I. by Picture Identification

intense
i. abandonment fear
anxiety reaction, i.
attack of intense fear
attack of intense terror
i. back pain
i. burning pain
chronic intense envy
i. concentration
i. confrontation
i. coughing
i. cramping
i. cycle of high-dose chemotherapy
i. effect
i. episodic dysphoria
i. euphoria
i. fear of fatness
i. feeling
i. headache pain
i. high
immediate intense need to void
i. inappropriate anger
inappropriate intense anger
i. interpersonal relationship
irritability, restlessness, and intense craving
i. itching
i. levels
i. motor agitation
i. need to void immediate
prolonged chest pain i.
i. psychoactive drug effect
i. pulsed light source
i. relationship
sensation of intense dread
short intense course
short-term anxiety i.
short-term irritability i.
short-term moodiness i.
i. stabbing pain
i. sweating
i. throbbing pain
unstable and intense relationships

intensely
small, intensely fluorescent ganglion

intensified
i. charge-coupled device
i. conventional insulin therapy
i. feeling
i. radiographic imaging system

intensifier
image i.

intensity
absolute dose i.
affect intensity measure
affect intensity problem
i. of contraction
i. difference limen
diminished intensity of movement
dolorimetric unit of pain i.
dose intensity analysis
drug dose i.
i. of electric field
electrosurgical current i.
fluorescent light i.
i. of headache
high beam i.
i. of impulse
i. of labor contractions
i. level
levels of shock i.
linear degenerative signal i.
luminous i.
mean fluorescent i.
microprobe analysis generalized intensity correction
moderate intensity exercise
Multivane I. Modulation Compensator
Numeric Pain I. Scale
i. of pain
pain intensity difference score
peak pain intensity difference score
percentage signal intensity loss
performance i.
performance versus intensity function for phonetically balanced words
point of maximum i.
present pain i.
radiant i.
radiation i.
relative dose i.
i. of roentgen ray
running frequency and i.
signal i.
Skin I. Score
sound i.
summed pain intensity difference
Visual Analogue Self Assessment Scales For Pain I.
Visual Analogue Self Assessment Scales For Pain I.
voice intensity controller

intensity-duration curve

intensity-modulated
i.-m. photon beam
i.-m. proton therapy
i.-m. radiation therapy

intensity/time
intensity/time duration of contractions

intensive
acute intensive treatment
i. antimicrobial therapy
cardiac surgery intensive care unit
cardiology intensive care unit
cardiothoracic intensive care unit
cardiovascular-thoracic intensive care unit
i. care facility
i. care medicine
i. care nursery
i. care, surgical
i. care unit psychosis
i. care ward
i. case management
i. chemotherapy treatment
i. colposcopy
i. combination chemotherapy
i. conventional therapy
i. coronary care unit
coronary intensive care unit
i. diabetes management
i. diabetes treatment
i. dietary therapy
i. exercise
fetal intensive care unit
i. group therapy
Hanover I. Score
infant intensive care unit
i. insight-oriented psychotherapy
i. insulin therapy
medical intensive care unit
medically managed intensive addiction treatment unit
mobile intensive care nurse
mobile intensive care unit
neonatal intensive care unit
neurologic intensive care unit

intensive *(continued)*
neurosurgery intensive care unit
neurosurgical intensive care unit
newborn intensive care unit
i. nursing care
i. observation
i. outpatient treatment program
Parental Stressor Scale: Neonatal I. Care Unit
pediatric intensive care unit
pediatric surgical intensive care
permission, limited information, specific suggestions, and intensive therapy
i. postnatal intervention
i. prenatal care
prenatal intensive care unit
prolonged intensive hyperventilation
psychiatric intensive care unit
pulmonary intensive care unit
regional neonatal intensive care unit
regional perinatal intensive care center
respiratory intensive care unit
respiratory-surgical intensive care unit
i. scientific investigation
i. special care nursery
i. special care unit
spinal intensive care unit
i. stimulation of senses
i. structured hospitalization
i. supportive care
i. supportive programs
surgical intensive therapy
surgical pulmonary intensive care unit
surgical respiratory intensive care unit
i. therapy observation unit
i. thoracic cardiovascular unit
thoracic intensive care unit
i. topical antibiotic therapy
transplant intensive care unit
trauma intensive care unit
i. treatment unit
i. use

intent
i. to control
homicidal i.
palliative i.
suicidal i.
volitional i.

intention
ataxia and intention tremor
delayed primary i.
delayed primary intention healing
healing by first, second, or third i.
healing by primary i.
healing by secondary i.
Health I. Scale
paradoxical i.
posthypoxic intention myoclonus
slight intention tremor
i. spasm
i. tremor of extremity
wound healed by first, second or third i.
wound healed by secondary i.

intentional
i. overdose
i. recall
i. replantation
i. termination of pregnancy
i. tremor
i. vomiting

intention-to-treat analysis

interactance
near-infrared i.

interacting
receptor interacting protein
weakly interacting massive particle

interaction
afferent stimulus i.
cell interaction molecule
child centered i.
chi-square automatic interaction detection
circular interaction between anxiety and pain
clinical interaction and detoxification
clinical and pharmacological i.
Clinical Test of Sensory I. & Balance
drug-drug i.
electron donor-acceptor i.
food-drug i.
hallucinogenic drug i.
herb drug i.
Hill Interaction Matrix
impaired social i.
intracortical interaction mapping
laser tissue i.
life-threatening drug i.
lipoxygenase interaction product
lymphocyte antibody lymphocytolytic i.
mind-body i.
mixed lymphocyte target i.
parent-child interaction evaluation
toxicity or drug i.

interactive
i. exercise
generalized linear interactive model
Swedish interactive thresholding algorithm

interarterial
i. communication
i. fluid
i. septum
i. shunt
i. volume

interarticularis
pars i.

interatrial
closure interatrial septal defect
i. communication
i. groove
i. pressure gradient
i. septal aneurysm
i. septal defect
i. septal defect closure
i. septum
i. shunting

interbody
anterior interbody fusion
anterior lumbar interbody fusion
anterior lumbar spine interbody fusion
anterior lumbar vertebral interbody fusion
posterior lumbar interbody fusion
posterolateral interbody fusion
unilateral posterior lumbar interbody fusion

intercalated
dorsal intercalated segment instability
dorsiflexed intercalated segment instability
volar flexed intercalated segment instability

intercanthal distance

intercarpal
attenuated intercarpal articular cartilage

intercarpal joint

intercavernous
anterior intercavernous sinus

intercellular
i. adhesion molecule-1, -2, -3
i. bridges
i. coupling
i. fluorescence
gap junction intercellular communication
i. junction
lateral intercellular space
obligate intercellular organisms
i. parasite
i. tissue space
i. water

intercept
pressure at slow component i.

interchange
extended binary-coded decimal interchange code

interclavicular
i. notch of occipital bone
i. notch of temporal bone

intercondylar
anterior intercondylar area
anterior intercondylar area of tibia
i. eminence
i. fracture of hip
i. groove
i. notch of femur
i. process

interconnection
neuronal i.

intercostal
i. anesthesia
anterior abdominal cutaneous branch of intercostal nerve
anterior cutaneous branch of intercostal nerve
anterior intercostal artery
anterior intercostal branch of internal thoracic artery
anterior intercostal vein
anterior pectoral cutaneous branch of intercostal nerve
anterolateral intercostal nerve
anterolateral intercostal perforator
anteromedial intercostal nerve
anteromedial intercostal perforator
i. artery
i. block
i. brachial nerve
i. catheter
i. drain
external intercostal muscle
fifth intercostal space
i. flap
i. groove
highest intercostal vein
innermost intercostal muscle
internal intercostal muscle
left intercostal margin
left intercostal space
left superior intercostal vein
i. ligament
i. lymph node
i. margin
medial cutaneous branch of dorsal branch of posterior intercostal artery
i. muscle
i. nerve block
i. nerve blockade
i. nerve cut
i. nerve resected
parasternal intercostal tenderness
pectoral and abdominal anterior cutaneous branch of intercostal nerve
point of maximum impulse fifth intercostal space
i. position for chest lead
posterior intercostal vein
right intercostal margin
right intercostal space
right superior intercostal vein
i. space retraction
sternal intercostal retraction
i. tenderness
i. tube
i. vein of hand
i. vessel ligated
i. zoster

intercourse
age at first i.
i. frequency
homosexual anal i.
involuntary deviate sexual i.
painful sexual i.
sexual i.

intercurrent diagnosis

interdental
i. gingival
i. groove
lingual interdental papilla

interdigestive
gastric interdigestive contraction
i. migrating contraction
i. migrating motor complex
i. motility complex
i. motor complex
i. myoelectric complex

interdigitating
i. cell
i. dendritic cell sarcoma

interdisciplinary
i. approach
i. group
physician directed interdisciplinary care

interest
activity interest and aptitude
apathy and lack of interest in personal goals
area of interest magnification
Campbell I. and Skill Survey
Crowley Occupational I.'s Blank
decline in interest of opposite sex
decreased sexual i.
enhanced interest and concentration
Guilford-Zimmerman I. Inventory
Jackson Vocational I. Survey
Kuder Occupational I. Survey
lack of interest in others
lack of reciprocal i.
Leisure I. Inventory
loss of interest, appetite and concentration
loss of interest in peer social activity
loss of interest in usual activity
loss of interest in personal grooming
loss of sexual i.
Milwaukee Academic I. Inventory
Minnesota Vocational I. Inventory
Occupational I.'s Explorer
Occupational I.'s Surveyor
Ohio Vocational I. Survey
patient's i.
Picture I. Exploration Survey
Reading-Free Vocational I. Inventory
region of i.
Safran Student's I. Inventory
special interest group
Strong Vocational I. Blank
Vocational I. Blank
Vocational I., Experience, and Skill Assessment
Vocational I. Questionnaire
Vocational I. and Sophistication Assessment
work and i.

interface
adjustment interface disorder
common gateway i.

interface *(continued)*
fat-blood i.
long-term bone-instrumentation i.
loss of distinction at gray/white matter i.
Monarch Mini Mask nasal i.
peripheral interface adapter
speech processor i.

interfacetal
unilateral interfacetal dislocation or subluxation

interfascicularis
fasciculus i.

interference
anterograde memory i.
electromagnetic interference/radiofrequency i.
laser interference acuity
noise interference level
Nomarsky interference contrast
preferred frequency speech interference level
proactive i.
reflection interference microscopy
retroactive i.
speech interference level
superconducting quantum interference device susceptometer
i. with intellectual and emotional growth
i. with judgment and decision making

interferenceradiofrequency
electromagnetic interference/radiofrequency interference

interferential
amplitude-summation interferential current therapy
i. current
frequency-difference interferential current therapy
i. stimulation

interfering
defective i.

interferometry
electronic speckle pattern i.

interferon
i. alfa
i. $alpha_1$
i. alpha 2-alpha
alpha interferon therapy
i. beta
consensus i.
gamma i.
human i.
human fibroblast i.
human leukocyte i.
human lymphoblastoid i.
human lymphocyte i.
immune i.
partially pure human leukocyte i.
recombinant human leukocyte interferon A
recombinant interferon alpha
recombinant interferon gamma
i. reference unit
i. regulatory factor-1
i. regulatory factor-2
tissue antagonist of i.
virus-induced i.

interferon-beta
i.-b. 1a
natural human i.-b.

interferon-gamma
natural human i.-g.
nucleocapsid antigen-stimulated i.-g.

interfollicular epidermis

interhemispheric
anterior interhemispheric approach
anterior interhemispheric cistern
anterior interhemispheric fissure
i. approach
arteriovenous interhemispheric angioma
basal interhemispheric approach
i. fissure
i. subarachnoid hemorrhage
i. subdural hematoma

interictal
spontaneous interictal spike

interim
i. glucose determination
i. progress note
i. treatment plan

interincisal
maximum interincisal distance

interior
paries interior orbitae

interlaminar
medial interlaminar nucleus

interleaved
continuous interleaved sampling

interleukin
recombinant human i.
i. regulation of immune system

interleukin-1
i.-1 alpha converting enzyme
i.-1 beta converting enzyme
i.-1 receptor antagonist protein

interleukin-2
p55 component of the high-affinity i.-2
polyethylene glycol-modified i.-2
i.-2 receptor
recombinant human interleukin-2, -3, 11

interleukin-3

interleukin-6
murine i.-6

interleukin-11

interline
Lisfranc articular i.

interlobar
i. artery
i. artery of kidney
i. duct
i. empyema
i. fissure
i. notch
i. pleurisy
i. vein
i. vein of kidney

interlobular
i. artery
i. artery of kidney
i. artery of liver
i. duct
i. emphysema
paucity of interlobular bile ducts
i. pleurisy
i. vein of kidney
i. vein of liver

intermaxillary
i. bone
i. elastic
i. fixation
i. suture

intermediary
fiscal i.
i. hemorrhage
key intermediary protein
i. letter
transcriptional intermediary factor 2

intermediate
anterior intermediate groove
anterior intermediate sulcus
i. bronchus
i. care area
i. care facility
i. care nursery

cartilage intermediate layer protein
i. cell column
i. circumflex artery
i. coronary artery syndrome
i. coronary care unit
i. density lipoprotein
i. dorsal cutaneous nerve
i. dose group
i. dose methotrexate
i. filament
i. filament protein
i. frequency
i. ganglion
i. hemorrhage
high-energy i.
i. host
i. low-density lipoprotein
i. lymphocytic lymphoma
malignant teratoma, i.
i. medical care unit
i. medicine unit
muscular coat of intermediate part of male urethra
muscular layer of intermediate part of male urethra
i. nucleus
nucleus arcuatus of intermediate hypothalamic area
peripheral indwelling intermediate infusion device
i. posterior curve
posterior intermediate curve
i. psychiatry
reactive nitrogen i.
reactive oxygen i.
replicative i.
i. restorative material
i. split-thickness skin graft
surgical intermediate care unit
i. surgical unit
transfer to i.

intermedius

nervus intermedius nerve
vastus i.
ventralis i.

intermenstrual

i. bleeding
i. fever
i. pain
i. spotting

intermetacarpal

i. joint
i. ligament

intermetatarsal

anatomic intermetatarsal angle
i. angle
i. articulation
i. joint

intermittent

i. abdominal pain
acute intermittent porphyria
acute intermittent primary angle-closure glaucoma
i. acute porphyria
i. affective disorder
i. androgen blockade
i. androgen deprivation
i. androgen suppression
i. angioneurotic edema
i. angle-closure glaucoma
i. aortic occlusion
i. assisted ventilation
i. asthma
i. attacks of severe vertigo
i. bladder irrigation
i. bleeding
i. catheterization
i. catheterization of bladder
i. catheterization protocol
i. catheter routine
i. cervical traction
i. cessation
i. chills and fever
chronic intermittent low back pain
chronic intermittent peritoneal dialysis
chronic low intermittent back pain
i. claudication
i. clean catheterization
clean intermittent bladder catheterization
clean intermittent self-catheterization
combined intermittent therapy
i. confusion
i. or continuous spasms
i. contraction
i. contracture
i. coronary sinus occlusion
i. cramps
daily intermittent peritoneal dialysis
i. demand ventilation
i. diarrhea
i. diplopia
i. diuretic therapy
i. double-step gait
i. double vision
i. elevation of blood pressure
i. episode of acute abdominal pain
i. episode of pain
i. esotropia
i. esotropia at near
expiration-synchronized intermittent mandatory ventilation
i. explosive personality disorder
i. facial contracture
i. flash of light
i. flow centrifugation leukapheresis
forced mandatory intermittent ventilation
frontal intermittent rhythmic delta activity
i. functional bowel problem
i. heart pain
i. hematuria
i. hemodialysis
i. hemoptysis
i. heparinization
i. hepatic fever
i. high-dose infusion
high intermittent suction
i. hydrosalpinx
i. hypertropia
i. infusion set
low intermittent wall suction
i. mechanical ventilation
mild intermittent asthma
minimal intermittent dosage of heparin
moderate intermittent suction
i. needle therapy
i. negative pressure-assisted ventilation
neurogenic peripheral intermittent claudication
nightly intermittent peritoneal dialysis
occipital dominant intermittent rhythmic delta activity
i. otorrhea
i. pain
painless intermittent hematuria
i. parasite
i. pelvic traction
i. percussive ventilation
i. periods of depression
i. peritoneal dialysis
i. photic stimulation
i. pigment darkening
i. pneumatic compression boot
i. porphyria
i. positive pressure breathing/inspiratory

intermittent *(continued)*
i. positive pressure inflation with oxygen
i. positive pressure respiration
i. positive pressure ventilation
pressure-controlled intermittent coronary sinus occlusion
psychosis, intermittent hyponatremia, polydipsia syndrome
i. pulse
i. radiation
i. reflux
i. rhythmic delta activity
i. self-catheterization
i. skilled nursing care
i. small bowel obstruction
spontaneous intermittent mandatory ventilation
i. spotting and cramping
i. sterilization
i. strabismus
i. straight catheterization
supervised intermittent ambulatory treatment
synchronized intermittent mandatory ventilation
synchronized nasal intermittent positive-pressure ventilation
i. therapy
i. tonic muscle contractions
i. tremor
i. vomiting

intermuscular
anal intermuscular septum
anterior intermuscular septum
anteromedial intermuscular septum
i. hernia
medial intermuscular septum
i. septum

intern
i. admission note
i. on call

internal
i. abdominal ring
i. absorbed dose
i. acoustic meatus
i. acoustic orifice
i. anal sphincter
anatomical internal os of uterus
i. anatomy
aneurysm of internal carotid artery
anterior intercostal branch of internal thoracic artery
anterior internal cerebellar artery
anterior internal fixation
anterior internal stabilization
anterior internal vertebral vein
anterior limb of internal capsule
anterosuperior internal ilium movement
AO internal fixator
AO spinal internal fixation
aponeurosis of internal oblique muscle
i. arousal insomnia
arteriovenous internal mammary fistula
artificial internal bladder
assisted reduction and internal fixation
i. auditory canal
i. auditory meatus
i. auricular vein
autologous internal jugular vein
automatic internal cardioverter-defibrillator
autopsy internal examination
i. awareness
backward internal rotation
bilateral internal carotid artery occlusion
bilateral internal mammary arteries
i. biliary drainage
i. biliary stent
i. bleeding
i. body heat
i. body temperature
i. borderzone infarct
i. branch of superior laryngeal nerve
i. canthal ligament
i. capsule
i. cardiac massage
i. cardioverter-defibrillator
i. carotid artery flow
i. carotid artery occlusion
i. carotid nerve
i. carotid stenosis
i. cerebral
i. cerebral vein
i. cervical device
i. cervical os
i. change
i. cholecystectomy
i. clock
closed reduction and internal fixation
common internal iliac artery
i. conflict
i. conjugate diameter
i. connection
i. conversion coefficient
i. derangement of knee joint
i. diameter
i. diameter to external diameter
differentiated internal structure
direct vision internal urethrotomy
i. disconnection
i. disorder
i. drainage
i. ear
i. elastica
i. elastic lamina
i. elastic membrane
i. electrode
i. emotional arousal
i. energy
European compression technique bone screw and internal fixation
i. event
expand internal components of knee
i. and external
i. eye pressure
i. factor
i. feeling
i. fetal heart rate monitoring
i. fetal monitoring
i. fetal scalp electrode
i. fistula
i. fixation of fracture
forced passive internal rotation
i. friction
i. hemorrhage
i. hemorrhoid
i. hemorrhoid of rectum
i. hernia
i. hydrocephalus
i. iliac adenopathy
i. iliac artery
i. iliac lymph node
i. iliac vein
i. inguinal ring
i. injury
i. insulin pump
i. integration
i. intercostal muscle
for internal use only
i. jugular catheter
i. jugular pressure
i. jugular vein cannulation
kidney internal splint/stent
knee of internal capsule
left anterior internal diameter
left internal carotid artery
left internal jugular vein
left internal thoracic artery

left internal mammary artery graft
left ventricular internal diameter
left ventricular internal diastolic diameter
left ventricular internal diastolic dimension
left ventricular internal dimension at end systole
left ventricular internal dimension diastole
left ventricular internal dimension systole
i. limiting membrane
male internal genitalia
i. mammary artery bypass
i. mammary artery catheterization
i. mammary artery graft
i. mammary artery implant
i. mammary lymph node
i. mammary lymphoscintigraphy
manual internal examination
marginal tentorial branch of internal carotid artery
i. maxillary artery
i. medial malleolus
mediastinal branch of internal thoracic artery
medical internal radiation dose
i. medicine
meningeal branch of cavernous part of internal carotid artery
meningeal branch of cerebral part of internal carotid artery
molecular internal layer
i. monitor
i. nares
i. node involvement
nuclear internal layer
i. oblique approximated
i. oblique muscle of abdomen
i. obstruction
i. obturator muscle
i. occipital nerve
occlusion of internal carotid artery
odontoid fracture internal fixation
opening of internal acoustic meatus
open reduction and internal fixation
optical internal urethrotomy
i. orifice
orifice of internal acoustic meatus
i. pacemaker
perforating artery of internal mammary
perforating artery of internal thoracic artery
perforating branch of internal thoracic artery
popliteal internal nerve
i. popliteal nerve
posterior limb of the internal capsule
posteroinferior i.
i. psychological conflict
i. pudendal vein
i. radiation therapy
i. reduction
relaxation internal sphincter
i. resistance
i. respiration
responding to internal stimuli
i. ribosome entry site
right internal capsule
right internal jugular vein
right internal mammary anastomosis
right internal mammary artery
right internal thoracic artery
right posterior internal carotid artery
right ventricle internal dimension diastole
right ventricular internal dimension
rigid internal fixation
i. rotation
i. rotation contracture of hip
i. rotation in extension
i. rotation in flexion
i. scar tissue
i. secretion
i. sensation
i. sense
i. shock
single internal mammary artery
i. spermatic fascia
i. spermatic vessel
i. sphincter muscle of anus
i. standard
i. strabismus
superior internal laryngeal nerve
i. surface area
i. tarsorrhaphy
i. telomerase standard
terminal internal carotid artery
i. thoracic artery graft
i. thoracic vein
i. tibial torsion
total hip articular replacement by internal eccentric shells
total internal reflection microscopy
i. transcribed spacer
i. transmission
i. urethral meatus
i. urethral orifice
velocity internal carotid artery
i. version
i. versus external
visual internal urethrotomy
i. visual reference

international

Arthur Adaptation of the Leiter I. Performance Scale
i. benzoate unit
i. calibrated ratio
I. Classification of Diseases
I. Classification of Diseases and Related Health Problems, 10th Edition
I. Classification of Diseases and Causes of Death
I. Classification of Diseases–Clinical Modification
I. Classification of Diseases 9th Ed. Injury Severity Score
I. Classification of Impairments, Disabilities, and Handicaps
I. Federation of Gynecology and Obstetrics classification of tumor staging
I. Index of Erectile Function
Leiter I. Performance Scale
i. milliunit
Mini I. Neuropsychiatric Interview
I. Nonproprietary Name
i. normalized ratio
one-millionth I. Unit
i. opacity unit
I. Pharmacopoeia
I. Prognostic Index
proposed international nonproprietary name
I. Prostate Symptom Score
i. protocol
Provisional I. Standard
recommended international nonproprietary name
I. Reference Preparation
Second I. Standard
I. Sensitivity Index
I. Slope Index
I. Table calorie
I. Unit

international *(continued)*
I. Unit per liter
I. Unit per minute
I. Workshop and Conference on Human Leukocyte Differentiation Antigens

internodal
anterior internodal pathway
anterior internodal tract of Bachmann
i. distance
i. ophthalmoplegia

internuclear
binocular internuclear ophthalmoplegia
i. bridging
i. ophthalmoplegia
wall-eyed bilateral internuclear ophthalmoplegia
wall-eyed monocular internuclear ophthalmoplegia

interocular
average interocular difference

interorbital
bony interorbital distance
medial osseous interorbital distance

interosseous
anterior interosseous artery
anterior interosseous nerve entrapment
anterior interosseous nerve of forearm
anterior interosseous nerve syndrome
anterior interosseous vein
i. artery
i. border of fibula
i. border of radius
i. border of tibia
i. border of ulna
i. cartilage
dorsal interosseous metacarpal vein
dorsal interosseous muscle of foot
dorsal interosseous muscle of hand
dorsal interosseous vein of foot
i. fascia
first digital interosseous muscle
first dorsal i.
i. groove
i. membrane
metatarsal interosseous ligament
microvascular free posterior interosseous flap
i. muscle
i. nerve of leg
oblique cord of interosseous membrane of forearm
palmar branch of anterior interosseous nerve
palmar interosseous artery
palmar interosseous muscle
perforating branch of anterior interosseous artery
plantar interosseous muscle
posterior interosseous artery
posterior interosseous nerve of forearm
posterior interosseous vein
i. talocalcaneal ligament
volar interosseous artery
volar interosseous muscle
volar interosseous nerve

interparoxysmal
migraine with interparoxysmal headache

interpeduncular
anterior recess of interpeduncular fossa
i. cistern
i. ganglion
i. nucleus

interpenetrating polymer network

interpersonal
I. Behavior Survey
I. Cognitive Problem Solving
I. Communication Inventory
i. conflict
i. contact
i. dependence
I. Dependency Inventory
disturbed interpersonal relationships
i. effectiveness
Fundamental I. Relations Orientation-Behavior
Fundamental I. Relations Orientation-Feelings
i. group therapy
history of interpersonal difficulty
impaired interpersonal relations
i. influences
intense interpersonal relationship
i. interaction
i. issue
I. Language Skills and Assessment
Life I. History Enquiry
limited interpersonal skills
other interpersonal problem
I. Perception Scale
i. problem
i. psychotherapy
i. reaction test
i. relations
i. skills
social or interpersonal situation
social interpersonal skills
Survey of I. Values
unstable interpersonal relationship

Inter-Person Perception Test

interphalangeal
i. amputation
i. articulation
i. dislocation
distal interphalangeal joint
hallux metatarsophalangeal interphalangeal scale
i. joint of foot
i. joint of hand
i. keratosis
palmar ligament of interphalangeal joint of hand
proximal interphalangeal/distal interphalangeal joints
terminal i.
i. width

interphalangeal/distal
proximal interphalangeal/distal interphalangeal joints

interpleural
i. analgesia
i. space

interpolation
full scan with interpolation projection

interposed
i. abdominal compression
i. abdominal compressions-cardiopulmonary resuscitation

interposition
antiperistaltic intestinal i.
autogenous cable graft interposition VII-VII neuroanastomosis
hepatodiaphragmatic interposition of colon
jejunal i.
ligament reconstruction with tendon i.

interpositional
alloplastic interpositional implant

autogenous interpositional shoulder arthroplasty

interpositus
anterior interpositus nucleus
nucleus i.

interpotential
mean interpotential interval

interpret
inability to interpret written word

interpretation
Figurative Language I. Test
i. of reality
mirror image i.
i. of reality
severe impairment in interpretation of reality
undisciplined interpretation and suggestion

interpupillary
i. distance
i. line

interrogation
Doppler i.

interrupted
i. aortic arch
i. black silk suture
i. chromic suture
i. cotton suture
evening interrupted suture
i. fashion
i. fine silk suture
i. lymphatic drainage
i. mattress suture
i. plain catgut
i. pledgeted suture
i. respiration
silk interrupted mattress suture
simple interrupted fashion
skin closed with interrupted silk
i. sleep
i. suture
i. tracing
i. urine flow
weak of interrupted urine stream

interrupter
ground-fault i.

interruption
i. of aortic arch
aortic arch i.
bitubal i.
i. of blood supply
i. in continuity of bone
duration of sleep i.
elective interruption of pregnancy
i. of flow of urination
infrahepatic interruption of inferior vena cava
pregnancy interruption service
i. of pregnancy for psychiatric indication
vaginal interruption of pregnancy with dilatation and curettage
voluntary interruption of pregnancy

interscalene
i. approach
i. blockade
i. brachial plexus

interscan
narrow interscan interval

interscapular
i. line
i. region

intersecting
copy intersecting pentagons test

intersegmental
i. muscle
i. range of motion palpation

intersomatic
lumbar intersomatic fusion expandable cage

interspace
narrowing of i.
second left i.
widening of i.

interspersed
long interspersed elements
short interspersed elements

intersphincteric
anal intersphincteric groove
per anum intersphincteric rectal dissection

interspinal
lumbar interspinal muscle

interspinous
bispinous or interspinous diameter
i. ligament
i. segmental spinal instrumentation technique

interstice
graft i.

interstitial
acute allergic interstitial nephritis
i. acute inflammatory cell
acute interstitial pneumonia
acute interstitial pneumonitis
acute interstitial tubular nephritis
allergic interstitial nephritis
i. atrophy
atypical interstitial pneumonia
autoimmune interstitial nephritis
i. brachytherapy
bronchiolitis with interstitial pneumonitis
i. cell
i. cell fluid
i. cells of Cajal
i. cell-stimulating hormone
i. cell tumor
i. change
chronic diffuse interstitial lung disease
chronic interstitial hepatitis
chronic interstitial inflammatory infiltrate
chronic interstitial lung disease
chronic interstitial nephritis
chronic interstitial salpingitis
chronic pulmonary interstitial fibrosis
classic interstitial pneumonitis with fibrosis
i. cleft
colloid osmotic pressure in interstitial fluid
i. congestion
i. cystitis
diffuse interstitial fibrosing pneumonitis
diffuse interstitial fibrosis of the lung
diffuse interstitial hemorrhage
diffuse interstitial lung disease
diffuse interstitial pneumonia
diffuse interstitial pulmonary calcification
diffuse interstitial pulmonary disease
diffuse interstitial pulmonary fibrosis
i. disease
i. duct
early interstitial fibrosis
i. edema
i. emphysema
extensive interstitial fibrosis
i. fat
i. fiber
i. fibrosis
i. fibrotic change
i. fluid
i. fluids and ground substance
i. fluid space
i. fluid volume
foamy interstitial plaque
focal interstitial fibrosis

interstitial *(continued)*
focal interstitial hemorrhage
focal interstitial scarring
focal subpleural interstitial fibrosis
i. gastritis
giant cell interstitial pneumonia
giant cell interstitial pneumonitis
i. gland
i. hemorrhage
i. hernia
i. hypersensitivity pneumonitis
i. hyperthermia
idiopathic interstitial pulmonary fibrosis
i. immaturity of lung
i. implant
i. implantation of radioactive isotope
i. infiltrate
i. inflammation
intrapulmonary interstitial emphysema
i. irradiation
i. keratitis
i. laser ablation of the prostate
i. laser coagulation of the prostate
i. laser photocoagulation
i. left ventricular myocardial fibrosis
lipoid interstitial pneumonitis
luetic interstitial keratitis
i. lung disease
lymphocytic interstitial pneumonia
i. lymphocytic pneumonia
lymphoid interstitial pneumonia
lymphoid interstitial pneumonitis
i. marking
Martinez Universal Perineal I. Template
i. mastitis
mild focal interstitial scarring
multiple interstitial pulmonary hemorrhage
i. myocarditis
necrotizing interstitial keratitis
i. nephritis
nonspecific chronic interstitial pneumonitis
nonspecific interstitial pneumonia-fibrosis
nonulcerative interstitial keratitis
i. nucleus of Cajal
i. organizing pneumonia
i. pancreatitis
patchy interstitial fibrosis
i. pattern
i. and perivascular collagen network
persistent interstitial pulmonary emphysema
plasma cell interstitial pneumonitis
i. pregnancy
progressive hypertrophic interstitial neuropathy
progressive interstitial pulmonary fibrosis
prostatic interstitial fluid
i. pulmonary edema
i. pulmonary emphysema
pulmonary interstitial disorder
pulmonary interstitial fibrosis
i. radiation pneumonitis
i. radiation therapy
i. radiofrequency
i. radiotherapy
renomedullary interstitial cell
respiratory bronchiolitis-associated interstitial lung disease
i. restrictive lung disease
i. scarring
i. substance
i. tabes
testicular interstitial fluid
i. therapy
i. tissue
transperineal interstitial permanent prostate brachytherapy
unusual interstitial pneumonitis
usual interstitial pneumonia
usual interstitial pneumonia of Liebow
usual interstitial pneumonitis
vascular congestion of interstitial vessel
i. water

interstitium
lung i.

intertransverse
anterior cervical intertransverse muscle
medial lumbar intertransverse muscle

intertriginous xanthoma

intertrigo
area of i.
candidal i.
eczema i.
i. labialis
monilial i.

intertrochanteric
i. crest
Dimon-Hughston intertrochanteric osteotomy technique
i. femoral fracture
femoral intertrochanteric fracture
i. fracture
i. line
i. plate
i. region fracture
i. ridge

interval
acromiohumeral i.
anterior atlantodental i.
anterior atlantoodontoid i.
atlantodens i.
background i.
biceps interval lesion
i. blood count
i. chemotherapy
i. clearing
confidence i.
critical coupling i.
defibrillation response i.
disease-free i.
electrocardiographic interval from the beginning of QRS complex to end of the T wave
electrocardiographic time-wave i.
electroencephalogram interval spectrum analysis
filtered atrial rate i.
fixed i.
fixed P-R i.
i. growth
heartrate-corrected OT i.
i. history
idiopathic long Q-T interval syndrome
i. improvement
induction-delivery i.
injection scan i.
isoelectric i.
joint interval histogram
longitudinal interval followup evaluation
mean interpotential i.
minimal time i.
narrow interscan i.
pacemaker escape i.
i. patency rate
i. platelet count
posterior atlantodental i.
preceding preparatory i.
predetermined interval of time
progression-free i.
prolonged QT i.

QKD i.
recurrence-free i.
reference i.
rupture-delivery i.
standard deviation i.
systolic time i.
temperature i.
time i.
time interval between cessation of contraception and conception
time interval between doses
time interval difference
time interval histogram
variable i.

intervening
i. peptide
i. sequence

intervention
acute medical management i.
cognitive behavioral i.
consent to i.
court-ordered obstetrical i.
crisis intervention center
disaster crisis i.
drug intervention program
early intervention in drug abuse
early intervention program
Epidemiology of Diabetes I.'s and Complications
evaluation, prediction, intervention, and control
expected intervention strategy
external i.
family intervention program
follow up intervention for normal development
Fracture I. Trial
i. indicator
innovative psychiatric nursing i.
intensive postnatal i.
Mental Health Early Intervention, Treatment, and Prevention Act of 2000
milieu management i.
Multiple Risk Factor I. Trial
myocardial infarction triage and i.
new approaches to coronary i.
Nursing Care I. Tool
Nursing I.'s Classification
percutaneous coronary i.
point of i.
postmenopausal estrogen/progestin i.
prevention and early i.
primary care i.
rape crisis intervention program
right to refuse i.
safety, monitoring, intervention, length of stay, and evaluation
Screening and Crisis I. Program
special i.
i. strategies
Therapeutic I. Scoring System

interventional
Advanced I. Systems
i. angiography
i. cardiac catheterization
i. cardiology
i. echocardiography
i. pain management
i. procedure
i. radiological technique
i. radiology
i. study
i. therapy

interventricular
anterior interventricular branch of left coronary artery
anterior interventricular groove
anterior interventricular sulcus
apical interventricular septal amplitude
i. artery
i. conduction delay
congenital defect interventricular septum of heart
i. foramen
i. groove
i. heart block
high membranous interventricular septum
ruptured interventricular septum
i. septal defect
i. septal excursion
i. septal motion
i. septal rupture
i. septal thickness
i. septum
i. septum aneurysm
i. sulcus of heart
Swiss cheese interventricular septum
i. veins

intervertebral
anterior intervertebral disc
anulus fibrosus of intervertebral disc
i. body
calcification intervertebral cartilage
i. cartilage
chondritis intervertebral cartilage
crushing of intervertebral disc
i. disc calcification
i. disc compression
i. disc disease
i. disc herniation
i. disc protrusion
i. disc rupture
i. disc space infection
extreme intervertebral disc collapse
i. fibrocartilage
i. foramen
herniated intervertebral disc
i. joint complex
juvenile intervertebral disc calcification
narrowing of intervertebral disc space
i. notch
painful minor intervertebral dysfunction
passive accessory intervertebral movements
passive intervertebral motion
passive physiological intervertebral movements
posterior intervertebral ganglion of head
prolapsed intervertebral disk
protruded intervertebral disk
ruptured intervertebral disc
rupture of intervertebral disc
i. vein
wide intervertebral space

interview
Adolescent Diagnostic I.
Amphetamine I. Rating Scale
Anxiety Disorder I. for Children
autism diagnostic i.
Children's I. for Psychiatric Disorders
Computerized Diagnostic I. for Children and Adolescents
Diagnostic I. for Children and Adolescents-Child Version
Diagnostic I. for Children and Adolescents-Parent Version
Diagnostic I. for Genetic Study
Diagnostic I. Schedule
Health Interview Survey
intake interview of family
Iowa Structured Psychiatric I.
Life Events and Difficulty Schedule I.
Mini International Neuropsychiatric I.
National Institute of Mental Health Diagnostic I. Schedule
psychiatric diagnostic i.

interview *(continued)*
Quality of Life I.
I. Schedule for Children and Adolescents
I. Schedule for Events and Difficulties
semistructured psychiatric i.
Simultaneous I. Technique
sodium amytal i.
structured clinical i.
Structured Clinical I. for DSM
Structured Clinical I. for DSM-IV Dissociative Disorders
structured interview for diagnosis of Alzheimer dementia
structured pain i.
Structured I. of Reported Symptoms
Structured and Scaled I. to Assess Maladjustment
Wing Autistic Disorder I. Checklist

Interview-Revised
Autism Diagnostic I.-R.

intestinal
i. abscess
acute intestinal infection
acute intestinal obstruction
i. adhesion
adynamic intestinal obstruction
i. anastomosis
i. angina
i. angiodysplasia
anterior intestinal portal
i. anthrax
antiperistaltic intestinal interposition
i. atony
i. atresia
i. bacteria
i. biopsy
i. bleeding
i. blockage
i. brush border
i. bypass surgery
i. candidiasis
chronic idiopathic intestinal pseudo-obstruction syndrome
chronic intestinal dysmotility
i. claudication
i. complaint
congenital intestinal aganglionosis
congenital intestinal atresia
constipation from intestinal obstruction
i. content
i. control in functional coitus
diarrhea from intestinal obstruction
i. disease
i. disorder
distal intestinal obstruction syndrome
i. disturbance
i. dyspepsia
i. epithelial cell
excessive intestinal gas
fasting intestinal contents
fasting intestinal flow rate
i. fatty acid-binding protein
fine intestinal needle
i. flora
i. flu
i. fluid
i. gas pattern
i. glycoprotein
gut intestinal cell
hemihypertrophy, intestinal web, preauricular skin tag, and congenital corneal opacity syndrome
i. hernia
i. herniation
human intestinal epithelium
i. hypermotility
idiopathic intestinal pseudo-obstruction
i. infarction
i. infection
i. inflammation
inflammatory intestinal disorder
i. intoxication
i. intoxification
i. ischemia
large intestinal descending colon
i. lining
liver and intestinal transplantation
i. loop
lower intestinal Crohn disease
i. lymphocyte
i. malrotation
massive intestinal bleeding
megalocystis microcolon intestinal hypoperistalsis syndrome
i. mucinous borderline tumor
i. mucosa
i. mucosal mast cell
i. neuronal dysplasia
i. neuropathy
nonocclusive intestinal ischemia
nonsteroidal antiinflammatory drug-induced intestinal stricture
i. obstruction
obstructive intestinal disease
overlying intestinal gas
painful intestinal contraction
i. parasite
i. parasites
partial intestinal obstruction
i. perforation
i. permeability
polyneuropathy, ophthalmoplegia, leukoencephalopathy, and intestinal pseudo-obstruction
i. polyp
porcine intestinal adenomatosis
portal hypertensive intestinal vasculopathy
primary intestinal lymphangiectasia
i. problem
i. pseudo-obstruction
i. queasiness
i. secretion
selective intestinal decontamination
i. serosa
severe intestinal infection
simulated intestinal fluid
small intestinal atresia
small intestinal submucosa
small intestinal wall
i. spasm
spasm of intestinal wall
specialized intestinal metaplasia
stapled intestinal anastomosis
i. stasis
i. stimulant
i. suture
i. tonsil
total small intestinal allotransplantation
i. tract carcinoid
i. tract gas
i. transplantation
i. upset
vasoactive intestinal peptide
vasoactive intestinal peptide-secreting tumor
vasoactive intestinal polypeptide immunoreactivity
vasoactive intestinal polypeptide tumor
i. villus
i. wall
i. wall perforation

intestine
benign polyps of large i.
carcinoid tumor of i.
distal portion of small i.
folds of large i.

human embryonic intestine cell
immunoproliferative small intestine disease
incision into i.
inflammation of i.
longitudinal layer of muscle coat of small i.
malignant histiocytosis of i.
mesentery
mucosa of large i.
mucosal surface of large i.
mucosal surface of small i.
muscular coat of large i.
muscular coat of small i.
muscular layer of large i.
muscular layer of small i.
nonrotation of i.
papillary adenoma of large i.
polyp of large i.
proximal i.
rent of i.
resection of i.
serosa of large i.
small intestine absorption
small intestine as a defense barrier
small intestine bacterial overgrowth
small intestine cancer
small intestine mesentery
small intestine transplant

in-the-canal hearing aid

intima
aortic tunica i.
arterial i.
pia i.

intimacy
Personal Assessment of I. in Relationships
Waring I. Questionnaire

intimal
aortic intimal dehiscence
i. arteriosclerosis
i. deformity
diffuse intimal thickening
i. elastic lamina
i. fibrosis
fibrous intimal thickening
i. flap
i. foamy plaques
i. hyperplasia
i. injury
i. layer
i. medial thickness
mesenchymal intimal cell
pulmonary intimal sarcoma
i. tear
i. thickening

intimidated
guilty, ashamed and i.

intolerance
abnormal intolerance to light
acquired monosaccharide i.
i. of being alone
bloating from lactose i.
i. to certain foods
i. to cold
i. of criticism
i. of defect
diarrhea from lactose i.
fatty food i.
food-chemical i.
formula protein i.
gestational carbohydrate i.
glucose i.
heat intolerance from alcohol
heat intolerance from diuretics
hereditary fructose i.
idiopathic environmental i.
lactose intolerance from antibiotic
lactose intolerance and galactosemia
milk protein i.
pregnancy-induced glucose i.
i. to specific drugs
i. to specific foods
i. and toxicity

intolerant
patient intolerant to aspirin therapy

intonation
melodic intonation therapy

intoxicants
driving under the influence of i.

intoxicated
driving while i.
operating motor vehicle while i.
patient i.
remove intoxicated driver

intoxication
acute alcohol i.
acute cocaine i.
acute intoxication with hallucinogen
acute treatment for acute drug i.
alcohol idiosyncratic i.
alcohol pathological i.
i. amaurosis
amphetamine or similarly acting sympathomimetic i.
cannabis intoxication, with perceptual disturbance
clinical manifestation of acute drug i.
differential diagnosis in acute drug i.
hallucinogenic drug i.
idiosyncratic alcohol i.
lead i.
mad honey i.
narcotic chemical i.
other or unspecified psychoactive substance i.
pathologic alcohol i.
pathologic drug i.
pathologic drug intoxication drug psychosis
self-induced water intoxication and psychosis
subacute treatment of acute drug i.
symptoms of acute drug i.
treatment of acute i.

intoxification
intestinal i.
metal i.

intraabdominal
i. abscess
i. adhesion
i. bleeding
i. carcinoma
i. hemorrhage
i. infection
i. injury
i. mass
i. metastasis
i. pressure
i. sepsis
i. surgery
i. varix
i. viscera

intraalveolar
i. hemorrhage
i. oxygen tension

intraamniotic
i. infection syndrome
i. saline infusion

intraaortic
i. balloon assistance
i. balloon catheter
i. balloon counterpulsation
i. balloon pulsation
i. balloon pump
i. balloon pumping assistance
i. counterpulsation
i. counterpulsation balloon
percutaneous intraaortic balloon counterpulsation

intraarterial
AT-II-induced intraarterial chemotherapy
i. blood pressure
i. catheterization
i. chemotherapy
i. digital subtraction angiogram
i. digital subtraction angiography
i. electrocardiogram
i. hepatic chemotherapy
i. hepatic infusion
i. infusion
i. injection
intraoperative intraarterial fibrinolytic therapy
local intraarterial fibrinolysis
i. secretin
i. thrombolytic therapy
i. vasopressin

intraarticular
comminuted intraarticular fracture
costal intraarticular cartilage

intraarticular cartilage

intraatrial
i. conduction defect
i. electrocardiogram
i. reentrant tachycardia
i. reentry tachycardia

intracapsular
i. cataract extraction
i. cataract extraction with peripheral iridectomy
combined intracapsular cataract extraction
i. fracture
i. incision
i. lens extraction
round pupil intracapsular cataract extraction

intracardiac
automatic intracardiac defibrillator
i. catheter recording
i. echocardiography
i. event
i. injection
i. lead
i. malformation
i. mapping
i. mass
i. medication
i. pacing
i. patch
i. pressure
i. pressure curve
i. shunt
i. thrombus
transthoracic intracardiac monitoring

intracarotid amobarbital procedure

intracaval endovascular ultrasound

intracavitary
i. application
i. brachytherapy
i. cesium therapy
i. container placement
i. gynecologic applicator
i. irradiation
multiplane intracavitary probe
i. pressure electrogram dissociation
i. pressure gradient
i. radiation
i. radiation sources
i. radiation therapy
i. radiotherapy
i. radium

intracavity
low-dose rate intracavity therapy

intracellular
i. activation
i. bacteria
i. binding protein
i. bridges
i. canaliculus
i. digestion
i. fluid volume
fungal intracellular pathogen
i. hydrogen ion concentration
killed intracellular bacteria
i. lipid
i. macroadenoma
i. magnesium test
obligate intracellular parasite
obligate intracellular protozoan
i. organism
i. proteolysis
soluble intracellular adhesion molecule
i. tachyzoite
T-cell-restricted intracellular antigen
i. toxin
i. water

intracerebral
i. aneurysm
atherosclerosis of intracerebral vessels
i. bleeding
delayed traumatic intracerebral hematoma
i. electrode
i. electroencephalogram
i. hematoma
i. hemorrhage
i. hypertension
hypertensive intracerebral hemorrhage
i. inoculation
massive intracerebral bleed
massive intracerebral hemorrhage
primary intracerebral hemorrhage
i. schwannoma
spontaneous intracerebral hemorrhage
i. and subarachnoid hemorrhage
i. tumor
vertebral arteries of intracerebral vessels

intracerebroventricular administration of morphine

intracisternal
human intracisternal A-type particle
i. A particle

intracompartment
solid-state transducer i.

intracorneal lens

intracoronary
i. aspiration thrombectomy
i. radiation therapy
selective intracoronary thrombolysis
i. thrombolysis balloon valvuloplasty
urokinase i.
i. vascular ultrasound

intracorporeal
i. electrohydraulic lithotripsy
heart i.
laparoscopic intracorporeal ultrasonography
laser-induced intracorporeal shock wave lithotripsy
i. laser lithotripsy
vasoactive intracorporeal pharmacotherapy

intracortical interaction mapping

intracranial
i. abnormality
i. abscess
i. anatomy
i. aneurysm clipped
angiographically occult intracranial vascular malformation

anterior circulation intracranial aneurysm
Arana-Iniquez intracranial cyst removal technique
i. arterial aneurysm
arteriosclerotic intracranial aneurysm
i. atherosclerotic disease
benign intracranial hypertension
berry intracranial aneurysm
i. bleeding
i. blood flow
i. blood pressure
i. bruit
i. calcification benign glandular tissue
i. cavity
coiled intracranial aneurysm
i. disease
dissecting intracranial aneurysm
electrical intracranial stimulation
i. electroencephalography
i. epidural pressure
familial intracranial aneurysm
i. ganglion
gyriform intracranial calcification
hemianopia in intracranial neoplasm
i. hemorrhage
high intracranial pressure
i. hypertension
idiopathic intracranial hypertension
increased intracranial pressure
i. injury
i. to intracranial anastomosis
i. lesion
i. mass
i. mass lesion
meningeal branch of intracranial part of vertebral artery
i. metastasis
i. monitor
multiple intracranial aneurysm
i. neoplasm
i. neoplasm headache
i. pressure catheter
i. pressure monitoring
i. pressure monitor in skull
primary intracranial neoplasm
i. reinforcement
relief of intracranial pressure
i. self-stimulation
severe intracranial lesion
i. sinus thrombosis
spontaneous intracranial hypotension
i. stimulation
thrombolysis-related intracranial hemorrhage
traumatic intracranial aneurysm
i. tumor
i. vascular abnormality
i. vascular evaluation
i. vascular malformation
i. vasospasm
i. venous malformation
Warfarin-Aspirin Symptomatic I. Disease

intractable
i. atopic dermatitis
i. bone pain
chronic intractable benign pain
chronic intractable shoulder pain
i. constipation
i. diarrhea of infancy
i. heart failure
i. junctional tachycardia
i. nausea
i. pelvic pain
i. plantar keratosis
i. postpartum hemorrhage
i. seizures
i. shock
i. skin rash

intracutaneous
i. reaction
i. test

intracytoplasmic
i. hyaline inclusion
i. immunoglobulin
i. membrane
i. sperm head injection
i. tuboreticular inclusion

intradermal
i. cancer test
Casoni intradermal test
cerebriform intradermal nevus
i. nevus
i. reaction
i. typhoid and paratyphoid vaccine

intradialytic
i. hypotension
i. parenteral nutrition

intradiscal
i. electrothermal coagulation
i. electrothermal therapy

intraductal
benign intraductal papilloma
i. brachytherapy
i. cancer
i. carcinoma of breast
extensive intraductal carcinoma
extensive intraductal component
noninfiltrating intraductal carcinoma
i. oncocytic papillary neoplasm
i. papillary carcinoma
i. papillary mucinous neoplasm
i. papillary mucinous tumor
i. papillary neoplasm of the pancreas
i. papilloma of breast
i. papillomatosis
i. secretin test
i. ultrasonography
i. ultrasound

intraduodenal stimulation

intradural
i. abscess
i. approach
i. dissection

intraepidermal
melanocytic intraepidermal neoplasia
neutrophilic intraepidermal IgA dermatosis

intraepithelial
anal intraepithelial neoplasia
anal squamous intraepithelial lesion
anogenital squamous intraepithelial neoplasia
i. carcinoma of cervix
i. cell
cervical intraepithelial neoplasia, grade 1–3
conjunctival intraepithelial neoplasia
crypt intraepithelial lymphocyte
i. cyst
i. dyskeratosis syndrome, hereditary benign
endometrial intraepithelial carcinoma
endometrial intraepithelial neoplasia
hereditary benign intraepithelial dyskeratosis
high-grade squamous intraepithelial lesion
laryngeal intraepithelial neoplasia
laser destruction of intraepithelial neoplasia
i. lesion
i. leukocyte
low-grade squamous intraepithelial lesion
i. lymphocyte

intraepithelial *(continued)*
mammary intraepithelial neoplasia
ovarian intraepithelial neoplasia
i. plexus
prostatic intraepithelial neoplasia
squamous intraepithelial cell
squamous intraepithelial lesion
squamous intraepithelial lesion/atypical squamous cell of undetermined significance
vaginal intraepithelial dysplasia
vaginal intraepithelial neoplasm
i. vesicles

intraesophageal
i. balloon distention
i. pH monitoring
i. variceal pressure

intrafallopian
embryo intrafallopian transfer
gamete intrafallopian tube transfer
transcervical intrafallopian tube transfer
transvaginal intrafallopian sperm transfer
zygote intrafallopian transfer

intragastric
i. cannula
i. titration

intrahepatic
i. abscess
i. atresia
benign recurrent intrahepatic cholestasis
i. bile duct
i. biliary calculus
i. cholangiocarcinoma
i. cholestasis
i. cholestasis of pregnancy
i. ductal dilation
i. portal hypertension
i. portal pressure
progressive familial intrahepatic cholestasia
recurrent intrahepatic obstructive jaundice
i. resistance
transjugular intrahepatic portosystemic stent shunt

intralesional
i. chemotherapy
i. laser photocoagulation

intralobar
i. fissure
i. nephrogenic rest

intraluminal
abnormal intraluminal pressure
i. adenocarcinoma
i. duodenal diverticulum
echogenic intraluminal thrombus
i. filling defect
i. gas
i. hemorrhage
i. mass
i. palliation
i. plaque
i. pressure
i. radiation therapy
i. somatostatin
i. stapler
i. stripper
i. typical bronchial carcinoid
i. ultrasound

intramammary
i. abscess
i. distance
i. lymph node

intramarginal
Minsky intramarginal splitting

intramedullary
i. arteriovenous malformation
i. bone graft
i. canal
i. catheter
i. device
elastic stable intramedullary nailing
i. fixation device
flexible intramedullary fixation
flexible intramedullary nail
gradual elongation intramedullary nailing
i. guide
i. hemorrhage
i. lesion
i. metatarsal decompression
i. nail
i. nailing
i. neoplasm
i. pin
i. rod fixation
Rush intramedullary nail
i. skeletal kinetic distractor
i. spinal cord metastasis
i. and spongiosa graft
i. supracondylar

intramembranous
dense intramembranous deposit disease

intramitochondrial
hepatic intramitochondrial crystalloid

intramucosal
i. hemorrhage
i. insert
i. hemorrhage and erosion
i. pH

intramural
i. abscess
aortic intramural hematoma
i. clot
i. duodenal hematoma
i. fibroid
i. hemorrhage
i. invasion
i. left anterior descending artery
i. microvessel density
i. protruding form
spontaneous intramural hematoma of the esophagus
i. thrombosis
i. thrombus
i. tumor

intramuscular
i. administration
i. anesthetic
i. antibiotic
i. artery of lower extremity
i. artery of upper extremity
i. bleeding
i. cocktail
i. compartment pressure
i. gamma globulin
i. immunoglobulin
i. injection
i. medication
occlusion of intramuscular artery
partial pressure of intramuscular carbon dioxide

intramyocardial coronary blood flow

intranasal
i. anesthesia
i. application
i. approach
i. block
cold-attenuated intranasal influenza vaccine
i. drug intake
endoscopic intranasal dacryocystorhinostomy
i. insulin
patient-controlled intranasal analgesia
i. spray
i. steroid

intranuclear
monkey intranuclear inclusion agent
neuronal intranuclear inclusion disease

intraoccipital
anterior intraoccipital joint
anterior intraoccipital synchondrosis
anterior synchondrosis i.

intraocular
anterior chamber intraocular lens
i. biopsy
cataract with intraocular lens
i. contact lens
i. disorder
i. fluid
foldable intraocular lens
i. foreign body
i. hemorrhage
heparin surface-modified intraocular lens
increased intraocular pressure
increased intraocular tension
insertion of intraocular lens
i. leaking wound
i. lens implant
i. lens implantation
i. lens power
i. lymphoma
i. metastasis
modified J-loop intraocular lens
i. muscle
normal intraocular tension
one-piece plate haptic silicone intraocular lens
optics of intraocular lens
posterior chamber intraocular lens
i. pressure
remove and replace intraocular lens
i. retinoblastoma
second stage of decreased intraocular tension
i. site
subcutaneous intraocular node
i. tension recorder
i. toxicity
i. transfer
i. tumor
i. ultrasound

intraoperative
i. arrhythmia
i. assessment
i. atrial ischemia
i. autologous transfusion
i. bleeding
i. blood loss
i. care
i. cholangiogram
i. cholangiography
i. conduction disturbance
i. digital subtraction angiography
i. echocardiography
i. electrical cortical stimulation
electron-beam intraoperative radiation therapy
electron-beam intraoperative radiotherapy
i. electron beam radiotherapy
i. electron beam therapy
i. endoscopic Congo red test
i. endoscopy
i. enteroscopy
i. fentanyl
i. fine-needle aspiration
heated intraoperative intraperitoneal chemotherapy
i. hemodynamics
i. hemorrhage
i. high dose rate
i. intraarterial fibrinolytic therapy
laparoscopic intraoperative ultrasound
i. mapping
i. neurophysiologic monitoring
no intraoperative complications
i. radiation surgery
i. radiation therapy
i. radiotherapy
i. recanalization
i. salvage
i. sonography
i. suture adjustment
i. transesophageal echocardiography
i. ultrasonography
i. ultrasound
i. vascular angiography

intraoral
i. anesthesia
i. cancer
i. cariogenicity test
i. cone for electron beam therapy
i. dental molds
i. device
i. lesion
i. projection
i. stent
i. vertical ramus osteotomy
i. vertical segmental osteotomy
i. wire

intraosseous
i. hemorrhage
i. infusion
i. infusion needle

intraparenchymal
i. cyst
i. hemorrhage
i. resistance

intraparietal sulcus

intrapartum
acute intrapartum fetal distress
i. antibiotic prophylaxis
i. blood loss
ex utero intrapartum tracheloplasty
ex utero intrapartum treatment
i. fetal distress
i. hemorrhage
i. period
selective intrapartum chemoprophylaxis
i. stillbirth
term delivery intrapartum death

intraperitoneal
i. abscess
i. adhesion formation
i. air
i. bleeding
direct intraperitoneal insemination
i. drug administration
exsanguinating intraperitoneal hemorrhage
free intraperitoneal air
i. glucose tolerance test
heated intraoperative intraperitoneal chemotherapy
i. hemorrhage
i. hyperthermic chemotherapy
i. hyperthermic perfusion
i. implant
i. insemination
i. lavage
metabolism in intraperitoneal chemotherapy
i. onlay mesh hernia repair
i. photodynamic therapy
i. pregnancy
i. rupture
i. shock
source of intraperitoneal bleeding
i. transfusion
i. viscus

intrapleural
i. catheter
i. chemotherapy
i. pressure

intrapleural *(continued)*
i. rupture
i. sealed drainage unit

intrapulmonary
i. artery
focal areas of intrapulmonary hemorrhage
focal intrapulmonary hemorrhage
i. hamartoma
i. interstitial emphysema
i. nodal metastases
i. percussive ventilation
i. shunt fraction
i. shunting
i. shunt ratio
i. vein

intrarenal
i. abscess
i. calculus
i. reflux

intraretinal
i. hemorrhage
i. microangiopathy
i. microvascular abnormality
peripheral intraretinal hemorrhage

intraspinal epidural pressure

intrasplenic transplantation

intrastent
i. minimal lumen cross-sectional area
i. recurrent disease
i. restenosis

intrastromal
i. corneal ring segments
laser-assisted intrastromal keratomileusis

intratesticular
i. cyst
i. hemorrhage

intrathecal
i. administration
i. anesthesia injection
i. baclofen
i. block
i. catheter
continuous intrathecal baclofen infusion
i. drug infusion
i. injection
i. therapy
i. *Treponema pallidum* antibody
triple intrathecal therapy

intrathoracic
i. artificial lung
i. blood volume
i. gas volume
i. goiter
mean intrathoracic pressure

intratracheal
i. magnesium
i. oxygen catheter
i. pulmonary ventilation
i. tube

intratrochanteric
femoral intratrochanteric fracture

intratubular
i. germ cell neoplasia, unclassified type
malignant intratubular germ-cell neoplasia

intrauterine
i. adhesion
ascending intrauterine infection
asymmetric intrauterine growth retardation
i. catheter
i. contraceptive device
i. contraction
i. death
i. device
i. dislocation
disseminated intrauterine clotting
i. distress
i. drug exposure
i. echocardiography
endometrial laser intrauterine thermal therapy
i. environment
i. fetal death
i. fetal demise
i. fetal distress
i. fetal growth retardation
i. fetal monitoring
i. fetal transfusion
i. fetus
i. foreign body
i. fracture
full-term intrauterine pregnancy
i. gas
i. gestation
i. gestational sac
i. growth rate
i. growth restriction
i. immunity
i. infection
i. insemination catheter
i. life
i. membrane
normotensive intrauterine growth restriction
i. pneumonia
i. polyp
poor intrauterine fetal growth
i. pregnancy at term
i. pregnancy, delivered
i. pregnancy, term birth, cesarean section
i. pregnancy, term birth, living infant
i. pressure catheter
i. pressure monitor
i. progesterone contraceptive system
i. respiration
term intrauterine pregnancy
total intrauterine volume
i. viral infection

intravaginal
artificial intravaginal insemination
i. cream
i. foam
i. insemination
i. ring
i. sponge
i. suppository

intravascular
adequacy of intravascular volume
i. agent
average intravascular pressure
balloon expandable intravascular stent
i. blood coagulation
i. catheter culture
i. coagulation and fibrinolysis syndrome
i. consumption coagulopathy
i. device infection
diffuse intravascular coagulopathy
disseminated intravascular blood coagulation
disseminated intravascular coagulation
disseminated intravascular coagulation syndrome
disseminated intravascular coagulopathy
i. erythrocyte aggregation
i. fetal air sign
i. fluid
i. foreign body retrieval
i. hydrostatic pressure
i. infection
i. mass
massive intravascular hemolysis
Masson intravascular endothelial proliferation
mean intravascular pressure
normal intravascular pressure

i. oxygenator
i. papillary endothelial hyperplasia
i. red cell aggregation
i. red light therapy
i. sclerosing bronchioloalveolar tumor
i. space
i. stent
i. thrombus
i. ultrasound
i. ultrasound catheter
i. volume expansion

intravenous
i. accurate control device
i. administration of medication
airway, breathing, circulation, intravenous crystalloid
i. alimentation
i. anesthesia
i. anesthetic agent
i. angiography
i. antibiotic
i. antioxidant therapy
arterial-selective intravenous vasodilator
bacterial intravenous protein
i. catheter
i. chemotherapy
i. cholangiogram
i. cholangiography
i. cholecystography
i. cocktail
continuous intravenous insulin infusion
continuous intravenous regional anesthesia
i. contrast material
i. contrast medium
curb intravenous use of drugs
digital intravenous angiography
i. digital subtraction angiography
dilute intravenous Pitocin
i. discontinued
i. diuretic
i. dose
i. drip
i. drug abuse
i. drug use
i. fat emulsion
i. feeding
i. fetal transfusion
i. fluid
i. fluids started
i. fluorescein angiography
i. gamma globulin
i. glucose tolerance test
high-dose intravenous methylprednisolone
i. histamine test
home intravenous antibiotic therapy
i. H2 receptor antagonist
i. hydration
i. hyperalimentation
illegal intravenous drug use
i. immune serum globulin
i. immunoglobulin
infected intravenous drug needle
i. infection site
i. injection
i. intubation
i. leiomyomatosis
limited intravenous pyelogram
i. line infection
i. loading dose
i. lock
low-dose intravenous insulin therapy
i. medication
i. methylprednisolone
i. needle site care
i. nutrition
i. nutritional fluid
i. nutritional therapy
patient treated initially with intravenous fluids
peripheral i.
peripheral intravenous administration
peripheral intravenous catheter
peripheral intravenous hyperalimentation
photoelectronic intravenous angiography
piggyback intravenous fluids
i. Pitocin drip
Pitocin intravenous drip
i. push dose
i. pyelogram
i. pyelography
i. radionuclide venography
rapid-sequence intravenous pyelography
i. regional anesthesia
i. regional sympathetic block
respiratory syncytial virus intravenous immunoglobulin
i. retrograde
i. retrograde access port
i. rider
Rous sarcoma virus immunoglobulin i.
i. sedation
i. sedative
self-controlled intravenous system
sharing infected intravenous drug needle
i. site of infection
slow intravenous drip
slow intravenous infusion
slow intravenous push
i. Soluset
subclavian intravenous line
subcutaneous i.
i. tension
i. therapy
i. tolbutamide tolerance test
total intravenous anesthesia
i. ultrasound catheter
i. urogram
i. urography
i. usage
i. vasopressin

intravenously enhanced computed tomography

intraventricular
i. aberration
accelerated intraventricular rhythm
acute intraventricular hemorrhage
i. bleed
i. catheter
i. conduction block
i. conduction defect
i. conduction delay
i. conduction pattern
i. delay
i. heart block
i. hematoma
i. hemorrhage grade 1–4
i. mass
nonspecific intraventricular conduction defect
i. pressure
preventricular intraventricular hemorrhage
i. septum
i. site
i. tumor

intravertebral foramen

intravesical
i. chemotherapy
i. electromotive drug administration
i. pressure
i. prostatic tissue
i. space

intravitreal
i. blood
i. hemorrhage

intravitreal *(continued)*
i. injection
i. neovascular frond

intrinsic
i. activity
i. factor concentrate
i. flow resistance
i. function
i. heart rate
hog intrinsic factor concentrate
i. muscle of foot
observed intrinsic frequency
optical intrinsic signal imaging
i. positive end-expiratory pressure
rat intrinsic factor concentrate
i. reflex
i. resistance to antibiotic
i. sphincter deficiency
i. sphincter dysfunction
i. stimulating activity
i. sympathomimetic activity

introitus
esophageal i.
marital i.
nonmarital i.
nulliparous i.
parous i.
patulous i.
relaxed i.
i. vaginae
vaginal i.
virginal i.
i. with good support

introversion
social i.

intrusion
alpha wave i.
NREM i.

intrusive
involuntary intrusive memories

intubate
do not i.

intubated
i. continuous positive-pressure
infant i.
patient rapidly i.

intubation
i. of airway
i. anesthesia
catheter-guided endoscopic i.
endobronchial intubation anesthetic technique
endoscopically assisted duodenal i.
endotracheal intubation and mechanical ventilation
esophageal intubation detection
general anesthesia with endotracheal i.
nasal endotracheal i.
nasotracheal i.
nasotracheal intubation anesthesia
oral endotracheal i.
rapid sequence i.
rapid sequence induction orotracheal i.
i. and suction
terminal ileum i.
total time to i.
tracheal intubation fiberscope
translaryngeal i.
i. tube

intussusception
apex of i.
hypoxia, intussusception, brain mass

invaginating
end-to-end i.

invagination
Oesch perforation invagination stripper

invalid chair

invariant
class II invariant chain-derived peptide

invasion
adenocarcinoma with myometrial i.
advanced local i.
benign pheochromocytoma with histological i.
blood vessel i.
i. depth radiography
lymphatic vessel i.
lymphovascular space i.
lymph vessel i.
metastasis, age, completeness of resection, local invasion, and tumor size
occipital condyle i.
perineural i.
seminal vesicle i.
severe invasion streptococcal syndrome
soft tissue i.
vascular i.

invasive
abusive invasive person
active invasive infectious process
i. activity test
i. adenocarcinoma
i. adenoma
i. aspergillosis
i. assessment
i. bacteremia
i. bladder cancer
i. brain surgery
i. breast cancer
i. carcinoma of breast
cardiac invasive procedure
cells consistent with invasive carcinoma
i. cervical cancer
i. cervical carcinoma
cervical invasive neoplasia
circumferential invasive carcinoma
continuous invasive monitoring
i. diagnostic evaluation
i. diagnostic procedure
i. ductal carcinoma
gonorrheal invasive peritonitis
i. growth of blood cell
i. growth of blood vessel
i. infection
i. lesion
i. lobular cancer
i. medical procedure
i. method
minimally invasive biopsy procedure
minimally invasive brain surgery
minimally invasive breast biopsy
minimally invasive cardiac surgery
minimally invasive coronary bypass grafting
minimally invasive direct coronary artery bypass graft
minimally invasive follicular carcinoma
minimally invasive laparoscopic surgery
minimally invasive spine surgery
minimally invasive valve repair
minimally invasive valve replacement surgery
minimally invasive video-assisted parathyroidectomy
i. mole
not invasive break-up time
i. pressure measurement
i. procedure
i. pulmonary aspergillosis
slow-growing invasive adenocarcinoma
slowly growing invasive adenocarcinoma

i. spinal surgery
subperiosteal minimally invasive laser endoscopic facelift
i. surgery
i. surgical staging
i. surgical technique
i. tendency
i. test
i. therapy
i. thymoma
i. thyroiditis
i. treatment
i. tumor
i. vulvar carcinoma
widely invasive follicular carcinoma

inventory

Adapted Sequenced I. of Communication Development
Adaptive Behavior I. for Children
Adult Career Concerns I.
Adult Personal Data I.
Adult Personality I.
alcohol use i.
I. of Anger Communications
Anorexia Nervosa I. for Self-Rating
Anxiety Status I.
Barclay Classroom Climate I.
Barclay Learning Needs Assessment I.
Basic Personality I.
Basic Personality i.
Basic Reading I.
Basic School Skills I.
Battelle Developmental I.
Beck Depression I.
Behavior Status I.
Bem Sex Role I.
Bipolar Psychological I.
Boston Diagnostic I. of Basic Skills
Brief Life History I.
Brief Pain I.
Brief Symptom I.
California Critical Thinking Dispositions I.
California Occupational Preference I.
California Personality I.
California Psychological I.
Career Assessment I.
Career Beliefs I.
Career Maturity I.
Caregiver's School Readiness I.
Caring Relationship I.
Carnegie Interest I.
Carrow Elicited Language I.
Cattell Infant Scale I.
I. of Childhood Memories and Imaginings
Children's Depression I.
Children's Perception of Support I.
Children's I. of Self-Esteem
Child Sexual Behavior I.
communal traumatic experiences i.
communicative development i.
Coping Health I. for Children
Coping Health I. for Parents
Coping Resources I.
Cornell Learning and Study Skills I.
I. for Counseling and Development
Cross-Cultural Adaptability I.
Cultural Attitude I.
Culture-Free Self-Esteem Inventories, Second Edition
defense mechanism i.
depression i.
Depression Status I.
Developmental Activities Screening I.
Diagnostic Mathematics Inventory
Discharge Readiness I.
Dizziness Handicap I.
Driver Risk I.
Dynamic Personality I.
Eating Disorder I.
Edinburgh Handedness I.
Ego State I.
Employee Reliability I.
Environmental Language I.
Environmental Response I.
Experiential World I.
Eyberg Child Behavior I.
Eysenck Personality I.
Family I. of Life Events and Changes
Family I. of Resources for Management
Foods and Moods I.
Freiburger Personality I.
functional assessment i.
I. of Functional Status After Childbirth
Global Severity Index of Brief Symptom I.
Golombok-Rust I. of Marital State
Gordon Personal I.
Gordon Personal Profile I.
Grief Experience I.
Group Styles I.
Guilford-Zimmerman Interest I.
Hall Occupational Orientation I.
Hearing Handicap I. for the Elderly
Heston Personality Inventory Test
Hutchins Behavior I.
Imagined Process I.
Impact Message I.
infertility perceptions i.
Institutional Functioning I.
Institutional Goals I.
Interpersonal Communication I.
Interpersonal Dependency I.
Jackson Personality I.
Jesness I.
Junior Eysenck Personality I.
Lazare-Klerman-Armour Personality Inventory
Learning I. of Kindergarten Experiences
Learning and Study Strategies I.
Leisure Interest I.
Leyton Obsessional I.
Maferr I. of Masculine Values
Marital Dyadic I.
Marriage Adjustment I.
Martin Suicide Depression I.
Maslach Burnout I.
Maudsley Obsessional Compulsive I.
Maudsley Personality I.
Medical I. Management System
Millon Adolescent Clinical I.
Millon Adolescent Personality I.
Millon Behavioral Health I.
Millon Clinical Multiaxial Inventory test
Milwaukee Academic Interest I.
Mini I. of Right Brain Injury
Minnesota Child Development I.
Minnesota Multiphasic Personality Inventory Depression Scale
Minnesota Multiphasic Personality I., Second Edition
Minnesota Teacher Attitude I.
Minnesota Vocational Interest I.
morbid anxiety i.
Multidimensional Fatigue Symptom I.
Multidimensional Pain I.
Multiscore Depression I.
Multivariate Personality I.
Narcissistic Personality I.
Neonatal Facial Pain I.

inventory *(continued)*
neonatal perception i.
Neonatal Withdrawal I.
Neuropsychiatric I.
Nuremberg Aging I.
obsessional compulsive inventory alpha
Obsessive-Compulsive I.
Ohio Work Values I.
Omnibus Personality I.
Oral Language Sentence Imitation Diagnostic I.
Organizational Culture I.
Orientation I.
Ostomy Assessment I.
Ostomy Assessment I.
Pain Appraisal I.
Pair Attraction I.
Parent as a Teacher I.
Partner Relationship I.
Pediatric Evaluation of Disability I.
Pediatric Evaluation of Disability I.
peer conformity i.
Peer Nomination I. for Depression
I. of Perceptual Skills
personality i.
Personality Assessment I.
Personal Orientation I.
Personal Relationship I.
Personal Style I.
Personal Values I.
Premarital Communication I.
Prescriptive Reading I.
Primary Self-Concept I.
Professional Sexual Role I.
Psoriasis Life Stress I.
I. of Psychic and Somatic Complaints in the Elderly
Psychological Screening I.
I. of Psychosocial Development
psychosomatic i.
Quality of Life I.
Quantitative I. of Alcohol Disorders
Racial Perceptions I.
Reading-Free Vocational Interest I.
Reading Miscue I.
Reasons for Living I.
Riley I. of Basic Learning Skills
Riley Preschool Developmental Screening I.
Risk-Taking, Attitude, Values I.
role perception picture i.
Safran Student's Interest I.
Salience I.
School Problem Screening I.
Self-Analysis I.
Self-Concept and Motivation I.
Self-Description I.
Self-Esteem I.
Self-Motivation I.
Self-Perception I.
Self-Rating Obsessive-Compulsive Personality I.
Senoussi Multiphasic Marital I.
Separation Anxiety Symptom I.
Sequenced I. of Language Development
sex i.
Sexual Arousability I.
Sexual Function I. Questionnaire
Shipley Personal I.
Singer-Loomis I. of Personality
Social Behavior Assessment I.
social stress and functionality i.
Spielberger State-Trait Anxiety I.
State-Trait Anger Expression I.
State-Trait Anxiety I.
State-Trait Personality I.
Strong-Campbell Interest I.
Student Adjustment I.
Student Opinion I.
Style of Mind I.
Substance Abuse Subtle Screening I.
I. of Suicide Orientation-30
i. of systems
Teacher School Readiness I.
Temperament and Values I.
Temple University Short Syntax I.
Test Anxiety I.
Urogenital Distress I.
Values I. for Children
Vocational Planning I.
Vocational Preference I.
Wakefield I.
Weinberger Adjustment I.
Westhaven Yale Multidimensional Pain I.
Wittenborn Psychiatric Symptoms I.

inverse
i. Fourier transform
pressure-controlled inverse ratio ventilation
i. treatment planning

inversion
ankle inversion injury
AP inversion stress vagina view
arrhythmia-insensitive flow-sensitive alternating inversion recovery
atrial inversion procedure
i. deformity
fluid attenuated inversion recovery
fluid attenuation inversion recovery
forced inversion film of ankle
infundibular arterial i.
i. instability
Mayo-Fueth inversion procedure
i. position
pressure inversion point
i. range
i. recovery spin-echo sequence
respiratory inversion point
saturation inversion projection
short inversion imaging recovery
short tau inversion recovery
short T1 inversion recovery
i. sprain
i. strain
i. strain x-ray
i. stress test
i. time
T-wave i.

inversus
blepharophimosis, ptosis, epicanthus inversus syndrome
complete situs i.
dextrocardia with situs i.
incomplete situs i.
situs inversus viscerum

invert
high-dose urea in invert sugar
low-dose urea in invert sugar
sodium bicarbonate in invert sugar
10% invert sugar injection in water
i. sugar 10% in saline
10% invert sugar in 0.9% sodium chloride saline injection
i. sugar 5% in water

inverted
cardiac stump i.
i. edge
i. hand position
i. horseshoe flap
i. insertion
i. nipple
i. polypoid hamartoma of rectum
i. radial reflex
i. repeats
i. testis

i. T incision
tonic labyrinthine i.
i. T wave
i. T-wave
i. wave
i. Y and spleen pedicle
i. Y-suspensor

inverted-T
i.-T. appearance
i.-T. fashion
i.-T. incision

inverting
continuous circular inverting suture
continuous inverting suture

investigation
clinical i.
Human I. Committee
intensive scientific i.

investigational
I. Device Exemption
i. drug data form
i. drug data sheet
i. new animal drug

investigator
clinical i.
digoxin investigators group
principal i.

investing
i. fascia
i. layer
i. tissues

investment
aponeurosis of i.
uterine positioning via ligament investment fixation truncation

invisible

involuntary
abnormal involuntary movement disorder
Abnormal I. Movement Scale
i. admission
bladder involuntary contraction
i. body function
i. body movement
i. commitment
i. contraction
court-ordered involuntary outpatient treatment
i. deviate sexual intercourse
i. discharge of feces
i. discharge of urine
i. dribbling of urine
drug-related involuntary movement
i. eye movement
i. facial expression
i. facial pain
i. function
i. general paroxysm
i. guarding
i. hospitalization
i. intrusive memories
irregular involuntary movement
i. jerk
i. jerking movements of legs
i. motor movement
i. motor tic
i. movement disorder
i. movements of chorea
i. muscle contraction
i. muscular contraction
i. muscular movement
i. repetitive movement
i. response
i. rhythmic oscillation
i. smoking
i. spasm of diaphragm
i. sterilization
i. trembling of body
i. trembling of limb
twitches and involuntary movements
i. twitching
verbal involuntary tic
i. verbal tic
voluntary control of involuntary utterances

involuting
angiomatous involuting nevus

involution
lymph node i.

involved
assessing severity: age of patient, systems involved, stage of disease, complications, response to therapy
i. field
fragment of immunoglobulin G involved in antigen binding
left i.

involvement
arcuate fiber i.
axillary lymph node i.
clinical manifestations, etiologic factors, anatomic involvement, pathophysiologic features
corneal epithelial i.
cranial nerve i.
dermal lymphatic i.
ectodermal and mesodermal dysplasia with osseous involvement ectodermal dysplasia-central
extensive metastatic i.
extent of skin i.
extrapyramidal i.
infection or bladder i.
internal node i.
left atrial i.
liver i.
lymphomatous bone marrow i.
lymphovascular i.
metastatic axillary i.
multisite lower genital tract i.
multivalvular i.
nasopharyngeal carcinoma with lymph node i.
nerve root i.
nervous system i.
nodal involvement in breast carcinoma
pagetoid epidermal i.
periaortic lymph i.
peripheral nerve i.
postponing sexual i.
primary node i.
i. in reckless activity
regional lymph i.
right atrial i.
soft tissue i.
survival relative to nodal involvement in breast carcinoma

involving
generalized infection involving fungus

iodide
apical iodide channel
cesium i.
emetine and bismuth i.
hydrogen i.
iodine potassium iodide
potassium iodide, saturated solution
saturated potassium iodide solution
saturated solution of potassium i.
sodium i.
supersaturated potassium i.
thallium-activated sodium iodide crystal

iodinated
i. bovine serum albumin
extravasated iodinated contrast material
i. human serum albumin
i. macroaggregated albumin
nonionic iodinated contrast

iodinated *(continued)*
radioactive iodinated human serum albumin
radioactive iodinated serum albumin
i. rat serum albumin

iodine
absolute iodine uptake
i. azide test
butanol-extractable i.
fetal iodine deficiency disorder
irradiated i.
lithium i.
i. lotion
Lugol iodine solution
Lugol iodine stain
merthiolate, iodine, formaldehyde concentration
merthiolate, iodine, formaldehyde method
merthiolate, iodine, formalin solution
plasma inorganic i.
i. potassium iodide
propidium i.
protein-bound i.
radioactive i.
radioactive iodine uptake
serum precipitable i.
serum protein-bound i.
thyroidal radioactive iodine uptake test
thyroxine i.
i. value

iodine-131
i.-131 therapy
i.-131 total body scan

iodization
universal salt i.

iodoform
bismuth iodoform paraffin
i. gauze
i. gauze packing
naphthalene creosote and i.

ion
argon ion plasma coagulation
i. conductance modulator
divalent ion metabolism
field ion microscopy
fluoride ion positron emission tomography
heavy ion irradiation
helium ion beam
high-energy ion scattering
high-performance ion exchange chromatography
histamine ion transfer
hydrogen i.
hydrogen ion concentration
integrated ion current
intracellular hydrogen ion concentration
i. kinetic energy
low-energy ion scattering
low-friction ion treatment
low potassium i.
mass-analyzed ion kinetic energy
multiple ion detection
phosphate i.
programmable multiple ion monitor
rutherford ion backscattering
secondary ion mass spectroscopy
selected ion flow tube
selected ion monitoring
i. surface scattering

ionic
i. charge number
low ionic strength
low ionic strength solution
i. strength

ionization
acid ionization dissociation constant
acute ionization detector
argon ionization detector
base ionization constant
chemical i.
chemical ionization mass spectrometry
desorption i.
electrohydrodynamic ionization mass spectrometry
electron i.
electron ionization mass spectrometry
electrospray ionization mass spectrometry
i. exposure rate
flame i.
flame ionization detector
matrix-assisted laser desorption and ionization mass spectrometry
multielectrode flame ionization detector
negative logarithm of acid ionization constant
i. potential
resonance ionization mass spectrometry
resonance ionization spectroscopy

ionized calcium

ionizing
biologic effects of ionizing radiation
health effects of ionizing radiation
high-energy ionizing radiation
low-dose of ionizing radiation
i. radiation unit

ionophore
calcium i.
potentiometric ionophore mediated immunoassay

ion-urea
phosphate i.-u.

Iowa
I. Achievement Test
I. Algebra Aptitude Test
I. Pressure Articulation Test
I. Structured Psychiatric Interview
I. Tests of Basic Skills

ipecac syrup

Ippy virus

iproniazid phosphate

ipsilateral
anisocoria with ipsilateral mydriasis
i. antegrade arteriography
i. aspect
i. breast tumor recurrence
i. competing message
i. contraction
i. ear
i. frontal routing of signals
i. head turning
i. hemidiaphragmatic paresis
i. instinctive grasp reaction
lower fossa active, lateral knee pain, and long leg on the side ipsilateral to the weak fossa
i. mentalis muscle
i. optic tectum
i. rhinorrhea
i. stroke
synchronous ipsilateral breast cancer
upper fossa active, medial knee pain, and short leg on the side ipsilateral to the weak fossa

iridectomy
argon laser i.
complete i.
intracapsular cataract extraction with peripheral i.
laser peripheral i.
Noyes iridectomy scissors

peripheral iridectomy operation
superior sector i.
surgical peripheral i.

iridis
ectasia i.
plicae i.
xanthomatosis i.

iridocorneal
angle of i.
i. endothelial syndrome
pectinate ligament of iridocorneal angle

iridocyclitis
Fuchs heterochromic i.

iridoplasty
argon laser peripheral i.

iridotomy
argon laser i.
laser i.
i. scissors

iris
angled iris hook and IOL dialer
angle of i.
anteflexion of i.
arterial circle of greater i.
arterial circle of lesser i.
atrophy of i.
blunt-tip iris scissors
i. ciliary body
closed iris forceps
i. cloudy
i. contraction reflex
craniofacial dysmorphism, absent corpus callosum, iris colobomas, connective tissue dysplasia syndrome
cyst of i.
i. dehiscence
i. diastasis
edema of i.
essential atrophy of i.
i. fixation lens
fold of i.
foreign body in i.
greater ring of i.
i. hamartoma
hemangioma of i.
hemorrhage of i.
i. hernia
herpes zoster of i.
i. hook
horizontal visible iris diameter
hyperemia of i.
implantation cyst of i.
major circulus arteriosus of i.
melanocytic iris tumor
melanoma of i.
minor arterial circle of i.
minor circulus arteriosus of i.
neovascularization of i.
neurogenic iris atrophy
notch of i.
outer border of i.
pectinate ligament of i.
peripheral iris roll
pigmented layer of i.
i. pigment epithelium
i. prolapse
prolapse of i.
protrusion of i.
i. and pupil
i. scissors
i. scraped free
segmental iris atrophy
i. stretching operation
stroma of i.
suture of i.
transfixation of i.
visible iris diameter

iritis
diabetic i.
follicular i.
Fuchs i.
gouty i.
nodular i.
i. papulosa
plastic i.
purulent i.
serous i.
spongy i.
sympathetic i.
tuberculous i.
uratic i.

iron
i. absorption
African iron overload
i. binding
bound serum i.
colloidal i.
i. deficiency anemia
i. deposits
erythroid iron turnover
i. hematoxylin
hepatic iron concentration
hepatic iron index
hepatic iron overload
high-potential iron protein
high serum-bound i.
histologically detectable i.
ineffective iron turnover
i. level
Lillie ferrous iron stain
liver and i.
liver, iron, and B complex
liver, iron, red bone marrow
i. low serum-bound
low serum-bound i.
i. lung
marrow iron turnover
mean plasma iron concentration
i. metabolism disease
monocrystalline iron oxides
oral iron therapy
paramagnetic iron species
parenteral iron dextran
plasma iron disappearance
plasma iron disappearance time
plasma iron turnover rate
polysaccharide iron complex
protein-bound i.
red blood cell iron turnover
red blood cell iron turnover rate
i. saturation level
i. saturation of serum transferrin
serum i.
Similac with i.
i. stain
i. storage disease
i. supplement
i. tolerance test
total i.
transferrin-bound i.
triple sugar iron agar
ultrasmall-particle superparamagnetic iron oxide
i. in urine
i. zone

iron-binding
i.-b. protein
total iron-binding capacity

iron-sufficient, not anemic

irradiance
high irradiance response

irradiated
i. bone
i. ergosterol
i. food
i. iodine
i. medium
i. red blood cell
i. surgical defects
i. victim
i. volume

irradiation
axillary irradiation therapy
biopsy after i.
i. and chemotherapy
convergent beam i.
elective neck i.

irradiation *(continued)*
electron beam scalp i.
endovascular i.
en face irradiation field
external beam i.
external cobalt i.
external irradiation therapy
extracorporeal irradiation of blood
extracorporeal irradiation of lymph
field size in half body i.
fractionated external beam i.
fractionated total body i.
generalized body i.
heavy ion i.
hemibody i.
high-dose external i.
i. injury
local i.
local tumor excision with i.
long wave i.
low-dose involved-field i.
low-dose rate i.
low-dose splenic i.
low-intensity laser i.
low LET external beam i.
minimal irradiation dose
paraaortic node i.
partial brain i.
photon irradiation technique in radiation therapy
i. process
prophylactic brain i.
prophylactic cranial i.
segmental sequential i.
selective lymphoid i.
sequential hemibody irradiation
stereotactic external-beam i.
i. sterilization
subtotal lymphoid i.
subtotal nodal i.
i. and surgery
i. therapy
thoracoabdominal i.
thymic i.
total axial node i.
total lymphoid i.
total lymphoid irradiation for allograft survival
total nodal i.
ultraviolet blood i.
ultraviolet germicidal i.
upper hemibody i.
volume treated in external i.
whole abdominopelvic i.
whole brain i.
whole skull i.

irrational
i. anxiety
i. behavior
i. beliefs
i. obsession with imagined ugliness
patient i.
i. rationality
i. thinking
i. thought
i. thoughts

irreducible
i. dislocation
i. fracture
i. hernia

irregular
i. astigmatism
i. bleeding
i. bone
i. border
i. bowel movements
i. brain function
i. breathing pattern
i. calcification
i. contraction
corneal irregular astigmatism
i. defect
i. disfigured cell
i. dopamine transmission
frontal irregular rhythmic delta activity
i. heart
i. heart action
i. heartbeat rhythm
i. heart rhythm
infiltrating irregular tumor mass
i. interval
i. involuntary movement
i.ly irregular pulse
i.ly irregular rhythm
i. jerky movements
i. menses
i. menstrual cycle
i. menstrual period
i. nystagmus
i. pulse
i. pupil
i. rate
i. rate and rhythm
regularly irregular rhythm
i. respirations
i. rhythm
i. spiking activity in electroencephalography
i. uterine bleeding
i. vaginal bleeding
violent and irregular jerking motion

irregularity
avulsive cortical i.
i. in brain chemistry
i. of pulse
sinus i.
i. of teeth

irregularly
i. irregular pulse
i. irregular rhythm
i. shaped bone

irresectable
carcinoma stage i.

irresistible impulse test

irreversible
i. brain death
i. catastrophic brain injury
i. coma
i. damage to brain cell
i. hereditary disease
i. hydrocolloid
i. loss rate
i. sickle cell

irrigated
anterior chamber irrigated with saline
bladder i.
operative area irrigated with antibiotic solution
operative area irrigated with normal saline
operative site i.
operative site irrigated with antibiotic solution
operative site irrigated with normal saline
pelvis i.
retroperitoneum i.
stoma i.
i. with saline
wound irrigated with normal saline

irrigating
i. and aspirating
contamination from irrigating solutions
i. solution

irrigating/aspirating
McIntyre irrigating/aspirating unit
Pearce coaxial irrigating/aspirating cannula

irrigation
i. and aspiration
bronchoscopy with i.

cold caloric i.
continuous bladder i.
copious antibiotic i.
i. and curettage
curettage and i.
i. and debridement
dilation and i.
i. and drainage
drainage, irrigation, fibrinolytic therapy
extravasation irrigation solution
flossing, brushing, and i.
intermittent bladder i.
nonsterile irrigation technique
pulsed irrigation for enhanced evacuation
salvarsan throat irrigation tube
i. techniques
tracheoscopy with i.
vaginal i.
whole-bowel i.

irrigator
olive-tip i.

irritability
i. and aggressiveness
agitation and i.
i., agitation and restlessness
i. and/or anxiety
anxiety and i.
atrial i.
i. and depression
i., depression and personality changes
disorientation and i.
duodenal i.
emotional i.
gastric outlet i.
hyperactivity and irritability anxiety
inappropriate i.
lapse into heightened i.
i. and mood swings
myotatic i.
nervousness and i.
patient has forgetfulness, irritability, and confusion
persistent i.
reflex i.
i., restlessness, and intense craving
short-term irritability intense
tension i.
i. and tremor
uterine i.

irritable
agitated, irritable and easily annoyed
i. bladder
bloating and irritable bowel syndrome
i. bowel syndrome with constipation
i. colon
i. colon syndrome
depressed or irritable mood
i. duodenal bulb
exhibits irritable negativism
heart i.
i. heart
increasingly i.
i. joint
i. and lightheaded
i. mood
moody, irritable and aggressive
patient i.
patient irritable and jumpy
i. stomach syndrome
i. stricture
i. voiding syndrome

irritant
i. contact dermatitis
mild i.
primary irritant contact dermatitis
i. reaction

irritation
acute nerve i.
acute throat i.
bursts of irritation and anger
constant skin irritation and rubbing
i. fever
gastrointestinal irritation and ulceration
i. of incision site
itching and i.
localized tissue i.
mild skin i.
nerve root i.
primary irritation index
total body i.
transient radicular i.
trigeminal nerve i.
vertebral irritation syndrome

Irvine
I. syndrome
I. viable organ-tissue transport system

ischemia
acute focal cerebral i.
acute myocardial i.
ambulatory ischemia monitoring
anterior wall i.
asymptomatic cardiac i.
Asymptomatic Cardiac I. Pilot
atherosclerosis-induced cavernosal i.
AVF-induced renal i.
cerebral basilar i.
cerebral ischemia steal
chemical indicator of i.
chorionic villus i.
chronic mesenteric i.
clandestine myocardial i.
cold ischemia time
critical limb i.
delayed cerebral i.
diaphragmatic myocardial i.
documented silent i.
donor-related warm i.
exercise-induced silent myocardial i.
hepatic ischemia and reperfusion
hypothermic i.
inferior wall i.
intraoperative atrial i.
lateral wall i.
left ventricular subendocardial myocardial i.
mesenteric i.
i. of myocardium
nonocclusive intestinal i.
nonocclusive mesenteric i.
plantar ischemia test
recurrent mesenteric i.
i. and reperfusion
segmental bronchus i.
silent myocardial i.
skeletal muscle i.
small bowel i.
total cerebral i.
transient brain stem i.
transient cerebral i.
transient episodes of myocardial i.
transient mesenteric i.
uteroplacental i.
vertebrobasilar territory i.

ischemia-guided medical therapy

ischemic
acute ischemic brain infarct
acute ischemic coronary syndrome
acute ischemic heart disease
acute ischemic stroke
i. acute renal failure
anterior ischemic optic neuritis
anterior ischemic optic neuropathy
i. arrhythmia
arteriolar ischemic ulcer

ischemic *(continued)*
arteriosclerotic ischemic optic neuropathy
arteritic anterior ischemic optic neuropathy
atherosclerotic ischemic neuritis
i. bone necrosis
i. bowel
i. brain infarction
i. brainstem infarction
i. burden
i. cardiomyopathy
i. cerebral infarction
cerebral ischemic event
i. cerebrovascular headache
i. change
chronic ischemic colonic lesion caused by phlebosclerosis
chronic ischemic heart disease
i. claudication
cold ischemic time
i. colitis
i. contracture
i. coronary heart disease
crescendo transient ischemic attack
i. damage to heart
delayed ischemic neurologic deficit
i. disease of the growing hip
donor organ ischemic time
early ischemic recurrence
i. event
i. foot
i. gangrene
gangrenous ischemic colitis
gangrenous ischemic enterocolitis
i. heart disease
i. heart failure
i. heart muscle
i. heart wall
i. hypoxia
hypoxic ischemic encephalopathy
i. left ventricle
i. leg disease
i. limb disease
i. mitral regurgitation
i. muscle contracture
i. muscle fiber
i. muscle necrosis
i. muscular atrophy
i. myocardial disease
myocardial ischemic disease
myocardial ischemic syndrome
i. myocardium
i. myopathy
i. necrosis of bone
i. necrosis of femoral head
nonarteritic anterior ischemic optic neuropathy
i. ocular inflammation
i. optic neuropathy
i. paralysis
i. paralysis and contracture
i. pattern
i. pericarditis
posterior ischemic optic neuropathy
i. preconditioning
i. pressure necrosis
prolonged reversible ischemic neurologic deficit
i. reflex
i. reperfusion injury
resolving ischemic neurologic deficit
i. rest angina
reversible ischemic attack
reversible ischemic neurologic deficit
reversible ischemic neurologic disability
i. score
silent ischemic brain damage
silent ischemic heart disease
i. skeletal muscle
i. stroke
i. sudden death
sudden death ischemic heart disease
i. sylvian wave
i. threshold
i. thrombotic cerebrovascular disease
i. time
i. tissue
i. tissue reperfusion
transient cerebral ischemic episode
transient ischemic attack and aging
transient ischemic attack, incomplete recovery
transient ischemic dilation
transient ischemic event
i. vascular disease

ischia
transverse diameter between i.

ischial
between ischial tuberosities
i. bone
i. brace
i. bursitis
i. ramus
i. spine
i. tuberosity
i. weight bearing leg brace
i. weightbearing prosthesis

ischiorectal
anterior recess of ischiorectal fossa
incision and drainage of ischiorectal abscess

ischium
ascending ramus of i.

island
antegrade island flap
artery island flap
Carey Island virus
erythroblastic i.
Great I. virus
life i.
Margarita Island type ectodermal dysplasia
myoepithelial cell i.
i. of Reil
reverse flow island flap
reverse forearm island flap
Rhode I. Pupil Identification Scale
vascularized double-sided preputial island flap and W flap glanuloplasty hypospadias repair

Isles
British Isles Lupus Assessment Group index

islet
alpha islet cell neoplasm
i. amyloid polypeptide
i. cell antigen
i. cell carcinoma
i. cell of pancreas
i. cell surface antibody
i. cell transplant
isolated pancreatic islet transplantation
malignant islet cell tumor
multicentric islet cell adenoma
pancreatic islet adenomatosis
pancreatic islet beta cell
pancreatic islet cell-specific enhancer sequence
pancreatic islet cell transplantation
pancreatic islet cell tumor

islets
i. of Langerhans
pancreatic i.

isobutyric acid

isocapnic
i. hyperventilation
i. hyperventilation with cold air
i. hyperventilation with room air

isocenter
linear accelerator isocenter motion

isocitrate
i. dehydrogenase
i. lyase
serum isocitrate dehydrogenase

isoelectric
i. focusing electrophoresis
i. focusing electrophoresis in polyacrylamide gel
i. focusing in polyacrylamide
i. interval
i. point
polyacrylamide gel isoelectric focusing

isoenzyme
alkaline phosphatase i.
alkaline phosphatase isoenzyme tumor marker
creatine kinase-BB i.
creatine kinase isoenzyme electrophoresis
creatine phosphokinase i.
lactate dehydrogenase i.
M and B isoenzyme of creatine kinase
muscle-brain isoenzyme of creative kinase
myocardial muscle creatine kinase i.

Isoflow
volume of I.

isoform
melanocortin receptor i.
prion protein normal i.

isohemagglutinin
anti-A i.
anti-B i.

isoimmunization
antepartum Rh i.

isolate
clinical isolates of bacteria
cluster of i.'s
nonsyncytia-forming i.

isolated
acute isolated myocarditis
i. angiitis of central nervous system
i. angiitis of the CNS
artery i.
i. asymmetric septal hypertrophy
ataxia with isolated vitamin E deficiency
i. brain
i. burst
i. cardiovascular malformation
clinically isolated syndrome
i. conduction defect
i. congenital folate malabsorption
i. cortical tubule
i. diffuse mesangial sclerosis
emotionally i.
i. episode
i. event
i. explosive disorder
familial isolated hypoparathyroidism
familial isolated primary hyperparathyroidism
i. flash of light
i. follicle-stimulating hormone deficiency syndrome
i. gastric varices type 1, 2
i. gland carcinoma in situ
i. gonadotropin deficiency
i. grand mal seizure
i. growth hormone deficiency
i. growth hormone deficiency type IB, II, III
i. heat perfusion
i. hepatic portal and arterial perfusion
highly addictive and i.
i. human growth deficiency
hyperthermic isolated limb perfusion
i. hyperthermic limb perfusion
i. hypogonadotropic hypogonadism
i. infusion
i. lactase deficiency
i. low high-density lipoprotein
muscles isolated and tagged
i. noncompaction of the ventricular myocardium
not i.
organ i.
organism isolated after 48 hours
organism isolated after 72 hours
i. pancreatic islet transplantation
i. pancreatitis
i. parietal endocarditis
patient feels i.
i. pelvic perfusion
i. perfused rabbit lung
i. perfused rat liver
i. phobia
i. postchallenge hyperglycemia
i. premature beat
i. proteinuria
socially i.
i. spike transients
superior pulmonary vein i.
syndrome of isolated diastolic dysfunction
i. systolic hypertension
i. thyroid-stimulating hormone deficiency
i. ultrafiltration
i. units
i. ventricular noncompaction
viruses isolated from patients
i. volume responder

isolation
alcoholism in i.
anterior horn cell i.
i. and asepsis
barrier isolation unit
i. bed
body substance i.
denial and i.
develop isolation technique
feeling of i.
germ-free isolation unit
hepatic vascular i.
hepatic venous isolation by direct hemoperfusion
i. hospital
i. and identification
left atrial isolation procedure
i. measures
negative-pressure isolation room
i. of patient
placed in i.
i. policies
posttransplant i.
i. precautions
respiratory isolation implementation efficiency
respiratory isolation implementation sensitivity
skin and wound i.
specific isolation precautions
standard isolation technique
stimulus isolation unit
strict i.
i. technique
total vascular i.
i. trash
update isolation technique
i. and withdrawal

isolette
out of i.
placed in i.
I. Servo control

isoleucine
peptide histidine i.

isomer
vicinal i.

isomerase
protein disulfide i.
triose i.
triosephosphate i.
uroporphyrin i.

isomerism
left atrial i.

isometric
angle isometric testing
i. contraction period
i. endurance time
i. exercise
i. hand grip test
integrated isometric tension
i. interval
neck i.
peak isometric torque
i. period of cardiac cycle
i. pressure
i. program
i. quad strengthening exercise
i. relaxation period
i. relaxation time
stretching and neck i.
i. systolic tension
i. transition
i. trunk stabilization

isomorphous
double isomorphous replacement
multiple isomorphous replacement
single isomorphous replacement

isonicotinic
i. acid
i. acid hydrazide

isonitrile
methoxyisobutyl isonitrile single-photon emission computed tomography

isoperistaltic
antecolic long-loop isoperistaltic gastrojejunostomy
side-to-side isoperistaltic strictureplasty

isopropyl
i. alcohol
i. chlorophenyl

isopter
nasal i.

isorrheic
limiting isorrheic concentration
minimal isorrheic concentration

isosexual
idiopathic isosexual puberty

isotachophoresis
capillary i.

isothiocyanate
fluorescein i.
rhodamine i.
rhodamine isothiocyanate conjugated
tetramethylrhodamine i.

isothionate
tetramethylrhodamine i.

isotonic
combination of i.'s
i. endurance test
i. reversal

isotope
blood isotope clearance
i. bone scan
carbon-14 i.
chromium i.
i. cisternography
cobalt i.
i. dilution-mass spectrometry
gas isotope ratio mass spectrometry
increased uptake of i.
interstitial implantation of radioactive i.
low LET i.
i. nephrogram
nonradioactive hydrogen i.
radioactive hydrogen i.
i. ratio mass spectrometry
i. scanning study
terminal half-life of isotopes
i. voiding cystourethrography

isotopic
myocardial isotopic perfusion scan
radioactive isotopic venogram, bilateral

isotopomer
mass isotopomer distribution analysis

isotropic
i. band striated muscle fiber
i. disc striated muscle fiber
effective isotropic radiated power
low temperature i.

isotype
light chain isotype suppression
M-component i.

isotypic
Oz isotypic determinant

isovelocity
proximal isovelocity surface area

isovolumetric
common peak developed isovolumetric pressure
i. relaxation
i. relaxation period

isovolumic
i. contraction
i. contraction time
external isovolumic contraction time
i. relaxation time

issue
aging i.
clinical practice i.
cross-cultural i.
damaged i.
end-of-life i.'s
ethical i.
family i.
family-oriented i.
impaired employee alcohol and drug treatment i.
inner child i.
interpersonal i.
key i.
legal i.
parenting i.
patient management i.
quality-of-life i.
sexual i.
sexuality i.
social i.
special teaching i.
underlying emotional i.

Issyk-Kul virus

isthmic
Mann isthmic cerclage

isthmus
i. of auditory tube
i. of His
Krönig i.
i. of thyroid gland

it
had it before, got it again
It Scale for Children
only handle it once rule
plug the lung until it grows

itch
diabolical i.
ground itch anemia
lumberman's i.
mad i.
Malabar i.

Moeller i.
Norway i.
Saint Ignatius i.
summer i.
vaginal i.
vulvar i.

itching

anal i.
anal itching and antibiotic
i. in anus
i. or burning sensation
chronic itching syndromes
control itching and sneezing
dandruff with i.
dry itching skin
fidgeting, aching, pulling, or itching feeling
i. generalized
intense i.
i. and irritation
lacrimation and i.
nasal i.
perianal i.
perineal i.
redness, dryness and i.
i. sensation
vaginal i.
vulvar i.

itchy

blister red, scaly, and i.
i. or chapped skin
i. lesion
red, swollen, and i.
runny itchy nose
runny nose and eyes i.
i. skin
i. skin rash
thick, red itchy patch of skin
i., watery eye
watery, itchy eyes
i., whitish vaginal discharge

item

parental environment i.
i. response theory

Ito

I. cell
hypomelanosis of I.
I. nevus
nevus of I.

itself

catheter coiled upon i.

ivy

poison i.

jabbing
severe, jabbing facial pain
sharp, jabbing or electrical pain

Jaccoud
J. arthritis
J. arthropathy

jacket
cardiac cooling j.
cuirass j.
fiberglass j.
flexion body j.
orthoplast j.
plaster of Paris j.
porcelain jacket crown
yellow jacket venom

Jackson
ankle scoring system of Baird and J.
J. Personality Inventory
J. rule
J. Vocational Interest Survey

jacksonian
j. attack
j. epilepsy
j. seizure

Jackson-Pratt
J.-P. to bulb suction
J.-P. drain

Jackson-Weiss syndrome

Jadassohn
anetoderma of J.
nevus of J.
J. nevus phakomatosis
nevus sebaceus of J.

jag
arousal j.
crying j.
j. drinker
j. drinking

Jakob-Creutzfeldt disease

Janus
J. family tyrosine kinase
J. kinase/signal transducer and activator of transcription

Japan
hemagglutinating virus of J.

Japanaut virus

Japanese
J. Accepted Name
J. B encephalitis
J. encephalitis virus vaccine
J. equine encephalitis
J. erection ring
J. spotted fever

jargon
j. agraphia
j. aphasia
medical j.
j. speech

Jarisch-Herxheimer reaction

jaundice
j. associated with sepsis
congenital hemolytic j.
extended jaundice of newborn
extrahepatic obstructive j.
homologous serum j.
j., chills and fever
j., lethargy and fever
j. and lethargy
neonatal cholestatic j.
j. of newborn
onset of j.
j. pruritus
rapid onset of j.
recurrent intrahepatic obstructive j.
j. without inflammation

jaundiced
infant j.
j. sclerae
skin j.

jaw
angle of j.
angled jaw rongeur
asymmetric j.'s
j. bone
broken j.
centric jaw relationship
chest pain radiating to jaw and shoulder
clenched j.
j. clenching
j. deformity
extreme jaw clenching
facial implant of j.
fractured j.
j. grinding
j. jerk reflex
j. joint
lower j.
lumpy jaw syndrome
misaligned j.
j. movement
multiple exostoses of j.
multiple nevoid, basal cell epithelioma, jaw cysts, bifid rib syndrome
j. muscle activity
nevoid basal cell epithelioma, jaw cysts, bifid rib syndrome
normal jaw function
j. pain
pain in chest, jaw, or extremity
pain radiating to j.
pain radiating to jaw and shoulder
parrot j.
partially edentulous j.
pincer j.
receding lower j.
j. strain
j. support
j. tension
j. thrust maneuver
tongue, jaw, neck dissection
upper j.
j. winking
j. wired
j. wiring

jawbone
denuded j.
j. loss
lower j.
upper j.

jaw-opening reflex

jealousy
alcoholic j.
delusion of jealousy and persecution

jejunal
j. artery
j. atresia
j. autotransplantation
j. bypass
j. diverticulitis
j. diverticulosis
j. diverticulum
j. extension tube
j. feeding tube
first jejunal vein
j. fistula
j. free flap
j. interposition
j. loop
j. mucosa
percutaneous endoscopic gastrostomy and jejunal extension tube
percutaneous endoscopic placement of jejunal tube
j. segment
j. tube through percutaneous endoscopic gastrostomy
j. ulcer
j. vein
j. villi

jejunitis
necrotizing j.
jejunoileal bypass
jejunostomy
direct percutaneous j.
fine-needle catheter j.
needle catheter j.
percutaneous endoscopic j.
j. tube feeding
jejunum
arterial arch of j.
j. and ileum adhesed
jelly
apple jelly nodule
apple jelly papule of lupus vulgaris
j. belly appearance
contraceptive j.
currant jelly sputum
Wharton j.
jerk
absent ankle j.
ankle j.
ankle jerk reflex
biceps j.
brachial radialis j.
elbow j.
increased knee j.
infantile myoclonic j.
jaw jerk reflex
macro square-wave j.
j. nystagmus
patellar j.
quadriceps j.
sudden body j.
tendon j.
timed repetitive ankle j.
triceps j.
wild limb j.
jerking
j. of body
discrete jerking musculature of face
j. of extremity
j. eye movements
head j.
involuntary jerking movements of legs
massive jerking movements
j. motions
rhythmic jerking movements
violent and irregular jerking motion
jerky
j. inspiration
irregular jerky movements
j. movements
j. pulse
j. respiration
j. step-wise movement
tremors and jerky movements
Jeryl
mumps virus vaccine Jeryl Lynn strain
Jesness
J. Behavior Checklist
J. Inventory
Jessner
lymphocytic infiltrate of J.
jet
anteriorly directed j.
j. area
Doppler color j.
high-frequency jet ventilator
j. humidifier
j. lavage
j. length
peak jet flow rate
percutaneous transtracheal jet ventilation
regurgitant jet area
transtracheal jet ventilation
twin jet nebulizer
j. ventilation
Jew
Ashkenazi J.
Jewish
Ashkenazi Jewish community
Ashkenazi Jewish heritage
jig
chamfer cut j.
drilling j.
femoral alignment j.
Joaquin
San Joaquin Valley disease
job
J. Attitude Scale
j. capacity evaluation
decline in job performance
J. Description Index
hatchet j.
j. hazardous to health
high-stress j.
j. task analysis
job-related injury
joining
variable diversity j.
joint
j. abnormality
accumulation of blood within j.
j. aches
j. aching
acromioclavicular j.
acromioclavicular joint injury
active ankle joint complex range of motion
acute joint syndrome
adjustable dynamic j.
j. alignment and motion
allograft joint replacement
alloplastic temporomandibular joint prosthesis
alumina bioceramic joint replacement
amputation of j.
ankle joint complex
ankle joint leg-curl
anterior intraoccipital j.
anterior joint capsule thickening
anterior joint impingement
anterior sacroiliac joint plate
anterior sternoclavicular j.
anterior tibiotalar part of medial ligament of ankle j.
anteromedial joint line
apophysial joint osteophyte
arthritic ankle joint narrowing
j. arthrocentesis
j. arthroplasty
articular disc of acromioclavicular j.
articular disc of distal radioulnar j.
articular disc of sternoclavicular j.
articular disc of temporomandibular j.
articular joint tissue catabolism
artificial hip j.
artificial joint implant material
artificial knee j.
j. aspiration
aspiration and injection of j.
asymmetric subtalar joint development
atlantooccipital joint dislocation
axial joint dissection
axial rotation j.
basal joint reflex
bleeding into j.
bone and joint examination
bone and joint infection
bone or joint pathology
j.'s and bones
bones, muscles, j.'s
bones, j.'s, and muscles
calcaneonavicular joint arthroscopy
j. capsule defect

j. cartilage
j. chondroma
chronic inflammation of j.
chronic joint pain
click heard at hip j.
computed tomography-guided percutaneous radiofrequency denervation of the sacroiliac j.
j. contracture and swelling
copious lavage of j.
cricoarytenoid joint ankylosis
customized joint repair
j. cyst
j. damage
j. debridement
j. debris
deformed gnarled j.
j. deformity
j. degeneration
j. destruction
j. disarticulation
j. disease
diseased joint with inflammation
j. dislocation
j. disorder
distal interphalangeal j.
distal radioulnar j.
j. distraction
dovetail joint osteotomy
j. effusion
elastic knee cage with medial and lateral contoured knee j.'s
j. examination
excessive joint play
excision of j.
exophytic joint disease
extensive manipulation of j.
facet joint arthropathy
facet joint block
facet joint disease
facet joint osteoarthritis
facial dysplasia, hyperextensibility of joints, clinodactyly, growth retardation, mental retardation syndrome
fact joint arthritis
failed joint replacement
femorotibial j.
finger joint size
j. flexibility
j. flexible
j. fluid analysis
fluid aspirated from j.
j. of foot
j. fracture
freely movable j.
full joint range of motion
full joint range of movement
j. function
fused apophyseal j.
j. fusion
general joint pain
glenohumeral j.
j. of hand
hand/wrist joint replacement
hip joint angle
inability to move a j.
incision into j.
indwelling prosthetic j.
infected joint lining
j. infection
inflamed swollen j.
j. inflammation
inflammation of j.
inflammatory joint disease
j. injection
j. injury
instability of lumbosacral j.
internal derangement of knee joint
interphalangeal joint of foot
interphalangeal joint of hand
j. interval histogram
intervertebral joint complex
knee joint alignment disorder
lateral joint line
limited joint mobility
limited joint motion
j. line
locking of j.
longitudinal midtarsal joint axis
loose body in j.
loss of appetite with joint swelling
manipulation of dislocated j.
MCP finger joint prosthesis
mechanical joint apparatus
medial joint of ankle
medial joint level
medial joint space
medial ligament of ankle j.
medial ligament of talocrural j.
medial ligament of temporomandibular j.
median atlantoaxial j.
membrane of j.
meniscus of acromioclavicular j.
mental retardation, coarse facies, epilepsy, joint contracture syndrome
mental retardation, overgrowth, craniosynostosis, distal arthrogryposis, sacral dimple, joint laxity
metacarpocarpal j.
metacarpophalangeal j.
metacarpophalangeal joint subluxation
metatarsophalangeal j.
middle atlantoepistrophic j.
middle carpal j.
midtarsal j.
mortise of j.
j. motion
MTP j.
multiple axis knee j.
narrowing of joint space
National J. Committee on Learning Disabilities
neural arch j.
neuropathic joint disease
neutrophil-mediated joint inflammation
oblique ligament of elbow j.
oblique midtarsal joint axis
open apophyseal j.
opening in j.
overuse of j.
j. pain and discomfort
painful inflammation of j.
pain in muscles and j.'s
j. pain and stiffness
j. pain and swelling
palmar ligament of interphalangeal joint of hand
palmar ligament of metacarpophalangeal j.
patellofemoral j.
patellofemoral joint syndrome
j. pathology
permanent joint damage
j. position sensation
j. position sense
pressure on toe j.
j. problems from arthritis
j. protection
proximal interphalangeal j.
proximal interphalangeal/distal interphalangeal j.'s
proximal radioulnar j.
radionuclide joint imaging
range of joint motion
j. range of motion
j. reconstruction
red swollen j.
reduced joint survey
relaxation of j.
repair of j.
repetitive motion in the j.
j. replacement center
j. rheumatoid arthritis

joint *(continued)*
sacroiliac j.
scapulothoracic j.
seeding of j.
septic finger j.
severe joint pain and fatigue
short stature, hyperextensibility of joints or hernia or both, ocular depression, Rieger anomaly, teething, delayed
silicone-based artificial j.
Smith subtalar joint arthroereisis peg
j. space
spondyloepimetaphyseal dysplasia with joint laxity
stabbing joint pain
j. stability
j. stabilized
j. stable
Staphylococcus aureus prosthetic joint infection
sternoclavicular j.
j. stiffening
j. stiffness
structural changes in j.
j. subluxation
subtalar joint axis
subtalar joint function
subtalar joint neutral position
j. surface
surgical immobilization of j.
Swanson wrist joint implant
j. swelling in hemodialysis
j. swollen and inflamed
swollen joint count
swollen and painful j.
swollen, stiff, inflamed j.
syndrome of limited joint mobility
synovial membrane of j.
temporomandibular joint dislocation
temporomandibular joint disorder
temporomandibular joint dysfunction
temporomandibular joint osteoarthritis
temporomandibular joint synovial fluid
tender joint count
j. tenderness
j. tissues
j. toilet
transient joint pain
j. trauma
j. treatment planning
twisting injury to j.
ulnar collateral ligament of elbow j.
ulnar collateral ligament of wrist j.
universal joint syndrome
weakness, dizziness and joint pain
worn facet j.

Jolly
J. body
J. reaction

Jones
Bence J.
Bence Jones protein
Bence Jones proteinuria
J. criteria

joule
j. equivalent
j. per coulomb
j. per kilogram
j. per tesla

Juan
San Juan virus

Jude
St. Jude annuloplasty ring
St. Jude valve

judgment
aberration of j.
automatic j.
change in j.
clinical j.
common sense j.
decreased j.
disintegration of j.
j. of distance
ethical j.
functioning, reasoning, orientation, memory, arithmetic, judgment, and emotion
impaired j.
impairment of j.
inflated judgment of accomplishments
interference with judgment and decision making
loss of j.
loss of recent memory, confusion and poor j.
mood, orientation, judgment, affect, content
moral j.
poor j.

jugular
abdominal jugular test
abnormal jugular reflex
anterior horizontal jugular vein
anterior jugular lymph node
aortic jugular test
autologous internal jugular vein
collapsed jugular vein
j. compression test
external j.
flat jugular vein
j. floor
j. foramen syndrome
j. ganglion of vagus nerve
high jugular bulb
inferior jugular ganglion
internal jugular catheter
internal jugular vein cannulation
left j.
left internal jugular vein
j. lymph nodes
j. neck vein distention
j. notch of temporal bone
occipital bone jugular incisure
right internal jugular vein
severed jugular vein
j. trunk
j. vein
j. venous arch
j. venous catheter
j. venous distention
j. venous oxygen saturation
j. venous pressure
j. venous pulsation
j. venous pulse
j. venous pulse tracing
j. wall

juice
gastric j.
grapefruit j.
normal human gastric j.
orange j.
pancreatic juice protein
pure pancreatic j.
secretes gastric j.

jumbo
fenestrated spiked open-span jumbo biopsy forceps

jump
primary antecubital jump bypass
j. walker

jump-start heart

jumpy
patient irritable and j.

junction
angular junction of eyelid
anomalous craniovertebral j.
anomalous junction of pancreaticobiliary ducts

anomalous junction of the pancreatobiliary duct
anomalous pancreatobiliary duct j.
anterior cervical approach to cervicothoracic j.
anterior cervicothoracic junction surgery
anterior junction line
aortic sinotubular j.
atrioventricular j.
atrioventricular junction anomaly
atrioventricular junction escape rhythm
autoimmune neuromuscular junction disorder
cardiac gap junction protein
cementoenamel j.
cortical medullary j.
costochondral j.
dentinoenamel j.
dermal-epidermal j.
dermal subcutaneous j.
j. of distal third
duodenojejunal j.
electrocardiographic junction between QRS complex and ST segment
esophagogastric j.
excitatory junction potential
j. field-effect transistor
gap j.
gap junction intercellular communication
gap junction protein
gastroesophageal j.
glossopalatal j.
ileocecal j.
inhibitory junction potential
ligation of esophagogastric j.
meatal advancement, glansplasty, penoscrotal junction meatotomy
meatal advancement, glanuloplasty, penoscrotal junction meatotomy
mucogingival j.
myoneural j.
neuroeffector j.
neuromuscular j.
original squamocolumnar j.
pancreaticobiliary ductal j.
patulous gastroesophageal j.
premature atrioventricular junction complex
tear in mucosa at cardioesophageal j.
tight j.
ureteropelvic j.
ureterovesical j.
uterotubal j.
vesicoureteral j.

junctional

accelerated junctional rhythm
j. arrhythmia
arteriovenous junctional rhythm
arteriovenous junctional tachycardia
atrioventricular junctional ablation
atrioventricular junctional bigeminy
atrioventricular junctional escape beat
atrioventricular junctional heart block
atrioventricular junctional pacemaker
atrioventricular junctional reentrant
atrioventricular junctional rhythm
atrioventricular junctional tachycardia
AV junctional rhythm
AV junctional tachycardia
j. axis
bigeminy j.
j. bradycardia
j. cavity
j. complex
j. contractions
j. depression
ectopic junctional beat
j. ectopic tachycardia
j. epidermolysis bullosa
j. escape beat
j. escape rhythm
j. extrasystole
j. fold
j. interspace
intractable junctional tachycardia
j. lymph node
j. nevus
j. pacemaker
paroxysmal junctional ventricular tachycardia
permanent junctional reciprocating tachycardia
j. premature beat
j. premature contraction
premature junctional complex
premature junctional contraction
premature junctional systole
j. reciprocating tachycardia
j. rhythm after cardiac surgery
j. slowing
j. tissue

jungle

j. fever
j. yellow fever

junior

j. baby food
j. clinician
J. Eysenck Personality Inventory

Junkman-Schoeller unit of thyrotropin

jurisprudence

medical j.

Jurona virus

just

j. noticeable difference
J. reflex

justo

pelvis justo major
pelvis justo minor

juvenile

j. absence epilepsy
j. acquired hypothyroidism
j. alcoholic
j. amaurotic idiocy
j. angiofibroma
j. ankylosing spondylitis
j. anxiety disorder
j. arrhythmia
j. arthritis
J. Arthritis Functional Assessment Report
j. atrophy
j. autoimmune myasthenia gravis
autosomal recessive juvenile parkinsonism
j. calcaneal fracture
j. cataract
j. cell
j. chorea
j. chronic arthritis
j. chronic myelocytic leukemia
j. chronic myelogenous leukemia
j. chronic polyarthritis
j. court
j. delinquent
j. dermatomyositis
j. dermatomyositis/polymyositis
j. diabetes mellitus
dominant juvenile optic atrophy
dominantly inherited juvenile optic atrophy
familial juvenile nephrophthisis
familial juvenile nephrophthisis-medullary cystic disease
familial juvenile polyposis
j. general paralysis
j. glaucoma

juvenile *(continued)*
j. granulosa cell tumor
j. hormone analog
j. idiopathic arthritis
idiopathic juvenile osteoporosis
j. idiopathic scoliosis
j. intervertebral disc calcification
j. laryngeal papilloma
j. macular degeneration
Meesman juvenile epithelial dystrophy
j. melanoma
j. memory deficit
j. muscular atrophy
j. myelomonocytic leukemia
j. myoclonic epilepsy
j. nasopharyngeal angiofibroma
j. neutrophil
j. open-angle glaucoma
j. osteomalacia
patient juvenile diabetic
j. pattern
pauciarticular juvenile chronic arthritis
pauciarticular juvenile rheumatoid arthritis
pedunculated juvenile polyp
j. periodontitis
j. pernicious anemia
j. pilocytic astrocytoma
j. plantar dermatitis
j. plantar dermatosis
polyarticular juvenile chronic arthritis
polyarticular juvenile rheumatoid arthritis
j. polyposis syndrome
j. polyps
j. reflex
j. residential care
j. rheumatoid arthritis rash
j. rheumatoid arthritis type I, II
Scheuermann juvenile kyphosis
systemic juvenile rheumatoid arthritis
j. tropical pancreatitis syndrome
j. wart
J. Wellness and Health Survey
j. xanthogranuloma
X-linked juvenile retinoschisis

juvenile-onset
j.-o. diabetes
j.-o. diabetes mellitus
j.-o. multisystem inflammatory disease
j.-o. neuronal ceroid lipofuscinosis
j.-o. rheumatoid arthritis

juvenilis
dementia paralytica j.
paralysis agitans j.
verruca plana j.

juxtaglomerular
j. apparatus
j. cell
j. cell hyperplasia
j. cell tumor
j. granulation index

juxtaposition
atrial appendage j.

Kabuki makeup syndrome

Kaeng Khoi virus

Kaes
line of K.

Kaes-Bechterew
band of K.-B.

Kahn
K. intelligence test
K. Test of Symbol Arrangement

kala-azar
canine k.-a.

kalium
extracellular k.
low kalium
k. potassium phosphate buffer
renal kalium wasting

kallikrein
basophil kallikrein of anaphylaxis
human urinary k.
k. inactivating unit
k. inactivation unit
k. inhibiting unit
potato kallikrein inhibitor
urinary k.

Kamese virus

Kammavanpettai virus

kanamycin-vancomycin
k.-v. blood agar
k.-v. laked blood agar

Kansas
Neonatal Behavioral Assessment Scale with Kansas Supplements

kansasii
Mycobacterium kansasii infection

Kaposi
acquired immunodeficiency syndrome with Kaposi sarcoma
African cutaneous Kaposi sarcoma
African lymphadenopathic Kaposi sarcoma
AIDS-related Kaposi sarcoma
appendiceal Kaposi sarcoma
Mediterranean Kaposi sarcoma
pulmonary Kaposi sarcoma
K. sarcoma
K. sarcoma herpesvirus
K. sarcoma human growth factor
K. sarcoma and opportunistic infection
K. varicelliform eruption
xeroderma of K.

Karmen unit

Karnofsky
K. performance score
K. performance status
K. rating scale

Kartagener
K. disease
K. syndrome
K. triad

Kartush

karyopyknotic index

karyotype
automatic karyotype system database
early prenatal k.
minor karyotype abnormality
sex k.'s
spectral k.

karyotypic
autosomal karyotypic disorder
major karyotypic abnormality

karyotyping
electrophoretic k.
fetal k.
spectral k.

katal per liter

Kaufman
K. Assessment Battery for Children
K. Development Scale
K. Survey of Early Academic and Language Skills
K. Test of Educational Achievement

Kawasaki
atypical Kawasaki disease
K. disease
K. syndrome

keeled chest

keep
to keep needle open
to keep open
to keep vein open
may keep at bedside
k. needle open
k. on
k. open
k. open rate
recognize, empathize, think, hear, integrate, notice, k.
k. vein open

keeping
married, keeping baby
not keeping baby
not married, keeping baby
not married, not keeping baby
out of wedlock and not keeping child
single parent keeping baby
single parent not keeping baby

Kehrer reflex

Kehr incision

Keith
K. bundle
K. node

Kell
K. blood group
K. blood system
K. factor

Keller
K. bunionectomy
Ganley modification of Keller arthroplasty
K. procedure

keloid
k. formation
k. scar

keloidalis
acne k.

Kenner-fecal medium

Kent
Fibers of K.
K. Infant Development Scale
K. State University Speech Discrimination Test

keratectomy
automated lamellar k.
excimer laser photorefractive k.
excimer laser phototherapeutic k.
no-touch transepithelial photorefractive k.
photoastigmatic refractive k.
radial k.
tracker-assisted photorefractive k.

keratic
mutton-fat keratic precipitate

keratin
antibody to k.

keratinocyte
allogenic keratinocyte graft
apoptotic k.
degeneration of k.
k. growth factor-2
k. growth factor receptor

keratitic precipitate

keratitis
amebic k.
artificial silk k.
Gram-positive bacterial k.
k. herpes

keratitis *(continued)*
herpes simplex k.
herpetic stromal k.
immune stromal k.
interstitial k.
luetic interstitial k.
Lyme disease k.
lymphogranuloma venereum k.
mixed bacterial-fungal k.
necrotizing interstitial k.
necrotizing stromal k.
necrotizing ulcerative k.
non-*Acanthamoeba* amebic k.
nonulcerative interstitial k.
ocular amoebic k.
onchocercal sclerosing k.
oyster shuckers' k.
peripheral ulcerative k.
k. punctata
stromal herpetic k.
superficial punctate k.

keratoacanthoma
subungual k.

keratoconjunctivitis
atopic dermatitis with k.
atopic eczema k.
epidemic k.
infectious bovine k.
limbic vernal k.
non-Sjögren keratoconjunctivitis sicca
k. sicca
superior limbic k.
vernal k.

keratocyst
odontogenic k.

keratocyte
guinea pig k.

keratoderma
k. hereditaria mutilans
lymphedematous k.
mutilating k.
mutilating keratoderma of Vohwinkel
nonepidermolytic palmoplantar k.
palmoplantar k.
senile k.

keratoma
indurated plantar k.

keratome
automated disposable k.
k. incision

keratometer
Marco manual k.

keratometric
k. power
k. readings
topographic simulated keratometric power

keratomileusis
automated laser k.
laser-assisted intrastromal k.
laser-assisted in situ k.
myopic k.

keratoneuritis
pathognomonic radial k.

keratopathy
aphakic bullous k.
bullous k.
climatic droplet k.
infectious crystalline k.
pearl diver's k.
peripheral anterior stent k.
pseudophakic bullous k.
punctate epithelial k.
striae k.

keratopharyngeus
musculus k.

keratoplasty
deep lamellar k.
hyperopic automated lamellar k.
lamellar k.
laser thermal k.
Magitot keratoplasty operation
manual lamellar k.
noncontact holmium:yttrium-argon-garnet laser thermal k.
partial penetrating k.
penetrating keratoplasty astigmatism
penetrating keratoplasty button
penetrating keratoplasty and glaucoma
photorefractive k.
thermal laser k.

keratosis
actinic k.
interphalangeal k.
intractable plantar k.
lichenoid k.
lichen planus-like k.
nevus follicularis k.
palmoplantar k.
precancerous actinic k.
seborrheic k.
senile k.
solar k.

keratotic
acute primary keratotic gingivostomatitis
carpet tack follicular keratotic plug
k. patch
k. scaling

keratotomy
arcuate transverse k.
astigmatic k.
astigmatic keratotomy enhancement
prospective evaluation of radial k.
radial and astigmatic k.

Kerckring
K. center
K. fold
folds of K.
nodules of K.
K. ossicle
valve of K.
K. valve

Kerley A, B, C line

ketamine
NMDA antagonist k.

Ketapang virus

ketoacid
branched-chain alpha ketoacid dehydrogenase

ketoacidosis
alcoholic k.
diabetes mellitus k.
diabetic k.

ketoaciduria
ataxia-deafness-retardation with k.

ketogenic
k. diet
k. steroid

ketogenic/antiketogenic ratio

17-ketogenic steroid

ketoglutarate
k. dehydrogenase
k. dehydrogenase complex

ketone
k. body ratio
chloromethyl k.
methyl butyl k.
methyl ethyl k.
urine glucose k.

17-ketosteroid reductase

key
foramen of Key and Retzius
k. integrative social system
k. intermediary protein
k. issue
k. pulse rate

keyhole
k. deformity
k. incision
MacCarty k.
k. pupil
k. surgery

keystone
k. ligament
K. Telebinocular Visual Survey
K. virus

Khan
Dera Ghazi Khan virus

Khoi
Kaeng Khoi virus

Ki
antibody K.

kick
k. count
knee k.

kicking
k. drug habit
k. the habit
k. smoking habit

kid
drug-affected k.
funny-looking k.

kidney
k. abscess
acquired cystic kidney disease
acute kidney inflammation
adipose capsule of k.
adult-onset polycystic kidney disease
adult polycystic kidney disease
adult-type polycystic kidney disease
allocating cadaveric k.
allogenic kidney transplant
anterior superior segmental artery of k.
arciform vein of k.
arcuate artery of k.
arcuate vein of k.
arterial segment of k.
arteriole of k.
arteriovenous kidney malformation
artery of anterior inferior segment of k.
artery of anterior superior segment of k.
artery of posterior segment of k.
artificial k.
atypical angiomyolipoma of the k.
atypical angiomyolipoma of k.
autosomal dominant medullary cystic kidney disease
autosomal-dominant polycystic kidney disease
autosomal recessive kidney disease
autosomal-recessive polycystic kidney disease
avascular kidney mass
baboon k.
baby hamster kidney cell
bovine embryonic kidney cell
bovine kidney cell
calf k.
chick embryo k.
childhood polycystic kidney disease
clear cell sarcoma of the k.
combined kidney and pancreas transplant
congenital multicystic k.
k. cortex
cortical arch of k.
cortical lobules of k.
cortical necrosis of k.
cortical scarring of k.
k. cyst
deer kidney virus
k. dialysis
diminished heart, kidney and brain function
k. disease
diseased k.
dog kidney cell
dog kidney tissue culture
k. donor
Dow Hollow Fiber k.
duplication of left k.
duplication of right k.
embryonic bovine k.
end-stage kidney disease
fatty liver and kidney syndrome
feline k.
k. function
glomerular capsule of k.
glomerular kidney disease
glomerulocystic k.
glomerulocystic kidney disease
granular atrophy of k.
guinea pig kidney absorption test
hamster k.
heart, kidney and brain function
heart, liver, and k.
hemisection of k.'s
heterotopic kidney transplant
high level of kidney protein rennin
hilum of k.
k. hilus
human embryo kidney cell
human embryonic k.
human fetal diploid kidney cell
human kidney cell
human kidney glandular kallikrein-1 gene
k.'s immature
immune kidney disease
impaired kidney function
increased kidney function
infantile polycystic kidney disease
interlobar artery of k.
interlobar vein of k.
interlobular artery of k.
interlobular vein of k.
k. internal splint/stent
k.s and urinary bladder
large white k.
lateral margin of k.
left k.
liver and kidney transplantation
liver, kidneys, and spleen
liver, kidneys, spleen, and bladder
liver, kidneys, and spleen not palpable
living donor k.
k. lobe
local bulge of kidney contour
long axis of k.
Madin-Darby bovine kidney cell
Madin-Darby canine k.
malignant neoplasm of k.
malignant rhabdoid tumor of k.
malpighian body of k.
medial border of k.
medulla of k.
medullary sponge k.
monkey k.
monkey kidney cell
monkey kidney fibroblast monolayer
monkey kidney tissue culture
multicystic dysgenetic k.
multicystic dysplasia k.
multicystic dysplastic k.
multilocular cystic k.
National K. and Urological Diseases Information Clearinghouse
necrotic kidney tissue
nonrotation of k.
normal human k.
normally functioning k.
normal rat k.

kidney *(continued)*
obstructed k.
palpable liver, spleen and k.'s
pancreas and k.
pancreas after kidney transplant
papillary foramina of k.
passing of kidney stone
permanent kidney damage
petechial hemorrhage of k.
piecemeal removal of kidney stone
pig k.
k. pole
pole of left k.
pole of right k.
polycystic k.
polycystic disease of k.
postmortem human k.
postmortem human kidney cell
primary African green monkey k.
primary rabbit k.
proliferative kidney disease
k. protein
ptosis of k.
k. punch
k. punch test
rabbit kidney vacuolating virus
relative medullary area of k.
renal kidney stone
retrograde kidney study
rhabdoid tumor of the k.
Rhesus monkey k.
right k.
segmental artery of k.
simultaneous double kidney transplantation
k. stone
swine k.
k. transplant
k. transplantation
k. transplant unit
k. treatment
k. ultrasound
k. ultrasound biopsy
upper pole of k.
k.'s, ureters, bladder x-ray
k.'s, ureters, and spleen x-ray
wearable artificial k.
k. weight

kidney-specific protein

Kienböck
K. disease
K. dislocation
K. unit of x-ray exposure

Kiesselbach
K. area
K. triangle

kill
log cell k.

killed
heat k.
k. intracellular bacteria
maximal number of microbes k.
k. measles virus vaccine
k. organism
poliomyelitis vaccine k.
k. polio vaccine

killer
autologous lymphokine activated killer cell
k. cell
k. cell inhibitory receptor
flow artifact k.
human natural killer cell
k. inhibitor receptors-human leukocyte antigen
low natural killer syndrome
lymphokine-activated killer cell
nasal T-cell/natural killer cell lymphoma
natural killer activity
natural killer cell
natural killer cell activation
natural killer cell antigen
natural killer cell leukemia
natural killer cell-stimulating factor
natural killer lymphocyte
natural killer target structure
natural killer T-cell
spontaneous killer cell
T/natural killer cell

killing
direct killing of incompetent individual
direct killing by lethal injection
infusoria killing unit
perforin killing pathway
phagocytosis and killing function

kilocalories
grams of nitrogen to nonprotein k.
nonprotein k.

kiloelectron volt

kilogram
amperes per k.
k. calorie
calories per kilogram per day
coulombs per k.
cubic centimeters per kilogram per day
joule per k.
microgram per kilogram per minute
milligram per k.
milligram per kilogram per day
milligram per kilogram per hour
milliliter per k.
milliosmoles per k.
mole per k.
osmoles per kilogram
patient's weight in k.'s
k. per liter
watt per k.

kilogram-meter per second squared

kilovolt
k. ampere
k. constant potential

kilovoltage
peak k.
k. peak
k. potential

Kimbrel unit

Kimmelstiel-Wilson
K.-W. disease
K.-W. syndrome

Kimray-Greenfield filter

kin
next of k.

kinase
adenosine k.
adenylate k.
adrenergic receptor k.
AMP-activated protein k.
beta-adrenergic receptor k.
Bruton tyrosine k.
calcium-calmodulin kinase II
calmodulin-dependent protein k.
choline k.
c-Jun N-terminal k.
conserved helix-loop-helix ubiquitous k.
creatine k.
creatine kinase fraction muscle
creatine kinase isoenzyme
creatine kinase isoenzyme electrophoresis
creatine kinase MB
creatine kinase MB fraction
creatine kinase myocardial band
cyclin-dependent k.
cyclin-dependent kinase inhibitor
cytokinin-regulated k.
cytokinin-regulated kinase I, II, L
cytosolic thymidine k.
extracellular regulated k.

focal adhesion k.
glycerol k.
glycerol kinase deficiency
glycogen synthetase k.
herpes simplex virus thymidine k.
k. inhibitory protein
Janus family tyrosine k.
liver pyruvate k.
MAP/ERK k.
MAP kinase pathway
M and B isoenzyme of creatine k.
MEK k.
mitogen-activated protein k.
mitogen-activated protein kinase cascade
mitogen-activated protein kinase pathway
MLC k.
muscle-brain isoenzyme of creative k.
myocardial muscle creatine kinase isoenzyme
myosin light-chain k.
neurotrophic tyrosine kinase receptor, type 1
nucleoside diphosphate k.
nucleoside 5′-diphosphate k.
periodically fluctuating protein k.
3-phosphoinositide-dependent protein k.
phosphorylation by the cellular double-stranded RNA-activated k.
protein kinase A, B, C, G
protein kinase activation ratio
protein tyrosine k.
rapid electrophoresis creatine k.
receptor protein tyrosine k.
receptor tyrosine k.
serine threonine kinase gene 11
serum creatine k.
serum pyruvate k.
thymidine k.
thymidine kinase deficiency
thymidine kinase, mitochondrial
thymidine kinase, soluble
tyrosine kinase activity
uridine monophosphate k.

kinase-2
tyrosine k.

kinase-3
glycogen synthase k.-3

kinase/signal
Janus kinase/signal transducer and activator of transcription

kind
error of the first k.

Kindergarten
K. Auditory Screening Test
K. Language Screening Test
Learning Inventory of Kindergarten Experiences
Phelps Kindergarten Readiness Scale
Phonetically Balanced K.
K. Readiness Test

kindling
limbic k.

kinematic
k. viscosity

kinesigenic
paroxysmal kinesigenic choreoathetosis
paroxysmal kinesigenic dyskinesia

kinesiology
applied k.

kinesis
color k.

kinesthetic
k. ability trainer
auditory and kinesthetic sensation
k. hallucination
visual, association, kinesthetic, tactile reading

kinetic
k. abrasion
k. ataxia
k. chain
closed kinetic chain
closed kinetic chain exercise
dialysate urea kinetic modeling
k. energy of a particle
k. energy released in the medium
K. Family Drawing
k. fibrinogen assay
k. hemolysis curve
intramedullary skeletal kinetic distractor
ion kinetic energy
manual kinetic perimetry
mass-analyzed ion kinetic energy
open kinetic chain exercises
k. perimetry
time-resolved imaging contrast k.'s
k. tremor
urea kinetic modeling

King-Armstrong unit

kininogen
high molecular weight k.

kinked
k. bowel
k. cord

kinking
aortic k.
arterial k.

kinky
k. hair disease
k. hair syndrome
Menkes kinky hair
Menkes kinky hair syndrome

Kinyoun
modified Kinyoun acid-fast stain

Kirschner wire

Kismayo virus

kiss
angel kisses lesion
angel's k.
angel's kiss capillary malformation

kissing
k. atherectomy technique
k. disease

kissing atherectomy technique

kit
Hardy-Rand-Ritter color vision test k.
home medical test k.
hyperalimentation k.
k. ligand
Massachusetts Vision K.
Melastatin test k.
M.O.M. basic k.
M.O.M. fluorescein k.
Moss G-tube PEG k.
mouse-on-mouse basic k.
mouse-on-mouse fluorescein k.
newborn screening k.
percutaneous access k.
Screening Kit of Language Development

Klamath virus

***Klebsiella* vaccine**

Kleihauer-Betke test

Kleijn
Magnus and de Kleijn tonic neck reflex

Klein-Levin syndrome

Klinefelter syndrome

Klippel disease

Klippel-Feil syndrome

Klumpke
K. brachial palsy
K. paralysis

knee
above k.
active knee extension
amputated above k.
anatomic modular k.
k. anatomy
anterior cruciate deficit of k.
anterior cruciate deficit k.
anterior translation of k.
anterolateral rotary knee instability
Apley knee test
k. arthrocentesis
k. arthrodesis
arthrometric knee laxity measurement
k. arthroplasty
arthroscopic knee surgery
k. arthroscopy
articular muscle of k.
articular surface of k.
articular vascular network of k.
artificial knee joint
4-bar linkage on knee prosthesis
4-bar linkage prosthetic knee mechanism
4-bar polycentric knee prosthesis
below k.
bicompartmental knee implant prosthesis
k. brace
buckling and/or locking of k.
cartilage-wearing knee bends
k.'s to chest
k. contracture
contralateral k.
cruciate condylar knee system
dashboard knee injury
deep knee bend
k. disarticulation
k. dislocation
dorsolateral surface of k.
double knee to chest
double-looped semitendinous and gracilis hamstring graft knee reconstruction technique
elastic knee cage orthosis
elastic knee cage with medial and lateral contoured knee joints
elastic knee sleeve brace
expand internal components of k.
k. extension
k. extension exercise
k. flexion
k. flexion-extension
flexion-rotation-drawer knee instability test
fluid aspirated from k.
full knee extension
hinged knee brace
k. holder
immobilized k.
k. immobilized
k. immobilizer
instability of k.
k. of internal capsule
internal derangement of knee joint
k. jerk reflex
k. joint alignment disorder
k. kick
ligament of k.
lower fossa active, lateral knee pain, and long leg on the side ipsilateral to the weak fossa
medial collateral ligament of k.
meniscus of k.
Milwaukee knee syndrome
multiple axis knee joint
k. orthosis
osteoarthritis of the k.
osteonecrosis of k.
k. pain
painful osteoarthritis of the k.
phased knee rehabilitation
posterior cruciate ligament of k.
posterior ligament of k.
prone knee bend
k. replacement
simple knee test
single-axis friction knee prosthesis
single-axis locking knee prosthesis
single knee to chest
k. sling exercises
spontaneous osteonecrosis of k.
k. sprain
terminal knee extension
through the k.
total knee arthroplasty
total knee arthroscopy
total knee prosthesis
total knee replacement, left
total knee replacement, right
total rotating k.
Translating and Congruent Mobile-Bearing Knee test
unicompartmental knee arthroplasty
upper fossa active, medial knee pain, and short leg on the side ipsilateral to the weak fossa
weight-activated locking knee prosthesis

knee-ankle
k.-a. orthosis
supracondylar knee-ankle orthosis

knee-ankle-foot orthosis

kneecap
grating sensation under k.

knee-foot-ankle orthosis

knee-heel test

knee-high socks

knife
arthroscopic k.
banana k.
beer k.
cautery k.
chemical k.
cleft palate k.
cold k.
cold knife cone aspiration
cold knife cone biopsy
cold knife conization
cold knife conization biopsy
diamond k.
diamond-dusted knife blade
electric k.
electrosurgical cutting k.
endarterectomy k.
k. and fork
forward-cutting k.
free-hand k.
full-radius resector k.
gamma k.
gamma knife stereotactic radiosurgery
goniopuncture k.
goniotomy k.
hernia k.
hot k.
micrometer k.
microsurgical k.
neurosurgical gamma k.
k. stab wound

knob
adenovirus fiber k.
aortic k.
malarial k.
notched aortic k.

knock
pericardial k.

knocked
not knocked out

knockout
insulin receptor k.

Knoop hardness number of solids

knot
arthroscopic k.
bow-tie k.
curved-needle surgeon's k.
endoscopic knot pusher
granny k.
Henry k.
k. holding capacity
modified Roeder k.
partial throw surgeon's k.
syncytial k.
syncytial knot formation
true knot in cord

knowledge
age-inappropriate knowledge of sexual behavior
k., aptitudes, and practices
k., attitude, behavior
k., attitude, behavior, and improvement in nutritional status
Crohn and Colitis K.
k. deficit
Diabetes: Basic K. Test
fund of k.
Medical Sciences K. Profile
Medical K. Self-Assessment Program
New Mexico K. of Occupations Test
K. of Occupations Test
Osteoporosis K. Questionnaire
k. of performance
Psychiatric K. and Skills Self-Assessment Program
k. of result
Sex K. and Attitude Test
k., skills, and abilities

known
all known allergies
also known as
k. drug allergies
hypersomnia related to a known organic factor
injury not k.
insomnia related to a known organic factor
no known basis
no known cure
no known diseases
no known drug allergies
no known food allergies
no known medication allergies

knuckle
aortic k.
k. cracking
k. of tube

knuckle-bender splint

Köbner
experimentally induced Köbner phenomenon
K. phenomenon

Koch
apex of Koch triangle

Kocher
K. fracture
K. incision

Koebner
linear Koebner reaction

koilonychia
occupational k.

Kölliker
membrana eboris of K.

Kolongo virus

koniocortex
auditory k.

Koplik
pathognomonic Koplik spot

Korean
K. conflict
K. hemorrhagic fever

Korsakoff
alcoholic Korsakoff psychosis
alcoholic Korsakoff syndrome
K. psychosis

Koshland-Némethy-Filmer model

Kovalevsky
canal of K.

Kowanyama virus

Krebs-Henseleit
K.-H. bicarbonate buffer
K.-H. cycle
K.-H. solution

Krebs-Ringer
K.-R. bicarbonate buffer
K.-R. bicarbonate buffer with glucose
K.-R. bicarbonate solution
K.-R. phosphate
K.-R. phosphate solution

Kreha
polysaccharide K.

Krönig isthmus

Krukenberg
K. amputation
K. tumor
K. vein

KUB
kidneys, ureters, bladder x-ray

Kuder
K. Occupational Interest Survey
K. Performance Test
K. Preference Record—Vocational

Kugel anastomosis

Kulchitsky cell carcinoma

Kunitz pancreatic trypsin inhibitor

Kunjin virus

Küntscher
K. nail
K. rod

Kupffer cell

Kurtzke Disability Status Scale

KUS
kidneys, ureters, and spleen x-ray

Kussmaul
K. coma
K. disease
K. respiration
K. sign

Kussmaul-Kien respiration

kwashiorkor
marasmic k.

kwashiorkor-marasmus syndrome

kymography
roentgen k.

kynurenic acid

kyphectomy
Sharrard-type k.

kyphoscoliosis
cataract, microcephaly, failure to thrive, k.

kyphosis
k. brace
cataract, microcephaly, arthrogryposis, k.
k. correction
Scheuermann juvenile k.

kyphotic
k. curvature
k. deformity

label
double label index
luminescent l.
not on l.

labeled
autologous labeled leukocyte
doubly labeled water
early labeled peak
l. lymphoblast
percentage of labeled mitoses
l. release experiment
l. streptavidin biotin

labeling
final printed l.
l. index
Nutrition L. and Education Act of 1990
peripheral blood labeling index
plasma cell labeling index
primed in situ l.
in situ end l.
thymidine labeling index
tritiated thymidine labeling index

labia (*pl. of* labium)

labial
anterior labial artery
anterior labial branch of deep external pudendal artery
anterior labial commissure
anterior labial nerve
anterior labial vein
l. cleft
l. hernia
posterior labial hernia
l. salivary gland
l. sulcus
superior labial region

labialis
herpes simplex l.
recurrent herpes l.

labile
l. aggregation stimulating substance
l. factor
l. hypertension
l. mood
l. peptide
l. personality
l. protein

lability
affective l.
exercise lability index
mood l.

labiodental sulcus

labioincisal edge

labioscrotal
partial labioscrotal fusion

labium, pl. **labia**
anterior commissure of labia
lingual labia
l. majus
l. minus

labor
accelerated painless l.
active phase of l.
arrest of l.
l. augmentation
contraction during l.
l. curve
l. and delivery
elective induction of l.
estimated date of l.
failure to progress in labor
first stage of l.
full-term uncomplicated pregnancy, labor, and delivery
induction of l.
l. inhibition
l. initiation
intensity of labor contractions
not in active l.
onset of spontaneous l.
patient in l.
Pitocin augmentation of l.
pregnancy, labor, and delivery
premature onset of l.
preterm l.
primary dysfunctional l.
spontaneous onset of l.
stages of l.
third stage of l.
l. trial
trial of l.
vaginal birth after cesarean—trial of l.
virtual labor monitor

laboratory
l. abnormality
l. admission baseline studies
l. animal dander allergy
associated laboratory finding
automated multitest l.
cardiac catheterization l.
cardiac exercise l.
Clinical L. Improvement Act
clinical vascular l.
colony-stimulating factor developed by Venereal Disease Research L.
composite clinical and laboratory index
l. data
drug analysis l.
Environmental Health L.
fasting laboratory work
l. findings
good laboratory practice
hygienic l.
independent l.
maximal containment l.
medical laboratory assay
mobile anaerobic l.
molecular genetics/oncology l.
neurovascular l.
no new laboratory test orders
noninvasive vascular laboratory studies
nuclear cardiology l.
pathology l.
peripheral vascular l.
preoperative laboratory workup
presurgical laboratory workup
l. procedure
radiation l.
l. reference
renal laboratory profile
l. report
routine admission laboratory test
routine laboratory work done
screening laboratory test
l. worker

laboratory-acquired infection

labored
increased and labored breathing
patient has labored breathing

labral
anterior labral avulsion
anterior labral disruption
inferior glenohumeral ligament labral complex

labroligamentous
anterior labroligamentous periosteal sleeve
anterior labroligamentous periosteal sleeve avulsion lesion

labrum
anterior glenoid l.
anterior labrum periosteal sleeve avulsion
anterior labrum periosteum shoulder arthroscopic lesion
superior labrum anterior and posterior

labyrinth
l. area hammer
artery of l.
l. of brain
Ludwig l.

labyrinth *(continued)*
membranous l.
osseous l.
renal l.
Santorini l.

labyrinthine
l. defect
optic labyrinthine righting
l. righting reflex
tonic labyrinthine inverted
tonic labyrinthine reflex
l. vein

laceration
abrasion and l.
anal sphincter l.
cardiac lacerations and hemopericardium
l. and contusion
flexor tendon l.
healed superficial l.
l. of heart
l. or hemorrhage
hemorrhage or l.
lid margin l.
partial-thickness corneal l.
soft tissue l.
spinal cord l.

Lachman test

lack
apathy and lack of interest in personal goals
l. of control
l. of energy
l. of feeling
l. of interest in others
l. of reciprocal interest

lacking
bacterial cell lacking an F plasmid

Lacks
Henrietta Lacks cell

lacrimal
ampulla of lacrimal canal
ampulla of lacrimal duct
anterior lacrimal crest
l. duct
l. fold
l. gland dysfunction
inferior lacrimal duct
l. lake
lids, lashes, l.'s, lymphatics
polyp in lacrimal sac
probing of lacrimal duct
l. sac
salivary and lacrimal secretion
superior lacrimal duct

lacrimale
os l.
punctum l.

lacrimalis
apparatus l.
avulsion of caruncula l.
canaliculus l.
papilla l.

lacrimation
gustatory l.
l. and itching
salivation, lacrimation, urination, defecation, gastrointestinal distress and emesis

lacrimoauriculoradiodental syndrome

lacrimonasal
catheterization lacrimonasal duct

lactalbumin
alpha l.
glucose, lactalbumin, serum, and hemoglobin
l. hydrolysate
hydrolysate lactalbumin Earle glucose

lactamase

lactase
isolated lactase deficiency
normal lactase activity
tissue lactase activity

lactate
l. arterial
arterial lactate level
blood l.
casein yeast lactate medium
cerebral metabolic rate of l.
l. dehydrogenase B
l. dehydrogenase elevating virus
l. dehydrogenase fraction 1–5
l. dehydrogenase isoenzyme
l. dehydrogenase, muscle
excess l.
l. extraction
liver lactate dehydrogenase
onset of blood lactate accumulation
potassium, sodium chloride, and sodium lactate solution
serum lactate dehydrogenase
sodium l.
l. threshold

lactated Ringer solution

lactating
breast firm and l.
l. rat serum factor

lactation
l. amenorrhea method
l. consultant

lactic
l. acid dehydrogenase
l. acid mineral medium
l. acidosis threshold
asymptomatic lactic acidemia
l. dehydrogenase total
l. dehydrogenase virus
heat-stable lactic dehydrogenase
mitochondrial myopathy, encephalopathy, lactic acidosis, strokelike episodes
myopathy, encephalopathy, lactic acidosis, strokelike episodes
l. peroxidase
plasma lactic dehydrogenase
polymer of lactic acid
procaine and lactic acid
salicylic and lactic acid paint

lactiferous
ampulla of lactiferous duct
l. duct

Lactobacillus
Lactobacillus acidophilus vaccine
Lactobacillus GG
Lactobacillus bulgaricus factor
Lactobacillus maintenance medium
Lactobacillus maintenance medium
Lactobacillus rhamnosus strain GG
L. viridescens

lactogen
animal placenta l.
immunoreactive human placental l.
ovine placental l.
platelet l.

lactogenic
l. hormone
ovine lactogenic hormone
placental lactogenic hormone

lactone
glucuronic acid l.
resorcylic acid l.

lactose
bloating from lactose intolerance
brilliant green lactose broth
bromothymol blue l.
l. coliform count
diarrhea from lactose intolerance
l. fermenting Gram-negative rod
l. hydrogen breath testing
l. intolerance from antibiotic
l. intolerance and galactosemia

l. malabsorption
milk lactose allergy
l. reduced diet
l. tolerance
l. tolerance test

lactose-free
l.-f. diet
l.-f. formula

lacuna
Morgagni l.
muscular l.
osseous l.
osteoclastic resorption l.
trophoblastic l.

lacunar
l. circulation infarct
l. dementia
l. infarction
medial lacunar lymph node
l. syndrome

ladder
l. incision
nucleosome l.

Laënnec cirrhosis

lag
compression lag screw
lid l.
mineralization lag time
mini lag screw system

Laimer
area of L.

lait
café au lait spot

lake
lacrimal l.
seminal l.
tear l.

Lambert
canal of L.

Lambert-Eaton myasthenic syndrome

lamella
anular l.
articular bone l.
articular lamella of bone
grand l.
ground l.
haversian l.
maximal number of l.

lamellar
automated lamellar keratectomy
autosomal dominant lamellar ichthyosis
l. body
l. body count
l. body density
deep lamellar keratoplasty
l. graft
l. granule
hyperopic automated lamellar keratoplasty
l. ichthyosis
l. keratoplasty
manual lamellar keratoplasty
osmiophilic lamellar inclusion body
partial lamellar sclerouvectomy

lamina
anterior limiting l.
basal l.
l. cortex
cricoid l.
dense fibrous l.
external elastic l.
follicular basal l.
glomerular basal l.
internal elastic l.
intimal elastic l.
limbus of osseous spiral l.
limiting lamina anterior
medial lamina of cartilage of pharyngotympanic auditory tube
membranous lamina of cartilage of pharyngotympanic auditory plate
orbital lamina of ethmoid bone
organum vasculosum of lamina terminalis
l. papyracea
l. propria lymphocyte
reticular l.

laminagraphy
cephalometric l.

laminar
l. air flow room
l. air flow unit
basal laminar deposit
horizontal laminar flow clean benches
l. tomography

laminate induration

lamination
carbon fiber lamination braid

laminectomy
cervical l.
decompressive lumbar l.
l. and fusion
lumbar l.

laminoplasty
open door l.

lamp
carbon arc l.
clamp l.
cold quartz mercury vapor l.
fixed slit l.
mercury arc l.
narrow band UVB l.
Nightingale examining l.

lance
heel l.

lancet
gum l.

lancinating pain

land
no-man's l.

landing zone

Landjia virus

landmark
anatomical l.
bony l.
Copying Drawings with L.'s
restriction landmark genomic scanning

Landry-Guillain-Barré syndrome

Lane
Arbuthnot Lane disease

Langat
L. encephalitis
L. virus

Lange
Brachmann-Cornelia de Lange syndrome
Cornelia de Lange syndrome

Langenbeck triangle

Langerhans
L. cell
L. cell granule
L. cell granulomatosis
L. cell histiocytosis
L. island
islets of L.
multifocal Langerhans cell

language
l. ability
l. acquisition device
adolescent language quotient
Adolescent L. Screening Test
l. age
algorithm-oriented l.
American Indian Sign L.
Aphasia L. Performance Scale
Appraisal of Language Disturbance
appraisal of language disturbances

language *(continued)*
l. assessment
Assessment of Children's L. Comprehension
attending to language stage
auditory comprehension of l.
Bankson Language Screening Test
Bristol L. Development Scale
Carrow Elicited L. Inventory
central language disorder
Clinical Evaluation of L. Function-Preschool
Clinical Evaluation of L. Functions
Coarticulation Assessment in Meaningful L.
common business-oriented l.
communication in sign l.
confused language syndrome
Del Rio L. Screening Test
l. development
developmental expressive language disorder
developmental language disorder
developmental receptive language disorder
Early L. Milestone Scale
English as a second l.
l. enrichment therapy
Environmental L. Inventory
l. experience approach
extensible markup l.
Fairview L. Evaluation Scale
Fairview L. Evaluation Test
Figurative L. Interpretation Test
Fluharty Preschool Speech and L. Screening Test
Fullerton L. Test for Adolescents
Grammatical Analysis of Elicited L.
hypertext markup l.
l. impairment
l. impediment
Interpersonal L. Skills and Assessment
Kaufman Survey of Early Academic and L. Skills
Kindergarten L. Screening Test
List Processing L.
mathetic function of l.
Mecham Verbal L. Scale
mixed receptive-expressive language disorder
L. Modalities Test for Aphasia
natural language processing
Oral L. Sentence Imitation Diagnostic Inventory
Oral L. Sentence Imitation Screening Test
Picture Articulation and L. Screening Test
Picture Story L. Test
Preschool L. Assessment Instrument
Preschool L. Scale
L. Proficiency Test
programming language 1
Right Hemisphere L. Battery
Riley Articulation and L. Test
L. Sampling Analysis
Screening Kit of L. Development
Screening Test for Auditory Comprehension of L.
Sequenced Inventory of L. Development
Sheffield Screening Test for Acquired L. Disorders
Slosson Articulation Language Test with Phonology
slow expressive language development
specific expressive language impairment
specific language disorder
speech and language impaired
speech and language pathologist
speech and language pathology
Speech and L. Screening Questionnaire
standard language test for aphasia
Stephens Oral L. Screening Test
String-Oriented Symbolic L.
Structure Photographic Expressive L. Test-II
STYCAR L. Test
Test of Adolescent L.
Test of L. Competence
Test of Early L. Development, Second Edition
Test of Pragmatic L.
Tests for Auditory Comprehension of L.
Test of Written L.
The Primary L. Screen
Unified Medical L. System
Utah Test of L. Development
Vane Evaluation of L. Scale
Verbal L. Development Scale
Zimmerman Preschool L. Scale

lanolin
anhydrous l.

lap
l. Nissen
l. sponge
sponge and lap count

laparoscope
flexible video l.

laparoscopic
l. adrenalectomy
l. antireflux surgery
l. appendectomy
l. approach
l. bilateral partial salpingectomy
l. bladder neck suspension
l. Burch procedure
l. cholecystectomy
l. common duct exploration
complete laparoscopic distal pancreatectomy
l. contact ultrasonography
l. donor nephrectomy
l. evaluation
l. examination
l. exploration of the common bile duct
extraperitoneal laparoscopic bladder neck suspension
l. fundoplication
l. gallbladder surgery
l. guidance
hand-assisted laparoscopic radical nephrectomy
hand-assisted laparoscopic surgery
l. inguinal herniorrhaphy
l. intracorporeal ultrasonography
l. intraoperative ultrasound
l. laser cholecystectomy
laser laparoscopic cholecystectomy
minimally invasive laparoscopic surgery
Munro and Parker classification for laparoscopic hysterectomy
l. Nissen fundoplication
l. orchiopexy
l. paraesophageal hernia repair
l. pelvic lymphadenectomy
l. pelvic lymph node dissection
l. radical nephrectomy
l. radical prostatectomy
l. repair of paraesophageal hernia
l. resection of the ureterosacral ligament
l. supracervical hysterectomy
l. technique
total extraperitoneal laparoscopic hernia repair
l. total occlusion
transabdominal preperitoneal laparoscopic hernia repair

l. transcystic common bile duct exploration
l. transcystic lithotripsy
transperitoneal laparoscopic adrenalectomy
transperitoneal laparoscopic nephrectomy
l. trocar
l. tubal banding
l. tubal cautery
l. tubal coagulation
l. tubal ligation
l. tubal sterilization

laparoscopically
l. assisted distal partial gastrectomy
l. assisted surgery

laparoscopic-assisted
l.-a. abdominal hysterectomy
l.-a. approach
l.-a. hepatectomy
l.-a. vaginal hysterectomy
l.-a. vaginal hysteroscopy

laparoscopy
diagnostic l.
hand-assisted l.
office laparoscopy under local anesthesia
standard l.

laparotomy
exploratory l.
second-look l.

Laplacian
body surface Laplacian mapping

lapse
l. into heightened irritability
momentary lapse of awareness
momentary lapse in normal breathing
time l.

large
l. amount
l. amplitude, slow wave activity
anaplastic large cell lymphoma
angiotropic large cell lymphoma
l. B-cell lymphoma
benign polyps of large intestine
l. bile duct
l. bowel obstruction
l. calorie
l. cell anaplastic lymphoma
l. cell calcifying Sertoli cell tumor
l. cell change
l. cell lung carcinoma
l. cell lymphoma
l. cell neuroendocrine carcinoma
l. cell non-Hodgkin lymphoma
l. chromophobe
l. cleaved cell
l. for date
l. dense-cored vesicle
diffuse large B-cell lymphoma
extra l.
l. field of view
folds of large intestine
follicular large cell lymphoma
full-term, large for gestational age
l. for gestational age
l. glucagon immunoreactivity
l. granular leukocyte
l. granular lymphocyte
l. granular vesicle
l. green soft stool
l. inguinal hernia sac
l. intestinal descending colon
large-base quad cane
limited-stage diffuse large cell lymphoma
l. local reaction
l. loop excision of transformation zone/loop electrosurgical excision procedure
l. loop excision of transition zone
l. lymphocyte
l. magnitude voluntary heart rate changes
mediastinal large B-cell lymphoma
l. and medium lymphocyte
mixed small cleaved and large cell lymphoma
l. motile cell
mucosa of large intestine
mucosal surface of large intestine
muscular coat of large intestine
muscular layer of large intestine
l. neuronal polypeptide
l. neutral amino acid
l. noncleaved
null cell anaplastic large cell lymphoma
l. number hypothesis
l. opaque vesicle
l. operable breast cancer
papillary adenoma of large intestine
patient vomited large quantities of blood
polyp of large intestine
primary cutaneous large B-cell lymphoma
primary mediastinal large cell lymphoma with sclerosis
rapid ingestion of large amounts of food
l. reticulocyte
secondary cutaneous large B-cell lymphoma
serosa of large intestine
l. transformed cell
undifferentiated large cell carcinoma
l. unilamellar vesicle
l. unstained cell
very large scale integration
l. vessel hematocrit
l. whirlpool
l. white kidney
l. yellow soft stools

large-core needle biopsy

large-needle aspiration biopsy

large-plaque
parapsoriasis l.-p.

large-scale integration

largest tumor dimension

large-vessel infarction

large-volume
l.-v. leukapheresis
l.-v. paracentesis
l.-v. parenteral infusion

larva
hookworm l.
neural larva migrans
ocular l.
visceral larva migrans

laryngeal
l. adductor reflex
allergic laryngeal edema
l. anesthesia
anomalous nonrecurrent right inferior laryngeal nerve
appendix of laryngeal ventricle
l. atresia
Composite L. Recurrence Staging System
l. cough reflex test
l. electromyography
epithelial hyperplastic laryngeal lesion
external branch of superior l.
l. fold
gastric laryngeal mask airway
l. granuloma
human laryngeal tumor cell

laryngeal *(continued)*
hyperemic laryngeal mucosa
l. infection
internal branch of superior laryngeal nerve
l. intraepithelial neoplasia
juvenile laryngeal papilloma
Luschka laryngeal cartilage
l. mask airway
maximum laryngeal height
l. melanosis
minimum laryngeal height
l. muscle
l. neoplasm
pharyngeal branch of recurrent laryngeal nerve
recurrent laryngeal nerve
l. saccule
sarcoma, breast and brain tumors, leukemia, laryngeal and lung cancer adenoma
l. squamous cell carcinoma
superior internal laryngeal nerve
l. tracheal anesthesia
transairway laryngeal control
l. vestibule

laryngectomy
anterior partial l.
subtotal supraglottic l.
supraglottic horizontal l.
total glottic transverse l.

laryngology
ophthalmology, otology, laryngology, and rhinology
otology, laryngology, and rhinology

laryngopharyngeal sensory stimulation

laryngopharyngectomy
partial l.
total l.

laryngoplasty
transnasal fiberoptic l.

laryngoscope
fiberoptic l.

laryngoscopy
direct l.
direct laryngoscopy and bronchoscopy
fiberoptic l.

laryngotomy
subhyoid l.
thyrohyoid l.

laryngotracheal
l. applicator
l. reconstruction
l. stenosis

laryngotracheitis
avian infectious l.
avian infectious laryngotracheitis virus

laryngotracheobronchitis
acute l.

larynx
anterior commissure of l.
appendix of ventricle of l.
atresia of l.
atrium of l.
electronic artificial l.
lymphatic follicle of l.
malignant neoplasm of l.
mucosa of l.
muscle of l.
polyp of l.
saccule of l.
verruca vulgaris of the l.
vestibule of l.

laser
l. ablation
l. adjustable silicone gastric banding
aggressive laser treatment
alexandrite laser lithotripsy
alexandrite long-pulsed l.
argon l.
argon-fluoride excimer l.
argon-krypton l.
argon laser coagulator
argon laser endophotocoagulation
argon laser iridectomy
argon laser iridotomy
argon laser peripheral iridoplasty
argon laser photocoagulation
argon laser therapy
argon laser trabeculectomy
argon laser trabeculopexy
argon laser trabeculoplasty
argon-pumped dye l.
argon-pumped tunable-dye l.
argon tuneable dye l.
arthroscopic laser instrument
arthroscopic laser surgery
arthroscopic lumbar laser diskectomy
Aurora diode soft-tissue l.
automated laser keratomileusis
carbon dioxide gas l.
carbon dioxide laser skin resurfacing
carbon dioxide laser vaporization
l. cell and flare meter
l. coagulation vaporization procedure
computed tomography laser mammography
computer assisted stereotactic laser microsurgery
computer guided laser beam
confocal laser scanning microscopy
contact laser ablation of prostate
contact laser vaporization of the prostate
contact transscleral laser cytophotocoagulation
continuous wave laser ablation
l. correlational spectroscopy
cryosurgery and laser therapy
l. desorption/ionization time-of-flight-mass spectrometer
l. destruction of intraepithelial neoplasia
diode laser trabeculoplasty
l. Doppler anemometry
l. Doppler flowmetry
l. Doppler flux
l. Doppler velocimetry
endometrial laser intrauterine thermal therapy
endonasal laser dacryocystorhinostomy
endoscopic laser foraminotomy
endoscopic laser recanalization
endoscopic laser therapy
endoscopic pulsed dye l.
endoscopic pulsed dye laser lithotripsy
excimer laser ablation
excimer laser coronary angioplasty
excimer laser photorefractive keratectomy
excimer laser phototherapeutic keratectomy
excimer laser, rotational atherectomy, and balloon angioplasty
face laser skin resurfacing
l. flare meter
flashlamp pulsed dye l.
flashlamp-pumped pulsed dye l.
l. gas
l. glaucoma surgery
grid laser photocoagulation
heart laser revascularization
l. heart surgery
high-energy pulsed ruby l.

holmium laser resection of the prostate
holmium YAG l.
holmium yttrium-aluminum garnet l.
hot tip laser probe
l. image custom arthroplasty
l. interference acuity
interstitial laser ablation of the prostate
interstitial laser coagulation of the prostate
interstitial laser photocoagulation
intracorporeal laser lithotripsy
intralesional laser photocoagulation
l. iridotomy
l. irradiation
l. laparoscopic cholecystectomy
laparoscopic laser cholecystectomy
light argon laser burn
liquid organic dye l.
l. lithotripsy
long-pulsed potassium-titanyl-phosphate l.
low-angle laser light scattering
low-energy l.
low-intensity laser irradiation
low-level laser therapy
March laser sclerostomy needle
matrix-assisted laser desorption and ionization mass spectrometry
matrix-assisted laser desorption ionization-time-of-flight mass spectrometry
MC-7000 multi-wavelength l.
MC-7000 ophthalmic l.
medical free electron l.
l. microprobe mass analyzer
mode-locked Nd:YAG l.
mucosal intact laser tonsillar ablation
Multipulse cosmetic treatment l.
MultiPulse laser system
myocardial laser revascularization
Nanolas Nd:YAG l.
Nd:YAG laser ablation
Nd:YAG laser cyclophotocoagulation
neodymium:yttrium aluminum garnet l.
neodymium: yttrium-lithium-fluoride laser
neodymium:yttrium lithium fluoride l.
neodymium:yttrium-lithium-fluoride photodisruptive l.
Nerve Fiber Analyzer laser ophthalmoscope
noncontact holmium:yttrium-argon-garnet laser thermal keratoplasty
normal-mode ruby l.
Nuvolase 660 laser system
OcuLight SL diode l.
l. office ventilation of ears with insertion of tubes
Ophthalas argon l.
ophthalmic laser microendoscope
orange dye l.
pancreatoscopic laser lithotripsy
panretinal argon laser photocoagulation
pediatric three-mirror laser lens
percutaneous excimer laser coronary angioplasty
percutaneous excimer laser coronary angioplasty system
percutaneous laser diskectomy
percutaneous transmyocardial laser revascularization
peripheral excimer laser angioplasty
l. peripheral iridectomy
peripheral laser angioplasty
l. photocoagulation of the communicating vessel
potassium titanyl phosphate l.
pulsed laser ablation
Q-switched neodymium:YAG l.
Q-switched ruby l.
quasielastic laser light-scattering spectroscope
red laser illumination
l. resection
l. resurfacing
scanning laser acoustic microscope
scanning laser ophthalmoscope
scanning laser tomography
selective laser trabeculoplasty
l. skin resurfacing
smooth excimer laser coronary angioplasty
Spectranetics laser sheath
surface enhanced laser desorption/ionization
l. surgery
l. therapy
l. therapy of hemorrhoid
l. thermal keratoplasty
thermal laser keratoplasty
l. tissue interaction
l. tomography scanner
l. trabeculoplasty
transconjunctival blepharoplasty laser resurfacing
transmyocardial laser revascularization
l. transmyocardial revascularization
l. uterosacral nerve ablation
l. uvulopalatoplasty
l. vaporization and excisional conization
vaporization laser ablation of prostate
l. vision correction
visual laser ablation of prostate
xenon arc l.
yttrium-aluminum-garnet laser

laser-assisted
l.-a. balloon angioplasty
l.-a. intrastromal keratomileusis
l.-a. microanastomosis
l.-a. myringotomy
l.-a. palatoplasty
same-day microsurgical arthroscopic lateral-approach l.-a.
l.-a. in situ keratomileusis
l.-a. spinal endoscopy
l.-a. uvulopalatoplasty
l.-a. vasal anastomosis
l.-a. vascular anastomosis

laser-capture microdissection

laser-indirect ophthalmoscope

laser-induced
l.-i. arterial fluorescence
l.-i. fluorescence
l.-i. fluorescence emission
l.-i. fluorescence spectroscopy
l.-i. intracorporeal shock wave lithotripsy
l.-i. thermography
l.-i. thermotherapy

laser-scanning confocal microscopy

lash
brows, lids, and lashes
lids, l.'s, and adnexa
lids, l.'s, lacrimals, lymphatics
l. margin
misdirected l.

L-asparaginase and methotrexate

Lassa fever virus

last
l. body mass index
l. bowel movement
date of last drink
date of last menstrual period

last *(continued)*
l. dose
first day of last menstrual period
l. living breath
l. menstrual period
l. normal vertebra
l. Pap smear
l. sexual contact
since last visit

lasting impression of impending failure

last-observation-carried-forward

lata
autogenous fascia lata sling procedure
falciform fold of fascia l.
fascia lata graft
pedicled fascia lata musculocutaneous flap
perianal condylomata l.

latae
tensor fasciae latae muscle

Latarjet
nerve of L.

late
l. abortion
l. ambulatory monitoring
l. antigen
l. asthmatic response
l. auditory evoked response
l. central nervous system toxicity
l. clamped umbilical cord
l. cortical cerebellar atrophy
l. cortical response
l. cutaneous anaphylactic reaction
l. deceleration
l. dedifferentiation
l. diastolic potential
l. distal cortical tubule
l. dumping syndrome
l. effects of normal tissue
l. fetal death
l. generalized tuberculosis
l. graft rejection
l. healed
l. immunoglobulin deficiency
l. infantile amaurotic familial idiocy
l. infantile neural ceroid lipofuscinosis
l. latent
l. luteal phase dysphoric disorder
metabolic toxemia of late pregnancy
l. neurological toxicity
nurse's late entry
l. positive component
l. postoperative suture adjustment
l. postpartum hemorrhage
l. progressing stroke
l. proximal cortical tubule
l. respiratory systemic syndrome
l. systolic click
l. systolic murmur
ventricular late potential
very late activation
very late antigen-4
Williams syndrome, late puberty

late-age
gait disorder, autoantibody, late-age onset, polyneuropathy

latency
absolute l.
auditory middle latency response
daytime multiple sleep latency test
distal motor l.
distal sensory l.
marked l.
mean latency time
middle latency response
motor l.
Multiple Sleep L. Test
peak latencies of pattern electroretinogram
l. period
pudendal-nerve terminal motor l.
l. reaction
l. relaxation
sensory l.
terminal l.
terminal motor l.
terminal sensory l.

latency-associated
l.-a. nuclear antigen
l.-a. peptide
l.-a. transcript

latent
Arracacha latent virus
l. autoimmune diabetes of adult
l. cardiomyopathy
l. class analysis
early l.
l. gout
l. homosexuality
l. hypermetropia
l. infection
l. iron-binding capacity
late l.
l. membrane protein-1
l. nuclear antigen
l. nystagmus
l. period
l. primary malignancy
l. schizophrenia
specific latent heat
l. syphilis

late-onset
l.-o. agammaglobulinemia
l.-o. Alzheimer disease
l.-o. hepatic failure

late-phase
l.-p. cutaneous reaction
l.-p. response

late progressing stroke

later
adjustment reaction of later life
l. onset nephrotic syndrome

lateral
l. abdominal region
acute lateral sclerosis
amyotrophic lateral sclerosis
l. amyotrophic sclerosis
angle of lateral eye
anterior lateral malleolar artery
anterior lateral myocardial infarct
anterior lateral myocardial infarction
anterior lateral nasal branch of anterior ethmoidal artery
anterior ramus of lateral sulcus of cerebrum
anteroposterior and l.
anteroposterior lateral sway
anteroposterior and lateral views
l. apical
AP and lateral view
articular facet of lateral malleolus
ascending ramus of lateral sulcus of cerebrum
l. atrial tunnel
atrium of lateral ventricle
Aufranc lateral approach
Axer lateral opening wedge osteotomy
l. basal
l. bending
l. border
l. cervical nucleus
cistern of lateral fossa of cerebrum
l. collateral ligament of ankle
l. collateral ligament complex

common palmar digital nerve of lateral plantar nerves
l. compartment reconstruction
l. compression
l. condylar fracture
l. condyle of femur
l. condyle of humerus
l. condyle of tibia
l. cortex
l. cricoarytenoid
cross-table lateral position
cross-table lateral view
l. crural steal
l. cutaneous branch
l. cutaneous nerve of calf
l. cutaneous nerve of forearm
l. cutaneous nerve of thigh
l. decubitus film
l. decubitus position
l. decubitus radiograph
l. deviation
l. disc attachment
l. distant view
L. Dominance Examination
dorsal lateral geniculate
elastic knee cage with medial and lateral contoured knee joints
l. electrical spine stimulation
l. electrical surface stimulation
elongation, derotation and lateral flexion
exaggerated craniocaudal lateral angle
exaggerated craniocaudal lateral view
excessive lateral pressure syndrome
extended lateral arm free flap
l. eye movement
l. facet syndrome
l. facial dysplasia
familial amyotrophic lateral sclerosis
far lateral inferior suboccipital approach
l. femoral cutaneous
l. femoral torsion
l. flank incision
l. force microscopy
l. frontal bone window
l. gaze
l. geniculate body
l. geniculate nucleus
l. giant fiber
gliosis of lateral column
l. ground
l. habenular
l. head displacement
l. head of malleolus
l. hemianopia
hemicentral, l.
l. hemisphere
high lateral tension
l. horn
l. hypothalamic area
l. hypothalamic nucleus
l. hypothalamic syndrome
l. hypothalamus
l. illumination
l. to the incision
inferior lateral angle
l. instability
l. intercellular space
l. joint line
left lateral bending
left lateral border
left lateral decubitus muscle
left lateral decubitus position
left lateral flexion
left lateral gaze
left lateral rectus eye muscle
left lateral thigh
left lateral ventricular preexcitation
long external lateral ligament
l. loop suspensor
lower fossa active, lateral knee pain, and long leg on the side ipsilateral to the weak fossa
lower lateral cutaneous nerve of arm
l. malleolus
l. margin of kidney
l. medullary infarction
l. medullary syndrome
l. meniscectomy
l. meniscus
l. motor column
l. nail fold
l. nasal fold
l. nuclear stratum
l. oblique x-ray view
l. olfactory tract
PA and lateral projection
Parkinson disease and lateral sclerosis-dementia complex
l. pharyngeal space
l. pharyngeal wall
l. plantar
popliteal lateral nerve
l. position test
l. posterior choroidal
posteroanterior and l.
l. preoptic area
primary lateral sclerosis
l. projection
l. pterygoid muscle
l. pterygoid plate
l. pylorus
l. recess stenosis
l. recess syndrome
l. rectus, both eyes
l. rectus eye muscle
l. rectus incision
l. reticular nucleus
right l.
right lateral bending
right lateral decubital position
right lateral femoral
right lateral gaze
right lateral position
right lateral thigh
right lateral rectus muscle
right upper l.
l. rotation
l. sacral vein
l. septal
l. sinus thrombophlebitis
slow lateral eye movement
l. spinothalamic tract
subcutaneous bursa of lateral malleolus
superficial branch of lateral plantar nerve
l. superior olive
l. suspensor ligament
l. talocalcaneal angle
l. talocalcaneal ligament
l. thoracic arteries
thoracolumbosacral orthosis—flexion, extension, lateral bending, and transverse rotation
l. tibial plateau
l. tibial torsion
torn lateral meniscus
l. ulnar collateral ligament
l. vaginal wall
l. venous sinus
l. ventricle
l. ventricular nerve
l. ventricular width to hemispheric width
l. ventromedial nucleus
l. vestibular nucleus
l. vestibulospinal tract
l. wall ischemia
l. wall pressure

laterality

atlas l.

laterality *(continued)*
cognitive laterality quotient
l. index

lateralization
PAC lateralization ratio

lateralized
l. headache
pseudoperiodic lateralized paroxysmal discharge

lateralizing
bilateral independent periodic lateralizing epileptiform discharge
l. and localizing
periodic lateralizing epileptiform discharge

lateral-opposed beam

lateral-view dual-energy radiography

laterothoracic
unilateral laterothoracic exanthem

late-stage heart failure

latex
l. agglutination
l. agglutination-inhibition test
l. allergy
l. condom
direct latex agglutination pregnancy test
l. direct agglutination reaction
l. ELISA for antigen protein
l. fixation
l. fixation test
l. flocculation test
monoclonal antibody-based latex agglutination
natural rubber latex allergy
l. particle
l. particle agglutination
l. particle agglutination inhibition
polystyrene latex particle
l. and resorcinol formaldehyde
reversed passive latex particle agglutination
severe latex allergy
slide latex agglutination

Latin
L. American female
L. American male

Latino virus

latissimus
anterior latissimus dorsi
l. dorsi
l. dorsi fasciocutaneous flap
l. dorsi muscle
l. dorsi musculocutaneous flap
l. dorsi myocutaneous flap
pedicled endoscopic latissimus dorsi harvest
posterior latissimus dorsi muscle
total autogenous l.

lattice
antigenic antibody lattice formation
l. corneal dystrophy
l. degeneration of retina
fibroblast-populated collagen l.

laughing
l. gas
inappropriate l.
l. out loud

laughs
patient laughs inappropriately

laughter
hysterical l.

laurel
oil of cherry l.

Laurence-Moon-Biedl-Bardet syndrome

Laurence-Moon-Biedl syndrome

Laurence-Moon syndrome

lavage
arthroscopic lysis and l.
bovine lavage extract surfactant
bronchial l.
bronchoalveolar l.
bronchoalveolar lavage fluid
continuous pericardial l.
continuous postoperative closed l.
copious lavage of joint
copious lavage performed
copious peritoneal l.
cow lung l.
diagnostic peritoneal l.
ductal lavage fluid
l. fluid
gastric l.
gastric lavage tube
nasocystic catheter l.
oral colonic l.
polyethylene glycol electrolyte lavage solution
protected bronchoalveolar l.

lavaged
area lavaged with sterile saline

law
all-or-none l.
Ångström l.
Arndt l.
assimilation l.
autonomic affective l.
common law marriage
l. of the heart
Henry l.
l. of initial value
Listing l.
Louis l.
Marey l.
Marfan l.
Mariotte l.
mass action l.
Mendel first l.
Mendel second l.
mental health l.
Müller l.
National Center on Poverty L., Inc.
Ohm l.
paradoxical l.
Poiseuille l.
Sherrington l.
Starling l.
wallerian l.
Weber l.

Lawrence Experimental Station agar

laxa
skeletal abnormalities, cutis laxa, craniostenosis, psychomotor retardation, facial abnormalities

laxative
l. abuse
l. abuse syndrome
aloin, belladonna, strychnine laxative
bath, laxative, enema, shampoo, and shower
l. of choice
l. dependence

laxity
arthrometric knee laxity measurement
collateral ligament l.
cruciate ligament l.
lower lid l.
mental retardation, overgrowth, craniosynostosis, distal arthrogryposis, sacral dimple, joint l.
pelvic muscle l.
spondyloepimetaphyseal dysplasia with joint l.

layer
abdomen closed in l.'s
anterior elastic l.
anterior layer of rectus abdominis sheath

anterior layer of thoracolumbar fascia
anterior limiting layer of cornea
aqueous layer of tear film
aqueous tear l.
cartilage intermediate layer protein
chest closed in anatomic l.'s
closed in anatomic l.'s
copper half-value l.
external muscle layer damaged
external plexiform l.
germinal layer hemorrhage
glomerular l.
granular l.
granular cell l.
half-value l.
hypertrophic smooth muscle l.
incision closed in l.'s
inner plexiform l.
leukocyte feeder l.
lining cell layer hyperplasia
lipid tear l.
longitudinal layer of muscle coat of small intestine
longitudinal layer of muscular coat
long pitch helicoidal l.
massive all layer liposuction
medial cartilaginous l.
membranous layer of subcutaneous tissue of abdomen
membranous layer of superficial fascia
membranous layer of superficial fascia of perineum
meningeal layer of dura mater
mesothelial cell l.
middle gray layer of superior colliculus
mitral cell l.
molecular l.
molecular external l.
molecular inner l.
molecular internal l.
molecular layer of cerebellar cortex
molecular layer of cerebral cortex
molecular layer of retina
molecular outer l.
mucous tear l.
muscle layer in fatty layer of subcutaneous tissue
muscular l.
muscular layer of bronchi
muscular layer of colon
muscular layer of ductus deferens
muscular layer of esophagus
muscular layer of female urethra
muscular layer of gallbladder
muscular layer of intermediate part of male urethra
muscular layer of large intestine
muscular layer of mucosa
muscular layer of pharynx
muscular layer of prostatic urethra
muscular layer of rectum
muscular layer of renal pelvis
muscular layer of seminal gland
muscular layer of small intestine
muscular layer of stomach
muscular layer of trachea
muscular layer of ureter
muscular layer of urinary bladder
muscular layer of uterine tube
muscular layer of vagina
nerve fiber bundle l.
nerve fiber layer analyzer
nerve fiber layer dropout
nerve fiber layer hemorrhage
nerve fiber layer infarct
nerve layer of retina
neural layer of optic part of retina
neuroepithelial layer of retina
nuclear external l.
nuclear inner l.
nuclear internal l.
nuclear outer l.
oblique fibers of muscular layer of stomach
olfactory nerve l.
orbital layer of ethmoid bone
outer fibrous l.
outer nuclear l.
outer plexiform l.
palisaded dentinoblastic l.
parabasal cell l.'s
parietal layer of leptomeninges
parietal layer of serous pericardium
parietal layer of tunica vaginalis of testis
perforated layer of sclera
periosteal cambium l.
periosteal layer of dura mater
peripapillary nerve fiber l.
pigmented layer of ciliary body
pigmented layer of iris
pigmented layer of retina
plexiform layer of cerebral cortex
porous layer bead
posterior collagenous l.
Purkinje l.
pyramidal cell l.
retinal nerve fiber l.
seromuscular l.
spongy layer of female urethra
spongy layer of vagina
tenth value layer radiation
turbid, no creamy l.
unstirred water l.
visceral layer of serous pericardium

4-layer bandage

laying

lay-on graft

Lazare-Klerman-Armour Personality Inventory

Lazaro

mal de San L.

lazy-H incision

lazy leukocyte syndrome

lazy-S incision

lazy-Z incision

LCx

automated LCx factor V Leiden assay

L-dopa

on-off effect of L.-d.

Le

L. Dantec virus
L. Fort classification
L. Fort fracture
L. Fort osteotomy

lead

acute lead poisoning
l. apron shield
augmented voltage unipolar left arm l.
augmented voltage unipolar left foot l.
augmented voltage unipolar right arm l.
aVF l.
aVL l.
aVR l.
blood lead level
chest and left leg lead in electrocardiography
electrocardiographic l.
elevation of blood lead level
endocardial balloon l.
fishhook l.
l. gout
high-velocity lead therapy

lead *(continued)*
indirect l.
intercostal position for chest l.
l. intoxication
intracardiac l.
l. level in blood
limb lead two
l. locking device
modified chest l.
l. monoxide
organic l.
pacemaker l.
pacemaker lead fracture
pacing l.
l. poisoning
poor progression of R wave in precordial l.'s
precordial l.
l. shielding in radiation
l. tetraacetate Schiff
tetraethyl l.
tetramethyl l.
transvenous defibrillation l.
tripolar l.
unipolar chest l.
unipolar limb l.
unipolar precordial l.

16-lead electrocardiogram

leader
authoritarian l.
L. Behavior Analysis II
L. Behavior Description Questionnaire

leading pole

leaf
ash leaf patch
ash leaf spot
l. of broad ligament
l. of diaphragm
maple leaf flap
palm leaf pattern

leaflet
anterior leaflet of the mitral valve
anterior leaflet prolapse
anterior mitral l.
anterior mitral valve l.
anterior motion of posterior mitral valve l.
anterior tricuspid l.
anterior tricuspid valve l.
aortic valve l.
aortic valve leaflet prolapse
apoon-like protrusion of l.
apposition of l.
arching of mitral valve l.
billowing mitral leaflet syndrome
bowing of mitral valve l.
flail mitral l.
incomplete mitral leaflet closure
medication information leaflet for seniors
mitral leaflet syndrome
mitral valve anterior l.
mitral valve leaflet excursion
patient information l.
posterior leaflet motion
posterior mitral valve l.
posterior tricuspid valve l.
prolapsing mitral l.
tricuspid valvular l.

leafspring
plastic l.
posterior leafspring orthosis

league
Little League elbow
Little League shoulder
National Urban L.
Older Women's L.

leak
air l.
anastomotic l.
anastomotic stump l.
aortic paravalvular l.
ascites due to bile l.
capillary leak syndrome
cerebrospinal fluid l.
Luschka duct l.
macular l.
neonatal air leak syndrome
perivalvular l.
l. point pressure
spinal fluid l.
systemic capillary leak syndrome
Valsalva leak point pressure
vascular leak syndrome

leakage
anastomotic l.
biliary l.
contrast media l.
microaneurysmal l.
parafoveal microvascular l.
perivalvular l.
placental l.
pulmonary capillary protein l.

leaking
arteriovenous l.
l. breast implant
l. of fluid
l. heart valve
intraocular leaking wound

leaky
l. heart valve
l. saline implant

lean
antalgic l.
l. body mass
l. body muscle mass
l. body weight
squarely face person, open posture, lean toward person, eye contact, relaxed
l. tissue

leaping atrophy

Learner
Self-Concept as a L.

learner
auditory l.

learning
l. ability
Adult Basic L. Examination
appropriate learning experience
arithmetical skills learning retardation
Assessment Program of Early L. Levels
avoidance and escape l.
Barclay Learning Needs Assessment Inventory
Blind Learning Aptitude Test
California Verbal L. Test
cataract, motor system disorder, short stature, learning difficulty, skeletal abnormalities syndrome
Children's Auditory Verbal L. Test-2
computer-assisted l.
Cornell L. and Study Skills Inventory
Detroit Tests of L. Aptitude - Primary, Second Edition
Detroit Tests of L. Aptitude, Third Edition
Developmental Indicators for Assessment of L.
developmental learning problem
l. disability
L. Disability Evaluation Scale
l. disabled
l. disorder
emotionally disturbed and learning disabled
Estimated L. Potential
l. handicap
Hawaii Early L. Profile
Health Evaluation and L. Program

heart rate control learning and awareness
Hiskey-Nebraska Test of L. Aptitude
l. impaired
Individual L. Disabilities Classroom Screening Instrument
L. Inventory of Kindergarten Experiences
Modified Word L. Test
Mullen Scales of Early L.
Names L. Test
National Joint Committee on L. Disabilities
paired associate l.
Paired Associate L. Subtest
Paired Associate L. Task
Rey Auditory Verbal L. Test
Rey Auditory Verbal L. Test
Riley Inventory of Basic L. Skills
Scales of Creativity and L. Environment
self-directed l.
L. and Study Strategies Inventory
L. Style Profile
Test of L. Accuracy in Children
Vocational L. Styles
Wide Range Assessment of Memory and L.

least
l. common factor
l. fatal dose
linear-nonlinear least squares
nonlinear least squares regression analysis
nonlinear least squares method
ordinary least squares
l. restrictive environment
l. significant change
l. significant difference
l. square
l. squares mean
weighted nonlinear least squares

leave
l. of absence
absent without l.
community leave for reorientation
Family and Medical Leave Act of 1993
l. on floor
l. on pass
temporary leave of absence
trial l.
unauthorized l.
l. without consent

leaving
quiescent phase of cells leaving the mitotic cycle

Leber
amaurosis congenita of L.
L. congenital amaurosis
L. hereditary optic neuropathy
L. optic atrophy

Lebombo virus

lecithin
cardiolipin natural l.
cardiolipin synthetic l.
egg l.
soybean l.
l. to sphingomyelin

lectin
mammalian binding lectin deficiency
mannan-binding lectin deficiency
mannose-binding l.
mitogenic adherence l.

LeDuc ureteral anastomosis

Lee
L. and Desus D test
L. double-loop locking suture

leech
American l.
artificial l.

Lee-White
L.-W. blood clotting method
L.-W. tritium clotting time

left
l. abdomen
abdominal left ventricular assist device
l. abdominal pain
abnormal left axis deviation
l. acromiodorsoanterior position of fetus
l. acromiodorsoposterior position of fetus
acute left ventricular heart failure
akinetic left ventricle
l. angle
l. angulation
anomalous left coronary artery
anomalous left coronary artery from pulmonary artery
anomalous left coronary artery from pulmonary artery syndrome
anomalous left main coronary artery
anomalous left pulmonary artery
anomalous origin of left coronary artery from pulmonary artery
l. antecubital
l. anterior bundle-branch block
anterior cusp of left atrioventricular valve
l. anterior descending coronary artery
l. anterior fascicular block
l. anterior hemiblock
l. anterior internal diameter
anterior interventricular branch of left coronary artery
l. anterior measurement
l. anterior oblique projection
l. anterior occipital
anterior portion of left medial segment IV of liver
l. anterior small thoracotomy
l. anterior spinal artery
l. anterior superior
l. anterior-superior fascicular block
l. anterior-superior hemiblock
l. anterior thigh
l. anterosuperior hemiblock
aortic impression of left lung
aortic and left ventricular tunnel
l. apexcardiogram, calibrated displacement
apex of left ventricle
apical left ventricular puncture
apical thickening of left ventricle
apicoposterior branch of left superior pulmonary vein
l. arm electrode for electrocardiogram
l. arm hemiparesis
l. arm, reclining
l. arm, recumbent
l. arm, sitting
artificial left heart pump
artificial left ventricular assist device
l. atrial abnormality
atrial anastomotic branch of circumflex branch of left coronary artery
l. atrial appendage
l. atrial ball-valve thrombus
l. atrial contraction
l. atrial diameter
l. atrial dimension
l. atrial emptying index
l. atrial end-diastolic pressure
l. atrial end-diastolic volume
l. atrial end-systolic volume
l. atrial enlargement
l. atrial function

left *(continued)*
l. atrial hypertension
l. atrial hypertrophy
l. atrial involvement
l. atrial isolation procedure
l. atrial isomerism
l. atrial myxoma
l. atrial neovascularization
l. atrial overloading
l. atrial posterior wall
l. atrial spontaneous echo contrast
l. atrial transesophageal pacing test
l. atrial transmural pressure
l. atrium of heart
augmented voltage unipolar left arm lead
augmented voltage unipolar left foot lead
l. auricle
auricle of left atrium
l. auricular appendage
axial left anterior oblique ventriculogram
l. axillary line
l. axis deviation, minimal
l. basal artery
l. and below
l. border of cardiac dullness
l. border dullness of heart to percussion
borderline left axis deviation
l. in bottle
l. brachial vein occlusion
l. brain damage
l. breast biopsy
l. breast biopsy examination
l. bundle
l. bundle-branch system block
l. buttock
cardiac notch of left lung
l. cardiac sympathetic ganglionectomy
l. carotid artery
l. carotid endarterectomy
l. caudal quarter ganglion
l. caudate nucleus
l. cerebral hemisphere
chest and left arm
chest and left leg lead in electrocardiography
l. circumflex artery
l. circumflex coronary artery
l. circumflex marginal
l. common carotid artery
l. common femoral artery
complete left bundle-branch block
complete left bundle branch block
concentric left ventricular hypertrophy
l. coronary angiography
l. coronary artery
l. coronary cusp
l. coronary sinus
l. coronary vein
l. costal border
l. costal margin
l. to count
l. deltoid
l. deviation of electrical axis
deviation to the l.
dextroduction of left eye
diaphragmatic surface of left lung
diastolic left ventricular index
l. direct inguinal hernia
l. dorsoanterior
l. dorsoposterior
l. dorsotransverse fetal position
dullness over left lung
duplication of left collecting system
duplication of left kidney
l. ear
easy normal l.
effective refractory period of the left ventricle
end-diastolic left ventricular pressure
l. end-expiratory pressure
end-systolic left ventricular pressure
l. esotropia
l. exotropia
l. eye
l. eye patched
l. femoral artery
l. femoral hernia
fixing left eye
l. foot
l. foot switch
l. forearm
l. frontal craniotomy
l. frontal hematoma
l. frontoanterior fetal position
l. frontolateral
l. frontoposterior position fetal
l. frontotransverse fetal position
l. gastric artery
l. gastric lymph node
l. gastric vein
l. giant cell
giant left atrium
global left ventricular ejection fraction
l. gluteal
l. gluteus
l. hand
heard best at left lower sternal border
heard best at left upper sternal border
l. heart blood volume
l. heart bypass
l. heart catheterization
l. heart failure
l. heart strain
l. heel strike
l. hemicolectomy
l. hemiplegia
l. hemisphere of brain
l. hemisphere brain damage
l. hemisphere damage
l. hemisphere deficit
l. hemisphere lesion
l. hemisphere stroke
l. hepatic artery
l. hepatic duct
l. hepatic lobe
l. hepatic vein
l. hilar lymph node
l. homonymous hemianopia
l. hyperphoria
l. hypertropia
hypesthesia of left leg
l. hypochondrium
hypoplasia of left heart
hypoplastic left atrium
hypoplastic left heart syndrome
hypoplastic left ventricle
hypoplastic left ventricular syndrome
l. iliac of abdomen
l. iliac artery
l. iliac crest
l. iliac fossa
impaired left discrimination
impaired left ventricular function
implantable left ventricular assist system
incomplete left bundle-branch block
l. index finger
l. inferior oblique muscle
l. inferior rectus
l. inferior vena cava
l. injured
l. innominate vein
l. intercostal margin

l. intercostal space
l. internal carotid artery
l. internal jugular vein
l. internal mammary artery graft
l. internal thoracic artery
interstitial left ventricular myocardial fibrosis
intramural left anterior descending artery
l. involved
ischemic left ventricle
l. jugular
l. kidney
l. lateral bending
l. lateral border
l. lateral decubitus muscle
l. lateral decubitus position
l. lateral flexion
l. lateral gaze
l. lateral rectus eye muscle
l. lateral thigh
l. lateral ventricular preexcitation
l. leg electrode for electrocardiogram
ligament of left superior vena cava
ligament of left vena cava
lingula of left lung
lingular division of the left lung
l. liver lobe
l. long leg
l. lower border of cardiac dullness
l. lower extremity
lower left quadrant
l. lower leg
lower lid, left eye
lower lid, oculus sinister
l. lower limb
l. lower lobe infiltrate
l. lower lobe of lung
l. lower lung
l. lower quadrant of abdomen
l. lower scapular border
l. lower sternal border
l. lung
l. main coronary artery disease
l. main stem bronchus
l. main stem coronary artery disease
l. main trunk
marginal branch of left circumflex coronary artery
marked left ventricular hypertrophy
l. mastoid
maximal l.
maximal left atrial dimension
maximal left ventricular developed pressure
maximal spatial vector to l.
l. maximal spatial voltage
mean diastolic left ventricular pressure
mean left atrial pressure
mean left ventricular systolic pressure
l. medial rectus eye muscle
l. median
l. mediolateral episiotomy
l. mentoanterior fetal position
l. mentoposterior fetal position
l. mentotransverse fetal position
l. midclavicular line
l. middle cerebral artery
l. middle cerebral artery thrombosis
l. middle ear exploration
l. middle finger
l. middle lobe
minor axis shortening of left ventricle
l. modified radical mastectomy
negative contrast left atriography
neonatal small left colon syndrome
neutral, sidebent right, rotated l.
nonweightbearing, l.
l. oblique inguinal hernia
l. occipitoanterior fetal position
l. occipitolateral fetal position
l. occipitoposterior position
l. occipitotransverse fetal position
l. occiput posterior fetal position
occlusion of left bronchus
occlusion of left carotid artery
opening of left parotid duct
l. otitis externa
l. otitis media
outer upper left quadrant
pain down left arm
l. parasternal impulse
percutaneous left heart bypass
phacoemulsification of the left eye
pole of left kidney
poorly contractile globular left ventricle
l. portal view
l. posterior descending artery
l. posterior fascicular block
l. posterior hemiblock
l. posterior-inferior fascicular block
l. posterior inferior hemiblock
l. posterior internal carotid artery
posterior leaf mitral valve
posterior left ventricular
l. posterior measurement
l. posterior oblique
l. posterior occipital
l. posterior ventricular preexcitation
posterior wall of left ventricle
l. posterolateral
proximal left anterior descending artery
l. pulmonary artery oxygen saturation
l. radial artery
l. radical neck dissection
rate-dependent left bundle-branch block
l. rectus femoris
l. renal artery
l. renal vein
l. ring finger
l. rostral quarter ganglion
l. rotation
rotation l.
l. sacroanterior position
l. sacroposterior fetal position
l. sacrotransverse
l. sacrum
l. salpingo-oophorectomy
l. scapuloanterior
l. scapuloposterior
scleral buckle, left eye
second left interspace
l. septum
l. short leg
l. somatosensory evoked potential
spontaneous left hemothorax
l. stellate ganglionic blockade
l. sternal border
l. sternal edge
l. subclavian artery
l. subclavian central venous pressure
l. subclavian vein
l. substantia nigra
l. superior intercostal vein
l. superior oblique
l. superior rectus
l. superior vena cava
l. sympathetic nerve
total knee replacement, l.
l. transatrial septal
l. transposition of great artery
transseptal left heart catheterization

left *(continued)*
l. triceps
triple vessel disease with abnormal left ventricle
tubular hypoplasia left aortic arch
l. uninjured
l. uninvolved
unpatched left eye
unprotected left main
upper l.
l. upper arm
l. upper extremity
l. upper eyelid
upper left quadrant
upper left sternal border
l. upper limb
l. upper lobe
l. upper lung
l. upper outer buttock
l. upper outer quadrant
l. upper quadrant of abdomen
l. upper scapular border
l. upper sternal border
l. ureteral
l. ureteral orifice
l. uterine displacement device
vaccination scar upper left arm
l. vastus lateralis muscle
l. ventricle
l. ventricle to aorta pressure gradient
l. ventricle bypass pump
l. ventricle of heart
l. ventricular
l. ventricular activation time
l. ventricular aneurysm
l. ventricular aneurysmectomy
l. ventricular angiogram
l. ventricular assist device
l. ventricular bundle-branch block
l. ventricular diastolic dimension
l. ventricular diastolic volume
l. ventricular dimension in end-diastole
l. ventricular dysfunction
l. ventricular ejection
l. ventricular ejection fraction
l. ventricular ejection time
l. ventricular ejection time index
l. ventricular end-diastole
l. ventricular end-diastolic area
l. ventricular end-diastolic circumference
l. ventricular end-diastolic diameter
l. ventricular end-diastolic dimension
l. ventricular end-diastolic pressure
l. ventricular end-diastolic volume
l. ventricular end-diastolic volume index
l. ventricular end-systolic area
l. ventricular end-systolic dimension
l. ventricular end-systolic volume
l. ventricular end-systolic volume index
l. ventricular enlargement
l. ventricular failure
l. ventricular fast filling time
l. ventricular filling pressure
l. ventricular free wall
l. ventricular function
l. ventricular functional shortening
l. ventricular heart failure
l. ventricular hemodynamic abnormalities
l. ventricular hypertrophy
l. ventricular infarct volume
l. ventricular inflow volume
l. ventricular initial diastolic pressure
l. ventricular injection
l. ventricular insufficiency
l. ventricular internal diameter
l. ventricular internal diastolic diameter
l. ventricular internal diastolic dimension
l. ventricular internal dimension at end systole
l. ventricular internal dimension diastole
l. ventricular internal dimension systole
l. ventricular mass
l. ventricular mass index
l. ventricular minute flow
l. ventricular muscle mass
l. ventricular outflow
l. ventricular outflow tract obstruction
l. ventricular outflow volume
l. ventricular overactivity
l. ventricular peak filling rate
l. ventricular peak systolic pressure
l. ventricular posterior wall
l. ventricular posterior wall thickness
l. ventricular preejection period
l. ventricular reduction
l. ventricular septal wall
l. ventricular slow filling time
l. ventricular strain
l. ventricular stroke volume index
l. ventricular stroke work
l. ventricular stroke work index
l. ventricular subendocardial myocardial ischemia
l. ventricular systolic diameter
l. ventricular systolic dimension
l. ventricular systolic dysfunction
l. ventricular systolic index
l. ventricular systolic output
l. ventricular tension
l. ventricular wall motion
l. ventricular wall motion abnormality
l. ventricular wall motion index
l. ventriculogram
l. ventrogluteal
l. vertebral artery
vision left eye
visual acuity, left eye
visual acuity, left eye, left perception with projection
l. visual field
l. without completing treatment

left-hand
l.-h. dominant
l.-h. grip
l.-h. side

left-handed
l.-h. individual
patient l.-h.

left/right
angled left/right cannula

left-right shunt

left-sided
l.-s. colon cancer
l.-s. heart failure
l.-s. weakness

left-to-right
l.-t.-r. ratio
l.-t.-r. shunting
l.-t.-r. shunt ratio

leg
adjustable leg and ankle repositioning mechanism
anatomic leg length inequality
anatomic short l.
anterior compartment of l.
anterior vein of the l.
back pain extends down l.'s
bilateral leg strength
bilateral short leg cane

chest and left leg lead in electrocardiography
chronic stasis leg ulcer
claudication in the l.
cold mottled insensate l.
l. com
l. cramp
creepy-crawly syndrome of l.'s
crossed straight leg raising
cruciate ligament of l.
double seated straight leg raise
l. edema
l.'s elevated higher than heart
extensor compartment of l.
face, legs, activity, cry, consolability
fidgety leg syndrome
heaviness in l.'s
hind leg paralysis
hypesthesia of left l.
hypesthesia of right l.
immobilization of injured l.
inequality in leg length
interosseous nerve of l.
involuntary jerking movements of l.'s
ischemic leg disease
ischial weight bearing leg brace
left leg electrode for electrocardiogram
left long l.
left lower l.
left short l.
l. length discrepancy
l. length inequality
long bent-knee leg cast
long leg brace with pelvic band
long leg fiberglass cast
long leg brace with free ankle
long leg cast
long leg cylinder cast
long leg posterior molded splint
long leg sitting
long leg walking cast
long leg weightbearing cast
long leg plaster cast
lower fossa active, lateral knee pain, and long leg on the side ipsilateral to the weak fossa
lower third of leg bone
medial cutaneous nerve of l.
moving toes, painful leg syndrome
negative straight leg raise
nighttime leg cramp
nocturnal leg cramp
nocturnal leg muscle cramp
numbness in lower l.
pain down l.
painful claudication of l.
painful leg cramp
pain radiating down l.'s
passive flexion of l.
peripheral pulses palpable both l.'s
posterior compartment of l.
potassium leg cramps
l. protection factor
restless leg syndrome
reverse straight leg raise
right l.
right short leg brace
short leg brace
short leg cylinder cast
short leg nonwalking cast
short leg nonweightbearing cast
short leg posterior-molded splint
short leg walking cast
straight leg raising tenderness
straight leg raising test
straight leg raise
l. strength
subischial leg length
l. transfer device
transverse ligament of l.
l. ulcer
upper fossa active, medial knee pain, and short leg on the side ipsilateral to the weak fossa

legal
l. commitment
ethical, legal, and social implications
l. issue
l. medicine

legally
l. committed
l. incompetent patient
l. separated

legally incompetent patient

leg-curl
ankle joint l.-c.

Legg-Calvé-Perthes disease

legholder
arthroscopic l.

Legionella
atypical *Legionella*-like organism
nosocomial *Legionella*

Legionnaire
L. disease
L. disease bacillus

legislation
mental health l.

Leibovitz-Emory medium

Leiden
automated factor V Leiden mutation test
automated LCx factor V Leiden assay
factor V L.
factor V deficiency Leiden mutation
factor V Leiden carrier
factor V Leiden gene
factor V Leiden mutation test
factor V Leiden thrombophilia

leiomyoma
angiolipoma, posttraumatic neuroma, glomus tumor, eccrine spiradenoma, and leiomyoma cutis
calcified leiomyoma of uterus
l. of uterus

leiomyomatosis
intravenous l.

leiomyosarcoma
epithelioid l.
uterine l.

Leishmania
localized *Leishmania* lymphadenitis

leishmaniasis
anthroponotic cutaneous l.
antimonial drug therapy for l.
cutaneous l.
diffuse cutaneous l.
disseminated cutaneous l.
localized cutaneous l.
mucocutaneous l.
New World l.
nondisseminated cutaneous l.
Old World l.
l. recidivans
l. vaccine
visceral l.
viscerotropic l.

leisure
L. Activities Blank
alternative leisure activity
l. counseling
L. Interest Inventory

Leiter
Arthur Adaptation of the Leiter International Performance Scale
L. International Performance Scale

Lembert suture

length
anal canal l.
anatomic leg length inequality
anterior arch l.
arch length deficiency
arch length index
atrial fibrillation cycle l.
available arch l.
l. of awareness of illness
axial l.
axial length of eye
basic cycle l.
basic drive cycle l.
l., breadth, height
cleavage fragment length polymorphism
l. complexity index
l. contraction compensation element
count median l.
l. of crown
crown-heel l.
crown-rump l.
cycle l.
cycle length, paced
diagnosis responsible for length of stay
diffusion l.
echo-train l.
effective focal l.
effective mandibular l.
effective path l.
effective refractory l.
end-diastolic segment l.
end-systolic segment l.
estimated length of program
extended length of utterance
femoral l.
fetal l.
fetal foot l.
focal l.
force, velocity, l.
fracture running length of bone
functional l.
functional urethral l.
gradual increase in length and complexity of utterance
head to rump l.
humerus l.
l. of illness
inequality in leg l.
jet l.
leg length discrepancy
leg length inequality
lesion l.
limb bone length ratio
limb length inequality
long bone l.
lumbar l.
lung l.
mandibular body l.
maximal force at rest l.
mean length of response
mean length of utterance
mean sac size and crown-rump l.
mutation-enriched restriction fragment length polymorphism assay
Nance analysis of arch l.
needle cord l.
l. of operation
pacing cycle l.
palpebral fissure l.
l. of path
percent stroke l.
peripheral capillary filtration slit l.
polymerase chain reaction-restriction fragment length polymorphism
pressure length loop
restriction fragment length polymorphism
rump heel l.
safety, monitoring, intervention, length of stay, and evaluation
sinus cycle l.
sinus node cycle l.
spinal l.
subischial leg l.
total arm l.
utterance l.
ventricular tachycardia cycle l.
wave lengths of rhythmic activity

length/corneal
axial length/corneal radius ratio

lengthening
Achilles tendon l.
Armistead ulnar lengthening operation
extensor tendon l.
heel cord l.
Lynn Achilles lengthening procedure
l. osteotomy
pelvic lengthening osteotomy
percutaneous heel cord l.
surgical Achilles tendon l.
tendo Achillis l.
tendo Achillis lengthening and toe flexor release

length-tension curve

length-to-diameter ratio

Lengyeh-Kerman-Vargar rating

lens
angled lens loupe
angled-vision lens system
annular bifocal contact l.
anterior chamber intraocular l.
anterior lens capsule
anterior pole of l.
aphakic contact l.
artificial lens implant
artificial lens implantation
aspheric contact l.
aspheric spectacle l.
aspiration of l.
axis of cylindric l.
ballasted contact l.
bandage contact l.
cast resin l.
cataract lens implantation
cataract with intraocular l.
contact l.
cylindrical l.
daily-wear contact l.
daily-wear soft contact l.
ectopia of l.
endoscope lens cleansing device
l. epithelial cell
extended-wear contact l.
extended-wear soft contact l.
l. extraction
first definite apical clearance l.
foldable intraocular l.
gas permeable contact l.
hard contact l.
heparin surface-modified intraocular l.
l. implant
implantable contact l.
insertion of intraocular l.
intracapsular lens extraction
intracorneal l.
intraocular contact l.
intraocular lens implant
intraocular lens power
iris fixation l.
ligament of l.
loose contact l.
luxation of l.
macular contact l.
Meditec bandage contact l.
meniscus concave l.
microbevel edge l.
microthin contact l.
minus carrier contact l.
minus spectacle l.
modified C-loop UV l.

modified J-loop intraocular l.
modified J-loop UV l.
multicurve contact l.
multifocal spectacle l.
negative meniscus l.
nuclear sclerosis of l.
nucleus of l.
one-piece multifocal l.
one-piece plate haptic silicone intraocular l.
L. Opacification Classification System
L. Opacities Classification System II
opaque contact l.
opening through l.
optical center of spectacle l.
optical contact l.
optical zone of contact l.
optics of intraocular l.
overall diameter of contact l.
panchamber UV l.
pediatric three-mirror laser l.
pediatric vitrectomy lens set
peripheral curve on contact l.
periscopic concave l.
periscopic convex l.
posterior chamber intraocular l.
posterior chamber lens implant
posterior pole of l.
pseudoexfoliation of lens capsule
l. removal
remove and replace intraocular l.
rigid contact l.
rigid gas-permeable contact l.
secondary focal point of lens
shagreen of the l.
single lens reflex
suspensory ligament of l.
tight lens syndrome
tinted contact l.
toric contact l.
transsclerally sutured posterior chamber l.

lensectomy
pars plana l.

lens-sparing external beam radiation therapy

lenticular
aspheric lenticular area
l. capsule
l. fossa
l. glaucoma
l. loop
l. nucleus
senile lenticular myopia

lentiform bone

lentiformis
nucleus l.

lentigines
l., atrial myxomas, cutaneous papular myxomas, blue nevi
l., electrocardiographic abnormalities, ocular hypertelorism, pulmonary stenosis, abnormalities of genitalia, retardation of growth, deafness syndrome
multiple lentigines syndrome

lentiginosis
multiple l.
periorificial l.

lentigo
l. maligna melanoma
malignant lentigo melanoma
nevoid l.
nevus spilus l.
senile l.
solar l.

lentis
ectopia l.
membrana capsularis lentis posterior
nucleus l.

lentiviral
live-attenuated lentiviral vaccine

Leonard
L. cathode ray unit

Leonard cathode ray unit

Leopold maneuver

Lepore
hemoglobin L.

lepromatous
borderline l.
l. leprosy

leprosus
lichen l.
pemphigus l.

leprosy
lepromatous l.
Lucio leprosy phenomenon

leptin
maternal plasma l.

leptomeningeal
l. arachnoid cyst
arterialized leptomeningeal vein
l. metastasis

leptomeninges
parietal layer of l.

leptomeningitis
mumps l.

lesbian
gay, lesbian, bisexual

lesion
abnormal anatomic l.
acute gastric mucosal l.
admixture lesion of heart
agenesis of corpus callosum-mental retardation-osseous lesions syndrome
anal squamous intraepithelial l.
anesthetic skin l.
angel kisses l.
angiocentric immunoproliferative l.
angiocentric lymphoproliferative l.
annular constricting l.
annular distribution of l.
anterior labroligamentous periosteal sleeve avulsion l.
anterior labrum periosteum shoulder arthroscopic l.
anterior parietal l.
anular constricting l.
aortic arch l.
aortic valve l.
aplastic bone l.
arciform distribution of l.
articular cartilage l.
atherosclerotic carotid artery l.
atrophic brain l.
atrophic hyperkeratotic l.
atrophic lesion of brain
atrophie blanche l.
benign lymphoepithelial l.
benign proliferative l.
biceps interval l.
bifurcation l.
blanchable red l.
central giant cell l.
chronic ischemic colonic lesion caused by phlebosclerosis
complete lower motor neuron l.
coronary artery l.
cortical bone l.
culprit lesion angioplasty
deep white matter l.
de novo l.
dorsomedial hypothalamic nucleus l.
dysplasia-associated lesion or mass
eczematous skin l.
enhancing brain l.
enhancing ring l.

lesion *(continued)*
eosinophilic fibrohistiocytic lesion of bone marrow
epileptogenic structural l.
epileptogenic temporal l.
epithelial hyperplastic laryngeal l.
erythematous satellite l.
exophytic skin l.
extent of cerebral l.
extracapillary l.
focal brain l.
focal hypoechoic l.
germ cell tumor with synchronous lesions in pineal and suprasellar region
glomerular tip l.
Gram stain of skin l.
granulomatous lesions of unknown significance
heart lesion cell
hemosiderotic fibrohistiocytic lipomatous l.
high-grade squamous intraepithelial l.
high thoracic cord l.
histocytoid hemangioma-like l.
hyperkeratotic verrucoid surfaced l.
hypoxic-ischemic l.
idiopathic minimal lesion nephrotic syndrome
idiopathic white matter l.
initial syphilitic l.
intracranial mass l.
left hemisphere l.
l. length
lichen planus-like l.
linear distribution of l.
linear streak l.
liver bull's eye l.
local glomerular l.
lower motor neuron l.
low-grade malignant cartilaginous l.
low-grade squamous intraepithelial l.
low-turnover bone l.
lumbosacral plexus l.
lumbosacral root l.
lymphoepithelial l.
lymphoproliferative skin l.
Lynch and Crues type 2 l.
lytic bone l.
maculopapular skin l.
malignant pituitary l.
marsupialization of l.
Meckel cave l.
melanocytic conjunctival l.
metachronous tissue l.
metaphyseal lesion of distal femur
metastatic bone l.
midline developmental l.
minimal change l.
minimal lesion disease
minimal lesion glomerulonephritis
minimal lesion nephrotic syndrome
minor glomerular l.
mixed bone l.
mixed fat-water density l.
Monteggia equivalent l.
mucocutaneous HSV l.
multifocal enhancing l.
multifocal white matter inflammatory l.
multilocular cystic l.
multiple bull's eye lesions bowel wall
multiple focal l.
multiple-ring-enhancing mass l.
nail bed l.
napkin ring annular l.
neoplastic pathologic l.
neurologic bladder l.
new lesion formation
nickel and dime l.
nodule-like alveolar l.
nonbacterial thrombotic endocardial l.
nonblanchable, abnormally colored l.
nondominant hemisphere l.
nonerosive gastric mucosal l.
nonneoplastic pathologic l.
Noonan-like giant cell l.
Noonan-like giant cell lesion syndrome
nucleus basalis l.
occipital lobe unilateral cerebral hemisphere l.
occupying space l.
ocular adnexal l.
oculomotor nerve l.
oil drop l.
l. on erythrocyte cell membrane at the site of complement fixation
optic chiasmal l.
optic nerve l.
optic radiation l.
optic tract l.
oral herpes l.
oral premalignant l.
organic cardiac l.
Osgood-Schlatter l.
osseous BA l.
osteochondral lesion of the talus
pagetic bone l.
papillomatous skin l.
papulosquamous skin l.
parenchymal brain l.
parietal cortex l.
parietal lobe bilateral cerebral hemisphere l.
parietal lobe unilateral cerebral hemisphere l.
parosteal bone l.
peripheral coin l.
peripheral nerve l.
periventricular hyperintense l.
photon-deficient bone l.
polypoid anorectal l.
precise lesion measuring
premalignant l.
rapidly growing l.
recurrent corneal l.
right hemisphere l.
segmental bronchus l.
severe intracranial l.
sharply demarcated circumferential l.
single enhancing CT l.
slowly developing l.
soft fleshy l.
soft fluctuant nodular l.
solitary bone l.
space-occupying l.
spontaneous l.
squamous intraepithelial l.
target lesion reintervention
target lesion revascularization
trabeculated bone l.
traumatic unidirectional Bankart lesion surgery
upper GI l.
upper motor neuron l.
white matter lesion cerebral

lesion/atypical
squamous intraepithelial lesion/atypical squamous cell of undetermined significance

less
bone conduction less than air conduction
l. than effective
particulate matter less than 10 micrometers diameter
pulmonic heart sound less than aortic second heart sound

second aortic sound less than second pulmonic sound

lessening

heat escape lessening posture

lesser

angulus on the lesser curve
arterial circle of lesser iris
l. cul-de-sac
l. curvature
l. esophageal sphincter
l. omentum
l. palatine artery
l. sac
l. trochanter
l. tubercle

let-down

milk l.-d.

lethal

acute lethal catatonia
l. antigen
aphid lethal paralysis virus
approximate lethal concentration
l. blow
l. concentration
direct killing by lethal injection
l. dose
l. dose in all exposed subjects
egg lethal dose
l. factor
l. graft-versus-host disease
incipient lethal concentration
l. injection
l. injury
median lethal dose
median lethal time
mental retardation, scapuloperoneal muscular dystrophy, lethal cardiomyopathy syndrome
l. midline granuloma
midline lethal granuloma
minimum lethal concentration
perinatal lethal osteogenesis imperfecta
potentially lethal arrhythmia
potentially lethal damage
repair of potentially lethal damage
l. time
tumor lethal dose

lethargic

dull and l.

lethargy

confusion and l.
hysteric l.
inactivity, lethargy and fatigue
jaundice and l.
jaundice, lethargy and fever
postictal l.

leucine

l. aminopeptidase
l. aminopeptidase test
l. enkephalin
l. flux
idiopathic leucine sensitivity
l. oxidation
l. rich repeat
serum leucine aminopeptidase
l. tolerance test

leucovorin

ara-C, VP-16, l.
calcium l.
methotrexate, leucovorin, Adriamycin, cyclophosphamide, Oncovin, prednisone, bleomycin
methotrexate, leucovorin, bleomycin, Adriamycin, cyclophosphamide, Oncovin, dexamethasone
methotrexate, Platinol, 5-fluorouracil, leucovorin, calcium
oxaliplatin with leucovorin and 5-fluorouracil

leukapheresis

autologous leukapheresis, processing, and storage
continuous-flow centrifugation l.
intermittent flow centrifugation l.
large-volume l.

leukemia

Abelson leukemia virus
Abelson murine leukemia virus
acute basophilic l.
acute granulocytic l.
acute leukemia protocol
acute lymphoblastic leukemia in children
acute lymphoblastic leukemia secondary to Burkitt lymphoma
acute lymphoblastic myelogenous l.
acute lymphocytic l.
acute lymphocytic leukemia antigen
acute megakaryoblastic l.
acute monoblastic l.
acute monocytic l.
acute myeloblastic l.
acute myelocytic l.
acute myeloid l.
acute myelomonoblastic l.
acute myelomonocytic l.
acute nonlymphoblastic l.
acute nonlymphocytic l.
acute nonlymphoid l.
acute progranulocytic l.
acute promyelocytic l.
acute undifferentiated l.
adult T-cell l.
adult T-cell leukemia antigen
adult T-cell leukemia virus
aleukemic granulocytic l.
aleukemic lymphocytic l.
aleukemic monocytic l.
amphotropic murine leukemia virus
l. antigen
atypical chronic myeloid l.
avian myeloblastosis leukemia virus reverse transcriptase
B-cell acute lymphoblastic l.
B-cell chronic lymphocytic l.
B-cell precursor lymphoblastic l.
B-cell prolymphocytic l.
bovine leukemia virus
cancer and leukemia group B
categories of acute nonlymphoblastic l.
central nervous system l.
chronic eosinophilic l.
chronic granulocytic l.
chronic lymphatic l.
chronic lymphocytic l.
chronic lymphocytic leukemia variant
chronic lymphosarcoma cell l.
chronic monoblastic l.
chronic monocytic l.
chronic myelocytic/myelogenous/myeloid leukemia accelerated phase
chronic myelocytic/myelogenous/myeloid leukemia blast crisis
chronic myelocytic/myelogenous/myeloid leukemia chronic phase
chronic myeloid l.
chronic myelomacrocytic l.
chronic myelomonocytic l.
chronic neutrophilic l.
chronic phase chronic myelogenous l.
chronic T-cell l.
common acute lymphoblastic leukemia antigen
common acute lymphocytic leukemia antigen
cutaneous T-cell l.
defective leukemia virus

leukemia *(continued)*
erythroblastic l.
erythroid leukemia virus
feline l.
feline leukemia virus
French-American-British leukemia classification system
Friend leukemia cell
Friend leukemia virus
gibbon ape leukemia virus
Gross leukemia antigen
Gross leukemia virus
hairy cell l.
hairy cell leukemia variant
hamster leukemia virus
human T-cell leukemia virus
human T-cell leukemia virus-associated membrane antigen
human T-cell leukemia virus type 1, 2, 3
human thymic l.
hypoplastic acute l.
l. inhibitory factor
juvenile chronic myelocytic l.
juvenile chronic myelogenous l.
juvenile myelomonocytic l.
lineage switch l.
lymphatic leukemia virus
lymphocytic l.
lymphoid l.
lymphoma syndrome l.
lymphosarcoma cell l.
Maloney leukemia virus
mast cell l.
mature cell l.
meningeal l.
microgranular acute promyelocytic l.
mixed cell l.
mixed lineage l.
Moloney murine leukemia virus
murine myeloid leukemia cell line
myeloid granulocytic l.
myeloid leukemia inhibitory factor
myelomonoblastic l.
myelomonocytic l.
myelomonocytic leukemia, subacute
Naegeli type of monocytic l.
natural killer cell l.
null cell acute lymphocytic l.
null cell lymphoblastic l.
oral hairy l.
Philadelphia chromosome-negative chronic myelogenous l.
Philadelphia chromosome-positive chronic myelogenous l.
plasma cell l.
prolymphocytic l.
promyelocytic l.
promyelocytic leukemia zinc finger
radiation leukemia protection
radiation leukemia virus
radiation myeloid l.
rat basophilic l.
Rauscher murine leukemia virus
Reider cell l.
resistant Friend leukemia cell
sarcoma, breast and brain tumors, leukemia, laryngeal and lung cancer adenoma
secondary l.
stem cell l.
T-cell acute lymphoblastic l.
T-cell chronic lymphatic l.
T-cell prolymphocytic l.
therapy-related acute myelogenous l.
therapy-related acute myeloid l.
thymus leukemia antigen
l. virus

leukemia-associated
l.-a. antigen
l.-a. inhibitory activity

leukemia-free survival

leukemia-inhibiting factor

leukemia-lymphoma
human T-cell leukemia-lymphoma virus

leukemia/lymphoma
adult T-cell l.

leukemia/small
B-cell chronic lymphocytic leukemia/small lymphocytic lymphoma

leukemic reticuloendotheliosis

leukemogenic
Moloney leukemogenic virus

leukemoid
lymphocytic leukemoid reaction
monocytic leukemoid reaction
myelocytic leukemoid reaction
neonatal leukemoid reaction

leukocidin
Neisser-Wechsberg l.
Panton-Valentine l.

leukoclastic angiitis

leukocyte
l. adherence inhibition factor
l. adhesion deficiency
l. adhesion deficiency type 1–4
l. adhesion inhibitor
l. adhesion molecule-1
l. alkaline phosphatase
l. alkaline phosphatase activity
alkaline phosphatase activity of granular l.
l. alkaline phosphatase stain
allogeneic mixed leukocyte culture
alpha-galactoside l.
l. antigen factor-3
antihuman leukocyte antigen antibody
l. ascorbic acid
autologous labeled l.
autologous mixed leukocyte reaction
automated differential leukocyte counter
l. automatic recognition computer
basophil granular l.
beta-hexosaminidase A l.
l. cell adhesion molecule
l. colony-forming unit
l. common antigen
dialyzable leukocyte extract
l. differential count
differential leukocyte count
donor leukocyte infusion
l. endogenous mediator
l. equivalent unit
l. esterase
l. esterase test
l. factor antigen-1
fecal leukocyte count test
l. feeder layer
l. function-associated antigen
l. histamine release test
histocompatibility leukocyte antigen
homologous leukocyte antibody
human l.
human leukocyte antigen system
human leukocyte antibody
human leukocyte antigen
human leukocyte antigen-A24
human leukocyte antigen allele
human leukocyte antigen restriction element
human leukocyte elastase
human leukocyte interferon
human peripheral blood l.
l. inclusion
indium-labeled leukocyte scan
l. infiltration factor

l. inhibitory factor
interferon
International Workshop and Conference on Human L. Differentiation Antigens
intraepithelial l.
killer inhibitor receptors-human leukocyte antigen
large granular l.
lazy leukocyte syndrome
localized leukocyte mobilization
l. migration enhancement
l. migration inhibition assay
l. migration inhibition factor
l. migration inhibition reaction
l. migration inhibition test
l. migration technique
l. mitogenic factor
mixed culture, l.
mixed leukocyte concentration
mixed leukocyte response
mixed skin cell leukocyte reaction
mononuclear l.
neutrophilic polymorphonuclear l.
neutrophil leukocyte count
nonadherent l.
nonfilament polymorphonuclear l.
nonhuman leukocyte antigen associated form
partially pure human leukocyte interferon
percent of polymorphonuclear l.
peripheral blood l.
polymorphonuclear leukocyte count
polymorphonuclear leukocyte infiltrate
polymorphonuclear leukocyte response
polymorphonuclear neutrophilic l.
l. poor
recombinant human leukocyte interferon A
secretory leukocyte protease inhibitor
small l.
soluble human leukocyte antigen
l. thromboplastin
umbilical cord blood l.
varieties of human leukocyte antigen

leukocyte-activating factor

leukocyte-antigen sensitivity testing

leukocyte-conditioned medium

leukocyte-poor
l.-p. packed cell
l.-p. red blood cell

leukocyte-specific
l.-s. activity
l.-s. antinuclear antibody

leukocytic pyrogen

leukocytoclastic
l. angiitis
l. vasculitis

leukocytosis
lymphocytic l.
mild l.
monocytic l.
neutrophilic l.
perinephrial l.
peripheral l.

leukocytosis-inducing factor

leukocytosis-promoting factor

leukoderma
occupational l.
patterned l.
periorbital l.

leukodystrophy
globoid l.
hereditary cerebral l.
metachromatic l.
metachronous l.
orthochromatic l.
progressive multifocal l.

leukoencephalitis
acute hemorrhagic l.
Montana myotis leukoencephalitis virus
necrotizing hemorrhagic l.

leukoencephalopathy
cerebral autosomal recessive arteriopathy with subcortical infarcts and l.
disseminated necrotizing l.
hereditary diffuse leukoencephalopathy with spheroids
perinatal telencephalic l.
polyneuropathy, ophthalmoplegia, leukoencephalopathy, and intestinal pseudo-obstruction
progressively diffused l.
progressive multifocal l.
reversible posterior l.
reversible posterior leukoencephalopathy syndrome
sclerosing l.

leukoerythroblastic reaction

leukokinesis-enhancing factor

leukoma

leukomalacia
cystic periventricular l.
periventricular l.

leukomyelitis
necrotizing hemorrhage l.

leukonychia
apparent l.
partial l.

leukopenia
alcoholism, leukopenia, pneumococcal sepsis
autoimmune l.
l. factor
lymphocytic l.

leukopheresis
plasma l.

leukoplakia
hairy l.
oral hairy l.
proliferative verrucous l.

leukoprotease
secretory leukoprotease inhibitor

leukoproteinase
secretory leukoproteinase inhibitor

leukoreduction filter

leukorrhea
menstrual l.

leukosis
avian l.
avian leukosis complex
avian leukosis virus
lymphoid leukosis virus

leukotactic
host leukotactic function
l. factor activity

leukotomy
transorbital l.

leukotriene
l. A
l. A_4
l. B
l. C
l. C4
l. C_4
l. E
l. E4
l. pathway inhibitor
l. receptor antagonist

leuteinizing
ovine leuteinizing hormone

levan
bacterial l.

levator
l. ani muscle
aponeurosis of superior levator palpebra
l. hernia
paradoxic levator excitation
paradoxic levator inhibition
tendinous arch of levator ani
l. veli palatini muscle

levatoris
musculi levatoris palpebrae superioris

LeVeen
L. dialysis shunt
L. valve

level
above level of heart
l. of achievement
l. of acuity
adaptation l.
Adult Performance L. Survey
airway, breathing, circulation, cervical spine, and consciousness l.
alpha antitrypsin l.
altered level of consciousness
alternate level of care
ammonia blood l.
l. of anger
annoyance l.
anterior midpapillary l.
anti-M2 antimitochondrial antibody l.
antithrombin III plasma l.
appropriate level of care
arachidonic acid l.
arterial lactate l.
aspartate aminotransferase l.
Assessment Program of Early Learning L.'s
attachment level gain
automatic phrase l.
l. of awareness
basal insulin l.
baseline level of functioning
below detectable l.'s
biosafety l.
blood alcohol l.
blood ethanol l.
blood glucose l.
blood glucose L.
blood lead l.
blood sugar l.
l. of care
cognitive awareness l.
l. of comfort
Comprehensive L. of Consciousness Scale
l. of concern
conditioned pitch l.
confidence l.
l. of consciousness
cord blood erythropoietin l.
criterion l.
critical carbohydrate l.
cumulative population doubling l.
decibels normal hearing l.
decibels sensation l.
decibels sound pressure l.
decreased level of consciousness
l. and degree of mental illness
developmental l.
difficulty functioning at normal ability l.
drug l.
effective perceived noise l.
elevation of blood lead l.
erratic blood glucose l.'s
examined hormone l.'s
factor l.
fasting gastrin l.
fasting glucose l.
fasting serum l.
l. of female gonadotropin
fluctuating hormone l.'s
fluctuating level of consciousness
free testosterone l.
l. of functioning
gentamicin peak l.
gentamicin trough l.
global level of functioning
glucose level control
glycosylated hemoglobin l.
graphic level recorder
health level seven
hearing l.
hearing threshold l.
high acid level in blood
high blood alcohol l.
high cholesterol l.
higher level skill
highest functional l.
highest level of activity
high level of anxiety
high level of arousal
high level of care
high level of function
high level of kidney protein rennin
l. of hopelessness
hormone l.'s
human chorionic gonadotropin l.
imbalance in neurotransmitter l.
l. of incompetence
increased level of blood sugar
l. of independent function
initial levels of alcohol intake
initial baseline l.
l. of injury
intense l.'s
intensity l.
iron saturation l.
lead level in blood
liver enzyme serum l.
loudness l.
loudness discomfort l.
low educational l.
low energy l.
lower circulating estrogen l.
lower level of care
lowest effect level of toxicity
lowest level term
lowest observed adverse effect l.
low liquid level monitor
maintain blood glucose l.
major image-distorting l.
masking level difference
maternal estriol l.
maternal serum l.
maximal comfort l.
maximal sustained level of ventilation
maximum level of independent mobility
medial joint l.
mental inhibition l.
metabolic equivalent l.
minimal bactercidal l.
minimal bactericidal l.
minimal response l.
minor image-distorting l.
most comfortable listening l.
most comfortable loudness l.
multiple air-fluid l.'s
muscle enzyme serum l.
narrowing at lumbosacral l.
noise interference l.
noise level monitor
Non-Reading Intelligence Test, Levels 1-3
no observed adverse effect l.
normal gonadal steroid l.
normalized hearing l.
normal triglyceride l.'s
optimal level of functioning
optimal level of independence
O2 saturation l.
output sound pressure l.
oxygen saturation l.
l. of pain

pain determined by level of anxiety
parathyroid hormone l.
peak blood l.
peak equivalent sound pressure l.
peak serum l.
peak and trough l.'s
perceived noise l.
pericardial air-fluid l.
peripheral hormone l.
plasma level monitoring
population doubling l.
preferred frequency speech interference l.
pressure pain tolerance l.
previous level of functioning
prior level of function
Reaction L. Scale
recommended exposure l.
reduction l.
L. of Rehabilitation Scale 1
resting expiratory l.
saturation sound pressure l.
Scaled Curriculum Achievement L.'s Test
l. of sedation
sensation level of hearing
sensorineural acuity l.
sensory acuity l.
serum alcohol l.
serum bactericidal l.
serum copper l.
serum digoxin l.
serum drug l.
serum-killing l.
serum lidocaine l.
serum methyl alcohol l.
serum protein l.
serum theophylline l.
serum triglyceride l.
l.'s of shock intensity
skin conductance l.
skin potential l.
sound l.
sound level meter
sound pressure l.
speech interference l.
sterility assurance l.
tolerance l.
tonic heart l.
total homocysteine l.
troponin I l.
uncomfortable listening l.
uncomfortable loudness l.
visual detection l.
vitamin B_{12} l.

level-dependent
blood oxygenation l.-d.

leverage
hemostatic occlusive leverage device

levonorgestrel
l. subdermal implant
subdermal levonorgestrel implant

levulinate

Lewandowsky

Lewis
L. a antibody
L. b antibody
L. blood group
L. lung carcinoma
L. triple response
L. X oligosaccharide
L. Y antigen

Lewisohn method

Lewis-Summer syndrome

Lewy
L. body
L. body dementia
L. body disease
cortical Lewy body
dementia with Lewy body
diffuse Lewy body dementia
diffuse Lewy body disease
incidental Lewy body

lexical
l. access
l. agraphia
l. ambiguity
l. category
l. cohesion
l. connotation
l. denotation

lexical-syntactic
l.-s. deficit
l.-s. syndrome

Leyden
L. ataxia
L. crystal
L. disease
L. hemophilia B

Leyden-Möbius muscular dystrophy

Leydig
L. cell adenoma
L. cell agenesis
L. cell aplasia
L. cell atrophy
L. cell embryology
L. cell hyperplasia
L. cell hypoplasia
L. cell insufficiency
L. cell secretion
L. cell secretory function
L. cells of the testis
L. cell stimulation
L. cell tumor
L. duct

Leyla
L. arm
L. bar

Leyton Obsessional Inventory

L/H
L. nodular pattern
L. type

Lhermitte
L. sign
L. syndrome

Lhermitte-Duclos
L.-D. disease
L.-D. syndrome

L'Homme rouge

LH-releasing hormone agonist therapy

liability
l. abuse
current l.'s
ergonomic assessment of risk and l.
hereditary neuropathy with liability for pressure palsy
other party l.
l. to pressure palsy

liaison
computer liaison nurse

lib
ad l.
ad lib feeding
patient up ad l.

liberal
l. cutoff score
l. doses of aspirin

libidinal
l. change
l. development
l. drive
l. energy
l. impulse

libido
l. analog
l. binding
diminished l.
l. fixation

libido *(continued)*
increased l.
normal libido, coitus, and climax

Libman-Sacks
L.-S. disease
L.-S. endocarditis
L.-S. syndrome

library
arrayed l.
l. ligation
National L. of Medicine
l. temple

lice
head l.
pubic l.

licensed
l. handgun
l. practical nurse
l. to practice
l. professional counselor
l. vocational nurse

Lich
L. extravesical technique
L. technique

lichen
anular lichen planus
atrophic lichen planus
l. aureus
l. chronicus simplex
genital lichen sclerosus
l. hemorrhagicus
l. infantum
l. iris
l. leprosus
linear lichen planus
l. myxedematosus
myxedematous l.
l. pilaris
l. planopilaris
l. planus anularis
l. planus follicularis
l. planus-like keratosis
l. planus-like lesion
l. planus overlap syndrome
l. planus pemphigoid
l. planus pigmentosus
l. planus verrucosus
l. ruber
l. ruber acuminatus
l. ruber moniliformis
l. ruber planus
l. ruber verrucosus
l. sclerosus
l. sclerosus et atrophicans
l. sclerosus scleroatrophy
l. scrofulosis
l. scrofulosorum
l. scrofulous
l. simplex
l. simplex chronicus
l. spinulosus
l. striatus
l. striatus epidermal nevus
l. strophulosus
l. syphiliticus
l. trichophyticus
l. tropicus
l. urticatus

lichenified
l. dermatitis
l. lesion
l. lid
l. plaque

lichenoid
l. acute pityriasis
l. amyloidosis
atypical lichenoid stomatitis
l. chronic dermatosis
l. contact dermatitis
l. dermatitis
l. dermatosis
distinctive exudative discoid and lichenoid dermatitis
l. drug eruption
l. dysplasia
l. eczema
l. eruption
l. graft-versus-host disease
l. keratosis
l. lesion
l. papule
parapsoriasis l.
l. phase
l. reaction

Lich-Gregoire
L.-G. anastomosis
L.-G. repair
L.-G. technique
L.-G. ureteroneocystostomy

Lichtenstein
L. hernial repair
L. herniorrhaphy

Lichtheim
L. aphasia
L. disease
L. plaques

Lichtman
L. aseptic necrosis classification
L. disease

licorice-induced
l.-i. hypermineralocorticoidism
l.-i. hypertension
l.-i. hypokalemia

lid
l. agglutination
Atkin lid block
Atkinson lid block
l. block
brows, lids, and lashes
l. closure reaction
l. closure reflex
l. crease
l. crusting
l. crutch spectacles
l. droop
l. ectropion
l. edema
l. eversion
external l.'s
l. fissure
l. forceps
l. imbrication syndrome
l. lag
l.'s and lashes
l.'s, lashes, and adnexa
l.'s, lashes, lacrimals, lymphatics
l. laxity
l. loading
lower lid laxity
lower lid, left eye
lower lid sling procedure
lower lid, oculus dexter
lower lid, oculus sinister
l. margin laceration
mechanical lid retraction
mesencephalic lid retraction
modified band lid method
l. notching
l. nystagmus
O'Brien lid block
pediatric lid speculum
l. plate
l. retraction
retrobulbar lid block
right lower l.
l. scurf
l. speculum
l. thrush
l. trephine
upper lid right eye
l. vesicle
warm compresses and lid scrubs

Liddle
L. dexamethasone suppression test
L. disease
L. syndrome

lidocaine
l., adrenaline, tetracaine
l. assay
l. blood concentration
l. hydrochloride
operative field anesthetized with 1% l.
serum lidocaine level
l. tissue concentration
l. toxicity

lie
anterior l.
l. detection
l. detector
longitudinal l.
oblique l.
occipitotransverse l.
posterior l.
transverse l.
transverse lie presentation

Lieberkühn
L. ampulla
L. crypt
L. follicle
L. gland

Lieberman
L. fragmentor
L. MicroFinger manipulator

Liebermeister
L. furrow
L. groove
L. rule

Liebow
usual interstitial pneumonia of Liebow

lienal
l. artery
l. vein

Lieutaud
L. body
L. triangle
L. trigone
L. uvula

life
active life expectancy
adjustment reaction of later l.
Adolescent L. Change Event Questionnaire
advanced cardiac life support
advanced pediatric life support
advanced trauma life support
L. After Cancer Care
altered life circumstance
appetite for l.
Arthritis Quality of L. Scale
Asthma Quality of L. Questionnaire
Atkinson L. Happiness
Atkinson L. Happiness Rating
autobiographical life chart
basic trauma life support
Brief Life History Inventory
calculated average l.
l. change unit
l. circumstance problem
l. course
l. crisis
l. cycle change
l. cycle of *Echinococcus*
l. cycle theory
Developmental Assessment of L. Experiences
diabetes quality of l.
l. difficulty
disability-adjusted life years
disability-free life expectancy
effective patient l.
end of l.
l. energy
l. event
l. events checklist
L. Events and Difficulty Schedule Interview
l. expectancy
expectation of l.
l. experience
L. Experiences Checklist
L. Experience Survey
extracorporeal life support
extra uterine l.
Family Index of L. Events
Family Inventory of L. Events and Changes
l. fear
Functional L. Scale
Gastrointestinal Quality of L. Index
gender identity disorder of adult l.
l. goal
L. Health Monitoring Program
health-related quality of l.
healthy years of l.
healthy years of life lost
Heroin Emergency L. Project
l. history
human development and family l.
l. impairment
improve quality of l.
increase in life span
L. Interpersonal History Enquiry
l. island
Life Satisfaction Index A, B
lost years of expected l.
marginal cost per year of life saved
mean effective l.
mean life span
median life span
Multidimensional Quality of L. Questionnaire for Persons with Human Immunodeficiency Virus
Multidimensional Student L. Satisfaction Scale
neonatal adjuvant life support
Parkinson Disease Quality of L. Scale
pediatric advanced life support
Pediatric Asthma Quality of L. Questionnaire
perceived quality of l.
potential years of life lost
preservation of quality of l.
Profile of Adaptation to L.
Psoriasis L. Stress Inventory
purpose in l.
quality of l.
quality-adjusted life expectancy
Quality of L. Index
Quality of L. Interview
Quality of L. Inventory
quality of life in epilepsy
Quality of L. Questionnaire-C30
Quality of L. Scale
quality of working l.
l. of radioisotope
recent life event
remission, relapse, and life expectancy
removal of life support
Respiratory Quality of L. Questionnaire
rhinoconjunctivitis-specific quality of life questionnaire
Salamon-Conte L. Satisfaction in the Elderly Scale
l. satisfaction
L. Satisfaction Rating
Self-Evaluation of Life Function scale
sex difference in life expectancy
L. Situation Questionnaire
Sleep Apnea Quality of L. Index
l. span
L. Span Study
l. stress
Stress From L. Experience
stroke-specific quality of l.
L. Study Sample

life *(continued)*
l. support unit
l. table
l. table method
l. table survival
threat to l.
total life expectancy
Transactional Analysis L. Position Survey
Vital Signs Quality of L.
World Health Organization Quality of Life 100-Item
years of healthy l.
years of life lost
years of life with disability
years of potential life lost before age 65

life-belt cataract

life-care at home

life-changing improvement

life-cycle adjustment

lifelong
l. abstinence
l. affiliation
l. obesity

lifelong-type dyspareunia

life-prolonging measures

lifesaving
denial of lifesaving medical treatment

lifespan
anticipated l.

lifestyle
active l.
l. adjustment
alternative l.
Alternative L. Checklist
alternative lifestyle community
antisocial l.
l. change
l. education
l. factor
gradual lifestyle modification
healthy l.
healthy lifestyle habit
heart-healthy l.
heart healthy l.
high-risk l.
inactive l.
independent l.
l. modification
physically inactive l.
therapeutic lifestyle change

life-support
l.-s. machine
l.-s. system

life-sustaining
l.-s. intervention
l.-s. medical treatment
l.-s. treatment

life-sustaining medical treatment

life-table analysis

life-terminating acts without the explicit request

life-threatening
l.-t. abnormal heartbeat
l.-t. asthma attack
l.-t. behavior
l.-t. blood clot
l.-t. brain injury
l.-t. cancer
l.-t. complication
l.-t. condition
l.-t. danger
l.-t. drug interaction
l.-t. event
l.-t. graft-versus-host disease
l.-t. heart arrhythmia
l.-t. heart rhythm
l.-t. heat stroke
l.-t. illness
l.-t. infection
l.-t. infectious agent
l.-t. injury
l.-t. ischemia

lifetime
l. aggression
l. anxiety disorder
average remaining l.
l. behavior
l. depression criterion
l. episode
l. expectancy
l. hierarchy
l. history
l. impulsivity

life-year
quality-adjusted l.-y.'s

Li-Fraumeni familial cancer syndrome

lift
cervicofacial face l.
chair l.
chin lift maneuver
endoforehead-endomidface l.
endoforehead-periorbital-cheek l.
head tilt and chin lift maneuver
head tilt with neck l.
heel l.
Hoyer l.
modified anterior hairline forehead l.
parasternal l.

lift-and-cut
l.-a.-c. biopsy
l.-a.-c. endoscopic mucosal resection

lifting
heavy l.

lift-off
l.-o. of heel in walk
l.-o. test

ligament
accessory collateral l.
allograft ligament replacement
allograft reconstruction of fibular collateral l.
ankle inferior transverse l.
ankle ligament protector
ankle ligament protector brace
anterior anular l.
anterior collateral l.
anterior commissure l.
anterior costotransverse l.
anterior cruciate l.
anterior cruciate ligament injury
anterior cruciate ligament reconstruction
anterior cruciate ligament repair
anterior cruciate ligament tear
anterior fibular l.
anterior-inferior capsular ligament dysfunction
anterior-inferior tibiofibular l.
anterior ligament of fibular head
anterior ligament of head of fibula
anterior ligament of Helmholtz
anterior ligament of malleus
anterior longitudinal l.
anterior mallear l.
anterior medial ankle l.
anterior meniscofemoral l.
anterior oblique l.
anterior platysma-cutaneous l.
anterior sacrococcygeal l.
anterior sacroiliac l.
anterior sacrosciatic l.
anterior sternoclavicular l.
anterior suspensory l.
anterior talocalcaneal l.
anterior talofibular ligament rupture
anterior talotibial l.

anterior tibiofibular l.
anterior tibiotalar part of deltoid l.
anterior tibiotalar part of medial ligament of ankle joint
anteroinferior glenohumeral l.
anterolateral femorotibial ligament tenodesis
anteromedial glenohumeral l.
anterosuperior glenohumeral l.
anular ligament entrapment
anular ligament of radius
anular ligament of radius
anular ligament of stapes
anular ligament of stapes
anular ligaments of trachea
anular ligament of trachea
apical dental l.
apical ligament of dens
arcuate ligament of Clifford
arcuate ligament of diaphragm
arcuate ligament of pubis
arcuate popliteal l.
arcuate pubic l.
artery of round ligament of uterus
arthroscopically assisted anterior cruciate ligament reconstruction
arthroscopic anterior cruciate ligament reconstruction
atlantal transverse l.
l. augmentation device
l. of auricle
autogenous patellar ligament graft
l. avulsion
l. of Bigelow
l. of Botallo
calcaneofibular l.
cardinal l.
collateral fibular l.
collateral ligament instability
collateral ligament laxity
collateral ligament rupture
collateral ligament stability
collateral radial l.
collateral tibial l.
collateral ulnar l.
coracoacromial l.
cruciate ligament injury
cruciate ligament laxity
cruciate ligament of leg
cruciate ligament reconstruction
cruciate ligament rupture
cruciate ligament tear
deltoid l.
dorsal radiocarpal l.
dorsoradial l.
l. elongation
l. of epididymis inferior and superior
fibular collateral l.
fibular collateral ligament of ankle
l. of foot
glenohumeral l.
l. graft
l. of head of femur
l.'s of head of fibula
l. of Henle
l. of Henry
humeral avulsion of the glenohumeral l.
l. of incus
inferior calcaneonavicular l.
inferior glenohumeral l.
inferior glenohumeral ligament labral complex
intermetacarpal l.
internal canthal l.
interosseous talocalcaneal l.
interspinous l.
l. of knee
laparoscopic resection of the ureterosacral l.
lateral collateral ligament of ankle
lateral collateral ligament complex
lateral suspensor ligament
lateral talocalcaneal l.
lateral ulnar collateral l.
leaf of broad l.
l. of left superior vena cava
l. of left vena cava
l. of lens
long calcaneocuboid l.
long external lateral l.
longitudinal bands of cruciform ligament of atlas
long plantar l.
l. of malleus
l. of Marshall
masseteric cutaneous l.
medial arcuate l.
medial canthal l.
medial capsular l.
medial check ligament of eyeball
medial collateral l.
medial collateral ligament degeneration
medial collateral ligament of elbow
medial collateral ligament of knee
medial collateral ligament tearing
medial ligament of ankle joint
medial ligament of talocrural joint
medial ligament of temporomandibular joint
medial ligament of wrist
medial palpebral l.
medial patellofemoral l.
medial ulnar collateral l.
median arcuate l.
median arcuate ligament of diaphragm
median cricothyroid l.
median cruciate l.
metatarsal interosseous l.
middle costotransverse l.
middle glenohumeral l.
Mueller anterolateral femorotibial ligament tenodesis
navicular cuneiform l.
oblique ligament of elbow joint
oblique retinacular l.
orbicular ligament of radius
ossification of anterior longitudinal l.
ossification of posterior longitudinal l.
outer anular/posterior longitudinal ligament complex
l. of ovary
palmar beak l.
palmar carpal l.
palmar carpometacarpal l.
palmar ligament of interphalangeal joint of hand
palmar ligament of metacarpophalangeal joint
pectinate ligament of iridocorneal angle
pectinate ligament of iris
periodontal l.
periodontal ligament fiber
peritoneal ligament of liver
posterior cruciate l.
posterior cruciate ligament of knee
posterior cruciate ligament tear
posterior ligament of knee
posterior longitudinal l.
posterior oblique l.
posterior talofibular l.
proximal collateral l.
pubourethral l.
radial collateral l.
radiate carpal l.
radiate ligament of head of rib

ligament *(continued)*
l. reconstruction with tendon interposition
l. reflecting edge
scapholunate l.
shelving border of inguinal l.
l. shelving edge
short plantar l.
l. of Struthers
superior ligament of epididymis
superior ligament of incus
superior ligament of malleus
suspensory ligament of axilla
suspensory ligament of breast
suspensory ligament of clitoris
suspensory ligament of Cooper
suspensory ligament of duodenum
suspensory ligament of esophagus
suspensory ligament of eye
suspensory ligament of gonad
suspensory ligament of lens
suspensory ligament of ovary
suspensory ligament of penis
suspensory ligament of testis
suspensory ligament of thyroid gland
tibial collateral l.
l. of Toldt
transverse carpal l.
transverse ligament of elbow
transverse ligament of leg
l. of Treitz
triangular ligament of liver
ulnar collateral l.
ulnar collateral ligament of elbow joint
ulnar collateral ligament of wrist joint
uterine positioning via ligament investment fixation truncation
volar carpal l.
l. of Wrisberg

ligament-bone
bone-patellar l.-b.
l.-b. complex

ligamentous
l. ankylosis
l. anterior dislocation
l. anterior dislocation composite graft
l. attachment
balanced ligamentous tension treatment
l. bouncing
l. box
l. calcification
l. and capsular repair
l. complex
l. control brace
l. disruption
l. ectopic pregnancy
l. facial fence
l. falx
l. injection
l. injury grade I–III
l. instability
l. joint
l. laxity
l. structure
l. tear

ligaments
l. of head of fibula

ligand
l. agent
antibody capture ligand assay
antigen capture ligand assay
l. assay
l. blotting
calcium-signal modulating cyclophilin B l.
CD 27 l.
CD 30 l.
CD 40 l.
l. concentration
crystal ligand field
Fas l.
kit l.
mixed ligand chelate
nuclear factor kappa B l.
osteoprotegerin l.
l. pathway
l. receptor
receptor activator of nuclear factor kappa B l.
TNF-related apoptosis inducing l.
tumor necrosis factor-related apoptosis-inducing l.
Western ligand blot

ligand-binding
l.-b. determinant
l.-b. domain

ligand-dependent action of thyroid hormone receptor

ligand-gated channel

ligand-independent
l.-i. action of thyroid hormone receptor
l.-i. stimulation

ligand-receptor
l.-r. complex
l.-r. interaction

ligand-to-metal charge transfer

ligase-chain
l.-c. reaction
l.-c. reaction assay
l.-c. reaction testing

ligated
appendix ligated and amputated
bleeder clamped and l.
doubly clamped, transected and stump l.
doubly ligated and sectioned
doubly ligated with transfixion suture
identified and l.
intercostal vessel l.
suture l.

ligation
aneurysm clip l.
l. of appendix
bilateral tubal l.
bilateral vas l.
cecal ligation and puncture
chronic bile duct l.
clip ligation of aneurysm
l. device
elastic band l.
endoscopic band l.
endoscopic hemorrhoid l.
endoscopic mucosal resection with l.
endoscopic variceal band l.
esophageal band l.
l. of esophagogastric junction
l. of Fas
femoral vein l.
l. of hemorrhoid
hemorrhoidal artery l.
l. hemorrhoidectomy
hepatic artery l.
high ligation of hernia sac
high ligation and stripping
high saphenous vein l.
laparoscopic tubal l.
modified Irving-type tubal l.
parotid duct l.
pelviscopic clip ligation technique
Pomeroy tubal l.
postpartum tubal l.
rubber band ligation of hemorrhoid
l. and stripping
tubal l.
varicose vein stripping and l.

ligator
multiple band l.
rubber band l.

ligature
anchor with suture l.
l. cutter
l. guide
linear in-line ligature carrier

light
abnormal intolerance to l.
l. absorption
l. and accommodation
accommodation l.
l. activation by stimulated emission of radiation
l. adaptation
l. amplification by stimulated emission of radiation
amyloid light chain
l. argon laser burn
l. around wire technique
autokinetic visible light phenomenon
axial ray of l.
l. bath
black l.
l. bulb appearance
l. cable
l. cast
l. cells of thyroid
l. chain deposition disease
l. chain isotype suppression
l. chain paraprotein
l. chain-related amyloidosis
l. coagulation
l. conductor
confusion with light sensitivity
consensual light reaction
consensual light reflex
constriction caused by l.
l. contact
l. contact assist
delayed light emission
l. diet
l. difference
l. differential threshold
l. differentiation
dim light melatonin onset
l. discrimination
l. and distance
l. drinking
l. duty
dynamic light scattering
early light breakfast
l. electrocautery
l. electrodesiccation
l. and electron immunoperoxidase observation
l. electron microscope
endoscopic light source
l. eruption
l. exposure
fiberoptic l.
flashing lights and/or scotoma
l. flow
fluorescent light intensity
free monoclonal urinary light chain
gamma light chain
glare around l.'s
l. guide
l. guide bundle
halo around l.'s
hand motion and light perception
high-intensity light source
high-resolution light microscopy
immunoglobulin light chain-origin amyloid deposit
infrared light
Integrated L. Control
intense pulsed light source
intermittent flash of l.
intravascular red light therapy
isolated flash of l.
kappa light chain
Lockwood light reflex
long-wavelength ultraviolet l.
low-angle laser light scattering
macular light reflex
marginal ray of l.
l. microscopy
midrange spectrum ultraviolet l.
midrange-wavelength ultraviolet l.
l. minimum
minimum light threshold
l. molecular weight meromyosin
monochromatic light source
monoclonal free light chain
morning bright light therapy
l. moving touch
narrow band UVB therapeutic light exposure
narrow-spectrum blue l.
near light reflex
near reaction to l.
normal light perception
normal pupillary reaction to l.
oblique ray of l.
ophthalmoscopy with reflected l.
l. optometer reflex
out of bilirubin l.
paraxial ray of l.
perception of l.
l. perception only
l. perception without projection
l. perception with projection
peripheral light detection
peripheral light loss
peripheral light scatter
peripheral ray of l.
persistent light reaction
persistent reactivity to l.
phototherapy l.'s
l. pipe pick
polarized light microscopy
l. projection test
psoralen plus ultraviolet light of A wavelength
pulsed light therapy
pupillary light reflex
pupils equal and reactive to light and accommodation
pupils equal, round, reactive to light and accommodation
pupils equal, round, reactive to light and accommodation directly and consensually
pupils react to light and accommodation
quantitative light induced fluorescence
l. reaction
reactive to light pupil
red light therapy
l. reflection rheography
l. reflex ring
relative light units
relative to rotation of a beam of polarized l.
l. response of pupil
l. scatter
l. scattering
l. scattering index
l. scatter technique
l. sensation
l. sense
l. sensitive
sensitivity to light and glare
shade response to light gray area
l. stimulus
swing light test
l. therapy
l. touch
l. touch testing
l. toxicity
l. transmission
l. treatment
ultraviolet l.
ultraviolet light, long wavelength
ultraviolet light, midrange-wavelength
l. urticaria
variable domain of light chain immunoglobulin

light *(continued)*
velocity of l.
Wood light examination of eye
xenon arc l.
light-adapted eye
light-cured
l.-c. cement
l.-c. dimethacrylate
light-dark
l.-d. cycle
l.-d. discrimination
light/dark amplitude ratio
light-emitting diode
lightheaded
irritable and l.
lightheadedness
dizziness or l.
orthostatic l.
positional l.
Lighthouse
L. Distance Visual Acuity Test
L. National Center for Vision and Aging
light-induced
l.-i. absorbance change
l.-i. fluorescence endoscopic bronchoscopy
l.-i. fluorescence endoscopy in combination with pharmacoendoscopy
lighting
paraxial l.
lightly
l. padded
l. staining coiled bacteria
light-near dissociation
lightning
l. attack
l. attacks in infantile spasm
l. cataract
l. eye movement
L. high-speed vitrectomy handpiece
Moore lightning streak
l. pain
l. seizure
l. streak
light-sparing effect
Lightspeed canal preparation technique
light-stress test
Lightwood-Albright syndrome
Lignac
L. disease
L. syndrome
Lignac-Fanconi
L.-F. disease
L.-F. syndrome
ligneous
l. conjunctivitis
l. thyroiditis
likelihood
maximal likelihood estimation
maximum likelihood estimator
maximum likelihood score
l. ratio
Likert scale
Likert-type response pattern
Liliequist membrane
Lillie
L. allochrome connective tissue stain
L. allochrome method
L. azure-eosin stain
L. ferrous iron stain
L. hematoxylin
lima bean trypsin inhibitor
limb
l. abnormality
l. abnormality syndrome
l. absence
l. accurate measurement
afferent ileal l.
alien limb phenomenon
alien limb sign
l. of anterior capsule
anterior limb of internal capsule
anterior limb of stapes
l. apraxia
artery of lower l.
artery of upper l.
artificial l.
asymmetric limb uptake
l. ataxia
l. atrophy
autosomal dominant mild short limb dwarfism
l. of bifurcation graft
l. blood flow
l. bone length ratio
l. brace
l. bud
claudication limb pain
congenital hemidysplasia with ichthyosiform erythroderma and limb defects syndrome
congenital limb deficiency
cortical thick ascending l.
critical limb ischemia
l. defect
l. deformity
l. disproportion
l. duplication
head, limbs, and body
heaviness of l.'s
l. of helix
l. holder
hyperthermic isolated limb perfusion
l. infarction
inflatable limb splint
involuntary trembling of l.
l. ischemia
ischemic limb disease
isolated hyperthermic limb perfusion
l. lead two
left lower l.
left upper l.
l. length inequality
long limb of incus
lower l.
lower limb orthosis
lower limb ossification center
lower limb prosthesis
lymph node of lower l.
lymph node of upper l.
mandibulofacial dysostosis with limb malformations syndrome
medullary thick ascending l.
medullary thick ascending limb of Henle
membranous limb of semicircular duct
mental retardation, spasticity, distal transverse limb defects syndrome
microcomputer upper limb exerciser
l. motion
multiple benign circumferential skin creases on l.
no spontaneous movement of l.'s
l. pain
paresthesia of l.
periodic limb movement disorder
periodic limb movements during sleep
periodic limb movement in sleep
phantom limb syndrome
posterior limb of the internal capsule
l. reanastomosis
l. reduction defects

l. reduction deformity
right lower l.
right upper l.
l. salvage
segmental limb systolic pressure
severed limb salvage technique
short limb dwarfism
single limb support
l. sparing surgery
stiffness or heaviness of l.'s
thick ascending l.
thick ascending limb of Henle loop
tonic hind limb extension
unipolar limb lead
unusual position of l.'s
upper l.
upper limb orthosis
upper limb prosthesis
upper limb tension test
l. vascular resistance

limbal
l. allograft
l. approach
l. arcade
l. autografting
l. autograft transplantation
l. bleeding
l. choristoma
l. compression
l. dermoid
l. follicle
l. girdle of Vogt
l. groove
l. guttering
l. incision
l. ischemia
l. neurofibroma
l. palisades of Vogt
l. papillae
l. parallel orientation
l. stem-cell deficiency
l. stem cell transplantation
l. stroma
l. suture
l. tissue
l. vasculitis
l. zone

limbal-based flap

limb-body wall complex

Limberg
L. flap
L. technique

limb-girdle
l.-g. dystrophy
l.-g. muscular dystrophy
l.-g. muscular weakness and atrophy
l.-g. syndrome

limbic
l. activation
anterior limbic association area
l. bands
l. center
l. circuit
l. circuitry
l. cortex
l. dopamine receptor
l. dysregulation
l. effect
l. encephalitis
endogenous limbic potential
l. epilepsy
l. forebrain
l. forebrain structure
l. GABAergic system
keratoconjunctivitis
l. kindling
l. lobe
l. midbrain area
paraneoplastic limbic encephalopathy
l. status epilepticus
l. structure
superior limbic keratoconjunctivitis
l. system
l. vernal keratoconjunctivitis

limb-kinetic
l.-k. apraxia
l.-k. dyspraxia

limb-length
l.-l. asymmetry
l.-l. discrepancy

Limbo
Gumbo Limbo virus

limbus
conjunctival l.
l. of cornea
l. corneae
cystoid cicatrix of l.
l. girdle
l. guttering
l. mass
nasal l.
l. of osseous spiral lamina
l. parallel orientation straddling tattoo mark
l. penicillatus
l. of perception
l. of sclera
l. of sphenoid bone
l. striatus
l. of tympanic membrane

lime
bone phosphate of l.
soda l.
triphosphate of l.

limen
difference limen threshold
intensity difference l.
l. nasi
temporal difference l.
terminal l.

liminal
l. sensation
l. sensitivity
l. stimulus

limit
allowable limits of error
below detectable l.'s
below lower l.
l. check
l. of detection
l. dextrans
l. dextrin
l. dextrinase
l. dextrinosis
l. dilution factor
elastic l.
exercise l.
expected upper l.
l. of flocculation
l. flocculation unit
l. of impurities
lower confidence l.
lower limit of detection
lower normal l.
maximum residue l.'s of veterinary drugs
metal endurance l.
normal l.'s
no time l.
permissible exposure l.'s
l.'s of quantitation
radiation dose l.
range of motion within normal l.'s
l. of reaction
l. salt intake
short-term exposure l.
threshold limit value
times upper limit of normal
upper confidence l.
upper and lower extremities within normal l.'s
upper limits of normal
within defined l.'s

limit *(continued)*
within full l.'s
within functional l.'s
within normal l.'s

limitans

limitation
chronic airflow l.
l. of exposure
flow l.
Functional L. Profile
Health and Activity L. Survey
l. of motion
l. of movement
no limitation of motion
swelling, tenderness, limitation of motion

limited
l. activity
l. anterior small thoracotomy
l. attention span
autopsy limited to abdomen
autopsy limited to brain
autopsy limited to heart and lungs
l. channel-capacity process
l. compression-dynamic compression plate
l. diet
l. disease
l. effect
l. examination
l. fasciectomy
l. fragment proteolysis
l. gallium scan
l. gastrectomy
l. hemorrhoidectomy
l. hepatectomy
l. hypothermia
l. intelligence
l. interpersonal skills
l. intravenous pyelogram
l. joint mobility
l. joint motion
l. neck motion
organ l.
permission, limited information, specific suggestions, and intensive therapy
l. progressive systemic sclerosis
l. quantity test performed on small specimen
l. resection
l. ROM
l. sampling model
l. scleroderma
l. support
syndrome of limited joint mobility
l. systemic scleroderma
time l.
l. toxicology screening
l. treadmill test
l. Wegener granulomatosis

limited-stage
l.-s. diffuse large cell lymphoma
l.-s. disease
l.-s. DLCL
l.-s. small cell lung cancer

limiter
motion control l.

limiting
l. alcohol intake
l. angle
anterior limiting lamina
anterior limiting layer of cornea
anterior limiting ring
assessment for limiting condition
l. decision
l. dilution analysis
l. dilution assay
l. dilution polymerase chain reaction
dose-intensity limiting criterion
external limiting membrane
internal limiting membrane
l. isorrheic concentration
l. lamina
l. lamina anterior
l. layer
l. layers of cornea
l. membrane
l. membrane of neural tube
l. membrane of retina
outer limiting membrane
patient with severe systemic disease limiting activity but not incapacitating
l. precursor cell
l. sulcus of Reil
l. sulcus of rhomboid fossa
l. viscosity number

limitus
hallux l.
hallux limitus deformity
McKeever arthrodesis for hallux l.

limp
antalgic l.
gluteal l.
l. hair from anemia
l. infant syndrome
psychogenic l.

Lindau
L. disease
L. tumor

Lindau-von Hippel disease

Lindemann
L. bur

Lindner
L. body
L. operation
L. sclerotomy

Lindsay operation

Lindstrom
L. Star
L. Star nucleus manipulator

line
aneuploid cell l.
l. angle
anterior axillary l.
anterior commissure-posterior commissure l.
anterior gluteal l.
anterior humeral l.
anterior junction l.
anterior median l.
anterior oblique line of radius
anterior spinal l.
anteromedial joint l.
antitension l.
aortic vent suction l.
arcuate line of Douglas
arcuate line of ilium
arcuate line of rectus sheath
Armstrong tube l.
arterial l.
arterial line culture
arterial line flush solution
arterial line insertion
arterial mean l.
l. artifact
axial line angle
l. of Bechterew
l. bisection error
l. of Blaschko
Burkitt lymphoma cell l.
carcinoma cell l.
cell repository l.
center line artifact
central line infection
central sacral l.
central venous l.
certified cell l.
cervical l.
l.'s of cleavage
continence l.
continuously cultured carcinoma cell line used for tissue cultures

cytotoxic T lymphocyte l.
l. of demarcation
l. of direction
distance between nasal l.'s
l. of Douglas
l. drawing
l. of duty
l.'s of expression
extended electron-loss line fine structure
l. of Farre
femoral arterial l.
femoral head l.
l. filter
l. of fixation
l. focus principle
fracture line consolidation
l. frequency noise dot
l. of Gennari
glabellolambda line craniometric point
glabellomeatal l.
glabelloopisthion l.
l. of gravity
hamster tumor l.
Hickman l.
human erythroleukemia l.
human lymphoblastoid cell l.
increased tension l.
indwelling venous l.
infected hyperalimentation l.
infraorbitomeatal l.
interpupillary l.
interscapular l.
intravenous line infection
l. of Kaes
Kerley A, B, C l.
lateral joint l.
left axillary l.
left midclavicular l.
l.ar in-line ligature carrier
lower anterior axillary l.
lower midclavicular l.
lumbar gravitational l.
lymphoblastoid cell l.
lymphoid cell l.
Maddox l.
major dense l.
male germ line tumor
mare's hair l.
mare's tail l.
marginal line calculus index
medial joint l.
Merkel cell carcinoma cell l.
methylene blue l.
midaxillary l.
midclavicular l.
midclavicular line to nipple
midcostal l.
middle axillary l.
middle cranial fossa l.
midsternal l.
milk l.'s
milk lines of abdomen
milk lines of thorax
MOLT-18, human T cell l.
monitoring lines inserted and positioned
Muehrcke l.
multiple line scan
multiple myeloma cell l.
multiple resistant cell l.'s
murine myeloid leukemia cell l.
neural cell l.
neuronal cell l.
no line of demarcation
oblique line of mandible
oblique line of thyroid cartilage
occipitomastoid suture l.'s
l. of Ogston
orbitomeatal l.
parallel line equal spacing
parasternal l.
pectineal line of femur
pectineal line of pubis
percutaneously inserted central line catheter
percutaneously placed l.
peripheral arterial l.
peripherally inserted catheter l.
l. placement
l. of pleural reflection
posterior axillary l.
L. printed per minute
l. probe assay
pubic hair l.
pulmonary artery l.
radial arterial l.
relaxed skin tension l.
l.'s of Retzius
right midclavicular l.
sacral horizontal plane l.
Schwalbe l.
l. sepsis
Sergent white l.
Serials on L.
skin tension l.
skull suture l.
l. for soleus muscle
l. spread function
straight line velocity
subclavian intravenous l.
l. test
thyroid T-cell l.
l. of Toldt
transverse l.
l.'s and tubes
umbilical arterial l.
umbilical artery l.
umbilical venous l.
upper midclavicular l.
vector cardiography electrode right midaxillary line
ventral venous l.
l. of vision
white line of Toldt
l. of Zahn
zygomaticofrontal suture l.

lineage
l. fidelity
l. heterogeneity
macrophage lineage antigen
monocyte lineage antigen
myeloid lineage antigen
neural crest-derived cell l.
l. promiscuity
l. restriction
l. switch
l. switch leukemia
ulcer-associated cell l.

lineage-associated
l.-a. antigen
l.-a. gene

linear
l. absorption coefficient
l. acceleration
l. accelerator-based radiosurgery
l. accelerator-based SRS
l. accelerator isocenter motion
l. actuator
l. alkyl sulfonate
l. amplification
l. amplifier
l. amputation
l. analog pain scale
l. analog pain score
l. analog self-assessment
l. array B-mode ultrasound transducer
l. array echoendoscope
l. array transrectal ultrasound probe
arterial linear density
l. artifact
l. atelectasis
l. atrophoderma of Moulin
l. atrophy
l. attenuation coefficient
l. band of maximal radiolucency
l. branching microcalcification
l. branching pattern

linear *(continued)*
l. calcification
l. capsulotomy
l. chromosome
l. closure
l. combination of atomic orbital-molecular orbital
l. combination of atomic orbitals
l. combination of fragment configuration
l. combination model software
constant linear velocity
l. correction factor
l. craniectomy
l. defect
l. degenerative signal intensity
l. density
l. dichroism
direct linear plotting
l. discriminant analysis
l. displacement analysis
l. distribution of lesion
l. echo
l. endotheliitis
l. energy transfer
l. epidermal nevus
l. epitope
l. erosion
l. extensor erythema
l. fluorescein
l. focal elastosis
l. fraction
l. fracture
l. free-energy relationship
generalized linear interactive model
general linear model
l. gingival erythema
l. graft
l. groove
l. growth
l. growth retardation
l. growth velocity
l. hearing aid
high-energy bent beam linear accelerator
high linear energy transfer radiation
l. hypocalcification
l. hypoplasia
l. IgA bullous dermatosis
l. IgA bullous disease
l. IgA dermatosis
l. IgA disease
l. IgM disease of pregnancy
l. incision
increased linear density
l. infiltration
inflamed linear verrucous epidermal nevus
inflammatory linear verrucous epidermal nevus
l. inflammatory verrucous epidermal nevus
l. in-line ligature carrier
l. keratopathy
l. Koebner reaction
l. lesion
l. lichen planus
low-energy linear accelerator
microphthalmia with linear skin defects
multiple linear regression analysis
l. opacity
opaque linear opacification
l. petechia
l. porokeratosis
l. probe
l. profile scan
l. programming
l. progressive systemic sclerosis
l. regression analysis
l. salpingostomy
l. scar
l. scarring
l. scleroderma variant
l. sebaceous nevus sequence
l. sebaceous nevus syndrome
l. skull fracture
l. streaking
l. streak lesion
l. subcutaneous atrophy
superficial linear array
l. telangiectasis
titanium linear cutter
transverse linear incision
l. variable differential transformer
l. vision
l. visual acuity test
l. visual analog scale
l. and whorled nevoid hypermelanosis

linearity
l. check
Mantel-Haenszel test for l.

linear-nonlinear least squares

linear-shaped hemorrhage

lined
seromuscular enterocystoplasty lined with urothelium

Linell-Ljungberg classification

liner
asbestos l.
bone l.

line-spread function

lingering hepatitis

Lin-Gettig syndrome

lingua
l. dissecta
l. fissurata
l. nigra
nigrities l.
nucleus fibrosus l.
l. plicata

lingual
l. airway dysfunction
l. alveolar bone
l. alveolar plate
l. alveolar ridge
l. alveolus
l. angle
anterior lingual gland
l. aponeurosis
l. appliance
l. approach
l. apron
l. arch
l. arch-forming pliers
l. artery
l. attachment
l. bar major connector
l. bone
l. bony expansion
l. branch of facial nerve
buccal of upper and lingual of lower
l. button
l. canine-to-canine retainer
l. cavity
l. clasp
l. corpuscle
l. crib
l. crossbite
l. crypt
l. cusp
l. cyst
l. delirium
l. developmental groove
l. dovetail
l. duct
l. embrasure
l. flange
l. folium
l. follicle
l. foramen
l. fossa
l. frenulum

l. frenum
l. ganglion
l. gingiva
l. gingival papilla
l. gland
l. gyrus
l. hemiatrophy
l. hemorrhoid
l. interdental papilla
l. labia
l. lipase
l. lobe
l. lymph node
l. margin
mesial incisal lingual surface
l. mucosa
l. muscle
l. nerve
l. plexus
progressive lingual hemiatrophy
l. root
l. sulcus
l. surface
l. surface of tooth
l. thyroid
l. thyroid gland
l. tongue flap
l. tonsil
l. ulcer
l. vein

linguapalatal
l. constriction
l. contact
l. contact pattern

linguine sign

linguistic
l. ambiguity
L. Analysis of Speech Samples
l. approach
l. aspect
Clinical Adaptive Test/Clinical L. and Auditory Milestone Scale
Clinical L. and Auditory Milestone Scale
l. competence
l. component
l. content of task
l. determinism
l. disorganization
l. disturbance

linguistics
anthropological l.
applied l.

lingula
l. cerebelli
l. of cerebellum
l. of left lung
lung l.
l. of mandible
l. mandibulae

lingular
l. artery
l. bronchus
l. division of the left lung
l. effusion
l. mandibular bony defect
l. segment
l. vein

linguogingival
l. fissure
l. groove

linguoincisal edge

linguomandibular reflex

lining
l. of abdominal cavity
cauterize lining of uterus
l. cell
l. cell layer hyperplasia
epithelial lining fluid
granulomatous l.
heart l.
hyaline membranes lining alveolar space
infected joint l.
inflammation of heart l.
intestinal l.
membranous l.
l. of nasal passage
pleural membrane l.
precancerous overgrowth of uterine l.
respiratory tract lining fluid
stomach l.
synovial lining cell
uterine l.

link
L. anatomical hip
l. antibody

linkage
l. analysis
antibody linkage method
associative l.
4-bar linkage on knee prosthesis
4-bar linkage prosthetic knee mechanism
disease linkage disequilibrium
l. disequilibrium
l. effector
l. equilibrium
l. group
l. map
partial l.
single nucleotide polymorphisms - linkage disequilibrium

linked
l. to dipalmitoyl phosphatidylethanolamine
radiation linked antibodies
radiation linked disease
l. suppression

linker
l. for activation of T cell
l. DNA

linoleic acid depression

Lint
modified Van Lint anesthesia
modified Van Lint block

Linton
L. flap
L. tube

lion
San Miguel sea lion virus

lion's claw grasper

lip
l. of acetabulum
l. adhesion operation
ankyloblepharon, ectodermal defect, and cleft lip and/or palate
anterior cervical l.
anterior lip of the acetabulum
anterior lip of the cervix
anterior lip of external os of uterus
anterior lip of uterine os
l. augmentation
bilateral cleft lip and palate
l. biting
l. border advancement
l. bumper
l. cancer
l. of cervix
cleft l.
cleft lip, cleft palate, lobster-claw deformity syndrome
cleft lip and alveolus
cleft lip and cleft palate
cleft lip deformity
l. closure
commissure of lips and mouth
l. competency
l. cosmetic
Cupid's bow upper l.
l. curtain
cyanosis of l.

lip *(continued)*
depressor muscle of lower l.
ectodermal dysplasia, cleft lip and palate, mental retardation, syndactyly syndrome I, II
l. elevator
l. enhancement
l. erotism
l. furrow band
l. of glenoid
l. habit appliance
lower l.
lower lip paralysis
medial cleft of l.
medial lip of linea aspera
median cleft l.
median cleft of lower lip and mandible
median cleft upper lip, mental retardation, pugilistic facies syndrome
Millard bilateral cleft lip repair
l.'s of mouth
navicular dorsal lip fracture
nodular blueberry l.'s
numbness of l.
osteophytic bone l.
outer lip of iliac crest
l. phenomenon
l. pit
posterior lip of acetabulum
posterior lip nerve
l. pseudocleft-hemangiomatous branchial cyst syndrome
l. reflex
l. scar revision
l. shave
l. sulcus
unilateral cleft of lip and palate
l. vermilion

lipase
l. assay
bile salt-stimulated l.
l. enzyme
hepatic triglyceride l.
hormone sensitive l.
lingual l.
lipoprotein l.
lipoprotein lipase activity
lipoprotein lipase deficiency
lipoprotein lipase gene
lysosomal acid lipase A, B
pancreatic l.
triglyceride l.
l. unit

lipectomy
hip l.
suction-assisted l.
ultrasound-assisted l.

lipedematous alopecia

lipemia
alimentary l.
postprandial l.
l. retinalis

lipemic
l. retina
l. retinopathy

lipid
l. accumulation
amphotericin B lipid complex
antihypertensive and lipid lowering
antihypertensive neural renomedullary l.'s
l. assay
l. bilayer
bilayer lipid membrane
black lipid membrane
l. body
l. cell neoplasm
l. cell ovarian tumor
l. cholecystitis
l. cholesterol
cholesterol-lowering l.
l. conjugate
l. content of storage fat
l. cyst
cytoplasmic lipid droplet
l. cytosome
l. degeneration
l. depletion
l. deposit
l. embolism
l. emulsion
l. envelope
l. exudate
fasting lipid profile
fasting plasma l.
l. fluidity unit
l. granulomatosis
l. hydrocarbon inclusion
l. hypothesis
ichthyosis and neutral lipid storage disease
l. inclusion
l. keratopathy
l. level
l. liquid crystal
membrane lipid cell
l. metabolism
l. metabolism disorder
mitochondria lipid glucogen
l. mobilization
l. moiety
monophosphoryl lipid A
l. myopathy
neutral lipid storage disease
nuclear aggregate l.
ovarian lipid cell neoplasm
l. panel
l. peroxidation
l. peroxide
l. pheresis
l. phosphorus
l. profile
l. reduction
skin surface l.
l. sphingomyelin
l. storage disease
l. synthesis
l. tail
l. tear layer
total l.'s
total lipid extract
l. tumor
vasodepressor l.

lipid-containing
l.-c. tumor
l.-c. vesicle

lipid-laden
l.-l. clear cell
l.-l. hepatocyte
l.-l. homogeneous adrenocortical carcinoma
l.-l. lysosome
l.-l. macrophage

lipid-lowering
l.-l. agent
l.-l. drug
l.-l. medication
l.-l. therapy

lipid-mobilizing hormone

lipidosis
neurovisceral l.

lipid-soluble secondary antioxidant

lipoamide
l. dehydrogenase
l. disulfide

lipoatrophic
l. diabetes
l. phenotype

lipoatrophy
anular l.
localized l.
partial l.
peripheral l.

lipochondral degeneration

lipochrome histiocytosis disease

lipocytic lesion

lipodystrophy
- partial face-sparing l.
- l. syndrome

lipodystrophy-acromegaloid gigantism syndrome

lipofuscin
- l. deposit
- l. granule

lipofuscinosis
- l. granular osmiophilic deposit
- juvenile-onset neuronal ceroid l.
- late infantile neural ceroid l.
- neural ceroid l.
- neuronal ceroid l.
- neuronal ceroid lipofuscinosis curvilinear body

lipogenic
- l. enzyme
- l. enzyme propensity

lipogenous diabetes

lipoglycan antigen

lipohypertrophy

lipoic acid

lipoid
- l. adrenal gland hypoplasia
- l. adrenal hyperplasia
- l. cell
- l. cell tumor
- congenital lipoid adrenal hyperplasia
- l. degeneration
- l. dermatoarthritis
- l. dystrophy
- exogenous lipoid pneumonia
- l. granuloma
- l. granulomatosis
- l. hyperplasia
- l. interstitial pneumonitis
- l. nephrosis
- l. ovarian neoplasm
- l. ovarian tumor
- l. pneumonia
- l. proteinosis
- l. theory of narcosis

lipolytic
- l. enzyme
- postheparin lipolytic activity

lipoma
- l. arborescens
- l. aspiration
- l. capsulare
- l. cavernosum
- l. of cord
- dorsal brain stem l.
- l. fibrosum
- macrocephaly, multiple lipomas, hemangiomata syndrome
- quadrigeminal cistern l.
- l. sarcomatosum
- spindle cell l.

lipomatosis
- benign symmetric l.
- encephalocraniocutaneous l.
- multiple symmetric l.

lipomatous
- l. hemangiopericytoma
- hemosiderotic fibrohistiocytic lipomatous lesion
- l. hypertrophy

lipomelanic reticulosis

lipomembranous
- polycystic lipomembranous osteodysplasia

lipoperoxidation
- hepatic l.

lipophagia granulomatosis

lipophagic
- l. granuloma
- l. intestinal

lipophilic
- l. cationic complex
- l. cationic diphosphine
- l. chloroethylnitrosourea
- l. compound
- l. *Corynebacterium*
- l. drug
- l. dye
- l. fungus
- l. hormone
- l. molecule
- l. prodrug
- l. topoisomerase I inhibitor
- l. yeast

lipophosphoprotein
- serum l.

lipoplasty
- external ultrasound-assisted l.
- suction-assisted l.
- ultrasonic-assisted l.

lipoplethoric diabetes

lipopolysaccharide
- l. binding protein
- l. coat
- l. endotoxin
- l. extract
- l. factor
- l. porins
- l. receptor
- l. vaccine

lipopolysaccharide-induced arthritis

lipoprotein
- abnormal l.
- apolipoprotein B-containing lipoprotein
- l. assay
- atherogenic low-density lipoprotein pattern B phenotype
- beta l.
- l. chylomicron
- l. concentration
- l. electrophoresis test
- familial high-density lipoprotein deficiency
- familial hypercholesterolemia, low-density l.
- l. glomerulopathy
- heparin-induced extracorporeal low-density lipoprotein precipitation
- high-density lipoprotein C
- intermediate density l.
- intermediate low-density l.
- isolated low high-density l.
- l. lipase
- l. lipase activity
- l. lipase deficiency
- l. lipase gene
- liver-specific membrane l.
- low-density lipoprotein apheresis
- low-density lipoprotein cholesterol
- low-density lipoprotein deficiency
- low-density lipoprotein receptor disorder
- low-density lipoprotein receptor-related protein
- malondialdehyde conjugated low-density l.
- malondialdehyde modified low-density l.
- microsomal l.
- non–high-density l.
- normal low-density l.
- oxidized low-density l.
- l. polymorphism
- l. receptor-related protein
- l. remnant
- remnant l.
- remnant-like lipoprotein particle
- triglyceride-rich l.
- very high density l.
- very low density l.
- very low density lipoprotein C

lipoprotein-associated coagulation inhibitor
lipoprotein-cholesterol
high-density l.-c.
l.-c. metabolism
lipoprotein-deficient fraction
lipoprotein-triglyceride
very low density l.-t.
lipoprotein-X
liposarcoma
myxoid l.
l. of uterus
liposclerosing myxofibrous tumor
liposculpture
three-dimensional superficial l.
liposomal
l. daunorubicin
l. doxorubicin
l. encapsulated anthracycline
l. amphotericin B
l. preparation
stealth liposomal doxorubicin
l. topoisomerase I inhibitor
liposomally
l. entrapped doxorubicin
l. entrapped second antibody
liposome
antibody-conjugated paramagnetic l.
l. drug delivery
liposome-encapsulated
l.-e. doxorubicin
l.-e. hemoglobin
l.-e. IL-2
l.-e. paclitaxel
l.-e. tetracaine
lipostatic
l. hypothesis
l. mechanism
liposuction
l. cannula
l. divot
l. fat fillant implant
four-pronged liposuction cannula
massive all layer l.
l. tube
tumescent l.
ultrasonic l.
ultrasonic-assisted l.
lipoteichoic acid
lipotrophic diabetes
lipotropic
l. factor
l. hormone
l. pituitary hormone
lipotropin
human l.
Lipovnik virus
Lipowitz metal
lipoxin
l. A4, B4
lipoxygenase
l. blockade
l. interaction product
l. pathway
12-lipoxygenase-generated lipid
5-lipoxygenase-generated lipid
lipoxygenase interaction product
lip/palate
arthrogryposis, ectodermal dysplasia, cleft lip/palate developmental delay syndrome
split hand-cleft lip/palate and ectodermal dysplasia
Lippe loop
lipping
arthritic l.
hypertrophic l.
narrowing and l.
posterior l.
Lipschütz
L. body
L. cell
L. disease
L. inclusion body
L. ulcer
lipuric diabetes
liquefaction
l. degeneration
l. necrosis
l. of subdural hematoma
l. of vitreous
liquefactive
basal cell liquefactive degeneration
l. degeneration
l. necrosis
liquefying
nodular liquefying panniculitis
liquid
l. air
l. antacid
l. barium suspension
bimolecular liquid membrane
l. cable
l. calcium
l. chemical germicide
l. chemical sterilization
l. chromatographic assay
l. chromatography coupled to tandem mass spectrometry
l. chromatography with electrochemical detection
clear l.
clear liquid diet
cold liquid diet
l. crystal contact thermography
l. crystal display projector
l. crystal thermogram
l. crystal thermography
denaturing high-performance liquid chromatography
l. diarrhea
l. diet
l. dram
l. emptying
l. ethyl chloride
l. extraction
l. feeding
l. food dysphagia
full liquid diet
high-performance liquid chromatography
high-power liquid chromatography
high-pressure liquid affinity chromatography
high-speed liquid chromatography
l. holding recovery
l. human serum
intake of l.
lipid liquid crystal
low liquid level monitor
low-pressure liquid chromatography
medium pressure liquid chromatography
l. membrane
micro liquid extraction
nectar-thick liquid diet consistency
l. nitrogen
l. organic compound
l. organic dye laser
l. ounce
l. oxygen
L. paraffin
l. perfluorocarbon
L. petrolatum
l. pint
predigested liquid protein
pudding-thick liquid diet consistency

l. quart
reversed phase high-performance liquid chromatography
reversed-phase liquid chromatography
l. scintillation counting
single-cell liquid cytotoxic assay
solidified l.
tidal liquid ventilation
time-resolved liquid scintillation counting
total liquid ventilation
l. ventilation
l. vitreous-aspirating cannula

liquid-assisted high-frequency oscillatory ventilation

liquidation of attachment

liquid-liquid
l.-l. chromatography
l.-l. distribution

liquid-solid chromatography

liquified
l. natural gas
l. petroleum gas
l. powder cocaine
l. vitreous

Liquimat lotion

liquor
l. cerebrospinalis
l. corneae
l. entericus
l. folliculi
meconium staining of l.

Lisch
L. nodule
L. spot

Lisfranc
L. amputation
L. arthrodesis
L. articular interline
L. articulation
L. disarticulation
L. dislocation
L. fracture
L. fracture-dislocation
L. joint
L. ligament
L. tubercle

Lison syndrome

Lissauer
L. bundle
L. column
L. fasciculus
L. marginal zone
L. tract

lissencephaly
Norman-Roberts lissencephaly syndrome

lissencephaly-pachygyria spectrum

list
Adjective Check L.
Amsterdam Depression L.
critical condition l.
Current L. of Medical Literature
danger l.
Depression Adjective Check L.
disabled l.
master drug l.
Multiple Affect Adjective Check L.
Personality Adjective Check L.
phonetically balanced percentage of word l.'s
phonetically balanced percentage of word lists
phonetically balanced word lists
problem l.
L. Processing Language
Rotterdam Symptom Check L.
Sales Attitude Check L.
seriously ill l.
symptom distress check l.
synthetic sentence l.
waiting l.

Listener
Equal Listener Response scale

listening
assistive listening device
l. attitude
auditory selective l.
L. Comprehension Test
directed l.
most comfortable listening level
Progressive Achievement Tests of L. Comprehension
Test of L. Accuracy in Children
uncomfortable listening level

Lister
L. corn
L. scissors
L. tubercle

Listeria
heat-killed *Listeria monocytogenes*
Listeria meningitis
L. monocytogenes
Listeria monocytogenes sepsis

listerial meningitis

listeriolysin O gene

listeriosis
neonatal l.

listhesis
anterior-posterior l.

listing
l. gait
L. law
L. plane
L. reduced eye
L. schematic eye

litem
guardian ad l.

liter
concentration in moles per l.
grams per l.
International Unit per l.
katal per l.
kilogram per l.
microgram per l.
milliequivalent per l.
milligram per l.
millikatal per l.
milliliters per l.
millimole per l.
mole per l.
nanomole per l.
oral airflow in liters per second
O2 saturation on three liters nasal cannula
O2 saturation on two liters nasal cannula
osmoles per l.
oxygen saturation on 2 liters nasal cannula
oxygen saturation on 3 liters nasal cannula
l.'s per centimeter of water
l.'s per minute
l. per minute per square meter
pulse oximetry on 2 liters of oxygen
unit per l.

literacy
l. deficiency
inadequate literacy skills
Test of Economic L.

literal
l. agraphia
l. alexia

literary
child-centered literary orientation

literature
Current List of Medical L.
Index to Dental L.

lithiasis
asymptomatic urinary l.
calcium phosphate urinary l.

lithiasis *(continued)*
l. conjunctivae
l. conjunctivitis
magnesium ammonium phosphate urinary l.

lithium
l. action on first messenger
l. action on membranes
l. action on second messenger
l. assay
l. bromide
l. carbonate
l. carmine
l. citrate
l. clearance
l. diluent
l. discontinuation
l. dose
l. fluoride
fractional excretion of l.
l. iodine
neodymium:yttrium lithium fluoride laser
l. resistance
l. salicylate
l. toxicity
yttrium lithium fluoride

lithium-induced
l.-i. hypothyroidism
l.-i. nephrogenic diabetes insipidus
l.-i. polydipsia

lithocholic acid-deoxycholic acid ratio

lithogenic
l. bile
l. index

litholysis
automatic computerized solvent l.

lithotomy
percutaneous cholangioscopic l.
percutaneous transhepatic cholangioscopic l.
l. position

lithotripsy
alexandrite laser l.
electrohydraulic l.
electrohydraulic extracorporeal l.
electrohydraulic shock wave l.
endoscopic pulsed dye laser l.
extracorporeal piezoelectric l.
extracorporeal shockwave l.
intracorporeal electrohydraulic l.
intracorporeal laser l.
laparoscopic transcystic l.
laser l.
laser-induced intracorporeal shock wave l.
pancreatoscopic laser l.
percutaneous ultrasonic l.
peroral shock wave l.
shock wave l.

litigious
l. delusional state
l. environment

little
l. ACTH
l. adrenocorticotrophic hormone
L. area
l. brown mushroom
L. disease
l. finger
l. fossa of cochlear window
l. fossa of oval vestibular window
l. growth hormone
l. head of humerus
l. head of mandible
L. League elbow
L. League shoulder
opposing muscle of little finger
l. toe

Littler-Cooley abductor digiti quinti transfer

littoral
l. cell
l. cell angioma

Littré
L. gland
L. hernia

Littré-Richter hernia

Litzmann obliquity

live
l. attenuated
l. birth
l. birth abortion
l. clinic
l. donor nephrectomy
l. embryo
full-term live birth
gravida, para, multiple births, abortions, live birth
influenza virus, attenuated live vaccine
monitored live voice
moribund patient not expected to l.
l. oak tree
l. oral poliovirus vaccine
poliomyelitis live vaccine
premature birth live infant
typhoid vaccine, attenuated l.
l. vaccine
l. vaccine strain
l. varicella vaccine
l. vector vaccine
Venezuelan equine encephalitis vaccine, attenuated l.
l. viral vector
l. virus
l. x-ray imaging
l. yeast cell derivative

live-attenuated
l.-a. HIV
l.-a. human immunodeficiency virus
l.-a. lentiviral vaccine
l.-a. recombinant *Salmonella typhi*
l.-a. virus
l.-a. virus vaccine

liveborn infant

livedo
l. annularis
lupus l.
l. pattern
l. racemosa
l. vasculitis

livedoid
l. dermatitis
l. vasculitis

livedo-patterned disease

liver
abnormal liver function test
l. abscess
l. acinus
active liver disease
acute fatty l.
acute fatty liver of pregnancy
acute liver failure
acute on chronic liver disease
adult polycystic liver disease
l. agenesis
l. alcohol dehydrogenase
alcoholic liver cirrhosis
alcoholic liver disease
alcoholic liver disease-type organic psychosis
alcohol-related liver disease
allogenic liver perfusion
l. allograft
l. allotransplantation
l. angiosarcoma
anhepatic stage of liver transplantation
anterior part of diaphragmatic surface of l.

anterior portion of left medial segment IV of l.
antifatty liver factor
atrial liver pulse
autologous liver cell
auxiliary heterotopic liver transplantation
auxiliary liver transplantation
auxiliary orthotopic liver transplantation
l. battery
l. bed
beef liver catalase
bioartificial l.
bioartificial extracorporeal liver support system
l. biopsy
l. blood flow
l. breath
l. bud
l. bull's eye lesion
l. calcification
l. cancer
l. capillary hemangioma
l. capsule
caudate lobe of l.
l. cell adenoma
l. cell carcinoma
l. cell dysplasia
l. cell membrane autoantibody
l. cell plate
l. cell tumor
Chang liver cell
chronic active liver disease
chronic liver disease
chronic liver failure
cirrhosis of l.
l. cirrhosis
cirrhotic liver parenchyma
clear cell sarcoma of the l.
l. clinic
cod liver oil
compression of liver cords
cyanotic atrophy of l.
l. cyst
l. cyst infection
l. damage
l. death
decompensated liver cirrhosis
decompensated liver disease
l. deposit
l. dialysis unit
l. diet
diffuse liver disease
diffuse liver enlargement
l. disease
l. disease organic psychosis
l. distention
l. distribution
l. dome
drug-induced liver disease
l. dullness
l. dysfunction
l. eater
l. echinococcosis
l. edge
l. encephalopathy
end-stage heart and liver disease
end-stage liver disease
end-stage liver failure
l. engorgement
l. enzyme
l. enzyme elevation
l. enzyme serum level
l. enzyme test
estimated liver blood flow
extracorporeal liver assist device
extracorporeal liver perfusion
l. failure
fatty l.
fatty liver cell
fatty liver disease
fatty liver and kidney syndrome
fetal liver cell
l. fibrosis
l. flap
l. flap sign
l. flocculation test
l. fluke
focal infarct of l.
focal nonfatty infiltration of l.
l. fraction elevated
fulminant liver disease
l. function
l. function profile
l. function series
l. function tests
gallbladder and liver scan
l. graft
l. hanging maneuver
heart and liver damage
heart, liver, and kidney
hemangioma of l.
hemolysis, elevated liver enzymes, and low platelet count
hepatitis-induced liver cancer
hepatocellular liver disease
hepatosplenomegaly with liver metastases
l. hilus
l. homogenate
horse liver alcohol dehydrogenase
hyperacute liver failure
hyperplastic liver nodule
l. imaging
l. imbalance
impaired liver function
impairment of liver function
impairment in liver function
inferior margin of l.
l. infiltrate
infrared liver scanner
l. injury
l. injury test
interlobular artery of l.
interlobular vein of l.
l. and intestinal transplantation
l. involvement
l. and iron
l., iron, and B complex
l., iron, red bone marrow
isolated perfused rat l.
l., kidneys, and spleen
l., kidneys, spleen, and bladder
l., kidneys, and spleen not palpable
l. and kidney transplantation
l. lactate dehydrogenase
left liver lobe
living donor liver transplantation
living-related liver transplantation
lobe of l.
lobular architecture of l.
lobule of l.
macrovesicular fatty l.
major liver resection
l. membrane antibody
metabolic liver disease
l. metastasis
metastatic liver cancer
micronodular liver cirrhosis
l. migration inhibitory factor
muscle, liver, brain, eye
muscle, liver, brain, eye disease
muscle, liver, brain, eye nanism
necrosis of l.
needle biopsy of l.
needle liver biopsy
nodular regenerative hyperplasia of liver
non-A–G chronic liver disease
nonalcoholic fatty liver disease
non-B, non-C chronic liver disease
noncolorectal liver metastasis
non-heart-beating donor liver transplantation
nonparasitic cyst of l.
nonparenchymal liver cell
obstructive liver disease
occlusive disease of l.

liver *(continued)*
omental tuberosity of l.
open liver biopsy
orthotopic liver transplant
l. palm
palpable liver edge
palpable liver, spleen and kidneys
l. parenchyma
parenchymatous liver disease
partial auxiliary orthotopic liver transplantation
Pediatric L. Transplant-Specific Scale
percutaneous transhepatic liver biopsy with tract embolization
peritoneal ligament of l.
l. phosphorylase
l. phosphorylase deficiency
l. plasma flow
l. plasma membrane
polycystic disease of l.
polycystic liver disease
portal hypertension of the l.
primary liver cell
primary liver cell cancer
pyogenic abscess of l.
l. pyruvate kinase
radiation-induced liver disease
reduced liver transplant
reduced-size liver transplant
l. regenerating serum factor
l. residue factor
right liver lobe
l. rupture
l. scan
segmental artery of l.
segments of l.
serosa of l.
l. shadow
shark liver oil
l. smear
soluble liver antigen
l. span
l., spleen masses
l. spot
stellate cell of l.
subacute liver failure
subcapsular hematoma of l.
l. tissue abnormality
l. toxicity
l. transaminase
l. transplant
l. transplantation
l. transplant rejection
triangular ligament of l.
l. tumor
l. volume
l. volume replaced by tumor

liver-directed therapy

liver-enriched
l.-e. activating protein
l.-e. inhibiting protein

liver-kidney-microsomal
l.-k.-m. antibody
l.-k.-m. type 1 antibody target assay

Liverpool Seizure Severity Scale

liver-specific
l.-s. antigen
l.-s. membrane lipoprotein
l.-s. protein

live-virus vaccine

livida
asphyxia l.

lividity
postmortem l.

Livierato sign

living
activities of daily l.
activities of daily living scale
adult congregate living facility
adult congruent living facility
adult living facility
adult-to-adult living related donor living transplant
alveolar living material
l. anatomy
Assisted L. Federation of America
assisted living facility
assisted living setting
auxiliary partial orthotopic living donor transplantation
l. bank
capable of independent l.
capacity for independent l.
center for independent l.
Checklist of Adaptive L. Skills
l. children
Communicative Abilities in Daily L.
community living arrangements
L. Conditions Rating Scale
cost of l.
daily living skills
l. death
l. donor
l. donor bilobar transplant
l. donor kidney
l. donor liver transplantation
l. donor nephrectomy
l. donor partial hepatectomy
extended activities of daily l.
l. female child
full-term deliveries, premature deliveries, abortions, living children
full-term living female child
full-term living male child
Functional L. Index-Cancer
Functional L. Index-Emesis
l. host cell
immature living female child
immature living male child
impairment of activities of daily l.
independent in activities of daily l.
independent living needs
independent living skills
intrauterine pregnancy, term birth, living infant
last living breath
l. male child
memory impaired assisted l.
mobility activities of daily l.
modify stressful living habits
patient independent in activities of daily l.
physical daily living skills
postures of daily l.
pregnancy, term, complicated delivered, living female
pregnancy, term, complicated delivered, living male
pregnancy, term, uncomplicated delivered, living female
pregnancy, term, uncomplicated delivered, living male
premature living female child
premature living male child
prudent living heart
Reasons for L. Inventory
l. relative transplant donor
l. renal donor
l. renal transplant
l. segmental donor pancreas transplantation
Shipley Institute of L. Scale
simulated activities of daily l.
skills of daily l.
l. skin equivalent
term birth, living child
term birth, living female
term birth, living infant
term birth, living male
term living newborn

transitional living program
l. unit
l. unrelated donor
l. and well
white female living child
white male living child
l. will
L. with Asthma Questionnaire
l. with disease
youngest living child

living-related
l.-r. donor
l.-r. donor transplantation
l.-r. liver transplantation

Livingston
L. insomnia scale
L. peribulbar wedge

Livingstone-Wheeler regimen

livor mortis

lizard
l. bite
l. skin

LKM1
LKM1 antibody
LKM1 assay

Llano Seco virus

Lloyd
L. Davies Trendelenburg position
L. stereocampimeter
L. syndrome

Lloyd-Roberts
L.-R. fracture
L.-R. fracture technique

Lloyd-Still index

load
average daily patient l.
axial compression l.
axial load teardrop fracture
axial load test
axial load 3-part, 2-plane fracture
l. beam
end-diastolic l.
expiratory threshold l.
l. factor
filtered l.
indentation load deflection
inspiratory threshold l.
metabolic heat load stimulator
plasma viral l.
potential renal solute l.
renal solute l.
resistive l.
resistive load detection
tryptophan load test
viral l.
volume load hypertrophy

load-deflection curve

load-displacement curve

loaded
l. breathing sensation
l. breathing test

loading
axial loading fracture
axial loading injury
axial loading of spine
axial weight l.
l. buffer
complex l.
dihydroepiandrosterone loading test
l. dose
functional and anatomic l.
inspiratory l.
intravenous loading dose

loafer temple

lobar
apical branch of inferior lobar branch of right pulmonary artery
apical segmental artery of superior lobar artery of right lung
l. atelectasis
l. atrophy
l. breast anatomy
l. bronchus
l. cavitation
l. cerebral atrophy
congenital lobar overinflation
l. consolidation
dense lobar infiltrate
l. division
l. dysfunction
l. dysmorphism
l. emphysema
frontotemporal lobar degeneration
l. gliosis
l. hemorrhage
l. holoprosencephaly
l. hyperplasia
infantile lobar emphysema
middle lobar artery
middle lobar artery of right lung
multiple lobar hemorrhage
l. panniculitis
l. pneumonia
recurrent lobar hemorrhage
l. sclerosis

lobe
anterior lobe hormone
anterior lobe of hypophysis
anterior lobe of pituitary
anterior pituitary l.
anterior tip of temporal l.
anteromedial temporal lobe resection
apical lobe fibrosis
artery of caudate l.
association cortex of parietal l.
autosomal dominant nocturnal frontal lobe epilepsy
autosomal dominant temporal lobe epilepsy
l. of azygos vein
bilateral lower l.'s
bilateral occipital lobe infarct
l. of brain
caudate lobe of liver
l. of cerebrum
deep l.
l. dysfunction
extratemporal lobe epilepsy
frontal l.
frontal lobe epilepsy
frontal lobe seizure
inferior frontal l.
inferior parietal and superior temporal l.
kidney l.
left hepatic l.
left liver l.
left lower lobe infiltrate
left lower lobe of lung
left middle l.
left upper l.
l. of liver
lower l.
lower lobe bronchus
lower lobe of lung
l. of lung
main lobe of lung
l. of mammary gland
medial frontal lobe syndrome
mesial aspect of temporal l.
mesial temporal l.
middle l.
middle lobe branch of right superior pulmonary vein
middle lobe bronchus
middle lobe of heart
middle lobe of prostate
middle lobe of right lung
middle lobe vein
native caudate l.
neural l.
neutrophil lobe count
nonlingular branch of upper lobe bronchus

lobe *(continued)*
occipital lobe of brain
occipital lobe unilateral cerebral hemisphere lesion
olfactory lobe of brain
orbital aspect of frontal l.
parietal lobe battery
parietal lobe bilateral cerebral hemisphere lesion
parietal lobe of brain
parietal lobe field defect
parietal lobe function
parietal lobe unilateral cerebral hemisphere lesion
parotid deep l.
l. of pituitary gland
l. of prostate
pyramidal lobe of thyroid gland
right frontal l.
right hepatic l.
right liver l.
right lower l.
right lower lobe infiltrate
right middle l.
right middle lobe bronchus
right middle lobe of lung
right middle lobe syndrome
right upper l.
superior lobe of heart
temporal l.
temporal lobe seizure
l. of thyroid gland
upper l.
upper lobe pulmonary edema

lobectomy
anterior temporal l.
anteromesial temporal l.
video-assisted thoracic surgical non-rib-spreading l.

Lobo disease

lobotomy
prefrontal l.

Lobstein
L. disease
L. ganglion
L. syndrome

lobster
l. clawhand
l. hand deformity

lobster-claw
cleft lip, cleft palate, lobster-claw deformity syndrome
l.-c. deformity
l.-c. foot
l.-c. hand

lobular
l. acinus
l. adenocarcinoma
l. alveolar pattern
l. architecture
l. architecture of liver
l. atelectasis
atypical lobular breast hyperplasia
atypical lobular hyperplasia
l. breast calcification
l. breast microcalcification
l. bronchiole
l. capillary hemangioma
l. carcinoma
l. carcinoma in situ
chronic lobular hepatitis
l. disarray
l. epithelial hyperplasia
l. glomerulonephritis
l. hepatitis
infiltrating lobular cancer
infiltrating lobular carcinoma
l. inflammation
l. neoplasia
pancreatic lobular panniculitis
l. panniculitis
l. patch of atelectasis
pleomorphic lobular carcinoma
terminal ductal lobular unit

lobulated
l. border
l. contour
l. filling defect
l. goiter
l. submucosal mass

lobulation
l. defect
microcephalus, imperforate anus, syndactyly, hamartoblastoma, abnormal lung lobulation, polydactyly

lobulation-polydactyly syndrome

lobule
ansiform l.
anterior lunate l.
anterior paracentral l.
l. of auricle
l. breast
central vein of hepatic l.
cortical lobule of kidney
l. of epididymis
falciform l.
hepatic l.
l. of liver
l. of mammary gland
medial l.
paracentral l.
quadrate l.
superior parietal l.
l. of testis
l. of thymus
l. of thyroid gland

lobuloalveolar tumor

local
l. abscess
l. adaptation syndrome
advanced local invasion
l. alcohol instillation effect
l. analgesia
l. anaphylaxis
l. anemia
l. anesthesia
l. anesthetic reaction
l. area communications network
l. argyria
l. asphyxia
l. bloodletting
l. bone blood flow
l. bulge of kidney contour
l. bulge renal contour
l. cavus
l. cementoosseous dysphasia
l. cerebral blood flow
l. cerebral glucose utilization
l. circuit theory
l. coil
l. compression fracture
contralateral local anesthesia
l. control
control of local and systemic disease
l. convulsion
l. death
l. decompression fracture
l. decongestion
l. depot injection
l. diagnostic block
l. disease
l. electroretinogram
l. epilepsy
l. epineurotomy
eutectic mixture of local anesthetics
l. excision
l. excitatory state
l. exhaust ventilation
l. field distortion
l. flap
florid local cementoosseous dysplasia
full-thickness local excision
l. glomerular lesion
l. hepatectomy

l. hormone
l. hypothermia
l. immunity
increased local heat
l. infection
l. infiltrative anesthesia
l. inflammation
l. inflammatory response
l. intraarterial fibrinolysis
l. invasion
l. irradiation
l. irrigation
l. isolation
large local reaction
Lotze local sign
l. lymph-node assay
l. medical doctor
l. medical review policy
metastasis, age, completeness of resection, local invasion, and tumor size
l. methotrexate injection
minimum local analgesic concentration
office laparoscopy under local anesthesia
l. outgrowth
l. ovarian condition
l. radiation
l. reaction
l. recurrence
l. recurrence after radiation therapy
l. recurrence-free survival
l. regional metastases
l. seizure
Shwartzman local reaction
l. side effect
l. sign
l. stimulant
l. surgery
l. symptom
l. tic
time to local failure
l. tissue advancement flap
l. tonic pupil
l. tracheal anesthesia
l. tumor excision
l. tumor excision with irradiation
l. tumor hyperthermia
l. twitch response
whole brain versus local brain radiation therapy
wide local excision

local-acting radioisotope

localization

l. agnosia
auditory l.
autologous white cell l.
autoradiographic l.
l. of behavior
l. of disease
l. of function
needle l.
neural crest tumor localization study
nuclear localization signal motif
percutaneous l.
l. of prostate cancer
simultaneous binaural midplace l.
stone imaging and l.
tumor localization scan

localization-related epilepsy seizure

localized

l. abdominal sign
l. abscess
l. acquired cutaneous pseudoxanthoma elasticum
l. adenopathy
l. adiposity
l. albinism
l. amnesia
l. amyloidosis
l. angiofollicular lymph node hyperplasia
l. angiokeratoma
l. bone destruction
l. brain activity
l. caliectasis
l. coarctation
l. collagen dystrophy
congenital localized absence of skin
l. cutaneous
l. cutaneous amyloidosis
l. cutaneous leishmaniasis
l. electroencephalographic seizure pattern
l. epidermolysis bullosa simplex
l. epilepsy
l. evoked potential
l. fibrous mesothelioma
l. fibrous tumor
l. function
l. gingivitis
l. granuloma annulare
l. headache
healthy patient with localized pathological process
healthy patient with localized pathologic process
l. hemolysis in gel
l. immune reaction
l. infection
l. infiltrate
l. inflammation
l. irritation
l. *Leishmania* lymphadenitis
l. leukocyte mobilization
l. lipoatrophy
l. lipodystrophy
l. magnetic resonance
marked localized reaction
l. molecular orbital
l. mucocutaneous candidiasis
l. myositis
l. neurodermatitis
l. nodular synovitis
l. pachygyria
l. pagetoid reticulosis
pain primarily l.
paroxysmal localized hyperhidrosis
l. pemphigoid of Brunsting-Perry
l. peritonitis
l. plaque formation
l. pretibial myxedema
l. progressive systemic sclerosis
l. prostate carcinoma
l. pustular psoriasis
l. scleroderma
l. tetanus
l. tissue irritation
l. tuberculous meningitis
l. tumor
l. vitiligo
l. vulvar pemphigoid of childhood

localizer

axial l.
breast l.

localizing

lateralizing and l.
l. sign
l. symptom

locally

l. acting paracrine effector
l. advanced breast cancer
l. advanced cancer
l. advanced cervical carcinoma
l. advanced esophageal cancer
l. advanced and inflammatory breast carcinoma
l. advanced melanoma
l. advanced non-small-cell lung cancer
l. advanced prostate cancer
l. made rapid urease test

local-regional failure

locate
unable to l.

location
abnormal location of immature myeloid precursor
l. anomaly
breast needle l.
character, onset, location, duration, exacerbation, remission
complement receptor l.
l. constancy
noncornual placental l.
normal size, shape, and l.
ostium primum l.

locator
driver tunnel locator apparatus
electronic apex l.
lower esophageal sphincter l.
point locator stimulator

lochia
l. alba
l. cruenta
moderate rubra l.
l. rubra
l. serosa

lock
axle lock and bumper
continuous running lock suture
dual lock total hip replacement
l. finger
flush heparin l.
friction lock pin
gait lock splint
heparin l.
intravenous l.
L. solution

Locke
L. bone clamp
L. egg serum medium
L. elevator
L. solution

locked
l. bite
l. cell
l. door seclusion
l. facet
l. hospital unit
l. twins

locked-in syndrome

Locke-Wallace Marital Adjustment test

lock-in amplifier

locking
anatomic medullary l.
anatomic medullary locking hip system
anterior locking plate system
l. bar
buckling and/or locking of knee
continuous locking manner
curved cannula with locking dilator
l. disk
dynamic locking nail
en bloc running locking suture
gamma locking nail
l. gate
gravity extension locking system
l. hook instrumentation
l. horizontal mattress suture
l. of joint
lead locking device
single-axis locking knee prosthesis
l. twins
weight-activated locking knee prosthesis

locking/grasping
atraumatic locking/grasping forceps

Lockwood
L. ligament
L. light reflex
L. tendon

locomotor
l. activity
l. arrest
l. ataxia

locomotor-respiratory coupling

locoregional
l. breast cancer
l. breast carcinoma
l. control
l. disease
l. failure
l. field radiotherapy
l. infusion
l. node
l. radiotherapy
l. recurrence-free survival
l. relapse
l. spread
l. transfection

loculated
l. abscess
l. architecture
l. empyema
l. pleural effusion
l. pleural fluid
l. pus

loculation
arachnoid loculation of the spine
l. of fluid

locus
l. of control
L. of Control-Chance
L. of Control-External
L. of Control-Internal
L. of Control-Powerful Others
L. of Control Scale
l. ferrugineus
l. of fixation
hereditary prostate cancer 1 l.
l. heterogeneity
l. heterogenicity
histocompatibility l.
histocompatibility locus antigen
l. niger
nonhistocompatibility locus antigen-associated form
personal locus of control
preferred retinal l.
quantitative trait l.
single major l.
Sociopolitical L. of Control

locus-specific probe

locutionary stage

lode
viral lode testing

Lodge
Gray Lodge virus

lodgepole pine tree

lodoxamide tromethamine

Loeb deciduoma

Loeffler, Löffler
L. agar
L. bacillus
L. blood culture medium
L. caustic stain
L. disease
L. endocarditis
L. eosinophilia
L. methylene blue dye
L. methylene blue stain
L. syndrome

Loehlein diameter

Loesche classification

Loevit cell

Loewenthal
L. bundle
L. reaction
L. tract

Loewi
L. reaction
L. sign
Löffler (*var. of* Loeffler)
Löfgren syndrome
log
l. cell kill
l. dose-response relationship
drug information l.
l. effect
l. infectious virus titer
l. magnitude ratio
motor activity l.
l. reduction value
l. roll maneuver
l. unit
logarithm
base of natural l.'s
negative logarithm of acid ionization constant
l. neutralization index
l. of odds
logarithmic
l. amplifier
l. curve
l. Minimum Angle of Resolution
l. phase
2-log decrease
1-log decrease
logic
arithmetic and logic unit
complementary metal-oxide semiconductor l.
emitter-coupled l.
undedicated logic array
logical
l. analysis of automatic thought
l. functioning
l. inference
mathematical optimization and logical dimensioning for radiotherapy
logistic
l. curve
l. discriminant analysis
multinomial polytomous logistic regression method
multiple logistic regression
multivariate logistic regression
multivariate logistic regression analysis
L. Organ Dysfunction Score
log-kill
l.-k. hypothesis
l.-k. model
log-rank test
Löhlein operation
loin pain hematuria syndrome
Lokern virus
***Lolium perenne* allergen**
lollipop
l. follicle
narcotic l.
Lombard-Dowell agar
Lombardy
L. leprosy
L. poplar tree
Lombart
L. radioscope
L. tonometer
Londermann
L. corneal trephine
L. operation
London
L. force
L. Psychogeriatric Scale
Tower of L.
lone
l. atrial fibrillation
l. episode
L. Star fever
L. Star tick
L. Star virus
long
l. abductor muscle of thumb
l. abductor tendon
l. adductor muscle
l. alignment rod
l. anal sphincter
anterior long fiber
anterior long toe flexor
apical long axis
l. arm brace
l. arm cast
l. arm of chromosome
l. arm of chromosome X
l. arm finger cast
l. arm navicular cast
l. arm posterior-molded splint
l. arm of Y chromosome
l. association fiber
l. axial oblique view
l. axis
l. axis acquisition
l. axis of body
l. axis of bone
l. axis of kidney
l. axis parasternal view
l. axis ray
l. axis of spleen
l. axis technique
l. axis traction chiropractic table
l. back board
l. below-elbow cast
l. bent-knee leg cast
l. bone deficiency
l. bone fracture
l. bone length
l. bone osteomyelitis
l. bone pseudoarthrosis
l. bone survey
l. buccal nerve
l. calcaneocuboid ligament
l. central artery
l. centric
cervix long, thick and closed
chronic long term illness
l. ciliary artery
l. ciliary nerve
l., closed, posterior cervix
L. coefficient
l. cone technique
l. course
l. crus of incus
l. curette
deletion of long arm of chromosome X
l. deltopectoral approach
l. double upright brace
l. dural tail
l. extensor muscle of great toe
l. extensor muscle of thumb
l. external lateral ligament
l. external rotator
l. face syndrome
l. fibular muscle
l. finger
l. flexor muscle of great toe
l. flexor muscle of thumb
L. formula
l. head of biceps
idiopathic long Q-T interval syndrome
l. incubation hepatitis
l. interspersed elements
left long leg
l. leg brace with free ankle
l. leg brace with pelvic band
l. leg cast
l. leg cylinder cast
l. leg fiberglass cast
l. leg plaster cast
l. leg posterior molded splint
l. leg sitting
l. leg walking cast
l. leg weightbearing cast
l. limb of incus

long *(continued)*
l. line
lower fossa active, lateral knee pain, and long leg on the side ipsilateral to the weak fossa
middle third of long bone
Mullins long transseptal sheath
l. muscle of head
l. muscle of neck
l. nerve of Bell
l. palmar muscle
parasternal long axis
l. peroneal muscle
l. pitch helicoidal layer
l. plantar ligament
l. posterior ciliary artery
l. posterior ciliary axis
l. process of incus
l. process of malleus
l. radial extensor muscle of wrist
l. radiolunate
l. root of ciliary ganglion
l. rotator muscle
l. R-P tachycardia
l. saphenous nerve
l. saphenous vein
l. seal
l. smoking history
l. spike burst
l. stem
subcostal long axis
l. subscapular nerve
l. terminal repeat sequence
l. thin extremity
l. thoracic artery
l. thoracic nerve entrapment
l. thoracic nerve palsy
l. thoracic vein
l. time dialysis
l. tract
l. tract sign
ultraviolet light, long wavelength
upper third of long bone
very long chain acyl-CoA dehydrogenase
very long chain fatty acid
l. vinculum
l. wave irradiation
l. weighted speculum

long-acting
l.-a. antirheumatic drug
l.-a. barbiturate
l.-a. beta agonist
l.-a. contraception
l.-a. contraceptive steroid
l.-a. drug
l.-a. gas
l.-a. inhaled beta-agonist
l.-a. injectable medication
l.-a. injection
l.-a. insulin
medium l.-a.
l.-a. neuroleptic
non-ergot long-acting prolactin inhibitor
octreotide long-acting release
l.-a. oxycodone
l.-a. release
l.-a. sulfonamide
l.-a. testosterone ester
l.-a. thyroid-stimulating hormone
l.-a. thyroid stimulator protector
l.-a. transmural stimulator

long-acting testosterone ester

long-axis
l.-a. fractional shortening
l.-a. view

long-bone radiograph

long-chain
l.-c. acyl-CoA dehydrogenase
l.-c. acyl-CoA dehydrogenase deficiency
l.-c. acyl-coenzyme A dehydrogenase
l.-c. fatty acid
l.-c. fatty acid oxidation
l.-c. 3-hydroxyacyl-CoA dehydrogenase deficiency
l.-c. hydroxyacyl-coenzyme A dehydrogenase
l.-c. monoglyceride
l.-c. polyunsaturated fatty acid
l.-c. triglyceride
l.-c. very long-chain acyl-CoA dehydrogenase deficiency

long-distance group

long-duration response

longevity quotient

long-handled
l.-h. dressing reacher
l.-h. foil condenser
l.-h. shoe horn
l.-h. sock donner
l.-h. sponge

longi

longissimus
l. capitis muscle
l. cervicis muscle
l. colli
l. dorsi
l. muscle of head
musculus l.
musculus longissimus capitis
musculus longissimus cervicis
musculus longissimus thoracis
l. thoracis muscle

longitudinal
l. aberration
l. acoustic wave
anterior longitudinal ligament
l. arch of foot
l. arch support
l. arc of skull
l. arteriography
l. assessment
l. axis of Fick
l. band of colon
l. bands of cruciform ligament of atlas
l. blood supply
l. B-mode
l. canal of modiolus
l. cerebral fissure
l. choledochotomy
l. ciliary muscle
l. colostomy
l. course specifier
curved longitudinal incision
l. data
l. deficiency
l. dense striation
l. diameter of heart
l. displaced complete tear
l. dissociation
l. distraction
l. duct of epoophoron
l. enterotomy
l. epiphysial bracket
l. epiphysial bracket
l. esophageal stricture
l. experimental study design
l. expert evaluation using all available data
l. fasciculi of colon
l. fasciculus
l. fiber
l. fissure of cerebrum
l. fold of duodenum
l. fracture
l. growth
l. hyperpigmented band
l. incision
l. interval followup evaluation
l. layer of muscle coat of small intestine
l. layer of muscular coat
l. layers of muscular tunic
l. lie
l. ligament

MacArthur Longitudinal Twin Study
l. magnetization
l. medial bundle
medial longitudinal arch
medial longitudinal bundle
medial longitudinal stria
median longitudinal raphe of tongue
median longitudinal section
l. melanonychia
midpapillary l.
l. midtarsal joint axis
l. muscle
l. nail hyperpigmentation
National Educational L. Survey
l. nerve
ossification of anterior longitudinal ligament
ossification of posterior longitudinal ligament
outer anular/posterior longitudinal ligament complex
l. oval pelvis
l. pharyngeal muscle
l. plane
l. pontine bundle
l. presentation
l. proton MR spectroscopy
l. random coefficient model
l. relaxation time
l. relaxivity
l. scan
l. section
spin-lattice or longitudinal relaxation time
l. study
l. sulcus
l. sulcus of heart
l. vertebral venous sinus

longitudinalis
arcus pedis l.
fasciculus longitudinalis medialis
musculus longitudinalis superior

long-lasting
l.-l. depolarization
l.-l. insulin
l.-l. potentiation

long-lived memory T cell

long-loop feedback signal

long-pulsed potassium-titanyl-phosphate laser

long-range
l.-r. objective
l.-r. planning

long-scale contrast

long-segment
l.-s. aganglionosis
l.-s. Barrett esophagus
l.-s. CLE
l.-s. congenital tracheal stenosis

long/short occluder

long-term
l.-t. abstinence
l.-t. acute care
l.-t. aftercare treatment
l.-t. antibiotic
l.-t. aspirin therapy
l.-t. associative memory
l.-t. bone-instrumentation interface
l.-t. care
l.-t. care facility
l.-t. care insurance
l.-t. catheter use
l.-t. central venous access catheter placement
l.-t. commitment
l.-t. consequence
l.-t. course
l.-t. course of abuse
l.-t. culture-initiating cell
l.-t. data
l.-t. declarative memory
l.-t. dependence
l.-t. detoxification program
l.-t. disability
l.-t. disease
l.-t. effect
l.-t. effectiveness
l.-t. effects of trauma
l.-t. electrocardiography
l.-t. epidural catheterization
l.-t. estrogen deprivation
l.-t. followup
l.-t. followup data
l.-t. goal
l.-t. healthcare facility
l.-t. heavy drinking
l.-t. heavy use
l.-t. hospitalization
l.-t. illness
l.-t. individual counseling
l.-t. inhalation
l.-t. injection sclerotherapy
l.-t. low-level white noise
l.-t. mechanical assistance
l.-t. memory
l.-t. monitoring
l.-t. nonprogressive disease
l.-t. oxygen therapy
l.-t. plan
l.-t. potentiation
l.-t. RBC transfusion therapy
l.-t. sequelae
l.-t. support group
l.-t. survival
l.-t. surviving
l.-t. survivor
l.-t. survivor of heart transplant
l.-t. variability
l.-t. variability-absent
l.-t. variability-average to moderate
l.-t. venous catheter

long-term detoxification program

longus
abductor pollicis l.
adductor hallucis l.
adductor longus muscle
l. capitis
l. capitis muscle
l. cervicis colli muscle
l. colli muscle
extensor carpi radialis l.
extensor carpi radialis longus flap
extensor carpi radialis longus muscle
extensor carpi radialis longus tendon
extensor digitorum l.
extensor hallucis l.
extensor pollicis l.
flexor digitorum l.
flexor hallucis l.
flexor pollicis l.
musculus abductor pollicis l.
musculus adductor l.
musculus extensor carpi radialis l.
musculus extensor hallucis l.
musculus extensor longus digitorum
musculus extensor longus pollicis
musculus extensor pollicis l.
musculus fibularis l.
musculus flexor hallucis l.
musculus flexor pollicis l.
musculus longus capitis
musculus longus colli
nervus ciliaris l.
palmaris l.
palmaris longus muscle
peroneus longus muscle
peroneus longus muscle avulsion
peroneus longus tendinopathy
pollicis longus abductor muscle
pollicis longus brevis
pollicis longus extensor muscle

longus *(continued)*
pollicis longus flexor muscle
rectus and longus capitis muscle

long-wavelength ultraviolet light

look
anxious l.
glazed l.

look-alike
amphetamine l.-a.

looking
preferential l.

loop
advanced insulin infusion with a control l.
afferent loop syndrome
Alden loop gastric bypass
alpha sigmoid l.
anastomosed to loop of bowel
anterior loop traction
articulatory loop component
ascending loop of Henle
attachable cerumen l.
autocrine-paracrine growth l.
bipolar cutting l.
blind l.
l. of bowel
l. caliber
capillary loop in dermal papilla
capillary loop in hair papilla
l. choledochojejunostomy
cine loop recording
l. circumferential wire
l. colostomy
continuous loop exercise echocardiogram
continuous loop wire
continuous loop wiring
l. diathermy cervical conization
dilated bowel l.
dilated bowel loop resection
distended afferent l.
l. distribution
l. diuretic
l. diversion
diverting loop colostomy
diverting loop ileostomy
efferent loop syndrome
l. electrode
l. electrosurgical excisional procedure
l. electrosurgical excision procedure
l. electrosurgical excision procedure conization
electrosurgical loop excision
l. end ileostomy
l. esophagojejunostomy
l. excision of the transformation zone
exercise tidal flow-volume l.
figure-of-eight wire l.
l. fixation
flow-volume l.
fluid-filled loop of bowel
l. forearm graft
l. gastric bypass method
l. gastric bypass procedure
l. gastric bypass technique
gastric loop bypass
l. gastrojejunostomy
l. of Henle
l. and hook strapping
l. of hypoglossal nerve
ileal loop stoma
l. ileostomy
large loop excision of transformation zone/loop electrosurgical excision procedure
large loop excision of transition zone
lateral loop suspensor
low-voltage diathermy l.
malrotation of bowel l.
matted bowel l.
maximum flow-volume l.
modified J l.
nail fold capillary loop abnormality
negative feedback l.
neuroendocrine control l.
neuronal feedback l.
neuronal feed-forward l.
nonrotation of bowel l.
peripheral chemoreflex l.
physiologic endometrial ablation/resection l.
pressure length l.
rabbit ileal loop test
l. recorder
self-emptying blind l.
self-filling blind l.
sigmoid loop colostomy
small bowel l.
stagnate loop syndrome
terminal ileal l.
thick ascending limb of Henle l.
thickened bowel l.
tidal breathing flow-volume l.
tidal flow-volume l.
l. of Vieussens

loose
l. anagen hair syndrome
ankle loose body
l. areolar plane
l. association
l. body
l. body in joint
l. bowel movement
l. cartilage
l. contact lens
l. debris
l. fibroelastic connective tissue
l. fracture
l. fragment
l. joint
l. junction
l. lens
medium brown loose stool
l. skin

loose-leaf tobacco

loosely
l. closed incision
wound loosely approximated

loosening
aseptic l.
l. of associations
l. joint

Looser
L. fissure
L. line
L. pseudofracture
L. zone

Loosett maneuver

lop ear

Lopez-Enriquez
L.-E. operation
L.-E. scleral trephine

Lorain
L. disease
L. dwarfism
L. infantilism

Lorain-Lévi
L.-L. dwarfism
L.-L. infantilism
L.-L. syndrome

Lorber criteria

Lord
L. dilation
L. dilation of hemorrhoid
L. hemorrhoidectomy

lordosis
l. cervicis
l. colli
compensatory l.
l. creation
l. lumbalis
lumbar l.
l. quotient

lordotic
l. albuminuria
anteroposterior lordotic projection
apical lordotic projection
apical lordotic view
l. aspect
cervical lordotic curvature
l. curve
l. deformity
flattening of normal lordotic curve
lumbar lordotic curve

lorentzian curve

Lorenz
L. cast
L. hip reduction
L. night splint
L. sign

Lorenzo
L. oil
L. oil diet

lorgnette
main en l.
l. occluder

Lortat-Jacobs disease

Los
L. Angeles classification
L. Angeles classification of GERD
L. Angeles Classification grade A, B, C, D esophagitis
L. Angeles preservation solution 1
L. Angeles variant galactosemia

Loschmidt's number

loser
nonsalt l.
salt l.

losing control

loss
abdomen showed evidence of weight l.
abdominal pain associated with blood l.
l. of ability to hold head up
abrupt loss of consciousness
Activity L. Assessment
l. of acuity
acute blood l.
age-related hearing l.
amnesia loss of memory
anemia secondary to blood l.
anterograde loss of memory
anticipated blood l.
l. of appetite from gastritis
l. of appetite from heart failure
l. of appetite from hepatitis
appetite loss from pernicious anemia
l. of appetite with indigestion
l. of appetite with joint swelling
articular bone l.
autism, dementia, ataxia, loss of purposeful hand use syndrome
autoimmune hearing l.
autoimmune sensorineural hearing l.
l. of autonomy
autosomal dominant nonsyndromic hearing l.
autosomal recessive nonsyndromic hearing l.
l. of balance
l. of belief
bilateral progressive hearing l.
l. of biographical memory
l. of bladder control
blood l.
blood loss anemia
l. of bone mass
l. of boundaries of ego
l. of bowel control
l. of breadwinner
central vision l.
chronic blood l.
l. coincidence
conductive hearing l.
l. of consciousness
l. of contact point
l. of control of bladder function
l. of correction
cortical sensory l.
cutaneous water l.
decreased appetite and loss of energy
l. of definition
delayed hearing l.
dialysate protein l.
dimness or loss of vision
l. discrimination
l. of distinction at gray/white matter interface
early pregnancy l.
l. of effect
l. of ego boundary
electron energy loss spectroscopy
l. of energy metabolism
estimated blood l.
estimated weight l.
evaporation water l.
excessive blood l.
excessive bone l.
excessive weight l.
l. experience
external fluid l.
fatigue and loss of appetite
fecal daily blood l.
female pattern hair l.
fluctuating hearing l.
fluctuating sensorineural hearing l.
l. of freedom
l. of function
functional hearing l.
gaze-evoked visual l.
glaucomatous visual field l.
l. of gloss
gradual loss of alertness
gradual loss of auditory discrimination
gradual loss of bone tissue
gradual loss of mental faculties
gradual memory l.
gravity induced loss of consciousness
hair loss from antidepressant
hair loss from birth control pill
hair loss from childbirth
hair loss and nausea
hallucinations and loss of reality
hearing l.
hearing loss from aging
hearing loss from antibiotic
hearing loss from aspirin
hearing loss from diuretics
hearing loss from infection of ear
hearing loss studies
heat loss center
heat loss by radiation
l. of heterogeneity
l. of heterozygosity
l. of heterozygosity chromosome 10
high-frequency sensorineural hearing l.
high-tone hearing l.
hippocampal volume l.
l. of identity
idiopathic sudden sensorineural hearing l.
idiopathic sudden sensory hearing l.
impaired hearing l.
l. of imprinting
l. of independence
infant weight l.
inner ear hearing l.
insensible water l.

loss *(continued)*
l. of intellectual faculties
l. of interest, appetite and concentration
l. of interest in peer social activity
l. of interest in personal grooming
l. of interest in usual activity
intraoperative blood l.
intrapartum blood l.
irreversible loss rate
l. of judgment
low air l.
low air loss therapy mattress
low-frequency sensorineural hearing l.
macrocephaly, hypertelorism, short limbs, hearing loss, developmental delay syndrome
male pattern hair l.
mechanical functional l.
memory loss from anemia
menstrual blood l.
migrainous vision l.
mild hearing l.
minimal blood l.
minor hearing l.
minoxidil and hair l.
mixed hearing l.
moderate hearing l.
monaural hearing l.
l. of motion
l. of movement
nasal field l.
natural hearing l.
negligible blood l.
l. of nerve impulse
neural hearing l.
noise-induced hearing l.
noise-reduced hearing l.
nonorganic visual l.
nonphysiologic visual field l.
nonrenal potassium l.
nonrenal water l.
nonsyndromic hearing l.
l. of normal architecture
normal blood l.
occult blood l.
occupational hearing l.
operative blood l.
painless progressive loss of vision
pain, pallor, pulse loss, paresthesia, and paralysis
partial hearing l.
percentage signal intensity l.
perceptive hearing l.
percutaneous anesthetic l.
peripheral light l.
peripheral visual field l.
periprosthetic bone l.
permanent childhood hearing l.
permanent hearing l.
postmenopausal bone l.
powered air l.
profound hearing l.
progressive hearing l.
progressive unilateral hearing l.
l. of protective sensation
protein loss in hepatic disease
psychogenic hearing l.
rapid bone l.
rapid loss of bone
rapidly progressing bilateral hearing l.
rate of energy l.
l. of recent memory, confusion and poor judgment
recurrent early pregnancy l.
recurrent fetal l.
l. of resistance
retrocochlear hearing l.
l. of righting reflex
segmental bone l.
selective hearing l.
sensorineural hearing l.
sensory neural hearing l.
separation or loss abandonment
severe bone l.
severe hearing l.
severe sensorineural hearing l.
severe visual l.
l. of sexual interest
l. of sight
slight hearing l.
soft tissue l.
speech discrimination l.
sponge blood l.
sudden hearing l.
symptomatic hearing l.
temporary hair l.
temporary hearing l.
Totman L. Index
transepidermal water l.
transient loss of consciousness
transient visual l.
treatment for hair l.
unilateral hearing l.
vertebral bone l.
l. of vision
l. of visual acuity
visual acuity l.
visual field l.
visual hearing l.
l. of vitreous
warning signs of hearing l.
weight l.
weight loss from anxiety
weight loss from pernicious anemia

Lossen rule

loss-of-function
l.-o.-f. disorder
l.-o.-f. mutation

loss-of-resistance technique

lost
L. Cord Club
l. to followup
healthy years of life l.
potential years of life l.
l. privileges
restore lost or thinning hair
l. surgical specimen
l. years of expected life
years of life l.
years of potential life lost before age 65

Lostorfer
L. body
L. corpuscle

Lotheissen hernia repair

lotion
iodine l.
nonalcoholic white shake l.
triamcinolone l.

Lottes reduction technique

Lotze local sign

loud
apneic spell associated with loud snoring
laughing out l.

loudness
alternate binaural loudness balance
alternate monaural loudness balance test
Békésy comfortable l.
binaural alternate loudness balance
l. discomfort level
l. equivalent
l. growth perception
l. level
monaural loudness balance test
monaural bifrequency loudness balance
most comfortable l.
most comfortable loudness level

most comfortable loudness range
range of comfortable l.
uncomfortable loudness level
l. unit

Louis
angle of L.
L. angle
L. law
St. Louis encephalitis virus

Louis-Bar syndrome

Louisiana ankle wrap technique

loupe
angled lens l.
angled nucleus removal l.
l. magnification
magnifying l.
nucleus removal l.
operating l.
panoramic l.

louping ill virus

louse
l. fly
head l.
l. infestation
scalp l.

louse-borne
l.-b. relapsing fever
l.-b. typhus

louse-borne relapsing fever

Lovaas
L. method
L. program
L. training

love
anal-sadistic l.
l. child
l. handle
sex and love addictions

Lovén reflex

Lovett clinical scale of strength

Lovibond
L. angle
L. profile sign

Lovset maneuver

low
abnormally low content
l. absolute glomerular filtration rate
Acute L. Back Pain Screening Questionnaire
acute low back syndrome
l. affinity antigen receptor
l. air loss
l. air loss bed
l. air loss therapy mattress
l. alpha coefficient
l. amplitude
l. anger threshold
l. animal fat
l. anion gap
l. anterior resection
l. anterior resection in combination with coloanal anastomosis
l. anxiety
as low as reasonably achievable radiation exposure
as low as readily practicable
l. atmospheric pressure
l. attenuation
atypical polypoid adenomyofibroma of low malignant potential
l. available carbohydrate diet
l. avidity
l. back
l. back bend
l. back disability
l. back injury
l. back neurosis
l. back pain
l. back pain psychogenic disorder
L. Back Pain Questionnaire
L. Back Pain Symptom Checklist
l. back syndrome
l. back tenderness
l. back trouble
l. bacteria diet
l. biological value
l. birth weight
l. birth weight infant
l. biscuit
l. biscuit firing
l. bisque firing
l. blood gas partition
l. blood pressure
l. blood sugar
l. body mass index
l. bone density
l. bone mass
l. bone turnover disease
l. breakage
l. calcium
l. calorie
l. carbohydrate
l. cardiac output
l. cardiac output syndrome
l. central venous pressure anesthesia
l. cervical approach
l. cervical transverse
l. cervical transverse cesarean section
l. cervical vertical incision
l. cholesterol
chronic intermittent low back pain
chronic low back strain
chronic low intermittent back pain
chronic low self-esteem
l. coloanal anastomosis
l. columnar cell
l. constant suction
l. continuous wall suction
l. contrast
l. conus medullaris
l. convex
l. cyclosporine
l. delirium
delta activity of low amplitude
differential reinforcement of low response rates
diffuse low attenuation
l. education
l. educational level
elective low forceps delivery
l. energy direct current
l. energy level
l. energy transfer
excessive diffuse low and medium wave beta activity
l. excitatory state
extremely low birth weight
extremely low frequency
l. fat and cholesterol diet
l. fever
l. flap cesarean section
l. flap transverse
l. flow principle
l. flow rate
l. forceps delivery
l. frequency alternating current
l. frequency band
l. friction arthroplasty
l. frustration tolerance
giant cell tumor of low malignant potential
l. glaze
l. glucose
l. glycemic index diet
l. Gomco suction
l. grade
heart disease, low risk
hemolysis, elevated liver enzymes, and low platelet count
high impulsiveness, low anxiety
high titer, low acidity

low *(continued)*
l. imperforate anus
l. impulsiveness
l. impulsiveness, high anxiety
l. impulsiveness, low anxiety
l. incision
l. income
l. inner quadrant
l. insertion of placenta
l. insulin therapy
l. intermittent wall suction
l. ionic strength
l. ionic strength solution
iron low serum-bound
isolated low high-density lipoprotein
l. kalium
l. LET external beam irradiation
l. LET isotope
l. liquid level monitor
l. malignant potential epithelial ovarian tumor
mechanical low back pain
mental retardation, congenital contracture, low fingertip arches syndrome
l. mobility group
moderately low birth weight
l. molecular weight
l. molecular weight dextran
l. molecular weight heparin
l. molecular weight oxidizing agent
l. molecular weight proteinuria
l. muscle tone
mutant hemoglobin with low affinity for oxygen
l. nasal bridge
l. natural killer syndrome
l. occipital hairline
l. outlet forceps
l. outlet forceps delivery
l. output
l. oxyhemoglobin saturation
physiologic low stress angioplasty
l. plasma albumin
postoperative low cardiac output
postpartum low back pain
postperfusion low flow
l. potassium dextran
l. potassium ion
l. potency
l. power microscopy
l. pressure bladder
l. probability, high consequence event
l. profile R-K marker
l. protein
l. rectal resection
l. renin, normal aldosterone
repeat low transverse cesarean section
l. right atrium
l. salt
l. saturated fat
l. segment transverse incision
l. self-esteem or guilt
l. sensory threshold
l. septal right atrium
l. serum-bound iron
severely low birth weight
slow low-efficiency dialysis
l. sodium intake
sterile elective low forceps vaginal delivery
sterile indicated low forceps vaginal delivery
sterile low midforceps vaginal delivery
l. steroid content combined oral contraceptive
l. temperature isotropic
l. tension
l. thyroid function
toxic dose, l.
l. transverse cesarean
l. transverse hysterotomy
l. transverse uterine incision
l. T3 syndrome
l. urethral pressure
l. urine pH
l. vertical
l. vertical cesarean section
l. vertical uterine incision
very low birth rate
very low birth weight
very low birth weight infant
very low birth weight preterm neonate
very low calorie diet
very low density
very low density lipoprotein
very low density lipoprotein C
very low density lipoprotein-triglyceride
very low frequency
l. virulence vaccine
l. vision
l. vision aid
l. vision clinic
l. volume
l. volume disease

low-affinity
l.-a. hemoglobin
l.-a. platelet factor

low-amplitude
l.-a. contraction
high-velocity l.-a.
l.-a. signal

low-angle
l.-a. laser light scattering

low-back pain

low-branched-chain amino acid diet

low-calcium
l.-c. dialysate
l.-c. diet
l.-c. test diet

low-calorie diet

low-compliance
l.-c. balloon
l.-c. bladder

low-contact
l.-c. dynamic compression plate
l.-c. stress

low-current electrocautery

low-density
l.-d. area
l.-d. lipoprotein apheresis
l.-d. lipoprotein cholesterol
l.-d. lipoprotein deficiency
l.-d. lipoprotein receptor disorder
l.-d. lipoprotein receptor-related protein
l.-d. lymphocyte

low-dose
l.-d. anesthetic
l.-d. arm
l.-d. aspirin therapy
l.-d. chemotherapy
l.-d. combination oral contraceptive
l.-d. continuous infusion
l.-d. CT scan
l.-d. danazol
l.-d. dexamethasone suppression test
l.-d. dobutamine stress radionuclide ventriculography
l.-d. dopaminergic agonist
l.-d. estrogen replacement
l.-d. group
l.-d. helical scanning technique
l.-d. heparin
l.-d. infusion
l.-d. intravenous insulin therapy
l.-d. involved-field irradiation

l.-d. of ionizing radiation
l.-d. mediastinal radiation therapy
l.-d. oral contraceptive
l.-d. rate
l.-d. rate intracavity therapy
l.-d. rate irradiation
l.-d. short synacthen test
l.-d. splenic irradiation
l.-d. steroids
l.-d. unfractionated heparin
l.-d. urea in invert sugar
l.-d. vaginal estrogen
l.-d. VV therapy

Lowe
L. disease
oculocerebrorenal disease of L.
L. oculocerebrorenal syndrome
L. ring

Löwe disease

low-egg-passage vaccine

Löwenberg
L. canal
L. scala

low-energy
l.-e. charged particle
l.-e. electron diffraction
l.-e. electron diffraction spectroscopy
l.-e. fracture
l.-e. ion scattering
l.-e. laser
l.-e. linear accelerator
l.-e. transurethral microwave thermotherapy

Löwenstein-Jensen
L.-J. agar
L.-J. medium

Löwenstein operation

lower
l. abdomen
l. abdominal flap
l. abdominal pain
l. abdominal periosteal reflex
l. abdominal surgery
l. abdominal tenderness
l. abdominal transverse incision
l. airway
l. airway disease
l. alveolar point
l. alveolar ridge
l. anterior axillary line
l. anterior dental height
l. anterior forceps
anterior lower cervical spine surgery
l. arch
arched lower back
arterial arch of lower eyelid
artery of lower limb
l. basilar aneurysm
below lower limit
bilateral lower lobes
l. blepharoplasty
l. body negative pressure
both lower extremities
l. brachial plexopathy
buccal of upper and lingual of l.
l. cervical cesarean section
l. cervical spine fusion
l. cervical spine posterior stabilization
l. chamber of heart
l. cheek flap
l. circulating estrogen level
l. clivus
l. collecting system
color and temperature normal, both lower extremities
columnar-lined lower esophagus
l. completely edentulous
complete lower motor neuron lesion
complete upper and lower dentures
l. confidence limit
l. costal margin
l. dental arcade
depressor muscle of lower lip
diagonal 1, 2 lower extremity
l. esophageal B ring
l. esophageal contraction ring
l. esophageal high-pressure zone
l. esophageal mucosal ring
l. esophageal ring
l. esophageal segment
l. esophageal sphincter
l. esophageal sphincter circular muscle
l. esophageal sphincter locator
l. esophageal sphincter pressure
l. esophageal sphincter relaxation
l. esophageal sphincter tone
l. esophageal stricture
l. esophageal transection
l. extremity
l. extremity amputation
l. extremity arterial
l. extremity arterial disease
l. extremity bypass graft
l. extremity edema
l. extremity equipment related
l. extremity fracture
L. Extremity Functional Scale
l. extremity nerve block
l. extremity noninvasive
l. extremity occlusive disease
l. extremity prosthesis
l. extremity reconstruction
l. extremity revascularization
l. extremity somatosensory evoked potential
l. extremity surgery
l. extremity venous
l. eyelid
l. fossa active, lateral knee pain, and long leg on the side ipsilateral to the weak fossa
l. frontal bone fracture
full lower denture
full upper denture, partial lower denture
l. ganglion
l. ganglion of glossopharyngeal nerve
l. ganglion of vagus nerve
l. gastrointestinal
l. gastrointestinal bleeding
l. gastrointestinal hemorrhage
l. genital tract infection
l. GI bleeding
l. GI tract foreign body
l. half
l. half headache of Sluder
heard best at left lower sternal border
l. hemianopia
l. hemianopsia
l. hook trial
horizontal incision across lower abdomen
hospital-acquired lower respiratory infection
l. impression
l. intestinal Crohn disease
intramuscular artery of lower extremity
l. jaw
l. jawbone
l. lateral cutaneous nerve of arm
left lower border of cardiac dullness
left lower extremity
left lower leg
left lower limb
left lower lobe infiltrate
left lower lobe of lung
left lower lung
left lower quadrant of abdomen

lower *(continued)*
left lower scapular border
left lower sternal border
l. left quadrant
l. level of care
l. lid laxity
l. lid, left eye
l. lid, oculus dexter
l. lid sling procedure
l. limb
l. limb orthosis
l. limb ossification center
l. limb prosthesis
l. limit of detection
l. lip
l. lip paralysis
l. lobe
l. lobe bronchus
l. lobe of lung
lymph node of lower limb
maximum assistance for lower body dressing
median cleft of lower lip and mandible
l. midclavicular line
l. midline
l. midline scar with hernia
minimal assistance for lower body dressing
l. motor neuron
l. motor neuron disease
l. motor neuron lesion
l. motor neuron palsy
multicentric lower genital tract neoplasia
multisite lower genital tract involvement
l. normal limit
numbness in lower back
numbness in lower leg
l. obstructive uropathy
l. outer quadrant
partial lower denture
l. partially edentulous
partial upper and lower dentures
patient independent in lower body dressing
pitting edema of lower extremity
l. pole
l. pole of incision
l. pole of testis
l. punctum
pyorrhea around lower and upper teeth
l. radicular obstetrical paralysis
receding lower jaw
recurrent lower respiratory tract disease
l. respiratory tract
l. respiratory tract illness
l. respiratory tract infection
l. respiratory tract inflammation
l. retina
right l.
right lower arm
right lower border of cardiac dullness
right lower extremity
right lower lid
right lower limb
right lower lobe infiltrate
right lower quadrant of abdomen
right lower quadrant defect
right lower scapular border
right lower sternal border
l. right quadrant
L. ring
l. risk of heart disease
l. sacral nerve root compression
l. segment
segmental bronchus lower extremity Doppler pressure
l. segment cesarean
somatic dysfunction lower extremity
l. sternal border
stimulation of lower bowel
l. third of leg bone
transient lower esophageal relaxation
l. transverse abdominal incision
l. trunk rotation
L. tubercle
upper and l.
upper body segment to lower body segment ratio
l. and upper extremities
upper and lower extremities within normal limits
l. urinary tract
l. urinary tract cancer
l. urinary tract dysfunction
l. urinary tract infection
l. urinary tract obstruction
l. urinary tract symptom
l. urinary tract tumor
l. uterine segment
l. uterine segment transverse cesarean section
l. yield point

lowered
progressively lowered stress threshold
l. resistance to infection
l. tumor antigenicity

lowering
antihypertensive and lipid l.
pressure lowering drug

lowest
l. common multiple
l. effective dose
l. effective toxic dose
l. effect level of toxicity
l. empty molecular orbital
l. level term
l. lumbar artery
l. observed adverse effect level
l. quadrant
l. splanchnic nerve
l. thyroid artery
l. unoccupied molecular orbital

Lowe-Terrey-MacLachlan syndrome

low-fat diet

low-fiber
l.-f. diet
high-carbohydrate, low-fiber diet

low-field magnetic resonance imaging

low-filter frequency

low-flow
l.-f. anesthetic
l.-f. anesthetic technique
l.-f. cardiopulmonary bypass
l.-f. sidestream capnography

low-flow sidestream capnography

low-flux
l.-f. cellulose-based membrane
l.-f. dialysis membrane

low-frequency
l.-f. activity
l.-f. blood group
l.-f. blood group antigen
l.-f. current field
l.-f. filter
l.-f. head-only rotational testing
l.-f. positive pressure ventilation
l.-f. sensorineural hearing loss
l.-f. tetanic stimulation
l.-f. tetanus
l.-f. transduction
l.-f. transfer

low-friction
l.-f. arthroplasty
l.-f. ion treatment

low-fusing alloy

low-grade
l.-g. astrocytoma
l.-g. B-cell lymphoma
l.-g. B-cell lymphoma of MALT type
l.-g. carcinoma
l.-g. CD20 positive lymphoma
l.-g. central osteogenic sarcoma
l.-g. diffuse astrocytoma
l.-g. disease
l.-g. dysplasia
l.-g. fever
l.-g. fibrillary astrocytoma
l.-g. fibromyxoid sarcoma
l.-g. glioma
l.-g. heroin
l.-g. intraosseous-type osteosarcoma
l.-g. malignant cartilaginous lesion
l.-g. mosaicism
l.-g. non-Hodgkin lymphoma
l.-g. non-Hodgkins lymphoma
l.-g. oligodendroglioma
l.-g. positive smear
l.-g. squamous intraepithelial lesion
l.-g. temperature

low-hepatic clearance drug

low-impact
l.-i. aerobic dance
l.-i. aerobic exercise
l.-i. aerobics
l.-i. exercise
l.-i. movement

low-intensity
l.-i. direct current
l.-i. exercise
l.-i. laser irradiation
l.-i. preparative regimen
l.-i. stimulation

low-level
l.-l. graded exercise test
l.-l. laser therapy
l.-l. radioactive tracer
l.-l. viral replication
l.-l. waste

low-linear energy transfer radiation

low-load
l.-l. prolonged stress
l.-l. prolonged stretch

Lown classification

Lown-Ganong-Levine syndrome

low-osmolality
l.-o. contrast agent
l.-o. contrast material
l.-o. contrast media

low-osmolar contrast medium

low-output heart failure

low–pass-filtered
l.-f. noise
l.-f. signal

low-phenylalanine diet

low-phosphorus diet

low-placed conus medullaris

low-power field

low-pressure
l.-p. baroreceptor
l.-p. breast pump
l.-p. cardiac tamponade
l.-p. cardiopulmonary baroreceptor
l.-p. glaucoma
high-volume, l.-p.
l.-p. liquid chromatography
l.-p. plasma spray
l.-p. plasma-sprayed
l.-p. urethra

low-profile
l.-p. bioprosthesis
l.-p. cup
l.-p. dorsal plate
l.-p. femoral prosthesis
l.-p. halo traction

low-protein diet

low-purine diet

low-renin essential hypertension

low-residue
l.-r. diet
l.-r. feeding

low-resolution banding

low-risk tumor

Lowry
L. assay
L. syndrome

Lowry-Maclean syndrome

Lowry-Wood syndrome

low-salt
l.-s. diet
l.-s. syndrome

low-saturated fatty acid diet

low-set ears

low-sodium
l.-s. diet
l.-s., high-potassium diet
l.-s., low-fat diet
l.-s. syndrome

low-speed handpiece

low-temperature
l.-t. holding pasteurization

low-tension glaucoma

low-titer viremia

low-turnover
l.-t. bone lesion
l.-t. disease
l.-t. osteoporosis

low-tyrosine diet

low-viscosity cement

low-voltage
l.-v. activity
l.-v. brain wave
l.-v. calibration
l.-v. diathermy loop
l.-v. electrocortical activity
l.-v. fast activity
l.-v. foci

loxoscelism
necrotic cutaneous l.

L-phenylalanine
L-p. mustard
L-p. mustard, vinblastine

L-selectin molecule

L-shaped
L-s. capsular incision
L-s. capsulotomy

L-triiodothyronine uptake

L-tryptophan-containing product

L-tryptophan ingestion

L-type calcium channel

Lu
L. antigen
L. blood group

lubricant
vaginal l.

lubricating drops

Lub syndrome

Lucas
L. and Drucker Motor Index
L. groove
L. sign

lucent
l. band
l. calculus
l. center
l. cleft
l. defect
metaphyseal lucent band
l. zone

Lucey-Driscoll syndrome

lucid layer

luciferase
l. assay
l. enzyme-based luminescence system
l. reporter gene

Lucio
L. leprosy phenomenon
L. phenomenon
L. reaction

lucite
l. beam spoiler
L. dilator
l. form
L. frame

Lucké
L. adenocarcinoma
L. carcinoma
L. tumor virus

Luck hand procedure

Ludloff bunionectomy

Ludwig
L. angina
angle of L.
L. angle
L. ganglion
L. labyrinth
L. nerve
L. stromuhr
L. Trial

Luebering-Rapaport pathway

Luedde
L. exophthalmometer
L. transparent rule

Luekens trap

lues
l. ascites
l. nervosa
l. tarda
l. test
l. venerea

Lues I, II

luetic
l. aneurysm
l. aortic aneurysm
l. aortitis
l. arteritis
l. chorioretinitis
l. diaphysitis
l. interstitial keratitis
l. mask
l. neuropathy

Luft
L. disease
L. syndrome

Lugano classification for testicular tumor

Lugol
L. chromoendoscopy
L. dye esophagoscopy
L. iodine solution
L. iodine stain

Lujan-Fryns syndrome

Lukes-Butler classification

Lukes-Collins
L.-C. classification
L.-C. classification of non-Hodgkin lymphoma
L.-C. non-Hodgkin lymphoma classification

Lukuni virus

Lumadex-FSI test

lumbar
l. abscess
l. accessory movement technique
acute lumbar trauma syndrome
l. agenesis
Albee lumbar spinal fusion
l. anesthesia
l. anesthetic technique
anterior lumbar interbody fusion
anterior lumbar spine interbody fusion
anterior lumbar vertebral interbody fusion
anterior ramus of lumbar nerve
l. anterior-root stimulator implant
l. aortography
l. appendicitis
l. approach
l. arachnoid peritoneal shunt
l. arcade
l. arteriography
l. artery
arthroscopic lumbar laser diskectomy
ascending lumbar vein
automated percutaneous lumbar discectomy
automated percutaneous lumbar diskectomy
l. brace
l. branch of iliolumbar artery
l. canal
l. canal stenosis
l. catheter
l. cerebrospinal fluid catheter
cervical, thoracic, and l.
l. cistern
continuous lumbar epidural anesthesia
l. curvature
l. curve
decompressive lumbar laminectomy
l. disc disease
l. discectomy
l. disc herniation
l. disc rupture
l. disc syndrome
l. diskectomy
l. diskography
l. distraction manipulation
dorsal root, l.
l. drain
l. drainage
l. enlargement of spinal cord
l. epidural abscess
l. epidural anesthesia
l. epidural block
l. epidural endoscopy
l. epidural steroid
l. epidural steroid injection
l. extension
l. extension test
l. extensor muscle
extraforaminal lumbar disc herniation
l. facet disease
l. facet injection
l. fascia
l. fifth vertebra to sacral first vertebra
first through fifth lumbar vertebrae or lumbar nerve
first lumbar ventral nerve root
l. flat back syndrome
l. flexure
fluoroscopic-assisted lumbar puncture
l. ganglion
l. ganglionectomy
l. gibbus
l. gravitational line
gravity lumbar reduction
l. hemangioma
l. hemilaminectomy
l. hernia
herniated lumbar disc
l. iliocostal muscle
increased lumbar curve
l. intersomatic fusion expandable cage
l. interspace
l. interspinal muscle
l. laminectomy
l. length
l. lordosis

l. lordotic curve
lowest lumbar artery
l. lymphatic plexus
l. lymph node
mammillary process of lumbar vertebra
medial lumbar intertransverse muscle
l. meningocele
microsurgical lumbar diskectomy
mid lumbar region
l. musculature
l. nervous plexus
l. orthosis
pain from lumbar disk
l. part
l. part of diaphragm
percutaneous endoscopic lumbar diskectomy
percutaneous lumbar diskectomy
posterior lumbar interbody fusion
l. puncture
l. puncture headache
l. puncture manometry
l. quadrate muscle
l. reflex
l. region
l. rib
l. root disease
l. rotator muscle
ruptured lumbar disc
second lumbar ventral nerve root
l. spinal block
l. spinal stenosis
l. spine
l. spine bone density
l. spine bone mineral density
l. spine index
l. splanchnic nerve
spurring of lumbar spine
l. suture
l. sympathetic block
l. sympathetic blockade
l. syringomyelia
l. theca
l. traction
l. triangle
l. trunks
unilateral posterior lumbar interbody fusion
l. vein
ventral root, l.

lumberman's itch

lumbocostal
l. ligament
medial lumbocostal arch
l. triangle of diaphragm

lumbocostoabdominal triangle

lumbodorsal
l. fascia
l. pain

lumboinguinal nerve

lumbopelvic complex

lumboperitoneal
l. shunt
Spetzler lumboperitoneal shunt

lumboradicular syndrome

lumbosacral
l. agenesis
l. angle
l. brace
l. canal
l. cartilaginous system
chairback lumbosacral orthosis
l. curve
l. dermal sinus
l. dimple
l. disk
l. dislocation
l. enlargement
l. enlargement of spinal cord
l. fascia
l. flexion
l. fusion
l. fusion elevator
l. instability
instability of lumbosacral joint
l. joint
l. junction
l. lipoma
narrowing at lumbosacral level
l. nerve trunk
l. nervous plexus
l. orthosis
l. plexopathy
l. plexus injury
l. plexus lesion
protruding lumbosacral disk
l. root lesion
l. sinus
l. skin pigment change
l. spine
l. tuft of hair

lumbrical
l. bar
l. canal
l. of foot
l. of hand
l. muscle
l. muscle of foot
l. muscle of hand

lumen
l. of appendix
artificial lumen narrowing
l. assessment
automatic lumen edge segmentation
l. of bowel
l. of bronchial artery
capillary l.
l. delineation
l. diameter
double l.
double lumen subclavian catheter
esophageal-tracheal double lumen airway
l. of the gut
l. of gut
l. hour
intrastent minimal lumen cross-sectional area
minimum lumen diameter
narrowing of l.
l. per square foot
l. per square meter
l. per watt
pharyngeotracheal l.
triple lumen catheter
l. of vein

luminal
l. acid
l. acid clearance
angiitic luminal compromise
l. antigen
l. antigliadin
l. area
l. brush-border membrane
l. bulge
l. caliber
l. CCK-releasing factor
l. compartment
l. content
l. contrast study
l. Crohn disease
l. defect
l. diameter
l. dimension
l. distention
l. EGF
l. endothelium
l. epithelium
l. factor
l. glucose
l. HCO^{3-}
l. infection
l. irregularity
l. narrowing
l. pH

luminal *(continued)*
l. stent
l. surface

luminance setting

luminescence
luciferase enzyme-based luminescence system

luminescent
l. label
l. paint

luminosity curve

luminous
l. efficiency
l. flux
l. flux density
l. intensity
l. retinoscope

lump
l. at site of injection
l. in breast does appear enlarged
l. growing in bone

lumpectomy
l. bed
endoscopic aspiration l.
l. and radiation

lumpy
bovine lumpy skin disease
l. jaw syndrome
l. skin disease

Lumsden center

Luna-Parker acid fuscin stain

lunar
l. caustic
l. hymen
l. periodicity

lunate
l. acrylic cement wrist prosthesis
anterior lunate lobule
avascular necrosis l.
l. bone
carpal lunate implant prosthesis
l. dislocation
l. excision
l. facet
l. facet dye punch injury
l. fissure
l. fossa
l. fossa depression
l. fracture
l. sulcus
l. surface of acetabulum
Swanson carpal lunate implant

Lund
L. and Broden method

Lund and Broden method

Lund-Browder
L.-B. burn diagram
L.-B. burn scale
L.-B. chart for burn estimation
L.-B. classification

Lundh test

lung
l. abscess
actual volume of l.
acute lung injury
acute lung rejection
l. adenocarcinoma cell
l. aeration
l. agenesis
AIDS-related lymphoma of the l.
allergic lung disorder
l. allograft
alveolar-interstitial lung disease
American L. Association
l. amyloidosis
ankylosing spondylitis, l.
l. ankylosis spondylitis
anterior border of l.
aortic impression of left l.
l. apex
apex of l.
apical segmental artery of superior lobar artery of right l.
apical segment of l.
l. aplasia
l. arch
l. architecture
arc welder's l.
asbestos-related lung carcinoma
l. aspiration
asymmetric lung opacity
atelectatic and edematous l.
atrium of l.'s
autopsy limited to heart and l.'s
l. base
l. base infiltrate
l. basement membrane
bauxite fibrosis of l.
beryllium lung disease
bilateral lung transplant
Bimodality L. Oncology Team
l. biopsy
l. biopsy tissue
bird fancier's l.
l. blast
l. block
blood from flow heart to l.'s
l. blood volume
bovine embryonic l.
brown induration of l.
l. bud
l. calculus
calf lung surfactant extract
l. cancer
L. Cancer Symptom Scale
L. Cancer Symptom Score
l. capacity
l. capillary time
carbon dioxide diffusing capacity of the l.
l. carcinoid
l. carcinoma
cardiac notch of left l.
l. cavity
l. cell
central lung distance
Chinese hamster l.
cholinergic innervation of l.
chronic diffuse interstitial lung disease
chronic hypoxic lung disease
chronic interstitial lung disease
chronic lung disease
chronic nonspecific lung disease
chronic obstructive lung disease
chronic suppurative lung disease
l. cirrhosis
l. clearance index
l.'s clear to auscultation
l.'s clear to auscultation and percussion
clear lung field
coal miner's l.
coal worker's l.
l.'s coarsely granular
l. coccidioidomycosis
l. compliance
compliance of l.
l. connectivity test
consolidation of l.'s
l. contusion
l. count curve
cow lung lavage
crackling sounds in l.'s
l. cylindroma
l. cyst
l. decortication
l. density
l. destruction
diabetic gangrene of l.
diaphragmatic surface of left l.
diaphragmatic surface of right l.
diffused lung uptake
diffuse infiltrative lung disease
diffuse interstitial fibrosis of the l.
diffuse interstitial lung disease
diffuse lung injury

diffusing capacity of l.
diffusing capacity of lung for carbon monoxide
diffusing capacity of lungs for oxygen
diminished lung volume
direct lung aspirate
dirty lung appearance
l. disease
l. donor
double lung transplant
dullness over left l.
dullness over right l.
dynamic compliance of l.
l. dysplasia
l. echinococcosis
l. edema
effect of asthma on l.
l. elastic recoil pressure
elastic recoil pressure of l.
en bloc bilateral lung transplant
end-expiratory lung volume
end-inspiratory lung volume
end-stage lung disease
eosinophilic granuloma of l.
extracorporeal lung assist
extravascular lung density
extravascular lung mass
extravascular lung water
failing lung sign
farmer's lung disease
fetal lung maturity
fibrotic lung disease
l. field
l. fluke disease
functional reserve capacity of l.'s
functional residual capacity of l.'s
l. function testing
gangrene of l.
granuloma of l.
l. growth and development
guinea pig lung strip
l. Hageman factor activator
hamartoma of l.
harvester's l.
heart and l.
heart, lungs, and abdomen
heart and lung function
heart and lungs normal
l. hemorrhage
l. hernia
hernia of l.
high lung volume
hilar substance of l.
hilum of l.
l. hilus
histoplasmosis of l.
l. homogenate
human embryoic lung fibroblast
human embryo lung cell culture
human embryonic lung fibroblast
human fetal diploid lung cell
human fetal lung fibroblast
human lung fibroblast
human lung field
human lung fluid
human lung surfactant
hyperlucent lung syndrome
hypersensitivity lung disease
hypoplastic lung syndrome
l. imaging fluorescence endoscope
l. imaging fluorescent endoscopy
immature l.
immature fetal l.
immature lung disease
immaturity of l.
improve efficiency of heart and l.'s
increased lung permeability
l. infarct
inflammatory lung disease
inhalational lung disease
l. injury
l. injury score
inoperable metastatic lung cancer
interstitial immaturity of l.
interstitial lung disease
interstitial restrictive lung disease
l. interstitium
intrathoracic artificial l.
l. involvement
isolated perfused rabbit l.
large cell lung carcinoma
left l.
left lower l.
left lower lobe of l.
left upper l.
l. length
l. lesion
Lewis lung carcinoma
limited-stage small cell lung cancer
l. lingula
lingula of left l.
lingular division of the left l.
lobe of l.
locally advanced non-small-cell lung cancer
lower lobe of l.
1-2-3 lung sign
lymphangiomyomatosis of l.
malt worker's l.
maximum expiratory airflow-static lung elastic recoil pressure
Mayo Lung Project
mesalamine-related lung toxicity
mesentery of l.
l. metastases
metastatic lung cancer
microcephalus, imperforate anus, syndactyly, hamartoblastoma, abnormal lung lobulation, polydactyly
microphallus, imperforate anus, syndactyly, hamartoblastoma, abnormal l.
middle lobar artery of right l.
middle lobe of right l.
l. morphogenesis
mushroom picker's l.
mushroom worker's l.
National Heart, L.'s, and Blood Institute Information Center
National L. Transplant Patient Association
needle aspiration lung biopsy
neonatal chronic lung disease
neonatal lung fibroblast
neuroepithelial body in l.
non-small-cell lung cancer
non-small-cell lung carcinoma
normal sheep lung fibroblast
NSE lung cancer tumor marker
oat cell lung cancer
oblique fissure of l.
occupational immunologic lung disease
occupational lung disease
occupational lung disorder
l. overdistention
overinflation of l.'s
oxygen toxicity in immature l.
l. parenchyma
parenchymal lung disease
parenchymal lung morphogenesis
partial collapse of l.
passively congested lung tissue
pediatric lung surgery
pedicle of l.
percutaneous lung tap
percutaneous needle lung aspiration
l. perfusion
perfusion lung scan
pigeon breeder l.
plug the lung until it grows
poorly differentiated lung cancer
poorly expanded l.'s

lung *(continued)*
premature accelerated lung maturation
primary lung disease
l. profile
radiographic lung area
rat lung strip
l. recruitment
residual volume/total lung capacity ratio
resistance to movement of lung tissue
l. resistance-related protein
respiratory bronchiolitis-associated interstitial lung disease
retained fetal lung fluid
retained lung fluid
l.'s revealed hyperresonance to percussion
right l.
right middle lobe of l.
right single lung transplant
right upper l.
roentgenographically occult lung cancer
root of l.
rounded border of l.
sarcoma, breast and brain tumors, leukemia, laryngeal and lung cancer adenoma
l. scan
l. shielding
shrinking lungs syndrome
sickle cell chronic lung disease
sickle cell lung disease
simultaneous independent lung ventilation
single-breath carbon monoxide diffusing capacity of l.
single lung reduction surgery
small cell carcinoma of l.
smoke-induced lung injury
l. sounds
squamous cell lung tumor
static lung compliance
steady-state carbon monoxide diffusing capacity of l.
l. strip
superior segment of l.
l. surgery
surgical lung biopsy
sustained maximal inspiratory lung exercise
l. tap
l. thermal volume
l. tissue
total capacity of l.
total lung capacity
total lung compliance
total lung water
training and test l.
transbronchial lung biopsy
transfusion-associated lung injury
transfusion-related acute lung injury
l. transplant
l. transplantation
l. transplant rejection
true total lung capacity
unilateral lung reduction surgery
l. unit
vanishing lung syndrome
ventilation/perfusion lung scan
ventilator-associated lung injury
ventilator-induced lung injury
l. volume reduction
l. volume reduction surgery
volumetric lung depth
V/Q lung scan
l. weight
wet lung syndrome
l. width
wood pulp worker l.
xenon lung ventilation imaging

lung-body weight ratio

lung-derived neurotrophic factor

lung-protective pressure-targeted ventilation

lung-to-finger circulation time

lungworm vaccine

lunocapitate bone

lunotriquetral
l. arthrodesis
l. dissociation
l. fusion

Luntz-Dodick punch

lunule of nail

Lunyo virus

lupoid
l. acne
chronic active lupoid hepatitis
l. hepatitis
l. leishmaniasis
l. sclerosis
l. sycosis
l. ulcer

lupus
acute cutaneous lupus erythematosus
acute lupus pericarditis
acute lupus pneumonitis
acute systemic lupus erythematosus
l. alopecia
l. angiitis
anticardiolipin lupus anticoagulant
l. anticoagulant activity
l. anticoagulant antibody
L. Anticoagulant Positive Control
l. anticoagulant syndrome
apple jelly papule of lupus vulgaris
l. band test
British Isles Lupus Assessment Group index
bullous systemic lupus erythematosus
l. cerebritis
chronic cutaneous lupus erythematosus
chronic discoid lupus erythematosus
l. crisis
discoid lupus erythematosus
disseminated lupus erythematosus
drug-induced l.
drug-induced lupus erythematosus
drug-induced lupus syndrome
drug-related l.
l. erythematosus
l. erythematosus body
l. erythematosus cell
l. erythematosus cell test
l. erythematosus discoides
l. erythematosus factor
l. erythematosus inhibitor
l. erythematosus, neonatal
l. erythematosus panniculitis
l. erythematosus peripheral neuropathy
l. erythematosus phenomenon
l. erythematosus preparation
l. erythematosus profundus
l. erythematosus, systemic
l. erythematosus tumidus
l. erythematous-like rash
l. fibrosus
l. glomerulonephritis
l. inhibitor
l. livedo
l. lymphaticus
membranous lupus nephritis
membranous lupus nephropathy
mesangial lupus nephritis
l. mutilans
neonatal lupus syndrome
l. nephritis

neuropsychiatric syndrome of systemic lupus erythematosus
l. obstetric syndrome
l. oculopathy
l. papillomatosus
pediatric lupus nephropathy
l. pernio
l. profundus
l. profundus/panniculitis
l. sebaceous
l. sebaceus
l. serpiginosus
subacute cutaneous lupus erythematosus
subcutaneous lupus erythematosis
l. superficialis
l. syndrome
Systemic L. Activity Measure
Systemic L. Erythematosus Disease Activity Index
l. thrombophilia
l. tuberculosus
l. vasculopathy
l. verrucosus
l. vorax
l. vulgaris
World Health Organization classification of lupus nephritis I, IIA, IIB, III, IV, V

lupus-like
l.-l. anticoagulant
l.-l. syndrome

lupus-scleroderma overlap syndrome

lupus-type inclusion

Luria-Delbruck
L.-D. fluctuation test
L.-D. model

Luria-Nebraska Neuropsychological Battery

Luride
L. acidulated phosphate fluoride paste
L. Drops

Luscher Color Test

Luschka
atresia of the foramen of Luschka and Magendie
L. bursa
L. cartilage
L. crypt
L. cystic gland
L. duct
L. duct leak
L. ducts
fibers of L.
L. gland
L. joint
L. laryngeal cartilage
L. ligament
L. and Magendie foramen
L. nerve
L. sinus
L. tonsil

Luse
L. bodies
L. body

LUST C-section

lust dynamism

lustrous central yellow point

lutea
macula l.

luteal
l. cell
l. cyst
l. dysfunction
dysharmonic luteal phase
l. function
inadequate luteal phase
late luteal phase dysphoric disorder
normal luteal phase
l. ovarian cyst
l. phase
l. phase defect
l. phase deficiency
l. phase inadequacy
l. phase insufficiency
l. phase support
l. phase therapy
short luteal phase

lutein cell

luteinization
l. inhibition
l. inhibitor
l. stimulant
l. stimulator

luteinization-inhibiting factor

luteinized
l. theca cell
l. thecoma
l. thecoma of ovary
l. unruptured follicle
l. unruptured follicle syndrome

luteinizing
bioassay of luteinizing hormone
biologically active luteinizing hormone
follicle-stimulating hormone and luteinizing hormone-releasing hormone
heterodimeric luteinizing hormone
l. hormone
l. hormone-beta
l. hormone beta core fragment
l. hormone-chorionic gonadotropin hormone
l. hormone-dependent androgen excess
l. hormone-follicle-stimulating hormone
l. hormone/follicle-stimulating hormone-releasing
l. hormone/follicle-stimulating hormone-releasing factor
l. hormone/human chorionic gonadotropin
l. hormone receptor
l. hormone receptor-binding inhibitor
l. hormone-releasing factor agonist
l. hormone-releasing hormone
l. hormone-releasing hormone agonist
l. hormone-releasing hormone analog
l. hormone-releasing hormone deficiency
l. hormone-secreting tumor
l. hormone secretion
l. principle
urinary luteinizing hormone

lutein-stimulating hormone

Lutembacher
L. complex
L. syndrome

luteolytic action

luteomammotrophic hormone

luteoplacental shift

luteotropic hormone

luteum
atretic corpus l.
l. cell
corpus l.
corpus luteum cyst
corpus luteum deficiency syndrome
corpus luteum dysfunction
corpus luteum function
corpus luteum hormone
corpus luteum insufficiency
corpus luteum of pregnancy

luteum *(continued)*
corpus luteum stimulating hormone
hemorrhagic corpus l.
persistent corpus l.
prolapse of corpus l.

luteus

Lutheran
L. blood antibody type
L. blood group system

luting
l. agent
l. cement

Lutz-Jeanselme nodule

Lutz-Miescher disease

Lutz-Splendore-Almeida
L.-S.-A. blastomycosis
L.-S.-A. disease

luxated lens

luxatio
l. erecta
l. erecta shoulder dislocation

luxation
atlantoaxial l.
l. of eyeball
l. of globe
l. of lens

Luxol fast blue stain

Luxtec coaxial illumination

luxury perfusion

luxus heart

Luys
L. body syndrome
nucleus of L.

lyase
adenylosuccinate lyase deficiency
argininosuccinate lyase assay
argininosuccinic acid l.
arginosuccinate lyase deficiency
ATP citrate l.
isocitrate l.

Lyb antigen

Lyda-Ivalon-Lucite implant

Lyell
L. disease
L. syndrome

lye stricture

lying
back l.
face lying position

***lyl-1* oncogene activation**

Lyle syndrome

Lyman model

Lyme
L. arthritis
L. arthritis serology
L. borreliosis antibody
L. carditis
L. disease
L. disease antibody test
L. disease arthritis
L. disease DNA detection
L. disease immunoblot
L. disease keratitis
L. disease serology
L. disease stage 1–3
L. disease vaccine
L. encephalopathy
L. enzyme-linked immunosorbent assay
L. meningitis
L. radiculoneuritis
L. titer

Lyme-associated peripheral facial nerve palsy

lymph
abdominal lymph node
abdominal lymph node biopsy
angiofollicular hyperplasia lymph node
angiofollicular lymph node hyperplasia
angiofollicular mediastinal lymph node hyperplasia
anorectal lymph node
anterior axillary lymph node
anterior deep cervical lymph node
anterior jugular lymph node
anterior mediastinal lymph node
anterior superficial cervical lymph node
anterior tibial lymph node
aortic lymph node
apical axillary lymph node
apical lymph node
appendicular lymph node
auricular lymph node
axillary lymph node
axillary lymph node dissection
axillary lymph node involvement
axillary lymph node metastasis
bilateral pelvic lymph node
bilateral pelvic lymph node dissection
bronchial lymph node
l. capillary
celiac lymph node metastasis
l. cell
l. channel
l. circulation
common iliac lymph nodes
complete lymph node dissection
l. cord
l. corpuscle
deep inguinal lymph node
draining lymph node
l. duct
elective lymph node dissection
elective regional lymph node dissection
l. embolism
external iliac lymph nodes
extracorporeal irradiation of l.
extraperitoneal endoscopic pelvic lymph node dissection
l. follicle
giant lymph node hyperplasia
l. gland
l. heart
hemorrhagic omental lymph nodes
hepatic lymph node
hilar lymph node
histiocytic hyperplasia of lymph node
histocytic hyperplasia of lymph nodes
ileocolic lymph node
iliac lymph nodes
infected lymph gland
inguinal lymph nodes
intercostal lymph node
internal iliac lymph node
internal mammary lymph node
intramammary lymph node
jugular lymph nodes
junctional lymph node
laparoscopic pelvic lymph node dissection
left gastric lymph node
left hilar lymph node
lingual lymph node
localized angiofollicular lymph node hyperplasia
lumbar lymph node
malar lymph node
malignant l.
mandibular lymph node
mastoid lymph node
medial lacunar lymph node
mediastinal lymph node
mediastinal lymph node hyperplasia
medulla of lymph node
mesocolic lymph node
mesorectal lymph node

metastatic lymph node tumor
middle colic lymph node
middle group of mesenteric lymph node
mucocutaneous lymph node
mucocutaneous lymph node syndrome
mucosa-associated lymph tissue
multicentric angiofollicular lymph node
nasolabial lymph node
nasopharyngeal carcinoma with lymph node involvement
neck lymph node
l. node basin
node bearing area of lymph nodes
l. node biopsy
l. node cell
l. node culture
l. node dissection
l. node drainage
l. node of elbow
l. node endometriotic adenoacanthoma
l. node enlargement
l. node excision
l. node fibrosis
l. node of head and neck
l. node histology
l. node hyperplasia
l. node involution
l. node of lower limb
l. node lymphocyte
l. node metastasis
l. node mononuclear cell
l. node permeability factor
l. node positivity
l. node revealing solution
l. node sampling
l. node seeking equivalent
l. node staging
l. node station
l. node of upper limb
l. nodule
obturator lymph node
occipital lymph node
occult lymph node metastasis
osmotic pressure of proteins in l.
pancreatic lymph node
pancreaticoduodenal lymph node
pancreaticosplenic lymph node
parapharyngeal lymph node
pararectal lymph node
parasternal lymph nodes
paravesical lymph node
parietal lymph node
parotid lymph node
pectoral axillary lymph node
pelvic lymph node dissection
periaortic lymph involvement
periaortic lymph node
periaortic lymph node metastasis
pericolonic lymph node
perihilar lymph node
peripancreatic lymph node
peripheral lymph node
perivascular lymph space
peroneal lymph node
pharyngeal lymph node
phrenic lymph node
pleural lymph node
prevertebral lymph node
primary tumor, regional lymph node, remote metastases classification, staging
pyloric lymph node
regional lymph involvement
regional lymph node
regional lymph node cell
regional lymph node dissection
regional lymph nodes cannot be addressed
retrocecal lymph node
retroperitoneal pelvic lymph node dissection
retropharyngeal lymph node
right gastric lymph node
right hilar lymph node
l. sac
sacral lymph node
scalene lymph node biopsy
selective complete lymph node dissection
sentinel lymph node detection
sentinel lymph node mapping
sentinel lymph node biopsy
shotty lymph node
l. sinus
solitary lymph node
l. space
splenic lymph node
submental lymph node
superficial inguinal lymph node
supraclavicular lymph node
therapeutic lymph node dissection
thymus-dependent zone of lymph node
tumor-draining lymph node
tumor-draining lymph node cell
tumor with lymph node metastases
l. varices
l. varix
l. vessel
l. vessel invasion

lymphadenectomy
endocavitary pelvic l.
laparoscopic pelvic l.
Meigs pelvic l.
retroperitoneal l.
sentinel l.

lymphadenitis
histiocytic necrotizing l.
localized *Leishmania* l.
necrotizing granulomatous l.

lymphadenoid
l. thyroiditis
l. tissue

lymphadenoma cell

lymphadenopathic
African lymphadenopathic Kaposi sarcoma

lymphadenopathy
angioblastic l.
angioimmunoblastic l.
angioimmunoblastic lymphadenopathy with dysproteinemia
angioimmunoblastic lymphadenopathy with dysproteinemia-like T-cell lymphoma
bilateral hilar l.
extended lymphadenopathy syndrome
generalized lymphadenopathy syndrome
idiopathic lymphadenopathy syndrome
immunoblastic l.
persistent generalized l.
sinus histiocytosis with massive l.
l. syndrome

lymphadenopathy-associated virus

lymphangiectasia
congenital pulmonary l.
congenital pulmonary cystic l.
primary intestinal l.

lymphangiectatic elephantiasis

lymphangioendothelial sarcoma

lymphangiography effect

lymphangioma
acquired progressive l.
l. cavernosum
l. circumscriptum
pancreatic cystic l.

lymphangioma *(continued)*
l. tuberosum multiplex
l. xanthelasmoideum
lymphangiomatous polyp
lymphangiomyomatosis of lung
lymphangitic
l. carcinomatosis
l. spread
l. spread of prostatic adenocarcinoma
lymphangitis
ascending l.
l. carcinomatosa
l. epizootica
lymphatic
l. abscess
afferent lymphatic drainage
afferent lymphatic vessel
l. angina
aortic lymphatic plexus
blood and lymphatic system
l. canal
l. capillary
l. carcinomatosis
l. chain
l. channel
l. choriomeningitis
chronic lymphatic leukemia
l. cisterna
l. corpuscle
l. cortex
dermal lymphatic involvement
l. development
l. disease
l. dissection
l. dissemination theory of endometriosis
l. drainage of genitalia
l. drainage pattern
draining lymphatic bed
l. duct
l. dyscrasia
l. dysplasia
l. edema
l. filariasis
l. filariasis granuloma
l. fistula
l. follicle
l. follicle of larynx
l. follicle of tongue
l. formation
l. grafting
interrupted lymphatic drainage
l. leukemia
l. leukemia virus
lids, lashes, lacrimals, l.'s
lumbar lymphatic plexus
l. malformation
l. mapping
l. metastasis
nerve, artery, vein, empty space, l.'s
l. nevus
l. nodule
l. obstruction
paracervical l.'s
periarterial lymphatic sheath
l. permeation
l. plexus
l. reconstruction
l. return rate
l. ring of cardia
l. ring of cardiac part of stomach
l. sarcoma
secondary lymphatic tissue
l. shunt
l. sinus
solitary lymphatic nodule
l. spread
l. stroma
l. system
T-cell chronic lymphatic leukemia
thoracic lymphatic duct
l. tissue
l. tracking
l. trunk
l. tuberculosis
l. valvule
l. vessel
l. vessel invasion
lymphaticovenous
l. anastomosis
l. bypass
l. communication
l. malformation
l. shunt
lymphaticus
lupus l.
nevus l.
nodulus l.
nodus l.
nodus lymphoideus malaris
lymphatic-venous malformation
lymphatolytic serum
lymphedema
l. alert bracelet
l. complex
l. grade II, III
manual lymphedema treatment
l. praecox
l. pump
l. tarda
lymphedema-distichiasis syndrome
lymphedematous keratoderma
lymphoablative technique
lymphoblast
Annapolis lymphoblast globulin
equine antihuman lymphoblast globulin
equine antihuman lymphoblast serum
human cultured l.
labeled l.
lymphoblastic
acute lymphoblastic leukemia in children
acute lymphoblastic leukemia secondary to Burkitt lymphoma
acute lymphoblastic lymphoma
acute lymphoblastic myelogenous leukemia
B-cell acute lymphoblastic leukemia
B-cell precursor lymphoblastic leukemia
common acute lymphoblastic leukemia antigen
diffuse and l.
l. leukemia
l. lymphoma
l. lymphoma-leukemia
malignant lymphoma, lymphoblastic type
null cell lymphoblastic leukemia
T-cell acute lymphoblastic leukemia
l. transformation
l. transformation test
lymphoblastoid
l. cell
l. cell line
human lymphoblastoid cell line
human lymphoblastoid interferon interferon
l. interferon
lymphocele aspiration
LymphoCide antibody
lymphocutaneous
l. nodule
l. pattern
l. sporotrichosis
lymphocyst omentum
lymphocyte
absolute lymphocyte count

l. activation
l. activation factor
l. activator
allodonor lymphocyte infusion
allogeneic lymphocyte cytotoxicity
allograft-bound l.
l. antibody
l. antibody lymphocytolytic interaction
antigen-binding l.
antihuman lymphocyte globulin
antihuman lymphocyte serum
antimouse lymphocyte serum
antitumor cytotoxic l.
antiviral lymphocyte serum
atypical l.
autologous mixed lymphocyte culture
autologous mixed lymphocyte reaction
autologous T l.
average lymphocyte output
bare lymphocyte syndrome
l. blastogenic factor
bone marrow l.
bursa-equivalent l.
l. cell
l. chemoattractant activity
l. chemoattractant factor
circulating blood l.
complement receptor l.
l. costimulatory molecule
l. count
crypt intraepithelial l.
l. culture fluid
cutaneous lymphocyte antigen
cytolytic T l.
cytotoxic l.
l. cytotoxicity
cytotoxic lymphocyte activation antigen 4 immunoglobulin
cytotoxic T l.
cytotoxic T-cell lymphocyte response
cytotoxic T lymphocyte antigen-4
cytotoxic T lymphocyte line
cytotoxic T lymphocyte precursor
daily replacement factor of l.'s
l. defined
l. depleted
l. depletion
l. detected membrane antigen
donor lymphocyte infusion
drug-induced lymphocyte stimulation test
l. dysfunction
l. enzyme stain
fowl antimouse lymphocyte globulin
l. function antigen
l. function assay
l. function-associated antigen
l. gene rearrangement
gut mucosal l.
Hodgkin disease of diffuse histiocytic lymphocyte depleted type
l. homing receptor
horse anti-Rhesus lymphocyte globulin
human l.
human lymphocyte antigen
human lymphocyte antigen-lymphocyte defined
human lymphocyte antigen-serologically defined
human lymphocyte interferon
human lymphocyte transformation
human peripheral l.
l. immune globulin
l. immunofluorescence test
interaction
intestinal l.
intraepithelial l.
lamina propria l.
large l.
large granular l.
large and medium l.
low-density l.
lymph node l.
marginal zone l.
matched lymphocyte transfusion
l. microcytotoxicity
l. migration
l. mitogenic factor
mitogen-induced lymphocyte proliferation
mixed lymphocyte concentration
mixed lymphocyte culture reaction
mixed lymphocyte culture test
mixed lymphocyte culture, weak
mixed lymphocyte reaction blocking factor
mixed lymphocyte response
mixed lymphocyte target interaction
monocytoid l.
mouse-specific bone marrow-derived lymphocyte antigen
natural killer l.
normal lymphocyte supernatant
normal lymphocyte transfer test
peptide activated l.
percentage of lymphocytes in differential count
periarteriolar lymphocyte sheath
peripheral blood l.
peripheral blood lymphocyte analysis
peripheral blood lymphocyte transformation
peripheral lymphocyte count
peritoneal exudate l.
plasmacytoid l.
l. predominance Hodgkin disease
l. predominant
primed lymphocyte test
primed lymphocyte typing
product of activated l.
l. proliferation
l. proliferation assay
l. proliferation/regression index
l. reactivity index
l. recirculation
l. recombinase
l. recruitment
residual lymphocyte output
salivary gland l.
l. separation medium
l. serine esterase
small l.
splenic lymphoma with villous l.
l. subpopulation
l. subset
l. subset count
l. subset panel
synovial fluid l.
thoracic duct l.
thymic lymphocyte antigen
thymus-dependent l.
thymus-derived l.
total l.
total lymphocyte count
l. transfer reaction
l. transformation test
l. transitional
tumor-associated l.
tumor-infiltrating l.
tumor-infiltrating lymphocyte technique
virus entry mediator, a receptor expressed by T l.
whole lymphocyte fraction

lymphocyte-activating
l.-a. determinant
l.-a. factor

lymphocyte-dependent antibody

lymphocyte detected membrane antigen

lymphocyte-detected membrane antigen

lymphocyte-induced angiogenesis factor

lymphocyte-mediated
l.-m. cytolysis
l.-m. cytotoxic
l.-m. cytotoxicity
l.-m. response

lymphocyte-predominant
l.-p. Hodgkin disease
l.-p. thymoma

lymphocyte-rich classic Hodgkin

lymphocyte-stimulating
l.-s. factor
l.-s. hormone

lymphocyte-transforming
l.-t. activity
l.-t. factor

lymphocytic
acute lymphocytic leukemia
acute lymphocytic leukemia antigen
l. adenohypophysitis
aleukemic lymphocytic leukemia
l. angiitis
l. angiitis and granulomatosis
antithoracic duct lymphocytic globulin
l. apoptosis
B-cell chronic lymphocytic leukemia
B-cell chronic lymphocytic leukemia/small lymphocytic lymphoma
l. blood cell
l. bronchitis
l. choriomeningitis
l. choriomeningitis virus
l. choriomeningitis virus encephalitis
l. choriomeningitis virus group
chronic lymphocytic leukemia variant
chronic lymphocytic thyroiditis
l. colitis
common acute lymphocytic leukemia antigen
l. cuffing
diffuse lymphocytic poorly differentiated
diffuse well-differentiated lymphocytic lymphoma
l. disease
endomyocardial lymphocytic infiltrates
l. enterocolitis
l. gastritis
l. granulomatosis
hypertrophic lymphocytic gastritis
l. hypophysitis
l. infiltrate of Jessner
l. infiltration
l. infiltration of the skin
l. infiltrative disease
intermediate lymphocytic lymphoma
interstitial lymphocytic pneumonia
l. interstitial pneumonia
l. leukemia
l. leukemoid reaction
l. leukocytosis
l. leukopenia
l. lymphoma
l. lymphosarcoma
malignant lymphocytic proliferation disease
malignant lymphoma, poorly differentiated l.
mantle cell lymphocytic lymphoma
l. meningitis
murine lymphocytic choriomeningitis virus
l. nodular Hodgkin disease
nodular poorly differentiated lymphocytic lymphoma
nonspecific chronic lymphocytic thyroiditis
null cell acute lymphocytic leukemia
pancreatic lymphocytic infiltration
l. pleocytosis
poorly differentiated lymphocytic lymphoma
l. series
signaling lymphocytic activation molecule
small lymphocytic lymphoma
l. thyroiditis
l. thyroiditis neoplasia
l. vasculitis
well-differentiated l.

lymphocytically determined

lymphocytolytic
lymphocyte antibody lymphocytolytic interaction

lymphocytoma cutis

lymphocytopenia
idiopathic CD4+ l.
idiopathic CD4 T-cell l.

lymphocytosis
acute infectious l.
benign monoclonal B-cell l.
bone marrow l.
diffuse infiltrative lymphocytosis syndrome
peripheral blood $CD8^+$ l.
l. syndrome

lymphocytosis-promoting factor

lymphocytotoxic antibody

lymphocytotoxicity test

lymphoepithelial
benign lymphoepithelial disease
benign lymphoepithelial lesion
l. carcinoma
l. cyst
l. endocrine gland
l. lesion
l. tumor

lymphoepithelioid
atypical lymphoepithelioid cell proliferation
l. cell lymphoma
l. lymphoma

lymphoepithelioma-like
l.-l. carcinoma
l.-l. carcinoma of skin
l.-l. thymic carcinoma

lymphogenous
l. dissemination
l. embolism
l. leukemia
l. metastasis

lymphogranuloma
l. malignum
psittacosis, lymphogranuloma venereum, trachoma
Schaumann benign l.
l. venereum
l. venereum antigen
l. venereum complement fixation test
l. venereum conjunctivitis
l. venereum infection
l. venereum keratitis
l. venereum-trachoma inclusion conjunctivitis
l. venereum virus

lymphogranulomatosis
l. maligna
l. X

lymphohematogenous disease

lymphohistiocytic
l. infiltration
l. variant

lymphohistiocytoid mesothelioma

lymphohistiocytosis
familial erythrophagocytic l.
familial hemophagocytic l.
hemophagocytic l.

lymphoid
l. aggregate
angiofollicular lymphoid hyperplasia
angiomatous lymphoid hamartoma
asymmetric nasopharyngeal lymphoid hyperplasia
l. body
bronchus-associated lymphoid tissue
l. cell
l. cell line
l. cholangitis
l. component
l. corpuscle
cutaneous lymphoid hyperplasia
l. dendritic cell
focal areas of lymphoid infiltrate
focal lymphoid hyperplasia
l. follicle
l. follicular reticulosis
gastrointestinal-associated lymphoid tissue
l. gland
gut-associated lymphoid disease
gut-associated lymphoid tissue
l. hemoblast
l. hemoblast of Pappenheim
l. hyperplasia
l. hypertrophy
l. hypophysitis
l. hypoplasia
l. infiltrate
l. infiltration
l. inflammatory pseudotumor
l. interstitial pneumonia
l. interstitial pneumonitis
l. leukemia
l. leukosis virus
marginal zone/mucosa-associated lymphoid tissue
l. marker
mucosa-associated lymphoid tissue function
mucosa-associated lymphoid tissue lymphoma
mucosa-associated lymphoid tumor
multicentric angiofollicular lymphoid hyperplasia
l. neoplasm
nodular lymphoid hyperplasia
non–mucosa-associated lymphoid tissue lymphoma
ocular adnexal lymphoid proliferation
l. organ
peripheral lymphoid cell
l. plasma
l. precursor B-cell
l. precursor T-cell
l. predominance
l. proliferation
l. pseudotumor
pulmonary lymphoid hyperplasia
reactive lymphoid hyperplasia
reactive lymphoid tissue
residual lymphoid tissue
Revised European-American Classification of Lymphoid Neoplasms
l. ring
selective lymphoid irradiation
l. series
skin-associated lymphoid tissue
l. stem cell
subtotal lymphoid irradiation
l. system
l. tissue
l. tissue lymphoma
total lymphoid irradiation for allograft survival
total lymphoid radiation
l. tumor
tumor-assisted lymphoid proliferation

lymphokine
autologous lymphokine activated killer cell
l. production

lymphokine-activated
l.-a. killer
l.-a. killer cell

lympholymphatic anastomosis

lympholytic agent

lymphoma
acute lymphoblastic leukemia secondary to Burkitt l.
acute lymphoblastic l.
adult T-cell l.
African Burkitt l.
aggressive good prognosis non-Hodgkin l.
aggressive histology l.
AIDS-related l.
AIDS-related lymphoma of the lung
AIDS-related non-Hodgkin l.
AIDS-related primary central nervous system l.
anaplastic large cell l.
angiocentric NK-cell l.
angiocentric T-cell l.
angioimmunoblastic l.
angioimmunoblastic lymphadenopathy-like T-cell l.
angioimmunoblastic lymphadenopathy with dysproteinemia-like T-cell l.
angioimmunoblastic T-cell l.
angiotropic large cell l.
Ann Arbor Hodgkin lymphoma stage I, IE, II, IIE, IIIE, IIIS, IIISE, IV
anterior chamber l.
B-cell l.
B-cell chronic lymphocytic leukemia/small lymphocytic l.
B-cell non-Hodgkin l.
blastoid variant of mantel cell l.
blastoma mantel cell l.
body cavity-based l.
Burkitt l.
Burkitt-like l.
Burkitt lymphoma cell line
centrocytic/mantle-cell l.
classic Hodgkin l.
composite l.
l. culture
cutaneous B-cell l.
cutaneous T-cell l.
diffuse l.
diffuse aggressive l.
diffuse histiocytic l.
diffuse histiocytic lymphoma of stomach
diffuse large B-cell l.
diffuse mixed l.
diffuse nodular l.
diffuse non-Hodgkin l.
diffuse poorly differentiated l.
diffuse undifferentiated l.
endemic Burkitt l.
enteropathy-associated T-cell l.
floral variant of follicular l.
follicle center lymphoma cell
follicular l.
follicular center cell l.
follicular large cell l.
follicular non-Hodgkin l.
gastrointestinal tract l.
giant follicular l.
hepatic non-Hodgkin l.
histiocytic l.
Hodgkin l.

lymphoma *(continued)*
human immunodeficiency virus-associated non-Hodgkin l.
human T-cell lymphoma virus
immunoblastic l.
l. implant
indolent follicular l.
intermediate lymphocytic l.
large B-cell l.
large cell l.
large cell anaplastic l.
large cell non-Hodgkin l.
limited-stage diffuse large cell l.
low-grade B-cell l.
low-grade B-cell lymphoma of MALT type
low-grade CD20 positive l.
low-grade non-Hodgkin l.
Lukes-Collins classification of non-Hodgkin l.
Lukes-Collins non-Hodgkin lymphoma classification
lymphoblastic l.
lymphocytic l.
lymphoepithelioid cell l.
lymphoid tissue l.
lymphoplasmacytoid l.
lymphoplasmacytoid lymphoma cell
malignant l.
malignant histiocytic l.
malignant lymphoma, lymphoblastic type
malignant lymphoma, histiocytic
malignant lymphoma, poorly differentiated lymphocytic
MALT/marginal zone l.
mantle cell lymphocytic l.
mantle zone l.
marginal zone B-cell l.
marginal zone cell l.
marginal zone l.
mediastinal B-cell lymphoma with sclerosis
mediastinal large B-cell l.
Mediterranean abdominal l.
Memorial Sloan-Kettering staging of childhood l.
mesencephalic cerebral l.
mesenterial Castleman l.
metastatic lymphoma of CNS
mixed cell nodular l.
mixed large- and small-cell non-Hodgkin l.
mixed lymphocytic-histiocytic l.
mixed small cleaved and large cell l.
monocytoid B-cell l.
mucosa-associated lymphoid tissue l.
multiclonal follicular l.
multilobated T-cell l.
nasal angiocentric l.
nasal T-cell/natural killer cell l.
natural killer-like T-cell l.
NK cell l.
nodal marginal zone B-cell l.
nodular l.
nodular histiocytic l.
nodular mixed l.
nodular, mixed cell l.
nodular non-Hodgkin l.
nodular poorly differentiated lymphocytic l.
nonhistiocytic type l.
non-Hodgkin l.
non-Hodgkin malignant l.
non–mucosa-associated lymphoid tissue lymphoma
null cell anaplastic large cell l.
null cell l.
null-type non-Hodgkin l.
l. of ocular adnexa
ocular adnexal l.
l. of ovary
parafollicular B-cell l.
paranasal sinus l.
peripheral T-cell l.
poorly differentiated lymphocytic l.
poorly differentiated lymphoma, diffuse
postthymic T-cell l.
primary bone l.
primary brain l.
primary central nervous system l.
primary cerebral non-Hodgkin l.
primary cutaneous large B-cell l.
primary effusion l.
primary extranodal l.
primary gastric l.
primary gastric non-Hodgkin l.
primary hepatosplenic l.
primary lymphoma of bone
primary mediastinal large-cell l.
primary mediastinal large cell lymphoma with sclerosis
primary non-Hodgkin lymphoma of bone
primary pulmonary non-Hodgkin l.
prostate gland l.
Rappaport classification of l.
l. screen
secondary cutaneous large B-cell l.
small cell malignant l.
small lymphocytic l.
small noncleaved cell l.
small noncleaved cell, non-Burkitt l.
splenic lymphoma with villous lymphocyte
splenic marginal zone l.
subcutaneous panniculitis-like T-cell l.
l. syndrome leukemia
T-cell-rich B-cell l.
thymus l.
true histiocytic l.
undifferentiated B-cell l.

lymphoma-leukemia
adult T-cell l.-l.
lymphoblastic l.-l.

lymphoma-nodular
poorly differentiated lymphocytic l.-n.

lymphomatoid
l. granulomatosis
l. panniculitis
l. papulosis

lymphomatosa
angina l.

lymphomatosis
avian l.
avian lymphomatosis virus
ocular l.

lymphomatosum
papillary adenocystoma l.
papillary cystadenoma l.

lymphomatous
AIDS-related lymphomatous meningitis
l. bone marrow involvement
l. erythroderma
l. mass
l. meningitis
l. polyposis
l. type

lymphomyeloid complex

lymphonodular
l. hyperplasia
l. pharyngitis

lymphopathia venereum

lymphopenic thymic dysplasia

lymphoplasmacytic
l. immunocytoma
l. infiltrate
l. lymphoma

lymphoplasmacytoid
l. cell
l. immunocytoma
l. lymphoma
l. lymphoma cell
l. morphology
lymphopoietic differentiation
lymphoproliferative
l. activity
angiocentric lymphoproliferative lesion
l. assay
atypical lymphoproliferative disorder
autoimmune lymphoproliferative syndrome
B-cell chronic lymphoproliferative disorder
B-cell lymphoproliferative disorder
chronic lymphoproliferative disorder
l. disease
l. disorder
l. lesion
l. malignancy
malignant lymphoproliferative disorder
monoclonal lymphoproliferative syndrome
node-based malignant lymphoproliferative disease
posttransplantation lymphoproliferative disease
prison-acquired lymphoproliferative syndrome
l. skin lesion
l. syndrome
l. tumor
l. virus group
X-linked lymphoproliferative disease
X-linked recessive lymphoproliferative syndrome
lymphoproliferative/myeloproliferative disease
lymphoreticular
l. cell
l. disease
l. disorder
l. malignancy
l. neoplasia
l. neoplasm
l. tumor
lymphosarcoma
l. cell
l. cell leukemia
chronic lymphosarcoma cell leukemia
follicular l.
gibbon ape lymphosarcoma virus
lymphocytic l.
lymphosarcoma-reticulum cell sarcoma
lymphoscintigraphy
axillary l.
gamma probe-guided l.
gamma probe guided l.
internal mammary l.
radionuclide functional l.
lymphostatic verrucosis
lymphotoxic antibody
lymphotoxin antitumor activity
lymphotrophic
human T-cell lymphotrophic virus type I–III
lymphotropic
human B lymphotropic virus
human T-cell lymphotropic virus
human T-cell lymphotropic virus I
human T-cell lymphotropic virus II
human T-cell lymphotropic virus III
l. papovavirus
l. retrovirus
simian T-cell lymphotropic virus
l. virus
lymphovascular
l. involvement
l. space
l. space invasion
lymphovenous
l. anastomosis
l. bypass
l. hemangioma
Lynch
L. approach
L. cancer family syndrome I, II
L. and Crues type 2 lesion
L. frontoethmoidectomy procedure
L. medial canthal incision
L. syndrome
***Lynghya* dermatitis**
Lynn
L. Achilles lengthening procedure
L. Achilles tendon repair technique
mumps virus vaccine Jeryl Lynn strain
Lyon
L. effect
L. hypothesis
L. phenomenon
lyophilized
allogenic lyophilized bone graft implant material
l. anterior pituitary
l. bone graft
l. cartilage
l. dura graft
l. dural patch
l. extract
l. human AT-III
lyophilized bone graft
lyre of David
lysate
argininosuccinate l.
melanoma cell l.
staphylococcal phage l.
whole-cell l.
lysed
clot l.
l. horse blood
l. tumor cell
lysergic
l. acid
l. acid amide
l. acid diethylamide
l. acid diethylamide assay
l. acid diethylamide and strychnine
lysine
l. decarboxylase
l. decarboxylase test
l. dehydrogenase
l. malabsorption syndrome
phenylalanine, lysine, and vasopressin
l. vasopressin
l. vasotonin
lysinuric protein intolerance
lysis
acute tumor l.
acute tumor lysis syndrome
l. of adhesion
arthroscopic lysis and lavage
ascites euglobulin lysis time
l. bladder neck adhesions
blood-clot lysis time
l. buffer
cell-mediated l.
l. centrifugation method
l. centrifugation technique
euglobulin clot l.

lysis *(continued)*
euglobulin clot lysis time
euglobulin lysis test
fibrin plate lysis area
follicle l.
hypotonic lysis buffer
immune l.
NK cell l.
l. of restricting strand
l., storage, and transportation
l. test
tumor lysis syndrome

lysogenic
l. bacterium
l. conversion
l. induction
l. strain

lysolecithin hemolytic anemia

lysosomal
l. accumulation
l. acid lipase A, B
l. dense body
l. disease
l. enzymatic activity
l. enzyme
l. enzyme disorder
l. glycoprotein
l. hydrolase enzyme assay
l. membrane
l. membrane glycoprotein-1
l. membrane glycoprotein-2
l. metabolite
l. proteinase
l. storage disease
l. storage disorder
l. trafficking regulator protein

lysosome
Golgi endoplasmic reticulum l.
l. trafficking regulator

lysostaphin susceptibility test

lysozymal enzyme release

lysozyme
l. assay
egg-white l.
l. F_2 element
hen egg l.
hen egg-white l.
human milk l.
human parotid l.
polymyxin, lysozyme, EDTA, and thallous acetate in heart infusion agar
serum l.
l. test

lysozyme-associated amyloidosis

lyssavirus
European bat lyssavirus 1

lysyl oxidase

Lyt antigen

Lythgoe effect

lytic
l. area
l. area bone flap
l. blastic changes
l. blockade
l. bone lesion
l. change
l. cocktail
l. enzyme
l. Epstein-Barr virus
l. infection
l. lesion
l. nephritic factor
l. unit
l. viral replication
l. virus

lytic-associated nuclear antigen

Lytico-Bodig syndrome

Lytren formula

***Lytta vesicata* sting**

M
M. antibody
M. antigen
M. band
M. and B isoenzyme of creatine kinase
M. cell
M. colony
M. component
M. concentration
M. cone excitation
M. line
M. phase
M. protein
M. protein factor
M. spike
M. virus

M2
M. artery segment
M. branch
M. inhibitor
M. segment of middle cerebral artery

3M
3M scanner
3M syndrome

M344
M. antibody
M. antigen

M_1
M_1 antigen
M_1 virus

Maastricht History and Advice Checklist-Revised

MAb-170 monoclonal antibody

MabThera monoclonal antibody

Mac-1 antigen

MacAndrew Addiction Scale

MacArthur
M. Longitudinal Twin Study
M. Story Stem Battery

Macaua virus

Macbeth
M. ColorChecker
M. illumination

MacCallan classification

MacCallum-Goodpasture stain

MacCallum patch

MacCarty keyhole

Macchiavellos stain

MacConkey
M. broth
M. II agar
sorbitol MacConkey agar

MacDermot-Winter syndrome

MacDonald sign

macerated
m. fetus
m. infant

maceration
m. of epithelium
plantar m.

Macewen
M. classification
M. hernia operation
M. herniorrhaphy
M. sign
M. triangle

MacFarlane serum method

Mach
M. band
M. band effect
M. number

Machado-Guerreiro test

Machado-Joseph
M.-J. ataxia
M.-J. Azorean disease

Machado test

Machek-Blaskovics operation

Machek-Brunswick operation

Machek-Gifford operation

Machek ptosis operation

Macherey-Nagel strep test

Mache unit

Machida
M. choledochoscope
M. scope

machine
air filtration m.
ankle exercise m.
m. artifact
cardiopulmonary bypass m.
computerized visual field m.
constant passive-motion m.
continuous passive motion m.
electric casting m.
m. error
focused segmented ultrasound m.
neutron therapy m.
Northland bone density m.
parallel virtual m.
m. preservation
smoke exposure m.
spinal analysis m.
m. worker dermatitis

machine-based intervention

machinery murmur

Machover Draw-A-Person Test

Machupo virus

MacIntosh
M. extraarticular tenodesis
McKeever and MacIntosh hemiarthroplasty

Mackay-Marg principle

Mack-Brunswick operation

Mackenrodt ligament

Mackenzie
M. amputation
M. disease

Mackinnon-Dellon criteria

Mackool system

Maclagan thymol turbidity test

Macleod
M. capsular rheumatism
M. syndrome

MacMARCKS protein

MacNeal
Novy and MacNeal blood agar

macroadenoma
intracellular m.

macroaggregated
m. albumin
m. albumin arterial perfusion
m. ferrous hydroxide
iodinated macroaggregated albumin
m. radioiodinated albumin
technetium-99m macroaggregated albumin

macrobiotic diet

macrobroth dilution

macrocephaly
autosomal dominant macrocephaly syndrome
benign familial m.
m., facial abnormalities, disproportionate tall stature mental retardation syndrome
m., hypertelorism, short limbs, hearing loss, developmental delay syndrome
m. lipoma
macrosomia, obesity, macrocephaly, ocular abnormality syndrome

macrocephaly *(continued)*
m., multiple lipomas, hemangiomata syndrome
m., pseudoepithelioma, multiple hemangiomas syndrome
m. with feeblemindedness and encephalopathy with peculiar deposits

macrocephaly-hamartomas syndrome

macrocyclic polyamine

macrocystic
m. adenoma
m. cystadenoma

macrocytic
m. achylic anemia
m. anemia of pregnancy
m. anemia tropical
m. erythrocyte
m. hyperchromatism
m. hyperchromic anemia
nonmegaloblastic macrocytic anemia
m. normochromic anemia
nutritional macrocytic anemia

macrodactylia fibrolipomatosis

macrofollicular
m. adenoma
m. pattern
m. thyroid papillary carcinoma

macrogenitosomia
m. praecox

macroglia cell

macroglobulin
a-2 m.
m. assay
a-2 macroglobulin coagulation inhibitor

macroglobulinemia
essential m.
myeloma or macroglobulinemia component
Waldenström m.

macroglobulin-trypsin

macroglossia
exomphalos, macroglossia, gigantism syndrome

macroglossia-omphalocele-visceromegaly syndrome

macrolide
m. antibiotic
m. antimicrobial
m. antimicrobial agent
m.'s, lincosamides, and streptogramins
m. therapy

macromolecular
m. content
m. contrast-enhanced MR imaging
m. contrast medium
m. drug
m. insoluble cold globulin
m. nonlipid compound
m. polar compound
m. uronate

macronodular
ACTH-independent bilateral macronodular hyperplasia
m. adrenal hyperplasia
m. cirrhosis
massive macronodular hyperplasia

macronutrient
m. balance
m. deficiency syndrome
m. supplementation

macroorchidism
m. marker X syndrome
mental retardation, macroorchidism syndrome

macrophage
m. activation factor
m. activation syndrome
m. agglutination factor
alveolar m.
m. chemotactic factor
chemotactic factor for m.
colony-forming unit-granulocyte, erythrocyte, megakaryocyte, m.
m. colony-stimulating factor
cultured m.'s
m. cytotoxicity factor
m. electrophoretic mobility
m. fibroblast
m. and granulocyte inducer
hemosiderin-laden m.'s
human alveolar m.
m. immunogenic antigen-recruiting factor
m. infectivity potentiator
m. infectivity potentiator protein
m. inflammatory protein
m. inflammatory protein-1
m. inflammatory protein alpha-1
m. inflammatory protein-1-alpha
m. inflammatory protein-1-beta
m. inflammatory protein I, II
m. lineage antigen
marginal metallophilic m.
marginal zone m.
m. migration index
m. migration-inhibiting factor
m. migration inhibition
m. migration inhibition test
m. migration inhibitory factor
m. oxidative burst
peritoneal m.
peritoneal exudate m.
m. phagocytic activity
pulmonary alveolar m.
m. slowing factor
splenic m.
m. spreading factor
tissue-infiltrating m.
m. tropic
m. tropism
tumor-associated m.
m. tumoricidal activity
m. variant

macrophage-activating factor

macrophage-agglutinating factor

macrophage-derived
m.-d. chemokine
m.-d. growth factor
m.-d. tumor necrosis factor

macrophage-inhibiting factor

macrophage-inhibition factor

macrophage-like synoviocyte

macrophage-targeted glucocerebrosidase

macrophage-tropic
m.-t. HIV strain
m.-t. human immunodeficiency virus strain
m.-t. virus

macrophagic myofasciitis

MacroPore distraction mesh

macrorestriction map

macroreticular dystrophy

macrosaccadic oscillation

macroscopic
m. agglutination
m. agglutination test
m. anatomy
m. appearance
m. BPH
m. broth dilution test
m. dysgenesis
m. evidence
m. examination
m. hematuria
m. lesion
m. magnetic moment

m. residual disease
m. sphincter

macrosomatia adiposa congenita

macrosomia
m. adiposa congenita
fetal m.
m., obesity, macrocephaly, ocular abnormality syndrome

macrosomia-mental retardation syndrome

macro square-wave jerk

macrostomia
ablepharon macrostomia syndrome

macrovascular disease

macrovesicular
m. fat
m. fat droplet
m. fatty liver
m. steatosis

Macro-Vue RPR Card Test

macula, pl. **maculae**
maculae acusticae
m. adherens
m. atrophica
m. communicans
m. communis
m. corneae
m. cribrosa
m. cribrosa inferior
m. cribrosa media
m. cribrosa quarta
m. cribrosa superior
m. densa
m. densa cell
m. densa chemoreceptor
m. densa receptor
disc, macula, vessels, periphery
m. flava
m. lutea
mongolian m.
neuroepithelium of m.
parafoveal m.
m. pellucida
m. of retina
m. sacculi
m. solaris
m. of utricle
maculae of utricle and saccule
m. utriculi
maculae utriculosaccularis

macula-off rhegmatogenous retinal detachment

macular
acquired immune deficiency syndrome-related macular degeneration
age-related macular degeneration
m. amyloidosis
annular macular dystrophy
aphakic cystoid macular edema
m. aplasia
m. area
m. arteriole
m. arteriole occlusion
m. artery
ataxia, myoclonic encephalopathy, macular degeneration, recurrent infections syndrome
atrophic age-related macular degeneration
m. atrophy
m. binocular vision
m. branch retinal vein occlusion
m. cherry-red spot
m. choroiditis
m. cluster
m. CMV
m. coloboma
m. contact lens
m. corneal dystrophy
cotton-spot macular edema
cystoid macular degeneration
cystoid macular edema
m. cytomegalovirus
m. degeneration
m. detachment
diabetic macular edema
m. disciform degeneration
disciform macular degeneration with subretinal neovascular membrane
m. disease
m. displacement
m. dragging
m. drusen
dry macular degeneration
m. dysplasia
m. dystrophy
ectodermal dysplasia, ectrodactyly, macular dystrophy syndrome
m. ectopia
m. edema
m. electroretinogram
epidermolysis bullosa, macular type
m. epiretinal membrane
m. eruption
m. erythema
erythematous macular dermatitis
m. evasion
m. fasciculus
focal macular choroidopathy
m. graying
m. hair cell
m. hemangioma
m. hemianopia
m. hemorrhage
m. heredodegeneration
m. hole
m. hole surgery
m. hypoplasia
juvenile macular degeneration
m. leak
m. leprosy
m. light reflex
middle macular arteriole
m. neuroretinopathy
nondescript m.
nonexudative macular degeneration
nonneovascular age-related macular degeneration
North Carolina macular dystrophy
m. ocular histoplasmosis syndrome
optic disc edema with a macular star
m. photocoagulation
M. Photocoagulation Study
m. photostress
polymorphous macular rash
m. pseudocoloboma
m. pucker
m. puckering
m. purpura
m. rash
m. retinoblastoma
m. retinopathy
Saenger m.
senile choroidal macular degeneration
senile macular chorioretinal degeneration
simultaneous macular perception
Sorsby pseudoinflammatory macular degeneration
m. sparing
m. splitting
m. stain
m. star
m. star formation
m. stereopsis
m. suppression
m. surface wrinkling
m. syphilid
m. target
m. traction

macular *(continued)*
m. translocation
m. venule
vitelliform macular degeneration

macular-papular-vesicular lesion

maculary fasciculus

maculata
parapsoriasis m.

maculatum
atrophoderma m.
atrophoderma striatum et m.

macule
café au lait m.

maculoanesthetic leprosy

maculopapillary bundle

maculopapular
m. bundle
m. eruption
erythematous maculopapular rash
m. exanthem
m. nodosa
m. rash
m. skin lesion

maculopathy
age-related m.
atrophic degenerative m.
nicotinic acid m.
operating microscope-induced phototoxic m.
soft drusen m.

maculosa
atrophia strata et m.

maculosus
morbus maculosus neonatorum

mad
m. cow disease
M. Hatter syndrome
m. honey intoxication
m. itch

Madden technique

MADDOC chemotherapy

Maddox
M. line
M. prism
M. rod hyperphoria
M. rod method
M. rod occluder
M. rod test
M. wing test

made
card made out
locally made rapid urease test
slip made out

Madelung
M. collar
M. deformity
M. disease
M. lipoma
M. neck
M. syndrome

Madin-Darby
M.-D. bovine kidney
M.-D. bovine kidney cell
M.-D. canine kidney

Madlener operation

Madonna finger

Madrid virus

Madura
M. boil
M. foot
M. skull

Madureira
Sena Madureira virus

Maeder-Danis dystrophy

Maertel regimen

Maestre de San Juan-Kallmann-de Morsier syndrome

mafenide
m. acetate
m. acetate for burn

Maferr Inventory of Masculine Values

Maffucci
M. disease
M. syndrome

magaldrate and simethicone

Magano classification

Magendie
atresia of the foramen of Luschka and M.
M. foramen
Luschka and Magendie foramen
median foramen of M.
M. sign
M. space
M. symptom

Magendie-Hertwig
M.-H. sign
M.-H. syndrome

magenta
m. I–III
m. tongue

maggot debridement therapy

magic
m. angle effect artifact
m. angle phenomenon
m. angle spinning NMR
m. bone
m. fantasy
m. helper
m. mouthwash

magis
OPMI PRO magis microscope

Magitot keratoplasty operation

magma reticulare

magna
arteria anastomotica m.
arteria anastomotica auricularis m.
arteria pancreatica m.
arteria radicularis m.
arteria radicularis anterior m.
arteria radicularis magna of Adamkiewicz
cisterna m.
mega cisterna m.

magnesia
m. and alumina oral suspension
milk of m.

magnesium
m. aluminum hydroxide
m. aluminum silicate
m. ammonium phosphate stone
m. ammonium phosphate urinary lithiasis
anhydrous magnesium sulfate
m. assay
m. balance
m. benzoate
m. carbonate
m. chloride
m. citrate
m. contrast medium
m. deficiency
m. deficiency infantile tremor syndrome
m. depletion
m. gluconate
m. hydroxide
m. hydroxide and mineral oil emulsion
m. hydroxide suspension
intracellular magnesium test
intratracheal m.
m. level
m. oxide
potassium and m.
m. salt
m. sulfate
m. sulfate, glycerin, and water enema
total-body m.
urinary magnesium volume

magnet
- ankle m.
- beam-bending m.
- main field m.
- m. operation
- m. reaction
- m. reflex
- m. therapy

magnetic
- m. anisotropy
- m. apraxia
- m. attraction
- auditory-evoked magnetic field
- axial breath-hold gradient-echo cine magnetic resonance imaging
- axial magnetic resonance image
- m. bolus tracking
- m. bore
- cervical magnetic resonance phlebography
- cine magnetic resonance imaging
- m. circuit
- m. circular dichroism
- constant magnetic field in nuclear magnetic resonance
- continuous arterial spin-labeled perfusion magnetic resonance imaging
- contrast-enhanced magnetic resonance angiography
- contrast medium-enhanced magnetic resonance imaging
- m. control suturing
- conventional magnetic resonance imaging
- m. core
- m. core memory
- m. crisis
- diffusion-weighted magnetic resonance imaging
- m. dipole
- m. dipole-dipole coupling
- m. dipole moment
- m. disk
- m. domain
- doxorubicin adsorbed to magnetic targeted carrier
- dynamic contrast-enhanced magnetic resonance imaging
- dynamic enhanced magnetic resonance imaging
- endoesophageal magnetic resonance imaging
- endoesophageal magnetic resonance imaging coil
- endorectal magnetic resonance imaging
- endoscopic magnetic resonance
- enhancement of magnetic resonance imaging
- m. extraction
- fast-frequency repetitive transcranial magnetic stimulation
- fast imaging steady precession sequence three-dimensional magnetic resonance imaging
- m. field
- field focused nuclear magnetic resonance
- m. field gradient
- m. field-search coil test
- m. field strength
- m. field vector
- m. flux
- m. flux density
- functional magnetic resonance angiography
- functional magnetic resonance imaging
- gadolinium-enhanced magnetic resonance imaging
- m. gait
- gated sweet magnetic imaging
- gradient magnetic field
- m. heart vector
- m. implant
- m. induction
- m. induction device
- m. inertia
- localized magnetic resonance
- low-field magnetic resonance imaging
- macroscopic magnetic moment
- magnetization transfer magnetic resonance imaging
- m. microsphere
- minimum basis set magnetic resonance angiography
- m. moment
- multisection diffuse-weighted magnetic resonance imaging
- nuclear magnetic resonance imaging
- nuclear magnetic resonance spectroscopy
- m. operation
- m. optical rotatory dispersion
- perfusion-weighted magnetic resonance imaging
- phase-contrast cine magnetic resonance imaging
- phosphorus magnetic resonance imaging
- phosphorus magnetic resonance spectroscopy
- phosphorus-31 magnetic resonance spectroscopy
- phosphorus nuclear magnetic resonance spectroscopy
- m. polarization
- proton magnetic resonance
- proton magnetic resonance spectroscopy
- m. quantum number
- radiofrequency magnetic field in nuclear magnetic resonance
- ratio of magnetic moment of a particle to Bohr magneton
- m. resonance
- m. resonance angiography
- m. resonance arteriography
- m. resonance arthrography
- m. resonance cholangiogram
- m. resonance cholangiography
- m. resonance cholangiopancreatography
- m. resonance colonography
- m. resonance coronary angiography
- m. resonance elastography
- m. resonance flowmetry
- m. resonance imaging
- m. resonance imaging thermometry
- m. resonance mammography
- m. resonance pancreatography
- m. resonance spectroscopic imaging-guided brachytherapy
- m. resonance spectroscopy
- m. resonance tomographic angiography
- m. resonance tomography
- m. resonance urography
- m. resonance venography
- m. source imaging
- m. starch microspheres
- m. stirrer
- m. susceptibility
- three-dimensional contrast-enhanced magnetic resonance angiography
- topical magnetic resonance
- transcranial cortical magnetic stimulation
- tritium nuclear magnetic resonance

magnetically
- m. activated cell sorter

magnetically *(continued)*
m. influenced homeopathic remedy
m. responsive microsphere

magnetite in tumor targeting

magnetization
longitudinal m.
spatial modulation of m.
m. transfer imaging
m. transfer magnetic resonance imaging
m. transfer ratio
transverse m.

magnetization-prepared
m.-p. 3D gradient-echo sequence
m.-p. rapid gradient echo-water excitation

magnetomotive force

magneton
Bohr m.
ratio of magnetic moment of a particle to Bohr m.

magnification
m. angiography
area of interest m.
cortical magnification factor
m. factor
Littmann Galilean magnification changer
m. mammography
microfocal direct magnification in vitro x-ray tube
ultrahigh magnification mammography

magnifying
m. colonoscopy
m. endoscope
m. enteroscope
m. glasses
m. lens
m. loupe
m. power

magnitude
average pulse m.
m. calculation
m. estimation
large magnitude voluntary heart rate changes
log magnitude ratio
m. preparation-rapid acquisition gradient echo
vector m.

magnocellular
m. basal forebrain
m. cholinergic neuron
m. deficit
m. dysfunction
m. hormone
m. neuroendocrine cell
m. neurosecretory neuron
m. neurosecretory system
m. nucleus
m. perikaryon
m. visual pathway

magnum
asymmetric small foramen m.
foramen magnum decompression

Magnus
M. and de Kleijn tonic neck reflex
M. operation
M. sign

magnus
auricularis m.
musculus adductor m.
nervus auricularis m.
nucleus raphe m.

Magnuson
M. debridement
M. reduction technique

Magnuson-Stack arthroplasty

Magpi
M. hypospadias repair
M. procedure

Magrath-modified regimen

Ma-Griffith end-to-end anastomosis

Maguari virus

Mahaim
M. bundle in heart
M. fiber

Maher disease

mahogany
m. cofactor
m. flush
M. Hammock virus

mai
ren mai channel

Maier sinus

Maillard
M. product
M. reaction
M. site

main
anomalous left main coronary artery
m. arteriole
m. bronchus
m. bundle
m. cuneate nucleus
m. d'accoucheur
distal portion main circumflex
M. Drain virus
m. duct
m. duct of Wirsung
m. effect
m. en crochet
m. en griffe
m. en griffe deformity
m. en lorgnette
m. en singe
m. fiber
m. field
m. field magnet
m. frame
left main coronary artery disease
left main stem bronchus
left main stem coronary artery disease
left main trunk
m. lobe of lung
m. pancreatic duct
m. papillary duct
m. portal vein peak velocity
m. pulmonary artery
m. renal artery
m. renal artery stenosis
m. renal vein
right main bronchus
right main coronary artery
m. sensory nucleus
m. stem bronchus
m. timing event
unprotected left m.
m. venule

mainstem
m. bronchus
m. carina
m. coronary artery
occlusion of mainstem bronchus

Mainstreaming
Attitudes Toward Mainstreaming Scale

maintain
inability to maintain attention
m. blood glucose level

maintained
adequate hemostasis m.
central, steady and maintained fixation
sympathetic maintained plan

maintainer
band and bar space m.
band and crib space m.
bonded space m.

cantilever space m.
m. cast space

maintaining

apparatus for maintaining pH of solution
disorders of initiating and maintaining sleep

maintenance

altered health m.
around-the-clock oral maintenance bronchodilator therapy
m. chemotherapy
continuing maintenance chemotherapy
m. cyclosporine monotherapy
m. dialysis
m. dialysis unit
m. dose
m. drug
m. drug therapy
m. electrolyte solution
Employee Health M. Examination
m. fluid
m. function
functional maintenance program
health care m.
health maintenance cooperative
health maintenance plan
m. hemodialysis
impaired home maintenance management
inadequate tissue m.
Lactobacillus maintenance medium
medical maintenance unit
m. medication
methadone m.
methadone maintenance and aftercare treatment program
methadone maintenance treatment
Physical Self M. Scale
protoplast maintenance medium
sleep maintenance insomnia
m. of wakefulness test

Mainz pouch

Maisonneuve

M. amputation
M. fibular fracture

Maissiat band

maitake mushroom

Maixner cirrhosis

Majewski

M. short rib polydactyly
M. syndrome

Majewsky operation

Majocchi

M. disease
M. granuloma
M. purpura

major

m. abdominal surgery
adult major depression
m. adverse cardiac event
m. affective disorder
m. agglutinin
m. alar cartilage
m. amblyoscope
m. amblyoscope test
m. amputation
m. anchorage
anterior palatal major connector
anterosuperior ilium m.
m. aorticopulmonary collateral arteries
m. aortopulmonary collateral artery
m. aphthae
m. arcade
m. arterial circle of iris
arteria palatina m.
m. artery
m. attachment figure
m. basic protein
m. break
m. breakpoint region
m. bronchus
m. calix
m. capsid protein gene
m. causalgia
m. circulus arteriosus of iris
m. component of adult hemoglobin
m. connector
m. coronary artery
m. coronary event
m. curve
m. deceleration injury
m. dense line
m. depression
m. depressive affective psychosis
m. depressive disorder
m. depressive episode
m. detoxification enzyme
m. diagnostic category
m. duodenal papilla
m. dysmorphism
m. epilepsy
erythema multiforme m.
m. fissure
m. forceps
m. form
m. fracture fragment
m. functional impairment
m. gangrene
m. gene
m. GI surgery
m. histocompatibility
m. histocompatibility complex
m. histocompatibility complex antigen
m. histocompatibility complex haplotype
m. histocompatibility complex restriction
m. histocompatibility region
m. histocompatibility system
m. histocompatibility type
m. hypnosis
m. hysteria
m. image-distorting level
m. impairment
m. impairment of functioning
m. injury vector
m. karyotypic abnormality
lingual bar major connector
m. liver resection
m. histocompatibility complex class I
medial crus of major alar cartilage of nose
m. medical insurance
m. mental illness
m. meridian
m. motor seizure
obstruction of major organs
m. organ profile
m. outer membrane protein
pectoralis m.
pectoralis major muscle
pectoralis major myocutaneous flap
pelvis justo m.
peptide major histocompatibility complex
m. proglucagon fragment
psoas major muscle
rhomboid major muscle
m. role therapy
m. salivary gland
Santorini major caruncle
m. serologic antigen
single major locus
subcutaneous bursa of teres m.
m. sublingual duct
m. symptom complex
teres major muscle
thalassemia m.
m. tranquilizer

major *(continued)*
trapezoidal paddle pectoralis major myocutaneous flap
m. urinary protein

majoris

majus
labium m.
omentum m.

MAK-6 cocktail

make
M. A Picture Story test
inability to make decisions
Inquiry Mode Questionnaire: A Measure of How You Think and make Decisions

Makeham hypothesis

makeup
Kabuki makeup syndrome

making
Assessment of Career Decision M.
m. change test
difficulty in decision m.
evidence-based decision m.
incapacitated of making decisions
interference with judgment and decision m.

Maklakoff tonometer

Makler insemination

Makonde virus

Malabar
M. itch
M. leprosy
M. ulcer

malabsorption
alcoholic malabsorption syndrome
m. disease
glucose-galactose m.
idiopathic bile acid m.
isolated congenital folate m.
lactose m.
lysine malabsorption syndrome
methionine malabsorption syndrome
m. symptom
m. syndrome
m. workup

malabsorptive diarrhea

Malacarne
M. pyramid
M. space

malachite green

maladaptive
m. behavioral change
continued maladaptive behavior
m. coping
m. coping mechanism
m. coping strategy
m. defense mechanism
m. feeling
m. impulse

maladie
m. de plongeurs
m. de roger

maladjustment
history of m.
occupational maladjustment syndrome
m. score
Structured and Scaled Interview to Assess M.

Malakal virus

malalignment
patellofemoral m.
patellofemoral malalignment pain
m. syndrome

malar
m. alloplastic augmentation
m. arch
m. area
m. bag suctioning
m. bone
m. butterfly rash
m. cheek pad
m. complex fracture
m. crescent
m. crest of great wing of sphenoid bone
m. deficiency
m. distribution
m. elevator
m. eminence
m. erythema
m. facial augmentation
m. fat pad
finger-assisted malar elevation
m. flatness
m. flush
m. fold
m. foramen
m. fracture
m. gland
m. groove
m. hypoplasia
m. lymph node
m. point
m. process
m. rash
zygomatic malar complex

malaria
benign tertian m.
cerebral m.
m. comatosa
m. control unit
m. endemic
m. film test
m. immunoglobulin
malignant tertian m.
m. prevention
m. prophylaxis
recurrent induced m.
m. smear
m. therapy
m. vaccine

malarial
m. anemia
m. cachexia
m. crescent
m. deposition pigment
m. dysentery
m. fever
m. granuloma
m. hemoglobinuria
m. hepatitis
hyperactive malarial splenomegaly syndrome
m. knob
malignant tertian malarial parasite
m. parasite
m. parasites
m. paroxysm
m. periodicity
m. pigment
remittent malarial fever
m. rosette
m. therapy

Malassez
M. debris
M. epithelial rests

Malassezia
Malassezia folliculitis

malate dehydrogenase

Malawer excision technique

Malayan filariasis

malayi
Brugia malayi adult antigen

Malaysian typhoid

Malbec operation

Malbran operation

mal del pinto

maldescended testis

male
m. accessory gland fluid

adult m.
m. alcoholism subtype
m. biological status
black m.
m. bond
m. breast
m. breast cancer
m. breast carcinoma
m. castration
Caucasian m.
m. child
m. circumcision
m. climacteric
m. climacteric syndrome
dysgenetic male pseudohermaphroditism
m. dyspareunia
m. dyspareunia male erectile disorder
m. epispadias
m. equivalent
m. erectile disorder
m. erectile dysfunction
m. escutcheon
m. external genitalia
m. factor
m. factor infertility
m. flank
m. foreheadplasty
m. frog test
full-term living male child
m. gender identity
m. genital duct
m. genital duct development
m. genitalia
m. genitalia melanoma
m. germ line tumor
m. gonad
m. hermaphroditism
Hispanic m.
homosexual m.
m. homosexual contact
m. homosexuality
m. hormone production
m. hormone testosterone
m. hypoactive sexual desire disorder
m. hypogonadism
immature dead male child
immature living male child
m. impotence after childbirth
m. impotence test
incomplete male pseudohermaphroditism
m. infertility
m. infertility problem
m. internal genitalia
m. karyotype
Latin American m.
living male child
Mexican American m.
mucosa of male urethra
muscular coat of intermediate part of male urethra
muscular coat of spongy part of male urethra
muscular layer of intermediate part of male urethra
navicular fossa of male urethra
newborn, term, normal, m.
nonwhite m.
normal adult m.
normal male adult genitalia
normal male infant
normal male sex chromosome type
Norwood Classification of M. Pattern Baldness
m. orgasm
m. pattern androgenetic alopecia
m. pattern baldness
m. pattern hair loss
m. pattern hirsutism
m. pattern obesity
m. phenotype
m. precocious puberty
pregnancy, term, complicated delivered, living m.
pregnancy, term, uncomplicated delivered, living m.
premature dead male child
premature living male child
m. pronucleus
m. pseudohermaphrodites
m. pseudohermaphroditism
m. reproductive organ
m. reproductive tract
m. sex chromosome
m. sex differentiation
m. sex hormone
m. sexual dysfunction
Spanish American m.
m. specific antigen
m. sperm
m. sterility
synthetic male hormone
term birth, living m.
m. Turner syndrome
unknown black m.
unknown white m.
viable male infant
well-nourished m.
white male living child
young male Caucasian

maleate
brompheniramine m.
chlorpheniramine m.
ergonovine m.
ergonovine maleate provocation angina

maleated bovine serum albumin

Malecot catheter

Malecot-type catheter

male-limited familial precocious puberty

male-to-female transmission

malevolent
m. behavior
m. concern
m. distrust

maleylacetoacetate
m. hydrolase
m. hydrolase, type Ib

malformation
angel's kiss capillary m.
angiographically occult intracranial vascular m.
angiographically occult vascular m.
angiographically visualized vascular m.
aortic arch m.
Arnold-Chiari m.
arterial m.
arteriovenous brain m.
arteriovenous colon m.
arteriovenous cord m.
arteriovenous fistula m.
arteriovenous fistulous m.
arteriovenous kidney m.
arteriovenous malformation of brain
arteriovenous malformation nidus
arteriovenous malformation nidus definition
arteriovenous malformation radiosurgery
auditory arteriovenous m.
capillary-lymphatic m.
cardiovascular m.
cerebral arteriovenous m.
cerebral venous m.
complex-combined vascular m.
congenital cardiovascular m.
congenital cystic adenomatoid m.
congenital malformation of heart
congenital vascular m.
m. of cortical development
craniocervical m.

malformation *(continued)*
cryptic vascular m.
cystic adenomatous m.
dural arteriovenous m.
extramedullary arteriovenous m.
gastric arteriovenous m.
intracranial vascular m.
intracranial venous m.
intramedullary arteriovenous m.
isolated cardiovascular m.
lymphatic m.
lymphaticovenous m.
lymphatic-venous m.
mandibulofacial dysostosis with limb malformations syndrome
medial hemispheric arteriovenous m.
medullary venous m.
mental retardation, blepharonasofacial abnormalities, hand malformations syndrome
minimal dose causing 100% death or m.
neural axis vascular m.
neural crest m.
obliterated arteriovenous m.
occult cerebral vascular m.
occult cerebrovascular m.
orbital arteriovenous m.
orofacial m.
osseous craniofacial arteriovenous m.
pelvic arteriovenous m.
pulmonary arteriovenous m.
split-cord m.
split spinal cord m.
urinary tract m.
vein of Galen aneurysmal m.
venous m.

malformed
m. ear
m. heart or heart valve
m. pinna
m. radial head

malfunction

malfunctioning
clicking of malfunctioning valve
m. immune system
m. insulin receptor cells

Malgaigne
M. amputation
M. fossa
M. fracture
M. hernia
M. triangle

Malherbe
M. calcifying epithelioma
M. disease
M. tumor

malic
m. acid
m. acid dehydrogenase
m. dehydrogenase
m. enzyme
m. enzyme gene

maligna
lentigo maligna melanoma
lymphogranulomatosis m.
onychia m.
papulosis atrophicans m.

malignancy
anterior skull base m.
m. associated cellular marker
m. associated neutropenia
borderline m.
extracolonic m.
humoral hypercalcemia of m.
hypercalcemia of m.
inoperable bladder m.
latent primary m.
lymphoproliferative m.
mimicker of m.
multiple primary m.
myositis with m.
no evidence of m.
occult primary m.
pelvic malignancy in pregnancy
there is no evidence of m.

malignancy-associated
m.-a. change
m.-a. hypercalcemia

malignant
m. acanthosis nigricans
m. acetabular osteolysis
m. acini prostate gland
m. adenoma
m. adrenal mass
m. airway obstruction
m. ameloblastoma
m. anemia
m. angioendotheliomatosis
angiomatoid malignant fibrous histiocytoma
m. angiomyolipoma
anthrax malignant pustule
m. arrhythmia
m. ascites fluid
m. astrocytoma
m. atrophic papulosis
atypical polypoid adenomyofibroma of low malignant potential
m. B-cell syndrome
m. biliary obstruction
m. biliary obstructive disease
m. blue nevus
m. bone aneurysm
m. brachial plexopathy
m. brain edema
m. brain neoplasm
m. brain tumor
m. breast calcification
m. breast tumor
m. bubo
m. cachexia
m. calcification
m. carbuncle
m. carcinoid syndrome
m. catarrhal fever
m. catarrhal fever disease
m. catarrhal fever virus
m. cell
m. chondroid syringoma
m. chondroma
m. chondrosarcoma
m. choroidal melanoma
m. ciliary epithelioma
classification of malignant tumors
m. clear cell acrospiroma
conventional cutaneous malignant melanoma
cutaneous malignant melanoma
cutaneous malignant melanoma of head and neck
m. cytotrophoblast
m. degeneration
diffuse malignant mesothelioma
diffuse malignant pleural mesothelioma
m. down
m. duodenal tumor
m. dysentery
m. dyskeratosis
m. dysphagia
m. dysplasia
m. eccrine poroma
m. eccrine spiradenoma
m. edema
m. effusion
elder malignant melanoma classification
m. endocarditis
m. endovascular papillary angioendothelioma
m. ependymoma

epidermotropic metastatic
malignant melanoma
m. epithelial tumor
m. epithelioid mesothelioma
m. etiology
m. exophthalmos
m. external otitis
m. external otitis syndrome
m. extrarenal rhabdoid tumor
familial atypical mole malignant
melanoma
m. familial myoclonic epilepsy
m. fasciculation
m. fibrohistiocytoma
m. fibroma
m. fibrous histiocytoma
m. fibrous histiocytoma of bone
m. fibrous histiocytoma of soft
tissue
m. fibrous xanthoma
first malignant neoplasm
m. giant cell tumor
giant cell tumor of low
malignant potential
m. glandular cell tumor
m. glandular schwannoma
m. glaucoma
m. glioma
m. glomus tumor
m. granular cell myoblastoma
m. granuloma
m. granulomatosis
m. growth
m. hemangioendothelioma
m. hemangiopericytoma
m. hepatic neoplasm
m. hepatoma
hereditary cutaneous malignant
melanoma
m. histiocytic lymphoma
m. histiocytosis
m. histiocytosis of intestine
histologically m.
m. hypercalcemia
m. hyperphenylalaninemia
m. hyperpyrexia
m. hypertension
m. hyperthermia
m. hyperthermia resistance
m. hyperthermia syndrome
m. hyperthermic rhabdomyolysis
m. hypothermia susceptibility
m. insulinoma
m. intratubular germ-cell
neoplasia
m. islet cell tumor
m. jaundice
m. lentigo melanoma
low-grade malignant cartilaginous
lesion
low malignant potential epithelial
ovarian tumor
m. lymph
m. lymphocytic proliferation
disease
m. lymphoma
m. lymphoma, histiocytic
m. lymphoma, lymphoblastic type
m. lymphoma, poorly
differentiated lymphocytic
m. lymphoproliferative disorder
m. malnutrition
m. melanoma
m. melanoma of choroid
m. melanoma in situ
m. mesenchymal tumor
m. mesothelioma
m. mesothelioma of the tunica
vaginalis
m. metastatic disease
metastatic malignant melanoma
metastatic malignant
pheochromocytoma
m. middle cerebral artery
infarction
m. mixed mesodermal tumor
m. mixed müllerian tumor
m. mixed oligoastrocytoma
m. mole syndrome
multicentric malignant glioma
m. myeloma
m. myoepithelioma
m. myopia
m. necrotizing otitis externa
m. neoplasia
m. neoplasm of bladder
m. neoplasm of bone
m. neoplasm of bronchus
m. neoplasm of kidney
m. neoplasm of larynx
m. neoplasm of scrotum
m. neoplastic disease
m. nephrosclerosis
nerve sheath malignant tumor
m. nerve sheath tumor
m. neurilemoma
m. neuroleptic syndrome
m. neutropenia
node-based malignant
lymphoproliferative disease
m. nodular hidradenoma
no malignant cell
non-Hodgkin malignant lymphoma
North American Malignant
Hyperthermia protocol
m. osteoid
m. otitis externa
m. ovarian germ cell tumor
ovarian malignant epithelial
neoplasm
ovarian malignant germ cell
tumor
m. ovarian neoplasm
m. ovarian teratoma
m. papillary mesothelioma
m. papillomatosis
m. papillomatosis of Degos
m. paraganglioma
m. pericardial effusion
m. peripheral nerve sheath tumor
m. persistent positional nystagmus
m. pheochromocytoma
m. pilocytic astrocytoma
m. pituitary lesion
m. pleural effusion
m. pleural mesothelioma
m. potentially fatal asthma
primary malignant melanoma of
the esophagus
primary malignant tumor
m. primary pheochromocytoma
m. progression
prostatic stromal proliferation of
uncertain malignant potential
m. pustule
m. pyoderma
m. rabbit fibroma virus
m. renal neoplasm
m. reticulopathy
m. reticulosis
m. rhabdoid tumor of kidney
m. rhabdoid tumor of soft tissue
m. scleritis
second malignant neoplasm
small cell malignant lymphoma
m. smallpox
m. small round cell tumor
m. spinal disease
stromal tumor of unknown
malignant potential
m. syncytiotrophoblast
m. systemic mastocytosis
m. teratoma, anaplastic
m. teratoma, intermediate
m. teratoma, trophoblastic
m. teratoma, undifferentiated
teratoma with malignant
transformation
m. tertian fever
m. tertian malaria

malignant *(continued)*
m. tertian malarial parasite
m. thrombocytopenia
m. thyroid nodule
m. transformation
m. trichilemma tumor
m. triton tumor
trophoblastic malignant tumor
m. trophoblastic teratoma
m. tumor
m. tumor of cervix
undetermined malignant potential
m. ventricular arrhythmia
m. ventricular tachycardia

malignum
m. adenoma
lymphogranuloma m.

Malin syndrome

Malis
M. hinge clamp

Mall
M. formula
M. ridge

malleable
m. endoscope
m. facial implant
m. splint
structural aluminum m.

mallear
anterior mallear fold
anterior mallear ligament
m. fold
m. ligament
m. process
m. prominence
m. stripe

malleatory chorea

mallei (*pl. of* malleus)

malleoincudal joint

malleolar
anterior lateral malleolar artery
anterior medial malleolar artery
AP malleolar bisection
arteriae malleolares posteriores mediales
m. artery
m. articular surface of fibula
m. articular surface of tibia
m. chip fracture
m. facet
m. fold
m. gel sleeve
m. groove
medial malleolar branch of posterior tibial artery
medial malleolar facet of talus
medial malleolar network
medial malleolar subcutaneous bursa
medial malleolar surface of talus
m. ossification center
m. plexus
m. stria
m. sulcus

malleolaris
arteria malleolaris anterior lateralis
arteria malleolaris anterior medialis
m. anterior medialis

Malleoloc ankle orthosis

malleolus
articular facet of lateral m.
articular facet of medial m.
belly button to medial m.
m. bone
m. externus
internal medial m.
lateral head of m.
m. lateralis
manubrium of m.
medial m.
medial anterior malleolus artery
m. medialis
medial malleolus of tibia
m. muscle
m. stasis ulcer
subcutaneous bursa of lateral m.
subcutaneous bursa of medial m.

mallet
anger m.
m. deformity
m. finger
m. finger deformity
m. finger orthotic
m. fracture
m. toe

malleus, pl. **mallei**
anterior ligament of m.
anterior process of m.
m. bone
hallux m.
m. handle
m. head
head of m.
ligament of m.
long process of m.
manubrium of m.
neck of m.
superior ligament of m.

Mallinckrodt
M. Institute guidelines
M. radioimmunoassay

Mallory
M. aniline blue stain
M. body
M. collagen stain

Mallory-Weiss
M.-W. syndrome
M.-W. tear

malnourished
m. child
dehydrated and m.
intrauterine fetally m.

malnutrition
energy-protein m.
fluid-electrolyte m.
protein-calorie m.
protein-energy m.

malnutrition-related
m.-r. diabetes mellitus

malocclusion
closed-bite m.
open-bite m.

malodorous
m. breath
m. discharge
m. fluid
m. sweat
m. urine

malomaxillary suture

malonaldehyde generation

malonate
oxyacetate m.
m. utilization test

malondialdehyde
m. conjugated low-density lipoprotein
m. modified low-density lipoprotein

Malone
M. ACE procedure
M. antegrade colonic enema stoma procedure
M. antegrade continence enema procedure
M. antegrade continent enema channel
M. cecostomy
M. continent appendicostomy

Maloney
M. bougie
M. dilation
M. leukemia virus

M. murine sarcoma
M. stain for aluminum

Malouf syndrome

Malpais Spring virus

mal perforant du pied

malpighian
m. body
m. body of kidney
m. body of spleen
m. capsule
m. cell
m. corpuscle
m. gland
m. glomerulus
m. layer
m. nodule
m. pyramid
m. rete
m. stigma
m. stratum
m. tubule
m. tuft
m. vesicle

Malpighi vesicle

malposition
m. of the branch pulmonary artery
crisscross heart m.
m. of great arteries
uterine m.

malpositioned wisdom teeth

malrotation
m. of bowel
m. of bowel loop
congenital malrotation of the gut
m. of duodenum
intestinal m.
multiple organ malrotation syndrome
m. with midgut volvulus

malt
m. agar
m. extract broth
m. soup extract
m. worker's lung

Malta fever

maltase
acid maltase deficiency
adult acid maltase deficiency

Maltese cross

MALT/marginal zone lymphoma

maltodextrin

maltose-binding protein

maltose fermentation test

malunion
angulatory m.
femoral shaft m.
fracture with m.

malunited
m. acetabulum
m. calcaneus fracture
m. forearm fracture

mamillary
m. body
m. body volume
m. duct
m. line
m. nuclei receptor
nucleus of mamillary body
peduncle of mamillary body
m. process
m. tubercle
m. tubercle of hypothalamus

mamillotegmental fasciculus

mamillothalamic
m. fasciculus
m. tract

mamma, pl. **mammae**
areola mammae
m. erratic
papilla mammae
m. virilis

mammaglobin
human mammaglobin RNA
m. breast cancer protein

mammalian
m. achaete-scute homologous protein-2
m. adenovirus
m. binding lectin deficiency
m. bombesin
m. cell
m. cell culture
m. cell membrane
m. diving response
m. hippocampus
m. orthoreovirus
m. rotavirus
m. target of rapamycin
m. transgenesis
m. type B, C, D oncovirus group

mammaplasty
Aries-Pitanguy m.
augmentation m.
Goulian m.

mammary
m. abscess
arteriovenous internal mammary fistula
m. artery
m. artery graft
m. aspiration specimen
m. aspiration specimen cytology test
m. atrophy
bilateral internal mammary arteries
m. body
m. branch
m. calculus
m. cancer virus of mice
m. crest
m. cyst
m. duct
m. duct ectasia
m. duct obstruction
m. ductogram
m. ductogram imaging
m. dysplasia
m. fibroadenoma
m. fistula
m. fold
m. gangrene
m. gland
m. gland mass
human mammary carcinoma cell membrane proteinase
human mammary tumor virus
internal mammary artery bypass
internal mammary artery catheterization
internal mammary artery graft
internal mammary artery implant
internal mammary lymph node
internal mammary lymphoscintigraphy
m. intraepithelial neoplasia
left internal mammary artery graft
m. line
lobe of mammary gland
lobule of mammary gland
medial mammary branch
mouse mammary epithelium
mouse mammary oncovirus
mouse mammary tumor
mouse mammary tumor virus
multicentric mammary carcinoma
murine mammary tumor virus
m. neuralgia
m. Paget disease
m. parenchymal stimulation
perforating artery of internal m.
m. plexus

mammary *(continued)*
m. region
m. ridge
right internal mammary anastomosis
right internal mammary artery
m. serum antigen
silicone gel-filled mammary implant
single internal mammary artery
m. souffle
spontaneous mammary tumor
m. tumor
m. tumor agent
m. tumorigenesis
m. tumor virus
m. tumor virus of mice
m. vein
m. vessel

mammary-derived growth inhibitor

mammillary
m. artery
m. body
m. fasciculus
m. peduncle
m. process of lumbar vertebra
m. region

mammillotegmental fasciculus

mammillothalamic tract

mammogram
abnormal m.
x-ray m.

mammographic
m. abnormality
m. appearance
m. detection
m. evaluation
m. finding
m. screening

mammography
computed tomography laser m.
computerized digital m.
contrast subtraction m.
high-resolution CT m.
magnetic resonance m.
Mammomat B m.
Trex digital mammography system
ultrahigh magnification m.
Xonics electron m.

Mammomat B mammography

mammoplasty
augmentation m.
McKissock m.

MammoSite RTS

mammosomatotroph
m. cell
m. cell adenoma

mammotropic
m. factor
m. hormone

man
Mendelian Inheritance in M.
milliroentgen equivalent m.
radiation equivalent in m.
stiff man syndrome
well-nourished m.

managed
m. behavioral health plans
m. care
M. Care Appropriateness Protocol
m. care environment
m. care organization
medically managed intensive addiction treatment unit
m. mental health
patient managed medically

management
Access M. Survey
acute medical management intervention
adolescent anger m.
m. algorithm
alternatives of m.
m. of anesthesia
anesthetic and fluid m.
anger management skill
anxiety management training
M. Appraisal Survey
m. of assaultive behavior
behavioral management technique
behavior management plan
m. of cardiac arrhythmia
care management continuity
care management integration
Childhood Asthma M. Program
community health management information system
computer-patient management problem
Conflict M. Appraisal
Conflict M. Survey
continue present m.
critical incident stress m.
diabetes disease management clinic
diabetes management center
diabetic m.
evaluation and management codes
facilities m.
failure of conservative m.
Family Inventory of Resources for M.
geriatric evaluation and management unit
health care m.
health information m.
healthy conflict m.
home m.
hospital m.
hospital-based stress m.
hospital management committee
impaired home maintenance m.
m. information system
m. of insomnia
integrated anger m.
Integrated M. of Childhood Illness
intensive case m.
intensive diabetes m.
interventional pain m.
Management Philosophies Scale I-V
mechanical endoscopic m.
Medical Inventory M. System
Menstrual Distress M. Questionnaire
milieu management intervention
multidisciplinary pain management center
needle management system
nonpharmacologic behavior m.
Pain M. Index
pain management center
pain management program
Patient Data M. Systems
patient management issue
patient management problem
physician practice m.
postoperative pain m.
primary care case m.
quality assurance/risk m.
real-time position m.
risk m.
routine health m.
stress management and imagery
subjective, objective, management, and analytic
total quality m.
M. Transactions Audit
Utilization M.
venous/arterial management protection
weight management program

Managerial Style Questionnaire

Manawatu virus

Manawa virus

Manchester
M. operation
M. ovoid
M. and Oxford Universities Scale for the Psychopathological Assessment of Dementia
M. system for brachytherapy
M. system for radium therapy

Manchester-Fothergill operation

Manchurian
M. hemorrhagic fever
M. typhus

Mancini
M. plate
M. technique

mandated
government mandated guideline
m. mental health coverage

mandatory
acquired immune deficiency syndrome mandatory testing
m. acquired immune deficiency syndrome testing
m. celiotomy
continuous mandatory ventilation
expiration-synchronized intermittent mandatory ventilation
extended mandatory minute ventilation
forced mandatory intermittent ventilation
m. immunization
m. minute ventilation
m. minute volume
spontaneous intermittent mandatory ventilation
synchronized intermittent mandatory ventilation

mandelic acid

Mandel Social Adjustment Scale

mandible
alveolar arch of m.
angle of m.
articular fossa of m.
ascending ramus of m.
m. body
condyle of m.
m. coronoid
fibrous dysplasia of the m.
m. head
head of m.
lingula of m.
little head of m.
median cleft of lower lip and m.
m. mentum
neck of m.
oblique line of m.
orbit, mandible, ear, cranial nerves, soft tissue syndrome
m. ramus
ramus of m.

mandibular
m. advancement
m. advancement appliance
m. advancement device
m. advancing device
m. alveolar mucosa
m. alveolus
m. angle
anterior horizontal mandibular osteotomy
anterior mandibular posturing
m. anteroposterior ridge slope
m. arch
m. arch bar
m. artery
articular surface of mandibular fossa
articular surface of mandibular fossa of temporal bone
m. articulation
augmentation of mandibular angle
m. axis
m. base
m. bicuspid
m. body fracture
m. body length
m. bone
m. border
m. branchial arch
m. canal
m. canine
m. cartilage
center of mandibular autorotation
m. central incisor
m. centric relation
composite mandibular reconstruction
m. condylar hypoplasia
m. condyle
m. condylectomy
m. condyle fracture
m. contour
m. coronoid graft
m. crest
curved, reformatted mandibular image
m. cuspid
m. cuspid-first bicuspid radiograph
m. cuspid radiograph
m. defect
m. dental arcade
m. dentition
m. dentition odontectomy
m. depth
m. deviation
m. disk
m. dislocation
m. distraction
m. distraction osteogenesis
m. distractor
m. division
m. dysostosis and peromelia
effective mandibular length
m. equilibration
m. excess
m. fissure
m. fixation
fixed mandibular implant
m. foramen
m. forceps
m. fossa
m. fracture
Frankfort mandibular incisor angle
Frankfort mandibular plane angle
m. functional reconstruction
m. gland
m. glide
m. gliding movement
m. guide-plane prosthesis
m. guide prosthesis
m. head
m. height
m. hemisection
m. hypoplasia
immobilization mandibular fracture
m. impression
incisal mandibular plane angle
m. joint
lingular mandibular bony defect
m. lymph node
marginal mandibular branch of facial nerve
maxillary mandibular odentectomy alveolectomy
meningeal branch of mandibular nerve
m. nerve
m. notch
orbital, mandibular, ear, neural, soft tissue
m. orthopedic repositioning appliance

mandibular *(continued)*
m. pain dysfunction syndrome
posterior mandibular depth
m. process
m. prognathism
m. ramus
m. reconstruction plate
m. reflex
m. ridge
sternal occipital mandibular immobilization
m. symphysis
m. tongue
m. tooth
m. torus
trigeminal nerve, mandibular division
m. tuberculosis
m. vestibulolingual sulcoplasty

mandibular-acral dysplasia

mandibularis
articulatio m.
glenoid fossa m.
nervus m.
nodus lymphoideus m.

mandibulectomy
anterior m.
marginal m.

mandibuloacral
m. dysostosis
m. dysplasia

mandibulofacial
m. dysostosis with epibulbar dermoids syndrome
m. dysostosis with limb malformations syndrome
m. dysotosis syndrome
m. dysplasia

mandibulomaxillary fixation

mandibulo-oculofacial dysmorphia

mandibulo-oculofacialis

maneuver
alerting maneuver on electroencephalogram
all-fours maneuver for shoulder dystocia
Apley compression m.
arm duration m.
arm raises m.
arm straighten m.
canalith repositioning m.
cast stroking maneuver during massage
chin lift m.
circular pressure maneuver during massage
fan stroking maneuver during massage
head tilt and chin lift m.
heat, steam, gum, yawn, and Valsalva m.
hyperextension postures and m.'s
jaw thrust m.
liver hanging m.
log roll m.
maximal forced expiratory m.
McKenzie extension m.
McMurray circumduction m.
military brace m.
modified Miller m.
modified Ritgen m.
Moore head-tilt m.
Muller m.
Murphy punch maneuver test
nasal airflow-inducing m.
Patrick cross-leg m.
relative response attributable to the m.
scaphoid shift m.
Valsalva m.

manganese
m. assay
m. chloride
m. chloride contrast medium
m. citrate
m. dioxide aerosol
m. dipyridoxyl diphosphate
m. intoxication
orthotoluidine manganese sulfate
m. poisoning
m. superoxide dismutase gene
m. tetrasodium-meso-tetra

mangled
M. Extremity Severity Score
m. extremity syndrome index

mango dermatitis

Mangoldt epithelial grafting

mangrove fly

mania
acute hallucinatory m.
adolescent m.
akinetic m.
alcoholic m.
anxious m.
atypical m.
compulsive m.
grandiose m.
hysterical m.
m. rating scale
Young M. Rating Scale

manic
acute manic episode
m. agitation
m. bipolar disorder
m. child
m. delirium
m. depression
m. depressive
m. episode
m. excitement
m. feature
full-blown manic depressive illness
m. hebephrenia

manic-depressive
m.-d. disorder
m.-d. illness
m.-d. insanity
National Depressive and M.-d. Association
m.-d. psychosis

manie
m. de perfection
m. de rumination

manifest
m. achievement
m. anxiety
M. Anxiety Scale
Children's M. Anxiety Scale
m. content
m. destiny
m. deviation
m. dream
m. goal
m. hyperopia
m. ischemia
m. latent nystagmus
no manifest improvement
m. refraction
Revised Children's M. Anxiety Scale
m. strabismus
Taylor M. Anxiety Scale

manifestation
clinical m.'s, etiologic factors, anatomic involvement, pathophysiologic features
clinical manifestation of acute drug intoxication
clinical manifestation of drug reaction
clinical manifestation of panic reaction
clinical manifestation of withdrawal
m. of depression

m. of emotion
extraglandular m.
extraintestinal m.
hemorrhagic m.
neuro-ophthalmologic m.

manifesting
m. carrier

manipulates
m. to gain power
m. to gain profit

manipulation
articulation m.
m. of articulation
biliary manipulation catheter
m. board
m. communication pattern
m. of dislocated joint
endoscopic stone m.
extensive manipulation of joint
genetic m.
lumbar distraction m.
osteopathic m.
osteopathic manipulation treatment
pancreatic duct m.
percutaneous stone m.
m. under anesthesia
urethral manipulation syndrome

manipulative
M. Aptitude Test
attention-seeking manipulative behavior
m. behavior
chiropractic manipulative reflex technique
m. device
m. drive
osteopathic manipulative medicine
osteopathic manipulative technique
osteopathic manipulative therapy
spinal manipulative therapy
visceral manipulative treatment

manipulator
angled m.
Lieberman MicroFinger m.
Lindstrom Star nucleus m.

manipulator-injector
Rowden uterine m.-i.
uterine m.-i.
Zinnanti uterine m.-i.

Mankin histologic/histochemical scale

man-made
m.-m. mineral fiber
m.-m. vitreous fiber

Mann
M. bunionectomy
M. isthmic cerclage
M. sign

manna
m. cannellata
m. communis

mannan-binding
m.-b. lectin deficiency
m.-b. protein

Mann-Bollman fistula

Mann-Coughlin arthrodesis

manner
allosteric m.
authoritative m.
continuous locking m.
m.'s deterioration
guarded m.
McLean m.
paracrine m.

Manning
M. criteria
M. score of fetal activity

Mannis
M. probe
M. suture

mannitol
m. administration
m. fermentation test
m. salt agar
sodium chloride, adenine, glucose, m.
yeast and m.

mannose
m. binding molecule
m. fermentation test
m. monooleate

mannose-binding
m.-b. lectin
m.-b. protein

mannose-resistant hemagglutination

mannose-sensitive hemagglutination

mannose-type sugar

Mann-Whitney
M.-W. rank sum statistic
M.-W. U test

manometer
aneroid m.
ventilator pressure m.

manometric
m. criteria
m. data
esophageal manometric sequence
m. evaluation
m. feature
m. finding
m. testing

manometry
anorectal m.
balloon reflex m.
m. catheter
esophageal m.
lumbar puncture m.
sphincter of Oddi m.

Manson
M. disease
M. eye worm
M. hemoptysis
M. pyosis
M. schistosomiasis

Manson-Aebli corneal section scissors

Mansonella
Mansonella ozzardi infection
Mansonella perstans infection
Mansonella streptocerca infection

mantel
blastoid variant of mantel cell lymphoma
blastoma mantel cell lymphoma

Mantel-Cox test

Mantel-Haenszel
M.-H. method
M.-H. procedure
M.-H. test
M.-H. test for linearity
M.-H. weighted odds ratio

mantle
m. block
m. cell
m. cell lymphocytic lymphoma
cement mantle grade classification
cerebral m.
m. complex
m. irradiation
m. islet
m. layer
m. radiotherapy
m. sclerosis
m. zone
m. zone hyperplasia
m. zone lymphoma
m. zone nodule
m. zone pattern

Mantoux
M. conversion
M. diameter

Mantoux *(continued)*
M. method
M. pit
M. reaction
M. technique
M. testing
M. tuberculin skin test

manual
m. active-resistive exercise
m. adjustment
m. arts therapist
axial manual traction test
m. breast pump
m. cavitation
m. cervical traction
m. cleavage
m. communication
m. compression
Consolidated Standards M.
m. contact
m. counting
Crime Classification M.
m. dexterity
m. differential
m. dilatation of anus
m. dominance
m. English
m. exploration of abdomen
m. extraction
m. fracture reduction
m. healing method
m. internal examination
m. keratometer
m. kinetic perimetry
m. lamellar keratoplasty
m. lymph drainage
m. lymphedema treatment
Marco manual keratometer
m. muscle test
m. muscle testing
m. organ stimulation technique
m. pelvimetry
rapid manual processing
m. reduction
m. resistance exercise
m. rotation
m. splinting of thoracic cage
m. thrust
m. vacuum aspiration
m. ventilation bag

manually
m. operated
placenta delivered m.
placenta removed m.

manubrial
right manubrial dullness

manubriogladiolar junction

manubriosternal
m. joint
m. junction
m. symphysis

manubrium
m. mallei
m. of malleolus
m. of malleus
m. of sternum

manus
m. cava
musculus abductor digiti minimi m.
musculus flexor digiti minimi brevis m.
opponens digiti minimi m.
palma m.

many
too many to count

Manz gland

map
axial curvature m.
brain electrical activity m.
computerized electroencephalographic m.
m. distance
m. dystrophy
m. pattern

map-dot corneal dystrophy

map-dot-fingerprint corneal epithelial dystrophy

MAP/ERK kinase

maple
m. leaf flap
m. bark stripper disease
m. syrup urine disease
m. tree
m. tree pollen

maplike skull

mapping
advanced cardiac m.
m. algorithm
arrhythmia mapping system catheter
atrial activation m.
auditory brain m.
axial curvature m.
body surface Laplacian m.
body surface potential m.
brain electrical activity m.
m. of cerebral sulcus
color-coded flow m.
color flow m.
m. of cortical function
cortical mapping of memory function
m. the defect
m. of defect
dementia care m.
digital phase m.
Doppler color-flow m.
electrical stimulation m.
endocardial activation m.
fluorescence overlay antigen m.
intracortical interaction m.
parallel analog m.
precordial electrocardiographic m.
pulsed-wave Doppler m.
sentinel lymph node m.
significance probability m.

Mapputta virus

Maprik virus

Mapuera virus

Maquet
M. advancement
M. anteromedial osteoplasty
M. dome osteotomy

Marañón
M. sign
M. syndrome

marantic
m. atrophy
m. clot
m. edema
m. endocarditis
m. thrombosis
m. thrombus

marasmic
m. female
m. kwashiorkor

marasmus
nutritional m.
m. syndrome

marathon group psychotherapy

marble
m. bone
m. bone disease
m. bone pattern
m. bone pin
m. cake hyperpigmentation
m. skin

marbled
m. hypopigmented streak
m. pure tone

Marburg
M. agent
M. hemorrhagic fever
M. virus

M. virus disease
M. virus group

Marburg-like viruses

Marburg-type MS

Marcacci muscle

march

m. albuminuria
m. anemia
M. disease
m. foot
m. fracture
m. hematuria
m. hemoglobinuria
M. laser sclerostomy needle
M. technique

Marchac

M. and Chiari short scar technique
M. dorsal nasal flap
M. glabella flap

Marchand

M. adrenals
M. cell
M. rest
M. wandering cell

Marchant zone

Marchetti test

Marchi

M. ball
M. degeneration
M. globule
M. tract

Marchiafava-Bignami

M.-B. aminoaciduria
M.-B. disease
M.-B. syndrome

Marchiafava-Micheli

M.-M. anemia
M.-M. disease
M.-M. syndrome

Marcille triangle

Marckwald operation

Marco

M. manual keratometer
M. perimeter
M. prism exophthalmometer
M. virus

Marcus

M. grading scale for avascular necrosis
M. Gunn
M. Gunn classification
M. Gunn dot
M. Gunn jaw-winking phenomenon
M. Gunn jaw-winking ptosis
M. Gunn jaw-winking syndrome
M. Gunn pupil
M. Gunn pupillary sign
M. Gunn relative afferent defect
M. Gunn test

Marcus-Balourdas-Heiple ankle fusion technique

Marcy hernia repair

Marden-Walker syndrome

mare

pregnant mare serum
pregnant mare serum gonadotropin

Marek

M. associated tumor-specific antigen
M. disease-like viruses
M. disease virus
M. herpesvirus disease

mare's

m. hair line
m. tail line

Marey law

Marfan

M. disease
M. epigastric puncture
M. law
neonatal Marfan syndrome
M. sign
M. syndrome

marfanoid

m. body habitus
m. craniosynostosis syndrome
m. habitus-mental retardation syndrome
m. habitus-microcephaly-glomerulonephritis syndrome
m. hypermobility syndrome
m. hypermobility syndrome

margarine disease

Margarinos-Torres lesion

Margarita Island type ectodermal dysplasia

margin

m. of acetabulum
anterior palpebral m.
anterior tibial m.
anterior vertebral body m.
m. of apposition
below right costal m.
buccal m.
costal m.
m. crease distance
m. of eyelid
fingerbreadth below right costal m.
m. of fossa ovalis
gingival m.
gingival margin trimmer
inferior margin of liver
infracostal m.
infraorbital m.
intercostal m.
lateral margin of kidney
left costal m.
left intercostal m.
lid margin laceration
lingual m.
lower costal m.
mastoid margin of occipital bone
mesovarian margin of ovary
metal crown m.
nasal margin of frontal bone
occipital margin of temporal bone
m. of orbit
orbital margin of eyelid
parietal margin of frontal bone
parietal margin of greater wing of sphenoid
m. of piriform aperture
posterior disc m.
m. reflex distance
m. of resection
right costal m.
right intercostal m.
right margin of heart
m. of safety
superior margin of cerebral hemisphere
supraorbital m.
m. of tongue
m.'s of wound brought into apposition
wound margin undermined

marginal

m. adaptation
m. alopecia
m. arcade
m. artery
m. artery of colon
m. artery of Drummond
m. atrial branch of right coronary artery
m. band
m. bevel
m. blepharitis
m. branch

marginal *(continued)*
m. branch of cingulate sulcus
m. branch of left circumflex coronary artery
m. branch of parietooccipital sulcus
m. branch of right coronary artery
callosal marginal branch
m. catarrhal ulcer
m. circumflex artery
m. consciousness
m. corneal degeneration
m. corneal ulcer
m. cost per year of life saved
m. crest
m. crest of tooth
m. crystalline dystrophy
m. degeneration of cornea
distal marginal ridge
m. donor
m. entropion
m. excess
m. excision
m. exostosis
m. fasciculus
first obtuse marginal artery
first obtuse marginal branch
m. fracture
m. function
m. furrow
m. furrow degeneration
m. gingiva
m. gingivitis
m. granulocyte pool
m. gyrus
m. heart failure
m. insertion
m. keratitis
m. layer
left circumflex m.
m. line calculus index
Lissauer marginal zone
m. mandibular branch of facial nerve
m. mandibulectomy
m. zone lymphoma
mesial marginal developmental groove
mesial marginal ridge
m. metallophilic macrophage
m. myotomy
m. nevus
nodal marginal zone B-cell lymphoma
obtuse m.
obtuse marginal artery
m. part
m. part of orbicularis oris muscle
pellucid marginal corneal degeneration
pellucid marginal retinal degeneration
m. ray of light
m. reflex distance
m. resection
m. ridge
m. ring ulcer of cornea
second obtuse marginal artery
second obtuse marginal branch
m. sinus
m. sinus of placenta
m. sinus rupture
m. sphincter
splenic marginal zone lymphoma
m. tear strip
m. tentorial branch of internal carotid artery
m. tubercle
m. tubercle of zygomatic bone
m. zone
m. zone B-cell lymphoma
m. zone cell
m. zone cell lymphoma
m. zone lymphocyte
m. zone macrophage
m. zone/mucosa-associated lymphoid tissue
m. zone pattern

marginalis
arcus m.
arcus marginalis coli
arteria marginalis coli
pars m.
pars marginalis musculi orbicularis oris
placenta previa m.

marginated
m. chromatin
m. granulocyte pool

margination of placenta

marian lithotomy

Marie
M. ataxia
M. disease
M. hypertrophy
M. sign
M. syndrome

Marie-Bamberger
M.-B. disease
M.-B. syndrome

Marie-Foix-Alajouanine
M.-F.-A. cerebellar atrophy
M.-F.-A. disease

Marie-Robinson syndrome

Marie-Sainton syndrome

Marie-Strümpell
M.-S. arthritis
M.-S. disease
M.-S. encephalitis
M.-S. spondylitis
M.-S. syndrome

marijuana
crude marijuana extract
m. delirium
m. delusional disorder
m. dependence
m. effect
m. flashback
grade of m.
m. intoxication

marimastat
matrix metalloproteinase inhibitor, m.

Marin Amat syndrome

marine
m. animal sting
m. dermatitis
m. envenomation
m. oxidation/fermentation
m. protein concentrate
m. vibrios

Marine-Lenhart syndrome

Marinesco-Garland syndrome

Marinesco-Radovici
palmomental reflex of M.-R.

Marinesco-Sjögren-Garland syndrome

Marinesco-Sjögren-like syndrome

Marinesco succulent hand

marinum
Mycobacterium marinum infection

Marion
Hoechst Marion Roussel stain

marionette line

Marion-Moschcowitz culdoplasty

Mariotte
M. blind spot
M. bottle
M. experiment
M. law
M. scotoma

marital
m. adjustment

M. Attitudes Evaluation
behavioral marital therapy
m. conflict
m. counseling
m. counselor
m. couples group therapy
m. discord
m. disharmony
m. disruption
m. dissatisfaction
M. Dyadic Inventory
Golombok-Rust Inventory of M. State
m. history
m. infidelity
m. introitus
Locke-Wallace Marital Adjustment test
M. Satisfaction Scale
Senoussi Multiphasic M. Inventory
m. status

Marituba virus

Marjolin ulcer

mark
alignment m.
limbus parallel orientation straddling tattoo m.
paddle marks from defibrillation
port wine m.
Tanner-Whitehouse Mark 2 bone-age assessment

marked
m. anger
m. anxiety
m. ascites
m. asynchrony
m. cocontraction
m. decline in academic functioning
m. degenerative change of hip
m. depression
m. hyaline deposition
m. icterus
m. impairment
m. impulsivity
m. latency
m. left ventricular hypertrophy
m. localized reaction
slightly more marked since

markedly
cardiac output markedly reduced
m. decreased reflex
m. dilated heart
m. increased
sclerae markedly icteric
m. tender
trachea markedly inflamed

marker
adrenal hyperandrogenism m.
alkaline phosphatase isoenzyme tumor m.
AP marker enzyme
m. chromosome
m. gene
6-HIAA tumor m.
human immunodeficiency virus quality audit m.
m. lesion
low profile R-K m.
macroorchidism marker X syndrome
malignancy associated cellular m.
MCA tumor m.
McDonald optic zone m.
MIB-1 cell proliferation m.
MSA tumor m.
multiple marker reverse transcriptase-polymerase chain reaction assay
multiple marker screening
Neumann-Shepard corneal m.
Neumann-Shepard oval optical center m.
neuron-specific enolase tumor m.
Nordin-Ruiz trapezoidal m.
NSE lung cancer tumor m.
olfactory marker protein
optical zone m.
Osher-Neumann corneal m.
p-ANC genetic m.
pancreatic cancer m.
peripheral androgen activity m.
polymorphic genetic m.
serological marker of disease
supernumerary marker chromosome
m. X
m. X chromosome
m. X syndrome
zinc glycinate m.
m.'s for zone

market men disease

marking
bronchovascular m.'s
chevron marking technique
m. clamp
haustral m.
interstitial m.
m. pen
peribronchial m.'s
perihilar m.
prominence of pulmonary m.'s
pulmonary m.'s
m. technique
m. time pattern

Markov
M. chain
M. chain Monte Carlo technique
multistage Markov model
M. process
M. state-transition model

Markwell
method of M.

Marlen double-faced adhesive disc

Marlex
M. closure
M. graft
M. hernial repair
M. mesh

Marlow
M. test

Marlowe-Crown Social Desirability Scale

Marmo method

marmoset virus

Maroteaux-Lamy
M.-L. disease
M.-L. mucopolysaccharidosis
mucopolysaccharidosis type VI M.-L.
M.-L. syndrome

Maroteaux-Malamut syndrome

Marquardt angulation osteotomy

Marquez-Gomez
M.-G. conjunctival graft
M.-G. operation

Marrakai virus

marriage
M. Adjustment Inventory
arranged m.
California M. Readiness Evaluation
common law m.
Conflict in M. Scale
m. contract
m. counseling
m. counselor
m. encounter
m. fear
open-end m.
M. Skills Analysis

married
m., keeping baby
not married, keeping baby

married *(continued)*
not married, not keeping baby
single, divorced, m.

marrow
m. ablation
adult bone m.
aerobic bone marrow culture
m. agent bone scintigraphy
allogeneic bone marrow cell
allogeneic bone marrow transplant
allogeneic bone marrow transplantation
allogeneic marrow transplantation
allogenic bone m.
allogenic bone marrow cell infusion
allogenic bone marrow transplantation
m. aplasia
aplastic bone m.
autologous and allogeneic marrow transplantation
autologous blood and marrow transplantation
autologous bone m.
autologous bone marrow cell
autologous bone marrow reinfusion
autologous bone marrow rescue
autologous bone marrow support
autologous bone marrow transplant
autologous peripheral blood stem cell bone marrow transplantation
m. blush
bone m.
bone marrow acid phosphatase
bone marrow arrest
bone marrow aspirate
bone marrow biopsy
bone marrow cell
bone marrow culture
bone marrow depression
bone marrow failure
bone marrow infection
bone marrow infusion
bone marrow lymphocyte
bone marrow lymphocytosis
bone marrow micrometastasis
bone marrow myeloid precursor
bone marrow necrosis
bone marrow neutrophil reserve
bone marrow pressure
bone marrow removed and stored
bone marrow stem cell
bone marrow suppression
bone marrow tap
bone marrow toxicity
bone marrow transplant
bone marrow transplant neutropenia
bone marrow transplant rejection
bone marrow transplant unit
m. canal
cancellous hematopoietic m.
m. cavity
m. cavity formation
m. cell
m. cell vacuolization
m. change
cryopreserved bone m.
degenerative bone marrow disease
m. disease
displacement bone marrow transplantation
donor bone m.
donor bone marrow engraftment
m. dosimetry
m. edema
eosinophilic fibrohistiocytic lesion of bone m.
m. failure syndrome
fetal bone m.
m. fibrosis
m. graft rejection
m. harvest
harvest bone m.
m. hematopoietic stem cell
human bone m.
m. hypoplasia
idiopathic aplastic bone m.
incompatible bone m.
index of marrow conversion
m. infiltration
m. injection
m. iron turnover
liver, iron, red bone m.
lymphomatous bone marrow involvement
mean marrow dose
metacarpophalangeal bone marrow development
metatarsophalangeal bone marrow development
mildly hyperplastic bone m.
m. monocyte
m. mononuclear cell
MPO bone marrow stain
myeloperoxidase bone marrow stain
National M. Donor Program
m. neutrophil reserve
normal bone m.
normal bone marrow extract
particulate cancellous bone and m.
pediatric fatty m.
percutaneous bone marrow infection
percutaneous bone marrow injection
porcine bone marrow transplantation
m. production rate
m. progenitor
m. recovery
red m.
regenerating bone marrow extract
m. release rate
m. repopulation activity
m. space
m. suppression
m. toxic drug
m. transplant
m. transplantation
tumor-induced marrow cytotoxicity
unidentified endosteal marrow cell
vascularized bone marrow transplantation
yellow bone m.

marrow-ablative
m.-a. chemoradiation
m.-a. chemotherapy

marrow-lymph gland

Marschalko-type plasma cell

Marseilles fever

marsh
M. disease
m. elder
m. fever

Marshall
M. Hall facies
ligament of M.
M. oblique vein
M. syndrome
M. and Tanner pubertal stage
M. test
M. vestigial fold

Marshall-Jewett-Strong classification

Marshall-Marchetti-Krantz
M.-M.-K. cystourethropexy
M.-M.-K. operation
M.-M.-K. procedure

Marshall-Marchetti procedure

Marshall-Smith syndrome

Marshall-Taylor vacuum extraction

Marshall-White syndrome

Marsh-Bendall factor
marshmallow bolus
marsupialization
m. of lesion
m. technique
marsupial notch
MART-1
M. melanoma antigen
M. peptide
Martegiani
area M.
M. area
M. funnel
Martin
M. anoplasty
M. broth
M. disease
M. gastrostomy
M. modification
M. reduction technique
M. Suicide Depression Inventory
Martin-Albright syndrome
Martin-Bell-Renpenning syndrome
Martin-Bell syndrome
Martinez
M. keratome
M. technique
M. Universal Perineal Interstitial Template
Martin-Gruber
M.-G. anastomosis
M.-G. connection
M.-G. phenomenon
Martin-Lewis medium
Martinotti cell
Martius
M. bulbocavernosus fat flap
M. fat pad
M. flap and fascial sling
M. graft
M. procedure
M. scarlet blue
Martorell aortic arch syndrome
Marx classification of microtia
Mary
angle of M.
Maryland
M. coma scale
M. Foot Score
M. Foot Score Profile
Marzola
M. flap
M. hair restoration surgery
mas
mas oncogene
mas protooncogene/oncogene
Masaoka
M. classification
M. staging system for thymoma
mascara particle inclusion
masculine
m. attitude
m. attitude in female neurotic
m. identity
Maferr Inventory of Masculine Values
m. pelvis
m. pubic hair
m. uterus
masculinum
ovarium m.
Masimo
M. SET home monitor
M. SET signal extraction pulse oximetry
mask
aerosol m.
anterior active mask rhinomanometry
m. of atopic dermatitis
bag, valve, m.
m. and bag ventilation
m. burn
close-fitting m.
m. data
double aerosol face m.
emergency oxygen mask assembly
m. face
face m.
m. facies
gastric laryngeal mask airway
high-humidity face m.
high-humidity tracheostomy m.
humidity m.
m. inhalation anesthesia
mist m.
Monarch Mini Mask nasal interface
nonrebreather face m.
nonrebreathing m.
open face m.
oxygen m.
partial nonrebreather oxygen m.
partial rebreathing m.
m. of pregnancy
m. sign
sterilized gown and m.
tracheostomy mask anesthesia
ventilated m.
ventilation by m.
Venturi m.
masked
m. affection
m. anxiety
m. audiology
m. depression
m. deprivation
m. diabetes
m. epilepsy
m. facies
m. gout
m. homosexuality
m. hyperthyroidism
opposite ear m.
m. thyroid autonomy
m. virus
masking
continuous tone m.
contralateral remote m.
decibel effective masking contralateral
m. dilemma
effective m.
m. efficiency
m. fear
m. level difference
overt compliance masking covert resistance
Speech with Alternating M. Index
masklike
m. face
m. facies
mask-mode cardiac imaging
Maslach Burnout Inventory
masochistic
m. behavior
m. character
m. character defense
m. component
Mason
M. fracture
M. fracture classification system
Mason-Pfizer monkey virus
mason's lung
masquerade
m. syndrome
m. technique
mass
abnormal mass of tissue growth
abnormal tissue m.

mass *(continued)*
m. absorption coefficient
accelerator mass spectrometry
m. accretion
m. action law
m. action principle
m. action theory
adjusted body m.
aerodynamic mass diameter
angiographic muscle mass index
anterior mediastinal m.
aortopulmonary window m.
apparent distribution m.
appendicular bone mass measurement
articular mass separation
articular mass separation fracture
m. of atom
atomic mass unit
m. attenuation coefficient
avascular brain m.
avascular kidney m.
avascular renal m.
m. balance
m. behavior
benign ovarian m.
body m.
body cell m.
body mass index
bone mineral m.
buccal m.
m. casualty
center of m.
chemical ionization mass spectrometry
m. collision stopping power
m. concentration
cystic fluid-filled m.
m. defect
m. density
density of the fat m.
density of the fat-free m.
density and strength of bone m.
m. doubling time
dysplasia-associated lesion or m.
m. effect
electrohydrodynamic ionization mass spectrometry
electron ionization mass spectrometry
electron rest m.
electrospray ionization mass spectrometry
erythrocyte m.
m. excision
excisional biopsy of tumor m.
excreted m.
extracellular mass to body cell mass ratio
extravascular m.
extravascular lung m.
fast atom bombardment mass spectrometry
fat and fat-free m.
filtered m.
floating mass transducer
m. fragmentography
gas isotope ratio mass spectrometry
hard, indurated colon m.
high-dose radiation to tumor m.
hypoxia, intussusception, brain m.
m. hysteria
ideal body m.
increased bone m.
increased muscle m.
m., induration, or tenderness
m. infection
infiltrating irregular tumor m.
initial body mass index
m. injection
inner cell m.
inner ear m.
intracranial mass lesion
intravascular m.
isotope ratio mass spectrometry
m. isotopomer distribution analysis
laser microprobe mass analyzer
last body mass index
lean body m.
lean body muscle m.
left ventricular m.
left ventricular mass index
left ventricular muscle m.
m. lesion
liquid chromatography coupled to tandem mass spectrometry
liver, spleen m.'s
lobulated submucosal m.
loss of bone m.
low body mass index
low bone m.
malignant adrenal m.
mammary gland m.
matrix-assisted laser desorption and ionization mass spectrometry
matrix-assisted laser desorption ionization-time-of-flight mass spectrometry
m. media
m. median aerodynamic diameter
m. median diameter of particles
mediastinal high-attenuation m.
Medicare Bone Mass Measurement Standardization M.
middle ear m.
m. miniature radiography
m. miniature roentgenography
mixed attenuation m.
mixed density m.
mixed echogenic solid m.
mobile mass x-ray
m. movement
multiple-ring-enhancing mass lesion
neonatal abdominal m.
noncalcified nodular m.
m. number
palpable abdominal m.
palpable neck m.
pancreatic acinar m.
parasellar brain m.
peak adult bone m.
peak bone m.
pelvic cystic m.
m. peristalsis
petrous apex m.
postmenopausal body m.
m. psychogenic illness
pulsatile epigastric m.
m. radiative stopping power
m. radiography unit
red blood cell m.
reduced renal m.
regional bone m.
relative molecular m.
resonance ionization mass spectrometry
retroperitoneal residual tumor m.
Riddoch mass reflex
right ventricular m.
sclerotic cemental m.
m. screening
secondary ion mass spectroscopy
m. sociogenic illness
soft tissue m.
solid bone m.
specimen mass measurement device
m. spectrometer
m. spectrometric analysis
m. spectrometry
m. spectrophotometer
m. spectrophotometric detector
m.'s or tenderness
time-of-flight mass spectometry
total body m.
total fat m.
total heme m.
total muscle m.

total tumor m.
m. transfer area coefficient
m. transfer coefficient
m. transfer factor
unified atomic mass unit
urinary bladder wall m.
venous distention or m.
ventricular m.
vertebral bone m.
weapons of mass destruction

massa
m. intermedia
m. lateralis atlantis

Massachusetts
M. General Hospital Utility Multi-Programming System
M. Vision Kit

massage
aqua PT water m.
m. ball
carotid sinus m.
m. of the carotid sinus
cast stroking maneuver during m.
circular pressure maneuver during m.
closed chest cardiac m.
closed chest m.
connective tissue m.
deep friction m.
deep tissue m.
diathermy and m.
diathermy, massage, and exercise
external cardiac m.
fan stroking maneuver during m.
heat, massage, and exercise
heat and massage therapy
heat, ultrasound, and m.
ice m.
internal cardiac m.
open chest cardiac m.
prostatic m.
qigong meridian m.
m. therapy
transverse friction m.
urine specimen after prostate m.
urine specimen before prostate m.
whirlpool, massage, exercise

mass-analyzed ion kinetic energy

Masselon
M. glasses
M. spectacles

masseter
m. abscess
m. muscle
musculus m.
m. reflex
m. tendon

masseteric
m. area
m. artery
m. cutaneous ligament
m. fascia
m. nerve
m. reflex

mass-forming pancreatitis

Massini maneuver

massive
m. all layer liposuction
m. aortic regurgitation
m. ascites
m. atelectasis
m. autotransfusion
m. bowel resection
m. bowel resection syndrome
m. breast hypertrophy
m. cerebral edema
m. collapse
m. embolus
m. fibrolipoma
m. gastrointestinal hemorrhage
m. genital prolapse
m. granuloma of sclera
m. granulomatous orchitis
m. heart attack
m. hemoptysis
m. hemorrhage
m. hepatic failure
m. hepatic necrosis
m. herniated disc
m. herniation
m. infarct of brain stem
m. infection
m. intestinal bleeding
m. intracerebral bleed
m. intracerebral hemorrhage
m. intravascular hemolysis
m. involvement
m. jerking movements
m. lymphadenopathy
m. macronodular hyperplasia
m. midbrain hemorrhage
m. ovarian cyst
m. parallel processing system
m. periretinal proliferation
m. pneumonia
m. preretinal retraction
progressive massive fibrosis
m. pulmonary embolus
m. pulmonary hemorrhage
sinus histiocytosis with massive lymphadenopathy
m. sliding graft
strongyloidiasis with massive hyperinfection
m. transfusion
m. variceal hemorrhage
m. vitreous hemorrhage
m. vitreous reaction
m. vitreous retraction
weakly interacting massive particle

massive-dose desensitization

massively
m. dilated abdomen
m. parallel signature sequencing

mass-like configuration

Masson
M. argentaffin stain
M. body
M. hemangioma
M. intravascular endothelial proliferation
M. nevus
M. pseudoangiosarcoma
M. trichrome
M. trichrome stain

Masson-Fontana ammoniac silver stain

mass-to-charge ratio

mast
bone marrow-derived cultured mast cell
m. cell
m. cell containing both tryptase and chymase
m. cell containing tryptase but not chymase
m. cell degranulating peptide
m. cell degranulation
m. cell degranulation test
m. cell disease
m. cell-enhancing activity
m. cell growth factor
m. cell hyperplasia
m. cell inhibitor
m. cell leukemia
m. cell nevus
m. cell proteinase
m. cell reticulosis
m. cell sarcoma
m. cell stabilizer
m. cell staining
m. cell tryptase
m. cell tumor
intestinal mucosal mast cell

mast *(continued)*
m. leukocyte
rat mast cell protease
rat mast cell technique
systemic mast cell disease

mastectomy
Auchincloss modified radical m.
axillary node dissection m.
bilateral mastectomy scar
breast reconstruction after m.
m. closure
complete simple m.
ductal glandular m.
extended radical m.
m. for gynecomastia
left modified radical m.
modified radical m.
non-skin-sparing m.
Patey radical m.
radical m.
right modified radical m.
simple m.
skin-sparing m.
Willy Meyer radical m.

master
aluminum master rod
m. apical file
m. of avoidance
m. cast
change description m.
m. cone
Drug M. File
m. drug list
m. duodenoscope
m. eye
m. file
m. gland
m. patient index
m. regulator gene
temporary master apical file
m. treatment plan

master-dominant eye

Masters-Allen syndrome

mastery
Concept Mastery Test
m. imagery
Woodcock Reading Mastery Test

masticating
m. apparatus
m. cycle

mastication disorder

masticatory
m. adaptation
m. apparatus
m. attack
m. bone
m. diplegia
m. efficiency
m. fat pad
m. force

mastitis
California mastitis test
cystic m.
fibrocystic m.
glandular m.
granulomatous m.
interstitial m.
m., metritis, agalactia syndrome
m. neonatorum
puerperal m.
submammary m.
suppurative m.
m. with breast-feeding

mastocytosis
malignant systemic m.
nasal m.
papular m.
m. syndrome

mastoid
m. abscess
m. air cell
m. angle of parietal bone
m. antrum
aperture of mastoid antrum
artificial m.
m. bone fracture
m. border of occipital bone
m. bowl
m. branch
m. branch of occipital artery
m. branch of posterior auricular artery
m. branch of posterior tympanic artery
m. canal
m. canaliculus
m. cavity
m. cell
m. complex
m. cortex
m. drainage
m. emissary vein
m. empyema
endaural mastoid incision
m. fascia
m. fontanelle
m. fontanelle
m. foramen
m. fossa
m. groove
left m.
m. lymph node
m. margin of occipital bone
m. osteitis
m. process
right m.
m. tip

mastoidectomy
canal wall down m.
canal wall up m.
tympanoplasty with m.
tympanoplasty without m.

mastoideum
antrum m.
os m.

mastoideus
angulus mastoideus ossis parietalis

mastopexy
simultaneous areolar mastopexy and breast augmentation
Wise areola mastopexy breast augmentation

masturbation
anal m.
m. behavior
compulsive m.
m. equivalent
m. fantasy

masturbatory activity

Masuda-Kitahara disease

Masugi nephritis

mat
m. burn
children's m.
m. foil
m. gold
mycelial m.

Matas aneurysmectomy

match
organ and recipient m.
Snider M. Test

matchbox sign

matched
m. lymphocyte transfusion
m. pairs signed rank test
m. peripheral dose
m. related donor
m. unrelated donor
m. unrelated donor stem cell transplant

Matchett-Brown hip arthroplasty

matching
blind m.
m. familiar figures

M. Familiar Figures Test
m. hypothesis

matchline technique

matchstick graft

mate

thread mate system

Mateer-Streeter ovum

mater

arachnoid m.
arachnoidea m.
arachnoidea mater cranialis
arachnoidea mater et pia m.
arachnoid mater cranialis
arachnoid mater and pia m.
arterial branch to dura m.
dura m.
dura mater prosthesis
meningeal layer of dura m.
periosteal layer of dura m.
pia m.
pia mater of brain

materia

m. alba
m. dentica

material

absorbent gelling m.
adrenergic receptor m.
allogenic lyophilized bone graft implant m.
alloplastic donor m.
alpha bone substitute m.
alpha-BSM bone repair m.
alpha-BSM bone substitute m.
aluminum oxide arthroplasty m.
alveolar living m.
amorphous m.
Aquaplast alloplastic m.
artificial joint implant m.
aspirated foreign m.
aspiration of blood m.
aspiration of bloody m.
attaching material implant superstructure
autogenous donor m.
autophagocytosed cellular m.
bone implant m.
celluloid implant m.
central material section
central material supply
coffee-ground m.
copious mucoid m.
core of atheromatous m.
cross-reacting m.
dark bloody m.
drainage of purulent m.
electron-dense amorphous m.
endodonic m.
excitability-inducing m.
extracellular m.
extracellular granular m.
extravasated iodinated contrast m.
m. failure break point
fibrillar absorbable hemostat m.
foreign material artifact
m. gain
gallium citrate contrast m.
gold implant m.
gonadotropin-inhibiting m.
gonadotropin-inhibitory m.
Gore-Tex augmentation m.
granular osmiophilic m.
m. gratification
Hazardous M.'s Response Unit
hollow-sphere implant m.
homograft implant m.
human genetic m.
impacted fecal m.
injection of radiopaque m.
insulin-like m.
intermediate restorative m.
intravenous contrast m.
low-osmolality contrast m.
medical materials account
metal suture m.
necrotic purulent m.
neurosecretory m.
nonionic contrast m.
nylon suture m.
oozing of purulent m.
osteoconductive bone grafting m.
other potentially infectious m.
paraffin implant m.
particulate crystalline m.
particulate crystalline material deposition
passing fecal m.
periodic acid-Schiff-positive m.
plastic implant m.
polyethylene implant m.
m.'s primary dye
Primary Reference M.
principal outer material protein
prompt excretion of contrast m.
PTFE graft m.
radar absorbent m.
radioactive m.
radiocontrast m.
Raji cell-binding m.
reference m.
retention of contrast m.
m. safety data sheet
silicone implant m.
specified risk m.'s
Standard Reference M.
subcutaneous augmentation m.
subdermal implant m.
subperiosteal implant m.
surface-active m.
synthetic graft m.
tantalum mesh implant m.
temporary endodontic restorative m.
M.'s Testing System
ureteral implant m.
vasodepressor m.
vasoexcitor m.
wire mesh implant m.

maternal

m. abdominal pressure
m. abuse
advanced maternal age
m. age
m. age-related risk
m. alcohol consumption
m. alcoholism
m. alpha fetoprotein
m. anesthesia
m. antiplatelet antibody
m. antithyroid antibody
m. asthma
m. attachment
m. attitude
M. Attitude Scale
M. Attitudes Evaluation
m. aunt
m. behavior
m. Bernard-Soulier syndrome
m. birthing position
m. blood clot patch therapy
m. blood type
m. central hemodynamics
m. and child health
m. and child health care
m. and child health service
m. cholestasis
m. chorioamnionitis
m. coagulopathy
m. cocaine use
m. competency
m. condition
m. contribution
m. cortical vein
m. cortical vein thrombosis
m. cotyledon
m. cyanotic heart disease
m. death
m. death rate
m. depression
m. deprivation
m. deprivation syndrome

maternal *(continued)*
m. desertion
m. diabetes
m. douche
m. drive
m. drug abuse
m. dysfunction
m. dystocia
m. electrocardiogram
emergency maternal and infant care
m. estradiol rhythm
m. estriol level
m. exercise
external fetal maternal monitor
m. factor
m. febrile morbidity
m. fetal hemorrhage
m. fetal medicine
first-trimester maternal seizure
m. fitness
m. floor infarction
m. fracture
full maternal behavior
gestational sac and maternal date
m. gonad
m. grandfather
m. health program
m. health risk factor
m. hemopathy
m. hepatitis
m. HLA haplotype
m. humoral immune response
m. hydramnios
m. hydration
m. hydrops
m. hydrops fetalis
m. hydrops syndrome
m. hypercalcemia
m. hyperglycemia-induced fetal hyperinsulinemia
m. hyperparathyroidism
m. hyperphenylalaninemia
m. hypertension
m. hypotension
m. hypothyroidism
m. hypothyroxinemia
m. IgG antibody
m. immunity
m. immunology
m. indication
m. indifference
m. and infant care
m. infection
m. inflammatory response
m. inheritance
m. insulin
m. karyotype
mean maternal glucose
m. meiosis I, II
m. mercury exposure
m. mortality
m. mortality rate
m. nutrition
m. ocular adaptation
older maternal age
m. outcome
m. parvovirus fetalis
m. pediatric unit
m. peripheral blood
m. phenylketonuria
m. physiology
m. plasma leptin
m. postpartum thyroid dysfunction
m. pulse
m. pyrexia
m. screening
m. serum
m. serum alpha-fetoprotein
m. serum level
m. size
m. smoking
m. sperm antibody
m. stature
m. steroid concentration
m. stress
strong partial maternal behavior
m. substance abuse
m. surveillance
m. tachycardia
m. thyrotropin receptor blocking antibody-induced congenital hypothyroidism
m. tissue
m. titer
m. toxic effect
M. Trait Anxiety Score
m. trauma
umbilical vein to maternal vein
m. uncle
m. undernourishment
m. uniparental heterodisomy
m. vascular response
m. venous
m. viremia
m. weight
m. weight gain

maternal-fetal
m.-f. hemorrhage
m.-f. histocompatibility
m.-f. histoincompatibility
m.-f. HIV
m.-f. HLA compatibility
m.-f. medicine
m.-f. microtransfusion
m.-f. transmission
m.-f. transmission of antibody

maternal-infant
m.-i. attachment
m.-i. bonding

maternally
m. inherited diabetes and deafness
m. inherited myopathy and cardiomyopathy

maternal-placental-fetal unit

maternal-placental unit

maternity
family-centered maternity care
family-centered maternity nursing
m. hospital

maternofetal transfusion

mathematical
m. ability
m. chaos
declining mathematical ability
m. determinant
m. expectation
m. modeling technique
m. optimization and logical dimensioning for radiotherapy

mathematics
assessment in m.
Diagnostic Mathematics Inventory
m. disorder
Individualized Criterion Reference Testing M.
Test of Cognitive Style in M.

mathetic function of language

Mathieu disease

Matie-Unna hypotrichosis

mating
assortative m.
assortive m.
m. behavior
negative assortative m.
nonrandom m.
m. type

MAT-LyLu variant

matrix, pl. **matrices**
m. adhesion
allograft dermal matrix graft
m. antigen
antinuclear matrix antibody
m. breakdown
m. calculus

cartilage oligomeric matrix protein
M. collagen
Colored Progressive Matrices
m. component
demineralized bone m.
m. deposition
drug evaluation m.
dural graft m.
euclidean distance matrix analysis
extracellular m.
extracellular matrix metalloproteinase inducer
fibrin matrix gel
germinal matrix hemorrhage
m. Gla protein
Hill Interaction Matrix
m. metalloprotease
m. metalloproteinase
m. metalloproteinase inhibitor
m. metalloproteinase inhibitor, marimastat
m. mineralization
nail matrix phenolization
noncollagen bone m.
nuclear m.
Odorant Confusion Matrix scale
Odorant Confusion Matrix score
pericellular m.
perilacunar mineral m.
predentin m.
proximal nail m.
quantization m.
Raven Colored Progressive Matrices Test
Raven Standard Progressive Matrices
reduced-acquisition m.
structure of the cytoplasmic m.
m. synthesis
total matrix formation rate
m. transdermal system
Treatment Rating Assessment M.
m. unguis
m. vesicle
wedge matrix resection

matrix-assisted
m.-a. laser desorption and ionization mass spectrometry
m.-a. laser desorption ionization-time-of-flight mass spectrometry

matrix-dissolution product

matroclinous inheritance

Matruh virus

matte
m. black forceps
m. black instrument

matted
m. bowel loop
m. omentum
m. peritoneum

matter
anisotropy of white m.
anterolateral white matter of cord
deep white matter hyperintensity
deep white matter infarct
deep white matter lesion
dissolved organic m.
dry m.
echogenicity of periventricular white m.
generalized white matter atrophy
gray m.
gray matter of brain
gray matter of spinal cord
idiopathic white matter lesion
loss of distinction at gray/white matter interface
microcephaly-calcification of cerebral white matter syndrome
multifocal white matter inflammatory lesion
nonvolatile m.
normal-appearing white m.
normal human white m.
occipital gray m.
particulate m.
particulate matter less than 10 micrometers diameter
periaqueductal gray m.
periventricular gray m.
pontine gray m.
scalloped appearance of white m.
suspended particulate m.
temporoparietal white m.
total particulate m.
white m.
white matter lesion cerebral
white matter damage
white matter edema
white matter hyperintensity
white matter signal abnormality
white matter thinning

Matti-Russe bone graft

Mattis
M. corneal scissors
M. Dementia Rating Scale

mattress
alarm mattress apnea
alternating pressure m.
chromic catgut mattress suture
continuous mattress suture
double-armed mattress suture
egg crate foam m.
horizontal mattress stitch
horizontal mattress suture
interrupted mattress suture
locking horizontal mattress suture
low air loss therapy mattress
silk interrupted mattress suture
subannular mattress suture
m. suture

Matucare virus

Matuhasi-Ogata phenomenon

maturation
m. arrest
band form in sixth stage of myelocyte m.
m. B cell
m. of breast cell
complete maturation arrest
m. division
erythrocyte maturation factor
glia maturation factor
growth and maturation of new skin
m. hypothesis
m. immunity
m. index
mucosal barrier m.
myelocyte at fourth stage of m.
myelocyte at third stage of m.
ovum m.
premature accelerated lung m.
pulmonary m.
skeletal m.
m. value

maturational
m. change
m. crisis

maturation-promoting factor

mature
m. abnormal chorionic villus
m. abnormal placenta
aspiration of mature oocyte
m. bacteriophage
m. B cell
m. bite
m. bone
m. burst-forming unit erythroid
m. cataphoria
m. cataract
m. cell leukemia
m. cystic ovarian teratoma
m. defense
m. dentin

mature *(continued)*
m. fibrosis
m. follicle
m. infant
m. lens
m. mediastinal teratoma
m. neutrophil
m. ovarian teratoma

mature-onset
m.-o. diabetes of the young
m.-o. diabetes of youth

maturity
Career M. Inventory
Columbia Mental M. Scale
m. fear
fetal lung m.
neonatal maturity classification of Dubowitz
neuromuscular maturity assessment
newborn maturity rating
m. onset deafness
sexual maturity rating
Vineland Social M. Scale

maturity-onset
m.-o. diabetes
m.-o. diabetes mellitus
m.-o. diabetes of the young
m.-o. diabetes of youth

matutinal
diurnal and matutinal variation
m. epilepsy
m. headache

Maudsley
M. Mentation Test
M. Obsessional Compulsive Inventory
M. Personality Inventory

Mauksch-Maumenee-Goldberg operation

Mauksch operation

Mauldsley Medical Questionnaire

Maumenee
M. vitreous-aspirating needle

Maumenee-Goldberg operation

Maunoir hydrocele

Maurer
M. cleft
M. dot
M. optimization test

Mauriac syndrome

Mauriceau-Levret maneuver

Mauriceau maneuver

Mauriceau-Smellie-Veit maneuver

Maurice corneal depot technique

Mauthner
M. cell
M. fiber
M. test

Max
M. protein

maxilla, pl. **maxillae**
alveolar arch of m.
anterior nasal spine of m.
ethmoidal crest of m.
nasal crest of m.
nasal crest of palatine process of m.
nasal notch of m.
notch of m.
palatine groove of m.

maxillaris
arcus dentalis m.
arteria m.
nervus m.

maxillary
acute maxillary sinusitis
m. advancement
m. alveolar buttress
m. alveolar protrusion
m. alveolar ridge
m. angle
anterior alveolar branch of maxillary nerve
anterior maxillary spine
m. anterior tooth
m. antrostomy
m. antrum
m. antrum closure
m. arch
m. artery
m. articulation
m. bicuspid
m. bicuspid radiograph
m. bite plate
m. bone
m. canal
m. canine
m. canine cusp
m. canine eminence
m. central incisor
m. corticotomy
m. crest
m. cuspid
m. cuspid radiograph
m. deficiency
m. deformity
m. dental arcade
m. dentition
m. depth
m. distraction osteogenesis
m. division
m. downgrafting
m. eminence
m. excess
m. expansion
m. first molar alveolus
m. fissure
m. foramen
m. fossa
m. fracture
m. ganglion
m. gland
m. hiatus
m. hypoplasia
m. impression
internal maxillary artery
m. mandibular odentectomy alveolectomy
median anterior maxillary cyst
meningeal branch of maxillary nerve
m. nerve
orbital branch of maxillary nerve
m. osteomyelitis
pterygoid branch of maxillary artery
rapid maxillary expansion
single central maxillary incisor
m. sinus
m. sinus aspiration
m. sinus carcinoma
m. sinusitis
surgically assisted rapid maxillary expansion
trigeminal nerve, maxillary division
vertical maxillary deficiency
vertical maxillary excess
zygomatic maxillary complex

maxillectomy cheek flap

maxilloalveolar breadth

maxillofacial
m. abnormality
m. anomaly
m. application
m. dysostosis
m. fracture
oral and maxillofacial surgery

maxillomandibular
m. advancement
m. advancement procedure
m. anchorage
asymmetric maxillomandibular growth

m. complex
m. disharmony
m. dysplasia
m. elastic
m. fixation
m. osteotomy

maxillonasal dysplasia

maximal

m. acid concentration
m. aerobic power
m. aggregation index
m. aggregation ratio
m. allowable concentration
m. allowable cost
m. allowable dose
m. androgen blockade
m. bactericidal dilution
m. benefit from hospitalization
brief maximal effort
Bruce maximal stress test
m. cardiac width
m. care unit
m. chest width
m. clearance
m. closure pressure
m. comfort level
m. concentration
m. containment laboratory
m. contrast
m. daily permissible intake
m. dose
m. drug concentration
m. effect
50% maximal effect
m. effort
m. electroshock
m. electroshock-induced seizure
m. electroshock model
m. electroshock seizure
m. esophageal pressure
m. exercise systolic pressure
m. exercise tolerance test
m. exercise ventilation
m. expiratory flow
m. expiratory flow rate
m. expiratory flow-static recoil curve
m. expiratory flow volume
m. expiratory flow volume curve
m. expiratory mouth pressure
m. extrapolated clotting time
m. flow per unit of time
m. flow-volume envelope
m. force at rest length
m. forced expiratory flow
m. forced expiratory maneuver
full width of photopeak measured at half maximal count
m. glucose disposal
m. hospital benefit
m. human dose
m. hydrocephalus
m. increment in growth and weight
indirect maximal breathing capacity
m. inspiratory flow
m. inspiratory flow rate
m. inspiratory force
m. inspiratory mouth pressure
m. intensity
m. left
m. left atrial dimension
left maximal spatial voltage
m. left ventricular developed pressure
m. likelihood estimation
linear band of maximal radiolucency
mean maximal expiratory flow
m. medical improvement
m. midexpiratory flow
m. midexpiratory flow rate
m. midexpiratory flow volume
m. midflow rate
m. mouth opening
m. noise area
m. number of lamella
m. number of microbes killed
m. oxygen consumption
m. oxygen intake
m. perfusion pressure
m. permissible concentration
m. permissible concentration of unidentified radionuclides
m. permissible dose
m. permitted intake
m. point of impulse
point of maximal impulse
m. possible effect
m. possible error
m. predicted heart rate
predicted maximal heart rate
m. predicted phonation time
m. print position
m. pulse rate
m. rate of urea synthesis
ratio of basal acid output to maximal acid output
m. recommended human dose
m. recycling capacity
m. reimbursement point
m. relation rate
m. relaxation rate
m. resting anal pressure
m. restrictive exercise
m. right
m. risk estimate
schedule of maximal allowance
m. sniff-induced esophageal pressure
m. sniff-induced gastric pressure
m. sniff-induced transdiaphragmatic pressure
m. spatial vector to left
m. specific binding capacity
m. static response assay
m. surgical blood order schedule
m. sustainable ventilatory capacity
m. sustained level of ventilation
sustained maximal inspiration
sustained maximal inspiratory lung exercise
m. sustained ventilatory capacity
m. terminal flow
time of maximal concentration
m. tolerable daily intake
m. tolerated concentration
m. tolerated dose
m. tolerated pressure
m. toleration
m. toleration volume
m. treadmill stress test
m. treadmill testing
m. tubular reabsorption rate for glucose
m. urethral pressure
m. urinary concentration
m. urinary flow rate
m. urinary osmolality
m. velocity
m. venous outflow
m. venous oxygen consumption
m. ventilation rate
m. ventilation time
m. ventilatory volume
m. voluntary contraction
m. voluntary ventilation

maximization

guinea pig maximization test

maximum

m. accumulated dose
m. acid output
m. acoustic output
m. allowable cost
m. amplitude
m. amplitude constant
m. anteroposterior diameter
m. assistance for lower body dressing

maximum *(continued)*
m. assistance for upper body dressing
m. assisted transfer
m. bactericidal dilution
m. bite force
m. bladder capacity
m. breathing capacity
m. coagulative necrosis
m. conduction velocity
m. contrast method
m. control
m. cystometric capacity
m. cytoreductive benefit
m. density
m. depth
m. determined heart rate
m. diameter
m. diameter to minimum diameter ratio
diastolic transmembrane voltage, m.
m. dose permissible dose
m. duration of phonation
m. duration of sustained blowing
m. eversion velocity
m. expiratory airflow-static lung elastic recoil pressure
m. expiratory flow
m. expiratory flow at 50% vital capacity
m. expiratory flow rate
m. expiratory flow volume
m. flow-volume loop
m. free flow rate
m. frequency range
full width at half m.
m. hospital benefit
m. inhibiting dilution
m. inhibiting duration
m. inspiratory pressure
m. interincisal distance
m. isolation
m. laryngeal height
m. level of independent mobility
m. likelihood estimator
m. likelihood score
m. loose-packed position
m. midexpiratory flow rate
m. observation nursery
one-repetition m.
m. oxygen consumption
m. oxygen uptake
patient reached maximum hospital benefit
peak maximum serum concentration
m. permissible concentration
m. permissible dose
point of maximum amplitude of wave
point of maximum impulse
point of maximum impulse fifth intercostal space
point of maximum intensity
point of maximum tenderness
m. power output
m. predicted heart rate
m. pressure picture
reached maximum hospital benefit
m. recommended daily dose
m. recommended human dose
repetition m.
m. residue limits of veterinary drugs
m. squeeze pressure
m. stimulation test
m. target absorbed dose
m. temperature
m. tolerable volume
m. tolerated dose
m. tolerated medical therapy
transport m.
tubular transport m.
m. urethral closure pressure
m. urinary concentration
m. vasal pressure
m. venous outflow
m. ventricular elastance
m. voluntary contraction
m. voluntary ventilation
m. walking distance
m. walking time

maximum-intensity pixel

maximum-intensive phototherapy

maximum-security forensic psychiatric hospital

maximus
gluteus m.
gluteus maximus muscle
gluteus maximus musculocutaneous flap
musculus gluteus m.
right gluteus m.

Maxon delayed-absorbable suture

Maxwell
M. coil
M. ring
M. spot

Maxwell-Brancheau arthroereisis

Maxwell-Lyons sign

may
M. apple
M. apple root
m. be elevated
m. fly
m. keep at bedside
m. repeat
m. repeat one time
M. sign

Mayaro virus disease

Maydl hernia

Mayer
M. acid alum hematoxylin stain
M. hemalum
M. hematoxylin
M. mucicarmine stain
M. pessary
M. wave

Mayfield
M. adapter
M. aneurysm clip
M. classification
M. head clamp
M. horseshoe headrest

Mayfield-Kees
M.-K. headholder
M.-K. headrest

May-Giemsa-Grünwald stain

May-Grünwald-Giemsa staining

May-Hegglin
M.-H. anomaly
M.-H. body
M.-H. syndrome

Maylard incision

Mayneord F factor

Mayo
M. abdominal clamp
M. ankle arthroplasty
M. approach
M. Asymptomatic Carotid Endarterectomy Study
M. bladder
M. block anesthesia
M. bunionectomy
M. carpal instability classification
M. classification of rheumatoid elbow
M. Clinic forefoot score
M. Clinic hip scoring system
M. Clinic system test for primary biliary cirrhosis
M. culdoplasty
M. elbow fracture classification
M. elbow performance score

M. hallux valgus modified operation
M. hysterectomy
M. Lung Project
M. modified total elbow arthroplasty
M. scissors
M. stand

Mayo-Fueth inversion procedure

Mayo-Robson point

Mayor sign

maze
m. behavior
catheter-based Maze procedure
Porteus maze test
M. procedure

Mazet disarticulation

Mazur
M. ankle elevation classification
M. ankle evaluation
M. ankle rating

Mazzini test

Mazzotti
M. reaction
M. test

MB-35 peptide

MC-7000
M. multi-wavelength laser
M. ophthalmic laser

McAllister grading system

McAndrews Alcoholism Scale

McArdle
M. disease
M. syndrome

McArdle-Schmid-Pearson disease

McBride
M. bunionectomy
M. bunion hallux valgus operation
M. hallux abductovalgus reduction
M. hallux valgus reduction

McBurney
M. appendectomy
M. appendectomy incision
M. point
M. sign

McCabe-Fletcher classification

McCall
M. culdoplasty
M. festoon
M. stitch

McCall-Schumann procedure

McCannel
M. implant
M. lens
M. ocular pressure reducer
M. suture
M. suture technique

McCarey-Kaufman transport medium

McCarthy
M. electrode
M. evacuator
M. Memory Scale
M. panendoscope
M. reflex

McCash
M. hand procedure
M. hand surgery

***MCC* gene**

McConnell extensile approach

McCoy
M. antibody
M. cell
M. culture medium

McCraw gracilis myocutaneous flap

McCune-Albright syndrome

McDonald
M. cervical cerclage
M. Deep Test of Articulation
M. maneuver
M. measurement
M. optic zone marker
M. procedure

McDonough
M. feline sarcoma virus
M. syndrome

McDowell Impairment Index

McElvenny foot procedure

MCF-7 breast cancer cell

McFarlane skin flap

McGavic operation

McGill-Melzack
M.-M. Pain Index
M.-M. Pain Score

McGlamry
M. elevator
M. and Feldman modification

McGoon index

McGregor forehead flap

McGuire
M. I/A system
M. operation

***MCH* gene**

McIndoe
M. bone rongeur
M. operation
M. procedure

McIndoe-Hayes
M.-H. construction
M.-H. procedure

McIntyre
M. I/A needle
M. I/A system
M. irrigating/aspirating unit
M. nylon cannula connector
M. reverse cystitome
M. truncated cone

McKay hip procedure

McKay-Marg tension

McKay-Simons clubfoot operation

McKee-Farrar
M.-F. prosthesis
M.-F. technique

McKeever
M. arthrodesis for hallux limitus
M. bunionectomy
M. and MacIntosh hemiarthroplasty

McKeever-Buck
M.-B. elbow operation
M.-B. elbow technique
M.-B. fragment excision

McKenzie
M. extension exercise
M. extension maneuver
M. hemostasis clip
M. test

McKissock mammoplasty

McKrae
M. herpes simplex virus
M. herpesvirus

McKusick
oculocerebral syndrome of Cross and M.
M. syndrome

McKusick-Kaufman syndrome

McLaughlin
M. acromioplasty
M. approach
M. arthroplasty
M. operation

McLean
Body Dysmorphic Disorder Modification of Yale-Brown Obsessive-Compulsive Scale, McLean version
M. classification of melanoma
M. fashion
M. manner
M. operation
M. suture
M. technique
M. tonometer

McLeod
M. phenotype
M. syndrome

McMaster
M. bone graft
M. Overall Treatment Evaluation
Western Ontario and McMaster Universities Osteoarthritis Index Physical Functioning subscale and chair-stand performance

McMaster-Toronto Arthritis Patient Reference

McMurray
M. circumduction maneuver
M. sign
M. test

McNeer classification

McNemar
M. test
M. test of significance

M-component
M.-c. hypergammaglobulinemia
M.-c. isotype

McPherson
M. needle holder
M. trabeculotome

McReynolds
M. keratome
M. operation
M. pterygium scissors
M. pterygium transplant
M. technique

McRoberts maneuver

McSpadden
M. compactor
M. endodontic technique

McVay
M. herniorrhaphy
M. operation
M. repair of hernia

McWhirter
M. mastectomy
M. technique

M.D.
M.D. Anderson Cancer Center
M.D. Anderson cancer staging
M.D. Anderson grading system
M.D. Anderson tumor score system

***MDM2* oncogene**

M'Dowel
frenulum of M.

mdr-1
mdr-1 gene
mdr-1 oncogene

***mdr* gene**

Meaban virus

meadow
m. dermatitis
m. fescue
m. fescue grass
m. foxtail grass

meadow-grass
m.-g. dermatitis
m.-g. dermatosis

Meadows syndrome

meal
after m.
after meal and at bedtime
barium m.
before every m.
dumping of barium m.
fatty meal sonogram
follow-through after barium m.
fractional test m.
home-delivered m.
mean indices of meal excursion
motor m.
multipurpose m.
M.'s on Wheels
M.'s on Wheels Association of America
m. planning
Riegel test m.
soybean oil m.
three times daily with m.
m. timing
m. tolerance test
trichloroethylene-extracted soybean-oil m.
with m.
m. worm

meal-related
m.-r. buffering
m.-r. treatment

meal-stimulated acid output

meal-time skill

mean
m. absorption time
m. acuity
m. age
m. airway pressure
m. airway resistance
m. allograft survival
m. alpha frequency
m. amplitude of glycerine excursion
m. ankle-brachial systolic pressure index
m.'s for anxiety
m. aortic flow velocity
aortic mean pressure
m. aortic pressure
arithmetic m.
m. arm muscle circumference
arterial m.
m. arterial
m. arterial blood pressure
arterial mean line
m. atrial pressure
m. atrial rate
average mean pressure
m. axillary count rate
m. birth weight
m. blood glucose
m. brachial artery pressure
brachial artery mean pressure
calculated mean organism
m. calorie
m. cardiac index
m. cardiac vector
m. carotid pressure
m. cell diameter
m. cell hemoglobin
m. cell hemoglobin concentration
m. cell thickness
m. cell threshold
m. cell volume
m. central dose
m. cerebral blood flow
m. circulating filling pressure
m. circulating time
m. circulation time
m. circulatory hematocrit
m. clinical value
m. colonic transit
m. consecutive difference
m. of consecutive differences
m. corneal power
m. corpuscular diameter
m. corpuscular hemoglobin

m. corpuscular hemoglobin concentration
m. corpuscular hemoglobin count
m. corpuscular thickness
m. corpuscular volume
m. daily dose
m. daily erect blood pressure
m. daily nitrogen balance
m. daily supine blood pressure
m. developmental quotient
m. deviation
m. diameter-thickness ratio
m. diastolic
m. diastolic gradient
m. diastolic left ventricular pressure
m. diffusivity
m. disintegration time
m. dissolution time
m. distal contraction amplitude
distal mean wave pressure
m. dominant frequency
m. dose
m. dose per unit cumulated activity
m. effective life
m. effective pressure
m. energy
m. episcleral heat dose
equivalent mean age at death
feeding mean arterial pressure
m. fluorescent intensity
m. fraction absorption
m. free path
m. frequency of compensation
m. generation time
geometric m.
geometric mean concentration
geometric mean diameter
geometric mean titer
m. gestational sac diameter
m. gradient
harmonic m.
m. hearing
m. hemoglobin concentration
m. hemolytic dose
m. horizontal candle power
hypothetical mean organism
hypothetical mean strain
m. indices of meal excursion
m. input time
m. inspiratory flow
m. intercriterion correlation
m. interpotential interval
m. intrathoracic pressure
m. intravascular pressure
m. latency time
least squares m.
m. left atrial pressure
m. left ventricular systolic pressure
m. length of response
m. length of utterance
m. life span
m. marrow dose
m. maternal glucose
m. maximal expiratory flow
m. menstrual cycle hematocrit
m. midexpiratory flow rate
normalized mean square root
m. normalized systolic ejection rate
m. optical density
m. particle size
m. percentage of desirable weight
m. perfusate temperature
m. plasma iron concentration
m. plasma volume
m. platelet volume
m. population doubling
m. power frequency
m. prediction error
m. pulmonary artery wedge pressure
m. pulmonary-blood-flow velocity
m. pulmonary capillary wedge pressure
pulmonary mean transit time
m. pulmonary transit time
m. QRS axis
reciprocal geometric mean titer
m. reference diameter
m. rejection grading
m. relational utterance
m. renal blood flow
m. residence time
m. residual gap
m. resistance time
m. resting diastolic blood pressure
m. resting potential
reticulocyte mean corpuscular volume
m. right atrial pressure
m. right ventricular pressure
root mean square residue
m. sac size
m. sac size and crown-rump length
sample m.
m. scale value
m. sitting diastolic blood pressure
m. sorted difference
m. spherical candle power
m. spherical equivalent
m. square deviation
m. square error
standard deviation of m.
standard error of the m.
standardized response m.
m. survival time
m. swell time botulism test
m. systemic arterial pressure
systemic mean arterial pressure
systolic, diastolic, mean blood pressure
m. systolic ejection rate
m. time between or before failures
m. total dose
m. transit time
m. tubular diameter
m. venous outflow
m. venous pressure
weighted mean index

meaning
affect-related m.
grammatical m.
hidden m.

meaningful
Coarticulation Assessment in Meaningful Language
m. conversation

Means-Lerman
M.-L. scratch
M.-L. scratch murmur

measles
m. antibody
atypical m.
atypical measles pneumonia
atypical measles syndrome
m. convalescent serum
diphtheria, pertussis, tetanus, poliomyelitis, and measles vaccine
m. encephalitis
m. exanthem
m. giant cell pneumonia
hemorrhagic m.
m. immune globulin
m. immunoglobulin
m. inclusion body encephalitis
killed measles virus vaccine
modified m.
m., mumps, rubella immunization
m., mumps, and rubella vaccine
m. and rubella
m. and rubella vaccine

measles *(continued)*
m., rubella and zoster
typical m.
m. vaccine
m. virus

measles-rinderpest-distemper virus group

measurable
m. disease
immunologically measurable insulin
not m.
m. undesirable respiratory contaminants

measure
m. of acid strength
affect intensity m.
APACHE II measure of disease severity
Assessment M. for Atopic Dermatitis
m. of balance
Bilingual Syntax M. II Test
m. of central tendency
comfort measures only
m. of competence
empty, measure, and record
functional assessment m.
Functional Independence M. for Children
functional status m.'s
m. of general cognitive functioning
Gross Motor Function M.
Inquiry Mode Questionnaire: A M. of How You Think and Make Decisions
isolation m.'s
life-prolonging m.'s
m. mucociliary clearance
no heroic m.'s
overall cognitive m.
parallel goniometric m.
Parents' Postoperative Pain M.
Prematurity Risk Evaluation M.
M.'s of Psychosocial Development
m. and record
relative-intensity m.
m. of resource use
Systemic Lupus Activity M.
x-ray immunosuppressive m.

measured
m. beam data
m. capacity
m. dose
m. energy expenditure
full width of photopeak measured at half maximal count
not m.
oxygen saturation as measured using pulse oximetry
serum thyroxine measured by column chromatography
serum thyroxine measured by displacement analysis

measurement
anatomic m.
ankle-brachial pressure m.
antegrade perfusion pressure m.
appendicular bone mass m.
Arthritis Impact M. Scale
arthrometric knee laxity m.
aural immittance m.
automated cardiac flow m.
automated cardiac flow measurement ultrasound
automated cardiac output m.
blood gas m.
cardiac output m.
Cardiovascular M. system
computer-automated measurement and control
m. control handle
crown-rump m.
m. effect
end-diastolic velocity m.
m. error
error of m.
m. of exposure
m. film
gas clearance m.
head circumference m.
home blood pressure m.
Home Observation for M. of the Environment
invasive pressure m.
left anterior m.
left posterior m.
limb accurate m.
Medicare Bone Mass M. Standardization Act
Mental M.'s Yearbook
microbubble concentration m.
midluteal progesterone m.
MPH distance m.
multicolor immunofluorescence m.
noninvasive blood pressure m.
nuchal translucency m.
nutation angle m.
optical density m.
peak flow m.
performance measurement system
peripheral blood mononuclear cell hepatitis B virus m.
probable error of m.
right anterior m.
segmental correction using x-ray m.
simulated real ear m.
skin fold m.
specimen mass measurement device
speech-controlled respirometer for ambulatory m.
transcutaneous oxygen pressure m.
Vineland M. of Social Competence
voiding urethral pressure m.

measure of resource use

measuring
anthropometric measuring tape
blood plasma measuring system
eye movement measuring apparatus
m. gauge
m. hat
m. heart function
indirect blood pressure measuring system
precise lesion m.
urine specimen volume measuring device
urine specimen volume measuring system

measuring-mounting catheter

meat
m. base formula
chopped meat medium
Ewald test m.
m. free

meatal
m. advancement
m. advancement and glanduloplasty procedure
m. advancement glans-phalloplasty
m. advancement and glansplasty
m. advancement, glansplasty, penoscrotal junction meatotomy
m. advancement, glanuloplasty, penoscrotal junction meatotomy
m. atresia
m. care
m. cartilage
m. stenosis
urethral meatal stenosis

meati (*pl. of* meatus)

meatoplasty and glanuloplasty

meatotomy
meatal advancement, glansplasty, penoscrotal junction m.
meatal advancement, glanuloplasty, penoscrotal junction m.

meatus, pl. **meati**
m. acusticus externus
anterior middle m.
anterior nasal m.
atrium of middle nasal m.
external auditory m.
external urethral m.
fishmouth m.
internal acoustic m.
internal auditory m.
internal urethral m.
middle meatus nasal antral window
nerve of external acoustic m.
notch in cartilage of acoustic m.
opening of external acoustic m.
opening of internal acoustic m.
orifice of external acoustic m.
orifice of internal acoustic m.

***mecA* gene**

Mecca balsam

MeCCNU
M. and Adriamycin
M., Oncovin, 5-fluorouracil
M., Oncovin, 5-fluorouracil plus streptozotocin

mechanical
m. abrasion
m. acne
m. acquired ptosis
actual mechanical advantage
m. agent
m. alopecia
alternating failure of response mechanical to electrical depolarization
m. alternation of the heart
m. amalgamator
m. anastomosis
m. anosmia
m. antidote
m. aptitude
assist-controlled mechanical ventilation
assisted mechanical ventilation
m. augmentation
m. auxiliary ventricle
m. avulsion
axial closed-loop hydraulic mechanical testing
m. axis
m. biliary obstruction
m. birth injury
m. bladder outlet resistance
m. blepharoptosis
m. bowel obstruction
breathing supported by mechanical respirator
m. cervical dilator
combined m.
m. compound scan
m. condenser
continuous mechanical ventilation
continuous mechanical ventilatory assistance
controlled mechanical ventilation
conventional mechanical ventilation
m. corepraxy
m. counterpulsation
m. creep of skin
m. cystitis
m. dead space
m. dermatome
m. diarrhea
direct mechanical ventricular actuation
m. diuretic
m. duct obstruction
m. dysfunction
m. dysmenorrhea
m. ectropion
emergency mechanical restraint
m. endoscopic management
endotracheal intubation and mechanical ventilation
m. esophageal obstruction
m. esophagojejunostomy
m. expiratory flow volume curve
m. extrahepatic obstruction
m. fragility
m. functional loss
m. heart
m. heart pump
m. heart valve
m. ileus
m. insulin pump
intermittent mechanical ventilation
m. jaundice
m. joint apparatus
m. lid retraction
m. loading
long-term mechanical assistance
m. low back pain
Minnesota M. Assembly Test
minor mechanical debridement
m. obstruction
m. pain threshold
m. percussion
m. percussor
percutaneous mechanical thrombectomy
m. pleurodesis
m. pressure
pureed, mechanical, soft diet
m. respirator
m. stimulation
m. strabismus
m. suffocation
m. tidal volume
m. vector
m. ventilation
m. ventilator
m. ventricular assistance
m. vessel blockage
m. vitrector
volume of mechanical dead space

mechanically
m. activated implant
m. assisted
m. detachable platinum coil
paralyzed and mechanically ventilated

mechanism
m. of action
adjustable leg and ankle repositioning m.
antireflux flap-valve m.
arousal boost m.
arousal reduction m.
autonomic cooling m.
4-bar linkage prosthetic knee m.
blood-clotting mechanism effects
body's natural defense m.
calcium homeostatic m.
central extensor m.
copulatory m.
coronary steal m.
m. of correction
cranial-sacral respiratory m.
defense mechanism inventory
endogenous brain m.
extensor mechanism dysfunction
feedback m.
immune defense m.
individual defense m.
inherited releasing m.
m. of injury
innate releasing m.
maladaptive coping m.
maladaptive defense m.
natural defense m.

mechanism *(continued)*
normal flap-valve m.
patient-operated selector m.
peptide growth factor signaling m.
perceptual cognitive m.
radical pair m.
sex arousal m.
terminal extensor m.
transport m.

mechanized scissors

mechanobullous disease

mechanoreceptor
m. activity
m. fiber
m. Golgi tendon organ

Mecholyl skin test

Meckel
M. arch
M. band
M. cartilage
M. cave
M. cave lesion
M. cavity
M. diverticulectomy
M. diverticulitis
M. diverticulum
M. ganglion
M. ligament
M. scan
M. syndrome

Meckel-Gruber syndrome

meconial colic

meconium
m. aspiration
m. aspiration syndrome
m. blockage syndrome
m. corpuscle
m. ileus
m. ileus appearance
m. ileus equivalent
m. obstruction
m. peritonitis
m. plug
m. plug syndrome
m. stain
m. stained
m. staining
m. staining of liquor
m. in trachea

meconium-stained
m.-s. amniotic fluid
m.-s. skin

Medani
Wad Medani virus

media
acute otitis m.
aortic tunica m.
arteria cerebri m.
arteria collateralis m.
arteria meningea m.
arteria temporalis m.
attenuated media raphe
bilateral otitis media, acute
bilateral otitis media with effusion
bilateral serous otitis m.
captioned media program
Chlamydia transport m.
chronic adhesive otitis m.
chronic otitis media with effusion
chronic suppurative otitis m.
m. clearing
contrast media excretion
contrast media leakage
contrast media nephrotoxicity
dermatophyte test m.
draining otitis m.
external otitis m.
gastric pars m.
Health M. Education
m. history
m. influence
injection of contrast m.
left otitis m.
low-osmolality contrast m.
macula cribrosa m.
mucoid otitis m.
nonsuppurative otitis m.
m. opacity
otitis m.
otitis media, acute, catarrhal
otitis media, acute, suppurating
otitis media, catarrhal, acute
otitis media, catarrhal, chronic
otitis media, chronic, suppurating
otitis media, purulent, acute
otitis media with effusion
otitis media without effusion
otitis media with perforated tympanic membrane
Oxgall media culture
pupils, tension, media, disc, and fundus
purulent otitis m.
radiographic contrast m.
resorbable blast m.
right otitis m.
right otitis media, suppurative, acute
right otitis media, suppurative, chronic
secretory otitis m.
serous otitis m.
m. tunica

mediae

medial
m. accessory olivary nucleus
m. amygdaloid nucleus
m. angle
m. angle of eye
angle of medial eye
m. anlage
m. antebrachial cutaneous nerve
m. anterior malleolus artery
anterior medial ankle ligament
anterior medial malleolar artery
anterior portion of left medial segment IV of liver
m. anterior thoracic nerve
anterior tibiotalar part of medial ligament of ankle joint
m. arch
m. arcuate ligament
m. arteriole of retina
m. arteriosclerosis
articular facet of medial malleolus
m. articular nerve
m. aspect
m. aspiration
m. atrial vein
m. basal branch of pulmonary artery
m. basal bronchopulmonary segment S VII
m. basal hypothalamus
m. basal segment
m. basal segmental artery
m. basal segmental bronchus
belly button to medial malleolus
m. bicipital groove
m. bicipital sulcus
m. border
m. border of foot
m. border of forearm
m. border of kidney
m. border of scapula
m. border of suprarenal gland
m. border of tibia
m. brachial cutaneous nerve
m. brachial fascial compartment
m. brachial nerve
m. branch
m. branch of artery of tuber cinereum
m. branch C2
m. branch of pontine artery

m. branch of posterior branch of spinal nerve
m. branch of posterior rami of spinal nerve
m. calcaneal branch of tibial nerve
m. calcaneocuboid
m. calcification
m. calcific sclerosis
m. canaliform dystrophy
m. canthal fissure
m. canthal incision
m. canthal ligament
m. canthal repair
m. canthal tendon
m. canthic fold
m. canthopexy
m. canthoplasty
m. canthus
m. canthus area
m. capsular imbrication
m. capsular ligament
m. capsule
m. capsulorrhaphy
m. carpal capsule
m. cartilaginous layer
m. cartilaginous plate
m. cell column
m. central nucleus of thalamus
m. central tegmental field
m. cerebral surface
m. check ligament of eyeball
m. circumflex artery of thigh
m. circumflex femoral artery
m. circumflex femoral vein
m. clear space
m. cleft of lip
m. cleft of palate
m. closing wedge phalangeal osteotomy
m. cluneal nerve
m. collateral artery
m. collateral ligament
m. collateral ligament degeneration
m. collateral ligament of elbow
m. collateral ligament of knee
m. collateral ligament tearing
m. collateral sprain
m. column calcaneal fracture
m. column instability
m. commissural artery
m. commissure of eyelid
common palmar digital nerve of medial nerve
common plantar digital nerve of medial plantar nerve
m. compartment
m. compartment disruption
m. compartment injury
m. compartment of thigh
m. component
m. condyle
m. condyle of femur
m. condyle of humerus
m. condyle of tibia
m. cord of brachial plexus
m. cortical overlap technique
m. crest of fibula
m. crossover toe
m. crural cutaneous branch of saphenous nerve
m. crural cutaneous nerve
m. crural strut graft
m. crural suture
m. crus
m. crus of facial canal
m. crus foot plate
m. crus of the horizontal part of the facial canal
m. crus of major alar cartilage of nose
m. crus of the superficial inguinal ring
m. cuneiform bone
m. cutaneous branch
m. cutaneous branch of dorsal branch of posterior intercostal artery
m. cutaneous nerve
m. cutaneous nerve of arm
m. cutaneous nerve of forearm
m. cutaneous nerve of leg
m. cutaneous thigh flap
cystic medial necrosis
cystic medial necrosis of ascending aorta
m. cystic necrosis
detachment of medial meniscus
m. deviation of the second toe
m. disc protrusion
m. displacement
m. displacement osteotomy
m. dissection
m. distally based fasciocutaneous flap
m. dog ear
m. dorsal cutaneous nerve
m. dorsal nucleus of thalamus
m. drainage
m. dysplasia
m. ectropion
elastic knee cage with medial and lateral contoured knee joints
m. elevation
m. eminence
m. eminence resection
m. eminence of rhomboid
m. end
m. epicanthal scar band
m. epicondylar apophysis
m. epicondylar crest
m. epicondylar fracture
m. epicondylar ridge
m. epicondyle
m. epicondylectomy
m. epicondyle of femur
m. epicondyle humeral fracture
m. epicondyle of humerus
m. epicondylitis
m. exostectomy
m. extended facial translocation
m. extensor expansion
m. extradural approach
m. femoral circumflex artery
m. femoral condyle
m. femoral torsion
m. femoral tuberosity
m. fibroplasia
m. fillet
m. flap
m. flexor muscle of forearm
m. foramen
m. forebrain bundle
m. frontal cortex
m. frontal gyrus
m. frontal lobe syndrome
m. frontobasal artery
m. gastrocnemius bursitis
m. gastrocnemius muscle
m. gastrocnemius muscle
m. genicular vein
m. geniculate
m. geniculate artery
m. geniculate body
m. geniculate fascia
m. geniculate nucleus
m. graft technique
m. great muscle
m. habenular
m. habenular nucleus
m. hamstring
m. hamulus
m. head
m. head of the gastrocnemius rupture
m. head-stem offset
m. heel-and-sole wedge
m. heel skive technique
m. heel wedge
m. heel wedge orthosis

medial *(continued)*
m. hemijoint articular space
m. hemispheric arteriovenous malformation
m. hip rotation
m. hip rotation in extension
m. horn
m. humeral condyle
m. hypothalamus
m. incisor tooth
m. inferior genicular artery
m. inguinal fossa
m. interlaminar nucleus
m. intermuscular septum
internal medial malleolus
intimal medial thickness
m. joint of ankle
m. joint level
m. joint line
m. joint space
m. lacunar lymph node
m. lamina of cartilage of pharyngotympanic auditory tube
left medial rectus eye muscle
m. ligament of ankle joint
m. ligament of talocrural joint
m. ligament of temporomandibular joint
m. ligament of wrist
m. limb
m. lip of linea aspera
m. lobule
m. longitudinal arch
m. longitudinal bundle
m. longitudinal fasciculus
longitudinal medial bundle
m. longitudinal stria
m. lumbar intertransverse muscle
m. lumbocostal arch
Lynch medial canthal incision
m. malleolar branch of posterior tibial artery
m. malleolar facet of talus
m. malleolar network
m. malleolar subcutaneous bursa
m. malleolar surface of talus
m. malleolus
m. malleolus of tibia
m. mammary branch
m. margin
m. hemispheric dynamics
m. medullary infarction
m. meniscectomy
m. meniscus
m. meniscus detachment
m. metaphyseal beak
m. necrosis
neurosensorial free medial plantar flap
m. nuclear stratum
m. nucleus of trapezoid body
m. oblique view
m. oblique x-ray view
m. olivocochlear
m. orbital sulcus
m. osseous interorbital distance
m. palpebral ligament
parietal branch of medial occipital artery
m. patellofemoral ligament
m. plantar
popliteal medial nerve
posterior branch of medial cutaneous nerve of forearm
m. posterior choroidal
posterior horn of medial meniscus
m. preoptic area
m. pterygoid muscle
m. pterygoid plate
m. rectus, both eyes
m. rectus extraocular muscle
m. rectus function
m. rectus muscle
m. rectus palsy
m. rectus transposition
right medial rectus muscle
right upper m.
m. rotation clubfoot
m. septal nucleus
significant medial event
m. snapping hip syndrome
subcutaneous bursa of medial malleolus
superficial branch of medial circumflex femoral artery
superficial branch of medial plantar artery
m. superior olive
m. superior temporal visual area
m. surface of cerebral hemisphere
m. talocalcaneal facet
m. temporal
m. temporal-lobe epilepsy
m. temporal visual area
m. thickening
m. tibial plateau
m. tibial stress syndrome
m. tibial torsion
torn medial meniscus
m. transplantation of patellar tendon insertion
ulnar branch of medial antebrachial cutaneous nerve
m. ulnar collateral ligament
upper fossa active, medial knee pain, and short leg on the side ipsilateral to the weak fossa
m. ventromedial nucleus
m. venulae of retina
m. vestibular nucleus
m. zone

medialization
anterior and posterior medialization thyroplasty

median
m. alveolar cyst
m. alveolar notch
m. anlage
m. antebrachial vein
m. anterior maxillary cyst
anterior median fissure
anterior median fissure of medulla oblongata
anterior median fissure of spinal cord
anterior median line
anterior median nucleus
m. aperture
m. aperture of fourth ventricle
m. arcuate ligament
m. arcuate ligament of diaphragm
m. artery
m. atlantoaxial joint
m. bar
m. bar formation
m. bar of Mercier
m. basilic vein
m. biopsy volume
m. callosal artery
m. canaliform dystrophy
m. cephalic vein
m. cleft face
m. cleft face syndrome
m. cleft lip
m. cleft of lower lip and mandible
m. cleft upper lip, mental retardation, pugilistic facies syndrome
comitant artery of median nerve
m. commissural artery
m. conjugate
m. corpectomy
count median aerodynamic diameter
count median diameter of particles

count median length
m. cricothyroid ligament
m. cruciate ligament
m. cubital vein
m. curative dose
m. detection threshold
distribution of median nerve
m. duration of response
m. effective concentration
m. effective dose
m. eminence
m. episiotomy
m. erythrocyte diameter
m. face syndrome
m. facial cleft
m. facial cleft syndrome
m. fatal dose
m. fissure
m. foramen of Magendie
m. frontal sulcus
m. furrow of prostate
m. glossoepiglottic fold
gray-scale m.
m. groove
m. groove of tongue
m. harelip
m. incision
left m.
m. lethal dose
m. lethal time
m. life span
m. line
m. longitudinal raphe of tongue
m. longitudinal section
mass median aerodynamic diameter
mass median diameter of particles
multiples of the appropriate gestational m.
m. nail dystrophy
m. nerve
m. nerve hypesthesia
m. nerve somatosensory evoked potential
m. palatine suture
palmar cutaneous branch of the median nerve
m. paralyzing dose
m. plane
m. range score
m. raphe
m. raphe cyst of the penis
m. reaction time
m. recognition threshold
m. relapse time
m. rhomboid glossitis
right m.
m. sternotomy incision
m. sulcus
m. survival time
tethered median nerve stress test
m. tissue culture infective dose
m. toxic concentration
m. toxic dose

mediastinal

m. abscess
m. adenoma
m. adenopathy
m. air
m. amyloidosis
angiofollicular mediastinal lymph node hyperplasia
m. angiolipoma
anterior mediastinal artery
anterior mediastinal compartment
anterior mediastinal lymph node
anterior mediastinal mass
aortopulmonary mediastinal stripe
m. arterial variant
m. artery
m. aspiration
m. B-cell lymphoma with sclerosis
m. border
m. branch
m. branch of internal thoracic artery
m. branch of thoracic aorta
m. bronchogenic cyst
m. bulk
caudal mediastinal node
cervical mediastinal exploration
m. collagenosis
m. cross-sectional imaging
m. crunch
m. CTD
m. deviation
m. disease
m. dissection
m. dorsal enteric cyst
m. duplication cyst
m. elastofibroma
m. enlargement
m. esophagojejunostomy
m. fibrosis
m. germ cell tumor
m. granuloma
m. hemorrhage
m. high-attenuation mass
m. histoplasmosis
m. irradiation
m. large B-cell lymphoma
m. lipoma
m. lipomatosis
low-dose mediastinal radiation therapy
m. lymphadenitis
m. lymphadenopathy
m. lymph node
m. lymph node hyperplasia
m. mass
mature mediastinal teratoma
m. mesenchymal tumor
myasthenia gravis and mediastinal tumors
narrow mediastinal waist
m. neoplasm
m. nodal station
m. node
m. parathyroid adenoma
m. pathology
periaortic mediastinal hematoma
m. pleura
m. pleura incised
m. pleurisy
primary mediastinal germ-cell tumor
primary mediastinal large-cell lymphoma
primary mediastinal large cell lymphoma with sclerosis
m. seminoma
m. shed blood
m. teratoma
m. tube
tuberculous mediastinal adenopathy
m. widening
m. yolk sac tumor

mediastinales

arteriae mediastinales anteriores
nodi lymphoidei mediastinales anteriores
nodi lymphoidei mediastinales posteriores

mediastinum

m. cerebelli
m. cerebri
m. dermoid
m. displacement
m. dysgerminoma
extraosseous plasmacytoma of the m.
m. inferius
secondary carcinoma of the upper m.
m. testis

mediate

m. agglutination
m. auscultation

mediate *(continued)*
m. contagion
m. percussion

mediated
m. cell death
cell mediated antibody
cell mediated cytotoxicity
cell mediated immunity
cellular mediated immune response
chromosomally mediated resistant *Neisseria gonorrhoeae*
chromosomal mediated resistance
electric field mediated transfer
m. function
immunologically mediated disease
neurally mediated vasovagal syncope
potentiometric ionophore mediated immunoassay
sympathetically mediated pain syndrome

mediating
m. action
m. effect

mediation
autoimmune immunoglobulin m.
conflict m.

mediator
m. cell
m. chemical released in the tissues
m. complex
leukocyte endogenous m.
nonantigenic specific m.
silencing mediator of retinoic acid and thyroid hormone receptor
virus entry mediator, a receptor expressed by T lymphocyte

mediator-related symptom

medical
m. abbreviation
acute medical illness
acute medical management intervention
m. adenomectomy
m. adhesive
adjuvant medical therapy
m. advice
aggressive medical care
m. air evacuation
air medical transportation
m. alert bracelet
m. alert center
m. alert necklace
m. anatomy
m. ankle orthosis
m. anthropology
m. antishock trousers
appropriate medical attention
m. assistance
assisted medical procreation
m. attention
M. Audiologic Tinnitus Patient Protocol
m. audit
auditory and medical evaluation
m. authorization
automated medical history
m. bacteriology
m. biophysics
m. board
m. care
m. care administration
m. care evaluation
m. care organization
m. castration
m. center
m. chemoprevention
chronic medical illness
coexisting medical condition
M. College Admission Test
m. comorbidity
comorbid medical problem
complementary medical practice
m. complications of obesity
comprehensive medical history
comprehensive medical plan
computer-based continuing medical education
m. condition
m. consultant
continuing medical education
m. contraindication
m. control physician
Cornell M. Index
court-ordered medical treatment
Current List of M. Literature
current medical evidence of record
current medical information and terminology
m. data screen
m. data system
m. decision-maker
m. deliberation
denial of lifesaving medical treatment
m. department
detailed medical history
diagnostic medical sonography
m. diathermy
m. dilation
disaster medical assistance team
m. discharge
discharged against medical advice
m. doctor
durable medical equipment
m. economic index
m. education
M. Education for National Defense
m. effect
electronic patient medical record
m. emergency
emergency medical attendant
emergency medical care
emergency medical care and rescue
emergency medical information
emergency medical team
emergency medical trauma center
emergency medical treatment
m. emergency treatment
m. ethics
m. etiology
m. evaluation
m. events
m. evidence
M. Examination and Diagnostic Coding System
m. examiner
extreme medical emergency
Family and M. Leave Act of 1993
family medical doctor
family medical history
m. fee schedule
focused medical review
m. followup
m. food
m. free electron laser
m. futility
m. gas analyzer
general medical clinic
general medical condition
general medical floor
general medical panel
m. geneticist
m. genetics
graduate medical education
m. group practice
m. healthcare
high-quality medical care
m. history
m. history as screening device for drug abuse
history of medical illness
m. history review

home medical equipment
home medical test kit
m. house officer
m. illness
m. impairment
m. implant
important medical event
m. improvement expected
m. improvement not expected
m. improvement possible
increased medical risk
independent medical examination
indirect medical education
individual medical record
m. induction
indwelling prosthetic medical device
inpatient non-psychiatric medical facilities
m. inspection
integrated medical services
m. intensity
m. intensive care unit
m. interaction
intermediate medical care unit
m. internal radiation dose
m. intervention
invasive medical procedure
ischemia-guided medical therapy
m. jargon
m. jurisprudence
M. Knowledge Self-Assessment Program
m. laboratory assay
life-sustaining medical treatment
local medical doctor
local medical review policy
m. maintenance unit
major medical insurance
m. materials account
Mauldsley M. Questionnaire
maximal medical improvement
maximum tolerated medical therapy
Medical Walk-In Clinic
mental disorder due to a general medical condition
mood disorder due to a general medical condition
multiple medical problem
m. mycology
National Ambulatory M. Care Survey
National Institute of General M. Sciences
Newport medical instrument
no medical health history
no medical ocular history
noncompliance with medical treatment
noncontributory past medical history
m. office assistant
m. office building
m. officer
m. oncologist
m. oncology
m. oncology unit
m. ophthalmoscopy
m. optical spectroscopy
m. optimal imaging
M. Outcomes Study
m. outpatient
m. outpatient program
past medical history
past medical history noncontributory
past medical history unremarkable
past medical illness
patient medical instruction
patient released against medical advice
patient's medical history
periodic medical review
m. personnel pool
present medical illness
previous medical illness
Primary Children's M. Center
prior medical record
private medical doctor
problem-oriented medical record
programmed medical history
m. progressive care unit
m. receiving station
refusal of medical aid
m. rehabilitation
m. reimbursement plan
m. resource utilization
routine medical care
Safe M. Device Act
M. Sciences Knowledge Profile
m. self-help
m. short procedure unit
signed out against medical advice
m. special care unit
state medical facilities plan
m. studies unit
m. subspecialist
supplementary medical insurance
m. support equipment
m. survey
m. tattooing
m. termination of pregnancy
m. therapy
m. therapy unit
m. thyroidectomy
m. toxic environment
m. training center
m. transcriptionist
m. treatment facility
Tri-Service M. Information System
m. ultrasound 3D portable, with advanced communication
Unified M. Language System
unit of medical time
m. unit, self-contained and transportable
World M. Association

medical-legal interaction

medically

m. fragile
m. inactive placebo
m. indigent adult
m. managed intensive addiction treatment unit
m. necessary
patient managed m.
patient treated m.
m. restricted diet

medical/surgical

other medical/surgical facility

medicamentosa dermatitis

Medicare

M. Bone Mass Measurement Standardization Act
certified for M.
Explanation of Medicare Benefits
qualified Medicare beneficiary

medicated urethral system

medication

m. abuse
m. administration guideline
m. administration record
m. administration team
adverse medication effect
m. allergy
antianxiety and antidepressant m.
antiepileptic m.
attitude to m.
m. bezoar
birth control m.
m. change
m. compliance
condition induced by m.
consistent medication compliance

medication *(continued)*
m. contraindication
deteriorating effect of m.
discontinue previous m.
m. dosage
m. guide
hormone replacement m.
m. incompatibility
m. information leaflet for seniors
intravenous administration of m.
long-acting injectable m.
m. management
monitored administration of m.
m. monitoring event system
no known medication allergies
noncompliant with m.
nonsteroidal antiinflammatory m.
oral antibiotic m.
oral contraceptive m.
oral pain m.
overuse of narcotic m.
parenteral analgesic m.
patient guide to m.
patient medication instruction
patient medication profile
patient noncompliant with m.
peripherally acting anticholinergic m.
programmable implantable medication system
psychotropic medication plan
m. rebound syndrome
m. regimen
m. release consent
relief medication unit index
m. responder
self-administered m.
sustained release m.
m. use evaluation

medication-assisted detoxification

medication-induced
m.-i. angioedema
m.-i. depressive syndrome
m.-i. esophageal injury
m.-i. headache
m.-i. hyperlipoproteinemia
m.-i. stuttering

medicinal
m. charcoal
m. chemistry
m. eruption

medicine
administrative m.
adolescent m.
aerospace m.
allergy relief m.
alternative m.
anesthesiology critical care m.
anticholinergic medicine therapy
artificial intelligence in m.
aviation m.
m. ball
clinical m.
complementary and alternative m.
m. concept
critical care m.
critical care medicine unit
emergency m.
engineering in medicine and biology
evidence-based m.
family medicine center
flight medicine clinic
forensic m.
general medicine and surgery
general preventive m.
industrial m.
integral traditional Chinese m.
intensive care m.
intermediate medicine unit
internal m.
legal m.
maternal fetal m.
National Library of M.
no regular m.'s
nuclear m.
nuclear medicine information system
nuclear medicine scan
occupational and environmental m.
Office of Alternative M.
osteopathic manipulative m.
osteopathic medicine and surgery
patent m.
pediatric emergency m.
physical m.
physical medicine and rehabilitation
prescription-only m.
preventive m.
psychosomatic m.
radioisotope m.
Rapid Estimation of Adult Literacy in M.
rehabilitation m.
research aviation m.
space m.
Standardized Nomenclature of M.
m. and surgery
Systematized Nomenclature of M. Clinical Terms
Systematized Nomenclature of M. Reference Terminology
Systemized Nomenclature of M.
traditional Chinese m.
tropical m.

Medicus
Cumulated Index M.
Index M.

Medi-Facts system

Medifil collagen

Medi-Mist nebulizer

Medin poliomyelitis

mediobasal brain structure

mediocarpal articulation

mediolateral
m. aspect
m. episiotomy
left mediolateral episiotomy
m. oblique
right m.
right mediolateral episiotomy
m. view

medionecrosis
m. of the aorta

mediorenal tumor

MediSense
M. Precision meter
M. Sof-Tact monitor

Meditec
M. bandage contact lens
M. laser

Medi-Tech catheter

Mediterranean
M. abdominal lymphoma
M. anemia
M. erythematous fever
M. exanthematous fever
familial Mediterranean fever
M. fever
M. Kaposi sarcoma
M. lymphoma
M. myoclonus
M. spotted fever

medium
acid bismuth yeast m.
Apathy gum syrup m.
aqueous mounting m.
m. artery
Barbour-Stoenner-Kelly m.
basal m.
m. below-elbow cast
Bergersen m.
m. biscuit
m. biscuit firing

m. bisque firing
Brinster medium for ovum culture
m. brown loose stool
m. caliber
m. callus Podi-Burr
m. carbide cone bur
casein yeast lactate m.
charcoal blood medium culture
charcoal viral transport m.
charcoal yeast extract m.
chemically defined m.
chopped meat m.
chopped meat-glucose-starch m.
complete m.
conditioned m.
contrast m.
m. corpuscular fragility
culture m.
cystine-tellurite m.
m. disk
m. dosage
Dulbecco modified Eagle medium
Eagle basal m.
Eagle minimal essential m.
Ethiodane contrast m.
Ethiodol contrast m.
excessive diffuse low and medium wave beta activity
extravasation of contrast m.
fibroblast-conditioned m.
m. fine bur
fluid thioglycolate m.
fluorescence-lactose-denitrification m.
m. frequency
gallium-67 citrate contrast m.
gelatin infusion medium
growth m.
Haemophilus test m.
high-osmolar contrast m.
high-osmolarity contrast m.
hypertonic buffered m.
improved minimal essential medium, hormone supplemented
infection m.
inhibitor-containing minimal m.
m. inspiratory
intravenous contrast m.
Kenner-fecal medium
kinetic energy released in the m.
lactic acid mineral m.
Lactobacillus maintenance m.
large and medium lymphocyte
Leibovitz-Emory m.
m. lesion
leukocyte-conditioned m.
Locke egg serum medium
Loeffler blood culture m.
Löffler coagulated serum m.
m. long-acting
Löwenstein-Jensen m.
low-osmolar contrast m.
lymphocyte separation m.
macromolecular contrast m.
magnesium contrast m.
manganese chloride contrast m.
Martin-Lewis medium
McCarey-Kaufman transport m.
McCoy culture m.
meglumine diatrizoate contrast m.
methylglucamine contrast m.
methyl red, Voges-Proskauer medium
Middlebrook 7H10, 7H11 m.
mineral basal m.
mineral salts m.
minimal m.
minimum essential m.
moderate number of medium rales
modified whole-egg slant m.
molybdenum-conditioned m.
motility test m.
Neuman-Tytell m.
New York City m.
Nicolle-Novy-MacNeal medium culture
NNN culture m.
nonionic contrast m.
nonionic dimer contrast m.
nutrient sporulation m.
outgrowth m.
oxidation-fermentation basal m.
Pantopaque contrast m.
peptone, glucose, and yeast extract m.
pokeweed activated spleen conditioned m.
potassium-containing minimal capacitation m.
prereduced anaerobically sterilized m.
m. pressure liquid chromatography
primary enrichment m.
proteose-yeast castione m.
protoplast maintenance m.
purple agarbase m.
radiographic contrast m.
radiopaque contrast m.
m. rales
m. range
reinforced clostridial m.
replacement culture m.
Roux conditioned m.
Salpix contrast m.
secondary enrichment m.
selective broth m.
Sertoli cell culture m.
serum, casein, glucose, yeast extract m.
Sinografin contrast m.
soluble in alkaline m.
soluble cytotoxic m.
soybean-casein digest m.
spleen cell conditioned m.
staphylococcus m.
sucrose m.
sulfide, indole, motility medium
supplemented Eagle minimal essential m.
synthetic medium old tuberculin trichloroacetic acid precipitated
tissue culture m.
transport m.
trypticase-peptone-glucose-yeast extract-trypsin medium
virus transport m.
Voges-Proskauer medium, test
m. voltage activity
m. yellow soft stools

medium-chain
m.-c. acyl-CoA dehydrogenase
m.-c. acyl-CoA dehydrogenase deficiency
m.-c. acyl-coenzyme A dehydrogenase
m.-c. fatty acid
m.-c. triglyceride
m.-c. triglyceride
m.-c. triglyceride oil

medi virus

Medlar body

Medpor

Medralone Injection

medroxyprogesterone
m. acetate
depot medroxyprogesterone acetate
m. injection

medulla
adrenal m.
m. of adrenal gland
anterior column of medulla oblongata
anterior median fissure of medulla oblongata
hemorrhage in m.
m. of kidney
m. lesion

medulla *(continued)*
m. of lymph node
microcystic disease of renal m.
nucleus arcuatus of medulla oblongata
m. oblongata
m. pons
pons and m.
rostral ventrolateral m.
ventrolateral m.

medullaris
artery of the conus m.
conus m.
low conus m.
low-placed conus m.

medullary
m. adenocarcinoma
adrenal medullary autograft
anatomic medullary locking
anatomic medullary locking hip system
anterior medullary velum
AO slotted medullary nail
m. arteries of brain
m. artery
ascending medullary vein thrombosis
atypical medullary carcinoma
autologous adrenal medullary tissue
autosomal dominant medullary cystic kidney disease
m. blood flow
m. body of cerebellum
m. body of vermis
m. bone
m. bone graft
m. bone infarct
m. bone pain
m. breast carcinoma
m. calcification
m. callus
m. canal
m. carcinoma
m. carcinoma of breast
m. carcinoma flush
m. carcinoma of thyroid
m. cavity
m. cell
m. center
m. chemoreceptor
m. chromaffinoma
closed medullary nailing
m. collecting duct
m. collecting tubule
m. cone
m. cords
cortical medullary junction
m. cyst
m. cystic disease
diamond-shaped medullary nail
m. dorsal horn
dorsal medullary reticular formation
m. duct epithelium
m. ducts of Bellini
m. dysplasia
familial medullary thyroid cancer
familial medullary thyroid carcinoma
m. fibrosarcoma
m. fixation
flexible medullary nail
flexible medullary reamer
fluted medullary rod
m. fold
m. glioma
m. groove
histiocytic medullary reticulosis
m. infarct
inner medullary collecting duct
lateral medullary infarction
lateral medullary syndrome
m. layers of thalamus
medial medullary infarction
m. artery of brain
m. carcinoma of the thyroid
minimal medullary concentration
multiple flexible medullary nail
m. nailing of tibia
m. necrosis
m. optic disease
m. parenchyma
patchy infiltration of medullary parenchyma
m. ray
m. recycling
relative medullary area of kidney
relative medullary thickness
m. renal carcinoma
m. reticulosis
m. sarcoma
m. sinus
m. sponge kidney
m. thick ascending limb
m. thick ascending limb of Henle
m. thymoma
m. thyroid cancer
m. thyroid carcinoma
uremic medullary cystic disease
m. venous malformation

medullated nerve fiber

medulloblastoma
melanotic m.
m. tumor

medulloepithelioma
adult m.
orbital m.

Medusa head

MedWatch form

Meek operation

Mees
M. line
M. stripe

Meesman
M. epithelial corneal dystrophy
M. juvenile epithelial dystrophy

meeting
community m.
M. Street School Screening Test

mefloquine prophylaxis

mega
m. ampere
m. cisterna magna

***Megabombus* sting**

megacolon
acquired functional m.
aganglionic m.
m. congenitum
m. dilatation
idiopathic m.
toxic m.

megacystic microcolon syndrome

megacystis-megaureter
m.-m. association
m.-m. syndrome

megaelectron volt

megaesophagus of achalasia

megakaryoblastic leukemia

megakaryocyte
m. colony-forming unit
colony-forming unit-granulocyte, erythrocyte, megakaryocyte, macrophage
m. colony-stimulating factor
m. growth and development factor
m. progenitor

megakaryocytic
m. aplasia
m. blastic phase
m. blood cell
idiopathic megakaryocytic aplasia

m. leukemia
m. marker
megaloblastic
m. anemia
m. anemia of pregnancy
m. crisis
m. erythropoiesis
megalocornea
m., developmental retardation, dysmorphic syndrome
megalocornea-mental retardation syndrome
megalocystis microcolon intestinal hypoperistalsis syndrome
megalocytic anemia
megalopia
m. hysterica
m. hysterics
***Megalopyge opercularis* sting**
megameatus-intact prepuce
meganewton per square meter
megaureter
m. classification
obstructive m.
megavitamin therapy
megavoltage
m. computed tomography
m. computed tomography-assisted stereotactic radiosurgery
m. computed tomography scanner
m. CT
m. CT-assisted stereotactic radiosurgery
m. CT scanner
m. external radiotherapy
m. machine
m. radiation
m. radiography
megavolt-ampere
megestrol acetate
meglumine
m. diatrizoate
m. diatrizoate contrast medium
m. diatrizoate enema study
meibomian
m. blepharitis
m. conjunctivitis
m. cyst
m. disease
m. duct
m. gland
m. gland carcinoma
m. gland dysfunction
m. gland expressor
m. gland obstruction
m. gland orifice metaplasia
m. secretion
m. sty
Meier-Gorlin syndrome
Meige
M. disease
M. syndrome
Meigs
M. capillary
M. pelvic lymphadenectomy
M. syndrome
Meigs-Kass syndrome
Meigs-Okabayashi procedure
Meigs-Werthein hysterectomy
Meinecke-Peper syndrome
Meinicke
M. test
M. turbidity reaction
meiosis
m. I, II
maternal meiosis I, II
oocyte m.
paternal meiosis I, II
meiosis-inducing substance
meiotic
m. division
m. drive
oocyte meiotic inhibitor
Meirowsky phenomenon
Meischer syndrome
Meissner
Auerbach and Meissner plexus
M. corpuscle
M. ganglion
M. plexus
Mel1a melatonin receptor
Mel1b melatonin receptor
melaleuca tree
melamine-formaldehyde resin
melancholia
affective m.
m. affective psychosis
agitated m.
m. attonita
melancholic
m. constitutional type
m. depression
m. feature
mood disorder with melancholic features
melanin
artificial m.
m. bleaching method
m. synthesis
m. transfer
melanin-concentrating hormone
melanin-like pigment
melanocortin
m. receptor isoform
melanocortin-2, -3, -4 receptor
melanocyte
m.-stimulating hormone-releasing hormone
m. release-inhibiting factor
m. release-inhibiting hormone
melanocyte-concentrating hormone
melanocyte-inhibiting
m.-i. factor
m.-i. hormone
melanocyte-releasing
m.-r. factor
m.-r. hormone
melanocyte-stimulating
m.-s. hormone
m.-s. hormone-inhibiting factor
m.-s. hormone-releasing factor
m.-s. hormone sequence
melanocytic
acquired melanocytic nevus
m. atypia
atypical melanocytic hyperplasia
atypical melanocytic nevus
congenital melanocytic nevus
m. conjunctival lesion
giant congenital melanocytic nevus
m. hamartoma
m. intraepidermal neoplasia
m. iris tumor
m. lesion
m. nevus
melanocytosis
meningeal m.
ocular m.
oculodermal m.
pagetoid m.
melanoderma
m. cachecticorum
parasitic m.
melanodermic leukodystrophy
melanoma
m. antigen-encoding gene family
m. antigen reacting to T cell

melanoma *(continued)*
m. antigen recognized by T cell
asymmetry, border, color, and diameter of m.
autologous melanoma system
m. cell
m. cell adhesion molecule
m. cell lysate
conventional cutaneous malignant m.
cutaneous malignant m.
cutaneous malignant melanoma of head and neck
desmoplastic neurotropic m.
elder malignant melanoma classification
epidermotropic metastatic malignant m.
m. of eyelid
familial atypical mole malignant m.
familial atypical multiple m.
familial atypical multiple-mole melanoma syndrome
m. growth-stimulating activity
Harding-Passey m.
hereditary cutaneous malignant m.
m. of iris
lentigo maligna m.
locally advanced m.
male genitalia m.
malignant m.
malignant choroidal m.
malignant lentigo m.
malignant melanoma of choroid
malignant melanoma in situ
MART-1 melanoma antigen
McLean classification of m.
m. metastasis
metastatic m.
metastatic malignant m.
minimal deviation m.
multiple primary m.
nail-apparatus m.
nevoid malignant m.
nodular m.
nodular malignant m.
ocular m.
primary cutaneous m.
primary malignant melanoma of the esophagus
m. in situ
m. specific antigen
superficial spreading m.
thick cutaneous m.
m. warning sign
m. whole-cell vaccine

melanoma-associated
m.-a. antigen
m.-a. antigen GD2
m.-a. antigen GD3
m.-a. antigen GM2
m.-a. gene
m.-a. retinopathy

melanoma/astrocytoma syndrome

melanomalytic glaucoma

melanonychia
longitudinal m.

melanophore-expanding principle

melanophore index

melanophore-stimulating hormone

melanosis
m. bulbi
m. cachecticorum
m. circumscripta precancerosa
m. coli
diabetic melanosis of cornea
laryngeal m.
neonatal pustular m.
neurocutaneous m.
neurocutaneous melanosis syndrome
m. oculi
oculodermal m.
primary acquired m.
Riehl m.
m. sclerae
transient neonatal pustular m.

melanosome
giant m.
giant pigment m.

melanotic
m. ameloblastoma
m. cancer
m. carcinoma
m. freckle
m. freckle of Hutchinson
m. lesion
m. medulloblastoma
m. melanoma
m. neuroectodermal tumor
m. neuroectodermal tumor of infancy
m. pigment
m. progonoma
m. protoporphyria
m. prurigo of Hebra
m. prurigo of Pierini
m. sarcoma
m. schwannoma
m. whitlow

melanotropic cell

melanotropin
m. release-inhibiting hormone

melanotropin release-inhibiting hormone

melanotropin-releasing hormone

Melao virus

melas
icterus m.

melasma
m. gravidarum
m. suprarenale
m. universale

Melastatin
M. gene
M. test kit

melatonin
dim light melatonin onset
Mel1a melatonin receptor
Mel1b melatonin receptor
m. rhythm
m. secretion

Melcher acid-soluble fraction

***Meleagris* adenovirus 1–3**

Meleda
M. disease
mal de M.

melena
hematemesis and m.
m., hematochezia or hematemesis
m. neonatorum
m. spuria
m. vera

Meleney
M. chronic undermining ulcer
M. synergistic gangrene
M. ulcer

melenic stool

melezitose fermentation test

melibiose fermentation test

Melinck-Needles syndrome

melioidosis *Pseudomonas pseudomallei* vaccine

Melkersson-Rosenthal syndrome

Meller operation

mellifera
Apis mellifera sting

mellitus
adult-onset diabetes m.
atypical diabetes m.

autoimmune diabetes m.
autosomal dominant diabetes m.
diabetes insipidus, diabetes mellitus, progressive bilateral optic atrophy, and sensorineural deafness
diabetes mellitus ketoacidosis
diabetes mellitus out of control
diabetes mellitus, pregnancy classification, class A–F
diabetes mellitus type 1
diabetes mellitus type 2
gestational diabetes m.
gestational diabetes mellitus, diet controlled, type 2
gestational diabetes mellitus, insulin controlled, type 1
infant of mother with gestational diabetes m.
insulin-dependent diabetes m.
insulin-independent diabetes m.
insulin-resistant diabetes m.
juvenile diabetes m.
juvenile-onset diabetes m.
malnutrition-related diabetes m.
maturity-onset diabetes m.
multiple epiphysial dysplasia-early onset diabetes mellitus syndrome
neonatal diabetes m.
new-onset diabetes m.
non-insulin-dependent diabetes m.
non-insulin-dependent diabetes mellitus type 1, 2
obese type 2 noninsulin-dependent diabetes m.
overt insulin-dependent diabetes m.
posttransplant diabetes m.
transient neonatal diabetes m.
type 1, 2 diabetes m.

Melnick

Melnick-Fraser syndrome

Melnick-Needles

M.-N. disease
M.-N. syndrome

melodic intonation therapy

melolabial flap

melting

m. point
m. temperature

Meltzer-Lyon test

Melzer reagent

member

adolescent gang m.
m. of a coven
cult m.
family member presence
m. months
per member per month
per member per year

membrana

m. abdominis
m. adventitia
m. atlantooccipitalis anterior
m. atlantooccipitalis posterior
m. basilaris
m. capsularis
m. capsularis lentis posterior
m. capsulopupillaris
m. cerebri
m. choriocapillaris
m. cordis
m. eboris
m. eboris of Kölliker
m. flaccida
m. fusca
m. granulosa
m. granulosa cell
m. granulosa externa
m. limitans
m. nictitans
m. pupillaris
m. ruyschiana
m. tympani
m. vitrea

membranae

limbus membranae tympani

membrane

adult familial hyaline membrane disease
alveolar basement m.
alveolar capillary m.
alveolar-capillary membrane permeability
alveolar wall basement m.
anterior atlantooccipital m.
anterior basement membrane dystrophy
anterior hyaloid m.
anterior membrane dystrophy
anterior recess of tympanic m.
antibasement membrane antibody
antibasement membrane antibody-induced glomerulonephritis
antibasement membrane nephritis
antibasement membrane zone autoantibody
antiepithelial membrane antigen antibody
m. antigen
antiglomerular basement m.
antiglomerular basement membrane antibody
antiglomerular basement membrane antibody disease
antiglomerular basement membrane antibody nephritis
antiglomerular basement membrane disease
antiglomerular basement membrane glomerulonephritis
antithyroid plasma membrane antibody
antitubular basement m.
antitubular basement membrane antibody
apical membrane of proximal convoluted tubule cell
artificial membrane rupture
artificial rupture of m.'s
asymmetric unit m.
atlantooccipital anterior m.
m. attack complex
basal m.
basement m.
basement membrane thickness
basement membrane zone
basilar m.
basolateral m.
benign mucous membrane pemphigoid
bilateral tympanic m.'s
bilayer lipid m.
bimolecular liquid m.
black lipid m.
m. bleb formation
m. bone
m. of bone
m. of brain
m. bridge
brush border m.
bulging tympanic m.
m. capacitance
capillary basement m.
capillary basement membrane thickness
capillary basement membrane width
m. catheter technique
cell m.
m. of cervix uterus
chorioallantoic m.
choroidal neovascular m.
chronic benign mucous membrane pemphigus
clinical hyaline membrane disease
m. closure time
m. coating granule

membrane *(continued)*
m. cofactor protein
collagenase soluble glomerular basement m.
m. component of diffusion
m. current
cytoplasmic m.
demarcation membrane system
Descemet m.
m. of Descemet
m. diffusing capacity
disciform macular degeneration with subretinal neovascular m.
double m.
m. effect
electrical membrane property
epiretinal m.
epiretinal membrane proliferation
epithelial membrane antigen
erythrocyte membrane protein
m. excitability
m. expansion theory
extensive hyaline membrane disease
external elastic m.
external limiting m.
external membrane protein
extracorporeal membrane oxygenation
extracorporeal membrane oxygenation affecting cognitive function
extracorporeal membrane oxygenator
feline oncornavirus-associated cell membrane antigen
fibrocartilaginous ring of tympanic m.
m. filter
m. filter technique
m. filtration method
fluorescent antibody to membrane antigen test
m. focal coli broth
glomerular basement m.
glomerular basement membrane disease
glomerular membrane antibodies
m. glycoprotein IB/IX
Gore-Tex augmentation m.
m. granulosa
Henle elastic m.
Henle fenestrated m.
Herpesvirus hominis membrane antigen
heterogeneous cation-exchange m.
high-performance membrane chromatography
hippocampal synaptic plasma m.
human mammary carcinoma cell membrane proteinase
human mesothelial cell m.
human T-cell leukemia virus-associated membrane antigen
hyaline membranes lining alveolar space
hyaline membrane disease
hydration of mucous m.'s
hyperplastic persistent pupillary m.
idiopathic epiretinal m.
m. immunoglobulin
indirect membrane immunofluorescence
inner m.
m. intact
m. integral protein
internal elastic m.
internal limiting m.
interosseous m.
intracytoplasmic m.
intrauterine m.
m. of joint
latent membrane protein-1
lesion on erythrocyte cell membrane at the site of complement fixation
limbus of tympanic m.
limiting membrane of neural tube
limiting membrane of retina
m. lipid cell
liquid m.
lithium action on m.'s
liver cell membrane autoantibody
liver membrane antibody
liver plasma m.
liver-specific membrane lipoprotein
low-flux cellulose-based m.
low-flux dialysis m.
luminal brush-border m.
lung basement m.
lymphocyte detected membrane antigen
lymphocyte-detected membrane antigen
lysosomal membrane glycoprotein-1
lysosomal membrane glycoprotein-2
macular epiretinal m.
major outer membrane protein
mammalian cell m.
m. marker
microvillous m.
milk fat globule m.
mitochondrial membrane potential
monoclonal antiepithelial membrane antigen
mucosal membrane graft
mucous m.
mucous membrane chancre
mucous membrane chancroid
mucous membrane exposure
mucous membrane graft
mucous membrane pemphigoid
mucous membrane provocation
mucous membrane ulceration
mucous membrane wart
mucous membranes moist
mucus membranes dry
muscle capillary basement m.
muscle capillary basement membrane thickening
nasal mucous m.
neonatal extracorporal membrane oxygenation
neonatal hyaline membrane disease
neovascular m.
nephrotoxic antiglomerular basement membrane antibody nephritis
nictitating m.
nictitating membrane response
nuclear m.
nuclear membrane abnormality
oblique cord of interosseous membrane of forearm
ocular-mucous membrane syndrome
oculomucous membrane syndrome
onion skin-like m.
opioid cell membrane receptor
oral mucous m.
oral mucous membrane dry
oral mucous membrane graft
oral mucous membrane moist
oral mucous membrane pink
oral mucous membrane pink and moist
osteocytic membrane system
otitis media with perforated tympanic m.
outer acrosomal m.
outer limiting m.
outer membrane protein
outer mitochondrial m.
parathyroid cell m.
m. peeler-cutter

m. peeling
perforated tympanic m.
perforation of tympanic m.
pericolic membrane syndrome
perifoveolar vitreoglial m.
periodontal m.
peripheral basement m.
m. permeability
persistent pupillary m.
persistent pupillary membrane remnant
photoreceptor m.
pigmented pupillary m.
pink, moist, and warm mucous membranes
placental m.'s
plasma m.
plasma membrane fatty acid binding protein
platelet m.
pleural membrane lining
posterior hyaloid m.
m. potential difference
prelabor rupture of the m.'s
prematurely ruptured m.
premature rupture of fetal m.'s
preterm premature rupture of m.'s
preterm spontaneous rupture of m.'s
prolonged premature rupture of m.'s
prolonged rupture of fetal m.'s
prostate-specific m.
m. protein
pulmonary endothelial m.
pulmonary hyaline m.
pulmonary hypoplasia membrane disease
reciprocal tension m.
renal glomerular basement membrane thickness
resting membrane potential
rod disc m.
m. ruffling
m. rupture
rupture of m.'s
ruptured m.'s
ruptured tympanic m.
Sarns membrane oxygenator
Schwann cell m.
self-contained enzymatic membrane immunoassay
senile retinal neovascular m.
serous m.
spontaneous premature rupture of m.'s
m. stabilizing action
streptococcal cell m.
m. stripping
subbasement m.
subepithelial basement m.
subretinal neovascular m.
subsynaptic m.
surface-connecting m.
surface membrane immunoglobulin
synaptic m.
synaptic plasma m.
syncytiotrophoblast microvillar plasma m.
syncytiovascular m.
synovial m.
synovial membrane of joint
tectorial m.
m. thickness
thin basement m.
thin basement membrane disease
m. transport defect
tubular basement m.
tympanic m.
tympanic membrane gray
tympanic membrane inflammation
tympanic membrane injected
tympanic membrane perforation
tympanic membrane thermometer
m. type 1–6
urothelial basement m.
vestibular m.
yellow hyaline membrane disease

membrane-associated estrogen receptor

membrane-bound
m.-b. membrane-type metalloproteinase
m.-b. receptor
m.-b. receptor molecule

membrane-coating granule

membrane-free hemolysate

membrane-spanning domain

membrane-stabilizing activity

membranolytic attack complex

membranoproliferative
chronic membranoproliferative glomerulonephritis
m. glomerulonephritis type I, II

membranous
m. acute inflammation
m. adhesion
m. ampulla
m. ampullae of the semicircular duct
aneurysm of membranous ventricular septum
m. aplasia cutis
m. bone
m. bronchiole
m. canal
m. cataract
chronic membranous glomerulonephritis
m. cochlea
m. conjunctivitis
m. croup
m. cytoplasmic body
m. deciduitis
m. desquamation
m. dysmenorrhea
m. gingivostomatitis
m. glomerulonephritis
m. glomerulonephropathy
m. glomerulopathy
high membranous interventricular septum
m. labyrinth
m. lamina of cartilage of pharyngotympanic auditory plate
m. laryngotracheobronchitis
m. layer
m. layer of subcutaneous tissue of abdomen
m. layer of superficial fascia
m. layer of superficial fascia of perineum
m. limb of semicircular duct
m. lining
m. lipodystrophy
m. lupus nephritis
m. lupus nephropathy
m. nephropathy
m. neuropathy
m. obstruction of the inferior vena cava
m. pattern
m. rhinitis
m. septum
m. stenosis
m. stomatitis
m. twins
m. urethra

memorandum of understanding

Memorial
M. Delirium Assessment Scale
M. dimension averaging method
M. Pain Assessment Card
M. Sloan-Kettering Cancer Center
M. Sloan-Kettering protocol
M. Sloan-Kettering staging of childhood lymphoma

Memorial *(continued)*
M. Symptom Assessment Scale-Physical
M. Symptom Assessment Scale-Psychological
M. University of Newfoundland Scale of Happiness

memory
m. ability
m. afterimage
age-associated memory impairment
age-related memory impairment
alteration of memory structure
amnesia loss of m.
m. amplification
anterograde loss of m.
anterograde memory interference
M. Assessment Scale
auditory memory span
auditory verbal m.
m. bias
m. B, T cell
m. buffer
Buschke M. Test
m. cell
concentration and m.
m. consolidation
continuous and confirmed memories of abuse
Continuous Visual M. Test
cortical mapping of memory function
m. defect
m. for design
M. for Designs test
m. deterioration
m. deviation quotient
m. difficulty
m. disability
m. disorder
m. distortion
m. disturbance
dynamic random access m.
m. dysfunction
early m.
m. by emotion
m. encoding
erasable programmable read-only m.
m. falsification
m. function
m. function deficit
functioning, reasoning, orientation, memory, arithmetic, judgment, and emotion
m. gap
gradual memory loss
Graham-Kendall M. for Designs Test
m. guidance saccade test
m. hallucination
m. illusion
m. image
immediate auditory m.
immediate visual m.
m. impaired assisted living
impaired memory for recent events
impaired memory of unknown cause
impaired short-term m.
m. impairment
impairment of m.
m.'s of incest
m. index
information memory concentration
intellectual function or m.
Inventory of Childhood Memories and Imaginings
involuntary intrusive m.'s
juvenile memory deficit
long-lived memory T cell
long-term m.
long-term associative m.
long-term declarative m.
loss of biographical m.
m. loss from anemia
loss of recent memory, confusion and poor judgment
magnetic core m.
McCarthy M. Scale
m., and distortion hypnosis
Monotic Word M. Test
Oliphant Auditory Discrimination M. Test
m. phenomenon
poor attention and m.
programmable read-only m.
random-access m.
read-only m.
recent event m.
recent memory impairment and confabulation
Revised M. and Behavior Problems Checklist
Rivermead Behavioral M. Test
shape memory alloy
short-term m.
Spatial Orientation M. Test
static random access m.
m. for symbolic unit
m. T cell
unverifiable memories of incest
visual memory span
Visual M. Score
Wechsler M. Scale
Wide Range Assessment of M. and Learning

men
market men disease
sexually active homosexual m.
m. who have sex with men
m. and women

***MEN1* gene**

menadione
Penassay broth plus glucose plus m.

menaquinone-6, -7

menaquinone vitamin K_2

menarche
m. factor
onset of m.

Mendel
M. dorsal foot reflex
M. first law
M. second law

mendelian
m. character
m. genetic disorder
m. genetics
m. inheritance
M. Inheritance in Man
m. syndrome
m. trait

Mendelson syndrome

Ménétrier disease

Menge pessary

Mengert
M. index
M. shock syndrome

Menghini biopsy technique

Mengo
M. encephalitis
M. virus

menhaden oil

Ménière
M. disease
M. syndrome
M. vertigo

meningea
m. anterior
arteria meningea anterior
arteria meningea media
arteria meningea posterior

meningeal
m. angiomatosis
anterior meningeal artery

anterior meningeal branch of anterior ethmoidal artery
m. anthrax
m. artery
m. artery groove
aseptic meningeal reaction
m. biopsy
m. branch
m. branch of cavernous part of internal carotid artery
m. branch of cerebral part of internal carotid artery
m. branch of intracranial part of vertebral artery
m. branch of mandibular nerve
m. branch of maxillary nerve
m. branch of occipital artery
m. branch of ophthalmic nerve
m. branch of spinal nerve
m. branch of vagus nerve
m. capillary angiomatosis
m. carcinoma
m. carcinomatosis
m. cell
m. cell tumor
m. diverticulum
m. fibrosis
m. filament
m. gliomatosis
m. granule
m. groove
m. headache
hemangioma of meningeal vessels
m. hemangiopericytoma
m. hemorrhage
m. hernia
m. hydrops
hypertensive meningeal hydrops
m. inflammation
m. involvement
m. irritation
m. layer of dura mater
m. leukemia
m. malignancy
m. melanocytosis
orbital branch of middle meningeal artery
parietal branch of middle meningeal artery
petrosal branch of middle meningeal artery
m. plague
m. prophylaxis
m. relapse
m. sarcoma
m. sign
m. stage
m. tick-borne encephalitis

menin gene

meninges (*pl. of* meninx)

meningioma
angioblastic m.
angiomatous m.
angioplastic m.
angle m.
atypical m.
m. of cribriform plate
m. en plaque
m. formation
m. growth
nerve sheath m.
ocular m.
olfactory groove m.
oncocytic m.
optic nerve sheath m.
orbital m.
parasagittal m.
parasellar m.
perioptic sheath m.
pituitary m.
psammomatous m.

meningitic
m. hydrocephalus
m. streak

meningitis
acute aseptic m.
acute aseptic meningitis syndrome
acute bacterial m.
acute cerebrospinal m.
AIDS-related cryptococcal m.
AIDS-related lymphomatous m.
aseptic meningitis syndrome
aseptic uremic m.
bacterial m.
m. of the base
m. carcinomatosa
cerebrospinal m.
coccidioidal m.
m. or encephalitis, metabolic, Reye syndrome
Gram-negative bacillary m.
group B streptococcal m.
localized tuberculous m.
meningococcic m.
m. necrotoxica reactiva
nosocomial bacterial m.
posttraumatic m.
thyroxine-binding m.
tuberculous m.

meningocele
anterior sacral m.
anterior thoracic m.
atretic m.
lumbar m.

meningococcal
m. arthritis
m. bacteremia
m. carrier state
m. conjugate
m. conjunctivitis
m. disease
m. embolus
m. endotoxin
Glasgow M. Septicemia Prognostic Score
m. meningitis
m. multifocal osteomyelitis
m. *Neisseria meningitidis* serogroups unspecified vaccine
m. polysaccharide
m. polysaccharide vaccine
m. sepsis
m. septicemia
serogroup C meningococcal vaccine
m. vaccine

meningococcic meningitis

***Meningococcus* vaccine**

meningocutaneous angiomatosis

meningoencephalitic stage

meningoencephalitis
aseptic m.
biundulant m.
diphasic m.
Frühsommer m.
nonvasculitic autoimmune inflammatory m.
primary amebic m.
m. syndrome

meningohypophyseal
m. artery
m. branch
m. trunk

meningooculofacial angiomatosis

meningothelial
m. appearance
m. arachnoid cell

meningotyphoid fever

meningovascular
m. involvement
m. neurosyphilis
m. syndrome
m. syphilis

meninx, pl. **meninges**
meninges of brain
m. fibrosa

meniscal
anterior horn meniscal tear
anterior oblique meniscal tear
m. aponeurosis
m. arrow
autogenous meniscal cartilage replantation
m. autograft transplantation
m. cleft
m. cyst
m. degeneration
m. excision
m. fibrocartilage
m. flounce
m. injury
m. tear
m. tearing

meniscectomy
lateral m.
medial m.
partial m.

meniscocapsular attachment

meniscocytic anemia

meniscofemoral
anterior meniscofemoral ligament
m. attachment
m. capsule

meniscoid entrapment

meniscotibial
m. attachment
m. capsule

meniscus
m. of acromioclavicular joint
articular m.
m. articularis
bucket-handle meniscus tear
bucket-handle tear of m.
m. concave lens
detachment of medial m.
m. floater
m. forceps
frayed m.
fraying of m.
m. graft
m. homolog
m. hook
m. of knee
lateral m.
m. lateralis
medial m.
medial meniscus detachment
negative m.
negative meniscus lens
periscopic m.
posterior horn of medial m.
slipped m.
m. tear
torn lateral m.
torn medial m.

Menkes
M. disease
M. disease gene
M. kinky hair
M. kinky hair syndrome
M. syndrome

Menkes-Kaplan syndrome

menopausal
m. depression
m. distress
m. estrogen
m. estrogen replacement therapy
m. flushing
m. gonadotropin
m. hot flash
human menopausal gonadotropin
patient is m.
m. symptom
m. syndrome
m. urinary gonadotropin

menopause
adjustment reaction of m.
onset of m.
premature m.
surgical m.

MenPS vaccine

menses
absent m.
irregular m.
m. [L. *catamenia*]
oligomenorrhea with anovulatory m.
onset of m.
m. phase

Mensor-Scheck hanging hip operation

menstrual
absence of menstrual periods
absent menstrual period from diabetes
m. acne
m. age
m. aspiration
m. blood loss
cessation of menstrual cycle
m. colic
m. cramp
m. cycle
m. cycle hemodynamic response
m. cycle induction
m. cycle regulation
m. cycle resumption
date of last menstrual period
m. dermatosis
diarrhea with menstrual cramps
M. Distress Management Questionnaire
m. edema
m. endometrium
m. epilepsy
m. extraction
m. extraction abortion
first day of last menstrual period
first menstrual period
m. flow
m. formula
m. function
heavy menstrual flow
heavy menstrual periods
heavy menstrual periods from anemia
m. history
m. irregularity
irregular menstrual cycle
irregular menstrual period
m. leukorrhea
mean menstrual cycle hematocrit
m. migraine
m. molimina
ovulatory menstrual cycle
m. pain
past menstrual period
m. pattern
m. period
m. phase
m. reflux
scanty menstrual flow
m. sclerosis
m. state
m. toxic shock syndrome

menstruation
anovular m.
m. induction
onset of early m.

mental
m. aberration
m. ability
m. abnormality
m. abuse
accelerated mental processes
m. act
m. activity
m. acuity
acute change in mental status
M. Adjustment to Cancer scale
affective schematic mental model
affect-related schematic mental model
m. age

m. agility
m. agitation
agonadism, mental retardation, short stature, retarded bone age syndrome
m. agraphia
alcoholic organic mental disorder
alcohol-induced organic mental syndrome
m. alertness
alopecia, contracture, dwarfism, mental retardation syndrome
alopecia, mental retardation, epilepsy, microcephaly syndrome
alpha-thalassemia mental retardation
altered mental state
altered mental status
M. Alternation Test
m. anesthesia
aniridia, ambiguous genitalia, mental retardation
aniridia, ambiguous genitalia, mental retardation triad syndrome
anxiety-related mental disorder
aortic arch anomaly-peculiar facies mental retardation syndrome
aortic stenosis, corneal clouding, growth and mental retardation syndrome
m. apparatus
m. arithmetic test
m. arousal
m. artery
m. asthenia
m. asymmetry
m. ataxia
m. audition
m. blind spot
m. block
m. block injection
brachydactyly, mesomelia, mental retardation, aortic dilation, mitral valve prolapse, characteristic facies syndrome
m. branch
m. branch of inferior alveolar artery
m. branch of mental nerve
Brief Neuropsychological Mental Status Examination
California Test of M. Maturity-Short Form
Cambridge M. Disorders in Elderly Examination
m. canal
cannabis-induced mental changes
cannabis organic mental disorder
m. capacity
m. capacity evaluation
cardiac rehabilitation mental stress
cataract, hypertrichosis, mental retardation
caudal appendage, short terminal phalanges, deafness, cryptorchidism, mental retardation syndrome
Charcot-Marie-Tooth syndrome, X-linked type II with deafness and mental retardation
chemical dependency and mental illness
m. chemistry
chronic organic mental syndrome
m. chronometry
m. claudication
clearing of mental symptoms
m. clouding
coloboma, heart anomaly, ichthyosis, mental retardation, and ear abnormality syndrome
Columbia M. Maturity Scale
community-based mental health treatment
community mental health center
comorbidity of mental disorder
comorbid mental disorder
m. competence
m. competency
complexity of mental processes
M. Component Summary
comprehensive mental health
concentrated mental activity
m. concept
m. confusion
congenital cataracts, sensorineural deafness, Down syndrome facial appearance, short stature, mental retardation syndrome
congenital emphysema, cryptorchidism, penoscrotal web, deafness, mental retardation syndrome
conscious mental control
m. control
m. coprolalia
m. data
deafness, onychoosteodystrophy, and mental retardation syndrome
decline in mental function
m. defect
m. deficiency
m. deficiency, spasticity, congenital ichthyosis syndrome
m. deficit
m. degradation
m. depression
m. derangement
m. deterioration
M. Deterioration Battery
m. development
m. development index
m. disability
disabling mental illness
m. discipline
m. disease
dislocated elbow, bowed tibiae, scoliosis, deafness, cataract, microcephaly, mental retardation syndrome
m. disorder
m. disorder due to alcoholism
m. disorder due to a general medical condition
m. disorganization
distal arthrogryposis, hypopituitarism, mental retardation, facial anomalies syndrome
m. distress
m. disturbance
disturbance of mental equilibrium
m. dynamism
m. eclipse
ectodermal dysplasia, cleft lip and palate, mental retardation, syndactyly syndrome I, II
effective mental health care
m. ego
employee mental illness
m. energy
m. evolution
m. examination
m. excitement
m. exercise
m. exhaustion
m. extraoral radiography
facial dysplasia, hyperextensibility of joints, clinodactyly, growth retardation, mental retardation syndrome
m. faculty
family history of mental illness
m. fatigue
m. flexibility
fluctuating mental status
m. fog
m. foramen
fragile site mental retardation 1

mental *(continued)*
fragile site mental retardation 2
fragile X mental retardation protein
m. function
general mental health
gingival fibromatosis, hypertrichosis, cherubism, mental retardation, epilepsy syndrome
gonadal failure, short stature, mitral valve prolapse, mental retardation syndrome
goniodysgenesis, mental retardation, short stature
gradual loss of mental faculties
Griffiths M. Developmental Scale
m. growth
m. and growth retardation-amblyopia syndrome
m. handicap
m. healing
m. health
m. health advocate
M. Health Association
m. health benefit
m. health care
m. health care professional
m. health care unit
m. health center
m. health clinic
m. health community
m. health counseling
m. health counselor
m. health department
m. health expert
m. health hold
m. health inpatient
m. health insurance benefit
m. health law
m. health legislation
m. health and mental retardation
m. health patient
m. health practitioner
m. health professional
m. health provider
m. health reform
m. health resource
m. health status
m. health system
m. health treatment
m. health treatment facility
m. health worker
m. height
higher mental function
Hodkinson M. Test
m. hospital
m. hygiene
m. hygiene clinic
hypersomnia related to another mental disorder
idiopathic mental deficiency
m. illness
m. image
m. imagery
impaired mental functioning
m. impairment
m. impression
m. inactivity
increased mental tension
m. inhibition level
m. inquest warrant
insomnia related to mental disorder
m. institution
insulin-resistant diabetes, acanthosis nigricans, hypogonadism pigmentary retinopathy, deafness, mental retardation syndrome
level and degree of mental illness
macrocephaly, facial abnormalities, disproportionate tall stature mental retardation syndrome
major mental illness
managed mental health
mandated mental health coverage
M. Measurements Yearbook
median cleft upper lip, mental retardation, pugilistic facies syndrome
m. Health Early Intervention, Treatment, and Prevention Act of 2000
m. Health Parity Act of 1998
Merrill-Palmer Scale of M. Tests
Methods for Epidemiology of Child and Adolescent M. Disorders
microcephaly, mental retardation, cataract, hypogonadism syndrome
microcephaly, mental retardation, retinopathy syndrome
microcephaly, mild mental retardation, short stature, skeletal anomalies syndrome
microcephaly, sparse hair, mental retardation, seizures syndrome
mixed sclerosing bone dysplasia, small stature, seizures, mental retardation syndrome
moderate mental retardation
modified version of the mini mental status examination
motor-sensory neuropathy, X-linked Type II, with deafness and mental retardation
multiple exostosis mental retardation syndrome
nasal hypoplasia, peripheral dysostosis, mental retardation syndrome
National M. Health Association
National Institute of M. Health
National Institute of M. Health Diagnostic Interview Schedule
National Institute of M. Health-Global Obsessive Compulsive Scale
no mental illness
nonprogressive cerebellar disorder with mental retardation
nonspecific mental retardation
Northern epilepsy with mental retardation
obesity, short stature, mental deficiency, hypogonadism, micropenis, finger contracture, cleft lip-palate syndrome
organic mental disorder
Otis-Lennon M. Ability Test
Otis Quick Scoring M. Abilities Test
parietal foramina, brachymicrocephaly, mental retardation syndrome
peripheral dysostosis, nail hypoplasia, mental retardation syndrome
persistent mental illness
petition of mental illness
m. and physical retardation, speech disorders, peculiar facies syndrome
plea of mental incompetence
positive mental attitude
prevention of mental illness
previously unrecognized mental illness
Primary M. Abilities Test
Primary Care Evaluation of M. Disorders
primary mental ability
profound mental retardation
m. retardation
m. retardation-adducted thumbs syndrome
m. retardation, ataxia, hypotonia, hypogonadism, retinal dystrophy syndrome

m. retardation, blepharonasofacial abnormalities, hand malformations syndrome
m. retardation, cerebral palsy
m. retardation-clasped thumb syndrome
m. retardation, coarse face, microcephaly, epilepsy, skeletal abnormalities syndrome
m. retardation, coarse facies, epilepsy, joint contracture syndrome
m. retardation, congenital contracture, low fingertip arches syndrome
m. retardation, congenital heart disease, blepharophimosis, blepharoptosis, hypoplastic teeth
M. Retardation and Development Disabilities
m. retardation-distal arthrogryposis syndrome
m. retardation, dysmorphism, cerebral atrophy syndrome
m. retardation, dystonic movements, ataxia, seizures syndrome
m. retardation, epilepsy, short stature, skeletal dysplasia syndrome
m. retardation, facial anomalies, hypopituitarism, distal arthrogryposis syndrome
m. retardation, gynecomastia, obesity syndrome
m. retardation, hearing impairment, distinct facies, skeletal anomalies syndrome
m. retardation, macroorchidism syndrome
m. retardation, microcephaly, blepharochalasis syndrome
m. retardation, mitral valve prolapse, characteristic face syndrome
m. retardation, optic atrophy, deafness, seizures syndrome
m. retardation, overgrowth, craniosynostosis, distal arthrogryposis, sacral dimple, joint laxity
m. retardation-overgrowth sequence
m. retardation-overgrowth syndrome
m. retardation, polydactyly, phalangeal hypoplasia, syndactyly, unusual face, uncombable hair
m. retardation, pre-and postnatal overgrowth, remarkable face, acanthosis nigricans syndrome
m. retardation-psoriasis syndrome
m. retardation, retinopathy, microcephaly syndrome
m. retardation, scapuloperoneal muscular dystrophy, lethal cardiomyopathy syndrome
m. retardation, short stature, hypertelorism syndrome
m. retardation, short stature, obesity, hypogonadism syndrome
m. retardation, skeletal dysplasia, abducens palsy syndrome
m. retardation-sparse hair syndrome
m. retardation, spasticity, distal transverse limb defects syndrome
m. retardation, spastic paraplegia, palmoplantar hyperkeratosis syndrome
m. retardation-spastic paraplegia syndrome
m. retardation, typical facies, aortic stenosis syndrome
m. scale
Scale for the Assessment of Unawareness of M. Disorder
severe mental illness
severe mental retardation
severe and persistent mental illness
Short Portable M. Status Questionnaire
slowness of mental action
state mental hospital
m. status change
m. status evaluation
m. status examination
M. Status Examination Record
m. status examination report
m. status, oriented
m. status questionnaire
m. status schedule
m. stress test
m. subnormality
treatment of mental illness
m. treatment rules
undifferentiated mental retardation
X-linked mental retardation-aphasia syndrome
X-linked mental retardation-blindness-deafness-multiple congenital anomalies syndrome
X-linked mental retardation, microphthalmia, microcornea, cataract, hypogenitalism-mental retardation-spasticity syndrome
X-linked mental retardation/multiple congenital anomaly
X-linked mental retardation, seizures, acquired microcephaly, agenesis of corpus callosum
X-linked mental retardation syndrome 1–6
X-linked mental retardation-fragile site 1, 2

mentale

mentalis
arteria m.
m. band
m. habit
ipsilateral mentalis muscle

mentality

mentally
chronically mentally ill
m. competent
conscious and mentally competent
m. defective
m. deficient
m. deranged
m. disabled
m. disordered sex offender
educable mentally handicapped
educable mentally retarded
educationally mentally handicapped
elderly and mentally infirm
guilty but mentally ill
m. handicapped
m. ill
m. ill chemical abuser
m. impaired
m. incompetent
National Alliance for the M. Ill
patient mentally alert
patient mentally ill
profoundly mentally retarded
m. retarded
m. retarded and developmentally disabled
severely mentally impaired
m. stable and oriented
trainable mentally retarded

Mentation
Maudsley Mentation Test

mentis

mentoanterior
left mentoanterior fetal position

mentoanterior *(continued)*
m. position
m. presentation
right mentoanterior fetal position

mentolabial furrow

mentolateral
right mentolateral fetal position

mentoposterior
left mentoposterior fetal position
persistent mentoposterior fetal position
m. position
m. presentation
right mentoposterior fetal position

Mentor
M. booklet
M. catheter
M. gun
M. pre-cut drain
M. wet-field electrocautery

mentotransverse
left mentotransverse fetal position
m. position
right mentotransverse position

mentum
m. anterior position
mandible m.
m. posterior fetal position
m. transverse position

menu
computer assisted menu planning

meperidine
m. analog
analog of m.
m. conscious sedation
m. hydrochloride
m. and promethazine

Mephyton Oral

mepivacaine intoxication

meralgia paresthetica

2-mercaptoethane
-m. sulfonate
-m. sulphonate sodium

2-mercaptoethanesulfonic acid

mercaptoimidazole

mercapturic acid pathway

Mercedes
M. cannula
M. pattern

Mercedes-Benz
M.-B. incision
M.-B. sign

Merchant
M. angle
M. congruence angle
M. and Dietz ankle score
M. view

Mercier
M. bar
median bar of M.

mercurial
m. behavior
m. diuretic
m. necrosis
m. stomatitis

mercuric
m. chloride
m. chloride-induced ARF
m. chloride-induced nephritis
m. chloride nephrotoxicity
m. cyanide
m. fixative
m. oxide

1-mercuri-2-hydroxypropane

mercurous chloride

mercury
alloy of m.
ammoniated m.
m. arc
m. arc lamp
m. artifact
m. assay
m. bichloride
m. biniodide
m. bougie
m. bougienage treatment
m. chloride
cold quartz mercury vapor lamp
m. deutoiodide
m. granuloma
m. hyperpigmentation
maternal mercury exposure
micrometer of m.
millimeters of m.
organic mercury poisoning
m. poisoning
m. pressure
m. sphygmomanometer
m. vapor poisoning

mercury-free vaccine

meridian
m. of cornea
extraordinary m.
m. of eyeball
propagated sensation along the m.
qigong meridian massage

meridional
m. aberration
m. amblyopia
m. balance
m. ciliary muscle fiber
m. cleavage
m. end-systolic stress
m. fibers
m. fibers of ciliary muscle
m. fold
m. implant
m. refractometer

Mering
von Mering reflex

merit
figure of m.

Merkel
M. cell
M. cell cancer
M. cell carcinoma
M. cell carcinoma cell line
M. cell neoplasm
M. cell tumor
M. corpuscle
M. filtrum ventriculi
M. fossa

Merkel-cell-neurite complex

Merle
M. d'Aubigné hip score
M. d'Aubigné and Postel hip rating scale

mermaid deformity

Mermet virus

Merocel
M. epistaxis packing
M. sponge
M. surgical spear

merocrine gland

meromyosin
heavy meromyosin of muscle
light molecular weight m.

merosin
m. deficiency
m. deficiency dystrophy

Merrill

Merrill-Palmer Scale of Mental Tests

Merrill program

mersalyl
m. acid
m. exchange assay
m. exchange method

mersalyl exchange assay

mersalyl exchange method
Merseburg triad
Mersilene
M. fascial strip
M. graft
M. mesh sling
M. suture
Mertens Visual Perception Test
merthiolate
m. formaldehyde solution
m., iodine, formaldehyde concentration
m., iodine, formaldehyde method
m., iodine, formaldehyde technique
m., iodine, formaldehyde technique
m., iodine, formalin solution
m., iodine, formaldehyde technique
merthiolate, iodine, formaldehyde method
Merzbacher-Pelizaeus disease
mesalamine enema
mesalamine-related lung toxicity
mesangial
m. angle
m. cell
m. cell proliferation
m. complex formation
m. deposit
diffuse mesangial hypercellularity
diffuse mesangial proliferation
diffuse mesangial sclerosis
m. glomerulonephritis
m. hypercellularity
m. immune injury
isolated diffuse mesangial sclerosis
m. lupus nephritis
m. matrix
murine mesangial cell
m. proliferation
m. proliferative glomerulonephritis
m. sclerosis
segmental mesangial hypercellularity
m. thickening
mesangiopathic glomerulonephritis
mesangioproliferative glomerulonephritis
mesatipellic pelvis
mescaline unit
mesectodermal dysplasia
mesencephali
aqueductus m.
mesencephalic
m. artery
m. central gray
m. cerebral lymphoma
m. cistern
m. cistern effacement
m. corticonuclear fiber
fetal mesencephalic tissue
m. flexure
m. hemorrhage
m. lesion
m. lid retraction
m. raphe
m. reticular formation
stereotactic mesencephalic tractotomy
m. tectum
mesencephalic-diencephalic junction
mesencephalon
m. aqueduct
m. lesion
mesenchymal
m. abnormality
benign mesenchymal tumor
m. bone tumor
m. cell
m. cells
m. change
m. chondrosarcoma
m. cleft
m. differentiation
m. dysgenesis
m. epithelium
m. hamartoma
human embryonic palatal mesenchymal cell
human mesenchymal stem cell
m. intimal cell
m. lesion
malignant mesenchymal tumor
mediastinal mesenchymal tumor
m. neoplasm
m. precursor
m. progenitor
m. progenitor cell
m. ridge
m. sex cord stromal tumor
m. stem cell
m. stromal cell
m. tissue
mesenchyme
Sertoli cell mesenchyme tumor
mesenterial Castleman lymphoma
mesenteric
acute mesenteric vascular insufficiency
m. adenitis
m. adenitis-ileitis complex
m. adenopathy
m. angiogram
m. angiography
anomalous mesenteric adhesion
aortic-superior mesenteric artery bypass
m. apoplexy
m. arcade
m. arterial embolism
m. arterial system
m. arterial thrombosis
m. arteriography
arteriosclerotic mesenteric vascular occlusive disease
m. arteriovenous fistula
m. artery
m. artery aneurysm
m. artery constriction
m. artery occlusion
m. artery syndrome
ascending branch of the inferior mesenteric artery
m. attachment
m. attachments of colon
Auerbach mesenteric plexus
m. blood flow
m. border
m. bypass graft
m. calcification
chronic mesenteric ischemia
m. circulation
m. collateral
m. cyst
m. defect
m. fibromatosis
m. gland
m. hematoma
m. hernia
inferior mesenteric artery
inferior mesenteric ganglion
inferior mesenteric vein
m. inflammatory venoocclusive disease
m. insufficiency
m. ischemia

mesenteric *(continued)*
m. lymphadenitis
m. lymph node
m. mass
m. microcirculation
middle group of mesenteric lymph node
narrow mesenteric stalk
nonocclusive mesenteric infarction
m. panniculitis
partial pressure of mesenteric venous carbon dioxide
m. phlegmon
recurrent mesenteric ischemia
m. root
shunt index via the inferior mesenteric vein
shunt index via superior mesenteric vein
m. stalk
superior m.
superior mesenteric artery blood flow
superior mesenteric artery blood velocity
superior mesenteric artery embolus
superior mesenteric artery occlusion
superior mesenteric artery syndrome
superior mesenteric ganglion
superior mesenteric vein
transient mesenteric ischemia
m. vascular occlusive disease
m. vasculitis
m. vein
m. vein thrombosis
m. venous thrombosis

mesenterica
arteria mesenterica superior
m. inferior
tabes m.

mesentericography

mesentericoparietal fossa

mesenteroaxial volvulus

mesentery
m. abscess
appendiceal m.
m. of appendix
m. of cecum
m. of lung
small intestine m.
soft tissue hemorrhage into m.
ventral m.

mesh
absorbable m.
m. erosion
fine mesh gauze
m. graft
m. grafting
m. graft urethroplasty
m. herniorrhaphy
intraperitoneal onlay mesh hernia repair
MacroPore distraction m.
Marlex m.
Mersilene mesh sling
moistened fine mesh gauze dressing
tantalum mesh graft
tantalum mesh implant material
titanium m.
wire mesh implant
wire mesh implant material

meshed ball implant

mesh graft urethroplasty

meshwork
posterior trabecular m.
trabecular m.

mesial
m. angle
m. angulation
anterior mesial temporal resection
m. aspect
m. aspect of temporal lobe
m. caries
m. cerebral structure
m. contact area
m. curvature
m. cusp ridge
m. developmental depression
m. displacement
m. distal
m. drift
m. epileptogenic cortex
m. hemisphere
m. incisal lingual surface
m. marginal developmental groove
m. marginal ridge
m., occlusal, distal
m. occlusal facial
m. occlusion
m. pit
m. temporal lobe
m. temporal sclerosis
m. triangular fossa

mesiobuccal
m. alveolus
m. canal
m. cusp
m. cusp ridge
m. developmental groove
m. root

mesiocervical

mesiodens-cataracts syndrome

mesiodistal
m. clasp
m. diameter of crown
m. fracture

mesiolabial bilobed transposition flap

mesiolingual
m. corner
m. cusp
m. cusp ridge
m. developmental groove
m. fossa

mesoatrial shunt

mesoblastic
congenital mesoblastic nephroma
m. nephroma
m. tissue

mesoblastoma ovarii

mesobrachyphalangy
microcephaly, mesobrachyphalangy, tracheoesophageal fistula syndrome

mesocaval
m. anastomosis
m. H-graft
m. H-graft shunt

mesocephalic hemianesthesia

mesocolic
m. band
m. hernia
m. lymph node

mesocolici
nodi lymphoidei m.

mesocolon
m. ascendens
ascending m.
sigmoid m.

mesocortical
m. dopamine pathway
m. dopaminergic system

mesodermal
axial mesodermal dysplasia complex
m. cell
m. core
m. dysgenesis
m. dysgenesis of anterior segment

m. dysplasia
ectodermal and mesodermal dysplasia with osseous involvement ectodermal dysplasia-central
m. heterotopia
malignant mixed mesodermal tumor
mixed mesodermal tumor
mixed ovarian mesodermal sarcoma
m. nevus
m. sarcoma
m. tumor

mesodermogenic neurosyphilis

mesodiencephalic junction

mesolateral fold

mesolimbic
m. dopamine
m. dopamine pathway
m. dopamine system
m. dopamine tract

mesomelia
brachydactyly, mesomelia, mental retardation, aortic dilation, mitral valve prolapse, characteristic facies syndrome
costovertebral segmentation defect with mesomelia syndrome

mesomelic
m. dwarfism
m. dwarfism-small genitalia syndrome
m. dysplasia
m. shortening

mesometanephric carcinoma

mesometric
m. dysplasia
m. pregnancy

meson
negative pi m.

mesonephric
m. adenocarcinoma
m. adenoma
m. carcinoma
m. cyst
m. duct
m. fold
m. rest
m. ridge
m. tubule

mesonephroid
m. clear cell carcinoma
m. tumor

mesopic perimetry

mesorectal
m. excision
m. lymph node
total mesorectal excision

mesoridazine besylate

mesostructure conjunction bar

mesothelial
m. cell
m. cell inclusion
m. cell layer
m. cyst
human mesothelial cell membrane
m. hyperplasia
peritoneal mesothelial cyst
pleural mesothelial cell
m. tissue

mesothelioma
atrioventricular nodal node m.
m. cancer
cystic m.
diffuse malignant m.
diffuse malignant pleural m.
localized fibrous m.
lymphohistiocytoid m.
malignant m.
malignant epithelioid m.
malignant mesothelioma of the tunica vaginalis
malignant papillary m.
malignant pleural m.

mesovarian
m. border of ovary
m. margin
m. margin of ovary

mesquite tree

message
competing m.
m. competition ratio
contralateral competing m.
end of m.
Impact Message Inventory
ipsilateral competing m.
transmitting electrochemical messages to the brain

message-2
testosterone repressed prostate m.

message competition ratio

messenger
external chemical m.
lithium action on first m.
lithium action on second m.
m. ribonucleic acid
m. ribonucleoprotein
m. ribonucleoprotein acid
m. RNA

messenger-like RNA

mesylate
m. salt
tirilazad m.

met
met gene
met protooncogene/oncogene

metabolic
m. aberration
m. abnormality
m. acidemia
m. acidosis
m. acidosis syndrome
m. action
m. activation
m. activity
m. activity factor
activity metabolic rate
m. alkalosis
m. alteration
amino acid metabolic disorder
anion gap metabolic acidosis
m. anomaly
m. anoxia
m. antagonism
m. antagonist
m. asymmetry
average daily metabolic rate
m. balance
m. balance of heart
basal metabolic rate
basic metabolic panel
basic metabolic profile
m. bone disease
m. bone disorder
m. bone series
m. bone survey
m. calculus
Candida metabolic antigen
m. capability
m. cardiomyopathy
cerebral metabolic function
cerebral metabolic rate
cerebral metabolic rate of glucose
cerebral metabolic rate of lactate
cerebral metabolic rate of oxygen
m. change
chronic metabolic acidosis
m. cirrhosis
m. clearance rate
m. coma
m. complication
m. condition
m. control
m. conversion
m. coronary dilation

metabolic *(continued)*
m. craniopathy
m. defect
m. dementia
m. derangement
m. detoxification
m. difference
m. disease
m. disease in newborn
m. disease organic psychosis
m. disorder
m. disorder screening
m. disorder with hepatic dysfunction
m. disorder with neurologic dysfunction
m. disturbance
m. dysperception
m. effect
m. and electrolyte disorder
m. emergency
m. encephalitis
m. encephalopathy
endocrine and m.
m., endocrine, and gastrointestinal
m., endocrine, and gastrointestinal disorders
m. energy
m. enthesopathy
Entner-Doudoroff metabolic pathway
m. equivalent
m. equivalent level
m. equivalent of task
m. error
ethanol metabolic rate
m. evaluation
fasting metabolic panel
flavin-containing mono-oxygenase metabolic system
m. headache
m. heat load stimulator
m. heat production
m. hemostasis
hyperchloremic metabolic acidosis
m. hypoglycemia
m. imbalance
m. increase
m. index
inherited metabolic disorder
m. liver disease
m. management
meningitis or encephalitis, metabolic, Reye syndrome
m., endocrine, and gastrointestinal
m. syndrome X
myocardial metabolic rate
myonephropathic metabolic syndrome
m. myopathy
National Institute of Arthritis and M. Diseases
nonunion gap metabolic acidosis
m. organ transplant complication
m. products test
regional cerebral metabolic rate for oxygen
m. remission
m. respiratory quotient
m. response
resting metabolic expenditure
resting metabolic rate
m. screening disorder
m. signal
somnolent metabolic rate
standardized metabolic rate
steroid metabolic clearance rate
m. stone workup
m. stress episode
m. study
m. syndrome cataract
m. test
m. toxemia of late pregnancy
toxic metabolic encephalopathy
toxic metabolic etiology
m. web
work metabolic rate

metabolic/endocrine

metabolic, endocrine, and gastrointestinal disorders

metabolism
absorption, distribution, metabolism, and excretion
amino acid m.
arachidonic acid m.
m. at rest
basal m.
bile salt m.
carbohydrate metabolism disorder
carbohydrate metabolism index
cerebral rate of glucose m.
m. disorder
divalent ion m.
essential metabolism ratio
first-pass m.
gastric first-pass metabolism
glucose m.
glucose metabolism in brain
hepatic m.
hepatic drug m.
inborn error of m.
m. inhibition test
m. in intraperitoneal chemotherapy
iron metabolism disease
lipid metabolism disorder
loss of energy m.
metal metabolism disorder
organic acid m.
peripheral thyroid hormone m.
respiratory m.
retinoic acid metabolism blocking agent

metabolite
arachidonic acid m.
cocaine metabolite assay
m. image
prostaglandin E m.
substituted m.

metabolizable
m. energy
total metabolizable energy

metabotropic
m. glutamate
m. glutamate receptor

metabotropic glutamate receptor

metacarpal
m. amputation
m. base
m. beak
m. block
m. bone
m. cortical density
dorsal interosseous metacarpal vein
m. fracture
m. hand
m. head
m. head fracture
m. index
m. ligament
neck of m.
perforating branch of palmar metacarpal artery
m. shortening

metacarpale

metacarpalia

metacarpalis
arteria metacarpalis palmaris

metacarpea
arteria metacarpea palmaris

metacarpi
musculus extensor ossis metacarpi pollicis

metacarpocarpal joint

metacarpophalangeae

metacarpophalangeal
m. arthroscopy

m. articulation
m. bone marrow development
m. dislocation
m. joint
m. joint subluxation
palmar ligament of metacarpophalangeal joint
m. profile

metacarpophalangeal joint subluxation

metacentric
m. chromosome
m. metaphase

metacercarial antigen

metacerebral giant cell

metachromatic
m. body
m. dye
m. granule
m. leukodystrophy

metachronous
m. adenoma
m. carcinoma
m. collagenous colitis
m. colon cancer
m. contralateral hernias
m. disease
m. lesion
m. leukemia
leukodystrophy
m. leukodystrophy
m. malignancy
m. metastasis
m. presentation
m. testicular germ cell tumor
m. tissue lesion

metaherpetic
m. keratitis
m. ulcer
m. ulceration of the cornea

metahypophysial diabetes

metal
m. alloy
m. base
m. base denture
base metal crown and bridge alloy
m. chelate complex
m. clamp
m. coil
m. crown
m. crown margin
m. dermatitis
m. endurance limit
m. failure
m. fatigue
ferromagnetic metal plate
m. foot plate
m. frame reinforced plastic bracket
m. fume fever
m. handle mixing spatula
hard metal disease
m. heart valve
heavy m.
heavy metal poisoning
heavy metal screen
heavy metal stain
m. hemi-toe implant
m. hyperpigmentation
immobilized metal affinity chromatography
m. intoxication
m. intoxification
Lipowitz m.
m. metabolism disorder
N-type metal oxide semiconductor
m. oxide semiconductor field effect transistor
paramagnetic m.
m. poisoning
m. suture material
trace metal elements injection
void metal composite
m. working fluid

metal-backed
m.-b. acetabular component
m.-b. acetabular cup

metal-catalyzed oxidative cleavage

metal-ceramic crown

metalinguistic assessment

metallic
anterior metallic fixation
m. artifact
m. bead
m. bead-chain cystourethrograph
m. bead-chain cystourethrography
m. biliary endoprosthesis
m. biliary stent
m. biliary stent migration
m. bond
m. cage
m. compound inhalation
m. cranioplasty
m. debris
m. density
m. distal end of tube
m. echo
m. embolus
m. foreign body
foreign body, m.
m. fragment
m. frontal needle
m. implant
open reduction metallic fixation
m. rale
self-expanding metallic stent
m. skin staple
m. taste

metalloendopeptidase
thermolysin-like m.

metallopeptidase
neutral m.

metallophilic
marginal metallophilic macrophage

metalloproteinase
extracellular matrix metalloproteinase inducer
matrix m.
matrix metalloproteinase inhibitor
matrix metalloproteinase inhibitor, marimastat
membrane-bound membrane-type m.
tissue inhibitor of m.

metalloproteinase-2
matrix m.

metalloproteinase-3
matrix m.

metalloproteinase-7
matrix m.

metalloproteinase-8
matrix m.

metalloproteinase-9
matrix m.

metalloproteinase-10
matrix m.

metalloproteinase-12
matrix m.

metalloproteinase-like, disintegrin-like, cysteine-rich protein

metalloproteinase-proteolytic enzyme

metalloproteinases-1

metal-on-metal hip replacement

metal-on-plastic hip replacement

metal-to-ligand charge transfer

metameric color

metamorphopsia varians

metamyelocyte cell

metanephric
m. adenofibroma
m. adenoma
m. blastema
m. bud
m. cap
m. diverticulum
m. duct

metanephrine assay

metaphase
m. cell
m. chromosome
metacentric m.

metaphoric dysplasia

metaphyseal

metaphyseal-diaphysial angle

metaphyseal lesion of distal femur

metaphyseal lucent band

metaphysial
m. abscess
m. abscess
m. aclasis
m. angiodysplasia
m. artery
m. aspiration
m. band
m. chondrodysplasia
m. chondrodysplasia
m. cortex
m. to diaphysial width ratio
m. dysostosis
m. dysplasia
m. dysplasia
m. exostosis
m. fibrous cortical defect
m. fibrous defect
m. fibrous defect
m. flaring
m. fracture
m. head resection with prosthesis
m. lesion
m. lesion of distal femur
m. lucent band
medial metaphyseal beak
m. sclerosis

metaphysis
m. angulation
autoparenchymatous m.
fibular m.
spondylar changes, nasal anomaly, striated m.'s

metaplasia
agnogenic myeloid m.
cardia-intestinal m.
meibomian gland orifice m.
mucinous columnar m.
myelofibrosis with myeloid m.
myeloid m.
myeloid metaplasia with myelofibrosis
myelosclerosis with myeloid m.
pancreatic acinar m.
polycythemia vera with myeloid m.
postpolycythemia myeloid m.
specialized intestinal m.
squamous m.

metaplastic
m. anemia
m. atrophic gastritis
autoimmune metaplastic atrophic gastritis
m. carcinoma
m. cell
m. columnar epithelium
environmental metaplastic atrophic gastritis
m. epithelial cell
m. epithelium
m. gastric fundic gland
m. mucus-secreting cell
m. pyloric gland

metapneumonic emphysema

metaproterenol inhaler

metasepithelial
ovarian epithelial m.

metastases
age, distant metastases, extent and size
age, metastases, extent and size risk criteria
at autopsy tumor, nodes, and m.
clinical staging of tumors, nodes, and metastases as determined by noninvasive examination
distant m.
freedom from m.
freedom from distant m.
free from distant m.
hepatosplenomegaly with liver m.
intrapulmonary nodal m.
local regional m.
lung m.
multiple brain m.
multiple synchronous subcutaneous m.
no evidence of distant m.
pathological tumor, nodes, metastases staging of cancer
primary tumor, regional lymph node, remote metastases classification, staging
tumor with lymph node m.

metastasis
aortic node m.
axillary lymph node m.
axillary nodal metastasis in breast carcinoma
carcinoma with m.
celiac lymph node m.
contralateral axillary m.
extrahepatic m.
m. gene
hemorrhagic tumor m.
hilar node m.
intramedullary spinal cord m.
leptomeningeal m.
lymph node m.
melanoma m.
m., age, completeness of resection, local invasion, and tumor size
miliary brain m.
MR discriminator of osseous m.
nodal metastasis in breast carcinoma
noncolorectal liver m.
occult bone m.
occult lymph node m.
ovarian cancer m.
parenchymal brain m.
periaortic lymph node m.
peritoneal implant m.
primary ovarian carcinoma with m.
soft tissue m.
m. of tumor
tumor, nodes, m.

metastasizing
m. septicemia

metastatic
m. abscess
m. adenocarcinoma
m. adenocarcinoma serosal surfaces
m. adenopathy
anthracycline-nave metastatic breast cancer
anthracycline-refractory metastatic breast carcinoma
m. arthritis
asymptomatic metastatic hormone-refractory prostate cancer
m. axillary involvement
m. basal cell carcinoma
m. bone lesion

m. bone survey
m. brain disease
m. brain tumor
m. breast cancer
m. breast carcinoma
m. calcification
m. calcinosis cutis
m. cancer of spinal fluid
m. carcinoid syndrome
m. carcinoma
m. carcinoma of unknown primary origin
m. cardiac tumor
m. cascade
m. cholangiocarcinoma
m. choroidal tumor
m. choroiditis
clinical evidence of metastatic disease
m. colon cancer
m. colorectal cancer
m. colorectal carcinoma
m. complication
m. contamination
m. cord compression
m. Crohn disease
m. deposit
m. disease
m. dissemination
distant metastatic disease
m. efficiency index
m. endophthalmitis
epidermotropic metastatic malignant melanoma
m. epidural spinal cord compression
extensive metastatic involvement
m. fat necrosis
m. granuloma
hormone-refractory metastatic prostate cancer
m. implant
m. infection
inoperable metastatic lung cancer
m. involvement
m. lesion
m. liver cancer
m. lung cancer
m. lymph node tumor
m. lymphoma
m. lymphoma of CNS
m. malignancy
m. malignant melanoma
malignant metastatic disease
m. malignant pheochromocytoma
m. melanoma
m. mixed müllerian tumor
m. mumps
m. myonecrosis
occult metastatic disease
m. ophthalmia
m. pneumonia
m. prostate cancer
m. renal cell carcinoma
m. retinitis
m. sarcoma
m. squamous carcinoma of head and neck
m. trophoblastic disease
m. tuberculous abscess
m. tumor
m. tumor of unknown origin

metatarsal
m. angle
angle of declination of m.
anterior metatarsal arch
m. artery
m. axis
m. bar shoe modification
m. block
m. bone
m. callosity
m. cuneiform exostosis
distal metatarsal articular angle
first dorsal metatarsal artery
first metatarsal head
first plantar metatarsal artery
m. flatfoot bar
m. flat head
m. fracture
m. free vascularized graft
m. head
m. head extractor
m. head osteochondritis
m. head osteotomy
m. head resection
m. interosseous ligament
intramedullary metatarsal decompression
navicular to first metatarsal angle
perforating branch of plantar metatarsal artery
plantar m.
m. shortening
m. stress fracture
talar axis–first metatarsal base angle
tuberosity of fifth m.
tuberosity of fifth metatarsal bone

metatarsalia

metatarsalis
arteria m.
arteria metatarsalis plantaris

metatarsea
arteria metatarsea plantaris

metatarsocuneiform
m. angle
m. arthrodesis
m. articulation

metatarsophalangeae

metatarsophalangeal
m. arthroplasty
m. articulation
m. articulations
m. bone marrow development
m. capsule
m. capsulotomy
m. creaking
m. crease
hallux metatarsophalangeal interphalangeal scale
m. implant
m. joint

metatarsus
m. abductus
m. adductocavus
m. adductocavus deformity
m. adductovarus
m. adductovarus deformity
m. adductus
m. adductus deformity
m. atavicus
m. atavicus deformity
m. cavus
Ganley and Ganley metatarsus adductus procedure
m. primus adductus
m. primus varus
true metatarsus adductus

metatrophic
m. dwarfism
m. dysplasia

metatropic
m. dwarfism
m. dysplasia

metatypical carcinoma

metazoal parasite

metazoan infection

Metchnikoff cellular immunity theory

Metenier sign

metenkephalin-like immunoreactivity

meter
amperes per m.
ampere-square m.
m. angle

meter *(continued)*
cubic m.
esotropia at 6 meters
home blood glucose m.
laser cell and flare m.
laser flare m.
m. lens
liter per minute per square m.
lumen per square m.
MediSense Precision m.
meganewton per square m.
milliroentgens per hour at one m.
mole per cubic m.
newton per m.
newton per square m.
newton-second per square m.
noise exposure m.
One Touch Ultra m.
oxygen saturation m.
peak flow m.
peak flow meter monitor
potential acuity m.
potential visual acuity m.
reciprocal ohm m.
roentgen m.
roentgen per hour at one m.
sound level m.
volt per m.
volume unit m.

meter-angle

metered-dose
m.-d. inhaler
inhaler
m.-d. inhaler-spacer device

metered solution inhaler

methacholine
m. bronchoprovocation challenge
m. challenge
m. challenge test
m. chloride
m. chloride skin test
high methacholine sensitivity
m. inhalation challenge
m. inhalation challenge response
m. provocative testing
reversal speed of bronchoconstriction in response to m.
speed of bronchoconstriction in response to m.

methacrylate
aminoglycoside-impregnated methyl methacrylate bead
glyceral m.
glycol m.
2-hydroxyethyl m.
methyl m.
methyl methacrylate cement
methyl methacrylate glue
methyl methacrylate implant
passivated polymethyl m.

methadone
m. addiction
m. assay
m. block
m. center
m. dependence
m. HCl
m. hydrochloride
m. maintenance
m. maintenance and aftercare treatment program
m. maintenance treatment
outpatient methadone program

methamphetamine
m. abuse
m. addiction
m. base
cardiovascular effects of m.
centrally active phenethylamine derivative related to amphetamine and m.
m. dependence
m. exposure
m. hydrochloride
neurotoxicity of m.

methane
m. monooxygenase
tricaine methane sulfonate

methanesulfonate
ethyl m.
methyl m.

methanol
m. assay
m. extraction residue
m. fixative
m. freezing method
m. toxicity

methantheline bromide

methasone-suppressed corticotropin-releasing hormone test

methemalbumin
m. assay

methemoglobin
m. level
m. reductase
m. reduction test

methenamine
Gomori methenamine silver
Grocott-Gomori methenamine silver nitrate
Grocott methenamine silver stain
m. hexamethylenetetramine
m. hippurate
periodic acid-silver m.
periodic acid-silver methenamine stain
m. silver stain

methicillin
factor essential for resistance to m.
m. sodium

methicillin-aminoglycoside-resistant *Staphylococcus aureus*

methicillin-resistant
m.-r. coagulase-negative *Staphylococcus*
m.-r. *Staphylococcus aureus*
m.-r. *Staphylococcus epidermidis*
m.-r. *Staphylococcus* species

methicillin-resistant *Staphylococcus* species

methicillin-susceptible
m.-s. coagulase-negative *Staphylococcus*
m.-s. *Staphylococcus aureus*

methiodide
pyridine aldoxime m.

methioninase
recombinant m.

methionine
m. enkephalin
m. malabsorption
m. malabsorption syndrome
m. metabolism
peptide histidine m.
m. synthase
m. synthase deficiency

methionine-enkephalin
immunoreactive m.-e.

method
acid-fast staining m.
m. of administration
adoptee family m.
aerosol rebreathing m.
agar/agarose-gel diffusion m.
alternative method of treatment
m.'s analysis
antialkaline phosphatase m.
antibody linkage m.
m. of approximation
area-length method for ejection fraction

ARM method of physical examination
Arvidsson dimension-length method for ventricular volume
m. of ascertainment
Ashby differential agglutination m.
Astrand 30-beat stopwatch m.
atrial extrastimulus m.
Attwood staining m.
Autenrieth and Funk m.
autoattenuation correction m.
automated airway tree segmentation m.
avidin-biotin-peroxidase m.
avidin-biotin-peroxidase complex m.
m. of Bernie Siegel
Bessey-Lowry-Brock method or unit
bone healing m.
border detection m.
Brunauer-Emmet-Teller m.
cable cerclage m.
m. of Cleary
computer tomographic methods of axial skeleton
computer tomographic methods of peripheral skeleton
Confusion Assessment M.
m. of constant stimuli
controlled partial rebreathing anesthesia m.
m. of defining criterion
m. of delivery
m. of Dickman
dilute blood clot lysis m.
Distress Risk Assessment M.
electrochemical relaxation m.
endoscopic mucosal resection, cap m.
endoscopic mucosal resection, tube m.
M.'s for the Epidemiology of Child and Adolescent Disorders T score
M.'s for Epidemiology of Child and Adolescent Mental Disorders
equal probability of selection m.
m. of Fabian
m. factor
finite element m.
Fisher-John melting point method
Folin-Wu m.
m. of Glees
glucose oxidase-perioxidase m.
goal attainment m.
head tilt m.
heparin assay rapid easy m.
immunosuppression m.
indirect m.
lactation amenorrhea m.
Lee-White blood clotting m.
life table m.
Lillie allochrome m.
loop gastric bypass m.
Lund and Broden m.
lysis centrifugation m.
Maddox rod m.
manual healing m.
maximum contrast m.
melanin bleaching m.
membrane filtration m.
Memorial dimension averaging m.
mersalyl exchange m.
merthiolate, iodine, formaldehyde method
methanol freezing m.
m. of Markwell
microtube dilution m.
millipore filter m.
modified band lid m.
modified Frost m.
modified Powell m.
monocular estimate m.
multinomial polytomous logistic regression m.
multiple cone root canal filling m.
natural healing m.
neck region-lifting m.
Neufeld dynamic m.
neutralization index m.
Nissen fundoplication m.
Nissen-Rosseti fundoplication m.
nonlinear least squares m.
numerical cipher m.
online assessment m.
open circuit m.
optical density m.
oral auditory m.
Paris method for radium therapy
Parker-Kerr closed method of end-to-end enteroenterostomy
Payr clamp m.
peracetic acid-based m.
periodic acid-Schiff m.
m. of Politzer
m. of rapid determination
rapid identification m.
rapid micromedia m.
repetitive excess mixed anhydride method
Roche, Wainer, and Thissen method of height prediction
Schafer method of artificial respiration
self-applied health enhancement m.
sensitivity of m.
sensory detection m.
sperm-washing insemination m.
m. of the sphere
standard method agar
Stanford biopsy m.
Study Attitudes and M.'s Survey
suction m.
Treatment Response Assessment M.
variable projection m.
verbal sample evaluation m.

method-*Neisseria*
rapid identification m.

methodology
assay m.
hemapheresis m.
m. study

methosulfate
phenazine m.

methoxyisobutylisonitrile
technetium-99m m.

methoxyisobutyl isonitrile single-photon emission computed tomography

methoxypsoralen

methydiphosphonate bone scan

methyl
m. acceptor protein
m. acetate
m. alcohol peripheral neuropathy
m. alcohol poisoning
m. alcohol toxicity
m. alcohol toxin
m. aldehyde
aminoglycoside-impregnated methyl methacrylate bead
angular m.
aqueous methyl cellulose
m. benzoate
benzoylarginine methyl ester
m. blue
m. bromide
m. butyl ketone
m. CCNU
m. cellulose paste
m. chloride
m. chloroform
corticosterone methyl oxidase

methyl *(continued)*
m. cysteine hydrochloride
m. dopa
m. ethyl ketone
fatty acid methyl ester
m. fluoracetate
m. green pyronin dye
m. indole
indole, methyl red, Voges-Proskauer, and citrate test
m. methacrylate
m. methacrylate cement
m. methacrylate glue
m. methacrylate implant
m. methanesulfonate
m. nitrosourea
m. oxidase
m. red
m. red test
m. red, Voges-Proskauer medium
serum methyl alcohol level
m. tertiary butyl ether
m. tetrahydrofolic acid
tosylarginine methyl ester

methyl-accepting chemotaxis protein

methylated
industrial methylated spirit
m. bovine serum albumin

methylation
MLH1 promoter m.

methylazoxymethanol acetate

methylbenzyl
m. alcohol
m. linoleic acid

methylbromide
homatropine m.

methylbutyrate
hydroxy beta m.

2-methylbutyric acid

methylcellulose
hydroxypropyl m.

methylcholanthrene-induced sarcoma

2-methyl citric acid

methyl-CpG-binding protein 2

methylcrotonyl

3-methylcrotonyl carboxylase

3-methylcrotonyl-CoA carboxylase deficiency

methyl cysteine hydrochloride

methyldopa
alpha m.
m. and hydrochlorothiazide

methylene
m. azure
m. blue
m. blue active substance
m. blue dye
m. blue enema
m. blue instillation
m. blue line
m. blue, reduced
m. blue reduction time
m. blue stain
m. blue test
carbolic methylene blue
m. chloride
m. dimethane sulfonate
m. diphenyl diisocyanate
m. diphosphate
m. diphosphonate
m. diphosphonate concentration
Loeffler methylene blue dye
Loeffler methylene blue stain
Nair buffered methylene blue stain
new methylene blue N stain
polychrome methylene blue stain
m. tetrahydrofolate reductase
m. tetrahydrofolate reductase thermolability

methylenedianiline
starch m.

3,4-methylenedioxymethamphetamine toxicity

methylenetetrahydrofolate
m. reductase
m. reductase gene

methylesterase
protein m.

methyl G

methylglucamine
m. contrast medium
m. diatrizoate

methyl green pyronin dye

methylguanidine
serum m.

methylhydrazine methylisopropylbenzamide

methylisopropylbenzamide
methylhydrazine m.

methylmalonic
m. acid
m. acidemia
m. acidemia with homocystinemia
adult-onset combined methylmalonic aciduria and homocystinuria
m. aminoaciduria

6-methylmercaptopurine riboside

methylmercaptopurine riboside

methylmercury intoxication

methylmethacrylate
m. block
m. cranioplastic plug
m. cranioplasty
temporary articulating methylmethacrylate antibiotic spacer

methylnitrate
atropine m.

methylphenidate
m. administration
m. challenge test
m. hydrochloride

methyl-phenyl-tetrahydropyridine
m.-p.-t. parkinsonism
m.-p.-t. poisoning

methylprednisolone
m. acetate
high-dose m.
high-dose intravenous m.
intravenous m.
m., Oncovin, procarbazine
m. pulse therapy
m. sodium succinate

15-methylprostaglandin $F_{2\alpha}$

methylrosaniline chloride

methyl-*tert*-butyl ether therapy

methyl tertiary butyl ether

methyltestosterone

methyl tetrahydrofolic acid

methylthymol
m. blue
m. blue complex

methyltransferase
catechol m.
guanidinoacetate m.
histamine m.
thiopurine m.

4-methylumbelliferyl-beta-D-glucoronidase test

methysergide maleate

meticulous hemostasis

metoclopramide
m. hydrochloride

m., dexamethasone, lorazepam, ondansetron

metopic
m. craniectomy
m. craniosynostosis
m. ridging

metoprolol tartrate

Metrazol-electroshock seizure

metric
m. data
m. ophthalmoscope
m. ophthalmoscopy

metritis
mastitis, metritis, agalactia syndrome

metrizamide
m. computed tomographic cisternography
computed tomographic metrizamide myelography
m. computed tomography cisternography
m. contrast study
m. CT cisternogram

metrizamide-assisted computed tomography

metronidazole
bismuth, metronidazole, tetracycline
bismuth subsalicylate, metronidazole, and amoxicillin
m., amoxicillin, clarithromycin, *H. pylori*, one-week therapy
m., omeprazole, amoxicillin
m., omeprazole, clarithromycin
omeprazole, amoxicillin, m.
omeprazole, bismuth subcitrate, tetracycline, and m.
omeprazole, metronidazole, clarithromycin
ranitidine bismuth citrate, metronidazole, tetracycline

metropathia hemorrhagica

metroperitoneal fistula

metropolitan
M. Achievement Test, Seventh Edition
M. Atlanta Congenital Defects Program
m. statistical area
M. Readiness Test
standard metropolitan statistical area

metrorrhagia myopathica

metyrapone
overnight metyrapone test
m. test
m. testing
m. therapy

metyrapone-induced hypercortisolism

Metzenbaum
blunt Metzenbaum scissors
M. scissors

Meulengracht diet

Meurmann
M. classification
M. external ear anomaly grade

Meuse fever

Mevacor Atherosclerosis Regression Study

mevalonic
m. acid
m. acidemia

MEVA probe

Mexican
M. American
M. American female
M. American male
M. hat cell
M. hat erythrocyte
M. hat sign
M. spotted fever
M. tea
M. typhus

Mexico
New Mexico Attitude Toward Work Test
New Mexico Career Planning Test
New Mexico Knowledge of Occupations Test
M. virus

Meyenburg
M. complex
M. disease
von Meyenburg complex

Meyer
M. cartilage
M. dysplasia
Willy Meyer radical mastectomy

Meyer-Archambault loop

Meyer-Betz
M.-B. disease
M.-B. syndrome

Meyer-Kendall Assessment Survey

Meyer-Schwickerath
M.-S. coagulator
M.-S. operation
M.-S. and Weyers syndrome

Meyerson nevus

Meynert
M. cell
M. cells
M. commissure
M. decussation
M. fasciculus
M. fountain decussation
M. layer
nucleus basalis of M.

mezlocillin sodium

MFG-IRAP retrovirus

M1G8
monoclonal antibody M.

MHC-restricted cytotoxic T cell

9- to 5-MHz convex array

30-mHz transducer-tipped catheter

Mi-2 antibody

Miami
M. Acute Care
M. fracture brace
M. STAR tissue expander

MIB-1
M. antibody
M. antigen
M. cell proliferation marker
M. expression
monoclonal antibody M.

Mibelli
angiokeratoma of M.
M. angiokeratoma
M. disease
M. porokeratosis
porokeratosis of M.
M. syndrome

MIBG-negative pelvic pheochromocytoma

mibuna temperate virus

micaceous scale

MICB gene

mice
epidemic disease of infant m.
epizootic diarrhea of infant m.
mammary cancer virus of m.
mammary tumor virus of m.
minute virus of m.
New Zealand m.
pneumonia virus of m.

mice *(continued)*
severe combined immunodeficient m.
tumor-bearing m.

micellar
critical micellar concentration
m. electrokinetic capillary chromatography
m. electrokinetic chromatography

micelle
critical micelle concentration
m.'s in vitreous

Michaelis
M. buffer
M. complex
M. constant

Michaelis-Menten dissociation constant

Michaelson
M. counter pressure
M. operation

Michel
M. anomaly
M. aplasia
M. clip
M. deformity
M. pick
M. solution
M. spur

Micheli
microelliptopoikilocytic anemia of Rietti, Greppi, and M.

Michelin tire baby syndrome

Michels syndrome

Michigan
M. Abuse Screening Test
M. Alcoholism Screening Test
M. Bone Health Study
M. Diabetic Neuropathy Score
M. Hand Outcomes Questionnaire
M. Neuropathy Screening Test
M. Picture Stories
M. Picture Test, Revised
Short Michigan Alcoholism Screening Test

Mickety-Wilson syndrome

miconazole nitrate

Micral
M. urine dipstick test
M. urine test strip

microabscess
Munro m.
m. of mycosis fungoides
Pautrier m.
m. of psoriasis

microadenoma
nonfunctioning m.
nonsecretory m.
pituitary m.

microagglutination test

microaggregate
centrifuged microaggregate filter

microaggregated
m. albumin
m. human serum albumin

microamperage
m. electrical nerve stimulation
m. neural stimulation

microanalysis
electron-probe m.

microanalytical reagent

microanalyzer
electronic m.
electron probe x-ray m.

microanastomosis
laser-assisted m.

microaneurysm
hemorrhage and m.
retinal capillary m.

microaneurysmal leakage

microangiopathic
m. anemia
m. hemolysis
m. hemolytic anemia
m. hemolytic uremic syndrome
m. process

microangiopathy
cerebral m.
intraretinal m.
thrombotic m.

microaspiration
sperm microaspiration retrieval technique

microassisted fertilization

microatomized protein food

microbe
maximal number of microbes killed
transmission of microbe to host

microbevel
m. edge lens

microbevel edge lens

microbial
aerobic microbial flora
m. alkaline protease inhibitor
m. antagonism
m. antigenic phase shift
m. approach
m. associate
m. associates
m. biofilm
m. collagenase
m. ecology
m. factor
m. flora
m. genetics
m. keratitis
m. persistence
m. sensitivity
m. susceptibility test
m. vitamin

microbiologic
m. assay
m. quality control

microbiology
m. automation
Cumulative Techniques and Procedures in Clinical M.

microbroth dilution

microbubble
m. concentration measurement
m. contrast enhancement

microcalcification
m. cluster
linear branching m.
lobular breast m.

microcatheter
ball-tip m.

microcautery unit

microcephalic
m. dwarfism
m. idiocy
m. primordial dwarfism 1
m. primordial dwarfism-cataracts syndrome

microcephaly
alopecia, mental retardation, epilepsy, microcephaly syndrome
cataract, microcephaly, arthrogryposis, kyphosis
cataract, microcephaly, failure to thrive, kyphoscoliosis
dislocated elbow, bowed tibiae, scoliosis, deafness, cataract, microcephaly, mental retardation syndrome
growth retardation, ocular abnormalities, microcephaly, brachydactyly, oligophrenia

mental retardation, coarse face, microcephaly, epilepsy, skeletal abnormalities syndrome
mental retardation, microcephaly, blepharochalasis syndrome
mental retardation, retinopathy, microcephaly syndrome
m., hiatus hernia, nephrotic syndrome
m., hypergonadotropic hypogonadism, short stature syndrome
m., infantile spasm, psychomotor retardation, nephrotic syndrome
m., mental retardation, cataract, hypogonadism syndrome
m., mental retardation, retinopathy syndrome
m., mesobrachyphalangy, tracheoesophageal fistula syndrome
m., microphthalmia, ectrodactyly, prognathism syndrome
m., mild developmental delay, short stature, distinctive face syndrome
m., mild mental retardation, short stature, skeletal anomalies syndrome
m., muscular build, rhizomelia-cataracts syndrome
m., oculodigital, esophageal, duodenal syndrome
m., sparse hair, mental retardation, seizures syndrome
nephrosis, microcephaly, hiatus hernia syndrome
X-linked mental retardation, seizures, acquired microcephaly, agenesis of corpus callosum

microcephaly-calcification of cerebral white matter syndrome

microcephaly-cardiomyopathy syndrome

microcephaly-cervical spine fusion anomalies

microcephaly-chorioretinopathy syndrome

microcephaly-deafness syndrome

microcephaly-digital anomalies syndrome

microcephaly-oculo-digito-esophageal-duodenal syndrome

microcephaly-spastic diplegia syndrome

microchip DNA array

microciliary clearance

microcirculation
m. abnormality
mesenteric m.

microcirculatory
m. compromise
m. disturbance
m. dysfunction
m. failure

microclip
dural m.

microcolon
megacystic microcolon syndrome
megalocystis microcolon intestinal hypoperistalsis syndrome

microcomplement fixation

microcomputer upper limb exerciser

microcornea
X-linked mental retardation, microphthalmia, microcornea, cataract, hypogenitalism-mental retardation-spasticity syndrome

microculture
m. and sensitivity
m. tetrazolium dye assay

microcurrent electrode

microcyst
milk of calcium m.

microcystic
m. adenoma
m. adnexal carcinoma
m. corneal dystrophy
m. degeneration
m. disease of renal medulla
m. eccrine carcinoma
m. edema
m. epithelial dystrophy
m. formation

microcystica

microcytic
m. anemia
m. erythrocyte
m. hypochromic anemia
m. red cell

microcytic/normochromic anemia

microcytotoxicity
m. assay
lymphocyte m.

microdeletion syndrome

microdialysis probe

microdilution
m. broth dilution test
m. broth susceptibility test
m. serum bactericidal test
m. susceptibility testing
m. system

microdiskectomy
arthroscopic m.

microdissection
laser-capture m.

microdontia-microcephaly-short stature syndrome

microdrepanocytic
m. anemia
m. disease

microdysgenesis
neuronal m.

microelliptopoikilocytic anemia of Rietti, Greppi, and Micheli

microemboli (*pl. of* microembolus)

microembolic signal

microembolism
delayed microembolism syndrome

microembolus, pl. **microemboli**
circulating microemboli index
gaseous m.

microencapsulation assay

microendoscope
ophthalmic laser m.

microendoscopic
m. discectomy system
m. foraminotomy
m. optical catheter
m. test card

microenvironment
hemopoietic inductive m.

microepididymal sperm aspiration

microextraction
solid-phase m.

micro eye movement

microfibrillar
m. collagen
m. collagen hemostat
m. protein

microfilament-mediated process

microfilaria, pl. **microfilariae**
nocturnal m.
peripheral blood preparation for microfilariae

microfilarial sheath
microfil-associated glycoprotein
microfilled
m. composite
m. composite resin
microfilm
computer output on m.
MicroFinger
Lieberman MicroFinger manipulator
microfluorometry
flow m.
microfocal direct magnification in vitro x-ray tube
microfold cell
microfollicular
m. adenoma
m. pattern
Microfuge tube
microglandular
m. adenosis
m. cervical hyperplasia
m. dysplasia
m. hyperplasia
microglia cell
microglial
m. cell
m. cluster
m. rod cell
microglobulin
2-microglobulin-origin amyloid deposit
micrognathia
adult acquired m.
micrognathia-glossoptosis syndrome
microgram
m. per kilogram per minute
m. per liter
microgranular acute promyelocytic leukemia
micrograph
electron m.
scanning electron m.
microhemagglutination
m. assay
m. assay for antibodies to *Treponema pallidum*
indirect microhemagglutination test
m. test for *Treponema pallidum*
microhematocrit
m. capillary tube
m. centrifugation
m. concentration
Micro-ID system
microimmunofluorescence test
microinfusion pump
microinvasive
m. adenocarcinoma
m. carcinoma classification
m. cervical cancer
microkeratome
automated m.
microlaparoscopic
m. cholecystectomy
m. sterilization
microlatex particle-mediated immunoassay
micro liquid extraction
microliter
m. 1/1,000 of an mL
microlithiasis
common bile duct m.
occult biliary m.
pulmonary alveolar m.
microlumbar
m. disc excision
m. diskectomy
m. diskography
microlymphaticovenous anastomosis
microlymphocytotoxicity
m. assay
m. test
micromanipulation
gamete m.
micromedia
rapid micromedia method
micromelia
disproportionate m.
micromelic
m. dwarfism
m. dysplasia
micromesh sheeting
micrometastasis, pl. **micrometastases**
bone marrow m.
micrometastases clonogenic assay
micrometastases detection assay
micrometastatic disease
micrometer
caliper m.
cubic m.
m. disk
m. knife
m. of mercury
ocular m.
particulate matter less than 10 micrometers diameter
micromillimeter
micromirror
digital micromirror device
micromultileaf
m. collimator
m. collimator system
micromyeloblastic leukemia
microneedle
curved microneedle holder
micronized
m. AlloDerm tissue
m. 17beta estradiol
m. diosmin
m. estradiol
m. flavonidic fraction
m. progesterone
m. purified flavonoid fracture
micronodular
m. adrenal disease
m. gastritis
m. hyperplasia
m. liver cirrhosis
m. pneumocyte hyperplasia
primary adrenocortical micronodular dysplasia
m. tuberculid
micronutrient
m. deficiency
m. supplementation
microorganism
enterococcus m.
fusobacteria m.'s
Gram-negative m.
Gram-positive m.
pathogenic m.
micropapillary
m. carcinoma
m. component
m. DCIS
m. serous carcinoma
m. serous ovarian carcinoma
micropapular tuberculid
microparticle
m. capture enzyme immunoassay
m. enzyme immunoassay
microparticulate enzyme immunoassay

micropenis
obesity, short stature, mental deficiency, hypogonadism, micropenis, finger contracture, cleft lip-palate syndrome

microperforate hymen

microphallus, imperforate anus, syndactyly, hamartoblastoma, abnormal lung

microphone
cardiac catheter m.
hearing aid m.
pressure zone m.

microphonic
cochlear m.

microphotoelectric plethysmography

microphthalmia
m. or anophthalmos with associated anomalies
anterior m.
arrhinia, choanal atresia, microphthalmia syndrome
microcephaly, microphthalmia, ectrodactyly, prognathism syndrome
m., dermal aplasia, sclerocornea syndrome
m. with linear skin defects
X-linked mental retardation, microphthalmia, microcornea, cataract, hypogenitalism-mental retardation-spasticity syndrome

microphthalmic
m. cyst
osteopetrotic m.

micropigmentation system

micropituitary rongeur

microplate
m. fixation
m. plasma methotrexate assay
m. plasma MTX assay

MicroPlus spirometer

micropoint
m. needle
m. suture

micropolycystic ovary syndrome

micropolygyria with muscular dystrophy

Micropore dressing

microporous
self-expanding microporous stent

microprecipitin
radioactive antigen m.

microprobe
m. analysis generalized intensity correction
laser microprobe mass analyzer

microptic
m. delirium
m. hallucination

micropuncture
anterior stromal m.

Microputor II

micro round-tip needle

microsatellite
m. analysis
m. instability
m. instability screening
m. instability testing
m. locus
m. marker
m. polymorphism
m. stable

MicroScan
M. gram-negative ID panel
M. System

microscope
analytical electron m.
analytic transmission electron m.
binocular dissecting m.
conventional transmission electron m.
electron m.
endothelial specular m.
high-power field microscope
high-voltage electron m.
light electron m.
near field scanning optical m.
OPMI PRO magis m.
OPMI VISU 200 m.
scanning laser acoustic m.
scanning transmission electron m.
scanning tunneling m.
m. slide
surgical microscope navigation
tonsillectomy with operating m.
transmission electron m.
two-photon laser-scanning m.
universal electron m.
x-ray tomographic m.

microscopic
m. absence
m. agglutination
m. agglutination test
m. aggregation index
m. air bubble
m. anatomy
m. angiogenesis grading system
autopsy microscopic examination
m. benign prostatic hyperplasia
m. BPH
m. colitis
m. colitis syndrome
m. cortical dysplasia
m. diagnosis
direct microscopic clump count
m. disease
electron microscopic examination
m. endoscopy surgery
m. epididymal sperm aspiration
m. factor
m. fat
m. field
filter paper microscopic test
m. foraminotomy
m. glasses
m. granular cell tumor
gross and m.
m. hematuria
m. hyphema
m. metastasis
m. polyangiitis
m. polyarteritis
m. polyarteritis nodosa
m. residuum
routine and m.
m. seeding
urinalysis, routine and m.

microscopically
m. controlled surgery
m. immature brain
m. normal tissue
m. positive, culturally negative

microscopy
analytical electron m.
atomic force m.
atomic resolution m.
confocal laser scanning m.
conventional transmission electron m.
electron m.
electron microscopy of stool
epiluminescent m.
field emission scanning electron m.
field ion m.
fluorescent m.
freeze fracture electron m.
high-resolution light m.
high-resolution transmission electron m.
high-voltage transmission electron m.

microscopy *(continued)*
immune electron m.
immunoelectron m.
laser-scanning confocal m.
lateral force m.
light m.
low power microscopy
low-voltage high-resolution scanning electron m.
oil immersion field microscopy
photoemission electron m.
polarized light m.
projection x-ray m.
reflection interference m.
scanning electron m.
scanning force m.
scanning photoacoustic m.
scanning probe m.
skin surface m.
total internal reflection m.
transmission electron m.
transmission scanning electron m.
ultrasound backscatter m.
urinalysis and m.
video-intensification m.
whole mount microscopy

microsection
submitted for m.

microslide culture

microsomal
m. antibody titer
m. antigen
antiliver microsomal antibody detection
antithyroid microsomal antibody
m. autoantibodies
m. damage
m. enzyme system
m. ethanol oxidizing system
m. heme oxygenase
m. hydroxylation
m. lipoprotein
liver/kidney microsomal antibody
thyroid microsomal antibody
m. triglyceride transfer protein

microsome
m. antibody
calf aortic m.
platelet m.
seminal vesicle m.

microsome-mediated mutagenesis

microsomia
craniofacial m.
hemifacial m.

microsphere
degenerative dense m.
degradable starch m.
dense m.
enterocoated microspheres of pancrelipase
human albumin m.
magnetically responsive m.
magnetic starch m.'s

microsporidia
m. infection
Microsporidia diagnostic procedure

microsporidial
m. infection
m. keratoconjunctivitis

microsporidian keratoconjunctivitis

microsporon
Audouin m.

microstomia prevention appliance

microstrabismic amblyopia

microstructured implant

microsurgery
computer assisted stereotactic laser m.
m. discectomy
endoscope-controlled m.
m. forceps
frameless stereotactic m.
rectal-expander-assisted transanal endoscopic m.
transanal endoscopic m.

microsurgical
m. denervation of the spermatic cord
m. discectomy
m. diskectomy
m. DREZotomy
m. drill system
m. epididymal sperm aspiration
m. epididymal sperm aspiration procedure
m. epididymovasostomy
m. extraction of ductal sperm
m. extraction of sperm from epididymis
m. free flap
m. free pulp flap
m. knife
m. lumbar diskectomy
Millennium LX microsurgical system
Mohs microsurgical resection
m. resection
same-day microsurgical arthroscopic lateral-approach laser-assisted
m. tubocornual anastomosis

microthin contact lens

microtia
aural m.
Marx classification of m.

microtia-absent patellae-micrognathia syndrome

Microtip catheter

microtiter
colorimetric microtiter plate
m. blood typing system

microtrabecular hepatocellular carcinoma

MicroTrak
M. direct fluorescent antibody staining
M. direct fluorescent antibody test

microtransfusion
maternal-fetal m.

microtremor
ocular m.

microtropic syndrome

microtube
m. dilution
m. dilution method
m. dilution test

microtubule
m. assembly
m. inhibitor
m. organizing center
m. protein
spindle m.

microtubule-associated protein

microtubule-binding domain

microunits per milliliter

microvascular
m. abnormality
m. anastomosis
m. angiopathy
m. bone transfer
m. circulation
m. compression syndrome
m. decompression
m. disease
m. Doppler ultrasonography
m. flap
m. forceps
m. free flap
m. free flap transfer
m. free muscle flap

m. free posterior interosseous flap
m. free tissue transfer
m. free toe transfer
m. graft
human dermal microvascular endothelial cell
intraretinal microvascular abnormality
m. lesion
parafoveal microvascular leakage
m. pressure
pulmonary microvascular permeability to protein
m. thrombosis

microvenous
m. anatomy
m. graft

microvenular hemangioma

microvesicular
m. fat
m. hepatic steatosis

microvessel
m. count
m. density
intramural microvessel density
optimized microvessel density analysis

microvillar
syncytiotrophoblast microvillar plasma membrane

microvillous membrane

microvillus
m. atrophy
m. inclusion disease

microvitreoretinal
m. spatula

Microvit vitrector

microwave
m. ablation
adjuvant microwave thermotherapy
m. amplification by stimulated emission of radiation
m. antenna design
m. applicator
m. cardiac ablation system
m. coagulation
m. coagulation therapy
m. diathermy
m. diathermy treatment
m. endometrial ablation
m. epitope retrieval technique
m. fixation
hazards from microwave radiation
high-energy transurethral microwave thermotherapy
m. hyperthermia
m. hyperthermia of the prostate
low-energy transurethral microwave thermotherapy
percutaneous microwave coagulation therapy
periurethral transurethral microwave thermotherapy
m. plaque thermotherapy
m. radiation injury
m. therapy
transurethral m.
transurethral microwave thermotherapy

micro Westcott scissors

micturating
m. cystogram
m. cystourethrogram
m. cystourethrography
m. urogram

micturition
m. center
m. cystourethrogram
detrusor muscle pressure-flow micturition study
nocturnal m.
pontine micturition center
m. syncope
m. urinary incontinence

midabdominal abscess

midaortic arch

midarm
m. circumference
m. fat area
m. muscle area
m. muscle circumference

Midas alloy

midaxillary
m. line
vector cardiography electrode right midaxillary line

midazolam conscious sedation

midbody
anterior midbody of corpus callosum

midbrain
m. abnormality
aqueduct of m.
m. aqueduct
m. corectopia
m. deafness
diminished attenuation midbrain and pons
m. disease
dissecting hemorrhage of m.
m. dysfunction
limbic midbrain area
massive midbrain hemorrhage
opening of aqueduct of m.
m. ptosis
m. raphe nucleus
m. reticular formation

midcarpal
m. arthrodesis
m. arthroscopy
m. capsule
m. compartment
m. dislocation
m. instability
m. radial
m. ulnar

midcavity forceps

midclavicular
left midclavicular line
m. line
m. line to nipple
lower midclavicular line
right midclavicular line
upper midclavicular line

mid-coquille lens

midcostal line

midcycle
m. bleeding
m. cervical mucus
m. spotting
m. surge

Middelburg virus

Middeldorpf tumor

middermal elastolysis

mid-diastolic
apical m.-d.
m.-d. murmur
m.-d. rumble

middle
adjustment reaction of middle age
m. adolescence
m. adulthood
m. age
m. age pedophilia
aggressive papillary middle ear tumor
alternative occipital artery middle cerebral artery
m. alveolar artery
anterior middle meatus
anterior middle superior alveolar
anterior wall of middle ear

middle *(continued)*
m. aortic syndrome
arachnoid cyst of the middle fossa
atelectasis of middle ear
m. atlantoepistrophic joint
atrium of middle nasal meatus
auditory middle latency response
m. axillary line
m. cardiac cervical nerve
m. cardiac vein
m. carpal joint
m. cell
m. cerebellar peduncle
m. cerebral aneurysm
m. cerebral artery
m. cerebral artery bifurcation
m. cerebral artery fenestration
m. cerebral artery infarct
m. cerebral artery occlusion
m. cerebral artery pressure
m. cerebral artery syndrome
m. cerebral artery thrombosis
m. cervical cardiac nerve
m. cervical fascia
m. cervical ganglion
m. cervical peduncle
m. chamber bubbling
chronic middle ear infection
m. class
m. class community
m. clinoid process
m. cluneal nerve
m. colic artery
m. colic lymph node
m. colic vein
m. collateral artery
m. constrictor muscle of pharynx
m. constrictor pharyngeal muscle
m. coronary sinus
m. costotransverse ligament
m. cranial fossa
m. cranial fossa approach
m. cranial fossa cyst
m. cranial fossa line
m. cuneiform bone
m. ear canal
m. ear cell
m. ear choristoma
m. ear cleft
m. ear disease
m. ear effusion
m. ear endoscopy
m. ear exploration
m. ear fluid
m. ear impedance
m. ear implantable
m. ear implantable system
m. ear infection
m. ear mass
m. ear muscle reflex
m. ear neoplasm
m. ear segment
m. ear space
m. ear surgery
m. esophageal constriction
m. ethmoidal air cell
m. extrahepatic bile duct
m. fascia
m. finger
m. finger amputation
m. fossa approach
m. fossa craniotomy approach
m. fossa exposure
m. fossa plate
m. fossa syndrome
m. fossa transtentorial translabyrinthine approach
m. fossa vestibular nerve section
m. fossa vestibular neurectomy
m. frontal convolution
m. frontal gyrus
m. frontal sulcus
m. game
m. genicular artery
m. genicular vein
m. gland
m. glenohumeral ligament
m. glial cell line-derived neurotrophic factor
m. glossoepiglottic fold
m. gluteal muscle
m. gluteal nerve
m. gray layer of superior colliculus
m. greater tubercle of facet of humerus
m. ground
m. group of mesenteric lymph node
m. hemorrhoidal artery
m. hemorrhoidal plexus
m. hemorrhoidal vein
m. hepatic artery
m. hepatic vein
hyperdense middle cerebral artery sign
implantable middle ear hearing device
m. insomnia
m. kidney
m. latency response
left middle cerebral artery
left middle cerebral artery thrombosis
left middle ear exploration
left middle finger
m. lobar artery
m. lobar artery of right lung
m. lobe
m. lobe branch of right superior pulmonary vein
m. lobe bronchus
m. lobe of heart
m. lobe of prostate
m. lobe of right lung
m. lobe syndrome
m. lobe vein
m. macular arteriole
malignant middle cerebral artery infarction
m. meatus
m. meatus nasal antral window
m. molecule
M2 segment of middle cerebral artery
no middle initial
no middle name
m. one-third of face underdevelopment
orbital branch of middle meningeal artery
parietal branch of middle meningeal artery
petrosal branch of middle meningeal artery
right middle cerebral artery thrombosis
right middle ear exploration
right middle finger
right middle lobe
right middle lobe bronchus
right middle lobe of lung
right middle lobe syndrome
right middle sternal border
m. sacral artery
scalene muscle, anterior, posterior, m.
superficial occipital artery to middle cerebral artery
m. temporal visual area
m. third of long bone
m. turbinate
m. upper arm circumference
m. uterine artery

Middlebrook
M. agar
M. broth
M. 7H10, 7H11 medium

Middlebrook-Dubos hemagglutination test

midepigastric tenderness

midexpiratory
m. flow
forced midexpiratory flow
maximal midexpiratory flow
maximal midexpiratory flow rate
maximal midexpiratory flow volume
maximum midexpiratory flow rate
mean midexpiratory flow rate
m. time

midface
m. alloplastic augmentation
anteriorization of m.
m. avulsion flap
m. degloving
m. degloving incision
m. degloving procedure
m. degloving technique
m. depth
m. fracture
m. hypoplasia
m. hypoplasia syndrome

midfacial
m. breadth
m. defect
m. degloving
m. fracture
m. hypoplasia

midflow
maximal midflow rate

midfoot
m. abductus
m. adductus
m. arthritis
m. arthrodesis
m. arthropathy
m. breech
m. cavus
m. fracture
guillotine midfoot amputation

midforceps
m. delivery
elective m.
m. maneuver
m. rotation
sterile low midforceps vaginal delivery
m. vaginal delivery

midge
m.t system

midge bite

midgut
malrotation with midgut volvulus

midgut volvulus

midinspiratory
m. flow
m. flow at 50% of vital capacity
m. flow rate

midlateral
m. approach
m. capsule

midlevel provider

midlife depression

midline
m. abdominal crease
m. aponeurotic closure
m. of brain cyst
carina midline sharp and mobile
central midline placement of electrodes in electroencephalography
m. central neuraxis
m. cerebellum
m. cleft palate
m. cleft syndrome
m. of columella
m. craniofacial tumor
m. cranioorbital clefting
cross m.
m. cross-lip Abbe flap
m. cystic structure
m. developmental lesion
m. disc herniation
m. disharmony
m. echoencephalograph
m. episiotomy
m. exposure
m. facial defect
firm and midline uterus
m. forehead flap
frontal midline placement of electrodes in electroencephalography
m. fusion defect
m. granuloma
m. granulomatosis
m. heart
idiopathic midline destructive disease
m. incision
m. lethal granuloma
lethal midline granuloma
lower m.
lower midline scar with hernia
m. malignant reticulosis
parietal midline zero electrode placement in electroencephalography
m. position
m. position of gaze
protrudes in m.
m. shift
m. skin incision
tongue m.
tongue protrudes in m.
m. vertical uterine extension
well-healed midline scar
m. zone

mid lumbar region

midluteal progesterone measurement

midmarginal branch of artery

mid-molecule parathyroid hormone

midnight plasma cortisol concentration

midpalmar
m. abscess
m. fascia

midpapillary
anterior m.
anterior midpapillary level
m. longitudinal
m. transverse

midparental height

midpelvis
plane of m.

midplace
simultaneous binaural midplace localization

midplane
m. depth
m. dose
identical midplane doses

midpoint
m. of sella turcica
m. skin test
temperature midpoint Celsius

midrange spectrum ultraviolet light

midrange-wavelength ultraviolet light

midright atrium

midsagittal
m. diameter
m. image
Pena midsagittal anorectoplasty
ratio of midsagittal diameter

midshaft fracture
midshunt peak velocity
midsigmoid colon
midsleep disturbance
mid-small bowel
midsternal
m. area
m. incision
m. line
midstream
clean-catch midstream urinalysis
clean-catch midstream urine
m. clean-catch urine
m. clean-catch urine culture
clean, midstream urine
second midstream bladder specimen
m. specimen of urine
third midstream bladder specimen
m. urinalysis
m. urine sample
m. urine specimen
midsystolic
m. buckling of mitral valve
m. click
m. murmur
midtarsal
Akron midtarsal osteotomy
m. dome osteotomy
m. joint
longitudinal midtarsal joint axis
oblique midtarsal joint axis
midtemporal
m. epilepsy
rhythmical midtemporal discharge
midthigh girth
midureteral stricture
midvaginal transverse septum
midvoid
culture m. specimen
m. urine specimen
midwife
auxiliary nurse m.
Miege disease
Miescher
M. actinic granuloma
M. cheilitis granulomatosa
M. elastoma
M. granulomatous cheilitis
M. syndrome
M. tube
Miescher-Leder granulomatosis
Mietens syndrome
Mietens-Weber syndrome
mifepristone RU 486; Mifeprex
migraine
m. abortive therapy
acute confusional m.
affective prodrome of m.
aphasic migraine headache
autosomal dominant m.
basilar hemiplegic m.
childhood migraine headache
chronic migraine headache
common m.
confusion from migraine headache
M. Disability Assessment Scale
m. equivalent
familial hemiplegic m.
m. headache
hemiplegic m.
m. hormone
m. ophthalmoplegia
ophthalmoplegic m.
m. sine hemicrania
syncopal migraine headache
m. syndrome
m. variant
m. with aphasia
m. with aura
m. with interparoxysmal headache
m. without aura
migraine-type headache
migrainous
m. attack
m. aura
m. cranial neuralgia
m. hallucination
m. headache
m. neuralgia
m. ophthalmoplegia
m. vision loss
migrans
erythema m.
neural larva m.
ocular larva m.
thrombophlebitis m.
visceral larva m.
migrant
m. erysipelas
m. pattern
migrated tumor
migrating
m. abscess
m. action potential complex
m. angioedema
m. cheilitis
m. epithelium
giant migrating contraction
interdigestive migrating contraction
interdigestive migrating motor complex
m. motor complex
m. myoelectric complex
m. phlebitis
migration
m. abnormality
m. of acetabular cup
m. adaptation
adjustment following m.
chemotactic m.
direct migration inhibition
m. disorder
m. enhancement factor
gastrostomy tube m.
m. index
m. inhibition
m. inhibition test
leukocyte migration inhibition assay
leukocyte migration enhancement
leukocyte migration inhibition factor
leukocyte migration inhibition reaction
leukocyte migration inhibition test
leukocyte migration technique
liver migration inhibitory factor
macrophage migration index
macrophage migration inhibition
macrophage migration inhibition test
macrophage migration inhibitory factor
metallic biliary stent m.
neural crest m.
neuroepithelial cell m.
neuronal migration disorder
neuronal migration disorders
random m.
m. theory
migrational
m. abnormality
m. anomaly
m. disorder
migration-inhibitory factor
migratory
m. arthralgia
m. cell
m. deep vein thrombophlebitis

m. glossitis
m. necrolytic erythema
nodular migratory panniculitis
m. ophthalmia
m. panniculitis
m. path
m. peripheral arthritis
m. pneumonia
m. polyarthritis
m. tumor

Miguel
San Miguel sea lion virus

Mikamo double-eyelid operation

Mikity-Wilson syndrome

Mikulicz
M. angle
M. aphthae
M. bag
M. cell
M. cells
M. clamp
M. colostomy
M. disease
M. drain technique
M. procedure
M. syndrome

Mikulicz-Radecki syndrome

Mikulicz-Sjögren syndrome

Milan Cancer Institute

Milch
M. classification of humeral fracture
M. condylar fracture classification
M. cuff resection of ulna technique
M. elbow fracture classification
M. elbow operation
M. elbow technique
M. fracture classification syndrome

mild
m. acetabular dysplasia
m. anemia
m. anorexia nervosa
m. anxiety reaction
apnea/bradycardia mild stimulation
asymptomatic mild endometriosis
m. ataxia
autosomal dominant mild short limb dwarfism
m. biventricular dilatation hypertrophy
m. chromic suture
m. chronic hepatitis
m. cognitive impairment
m. colloid depletion
m. dehydration
m. delusion
m. dementia
m. depression
m. disability
m. distress
m. down-slant to palpebral fissure
m. eccentricity in demeanor
m. focal chronic inflammatory infiltrate
m. focal cortical nodular hyperplasia
m. focal interstitial scarring
m. head injury
m. hearing impairment
m. hearing loss
m. hemophilia
m. hyperphenylalaninemia
m. hypertension
m. illness
m. intermittent asthma
m. irritant
m. leukocytosis
m. mental retardation
microcephaly, mild developmental delay, short stature, distinctive face syndrome
microcephaly, mild mental retardation, short stature, skeletal anomalies syndrome
m. to moderately impaired
m. overt thyrotoxicosis
patient with mild to moderate systemic disease
m. persistent asthma
m. pulmonic stenosis
m. scoliosis
m. sickle cell disease
m. skin irritation
m. spastic diplegic cerebral palsy
m. systemic atherosclerosis
m. thyroid failure
m. trabeculation
m. traumatic brain injury
m. ulcerative colitis
m. X-linked recessive muscular dystrophy

mildly
m. dilated congestive cardiomyopathy
m. hyperplastic bone marrow
m. icteric infant
infant mildly icteric
m. subnormal

mild-to-moderate obesity

miles
M. abdominoperineal resection
m. per hour
M. syndrome

Miles-Carpenter syndrome

milestone
Clinical Adaptive Test/Clinical Linguistic and Auditory M. Scale
Clinical Linguistic and Auditory M. Scale
Early Language M. Scale
m. event

milia
m. cyst
m. en plaque
multiple m.
multiple eruptive m.
m. neonatorum
periocular m.

Milian
M. citrine skin
M. disease
M. erythema
M. sign
M. syndrome

miliaria
m. alba
apocrine m.
m. crystalloid
occlusion m.
m. papulosa
m. profunda
m. propria
m. pustulosa
m. rubra
m. vesiculosa

miliaris

miliary
m. abscess
m. acne
acute miliary tuberculosis
m. aneurysm
m. brain metastasis
m. calcified necrosis
m. embolism
m. fever
m. granulomatosis
m. granulomatous inflammation
m. infiltrate
m. lesion
m. metastasis
m. nodule
m. papular syphilid
m. pulmonary aspergillosis
Redlich-Fisher miliary plaque

miliary *(continued)*
m. sarcoid
m. sudamina
m. tuberculosis
milieu
m. environment
m. management intervention
m. therapy
military
m. antishock trousers
m. brace maneuver
m. brace position
foreign m.
m. forensic psychiatry
full-jacketed military round
m. history
m. medicine
sick in quarters m.
milium
m. cyst
m. neonatorum
milk
m. abscess
alcohol in breast m.
m. alkali syndrome
m. allergy
ampulla of milk duct
m. anemia
banked breast m.
m. of bismuth
m. bolus obstruction
breast m.
m. of calcium microcyst
m. of calcium urinary tract cyst
certified raw m.
cornmeal, soybean, m.
m. corpuscle
cow's m.
cow's milk allergy
cow's milk anemia
cow's milk protein
cow's milk protein allergy
m. crust
m. cyst
m. diet
diphasic milk fever
dried skim m.
m. drinker's syndrome
m. duct
m. ejection reflex
expressed breast m.
m. factor
m. fat globule
m. fat globule membrane
m. fat globule protein
m. fever
full-strength breast m.
m. gland
human breast m.
human milk fat globule
human milk fortifier
human milk lysozyme
human milk reverse transcriptase enzyme
m. intolerance
m. lactose allergy
m. leg
m. let-down
m. let-down reflex
m. lines
m. lines of abdomen
m. lines of thorax
m. of magnesia
m. and molasses
mother's breast m.
mouse milk fat globule
m. precipitin disease
preterm m.
m. protein allergy
m. protein hydrolysate
m. protein intolerance
m. proteolysis test
m. ring
m. ring test
m. scall
m. scan
m. sickness
skim m.
m. stool
m. teeth
term m.
m. tetter
m. thistle
m. triglyceride
whole m.
whole boiled m.
whole cow's m.
woman m.
milk-based formula
milkers'
m. node
m. nodule virus
milk-free diet
milk-induced colitis
milking of umbilical cord
milkmaid's
m. elbow dislocation
m. grip
m. hand
m. sign
Milkman syndrome
milk-of-calcium calcification
milk-plasma ratio
milkshake
vanilla m.
milk/soy-protein allergy
milky
m. ascites
m. cataract
m. fluid
mill
bone m.
m. fever
paper mill worker's disease
m. wheel murmur
Millar
M. asthma
M. catheter
Millard
M. advancement rotation flap reconstruction
M. bilateral cleft lip repair
M. flap
M. forked flap technique
M. graft augmentation
Millard-Gubler syndrome
milled-in curves
Millennium LX microsurgical system
Millen-Read modification
Millen technique
miller
M. Analogies Test
M. Assessment for Preschoolers
m. asthma
M. Behavioral Style Scale
M. blade
M. chemicoparasitic theory
M. collutory
M. Fisher syndrome
M. flatfoot operation
M. foot procedure
M. index
modified Miller maneuver
Norman Miller vaginopexy
M. ovum
M. syndrome
Miller-Abbott tube
Miller-Dieker lissencephaly syndrome
Miller-Fisher
M.-F. test
M.-F. variant
Miller-Galante I hemiarthroplasty

Miller-Yoder Test of Grammatical Comprehension

Milles syndrome

millet seed nodule

Millex filter

milliampere
- atrial m.
- m. impulse

millicuries destroyed

milliequivalent
- m.'s per 24 hours
- m. per liter

Milligan-Morgan hemorrhoidectomy

milligram
- femtomoles per m.
- m.'s percent
- m. per deciliter
- m. per hour
- m. per kilogram
- m. per kilogram per day
- m. per kilogram per hour
- m. per liter

milli-International unit one-thousandth of an International Unit

millikatal per liter

milliliter
- colonies per m.
- curies per m.
- grams per m.
- microunits per m.
- m. per deciliter
- m. per kilogram
- m.'s per liter
- m.'s per minute
- 100 units per m.

millimass unit

millimeter
- cubic m.
- m.'s of mercury
- m.'s partial pressure
- m.'s of water

millimole per liter

million
- m. electron volts
- infectious units per m.
- m. international units
- m.'s of particles per cubic foot of air
- parts per hundred m.
- m. units

millionth

milliosmoles per kilogram

millipede sting

millipore
- m. filter method
- single antibody millipore filtration

milliroentgen
- m. equivalent man
- m. equivalent physical
- m.'s per hour at one meter

milliunit
- international m.

Millon
- M. Adolescent Clinical Inventory
- M. Adolescent Personality Inventory
- M. Behavioral Health Inventory
- M. Clinical Multiaxial Inventory test

Mills-Reincke phenomenon

mill wheel murmur

***mil/raf* protooncogene/oncogene**

Milroy
- M. disease
- M. edema

Miltner rotary bone rasp

Milton
- M. disease
- M. edema
- M. urticaria

Milwaukee
- M. Academic Interest Inventory
- M. brace
- M. knee syndrome
- M. shoulder syndrome

mimetic
- m. chorea
- m. convulsion
- m. labor

mimic convulsion

mimicker of malignancy

mimicry
- antigenic m.
- molecular m.

Mims
- nevus sebaceous of Feuerstein and M.

MiMyCA syndrome

Minaar
- M. classification of coalition
- M. classification system
- M. coalition classification

Minamata disease

Minatitlan virus

mind
- m. blindness
- m. control
- Style of M. Inventory

mind-altering
- m.-a. drug

mind-body
- m.-b. dualism
- m.-b. interaction
- m.-b. intervention
- m.-b. medicine

mineral
- apparent mineral corticoid excess syndrome
- m. apposition rate
- areal bone mineral density
- m. balance study
- m. basal medium
- bone mineral content
- bone mineral densitometry
- bone mineral density
- bone mineral mass
- decreased bone mineral density
- m. deficiency
- m. dust airway disease
- m. fiber
- m. flux
- m. homeostasis
- lactic acid mineral medium
- lumbar spine bone mineral density
- magnesium hydroxide and mineral oil emulsion
- man-made mineral fiber
- matrix
- m. metabolism
- m. oil
- perilacunar mineral matrix
- proteins, vitamins, and m.'s
- m. requirement
- m. salts medium
- standard mineral base
- m. supplementation
- total body bone m.
- total body bone mineral density
- m. trioxide aggregate
- volumetric bone mineral density

mineralization
- bone m.
- m. defect
- m. front
- m. impairment
- m. lag time
- matrix m.

mineralized
m. bone histology
m. matrix
mineralizing microangiopathy
mineralocorticoid
m. agonist
apparent mineralocorticoid excess syndrome
apparent mineralocorticoid excess
m. deficiency
m. excess
m. hormone
m. receptor
m. replacement
m. replacement therapy
mineralocorticoid-deficiency RTA
mineral-related nutritional disorder
miner's
m. anemia
m. blindness
coal miner's lung
m. cramp
m. cramps
m. disease
m. headache
m. lung
m. nystagmus
Minerva
M. fixation
Ming criteria
mini
Assura closed mini pouch
m. condylar plate
m. hormone
M. International Neuropsychiatric Interview
M. Inventory of Right Brain Injury
m. lag screw system
modified version of the mini mental status examination
Monarch Mini Mask nasal interface
m. object test
m. Vidas automated immunoassay system
miniature
m. carrier
m. centrifugal fast analyzer
m. endplate current
m. endplate potential
m. forceps
giant miniature endplate potential
mass miniature radiography
mass miniature roentgenography
reversed passive hemagglutination by miniature centrifugal fast analysis
m. scarlet fever
miniature-type congenital adrenal hypoplasia
minicircular capsulorrhexis
minicore myopathy
mini-dose heparin
minidrop 60 minidrops = 1 mL
mini-exon-derived
m.-e.-d. ribonucleic acid gene
m.-e.-d. RNA gene
minifixator
articulate m.
mini-functional
m.-f. endoscopic sinus surgery
mini-invasive vascular study
mini-keratoplasty stitch scissors
minilaparoscope cholecystectomy
minilaparotomy cholecystectomy
minimal
m. acceptable height
m. access general surgery
m. access spinal technology
m. active muscle tendon tension
m. air
m. allergies
m. alveolar concentration
ambulates with minimal assist
ambulates with minimal assistance
m. amplitude nystagmus
m. anchorage
m. anesthetic concentration
m. angle resolution
m. antibiotic concentration
m. apparent viscosity
m. assistance for lower body dressing
m. assistance for transfers
m. assistance for upper body dressing
m. assisted transfer
m. audible field
m. audible pressure
m. average dose
m. bactercidal level
m. bacterial concentration
m. bactericidal concentration
m. bactericidal level
m. blood loss
m. brain damage
m. brain dysfunction
m. brain dysfunction syndrome
m. cerebral dysfunction
m. change
m. change disease
m. change idiopathic nephrotic syndrome
m. change lesion
m. change nephropathy
m. change nephrotic syndrome
m. complete-killing concentration
m. concentration of bilirubin
m. contrast
m. coronary vascular resistance index
m. cross-sectional area
m. cue
m. cumulative cardiotoxic dose
m. cytotoxic epitope
m. daily requirement
m. deformation target
m. detectable concentration
m. detectable quantity
m. deviation adenocarcinoma
m. deviation melanoma
m. differentiation
m. dosage
m. dose
m. dose causing 100% death or malformation
m. dose possible
Eagle minimal essential medium
m. effective diameter
m. effective dose
m. erythema dose
m. essential solution
m. euthyroid Graves disease
m. fatal dose
m. forearm vascular resistance
m. fungicidal concentration
m. glomerular change
m. height velocity
m. hemolytic dilution
m. hemolytic dose
m. identifiable odor
idiopathic minimal lesion nephrotic syndrome
improved minimal essential medium, hormone supplemented
m. infecting dose
inhibitor-containing minimal medium
m. inhibitory concentration
m. inhibitory dilution
m. inhibitory dose
m. inspiratory pressure
m. intermittent dosage of heparin

intrastent minimal lumen cross-sectional area
m. irradiation dose
m. isorrheic concentration
left axis deviation, m.
m. lesion disease
m. lesion glomerulonephritis
m. lesion nephrotic syndrome
m. lethal dose
m. medium
m. medullary concentration
m. morbidostatic dose
m. mycoplasmacidal concentration
m. necrosing dose
patient needs minimal assistance for wheelchair mobility
m. perceptible color difference
m. perceptible difference
m. perceptible odor
m. peripheral dose
m. phototoxic erythema dose
m. pigment
m. pigment oculocutaneous albinism
m. popular dose
m. port diameter
potassium-containing minimal capacitation medium
m. protozoacidal concentration
m. pure radium equivalent
m. reacting dose
m. recognizable odor
M. Record of Disability
m. renal disease
m. reproductive unit
m. residual disease
m. response level
stroke with minimal residuum
supplemental minimal sodium
supplemented Eagle minimal essential medium
m. support
m. threshold
m. time interval
m. transurethral resection of prostate
m. urticarial dose
m. venous oxygen consumption
m. weight bearing

minimal-change
m.-c. disease
m.-c. glomerulonephritis

minimal-incision pubovaginal suspension

minimally
m. active infant
m. attenuating medical-grade foam
m. displaced fracture
m. invasive biopsy procedure
m. invasive brain surgery
m. invasive breast biopsy
m. invasive cardiac surgery
m. invasive coronary bypass grafting
m. invasive direct coronary artery bypass graft
m. invasive follicular carcinoma
m. invasive laparoscopic surgery
m. invasive spine surgery
m. invasive valve repair
m. invasive valve replacement surgery
m. invasive video-assisted parathyroidectomy
subperiosteal minimally invasive laser endoscopic facelift
m. symptomatic hypothyroidism

minimal-pigment oculocutaneous albinism

MiniMed

Mini-Med tubing

Mini-Mental State Examination of Folstein

minimi
abductor digiti minimi muscle
extensor digiti m.
extensor digiti minimi muscle
extensor digiti minimi tendon
extensor digit m.
flexor digiti minimi muscle
musculus abductor digiti minimi manus
musculus abductor digiti minimi pedis
musculus extensor digiti m.
musculus extensor minimi digiti
musculus flexor digiti minimi brevis manus
musculus flexor digiti minimi brevis pedis
opponens digiti m.
opponens digiti minimi manus
opponens digiti minimi muscle

mini-microaggregated albumin colloid

minimicrosphere
human albumin m.

minimize
m. or delay urinary incontinence

minimize or delay urinary incontinence

minimum
m. acceptable field
m. alveolar anesthetic concentration
m. alveolar concentration
m. audible field
m. audible pressure
M. Auditory Capabilities Test
m. bactericidal concentration
m. bactericidal concentration test
m. basis set magnetic resonance angiography
m. blood pressure
m. clinically important difference
m. complete-killing concentration
m. concentration of bilirubin
m. daily requirement
m. data set
demand minimum functional capacity
m. detectable concentration
m. deviation
m. duration
m. effective analgesic concentration
m. effective concentration
m. effective dose
m. effective naproxen dose
m. elicitation threshold
m. essential medium
M. Essentials Test
m. flow rate
m. hemolytic dose
m. incision surgery
m. infective dose
m. inhibitory concentration
m. inhibitory concentration susceptibility test
m. isolation
m. laryngeal height
m. lethal concentration
m. lethal dose
light m.
m. light
m. light threshold
m. local analgesic concentration
logarithmic M. Angle of Resolution
m. lumen diameter
maximum diameter to minimum diameter ratio
m. mycoplasmacidal concentration
m. obstructive volume
m. perceptible acuity
m. reacting dose

minimum *(continued)*
m. separable acuity
m. separable angle
suggested minimum increment
m. target absorbed dose
m. temperature
time above minimum inhibitory concentration
m. tolerance dose
m. toxic dose
trough minimum serum concentration
m. visible angle
m. visual angle

minimum-access surgery

minimus
digitus m.
gluteus m.
gluteus minimus muscle
musculus adductor m.

minin ray

mini-open approach

MiniOX
M. 1A oxygen analyzer
M. I, II, III, 100-IV oxygen monitor

mini-Pena procedure

miniplate fixation

minipuberty of infancy

minipump
osmotic m.

minisatellite
m. allele
m. DNA

Miniscope MS-3

mini-Sugita clip

Minitran Patch

mini Vidas automated immunoassay system

mink
Aleutian mink disease
Aleutian mink disease virus
m. enteritis virus
transformed mink fibroblast
transmissible mink encephalopathy

Minkowski-Chauffard syndrome

Minnal virus

Minnesota
M. antilymphoblast globulin
M. antilymphocyte globulin
M. Child Development Inventory
M. Clerical Aptitude Test
M. Clerical Assessment Battery
M. Cocaine Craving Scale
M. Comprehensive Epilepsy Program
M. Differential Diagnosis of Aphasia
M. Engineering Analogies Test
M. Importance Questionnaire
M. Mechanical Assembly Test
M. Multiphasic Personality Inventory Depression Scale
M. Multiphasic Personality Inventory, Second Edition
M. Occupational Classification System
M. Paper Form Board Test
M. Percepto-Diagnostic Test
M. Satisfaction Scale
M. Scholastic Aptitude Test
M. Spatial Relations Test
M. Teacher Attitude Inventory
M. Test for Differential Diagnosis of Aphasia
M. Vocational Interest Inventory

Minnesota-Hartford Personality Assay

minocycline
m. hyperpigmentation
m. periodontal therapeutic system
m. pleurodesis

minocycline-associated pigment

minor
m. acute illness
m. agglutinin
m. alar cartilage
m. alpha asymmetry
alpha-thalassemia m.
m. amputation
m. analysis
angry reaction to minor stimuli
aphthae m.
m. arterial circle
m. arterial circle of iris
arteria palatina m.
m. axis shortening of left ventricle
m. calix
m. causalgia
m. cerebral dysfunction
m. circulus arteriosus
m. circulus arteriosus of iris
m. cluster region
m. connector
m. curve
m. depressive disorder
M. disease
m. duodenal papilla
m. dysmorphism
m. epilepsy
m. fissure
m. forceps
m. form
m. fraction of adult hemoglobin
m. gland obstruction
m. glomerular lesion
m. group antigen incompatibility
m. hallucination
m. head injury
m. hearing loss
m. hippocampus
hippocampus m.
m. histocompatibility antigen
m. histocompatibility complex
m. hypertensive infant
m. hypnosis
m. hysteria
m. image-distorting level
m. impairment
M. iodine-starch test
m. karyotype abnormality
m. lymphadenopathy
m. mechanical debridement
a minor blood group
m. motor seizure
musculus iliacus m.
m. neurologic dysfunction
painful minor intervertebral dysfunction
pectoralis minor muscle
pelvis justo m.
m. physical anomaly
m. surgery suite
thalassemia m.
m. tranquilizer

minor-determinant mixture

minoris
apertura pelvis m.

minority
m. community
m. discrimination
m. group
m. group psychiatry
National Center on M. Health and Health Disparities

minor neurologic dysfunction

Minot disease

Minot-Murphy diet

Minot-von Willebrand syndrome

minoxidil and hair loss

Minsky
M. circle
M. intramarginal splitting
M. operation

minus
m. carrier contact lens
m. cylinder
labium m.
m. sense-RNA genome
m. spectacle lens
standard observed minus expected
m. two hours two hours prior to treatment

minute
alveolar minute ventilation
alveolar ventilation per m.
m. alveolar volume
m. anatomy
beats per m.
births per m.
m. bleeding
m. bleeding ulcer
breaths per m.
counts per m.
cubic feet per m.
cycles per m.
disintegrations per m.
double minute chromosome
double minute sphere
drops per m.
extended mandatory minute ventilation
feet per m.
gallons per m.
heart minute output
impulses per m.
International Unit per m.
left ventricular minute flow
lines printed per m.
liter per minute per square meter
liters per m.
mandatory minute ventilation
mandatory minute volume
microgram per kilogram per m.
milliliters per m.
multiple minute digitate hyperkeratosis
m. output
oxygen consumption per m.
m. oxygen uptake
pressure time per m.
pulses per m.
respiratory rate per m.
m. respiratory volume
shocks per m.
m. ventilation
ventilation per minute of dead space
m. ventilatory volume
vibration per m.
m. virus of canines
m. virus of mice
m. volume of air or blood
volume of inspired gas per m.

7-minute
-m. neurocognitive battery
-m. screen

6-minute walking test

Minx
Ohmeda Minx pulse oximeter

miosis
paralytic m.
pupil m.

miostagmin reaction

miotic
m. alkaloid
m. division
m. pupil
m. therapy

Mira
M. cautery
M. diathermy unit

miracidial immobilization test

miracidium-hatching test

Miraluma test

Mirchamp sign

mires of ophthalmometer

Mirhosseini-Holmes-Walton syndrome

Mirim virus

mirror
Apfelbaum m.
m. area
m. coating
m. drawing
m. duplication
m. examination
m. exercise
m. fear
m. focus
m. hand
m. haploscope
m. image
m. image breast biopsy
m. image interpretation
m. laryngoscopy
m. rocking test
m. syndrome

mirror-image
m.-i. artifact
m.-i. brachiocephalic branching
m.-i. cell
m.-i. complementary antibody
m.-i. dextrocardia

misaligned jaw

miscarriage
recurrent m.
spontaneous m.
threatened m.

miscellaneous reaction

miscible
rapidly miscible pool

Miscue
Reading Miscue Inventory

misdirected
aqueous misdirected glaucoma
m. lash

misdirection
aqueous m.
oculomotor nerve m.
m. phenomenon

misery perfusion syndrome

misfolded protein

Mishima-Hedbys method

mismatch
immobilized mismatch binding protein
mutation mismatch repair
m. negativity
m. repair

mismatched related donor

misoprostol
oral m.

misplaced
m. exocytosis
m. gout
m. hope

misregistration
m. artifact
chemical shift misregistration artifact
oblique flow m.

missed
m. abortion
m. bronchogenic carcinoma
m. diagnosis
m. dose
m. labor

missed *(continued)*
m. ostium sequence
m. period

missense
m. mutation
novel missense mutation

missing
m. block
decayed, missing, and filled teeth
m. self hypothesis
m. teeth

missionary position

mist
m. bacillus
child-adult m.
cold mist humidifier
cool mist vaporizer
m. mask
nebulized mist treatment
m. tent
m. therapy
ultrasonic m.
warm mist humidifier

mistreatment history

misty vision

misuse
alcohol m.

Mital
M. elbow release
M. elbow release operation
M. elbow release technique

Mitchell
M. bunionectomy
M. disease
M. distal osteotomy
M. hallux valgus procedure
M. River virus
Weir Mitchell treatment

MIT:DIT ratio

mite
avian mite dermatitis
m. bite
cat mite dermatitis
m. control
harvest m.'s
house dust m.
m. infestation
northern fowl m.
onion mite dermatitis
m. typhus

mite-borne typhus

Mitek absorbable anchor

Mitis-type Ehlers-Danlos syndrome

mitochondria
m. lipid glucogen

mitochondrial
m. antibody
m. aspartate aminotransferase
m. ataxia
m. ATP production
m. biogenesis
m. cardiomyopathy
m. chromosome
m. complex
m. condensation
m. cristae alteration
m. cytopathy
m. defect
m. deoxyribonucleic acid analysis
m. deoxyribonucleic acid polymerase gamma
m. disease
m. disorder
m. DNA
m. DNA mutation
m. DNA polymerase gamma
m. DNA syndrome
m. dysfunction
m. encephalomyopathy
m. encephalomyopathy with sensorimotor polyneuropathy
m. encephalomyopathy with sensorimotor polyneuropathy, ophthalmoplegia, and paralysis
m. encephalopathy
m. enzyme
m. ethanol oxidase system
m. fatty acid beta-oxidation
m. free radical generation
fumarate hydratase, m.
m. glutamate dehydrogenase pathway
glutamic-oxaloacetic transaminase, m.
m. glycine cleavage system
m. hydroxylase enzyme
m. inheritance
m. injury
m. matrix
m. membrane potential
m. myopathy
m. myopathy, encephalopathy, lactic acidosis, strokelike episodes
m. neurogastrointestinal encephalomyopathy
nucleoside-associated mitochondrial toxicity
outer mitochondrial membrane
m. oxidative phosphorylation
m. P450 monooxygenase
m. porin
m. respiratory chain defect
m. respiratory chain enzyme
m. respiratory chain enzyme complex
m. targeting sequence
thymidine kinase, m.
m. toxicity

mitochondrion of hemoflagellate

mitogen
m. activation
pokeweed m.
m. response

mitogen-activated
m.-a. protein
m.-a. protein kinase
m.-a. protein kinase cascade
m.-a. protein kinase pathway

mitogen-activating
m.-a. protein

mitogenic
m. activity
m. adherence lectin
m. effect
m. factor
leukocyte mitogenic factor
m. peptide

mitogen-induced lymphocyte proliferation

mitomycin
Adriamycin, vincristine, mitomycin C
m. adsorbed onto activated charcoal
m. C, Adriamycin, cyclophosphamide
m. C, Adriamycin, Platinol
m. cardiotoxicity
m. C, etoposide, Platinol
m. C and 5-FU Nigro protocol
m. C, Oncovin, bleomycin, cisplatin
m. and 5-fluorouracil
m., 5-fluorouracil, Adriamycin
m., vinblastine, Platinol

mitosis, pl. **mitoses**
percentage of labeled mitoses
m. phase
phase of mitosis in cell growth cycle

mitosis-karyorrhexis index

mitosis-promoting
m.-p. factor

mitotic
m. activity
m. apparatus
m. arrest
m. chromosome
m. cycle
m. division
m. figure
m. index
m. inhibitor
nuclear mitotic apparatus
m. organizing center
quiescent phase of cells leaving the mitotic cycle
m. spindle apparatus
m. spindle inhibitor

mitotic-control protein

mitotic-karyorrhectic index

mitotic-karyorrhexis
m.-k. index

mitral
acute mitral regurgitation
m. annular calcification
m. annular calcium
m. annulus calcification
anomalous mitral arcade
anterior cusp of mitral valve
anterior leaflet of the mitral valve
anterior mitral leaflet
anterior mitral valve leaflet
anterior motion of posterior mitral valve leaflet
m. anuloplasty
m. and aortic valve replacement
m. apparatus
m. arcade
arching of mitral valve leaflet
m. area
m. atresia
m. balloon commissurotomy
balloon mitral commissurotomy
balloon mitral valvotomy
balloon mitral valvuloplasty
m. balloon valvotomy
billowing mitral leaflet syndrome
bowing of mitral valve leaflet
brachydactyly, mesomelia, mental retardation, aortic dilation, mitral valve prolapse, characteristic facies syndrome
calcific mitral stenosis
m. cell layer
m. cells
m. click
combined mitral stenosis and regurgitation
m. commissurotomy
m. component
m. configuration of cardiac shadow
congenital anomaly of mitral valve
congenital mitral regurgitation
m. deceleration slope
m. disease
early mitral valve closure
fishmouth configuration of mitral valve
flail mitral leaflet
floppy mitral valve
gonadal failure, short stature, mitral valve prolapse, mental retardation syndrome
m. gradient
idiopathic mitral valve prolapse
m. incompetence
incomplete mitral leaflet closure
m. insufficiency
ischemic mitral regurgitation
m. leaflet
m. leaflet syndrome
mental retardation, mitral valve prolapse, characteristic face syndrome
midsystolic buckling of mitral valve
mitral pressure half-time Doppler
mixed mitral disease
opening mitral valve snap
m. opening snap
open mitral commissurotomy
open mitral valve commissurotomy
parachute deformity of mitral valve
percutaneous mitral balloon commissurotomy
percutaneous mitral balloon valvotomy
percutaneous mitral balloon valvuloplasty
percutaneous mitral balloon valvulotomy
percutaneous mitral valvoplasty
percutaneous transatrial mitral commissurotomy
percutaneous transvenous mitral commissurotomy
posterior m.
posterior leaf mitral valve
posterior mitral valve leaflet
premature mitral closure
mitral pressure half-time Doppler
prolapsed mitral valve syndrome
prolapse of mitral valve
prolapsing mitral leaflet
quadricusp mitral valve
m. reflux
m. regurgitant flow
m. regurgitant murmur
rheumatic mitral stenosis
silent mitral stenosis
m. stenoregurgitation
m. stenosis in pregnancy
supraannular mitral valve replacement
systolic anterior motion of mitral valve
thickened mitral valve
m. valve
m. valve aneurysm
m. valve anterior leaflet
m. valve, aorta, skeleton, skin
m. valve area
m. valve atresia
m. valve closure
m. valve disease
m. valve echo
m. valve endocarditis
m. valve gradient
m. valve hypoplasia
m. valve insufficiency
m. valve leaflet excursion
m. valve opening
m. valve orifice
m. valve orifice area
m. valve prolapse
m. valve prolapse, aortic anomalies, skeletal changes, and skin changes syndrome
m. valve prosthesis
m. valve regurgitation
m. valve repair
m. valve stenosis
m. valve surgery
m. valve-transverse
m. valvular disease
m. valvulotomy

mitral valvular disease

Mitrofanoff
M. appendicovesicostomy
M. catheterizable channel
M. conduit
M. continent urinary stoma
M. principle
M. technique

Mitsuda
M. antigen

Mitsuda *(continued)*
M. radiation
M. reaction
M. test
Mitsuyasu staging system
mitten
slow mitten pattern
Mittendorf dot
Mittendorf-Williams rule
mitten hand
mitten-hand deformity
Mittlemeir broach
Mitutoyo digital caliper
Mity engine T-file
Mitzuo phenomenon
mix
fragrance m.
mixed
m. abscess
m. acid-base disorder
m. acid fermentation
adjustment disorder with mixed anxiety and depressed mood
adjustment disorder with mixed disturbance of emotions
m. aerobic and anaerobic abscess
m. aerobic and anaerobic flora
m. agglutination test
m. agonist-antagonist
allogeneic mixed leukocyte culture
m. amputation
m. aneurysm
m. antiglobulin reaction
m. antiinflammatory syndrome
m. anxiety depression disorder
m. aortic valve disease
m. aphasia
m. apnea
m. asthma
m. astigmatism with myopia predominating
m. attenuation mass
atypical or mixed organic brain syndrome
atypical mixed or other personality disorder
autologous mixed leukocyte reaction
autologous mixed lymphocyte culture
autologous mixed lymphocyte reaction
m. bacterial-fungal keratitis
m. bacterial toxin
m. bag
m. beat
m. bipolar affective psychosis
m. bipolar state
m. bone lesion
m. calculus
m. capillary cavernous hemangioma
m. cataract
m. cell agglutination reaction
m. cell leukemia
m. cell nodular lymphoma
m. cell sarcoma
m. cellular Hodgkin disease
m. cellularity Hodgkin disease
m. cerebral dominance
m. cerebral palsy
m. chancre
m. cirrhosis
m. compulsive states psychasthenia
m. connective-tissue disease
m. connective tissue disease
m. connective tissue disorder
conversion disorder, mixed type
m. cord syndrome
m. cryoglobulinemia
m. cryoglobulinemia with glomerulonephritis
m. cryoglobulin syndrome
m. culture, leukocyte
m. deafness
m. density mass
m. dentition analysis
m. design
m. development developmental delay disorder
m. diet
difference in nitrogen tension between mixed alveolar gas and mixed arterial blood
difference in partial pressures of oxygen in mixed alveolar gas and mixed arterial blood
diffuse mixed lymphoma
m. discrete-continuous random variable
m. disturbance stress reaction
m. disulfide
m. donor-host hematopoietic chimerism
m. echogenic solid mass
m. epithelial-mesenchymal tumor
m. esotropia
m. essential cryoglobulinemia
essential mixed cryoglobulinemia
m. expired carbon dioxide tension
m. expired gas
m. failure
m. fat-water density lesion
m. feather
m. feature
m. flexor/extensor fit
m. follicular hyperplasia
m. foot dominant
m. form cerebral palsy
m. function oxidase system
m. fungal/bacterial infection
m. fungal organism
m. germ cell-sex cord stromal tumor
m. germ cell tumor
m. GH-PRL cell adenoma
m. GH- and prolactin-secreting adenoma
m. gland
m. glioma
m. gonadal dysgenesis
m. growth hormone-prolactin cell adenoma
m. growth hormone- and prolactin-secreting adenoma
m. growth on culture
m. headache
m. hearing impairment
m. hearing loss
m. hemadsorption
m. hemangioma
m. hematopoietic chimerism
m. hemorrhoid
m. hemorrhoids
m. hepatic porphyria
m. histology tumor
Hodgkin disease, mixed nodular type
m. hyperlipemia
m. hyperlipidemia
m. hyperlipoproteinemia familial type 5 hyperlipidemia
m. hypoglycemia
m. hypothyroidism
m. immunity
m. immunofluorescence
m. infantile spasm
m. inflammatory granuloma
m. joint
m. large- and small-cell non-Hodgkin lymphoma
m. leprosy
m. leukocyte concentration
m. leukocyte culture
m. leukocyte response

m. leukocyte-trophoblast culture
m. ligand chelate
m. lineage leukemia
m. lymphocyte concentration
m. lymphocyte culture
m. lymphocyte culture reaction
m. lymphocyte culture test
m. lymphocyte culture, weak
m. lymphocyte reaction blocking factor
m. lymphocyte response
m. lymphocyte target interaction
m. lymphocytic-histiocytic lymphoma
malignant mixed mesodermal tumor
malignant mixed müllerian tumor
malignant mixed oligoastrocytoma
m. mesodermal tumor
metastatic mixed müllerian tumor
m. mitral disease
m. monitor
müllerian mixed tumor
m. müllerian sarcoma
m. müllerian tumor
m. nail infection
m. nerve action potential
m. neutron and photon radiotherapy
nodular, mixed cell lymphoma
nodular mixed lymphoma
m. obstructive apnea-hypopnea index
m. oligoastrocytoma
m. opioid agonist-antagonist
m. ovarian mesodermal sarcoma
oxygen content of mixed venous blood
partial oxygen pressure in mixed venous blood
partial pressure of carbon dioxide in mixed venous blood
m. pattern
m. phenotype tumor
m. photon-electron technique
m. pituitary adenoma-gangliocytoma
m. porphyria
m. receptive-expressive language disorder
repetitive excess mixed anhydride method
m. respiratory
m. respiratory failure
m. respiratory vaccine
m. reverse passive antiglobulin hemagglutination
m. rheumatoid and degenerative arthritis
m. sclerosing bone dysplasia, small stature, seizures, mental retardation syndrome
m. sclerosing bone dystrophy
m. seborrheic-staphylococcal blepharitis
m. sensorimotor polyneuropathy
m. sensory polyneuritis
m. sex cord-stromal tumor
m. skin cell leukocyte reaction
m. sleep apnea
m. small cleaved and large cell lymphoma
m. sore
m. strabismus
suppertime mixed insulin and daytime sulfonylureas
m. thymoma
m. tissue tumor
m. tumor of salivary gland
m. tumor of skin
m. type of incontinence
m. umbilical arterial acidemia
m. uremic osteodystrophy
m. uterine tumor
m. vaccine, respiratory infection
m. venous
m. venous blood
m. venous hypoxia
m. venous oxygen
m. venous oxygen content
m. venous oxygen saturation
m. vespid antigen
m. vespid venom
m. virus respiratory infection
X-linked progressive mixed deafness with perilymphatic gusher

mixed-cellularity type

mixed-density mass

mixed-function oxygenase

mixed-linker PCR

mixed-type

m.-t. carcinoma
m.-t. cerebral palsy
m.-t. delusion
m.-t. epilepsy

mixing

m. lesion
metal handle mixing spatula
pulmonary blood mixing volume
right heart mixing volume

Mixter clamp

mixture

alcohol, chloroform, and ether m.
amino acid m.
anesthetic gas m.
m. approach
automated mixture control
ether-chloroform mixture
eutectic mixture of local anesthetics
helium-oxygen m.
toxoid-antitoxoid m.
toxoid-antitoxoid mixture esterase
xylene-alcohol m.

Miyagawa body

Miyake technique

Miyazaki-Bonney

M.-B. test
M.-B. test for stress incontinence

Miyazaki technique

Miyoshi myopathy

Mizuo-Nakamura

M.-N. effect
M.-N. phenomenon

M-K medium

Mladick

M. abdominoplasty
M. ear reconstruction

MLH1 **gene**

MLH1 promoter methylation

MLM **gene**

10-mm

-m. trocar
-m. umbilical port

2-mm/3-cm coil

2-mm/6-cm coil

5-mm suprapubic trocar

10-mm umbilical port

Mn936-77 virus

mnemic hypothesis

mnemonic dementia

MNSs

M. antigen
M. blood group

MO1 antigen

Mobala virus

mob behavior

Moberg
M. advancement flap
M. arthrodesis
M. deltoid muscle transfer
M. deltoid-to-triceps transfer
M. flap
M. free tendon graft

Moberg-Gedda fracture

Mobetron mobile, self-shielded electron accelerator

mobile
m. advanced real-time image
m. anaerobic laboratory
m. arc
m. arm support
m. artery and vein imaging system
carina midline sharp and m.
m. coronary care unit
m. crisis outreach team
m. duodenum
m. electroconvulsive therapy apparatus
m. end
fundus anterior, normal size and shape, and m.
m. gene
healthy mobile sperm
m. hospital
Immediate Response M. Analysis
m. intensive care nurse
m. intensive care unit
m. mass x-ray
Mobetron mobile, self-shielded electron accelerator
m. surgical unit

mobile advanced real-time image

mobility
m. activities of daily living
m. aid
assistance and m.
bed mobility skill
circulation, sensation, m.
delirium, infection, atrophic urethritis and vaginitis, pharmaceuticals, psychological disorders, excessive urine output, restricted mobility, stool impaction
m. disability
electrophoretic m.
electrophoretic mobility shift analysis
electrophoretic mobility shift assay
gait and m.
heteroduplex mobility assay
high mobility group
impaired physical m.
limited joint m.
low mobility group
macrophage electrophoretic m.
maximum level of independent m.
patient needs minimal assistance for wheelchair m.
Performance-Oriented M. Assessment
relative m.
restore mobility and reduce pain
Rivermead M. Index
m. shift assay
m. specialist
syndrome of limited joint m.
tanned erythrocyte electrophoretic m.

mobilization
ASTM augmented soft tissue m.
augmented soft tissue m.
lipid m.
localized leukocyte m.

mobilizing agent

Mobin-Uddin filter

Mobitz
M. atrioventricular block
M. I heart block
M. I, II block
M. type I, II block

Möbius-von Graefe-Stellway sign

MOC-31 antibody

moccasin
m. appearance
m. foot
m. snake bite

moccasin-type tinea pedis

modal
m. adaptive task
m. auxiliary
m. dose
m. frequency
m. sensitivity

modality
adjuvant diagnostic m.
atypical sensory m.
auditory m.
combined drug and radiation m.
combined modality therapy
immune response and combined modality treatment
independent toxicity in combined modality therapy
individual sensory m.
Language Modalities Test for Aphasia
pacing m.
Symbol Digit Modalities Test

Modane
M. Bulk
M. Soft

mode
m. abandonment
m. of action
m. of administration with hallucinogen
amplitude m.
assist-control mode ventilation
asynchronous transfer m.
automatic mode conversion
automatic mode switching
autosomal recessive m.
Bernse Coping M.'s
common mode rejection
control mode ventilation
m. of death
m. of inheritance
Inquiry M. Questionnaire: A Measure of How You Think and Make Decisions
motion m.
pulse-inversion mode ultrasound
rapid processing m.
stimulated echo acquisition m.
time-motion m.
transverse electromagnetic m.
ventricular pacing, atrial sensing, triggered mode, pacemaker

model
affective schematic mental m.
affect-related schematic mental m.
affect trauma m.
AIDS risk-reduction m.
autoregressive model for signal analysis
awareness training m.
Clinical Practice M.
m. denture wax
discriminant analytic m.
Emory Pain Estimate M.
m. game
generalized linear interactive m.
general linear m.
Health Belief M.
high-risk model of threat perception
m. of illness
m. immune complex

Koshland-Némethy-Filmer m.
limited sampling m.
linear combination model software
longitudinal random coefficient m.
Markov state-transition m.
maximal electroshock m.
Monod-Wyman-Changeux model
Mortality Probability M.
multifactorial m.
multistage Markov m.
nonlinear mixed-effects model
Ogawa model for hematopoiesis
Preventive Health M.
risk m.
risk-screening m.
Schmitt-Erlanger model of reentry
subhuman primate m.
m. system

model-based image processing

modeling

m. compound
cortical bone m.
m. derivation
dialysate urea kinetic m.
m. exercise
mathematical modeling technique
Monte Carlo m.
urea kinetic m.

mode-locked Nd:YAG laser

moderate

m. allergies
m. amplitude
m. arthritic condition
m. ataxia
m. atherosclerosis with calcification
m. atopic dermatitis
m. category
m. chronic hepatitis
m. constant suction
m. dehydration
m. depression
m. difficulty
m. disability
m. hearing impairment
m. hearing loss
m. hirsutism
m. hypothermia
m. infiltrate
m. intensity exercise
m. intermittent suction
long-term variability-average to m.
m. mental retardation
m. number of medium rales
patient with mild to moderate systemic disease
m. persistent asthma
m. renal failure
m. renal insufficiency
m. resistance
m. rubra lochia
m. tactile stimulus
m. ulcerative colitis

moderate-dose methotrexate, bleomycin, Adriamycin, cyclophosphamide, Oncovin, dexamethasone

moderately

m. advanced
m. constricted and equally reactive pupil
m. constricted and slightly reactive pupil
m. differentiated
m. differentiated adenocarcinoma
m. differentiated adenoma
m. differentiated neuroendocrine carcinoma
m. dilated and equally reactive pupil
m. dilated and slightly reactive pupil
m. dilated ureter
m. disabled
m. low birth weight
mild to moderately impaired
m. narrow anterior chamber angle
m. susceptible
m. wide open anterior chamber angle

moderate-severe allergies

moderator band

modern

m. genetics
M. Occupational Skills Test

modification

Allman modification of Evans ankle reconstruction
Anderson modification of Berndt-Harty classification
Astler-Coller modification of Dukes classification
behavior m.
behavior modification technique
Biological Response M. Program
Body Dysmorphic Disorder M. of Yale-Brown Obsessive-Compulsive Scale, McLean version
cardiac risk factor m.
chromosome modification site
Cooley modification of Waterson anastomosis
dose m.
electrophysiologic behavior m.
Ganley modification of Keller arthroplasty
gradual lifestyle m.
International Classification of Diseases–Clinical M.
lifestyle m.
McGlamry and Feldman m.
metatarsal bar shoe m.
Nottingham modification of Scarff-Bloom-Richardson grading
oxidative modification of LDL
pylorus-preserving Whipple m.
Rossetti modification of Nissen fundoplication
thematic content modification program

modified

m. acid
m. acid-fast stain
m. amino acid
aniline blue modified trichrome stain
m. anterior hairline forehead lift
m. anterior scoring technique
antrum-sparing modified Whipple procedure
Auchincloss modified radical mastectomy
M. Autonomic Perception Questionnaire
m. Bagshawe protocol
m. band lid method
m. barbital buffer
m. Bardach repair
m. barium swallow
m. barium swallow with videofluoroscopy
m. Barthel degree of disability index
m. Bassini herniorrhaphy
m. Becker repair
m. Beighton criteria
m. Belsey fundoplication
m. Belsey fundoplication procedure
m. Belsey fundoplication technique
m. Bernard-Burow procedure
m. Bernard-Burow technique

modified *(continued)*
m. Bernoulli equation
m. Blalock-Taussig
m. Blalock-Taussig shunt
m. Boyd amputation
m. Boyd amputation of ankle and distal tibial physis
m. Boyd ankle arthrodesis
m. brachial technique
m. Broström-Evans procedure
m. Burch colpourethropexy
m. Cantwell technique
m. cast
chemically modified protein
m. chest lead
m. Child technique
m. Chopart amputation
m. Chrisman-Snook ankle reconstruction
M. Clinical Technique test
m. C-loop UV lens
m. Cocklin toe operation
m. Cotrel cast
m. Crawford Campbell inlaid bone-grafting technique
m. Dallas classification of disc morphology grades 0–7
m. Darrach-type elevator
m. desmosome
m. Dieterle stain
m. directly observed therapy
m. double-opposing tab flap nipple reconstruction
m. double-opposing tablet
m. Draize test
Dulbecco modified Eagle medium
m. Essed-Schroeder corporoplasty
m. Fischer classification
m. fishtail excision
m. flap operation
m. Fontan operation
m. Fontan procedure
m. Frankel classification
m. Frost method
m. Frost suture
m. gain ratio
Gait Abnormality Rating Scale M.
m. Gait Abnormality Rating Scale
genetically m.
genetically modified organisms
m. Gibson incision
m. Gilsbach technique
glycopeptide moiety modified derivative
m. Gomori trichrome reaction
m. gull wing incision
m. Hanks balanced salt solution
m. Harrington rod
m. Harris hip score
m. Hassan open technique
M. Health Assessment Questionnaire
m. heat-degraded gelatin
m. Heller esophagomyotomy
m. Hohmann bunionectomy
m. Hoke-Miller flatfoot procedure
m. immune serum globulin
M. Injury Severity Score
m. innervated antral pouch
m. Irving-type tubal ligation
m. J loop
m. J-loop intraocular lens
m. J-loop UV lens
m. Kinyoun acid-fast stain
left modified radical mastectomy
malondialdehyde modified low-density lipoprotein
Mayo hallux valgus modified operation
Mayo modified total elbow arthroplasty
m. measles
m. Miller maneuver
M. Mini-Mental State Examination
m. monovision
m. neck dissection
m. oxidase test
m. Peyronie bladder neck suspension
m. piggyback
m. Pomeroy technique
m. Powell method
protein-sparing modified fast
m. radical hysterectomy
m. radical mastectomy
m. rapid fermentation test
m. rhyme hearing test
M. Richardson technique
right modified radical mastectomy
m. Ritgen maneuver
m. Rodman skin thickness score
m. Roeder knot
m. sea water yeast extract agar
m. sham feeding
m. Simpson rule
m. sling
m. smallpox
M. Somatic Perception Questionnaire
m. systemic Berlin-Frankfurt-Munster therapy
Thayer-Martin, modified agar
thermoacidurans agar m.
m. tone decay test
m. treadmill exercise testing
m. trichrome stain
m. University of Wisconsin solution
m. vaccine virus Ankara
m. Van Lint anesthesia
m. Van Lint block
m. varicella-like syndrome
m. version of the mini mental status examination
m. whole-egg slant medium
m. Wies procedure
M. Word Learning Test

modified double-opposing tab flap nipple reconstruction

modifier
biologic response m.
multidimensional analysis beam m.
selective estrogen response m.

modify
m. hearing patterns
m. stressful living habits

modifying
m. gene
time and m.

modiolus
m. of angle of mouth
m. anguli oris
longitudinal canal of m.
spiral vein of m.

Modoc virus

modular
M. Acetabular Revision System
anatomic modular knee
catabolite modular factor
knee
M. One pneumatonometer

modulated
Rate M. Pacing

modulating
calcium-signal modulating cyclophilin B ligand
immune modulating Nutrition

modulation
amplitude m.
attenuation-based on-line modulation of the tube current
brightness m.
frequency m.
immune modulation procedure

Multivane Intensity M. Compensator
m. potential
pulse code m.
m. rate
rheumatic pain modulation disorder
self-phase m.
spatial modulation of magnetization
m. transfer factor
m. transfer function

modulator
m. of adenylate cyclase
cAMP-response element m.
downstream regulatory element antagonistic modulator gene
full allosteric m.'s
ion conductance m.
multidrug resistance m.
partial allosteric m.'s
m. protein
selective androgen-receptor m.
selective estrogen receptor m.

modulator/demodulator

module
Peak gait m.
Testing-Teaching M. of Auditory Discrimination
venous pressure m.

modulus
m. blipped echo-planar single-pulse technique
M. CD anesthesia system
m. of compression
m. of elasticity
section m.

MODY3 HNF-1-alpha mutation

Moeller
M. decarboxylation test
M. glossitis
M. itch

Moeller-Barlow disease

Moersch-Woltman syndrome

mofetil
mycophenolate m.

Mogen
M. circumcision
M. clamp

Mohr-Claussen syndrome

Mohrenheim fossa

Mohr syndrome

Mohr-Tranebjaerg syndrome

Mohs
M. chemosurgery
M. defect
M. fresh tissue chemosurgery technique
M. fresh-tissue technique
M. hardness
M. hardness number
M. hardness scale
M. hardness test
M. micrographic surgery
M. microsurgical resection
M. procedure

moiety
asparagine-linked glycosylation m.
glycopeptide moiety modified derivative
lipid m.

moist
m. desquamation
m. gangrene
m. heat
m. heat therapy
m. heat treatment
hot moist compresses
hot moist packs
hot moist poultice
mucous membranes m.
oral mucosa pink and m.
oral mucous membrane m.
oral mucous membrane pink and m.
m. pack
m. papule
pink, moist, and warm mucous membranes
m. rale
m. snuff
m. tetter
warm moist heat
warm moist pack unsterile
m. wart

moistened fine mesh gauze dressing

moisture
m. fear-molar approach
heat and moisture exchanging filter
synthetic, adhesive, moisture vapor permeable
m. vapor transmission rate

moisturizer
occlusive m.
topical m.

Moju virus

Mokola virus

molar
m. absorbancy index
m. absorption coefficient
m. absorptivity
m. band
m. behavior
m. bite position
m. bracket
m. concentration
m. crowding
m. degeneration
m. esterification rate
m. evacuation
m. extinction coefficient
m. gland
m. heat capacity
human molar thyrotropin
hundredth molar solution
impacted m.
maxillary first molar alveolus
mulberry m.
m. permanent tooth
m. pregnancy
m. solution
tenth molar solution

molasses
milk and m.

mold
m. acetabular arthroplasty
m. aeroallergen
Aufranc concentric hip m.
m. control
ear m.
endolaryngeal brachytherapy m.
m. guide
intraoral dental m.'s
m. spore
m. therapy

molded
m. ankle-foot orthosis
m. frame
long leg posterior molded splint

molding
atheroma m.
m. of head
passive alveolar molding appliance

mold-injected lens

Moldite
Ophthalmic Moldite Powder

mole
amniography in hydatidiform m.
atypical mole syndrome
concentration in moles per liter
familial atypical mole malignant melanoma

mole *(continued)*
m. fraction
hydatidiform m.
invasive m.
malignant mole syndrome
partial hydatidiform m.
m. per cubic meter
m. per kilogram
m. per liter

molectron laser

molecular
m. adsorbent recirculating system
m. allelotyping
m. anemia
m. approach
m. assay
m. behavior
m. biology
m. biophysics
m. cell biology
m. chaperone
m. clone
m. cloning
m. cloning and sequencing
m. coincidence detection
m. diagnostic technique
m. diffusion
m. disease
m. dispersed solution
m. dispersion
m. dissociation theory
m. distillation
m. dualism
electromagnetic molecular electronic resonance
m. epidemiology
m. exclusion chromatography
m. external layer
m. and general genetics
m. genetic alteration
m. genetic analysis
m. genetics
m. genetics/oncology laboratory
m. genetic study
m. genetic technique
highest occupied molecular orbital
high molecular weight
high molecular weight component
high molecular weight dextran
high molecular weight glycoprotein
high molecular weight hemoglobin
high molecular weight kininogen
high molecular weight melanoma-associated antigen
high molecular weight polyethylene
human molecular genetics
m. hybridization study
m. inner layer
m. internal layer
m. latency
m. layer
m. layer of cerebellar cortex
m. layer of cerebral cortex
m. layer of retina
m. layers of olfactory bulb
light molecular weight meromyosin
localized molecular orbital
lowest empty molecular orbital
lowest unoccupied molecular orbital
low molecular weight dextran
low molecular weight heparin
low molecular weight oxidizing agent
low molecular weight proteinuria
m. marker
m. mimicry
new molecular entity
m. orbital
m. outer layer
m. probe hybridization
m. probe testing
m. recognition unit
m. regulation
relative molecular mass
m. target-based screen
type of molecular bond
m. typing
ultrahigh molecular weight
ultrahigh molecular weight polyethylene
m. weight
m. weight distribution
m. weight ratio

molecular-based conceptual therapy

molecular and general genetics

molecule
adhesion molecule cascade
antiplatelet endothelial cell adhesion m.
cell adhesion m.
cell-cell adhesion m.
cell interaction m.
cellular adhesion m.
circulating adhesion m.
cleaved polyprotein precursor m.
cleaved polyprotein precursor molecule product
endothelial-leukocyte adhesion m.
m. hapten
highly reactive oxygen m.'s
leukocyte cell adhesion m.
L-selectin m.
lymphocyte costimulatory m.
mannose binding m.
melanoma cell adhesion m.
membrane-bound receptor m.
MHC class I m.
middle m.
monocyte adhesion m.
nascent collagen m.
nerve cell adhesion m.
neural cell adhesion m.
neural cell adhesive m.
neurotrophic enhancing m.
number of m.'s
number of density of m.
signaling lymphocytic activation m.
soluble intracellular adhesion m.
vascular cell adhesion m.

molecule-1
endothelial-leukocyte adhesion m.
intercellular adhesion molecule-1, -2, -3
leukocyte adhesion m.
mucosal addresin cell adhesion m.
platelet endothelial cell adhesion m.
vascular cell adhesion m.

molecule-2

molecule-3

molestation
sexual m.

molested
adults molested as children

molester
child m.

molimina
menstrual m.
m. of puffiness

molindone hydrochloride

Moll
adenocarcinoma of M.
apocrine gland of M.
M. gland cystadenoma

Mollaret
M. HSV
M. meningitis

molle
fibroma m.

heloma m.
papilloma m.

Moller microscope

Mollica-Pavone-Anterer syndrome

Mollica syndrome

mollusciformis
nevus m.

molluscoid neurofibroma

molluscum
m. body
m. conjunctivitis
m. contagiosum
m. contagiosum virus
m. corpuscle
m. fibrosum
m. fibrosum gravidarum
m. fibrosum pendulum
m. giganteum
m. sebaceum
m. varioliformis
m. verrucosum
m. virus

Moloney
M. cell surface antigen
M. hernia repair
M. leukemogenic virus
M. murine leukemia virus
M. murine sarcoma virus
M. strain
M. test
M. virus

MOLT-18, human T cell line

Molteno
M. episcleral explant
M. implant
M. shunt tube

Molulsky dye reduction test

molybdenum
m. cofactor
m. cofactor deficiency
m. rotating anode x-ray tube
stainless steel and m.
m. target

molybdenum-99 breakthrough test

molybdenum-conditioned medium

moment
m. of aggression
anterior bending m.
m. arm
central principal moments of inertia
m. of death
electromagnetic m.
m. of force
gradient moment nulling
gradient moment reduction
gradient moment rephasing
m. of inertia
macroscopic magnetic m.
magnetic m.
magnetic dipole m.
product m.
ratio of magnetic moment of a particle to Bohr magneton

momentary
m. lapse of awareness
m. lapse in normal breathing

momentum
angular m.
atomic orbital with angular momentum quantum number zero
nuclear angular m.

mometasone

Momose lens

Monaghan respirator

Monakow
accessory nucleus Monakow nucleus
M. bundle
M. fascia
M. fiber
M. syndrome

monarticular arthritis

Monas-Nitz Neuropsychological Battery

monaural
alternate monaural loudness balance test
m. bifrequency loudness balance
m. hearing
m. hearing aid
m. hearing loss
m. loudness balance test

Mönckeberg
M. arrhythmia
M. arteriosclerosis
M. calcification
M. degeneration
M. sclerosis

Moncrieff
M. cannula
M. discission
M. operation

Monday
M. morning colic
M. morning headache
M. morning heart attack

Monday-Wednesday-Friday

Mondini
M. anomaly
M. aplasia
M. deafness
M. deformity
M. dysplasia
M. hearing impairment
M. malformation

Mondor
M. disease
M. syndrome

Monfort abdominoplasty

Monge
M. disease
M. syndrome

mongolian
m. fold
m. idiot
m. macula
m. macule
m. spot

mongoloid
m. features
m. slant

monilial
m. diaper dermatitis
m. diaper rash
m. esophagitis
m. granuloma
m. infection
m. intertrigo
m. onychia
m. paronychia
m. rash
m. vaginitis

moniliasis
oral m.

moniliform hair

moniliformis
lichen ruber m.

Monistat-3 vaginal suppository

Monistat-Derm Topical

Monistat IV Injection

monitor
aerosol inhalation m.
ambulatory blood pressure m.
ambulatory electrogram m.
ambulatory Holter m.
automatic single-needle m.
blood glucose m.
blood perfusion m.

monitor *(continued)*
blood pressure m.
cardiac m.
cardiac-apnea m.
cardiac event m.
cardiovascular m.
cerebral function m.
3-channel Holter m.
channel 3 Holter m.
electronic glucose m.
endotracheal cardiac output m.
esophageal Doppler m.
external fetal maternal m.
fetal heart m.
fetal heart monitor tracing
m. fluid intake and output
heart rate m.
Holter m.
Holter monitor evaluation
home blood glucose m.
home cardiorespiratory m.
home uterine activity m.
internal m.
intracranial pressure monitor in skull
intrauterine pressure m.
low liquid level m.
Masimo SET home m.
MediSense Sof-Tact m.
MiniOX I, II, III, 100-IV oxygen m.
mixed m.
Neo-trak 515A neonatal m.
Nerve Integrity Monitor 2
Nicolet Nerve Integrity M.
nocturnal tumescence m.
noise level m.
noninvasive cardiac output m.
noninvasive glucose m.
occlusion dose m.
m. pattern
peak flow meter m.
m. peptide
portable monitor of respiratory parameters
programmable multiple ion m.
quality assurance m.
return electrode m.
sleep apnea m.
transcutaneous carbon dioxide m.
transcutaneous oxygen m.
transtelephonic exercise m.
m. unit
Vantage Performance m.
ventricular arrhythmia m.
virtual labor m.

monitored
m. administration of medication
m. anesthesia care
m. anesthesia care anesthesia
m. anesthesia care anesthetic technique
m. anesthesia control
apnea monitored baby
m. baby apnea
m. bed
heart rate m.
m. live voice
multiple monitored electroconvulsive therapy
patient m.
m. self-care evaluation

monitoring
ambulatory electrocardiographic m.
ambulatory Holter m.
ambulatory ischemia m.
ambulatory oximetry m.
anticoagulation monitoring requirement
m. audiometry
biomedical monitoring system
Birth Defects M. Program
blood coagulation m.
blood glucose m.
cardiac ambulatory monitoring unit
cardiac hemodynamic m.
Collaborative Home Infant M. Evaluation
continuous glucose monitoring system
continuous invasive m.
continuous long-term m.
coronary arrhythmia monitoring unit
data monitoring board
direct eighth nerve m.
Doppler monitoring of fetus
drowsiness monitoring device
drug use m.
electronic fetal m.
end-tidal carbon dioxide m.
end-tidal CO2 m.
epilepsy monitoring unit
external fetal m.
external fetal heart rate monitoring
fetal heart rate m.
growth monitoring, oral rehydration, breast feeding, and immunization
m. heartbeat
home blood glucose m.
home blood pressure m.
home blood sugar m.
home prothrombin time m.
home uterine m.
home uterine activity m.
human glucose m.
internal fetal m.
internal fetal heart rate m.
intracranial pressure m.
intraesophageal pH m.
intraoperative neurophysiologic m.
intrauterine fetal m.
late ambulatory m.
Life Health M. Program
m. lines inserted and positioned
long-term m.
medication monitoring event system
neuromuscular blockade m.
nocturnal penile erection m.
nonstress test fetal monitoring
observation and m.
pacemaker monitoring transtelephonic
plasma level m.
Pregnancy Risk M. System
prescription event m.
pressure monitoring device
prospective outcomes monitoring evaluation system
pulmonary artery pressure m.
pulse oximetry m.
quality information monitoring system
remote study m.
safety, monitoring, intervention, length of stay, and evaluation
selected ion m.
self blood-glucose m.
self-blood sugar m.
serum glucose m.
socially acceptable monitoring instrument
m. technique
therapeutic drug m.
therapeutic outcomes m.
thermometer monitoring in hyperthermia
transtelephonic m.
transtelephonic ambulatory monitoring system
transtelephonic arrhythmia m.
transtelephonic electrocardiographic m.
transthoracic intracardiac m.

monkey
antiserum, m.
m. B virus
m. cell
enterocytopathogenic monkey orphan virus
m. epithelium
m. facies
grivet monkey cell
m. hand
m. intranuclear inclusion agent
m. kidney
m. kidney cell
m. kidney fibroblast monolayer
m. kidney tissue culture
m. malaria
m. polyoma virus
m. pox
primary African green monkey kidney
m. red blood cell
Rhesus monkey kidney
Yaba monkey virus

monkeypox virus

monoallelic
m. expression
m. transcription

monoamine
m. hypothesis
m. oxidase
m. oxidase A deficiency
m. oxidase B inhibitor
m. oxidase inhibitor
m. oxidase type A, B
m. pathway
reversible inhibitor of monoamine oxidase-type A
m. serotonin
serum monoamine oxidase
vesicular monoamine transporter

monoaminergic fiber

monoamniotic
monochorionic monoamniotic placenta
monochorionic, monoamniotic twins
m. twins

monoarticular
m. antigen-induced arthritis
m. arthritis
m. arthritis of unknown etiology
m. synovitis

monobasic acid

monoblastic
acute monoblastic leukemia
chronic monoblastic leukemia

monoblast predominance

monoblock
m. femoral component
m. femoral stem prosthesis

monoblock femoral stem prosthesis

monobromated camphor

monocanalicular intubation

monocarboxylate/proton cotransporter

monocarboxylate transporter

monocellular suspension

monochloroacetic acid

monochlorobenzidine

monochorial twins

monochorionic
m. diamnionic placenta
m. diamniotic placenta
m. diamniotic placenta twins
m. diamniotic twin pregnancy
m. monoamniotic placenta
m., monoamniotic twins
m. placentation
m. twins

monochromatic
m. aberration
m. cone
m. eye
m. light source
m. photography
m. ray

Monoclate P

monoclonal
m. adenoma
m. antibodies against gastric mucins
m. antibody
m. antibody ABX-CBL
m. antibody A103 fine-needle aspiration biopsy
m. antibody anticancer vaccine
m. antibody B291
m. antibody-based latex agglutination
m. antibody BR96
m. antibody coagglutination test
m. antibody-defined antigen
m. antibody ED1
m. antibody imaging
m. antibody M1G8
m. antibody MIB-1
m. antibody PC10
m. antibody scintigraphic scan
m. antibody staining
m. antibody therapy
anticarcinoembryonic antigen monoclonal antibody
anti-CD11a humanized monoclonal antibody for psoriasis
anti-CD31 monoclonal antibody
anti-CEA monoclonal antibody
m. anticytokeratin
anticytokeratin monoclonal antibody
anti-DCP monoclonal antibody
antidesmin monoclonal antibody
anti-E-cadherin monoclonal antibody
m. antiendothelial cell antibody
m. antiendotoxin antibody
antiepidermal growth factor receptor monoclonal antibody
m. antiepithelial membrane antigen
m. antigen
m. antiglial fibrillary acidic protein
m. anti-HBc
anti-HER2 monoclonal antibody
m. anti-IgE antibody
anti-IgE humanized monoclonal antibody
antiimmunoglobulin E humanized monoclonal antibody
anti-interleukin-2 receptor alpha monoclonal antibody
m. antimalignin antibody
antispermicidal monoclonal antibody
anti-tau monoclonal antibody
m. anti-T-cell antibody
antivascular endothelial growth factor monoclonal antibody
m. autoantibody
m. band
m. B-cell neoplasm
m. B-cell pattern
benign monoclonal B-cell lymphocytosis
benign monoclonal gammopathy
bispecific monoclonal antibody
m. component
essential monoclonal gammopathy
m. expansion
m. free light chain
free monoclonal urinary light chain
m. gammopathy

monoclonal *(continued)*
m. gammopathy of undetermined significance
m. gammopathy of unknown significance
m. growth
IgA monoclonal gammopathy
m. immunoglobulin
m. integration
m. lymphoproliferative syndrome
MAb 12C3 monoclonal antibody
MAb-170 monoclonal antibody
MabThera monoclonal antibody
m. mouse anti-ICAM-1
m. mouse anti-VCAM-1
neutralizing murine monoclonal antitumor necrosis factor antibody
OKT3 anti-CD3 monoclonal antibody
OKT3 murine monoclonal antibody
Oncolym radiolabeled monoclonal antibody
m. origin
osteosarcoma antigen-associated monoclonal antibody
m. peak
polyneuropathy, organomegaly, endocrinopathy, monoclonal gammopathy, and skin changes syndrome
m. protein, skin
m. rheumatoid factor
m. spike

monocomponent highly purified pork insulin

Monocryl suture

monocrystalline
antimony monocrystalline electrode
m. iron oxides

monocular
m. aphakia
m. blindness
m. bobbing movement
m. confrontation visual field test
m. deprivation
m. depth perception
m. diplopia
m. dressing
m. electro-oculogram
m. estimate method
m. field defect
m. fixation
m. glaucoma
m. heads-up display imaging system
m. heterochromia
m. indirect ophthalmoscope
m. indirect ophthalmoscopy
m. nystagmus
m. occlusion
m. oscillopsia
m. patch
m. strabismus
m. telescope
m. temporal arcuate defect
m. temporal crescent
total monocular blindness
transient monocular blindness
m. vision
wall-eyed monocular internuclear ophthalmoplegia

monocular-estimate-method dynamic retinoscopy

monocyte
m. adhesion molecule
adult m.
blood m.
m. cell
m. chemoattractant and activity factor
m. chemoattractant protein
m. chemoattractant protein-1
m. chemotactic and activating factor
m. chemotactic factor
m. chemotactic peptide-1
m. chemotactic protein
m. chemotactic protein-1
circulating m.
m. colony-stimulating factor
m. function test
m. lineage antigen
m. monolayer assay
peripheral blood m.
peripheral monocyte count
m. presenting
surface adherent m.
m. tissue factor
m. tropic virus

monocyte-derived
m.-d. dendritic cell
m.-d. macrophage
m.-d. neutrophil chemotactic factor

monocyte-lymphocyte ratio

monocyte-macrophage
m.-m. progenitor
m.-m. system

monocyte-tropic strain

monocytic
acute monocytic leukemia
aleukemic monocytic leukemia
m. angina
m. blood cell
chronic monocytic leukemia
m. ehrlichiosis
human monocytic ehrlichiosis
m. leukemia
m. leukemoid reaction
m. leukocytosis
m. marker
Naegeli type of monocytic leukemia
m. sarcoma

monocytic blood cell

monocytic leukemoid reaction

monocytogenes
m. bacterium
heat-killed *Listeria monocytogenes*
Listeria monocytogenes sepsis

monocytoid
m. B-cell
m. B-cell lymphoma
m. B-lymphocyte
m. cell
m. lymphocyte

monocytosis
avian m.

monodeiodinase

5′-monodeiodinase activity

monodeiodinase activity

monodeiodination activity

monodermal tumor

monodisperse aerosol

Monod-Wyman-Changeux model

monofactorial inheritance

monofilament
calibrated m.
continuous running monofilament suture
m. nylon suture
m. pressure esthesiometer
Semmes-Weinstein m.

monofixation
m. syndrome

monofluoroacetate
sodium m.

monogamous
m. bivalency
mutually monogamous relationship

monogenic disorder

monoglyceride
m. hydrolase
long-chain m.
monohybrid cross
monohydrate
monosodium urate m.
monosodium urate monohydrate crystal
nitrofurantoin m.
monohydric alcohol
monohydrochloride
arginine m.
monohydrolase
orthophosphoric ester m.
monoiodinated tyrosine
monoisocentric technique
Mono Lake virus
monolateral strabismus
monolayer
m. culture
monkey kidney fibroblast m.
monocyte monolayer assay
monolayered endothelium
monoleptic fever
monomania
affective m.
monomelica
monomelic amyotrophy
monomer
m. in fetal hemoglobin
fibrin m.
soluble fibrin m.
soluble fibrin monomer complex
vinyl chloride m.
monomeric precursor
monomethanearsonate
disodium m.
monomicrobial necrotizing cellulitis
monomorphic
m. adenoma
m. lymphoma
nonsustained monomorphic ventricular tachycardia
sustained monomorphic ventricular tachycardia
m. ventricular tachycardia
monomorphous papular eruption
mononeuritis
m. multiplex
m. with paralysis
mononeuropathies
multiple m.
mononeuropathy
m. electrodiagnosis
entrapment m.
m. multiplex
musculocutaneous m.
peripheral m.
mononuclear
blood mononuclear cell
m. cell infiltrate
m. cell infiltration
m. cell pleocytosis
m. cell recruitment
m. cell tissue factor
cord blood mononuclear cell
m. dyspepsia
m. histiocytic portal infiltrate
human peripheral mononuclear cell
m. leukocyte
lymph node mononuclear cell
marrow mononuclear cell
peripheral blood mononuclear cell
peripheral blood mononuclear cell hepatitis B virus measurement
m. phagocyte
m. phagocyte system
m. reaction
m. Reed-variant cell
m. response
mononucleosis
acute infectious m.
cytomegaloviral m.
hepatitis-infectious m.
m. infectiosa
infectious m.
infectious mononucleosis receptor
posttransfusion m.
m. syndrome
mononucleosis-like
m.-l. illness
m.-l. symptom
m.-l. syndrome
mononucleosis-type syndrome
mononucleotide
flavin m.
nicotinamide m.
nicotinic acid m.
reduced form of flavin m.
monooleate
mannose m.
monooxygenase
methane m.
mitochondrial P450 m.
m. pathway
monophasic
m. action potential
m. action potential duration
acute monophasic experimental autoimmune encephalomyelitis
m. choriocarcinoma
m. endplate activity
m. oral contraceptive
m. regimen
m. R wave
m. synovial sarcoma
monophonic
m. wheeze
m. wheezing
monophosphate
adenine arabinoside m.
adenosine 3′,5′-cyclic m.
adenosine 5′ m.
adenosine monophosphate deaminase deficiency
azidothymidine m.
carbovir m.
concentration of adenosine m.
cyclic adenosine m.
cyclic arginine m.
deoxycytidine m.
deoxyguanosine m.
deoxyuridine m.
fluorouridine m.
hexose m.
hexose monophosphate pathway
hexose monophosphate shunt
inosine monophosphate dehydrogenase
muscle adenosine monophosphate deaminase deficiency
nephrogenous cyclic adenosine m.
thymidine m.
uridine monophosphate kinase
xanthine m.
3,′5′-monophosphate
cyclic uridine -m.
3,5-monophosphate
5′-monophosphate
adenosine -m.
inosine -m.
thymidine -m.
uridine -m.
xanthosine -m.
5'-monophosphate
nucleoside -m.
monophosphoryl lipid A
monophyletic cluster

monopolar
arthroscopic monopolar thermal stabilization forefoot compression sleeve
m. cathodal stimulator
m. coagulation
m. electrocoagulation

Monopty core biopsy

monorecidive chancre

monorhythmic
m. frontal delta
m. frontal delta activity

monosaccharide
acquired monosaccharide intolerance

monosaturated fatty acid

monosodium
m. glutamate
m. glutamate-induced headache
m. glutamate poisoning
m. urate
m. urate monohydrate
m. urate monohydrate crystal

monosomy
m. 1–22
autosomal m.
m. G
m. G syndrome
mosaic autosomal m.
partial monosomy 1p–22p
partial monosomy XP21, XP22
partial monosomy Xq
m. 7 syndrome
m. x
m. Xq

monospecific antiserum

Monospot
M. screen
M. test
M. test

monostearate
glyceryl m.
penicillin aluminum m.

Monosticon Dri-Dot test

monostotic
m. disease
m. fibrous dysplasia
m. form

monosymptomatic
m. circumscription
m. delusional pseudocyesis
m. hyperthyroidism
m. hypochondriacal
m. hypochondriacal psychosis
m. hypochondriasis
m. nocturnal enuresis

monosynaptic
m. connection
m. reflex

mono test

monotherapy
androgen ablative m.
estrogen m.
maintenance cyclosporine m.
nonsteroidal antiandrogen m.
nucleoside m.
nucleoside analog m.
perindopril m.

Monotic Word Memory Test

monotypic effect

monounsaturated fatty acid

Mono-Vac test

monovalent
m. antiserum
m. oral polio virus vaccine
poliovirus vaccine monovalent oral

monovision
modified m.

monovular twins

monoxenic culture

monoxide
carbon m.
carbon monoxide hemoglobin
carbon monoxide myoglobin
carbon monoxide oximetry
carbon monoxide pressure or tension
carbon monoxide transfer factor
diffusing capacity for carbon m.
diffusing capacity of lung for carbon m.
functional uptake of carbon m.
lead m.
single-breath carbon monoxide diffusing capacity of lung
steady-state carbon monoxide diffusing capacity of lung

monozygotic twins

Monro
M. aqueduct
M. bursa
M. doctrine
M. fissure
foramen of M.
M. foramen
M. line

mons pubis

monster
m. cell
Gila monster bite

montage
circumferential bipolar m.
referential m.

Montana myotis leukoencephalitis virus

Monte
M. Carlo calculation
M. Carlo modeling
M. Carlo photon transport
M. Carlo photon transport simulation
M. Carlo technique
M. Dourado virus
Markov chain Monte Carlo technique

Montefiore syndrome

Monteggia
M. dislocation
M. equivalent lesion
M. forearm fracture
M. fracture-dislocation
M. fracture-dislocation of ulna

Montenegro
M. reaction
M. skin test
M. test

Monterey cypress tree

Montevideo unit

Montezuma's revenge

Montgomery
M. follicle
M. gland
M. glands
M. strap
M. tubercle

Montgomery-Asberg Depression Rating Scale

month
member m.'s
m., date, year
m.'s old
per member per m.
per patient per m.
work-level m.

monthly
m. interval
m. progress note
special monthly compensation
special monthly pension

Monticelli-Spinelli
M.-S. distraction
M.-S. distraction technique
M.-S. fixator
M.-S. frame
monticulus
m. cerebelli
Montreal platelet syndrome
mood
abrupt mood change
adjustment disorder with angry m.
adjustment disorder with anxious m.
adjustment disorder with mixed anxiety and depressed m.
alcohol mood disorder
alpha-methyldopa-induced mood disorder
altered mood and perception
amitriptyline-induced mood disorder
m. and/or affect
anxious m.
anxious mood adjustment reaction
appearance, mood, sensorium, intelligence, and thought process
behavioral, anxiety, mood, and other types of disorders
bereavement-related mood disorder
m. brightening
m. change
m. chart
Claude M. Scale
m. cluster score
Clyde M. Scale
cocaine mood disorder
m. congruent
co-occurring mood disorder
delusional mood disorder
Dementia M. Assessment Scale
depressed or irritable m.
m. deterioration
m. disorder
m. disorder due to a general medical condition
m. disorder patient
m. disorder with atypical features
m. disorder with catatonic features
m. disorder with melancholic features
m. disorder with postpartum onset
m. disorder with rapid cycling
m. disorder with seasonal pattern
m. disturbance
electroconvulsive therapy-induced mood disorder
m. elevation
m. elevator
m. episode
erratic m.
euphoric m.
euthymic m.
expansive m.
Fatigue-Inertia Subscale of the Profile of M. States
fluctuating mood disturbance
Foods and M.'s Inventory
hallucinogen mood disorder
m. induction
m. instability
irritability and mood swings
irritable m.
labile m.
m. lability
m., orientation, judgment, affect, content
organic mood disorder
organic mood syndrome
M. and Physical Symptoms Scale
Profile of M. States
m. stabilizer
m. state
Visual Analogue M. Scale
mood-altering
m.-a. capacity
m.-a. drug
m.-a. substance
mood cluster score
mood-congruent
m.-c. delusion
m.-c. hallucination
m.-c. psychotic feature
mood-incongruent
m.-i. delusion
m.-i. hallucination
moodiness
short-term moodiness intense
moody, irritable and aggressive
moon
m. blindness
M. boot
m. face
m. facies
M. molars
M. teeth
Mooney
M. brace
M. cast
M. Problem Checklist
moon-shaped
m.-s. face
m.-s. facies
Moore
Austin Moore arthroplasty
Austin Moore chisel
Austin Moore hemiarthroplasty
Austin Moore reamer
M. classification for vascular anomalies of the gastrointestinal tract
M. fracture
M. gallstone scoop
M. head-tilt maneuver
M. hip endoprosthesis system
M. lightning streak
M. prosthesis
M. syndrome
Moore-Federman syndrome
Mooren corneal ulcer
Moore-Troutman corneal scissors
Mooser
M. body
M. cell
mop
Mopeia virus
mop-end
m.-e. Achilles tendon tear
m.-e. appearance
MOPP chemotherapy protocol
Mor
Clo Mor virus
mor1 virus
morado
mal m.
moral
m. anxiety
m. assessment
m. ataxia
m. behavior
m. code
m. conduct
m. consistency
m. deficiency
m. deficiency personality disorder
m. development
m. emotion
m. hazard
m. idiocy
m. imbecile
m. independence
m. insanity
m. judgment

moral deficiency personality disorder

morale
Philadelphia Geriatric Center Morale Scale

morality
m. of constraint
m. of conventional role conformity
m. of cooperation

Moran
M. operation
M. proptosis

Morand foot

Morax
M. keratoplasty
M. operation

Morax-Axenfeld
M.-A. bacillus
M.-A. conjunctivitis
M.-A. diplococcus

Moraxella
M. catarrhalis
Moraxella catarrhalis vaccine
Moraxella conjunctivitis
Moraxella keratitis

morbid
m. anxiety
m. anxiety inventory
m. dependence
m. desire
m. doubt
m. fear
m. idea
m. imitation
m. impulse
m. obesity
m. thirst

morbidity
cardiovascular morbidity and mortality
drug-related m.
m. excess
infant morbidity and mortality
maternal febrile m.
m. and mortality
operative morbidity and mortality
perinatal morbidity rate
m. predictor
proportional morbidity ratio
proportionate morbidity ratio
m. rate
standard morbidity ratio

morbidity-mortality rate

morbidly obese

morbidostatic
minimal morbidostatic dose

morbilli
equine morbilli virus

morbilliform
m. basal cell carcinoma
m. eruption
m. erythema
m. rash
m. skin rash

morbus
m. Darier
m. Down
m. hemolyticus neonatorum
m. maculosus neonatorum

morcellation operation

morcellator
motorized m.

morcellized
m. bone
m. bone graft
m. cancellous graft

Morch respirator

Morck
M. cement
M. cement bifocal

more
frequency of the more common allele of a pair
no more information
slightly more marked since

Moreira bolt

Morel
M. disease
M. ear
M. syndrome

morel
false m.

Morel-Fatio-Lalardie operation

Morel-Wildi syndrome

MORE trial

Morgagni
anterior retrosternal hernia of M.
appendix of M.
M. appendix
M. cartilage
M. caruncle
M. cataract
M. column
column of M.
M. columns
M. concha
crypt of M.
M. crypt
M. cyst
M. disease
foramen of M.
M. foramen
foramen of Morgagni hernia
M. fossa
M. fovea
M. frenum
M. globule
M. hernia
M. humor
hydatid of M.
M. hydatid
M. hyperostosis
M. lacuna
M. liquor
prolapse of M.
M. sphere
M. syndrome
M. tubercle

Morgagni-Adams-Stokes syndrome

morgagnian
m. cataract
m. globule

Morgagni-Turner-Albright syndrome

Morgagni-Turner syndrome

morgan
M. bacillus
M. dot
M. fold
Fort Morgan virus
M. line

Moria
M. obturator
M. trephine

Moria-France dacryocystorhinostomy clamp

moribund patient not expected to live

Moriche virus

Morison pouch

Morley peritoneocutaneous reflex

morning
m. admission
m. after
m. after pill
m. bright light therapy
m. corticotropin-releasing hormone test
m. cortisol
m. diarrhea
m. drinking

drug-induced morning drowsiness
early morning awakening
early morning specimen of urine
first morning urine
m. glory disc
m. glory disc anomaly
m. glory optic atrophy
m. glory optic disk anomaly
m. glory retinal detachment
m. glory syndrome
m. headache
Monday morning colic
Monday morning headache
Monday morning heart attack
m. [L. *mane*]
m. and night
night and m.
m. osmolality
m. ptosis
m. sickness
m. stiffness
stitches out in m.

morning-after
m.-a. contraception
m.-a. pill

Moro
incomplete Moro reflex
M. reaction
M. reflex
M. response

Moro-Heisler diet

morpheaform
m. basal cell
m. basal cell carcinoma
m. pattern
m. sarcoid

morphea-type basal cell carcinoma

morphemes

morphine
m. addiction
m. cholescintigraphy
cocaine and m.
m. and cocaine
m. controlled-release
m. dependence
hemagglutination inhibition morphine test
heroin, morphine, and cocaine
high-dose m.
M. HP
hypodermic morphine sulfate
m. injector's septicemia
intracerebroventricular administration of m.
nebulized preservative-free morphine sulfate
neonatal morphine solution
oral morphine sulfate
rectal morphine sulfate suppository
subcutaneous morphine pump
substitute for m.
m. sulfate
m. sulfate controlled-release suppository
m. sulfate immediate release
sustained-release morphine sulfate

Morphine-Benzedrine Group Scale

morphine-controlled release

morphine-like
m.-l. compound
m.-l. factor

morphine-potentiated
m.-p. HIV replication
m.-p. human immunodeficiency virus replication

morphogenesis
lung m.
parenchymal lung m.

morphogenetic
bone morphogenetic protein
bone morphogenetic protein type 2
m. lesion
m. protein
recombinant human bone morphogenetic protein

morphogenic protein 6

morpholino anthracycline

morpholinoethanesulfonic acid

morphologic
m. abnormality
m. analysis
m. assessment
m. change
m. classification
m. criterion
m. differentiation
m. element
m. examination
m. feature
m. manifestation
m. pattern

morphological
m. characteristic
m. correlation
m. deformation
m. difference
pancreatic ductal morphological change
m. sex

morphology
Antoni classification of schwannoma m.
Gram-stain m.
histologic m.
m. index
lymphoplasmacytoid m.
modified Dallas classification of disc morphology grades 0–7
QRS m.
red cell morphology index
m. system CAS-200
Test for Examining Expressive M.
yeast morphology agar

morphometric
m. abnormality
m. analysis

morphometry
aerosol-derived airway m.
m. analysis
computerized nuclear m.

Morquio
M. disease
M. mucopolysaccharidosis
mucopolysaccharidosis type IV M.
M. sign
M. syndrome

Morquio-Brailsford
M.-B. disease
M.-B. syndrome

Morquio-Ullrich
M.-U. disease
M.-U. syndrome

Morrey-Coonrad design

Morrison donor site design

Morris syndrome

Morrow Assessment of Nausea and Emesis

Morrow-Brown needle

Morsch-Retec respirator

Morse code pattern

morselized
cancellous morselized bone graft
m. cartilage
m. cartilage onlay radix graft

Morsier
Maestre de San Juan-Kallmann-de Morsier syndrome

Morsier *(continued)*
Maestre-Kallmann-de Morsier syndrome
mors thymica
mortality
age-standardized mortality ratio
cardiovascular morbidity and m.
corrected perinatal m.
crude mortality ratio
m. data
infant morbidity and m.
infant mortality rate
morbidity and m.
neonatal m.
operative morbidity and m.
operative mortality rate
Pediatric Risk of Mortality Score
perinatal m.
perinatal mortality counseling program
perinatal mortality counseling team
postneonatal mortality syndrome
postperinatal infant m.
m. predictor
M. Probability Model
proportional mortality ratio
m. rate
m. rate doubling time
m. rate ratio
relative standardized mortality ratio
Risk-Adjusted M. Index
m. risk factor
risk factor for m.
standardized mortality ratio
standardized proportionate m.
standard mortality ratio
transplant-related m.
treatment-related m.
mortis
livor m.
rigor m.
mortise
ankle m.
ankle mortise axis
ankle mortise diastasis
ankle mortise fracture
ankle mortise widening
ball-and-socket ankle m.
bone m.
m. of bone
m. joint
m. of joint
tibiofibular m.
m. view
Morton
M. disease
M. foot
M. neuroma
M. toe
morula cell
morular cell
morus
nevus m.
Morvan
M. chorea
M. disease
mos
mos protooncogene
mos protooncogene/oncogene
mosaic
m. aneuploidy
anterior mosaic crocodile shagreen
m. arthroplasty
m. artifact
m. attenuation pattern
m. autosomal monosomy
bean golden mosaic virus
cauliflower mosaic virus
cucumber mosaic virus
m. detector configuration
m. duodenal mucosal pattern
m. fungus
m. genome
m. genome structure
m. trisomy 14
NBT mosaic pattern
Paget disease-like mosaic appearance
Pallister mosaic aneuploidy
Pallister mosaic syndrome
m. pattern
m. perfusion
m. skin
m. tetrasomy 8p syndrome
tobacco mosaic virus
m. translocation
m. Turner syndrome
m. verruca
m. wart
yam mosaic virus
mosaicism
confined placental m.
variegated translocation m.
m. for XXX
mosaicplasty
arthroscopic m.
moschata
nux moschata nutmeg
Moschcowitz
M. sign
M. test
M. thrombotic thrombocytopenic purpura disease
Moschowitz
M. fashion
M. procedure
Moscow typhus
Mose
M. concentric rings
Moseley
M. bone age graph
M. fasciotome
Mosher
M. air cell
M. operation
Mosher-Toti operation
Mosler
M. diabetes
M. sign
Mosqueiro virus
mosquito
anopheline m.
m. bite
m. bite infection
m. forceps
m. hemostat
m. hemostatic clamp
m. hemostatic forceps
mosquito-borne
m.-b. disease
Southeast Asia mosquito-borne hemorrhagic fever
Moss
M. classification
M. G-tube
M. G-tube PEG kit
M. operation
M. traction
Mosse syndrome
Mossman fever
Mossuril virus
mossy
m. cell
m. fibers
m. fiber sprouting
m. foot
most
m. anterior point of anterior contour of the sella turcica
m. comfortable frequency
m. comfortable listening level
m. comfortable loudness

m. comfortable loudness level
m. comfortable loudness range
m. posterior point on posterior contour of sella turcica
m. probable number
m. recent episode
m. significant bit
m. significant digit
m. significant other

Mostofi
M. classification
M. classification of testicular tumor
M. histologic typing

Motais operation

moth
m. dermatitis
m. patch

mothball
naphthalene m.

moth-eaten
m.-e. alopecia
m.-e. appearance
m.-e. baldness
m.-e. bone destruction

mother
M.'s Assessment of the Behavior of Her Infant
m. and baby endoscope
m. breast milk
m. burnout
m. card
m. cell
m. of child
m. colony
m. complex
m. confessor
m. cyst
m. dermatitis
diabetic m.
m. endoscopic retrograde cholangiopancreatoscopy system
m. and father
fetus of diabetic m.
m. figure
m. fixation
foster m.
m. hypnosis
identified high-risk m.
m. image
infant of diabetic m.
infant of drug abusing m.
infant of high-risk m.
infant of infected m.
infant of mother with gestational diabetes mellitus
infant of nondiabetic m.
infant of substance-abusing m.
m. infected with acquired immune deficiency syndrome
m. lesion
teenage m.
transmission of infected mother to infant
unwed m.
m. yaw

mother-child
m.-c. attachment
m.-c. bond
m.-c. dyad
m.-c. experience
m.-c. interaction
m.-c. relationship

Mother-Child Relationship Evaluation

motherhood

mother-infant
m.-i. attachment
m.-i. bonding
m.-i. interaction
m.-i. transmission

Mother/Infant Communication Screening

mother-to-child
m.-t.-c. transmission

mother-to-fetus/infant transmission

motif
immunoreceptor tyrosine-based activation m.
nuclear localization signal m.
ribonucleic acid-binding m.
RNA-binding m.
Y chromosome RNA recognition m.

motile
m. cell
large motile cell
m. leukocyte
not m.
m. scotoma
m. sperm

motilin
m. effect
m. receptor agonist

motilin-like immunoreactivity

motility
m. adhesion
m. agent
altered gastric m.
altered sperm m.
autocrine motility factor
autocrine motility factor of the bladder
autocrine motility factor receptor
automated motility factor
m. disorder
m. disturbance
esophageal m.
esophageal motility disorder
m. examination
m. implant
m. index
ineffective esophageal m.
interdigestive motility complex
neurohumoral control of m.
nonspecific esophageal motility disorder
ocular motility disorder
ocular motility effect
ocular motility test
postoperative gastrointestinal m.
receptor for hyaluronan-mediated m.
small bowel m.
sulfide, indole, motility medium
m. test
m. test medium

motility-related dysphagia

motion
acoustic respiratory motion sensor
active ankle joint complex range of m.
active-assisted range of m.
active integral range of m.
active motion testing
active and passive range of m.
active resistive range of m.
m. activity
advanced real-time motion analysis
akinetic segmental wall motion abnormality
alternate motion rate
alternating motion rate
alternating range of m.
m. analysis system
ankle dorsiflexion range of m.
ankle inversion-eversion range of m.
anterior motion of posterior mitral valve leaflet
anterior wall m.
aortic motion artifact
apical wall m.
AP translatory m.
arc of m.
articular motion device

motion *(continued)*
m. artifact
m. artifact rejection system
m. artifact suppression technique
asymmetry, range of motion abnormality, tissue texture abnormality
m. automated perimetry
automatic motion correction
m. averaging
back range of m.
m. barrier
m. blur
brisk wall m.
cardiac wall m.
cervical motion tenderness
cervical range of m.
m. compensation gradient pulse
complete and pain-free range of m.
m. concentration
continuous passive motion device
continuous passive m.
continuous passive motion machine
contrast threshold for motion perception
m. control
controlled ankle m.
m. control limiter
m. control procedure
m. degradation
m. demand
m. detection threshold
m. and displacement perimetry
ejection fraction/wall m.
embryonic heart m.
end range of m.
extraocular m.
m. fear
fetal cardiac m.
fetal heart m.
full extraocular m.
full, free range of m.
full joint range of m.
gradient motion rephasing
hand m.
hand motion at 3 feet vision test
hand motion and light perception
head and neck m.
helical axis of m.
high regional wall motion velocity
intersegmental range of motion palpation
interventricular septal m.
jerking m.'s
joint alignment and m.
joint range of m.
left ventricular wall m.
left ventricular wall motion abnormality
left ventricular wall motion index
limitation of m.
limited joint m.
limited neck m.
linear accelerator isocenter m.
loss of m.
m. mode
navigator echo motion correction technique
neck full range of m.
neurologic/circulatory/range of m.
no limitation of m.
normal range of m.
pain aggravated by m.
pain-free range of m.
pain on m.
paradoxical chest wall m.
paradoxical vocal cord m.
m. parallax
passive accessory motion test
passive assistance range of m.
passive intervertebral m.
m. perception disorder
posterior leaflet m.
quality of m.
quantitative wall motion score
range of joint m.
range of motion complete and pain-free
range of motion within normal limits
regional wall m.
regional wall motion abnormality
repetitive hand m.
repetitive motion disorder
repetitive motion injury
repetitive motion in the joint
repetitive motion syndrome
resistive range of m.
restricted range of m.
segmental wall m.
segmental wall motion abnormality
sensation, circulation, m.
short arc m.
m. sickness
m. sickness susceptibility
simple harmonic m.
spinal range of m.
swelling, tenderness, limitation of m.
systemic anterior m.
systolic m.
systolic anterior motion of mitral valve
systolic wall motion velocity
tenderness, asymmetry, restricted motion, and tissue texture changes
time m.
tissue texture changes, asymmetry, restriction of motion, tenderness
total active m.
total passive m.
total range of m.
tricuspid annular m.
ventricular wall m.
ventricular wall motion abnormality
vertebral motion unit
violent and irregular jerking m.
m. vision
voluntary range of m.
wall m.
wall motion index
wall motion score index

motion-resistant pulse oximetry

motivated
m. error
m. forgetting
highly m.
m. individual

motivation
adult m.
m. analysis
m. analysis test
m. analysis testing
m. for cross dressing
m. deterioration
m. factor
m. impairment
primary m.
m. research
School M. Analysis Test
Self-Concept and M. Inventory

motivational
m. enhancement therapy
m. factor
m. hierarchy
m. impairment

motive
m. achievement
aroused m.
autonomy of m.'s
proton motive force

motoneuron
gamma m.
heteronymous m.'s
homonymous m.'s
ocular m.

motor
m. ability
m. abnormality
m. abreaction
m. activity
m. activity log
adventitious motor flow
afferent motor aphasia
afferent motor unit
m. agraphia
aimless motor activity
Alberta Infant M. Scale
m. alexia
alpha motor neuron
m. amusia
anterior horn cell motor impairment
m. aphasia
m. aphasia transcortical
m. apraxia
m. area
M. Assessment Scale
asymmetric motor neuropathy
m. ataxia
m. aura
m. automatism
autonomic motor neuron
autonomic motor pool
autonomic visceral motor nucleus
m. axon
m. behavior
best motor response
m. branch
California Infant Scale for M. Development
capillary refill, sensation, motor function, temperature
cataract, motor system disorder, short stature, learning difficulty, skeletal abnormalities syndrome
m. cell
central motor conduction time
m. change
chronic motor or vocal tic disorder
circulation, motor ability, sensation, and swelling
circulation, respiration, abdomen, motor, and speech
cognitive and motor changes
cognitive perceptual motor skills
complete lower motor neuron lesion
complex motor seizure
complex motor tic
complex motor unit
m. compliance
compound motor action potential
m. conduction
m. conduction block
congenital ocular motor apraxia
conscious control of motor units
continuous motor unit activity
m. control
m. control of the ego
control motor skills
m. control test
conversion disorder, motor type
m. conversion symptom
m. coordination
m. coordination test
m. cortex
m. cortex unit
m. cortical center
cortical motor area
cortical motor output
cranial motor nuclei
m. dapsone neuropathy
m. deconditioning
m. decussation
m. deficit
deficits in attention, motor control, perception
m. depressant
detrusor motor instability
m. development
developmental motor quotient
m. development examination
m. disability
m. discriminative acuity
m. disinhibition
m. disorder
distal motor latency
m. disturbance
dorsal motor nucleus of vagus
m. dysfunction
efferent motor aphasia
m. end-organ
m. endplate
m. evoked potential
m. examination
excessive motor activity
eyes, motor, verbal
m. fascicle
m. fiber
m. finding
fine m.
fine motor activity
fine motor coordination
fine motor development
fine motor function
fine motor movement
fine motor skill
m. fluctuation
Frostig Developmental Test of Visual M. Perception
m. function
m. function assessment
m. function deficit
m. fusion
Gross M. Function Measure
gross motor activity
gross motor deficit
gross motor development
gross motor skill
m. habit
m. hemideficit
m. hemiplegia
hereditary motor sensory neuropathy II-deafness-mental retardation
hereditary sensory motor neuropathy type I–III
human immunodeficiency virus associated motor cognitive disorder
m. hyperactivity
m. image
m. immobility
impaired motor coordination
impaired motor function
m. impairment
m. impersistence
M. Impersistence Test
m. impulse
individual motor unit action potential
m. inertia
m. inhibition
intact motor skills
intact motor tract
intellectual and motor skills
intense motor agitation
interdigestive migrating motor complex
interdigestive motor complex
involuntary motor movement
involuntary motor tic
m. latency
lateral motor column
lower motor neuron disease
lower motor neuron lesion
lower motor neuron palsy
Lucas and Drucker M. Index
macro motor unit action potential

motor *(continued)*
major motor seizure
m. meal
migrating motor complex
minor motor seizure
multifocal acquired motor axonopathy
multifocal demyelinating motor neuropathy
muscular response to electrical stimulation of motor nerve
m. nerve
m. nerve conduction velocity
neurogenic motor evoked potential
m. neuron
m. neuron disease
m. neuron palsy
m. neuron sign
m. neuron weakness
m. neuropathy
m. neuropathy with multifocal conduction block
nonprogressive motor impairment syndrome
nonspecific esophageal motor dysfunction
ocular motor apraxia
ocular motor cranial nerve
ocular motor dysmetria
ocular motor syndrome
ocular motor system
m. oculi
operating motor vehicle while intoxicated
oral m.
m., pain, touch, reflex deficit
partial motor seizure
m. pattern
Peabody Developmental M. Activity Cards
Peabody Developmental M. Scale
pedestrian hit by motor vehicle
m. perception
m. perception dysfunction
perceptual cognitive motor function
perceptual motor development
perceptual motor skills
m. planning
Primary Visual M. Test
pudendal-nerve terminal motor latency
pulse, motor, and sensory
pure motor hemiparesis
m. radiculopathy
m. response
m. restlessness
Rivermead motor assessment
m. root
m. root of ciliary ganglion
m. scale
m. seizure
sensation and motor function
sensory motor integration
m. skill
spontaneous motor activity
supplemental motor area
supplementary motor area
survival motor neuron telomeric gene
terminal motor latency
Test of Infant M. Performance
m. tic
toddler and infant motor evaluation
transcortical motor aphasia
unimpaired motor function
m. unit action potential
upper motor neurogenic bladder
upper motor neuron lesion
m., vascular, and sensory
m. vehicle accident
m. vehicle collision
m. vehicle injury
Wolf M. Function Test

motor-axonal neuropathy

motorcycle accident

motor-evoked
m.-e. response
m.-e. response to transcranial stimulation

motoric
m. abnormality
m. hyperactivity
m. immobility

motorized
m. bur
m. cutter
m. morcellator

motor-output disability

motor-sensory
m.-s. axonal neuropathy
m.-s. neuropathy, X-linked Type II, with deafness and mental retardation

Mot-R-Pak vitrectomy system

Mott
M. body
M. cell

mottled
m. appearance
m. calcification
cold mottled insensate leg
m. density
m. distribution
m. enamel
hemorrhagic appearance, m.
hemorrhagic area, m.
m. opacity
m. rarefaction
m. retina

mottling
early receptor potential m.
m. of fundus
m. pattern
m. of skin

moubata
Ornithodoros m.

Mouchet
M. disease
M. fracture

Moulin
linear atrophoderma of M.

mound
breast mound reduction and nipple reconstruction with wraparound flap
pearl white m.'s

mount
M. Elgon bat virus
nigrosin m.
wet m.
whole mount microscopy

mountain
acute mountain sickness
m. anemia
m. balm
m. cedar
m. cedar tree
m. disease
Great Smoky Mountains Study of Youth
m. sickness

mounted
m. diamond points

mounting
aqueous mounting medium

mouse
m. amniotic fluid
m. antialopecia factor
m. antibody production test
m. antirat serum
m. bed sign
m. cancer
m. cytomegalovirus
m. ear erosion

m. embryo
m. embryo fibroblast
m. encephalomyelitis
m. encephalomyelitis virus
m. epidermal growth factor
m. epithelial cell
m. epithelium
m. erythroleukemia
m. fear
m. gamma globulin
m. hepatitis
m. hepatitis virus
m. leukemia virus
m. mammary epithelium
m. mammary oncovirus
m. mammary tumor
m. mammary tumor virus
m. milk fat globule
monoclonal mouse anti-ICAM-1
monoclonal mouse anti-VCAM-1
m. neutralization test
newborn m.
newborn mouse brain
New Zealand obese m.
New Zealand white m.
normal mouse serum
m. ovarian tumor
m. parotid tumor virus
m. poliomyelitis
m. poliomyelitis virus
m. red blood cell
m. rosette-forming cell
m. salivary gland virus
m. serum
m. serum albumin
m. serum protein
m. stem cell-like cell
suckling m.
suckling mouse brain
Swiss Webster mouse
m. thymic virus
m. thyroglobulin
m. urine
m. urine protein
m. uterine weight unit
m. vas deferens

mouse-on-mouse
m.-o.-m. basic kit
m.-o.-m. fluorescein kit

mousepox virus

mouse-specific
m.-s. B-lymphocyte antigen
m.-s. bone marrow-derived lymphocyte antigen

moustache dressing

mousy odor

mouth
angle of m.
m. breathing
burning mouth from aspirin
burning mouth from cold sore
burning mouth from depression
burning mouth from diabetes
burning mouth syndrome
by m.
m. care
closed mouth impression
commissure of lips and m.
cracked mouth corners from sagging cheek
m. denture wax
depressor muscle of angle of m.
down-turned mouth corners
dry mouth from antihistamine
m. erythema multiforme
fish mouth incision
m. fistula
floor of m.
m. flora
full mouth dentures
m. gag
m. gag frame
m. guard
lips of m.
maximal expiratory mouth pressure
maximal inspiratory mouth pressure
maximal mouth opening
modiolus of angle of m.
by mouth feeding
by mouth per os
nothing by m.
nothing by mouth at bedtime
nothing by mouth nil per os
nothing per m.
numbness and tingling around m.
orbicular muscle of m.
m. pressure
scalded mouth syndrome
special mouth care
temperature by m.
time of peak emptying rate of m.
trench mouth from anxiety

Mouth-Aid
Orajel M.-A.

mouth-and-hand synkinesis

mouthpiece
sip-and-puff m.

mouthrinse

mouthstick appliance

mouth-to-mask breathing

mouth-to-mouth resuscitation

mouth-to-nose/mouth resuscitation

mouthwash
antibacterial m.
astringent m.
magic m.

movable
carina freely m.
freely movable joint
m. heart
m. joint

Movat
M. stain
M. technique

move
m.'s all extremities
m.'s all extremities equally well
cord moves normally
inability to move a joint
inability to move tongue

movement
abnormal eye m.'s
abnormal involuntary movement disorder
Abnormal Involuntary M. Scale
m. abnormality
abnormal muscle m.
absence of voluntary muscle m.
active hip m.
adventitious choreiform m.
m. after effect
alpha-nonrapid eye m.
alpha-nonrapid eye movement sleep
altered bowel m.
anteroposterior m.
anterosuperior external ilium m.
anterosuperior internal ilium m.
m. arm vector
m. arousal index
m. artifact
m. assessment of infant
athetotic movement disorder
atypical stereotyped movement disorder
automatic movement reaction
autosomal dominant movement disorder
Awareness Through M.
bowel m.
caliper rib m.
chaotic eye m.
choreic athetoid m.'s
clumsy hand m.

movement *(continued)*
color, warmth, movement sensation
complex rotational m.
conjugate eye m.
conjugate movement of eyes
conjugate ocular m.
constraint-induced m.
control head m.
daily fetal movement count
daily fetal movement record
decreased fetal m.
Developmental Eye M.
diminished bowel m.
diminished intensity of m.
disconjugate movement of eye
disconjugate roving eye m.
disjointed agitated m.
m. disorder
m. disorder effect
drug-induced movement disorders
drug-related involuntary m.
m. duration
dynamic movement of inertia
equal ocular m.
external m.
extraocular m.
extraocular eye movements normal
extraocular movements full and conjugate
extraocular movements intact
extraocular movements full and conjugate
m. of extremities
eye movement desensitization reprocessing
eye movement gauge
eye movement measuring apparatus
eye movement recording
fetal breathing m.
fetal movement acceleration test
fetal movement count
fetal movement felt
fetal movement record
fine hair m.
fine motor m.
five-finger m.
fluid m.
frequent bowel m.
Frostig M. Skills Test Battery
full extraocular m.
full joint range of m.
full passive m.'s
full passive m.'s
functional m.
good fetal m.
hand m.
head m.
m. of heart
horizontal eye m.
m. illusion
impairment of power of voluntary m.
inability to perform purposeful m.'s
increased rapid eye movement sleep
infant tracks m.
m. injury
intact m.
involuntary body m.
involuntary movements of chorea
involuntary eye m.
involuntary jerking m.'s of legs
involuntary motor m.
involuntary movement disorder
involuntary muscular m.
involuntary repetitive m.
irregular bowel m.'s
irregular involuntary m.
irregular jerky m.'s
jerking eye m.'s
jerky step-wise m.
last bowel m.
lateral eye m.
lightning eye m.
limitation of m.
loose bowel m.
loss of m.
lumbar accessory movement technique
mandibular gliding m.
massive jerking m.'s
mental retardation, dystonic movements, ataxia, seizures syndrome
micro eye m.
monocular bobbing m.
multifocal clonic m.
muscle m.
neuroleptic-induced acute movement disorder
no bowel m.
nonoptic reflex eye m.
nonrapid eye m.
nonrapid eye movement sleep
normal bowel m.
normal extraocular m.'s
normal retinal m.
no spontaneous movement of limbs
oral commissure m.
orofacial m.
overhead movement of arm
pain aggravated by m.
painful and restricted m.
paradoxical abdominal m.
paradoxical movement of eyelids
parkinsonian movement disorder
passive accessory intervertebral m.'s
passive accessory intervertebral m.'s
passive physiological intervertebral m.'s
patient has no purposeful m.
peak-dose choreoathetoid dyskinetic m.
pelvic floor m.
periodic leg m.
periodic limb m.
periodic limb movements during sleep
periodic limb movement disorder
periodic limb movement in sleep
periodic movement disorder
pursuit eye m.
quality of m.
range of m.
rapid alternating m.'s
rapid eye m.
rapid eye movement sleep
rapid head m.
rapid movement disorder
rapid rhythmic alternating m.'s
resistance to movement of lung tissue
resistive m.
respiratory m.
restricted eye m.
rhythmic jerking m.'s
saccadic eye m.
sequential volitional oral m.
sleep-onset rapid eye movement period
slow eye m.
slow lateral eye m.
smooth pursuit eye m.
stereotypic movement disorder
straining on bowel m.
tarry black bowel m.
therapeutic humor m.
m. therapy
total fluid m.
tremors and jerky m.'s
twitches and involuntary m.'s
vergence eye m.'s
vocal cord m.
water bowel m.

movement-associated fetal heart rate accelerations

movement-produced stimulus

movement-related cortical potential

moving
autoregressive moving average
m. boundary electrophoresis
light moving touch
simulated moving bed chromatography
slowest moving protease
m. toes, painful leg syndrome

moving-strip technique

Mowlem-Jackson technique

Mowrey
M. 695 amalgam
M. B inlay
M. gold

moyamoya
m. collateral enlargement
m. disease
m. syndrome

Moynahan alopecia syndrome

Moynihan
M. clamp
M. gallstone scoop
M. respirator
M. syndrome

Mozart ear

MP13 virus

MP15 virus

M-phase-promoting factor

MPL-containing liposome

M-Prednisol Injection

mps1-induced arrest

MPTP-induced parkinsonism

MpV virus

Mr. Color test

MRI-based stereotactic biopsy

MRI-compatible hollow-fiber bioreactor

MRI-guided breast biopsy

MR-VP broth

MS-3
Miniscope M.

MS-1, -2 agent

MS-1 hepatitis

Mseleni disease

MSH_2 gene

MSP8 virus

MS2 virus

MT-2 cell

MTN blot

MTS1 gene

MTX
microplate plasma MTX assay

MTX/ara-C regimen

M-type
M.-t. extractor
M.-t. genetic group

Mu
Mu antigen
Mu virus

Mubarak-Hargens
M.-H. decompression
M.-H. decompression technique

Mucambo virus

mucate fermentation test

much
as much as needed
as much as possible

Mucha disease

Mucha-Habermann
M.-H. disease
M.-H. syndrome

Much granule

mucicarmine
Mayer mucicarmine stain
m. stain

mucigen granule

mucilloid
psyllium hydrophilic m.

mucin
m. clot prevention test
m. clot test
m. core protein
m. core protein-1
m. depletion
m. granule
hog gastric m.
m. layer
monoclonal antibodies against gastric m.'s
ovine submaxillary m.
polymorphic epithelial m.
m. strand
m. of tear

mucinglycoprotein

mucin-hypersecreting carcinoma

mucin-like carcinoma-associated antigen

mucinoid degeneration

mucinosafollicular
alopecia mucinosa/follicular mucinosis

mucinosis
alopecia mucinosa/follicular m.
oral focal m.
papular m.
reticular erythematous m.

mucinous
m. adenocarcinoma of ovary
m. adenocarcinoma tumor
m. adenoma
m. ascites
m. atrophy
m. borderline ovarian tumors
m. breast carcinoma
m. bronchogram
m. carcinoma
m. cell adenocarcinoma
m. columnar metaplasia
m. cyst
m. cystadenocarcinoma
m. cystadenoma
m. cystadenoma of ovary
m. cystic neoplasm
m. cystic tumor
m. degeneration
m. ductal ectasia
m. ductal ectasia of the pancreas
m. duct ectasia
m. ductectatic tumor of pancreas
m. eccrine carcinoma
m. edema
endocervical mucinous borderline tumor
intestinal mucinous borderline tumor
intraductal papillary mucinous neoplasm
intraductal papillary mucinous tumor
m. ovarian neoplasm
m. tumor

mucin-producing
m.-p. adenocarcinoma
m.-p. cancer
m.-p. carcinoma
m.-p. tumor
m.-p. tumor of the pancreas

mucin-secreting adenocarcinoma

Muckle-Wells syndrome

mucoadhesive
bioerodible m.

mucobuccal fold

mucocele
appendiceal m.
appendix m.
m. formation
m. of gallbladder

mucociliary
m. clearance
m. clearance rate
m. clearance time
m. drainage pathway
m. flow
m. function
m. transport

mucocutaneous
autoimmune blistering mucocutaneous disease
m. border
m. candidiasis
m. candidosis
chronic mucocutaneous candidiasis
m. disease
m. hemorrhoid
m. herpes simplex
m. HSV lesion
hypoparathyroidism, Addison disease, and mucocutaneous candidiasis syndrome
hypoparathyroidism, adrenal insufficiency, mucocutaneous candidiasis syndrome
m. junction
m. leishmaniasis
m. lesion
localized mucocutaneous candidiasis
m. lymph node
m. lymph node syndrome
m. manifestation
m. ocular syndrome
m. pigmentation
m. rash
m. reaction
m. relapse
skin, eye, m.
m. sporotrichosis
m. transmission
m. vesicle

mucoepidermoid
m. carcinoma
m. carcinoma of parotid
m. carcinoma of tongue
central mucoepidermoid carcinoma
sclerosing mucoepidermoid carcinoma with eosinophilia
m. tumor

mucogingival
apically repositioned flap in mucogingival surgery
m. junction

mucoid
m. adenocarcinoma
m. colony
copious mucoid material
m. degeneration
m. degeneration of umbilical cord
m. diarrhea
m. discharge
m. exopolysaccharide
m. impaction
m. impaction of bronchus
m. myoma degeneration
m. otitis media
m. sputum
m. wedge

mucolipidosis, pl. **mucolipidoses**
m. I–IV
m. type II, III

mucomembranous enteritis

mucoperichondrial
m. elevation
m. flap

mucoperiosteal
m. flap
m. flap technique
m. flap trimming
m. implant placement

mucopolysaccharide
acid m.
m. pattern
m. protein
m. storage disease I–VIII
sulfated acid m.

mucopolysaccharidosis
m. F
m. IH
m. I, II
m. IS
Maroteaux-Lamy m.
Morquio m.
m. MPS I, II
m. MPS III A, B, C, D
m. MPS VI–VIII
m. IV A, B
m. type I Hurler
m. type I Hurler-Scheie
m. type III Sanfilippo A, B, C
m. type I Scheie
m. type IV Morquio
m. types I, II, III, IIIB, III, IIID, IVA, IVB, VI, VII
m. type VII Sly
m. type VI Maroteaux-Lamy

mucopolysacchariduria

mucoprotein
m. assay
swine-associated m.
Tamm-Horsfall m.

mucopurulent
m. cervicitis
m. conjunctivitis
m. discharge
m. endocervical exudate
m. hemorrhagic effusion
m. sputum

mucopyocele of the clivus

***Mucor* mold**

mucormycosis
cardiac m.
m. esophagitis
gastrointestinal m.
m. sinusitis

mucosa
alveolar m.
m. appeared inflamed
atrophic gastric m.
atrophic vaginal m.
m. of bronchi
m. of colon
congestion of bladder m.
m. of ductus deferens
duodenal m.
effacement of m.
endocervical columnar m.
m. of esophagus
extensive bronchial mucosa hemorrhage
m. of female urethra
m. of gallbladder
gastric m.
hyperemic laryngeal m.
hyperemic nasal m.
m. of large intestine
m. of larynx
m. of male urethra
mandibular alveolar m.
multifocal ectopic gastric m.
muscular layer of m.
necrotic bladder m.
Neisseria mucosa endocarditis
nevus spongiosus albus m.
oral mucosa cyanosis
oral mucosa dry
oral mucosa pink
oral mucosa pink and moist
small bowel m.

tear in mucosa at cardioesophageal junction
transitional m.

mucosa-associated
m.-a. lymphoid tissue
m.-a. lymphoid tissue function
m.-a. lymphoid tissue lymphoma
m.-a. lymphoid tumor
m.-a. lymph tissue

mucosae
muscularis m.

mucosal
m. ablation
m. abnormality
m. abrasion
acute gastric mucosal lesion
m. addresin cell adhesion molecule-1
m. adenocarcinoma
m. advancement
m. aneuploidy
m. angiography
anorectal mucosal prolapse
antral mucosal cyst
antral mucosal diaphragm
antral mucosal thickening
m. atrophy
m. background
m. barrier
m. barrier maturation
m. biopsy
m. bipedicle flap
bladder mucosal hemorrhage
m. bleeding
m. blood flow
m. blood hemoglobin
m. blood vessel
m. border
bovine mucosal disease
bovine viral diarrhea mucosal disease
m. break
m. bridge
m. bridging
m. candidiasis
m. cell proliferation
m. coat
m. cobblestoning
m. collar
m. crinkling
cutting endoscopic mucosal resection
m. cyst
m. destruction
m. detachment
m. disease
m. disease virus
m. disease virus group
m. diverticulum
m. dysplasia
m. ecology
m. electrosensitivity
m. elevation
endoscopic mucosal ablation
endoscopic mucosal resection
endoscopic mucosal resection, cap method
endoscopic mucosal resection, tube method
endoscopic mucosal resection with ligation
m. erosion
m. erythema
esophageal mucosal ring
m. esophageal ring
m. excision
m. fatty acid
m. fluid
focal inflammatory mucosal change
m. fold
m. fold of gallbladder
gastric mucosal atrophy
gastric mucosal barrier
gastric mucosal blood flow
gastric mucosal ectopia in rectum
gastric mucosal erosion
gastric mucosal hemorrhage
m. gastric ulcer
m. graft
m. grafting
m. guideline pattern
gut mucosal lymphocyte
m. hemorrhage
m. hernia
m. hexosamine content
hyperemic mucosal pattern
m. hyperkeratosis
hyperplastic-like mucosal change
m. IgA
m. immune response
m. immunity
m. inflammation
m. inflammatory hyperplasia
m. intact laser tonsillar ablation
intestinal mucosal mast cell
m. irregularity
m. leishmaniasis
m. lesion
lift-and-cut endoscopic mucosal resection
lower esophageal mucosal ring
m. mast cell
m. melanoma
m. membrane graft
mosaic duodenal mucosal pattern
multiple mucosal neuroma syndrome
nasal mucosal ulceration
m. neurolysis
m. neuroma
m. neuroma syndrome
nonerosive gastric mucosal lesion
oral mucosal epithelia
oral mucosal transudate
m. oral therapeutic system
m. pemphigoid
m. rosette
selected mucosal biopsy
m. sloughing
stress-related mucosal damage
m. surface of large intestine
m. surface of small intestine
m. toxicity
m. transudate
m. ulcerative colitis
m. wave

mucosa-to-mucosa anastomosis

mucosectomy
endoscopic aspiration m.

mucoserous cell

mucositis
m. necroticans agranulocytica
oral m.
oropharyngeal m.

mucous
m. alveolus
m. assay
benign mucous membrane pemphigoid
bronchial mucous proteinase inhibitor
m. bronchogram
m. bronchogram sign
m. carcinoid
m. carcinoma
m. cast
m. cell
m. cell hyperplasia
cervical mucous basal body temperature
cervical mucous extract
cervical mucous plug
cervical mucous solution
chronic benign mucous membrane pemphigus
m. colic
m. colitis
m. connective tissue
m. crypt

mucous *(continued)*
m. crypt of duodenum
m. cyst
m. degeneration
m. depletion
m. desiccation
m. diarrhea
m. discharge
m. enteritis
m. escalator
m. fistula
m. gel thickness
m. gland
m. gland adenoma of bronchus
m. gland of auditory tube
m. glycoprotein
m. granule
hydration of mucous membranes
m. inspissation
m. membrane
m. membrane chancre
m. membrane chancroid
m. membrane exposure
m. membrane graft
m. membrane pemphigoid
m. membrane provocation
m. membranes moist
m. membrane ulceration
m. membrane wart
nasal mucous membrane
m. ophthalmia
oral mucous membrane
oral mucous membrane dry
oral mucous membrane graft
oral mucous membrane moist
oral mucous membrane pink
oral mucous membrane pink and moist
m. papule
m. patch
pink, moist, and warm mucous membranes
m. plaque
m. plug
m. plugging
m. rale
m. retention cyst
m. stool
m. tear layer
m. thread
tracheal mucous velocity

mucro cordis

mucus
m. blanket
cervical m.
cervical mucus penetration test
m. escape reaction
m. extractor
m. extravasation
m. flow rate
m. hypersecretion
m. impaction
m. membranes dry
midcycle cervical m.
overproduction of m.
sperm-cervical mucus contact
m. strand
m. thread

mucus-producing adenopapillary carcinoma

mucus-secreting
m.-s. cell
m.-s. gland

mucus-stimulating substance

mud
m. bed
biliary m.
m. fever

Mudjinbarry virus

Muehrcke
M. bands
M. line
M. sign

Mueller
M. anterolateral femorotibial ligament tenodesis
M. arthrodesis
M. cautery
cells of M.
M. compression apparatus
M. cup
M. distractor
M. eye shield
M. femoral supracondylar fracture classification
M. gland
M. hip arthroplasty
M. humerus fracture classification
M. implant
M. method
M. muscle
M. operation
M. trigone

Mueller-Hinton
M.-H. agar
M.-H. broth
M.-H. medium

Muenster
M. cast
M. protocol

Muerto Canyon virus

muffled heart sound

MUG test

mugwort weed pollen

mu-heavy-chain disease

mu-heavy chain disease

Muhlmann appliance

Muir Springs virus

Muir-Torre
M.-T. syndrome
M.-T. syndrome of hereditary nonpolyposis colon cancer

mulaire lesion

mulberry
m. calculus
m. gallstone
m. molar
m. ovary
paper m.
paper mulberry tree
m. pattern
m. rash
m. spot
m. tumor

mulberry-shaped mass

mulberry-type papilloma

Mulder
angle of M.
M. click

mule deer poxvirus

Mules
M. graft
M. implant
M. operation
M. scoop
M. vitreous sphere

mule-spinners' cancer

Mullen Scales of Early Learning

Müller
M. canal
M. capsule
M. cell
M. cell footplate
M. duct
M. duct body
M. empyema
M. empyema catheter
M. fibers
M. ganglion
M. law
M. maneuver
M. muscle
M. sign
M. syndrome
M. tubercle

Muller-Hermelink
M.-H. criteria
Müller-Hillis maneuver
müllerian
m. abnormality
m. adenosarcoma
m. agenesis
m. capsule
m. cyst
m. derivative
m. duct
m. duct anomaly
m. duct cyst
m. duct derivation syndrome
m. duct derived structure
m. duct fusion
m. duct inhibitory factor
m. duct, unilateral renal agenesis, and anomalies of the cervicothoracic somites
m. fusion defect
m. hypoplasia
m. inhibiting factor
m. inhibiting hormone
m. inhibitory hormone
malignant mixed müllerian tumor
metastatic mixed müllerian tumor
mixed müllerian sarcoma
m. mixed tumor
m., renal, cervicothoracic, somite abnormalities
m., renal, cervicothoracic, somite abnormalities syndrome
persistent müllerian duct syndrome
m. regression factor
müllerian-inhibiting
m.-i. hormone
m.-i. substance
m.-i. substance receptor
Muller maneuver
Mullins
M. blade technique
M. long transseptal sheath
multangular
m. bone
Multi
M. Axis Ankle
M. Balance System
multiaccess catheter
multiagent chemotherapy
multiangle polarized scatter separation
multiantigenic peptide
multiaxial
M. Assessment of Pain
m. classification
m. classification system
m. evaluation
m. fashion
Millon Clinical Multiaxial Inventory test
multiaxis foot
multibacillary leprosy
multibanded appliance
multicapsin
multicelled embryo
multicellular
basic multicellular unit
m. helminth
m. tumor spheroid
multicenter
M. AIDS Cohort Study
M. Myocarditis Treatment Trial
M. Oral Carvedilol Heart Failure Assessment
m. trial
multicentric
m. angiofollicular lymph node
m. angiofollicular lymphoid hyperplasia
m. basal cell carcinoma
m. carcinoid tumor
m. Castleman disease
m. disease
m. foci
m. islet cell adenoma
m. lower genital tract neoplasia
m. malignant glioma
m. mammary carcinoma
m. reticulohistiocytosis
***Multiceps* infection**
multichannel
m. analyzer
m. cystometrogram
m. cystometry
m. implant
m. recorder
sequential multichannel autoanalyzer
m. signed averager
simultaneous multichannel autoanalyzer
multiclonal follicular lymphoma
multicoil array technique
multicolony-stimulating factor
multicolor
m. data analysis
m. FISH cytogenetic technique
m. immunofluorescence measurement
multicomponent behavioral treatment
multicopy suppressor screen
multicore
m. disease
m. myopathy
multicrystal gamma camera
multicultural
System of Multicultural Assessment
System of Multicultural Pluralistic Assessment
multicurve contact lens
multicystic
m. acoustic neuroma
m. ameloblastoma
congenital multicystic kidney
m. disease
m. dysgenetic kidney
m. dysplasia
m. dysplasia kidney
m. dysplastic kidney
m. encephalomalacia
m. encephalopathy
m. kidney disease
m. renal dysplasia
multidermatomal herpes zoster
multidetector
m. computed tomography
m. CT
m. CTA
m. CT scanner
multideterminant molecule
Multidex filler
multidigit dactylitis
multidimensional
m. actuarial classification
m. analysis beam modifier
m. assessment
m. assessment of outcome
M. Assessment of Philosophy of Education
m. construct
Endler M. Anxiety Scale
m. family therapy
M. Fatigue Symptom Inventory
m. flow cytometry
m. Fourier transform
m. framework
Inpatient M. Psychiatric Scale

multidimensional *(continued)*
OARS M. Functional Assessment Questionnaire
M. Pain Inventory
M. Personality Questionnaire
M. Quality of Life Questionnaire for Persons with Human Immunodeficiency Virus
M. Scale of Perceived Social Support
m. scaling
M. Scalogram Analysis
M. Self Concept Scale
M. Student Life Satisfaction Scale
Westhaven Yale M. Pain Inventory

Multi-Dimensional Voice Program 4305

multidirectional
atraumatic, multidirectional, bilateral rehabilitation inferior capsular shift
atraumatic, multidirectional, bilateral radial instability
atraumatic multidirectional instability
m. instability

multidisciplinary
m. approach
m. group psychiatry
m. pain management center
m. pain treatment
m. team approach
m. treatment plan

multidose
m. activated charcoal
m. insulin treatment

multidrug
m. abuse
m. chemotherapy
m. regimen
m. resistance
m. resistance-associated mutation
m. resistance associated protein
m. resistance detoxification
m. resistance gene
m. resistance modulator
m. resistance protein
m. resistant
m. therapy

multidrug-resistant
m.-r. *Streptococcus pneumoniae*
m.-r. tuberculosis

multiecho
m. axial
m. axial image
m. coronal image
preinversion m.

multielectrode flame ionization detector

Multi-Environment Scheme

multifactorial
m. disease
m. disorder
m. etiology
m. event
m. inheritance
m. model
m. trait

multi-family group counseling

multifetal
m. gestation
m. pregnancy
m. pregnancy reduction

multifidus muscle

multifield beam

Multifire clip applicator

MULTIFIT trial

multifocal
m. acquired motor axonopathy
acute multifocal posterior placoid pigment epitheliopathy
acute posterior multifocal placoid pigment epitheliopathy
m. aggressive infiltrate
m. anaplastic astrocytoma
m. area
m. area of hyperintensity
m. atrial tachycardia
m. atrophic gastritis
m. autonomic adenoma
m. bladder tumor
m. brain tumor
m. breast carcinoma
m. change
m. chorioretinal disease
m. choroiditis
chronic recurrent multifocal osteomyelitis
m. clonic convulsion
m. clonic movement
m. clonic seizure
m. demyelinating motor neuropathy
m. ectopic gastric mucosa
m. electroretinogram
m. enhancing lesion
m. eosinophilic granuloma
m. fibrosclerosis
m. fibrosis
m. functional autonomy
m. giant cell encephalitis
m. glioma
m. heartbeat
m. hemorrhagic sarcoma
hereditary multifocal relapsing inflammation
m. histiocytosis
m. infiltrated duct cell carcinoma
m. Langerhans cell leukodystrophy
m. leukoencephalopathy
meningococcal multifocal osteomyelitis
m. motor neuropathy
motor neuropathy with multifocal conduction block
m. myoclonus
one-piece multifocal lens
m. osteomyelitis
peripheral multifocal chorioretinitis
m. posterior pigment epitheliopathy
m. premature ventricular contraction
progressive multifocal leukodystrophy
progressive multifocal leukoencephalopathy
progressive multifocal leuko-J encephalopathy
m. and recurrent choroidopathy
m. spectacle lens
m. spike
m. white matter inflammatory lesion

multifocal-extensive
m.-e. DCIS
m.-e. disease

multifollicular ovary

multiforme
atypical erythema m.
erythema multiforme major
generalized erythema m.
glioblastoma m.
m. granuloma
herpes-associated erythema m.
mouth erythema m.
oral erythema m.
recurrent glioblastoma m.

multiforme-like

multiforme/toxic
erythema multiforme/toxic epidermal necrolysis

multifunctional
m. acrylic
m. extracellular glycoprotein

multigas
smart anesthesia m.

multigated
m. angiogram
m. angiography
m. blood pool image at rest
m. blood pool image during exercise
m. cardiac blood pool scanning

multigene transcript

multigenic disorder

multigland disease

multiglandular disease

multigravida
patient m.

multiheteronodular toxic goiter

multihormonal system disorder

multihospital system

multiinfarct
m. dementia
m. dementia, uncomplicated
m. dementia with delirium
m. dementia with delusions
m. dementia with depression
m. disease

multiinstitutional arrangement

multi-item index

multilamellar cytosome

multilaminar vesicle

multilaminated structure

multilanguage aphasia

multileaf
m. collimator
segmental multileaf collimator

multilevel
m. atherosclerotic arterial occlusive disease
m. care
m. fracture
m. fusion

MultiLight system

multilineage
m. colony-stimulating factor
m. origin
m. reconstitution

Multilingual
M. Aphasia Battery
M. Aphasia Examination

multilobated
m. nucleus
m. T-cell lymphoma

multilobe infiltrate

multilobular
m. cirrhosis
m. configuration

multilocal genetics

multilocular
m. adipose tissue
m. crypt
m. cystic kidney
m. cystic lesion
m. cystic nephroma
m. fat
m. hydatid cyst
m. peritoneal inclusion cyst
m. thymic cyst
m. vesicle

multiloculated cyst

multilocus
m. enzyme electrophoresis
m. enzyme electrophoresis analysis
m. sequence typing

multilog effect

multilumen
m. catheter
m. central venous pressure

multimammate
m. papilloma virus
m. rate

multimembrane spanner

multimeric molecule

multimodal
m. adjuvant therapy
m. analgesia
m. association cortex
m. behavior therapy
m. code
m. physical therapy
m. treatment
m. treatment plan

multimodality
m. evoked potential
m. evoked response
m. therapy
m. treatment program

multimonitored
m. electroconvulsive treatment

multimonitored electroconvulsive treatment

multinodular
benign multinodular goiter
m. euthyroid goiter
nontoxic multinodular goiter
m. thyroid gland
m. thyroid nodule
toxic multinodular goiter

multinomial polytomous logistic regression method

multinuclear leukocyte

multinucleate
m. cell angiohistiocytoma

multinucleate cell angiohistiocytoma

multinucleated
m. atypia of the vulva
m. cell encephalitis
m. dentinoblastic cell
m. giant epithelial cell
m. osteoclastic giant cell
percentage of multinucleated cells

Multi-Optics lens

multiorgan
drug-induced delayed multiorgan hypersensitivity syndrome
m. dysfunction
m. dysfunction syndrome
m. hernia
m. system failure

multiorgan system failure

multiparameter
m. intraarterial sensor
Neurotrend continuous multiparameter system

multiparity
grand m.

multipartita
placenta m.

multipartite fracture

multiphase
m. appliance
m. attachment
m. bracket

multiphasic
automated multiphasic health testing
automated multiphasic screening
m. CT
M. Environmental Assessment Procedure
m. health checkup
m. health screen test
m. health testing
Minnesota Multiphasic Personality Inventory Depression Scale

multiphasic *(continued)*
Minnesota M. Personality Inventory, Second Edition
m. screening
Senoussi M. Marital Inventory

multiphoton excitation

multiplanar
axial multiplanar reformation technique
m. compression
m. computed tomography scan
computed tomography with multiplanar reconstructions
m. CT scan
m. deformity
m. display
m. distraction
m. endoscopic facial rejuvenation technique
fast multiplanar spoiled gradient-recalled imaging
m. gradient recall
m. gradient refocused
m. imaging
m. MRI
phase-offset m.
phase-ordered m.
m. reconstruction
m. reformatting view

multiplane
m. dosage calculation
m. intracavitary probe

multiple
m. abrasions
m. abscesses
m. abstract variance analysis
m. abutment
m. abutment support
m. access
m. accessory spleens
m. action
m. action cutter
acute multiple brain infarct
m. acute rejection episode
m. acyl-coenzyme A dehydrogenase deficiency
m. adenoma
m. adenomatous polyps
m. adjuvant
m. admission
M. Affect Adjective Check List
m. agent therapy
m. air-fluid levels
m. alcohol
m. allele
m. amputation
m. anal sphincterotomies
m. analysis
m. analysis of variance
m. anchorage
m. anterior pituitary hormone deficiency
m. antigen stimulation test
m. anxiety comorbidity
m. aortopulmonary collateral artery
m.'s of the appropriate gestational median
m. arbitrary amplicon profiling
Arizona Cancer Center multiple myeloma staging system
m. articular contracture
m. articular rigidity
m. association
automated multiple analysis
m. automated sample harvester
m. axis knee joint
m. band ligator
m. basal cell carcinoma syndrome multiple basal cell nevus syndrome
m. basal cell neuroma syndrome
m. basal cell nevoid syndrome
m. baseline design
m. benign circumferential skin creases on limb
m. benign cystic epithelioma
m. biopsies taken
m. biopsy
m. biotin-avidin amplification
m. birth
bleeding from multiple sites
m. blocks
m. blunt trauma
m. bone enchondromata
m. bone myeloma
m. brain metastases
m. buccal frenula
m. bull's eye lesions bowel wall
m. calcification
m. calices
m. cancellous chip graft
m. carboxylase deficiency
m. cartilaginous exostoses
m. cartilaginous exostosis
m. cervix
m. chemical sensitivity
m. chemical sensitivity syndrome
m. choice discrimination test
m. choice question
m. cholesterol emboli syndrome
m. chords
chronic progressive multiple sclerosis
m. clasp
m. cognitive deficits
m. coil array
m. colon filling defect
m. combined sclerosis
m. complex developmental disorder
m. compressed tablet
m. concentric GI rings
m. concentric ring sign
m. cone root canal filling method
m. congenital abnormalities
m. congenital anomalies
m. congenital anomalies/mental retardation syndrome
m. congenital fibromatosis
m. core biopsies
m. correlation
m. cortical infarction
m. cortical infarcts
m. cyst
m. daily fraction
m. daily injection
m. daily insulin injection
daytime multiple sleep latency test
m. deficiency
m. delusions
dementia due to multiple etiologies
m. digits
m. discharge
m. dislocations
m. distinct identities
m. domains of self
m. dosage insulin
m. dose
m. dose vial
m. drug-resistant
m. ego state
m. enchondroma
m. enchondromatosis
m. endochondromatosis
m. endocrine abnormalities
m. endocrine adenomatosis
m. endocrine adenomatosis type I, II
m. endocrine adenopathy
m. endocrine deficiency, Addison disease, and candidiasis syndrome
m. endocrine deficiency-autoimmune candidiasis

m. endocrine neoplasia syndrome, type 1, 2A, 2B, 3
m. endocrine neoplasia type 1, 2, 2a, 2b, 3
m. endocrine neoplasm
m. endocrinoma
m. endocrinopathy
m. endocrinoplasia
m. endpoints
epilepsy with multiple independent spike focus
m. epiphysial dysplasia
m. epiphysial dysplasia-early onset diabetes mellitus syndrome
m. epiphysial dysplasia tarda syndrome
m. eruptive milia
m. evanescent white dot syndrome
m. event curve
exacerbating-remitting multiple sclerosis
m. exostoses
m. exostoses of jaw
m. exostoses-mental retardation syndrome
m. exostosis
m. exostosis mental retardation syndrome
m. factor analysis
familial atypical multiple melanoma
familial multiple endocrine neoplasia
familial multiple factor deficiency 1
m. familial polyposis
m. family therapy
fast acquisition multiple excitation
m. finger
m. fission
m. flexible medullary nail
m. focal lesion
m. focus
m. foramina
m. fracture
m. fragment wounds
m. gallstones
m. gas rebreathing
m. gastrointestinal polyps
m. gated acquisition
m. gated acquisition scan
m. gated equilibrium scintigraphy
m. gestation
m. gland hyperplasia
m. glandular deficiency syndrome
gravida, para, multiple births, abortions, live birth
m. gumma
m. gunshot wound
m. hamartoma syndrome
m. handicap
m. handicapped
m. health screening
m. hepatitis virus infection
m. hereditary cutaneomandibular polyoncosis
m. hereditary exostosis
m. hereditary hemorrhagic telangiectasis
m. hereditary osteochondral exostosis
m. hook assembly
m. hook assembly C-D instrumentation
m. hospitalizations
iatrogenic multiple pregnancy
m. identification
m. idiopathic hemorrhagic sarcoma
m. inert gas elimination technique
m. infarct
m. injection regimen
m. injection therapy of insulin
m. interstitial pulmonary hemorrhage
m. intestinal neoplasia
m. intracranial aneurysm
m. ion detection
m. isomorphous replacement
m. keratoacanthoma
m. lentigines syndrome
m. lentiginosis
m. linear regression analysis
m. line scan
m. line-scan imaging
m. lobar hemorrhage
m. logistic regression
m. loops of small bowel
lowest common m.
m. luteinized theca cyst
m. lymphomatous polyposis
macrocephaly, multiple lipomas, hemangiomata syndrome
macrocephaly, pseudoepithelioma, multiple hemangiomas syndrome
m. marker reverse transcriptase-polymerase chain reaction assay
m. marker screening
m. medical problem
m. milia
m. minute digitate hyperkeratosis
m. monitored electroconvulsive therapy
m. mononeuropathies
m. mucosal neuroma
m. mucosal neuroma syndrome
m. myeloma
m. myeloma cell line
m. myeloma staging
m. myelomatosis
m. myofibromatosis
m. myositis
m. nevoid-basal cell carcinoma
m. nevoid-basal cell carcinoma syndrome
m. nevoid, basal cell epithelioma, jaw cysts, bifid rib syndrome
nitrogen washout, multiple breath
m. noninguinal sites
nuclear multiple gaited acquisition
m. nucleocapsid virus
m. nucleopolyhedrovirus
m. occurrence of unexplained symptoms
m. ocular coloboma
m. opportunistic pathogen infection
m. oral frenula
m. oral vitamin
m. organ dysfunction
m. organ dysfunction syndrome
m. organ failure
m. organ failure syndrome
m. organ malrotation syndrome
m. organ system dysfunction
m. organ system failure
m. osteomas
m. outcomes of raloxifene evaluation trial
overdosed with multiple drugs
m. overlapping thin-slab acquisition
m. parasitism
m. personality disorder
m. pituitary hormone deficiencies
m. planar gradient-recalled
m. polyposis
m. pregnancy
m. presentation phenotype
m. primary malignancy
m. primary melanoma
m. primary neoplasm
m. primary neoplasms
primary-progressive multiple sclerosis
programmable multiple ion monitor
programmed multiple development

multiple *(continued)*
m. pterygium syndrome
m. pulmonary infarct
m. punctuate hemorrhage
m. puncture tuberculin test
relapsing-remitting multiple sclerosis
m. resistant cell lines
M. Risk Factor Intervention Trial
m. scan average dose
m. sclerosis-associated agent
m. sclerosis susceptibility gene
m. self-healing squamous carcinoma
m. sensory defect dizziness
m. sensory deficit
sequential multiple analysis
sequential multiple analyzer
serial multiple analysis
m. serositis
M. Severity of Illness System
m. sib case
simultaneous multiple analyzer
m. in situ hybridization
M. Sleep Latency Test
m. soft tissue injuries
m. stab wounds
m. subcortical infarction
m. subpial transection
m. sulfatase deficiency
m. sulfatase deficiency syndrome
m. symmetric lipomatosis
m. synchronous subcutaneous metastases
m. synostoses syndrome
m. system atrophy
m. tic disorder
m. tics
m. trace elements
tracheoesophageal fistula, esophageal atresia, multiple congenital anomaly syndrome
traumatic multiple hemorrhages
m. trichoepithelioma
tricho-rhino-auriculo-phalangeal multiple exostoses
trichorhinophalangeal multiple exostoses
m. unit activity
m. villous infarcts
m. vision
m. vitamin injection
volumetric multiple exposure transmission holography
m. X syndrome

multiple-allele-specific diagnostic assay

multiple-breath nitrogen washout

multiple coil array

multiple-drug
m.-d. regimen
m.-d. resistance gene
m.-d. resistant tuberculosis

multiple-drug-resistant enterococci

multiple-frequency bioimpedance

multiple gated
m. g. equilibrium scintigraphy

multiple-punch resection

multiple-ring-enhancing mass lesion

multiple-site perineal applicator technique

multiple-type hyperlipoproteinemia

multiplex
arthrochalasis multiplex congenita
arthrochalasis multiplex congenita Ehlers-Danlos syndrome
arthrogryposis congenita m.
arthrogryposis multiplex congenita
BCR-ABL multiplex reverse transcriptase polymerase chain reaction assay
m. dysostosis
lymphangioma tuberosum m.
mononeuritis m.
mononeuropathy m.
myeloma m.
myelomatosis m.
myodysplasia fibrosa m.
myopathic arthrogryposis multiplex congenita
neuropathic arthrogryposis multiplex congenita
m. nevus
m. polymerase chain reaction
steatocystoma m.
m. steatocystoma
xanthoma m.
xanthoma tuberosum m.

multiplication
cell multiplication inhibition
countercurrent m.
m. factor
m. rate

multiplication-stimulating activity

multiplicative division

multiplicities

multiplicity
m. of infection
m. reactivation

multiplied
m. by
concentration multiplied by time

multiplier
countercurrent m.
countercurrent multiplier principle
m. effect
photoelectric multiplier tube

multiploid tumor

multiplying digital-to-analog converter

multipolar
m. cell
m. coagulation
m. electrocautery
m. electrocoagulation

multiport collimated cobalt-60 therapy

multipotent
m. hematopoietic cell
m. hematopoietic progenitor

multipotential progenitor

Multi-Pro biopsy needle

MultiPulse
M. cosmetic treatment laser
M. laser system
M. laser system

multipuncture
m. battery
m. device
m. method
percutaneous multipuncture technique
m. technique
m. test

multipurpose
m. access port
m. angled clamp
m. curved clamp
m. meal

multiresistant bacteria

multirooted abutment

multisample

multiscope
roaming optical access m.

Multiscore Depression Inventory

multisection
combined multisection diffuse-weighted and hemodynamically weighted echoplanar MR

m. diffuse-weighted magnetic resonance imaging

multisite lower genital tract involvement

multislice

m. acquisition

m. computed tomography

m. CT

multispecific

canicular multispecific organic anion transporter

multispectral fluorescent in situ hybridization

multistage

m. graded exercise test

m. Markov model

Multistar angiographic unit

multistate

m. drug distribution ring

m. information system

multistep

cancer multistep therapy

multisweep

high-resolution m.

multisynaptic pathway

multisystem

m. atrophy

m. disorder

juvenile-onset multisystem inflammatory disease

m. organ failure

m. trauma

multisystemic therapy

multitargeted

m. antifolate

m. chemotherapy

multitest

automated multitest laboratory

M. CMI device

M. CMI system

m., mycology plate

M. test

m. yeast plate

multithread allergosorbent test

multivalent

m. antigen

m. antiserum

m. vaccine

multi-valve insufficiency

multivalvular involvement

Multivane Intensity Modulation Compensator

multivariant

m. analysis

m. discriminant analysis

multivariate

m. analysis of covariance

m. analysis of variance

m. logistic regression

m. logistic regression analysis

M. Personality Inventory

multivesicular body

multivessel coronary disease

multivitamin

m. infusion

pediatric multivitamin infusion

multivitamin-mineral formula

multivoxel spectroscopy

multiwire proportional chamber

multocida

Pasteurella multocida osteomyelitis

Mulvihill-Smith syndrome

Muma Assessment Program

Mumford-Gurd arthroplasty

mummification

m. necrosis

stillbirth, mummification, embryonic death, infertility syndrome

mummified

m. cell

m. fetus

mummy wrap

mumps

m. antibody titer

m. arthritis

attenuated mumps virus

m. encephalitis

m. epididymitis

m. facial nerve palsy

m. keratitis

m. leptomeningitis

measles, mumps, rubella immunization

measles, mumps, and rubella vaccine

m. meningitis

m. meningoencephalitis

metastatic m.

m. orchitis

m. sensitivity test

m. serology

m. skin test antigen

m. vaccine

m. virus

m. virus culture

m. virus vaccine

m. virus vaccine Jeryl Lynn strain

mumu fever

Münchausen

M. disease

M. disease by proxy

M. by proxy syndrome

munching pattern

Munguba virus

municipal hospital

Munro

M. abscess

M. microabscess

M. and Parker classification for laparoscopic hysterectomy

M. point

Munro-Kerr maneuver

Munsell color

Munson sign

mupirocin ointment

mupirocin-resistant

m.-r., methicillin-resistant *Staphylococcus aureus*

m.-r. MRSA

m.-r. *Staphylococcus aureus*

mural

m. aneurysm

m. arch

m. architecture

calcific mural atherosclerosis

m. cell

m. change

m. clot

m. CNS nodule

m. defect

m. degeneration

m. dilatation

m. endocarditis

m. endocardium

m. pregnancy

sarcoma-like mural nodule

m. thrombosis

m. thrombus

m. trophectoderm

muramic acid

muramidase

urinary muramidase activity

muramyl

m. dipeptide

m. tripeptide

Murdoon eye speculum

Murex
M. *Candida albicans* test

murine
Abelson murine leukemia virus
amphotropic murine leukemia virus
antibody to murine cardiac myosin
m. B16 cell
m. colony-forming unit
m. erythroblastosis virus
m. erythroleukemia
m. erythroleukemia cell
m. fibroblast transformation
Friend murine erythroleukemia
m. gene
m. graft
m. granulocyte-macrophage colony-stimulating growth factor
Harvey murine sarcoma virus
m. hepatitis
m. homolog
m. interleukin
m. interleukin-6
m. L cell
m. leukemia
m. leukemia virus
m. lymphocytic choriomeningitis virus
m. macrophage
Maloney murine sarcoma
m. mammary tumor virus
m. melanoma
m. mesangial cell
m. model
Moloney murine leukemia virus
Moloney murine sarcoma virus
m. myeloid leukemia cell line
m. neuroblastoma
neutralizing murine monoclonal antitumor necrosis factor antibody
nonimmunogenic murine tumor cell
OKT3 murine monoclonal antibody
m. osteopetrosis mutation
Rauscher murine leukemia virus
m. retina
m. sarcoma virus
Theiler murine encephalomyelitis virus
m. thymoma
m. tumor cell
m. typhus

murine-acquired
m.-a. immunodeficiency syndrome

murmur
aortic regurgitation m.
aortic stenosis and aortic insufficiency m.'s
aortic systolic ejection m.
apical mid-diastolic heart m.
apical presystolic m.
apical systolic heart m.
Austin Flint m.
benign heart m.
blowing systolic m.
cardiac m.
continuous heart m.
diamond ejection m.
diastolic m.
early diastolic m.
ejection m.
Eustace Smith m.
functional heart m.
m.'s, gallops, or rubs
goose honk m.
grade 1–6 heart m.
harsh systolic m.
heart m.
holosystolic m.
incompetent aortic m.
innocent heart m.
late systolic m.
Means-Lerman scratch m.
mid-diastolic m.
midsystolic m.
mill wheel m.
mitral regurgitant m.
presystolic m.
primary pulmonary hypertension m.
regular rate, clear tones, no m.'s
m.'s, rubs, and gallops
systolic click murmur syndrome
systolic ejection m.
systolic heart m.
m. of valvulitis

Murphy
M. Achilles tendon advancement
M. drip
M. heel cord advancement
M. hole
M. percussion
M. punch maneuver test
M. sign
M. staging system
M. unit

Murphy-Meisgeier Type Indicator for Children

Murray
M. fixation
M. test
M. Valley encephalitis
M. Valley encephalitis virus
M. Valley rash

Murre virus

Murri disease

Murutucu virus

Mus
Mus adenovirus 1–2

muscae volitantes

muscarinic
m. acetylcholine receptor
m. action
m. activity
m. agonist
m. agonist carbamylcholine
m. antagonist
m. blockade
m. cholinergic agonist
m. cholinergic blockade
m. cholinergic receptor
m. cholinergic side effect
m. receptor autoantibody

muscle
m. of abdomen
abdominal muscle guarding
abdominal muscle strength
abdominal muscle tone
abductor digiti minimi m.
abductor digiti quinti m.
abductor hallucis brevis m.
abductor pollicis brevis m.
abductor pollicis longus m.
m. ability
abnormal muscle movement
abnormal muscle response
abnormal muscle tone
m. absence
absence of voluntary muscle movement
accessory muscles of respiration
acoustic muscle reflex
m. actin
m. activity
acute heart muscle degeneration
adductor brevis m.
adductor hallucis m.
adductor longus m.
adductor pollicis m.
adductor pollicis obliquus m.
m. adenosine monophosphate deaminase deficiency
m. adenylate deaminase
airway smooth m.
alcoholic heart muscle disease
alpha smooth muscle actin
m. of anal triangle

m. analysis
angiographic muscle mass index
anisotropic band in striated m.
anomalous muscle band
anomalous muscle bundle
ansa hypoglossus m.
antagonistic muscle strength
anterior auricular m.
anterior belly of digastric m.
anterior cervical intertransverse m.
anterior fascicle of palatopharyngeus m.
anterior papillary m.
anterior rectus m.
anterior rectus muscle of head
anterior scalene m.
anterior scalenus m.
anterior serratus m.
anterior tibial m.
antiheart muscle autoantibody
antismooth muscle actin
antismooth muscle antibody
antismooth muscle antibody assay
antismooth muscle antigen
m. of antitragus
antropyloric muscle thickness
anulospiral ending of muscle spindle
aplastic abdominal muscle syndrome
aponeurosis of abdominal oblique m.
aponeurosis of external oblique m.
aponeurosis of internal oblique m.
aponeurosis of vastus m.
appendicular skeletal m.
arm muscle circumference
arrector muscle of hair
arrector pili m.
arterial smooth muscle cell
articular muscle of elbow
articular muscle of knee
m. artifact
aryepiglottic part of oblique arytenoid m.
ascending part of trapezius m.
Ashworth score of muscle spasticity
m. asthenia
m. atonia
atonic sclerotic muscle dystrophy
atrophied abdominal m.'s
m. atrophy
atrophy of abdominal m.
m. atrophy-contracture-oculomuscle apraxia syndrome
m.'s of auditory ossicles
auricularis anterior m.
auricularis posterior m.
auricularis superior m.
axillary arch m.
m. of back
m. of back proper
m. balance
beating heart m.
m. belly
biceps femoris m.
m. biopsy
blood diffuses into heart m.
m. blood flow
blood-starved heart muscle tissue
bones, m.'s, joints
bones, joints, and m.'s
bovine embryo skeletal m.
m. breakdown
m. bulk
m. bundle
m. cachexia
m. capillary basement membrane
m. capillary basement membrane thickening
cardiac m.
cardiac muscle wrap
m. carnitine deficiency
m. carnitine palmitoyltransferase deficiency
m. catabolism
cataplexy muscle weakness
chronic alcoholic heart muscle disease
chronic muscle pain syndrome
circular m.
circular Santorini m.'s
m. clamp
clenched muscles in head and neck
m. of coccyx
cognition and muscle control
m. of common bile duct
compensatory hypertrophy of heart m.
compound muscle action potential
compressor muscle of naris
condition muscles with aerobic exercise
m. cone
congenital muscle fiber-type disproportion
m. contractile protein
m. contractility
contractility of heart m.
m. contraction
m. contraction headache
contraction of heart m.
m. contracture
m. contusion
m. cramp
creatine kinase fraction muscle
cricothyroid m.
m. crushing injury
m. curve
m. cylinder
dartos muscle of scrotum
dead area of heart m.
death of heart muscle tissue
de-epithelialized rectus abdominis muscle graft
m. of deglutition
delayed muscle soreness
delayed-onset muscle soreness
deltoid m.
m. denervation
m. depressor
depressor muscle of angle of mouth
depressor muscle of lower lip
depressor muscle of septum of nose
deterioration of heart m.
detrusor muscle instability
detrusor muscle leak-point pressure
detrusor muscle pressure-flow micturition study
diabetic muscle infarction
diastasis of m.
diffuse muscle atrophy
m. dilator
m. disease
disintegration of m.
m. disorder
m. dissection
m. distraction
dorsal interosseous muscle of foot
dorsal interosseous muscle of hand
m. dystonia
m. effect
electrical muscle stimulation
m. in elongated state
embryonic chick m.
endoscopic muscle plication
m. endplate
m. energy
m. energy technique
enlarged heart m.
m. enlargement

muscle *(continued)*
m. enzyme
m. enzyme serum level
m. enzyme test
m. epithelium
m. erotism
evoked muscle action potential
m. examination
extensor carpi radialis brevis m.
extensor carpi radialis longus m.
extensor carpi ulnaris m.
extensor digiti minimi m.
extensor digiti quinti m.
extensor digitorum communis m.
extensor hallucis brevis m.
external intercostal m.
external muscle layer damaged
external oblique m.
external oblique muscle of abdomen
extraocular m.
extraocular muscles intact
m. of eye
m. of eyeball
eye muscle imbalance
m.'s of facial expression
m. fascia
m. fascicle
m. fasciculation
fast-glycolytic muscle fiber
m. fiber
m. fiber action potential
m. fiber conduction velocity
m. fiber type disproportion
m. fibrosis
m. filling
m. filter
first digital interosseous muscle
m. flap
flexor digiti minimi muscle
flexor digiti quinti muscle
flexor digitorum profundus m.
flexor hallucis brevis m.
m. force
m. forceps
m. fraction enzyme of creatine phosphokinase
functional muscle test
m. function test
galvanic muscle stimulation
gastrocnemius and soleus m.'s
gastrointestinal smooth muscle tumor
generalized muscle aches
gluteus maximus m.
gluteus minimus m.
m. graft
great adductor m.
greater psoas m.
greater rhomboid m.
greater trochanter m.
greater zygomatic m.
greatest gluteal m.
m. group
m. guarding
guinea pig tracheal smooth m.
m. of head
heart muscle abnormality
heart muscle cell
heart muscle damage
heart muscle death
heart muscle disease
heart muscle fiber
heart muscle tissue
heart muscle weakness
heavy meromyosin of m.
m. hemoglobin
m. hernia
m. herniation
herniation of m.
m. hook
human aortic smooth muscle cell
m.'s of hyoid bone
hyperplastic muscle fiber
hypertrophic smooth muscle layer
m. hypertrophy
m. hypotonia
m. imbalance
impaired contractility of hypertrophied m.
improved muscle tone
increased blood flow to heart m.
increased muscle mass
increased muscle strength
increased muscle tone
inferior oblique eye m.
inferior rectus muscle
inferior tarsal m.
inflammation of heart m.
injured heart m.
innermost intercostal m.
inspiratory m.
inspiratory muscle training
intact chest m.'s
intercostal m.
intermittent tonic muscle contractions
internal intercostal m.
internal oblique muscle of abdomen
internal obturator m.
internal sphincter muscle of anus
intersegmental m.
intraocular m.
intrinsic muscle of foot
involuntary muscle contraction
ipsilateral mentalis m.
m. ischemia
ischemic heart m.
ischemic muscle contracture
ischemic muscle fiber
ischemic muscle necrosis
ischemic skeletal m.
m.'s isolated and tagged
isotropic band striated muscle fiber
isotropic disc striated muscle fiber
jaw muscle activity
lactate dehydrogenase, m.
laryngeal m.
m. of larynx
lateral pterygoid m.
lateral rectus eye m.
latissimus dorsi m.
m. layer in fatty layer of subcutaneous tissue
lean body muscle mass
left inferior oblique muscle
left lateral decubitus muscle
left lateral rectus eye m.
left medial rectus eye m.
left vastus lateralis m.
left ventricular muscle mass
m. lengthening
levator ani m.
levator veli palatini muscle
line for soleus m.
m., liver, brain, eye disease
long abductor muscle of thumb
long adductor m.
long extensor muscle of great toe
long extensor muscle of thumb
long fibular m.
long flexor muscle of great toe
long flexor muscle of thumb
longissimus capitis m.
longissimus cervicis m.
longissimus muscle of head
longissimus thoracis m.
longitudinal m.
longitudinal ciliary m.
longitudinal layer of muscle coat of small intestine
longitudinal pharyngeal m.
long muscle of head
long muscle of neck
long palmar m.
long peroneal m.

long radial extensor muscle of wrist
long rotator m.
longus capitis m.
longus cervicis colli m.
longus colli m.
lower esophageal sphincter circular m.
low muscle tone
lumbar extensor m.
lumbar iliocostal m.
lumbar interspinal m.
lumbar quadrate m.
lumbar rotator m.
lumbrical muscle of foot
lumbrical muscle of hand
manual muscle test
manual muscle testing
marginal part of orbicularis oris m.
m. mass
mean arm muscle circumference
medial flexor muscle of forearm
medial gastrocnemius m.
medial gastrocnemius m.
medial great m.
medial lumbar intertransverse m.
medial pterygoid m.
medial rectus extraocular m.
medial rectus m.
meridional ciliary muscle fiber
meridional fibers of ciliary m.
microvascular free muscle flap
midarm muscle area
middle constrictor muscle of pharynx
middle constrictor pharyngeal m.
middle ear muscle reflex
middle gluteal m.
minimal active muscle tendon tension
Moberg deltoid muscle transfer
m. movement
multifidus m.
m., liver, brain, eye
m., liver, brain, eye nanism
muscular fascia of extraocular m.
myocardial muscle creatine kinase isoenzyme
myometrial smooth m.
m. necrosis
nerves and m.'s
neurogenic muscle weakness, ataxia, and retinitis pigmentosa
nocturnal leg muscle cramp
nonocular muscle group
normal muscle development
oblique abdominal m.
oblique arytenoid m.
oblique auricular m.
oblique capitis m.
oblique muscle of abdomen
oblique muscle of eyeball
oblique muscle hook
obliquity superior m.
obliquus abdominis externus m.
obliquus capitis superior m.
obturator externus m.
occipital belly of occipitofrontalis m.
ocular muscle dystrophy
ocular muscle palsy
ocular muscle paralysis
ocular muscle transplant
opponens digiti minimi m.
opponens digiti quinti m.
opposing muscle of little finger
opposing muscle of thumb
optic muscle recession
orbicularis oculi m.
orbicularis oris m.
orbicular muscle of eye
orbicular muscle of mouth
overuse of m.
oxygen-starved heart m.
m. pain, allergy, tachycardia and tiredness, headache syndrome
painful muscle contraction
painful muscle spasm
pain in m.'s and joints
pain and spasm of m.'s
palmar interosseous m.
palmaris brevis m.
palmaris longus m.
palpebrae superioris m.
palsy of m.
panniculus carnosus m.
papillary m.
papillary muscle fibrosis
papillary muscle rupture
parallel elastic component of m.
m. paralysis
paraspinal muscle spasm
paravertebral m.
paravertebral muscle spasm
m. paretic nystagmus
patient exhibited muscle guarding
pectoralis major m.
pectoralis minor m.
pelvic floor m.
pelvic floor muscle exercise
pelvic muscle laxity
peripheral muscle strength
peroneal muscle atrophy
peroneus brevis m.
peroneus longus m.
peroneus longus muscle avulsion
m. phosphofructokinase deficiency
m. phosphorylase deficiency
piriformis muscle spasm
plantar interosseous m.
pollicis adductor m.
pollicis brevis abductor m.
pollicis brevis extensor m.
pollicis brevis flexor m.
pollicis longus abductor m.
pollicis longus extensor m.
pollicis longus flexor m.
poor muscle tone
posterior auricular m.
posterior latissimus dorsi muscle
posterior papillary m.
posterior tibial m.
preclinical heart muscle disease
profundus flexor digitorum m.
progressive muscle relaxation
progressive postpolio muscle atrophy
pronator quadratus m.
pronator teres m.
m. proprioceptor
proximal muscle weakness
psoas major m.
pterygoid m.
pubococcygeal m.
pupillary sphincter m.
quadratus femoris m.
quadratus lumborum m.
quadriceps femoris m.
quantitative muscle testing
radial extensor m.
rapid muscle growth
m. receptor
m. receptor organ
reconstruct heart m.
rectus abdominis m.
rectus abdominis muscle flap
rectus abdominis muscle transfer
rectus femoris m.
rectus femoris muscle flap
rectus and longus capitis muscle
rectus muscle splitting incision
m. reflected from insertion
m. relaxant
relaxation of heart m.
m. resection
resection of m.
respiratory muscle strength
m. response test
resting muscle activity
rhomboid major m.

muscle *(continued)*
right deltoid m.
right inferior oblique muscle
right lateral rectus m.
right medial rectus muscle
right superior oblique m.
right superior rectus m.
m. rigidity
rippling muscle disease
m. sarcoma
scalene m.
scalene muscle, anterior, posterior, middle
scalenus anterior m.
scarring of heart m.
semispinalis capitis m.
semispinalis cervicis m.
semispinal muscle of head
sensitize heart muscle to digitalis toxicity
series elastic component of muscles
serratus anterior muscle flap
m. sheath
m. shortening
silent heart muscle distress
skeletal muscle ischemia
skeletal muscle protein
skeletal muscle relaxant
small muscle atrophy
smooth m.
smooth muscle actin
smooth muscle activating factor
smooth muscle antibody
smooth muscle autoantibody
smooth muscle cell
smooth muscle contracting agent
smooth muscle contraction
smooth muscle tumors
m. sound
m. spasm
spastic muscle activity
m. splitting
m. splitting incision
stapedius m.
stimulate heart m.
m. strength
m. stretch reflex
striated m.
superior constrictor muscles of pharynx
superior gemellus m.
superior rectus m.
superior tarsal m.
supraclavicular m.
m. surgery
m. sympathetic nerve activity
symptomatic alcohol heart muscle disease
systematic nutritional muscle testing
temperature, m.
temporalis m.
temporalis muscle temperature
temporal muscle wasting
tendinous arch of soleus m.
m. and tendon
m. tension headache
tensor fasciae latae m.
teres major m.
m. testing
thenar muscle atrophy
thenar muscle contraction
thickened heart m.
tibialis anterior m.
toe extensor m.
m. tone
m. tonicity
total muscle mass
transferring immature muscle cell
m. transposition
transverse arytenoid m.
transverse muscle of abdomen
transverse rectus abdominis m.
transversus abdominis m.
uninhibited detrusor muscle capacity
m. of upper extremity atrophic
uterine muscle tone
vascular smooth muscle cell
vastus lateralis m.
vastus medialis m.
vastus medialis oblique m.
ventilatory muscle training
volar interosseous m.
voluntary muscle action
m. wasting
weakened heart m.
m. weakening myasthenia gravis
m. weakness

muscle-brain
m.-b. isoenzyme
m.-b. isoenzyme of creative kinase

muscle carnitine palmitoyltransferase deficiency

muscle-eye-brain
m.-e.-b. disease
m.-e.-b. disease of Santavuori
m.-e.-b. syndrome

muscle-relaxant
m.-r. drug

muscle/ribonucleoprotein
antibody-smooth m.

muscle-specific
m.-s. actin
m.-s. enolase

muscle-strengthening exercise

muscle-tendon
m.-t. attachment
m.-t. junction

Muscle-Wells syndrome

muscular
adult-onset spinal muscular atrophy
m. anesthesia
Aran-Duchenne muscular atrophy
Aran-Duchenne muscular dystrophy
m. artery of ophthalmic artery
m. asthenopia
m. atrioventricular septum
atrophic muscular paralysis
m. atrophy
m. atrophy and cyanosis
m. attachment
m. balance
Becker muscular dystrophy
m. body
m. bolster
m. branch
m. branch of deep fibular nerve
m. bridge
m. change
chronic spinal muscular atrophy
m. clamp
clofibrate-induced muscular syndrome
m. coat
m. coat of bronchi
m. coat of colon
m. coat of ductus deferens
m. coat of esophagus
m. coat of female urethra
m. coat of gallbladder
m. coat of intermediate part of male urethra
m. coat of large intestine
m. coat of pharynx
m. coat of prostatic urethra
m. coat of rectum
m. coat of small intestine
m. coat of spongy part of male urethra
m. coat of stomach
m. coat of trachea
m. coat of ureter
m. coat of urinary bladder

m. coat of uterine tube
m. coat of uterus
m. coat of vagina
congenital atonic sclerotic muscular dystrophy
congenital muscular dystrophy
m. contraction
m. coordination
m. cramp
m. crus
m. crus of diaphragm
m. cuff
m. cushion
deep muscular aponeurotic system
m. degeneration
m. diaphragm
m. diastasis
disuse muscular atrophy
Duchenne-Aran muscular atrophy
Duchenne de Boulogne muscular dystrophy/Becker muscular dystrophy
Duchenne de Boulogne muscular dystrophy
Duchenne muscular atrophy
Duchenne muscular dystrophy
m. dystrophy
m. dystrophy, progressive
Emery-Dreifuss muscular dystrophy
esophageal muscular ring
m. esophageal ring
facioscapulohumeral muscular dystrophy
m. fascia
m. fascia of extraocular muscle
m. fibril
Fukuyama congenital muscular dystrophy
m. funnel
m. graft
m. hyperalgesia
m. hyperesthesia
hypertrophic muscular subaortic stenosis
m. hypertrophy
m. hypertrophy syndrome
m. hypotonia
idiopathic muscular dystrophy
m. imbalance
improve muscular contraction
m. incompetence
induced muscular tension
infantile spinal muscular atrophy
m. infantilism
m. injury
m. insufficiency
involuntary muscular contraction
involuntary muscular movement
ischemic muscular atrophy
m. jerk
juvenile muscular atrophy
m. lacuna
m. layer
m. layer of bronchi
m. layer of colon
m. layer of ductus deferens
m. layer of esophagus
m. layer of female urethra
m. layer of gallbladder
m. layer of intermediate part of male urethra
m. layer of large intestine
m. layer of mucosa
m. layer of pharynx
m. layer of prostatic urethra
m. layer of rectum
m. layer of renal pelvis
m. layer of seminal gland
m. layer of small intestine
m. layer of stomach
m. layer of trachea
m. layer of ureter
m. layer of urinary bladder
m. layer of uterine tube
m. layer of vagina
Leyden-Möbius muscular dystrophy
limb-girdle muscular dystrophy
limb-girdle muscular weakness and atrophy
longitudinal layer of muscular coat
longitudinal layers of muscular tunic
mental retardation, scapuloperoneal muscular dystrophy, lethal cardiomyopathy syndrome
microcephaly, muscular build, rhizomelia-cataracts syndrome
micropolygyria with muscular dystrophy
mild X-linked recessive muscular dystrophy
neuritic muscular atrophy
neuropathic muscular atrophy
oblique fibers of muscular layer of stomach
ocular muscular dystrophy
oculogastrointestinal muscular dystrophy
ophthalmoplegic muscular dystrophy
m. pain-fasciculation syndrome
para muscular incision
partially m.
postpoliomyelitis muscular atrophy
progressive muscular atrophy
progressive muscular dystrophy
progressive postmyelitis muscular atrophy
progressive spinal muscular atrophy
proximal spinal muscular atrophy
m. response to electrical stimulation of motor nerve
m. rheumatism
severe childhood autosomal recessive muscular dystrophy
spinal muscular atrophy
spinal progressive muscular atrophy
m. strabismus
m. subaortic stenosis
tardive muscular dystrophy
m. torticollis
m. vein
m. ventricular septal defect
m. ventricular septum
m. weakness
Werdnig-Hoffmann muscular atrophy

musculares

arteriae musculares arteriae ophthalmicae

muscularis

m. externa
m. mucosae
m. propria

musculature

aponeurotic m.
axial m.
discrete jerking musculature of face
hip m.
lumbar m.
paravertebral m.
pharyngeal m.

musculi (*pl. of* musculus)

musculoaponeurotic

m. control
skin-adipose superficial musculoaponeurotic system
m. structure
superficial musculoaponeurotic system

musculocutaneous

m. amputation
anterior quadriceps musculocutaneous flap technique

musculocutaneous *(continued)*
m. artery
m. flap harvest
m. free flap
free transverse rectus abdominis musculocutaneous flap
gluteus maximus musculocutaneous flap
latissimus dorsi musculocutaneous flap
m. mononeuropathy
m. nerve
pedicled fascia lata musculocutaneous flap
rectus abdominis musculocutaneous flap
transverse rectus abdominis musculocutaneous flap

musculofascial
m. flaccidity
m. flap
m. layer

musculofascially
incision closed m.

musculoligamentous

musculomucosal
facial artery m.

musculoperitoneal
transverse rectus abdominis musculoperitoneal flap

musculophrenic
m. artery
m. branch

musculophrenica
arteria m.

musculoskeletal
m. adaptation
m. chest wall pain
chronic musculoskeletal pain syndrome
m. deformity
m. disorder
m. evaluation, rehabilitation and conditioning
M. Function Assessment
m. impairment
m. infection
m. manifestation
m. mass
m. pain
m. pain syndrome
physiological musculoskeletal reaction
psychophysiologic musculoskeletal reaction
Short Musculoskeletal Function Assessment
m. system
m. tuberculosis

musculospiral groove

musculotendinous
m. aponeurosis
m. cuff
m. damage
m. flap
m. unit

musculus, pl. **musculi**
m. auricularis anterior
m. auricularis posterior
m. constrictor urethrae
m. extensor pollicis brevis
m. flexor carpi radialis
m. flexor carpi ulnaris
m. flexor digiti minimi brevis manus
m. flexor digiti minimi brevis pedis
m. flexor hallucis brevis
m. flexor hallucis longus
m. flexor pollicis brevis
m. flexor pollicis longus
m. gluteus maximus
m. gluteus quartus
m. iliacus minor
m. iliocostalis cervicis
m. iliocostalis lumborum
m. iliocostalis thoracis
m. iliocostalis thoracis
m. longissimus capitis
m. longissimus cervicis
m. longissimus thoracis
m. longitudinalis superior
m. longus capitis
m. obliquus superior bulbi
m. obliquus superior oculi
m. orbicularis oculi
m. rectus lateralis bulbi
m. rectus lateralis oculi
m. rectus medialis bulbi
m. rectus medialis oculi
m. sphincter pupilla

Musgrave
M. footprint pedobarograph
M. Footprint System

mushroom
Amanita mushroom hepatotoxicity
m. appearance
autumn skullcap m.
m. corneal graft
m. dust
m. gyrus
little brown m.
pepper bolete m.
m. picker's lung
m. poisoning
Silastic mushroom catheter
m. worker's lung

mushroom-hook layer

mushrooming of fimbria

music
m.'s Achievement Test 1-4
m. blindness
m. deafness
m. therapy
m. therapy/audiokinetics

musical
m. agraphia
m. alexia
M. Aptitude Profile
m. bruit
m. murmur
m. rales

musician's overuse syndrome

mussel
New Zealand green-lipped m.

Musshoff modification

mustache technique

mustard
M. atrial baffle repair
M. atrial switch procedure
m. chlorohydrin
chloroquine m.
m. gas
L-phenylalanine m.
L-phenylalanine mustard, vinblastine
nitrogen m.
nitrogen mustard, Adriamycin, CCNU
nitrogen mustard, Oncovin, procarbazine, bleomycin, Adriamycin, prednisone
nitrogen mustard oxide
nitrogen mustard therapy
nitrogen mustard, vincristine, procarbazine, prednisone/doxorubicin, bleomycin, vinblastine
M. operation
L-phenylalanine m.
M. procedure
quinacrine m.
M. technique
uracil m.

Mustardé
M. graft

M. operation
M. procedure
M. rotational cheek flap

Mustargen
M., Adriamycin, bleomycin, Oncovin, prednisone
M., Oncovin, bleomycin
M., Oncovin, procarbazine, prednisone

musty odor

mutagenesis
m. assay
cell-mediated m.
microsome-mediated m.

mutagenic
m. activity
m. treatment

mutans streptococci

mutant
m. allele
m. allele-specific amplification
auxotrophic m.
m. cell
m. gene
m. hemoglobin with low affinity for oxygen
m. homoplasmy
human genetic mutant cell repository
m. hybrid
m. Ras peptide-pulsed dendritic cell therapy
Shigella m.

mutase

mutated
autologous T lymphocytes stimulated with the patient's tumor-specific mutated RAS peptides
m. in colon cancer
m. colorectal carcinoma

mutation
amplification refractory mutation system
amplification refractory mutation system-polymerase chain reaction
m. analysis
androgen receptor gene m.
APC gene mutation assay
A-T m.
A-T mutation gene
automated factor V Leiden mutation test
autosomal recessive m.
auxotrophic m.
m. carrier
m. carrier status
m. cluster region
factor V deficiency Leiden m.
factor V Leiden mutation test
m. frequency
m. in hematopoietic tissue
loss-of-function m.
m. mismatch repair
missense m.
mitochondrial DNA m.
MODY3 HNF-1-alpha m.
multidrug resistance-associated m.
murine osteopetrosis m.
mutator m.
new m.
nonsense m.
novel missense m.
ochre suppressor genetic m.
osteopetrotic m.
m. rate
suppression and m.
testicular feminization m.
m. testing

mutational
m. dysostosis
m. spectrum
m. strategy

mutation-enriched restriction fragment length polymorphism assay

mutator mutation

Mutchinick syndrome

mutilans
m. arthritis
keratoderma hereditaria m.

mutilating
m. acropathy
m. keratoderma
m. keratoderma of Vohwinkel
m. leprosy

mutilation
female genital m.
female genital tract m.

mutiresistant *Staphylococcus aureus*

mutism
akinetic m.
apathetic akinetic m.
hysterical m.

mutton-fat
m.-f. deposit
m.-f. keratic precipitate

mutton fat

mutual
m. affective responsiveness
m. aid group
m. consent
m. grief
m. resistance
m. self-help course

mutually monogamous relationship

muzzled sperm

MVF chemotherapy protocol

MVG-51 virus

Myà disease

myalgia
m. thermica

myalgic
m. asthenia
m. encephalomyelitis

myasthenia
adult-onset myasthenia gravis
m. angiosclerotica
autoimmune myasthenia gravis
congenital myasthenia gravis
double vision from myasthenia gravis
experimental autoimmune myasthenia gravis
m. gravis
m. gravis and mediastinal tumors
m. gravis pseudoparalytica
m. gravis syndrome
juvenile autoimmune myasthenia gravis
muscle weakening myasthenia gravis
neonatal m.
neonatal myasthenia gravis
ocular m.
ocular myasthenia gravis
pediatric m.
penicillamine-induced m.
persistent neonatal myasthenia gravis

myasthenia-like syndrome

myasthenic
m. crisis
m. facies
Lambert-Eaton myasthenic syndrome
neonatal myasthenic syndrome
m. nystagmus
slow-channel congenital myasthenic syndrome
m. syndrome of Eaton-Lambert

myatonia congenita

myb
myb oncogene
myb protein
myb protooncogene/oncogene
myc
myc oncogene
myc protein
myc protooncogene/oncogene
Mycelex-G topical
Mycelex Troche
mycelia-derived antigen
mycelial
m. antibody
m. fungus
m. mass
m. mat
m. phase of fungus
mycelium
nonseptate m.
myc epitope
mycetismus
mycetoma
Nicolle white m.
Mycifradin Sulfate
***MYCN* protooncogene**
mycobacteria, sing. **mycobacterium**
m. antibiotic supplement
atypical m.
atypical mycobacteria infection
m. culture
m. growth indicator tube
m. growth indicator tube system
nontuberculous m.
m. other than *Mycobacterium tuberculosis*
mycobacterial
m. abscess
m. antibody
m. arthritis
atypical mycobacterial arthritis
atypical mycobacterial colonization
atypical mycobacterial infection
m. choroiditis
m. culture
m. disease
disseminated nontuberculous mycobacterial infection
m. infection
m. lymphadenitis
m. necrotizing pneumonia
nontuberculin mycobacterial disease
nontuberculous mycobacterial disease
nontuberculous mycobacterial infection
m. organism
potentially pathogenic environmental m.
m. protein
mycobacterial necrotizing pneumonia
mycobacteriosis
atypical m.
mycobacterium
M. abscessus infection
amplified *Mycobacterium tuberculosis* direct test
atypical m.
M. avium
M. avium complex
M. avium complex infection
M. avium infection
M. avium-intracellulare
M. avium-intracellulare bacteremia
M. avium-intracellulare complex
M. avium-intracellulare infection
M. bovis BCG
M. chelonae abscess
M. chelonea infection
disseminated *Mycobacterium avium-intracellulare* complex
disseminated *Mycobacterium avium-intracellulare* complex
M. fortuitum-chelonae complex
M. fortuitum complex
M. fortuitum infection
M. fortuitum third biovar complex
M. haemophilum infection
M. kansasii infection
M. keratitis
M. marinum infection
mycobacteria other than *Mycobacterium tuberculosis*
Mycobacterium cell wall complex
Mycobacterium Tuberculosis Direct
M. phage Leo
M. terrae-triviale complex
M. tuberculosis
M. tuberculosis detection
M. xenopi infection
mycobiotic agar
Mycogen II Topical
mycolic acid
mycological
standard mycological identification technique
Mycolog-II Topical
mycology
medical m.
multitest, mycology plate
Myconel topical
mycophenolate mofetil
mycophenolic acid
Mycoplasma
M. arthritidis
M. arthritidis mitogen
M. hominis bacteremia
indirect enzyme immunoassay for anti-*M.* pneumoniae IgM
M. infection
M. pneumonia
M. serology
M. T-strain
M. T-strain culture
mycoplasma
m. disease
M. IgM titer
m. pneumonia of pig
mycoplasmacidal
minimal mycoplasmacidal concentration
minimum mycoplasmacidal concentration
mycoplasmal
m. antibody
m. encephalitis
m. pharyngitis
m. pneumonia
Mycosel agar
mycosis
allergic bronchopulmonary m.
m. favosa
m. fungoides palmaris et plantaris
m. fungoides/Sézary syndrome
microabscess of mycosis fungoides
opportunistic systemic m.
mycotic
m. abscess
m. aortic aneurysm
m. brain aneurysm
m. club nail
m. corneal ulcer disease
m. dermatitis
m. disease
m. gastritis
m. infection
m. keratitis
m. snowball opacity
m. stomatitis
m. vaginosis

Myco-Triacet II

Mydfrin Ophthalmic

Mydriacyl
- tropicamide 1% ophthalmic solution M.

mydriasis
- alternating m.
- amaurotic m.
- anisocoria with ipsilateral m.
- paralytic m.
- spastic m.

mydriatic
- m. provocative test
- m. rigidity
- m. test for angle-closure glaucoma

mydriatic-cycloplegic therapy

myectomy
- anorectal m.
- m. operation
- orbicularis m.
- septal m.

myelin
- abnormal tubular m.
- antiperipheral nerve myelin antibody
- m. ball
- m. ball formation
- m. base protein
- m. basic protein
- m. basic protein assay
- m. basic protein deficiency
- m. body
- m. breakdown
- m. degeneration
- m. degradation
- m. disorder
- m. figure
- oral bovine m.
- m. pallor
- peripheral myelin protein
- peripheral myelin protein 22 gene
- peripheral nerve m.
- serum myelin basic protein
- m. sheath
- tubular m.

myelin-associated
- m.-a. glycoprotein
- m.-a. glycoprotein antibody detection

myelinated
- m. axon
- m. fiber bundle
- m. retinal nerve fiber

myelination
- m. of axon
- nerve fiber m.
- optic nerve m.
- m. of retinal nerve

myelinic degeneration

myelinoclastic
- m. diffuse cerebral sclerosis
- m. disease

myelin-oligodendrocyte
- m.-o. glycoprotein

myelin/oligodendrocyte-specific protein

myelinolysis
- central pontine m.

myelitic enterovirus

myelitis
- acute necrotizing m.
- acute transverse m.
- amyotrophic syphilitic m.
- transverse m.

myeloablative
- m. chemoradiotherapy
- m. chemotherapy
- m. conditioning

myeloblast
- m. cell
- refractory anemia with excess m.'s

myeloblastic
- acute myeloblastic leukemia
- m. leukemia
- m. protein

myeloblastoma
- granular cell m.

myeloblastosis
- avian m.
- avian myeloblastosis leukemia virus reverse transcriptase
- avian myeloblastosis virus reverse transcriptase
- refractory anemia with partial m.

myeloblastosis-associated virus

myeloblast-promyelocyte compartment

myelocyte
- m. at fourth stage of maturation
- m. at third stage of maturation
- band form in sixth stage of myelocyte maturation
- m. cell
- m. A, B, C
- neutrophil m.
- neutrophilic m.

myelocytic
- acute myelocytic leukemia
- m. crisis
- juvenile chronic myelocytic leukemia
- m. leukemia
- m. leukemoid reaction

myelocytic/myelogenous/myeloid
- chronic myelocytic/myelogenous/myeloid leukemia accelerated phase
- chronic myelocytic/myelogenous/myeloid leukemia blast crisis
- chronic myelocytic/myelogenous/myeloid leukemia chronic phase

myelocytomatosis
- avian myelocytomatosis virus

myelodysplasia
- occult m.
- pediatric m.
- therapy-related m.

myelodysplastic
- m. cancer
- chronic myelodysplastic syndrome
- primary myelodysplastic syndrome
- secondary myelodysplastic syndrome
- m. syndrome
- therapy-related myelodysplastic syndrome

myelofibrosis
- acute m.
- m. anemia
- chronic idiopathic m.
- idiopathic m.
- myeloid metaplasia with m.
- m. osteosclerosis
- m. proliferation/regression index
- m. with myeloid metaplasia

myelogenic
- m. leukemia
- m. sarcoma

myelogenous
- acute lymphoblastic myelogenous leukemia
- m. callus
- chronic phase chronic myelogenous leukemia
- juvenile chronic myelogenous leukemia
- m. leukemia
- Philadelphia chromosome-negative chronic myelogenous leukemia

myelogenous *(continued)*
Philadelphia chromosome-positive chronic myelogenous leukemia
therapy-related acute myelogenous leukemia

myelographic block

myelography
computed tomographic m.
computed tomographic metrizamide m.
computer-aided m.
computer-assisted m.
delay computer tomographic m.

myeloid
abnormal location of immature myeloid precursor
acute myeloid leukemia
agnogenic myeloid metaplasia
m. associated antigen
atypical chronic myeloid leukemia
m. basic protein
m. blood element
bone marrow myeloid precursor
m. cell
m. cell infiltration
chronic myeloid leukemia
m. colony
m. colony-forming capacity
m. dendritic cell
m. depletion
m. depression
m. disease
m. engraftment
m. to erythroid
m. to erythroid ratio
m. granulocytic leukemia
m. growth factor
idiopathic myeloid proliferation
m. leukemia inhibitory factor
m. lineage antigen
m. marker
m. metaplasia
m. metaplasia with myelofibrosis
murine myeloid leukemia cell line
myelofibrosis with myeloid metaplasia
m. progenitor factor 1
myelosclerosis with myeloid metaplasia
pluripotent myeloid stem cell
polycythemia vera with myeloid metaplasia
m. pool
postpolycythemia myeloid metaplasia
m. precursor
m. precursor cell
m. progenitor
m. progenitor inhibitory factor
m. progenitor inhibitory factor-1
radiation myeloid leukemia
m. sarcoma
m. stem cell
therapy-related acute myeloid leukemia

myeloma
Arizona Cancer Center multiple myeloma staging system
m. cast nephropathy
m. cell
m. growth factor
m. kidney
m. or macroglobulinemia component
malignant m.
multiple bone m.
multiple myeloma cell line
multiple myeloma staging
m. multiplex
osteosclerotic m.
phosphorylcholine-binding myeloma protein
m. protein
smoldering m.

myelomacrocytic
chronic myelomacrocytic leukemia

myelomalacia
angiodysgenetic m.

myelomatosis
multiple m.
m. multiplex

myelomonoblastic
acute myelomonoblastic leukemia
m. leukemia

myelomonocytic
acute myelomonocytic leukemia
m. antigen
m. cell
chronic myelomonocytic leukemia
juvenile myelomonocytic leukemia
m. leukemia
m. leukemia, chronic
m. leukemia, subacute

Myelo-Nate
M.-N. needle
M.-N. set

myeloneuropathy

myelo-optic neuropathy

myelopathic
m. anemia
m. polycythemia

myelopathy
acute transverse m.
AIDS-associated vacuolar m.
cervical spondylotic m.
human T-cell lymphotropic virus type I associated m.
posttraumatic progressive m.
rheumatoid cervical m.
spondylotic caudal m.
tropical spastic paraparesis/HTLV-I associated m.

myeloperoxidase
m. bone marrow stain
m. deficiency
m. system

myelophthisic
m. anemia
m. splenomegaly

myelophthisis marrow

myelopoiesis
transient abnormal m.

myeloproliferative
chronic myeloproliferative disorder
m. disease
m. disorder
m. leukemia virus
m. reaction
m. sarcoma virus
m. syndrome

myelosclerosis with myeloid metaplasia

myelosclerotic anemia

myelosis
aleukemic m.
aplastic m.
nonleukemic m.

myelosuppression chemotherapy

myelosuppressive
m. agent
m. chemotherapy
m. therapy

myelotoxic drug

myenteric
m. ganglion cell
m. plexus
m. plexus neuropathy
m. reflex

Myers-Briggs Type Indicator psychologic test

Myers bunching technique

Myerson sign

myf-5 gene

Myhre syndrome

myiasis
African furuncular m.
aural m.
nasal m.
nosocomial m.
obligate m.
ocular m.
m. oestruosa
Mykines virus
myl
myl oncogene
myl protooncogene/oncogene
mylohyoid
m. branch
m. branch of inferior alveolar artery
m. bridge
m. fossa
m. groove
m. line
m. muscle
myoablative therapy
myoadenylate
m. deaminase
m. deaminase deficiency
myoblastoma
granular cell m.
malignant granular cell m.
myoblast transfer therapy
Myobock artificial hand
myocardia (*pl. of* myocardium)
myocardial
m. abscess
acute myocardial ischemia
acute subendocardial myocardial infarction
m. anoxia
anterior atrial myocardial bundle
anterior lateral myocardial infarct
anterior lateral myocardial infarction
anterior myocardial infarct
anterior myocardial infarction
anterior wall myocardial infarct
anterior wall myocardial infarction
anteroinferior myocardial infarct
anteroinferior myocardial infarction
anterolateral myocardial infarct
anterolateral myocardial infarction
anteroseptal myocardial infarct
anteroseptal myocardial infarction
apical-lateral wall myocardial infarct
apical myocardial infarct
apical myocardial infarction
arrhythmic myocardial infarct
arrhythmogenic myocardial tissue ablation
m. band
m. band enzymes of creatine phosphokinase
m. beta-adrenergic receptor
m. blood flow
m. blush
m. bridge
m. bridging
m. calcification
m. cell
m. cellular degeneration
m. cellular hypertrophy
m. centroid
chills from myocardial infarction
clandestine myocardial ischemia
complete myocardial infarction
conduction defect in acute myocardial infarction
m. contractile force
m. contractile function
m. contractile state
m. contractility
m. contraction
m. contracture
m. contrast appearance time
m. contrast echocardiography
m. contusion
creatine kinase myocardial band
m. cytochrome
m. damage
m. depressant factor
m. depressant substance
m. depression
diaphragmatic myocardial infarct
diaphragmatic myocardial ischemia
m. dilatation
dipyridamole myocardial scintigraphy
direct acute myocardial infarction angioplasty
direct myocardial revascularization
m. disarray
m. disease
m. disease of unknown origin
m. Doppler velocity
m. dysfunction
evolving myocardial infarction
exercise-induced silent myocardial ischemia
m. fiber degeneration
m. fibrosis
m. fractional flow reserve
m. function
m. hamartoma
m. hibernation
m. hypertrophy
m. idiopathic hypertrophy
idiopathic myocardial hypertrophy
m. imaging
impending myocardial infarction
m. infarct
infarct avid myocardial scintigraphy
m. infarction
m. infarction recovery index
m. infarction rehabilitation program
m. infarction research unit
m. infarction triage and intervention
inferior myocardial infarct
inferior wall myocardial infarction
inferoposterior myocardial infarction
m. infundibular stenosis
inherent strength of myocardial contraction
m. injury
m. insufficiency
interstitial left ventricular myocardial fibrosis
m. ischemic disease
ischemic myocardial disease
m. ischemic syndrome
m. isotopic perfusion scan
m. laser revascularization
left ventricular subendocardial myocardial ischemia
m. metabolic rate
m. muscle creatine kinase isoenzyme
m. necrosis
non–Q-wave myocardial infarction
non-ST-elevation myocardial infarction
nontransmural myocardial infarction
old healed myocardial infarction
old inferior wall myocardial infarction
m. oxygen consumption
percutaneous transluminal myocardial revascularization
percutaneous transluminal septal myocardial ablation
m. perfusion
m. perfusion imaging
m. perfusion reserve
perioperative myocardial infarction

myocardial *(continued)*
planar myocardial imaging
posterior wall myocardial infarction
previous posterior myocardial infarction
primary myocardial disease
m. protection system
Q-wave myocardial infarction
radiofrequency percutaneous myocardial revascularization
recurrent myocardial infarction
regional myocardial blood flow
m. resection
rule out myocardial infarct
rule out myocardial infarction
m. siderosis
silent myocardial infarction
silent myocardial ischemia
status post myocardial infarction
m. steal syndrome
stress myocardial image
m. stress perfusion scintigraphy
striped tag myocardial tagging system
m. stunning
subendocardial myocardial injury
m. substrate uptake
thallium myocardial perfusion
thallium myocardial scintigraphy
threatened myocardial infarction
m. toxicity
transient episodes of myocardial ischemia
transmural myocardial infarction
unstable angina/non-Q-wave myocardial infarction
m. vascular capacity
m. vasodilation
m. ventilation, oxygen rate
m. wall thickness

myocardiopathy
congestive m.
m. of unknown origin

myocarditis
acute bacterial m.
acute isolated m.
cardiac sarcoidosis m.
clostridial m.
Coxsackie virus m.
echovirus m.
hypersensitivity m.
idiopathic m.
infectious m.
interstitial m.
Multicenter Myocarditis Treatment Trial
protozoal m.
toxic m.
viral m.

myocardium, pl. **myocardia**
contractile function in cells of m.
idiopathic disease of m.
infarct of m.
ischemia of m.
isolated noncompaction of the ventricular m.

myoclin gene

myoclonal jerk

myoclonic
m. absence
m. alien hand syndrome
m. astatic epilepsy
m. ataxia
ataxia, myoclonic encephalopathy, macular degeneration, recurrent infections syndrome
m. convulsion
m. dystonia
m. encephalopathy
m. encephalopathy syndrome
m. epilepsy
m. epilepsy of adolescence
epilepsy with myoclonic absence
infantile myoclonic jerk
infantile myoclonic seizure
m. jerk
juvenile myoclonic epilepsy
malignant familial myoclonic epilepsy
m. petit mal
m. seizure
severe myoclonic epilepsy
severe myoclonic epilepsy in infancy
m. spasm
m. twitch activity
m. twitching

myoclonus
cherry-red spot m.
degenerative myoclonus epilepsy
m. epilepsy
m. nystagmus
oculopalatal myoclonus syndrome
posthypoxic intention m.
progressive encephalomyelitis with rigidity and m.
progressive myoclonus epilepsy
m. syndrome

myocutaneous
anterior myocutaneous flap
m. flap
free transverse rectus abdominis myocutaneous flap
gracilis myocutaneous unit
m. graft
latissimus dorsi myocutaneous flap
McCraw gracilis myocutaneous flap
pectoralis major myocutaneous flap
rectus abdominis myocutaneous flap
trapezoidal paddle pectoralis major myocutaneous flap

myocyte
Anitschkow m.
m. necrosis

myocytic hypertrophy

myocytolysis of heart

myoD
myoD gene
myoD protein

myodysplasia
m. fibrosa multiplex

myoelectric
m. hand
interdigestive myoelectric complex
migrating myoelectric complex
m. signal

myoepithelial
m. cell
m. cell island
m. cell process
m. differentiation
m. flap
m. sialadenitis

myoepithelioma
malignant m.

myofascial
associated myofascial trigger point
m. closure
m. disruption
m. dysfunction
m. flap
galeal myofascial flap
m. pain
m. pain-dysfunction
m. pain-dysfunction syndrome
m. release

myofasciitis
macrophagic m.

myofiber
m. diameter

m. disarray
perifascicular myofiber necrosis

myofibrillar dropout

myofibroblast
m. cell
m. contraction

myofibroblastic
m. differentiation
m. feature
inflammatory myofibroblastic tumor
pseudosarcomatous myofibroblastic tumor
m. tumor

myofibrohistiocytic proliferation

myofibromatosis
multiple m.
periorbital infantile m.

myogenic
m. acquired ptosis
m. cell
m. paralysis
postauricular m.
m. regeneration

myoglobin
carbon monoxide m.
m. clearance test
m. release

myoglobinuria
idiopathic m.

myoglobinuric rhabdomyolytic acute renal failure

myoglobulin
human myoglobulin radioimmunoassay

myography
acoustic m.

myoid visual cell

myointimal hyperplasia

myokymic discharge

myolysis

myoma, pl. **myomes, myomata**
asymptomatic m.
calcified m.
m. fixation instrument
mucoid myoma degeneration
parasitic m.
m. screw
myomata uteri
uterine m.

myomectomy
surgical myomectomy as reproductive therapy
uterine m.

myometrial
adenocarcinoma with myometrial invasion
m. arcuate artery
m. contraction
m. coring
m. neurofibroma
m. oxytocin receptor
m. relaxation
m. smooth muscle

myomucosal
facial artery m.
m. flap

myonecrosis
metastatic m.
nonclostridial anaerobic m.
m. syndrome

myonephropathic metabolic syndrome

myoneural
m. blockade
m. junction

myoneuro-gastrointestinal encephalopathy

myopathic
m. arthrogryposis
m. arthrogryposis multiplex congenita
m. atrophy
m. carnitine deficiency
m. disorder
m. eyelid retraction
m. facies
m. gait
m. limb-girdle syndrome
m. ptosis

myopathica
metrorrhagia m.

myopathy
centronuclear m.
childhood visceral m.
familial visceral m.
m. hand
idiopathic inflammatory m.
maternally inherited myopathy and cardiomyopathy
mitochondrial myopathy, encephalopathy, lactic acidosis, strokelike episodes
m., encephalopathy, lactic acidosis, strokelike episodes
proximal myotonic m.
X-linked myotubular m.

myopathy-lactic acidosis-sideroblastic anemia syndrome

myopathy-myxedema syndrome

myopharyngeal stricture

myophosphorylase
m. deficiency
m. deficiency glycogenosis

myopia
axial m.
high m.
m. index
malignant m.
mixed astigmatism with myopia predominating
night m.
nyctalopia with congenital m.
pathologic m.
physiologic m.
progressive m.
senile lenticular m.
severe m.
simple m.

myopic
m. anisometropia
m. astigmatism
m. choroidal atrophy
m. choroidopathy
compound myopic astigmatism
m. conus
m. crescent
m. degeneration
m. error
m. keratomileusis
m. maculopathy
m. reflex
m. regression
m. retinal degeneration

myorelaxant
m. drug
m. property

myorhythmia
oculomasticatory m.

myosarcoma
angiomatoid m.

myosin
antibody to murine cardiac m.
anticardiac m.
m. ATPase inhibitor
m. crossbridge
m. filament
m. heavy chain
m. light chain

myosin *(continued)*
m. light-chain kinase
m. light-chain phosphatase
m. light-chain phosphorylation
region of sarcomere containing only myosin filaments

myosin-binding protein-C

myosis
endolymphatic stromal m.

myositis
cervical tension m.
Childhood Myositis Assessment Scale
m. fibrosa
inclusion body m.
necrotizing myositis fasciitis
m. ossificans
m. ossificans circumscripta
m. ossificans progressiva
overlap m.
m. purulenta
m. purulenta tropica
m. with malignancy

myositis-associated autoantibody

myositis-specific
m.-s. antibody
m.-s. autoantibody

myotactic reflex

myotatic
m. contraction
m. contracture
m. irritability

myotis
Montana myotis leukoencephalitis virus

myotomy
extramucosal duodenal m.
Heller myotomy with Dor fundoplication
m. operation

myotonia
m. acquisita
m. atrophica
m. chondrodystrophia
m. congenita
m. hereditaria
m. neonatorum
percussion m.

myotonic
m. afterdischarge
m. cataract
m. chondrodystrophy
m. discharge
m. dystrophy
m. dystrophy cataract
m. dystrophy effect
m. dystrophy gene
m. facies
m. muscular dystrophy
proximal myotonic myopathy
m. pupil

MyoTrac
M. device

myotropic hormone

myotubular
m. myopathy
X-linked myotubular myopathy

myovascular insufficiency

myringitis bulbosa

myringotomy
bilateral myringotomy and tubes
m. blade
m. and grommet insertion
laser-assisted m.
OtoScan laser-assisted m.
m. tube
m. with aspiration

myristic acid

myristoyl-coenzyme A

myrmecia wart

myrtiform caruncle

myself
How I See Myself Scale

Mysoline

mystery syndrome

mystical
m. experience
m. influence

myths
Sexual Myths Scale

Mytrex F Topical

myxadenitis labialis

myxedema
m. ascites
m. ataxia
m. coma
m. depression
exophthalmos, myxedema circumscriptum praetibiale, and osteoarthropathia hypertrophicans syndrome
m. heart
m. ileus
localized pretibial m.
operative m.
pituitary m.
pretibial m.

myxedema-myotonic dystrophy syndrome

myxedematosus
lichen m.

myxedematous
m. arthropathy
m. dementia
m. endemic cretinism
m. face
m. facies
m. goiter
m. infantilism
m. lichen
m. neuropathy

myxofibrous
liposclerosing myxofibrous tumor

myxoid
m. cell pattern
m. chondrosarcoma
m. crystal
m. cyst
m. degeneration
m. degenerative change
m. dysplasia
extraskeletal myxoid chondrosarcoma
m. fibrolipoma
m. fibroma
m. histopathologic subtype
m. liposarcoma
m. matrix
nevi, atrial myxoma, myxoid neurofibroma, and ephelides syndrome
m. pseudocyst
skeletal myxoid chondrosarcoma
m. stroma

myxoma
atrial m.
cardiac m.
m. enchondromatosum
m. fibrosum
left atrial m.
lentigines, atrial myxomas, cutaneous papular myxomas, blue nevi
m. nabothian
nerve sheath m.
nevi, atrial myxoma, myxoid neurofibroma, and ephelides syndrome
m. sarcomatosum
m. virus
m. virus subgroup

myxomatosis
m. virus

myxomatous
m. cell
m. change
m. degeneration
degeneration of myxomatous heart valve
m. soft connective tissue
m. tissue

myxomembranous
m. colitis
m. enteritis

myxopapillary ependymoma

N1 virus

N4 virus

N5 virus

N=1 trial

Na

$N.^{+}$-K^{+} ATPase pump
ouabain-sensitive Na^{+}-K^{+} ATPase
N. Pent

nave T cell

Naboth

N. cyst
N. follicle
N. gland
N. ovule
N. vesicle

nabothian

n. cyst
n. follicle
n. gland
myxoma n.
n. ovule
n. vesicle

***N*-acetylaspartate/creatine ratio**

***N*-acetylaspartylglutamate**

***N*-acetylation polymorphism**

***N*-acetyl-beta-glucosaminidase**

***N*-acetyl-D-galactosamine**

***N*-acetylgalactosamine-4-sulfatase deficiency**

***N*-acetyl-β-D-glucosamidase**

***N*-acetylglucosamine**

-a. fermentation test
-a. receptor

***N*-acetyl-p-benzoquinoneimine**

***N*-acetyl procainamide**

nacreous ichthyosis

n-acylamino acid

Nadbath

N. akinesia
N. block
N. facial block

NADH

nadh dehydrogenase

nadir

n. blood count
n. hypoglycemia

Nadler superior radial scissors

NADPH

N. dehydrogenase
N. dehydrogenase quinone

NADPH-cytochrome

NADPH-dependent oxidase

Naegeli

N. leukemia
N. syndrome
N. type
N. type of monocytic leukemia

Naegeli-Franceschetti-Jadassohn syndrome

Naegleria

Naegleria cyst
Naegleria infection

nafcillin sodium

Naffziger operation

Naftin cream

Naga sore

Nagel

N. anomaloscope
N. test

Nägele

N. obliquity
N. pelvis
N. rule

Nageotte

N. bracelet
N. cell

Nager

N. acrofacial dysostosis
N. anomaly
N. sign
N. syndrome

Nager-de Reynier syndrome

nagging

n. cough
n. cough and hoarseness

Nagler

N. reaction
N. test

Nahai-Mathes flap

Na^{+}/H^{+}-ion exchanger

nail

alopecia, nail dystrophy, ophthalmic complication, thyroid dysfunction, hypohidrosis, ephelides and enteropathy, and respiratory tract infection
antegrade femoral n.
AO slotted medullary n.
n. assembly
Atasoy-type flap for nail injury repair
n. avulsion
avulsion of nail plate
n. bed
n. bed cancer
n. bed cyanosis
n. bed graft
n. bed hematoma evacuation
n. bed infection
n. bed lesion
n. bed lesion
n. biter
n. biting
n. breaking from athlete foot
n. breaking from circulatory problem
n. change
closed unlocked n.
n. clubbing
cyanosis of nail bed
n. defect
dermatophyte infection of n.'s
diamond-shaped medullary n.
n. disorder
n. driver
n. dust
dynamic locking n.
n. dystrophy
n. extender
n. extension
femoral neck n.
flexible intramedullary n.
flexible medullary n.
fluted titanium n.
n. fold
n. fold capillarioscopy
n. fold capillarioscopy abnormality
n. fold capillary loop abnormality
n. fold removal
n. fungus
fungus infected n.
gamma locking n.
n. groove
Hansen-Street n.
n. horn
n. hyperpigmentation
improper nail trimming
n. infection
n. infection and care
n. inserted into neck and head of femur
n. keratin
Küntscher n.
lateral nail fold

N

nail *(continued)*
longitudinal nail hyperpigmentation
lunule of n.
n. matrix
n. matrix phenolization
median nail dystrophy
mental retardation-absent nails of hallux and pollex syndrome
mixed nail infection
multiple flexible medullary n.
mycotic club n.
occult border of n.
pachyonychia congenita syndrome of n.
pale nail bed
n. patella syndrome
peripheral dysostosis, nail hypoplasia, mental retardation syndrome
n. pit
n. pitting
n. plate
n. plate of nailbed
n. polish
proximal nail matrix
n. pulse
n. ringworm
n. root
Rush intramedullary n.
n. shedding
shedding of n.'s
n. skin
Suppan nail technique
n. trephination
n. wall
n. wart
white or pale nails from anemia
yellow nail syndrome

nail-apparatus melanoma

nail-biting
severe nail-biting habit

nail-fold
n.-f. capillary
n.-f. infection

nailing
closed medullary n.
crutch and belt femoral closed n.
elastic stable intramedullary n.
gradual elongation intramedullary n.
intramedullary n.
medullary nailing of tibia
titanium elastic n.

20-nail involvement

nail-patella-elbow syndrome

nail-patella syndrome

nail-plate fixation

nail-to-nail bed angle

Nair buffered methylene blue stain

Nairobi
N. eye
N. sheep disease

naive
n. B cell
n. T cell

Najjar syndrome

Nakalanga
N. dwarfism
N. syndrome

Na/K-ATPase activity

naked
n. DNA encoding
n. DNA vector vaccine
n. plasmid DNA
n. tubercle
n. virus
n. vision
n. weight

Nalebuff classification

nalidixic
n. acid
n. acid agar
n. acid test

Nama keratopathy

name
British approved n.
International Nonproprietary N.
Japanese Accepted N.
N.'s Learning Test
no middle n.
Pharmacy Equivalent N.
proposed international nonproprietary n.
recommended international nonproprietary n.
n. unknown

naming
Boston Naming Test
color n.
Hundred Pictures Naming Test
online cross-modal n.
n. speed deficit
visual n.

naming speed deficit

NANB hepatitis

Nance analysis of arch length

Nance-Horan syndrome

nandrolone decanoate

nanism
mulibrey n.
mulibrey nanism or dwarfism
muscle, liver, brain, eye n.

nanism-constrictive pericarditis syndrome

nanocephalic
n. dwarf
n. dwarfism

nanogram
n. per cubic centimeter
n. per mL

Nanolas Nd:YAG laser

nanomolar concentration

nanomole per liter

Nantucket knee

nanukayami fever

nap behavior

nape
n. of neck
n. nevus

Na^+-phosphate cotransporter

naphthalene
n. acetic acid
n. creosote and iodoform
n. diisocyanate
n. mothball

naphthaline cataract

naphthol
fuchsin, amido black, and naphthol yellow

naphthoxylactic acid

napkin
n. dermatitis
n. psoriasis
n. rash
n. ring annular lesion
n. ring anular stenosis
n. ring anular tumor
n. ring calcar allograft
n. ring carcinoma
n. ring compression
n. ring compression
n. ring defect
sanitary n.

Naples
sandfly fever Naples virus

nappy test

naproxen
minimum effective naproxen dose
n. sodium

Na^+ pump

Naranjal virus

naratriptan
n. HCl
n. hydrochloride

narcissistic
n. character
n. character structure
n. composite
n. diagnosis
n. disturbance
n. dynamics
n. ego ideal
n. equilibrium
n. feature
n. personality
n. personality disorder
N. Personality Inventory
n. rage
n. trait

narcolepsy
n. cataplexy syndrome
n. experience
n. syndrome

narcoleptic
n. attack
n. sleep

narcosis
continuous n.
lipoid theory of n.
nitrogen n.
oxygen deprivation theory of n.
n. paralysis

narcotic
n. abuse
n. addict
n. addiction
n. agent
n. agonist drug
n. analgesia
n. analgesic
N.'s Anonymous
n. antagonist
n. antagonist drug
n. blockade
n. blockade drug
n. blocking drug
n. bowel syndrome
n. chemical intoxication
n. dependence
n. depression
n. detoxification
n. drug
n. drug dependence
n. effect
n. habit
n. hunger
n. lollipop
neonatal narcotic abstinence syndrome
neonatal narcotic pack
Neonatal N. Withdrawal Index
oral narcotic agent
n. overdose
overuse of n.'s
overuse of narcotic medication
n. poisoning
postoperative narcotic infusion
prescription n.
n. reversal
n. sedative
n.'s treatment center
n. treatment facility
n. treatment program
n. withdrawal
n. withdrawal scale
n. withdrawal syndrome

narcotic-addicted mother

narcotic-induced respiratory depression

narcotine analog

naris, pl. **nares**
anterior n.
anteverted n.
compressor muscle of n.
n. constriction
internal nares
musculus dilator n.
n. not obstructed
obstructed nares
packed nares
n. packed
posterior nares
right nostril naris

narrative
n. account
n. data
n. description
n., assessment, and plan
n. notes

narrow
acute narrow angle glaucoma
n. albumin gradient ascites
n. anteroposterior diameter
n. band noise
n. band spectrophotometer
n. band UVB
n. band UVB lamp
n. band UVB therapeutic light exposure
n. beam
n. beam half-thickness
n. bifrontal diameter
n. caliber
n. chest
n. collimation
n. complex supraventricular tachycardia
n. complex tachycardia
n. cone
n. duodenal opening
duodenal opening n.
n. field
n. fissure bur
n. foot
n. frequency band
n. gauze roll
n. hand
n. interscan interval
n. mediastinal waist
n. mediastinum
n. mesenteric stalk
moderately narrow anterior chamber angle
n. nasal bridge
n. palate
n. pubic arch
n. pulmonary outflow tract
n. rim of cytoplasm
n. spinal channel
n. therapeutic index
very narrow anterior chamber angle

narrow-angle
chronic narrow-angle glaucoma
n.-a. glaucoma

narrow-base quad cane

narrowed
n. arteriole
n. atrial ventricular valve
n. blood vessel
n. coronary artery
n. disc space
n. duct
n. outlet
n. pulse
n. urethra

narrowing
antral stomach n.
n. of aortic valve
arterial n.
arteriolar n.
n. of artery
arthritic ankle joint n.

narrowing *(continued)*
artificial lumen n.
n. asymmetry
atherosclerotic n.
n. at lumbosacral level
n. of blood vessel
n. of bronchiolar passages
n. of carotid artery
Carotid Artery Stenosis with Asymptomatic N.: Operation Versus Aspirin Study
n. of common duct
n. of coronary artery
disc space n.
eccentric n.
esophageal n.
n. of esophagus
n. of forefoot
n. of gastric outlet
n. of heart valve
n. of interspace
n. of intervertebral disc space
n. of joint space
n. and lipping
n. of lumen
luminal n.
n. of ostia of coronary artery
n. of outlet
n. of perceptions
retinal arterial narrowing and straightening
n. of retinal arteriole
scarring and narrowing of esophagus
segmental bronchus n.
severe heart valve n.
n. of spinal canal
systolic coronary artery n.
n. of visual field

narrow-slit illumination

narrow-spectrum
n.-s. agent
n.-s. blue light

Narula method

Nasahist B

nasal
n. accessory artery
n. air emission
n. airflow-inducing maneuver
n. airstream
n. airway
n. airway clear
n. airway obstructed
n. airway obstruction
n. airway resistance
n. ala
n. alar cartilage cleft
n. alar rim
n. alar rim reconstruction
n. allergen challenge
allergen specific nasal challenge
n. allergic disorder
n. allergy
n. angiocentric lymphoma
angiomatous nasal polyp
angular nasal artery
anterior lateral nasal branch of anterior ethmoidal artery
anterior nasal discharge
anterior nasal meatus
anterior nasal packing
anterior nasal septum
anterior nasal spine
anterior nasal spine of maxilla
anterior nasal valve
n. antigen challenge test
n. antral window
n. antrostomy
n. antrum
n. aperture
n. arch
n. architecture
n. arteriole of retina
artery of angular nasal branch
n. assimilation
n. asthma
n. atrium
atrium of middle nasal meatus
n. bilevel biphasic positive airway pressure
n. blockage
blocked nasal passage
n. bone
n. bone fragment
n. border
n. border of frontal bone
n. border of optic disc
n. branch
n. breathing
n. bridge
broad nasal bridge
budesonide aqueous nasal spray
bulbous nasal tip
bulldog nasal scissors
n. burning
n. buttonhole incision
n. calculus
n. canal
n. cannula
n. cannula dermatitis
n. canthus
n. capsule
n. cartilage
n. catarrh
n. cauterization
n. cavity
n. cavity cancer
n. cavity wall
n. cell
n. chamber
n. chondritis
n. chondroma
chronic hyperplastic sinusitis with nasal polyposis
n. clearance
n. concha
congenital nasal pyriform aperture stenosis
n. congestion
n. congestion score
n. consonant
n. continuous positive airway pressure
n. contour
contour of nasal bone
cosmetic nasal surgery
n. coupling
n. CPAP
n. crest
n. crest of horizontal plate of palatine bone
n. crest of maxilla
n. crest of palatine process of maxilla
n. cross-sectional area
n. culture
culture of nasal washing
n. cytology
n. decongestant
deflection of nasal septum
n. deformity
n. degloving
depression of nasal bone
deviated nasal septum
difficulty in nasal breathing
n. diphtheria
n. discharge
n. dissection
distance between nasal lines
n. dome
n. dome cartilage
n. dorsum
n. douche
n. drip pad
n. duct
n. duodenostomy tube
n. duplication
n. dysplasia
n. ectropion
n. elevator

n. eminence
n. emission
n. encephalocele
n. endoscope
n. endoscopic surgery
n. endoscopy
n. endotracheal intubation
n. endotracheal tube
enzootic nasal tumor
n. escape
ethmoidal process of inferior nasal concha
n. feeding
n. field loss
n. flaring
flat-bladed nasal speculum
n. floor
n. foramen
n. fossa
n. fracture
n. Fraser suction technique
n. ganglion
n. gavage
n. gland
n. glioma
n. hair
n. height
n. hemianopia
n. hemianopsia
n. hemifield
n. hemorrhage
n. herpes
high-flow nasal cannula
hyperemic nasal mucosa
n. hypoplasia, peripheral dysostosis, mental retardation syndrome
n. index
infant nasal cannula assembly
n. infection
inferior nasal artery
inferior nasal quadrant
inferior nasal vein
inflamed nasal passage
n. injection
n. insulin
n. intubation
n. irritation
n. isopter
n. itching
n. laceration
lateral nasal fold
n. lavage
n. limbus
lining of nasal passage
low nasal bridge
Marchac dorsal nasal flap
n. margin of frontal bone
n. mask
n. mastocytosis
n. meatus
n. membrane
middle meatus nasal antral window
Monarch Mini Mask nasal interface
n. mucosa
n. mucosal ulceration
n. mucous membrane
n. mucus
n. myiasis
narrow nasal bridge
n. nicotine spray
n. nocturnal ventilation
n. notch of maxilla
obstructed nasal passage
n. obstruction
olfactory groove of nasal cavity
O2 by nasal cannula
O_2 by nasal cannula
n. ora serrata
O2 saturation on three liters nasal cannula
O2 saturation on two liters nasal cannula
n. oxygen
oxygen by nasal cannula
oxygen saturation on 2 liters nasal cannula
oxygen saturation on 3 liters nasal cannula
n. pack
n. packing
n. papillomatosis
n. passage
n. passage inflammation
peak nasal inspiratory flow
n. periphery
n. pillow
n. polyp
n. polypectomy
n. polyposis
n. positive pressure ventilation
posterior nasal spine
posterior nasal spine to soft palate
n. prong continuous positive airway pressure
n. prongs
n. provocation test
purulent nasal drainage
n. pyramid
n. pyriform aperture stenosis
n. recess
n. reconstruction
reduced nasal fracture
n. refinement
n. reflex
n. region
n. regurgitation
n. resonance
n. respiration
n. root
n. scraping
n. secretion
n. septal deviation
n. septal perforation button
n. septoplasty
n. septum
n. sinus
n. sinus disease
n. smear
n. solar dermatitis
n. speculum
n. speech
n. spine
spondylar changes, nasal anomaly, striated metaphyses
n. spray
n. spray insulin
n. step defect
n. steroid
n. steroid spray
n. stuffiness
superior n.
superior nasal artery
superior nasal quadrant
superior nasal vein
n. suture
n. swab
n. swab culture
n. swelling
n. symptom score
synchronized nasal intermittent positive-pressure ventilation
n. tampon
n. T-cell/natural killer cell lymphoma
n. tip cautery
n. tip thermistor
n. turbinate
n. venule of retina
n. verge
n. vestibular stenosis
n. vestibule
n. vestibule cancer
n. voice
n. wash
n. washing

nasalis

angulus oculi n.

nasalis *(continued)*
arteria nasalis posterior septi
n. flap
nascent
n. collagen molecule
n. protein
n. protein chain
nasi
agger nasi cell
apex n.
flaring of ala n.
flaring of alae n.
limen n.
plica n.
Nasik ***Vibrio***
nasion pogonion
Nasmyth cuticle
nasoantral window
nasobiliary
n. drain
n. drainage
n. drainage catheter
n. drain cholangiography
endoscopic nasobiliary drainage
n. tube
nasobronchial reflex
nasociliary
n. branch
n. branches of ophthalmic nerve
n. ganglion
n. neuralgia
nasocystic catheter lavage
nasoduodenal feeding
nasoendotracheal tube
nasoenteric feeding
nasoethmoidal
n. encephalocele
n. fracture
nasofacial
n. analysis
n. groove
nasofrontal
n. angle
n. buttress
n. duct
n. suture
n. vein
nasogastric
n. aspirate
n. aspiration
n. decompression
n. drainage
n. drip feeding
n. feedings
n. feeding tube
n. intubation
n. lavage
n. replacement
n. suction
n. tube feeding
n. tube suctioning
nasogastrojejunal tube
nasogastrojejunostomy
nasogram curve
nasointestinal tube
nasojejunal
n. feeding
n. feeding tube
n. tube
nasojugal
n. fold
n. groove
nasolabial
n. angle
n. complex
n. crease
n. cyst
n. droop
n. fistula
n. fold
n. fold asymmetry
n. furrow
n. groove
n. junction
n. lymph node
n. reflex
n. sulcus
nasolacrimal
n. blockade
n. canal
congenital nasolacrimal duct obstruction
n. cyst
n. drainage system
n. duct
n. duct obstruction
n. duct probe
n. dysfunction
n. gland
n. groove
n. occlusion
primary acquired nasolacrimal duct obstruction
n. reflex
n. sac
nasomandibular fixation
nasomaxillary
n. balloon
n. buttress
n. dysplasia
n. fracture
n. groove
n. suture
nasomental reflex
naso-orbital fracture
nasopalatine
n. canal
n. duct
n. duct cyst
n. foramen
n. groove
n. injection
n. nerve
n. recess
nasopancreatic
n. catheter
n. drainage
nasopharyngeal
n. abscess
n. airway
n. airway obstruction
n. angiofibroma
n. applicator
n. area
n. aspirate
asymmetric nasopharyngeal lymphoid hyperplasia
n. atresia
n. biopsy
n. blastomycosis
n. bursa
n. cancer
n. carcinoma
n. carcinoma in situ
n. carcinoma with lymph node involvement
n. cooling
n. craniopharyngioma
n. culture
n. cyst
n. electrode
n. electrode placement
n. electrode placement in electroencephalography
Epstein-Barr nasopharyngeal carcinoma
n. fiberscope
n. fibroma
n. flora
n. fold
n. groove
n. hematoma
n. hemorrhage

juvenile nasopharyngeal angiofibroma
n. leishmaniasis
n. neoplasm
n. reflux
n. smear
n. specimen
n. stenosis
n. suction
n. suctioning
n. swab
n. tissue
n. ulcer
n. wall
n. wash
n. washing

nasopharyngeal-associated lymphoid tissue

nasopharyngoscopy biofeedback therapy

nasopharynx
n. cancer
posterior n.

nasoseptal
n. deviation
n. reconstruction
n. repair

nasotracheal
n. aspiration
n. catheter
n. intubation
n. intubation anesthesia
n. suction
n. suctioning
n. tube

nasoturbinal concha

Nasoule virus

nasovesicular
n. catheter
n. catheter technique

NASTRA study

Nasu-Hakola disease

natal
n. cleft
n. sore
n. teeth

natatory cord

natiform skull

national
N. Adult Reading Test
N. Alliance of Breast Cancer Organization
N. Alliance for Hispanic Health
N. Alliance for the Mentally Ill
N. Ambulatory Medical Care Survey
N. Aphasia Association
N. Arthritis Action Plan
N. Arthritis Data Workgroup
N. Asian Pacific Center on Aging
N. Association of Activity Professionals
N. Association of Anorexia Nervosa and Associated Disorders
N. Association of Area Agencies on Aging
N. Association of the Deaf
N. Association for Health & Fitness
N. Association for Hispanic Elderly
N. Association for Home Care
N. Association of Pediatric Nurse Associates and Practitioners
N. Association of Progressional Geriatric Care Managers
N. Association of Psychiatric Health Systems
N. Asthma Education Program
N. Attention Test
N. Bar Association
N. Biomedical Tracer Facility
N. Cancer Data Base
N. Cancer Institute
N. Cancer Institute Cooperative Group
N. Cancer Institute Protocol 89-C-41
N. Caucus and Center on Black Aged, Inc.
N. Center for Child Abuse and Neglect
N. Center on Elder Abuse
N. Center on Minority Health and Health Disparities
N. Center on Poverty Law, Inc.
n. character
N. Cholesterol Education guidelines
N. Cholesterol Education Program
N. Cholesterol Education Program criteria
N. Cholesterol Evaluation Program
N. Collegiate Athletic Association drug testing policy
N. Collegiate Athletic Association prohibited drug
N. Comorbidity Study
N. Comprehensive Cancer Network
N. Cooperative Dialysis Study
N. Cooperative Growth Study
N. Death Index
N. Depressive and Manic-Depressive Association
N. Diabetes Data Group
N. Diabetes Information Clearinghouse
N. Digestive Diseases Information Clearinghouse
N. Educational Longitudinal Survey
n. emergency
n. epithet
N. Eye Institute Visual Function Questionnaire
N. Family Caregivers Association
N. Formulary
N. Health Information Center
n. health insurance
N. Health and Nutrition Examination Follow-Up Study
N. Health and Nutrition Examination Survey
N. Heart, Lungs, and Blood Institute Information Center
N. Immunization Program
N. Institute of Acquired Immune Deficiency
N. Institute of Allergy and Infectious Disease
N. Institute of Arthritis and Metabolic Diseases
N. Institute of General Medical Sciences
N. Institute of Mental Health
N. Institute of Mental Health Diagnostic Interview Schedule
N. Institute of Mental Health-Global Obsessive Compulsive Scale
N. Institute for Occupational Safety and Health
N. Institute on Aging
N. Institute on Alcohol Abuse and Alcoholism
N. Institutes of Health
N. Institutes of Health Chronic Prostatitis Symptom Index
N. Joint Committee on Learning Disabilities
N. Kidney and Urological Diseases Information Clearinghouse
N. Library of Medicine

national *(continued)*
Lighthouse N. Center for Vision and Aging
N. Lung Transplant Patient Association
N. Marrow Donor Program
Medical Education for N. Defense
N. Mental Health Association
N. Organization of Victim Assistance
n. outpatient profile
N. Prevention Information Network
N. Prostatic Cancer Project criteria
N. Self-Help Clearinghouse
N. STD and AIDS Hotlines
N. Type Culture Collection
N. Urban League
N. Wilms Tumor Study
N. Women's Health Information Center
N. Women's Health Network

native
n. albumin
N. American
n. anergy
n. aorta
n. aortic valve
n. aortic valve closure
n. atherosclerosis
n. caudate lobe
n. condyle
n. coronary anatomy
n. coronary artery
n. deoxyribonucleic acid
n. immunity
n. LDL
n. pancreas
n. squamous epithelium
n. tissue harmonic imaging
n. type anti-DNA antibody
n. valve endocarditis
n. vessel

natriuretic
atrial natriuretic factor
atrial natriuretic factor receptor
atrial natriuretic hormone
atrial natriuretic peptide
atrial natriuretic polypeptide
brain natriuretic peptide
B-type natriuretic peptide
C-type atrial natriuretic peptide
n. hormone
human atrial natriuretic peptide
N-terminal atrial natriuretic peptide
n. peptide
n. peptide receptor
n. plasma dialysate
n. polypeptide
proatrial natriuretic factor

natural
n. agglutinin
n. aging process
n. anergy
n. antibody
n. anticancer agent
n. apophysial glide
n. bacterial flora
n. barrier
base of natural logarithms
body's natural balance bacteria
body's natural healing ability
body's natural defense mechanism
n. bristle
cardiolipin natural lecithin
n. cell-mediated cytotoxicity
n. chemotherapy agent
n. childbirth
n. conception
n. cytotoxicity
n. cytotoxicity receptor
n. death
n. defense mechanism
n. delivery
n. dentition
designed after natural anatomy
died a natural death
n. disaster
n. disease
n. displacement
n. dye
n. emotion
n. environment
exogenous natural surfactant
n. family planning
n. fecundity
n. focus of infection
n. frequency
n. group
n. growth hormone
n. healing method
n. hearing loss
n. hemolysin
n. hemostatic process
n. history
n. history of congestive heart failure
n. holistic technique
n. hormone
n. human interferon-beta
n. human interferon-gamma
human natural killer cell
n. immunity
n. joint
n. killer
n. killer activity
n. killer cell
n. killer cell activation
n. killer cell antigen
n. killer cell leukemia
n. killer cell-stimulating factor
n. killer-like T-cell lymphoma
n. killer lymphocyte
n. killer-mediated cytotoxicity
n. killer target structure
n. killer T-cell
n. language processing
liquified natural gas
low natural killer syndrome
pathophysiology and natural history
patient has natural immunity to hepatitis B virus
n. resistance macrophage-associated protein
n. rubber latex allergy
n. selection
n. selection theory
sustained natural apophysial glide
n. or synthetic hormone
n. thymocytotoxic autoantibody
n. UV radiation
n. variation
xenoreactive natural antibody

naturalistic
n. design
n. followup study

nature
n. of illness
n. of specimen

naturopathic
n. doctor
n. physician

Nauheim
N. bath
N. treatment

nausea
chemotherapy-induced nausea and emesis
n. and diarrhea
dizziness and n.
n. and emesis
fever, chills, sweating, nausea, vomiting, and diarrhea
fever, cough, nausea, and vomiting

n. gravidarum
hair loss and n.
intractable n.
Morrow Assessment of N. and Emesis
n., vomiting, diarrhea, and constipation
no nausea or vomiting
no nausea, vomiting, diarrhea or constipation
no nausea, vomiting, or diarrhea
onset of n.
pain and n.
postchemotherapy nausea and vomiting
postoperative n.
postoperative nausea and vomiting
radiation-induced nausea and vomiting
n. and vomiting
n., vomiting, and diarrhea
n. and vomiting of pregnancy

Navajo
N. brainstem syndrome
N. neuropathy

Naval Hospital

Navarre catheter

Navarro virus

navicular
n. abdomen
n. arthritis
n. articular surface of talus
n. body
n. body fracture
n. bone
n. bone of hand
carpal navicular bone
n. cell
n. cookie in shoe
n. cuneiform ligament
n. dorsal lip fracture
n. drop test
n. to first metatarsal angle
n. fossa
n. fossa of male urethra
n. fracture
long arm navicular cast
short arm navicular cast

naviculocapitate
n. fracture
n. fracture syndrome

naviculocuneiform
n. breach
n. coalition
n. fusion

navigated brain tumor surgery

navigation
surgical microscope n.

navigator
n. echo
n. echo-based real-time respiratory gating and triggering
n. echo motion correction technique

Navio
Serra do Navio virus

Naylor-Harwood Adult Intelligence Scale

N-butyl
N.-b. cyanoacrylate

N-butyl-deoxynojirimycin

n-capric acid

n-caproic acid

n-carbamoylaspartic acid

n-carbamoylglutamic acid

NCEP criteria

Nck protein

NCoA-1 coactivator

NCoA-2 coactivator

n-decanoic acid

Ndelle virus

n-docosanoic acid

n-dodecanoic acid

Ndumu virus

NdYAG
mode-locked Nd:YAG laser
Nanolas Nd:YAG laser
Nd:YAG laser ablation
Nd:YAG laser cyclophotocoagulation

NE-8D virus

Neale Reading Analysis

near
n. acuity testing
brought out near edge of incision
n. death experience
distance and near vision
n. drowning
N. East equine encephalomyelitis
esophoria for n.
n. esotropia
esotropia for n.
esotropia at n.
exophoria, near viewing
n. field scanning optical microscope
n. fixation
n. fixation position of gaze
n. gaze
n. gaze reflex
illuminated near card
intermittent esotropia at n.
n. light reflex
n. patient test
n. reaction
n. reaction to light
n. response
n. syncope
n. triad
n. vision
n. vision test
n. vision testing
n. visual acuity
n. visual point

near-death experience

near-fatal asthma

near gaze reflex

near-infrared
n.-i. interactance
n.-i. spectroscopy

nearly
n. ideal binary solvent
N. Me breast form
n. total thyroidectomy

nearly ideal binary solvent

near-miss sudden infant death syndrome

near-point
n.-p. accommodation
n.-p. esophoria
n.-p. exophoria
n.-p. phoria
n.-p. relative

near-reflex spasm

near-term
n.-t. gestation
n.-t. pregnancy

near-total
n.-t. esophagectomy
n.-t. gastrectomy
n.-t. thyroidectomy

near-ultraviolet

near-UV excited autofluorescence diagnosis system

near-viable fetus

near-water
n.-w. attenuation
n.-w. density

Nebcin Injection

Nebraska
N. calf diarrhea virus
N. calf scours virus

Nebuhaler inhaler

nebular stromal opacity

nebulization
continuous albuterol n.
continuous nebulization therapy
n. ventilator

nebulized
n. bronchodilator
n. isoproterenol
n. mist treatment
n. preservative-free morphine sulfate
n. solution

nebulizer
compressed air-driven n.
compressor-generated n.
handheld n.
high-density n.
Puritan heated n.
side-arm n.
small-volume n.
twin jet n.
ultrasonic n.
updraft n.

necessary
administratively necessary days
n. condition
medically n.
no special preparation necessary for test
no treatment n.

neck
adenoid cystic carcinoma of head and n.
advanced resected head and neck cancer
anatomical neck of humerus
n. of aneurysm
aneurysm remnant n.
anterior triangle of n.
asymmetric tonic neck reflex
asymptomatic neck bruit
n. of bladder
bladder n.
bladder neck contracture
bladder neck obstruction
bladder neck resection
bladder neck suspension
n. brace
n. of cervix
n. circumference
clenched muscles in head and n.
n. coil
n. complaint
n. of condyle
congenital cartilaginous rest of n.
cord around infant n.
cutaneous malignant melanoma of head and n.
deep space neck infection
n. dermatitis
n. diameter
N. Disability Index
n. dissection
n. droop
elective neck dissection
elective neck irradiation
endoscopic bladder neck suspension
n. exploration
n. extension position
extraperitoneal laparoscopic bladder neck suspension
extrathyroidal neck radioactivity
femoral n.
femoral neck fracture
femoral neck nail
femoral neck prosthesis
femoral neck version
n. of femur
n. of fibula
n. flap
n. flexion
n. flexor
n. flexor tendon
n. fracture
n. full range of motion
Functional Assessment of Cancer Therapy–Head and N.
Functional Assessment of Cancer Therapy–Head and N.
functional neck dissection
n. of gallbladder
glands, goiter, or stiffness of n.
glandular neck cell
n. of glans
n. of glans penis
n. of hair follicle
head and n.
n. and head of femur
head and neck cancer
head and neck in extended position
head and neck motion
head and neck normal
head, neck, and shaft
head and neck squamous cell carcinoma
head and neck tremor
head tilt with neck lift
n. of humerus
immobilization of neck injury
n. infection
n. injury
innervation of head and n.
n. irradiation
n. isometric
jugular neck vein distention
laparoscopic bladder neck suspension
left radical neck dissection
n. lesion
limited neck motion
long muscle of n.
n. lymphadenopathy
n. lymph node
lymph node of head and n.
lysis bladder neck adhesions
Magnus and de Kleijn tonic neck reflex
n. of malleus
n. of mandible
n. mass
n. of metacarpal
n. metastasis
metastatic squamous carcinoma of head and n.
modified neck dissection
modified Peyronie bladder neck suspension
n. motion
n. muscles
nail inserted into neck and head of femur
nape of n.
needle bladder neck suspension
Newman classification of radial neck and head fracture
normal head and n.
nuchal cord around infant's n.
ophthalmology, otorhinolaryngology, and head and neck surgery
osteotomy of condylar n.
n. pain
pain spreading to n.
palpable neck mass
n. of pancreas
partial neck dissection
n. passively flexed
Pauwels femoral neck fracture classification
penetrating neck wound
percutaneous bladder neck stabilization
percutaneous bladder neck suspension

Pereyra bladder neck suspension
performance status scale for head and neck cancer
pulsating neck vein
n. pushup
radiation-induced sarcoma of the head and n.
n. of radius
n. reflex
n. region-lifting method
rhabdomyosarcoma of head and n.
right radical neck dissection
n. of scapula
selective neck dissection
n. and shoulder pain
squamous cell carcinoma of head and n.
squamous cell head and neck cancer
n. strain
stretching and neck isometric
n. supple
n. surgery
surgical neck of humerus
symmetric tonic neck reflex
tight nuchal cord around infant's n.
tongue, jaw, neck dissection
tonic neck reflex
transurethral incision of bladder n.
transurethral resection of vesical n.
transvaginal bladder neck suspension
n. vein distended
n. vein distention
vesical n.
vesical neck contracture
Wookey neck flap

Neckar river virus

neck-capsule distance

necklace
medical alert n.
n. of pearls
n. of Venus

neck-righting reflex

neck-shaft angle

neck-to-thigh ratio

necrobiotic
n. coagulum
n. granuloma
n. xanthogranuloma

necrogenic
n. tubercle
n. wart

necrogranulomatous keratitis

necrolysis
erythema multiforme/toxic epidermal n.
total epidermal n.
toxic epidermal n.

necrolytic
n. migratory erythema
migratory necrolytic erythema

necropsy specimen

necrosing
minimal necrosing dose

necrosis
acute hepatocellular n.
acute renal n.
acute sclerosing hyaline n.
acute tubular n.
anterior segment n.
antitumor necrosis factor-based therapy
aortic idiopathic n.
aortic wall n.
areas of hemorrhage and n.
n. of ascending aorta
aseptic epiphysial n.
aseptic necrosis of bone
asphyxia-related renal n.
aspirin-induced papillary n.
avascular bone n.
avascular cortical infarction n.
avascular femoral head n.
avascular necrosis of bone
avascular necrosis of the femoral head
avascular necrosis lunate
avascular scaphoid n.
avascular tarsal scaphoid n.
avascular vertebral body n.
n. bacillus
bilateral acute retinal n.
bilateral cortical n.
bone marrow n.
n. of bowel
n. of brain
central hemorrhagic n.
centrilobar n.
cerebral radiation n.
cortical necrosis of brain
cortical necrosis of kidney
cystic medial n.
cystic medial necrosis of ascending aorta
cystic suppurative n.
delayed conditioned n.
disseminated fat n.
electrolyte and steroid cardiopathy with n.
ethanol-induced tumor n.
n. factor
gangrenous pulp n.
idiopathic aseptic n.
infantile bilateral striatal necrosis syndrome
infected pancreatic n.
infectious hematopoietic necrosis virus
infectious pancreatic necrosis virus
ischemic bone n.
ischemic muscle n.
ischemic necrosis of bone
ischemic necrosis of femoral head
ischemic pressure n.
Lichtman aseptic necrosis classification
n. of liver
macrophage-derived tumor necrosis factor
Marcus grading scale for avascular n.
massive hepatic n.
maximum coagulative n.
medial cystic n.
metastatic fat n.
miliary calcified n.
neutralizing murine monoclonal antitumor necrosis factor antibody
Paget quiet n.
n. of pancreas
pancreatic glandular n.
papillary n.
perifascicular myofiber n.
pontosubicular neuron n.
postischemic acute tubular n.
n. progrediens
progressive outer retinal n.
pulmonary hemorrhagic n.
recombinant tumor necrosis factor alpha
renal papillary n.
renal tubular n.
satellite tobacco necrosis virus
scrotal fat n.
small focus of hepatic n.
soluble tumor necrosis factor-a receptor type I
spleen necrosis virus
spontaneous hemorrhagic n.

necrosis *(continued)*
subacute hepatic n.
subcutaneous fat n.
tobacco necrosis virus
toxic epidermal n.
traumatic fat n.
n. of tumor
tumor necrosis factor-alpha
tumor necrosis factor
tumor necrosis factor-beta
tumor necrosis factor-binding protein
tumor necrosis factor receptor
tumor necrosis factor receptor-associated periodic syndrome
tumor necrosis factor-related activation-induced cytokine
tumor necrosis factor-related apoptosis-inducing ligand
tumor necrosis serum
n. and ulceration

necrotic
n. abscess
n. adipocyte
n. angina
n. arachnidism
n. area
n. bladder mucosa
n. bone
n. bone pseudocyst
n. caries
n. cell death
n. cementum
n. center
n. cirrhosis
n. coagulum
n. core
n. cutaneous loxoscelism
n. cyst
débrided necrotic tissue
debridement of necrotic tissue
n. debris
n. enteritis
n. excoriation
n. facial dysplasia
n. flap
n. focus
n. follicle
friable necrotic tissue
n. gangrene tissue
n. gangrenous tissue
n. granuloma
n. hemorrhagic colitis
n. hemorrhoid
n. infectious conjunctivitis
n. inflammatory cell
n. kidney tissue
n. lesion
n. palatal ulcer
n. placenta
n. placental tissue
n. pocket
posterior necrotic zone
n. purulent material
residual necrotic tissue
n. toe
n. tumor
n. ulcer
n. ulceration

necrotisans

necrotized chilblain

necrotizing
acute necrotizing myelitis
acute necrotizing pancreatitis
acute necrotizing ulcerative gingivitis
n. adrenalitis
n. amebic enterocolitis
n. angiitis
n. arteriolitis
n. aspergillosis
benign necrotizing otitis externa
n. bowel disease
n. bowel vasculitis
n. bronchopneumonia
n. cellulitis
n. colitis
n. crescentic glomerulonephritis
cutaneous necrotizing vasculitis
n. cystitis
disseminated necrotizing leukoencephalopathy
n. encephalitis
n. encephalomyelitis
n. encephalomyelopathy
n. encephalopathy
n. enterocolitis
n. erysipelas
n. external otitis
n. factor
n. fasciitis of the scrotum
focal hemorrhagic necrotizing cystitis
n. funisitis
n. gingivostomatitis
n. granuloma
n. granulomatous inflammation
n. granulomatous lymphadenitis
n. granulomatous systemic arteritis
n. granulomatous vasculitis
n. hemorrhage leukomyelitis
n. hemorrhagic leukoencephalitis
histiocytic necrotizing lymphadenitis
infantile necrotizing encephalomyelopathy
n. inguinal adenopathy
n. interstitial keratitis
n. jejunitis
lymphadenitis
malignant necrotizing otitis externa
monomicrobial necrotizing cellulitis
mycobacterial necrotizing pneumonia
n. myositis
n. myositis fasciitis
neonatal necrotizing enterocolitis
n. nodular scleritis
odontogenic cervical necrotizing fasciitis
n. pancreatitis
n. papillitis
peripheral necrotizing retinitis
n. pneumonia
n. pseudomembranous colitis
pseudomembranous necrotizing enterocolitis
rapidly progressive necrotizing glomerulonephritis
n. respiratory granulomatosis
n. retinitis
n. retinopathy
n. sarcoid granulomatosis
n. scleritis with adjacent inflammation
n. scleritis without adjacent inflammation
n. sclerocorneal ulceration
n. sialometaplasia
n. soft-tissue infection
n. stromal keratitis
subacute necrotizing encephalomyelopathy
n. superficial tracheobronchitis
systemic necrotizing vasculitis
n. tonsillitis
n. ulcerative gingivitis
n. ulcerative keratitis
n. ulcerative periodontitis
n. ulcerative stomatitis

necrotoxica
meningitis necrotoxica reactiva

nectar-thick liquid diet consistency

nectary
n. of floral unit

nectary of floral unit

need

n. for admiration
assessing needs of hallucinogen abuser
n. for care
certificate of n.
Children with Special Health Care N.'s
community periodontal index of treatment n.'s
n. for constant attention
n. to control
create physical n.
decreased need for sleep
estimated energy n.'s
estimated protein n.'s
Functional N.'s Assessment
immediate intense need to void
independent living n.'s
intense need to void immediate
patient needs minimal assistance for wheelchair mobility
patient's n.'s identified
person in need of supervision
Screening Children for Related Early Educational N.'s
unmet dependency n.

needed

as n.
as much as n.
home, no services n.
number needed to treat

needle

n. ablation
adjustable-length gauge n.
n. arthroscopy
n. aspirate
n. aspiration
n. aspiration biopsy
n. aspiration cytology
n. aspiration lung biopsy
aspiration needle biopsy
n. bath
n. biopsy diagnosis
n. biopsy of liver
n. biopsy of prostate
n. biopsy specimen
bipolar needle recording electrode
n. bladder neck suspension
blunt-tipped epidural n.
bone biopsy n.
breast needle location
bronchoscopic needle aspiration
n. catheter jejunostomy
clean needle technique
closed core needle biopsy
concentric needle electromyography
n. cord length
n. core biopsy
core biopsy n.
core needle biopsy
correct sponge and needle count
n. count
n. cricothyroidotomy
n. cricothyrotomy
n. culture
curved needle biopsy
cutting needle biopsy
n. cystourethropexy
n. deviation
diamond point n.
n. diathermy excision of the transformation zone
double needle operation on cataract
n. electrode
n. electrode electromyography
n. electrode examination
n. electromyography
endoscopic in-line needle holder
n. exchange program
fine intestinal n.
gauge of n.
guided needle biopsy
guillotine needle biopsy
history of needle sharing
n. holder
n. holder clamp
infected intravenous drug n.
intermittent needle therapy
intraosseous infusion n.
intravenous needle site care
keep needle open
to keep needle open
large-core needle biopsy
n. liver biopsy
n. localization
n. management system
March laser sclerostomy n.
Maumenee vitreous-aspirating n.
McIntyre I/A n.
McPherson needle holder
metallic frontal n.
micro round-tip n.
Multi-Pro biopsy n.
neurosurgery needle holder
noncoring Huber n.
Nottingham colposuspension n.
nucleus hydrolysis n.
number of needle passes
Paton needle holder
percutaneous needle aspiration
percutaneous needle aspiration biopsy
percutaneous needle cholangiogram
percutaneous needle lung aspiration
percutaneous needle puncture
percutaneous transthoracic needle biopsy
Pereyra needle suspension
n. probe
prostate needle biopsy
prostatic needle biopsy
protected transbronchial needle aspirate
n. sharing
sharing infected intravenous drug n.
n. shower
Silverman needle biopsy
single needle device
skinny needle aspiration
n. spatula
n. and sponge count
n. and sponge count correct times three
n. and sponge count correct times two
n., sponge, and instrument count correct times three
n., sponge, and instrument count correct times two
sponge and needle count
n. spoon
n. spud
stereotactically guided core needle biopsy
stereotactic needle biopsy
n. stick
n. stick injury
n. suspension
n. tip
n. track
transbronchial needle aspiration
transrectal needle biopsy
transrectal needle biopsy of prostate
transthoracic needle aspiration
transthoracic needle aspiration biopsy
transurethral needle biopsy of the prostate

needle *(continued)*
Tru-Cut needle biopsy
ultrasonically guided needle biopsy
needle-free injection system
needle-knife
n.-k. electrocautery
n.-k. endoscopic pancreatic sphincterotomy
n.-k. fistulotomy
n.-k. precut papillotomy
needle-localized open biopsy
Needleman-Wunsch algorithm
needle-marked arm
needlepoint electrocautery
needles-and-pins sensation
needlescopic procedure
need-persistence
Neer
N. acromioplasty
N. acromioplasty for rotator cuff tear
N. capsular shift procedure
N. classification of shoulder fracture
N. femur fracture classification
N. hemiarthroplasty
N. humerus fracture classification
N. II humeral component
N. test
Neer-Horowitz
N.-H. classification of humeral fracture
Neethling virus
nef
n. gene
n. gene-deleted virus
n. protein
nef-deleted virus
negation
n. delusion
n. of the ego
negative
n. abdominal pressure
AB negative blood type
n. accommodation
additional cost of false n.'s
adverse negative immunosuppressive effect
n. aerobe
n. aerobic bacillus
n. affect
n. affectivity
n. afterimage
n. afterpotential
n. anergy
n. antigenemia
n. appendectomy
n. arterial-portal glucose gradient
n. aspiration
n. assortative mating
asymmetric negative T-wave
n. attitude
axillary node n.
n. bacteremia
n. bacteria
n. balance
n. balance of body fluid
n. base excess
n. behavior
blood type A n.
blood type O n.
B negative blood type
n. body image
n. bone scan
n. brain scan
breakpoint cluster region n.
n. breast biopsy
n. cardiogram
n. casting
n. catalyst
n. celiotomy
n. change
n. chemotaxis
n. chronotropism
n. command
conative negative variation
n. conditioning
n. conditioning for sleep
n. congruence angle
contingent negative variation
continuous negative airway pressure
continuous negative extrathoracic pressure
n. contrast
n. contrast echocardiography
n. contrast imaging agent
n. contrast left atriography
n. control
n. control enzyme induction
n. control repression
n. control test
n. convergence
n. cooperativity
n. correlation
n. crossmatch
n. culture
culture negative for growth
culture negative for pathogens
n. cytology
n. cytotaxis
cytotoxicity negative, absorption positive
n. to date
n. delta sign
n. delusion
n. diagnosis
distorted negative thinking
n. dromotropism
Duffy antigen A negative phenotype
Duffy antigen B negative phenotype
n. effect
n. electrocardiogram
n. electron
n. electrotaxis
n. emotion
n. emotionality
n. end-expiratory pressure
essentially n.
n. eugenics
n. evaluation
n. expectation
n. expiratory force
n. expiratory pressure
n. factor
false n.
family history n.
n. feedback
n. feedback loop
n. feedback regulation
n. feeling
n. finding
Gram stain negative bacteremias
guaiac n.
Hemoccult negative stools
n. hero
n. image
n. imagery
n. immunosuppressive effect
n. inspiratory force
n. inspiratory pressure
n. interference
intermittent negative pressure-assisted ventilation
n. logarithm of acid ionization constant
lower body negative pressure
n. meniscus
n. meniscus lens
microscopically positive, culturally n.
n. pi meson
n. nevus
number of similar n.'s
n. patch test

peak negative pressure
n. peritoneal cytology
n. phase
positive to negative ratio
Positive and N. Stroke Scale
Positive and N. Syndrome Scale
postimperative negative variation
n. predictive value
predictive value of a negative test
n. pressure device
n. pressure respirator
n. punch biopsy
n. reaction
replication error n.
n. Rh blood
Rhesus n.
Rinne test n.
Scale for the Assessment of N. Symptoms
schedule for negative symptoms
n. Schick test
n. scotoma
n. sedimentation Svedberg unit
n. selection
n. selection procedure
n. self-image
n. straight leg raise
n. strand virus
n. symptom
n. therapeutic reaction
total n.'s
n. T_3 response element
n. triiodothyronine response element
true n.
true negative fraction
true negative rate
n. ulnar variance
n. variation
n. vertical divergence
n. vertical vergence
n. visual phenomenon

negatively
n. bathmotropic
n. correlated region
n. dromotropic
n. inotropic
n. staining region of chromosome

negative-pressure
n.-p. box
n.-p. isolation room
n.-p. respirator
n.-p. ventilation

negative-sense genome

negativism
adolescent n.
exhibits irritable n.

negativistic
n. behavior
n. bias

Negishi virus

neglect
adult survivor of n.
n. of child
child abuse and n.
n. of duty
n. dyslexia
history of n.
National Center for Child Abuse and N.
suspected child abuse or n.
unilateral spatial n.

negligible blood loss

negotiable order of withdrawal

negotiating goals skills

Negri
N. body
N. corpuscle

Neher operation

Nehra-Mack operation

neighborhood
n. family care center
n. health center

Neill-Dingwall syndrome

Neill-Mooser
N.-M. body
N.-M. reaction

Neisser
N. coccus
N. granule

Neisseria
chromosomally mediated resistant *Neisseria gonorrhoeae*
Neisseria gonorrhoeae culture
Neisseria gonorrhoeae DNA detection test
Neisseria gonorrhoeae susceptibility testing
Neisseria gonorrhoeae urethritis
Neisseria meningitidis B
meningococcal *Neisseria meningitidis* serogroups unspecified vaccine
Neisseria mucosa endocarditis
Neisseria meningitidis B
non–penicillinase-producing *Neisseria gonorrhoeae*
quinolone-resistant *Neisseria gonorrhoeae*
rapid identification method-*Neisseria*
tetracycline-resistant *Neisseria gonorrhoeae*

Neisseria gonorrhoeae
chromosomally mediated resistant g.
penicillinase-producing g.
quinolone-resistant g.
tetracycline-resistant g.

neisserial
n. conjunctivitis
n. infection

Neisser-Wechsberg leukocidin

Nélaton
N. ankle dislocation
N. catheter
N. fiber
N. fold
N. line

Nelson
N. Bay orthoreovirus
N. finger exerciser
N. grading system
N. sign
N. syndrome
N. tumor

nemaline myopathy

nematode
anisakid n.
n. dermatitis

neoadjuvant
n. androgen deprivation
n. androgen derivation therapy
n. antiandrogenic treatment
n. chemoradiation
n. chemotherapy
n. hormonal therapy

neoanal function

Neo-Cobefrin

neocortex atrophy

neocortical
n. association area
n. coverage
n. temporal-lobe epilepsy

neodymium:YAG laser

neodymium:yttrium
n. lithium fluoride laser

neodymium:yttrium-aluminum-garnet
n.-a.-g. laser

neodymium:yttrium-lithium-fluoride
n.-l.-f. photodisruptive laser

neodymium:yttrium lithium fluoride laser

neodymium: yttrium-lithium-fluoride laser

neoelectroencephalography

Neo-Gen screening

neointimal hyperplasia

Neolens lens

neomycin

bacitracin, polymyxin B, neomycin sulfate
n. dermatitis
n. egg yolk agar
fluorometholone and neomycin sulfate
n. and polymyxin B
polymyxin B sulfate, bacitracin, and n.
n. sulfate

neonatal

n. abdominal mass
N. Abstinence Scoring System
n. abstinence sign
n. acne
n. adjuvant life support
n. adrenal gland hemorrhage
n. adrenal ultrasound
n. adrenoleukodystrophy
n. air leak syndrome
Albert Einstein N. Developmental Scale
alloimmune neonatal neutropenia
alloimmune neonatal thrombocytopenic purpura
n. alloimmune thrombocytopenia
n. alloimmune thrombocytopenic purpura
n. amblyogenic stimulus
n. anemia
n. anesthesia
n. apnea
n. apoplexy
n. arginine vasopressin
n. ascites
n. asphyxia
n. auditory response cradle
autoimmune neonatal thrombocytopenia
n. autoimmune neutropenia
n. autoimmune thrombocytopenia
automatic neonatal walking reflex
n. Bartter syndrome
N. Behavioral Assessment Scale
N. Behavioral Assessment Scale with Kansas Supplements
benign familial neonatal convulsions
n. biliary function
n. bilirubin
n. biotin deficiency
n. blood volume
n. botulism
n. brain injury
Brazelton N. Behavioral Assessment Scale
n. breast hyperplasia
n. breath-holding spell
n. bullous dermatitis
n. calf diarrhea virus
n. candidiasis
n. cardiac failure
n. cerebral hemorrhage
n. cerebrovascular accident
n. chest disease
n. cholestasia
n. cholestasis
n. cholestasis workup
n. cholestatic hepatitis
n. cholestatic jaundice
n. choroid plexus hemorrhage
n. chronic idiopathic neutropenia
n. chronic lung disease
n. citrullinemia
n. cold injury
n. complications of drug abuse
n. condition
n. conjugated hyperbilirubinemia
n. conjunctivitis
n. convulsion
n. CVA
n. cyanotic congenital heart disease
n. cystic pulmonary emphysema
n. death
n. death rate
n. dentition
n. dermatology
n. diabetes mellitus
n. diagnosis
n. distress
n. drug addiction seizure
early neonatal death
Early N. Neurobehavior Scale
Einstein N. Neurobehavioral Assessment Scale
n. elastin deposition
n. encephalopathy
n. enterovirus infection
n. exchange transfusion
n. exstrophic bladder repair
n. extracorporal membrane oxygenation
N. Facial Coding System
N. Facial Pain Inventory
n. flatfoot
n. gastrointestinal hemorrhage
n. giant cell hepatitis
n. gliosis
n. goiter
n. gonococcal disease
n. Graves hyperthyroidism
n. Guillain-Barré syndrome
n. Guthrie card
n. gynecomastia
n. hemochromatosis
n. hemorrhagic disease
n. hepatitis syndrome
n. herpes
n. herpes simplex
n. herpes simplex virus
n. herpes simplex virus infection
n. HMD
n. HSV-1, -2 encephalitis
n. hyaline membrane disease
n. hydrocephalus
n. hyperbilirubinemia
n. hypercalcemia
n. hyperparathyroidism
n. hypertension
n. hyperthermia
n. hypocalcemia
n. hypoglycemia
n. hypoglycemic seizure
n. hypomagnesemia
n. hypothyroidism
n. hypotonia
n. hypoxia
n. hypoxic-ischemic encephalopathy
n. inclusion blennorrhea
n. inclusion conjunctivitis
N. Infant Pain Scale
n. infection
n. intensive care unit
n. intubation
n. iron-storage disease
n. isoimmune thrombocytopenia
n. jaundice
n. leukemoid reaction
n. line
n. listeriosis
n. lung fibroblast
n. lupus
n. lupus erythematosus
lupus erythematosus, n.
n. lupus syndrome
n. Marfan syndrome
n. marker

n. maturity classification of Dubowitz
n. medicine
n. meningitis
n. metabolism
n. monitor
n. morbidity
n. morphine solution
n. mortality
n. mortality rate
n. mortality risk
n. myasthenia
n. myasthenia gravis
n. myasthenic syndrome
n. narcotic abstinence syndrome
n. narcotic pack
N. Narcotic Withdrawal Index
n. necrotizing enterocolitis
Neo-trak 515A neonatal monitor
n. neutropenia
normal neonatal nursery
n. ocular prophylaxis
n. olivopontocerebellar atrophy
n. ophthalmia
n. opium solution
n. osseous dysplasia
n. outcome
Parental Stressor Scale: N. Intensive Care Unit
n. perception inventory
persistent neonatal myasthenia gravis
n. phototherapy
n. placing
n. pseudohydrocephalic progeroid syndrome
N. Pulmonary Insufficiency Index
n. pustular melanosis
regional neonatal intensive care unit
n. respiratory distress syndrome
n. resuscitation
n. ring
Score for Neonatal Acute Physiology-Perinatal Extension
n. screening
n. seizure
n. sepsis
n. septicemia
n. serum
n. severe hyperparathyroidism
simple neonatal procedure
n. skin allograft
n. small left colon syndrome
spontaneous neonatal chylothorax
n. staphylococcal disease
n. stepdown unit
n. systemic candidiasis
n. teeth
n. tetanus
n. tetany
n. thymectomy
n. thyroid dysfunction
n. toxoplasmosis
transient neonatal diabetes
transient neonatal diabetes mellitus
transient neonatal hyperammonemia
transient neonatal pustular melanosis
n. tuberculosis
n. tyrosinemia
Universal N. Hearing Screening
N. Withdrawal Inventory

neonatal/high risk

neonatally tolerant

neonatal/medium risk

neonate

athyrotic n.
n. examination
preterm n.
very low birth weight preterm n.

neonatology

pediatric n.

neon particle

neopentyl glycol succinate

neoplasia

anal intraepithelial n.
anogenital squamous intraepithelial n.
cervical epithelial n.
cervical intraepithelial neoplasia, grade 1–3
cervical invasive n.
conjunctival intraepithelial n.
endometrial intraepithelial n.
familial multiple endocrine n.
intratubular germ cell neoplasia, unclassified type
laryngeal intraepithelial n.
laser destruction of intraepithelial n.
lobular n.
lymphocytic thyroiditis n.
malignant intratubular germ-cell n.
mammary intraepithelial n.
melanocytic intraepidermal n.
multicentric lower genital tract n.
multiple endocrine neoplasia syndrome, type 1, 2A, 2B, 3
multiple endocrine neoplasia type 1, 2, 2a, 2b, 3
multiple intestinal n.
ovarian intraepithelial n.
prostatic intraepithelial n.
vaginal intraepithelial n.
vulvar intraepithelial n.

neoplasm

alpha islet cell n.
benign vascular n.
central benign n.
n. embryonic antigen
epithelioid soft-tissue n.
first malignant n.
gestational trophoblastic n.
gonadal germ cell n.
hemianopia in intracranial n.
intracranial neoplasm headache
intraductal oncocytic papillary n.
intraductal papillary mucinous n.
intraductal papillary neoplasm of the pancreas
lipid cell n.
lipoid ovarian n.
malignant brain n.
malignant hepatic n.
malignant neoplasm of bladder
malignant neoplasm of bone
malignant neoplasm of bronchus
malignant neoplasm of kidney
malignant neoplasm of larynx
malignant neoplasm of scrotum
malignant ovarian n.
malignant renal n.
Merkel cell n.
middle ear n.
monoclonal B-cell n.
mucinous cystic n.
mucinous ovarian n.
multiple endocrine n.
multiple primary n.'s
multiple primary n.
nonseminomatous germ cell n.
ovarian lipid cell n.
ovarian malignant epithelial n.
pancreatic endocrine n.
papillary cystic n.
parenchymal brain n.
peripheral benign n.
primary intracranial n.
radiation-induced n.
renal epithelioid oxyphilic n.
Revised European-American Classification of Lymphoid Neoplasms
second malignant n.
slow-growing cortical n.

neoplasm *(continued)*
- n. staging
- vaginal intraepithelial n.

neoplastic
- n. adenohypophysial cell
- n. aneurysm
- n. angioendotheliomatosis
- n. angiogenesis
- angiomatous neoplastic tissue
- n. arachnoiditis
- n. brachial plexopathy
- n. calcification
- n. cell proliferation
- n. change
- n. clone
- n. cyst
- n. destruction of spinal element
- n. dissemination
- n. follicle
- n. fracture
- n. growth
- n. hyperplasia
- n. lymphocyte
- malignant neoplastic disease
- n. meningitis
- n. pathologic lesion
- n. pathology
- n. pericardial effusion
- n. polyp
- n. process
- n. proliferating angioendotheliomatosis
- n. sequela
- n. state
- n. trophoblastic disease
- n. urothelium

Neo-Polycin ointment

neoprecipitin test

neoprene
- n. brace
- n. fabric

neopterin to biopterin ratio

neopyrithiamin hydrochloride

Neosar Injection

neospinothalamic tract

Neosporin ointment

neostigmine test

Neo-Synephrine

NeoTect imaging agent

Neo-trak 515A neonatal monitor

neotype
- n. culture
- n. strain

neovagina construction

neovaginal cavity

neovascular
- n. angle-closure glaucoma
- n. bundle
- choroidal neovascular membrane
- disciform macular degeneration with subretinal neovascular membrane
- n. glaucoma
- intravitreal neovascular frond
- n. membrane
- n. net
- senile retinal neovascular membrane
- subretinal neovascular membrane
- n. tuft

neovascularization
- choroidal or subretinal n.
- n. of disc
- n. elsewhere on retina
- n. of iris
- left atrial n.
- n. of new vessels elsewhere
- occult choroidal n.
- n. of optic disc
- peripapillary subretinal n.
- n. of retina
- subretinal n.

nephelometric
- n. immunoassay
- n. inhibition assay
- n. turbidity units

nephrectomy
- n. allograft
- apical polar n.
- hand-assisted laparoscopic radical n.
- laparoscopic donor n.
- laparoscopic radical n.
- live donor n.
- living donor n.
- transperitoneal laparoscopic n.

nephric
- n. blastema
- n. duct

nephritic
- n. calculus
- n. colic
- n. edema
- n. factor
- hereditary nephritic protein
- lytic nephritic factor
- n. syndrome

nephritis
- acute allergic interstitial n.
- acute focal bacterial n.
- acute interstitial tubular n.
- allergic interstitial n.
- antibasement membrane n.
- antiglomerular basement membrane antibody n.
- antiglomerular basement membrane-negative crescentic glomerular n.
- antikidney serum n.
- arteriosclerotic n.
- autoimmune interstitial n.
- n. caseosa
- chronic interstitial n.
- n. dolorosa
- n. gravidarum
- Henoch-Schönlein purpura n.
- hereditary chronic n.
- Heymann nephritis antigenic complex
- ICR strain-derived glomerular n.
- interstitial n.
- lupus n.
- membranous lupus n.
- mercuric chloride-induced n.
- mesangial lupus n.
- nephrotoxic antiglomerular basement membrane antibody n.
- nephrotoxic serum n.
- passive Heymann n.
- pauciimmune glomerular n.
- tubulointerstitial n.
- tubulointerstitial nephritis and uveitis syndrome
- World Health Organization classification of lupus nephritis I, IIA, IIB, III, IV, V

nephritogenic
- n. antigen
- n. effector
- n. epitope
- n. process

nephroblastoma
- cystic, partially differentiated n.
- fetal rhabdomyomatous n.

nephroblastomatosis complex

nephrogenic
- n. ascites
- n. bladder adenoma
- congenital nephrogenic diabetes insipidus
- n. cord
- n. diabetes
- n. diabetes insipidus
- intralobar nephrogenic rest
- lithium-induced nephrogenic diabetes insipidus

n. metaplasia
perilobar nephrogenic rest
n. rest

nephrogenous
n. albuminuria
n. cAMP
n. cyclic adenosine monophosphate
n. dialysis ascites
n. proteinuria

nephrogram
isotope n.

nephrographic
generalized n.
n. phase

nephrolithiasis
autosomally inherited forms of n.
N. Clinical Guidelines Panel
X-linked hypercalciuric n.
X-linked recessive n.

nephrolithotomy
percutaneous n.
simultaneous bilateral percutaneous n.

nephrolithotripsy
percutaneous ultrasonic n.

nephrology
pediatric n.

nephrolumbar ganglion

nephroma
congenital mesoblastic n.
multilocular cystic n.
rat nephroma tissue culture

nephron
n. loss
single n.

nephronophthisis type 1

nephron-sparing surgery

nephropathic
n. cardiopathy
n. cystinosis
n. immune response
n. immunoglobulin

nephropathy
acute vasomotor n.
AIDS-associated n.
analgesic-associated n.
chronic allograft n.
chronic transplant n.
cisplatin n.
contrast media-induced n.
diabetic n.
heroin-associated n.
human immunodeficiency virus-associated n.
membranous n.
membranous lupus n.
minimal change n.
myeloma cast n.
pediatric lupus n.
puromycin aminonucleoside n.
reflex n.
tubulointerstitial n.

nephrophthisis-medullary cystic disease

nephrosclerosis
benign n.
hyperplastic arteriolar n.
hypertensive n.
malignant n.

nephroscope
flexible n.
percutaneous n.

nephroscopy
antegrade n.
percutaneous n.

nephrosis
congenital n.
lipoid n.
n., microcephaly, hiatus hernia syndrome

nephrosis-microcephaly syndrome

nephrosis-neuronal dysmigration syndrome

nephrostomy
n. drain
n. drainage
percutaneous n.
percutaneous nephrostomy catheter
percutaneous nephrostomy tube
pigtail nephrostomy tube
n. tube

nephrotic
congenital nephrotic syndrome
n. edema
frequently relapsing nephrotic syndrome
idiopathic minimal lesion nephrotic syndrome
idiopathic nephrotic syndrome
infantile nephrotic syndrome
later onset nephrotic syndrome
microcephaly, hiatus hernia, nephrotic syndrome
microcephaly, infantile spasm, psychomotor retardation, nephrotic syndrome
minimal change idiopathic nephrotic syndrome
minimal change nephrotic syndrome
minimal lesion nephrotic syndrome
steroid-responsive nephrotic syndrome
steroid-sensitive idiopathic nephrotic syndrome
n. syndrome

nephrotic-range proteinuria

nephrotoxic
n. acute renal failure
n. agent
n. antibody
n. antiglomerular basement membrane antibody nephritis
n. antiserum
n. drug
n. serum
n. serum nephritis

nephrotoxicity
aminoglycoside n.
contrast media n.
mercuric chloride n.

Nepuyo virus

Neri-Barré syndrome

Nernst equation

nerve
abducens nerve sign
accompanying vein of hypoglossal n.
acoustic nerve damage
n. activity
acupuncture and transcutaneous electrical nerve stimulation
acute idiopathic peripheral facial nerve palsy
acute nerve irritation
afferent digital n.
all-median nerve hand
n. allografting
all-ulnar nerve hand
alpha nerve fiber
n. anastomosis
anomalous nonrecurrent right inferior laryngeal n.
ansa cervicalis n.
ansa hypoglossal n.
antebrachial cutaneous n.
anterior abdominal cutaneous branch of intercostal n.
anterior alveolar branch of maxillary n.
anterior alveolar n.

nerve *(continued)*
anterior ampullar n.
anterior ampullary n.
anterior antebrachial n.
anterior auricular n.
anterior branch of axillary n.
anterior branch of thoracic n.
anterior crural n.
anterior cutaneous branch of femoral n.
anterior cutaneous branch of iliohypogastric n.
anterior cutaneous branch of intercostal n.
anterior cutaneous n.
anterior cutaneous nerve of abdomen
anterior ethmoidal n.
anterior femoral cutaneous n.
anterior interosseous nerve entrapment
anterior interosseous nerve of forearm
anterior interosseous nerve syndrome
anterior labial n.
anterior nerve root
anterior palatine n.
anterior pectoral cutaneous branch of intercostal n.
anterior pulmonary branch of vagus n.
anterior ramus of cervical n.
anterior ramus of lumbar n.
anterior ramus of sacral n.
anterior ramus of spinal n.
anterior ramus of thoracic n.
anterior root of spinal n.
anterior scrotal n.
anterior superior alveolar branch of infraorbital n.
anterior supraclavicular n.
anterior thoracic n.
anterior tibial n.
anterior tibial nerve dermatome
anterolateral intercostal n.
anteromedial intercostal n.
antiperipheral nerve myelin antibody
aortic depressor n.
aplasia of optic n.
n. approximator
arachnoid nerve root sheath dilation
arcuate nerve fiber bundle
area of facial n.
Arnold nerve reflex cough syndrome
artery and/or n.
artery to sciatic n.
articular branch of deep fibular n.
articular recurrent n.
atrophy of optic n.
auditory tube n.
auricular branch of vagus n.
auricular nerve of Arnold
auriculotemporal nerve syndrome
autogenous nerve graft
autonomic nerve block
autonomic nerve fiber
autonomic nerve preservation
autonomic nerve tumor
autonomic postganglionic nerve terminal
n. avulsion
avulsion of n.
axillary nerve palsy
n. biopsy
n. block
n. block anesthesia
n. block infusion
n. blocking anesthesia
brachial cutaneous n.
n. branch
n. bundle
n. canal
n. cap
cardiac sympathetic n.
carotid sinus n.
n. to carotid sinus
carotid sinus nerve stimulation
n. cell
n. cell adhesion molecule
n. cell body
n. cell death
n. cell degeneration
n. cell disorder
n. cell growth
n. cell survival
n. cell tumor
n. center
cerebral nerve ganglionectomy
cervical nerves 1–8
choking of optic nerve head
n.'s and circulation
n. coaptation
collateral nerve sprouting
comitant artery of median n.
common palmar digital n.
common palmar digital nerve of lateral plantar nerves
common palmar digital nerve of medial nerve
common palmar digital nerve of ulnar nerve
common peroneal n.
common plantar digital nerve of medial plantar nerve
communicating branch of glossopharyngeal nerve with auricular branch of vagus nerve
compound nerve action potential
n. compression
n. compression anesthesia
n. compression-degeneration syndrome
compression of spinal n.
n. compression syndrome
n. compression test
n. conduction
n. conduction deafness
conduction of nerve impulse
n. conduction velocity
n. conduction velocity study
n. conduction velocity test
conjoined nerve root anomaly
n. cooling
n. core
n. of Cotunnius
cranial n.'s
cranial nerves grossly intact
cranial nerves I–XII
cranial nerve distribution
cranial nerve impairment
cranial nerve involvement
cranial nerve palsy
cranial nerve sign
cranial nerve transection
cross-facial nerve grafting
n. crossing
n. cross section
n. crush injury
n. damage
n. deafness
n. decompression
degenerative of dopamine-producing nerve cell
diaphragmatic nerve stimulation
digital nerve block
direct eighth nerve monitoring
direct electrical nerve stimulation
N. Disability Score
n. discontinuity
disposable pudendal nerve electrode
n. distribution
distribution of median n.
dorsal cutaneous n.

dorsal nerve root
dorsal penile nerve block
n. dysplasia
efferent nerve impulse
efferent renal sympathetic nerve activity
eighth cranial n.
eighth nerve action potential
eighth nerve activity
electrical nerve stimulation
n. ending
n. entrapment
n. entrapment neuralgia
n. entrapment site
n. entrapment syndrome
n. entubulation
evoked sensory nerve action potential
n. evulsion
n. excitability test
n. of external acoustic meatus
facial n.
facial nerve block
facial nerve injury
n. factor
n. fascicle
femoral cutaneous n.
femoral nerve block
n. fiber
n. fiber action potential
N. Fiber Analyzer
N. Fiber Analyzer laser ophthalmoscope
n. fiber axon
n. fiber bundle
n. fiber bundle defect
n. fiber bundle layer
n. fiber layer analyzer
n. fiber layer dropout
n. fiber layer hemorrhage
n. fiber layer infarct
n. fiber myelination
n. fibril
n. field
n. filament
first to fifth sacral n.'s
first lumbar ventral nerve root
first through fifth lumbar vertebrae or lumbar n.
first to twelfth thoracic n.'s
n. force
functional transcutaneous nerve stimulation
n. function impairment
n. ganglion
n. gap
n. gas
n. gas poisoning
gastrointestinal autonomic nerve tumor
general somatic afferent nerve
general somatic efferent n.
general visceral afferent n.
general visceral efferent n.
glaucomatous optic nerve atrophy
glaucomatous optic nerve damage
glioma of optic n.
glossopharyngeal nerve sign
n. graft
n. of Grassi
greater palatine n.
greater splanchnic n.
n. growth factor
n. growth factor antiserum
n. growth factor receptor
n. growth inhibitor
n. growth stimulating activity
n. head angioma
n. head drusen
healthy nerve cell
hereditary atrophy optic n.
n. hook
hypogastric n.
hypoglossal nerve sign
iliohypogastric nerve block
ilioinguinal-iliohypogastric nerve block
n. impingement
impingement on spinal n.
n. implant
n. implantation
n. impulse
indirect optic nerve injury syndrome
inferior alveolar n.
inferior ganglion of vagus n.
inferior gluteal n.
n. injection
n. injury
n. input
N. Integrity Monitor 2
intercostal brachial n.
intercostal nerve block
intercostal nerve blockade
intercostal nerve cut
intercostal nerve resected
intermediate dorsal cutaneous n.
internal branch of superior laryngeal n.
internal carotid n.
internal occipital n.
internal popliteal n.
interosseous nerve of leg
n. involvement
n. irritation
jugular ganglion of vagus n.
n. junction
laser uterosacral nerve ablation
n. of Latarjet
lateral cutaneous nerve of calf
lateral cutaneous nerve of forearm
lateral cutaneous nerve of thigh
lateral ventricular n.
n. layer of retina
left sympathetic n.
lingual branch of facial n.
long buccal n.
long ciliary n.
long nerve of Bell
long saphenous n.
long subscapular n.
long thoracic nerve entrapment
long thoracic nerve palsy
n. loop
loop of hypoglossal n.
loss of nerve impulse
lower extremity nerve block
lower ganglion of glossopharyngeal n.
lower ganglion of vagus n.
lower lateral cutaneous nerve of arm
lower sacral nerve root compression
lowest splanchnic n.
lumbar splanchnic n.
lumbosacral nerve trunk
Lyme-associated peripheral facial nerve palsy
malignant nerve sheath tumor
malignant peripheral nerve sheath tumor
marginal mandibular branch of facial n.
medial antebrachial cutaneous n.
medial anterior thoracic n.
medial articular n.
medial brachial cutaneous n.
medial brachial n.
medial branch of posterior branch of spinal n.
medial branch of posterior rami of spinal n.
medial calcaneal branch of tibial n.
medial cluneal n.
medial crural cutaneous branch of saphenous n.
medial crural cutaneous n.
medial cutaneous n.

nerve *(continued)*
medial cutaneous nerve of arm
medial cutaneous nerve of forearm
medial cutaneous nerve of leg
medial dorsal cutaneous n.
median n.
median nerve hypesthesia
median nerve somatosensory evoked potential
medullated nerve fiber
meningeal branch of mandibular n.
meningeal branch of maxillary n.
meningeal branch of ophthalmic n.
meningeal branch of spinal n.
meningeal branch of vagus n.
mental branch of mental n.
microamperage electrical nerve stimulation
middle cardiac cervical n.
middle cervical cardiac n.
middle cluneal n.
middle fossa vestibular nerve section
middle gluteal n.
mixed nerve action potential
motor nerve conduction velocity
mumps facial nerve palsy
n.'s and muscles
muscle sympathetic nerve activity
muscular branch of deep fibular n.
muscular response to electrical stimulation of motor n.
myelinated retinal nerve fiber
myelination of retinal n.
nasociliary branches of ophthalmic n.
n., artery, vein, empty space, lymphatics
nervus intermedius n.
n. net pulse
neurohypophysial nerve terminal
neurolytic nerve block
neurosurgical nerve block
Nicolet N. Integrity Monitor
ninth cranial n.
nuclear-fascicular trochlear nerve palsy
nucleus of abducens n.
nucleus of abducent n.
nucleus of accessory n.
nucleus of acoustic n.
nucleus of cranial n.
nucleus of hypoglossal n.
obturator nerve damage
ocular motor cranial n.
oculomotor n.
oculomotor cranial nerve palsy
oculomotor nerve fascicle
oculomotor nerve lesion
oculomotor nerve misdirection
oculomotor nerve synkinesis
old nerve injury
olfactory cranial n.
olfactory nerve layer
opening for dorsal nerve of penis
ophthalmic recurrent n.
optic n.
optical nerve atrophy
optic nerve aplasia
optic nerve atrophy
optic nerve coloboma
optic nerve cupping
optic nerve damage
optic nerve disease
optic nerve disorder
optic nerve drusen
optic nerve dysfunction
optic nerve dysplasia
optic nerve fiber
optic nerve glioma
optic nerve head analysis
optic nerve hemangioblastoma
optic nerve injury
optic nerve lesion
optic nerve myelination
optic nerve pit
optic nerve sheath
optic nerve sheath decompression
optic nerve sheath fenestration
optic nerve sheath meningioma
optic nerve tumor
opticoacoustic nerve atrophy
orbital branch of maxillary n.
orbital optic n.
orbit, mandible, ear, cranial nerves, soft tissue syndrome
painful nerve disorder
palmar branch of anterior interosseous n.
palmar cutaneous branch of the median n.
palmar cutaneous branch of the ulnar n.
palmar digital n.
palpebral branch of infratrochlear n.
n. palsy
papilla of optic n.
papillomacular nerve fiber bundle
paracentral nerve fiber bundle
n. paralysis
parasympathetic nerve system
n. pathway
peak phrenic nerve activity
pectoral and abdominal anterior cutaneous branch of intercostal n.
pelvic autonomic n.
pelvic autonomic nerve preservation
pelvic floor n.
pelvic nerve injury
percutaneous electrical nerve stimulation
percutaneous epidural nerve stimulator
percutaneous radiofrequency facet nerve block
perforating cutaneous n.
pericardial branch of phrenic n.
perineal branch of posterior cutaneous nerve of thigh
perineal branch of posterior femoral cutaneous n.
peripapillary nerve fiber layer
peripapillary retinal n.
peripapillary retinal nerve fiber
peripheral n.
peripheral facial nerve palsy
peripheral nerve block
peripheral nerve conduction
peripheral nerve damage
peripheral nerve evaluation
peripheral nerve injury
peripheral nerve involvement
peripheral nerve lesion
peripheral nerve myelin
peripheral nerve root syndrome
peripheral nerve sheath tumor
peripheral oculomotor n.
permanent cranial nerve deficit
peroneal nerve entrapment
peroneal nerve palsy
pharyngeal branch of glossopharyngeal n.
pharyngeal branch of recurrent laryngeal n.
pharyngeal branch of vagus n.
phrenic n.
phrenic nerve stimulation
pinched sciatic n.
plantar digital n.
plexus nerve block
popliteal external n.
popliteal internal n.
popliteal lateral n.

popliteal medial n.
popliteal nerve block
posterior ampullary n.
posterior auricular n.
posterior branch of great auricular n.
posterior branch of medial cutaneous nerve of forearm
posterior branch of obturator n.
posterior branch of spinal n.
posterior cutaneous nerve of arm
posterior cutaneous nerve of forearm
posterior cutaneous nerve of thigh
posterior interosseous n.
posterior interosseous nerve of forearm
posterior lip n.
posterior tibial n.
n. pressure
n. receptor
recurrent laryngeal n.
n. reflex
n. regeneration
regeneration of n.
n. repair
repetitive nerve stimulation
retinal nerve fiber layer
n. root anomaly
n. root compression
n. root involvement
n. root irritation
n. root stimulation
n. root syndrome
sacral nerve stimulation
sciatic nerve compression
sciatic nerve entrapment
sciatic nerve syndrome
second lumbar ventral nerve root
Seddon nerve graft
selective nerve root block
n. sensation
sensory branch of radial n.
sensory nerve action potential
sensory nerve conduction velocity
seventh cranial n.
sham transcutaneous nerve stimulation
n. sheath
n. sheath malignant tumor
n. sheath meningioma
n. sheath myxoma
n. sign
n. signal
spinal accessory n.
spinal accessory nerve palsy
n. sprouting
stellate ganglion nerve block
n. stimulant
stimulate nerve impulse
n. stimulation
n. stimulator
Stoller afferent nerve stimulation
n. structure
subcutaneous nerve stimulation
superficial branch of lateral plantar n.
superficial branch of ulnar n.
superficial radial n.
superior ganglion of vagus n.
superior gluteal n.
superior internal laryngeal n.
supracapsular nerve entrapment syndrome
supraclavicular nerve block
suprascapular nerve compression
n. suture
sympathetic efferent nerve activity
sympathetic nerve block
N. Symptom Score
n. tabes
tenth cranial n.
terminal nerve ending
tethered median nerve stress test
third cranial n.
third nerve palsy
n. tissue
n. tissue regrowth
total nerve deafness
n. toxicity
toxic optic nerve atrophy
transcutaneous electrical nerve stimulation
transcutaneous electrical nerve stimulator
n. transplant
trigeminal n.
trigeminal nerve, mandibular division
trigeminal nerve, maxillary division
trigeminal nerve irritation
trigeminal nerve, ophthalmic division
n. trunk
n. tumor
twelfth cranial n.
twelfth nerve palsy
ulnar branch of medial antebrachial cutaneous n.
ulnar nerve compression
ulnar nerve conduction velocity
ulnar nerve distribution
ulnar nerve entrapment
ulnar nerve palsy
upper extremity nerve block
vagal accessory n.
vagus nerve palsy
vagus nerve paralysis
vein, artery, n.
ventral nerve root
vestibulocochlear n.
volar interosseous n.
n. of Willis

nerve-approximating clamp

nerve-muscle junction

nerve-numbing drug

nerve-sparing

n.-s. cryosurgery
n.-s. dissection
n.-s. surgery

nerve-to-soleus

nervi (*pl. of* nervus)

nervorum

arteriae n.

nervosa

anorexia n.
anorexia nervosa and associated disorders
Anorexia Nervosa Inventory for Self-Rating
bulimia n.
mild anorexia n.
National Association of Anorexia Nervosa and Associated Disorders

nervous

AIDS-related primary central nervous system lymphoma
n. and apprehensive
n. asthenopia
n. asthma
autonomic division of nervous system
autonomic nervous system disorder
autonomic nervous system dysfunction
autonomic part of peripheral nervous system
n. bladder
n. breakdown
central auditory nervous system
central nervous system
central nervous system depression
central nervous system leukemia
n. chill

nervous *(continued)*
chronic nervous degenerative disease
chronic nervous exhaustion syndrome
n. clucking
n. colon
n. consumption
n. cough
n. damage
n. debility
n. depression
development and/or central nervous system anomalies, genital hypoplasia, ear anomalies
n. discharge
n. disease
n. disorder
n. distribution
n. disturbance
n. dyspepsia
n. dysphagia
n. energy
enteric nervous system
n. eructation
n. exhaustion
n. fatigability
n. fatigue
n. force
n. gastritis
n. giggling
granulomatous angiitis of the central nervous system
n. gut
hereditary disease of nervous system
idiopathic central nervous system hypersomnolence
n. impulse
incomplete development of autonomic nervous system
n. indigestion
information processing in central nervous system
n. instability
isolated angiitis of central nervous system
late central nervous system toxicity
n. lobe
lumbar nervous plexus
lumbosacral nervous plexus
organic central nervous system deterioration
parasympathetic division of antonomic nervous system
peripheral nervous stimulator
peripheral nervous system disorder
n. personality
primary angiitis of the central nervous system
primary central nervous system
primary central nervous system lymphoma
n. respiration
n. response
n. stimulant
sympathetic autonomic nervous system
n. symptoms
n. system
n. system effect
n. system involvement
n. tachypnea
n. tension
n. tension headache
n. tic
n. tinnitus
n. tissue vaccine
n. vomiting

nervousness
n. from caffeine
n. from depression
n. from pain in back
n. and irritability
tension and n.

nervus, pl. **nervi**
n. acusticus
nervi anales inferiores
n. auricularis magnus
n. auricularis posterior
n. canalis pterygoidei
n. cervicalis superficialis
n. communicans peroneus
n. ethmoidalis anterior
n. ethmoidalis posterior
n. gluteus superior

Nesbit corporeal

nest
n.'s of nevus cells
n.'s and strands of cells
n. of von Brunn

nested
one-step nested PCR
n. PCR
n. primer
two-step nested PCR

net
n. acid excretion
n. acid flux
n. acid input
n. anabolism
apparent net transfer rate
n. calcium absorption
n. calcium influx
n. catabolism
n. dietary protein
n. efflux
n. electrochemical potential gradient
n. flux
n. gradient of fluid outflow
n. hepatic glucose uptake
n. histocompatibility ratio
neovascular n.
nerve net pulse
n. nitrogen utilization
Pap N.
parafoveal capillary n.
n. protein ratio
n. protein utilization
n. reproduction rate
total net positive
urine net charge

Netherton syndrome

N-ethylmaleimide

N-ethyl-3,4-methylenedioxyamphetamine

Netivot virus

netlike mottling

netted pattern

nettle rash

Nettleship
N. disease
N. syndrome

Nettleship-Falls-type ocular albinism

Nettleship-Falls X-linked ocular albinism

Nettleship-Wilder dilator

nettling hair

network
articular vascular n.
articular vascular network of elbow
articular vascular network of knee
artificial neural n.
artificial neural network algorithm
augmented transition n.
capitated primary care n.
community health n.
Cooperative Human Tissue N.
Drug Abuse Warning N.

n. of heel
Human Genome Epidemiology N.
hybrid neural n.
integrated health delivery n.
interpenetrating polymer n.
interstitial and perivascular collagen n.
local area communications n.
medial malleolar n.
National Comprehensive Cancer N.
National Prevention Information N.
National Women's Health N.
neural n.
n. operating system
primary care n.
probabilistic neural n.
systems network architecture
terminal capillary n.
n. theory
Toxicology Information Conversational On-Line N.

neu
n. differentiation factor

Neubauer
N. chamber
N. hemocytometer

Neufeld
N. capsular swelling
N. capsular test
N. dynamic method
N. reaction

Neugebauer-LeFort procedure

Neuhauser syndrome

neu/HER2 oncogene

Neu-Laxova syndrome

Neumann
N. cells
N. disease

Neumann-Shepard
N.-S. corneal marker
N.-S. oval optical center marker

Neuman-Tytell medium

***neu* oncogene**

Neurairtome drill

neural
n. activation
n. activity
anterior neural tube closure
anterior neural tube defect
antihypertensive neural renomedullary lipids
n. arc
n. arch
n. arch cleft
n. arch defect
n. arch fracture
n. architecture
n. arch joint
n. arch resection technique
n. arch of vertebra
artificial neural network
artificial neural network algorithm
n. atrophy
n. axis
n. axis vascular malformation
n. block
n. canal
n. capacity
cardiac neural chest
n. cell adhesion molecule
n. cell adhesive molecule
n. cell line
n. ceroid lipofuscinosis
n. claudication
n. control
n. crest
n. crest cell
n. crest-derived cell lineage
n. crest malformation
n. crest migration
n. crest origin
n. crest precursor
n. crest syndrome
n. crest tissue
n. crest tumor
n. crest tumor localization study
cutaneous neural tumor
n. cyst
n. cytoarchitecture
n. darwinism
n. deafness
n. deficit
n. discharge
n. ectoderm
n. efficiency
n. element
epidural neural blockade
n. excitation
field-electrical neural stimulation
n. filament
n. fold
n. foramen
n. foramen remodeling
n. foramina
n. foraminal canal
n. foraminal stenosis
n. foraminotomy
n. function
n. ganglion
n. groove
n. growth factor
n. growth factor receptor
n. hamster cell
n. hearing loss
hybrid neural network
n. impulse
n. index
n. larva migrans
late infantile neural ceroid lipofuscinosis
n. layer of optic part of retina
n. leprosy
n. lesion
limiting membrane of neural tube
n. lobe
n. mechanism
microamperage neural stimulation
n. neoplasm
n. network
n. nevus
orbital, mandibular, ear, neural, soft tissue
n. parenchyma
patent neural foramina
n. pathway
n. plate
probabilistic neural network
n. reflex
n. relationship
n. rim
sensory neural hearing loss
n. stalk
n. stimulus
n. structure
n. theory
n. therapy
n. thread protein
n. tissue
n. transmission
n. transmitter
n. transplantation
n. tube
n. tube defect
n. tumor

neuralgia
atypical facial n.
atypical trigeminal n.
n. of bladder
n. facialis vera
glossopharyngeal n.
idiopathic trigeminal n.
migrainous cranial n.
nerve entrapment n.
postherpetic n.
trigeminal n.

neuralgia-inducing cavitational osteonecrosis

neuralgic
n. amyotrophy
n. headache
short duration, unilateral, neuralgic, conjunctival injection and tearing

neurally
n. mediated hypotension
n. mediated vasovagal syncope

neural-mediated flushing

neuraminidase
n. deficiency
n. and galactose oxidase
hemagglutinin n.
n. inhibition
n. inhibitor
n. treatment
Vibrio cholerae n.

neurasthenia
angioparalytic n.
angiopathic n.
aviator's n.
n. gravis

neurasthenic
n. asthenopia
n. helmet
n. vertigo

neuraxial
n. desmoplastic neuroepithelial tumor
n. opioid infusion

neuraxis
midline central n.
n. radiation
n. radiotherapy
n. staging
n. tumor

neurectomy
adductor tenotomy and obturator n.
cochleovestibular n.
greater superficial petrosal n.
middle fossa vestibular n.
retrolabyrinthine vestibular n.
vestibular n.

neurenteric
n. canal
n. cyst

neurilemma cell

neurilemoma
Antoni n.
Antoni type A, B n.
malignant n.

neurinomatosis
n. centralis
n. universalis

neurite
n. extension
n. growth
n. outgrowth

neuritic
n. atrophoderma
n. cytoskeletal abnormality
n. muscular atrophy
n. plaque

neuritis
anterior ischemic optic n.
asymptomatic optic n.
atherosclerotic ischemic n.
brachial n.
experimental allergic n.
greater occipital n.
n. nodosa
optic demyelinating n.
Optic Neuritis Treatment Trial
parainfectious optic n.
paralytic brachial n.
paraneoplastic optic n.
n. plaque
retrobulbar n.
retrobulbar optic n.
n. senile plaque

neuroablative technique

neuroadenolysis of pituitary

neuroallergic syndrome

neuroanastomosis
autogenous cable graft interposition VII-VII n.
hypoglossal-facial n.
spinal accessory-hypoglossal n.

neuroanatomic
n. change
n. circuit
n. connection
n. technique

neuroanatomy of aging

neuroarticular dysfunction

neuroaxonal
infantile neuroaxonal dystrophy

neurobehavioral
n. abnormality
n. approach
n. assessment
N. Cognitive Status examination
n. consequence
n. deficit
Early Neonatal Neurobehavioral Scale
Einstein Neonatal N. Assessment Scale
n. feature
n. function
n. impairment
integrative neurobehavioral approach
N. Rating Scale
n. therapy

neuro-Behçet disease

neurobiological
n. cause
n. factor
Nursery Neurobiological Risk Score

neurobiology of early childhood development

neuroblast
olfactory n.

neuroblastoma
n. cell
human n.
murine n.
n. and opsoclonus-myoclonus

neurocardiogenic syncope

NeuroCell-HD, -PD

neurocentral joint

neurochemical
autopsy-based neurochemical study
n. change
n. disequilibrium
n. effect
false neurochemical transmitter
n. imbalance
n. impulse

neurocirculatory
n. asthenia
n. disorder
n. dystonia

neurocognitive
n. alteration
n. deficit
n. disorder
n. function
n. impairment
n. index
n. information
7-minute neurocognitive battery

neuro convex transducer

neurocristic hamartoma

neurocutaneous
n. angiomatosis
n. disorder
n. flap

n. melanosis
n. melanosis syndrome

neurodegenerative
n. disease
n. disorder
n. syndrome

neurodermatitis
localized n.
nodular n.
nummular n.

neurodevelopmental
alcohol-related neurodevelopmental disorder
n. approach
n. assessment
Bayley Infant Neurodevelopmental Screener
n. deficit
n. delay
n. disability
n. disorder
n. dysfunction
n. screening test
n. techniques
n. treatment physical therapy

neurodevelopment testing

neurodiagnostic
n. evaluation
n. procedure
n. scanner
n. study

neuroectodermal
central primitive neuroectodermal tumor
n. defect
n. dysplasia
Ewing sarcoma/peripheral neuroectodermal tumor
n. hamartoma
melanotic neuroectodermal tumor
melanotic neuroectodermal tumor of infancy
n. origin
peripheral primitive neuroectodermal tumor
primary neuroectodermal tumor
primitive neuroectodermal tumor-medulloblastoma
n. tumor

neuroeffector junction

neuroendocrine
n. body
n. cancer
n. carcinoma
n. cell
n. control
n. control loop
n. differentiation
diffuse neuroendocrine system
n. ductal carcinoma in situ
large cell neuroendocrine carcinoma
magnocellular neuroendocrine cell
moderately differentiated neuroendocrine carcinoma
n. neoplasm
primary neuroendocrine carcinoma of skin
n. programming
pulmonary neuroendocrine cell
n. reflex
n. small cell carcinoma
small cell undifferentiated neuroendocrine carcinoma
n. system
n. theory
n. tumor

neuroendocrinological disease

neuroepithelial
Askin thoracopulmonary neuroepithelial tumor
n. body
n. body in lung
n. cell
n. cell migration
n. cell proliferation
n. cells
n. cyst
dysembryoplastic neuroepithelial tumor
n. element of retina
n. layer of retina
neuraxial desmoplastic neuroepithelial tumor
pulmonary neuroepithelial endocrine
n. tumor

neuroepithelioma
orbital n.
peripheral n.

neuroepithelium
n. of ampullary crest
n. of macula

neurofacial-digitorenal syndrome

neurofeedback training

neurofibrae
n. efferentes

neurofibrillary
n. degeneration
n. tangle

neurofibroma
aryepiglottic fold n.
limbal n.
molluscoid n.
myometrial n.
nevi, atrial myxoma, myxoid neurofibroma, and ephelides syndrome
orbital n.
ovarian n.
n. of pleura
plexiform n.

neurofibromas

neurofibromatosis
n. 2 gene
n., type I
n., type II
n., type 1 syndrome
n. type 1, 2
n. with Noonan phenotype

neurofibromatosis-Noonan syndrome

neurofilament
n. promoter
n. protein
n. triplet polypeptide
n. triplets antibody

neurogastrointestinal
mitochondrial neurogastrointestinal encephalomyopathy
n. peptide

neurogenic
n. abnormality
n. acquired ptosis
n. airway
n. arthrogryposis
n. arthropathy
autonomic neurogenic bladder
axonopathic neurogenic thoracic outlet syndrome
n. bladder
n. bladder disorder
n. bladder dysfunction
n. blepharoptosis
n. bowel
n. cachexia
central neurogenic hyperventilation
n. claudication
n. clubfoot
n. component
n. diabetes insipidus
n. disease
n. disorder
n. dysarthria
n. dysphagia
n. dysplasia of hip

neurogenic *(continued)*
n. equinus deformity
n. erectile dysfunction
n. factor
n. fiber type group
n. fracture
n. hip disease
n. hip dysplasia
n. hypertension
n. hyperventilation
n. hypogonadism
n. iris atrophy
n. mesenchyme
n. motor evoked potential
n. muscle weakness, ataxia, and retinitis pigmentosa
n. muscular atrophy
n. orthostatic hypotension
n. peripheral intermittent claudication
n. precocious puberty
n. pulmonary edema
n. sarcoma
n. shock
n. theory
n. tonus
n. tumor
uninhibited neurogenic bladder
upper motor neurogenic bladder

neuroglia
n. cell
peripheral n.

neuroglial
n. cell
n. fiber

neuroglycopenic symptom

neurohormonal
n. abnormality
n. cell
n. function
n. stimulation

neurohumoral
n. control of motility
n. disease
n. excitation state
n. factor
n. hypothesis

neurohypophyseal hormone

neurohypophysial
n. diabetes insipidus
n. hormone
n. nerve terminal
n. peptide
n. stalk

neurohypophysis
infundibulum of n.

neuroichthyosis-hypogonadism syndrome

neuroid
n. cell
n. nevus

neuroimaging
n. approach
n. assessment
n. study

neuroimmune dysfunction

neurointermediate nursing unit

neurokinin-1 receptor antagonist

neurokinin A, B

neuroleptanalgesia
n. anesthesia
n. anesthetic technique

neuroleptic
n. adjunct
n. agent
n. anesthesia
n. antipsychotic drug
n. dosage
n. dose
n. dose-dependent akathisia
n. dosing
n. exposure
long-acting n.
malignant neuroleptic syndrome
n. malignant syndrome
n. medication
n. therapy
n. toxicity
n. withdrawal

neuroleptic-induced
n.-i. acute dystonia
n.-i. acute movement disorder
n.-i. akathisia
n.-i. akinesia
n.-i. dysphoria
n.-i. tardive dyskinesia

neurolinguistic
n. assessment
n. deficit
n. program

neurolipomatosis dolorosa

neurologic
n. abnormality
N. and Adaptive Capacity Score
n. adverse effect
adverse neurologic complication
n. age
n. assessment
bilirubin-induced neurologic dysfunction
n. bladder dysfunction
n. bladder lesion
n. check
n. cognition
n. company
n. complication
n. complication of systemic cancer
n. control
n. defect
n. deficit
degenerative neurologic disease
delayed ischemic neurologic deficit
n. demyelinating disease
n. deterioration
n. development
n. diagnosis
n. disability
N. Disability Score
n. disorder
n. disturbance
n. dysfunction
n. dysregulation
n. endemic cretinism
n. evaluation
n. event
n. examination
n. feature
focal neurologic deficit
focal neurologic disturbance
n. function
n. genodermatosis
n. geriatrics
global neurologic dysfunction
gross neurologic deficit
n. handicap
high-pressure neurologic syndrome
n. impairment
n. improvement
n. instability
n. intensive care unit
n. involvement
metabolic disorder with neurologic dysfunction
n. migraine
minor neurologic dysfunction
objective neurologic signs
other neurologic disease
other neurologic disorder
paraneoplastic neurologic syndrome
n. paraneoplastic syndrome
peripheral neurologic adverse effect

physical and neurologic examination for soft signs
prolonged reversible ischemic neurologic deficit
n. rehabilitation
resolving ischemic neurologic deficit
reversible ischemic neurologic deficit
reversible ischemic neurologic disability
n. specialist
n. status
n. symptom
n. symptomatology
n. syndrome
transient focal neurologic event
transient neurologic symptoms
n. vital signs

neurological
n. amnesia
n. apnea
n. assessment
awake neurological assessment
n. basis
chronic infantile neurological, cutaneous, and articular
n. complication
n. condition
n. control
n. damage
n. defect
n. deficit
deteriorating neurological disorder
n. disability
n. disease
n. disease syndrome
n. disorder
n. disturbance
n. dysfunction
n. effect
n. emergency
n. evaluation
n. evoked response
n. examination
N. Examination for Children
n. examination of extremities
focal neurological impairment
n. footdrop
n. function
n. functioning
n. hammer
n. handicap
n. illness
impaired neurological function
n. impairment
n. injury
n. irregularity
late neurological toxicity
n. parameter
postmalarial neurological syndrome
progressive intellectual and neurological deterioration
n. rehabilitation
severe neurological impairment
n. sign
n. signs stable
n. symptom
n. syndrome
n. testing
n. trauma
Yasargil neurological instrument

neurologically
n. evoked response
n. handicapped
n. impaired
n. intact

neurologiccirculatoryrange
neurologic/circulatory/range of motion

neurologic/circulatory/range of motion

neurology
child n.
psychiatry and n.

neuroloptic drug

neurolymphomatosis
avian neurolymphomatosis virus

neurolysis
celiac plexus n.
mucosal n.

neurolytic
n. celiac plexus block
n. drug
n. nerve block

neuroma
acoustic n.
amputation stump n.
angiolipoma, posttraumatic neuroma, glomus tumor, eccrine spiradenoma, and leiomyoma cutis
n. in continuity
n. cutis
n. excision
mucosal neuroma syndrome
multicystic acoustic n.
multiple basal cell neuroma syndrome
multiple mucosal n.
multiple mucosal neuroma syndrome
palisaded encapsulated n.
slow-growing acoustic n.

neuromatosis elephantiasis

neuromechanical correction

neuromediated syncope

neurometric test battery

neuromodulatory
percutaneous neuromodulatory therapy

Neuromotor
Harris Infant Neuromotor Test

neuromuscular
n. atrophy
autoimmune neuromuscular junction disorder
n. block
n. blockade
n. blockade monitoring
n. blockage
n. blocking agent
n. blocking drug
body oscillation neuromuscular gain
n. cell
n. choristoma
chronic neuromuscular disease
n. complication of drug abuse
n. component
n. condition
n. contractility
n. control
n. control exercise
n. deficit
n. development of speech
n. disease
n. disorder
n. disorder-causing drug
n. effect
n. electrical stimulation therapy
n. electrical stimulator
n. eyelid retraction
n. facilitation
n. feedback training
n. firing
n. firing in normal subject
n. firing in spastic subject
n. function
functional neuromuscular stimulation
n. gait pattern change
n. hamartoma
n. hypertension
n. imbalance
n. integration

neuromuscular *(continued)*
n. junction
n. maturity
n. maturity assessment
n. pacification
n. paralysis
progressive idiopathic neuromuscular disease
proprioceptive neuromuscular facilitation
proprioceptive neuromuscular fasciculation reaction
n. ptosis
n. reeducation technique
n. spindle
submaximal neuromuscular block
n. tension
n. tension state
n. therapy
n. toxicity
n. transmission
n. transmission blockade
n. unit
n. weakness

neuromuscularly handicapped

neuromyelitis optica

neuromyoarterial glomus

neuromyopathic
n. disease
n. disorder

neuron
alpha motor n.
argyrophilic and argyophobic n.
autonomic motor n.
n. body
n. of brain
complete lower motor neuron lesion
n. doctrine
fast component of n.
giant serotonin-containing n.
histamine-containing n.
n. in spinal cord
n. II
lower motor n.
lower motor neuron disease
lower motor neuron lesion
lower motor neuron palsy
magnocellular cholinergic n.
magnocellular neurosecretory n.
motor n.
motor neuron palsy
motor neuron sign
motor neuron weakness
noncholinergic n.
pain transmission n.
pontosubicular neuron necrosis
primary afferent nociceptor n.
sensory n.
shrunken atrophied n.'s
n. in spinal cord
survival motor neuron telomeric gene
sympathetic preganglionic n.
thalamic projection n.
tuberohypophyseal dopaminergic n.
tuberoinfundibular dopaminergic n.
upper motor n.
upper motor neuron lesion
ventromedial hypothalamic neuron, nucleus

neuronal
n. achromasia
n. activation
n. activity
adenohypophysial neuronal choristoma
n. adhesion
n. aggregate
n. apoptosis inhibitory protein
n. apoptotic process
n. cell
n. cell apoptosis
n. cell line
n. cell origin tumor
n. ceroid lipofuscinosis
n. ceroid lipofuscinosis curvilinear body
n. circuit
n. connection
n. cytoplasm
n. cytosol
n. cytotoxic edema
n. damage
n. death
n. degeneration
n. differentiation
n. discharge
n. dysplasia
n. element firing
n. excitability
n. feedback loop
n. feed-forward loop
n. function
n. GM1 gangliosidosis
n. hamartoma
n. heterotopia
n. hyperexcitability
hypoxic-ischemic neuronal injury
n. impulse
n. interconnection
intestinal neuronal dysplasia
n. intranuclear inclusion disease
juvenile-onset neuronal ceroid lipofuscinosis
large neuronal polypeptide
n. metabolism
n. microdysgenesis
n. migration disorder
n. migration disorders
pituitary adenoma-adenohypophysial neuronal choristoma
n. shock
n. somata
n. vacuolation

neuronal-glial tumor

neuron-specific
n.-s. cytoskeletal protein
n.-s. enolase
n.-s. enolase stain
n.-s. enolase tumor marker

neuro-ophthalmic manifestation

neuro-ophthalmologic
n.-o. case history
n.-o. diagnosis
n.-o. examination
n.-o. manifestation

neuroparalytic
n. keratitis
n. keratopathy
n. ophthalmia

neuropathic
n. albuminuria
n. amyloidosis
n. anhidrosis
n. ankle
n. arthritis
n. arthrogryposis multiplex congenita
n. arthropathy
n. atrophy
n. bladder
n. cachexia
chronic diabetic neuropathic pain
chronic infectious neuropathic agent
n. collapse
n. cystinosis
diabetic neuropathic osteoarthropathy
n. diathesis
n. disease
n. disorder
n. edema
n. eschar

n. eyelid retraction
n. foot
n. foot deformity
n. forefoot ulceration
n. fracture
n. hyperkyphoscoliosis
n. joint disease
n. muscular atrophy
n. pain
n. tonic pupil
n. ulcer

neuropathy
acute motor-axonal n.
acute motor-sensory axonal n.
alcoholic peripheral n.
alcohol-induced peripheral n.
anterior compressive optic n.
anterior ischemic optic n.
anterograde fast component n.
arsenic peripheral n.
arteriosclerotic ischemic optic n.
arteritic anterior ischemic optic n.
asymmetric motor n.
autonomic n.
autosomal dominant hereditary optic n.
autosomal recessive hereditary optic n.
autosympathectomy secondary to n.
avitaminosis B_{12} peripheral n.
brachial plexus n.
n. of chemotherapy
chronic sensorimotor n.
congenital hypomyelinating n.
diabetic autonomic n.
diabetic peripheral n.
distal acquired demyelinating symmetrical n.
distal symmetric sensory n.
familial visceral n.
n. of feet
giant axonal n.
griseofulvin peripheral n.
hereditary motor sensory neuropathy II-deafness-mental retardation
hereditary motor-sensory neuropathy type IA, II, III–VII
hereditary neuropathy with liability for pressure palsy
hereditary sensory n.
hereditary sensory and autonomic neuropathy types I-IV
hereditary sensory motor neuropathy type I–III
hereditary neuropathy with susceptibility to pressure palsy
hypertensive optic n.
hypertrophic n.
ischemic optic n.
Leber hereditary optic n.
lupus erythematosus peripheral n.
membranous n.
methyl alcohol peripheral n.
Michigan Diabetic N. Score
Michigan N. Screening Test
motor dapsone n.
motor neuropathy with multifocal conduction block
motor-sensory axonal n.
motor-sensory neuropathy, X-linked Type II, with deafness and mental retardation
multifocal demyelinating motor n.
multifocal motor n.
myenteric plexus n.
Navajo n.
nonarteritic anterior ischemic optic n.
nondiabetic immune-mediated n.
nutritional optic n.
onion bulb n.
optic n.
optic and chiasmal n.
n. pain
painful diabetic n.
parainfectious optic n.
peripheral autonomic n.
peripheral diabetic n.
peroneal entrapment n.
posterior ischemic optic n.
progressive hypertrophic interstitial n.
radiation optic n.
sensory ataxic neuropathy with dysarthria and ophthalmoplegia
subacute sensory n.
tropical ataxic n.
ulnar compression n.

neuropeptide
n. change
n. gamma
n. gene
n. immunocytochemistry

neuropeptide B, K, Y

neurophysin
n. associated with vasopressin
estrogen-stimulated n.
human n.
n. II
n. I, II
nicotine-stimulated n.
oxytocin-associated n.
n. protein

neurophysin I

neurophysin-positive varicosity

neurophysiologic
n. change
n. factor
intraoperative neurophysiologic monitoring

neurophysiological
n. assessment
n. finding
n. heterogeneity

neuropilin
n. 1 assay
n. 2 assay

neuroprotective
n. drug
n. therapy

neuropsychiatric
n. acquired immunodeficiency syndrome rating scale
n. condition
n. disease
n. disorder
n. drug
n. effect
n. feature
N. Inventory
Mini International N. Interview
pediatric autoimmune neuropsychiatric diseases associated with streptococcal infection
pediatric autoimmune neuropsychiatric disorders associated with streptococcal infection
n. symptom
n. syndrome of systemic lupus erythematosus

neuropsychologic
n. area
n. assessment
n. battery
n. characteristic
n. deficit
n. disorder
n. domain
n. evaluation
n. examination
n. finding
n. functioning
n. impairment
n. testing

neuropsychological
Adult Neuropsychological Questionnaire
n. assessment
Brief Neuropsychological Mental Status Examination
Child Neuropsychological Questionnaire
n. defect
n. deficiency
n. deficit
delayed neuropsychological sequela
n. evaluation
n. function
Halstead-Reitan Neuropsychological Battery
Halstead-Reitan Neuropsychological Test Battery
n. impairment
Luria-Nebraska Neuropsychological Battery
Monas-Nitz Neuropsychological Battery
Reitan-Indiana Neuropsychological Battery
n. test
n. test battery
n. testing
n. test profile
n. test Z score

neuroradiological findings

neuroradiologic imaging procedure

neurorehabilitation strategy

neuroretinal rim

neuroretinopathy
hypertensive n.
macular n.

neurosecretory
n. cell
n. gland
n. granule
magnocellular neurosecretory neuron
magnocellular neurosecretory system
n. material
n. vessel

Neurosector
ATL real-time Neurosector scan imaging
ATL real-time Neurosector scanner

neurosensorial free medial plantar flap

neurosensory
n. deafness
n. deficit
n. flap
n. impairment
n. retina
n. retinal detachment

neurosis, pl. **neuroses**
acute conditioned n.
anxiety n.
Freeman Anxiety N. and Psychosomatic Test
generalized anxiety n.
low back n.
obsessive-compulsive n.
Obsessive-Compulsive N. Scale
occlusal habit n.
pain-type anxiety n.
Psychiatric Questionnaire Obsessive-Compulsive N.

neuro-specific enolase antibody

neurostimulating procedure

neurostimulator
percutaneous epidural n.

neurosurgery
n. intensive care unit
n. needle holder

neurosurgical
n. anesthesia
n. approach
N. Cervical Spine Scale
n. closure
n. continuous care unit
n. evaluation
n. examination
n. gamma knife
n. headrest
n. intensive care unit
n. intervention
n. nerve block

neurosyphilis
asymptomatic n.
n. cryptomeningitis
ectodermogenic n.
meningovascular n.
mesodermogenic n.
parenchymatous n.
paretic n.

neurotensin
radioassayable n.
n. receptor type 1, 2

neurotensin-like immunoreactivity

neurotic
n. acting out
adolescent neurotic delinquency
affective neurotic personality disorder
antisocial neurotic personality
antisocial neurotic personality disorder
n. anxiety state
anxiety state neurotic disorder
n. atrophy
atypical neurotic anxiety state
avoidant neurotic personality disorder
n. delinquency
n. depression
n. depressive reaction
n. depressive state
n. direction profile
n. excoriation
n. factor
n. fatigue
n. feature
n. guilt
n. hysteric disorder
n. illness
masculine attitude in female n.
n. obsessive
obsessive n.
n. overlay
panic attack neurotic anxiety state
n. patient
N. Personality Factor Test
reactive neurotic depression
n. score
n. syndrome

neuroticism
N. Scale Questionnaire

neuroticum
papilloma n.

neurotized melanocytic nevus

neurotologic
n. complication
n. examination

neurotomy
glossopharyngeal n.
opticociliary n.

neurotonic
n. congestion
n. pupil
n. reaction

neurotoxic
n. cascade
n. drug
n. effect

n. esterase
n. shellfish poisoning

neurotoxicity
antibiotic n.
antihistamine n.
n. of chemotherapy
codeine n.
n. of methamphetamine
peripheral n.

neurotoxin
eosinophil-derived n.

neurotransmitter
n. action
n. activity
ascending neurotransmitter system
brain n.
n. change
n. depletion
imbalance in neurotransmitter level
n. release

neurotrauma center

Neurotrend continuous multiparameter system

neurotrophic
n. atrophy
brain-derived neurotrophic factor
ciliary-derived neurotrophic factor receptor
ciliary neurotrophic factor
n. enhancing molecule
n. factor
n. factor expression
n. food ulcer
n. fracture
glial-derived neurotrophic factor
heparin-binding neurotrophic factor
n. hormone
n. keratitis
n. keratopathy
lung-derived neurotrophic factor
middle glial cell line-derived neurotrophic factor
n. tyrosine kinase receptor, type 1
n. therapy
n. ulcer
n. virus

neurotropic
n. attraction
brain-derived neurotropic factor
desmoplastic neurotropic melanoma
n. effect
n. environment
glial cell line-derived neurotropic factor
n. virus

neurovascular
n. anatomy
n. bundle
n. bundle of Walsh
n. check
n. complication
n. compression
n. compression syndrome
n. compromise
n. corn
n. cross compression
n. dystrophy
n. free flap
n. hilus
n. laboratory
noninvasive neurovascular studies
n. sheath
n. status
n. structure

neurovegetative functioning or symptom

neurovesicle dysfunction

neurovisceral lipidosis

neurovisual manifestation

neutral
n. amino acid
n. amyloid probe
n. angle
n. anteversion
articulatory specified neutral reference
n. attitude
n. axis
n. axis of straight beam
n. buffered formalin fixative
calcium-activated neutral protease
n. density
n. density filter test
n. detergent fiber
n. endopeptidase
n. endopeptidase inhibition
n. fraction
n. or gray area
n. hip position
n. hook
ichthyosis and neutral lipid storage disease
n. image
large neutral amino acid
n. lipid storage disease
n. metallopeptidase
n., sidebent right, rotated left
n. point
n. protamine Hagedorn insulin
n. protease
n. proteinase
quadriceps neutral angle
n. red
n. regular insulin
subtalar joint neutral position
n. thermal environment
n. zone

neutralization
acid neutralization capacity
anterior n.
n. epitope
focus-reduction neutralization test
n. index
n. index method
logarithm neutralization index
mouse neutralization test
plaque n.
platelet neutralization procedure
serum n.
n. technique
n. test
toxin n.
virus n.

neutralized
heparin neutralized thrombin time

neutralize stomach acidity

neutralizing
n. acid in stomach
n. antibody
n. antibody to vascular endothelial growth factor
n. murine monoclonal antitumor necrosis factor antibody
parvovirus B19 neutralizing antibody assay

neutrocytic
culture-negative neutrocytic ascites

neutrogenic precautions

neutron
n. absorption process
n. activation analysis
n. beam
n. beam radiation
n. beam therapy
n. bombardment
boron neutron capture therapy
n. capture therapy
instrumental neutron activation analysis
mixed neutron and photon radiotherapy
n. number
number of neutrons in an atomic nucleus

neutron *(continued)*
n. number density
partial body neutron activation
radiochemical neutron activation analysis
n. radiography
n. technique
n. therapy machine
total body neutron activation
total body neutron activation analysis
unit of neutron dosage

neutropenia
alloimmune neonatal n.
autoimmune n.
autoimmune neutropenia of infancy
bone marrow transplant n.
chemotherapy-induced n.
chronic benign n.
drug-related n.
febrile n.
idiopathic n.
malignancy associated n.
neonatal autoimmune n.
neonatal chronic idiopathic n.
severe chronic n.
severe congenital n.

neutropenia-related bacterial infection

neutropenic
n. colitis
n. enterocolitis
n. fever
n. host
n. patient

neutrophil
absolute neutrophil count
n. actin deficiency
n. actin dysfunction
n. activating factor
n. activation
afunctional n.
n. aggregation activity
n. alkaline phosphatase
n. antibody
n. antibody and transfusion reaction
n. apoptosis
assay neutrophil cytoplasmic antibody
n. bactericidal index
band n.
n. band
bone marrow neutrophil reserve
n. chemotactant factor
n. chemotactic activity
n. chemotactic deficiency
n. chemotactic factor
n. chemotactic peptide
n. chemotactic response
n. chemotaxis
n. defect
n. diffraction factor
n. dysfunction
n. dysplasia
n. egress
n. elastase
n. engraftment
n. functional disorder
n. granule
n. granulopoiesis
human neutrophil collagenase
human neutrophil elastase
human neutrophil peptide-4
hypersegmented n.
n. ingress
n. leukocyte count
n. lobe count
marrow neutrophil reserve
n. migration
n. migration-inhibition factor
monocyte-derived neutrophil chemotactic factor
n. myelocyte
nonsegmented n.'s
partially functional n.
polymorphonuclear n.
polymorphonuclear neutrophil chemotactic factor
n. polynucleosis
n. pooling
n. recovery
n. reserve
n. respiratory burst activity
segmented n.'s
stab n.
stabkernige band n.
totally functional n.

neutrophil-activating
anionic neutrophil-activating peptide
n.-a. factor
n.-a. peptide
n.-a. peptide-1
n.-a. protein

neutrophilic
acute febrile neutrophilic dermatosis
n. cell
n. chemotactic factor
chronic neutrophilic leukemia
n. cryptitis
n. dermatosis
n. eccrine hidradenitis
febrile neutrophilic dermatosis
n. gastroduodenitis
n. infiltration
n. inflammation
n. intraepidermal IgA dermatosis
n. leukemia
n. leukocyte
n. leukocytosis
n. myelocyte
n. necrosis
n. pleocytosis
n. polymorphonuclear leukocyte
polymorphonuclear neutrophilic granulocyte
polymorphonuclear neutrophilic leukocyte
n. xanthoma

neutrophil-immobilizing factor

neutrophil-inducing activity

neutrophil-mediated joint inflammation

neutrophils

neutrophil-specific secondary granule deficiency

neutropic drug

never exposed

nevi (*pl. of* nevus)

Neviaser
N. acromioclavicular technique
N. arthroplasty
N. frozen shoulder classification

Neville upper reservoir buffer

Nevin staging

nevocellular nevus

nevocytic
congenital nevocytic nevus
n. nevus

nevoid
n. amentia
n. anomaly
n. basal cell carcinoma syndrome
n. basal cell epithelioma, jaw cysts, bifid rib syndrome
n. elephantiasis
n. hyperkeratosis of nipple and areola
n. hypermelanosis
n. hypertrichosis
n. keratosis
n. lentigo
linear and whorled nevoid hypermelanosis

n. malignant melanoma
multiple basal cell nevoid syndrome
multiple nevoid, basal cell epithelioma, jaw cysts, bifid rib syndrome
n. telangiectasia

Nevo syndrome

nevus, pl. **nevi**

n. acneiformis unilateralis
acquired melanocytic n.
n. anemicus
angiomatoid Spitz n.
angiomatous involuting n.
n. arachnoideus
n. araneus
nevi, atrial myxoma, myxoid neurofibroma, and ephelides syndrome
A-type nevus cell
atypical melanocytic n.
basal cell n.
basal cell nevus syndrome
n. cavernosus
n. cell
n. cell, A-, B-, C-type
cellular blue n.
cerebriform intradermal n.
congenital melanocytic n.
congenital nevocytic n.
deep penetrating n.
n. depigmentosus
dysplastic n.
dysplastic nevus syndrome
epithelioid combined nevi
epithelioid combined nevi deep penetrating n.
n. epitheliomatocylindromatosus
familial dysplastic nevus syndrome
n. fibrosus
n. follicularis keratosis
giant congenital melanocytic n.
giant pigmented hairy n.
hair follicle n.
inflamed linear verrucous epidermal n.
inflammatory linear verrucous epidermal n.
n. of Ito
n. of Jadassohn
Jadassohn nevus phakomatosis
lentigines, atrial myxomas, cutaneous papular myxomas, blue nevi
lichen striatus epidermal n.
linear epidermal n.
linear inflammatory verrucous epidermal n.
linear sebaceous nevus sequence
linear sebaceous nevus syndrome
n. lymphaticus
malignant blue n.
mast cell n.
melanocytic n.
n. mollusciformis
n. morus
multiple basal cell carcinoma syndrome multiple basal cell nevus syndrome
n. nervosus
nests of nevus cells
nevocellular n.
nodular connective tissue disease n.
oral epithelial n.
n. of Ota
Ota nevus syndrome
n. papillaris
n. papillomatosus
n. pigmentosus
n. pigmentosus et pilosus
plexiform spindle cell n.
n. profundus
n. sanguineus
n. sebaceous
n. sebaceous of Feuerstein and Mims
n. sebaceus
n. sebaceus of Jadassohn
n. simplex
n. spilus
n. spilus lentigo
spindle cell n.
n. spongiosus albus mucosa
n. sudoriferous
n. syndrome
n. unius lateralis
n. varicosus osteohypertrophicus
n. vascularis
n. vasculosus
n. vasculosus osteohypertrophicus
n. venosus
n. verrucosis
n. vinosus
n. of vulva

nevus-cell nevus

new

n. admission
n. age
n. age suicide prevention
n. antigenic determinant
n. approaches to brain tumor therapy
n. approaches to coronary intervention
assumption of new identity
n. bag hung
N. Ballard Score
n. bone formation
n. chemical entity
n. column of bone
n. combination
n. dermis
n. device angioplasty
n. differentiation factor
n. dosage form
n. drug
n. drug therapy
elevated new vessels elsewhere
elevated new vessels on the disc
n. evidence
extensive new bone formation
n. fuchsin
growth and maturation of new skin
N. Hampshire rule
n. happy bur
N. Haven study
n. host cell
n. identity
N. Injury Severity Score
investigational new animal drug
n. lesion formation
n. methylene blue N stain
N. Mexico Attitude Toward Work Test
N. Mexico Career Planning Test
N. Mexico Knowledge of Occupations Test
N. Minto virus
n. molecular entity
n. mutation
neovascularization of new vessels elsewhere
New York City medium
New Zealand obese mouse
New Zealand white mouse
no new laboratory test orders
no new order
N. and Nonofficial Drugs
n. patient
n. patient set-up
replaced with new bone
retaining new information
n. skin growth
stimulate new vessel growth
n. tuberculin
tuberculin R new tuberculin
tuberculin Ruckland new tuberculin

new *(continued)*
n. variant Creutzfeldt-Jakob disease
n. vessel
n. vessel disc
n. vessels elsewhere
n. working formulation
N. World hemorrhagic fever
N. World leishmaniasis
N. World screwworm
N. York erysiphake
N. York Heart Association classification of heart disease
N. York vaccinia virus
N. Zealand green-lipped mussel
N. Zealand mice

newborn
n. abuse
alloimmune hemolytic disease of n.
n. anesthesia
n. Apgar score
n. aspiration
aspiration of n.
B-cytomegalic inclusion disease of n.
N. Behavior Assessment Scale
n. calf serum
n. care
n. center
n. circumcision
congenital anemia of n.
n. conjunctivitis
n. convalescent care unit
n. crossmatch
Distress Scale for Ventilated N. Infants
drowned newborn syndrome
n. drug toxicity
n. drug withdrawal
n. examination
extended jaundice of n.
full-term n.
n. helpful hints
hemolytic anemia of n.
hemolytic disease of n.
hemorrhage of n.
hemorrhagic disease of n.
n. hepatitis
hyperthermia in n.
idiopathic respiratory distress of n.
n. infant
n. infant care
n. intensive care
n. intensive care unit
jaundice of n.
n. maturity rating
metabolic disease in n.
n. mouse
n. mouse brain
n., term, normal, female
n., term, normal, male
normal n.
normal newborn nursery
n. nursery
Parrot atrophy of n.
persistent pulmonary hypertension of n.
premature n.
preterm n.
n. respiratory distress syndrome
n. resuscitation
resuscitation of depressed n.
n. screening kit
n. screening program
n. screen serum thyroxine and phenylketonuria
n. special care unit
tachypnea of n.
term n.
term living n.
transient hyperammonemia of n.
transient respiratory distress of the n.
transient tachypnea of n.
universal newborn hearing screening program

Newcastle
N. bone disease
N. classification
N. disease virus
N. disease virus therapy
enhancement Newcastle disease
N. virus disease

Newcastle-Manchester bacillus

newer rifamycin

Newfoundland
Memorial University of Newfoundland Scale of Happiness

new-generation
n.-g. antipsychotic
n.-g. antipsychotic drug

Newington brace

newly
n. abstinent alcoholic
n. acquired disease
n. diagnosed
n. diagnosed diabetes
n. emergent categorical change
n. presented
n. reformulated

Newman classification of radial neck and head fracture

Newman-Keuls
N.-K. procedure
N.-K. test

new-onset
n.-o. diabetes mellitus
n.-o. hydrocephalus
n.-o. JDM
n.-o. seizures

Newport
N. hip system
N. medical instrument

newton
N. disk
N. force
n. per meter
n. per square centimeter
n. per square meter

newtonian
n. aberration
n. body
n. constant of gravitation
n. flow
n. fluid

newton-meter

newton-second per square meter

NewVues lens

Nexacryl
N. tissue adhesive

NexGen component

next
n. generation
n. of kin
n. time
n. visit

Neyman-Pearson statistical hypothesis

Nezelof
N. syndrome
N. type of thymic alymphoplasia

Nezhat-Dorsey suction-irrigator

***NF-1* gene**

NF-1 transcription factor

***NF-2* gene**

NF-ATc protein

NF-κB
receptor activator of N.

NF-kappa-B element

N-formylglycinamide ribotide

Ngaingan virus

Ngari virus

ni
- *Trichoplusia ni* SNPV

niacin
- n. accumulation test
- n. deficiency
- n. maculopathy

Niamtu video imaging system

Nicholas
- N. five-in-one reconstruction
- N. five-in-one reconstruction technique

Nichols
- N. procedure
- N. radioimmunoassay

nicked free beta subunit of human chorionic gonadotropin

nickel
- n. allergy
- arsenic nickel silicon
- n. dermatitis
- n. and dime lesion
- n. hand dermatitis
- n. sensitivity
- n. sulfate

nickel-cadmium

nickel-titanium
- n.-t. alloy
- n.-t. file

Nickerson medium

nicking
- arteriovenous n.
- hemorrhages, exudates, and/or n.
- Nida nicking operation
- n. of retinal vein

nick translation

Nicola arthroplasty

Nicolas-Favre disease

Nicolau syndrome

Nicolet Nerve Integrity Monitor

Nicoll
- N. bone
- N. cancellous bone graft
- N. cancellous insert graft
- N. classification
- N. fracture operation
- N. fracture repair procedure

Nicolle-Novy-MacNeal medium culture

Nicolle white mycetoma

Nicol prism

nicotinamide
- n. adenine dinucleotidase
- n. adenine dinucleotide
- n. adenine dinucleotide glycohydrolase
- n. adenine dinucleotide phosphate positive
- n. mononucleotide
- oxidized form of nicotinamide adenine dinucleotide
- oxidized form of nicotinamide adenine dinucleotide phosphate

nicotinamide-adenine dinucleotide

nicotine
- n. abstinence
- n. abuse
- n. addict
- n. addiction
- n. administration
- n. craving
- n. dependence
- Fagerstrom Test for Nicotine Dependence
- n. gum
- n. habit
- n. inhaler
- n. nasal spray
- n. patch
- n. patch therapy
- physical dependence on nicotine gum
- n. replacement therapy
- n. skin patch
- n. stomatitis
- tar and n.
- n. tartrate
- transdermal nicotine patch
- n. transdermal patch
- n. transdermal system
- n. withdrawal

nicotine-related
- n.-r. disorder NOS
- n.-r. disorder, not otherwise specified

nicotine-stimulated
- n.-s. neurophysin
- n.-s. pathway

nicotinic
- n. acetylcholine receptor
- n. acid
- n. acid deficiency
- n. acid dehydrogenase
- n. acid maculopathy
- n. acid mononucleotide
- n. agonist
- n. cholinergic receptor
- n. receptor blockade therapy

nicotinic-type receptor

nictitans
- membrana n.

nictitating
- n. membrane
- n. membrane response
- n. spasm

Nida nicking operation

nidus
- n. angle
- arteriovenous malformation n.
- arteriovenous malformation nidus definition
- n. avis
- AVM nidus definition
- n. definition
- n. demarcation

Nieden syndrome

Niemann
- N. disease
- N. splenomegaly

Niemann-Pick
- N.-P. C disease
- N.-P. C1 disease
- N.-P. cell
- N.-P. disease
- N.-P. disease, type A, B, C, D
- N.-P. disease type I, II

Niemeier
- N. classification
- N. gallbladder perforation

Nievergelt disease

niger
- locus n.

night
- all night sleep recording
- n. blindness
- n. brace
- n. care facility
- chills, fever, and night sweats
- congenital stationary night blindness
- n. cramp
- current night terrors
- drenching night sweats
- each bedtime, every n.
- n. eating syndrome
- every n.
- n. fantasy
- n. fear
- fever and night sweats

night *(continued)*
n. frequency of voiding
n. grinding of teeth
n. hospital
Lorenz night splint
morning and n.
n. and morning
n. myopia
shaking chills and night sweats
n. sight
n. sleep deprivation
n. sleep recording
n. soil
n. sweats
tension night splint
n. terrors
n. vision
n. wandering

night-day rhythm

Nightingale examining lamp

nightly intermittent peritoneal dialysis

nightmare
n. disorder
insomnia and n.'s
rescripting n.

nighttime
n. activity
n. agitation
alcohol-induced nighttime sleep
n. awakening
n. calf cramp
n. heartburn
n. leg cramp
n. urination
n. voiding

nigra
dermatosis papulosa n.
left substantia n.
papulosa nigra dermatosis
right substantia n.

nigricans
acanthosis n.
hirsutism, androgen excess, insulin resistance, acanthosis nigricans syndrome
hyperandrogenism, insulin resistance, and acanthosis nigricans syndrome
insulin-resistant diabetes, acanthosis nigricans, hypogonadism pigmentary retinopathy, deafness, mental retardation syndrome
malignant acanthosis n.
mental retardation, pre-and postnatal overgrowth, remarkable face, acanthosis nigricans syndrome
n. syndrome

nigricans-hyperinsulinemia syndrome

nigrities lingua

Nigro
mitomycin C and 5-FU Nigro protocol

nigroid body

Nigro protocol

nigrosin
n. mount
n. preparation

nigrostriatal
n. bundle
n. dopaminergic system
n. dopamine system

nigrostriate fiber

NIH
N. Classification Category I acute bacterial prostatitis
N. Classification Category II chronic bacterial prostatitis
N. Classification Category III inflammatory and noninflammatory chronic pelvic pain
N. Classification Category IV asymptomatic inflammatory prostatitis
N. Classification System for Prostatitis

Niikawa-Kuroki syndrome

Nijmegen breakage syndrome

Nikiforoff method

Nikolsky sign

Nikon
N. Auto Refractometer NR-1000F

nil
n. disease
nothing by mouth nil per os
n. per os

Nile
N. blue
N. blue fat stain
N. blue A
West Nile encephalitis
West Nile encephalitis virus
West Nile fever

Nimbus test

NIMH
N. global scale

nine
factor IX nine
protoporphyrin n.
rule of n.'s
n.'s rule

nine-mile fever

ninety hue discrimination test

ninth
n. cranial nerve
n. nerve

ninth-day erythema

Nipah virus

Niplette device

Nippe test

nipple
n. abnormality
accessory n.
n. adenoma
antireflux n.
antirefluxing n.
antral nipple sign
aortic n.
aortic nipple sign
areola of n.
Ashford retracted nipple operation
n. aspirate fluid
n. aspiration cytology
n. asymmetry
breast mound reduction and nipple reconstruction with wraparound flap
darkening of n.
n. discharge
n. discharge cytology
n. discharge from antidepressant
n. discharge from breast injury
distortion or retraction of n.
n. eczema
n. fed
n. feeding
n. flow rate
n. grafting
inverted n.
n. involvement
n. line
n. marker
midclavicular line to n.
modified double-opposing tab flap nipple reconstruction
nevoid hyperkeratosis of nipple and areola
O_2 flowmeter n.
premie n.

n. resection
n. retraction
n. shadow
n. shield
sternal notch to n.
n. stimulation
n. stimulation contraction stress test
supernumerary n.

nipple-areola complex

nipple-areolar
n.-a. amputation
n.-a. reconstruction

nipple-fed baby

Nique virus

Nisbet
N. chancre
N. disease

Nissen
N. antireflux operation
N. 360-degree wrap fundoplication
N. fundoplasty
N. fundoplication method
N. fundoplication operation
N. fundoplication procedure
N. fundoplication technique
N. fundoplication wrap
laparoscopic Nissen fundoplication
open Nissen fundoplication
Rossetti modification of Nissen fundoplication

Nissen-Rosseti
N.-R. fundoplication method
N.-R. fundoplication procedure
N.-R. fundoplication technique

Nissl
N. bodies
N. degeneration
N. granule
N. substance

Nitabuch layer

Nite

niter paper

nitinol
N. arch
n. basket

Nitra lamp

nitrate
n. agar
amyl n.
amyl nitrate abuse
amyl nitrate inhalant
n. broth
cellulose n.
n. disc test
n. to gas
Grocott-Gomori methenamine silver n.
n. reducer
n. reductase
n. reduction test
silver n.
silver nitrate immunoperoxidase
silver nitrate solution

nitrate-negative strain

Nitrazine
fern-positive N.
N. fern test

nitric
n. acid
n. acid test
constitutive nitric oxide synthase
endothelial constitutive nitric oxide synthase
endothelial constitutive nitric oxide synthetase
endothelial nitric oxide synthase
endothelium-derived nitric oxide
exhaled nitric oxide
induced nitric oxide synthase
inducible nitric oxide synthase
inducible nitric oxide synthetase
inhaled nitric oxide
n. oxide
n. oxide hemoglobin
n. oxide/nitrogen
n. oxide-releasing NSAID
n. oxide synthase gene
n. oxide synthase inhibitor

nitrilotriacetic acid

nitrite
amyl n.
n. headache
n. inhalant
n. positive
n. reductase
n. reduction test

nitritoid reaction

***P*-nitro-alpha-acetylamino-beta-hydroxypropiophenone**

Nitro-Bid Ointment

nitroblue
n. tetrazolium
n. tetrazolium dye
n. tetrazolium dye test
n. tetrazolium-paraaminobenzoic acid

nitroblue tetrazolium-paraaminobenzoic acid

nitrocellulose membrane

Nitrodisc Patch

Nitro-Dur Patch

nitrofurantoin monohydrate

Nitrogard Buccal

nitrogen
alkali-soluble n.
alpha-amino n.
amino acid n.
antibody n.
n. autotrophy
n. balance
blood urea n.
carbon, hydrogen, and n.
n. clearance delay
n. cycle
dialysate urea n.
difference in nitrogen tension between mixed alveolar gas and mixed arterial blood
n. dilution
n. dioxide
n. dioxide inhalation
n. distribution
electrolytes, blood urea nitrogen, and serum creatinine
n. equivalent
n. excretion
final n.
grams of nitrogen to nonprotein kilocalories
high calorie and n.
n. lag
liquid n.
mean daily nitrogen balance
multiple-breath nitrogen washout
n. mustard
n. mustard, Adriamycin, CCNU
n. mustard, Oncovin, procarbazine, bleomycin, Adriamycin, prednisone
n. mustard oxide
n. mustard therapy
n. mustard, vincristine, procarbazine, prednisone/doxorubicin, bleomycin, vinblastine
n. narcosis
net nitrogen utilization
Nocardia water-soluble n.
nonprotein n.
nonurea n.
normalized protein nitrogen appearance

nitrogen *(continued)*
partial pressure of n.
n. partial pressure
particulate organic n.
plasma urea n.
protein nitrogen unit
reactive nitrogen intermediate
n. retention
serum urea n.
single-breath nitrogen washout
single-breath nitrogen test
total ammonia n.
total body n.
total excretory n.
total fecal n.
total urinary n.
urea n.
uric acid n.
urinary n.
urinary nitrogen appearance
urinary urea nitrogen excretion
urine urea n.
n. washout
n. washout, multiple breath
n. washout, single breath
n. washout test
n. wasting
yeast nitrogen base

nitrogen/creatinine
blood urea nitrogen/creatinine ratio

nitrogenous base

nitrogen-phosphorus
n.-p. detector
n.-p. detector in gas chromatography

nitrogen-specific detector

nitroglycerin
n. headache
n. ointment
oral n.
n. patch
sublingual n.
sustained-release n.
n. therapy
transdermal n.
trinitroglycerol nitroglycerin

Nitroglyn Oral

nitroid shock

nitroimidazole compound

Nitrol
N. ointment
N. paste

Nitrolingual Translingual Spray

Nitrong SR

nitron radical trap

nitroprusside
n. infusion
n. poisoning
sodium n.

4-nitroquinolin-1-oxide-induced tumor

nitrosamine
tobacco-specific n.

nitrosourea
n. hydrochloride
methyl n.

nitrous
n. acid
inhaled nitrous oxide
n. oxide
n. oxide barbiturate
n. oxide-donor drug
n. oxide-oxygen-opioid anesthetic technique
n. oxide to oxygen ratio
n. oxide tank

Nizetic operation

NJ
N. feeding
N. feeding tube

NK1 receptor

NK2 receptor

NK3 receptor

Nkolbisson virus

N-linked
N.-l. glycosylated site
N.-l. glycosylation
N.-l. pattern

NLite laser

NM1 virus

nm23 gene

nm23-H1 protein

NMDA
N. antagonist ketamine
N. inhibitor

N-methyl-D-aspartate inhibitor

N-methyl D-aspartic acid

N-methyl-D-glucamide

N1-methylnicotinamide

N-methyl-4-phenyl-1,2,3,6-tetrahydropyridine

N-methylspiperone

N-methyltransferase

N-myc
-m. oncogene

N-myristoyl
N.-m. glycine
N.-m. transferase

N-nitroso compound

no
no abnormal discovery
no abnormality
no abnormality demonstrable
no abnormality of fetus
no action indicated
no active disease
no active pulmonary disease
no acute change
no acute disease
no acute distress
no acute inflammation
no acute trauma
no added salt
no adverse reaction
no alternative
no anatomical cause of death
anterior displacement no reduction
no apparent abnormalities
no apparent anesthetic complication
no apparent disease
no apparent disease seen in chest
no apparent distress
no appreciable change
no appreciable disease
no blood return
no bone injury
no bone pathology
no bowel movement
no brain damage
no caffeine or pepper
no cardiopulmonary resuscitation
no casualty
no change
no clubbing, cyanosis, or edema
no code blue
no complaints
no complaints offered
no concentrated carbohydrates
no concentrated sweets
no congenital abnormalities
no congenital deformities
no data
no data available
no date
no defects
no demonstrable antibodies
no detectable activity
no detectable antibody

no deviation of electrical axis
no discernible finding
no disease
no disease found
no ectopia
no effect
en bloc no touch technique
no enlargement
no essential abnormalities
no essential change
no evidence of abnormality
no evidence of active disease
no evidence of disease
no evidence of disease-stationary disease
no evidence of distant metastases
no evidence of malignancy
no evidence of pathology
no evidence of primary tumor
no evidence of pulmonary disease
no evidence of recurrence
no evidence of recurrent disease
no expiration date
no facies
no family doctor
no family physician
finding of no significant impact
no further action required
no further information
no further treatment
no gammopathy detected
no good
no heroic measures
no histologic abnormalities
no histopathologic abnormality
home, no services needed
no identifiable disease
no improvement
no improvement with pinhole
no infection-no rejection
no infection present
no inflammation present
no inflammatory signs
no information available
no intraoperative complications
no known allergies
no known basis
no known cure
no known diseases
no known drug allergies
no known food allergies
no known medication allergies
no light perception
no limitation of motion
no line of demarcation
no malignant cell
no manifest improvement
no medical health history
no medical ocular history
no mental illness
no middle initial
no middle name
no more information
no nausea or vomiting
no nausea, vomiting, or diarrhea
no nausea, vomiting, diarrhea or constipation
no new laboratory test orders
no new order
in no apparent distress
no regular medicines
no observed adverse effect level
no observed effect dose
no palpable enlargement
no palpable thrill
no pathologic diagnosis
patient has no purposeful movement
no phone
pinhole no improvement
no predisposing factor
no prenatal care
no present illness
no previous admission
no previous complaint
no previous history
no prior tracings
no progression
no radiographically visible recurrence
no recent illnesses
no refill
regular rate, clear tones, no murmurs
no report
no response
no sample
no sequelae
no serious abnormality
no significant abnormality
no significant anomaly
no significant change
no significant change from previous tracing
no significant defect
no significant deficiency
no significant deviation
no significant difference
no significant disease
no significant findings
no sign of infection
no sign of inflammation
no signs of acute disease
sinus rhythm, no ectopy
no special preparation necessary for test
no spontaneous movement of limbs
strict no information in paper
no test
there is no evidence of malignancy
no time limit
no treatment indicated
no treatment necessary
turbid, no creamy layer
no venereal disease
no venous distention
no voluntary activity
no weightbearing
well-healed, no residuals
well-healed, no sequelae

Noack syndrome

noble
N. bowel plication
n. gold alloy

Noble-Mengert perineal repair

Nocard bacillus

Nocardia
Nocardia brain abscess
Nocardia water-soluble nitrogen

Nocardia
N. brain abscess
N. culture
N. dacryolith
N. keratitis
N. pneumonia
N. water-soluble nitrogen

nocardial endophthalmitis

nocardioform bacteria

nocardiosis

nociceptin/orphanin
n. FQ
n. FQ peptide

nociceptive
n. circuit
n. impulse
n. neurotransmitter
n. pain
n. pathway

nociceptor
n. activation
n. agent
angry backfiring C n.
primary afferent nociceptor neuron

nociceptor-induced inflammation

nocturia
age-related n.
patient has n.

nocturnal
n. acid reflux
n. agitation
n. amaurosis
n. amblyopia
n. angina
n. arrhythmogenesis
n. asthma
autosomal dominant nocturnal frontal lobe epilepsy
n. awakening
n. caffeine
complex partial nocturnal seizure
n. confusion
n. confusional episode
n. diarrhea
n. drinking syndrome
n. dyspnea
n. eating syndrome
n. emission
n. enuresis
n. epilepsy
episodic nocturnal wandering
n. erection
n. gastric reflux
n. groaning
n. hallucination
n. heartbeat
n. heartburn
n. hemiplegia
n. hemodialysis
n. hemoglobinuria
n. hypoglycemia
n. hypotensive episode
n. hypoxemia
n. leg cramp
n. leg muscle cramp
n. microfilaria
n. micturition
monosymptomatic nocturnal enuresis
n. myoclonus
nasal nocturnal ventilation
Oriental nocturnal death syndrome
n. oxygen therapy
n. oxygen therapy trial
n. painful tonic spasm
n. paroxysmal dystonia
paroxysmal nocturnal hemoglobinuria
paroxysmal nocturnal hemoglobinuria cell
n. penile erection monitoring
n. penile tumescence
n. penile tumescence testing
n. periodicity
n. polysomnogram
n. polysomnography
primary nocturnal enuresis
psychogenic nocturnal polydipsia
n. regurgitation
n. rhythm
n. seizure
simplified nocturnal home hemodialysis
n. sleep
n. symptom
n. thyroid-stimulating hormone surge
n. tidal peritoneal dialysis
n. TSH surge
n. tumescence monitor
n. urinary frequency
n. urinary incontinence
n. vasopressin release
n. wheezing

nodal
apical cardiac nodal enlargement
n. arrhythmia
n. artery
atrioventricular nodal conduction
atrioventricular nodal branch
atrioventricular nodal bypass tract
atrioventricular nodal function
atrioventricular nodal node mesothelioma
atrioventricular nodal orifice
atrioventricular nodal ostium
atrioventricular nodal reentrant tachycardia
atrioventricular nodal reentry
atrioventricular nodal rhythm
atrioventricular nodal septal defect
atrioventricular nodal septum
atrioventricular nodal valve
atypical atrioventricular nodal reentrant tachycardia
AV nodal reentrant tachycardia
AV nodal reentry tachycardia
axillary nodal metastasis in breast carcinoma
n. basin
n. beat
n. bigeminy
n. bradycardia
n. cell
n. conduction
coronary nodal rhythm
corrected sinus nodal recovery time
n. disease
n. drainage
n. dysfunction
enhanced atrioventricular nodal conduction
n. escape
n. escape rhythm
n. extirpation
n. extrasystole
n. fever
n. hypodensity
intrapulmonary nodal metastases
n. involvement
n. involvement in breast carcinoma
n. irradiation
n. marginal zone B-cell lymphoma
mediastinal nodal station
n. metastasis
n. metastasis in breast carcinoma
nonparoxysmal nodal rhythm
nonparoxysmal nodal tachycardia
optical nodal point
paroxysmal atrioventricular nodal reciprocal tachycardia
paroxysmal nodal rhythm
n. paroxysmal tachycardia
n. pathway
n. plane
n. point
n. premature beat
n. premature contraction
premature nodal beat
premature nodal contraction
n. reentrant paroxysmal tachycardia
n. sampling
sinoatrial nodal reentry
n. staging procedure
subtotal nodal irradiation
survival relative to nodal involvement in breast carcinoma
n. tissue

Nodamura virus

nodding
n. of head
n. spasm

node
abdominal lymph n.
abdominal lymph node biopsy
n. ablation
angiofollicular hyperplasia lymph n.
angiofollicular lymph node hyperplasia
angiofollicular mediastinal lymph node hyperplasia

anorectal lymph n.
anterior axillary lymph n.
anterior deep cervical lymph n.
anterior jugular lymph n.
anterior mediastinal lymph n.
anterior superficial cervical lymph n.
anterior tibial lymph n.
anthracotic hilar n.
aortic lymph n.
aortic node metastasis
aortic window n.
apical axillary lymph n.
apical lymph n.
appendicular lymph n.
artery to atrioventricular n.
artery to the sinoatrial n.
n. of Aschoff and Tawara
at autopsy tumor, nodes, and metastases
atrioventricular n.
atrioventricular nodal node mesothelioma
atrioventricular node artery
atrioventricular node dysfunction
atrioventricular node function
atrioventricular node of His
auricular lymph n.
AV node ablation
AV node dysfunction
axillary lymph n.
axillary lymph node dissection
axillary lymph node involvement
axillary lymph node metastasis
axillary node dissection mastectomy
axillary node negative
axillary node positive
n. of azygos arch
n. bearing area of lymph nodes
bilateral pelvic lymph n.
bilateral pelvic lymph node dissection
n. biopsy
bronchial lymph n.
n. calcification
calcified hilar n.
caudal mediastinal n.
celiac lymph node metastasis
clinical staging of tumors, nodes, and metastases as determined by noninvasive examination
clinical status of n.
n. of Cloquet
common iliac lymph n.'s
complete lymph node dissection
corrected adjusted sinus node recovery time
corrected time of sinoatrial node function recovery
deep inguinal lymph n.
n. dissection
n. distribution
draining lymph n.
elective lymph node dissection
elective regional lymph node dissection
external iliac lymph n.'s
extraperitoneal endoscopic pelvic lymph node dissection
giant lymph node hyperplasia
n. group
hemorrhagic omental lymph n.'s
hepatic lymph n.
hilar lymph n.
hilar node metastasis
histiocytic hyperplasia of lymph n.
histocytic hyperplasia of lymph n.'s
ileocolic lymph n.
iliac lymph n.'s
inguinal lymph n.'s
intercostal lymph n.
internal iliac lymph n.
internal mammary lymph n.
internal node involvement
intramammary lymph n.
n. involvement
jugular lymph n.'s
junctional lymph n.
laparoscopic pelvic lymph node dissection
left gastric lymph n.
left hilar lymph n.
lingual lymph n.
localized angiofollicular lymph node hyperplasia
lumbar lymph n.
lymph node basin
lymph node cell
lymph node culture
lymph node drainage
lymph node of elbow
lymph node endometriotic adenoacanthoma
lymph node excision
lymph node fibrosis
lymph node of head and neck
lymph node histology
lymph node hyperplasia
lymph node involution
lymph node of lower limb
lymph node lymphocyte
lymph node mononuclear cell
lymph node permeability factor
lymph node positivity
lymph node revealing solution
lymph node sampling
lymph node seeking equivalent
lymph node staging
lymph node station
lymph node of upper limb
malar lymph n.
mandibular lymph n.
mastoid lymph n.
medial lacunar lymph n.
mediastinal lymph n.
mediastinal lymph node hyperplasia
medulla of lymph n.
mesenteric lymph n.
mesocolic lymph n.
mesorectal lymph n.
metastatic lymph node tumor
middle colic lymph n.
middle group of mesenteric lymph n.
mucocutaneous lymph n.
mucocutaneous lymph node syndrome
multicentric angiofollicular lymph n.
nasolabial lymph n.
nasopharyngeal carcinoma with lymph node involvement
neck lymph n.
obturator lymph n.
occipital lymph n.
occult lymph node metastasis
pancreatic lymph n.
pancreaticoduodenal lymph n.
pancreaticosplenic lymph n.
paraaortic lymph n.
paraaortic node irradiation
paraaortic node sampling
parapharyngeal lymph n.
pararectal lymph n.
parasternal lymph n.'s
paratracheal node chain
paravesical lymph n.
parietal lymph n.
parotid lymph n.
pathological tumor, nodes, metastases staging of cancer
pectoral axillary lymph n.
pelvic lymph n.
pelvic lymph node dissection
pelvic node sampling
periaortic infrarenal n.

node *(continued)*
periaortic lymph n.
periaortic lymph node metastasis
periaortic node sampling
pericolonic lymph n.
perihilar lymph n.
peripancreatic lymph n.
peripheral lymph n.
peroneal lymph n.
pharyngeal lymph n.
phrenic lymph n.
pleural lymph n.
popliteal lymph n.
popliteal node area
posterior cervical n.'s
prevertebral lymph n.
primary node involvement
primary tumor, regional lymph node, remote metastases classification, staging
pyloric lymph n.
n. of Ranvier
regional lymph n.
regional lymph nodes cannot be addressed
regional lymph node cell
regional lymph node dissection
n. resection
retrocecal lymph n.
retroperitoneal pelvic lymph node dissection
retropharyngeal lymph n.
right gastric lymph n.
right hilar lymph n.
n.'s of Rouviere
sacral lymph n.
n. sampling
scalene lymph node biopsy
selective complete lymph node dissection
sentinel lymph n.
sentinel lymph node biopsy
sentinel lymph node detection
sentinel lymph node mapping
shotty lymph n.
sinoatrial n.
sinoatrial node artery
sinuatrial n.
sinus n.
sinus node cycle length
sinus node dysfunction
sinus node electrogram
sinus node formation
sinus node impulse
sinus node potential
sinus node recovery time
solitary lymph n.
splenic lymph n.
subcutaneous intraocular n.
submental lymph n.
superficial distal axillary n.
superficial inguinal lymph n.
supraclavicular lymph n.
supraclavicular node biopsy
therapeutic lymph node dissection
thymus-dependent zone of lymph n.
total axial node irradiation
tumor-draining lymph n.
tumor-draining lymph node cell
tumor, nodes, metastasis
tumor with lymph node metastases

node-based malignant lymphoproliferative disease

node-negative
n.-n. carcinoma
n.-n. disease
n.-n. melanoma
n.-n. patient
n.-n. primary tumor

node-positive
n.-p. breast cancer
n.-p. disease

nodi (*pl. of* nodus)

no-dialysis days

NO-donor drug

nodosa
infantile periarteritis n.
infantile polyarteritis n.
microscopic polyarteritis n.
periarteritis n.
n. phthisis
polyarteritis n.

nodose
n. arteriosclerosis
n. ganglion

nodosum

nodoventricular bypass fiber

nodular
n. adenosis
n. adrenal hyperplasia
n. adrenocortical hyperplasia
n. amyloidoma
n. amyloidosis
n. aneurysm
n. appearance
n. arteriosclerosis
autonomous nodular hyperplastic gland
n. autonomy
n. basal cell carcinoma
n. blastema
n. blueberry lips
n. body
n. bronchiectasis
n. calcific aortic stenosis
calcific nodular aortic stenosis
n. chondrodermatitis
chronic rheumatoid nodular fibrositis
n. colloid goiter
n. complete response
n. conjunctivitis
n. connective tissue disease nevus
n. corneal degeneration
n. cortical adrenal hyperplasia
n. cortical sclerosis
n. density
n. and diffuse fibrous proliferation
n. and diffuse lymphoma
diffuse nodular hyperplasia
diffuse nodular lymphoma
n. disease
n. disorder
n. elastosis
n. embryo
n. enhancement
n. eosinophilic panniculitis
n. episcleritis
n. fasciitis
focal nodular hyperplasia
follicular nodular hyperplasia
n. gastritis
n. granulomatous vasculitis
n. growth of tissue
n. headache
n. heterotopia
n. hidradenoma
n. and histiocytic
n. histiocytic lymphoma
Hodgkin disease, mixed nodular type
Hodgkin disease, nodular sclerosis
n. hyperintense focus
n. hyperplasia of ovary
n. hyperplasia of prostate gland
hypertrophic nodular gliosis
n. infiltrate
n. infiltration
n. iritis
n. leprosy
n. lesion
L/H nodular pattern
n. liquefying panniculitis
n. liver
localized nodular synovitis

lymphocytic nodular Hodgkin disease
n. lymphoid hyperplasia
n. lymphoma
n. malignant melanoma
malignant nodular hidradenoma
n. melanoma
n. metastases
n. metastasis
n. migratory panniculitis
mild focal cortical nodular hyperplasia
n., mixed cell lymphoma
mixed cell nodular lymphoma
n. mixed lymphoma
n. myositis
necrotizing nodular scleritis
n. neurodermatitis
noncalcified nodular mass
n. non-Hodgkin lymphoma
n. nonsuppurative panniculitis
nontoxic nodular goiter
n. non-X histiocytosis
n. panencephalitis
n. panniculitis
n. paragranuloma
partial nodular transformation
n. pattern
pigmented nodular adrenocortical disease
n. poorly differentiated lymphocytic lymphoma
primary adrenocortical nodular dysplasia
primary pigmented nodular adrenocortical disease
n. prostatic hypertrophy
n. pseudosarcomatous fasciitis
n. pulmonary amyloidosis
n. regenerative hyperplasia
n. regenerative hyperplasia of liver
n. renal blastoma
Salzmann nodular corneal dystrophy
n. scabies
n. scleritis
n. sclerosing Hodgkin disease
n. shadow
soft fluctuant nodular lesion
n. subepidermal fibrosis
n. synovitis
n. syphilid
n. thickening
n. thyroid
toxic nodular goiter
n. tuberculid
n. vasculi
n. xanthoma

nodular/diffuse non-Hodgkin lymphoma

nodularis

nodularity
antral n.

nodular-lymphocytic, poorly differentiated

nodule
adenomatous hyperplastic n.
aortic valve n.
apple jelly n.
autonomously functioning thyroid n.
autonomous thyroid n.
autonomous toxic n.
calcareous n.'s
colloid nodule of thyroid
confluence of n.'s
cortical hyperplastic n.
n.'s, eosinophilia, rheumatism, dermatitis, and swelling syndrome
granular inflammatory n.
hard subcutaneous n.
hyperplastic alveolar n.
hyperplastic liver n.
n.'s of Kerckring
malignant thyroid n.
mantle zone n.
milkers' nodule virus
millet seed n.
multinodular thyroid n.
mural CNS n.
noncavitating pulmonary n.
n. palpable
peritoneum studded with tumor n.'s
reactive spindle cell n.
sarcoma-like mural n.
soft fleshy n.
soft tissue n.
solitary autonomous n.
solitary lymphatic n.
solitary pulmonary n.
n.'s in sparganosis
studded with numerous tumor n.'s
thyroid nodule ablation
toxic thyroid n.
vocal cord n.

nodule-inducing virus

nodule-in-nodule lesion

nodule-like alveolar lesion

noduli (*pl. of* nodulus)

nodulocystic acne

noduloulcerative
n. basal cell carcinoma
n. syphilis
n. tertiary syphilis

noduloulcerative basal cell carcinoma

noduloulcerative tertiary syphilis

nodulus, pl. **noduli**
n. cerebelli
n. conjunctivalis
n. lymphaticus
noduli lymphoidei solitarii
n. syndrome

nodus, pl. **nodi**
nodi lymphatici mesenterici inferiores
nodi lymphatici mesenterici superiores
nodi lymphatici pancreatici superiores
nodi lymphatici paravesiculares
nodi lymphatici postcavales
nodi lymphatici postvesiculares
nodi lymphatici prevesiculares
nodi lymphoidei abdominis
nodi lymphoidei appendiculares
nodi lymphoidei mastoidei
nodi lymphoidei mediastinales anteriores
nodi lymphoidei mediastinales posteriores
nodi lymphoidei mesenterici
nodi lymphoidei mesenterici inferiores
nodi lymphoidei mesenterici superiores
nodi lymphoidei mesocolici
nodi lymphoidei obturatorii
nodi lymphoidei occipitales
nodi lymphoidei pancreatici
nodi lymphoidei pancreaticoduodenales
nodi lymphoidei pancreaticolienales
nodi lymphoidei pancreaticosplenales
nodi lymphoidei paracolici
nodi lymphoidei paramammarii
nodi lymphoidei pararectales
nodi lymphoidei parasternales
nodi lymphoidei paratracheales
nodi lymphoidei parauterini
nodi lymphoidei paravaginales
nodi lymphoidei parietales

nodus *(continued)*
nodi lymphoidei parotidei profundi
nodi lymphoidei parotidei profundi preauriculares
nodi lymphoidei pelvis
nodi lymphoidei phrenici inferiores
nodi lymphoidei phrenici superiores
nodi lymphoidei popliteales
nodi lymphoidei precaecales
nodi lymphoidei prelaryngeales
nodi lymphoidei prepericardiaci
nodi lymphoidei pretracheales
nodi lymphoidei prevertebrales
nodi lymphoidei promontorii
nodi lymphoidei pylorici
nodi lymphoidei rectales superiores
nodi lymphoidei retrocecales
nodi lymphoidei retropharyngeales
nodi lymphoidei retropylorici
nodi lymphoidei sacrales
nodi lymphoidei sigmoidei
nodi lymphoidei subaortici
nodi lymphoidei subpylorici
nodi lymphoidei thoracis
nodi lymphoidei thyroidei
nodi lymphoidei tracheobronchiales inferiores
nodi lymphoidei tracheobronchiales superiores
n. lymphoideus mandibularis
n. lymphoideus proximalis profundus
n. lymphoideus suprapyloricus
n. lymphoideus tibialis posterior

NOE fracture

no-fault insurance

Noguchi test

Noiles hinge

noire
atrophie n.

noise
acoustic noise test
n. analyzer
automobile airbag impulse n.
average peak n.
broadband n.
n. condition
n. count
n. criterion
n. detection threshold
effective perceived noise level
n. equivalent counts
n. equivalent power
n. exposure
n. exposure meter
n. factor
n. figure
n. generator
n. induced
n. interference level
n. level
n. level monitor
line frequency noise dot
long-term low-level white n.
low–pass-filtered n.
maximal noise area
narrow band n.
n. and number index
perceived n.
perceived noise level
n. reduction
n. reduction coefficient
N. Reduction Rating
signal-difference to noise ratio
n. spike artifact
n. tone difference
Tone in N. test
wide band n.

noise-induced
n.-i. damage
n.-i. deafness
n.-i. error
n.-i. hearing damage
n.-i. hearing loss
n.-i. permanent threshold shift
n.-i. temporary threshold shift

noise-reduced hearing loss

noise-to-harmonic ratio

noisy chest

No-Kor needle

Nokrome bifocal

Nola virus

No-Lok bolt

noma
n. neonatorum
in noma ulcer
n. pudendi
n. vulvae

no-man's land

Nomarski microscopy

Nomarsky interference contrast

Nombre
Sin Nombre virus

nomegestrol acetate

nomenclatural type

nomenclature
Anglo-Saxon n.
anorectal n.
Standard N. of Athletic Injuries
Standard N. of Diseases and Operations
Standardized N. of Medicine
Standard Units and N.
Systematized N. of Medicine Clinical Terms
Systematized N. of Medicine Reference Terminology
Systematized N. of Pathology
Systemized N. of Medicine

nominal
n. allotype
n. aphasia
n. compound
n. single dose
n. standard dose

nomination
Peer Nomination Inventory for Depression

nomogram
heparin dosing n.
n. system

nomothetic approach

non.

non-A
n.-A. hepatitis
n.-A. hepatitis virus
n.-A., non-B hepatitis
n.-A., non-B hepatitis virus
n.-A., non-B, non-C hepatitis
n.-A. non-B
n.-A. non-B hepatitis
n.-A., non-B, non-C
n.-A. syndrome

non-ABC hepatitis

nonabsorbable
n. disaccharide
n. surgical suture

nonabsorbent material

non-*Acanthamoeba* amebic keratitis

nonaccidental
n. injury
suspected nonaccidental trauma
n. trauma

nonaccommodative
n. esodeviation
n. esophoria
n. esotropia

nonacetylated salicylate

nonacute
n. profile
n. total occlusion

nonaddictive painkiller

nonadherence index

nonadherent
n. cell
n. leukocyte

nonadrenergic
n. inhibitory response
n. noncholinergic

non-A-E hepatitis

non-*Aeruginosa* pseudomonad

nonaffective psychotic disorder

non-A–G
n.-A. chronic liver disease
n.-A. fulminant hepatitis

nonaggressive tumor

nonalcoholic
n. fatty liver disease
n. steatohepatitis
n. white shake lotion

nonalkylating agent

nonallergic
n. asthma
blood eosinophilic nonallergic rhinitis
n. contact urticaria
eosinophilic nonallergic rhinitis
noneosinophilic nonallergic rhinitis
n. noninfectious perennial rhinitis
n. rhinitis
n. rhinitis with eosinophilia syndrome

non-Alzheimer disease-related pattern

nonambulatory restraint

nonanaphylactic reaction

nonandrogenic progestin

nonaneurysmal
perimesencephalic nonaneurysmal subarachnoid hemorrhage

nonangiogenic cell

nonanion gap acidosis

nonan malaria

nonantigenic specific mediator

nonappendiceal carcinoid

nonarteriosclerotic
familial idiopathic nonarteriosclerotic cerebral calcification

nonarteritic
n. anterior ischemic optic neuropathy

nonarticular
n. arthritis
n. distal radial fracture
n. rheumatism
n. syndrome

nonaspirating
n. ultrasonic phaco chopper tip

nonatopic allergic conjunctivitis

nonautoimmune
n. familial hyperthyroidism
n. nontoxic diffuse goiter

nonaxial
n. beam technique
n. fashion
n. format

non-B
n.-B. cell
chronic active viral hepatitis, non-A, n.-B.
n.-B. hepatitis
n.-B. hepatitis virus
non-A, non-B hepatitis
non-A, non-B hepatitis virus
non-A, non-B, non-C hepatitis
n.-B., non-C chronic liver disease
persistent viral hepatitis, non-A, n.-B.

nonbacterial
acute infectious nonbacterial gastroenteritis
chronic nonbacterial prostatitis
n. cystitis
n. diarrhea
epidemic acute nonbacterial gastroenteritis
n. gastroenteritis
n. gastroenteritis virus
n. infantile gastroenteritis
n. infection
n. infectious arthritis
n. prostatitis
n. thrombotic endocardial lesion
n. thrombotic endocarditis
n. thrombotic vegetation
n. verrucous endocarditis

nonbarbiturate therapy

nonbattle
n. casualty
n. injury

non-B-cell leukemia

nonbed
n. care
n. occupancy

non-beta cell tumor

nonbizarre delusion

nonblanchable, abnormally colored lesion

nonblanching purpura

nonbleeding visible vessel

nonbreathing pressure relieving

nonbullous
n. congenital erythrodermic ichthyosis
n. congenital ichthyosiform erythroderma
n. impetigo

non-Burkitt subtype

non-C
n.-C. hepatitis
non-A, non-B, n.-C.
non-A, non-B, non-C hepatitis

noncalcareous stone

noncalcemic analog

noncalcified
n. carcinoma
n. coronary stenosis
n. nodular mass
n. valve

noncancerous
n. enlargement of prostate gland
gastric noncancerous area
n. polyp
n. skin growth

noncapsulated
rough, noncapsulated, avirulent bacterial culture

noncarbonic acid

noncardiac
n. angiography
n. chest pain
n. pulmonary edema
n. surgery
n. syncope

noncardiogenic
n. origin
n. pulmonary edema

noncaseating
n. conjunctival granuloma
n. granulomatous disease

noncausal association

noncavitating
n. pulmonary nodule

noncavitating pulmonary nodule
noncentral ulcer
nonceruloplasmin plasma copper
nonchild-resistant container
noncholecystokinin substance
noncholera *Vibrio*
noncholinergic
n. neuron
nonadrenergic n.
nonchromaffin paraganglioma
noncicatrizing alopecia
noncircumferential stenosis
noncirrhotic portal fibrosis
nonclassic
n. congenital adrenal hyperplasia
nonclassical
n. adrenal hyperplasia
n. hydroxylase deficiency
n. 21-hydroxylase deficiency
noncleaved
n. follicular center cell
large n.
small noncleaved cell lymphoma
small noncleaved cell, non-Burkitt lymphoma
noncleaved-cell lymphoma
nonclinical manager
nonclonogenic proliferating cell
nonclostridial
n. anaerobic cellulitis
n. anaerobic myonecrosis
n. infection
noncohesive
n. gold
n. gold foil
noncolicky epigastric pain
noncollagen
n. bone matrix
n. protein
noncolorectal liver metastasis
noncomitant
n. heterotropia
n. squint
n. strabismus
noncommunicating
n. biliary cyst
n. diverticulum
n. hydrocele
n. hydrocephalus
n. uterine horn
noncompaction
isolated noncompaction of the ventricular myocardium
isolated ventricular n.
noncompetitive assay
noncomplex PSA
noncompliance with medical treatment
noncompliant
patient n.
n. patient
patient noncompliant with medication
n. with medication
nonconcomitant strabismus
nonconducted premature atrial contraction
nonconfluent plaque
nonconfrontational communication skills
noncongestive glaucoma
nonconjugative plasmid
nonconsenting adult
noncontact
air-puff noncontact tonometer
n. holmium:yttrium-argon-garnet laser thermal keratoplasty
n. supervision
n. tonometer
n. tonometry
noncontained
n. disc
n. disc herniation
noncontraceptive estrogen
noncontractile
n. area
n. cell
noncontrast
n. CT scan
n. helical computed tomography
n. phase
noncontributory
family history n.
n. family history
past history n.
n. past history
past medical history n.
n. past medical history
n. to present illness
nonconvoluted type
nonconvulsive
n. epilepsy
n. status epilepticus
noncoplanar
n. arch technique
n. arc technique
n. beam
n. beam technique
noncoring Huber needle
noncornified cell
noncornual placental location
noncoronary
n. cause
n. cusp
n. sinus
noncorticosteroid antiinflammatory agent
noncosmetic panniculectomy
noncovalent bond
noncovalently bonded dimer of C-terminal immunoglobulin of Fc fragment
noncross-reactive drug
noncurative resection
noncured sarcoidosis
noncurrent serum
noncycloplegic distance static retinoscopy
noncytolytic virus
nondeciduous placenta
nondefinitive pattern
nondeforming arthritis
nondenaturing condition
nondepolarizing
n. block
n. blockade
nondermatomal sensory abnormality
nondermatophyte
n. fungal infection
n. fungus
nondermatophytic mold
nondescript macular
nondestructive testing
nondetachable
n. balloon
n. balloon catheter
nondetectable
not n.
time to n.
nondiabetic
n. extremity
n. gastroparesis
n. glycosuria

n. immune-mediated neuropathy
infant of nondiabetic mother

nondiagnostic culdocentesis

nondifferentiated cell

nondihydropyridine calcium channel blocker

nondirective approach

nondisabling
nonsymptomatic, n.

nondispersive
n. infrared analyzer
n. infrared spectrometer

nondisplaced fracture

nondisseminated cutaneous leishmaniasis

nondissociated acid

nondissociative
carpal instability n.

nondistended/nontender

nondominant
n. hemisphere
n. hemisphere lesion

nondrug-related reaction

none
all or n.
n. detectable
n. detected
n. found
n. obtained

noneczematous persistent papular gold eruption

noneloquent
eloquent versus noneloquent area

nonemotional
verbal nonemotional stimuli

nonencapsulated sclerosing tumor

nonendocrine disease

nonenhanced
n. computed tomography
n. CT
n. CT scan

nonenhancing lesion

nonenteropathogenic virus

nonenveloped virus

nonenzymatic
n. glycation
n. photolysis
n. protein glycation

noneosinophilic nonallergic rhinitis

nonepidermolytic palmoplantar keratoderma

nonepileptic
n. attack disorder
n. event
n. myoclonus
n. seizure

nonepithelial tumor

nonequilibrium pH gradient gel electrophoresis

non-ergot long-acting prolactin inhibitor

nonerosive
n. esophagitis
n. gastric mucosal lesion
n. gastroesophageal reflux disease
nonspecific nonerosive duodenitis
nonspecific nonerosive gastritis

nonessential amino acid

nonesterified
n. cholesterol
n. fatty acid

nonestrogen drug

nonestrogenic

nonestrogen-regulated growth

nonexercise
n. activity thermogenesis

nonexercise activity thermogenesis

nonexertional
n. angina
n. dyspnea

nonexpansile lung

nonexudative macular degeneration

nonfamilial
n. aniridia
n. gastrointestinal polyposis
n. hematuria
n. hyperinsulinemic hypoglycemia
n. hyperinsulinism of infancy
n. parathyroid adenoma

nonfasting glucose

nonfatal
n. attempt at suicide
n. complication
n. heart attack
n. injury
n. stroke

nonfatty
focal nonfatty infiltration of liver

nonfenestrated
n. capillary
n. forceps

nonfermentative
n. gram-negative bacilli

nonfermenting bacteria

nonferromagnetic MR-compatible frame

nonferrous extract

nonfilament polymorphonuclear leukocyte

nonfilarial elephantiasis

non-fire setter

nonfixed tissue

nonfluent
n. aphasia
n. aphasic seizure
n. aphasic speech

nonfollicular pustulosis

nonfrank breech

nonfrosted tip

nonfunction
primary n.

nonfunctional
n. grinding
n. pituitary adenoma
n. pituitary tumor
n. streak

nonfunctioning
n. adrenal carcinoma
n. catheter
clinically nonfunctioning pituitary adenoma
n. gallbladder
n. kidney
n. lung
n. microadenoma
n. pheochromocytoma
n. pituitary adenoma
n. pituitary tumor

nongenital
n. pelvic organ
n. skin fibroblast

nongenomic
n. action
n. factor
n. glucocorticoid effect

nongerminoma
n. germ cell tumor

nongerminoma germ cell tumor

nongestational choriocarcinoma

nonglucogenic/glucogenic ratio

nonglycoside inotropic agent

nongonococcal
n. bacterial arthritis
n. cervicitis
n. septic arthritis
n. urethritis

nongovernmental organizations

nongranular
n. clear chromophobe cell
n. leukocyte

nongranulomatous
n. anterior uveitis
n. choroiditis
n. ileojejunitis
n. iridocyclitis
n. salpingitis

non-Graves disease hyperthyroidism

nongrowth hormone deficient short stature

nonhealing
n. sore
n. ulcer
n. ulceration
n. wound

non-heart-beating
n.-h.-b. donor
n.-h.-b. donor liver transplantation

nonhematologic toxicity

nonhematopoietic
n. element
n. growth factor

nonhemoglobin protein

nonhemolytic
n. aerobic organism
febrile nonhemolytic transfusion react
n. febrile transfusion reaction
n. jaundice
n. streptococcus

nonhemophiliac patient

nonhemorrhagic
acute nonhemorrhagic infarct

nonhereditary breast cancer

non–high-density lipoprotein

nonhistiocytic type lymphoma

nonhistocompatibility locus antigen-associated form

nonhistone
n. chromatin
n. chromosomal
n. chromosomal protein
n. protein

non-HIV chronic gingivitis

non-HLA-associated form

non-Hodgkin
hepatic non-Hodgkin lymphoma
n.-H. leukemia
n.-H. lymphoma
n.-H. malignant lymphoma

nonhomogeneous consolidation

nonhomologous
n. chromosome
n. recombination

nonhormonal regulator

nonhuman leukocyte antigen associated form

nonhydrostatic pulmonary edema

nonhyperglycemic glycosuria

nonicteric
n. hepatitis
n. sclerae

nonidentical twins

nonimmediate-type immunologic drug reaction

nonimmune
n. agglutination
n. fetal hydrops
n. hemolysis
n. hydrops fetalis
n. renal disease
n. serum
n. sheep serum

nonimmunized
n. rabbit serum

nonimmunized rabbit serum

nonimmunocompromised host

nonimmunogenic murine tumor cell

nonimmunologic
n. basis
n. complication
n. contact urticaria
n. drug reaction

noninfarct zone

noninfectious
n. aortitis
n. chronic cystitis
n. diarrheal disease
n. disease complication
nonallergic noninfectious perennial rhinitis
n. urethritis

noninfiltrating intraductal carcinoma

noninflammatory
n. arthritis
n. diarrhea
n. edema
n. myopathy
NIH Classification Category III inflammatory and noninflammatory chronic pelvic pain

noninguinal
multiple noninguinal sites

noninherited
n. factor
n. maternal antigen
n. paternal antigen

noninhibitory media

non-insulin-dependent
n.-i.-d. diabetes
n.-i.-d. diabetes mellitus
n.-i.-d. diabetic

nonintestinal fibroblast

noninvasive
arterial noninvasive vascular assessment
n. aspergillosis
n. assessment of urinary flow
n. blood pressure
n. blood pressure measurement
n. brain imaging study
n. breast carcinoma
n. cardiac evaluation
n. cardiac output monitor
n. cardiac testing
n. carotid baroceptor stimulation
n. carotid examination
n. carotid study
n. cervical cancer
clinical staging of tumors, nodes, and metastases as determined by noninvasive examination
n. corneal redox fluorometry
n. coronary angiography
n. diagnosis
n. diagnostic procedure
n. diagnostic test
n. evaluation
n. evaluation of radiation output
n. examination
n. extrathoracic ventilator
n. flow study
n. glucose monitor
lower extremity n.
n. management
n. motion ventilation
n. neurovascular studies
n. detection of trisomy 18

n. positive pressure ventilation
n. procedure
n. programmed stimulation
n. surgery
n. tear film break-up time
n. technique
n. thymoma
n. vascular assessment
n. vascular laboratory studies
n. ventilatory support

noninvolved
n. bone
n. psoriatic skin

nonionic
n. contrast agent
n. contrast material
n. contrast medium
n. contrast radiography
n. detergent soluble
n. dimer
n. dimer contrast medium
n. iodinated contrast
n. surfactant vesicle

nonionized hemoglobin

nonionizing
n. electromagnetic radiation
n. nonthermal application
n. radiation

nonirrigating descending colostomy

nonirritating test substance

nonischemic
n. chest pain
n. CRVO

non-islet cell tumor hypoglycemia

nonislet-cell tumor-induced hypoglycemia

nonisolated proteinuria

nonisotopic
n. detection system
n. RNase cleavage assay
n. in situ hybridization

nonkeratinizing epidermoid carcinoma

nonketotic
n. coma
n. glycine
n. hyperglycemia
hyperglycemic hyperosmolar nonketotic syndrome
n. hyperglycinemia
n. hyperglycmic-hyperosmolar coma
n. hyperosmolar
n. hyperosmolar acidosis
n. hyperosmolar coma
hyperosmolar hyperglycemic nonketotic coma
hyperosmolar hyperglycemic nonketotic syndrome
hyperosmolar nonketotic diabetic coma
hyperosmolar nonketotic diabetic state
n. hyperosmolar state
n. hyperosmolar syndrome
n. hyperosmotic
n. hypoglycemia
n. hypoglycemic acidosis
n. state

nonkinesigenic
paroxysmal nonkinesigenic dyskinesia

nonlactating breast

nonlactose
n. fermentation
n. fermenting gram-negative rod

nonleaking bleb

nonlethal
n. dwarfism
n. dysplasia

nonleukemic myelosis

nonlinear
n. developmental curve
n. distortion
n. IgA deposition
n. least squares method
n. least squares regression analysis
n. mixed-effects model
weighted nonlinear least squares

nonlingular
n. branch
n. branch of upper lobe bronchus

nonlipid
macromolecular nonlipid compound

nonlocalized inflammation

nonlocking closure

nonlymphocytic
acute nonlymphocytic leukemia
n. cell
n. leukemia

nonlymphoid
acute nonlymphoid leukemia
n. leukemia

nonmalignant
n. adenoidal hypertrophy
n. disease

nonmarital introitus

nonmatching donor relative

nonmaternal death

nonmechanical trephination

nonmedullary
familial nonmedullary thyroid carcinoma

nonmedullated fiber

nonmegaloblastic macrocytic anemia

nonmelanoma skin cancer

nonmenstrual toxic shock syndrome

nonmetastatic
n. gestational trophoblastic disease
n. trophoblastic disease

nonmetric principal component analysis

nonmonogamous partner

nonmotile
n. bacteria
n. organism
n. pleomorphic bacillus
n. sperm

nonmucinous adenocarcinoma

non–mucosa

non–mucosa-associated lymphoid tissue lymphoma

nonmydriatic retinal photography

nonmyelinated axon

nonmyeloablative
n. allogeneic stem cell transplant
n. allogenic transplant
n. conditioning
n. conditioning regimen
n. HSCT

nonmyelosuppressive agent

nonnarcotic
n. analgesic
n. medication

nonnecrotizing angiitis

Nonne-Milroy disease

Nonne-Milroy-Meige syndrome

nonneoplastic
n. cyst
n. disease

nonneoplastic *(continued)*
n. lymphadenopathy
n. pathologic lesion
n. syndrome
nonneovascular age-related macular degeneration
nonnephrotic proteinuria
nonnephrotic-range proteinuria
nonneurogenic dysphagia
nonneuronal enolase
nonneuropathic systemic amyloidosis
nonnociceptive pain
nonnucleoside
n. reverse transcriptase inhibitor
n. RT inhibitor
nonnutrient agar plate
nonnutritive
n. sucking
n. sucking opportunity
nonobese
n. diabetic
n. type 2 NIDDM
nonobstructive
n. atelectasis
n. cardiomyopathy
n. hepatic parenchymal disease
n. jaundice
nonoccluded
n. baculovirus
n. virus
nonocclusive
n. dressing
n. intestinal ischemia
n. mesenteric infarction
n. mesenteric ischemia
nonocular muscle group
nonodontogenic cyst
nonofficial
New and Nonofficial Drugs
nonopaque
n. calculus
radio nonopaque stone
nonoperable
n. cancer
n. tumor
nonoperative
n. approach
n. biopsy technique
n. closure
n. diagnosis
nonoptic reflex eye movement
nonoral estradiol delivery system
nonorganic
n. blepharospasm
n. disorder diagnosis
n. failure to thrive
n. paresis
n. visual loss
nonosmotic stimulus
nonossifying fibroma
nonoxynol-9 cream
nonpalpable
n. abnormality
n., nontender
n. purpura
n. thyroid
nonpapillary
n. hyperplasia
n. thyrogenic carcinoma
nonparalytic
n. hypotonia
n. polio
n. poliomyelitis
n. strabismus
nonparasitic
n. cyst of liver
n. sycosis
nonparathyroid-related hypercalcemia
nonparenchymal
n. liver cell
nonparoxysmal
n. atrial tachycardia
n. atrioventricular junctional tachycardia
n. nodal rhythm
n. nodal tachycardia
nonpathogenic
n. fungus
n. spirochetal
nonpathological
n. amnesia
n. anxiety
n. dissociation
nonpatient contact
nonpenetrant gene
nonpenetrating
n. head trauma
n. keratoplasty
n. rupture
n. wound
non–penicillinase
nonpeptide antagonist
nonperforated
n. appendicitis
n. appendix
n. ulcer
nonpharmacologic
n. behavior management
n. therapy
nonpharmacological intervention
nonphotic
n. cue
n. entrainment
nonphysician surgical assistant
nonphysiologic visual field loss
nonpigmented
n. ciliary epithelium
n. endometriosis
n. nevus
nonpigment-producing acid-fast bacillus
nonpitting edema
nonpituitary thyrotropin
nonplacental blood flow
nonplague yersiniosis
nonpolar
n. amino acid
n. compound
nonpolio enterovirus
nonpolyposis
hereditary nonpolyposis colon cancer
hereditary nonpolyposis colon carcinoma
hereditary nonpolyposis colorectal cancer
hereditary nonpolyposis colorectal carcinoma
Muir-Torre syndrome of hereditary nonpolyposis colon cancer
n. colorectal cancer
nonprecipitable antibody
nonprecipitating antibody
nonprecipitation antibody
nonpregnant endometrium
nonprescription
n. drug
n. drug abuse
n. drug addiction
n. medication
over-the-counter nonprescription drug
n. pain reliever
nonpreserved artificial tears

nonprimary
n. first episode
n. infection

nonproductive
n. activity
n. behavior
n. cough

nonprogressive
n. cerebellar disorder with mental retardation
n. hypoplastic syndrome
long-term nonprogressive disease
n. motor impairment syndrome
partial nonprogressive stroke

nonproliferative
n. diabetic retinopathy
n. retinopathy

nonproprietary
International Nonproprietary Name
proposed international nonproprietary name
recommended international nonproprietary name

nonprotein
n. bound
n. carbohydrate calorie
n. kilocalories
n. nitrogen

nonpsychotic
n. Alzheimer patient
n. anxiety
n. hallucination

nonpulmonary route of elimination

nonpurgeable organic carbon

nonpurulent fluid

nonpyknotic nucleus

non-Q MI

non–Q-wave myocardial infarction

nonradioactive
n. hydrogen isotope
n. immunoassay
n. in situ hybridization

nonrandom
n. mating
n. X chromosome inactivation

nonrandomized
n. study
n. trial

nonrapid
n. eye movement
n. eye movement-rapid eye movement cycle
n. eye movement sleep

nonreactive
n. dermatitis
n. immunoassay
n. NST
n. pupil
pupil n.
n. RPR
serology n.
n. serology
n. tuberculosis
n. VDRL

Non-Reading
N.-R. Aptitude Test Battery
N.-R. Intelligence Test, Levels 1-3

nonreassuring
n. fetal heart beat pattern
n. fetal status
n. fetal testing
n. FHR

nonrebreather face mask

nonrebreathing
n. anesthesia
n. mask
n. system

nonrecurrent
anomalous nonrecurrent right inferior laryngeal nerve

nonreflective glass screen

nonrefractive accommodative esotropia

nonrehydrated guaiac examination

non-REM sleep

nonrenal
n. azotemia
n. clearance
n. death
n. potassium loss
n. water loss

nonresorbable
n. fixation
n. resin

nonrespiratory
n. acidosis
n. infection

nonresponder tolerance

nonresponsive
n. to antibiotic
n. patient
patient n.
n. tumor

nonrestorative sleep

nonrhabdomyosarcoma soft tissue sarcoma

nonrhegmatogenous retinal detachment

nonrheumatic
n. aortic insufficiency
n. atrial fibrillation

nonrheumatoid
n. episcleritis
n. scleritis

nonrhythmic electroencephalogram activity

non–rosette-forming cell

nonrotation
n. of bowel loop
n. of intestine
n. of kidney

nonsalt loser

nonsalt-losing adrenogenital syndrome

nonsalt-wasting congenital adrenal hyperplasia

nonsaturating
tilted optimized nonsaturating excitation

nonscarring alopecia

nonsclerosing ileitis

nonseasonal hay fever

nonsecreting
n. pituitary adenoma
n. pituitary tumor

nonsecretory
n. adrenal adenoma
n. glucagonoma
n. microadenoma

nonsedating antihistamine

nonsegmented neutrophils

nonselective
n. adenosine receptor antagonist
n. arterial digital angiography

nonseminomatous
n. germ cell neoplasm
n. germ cell testicular tumor

nonsense
n. codon
n. mutation
n. triplet

nonseptate mycelium

non–service-connected disability

nonsex hormone-binding globulin bound testosterone
nonsexual generation
nonsexually transmitted disease
nonshedding dog
nonshivering thermogenesis
nonsignificant difference
non-Sjögren keratoconjunctivitis sicca
non-skin-sparing mastectomy
non-small
non-small-cell
n.-s.-c. lung cancer
n.-s.-c. lung carcinoma
nonspecific
n. abdominal pain
n. abnormality
n. abnormality of ST segment and T wave
n. absorption
n. accumulation
n. anergy
n. arousal
n. arrhythmia
n. arthralgia
n. benefit
n. binding
n. bowel gas pattern
n. building-related illness
n. cardiomyopathy
cell-cycle nonspecific agent
n. change
n. cholinesterase
n. chronic interstitial pneumonitis
n. chronic lymphocytic thyroiditis
chronic nonspecific diarrhea
chronic nonspecific diarrhea of childhood
chronic nonspecific lung disease
n. climatic change
n. colitis
n. complaint
n. conglomerate
n. cross-reacting antigen
n. dermatitis
n. effect
n. effector cell
n. encephalomyeloneuropathy
n. encephalopathy
n. erosive gastritis
n. esophageal motility disorder
n. esophageal motor dysfunction
n. esophagitis
n. esterase
n. esterase stain
n. etiology
n. gingivitis
n. granulomatous disease
n. granulomatous orchitis
n. hepatocellular abnormality
n. histologic pattern
n. ileitis
n. immunity
n. immunotherapy
n. interstitial pneumonia-fibrosis
n. interstitial pneumonitis
n. intraventricular conduction defect
n. mental retardation
n. mesenchyme
n. nonerosive duodenitis
n. nonerosive gastritis
n. protein
n. reaction
n. ST change
n. stomatitis
n. ST and T wave
n. ST-T wave abnormality
n. ST-T wave change
n. ST wave segment changes on electroencephalogram
subtle and nonspecific symptom
n. suppressor cell
n. tachycardia
n. therapy
n. urethritis
n. vaginitis
n. vaginosis
nonspherocytic
congenital nonspherocytic hemolytic anemia
congenital nonspherocytic hemolytic disease
hereditary n.
hereditary nonspherocytic hemolytic anemia
non-spore-forming bacteria
nonstandard electrolyte solution
nonstarch polysaccharides
non-ST-elevation myocardial infarction
nonsterile irrigation technique
nonsteroidal
n. antiandrogen
n. antiandrogen monotherapy
n. antiestrogen
n. antiinflammatory
antiinflammatory nonsteroidal agent
n. antiinflammatory agent
n. antiinflammatory compound
n. antiinflammatory drug
n. antiinflammatory drug gastropathy
n. antiinflammatory drug-induced intestinal stricture
n. antiinflammatory medication
n. aromatase inhibitor
n. estrogen
nonsteroid-dependent asthmatic
nonstick gauze
nonstrenuous activity
nonstreptococcal pharyngitis
nonstress
fetal heart rate nonstress test
perinatal nonstress test
reactive nonstress test
n. test fetal monitoring
nonstressed fetus
nonstructural
n. gene
n. protein 4
n. protein
nonstruvite calculus
nonsuction grasper
nonsupported arm exercise
nonsuppressible
n. insulinlike activity
n. insulinlike activity factor
n. insulin-like protein
nonsuppurative
n. ascending cholangitis
chronic nonsuppurative destructive cholangitis
n. destructive cholangitis
nodular nonsuppurative panniculitis
n. otitis media
n. panniculitis
nonsurgeon, emergency department
nonsurgical
n. clinician
n. septal reduction therapy
n. therapeutic abortion
nonsusceptible
nonsustained
n. erection
n. monomorphic ventricular tachycardia
n. polymorphic ventricular tachycardia
ventricular tachycardia n.

nonsymptomatic
n. hemorrhoid
well-healed, n.
nonsymptomatic, nondisabling
nonsynchronous budding
nonsyncytia-forming
n.-f. HIV
n.-f. human immunodeficiency virus
n.-f. isolate
nonsyncytium-inducing chemokine
non-syncytium-inducing variant of AIDS virus
nonsyndromic
autosomal dominant nonsyndromic hearing loss
n. autosomal recessive disorder
autosomal recessive nonsyndromic hearing loss
n. bicoronal synostosis
n. bile duct paucity
n. coronal craniosynostosis
n. deafness
n. familial enlarged vestibular aqueduct
n. hearing loss
n. hereditary hearing impairment
nonsyphilitic treponematosis
nonsystemic reaction
nontender
breasts soft and n.
n. incarcerated inguinal hernia
nonpalpable, n.
nontest ear
nonthermal
nonionizing nonthermal application
nonthrombocytopenic
allergic nonthrombocytopenic purpura
n. preterm infant
n. purpura
nonthyroid
n. illness
n. index
nonthyroidal
n. disease
n. illness
n. illness syndrome
nontoxic
highest nontoxic dose
n. multinodular goiter
n. nodular goiter
nonautoimmune nontoxic diffuse goiter
n. sporadic goiter
n. thyroid adenoma
nontransmural
n. infarction
n. myocardial infarction
nontranssexual
gender identity disorder of adolescence or adulthood, nontranssexual type
nontraumatic
n. cardiac arrest
n. cardiac tamponade
n. coma
n. spinal tap
nontreatment group
nontreponemal
n. flocculation test
n. genital ulcer disease
n. serologic test
n. serology
n. syphilis test
non-*Treponema* titer
nontropical sprue
nontubed closed distant flap graft
nontuberculin mycobacterial disease
nontuberculous
disseminated nontuberculous mycobacterial infection
n. meningitis
n. mycobacteria
n. mycobacterial disease
n. mycobacterial infection
n. pneumonia
n. species
nontumorous
n. hypergastrinemic hyperchlorhydria
nontumorous hypergastrinemic hyperchlorhydria
nonturning against self psychology
nontypeable *Haemophilus influenzae*
non-typhi *Salmonella*
nontyphoid
n. salmonella
n. *Salmonella* bacteremia
nontyphoidal
n. salmonella infection
n. *Salmonella* species
n. salmonellosis
nontyphoid *Salmonella* bacteremia
nonulcer
n. dyspepsia
n. dysplasia
recurrent nonulcer dyspepsia
nonulcerative
n. blepharitis
n. disease
n. interstitial keratitis
nonuniform
n. attenuation
n. rotational defect
nonuniformity
dose nonuniformity ratio
nonunion
ankylosis n.'s
atrophic n.
avascular n.
bony n.
draining infected n.
n. fracture
n. of fracture
n. of fracture site
n. fracture trauma
fracture with n.
gap n.
n. gap metabolic acidosis
n. horse-hoof fracture
scaphoid nonunion advanced collapse
nonunited olecranon
nonurea
distillable nonurea adductable
n. nitrogen
nonurgent problem
nonuser
tobacco n.
nonvaccine serotype
nonvalent pneumococcal conjugate vaccine
nonvalved conduit
nonvalvular
n. atrial fibrillation
chronic nonvalvular atrial fibrillation
n. heart disease
nonvariceal bleeding
nonvascular abdominal surgery

nonvascularized
n. bone graft
n. fibular strut graft

nonvasculitic autoimmune inflammatory meningoencephalitis

nonvenereal
n. bubo
n. syphilis
n. treponematosis

nonventilated group

nonverbal
N. Ability Test
n. abstractive ability
n. behavior
n. communication
n. communication skill
n. cue
n. developmental index
n. expression
n. information
n. learning disability
Profile of N. Sensitivity
Test of N. Auditory Discrimination
Test of N. Intelligence
Toronto Biculture Test of N. Reasoning

nonvertex fetus

nonviable fetus

nonviolent
n. behavior
n. crime
n. delinquent

nonviral chronic hepatitis

nonvisualization of gallbladder

nonvital
n. bleaching
n. hepatitis

nonvolatile
n. acid
n. matter

nonwalking
short leg nonwalking cast

nonweightbearing
n. ambulation
n. brace
n. crutch walk
n. crutch walking
n. exercise
n., left
n., right
short leg nonweightbearing cast
touchdown n.

nonwhite
n. female
n. male

Noon
N. pollen unit

Noonan
neurofibromatosis with Noonan phenotype
N. syndrome

Noonan-like
N.-l. giant cell lesion
N.-l. giant cell lesion syndrome

noradrenaline
n. acid tartrate
n. bitartrate
n. reuptake inhibitor

noradrenergic
n. afferent
n. blocker
dorsal noradrenergic bundle
n. drug
n. effect
n. receptor
serotonin noradrenergic reuptake inhibitor
n. and specific serotonergic antidepressant

noradrenergic and specific serotonergic antidepressant

Nord appliance

nor-derivative progestin

NordiCare Back Therapy System

Nordic Track

nordihydroguaiaretic acid

Nordin-Ruiz trapezoidal marker

norepinephrine
apparent norepinephrine secretion rate
n. perikaryon
plasma n.
n. reuptake inhibitor
titrated norepinephrine excretion
n. transporter
urinary n.

norepinephrine-selective

norethindrone acetate

norgestrel
conjugated equine estrogen plus n.

norgestrel/ethinyl estradiol combination

Norio syndrome

norma
n. anterior
n. basilaris
n. facialis
n. frontalis
n. inferior
n. lateralis

normal
n. abdomen
absorbed normal pooled plasma
n. and active
adult, n.
n. adult female
n. adult male
n. affect
n. affective processing
affect within normal range
n. aging
n. alpha rhythm
aminooxypentane regulated-on-activation normal T-expressed and secreted
n. anatomic alignment
n. anatomic position
n. anatomic variation
n. animal
n. anteroposterior view
n. antibody
n. antithrombin
n. antitoxin
n. anxiety
n. in appearance
n. appendix
n. AP view
n. atmosphere
n. autistic phase
n. axis
n. axis deviation
n. base deficit
n. birth weight
n. bite
n. bladder caliber
n. blood index
n. blood indices
n. blood loss
n. blood pressure
n. blood serum
n. body temperature
n. bone marrow
n. bone marrow extract
n. bowel action
n. bowel function
n. bowel movement
n. bowel sounds

bowel sounds n.
bowel sounds normal and active
n. brain stem
n. breast tissue
n. burro serum
n. calcification
n. caliber duct
n. cardiac sound
cardiac sounds n.
n. carrier hepatitis
n. chest
n. chest film
n. child
n. childhood development
n. childhood diseases
n. childhood disorders
n. cholesteremic xanthomatosis
n. CI
n. circuitry
citrated normal rabbit serum
n. clonal CD4+ T cell
n. colon
color and temperature normal, both lower extremities
color and texture n.
n. color vision
n. complement of cells
n. concentration
conforms to social n.
n. contour of heart
n. control
cord normal in appearance
n. cornification
n. coronary arteries
n. curve
decibels normal hearing level
n. delivery
n. deposition
n. detrusor contractility
n. detrusor reflex
n. development
n. differential
difficulty functioning at normal ability level
diphtheria toxin n.
n. distribution
n. distribution of hair
n. dog serum
n. dose
easy n.
easy normal left
easy normal right
n. echogenicity
n. ejection fraction
n. electrical axis
n. electroencephalogram
n. electroencephalogram activity
n. emptying
enhancing normal breathing
n. equivalent deviation
n. evacuation of barium
n. exercise study
extension 50% of n.
n. external female genitalia
n. extracellular fluid volume
extraocular eye movements n.
n. extraocular movements
n. fecal antigen
n. female adult genitalia
n. female sex chromosome type
n. fetal development
n. fetal growth
n. flap-valve mechanism
flattening of normal lordotic curve
n. flexion of great toe
n. flora
n. flow
follow up intervention for normal development
n. full-term delivery
full-term normal delivery
full-term, normal, spontaneous delivery
n. functioning ileal transverse colostomy
n. fundus
fundus anterior, normal size and shape, and mobile
n. gastroesophageal reflux of infancy
n. glandularity
glucose in normal saline
n. glucose tolerance
n. goat serum
n. gonadal steroid level
n. growth and development
n. gut flora
n. hair distribution
hair normal texture
n. head and neck
head and neck n.
n. hearing
n. heart activity
n. heartbeat
n. heart function
heart and lungs n.
heart reduced to normal size
n. heart rhythm
n. heart size
heart sounds n.
n. heat defense
n. hematopoietic cell
n. histology
n. hormonal balance
n. horse serum
n. hospital air
n. host
n. human development
n. human diploid fibroblast
n. human gastric juice
n. human globulin
n. human kidney
n. human pooled plasma
n. human serum
n. human white matter
n. hydration
n. hypertrophic changes
n. immature brain tissue
n. immune system function
impaired normal activity
n. inactivated rabbit serum
n. individual
n. intelligence
n. intraocular tension
n. intravascular pressure
n. jaw function
n. Krebs-Henseleit solution
n. lactase activity
last normal vertebra
late effects of normal tissue
n. libido, coitus, and climax
n. light perception
n. limits
loss of normal architecture
n. low-density lipoprotein
lower normal limit
low renin, normal aldosterone
n. luteal phase
n. lymphocyte supernatant
n. lymphocyte transfer test
n. male adult genitalia
n. male infant
n. male sex chromosome type
n. menstrual period
microscopically normal tissue
momentary lapse in normal breathing
n. mouse serum
n. muscle development
n. neonatal nursery
neuromuscular firing in normal subject
n. newborn
n. newborn nursery
newborn, term, normal, female
newborn, term, normal, male
n. nursery
operative area irrigated with normal saline

normal *(continued)*
operative site irrigated with normal saline
n. opsonin
n. ovarian surface epithelium
n. ovariotomy
n. palate and pharynx
palate and pharynx n.
patient delivered normal infant
n. pelvic examination
percentage of n.
n. perfusion pressure breakthrough
n. pilosebaceous apparatus
n. placentation
n. plantar response
n. pool plasma
postoperative course n.
n. postpartum
predicted n.
n. pregnancy
n. pregnancy and delivery
n. prenatal care
n. pressure and temperature
prion protein normal isoform
n. pulmonary function
n. pupillary reaction to light
n. P wave
n. range
n. range of motion
range of motion within normal limits
n. rat kidney
n. reaction
n. record
reference normal serum
n. reference serum
reflux into terminal ileum n.
regulated upon activation, normal T-cell expressed and secreted
n. renal function
n. renin essential hypertension
replacement normal saline
n. resting pulse
n. resting pulse rate
restoration of normal anatomic alignment
resumption of normal sinus rhythm
n. retinal correspondence
n. retinal movement
n. rhythm of heart
n. saline
n. saline bolus
n. saline enema
n. saline solution
n. serum
n. serum albumin
serum normal agglutinator
n. serum thyroxine
n. sheep lung fibroblast
n. sheep red blood cell
shock heart into normal rhythm
n. single dose
n. sinus heart rhythm
n. sinus rate and rhythm
n. size and configuration
n. size heart
n. size and shape
n. size, shape, and consistency
n. size, shape, and location
n. size, shape, and position
n. size, shape, and position, anteverted and anteflexed uterus
n. sodium diet
n. sphincter tone
n. spinal fluid
n. spontaneous full-term delivery
n. spontaneous vaginal birth
standard normal deviation
sterile normal saline
n. temperature and pressure
n. tension
term normal delivery
n. throat flora
times upper limit of n.
n. toxin
n. transformation zone colposcopy
n. triglyceride levels
n. triglyceridemia
n. triglycerides
upper limits of n.
upper and lower extremities within normal limits
n. urinary function
n. urination
n. urine flow
n. urine output
n. vaginal delivery
n. value
n. variant short stature
n. visual acuity
n. vital capacity
n. vital signs
vital signs n.
n. volunteer
n. waking activity
n. waking electroencephalogram
n. waking electroencephalogram pattern
n. well developed
within normal range
wound irrigated with normal saline

normal-appearing
n.-a. stomach
n.-a. white matter

normal-finger tension

normalization
assay n.

normalized
n. alignment score
n. area under the curve
n. average glandular dose
n. cross-section
n. hearing
n. hearing level
international normalized ratio
mean normalized systolic ejection rate
n. mean square root
n. protein catabolic rate
n. protein nitrogen appearance

normalized alignment score

normally
bladder empties n.
cord moves n.
n. functioning kidney
n. nourished
n. progressing pregnancy
round, regular, react n.

normally functioning kidney

normal-mode ruby laser

normal-pressure
n.-p. glaucoma
n.-p. hydrocephalus

normal-tension glaucoma

Norman-Landing syndrome

Norman Miller vaginopexy

Norman-Roberts lissencephaly syndrome

Norman-Wood syndrome

normative
n. aging process
n. aspect
n. behavior
n. crisis
n. data
n. ethics

normetanephrine

normoactive
n. bowel sounds
n. bowel tone

normoblast
polychromatic n.

normocalcemic
n. hypercalciuria
n. primary hyperparathyroidism

normocapnic
hyperoxic n.

normocephalic
atraumatic n.
n. and atraumatic
n. head

normocholesteremic xanthoma

normochromic
n. anemia
n. erythrocyte
macrocytic normochromic anemia
n., normocytic anemia
n. normocytic erythrocyte
normocytic normochromic anemia

normocytic
n. erythrocyte
n. hypochromic anemia
n. normochromic anemia
normochromic normocytic erythrocyte

normoglycemic glycosuria

normokalemic
n. periodic paralysis

normokalemic periodic paralysis

normolipemic xanthomatosis

normolipoproteinemic xanthomatosis

normoprolactinemic woman

normospermatogenic sterility

normotensive
n. hydrocephalus
n. intrauterine growth restriction
n. Wistar rat

normovolemic
acute normovolemic hemodilution

norm physiological reflex

Norrie
N. disease
N. syndrome

Norrie-Warburg syndrome

Norris-Carrol criteria

Norris Educational Achievement Test

19-nortestosterone derivative

North
N. American antisnakebite serum
N. American blastomycosis
N. American Brain Tumor Consortium
N. American Malignant Hyperthermia protocol
N. American Nursing Diagnosis Association
N. Asian tick typhus
N. Carolina macular dystrophy
N. Queensland tick fever
N. Queensland tick typhus

Northbent scissors

Northeast Organ Procurement Organization

northern
n. bean extract
N. blot
N. blot analysis
N. blot technique
N. blot test
N. epilepsy with mental retardation
n. fowl mite
N. hybridization
n. rat flea
n. rat flea bite

Northland bone density machine

Northway
N. staging
N. virus

Northwestern
N. Syntax Screening Test
N. University Children's Perception of Speech Test

Norton operation

nortriptyline HCl

Norwalk
N. agent
N. disease
N. gastroenteritis
recombinant Norwalk virus
N. virus

Norwalk-like
N.-l. agent
N.-l. agent virus

Norway itch

Norwegian scabies

Norwood
N. classification
N. Classification of Male Pattern Baldness
N. classification system
N. donor site design

no-scalpel vasectomy

nose
ala of n.
n. anesthesia
anteater n.
apex of n.
artery of n.
artificial n.
blunt nose hemostat
n. bolus
n. clamp
n. cleft
n. clip
n. cone
depressor muscle of septum of n.
n. drops
ears, nose, and throat
n. to ear to xiphoid
eyes, ears, nose and throat
hair of n.
hammer n.
head, eyes, ears, nose, and throat
head, eyes, ears, nose, and throat unremarkable
n. height
medial crus of major alar cartilage of n.
oozing of blood from n.
packed n.
n. piercing
runny itchy n.
runny nose and eyes itchy
saddle n.
saddle nose deformity
sinuses, nose, throat
skin, head, eyes, ears, nose, and throat
n. stuffiness
whistling in nose while breathing

nose-breather
obligate n.-b.

nosed
end-biting blunt nosed rongeur

nosema disease

nose-pad dermatitis

nosocomial
n. acquired pneumonia
n. anemia
n. aspergillosis
n. bacteremia
n. bacterial infection
n. bacterial meningitis
n. and cross infection
n. diarrhea
n. eye infection
fatal nosocomial infection
n. fire

nosocomial *(continued)*
n. fungal infection
n. gangrene
n. gastroenteritis
n. gastrointestinal infection
n. Gram-negative infection
n. Gram-negative organism
Gram-positive nosocomial infection
n. Gram-positive infection
n. Gram-positive organism
n. gynecological infection
n. infective endocarditis
n. keratitis
n. *Legionella*
n. meningitis
n. myiasis
n. pathogen
n. postpartum endometritis
n. respiratory tract infection
n. retinochoroiditis
n. rotavirus infection
n. salmonellosis
n. septicemia
n. urinary tract infection
n. viral conjunctivitis
n. wound infection

nosologic black hole

nosotropic
n. drug
n. drug dementia of Alzheimer type

no-stitch phacoemulsification surgery

nostras
n. elephantiasis
influenza n.

nostril
anteverted n.
oozing of blood from n.
packed n.
right nostril naris

not
n. acidified
n. in active labor
n. admitted
n. at bedside
n. at risk
n. attempted
n. available
n. available at the present time
n. to be resuscitated
n. breastfed
n. classified
n. completed
n. considered disabling
n. considered disqualifying
n. cultured
n. detected
n. determined
n. diagnosed
n. in distress
n. done
n. elevated
n. elsewhere classifiable
n. elsewhere classified
n. elsewhere coded
n. elsewhere specified
n. enlarged
n. enough cells
n. equal
n. evaluated
n. examined
n. to exceed
n. favorably considered
n. filtered
n. fit for duty
n. found
n. found this examination
n. guilty by reason of insanity
has not voided
n. identified
n. invasive break-up time
n. isolated
n. keeping baby
n. knocked out
n. married, keeping baby
n. married, not keeping baby
n. measurable
n. measured
n. motile
n. nondetectable
n. on label
n. on patient
n. on unit
n. otherwise provided for
n. out of bed
n. palpable
n. perceptible
n. performed
n. pregnant
n. present
n. prisoner of war
n. for publication
n. reached
n. reacting
n. remarkable
n. resolved
n. routine care
n. sufficient quantity
n. symptomatic
n. tested
n. vaccinated
n. venereal
n. volatile
n. weighed
n. yet diagnosed
n. yet discovered
n. yet published

notalgia paresthetica

notariorum
paralysis n.

notation
computerized notation system
Fisher-Race notation

notch
n. of acetabulum
angular notch of stomach
anterior cerebellar n.
anterior notch of auricle
anterior notch of cerebellum
anterior notch of ear
aortic dicrotic notch pressure
n. of apex of heart
arterial dicrotic notch pressure
n. of cardiac apex
cardiac notch of left lung
cardiac notch of stomach
n. in cartilage of acoustic meatus
n. chest sign
clavicular notch of sternum
n. correction
costal notches of sternum
n. cut
dicrotic n.
n. of femur
n. filter
n. of gallbladder
n. gene family
greater sacrosciatic n.
greater sciatic n.
inferior thyroid n.
interclavicular notch of occipital bone
interclavicular notch of temporal bone
intercondylar notch of femur
n. of iris
jugular notch of temporal bone
n. for ligamentum teres
N. ligand
maxilla
n. of maxilla
median alveolar n.
nasal notch of maxilla
n. of radius

sciatic n.
N. signaling pathway
sternal notch to nipple
n. of sternum
superior thyroid n.
suprasternal n.
ulnar notch of radius
n. width index

notch-and-roll maneuver

notching
alar n.
antegonial n.
lid n.

notchplasty blade

note
attending's admission n.'s
n. blindness
followup n.
n. has been dictated/look for report
interim progress n.
intern admission n.
monthly progress n.
narrative n.'s
n., record, report
nurse's n.'s
off-service n.
percussion n.
postoperative n.
progress n.
resident's admission n.'s
resident's progress n.

nothing
n. abnormal detected
n. abnormal discovered
n. done
n. by mouth
n. by mouth at bedtime
n. by mouth nil per os
n. per mouth
n. per rectum
n. per vagina

Nothnagel
N. sign
N. syndrome

Nothnagel-type acroparesthesia

no-threshold
n.-t. body
n.-t. concept

notice
advance beneficiary n.
n. of disagreement
n. of proposed rulemaking
recognize, empathize, think, hear, integrate, notice, keep
until further n.

noticeable
barely noticeable difference
just noticeable difference

notifiable
n. disease
n. infectious disease

notification
funeral home n.
premarket n.

notify
n. of death
n. house officer

notion
grandiose n.

notochordal canal

no-touch transepithelial photorefractive keratectomy

Nottingham
N. colposuspension needle
N. Health Profile
N. modification of Scarff-Bloom-Richardson grading
N. Prognostic Index

nourished
normally n.
patient well n.
patient well developed, well n.
poorly n.

Novafil suture

NovaPulse

Nova Rectal

novel
n. antipsychotic
n. antipsychotic drug
n. diet
N. erythropoiesis
N. erythropoiesis-stimulating hormone
N. erythropoiesis-stimulating protein
n. form
n. form of consolidation chemotherapy
n. glycoprotein tapasin
n. missense mutation
n. pathogen

novo
de novo lesion
de novo thymidylate synthesis
saphenous vein graft de n.

novobiocin susceptibility test

Novoste Beta-Cath System

nov-ovalis

novum
new [L. *novum*]

Novus
N. 2000 ophthalmoscope

Novy and MacNeal blood agar

Novy-McNeal-Nicolle
N.-M.-N. biphasic blood agar
Novy-MacNeal-Nicolle medium

now

NoxBOX monitor

noxious
n. agent
diffuse noxious inhibitory control
patient responsive to noxious stimuli
n. stimulus
n. substance

Noyes
N. iridectomy scissors

NP-59
N. isotope
N. scintigraphy

N-phosphoacetate-L aspartate

***N*-phosphonoacetyl-*l*-aspartic acid**

***N-Ras* gene**

NREM-REM cycle

NR-1000F
Nikon Auto Refractometer N.

NSAID-induced gastric injury

nt-1, -2 virus

Ntaya virus

N-telopeptide
N.-t. collagen
N.-t. urine test

***N*-terminal**
-t. atrial natriuretic peptide
-t. fragment
-t. peptide
-t. telopeptide of type I collagen

N-type metal oxide semiconductor

nuchal
n. arm
n. cord
n. cord around infant's neck
n. cyst
n. cystic hygroma
n. dystonia
n. fascia
n. fibrocartilaginous pseudotumor
n. fibroma
n. fold
n. hemangioma
n. ligament
n. line
n. nevus
n. rigidity
tight nuchal cord around infant's neck
n. translucency
n. translucency in a fetus
n. translucency measurement
n. translucency screening
n. translucency thickness

Nuck
canal of N.
N. canal
N. diverticulum
N. hydrocele
patent canal of N.

nuclear
n. accessory hormone
n. agenesis
n. aggregate lipid
n. aggregation
n. angiography
n. angular momentum
n. antibody
anti-Epstein-Barr nuclear antigen
antiextractable nuclear antibody
n. antigen
anti-Mi-2 nuclear antibody
antineuronal nuclear antibody
antiproliferating cell nuclear antigen
n. anular differentiation
n. aplasia
apoptic nuclear fragment
n. arc
n. arthrogram
aryl hydrocarbon receptor nuclear translocator
n. atom
n. atypia
n. bag
n. bag fiber
n. bleeding scan
n. bone imaging
n. bronzing
n. bubbling artifact
cardiac nuclear probe scan
n. cardiac scan
n. cardiology laboratory
n. cardiovascular imaging
n. cataract
n. cell
n. cerebral angiogram
n. cerebral angiography
n. chain
n. chain fiber
n. change
chemical, biological, radiological or nuclear weapons
n. chemistry
n. chromation
n. complex
computerized nuclear morphometry
n. condensation
constant magnetic field in nuclear magnetic resonance
n. contour index
n. convolution
n. crystalline aggregate
n. debris
n. decay
n. degeneration
n. depression
n. developmental cataract
n. disintegration
n. DNA
n. dot pattern
n. dust
dynamic nuclear polarization
electron nuclear double resonance
embryonal nuclear cataract
n. enema
n. envelope
Epstein-Barr virus nuclear antigen
n. excision repair instability
n. expression
n. external layer
extractable nuclear antibody
extractable nuclear antigen
n. factor
n. factor of activated T cell
n. factor kappa B ligand
n. factor kappa B transcription factor protein
n. family
n. fast red stain
field focused nuclear magnetic resonance
first-pass nuclear angiocardiography
n. fragment
n. fragmentation
n. globulin inclusion
n. grade
n. hepatobiliary imaging
hepatocyte nuclear factor
hepatocyte nuclear factor-3
hepatocyte nuclear factor-4
hepatocyte nuclear factor-4a
heterogeneous nuclear ribonucleic acid
heterogeneous nuclear ribonucleoprotein
n. horizontal gaze paralysis
n. hormone receptor
n. hyaloplasm
n. imaging
n. inclusion body
infantile nuclear cerebral degeneration
n. inner layer
n. internal layer
n. jaundice
latency-associated nuclear antigen
latent nuclear antigen
lateral nuclear stratum
n. layers of retina
n. localization signal
n. localization signal motif
lytic-associated nuclear antigen
n. magnetic resonance
n. magnetic resonance imaging
n. magnetic resonance spectroscopy
n. matrix
n. matrix protein
medial nuclear stratum
n. medicine
n. medicine information system
n. medicine scan
n. membrane
n. membrane abnormality
n. milk
n. mitotic apparatus
n. morphometry
n. multiple gaited acquisition
n., biologic, chemical
n. ophthalmoplegia
n. outer layer
outer nuclear layer
n. palsy
paraventricular nuclear stratum
Pelger-Huët nuclear anomaly
Pelger-Huët nuclear anomaly
n. pharmacist
n. pharmacy

phosphorus nuclear magnetic resonance spectroscopy
n. polyhidrosis virus
n. pore complex
progressive nuclear palsy
proliferating nuclear cell antigen
n. quadruple resonance
n. radiation
radiofrequency magnetic field in nuclear magnetic resonance
receptor activator of nuclear factor-kappa B
receptor activator of nuclear factor kappa B ligand
n. receptor corepressor
rheumatoid arthritis nuclear antigen
n. ribonucleic acid
n. ribonucleoprotein
n. ring
round spermatid nuclear injection
n. runoff assay
n. scan
n. scintigraphy
n. sclerosis
n. sclerosis of lens
n. sex
small nuclear ribonucleic acid
small nuclear ribonucleoprotein
small nuclear ribonucleoprotein-associated polypeptide
n. stress test
n. tissue
total nuclear score
n. tracer
n. track emulsion
n. transcription factor
n. translocation
tritium nuclear magnetic resonance
n. venogram
n. ventricular function study
n. zone

nuclear-cytoplasmic
n.-c. ratio

nuclear-fascicular trochlear nerve palsy

nuclear-tagged cell

nuclease

nucleated
absolute nucleated red blood cell
n. cell count
n. endothelial cell
n. erythrocyte
peripheral nucleated cell
n. RBC
n. red blood cell mass
n. red cell

nucleation time

nuclei (*pl. of* nucleus)

nucleic
n. acid
n. acid amplification
n. acid amplification technique
n. acid amplification test
n. acid amplification testing
n. acid base
n. acid-binding protein
n. acid construct
n. acid detection
n. acid hybridization
n. acid hybridization analysis
n. acid hybridization test
n. acid immunization
n. acid phosphatase
n. acid probe
n. acid probe assay
n. acid sequence-band amplification
n. acid sequence-based amplification
n. acid sequence-based analysis
n. acid sequencing
n. acid vaccination
n. acid vector
infectious nucleic acid
pentose nucleic acid
peptide nucleic acid

nucleocapsid
n. antigen-specific
n. antigen-stimulated interferon-gamma
HIV nucleocapsid protein
multiple nucleocapsid virus

nucleolar
argyrophilic nucleolar organizer region
argyrophilic nucleolar organizer region staining
n. chromosome
n. organizing region
n. pattern
silver-staining nucleolar organizer region
n. staining

nucleolus, pl. **nucleoli**
chromatin clumps and nucleoli

nucleolus-organizing region

nucleoplasmic index

nucleopolyhedrovirus
multiple n.
single n.

nucleoprotein
extractable n.

nucleoside
n. analog
n. analog monotherapy
n. analog reverse transcriptase inhibitor
n. analog RT inhibitor
n. bisphosphate
n. diphosphate
n. diphosphate kinase
n. 5′-diphosphate kinase
n. diphosphate sugar
n. monophosphate
n. 5’-monophosphate
n. monotherapy
n. pair
n. reverse transcriptase inhibitor
n. triphosphate

nucleoside-associated mitochondrial toxicity

nucleosome
n. antibody
n. ladder

nucleotidase
diphosphopyridine n.

nucleotide
adenosine nucleotide translocator
n. analog
n. deletion
diphosphopyridine n.
guanine nucleotide regulatory protein
n. pair
n. polymorphism
purine nucleotide cycle
pyridine n.
n. residue
n. reverse transcriptase inhibitor
n. sequence
n. sequence analysis
single nucleotide polymorphism
single nucleotide polymorphisms - linkage disequilibrium
total adenine n.
n. triphosphate
triphosphopyridine n.

nucleotide-binding domain

nucleotomy
percutaneous n.

Nuclepore filter

nucleus, pl. **nuclei**

nucleus *(continued)*
n. of abducens nerve
n. of abducent nerve
n. of accessory nerve
accessory nucleus Monakow n.
n. of acoustic nerve
n. acusticus
n. ambiguus
n. amygdalae
n. amygdalae centralis
n. amygdalae corticalis
n. amygdalae lateralis
n. amygdalae medialis
angled nucleus removal loupe
angular vestibular n.
n. anterior
anterior dorsal n.
nuclei anteriores thalami
anterior extremity of caudate n.
anterior hypothalamic n.
anterior interpositus n.
anterior median n.
anterior nucleus of thalamus
anterior nucleus of trapezoid body
anterior olfactory n.
anterior periventricular n.
anterodorsal nucleus of thalamus
anterodorsal thalamic n.
n. anteroinferior thalami
anteromedial caudate n.
anteromedial nucleus of thalamus
anteromedial thalamic n.
n. anterosuperior thalami
n. anteroventralis
n. anteroventralis thalami
anteroventral nucleus of thalamus
anteroventral thalamic n.
arcuate n.
arcuate nucleus of brain
arcuate nucleus of the hypothalamus
arcuate nucleus of thalamus
n. arcuatus
n. arcuatus of intermediate hypothalamic area
n. arcuatus medullae oblongatae
n. arcuatus of medulla oblongata
n. arcuatus thalami
autonomic oculomotor n.
autonomic visceral motor n.
n. basalis
n. basalis of Ganser
n. basalis lesion
n. basalis of Meynert
n. caeruleus
n. of Cajal
caudal central n.
nuclei of caudal colliculus
n. caudalis centralis
caudate n.
n. caudatus
n. centralis
n. centralis lateralis
n. centralis lateralis thalami
n. centralis medialis thalami
n. centralis superior raphe
n. centralis tegmenti superior
nuclei cerebelli
n. cervicalis lateralis
cochlear n.
n. cochlearis anterior
n. cochlearis posterior
corticomedial amygdaloid n.
cranial motor nuclei
cranial motor nuclei
nuclei of cranial nerve
n. of cranial nerve
nuclei of cranial nerve
n. of cuneate fasciculus
n. cuneatus
n. cuneatus, pars centralis
n. cuneatus pars, rostralis
n. cuneatus tubercle
Deiters n.
dorsal column n.
nuclei dorsales thalami
n. dorsales thalami
n. of dorsal field
n. dorsalis
n. dorsalis of Clarke
dorsal motor nucleus of vagus
dorsal raphe n.
dorsal vagal n.
dorsomedial n.
dorsomedial hypothalamic nucleus lesion
n. dorsomedialis-ventromedialis
n. endopeduncularis
n. facialis
n. fasciculi gracilis
fastigial n.
n. fibrosus lingua
fully resonant n.
n. gigantocellularis medullae oblongatae
n. of Goll
n. gracilis tubercle
n. habenula
n. habenularis lateralis
n. habenularis medialis
herniation of nucleus pulposus
n. hydrolysis needle
n. hypoglossalis
n. of hypoglossal nerve
hypothalamic ventromedial n.
n. implant
infundibular n.
intermediate n.
interpeduncular n.
n. interpositus
interstitial nucleus of Cajal
lateral cervical n.
lateral geniculate n.
lateral hypothalamic n.
n. lateralis medullae oblongatae
nucleus lateralis posterior
n. lateralis tuberis
lateral reticular n.
lateral ventromedial n.
lateral vestibular n.
left caudate n.
n. of lens
n. lentiformis
n. lentis
Lindstrom Star nucleus manipulator
n. of Luys
magnocellular n.
main cuneate n.
n. of mamillary body
mamillary nuclei receptor
medial accessory olivary n.
medial amygdaloid n.
medial central nucleus of thalamus
medial dorsal nucleus of thalamus
medial geniculate n.
medial habenular n.
medial interlaminar n.
medial nucleus of trapezoid body
medial septal n.
medial ventromedial n.
medial vestibular n.
midbrain raphe n.
nuclei nervi trigemini
nucleus lateralis posterior
number of neutrons in an atomic n.
oculomotor n.
n. of optic tract
Orphan Annie-eyed clear n.
oval hyperchromatic n.
owl's eye n.
parafascicular n.
paramedian reticular n.
n. paraventricularis
paraventricular nucleus of the hypothalamus
paraventricular thalamic n.

Pearce nucleus hydrodissector
pedunculopontine n.
periaqueductal gray n.
periventricular n.
nuclei periventriculares
pontine n.
n. of posterior commissure
premamillary n.
n. preopticus
n. of pretectal area
prosthetic disk n.
n. pulposus
n. pulposus herniation
quasiresonant n.
n. raphe magnus
red n.
n. removal loupe
reticular n.
n. retroambigualis
rhombencephalic gustatory n.
right caudate n.
sexually dimorphic n.
n. spatula
sublentiform n.
subthalamic n.
subthalamic nucleus implant
suprachiasmatic n.
supramamillary n.
supraoptic hypothalamic n.
n. supraopticus
supratrochlear n.
thalamic gustatory n.
trigeminal n.
trochlear n.
n. ventralis anterior of thalamus
ventral posterolateral n.
ventrocaudal n.
ventrolateral nucleus of hypothalamus
ventromedial n.
ventromedial hypothalamic neuron, nucleus
ventromedial nucleus of the hypothalamus
vestibular n.
visceral n.

nuclide analysis

nuda

nude
n. bone graft transplantation
n. mouse

Nu-Derm
N.-D. hydrocolloid
Obagi N.-D.
N.-D. System

nudge test

Nugent
N. criteria
N. score

Nugent-Gradle scissors

Nugent-Green-Dimitry erysiphake

Nugget virus

null
n. allele
n. cell
n. cell acute lymphocytic leukemia
n. cell adenoma
n. cell anaplastic large cell lymphoma
n. cell lymphoblastic leukemia
n. cell lymphoma
n. cell tumor
n. condition
n. hypothesis
n. lymphocyte
n. point
n. zone

nulligravida
n. female
patient n.
n. patient

nulling
gradient moment n.

nullipara

nulliparous
n. introitus
patient n.

null-type non-Hodgkin lymphoma

numb
n. cheek syndrome
n. chin syndrome
n. finger
n. hand

number
atomic n.
atomic orbital with angular momentum quantum number zero
n. of atoms
average gradient n.
Brinell hardness n.
computed tomography n.
n. concentration
n. connection test
n. of degrees of freedom
n. of density of molecule
n. of different words
diploid chromosome n.
n. dysgnosia
n. equal to one; single patient trial
n. of excitation
fluoride n.
haploid chromosome n.
Hedstrom n.
hospital day n.
incompatibility n.
ionic charge n.
Knoop hardness number of solids
large number hypothesis
limiting viscosity n.
linking n.
Loschmidt's n.
magnetic quantum n.
mass n.
maximal number of lamella
maximal number of microbes killed
moderate number of medium rales
Mohs hardness n.
n. of molecules
most probable n.
n. needed to treat
n. of needle passes
neutron n.
neutron number density
n. of neutrons in an atomic nucleus
noise and number index
n. of dissimilar matches
n. of observations
organism identification number
Peclet n.
personal identification n.
plasma exchange number three
n. of pregnancies producing viable offspring
principal quantum n.
proton n.
Rayleigh n.
Reynolds n.
Rockwell hardness n.
n. of similar negatives
n. of similar positives
spin quantum n.
stoichiometric n.
suicide precautions number 1, 2
time required to double number of cells in given population
Treatment Authorization N.
triploid chromosome n.
turnover n.
unique patient n.
n. user identification

number *(continued)*
variable numbers of tandem repeats
Vickers hardness n.
wave n.
n. of words chosen

numbness
aching and n.
n. in arm
n. of arm
n. in back
cold burning, pain and n.
n. in extremity
n. of face
n. in feet
n. of finger
n. in foot
n. and hypesthesia
n. of lip
n. in lower back
n. in lower leg
n., weakness and paralysis of arm
pain and n.
periodic hemilingual n.
n. and tingling
n. or tingling
n. and tingling around mouth
n., tingling, and burning
n. and tingling in finger
tingling and numbness in feet
n., tingling, and pain
n. in toe
n. of tongue
n. or weakness

numeric
n. aperture
n. hypertrophy
N. Pain Intensity Scale
n. rating scale

numerical
n. aperture
N. Attention Test
n. cipher method
n. taxonomy
verbal, numerical, and reasoning
n. visual acuity
Visual N. Discrimination Pretest

numeric rating scale

numerous
n. coarse rales
red cells too numerous to count
studded with numerous tumor nodules
too numerous to count

nummular
n. atrophy
n. dermatitis
n. eczema
n. eczematous dermatitis
n. erythema
n. keratitis
n. lesion
n. neurodermatitis
n. syphilid

nummularis
psoriasis n.

Nunn engorged corpuscles

Nuremberg Aging Inventory

Nurick classification of spondylosis

Nurolon suture

nurse
n. aide
American N.'s Association
auxiliary nurse midwife
n. cell
n. cell environment
charge n.
computer liaison n.
diabetes nurse educator
n. diagnosis
did not n.
flight n.
head n.
home health n.
human skin nurse cell
n. late entry
licensed practical n.
licensed vocational n.
n. manager
mobile intensive care n.
National Association of Pediatric N. Associates and Practitioners
n. notes
oncology certified n.
ophthalmic n.
n. practitioner
primary n.
private day n.
private duty n.
public health n.
quality control n.
scrub n.
sexual assault nurse examiner
N. Training Act
visiting registered n.

nurse cell environment

nursed
n. fair
n. fairly well
n. poorly

nursed fairly well

nurse-managed center

nurse-midwife
certified n.-m.

nursery
convalescent growing n.
extended-care n.
full-term n.
hand washing in n.
intensive care n.
intensive special care n.
intermediate care n.
maximum observation n.
N. Neurobiological Risk Score
newborn n.
normal n.
normal neonatal n.
normal newborn n.
premature n.
special care n.
well-baby n.
well-born n.

Nurses'
N. Observation Scale for Inpatient Evaluation

Nurse's
N. Global Impressions

nurse's

nurse-to-nurse orders

nursing
n. action
n. assignment
n. assistant
n. audit
n. bottle caries
n. care
n. care card
n. care continuity
n. care integration
N. Care Intervention Tool
n. care plan
certified skilled nursing facility
clinical n.
community nursing home
contract nursing home
n. coordination
coronary care n.
critical care n.
n. facility
n. facility-acquired pneumonia
family-centered maternity n.

general nursing assistance
general nursing care
n. goal
home n.
n. home
n. home care
n. home care unit
home nursing care
n. home placement
n. home transfer
innovative psychiatric nursing intervention
intensive nursing care
intermittent skilled nursing care
n. intervention
N. Interventions Classification
neurointermediate nursing unit
North American N. Diagnosis Association
n. office
operating nursing procedure
patient discharged to nursing home
patient discharged to skilled nursing facility
patient transferred to nursing home
patient transferred to skilled nursing facility
n. practice
primary care n.
n. procedure
n. quality assurance
regular nursing floor
restorative nursing program
scheduled nursing activities program
skilled nursing extended care facility
skilled nursing care
skilled nursing visit
n. station
Systematic N. Observation of Psychopathology
transfer to nursing home
n. triage

Nursing-Care Dependency scale

Nursoy formula

nurturing environment

Nussbaum experiment

nut
areca n.

nutation
n. angle
n. angle measurement

nutcracker
n. esophagus
n. fracture

nutmeg
n. appearance
nux moschata n.

nutraceutical data

nutricia
arteria nutricia tibiae
arteria nutricia ulnae

nutriciae

nutrient
absorption of n.'s
n. absorption
n. agar
anomalous fibular nutrient artery
n. artery
n. artery of femur
n. artery of fibula
n. artery growth
n. artery of humerus
n. artery of radius
n. artery of the tibia
n. artery of tibia
n. artery of ulna
n. broth
calcium nutrient agar
n. canal
n. canal of bone
n. deficiency
diffusion of oxygen and n.'s
n. enema
n. flap
n. foramen
n. gelatin agar
oxygenated fluorocarbon nutrient emulsion
recommended nutrient intake
n. requirement
n. sporulation medium
total digestible n.'s
total nutrient admixture

nutrition
alteration in nutrition intake
artificial nutrition and hydration
cachexia and n.
central venous n.
child n.
cyclic total parenteral n.
diet and n.
enteral n.
enteral nutrition solution
n. and exercise
fluids and n.
fluids, aeration, nutrition, communication, activity, and pain
fluids, aeration, nutrition, communication, activity, and stimulation
fluids, electrolytes, n.
Food and N. Information Center
health and nutrition examination survey
hemodialysis prognostic nutrition index
home enteral n.
home nutrition therapy
home total parenteral n.
immune modulating nutrition
n. intake
intradialytic parenteral n.
intravenous n.
N. Labeling and Education Act of 1990
National Health and N. Examination Follow-Up Study
National Health and N. Examination Survey
parenteral and enteral n.
partial parenteral n.
peripheral parenteral n.
peripheral vein total parenteral n.
peripheral venous n.
n. plan
n. ratio
n. repletion
n. status
supplementary parenteral n.
support parenteral n.
total enteral n.
total peripheral parenteral n.
n. and weight control

nutritional
n. adequacy
n. amblyopia
n. amenorrhea
n. anemia
appropriate nutritional supplementation
n. blindness
n. change
n. characteristic
n. cirrhosis
n. consultation
n. counseling
n. deficiency
n. deficiency cataract
n. deficiency dermatitis
n. deficiency disorder
n. deficiency eczema

nutritional *(continued)*
n. deficit
n. deprivation syndrome
n. dropsy
n. edema
enteral nutritional supplement
enteral nutritional support
enteral nutritional therapy
fatty nutritional cirrhosis
n. hemosiderosis
n. hepatotoxicity
n. imbalance
n. immunity
n. immunology
n. intervention
intravenous nutritional fluid
intravenous nutritional therapy
knowledge, attitude, behavior, and improvement in nutritional status
n. macrocytic anemia
n. marasmus
mineral-related nutritional disorder
n. neuropathy
n. optic neuropathy
physician's nutritional recommendation
n. polyneuropathy
n. problem
prognostic nutritional index
n. rickets
n. secondary hyperparathyroidism
n. state
n. status
n. status assessment
n. status type
n. supplementation
n. support
n. support service
n. support team
n. surveillance
systematic nutritional muscle testing
therapeutic nutritional intake
n. therapy

nutritionally
n. balanced diet
n. deprived
n. variant streptococcus

nutritive
n. enema
n. equilibrium
n. sucking

nutures
caregiver nutures patient

Nuvita lens

Nuvolase 660 laser system

nux moschata nutmeg

Nyando virus

nyctalopia with congenital myopia

nyctohemeral rhythm

NYHA
N. congestive heart failure classification
N. functional classification

Nyhan-Lesch syndrome

Nylen-Bárány maneuver

nylidrin hydrochloride

nylon
n. bristle
n. catheter
n. fiber
n. frame
n. loop
McIntyre nylon cannula connector
monofilament nylon suture
n. retention suture
n. stocking dermatitis
n. suture material

Nyquist
N. criterion
N. frequency

nystagmoid-like oscillation

nystagmoid movement

nystagmus
benign paroxysmal positioning n.
n. blockage syndrome
congenital n.
direction-changing positional n.
end-gaze physiologic n.
endpoint n.
n. examination
fine rapid n.
gaze n.
horizontal gaze n.
latent n.
malignant persistent positional n.
manifest latent n.
minimal amplitude n.
muscle paretic n.
ocular bobbing n.
ocular dysmetria n.
ocular flutter n.
n. on upward gaze
optokinetic after n.
periodic alternating windmill n.
peripheral vestibular n.
positional alcohol n.
refractory convergence n.
rotatory n.
Southern California Postrotary N. Test
spontaneous n.
sustained horizontal n.
n. test
upbeat torsional n.
n. with demyelination

nystatin
gentamicin, vancomycin, and n.
triamcinolone and n.

oak
live oak tree
poison o.
o. tree
o. tree pollen

Oaks straight cannula

Oak-Vale virus

o-aminobenzoic acid

OARS Multidimensional Functional Assessment Questionnaire

oasthouse urine disease

oat
o. cell
o. cell carcinoma
o. cell lung cancer
o. cell tumor

oath
Hippocratic o.

oatmeal-tomato paste agar

oatmeal treatment

OAV dysplasia

Obagi
O. chemical peel
O. controlled variable-depth peel
O. Nu-Derm

obedience
automatic o.

Ober
O. anterior transfer
O. test

Obermeier spirillum

Obersteiner-Redlich line

obese
o. abdomen
o. adolescent
o. bed
o. body
o. child
o. hypertensive patient
morbidly o.
New Zealand obese mouse
o. pannus
o. patient
o. type 2 noninsulin-dependent diabetes mellitus

obesity
cardiorespiratory syndrome of obesity in child
o. care
Central O. Index
o. in endometrial sarcoma
family history of o.
o. of hyperinsulinism
hypotonia, hyperphagia, hypogonadism, o.
hypotonia, hypomentia, hypogonadism, and obesity syndrome
o. hypoventilation syndrome
o. and inactivity
o. index
macrosomia, obesity, macrocephaly, ocular abnormality syndrome
male pattern o.
medical complications of o.
mental retardation, gynecomastia, obesity syndrome
mental retardation, short stature, obesity, hypogonadism syndrome
o., short stature, mental deficiency, hypogonadism, micropenis, finger contracture, cleft lip-palate syndrome

obesity-associated diabetes

obesity-hypotonia syndrome

obesity-related hyposomatotropism

obesity/type 2 diabetes syndrome

object
o. addict
o. addiction
agent, action, and o.
o. agnosia
o. of arousal
o. assembly
o. assembly test
o. attachment
o. attitude
o. blindness
o. cathexis
o. choice
O. Classification Test
o. code
o. concept
o. consistency
o. constancy
o. coordinate system
o. of a delusion
o. displacement
o. distance
distant objects blurry
distant objects fuzzy
o. finding
focus object distance
foreign o.
o. halos
o. identification
o. ill
inability to recognize o.'s
mini object test
oriented to time, place, person, and objects watch, pen, book
o. of regard
o. size
O. Sorting Scales psychologic test
O. Sorting Test
o. space
o. test
turning against o.
unidentified bright o.
unidentified foreign o.

object/body
foreign o.

object/image
o. conjugacy
o. relationship

objectionable
aggressive objectionable behavior

objective
o. angle
o. anxiety
o. assessment
behavior o.
o. benefit
o. complement
o. correlative
o. criticism
o. examination
o. findings
o. improvement
long-range o.
o. neurologic signs
o. optometer
O. Pain Scores
o. perimetry
o. prism-neutralized cover test
o. refractor
o. structural clinical examination
subjective, objective, management, and analytic
surgical treatment o.
o. swelling
o. symptom
systematic, complete, objective, practical, empirical
o. tinnitus
o. vertigo
visualized treatment o.

Objective-Analytic Anxiety Battery

object-space focus

obligate
o. aerobe
o. anaerobe
o. autotroph
o. carrier
o. heterozygote
o. intercellular organisms
o. intracellular parasite
o. intracellular protozoan
o. myiasis
o. nose-breather

obligations fear

obligatory
o. heel valgus
o. suppression
o. thermogenesis

oblique
o. abdominal muscle
o. aberration
o. amputation
o. annihilation photon pair
anterior o.
anterior oblique ligament
anterior oblique line of radius
anterior oblique meniscal tear
anterior oblique position
anterior oblique projection
aponeurosis of abdominal oblique muscle
aponeurosis of external o.
aponeurosis of external oblique muscle
aponeurosis of internal oblique muscle
aryepiglottic part of oblique arytenoid muscle
o. arytenoid
o. arytenoid muscle
o. astigmatism
astigmatism of oblique pencils
o. auricular muscle
axial left anterior oblique ventriculogram
o. axial MR imaging
o. base-wedge osteotomy
o. bundle of pons
o. capitis muscle
o. closing wedge osteotomy
o. cord
o. cord of interosseous membrane of forearm
o. coronal plane
o. crest
o. diameter
o. displacement
o. displacement osteotomy
distal oblique groove
o. dysfunction
external oblique aponeurosis
external oblique fascia
external oblique muscle
external oblique muscle of abdomen
o. facet wiring
o. facial cleft
o. fibers of muscular layer of stomach
o. fissure
o. fissure of lung
o. flap
o. flow misregistration
o. fluoroscopy
o. forward-viewing instrument
o. fracture
o. gastric fiber
o. head
o. hernia
o. illumination
o. incision
inferior oblique eye muscle
inferior oblique overaction
inferior oblique recession
internal oblique approximated
internal oblique muscle of abdomen
lateral oblique x-ray view
left anterior oblique projection
left inferior oblique muscle
left oblique inguinal hernia
left posterior o.
left superior o.
o. lie
o. ligament of elbow joint
o. line
o. line of mandible
o. line of thyroid cartilage
long axial oblique view
Marshall oblique vein
medial oblique view
medial oblique x-ray view
mediolateral o.
o. midtarsal joint axis
o. muscle
o. muscle of abdomen
o. muscle of eyeball
o. muscle hook
o. nystagmus
overactive superior o.
o. palsy
o. position
posterior oblique ligament
o. presentation
o. prism
o. prism device
o. ray of light
o. retinacular ligament
o. ridge
right anterior o.
right anterior caudocranial o.
right anterior oblique position
right anterior oblique projection
right anterior oblique view
right inferior oblique muscle
right oblique inguinal hernia
right posterior oblique radiologic view
right superior oblique muscle
right superior oblique palsy
o. study
superior o.
o. talus
transverse groove of oblique ridge
vastus medialis oblique muscle
vertical subcondylar o.
o. view

obliquity
Litzmann o.
Nägele o.
o. superior muscle

obliquus
o. abdominis externus muscle
adductor pollicis obliquus muscle
o. capitis superior
o. capitis superior muscle
o. externus abdominis
musculus arytenoideus o.
musculus obliquus superior bulbi
musculus obliquus superior oculi
o. vastus
vastus medialis obliquus musculus

obliterans
arteriosclerosis o.
atherosclerosis o.
balanitis xerotica o.
bronchiolitis o.
bronchiolitis obliterans syndrome
thromboangiitis o.

obliterated
o. arteriovenous malformation
o. basal cistern

obliterating
o. arteritis
o. endarteritis

obliteration
o. of apophyseal space
balloon-occluded retrograde transvenous o.
percutaneous transhepatic o.
terminal hepatic vein o.

obliterative
o. airway disease
o. arachnoiditis
o. arteriosclerosis
o. arteritis
o. bronchitis
o. cardiomyopathy
o. coronary artery disease
o. endarteritis
o. fibroproliferative bronchiolitis
o. granulomatous fibrosis
o. pleuritis
o. pulmonary hypotension
o. vascular disease

oblongata
anterior column of medulla o.
anterior median fissure of medulla o.
medulla o.
nucleus arcuatus of medulla o.
pons o.

oblongatae
nucleus arcuatus medullae o.
nucleus gigantocellularis medullae o.
nucleus lateralis medullae o.

oblong fovea of arytenoid cartilage

Obodhiang virus

O'Brien
O. actinic granuloma
O. akinesia technique
O. anesthesia
O. capsular shift procedure
O. cataract
O. classification of radial fracture
O. goniometer
O. lid block
O. marker
O. spud
O. stitch scissors

Obrinsky syndrome

obscene
o. expression
o. gesture

obscured fovea

obscure vision

observation
o. and assessment
Autism Diagnostic O. Schedule
behavioral observation audiometry
cardiac observation unit
o. care unit
Cognitive O. Guide
o. commitment
coronary observation ratio
daily observation for rejection
o. delusion
direct observation evaluation
direct observation unit
discharge patient after period of o.
emergency observation bed
epidemic observation unit
evaluation and o.
o. and examination
o. hip
Home O. for Measurement of the Environment
24-hour period of observation and hydration
o. and hydration
intensive o.
intensive therapy observation unit
light and electron immunoperoxidase o.
maximum observation nursery
o. and monitoring
number of o.'s
Nurses' O. Scale for Inpatient Evaluation
Pain O. Scale for Young Children
patient admitted for o.
patient admitted for observation and treatment
prelinguistic autism diagnostic o.
Receptive-Expressive Observation Scale
special o.
suicidal observation status
Systematic Nursing O. of Psychopathology
o. and treatment
treatment and o.
under o.
visual observation shivering score

observational study

observed
clinically observed seizure
directly observed therapy
directly observed treatment, short course
heart o.
o. intrinsic frequency
lowest observed adverse effect level
modified directly observed therapy
no observed adverse effect level
no observed effect dose
standard observed minus expected

observer
O. Assessment of Alertness and Sedation
o. drift
o. variation

obsession
aggressive o.
alien o.
idiosyncratic obsessions and rituals
irrational obsession with imagined ugliness

obsessional
o. anxiety
o. brooding
o. character
o. compulsive inventory alpha
o. fascination
o. feature
o. idea
o. impulse
Leyton Obsessional Inventory
Maudsley Obsessional Compulsive Inventory
overvalued obsessional ideas
o. thought
vague obsessional thoughts

obsessive
o. attack
o. behavior
Children's Yale-Brown O. Compulsive Scale
o. dieting
o. doubt
o. exercise
o. fantasy
o. fear
o. feeling
o. feelings of responsibility
o. impulse
National Institute of Mental Health-Global O. Compulsive Scale
o. neurotic
neurotic o.
o. personality
o. rumination
o. symptoms

obsessive-compulsive
o.-c. behavior
o.-c. conduct disorder
o.-c. disorder with poor insight type
O.-c. Drinking Scale
o.-c. feature
O.-c. Inventory

obsessive-compulsive *(continued)*
- o.-c. neurosis
- O.-c. Neurosis Scale
- o.-c. overeating
- o.-c. personality
- o.-c. personality disorder
- o.-c. reaction

obsessive feelings of responsibility

obsessive-type personality

obsolete

obstacle-dominance

Obstbaum synechia spatula

obstetric
- o. accident
- o. anesthesia
- o. binder
- o. brachial plexus injury
- o. brachial plexus palsy
- o. care
- clinical obstetrics and gynecology
- o. complication
- o. conjugate
- o. conjugate diameter
- o. conjugate of outlet
- o. conjugate of pelvic outlet
- o. damage
- o. factor
- International Federation of Gynecology and O. classification of tumor staging
- o. forceps
- o.'s and gynecology
- o. hand
- o. history
- o. hysterectomy
- lupus obstetric syndrome
- o. neuropathy
- o. operation
- o. outcome
- o. paralysis
- o. position
- postpartum o.'s
- o. prediabetes
- o. risk factor
- surgery, gynecology, and o.'s
- o. traction injury
- o. ultrasound

obstetrical
- o. complication
- o. conjugate
- court-ordered obstetrical intervention
- o. hand
- o. history
- o. injury
- lower radicular obstetrical paralysis
- o. ultrasound

obstetrician-gynecologist

obstetrician's hand

obstetrics

obstetrics-aborted

obstetrics-delivered

obstetrics-not delivered

obstructed
- o. airway
- o. blood flow
- o. bowel
- o. by foreign body
- o. kidney
- o. nares
- naris not o.
- nasal airway o.
- o. nasal passage
- o. throat

obstructing
- o. adhesions
- o. bolus of food
- o. bronchial aspergillosis
- o. cancer
- o. colorectal cancer
- o. mass

obstruction
- acute abdominal o.
- acute intestinal o.
- adynamic intestinal o.
- o. of airflow
- o. of air passage
- airway o.
- o. of airway
- airway obstruction in conscious patient
- airway obstruction in unconscious patient
- anorectal outlet o.
- aortic arch o.
- aortic outflow o.
- aortic valve o.
- o. of appendix
- arachnoid villi o.
- benign prostatic o.
- bilateral ureteral o.
- o. of bile flow
- biliary tract o.
- bladder neck o.
- bladder outflow o.
- bladder outlet o.
- bowel o.
- o. box
- cardiac obstruction in syncope
- chronic airflow o.
- chronic airway o.
- chronic obstruction of biliary tract
- chronic thrombotic pulmonary vascular o.
- common bile duct o.
- complete bowel o.
- complete obstruction of airway
- complete small bowel o.
- congenital duodenal o.
- congenital high airway obstruction syndrome
- congenital nasolacrimal duct o.
- constipation from intestinal o.
- coronary artery o.
- diarrhea from intestinal o.
- distal ileal obstruction syndrome
- distal intestinal obstruction syndrome
- o. drive
- o. of duct
- o. duodenum
- o. of esophagus
- eustachian tube o.
- extrahepatic portal vein o.
- o. of fallopian tube
- gastric outlet o.
- hepatic venous outflow o.
- incomplete bowel o.
- intermittent small bowel o.
- intestinal o.
- large bowel o.
- left ventricular outflow tract o.
- lower urinary tract o.
- o. of major organs
- malignant airway o.
- malignant biliary o.
- mammary duct o.
- mechanical biliary o.
- mechanical bowel o.
- mechanical duct o.
- mechanical esophageal o.
- mechanical extrahepatic o.
- meibomian gland o.
- membranous obstruction of the inferior vena cava
- milk bolus o.
- minor gland o.
- nasal airway o.
- nasolacrimal duct o.
- nasopharyngeal airway o.
- outflow tract o.
- pancreatic duct o.
- paralytic colonic o.
- partial bile outflow o.
- partial bowel o.

partial intestinal o.
partial obstruction of bladder
partial small bowel o.
peripheral airway o.
portal vein o.
primary acquired nasolacrimal duct o.
prostatic outlet o.
proximal tubal o.
pulmonary artery o.
pulmonary vascular o.
pulmonary venous o.
o. of renal artery
salivary duct o.
segmental biliary o.
sleep apnea-hypersomnolence syndrome associated with upper airway o.
small airway o.
small bowel o.
splenic vein o.
strangulated bowel o.
superior vena cava o.
o. of syndrome
total o.
unilateral ureteral o.
upper airway o.
upper respiratory o.
o. of ureter
o. of urethra
vas deferens o.
o. with ascites

obstruction/incompetence

obstructive

o. abnormality
acute obstructive suppurative cholangitis
o. adenoids
o. airflow disease
o. airway defect
o. airway disease
o. anuria
o. apnea
o. appendicitis
o. atelectasis
o. azoospermia
o. biliary cirrhosis
o. bronchitis
o. calculus
o. cardiomyopathy
cerebrovascular obstructive disease
o. cholangitis
chronic obstructive airway disease
chronic obstructive bronchitis
chronic obstructive bullous emphysema
chronic obstructive lung disease
chronic obstructive outflow disease
chronic obstructive pulmonary disease
chronic obstructive pulmonary emphysema
chronic obstructive respiratory disease
o. cirrhosis
o. colorectal cancer
combined central and obstructive sleep apnea
o. component
o. coronary disease
o. defecation
o. defect
diffuse obstructive pulmonary syndrome
o. diverticulitis
o. dysfunctional ileitis
o. dysmenorrhea
o. element
o. emphysema
o. esophagogastric cancer
extrahepatic obstructive jaundice
familial hypertrophic obstructive cardiomyopathy
o. gastroduodenal Crohn disease
o. glaucoma
o. hydrocephalus
hypertrophic obstructive cardiomyopathy
o. hypopnea
o. intestinal disease
o. jaundice
o. liver disease
lower obstructive uropathy
o. lung disease
o. malformation
malignant biliary obstructive disease
o. megaureter
minimum obstructive volume
mixed obstructive apnea-hypopnea index
o. nephropathy
o. phlebitis
o. pneumonia
o. pulmonary disease
o. pulmonary emphysema
pulmonary vascular obstructive disease
o. purpura
recurrent intrahepatic obstructive jaundice
o. respiratory disease
o. retinal vasculitis
reversible obstructive airways disease
o. shock
o. sleep apnea
o. sleep apnea-hypopnea syndrome
o. sleep apnea syndrome
o. sleep disorder
O. Sleep Disorders-6 test
o. thrombus
o. uropathy
o. voiding symptom

obtain

unable to o.

obtained

o. coefficient
good exposure o.
hemostasis o.
none o.
o. under test conditions

obtundation

increased o.

obtunded

patient o.
somnolent and o.

obturator

adductor tenotomy and obturator neurectomy
o. artery
o. avulsion fracture
o. branch of pubic branch of inferior epigastric vein
o. bypass
o. canal
core biopsy o.
o. crest
esophageal obturator airway
o. externus muscle
o. fascia
o. foramen
o. groove
o. hernia
internal obturator muscle
o. lymph node
o. muscle
o. nerve
o. nerve damage
posterior branch of obturator artery
posterior branch of obturator nerve
o. sign
o. vein

obturatoria

arteria o.

obturatorii
nodi lymphoidei o.

obtuse
first obtuse marginal artery
first obtuse marginal branch
o. marginal
o. marginal artery
o. marginal branch
second obtuse marginal artery
second obtuse marginal branch

obvious physical exhaustion

Oc1r virus

occasional
o. auditory hallucination
o. gambler
o. tactile hallucination

occipital
o. alpha
alternative occipital artery middle cerebral artery
o. anchorage
o. angle
o. angle of parietal bone
anterior condyloid canal of occipital bone
anterior occipital artery-middle cerebral artery bypass
o. apoplexy
o. artery
o. aspect
o. association
o. association cortical area
auricular branch of occipital artery
o. belly
o. belly of occipitofrontalis muscle
bilateral occipital lobe infarct
o. bone jugular incisure
o. border
o. border of parietal bone
o. border of temporal bone
o. bossing
o. brachycephaly
o. branch
o. cephalocele
o. cerebral vein
o. condyle
o. condyle fracture
o. condyle hypoplasia
o. condyle invasion
o. condyle syndrome
o. cortex
o. cortex damage
o. cortex tissue
o. cortical dysplasia of Taylor
o. corticectomy
o. diploic vein
o. dominant intermittent rhythmic delta activity
o. dysplasia
o. emissary vein
o. encephalocele
o. eye field
o. flattening
o. fontanelle
o. foramen
o. forceps
o. forelock
galeal occipital flap
o. glioblastoma
o. gray matter
greater occipital neuritis
o. groove
o. gyri
o. gyrus
o. headache
o. hematoma
o. horn
o. horn syndrome
interclavicular notch of occipital bone
internal occipital nerve
left anterior o.
left posterior o.
o. lobe
o. lobe of brain
o. lobe unilateral cerebral hemisphere lesion
low occipital hairline
o. lymph node
o. margin
o. margin of temporal bone
mastoid border of occipital bone
mastoid branch of occipital artery
mastoid margin of occipital bone
meningeal branch of occipital artery
o. muscle
o. nerve
parietal branch of medial occipital artery
positive occipital sharp transients of sleep
o. protuberance
o. region
o. regions of head
right anterior o.
sternal occipital mandibular immobilization
superficial occipital artery to middle cerebral artery
temporal, occipital, parietal
o. temporal sulcus
o. vein

occipitale
os o.

occipitales
nodi lymphoidei o.

occipitalization
o. of atlas
atlas o.

occipitoanterior
left occipitoanterior fetal position
o. position

occipitoatlantoaxial
o. anomaly
o. complex
o. fusion

occipitoaxial joint

occipitocervical
o. angle
anterior occipitocervical arthrodesis
anterior occipitocervical spine
o. arthrodesis
o. articulation
o. fixation
o. fusion

occipito-faciocervico-thoraco-abdomino-digital dysplasia

occipitofrontal
o. circumference
o. diameter
o. fasciculus
o. headache
o. muscle
o. radiation

occipitolateral
left occipitolateral fetal position
right occipitolateral fetal position

occipitomastoid
o. suture
o. suture lines
o. suture lines

occipitomental diameter

occipitonuchal

occipitoparietal
bilateral o.
o. suture

occipitopontine fiber

occipitoposterior
left occipitoposterior position
persistent occipitoposterior fetal position
o. position

right occipitoposterior position
right occipitoposterior presentation

occipitosacral fetal position

occipitosphenoidal suture

occipitotectal fiber

occipitotemporal
o. convolution
o. cortex
o. gyrus

occipitotemporalis
o. lateralis
o. medians

occipitothalamic radiation

occipitotransverse
left occipitotransverse fetal position
o. lie
o. position
right occipitotransverse fetal position

occiput
o. anterior
left occiput posterior fetal position
persistent occiput posterior position
persistent occiput posterior presentation
o. posterior
o. presentation
o. right anterior
o. right posterior
o. transverse

occluded
o. artery
o. baculovirus
o. carotid vessel
o. common bile duct
o. common bile duct stone
o. coronary vessel
o. pupil
salpingitis in previously occluded tubes
splanchnic occluded portal pressure
o. virus

occludens
zonula o.
zonula occludens toxin

occluder
lorgnette o.
Maddox rod o.

occluding
o. agent
o. centric relation record
o. frame

occlusal
o. adjustment
o. adjustment armamentarium
o. adjustment instrument
alveolar occlusal border
alveolar occlusal plane
o. amalgam
o. analysis
o. appliance therapy
auxiliary occlusal rest
o. balance
o. bite force
o. cant
o. canting
o. caries
o. cavity
o. cephalometric analysis
o. clearance
o. climate
o. contouring
o. correction
o. cross-section radiograph
o. curvature
o. curve
o. cusp
o. disharmony
o. disturbance
o. dovetail
o. embrasure
o. equilibration
o. facet
o. film
o. film radiography
o. force
o. form
o. function
o. glide
o. groove
o. guard
o. habit neurosis
o. harmony
mesial, occlusal, distal
mesial occlusal facial
o. pattern
o. position
reconstruction occlusal surface
o. surface
o. surface of tooth
o. vertical dimension

occlusion
acute abdominal aortic o.
acute coronary o.
o. amblyopia
o. analysis
o. angiography
angioplasty-related vessel o.
anterior determinants of cusp o.
o. aorta
arterial occlusion sign
o. of artery
atrial septal defect o.
atrial septal defect occlusion system
o. balance
o. balloon catheter with silicone balloon
balloon coronary o.
balloon test o.
bilateral internal carotid artery o.
bilateral tubal o.
bradycardia after arteriovenous fistula o.
braided occlusion device
branch retinal artery o.
branch retinal vein o.
o. of branch vein
branch vein o.
o. of bronchus
central retinal artery o.
central retinal vein o.
centric relation o.
centric relation-centric o.
o. cholangiogram
chronic total o.
component of o.
coronary sinus occlusion pressure
deep venous o.
o. dermatitis
disturbance of function occlusion syndrome
o. dose monitor
o. effect
embolic o.
end-inspiratory airway o.
endovascular balloon o.
femoropopliteal artery o.
height of o.
hepatic vein o.
iliac artery o.
intermittent aortic o.
intermittent coronary sinus o.
internal carotid artery o.
o. of internal carotid artery
o. of intramuscular artery
laparoscopic total o.
left brachial vein o.
o. of left bronchus
o. of left carotid artery
macular arteriole o.
macular branch retinal vein o.
o. of mainstem bronchus
mesenteric artery o.

occlusion *(continued)*
middle cerebral artery o.
o. miliaria
nasolacrimal o.
nonacute total o.
o. nystagmus
ophthalmic artery o.
parent artery o.
part-time occlusion eye patch
peripheral arterial o.
peripheral branch retinal vein o.
peripheral vascular o.
persistent withdrawal o.
portal vein o.
pressure-controlled intermittent coronary sinus o.
pulmonary artery occlusion pressure
pulmonary venous o.
o. of pupil
o. of retinal arteriole
retinal vein o.
o. of retinal vein
right brachial vein o.
o. of right carotid artery
salpingitis after previous tubal o.
selective tubal occlusion procedure
splanchnic artery o.
superior mesenteric artery o.
o. therapy
o. time
total occlusion of basilar artery
tubal occlusion device
tuboovarian abscess after previous tubal o.
unilateral ureteral o.
venous occlusion plethysmography
vertebral artery o.

occlusive
aortic occlusive disease
aortoiliac occlusive disease
o. arterial disease
arterial occlusive change
arterial occlusive disease
o. arterial thrombus
arteriolar occlusive disease
arteriosclerotic mesenteric vascular occlusive disease
o. artery disease
o. atherosclerosis
atherosclerotic occlusive syndrome
o. azoospermia
o. carotid artery disease
o. carotid disease
carotid occlusive disease
carotid occlusive disease retinopathy
o. cerebrovascular disease
o. cerebrovascular insult
o. clamp
o. coronary artery disease
coronary artery occlusive disease
o. coronary disease
o. disease
o. disease of liver
o. dressing
o. and dry dressing
dry and occlusive dressing
femoropopliteal occlusive disease
o. heart disease
hemostatic occlusive leverage device
o. hyperemia
o. ileus
lower extremity occlusive disease
o. meningitis
mesenteric vascular occlusive disease
o. microangiopathy
o. moisturizer
multilevel atherosclerotic arterial occlusive disease
o. patch test
peripheral arterial occlusive disease
peripheral arteriosclerotic occlusive disease
peripheral occlusive arterial disease
peripheral vascular occlusive disease
o. phase
popliteal artery occlusive disease
popliteal occlusive disease
o. retinal arteritis
o. sheeting
sinovenous occlusive disease
o. therapy
o. thrombus
o. vascular disease
vascular occlusive episode
o. vasculitis
vertebrobasilar occlusive disease

occuloglandular syndrome

occult
o. abscess
acute zonal occult outer retinopathy
angiographically occult intracranial vascular malformation
angiographically occult vascular malformation
angiographically occult vessel
o. annular ciliary body
o. bacteremia
o. biliary microlithiasis
o. bleeding
o. blood
o. blood loss
o. blood-negative
o. blood-positive
o. blood in stool
o. blood test
o. blood testing
o. bone metastasis
o. border of nail
o. cancer
o. carcinoma
o. cerebral vascular malformation
o. cerebrovascular malformation
o. choroidal neovascularization
o. cleft palate
o. clonal B-cell population
o. cord prolapse
o. detection
o. diabetes
o. diaphragmatic injury
o. dysraphism
o. enterotomy
o. extrahepatic disease
fecal occult blood
fecal occult blood test
o. filariasis
o. focus
o. fracture
o. frontal focus
o. gastrointestinal bleeding
o. head trauma
o. hepatic disease
o. hepatitis
o. hydrocephalus
o. immunization
immunological fecal occult blood test
o. infection
o. lymph node metastasis
o. metastasis
o. metastatic disease
o. myelodysplasia
o. neuroblastoma
o. pericarditis
o. primary malignancy
o. pulmonary embolus
roentgenographically occult lung cancer
stool positive for occult blood
o. temporal arteritis of Simmons
trace occult blood

o. trauma, postanoxia, ventriculoperitoneal

occulta
spina bifida o.

occupancy
absent bed o.
completion bed occupancy care
nonbed o.
peak occupancy time

occupation
Knowledge of O.'s Test
New Mexico Knowledge of O.'s Test

occupational
o. ability
o. ability pattern
o. abrasion
o. acne
o. activity
o. adjustment
o. airway disease
o. allergen
o. allergic alveolitis
o. analysis
o. asthma
Basic O. Literacy Test
o. behavior
California O. Preference Inventory
California O. Preference Survey
o. checklist
o. choice
o. cramp
o. crisis
Crowley O. Interests Blank
o. deafness
o. delirium
o. dermatitis
o. dermatosis
o. drinking
o. dysfunction
o. and environmental medicine
o. exposure
o. exposure to chemicals
o. family
o. function
o. functioning
Gordon Occupational Checklist-II
Hall O. Orientation Inventory
o. hazard
o. health
o. health center
o. health risk
o. health and safety
o. hearing loss
o. hierarchy
o. history
o. immunologic lung disease
o. impairment
impairment in occupational functioning
o. inhibition
O. Interests Explorer
O. Interests Surveyor
o. koilonychia
Kuder O. Interest Survey
o. lens
o. leukoderma
o. lung disease
o. lung disorder
o. maladjustment syndrome
Minnesota O. Classification System
Modern O. Skills Test
National Institute for O. Safety and Health
o. non-IgE-dependent asthma
Occupational Check List
o. ophthalmology
outpatient occupational therapy
o. paralysis
o. parenchymal disease
o. radiation
o. rehabilitation
remedial occupational therapy
O. Roles Questionnaire
o. rubber dermatitis
Social and O. Functioning Assessment
o. and social impairment
O. Stress Indicator
o. stress syndrome
o. therapist
o. therapy/recreational therapy
o. vitiligo

occupationally induced asthma

occupation-related syndrome

occupied
highest occupied molecular orbital

Occup Rx

occupying space lesion

occurrence
adverse patient o.'s
multiple occurrence of unexplained symptoms
spike occurrence density

Oceanside virus

Ochoa syndrome

ochre
o. codon
o. hemorrhage
o. mass
o. membrane
o. suppressor genetic mutation

ochronosis
ocular o.

ochronotic
o. arthritis
o. arthropathy
o. spondylosis

Ochsner
O. clamp
O. method

Ockelbo
O. disease
O. virus

o'clock
Frimberger-Karpiel 12 o'clock papillotome

o'clock position

1-o'clock position

2-o'clock position

3-o'clock position

4-o'clock position

5-o'clock position

6-o'clock position

7-o'clock position

8-o'clock position

9-o'clock position

10-o'clock position

11-o'clock position

12-o'clock position

O'Connor
O. depressor
O. finger dexterity test
O. marker
O. operation

O'Connor-Peter operation

octacalcium phosphate

octafluoropropane gas

octamer-binding transcription factor

octapeptide
cholecystokinin o.

octave
o. band analyzer
o. frequency

Octopus
O. automated perimetry

Octopus *(continued)*
O. 500 EZ
O. 201 perimeter test
octreotide
o. acetate
o. effect
o. long-acting release
o. scan
o. therapy
octulosonic acid
Oculab Tono-Pen
Oculaid lens
ocular
o. abnormality
abridged ocular chart
o. adnexa
o. adnexal inflammatory pseudotumor
o. adnexal lesion
o. adnexal lymphoid proliferation
o. adnexal lymphoma
o. adnexal tumor
o. albinism
o. albinism with late-onset sensorineural deafness
o. alignment
o. allergy
o. amoebic keratitis
o. angle
anterior ocular segment
o. apraxia
o. aspergillosis
o. ataxia
o. atopic dermatitis
autosomal recessive ocular albinism
autosomal recessive ocular Ehlers-Danlos syndrome
o. axis
o. ballottement
o. barrier
o. bartonellosis
o. blepharospasm
o. bobbing
o. bobbing nystagmus
o. calcification
o. capsule
cerebral, ocular, dental, auricular, skeletal syndrome
o. chemical burn
cicatricial ocular pemphigoid
o. cicatricial pemphigoid
o. coherence tomography
o. coloboma
o. coloboma-imperforate anus syndrome
o. complication
o. complications of diabetes
o. cone
congenital ocular motor apraxia
conjugate ocular movement
o. convergence
o. counterrolling
o. countertorsion reflex
o. crisis
o. cryptococcal infection
o. cul-de-sac
o. cytology
o. density
o. deviation
o. dipping
o. disorder
o. dominance
o. dominance column
o. duction
o. dyskinesia
o. dysmetria
o. dysmetria nystagmus
o. dysmetria test
o. dysmotility
o. echography
equal ocular movement
o. etiology of headache
family ocular history
o. flora
o. flutter
o. flutter nystagmus
o. fundus
o. globe
growth retardation, ocular abnormalities, microcephaly, brachydactyly, oligophrenia
o. gymnastics
o. headache
o. hemodynamic assessment
o. hemodynamic value
o. herpes
o. herpes infection
o. herpes simplex
herpetic ocular disease
o. histidinemia
o. histoplasmosis
o. histoplasmosis syndrome
o. history
o. humor
o. hypertelorism
o. hypertension
o. hypertension glaucoma
o. hypertension indicator
o. hypertensive glaucoma
hypertensive ocular disease
o. hypoperfusion syndrome
o. hypotelorism
o. hypotony
o. image
o. immune disease
o. immunology
o. inflammation
o. inflammatory disease
o. inflammatory disorder
o. injury
o. involvement
o. irritation
ischemic ocular inflammation
o. ischemic syndrome
o. larva
o. larva migrans
o. lens
lentigines, electrocardiographic abnormalities, ocular hypertelorism, pulmonary stenosis, abnormalities of genitalia, retardation of growth, deafness syndrome
o. lymphoma
lymphoma of ocular adnexa
o. lymphomatosis
macrosomia, obesity, macrocephaly, ocular abnormality syndrome
macular ocular histoplasmosis syndrome
o. malformation
o. manifestation
o. marker
o. massage
maternal ocular adaptation
McCannel ocular pressure reducer
o. medium
o. melanocytosis
o. melanoma
o. meningioma
o. micrometer
o. microtremor
o. migraine
o. motility
o. motility disorder
o. motility effect
o. motility test
o. motoneuron
o. motor apraxia
o. motor cranial nerve
o. motor dysmetria
o. motor syndrome
o. motor system
o. movement
mucocutaneous ocular syndrome
multiple ocular coloboma
o. muscle
o. muscle dystrophy

o. muscle palsy
o. muscle paralysis
o. muscle transplant
o. muscular dystrophy
o. myasthenia
o. myasthenia gravis
o. mycosis
o. myiasis
o. myoclonus
o. myopathy
neonatal ocular prophylaxis
Nettleship-Falls-type ocular albinism
Nettleship-Falls X-linked ocular albinism
no medical ocular history
o. nystagmus
o. ochronosis
o. albinism 1, 2, 3
o. onchocerciasis
o. oscillation
o. pain
o. palsy
o. paresis
o. pathology
pediatric ocular sarcoidosis
o. pemphigus
o. perfusion pressure
o. phthisis
o. plethysmodynamography
o. plethysmography
o. pneumoplethysmography
o. pressure reducer
presumed ocular histoplasmosis syndrome
o. prophylaxis
o. prosthesis
pseudopresumed ocular histoplasmosis syndrome
o. radiation therapy
o. refraction
o. region
o. rigidity
o. rosacea
o. saccade
o. sarcoidosis
short stature, hyperextensibility of joints or hernia or both, ocular depression, Rieger anomaly, teething, delayed
o. siderosis
o. sign
o. sparganosis
o. spectrum
superficial ocular trauma
o. surface
o. surface disease
o. syphilis
o. syphilitic disease
o. tension
o. tilt reaction
o. torticollis
o. toxicity
o. toxocariasis
o. toxoplasmosis
o. trachoma
o. trauma
o. tuberculosis
o. vaccinial conjunctivitis
o. vergance and accommodation sensor
o. vertigo
o. vesicle
X-linked ocular albinism
o. zoster

ocular-mucous membrane syndrome

ocular-scoliotic type Ehlers-Danlos syndrome

oculi (*pl. of* oculus)

OcuLight SL diode laser

oculoauditory syndrome

oculoauricular dysplasia

oculoauriculofrontonasal syndrome

oculoauriculovertebral
o. dysplasia
o. spectrum

oculobuccogenital syndrome

oculocardiac reflex

oculocephalic
o. maneuver
o. reflex
o. synkinesis
o. test
o. vascular anomaly

oculocephalogyric
o. crisis
o. reflex

oculocerebral
o. dystrophy
o. hypopigmentation syndrome
o. lymphoma
o. syndrome of Cross and McKusick

oculocerebrocutaneous syndrome

oculocerebrofacial syndrome

oculocerebrorenal
o. disease of Lowe
o. dystrophy
Lowe oculocerebrorenal syndrome
o. syndrome

oculocutaneous
o. albinism
o. albinoidism
autosomal dominant oculocutaneous albinism
o. hypopigmentation
o. laser
o. lesion
minimal pigment oculocutaneous albinism
minimal-pigment oculocutaneous albinism
o. albinism type I
o. syndrome
o. telangiectasia
tyrosinase-negative oculocutaneous albinism
o. tyrosinemia or tyrosinosis

oculodental syndrome

oculodentodigital
o. dysplasia
o. syndrome

oculodentoosseous dysplasia

oculodermal
o. disorder
o. melanocytosis
o. melanosis

oculodigital
microcephaly, oculodigital, esophageal, duodenal syndrome
o. reflex
o. sign of Franchesseti

oculodynamic test

oculofacial paralysis

oculogastrointestinal muscular dystrophy

oculogenital
o. disease
o. infection

oculogenitolaryngeal syndrome

oculoglandular
o. conjunctivitis
o. disease
Parinaud oculoglandular conjunctivitis
Parinaud oculoglandular syndrome
o. syndrome
o. tularemia

oculogravic illusion

oculogyral illusion

oculogyric
auditory oculogyric reflex

oculogyric *(continued)*
auditory oculogyric response
o. auricular reflex
o. crisis
o. mechanism
palpebral oculogyric reflex
oculoleptomeningeal amyloidosis
oculomandibulodyscephaly-hypotrichosis syndrome
oculomandibulofacial syndrome
oculomasticatory myorhythmia
oculomelic amyoplasia
oculomotor
o. abnormality
alternating oculomotor hemiplegia
o. apparatus
o. apraxia
autonomic oculomotor nucleus
o. cranial nerve palsy
o. decussation
o. deficit
o. disorder
o. disturbance
o. dysfunction
external oculomotor ophthalmoplegia
o. foramen
o. nerve
o. nerve fascicle
o. nerve lesion
o. nerve misdirection
o. nerve synkinesis
o. nucleus
o. paresis with cyclic spasm
peripheral oculomotor nerve
o. root
o. root of ciliary ganglion
o. system
oculomotorius
nervus o.
oculomucous membrane syndrome
oculo-oral-genital syndrome
oculopalatal
o. myoclonus
o. myoclonus syndrome
oculopalatocerebral syndrome
oculopalatoskeletal syndrome
oculoparalytic illusion
oculopathy
lupus o.
oculopharyngeal
o. muscular dystrophy
o. reflex
o. syndrome
oculoplastic
o. reconstruction
o. surgery
oculoplethysmography/carotid phonoangiography
oculopupillary reflex
oculorenal syndrome
oculorespiratory reflex
oculorotatory muscle
oculosensory cell reflex
oculosympathetic
o. dysfunction
o. paresis
o. pathway
o. syndrome
oculovertebral dysplasia
oculovestibular reflex
oculus, pl. **oculi**
albuginea oculi
angulus oculi lateralis
angulus oculi medialis
angulus oculi nasalis
aqua oculi
o. dexter
lower lid, oculus dexter
lower lid, oculus sinister
melanosis oculi
motor oculi
musculi oculi
musculus obliquus superior oculi
musculus orbicularis oculi
musculus rectus lateralis oculi
musculus rectus medialis oculi
orbicularis oculi
orbicularis oculi muscle
pars orbitalis musculi orbicularis oculi
pars palpebralis musculi orbicularis oculi
retinal detachment, oculus dexter
retinal detachment, oculus sinister
retroorbicularis oculi fat
o. sinister
suborbicularis oculi fat
tension oculus sinister
tunica albuginea oculi
o. unitas
oculi unitas
oculi uterque
visio oculus uterque
oculus]
Ocuscan
O. 400 transducer
Ocusert device
Ocusoft scrub
Ocutome
O. II fragmentation system
O. vitrectomy unit
odd
o. behavior
o. belief
o. chromosome
logarithm of o.'s
Mantel-Haenszel weighted odds ratio
o.'s ratio
relative o.'s
oddball
auditory 3-stimuli oddball task
Oddi
O. manometry
O. muscle
O. spasm
sphincter of O.
O. sphincter
sphincter of Oddi dysfunction
sphincter of Oddi manometry
sphincter of Oddi pressure
sphincter of Oddi spasm
ODED syndrome
odentectomy
maxillary mandibular odentectomy alveolectomy
***o*-desmethylencainide**
o-diethylaminoethyl cellulose
Odland body
O'Donnell operation
O'Donoghue
O. ACL reconstruction
O. facetectomy
odontalgia dentalis
odontectomy
o. and alveoloplasty
mandibular dentition o.
odontogenic
adenomatoid odontogenic tumor
o. adenomatoid tumor
calcifying epithelial odontogenic tumor
central granular cell odontogenic tumor
o. cervical necrotizing fasciitis
clear cell odontogenic tumor
o. cyst
o. dysplasia

o. epithelium
o. facial pain
o. fiber
o. fibroma
o. fibrosarcoma
o. gingival epithelial hamartoma
o. infection
o. keratocyst
o. keratocytosis-skeletal anomalies syndrome
orofacial odontogenic infection
squamous odontogenic tumor

odontoid
o. agenesis
atlas odontoid distance
o. bone
o. condyle
o. condyle fracture
o. dysplasia
o. fracture internal fixation
o. fracture stabilization
o. ligament
pannus deformity of o.
o. process displacement

odontoma adamantinum

odontoonychodermal dysplasia

odonto-tricho-ungual-digital-palmar syndrome

odor
apocrine body o.
o. blindness
body o.
o. control
o. event-related potential
o. fear
heightened sensitivity to o.'s
minimal identifiable o.
minimal perceptible o.
minimal recognizable o.

Odorant
O. Confusion Matrix scale
O. Confusion Matrix score

odotogenic
calcifying odotogenic cyst

Odrenisrou virus

O'Driscoll report

O'Duffy criteria

oedema

oedipal
o. behavior
o. complex
o. conflict

Oedipus complex

OEIS
O. abnormality
O. complex

oersted centimeter-gram-second unit of magnetic field strength

Oesch perforation invagination stripper

oesophageal
anterior oesophageal sensor

Oestreicher-Turner syndrome

oestrogen estrogen-replacement therapy

oestruosa
myiasis o.

of
in care of
died of
history of
on account of
out of
patient complains of
removal of
report of
under care of
by way of

off
aortic cross clamp o.
o. balance
cast off, to x-ray
o. effect
o. glide
o. guard
o. and on
personal time o.
right toe o.
rotating delivery of excitation off resonance
time o.
o. work

offals
specified bovine o.

off-axis
o.-a. dose inhomogeneity
o.-a. factor
o.-a. imaging
o.-a. ratio

off-center
o.-c. cut
o.-c. ratio

offender
adolescent sex o.
habitual o.
mentally disordered sex o.
sex o.

offense
alcohol o.
alcohol-related o.

offensive chat-room dialogue

offered
no complaints o.

Offer Self-Image Questionnaire for Adolescents

office
O. of Alternative Medicine
o. blood pressure
o. call
o. cystometrics
follow-up office visit
o. hypertension
initial office visit
o. laparoscopy under local anesthesia
laser office ventilation of ears with insertion of tubes
medical office assistant
medical office building
nursing o.
O. on Smoking and Health
patient discharged to office followup
postoperative office visit
o. treatment
o. visit
will follow in o.

office-based anesthesia

officer
duly authorized o.
house o.
medical o.
medical house o.
notify house o.

official
public health o.

off-pump
o.-p. coronary artery bypass

off-service note

offset
o. drill hole
o. frequency
o. hinge
medial head-stem o.

offside
high-frequency contralateral routing of offside signals

off-site anesthesia

offspring
o. of diabetic parents

offspring *(continued)*
number of pregnancies producing viable o.

off-time
critical o.-t.

Ofuji disease

Ogawa
O. model
O. model for hematopoiesis

O'Gawa two-way aspirating cannula

Ogden
O. epiphysial fracture classification
O. fracture classification system

Ogilvie syndrome

Ogino-Knaus rule

Ogita test

Ogston
line of O.
O. line

Ogston-Luc operation

Oguchi disease

Ogura operation

Ohara disease

Ohdo blepharophimosis syndrome

Ohio
O. humidifier
O. pediatric tent with compressed air
O. pediatric tent with oxygen
O. Tests of Articulation and Perception of Sounds
O. Vocational Interest Survey
O. warmer
O. Work Values Inventory

ohm
O. law
reciprocal o.
reciprocal ohm centimeter
reciprocal ohm meter
o. resistance

ohm-centimeter

Ohmeda
O. hand-held oximeter
O. Minx pulse oximeter

Ohtahara syndrome

"oid-oid" disease

oil
o. acne
o. of American wormseed
o. of anise
aromatic castor o.
o. bath
o. of bay
o. of bergamot
o. of bitter almond
o. of bitter orange
brominated vegetable o.
o. of cardamom
castor o.
o. of chenopodium
o. of cherry laurel
o. of cinnamon
o. of citronella
o. of clove
cod liver o.
o. of coriander
o. cyst
o. drop change
o. drop lesion
o. drop sign
o. embolism
o. enema
ethiodized oil emulsion
evening primrose o.
o. of evening primrose
o. folliculitis
o. gland
o. granuloma
o. immersion
o. immersion field microscopy
o. layer
Lorenzo oil diet
magnesium hydroxide and mineral oil emulsion
MCT oil formula
medium-chain triglyceride o.
menhaden o.
mineral o.
o. red O
penicillin in beeswax and o.
penicillin, oil, and beeswax
o. pneumonia
progesterone in o.
o. retention enema
shark liver o.
soybean oil meal
sulfated hydrogenated caster o.
tea tree o.
toxic oil epidemic syndrome
o. vaccine
water in o.
o. in water emulsion

oil-associated pneumoparalytic eosinophilic syndrome

oil-immersion microscopy

oil-spot discoloration

oil-water ratio

oily
o. granuloma
o. secretion
o. skin
o. stool
transcatheter oily chemoembolization

ointment
o. base
o. granuloma
hydrophilic o.
Neosporin o.
Nitro-Bid O.
nitroglycerin o.
ophthalmic o.
o. of tar
triamcinolone o.

okadaic acid

Okamura technique

Okazaki fragment

Okhotskiy virus

Okola virus

Okuma plate

olanzapine toxicity

old
o. age
O. Age Assistance
o. age benefits
o. age dementia
o. age imbecility
o. age pension
o. age pensioner
o. cystic infarct
debilitating effects of old age
o. dislocation
o. ecchymosis
o. eye
o. fracture
good old boy
o. guard
o. healed fracture
o. healed myocardial infarction
human old tuberculin
o. incision excised
o. infarct
o. inferior wall myocardial infarction
o. man's pemphigus
months o.
o. nerve injury
synthetic medium old tuberculin
trichloroacetic acid precipitated o. tuberculin [Tuberkulin]
weeks o.

O. World leishmaniasis
years o.
o. yellow enzyme

older
o. maternal age
O. Women's League

older maternal age

Oldfield syndrome

oleandomycin phosphate

olecranon
o. apophysitis
o. bursa
o. bursitis
o. fossa
o. fracture
o. ligament
nonunited o.
Papavasiliou classification of olecranon fracture
o. procedure
o. process
o. spur

oleic
o. acid
o. acid uptake test
Dubois oleic albumin complex
Dubois oleic serum complex
o. acid I 125

oleoresin
aspidium o.

olfacto-ethmoidohypothalamic dysplasia

olfactogenital
o. dysplasia
o. syndrome

olfactorial ability

olfactory
accessory olfactory bulb
o. acuity
o. agnosia
o. amnesia
o. anesthesia
o. angle
anterior olfactory nucleus
o. area
o. aura
o. axonal growth
o. brain
o. bulb
o. bundle
o. canal
o. cell
o. cilium
o. cleft
o. coefficient
o. cortex
o. cranial nerve
o. deficit
o. disorder
o. epithelium
o. erotism
o. esthesioneuroblastoma
o. fatigue
o. filum
o. foramen
o. ganglion
o. gland
o. glomerulus
o. groove
o. groove meningioma
o. groove of nasal cavity
o. groove tumor
o. gyrus
o. hair
o. hallucination
o. hyperesthesia
o. hypesthesia
lateral olfactory tract
o. lobe of brain
o. marker protein
molecular layers of olfactory bulb
o. nerve layer
o. neuroblast
o. neuroblastoma
o. peduncle
o. placode
o. reference syndrome
o. region
o. spread
o. threshold
o. tubercle
vivid visual, auditory and olfactory hallucinations

Olifantsvlei virus

oligoadenylate synthase

oligoarthritis
asymmetric o.

oligoarthropathy
asymmetric o.

oligoarticular
o. disease
o. seronegative rheumatoid arthritis

oligoasthenoteratozoospermia syndrome

oligoastrocytoma
malignant mixed o.
mixed o.

oligoclonal
o. band
o. banding
o. immunoglobulin

oligodendrocyte
o. destruction
o. injury

oligodendroglia cell

oligodendroglial cell

oligodendroglialike cell

oligodendroglioma
low-grade o.

oligodeoxynucleotide
o. antisense probe
immunostimulatory o.

oligogenic inheritance

oligo man

oligomenorrhea with anovulatory menses

oligomenorrheic
o. polycystic ovary syndrome

oligomenorrheic polycystic ovary syndrome

oligomer
procyanidol o.

oligomeric
cartilage oligomeric matrix protein
o. proanthocyanidin

oligonucleotide
allele-specific o.
antisense oligonucleotide viral therapy
antitelomerase antisense o.
o. inhibition
o. probe
sequence-specific oligonucleotide probe hybridization
triplex-forming o.

oligophrenia
alopecia, epilepsy, oligophrenia syndrome
cerebellar vermis hypoplasia, oligophrenia, congenital ataxia, coloboma, hepatic fibrosis
growth retardation, ocular abnormalities, microcephaly, brachydactyly, o.

oligophrenia-ichthyosis syndrome

oligosaccharide
o. chain
fructose-terminated o.

oligosaccharide *(continued)*
Lewis X o.
o. transferase enzyme
oligoteratoasthenozoospermia syndrome
O-linked
O.-l. pattern
O.-l. saccharide
Oliphant
O. Auditory Discrimination Memory Test
O. Auditory Synthesizing Test
oliva inferior
olivary
o. body
o. degeneration
o. eminence
medial accessory olivary nucleus
olive
inferior o.
lateral superior o.
medial superior o.
o. tree
o. tree pollen
Olivecrona
O. clip
O. dura scissors
Oliver
O. sign
O. syndrome
Oliver-McFarlane syndrome
olive-tip
o.-t. cannula
o.-t. capsule polisher
o.-t. irrigator
olive-tipped catheter
Olivier-Bertrand-Tipal frame
olivocerebellar
o. fiber
o. tract
olivocochlear
o. bundle
o. bundle of Rasmussen
medial o.
olivopontocerebellar
o. atrophy
o. degeneration
neonatal olivopontocerebellar atrophy
sporadic olivopontocerebellar ataxia
X-linked olivopontocerebellar ataxia
olivospinal fiber
Ollendorf syndrome
Ollier
O. arthrodesis approach
O. disease
O. dyschondroplasia
O. graft
O. syndrome
Ollier-Klippel-Trenaunay-Weber syndrome
Olmsted syndrome
Olshausen
O. procedure
O. sign
O. suspension
olympian forehead
Olympus
O. adapter
O. endoscopy system
O. videoscope
O'Malley-Pearce-Luma lens
omega
O. Cohort
o. nail
omega-3, -6 fatty acid
omega-conotoxin-sensitive pathway
omega-3 fatty acid
omega-3 polyunsaturated fatty acid
omen formation
Omenn syndrome
omental
o. adhesion
o. adhesive band
o. appendage
o. appendix
o. apron
o. band
o. biopsy
o. branch
o. bursa
o. bursitis
o. cake
o. cyst
o. eminence of pancreas
o. enterocleisis
o. fat
o. filler
o. flap
o. foramen
o. graft
o. hammock
hemorrhagic omental lymph nodes
o. hernia
o. tuberosity
o. tuberosity of liver
o. tuberosity of pancreas
omentales
omentectomy
partial o.
omentum
bowel adherent to o.
greater o.
lesser o.
lymphocyst o.
o. magnum
o. majus
matted o.
pancreaticosplenic o.
omeprazole
metronidazole, omeprazole, amoxicillin
metronidazole, omeprazole, clarithromycin
o., amoxicillin, clarithromycin
o., amoxicillin, metronidazole
o., bismuth subcitrate, tetracycline, and metronidazole
o., metronidazole, clarithromycin
Omer-Capen carpectomy
OMF syndrome
omicron-nitrophenyl-beta-galactosidase
omission of duty
Ommaya reservoir
Omni clip gun
OmniFlex
omnifocal lens
omoclavicular fossa
omohyoid muscle
Omo virus
omphaloangiopagous twins
omphalocele
omphalocele-cleft palate syndrome
omphalomesenteric
o. artery
o. cord
o. duct
o. duct cyst
o. duct remnant
o. vein
Omsk
O. hemorrhagic fever
O. hemorrhagic fever virus

on

absolute temperature on the Rankine scale
on account of
acute on chronic liver disease
acute on chronic renal failure
on admission
alcohol effect on brain
alcohol on breath
alerting maneuver on electroencephalogram
alerting stimulus on electroencephalogram
ambulates on parallel bars
angulus on the lesser curve
aortic cross clamp on
apolipoprotein E epsilon 4 gene on chromosome 19
on arrival
articular surface on calcaneus for cuboid bone
artifact on x-ray
associative response to a white space on a card
attenuation coefficient on MRI scan
attenuation value on MRI scan
ball on back
bladder emptied on voiding
bleeding on touch
bordering on insanity
born on arrival
burning on urination
calcium deposit on heart valves
on call
callus on hand
chest pain on deep breathing
chest pain on exertion
computer output on microfilm
concentric circle pattern on breast self-examination
condition on admission
condition on discharge
dead on arrival
dead on arrival despite resuscitative attempts
dependence on hallucinogen
derived value on apex cardiogram
diagnosis or condition deferred on Axis I, II
on direct questioning
discharged on visit
distal tingling on percussion
double needle operation on cataract
dribbling on urination
dullness on percussion
dull on questioning
on duty
dyspnea on exercise
on edge
on effect
effect of asthma on lung
electrodes placed on the surface of head
elements on urinalysis
entry on duty
epilepsy with grand mal seizures on awakening
on examination
fell on outstretched hand
hair on head
on hand
impact on fetus
impingement on spinal nerve
impulse on coughing
increased dyspnea on exertion
injured on duty
intact on admission
International Workshop and Conference on Human Leukocyte Differentiation Antigens
intern on call
leave on floor
leave on pass
lesion on erythrocyte cell membrane at the site of complement fixation
limited quantity test performed on small specimen
lithium action on first messenger
lithium action on membranes
lithium action on second messenger
lower fossa active, lateral knee pain, and long leg on the side ipsilateral to the weak fossa
Meals on Wheels
Meals on Wheels Association of America
mixed growth on culture
most posterior point on posterior contour of sella turcica
multiple benign circumferential skin creases on limb
National Asian Pacific Center on Aging
National Association of Area Agencies on Aging
National Caucus and Center on Black Aged, Inc.
National Center on Elder Abuse
National Center on Minority Health and Health Disparities
National Center on Poverty Law, Inc.
National Institute on Aging
National Institute on Alcohol Abuse and Alcoholism
National Joint Committee on Learning Disabilities
neovascularization elsewhere on retina
not on label
not on patient
not on unit
nonspecific ST wave segment changes on electroencephalogram
nystagmus on upward gaze
off and on
Office on Smoking and Health
orders accompanying patient on admission
O2 saturation on three liters nasal cannula
O2 saturation on two liters nasal cannula
out on pass
oxygen saturation on 2 liters nasal cannula
oxygen saturation on 3 liters nasal cannula
pacing on demand
pain on chewing
pain on deep breathing
pain on defecation
pain on exertion
pain on a scale from 1 to 10
pain on swallowing
pain on urination
pain on walking
paroxysmal dyspnea on exertion
patient education on drug abuse
patient on a high
patient on ventilator
patient released on overnight pass
peripheral curve on contact lens
phosphatase and tensin homologue deleted on chromosome
physical dependence on nicotine gum
pressure on the brain
pressure on expiration
pressure on inspiration
pressure on spinal cord
pressure on toe joint

on *(continued)*
progressive weakness on one side of the body
prone on elbows
pulse oximetry on 2 liters of oxygen
purplish hemorrhagic spot on skin
radiation assault on tumor
radiation therapy on prophylactic basis
red patch or blister on arm
red spot on breast
Serials on Line
shortness of breath on exertion
simultaneous peripheral operation on-line
slipped on ice
straining on bowel movement
tenderness on palpation
thorax resonant on percussion
Tinel sign distal tingling on percussion
treated on an outpatient basis
upper fossa active, medial knee pain, and short leg on the side ipsilateral to the weak fossa
upstroke pattern on apex cardiogram
urine sterile on culture
wave on electrocardiogram
wave on phlebogram
waxy deposit on brain
wearing patch on arrival
wheezing on inspiration

Onat syndrome

on-axis imaging

on-call
o.-c. to operating room
physician o.-c.

once
only handle it once rule
o. a week
o. weekly

once-daily
o.-d. aminoglycoside
o.-d. dosing

onchocercal sclerosing keratitis

onchocerciasis
O. Control Program
ocular o.

oncocytic
o. adenocarcinoma
o. adenoma
o. carcinoma
o. cell
o. epithelial cell
o. hepatocellular tumor
intraductal oncocytic papillary neoplasm
o. meningioma
o. schneiderian papilloma
o. variant

oncocytoid
o. carcinoid
o. change

oncofetal
o. antigen
o. fibronectin
o. marker

oncogene ribonucleic acid

oncogenic
o. agent
o. osteomalacia
o. rickets
o. virus

oncogenous osteomalacia

oncologic
o. clearance
complex oncologic therapy protocol
o. consideration
o. emergency
o. imaging
o. therapy protocol

oncologist
medical o.

oncology
Bimodality Lung O. Team
o. certified nurse
gynecologic o.
human o.
medical o.
medical oncology unit
radiation o.
radiation therapy oncology group
sonographic planning of oncology treatment
surgical diagnostic o.

Oncolym radiolabeled monoclonal antibody

oncolysate

On-Command catheter

oncoprotein
o. antigen
HER-2/neu o.

oncosphere embryo

oncotic
colloid oncotic pressure
o. force
increasing oncotic pressure
plasma oncotic pressure
o. pressure
tissue oncotic pressure

oncovirus
mammalian type B, C, D oncovirus group
mouse mammary o.

ondansetron
metoclopramide, dexamethasone, lorazepam, o.

on-demand analgesia computer

Ondine
O. curse
O. curse, periodic breathing
O. curse syndrome

one
American Heart Association Step O. Diet
blurred vision in one eye
dangerous to one's self
o. day at a time
direct vision times o.
o. fingerbreadth above umbilicus
o. fingerbreadth below umbilicus
forced expiratory volume at one second
forced expiratory volume in one second as percent of FVC
forced expiratory volume in one second to forced vital capacity ratio
forced inspiratory volume in one second
o. hand-two foot syndrome
may repeat one time
Micro O. pneumatonometer
milliroentgens per hour at one meter
Modular O. pneumatonometer
number equal to one; single patient trial
oriented times o.
postoperative day o.
presence of only one sex chromosome
progressive weakness on one side of the body
roentgen per hour at one meter
O. Touch glucometer
O. Touch Profile
O. Touch Ultra meter
o. ventricle heart

one-and-a-half syndrome

one-block claudication
one-child sterility
one-dimensional chemical-shift imaging
one-egg twins
one-horned uterus
one-hour
o.-h. glucose tolerance test
o.-h. PG
o.-h. prostaglandin
O'Neil cup
oneiric
o. delirium
o. hyperesthesia
oneirodynia
o. activa
o. gravis
one-leg hop for distance test
one-lung
o.-l. anesthesia
o.-l. ventilation
one-millionth International Unit
one-piece
o.-p. bifocal
o.-p. disposable plug
o.-p. multifocal lens
o.-p. plate haptic silicone intraocular lens
one-pillow orthopnea
one-plane
o.-p. bilateral external fixator
o.-p. bilateral frame
o.-p. deformity
o.-p. lens
one-repetition maximum
one-sided
o.-s. chorea
o.-s. headache
one-snip
o.-s. punctum
o.-s. punctum operation
one-stage
o.-s. amputation
o.-s. esthetic correction
o.-s. grafting
o.-s. reconstruction of eye socket and eyelids
One-Step
one-step nested PCR
one-stitch
o.-s. cataract procedure
o.-s. technique
one-tail test
one-time only
one-year survival rate
on-eye predicted power
ongoing
o. clinical trial
o. cognitive process
complete and ongoing assessment
o. monitoring
onion
o. body
o. bulb change
o. bulb formation
o. bulb neuropathy
o. mite dermatitis
o. skin-like membrane
onionskin
o. appearance
o. change
o. configuration of collagenous fiber
***o*-nitrophenyl-beta-galactosidase**
onlay
o. bone graft
o. bone graft cast
o. bone grafting
o. cancellous iliac graft
composite o.
o. cortical graft
o. denture
gingival onlay graft
intraperitoneal onlay mesh hernia repair
morselized cartilage onlay radix graft
o. patch anastomosis
On-Line
Bioethical Information O.-L.
Chemical Dictionary O.-L.
Documents O.-L.
MEDLARS O.-L.
online
o. assessment method
audiovisuals o.
o. counseling
o. cross-modal naming
o. education
o. encounter
Giannetti O. Psychosocial History
patient-centered access to secure systems o.
o. prospective drug utilization review
simultaneous peripheral operation o.
o. transaction processing
only
o. child
comfort measures o.
drugs o.
for external use o.
o. handle it once rule
for internal use o.
light perception o.
one-time o.
patient treated with comfort care o.
physician o.
presence of only one sex chromosome
region of sarcomere containing only myosin filaments
Spanish-speaking o.
on-off
o.-o. effect of L-dopa
o.-o. flushing reservoir
onset
age at o.
age at onset of use
o. of agitation
alleged onset date
o. of atrial fibrillation
o. of blood lactate accumulation
character, onset, location, duration, exacerbation, remission
o. of chills and fever
o. of contractions
o. and course of disease
dim light melatonin o.
o. of dyspnea
o. of early menstruation
early onset Parkinsonism-mental retardation syndrome
o. of facial weakness
o. of fever
o. of flashes and floaters
o. frequency
gait disorder, autoantibody, late-age onset, polyneuropathy
hospital onset of infection
immediately after o.
o. of jaundice
later onset nephrotic syndrome
maturity onset deafness
o. of menarche
o. of menopause
o. of menses
mood disorder with postpartum o.

onset *(continued)*
multiple epiphysial dysplasia-early onset diabetes mellitus syndrome
o. of nausea
o. of overt heart failure
o. of pain
o. of paralysis
period of o.
premature onset of labor
rapid onset of jaundice
o. of senility
sleep onset insomnia
o. of spontaneous labor
spontaneous onset of labor
sudden-dosage o.
o. of symptoms
o. of unconsciousness
o. of ventricular depolarization
very early onset schizophrenia
voice onset time
wake after sleep o.
wake after sleep onset time
wakefulness after sleep o.

on-site
eligibility o.-s.
o.-s. intervention

Ontak protein

Ontario
Western Ontario Instability Index
Western Ontario and McMaster Universities Osteoarthritis Index Physical Functioning subscale and chair-performance
Western Ontario and McMaster Universities Osteoarthritis Index Physical Functioning subscale and chair-stand performance
Western Ontario Rotator Cuff

onto
mitomycin adsorbed onto activated charcoal

ontogeny
osteoblast o.

onychalgia nervosa

onychia
o. lateralis
o. maligna
monilial o.
o. parasitica
o. periungualis
o. piannic
o. punctata
o. sicca

onychodysplasia
brachymorphism, onychodysplasia, dysphalangism
congenital onychodysplasia of the index finger

onychodystrophy-congenital deafness syndrome

onychomycosis
candidal o.
distal subungual o.
proximal subungual o.
superficial white o.

onychoosteodysplasia
hereditary onychoosteodysplasia syndrome

onychoosteodystrophy
deafness, onychoosteodystrophy, and mental retardation syndrome

onychopachydermoperiostitis
psoriatic o.

O'nyong-nyong
O.-n. fever
O.-n. virus

oocyst
prepatient periods to o.

oocyte
aspiration of mature o.
o. atresia
o. collection
o. cryopreservation
o. culture
direct oocyte sperm transfer
o. donation
o. donor
o. extrusion
follicle puncture for oocyte retrieval
hamster oocyte penetration test
immature oocyte retrieval
o. maturation-inhibiting factor
o. maturation inhibitor
o. meiosis
o. meiotic inhibitor
peritoneal oocyte and sperm transfer
o. production
o. recovery
o. retrieval
transvaginal ultrasound-directed oocyte retrieval

oophorectomy
bilateral partial o.

oophoritic cyst

oophoritis
autoimmune o.
o. parotidea

oozing
o. about shunt site
active oozing from site
active oozing from wound
bleeding and o.
o. of blood
o. of blood from nose
o. of blood from nostril
blood oozing from os
o. dermatitis
o. of fistula
o. of fluid
o. from dermatitis
o. from eczema
o. from os
o. from site
o. from wound
o. of purulent material
venous o.

Opa
O. protein
O. typing

opacification
o. cherry-red spot
ground-glass o.
Lens Opacification Classification System
opaque linear o.
pedal artery o.
posterior capsular o.
posterior capsule o.

opacified cuff

opacity
asymmetric lung o.
Caspar ring o.
corneal o.
ground-glass o.
hemihypertrophy, intestinal web, preauricular skin tag, and congenital corneal opacity syndrome
international opacity unit
Lens Opacities Classification System II
mycotic snowball o.
nebular stromal o.
patchy alveolar o.
peripheral corneal o.
o. protein

opal codon

opalescent
o. cornea

o. dentin
hereditary opalescent dentin

opaline patch

opaque

o. arthrography
o. branching structure
o. calculus
o. contact lens
o. enamel
o. foreign body
large opaque vesicle
o. linear opacification
o. material
o. medium
o. shadow

open

o. access endoscopy
o. adjustable silicone gastric banding
o. adrenalectomy
o. to air
o. air factor
o. airway
o. amputation
o. anesthesia system
o. angiography
o. anti-reflux surgery
o. apex
o. apophyseal joint
o. appendectomy
o. application test
o. approach
o. awareness
o. base wedge osteotomy
o. base wedge osteotomy/bunionectomy
o. beam
o. bed warmer
o. bite
o. bladder brachytherapy implant
o. bone graft epiphysiodesis
o. book fracture
bowels o.
o. brain biopsy
o. bronchus sign
o. canalicular system of platelets
o. capsulotomy
o. care area
o. carpal tunnel release
o. cavity
o. cell foam
o. chain compound
o. chest cardiac massage
o. chest cardiac resuscitation
o. cholecystectomy
o. circuit
o. circuit method
o. clam-shell MRI
o. class
o. colectomy
o. comedo
o. common bile duct exploration
o. cordotomy
o. coronal browlift
o. crib
o. cystotomy
o. debridement
o. dermal sinus
o. disc surgery
o. discussion
o. dislocation
o. diverticulectomy
o. door laminoplasty
o. double-decked hook cervical system
o. drainage
o. dressing
o. drop anesthesia
o. drop technique
o. duct
o. earmold
o. endarterectomy
o. end flow-through radiopaque tip
o. endotracheal suction
o. endotracheal suctioning
o. epicutaneous test
o. esophagectomy
o. esophagomyotomy
o. exit foramen
eyes o.
o. face mask
o. flap
o. flap drainage
o. flap technique
o. foreheadplasty
o. fracture
o. fracture wound drain
o. fundoplication
o. gastrostomy tube placement
o. group
o. harvesting technique
o. Hasson technique
o. head injury
o. hemorrhoidectomy
o. hernia operation
o. herniorrhaphy
o. horizon
o. hospital
o. hostility
imaging-guided open biopsy
o. injury
keep o.
keep needle o.
to keep needle o.
to keep open
keep open rate
to keep vein o.
keep vein open
o. kinetic chain exercises
o. lens
o. liver biopsy
o. loop
o. lung biopsy
o. mitral commissurotomy
o. mitral valve commissurotomy
moderately wide open anterior chamber angle
modified Hassan open technique
o. mouth
needle-localized open biopsy
o. Nissen fundoplication
o. patch test
o. posterior fontanelle
postoperative open heart surgery
o. prostatectomy
o. psychiatry
o. reading frame
o. reduction
o. reduction and external fixation
o. reduction of humerus
o. reduction and internal fixation
o. reduction metallic fixation
o. reduction of radius and ulna
o. reduction of skull fracture
o. sore
squarely face person, open posture, lean toward person, eye contact, relaxed
o. surgical biopsy
o. technique
transfer to o.
o. tuberculosis
wall coated open tubular
o. wedge
o. wedge osteotomy
o. wet dressing
wide o.
wide open anterior chamber angle
o. wound

open-air drying

open-angle

chronic open-angle glaucoma
o.-a. glaucoma
juvenile open-angle glaucoma
primary open-angle glaucoma

open-bite malocclusion

open-book fracture

open-chest
o.-c. cardiac compression
o.-c. cardiopulmonary resuscitation

open-door hospital

opened
o. anteriorly
bowels not o.
o. infraumbilically
o. posteriorly
o. suprapubically
o. transversely
o. vertically

open-ended vasectomy

open-end marriage

opener
can opener capsulotomy

open-funnel detachment

open-heart
o.-h. rehabilitation program

opening
o. abductory wedge osteotomy
anodal o.
anodal opening clonus
anodal opening contraction
anodal opening picture
anodal opening sound
anodal opening tetanus
aortic o.
aortic opening click
aortic opening of heart
o. of aortic valve
aortic valve o.
aortic valve opening to aortic valve closing ratio
apraxia of eyelid o.
o. of aqueduct of midbrain
atrioventricular opening of His
atrioventricular valve o.
auriculoventricular valve o.
Axer lateral opening wedge osteotomy
o. axis
calculated opening area
o. of carotid canal
cathodal opening contraction
o. of cerebral aqueduct
o. contraction
o. of coronary sinus
o. for dorsal artery of penis
o. for dorsal nerve of penis
duodenal opening narrow
early opening of valve
effect of opening eyes
o. of external acoustic meatus
o. flap
o. of frontal sinus
incisal o.
o. of inferior vena cava
initial opening pressure
o. of internal acoustic meatus
o. in joint
o. of left parotid duct
maximal mouth o.
mitral opening snap
mitral valve o.
o. mitral valve snap
narrow duodenal o.
o. of orbital cavity
patent opening for bile drainage
o. pressure
pressure at airway o.
pulmonary valve o.
o. snap ejection systolic click
o. through lens
o. tricuspid valve snap
upper airway opening pressure
velopharyngeal o.
voluntary o.

open-loop
o.-l. accommodation
o.-l. insulin delivery system
o.-l. pump therapy

open-sky
o.-s. cataract wound
o.-s. cryoextraction
o.-s. cryoextraction operation
o.-s. dissection
o.-s. technique
o.-s. trephination
o.-s. vitrectomy

open-wedge biopsy specimen

operable
o. breast cancer
large operable breast cancer
o. pancreatic carcinoma
primary operable breast cancer

operable breast cancer

operable pancreatic carcinoma

opera-glass
o.-g. deformity
o.-g. hand

operant
o. acceleration of heart rate
autoclitic o.
o. behavior
o. behaviorism
o. behavior theory
o. conditioning
o. conditioning audiometry
o. deceleration of heart rate
human operant heart rate conditioning
Schedule-Controlled Operant Behavior
tangible reinforcement of operant conditioned audiometry

OPERA procedure

operated
manually o.

operating
cardiovascular operating room
o. cycle
exclusive operating room
o. field
o. frequency
o. loupe
o. microscope
o. microscope-induced phototoxic maculopathy
o. motor vehicle while intoxicated
network operating system
o. nursing procedure
on-call to operating room
receiver operating characteristic
receiver operating characteristic curve
relative operating characteristic
o. scope
standard operating procedure
o. suite
o. theatre sterile supply unit
tonsillectomy with operating microscope
total operating time
void on-call to operating room

operation
O. Anaconda
aneurysmal clipping o.
anterior ankle shift o.
anular corneal graft o.
Armistead ulnar lengthening o.
arterial switch o.
Ashford retracted nipple o.
atrial baffle o.
atrial switch o.
before time of o.
cardiopulmonary bypass o.
Carotid Artery Stenosis with Asymptomatic Narrowing: O. Versus Aspirin Study
cataract flap o.
cautery-assisted palatal stiffening o.
o. code
Coping O.'s Preference Enquiry

double needle operation on cataract
Emergency O.'s Center
encircling of scleral buckle o.
enucleation of eyeball o.
exenteration of orbital contents o.
gastric bypass o.
iris stretching o.
length of o.
lip adhesion o.
Macewen hernia o.
Machek ptosis o.
Magitot keratoplasty o.
Mayo hallux valgus modified o.
McBride bunion hallux valgus o.
McKay-Simons clubfoot o.
McKeever-Buck elbow o.
Mensor-Scheck hanging hip o.
Mikamo double-eyelid o.
Milch elbow o.
Miller flatfoot o.
Mital elbow release o.
modified Cocklin toe o.
modified flap o.
modified Fontan o.
Nicoll fracture o.
Nida nicking o.
Nissen antireflux o.
Nissen fundoplication o.
one-snip punctum o.
open hernia o.
open-sky cryoextraction o.
orbital implant o.
orthotopic hemi-Koch o.
Osborne-Cotterill elbow dislocation o.
pars plana o.
pattern-cut corneal graft o.
pedicle flap o.
peripheral iridectomy o.
o.'s research
second-look o.
sham operation
Silva-Costa o.
simultaneous peripheral operation on-line
sphincter-preserving o.
Standard Nomenclature of Diseases and O.'s
total hip replacement o.

operational
o. definition
o. evaluation
o. fatigue
o. taxonomic unit
o. technique

operative
o. ablation
o. ankylosis
o. approach
o. area irrigated with antibiotic solution
o. area irrigated with normal saline
o. arteriography
o. arthroscopy
o. arthrotomy
o. biliary bypass
o. blood loss
o. bronchoscopy
o. cholangiogram
o. cholangiography
cholecystectomy and operative cholangiogram
o. choledochoscopy
o. consent
contaminated operative wound classification
o. correction
o. decompression
delayed closure of operative wound
o. delivery with forceps
o. dentistry
o. diagnosis
diagnostic arthroscopy, operative arthroscopy, and possible operative arthrotomy
diagnostic and operative arthroscopy
dirty operative wound classification
o. drainage
o. excision
o. exposure
o. field
o. field anesthetized
o. field anesthetized with 1% lidocaine
o. field prepared and draped
o. field prepped and draped
o. finding
o. incision
o. informed consent
o. laparoscopy
o. morbidity and mortality
o. mortality rate
o. myxedema
o. pancreatography
o. permit signed
o. procedure
o. region
o. repair
o. risk
o. scar
o. site
o. site complication
o. site infection
o. site irrigated
o. site irrigated with antibiotic solution
o. site irrigated with normal saline
o. suite
o. technique
o. therapy
o. vaginal delivery
o. wound
o. wound clean and healed

operator
o. certification
Computer O. Aptitude Battery
o. gene
o. locus

opercula (*pl. of* operculum)

opercular
o. cortex
o. epilepsy

opercularis
Megalopyge opercularis sting

operculated
o. hole
o. tear

operculate egg

operculum, pl. **opercula**
o. frontale
parietal o.
peripheral retinal o.

operon
arabinose o.
o. promoter sequence

ophiasic alopecia areata

Ophthalas
O. argon laser

ophthalmia
Egyptian o.
gonococcal o.
gonococcal ophthalmia neonatorum
o. hepatica
metastatic o.
migratory o.
mucous o.
neonatal o.
o. neonatorum
neuroparalytic o.
nivalis o.
o. nivalis

ophthalmia *(continued)*
o. nodosa
periodic o.
sympathetic o.

ophthalmic
o. acid
o. administration of insulin
alopecia, nail dystrophy, ophthalmic complication, thyroid dysfunction, hypohidrosis, ephelides and enteropathy, and respiratory tract infection
o. anesthesia
o. aneurysm
anterior ethmoidal branch of ophthalmic artery
o. artery
o. artery aneurysm
o. artery occlusion
o. artery pressure
o. biometry by ultrasound echography
o. cautery
O. Confidence Index
o. corticosteroid
o. cul-de-sac
o. cup
o. disorder
Doppler ophthalmic test
o. Doppler sonogram
o. drug
o. examination
o. ganglion
o. glucocorticoid
o. Graves disease
o. herpes
o. hook
o. hyperthyroidism
o. laser microendoscope
MC-7000 ophthalmic laser
meningeal branch of ophthalmic nerve
o. migraine
O. Moldite Powder
muscular artery of ophthalmic artery
Mydfrin O.
nasociliary branches of ophthalmic nerve
o. nerve
o. nurse
o. ointment
palladium 103 ophthalmic plaque brachytherapy
palladium 103 ophthalmic plaque radiotherapy
physostigmine salicylate o.
pilocarpine 1% ophthalmic solution
o. plexus
o. reaction
o. recurrent nerve
reversed ophthalmic artery flow
o. segment
o. solution
o. sponge
o. test
trigeminal nerve, ophthalmic division
tropicamide 1% ophthalmic solution Mydriacyl
o. tumor
o. vein
o. vesicle
o. vitreous surgical technique
o. zoster

ophthalmica
arteria o.

ophthalmicae
arteriae musculares arteriae o.

ophthalmicus
herpes zoster o.

ophthalmology
occupational o.
o., otology, laryngology, and rhinology
o., otorhinolaryngology, and head and neck surgery

ophthalmomandibulomelic dysplasia

ophthalmomeningeal vein

ophthalmometer
mires of o.

ophthalmoparesis
progressive external o.

ophthalmopathy
Graves o.
thyroid-associated o.
thyroid-related o.

ophthalmoplegia
binocular internuclear o.
chronic progressive external o.
o. externa
external oculomotor o.
internodal o.
internuclear o.
mitochondrial encephalomyopathy with sensorimotor polyneuropathy, ophthalmoplegia, and paralysis
polyneuropathy, ophthalmoplegia, leukoencephalopathy, and intestinal pseudo-obstruction
o. progressiva
progressive external o.
sensory ataxic neuropathy with dysarthria and o.
o. totalis
wall-eyed bilateral internuclear o.
wall-eyed monocular internuclear o.

ophthalmoplegia-hypotonia-ataxia-hypacusis-athetosis syndrome

ophthalmoplegic
o. exophthalmos
o. migraine
o. muscular dystrophy

ophthalmoscope
AO binocular indirect o.
binocular indirect o.
laser-indirect o.
monocular indirect o.
Nerve Fiber Analyzer laser o.
Novus 2000 o.
scanning laser o.

ophthalmoscopic examination

ophthalmoscopy
indirect o.
medical o.
metric o.
monocular indirect o.
o. with reflected light

Ophthalon suture

Ophthimus
O. High-Pass Resolution perimeter
O. ring perimeter

opiate
o. abstinence
o. abstinence syndrome
o. abuse
o. addict
o. addiction
o. analgesia
o. analgesic
o. antagonist
o. antispasmodic
o. detoxification
o. drug
o. intoxication
rapid opiate detoxification under anesthesia
o. receptor
o. receptor agonist

o. use
o. withdrawal
o. withdrawal symptom
o. withdrawal syndrome

opiate-dependent patient

opiate-directed behavior

opinion
examination, opinion, and advice
second o.
Student O. Inventory
Suicide O. Questionnaire
O.'s toward Adolescents
Vocational O. Index

Opinionnaire
Purdue Student-Teacher O.

opioid
o. abuse
o. abuser
o. activity
o. addict
o. addiction
o. agonist
o. analgesia
o. analgesic
o. anesthesia
o. antagonist
o. antidiarrheal
antisecretory o.
o. cell membrane receptor
chronic opioid analgesic therapy
o. dependence
endogenous opioid peptide
o. escalation index
o. growth factor
o. intoxication
o. maintenance
o. medication
mixed opioid agonist-antagonist
o. mortality
neuraxial opioid infusion
o. overdose
overdosed with o.
o. peptide
pituitary opioid peptide
rapid opioid detoxification
o. receptor agonist
o. receptor antagonist
spinal opioid analgesia
o. toxicity
o. withdrawal

opipramol hydrochloride

opisthotonic
o. posture
o. posturing

opisthotonos fetalis

Opitz
autosomal dominant Opitz syndrome
O. BBB syndrome
O. disease
X-linked Opitz syndrome

Opitz-Christian syndrome

Opitz-Frias syndrome

Opitz-Kaveggia syndrome

opium
o. addiction
o. alkaloid
o. and belladonna
belladonna and o.
o. deodoratum
deodorized tincture of o.
o. dependence
o. granulatum
o. habit
neonatal opium solution
o. smoking
tincture of o.

O-plasty to Z-plasty

OPMI
O. PRO magis microscope
O. VISU 200 microscope

Oppenheim
O. amyotonia
O. brace
O. congenital hypotonia
O. disease
O. gait
O. reflex
O. sign

opponens
o. bar
o. digiti minimi
o. digiti minimi manus
o. digiti minimi muscle
o. digiti quinti
o. digiti quinti muscle
o. weakness

opponent
o. color
o. colors theory

opportunistic
antifungal-resistant opportunistic infection
o. complication
o. disease
o. fungus
o. illness
o. infection
Kaposi sarcoma and opportunistic infection
multiple opportunistic pathogen infection
o. organism
o. pathogen
o. pneumonia
o. systemic fungal infection
o. systemic mycosis

opportunity
nonnutritive sucking o.

opposed
sequential paired opposed plaque

opposing
anterior and posterior opposing portals
o. articular surfaces
o. muscle of little finger
o. muscle of thumb

opposite
o. affect state
o. biological sex
cold to the opposite, warm to the same
decline in interest of opposite sex
o. ear masked

opposition
o. breathing
o. contracture
o. defiance disorder
o. exercise
o. movement

oppositional
o. attitude
o. behavior
o. defiance
o. defiant disorder
o. disorder
o. disorder of adolescence
o. disorder of childhood
o. movement

opposition-versus-pressure relation

Opraflex drape

opsoclonus
paraneoplastic o.

opsoclonus-myoclonus
o.-m. diarrhea
o.-m. etiology
neuroblastoma and o.-m.
o.-m. syndrome

opsonic
o. action
o. activity
o. defect
o. deficiency

opsonic *(continued)*
o. index
o. receptor

opsonin
normal o.

opsonization
antigen-reactive cell o.

opsonizing antibody

opsonophagocytic defect

opsonophagocytosis assay

Optaloy amalgam alloy

Opthascan Mini-A scan

optic
o. aberration
accessory optic tract
o. activity
o. agnosia
o. agraphia
o. alexia
o. angle
anterior compressive optic neuropathy
anterior ischemic optic neuritis
anterior ischemic optic neuropathy
anterior optic chiasmal syndrome
o. antipode
o. aphasia
aplasia of optic nerve
o. apparatus glioma
arteriosclerotic ischemic optic neuropathy
arteritic anterior ischemic optic neuropathy
o. artery
asymptomatic optic neuritis
o. ataxia
o. atrophy
o. atrophy-ataxia syndrome
atrophy of optic nerve
o. atrophy tremor
autosomal dominant hereditary optic neuropathy
autosomal-dominant optic atrophy
autosomal recessive hereditary optic neuropathy
autosomal-recessive optic atrophy
o. axis
back optic zone radius
basal optic root
o. canal
o. capsule
o. center
o. chiasm
o. chiasmal lesion
o. and chiasmal neuropathy
o. chiasmal syndrome
o. chiasm compression
o. chiasm disease
o. chiasm tumor
choking of optic nerve head
o. coloboma
o. commissure
o. complex tumor
contralateral optic tectum
o. cul-de-sac
o. cup
o. cupping
o. cup-to-disk ratio
o. decussation
o. demyelinating neuritis
o. density
diabetes insipidus, diabetes mellitus, progressive bilateral optic atrophy, and sensorineural deafness
o. diaphragm
o. disc anomaly
o. disc atrophy
o. disc cupping
o. disc dragging
o. disc drusen
o. disc drusen calcification
o. disc drusen retinopathy
o. disc dysplasia
o. disc edema
o. disc edema with a macular star
o. disc hyperemia
o. disc pallor
o. disc pit
o. disc swelling
o. disc topography
o. disc tubercle
dominant juvenile optic atrophy
dominantly inherited juvenile optic atrophy
dominant optic atrophy
o. evagination
o. fissure
o. foramen
front optic zone radius
o. fundi and peripheral fields
o. fundus
o. ganglion
glaucomatous optic nerve atrophy
glaucomatous optic nerve damage
o. glioma
glioma of optic chiasm
glioma of optic nerve
o. groove
growth retardation, alopecia, pseudoanodontia, and optic atrophy syndrome
hereditary atrophy optic nerve
hereditary optic atrophy
o. hyperesthesia
hypertensive optic neuropathy
o. hypocalcemia
o. illusion
o. implant
indirect optic nerve injury syndrome
inner optic anlage
o.'s of intraocular lens
ipsilateral optic tectum
o. iridectomy
o. keratoplasty
o. labyrinthine righting
o. layer
Leber hereditary optic neuropathy
Leber optic atrophy
McDonald optic zone marker
medullary optic disease
mental retardation, optic atrophy, deafness, seizures syndrome
morning glory optic atrophy
morning glory optic disk anomaly
o. muscle recession
nasal border of optic disc
neovascularization of optic disc
o. nerve
o. nerve aplasia
o. nerve atrophy
o. nerve coloboma
o. nerve cupping
o. nerve damage
o. nerve disease
o. nerve disorder
o. nerve drusen
o. nerve dysfunction
o. nerve dysplasia
o. nerve fiber
o. nerve glioma
o. nerve head
o. nerve head analysis
o. nerve hemangioblastoma
o. nerve hypoplasia
o. nerve injury
o. nerve lesion
o. nerve myelination
o. nerve pit
o. nerve sheath
o. nerve sheath decompression
o. nerve sheath fenestration
o. nerve sheath meningioma
o. nerve tumor

neural layer of optic part of retina
O. Neuritis Treatment Trial
o. neuropathy
nonarteritic anterior ischemic optic neuropathy
nucleus of optic tract
nutritional optic neuropathy
orbital optic nerve
osteogenesis imperfecta, optic atrophy, retinopathy, developmental delay syndrome
outer optic anlage
pale optic disc
pallor of optic disc
o. papilla
o. papilla cavity
papilla of optic nerve
parainfectious optic neuritis
parainfectious optic neuropathy
paraneoplastic optic neuritis
o. perineuritis
o. pit
posterior ischemic optic neuropathy
primary optic atrophy
o. primordium
progressive encephalopathy, edema, hypsarrhythmia, optic atrophy
o. radiation
o. radiation lesion
radiation optic neuropathy
o. recess
o. reflex
retrobulbar optic neuritis
o. stalk
o. strut
o. sulcus
o. tectum
o. thalamus
toxic optic nerve atrophy
o. tract
o. tract compression
o. tract damage
o. tract lesion
o. tract pituitary tumor
o. tract syndrome
o. vesicle

optica
neuromyelitis o.

optical
o. aberration
o. activity
o. alexia
o. allachesthesia
American O.
anterior optical zone
average optical density
o. axis
o. bench
o. biopsy
O. Biopsy System
o. blur
o. breakdown
o. cavity
o. center
o. centering instrument
o. center of spectacle lens
o. character recognition
o. chromatography
o. clarity
o. coherence tomography
o. coherence tomography in uveitis
o. coherent tomography
computerized optical densitometry
o. contact lens
o. correction
o. cross
o. crystallography
o. densitometry
o. density
o. density measurement
o. density method
density optical standard
o. density unit
density optical unknown
o. device
o. disc anomaly
o. disc swelling
dynamic optical breast imaging system
o. emission spectroscopy
o. fiber
o. fossa
o. frame
o. glass
gold-labeled optical rapid immunoassay
o. heterogeneity
hypertension optical treatment study
o. illusion
o. image
o. immunoassay
integrated optical density
o. internal urethrotomy
o. intrinsic signal imaging
o. iridectomy
o. keratoplasty
magnetic optical rotatory dispersion
o. mammography
microendoscopic optical catheter
near field scanning optical microscope
o. nerve atrophy
Neumann-Shepard oval optical center marker
o. nodal point
o. pachymeter
o. parametric oscillator
o. path difference
o. penetration depth
posterior optical zone
o. power
o. ray tracing
o. rehabilitation
roaming optical access multiscope
o. rotation
o. rotatory dispersion
o. scanning
specific optical rotation
o. surface imaging
o. system
in vivo optical spectroscopy
o. zone
o. zone centration
o. zone of contact lens
o. zone diameter
o. zone marker

optically
o. empty
o. inactive
o. inactive chemical
o. transparent electrode

Opticians Association of America

opticoacoustic nerve atrophy

opticocerebral syndrome

opticochiasmatic
o. arachnoiditis
arachnoiditis of opticochiasmatic cistern
o. glioma

opticociliary
o. neurectomy
o. neurotomy
o. shunt
o. shunt vein
o. shunt vessel

opticocochleodentate degeneration

opticofacial winking reflex

opticokinetic nystagmus

opticopyramidal syndrome

optics of intraocular lens

opticus
nervus o.

Optiflex lens

optimal
automated endoscopic system for optimal positioning
automatic endoscopic system for optimal positioning
o. care
o. cutting temperature
o. cytoreduction
o. development
o. diastolic pressure
o. diet
o. dose
o. dose of chemotherapy
o. dose selection
o. group size
hypertension optimal treatment
o. immunoassay
o. immunomodulating dose
o. intensity
o. level of functioning
o. level of independence
o. management
o. sampling theory
o. therapeutic dose

OptiMed device

Optimism-Pessimism Scale, revised

optimistic
o. atmosphere
o. expectation

optimization
mathematical optimization and logical dimensioning for radiotherapy
Maurer optimization test

optimized
o. microvessel density analysis
tilted optimized nonsaturating excitation

optimizing
Spofford-Christopher oxygen optimizing program

optimum
o. biologic dose
o. calorie intake
o. dose
o. information size
o. temperature

option
adjuvant treatment o.
initial planning o.
volume-guaranteed pressure o.

Opti-Pure System

Optiray contrast

Optisol medium

Opti-Vu lens

optochiasmatic
o. arachnoiditis
o. tuberculoma

Optochin-resistant ***Streptococcus pneumoniae***

Optochin susceptibility test

optokinetic
o. after nystagmus
o. disorder
o. drum
o. reflex
o. stimulator
o. stimulus
o. system
o. tape

optometer
automatic infrared o.
light optometer reflex
objective o.

optomotor reflex

Optyl frame

O-R
O.-R. system

or
ability to think or concentrate
acute cervical traumatic sprain or syndrome
adjuvant hormonal or chemotherapy treatment
aggressive or violent behavior
alcohol or drug abuse
algebraic unknown or space coordinate
all or none
alternating current or direct current
amphetamine or similarly acting sympathomimetic intoxication
anomalous pulmonary venous connection, total or partial
Assessment for Persons Profoundly or Severely Impaired
atypical or mixed organic brain syndrome
atypical mixed or other personality disorder
Bessey-Lowry-Brock method or unit
bispinous or interspinous diameter
bloating or belching
bloating or diarrhea
blocking or attenuation
blunted or flat affect
blurred or fuzzy vision
blurring or dimming of vision
bone or joint pathology
bone marrow-derived cell or lymphocyte
breasts ropy or granular
carbon monoxide pressure or tension
ceramic or plastic brace
choroidal or subretinal neovascularization
chronic or incurable disease
chronic motor or vocal tic disorder
clubbing or tremor
cold or ice whirlpool treatment
confused or impoverished thought and speech
constriction or spasm of blood vessel
cyanosis, clubbing or edema
damaged or blocked fallopian tubes
decimal scale of potency or dilution
decrease in coordination or equilibrium
decrease in energy or fatigue
delayed or impaired speech
delusional or ideas of reference
delusion, hallucination, or illusion
depersonalization or derealization
depressed or irritable mood
dermal or oral herpes
diagnosis or condition deferred on Axis I, II
difficulty or inability to speak
diminished ability to think or concentration
dimness or loss of vision
disoriented or slow thought process
distortion or retraction of nipple
dizziness or lightheadedness
dysplasia-associated lesion or mass
evaluate extent of injury or illness
excessive or inappropriate guilt
exposure to blood or body fluid
fidgeting, aching, pulling, or itching feeling
fight, flee, freeze, or faint
fight or flight reaction
first in alpha series or group

first through fifth lumbar vertebrae or lumbar nerve
fourth in a series or group
gender identity disorder of adolescence or adulthood, nontranssexual type
glands, goiter, or stiffness of neck
goiter or stiffness of glands
grunting or retraction
healing by first, second, or third intention
heat, reddening, swelling, or tenderness
heightened awareness of touch or taste
hemorrhage or laceration
hot or cold flash
hydrocephalus, agyria, retinal dysplasia with or without encephalocele syndrome
ichthyosis, follicularis, atrichia or alopecia, photophobia syndrome
illness or injuries
illusion or perceptual distortions
immunoreactive insulin to serum or plasma glucose ratio
impaired thinking or concentration
inability to chew or swallow
infection or bladder involvement
inflammatory carcinoma or breast
intellectual function or memory
intermittent or continuous spasms
itching or burning sensation
itchy or chapped skin
laceration or hemorrhage
low self-esteem or guilt
malformed heart or heart valve
masses or tenderness
mean time between or before failures
melena, hematochezia or hematemesis
meningitis or encephalitis, metabolic, Reye syndrome
minimal dose causing 100% death or malformation
minimize or delay urinary incontinence
minute volume of air or blood
mulibrey nanism or dwarfism
murmurs, gallops, or rubs
myeloma or macroglobulinemia component
nagging cough or hoarseness
natural or synthetic hormone
neurovegetative functioning or symptom
neutral or gray area
no caffeine or pepper
no clubbing, cyanosis, or edema
no nausea or vomiting
no nausea, vomiting, or diarrhea
no nausea, vomiting, diarrhea or constipation
numbness or tingling
numbness or weakness
oculocutaneous tyrosinemia or tyrosinosis
other or unspecified psychoactive substance intoxication
outstretched hand or tongue
pain in chest, jaw, or extremity
partial seizures with or without generalized tonic-clonic seizures
patient in cardiac or respiratory distress
persistent vomiting or confusion headache
physical harm or violence
physically or otherwise health-impaired
placebo capsule or tablet
posttraumatic signs or symptoms
prothrombin induced by vitamin K absence or antagonist-II
quality-adjusted time without symptoms or toxicity
rales, rhonchi or, wheezes
rebound guarding or rigidity
red patch or blister on arm
restore lost or thinning hair
retraction or grunting
R or L
separation or loss abandonment
sharp, jabbing or electrical pain
significant sharp spike or delta wave
social or interpersonal situation
spin-spin or transverse relaxation time MRI scan
stiffness or heaviness of limbs
suicidal or homicidal feeling
suspected child abuse or neglect
swelling of hands or feet
tenderness to palpation or percussion
terminal or end
threat to self or others
time without symptoms of progression or toxicity
toxicity or drug interaction
unilateral interfacetal dislocation or subluxation
unusually hostile or aggressive behavior
VD or M
venous distention or mass
vertebral abnormality, anal imperforation, tracheoesophageal fistula, and radial, ray, or renal anomalies
visual or auditory stimulation
W or A
weakness or atrophy
white or pale nails from anemia
without redness or swelling
wound healed by first, second or third intention

ora
o. globule
nasal ora serrata
scope passed per o.

Oragrafin

Orajel
O. Mouth-Aid

oral
o. administered drug
o. administration
o. administration of insulin
o. aggressive
o. airflow in liters per second
o. airway
o. alimentary automatism
o. alimentation
o. allergy syndrome
o. anal fistula
o. analgesic
O. Analogue Scale
o. anesthesia
o. anesthetic
o. anesthetic technique
o. anomaly
o. antiarrhythmic therapy
o. antibiotic
o. antibiotic medication
o. anticoagulant
o. anticoagulant therapy
o. anticoagulation
o. antidiabetic agent
o. antifungal
o. antifungal agent
o. antihistamine
o. antimicrobial prophylaxis
o. antimotility agent
o. antiviral agent
o. anxiety
aphthous oral ulcer

oral *(continued)*
o. aphthous ulcer
o. appliance
o. appliance therapy
o. apraxia
o. arch
around-the-clock oral maintenance bronchodilator therapy
o. atresia
o. attenuated poliomyelitis virus vaccine
o. attenuated poliovirus vaccine
o. attenuated *Salmonella typhi* vaccine
o. auditory method
o. bacteria
o. barium suspension
o. behavior
o. bile acid
o. bioavailabilty
o. biology
o. birth control pill
o. biting period
o. bleeding
o. blister
o. bovine myelin
o. bronchodilator
o. cancer
o. cancer examination
o. cancer screening
o. candidiasis
o. candidosis
o. canker
o. carcinoma
o. care
o. cavity
o. cavity abnormality
o. cavity cancer
o. cavity cytology
o. cavity proper
o. cavity tuberculosis
o. cavity tumors
o. cephalocele
o. challenge
o. character
o. chemotherapy
o. cholecystogogic
o. cholecystogram
o. cholecystogram imaging
o. cholecystographic dye
o. cholecystography
chronic oral, facial, head pain
o. cleft
o. coitus
o. colonic lavage
combination oral contraceptive
combined oral contraceptive
o. commissure
o. commissure movement
o. commissuroplasty
o. communication
o. complication
o. condyloma planus
o. conjugated estrogen
o. contraception
o. contraceptive
o. contraceptive agent
o. contraceptive efficacy
o. contraceptive hormone
o. contraceptive-induced chorea
o. contraceptive-induced hypertension
o. contraceptive medication
o. contraceptive pill
o. contraceptive steroid
o. contraceptive therapy
o. contraceptive use
o. contrast
o. contrast imaging agent
Controlled O. Word Association Test
o. copulation
o. corticosteroid
cortisone-primed oral glucose tolerance test
o. crisis
o. Crohn disease
daily oral hygiene
o. debris
o. decongestant
o. dependence
dermal or oral herpes
o. diabetes drug
o. diaphragm
o. disease
o. disease control
o. donovanosis
o. dosage
o. dose
o. drug therapy
o. dyskinesia
o. ego
o. enanthem
o. endotracheal intubation
o. endotracheal tube
o. environment
o. epithelial cell genetic fingerprinting
o. epithelial cell genotyping
o. epithelial nevus
o. epithelium
o. erotism
o. erythema multiforme
o. esophageal stethoscope
o. esophageal tube
o. estrogen therapy
o. estrone
o. evacuator
o. exploration
o. feeding
o. fissure
o. fixation
o. flora
o. florid papillomatosis
o. fluid
o. focal mucinosis
o. form recognition
o. fossa
o. frowning
o. gangrene
o. gastric
o. gastric tube
Gilmore O. Reading Test
o. glucose challenge test
o. glucose tolerance
o. glucose tolerance test
o. glucose tolerance testing
o. gold
o. gratification
Gray O. Reading Test-Revised
Gray O. Reading Test, Third Edition
growth monitoring, oral rehydration, breast feeding, and immunization
o. habit
o. hairy leukemia
o. hairy leukoplakia
o. hamartoma
o. health care
o. health status
o. hemangioma
o. herpes
o. herpes lesion
o. history
o. hormone replacement therapy
human oral epidermoid carcinoma cell
o. hydration
o. hygiene
O. Hygiene Index-Simplified
o. hygiene instruction
o. hyperpigmentation
o. hypoglycemic
o. hypoglycemic agent
o. hyposensitization
o. impulse
o. infection
o. ingestion
o. insulin
o. intake

o. intubation
o. iron
o. iron therapy
o. keratosis
O. Language Sentence Imitation Diagnostic Inventory
O. Language Sentence Imitation Screening Test
o. lesion
o. lesions
o. leukoplakia
live oral poliovirus vaccine
low-dose combination oral contraceptive
low-dose oral contraceptive
low steroid content combined oral contraceptive
magnesia and alumina oral suspension
o. manifestation
o. and maxillofacial surgery
o. medication
Mephyton O.
o. misoprostol
o. moniliasis
monophasic oral contraceptive
monovalent oral polio virus vaccine
o. morphine sulfate
o. motor
o. mucosa
o. mucosa cyanosis
o. mucosa dry
o. mucosal epithelia
mucosal oral therapeutic system
o. mucosal transudate
o. mucosa pink
o. mucosa pink and moist
o. mucositis
o. mucous membrane
o. mucous membrane dry
o. mucous membrane graft
o. mucous membrane moist
o. mucous membrane pink
o. mucous membrane pink and moist
Multicenter O. Carvedilol Heart Failure Assessment
multiple oral frenula
multiple oral vitamin
o. narcotic agent
o. nitroglycerin
Nitroglyn O.
o. order
oropharynx, oral cavity
o. osmotic
ostomotic release oral system
o. pain medication
o. passage
o. peripheral examination
personal oral hygiene
o. pharyngeal airway
o. phosphate
placebo-controlled oral challenge testing
o. polio immunization
o. polio vaccine
o. poliovirus vaccine
poliovirus vaccine monovalent o.
poliovirus vaccine trivalent o.
poor oral intake
o. postinflammatory hyperpigmentation
postoperative regimen for oral early feeding
o. premalignant lesion
o. radiation
o. radiation death
recurrent oral ulcer
o. region
o. rehabilitation
o. rehydration
o. rehydration salt
o. rehydration solution
o. rehydration therapy
repeated oral doses of activated charcoal
o. route
o. secretion
o. sedative
sequential oral contraceptive
sequential volitional oral movement
Simplified O. Hygiene Index
Slosson Oral Reading Test-Revised
spheroidal oral drug absorption system
o. squamous cell carcinoma
Stephens O. Language Screening Test
o. steroid
o. steroid drug
o. stomatitis
o. submucous fibrosis
o. supplement
o. surgery handpiece
o. suspension
sustained-release o.
o. tattoo
o. temperature
temperature, o.
o. temperature device
o. tetravalent rotavirus vaccine
o. thermometer
thrombosed oral varix
o. thrush
o. tissue
o. tolerance
o. transfer factor
o. transmission of saliva
o. transmission of viral hepatitis
o. transmucosal
o. transmucosal fentanyl citrate
o. treatment
o. triphasic tablets
trivalent oral poliovirus vaccine
o. tuberculosis
o. ulcer
o. ulceration
o. vasodilator
O. Verbal Intelligence Test
o. virus
o. yeast infection

oral Crohn disease

oral-duodenal

oral-facial-digital syndrome

oral-hairy leukoplakia

oralis
ventralis oralis anterior
ventralis oralis posterior

orally
o. disintegrating tablet
o. ingested

oral-nasal acoustic ratio

oral-ocular-genital syndrome

orange
Agent O.
o. blossom
o. cast
o. dye laser
o. green stain
o. indicator color
o. juice
oil of bitter o.
o. peel appearance
o. punctate pigmentation

orange G

OraSure
O. device
O. test

Oratec
O. chisel
O. device

Orban file

orbicular
o. alignment
o. bone

orbicular *(continued)*
o. eczema
o. ligament
o. ligament of radius
o. muscle
o. muscle of eye
o. muscle of mouth
o. reflex
o. zone of hip

orbiculare
os o.
Pityrosporon o.

orbicularis
o. ciliaris
marginal part of orbicularis oris muscle
musculus o.
musculus orbicularis oculi
o. myectomy
o. oculi
o. oculi muscle
o. oris
o. oris muscle
pars marginalis musculi orbicularis oris
pars orbitalis musculi orbicularis oculi
pars palpebralis musculi orbicularis oculi
o. phenomenon
psoriasis o.
o. pupillary reflex
o. reaction
o. reflex
o. sign
o. strength

orbiculoanterocapsular fiber

orbiculociliary fiber

orbiculoposterocapsular fiber

Orbis-Sigma cerebrospinal fluid shunt valve

orbit
aneurysm of o.
angular process of o.
anophthalmic orbit syndrome
aperture of o.
apex of o.
o. artifact
o. blade
exenterated o.
filariasis of o.
fracture of o.
granuloma of o.
o. hamartoma
hemangioma of o.
hematoma of o.
hemorrhage in o.
o., mandible, ear, cranial nerves, soft tissue syndrome
margin of o.

orbitae
paries interior o.
paries lateralis o.
paries medialis o.
paries superior o.

orbital
o. abscess
o. adipose tissue
o. akinesia
o. amyloidosis
o. anesthesia
o. aneurysm
o. angiography
o. angioma
o. angiosarcoma
anterior retinal orbital canal
o. aperture
o. apex
o. apex syndrome
o. arch
o. arch of frontal bone
o. arteriovenous malformation
o. artery
o. aspect of frontal lobe
atomic o.
atomic orbital with angular momentum quantum number zero
o. axis
o. bar
o. base
bilateral orbital decompression
o. blood cyst
o. blood flow
o. blow-in fracture
o. blow-out fracture
o. bone
o. bone hypoplasia
o. border of sphenoid bone
o. box osteotomy
o. branch
o. branch of maxillary nerve
o. branch of middle meningeal artery
o. branch of pterygopalatine ganglion
o. canal
o. capillary hemangioma
o. cavity
o. cellulitis
o. cephalocele
o. chemosis
o. childhood tumor
o. chocolate cyst
o. coke-bottle sign
comminuted orbital fracture
o. compartment syndrome
o. content
o. crest
o. CT scan
o. cyst
o. decompression
o. depression
o. dermoid
o. dermoid cyst
o. disease
o. dysmorphology
o. dystopia
o. echography
o. eminence
o. eminence of zygomatic bone
o. emphysema
o. encephalocele
o. enlargement
o. enucleation
o. enucleation compressor
o. exenteration
o. exenteration gastroscopic access technique
exenteration of orbital contents operation
o. extension
o. fascia
o. fasciae
o. fasciitis
o. fat
o. fat body
o. fat pad
o. fat suppression
o. fibroblast
o. fibroma
o. fibromatosis
o. fibrosarcoma
o. fissure
o. fissure width
floating spherical gaussian o.
o. floor
o. floor blow-out
o. floor fracture
o. floor implant
o. floor plate
o. floor prosthesis
o. floor syndrome
o. fracture
o. ganglion
o. glioma
o. granulocytic sarcoma
o. granuloma
o. gyri
o. hamartoma
o. height

o. hemangioendothelioma
o. hemangioma
o. hemangiopericytoma
o. hematoma
o. hemorrhage
o. hernia
highest occupied molecular o.
o. hypertelorism
o. hypotelorism
o. hypoxia
idiopathic orbital inflammatory syndrome
o. implant
o. implant operation
o. index
o. infarction
o. infection
inferior orbital rim
o. inferior rim
o. inflammation
o. inflammatory disease
o. lamina
o. lamina of ethmoid bone
o. layer of ethmoid bone
o. lens
o. lesion
linear combination of atomic o.'s
linear combination of atomic orbital-molecular o.
o. lipoma
localized molecular o.
lowest empty molecular o.
lowest unoccupied molecular o.
o. lymphoma
o. margin
o. margin of eyelid
medial orbital sulcus
o. medulloepithelioma
o. melanoma
o. meningioma
o. mesenchyme
o. metastasis
molecular o.
o. muscle
o. myositis
o. neoplasm
o. neuritis
o. neuroepithelioma
o. neurofibroma
o. neuroma
o. opening
opening of orbital cavity
o. ophthalmoplegia
o. optic nerve
o., mandibular, ear, neural, soft tissue
o. osteomyelitis
palisading orbital granuloma
o. palsy
o. pathology
o. periosteum
o. periostitis
o. pit
o. plane
o. plane of frontal bone
o. plaque brachytherapy
o. plate of ethmoid bone
o. plate of frontal bone
o. polymyositis
o. portion of eyelid
o. pseudotumor
o. radiology
o. radiotherapy
o. region
o. resilience
o. rhabdomyosarcoma
o. ridge
o. rim fracture
o. roentgenogram
o. roof
o. section
o. septum
subperiosteal orbital abscess
o. sulcus
o. superior fissure
superior orbital fissure syndrome
o. surgery
o. tissue
o. tomography
o. trauma
o. tuberculosis
o. tumor
o. varix
o. vasculitis
o. vein thrombosis
o. venography
o. vessel
o. wall fracture
o. width
o. wing of sphenoid bone
o. x-ray

orbitale inferius

orbitalis
musculus o.
pars orbitalis musculi orbicularis oculi
pars orbitalis ossis frontalis

orbitofacial cleft

orbitofrontal
o. activity
o. approach
o. area
o. artery
o. cortex
o. dominance
o. epilepsy

orbitofrontalis
arteria orbitofrontalis lateralis
arteria orbitofrontalis medialis

orbitomalar foramen

orbitomeatal line

orbitonasal dislocation

orbitopalpebral furrow

orbitozygomaticomaxillary
o. complex
o. fibrous dysplasia

orchard
o. grass
o. grass pollen

orchiectomy
inguinal o.

orchiopexy
laparoscopic o.

orchitis
experimental allergic o.
massive granulomatous o.
nonspecific granulomatous o.
o. parotidea
o. variolosa

order
o.'s accompanying patient on admission
asymmetry and order effect
automatic stop o.
o. blank
check doctor's o.
copied standing o.
diet o.
doctor's o.
doctor's order book
o. of extinction
future order screen
Hospital Indicator for Physicians Orders
hospital transfer o.
maximal surgical blood order schedule
negotiable order of withdrawal
no new o.
no new laboratory test o.'s
o.'s not to resuscitate
nurse-to-nurse orders
oral o.
outpatient commitment o.
phone o.
physician's o.
physician's order form
physician supplemental o.

order *(continued)*
postoperative o.'s
provider order entry
routine o.
standing o.
surgical blood order equation
trial prescription o.
unflagged o.
verbal o.
written o.

ordered
o. array
respiratory ordered phase encoding

order/results communication

ordinal
Assessment in Infancy Ordinal Scales of Psychological Development
o. designation of the exanthemata

ordinal designation of the exanthemata

ordinary
o. conversational voice
o. disease of childhood
o. least squares
o. warfare

Oregon
O. Adolescent Depression Project-Conduct Disorder Screener
O. ash

Orentreich punch

orexigenic
o. agent
o. peptide

Orexin A, B

orf
o. virus
o. virus subgroup

3′orf gene

organ
o. ablation
o. activity
acute organ rejection
o. allocation policy
o. allograft
o.'s at risk
o. blood flow
blood-forming o.
cadaveric whole organ transplant
o. capsule
chronic organ rejection
circumventricular o.
combat rejection of transplanted o.
o. compromise
o. confined
consent for organ donation
o. of Corti
criteria for organ donation
critical organ shielding blocks
o. culture
o. damage
donated human o.'s
o. donation
o. donor
o. donor candidate
o. donor card
donor organ ischemic time
o. dysfunction
electrical organ discharge
endocrine organ transplant complication
end organ damage
end organ dysfunction
end-stage organ disease
o. erotism
extralymphatic organ site
o. failure
o. failure criteria
fetal thymus organ culture
o. function
o. of Giraldes
Golgi tendon o.
o. graft
o. harvest
o. harvesting
healthy appearing o.
o. of hearing
hollow viscus o.
o. hypoperfusion
infected organ donor
o. inferiority
o. inferiority complex
O. Injury Scaling
o. isolated
o. limited
Logistic O. Dysfunction Score
major organ profile
male reproductive o.
o. malformation
o. malfunction
manual organ stimulation technique
mechanoreceptor Golgi tendon o.
metabolic organ transplant complication
multiple organ failure syndrome
multiple organ dysfunction
multiple organ dysfunction syndrome
multiple organ failure
multiple organ malrotation syndrome
multiple organ system dysfunction
multiple organ system failure
muscle receptor o.
nongenital pelvic o.
Northeast O. Procurement Organization
obstruction of major o.'s
palpable o.'s
parapineal o.
o. parking
pelvic organ prolapse
o. perfusion
pillar of Corti o.
o. preservation
o. procurement
procurement of cadaver organs for transplantation
procurement of donor organs and tissue
o. procurement organization
receptor organ of hearing
o. recipient
o. recipient candidate
o. and recipient match
o. recovery coordinator
o. recovery team
regional organ procurement
o. rejection
o. rejection of transplantation
o. replacement
o. retrieval
o. retrieval and preservation
sepsis-related organ failure assessment
sequential organ failure assessment
o. sharing
soft organs not palpable
solid organs not palpable
solid organ transplant
o. source
special sense o.'s
subcommissural o.
subfornical o.
o. system
o. system failure index
target o.
target organ disease
o. and tissue distribution
o. and tissue recovery
o. tolerance dose
o. transplant
o. for transplantation
o. transplantation
o. transplant center

o. transplant infection
o. transplant recipient
o. viability
o. of vision
vomeronasal o.
o. xenograft
o. of Zuckerkandl

organa genitalia

organ-cultured corneal tissue

organelles
paired o.

organic
o. acid
o. acidemia
o. acid-labile fluoride
o. acid metabolism
o. acidosis
o. acid screen
o. acid-soluble phosphorus
o. aciduria
acute organic brain syndrome
affective paranoid organic psychosis
o. affective syndrome
alcoholic liver disease-type organic psychosis
alcoholic organic mental disorder
alcohol-induced organic mental syndrome
alcoholism organic psychosis
o. amblyopia
o. amnesia
o. amnestic syndrome
anergastic organic psychosis
o. anion-binding protein
o. anionic dye
o. anion transporter polypeptide
o. anxiety
o. anxiety disorder
o. anxiety syndrome
o. approach
o. arsenical
arteriosclerotic brain disease-type organic psychosis
o. articulation disorder
atypical or mixed organic brain syndrome
o. brain changes
o. brain disease
o. brain disorder
o. brain dysfunction
o. brain syndrome with hallucinogen
canicular multispecific organic anion transporter
cannabis organic mental disorder
o. carbon
o. cardiac lesion
o. catalyst
o. cause
o. central nervous system deterioration
o. chemistry
childbirth organic psychosis
chronic organic brain syndrome
chronic organic mental syndrome
o. CNS deterioration
o. colon pathology
o. compound
o. conditioning film
o. contracture
o. damage to brain
o. deafness
o. defect
o. delirium
o. delusion
o. delusional disorder
o. delusional syndrome
delusional transient organic psychosis
o. dementia
o. deterioration
o. disease
dissolved organic matter
o. drivenness
o. dust toxic syndrome
o. dyscontrol
o. dysfunction
o. dyslalia
endocrine disease organic psychosis
o. epilepsy
o. etiology
o. factor
o. failure to thrive
o. hallucination
o. hallucinosis
o. hallucinosis syndrome
o. headache
o. hearing impairment
o. heart disease
o. hyperkinetic syndrome
hypersomnia related to a known organic factor
o. impairment
o. impotence
insomnia related to a known organic factor
O. Integrity Test
o. lead
liquid organic compound
liquid organic dye laser
liver disease organic psychosis
o. matrix
o. mental disorder
o. mental syndrome
o. mercury poisoning
metabolic disease organic psychosis
o. mood disorder
o. mood syndrome
o. murmur
nonpurgeable organic carbon
o. osmolyte
particulate organic carbon
particulate organic nitrogen
persistent organic pollutants
o. personality disorder
o. personality syndrome
o. psychosis
o. radical
residual organic carbon
o. solvent poisoning
total organic carbon
volatile organic compound
volatile organic compounds

organica

organically
o. impaired brain activity
o. impaired brain function

organics-in-water analyzer

organification defect

organism
Aerococcus-like o.
antibiotic-resistant gram-negative o.
atypical *Legionella*-like o.
beta-lactamase-producing o.
calculated mean o.
Campylobacter-like o.
o. carriage
causative organism identified
o. embolus
Escherichia coli o.
genetically modified o.'s
Gram-negative aerobic o.
Helicobacter pylori-like o.
hospital-acquired organism infection
hypothetical mean o.
o. identification
o. identification number
intracellular o.
o. isolated after 48 hours
o. isolated after 72 hours
killed o.
mixed fungal o.
nonhemolytic aerobic o.
nonmotile o.

organism *(continued)*
nosocomial Gram-negative o.
nosocomial Gram-positive o.
obligate intercellular o.'s
penicillinase-producing organisms susceptibility testing
o.'s per high power field
pleuropneumonia-like o.
predominating o.
replicate organism detection and counting
replicate organism direct agar contact

organism-host interaction

organism/hpf

organismic causation

organism-specific antibody index

organization
Assessment of Conceptual O.
O. of Chinese Americans
community o.
o. development
exclusive provider o.
health insuring o.
health maintenance o.
Hooper Visual O. Test
managed care o.
medical care o.
National Alliance of Breast Cancer O.
National O. of Victim Assistance
nongovernmental o.'s
Northeast Organ Procurement O.
organ procurement o.
Pan American Health Organization grade 0–2
perceptual o.
Perceptual O. Deviation Quotient
preferred provider o.
Sensory O. Test
Visual O. Test
World Health Organization classification of lupus nephritis I, IIA, IIB, III, IV, V
World Health Organization Quality of Life 100-Item

organizational
o. chaos
O. Culture Inventory
o. entry
O. Value Dimensions Questionnaire

organized
o. activity
o. care psychiatry
o. clot
o. delivery system
o. hematoma
o. thrombus
o. vitreous

organizer
argyrophilic nucleolar organizer region
argyrophilic nucleolar organizer region staining
argyrophil organizer region protein
o. gene
silver-staining nucleolar organizer region

organizing
o. aspiration pneumonia
cryptogenic organizing pneumonia
o. hemorrhagic cyst
interstitial organizing pneumonia
o. interstitial pneumonia
mitotic organizing center
nucleolar organizing region
o. pneumonitis
o. thrombus

organochlorine insecticide

organoid nevus

organomegaly
polyneuropathy, organomegaly, endocrinopathy, monoclonal gammopathy, and skin changes syndrome
polyneuropathy, organomegaly, endocrinopathy, M protein, and skin changes syndrome

organophosphate
o. compound
o. ingestion
o. insecticide
o. toxicity

organophosphorous compound poisoning

organotypic culture

organs at risk

organ-specific
o.-s. antigen
o.-s. illness

organum
o. vasculosum of lamina terminalis
o. visus

orgasm
coital o.
o. delay
o. dysfunction
male o.

orgasmic
o. anhedonia
o. capacity
o. cephalalgia
o. deficiency
o. deficiens
o. disorder
o. dysfunction
o. flush
o. impairment

orgastic impotence

***Orgyia pseudotsugata* MNPV**

Oriboca virus

oriental
O. blood fluke
O. boil
O. button
O. cholangiohepatitis
o. hemoptysis
O. nocturnal death syndrome
O. ringworm
O. schistosomiasis
o. sore
o. ulcer

Orientation-30
Inventory of Suicide O.

orientation
academic o.
achievement o.
angle of o.
child-centered literary o.
Children's O. and Amnesia Test
conditioned orientation reflex audiometry
condition orientation reflex audiometry
Coping O.'s to Problems Experienced
o. cue
o. disorder
evaluate orientation, attention, and recent recall
functioning, reasoning, orientation, memory, arithmetic, judgment, and emotion
Galveston O. and Amnesia Test
Galveston O. and Awareness Test
Hall Occupational O. Inventory
hard food o.
hearing aid o.
o. to hospital
O. Inventory
limbal parallel o.

limbus parallel orientation straddling tattoo mark
mood, orientation, judgment, affect, content
Personal O. Inventory
phalangeal articular o.
reality o.
Right-Left O. Test
Spatial O. Memory Test
Student O.'s Survey
o. test
testing, orientation, work, evaluation, rehabilitation
test orientation procedure

orientation/alertness remediation

Orientation-Behavior
Fundamental Interpersonal Relations O.-B.

Orientation-Feelings
Fundamental Interpersonal Relations O.-F.

oriented
alert and o.
o. and alert
alert, cooperative, and o.
alert and oriented to person, place, and time
alert and oriented to person, place, time, and date
o. in all spheres
awake, alert, o.
goal oriented task
mentally stable and o.
mental status, o.
oriented
patient alert and o.
patient oriented to person, place and time
o. to person, place, and time
reality o.
sexually oriented hallucination
o. to time
o. to time and place
o. to time, place, and person
o. to time, place, person, and objects watch, pen, book
o. times one
o. times two

orienting
o. reflex
o. response
skin conductance orienting response

orifice
atrioventricular nodal o.
average orifice area
common atrioventricular o.
effective orifice area
effective regurgitant o.
o. of external acoustic meatus
external urethral o.
o. flow
o. of ileal papilla
o. of inferior vena cava
o. of internal acoustic meatus
internal acoustic o.
internal urethral o.
left ureteral o.
meibomian gland orifice metaplasia
mitral valve o.
mitral valve orifice area
regurgitant orifice area
right ureteral o.
segmental bronchus o.
ureteral o.

orificial tuberculosis

origin
amyloid of immunoglobulin o.
amyloid of unknown o.
anatomic origin and distribution
anomalous origin of left coronary artery from pulmonary artery
aponeurosis of o.
o. of artery
O. balloon
bilirubin of undetermined o.
bleeding of undetermined o.
bruising of undetermined o.
chick embryo o.
duck embryo origin vaccine
female adnexal tumor of probable wolffian o.
fever of undetermined o.
fever of unknown o.
illness of emotional o.
metastatic carcinoma of unknown primary o.
metastatic tumor of unknown o.
myocardial disease of unknown o.
myocardiopathy of unknown o.
neural crest o.
neuronal cell origin tumor
pancreatic head o.
paternal o.
prolonged fever of unknown o.
pyrexia of undetermined o.
pyrexia of unknown o.
site of o.
syncope of unknown o.
undetermined o.
unknown o.

original
o. claim
o. host cell
o. incident
o. incision
o. injection site
o. package
o. squamocolumnar junction
o. tuberculin
o. tumor site
o. University of Wisconsin solution

originally derived

Orion
O. electrode
O. inhaler

oris
buccinator-orbicularis o.
marginal part of orbicularis oris muscle
modiolus anguli o.
orbicularis oris muscle
pars marginalis musculi orbicularis o.

Oriximina virus

ORL-1 receptor

Ormond disease

ornithine
o. acetyltransferase
o. aminotransferase
o. carbamoyltransferase
o. carbamoyltransferase assay
o. carbamoyl transferase deficiency
o. carbamoyltransferase deficiency
o. cycle
o. decarboxylase
heterozygous ornithine transcarbamylase
serum ornithine carbamoyltransferase
o. test
o. tolerance test
o. transcarbamylase
o. transcarbamylase deficiency

ornithine-ketoacid
o.-k. aminotransferase deficiency
o.-k. transaminase

Ornithodoros moubata

ornithosis virus

oroanal contact

oroantral
o. communication
o. fistula
orocecal transit time
orodigitofacial
o. dysostosis
o. dysplasia
oroendotracheal tube
orofacial
o. carcinoma
o. chorea
o. cleft
o. dysfunction syndrome
o. dyskinesia
o. fistula
o. herpes simplex
o. malformation
o. movement
o. odontogenic infection
orofaciodigital syndrome
orogastric
o. feeding
o. gonococcal aspirate
o. tube
orogenital activity
orolabial herpes
oromandibular
o. defect
o. dystonia
oronasal
o. acoustic ratio
o. communication
o. fistula
o. junction
oropharyngeal
o. airway
o. airway space
o. anesthesia
o. anthrax
o. aphthae
o. approach
o. aspiration
o. cancer
o. candidiasis
o. carcinoma
o. configuration
o. cyst
o. damage
o. defect
o. disease
o. dysfunction
o. dysphagia
o. dystonia
o. esophagram
o. flora
o. gonorrhea
o. hemorrhage
o. infection
o. isthmus
o. lesion
o. mucosa
o. mucositis
o. pack
topical oropharyngeal anesthesia
o. tube
o. tularemia
o. tumor
oropharynx
o., oral cavity
posterior o.
Oropouche virus
orotic
o. acid
o. acidemia
o. aciduria
orotidylate decarboxylase deficiency
orotidylic
o. acid
o. acid decarboxylase
orotracheal
o. intubation
rapid sequence induction orotracheal intubation
o. suction
o. tube
Oroya fever
orphan
O. Annie eye
O. Annie-eyed clear nucleus
chicken-embryo-lethal o.
o. disease
o. drug
enterocytopathogenic avian orphan virus
enterocytopathogenic bovine orphan virus
enterocytopathogenic cat orphan virus
enterocytopathogenic dog orphan virus
enterocytopathogenic equine orphan virus
enterocytopathogenic human o.
enterocytopathogenic human orphan virus
enterocytopathogenic monkey orphan virus
enterocytopathogenic porcine orphan virus
enterocytopathogenic rodent orphan virus
enterocytopathogenic swine orphan virus
o. receptor
respiratory enteric orphan virus
retinoic acid-related orphan receptor
o. virus
Orpington prognostic scale
Ortho
O. DX electromedical stimulator
orthochromatic leukodystrophy
orthochromic erythrocyte
orthoclase ceramic feldspar
orthocresolphthalein complex
orthodontic
o. appliance
o. attachment
o. camouflage
corrective o.'s
cosmetic o.'s
o. force
o. treatment
orthodromic reciprocating tachycardia
Orthofix apparatus
Ortho-Foam elbow/heel pad
orthoglycemic glycosuria
orthognathic correction
orthogonal
o. analysis
o. angiographic projection
o. angiography
o. axis
o. C-arm fluoroscopy
o. combination
o. depression factor
holistic orthogonal parameter estimation
o. plane
o. polarization spectral
o. radiography
right-handed orthogonal coordinate system
orthogonal-hole test pattern
Orthogon lens
orthograde conduction
orthoiodohippuric acid
orthokeratinized cyst
Ortho-Kung T cell
orthomolecular therapy

orthonasal perception

orthopaedic
- o. anomaly
- AO-ASIF orthopaedic implant
- o. bed
- o. bone file
- o. broach
- o. bur
- o. cement
- o. chisel
- o. condition
- o. curette
- o. cutting instrument
- o. depth gauge
- o. dynamometer
- o. evaluation
- o. felt
- o. force
- o. forceps
- o. goniometer
- o. gouge
- o. hammer
- o. hardware
- o. hemostat
- soft ankle, cushioned heel orthopaedic appliance

Orthopantomograph-3, -10

orthopedic
- o. anesthesia
- o. anomaly
- chronic orthopedic impairment
- computer-assisted orthopedic surgery
- craniomandibular orthopedic repositioning device
- o. examination
- o. examination, special
- o. grafting
- o. implant
- o. implant infection
- mandibular orthopedic repositioning appliance
- pediatric orthopedic examination
- presurgical orthopedic correction
- o. rehabilitation
- o. research
- o. treatment

orthophoria
- asthenic o.

orthophosphate
- inorganic o.

orthophosphoric
- o. acid
- o. acid etch gel
- o. ester monohydrolase

orthoplast
- O. fracture brace
- o. jacket

orthopnea
- breathlessness, insomnia and o.
- one-pillow o.
- o. position

orthopneic position

orthoptic biventricular artificial heart

orthoreovirus
- avian o.
- mammalian o.
- Nelson Bay o.

orthorhythmic pacemaker

orthoscopic
- o. lens
- o. spectacles

orthosis
- Adjustable Advanced Reciprocating Gait O.
- airplane splint o.
- ambulation training o.
- ankle contracture o.
- ankle-foot o.
- ankle-foot orthosis brace sock
- ankle-foot plastic o.
- ankle stabilizing o.
- ankle stabilizing orthosis support
- anteroposterior control o.
- Atlanta brace o.
- Atlanta-Scottish Rite abduction o.
- balanced forearm o.
- ball-bearing forearm o.
- below-knee o.
- cervical o.
- cervicothoracic o.
- chairback lumbosacral o.
- cock-up splint o.
- o. drop-lock ring
- dynamic tone-reducing o.
- elastic knee cage o.
- elastic twister o.
- elbow o.
- elbow-wrist-hand o.
- electrospinal o.
- flexion-extension control cervical o.
- flexor hinge o.
- foot o.
- four-poster cervical o.
- hallux valgus o.
- hand o.
- hip o.
- hip guidance o.
- hip-knee-ankle o.
- hip-knee-ankle-foot o.
- hip-knee orthosis splint
- knee o.
- knee-ankle o.
- knee-ankle-foot o.
- knee-foot-ankle o.
- lower limb o.
- lumbar o.
- lumbosacral o.
- Malleoloc ankle o.
- medial heel wedge o.
- medical ankle o.
- molded ankle-foot o.
- passive prehension o.
- patellar tendon-bearing o.
- pelvic stabilization o.
- plantar arch support o.
- plantar fasciitis o.
- polypropylene glycol-ankle-foot o.
- polypropylene glycol-thoracolumbosacral o.
- posterior leafspring o.
- pressure-relief ankle-foot o.
- prosthesis and o.
- reciprocating gait o.
- sacroiliac o.
- shoulder, elbow, wrist, hand o.
- spinal o.
- sternooccipital-mandibular immobilization o.
- supracondylar knee-ankle o.
- supramalleolar o.
- Therapy Carrot finger contracture o.
- thoracic o.
- thoracolumbar spinal o.
- thoracolumbosacral spinal o.
- tone-reducing ankle-foot o.
- total contact o.
- trunk-hip-knee-ankle-foot o.
- upper limb o.
- wrist-hand o.

orthosis—flexion
- thoracolumbosacral orthosis—flexion, extension, lateral bending, and transverse rotation

orthostatic
- o. acrocyanosis
- o. albuminuria
- o. blood pressure
- o. change
- chronic idiopathic orthostatic hypotension
- chronic orthostatic hypotension
- o. dizziness
- o. dyspnea

orthostatic *(continued)*
o. edema
o. epileptoid
o. fluctuation
o. hypertension
o. hypotension
idiopathic orthostatic hypotension
instantaneous orthostatic hypotension
o. intolerance
o. lightheadedness
neurogenic orthostatic hypotension
postural orthostatic tachycardia syndrome
o. proteinuria
o. purpura
o. stress
sympathetic orthostatic hypotension
o. syncope
o. tachycardia

orthotic
Charcot restraint orthotic walker
o. device
dynamic orthotic cranioplasty
mallet finger o.
pressure-relief ankle-foot o.
prosthetic and o.
o. shoe
Universal plantar fasciitis o.

orthotoluidine
o. arsenite
o. manganese sulfate

orthotopic
o. appendicocystostomy
auxiliary orthotopic liver transplantation
auxiliary partial orthotopic living donor transplantation
o. bladder
o. bladder augmentation
o. bladder substitution
o. colonic reservoir
o. continent reservoir
o. diversion
o. glioma
o. graft
o. heart transplant
o. heart transplantation
o. hemi-Koch operation
o. hepatic transplant
o. liver transplant
o. liver transplantation
partial auxiliary orthotopic liver transplantation
surgical orthotopic implantation
o. univentricular artificial heart

Ortho-Vent bandage

orthovoltage beam

Orticochea flap

Ortolani
Barlow and Ortolani test
O. click
O. maneuver
O. sign
O. test

Orungo virus

os
os calcis bone
os calcis osteotomy
os calcis pin fixation

Osborne-Cotterill elbow dislocation operation

Osborne operation

oscillating
air-driven oscillating saw
o. gouge
o. nystagmus
tomogram with oscillating Bucky
o. vision

oscillation
body oscillation neuromuscular gain
Finger O. Test
forced o.
forced oscillation technique
high-frequency chest wall o.
high-frequency oscillation ventilation
high-frequency oscillation ventilator
involuntary rhythmic o.
rhythmic horizontal oscillation of eyeball

oscillator
bone-conduction o.

oscillatory
o. behavior
high-frequency o.
high-frequency oscillatory ventilation
liquid-assisted high-frequency oscillatory ventilation
postocclusive oscillatory response
o. potential

oscillometric method

oscillopsia
gait imbalance and o.
monocular o.

oscilloscope
cathode ray o.

Osgood operation

Osgood-Schlatter
O.-S. disease
O.-S. lesion
O.-S. syndrome

OSHA blood-borne pathogen standard

O'Shea lens

Osher-Neumann corneal marker

Osiander sign

Osier
O. disease
O. node
O. phenomenon
O. sign
O. syndrome

Osier-Vaquez disease

Osier-Weber
O.-W. disease
O.-W. syndrome

Osler
O. disease
O. erythema
O. hemangiomatosis
O. node
O. sign
O. syndrome II
O. triad

Osler-Rendu-Weber disease

Osler-Vaquez disease

Osler-Weber-Rendu
O.-W.-R. disease
O.-W.-R. syndrome

osmic
o. acid
o. acid fixative

osmiophilic lamellar inclusion body

osmolal gap

osmolality
calculated serum o.
o. dehydration test
increased urine o.
maximal urinary o.
morning o.
plasma o.
serum o.
o. serum
urinary o.
o. urine
urine o.
o. urine spot test

osmolar
o. clearance
o. dehydration
o. gap

osmolarity
o. of blood
o. of blood and urine
o. gap

osmole
osmoles per kilogram
osmoles per liter

Osmolite feeding

osmolyte
organic o.

osmometer
freezing point o.

Osmond-Clarke foot procedure

osmoregulatory defect

osmosis
reverse o.

osmotic
capillary osmotic pressure
o. cataract
o. cathartic
o. cell injury
o. clearance
o. coefficient
colloid osmotic pressure in interstitial fluid
colloid osmotic pressure in plasma
o. demyelination
o. demyelination syndrome
o. diarrhea
o. dilator
o. diuresis
o. diuretic
o. driving agent
o. equilibrium
o. erythrocyte enrichment
o. fragility
o. fragility test
o. gap
o. hemostasis
o. homeostasis
o. minipump
o. nephrosis
oral o.
plasma osmotic pressure
o. pressure
o. pressure of plasma
o. pressure of proteins in lymph
o. regulation
o. stimulus
o. threshold

osmotically
o. active substance
o. induced asthma

osmotically active substance

osmotically induced asthma

ossa
o. carpi
o. digitorum
O. virus

osseocartilaginous
o. arch
o. craniofacial skeleton

osseocutaneous flap

osseointegrated
o. cylinder implant
o. dental implant
o. fixture

osseointegrating
titanium hollow-screw osseointegrating reconstruction plate

osseoligamentous arch

osseous
o. abnormality
o. activity
o. adjustment
o. ampulla
o. ankylosis
o. anomaly
o. attachment
o. BA lesion
o. bone contusion
o. bridge
o. bridge prevention
o. cell
o. cervical spine injury
o. choristoma
o. choristoma of the tongue
o. cleft
o. coagulum trap
o. coalition
o. craniofacial arteriovenous malformation
o. defect
o. destructive process
o. drift
o. dysplasia
o. dystrophy
ectodermal and mesodermal dysplasia with osseous involvement ectodermal dysplasia-central
o. equinus
o. fixation
o. flap
o. foraminal encroachment
o. fragment
o. fragmentation
o. genioplasty
o. graft
o. grafting
o. heteroplasia
o. homeostasis
o. hydatid cyst
o. labyrinth
o. lacuna
o. lesion
limbus of osseous spiral lamina
o. matrix
medial osseous interorbital distance
o. metastasis
MR discriminator of osseous metastasis
neonatal osseous dysplasia
o. pain
o. system
o. tissue

ossicle
Andernach o.
anlagen of the auditory o.
auditory o.
o. chain
Kerckring o.
muscles of auditory o.'s

ossicular
o. chain
o. chain reconstruction
o. discontinuity
o. disruption
partial ossicular replacement prosthesis
total ossicular chain replacement prosthesis
total ossicular reconstruction prosthesis
vibrating ossicular prosthesis

ossiculoplasty
Austin-Kartush group C patient related to o.

ossiculorum

ossificans
fibrodysplasia ossificans progressiva
myositis o.
myositis ossificans circumscripta
myositis ossificans progressiva
osteitis o.
periostitis ossificans toxica
polymyositis ossificans progressiva

ossification
abnormal endochondral o.
o. of anterior longitudinal ligament
o. of cartilaginous structure
o. center
heterotopic o.
heterotropic o.
hypertrophic o.
lower limb ossification center
malleolar ossification center
paraarticular heterotopic o.
periarticular heterotopic o.
o. of posterior longitudinal ligament

ossific center

ossified
o. body
o. cartilage

ossifying
o. arachnoiditis
o. bone fibroma
o. cartilage
o. cochleitis
o. epiphysis
o. fibroma

ossis
angulus frontalis ossis parietalis
angulus mastoideus ossis parietalis
angulus occipitalis ossis parietalis
articulatio ossis pisiformis
musculus extensor ossis metacarpi pollicis
pars basilaris ossis occipitalis
pars orbitalis ossis frontalis

ossium

osteitis
o. distal phalanx
o. fibrosa
mastoid o.
o. ossificans
o. symphysis pubis

osteoarthritic
o. cartilage
o. change
o. hypertrophic spur formation

osteoarthritis
erosive o.
facet joint o.
generalized o.
o. grading classification
o. of the hip
hip o.
hypertrophic pulmonary o.
o. of the knee
painful osteoarthritis of the knee
phalangeal o.
radiologic o.
o. of the spine
sports-related o.
temporomandibular joint o.
Western Ontario and McMaster Universities O. Index Physical Functioning subscale and chair-performance
Western Ontario and McMaster Universities O. Index Physical Functioning subscale and chair-stand performance

osteoarthropathia
exophthalmos, myxedema circumscriptum praetibiale, and osteoarthropathia hypertrophicans syndrome

osteoarthropathy
diabetic neuropathic o.
hypertrophic pulmonary o.
idiopathic hypertrophic o.
pulmonary hypertrophic o.
secondary hypertrophic o.

osteoarthroscopy

osteoarticular
o. allograft
o. allograft transplantation
o. candidiasis
o. defect
o. destruction
o. graft
peripheral osteoarticular tuberculosis
o. sporotrichosis
o. tuberculosis

osteoblast
o. heterogenicity
o. ontogeny
o. phenotype
o. progenitor proliferation

osteoblastic
o. activity
o. bone regeneration
o. lesion
o. phenotype
o. resorption
o. tumor

osteoblast-mediated bone formation

osteocalcin
O. level
O. secretion

osteocartilage
autogenous osteocartilage transfer

osteocartilaginous
o. body
o. defect
o. excision
o. exostosis
o. framework
o. graft
o. growth

osteochondral
o. allograft
o. autograft transfer system
o. contusion
o. defect
o. exostosis
o. fracture arthrography
o. fracture of the dome of the talus
o. fragment
o. graft
o. grafting
o. junction
o. lesion of the talus
multiple hereditary osteochondral exostosis

osteochondritis
o. of capitellum
o. dissecans
metatarsal head o.

osteochondromatous
bizarre parosteal osteochondromatous proliferation

osteochondrosis
o. dissecans

osteoclast
o. activity
o. apoptosis
o. differentiation factor
o. dysfunction
o. precursor
o. ultrastructure

osteoclast-activated bone resorption

osteoclast-driven bone resorption

osteoclastic
o. activity
o. bone
o. bone resorption
o. erosion
o. function
o. giant cell
multinucleated osteoclastic giant cell

o. nucleus
o. osteolysis
o. resorption lacuna
o. stimulation

osteoclast-like giant cell

osteoclast-mediated
o.-m. bone
o.-m. bone resorption

osteoclastogenesis inhibitory factor

osteoconductive bone grafting material

osteocutaneous
o. fillet flap

osteocytic
o. membrane system
o. osteolysis

osteodental dysplasia

osteodysplasia
polycystic lipomembranous o.

osteodysplastica

osteodysplastic primordial dwarfism

osteodystrophy
Albright hereditary o.
aplastic uremic o.
mixed uremic o.
parathyroid o.
pediatric renal o.
renal o.

osteoectasia with hyperphosphatasia

osteogenesis
distraction o.
o. imperfecta
o. imperfecta congenita
o. imperfecta congenita syndrome
o. imperfecta, optic atrophy, retinopathy, developmental delay syndrome
o. imperfecta tarda
o. imperfecta type I–IV
mandibular distraction o.
maxillary distraction o.
perinatal lethal osteogenesis imperfecta

osteogenetic
o. fiber
o. layer

osteogenic
o. bone fibroma
o. cell
determined osteogenic precursor cell
o. differentiation
o. fibroma
human osteogenic sarcoma
o. imperfecta
low-grade central osteogenic sarcoma
o. protein-1
o. protein-2
o. sarcoma
o. tissue

osteoglophonic
o. dwarfism
o. dysplasia

Osteograf binder

Osteograf/N HA

osteohypertrophicus
nevus varicosus o.
nevus vasculosus o.

osteoid
o. accumulation
o. area
o. carcinoma
fractional osteoid surface
malignant o.
o. osteoma
o. seam thickness
o. surface
o. volume

Osteolock
O. acetabular component

osteolysis
atraumatic osteolysis of distal clavicle
familial expansile o.
malignant acetabular o.

osteolytic
o. flame
o. lesion

osteoma
calcinosis cutis, osteoma cutis, poikiloderma, and skeletal abnormalities syndrome
cavalryman's o.
o. cutis
o. dentale
o. durum
multiple o.'s
osteoid o.

osteomalacia
aluminum-associated o.
aluminum-induced o.
axial o.
juvenile o.
oncogenic o.
oncogenous o.
o. syndrome

osteomanipulative therapy

Osteomark
O. NTx assay
O. NTx serum test

Osteomin freeze-dried bone

osteomusculocutaneous
o. deep circumflex iliac groin flap
pedicled compound rib-latissimus dorsi osteomusculocutaneous flap

osteomyelitic cloaca formation

osteomyelitis
acute hematogenous o.
chronic recurrent multifocal o.
diffuse sclerosing o.
long bone o.
meningococcal multifocal o.
Pasteurella multocida o.
posttraumatic chronic o.
synovitis, acne, pustulosis, hyperostosis, osteomyelitis syndrome

osteomyocutaneous
o. free flap
o. free-tissue transfer

osteonal bone union

osteonecrosis
o. of femur
o. of knee
neuralgia-inducing cavitational o.
spontaneous osteonecrosis of knee

osteoonychodysplasia
hereditary o.

osteopathic
o. hospital
o. manipulation
o. manipulation treatment
o. manipulative medicine
o. manipulative technique
o. manipulative therapy
o. medicine
o. medicine and surgery
o. physician

osteopathy
o. in the cranial field
hypovitaminosis D o.

osteopenic
o. bone
o. bone stock
o. halo

osteoperiosteal
o. bone graft

osteoperiosteal *(continued)*
o. flap
o. iliac bone graft
o. production

osteoperiostitis
alveolodental o.

osteopetrosis
autosomal-dominant benign form of o.
murine osteopetrosis mutation

osteopetrotic
o. microphthalmic
o. mutation
o. phenotype

osteophyte
anterior o.
apophysial joint o.
bridging o.
o. elevator
o. formation

osteophytic
o. bone lip
o. bridge
o. defect

osteoplastic
o. amputation
o. bone flap
o. craniotomy
o. flap clamp
o. frontal sinus procedure
o. genioplasty

osteoplasty
Maquet anteromedial o.

osteoporosis
o. of bone
o. circumscripta
glucocorticoid steroid-induced o.
idiopathic juvenile o.
O. Knowledge Questionnaire
postmenopausal o.
o. screening
Simple Calculated O. Risk Estimation
transient osteoporosis of hip

osteoporosis-pseudolipoma syndrome

osteoporotic
o. bone
o. compression fracture
o. cytokine
o. fracture
spontaneous osteoporotic fracture of sacrum

osteoprogenitor cell

osteoprotegerin
o. factor
o. ligand

osteosarcoma
o. antigen
o. antigen-associated monoclonal antibody
o. of bone
human o.
low-grade intraosseous-type o.
paraosteal o.
small cell o.
undifferentiated o.

osteosclerosis
autosomal dominant o.
myelofibrosis o.

osteosclerotic
o. anemia
o. myeloma

osteosis
o. cutis

osteosynthesis
anterior column o.

osteotome
air compression o.
alar o.
arthroscopic o.
Aufranc o.
backcutting o.
box o.
disposable one-piece o.

osteotomy
Akin proximal phalangeal o.
Akron midtarsal o.
Amspacher-Messenbaugh closing wedge o.
o. analysis simulation software
Anderson-Fowler calcaneal displacement o.
anterior calcaneal o.
anterior horizontal mandibular o.
anterior innominate o.
anterior segmental dentoalveolar o.
Axer lateral opening wedge o.
Axer varus derotational o.
ball-and-socket trochanteric o.
barrel stave osteotomy procedure
bilateral sagittal split ramus o.'s
bilateral vertical ramus o.
o. bunionectomy
chevron osteotomy with rigid screw fixation
closed base wedge o.
closing abductory wedge o.
o. of condylar neck
controlled depth osteotomy cutter
cranioorbitozygomatic o.
crescentic shelf o.
derotational varus o.
derotation femoral o.
Dimon-Hughston intertrochanteric osteotomy technique
dorsiflexory wedge o.
dovetail joint o.
femoral derotation o.
greater tuberosity o.
high tibial o.
intraoral vertical ramus o.
intraoral vertical segmental o.
Le Fort o.
Maquet dome o.
Marquardt angulation o.
maxillomandibular o.
medial closing wedge phalangeal o.
medial displacement o.
metatarsal head o.
midtarsal dome o.
Mitchell distal o.
oblique base-wedge o.
oblique closing wedge o.
oblique displacement o.
open base wedge o.
opening abductory wedge o.
open wedge o.
orbital box o.
os calcis o.
palatal bone o.
pelvic lengthening o.
Potts eversion o.
Potts tibial o.
power-oriented depth controlled osteotomy cutter
sagittal split ramus o.
segmental alveolar o.
o. site
transtrochanteric valgus o.
upper tibial o.
varus derotational o.
varus rotational o.
vertical sagittal split o.

osteotomy/bunionectomy
closed wedge o.
open base wedge o.

ostia (*pl. of* ostium)

ostial
aortic ostial stenosis
o. artery atherosclerosis
o. atherosclerotic plaque
o. cannulation
coronary ostial dimple
uterine ostial access catheter

ostiomeatal
o. complex
o. unit

ostium, pl. **ostia**
o. anatomicum
aneurysmal o.
anterior ethmoidal o.
o. aortae
aortic o.
artery o.
atrial ostium primum defect
atrioventricular nodal o.
o. cardiacum
o. ileocecale
missed ostium sequence
narrowing of ostia of coronary artery
o. primum
o. primum location

ostomotic release oral system

ostomy
O. Assessment Inventory
o. care
closed-end ostomy pouch
o. rehabilitation

ostrum
backward-biting ostrum punch

Ostrum-Furst syndrome

Ostrup harvesting technique

Ostwald solubility coefficient

O'Sullivan operation

Oswestry Disability Score

Ota
nevus of O.
O. nevus
O. nevus syndrome

otalgia dentalis

Othello delusion

other
o. administrative reasons
alcohol and other drug abuse
alcohol, tobacco, and other drugs
atypical mixed or other personality disorder
avoidance of o.'s
behavioral, anxiety, mood, and other types of disorders
carbon separated from the carboxyl group by 2 other carbon atoms
o. cerebral palsy
death of other cause
differential reinforcement of other behavior
every other day
o. febrile illness
o. interpersonal problem
Locus of Control-Powerful O.'s
o. medical/surgical facility
most significant o.
mycobacteria other than *Mycobacterium tuberculosis*
Mycobacteria other than tuberculosis
o. neurologic disease
o. neurologic disorder
o. party liability
o. potentially infectious material
syphilis, toxoplasmosis, other agents, rubella, cytomegalovirus, herpes simplex virus
o. than psychotic
toxoplasmosis, other infections, rubella, cytomegalovirus infection, herpes simplex syndrome
o. or unspecified psychoactive substance intoxication

otherwise
alcohol-related use disorder, not otherwise specified
cannabis-related disorder, not otherwise specified
dissociative disorder not otherwise specified
nicotine-related disorder, not otherwise specified
not otherwise specified
not otherwise provided for
not otherwise provided for
pervasive developmental disorder not otherwise specified
physically or otherwise health-impaired
typhoid vaccine, not otherwise specified

otic
o. abscess
o. barotrauma
o. capsule
o. depression
o. ganglion
o. hydrocephalus

oticus
herpes o.

Otis Quick Scoring Mental Abilities Test

otitic
o. abscess
o. hydrocephalus

otitis
acute otitis media
benign necrotizing otitis externa
bilateral otitis externa
bilateral otitis media, acute
bilateral otitis media with effusion
bilateral serous otitis media
chronic adhesive otitis media
chronic otitis media with effusion
chronic suppurative otitis media
o. desquamativa
o. diphtheritica
draining otitis media
endotoxin-mediated otitis media with effusion
o. externa
external otitis media
left otitis externa
malignant external o.
malignant external otitis syndrome
malignant necrotizing otitis externa
malignant otitis externa
o. media
o. media, acute, catarrhal
o. media, acute, suppurating
o. media, catarrhal, acute
o. media, catarrhal, chronic
o. media, chronic, suppurating
o. media, purulent, acute
o. media with effusion
o. media without effusion
o. media with perforated tympanic membrane
necrotizing external o.
nonsuppurative otitis media
right otitis externa
right otitis media
right otitis media, suppurative, acute
right otitis media, suppurative, chronic
seborrheic external o.
secretory otitis media

otoacoustic
distortion-product otoacoustic emission
o. emission
o. emission test
o. emission testing
evoked otoacoustic emission
spontaneous otoacoustic emission
transient evoked otoacoustic emission

otodental dysplasia

Oto-Flex
O.-F. carbide bur
O.-F. crura saw
O.-F. drill
Otofuke agent
otolithic crisis
otolithic-ocular reflex
otology, laryngology, and rhinology
otomandibular
o. dysostosis
o. facial dysmorphogenesis
o. syndrome
otomastoiditis
Aspergillus o.
otopalatodigital syndrome
otoplasty
anterior-posterior o.
Crieklair o.
otorhinolaryngology
ophthalmology, otorhinolaryngology, and head and neck surgery
otorrhea
intermittent o.
otospondylometaphyseal dysplasia
ototoxic drug
ototoxicity
aminoglycoside o.
gentamicin o.
Ottawa School Behavior Checklist
Otto
O. disease
O. pelvis
ouabain
o. insensitive
o. sensitive
ouabain-like
o.-l. compound
o.-l. factor
o.-l. hormone
o.-l. substance
ouabain-sensitive Na^+-K^+ ATPase
Ouango virus
Oubi virus
Ouchterlony
O. double diffusion
O. double diffusion technique
O. gel diffusion technique
O. method
ounce
apothecary's o.
calories per o.
fluid o.
liquid o.
o. troy
our
in our culture
Ourem virus
out
asocial acting o.
base o.
o. of bed with bathroom privileges
o. of bilirubin light
o. of the blue
born out of asepsis
o. of bounds
brought out near edge of incision
carcinoma to be ruled o.
card made o.
o. of cast
o. of character
check o.
o. of control
criminal acting o.
dangle out of bed
diabetes mellitus out of control
o. the door
drain brought out through stab wound
feet out of bed
fell out of bed
focus o.
gallbladder shelled out from the gallbladder bed
o. of hospital
impulsive acting o.
o. of isolette
laughing out loud
neurotic acting o.
not knocked o.
not out of bed
o. of
o. on pass
passive-aggressive acting o.
o. of pelvis
o. of plaster cast
pulled catheter o.
o. of radiant warmer
regloving and regowning carried o.
O. rule
rule o.
rule out appendicitis
rule out myocardial infarct
rule out myocardial infarction
o. of sequence
signed out against medical advice
slip made o.
o. of specification deviation from standard
o. of splint
step out, turn o.
stitches out in afternoon
stitches out in morning
o. of stock
to take o.
time o.
o. of town
transfer o.
up out of bed as tolerated
urethral catheter o.
urinary catheter o.
o. of wedlock
o. of wedlock and not keeping child
x-ray out of plaster
outbreak
common source o.
Ebola virus o.
food-borne illness o.
prevent further o.
waterborne illness o.
outburst
aggressive o.
o. of anger
anger o.
angry o.
autosomal dominant compelling helioophthalmic outburst syndrome
explosive o.
outcome
American Heart Association Stroke O. Classification
o. assessment
O.'s and Assessment Information Set
o. domain
evidence-based o.'s
Functional O.'s of Sleep Questionnaire
Glasgow O. Scale
Glasgow O. Score
o. goal
Hemiballism/Hemichorea O. Rating Score
o. of illness
improved pregnancy o.

Medical O.'s Study
Michigan Hand O.'s Questionnaire
multidimensional assessment of o.
multiple outcomes of raloxifene evaluation trial
Patient O.'s Research Team
prospective outcomes monitoring evaluation system
Sinonasal O. Test-16
therapeutic outcomes monitoring
Treatment Outcome PTSD scale
voice outcome survey

outdated
tetanus toxoid o.

outer
o. acrosomal membrane
acute zonal occult outer retinopathy
o. anular/posterior longitudinal ligament complex
o. aspect
o. band of Baillarger
o. border of iris
o. border of the uterus
o. canthal distance
o. canthus
o. canthus of eye
o. cone fiber
o. convexity
o. cortical blood flow
o. crossbar
o. dense fibers of spermatozoon
o. diameter
o. ear
o. ear canal
o. enamel epithelium
o. fibrous layer
o. hair cell
o. hamstring
intact outer rim
o. layer
left upper outer buttock
left upper outer quadrant
o. limiting membrane
o. lip of iliac crest
lower outer quadrant
major outer membrane protein
o. malleolus
o. membrane protein
o. mitochondrial membrane
molecular outer layer
o. nuclear layer
nuclear outer layer
o. optic anlage
o. plexiform layer
principal outer material protein
progressive outer retinal necrosis
recombinant outer surface protein A
o. retina
right upper outer quadrant
rod outer segment
o. segment
o. spiral fibers of cochlea
o. surface protein
universal frame outer socket
o. upper left quadrant
o. upper right quadrant
o. wall

Outerbridge
O. classification
O. degenerative arthritis staging

outermost
o. covering
o. layer

outflow
aortic outflow gradient
aortic outflow obstruction
atretic outflow tract
o. of bile
o. biliary tract
bladder outflow obstruction
chronic obstructive outflow disease
o. conduit
o. control
o. disorder
frontal outflow tract
hepatic o.
hepatic venous outflow obstruction
information outflow rate
left ventricular o.
left ventricular outflow tract obstruction
left ventricular outflow volume
maximal venous o.
maximum venous o.
mean venous o.
narrow pulmonary outflow tract
net gradient of fluid o.
o. obstruction
partial bile outflow obstruction
o. rate
o. resistance
right ventricular o.
right ventricular outflow tract
o. tract
o. tract obstruction
ventricular outflow tract
o. volume

outgrowth
local o.
o. medium
neurite o.

outlet
anorectal outlet obstruction
arterial thoracic outlet syndrome
axonopathic neurogenic thoracic outlet syndrome
bladder outlet obstruction
creative o.
o. decompression
deformity of gastric o.
o. delay
o. dysfunction
o. foramina
o. forceps delivery
gastric o.
gastric outlet irritability
gastric outlet obstruction
low outlet forceps
low outlet forceps delivery
mechanical bladder outlet resistance
narrowed o.
narrowing of o.
narrowing of gastric o.
obstetric conjugate of o.
obstetric conjugate of pelvic o.
o. obstruction
pelvic o.
prostatic outlet obstruction
relaxed vaginal o.
repair relaxed vaginal o.
o. strut fracture
o. syndrome
thoracic outlet decompression

outlier threshold

outline
o. form
heart size and o.

out-of-control
o.-o.-c. adolescent
o.-o.-c. behavior

out-of-pocket expense

outpatient
o. anesthesia
o. basis
o. biopsy
o. care
o. catheterization
o. clinic
o. clinic substation
o. code editor
o. commitment order

outpatient *(continued)*
comprehensive outpatient treatment
comprehensive outpatient rehabilitation facility
court-ordered involuntary outpatient treatment
o. department
o. detoxification
o. diagnostic center
o. dialysis
o. dialysis clinic
o. dispensary
o. drug treatment
emergency o.
o. endometrial resection/ablation procedure
o. endoscopy
o. evaluation
o. facility
o. followup
full outpatient rate
o. hospital
hospital outpatient department
inpatient to outpatient transfer
intensive outpatient treatment program
medical o.
medical outpatient program
o. medication
o. methadone program
national outpatient profile
o. occupational therapy
o. parenteral antibiotic therapy
patient to be followed as an o.
patient followed on an outpatient basis
o. physical therapy
place outpatient in inpatient bed
o. procedure
O. Prospective Payment System
o. rehabilitation center
o. renal dialysis unit
o. speech therapy
o. surgical unit
o. therapy
treated on an outpatient basis
o. treatment, nonservice-connected
o. treatment, service-connected
o. visit

outpouching
aneurysmal o.

output
acid o.
adequate cardiac o.
adequate urine o.
o. amplitude
augmented cardiac o.
automated cardiac output measurement
average lymphocyte o.
basal acid o.
basal pepsin o.
bile phospholipid o.
bile salt o.
biliary cholesterol o.
brachial artery o.
o. capacitor
carbon dioxide o.
cardiac minute o.
cardiac output index
cardiac output markedly reduced
cardiac output measurement
cardiac output recorder
cardiac output by thermodilution
chest tube o.
computer output on microfilm
continuous cardiac o.
continuous cardiac output with SvO_2
cortical motor o.
delirium, infection, atrophic urethritis and vaginitis, pharmaceuticals, psychological disorders, excessive urine output, restricted mobility, stool impaction
o. disability
endotracheal cardiac output monitor
gastric fluid, basal acid o.
heart minute o.
hepatic glucose o.
hourly o.
human glucose o.
immunoreactive trypsin o.
o. impedance
impedance cardiac o.
inadequate cardiac o.
insulin-induced peak acid o.
intake and o.
o. and intake
left ventricular systolic o.
low cardiac o.
low cardiac output syndrome
maximum acid o.
maximum acoustic o.
maximum power o.
meal-stimulated acid o.
minute o.
monitor fluid intake and o.
o. nerve
noninvasive cardiac output monitor
noninvasive evaluation of radiation o.
normal urine o.
peak acid o.
peak acid output after gastrin-releasing peptide
peak acid output after pentagastrin stimulation
peak acid output insulin-induced
peak pepsin o.
postoperative low cardiac o.
predicted cardiac o.
ratio of basal acid output to maximal acid o.
residual lymphocyte o.
resting cardiac o.
right ventricle stroke o.
o. signal processor
o. sound pressure level
thermodilution cardiac o.
urinary o.
urine acid o.
o. voltage

outreach
assertive o.
mobile crisis outreach team

outrigger
o. arm
o. cast
o. splint

outside
o. activity
o. activity avoidance
o. control
o. density
o. diameter
o. doctor
o. force
o. hospital
o. influence
o. pass
review of outside film

outstretched
fell on outstretched hand
o. fingertips
o. hand
o. hand or tongue

outward
o. expression of anger with impulsive feature
o. focus

ova (*pl. of* ovum)

Ovadia-Beals classification of tibial plafond fracture

oval
o. amputation
o. aneurysm
o. aneurysm with bleb
o. arch
o. area of Flechsig
o. bur
o. cornea
o. corpuscle
o. curved-cup curette
Dameshek oval target cell
o. eye patch
o. fasciculus
o. fat body
fenestration of oval window
o. foramen
o. foramen of heart
o. forceps
o. fossa
o. hyperchromatic nucleus
little fossa of oval vestibular window
longitudinal oval pelvis
o. macrocyte
Neumann-Shepard oval optical center marker
o. target cell
o. window
o. window defect
o. window reflex

ovalbumin
o. antigen
chicken o.
chicken ovalbumin upstream promoter

ovale
anatomically patent foramen o.
foramen o.
foramen ovale cordis
foramen ovale of heart
o. malaria
patent foramen o.

ovalis
annulus o.
anulus o.
margin of fossa o.

ovalocytary anemia

ovalocytosis
Southeast Asian o.

ovaria (*pl. of* ovarium)

ovarian
o. ablation
o. abnormality
o. abscess
o. activity
advanced ovarian cancer
o. agenesis
o. amenorrhea
o. anatomy
o. androgenic hyperfunction
o. androgen secretion
anovular ovarian follicle
o. antibody
o. aplasia
o. artery
o. ascorbic acid depletion test
atretic ovarian follicle
o. atrophy
autologous ovarian transplantation
benign ovarian mass
o. borderline tumor
o. branch
o. branch of uterine artery
o. bursa
o. cancer
o. cancer metastasis
o. carcinoid tumor
o. carcinoma
o. carcinoma antigen
o. carcinoma debulking
o. carcinoma with ascites
o. cautery
o. cholesterol depletion test
o. choriocarcinoma
chromosomally competent ovarian failure
chromosomally incompetent ovarian failure
o. clear cell adenocarcinoma
o. clear cell carcinoma
o. colic
o. cortex
o. cycle
o. cycle change
o. cystadenocarcinoma
o. cystadenofibroma
o. cystadenoma
o. cystectomy
o. cystic teratoma
o. cyst torsion
o. dermoid
o. dermoid cyst
o. disease
o. disorder
o. Doppler signal
o. duct
o. dwarfism
o. dysfunction
o. dysgenesis
o. dysgenesis-sensorineural deafness syndrome
o. dysgerminoma
o. dysmenorrhea
o. embryonal teratoma
o. endometrioid carcinoma
o. endometrioma
o. endometriosis
o. endometriosis cyst
o. enlargement
o. epithelial cancer
o. epithelial carcinoma
o. epithelial metasepithelial
epithelial ovarian cancer
o. epithelial tumor
o. estrogen
o. estrogen synthesis
o. factor
o. failure
o. fibroma
o. fibromatosis
o. fimbria
fimbriae of ovarian tube
o. follicle
o. follicle exhaustion
o. fossa
o. function
o. gametogenesis
o. germ cell tumor
o. germinal epithelium
o. goiter
o. gonadoblastoma
o. granulosa cell
o. granulosa-stromal cell tumor
o. granulosa-theca cell tumor
o. growth factor
hereditary breast and ovarian cancer
o. hernia
o. hilar cell tumor
o. hormone
human ovarian cancer
o. hyperandrogenism
o. hyperstimulation
o. hyperstimulation syndrome
o. hyperthecosis
o. hypertrophy
o. hypoandrogenism
immature ovarian teratoma
o. immature teratoma
o. inflammatory cyst
inoperable ovarian cancer
o. intraepithelial neoplasia
o. leiomyoma
o. ligament
o. lipid cell neoplasm
lipid cell ovarian tumor
lipoid ovarian neoplasm
lipoid ovarian tumor
local ovarian condition

ovarian *(continued)*
low malignant potential epithelial ovarian tumor
luteal ovarian cyst
o. lymphoma
o. malignancy
o. malignant epithelial neoplasm
o. malignant germ cell tumor
malignant ovarian germ cell tumor
malignant ovarian neoplasm
malignant ovarian teratoma
o. mass
massive ovarian cyst
mature cystic ovarian teratoma
mature ovarian teratoma
micropapillary serous ovarian carcinoma
mixed ovarian mesodermal sarcoma
mouse ovarian tumor
mucinous borderline ovarian tumors
mucinous ovarian neoplasm
o. neurofibroma
normal ovarian surface epithelium
o. papillary serous adenocarcinoma
pelvic ovarian vein thrombosis
o. pregnancy
primary ovarian carcinoma
primary ovarian carcinoma with metastasis
primary ovarian failure
puerperal ovarian vein thrombophlebitis
puerperal ovarian vein thrombosis
rabbit ovarian antitumor serum
rat ovarian weight
o. remnant
o. serous borderline tumor
serous epithelial ovarian carcinoma
severe ovarian hyperstimulation syndrome
o. steroidogenesis
o. steroidogenic dysfunction
o. stroma
o. stromal hyperplasia
o. surface epithelium
o. tuberculosis
o. tumor registry
ureteric branch of ovarian artery
uterine tumor resembling an ovarian sex-cord tumor
o. varicocele
o. vein
o. vein thrombosis
o. venous plasma oxytocin
o. wedge resection

ovarii
mesoblastoma o.

ovariotomy
normal o.

ovaripriva
cachexia o.

ovarium, pl. **ovaria**
o. gyratum
o. masculinum

ovary
autoamputation of o.
Chinese hamster o.
failing ovary syndrome
gonadotrophin-resistant ovary syndrome
hilum of o.
o. in inguinal hernia
ligament of o.
luteinized thecoma of o.
lymphoma of o.
mesovarian border of o.
mesovarian margin of o.
micropolycystic ovary syndrome
mucinous adenocarcinoma of o.
mucinous cystadenoma of o.
nodular hyperplasia of o.
oligomenorrheic polycystic ovary syndrome
papillary cystadenocarcinoma of o.
placenta, o.'s, uterus
polycystic o.
postmenopausal palpable o.
rabbit antibody to human o.
rabbit antibody to pig o.
o. reserve
sclerocystic disease of the o.
suspensory ligament of o.
tubes and o.'s

Ovenstone factor

over
closed over wound
o. the counter
delta over baseline
o. diagnose
dullness over left lung
dullness over right lung
electrodes applied over cerebral cortex
feet over edge of bed
guilt over disloyalty
please turn the patient o.
weak and dizzy all o.
o. the wire

overaction
inferior oblique o.

overactive
o. bladder
o. gland
o. immune system
o. superior oblique
o. superior rectus
o. thyroid
o. thyroid disorder
o. thyroid gland
uninhibited overactive bladder

overactivity
augmentation agent overactivity in OCD
detrusor o.
left ventricular o.
right ventricular o.
thyroid o.

overall
o. alignment
o. assessment
o. cognitive functioning
o. cognitive measure
o. depressive symptom
o. diameter
o. diameter of contact lens
o. disability
improved overall functioning
increased overall treatment of duration
Pediatric O. Performance Category scale
o. survival
o. therapeutic goal
o. treatment time

overanxious
o. disorder
o. disorder of adolescence
o. disorder of childhood

overcontrolled hostility scale

overdistension of bladder

overdistention
o. of alveolar populations
lung o.

overdose
alcohol, epilepsy, insulin, overdose, uremia, trauma, infection, psychiatric, stroke
drug o.
o. toxicity
o. with hallucinogen

overdosed
patient overdosed with hallucinogen
o. with antidepressant
o. with cannabinoid
o. with inhalant
o. with multiple drugs
o. with opioid

overdrive
atrial overdrive stimulation rate

overeating
obsessive-compulsive o.

overexposed to sun

overexposure
o. to heat
o. to sunlight

overflow
o. aminoaciduria
o. diabetes
o. encopresis
o. fecal incontinence

overgrafting
dermal o.

overgrowth
adenocarcinoma of the uterus with sarcomatous o.
bacterial o.
gastric bacterial o.
mental retardation, overgrowth, craniosynostosis, distal arthrogryposis, sacral dimple, joint laxity
mental retardation, pre-and postnatal overgrowth, remarkable face, acanthosis nigricans syndrome
precancerous overgrowth of uterine lining
small bowel bacterial o.
small intestine bacterial o.

overhead
o. exercise test
o. frame
o. frame trapeze
o. movement of arm
surgical overhead canopy

overhinge
variable flexion o.

Overholt operation

overinflation
congenital lobar o.
o. of lungs

overlap
bivalve overlap brace
o. disease
horizontal o.
lichen planus overlap syndrome
lupus-scleroderma overlap syndrome
medial cortical overlap technique
o. myositis
o. syndrome
zero differential o.

overlapping
o. biphasic impulse
o. clones
o. closure of peritoneum
multiple overlapping thin-slab acquisition
o. suture

overlay
o. cantilevered bone graft
colony overlay test
o. crown
o. denture
o. drafting
fluorescence overlay antigen mapping
neurotic o.

overload
African iron o.
fluid volume o.
hepatic iron o.
information overload testing aid
right ventricular diastolic o.
volume o.

overloading
left atrial o.

overlying
o. attenuation artifact
o. bowel content
o. bowel gas
o. bowel shadows
o. branching pattern
o. gas shadow
o. intestinal gas

overnight
o. Giemsa stain
o. high-dose dexamethasone suppression test
o. metyrapone test
o. 1-mg dexamethasone suppression test
o. oximeter
o. oximetry
o. pass
patient released on overnight pass
o. sleep evaluation

overproduction
o. of mucus
o. of saliva

overrepresented
o. characteristic
o. experience

override
aortic o.

overriding
o. aorta
o. finger

overripe cataract

overseas duty

over-shoulder strap

overside drainage

overstimulation and resulting confusion

overt
O. Aggression Scale
o. agitation
O. Agitation Severity Scale
o. behavior
o. behavior consequences of divorce
o. bilirubin encephalopathy
o. compliance
o. compliance masking covert resistance
o. criticism
o. diabetes
o. gesture
o. glycosuria
o. hallucination
o. heart failure
o. homosexuality
inappropriate overt anger
o. insulin-dependent diabetes mellitus
o. loss
mild overt thyrotoxicosis
onset of overt heart failure
patient exhibits overt hostility
o. response
o. symptom of heart disease

over-the-counter
o.-t.-c. agent
o.-t.-c. drug
o.-t.-c. drug abuse
o.-t.-c. drug addiction
o.-t.-c. drug-related disorder
o.-t.-c. medication
o.-t.-c. nonprescription drug
o.-t.-c. prescription

overture
suicidal o.

overuse
o. of drugs
o. injury
o. of joint
o. of muscle
musician's overuse syndrome
o. of narcotic medication
o. of narcotics
o. strain injury
o. syndrome
o. tendinitis
overvalued
o. false ideas
o. ideation
o. obsessional ideas
overview
human immunodeficiency virus overview of problems evaluation system
overwear syndrome
overwhelming
o. anxiety
o. childhood experience
o. depression
o. fatigue
o. postsplenectomy infection
o. sense of panic
overworked B-cell hypothesis
oviduct
ampulla of o.
angiomyoma of o.
fimbriated end of o.
human oviduct fluid
ovine
o. AAV virus
o. adenovirus 1–6
o. corticotropin-releasing factor
o. corticotropin-releasing hormone
o. growth hormone
o. lactogenic hormone
o. leuteinizing hormone
o. pancreatic polypeptide
o. placental lactogen
o. prolactin
o. submaxillary mucin
ovoid
afterloading tandem and o.'s
o. arch
Fletcher-Suit afterloading o.'s
Manchester o.
o. mass
tandem and o.'s
ovoidalis
articulatio o.
ovomucoid trypsin inhibitor
ovulation
o. cycle
o. disorder
estimated time of o.
o. induction
o. number
pituitary hormone trigger o.
post ovulation hormone change
ovulatory
o. age
o. bleeding
o. defect
o. disturbance
o. failure
o. follicle
o. menstrual cycle
o. menstruation
o. mucus
ovule
Naboth o.
nabothian o.
ovulocyclic porphyria
ovum, pl. **ova**
aspiration of ova
ova, blood, and parasites
Brinster medium for ovum culture
o. capture
o. donation
o. forceps
hamster zona-free ovum test
implantation of fertilized o.
Mateer-Streeter o.
o. maturation
Miller o.
ova, cysts, and parasites
ova and parasites examination
ripe o.
ova weight
ovum-capture inhibitor
Owen line
Owestry Disability Questionnaire
owl's
o. eye appearance
o. eye cell
o. eye inclusion body
o. eye nucleus
o. eyes view of hydrocele
own
o. bed bath
o. recognizance
sign own release
Owren
O. deficiency
O. disease
ox
ox heart
ox red blood cell
ox warble
oxacillin
o. aminoglycoside-resistant *Staphylococcus aureus*
o. disc diffusion test
o. sodium
oxacillin-resistant
o.-r. *Staphylococcus aureus*
oxalate
calcium o.
calcium oxalate calculus
calcium oxalate crystal
calcium oxalate renal stone
calcium oxalate stone former
o. calculus
o. crystal
o. crystals
o. stone
oxalated
Veronal-buffered oxalated saline
oxalic
o. acid
o. acid assay
o. acid stain
o. gout
oxaliplatin
o. with leucovorin and 5-fluorouracil
oxaloacetic
o. acid test
erythrocyte glutamic oxaloacetic transaminase
Oxford
O. fixator
Manchester and Oxford Universities Scale for the Psychopathological Assessment of Dementia
O. operation
Oxgall media culture
oxidase
acylcoenzyme A o.
amino acid o.
choline o.
corticosterone methyl o.
cytochrome c o.
o. cytosolic factor
glucose o.
glucose oxidase test
hydroxyphenylpyruvate o.

mitochondrial ethanol oxidase system
mixed function oxidase system
modified oxidase test
monoamine o.
monoamine oxidase A deficiency
monoamine oxidase B inhibitor
monoamine oxidase type A, B
NADPH oxidase system
neuraminidase and galactose o.
plasma amine o.
polyamine o.
o. reaction
serum monoamine o.
serum xanthine o.
xanthine o.
xanthine oxidase reaction

oxidation
advanced oxidation protein product
arachidonic acid o.
o. disorder
fatty acid o.
o. of fatty acid
glucose oxidation quotient
leucine o.
long-chain fatty acid o.
pyruvate oxidation factor
o. of solution

oxidation/fermentation
marine o.

oxidation-fermentation basal medium

oxidation-reduction
o.-r. potential
o.-r. system

oxidative
o. brain injury
o. burst
o. cell injury
o. cellular injury
o. damage
o. deamination
o. decarboxylation
o. degeneration
fast o.
macrophage oxidative burst
metal-catalyzed oxidative cleavage
mitochondrial oxidative phosphorylation
o. modification of LDL
o. phosphorylation
o. phosphorylation ratio
slow o.
o. stress

oxide
aluminum bismuth o.
aluminum oxide abrasive
aluminum oxide arthroplasty material
aluminum oxide ceramic coating
aluminum oxide ceramic core
chloroethylene o.
constitutive nitric oxide synthase
endothelial constitutive nitric oxide synthase
endothelial constitutive nitric oxide synthetase
endothelial nitric oxide synthase
endothelium-derived nitric o.
ethylene o.
ethylene oxide gas
exhaled nitric o.
induced nitric oxide synthase
inducible nitric oxide synthase
inducible nitric oxide synthetase
inhaled nitric o.
inhaled nitrous o.
magnesium o.
metal oxide semiconductor field effect transistor
monocrystalline iron o.'s
nitric o.
nitric oxide hemoglobin
nitric oxide synthase gene
nitric oxide synthase inhibitor
nitrogen mustard o.
nitrous o.
nitrous oxide barbiturate
nitrous oxide to oxygen ratio
nitrous oxide tank
N-type metal oxide semiconductor
tin o.
trimethylamine o.
ultrasmall-particle superparamagnetic iron o.
zinc o.

oxide-barbiturate

oxide/nitrogen
nitric o.

oxidized
o. adenosine
o. cellulose
o. cotton
o. form of nicotinamide adenine dinucleotide
o. form of nicotinamide adenine dinucleotide phosphate
o. glutathione
o. gluthathione
o. hemoglobin
inosine, o.
o. low-density lipoprotein

oxidized-reduced

oxidizing
o. agent
o. gas
low molecular weight oxidizing agent
microsomal ethanol oxidizing system

oxime
hexamethylpropyleneamine o.
^{99m}Tc-hexamethylpropyleneamine o.
technetium-99m hexamethylpropylene amine oxime single-photon emission computed tomography

oximeter
finger o.
Ohmeda hand-held o.
Ohmeda Minx pulse o.
overnight o.
pulse o.
tissue reflectance o.

oximeter/end
pulse oximeter/end tidal CO_2

oximetry
ambulatory oximetry monitoring
arterial blood o.
carbon monoxide o.
ear o.
MARS pulse o.
Masimo SET signal extraction pulse o.
motion-resistant pulse o.
oxygen saturation as measured using pulse o.
pulse o.
pulse oximetry on 2 liters of oxygen
pulse oximetry waveform systolic blood pressure
reflectance pulse o.
o. sensor

3-oxoacid-CoA transferase

oxolinic acid

oxyacetate malonate

oxybutynin chloride

oxycodone
o. and acetaminophen
o. and aspirin
long-acting o.

oxygen
abnormal oxygen affinity
o. acceptor

oxygen *(continued)*
o. administration
o. affinity anoxia
o. affinity hypoxia
o. in air
alveolar-arterial difference in partial pressure of o.
alveolar-arterial oxygen gradient
alveolar-arterial oxygen tension difference
alveolar-arterial oxygen tension gradient
alveolar oxygen partial pressure
alveolar-to-arterial oxygen difference
aortic oxygen content
aortic oxygen saturation
apparent oxygen utilization
arterial to alveolar oxygen tension ratio
arterial oxygen concentration
arterial oxygen desaturation
arterial oxygen partial pressure
arterial oxygen saturation
arterial oxygen tension
arteriovenous oxygen content difference
arteriovenous oxygen difference
o. at atmospheric pressure
o. availability
biochemical oxygen demand
biological oxygen demand
blood oxygen capacity
blood oxygen release rate
brain tissue partial pressure of o.
o. capacity
o. capacity of blood
carbon dioxide with o.
central venous o.
cerebral glucose oxygen quotient
cerebral metabolic rate of o.
chemical oxygen demand
o. cisternography
o. concentration
o. concentration in pulmonary capillary blood
concentration of total o.
o. consumed
o. consumption
o. consumption index
o. consumption per minute
o. content
o. content of blood
o. content of blood decreases
o. content determination
o. content of mixed venous blood
continuous oxygen therapy
control of heart rate during oxygen deprivation
crying, requirement for oxygen supplementation, increases in heart rate and blood pressure
o. debt
decreasing consumption of o.
o. deficiency
o. deficit
o. delivery
o. delivery index
o. demand
demand oxygen delivery device
o. deprivation
o. deprivation theory of narcosis
o. desaturation
o. desaturation index
difference in partial pressures of oxygen in mixed alveolar gas and mixed arterial blood
diffusing capacity of lungs for o.
o. diffusion
diffusion of oxygen and nutrients
o. disposable boot device
o. dissociation curve
dissolved o.
dissolved oxygen deficit
o. effect
effective oxygen transport
electrolyte biochemical oxygen demand
emergency oxygen mask assembly
o. enhancement ratio
equivalent oxygen performance
o. and ether gas
o. extraction fraction
o. extraction index
o. extraction rate
o. extraction ratio
fetal arterial oxygen saturation
flow of blood and oxygen to heart
o. flux
forced inspiratory o.
fractional concentration of inspired o.
fractional concentration of oxygen in expired gas
fractional inspired oxygen concentration
fractional percentage of inspired o.
fraction of inspired o.
o. free radical
o. gain factor
gas and o.
gas, oxygen, and ether anesthesia
o. half-saturation pressure of hemoglobin
helium and o.
hemoglobin-based oxygen carrier
hemoglobin oxygen dissociation curve
high o.
high air flow with oxygen entrainment
high-flow oxygen conserver
highly reactive oxygen molecules
high oxygen concentrate
high oxygen percentage
high oxygen percentage in retinopathy of prematurity
high oxygen pressure
high partial pressure of o.
high-pressure o.
home oxygen therapy
o. hood
humidifier and o.
hyperbaric o.
hyperbaric oxygen chamber
hyperbaric oxygen drenching
hyperbaric oxygen therapy
hyperbaric oxygen treatment
hypothermia oxygen warmer
imbalance of o.
o. income
infant with o.
o. inhalation
inspired oxygen tension
o. insufficiency
o. intake
intermittent positive pressure inflation with o.
intraalveolar oxygen tension
intratracheal oxygen catheter
jugular venous oxygen saturation
left pulmonary artery oxygen saturation
o. level
liquid o.
long-term oxygen therapy
o. mask
maximal venous oxygen consumption
maximum oxygen consumption measurement
o. metabolite
minimal venous oxygen consumption
MiniOX 1A oxygen analyzer
MiniOX I, II, III, 100-IV oxygen monitor
minute oxygen uptake

mixed venous o.
mixed venous oxygen content
mixed venous oxygen saturation
o. monitor
mutant hemoglobin with low affinity for o.
myocardial oxygen consumption
myocardial ventilation, oxygen rate
nasal o.
o. by nasal cannula
nitrous oxide to oxygen ratio
nocturnal oxygen therapy
nocturnal oxygen therapy trial
Ohio pediatric tent with o.
partial nonrebreather oxygen mask
partial oxygen pressure in mixed venous blood
partial pressure of o.
o. partial pressure
partial pressure alveolar o.
partial pressure arterial o.
partial pressure of inspiratory o.
partial pressure tension of oxygen, vein
partial venous gas tension of o.
peak exercise oxygen consumption
peak oxygen uptake
peripheral fractional oxygen extraction
o. permeability
o. poisoning
portable oxygen tank
pressure of o.
pulse oximetry on 2 liters of o.
o. quotient
rapid recompression-high pressure o.
reactive oxygen intermediate
reactive oxygen species
real oxygen transport
regional cerebral metabolic rate for o.
regional oxygen saturation
o. saturation as measured using pulse oximetry
o. saturation index
o. saturation level
o. saturation meter
o. saturation on 2 liters nasal cannula
o. saturation on 3 liters nasal cannula
saturation of oxygen in arterial blood
singlet o.
Spofford-Christopher oxygen optimizing program
supplemental oxygen system
o. supply
systemic hyperbaric oxygen therapy
systemic oxygen transport
o. tent
o. therapy
o. toxicity
o. toxicity in immature lung
transcutaneous oxygen monitor
transcutaneous partial pressure of o.
transcutaneous oxygen pressure measurement
o. transport rate
transtracheal o.
transtracheal oxygen therapy
o. under high pressure
o. uptake efficiency slope
o. utilization
o. ventilation equivalent
volume oxygen consumption
volume of oxygen consumption per unit of time

oxygenase
heme o.
microsomal heme o.

oxygenated
o. blood
o. blood supply
o. fluorocarbon nutrient emulsion
o. hemoglobin

oxygenation
o. before recirculation
blood oxygenation level-dependent
compliance, rate, oxygenation, and pressure
compliance, rate, oxygenation, and pressure index
extracorporeal membrane o.
extracorporeal membrane oxygenation affecting cognitive function
hyperbaric o.
o. index
neonatal extracorporal membrane o.

oxygenator
extracorporeal membrane o.
intravascular o.
plasma-resistant fiber o.
Sarns membrane o.

oxyhemoglobin
arterial oxyhemoglobin saturation
o. curve
low oxyhemoglobin saturation
total o.

oxymorphone hydrochloride

oxyntic
o. cell
o. gland

oxyphil
o. adenoma
o. cell
o. chromatin
o. granule

oxyphilic
o. adenoma
o. carcinoma
o. change
o. cytoplasm
o. endometrioid adenocarcinoma
o. leukocyte
o. metaplasia
renal epithelioid oxyphilic neoplasm

oxytalan
o. fiber
o. fiber stain

oxytocic fraction

oxytocin
o. analog
arginine o.
o. augmentation
o. challenge test
myometrial oxytocin receptor
ovarian venous plasma o.
Pitocin o.
o. secretion

oxytocin-associated neurophysin

oxytocinergic
o. cell body
o. neuron

oxyuris nodule

oyster
o. shuckers' keratitis
o. virus

Oz
Oz antigen
Oz isotypic determinant

ozzardi
Mansonella ozzardi infection

P450
P. aromatase placental deficiency
P. cytochrome
cytochrome P450 enzyme 19, 27
cytochrome P450 11-beta-hydroxylase
cytochrome P450 21-beta-hydroxylase
cytochrome P450 enzyme 1A1
cytochrome P450 enzyme 11A
cytochrome P450 enzyme 21B
P. metabolism
mitochondrial P450 monooxygenase

p53
p. allelotyping
p. analysis
p. antibody
p. assay
p. expression
p. gene
p. immunoreactivity

pacchionian
p. bodies
p. corpuscles
p. depression
p. foramen
p. gland
p. granulation

pace
atrium p.

paced
P. Auditory Serial Addition Test
p. breathing
cycle length, p.
p. rhythm
p. ventricular evoked response
ventricular paced rhythm

pacemaker
p. adaptive rate
p. afterpotential
antitachycardia p.
p. artifact
atrial demand-inhibited p.
atrial inhibited p.
atrial-synchronous ventricular-inhibited p.
atrial tracking p.
atrioventricular junctional p.
automated external defibrillator p.
p. breathing
p. burst pacing
p. capture
cardiac pacemaker artifact
cardiac pacemaker battery change
p. cell
p. check
p. circus-movement tachycardia
p. current
p. damage
dual chamber p.
dual chamber pacemaker implantation
dual demand p.
dual-mode, dual-pacing, dual-sensing p.
electronic p.
p. endocarditis
p. end-of-life
endogenous circadian p.
p. escape interval
p. failure
fixed rate p.
p. function
gastrointestinal pacemaker cell tumor
p. of heart
p. impedance
p. implant
implantation of p.
p. implanted under skin
p. infection
p. insertion
p. lead
p. lead fracture
p. malfunction
p. monitoring
p. monitoring transtelephonic
orthorhythmic p.
p. output
permanent cardiac p.
permanent demand ventricular p.
permanent pacemaker implantation
permanent pacemaker placement
permanent transvenous demand p.
p. placement
p. pocket
p. potential
p. pulse generator
p. replacement
p. rhythm
P. Selection in the Elderly
p. sensitivity
p. sound
p. spike
p. stimulus
p. syndrome
temporary p.
temporary pacemaker implant
temporary transvenous p.
p. threshold
transvenous p.
transvenous catheter p.
p. undersensing
p. unit
ventricular asynchronous p.
ventricular pacing, atrial sensing, triggered mode, p.
wandering atrial p.
p. wire

pacer
p. cardioverter-defibrillator
p. spike

pacer-cardioverter defibrillator

pacesetter potential

pachyderma circumscripta

pachygyria
localized p.

pachymeningitis
adhesive chronic p.
chronic hypertrophic p.
p. externa

pachymeter
optical p.

pachyonychia
p. congenita
p. congenita syndrome of nail

Pacific
P. Coast demineralized cortical bone powder
P. Coast Tissue Bank
National Asian Pacific Center on Aging

pacification
neuromuscular p.

pacing
antitachycardia p.
arterial demand p.
p. artifact
atrial synchronous ventricular inhibited p.
atrioventricular sequential p.
p. behavior
burst of rapid atrial p.
burst of ventricular p.
cardiac p.
cardiac pacing electrode
cardioventricular p.
p. catheter
p. code
continuous ventricular asynchronous p.
coupled atrial p.
p. cycle length
p. digital ventriculography
direct His bundle p.
p. electrode
p. electrode wire

P

pacing *(continued)*
p. esophageal stethoscope
p. function
implantable cardioverter-defibrillator/atrial tachycardia p.
p. impulse
p. lead
left atrial transesophageal pacing test
p. modality
p. mode
p. on demand
pacemaker burst p.
rapid straight p.
Rate Modulated P.
p. and sensing threshold
sequential atrioventricular p.
sequential ventriculoatrial p.
p. stimulus
p. stress test
p. system analyzer
p. threshold
transcutaneous p.
transesophageal atrial p.
transesophageal echocardiography with p.
transesophageal ventricular p.
ventricular pacing, atrial sensing, triggered mode, pacemaker
ventricular demand p.
ventricular synchronous p.

pacinian corpuscle

Paci operation

Pacis BCG

pack
chemical snap p.
p. of cigarettes
heat, ultrasound, and massage
hot packs and bed rest
hot moist p.'s
hot wet p.
ice p.
moist p.
neonatal narcotic p.
packs per day
p.'s per year cigarettes
p.'s per year history
p. removal
take home p.
ward p.
warm moist pack unsterile
wet p.

package
cocaine package ingestion
Cognitive Behavior Therapy P.
p. insert
original p.
patient package insert
tapered steroid dosing p.

Packard radioimmunoassay system

packed
p. cells
p. cell volume
p. erythrocytes
frozen packed cell
p. human blood cell
leukocyte-poor packed cell
p. nares
naris p.
p. nose
p. nostril
Pall-filtered packed cell
p. RBC
p. red blood cell
p. red blood cell transfusion
super packed platelet
total packed cell volume
unit of packed red blood cells
volume of packed red blood cells
washed packed cells
water p.
p. with gauze

packer tunnel silicone sponge

packing
anterior nasal p.
p. for bleeding
p. chamber
p. forceps
p. fraction
gauze p.
iodoform gauze p.
Merocel epistaxis p.
nasal p.
Nu Gauze p.
p. of paracolic gutter

Packo pars plana cannula

pack-year

paclitaxel
liposome-encapsulated p.

Pacora virus

Pacui virus

pad
alternating pressure p.
antimesenteric fat p.
arch insole p.
artificial fat p.
axillary fat p.
p. cover
epicardial fat p.
epicardial fat pad sign
eye pad and shield applied
herniated fat p.
Hoffa fat p.
hot p.
infrapatellar fat p.
malar cheek p.
malar fat p.
Martius fat p.
masticatory fat p.
nasal drip p.
orbital fat p.
Ortho-Foam elbow/heel p.
painful heel p.
parapharyngeal fat p.
patellar fat p.
pedicled buccal fat pad flap
pericardial fat p.
perineal p.'s
pre-Achilles fat p.
protective eye p.
retropatellar fat p.
scalene fat pad biopsy
submental fat p.
supraclavicular fat p.
urine collection p.'s

padded
p. bolster
p. button
p. cell
lightly p.
thickly p.

padding
antral p.
displacement of cartilage p.
felt p.

paddle
cardioversion p.
compression p.
defibrillator p.
p. marks from defibrillation
p. temple
trapezoidal paddle pectoralis major myocutaneous flap

paddy keratitis

Page
P. ameba saline
P. grade for breast tumor
P. medium

Pagenstecher
P. circle
P. operation

Paget
P. abscess

P. abscess syndrome
P. carcinoma
P. cell
P. disease of anus
P. disease of bone
P. disease of breast
P. disease-like mosaic appearance
P. disease of perianal area
P. disease of vulva
P. extramammary disease
extramammary Paget disease
mammary Paget disease
P. quiet necrosis

pagetic
p. bone
p. bone lesion

pagetoid
p. bone
p. cell
p. epidermal involvement
localized pagetoid reticulosis
p. melanocytosis
p. melanoma

Paget-von Schroetter syndrome

Pahayokee virus

PAHO
PAHO grade 0, 1, 2
PAHO stage 0, 1a, 1b, 2, 3

Pahvant
P. Valley fever
P. Valley plague

pain
p. in abdomen with constipation
p. in abdomen with diarrhea
p. in abdomen with vomiting
abdominal cramping p.
abdominal pain associated with blood loss
abdominal pain with colitis
abdominal pain with Crohn disease
abdominal swelling and p.
aches and p.'s
Achilles tendon p.
acute flank p.
Acute Low Back P. Screening Questionnaire
acute pelvic p.
Adolescent and Pediatric P. Tool Scale
p. aggravated by motion
p. aggravated by movement
alertness, response to voice, response to pain, unresponsive
amputation-related bone p.
P. Anxiety Symptoms Scale
P. Apperception Test
P. Appraisal Inventory
ascending pathway of pain projection
associated with abdominal p.
p. asymbolia
asymbolia to p.
p. at incision site
p. at rest
atypical facial p.
p. avoidance
p. in back
back pain after childbirth
back pain extends down legs
back pain and weakness
p. behavior
Behavioral Assessment of P. Questionnaire
Berne pain questionnaire
p. between shoulders
biliary tract p.
blinding head p.
p. blocking illusion
block pain impulse
brain-based pain control
breast pain from breast-feeding
Brief Pain Inventory
p. and burning
burning abdominal p.
calf pain from arteriosclerosis
cardiac chest p.
p. cascade
p. catastrophizing scale
central poststroke p.
chest p.
p. in chest, jaw, or extremity
chest pain center
chest pain from heart problem
chest pain on deep breathing
chest pain on exertion
chest pain radiating to jaw and shoulder
chest pain and tightness
chest pain of unknown etiology
chest pain with hoarseness
childbirth without p.
Children's Comprehensive P. Questionnaire
p. and chills
chronic p.
chronic aches and p.'s
chronic benign p.
chronic bone p.
chronic diabetic neuropathic p.
chronic headache p.
chronic heel pain syndrome
chronic intermittent low back p.
chronic intractable benign p.
chronic intractable shoulder p.
chronic joint p.
chronic low intermittent back p.
chronic muscle pain syndrome
chronic musculoskeletal pain syndrome
chronic oral, facial, head p.
chronic pelvic p.
chronic pelvic pain syndrome
chronic prostatitis/pelvic pain syndrome
chronic widespread p.
circular interaction between anxiety and p.
claudication limb p.
p. clinic
p. clinic program
p. cocktail
cold burning, pain and numbness
p. complaint
complex regional pain syndrome
constant abdominal p.
constant, harsh p.
p. control
p. control infusion pump
p. control unit
P. Coping Questionnaire
coughing up blood with chest p.
cramping abdominal p.
cramp-like pelvic p.
crampy abdominal p.
p. crisis
cumulative pain score
p. cycle
cycle of pain and inactivity
debilitating back p.
debility and/or p.
decondition pain behavior
p. determined by level of anxiety
diarrhea with abdominal pain and swelling
P. Disability Index
p. and discomfort
p. disorder
p. disorder, chronic
p. and distress score
dolorimetric unit of pain intensity
p. down left arm
p. down leg
p. down right arm
p. drawing
dull abdominal p.
dull aching p.
dull epigastric p.
p. during urination

pain *(continued)*
dysesthetic pain syndrome
p. dysfunction syndrome
electronic pain control
Emory P. Estimate Model
esophageal chest p.
p. exacerbation
exertional chest p.
facial pain from arthritis
p. and fatigue
p., fatigue, and insomnia
p. and fever
p. fiber
fluids, aeration, nutrition, communication, activity, and p.
p. from arthritis
p. from cancer
p. from conjunctivitis
p. from heart problem
p. from herniated vertebral disc
p. from lumbar disc
p. from TMJ
generalized abdominal p.
general joint p.
hammering head p.
p. of heart attack
heat, absence of use, redness, pain, pus, swelling
heel stick p.
Hendler Test for Chronic P.
herpes zoster p.
p. history
p. impulse
impulse transmitted p.
incisional p.
increased pain threshold
increased pain tolerance
increased tolerance of p.
p. increasing in severity
intense back p.
intense burning p.
intense headache p.
intense stabbing p.
intense throbbing p.
p. intensity difference score
intensity of p.
intermittent abdominal p.
intermittent episode of acute abdominal p.
intermittent episode of p.
intermittent heart p.
interventional pain management
intractable bone p.
intractable pelvic p.
involuntary facial p.
joint pain and discomfort
joint pain and stiffness
joint pain and swelling
left abdominal p.
level of p.
linear analog pain scale
linear analog pain score
loin pain hematuria syndrome
low back p.
low back pain psychogenic disorder
Low Back P. Questionnaire
Low Back P. Symptom Checklist
lower abdominal p.
lower fossa active, lateral knee pain, and long leg on the side ipsilateral to the weak fossa
lumbodorsal p.
p. management
p. management center
P. Management Index
p. management program
mandibular pain dysfunction syndrome
McGill P. Assessment Questionnaire
McGill-Melzack P. Index
McGill-Melzack P. Score
p. measurement
mechanical low back p.
mechanical pain threshold
p. medication
medullary bone p.
Memorial P. Assessment Card
motor, pain, touch, reflex deficit
Multiaxial Assessment of P.
Multidimensional P. Inventory
multidisciplinary pain management center
multidisciplinary pain treatment
muscle pain, allergy, tachycardia and tiredness, headache syndrome
p. in muscles and joints
musculoskeletal chest wall p.
myofascial p.
p. and nausea
neck and shoulder p.
Neonatal Facial P. Inventory
Neonatal Infant P. Scale
nervousness from pain in back
NIH Classification Category III inflammatory and noninflammatory chronic pelvic p.
noncardiac chest p.
noncolicky epigastric p.
nonischemic chest p.
nonnociceptive p.
nonprescription pain reliever
nonspecific abdominal p.
p. and numbness
numbness, tingling, and p.
Numeric P. Intensity Scale
Objective P. Scores
P. Observation Scale for Young Children
odontogenic facial p.
p. on chewing
p. on deep breathing
p. on defecation
p. on exertion
p. on motion
p. on palpation
onset of p.
p. on swallowing
p. on urination
p. on walking
oral pain medication
p., fatigue, and insomnia
p. on a scale from 1 to 10
p., pallor, pulse loss, paresthesia, and paralysis
pancreatic cancer p.
Parents' Postoperative P. Measure
paroxysmal evoked p.
paroxysmal pain disorder
patellofemoral malalignment p.
patellofemoral pain syndrome
patient in chronic p.
P. Patient Profile
peak pain intensity difference score
pediatric back p.
P. Perception Profile
periodic bone p.
peripheral deafferentation p.
phantom breast p.
phantom foot p.
phantom limb p.
pleuritic chest p.
postmastectomy pain syndrome
postoperative pain management
Postoperative P. Questionnaire
postpartum low back p.
precordial chest p.
pre-heart attack p.
Premature Infant P. Profile
present pain intensity
pressure pain threshold
pressure pain tolerance level
p. prevention
p. primarily localized
p. profile
prolonged chest pain intense
psychogenic chest p.

psychogenic pelvic p.
psychosomatic aches and p.'s
quadrant p.
p. radiating to back
radiating chest p.
p. radiating down legs
p. radiating into back
p. radiating to jaw
p. radiating to jaw and shoulder
p. radiation
P. Rating Index
p. reaction
recurrent abdominal p.
recurrent abdominal pain syndrome
p. reflex
p. rehabilitation
p. related to exertion
p. relief
p. reliever
p. relieving injection
p. response
rest p.
restore mobility and reduce p.
retropatellar pain syndrome
retrosternal chest p.
rheumatic pain modulation disorder
right abdominal p.
p. sensation
p. sensitive
p. sensitivity range
severe, jabbing facial p.
severe joint pain and fatigue
sharp, jabbing or electrical p.
shoulder pain and stiffness
p. and soreness
p. and spasm of muscles
spinal cord p.
p. spreading to arm
p. spreading to neck
p. spreading to shoulder
stabbing joint p.
structured pain interview
p. study
substernal chest p.
p. and suffering
summed pain intensity difference
p. support group
Survey of P. Attitudes
p. and swelling
sympathetically independent pain syndrome
sympathetically mediated pain syndrome
p. syndrome
temporary relief of headache p.
p. and tenderness
p. therapy
p. threshold
throbbing pain in head
Toddler-Preschooler Postoperative P. Scale
p. tolerance
total pain relief
transient joint p.
p. transmission neuron
p. and trauma
p. treatment unit
p. and twitching
unilateral head p.
upper abdominal p.
upper fossa active, medial knee pain, and short leg on the side ipsilateral to the weak fossa
vague abdominal p.
visual analog pain score
Visual Analogue Self Assessment Scales For P. Intensity
weakness, dizziness and joint p.
p. well controlled
Westhaven Yale Multidimensional P. Inventory
p. with breathing difficulty
p. with hoarseness
p. with palpitation
p. with vomiting
zoster-associated p.

Paine carpal tunnel retinaculotome

pain-free

complete and pain-free range of motion
p.-f. range of motion
range of motion complete and p.-f.
p.-f. walking time

painful

p. adiposity
p. affect
alert, verbal stimulus response, painful stimulus response, unresponsive
alert, vocal stimulus, painful stimulus, unresponsive
p. anesthesia
p. arc sign
p. arc syndrome
p. area
p. arthritis
p. articular syndrome
p. bruising syndrome
p. burning of feet
p. burning sensation in chest
chronic, painful arthritis
p. claudication of leg
p. consequence
p. and debilitating
p. defecation
p. diabetic neuropathy
p. disc derangement
p. feeling
p. femoral head prosthesis
p. gait
p. heel pad
p. heel spur
p. heel syndrome
p. hematuria
p. hemorrhagic glaucoma
p. inability to urinate
p., inflamed area
p. inflammation
p. inflammation of joint
p. intercourse
p. intestinal contraction
p. joint
p. leg cramp
p. menstruation
p. minor intervertebral dysfunction
p. mouth
moving toes, painful leg syndrome
p. muscle contraction
p. muscle spasm
p. nerve disorder
p. neuroma
nocturnal painful tonic spasm
p. ophthalmoplegia
p. osteoarthritis of the knee
p., inflamed area
patient responsive to painful stimuli
p. and restricted movement
p. sensation
p. sexual intercourse
p. shoulder syndrome
p. stimulus
p. subacute thyroiditis
p. swallowing
p. swelling of breast
p. swollen gland
swollen and painful joint
p. symptom
p. thyroiditis
p. tonic seizure
p. ulcer
p. urination
p. vision
p. withdrawal reaction

painkiller
nonaddictive p.

painless
accelerated painless labor
p. cold-sensitive digital vasospasm
p. hematuria
p. hyperthyroidism
p. intermittent hematuria
p. jaundice
p., small intact blister
p. postpartum thyroiditis
postpartum painless thyroiditis with transient thyrotoxicosis
p. progressive loss of vision

paint
p. brushing
p. gun injury
luminescent p.
salicylic and lactic acid p.
whole chromosome p.

painter's colic

pain-type
p.-t. anxiety
p.-t. anxiety neurosis

pair
P. Attraction Inventory
base p.
p. bond
p.'s and chains
forced pair copulation
frequency of the more common allele of a p.
frequency of rarer allele of a gene p.
Gram-positive cocci in p.'s and chains
matched p.'s signed rank test
nucleotide p.
oblique annihilation photon p.
radical pair mechanism

paired
p. associate learning
P. Associate Learning Subtest
P. Associate Learning Task
p. associates
p. beats
p. box
p. box homeotic 3 gene
p. box homeotic 8 gene
p. cocci
p. discharge
p. electrical stimulation
p. electrode recording
p. gene
p. helical filaments
p. organelles
sequential paired opposed plaque

pair-fed
zinc adequate p.-f.

pajaroello tick

palatal
p. abscess
p. alveolar fracture
anterior palatal bar
anterior palatal major connector
p. aponeurosis
p. arch
p. area
asymmetric palatal paresis
p. bone
p. bone osteotomy
cautery-assisted palatal stiffening operation
p. cleft
p. clicking
p. closure
p. connector
p. dimple
p. distraction
p. edema
p. expansion
p. expansion appliance
p. fistula
p. fistula closure
p. flap
p. fronting
p. gland
p. height index
human embryonic palatal mesenchymal cell
p. index
p. mucosa
necrotic palatal ulcer
p. petechiae
p. reflex
surgically assisted rapid palatal expansion

palate
ankyloblepharon, ectodermal defect, and cleft lip and/or p.
arch of p.
bilateral cleft lip and p.
p. bone
bony hard p.
carcinoma of hard p.
cardiac abnormality, abnormal facies, thymic hypoplasia, cleft palate, hypocalcemia
cleft lip and cleft p.
cleft lip, cleft palate, lobster-claw deformity syndrome
cleft palate knife
cleft palate tenaculum
conotruncal cardiac defect, abnormal face, thymic hypoplasia, cleft p.
cutaneous suture of p.
ectodermal dysplasia, cleft lip and palate, mental retardation, syndactyly syndrome I, II
ectrodactyly-cleft palate syndrome
p. fracture
hard and soft p.'s
height of p.
inflammatory papillary hyperplasia of the p.
medial cleft of p.
midline cleft p.
normal palate and pharynx
occult cleft p.
omphalocele-cleft palate syndrome
partial cleft p.
p. and pharynx normal
posterior nasal spine to soft p.
ramus, body, symphysis, p.
soft p.
submucous cleft p.
unilateral cleft of lip and p.

palati

palatine
anterior palatine arch
anterior palatine foramen
anterior palatine groove
anterior palatine nerve
anterior palatine suture
p. aponeurosis
p. arch
p. artery
ascending palatine artery
p. block anesthesia
p. bone fissure
p. canal
p. crest of horizontal process of palatine bone
descending palatine artery
p. durum
ethmoidal crest of palatine bone
p. fold
p. foramen
p. gland
greater palatine artery
greater palatine canal
greater palatine foramen
greater palatine groove
greater palatine nerve
p. groove of maxilla
p. index
lesser palatine artery

median palatine suture
nasal crest of horizontal plate of palatine bone
nasal crest of palatine process of maxilla
p. nerve
palatomaxillary groove of palatine bone
pharyngeal branch of descending palatine artery
p. suture
p. tonsil
transverse palatine suture
p. uvula
p. velum

palatini
arcus p.
levator veli palatini muscle
tensor veli p.

palatinum
os p.

palatinus major

palatoglossal
p. arch
p. band
p. fold

palatoglossus
arcus p.

palatomaxillary
p. arch
p. canal
p. cleft
p. groove
p. groove of palatine bone
p. index
p. suture

palatopharyngeal
p. arch
p. closure
congenital palatopharyngeal incompetence
p. flap
p. fold
p. muscle

palatopharyngeus
anterior fascicle of palatopharyngeus muscle
arcus p.
p. flap

palatoplasty
laser-assisted p.

palatovaginal
p. canal
p. groove

palatum
p. durum

pale
p. cell acanthoma
p. and clammy skin
p. color
p. and diaphoretic
p. facial appearance
p. hypertension
p. nailbed
p. optic disc
skin pale and diaphoretic
white or pale nails from anemia

Palestina virus

palindromic
p. arthropathy
p. DNA
repetitive extragenic palindromic polymerase chain reaction
p. rheumatism

palisade
p. cell
p. formation
p. layer
limbal palisades of Vogt
p.'s of Vogt

palisaded
p. dentinoblastic layer
p. encapsulated neuroma

palisading
p. epithelioid cell
p. granuloma
p. histiocyte
p. orbital granuloma
p. rod

palladium
p. 103 ophthalmic plaque brachytherapy
p. 103 ophthalmic plaque radiotherapy

Pall-filtered
P.-f. packed cell
P.-f. whole blood

palliation
p. of great vessels
p. index
intraluminal p.
p., quality, radiation, severity, time

palliative
p. bypass
p. care service
p. care unit
p. cerebrospinal shunt procedure
p. chemotherapy
p. cystectomy
p. decompression
p. drug
elected palliative care
p. esophagostomy
p. exeresis
p. gastrojejunostomy
p. gastrostomy
p. hepatojejunostomy
p. home care
p. intent
p. management
p. radiation therapy
p. radiation treatment
p. radiotherapy
p. resection
p. shunt

pallid
p. breath-holding spell
p. and shocky

pallidal
p. atrophy
p. cell
p. degeneration
p. index

pallidotomy
posteroventral p.

pallidum
colony-stimulating factor microhemagglutination-*Treponema pallidum* test
direct fluorescent antibody examination for *Treponema pallidum*
intrathecal *Treponema pallidum* antibody
microhemagglutination assay for antibodies to *Treponema pallidum*
microhemagglutination test for *Treponema pallidum*
Treponema pallidum immobilization immune adherence
Treponema pallidum agglutination
Treponema pallidum complement
Treponema pallidum complement fixation
Treponema pallidum cryolysis complement
Treponema pallidum hemagglutination
Treponema pallidum hemagglutination assay
Treponema pallidum hemagglutination test
Treponema pallidum immobilization
Treponema pallidum immobilization test

pallidus
globus p.

Pallister
P. mosaic aneuploidy
P. mosaic syndrome

Pallister-Hall syndrome

pallor
p. and cyanosis
p. of disc
p. from anemia
myelin p.
p. of optic disc
optic disc p.
pain, pallor, pulse loss, paresthesia, and paralysis
skin p.
p. of skin

palm
p. guard
p. of hand
p. leaf pattern
liver p.
simian crease of p.

palma manus

palmar
p. advancement flap
p. angulation
p. aponeurosis
p. approach
p. arterial arch
Atasoy palmar flap
p. beak ligament
p. branch
p. branch of anterior interosseous nerve
p. carpal branch of radial artery
p. carpal branch of ulnar artery
p. carpal ligament
p. carpal tendinous sheath
p. carpometacarpal ligament
p. cock-up splint
common palmar digital nerve
common palmar digital nerve of lateral plantar nerves
common palmar digital nerve of medial nerve
common palmar digital nerve of ulnar nerve
p. contraction
p. contracture
p. creaking
p. crease
p. cross-finger flap
p. cutaneous branch of the median nerve
p. cutaneous branch of the ulnar nerve
p. cutaneous vein
p. digital artery
p. digital nerve
p. digital vein
p. displacement
distal palmar crease
p. and dorsal aspects
p. dysesthesia
p. erythema
p. fascia
p. fasciitis
p. fasciitis and polyarthritis syndrome
p. fasciotomy
p. fibromatosis
p. flexion
p. grasp reflex
p. hyperhidrosis
p. hyperlinearity
p. interosseous artery
p. interosseous muscle
p. keratosis
p. lesion
p. ligament of interphalangeal joint of hand
p. ligament of metacarpophalangeal joint
long palmar muscle
perforating branch of deep palmar arch
perforating branch of palmar metacarpal artery
proximal palmar crease
p. rash
p. reflex grasp
single palmar crease
p. space
p. surface
p. surface desensitization
thenar palmar crease
p. xanthoma

palmare
xanthoma striatum p.

palmares

palmaris
aponeurosis p.
arcus venosus palmaris profundus
arteria digitalis palmaris communis
arteria digitalis palmaris propria
arteria metacarpalis p.
arteria metacarpea p.
p. brevis
p. brevis muscle
p. brevis tendon
p. longus
p. longus muscle
mycosis fungoides palmaris et plantaris
pustulosis palmaris et plantaris

palmar-plantar
p.-p. erythrodysesthesia
p.-p. erythrodysesthesia syndrome

palmatae
plicae p.

palmate
p. fold
p. fold of cervical canal

Palmer
P. acid test for peptic ulcer
P. classification
P. classification of trapezial ridge fracture

palmetto
saw palmetto berry extract

palmin test

palmitate
ascorbyl p.

palmitic acid

palmitoleic acid

palmitoyl carnitine

palmitoyltransferase
carnitine p.
carnitine palmitoyltransferase I, II deficiency
muscle carnitine palmitoyltransferase deficiency

palmomental reflex of Marinesco-Radovici

palmoplantar
p. eccrine hidradenitis
p. erythrodysesthesia
p. erythrodysesthesia syndrome
p. fibromatosis
p. keratoderma
keratoderma
p. keratosis
mental retardation, spastic paraplegia, palmoplantar hyperkeratosis syndrome
nonepidermolytic palmoplantar keratoderma
p. pustulosis

palpable
p. abdominal mass
p. abnormality
p. adenopathy
p. aortic ejection sound
p. bony abnormality

p. carotid pulse
p. cord
p. femoral pulse
p. gallbladder
p. gonad
p. kidney
p. liver edge
liver, kidneys, and spleen not p.
p. liver, spleen and kidneys
p. lymphadenopathy
p. mass
p. neck mass
p. node
p. nodule
no palpable enlargement
no palpable thrill
not p.
p. organs
pedal pulse not p.
pedal pulse p.
peripheral pulse p.
peripheral pulses palpable both legs
postmenopausal palpable ovary
p. purpura
p. radial pulse
p. rale
soft organs not p.
solid organs not p.
p. spleen
p. stone
p. thrill
p. thyromegaly

palpating finger

palpation
abdomen tender to p.
p. of anterior superior iliac spine
auscultation and p.
inspection, palpation, percussion, and auscultation
intersegmental range of motion p.
pain on p.
p., percussion, and auscultation
tender to p.
tenderness to digital p.
tenderness on p.
tenderness to palpation or percussion
p. thyroiditis

palpatory
p. diagnosis
p. examination
p. percussion

palpebra, pl. **palpebrae**
aponeurosis of superior levator p.
p. inferior
musculi levatoris palpebrae superioris
paraphimosis palpebrae
palpebrae superioris muscle

palpebral
p. adipose bag
anterior palpebral margin
p. aperture
p. artery
p. blotch
p. branch
p. branch of infratrochlear nerve
p. cartilage
p. commissure
p. conjunctiva
p. conjunctivitis
digital anomalies, short palpebral fissures, atresia of esophagus or duodenum syndrome
downsloping palpebral fissure
p. edema
p. fascia
p. fissure
p. fissure height
p. fissure inclination
p. fissure length
p. fissure widening
p. fold
p. furrow
p. gland
p. ligament
p. lobe
p. margin
medial palpebral ligament
mild down-slant to palpebral fissure
p. oculogyric reflex
p. opening
p. raphe
p. slant
p. vein

palpebrales
arteriae p.
p. inferiores

palpebralis
arcus palpebralis superior
pars palpebralis musculi orbicularis oculi

palpebrarum
pediculosis p.
xanthelasma p.
xanthoma p.

palpebromandibular reflex

palpebronasal fold

palpebronasalis
plica p.

palpitation
p.'s from anxiety
heart p.'s
pain with p.
paroxysmal p.
premonitory p.
p. and shortness of breath

palsy
acute idiopathic peripheral facial nerve p.
ataxic cerebral p.
athetoid cerebral p.
atonic cerebral p.
axillary nerve p.
Bell p.
cerebral p.
cerebral palsy clinic
conjugate gaze p.
cranial nerve p.
deltoid p.
hemiplegic form of cerebral p.
hereditary neuropathy with liability for pressure p.
hereditary neuropathy with susceptibility to pressure p.
horizontal gaze p.
Klumpke brachial p.
liability to pressure p.
long thoracic nerve p.
lower motor neuron p.
Lyme-associated peripheral facial nerve p.
medial rectus p.
mental retardation, cerebral p.
mental retardation, skeletal dysplasia, abducens palsy syndrome
mild spastic diplegic cerebral p.
mixed cerebral p.
mixed form cerebral p.
mixed-type cerebral p.
motor neuron p.
mumps facial nerve p.
p. of muscle
nerve p.
nuclear-fascicular trochlear nerve p.
obstetric brachial plexus p.
ocular muscle p.
oculomotor cranial nerve p.
other cerebral p.
peripheral facial nerve p.
peroneal nerve p.
persistent facial p.
progressive bulbar p.

palsy *(continued)*
progressive nuclear p.
progressive supranuclear p.
pseudobulbar p.
right superior oblique p.
spinal accessory nerve p.
supranuclear gaze p.
third nerve p.
twelfth nerve p.
ulnar nerve p.
vagus nerve p.
vertical gaze p.
vocal cord p.

Paltauf dwarf

paludal fever

Palyam virus

pamaquine

***p*-aminohippurate clearance**

***p*-aminohippuric acid**

p-aminophenylarsonate

p-aminopropiophenone

p-aminosalicylic acid

pampiniform
p. body
p. plexus

panacinar
p. disease
p. emphysema

Pan American Health Organization grade 0–2

panaritium digiti

Panas operation

panatrophy of Gower

panbronchiolitis
diffuse p.

pancake
p. appearance
bivalved pancake plaster hand cast
p. compression

p-ANC genetic marker

panchamber UV lens

Pancoast
P. operation
P. superior sulcus syndrome
P. suture
P. tumor

pancreas
p. accessorium
adenocarcinoma in head of p.
p. after kidney transplant
amount of insulin extractable from p.
anlage of p.
anterior border of body of p.
p. antigen retrieval
artery to tail of p.
artificial endocrine p.
p. cancer
carcinoma head of p.
combined kidney and pancreas transplant
p. cystadenoma
p. divisum
endoscopic retrograde parenchymography of p.
p. enzyme
excision head of p.
fibrocystic disease of the p.
head of p.
human fetal pancreas transplant
incomplete pancreas divisum
intraductal papillary neoplasm of the p.
islet cell of p.
p. and kidney
living segmental donor pancreas transplantation
mucinous ductal ectasia of the p.
mucinous ductectatic tumor of p.
mucin-producing tumor of the p.
neck of p.
necrosis of p.
omental eminence of p.
omental tuberosity of p.
pseudocyst of p.
resection head of p.
segmental pancreas donation
solid and cystic tumor of the p.
stomach, duodenum, and p.
p. sufficient
superior border of body of p.
p. transplantation alone

pancreatectomy
complete laparoscopic distal p.
distal p.

pancreatic
p. abscess
p. acinar cell
p. acinar cell carcinoma
p. acinar mass
p. acinar metaplasia
p. acinus
p. agenesis
alcoholic possible pancreatic encephalopathy
p. allograft
p. alpha-amylase
p. alpha-cell tumor
p. amylase
p. anastomosis
p. angiography
antecedent pancreatic injury
p. arteriography
p. arteriole
p. artery
p. artery aneurysm
artery of the pancreatic tail
p. ascariasis
p. ascites
p. atrophy
p. autotransplantation
avian pancreatic polypeptide
p. bacterial infection
p. biopsy
p. bladder
p. blood flow
p. body
bovine pancreatic polypeptide
bovine pancreatic trypsin inhibitor
p. branch
p. bypass
p. calcification
p. calculus
p. cancer marker
p. cancer pain
canine pancreatic polypeptide
p. capsule
p. cholera
p. cholera syndrome
p. colic
p. colipase
p. complication
p. cutaneous fistula
p. cyst
p. cystadenocarcinoma
p. cystic fibrosis
p. cystic lymphangioma
p. cystoduodenostomy
p. degeneration
p. denervation
p. deoxyribonuclease
p. diabetes
p. diarrhea
p. diastase
p. digestion
p. digestive zymogen
p. disease
p. disorder
p. diverticulum
p. divisum
p. dornase
p. dorsal anlage
p. duct
p. ductal adenocarcinoma

p. ductal hypertension
p. ductal morphological change
p. duct branch
p. duct cell carcinoma
p. duct-choledochus channel
p. duct dilatation
p. duct disruption
p. ductectatic-type carcinoma
p. duct encasement
p. duct hyperplasia
p. duct manipulation
p. duct obstruction
p. ductogram
p. duct pressure
p. duct sphincter
p. duct sphincterotomy
p. duct stone
p. duct stricture
duodenum-preserving pancreatic head resection
p. dysfunction
p. edema
p. encephalopathy
p. endocrine neoplasm
p. endocrine tumor
p. endopeptidase
endoscopic pancreatic sphincterotomy
endoscopic pancreatic stenting
p. endoscopy
p. enema
enzymatic pancreatic secretion
p. enzyme replacement therapy
p. enzyme secretion
p. exocrine
p. exocrine deficiency
p. exocrine deficit
p. exocrine dysfunction
p. exocrine function insufficiency
p. exocrine function test
p. exocrine insufficiency
exocrine pancreatic insufficiency
p. exopeptidase
p. extract
p. fascia
fibrocalculous pancreatic diabetes
p. fibrosis
p. fistula
p. flare
p. fluid collection
p. functioning diagnostant
p. fungal detection
p. fungus
p. gland
p. glandular necrosis
glicentin-related pancreatic polypeptide
p. hamartoma
p. head cancer
p. head origin
p. head resection
high-strength pancreatic enzymes
human pancreatic amylase
human pancreatic polypeptide
human pancreatic trypsin inhibitor
p. hypoplasia
p. imaging
p. infantilism
infected pancreatic necrosis
infectious pancreatic necrosis virus
p. inflammation
inoperable pancreatic cancer
p. insufficiency syndrome
integrated pancreatic polypeptide response
p. islet adenomatosis
p. islet beta cell
p. islet cell-specific enhancer sequence
p. islet cell transplantation
p. islet cell tumor
p. islets
isolated pancreatic islet transplantation
p. juice protein
Kunitz pancreatic trypsin inhibitor
p. lesion
p. lipase
p. lobular panniculitis
p. lymph node
p. lymphocytic infiltration
p. necrosis
needle-knife endoscopic pancreatic sphincterotomy
p. neoplasm
p. oncofetal antigen
operable pancreatic carcinoma
ovine pancreatic polypeptide
p. parenchyma
p. parenchymal perfusion
patent pancreatic duct
percutaneous fine-needle pancreatic biopsy
p. polypeptide
p. polypeptide-secreting tumor
porcine p.
porcine pancreatic elastase
porcine pancreatic polypeptide
p. pseudocyst
pure pancreatic juice
p. scan
p. secretion
p. secretory flow rate
p. secretory trypsin inhibitor
p. sepsis
severe pancreatic insufficiency
p. spasmolytic peptide
p. steatorrhea
p. stone protein
p. suppression test
p. tissue
p. transplantation
p. transplantation alone
tropical pancreatic diabetes
p. trypsin inhibitor
p. tuberculosis
p. vein

pancreatica

ansa p.
arteria pancreatica magna
magna

pancreatici

lymphonodus pancreatici inferiores
lymphonodus pancreatici superiores
nodi lymphatici pancreatici superiores
nodi lymphoidei p.

pancreaticobiliary

anomalous arrangement of pancreaticobiliary ductal system
anomalous junction of pancreaticobiliary ducts
anomalous pancreaticobiliary communication
anomalous pancreaticobiliary ductal union
p. common channel
p. disease
p. disorder
p. duct
p. ductal junction
p. ductal system
p. ductography
p. endoscopy
p. tract

pancreaticoduodenal

p. allograft
anterior and posterior superior pancreaticoduodenal artery
anterior superior pancreaticoduodenal artery
p. arcade vessel
p. arterial arcade
p. arteriography
p. artery
p. artery aneurysm
p. lymph node

pancreaticoduodenal *(continued)*
posterior superior pancreaticoduodenal vein
p. vein

pancreaticoduodenales
nodi lymphoidei p.

pancreaticoduodenalis
arteria p.
arteria pancreaticoduodenalis superior
arteria pancreaticoduodenalis superior anterior
arteria pancreaticoduodenalis superior posterior

pancreaticogastrostomy anastomosis

pancreaticohepatic syndrome

pancreaticojejunostomy anastomosis

pancreaticolienales
nodi lymphoidei p.

pancreaticosplenales
nodi lymphoidei p.

pancreaticosplenic
p. ligament
p. lymph node
p. omentum

pancreaticus
ansa p.

pancreatis insufficiency

pancreatitis
acute edematous p.
acute gallstone p.
acute hemorrhagic p.
acute necrotizing p.
acute recurrent p.
alcohol-related chronic p.
chronic alcoholic p.
chronic calcific pancreatitis of the tropics
chronic calcifying p.
chronic relapsing p.
drug-associated primary acute p.
p. dysfunction
hereditary p.
idiopathic recurrent p.
juvenile tropical pancreatitis syndrome
necrotizing p.
p. secondary to gallstones
severe acute p.
severe hemorrhagic p.
tropical calcific p.

pancreatitis-associated
p.-a. ascites fluid
p.-a. protein

pancreatitis-related
p.-r. bleeding
p.-r. hemorrhage

pancreatobiliary
anomalous junction of the pancreatobiliary duct
anomalous pancreatobiliary duct junction
p. canal

pancreatocholangiography
endoscopic p.

pancreatocholangitis
sclerosing p.

pancreatoduodenectomy
pylorus-preserving p.

pancreatogenic diarrhea

pancreatogenous fatty diarrhea

pancreatogram
endoscopic retrograde p.

pancreatography
computed tomography under endoscopic retrograde p.
endoscopic digital p.
endoscopic retrograde p.
magnetic resonance p.
three-dimensional computed tomography p.

pancreatorenal syndrome

pancreatoscope
peroral electronic p.

pancreatoscopic laser lithotripsy

pancreatoscopy
peroral p.

pancrelipase
enterocoated microspheres of p.

pancreolauryl test

pancreozymin
p. secretin
secretin p.
secretin, cholecystokinin, p.
p. secretin test

pancreozymin-cholecystokinin

pancreozymin secretin test

pancuronium
p. bromide
p. Pavulon

pancytokeratin antibody

pancytopenia
aplastic p.
autoimmune p.
Fanconi p.

panda appearance

pandemic
p. disease
p. epidemiology
p. flu
p. influenza

pandevelopmental retardation

panduriformis
placenta p.

panel
basic metabolic p.
chemistry p.
coagulation p.
electrolyte p.
Farnsworth panel D-15 color vision test
fasting metabolic p.
general medical p.
hepatic functional p.
hypersensitivity pneumonitis p.
independent adjudicating p.
lipid p.
lymphocyte subset p.
MicroScan gram-negative ID p.
Nephrolithiasis Clinical Guidelines P.
p. of reactive antibodies
renal function p.
Testicular Tumor P.
urine drug p.
viral hepatitis p.

panencephalitis
nodular p.
progressive rubella p.
subacute sclerosing p.

panendoscope
flexible forward-viewing p.
McCarthy panendoscope

Paneth
P. cell
P. cell-like change

pang
hunger p.

pangastritis
atrophic p.

Pangola stunt virus

panhypopituitarism
autoimmune p.

panic
active panic attack

acute homosexual p.
agoraphobia without history of panic disorder
agoraphobia with panic attack
p. and anxiety disorder
anxiety and panic disorder clinic
anxiety panic reaction
p. attack
p. attack neurotic anxiety state
p. button
clinical manifestation of panic reaction
p. delirium
p. diathesis
p. disorder
p. disorder with agoraphobia
p. disorder without agoraphobia
p. episode
full-blown panic attack
homosexual p.
overwhelming sense of p.
p. reaction
p. reactions with hallucinogen

pankeratin antibody

panleukopenia
feline panleukopenia virus
p. virus

panlobular emphysema

panmetatarsal head resection

panmyelopathy
Döhle body p.

panni (*pl. of* pannus)

panniculectomy
noncosmetic p.

panniculitis
annular atrophic connective tissue panniculitis of the ankle
histiocytic cytophagic p.
lupus erythematosus p.
mesenteric p.
nodular eosinophilic p.
nodular liquefying p.
nodular migratory p.
nodular nonsuppurative p.
pancreatic lobular p.

panniculus, pl. **panniculi**
abdominal p.
p. adiposus
p. carnosus
p. carnosus muscle

pannus, pl. **panni**
allergic p.
p. carnosus
p. cell
p. deformity
p. deformity of odontoid
eczematous p.
p. formation
obese p.
p. siccus
trachomatous p.

Panoptic bifocal

panoral
p. radiography
p. x-ray examination

panoramic
p. CT scan
p. extraoral radiography
p. loupe
p. radiograph
p. tomography
p. view
p. visualization

Panoview
P. arthroscope
P. arthroscopic system

panretinal
p. ablation
p. argon laser photocoagulation
p. membrane

pansystolic murmur

pantalar
p. arthrodesis
p. fusion

pantalocrural
p. arthritic destruction
p. arthritis

pantaloon
p. brace
p. embolism
p. inguinal hernia
p. patch

pantetheine

p24 antigen testing

Pantomime Recognition Test

Panton-Valentine leukocidin

Pantopaque
cervical Pantopaque column
P. cisternography
P. contrast medium

pantoscopic
p. angle
p. angling
p. effect
p. spectacles
p. tilt

pantothenic
p. acid
p. acid assay
p. acid deficiency-induced colitis
p. acid unit

pants-over-vest
p.-o.-v. capsulorrhaphy
p.-o.-v. hernial repair
p.-o.-v. herniorrhaphy

Panum fusion area

panuveitis
granulomatous p.

Papanicolaou
P. smear
P. stain
P. stain of sputum
P. test

Papavasiliou
P. classification
P. classification of olecranon fracture

papaverine hydrochloride

paper
p. autoradiography
p. capacitor
carbonless paper syndrome
p. chromatography
p. dermatitis
p. electrophoresis
p. enzyme-linked immunosorbent assay
filter p.
filter paper microscopic test
filter paper activity
high-voltage paper electrophoresis
p. mill worker's disease
Minnesota P. Form Board Test
p. mulberry
p. mulberry tree
p. radioimmunosorbent technique
p. radioimmunosorbent test
strict no information in p.

Papez
P. circle
P. circuit

papilla, pl. **papillae**
anal p.
anogenital vestibular p.
area cribrosa papillae renalis
atrophied p.
p. of Bergmeister
p. of breast
capillary loop in dermal p.
capillary loop in hair p.
p. of columnar epithelium
papillae of corium
p. dentis
p. dermatis

papilla *(continued)*
p. of dermis
papillae dermis
p. diameter
p. ductus parotidei
p. gingivalis
p. graft
hair p.
hypertrophied p.
p. lacrimalis
limbal papillae
lingual gingival p.
lingual interdental p.
major duodenal p.
p. mammae
minor duodenal p.
optic p.
p. of optic nerve
optic papilla cavity
orifice of ileal p.
renal p.
p. of Vater

papillaris
areola p.
nevus p.

papillary
p. adenocystoma lymphomatosum
p. adenoma of large intestine
p. adenomatous polyp
aggressive digital papillary adenocarcinoma
aggressive digital papillary adenoma
aggressive papillary middle ear tumor
anterior papillary muscle
p. apocrine change
p. area
aspirin-induced papillary necrosis
p. atrophy
p. bile duct stenosis
p. blush
p. breast carcinoma
p. carcinoma of thyroid
p. collecting duct
p. conjunctival hypertrophy
p. conjunctivitis
conventional papillary carcinoma
p. craniopharyngioma
p. cyst
p. cystadenocarcinoma of ovary
p. cystadenoma lymphomatosum
p. cystic adenoma
p. cystic neoplasm
p. cystitis
p. DCIS
p. dermal peel
p. dermis
p. duct
p. duct of Bellini
p. eccrine adenoma
p. ectasia
p. endometrial carcinoma
endoscopic papillary balloon dilation
p. ependymoma
p. epididymal cystadenoma
p. excrescence
p. fibroelastoma
follicular variant of papillary thyroid carcinoma
p. foramen
p. foramina of kidney
p. frond
p. gastric carcinoma
giant papillary conjunctivitis
giant papillary hypertrophy
p. gingivitis
p. hemangioma
hereditary papillary renal cancer
hereditary papillary renal cell carcinoma
p. hidradenoma
p. hyperplasia
p. hypertrophy
inflammatory papillary hyperplasia
inflammatory papillary hyperplasia of the palate
intraductal oncocytic papillary neoplasm
intraductal papillary carcinoma
intraductal papillary mucinous neoplasm
intraductal papillary mucinous tumor
intraductal papillary neoplasm of the pancreas
intravascular papillary endothelial hyperplasia
p. layer
macrofollicular thyroid papillary carcinoma
malignant endovascular papillary angioendothelioma
malignant papillary mesothelioma
p. mesothelioma
p. muscle
p. muscle dysfunction
p. muscle fibrosis
p. muscle rupture
p. necrosis
p. nephrocalcinosis
ovarian papillary serous adenocarcinoma
posterior p.
posterior papillary muscle
p. renal cell carcinoma
renal papillary necrosis
p. response
p. ruff
p. serous carcinoma of the peritoneum
p. serous cystadenocarcinoma
p. stasis
p. thyroid cancer
p. thyroid carcinoma
p. tumor
p. tumor projection
usual type papillary carcinoma
uterine papillary serous carcinoma

papilledema
asymmetric p.
hemorrhage, papilledema, exudate

papilliform
p. rash
p. tumor

papillitis
necrotizing p.

papilloma
p. acuminatum
anal human papilloma virus infection
benign intraductal p.
p. of bladder
p. of breast
p. breast
p. canaliculum
choroid plexus p.
p. durum
p. forceps
human papilloma virus
infectious papilloma virus
intraductal papilloma of breast
juvenile laryngeal p.
p. molle
multimammate papilloma virus
p. neuroticum
oncocytic schneiderian p.
p., inner canthus
recurrent respiratory p.
squamous cell p.
transitional cell p.
p. virus, polyoma virus, vacuolative virus

papillomacular nerve fiber bundle

papillomatosis
p. of breast
confluent, reticulate p.
p. coronae

florid cutaneous p.
p. of Gougerot-Carteaud
malignant papillomatosis of Degos
oral florid p.
recurrent respiratory p.
subareolar duct p.

papillomatosus
lupus p.
nevus p.

papillomatous
p. goiter
p. papule
p. skin lesion

papillomavirus
bovine p.
human p.
human papillomavirus type 16
p. hybridization
p. infection
Shope p.
subclinical papillomavirus infection

papillotome
Frimberger-Karpiel 12 o'clock p.

papillotomy
endoscopic p.
needle-knife precut p.

Papineau
P. bone graft
P. cancellous graft
P. grafting

papovavirus
lymphotropic p.

pappataci
p. fever
p. fever virus

Pappenheim
lymphoid hemoblast of P.

Pappenheimer body

papular
p. acne
p. acrodermatitis
p. acrodermatitis of childhood
bovine papular stomatitis
p. dermatitis
p. dermatitis of pregnancy
p. eruption
p. exanthem
p. fever
p. fibroplasia
lentigines, atrial myxomas, cutaneous papular myxomas, blue nevi
p. lesion
p. mastocytosis
miliary papular syphilid
monomorphous papular eruption
p. mucinosis
noneczematous persistent papular gold eruption
pruritic papular eruption
p. rash

papule
apple jelly papule of lupus vulgaris
erythematous p.
erythematous hyperpigmented p.
indolent p.
indurated p.
lichenoid p.
moist p.
mucous p.
papillomatous p.
pearly coronal p.
pearly penile p.
pruritic urticarial p.'s and plaques
pruritic urticarial p.'s and plaques of pregnancy

papulonecrotic tuberculid

papulonodular rash

papulosa
dermatosis papulosa nigra
iritis p.
miliaria p.
p. nigra dermatosis

papulosis
atrophic p.
p. atrophicans maligna
malignant atrophic p.

papulosquamous
p. dermatitis
p. dermatosis
p. disease
p. disorder
p. eruption
p. skin lesion

papulovesicular
p. acrodermatitis
p. acrolocated syndrome
p. lesion

papyracea
lamina p.

papyraceus
fetus p.

paraaminobenzoic acid

paraaminohippurate clearance

paraaminohippuric acid

paraaminomethylbenzoic acid

paraaminosalicylic acid

paraaortic
p. body
p. hematoma
p. lymphadenectomy
p. lymphadenopathy
p. lymph node
p. node irradiation
p. node sampling

paraaortica

paraarticular
p. arthrodesis
p. bone remodeling
p. calcification
p. heterotopic ossification

parabasal
p. body
p. cell
p. cell layers
p. filament

parabolic
p. curve
p. flow
p. reflector

parabulbar anesthesia

paracarcinomatous encephalomyelopathy

paracardiac metastasis

paracellular calcium resorption

paracelsian method

paracentesis
abdominal p.
p. abdominis
anterior chamber p.
aqueous p.
p. fluid cytology
large-volume p.
p. and suction
therapeutic p.
p. and tubing of ears

paracentral
anterior paracentral gyrus
anterior paracentral lobule
p. branch of callosomarginal artery
p. branch of pericallosal artery
p. cell
p. defect
p. fissure
p. gray area
p. gyrus
p. hemianopia
p. lobe

paracentral *(continued)*
p. lobule
p. nerve fiber bundle
p. ring scotoma
p. visual field

paracentralis
arteria p.

paracervical
p. anesthetic
p. block
p. blockade
p. block anesthesia
p. ganglion
p. injection
p. lymphatics

paracetamol
p. absorption
p. absorption test

parachordal cartilage

parachute
p. deformity
p. deformity of mitral valve

paracoagulation
protamine paracoagulation phenomenon

paracoccidioidal granuloma

Paracoccidioides
anti-*Paracoccidioides brasiliensis* antibody

paracolic
p. abscess
p. groove
p. gutter
packing of paracolic gutter

paracolici
nodi lymphoidei p.

paracolon bacillus

paracolostomy
p. hernia
p. herniation

paracorporeal heart

paracostal incision

paracrine
p. action
p. agent
p. cell
p. communication
p. cytokine
p. effect
p. factor
locally acting paracrine effector
p. loop
p. manner
p. regulation
p. secretion
p. suppressor
p. system

paracyclic ovulation

paradental cyst

paradigm
p. clash
gap p.
simple response p.

paradox
early systolic p.

paradoxic
p. gustolacrimal reflex
p. levator excitation
p. levator inhibition
p. splitting

paradoxical
p. abdominal movement
p. aciduria
p. air embolism
p. ankle reflex
p. anxiety
p. breathing
p. bronchospasm
p. cerebral embolism
p. cerebral embolus
p. chest wall motion
p. cold
p. cold response
p. colon dilatation
p. combination
p. contraction
p. darkness reaction
p. depression
p. diaphragm phenomenon
p. diarrhea
p. diplopia
p. effect
p. extensor reflex
p. flexor reflex
p. incontinence
p. injunction
p. intention
p. law
p. movement of eyelids
p. pulse
p. pupil
p. pupillary phenomenon
p. pupillary reflex
p. response
p. rocking impulse
p. sleep
p. systolic expansion
p. vocal cord motion
p. vocal fold dysfunction

paradoxus
pulsus p.

paraduodenal
p. fold
p. fossa
p. hernia

paradysentery bacillus

paraesophageal
p. collateral vein
p. diaphragmatic hernia
p. hernia type I, II
p. hiatal hernia
p. hiatus hernia
laparoscopic paraesophageal hernia repair
laparoscopic repair of paraesophageal hernia

parafascicular
p. nucleus
p. thalamotomy

paraffin
p. bath
bismuth iodoform p.
p. block
p. block embedding
p. breast augmentation
p. cancer
p. embedding
p. granuloma
p. heat therapy
p. immunoperoxidase
p. implant
p. implant material
p. section

paraffin-embedded
formalin-fixed p.-e.
p.-e. semithin section
p.-e. tissue

paraflocculus syndrome

parafollicular
p. B-cell lymphoma
p. calcitonin-producing cell
p. duct

paraformaldehyde-lysine-periodate

parafoveal
p. capillary net
p. cystic space
p. fluorescein
p. halo
p. macula
p. microvascular leakage

parafrenal abscess

paraganglia
aorticosympathetic p.

paraganglioma
aorticopulmonary p.
malignant p.
paravertebral p.
paraganglion
aortic p.
paraganglionic cell
paragigantocellularis
paraglenoid groove
paraglottic area
Paragonimus **granuloma**
paragranuloma
nodular p.
parahippocampal
p. activation
p. gyrus
parainfectious
p. optic neuritis
p. optic neuropathy
parainfluenza
p. antibody test
p. antigen
p. culture
p. paramyxovirus vaccine
p. type 1, 2, 3, 4A, 4B
p. viral disease
p. virus antigen
p. virus culture
p. virus serology
p. virus type 1–4, 4B
parainfluenzae
Haemophilus p.
paraisopropyliminodiacetic acid scan
parakeratinized
p. cyst
p. epithelium
paralabral cyst
paralaryngeal space
paraldehyde assay
paralimbic
p. cortex
p. region
paralingual extension
parallax
heteronymous p.
homonymous p.
motion p.
p. and refraction
stereoscopic p.
p. test
parallel
ambulates on parallel bars
p. analog mapping
p. arrays
p. attachment
p. bars
p. beam
p. blockout
p. bone
p. channel sign
p. cine
p. circuit
p. circulation
p. data acquisition coil
p. development of axillary hair
p. development of pubic hair
p. distribution
p. dream
p. elastic component of muscle
p. elastic element
p. fiber
p. goniometric measure
p. hole collimation
p. incision
p. interface
limbal parallel orientation
limbus parallel orientation straddling tattoo mark
p. line equal spacing
massively parallel signature sequencing
massive parallel processing system
p. ray
p. virtual machine
parallel-hole collimator
paralleling
p. cone position
p. coping
parallelism
p. of articular surface
p. of gaze
parallel-opposed
p.-o. beam
p.-o. fields
parallel-plate flow chamber
paralysis, pl. **paralyses**
p. of accommodation
acute atrophic spinal p.
acute flaccid p.
p. agitans
p. agitans juvenilis
aphid lethal paralysis virus
ascending flaccid p.
atrophic muscular p.
bilateral abductor vocal cord p.
bilateral diaphragm p.
bilateral vocal fold p.
p. and coma
congenital abducens-facial p.
p. of conjugate upward gaze
p. of diaphragm
familial periodic p.
general p.
general paralysis of the insane
hind leg p.
hypesthesia and p.
idiopathic facial p.
incomplete facial p.
ischemic paralysis and contracture
juvenile general p.
lower lip p.
lower radicular obstetrical p.
mitochondrial encephalomyopathy with sensorimotor polyneuropathy, ophthalmoplegia, and p.
mononeuritis with p.
normokalemic periodic p.
p. notariorum
nuclear horizontal gaze p.
numbness, weakness and paralysis of arm
ocular muscle p.
onset of p.
pain, pallor, pulse loss, paresthesia, and p.
paralytic infantile p.
partial facial p.
peripheral facial p.
sleep p.
Todd p.
unilateral vocal cord p.
vagus nerve p.
vocal cord p.
p. of vocal cord
paralytic
p. abasia
p. bladder
p. brachial neuritis
p. chest
p. chorea
p. colonic obstruction
congenital syphilitic paralytic dementia
p. contracture
p. dementia
p. ectropion
p. foot
p. heterotropia
p. hypotonia
p. idiocy
p. ileus
p. incontinence
p. infantile paralysis

paralytic *(continued)*
p. miosis
p. mydriasis
p. polio
p. poliomyelitis
p. pontine exotropia
severe paralytic illness
p. shellfish poisoning
p. strabismus
vaccine-associated paralytic polio
vaccine-associated paralytic poliomyelitis

paralytica
aphonia p.
p. aphonia
dementia paralytica juvenilis

paralyzed
p. and mechanically ventilated
p. muscle
p. vocal cord

paralyzing
p. depression
p. dose
p. injury
median paralyzing dose

paramagnetic
antibody-conjugated paramagnetic liposome
p. artifact
p. cation
p. contrast
p. contrast agent
p. contrast-enhanced MR study
p. contrast enhancement
p. contrast injection
electron paramagnetic resonance
electron paramagnetic response
p. enhancement
p. enhancement accentuation by chemical shift imaging
p. iron species
p. metal
p. microsphere
p. nucleus

paramagnetism
apparent p.

paramammarii
nodi lymphoidei p.

Paramatta agent

paramedian
p. approach
p. artery
p. clefting syndrome
p. durotomy
p. forehead flap
p. frontal bone window
p. incision
pontine paramedian reticular formation
p. pontine reticular formation
p. reticular nucleus

paramedical staff

paramesonephric
p. duct
p. duct cyst

parameter
body segment p.
hematologic p.'s
hemodynamic p.'s
holistic orthogonal parameter estimation
portable monitor of respiratory p.'s
systemic hemodynamic p.'s
total radical-trapping antioxidant p.

parametrial
p. mass
p. thickening

parametric
p. abscess
p. imaging
optical parametric oscillator

parametritic abscess

paramnesia
reduplicative p.

Paramushir virus

paramyotonia
ataxic p.
p. congenita

paramyxovirus
avian paramyxovirus virus 1–9
P. infection
parainfluenza paramyxovirus vaccine

paranasal
p. cancer
p. cell
p. sinus
p. sinusitis
p. sinus lymphoma
p. sinus tumor

Paraná virus

paraneoplastic
p. acrokeratosis
p. amyloidosis
p. anemia
p. anorexia
p. antiphospholipid syndrome
autoimmune paraneoplastic syndrome
p. basophilia
p. cachexia
p. cerebellar degeneration
p. cerebral degeneration
p. complication
p. dermatomyositis
p. disease
p. ectopic ACTH production
p. encephalomyelitis
p. encephalomyelopathy
p. endocarditis
p. eosinophilia
p. erythema
p. erythrocytosis
p. granulocytosis
p. growth hormone
p. hepatopathy
p. hypercalcemia
p. hypercoagulability
p. hypocalcemia
p. limbic encephalopathy
p. malabsorption
neurologic paraneoplastic syndrome
p. neurologic syndrome
p. opsoclonus
p. optic neuritis
p. pemphigus
p. retinopathy
p. tumor

paranephric
p. abscess
p. body
p. fat

paraneural
p. anesthesia
p. block

paranoia
acute hallucinatory p.
affect-laden p.
alcoholic p.
amorous p.
p. and delusions psychiatric syndrome
p. dementia gravis
erotic p.
hallucinatory p.
insomnia and p.
querulous p.

paranoiac character

paranoica
aphonia p.
aphrasia p.

paranoid
acute paranoid schizophrenic reaction
affective paranoid organic psychosis
affective and paranoid state
alcoholic paranoid psychosis
alcoholic paranoid state
alcohol-induced paranoid state
arteriosclerotic paranoid state
atypical paranoid disorder
p. behavior
p. belief system
chronic paranoid schizophrenic reaction
p. condition
p. delusion
p. delusional belief
delusional paranoid disorder
p. dementia
p. depression
p. disorder
p. erotism
p. fear
p. feature
p. grandiose delusion
p. hostility
p. ideation
p. individual
p. insomniac
p. personality disorder
p. psychosis
p. schizophrenia
schizophrenia, paranoid type, subchronic
schizophrenic reaction, acute, p.
schizophrenic reaction, chronic, p.
transient paranoid ideation

paranoid-type
p.-t. alcoholic psychosis
p.-t. arteriosclerotic
p.-t. arteriosclerotic dementia
p.-t. arteriosclerotic psychosis

paranormal
p. capacity
p. cognition
subjective paranormal experience

paranuclear
p. body
p. cytoplasm

paraosteal osteosarcoma

paraparesis
hereditary spastic p.
tropical spastic p.

paraparesis/HTLV
tropical spastic paraparesis/HTLV-I associated myelopathy

parapatellar arthrotomy

parapelvic cyst

paraperitoneal hernia

parapharyngeal
p. abscess
p. fat
p. fat pad
p. lymph node
p. space

paraphasic
fluent paraphasic speech

paraphenylenediamine dermatitis

paraphilia
atypical p.

paraphiliac
p. behavior
p. coercive disorder
p. fantasy
p. focus
p. imagery

paraphimosis palpebrae

paraphrenia
p. confabulans
p. fantastica

paraphrenic dementia

paraphysial
p. body
p. cyst

parapineal organ

parapituitary area

paraplegia
p. dolorosa
p. in extension
familial spastic p.
p. in flexion
hereditary spastic p.
mental retardation, spastic paraplegia, palmoplantar hyperkeratosis syndrome
mental retardation-spastic paraplegia syndrome
spastic p.

paraplegic
p. headache
p. pain
p. rehabilitation

parapneumonic
p. effusion
p. empyema
p. infiltrate

Parapost bur

paraprotein
light chain p.

parapsoriasis
p. acuta et varioliformis
p. en plaque
p. en plaques
p. guttata
p. large-plaque
p. lichenoid
p. maculata

paraquat
p. ingestion
p. lung

pararectal
p. abscess
p. fistula
p. fossa
p. lymph node
p. space

pararectales
nodi lymphoidei p.

pararectus
p. approach
p. incision

pararenal
p. abscess
anterior pararenal space
p. aortic aneurysm
p. aortic atherosclerosis

parareticular
pontine parareticular formation

parasaccular hernia

parasacral block

parasagittal
p. cerebral injury
p. cortical infarction
p. depression
p. falx
p. groove
p. lesion
p. meningioma
p. plane
p. zone

parascapular flap

parasellar
p. brain mass
p. cistern
p. dermoid tumor
p. dysgerminoma
p. lesion
p. meningioma
p. metastasis
p. region

parasellar *(continued)*
p. syndrome
p. tissue
p. tumor

paraseptal cartilage

parasite
apicomplexan p.
autistic p.
autochthonous p.
ectophytic p.
endophytic p.
entozoic p.
eurytrophic p.
p. examination
facultative p.
incidental p.
intercellular p.
intermittent p.
intestinal p.'s
intestinal p.
malarial p.
malarial p.'s
malignant tertian malarial p.
metazoal p.
obligate intracellular p.
ova, blood, and p.'s
ova and p.'s examination
protozoan p.
sporozoan p.
spurious p.
tertian p.

parasite-host ecosystem

parasitemia stage

parasitic
p. blepharitis
p. brain abscess
p. cardiomyopathy
p. castration
p. chylocele
p. cyst
p. disease
p. ectopic pregnancy
p. embolus
p. endophthalmitis
p. fetus
p. flap
p. flatworm
p. fungus
p. gastroenteritides
p. gastroenteritis
p. granuloma
p. hemoptysis
p. infection
p. infestation
p. keratitis
p. leiomyoma
p. melanoderma
p. myoma
p. thyroiditis
p. uveitis
p. worm

parasitica
onychia p.

parasitism
multiple p.

parasitized erythrocyte

parasitophorous vacuole

parasomnia
NREM arousal p.

parasomniac
p. consciousness
p. conscious state

paraspinal
p. abnormality
p. abscess
p. approach
p. calcification
p. muscle
p. muscle spasm

paraspinous
p. aspect
p. fascia
p. muscle

parasternal
p. bulge
p. chondrodynia
p. examination
p. heave
p. hernia
high right parasternal view
p. intercostal tenderness
left parasternal impulse
p. lift
p. line
p. long axis
long axis parasternal view
p. lymph nodes
p. node
right parasternal impulse
p. short axis

parasternales
nodi lymphoidei p.

parastomal hernia

parastriate
p. area
p. cortex

parasuicidal
p. behavior
p. event
p. incident

parasympathetic
p. division of antonomic nervous system
p. drug
p. epilepsy
p. fiber
p. ganglion
p. innervation
p. nerve
p. nerve system
p. outflow
p. pathway

parasympatholytic drug

parasympathomimetic
p. agent
p. anticholinesterase
p. drug

parasymphysial fracture

parasymphysis
p. area
p. fracture

parasystolic ventricular tachycardia

parataxic distortion

paratenic host

paraterminal
p. body
p. gyrus

paratesticular
p. fat
p. rhabdomyosarcoma

parathyroid
p. adenoma
p. artery
asymmetric parathyroid enlargement
p. autograft
autonomous parathyroid chief cell proliferation
p. autotransplantation
p. biopsy
bovine parathyroid hormone
p. carcinoma
p. cell membrane
p. chief cell
p. computed tomography
p. crisis
p. cyst
p. disease
p. disorder
ectopic parathyroid adenoma
p. extracellular calcium-sensing receptor
p. extract
p. gland

p. gland dysfunction
p. gland enlargement
p. gland hyperplasia
p. gland immaturity
p. hormone
p. hormone assay
p. hormone excess
p. hormone gene transcription
p. hormone level
p. hormonelike polypeptide
p. hormonelike protein
p. hormone-mediated calcium efflux
p. hormone-related peptide
p. hormone-related protein
p. hormone-related protein-transfected RIN-141 cell
p. hormone resistance syndrome
p. hormone secretion
p. hormone secretion rate
human parathyroid hormone
p. insufficiency
intact parathyroid hormone
mediastinal parathyroid adenoma
mid-molecule parathyroid hormone
nonfamilial parathyroid adenoma
p. osteodystrophy
pathologic parathyroid disease
plasma parathyroid hormone
p. scintigraphy
p. secretory protein
serum immunoreactive parathyroid hormone
p. tetany
total parathyroid hormone secretion
p. ultrasound

parathyroidal abscess

parathyroidectomy
acute p.
p. and autotransplantation
chronic p.
minimally invasive video-assisted p.

parathyroprival tetany

paratracheal
p. adenopathy
p. convexity
p. lymphadenopathy
p. node chain
p. region

paratracheales
nodi lymphoidei p.

paratuberculous lymphadenitis

paratyphoid
p. A, B
p. bacillus
p. bacteria
p. fever
p. infection
intradermal typhoid and paratyphoid vaccine
p. fever, types A, B, C
typhoid, paratyphoid A, B, C vaccine
typhoid, paratyphoid A, B, tetanus toxoid, and diphtheria toxoid vaccine

paraumbilical
p. anterior abdominal wall
p. hernia
p. vein
p. vein tumor

paraurethral
p. canal
p. cyst
p. duct
p. gland

parauterini
nodi lymphoidei p.

paravaccinia
p. virus
p. virus infection

paravaginal
p. cystocele
p. cystocele repair
p. defect
p. defect repair
p. fascial repair
p. hysterectomy
p. incision

paravaginales
nodi lymphoidei p.

paravalvular
aortic paravalvular leak

paravariceal fibrosis

paraventricular
p. cyst
p. fiber
p. neuron
p. nuclear stratum
p. nucleus of the hypothalamus
p. thalamic nucleus

paraventricularis
nucleus p.

paravertebral
p. abscess
p. anesthesia
p. block
p. ganglion
p. gutter
p. line
p. mass
p. muscle
p. muscle spasm
p. musculature
p. paraganglioma
p. triangle

paravesical
p. fossa
p. lymph node
p. space

paravesiculares
nodi lymphatici p.

paraxial
p. fibular hemimelia
p. lighting
p. ray
p. ray of light

parchment
p. crackling
p. induration

Pardue flap

parenchyma
acinar p.
cirrhotic liver p.
p. congested
dense p.
p. edematous
p. extremely congested
p. glandulae thyroideae
incised renal p.
p. infiltration
lung p.
patchy infiltration of medullary p.

parenchymal
p. abscess
p. amyloidosis
p. atrophy
p. bacillary peliosis
p. blastoma
p. blood
p. brain injury
p. brain lesion
p. brain metastasis
p. brain neoplasm
breast parenchymal pattern
p. breast pattern
p. cell
p. cerebral hemorrhage
p. change
p. collapse
p. cone
p. consolidation
p. cyst
p. density

parenchymal *(continued)*
p. disease
p. dissection
p. echogenicity
p. fibrosis
fixed parenchymal turnover
p. granuloma
p. hematoma
p. hemorrhage
p. infiltrate
p. lung disease
p. lung morphogenesis
mammary parenchymal stimulation
nonobstructive hepatic parenchymal disease
occupational parenchymal disease
p. opacification
pancreatic parenchymal perfusion
pulmonary parenchymal disease
pulmonary parenchymal tissue volume
pulmonary parenchymal window
p. scarring

parenchymatosus
xerosis p.

parenchymatous
p. acute renal failure
p. atrophy
p. cartilage
p. cell of corpus pineale
p. cerebellar degeneration
p. congenital syphilis
p. corneal dystrophy
p. degeneration
p. disease
p. form
p. glossitis
p. goiter
p. hematoma
p. hemorrhage
p. hepatitis
p. involvement
p. keratitis
p. liver disease
p. neurosyphilis

parenchymography
endoscopic retrograde parenchymography of pancreas

parent
Abbreviated P. Symptom Questionnaire
p. abuse
Ackerman-Schoendorf Scales for P. Evaluation of Custody
adoptive p.
alcoholic p.
P.'s Anonymous
p. anxiety rating scale
p. artery
p. artery occlusion
P. as a Teacher Inventory
p.'s at risk
P. Attitude Scale
authoritarian rejecting-neglecting p.
P. Awareness Skills Survey
p. burnout
p. cell
p. to child
p. child
Children of Aging P.'s
children of incarcerated p.'s
Conners P. Questionnaire
controlling p.
Coping Health Inventory for P.'s
custodial p.
p. cyst
p. drug
p. effectiveness training
p. ego state
Eidetic P.'s Test
p. fixation
p. guidance work
p. image
impaired p.
offspring of diabetic p.'s
P. Perception of Child Profile
p. rating scale
single parent keeping baby
single parent not keeping baby
P. Symptom Questionnaire

parentage determination

parental
p. abuse
anomalous parental vocal pattern
p. attitudes toward sex
p. behavior
p. bonding instrument
p. care
p. consent
p. control
p. control problem
p. criticism
p. custody
p. death
p. denial
p. development questionnaire
p. divorce
p. dysfunction
p. environment
p. environment characteristic
p. environment item
p. failure to guide
p. feeding practice
first parental generation
p. fit
p. generation
p. habits of blame
p. habits of praise
Hereford P. Attitude Survey
p. indecisiveness
p. indifference
p. karyotype
p. Rh incompatibility
P. Stress Index
P. Stressor Scale: Neonatal Intensive Care Unit

parent-child
p.-c. bond
p.-c. communication schedule
p.-c. conflict
p.-c. conflict counseling
p.-c. dyad
p.-c. group therapy
p.-c. interaction
p.-c. interaction evaluation

parenteral
p. absorption
p. administration
p. alimentation
p. analgesia
p. analgesic
p. analgesic medication
p. anesthesia
p. antibiotic
p. anticonvulsant
p. antigen
p. antihypertensive agent
p. antimicrobial agent
p. chemotherapy
p. corticosteroid
cyclic total parenteral nutrition
p. diarrhea
p. diphenhydramine
p. diuretic
p. drug
p. drug abuser
p. drug administration
p. and enteral nutrition
p. feeding
p. fluids
p. formula
p. guanethidine
home parenteral antibiotic therapy
home total parenteral nutrition
p. hyperalimentation
p. injection
p. inoculation
intradialytic parenteral nutrition
p. iron dextran

large-volume parenteral infusion
p. nutrition-associated cholestatic
outpatient parenteral antibiotic therapy
penicillin G, parenteral, aqueous
peripheral vein total parenteral nutrition
small volume parenteral infusion
supplementary parenteral nutrition
support parenteral nutrition
p. therapy
total parenteral alimentation
total peripheral parenteral nutrition
p. vasodilator

parenteral-controlled analgesia

parenterally transmitted non-A non-B hepatitis

parenteric fever

parenthood
planned p.

parent-infant traumatic stress

parenting
p. ability
attachment p.
dysfunctional parenting style
p. issue
P. Stress Index

parent-metabolite ratio

Parents'
P. Postoperative Pain Measure

Parent's Choice formula

Parent-Teacher Questionnaire

parenzyme, buccal

paresis
asymmetric palatal p.
cerebral gaze p.
general p.
general paresis of insane
ipsilateral hemidiaphragmatic p.
oculomotor paresis with cyclic spasm

paresthesia
p. of extremity
p. of feet
p. of limb
pain, pallor, pulse loss, paresthesia, and paralysis
perioral p.

paresthetica
meralgia p.
notalgia p.

paretic
p. agraphia
p. analgesia
p. curve
p. dementia
p. eye
p. impotence
muscle paretic nystagmus
p. neurosis
p. neurosyphilis
p. nystagmus

paries, pl. **parietes**
p. anterior vaginae
p. anterior ventriculi
p. interior orbitae
p. lateralis orbitae
p. medialis orbitae
p. superior orbitae

parietal
p. abdominal fascia
p. abscess
p. angle
p. angle of sphenoid
anterior parietal artery
anterior parietal artery aneurysm
anterior parietal lesion
p. area
ascending frontal p.
ascending parietal convolution
ascending parietal gyrus
p. association area
association cortex of parietal lobe
p. band
p. body
p. bone flap
p. bone thickness
p. bone thinning
p. border
p. border of frontal bone
p. border of sphenoid bone
p. border of squamous part of temporal bone
p. boss
p. branch
p. branch of medial occipital artery
p. branch of middle meningeal artery
p. branch of superficial temporal artery
p. bulge
p. cell
p. cell antibody
p. cell hyperplasia
p. cell index
p. cell vagotomy
p. cephalohematoma
p. convexity
p. cortex
p. cortex damage
p. cortex lesion
p. corticectomy
craniosynostosis, ataxia, trigeminal anesthesia, parietal anesthesia and pons, vermis fusion syndrome
p. craniotomy
p. defect
p. diameter
p. eminence
p. emissary vein
p. encephalocele
p. epithelium
p. eye
p. fistula
p. foramen
p. foramina, brachymicrocephaly, mental retardation syndrome
gastric parietal cell
p. gyrus
p. headache
p. hernia
p. hump
inferior parietal and superior temporal lobe
isolated parietal endocarditis
p. lamina
p. layer
p. layer of leptomeninges
p. layer of serous pericardium
p. layer of tunica vaginalis of testis
p. lobe
p. lobe battery
p. lobe bilateral cerebral hemisphere lesion
p. lobe of brain
p. lobe field defect
p. lobe function
p. lobe unilateral cerebral hemisphere lesion
p. lymph node
p. margin
p. margin of frontal bone
p. margin of greater wing of sphenoid
mastoid angle of parietal bone
p. midline zero electrode placement in electroencephalography
occipital angle of parietal bone
occipital border of parietal bone
p. operculum
p. pain

parietal *(continued)*
p. peritoneal inflammation
p. peritoneum
p. pleura
p. pleural tissue
p. shunt
superior parietal lobule
temporal, occipital, p.

parietale
os p.

parietales
arteriae p.
nodi lymphoidei p.

parietes (*pl. of* paries)

parietooccipital
p. aphasia
p. approach
p. area
p. artery
p. branch of anterior cerebral artery
p. branch of posterior cerebellar artery
p. branch of posterior cerebral artery
p. craniotomy
p. dysfunction
p. fissure
p. hypoperfusion
marginal branch of parietooccipital sulcus
p. region
p. suture

parietooccipitalis
arcus p.
arteria p.
arteriae p.

parieto-occipital-temporal junction

parietopontine fiber

parietotemporal area

Parinaud
P. oculoglandular conjunctivitis
P. oculoglandular syndrome
P. ophthalmoplegia

Parinaud-plus syndrome

Paris
P. classification
P. method
P. method for radium therapy
plaster of P.
plaster of Paris cast
plaster of Paris jacket

parity
p. bit
p. check
Mental Health Parity Act of 1998

park
P. aneurysm
p. bench position
Hart Park virus

Parker
Munro and Parker classification for laparoscopic hysterectomy

Parker-Kerr
P.-K. closed method of end-to-end enteroenterostomy

Parkes-Weber syndrome

parking
p. for handicapped
organ p.

Parkinson
P. crisis
P. dementia
P. dementia complex
P. disease
P. disease and lateral sclerosis-dementia complex
P. Disease Quality of Life Scale
P. Disease Questionnaire
early-onset Parkinson disease
P. facies
idiopathic Parkinson disease
P. mask
P. rigidity
P. sign
P. syndrome
P. tremor disorder
Unified Parkinson Disease Rating Scale

parkinsonian
p. crisis
p. dementia
p. dysarthria
p. facies
p. gait
p. movement disorder
p. reaction
p. syndrome

parkinsonism
autosomal recessive juvenile p.
drug-induced p.
postencephalitic p.
senile p.

parkinsonism-dementia complex

Parkinson-like
P.-l. facies
P.-l. tremor

Parkland
P. burn resuscitation formula
P. fluid requirement formula for burn patients
P. formula for fluid resuscitation for burn trauma
P. Hospital technique
P. Rapid Exam

Parks-Bielschowsky three-step head-tilt test

Parks hemorrhoidectomy

Park-Williams bacillus

parolfactory
anterior parolfactory sulcus
p. area
p. gyrus

paronychia
incision and drainage of p.
monilial p.

Paroo River virus

parosteal
bizarre parosteal osteochondromatous proliferation
p. bone lesion
p. chondrosarcoma
p. fasciitis

parotid
p. adenocarcinoma
p. bed
p. body
p. branch
p. bubo
p. cancer
p. capsule
p. carcinoma
p. collector
p. cyst
p. deep lobe
p. dissection
p. duct
p. duct ligation
p. duct transposition
p. enlargement
p. fascia
p. flow rate
p. fluid
p. gland
p. gland abscess
p. gland enlargement
p. gland exposure guideline
p. gland tuberculosis
p. hormone
human parotid lysozyme
p. lymph node
mouse parotid tumor virus

mucoepidermoid carcinoma of p.
opening of left parotid duct
pretragal parotid gland
p. sialography
p. tenderness
p. tumor
p. vein

parotidea
oophoritis p.
orchitis p.

parotis

parotitis
acute suppurative p.
p. phlegmonosa

parous
p. cervix
p. introitus

parovarian
p. cyst
p. cystadenocarcinoma

paroxysm
febrile p.
involuntary general p.
malarial p.

paroxysmal
p. aciduria
p. alpha activity
p. anal hyperkinesis
p. ataxia
p. atrial fibrillation
atrial paroxysmal tachycardia
p. atrial tachycardia
p. atrioventricular nodal reciprocal tachycardia
atrioventricular reentrant paroxysmal tachycardia
p. auricular fibrillation
p. auricular tachycardia
p. AV block
benign paroxysmal positional vertigo
benign paroxysmal positioning nystagmus
benign paroxysmal torticollis
p. blinking
p. bursting
p. cerebral dysrhythmia
p. change
chronic paroxysmal hemicrania
p. cold hemoglobinuria
p. contraction
p. convulsion
p. cough
p. coughing
p. depolarization shift
p. depolarizing shift
p. discharge
p. drinking
p. dyspnea on exertion
p. dystonia
p. emotional state
p. epileptiform discharge
episodic paroxysmal hemicrania
p. evoked pain
p. exertional dyskinesia
p. exertion-induced dyskinesia
familial paroxysmal polyserositis
p. flushing
p. hand hematoma
p. hemicrania
p. high-voltage discharge
p. high-voltage slow wave
p. hypercyanotic attack
p. hypersexuality
p. hypersomnia
p. hypertension
p. hyperthermia
p. hypnogenic dyskinesia
p. hypothermia
p. hypoxic spell
idiopathic paroxysmal cerebral dysrhythmia
p. junctional ventricular tachycardia
p. kinesigenic choreoathetosis
p. kinesigenic dyskinesia
p. localized hyperhidrosis
p. nocturnal dyspnea
p. nocturnal hemoglobinuria
p. nocturnal hemoglobinuria cell
nocturnal paroxysmal dystonia
nodal paroxysmal tachycardia
nodal reentrant paroxysmal tachycardia
p. nodal rhythm
p. nodal tachycardia
p. nonkinesigenic dyskinesia
p. pain disorder
p. palpitation
p. peritonitis
p. positional vertigo
pseudoperiodic lateralized paroxysmal discharge
recalcitrant benign paroxysmal positional vertigo
p. reentrant supraventricular tachycardia
p. rhabdomyolysis
p. sinus tachycardia
slow paroxysmal atrial tachycardia
specific paroxysmal discharge
p. stage
p. supraventricular arrhythmia
p. tachyarrhythmia

parrot
P. artery
P. atrophy
P. atrophy of newborn
Australian parrot feather
Australian parrot protein
p. beak
p. beak deformity
P. disease
p. feather
p. fever
p. foot
p. jaw
P. node
P. sign
p. tongue
P. ulcer

Parry
P. Creek virus
P. disease

Parry-Romberg disease

Parsonage-Turner disease

part
p. affected
affected p.'s
alveolar soft part sarcoma
anterior part of anterior commissure of brain
anterior part of diaphragmatic surface of liver
anterior part of pons
anterior part of tongue
anterior tibiotalar p.
anterior tibiotalar part of deltoid ligament
anterior tibiotalar part of medial ligament of ankle joint
anular part of fibrous digital sheath of digits of hand and foot
apex of petrous part of temporal bone
aryepiglottic part of oblique arytenoid muscle
ascending part of aorta
ascending part of duodenum
ascending part of trapezius muscle
atlantic part of vertebral artery
autonomic part of peripheral nervous system
body p.
certified distinct p.

part *(continued)*
p. of the electrocardio-graphic cycle representing atrial depolarization
p.'s of human body
human figure parts response
lumbar part of diaphragm
lymphatic ring of cardiac part of stomach
marginal part of orbicularis oris muscle
medial crus of the horizontal part of the facial canal
meningeal branch of cavernous part of internal carotid artery
meningeal branch of cerebral part of internal carotid artery
meningeal branch of intracranial part of vertebral artery
muscular coat of intermediate part of male urethra
muscular coat of spongy part of male urethra
muscular layer of intermediate part of male urethra
neural layer of optic part of retina
parietal border of squamous part of temporal bone
p.'s per billion
p.'s per hundred million
p.'s per trillion
presenting p.
presenting part of fetus
protrusion of fetal p.
soft parts giant cell tumor
spongy part of bone

partial
activated partial thromboplastin time
p. adactyly
p. adjustment
p. adrenalectomy
p. adrenocortical insufficiency
p. agenesis
p. agenesis of vermis
p. agglutinin
p. agonist
p. agonist activity
p. agonist-partial antagonist
p. aim
p. albinism
p. albinism with immunodeficiency
p. allosteric modulators
alveolar-arterial difference in partial pressure of oxygen
alveolar oxygen partial pressure
alveolar partial pressure of inhalational anesthetic
p. alveolectomy
alveolocapillary partial pressure gradient
p. amnesia
p. amputation
p. androgen insensitivity
p. androgen insensitivity
p. androgen insensitivity syndrome
p. androgen sensitivity
p. anencephaly
p. aneuploidy
p. ankylosis
p. anodontia
p. anomalous pulmonary veins
p. anomalous pulmonary venous connection
anomalous pulmonary venous connection, total or p.
p. anomalous pulmonary venous drainage
p. anomalous pulmonary venous return
p. anterior cerebral infarct
p. anterior circulation infarct
p. anterior circulation syndrome
anterior partial laryngectomy
p. antigen
p. aphalangia
p. arterial gas tension of carbon dioxide
arterial oxygen partial pressure
arterial partial pressure of CO_2
articulated partial denture
p. atrioventricular canal
p. atrioventricular canal defect
automated activated partial thromboplastin
p. auxiliary orthotopic liver transplantation
auxiliary partial orthotopic living donor transplantation
axial partial childhood cataract
p. baldness
benign partial epilepsy with centrotemporal spike
bilateral partial oophorectomy
bilateral partial salpingectomy
p. bile outflow obstruction
p. birth abortion
p. bladder denervation
p. blindness
p. blocking
p. body neutron activation
p. bony impaction
p. bowel obstruction
p. brain irradiation
brain tissue partial pressure of oxygen
p. breech extraction
p. bursal surface tear
cantilever fixed partial denture
p. cataract
p. central hypophysectomy
p. cleft palate
clinical partial response
p. colectomy
p. collapse of lung
p. combined immunodeficiency disorder
p. complex epilepsy
complex partial epilepsy
complex partial nocturnal seizure
complex partial status epilepticus
p. complex seizure
p. conjunctival flap
controlled partial rebreathing anesthesia method
p. corpus callosum agenesis
p. correlation
p. cricoid cleft
p. cricotracheal resection
p. cross dressing
p. cystectomy
p. delirium
p. delusion
p. denture
p. denture, distal extension
p. denture impression
p. denture prosthesis
p. denture prosthetics
p. denture retention
p. dentures
p. denture unit
difference in partial pressures of oxygen in mixed alveolar gas and mixed arterial blood
p. DiGeorge anomaly
p. disability
p. diskectomy
p. dislocation
p. dislodgement
p. duodenopancreatectomy
p. duplication
p. dural resection
p. emptying of stomach
p. encircling endocardial ventriculotomy
p. enterocele
p. epileptic seizure
p. epileptogenic discharge

p. ethmoidectomy
p. exchange transfusion
p. expiratory flow-static recoil curve
p. expiratory flow volume
p. external biliary diversion
p. face-sparing lipodystrophy
p. facetectomy
p. facial paralysis
p. fasciectomy
p. fasting
p. fibulectomy
fixed partial denture
p. flip angle imaging
p. form of DiGeorge syndrome
p. Fourier imaging
full upper denture, partial lower denture
p. fundoplication
gas partial pressure
p. gastrectomy
p. gastric resection
p. glossectomy
p. gonadal dysgenesis
good partial response
p. hand amputation
p. hearing loss
p. heart block
p. hemianopia
p. hemilaminectomy
p. hemimelia
p. hepatectomy
p. hepatic vascular exclusion
high partial pressure of oxygen
p. homonymous field defect
p. hospitalization
p. hospitalization program
p. hospital patient population
p. hospital setting
p. hospital treatment program
p. hydatidiform mole
p. 21-hydroxylase deficiency
p. hypopituitarism
p. hysterectomy
p. ileal bypass
p. impairment of conduction
p. insulin resistance
p. intestinal obstruction
p. isolation
p. keratoplasty
p. labioscrotal fusion
p. lamellar sclerouvectomy
laparoscopically assisted distal partial gastrectomy
laparoscopic bilateral partial salpingectomy
p. laryngopharyngectomy
p. leukonychia
p. linkage
p. lipoatrophy
p. lipodystrophy
p. liquid ventilation
living donor partial hepatectomy
p. lower denture
p. meniscectomy
millimeters partial pressure
p. monosomy 1p–22p
p. monosomy XP21, XP22
p. monosomy Xq
p. motor seizure
p. neck dissection
p. nodular transformation
p. nonprogressive stroke
p. nonrebreather oxygen mask
p. obstruction of bladder
p. omentectomy
p. ophthalmoplegia
p. ossicular replacement prosthesis
oxygen partial pressure
p. oxygen pressure in mixed venous blood
p. parenteral nutrition
patient in partial restraint
p. penetrating keratoplasty
permanent p.
p. permanent impairment
permanent partial disability
p. placenta previa
p. plasma exchange
poor partial response
p. pressure
p. pressure alveolar oxygen
p. pressure of arterial carbon dioxide
p. pressure arterial oxygen
p. pressure of carbon dioxide in arterial gas
p. pressure of carbon dioxide in mixed venous blood
p. pressure of end-tidal CO_2
p. pressure of inspiratory oxygen
p. pressure of intramuscular carbon dioxide
p. pressure of mesenteric venous carbon dioxide
p. pressure of nitrogen
p. pressure of oxygen
p. pressure tension of carbon dioxide, vein
p. pressure tension of oxygen, vein
p. pressure of water vapor
p. prophylaxis
p. prothrombin time
prothrombin time and partial thromboplastin time
p. quadriplegia
p. reaction of degeneration
p. rebreathing mask
refractory anemia with partial myeloblastosis
p. reinforcement
p. reinforcement extinction effect
p. remission
removable partial denture
repeated partial asphyxia
p. resection
p. resection of stomach
p. response
p. saturation spin echo
p. sclerectasia
p. seizures with or without generalized tonic-clonic seizures
p. shoulder
p. small bowel obstruction
p. splenic embolization
strong partial maternal behavior
p. subligamentous calcification
temporary partial disability
p. thromboplastin time
p. thromboplastin time control
p. throw surgeon's knot
p. thyroidectomy
p. thyroid-stimulating hormone hyporesponsiveness
touchdown partial weightbearing
transcutaneous partial pressure of oxygen
p. TSH hyporesponsiveness
p. upper and lower dentures
p. veneer crown
p. venous gas tension of oxygen
p. villous atrophy
p. weightbearing
whole-blood partial thromboplastin time
p. zona dissection
p. zona drilling
p. zonal dissection

partially

p. amputated
cystic, partially differentiated nephroblastoma
p. dissolved gutta-percha
p. duplicated ureter
p. edentulous dental arch
p. edentulous jaw
p. follicular
p. functional neutrophil
p. impacted wisdom teeth

partially *(continued)*
lower partially edentulous
p. muscular
patient partially improved
p. pure human leukocyte interferon
p. sighted
p. unexplained sudden infant death syndrome
upper partially edentulous

partial-reinforcement effect

partial-thickness
p.-t. burn
p.-t. corneal laceration
p.-t. craniectomy
p.-t. flap
p.-t. trephination

participating
trained participating father birth
trained participating husband birth

participation
condition of p.
family participation unit
hospital p.

particle
p. accelerator
p. agglutination test
alpha p.
antisignal recognition particle antibody
p. approach
aspiration of food p.
p. beam
p. beam radiation therapy
p. beam radiosurgery
ciliary particle transport
p. concentration fluorescence immunoassay
coronavirus-like p.
count median diameter of p.'s
degree of fineness of abrasive p.'s
p. domain
electron-dense iron-containing p.
electron transport p.
human intracisternal A-type p.
intracisternal A p.
kinetic energy of a p.
latex p.
latex particle agglutination inhibition
low-energy charged p.
mascara particle inclusion
mass median diameter of p.'s
mean particle size
millions of particles per cubic foot of air
polystyrene latex p.
ratio of magnetic moment of a particle to Bohr magneton
remnant-like lipoprotein p.
reversed passive latex particle agglutination
ribosome-like p.
sickle-shaped particle cell
signal recognition p.
p. size distribution
small spherical p.
p. transport time
virus-like p.
weakly interacting massive p.

particle-enhanced turbidimetric inhibition immunoassay

particle-induced x-ray emission

particular complex

particulate
p. arterial embolization
p. cancellous bone graft
p. cancellous bone and marrow
p. component
p. crystalline material
p. crystalline material deposition
p. debris
p. echo
p. embolization
fine suspended p.
high-efficiency particulate air filter
high-efficiency particulate arresting
p. matter
p. matter less than 10 micrometers diameter
p. organic carbon
p. organic nitrogen
p. retinopathy
suspended particulate matter
total particulate matter
total suspended p.
ultralow particulate air

Partington syndrome

partita
patella p.

partition
atrial p.
p. chromatography
p. coefficient
low blood gas p.
reversed phase ion-pair p.

partly soluble

partner
p. gene
nonmonogamous p.
P. Relationship Inventory

Partnership for Caring

Partridge band

Partsch chisel

part-time occlusion eye patch

parturient
p. apoplexy
p. canal
p. fever

parturition
after p.

party
cocktail party patter
other party liability

parvilocular
p. cyst
p. cystoma

Parvin gravity technique

parvo
serum parvo virus-like virus

parvocellular
p. cell
p. division
p. neuron
p. pathway

parvo-like virus

parvovirus
p. B19 DNA
p. B19 IgG antibody
p. B19 IgM antibody
p. B19 infection
p. B19 neutralizing antibody assay
p. B19 red cell aplasia
p. B19 serology
canine p.
human p.
p. infection
maternal parvovirus fetalis
porcine p.

parvovirus-associated arthritis

parvus alternans

Pascal-Suttle Test psychiatry

Pascheff conjunctivitis

Pasini
atrophoderma of Pasini and Pierini

Pasini-Pierini idiopathic atrophoderma

pass
assessment adjustment p.
p. coaxially
family assessment adjustment p.
first p.
high pass filter
inability to pass urine
leave on p.
number of needle p.'s
out on p.
outside p.
patient released on overnight p.
recirculating single p.
therapeutic p.
therapeutic home p.
weekend p.

passage
adiabatic fast p.
air passage become inflamed
arteriovenous passage time
attempted passage of instrument
p. of bile
blocked breathing p.
blocked nasal p.
block passage of bile
p. of blood
p. of catheter
p. of clot
p. comprehension
constriction of breathing p.'s
p. of dark brown urine
p. of flatus
p. of flatus per vagina
foreign body in air p.
free air p.
high cell p.
inflamed nasal p.
lining of nasal p.
narrowing of bronchiolar p.'s
nasal passage inflammation
obstructed nasal p.
obstruction of air p.
p., power, and passenger
p. of sound
p. of stone
p. of tissue

passaged
cell p.

Passavant fold

passed
barium passed through esophagus into stomach
catheter passed with ease
forceps passed up through incision
scope passed per ora
p. through esophagus into stomach
p. with ease
p. without difficulty

passenger
passage, power, and passenger

passer
curved p.

passing
closed-loop system passing electrode
p. fecal material
p. flatus
p. gas
p. of kidney stone

passion
crime of p.

passionelle
attitude p.

passivated polymethyl methacrylate

passive
p. accessory intervertebral movements
p. accessory motion test
p. accommodation
active and passive range of motion
p. administration
p. agglutination
p. aggression
p. aggressive
p. algolagnia
p. alloimmune thrombocytopenia
p. alveolar molding appliance
p. analysis
p. anaphylaxis
p. Arthus reaction
artificial passive immunity
p. assistance exercise
p. assistance range of motion
p. atelectasis
p. avoidance
p. avoidance reaction
p. behavior
p. bilingualism
p. castration complex
p. chest drainage
p. chest expansion
p. clot
p. congestion
p. congestive failure
continuous anatomical passive exerciser
continuous passive motion device
continuous passive motion
continuous passive motion machine
p. cutaneous anaphylactic reaction
p. cutaneous anaphylaxis
p. cutaneous anaphylaxis test
p. dependence
p. diffusion
p. dorsiflexion
p. duction
p. eruption
p. euthanasia
p. exercise
p. extension
p. external rewarming
p. flexion
p. flexion of leg
p. forced duction test
forced passive full forward flexion
forced passive internal rotation
full passive movements
p. gliding technique
p. head-up tilt test
p. hemagglutination
p. hemagglutination inhibition
p. hemagglutination test
p. Heymann nephritis
p. humoral immunotherapy
p. hyperemia
p. hyperemia of retina
p. hyperpolarizing potential
p. illusion
p. immunity
p. immunization
p. immunization therapy
p. immunoprophylaxis
p. immunotherapy
p. incontinence
infant passive hand
p. influence
p. intervertebral motion
p. length-tension curve
mixed reverse passive antiglobulin hemagglutination
p. movement
p. physiological intervertebral movements
p. prehension orthosis
p. pulmonary hypertension
p. resistance exercise
reversed passive hemagglutination
reversed passive hemagglutination by miniature centrifugal fast analysis
reversed passive hemagglutination reaction

passive *(continued)*
reversed passive latex particle agglutination
reverse passive anaphylaxis
p. ROM
p. smoke exposure
p. therapy
p. tobacco smoke
total passive motion
p. treatment
p. tremor
p. venous congestion

passive-aggressive
p.-a. acting out
p.-a. behavior
p.-a. feature
p.-a. personality
p.-a. personality disorder

passive-dependent personality

passively
neck passively flexed
p. congested lung tissue

passive-motion

passivity
p. in anger expression
p. delusion
p. and inaction

passover humidifier

Passport disposable injection system

past
p. alcoholism
p. behavior
Current and P. Psychopathology Scales
p. dental history
p. event
p. experience
p. head injury
p. history noncontributory
p. history not remarkable
p. medical history
p. medical history noncontributory
p. medical history unremarkable
p. medical illness
p. menstrual period
noncontributory past history
noncontributory past medical history
p. ocular history
p. pertinent history
p. pointing
p. relevant history
p. relevant work
p. sleepwalker
p. social history
p. surgical history

paste
absorbable collagen p.
anchovy paste abscess
bismuth-iodoform-paraffin p.
p. carrier
Luride acidulated phosphate fluoride p.
methyl cellulose p.
oatmeal-tomato paste agar
skin exposure reduction paste against chemical warfare agent

Pasteur
P. Culture Collection
P. effect
P. Institute bacillus Calmette-Guérin vaccine

Pasteurella
Pasteurella multocida osteomyelitis
Pasteurella species taxon 16

pasteurization
high temperature-short time pasteurization
low-temperature holding pasteurization

Pastia
P. line
P. sign

pastoral
p. care
p. counseling
p. counselor
p. help

past-pointing test

pasty-looking patient

Pata virus

patch
alkali patch test
p. amnesia
anterior sandwich patch technique
p. aortoplasty
aortoplasty with patch graft
ash leaf p.
p. of atelectasis
atopy patch test
autologous patch graft
autologous pericardial p.
binocular eye p.
blood patch injection
cardiovascular patch graft
p. clamp
p. clamp electrophysiology
p. clamping
p. clamp technique
p. crinkling
dynamic aortic p.
p. electrode
epidural blood p.
epidural blood patch anesthetic technique
p. esophagoplasty
p. Gore-Tex graft
p. graft angioplasty
p. graft urethroplasty
gray p.'s
keratotic p.
lobular patch of atelectasis
lyophilized dural p.
maternal blood clot patch therapy
Minitran P.
negative patch test
nicotine patch therapy
nicotine skin p.
nicotine transdermal p.
Nitrodisc P.
Nitro-Dur P.
occlusive patch test
onlay patch anastomosis
open patch test
oval eye p.
part-time occlusion eye p.
peau d'orange p.
Peyer p.
p. prosthesis
red patch or blister on arm
p. skin test
TB patch test
p. technique
p. test for allergy
p. test for tuberculosis
thick, red itchy patch of skin
transdermal nicotine p.
tuberculosis patch test
wearing patch on arrival
white patches from anemia

patched
both eyes p.
left eye p.
right eye p.

patching
pressure p.

patchy
p. alveolar opacity
p. anterior stromal infiltrate
p. area
p. area of bronchopneumonia
p. area of consolidation
p. area of density
p. area of fibrosis
p. area of pneumonia

p. area of pneumonic consolidation
p. atelectasis
p. atrophy
p. atrophy of renal cortex
p. baldness
p. chronic inflammatory infiltrate
p. colitis
p. colonic ulcer
p. colonic ulceration
p. distribution of tracer
p. infiltration
p. infiltration of medullary parenchyma
p. infiltrative process
p. interstitial fibrosis
p. pneumonia
p. pneumonic infiltrate
p. purpuric hemorrhage
p. window defect

patella, pl. **patellae**
p. alta
apex of head of p.
articular surface of p.
p. baja
p. ballottement
p. bone
chondromalacia patellae
p. cup
p. disease
dislocation of p.
ear, patella, short stature syndrome
nail patella syndrome
p. partita
subluxation of p.
p. tendon socket
tripartite fracture of p.

patellar
p. advancement
p. affection
p. alignment
p. anastomosis
p. apprehension sign
p. apprehension test
arthroscopy-assisted patellar tendon substitution
autogenous patellar ligament graft
autogenous patellar tendon reconstruction
p. bar
p. bone-tendon-bone autograft
p. bursa
p. bursitis
p. cartilage thickness
p. chondromalacia
p. clonus
p. clunk syndrome
p. contour
p. dislocation
p. dislocation cast
p. dome
p. edge
p. facet cartilage
p. fat pad
p. femoral syndrome
p. fossa
p. fossa of vitreous
p. fracture
p. glide
p. glide test
p. groove
p. inhibition test
p. jerk
p. ligament
medial transplantation of patellar tendon insertion
p. prosthesis
p. reflex
p. release
p. stabilizing brace
p. synovial fold
p. tenderness
p. tendon
p. tendon advancement
p. tendon autograft
p. tendon bearing
p. tendon-bearing cast prosthesis
p. tendon-bearing orthosis
p. tendon-bearing–supracondylar-suprapatellar prosthesis
p. tendon-bearing suspension
p. tendon graft donor site
p. tendon insertion
p. tendon reflex
p. tendon stabilization
p. tendon suspension
p. tendon transfer
p. tendon transplant
p. tendon transposition
vascularized patellar tendon

patellofemoral
p. alignment
p. angle
p. articular cartilage
p. articulation
p. brace
p. compartment
p. congruence
p. crepitation
p. degenerative arthritis
p. disease
p. disorder
p. dysarthrosis
p. dysfunction
p. dysplasia
p. groove
p. groove cartilage
p. joint
p. joint syndrome
p. malalignment
p. malalignment pain
medial patellofemoral ligament
p. pain syndrome

patency
arterial p.
p. of artery
catheter p.
coronary artery bypass graft p.
graft p.
interval patency rate
p. of vein

patent
p. airway
anatomically patent foramen ovale
p. anus
p. bifurcation
p. blue V dye
p. branch
p. bronchus sign
p. canal of Nuck
p. ductus
p. ductus arteriosus
p. ductus venosus
p. fallopian tube
p. foramen ovale
p. gastrojejunostomy
p. iridectomy
p. medicine
p. neural foramina
p. opening
p. opening for bile drainage
p. orifice
p. os
p. pancreatic duct
p. blue V
p. processus vaginalis
p. renal agenesis
p. urachus
p. ureter
p. vessel
p. vitelline duct
widely p.

paternal
p. abuse
p. age
p. attitude
p. aunt
p. behavior
p. care
p. competency

paternal *(continued)*
p. deprivation
p. desertion
p. drive
p. grandfather
p. grandmother
p. great-grandfather
p. great-grandmother
p. indifference
p. karyotype
p. meiosis I, II
noninherited paternal antigen
p. origin

paternally contributing

paternity
p. blues
p. index
p. testing

Paterson-Brown-Kelly syndrome

Paterson-Kelly syndrome

Paterson syndrome

Patey radical mastectomy

path
p. analysis
effective path length
length of p.
mean free p.
optical path difference

pathogen
acquired immune deficiency syndrome primary p.
airborne p.
culture negative for p.'s
enteric p.
fungal intracellular p.
Gram-positive surgical p.
multiple opportunistic pathogen infection
nosocomial p.
novel p.
opportunistic p.
OSHA blood-borne pathogen standard
specific pathogen free
Surveillance and Control of P.'s of Epidemiologic Importance

pathogenesis dynamic

pathogenic
p. care
p. dystonia
p. factor
p. family pattern
grossly pathogenic care
p. microorganism
potentially pathogenic environmental mycobacterial
p. strain

pathognomonic
p. Askanazy cell
p. black eschar
p. fantasy
p. Koplik spot
p. radial keratoneuritis
p. symptom

pathologic
p. abnormality
p. absorption
p. alcohol intoxication
p. amenorrhea
p. amputation
p. anatomy
p. anthropology
p. apnea
p. atrophy
p. barrier
p. behavior
p. breast discharge
p. calcification
p. care
p. cause
p. cell
p. cell death
p. character formation
p. characteristic
p. classification
p. communication
p. compression fracture
p. condition
p. consultation
p. correlation
p. cupping
p. diagnosis
p. dislocation
p. drowsiness
p. drug intoxication
p. drug intoxication drug psychosis
p. drunkenness
p. emotionality
p. entity
p. examination
p. fallacy
p. feature
p. finding
p. gambler
p. gambling
p. gambling disorder
p. glycosuria
p. grief reaction
p. grieving
p. guilt
healthy patient with localized pathologic process
p. histology
p. hypercortisolemia
p. hyperreflexia
p. insult
p. myopia
neoplastic pathologic lesion
nonneoplastic pathologic lesion
no pathologic diagnosis
p. parathyroid disease
p. secondary erythrocytosis
p. spontaneous activity

pathological
alcohol pathological intoxication
p. apnea
p. cavus
p. change
p. characteristic
p. communication
p. crying
p. depression
p. diagnosis
p. dissociation
p. drowsiness
p. emotionality
p. endocrine tissue
p. examination
p. feature
p. finding
p. gambling
p. gynecomastia
p. habit disorder
p. hair pulling
healthy patient with localized pathological process
history of pathological use
p. homophobia
p. report
p. specimen
p. tissue examination
p. tumor, nodes, metastases staging of cancer

pathologically confirmed complete remission

pathologist
speech and language p.
speech-language p.

pathology
association deficit p.
bone or joint p.
clinical p.
p. examination
forensic p.
p. laboratory
no bone p.

no evidence of p.
organic colon p.
p. point
speech and language p.
speech pathology and audiology
p. and staging
Systematized Nomenclature of P.

pathometer attachment

pathophysiologic

clinical manifestations, etiologic factors, anatomic involvement, pathophysiologic features
p. factor
p. mechanism

pathophysiological

p. basis
p. cascade
p. condition

pathophysiology

p. of delirium
p. and natural history

pathosis

apical p.
attitudinal p.

Pathum Thani virus

pathway

accessory conduction p.
afferent visual p.
alternative pathway of complement cascade
antegrade fast p.
anterior cingulate p.
anterior internodal p.
anterior visual p.
anterior visual pathway dysfunction
antiapoptotic signaling p.
arachidonic acid p.
ascending pathway of pain projection
atrioventricular p.
classical p.
Embden-Meyerhof glycolytic p.
Entner-Doudoroff metabolic p.
final common p.
hexose monophosphate p.
leukotriene pathway inhibitor
magnocellular visual p.
MAP kinase p.
mercapturic acid p.
mesocortical dopamine p.
mesolimbic dopamine p.
mitochondrial glutamate dehydrogenase p.
mitogen-activated protein kinase p.
mucociliary drainage p.
Notch signaling p.
pentose phosphate p.
perforin killing p.
porphyrin biosynthetic p.
purified alternate p.
recombinant human tissue factor pathway inhibitor
reentrant p.
tissue factor pathway inhibitor

patient

p. ability to perform
p. abuse
p. abusive and hostile
abusive and hostile p.
p. acting inappropriately
p. acutely ill
adequate patient care
p. admitted for evaluation and workup
p. admitted for observation
p. admitted for observation and treatment
p. admitted and transfused with whole blood
p. admitted with active infection
adverse patient occurrences
p. advocate
p. afebrile
AIDS patient care
airway obstruction in conscious p.
airway obstruction in unconscious p.
p. alert and cooperative
p. alert and oriented
p. alert to space, time, and person
p. ambulates with assistance
p. ambulates with walker
ambulatory patient group
ambulatory peritoneal dialysis p.
p. analgesia
p. anesthetized
p. anorectic
p. anorexic
p. appetite is good
p. appetite is poor
artery-clogging plaque in atherosclerosis p.
ARTMA virtual p.
assessing severity: age of patient, systems involved, stage of disease, complications, response to therapy
P. Assessment Program
asymptomatic hemodialysis p.
p. at complete bed rest
p. at high-risk of exposure
Austin-Kartush group C patient related to ossiculoplasty
p. authentication
authorized walk-in p.
autologous patient donor
autologous T lymphocytes stimulated with the p. tumor-specific mutated RAS peptides
p. autonomy
average daily patient load
p. awake, alert, and cooperative
p. bedridden
p. to be followed as an outpatient
p. bill of rights
p. brain dead
p. burned beyond recognition
p. to call
caloric requirements for burn p.'s
p. in cardiac arrest
p. in cardiac or respiratory distress
p. in cardiogenic shock
p. care
p. care aide
p. care assistant
p. care coordinator
caregiver abandoning p.
caregiver nutures p.
P. Care Information System
p. care plan
p. care report
p. care unit
p. in catatonic state
centralized cancer patient data system
central patient station
p. chemical history
p. chronically ill
p. in chronic pain
p. combative and agitated
p. complains of
p. in complete restraint
p. completes independent transfers
p. compliance
computer-based patient record
computerized patient record
p. concealed illness
p. condition deteriorated
p. condition stabilized
p. confused
p. constipated
p. contact record
p. continent
p. contract

patient *(continued)*
p. cooperative
p. cyanotic
p. data bank
P. Data Management Systems
p. data system
p. day
p. deeply comatose
p. defervesced
p. dehydrated
p. delay
p. delivered congenitally deformed infant
p. delivered normal infant
p. demonstration
p. denies complaints
depressed heart attack p.
p. dialyzed
p. diaphoretic
p. difficult to arouse
difficult-denture p.
direct patient care
p. discharged ambulatory
p. discharged from hospital
p. discharged in good condition
p. discharged to home care
p. discharged improved
p. discharged to nursing home
p. discharged to office followup
p. discharged to skilled nursing facility
p. discharged to SNF
discharge patient after period of observation
p. dismissed in good condition
p. disquietude
p. distress alarm
p. does ADL with supervision
p. drug history
drug-related adverse patient event
dual diagnosis p.
p. dysarthric
p. dysphagic
p. dyspneic
p. edentulous
p. education
p. education on drug abuse
p. education program
effective patient life
electronic patient medical record
p. emotionally ill
p. empirically treated
essential hypertensive p.
established p.
p. evaluated
p. evaluation center
P. Evaluation Grid
p. evaluation rating scale
p. examined
exercises for heart p.
exercises for patient in home
p. exhibited muscle guarding
p. exhibits overt hostility
p. expired
p. exposure guideline
p. expressed guilt feeling
p. failed to respond
p. faking illness
p. febrile
p. feeling hostile
p. feels guilty
p. feels isolated
p. file
p. followed on an outpatient basis
p. functional ability
p. gags reflexively
p. global assessment of disease activity
p. goal
p. guide to medication
p. has constipation
p. has diarrhea
p. has difficulty swallowing
p. has disorientation and hallucinations
p. has fear of hospital
p. has flat affect
p. has forgetfulness, irritability, and confusion
p. has good rapport with others
p. has headache
p. has heartburn
p. has indigestion
p. has insomnia
p. has labored breathing
p. has natural immunity to hepatitis B virus
p. has nocturia
p. has no purposeful movement
p. has polydipsia
p. has polyuria
p. has whiplash injury
healthy patient with localized pathological process
healthy patient with localized pathologic process
heart attack p.
heart transplant p.
p. heavy drinker
help patient achieve independence
p. hemiplegic
p. heparinized
p. hesitancy
p. highly compulsive
p. high-strung
p. history
p. home environment
p. hospital course turbulent
p. hospitalized
p. hospitalized for workup
p. hyperactive
p. hypersensitive
p. hypersensitive to aspirin
p. hyperventilating
p. hypoglycemic
p. hypotensive
p. hysterical
p. identification bracelet
p. immature
immediate patient care
p. immobilized
immune depressed p.
p. immune to hepatitis B infection
p. immune response
p. immunocompromised
immunocompromised cancer p.
p. immunodepressed
p. immunosuppressed
p. impacted
p. implant
p. improved
p. inappropriate
p. inarticulate
p. incapacitated of caring for self
p. inclusion criteria
p. incoherent
p. incompetent
p. incontinent of feces
p. incontinent of stool
p. incontinent of urine
p. incurably ill
p. independent in activities of daily living
p. independent in ADLs
p. independent in ambulation
p. independent in bathing with cueing
p. independent in boosting and rolling
p. independent in dressing
p. independent in feeding
p. independent in lower body dressing
p. independent in upper body dressing
p. independent with bathing
p. independent with small based quad cane

p. infectious
p. information leaflet
p. insomniac
p. intense
p. interest
p. intolerant to aspirin therapy
p. intoxicated
p. irrational
p. irritable
p. irritable and jumpy
p. is hypertensive
p. is hyperventilating
p. is hypoglycemic
p. is menopausal
isolation of p.
p. is a poor surgical risk
p. is postmenopausal
p. is prepped and draped
p. is prepped and draped for surgery
p. is prepped and draped in usual sterile fashion
p. juvenile diabetic
p. in labor
p. laughs inappropriately
p. left-handed
legally incompetent p.
p. managed medically
p. management issue
p. management problem
master patient index
McMaster-Toronto Arthritis P. Reference
Medical Audiologic Tinnitus P. Protocol
p. medical history
p. medical instruction
p. medication instruction
p. medication profile
mental health p.
p. mentally alert
p. mentally ill
p. monitored
mood disorder p.
moribund patient not expected to live
p. multigravida
National Lung Transplant P. Association
near patient test
p. needs identified
p. needs minimal assistance for wheelchair mobility
new p.
new patient set-up
p. noncompliant
p. noncompliant with medication
nonpsychotic Alzheimer p.
p. nonresponsive
p. not circumcised
not on p.
p. nulligravida
p. nulliparous
number equal to one; single patient trial
obese hypertensive p.
p. obeys commands
p. obtunded
p. on a high
p. on ventilator
orders accompanying patient on admission
p. oriented to person, place and time
P. Outcomes Research Team
p. overdosed with hallucinogen
p. package insert
Parkland fluid requirement formula for burn p.'s
partial hospital patient population
p. partially improved
p. in partial restraint
per patient per month
p. physically active
p. physically impaired
physical status patient classifications
please turn the patient over
postinfarct p.
Postural Assessment Scale for Stroke P.'s
p. prepped and positioned
p. previously hospitalized
private p.
professional simulated p.
p. profile
progressive patient care
p. progress record
p. pronounced dead
p. pulls hair
quality of patient care
p. rapidly intubated
P. Rated Anxiety Scale
Rating Form of IBD P. Concerns
p. reached maximum hospital benefit
p. receiving respiratory assistance
p. recovery plan
p. regained active status
p. rehydrated
p. relations
p. released against medical advice
p. released in care of relative
p. released on overnight pass
p. release form
renal impaired p.
renal transplant p.
p. report form
p. requesting admission
p. responded to treatment
p. responded verbally
p. responsive to noxious stimuli
p. responsive to painful stimuli
p. responsive to verbal command
p. restrained with vest
p. to return
p. right-handed
p. satisfaction questionnaire
secretion spills from hepatitis p.'s
p. serum
Sheehan P. Rated Anxiety Scale
single patient system
p. spiked a fever
p. spilled protein
p. spilled sugar
p. in stable condition
stress in hypertensive p.
p. suffered respiratory arrest
p. symptomatic
p. symptomatically improved
p. symptom-free
p. taught deep breathing
p. terminally ill
p. termination record
p. time
p. tolerated full course of radiation
p. tolerated the procedure well
p. tolerated traction well
p. totally inoperable
total patient care
p. transfer form
p. transferred to nursing home
p. transferred to skilled nursing facility
p. transferred to SNF
p. transfers with standby assistance
p. treated conservatively
p. treated empirically
p. treated in hospital
p. treated initially
p. treated initially with intravenous fluids
p. treated medically
p. treated for smoke inhalation
p. treated with comfort care only
p. treated with supportive care

patient *(continued)*
p. treatment file
p. under self-hypnosis
unique patient number
p. unknown acquired immune deficiency syndrome carrier
p. unsteady in gait
p. up ad lib
p. up in chair
upon arrival patient found
p. very disturbed
very important p.
virtual patient record
viruses isolated from p.'s
p. vomited large quantities of blood
p. vomiting blood
p. waiting
walk-in p.
p. weak, hypotensive and unresponsive
p. weaned from respirator
p. wears dentures
weighted patient care unit
p. weight in kilograms
p. well developed
p. well developed, well nourished
p. well hydrated
p. well nourished
p. wheezing
p.'s with diabetes
p. with incapacitating systemic disease
p. with mild to moderate systemic disease
p. with severe systemic disease limiting activity but not incapacitating
young adult chronic p.

patient-centered
p.-c. access to secure systems online
p.-c. approach

patient-controlled
p.-c. analgesia anesthetic technique
p.-c. analgesic
p.-c. epidural analgesia
p.-c. epidural anesthesia
p.-c. intranasal analgesia
p.-c. sedation

patient-focused care

patient-heated serum

patient-operated selector mechanism

patient-oriented evidence

patient-physician relationship

Patois virus

Paton
P. corneal trephine
P. line
P. transplant speculum

Patrick
P. cross-leg maneuver
P. drill
P. sign
P. test

patter
cocktail party p.

pattern
Activity P. Indicator
adipofascial axial pattern cross-finger flap
advanced sleep-phase p.
p. of aggression
alternative patterns of complement
p. analysis
anhaustral colonic gas p.
anomalous parental vocal p.
p. of antisocial behavior
anular tear p.
AO fracture p.
p. arborization
arterial deficiency p.
artery-like pattern of enhancement
atherogenic low-density lipoprotein pattern B phenotype
attritional pattern change
atypical vessel colposcopic p.
autosomal dominant p.
axial pattern scalp flap
axial pattern vascularized skin flap
behavior p.
binge eating p.
bizarre eating p.
bizarre gait p.
bowel gas p.
p. of brain electrical activity
brain wave p.
breast parenchymal p.
p. of breathing
p. of cancer spread
p. of care
p.'s of care study
change in bladder p.
change in bowel p.
circadian testosterone p.
computerized pattern generator
concentric circle pattern on breast self-examination
p. of conduct
cribriform growth p.
delusional thought p.
p. of destruction
destructive thought p.
p. of detachment
p. discrimination
p. discrimination perimetry
p. disruption point
p. distortion amblyopia
p. of distribution
disturbed sleep p.
p. of drainage
p. dystrophy
early repolarization p.
p. of electrical activity
electroencephalogram burst suppression p.
electronic speckle pattern interferometry
electrophoretic p.
p. electroretinogram
episodic pattern of binge eating
p. evoked retinal response
p. of expression
fasciocutaneous axial pattern flap
female pattern androgenetic alopecia
female pattern hair loss
fibrosing alopecia in a pattern distribution
fixed action p.
p. generator
habitual p.'s
p. of hallucinogen abuse
hyperemic mucosal p.
identical p.'s
image patterns of anxiety
p. of impulsivity
P.'s of Individual Change Scale
p. of inheritance
intestinal gas p.
intraventricular conduction p.
irregular breathing p.
L/H nodular p.
Likert-type response p.
linear branching p.
linguapalatal contact p.
lobular alveolar p.
localized electroencephalographic seizure p.
lymphatic drainage p.
male pattern androgenetic alopecia
male pattern baldness
male pattern hair loss
male pattern obesity
manipulation communication p.

mantle zone p.
marble bone p.
marginal zone p.
marking time p.
modify hearing p.'s
monitor p.
monoclonal B-cell p.
mood disorder with seasonal p.
Morse code p.
mosaic attenuation p.
mosaic duodenal mucosal p.
mucosal guideline p.
myxoid cell p.
NBT mosaic p.
neuromuscular gait pattern change
non-Alzheimer disease-related p.
nondefinitive p.
nonreassuring fetal heart beat p.
nonspecific bowel gas p.
nonspecific histologic p.
normal waking electroencephalogram p.
Norwood Classification of Male P. Baldness
nuclear dot p.
occupational ability p.
orthogonal-hole test p.
overlying branching p.
palm leaf p.
parenchymal breast p.
pathogenic family p.
peak latencies of pattern electroretinogram
pervasive pattern of instability
physiologic pattern release
plasmid pattern analysis
positive spike p.
precision encoder and pattern recognizer
preferred practice p.'s
p. recognition
reflex-inhibiting p.
p. reversal visual evoked potential
rhythmic inhibitory p.
scintillating speckled p.
Seasonal P. Assessment Questionnaire
segmental alveolar p.
shift in direction and pattern of brain electrical activity
sine wave p.
sleep patterns of insomniac
slow mitten p.
symmetrical sleep p.
tangential speech p.
upstroke pattern on apex cardiogram
variety of abuse patterns
p. visual-evoked response
wax p.

pattern-cut
p.-c. corneal graft
p.-c. corneal graft operation

patterned
p. alopecia
P. Elicitation Syntax Screening Test
p. homeopathy
p. leukoderma

pattern-evoked electroretinogram

patterning
Aston p.
p. exercise

pattern-shift visual-evoked response

patulous
p. anus
p. cardia
p. gastroesophageal junction
p. hiatus
p. introitus
p. urethral wall

pauciarticular
p. juvenile chronic arthritis
p. juvenile rheumatoid arthritis
p. onset

paucibacillary leprosy

paucicellular
p. area
p. collagen

pauciimmune
p. antineutrophil cytoplasmic antibody-associated glomerulonephritis
p. crescentic glomerulonephritis
p. glomerular nephritis

paucity
p. of bowel gas
congenital paucity of secondary synaptic clefts syndrome
p. of data
p. of expressive gestures
p. of findings
p. of gas
p. of interlobular bile ducts
nonsyndromic bile duct p.

Paufique
P. operation
P. synechiotomy
P. trephine

Paul
P. treatment

Paul-Bunnell
P.-B. antibody test
P.-B. test

Paul-Bunnell-Barrett test

Paulo
São Paulo fever
São Paulo typhus

pause
end-inspiratory p.
p. and squeeze technique

Pautler infusion cannula

Pautrier
P. abscess
P. microabscess

Pauwels
P. angle
P. femoral neck fracture classification
P. fracture

paving-stone degeneration

Pavlov reflex

Pavulon
pancuronium P.

Pavy disease

paw-like hand

***PAX2* gene**

***PAX8* gene**

Paxton disease

pay
did not p.

payment
ambulatory payment classification group
p. error prevention program
Outpatient Prospective P. System
request for p.

Payr
P. clamp method
P. disease
P. sign

PB-1 virus

PBCV-1 virus

PBHA
porous block hydroxyapatite

PBP1 virus

PBS1 virus

PC10
monoclonal antibody P.

PC84 virus

P.C.A. E-Series hip replacement
PCL-oriented placement
PCNA-labeling index
PC11NB
p55 component of the high-affinity interleukin-2
PCR-enzyme immunoassay
P4502D6
anticytochrome P4502D6 assay
-PD
NeuroCell-HD, -P.
4p deletion syndrome
PDGF
P. gene
P. protein
PDI-mediated disulfide bond reduction
PE1 virus
Peabody
P. Developmental Motor Activity Cards
P. Developmental Motor Scale
P. Individual Achievement Test
P. Picture Vocabulary Test-Revised
peace
serenity, tranquility, peace user's term for dimethoxymethylamphetamine
Peacekeeper cannula
peak
p. absorption spike
p. acid output
p. acid output after gastrin-releasing peptide
p. acid output after pentagastrin stimulation
p. acid output insulin-induced
p. acoustic gain
p. admittance
p. adult bone mass
p. airway pressure
p. amplitude
p. amplitude period
p. aortic flow velocity
aortic valve peak instantaneous gradient
arch peak area
p. area
arterial peak systolic pressure
automatic peak tracking
average peak noise
average peak velocity
baseline average peak velocity
p. behavioral effect
p. blood level
p. blood pressure
p. bone mass
p. broadening
p. clipping
common peak developed isovolumetric pressure
p. concentration
contraction peak force
p. cough flow
p. count density
Cupid's bow p.
p. diastolic filling rate
p. diastolic gradient
p. diastolic pressure
p. diastolic velocity
p. dP/dt
p. early diastolic filling velocity
early labeled p.
p. ejection rate
p. ejection time
p. ejection velocity
p. electron volt
p. emptying rate
p. end-expiratory pressure
p. equivalent sound pressure level
p. exercise
p. exercise oxygen consumption
p. exercise ventilation
p. experience
p. expiratory flow
p. expiratory flow rate
p. expiratory flow time
P. Fixation System
p. flow
p. flow measurement
p. flowmeter
p. flow meter
p. flow meter monitor
p. flow sensitivity
p. flow whistle
P. gait module
gentamicin peak level
p. growth velocity
p. heart rate
heart rate p.
p. height velocity
p. hyperemic average velocity
p. inflation pressure
p. inspiratory flow
p. inspiratory flow rate
p. inspiratory ventilator pressure
p. instantaneous gradient
insulin-induced peak acid output
p. isometric torque
p. jet flow rate
kilovoltage p.
p. kilovoltage
p. latencies of pattern electroretinogram
left ventricular peak filling rate
left ventricular peak systolic pressure
p. level
main portal vein peak velocity
p. maximum serum concentration
midshunt peak velocity
p. nasal inspiratory flow
p. negative pressure
p. occupancy time
p. oxygen uptake
p. pain intensity difference score
p. pepsin output
percent predicted peak expiratory flow
p. phrenic nerve activity
p. plasma concentration
p. reactive hyperemia blood flow
p. repetition frequency
p. respiratory ratio
right ventricular peak filling rate
p. scatter factor
p. secretory flow rate
p. serum level
sharp Bragg p.
spatial average temporal p.
spatial peak temporal average
spectral p.
spontaneous peak inspiratory force
standard peak dilution
p. systolic aortic pressure
p. systolic gradient pressure
p. systolic velocity
temporal p.
p. thyroid-stimulating hormone response
p. tidal expiratory flow
p. tidal inspiratory flow
time to p.
time to peak contrast
time of peak emptying rate of mouth
time of peak emptying rate of pharynx
time to peak expiratory flow
time to peak expiratory flow and total expiration time
time to peak filling rate
time of peak filling rate of esophagus
time to peak inspiratory flow

time to peak tension
time to peak tidal expiratory flow
p. transaortic valve gradient
p. and trough
p. and trough levels
p. TSH response
tumor peak systolic velocity
p. and valley
voltage p.
volume to peak expiratory flow and total expiratory volume
p. weight velocity
p. work capacity
p. work rate
Wright peak flowmeter

peak-dose
p.-d. choreoathetoid dyskinetic movement
p.-d. dyskinesia

peak-flow gauge

peak-to-peak
p.-t.-p. threshold

peak-to-resting-velocity ratio

peanut
p. agglutinin
p. implant

pear cataract

Pearce
P. coaxial irrigating/aspirating cannula
P. nucleus hydrodissector
P. trabeculectomy

pearl
autologous pearl fat graft
p. cell
p. cyst
p. diver's keratopathy
P. Drops
Elschnig p.
P. Index
necklace of p.'s
p. white mounds

pearly
p. body
p. CNS tumor
p. coronal papule
p. neoplasm
p. penile papule

pear-shaped
p.-s. body
p.-s. defect
p.-s. extension tube
p.-s. pupil

Pearson
P. attachment
P. attachment to Thomas splint
P. correlation
P. correlation coefficient
P. correlation coefficient pedantic
P. marrow-pancreas syndrome
P. syndrome

Pease-Allen Color test

Peaton virus

peau
p. de chagrin
p. d'orange
p. d'orange appearance
p. d'orange appearance of the breast
p. d'orange appearance in breast carcinoma
p. dórange in breast carcinoma
p. d'orange patch

Pebax counter unit

peccant humor

Peclet number

Pecquet
P. cistern
P. cisterna
P. duct
P. reservoir

pectate line

pecten
p. of anal canal
p. analis
p. band

pectinate
p. body
p. fiber
p. ligament
p. ligament of iridocorneal angle
p. ligament of iris
p. line
p. muscle
p. villi

pectineal
p. crural hernia
p. fascia
p. hernia
p. ligament
p. line
p. line of femur
p. line of pubis
p. muscle

pectineus muscle

pectin sugar

pectoral
p. and abdominal anterior cutaneous branch of intercostal nerve
anterior pectoral cutaneous branch of intercostal nerve
p. axillary lymph node
p. branch
p. branch of thoracoacromial artery
p. catheter
p. fascia
p. girdle
p. gland
p. groove
p. heart
p. muscle
p. reflex
p. region

pectoralis
p. fascia
p. major
p. major muscle
p. major myocutaneous flap
p. minor muscle
trapezoidal paddle pectoralis major myocutaneous flap

pectoriloquy
aphonic p.
whispering p.

pectoris
angina p.
stable angina p.
unstable angina p.
variant angina p.

pectus
p. bar
p. carinatum
p. carinatum deformity
p. deformity
p. excavatum
p. excavatum deformity
p. recurvatum

peculiar
p. behavior
macrocephaly with feeblemindedness and encephalopathy with peculiar deposits
mental and physical retardation, speech disorders, peculiar facies syndrome

Peczon
P. I/A cannula
P. I/A unit
P. I/A vectis

pedal
p. artery opacification
bilateral pedal pulses present
p. bone
carpal pedal spasm
p. control venography
p. disability benefit
p. edema
p. exerciser
foot pedal suction control
p. pulse
p. pulse not palpable
p. pulse palpable
p. pulse present
p. pulses equal and strong
p. pulse weak
p. spasm

pedantic
Pearson correlation coefficient p.

Pedersen hypothesis

pedestrian hit by motor vehicle

pediatric
p. acquired immunodeficiency syndrome
P. Acute Admission Severity classification
p. and adolescent epilepsy
Adolescent and P. Pain Tool Scale
p. advanced life support
advanced pediatric life support
P. AIDS Clinical Trial Group Protocol
p. airway
p. allergy
American P. Gross Assessment Record
p. analgesic
p. anesthesia system
p. anesthetic
p. aphakia
Assura pediatric pouch
P. Asthma Quality of Life Questionnaire
p. audiology
p. autoimmune neuropsychiatric diseases associated with streptococcal infection
p. autoimmune neuropsychiatric disorders associated with streptococcal infection
p. back pain
p. balloon
P. Behavior Scale
p. blade plate
p. bone rongeur
p. brain stem glioma
p. brainstem glioma
p. bronchiolitis
p. cancer
p. carcinoma
p. cardiology
p. cardiovascular surgery
p. cocktail
p. colonoscope
p. colonoscopy
p. critical care center
P. Crohn Disease Activity Index
p. cryptococcal epididymoorchitis
p. dentistry
p. dermatology
developmental p.'s
p. dose
p. dosing information
P. Early Elemental Examination
p. emergency department
emergency department approval for p.'s
p. emergency medicine
p. endocrinology
p. endoscopy
p. esophagogastroduodenoscopy
p. esophagoplasty
P. Evaluation of Disability Inventory
P. Examination of Educational Readiness
P. Extended Examination at Three
p. fatty marrow
p. feeding tube
p. fiberscope
p. fibroxanthoma
p. flatfoot
p. forceps
p. gastroscope
p. gonococcal conjunctivitis
p. gonococcal infection
p. gynecology
p. headrest
p. hemangioma
p. hematology-oncology
p. hepatojejunostomy
p. hernia
p. hypertension
p. infectious disease
developmental screening test
p. intensive care unit
p. lid speculum
P. Liver Transplant-Specific Scale
p. lung surgery
p. lupus nephropathy
p. lymphoma
p. mass
maternal pediatric unit
p. multivitamin infusion
p. myasthenia
p. myelodysplasia
National Association of P. Nurse Associates and Practitioners
p. neonatology
p. nephrology
p. ocular sarcoidosis
Ohio pediatric tent with compressed air
Ohio pediatric tent with oxygen
p. orthopedic examination
Pediatric Overall Performance Category scale
Pediatric Risk of Mortality Score
p. pneumogram
p. radiology
regional pediatric pulmonary center
p. renal osteodystrophy
p. sedation unit
p. special care unit
p. spectrum of disease
P. Speech Intelligibility Test
Standards for P. Immunization
p. surgical intensive care
P. Symptom Checklist
p. three-mirror laser lens
P. Trauma Scale
P. Trauma Score
p. urine collector
p. vitrectomy lens set
p. walk-in clinic

Pediatrician infant dietary supplement

pedicle
p. anatomy
p. of arch of vertebra
p. axis angle
p. bone graft
p. cone
p. cortex disruption
p. diameter
p. dimension
p. entrance point
p. erosion
p. evaluation
p. fat graft
p. flap
p. flap operation
p. flap urethroplasty
p. fracture
gastric augment and single pedicle tube
intact p.

inverted Y and spleen p.
p. of lung
p. tip amputation
tubed pedicle flap

pedicled
p. buccal fat pad flap
p. cartilage graft
p. colon transfer
p. compound rib-latissimus dorsi osteomusculocutaneous flap
p. endoscopic latissimus dorsi harvest
p. enteric donor site
p. fascia lata musculocutaneous flap
p. fibular transfer
p. galeal frontalis flap
p. groin flap

pedicular fixation

pediculated flap

pediculosis
capitis p.
p. capitis
p. corporis
p. corpus
p. palpebrarum
p. pubis
p. vestimenti

pediculous blepharitis

pediculus arcus vertebrae

pedigree
p. analysis
p. chart

pedis
arcus pedis longitudinalis
arcus pedis transversalis
arteria arcuata p.
dorsalis p.
dorsalis pedis pulse
malum perforans p.
moccasin-type tinea p.
musculus abductor digiti minimi p.
musculus flexor digiti minimi brevis p.

pedobarograph
Musgrave footprint p.

pedobarography
dynamic p.

pedodontic endodontics

pedodynographic examination

pedophilia
adolescent p.
middle age p.

pedophilic behavior

peduncle
anterior peduncle of thalamus
p. cerebral
p. of cerebrum
p. of corpus callosum
decussation of superior cerebellar p.'s
p. of flocculus
p. of hypophysis
p. of mamillary body
mammillary p.
middle cerebellar p.
middle cervical p.
olfactory p.
pineal p.
superior cerebellar p.

peduncular
p. ansa
p. hallucination
p. hallucinosis
p. loop
peduncularis ansa p.

peduncularis
ansa p.
p. ansa peduncular

pedunculated
p. adenoma
p. adenomatous polyp
p. fibroid
p. fibroma
p. growth
p. juvenile polyp
p. lesion
p. nodule
p. papilloma
small pedunculated adenomatous polyps

pedunculomamillaris

pedunculopontine
p. cholinergic group
p. nucleus

peek sign

peel
Obagi chemical p.
Obagi controlled variable-depth p.
orange peel appearance
papillary dermal p.
pleural p.

peeler-cutter
membrane p.-c.

peeling
chemical face p.
continual skin peeling syndrome
p. of feet and hands
membrane p.

peer
p. abuse
age p.
p. anxiety
p. censure
p. conformity inventory
p. criticism
drug-using peer group
p. group
hospital peer review
loss of interest in peer social activity
P. Nomination Inventory for Depression
p. review committee

peer-driven intervention

peer-support program

peg
p. base plate
p. bone graft
p. cell
p. device
p. flap
rete p.
Smith subtalar joint arthroereisis p.

pegademase bovine

peg-and-socket
p.-a.-s. articulation
p.-a.-s. joint

Pegboard
Tactile Reproduction P.

pegging
bone p.

peg-in-hole arthroereisis

pegorgotein
polyethylene glycol-conjugated superoxide dismutase p.

pegylated interferon

pejorative delusion

Pel-Ebstein
P.-E. disease
P.-E. fever
P.-E. pyrexia
P.-E. symptom

Pelger-Huët
P.-H. cell
P.-H. nuclear anomaly

peliosis
bacillary p.
p. hepatitis

peliosis *(continued)*
parenchymal bacillary p.
p. rheumatica

Pelizaeus-Merzbacher disease

pellagra
alcoholic pellagra encephalopathy
p. dementia
pellagra sine p.
p. preventive
p. preventive factor

pellagra-associated dermatitis

pellagroid
p. dermatitis
p. erythema

Pellegrini-Stieda
P.-S. calcification
P.-S. disease

pellet
p. artifact
p. extrusion
p. implantation

Pelli-Robson
P.-R. contrast sensitivity chart
P.-R. letter chart

Pellizzi syndrome

pellucid
p. marginal corneal degeneration
p. marginal retinal degeneration

pellucida
macula p.
zona p.
zona pellucida 1, 2, 3

pellucidi

pellucidum
anterior vein of septum p.
septum p.
septum pellucidum absent with porencephalia syndrome
syndrome of absence of septum pellucidum with poerencephaly

Pelosi hysterotomy

pelves (*pl. of* pelvis)

pelvic
p. abscess
p. actinomycosis
acute pelvic inflammatory disease
acute pelvic pain
p. adhesion
p. adhesive disease
p. aneurysm
p. angle
anterior pelvic exenteration
anterior pelvic tilt
anterior sagittal pelvic inlet
anteroposterior diameter of pelvic inlet
p. appendicitis
p. appendix
p. architecture
p. arterial embolization
p. arteriogram
p. arteriography
p. arteriovenous malformation
p. artery
p. aspiration biopsy
p. autonomic nerve
p. autonomic nerve preservation
p. autonomic plexus
p. avulsion fracture
p. axis
p. band
bilateral pelvic lymph node
bilateral pelvic lymph node dissection
p. bleeding
p. bone
p. boost radiotherapy
p. brace
p. brim
p. canal
p. cavity
p. C-clamp
p. cellulitis
p. chocolate cyst
chronic pelvic inflammatory disease
chronic pelvic pain
chronic pelvic pain syndrome
p. circumference
p. collateral vessel
p. colon
p. colonic surgery
p. colon of Waldeyer
p. congestion syndrome
p. contraction
p. cramp
cramp-like pelvic pain
p. cystic mass
p. diameter
p. diaphragm
p. direction
p. discontinuity
p. dissection
p. drainage
endocavitary pelvic lymphadenectomy
p. endometriosis
entrance of fetal head into superior pelvic strait
p. evisceration
p. examination under anesthesia
p. exenteration
exenterative surgery for pelvic cancer
p. exostosis
extraperitoneal endoscopic pelvic lymph node dissection
p. fascia
p. fibromatosis
p. finding
p. fixation
p. flexion contracture
p. floor
p. floor descent
p. floor disorder
p. floor dysfunction
p. floor dyssynergia
p. floor electrical stimulation
p. floor electromyography
p. floor exercise
p. floor movement
p. floor muscle
p. floor muscle exercise
p. floor nerve
p. floor pressure
p. floor relaxation
p. floor syndrome
p. floor weakness
p. forceps
p. fossa
p. fracture frame
p. ganglion
Ganz anti-shock pelvic fixator
p. girdle
p. girdle relaxation
good pelvic support
Gram stain of pelvic abscess
p. gutter
p. hematocele
p. hematoma
p. inclination
p. index
p. infection
p. infertility factor
p. inflammation
p. inflammatory disease
inflammatory pelvic disease
p. inlet
intermittent pelvic traction
intractable pelvic pain
p. involvement
p. irradiation
isolated pelvic perfusion
p. joint
p. kidney
laparoscopic pelvic lymphadenectomy

laparoscopic pelvic lymph node dissection
p. laparoscopy
p. laparotomy
p. lengthening osteotomy
p. limb
long leg brace with pelvic band
p. lymphadenectomy
p. lymphadenopathy
p. lymph node
p. lymph node dissection
p. malignancy
p. malignancy in pregnancy
p. mass
p. measurement
Meigs pelvic lymphadenectomy
p. metastasis
MIBG-negative pelvic pheochromocytoma
p. muscle exercise
p. muscle laxity
p. nerve injury
NIH Classification Category III inflammatory and noninflammatory chronic pelvic pain
p. node dissection
p. node sampling
nongenital pelvic organ
normal pelvic examination
obstetric conjugate of pelvic outlet
p. odor
p. organ prolapse
p. osteomyelitis
p. outlet
p. ovarian vein thrombosis
p. pain
p. phased-array coil
posterior pelvic tilt
psychogenic pelvic pain
p. and rectal examination
p. relaxation
relaxed pelvic floor
renal pelvic hemorrhage
retroperitoneal pelvic lymph node dissection
p. rhabdomyosarcoma
p. rock
septic pelvic thrombophlebitis
p. stabilization orthosis
static pelvic traction
p. support
p. support index
tendinous arch of pelvic fascia
p. thrombophlebitis
p. tilt exercise
total pelvic exenteration
p. tumor
p. ultrasound
p. venous incompetence
p. viscera
p. viscera surrounded by hematoma
p. wall
p. washings

pelvicaliceal
p. change
p. dilatation
p. distention

pelvici

pelvic-ureteric

pelvimetry
computed tomographic p.
manual p.
roentgenographic p.

pelvirectal
p. abscess
p. achalasia
p. fistula

pelvis, pl. **pelves**
apertura pelvis inferior
apertura pelvis minoris
apertura pelvis superior
p. and calix
p., calix and ureter
p. capsular dysplasia
dual drop p.
p. enlargement
p. fracture
p. of gallbladder
p. and hip
hip and p.
hyperthermia in p.
p. irrigated
p. justo major
p. justo minor
longitudinal oval p.
muscular layer of renal p.
nodi lymphoidei p.
out of p.

pelviscopic clip ligation technique

Pemberton
P. acetabuloplasty
P. sign

pemphigoid
antiepiligrin cicatricial p.
benign mucous membrane p.
bullous pemphigoid antigen
cicatricial ocular p.
lichen planus p.
localized pemphigoid of Brunsting-Perry
localized vulvar pemphigoid of childhood
mucous membrane p.
ocular cicatricial p.

pemphigus
p. antibody
bullous p.
chronic benign mucous membrane p.
p. contagiosum
p. contagiosus
p. crouposus
p. erythematosus
familial benign chronic p.
p. gangrenosus
p. hemorrhagicus
herpetiform p.
p. leprosus
p. neonatorum
paraneoplastic p.
p. syphiliticus
p. vegetans
p. vulgaris

pen
P. A/N
downward pen deflection
p. grasp
insulin pen pump
marking p.
oriented to time, place, person, and objects watch, pen, book

penal
halfway house for penal rehabilitation

penalty, frustration, anxiety, guilt, hostility

Pena midsagittal anorectoplasty

Penassay
P. broth plus glucose
P. broth plus glucose plus menadione

pencil
astigmatism of oblique p.'s
p. and cup deformity
p. dosimeter
electrosurgical p.
p. grip
p. method
p. tenderness

pencil-beam approach

penciling
p. deformity
p. of the distal clavicle

pencil-thin stool

Pendred
P. disease
P. syndrome
P. syndrome gene

pendrin protein

pendular
p. eye-tracking test
p. nystagmus

pendular-jerk waveform

pendulous
p. abdomen
p. breast
breast pendulous and atrophic
p. heart

pendulum
p. exercise
molluscum fibrosum p.

penes (*pl. of* penis)

penetrant gene

penetrated
infection penetrated bone

penetrating
p. abdominal trauma
p. abdominal trauma index
p. abdominal wound
aortic penetrating ulcer
p. aortic ulcer
p. atherosclerotic ulcer
p. brain injury
p. cardiac wound
p. corneal graft
p. corneal transplant
p. craniocerebral injuries
deep penetrating nevus
p. drill
epithelioid combined nevi deep penetrating nevus
p. fracture
p. full-thickness corneal graft
p. keratoplasty astigmatism
p. keratoplasty button
p. keratoplasty and glaucoma
p. neck wound
p. renal injury
p. rupture
p. trauma
p. wound of the abdomen
p. wound of heart

penetration
anterior cortex p.
cervical mucus penetration test
hamster egg penetration assay
hamster oocyte penetration test
hospital-acquired penetration contact
sperm penetration assay

Penfield hypothesis

penguinpox virus

penicillamine-induced myasthenia

penicillatus
limbus p.

penicillin
p. allergy skin testing
p. aluminum monostearate
p. amidase
p. aqueous
aqueous procaine p.
aqueous procaine penicillin G
p. b
p., bacitracin, streptomycin, caprylate
p. in beeswax and oil
p. desensitization
p. disc test
p. G
p. G benzathine
p. G benzathine and procaine combined
p. G, parenteral, aqueous
p. G procaine
hemagglutinating penicillin antibody
penicillinase-resistant p.
penicillinase-resistant synthetic p.
p., oil, and beeswax
p., streptomycin, tetracycline
postnatal penicillin prophylaxis
potassium penicillin G
sulfobenzyl p.
therapeutic continuous p.
p. V
p. V potassium

penicillin-allergic patient

penicillinase-producing
p.-p. *Neisseria gonorrhoeae*
p.-p. organisms susceptibility testing

penicillinase-resistant synthetic penicillin

penicillinase test

penicillin-binding protein

penicillin-inhibitor combinations

penicillin-nonsusceptible
Streptococcus pneumoniae

penicillin-resistant
p.-r. pneumococcus
p.-r. *Streptococcus pneumoniae*

penicillin-sensitive
p.-s. enzyme
p.-s. *Streptococcus pneumoniae*

Penicillium
Penicillium brevicompactum virus
Penicillium chrysogenum virus
Penicillium cyaneo-fulvum virus
Penicillium fungus
Penicillium roqueforti toxin
Penicillium stoloniferum F, S virus

penicilloyl
p. G, G/V, V
p. polylysine
p. polylysine skin test

penile
p. agenesis
p. amputation
p. arousal
p. arteriography
arteriosinusoidal penile fistula
p. artery
p. biothesiometry
p. block
p. blood flow
p. blood flow study
p. blood pressure
p. body
p. brachial index
p. bulb dosimetry
p. bulb imaging
p. cancer
p. carcinoma
p. chordee
p. condyloma
congenital penile deviation
p. crus
p. curvature
p. cyst
p. deformity
p. discharge
dorsal penile nerve block
p. duplex ultrasonography
p. duplication
p. dysgenesis
p. edema
p. epispadias
p. erection
p. extensibility
p. fibromatosis
p. fibrosis
p. flaccidity
p. flap
p. gangrene

p. girth enhancement
p. herpes
p. implant
p. impotence
p. induration
inflatable penile prosthesis
p. injury
p. ischemia
p. length
p. lesion
nocturnal penile erection monitoring
nocturnal penile tumescence
nocturnal penile tumescence testing
pearly penile papule
p. plethysmograph
p. prosthesis
pump-operated penile implant
p. reflex
p. self-injection
p. shaft
p. skin
Small-Carrion penile prosthesis
p. tuberculosis
p. urethra

penile-brachial
p.-b. pressure index
p.-b. pulse index

peninsula pupil

penis, pl. **penes**
albuginea p.
angiofibroma of p.
arteria bulbi p.
arteriae perforantes p.
arteria profunda p.
artery of bulb of p.
artificial p.
p. at twelve syndrome
autoamputation of p.
p. captivus
p. envy
p. fear
p. fracture
glans p.
median raphe cyst of the p.
musculus erector p.
neck of glans p.
opening for dorsal artery of p.
opening for dorsal nerve of p.
os p.
perforating artery of p.
prepuce of p.
septum of glans p.
suspensory ligament of p.

Pennsylvania
University of Pennsylvania Smell Identification Test

penopubic epispadias

penoscrotal
congenital emphysema, cryptorchidism, penoscrotal web, deafness, mental retardation syndrome
p. edema
p. hypospadias
meatal advancement, glansplasty, penoscrotal junction meatotomy
meatal advancement, glanuloplasty, penoscrotal junction meatotomy

Penrose drain

pension
compensation and p.
compensation, pension, and education
disability p.
old age p.
special monthly p.
P. and Welfare Benefits Administration

pensioner
old age p.

pensylvanicum
Xanthium p.

penta-acetylglucopyranosyl guanine

pentagastrin
p. gastric secretory test
peak acid output after pentagastrin stimulation
p. provocation test

pentagonal block excision

pentagons
copy intersecting pentagons test

pentalogy
p. of Cantrell
p. of Cantrell syndrome
p. of Fallot

pentamidine
aerosol p.

pentastomum

pentate
indium p.

pentavalent
p. botulism toxin
p. dimercaptosuccinate
p. form
p. gas gangrene antitoxin

pentobarbital
p. coma
p. sodium

pentolinium tartrate

pentose
p. assay
p. nucleic acid
p. phosphate cycle
p. phosphate pathway

pentosuria
alimentary p.

pent-up hostility

Pen-Vee K

people
aggression to people and animals
inability to relate to p.
p. with epilepsy

pepper
p. bolete mushroom
caffeine, alcohol, pepper, spicy foods
no caffeine or p.
P. syndrome
P. type
P. Visual Skills for Reading Test

pepper-and-salt fundus

peppermint camphor

pepsin
p. A
active p.
alkali-stable p.
basal pepsin output
fragment of immunoglobulin G after digestion with the enzyme p.
inactivated p.
peak pepsin output
p. unit

pepsinogen
p. 1
p. A-C ratio
plasma p.
total immunoreactive serum p.

peptic
p. aspiration pneumonia
p. aspiration pneumonitis
p. cell
p. cell receptor
p. digestion
duodenal peptic ulcer disease
p. esophageal stricture
p. esophagitis
p. gastritis
p. gland

peptic *(continued)*
p. inflammatory disease
Palmer acid test for peptic ulcer
perforated acid peptic ulcer
p. stricture
p. ulceration
p. ulcer disease

peptidase
p. A, C, D, S

peptide
p. activated lymphocyte
anionic neutrophil-activating p.
p. antibiotic
anticyclic citrullinated peptide antibody
p. antigen
atrial natriuretic p.
autologous T lymphocytes stimulated with the patient's tumor-specific mutated RAS p.'s
p. bond
bradykinin potentiating p.
brain natriuretic p.
B-type natriuretic p.
C p.
calcitonin gene-related p.
carboxyl terminal p.
class II invariant chain-derived p.
connective tissue-activating p.
p. cotransmitter
C-type atrial natriuretic p.
delta sleep-inducing p.
diabetes-associated p.
endogenous opioid p.
gastric inhibitory p.
gastrin-releasing p.
glucagon-like p.
glucose-dependent insulin-releasing p.
glucose insulinotropic p.
gonadotropin-releasing hormone-associated p.
p. growth factor
p. growth factor receptor signal
p. growth factor signaling mechanism
growth hormone-releasing p.
helix-bundle p.
p. HI
p. histidine isoleucine
p. histidine methionine
p. hormone
human atrial natriuretic p.
intervening p.
labile p.
latency-associated p.
p. ligand
p. major histocompatibility complex
mast cell degranulating p.
multiantigenic p.
neutrophil chemotactic p.
nociceptin/orphanin FQ p.
N-terminal atrial natriuretic p.
p. nucleic acid
pancreatic spasmolytic p.
parathyroid hormone-related p.
peak acid output after gastrin-releasing p.
pituitary opioid p.
procollagen type III aminoterminal p.
p. regulatory factor
solid phase peptide synthesis
thrombin receptor-activating p.
thrombin receptor-activating peptide 6
trypsin activation p.
trypsinogen-activating p.
urinary gonadotropin p.
vasoactive intestinal p.
vasoinhibitory p.
p. YY

peptide-1
glucagon-like p.
monocyte chemotactic p.

peptide-4
human neutrophil p.

peptidergic
p. fiber
p. neuron

peptide-secreting
vasoactive intestinal peptide-secreting tumor

peptide-specific T cell

peptidoglycan
p. rigid cell wall
p. synthesis

peptidomimetic inhibitor complex

peptone
duodenal peptone infusion
p., glucose, and yeast extract medium
tryptophan peptone glucose broth
yeast, peptone, and adenine sulfate

peptone-yeast extract

peptone-yeast-glucose-maltose broth

peracetic
p. acid-based method
p. acid-Schiff reaction

perborate
sodium p.

perceived
p. danger
effective perceived noise level
p. emotional abandonment
p. exertion
p. illness threat
Multidimensional Scale of P. Social Support
p. noise
p. noise level
p. quality of life
rated perceived exertion
rate of perceived exertion
rating of perceived breathing difficulty
rating of perceived exertion

percent
abnormal forms p.
p. body fat
forced expiratory volume in one second as percent of FVC
p. fractional shortening
gram p.
milligrams p.
p. of polymorphonuclear leukocyte
p. predicted peak expiratory flow
p. reactive antibody
p. reactive antibody/panel reactive antibody
p. reduction in urea
p. stroke length
volume p.

percentage
p. of acceleration time
p. classification
P. of Consonants Correct-Revised
p. depth dose
fractional percentage of inspired oxygen
p. of goblet cell
high oxygen p.
high oxygen percentage in retinopathy of prematurity
p. of labeled mitoses
p. of lymphocytes in differential count
mean percentage of desirable weight
p. of multinucleated cells
p. of normal

phonetically balanced percentage of word lists
shortening fraction p.
p. signal intensity loss
volume p.

percentile rank

percept
p. analysis
p. image

perceptible
p. acuity
minimal perceptible color difference
minimal perceptible difference
minimal perceptible odor
minimum perceptible acuity
not p.

perception
P. of Ability Scale for Students
alteration in time p.
altered mind-body p.
altered mood and p.
altered sensory p.
altered spatial p.
altered time p.
p. analysis
auditory perception of speech sounds
auditory space p.
blurred sensory p.'s
p. of body image
Children's P. of Support Inventory
color p.
contrast threshold for motion p.
current perception threshold
decreased sensory p.
p. deficiency
p. deficit
deficits in attention, motor control, p.
Developmental Test of Visual P.
Differentiation of Auditory P. Skill
p. disorder
p. dissociation
distorted depth p.
distorted sense of time and p.
distortion of sensory p.
p. disturbance
Early Speech P. Test
p. ego
p. of the environment
extrasensory p.
Frostig Developmental Test of Visual Motor P.
Frostig Program for the Development of Visual P.
General Health P. Questionnaire
hallucinogen persisting perception disorder
hand motion and light perception
heart rate p.
heightened perception of colors
high-risk model of threat p.
p. illusion
p. impaired
infertility perceptions inventory
Interpersonal P. Scale
Inter-Person P. Test
p. of light
light perception only
light perception without projection
light perception with projection
limbus of p.
loudness growth p.
Mertens Visual P. Test
Modified Autonomic P. Questionnaire
Modified Somatic P. Questionnaire
monocular depth p.
motion perception disorder
Motor-Free Visual P. Test
motor perception dysfunction
narrowing of p.'s
neonatal perception inventory
no light p.
normal light p.
Northwestern University Children's P. of Speech Test
Ohio Tests of Articulation and P. of Sounds
Pain P. Profile
Parent P. of Child Profile
Racial P.'s Inventory
Rapidly Alternating Speech P. Test
red-green color perception deficiency
P. of Relationships Test
role perception picture inventory
simultaneous foveal p.
simultaneous macular p.
single-electrode current perception threshold
Speech-Sound P. Test
spouse's perception of disease
subliminal p.
supersensitivity p.
Tests of P. of Scientists and Self
p., thought and recognition of information
vibration perception testing
vibration perception threshold
visual p.
visual acuity, left eye, left perception with projection
Weber Advanced Spatial P. test

perceptional insanity

perceptive
p. deafness
p. epilepsy
p. hearing impairment
p. hearing loss
progressive perceptive deafness

perceptual
p. abnormality
p. analysis
p. anchoring
p. aspect
auditory perceptual disability
auditory perceptual disorder
cannabis intoxication, with perceptual disturbance
p. closure
p. cognitive mechanism
p. cognitive motor function
cognitive perceptual motor skills
color and space perceptual disturbance
p. consciousness
p. consistency
p. constancy
p. cue
p. cycle
p. defect
p. defense
p. deficit
p. deprivation
p. disability
p. disorder
p. distortion
p. disturbance
p. domain
p. emotive stimulus
p. error
p. expansion
p. experience
p. extinction
p. field
p. filter
p. filtering
illusion or perceptual distortions
p. immaturity
p. induction
Inventory of P. Skills
p. motor development

perceptual *(continued)*
p. motor skills
p. organization
P. Organization Deviation Quotient
Rivermead P. Assessment Battery
Sensory P. Examination
p. span time
p. speed

perceptually
p. adequate sound
p. handicapped

perceptual-motor
p.-m. ability impairment
p.-m. disability

perceptual-spatial deficit

Percheron
artery of P.

perchlorate discharge test

Percoll gradient

percreta
placenta p.

percussion
p. of abdomen
p. and auscultation
auscultation and p.
p. and auscultation
chest clear to auscultation and p.
chest clear to percussion and auscultation
chest percussion and auscultation
chest percussion and postural drainage
chest percussion and vibration
clear to auscultation and p.
compression and p.
costovertebral angle tenderness to p.
distal tingling on p.
dullness on p.
dullness to p.
p. hammer
hyperresonance to p.
inspection, palpation, percussion, and auscultation
left border dullness of heart to p.
lungs clear to auscultation and p.
lungs revealed hyperresonance to p.
mechanical p.
p. myotonia
p. note
palpation, percussion, and auscultation
postural drainage and p.
p. and postural drainage
postural drainage, percussion and vibration
p. sound
p. of suprapubic area
p. tenderness
tenderness to palpation or p.
thorax resonant on p.
Tinel sign distal tingling on percussion
p. and vibration
p., vibration, and drainage
p., vibration, and suction

percussive
high-frequency percussive ventilation
intermittent percussive ventilation
intrapulmonary percussive ventilation

percussor
mechanical p.

percuss and vibrate

percutaneous
p. abscess drainage
p. abscess and fluid drainage
p. absorption
p. access
p. access kit
p. Achilles tendon repair
p. adductor tenotomy
p. alcohol injection
p. alcohol serotherapy
p. allergy testing
p. anesthetic loss
p. antegrade biliary drainage
p. antegrade pyelography
p. antegrade urography
p. anterior gastropexy
p. appendectomy
Arrow-Trerotola percutaneous thrombectomy device
p. arterial cannulation
p. arterial closure device
p. arteriogram
p. arteriography
p. aspirate
p. aspiration, instillation of hypertonic saline, respiration
p. aspiration thromboembolectomy
p. autogenous dowel bone graft
p. automated diskectomy
automated percutaneous diskectomy
automated percutaneous lumbar discectomy
automated percutaneous lumbar diskectomy
p. bacille Calmette-Guérin administration
p. balloon angioplasty
p. balloon aortic valvuloplasty
p. balloon aspiration
p. balloon commissurotomy
p. balloon dilation
p. balloon pericardiotomy
p. balloon pulmonic valvuloplasty
bilateral percutaneous cervical cordotomy
p. biliary bypass
p. biliary drainage
p. bladder aspiration
p. bladder neck stabilization
p. bladder neck suspension
p. bone marrow infection
p. bone marrow injection
p. breathing assister
p. cabling
p. cardiopulmonary bypass
p. cardiopulmonary bypass support
p. carotid arteriogram
p. catheter cecostomy
p. catheter drainage
p. catheter insertion
p. cecostomy
p. cecotomy
p. central venous catheter
p. cervical cordotomy
p. cholangiography
p. cholangioscopic lithotomy
p. cholecystectomy
p. cholecystolithotomy
p. cholecystostomy
p. cholecystotomy catheter
p. choledochoscopy
closed reduction and percutaneous pin fixation
closed reduction and percutaneous pin ring
p. coagulation of gasserian ganglion
computed tomography-guided percutaneous radiofrequency denervation of the sacroiliac joint
p. conchotome biopsy technique
p. cord cyst puncture
p. cordotomy
p. core bone biopsy
p. coronary angioplasty

p. coronary intervention
p. coronary revascularization
p. coronary rotational atherectomy
p. coronary transluminal angioplasty
p. corticotomy
p. CT-guided aspiration
p. cyst aspiration
p. debulking
p. dilatational tracheotomy
p. dilatation of biliary duct
p. dilational tracheostomy
p. dilational tracheotomy
direct percutaneous jejunostomy
direct percutaneous transhepatitic cholangiography
p. dissolution of thrombus
p. drain
p. drainage of epididymal abscess
dual percutaneous endoscopic gastrostomy
p. electrical nerve stimulation
p. electrode array
p. embolization therapy
p. endofluoroscopy
p. endoluminal gastrostomy
p. endoluminal gastrostomy tube
p. endopyeloureterotomy
p. endoscopic
p. endoscopic cecostomy
p. endoscopic gastrojejunostomy
p. endoscopic gastrostomy
p. endoscopic gastrostomy insertion
p. endoscopic gastrostomy and jejunal extension tube
p. endoscopic gastrostomy tube
p. endoscopic jejunostomy
p. endoscopic lumbar diskectomy
p. endoscopic placement of jejunal tube
p. endoscopic recanalization
p. endoscopic removal
p. endoscopy
p. endovascular treatment
p. enterostomy
p. epididymal sperm aspiration
p. epidural nerve stimulator
p. epidural neurostimulator
p. epiphysiodesis
p. ethanol ablation
p. ethanol ablation of tumor
p. ethanol injection
p. excimer laser coronary angioplasty
p. excimer laser coronary angioplasty system
p. excisional breast biopsy
p. exposure
p. exposure risk
p. external drainage
p. femoral approach
p. femoral vein
p. femoral vein catheter
p. femoral venous catheter
p. fetal cystoscopy
p. fetal tissue sampling
p. fetal transfusion
p. fine-needle aspiration
p. fine-needle aspiration biopsy
p. fine-needle ethanol injection
p. fine-needle pancreatic biopsy
fine-needle percutaneous cholangiogram
p. fixation
p. FNA
p. gastroenterostomy
p. glycerol rhizolysis
p. heel cord lengthening
p. hepatobiliary cholangiography
p. injury
p. intraaortic balloon counterpulsation
jejunal tube through percutaneous endoscopic gastrostomy
p. laser disc decompression
p. laser diskectomy
p. left heart bypass
p. line
p. liver biopsy
p. localization
p. low-stress angioplasty
p. lumbar diskectomy
p. lung tap
p. mechanical thrombectomy
p. microwave coagulation therapy
p. mitral balloon commissurotomy
p. mitral balloon valvotomy
p. mitral balloon valvuloplasty
p. mitral balloon valvulotomy
p. mitral commissurotomy
p. mitral valvoplasty
p. multipuncture technique
p. needle
p. needle aspiration
p. needle aspiration biopsy
p. needle cholangiogram
p. needle lung aspiration
p. needle puncture
p. nephrolithotomy
p. nephroscope
p. nephroscopy
p. nephrostomy
p. nephrostomy catheter
p. nephrostomy tube
p. neuromodulatory therapy
p. nucleotomy
p. on-surface stimulation
p. peritoneal biopsy
p. plantar fasciotomy
primary percutaneous transluminal coronary angioplasty
p. radiofrequency
p. radiofrequency denervation
p. radiofrequency facet nerve block
radiofrequency percutaneous myocardial revascularization
p. radiofrequency rhizolysis
renal percutaneous transluminal angioplasty
p. retrogasserian glycerol injection
retrograde percutaneous gastrostomy
p. rotational thrombectomy
p. rotational transluminal coronary angioplasty
simultaneous bilateral percutaneous nephrolithotomy
p. stenting
p. stereotactic radiofrequency rhizotomy
p. stone manipulation
p. stone removal
p. stricture dilatation
p. suprapubic cystostomy
p. thrombolytic device
p. transatrial mitral commissurotomy
p. transhepatic biliary drainage
p. transhepatic biliary drainage-enteric feeding
p. transhepatic catheterization
p. transhepatic cholangio-drainage
p. transhepatic cholangiogram
p. transhepatic cholangiography
p. transhepatic cholangioscopic lithotomy
p. transhepatic cholangioscopy
p. transhepatic cholecystolithotomy
p. transhepatic cholecystoscopy
p. transhepatic drainage
p. transhepatic gallbladder drainage
p. transhepatic liver biopsy with tract embolization
p. transhepatic obliteration
p. transhepatic portography
p. transluminal angioplasty

percutaneous *(continued)*
p. transluminal angioplasty with stent placement
p. transluminal angioscopy
p. transluminal balloon angioplasty
p. transluminal balloon dilatation
p. transluminal balloon valvuloplasty
p. transluminal coronary angioplasty
p. transluminal coronary arteriography
p. transluminal coronary recanalization
p. transluminal coronary revascularization
p. transluminal coronary rotational ablation
p. transluminal coronary rotational atherectomy
p. transluminal dilatation
p. transluminal endomyocardial revascularization
p. transluminal myocardial revascularization
p. transluminal renal angioplasty
p. transluminal septal myocardial ablation
p. transluminal ultrasonic coronary angioplasty
p. transmyocardial laser revascularization
p. transpedicular diskectomy
p. transthoracic needle biopsy
p. transtracheal jet ventilation
p. transvenous mitral commissurotomy
p. tumor ablation
p. ultrasonic lithotripsy
p. ultrasonic nephrolithotripsy
p. ultrasonic pyelolithotomy
p. umbilical blood sampling
p. ureteral dilatation
p. ureteral stent
venting percutaneous gastrostomy
p. vertebroplasty

percutaneously
cannulated p.
p. inserted central line catheter
p. inserted spinal cord electrical stimulation
p. placed line

perenne
Lolium perenne allergen

perennial
p. allergic conjunctivitis
p. allergic rhinitis
allergic rhinitis p.
p. allergic rhinoconjunctivitis
p. allergies
p. antigen
p. asthma
p. hay fever
nonallergic noninfectious perennial rhinitis

Pereyra
P. bladder neck suspension
P. needle
P. needle suspension

Perez sign

perfect
p. fungus
p. stage
p. state

perfection
manie de p.

perfilcon A

perfluorocarbon
p. gas
liquid p.

perfluorocarbon-associated gas exchange

perfluorochemical liquid

perfluoropropane gas

perforans
mal p.
malum p.
malum perforans pedis

perforant
mal p.
mal perforant du pied

perforantes
arteriae p.
arteriae perforantes anteriores
arteriae perforantes penis

perforated
p. acid peptic ulcer
anterior perforated substance
p. aortic cusp
p. appendicitis
p. cancer
p. carcinoma
p. cholecystitis
p. corneal ulcer
p. diverticulitis
p. diverticulum
p. duodenal ulcer
p. eardrum
p. gallbladder
p. gangrenous appendix
p. gastric ulcer
p. layer of sclera
otitis media with perforated tympanic membrane
p. peptic ulcer
p. retrocecal appendix
p. septum
p. tympanic membrane
p. uterus
p. viscus

perforating
p. abscess
acquired perforating dermatosis
p. alveolar artery
p. aneurysm
anterior perforating artery
p. appendicitis
p. arteries of peronea
p. artery of deep femoral artery
p. artery of foot
p. artery of hand
p. artery infarct
p. artery of internal mammary
p. artery of internal thoracic artery
p. artery of penis
p. branch
p. branch of anterior interosseous artery
p. branch of deep palmar arch
p. branch of fibular artery
p. branch of internal thoracic artery
p. branch of palmar metacarpal artery
p. branch of peroneal artery
p. branch of plantar metatarsal artery
p. calcific elastosis
p. canal
chronic perforating hyperplasia of pulp
p. colorectal carcinoma
p. cutaneous nerve
p. disease
p. disease of hemodialysis
p. disorder of uremia
p. diverticulitis
p. fiber
p. fibers of Sharpey
p. folliculitis
p. forceps
p. fracture
p. granuloma annulare
incompetent perforating vein
p. keratoplasty
reactive perforating collagenosis

perforation
apical root p.
appendiceal p.
p. and bleeding
p. of bowel
p. of colon
p. of common bile duct
duodenal ulcer p.
p. of esophagus
p. of gallbladder
intestinal wall p.
nasal septal perforation button
Niemeier gallbladder p.
Oesch perforation invagination stripper
spontaneous biliary p.
subsynaptic plate p.
p. of tympanic membrane
tympanic membrane p.

perforator
anterolateral intercostal p.
anteromedial intercostal p.
deep inferior epigastric artery p.
p. flap
incompetent perforator vein
rejuvenation with sparing of vascular p.'s
subfascial endoscopic perforator surgery
superior gluteal artery p.
p.'s and tributaries

perforatus

perforin killing pathway

perform
ability to p.
decline in ability to perform routine tasks
p. endoscopy
inability to perform purposeful movements
patient's ability to p.

performance
p. abnormality
Adult P. Level Survey
p. anxiety
Aphasia Language P. Scale
p. area
Arthur Adaptation of the Leiter International P. Scale
p. assessment
P. Assessment of Syntax Elicited and Spontaneous
auditory continuous performance task
automaticity of p.
cardiac p.
p. characteristic
clinical performance score
coefficient of p.
p. component
p. context
continuous performance task
continuous performance test
p. and cost efficiency
decline in job p.
equivalent oxygen p.
p. evaluation procedure
p. fear
Functional P. Record
p. goal
impaired cognitive p.
impairment of systolic and diastolic p.
improved performance and tolerance
p. improvement
p. index
P. Intelligence Quotient
p. intensity
Karnofsky performance score
Karnofsky performance status
knowledge of p.
Kuder P. Test
Leiter International P. Scale
Mayo elbow performance score
p. measurement system
Pediatric Overall Performance Category scale
Physical P. Test
Printing P. School Readiness Test
professional performance evaluation
p. status scale for head and neck cancer
Tactile P. Test
Test of Infant Motor P.
treadmill performance test
Vantage Performance monitor
p. versus intensity function for phonetically balanced words
Western Ontario and McMaster Universities Osteoarthritis Index Physical Functioning subscale and chair-stand p.

Performance-Diagnostic
Test of Articulation P.-D.

performance-intensity
p.-i. function
p.-i. function test

Performance-Oriented Mobility Assessment

Performance-Screen
Test of Articulation P.-S.

performed
appendectomy performed in routine fashion
copious lavage p.
limited quantity test performed on small specimen
not p.

performic
p. acid-Schiff
p. acid-Schiff reaction

performing scale

perfringens
Clostridium perfringens enterotoxin

perfusate
p. bag
p. drip
mean perfusate temperature

perfused
isolated perfused rabbit lung
isolated perfused rat liver

perfusion
p. abnormality
adenosine radionuclide perfusion imaging
adequate coronary p.
p. agent
allogenic liver p.
antegrade perfusion pressure measurement
Arndorfer capillary perfusion system
p. balloon catheter
blood perfusion monitor
brain perfusion study
cardioplegic perfusion solution
cerebral cortex perfusion rate
cerebral tissue perfusion pressure
p. computed tomography
continuous arterial spin-labeled perfusion magnetic resonance imaging
continuous hyperthermic peritoneal p.
p. cooling
cranial perfusion pressure
p. CT
p. defect
p. deficit
digital blood p.
diminished airway p.
distal perfusion system
Doppler perfusion index
dual balloon perfusion catheter
extracorporeal liver p.

perfusion *(continued)*
ex vivo p.
fallopian tube sperm p.
p. flow rate
hepatic arterial perfusion scintigraphy
hepatic perfusion index
hyperthermic antiblastic p.
hyperthermic isolated limb p.
intraperitoneal hyperthermic p.
isolated heat p.
isolated hepatic portal and arterial p.
isolated hyperthermic limb p.
isolated pelvic p.
lung p.
p. lung scan
macroaggregated albumin arterial p.
maximal perfusion pressure measurement
misery perfusion syndrome
myocardial p.
myocardial isotopic perfusion scan
myocardial perfusion reserve
myocardial stress perfusion scintigraphy
normal perfusion pressure breakthrough
pancreatic parenchymal p.
p. pressure
pulmonary capillary blood flow p.
pulmonary perfusion scanning
regional cerebral perfusion pressure
remote access p.
retrograde cerebral p.
p. scintigraphy
segmental bronchus perfusion abnormality
skin perfusion pressure
SPECT brain perfusion scintigraphy
spinal cord perfusion pressure
standard perfusion fluid
p. study
superficial renal cortical p.
thallium myocardial p.
thallium perfusion imaging
tubal perfusion pressure
twin reversed arterial p.
ventilation and p.
ventilation perfusion defect
ventriculolumbar p.

perfusion-assisted direct coronary artery bypass

perfusion-weighted magnetic resonance imaging

pergolide mesylate

Perheentupa syndrome

periadenitis aphthae

periadrenal hemorrhage

perialar
p. crescentic advancement flap
p. crescentic excision

periampullary
p. adenoma
p. cancer
p. carcinoma
p. diverticulum
p. duodenal diverticulum
p. duodenal tumor
p. malignancy

periamygdaloid
p. area
p. cortex

perianal
p. anorectal space
p. aphthosis
p. area
p. candidosis
p. condyloma
p. condyloma acuminatum
p. condylomata
p. condylomata lata
p. Crohn disease
P. Crohn Disease Activity Index
p. dermatitis
p. discomfort
p. disease
p. edema
p. erythema
p. fistula
p. fistula abscess
p. hematoma
p. herpes
p. hypopigmentation
p. irritation
p. itching
Paget disease of perianal area
p. reflex
p. skin
p. squamous cell carcinoma
p. streptococcal cellulitis
p. wart

periaortic
p. area
p. atelectasis
p. chain
p. infrarenal node
p. lymphadenopathy
p. lymph involvement
p. lymph node
p. lymph node metastasis
p. mediastinal hematoma
p. node sampling

periapical
p. abscess
p. access
p. cemental dysplasia
p. cementum
p. curettage
p. cyst
p. fibroma
p. film
full-mouth p.'s
p. granuloma
p. x-ray

periappendiceal abscess

periaqueductal
p. central gray
p. glioma
p. gray area
p. gray matter
p. gray nucleus
p. gray substance
p. hemorrhage
p. syndrome

periaqueductal-periventricular

periareolar
p. area
p. augmentation
p. de-epithelialization

periarterial
anterior coronary periarterial plexus
p. lymphatic sheath

periarteriolar
p. lymphocyte sheath
p. transudate

periarteritis
p. gummosa
infantile periarteritis nodosa
p. nodosa

periarticular
p. abscess
p. calcification
p. disorder
p. fibrositis
p. fluid collection
p. fracture
p. heterotopic ossification
p. margin
p. soft tissue

peribronchial
p. alveolar space
p. connective tissue
p. cuffing
p. desquamation
p. distribution
p. fibrosis
p. infiltration
p. inflammatory infiltrate
p. markings
p. pneumonia

peribulbar
p. anesthesia
p. anesthetic technique
p. injection
Livingston peribulbar wedge
p. needle

pericallosa
arteria p.

pericallosal
p. azygos artery
p. cistern
paracentral branch of pericallosal artery

pericanalicular connective tissue

pericapsular fat infiltration

pericardia (*pl. of* pericardium)

pericardiacophrenica
arteria p.

pericardiacophrenic artery

pericardiac tamponade

pericardial
p. air-fluid level
p. aorta
autologous pericardial patch
p. baffle
p. bioprosthetic tissue
p. biopsy
p. branch
p. branch of phrenic nerve
p. branch of thoracic aorta
p. calcification
p. cancer
p. cavity
p. chyle with tamponade
p. compliance
p. constriction-growth failure syndrome
continuous pericardial lavage
p. decompression
p. defect
p. diaphragmatic adhesion
p. disease
p. duplication cyst
p. effusion
p. fat pad
p. flap
p. fluid
p. fluid culture
p. fluid cytology
p. fluid examination
p. friction rub
p. friction sound
p. fusion
p. hemangioma
p. hematoma
p. knock
p. lavage
malignant pericardial effusion
p. mesothelioma
p. murmur
neoplastic pericardial effusion
p. tap
p. thickening
p. tuberculosis
p. window

pericardii
hydrops p.

pericardiocentesis
echo guided p.
p. procedure

pericardioperitoneal canal

pericardiophrenic artery

pericardiopleural fold

pericardiotomy
percutaneous balloon p.

pericarditis
acute idiopathic p.
acute lupus p.
p. calculosa
nanism-constrictive pericarditis syndrome
postoperative constrictive p.
purulent p.
p. sicca
p. with effusion

pericardium, pl. **pericardia**
adhesions of pericardium around heart
p. around heart
autologous p.
p. calcareous deposit
empyema of p.
p. fibrosa
p. fibrosum
heart with p.
p. meridian
parietal layer of serous p.
petechial hemorrhage of p.
serous p.
shaggy p.
thickened p.
visceral layer of serous p.

pericellular matrix

pericemental
p. abscess
p. attachment

pericementitis
apical p.

pericentral
p. cholestasia
p. fibrosis
p. rod-cone dystrophy
p. scotoma

pericholangiolitic cirrhosis

pericholecystic
p. abscess
p. edema
p. fluid collection

perichondral
p. bone
p. cell seeding
p. circulation

perichondrial
p. double cartilage block technique
p. elevator
p. flap
p. graft

perichondritis
arytenoid p.
auricular p.
peristernal p.

perichondrium
anterior p.

perichoroidal space

pericolic
p. abscess
p. membrane syndrome

pericolonic
p. abscess
p. fat
p. lymph node
p. penetration

pericolostomy
p. area
p. hernia

pericorneal plexus

pericoronal
p. abscess
p. flap

pericyte edema generation

peridental ligament

periductal
p. calcification
p. fibrosis
p. gland

peridural
p. analgesia
p. anesthesia
p. artery

periesophageal
p. abscess
p. blood vessel
p. fat
p. hemorrhage

perifascicular
p. atrophy
p. myofiber necrosis

periflexural
asymmetric periflexural exanthem of childhood

perifollicular
p. accentuation
p. fibroma
p. fibrosis
p. granuloma

perifornical
p. area
p. region

perifoveal arteriole

perifoveolar vitreoglial membrane

perigastric deformity

perihepatic
p. abscess
p. adhesion

perihilar
p. area
p. batwing infiltrate
p. calcification
p. density
p. lymph node
p. marking
p. mass
p. scarring

periinfarction
p. block
p. conduction defect

perikaryal
p. cytoplasm
p. group

perikaryon
magnocellular p.
norepinephrine p.

perilacunar mineral matrix

perilimbal
p. incision
p. stroma
p. suction
p. suction cup
p. ulceration
p. vitiligo

perilimbic circulation

perilobar
p. nephrogenic rest
p. pancreatitis

perilobular
p. connective tissue
p. duct
p. fibrosis

perilous
p. activity
p. course

perilunar dislocation

perilunate
p. carpal dislocation
p. fracture
p. fracture-dislocation

perilymph
p. fistula
p. fluid

perilymphatic
p. cavity
p. duct
p. fistula
p. fistula syndrome
p. fluid
p. gusher
X-linked progressive mixed deafness with perilymphatic gusher

perimacular vasculature

perimedial dysplasia

perimenarchal period

perimenopausal period

perimenstrual syndrome

perimesencephalic
p. cistern
p. nonaneurysmal subarachnoid hemorrhage

perimeter
arc and bowl p.
arch p.
arch perimeter analysis
p. corneal reflex test
p. earmold
Ferree-Rand p.
p. flap
Marco p.
Octopus 201 perimeter test
Ophthimus High-Pass Resolution p.
Ophthimus ring p.
Peritest p.
p. projection
visual fields by Goldmann-type p.

perimetric technique

perimetry
automated static threshold p.
kinetic p.
manual kinetic p.
motion automated p.
motion and displacement p.
Octopus automated p.
pattern discrimination p.
short wavelength automated p.

perimysial fibroblast

perinasal skin

perinatal
p. acidosis
p. anoxia
p. asphyxia
p. cerebral hemorrhage
p. clavicle fracture
Collaborative Perinatal Study
p. condition
corrected perinatal mortality
p. craniocerebral trauma
p. death
p. development
p. distress
p. distress prediction
p. effect
p. gangrene of buttock
p. hemochromatosis
p. herpes
p. HIV transmission
p. humerus fracture
p. hydronephrosis
p. hypoxemia
p. hypoxia
p. injury
p. insult
p. lethal osteogenesis imperfecta
p. medicine
p. monitor
p. morbidity
p. morbidity rate
p. mortality
p. mortality counseling program
p. mortality counseling team
p. mortality rate
p. nonstress test

regional perinatal intensive care center
p. stress test
p. substance abuse
p. telencephalic leukoencephalopathy
p. transmission

perindopril monotherapy

perinea (*pl. of* perineum)

perineal
abdominal and p.
p. abscess
p. analgesia
p. anesthesia
p. area
p. artery
p. artery axial flap
p. body
p. branch of posterior cutaneous nerve of thigh
p. branch of posterior femoral cutaneous nerve
p. candidiasis
p. Crohn disease
p. defect
p. descent
p. desquamation
p. drain
p. fascia
p. fistula
p. flexure
p. flexure of anal canal
p. flexure of rectum
p. hernia
p. hygiene
p. hypospadias
p. irritation
p. itching
p. laceration
p. lesion
Martinez Universal P. Interstitial Template
p. massage
p. MRSA colonization
multiple-site perineal applicator technique
p. nerve
Noble-Mengert perineal repair
p. pads
p. prep and drape
p. prostatectomy
p. pruritus
radical perineal prostatectomy
p. region
p. skin tag
p. support
p. support stitch
p. support suture
p. tear
p. tissue

perinealis
arteria p.

perineobulbar
p. detrusor facilitative reflex
p. detrusor inhibitory reflex

perineoplastic thyroiditis

perineoscrotal
p. hypospadias
pseudovaginal perineoscrotal hypospadias

perinephrial leukocytosis

perinephric
p. abscess
p. abscess drainage
p. air injection
p. capsule
p. fascia
p. fat
p. fluid collection
p. hematoma

Perinet virus

perineum, pl. **perinea**
anterior p.
p. care
membranous layer of superficial fascia of p.
os p.

perineural
p. anesthesia
p. arachnoid cyst
p. block
p. cell
p. channel
p. fibroblastoma
p. fibroma
p. fibrosis
p. infiltration
p. invasion

perineuritis
optic p.

perineuronal end foot

perinuclear
p. ANCA
p. antineutrophil cytoplasmic antibody
p. antineutrophil cytoplasmic autoantibody
p. cataract
p. CD15 antigen
p. cisterna
p. halo

periocular
p. area
p. bulge
p. capillary hemangioma
p. depigmentation
p. dermatitis
p. drug sensitivity
p. ecchymosis
p. festooning
p. infection
p. injection
p. milia
p. skin

period
absence of menstrual p.'s
absent menstrual period from diabetes
absolute refractory p.
p. of abstinence
active treatment p.
antegrade refractory p.
association p.
at-home recovery p.
atrial effective refractory p.
atrioventricular refractory p.
at-risk p.
cardiac refractory p.
corrected preejection p.
p.'s of crisis
date of last menstrual p.
diastolic filling p.
p. to discharge
discharge patient after period of observation
early postoperative p.
effective conduction p.
effective refractory p.
effective refractory period of the left ventricle
entire treatment p.
first day of last menstrual p.
first menstrual p.
fluctuating periods of remission and relapse
full p.
functional conduction p.
functional refractory p.
gap 0, 1, 2 p.
p. gene
heavy menstrual p.'s
heavy menstrual periods from anemia
24-hour period of observation and hydration
incubation p.
induction p.
initial dose p.

period *(continued)*
intermittent periods of depression
irregular menstrual p.
isometric contraction p.
isometric period of cardiac cycle
isometric relaxation p.
isovolumetric relaxation p.
last menstrual p.
latency p.
latent p.
left ventricular preejection p.
menstrual p.
normal menstrual p.
p. of onset
oral biting p.
past menstrual p.
peak amplitude p.
pitch period perturbation
postoperative period guarded
postventricular atrial refractory p.
preejection p.
preejection period index
prepatient periods to oocyst
previous menstrual p.
p. protein
rapid filling p.
refractory p.
refractory period of transmission
right preejection p.
right ventricular refractory p.
roentgen-equivalent-man p.
silent p.
sleep-onset rapid eye movement p.
sustained periods of grandiosity
systolic ejection p.
total atrial refractory p.
total infusion p.
ventricular effective refractory p.
vulnerable p.

periodic
p. abdominalgia
p. acid
p. acid-Schiff
p. acid-Schiff-Alcian blue
p. acid-Schiff-Alcian blue combination stain
p. acid-Schiff-hematoxylin stain
p. acid-Schiff method
p. acid-Schiff-positive
p. acid-Schiff-positive material
p. acid-Schiff reaction
p. acid-Schiff resistant
p. acid-Schiff stain
p. acid-Schiff technique
p. acid-Schiff test
p. acid-silver methenamine
p. acid-silver methenamine stain
p. acid staining
p. acid-thiocarbohydrazide-silver proteinate stain
Alcian blue and periodic acid-Schiff
p. alternating gaze
p. alternating gaze deviation
p. alternating windmill nystagmus
p. arthralgia
p. auscultation
autosomal-dominant periodic fever syndrome
bilateral independent periodic lateralizing epileptiform discharge
p. biopolymer
p. blood transfusion
p. bone pain
p. breathing
p. breathing cycle
p. breathing in infants
p. bursts of high voltage
p. catatonia
p. cessation of breathing
p. confusion
p. dilatation
p. dilatation of esophagus
p. disease
p. drinker
p. drinking
p. dropped beat
Early and Periodic Screening, Diagnosis, and Treatment program
p. edema
p. esotropia
p. evaluation record
p. exotropia
familial periodic paralysis
p. fever
p. fever, aphthous stomatitis, pharyngitis, cervical adenitis
p. fever syndrome
p. filariasis
p. health examination
p. hemilingual numbness
p. hypersomnia
p. inoculation
p. insanity
p. lateralizing epileptiform discharge
p. leg movement
p. limb movement
p. limb movement disorder
p. limb movements during sleep
p. limb movement in sleep
p. medical review
menstrual-associated periodic hypersomnia
p. movement disorder
p. neutropenia
normokalemic periodic paralysis
Ondine curse, periodic breathing
p. ophthalmia
p. paralysis
p. acid-concanavalin A
p. peritonitis
p. polyserositis
p. safety update reporting
p. sharp wave complex
p. short pulse
p. strabismus
p. swelling
p. synchronous discharge
tumor necrosis factor receptor-associated periodic syndrome
p. vomiting

periodic acid-concanavalin A

periodically fluctuating protein kinase

periodicity
lunar p.
malarial p.
nocturnal p.

period/left
preejection period/left ventricular ejection time

periodontal
p. abscess
p. anesthesia
apical periodontal abscess
apical periodontal cyst
p. armamentarium
p. atrophy
p. bony defect
p. cement
p. chart
p. chisel
community periodontal index of treatment needs
p. cyst
p. disease
P. Disease Index
p. disease rate
p. disease score
p. dressing
p. file
p. flap
p. graft
p. grafting
p. gum care
P. Index
p. infection

p. ligament
p. ligament fiber
p. membrane
minocycline periodontal therapeutic system
p. pockets
p. prophylactics

periodontitis
chronic destructive p.
p. complex
p. Ehlers-Danlos syndrome
human immunodeficiency virus-associated p.
juvenile p.
necrotizing ulcerative p.

periodontium alteration

perioperative
p. analgesia
p. anoxia
p. antibiotic
p. antibiotic prophylaxis
p. antibiotic therapy
p. bacteremia
p. cardiac complication
p. cisternography
p. complication
p. corneal abrasion
p. data
p. death
p. morbidity
p. myocardial infarction
p. respiratory therapy

perioptic
p. cerebrospinal fluid
p. hygroma
p. neuritis
p. sheath meningioma
p. subarachnoid space

perioral
p. area
p. dermatitis
p. fissure
p. flaw
p. paresthesia

periorbital
p. area
p. bidirectional Doppler
p. cellulitis
p. dermatitis
p. directional Doppler ultrasonography
p. Doppler imaging
p. ecchymosis
p. edema
p. erythema
p. fat
p. fat atrophy
p. freckling
p. fullness
p. hemangioma
p. hematoma
p. hyperpigmentation
p. infantile myofibromatosis
p. leukoderma
p. membrane
p. puffiness
p. soft tissue
p. swelling
p. volume augmentation

periorificial
p. dermatitis
p. lentiginosis

periostea (*pl. of* periosteum)

periosteal
anterior labroligamentous periosteal sleeve
anterior labroligamentous periosteal sleeve avulsion lesion
anterior labrum periosteal sleeve avulsion
p. artery
p. arthritis
p. band
p. bone
p. bone collar
p. bud
p. button
p. cambium layer
p. chondroma
p. chondrosarcoma
p. cloaking
p. creep
curved periosteal elevator
p. cyst
p. desmoid
p. dysplasia
p. elevation
p. elevator
p. envelope
p. fibroma
p. fibrosarcoma
fine periosteal elevator
p. flap
galeal periosteal flap
p. ganglion
p. graft
p. hypertrophy
p. implantation
p. irregularity
p. layer of dura mater
lower abdominal periosteal reflex
p. ossification
p. osteogenesis
p. procedure
p. sarcoma
p. thickening
p. transplantation

periosteocytic space

periosteum, pl. **periostea**
anterior labrum periosteum shoulder arthroscopic lesion
p. incised
p. incised and retracted
orbital p.

periostitis
alveolodental p.
orbital p.
p. ossificans toxica

periotic
p. bone
p. cartilage
p. duct

periovarian adhesion

periovulatory phase

peripancreatic
p. abdominal drainage
p. area
p. artery
p. fat plane
p. fibrosis
p. fluid
p. fluid collection
p. lymphadenopathy
p. lymph node
p. neoplasm
p. pseudoaneurysm

peripapillary
p. central serous choroidopathy
p. choroid
p. choroidal arterial system
p. choroidal atrophy
p. coloboma
p. nerve fiber layer
p. retinal height
p. retinal nerve
p. retinal nerve fiber
p. scar
p. sclerosis
p. scotoma
p. staphyloma
p. staphylomata
p. subretinal neovascularization

peripartum
p. cardiac failure
p. cardiomyopathy
p. endoscopy

peripatellar
p. incision
p. pain
peripelvic
p. collateral vessel
p. cyst
p. extravasation
p. fat
peripheral
p. ablative surgery
P. Access System
P. Access System Port catheter system
p. acinar vein
p. acrocyanosis
acute idiopathic peripheral facial nerve palsy
p. adrenergic agent
p. ageusia
p. agglutinin
p. airspace
p. air space disease
p. airway
p. airway obstruction
alcoholic peripheral neuropathy
alcohol-induced peripheral neuropathy
allogeneic peripheral cell transplant
p. ameloblastic fibroma
p. ameloblastoma
p. androgen activity
p. androgen activity marker
p. androgen blockade
p. anergy
p. anesthesia
p. aneurysm
p. angiography
anterior peripheral curve
p. anterior stent keratopathy
p. anterior synechia
anti-CD3 stimulated peripheral blood lymphocytes transduced with a gene encoding a chimeric
p. antimuscarinic side effect
antiperipheral nerve myelin antibody
p. apnea
argon laser peripheral iridoplasty
p. aromatization
arsenic peripheral neuropathy
p. arterial aneurysmal disease
p. arterial arcade
p. arterial catheter
p. arterial disease
p. arterial line
p. arterial occlusion
p. arterial occlusive disease
p. arterial tone
p. arterial vasodilation theory
p. arteriography
p. arteriosclerosis
p. arteriosclerotic occlusive disease
arteriosclerotic peripheral vascular disease
p. arteriovenous fistula
p. artery
p. artery disease
p. arthritis
p. atherosclerosis
p. atherosclerotic disease
p. auditory disorder
p. auditory function
autologous peripheral blood stem cell bone marrow transplantation
autologous peripheral hematopoietic stem cell support
p. autonomic neuropathy
autonomic part of peripheral nervous system
avascular peripheral retina
avitaminosis B_{12} peripheral neuropathy
p. avulsion
p. balloon angioplasty
p. basement membrane
p. basophilia
p. benign neoplasm
p. benzodiazepine receptor
p. bile duct
p. bladder denervation
p. blood
p. blood $CD8^+$ lymphocytosis
p. blood cell
p. blood cell count
p. blood circulation
p. blood count
p. blood eosinophilia
p. blood eosinophils
p. blood flow
p. blood labeling index
p. blood leukocyte
p. blood lymphocyte
p. blood lymphocyte analysis
p. blood lymphocyte transformation
p. blood monocyte
p. blood mononuclear cell
p. blood mononuclear cell hepatitis B virus measurement
p. blood preparation
p. blood preparation for microfilariae
p. blood pressure
p. blood progenitor cell
p. blood progenitor cell transplant
p. blood smear
p. blood stem cell
p. blood stem cell autografting
p. blood stem cell infusion
p. blood stem cell rescue
p. blood stem cell reserve
p. blood stem cell support
p. blood stem cell transplantation
p. blood studies
p. bolus chase
p. border
p. branch retinal vein occlusion
p. bruit
p. capillary filtration slit length
p. carcinoma
p. cataract
p. catecholamine
p. catecholamine receptor
p. cavity wall
p. cemental dysplasia
p. chemical sympathectomy
p. chemoreceptor
p. chemoreflex loop
p. cholangiocarcinoma
p. cholinergic activity
p. chondrosarcoma
p. chorioretinal atrophic spot
p. chorioretinal atrophy
chronic peripheral arterial disease
p. circulation
p. circulatory failure
p. circulatory vasoconstriction
p. coin lesion
computer tomographic methods of peripheral skeleton
p. consolidation
p. corneal opacity
p. corneal ulcer
p. coronary pressure
p. cue test
p. curve on contact lens
p. cutaneous vasoconstriction
p. cyanosis
p. cyanosis of extremities
p. cystoid degeneration
p. cytotrophoblast cell
p. deafferentation pain
decreasing peripheral vascular resistance
p. dentin
dependent peripheral edema

p. detection test
p. diabetes insipidus
p. diabetic neuropathy
diabetic peripheral neuropathy
p. diabetic retinopathy
p. directional atherectomy
p. disciform degeneration
p. dual-energy x-ray absorptiometry
p. dysarthria
p. dysostosis
p. dysostosis, nail hypoplasia, mental retardation syndrome
p. edema
p. electromyographic activity
p. endotheliitis
p. enhancement
p. eosinophil count
p. eosinophilia
p. epilepsy
p. examination
p. excimer laser angioplasty
p. extremity edema
p. exudative choroidal hemorrhagic retinopathy
p. facial nerve palsy
p. facial paralysis
p. fat wasting
p. fibrosis
p. field image
p. fields
p. fractional oxygen extraction
p. frame implant substructure
p. fusion
p. gangrene
p. giant cell reparative granuloma
p. giant cell tumor
p. glare
p. glioma
p. glucocorticoid deficiency
p. glucose uptake
p. glycerol injection
good peripheral circulation
griseofulvin peripheral neuropathy
p. hepatojejunostomy
p. hormone level
human peripheral blood leukocyte
human peripheral lymphocyte
human peripheral mononuclear cell
p. hypoperfusion
increased peripheral vasodilation and hypotension
p. indwelling intermediate infusion device
p. infusion
p. injection
p. insulin sensitivity
p. interface adapter
intracapsular cataract extraction with peripheral iridectomy
p. intraretinal hemorrhage
p. intravenous
p. intravenous administration
p. intravenous catheter
p. intravenous hyperalimentation
p. iridectomy operation
p. iris roll
p. jaundice
p. joint
p. laser angioplasty
laser peripheral iridectomy
p. leukocytosis
p. light detection
p. light loss
p. light scatter
p. lipoatrophy
p. lipodystrophy
lupus erythematosus peripheral neuropathy
Lyme-associated peripheral facial nerve palsy
p. lymph node
p. lymphocyte count
p. lymphoid cell
malignant peripheral nerve sheath tumor
maternal peripheral blood
methyl alcohol peripheral neuropathy
migratory peripheral arthritis
p. monocyte count
p. mononeuropathy
p. multifocal chorioretinitis
p. muscle strength
p. myelin protein
p. myelin protein 22 gene
nasal hypoplasia, peripheral dysostosis, mental retardation syndrome
p. necrotizing retinitis
p. nerve
p. nerve block
p. nerve conduction
p. nerve damage
p. nerve evaluation
p. nerve injury
p. nerve involvement
p. nerve lesion
p. nerve myelin
p. nerve root syndrome
p. nerve sheath tumor
p. nervous stimulator
p. nervous system
p. nervous system disorder
p. neuritis
p. neuroectodermal tumor
p. neuroepithelioma
neurogenic peripheral intermittent claudication
p. neuroglia
p. neurologic adverse effect
p. neuroma
p. neurotoxicity
p. neutropenia
p. nucleated cell
p. nystagmus
p. occlusive arterial disease
p. oculomotor nerve
optic fundi and peripheral fields
oral peripheral examination
p. organ
p. osteoarticular tuberculosis
p. parenteral nutrition
p. perfusion
p. polyneuropathy
p. posterior curve
posterior peripheral curve
p. primitive neuroectodermal tumor
p. proliferation
p. protein sparing solution
p. pulmonary artery stenosis
p. pulse
p. pulse palpable
p. pulses full and equal bilaterally
p. pulses intact
p. pulses palpable both legs
p. quantitative computed tomography
p. ray of light
p. reflex
p. resistance unit
p. retina
p. retinal ablation
p. retinal operculum
p. retinal vascular sheathing
p. ring of hemoglobin
p. ring infiltrate
p. rod function
p. root compression
p. scalloping
p. scotoma
simultaneous peripheral operation on-line
p. stem cell harvest
p. stem cell transplant
stenosing peripheral arterial disease
surgical peripheral iridectomy

peripheral *(continued)*
symmetrical peripheral gangrene
systemic peripheral vascular resistance
p. T_4
p. tapetochoroidal degeneration
p. T-cell lymphoma
p. thyroid hormone metabolism
p. thyroxine
p. tissue resistance to thyroid hormone
total peripheral parenteral nutrition
total peripheral resistance index
total peripheral vascular resistance
p. total resistance
p. ulcerative keratitis
upright peripheral plasma renin activity
p. uveitis
p. vascular
p. vascular disease
p. vascular insufficiency
p. vascular laboratory
p. vascular occlusion
p. vascular occlusive disease
p. vascular resistance
p. vascular resistance index
p. vascular surgery
p. vascular system
p. vein plasma
p. vein renin activity
p. vein total parenteral nutrition
p. venous disease
p. venous nutrition
p. venous pressure
p. vessel
p. vestibular deficit
p. vestibular nystagmus
p. vision
p. visual field
p. visual field loss
p. vitreoretinal traction
p. white blood cell
p. zone

peripherally
p. acting anticholinergic medication
p. inserted catheter line
p. inserted central venous catheter

peripheral-type benzodiazepine receptor

peripherin/RDS gene

periphery
p. of the anulus
p. of cornea
p. denture
disc, macula, vessels, p.
p. of eye
posterior pole and p.
p. of retina

periportal
p. area
p. carcinoma
p. cardiomyopathy
p. cirrhosis
p. collar
p. fibrosis
p. hepatocyte

periprostatic block

periprosthetic
p. bone loss
p. bone resorption
p. breast abscess
p. fibrous capsule
p. fluid
p. fracture

periradial
anular periradial recess

perirectal
p. abscess
p. cellulitis
p. disease
p. fat
p. fat infiltration
p. fistula
p. infection
p. inflammation

perirenal
p. abscess
p. air study
p. bleeding
p. compartment
p. fascia
p. fasciitis
p. fat
p. fat capsule
p. hematoma
p. space
p. tissue

periretinal edema

periscapular
curved periscapular incision
p. incision

periscleral space

periscopic
p. concave
p. concave lens
p. convex
p. convex lens
p. meniscus
p. spectacles

perisinusoidal
p. cell
p. fibrin deposition
p. fibrosis

peristalsis
p. of abdomen
antral p.
p. of bowel
p. of colon
high-amplitude p.
small bowel p.

peristaltic
abnormal peristaltic action of colon
p. activity
p. anastomosis
p. contraction
p. hyperemia
p. motion
p. movement
p. pump
p. rush
p. sound
p. wave

peristernal perichondritis

peristimulus time

peristomal area

peristriate
p. area
p. cortex
p. visual cortex

perisylvian
p. abnormality
p. cortex

peritarsal network

peritendinitis
p. calcarea
p. crepitans

peritendinous
p. adhesion
p. calcification
p. fibrosis

Peritest perimeter

perithymic fat

perithyroidal adventitia

peritonea (*pl. of* peritoneum)

peritoneal
p. access
p. adenocarcinoma
p. adhesion
ambulatory peritoneal dialysis patient

p. anatomy
p. aspiration
p. attachment
automated peritoneal dialysis
p. autoplasty
p. band
p. biopsy
p. blastomycosis
p. borderline tumor
p. cancer
p. carcinoma
p. carcinomatosis
p. cavity
p. cavity abscess
p. cavity fluid
p. cell
chronic ambulatory peritoneal dialysis
chronic intermittent peritoneal dialysis
continuous abdominal peritoneal dialysis
continuous ambulatory peritoneal dialysis
continuous cycler-assisted peritoneal dialysis
continuous cyclical peritoneal dialysis
continuous cyclic peritoneal dialysis
continuous cycling peritoneal dialysis
continuous hyperthermic peritoneal perfusion
copious peritoneal lavage
p. cytological assessment
p. cytology sample
daily intermittent peritoneal dialysis
p. defect
Denver peritoneal venous shunt
p. deposit
diagnostic peritoneal lavage
p. dialysate
p. dialysis
p. dialysis-associated peritonitis
p. dialysis catheter
p. dialysis creatinine clearance target
p. dialysis effluent
p. dialysis fluid
p. dialysis system
p. dialysis urea removal
p. disease
p. dissemination
p. drain
p. drainage
p. dropsy
p. encapsulation
p. envelope
p. equilibration test
equilibrium peritoneal dialysis
p. exudate
p. exudate cell
p. exudate lymphocyte
p. exudate macrophage
p. fibrosis
p. flap
p. fluid cytology
p. fluid examination
p. fossa
free peritoneal air
free peritoneal fluid
p. friction rub
p. fungal infection
Gram stain of peritoneal fluid
p. hernia
home-automated peritoneal dialysis
home peritoneal dialysis
p. implant
p. implant metastasis
p. incision
p. insufflation
intermittent peritoneal dialysis
p. irritation
p. lavage
p. ligament of liver
lumbar arachnoid peritoneal shunt
p. lymphoma
p. macrophage
p. mesothelial cyst
p. mesothelioma
p. metastasis
p. mouse
multilocular peritoneal inclusion cyst
negative peritoneal cytology
nightly intermittent peritoneal dialysis
nocturnal tidal peritoneal dialysis
p. oocyte and sperm transfer
parietal peritoneal inflammation
percutaneous peritoneal biopsy
positive peritoneal cytology
primary peritoneal carcinoma
primary peritoneal drainage
prolonged-dwell peritoneal dialysis
p. pseudomyxoma
subcutaneous peritoneal administration device
subdural p.
p. tap
title peritoneal dialysis
p. transudate
p. tuberculosis
ventricles to peritoneal cavity shunt
ventricular p.

peritonealis

peritonei
pseudomyxoma p.

peritoneocutaneous
Morley peritoneocutaneous reflex

peritoneojugular shunt

peritoneovenous shunt

peritoneum, pl. **peritonea**
abdominal p.
p. desmoid tumor
p. incised
matted p.
overlapping closure of p.
papillary serous carcinoma of the p.
parietal p.
petechial hemorrhage of p.
p. smooth and glistening
p. studded with tumor nodules

peritonitis
acute diffuse p.
p. carcinomatosa
p. encapsulans
Escherichia coli sepsis p.
feline infectious p.
feline infectious peritonitis virus
gonorrheal invasive p.
peritoneal dialysis-associated p.
sclerosing encapsulating p.
P. Severity Score
spontaneous acute bacterial p.
tuberculous p.

peritonsillar
p. abscess
p. cellulitis
p. edema
p. tag

peritracheal gland

peritrapezial arthritis

peritraumatic dissociation

peritubular
p. capillary
p. contractile cell
p. dentin
p. endothelial cell
p. fluid
p. HCO^{3-}

peritumoral
p. band

peritumoral *(continued)*
p. brain edema
p. cyst
peritumor glial reaction
periumbilical
p. abscess
p. hernia
p. incision
p. pain
p. staining
periungual
p. avascularity
p. desquamation
p. erythema
p. fibroma
p. flaking
p. wart
periungualis
onychia p.
periureteral
p. abscess
p. fibrosis
periurethral
p. abscess
p. bulking agent
p. collagen injection
p. duct carcinoma
p. gland
p. transurethral microwave thermotherapy
perivaginal fascia
perivalvular
p. abscess
p. dehiscence
p. disruption
p. leak
p. leakage
perivascular
axillary perivascular technique
p. calcification
p. canal
p. change
p. cloaking
p. cuff
p. cuffing
dilated perivascular spaces
p. distribution
p. end foot
p. epithelioid cell
p. fibroblast
p. gliosis
His perivascular space
p. infiltration
interstitial and perivascular collagen network
p. lymph space
p. pattern
p. sheathing
perivasculitis
granulomatous p.
perivenous encephalomyelitis
periventricular
anterior periventricular nucleus
p. border
p. calcification
cystic periventricular leukomalacia
p. disease
p. echogenicity
echogenicity of periventricular white matter
p. echolucency
p. encephalomalacia
p. fiber
p. gray matter
p. gray substance
p. hemorrhage
p. hyperintense lesion
p. hyperintensity
p. infarction
p. inhibitor
p. leukomalacia
p. nucleus
p. radiolucency
periventriculares
nuclei p.
periventricular-intraventricular hemorrhage
perivenular
progressive perivenular alcoholic fibrosis
perivesical
p. abscess
p. fascia
perizonalium
Perlita
San Perlita virus
permanent
p. blindness
p. brachytherapy
p. callus
p. cardiac pacemaker
p. childhood hearing impairment
p. childhood hearing loss
p. colostomy
p. cranial nerve deficit
p. demand ventricular pacemaker
p. dentition
p. diabetes insipidus
p. disability
P. Disability Rating Board
p. end colostomy
p. filling
p. flexure contracture
p. hearing loss
p. ileostomy
p. impairment
p. implant
p. implant therapy
p. incidence
p. joint damage
p. junctional reciprocating tachycardia
p. kidney damage
molar permanent tooth
noise-induced permanent threshold shift
p. pacemaker implantation
p. pacemaker insertion
p. pacemaker placement
p. partial
p. partial disability
partial permanent impairment
p. Disability Rating Board
p. threshold shift
p. and total
p. total disability
p. tracheotomy
transperineal interstitial permanent prostate brachytherapy
p. transvenous demand pacemaker
p. visual impairment
permanently
Aid to P. and Totally Disabled
p. implanted ventricular assist device
permanganate
potassium p.
permeability
alveolar p.
alveolar-capillary membrane p.
p. area
p. coefficient
p. constant
p. factor
high permeability edema
increased lung p.
increasing capillary p.
p. index
intestinal p.
lymph node permeability factor
p. pulmonary edema
pulmonary microvascular permeability to protein
p. quotient
p. surface
thymus permeability factor
p. of vacuum

vascular p.
vascular endothelial growth factor/vascular permeability factor

permeable
gas permeable contact lens
highly permeable transparent dressing
synthetic, adhesive, moisture vapor p.

permeation
gel permeation chromatography
lymphatic p.

permissible
daily permissible intake
p. dose
p. exposure limits
maximal daily permissible intake
maximal permissible concentration
maximal permissible concentration of unidentified radionuclides
maximum dose permissible dose
maximum permissible concentration

permission
p. for autopsy denied
p. for autopsy granted
p. for blood transfusion
p., limited information, specific suggestions, and intensive therapy
p. for surgery

permissive hypercapnia

permit
autopsy permit signed
operative permit signed

permitted
maximal permitted intake

permitting safe expression of anger

pernicious
p. anemia
p. anemia-like syndrome and immunoglobulin deficiency
appetite loss from pernicious anemia
dementia from pernicious anemia
juvenile pernicious anemia
p. malaria
tongue inflammation from pernicious anemia
p. vomiting
weight loss from pernicious anemia

pernio
lupus p.

peromelia
mandibular dysostosis and p.

peronea
arteria p.
perforating arteries of p.

peroneal
anterior peroneal artery
p. artery
p. atrophy
p. bone
p. border of foot
p. bypass
common peroneal nerve
p. communicating branch
p. compartment syndrome
p. entrapment neuropathy
functional electronic peroneal brace
p. groove
long peroneal muscle
p. lymph node
p. muscle
p. muscle atrophy
p. nerve
p. nerve entrapment
p. nerve palsy
perforating branch of peroneal artery
p. tendon
p. vein

peroneus
p. brevis
p. brevis elongation
p. brevis flap
p. brevis graft
p. brevis muscle
p. brevis split
p. brevis tendon
p. brevis transfer
p. brevis transplant
p. communis
p. longus
p. longus muscle
p. longus muscle avulsion
p. longus tendinopathy
nervus communicans p.

peroral
p. approach
p. cholangiopancreatoscopy
p. cholangioscopy
p. cone radiation therapy
p. electronic pancreatoscope
p. endoprosthesis
p. endoscopy
p. esophageal dilation
p. excision
p. pancreatoscopy
p. shock wave lithotripsy

peroxidase
airway p.
antithyroid peroxidase antibody
avidin-biotin p.
avidin-biotin-horseradish peroxidase complex
avidin-biotin peroxidase complex
concanavalin A-horseradish p.
glutathione p.
hepatocatalase p.
horseradish p.
lactic p.
peroxidase antibody to p.
platelet p.
reduced glutathione p.
streptavidin-biotin peroxidase complex
thyroid p.
tryptophan p.

peroxidase-antiperoxidase technique

peroxidase-labeled antibodies test

peroxidatic activity

peroxidation
lipid p.

peroxide
p. flush
p. hemolysis test
hydrogen peroxide ultrasound
red cell peroxide hemolysis
vaporized hydrogen p.
zinc p.

peroxisomal proliferator receptor

peroxisome
p. proliferator-activated receptor
p. proliferator-activated receptor gamma
p. proliferator response element

peroxyl
total peroxyl radical-trapping antioxidant potential

perpendicular
p. anterior wall
p. fashion
incised p.

Perroncito
apparatus of P.

persecution
p. delusion
delusion of jealousy and p.
p. ideation

persecutory
p. anxiety
p. delusion
p. delusional disorder
perseveration
clonic p.
p. deficit
p. of speech
perseverative error
Persian Gulf syndrome
persistence
p. of fetal circulation
hereditary persistence of fetal hemoglobin
microbial p.
persistent
aneurysm of persistent trigeminal artery
p. anovulation
p. anxiety
p. atrial standstill
p. bronchopleural fistula
p. chronic hepatitis
chronic persistent hepatitis
p. clonus
p. complete atrioventricular canal
p. corpus luteum
p. cough and phlegm
p. cough with hemoptysis
p. delusion
p. discomfort
p. ductus arteriosus
p. ectopic pregnancy
p. edema
p. emotional condition
p. epithelial defect
p. estrogen secretion
p. facial palsy
p. fetal circulation
p. fetal circulation with pulmonary hypertension
p. frontal suture
p. generalized lymphadenopathy
p. gross splenomegaly
p. hacking cough
p. headache
p. hoarseness
p. hyperinsulinemic hypoglycemia of infancy
p. hyperparathyroidism
p. hyperphenylalaninemia
p. hyperplasia of primary vitreous
hyperplastic persistent pupillary membrane
p. hyperplastic primary vitreous
p. hypersomnia
p. hypertrophic vitreous
p. identity disturbance
p. inappropriate idea
p. inappropriate image
p. inappropriate impulse
p. incontinence
p. indigestion
p. interstitial pulmonary emphysema
p. irritability
p. ischemia
p. light reaction
malignant persistent positional nystagmus
p. mental illness
p. mentoposterior fetal position
mild persistent asthma
moderate persistent asthma
p. müllerian duct syndrome
p. neonatal myasthenia gravis
noneczematous persistent papular gold eruption
p. occipitoposterior fetal position
p. occiput posterior position
p. occiput posterior presentation
p. organic pollutants
p. viral hepatitis, type B
p. polyuria
p. postdrainage hypotony
posttraumatic persistent pneumothorax
p. primary hyperplastic vitreous
primary persistent hyperplastic vitreous
p. proteinuria
p. pulmonary hypertension
p. pulmonary hypertension of newborn
p. pupillary membrane
p. pupillary membrane remnant
p. reactivity to light
severe and persistent mental illness
p. tolerant infection
p. trigeminal artery
p. trophoblastic disease
p. truncus arteriosus
p. vaginal cornification
p. varicose veins
p. vegetative state
p. viral hepatitis
p. viral hepatitis, non-A, non-B
p. viral hepatitis, type B
p. viral syndrome
p. vomiting or confusion headache
p. withdrawal occlusion
persisting
alcohol-induced persisting dementia
alcohol persisting dementia
anxiolytic-induced persisting dementia
chronic persisting hepatitis
p. dementia
p. galactorrhea-amenorrhea syndrome
hallucinogen persisting perception disorder
p. hepatitis
p. proteinuria
person
abusive invasive p.
alert and oriented to person, place, and time
alert and oriented to person, place, time, and date
Assessment for P.'s Profoundly or Severely Impaired
Attitudes Toward Disabled P.'s
displaced p.
p. gametocyte week
Genetically Handicapped P.'s Program
handicapped p.
Multidimensional Quality of Life Questionnaire for P.'s with Human Immunodeficiency Virus
p. in need of supervision
oriented to person, place, and time
oriented to time, place, and p.
oriented to time, place, person, and objects watch, pen, book
patient alert to space, time, and p.
patient oriented to person, place and time
place and p.
p., place, and time
place, time, and p.
place, person, and time
poor p.
squarely face person, open posture, lean toward person, eye contact, relaxed
p. with AIDS
p. with a disability
personal
p. abandonment

additional personal injury protection
p. adjustment
P. Adjustment and Role Skills Scale
adolescent personal identity
Adult P. Data Inventory
p. agenda
p. agony
altered personal behavior
apathy and lack of interest in personal goals
p. assault
P. Assessment for Continuing Education
P. Assessment of Intimacy in Relationships
p. belief
p. care
p. care attendant
p. care boarding home
p. care clinic
p. care home
p. care service
p. control
p. counselor
decline in personal grooming
p. desire for gain
p. development
direct personal contact
p. disposition
Edwards P. Preference Schedule
p. emergency response system
p. experience
P. Experience and Attitude Questionnaire
P. Experience Screening Questionnaire
fear of personal harm
p. function
p. goal
Gordon P. Inventory
Gordon P. Profile
Gordon P. Profile Inventory
p. growth
p. habit
p. health cost
p. heart device
p. history
p. history of depressive disorders
p. hygiene
p. hygiene facility
p. identification number
p. identity
p. identity disturbance
p. image
indirect personal contact
p. injury
p. injury accident
p. injury collision
p. injury protection
p. locus of control
loss of interest in personal grooming
p. oral hygiene
P. Orientation Inventory
p. portable stimulator
P. Preference Scale
P. Problems Checklist for Adolescents
Progress Assessment Chart of Social and P. Development
p. protective equipment
P. Relationship Inventory
P. and Role Skills
p. self-maintenance activity
Shipley P. Inventory
p. and social history
P. Strain Questionnaire
P. Style Inventory
p. time off
P. Values Abstract
P. Values Inventory
p. watercraft accident

personality

p. abnormality
addiction-prone p.
P. Adjective Check List
Adult P. Inventory
affective neurotic personality disorder
Allport personality trait theory
amoral psychopathic p.
antisocial neurotic p.
antisocial neurotic personality disorder
antisocial personality trait
antisocial trends psychopathic p.
anxiety-avoiding personality disorder
anxious-neurotic personality trait
apathetic-type personality disorder
asocial trends psychopathic p.
p. assessment
P. Assessment Inventory
p. assessment system
asthenic personality disorder
atypical mixed or other personality disorder
avoidant neurotic personality disorder
avoidant personality disorder
Basic Personality Inventory
borderline p.
borderline personality disorder
California P. Inventory
California Test of P.
p. change disorder
Children's P. Questionnaire
Child P. Scale
chronic depressive personality disorder
cognitive personality trait
compulsive personality disorder
Comrey P. Scale
cult of p.
dependent personality disorder
p. deterioration
p. development
p. deviation
P. Diagnostic Questionnaire-Revised
Dimensional Assessment of P. Pathology-Basic Questionnaire
p. disintegration
disintegration of p.
p. disorder
p. disorder diagnosis
p. disorder examination
p. disorder NOS
p. disorder profile
p. disorder score
disorientation and personality change
Dynamic P. Inventory
p. dynamics
p. dysfunction
Early School P. Questionnaire
explosive personality disorder
Eysenck P. Inventory
Eysenck P. Questionnaire
p. factor
16 P. Factor Questionnaire
p. factor questionnaire
p. feature
p. formation
Freiburger P. Inventory
p. functioning
Gardner Analysis of P. Survey
p. and gender
Guilford-Zimmerman P. Test
Heston P. Index
Heston Personality Inventory Test
High School P. Questionnaire
histrionic personality disorder
histrionic personality trait
increased personality disintegration
P. Index
intermittent explosive personality disorder
p. inventory

personality *(continued)*
irritability, depression and personality changes
Jackson P. Inventory
Junior Eysenck P. Inventory
Lazare-Klerman-Armour Personality Inventory
Maudsley P. Inventory
Millon Adolescent P. Inventory
Minnesota-Hartford P. Assay
Minnesota Multiphasic Personality Inventory Depression Scale
Minnesota Multiphasic P. Inventory, Second Edition
moral deficiency personality disorder
multiple personality disorder
Multivariate P. Inventory
Narcissistic P. Inventory
Neurotic P. Factor Test
Omnibus P. Inventory
organic personality disorder
organic personality syndrome
paranoid personality disorder
passive-aggressive p.
passive-aggressive personality disorder
passive-dependent p.
P. Rating Scale
P. Research Form
Sales P. Questionnaire
schizoid personality disorder
schizoid-schizotypal personality disorder
schizotypal personality disorder
Self-Rating Obsessive-Compulsive P. Inventory
Singer-Loomis Inventory of P.
Sixteen P. Factors Test
sociopathic personality disorder
State-Trait P. Inventory
p. trait
p. trait disorder
type A, B p.

personalized aerobics for cardiovascular enhancement

personnel
Hilson P. Profile/Success Quotient
medical personnel pool
P. Security Preview
P. Tests for Industry
unlicensed assistive p.

person-year
p.-y. rad

person-years of exposure

perspective
alternating p.
alternative p.
atmospheric p.
gain p.
holistic p.

perspiration
profuse p.

perstans
Mansonella perstans infection

pertechnetate

Perthes
P. disease
P. test

pertinent
past pertinent history
p. physical findings

perturbation
average perturbation quotient
pitch period p.
relative average p.

pertussis
p., acellular antigens, vaccine
acellular pertussis vaccine with diphtheria and tetanus toxoid
p. agglutination test
anti-*Bordetella pertussis* antibody
diphtheria, pertussis, and tetanus
diphtheria, pertussis, and tetanus immunization
diphtheria, tetanus, pertussis, *Haemophilus influenzae* type b vaccine
diphtheria, pertussis, tetanus, poliomyelitis, and measles vaccine
diphtheria, tetanus toxoid, and acellular pertussis vaccine
diphtheria, tetanus toxoids, whole-cell pertussis, and *Haemophilus influenzae* type b conjugate
diphtheria, tetanus toxoids, whole-cell pertussis vaccine
diphtheria, pertussis, and tetanus vaccine
Haemophilus pertussis vaccine
p. immune globulin
p. immunoglobulin
p., whole-cell antigens, vaccine
p. serology
p. syndrome
p. toxin
p. toxoid

pertussis-like syndrome

pervasive
p. affect
p. anhedonia
p. anxiety
atypical pervasive developmental disorder
p. developmental disorder
p. developmental disorder not otherwise specified
p. emotion
p. pattern of instability

pes
p. abductus
p. adductus
p. anserine transfer
p. anserinus
p. anserinus bursa
p. anserinus bursitis
anterior pes cavus
p. arcuatus
p. arcuatus clawfoot deformity
p. calcaneocavus
p. calcaneovalgus
p. calcaneus
p. cavovalgus
p. cavovarus
p. cavus
p. cavus clawfoot deformity
p. cavus deformity
p. equinovalgus
p. equinovarus
p. equinovarus adductus
equinovarus pes deformity
p. equinus
p. excavatum
p. planus
p. pronatus
p. tendonitis
p. valgus
p. varus

pessary
Mayer p.
Menge p.
ring p.
Wylie p.

pessimistic
p. attitude
p. rumination

Peste
la Peste vaccine

pesticides
health aspects of p.

pestis

pet-borne illness

petechia, pl. **petechiae**
- hemorrhagic petechiae
- linear p.
- palatal petechiae
- petechiae of tongue

petechial
- p. angioma
- diffuse petechial hemorrhage
- p. eruption
- p. exanthem
- focal petechial hemorrhage
- p. hemorrhage
- p. hemorrhage of bowel
- p. hemorrhage of kidney
- p. hemorrhage of pericardium
- p. hemorrhage of peritoneum
- p. hemorrhage of skin
- p. hemorrhaging
- p. purpura
- p. rash
- subendocardial petechial hemorrhage

petit
- P. aponeurosis
- atypical petit mal seizure
- P. canal
- P. hernia
- P. herniotomy
- P. ligament
- p. mal
- p. mal convulsion
- p. mal epilepsy
- p. mal seizure
- p. mal variant
- myoclonic petit mal

petition of mental illness

petroclival area

petrolatum
- hydrophilic p.
- red veterinary p.

petroleum
- crude coal tar in p.
- liquified petroleum gas
- scientifically treated p.

petrooccipital
- p. fissure
- p. joint

petrosal
- p. approach
- p. artery
- p. bone
- p. branch of middle meningeal artery
- p. foramen
- p. fossa
- p. ganglion
- greater superficial petrosal neurectomy
- inferior petrosal sinus sampling
- p. nerve

petrositis
- apical p.

petrous
- p. apex
- p. apex mass
- apex of petrous part of temporal bone
- apex of petrous portion of temporal bone
- p. apex tumor
- p. bone
- caries of petrous bone
- p. carotid canal
- p. ganglion
- p. osteomyelitis
- p. ridge
- p. tip

Pettigrew syndrome

Peutz-Jeghers syndrome

Peyer
- P. gland
- P. patch

Peyronie
- P. disease
- modified Peyronie bladder neck suspension
- P. plaque

Pfannenstiel incision

Pfeiffer
- P. disease
- P. syndrome

Pfuhl sign

pH4
- area under p.

phaco
- nonaspirating ultrasonic phaco chopper tip

phacoemulsification
- p. of the left eye
- no-stitch phacoemulsification surgery
- p. procedure
- p. of the right eye

phacogenic glaucoma

phacolytic glaucoma

phage
- immature p.
- staphylococcal phage lysate

phagedenic
- tropical phagedenic ulcer

phagocyte
- absolute phagocyte count
- p. dysfunction
- mononuclear p.

phagocytic
- p. deficiency
- p. dysfunction immunodeficiency
- p. function
- p. immunity
- p. index
- macrophage phagocytic activity
- reticuloendothelial phagocytic capacity

phagocytosis
- p. and killing function
- p. promoting factor

phakic eye

phakomatosis
- Jadassohn nevus p.

phalangeal
- Akin proximal phalangeal osteotomy
- p. articular orientation
- p. articulation
- p. bone
- p. condylectomy
- p. degloving
- p. diaphysial fracture
- p. dislocation
- distal phalangeal width
- p. fracture
- p. fracture fixation
- p. herniation
- p. joint
- medial closing wedge phalangeal osteotomy
- mental retardation, polydactyly, phalangeal hypoplasia, syndactyly, unusual face, uncombable hair
- p. osteoarthritis
- p. tuft

phalangoepiphyseal
- angel-shaped phalangoepiphyseal dysplasia

phalanx, pl. **phalanges**
- caudal appendage, short terminal phalanges, deafness, cryptorchidism, mental retardation syndrome
- clubbing of distal p.
- distal p.
- osteitis distal p.

phalanx *(continued)*
proximal p.
terminal p.

Phalen
P. maneuver
P. sign
P. test

phallus envy

phantom
p. aneurysm
p. arm
p. bone
p. breast pain
Brown-Roberts-Wells phantom base
p. corpuscle
p. extremity
p. foot pain
p. hand
p. illness
p. limb
p. limb pain
p. limb syndrome

pharmaceutical
delirium, infection, atrophic urethritis and vaginitis, p.'s, psychological disorders, excessive urine output, restricted mobility, stool impaction
p. research and testing

pharmacist
nuclear p.

pharmacocavemosometry
dynamic infusion p.

pharmacodynamic
age-related p.'s
age-related pharmacodynamic change
age-related pharmacodynamic response
altered p.'s

pharmacoelectroencephalography
quantitative p.

pharmacoendoscopy
light-induced fluorescence endoscopy in combination with p.

pharmacogenic confusional syndrome

pharmacokinetic
age-related pharmacokinetic change
p. change
clinical pharmacokinetics consulting service
clinical pharmacokinetics team
computerized pharmacokinetic model-driven drug infusion
p. drug-monitoring service

pharmacologic
p. agent
p. aid
p. atrial defibrillator
p. autonomic block
p. dosing
p. erection program
p. factor
p. impact
p. management
p. manipulation
p. method
sequential treatment employing pharmacologic support
p. therapy
p. treatment

pharmacological
p. approach
p. blockade
clinical and pharmacological interaction
p. difference
p. intervention

Pharmacopeia
United States Pharmacopeia Drug Information

Pharmacopoeia
International P.

pharmacotherapy
antipsychotic p.
p. for hyperactivity
vasoactive intracorporeal p.

pharmacy
p. to dose
P. Equivalent Name
nuclear p.
p. and therapeutics

pharyngea
aponeurosis p.
arteria pharyngea ascendens

pharyngeal
p. abscess
p. acid reflux
p. anesthesia
p. aperture
p. arch
p. area
ascending pharyngeal artery
ascending pharyngeal plexus
binasal pharyngeal airway
p. branch
p. branch of artery of pterygoid canal
p. branch of ascending pharyngeal artery
p. branch of descending palatine artery
p. branch of glossopharyngeal nerve
p. branch of inferior thyroid artery
p. branch of recurrent laryngeal nerve
p. branch of vagus nerve
p. candidiasis
p. cartilage
p. cleft
crypts of pharyngeal tonsil
p. diverticulum
p. exudate
p. fistula
p. groove
p. hypophysis
p. incompetence
p. injection
p. isthmus
lateral pharyngeal wall
longitudinal pharyngeal muscle
p. lymph node
middle constrictor pharyngeal muscle
p. mucosa
p. musculature
oral pharyngeal airway
posterior aspect of pharyngeal wall
p. pouch
p. tonsil

pharyngeotracheal lumen

pharynges (*pl. of* pharynx)

pharyngitis
acute p.
arcanobacterial p.
atrophic p.
candidal p.
gangrenous p.
glandular p.
granular p.
p. herpetica
hypertrophic p.
lymphonodular p.
mycoplasmal p.
nonstreptococcal p.
periodic fever, aphthous stomatitis, pharyngitis, cervical adenitis
purulent p.
pustular p.

pharyngobasilar
p. fascia
p. fold

pharyngoconjunctival
acute pharyngoconjunctival fever
p. fever
p. fever virus

pharyngoepiglottic
p. arch
p. fold

pharyngoesophageal
p. constriction
p. cushion
p. defect
p. diverticulum
p. function
p. reconstruction
Wookey pharyngoesophageal reconstruction

pharyngopalatine
p. arch
p. muscle

pharyngopalatinus
arcus p.

pharyngotympanic
p. groove
medial lamina of cartilage of pharyngotympanic auditory tube
membranous lamina of cartilage of pharyngotympanic auditory plate
p. tube

pharynx, pl. **pharynges**
middle constrictor muscle of p.
muscular coat of p.
muscular layer of p.
normal palate and p.
palate and pharynx normal
posterior pharynx not injected
superior constrictor muscles of p.
time of peak emptying rate of p.

phase
accelerated p.
active phase of labor
acute p.
acute phase reactant
acute phase reaction
acute phase response
acute phase response element
anal phase of infancy
p. analysis
p. angle
arrest of active phase dystocia
automaticity recovery p.
p. cancellation
chronic myelocytic/myelogenous/myeloid leukemia chronic p.
chronic phase chronic myelogenous leukemia
cumulative phase advancement
p. cycling
p. delay
delayed sleep p.
delayed sleep phase syndrome
p. difference
digital phase mapping
p. disparity
double antibody solid p.
dysharmonic luteal p.
early proliferative p.
end-expiratory p.
endogenous circadian rhythm p.
excretory p.
free fatty-acid p.
gap 0 p.
gas-liquid phase chromatography
growth phase of facial hair
harmonic p.
heart relaxed p.
hepatic arterial p.
hepatic arterial-dominant p.
p. imaging
immediate phase reaction
inadequate luteal p.
initial assessment p.
inspiratory phase gas
late luteal phase dysphoric disorder
luteal phase inadequacy
luteal phase insufficiency
luteal phase support
luteal phase therapy
megakaryocytic blastic p.
microbial antigenic phase shift
p. of mitosis in cell growth cycle
mycelial phase of fungus
nephrographic p.
noncontrast p.
normal autistic p.
normal luteal p.
portal venous p.
prolonged phase endometrium
quadrature phase detector
quiescent phase of cells leaving the mitotic cycle
respiratory ordered phase encoding
p. response curve
resting phase of facial hair
reverse p.
reversed phase high-performance liquid chromatography
reversed phase ion-pair partition
p. shift artifact
short luteal p.
solid p.
solid phase fluorescence immunoassay
solid phase peptide synthesis
solid phase radioimmunoassay
solid phase receptacle
time required to complete G_1 phase of cell cycle
time required to complete G_2 phase of cell cycle
time required to complete M phase of cell cycle
time required to complete S phase of cell cycle
p. transfer catalyst
yeast p.

phase-contrast
p.-c. cine magnetic resonance imaging
p.-c. microscopy

phased
annular phased array system
MRCP using HASTE with a phased array coil
p. knee rehabilitation

2.0-MHz phased-array probe

phase-invariant signature algorithm

phase-offset multiplanar

phase-ordered multiplanar

phase-sensitive gradient-echo MR imaging

phasic
p. activity
p. detrusor instability

Phelps Kindergarten Readiness Scale

phenacetin
p., aspirin, and caffeine
p. breath test
salicylamide, phenacetin, caffeine

phenazine methosulfate

phencyclidine
amphetamine/methamphetamine, opiates, and p.
p. hydrochloride

phenethylamine
centrally active phenethylamine derivative related to amphetamine and methamphetamine
phenethylbiguanide
phenobarbital
antenatal phenobarbital treatment
p. and belladonna
p. sodium
very high dose p.
phenododecinium bromide
phenol
p. alcohol
aqueous p.
p. red
typhoid vaccine, heat and phenol inactivated, dried
phenolic
aqueous synthetic dual phenolic disinfectant
phenolization
angular p.
nail matrix p.
phenol-lyase
tyrosine p.-l.
phenomenon, pl. **phenomena**
alien limb p.
angry back p.
aqueous influx p.
Ascher aqueous influx p.
Ascher glass-rod p.
Austin Flint p.
autokinetic visible light p.
baked brain p.
calcification, Raynaud phenomenon, scleroderma, telangiectasis syndrome
coronary steal p.
experimentally induced Köbner p.
gap conduction p.
Gunn jaw-winking p.
hastening p.
hypnagogic phenomena
Köbner p.
Lucio leprosy p.
lupus erythematosus p.
magic angle p.
Marcus Gunn jaw-winking p.
negative visual p.
paradoxical diaphragm p.
paradoxical pupillary p.
protamine paracoagulation p.
Raynaud p.
Sanarelli-Shwartzman p.
Wenckebach phenomena
phenotype
atherogenic low-density lipoprotein pattern B p.
cancer proneness p.
Duffy antigen A, B positive p.
Duffy antigen A negative p.
Duffy antigen B negative p.
hypoglossia-limb deficiency p.
mixed phenotype tumor
multiple presentation p.
neurofibromatosis with Noonan p.
single presentation p.
phenotyping
alpha$_1$-antitrypsin p.
phenylacetylisoglutamine
phenylalanine, lysine, and vasopressin
phenylketonuria
maternal p.
newborn screen serum thyroxine and p.
phenylmercuric
p. acetate
p. chloride
phenytoin assay
pheochromocytoma
benign p.
benign pheochromocytoma with histological invasion
malignant primary p.
metastatic malignant p.
MIBG-negative pelvic p.
p., thyroid carcinoma syndrome
pheresis
lipid p.
platelet p.
Philadelphia
P. chromosome
P. chromosome-negative
P. chromosome-negative chronic myelogenous leukemia
P. chromosome-positive
P. chromosome-positive chronic myelogenous leukemia
P. collar
P. Geriatric Center Morale Scale
P. Head Injury Questionnaire
Philippson reflex
philosophy
analytical p.
anthropological p.
Ayurveda p.
hospice p.
Management P.'s Scale I-V
Multidimensional Assessment of P. of Education
phimosis
adult p.
pHisoHex face wash
phlebectomy
greater saphenous p.
phlebitis
gouty p.
migrating p.
obstructive p.
postinfusion p.
septic p.
phlebogram
ascending contrast MR p.
wave on p.
phlebograph
impedance p.
phlebography
ascending contrast p.
ascending contrast phlebography imaging
cervical magnetic resonance p.
digital subtraction p.
phlebosclerosis
chronic ischemic colonic lesion caused by p.
phlegm
coughing with p.
increased p.
persistent cough and p.
phlegmon
mesenteric p.
phlegmonosa
parotitis p.
phlegmonous
p. abscess
p. adenitis
p. cellulitis
p. change
p. enteritis
p. erysipelas
p. gastritis
p. reaction
phlogistic corticoid
Phnom Penh bat virus
phobia
Brief Social P. Scale
generalized social p.
simple p.
phobic
p. anxiety
p. attitude

p. avoidance
p. avoidant behavior
total phobic anxiety

phonation
cine phonation study
maximal predicted phonation time
maximum duration of p.
p., respiration, articulation-resonance
speaking p.
p. time
p. volume

phone
no p.
p. order

phoneme
anterior feature English p.
Denver Auditory P. Sequencing Test

phonemic segmentation test

phonetic
applied p.'s
articulatory p.'s
auditory p.'s
p. babble
p. context

phonetically
p. balanced
P. Balanced Kindergarten
p. balanced percentage of word lists
p. balanced rhyme test
p. balanced word
p. balanced word lists
performance versus intensity function for phonetically balanced words

phonoangiogram
carotid p.

phonoangiography
carotid p.
oculoplethysmography/carotid p.

phonoangiography/oculoplethysmography
carotid p.

phonologic-acquisition device

phonological
aphasic phonological impairment
Assessment of P. Processes
assimilation phonological process

phonologic programming deficit syndrome

Phonology
Bankson-Bernthal Test of P.
Slosson Articulation Language Test with P.

phoria
monofixational p.
nearpoint p.

phosphatase
acid p.
p. acid serum
alkaline p.
alkaline phosphatase activity of granular leukocyte
alkaline phosphatase antialkaline p.
alkaline phosphatase isoenzyme tumor marker
alkaline phosphatase and pyrophosphate
alkaline phosphatase test
antialkaline phosphatase method
antidigoxigenin alkaline phosphatase antibody-conjugate
bacterial alkaline p.
bone alkaline p.
bone marrow acid p.
bone-specific alkaline p.
diphosphoglycerate p.
erythrocyte acid p.
glycogen synthetase p.
heat-stable alkaline p.
leukocyte alkaline p.
leukocyte alkaline phosphatase activity
leukocyte alkaline phosphatase stain
myosin light-chain p.
neutrophil alkaline p.
nucleic acid p.
placental acid p.
placental alkaline p.
polyclonal antiplacental alkaline p.
prostate-specific acid p.
prostatic acid p.
serum acid p.
serum alkaline p.
synthase p.
tartrate-resistant acid p.
p. and tensin homologue deleted on chromosome
total alkaline p.
total serum prostatic acid p.

phosphatase-1

phosphate
basic calcium p.
p. binder
p. binding
biodegradable calcium phosphate cement
bone phosphate of lime
calcium phosphate crystal deposition disease
calcium phosphate stone
calcium phosphate urinary lithiasis
p. carrier compound
p. clearance
p. crystals
p. cycle
p. deficiency
p. depletion
p. excretion index
filtered p.
flavin phosphate, reduced
high-energy p.
inorganic p.
inosine, pyruvate, and inorganic p.
p. ion
p. ion-urea
iproniazid p.
kalium potassium phosphate buffer
Krebs-Ringer p.
Krebs-Ringer phosphate solution
Luride acidulated phosphate fluoride paste
magnesium ammonium phosphate stone
magnesium ammonium phosphate urinary lithiasis
nicotinamide adenine dinucleotide phosphate positive
octacalcium p.
oxidized form of nicotinamide adenine dinucleotide p.
pentose phosphate cycle
p., saline, glucose
potassium titanyl phosphate laser
purified diphtheria toxoid precipitated by aluminum p.
pyruvate, inosine, glucose phosphate, and adenine
p. reabsorption index
p. restricted diet
p. retention
p., saline, glucose
p. supplemental diet
tryptone phosphate broth
tubular reabsorption of p.
urine diribose p.

phosphate-binding agent

phosphate-buffered
Dulbecco phosphate-buffered saline
p.-b. formalin
p.-b. saline
p.-b. sodium

phosphate-dependent glutaminase

phosphate-independent glutaminase

phosphatidylcholine
polyunsaturated p.
saturated p.

phosphatidylethanolamine
bacterial p.
linked to dipalmitoyl p.

phosphodiesterase
p. 5
p. III inhibition
p. type 5 inhibitor

phosphodiesterase-activating factor

phosphofructokinase
muscle phosphofructokinase deficiency

phosphohexokinase
platelet p.

phosphohydrolase

3-phosphoinositide-dependent protein kinase

phosphokinase
creatine p.
creatine phosphokinase isoenzyme
muscle fraction enzyme of creatine p.
myocardial band enzymes of creatine p.
serum creatine p.

phospholipid
p. assay
bile phospholipid concentration
bile phospholipid output
cholesterol to phospholipid ratio
essential p.

phosphor
photostimulable phosphor dental radiography

phosphorus
p. balance
p. binding
calcium to phosphorus ratio
p. content
deoxyribonucleic acid p.
p. distribution
halogen p.
inorganic p.
p. magnetic resonance imaging
p. magnetic resonance spectroscopy
p. nuclear magnetic resonance spectroscopy
organic acid-soluble p.
radioisotope of p.
theoretical renal phosphorus threshold
total body p.

phosphorus-31 magnetic resonance spectroscopy

phosphorus-dissolving bacteria

phosphorylase
brain-type glycogen p.
liver phosphorylase deficiency
muscle phosphorylase deficiency

phosphorylase-rupturing enzyme

phosphorylation
p. by the cellular double-stranded RNA-activated kinase
mitochondrial oxidative p.
myosin light-chain p.
oxidative p.
oxidative phosphorylation ratio

phosphorylcholine-binding myeloma protein

phosphotransferase system

phosphotungstic acid-hematoxylin stain

phosphotyrosine-binding domain

photic
critical frequency of photic driving
p. driving
p. epilepsy
intermittent photic stimulation
p. stimulation
p. stimulation procedure

photo
p. allergy
P. Articulation Test psychology
fundus p.

photoacoustic
scanning photoacoustic microscopy
p. spectroscopy

photoallergic
p. contact dermatitis
p. drug reaction

photoastigmatic refractive keratectomy

photobleaching
fluorescence photobleaching recovery
fluorescence recovery after p.

photochemotherapy
extracorporeal p.

photocoagulation
argon laser p.
grid laser p.
infrared p.
interstitial laser p.
intralesional laser p.
laser photocoagulation of the communicating vessel
Macular P. Study
panretinal argon laser p.
p. procedure
proliferative retinopathy p.
p. scatter

photocoagulator
xenon arch p.

photocontact allergic

photodiode
silicon p.

photodisruptive
neodymium:yttrium-lithium-fluoride photodisruptive laser

photodynamic
5-aminolevulinic acid photodynamic therapy
p. diagnosis
intraperitoneal photodynamic therapy
p. therapy

photoelectric
p. multiplier tube
p. registration device

photoelectron
angular resolved photoelectron spectroscopy
p. diffraction
single photoelectron counting
p. spectroscopy
ultraviolet photoelectron spectroscopy

photoelectronic intravenous angiography

photoemission
p. electron microscopy
x-ray photoemission spectroscopy

photograph
total body p.

photographic
p. effect

Structure P. Expressive Language Test-II

photography
endoscopic p.
monochromatic p.
nonmydriatic retinal p.
retinal fundus p.

photoionization detector

photolysis
nonenzymatic p.

photometric
flame photometric detector

photometry
colorimetry, including spectrophotometry and p.
ultraviolet p.

photomultiplier tube

photon
p. absorption densitometry
p. beam radiosurgery
p. densitometry
p. density
electron and photon therapy
equivalent effective p.
external beam photon therapy
p. gamma ray
intensity-modulated photon beam
p. irradiation technique in radiation therapy
mixed neutron and photon radiotherapy
Monte Carlo photon transport
Monte Carlo photon transport simulation
oblique annihilation photon pair
radial photon absorptiometry
p. therapy

photon-activated drug delivery system

photon-deficient bone lesion

photon-radiosurgical therapy

photon-stimulated desorption

photopalpebral reflex

photopeak
full width of photopeak measured at half maximal count

photopheresis
extracorporeal p.

photophobia
ichthyosis, follicularis, atrichia or alopecia, photophobia syndrome

photophoresis
extracorporeal p.

photoprotection
suntan photoprotection factor

photoradiation therapy

photoreacting enzyme

photoreactivating enzyme

photoreactive

photoreceptor membrane

photorefractive
excimer laser photorefractive keratectomy
p. keratoplasty
no-touch transepithelial photorefractive keratectomy
p. surgery
tracker-assisted photorefractive keratectomy

photosensitive
p. dermatitis
p. epilepsy
p. reaction

photosensitivity dermatitis

photostimulable phosphor dental radiography

photostress
macular p.
p. recovery test
p. recovery time

photosynthetically active radiation

photosynthetic unit

phototherapeutic
excimer laser phototherapeutic keratectomy

phototherapy
fiberoptic p.
p. lights

photothrombosis
arterial p.

phototoxic
p. contact dermatitis
p. lesion
p. maculopathy
minimal phototoxic erythema dose
operating microscope-induced phototoxic maculopathy
p. reaction

phrase
automatic phrase level
p. construction

phrenic
p. artery
p. ganglion
p. lymph node
p. nerve
p. nerve stimulation
peak phrenic nerve activity
pericardial branch of phrenic nerve
p. vein

phrenica
arteria phrenica superior

phrenici
nodi lymphoidei phrenici inferiores
nodi lymphoidei phrenici superiores

phrenitica
aphrodisia p.

phthisis
aneurysmal p.
nodosa p.
ocular p.

phyllodes
cystosarcoma p.

physeal
p. bony bridging
p. damage
p. injury

physical
p. abilities analysis
p. ability
P. Ability Test
p. abnormality
p. abuse
p. activity
P. Activity Readiness Questionnaire
adjustment reaction physical symptom
p. age
p. agent
p. agitation
alcohol-related physical problem
anxiety due to physical disorder
p. appearance
ARM method of physical examination
ASA physical status
Asher physical build assessment technique
p. assault
P. Assessment Center
p. assistance
associated physical examination finding
asthma of physical effort
atypical factitious disorder with physical symptoms
p. barrier

physical *(continued)*
p. and biochemical effect
p. bondage
p. capacity evaluation
p. change
p. change in brain
chest physical therapy
chronic factitious illness with physical symptoms
complete p.
complete physical examination
P. Component Summary
p. concern
create physical need
p. daily living skills
p. deconditioning
p. defect
degree of physical functioning
p. dependence
p. dependence capacity
p. dependence on nicotine gum
p. dependency
depression triggered by physical illness
p. diagnosis
p. disability
p. discipline
p. discomfort
dynamic physical activity
p. education
p. effect
p. effect of hallucinogen abuse
p. effects of drug abuse
p. efficiency index
emergency physical restraint
p. evaluation
p. examination
p. exercise
p. experience
Facial Disability Index P.
factitious disorder with physical symptoms
feeling of intellectual and physical power
p. finding
p. fitness
p. functioning
p. growth
p. half-life
p. handicap
p. harm
p. harm or violence
health-oriented physical education
history and p.
history and physical examination
history, physical, impression, and plan
p. hyperactivity
p. immaturity
impaired physical mobility
p. impairment
p. inactivity
increased physical activity
p. independence
industrial physical therapist
initial physical examination
p. injury
p. inoculation
p. maturity
p. medicine
p. medicine and rehabilitation
mental and physical retardation, speech disorders, peculiar facies syndrome
milliroentgen equivalent p.
minor physical anomaly
Mood and P. Symptoms Scale
multimodal physical therapy
neurodevelopmental treatment physical therapy
p. and neurologic examination for soft signs
obvious physical exhaustion
outpatient physical therapy
P. Performance Test
pertinent physical findings
primary physical dependence
programmed physical examination
p. reconditioning exercise
reduced tolerance for physical activity
P. Self Maintenance Scale
Smith physical capacities evaluation
sport p.
p. status patient classifications
p. symptoms
p. therapist
p. therapy
p. therapy assistant
p. therapy services
thermic effect of physical activity
P. Tolerance Profile
p. training
underlying physical illness
p. volume test
Western Ontario and McMaster Universities Osteoarthritis Index P. Functioning subscale and chair-performance
Western Ontario and McMaster Universities Osteoarthritis Index P. Functioning subscale and chair-stand performance
p. withdrawal symptoms
p. work capacity

physically
p. aggressive
p. disabled
halfway house for physically handicapped
p. handicapped
p. impaired
p. inactive
p. inactive lifestyle
p. or otherwise health-impaired
patient physically active
patient physically impaired
rehabilitation center for physically handicapped

physician
admitting p.
p. assistant
attending p.
attending p. statement
chest p.
consent form to delivery by alternative p.
P. Data Query
p. directed interdisciplinary care
disease-oriented physician education
p. drug abuse
emergency department p.
emergency room p.
family p.
p.'s forum
P.'s Health Study II
Hospital Indicator for P.'s Orders
medical control p.
no family p.
p. nutritional recommendation
p. on-call
p. only
p. order
p. order
p. order form
p. practice management
primary care p.
p. of record
p. referral service
referring p.
p. supplemental order
treating p.

physician-assisted suicide

physics
American Institute of P.
enthalpy physics

Physiognomic Cue Test

physiologic
p. age
p. aging rate
p. alopecia
p. amenorrhea
p. anatomy
p. anemia
p. aspect
p. atrophy
automated physiologic profile
p. barrier
p. blind spot
p. change
p. congestion
p. dead space
p. delay
p. dose
p. drift
p. drive
p. dwarfism
p. ecology
p. effect
end-gaze physiologic nystagmus
p. endometrial ablation/resection loop
p. epilepsy
p. equilibrium
p. excavation
p. flatfoot
p. full value
p. habit
p. homeostasis
p. hyaluronidase inhibitor
p. hypertrophy
p. icterus
p. incompatibility
p. jaundice
p. low stress angioplasty
p. monitoring
p. murmur
p. myopia
p. pattern release
p. reflux test
p. rest position
resultant physiologic acceleration
p. retina
p. saline solution
p. salt solution
p. shunt flow
p. splitting
p. squamocolumnar
p. stability index
p. third heart sound
p. vertigo

physiologica

physiological
p. age
anorectal physiological dysfunction
p. arousal
p. artifact
p. component
p. condition
p. drive
p. hyperarousal
p. musculoskeletal reaction
norm physiological reflex
passive physiological intervertebral movements

physiology
acute physiology and chronic health evaluation score
anatomy and p.
anorectal physiology testing
p. of heart contraction
Simplified Acute P. Score
Simplified Acute P. Score version II

physiotherapy
aqua PT dry p.
chest p.

physis
modified Boyd amputation of ankle and distal tibial p.

physostigmine salicylate ophthalmic

Phys Ther

phytobezoar
small bowel p.

phytoestrogen
soy phytoestrogen extract

phytohemagglutinin
p. activation
p. antigen

pia
p. arachnoid
arachnoidea mater et pia mater
arachnoid mater and pia mater
p. intima
p. mater
p. mater of brain

piannic
onychia p.

Pichinde virus

pick
apical p.
P. atrophy
P. body
P. bundle
P. cells
P. disease
light pipe p.
Michel p.
P. retinitis
P. syndrome
P. tubular adenoma

picker's
mushroom picker's lung

Pickford Projectives Picture

pick-up walker

pickwickian syndrome

Picola virus

picric acid turbidity

pictorial
p. anticipatory guidance
P. Instrument for Children and Adolescents
P. Test of Intelligence

picture
anodal closure p.
anodal opening p.
p. archival communication system
P. Arrangement psychology
P. Articulation and Language Screening Test
Beery P. Vocabulary Screening
p. completion
Discrimination by Identification of P.'s
p. element
Expressive One-Word P. Vocabulary Test
p. frustration study
Hundred P.'s Naming Test
P. Identification for Children-Standardized Index
P. Identification Test
P. Interest Exploration Survey
Make A P. Story test
maximum pressure p.
Michigan P. Stories
Michigan P. Test, Revised
Missouri Children's Picture Series
Peabody Picture Vocabulary Test-Revised
Pickford Projectives P.
Quick P. Vocabulary Test
P. Reasoning Test
Receptive One-Word P. Vocabulary Test
role perception picture inventory
Spondee P. Test
P. Story Language Test
p. symbols
Word Intelligibility by P. Identification

picture-frustration study, test

Pidgin Sign English

pie
buttress pie plate

piece
free secretory p.
secretory p.
T p.

piecemeal
p. degranulation
p. removal of kidney stone

pied
mal perforant du p.

piercing
nose p.

Pierini
atrophoderma of Pasini and P.
melanotic prurigo of P.

piety
filial p.

piezoelectric
extracorporeal piezoelectric lithotripsy

pig
antiserum, guinea p.
p. aortic endothelial cell
p. cell implant
guinea p.
guinea pig kidney absorption test
guinea pig lung strip
guinea pig albumin
guinea pig antiinsulin serum
guinea pig complement
guinea pig dander
guinea pig embryo
guinea pig gamma globulin
guinea pig ileum
guinea pig inoculation
guinea pig keratocyte
guinea pig maximization test
guinea pig myelin-basic protein
guinea pig spleen
guinea pig trachea
guinea pig tracheal smooth muscle
guinea pig unit
p. insulin
p. kidney
mycoplasma pneumonia of p.
rabbit antibody to pig ovary

pigeon
p. breast
p. breast deformity
p. breeder disease
p. breeder lung
p. chest
p. serum
p. toe

piggyback
p. intravenous fluids
modified p.

pigment
accumulation of bile p.
acute multifocal posterior placoid pigment epitheliopathy
acute posterior multifocal placoid pigment epitheliopathy
p. cell
p. cirrhosis
p. clumping
common duct pigment stone
congenital hypertrophy of retinal pigment epithelium
cytochrome p.
p. dispersion syndrome
p. epithelial detachment
p. epithelium
p. floater
gallbladder pigment stones
giant pigment melanosome
p. granule
immediate pigment darkening
p. implantation
p. inspiratory factor
intermittent pigment darkening
iris pigment epithelium
p. layer
lumbosacral skin pigment change
malarial deposition p.
minimal p.
minimal pigment oculocutaneous albinism
multifocal posterior pigment epitheliopathy
prone to developing pigment gallstones
reticular degeneration of pigment epithelium
retinal pigment epithelial cell
retinal pigment epithelium
retina pigment epithelium detachment

pigmental
chronic pigmental purpura

pigmentary
p. cirrhosis
p. degeneration
p. dysplasia
p. glaucoma
insulin-resistant diabetes, acanthosis nigricans, hypogonadism pigmentary retinopathy, deafness, mental retardation syndrome
p. retinopathy

pigmentation
amiodarone p.
area of increased p.
arsenic p.
hematogenous p.
mucocutaneous p.
orange punctate p.
retrocorneal p.
scleral p.

pigmented
p. basal cell carcinoma
diffuse pigmented villonodular synovitis
p. epithelium
p. gallstone
giant pigmented hairy nevus
p. growth
p. layer of ciliary body
p. layer of iris
p. layer of retina
p. lesion
p. mole
p. nevus
p. nodular adrenocortical disease
p. nodule
primary pigmented nodular adrenocortical disease
p. pupillary membrane
p. retina epithelial cell
p. spindle cell
p. villonodular bundle
p. villonodular synovitis
p. villonodular tenovagosynovitis

pigmenti
incontinentia p.

pigmentosa
neurogenic muscle weakness, ataxia, and retinitis p.
retinitis p.
retinitis pigmentosa GTPase regulator gene
X-linked retinitis p.

pigmentosum
atrophoderma p.
morphea p.
xeroderma p.
xeroderma pigmentosum group A, C

pigmentosus
lichen planus p.
nevus p.
nevus pigmentosus et pilosus

pigtail
p. curl of catheter
p. curl of stent tube
p. nephrostomy tube

pilar
anogenital pilar cyst

pilaris
lichen p.
pityriasis rubra p.

pili
arrector p.
arrector pili muscle
musculus arrector p.

pill
birth control p.
Chlamydia from birth control p.
p. counter
emergency contraceptive p.
hair loss from birth control p.
hepatitis from birth control p.
morning after p.
oral birth control p.
oral contraceptive p.
progestin-only p.

pillar
anterior faucial p.
anterior pillar of fauces
anterior pillar of fornix
anterior pillar tumor
anterior tonsillar p.
articular pillar fracture
p. of Corti organ
p. of diaphragm

pillow
antibacterial p.
cervical skull p.
p. inserted under shoulder
nasal p.

pilocarpine 1% ophthalmic solution

pilocystic cerebellar astrocytoma

pilocytic
malignant pilocytic astrocytoma

pilonidal
p. abscess
p. area
p. cyst
p. cystectomy
p. fistula
infected pilonidal cyst
p. sinus
p. sinus disease

pilorum
atrophia pilorum propria

pilosebaceous
normal pilosebaceous apparatus

pilosus
nevus pigmentosus et p.

pilot
Asymptomatic Cardiac Ischemia P.

Piltz reflex

pilus
arrector p.
errector p.

pin
alignment p.
apex p.
arum fixation p.
axial pin technique
closed reduction and percutaneous pin fixation
closed reduction and percutaneous pin ring
drill p.
freeze-dried bone p.
friction lock p.
friction-retained p.
p. guide
p. holder
p. implant
intramedullary p.
LIH hook p.
marble bone p.
os calcis pin fixation
p.'s and plaster
p. traction

pincer jaw

pinch
p. biopsy
Braun pinch graft technique
p. gauge
p. grasp
tail p.

pinched sciatic nerve

pinching pain

pine
Australian p.
Australian pine tree
lodgepole pine tree
p. tar

pineal
p. antigonadotropin
p. blastoma
p. body
p. cell
p. cell tumor
p. cyst
p. disease
germ cell tumor with synchronous lesions in pineal and suprasellar region
p. gland
p. gland tumor
p. gonadal syndrome
p. mass
p. peduncle
p. recess

pineale
parenchymatous cell of corpus p.

pinealis
pedunculus corpus p.

pineapple
p. test for butyric acid in stomach

pinhole
p. no improvement
no improvement with p.
p. pupil
p. vision

pink
p. eye
p. indicator color
p., moist, and warm mucous membranes
oral mucosa p.
oral mucosa pink and moist
oral mucous membrane p.
oral mucous membrane pink and moist
p. puffer sign of emphysema
sharp and p.

pink-eyed, tan-hooded rat

pinna, pl. **pinnae**
anteverted p.
malformed p.

pinned
p. femur
p. hip

pinning
Asnis p.
hip p.

pinocytotic vesicle

pinpoint
p. os
pupil p.
p. pupil

pinprick
p. analgesia
diminished sensation to p.
p. test

pins-and-needles sensation

pint
liquid p.
pinto
mal del p.
pintos
mal de los p.
pinworm infection
pipe
clay pipe cancer
p. dream
glass p.
p. light
light pipe pick
pipestem
Symmers clay pipestem fibrosis
pipette
air-displacement p.
blowout p.
piriform
p. angle
anterior piriform gyrus
p. aperture
p. aperture access
p. aperture stenosis
p. area
p. cortex
p. fossa
margin of piriform aperture
p. sinus
piriformis
apertura p.
p. muscle spasm
Piry virus
pisiform
articulation of pisiform bone
p. bone
p. bursa
p. fracture
p. joint
pisiformis
articulatio ossis p.
pisohamate ligament
pisotriquetral
p. arthritis
p. articulation
piston
cannulated expulsion p.
***Pisum sativum* agglutinin**
pit
articular pit of head of radius
central p.
distal p.
gastric p.'s
mesial p.
optic disc p.
optic nerve p.
pitch
ascending pitch break
calcaneal pitch angle
coal tar pitch volatiles
conditioned pitch level
dichotic pitch discrimination test
long pitch helicoidal layer
p. period perturbation
Pitocin
P. augmentation of labor
dilute intravenous P.
P. intravenous drip
intravenous Pitocin drip
P. oxytocin
pitting
anal p.
p. edema
p. edema of ankle
p. edema of lower extremity
nail p.
remitting seronegative symmetric synovitis with pitting edema
Pitt-Rogers-Danks syndrome
Pittsburgh pneumonia agent
pituitary
p. ablation
p. abscess
p. adenoma
p. adenoma-adenohypophysial neuronal choristoma
p. adenylate cyclase activating polypeptide
p. adiposity
adrenocorticotrophic hormone-secreting pituitary tumor
p. adrenotropic hormone
p. agenesis
p. amyloid
p. aneurysm
angled pituitary rongeur
animal pituitary gonadotropin
anterior p.
anterior lobe of p.
anterior pituitary extract
anterior pituitary function
anterior pituitary gland
anterior pituitary gonadotropin
anterior pituitary hormone
anterior pituitary insufficiency
anterior pituitary lobe
anterior pituitary resection
p. aplasia
apoplexy of p.
autoimmune pituitary disease
p. body
p. carcinoma
chorioretinopathy and pituitary dysfunction
circulating pituitary hormone
clinically nonfunctioning pituitary adenoma
combined pituitary hormone deficiency
p. cyst
p. deficiency
p. dwarfism
p. dysfunction
p. dystopia
p. endocrine disorder
endocrine inactive pituitary tumor
p. enlargement
p. eunuchism
p. fossa
p. function test
p. gigantism
p. gland
p. gland function
p. gland tumor
glycoprotein-secreting pituitary tumor
p. gonadotropic hormone
p. gonadotropin
p. gonadotropin effect
p. gonadotropin inhibition
gonadotropin-producing pituitary adenoma
p. gonadotropin secretion
p. gonadotropin suppression
p. grasper
p. growth hormone
p. hormone deficit
p. hormone function
p. hormone hypofunction
p. hormone release
hormone-secreting pituitary tumor
p. hormone trigger ovulation
human p.
human pituitary follicle-stimulating hormone
human pituitary gonadotropin
human pituitary growth hormone
p. hyperfunction
p. hyperplasia
p. hypersecretion
p. hypogonadism
p. hypoplasia
hypothalamic pituitary adrenocortical axis
hypothalamic, pituitary, thyroid
p. hypothyroidism
p. imaging

p. infantilism
p. infarction
p. insufficiency
p. irradiation
lipotropic pituitary hormone
lobe of pituitary gland
lyophilized anterior p.
lyophilized anterior pituitary tissue
malignant pituitary lesion
p. meningioma
p. metastasis
p. microadenoma
p. microsurgery
mixed pituitary adenoma-gangliocytoma
multiple anterior pituitary hormone deficiency
multiple pituitary hormone deficiencies
p. myxedema
p. necrosis
neuroadenolysis of p.
nonfunctional pituitary adenoma
nonfunctional pituitary tumor
nonfunctioning pituitary tumor
nonsecreting pituitary adenoma
nonsecreting pituitary tumor
p. opioid peptide
optic tract pituitary tumor
posterior p.
posterior pituitary hormone
prolactin-producing pituitary adenoma
prolactin secreting pituitary tumor
p. reproductive hormone
p. resistance to thyroid hormone
p. RTH
p. secretion
selective pituitary resistance to thyroid hormone
p. stalk
p. stalk distortion
p. stimulation
p. surgery
p. thyroid hormone resistance
transsphenoidal pituitary resection
TSH-secreting pituitary tumor
p. tumor transforming gene

pituitary-adrenal

pituitary-specific transcription factor-1

pityriasis
p. alba
atypical pityriasis rosea
p. capitis
p. folliculorum
lichenoid acute p.
p. nigra
p. rosea
rubra p.
p. rubra pilaris
p. simplex
p. versicolor

Pityrosporon
P. orbiculare
P. ovale

pivot
p. joint
p. point
reverse pivot shift
p. shift test
stand and p.
p. transfer
p. transfer from wheelchair

pivotal
standing pivotal transfer

Pixuna virus

place
alert and oriented to person, place, and time
alert and oriented to person, place, time, and date
p. of birth
catheter in p.
conditioned place preference
confusion about time and p.
p. of death
disorientation to time and p.
oriented to person, place, and time
oriented to time and p.
oriented to time, place, and person
oriented to time, place, person, and objects watch, pen, book
p. outpatient in inpatient bed
patient oriented to person, place and time
p. and person
person, place, and time
thoracotomy tube in p.
p. and time
p., time, and person
usual place of residence

placebo
p. capsule or tablet
p. control group
p. effect
inactive p.
p. injection
medically inactive p.

placebo-controlled
double-blind placebo-controlled randomized clinical trial
p.-c. drug study
p.-c. oral challenge testing

placed
p. at bedrest
drain placed into wound
electrodes placed on the surface of head
p. in incubation
infant placed in incubator
infant placed under Bili-Lite
infant placed in warmer
p. in isolation
p. in isolette
percutaneously placed line
sandbag placed for support
p. in traction
p. in warmer

placement
Advanced P. Examination
Advanced P. Program
anular p.
aortic graft p.
biliary sphincterotomy and stent p.
cartilage strut p.
central midline placement of electrodes in electroencephalography
chest tube p.
Comparative Guidance and P. Program
p. counseling
discharge p.
electrode placement device
endotracheal tube p.
feeding tube p.
fluoroscopic p.
foster home p.
frontal midline placement of electrodes in electroencephalography
frontal polar electrode placement in electroencephalography
graft p.
halfway house p.
implant p.
intracavitary container p.
line p.
long-term central venous access catheter p.
mucoperiosteal implant p.
nasopharyngeal electrode p.

placement *(continued)*
nasopharyngeal electrode placement in electroencephalography
nursing home p.
open gastrostomy tube p.
pacemaker p.
parietal midline zero electrode placement in electroencephalography
PCL-oriented p.
percutaneous endoscopic placement of jejunal tube
percutaneous transluminal angioplasty with stent p.
permanent pacemaker p.
training and placement service
variable screw p.

placenta, pl. **placentae**
ablatio placentae
abruptio placentae
p. accreta
animal placenta lactogen
annular p.
anterofundal p.
anular p.
p. biloba
p. bipartite
complete placenta previa
p. delivered
p. delivered intact
p. delivered manually
dichorionic p.
dichorionic-diamniotic p.
endotheliochorial p.
epitheliochorial p.
p. expelled
p. extracted
p. febrilis
p. fetalis
hematoma of p.
horseshoe p.
incarcerated p.
p. increta
p. inflamed
p. intact
low insertion of p.
marginal sinus of p.
margination of p.
mature abnormal p.
monochorionic diamnionic p.
monochorionic diamniotic p.
monochorionic diamniotic placenta twins
monochorionic monoamniotic p.
p. multipartita
necrotic p.
nondeciduous p.
p., ovaries, uterus
p. panduriformis
pars uterina placentae
partial placenta previa
p. percreta
premature separation of p.
p. previa
p. previa centralis
p. previa marginalis
p. reflexa
p. removed manually
p. reniformis
retained p.
p. spuria
total placenta previa
p. triloba
p. tripartita
tripartite p.
p. triplex
zonary p.
zonular p.

placental
p. abruption
p. acid phosphatase
p. alkaline phosphatase
p. barrier
p. biopsy
p. bleeding
p. bleeding site
p. blood flow
p. circulation
confined placental mosaicism
p. dysfunction
p. dysmaturity
p. dystocia
p. edema
p. extrusion
p. fragment
p. function test
p. grade biophysical profile
p. growth
p. growth factor
p. growth hormone
p. hemorrhage
human placental thyrotropin
human placental uterotropic hormone
p. hydrops
p. immunity
immunoreactive human placental lactogen
p. implantation
p. index
p. insufficiency
p. lactogenic hormone
p. leakage
p. lobe
p. membrane
p. membranes
p. migration
necrotic placental tissue
noncornual placental location
ovine placental lactogen
P450 aromatase placental deficiency
p. protein 5
p. presentation
p. protein
purified placental protein
purified placental protein, human
p. residual blood volume
retained placental tissue
p. site trophoblastic tumor
p. thrombosis
p. tissue
total placental estrogen
p. transfer

placentation
monochorionic p.
normal p.

placentofetal transfusion

placentogram
displacement p.

placing
neonatal p.

placode
auditory p.
olfactory p.

placoid
acute multifocal posterior placoid pigment epitheliopathy
acute posterior multifocal placoid pigment epitheliopathy

plafond
Ovadia-Beals classification of tibial plafond fracture

plagiocephaly
synostotic frontal p.

plague
aerosolized plague weapon
bubonic p.
fowl plague virus
meningeal p.
Pahvant Valley p.
squirrel plague conjunctivitis

plain
p. abdominal radiograph
p. catgut
catgut plain tie
p. catgut suture
p. 2-0 catgut suture

p. 3-0 catgut suture
p. 4-0 catgut suture
coastal p.'s virus
p. film of abdomen
p. gauze
p. gut
p. gut suture
high abdominal plain film
interrupted plain catgut
p. spine radiograph
p. view
p. x-ray

plan

assessment and p.
assessment, plan, implementation, and evaluation
assisted health insurance p.
behavior management p.
p.'s of care
comprehensive health insurance p.
comprehensive medical p.
comprehensive treatment p.
development of discharge p.
family health insurance p.
healthcare rationing p.
health maintenance p.
history, physical, impression, and p.
impulsivity to plan ahead
independent practice p.
individualized p.
Individualized Family Service P.
individual treatment p.
initial psychiatric treatment p.
interim treatment p.
long-term p.
managed behavioral health p.'s
master treatment p.
medical reimbursement p.
multidisciplinary treatment p.
multimodal treatment p.
narrative, assessment, and p.
National Arthritis Action P.
nursing care p.
patient care p.
patient recovery p.
prepaid health p.
psychotropic medication p.
respiratory care p.
standardized care p.
state medical facilities p.
sympathetic maintained p.
treatment p.
p.'s of treatment

plana

articulatio p.
lensectomy
Packo pars plana cannula
pars p.
pars plana approach
pars plana Baerveldt tube insertion with vitrectomy
pars plana lensectomy
pars plana operation
trans pars plana vitrectomy
verruca plana juvenilis

planar

anterior planar image
anterior planar imaging
axial echo planar diffusion weighted imaging
conventional planar imaging
dynamic planar reconstructor
p. imaging
multiple planar gradient-recalled
p. myocardial imaging
p. scintigraphy
single-photon planar imaging
single-photon planar scintigraphy
p. thallium scintigraphy
p. thallium test

Planck constant

plan-do integration

plane

alveolar occlusal p.
axial plane angular deformity biomechanics
axial plane imaging
p. of body
coordinate axis in p.
p. of dissection
extended supraplatysmal p.
fracture bilaterally in a horizontal p.
Frankfort horizontal plane of skull
Frankfort mandibular plane angle
horizontal p.
p. of incidence
incisal mandibular plane angle
p. joint
loose areolar p.
p. of midpelvis
oblique coronal p.
orbital plane of frontal bone
peripancreatic fat p.
p. polarization
p. of regard
root p.
sacral horizontal plane line
short axis p.
supracristal p.
temporal p.
transtrabecular p.
transumbilical p.

planimetry

radiographic p.

planing

p. curve
root planing and curettage
scaling and root p.

planitis

pars p.

planned

p. awakening
p. extracapsular cataract extraction
p. parenthood

planner

discharge p.

planning

career planning program
computer assisted menu p.
discharge p.
discharge planning coordinator
family p.
family planning clinic
family planning health assistant
initial planning option
initiate discharge p.
inverse treatment p.
joint treatment p.
long-range p.
natural family p.
New Mexico Career P. Test
population p.
radiation therapy p.
radiation therapy planning system
radiation treatment p.
sonographic planning of oncology treatment
p. target volume
treatment planning conference
Vocational P. Inventory

planoconcave lens

planoconvex lens

planopilaris

lichen p.

planovalgus

p. deformity
p. foot

plant

arum p.
p. protease test
wastewater treatment p.

plantar

p. angulation
apex plantar deformity

plantar *(continued)*
p. aponeurosis
aponeurosis of plantar transverse fasciculi
p. approach
p. arch
p. arch support orthosis
p. aspect
p. aspect of foot
p. bony prominence
p. bursa
p. calcaneal spur
p. capsule
common palmar digital nerve of lateral plantar nerves
common plantar digital nerve of medial plantar nerve
p. compartment
p. crease
p. dermatitis
p. dermatosis
p. desquamation
p. digital artery
p. digital nerve
endoscopic plantar fasciotomy
p. erythema
p. fascia
p. fascial release
p. fascia syndrome
p. fasciitis
p. fasciitis orthosis
p. fasciitis syndrome
p. fasciotomy
p. fibroma
first plantar metatarsal artery
p. flexed
p. flexion
p. flexion of foot
p. flexor
flexor plantar response
p. flexor reflex
p. foot
p. foot defect
forced plantar flexion
indurated plantar keratoma
p. interosseous muscle
intractable plantar keratosis
p. ischemia
p. ischemia test
juvenile plantar dermatitis
juvenile plantar dermatosis
lateral p.
p. ligament
p. maceration
medial p.
p. metatarsal
p. nerve
p. neuroma
neurosensorial free medial plantar flap
normal plantar response
percutaneous plantar fasciotomy
perforating branch of plantar metatarsal artery
p. puncture wound
radical posteromedial and plantar release
p. rash
p. reflex
p. response
p. response downgoing
p. response upgoing
short plantar ligament
superficial branch of lateral plantar nerve
superficial branch of medial plantar artery
p. surface
Universal plantar fasciitis orthotic
p. wart

plantaris
aponeurosis p.
arcus plantaris profundus
arcus venosus p.
arteria digitalis plantaris communis
arteria digitalis plantaris propria
arteria metatarsalis p.
arteria metatarsea p.
arteria plantaris lateralis
arteria plantaris medialis
arteria plantaris profundus
mycosis fungoides palmaris et p.
pustulosis palmaris et p.
verruca p.

planum
os p.
xanthoma p.

planus
anular lichen p.
atrophic lichen p.
lichen planus anularis
lichen planus follicularis
lichen planus overlap syndrome
lichen planus pemphigoid
lichen planus pigmentosus
lichen planus verrucosus
lichen ruber p.
linear lichen p.
oral condyloma p.
pes p.

plaque
annular erythematous p.
p. in artery
artery-clogging plaque in atherosclerosis patient
asbestos pleural p.
atherosclerotic p.
atherosclerotic plaque rupture
attachment p.'s
p. in blood vessel
p. in brain
costal p.
p. deposit
diaphragmatic p.
erythematous confluent p.
foamy interstitial p.
p. formation
hemolytic plaque assay
p. index
intimal foamy p.'s
Lichtheim p.'s
localized plaque formation
meningioma en p.
microwave plaque thermotherapy
milia en p.
neuritic p.
neuritis senile p.
p. neutralization
p. obstruction
orbital plaque brachytherapy
ostial atherosclerotic p.
palladium 103 ophthalmic plaque brachytherapy
palladium 103 ophthalmic plaque radiotherapy
parapsoriasis en p.'s
parapsoriasis en p.
posterior subcapsular cataractous p.
prion protein scrapie isoform-reactive p.
protein A hemolytic plaque assay
pruritic urticarial papules and p.'s
pruritic urticarial papules and plaques of pregnancy
Redlich-Fisher miliary p.
reverse hemolytic plaque assay
sclerose en p.'s
senile p.
sequential paired opposed p.
wheal and p.

plaque-forming
p.-f. cell
p.-f. unit

plaque-like lesion

plaquing
atherosclerotic p.
pleural p.

plasma
absolute plasma concentration
absorbed normal pooled p.
absorbed test p.
aged substrate p.
air plasma spray
p. aldosterone
p. aldosterone concentration
p. amine oxidase
p. antiendotoxin core antibody
antihemophilic plasma human
antihuman thymocyte p.
antiplatelet p.
anti-*Pseudomonas* human p.
antithrombin III plasma level
antithyroid plasma membrane antibody
p. appearance rate
argon beam plasma coagulation
argon ion plasma coagulation
argon plasma coagulator
arterial plasma input
arterial renal plasma flow
assay reference p.
p. bicarbonate
p. bilirubin concentration
blood plasma measuring system
bovine plasma albumin
p. catecholamine concentration
p. cell
p. cell count
p. cell dyscrasia
p. cell dyscrasia of unknown significance
p. cell granuloma
p. cell hepatitis
p. cell interstitial pneumonitis
p. cell labeling index
p. cell leukemia
p. clearance rate
p. clot diffusion chamber
p. clotting time
colloid osmotic pressure in p.
complement-activated p.
p. concentration
constituent of alpha protein plasma fraction
constituent of gamma protein plasma fraction
constituent of plasma protein fraction
contralateral renal plasma flow
p. cortisol
p. cytoma
p. defect
p. depletion
p. digoxin concentration
p. disappearance curve
donor's p.
effective renal plasma flow
p. equivalent unit
p. exchange
p. exchange number three
fasting plasma lipid
p. fibronectin
p. flow
fresh frozen p.
fresh frozen plasma transfusion
frozen p.
p. gastrin
glomerular plasma flow
p. glucose
p. glucose disappearance rate
p. glucose tolerance rate
p. growth hormone
hepatic plasma flow
hippocampal synaptic plasma membrane
human platelet-rich p.
human seminal plasma inhibitor
hypofibrinogenic p.
immunoblastic p.
immunoreactive p.
p. immunoreactive insulin
immunoreactive insulin to serum or plasma glucose ratio
p. immunoreactive secretion
p. infusion
p. inorganic iodine
p. insulin activity
p. iron disappearance
p. iron disappearance time
p. iron turnover rate
p. lactic dehydrogenase
p. leukopheresis
p. level monitoring
liver plasma flow
liver plasma membrane
low plasma albumin
low-pressure plasma spray
lymphoid p.
Marschalko-type plasma cell
maternal plasma leptin
mean plasma iron concentration
mean plasma volume
p. membrane
p. membrane fatty acid binding protein
microplate plasma methotrexate assay
microplate plasma MTX assay
midnight plasma cortisol concentration
natriuretic plasma dialysate
nonceruloplasmin plasma copper
p. norepinephrine
normal human pooled p.
normal pool p.
p. oncotic pressure
p. osmolality
osmotic pressure of p.
p. osmotic pressure
ovarian venous plasma oxytocin
p. parathyroid hormone
partial plasma exchange
peak plasma concentration
p. pepsinogen
peripheral vein p.
platelet adhesiveness plasma factor
platelet-depleted p.
platelet-poor p.
platelet-rich p.
p. polymorphonuclear elastase
pooled human p.
poor platelet p.
postheparin p.
postprandial plasma glucose
p. potassium
pregnancy-associated plasma protein
pregnancy-associated plasma protein A, C
p. prekallikrein
prostacyclin synthesis-stimulating plasma factor
p. protamine precipitating
p. protein fraction
p. protein globulin
protein plasma substitute
p. prothrombin conversion
p. prothrombin conversion accelerator
p. prothrombin conversion factor
rapid plasma reagent
rapid plasma reagin
rapid plasma reagin circle card test
rapid plasma reagin complement fixation
red blood cell to plasma ratio
renal vein plasma renin activity
p. renin concentration
p. renin substrate activity
single-donor frozen p.
single-nephron glomerular plasma flow
p. skimming
p. sodium
stable plasma protein solution
steady-state plasma glucose

plasma *(continued)*
steady-state plasma insulin
steroid-binding plasma protein
synaptic plasma membrane
syncytiotrophoblast microvillar plasma membrane
target plasma concentration
therapeutic plasma exchange
thromboplastic plasma component
p. thromboplastin
p. thromboplastin antecedent
p. thromboplastin component
p. thromboplastin factor
titanium plasma sprayed
total plasma catecholamines
total plasma cholesterol
p. transfusion
p. triglyceride
Universal Control Reference P.
upright peripheral plasma renin activity
p. urea nitrogen
venous renal plasma flow
p. viral load
p. viscosity
p. volume
zoster immune p.
zymosan-activated plasma rabbit

plasmacytic
angiofollicular and plasmacytic polyadenopathy

plasmacytoid lymphocyte

plasmacytoma
extramedullary solitary p.
extraosseous plasmacytoma of the mediastinum
solitary plasmacytoma of bone

plasma-free red cell

Plasma-Lyte A, M

plasma-mass
inductively-coupled plasma-mass spectrometer

plasmapheresis
double filtration p.
p. treatment

plasma-recognition-factor activity

plasma-resistant fiber oxygenator

plasma-sprayed
low-pressure p.-s.

plasmid
bacterial cell lacking an F p.
bacterial cell with an F p.
conjugative plasmid in F^+ bacterial cell
drug-resistant p.
hybrid F p.
naked plasmid DNA
p. pattern analysis
resistance p.

plasmin-inhibitor complex

plasminogen
p. activator
p. activator inhibitor
p. activator inhibitor type 1, 2
p. activator-releasing hormone
anisoylated plasminogen streptokinase activator complex
2-chain urokinase plasminogen activator
extrinsic plasminogen activator
recombinant plasminogen activator
recombinant, single-chain, urokinase-type plasminogen activator
recombinant tissue-type plasminogen activator
urokinase plasminogen activator
urokinase plasminogen activator receptor
urokinase-type plasminogen activator
vascular plasminogen activator

plasmin renin activity

Plasmodium

plasmon
surface plasmon resonance

plaster
p. bandage
below-knee walking p.
bivalved pancake plaster hand cast
p. boot
change of p.
p. dressing
immobilized in plaster cast
in p.
long leg plaster cast
out of plaster cast
p. of Paris
p. of Paris cast
p. of Paris jacket
pins and p.
short arm plaster splint
x-ray in p.
x-ray out of p.

plastic
acrylic p.
p. adhesive dressing
p. anatomy
ankle-foot plastic orthosis
p. bifocal
carbon fiber-reinforced p.
ceramic or plastic brace
p. closure
p. frame
p. heart valve
p. implant
p. implant material
p. induration
p. iritis
p. leafspring
p. lens
p. lymph
metal frame reinforced plastic bracket
p. reconstruction
p. and reconstructive surgery
p. repair
p. sphere implant

plasty
aqueductal p.
shape of incisions in V-Y p.

plate
agar plate count
angled blade plate fixation
anterior cervical p.
anterior cervical plate fixation system
anterior locking plate system
anterior plate fixation
anterior sacroiliac joint p.
athletic shoe carbon fiber p.
avulsion of nail p.
blade plate driver
blood agar p.
buttress pie p.
carbon fiber-reinforced p.
cast with dorsal toe plate extension
cast with volar toe plate extension
colorimetric microtiter p.
compression plate fixation
compression plate and screw
contoured anterior spinal p.
cortical bone p.
cribriform plate injury
dense p.
dynamic compression p.
dynamic compression plate fixation
Eddy hot plate test
epiphysial growth p.
ferromagnetic metal p.
fibrin plate lysis area
p. fixation

flat p.
flat plate of abdomen
flat plate radiography
p. fracture
glansplasty in situ tubularization of urethral p.
glanuloplasty in situ tubularization of urethral p.
gravity settling culture plate
growth plate fracture
growth plate injury
heterotopic plate count
hot plate reaction time
hot plate test
lateral pterygoid p.
limited compression-dynamic compression p.
lingual alveolar p.
liver cell p.
low-contact dynamic compression p.
low-profile dorsal p.
mandibular reconstruction p.
maxillary bite p.
medial cartilaginous p.
medial crus foot p.
medial pterygoid p.
membranous lamina of cartilage of pharyngotympanic auditory p.
meningioma of cribriform p.
metal foot p.
middle fossa p.
mini condylar p.
multitest, mycology plate
multitest yeast p.
nail plate of nailbed
nasal crest of horizontal plate of palatine bone
nonnutrient agar p.
one-piece plate haptic silicone intraocular lens
orbital floor p.
orbital plate of ethmoid bone
orbital plate of frontal bone
pediatric blade p.
peg base p.
polystyrene agglutination p.
quadrigeminal plate cistern
p. and screw fixation of fracture
subsynaptic plate perforation
thrust plate prosthesis
tibial base p.
titanium hollow-screw osseointegrating reconstruction p.
trimandibular p.
trypticase soy p.
tubularized incised plate
Universal bone p.
variable screw p.

plateau

condylar plateau angle
lateral tibial p.
medial tibial p.
positive expiratory pressure p.
tibial p.
tibial plateau fracture

platelet

p. abnormality
p. accumulation index
p. activating/aggregating factor
p. activation
p. activation defect
p. adhesion
p. adhesiveness
p. adhesiveness plasma factor
p. agglutination
p. agglutinin
p. aggregate ratio
p. aggregation
p. aggregation as a risk of diabetes
p. aggregation factor
p. aggregation test
p. alloimmunization
p. antibody
p. antigen
arachidonate-induced platelet aggregation
p. associated
autologous platelet gel
bizarre p.
blood platelet disorder
circulating platelet aggregate
p. clump
p. clumping
clumping of p.
p. complement fixation test
p. concentrate
p. concentration
p. count
p. count decreased
p. count increased
p. count increment
p. count posttransfusion
p. count pretransfusion
p. destruction
p. disorder
p. distribution width
p. dysfunction
p. endothelial cell adhesion molecule-1
p. estimate
p. factor 1–4
flow cytometric p.
p. function analysis
p. function study
p. function test
gel-filtered p.
giant p.
p. granule extract
gray platelet syndrome
p. hematocrit
hemolysis, elevated liver enzymes, and low platelet count
human platelet antigen
human platelet suspension
p. imaging
indirect platelet count
inherited giant platelet disorder
interval platelet count
p. lactogen
low-affinity platelet factor
p. membrane
p. microsome
Montreal platelet syndrome
p. neutralization procedure
open canalicular system of p.'s
p. peroxidase
p. pheresis
p. phosphohexokinase
p. ^{125}I-labeled staphylococcal protein A
pooled platelet concentrate
poor platelet plasma
preleukemia p.
pulmonary platelet trapping
random-donor p.
random single donor p.
recombinant platelet factor-4
ristocetin-induced platelet agglutination
side platelet aggregation test
single-donor apheresis p.
p. skimming
spontaneous platelet aggregation
p. stability
standard platelet count
super packed p.
p. survival time
p. suspension immunofluorescence test
p. thromboplastin antecedent
p. transfusion
p. transfusion therapy
tumor-cell-induced platelet aggregation
Ultegra rapid platelet function assay
in vivo adhesive p.
zoster immune p.

platelet-activating
p.-a. factor
p.-a. factor acetylhydrolase
p.-a. factor of anaphylaxis

platelet-aggregating factor

platelet-associated immunoglobulin G

platelet-depleted plasma

platelet-derived
p.-d. angiogenesis factor
p.-d. endothelial cell growth factor
p.-d. epidermal growth factor
p.-d. histamine-releasing factor
p.-d. wound healing factor

platelet-poor
p.-p. blood
p.-p. plasma

platelet-rich plasma

platelet-stimulating factor

plate-screw fixation

platform
computerized dynamic platform posturography

plating
anterior spinal p.
eccentric dynamic compression p.
p. efficiency
secondary plating efficiency
variable spinal p.

Platinol
Adriamycin and P.
Adriamycin, Platinol, etoposide
ara-C and P.
methotrexate, Platinol, 5-fluorouracil, leucovorin, calcium
mitomycin C, Adriamycin, P.
mitomycin C, etoposide, P.
Oncovin, dianhydrogalactitol, Adriamycin, P.

platinum
p. coil
electrodetachable platinum coil
mechanically detachable platinum coil

platysma
p. incised
p. muscle

play
analytical play therapy
associative p.
directive group play therapy
directive play therapy group
excessive joint p.
p. group therapy
Symbolic P. Test
therapeutic play group

Playas virus

playing
role p.

plea of mental incompetence

Pleasant Events Schedule

please turn the patient over

pleasing
esthetically p.

pleasure
aesthetic p.
inability to feel p.

pledget
alcohol p.
Betadine-soaked p.
cotton p.

pledgeted
interrupted pledgeted suture

pleiotrophic functional defect

pleiotrophin/midkine growth enhancer

pleiotropic drug resistance

pleocytosis
lymphocytic p.
mononuclear cell p.
neutrophilic p.

pleomorphic
p. adenocarcinoma
p. adenoma
p. cell
p. hyalinizing angiectatic tumor
p. lobular carcinoma
p. lymphoma
nonmotile pleomorphic bacillus
p. organism
recurrent pleomorphic adenoma
salivary gland pleomorphic adenoma
p. xanthoastrocytoma

plethysmodynamography
ocular p.

plethysmograph
penile p.
venous volume p.

plethysmography
body p.
impedance p.
microphotoelectric p.
ocular p.
respiratory inductance p.
respiratory inductive p.
segmental bronchus p.
surface inductive p.
venous impedance p.
venous occlusion p.

pleura, pl. **pleurae**
adipose fold of the p.
costodiaphragmatic recess of p.
costomediastinal recess of p.
hydrops of p.
p. incised
mediastinal p.
mediastinal pleura incised
neurofibroma of p.
parietal p.
pulmonary p.
visceral pleura incised

pleural
p. abrasion
p. adhesion
angled pleural tube
apical pleural stripping
apical pleural thickening
artificial pleural effusion procedure
asbestos-induced pleural fibrosis
asbestos pleural plaque
asbestos-related pleural disease
asbestos-related pleural effusion
asbestos-related pleural thickening
p. aspirate
aspiration of pleural cavity
bilateral pleural rub
p. biopsy
p. calcification
p. calculus
p. cavity
closed pleural biopsy
closed pleural drainage
p. crackles
culture of pleural effusion
p. cyst
p. density
diffuse malignant pleural mesothelioma
p. disease
p. drainage
p. effusion
p. empyema
extent of pleural carcinomatosis score
p. exudate
p. fibrosis
p. fluid
p. fluid aspiration
p. fremitus
p. friction rub
p. inflammatory change

p. lavage
line of pleural reflection
loculated pleural effusion
loculated pleural fluid
p. lymph node
p. mass
p. membrane lining
p. mesothelial cell
p. metastasis
p. opened
parietal pleural tissue
p. peel
p. pericarditis
p. plaquing
p. pressure
p. pressure gradient
p. rale
p. rate
p. sac
p. scarring
p. space
p. surface
p. tap
p. tear
p. thickening
transudative pleural effusion
p. tube
p. tuberculosis
ventricular pleural pressure gradient
p. villi
visual pleural space

pleurisy
encysted p.
hemorrhagic p.
interlobar p.
interlobular p.
mediastinal p.
pulmonary p.
tuberculous p.
p. with effusion

pleuritic
p. chest pain
p. effusion
p. pneumonia
p. respiration
p. rub

pleuritis
p. and emphysema
obliterative p.
reactive eosinophilic p.

pleurodesis
mechanical p.
minocycline p.
talc p.
thor scopic talc p.

pleuroesophageal fistula

pleuropericardial
p. adhesion
p. canal
p. cyst
p. hiatus
p. rub
p. window

pleuroperitoneal
p. canal
p. cavity
Denver pleuroperitoneal shunt
p. fold
p. foramen
p. hernia
p. hiatus

pleuropneumonia
contagious bovine p.

pleuropneumonia-like organism

pleuropulmonary
p. adhesion
p. blastoma
p. disease

plexiform
external plexiform layer
inner plexiform layer
p. layer
p. layer of cerebral cortex
p. layers of retina
p. neurofibroma
p. spindle cell nevus

plexogenic
primary plexogenic hypertension

plexopathy
lower brachial p.
lumbosacral p.
malignant brachial p.
neoplastic brachial p.

plexus
angular aqueous sinus p.
p. annularis
anterior cerebral artery p.
anterior coronary periarterial p.
anterior division of brachial p.
anterior pulmonary p.
anterocrural celiac plexus block
aortic lymphatic p.
areolar venous p.
articular vascular p.
ascending pharyngeal p.
Auerbach and Meissner p.
Auerbach mesenteric p.
p. block
brachial plexus block
brachial plexus injury
brachial plexus neuropathy
brachial plexus traction injury
celiac plexus neurolysis
choroid plexus carcinoma
choroid plexus cyst
choroid plexus papilloma
p. coccygeus
ganglion of sympathetic p.
inferior hypogastric p.
inferior spermatic p.
interscalene brachial p.
lumbar lymphatic p.
lumbar nervous p.
lumbosacral nervous p.
lumbosacral plexus injury
lumbosacral plexus lesion
medial cord of brachial p.
middle hemorrhoidal p.
myenteric plexus neuropathy
neonatal choroid plexus hemorrhage
p. nerve block
neurolytic celiac plexus block
obstetric brachial plexus injury
obstetric brachial plexus palsy
p. ophthalmicus
pelvic autonomic p.
posterior coronary p.
sacral p.
p. of Santorini
superficial vascular p.
superior hemorrhoidal p.
trunks of brachial p.

pliable
soft and p.

plica, pl. **plicae**
bucket-handle p.
plicae iridis
p. nasi
plicae palmatae
p. palpebronasalis
p. pubovesicalis
p. rectouterina
p. salpingopharyngea
p. stapedis
p. supratonsillaris
p. triangularis
plicae tubariae tubae uterinae
plicae vaginae
p. vesicalis transversa
p. vocalis

plicata
lingua p.
pars p.

plication
p. defect
endoscopic muscle p.
fundal p.
Noble bowel p.
p. sutures

pliers
debonding p.
lingual arch-forming p.

plongeurs
maladie de p.

plot
Scatchard p.

plotting
direct linear p.

plucking
p. at clothes
hair p.

plug
anorectal p.
bone-graft p.
bone plug cutter
bone plug extractor
bone plug setter
carpet tack follicular keratotic p.
cervical mucous p.
echogenic p.
p. the lung until it grows
meconium p.
meconium plug syndrome
methylmethacrylate cranioplastic p.
Micro punctum p.
mucous p.
one-piece disposable p.
punctal p.
removable silicone p.

plugged
p. artery
p. ear
telescoping plugged catheter
p. tube

plugger
automatic p.

plugging
p. of bronchial tree
mucous p.

Plummer disease

Plummer-Vinson
P.-V. radium applicator
P.-V. syndrome

plunging goiter

pluralistic
System of Multicultural P. Assessment

pluridirectional tomography

pluripotent
p. hemopoietic stem cell
p. myeloid stem cell

plus
ara-C plus 6-thioguanine
conjugated equine estrogen plus norgestrel
fluorescence plus Giemsa stain
four plus edema
Hanks balanced salt solution plus glucose
hypertension plus proteinuria
MeCCNU, Oncovin, 5-fluorouracil plus streptozotocin
Pap plus speculoscopy
Penassay broth plus glucose
Penassay broth plus glucose plus menadione
psoralen plus ultraviolet light of A wavelength
ticlopidine plus aspirin
truncal vagotomy plus antrectomy
truncal vagotomy plus pyloroplasty
vegetable protein diet plus fiber
vincristine, doxorubicin, cyclophosphamide, dactinomycin plus ifosfamide with mesna

PMP22 gene

PMPA

pneumatic
p. antiembolic stocking
p. antishock garment
p. bone
circumferential pneumatic compression
circumferential pneumatic compression suit
p. compression
p. compression boot
p. compression device
p. compression sleeve
p. compression stocking
p. compression therapy
p. cuff
p. dilator
external pneumatic calf compression
external pneumatic compression
p. garment
intermittent pneumatic compression boot
p. tourniquet
p. tourniquet control
p. tourniquet-controlled bleeding

pneumatonometer
Micro One p.
Modular One p.

pneumatosis

pneumococcal
alcoholism, leukopenia, pneumococcal sepsis
p. bacteremia
bacteremia-associated pneumococcal pneumonia
p. bacteria
p. capsular polysaccharide
p. conjugate vaccine
p. disease
p. empyema
p. infection
p. meningitis
nonvalent pneumococcal conjugate vaccine
p. pneumonia
p. polysaccharide vaccine
polyvalent pneumococcal polysaccharide
p. *Streptococcus pneumoniae* polysaccharide
p. vaccine
p. 7-valent conjugate vaccine
7-valent pneumococcal conjugate

pneumococcus, pl. **pneumococci**
penicillin-resistant p.
resistant p.
p. vaccine

pneumoconiosis
coal worker's p.

pneumocystic pneumonia

Pneumocystis
P. carinii
Pneumocystis carinii choroiditis
Pneumocystis carinii pneumonia

pneumocystosis
extrapulmonary p.

pneumocyte
fibroblast pneumocyte factor
micronodular pneumocyte hyperplasia

pneumoencephalitis
avian p.
avian pneumoencephalitis virus

pneumoenteric defect

pneumogram
pediatric p.

pneumonectomy
extrapleural p.
simultaneously stapled p.

pneumonia
acute fibropurulent p.
acute interstitial p.
atypical bronchial p.
atypical interstitial p.
atypical measles p.
atypical primary p.
bacteremia-associated pneumococcal p.
bronchiectasis, eosinophilia, asthma, p.
bronchiolitis obliterans-organizing p.
chronic eosinophilic p.
community-acquired p.
cryptogenic organizing p.
desquamative interstitial p.
diffuse interstitial p.
Eaton agent p.
eosinophilic p.
exogenous lipoid p.
giant cell interstitial p.
group B streptococcal p.
hospital-acquired p.
idiopathic acute eosinophilic p.
idiopathic interstitial p.
influenza virus p.
interstitial lymphocytic p.
interstitial organizing p.
lymphocytic interstitial p.
lymphoid interstitial p.
measles giant cell p.
mycobacterial necrotizing p.
mycoplasmal p.
mycoplasma pneumonia of pig
nosocomial acquired p.
nursing facility-acquired p.
organizing aspiration p.
organizing interstitial p.
patchy area of p.
peptic aspiration p.
Pittsburgh pneumonia agent
pneumocystic p.
Pneumocystis carinii p.
primary atypical p.
progressive pneumonia virus
Pseudomonas aeruginosa p.
P. Severity Index
Staphylococcus aureus p.
usual interstitial p.
usual interstitial pneumonia of Liebow
p. vaccination
p. vaccine
ventilator-associated p.
viral porcine p.
p. virus of mice

pneumoniae
drug-resistant *Streptococcus pneumoniae*
indirect enzyme immunoassay for anti-*Mycoplasma pneumoniae* IgM
multidrug-resistant *Streptococcus pneumoniae*
Optochin-resistant *Streptococcus pneumoniae*
penicillin-nonsusceptible *Streptococcus pneumoniae*
penicillin-resistant *Streptococcus pneumoniae*
penicillin-sensitive *Streptococcus pneumoniae*
pneumococcal conjugate vaccine
pneumococcal *Streptococcus pneumoniae* polysaccharide
Streptococcus p.

pneumonia-fibrosis
nonspecific interstitial p.-f.

pneumonic
p. consolidation
p. infiltrate
patchy area of pneumonic consolidation
patchy pneumonic infiltrate
p. process

pneumonitis
acute interstitial p.
acute lupus p.
acute radiation p.
aspiration p.
bronchiolitis with interstitial p.
chronic pneumonitis of infancy
chronic progressive coccidioidal p.
classic interstitial pneumonitis with fibrosis
desquamative interstitial p.
diffuse interstitial fibrosing p.
giant cell interstitial p.
herpes simplex p.
hypersensitivity p.
hypersensitivity pneumonitis panel
interstitial hypersensitivity p.
interstitial radiation p.
lipoid interstitial p.
lymphoid interstitial p.
nonspecific chronic interstitial p.
nonspecific interstitial p.
peptic aspiration p.
plasma cell interstitial p.
summer-type hypersensitivity p.
unusual interstitial p.
usual interstitial p.

pneumonoconiosis
silicotic p.

pneumoparalytic
oil-associated pneumoparalytic eosinophilic syndrome

pneumoperitoneal
extracorporeal pneumoperitoneal access bubble

pneumoplethysmography
ocular p.

pneumotaxic center

pneumothorax
artificial p.
closed chest p.
posttraumatic persistent p.
primary spontaneous p.
simultaneous bilateral spontaneous p.
spontaneous p.

PO2
alveolar-arterial PO_2 difference

pocket
abdominal p.
air p.
p. depth
expander p.
necrotic p.
pacemaker p.
periodontal p.'s
pus p.
p. of pus
Rathke p.
rheumatoid p.
tooth p.
p. of Zahn

pocketing of barium

pock-forming unit

Podi-Burr
medium callus P.-B.

poerencephaly
syndrome of absence of septum pellucidum with p.

pogonion
nasion p.

poikiloderma
p. atrophicans vasculare
calcinosis cutis, osteoma cutis, poikiloderma, and skeletal abnormalities syndrome
hereditary sclerosing p.

point
altered set p.
anterior commissure-posterior commissure reference p.

point *(continued)*
anterior focal p.
A point chart
p. of application
p. of articulation
associated myofascial trigger p.
p. of basal convergence
bleeding points secured
boiling p.
Bolton craniometric p.
Broadbent registration p.
cannulated drill p.
carbon steel drill p.
p. of care
critical point drying
diamond point needle
dilution end p.
electrodesiccated bleeding p.
electrosensitive p.
electrotherapeutic point stimulation
end p.
p. of entry
p. of entry, traction and twist
equal-pressure p.
p. estimation by sequential testing
extra p.
facial artery pressure p.
far point of accommodation
Fisher-John melting point method
p. of fixation
freezing p.
freezing point osmometer
fusion p.
glabellolambda line craniometric point
Hazard Analysis Critical Control P.'s
hemolysis end p.
hydrostatic indifference p.
p. of identical flow
inferior point of pubic bone
p. of intervention
isoelectric p.
p. locator stimulator
loss of contact p.
lower alveolar p.
lower yield p.
lustrous central yellow p.
material failure break p.
p. of maximal impulse
maximal point of impulse
maximal reimbursement p.
p. of maximum amplitude of wave
p. of maximum impulse
p. of maximum impulse fifth intercostal space
p. of maximum intensity
p. of maximum tenderness
melting p.
most anterior point of anterior contour of the sella turcica
most posterior point on posterior contour of sella turcica
mounted diamond p.'s
near visual p.
optical nodal p.
pathology p.
pattern disruption p.
pedicle entrance p.
point to p.
popliteal artery pressure p.
Precarious Point virus
pressure inversion p.
Quality P. of Service
reference point following QRS complex, at beginning of ST segment
p. of regard
remote point of convergence
respiratory inversion p.
sacrococcygeal to inferior pubic p.
secondary focal point of lens
p. of service
single reference p.
sperm entry p.
p. of subjective equality
Sudeck critical p.
supramentale craniometric point
p. of symmetry
tender p.
p. of tenderness
thermal death p.
thermal inactivation p.
transition p.
trigger p.
upper yield p.
Valsalva leak point pressure
working p.
yield p.
zero point of charge
z point pressure

pointer
hip p.

pointes
torsade de p.
torsade de pointes ventricular tachycardia

pointing
Auditory P. Test
past p.

point-of-care
arterial blood gas point-of-care test
p.-o.-c. testing

point-prevalent survey

point-resolved spectroscopy

58-point Scandinavian Stroke Scale

point-spread function

point-to-point protocol

Poiseuille
P. law
P. space

poison
absorbed p.
arrow p.
p. ivy
p. oak

poisoning
acute lead p.
amnesic shellfish p.
carbon tetrachloride p.
clostridial food p.
dehydration, poisoning, trauma
diarrheic shellfish p.
ethylene glycol p.
food p.
heavy metal p.
mercury vapor p.
methyl alcohol p.
monosodium glutamate p.
nerve gas p.
neurotoxic shellfish p.
organic mercury p.
organic solvent p.
organophosphorous compound p.
paralytic shellfish p.
zinc chloride p.

poisonous
p. gas
ingestion of poisonous substance
ingestion of potentially poisonous substance
p. substance

pokeweed
p. activated spleen conditioned medium
p. antiviral protein
p. mitogen

Poland syndrome

polar
anterior polar cataract
apical polar nephrectomy
p. body
p. cataract

frontal polar electrode placement in electroencephalography
p. hyperplasia
macromolecular polar compound

polaris
arteria polaris frontalis
arteria polaris temporalis

polarity
electrodialysis with reversed polarity

polarization
angle of p.
chemically induced dynamic electron p.
circular p.
delayed after p.
dynamic nuclear p.
fluorescence p.
fluorescence polarization immunoassay
fluorescent polarization immunoassay
magnetic p.
orthogonal polarization spectral
plane p.
transverse p.

polarized
multiangle polarized scatter separation
p. light microscopy
relative to rotation of a beam of polarized light

polarizing
p. lens
p. microscope
zone of polarizing activity

polarography
differential pulse p.

pole
animal p.
anterior p.
anterior pole cataract
anterior pole of eyeball
anterior pole of lens
barber pole sign
p. of calices
inferior p.
kidney p.
leading p.
p. of left kidney
lower p.
lower pole of incision
lower pole of testis
posterior p.
posterior pole of eye
posterior pole of lens
posterior pole and periphery
p. of right kidney
right upper p.
strength of p.
trailing p.
upper pole of kidney
upper pole of uterine incision

policy
hospital p.
infection control p.
isolation p.'s
local medical review p.
National Collegiate Athletic Association drug testing p.
organ allocation p.
p. and procedure
p. target adjustment factor

polio
enhanced inactivated polio vaccine
p. immunization
inactivated polio vaccine
killed polio vaccine
monovalent oral polio virus vaccine
nonparalytic p.
NP p.
oral polio immunization
paralytic p.
p. vaccine
vaccine-associated paralytic p.
p. virus

polioencephalitis
acute p.
superior hemorrhagic p.

poliomyelitis
anterior acute p.
ascending p.
diphtheria, pertussis, tetanus, poliomyelitis, and measles vaccine
p. immunization
p. immunoglobulin
p. live vaccine
Medin p.
mouse p.
mouse poliomyelitis virus
nonparalytic p.
oral attenuated poliomyelitis virus vaccine
paralytic p.
p. vaccine
vaccine-associated paralytic p.
p. vaccine inactivated
p. vaccine killed
p. virus

poliovirus
p. hominis
human p.
inactivated poliovirus vaccine
live oral poliovirus vaccine
oral attenuated poliovirus vaccine
p. sensitivity
trivalent oral poliovirus vaccine
p. vaccine
p. vaccine monovalent oral
p. vaccine trivalent oral

polish
nail p.

polished
collarless, polished, tapered

polisher
olive-tip capsule p.

polisher-stimulator

polishing
posterior capsular p.

***Polistes* wasp venom**

Politzer
method of P.

pollen
p. adherence factor
alder tree p.
alfalfa weed p.
p. allergy
p. antigen
ash tree p.
p. asthma
maple tree p.
mugwort weed p.
Noon pollen unit
oak tree p.
olive tree p.
orchard grass p.
ragweed p.

pollen-induced allergy

pollex
mental retardation-absent nails of hallux and pollex syndrome

pollicis
abductor p.
abductor pollicis brevis muscle
abductor pollicis brevis tendon
abductor pollicis longus
adductor p.
p. adductor muscle
adductor pollicis obliquus muscle
adductor pollicis brevis tendon
adductor pollicis muscle
arteria princeps p.
p. artery
articulatio carpometacarpalis p.

pollicis *(continued)*
p. brevis
p. brevis abductor muscle
p. brevis extensor muscle
p. brevis extensor tendon
p. brevis flexor muscle
extensor pollicis brevis
extensor pollicis brevis tendon
extensor pollicis longus
flexor p.
flexor pollicis brevis
flexor pollicis longus
p. longus
p. longus abductor muscle
p. longus brevis
p. longus extensor muscle
p. longus flexor muscle
musculus abductor pollicis brevis
musculus abductor pollicis longus
musculus adductor p.
musculus extensor brevis p.
musculus extensor longus p.
musculus extensor ossis metacarpi p.
musculus extensor pollicis brevis
musculus extensor pollicis longus
musculus flexor pollicis brevis
musculus flexor pollicis longus

Pollock operation

pollutant
aerosolized pollutant exposure
health effects of environmental p.'s
persistent organic p.'s

pollution
air pollution adaptation
air pollution index
air pollution syndrome
p. and environmental degradation

Pólya
anterior Pólya procedure

polyacrylamide
p. bead
p. gel
p. gel electrophoresis
p. gel electrophoresis with silver stain
p. gel isoelectric focusing
isoelectric focusing in p.
isoelectric focusing electrophoresis in polyacrylamide gel

polyadenopathy
angiofollicular and plasmacytic p.

polyamine
macrocyclic p.
p. oxidase

polyarteritis
infantile polyarteritis nodosa
microscopic p.
microscopic polyarteritis nodosa
p. nodosa

polyarthritis
acute symmetric p.
chronic p.
juvenile chronic p.
palmar fasciitis and polyarthritis syndrome
rheumatoid p.

polyarticular
p. gonococcal arthritis
p. gout
p. juvenile chronic arthritis
p. juvenile rheumatoid arthritis

polycentric
4-bar polycentric knee prosthesis
4-bar polycentric knee prosthesis

polychemotherapy
adjuvant p.

polychlorinated

polychondritis
atrophic p.
relapsing p.

polychromatic
p. cell
p. erythroblast
p. erythrocyte
p. normoblast

polychrome methylene blue stain

polychromic erythrocytes

polyclonal
p. activator
p. antibody
anti-GFP polyclonal antibody
p. antiplacental alkaline phosphatase
antithymidylate synthase polyclonal antibody
ATGAM polyclonal antibody
p. B-cell activity
p. carcinoembryonic antigen
p. gamma globulin
p. gammopathy
p. gammopathy identified
p. hypergammaglobulinemia
p. rheumatoid factor

polycyclic aromatic hydrocarbon

polycystic
acute polycystic disease
adult-onset polycystic kidney disease
adult polycystic kidney disease
adult polycystic liver disease
adult-type polycystic kidney disease
autosomal-dominant polycystic kidney disease
autosomal-recessive polycystic kidney disease
p. change
childhood polycystic kidney disease
congenital polycystic disease
p. cyst
p. disease of kidney
p. disease of liver
dysgenetic polycystic disease
infantile polycystic kidney disease
p. kidney
p. kidney disease
p. lipomembranous osteodysplasia
p. liver disease
p. lung
oligomenorrheic polycystic ovary syndrome
p. ovarian disease
p. ovarian syndrome
p. ovary
p. ovary disease
p. renal disease
p. tumor

polycythemia
Friend virus p.
p. hypertonica
p. rubra
p. rubra vera
p. vera with myeloid metaplasia

polycytidylic
copolymer of polyinosinic and polycytidylic acid

polydactyly
p., imperforate anus, vertebral anomalies syndrome
Majewski short rib p.
mental retardation, polydactyly, phalangeal hypoplasia, syndactyly, unusual face, uncombable hair
microcephalus, imperforate anus, syndactyly, hamartoblastoma, abnormal lung lobulation, p.

polydioxanone suture

polydipsia
lithium-induced p.
patient has p.
psychogenic nocturnal p.

psychosis, intermittent hyponatremia, polydipsia syndrome

polydrug
p. abuse
p. addiction
p. dependence
p. use

polyendocrine
autoimmune polyendocrine syndrome

polyendocrinopathy
autoimmune polyendocrinopathy, candidiasis, ectodermal dysplasia
autoimmune polyendocrinopathy, candidiasis, ectodermal dystrophy

polyester
sucrose p.
p. suture

polyethylene
p. glycol-adenosine deaminase
p. glycol-conjugated superoxide dismutase pegorgotein
p. glycol electrolyte lavage solution
p. glycol-modified adenosine deaminase
p. glycol-modified interleukin-2
high-density p.
high molecular weight p.
p. implant
p. implant material
insertion of polyethylene implant
porous high-density p.
recombinant polyethylene glycol
p. stent
p. strut
p. suture
p. tube
ultrahigh molecular weight p.
p. vacuum cup

polyglandular
adult-onset polyglandular syndrome
autoimmune polyglandular endocrinopathy
autoimmune polyglandular failure
autoimmune polyglandular hypofunction
autoimmune polyglandular syndrome
p. autoimmune syndrome type I, II

polyglycolide
auto-reinforced polyglycolide rod

polyhedrosis
cytoplasmic polyhedrosis virus

polyhidrosis
nuclear polyhidrosis virus

polyimmunoglobulin receptor

polyinosinic
copolymer of polyinosinic and polycytidylic acid

polylevolactic
self-reinforcing polylevolactic acid

poly-L-lactide
self-reinforced p.-L.-l.

polylysine
penicilloyl polylysine skin test

polymer
dehydrogenated p.
p. fume fever
glucose p.
interpenetrating polymer network
sulfonated p.
synthetic RNA p.

polymerase
allele-specific polymerase chain reaction
anti-RNA polymerase antibody
arbitrarily-primed polymerase chain reaction
arbitrary-primed polymerase chain reaction
BCR-ABL multiplex reverse transcriptase polymerase chain reaction assay
p. chain reaction
p. chain reaction analysis of prostate-specific antigen
p. chain reaction-restriction fragment length polymorphism
p. chain reaction–single-strand conformation polymorphism
p. chain reaction in situ hybridization
competitive polymerase chain reaction
deoxyribonucleic acid p.
limiting dilution polymerase chain reaction
mitochondrial deoxyribonucleic acid polymerase gamma
mitochondrial DNA polymerase gamma
multiplex polymerase chain reaction
primer-dependent deoxynucleic acid p.
primer-dependent deoxynucleic acid polymerase index
quantitative competitive polymerase chain reaction
repetitive extragenic palindromic polymerase chain reaction
reverse transcriptase polymerase chain reaction
ribonucleic acid-dependent deoxyribonucleic acid p.
in situ polymerase chain reaction

polymerase-inducing unit

polymerization
degree of p.

polymerized
p. human albumin
individually polymerized grass
p. ragweed

polymethyl
passivated polymethyl methacrylate

polymicrobial infection

polymorphic
p. delta activity
eosinophilic, polymorphic, and pruritic eruption associated with radiotherapy
p. epithelial mucin
p. genetic marker
nonsustained polymorphic ventricular tachycardia
posterior polymorphic dystrophy of cornea
random amplified polymorphic DNA
rapid amplification of polymorphic DNA
p. reticulosis

polymorphism
angiotensin-converting enzyme gene p.
cleavage fragment length p.
mutation-enriched restriction fragment length polymorphism assay
PCR combined with single-strand conformation p.
polymerase chain reaction-restriction fragment length p.
polymerase chain reaction–single-strand conformation p.
restriction fragment length p.
short tandem repeat p.
simple tandem repeat p.
single nucleotide p.

polymorphism *(continued)*
single nucleotide p.'s - linkage disequilibrium
single-stranded conformational p.

polymorphonuclear
p. basophil
p. eosinophil
p. granulocyte
p. leukocyte
p. leukocyte count
p. leukocyte infiltrate
p. leukocyte response
p. neutrophil
p. neutrophil chemotactic factor
p. neutrophilic granulocyte
p. neutrophilic leukocyte
neutrophilic polymorphonuclear leukocyte
nonfilament polymorphonuclear leukocyte
percent of polymorphonuclear leukocyte
p. per low-power field
plasma polymorphonuclear elastase

polymorphous
p. light eruption
p. low-grade adenocarcinoma
p. low-grade carcinoma
p. macular rash
p. posterior corneal dystrophy
posterior polymorphous corneal dystrophy

polymyalgia
p. rheumatica
p. rheumatica syndrome

polymyositis
p. and dermatomyositis
orbital p.
p. ossificans progressiva

polymyositis-dermatomyositis

polymyositis-scleroderma

polymyxin
p. B
bacitracin, polymyxin B, neomycin sulfate
p. B sulfate, bacitracin, and neomycin
gentamicin, clindamycin, and polymyxin topical preparation
p., lysozyme, EDTA, and thallous acetate in heart infusion agar
neomycin and polymyxin B

polyneuritic
alcoholic polyneuritic psychosis
p. insanity

polyneuritiformis

polyneuritis
acute idiopathic p.
acute infectious p.
mixed sensory p.

polyneuropathy
acute canine idiopathic p.
acute inflammatory demyelinating p.
autoimmune demyelinating p.
chronic relapsing demyelinating inflammatory p.
critical illness p.
demyelinated inflammatory chronic p.
diabetic p.
distal sensory p.
distal symmetrical p.
distal symmetric sensory p.
familial amyloid p.
familial amyloidotic p.
gait disorder, autoantibody, late-age onset, p.
mitochondrial encephalomyopathy with sensorimotor p.
mitochondrial encephalomyopathy with sensorimotor polyneuropathy, ophthalmoplegia, and paralysis
mixed sensorimotor p.
p., ophthalmoplegia, leukoencephalopathy, and intestinal pseudo-obstruction
p., organomegaly, endocrinopathy, monoclonal gammopathy, and skin changes syndrome
segmental demyelinating p.
sensorimotor p.

polynitroxyl albumin

polynuclear
p. aromatic hydrocarbon
p. eosinophil

polynucleosis
neutrophil p.

polyolefin copolymer

polyoma
monkey polyoma virus
papilloma virus, polyoma virus, vacuolative virus
p. virus

polyoncosis
multiple hereditary cutaneomandibular p.

polyostotic fibrous dysplasia

polyp
adenomatous p.
angiomatous nasal p.
Antioxidant P. Prevention Trial
antral choanal p.
p. of antrum of stomach
automated polyp detection
benign adenomatous p.
benign polyps of large intestine
p. of body of stomach
p. in canaliculus
p. of cervix
p. of colon
diminutive p.
p. of duodenal bulb
p. of duodenum
fundic gland p.
p. of fundus of stomach
gastric antral sessile p.
hyperplastic rectal p.
inflammatory cloacogenic p.
inflammatory colonic p.
inflammatory fibroid p.
juvenile p.'s
p. in lacrimal sac
p. of large intestine
p. of larynx
lymphangiomatous p.
multiple adenomatous p.'s
multiple gastrointestinal p.'s
papillary adenomatous p.
pedunculated adenomatous p.
pedunculated juvenile p.
4-pronged polyp grasper
small pedunculated adenomatous p.'s
sporadic adenomatous p.'s

polypectomy
electrosurgical snare p.
endocervical p.
nasal p.
p. procedure
saline-assisted p.

polypeptide
adrenocortical p.
adrenocorticotropic p.
atrial natriuretic p.
avian pancreatic p.
bovine pancreatic p.
canine pancreatic p.
endothelial-monocyte activating polypeptide II

Escherichia coli p.
gastric inhibitory p.
glicentin-related pancreatic p.
p. growth factor
human pancreatic p.
insulin-releasing p.
integrated pancreatic polypeptide response
islet amyloid p.
large neuronal p.
neurofilament triplet p.
organic anion transporter p.
ovine pancreatic p.
pancreatic p.
parathyroid hormonelike p.
pituitary adenylate cyclase activating p.
porcine pancreatic p.
serum tissue polypeptide antigen
small nuclear ribonucleoprotein-associated p.
thymic p.
tissue polypeptide antigen
tumor polypeptide antigen
vasoactive intestinal polypeptide immunoreactivity
vasoactive intestinal polypeptide tumor

polypeptide-1
apo B mRNA-editing catalytic p.

polyphasic
brief, small, abundant, polyphasic potential

polyphenol
green tea p.

polyphosphomolybdic
tannic acid, polyphosphomolybdic acid, and amido acid staining technique

polyphosphoric ester

polypoid
p. adenocarcinoma of colon
p. adenoma
p. anorectal lesion
atypical polypoid adenomyofibroma
atypical polypoid adenomyofibroma of low malignant potential
atypical polypoid adenomyoma
p. change
p. degeneration
p. dysplasia
p. excrescence
p. fibroma
p. hyperplasia
inverted polypoid hamartoma of rectum
p. tissue

polypoidal
idiopathic polypoidal choroidal vasculopathy

polyposis
adenoma familial p.
adenomatous p.
adenomatous polyposis coli
attenuated adenomatous polyposis coli
attenuated familial adenomatous p.
chronic hyperplastic sinusitis with nasal p.
p. coli
familial adenomatous p.
familial juvenile p.
familial polyposis coli
gastrointestinal p.
juvenile polyposis syndrome
lymphomatous p.
multiple familial p.
multiple lymphomatous p.
nonfamilial gastrointestinal p.
postinflammatory p.
segmental colonic adenomatous polyposis syndrome

polypous gastritis

polypropylene
p. glycol
p. glycol-ankle-foot orthosis
p. glycol-thoracolumbosacral orthosis
p. suture

polyprotein
cleaved polyprotein precursor molecule
cleaved polyprotein precursor molecule product

polyradiculitis
ascending p.

polyradiculoneuritis
acute idiopathic demyelinating p.

polyradiculoneuropathy
acute inflammatory demyelinating p.
chronic inflammatory demyelinating p.

polyradiculopathy
acute inflammatory demyelinating p.
chronic inflammatory demyelinating p.

polyribosylribitol phosphate-diphtheria toxoid conjugate

polysaccharide
anti-arteriosclerosis polysaccharide factor
antistreptococcal polysaccharide A test
p. egg antigen
Haemophilus influenzae type b polysaccharide vaccine
Histoplasma capsulatum polysaccharide antigen
p. iron complex
p. Kreha
meningococcal polysaccharide vaccine
nonstarch p.'s
pneumococcal capsular p.
pneumococcal polysaccharide vaccine
pneumococcal *Streptococcus pneumoniae* p.
polyvalent pneumococcal p.
protein p.
protein-bound p.
p. storage disease
p. substance
p. substance tumor
p. tetanus conjugate vaccine
tumor polysaccharide substance
typhoid vaccine, Vi capsular p.

polysaccharide-iron complex

polyserositis
familial paroxysmal p.

polysomnogram
nocturnal p.

polysomnographic study

polysomnography
ambulatory p.
nocturnal p.

polysplenia
situs ambiguus with p.

polystyrene
p. agglutination plate
p. latex particle

polystyrene-tube radioimmunoassay

polysubstance
p. abuse
p. dependence
p. use and abuse

polysulfone filter

polytetrafluoroethylene
expanded p.

polytomous
multinomial polytomous logistic regression method
polyunsaturated
fatty acids p.
p. free fatty acid
long-chain polyunsaturated fatty acid
omega-3 polyunsaturated fatty acid
p. phosphatidylcholine
short-chain polyunsaturated fatty acid
polyunsaturated-to-saturated fatty acids ratio
polyurethane
p. film
p. foam
p. foam dressing
p. implant
polyurethane-polyvinyl graphite
polyuria
patient has p.
persistent p.
polyvalent
p. pneumococcal polysaccharide
p. tolerance
polyvalvular
congenital polyvalvular disease
polyvinyl
p. acetate
p. alcohol fixative
p. alcohol foam
p. chloride
p. sponge implant
pomatia
Helix pomatia agglutinin
Pomeroy
modified Pomeroy technique
P. operation
P. technique
P. tubal ligation
pomonella
Cydia pomonella granulovirus
ponderal
p. index
somatotyping ponderal index
Pongola virus
pons
anterior part of p.
arteries of p.
p. cerebelli
p. and cerebellum
craniosynostosis, ataxia, trigeminal anesthesia, parietal anesthesia and pons, vermis fusion syndrome
diminished attenuation midbrain and p.
p. hypertrophy
p. lesion
medulla p.
p. and medulla
oblique bundle of p.
p. oblongata
Ponteves virus
pontile hemianesthesia
pontine
p. angle
p. artery
central pontine myelinolysis
p. cistern
p. flexure
p. gaze center
p. gray matter
p. hemorrhage
p. hyperintensity
p. infarct
p. junction
p. lesion
longitudinal pontine bundle
medial branch of pontine artery
p. micturition center
p. nucleus
paralytic pontine exotropia
paramedian pontine reticular formation
p. paramedian reticular formation
p. parareticular formation
p. reticular formation
pontis
arteriae p.
pars anterior p.
pars basilaris p.
pontocerebellaris
angulus p.
pontogeniculooccipital spike
pontomesencephalic
anterior pontomesencephalic vein
pontosubicular neuron necrosis
pool
aquatic therapy p.
autonomic motor p.
blood pool activity
blood pool imaging
cardiac p.
cardiac blood pool imaging
circulating granulocyte p.
equilibrium-gated blood pool study
gated blood pool angiography
gated blood pool scanning
gated blood pool scintigraphy
gated blood pool ventriculogram
gated blood pool study
gated cardiac blood p.
gated cardiac blood pool imaging
marginal granulocyte p.
marginated granulocyte p.
medical personnel p.
MUGA cardiac blood pool imaging
multigated blood pool image at rest
multigated blood pool image during exercise
multigated cardiac blood pool scanning
normal pool plasma
rapidly miscible p.
swimming pool granuloma
total blood granulocyte p.
total cellular receptor p.
pooled
absorbed normal pooled plasma
p. human plasma
p. human serum
normal human pooled plasma
p. platelet concentrate
pooling
dependent p.
p. of dye
neutrophil p.
poor
p. academic achievement
p. adaptability
p. air exchange
p. alignment
p. appetite
p. attention and memory
p. balance
p. bladder control
p. blood circulation
p. body image
p. bone stock
p. caloric intake
p. circulation
p. circulation in hand
p. clot
p. condition
p. dental hygiene
p. dental repair
p. dentition
dentition in poor repair
p. dietary habit

p. dietary intake
p. distal runoff
p. exercise tolerance
fatty acid p.
p. feeding
p. form response
p. health
p. historian
p. impulse control
infant suck is p.
p. intrauterine fetal growth
p. judgment
leukocyte p.
loss of recent memory, confusion and poor judgment
p. muscle tone
p. nutrition
obsessive-compulsive disorder with poor insight type
p. oral intake
p. partial response
patient is a poor surgical risk
patient's appetite is p.
p. person
p. platelet plasma
p. p.o. intake
p. posture
p. precordial R-wave progression
prognosis is p.
p. progression of R wave in precordial leads
p. respiratory effort
p. risk for anesthesia
p. R-wave progression electrocardiogram
p. wound healing

poorly
p. contractile globular left ventricle
p. developed
p. differentiated
p. differentiated adenocarcinoma
p. differentiated anaplastic carcinoma
p. differentiated defined
p. differentiated defined border
p. differentiated ductal carcinoma
p. differentiated embryonal cell tumor
p. differentiated large-cell carcinoma
p. differentiated lung cancer
p. differentiated lymphocytes
p. differentiated lymphocytic lymphoma
p. differentiated lymphocytic lymphoma-nodular
p. differentiated lymphoma, diffuse
p. differentiated small-cell carcinoma
p. differentiated squamous cell carcinoma
diffuse lymphocytic poorly differentiated
diffuse poorly differentiated lymphoma
p. expanded lungs
p. fitting dentures
p. groomed
malignant lymphoma, poorly differentiated lymphocytic
nodular-lymphocytic, poorly differentiated
nodular poorly differentiated lymphocytic lymphoma
p. nourished
nursed p.
p. reversible asthma
p. visualized gallbladder
p. visualizing gallbladder

poplar
Lombardy poplar tree

popliteal
p. arch
arcuate popliteal ligament
p. artery
p. artery aneurysm
p. artery occlusive disease
p. artery pressure point
p. bypass
p. cyst
p. external nerve
femoral above-knee popliteal bypass
p. fossa
p. fossa tumor
p. groove
infragenicular popliteal artery
p. internal nerve
internal popliteal nerve
p. joint
p. lateral nerve
p. ligament
p. line
p. lymph node
p. medial nerve
p. muscle
p. nerve block
p. node area
p. notch
p. occlusive disease
p. pulse
p. space
supragenicular popliteal artery
p. tibial bypass vein graft
p. vein

popliteales
nodi lymphoidei p.

popliteal-femoral bypass

popliteal-tibial artery bypass

popliteus tendon

popular
minimal popular dose
p. response

population
p. correlation coefficient
cumulative population doubling level
current population survey
p. doubling level
p. doubling time
high-risk adolescent p.
industrial p.
mean population doubling
occult clonal B-cell p.
overdistention of alveolar p.'s
partial hospital patient p.
p. pharmacokinetics
p. planning
p. sample
p. size
p. standard deviation
time required to double number of cells in given p.
total p.
zero population growth

Porak-Durante syndrome

porcelain
alumina-reinforced porcelain crown
aluminous p.
p. aorta
p. dentures
etched porcelain veneer
p. gallbladder
p. jacket crown
p. veneer
p. veneer bridge
p. veneer crown

Porch Index of Communicative Abilities in Children

porcine
p. aortic valve prosthesis
p. bioprosthesis
p. bone marrow transplantation
p. calcitonin
Carpentier-Edwards porcine bioprosthesis

porcine *(continued)*
p. endogenous retrovirus
enterocytopathogenic porcine orphan virus
p. graft
p. growth hormone
p. heart valve
p. heterograft
infectious porcine encephalomyelitis
p. intestinal adenomatosis
p. pancreatic
p. pancreatic elastase
p. pancreatic polypeptide
p. parvovirus
p. prosthesis
p. prosthetic valve
purified porcine insulin
stentless porcine valve
p. stress syndrome
p. trypsin
p. valve bioprosthesis
viral porcine pneumonia
p. xenograft

pore
auditory p.
nuclear pore complex
septal p.

porencephalia
septum pellucidum absent with porencephalia syndrome

porencephalic cyst

porencephaly
familial p.

porin
lipopolysaccharide p.'s
mitochondrial p.

pork
p. insulin
monocomponent highly purified pork insulin
purified pork insulin

pornography dependence

Porocoat material

porokeratosis
disseminated superficial actinic p.
p. of Mibelli

poroma
apocrine p.
malignant eccrine p.

porous
anatomic porous replacement
anatomic porous replacement hemispheric acetabular component
p. block hydroxyapatite
p. bone
p. high-density polyethylene
p. implant
p. layer bead
p. and spongy bone

porous-coated
p.-c. acetabular cup
p.-c. anatomic prosthesis

porphobilinogen
p. deaminase
p. synthase

porphobilinogen—quantitative

porphyria
acute intermittent p.
chronic erythropoietic p.
congenital erythropoietic p.
cutaneous hepatic p.
erythropoietic p.
p. hepatica
hepatoerythrocytic p.
hepatoerythropoietic p.
intermittent acute p.
mixed hepatic p.
South African type p.
variegate p.

porphyrin
p. biosynthetic pathway
boronated p.
free erythrocyte p.
p. screening
p. test
p. in urine

port
anterior port scalp excision
arterial port catheter system
endoscopic access p.
p. of entry
intravenous retrograde access p.
minimal port diameter
10-mm umbilical p.
multipurpose access p.
Peripheral Access System P. catheter system
venous access p.
p. wine hemangioma
p. wine mark

porta
p. hepatis
p. pulmonis

portable
AP supine portable view
p. cervical spine
p. chest radiograph
p. chest x-ray
p. defibrillator
p. dialysis unit
P. Document Format
p. film
p. film of abdomen
p. insulin dosage-regulating apparatus
p. insulin infusion pump
medical ultrasound 3D portable, with advanced communication
p. monitor of respiratory parameters
p. oxygen tank
personal portable stimulator
Short P. Mental Status Questionnaire

portacaval
p. anastomosis
p. bypass
end-to-side portacaval shunt
p. H graft
side-to-side portacaval shunt
temporary portacaval anastomosis
p. transportation
p. transposition

portal
acute portal inflammation
anterior intestinal p.
anterior and posterior opposing p.'s
anterocentral arthroscopic p.
anteroinferior p.
anterolateral p.
anteromedial p.
AP-PA p.
arterialization of portal vein
arthroscopic entry p.
aspiration p.
cavernous transformation of the portal vein
p. cirrhosis
p. drainage
electronic portal imaging device
p. embolization
extrahepatic portal hypertension
extrahepatic portal vein obstruction
free portal pressure
hepatic p.
hepatic-occluded portal pressure
hepatic portal vein
hepatic portal venous gas
hepatotropic portal blood factor
p. hypertension
p. hypertension of the liver
p. hypertension with ascites
p. hypertensive gastropathy

p. hypertensive intestinal vasculopathy
hypothalamohypophysial portal circulation
hypothalamohypophysial portal system
idiopathic portal hypertension
p. inflammation
p. insulin infusion system
intrahepatic portal hypertension
intrahepatic portal pressure
isolated hepatic portal and arterial perfusion
left portal view
main portal vein peak velocity
mononuclear histiocytic portal infiltrate
noncirrhotic portal fibrosis
right portal vein
p. shunt
p. shunt index
splanchnic occluded portal pressure
p. tract
transhepatic portal vein
tumor thrombus in the portal vein
p. vein
p. vein aneurysm
p. vein blood flow velocity
p. vein congestive index
p. vein dilation
p. vein infusion
p. vein obstruction
p. vein occlusion
p. vein thrombosis
p. vein tumor thrombus
p. venous access
p. venous and enteric drainage technique
p. venous flow
p. venous phase
p. venous pressure
p. venous sampling
p. venous velocity

portal-systemic
p.-s. anastomosis
p.-s. encephalopathy

portarenal shunt

Porter-Silber
P.-S. chromogen
P.-S. chromogen test

Porteus maze test

portio
cervical p.

portion
animo-terminal portion of heavy chain of immunoglobulin
anterior portion of left medial segment IV of liver
apex of petrous portion of temporal bone
apical portion of root
aponeurotic portion of diaphragm
avulsion of portion of finger
central apical p.
devitalized portion of bone
distal portion main circumflex
distal portion of small intestine
edible p.
fundal portion of uterus
orbital portion of eyelid
proximal and distal portion of vessel

portocaval
end-to-side portocaval shunt

portoenterostomy
hepatic p.

portography
computed tomography arterial p.
percutaneous transhepatic p.
transhepatic p.

portopulmonary hypertension

portosystemic
p. encephalopathy
p. gradient
p. shunting
transjugular intrahepatic portosystemic stent shunt

port-wine
p.-w. mark
p.-w. nevus
p.-w. stain birthmark

position
abnormal position of infant
p. and alignment
alignment and p.
anatomical position and alignment
anatomical position of duodenum
anatomic position and alignment
angle position potentiometer
angular position of ramus
anomalous tongue p.
anterior oblique p.
arch and slouch p.
asynclitic position of fetus
barber chair p.
beach chair p.
centric p.
claw toe p.
p. of comfort
controlled position brace
cornual position of uterus
cross-table lateral p.
decubitus p.
dorsal decubitus p.
dorsal elevated p.
dorsal recumbent p.
p. of ease
electrical heart p.
extraretinal eye position information
face lying p.
p. of fetus
final consonant p.
free position gravity
frontodextra anterior p.
frontodextra posterior position
frontooccipital fetal position
p. of function
functional resting position splint
hand held in position of extension
head dependent p.
head and neck in extended p.
impaired discriminatory, vibratory and position sensation
p. indicating device
p. of infant
intercostal position for chest lead
inverted hand p.
joint position sensation
lateral decubitus p.
lateral position test
left acromiodorsoanterior position of fetus
left acromiodorsoposterior position of fetus
left dorsotransverse fetal position
left frontoanterior fetal position
left frontoposterior position fetal
left frontotransverse fetal position
left lateral decubitus p.
left mentoanterior fetal position
left mentoposterior fetal position
left mentotransverse fetal position
left occipitoanterior fetal position
left occipitolateral fetal position
left occipitoposterior p.
left occipitotransverse fetal position
left occiput posterior fetal position
left sacroanterior p.
left sacroposterior fetal position
Lloyd Davies Trendelenburg p.
maternal birthing p.
maximal print p.

position *(continued)*
maximum loose-packed p.
mentum anterior p.
mentum posterior fetal position
mentum transverse p.
midline position of gaze
military brace p.
molar bite p.
near fixation position of gaze
neck extension p.
neutral hip p.
normal anatomic p.
normal size, shape, and p.
normal size, shape, and position, anteverted and anteflexed uterus
occipitosacral fetal position
paralleling cone p.
park bench p.
persistent mentoposterior fetal position
persistent occipitoposterior fetal position
persistent occiput posterior p.
physiologic rest p.
p., quality, radiation, severity, time
postural rest p.
real-time position management
p. response
resting calcaneal stance p.
retruded contact p.
right acromiodorsoanterior fetal p.
right acromiodorsoposterior fetal p.
right anterior oblique p.
right frontoanterior fetal position
right frontolateral fetal position
right frontoposterior fetal position
right frontotransverse fetal position
right lateral decubital p.
right lateral p.
right mentoanterior fetal position
right mentolateral fetal position
right mentoposterior fetal position
right mentotransverse p.
right occipitoanterior p.
right occipitolateral fetal position
right occipitoposterior p.
right occipitotransverse fetal position
right sacroanterior fetal position
right sacrolateral fetal position
right sacroposterior fetal position
semihorizontal heart p.
p. sense
sensor position indicator
subtalar joint neutral p.
tibial sesamoid p.
Transactional Analysis Life P. Survey
turn and p.
unusual position of limbs
usual anatomic p.

positional
p. alcohol nystagmus
benign paroxysmal positional vertigo
direction-changing positional nystagmus
disabling positional vertigo
p. dysfunction
p. dyspnea
facilitated positional release
p. feedback stimulation trainer
p. lightheadedness
malignant persistent positional nystagmus
paroxysmal positional vertigo
recalcitrant benign paroxysmal positional vertigo
p. vertigo

positioned
monitoring lines inserted and p.
patient prepped and p.

positioner
arm p.
gallbladder bag p.
head p.

positioning
automated endoscopic system for optimal p.
automatic endoscopic system for optimal p.
automatic positioning system
benign paroxysmal positioning nystagmus
four-in-one positioning block system
held after p.
tone and p.
uterine positioning via ligament investment fixation truncation

positive
p. activity
additional cost of false p.'s
p. airway pressure
p. airway pressure ventilation
p. alternative
p. antinuclear antibody
P. Attention Behavior
p. attention received
p. attitude
auto-titrating continuous positive airway pressure
axillary node p.
bilevel positive airway pressure
blood type A, O p.
p. bowel sounds
breakpoint cluster region p.
p. cardiac disease risk factors
constant positive airway pressure
continuous positive airway pressure
continuous positive airway pressure device
continuous positive pressure breathing
p. culture
p. cytology
cytotoxicity negative, absorption p.
p. distending pressure
Duffy antigen A, B positive phenotype
duration of positive pressure
p. end-airway pressure
p. end-expiratory pressure
p. end-expiratory pressure/continuous positive airway pressure
end positive pressure breathing
expiratory positive airway pressure
p. expiratory pressure
p. expiratory pressure plateau
p. family history
family history p.
p. feeling
p. findings
guaiac p.
Hemoccult positive stools
hereditary erythroblastic multinuclearity with positive acidified serum
high-frequency positive pressure
p. HIV
p. image
ingrown positive strain
inspiratory positive airway pressure
p. inspiratory pressure
inspiratory resistance and positive expiratory pressure
intermittent positive pressure breathing/inspiratory
intermittent positive pressure inflation with oxygen
intermittent positive pressure respiration

intermittent positive pressure ventilation
intrinsic positive end-expiratory pressure
late positive component
low-frequency positive pressure ventilation
low-grade CD20 positive lymphoma
low-grade positive smear
Lupus Anticoagulant P. Control
p. mental attitude
microscopically positive, culturally negative
nasal bilevel biphasic positive airway pressure
nasal continuous positive airway pressure
nasal positive pressure ventilation
nasal prong continuous positive airway pressure
p. to negative ratio
P. and Negative Stroke Scale
P. and Negative Syndrome Scale
nicotinamide adenine dinucleotide phosphate p.
nitrite p.
noninvasive positive pressure ventilation
number of similar p.'s
p. occipital sharp transients of sleep
p. peritoneal cytology
positron positive electron
p. predictive value
predictive value of a positive test
premenopausal hormone receptor p.
p. pressure breathing
p. pressure infusion device
replication error p.
Rhesus p.
Rinne test p.
p. risk factors for cardiac disease
p. rolandic spike
Scale for the Assessment of P. Symptoms
p. sharp wave fibrillations
p. spike pattern
spontaneous positive end expiratory pressure
stool positive for occult blood
p. support ventilator
P. Symptom Distress Index
p. symptom total
total p.'s
total net p.
treponemal false p.
true p.
true positive fraction
true positive rate
true positive stress test
p. ulnar variance
uniformly p.
variable positive airway pressure
variably p.
p. vertical divergence
P. Well-being scale

positive-negative
p.-n. ambivalent quotient
p.-n. pressure breathing
p.-n. pressure respiration

positive-pressure
intubated continuous p.-p.
synchronized nasal intermittent positive-pressure ventilation
p.-p. ventilation

positivity
differential time to p.
lymph node p.

positron
average positron energy
p. emission computed tomography
p. emission tomography balloon
p. emission tomography scan
p. emission tomography technique
p. emission transaxial tomography
p. emission transverse tomography
fluoride ion positron emission tomography
p. positive electron

possible
alcoholic possible pancreatic encephalopathy
p. allergic reaction
as much as p.
as often as p.
diagnostic arthroscopy, operative arthroscopy, and possible operative arthrotomy
p. hallucination
maximal possible effect
maximal possible error
medical improvement p.
minimal dose p.
p. source of bleeding
p. vertebrobasilar system

post
P. Anesthesia Discharge Scoring System
p. balloon angioplasty restenosis
p. coital headache
p. concussive headache
p. coronary artery bypass graft
p. delivery headache
p. heart attack apoptosis
p. history
p. ovulation hormone change
p. space preparation
status p.
status post myocardial infarction
status post surgery
status post transurethral resection of prostate
p. tib
p. treatment abstinence

postabortion healing

postanal gut

postanesthesia
p. care unit
p. hemodynamic
p. recovery area
p. recovery score
satisfactory postanesthesia course

postanesthetic
p. apnea
drug-induced postanesthetic depression
drug-induced postanesthetic respiratory depression
p. recovery unit
p. respiratory depression

postangioplasty
p. angiography
p. aortography
restenosis p.

postanoxia
occult trauma, postanoxia, ventriculoperitoneal

postanoxic encephalopathy

postantibiotic effect

postatrophic hyperplasia

postauricular
p. area
p. graft
p. incision
p. myogenic
p. and retroauricular scalping

postaxial acrofacial dysostosis syndrome

postbulbar
p. duodenum
p. ulcer

postburn
p. day
days p.

postcapillary venule

postcardiac
p. arrest
p. injury syndrome
p. surgery

postcardiotomy
p. shock
p. syndrome

postcavales
nodi lymphatici p.

postcaval shunt

postcentral
artery of postcentral sulcus

postcesarean hemorrhage

postchallenge
isolated postchallenge hyperglycemia

postchemotherapy nausea and vomiting

postcholecystectomy syndrome

postciliary artery

postcoital
p. bleeding
p. contraception
p. headache
p. pain
p. spotting
p. test

postconceptional age

postconcussion
p. amnesia
p. disorder
p. headache
p. syndrome

postconcussive syndrome

postcoronary care unit

postdecapitation convulsion

postdisaster trauma

postdrainage
persistent postdrainage hypotony

postdural puncture headache

Postel
Merle d'Aubigné and Postel hip rating scale

postencephalitic parkinsonism

postentry day

posterial tibial

posterior
acute multifocal posterior placoid pigment epitheliopathy
acute posterior multifocal placoid pigment epitheliopathy
p. airway space
p. ampullary nerve
aneurysm of posterior communicating artery
p. angle
angle of posterior rib
anterior and p.
anterior motion of posterior mitral valve leaflet
anterior and posterior fusion
anterior and posterior medialization thyroplasty
anterior and posterior opposing portals
anterior and posterior radicular artery
anterior and posterior repair
anterior and posterior superior pancreaticoduodenal artery
anterior and posterior vestibular veins
anterior release posterior fusion
anterior temporal branch of posterior cerebral artery
aortic posterior wall
apex posterior angulation
apex of posterior horn
apex of posterior horn of spinal cord
apical posterior artery
p. apical radius
aponeurosis of posterior superior serratus
p. approach
p. arch vein
arcus posterior atlantis
arteria auricularis p.
arteria cecalis p.
arteria cerebri p.
arteria choroidea p.
arteria communicans p.
arteria conjunctivalis p.
arteria ethmoidalis p.
arteria meningea p.
arteria nasalis posterior septi
arteria pancreaticoduodenalis superior p.
arteria parietalis p.
arteria temporalis p.
arteria tibialis p.
arteria tympanica p.
artery of posterior segment of kidney
ascending posterior branch
p. aspect
p. aspect of pharyngeal wall
p. atlantodental interval
auricular branch of posterior auricular artery
p. auricular flap
p. auricular groove
auricularis posterior muscle
p. auricular muscle
p. auricular nerve
p. auricular vein
p. axillary fold
p. axillary line
p. baffle
p. bite wing
p. border
p. border of eyelid
p. border of fibula
p. border of heart
p. branch
p. branch of great auricular nerve
p. branch of medial cutaneous nerve of forearm
p. branch of obturator artery
p. branch of obturator nerve
p. branch of recurrent ulnar artery
p. branch of renal artery
p. branch of spinal nerve
calcaneonavicular ligament-tibialis posterior tendon advancement
p. capsular cataract
p. capsular opacification
p. capsular polishing
p. capsule
p. capsule opacification
p. central curve
central posterior curve
p. cerebral artery
p. cervical
p. cervical nodes
p. chamber
p. chamber of eye
p. chamber intraocular lens
p. chamber lens implant
p. chest tube
p. circulation
p. circulation infarct
p. circulation syndrome
p. circumflex artery
p. collagenous layer
p. colporrhaphy
p. colpotomy

p. column
p. commissure
p. communicating aneurysm
p. communicating artery
p. communicating artery aneurysm
p. compartment
p. compartment of arm
p. compartment of forearm
p. compartment of leg
p. compartment of thigh
concave posterior surface
p. corneal deposit
p. coronary plexus
p. cortex
p. cranial fossa
p. cricoarytenoid
p. cruciate ligament
p. cruciate ligament of knee
p. cruciate ligament tear
p. cruciate sprain
p. crus
p. crus of stapes
p. cul-de-sac of vagina
p. curvature
p. cutaneous nerve of arm
p. cutaneous nerve of forearm
p. cutaneous nerve of thigh
p. decompression
deep posterior tibiotalar
p. descending artery
p. descending branch
p. descending coronary artery
p. disc margin
p. dislocation
p. dislocation injury
p. displacement
p. division
p. drainage
p. drawer test
p. endplate
p. ethmoid
exertional deep posterior compartment syndrome
p. facet dislocation
p. facet displacement
p. flap
flexion injury posterior atlantoaxial arthrodesis
p. fontanelle
p. fornix
p. fossa
p. fossa approach
p. fossa extra-axial arachnoid cyst
p. fossa tumor
p. fourchette
p. fracture
frontodextra posterior position
p. gastroenterostomy
p. glide
p. glottic stenosis
p. gutter
p. horn
p. horn of medial meniscus
p. hyaloid membrane
p. hypothalamic area
p. hypothalamus
p. iliac crest
p. impaction
p. incision
p. inferior cerebellar artery
p. inferior communicating artery
p. inferior iliac spine
p. intercostal vein
p. intermediate curve
intermediate posterior curve
p. interosseous artery
p. interosseous nerve
p. interosseous nerve of forearm
p. interosseous vein
p. intervertebral ganglion of head
p. ischemic optic neuropathy
p. labial hernia
lateral posterior choroidal
p. latissimus dorsi muscle
p. leaflet
p. leaflet motion
p. leaf mitral valve
p. leafspring orthosis
left atrial posterior wall
left occiput posterior fetal position
left posterior descending artery
left posterior fascicular block
left posterior hemiblock
left posterior inferior hemiblock
left posterior internal carotid artery
left posterior measurement
left posterior oblique
left posterior occipital
p. left ventricular
left ventricular posterior wall
left ventricular posterior wall thickness
left posterior ventricular preexcitation
p. lie
p. ligament of knee
p. limb of the internal capsule
p. lip of acetabulum
p. lip nerve
p. lipping
long, closed, posterior cervix
p. longitudinal ligament
long leg posterior molded splint
long posterior ciliary artery
long posterior ciliary axis
lower cervical spine posterior stabilization
p. lumbar interbody fusion
p. mandibular depth
mastoid branch of posterior auricular artery
mastoid branch of posterior tympanic artery
medial branch of posterior branch of spinal nerve
medial branch of posterior rami of spinal nerve
medial cutaneous branch of dorsal branch of posterior intercostal artery
medial malleolar branch of posterior tibial artery
membrana atlantooccipitalis p.
membrana capsularis lentis p.
mentum posterior fetal position
microvascular free posterior interosseous flap
p. mitral
p. mitral valve leaflet
most posterior point on posterior contour of sella turcica
multifocal posterior pigment epitheliopathy
musculus auricularis p.
p. myocardial infarction
p. nares
p. nasal spine
p. nasal spine to soft palate
p. nasopharynx
p. necrotic zone
p. nephrectomy
nervus auricularis p.
nervus ethmoidalis p.
nodus lymphoideus tibialis p.
nucleus cochlearis p.
nucleus lateralis p.
nucleus of posterior commissure
p. oblique ligament
p. occipitoatlantal hypermobility
occiput p.
occiput right p.
open posterior fontanelle
p. optical zone
p. oropharynx
ossification of posterior longitudinal ligament
p. papillary

posterior *(continued)*
p. papillary muscle
parietooccipital branch of posterior cerebellar artery
parietooccipital branch of posterior cerebral artery
p. pelvic tilt
perineal branch of posterior cutaneous nerve of thigh
perineal branch of posterior femoral cutaneous nerve
p. peripheral curve
persistent occiput posterior position
persistent occiput posterior presentation
p. pharynx not injected
p. pituitary
p. pituitary hormone
p. pole
p. pole of eye
p. pole of lens
p. pole and periphery
p. polymorphic dystrophy of cornea
p. polymorphous corneal dystrophy
polymorphous posterior corneal dystrophy
previous posterior myocardial infarction
pterygoid branch of posterior deep temporal artery
p. reduction device
reversible posterior leukoencephalopathy
reversible posterior leukoencephalopathy syndrome
right posterior oblique radiologic view
right posterior internal carotid artery
right posterior ventricular preexcitation
p. root
p. root entry zone
p. sacroiliac spine
sacrum p.
p. sagittal diameter
p. sagittal index
scalene muscle, anterior, posterior, middle
selective posterior rhizotomy
p. semicircular canal
p. spinal fusion
p. subcapsular cataract
p. subcapsular cataractous plaque
p. subcapsular precipitates
p. superior iliac spine
superior labrum anterior and p.
p. superior pancreaticoduodenal vein
p. surface
p. synechiae
p. synechiotomy
p. talofibular
p. talofibular ligament
p. terminal vein
p. tibial
p. tibial artery
p. tibial muscle
p. tibial nerve
p. tibial pulse
p. tibial tendinitis
p. tibial tendon
p. tibial tendon dysfunction
p. tibial transfer
p. tibial vein
p. trabecular meshwork
transsclerally sutured posterior chamber lens
p. tricuspid valve leaflet
unilateral posterior lumbar interbody fusion
p. urethra
p. urethral injury
p. urethral valve type I–IV
p. vaginal hernia
p. vaginal wall
ventralis oralis p.
ventral posterior inferior
p. view
p. vitreal detachment
p. vitreous
p. vitreous detachment
p. wall
p. wall excursion
p. wall of heart
p. wall infarct
p. wall of left ventricle
p. wall myocardial infarction
p. wall thickness
p. wall thickness at end-diastole
p. wall velocity
YAG posterior capsulotomy

posterioris

posteriorly
opened p.

posteroanterior
p. film
p. and lateral
p. position
p. study
p. view

posteroinferior
p. aspect
p. cerebellar artery
p. external
p. internal

posterolateral
p. approach
p. aspect
p. branch
p. coronary artery
p. drainage
p. fissure
p. fontanelle
p. groove
p. infarction
p. interbody fusion
left p.
p. spinal artery
ventral posterolateral nucleus

posteromedial
p. aspect
p. central artery
p. hypothalamus
radical posteromedial and plantar release
p. release

posteromedialis
ventralis p.

posteroseptal wall

posterotemporal region

posteroventral pallidotomy

postexercise
p. hypotension
immediate p.
p. index

postexertional dyspnea

postexposure
rabies postexposure prophylaxis
p. treatment

postextrasystolic potentiation

postgamma proteinuria

postganglionic
autonomic postganglionic nerve terminal
p. vagal stimulation

postgonococcal urethritis

post-head injury syndrome

posthemorrhagic
p. hydrocephalus
p. ventricular dilatation
p. ventricular dilation
p. ventriculomegaly

postheparin
p. esterase

p. lipolytic activity
p. plasma

postherpetic
p. neuralgia
p. neuropathy
p. pain

posthospital care

posthypnotic suggestion

posthypoxic intention myoclonus

postictal
p. activity
p. cognitive dysfunction
p. confusion
p. depression
epileptic postictal sleep
p. immobility
p. lethargy
prolonged postictal encephalopathy
p. psychosis
p. slowing
p. state
p. stupor

posticus

postimperative negative variation

postinfarction
p. angina
p. pericarditis

postinfarct patient

postinfection
p. encephalitis
p. encephalomyelopathy

postinfectious
acute postinfectious glomerulonephritis
p. arthritis
p. bradycardia
p. encephalitis
p. encephalomyelitis
p. glomerulonephritis
p. hydrocephalus

postinflammatory
p. adenopathy
p. corticoid
oral postinflammatory hyperpigmentation
p. polyposis

postinfluenzal encephalitis

postinfluenza-like hyposmia and hypogeusia

postinfusion phlebitis

postinhibition rebound

postinoculation
days p.

postinspiratory pressure

postirradiation fracture

postischemic
p. acute renal failure
p. acute tubular necrosis
p. atrophy
p. changes
p. myocardium
p. reperfusion injury
p. revascularization

postlaminectomy pain

postlaser day

postlumbar puncture headache

postmalarial neurological syndrome

postmarketing surveillance

postmastectomy pain syndrome

postmature
p. fetus
p. infant

postmaturity syndrome

postmenopausal
p. amenorrhea
p. bleeding
p. body mass
p. bone loss
p. breast cancer
p. estrogen
p. estrogen/progestin intervention
p. estrogen replacement
p. estrogen therapy
p. hirsutism
p. hormonal status
p. hormonal therapy
p. hormone therapy
p. hyperplasia
p. osteoporosis
p. palpable ovary
patient is p.
p. syndrome
p. weight gain

postmenstrual
p. stress
p. tension

postmicturition dribble

postmitochondrial supernatant

postmortem
p. cesarean delivery
p. diagnosis
p. examination
p. findings
p. human kidney
p. human kidney cell
p. intussusception
p. lividity
p. rigidity

postmyelitis
progressive postmyelitis muscular atrophy

postmyocardial
p. infarction
p. infarction syndrome

postnasal
p. bleeding
chronic postnasal drip
p. discharge
p. drainage
p. drainage syndrome
p. dressing
p. drip
p. drip due to rhinitis
p. drip due to sinusitis
p. drip syndrome

postnatal
p. care
p. course
p. depression
Edinburgh P. Depression Scale
p. followup
p. growth deficiency
p. infection
intensive postnatal intervention
mental retardation, pre-and postnatal overgrowth, remarkable face, acanthosis nigricans syndrome
p. penicillin prophylaxis

postnecrotic cirrhosis

postneonatal
p. death
p. mortality syndrome

postocclusive
p. oscillatory response
p. reactive hyperemia

postoncolytic immunity

postoperative
p. abdominal distention
acute postoperative renal failure
p. adhesion
adjustable postoperative protective prosthetic socket
p. analgesia
p. antibiotic
p. arrhythmia
p. atelectasis
p. atrial fibrillation
p. bladder dysfunction

postoperative *(continued)*
p. bleeding
p. care
p. casting
p. chronologic year
complicated postoperative course
p. complication
p. constrictive pericarditis
continuous postoperative closed lavage
p. course
p. course complicated
p. course normal
p. course uncomplicated
p. course uneventful
p. day
p. day one
p. death
p. deep venous thrombosis
p. diagnosis
p. dialysis
p. discomfort
early postoperative period
early postoperative suture adjustment
p. endophthalmitis
p. ERCP
p. exercise
p. extubation
p. fever
p. flexor tendon
p. followup
p. gastrointestinal motility
p. heart failure
p. hemorrhage
p. hepatic failure
p. holding area
p. ileus
immediate postoperative prosthesis
immediate postoperative prosthetic fitting
immediate postoperative stability
p. infection
p. inflammation
p. instruction
p. irradiation
p. irrigation
late postoperative suture adjustment
p. low cardiac output
p. morbidity
p. narcotic infusion
p. nausea
p. nausea and vomiting
p. note
p. office visit
p. open heart surgery
p. orders
p. pain
p. pain management
P. Pain Questionnaire
Parents' P. Pain Measure
p. period guarded
p. progress
p. pulmonary function
p. pulmonary problem
p. radiation
p. radiation therapy
p. radiotherapy
p. reaction
p. reactive hyperemia
p. recovery
p. regimen for oral early feeding
p. respiratory therapy
p. respiratory treatment
p. shock
status p.
Toddler-Preschooler P. Pain Scale
uncomplicated postoperative course
uneventful postoperative course
p. vomiting
p. wound infection

postoperatively stormy course

postorbital pain

postovulatory day

postparacentesis circulatory dysfunction

postpartum
p. alopecia
p. amenorrhea
p. atony
p. bleeding
p. breast engorgement
p. cardiomyopathy
p. care
p. day
p. depression
p. endometritis
p. examination
p. followup
p. hemorrhage
p. hypertension
p. incontinence
p. infection
intractable postpartum hemorrhage
late postpartum hemorrhage
p. low back pain
maternal postpartum thyroid dysfunction
mood disorder with postpartum onset
normal p.
nosocomial postpartum endometritis
p. obstetrics
painless postpartum thyroiditis
p. painless thyroiditis with transient thyrotoxicosis
primary postpartum hemorrhage
p. psychosis
p. reaction
p. renal failure
P. Self-Evaluation Questionnaire
p. sterilization
p. thyroid disease
p. thyroid dysfunction
p. thyroiditis
p. tubal ligation

postpeel
prolonged postpeel erythema

postperfusion
p. low flow
p. syndrome

postpericardiotomy syndrome

postperinatal infant mortality

postphlebitic syndrome

postpill amenorrhea

postpolio
p. atrophy syndrome
progressive postpolio muscle atrophy

postpoliomyelitis
p. muscular atrophy
p. syndrome

postpolycythemia myeloid metaplasia

postponing sexual involvement

postprandial
p. blood sugar
p. distention
p. fullness
glucose, p.
2-hour postprandial blood sugar
p. hypotension
idiopathic postprandial syndrome
p. lipemia
p. plasma glucose
p. state
p. syndrome

postprostatectomy incontinence

postpump syndrome

postradiation
p. cystitis
p. dysplasia
p. fistula

postreduction film

postrema
area p.

postremission
sequential postremission chemotherapy

postrenal
p. albuminuria
p. anuria
p. azotemia
p. proteinuria

postreplication repair

postrotary
Southern California P. Nystagmus Test

postseizure stupor

postshingles pain

postshunt encephalopathy

postspinal anesthetic headache

poststatic dyskinesia

poststenotic
p. dilatation
p. dilation

poststimulus
p. time
p. time histogram
p. time histograph

poststreptococcal
p. acute glomerulonephritis
acute poststreptococcal glomerulonephritis
p. glomerulonephritis
p. reactive arthritis

poststress ethanol consumption

poststroke
central poststroke pain
p. depression

postsurgical
p. abdomen
p. change
p. gastroparesis syndrome
p. healing
immediate postsurgical fitting of prosthesis
p. incontinence
p. infection
p. unit

postsynaptic
p. density
inhibitory postsynaptic current
inhibitory postsynaptic potential
p. membrane
p. potential
p. terminal

postterm infant

posttetanic
p. count
p. facilitation
p. potentiation

postthrombophlebitis syndrome

postthrombotic syndrome

postthymic T-cell lymphoma

posttonsillectomy hemorrhage

posttransfusion
p. hepatitis
p. mononucleosis
p. non-A, non-B hepatitis
platelet count p.
p. purpura
p. reaction
p. rejection
p. syndrome

posttransplant
p. acute renal failure
p. diabetes mellitus
p. lymphoproliferative disease
p. lymphoproliferative disorder

posttransplantation
p. lymphoproliferative disease

posttransplant isolation

posttraumatic
acute posttraumatic stress syndrome
p. acute renal failure
p. amnesia
angiolipoma, posttraumatic neuroma, glomus tumor, eccrine spiradenoma, and leiomyoma cutis
p. arthritis
p. brain syndrome
p. chronic osteomyelitis
chronic posttraumatic headache
chronic posttraumatic vertigo
early posttraumatic epilepsy
p. endophthalmitis
p. epilepsy
p. fibromyalgia syndrome
p. headache
p. hemorrhage
p. hyperirritability syndrome
p. meningitis
p. persistent pneumothorax
p. progressive myelopathy
p. pulmonary insufficiency
p. seizure
p. signs or symptoms
p. stress disorder
subjective posttraumatic syndrome

posttussive suction

postural
p. abnormality
anticonvulsant medication-induced postural tremor
P. Assessment Scale for Stroke Patients
p. back problem
p. balance
p. blood pressure
chest percussion and postural drainage
p. collapse
p. component
p. drainage
p. drainage and clapping
p. drainage and percussion
p. drainage, percussion and vibration
fine postural tremor
p. hypertension
p. hypotension
p. instability
p. insufficiency
p. orthostatic tachycardia syndrome
percussion and postural drainage
reactive extensor postural synergy
p. reflex
p. rest position
p. stimulation test
p. stress test
tonic postural epilepsy
p. vertical dimension
p. vertigo

posture
abnormal spinal p.
change in gait and p.
coordination and p.
p.'s of daily living
developmental sequence p.
forward flexion p.
forward head p.
heat escape lessening p.
hyperextension p.'s and maneuvers
squarely face person, open posture, lean toward person, eye contact, relaxed
upright p.

posturing
anterior mandibular p.
athetotic p.
axial p.
decerebrate p.
decorticate p.

posturing *(continued)*
equinovarus p.
opisthotonic p.

postvaccination encephalitis

postvagotomy diarrhea

postventricular
p. atrial blanking
p. atrial refractory period

postvesiculares
nodi lymphatici p.

post-Vietnam psychiatric syndrome

postviral
p. encephalitis
p. fatigue syndrome

postvoid
p. dribble
p. dribbling of urine
p. residual volume

postvoiding
p. cystogram
p. film
p. residual volume

potassium
p. bromide
p. cardioplegia
p. channel-interacting protein
p. chloride
cold potassium cardioplegia
crystalloid potassium cardioplegia
p. deficiency
p. deficit
p. depletion
p. diet
distal effective potassium secretion
exchangeable body p.
fractional excretion of p.
p., glucose, and insulin
glucose, insulin, and p.
glucose potassium insulin
p. hemoglobinate
p. in 24-hour urine
p. hydroxide stain
p. intake
p. iodide, saturated solution
iodine potassium iodide
kalium potassium phosphate buffer
p. leg cramps
p. level
p. loss
low potassium dextran
low potassium ion
p. and magnesium
nonrenal potassium loss
penicillin V p.
p. permanganate
plasma p.
p. chloride sustained release tablet
p. penicillin G
p. restriction
saturated potassium iodide solution
saturated solution of potassium iodide
p., sodium chloride, and sodium lactate solution
sodium and potassium spot urine test
p. solubility product
supersaturated potassium iodide
p. supplement
p. titanyl phosphate laser
total body potassium
total exchangeable p.
transtubular potassium concentration gradient
urinary potassium volume excretion rate
urine p.

potassium-39, -40, -42, -43

potassium-containing minimal capacitation medium

potato
p. kallikrein inhibitor
p. spindle tuber viroid

potency
cumulative potency rate
decimal scale of potency or dilution
extra high p.
high p.
homeopathic symbol for decimal scale of p.'s
low p.
p. ratio
relative p.
uterine-stimulating p.

potent hormone angiotensin II

potential
p. abnormality of glucose tolerance
action p.
action potential duration
p. acuity meter
antidromic p.
atypical polypoid adenomyofibroma of low malignant p.
auditory brainstem-evoked p.
auditory evoked p.
average evoked p.
biotic p.
body surface potential mapping
brain evoked p.
brainstem auditory evoked p.
p. for breakdown
brief, small, abundant motor-unit action p.
brief, small, abundant, polyphasic p.
Cancer P. Index
cell replication p.
cervical somatosensory evoked p.
chemical p.
cochlear p.
compound motor action p.
compound muscle action p.
compound muscle-motor action p.
compound nerve action p.
contact potential difference
corneal-retinal p.
cortical auditory evoked p.
cortical somatosensory evoked p.
dermatomal somatosensory-evoked p.
p. difference in volts
dorsal root p.
early receptor p.
early receptor potential mottling
eighth nerve action p.
elbow sensory p.
electrical evoked p.
electrical potential in volts
electrochemical potential gradient
electrode p.
electrodispersive skin p.
endocardial p.
endogenous limbic p.
endplate p.
p. energy
p. erythropoietin-responsive cell
Estimated Learning P.
event-related brain p.
event-related slow-brain p.
evoked muscle action p.
evoked potential response
evoked potential signal averaging
evoked potential study
evoked sensory nerve action p.
evoked synaptic p.
evoked visual p.
excitatory junction p.
excitatory postsynaptic p.
extreme somatosensory evoked p.
p. fetal hypertensive crisis

fibrillating action p.
fibrinolytic p.
galvanic skin p.
giant cell tumor of low malignant p.
giant miniature endplate p.
p. gradient
p. of hallucinogen abuse
high-risk potential victims
p. for human betterment
p. hypertensive crisis
individual motor unit action p.
induced p.
p. for infection
inhibitory junction p.
inhibitory postsynaptic p.
p. injury
p. inpatient admission
ionization p.
p. isolation
kilovoltage p.
kilovolt constant p.
late diastolic p.
left somatosensory evoked p.
localized evoked p.
lower extremity somatosensory evoked p.
low malignant potential epithelial ovarian tumor
mean resting p.
median nerve somatosensory evoked p.
membrane potential difference
migrating action potential complex
miniature endplate p.
mitochondrial membrane p.
mixed nerve action p.
monophasic action p.
monophasic action potential duration
motor evoked p.
motor unit action p.
movement-related cortical p.
multimodality evoked p.
muscle fiber action p.
nerve fiber action p.
net electrochemical potential gradient
neurogenic motor evoked p.
odor event-related p.
oscillatory p.
oxidation-reduction p.
pacesetter p.
passive hyperpolarizing p.
pattern reversal visual evoked p.
postsynaptic p.
prostatic stromal proliferation of uncertain malignant p.
readiness p.
redox p.
p. relation
p. renal solute load
repetitive bursts of action p.
repetitive fibrillation p.
reproductive p.
resting membrane p.
right somatosensory evoked p.
right ventricular endocardial p.
p. for self-harm
sensory evoked p.
sensory nerve action p.
short-latency somatosensory-evoked p.
short latent-evoked p.
single potential analysis cavernous electrical activity
sinus node p.
skin potential level
skin potential reflex
slow inhibitory p.
somatosensory brainstem evoked p.
somatosensory cortical evoked p.
p. source of infection
spike p.
spinal evoked p.
standard electrode p.
stress-generated p.
stromal tumor of unknown malignant p.
subminiature end-plate p.
summating p.
summation p.
threshold p.
p. tolerance to hallucinogen
total peroxyl radical-trapping antioxidant p.
transmembrane p.
transmembrane potential gradient
transmucosal potential difference
trigeminal evoked p.
triphasic action p.
undetermined malignant p.
upper extremity somatosensory evoked p.
ventricular late p.
vertex p.
p. visual acuity meter
visual-evoked cortical p.
visually evoked cortical p.
p. years of life lost
years of potential life lost before age 65

potentially
p. compensable event
p. fatal disease
p. harmful drug
p. infectious
p. infectious blood specimen
ingestion of potentially poisonous substance
p. lethal arrhythmia
p. lethal damage
p. life-threatening illness
malignant potentially fatal asthma
other potentially infectious material
p. pathogenic environmental mycobacterial
repair of potentially lethal damage

potentiated
enzyme potentiated desensitization

potentiating
bradykinin potentiating factor
bradykinin potentiating peptide

potentiation
alcohol p.
long-lasting p.
long-term p.
postextrasystolic p.
posttetanic p.

potentiator
macrophage infectivity p.
macrophage infectivity potentiator protein

potentiometer
angle position p.

potentiometric ionophore mediated immunoassay

Pott
P. abscess
P. aneurysm
P. ankle fracture
P. curvature
P. disease
P. gangrene
P. paralysis
P. puffy tumor
P. syndrome

Potter
P. disease
P. facies
P. syndrome

Potts
P. anastomosis
P. eversion osteotomy

Potts *(continued)*
P. splint
P. tibial osteotomy
pouch
antibiotic bead p.
arachnoid retrocerebellar p.
Assura closed mini p.
Assura convex drainable p.
Assura convex urostomy p.
Assura pediatric p.
banded gastroplasty with a divided p.
p. biopsy
closed-end ostomy p.
p. configuration
p. development
p. of Douglas
endorectal ileal p.
p. excision
p. of Hartmann
ileal pouch anal anastomosis
inlet p.
innervated antral p.
modified innervated antral p.
Rathke pouch homeobox transcription factor
suprapatellar p.
poultice
hot moist p.
pound
Bloembergen, Purcell, and P. theory
p. per cubic foot
poundal
foot p.
pound-force
foot p.-f.
p.-f. foot
pounding
p. heart
p. of heart
Poupart ligament
poverty
p. of content
p. of content of speech
p. of content of thought
p. of ideas
income poverty guideline
National Center on P. Law, Inc.
Powassan
P. encephalitis
P. virus
powder
acetone powder extract
p. bed
p. board
p. burn
demineralized bone p.
dry powder inhaler
liquified powder cocaine
Ophthalmic Moldite P.
Pacific Coast demineralized cortical bone p.
wettable p.
powdered extract
Powell
modified Powell method
power
apparent p.
p. of attorney
back vertex p.
battery-charging power supply
p. building
p. building exercise
p. bur
candle p.
carbon dioxide combing p.
combining p.
combining power test
delusion of p.
discriminating p.
p. Doppler imaging
durable power of attorney for health care
effective isotropic radiated p.
p. factor
feeling of intellectual and physical p.
healing power of warm baths
heart rate power spectral analysis
high definition p.
impairment of power of voluntary movement
intellectual power factor
intraocular lens p.
keratometric p.
low power microscopy
manipulates to gain p.
mass collision stopping p.
mass radiative stopping p.
maximal aerobic p.
maximum power output
mean corneal p.
mean horizontal candle p.
mean power frequency
mean spherical candle p.
noise equivalent p.
on-eye predicted p.
organisms per high power field
passage, power, and passenger
radiant p.
reactive p.
sound p.
p. spectral analysis
p. spectral density
spectral power distribution
spherical candle p.
topographic simulated keratometric p.
uninterruptible power supply
powered
p. air loss
p. endoscopic sinus surgery
power-oriented depth controlled osteotomy cutter
pox
African swine p.
poxvirus
attenuated poxvirus vector
mule deer p.
1p–22p
partial monosomy 1p–22p
pp′-dichlorodiphenyldichloroetene
p-p factor
P-R
P.-R. interval
P.-R. segment
practicable
as low as readily p.
practical
p. approach design
p. counseling
licensed practical nurse
p. nurse
systematic, complete, objective, practical, empirical
practice
Clinical P. Model
clinical practice guidelines
clinical practice issue
Code of P.
complementary medical p.
cultural belief and p.
current p.
family p.
family practice center
general p.
good laboratory p.
independent practice association
independent practice plan
knowledge, aptitudes, and p.'s
licensed to p.
medical group p.
nursing p.
parental feeding p.
physician practice management

preferred practice patterns
primary private practice insurance
private p.
standard p.
Supervisory P.'s Test

practitioner
family p.
general p.
mental health p.
National Association of Pediatric Nurse Associates and P.'s
rural general p.

Practitioners'
Dental Practitioners' Formulary

Prader-Willi syndrome

praecox
icterus p.

praeputialis
herpes p.

praetibiale
exophthalmos, myxedema circumscriptum praetibiale, and osteoarthropathia hypertrophicans syndrome

Pragmatic
Test of Pragmatic Language

Prague
P. strain Rous sarcoma virus

praise
parental habits of p.

Prausnitz-Küstner
P.-K. sclerosis
P.-K. test

Praxis
Sensory Integration and Praxis Tests

pre
p. contractile heart

preacher's hand

pre-Achilles fat pad

pre-acquired immune deficiency syndrome

preadipocyte factor-1

preadmission
p. certification
p. information
p. information
p. screening
p. screening and assessment team
p. screening summary
p. testing
p. testing program

pre-aid to the disabled

prealbumin
human serum p.
thyroid-binding p.
thyronine-binding p.
thyroxine-binding p.
tryptophan-rich p.

prealbumin-associated hyperthyroxinemia

preanesthetic medication

preauricular
hemihypertrophy, intestinal web, preauricular skin tag, and congenital corneal opacity syndrome

preauriculares
nodi lymphoidei parotidei profundi p.

prebed care

precaecales
nodi lymphoidei p.

precancerosa
melanosis circumscripta p.

precancerous
p. abnormality
p. actinic keratosis
p. cell
p. cervical growth
p. change
p. condition
p. dermatosis
p. disease
p. dysplasia
p. growth
p. keratosis
p. lesion
p. overgrowth of uterine lining
p. polyp
p. skin spot
p. spot

Precarious Point virus

precaution
blood and body fluid p.
cardiac p.'s
elopement p.
fall p.'s
isolation p.'s
neutrogenic p.'s
specific isolation p.'s
suicide precautions number 1, 2
universal p.'s

preceded
classic headache preceded by aura
headache preceded by classic aura

preceding
p. foreperiod
p. preparatory interval

precentral
p. area
p. artery
artery of precentral sulcus
p. cerebellar vein
p. fissure
p. gyrus

precession
fast imaging steady precession sequence three-dimensional magnetic resonance imaging
fast imaging with steady p.
fast imaging with steady-state free p.
reverse fast imaging with steady-state free p.
steady-state free p.

precipitable
p. fraction heparin
serum precipitable iodine

precipitate
immune p.
p. labor
mutton-fat keratic p.
posterior subcapsular p.'s
tuberculin p.

precipitated
p. calcium carbonate
purified diphtheria toxoid precipitated by aluminum phosphate
synthetic medium old tuberculin trichloroacetic acid precipitated
p. withdrawal diarrhea

precipitating
p. cause
emotional stress precipitating tremor
p. event
p. factor
plasma protamine p.

precipitation
agar gel precipitation test
diffuse p.
heparin-induced extracorporeal low-density lipoprotein p.
immune complex p.
Price precipitation reaction
p. thin-layer chromatography
tuberculin p.

precipitin
circumoval p.

precipitin *(continued)*
gel diffusion p.
immunodiffusion tube p.
milk precipitin disease
p. reaction
rheumatoid arthritis p.
p. test
tube p.

precise lesion measuring

precision
p. encoder and pattern recognizer
p. high dose
MediSense Precision meter

preclinical heart muscle disease

preclotted graft

precocious
central precocious puberty
male-limited familial precocious puberty
male precocious puberty
neurogenic precocious puberty
p. pubarche
p. puberty

preconditioning
ischemic p.

precordial
p. acceleration tracing
p. A wave
p. bulge
p. chest leads
p. chest pain
p. electrocardiographic mapping
p. heart rate
p. heave
p. honk
p. lead
p. pain
poor precordial R-wave progression
poor progression of R wave in precordial leads
p. pulse
p. stethoscope
p. thrill
unipolar precordial lead

precordium
anterior p.

precoronary
p. care
p. care area

precunealis
arteria p.

precursor
abnormal location of immature myeloid p.
adrenal steroid p.
Alzheimer precursor protein
amine precursor uptake and decarboxylation cell
amyloid precursor protein
arginine vasopressor p.
B-cell precursor lymphoblastic leukemia
bone marrow myeloid p.
cleaved polyprotein precursor molecule
cleaved polyprotein precursor molecule product
cytotoxic T lymphocyte p.
determined osteogenic precursor cell
effector cell p.
erythroid committed p.
p. fluid
lymphoid precursor B-cell
lymphoid precursor T-cell
myeloid precursor cell
neural crest p.
red blood cell precursor production rate
target-attaching globulin p.
thrombus precursor protein
p. uptake

precut
needle-knife precut papillotomy

PRED
ara-C + DNR + PRED + MP

predatory
aggressive predatory type

predentin matrix

predeposit
autologous predeposit donation

predetermined interval of time

prediabetes
genetic p.
obstetric p.

predialyzed
p. human albumin
p. human serum

predicted
p. adult height
p. blood volume
p. cardiac output
p. functional residual capacity
p. maximal heart rate
maximal predicted heart rate
maximal predicted phonation time
maximum predicted heart rate
p. normal
on-eye predicted power
percent predicted peak expiratory flow
total blood volume predicted from body surface
p. vital capacity

predicting
indices predicting response

prediction
Dropout P. and Prevention
evaluation, prediction, intervention, and control
mean prediction error
perinatal distress p.
sensitivity prediction by acoustic reflex

predictive
P. Ability Test
p. accuracy
positive predictive value
P. Salvage Index
p. value of a negative test
p. value of a positive test

predictor
independent p.
morbidity p.
mortality p.

predigested liquid protein

predischarge graded exercise test

predisposing
no predisposing factor

predisposition
fundamental p.
genetic p.
genetic predisposition to psychiatric illness
hereditary p.
p. towards illness

prednisolone
ara-C, daunorubicin, prednisolone, mercaptopurine
p. glucose tolerance test

prednisone/Adriamycin

predominance
anterior p.
lymphocyte predominance Hodgkin disease
lymphoid p.
monoblast p.

predominant
p. affect
p. feature

p. hyperparathyroid bone disease
lymphocyte p.

predominantly
attention deficit hyperactivity disorder, predominantly hyperactive-impulsive type
p. epithelial thymoma

predominating
mixed astigmatism with myopia p.
p. organism

preeclampsia of pregnancy

preeclamptic toxemia

preejection
corrected preejection period
left ventricular preejection period
p. period
p. period index
p. period/left ventricular ejection time
right preejection period

preemptive
p. analgesia
p. immunity

preepiglottic space

preexcitation
left lateral ventricular p.
left posterior ventricular p.
right posterior ventricular p.
p. syndrome
ventricular p.

preexisting
p. cognitive impairment
p. condition
p. coronary disease
p. dementia
p. discomfort
p. emotional problem
exacerbation of preexisting psychiatric illness
p. hepatic disease
p. illness

prefabricated
allogenically vascularized prefabricated flap

preference
Autonomy P. Index
California Occupational P. Inventory
California Occupational P. Survey
conditioned place p.
Coping Operations P. Enquiry
Edwards Personal P. Schedule
idiosyncratic food p.
Kuder Preference Record—Vocational
Personal P. Scale
p. record
Sexuality P. Profile
standard fixation preference test
Vocational P. Inventory

preferential looking

preferred
p. frequency speech interference level
p. practice patterns
p. provider
p. provider organization
p. retinal locus
p. treatment in cancer

prefrontal
anterior cingulate prefrontal syndrome
p. area
p. cortex
dorsolateral prefrontal cortex
p. lobotomy
p. region
p. sonic treatment

preganglionic
p. cell
sympathetic preganglionic neuron

pregnancy
acute fatty liver of p.
p. advisory service
p. alpha-2 glycoprotein
antiretroviral pregnancy registry
anxiety during p.
arrhythmia in p.
asthma and p.
p. at term
p. and birth complication
care and treatment during p.
cervical ectopic p.
cholestatic hepatosis of p.
p. complication
corpus luteum of p.
diabetes mellitus, pregnancy classification, class A–F
diabetes of p.
direct latex agglutination pregnancy test
early pregnancy factor
early pregnancy loss
early pregnancy test
early pregnancy wastage
ectopic p.
ectopic pregnancy and abortion
elective interruption of p.
elective termination of p.
extrauterine p.
fimbrial ectopic p.
first full-term p.
Friedman test for p.
full-term intrauterine p.
full-term uncomplicated pregnancy, labor, and delivery
heartburn of p.
high-risk p.
home pregnancy test
2-hour pregnancy test
hypertension in p.
hyperthyroidism in p.
iatrogenic multiple p.
improved pregnancy outcome
intentional termination of p.
interruption of pregnancy for psychiatric indication
p. interruption service
intrahepatic cholestasis of p.
intrauterine pregnancy at term
intrauterine pregnancy, delivered
intrauterine pregnancy, term birth, cesarean section
intrauterine pregnancy, term birth, living infant
ligamentous ectopic p.
linear IgM disease of p.
macrocytic anemia of p.
mask of p.
medical termination of p.
megaloblastic anemia of p.
metabolic toxemia of late p.
mitral stenosis in p.
monochorionic diamniotic twin p.
nausea and vomiting of p.
normally progressing p.
normal pregnancy and delivery
number of p.'s producing viable offspring
papular dermatitis of p.
parasitic ectopic p.
pelvic malignancy in p.
persistent ectopic p.
preeclampsia of p.
p., labor, and delivery
p., not delivered
p., term, complicated delivered, living female
p., term, complicated delivered, living male
p., term, uncomplicated
p., term, uncomplicated delivered, living female
p., term, uncomplicated delivered, living male

pregnancy *(continued)*
prognostically bad signs during p.
pruritic urticarial papules and plaques of p.
psychosis during p.
Quick Test psychology, pregnancy, prothrombin
radiation exposure in p.
radioreceptor assay pregnancy blood
p. rate
recurrent early pregnancy loss
P. Risk Monitoring System
ruptured ectopic p.
p. serum
surgical termination of p.
p. terminated
termination of p.
term intrauterine p.
p. test
third p.
time to p.
tubal ectopic p.
unruptured ectopic p.
p. urine hormone
urine pregnancy test
p. uterine, undelivered
vaginal interruption of pregnancy with dilatation and curettage
voluntary interruption of p.
voluntary termination of p.
willful exposure to unwanted p.
p. zone
p. zone protein

pregnancy-associated
p.-a. globulin
p.-a. plasma protein
p.-a. plasma protein A, C

pregnancy-induced
p.-i. glucose intolerance
p.-i. hypertension

pregnancy-related anemia

pregnanediol
p. glucuronide
sodium pregnanediol glucuronide

pregnant
p. abdomen
healthy pregnant women
p. mare serum
p. mare serum gonadotropin
not p.
p. uterus

pre-heart attack pain

prehension
Erhardt Developmental P. Assessment
passive prehension orthosis

prehospital index

preimplantation
p. embryo
p. genetic diagnosis

preinfarction angina

pre-intake interview

preinversion multiecho

prejudice
age p.

prekallikrein
p. activator
plasma p.

prelabor rupture of the membranes

prelaryngeales
nodi lymphoidei p.

preleukemia platelet

preleukemic
primary acquired preleukemic syndrome
p. syndrome

preliminary
p. anatomic diagnosis
p. diagnostic clinic
p. film of abdomen
p. findings
p. impression
p. studies

prelinguistic autism diagnostic observation

preload
LV p.
p. reduction

premalignant
p. condition
p. lesion
oral premalignant lesion

premamillary nucleus

Premarital Communication Inventory

premarket
p. approval application
p. notification

prematura

premature
p. accelerated lung maturation
p. aging
p. alopecia
p. appropriate for gestational age
p. atherosclerosis
p. atrial beat
p. atrial complex
p. atrial contraction
atrial premature beat
atrial premature complex
atrial premature contraction
atrial premature depolarization
p. atrial stimulus
p. atrioventricular junction complex
p. auricular beat
p. auricular contraction
auricular premature beat
p. auricular systole
p. birth
p. birth live infant
p. chromosome condensation
p. closure of valve
p. coronary disease
p. dead female child
p. dead male child
p. death
p. delivery
p. discharge
p. ductus arteriosus closure
p. ejaculation
p. eruption
p. excitation
extremely premature infant
full-term deliveries, premature deliveries, abortions, living children
p. gonadal failure
p. heart disease
p. infant
P. Infant Pain Profile
isolated premature beat
p. junctional beat
p. junctional complex
p. junctional contraction
junctional premature beat
junctional premature contraction
p. junctional systole
p. living female child
p. living male child
p. lung
membranes
p. menopause
p. mitral closure
multifocal premature ventricular contraction
p. newborn
p. nodal beat
p. nodal contraction
nodal premature contraction

nonconducted premature atrial contraction
p. nursery
p. onset of labor
p. ovarian failure
preterm premature rupture of membranes
prolonged premature rupture of membranes
pulmonary insufficiency of the p.
p. rupture of fetal membranes
p. separation of placenta
spontaneous premature rupture of membranes
p. spontaneous rupture of bag of waters
supraventricular premature beat
supraventricular premature contraction
p. systole
p. top codon
p. tricuspid closure
unifocal premature ventricular contractions
p. vascular disease
p. ventricular beat
p. ventricular complex
p. ventricular contraction
p. ventricular contraction with coupling
p. ventricular depolarization
p. ventricular extrasystole
ventricular premature activation
ventricular premature beat
ventricular premature complex
ventricular premature contraction
ventricular premature contraction threshold
ventricular premature depolarization
ventricular premature depolarization contraction
p. ventricular systole

prematurely ruptured membrane

prematurity
anemia of p.
anetoderma of p.
apnea of p.
chronic pulmonary insufficiency of p.
high oxygen percentage in retinopathy of p.
hypothyroxinemia of p.
p. index
pulmonary immaturity of p.
pulmonary insufficiency of p.
retinopathy of p.
P. Risk Evaluation Measure
threshold stage III of retinopathy of p.

premedication regimen

premenopausal
p. amenorrhea
p. hormone receptor positive

premenstrual
p. assessment form
p. asthma
P. Distress Questionnaire
p. dysphoric disorder
p. dysphoric syndrome
p. exacerbation of asthma
p. symptoms
p. tension
p. tension syndrome

premie nipple

premolar
p. band
p. crowding
incisors, canines, p.'s, and molars
p. teeth

premonitory
p. contraction
p. feeling
p. headache
p. pain
p. palpitation
p. symptom

premorbid
p. adjustment
p. dementia
p. functioning
p. inferiority feeling
schizophrenia with premorbid association

premotor cortex

prenatal
p. abuse of illicit drug
p. alcohol exposure
p. care
p. cocaine exposure
p. course
p. diagnosis
early prenatal karyotype
p. fluoride
good prenatal care
p. history
increased prenatal care
p. infection
p. injury
p. intensive care unit
intensive prenatal care
p. mortality
no prenatal care
normal prenatal care
p. screening test
p. testing
p. transplant
p. ultrasonography
p. vitamins

preoccupation with fantasies of grandeur

preocular tear film

preoperative
p. analgesia
p. anemia
p. anesthesia
p. angiogram
p. angiography
p. antibiotic
p. antimicrobial prophylaxis
p. assessment
p. autologous blood donation
p. autologous donation
p. biopsy
p. chemoradiotherapy
p. chemotherapy
p. contraindication to surgery
p. diagnosis
p. dose
p. enema
p. evaluation
p. examination
p. factor
p. fasting
p. gastric aspiration
p. holding area
p. irradiation
p. irrigation
p. laboratory workup
p. orders
p. radiation therapy
p. radiotherapy
p. screening
p. skin preparation
p. staging of cancer
p. ultrasound
p. visit

preoptic
anterior hypothalamic preoptic area
lateral preoptic area
medial preoptic area
p. anterior hypothalamic area

preoptica
area p.

preopticus
nucleus p.

preoral gut

prepaid health plan

prepancreatica
arteria p.

preparation
atypical antipsychotic p.
bowel p.
gentamicin, clindamycin, and polymyxin topical p.
inadequate bowel p.
International Reference P.
Lightspeed canal preparation technique
lupus erythematosus p.
no special preparation necessary for test
peripheral blood p.
peripheral blood preparation for microfilariae
post space p.
preoperative skin p.

preparative
low-intensity preparative regimen

preparatory
preceding preparatory interval
zone of preparatory calcification

prepared
p. childbirth
operative field prepared and draped

preparedness
anxiety p.

preparticipation sports examination

prepatellar
p. bursa
p. bursa inflammation
p. bursitis

prepatient periods to oocyst

prepericardiaci
nodi lymphoidei p.

preperitoneal
p. abscess
p. approach
p. distention balloon
p. space
transabdominal preperitoneal laparoscopic hernia repair

prephloric
erosive prephloric change

prepiriform cortex

preplaced suture

preponderance
directional p.

prepped
abdomen prepped and draped
abdomen scrubbed, prepped, and draped
operative field prepped and draped
patient is prepped and draped
patient is prepped and draped for surgery
patient is prepped and draped in usual sterile fashion
patient prepped and positioned
sterilely prepped and draped

preproliferative diabetic retinopathy

prepubertal
p. child
p. testicular tumor

prepubescent
p. female
p. male
p. schizophrenia

prepuce
p. of clitoris
megameatus-intact p.
p. of penis

prepulse inhibition

preputial
p. calculus
p. gland
vascularized double-sided preputial island flap and W flap glanuloplasty hypospadias repair

prepyloric
p. antrum
p. atresia
p. ulcer

Pre-Reading Expectancy Screening Scale

prereduced anaerobically sterilized medium

prerenal
p. acute renal failure
p. anuria
p. azotemia
p. uremia

prerequisite
Screening Test for Educational P. Skills

preretinal
p. hemorrhage
massive preretinal retraction

preschool
P. Behavior Questionnaire
California P. Social Competency Scale
P. Evaluation and Assessment for Children with Handicaps
Fluharty P. Speech and Language Screening Test
P. Language Assessment Instrument
P. Language Scale
p. Evaluation and Assessment for Children with Handicaps
Riley P. Developmental Screening Inventory
Wechsler P. and Primary Scale of Intelligence
Zimmerman P. Language Scale

preschool-age psychiatric assessment

preschooler
Miller Assessment for P.'s

prescreening
P. Development Questionnaire
Revised Denver P. Development Questionnaire

prescription
P. Analyses and Cost
p. bottle
p. drug
p. drug abuse
p. drug addiction
p. drug dependence
P. Drug User Fee Act
electronic p.
p. event monitoring
p. gum
has worn prescription glasses
improper use of p.
p. medication
p. narcotic
over-the-counter p.
signature prescription
treatment p.
trial prescription order

prescription-only medicine

Prescriptive Reading Inventory

presence
family member p.
p. of only one sex chromosome

presenile
Alzheimer presenile dementia
p. arteriosclerosis
p. cataract
p. dementia

presenilis

present
active and p.
p. and active reflexes
before p.
bilateral pedal pulses p.
bowel sounds present and active
chest tube present in abdomen
p. complaint
continue present management
p. distress
p. episode
p. examination
greatest single allergen p.
history of present complaint
history of present illness
p. medical illness
no infection p.
no inflammation p.
noncontributory to present illness
no present illness
not p.
not available at the present time
p. pain intensity
pedal pulse p.
p., active, equal
Schizophrenic Subscale of P. State Examination
P. State Examination

presentation
aleukemic p.
antigen p.
arm p.
atypical p.
cephalic p.
complete breech p.
euphoric p.
face p.
p. of fetus
footling breech p.
frank breech p.
full-breech p.
head-down p.
incomplete breech p.
incomplete foot p.
longitudinal p.
mentoanterior p.
mentoposterior p.
metachronous p.
multiple presentation phenotype
oblique p.
occiput p.
persistent occiput posterior p.
placental p.
right occipitoposterior p.
single presentation phenotype
singleton breech p.
transverse lie p.
vertex p.

presented
newly p.

presenting
p. characteristic
history of presenting problem
monocyte p.
p. part
p. part of fetus
p. symptom

preservation
anal ileostomy with preservation of sphincter
autonomic nerve p.
capsule cartilage articular p.
p. of health
Los Angeles preservation solution 1
machine p.
organ retrieval and p.
pelvic autonomic nerve p.
p. of quality of life

preservative
formaldehyde-releasing p.
p. free
stool p.

preservative-free solution system

preserved
amniotic fluid drained and p.

presexual youth

press
shoulder p.

Press-Fit component

pressor
p. agent
cold p.
cold pressor test
p. dose
p. drug
p. effect
effective pressor dose
fastigial pressor response
renal pressor substance
p. support

pressure
abdominal leak-point p.
abnormal intraluminal p.
acoustic pressure amplitude
adjustable pressure shunt
air pressure effect
air pressure enema reduction
air pressure splint
airway p.
airway pressure disconnect
airway pressure excursion
airway pressure release ventilation
p. alopecia
alternating pressure mattress
alternating pressure pad
alveolar p.
alveolar-arterial difference in partial pressure of oxygen
alveolar-arterial pressure difference
alveolar oxygen partial p.
alveolar partial pressure of inhalational anesthetic
alveolocapillary partial pressure gradient
ambient temperature and p.
ambient temperature and pressure, dry
ambulatory blood p.
ambulatory blood pressure monitor
ambulatory venous p.
p. amplitude
anal sphincter squeeze p.
ankle-arm pressure index
ankle-brachial blood p.
ankle-brachial blood pressure ratio
ankle-brachial pressure index
ankle-brachial pressure measurement
ankle systolic p.
antegrade perfusion pressure measurement
antegrade pressure study
antral pressure transducer
aortic blood p.
aortic dicrotic notch p.
aortic mean p.
aortic pressure gradient
aortic pullback p.
aortic root p.
aortic systolic p.
aortic valve pressure gradient
appropriate blood pressure cuff size
area diastolic p.
area systolic p.
arterial blood p.
arterial carbon dioxide p.
arterial dicrotic notch p.
arterial oxygen partial p.
arterial partial p.
arterial partial pressure of CO_2
arterial peak systolic p.
arterial pressure index
arteriovenous pressure gradient
ascending aortic p.

pressure *(continued)*
p. at airway opening
atmospheres of p.
atrial filling p.
p. atrophy
p. at slow component intercept
p. augmentation
automated blood pressure cuff
auto-positive end-expiratory p.
auto-titrating continuous positive airway p.
average diastolic p.
average intravascular p.
average mean p.
back p.
p. balanced
p. bandage
barometric p.
Bennett pressure ventilator
bilevel positive airway p.
bladder p.
blood p.
blood pressure assembly
blood pressure decreased
blood pressure monitor
blood pressure and pulse
blood pressure, pulse, respiration, and temperature
blood pressure recorder
blood pressure, right arm
body temperature, pressure, dry
bone marrow p.
borderline high blood p.
both end-expiratory p.'s
brachial arterial p.
brachial artery mean p.
brain tissue partial pressure of oxygen
p. breathing
p. breathing assister
capillary hydrostatic p.
capillary osmotic p.
capillary wedge p.
p. of carbon dioxide
carbon dioxide p.
carbon monoxide pressure or tension
carotid sinus p.
p. catheter
centimeters of water cuff p.
central venous p.
cerebral subarachnoid venous p.
cerebral tissue perfusion p.
cerebrospinal fluid p.
p. chamber
chronic high blood p.
circular pressure maneuver during massage
colloid hydrostatic pressure gradient
colloid oncotic p.
colloid osmotic p.
colloid osmotic pressure in interstitial fluid
colloid osmotic pressure in plasma
common peak developed isovolumetric p.
compliance, rate, oxygenation, and p.
compliance, rate, oxygenation, and pressure index
constant positive airway p.
continuous distending airway p.
continuous negative airway p.
continuous negative extrathoracic p.
continuous positive airway p.
continuous positive airway pressure device
continuous positive pressure breathing
p. control
p. to control bleeding
controlled high blood p.
p. control ventilation
coronary sinus occlusion p.
coronary wedge p.
cranial perfusion p.
crying, requirement for oxygen supplementation, increases in heart rate and blood p.
p. cuff
Cushing pressure response
p. cushion
decibels sound pressure level
decreased tension pressure
delayed pressure urticaria
detrusor muscle leak-point p.
developed p.
diastolic arterial p.
diastolic blood p.
diastolic pulmonary artery p.
difference in partial pressures of oxygen in mixed alveolar gas and mixed arterial blood
diffuse dull, aching pressure discomfort
diffusion p.
distal mean wave p.
distending airway p.
Doppler pressure gradient
downstream venous p.
p. dressing
p. dressing applied
duration of positive p.
effective filtration p.
effective systolic p.
elastic recoil pressure of lung
end-diastolic aortic-left ventricular pressure gradient
end-diastolic left ventricular p.
end-expiratory esophageal p.
endoneural fluid p.
end positive pressure breathing
end-systolic left ventricular p.
epidural pressure waveform
episcleral venous p.
p. equalization
p. equalization tube
equalize air p.
p. equalizing tube
erect diastolic blood p.
erratic blood p.
esophageal p.
esophageal-directed pressure support
eustachian tube p.
excessive lateral pressure syndrome
exercise pressure index
expiratory positive airway p.
external cardiac p.
external pressure circulatory assistance
extreme p.
facial artery pressure point
feeding mean arterial p.
femoral artery p.
femoral blood p.
filling p.
finger arterial blood p.
finger systolic blood p.
p. flow gradient
fluid p.
p. fracture
free hepatic venous p.
free portal p.
fundal p.
gas partial p.
gastric p.
gastric-intrapleural p.
gastroesophageal pressure gradient
gentle pressure bandage applied
p. gradient
p. gun injury
p. half-time
p. half-time technique
heart rate-systolic blood pressure product

hepatic-occluded portal p.
hepatic vein free p.
hepatic venous pressure gradient
hepatic wedge p.
hereditary neuropathy with liability for pressure palsy
hereditary neuropathy with susceptibility to pressure palsy
high bladder p.
high blood p.
higher air p.
high-frequency positive p.
high intracranial p.
high oxygen p.
high partial pressure of oxygen
home blood pressure measurement
home blood pressure monitoring
Honan pressure reducer
hydromotive p.
hydrostatic p.
inability to control blood p.
increased blood p.
increased central venous p.
increased intracranial p.
increased intraocular p.
increased pressure of blood
increased pressure inside the eye
increased pulmonary artery p.
increased venous p.
increasing oncotic p.
p. increment rate
indirect blood pressure measuring system
inferior vena cava p.
p. infusion device
initial opening pressure
p. in inspiration
inspiratory positive airway p.
inspiratory resistance and positive expiratory p.
instantaneous p.
instantaneous diastolic p.
interatrial pressure gradient
intermittent elevation of blood p.
intermittent positive pressure breathing/inspiratory
intermittent positive pressure inflation with oxygen
intermittent positive pressure respiration
intermittent positive pressure ventilation
internal eye p.
internal jugular p.
intraabdominal p.
intraarterial blood p.
intracardiac pressure curve
intracavitary pressure electrogram dissociation
intracavitary pressure gradient
intracranial blood p.
intracranial epidural p.
intracranial pressure catheter
intracranial pressure monitoring
intracranial pressure monitor in skull
intraesophageal variceal p.
intrahepatic portal p.
intramuscular compartment p.
intraocular p.
intrapleural p.
intraspinal epidural p.
intrauterine pressure catheter
intrauterine pressure monitor
intravascular hydrostatic p.
intraventricular p.
intravesical p.
intrinsic positive end-expiratory p.
invasive pressure measurement
p. inversion point
Iowa P. Articulation Test
ischemic pressure necrosis
jugular venous p.
lateral wall p.
leak point p.
left atrial end-diastolic p.
left atrial transmural p.
left end-expiratory p.
left subclavian central venous p.
left ventricle to aorta pressure gradient
left ventricular end-diastolic p.
left ventricular filling p.
left ventricular initial diastolic p.
left ventricular peak systolic p.
p. length loop
liability to pressure palsy
low atmospheric p.
low blood p.
low central venous pressure anesthesia
lower body negative p.
lower esophageal sphincter p.
p. lowering drug
low-frequency positive pressure ventilation
low pressure bladder
low urethral p.
lung elastic recoil p.
p. maintained
p. management
p. mapping
maternal abdominal p.
maximal closure p.
maximal esophageal p.
maximal exercise systolic p.
maximal expiratory mouth p.
maximal inspiratory mouth p.
maximal left ventricular developed p.
maximal perfusion p.
maximal resting anal p.
maximal sniff-induced esophageal p.
maximal sniff-induced gastric p.
maximal sniff-induced transdiaphragmatic p.
maximal tolerated p.
maximal urethral p.
maximum expiratory airflow-static lung elastic recoil p.
maximum inspiratory p.
maximum pressure picture
maximum squeeze p.
maximum urethral closure p.
maximum vasal p.
McCannel ocular pressure reducer
mean airway p.
mean ankle-brachial systolic pressure index
mean aortic p.
mean arterial blood p.
mean atrial p.
mean brachial artery p.
mean carotid p.
mean circulating filling p.
mean daily erect blood p.
mean daily supine blood p.
mean diastolic left ventricular p.
mean effective p.
mean intrathoracic p.
mean intravascular p.
mean left atrial p.
mean left ventricular systolic p.
mean pulmonary artery wedge p.
mean pulmonary capillary wedge p.
mean resting diastolic blood p.
mean right atrial p.
mean right ventricular p.
mean sitting diastolic blood p.
mean systemic arterial p.
mean venous p.
measurement
p. measurement
medium pressure liquid chromatography
Michaelson counter p.
microvascular p.
middle cerebral artery p.
millimeters partial p.

pressure *(continued)*
minimal audible p.
minimal inspiratory p.
minimum audible p.
minimum blood p.
mitral pressure half-time Doppler
p. monitoring device
monofilament pressure esthesiometer
mouth p.
multilumen central venous p.
nasal bilevel biphasic positive airway p.
nasal continuous positive airway p.
nasal positive pressure ventilation
nasal prong continuous positive airway p.
p. necrosis
negative abdominal p.
negative end-expiratory p.
negative expiratory p.
negative inspiratory p.
negative pressure device
negative pressure respirator
nitrogen partial p.
nonbreathing pressure relieving
noninvasive blood p.
noninvasive blood pressure measurement
noninvasive positive pressure ventilation
normal blood p.
normal intravascular p.
normal perfusion pressure breakthrough
normal pressure and temperature
normal temperature and p.
ocular perfusion p.
ocular pressure reducer
p. of CO_2
office blood p.
p. on the brain
p. one-half time
p. on expiration
p. on inspiration
p. on spinal cord
p. on toe joint
opening p.
ophthalmic artery p.
optimal diastolic p.
orthostatic blood p.
osmotic p.
osmotic pressure of plasma
osmotic pressure of proteins in lymph
output sound pressure level
p. of oxygen
oxygen at atmospheric p.
oxygen half-saturation pressure of hemoglobin
oxygen partial p.
oxygen under high p.
PA filling p.
p. pain threshold
p. pain tolerance level
p. palsy
pancreatic duct p.
partial p.
partial oxygen pressure in mixed venous blood
partial pressure alveolar oxygen
partial pressure of arterial carbon dioxide
partial pressure arterial oxygen
partial pressure of carbon dioxide in arterial gas
partial pressure of carbon dioxide in mixed venous blood
partial pressure of end-tidal CO_2
partial pressure of inspiratory oxygen
partial pressure of intramuscular carbon dioxide
partial pressure of mesenteric venous carbon dioxide
partial pressure of nitrogen
partial pressure of oxygen
partial pressure of water vapor
partial pressure tension of carbon dioxide, vein
partial pressure tension of oxygen, vein
p. patching
peak airway p.
peak blood p.
peak diastolic p.
peak end-expiratory p.
peak equivalent sound pressure level
peak inflation p.
peak inspiratory ventilator p.
peak negative p.
peak systolic aortic p.
peak systolic gradient p.
pelvic floor p.
penile blood p.
penile-brachial pressure index
perfusion p.
peripheral blood p.
peripheral coronary p.
peripheral venous p.
plasma oncotic p.
plasma osmotic p.
pleural p.
pleural pressure gradient
p. pneumothorax
p. point
popliteal artery pressure point
portal venous p.
positive airway p.
positive airway pressure ventilation
positive distending p.
positive end-airway p.
positive end-expiratory p.
positive end-expiratory pressure/continuous positive airway p.
positive expiratory p.
positive expiratory pressure plateau
positive inspiratory p.
positive-negative pressure breathing
positive-negative pressure respiration
positive pressure breathing
positive pressure infusion device
postinspiratory p.
postural blood p.
p., volume, temperature
primary high blood p.
prostatic pressure coefficient
proximal tubular p.
pulmonary arterial diastolic p.
pulmonary arterial pressure-pulmonary venous p.
pulmonary artery diastolic and wedge p.
pulmonary artery end-diastolic p.
pulmonary artery occlusion p.
pulmonary artery pressure monitoring
pulmonary artery systolic p.
pulmonary capillary wedge p.
pulmonary hypertension p.
pulmonary venous p.
pulse oximetry waveform systolic blood p.
quasistatic pressure volume
radial artery systolic p.
rapid recompression-high pressure oxygen
p. rate product
regional cerebral perfusion p.
relief of intracranial p.
renal artery p.
renovascular p.
resting ankle-arm pressure index
resting blood p.

resting head p.
resting venous p.
right atrial mean p.
right atrial pressure elevation
right end-expiratory p.
right ventricular diastolic p.
right ventricular end-diastolic p.
right ventricular filling p.
right ventricular initial diastolic p.
right ventricular systolic p.
saturation sound pressure level
p. score
screen filtration p.
seated diastolic blood p.
secondary high blood p.
segmental bronchus lower extremity Doppler p.
segmental limb systolic p.
p. sensation in chest
shunt p.
skin perfusion p.
small blood pressure cuff
small end-expiratory p.
p. sore
p. sore risk assessment
sound p.
sound pressure level
sphincter of Oddi p.
spinal cord perfusion p.
spinal fluid p.
splanchnic occluded portal p.
spontaneous positive end expiratory p.
standard temperature and pressure, dry
standing diastolic blood p.
standing venous p.
static volume p.
stopped flow p.
supine diastolic blood p.
p. supported ventilation
p. support ventilation
systemic arterial p.
systemic blood p.
systemic mean arterial p.
systolic arterial p.
systolic blood p.
systolic, diastolic, mean blood p.
systolic pressure time index
temperature and p.
tender to p.
thoracic duct p.
p. time index
p. time per minute
p. time product
tissue hydrostatic p.
tissue oncotic p.
toe blood p.
total p.
transcutaneous carbon dioxide p.
transcutaneous oxygen pressure measurement
transcutaneous partial pressure of oxygen
transdiaphragmatic p.
transmembrane hydrostatic p.
p. transmission ratio
transmural pressure airway
transpulmonary p.
transvalvular pressure gradient
transversely excited atmospheric p.
tubal perfusion p.
p. ulcer
P. Ulcer Scale for Healing
unassisted diastolic p.
unassisted systolic p.
uncontrolled high blood p.
upper airway closing p.
upper airway opening p.
upper esophageal sphincter p.
ureteral back p.
urethral closure p.
urethral closure pressure profile
urethral pressure profilometry
Valsalva leak point p.
vapor p.
variable positive airway p.
venous blood p.
venous dialysis p.
venous pressure gradient support stockings
venous pressure module
venous stop flow p.
ventilator pressure manometer
ventricular diastolic p.
ventricular end-diastolic p.
ventricular filling p.
ventricular fluid p.
ventricular pleural pressure gradient
voiding p.
voiding urethral pressure measurement
volume-assured pressure support
volume-guaranteed pressure option
p.'s and waves
wedged renal vein p.
wedge hepatic venous p.
yield p.
zero end-expiratory p.
zero-flow p.
p. zone microphone
z point p.

pressure-assisted
intermittent negative pressure-assisted ventilation

pressure/continuous
positive end-expiratory pressure/continuous positive airway pressure

pressure-controlled
p.-c. intermittent coronary sinus occlusion
p.-c. inverse ratio ventilation

pressured
p. behavior
p. speech

pressure-flow study

pressure-regulated volume control

pressure-relief
p.-r. ankle-foot orthosis
p.-r. ankle-foot orthotic

pressure-retaining flow-relieving

pressure-time integral

pressure-volume
p.-v. curve
elastic p.-v.

pressurized
p. air
p. metered-dose inhaler

presternal notch

prestress
compliant prestress system

presumed
p. circle area ratio
p. ocular histoplasmosis syndrome

presumptive
p. cause
p. diagnosis

presurgical
p. coagulation evaluation
p. laboratory workup
p. orthopedic correction
p. psychological screening
p. testing

presynaptic terminal

presystolic
apical presystolic murmur
p. gallop
p. murmur
p. thrill

pretectal
nucleus of pretectal area

pretectalis
area p.

preterm
Assessment of P. Infants Behavior
p. birth
p. delivery
p. infant
p. labor
p. milk
p. neonate
p. newborn
nonthrombocytopenic preterm infant
p. premature rupture of membranes
spontaneous preterm birth
p. spontaneous rupture of membranes
very low birth weight preterm neonate

pretest
Visual Numerical Discrimination P.

pretibial
p. bearing
p. buttress
p. edema
localized pretibial myxedema
p. myxedema
p. rash

Pretoria virus

pretracheales
nodi lymphoidei p.

pretracheal fascia

pretragal parotid gland

pretransfusion
platelet count p.
p. testing

pretreatment anxiety

prevailing
customary, prevailing, and reasonable

prevalence
amebic prevalence rate
p. of hallucinogen abuse

prevalent illness

prevent
Antihypertensive and Lipid-Lowering Treatment to P. Heart Attack Trial
p. further outbreak
p. heart disease
hepatitis C antiviral long-term treatment to prevent cirrhosis
p. spread of infection
p. transmission of disease
p. withdrawal symptom

prevention
acquired immune deficiency syndrome p.
p. of anginal attack
Antioxidant Polyp P. Trial
Diabetes P. Program
Dropout Prediction and P.
p. and early intervention
HIV prevention and control
p. of hospital infection
infection p.
p. of infection
infection prevention and control
Mental Health Early Intervention, Treatment, and Prevention Act of 2000
p. of mental illness
microstomia prevention appliance
mucin clot prevention test
National P. Information Network
new age suicide p.
osseous bridge p.
payment error prevention program
The Injury P. Program
p. and treatment of depression

preventive
p. allergy treatment
p. antibiotic
antigen-specific preventive therapy
p. aspirin therapy
p. dental health behavior
p. dose
general preventive medicine
p. health behavior
P. Health Model
p. medicine
pellagra p.
pellagra preventive factor
p. treatment

preventive aspirin therapy

preventricular intraventricular hemorrhage

prevertebral
p. fascia
p. ganglion
p. layer
p. lymph node
p. soft tissue
p. space

prevertebrales
nodi lymphoidei p.

prevesicle space

prevesiculares
nodi lymphatici p.

previa
complete placenta p.
partial placenta p.
placenta p.
placenta previa centralis
placenta previa marginalis
total placenta p.

preview
Personnel Security P.

previous
p. abnormality of glucose tolerance
compared with previous study
discontinue previous medication
p. history
p. infarction
p. level of functioning
p. medical illness
p. menstrual period
no previous admission
no previous complaint
no previous history
no significant change from previous tracing
p. posterior myocardial infarction
p. psychiatric history
salpingitis after previous tubal occlusion
p. seizure disorder
p. trouble
tuboovarian abscess after previous tubal occlusion
well-healed previous excisional scars

previously
patient previously hospitalized
p. unrecognized mental illness
salpingitis in previously occluded tubes

prevocational
P. Assessment and Curriculum Guide
Social and P. Information Battery

Preyer reflex

priapism
arterial p.

Price precipitation reaction

prick
histamine equivalent p.
p. skin test

prickling sensation

prickly
p., burning, and tingling feeling
p. heat
p. heat rash
p. sensation

Prieto syndrome

primam
incision healed per p.
per primam healing
wound healed per p.

primarily
pain primarily localized
p. respiratory alkalosis

primary
abnormal primary function
p. abscess
acquired immune deficiency syndrome primary pathogen
p. acquired melanosis
p. acquired nasolacrimal duct obstruction
p. acquired preleukemic syndrome
p. acquired sideroblastic anemia
acute intermittent primary angle-closure glaucoma
acute primary angle-closure glaucoma
acute primary keratotic gingivostomatitis
p. adenocarcinoma of the gallbladder
adrenal primary aldosteronism
p. adrenocortical micronodular dysplasia
p. adrenocortical nodular dysplasia
p. affective disorder
p. afferent nociceptor neuron
p. African green monkey kidney
AIDS-related primary central nervous system lymphoma
p. aldosteronism
p. amebic meningoencephalitis
p. amenorrhea
p. anastomosis
p. angiitis of the central nervous system
p. angiitis of CNS
p. angle-closure glaucoma
p. antecubital jump bypass
anterior primary division
p. antiphospholipid antibody syndrome
p. anxiety
p. atelectasis
p. atrial arrhythmia
p. atypical pneumonia
atypical primary pneumonia
p. biliary cirrhosis
p. bone cancer
p. bone lymphoma
p. bone sarcoma
p. brain lymphoma
p. brain tumor
p. cancer
p. cancer site
cancer of unknown p.
cancer of unknown primary site
capitated primary care network
carcinoma of uncertain primary site
carcinoma of unknown p.
p. carcinoma unknown
carcinoma of unknown primary site
p. care
p. care case management
p. care clinic
P. Care Evaluation of Mental Disorders
p. caregiver
p. care intervention
p. care network
p. care nursing
p. care physician
p. care provider
p. care unit
p. central nervous system
p. central nervous system lymphoma
p. cerebral non-Hodgkin lymphoma
p. cesarean section
p. chemotherapy
P. Children's Medical Center
p. choana
chronic primary angle-closure glaucoma
chronic primary headache
p. ciliary dyskinesia
p. cleavage
p. closure
p. colorectal cancer
community-oriented primary care
p. contraction
p. contribution
p. cutaneous large B-cell lymphoma
p. cutaneous melanoma
p. degenerative cerebral disease
p. degenerative dementia
p. degenerative dementia of Alzheimer type
delayed primary closure
delayed primary intention
delayed primary intention healing
delayed primary repair
p. dendrite
p. dental caries
p. dentition
p. dependence study
Detroit Tests of Learning Aptitude - P., Second Edition
p. diagnosis
drug-associated primary acute pancreatitis
p. drug resistance
p. dysfunctional labor
p. dysmenorrhea
p. effusion lymphoma
p. empty sella syndrome
p. enrichment medium
p. extranodal lymphoma
p. fallopian tube carcinoma
familial isolated primary hyperparathyroidism
familial primary pulmonary hypertension
p. fibromyalgia
p. fibromyalgia syndrome
p. flash distillate
p. ganglion
p. gangrene
p. gastric lymphoma
p. gastric non-Hodgkin lymphoma
p. generalized epilepsy
p. glaucoma
p. glaucoma triple procedure
p. glioma
p. goal
p. gouty arthritis
p. graft failure
p. growth
p. head vein
p. healing
healing by primary intention
p. health care
p. hemorrhage
p. hepatic carcinoma
p. hepatic disease
p. hepatocellular carcinoma
p. hepatosplenic lymphoma
p. high blood pressure
high-risk primary breast cancer
p. high-risk replacement surgery
p. human fetal glia
p. hydrocephalus
p. hyperparathyroidism
p. hypersomnia
p. hypertension

primary *(continued)*
p. hyperthyroidism
p. hypoadrenalism
p. hypogonadism
p. hypoparathyroidism
p. hypothyroidism
p. immune deficiency
p. immune response
p. immunodeficiency
p. immunodeficiency syndrome
p. implant
p. impression
p. infarction
p. infection
p. infertility
p. insanity
p. insomnia
p. integration
intention
p. interpretation
p. intestinal lymphangiectasia
p. intracerebral hemorrhage
p. intracranial neoplasm
p. irritant contact dermatitis
p. irritation index
latent primary malignancy
p. lateral sclerosis
p. lesion
p. liver cell
p. liver cell cancer
p. lung disease
p. lymphoma of bone
malignancy
p. malignant melanoma of the esophagus
malignant primary pheochromocytoma
p. malignant tumor
materials primary dye
Mayo Clinic system test for primary biliary cirrhosis
p. mechanism
p. mediastinal germ-cell tumor
p. mediastinal large-cell lymphoma
p. mediastinal large cell lymphoma with sclerosis
p. melanoma
P. Mental Abilities Test
p. mental ability
metastatic carcinoma of unknown primary origin
p. motivation
multiple primary malignancy
multiple primary neoplasm
multiple primary neoplasms
p. myelodysplastic syndrome
p. myocardial disease
p. neoplasm
p. neuroectodermal tumor
p. neuroendocrine carcinoma of skin
p. nocturnal enuresis
p. node involvement
node-negative primary tumor
no evidence of primary tumor
p. nonfunction
p. non-Hodgkin lymphoma of bone
normocalcemic primary hyperparathyroidism
p. nurse
occult primary malignancy
p. open-angle glaucoma
p. operable breast cancer
p. optic atrophy
p. ovarian carcinoma
p. ovarian carcinoma with metastasis
p. ovarian failure
p. percutaneous transluminal coronary angioplasty
p. peritoneal carcinoma
p. peritoneal drainage
p. peritonitis
persistent hyperplasia of primary vitreous
persistent hyperplastic primary vitreous
p. persistent hyperplastic vitreous
persistent primary hyperplastic vitreous
p. physical dependence
p. pigmented nodular adrenocortical disease
p. plexogenic hypertension
p. postpartum hemorrhage
p. private practice insurance
p. pulmonary hypertension
p. pulmonary hypertension murmur
p. pulmonary hypertension risk factor
p. pulmonary non-Hodgkin lymphoma
p. rabbit kidney
P. Reference Material
p. regimen
p. sampling unit
p. sclerosing cholangitis
Screening Assessment for Gifted Elementary Students, P.
P. Self-Concept Inventory
p. sensorimotor cortex
p. Sjögren syndrome
p. sleep disorder
p. spontaneous pneumothorax
spontaneous primary hypothyroidism
p. stem
p. surgical ward
p. symptomatic diffuse esophageal spasm
syndrome of primary aldosteronism
p. syphilis
p. systemic vasculitis
P. Test of Cognitive Skills
The P. Language Screen
p. thrombocythemia
p. thymic carcinoma
p. tumor, regional lymph node, remote metastases classification, staging
p. tumor site
p. tumor site unknown
p. union
unknown primary carcinoma
unknown primary tumor
p. ventricular fibrillation
p. ventricular tachycardia
p. visual cortex
P. Visual Motor Test
Wechsler Preschool and P. Scale of Intelligence

primary-acquired immunodeficiency

primary-progressive multiple sclerosis

primate
p. chorionic gonadotropin
subhuman primate model

primed
arbitrary primed PCR
p. lymphocyte test
p. lymphocyte typing
p. in situ labeling

5′-monodeiodinase type I

primer
PCR with arbitrary p.
reverse transcriptase primer extension
sequence-independent single primer amplification
sequence-specific DNA p.

primer-dependent
p.-d. deoxynucleic acid polymerase
p.-d. deoxynucleic acid polymerase index

primigravida
elderly p.

priming
cross-modal p.

primitive
central primitive neuroectodermal tumor
p. fetal hemoglobin
p. gut
p. hypoglossal artery
p. neuroectodermal tumor
p. neuroectodermal tumor-medulloblastoma
peripheral primitive neuroectodermal tumor
p. trigeminal artery
p. tumor cell

primordial
p. cartilage
p. cyst
p. dwarfism
p. germ cell
p. gigantism
microcephalic primordial dwarfism 1
microcephalic primordial dwarfism-cataracts syndrome
osteodysplastic primordial dwarfism

primordium
optic p.

primrose
evening primrose oil
oil of evening p.

primum
atrial ostium primum defect
ostium p.
ostium primum location

primus
digitus p.
metatarsus primus adductus
metatarsus primus varus

princeps
arteria princeps pollicis

principal
carbon atom farthest from principal functioning group
p. cell
central principal axis of inertia
central principal moments of inertia
p. components analysis
p. diagnosis
p. focus
p. investigator
nonmetric principal component analysis
p. outer material protein
p. quantum number
p. sulcus

principle
antianemia p.
antianemic p.
anticipatory-maturation p.
axial compression p.
countercurrent multiplier p.
Fick p.
hemodynamic p.
line focus p.
low flow p.
luteinizing p.
Mackay-Marg p.
mass action p.
melanophore-expanding p.
Mitrofanoff p.
transforming p.
tumor-inhibiting p.

print
maximal print position

printed
p. circuit
final printed labeling
lines printed per minute

Printing Performance School Readiness Test

Prinzmetal
P. effect
P. variant angina

prion
p. protein
p. protein normal isoform
p. protein scrapie isoform-reactive plaque

prior
p. to admission
p. to arrival
p. to birth
p. to conception
p. to delivery
did not exist prior to enlistment
p. to discharge
existed prior to enlistment
existed prior to service
p. to exposure
home evaluation prior to discharge
p. to hospitalization
p. level of function
p. medical record
minus two hours two hours prior to treatment
no prior tracings

priority
P. Counseling Survey
Treatment Priority Index

prism
p. adaptation test
p. and alternate cover test
AO rotary p.
apex of p.
base-down p.
base of prism in
base of prism down
base of prism out
base of prism up
base-up p.
p. diopter
p. glasses
Marco prism exophthalmometer
oblique prism device
refracting angle of p.
simultaneous prism and cover test

prison
p. fever typhus

prison-acquired lymphoproliferative syndrome

prisoner
not prisoner of war
p. of war

private
p. day nurse
p. diagnostic clinic
p. duty nurse
p. hospital
p. medical doctor
p. patient
p. practice
primary private practice insurance
p. psychiatric hospital

privileges
bathroom p.
lost p.
out of bed with bathroom p.

pro
p. arrhythmic effect
p. time

proactivator

proactive
p. inhibition
p. interference

proanthocyanidin
oligomeric p.

proatrial natriuretic factor

probabilistic neural network

probability

cumulative probability of success
p. curve
p. density function
equal probability of selection method
p. of having disease
high probability of survival
low probability, high consequence event
Mortality P. Model
p. of not having disease
sequential probability ratio test
significance probability mapping
significance probability value
p. of type I, II error

probable

p. allergic rhinitis
p. causal relationship
p. error
p. error of measurement
female adnexal tumor of probable wolffian origin
most probable number

probably

highly probably drunk

proband

adult-onset p.
autistic p.

probe

antisense RNA p.
biliary balloon p.
bipolar cautery p.
bipolar circumactive p.
cardiac nuclear probe scan
centromere enumeration p.
cervical p.
Clinical P.'s of Articulation Consistency
Doppler velocity p.
electromagnetic focusing field probe
electron probe x-ray microanalyzer
endolaser probe tip
p. excision
front-loading ultrasound p.
gamma probe guided lymphoscintigraphy
gamma probe radiolocalization
heater p.
heater probe cauterization
heater probe coagulation
heater probe therapy
heater probe unit
high-frequency ultrasound probe sonography
hot tip laser p.
injection gold p.
linear array transrectal ultrasound p.
line probe assay
2.0-MHz phased-array p.
molecular probe hybridization
molecular probe testing
multiplane intracavitary p.
nasolacrimal duct p.
neutral amyloid p.
nucleic acid p.
nucleic acid probe assay
oligodeoxynucleotide antisense p.
scanning probe microscopy
sequence-specific oligonucleotide probe hybridization
serial probe recognition
ultrasound catheter p.

probe-assisted

catheter probe-assisted endoluminal ultrasonography

probing

p. depth
p. finger
p. of lacrimal duct
p. of wound

problem

activity-related heart p.
Adolescent P. Severity Index
affect intensity p.
alcohol-related physical p.
alcohol-related psychiatric p.
p. behavior
Behavior Problem Checklist
cardiovascular problems related to drug abuse
chest pain from heart p.
p. child
chronic health p.
circulatory problem from diabetes
circulatory problem with cold sensitivity
clamminess from circulatory p.
clinical appraisal of psychosocial p.
comorbid medical p.
completion, arithmetic p.'s, vocabulary, following directions
computer-patient management p.
Coping Orientations to P.'s Experienced
cross generational p.
crush injury renal p.
developmental learning p.
p. drinker
p. drinking
drug-related p.
p. elicitation technique
Emotional and Behavior P. Scale
Everyday P. Checklist
p.'s from aging gums
p. gambler
general health p.
hearing p.
hearing aid p.
heart rhythm p.
hepatic problems related to drug abuse
history of presenting p.
human immunodeficiency virus overview of problems evaluation system
immune dysfunction p.
incurable problem drinker
intermittent functional bowel p.
International Classification of Diseases and Related Health P.'s, 10th Edition
Interpersonal Cognitive P. Solving
joint problems from arthritis
life circumstance p.
p. list
male infertility p.
means-end problem solving
Mooney P. Checklist
multiple medical p.
nail breaking from circulatory p.
other interpersonal p.
pain from heart p.
parental control p.
patient management p.
Personal P.'s Checklist for Adolescents
postoperative pulmonary p.
postural back p.
preexisting emotional p.
p. reporting program
Revised Memory and Behavior P.'s Checklist
School P. Screening Inventory
p. solving
p. solving information
p. status report
stress caused health p.
symptom problem index
weight-related health p.

problem-analysis report

problematic behavior

problem-oriented

p.-o. diagnosis
p.-o. medical record

P.-o. Screening Instrument for Teenagers
p.-o. system of charting

problem-solving
p.-s. ability
critical p.-s.
p.-s. skill

proboscis lateralis

procainamide
N-acetyl p.

procaine
aqueous procaine penicillin
aqueous procaine penicillin G
p. and lactic acid
penicillin G p.
penicillin G benzathine and procaine combined

procedural
Current P. Terminology
p. sedation and analgesia

procedure
abdominal pull-through p.
age correction p.
p. alternative
p.'s, alternatives, indications and complications
antegrade continence enema p.
anterior cricoid split p.
anterior Pólya p.
anterior stabilization p.
Antivirogram test p.
antrum-sparing modified Whipple p.
apron flap p.
arterial reconstructive p.
arterial switch p.
arthroscopic transglenoid suture stabilization p.
artificial divergence p.
artificial pleural effusion p.
atrial inversion p.
atrial septoplasty p.
atrial septostomy p.
atrial switch p.
autogenous fascia lata sling p.
barrel stave osteotomy p.
bidirectional Glenn p.
bladder chimney p.
canalith repositioning p.
cardiac invasive p.
cardiac revascularization p.
cardiac valve p.
carotid Amytal p.
catheter-based Maze p.
Clifton Assessment P.'s for the Elderly
clinical p.
comprehensive renal scintillation p.
coronary artery revascularization p.
crushing procedure skull of fetus
cryo destruction p.
Cumulative Techniques and P.'s in Clinical Microbiology
Damian graft p.
Damus-Kaye-Stansel procedure
definitive p.
diagnostic procedure and treatment
diagnostic test and p.
diverting colostomy with pull-through p.
Draw-A-Person Screening P. for Emotional Disturbance
egg retrieval p.
emergency p.
endocardial resection p.
endorectal ileoanal pull-through p.
extended endocardial resection p.
filed procedure in cardiac arrest
fixed-dose p.
frozen animal p.
Ganley and Ganley metatarsus adductus p.
gastric bypass p.
gastric emptying p.
gastric pull-through p.
gastric pull-up p.
gastric stapling p.
gastrointestinal procedure unit
general p.
glans approximation p.
Gram stain p.
heart trimming p.
Heller-Dor procedure
imaging p.
immune modulation p.
immunodiffusion p.
intracarotid amobarbital p.
invasive p.
invasive diagnostic p.
invasive medical p.
laboratory p.
laparoscopic Burch p.
large loop excision of transformation zone/loop electrosurgical excision p.
laser coagulation vaporization p.
left atrial isolation p.
loop electrosurgical excision p.
loop electrosurgical excisional p.
loop electrosurgical excision procedure conization
loop gastric bypass p.
lower lid sling p.
Luck hand p.
Lynch frontoethmoidectomy p.
Lynn Achilles lengthening p.
Malone ACE p.
Malone antegrade colonic enema stoma p.
Malone antegrade continence enema p.
maxillomandibular advancement p.
Mayo-Fueth inversion p.
McCash hand p.
McElvenny foot p.
McKay hip p.
meatal advancement and glanduloplasty p.
medical short procedure unit
Microsporidia diagnostic p.
microsurgical epididymal sperm aspiration p.
midface degloving p.
Miller foot p.
minimally invasive biopsy p.
Mitchell hallux valgus p.
modified Belsey fundoplication p.
modified Bernard-Burow p.
modified Broström-Evans p.
modified Fontan p.
modified Hoke-Miller flatfoot p.
modified Wies p.
motion control p.
Multiphasic Environmental Assessment P.
Mustard atrial switch p.
Neer capsular shift p.
negative selection p.
neuroradiologic imaging p.
Nicoll fracture repair p.
Nissen fundoplication p.
Nissen-Rosseti fundoplication p.
nodal staging p.
noninvasive diagnostic p.
nursing p.
O'Brien capsular shift p.
one-stitch cataract p.
operating nursing p.
operative p.
Osmond-Clarke foot p.
osteoplastic frontal sinus p.
outpatient endometrial resection/ablation p.
palliative cerebrospinal shunt p.
patient tolerated the procedure well

procedure *(continued)*
performance evaluation p.
photic stimulation p.
platelet neutralization p.
policy and p.
primary glaucoma triple p.
reverse filling p.
scleral buckling p.
selective tubal occlusion p.
shunt p.
simple neonatal p.
standard operating p.
surgical procedure for subarachnoid hemorrhage
surgical short procedure unit
test orientation p.
Thal fundoplication p.
total fundoplication p.
total hip replacement p.
transurethral prostate p.
transvaginal Burch p.
trial assessment procedure scale

procerus
musculus p.

process
abnormal growth p.
accelerated mental p.'s
active disease p.
active epileptic p.
active invasive infectious p.
age-related deterioration p.
age-related developmental p.
altered thought p.
angular process of orbit
antenatal disease p.
anterior calcaneal process fracture
anterior clinoid p.
anterior process of malleus
appearance, mood, sensorium, intelligence, and thought p.
articular process of vertebra
Assessment of Phonological P.'s
assimilation phonological p.
automatic psychological p.
basic adaptive p.
blocking of thought p.
chronic inflammatory granulomatous p.
complexity of mental p.'s
complex psychophysiological p.
comprehensive identification p.
concrete thought p.
coracoid p.
coronoid process of ramus
p. diagnostic
disoriented or slow thought p.
egocentric thought p.
p. of elimination
ethmoidal process of inferior nasal concha
foot p.
healthy patient with localized pathologic p.
healthy patient with localized pathological p.
highly activity epileptic p.
Imagined P. Inventory
immune destructive p.
improved thought p.
inflammatory p.
infundibular p.
inhibitor of radical p.'s
limited channel-capacity p.
long process of incus
long process of malleus
mammillary process of lumbar vertebra
middle clinoid p.
myoepithelial cell p.
nasal crest of palatine process of maxilla
natural aging p.
natural hemostatic p.
neuronal apoptotic p.
neutron absorption p.
normative aging p.
odontoid process displacement
ongoing cognitive p.
osseous destructive p.
palatine crest of horizontal process of palatine bone
patchy infiltrative p.
progressive degenerative disease p.
pterygoid p.
simulated fluorescence p.
P. Skills Rating Scale
staging process and imaging
stall the healing p.
superior articular p.
thinning process of bone
thought p.
topic-oriented process group

processed
sectionally processed antibody coated

processing
abbreviated rapid p.
altered tau p.
auditory processing disorder
autologous leukapheresis, processing, and storage
automatic data p.
automatic signal p.
automatic tissue p.
central auditory processing battery
central auditory processing disorder
central processing unit
data p.
digital imaging p.
digital signal p.
digital sound p.
distributed data p.
electronic claims p.
electronic data p.
p. information
information processing in central nervous system
List P. Language
massive parallel processing system
model-based image p.
natural language p.
normal affective p.
online transaction p.
psychological information, acquisition, processing, and control system
rapid manual p.
rapid processing mode
slow cognitive p.
supply, processing, and distribution department
Weidel Auditory P. Test

processor
data acquisition p.
input signal p.
output signal p.
speech processor interface
time domain signal p.
wearable speech p.
word p.

processus
patent processus vaginalis

procidentia
anal p.
p. of uterus

procoagulant activity

procollagen
carboxyterminal propeptide of type 1 p.
p. type III aminoterminal peptide
type II procollagen gene

proconvertin
prothrombin, proconvertin, Stuart factor, antihemophilic B factor
prothrombin and proconvertin test

procreation
assisted medical p.

proctitis
allergic p.
epidemic gangrenous p.
gonorrheal p.
ulcerative p.

proctocolectomy
restorative p.
totally stapled restorative p.

proctocolitis
aphthoid p.

proctoscopic examination

proctosigmoidoscopic
p. evaluation
p. examination

proctosigmoidoscopy
fiberoptic p.

procurement
p. of cadaver organs for transplantation
donor p.
p. of donor organs and tissue
Northeast Organ P. Organization
organ p.
organ procurement organization
regional organ p.

procursiva
aura p.

procyanidol oligomer

prodigy
child p.

prodromal
p. episode
p. illness
p. labor
p. period
p. phase
p. stage

prodrome
affective prodrome of epilepsy
affective prodrome of migraine
AIDS p.
epileptic p.

prodrug
antibody-directed enzyme prodrug therapy
tumor-activated p.

producing
number of pregnancies producing viable offspring

producing cell

product
p. of activated lymphocyte
advanced oxidation protein p.
anthrax-contaminated animal p.
approved drug p.
blood product contaminated by acquired immune deficiency syndrome
brightness area p.
cleaved polyprotein precursor molecule p.
combination p.
p.'s of conception
cross-linked fibrin degradation p.
cytotoxin-associated gene product A
degradation p.
p. development protocol
digoxin reduction p.
dose area p.
Drug P. Information File
enzyme p.
evacuation of retained products of conception
fibrin breakdown p.
fibrin degradation p.
fibrin/fibrinogen degradation p.
fibrinogen breakdown p.
fibrinogen degradation p.
fibrinogen split p.
fibrinolytic split p.
fibrin split p.
gene p.
heart rate-systolic blood pressure p.
hybridoma p.
lipoxygenase interaction p.
metabolic products test
p. moment
potassium solubility p.
pressure rate p.
pressure time p.
protein gene p.
radiopharmaceutical drug p.
rate-pressure p.
reaction p.
real-time dose area p.
resistive exercise p.
retained products of conception
p. selection allowed
split products of fibrin
Summary of P. Characteristics
L-tryptophan-containing p.

product-enhanced reverse transcriptase

production
antibody production assay
bilirubin p.
blood production rate
cortisol production rate
crypt cell production rate
ectopic hormone p.
endogenous glucose p.
estradiol production rate
excessive heat p.
glucose p.
glucose production rate
heat p.
hepatic glucose p.
p. hormone
hourly fetal urine production rate
humoral antibody p.
increase heart p.
insulin production rate
male hormone p.
marrow production rate
metabolic heat p.
mitochondrial ATP p.
mouse antibody production test
paraneoplastic ectopic ACTH p.
p. rate
red blood cell precursor production rate
p. of red blood cells
reticulocyte production index
reticulocytic production index
p. of sex hormone
sound production sample
sound production tasks
testosterone production rate
thyroid hormone p.
urinary production rate
venous carbon dioxide p.
ventilation/carbon dioxide p.
in vitro antibody production assay

productive
p. bronchitis
p. cough
p. cough and expectoration
cough productive of bloody sputum
p. sputum
p. tuberculosis

productivity to respiration ratio

product-line manager

professional
P. and Administrative Career Examination
allied health p.
p. association
p. counselor
P. Employment Test
p. ethics
p. gambler
health p.
p. help

professional *(continued)*
independent professional review
infection control p.
p. information brochure
licensed professional counselor
mental health care p.
mental health p.
National Association of Activity P.'s
p. performance evaluation
p. relations
P. Sexual Role Inventory
p. simulated patient

proficiency
Arizona Articulation P. Scale
P. Assessment Report
Language P. Test
Trainer's Assessment of P.

profile
P. of Adaptation to Life
analytical profile index
anatomic p.
aortic valve velocity p.
Aphasia Diagnostic P.'s
Apraxia P.: A Descriptive Assessment Tool for Children
ASTRA profile test
automated chemistry p.
automated physiologic p.
basic health p.
basic metabolic p.
Behavior Activity P.
Behavior Rating P., Second Edition
biochemical p.
biophysical p.
biophysical profile score
blood cell p.
blood chemistry p.
Burke Stroke Time-Oriented p.
cellular immunocompetence p.
cell volume p.
cerebral vascular profile study
cerebrovascular p.
chemical enzyme p.
chemistry screening p.
Child Health and Illness P., Adolescent Edition
cholesteric analysis p.
cholesteric analysis profile test
Diversity Awareness P.
Emotions P. Index
executive 22 chemistry p.
fasting chemistry p.
fasting lipid p.
Fatigue-Inertia Subscale of the P. of Mood States
fetal biophysical p.
Functional Limitation P.
Gordon Personal P.
Gordon Personal P. Inventory
Hawaii Early Learning P.
health illness p.
hemostatic screening p.
Hospital Admission Risk P.
hospital chemistry p.
humoral immunocompetence p.
Hypnotic Induction P.
Learning Style P.
linear profile scan
lipid p.
liver function p.
Lovibond profile sign
low profile R-K marker
major organ p.
Medical Sciences Knowledge P.
metacarpophalangeal p.
P. of Mood States
Musical Aptitude P.
national outpatient p.
neuropsychological test p.
neurotic direction p.
nonacute p.
P. of Nonverbal Sensitivity
Nottingham Health P.
One Touch P.
P. of Out-of-Body Experiences
Pain Patient P.
Pain Perception P.
Parent Perception of Child P.
patient medication p.
personality disorder p.
Physical Tolerance P.
placental grade biophysical p.
Premature Infant Pain P.
Psychiatric Evaluation P.
Psychoeducational P.
Psycho-Epistemological P.
Psychotic Inpatient P.
Psychotic Reaction P.
random chemistry p.
reduced p.
renal laboratory p.
Sexuality Preference P.
Sickness Impact P.
slice sensitivity p.
Thackray Reading Readiness P.
therapeutic class p.
thyroid function p.
ultralow p.
urethral closure pressure p.
Validity Indicator P.
Vocal P.'s Analysis

profile-based therapy

profile–diagnosis
coagulation p.

Profile-II
Developmental P.-I.

profile–presurgery
coagulation p.

Profile/Success
Hilson Personnel Profile/Success Quotient

profiling
ethnic p.
multiple arbitrary amplicon p.

profilometry
urethral pressure p.

profit
manipulates to gain p.

profound
p. amnesia
p. anemia
p. anxiety
p. change in affect
p. change in behavior
p. dementia
p. depression
p. hearing impairment
p. hearing loss
p. hypothermia
p. hypothermic circulatory arrest
p. mental retardation
p. thrombocytopenia
p. weakness

profoundly
Assessment for Persons P. or Severely Impaired
p. hypothermic circulatory arrest
p. mentally retarded
severely and profoundly handicapped

profunda
arteria auricularis p.
arteria cervicalis p.
arteria circumflexa ilium p.
arteria profunda brachii
arteria profunda penis
arteria temporalis p.
p. brachii artery
p. femoris
p. femoris artery
p. femoris vein

profundae

profundi
nodi lymphoidei parotidei p.
nodi lymphoidei parotidei profundi preauriculares

profundus
arcus plantaris p.
arcus venosus palmaris p.
arcus volaris p.
arteria plantaris p.
flexor p.
flexor digitorum profundus muscle
p. flexor digitorum muscle
flexor digitorum profundus tendon
p. flexor digitorum tendon
flexor profundus tendon
lupus erythematosus p.
nodus lymphoideus proximalis p.

profundus/panniculitis
lupus p.

profuse
p. bleeding
p. diarrhea
p. hemorrhage
p. menstruation
p. perspiration
p. sweating

progenitalis
herpes p.

progenitor
autoimmune progenitor cell
autologous hematopoietic progenitor cell transplantation
committed progenitor cell
granular progenitor cell
hematopoietic progenitor cell
marrow p.
megakaryocyte p.
mesenchymal p.
mesenchymal progenitor cell
monocyte-macrophage p.
multipotent hematopoietic p.
multipotential p.
myeloid p.
myeloid progenitor factor 1
myeloid progenitor inhibitory factor
myeloid progenitor inhibitory factor-1
osteoblast progenitor proliferation
peripheral blood progenitor cell
peripheral blood progenitor cell transplant

progeroid
neonatal pseudohydrocephalic progeroid syndrome

progestational hormone

progesterone
p. antagonist
autoimmune progesterone dermatitis
p. challenge test
p. effect
estrogen and p.
intrauterine progesterone contraceptive system
midluteal progesterone measurement
p. in oil
p. receptor
p. receptor assay
p. resistance
salivary p.
uterine progesterone system
p. withdrawal

progesterone-induced blocking factor

progestin
p. challenge test
nonandrogenic p.
nor-derivative p.
p. receptor

progestin-binding complement

progestin-only pill

progestogen

progestogen-dependent endometrial protein

prognathism
mandibular p.
microcephaly, microphthalmia, ectrodactyly, prognathism syndrome

prognosis, pl. **prognoses**
aggressive good prognosis non-Hodgkin lymphoma
grave p.
p. is good
p. is guarded
p. is poor

prognostic
coronary prognostic index
diagnostic and prognostic indicators
Duke treadmill prognostic score
p. finding
Glasgow Meningococcal Septicemia P. Score
hemodialysis prognostic nutrition index
initial prognostic score
International P. Index
Nottingham P. Index
p. nutritional index
Orpington prognostic scale
p. score

progonoma
melanotic p.

program
addiction treatment p.
adolescent day treatment p.
Advanced Placement P.
AIDS Drug Assistance P.
alcohol dependence treatment p.
alcohol rehabilitation p.
aquatic exercise p.
aquatic stabilization p.
Assessment P. of Early Learning Levels
Biological Response Modification P.
Birth Defects Monitoring P.
bowel training p.
Cancer Surveillance P.
captioned media p.
cardiac rehabilitation p.
career planning p.
Certified Hospital Admission P.
Child Health Assessment P.
Childhood Asthma Management P.
community-based psychiatric p.
Community-Oriented P.'s Environment Scale
Comparative Guidance and Placement P.
computer therapy p.
cooperative institutional research p.
coronary rehabilitation p.
correctional health care p.
crippled children's p.
Diabetes Prevention P.
drug abuse reporting p.
drug dependence treatment p.
drug intervention p.
dual diagnosis p.
early intervention p.
Early and Periodic Screening, Diagnosis, and Treatment p.
estimated length of p.
p. evaluation and review technique
family intervention p.
family risk assessment p.
fast track p.
federal immunization p.
Frostig P. for the Development of Visual Perception
functional exercise p.
functional maintenance p.

program *(continued)*
Genetically Handicapped Persons P.
graded exercise p.
group-living p.
Health Evaluation and Learning P.
hearing conservation p.'s
heart rehabilitation p.
home chemotherapy p.
home exercise p.
hospital inservice p.
hospital insurance p.
hospital residency p.
Hypertension Detection and Followup P.
hypertension screening p.
independent progressive home exercise p.
individualized education p.
infection surveillance and control p.
intensive outpatient treatment p.
Life Health Monitoring P.
long-term detoxification p.
maternal health p.
Medical Knowledge Self-Assessment P.
medical outpatient p.
methadone maintenance and aftercare treatment p.
MET 1 p.
Minnesota Comprehensive Epilepsy P.
Multi-Dimensional Voice Program 4305
multimodality treatment p.
Muma Assessment P.
myocardial infarction rehabilitation p.
narcotic treatment p.
National Cholesterol Education P. criteria
needle exchange p.
neurolinguistic p.
newborn screening p.
Onchocerciasis Control P.
open-heart rehabilitation p.
outpatient methadone p.
pain clinic p.
pain management p.
PAR Admissions Testing p.
partial hospitalization p.
partial hospital treatment p.
Patient Assessment P.
patient education p.
payment error prevention p.
perinatal mortality counseling p.
pharmacologic erection p.
preadmission testing p.
problem reporting p.
progressive home exercise p.
Psychiatric Knowledge and Skills Self-Assessment P.
public health education p.
quality assurance p.
rape crisis intervention p.
rest-exercise p.
restorative nursing p.
scheduled nursing activities p.
School Health Additional Referral P.
Screening and Crisis Intervention P.
Sibling Training P.
Spofford-Christopher oxygen optimizing p.
Stroke Education P.
substance abuse treatment p.
syringe exchange p.
The Injury Prevention P.
thematic content modification p.
transitional living p.
universal newborn hearing screening p.
vertical stabilization p.
Vietnam Veterans Evaluation and Treatment P.
vocational rehabilitation p.
vocational skills assessment and development p.
weight management p.
Women, Infants, and Children P.
work hardening p.
written home exercise p.

program/home
accreditation program/home health care

program/hospice
accreditation program/hospice care

program/long
accreditation program/long-term care

programmable
p. cardioverter-defibrillator
p. device
erasable programmable read-only memory
p. implantable medication system
p. multiple ion monitor
p. pacemaker
p. read-only memory

programmed
p. cell death
p. electrical stimulation
p. instruction
p. medical history
p. multiple development
noninvasive programmed stimulation
p. physical examination
p. symbols
p. ventricular stimulation

programmer
Computer P. Aptitude Battery

programming
articulation p.
p. language 1
linear p.
neuroendocrine p.
phonologic programming deficit syndrome
Rucker-Gable Educational P. Scale

progranulocytic
acute progranulocytic leukemia

progrediens
necrosis p.

progress
P. Assessment Chart of Social and Personal Development
failure to progress in labor
interim progress note
monthly progress note
resident's progress note
Sequential Tests of Educational P., Series III

progressed
disease progressed slowly

progressing
early progressing stroke
late progressing stroke
rapidly progressing bilateral hearing loss

progression
p. of activity
arithmetic p.
p. of atherosclerosis
p. of disease
double-limb p.
foot progression angle
freedom from p.
free from p.
geometric p.
gradual exercise p.
no p.
poor precordial R-wave p.

poor progression of R wave in precordial leads
poor R-wave progression electrocardiogram
single-limb p.
steady-state free p.
stroke in p.
symptomatic progression of disease
p. of symptoms
time to p.
time-to-disease p.
time to tumor p.
time without symptoms of progression or toxicity
vertical float progression aquatic therapy

Progressional

National Association of Progressional Geriatric Care Managers

progression-free

p.-f. interval
p.-f. survival

progressiva

fibrodysplasia ossificans p.
myositis ossificans p.
polymyositis ossificans p.

progressive

p. accumulated stress
P. Achievement Tests of Listening Comprehension
acquired progressive lymphangioma
p. ambulation
p. assistive exercise
bilateral progressive hearing loss
p. brain disease
p. bulbar palsy
p. cardiac care
p. care unit
p. cataract
chronic progressive coccidioidal pneumonitis
chronic progressive course
chronic progressive external ophthalmoplegia
chronic progressive headache
chronic progressive hereditary chorea
chronic and progressive illness
chronic progressive multiple sclerosis
Colored P. Matrices
p. condylar resorption
p. curvature of radius
p. decline in function
p. degeneration
p. degenerative disease process
p. dementia
p. deterioration
P. Deterioration Scale
diabetes insipidus, diabetes mellitus, progressive bilateral optic atrophy, and sensorineural deafness
p. dialysis encephalopathy
p. diet
p. disability
p. disease
disease incurable, p.
p. disorder
p. disseminated histoplasmosis
p. downhill course
p. dysarthria
early progressive resistance
p. encephalomyelitis with rigidity and myoclonus
p. encephalopathy, edema, hypsarrhythmia, optic atrophy
p. exercise test
p. external ophthalmoparesis
p. external ophthalmoplegia
p. familial intrahepatic cholestasia
familial progressive hyperpigmentation
p. fatigue and weakness
p. form of tick-borne encephalitis
p. gait imbalance
p. hearing loss
p. hemiparesis
hereditary progressive ataxia
p. hoarseness
p. home exercise program
p. hydrocephalus
p. hypertrophic interstitial neuropathy
p. idiopathic neuromuscular disease
idiopathic rapidly progressive glomerulonephritis
p. impairment of vision
p. inability to walk
independent progressive home exercise program
p. intellectual and neurological deterioration
p. interstitial pulmonary fibrosis
p. jaundice
limited progressive systemic sclerosis
linear progressive systemic sclerosis
p. lingual hemiatrophy
localized progressive systemic sclerosis
p. massive fibrosis
medical progressive care unit
p. multifocal leukodystrophy
p. multifocal leukoencephalopathy
p. multifocal leuko-J encephalopathy
p. muscle relaxation
p. muscular atrophy
p. muscular dystrophy
muscular dystrophy, p.
p. myoclonus epilepsy
p. myopia
p. nuclear palsy
p. outer retinal necrosis
painless progressive loss of vision
p. patient care
p. perceptive deafness
p. perivenular alcoholic fibrosis
p. pneumonia virus
p. postmyelitis muscular atrophy
p. postpolio muscle atrophy
posttraumatic progressive myelopathy
rapidly progressive necrotizing glomerulonephritis
rapidly progressive crescenting glomerulonephritis
Raven Colored P. Matrices Test
Raven Standard Progressive Matrices
p. relaxation for insomnia
p. relaxation training
p. relaxation under hyperactivity
p. renal failure
p. resistance
p. resistance exercise
p. rubella panencephalitis
slowly progressive hereditary disorder
p. spinal ataxia
p. spinal muscular atrophy
spinal progressive amyotrophy
spinal progressive muscular atrophy
p. supranuclear palsy
p. symmetric erythrokeratodermia
systemic progressive sclerosis
p. systemic scleroderma
p. systemic sclerosis
p. transformation of germinal center
p. unilateral hearing loss
p. weakness

progressive *(continued)*
p. weakness of extremity
p. weakness on one side of the body
X-linked progressive mixed deafness with perilymphatic gusher

progressively
p. diffused leukoencephalopathy
handwriting progressively shaky
p. lowered stress threshold

progressive-resistive exercise

progress note

prohibited
National Collegiate Athletic Association prohibited drug

prohormone
p. convertase 1, 2, 3

proinsulin
p. antibody
immunoreactive p.

proinsulin-like component

project
adolescent diversion p.
Breast Cancer Detection Demonstration P.
Children's Art P.
comprehensive hospital infections p.
Fort Bragg evaluation p.
Heroin Emergency Life P.
Hospital Utilization P.
Human Genome P.
National Prostatic Cancer P. criteria
Rochester Epidemiology P.

projectile vomiting

projection
Age P. Test
anterior oblique p.
anteroposterior lordotic p.
apical lordotic p.
applied extrasensory p.
ascending pathway of pain p.
auditory projection area
average pixel p.
axial calcaneal p.
axial sesamoid p.
coronal maximum-intensity p.
coronary maximum-intensity p.
effective sensory p.
erect posterior-anterior projection
full scan with interpolation p.
lateral p.
left anterior oblique p.
light perception with p.
light perception without p.
light projection test
orthogonal angiographic p.
PA and lateral p.
papillary tumor p.
right anterior oblique p.
saturation inversion p.
scanned projection radiography
scan projection radiography
specific thalamic projection system
stereotactic surface p.
thalamic projection neuron
variable projection method
visual acuity, left eye, left perception with p.
p. x-ray microscopy

projective
House-Tree-Person P. Technique psychologic test
Pickford P.'s Picture

projector
liquid crystal display p.
Ultramatic Project-O-Chart p.

prolactin
p. chronic growth hormone
decidual p.
p. deficiency
p. excess
human p.
p. inducible protein
p. inhibitor
p. inhibitory hormone
p. level
non-ergot long-acting prolactin inhibitor
ovine p.
p. release-inhibiting hormone
p. secreting pituitary tumor

prolactin-binding assay

prolactin-inhibiting
p.-i. factor
p.-i. hormone

prolactin-producing pituitary adenoma

prolactin-releasing
p.-r. factor
p.-r. hormone

prolapse
anorectal mucosal p.
anterior leaflet p.
aortic cusp p.
p. of aortic valve
aortic valve leaflet p.
brachydactyly, mesomelia, mental retardation, aortic dilation, mitral valve prolapse, characteristic facies syndrome
p. of cord
coronary spasm and p.
p. of corpus luteum
p. gastropathy syndrome
gonadal failure, short stature, mitral valve prolapse, mental retardation syndrome
idiopathic mitral valve p.
p. of iris
massive genital p.
mental retardation, mitral valve prolapse, characteristic face syndrome
mitral valve p.
p. of mitral valve
mitral valve prolapse, aortic anomalies, skeletal changes, and skin changes syndrome
p. of Morgagni
occult cord p.
pelvic organ p.
rectal p.
p. repair
symptomatic uterine p.
third-degree uterine p.
tricuspid valve p.
umbilical cord p.
p. of urethra and bladder
p. of uterus

prolapsed
p. bladder
p. bowel
p. cord
p. hemorrhoid
p. intervertebral disk
p. mitral valve
p. mitral valve syndrome
p. rectum
p. vaginal wall

prolapsing
p. hemorrhoid
p. mitral leaflet

Prolene suture

proliferans
angiocholitis p.
angioendotheliomatosis p.
retinitis p.

proliferating
p. bile ductules
endothelial proliferating factor
neoplastic proliferating angioendotheliomatosis

nonclonogenic proliferating cell
p. nuclear cell antigen

proliferation
anterior hyaloidal fibrovascular p.
appositional crystal p.
atypical lymphoepithelioid cell p.
atypical small acinar proliferation of prostate
autonomous parathyroid chief cell p.
bizarre parosteal osteochondromatous p.
p. of bone
diffuse mesangial p.
epimacular p.
epiretinal membrane p.
fibrous p.
hepatocyte proliferation inhibitor
idiopathic myeloid p.
p. inhibitory factor
malignant lymphocytic proliferation disease
massive periretinal p.
Masson intravascular endothelial p.
mesangial cell p.
MIB-1 cell proliferation marker
mitogen-induced lymphocyte p.
mucosal cell p.
neoplastic cell p.
neuroepithelial cell p.
nodular and diffuse fibrous p.
ocular adnexal lymphoid p.
osteoblast progenitor p.
prostatic stromal proliferation of uncertain malignant potential
stem cell proliferation factor
tumor-assisted lymphoid p.

proliferation-inhibiting factor

proliferation/regression
lymphocyte proliferation/regression index
myelofibrosis proliferation/regression index

proliferative
acute p.
acute proliferative glomerulonephritis
benign proliferative lesion
p. breast disease
p. capacity
chronic proliferative glomerulonephritis
p. diabetic retinopathy
p. diabetic retinopathy with vitreous hemorrhage
diffuse proliferative glomerulonephritis
early proliferative phase
p. endometrium
extracapillary proliferative glomerulonephritis
focal proliferative glomerulonephritis
p. glomerulonephritis
p. helper cell
p. hemorrhagic enteropathy
p. hyperplasia
p. index
p. kidney disease
relative proliferative capacity
p. retinopathy photocoagulation
p. sickle retinopathy
streptococcal proliferative factor
p. verrucous leukoplakia
p. vitreoretinopathy
p. zone

proliferator
peroxisomal proliferator receptor
peroxisome proliferator response element

proline
protocollagen proline hydroxylase

prolongata
alalia p.

prolongation
axillary p.
expiratory p.

prolonged
p. action
p. acute hepatitis
p. acute tissue expansion
p. antibiotic therapy
p. bleeding time
p. bradycardia
p. capillary refill
p. cerebral apnea
p. chest pain intense
p. contractile duration
p. and deep breathing
p. deep inspiration
p. diarrhea
p. exposure
p. febrile convulsions
p. fever of unknown origin
p. gestation
p. grief
p. heavy drinking
p. hospital care
p. hospitalization
p. hypotension
p. illness
p. inactivity
p. indigestion
p. indwelling catheter
p. intensive hyperventilation
p. jaundice
p. labor
low-load prolonged stress
low-load prolonged stretch
p. phase endometrium
p. postictal encephalopathy
p. postpeel erythema
p. premature rupture of membranes
p. QT interval
p. QT syndrome
p. remission
p. respiratory support
p. reversible ischemic neurologic deficit
p. rupture of fetal membranes
p. sleep apnea
p. symptomatic illness
p. venous access devices

prolonged-dwell peritoneal dialysis

prolymphocytic
B-cell prolymphocytic leukemia
p. leukemia
T-cell prolymphocytic leukemia

promethazine
meperidine and p.

prominence
aortic p.
p. of bone
hilar p.
mallear p.
plantar bony p.
p. of pulmonary markings
p. of pulmonary vasculature
p. of pulmonary vessel
p. of right hilum
sacral p.

prominent
p. bruit
p. forehead
p. hallucination
p. heel
p. murmur
p. shoulder blade

promiscuity
lineage p.

promontory
sacral p.
p. stimulation test

promoter
basal promoter element
chicken ovalbumin upstream p.
eosinophil stimulation p.
insulin promoter factor-1
MLH1 promoter methylation
operon promoter sequence

promoting
phagocytosis promoting factor
p. aphasics communicative effectiveness

prompt
p. excretion of contrast material
p. excretion of dye
p. spill into duodenum

promyelocytic
acute promyelocytic leukemia
p. leukemia
p. leukemia zinc finger
microgranular acute promyelocytic leukemia

pronated
p. foot
forearm p.
p. hand

pronation
p. contracture
p. of foot
hindfoot p.
p. spring control
p. and supination

pronation-eversion-external rotation

pronation-external rotation

pronation-lateral rotation fracture

pronator
anterior pronator teres
p. quadratus
p. quadratus muscle
p. teres
p. teres muscle

pronatus
pes p.

prone
accident p.
p. cranial support device
p. to developing pigment gallstones
highly prone to fantasy
p. knee bend
p. on elbows
p. position

proneness
cancer proneness phenotype
Suicide-Depression P. Checklist

prong
binasal p.'s
nasal p.'s
nasal prong continuous positive airway pressure

4-pronged polyp grasper

3-prong headrest

pronounced
p. dead
patient pronounced dead

pronouncement of brain death

pronuclear stage transfer

pronucleate
p. stage embryo transfer
p. stage tubal transfer

pronucleus
male p.

pronunciation
artifact p.

proof
p. of eligibility
p. of illness

propagated
p. sensation along the channel
p. sensation along the meridian
p. thrombus

propagating
p. clustered contraction
p. thrombosis

propagation
impulse p.

propensity
lipogenic enzyme p.

propeptide
carboxyterminal propeptide of type 1 procollagen
C propeptide of type II collagen

proper
p. alignment of fracture
p. lamina
muscle of back p.
oral cavity p.
temporalis fascia p.

properdin factor B

properitoneal
p. fat
p. hernia

properly
inability to arrange words p.

property
anisotropic bone p.
antiapoptotic p.'s
p. damage accident
p. damage collision
direct anticancer p.'s
dopamine receptor agonist p.
electrical membrane p.
lipid-independent anti-atherosclerotic p.
psychoactive p.'s of hallucinogen
segment inertial p.'s

prophylactic
p. antibiotic
p. antibiotic treatment
p. anticonvulsant
antiviral p.
p. brain irradiation
p. cranial irradiation
p. decompression
p. dentistry
p. drug
p. gamma globulin
p. mastectomy
p. medication
p. penicillin
periodontal p.'s
protected environment units and prophylactic antibiotic
radiation therapy on prophylactic basis
p. treatment
p. whole brain radiation therapy

prophylaxis
anaphylactic shock p.
deep venous thrombosis p.
dental p.
intrapartum antibiotic p.
neonatal ocular p.
oral antimicrobial p.
perioperative antibiotic p.
postnatal penicillin p.
preoperative antimicrobial p.
rabies postexposure p.
stress ulcer p.

propidium iodine

propionate
cellular acetate p.
dihydrotestosterone p.
testosterone p.

proportion
aneurysmal p.
p. free thyroxine
in proportion to age

proportional
p. assist ventilation

p. assist ventilator
p. counter spectrometry
p. morbidity ratio
p. mortality ratio
multiwire proportional chamber

proportional-integral-derivative

proportionate
p. morbidity ratio
standardized proportionate mortality

proposal
request for p.

proposed
notice of proposed rulemaking
p. international nonproprietary name

propria
arteria cochlearis p.
arteria digitalis palmaris p.
arteria digitalis plantaris p.
arteria hepatica p.
atrophia pilorum p.
lamina propria lymphocyte
miliaria p.
muscularis p.

proprioception
general p.

proprioceptive
p. discrimination
p. neuromuscular facilitation
p. neuromuscular fasciculation reaction
p. reflex
p. sense
p. stimuli

proprioceptor
muscle p.

proprius
anterior fasciculus p.
extensor digiti quinti p.
extensor indicis p.
extensor proprius hallucis
extensor quinti p.
musculus extensor digiti quinti p.
musculus extensor indicis p.

proprotein convertase

proptosis
axial p.
Moran p.

propulsion
electromolecular p.

propyldisulfide
thiamine p.

proserum prothrombin conversion accelerator

prosopagnosia
apperceptive p.
associative p.

Prospect Hill virus

prospective
p. drug review
p. evaluation of radial keratotomy
online prospective drug utilization review
p. outcomes monitoring evaluation system
Outpatient P. Payment System
randomized prospective trial
p. randomized trial

prostacyclin-stimulating factor

prostaglandin
p. E metabolite
endogenous inhibitor of prostaglandin synthase
endorphin, dopamine, and prostaglandin theory
p. F receptor
p. H synthase
immunoreactive prostaglandin E
p. inhibitor
one-hour p.
p. synthetase
p. synthetase inhibitor

prostaglandin-like substance

prostate
p. abscess
adenocarcinoma of prostate gland
p. anatomy
androgen-dependent prostate cancer
androgen-independent prostate cancer
androgen-independent prostate carcinoma
p. antigen
apex of p.
asymptomatic metastatic hormone-refractory prostate cancer
atypical small acinar proliferation of p.
benign hypertrophy of p.
p. brachytherapy
p. cancer
cancer of p.
cancer of the prostate and brain gene
p. cancer screening
p. cancer treatment
p. capsule
p. carcinoma
carcinoma of p.
p. chips
coagulation and hemostatic resection of p.
contact laser ablation of p.
contact laser vaporization of the p.
cryosurgical ablation of the p.
Danish P. Symptom Score
digital examination of p.
p. enlargement
fibroadenomatosis hyperplasia of prostate gland
p. gland
p. gland benign hyperplasia
p. gland biopsy
p. gland innervation
p. gland lymphoma
p. gland sarcoma
p. gland secretion
hereditary prostate cancer 1 locus
holmium laser resection of the p.
hormone-dependent prostate cancer
hormone-independent prostate cancer
hormone-refractory metastatic prostate cancer
hormone-refractory prostate cancer
hormone-resistant prostate cancer
p. hormone therapy
p. hyperplasia
International P. Symptom Score
interstitial laser ablation of the p.
interstitial laser coagulation of the p.
lobe of p.
localization of prostate cancer
localized prostate carcinoma
locally advanced prostate cancer
malignant acini prostate gland
median furrow of p.
metastatic prostate cancer
microwave hyperthermia of the p.
middle lobe of p.
minimal transurethral resection of p.
needle biopsy of p.
p. needle biopsy
p. neoplasm
nodular hyperplasia of prostate gland
p. nodule

prostate *(continued)*
noncancerous enlargement of prostate gland
p. puncture biopsy
radical prostate surgery
radioactive seeding of p.
p. screening
small cell undifferentiated carcinoma of the p.
soft and smooth prostate
status post transurethral resection of p.
testosterone repressed prostate message-2
p. tissue
total transurethral resection of p.
transperineal interstitial permanent prostate brachytherapy
transrectal needle biopsy of p.
transrectal ultrasound of p.
transurethral electrovaporization of p.
transurethral evaporation of p.
transurethral incision of p.
transurethral needle biopsy of the p.
transurethral prostate procedure
transurethral resection of p.
transurethral vaporization of p.
transurethral vaporization-resection of p.
p. tumor
urine specimen after prostate massage
urine specimen before prostate massage
vaporization laser ablation of p.
visual laser ablation of p.

prostate-binding protein

prostatectomy
laparoscopic radical p.
open p.
perineal p.
radical perineal p.
radical retropubic p.
retropubic p.
suprapubic p.
transurethral ultrasound-guided laser-induced p.
transurethral ultrasound-guided laser-induced prostatectomy system
transvesical p.
visual laser-assisted p.

prostate-specific
p.-s. acid phosphatase
age-adjusted prostate-specific antigen
p.-s. antigen bound to alpha-1 antichymotrypsin
p.-s. antigen density
p.-s. antigen doubling time
p.-s. antigen transition zone
p.-s. antigen velocity
p.-s. membrane
p.-s. membrane antigen

prostatic
p. abscess
p. acid phosphatase
p. adenocarcinoma
p. adenoma
alloplastic prostatic bladder
p. artery
p. balloon dilatation
p. bed
benign prostatic enlargement
benign prostatic hyperplasia
benign prostatic hypertrophy
benign prostatic obstruction
p. biopsy
p. calculus
p. cancer
p. carcinoma
p. chip
p. cyst
p. duct
p. echogram
p. enlargement
expressed prostatic secretions
p. fascia
p. fossa
p. ganglion
p. hyperplasia
p. hyperthermia
p. hypertrophy
p. infection
p. interstitial fluid
p. intraepithelial neoplasia
intravesical prostatic tissue
p. lobe
lymphangitic spread of prostatic adenocarcinoma
p. massage
microscopic benign prostatic hyperplasia
muscular coat of prostatic urethra
muscular layer of prostatic urethra
National P. Cancer Project criteria
p. needle biopsy
p. neoplasm
nodular prostatic hypertrophy
p. outlet obstruction
p. pressure coefficient
p. secretion
p. specific antigen
p. stromal proliferation of uncertain malignant potential
p. tissue
total serum prostatic acid phosphatase
transrectal prostatic hyperthermia
transurethral prostatic resection
p. urethra

prostatitis
allergic granulomatous p.
asymptomatic inflammatory p.
chronic bacterial p.
chronic nonbacterial p.
National Institutes of Health Chronic P. Symptom Index
NIH Classification Category I acute bacterial p.
NIH Classification Category II chronic bacterial p.
NIH Classification Category IV asymptomatic inflammatory p.
NIH Classification System for P.
nonbacterial p.

prostatitis/pelvic
chronic prostatitis/pelvic pain syndrome

prosthesis
advanced mobile-bearing p.
alloplastic temporomandibular joint p.
alumina-alumina total hip replacement p.
alumina cemented total hip p.
anatomic surface p.
aortic bifurcation p.
aortic valve p.
articulating disc p.
ball-type disc p.
4-bar linkage on knee p.
4-bar polycentric knee p.
bicompartmental knee implant p.
bipolar femoral head p.
bipolar hip replacement p.
blood vessel p.
bone-anchored p.
breast prosthesis rupture
cardiac valve p.
carpal lunate implant p.
collagen tape p.
computerized assisted design p.
cruciate condylar unconstrained p.
debonded femoral stem p.

debridement and prosthesis retention
dental p.
duckbill voice p.
dura mater p.
elastic-type disc p.
femoral neck p.
femoral prosthesis broach
femoral prosthesis fixation
forged cobalt-chromium alloy p.
great toe implant p.
heart valve p.
hollow sphere p.
homograft incus p.
immediate postoperative p.
immediate postsurgical fitting of prosthesis
incus replacement p.
inflatable penile p.
insertion of p.
ischial weightbearing p.
lower extremity p.
lower limb p.
low-profile femoral p.
lunate acrylic cement wrist p.
mandibular guide-plane p.
mandibular guide p.
MCP finger joint p.
metaphysial head resection with p.
mitral valve p.
monoblock femoral stem p.
orbital floor p.
p. and orthosis
painful femoral head p.
partial denture p.
partial ossicular replacement p.
patellar tendon-bearing cast p.
patellar tendon-bearing–supracondylar-suprapatellar prosthesis
porcine aortic valve p.
porous-coated anatomic p.
radius cap p.
single-axis friction knee prosthesis
single-axis locking knee prosthesis
Small-Carrion penile p.
stapes replacement p.
threaded titanium acetabular p.
thrust plate p.
total condylar prosthesis III
total hip p.
total knee p.
total ossicular chain replacement p.
total ossicular reconstruction p.
tracheoesophageal p.
trileaflet aortic p.
universal proximal femur p.
upper limb p.
vibrating ossicular p.
weight-activated locking knee p.
Zimaloy femoral head p.

prosthetic

adjustable postoperative protective prosthetic socket
p. antibiotic-loaded acrylic cement
p. aortic valve
p. appliance
p. ball valve
4-bar linkage prosthetic knee mechanism
bipolar prosthetic cup
p. bladder
caged-ball prosthetic valve
p. cardiac valve
p. dentistry
p. device
p. disk nucleus
p. femoral head
giant prosthetic reinforcement of the visceral sac
p. heart valve
p. heart valve surgery
immediate postoperative prosthetic fitting
p. implant
indwelling prosthetic joint
indwelling prosthetic medical device
p. infectious endocarditis
p. joint
p. joint infection
p. lens
p. limb
p. and orthotic
partial denture p.'s
porcine prosthetic valve
p. ring anuloplasty
Staphylococcus aureus prosthetic joint infection
p. valve dysfunction
p. valve endocarditis
p. valve regurgitation
p. valve stenosis
p. valve thrombosis
p. valve vegetation
p. vegetation

protamine

heparin protamine titration
neutral protamine Hagedorn insulin
p. paracoagulation phenomenon
plasma protamine precipitating
p. response test
p. sulfate
p. zinc insulin

protease

alkaline protease inhibitor
amyloid A-degrading p.
anti-HIV protease inhibitor
antihuman immunodeficiency virus protease inhibitor
aspartyl protease class
binding protein p.
calcium-activated neutral p.
p. inhibitor
microbial alkaline protease inhibitor
plant protease test
rat mast cell p.
secretory leukocyte protease inhibitor
serine protease inhibitor
slowest moving p.
slow-moving p.
staphylococcal p.
Staphylococcus aureus p.

protease-activated receptor

protease-antiprotease imbalance

protected

p. bronchoalveolar lavage
p. brush catheter
p. catheter aspirate
p. catheter brushing specimen
p. environment units and prophylactic antibiotic
flexible fiberoptic bronchoscopy with protected brush
p. specimen brushing
p. transbronchial needle aspirate

protection

additional personal injury p.
p. and advocacy
automated boundary p.
child protection team
critical infrastructure p.
environmental p.
p. factor
hearing protection device
joint p.
leg protection factor
myocardial protection system
personal injury p.
radiation leukemia p.
radiation protection guide
p., rest, ice, compression, elevation, support

protection *(continued)*
p., restricted activity, ice, compression, elevation
ribonuclease protection assay
Short Transitional Edge P.
skin protection factor
sun protection factor
topical skin p.
venous/arterial management p.

protective
adjustable postoperative protective prosthetic socket
p. agent
p. antigen
p. care unit
cerebral protective therapy
Child P. Services
p. dressing
p. eye pad
p. eye shield
p. eyewear
p. glove
p. inoculation
loss of protective sensation
personal protective equipment
p. services
total protective environment

protector
ankle ligament p.
ankle ligament protector brace
autogenous corneal p.
disposable elbow p.
disposable heel p.
long-acting thyroid stimulator p.

protein
p. absorption
acidic proline-rich p.
activated protein C
activated protein C resistance
activator p.
acute-phase p.
acute-phase reactant p.
acyl carrier p.
adenovirus E1A p.
advanced oxidation protein product
p. A-gold technique
p. A hemolytic plaque assay
p. A immobilized in collodion charcoal
aldosterone-induced p.
Alzheimer precursor p.
AMP-activated protein kinase
amyloid A p.
amyloid precursor p.
androgen binding p.
animal protein diet
animal protein factor
antibodies to the Epstein-Barr virus transactivator p.
p. antibody
antibody to c100 p.
anti-*Escherichia coli*-derived protein antibody
antigen binding p.
antiglial fibrillary acidic p.
antilens protein antibody
antiviral p.
argyrophil organizer region p.
ascitic fluid total p.
assimilation regulatory p.
Australia antigen p.
Australian parrot p.
autolyzed yeast p.
bacterial intravenous p.
bactericidal/permeability-increasing p.
basic p.
Bence Jones p.
beta-lactamase inhibiting p.
p. binding
p. binding abnormality
binding protein protease
biotin carboxyl carrier p.
bone Gla p.
bone morphogenetic p.
bone morphogenetic protein type 2
p. bound
bovine spinal cord p.
brain/muscle ARNT-like protein 1
brain protein solvent
p. breakdown
breast cyst fluid p.
calcium-binding p.
calmodulin-dependent protein kinase
cAMP receptor p.
carbohydrate-binding p.
p. carboxymethylase
cardiac gap junction p.
cartilage intermediate layer p.
cartilage oligomeric matrix p.
p. catabolic rate
catabolite activator p.
catabolite gene activator p.
CCAAT/enhancer binding p.
p. C deficiency
cell attachment p.
cell surface p.
cellular retinoic acid-binding p.
cellular retinol-binding p.
centromere p.
channel-forming integral p.
chemically modified p.
cholesteryl ester transfer p.
chymotrypsin-like p.
clottable p.
cobalamin-binding p.
coenzyme A-synthesizing protein complex
cold-inducible ribonucleic acid-binding p.
collagenase-digestible p.
colon-specific antigen p.
competitive protein binding
complement control p.
constituent of alpha protein plasma fraction
constituent of gamma protein plasma fraction
constituent of plasma protein fraction
contraction-associated p.
copper-binding p.
corticotropin-releasing hormone-binding p.
cow's milk p.
cow's milk protein allergy
C-reactive p.
C-reactive protein antiserum
cross-linked p.
cross-reactive p.
crude p.
cyclic AMP-binding p.
cystic fibrosis p.
cytochrome p.
cytosol p.
daily protein intake
D-binding p.
p. deficiency
p. degradation
delipidized serum p.
p. depletion
p. deposit
p. deprived
dialysate protein loss
p. diet
dietary protein intake
digestible p.
p. disulfide isomerase
p. efficiency ratio
elastase-like p.
p. electrophoresis
enhanced green fluorescent p.
eosinophil cationic p.
eosinophilic cationic p.
eosinophil protein X
epidermal cell surface p.
epidermal soluble p.
Epstein-Barr early region p.

erythrocyte membrane p.
estimated protein needs
estimated protein requirement
estradiol-binding p.
estramustine binding p.
estrogen receptor p.
p. excretion
external membrane p.
Fas-associating protein with death domain
fatty acid-binding p.
fatty acid-binding protein 2
fatty acid transport p.
fetal estrogen-binding p.
fibrous protein
fish protein concentrate
fixation p.
FK-binding protein 12
FK-binding protein rapamycin-associated p.
fluorescein-labeled serum p.
fluorescein to protein ratio
folic acid-binding p.
follicle regulatory p.
formula protein intolerance
fragile X mental retardation p.
galactose-binding p.
gap junction p.
p. gene product
G inhibiting p.
glial fibrillary acidic p.
globular protein
globular-fibrous protein
glycine-rich RNA-binding p.
glycosylated protein spanning viral envelope
glycosylated serum p.
G-myeloma p.
green fluorescent p.
gross cystic disease fluid p.
growth-associated p.
growth hormone-binding p.
G-stimulating p.
guanine nucleotide regulatory p.
guinea pig myelin-basic p.
heart fatty acid binding p.
heat shock p.
heavy-chain disease protein
hemopexin serum protein
hepatic binding p.
hereditary nephritic p.
high biological value p.
high level of kidney protein rennin
high-potential iron p.
high-resolution protein electrophoresis
histidine-rich calcium-binding p.
HIV nucleocapsid p.
human pancreas-specific p.
human serum p.
hydrolyzed animal p.
hydrophobic p.
hypocaloric protein feeding
IGF-binding p.
immobilized mismatch binding p.
p. immunoelectrophoresis
immunosuppressive acidic p.
increased excretion of p.
infectious cell p.
insulin growth factor-binding p.
p. intake
interleukin-1 receptor antagonist p.
intermediate filament p.
intestinal fatty acid-binding p.
p. intolerance
intracellular binding p.
iron-binding p.
key intermediary p.
kidney p.
kidney-specific p.
p. kinase A, B, C, G
p. kinase activation ratio
kinase inhibitory p.
labile p.
latex ELISA for antigen p.
LDL receptor-related p.
p. level
light chain of protein molecules
lipopolysaccharide binding p.
lipoprotein receptor-related p.
liver-enriched activating p.
liver-enriched inhibiting p.
liver-specific p.
p. loss
p. loss in hepatic disease
low p.
low-density lipoprotein receptor-related p.
lung resistance-related p.
lysinuric protein intolerance
lysosomal trafficking regulator p.
macrophage infectivity potentiator p.
macrophage inflammatory p.
macrophage inflammatory protein I, II
macrophage inflammatory protein alpha-1
major basic p.
major capsid protein gene
major outer membrane p.
major urinary p.
maltose-binding p.
mammaglobin breast cancer p.
mannan-binding p.
mannose-binding p.
marine protein concentrate
p. mass
matrix Gla p.
membrane cofactor p.
membrane integral p.
metalloproteinase-like, disintegrin-like, cysteine-rich protein
methyl-accepting chemotaxis p.
methyl acceptor p.
methyl-CpG-binding protein 2
p. methylesterase
microatomized protein food
microfibrillar p.
microsomal triglyceride transfer p.
microtubule p.
microtubule-associated p.
milk fat globule p.
milk protein allergy
milk protein intolerance
mitogen-activated p.
mitogen-activated protein kinase cascade
mitogen-activated protein kinase pathway
mitogen-activating p.
mitotic-control p.
modulator p.
monoclonal antiglial fibrillary acidic p.
monoclonal protein, skin
monocyte chemoattractant p.
monocyte chemotactic p.
morphogenic protein 6
mouse serum p.
mouse urine p.
M protein factor
mucin core p.
multidrug resistance p.
multidrug resistance associated p.
muscle contractile p.
myelin base p.
myelin basic p.
myelin basic protein assay
myelin basic protein deficiency
myelin/oligodendrocyte-specific p.
myeloid basic p.
nascent protein chain
natural resistance macrophage-associated p.
net dietary p.
net protein ratio
net protein utilization
neural thread p.

protein *(continued)*
neurofilament p.
neuronal apoptosis inhibitory p.
neuron-specific cytoskeletal p.
neutrophil-activating p.
p. nitrogen unit
noncollagen p.
nonenzymatic protein glycation
nonhemoglobin p.
nonhistone p.
nonhistone chromosomal p.
nonstructural p.
nonstructural protein 4
nonsuppressible insulin-like p.
normalized protein catabolic rate
normalized protein nitrogen appearance
Novel erythropoiesis-stimulating p.
nuclear factor kappa B transcription factor p.
nuclear matrix p.
nucleic acid-binding p.
olfactory marker p.
organic anion-binding p.
osmotic pressure of proteins in lymph
outer membrane p.
outer surface p.
pancreatic juice p.
pancreatic stone p.
pancreatitis-associated p.
parathyroid hormonelike p.
parathyroid hormone-related p.
parathyroid secretory p.
patient spilled p.
penicillin-binding p.
periodically fluctuating protein kinase
peripheral myelin p.
peripheral myelin protein 22 gene
peripheral protein sparing solution
3-phosphoinositide-dependent protein kinase
phosphorylcholine-binding myeloma p.
placental p.
placental protein 5
plasma membrane fatty acid binding p.
plasma protein fraction
plasma protein globulin
p. plasma substitute
platelet ^{125}I-labeled staphylococcal protein A
pokeweed antiviral p.
polyneuropathy, organomegaly, endocrinopathy, M protein, and skin changes syndrome
p. polysaccharide
potassium channel-interacting p.
predigested liquid p.
pregnancy-associated plasma p.
pregnancy-associated plasma protein A, C
pregnancy zone p.
principal outer material p.
prion p.
prion protein normal isoform
prion protein scrapie isoform-reactive plaque
p. profile
progestogen-dependent endometrial p.
prolactin inducible p.
prostate-binding p.
proteolipid p.
PTH-related p.
pulmonary capillary protein leakage
pulmonary microvascular permeability to p.
purified *Brucella* p.
purified fusion p.
purified placental p.
purified placental protein, human
purified protein derivative
purified protein derivative–Battey
purified protein derivative of tuberculin
purified protein derivative–standard
purified protein derivative test
p., quantity not sufficient
rat serum p.
rat urine p.
Rb protein expression
reactive p.
receptor-associated p.
receptor interacting p.
receptor protein tyrosine kinase
recombinant human activated protein C
recombinant human bone morphogenetic p.
recombinant outer surface protein A
regression-associated p.
regulatory p.
Reiter protein complement-fixation test
Reiter protein reagin
resistance activated protein C
retinoblastoma p.
retinoic acid-binding p.
retinol-binding p.
RFX-associated p.
riboflavin-binding p.
riboflavin carrier p.
p. S
p. S deficiency
selective protein index
serotonin-binding p.
serum protein and immunofixation electrophoresis system
serum myelin basic p.
serum protein electrolytes
serum protein electrophoresis
serum protein electrophoretogram
serum protein level
sex-limited p.
Siebert purified protein derivative of tuberculin
signal recognition p.
single-celled p.
single-chain antigen-binding p.
skeletal muscle p.
small p.
Sma- and Mad-related p.
soluble cytoplasmic p.
soluble ribonuclear p.
stable plasma protein solution
staphylococcal protein A
steroid acute regulatory p.
steroid acute respiratory p.
steroid-binding plasma p.
steroidogenic acute regulatory p.
steroid protein activity index
sterol regulatory element binding p.
stimulated protein synthesis
stratum corneum basic p.
stress-activated protein 1
Structural Classification of P.'s
surface binding p.
p. synthesis
synthesizing protein complex
Tamm-Horsfall p.
testis-specific binding p.
testosterone-binding p.
textured vegetable p.
thrombus precursor p.
thymus p.
thyroxine-binding p.
total body p.
total body protein turnover
total circulating p.
total protein tuberculin
total serum p.
toxic shock-associated p.

translation-inhibiting p.
transport-associated p.
trifunctional protein deficiency
triglyceride-rich p.
p. truncation testing
tumor amplified protein expression therapy
tumor necrosis factor-binding p.
type-specific M p.
p. tyrosine kinase
uncoupling p.
uncoupling protein 1, 2, 3
urinary excretion of p.
urine protein electrophoresis
vegetable protein diet plus fiber
viral p.
viral protein R
virus p.
vitamin D-binding p.
p.'s, vitamins, and minerals
in vitro protein digestibility
whole-body p.
Wiskott-Aldrich syndrome p.
zinc finger p.
zona glomerulosa p.

protein-1
endothelial PAS-domain p.
latent membrane p.
macrophage inflammatory p.
monocyte chemoattractant p.
monocyte chemotactic p.
osteogenic p.
sphingolipid activator p.
thyroid-specific enhancer binding p.

protein-2
mammalian achaete-scute homologous p.
sterol carrier p.

protein-6

protein-43
growth-associated p.

proteinaceous
p. coating
p. exudate
p. fluid
p. material

protein-1-alpha
macrophage inflammatory p.-a.

proteinase
bronchial mucous proteinase inhibitor
cysteine proteinase inhibitor
human mammary carcinoma cell membrane p.
p. K digestion
mast cell p.
serine p.

proteinate
periodic acid-thiocarbohydrazide-silver proteinate stain

protein-B
surfactant p.-B.

protein-1-beta
macrophage inflammatory p.-b.

protein-binding abnormality

protein-bound
p.-b. iodine
p.-b. iron
p.-b. polysaccharide
p.-b. thyroxine

protein-C
myosin-binding p.-C.
surfactant p.-C.

protein-calorie
p.-c. malnutrition
p.-c. undernutrition

protein-energy malnutrition

protein-free supernatant

protein-II
histidine-rich p.-I.

protein-induced eosinophilic colitis

protein-lipid complex

protein-losing enteropathy

proteinosis
lipoid p.
pulmonary alveolar p.

protein-sparing
p.-s. modified fast
p.-s. therapy

proteinuria
Bence Jones p.
edema, proteinuria, hypertension
hypertension plus p.
low molecular weight p.
orthostatic p.
persisting p.
postgamma p.

proteoglycan
human stromelysin aggregated p.
p. subunit

proteolipid protein

proteolysis
intracellular p.
limited fragment p.
milk proteolysis test

proteolytic activity

proteose-peptone beef extract

proteose-yeast castione medium

Proteus syndrome

prothoracotropic hormone

prothrombin
p. activity
p. complex
p. consumption index
p. consumption time
p. conversion factor
p. deficiency
p. fragment 1.2
home prothrombin time monitoring
p. induced by vitamin K absence or antagonist-II
plasma prothrombin conversion
plasma prothrombin conversion accelerator
plasma prothrombin conversion factor
p. and proconvertin test
proserum prothrombin conversion accelerator
p., proconvertin, Stuart factor, antihemophilic B factor
quick prothrombin time
Quick Test psychology, pregnancy, prothrombin
serum prothrombin conversion accelerator
serum prothrombin activity
p. test
p. time control
p. time fixing agent
p. time and partial thromboplastin time
p. time ratio

prothrombin-complex concentration

protocol
acute leukemia p.
AOPE chemotherapy p.
APO chemotherapy p.
appropriateness evaluation p.
axial T1-SE p.
Bruce treadmill p.
chronotropic exercise assessment p.
complex oncologic therapy p.
Cornell exercise p.
p. data query
Davidson protocol exercise test
Gliadel wafer treatment p.
immunosuppressed p.
inpatient treatment p.

protocol *(continued)*
Integrated Auricular Reconstruction P.
intermittent catheterization p.
international p.
Managed Care Appropriateness P.
Medical Audiologic Tinnitus Patient P.
Memorial Sloan-Kettering p.
mitomycin C and 5-FU Nigro p.
modified Bagshawe p.
MOPP chemotherapy p.
MVF chemotherapy p.
MVT chemotherapy p.
National Cancer Institute P. 89-C-41
North American Malignant Hyperthermia p.
oncologic therapy p.
PACE chemotherapy p.
per p.
point-to-point p.
product development p.
Reeves treadmill p.
resident assessment p.
Sheffield treadmill p.
telomere repeat amplification p.
telomeric repeat amplification p.
therapist-driven p.

protocollagen proline hydroxylase

protodiastolic gallop

proton
attached proton test
p. beam
p. beam radiation
p. beam radiosurgery
p. beam therapy
p. density
intensity-modulated proton therapy
longitudinal proton MR spectroscopy
p. magnetic resonance
p. magnetic resonance spectroscopy
p. motive force
p. number
p. pump blocker
p. pump inhibitor
p. relaxation enhancement
p. relaxation rate
single proton counting

proton-density axial image

proton-electron dipole-dipole

proton-induced x-ray emission

protooncogene
HER-2/neu p.
MOS p.
mos p.
MYCN p.

protooncogene/oncogene
lyt-1 p.
lyt-10 p.
mas p.
met p.
mil/raf p.
mos p.
myb p.
myc p.
myl p.

protoplasm
granular p.

protoplasmaticum
astrocytoma p.

protoplasmic
p. astrocyte
p. astrocytoma

protoplast
P. material
p. maintenance medium

protoporphyria
erythropoietic p.

protoporphyrin
erythrocyte p.
free erythrocyte p.
p. IX
p. nine
tin p.
zinc p.

protoporphyrin/heme
zinc p.

protozoacidal
minimal protozoacidal concentration

protozoal
p. dysentery
p. infection
p. myocarditis
p. organism

protozoan
p. cyst
p. enteritis
p. infection
obligate intracellular p.
p. parasite

protracted
p. diarrhea
p. diarrhea of infancy
idiopathic protracted diarrhea
p. venous infusion

protractor
arthrodial p.

protruded
p. eyeball
p. intervertebral disk

protrudes
p. in midline
tongue protrudes in midline

protruding
p. cystocele
p. ear
exposed protruding form
p. growth
intramural protruding form
p. lumbosacral disk
p. spine
p. tongue

protrusion
abnormal p.
anal p.
apoon-like protrusion of leaflet
conical protrusion of center of cornea
p. of disc
disc p.
p. of eye
p. of eyeball
p. of fetal part
forward p.
hernial p.
intervertebral disc p.
p. of iris
maxillary alveolar p.
medial disc p.
tongue p.
p. of tongue

protrusive relationship

protuberance
occipital p.

protuberans
dermatofibrosarcoma p.
fibrosarcomatous variant of dermatofibrosarcoma p.

protuberant abdomen

provided
not otherwise provided for

provider
dental health care p.
emergency care p.
exclusive provider organization
healthcare p.
mental health p.
midlevel p.
p. order entry
preferred p.

preferred provider organization
primary care p.
usual provider continuity

provisional
p. amputation
p. cortex
p. denture
p. diagnosis
p. fixation
P. International Standard

provocateur
agent p.

provocation
aggression without p.
bronchial provocation challenge
conjunctival provocation test
p. dose
dumping provocation test
ergonovine maleate provocation angina
ergonovine provocation test
histamine provocation test
hyperventilation provocation test
mucous membrane p.
nasal provocation test
pentagastrin provocation test

provocative
p. behavior
inappropriate sexually provocative behavior
methacholine provocative testing
mydriatic provocative test
p. test
p. testing
p. use test

provoked
electronically provoked response

proximal
absolute proximal reabsorption
Akin proximal phalangeal osteotomy
p. alveolar region
p. aorta
apical membrane of proximal convoluted tubule cell
p. articular set angle
p. aspect
autosomal recessive renal proximal tubulopathy and hypercalciuria
p. bile duct
p. bowel
p. bowel distention
p. brain shift
p. bronchiectasis
p. cavity
p. circumflex artery
p. clipping
p. clot
p. coil
p. collateral ligament
p. colon
p. communicating branch
p. contour
p. convoluted tubule
p. coronary
p. coronary sinus
p. dilation
distal and p.
p. and distal portion of vessel
diverting proximal colostomy
p. duodenum
early distal proximal tubule
p. end
p. end of rib
p. end of ulna
p. enterostomy
p. esophagus
feathered edge proximal finishing
p. femoral focal deficiency
p. femoral fracture
p. femur
p. femur focal deficiency
p. fibula
p. focal femoral deficiency
fractional proximal resorption
p. gastrectomy
p. gastric exclusion
p. gastric resection
p. gastric vagotomy
His bundle electrogram, p.
human proximal tubule
p. humeral fracture
p. humerus
identified proximal ends of tendon
p. interphalangeal/distal interphalangeal joints
p. interphalangeal joint
p. intestine
p. isovelocity surface area
p. jejunum
late proximal cortical tubule
p. left anterior descending artery
p. muscle weakness
p. myotonic myopathy
p. nail matrix
p. obstruction
p. occlusion
p. over-shoulder strap
p. palmar crease
p. phalanx
p. radioulnar joint
p. reference axis
selective proximal vagotomy
p. shaft
p. small bowel
p. spinal muscular atrophy
p. straight tubule
p. subcontact area
p. subungual onychomycosis
p. third of bone
p. tibia
p. tibial epiphysis
tibial fracture brace proximal support
p. tubal obstruction
p. tubular pressure
universal proximal femur prosthesis
p. ureter
p. ureterolithiasis
p. ureterolithotomy
p. vein thrombosis
ventricular atrial proximal coronary sinus

proximalis
articulatio radioulnaris p.
nodus lymphoideus proximalis profundus

proximum
punctum p.

proxy
factitious disorder by p.
Münchausen disease by p.
Münchausen by proxy syndrome

PrP^{Sc}-reactive plaque

prudent
p. living heart
p. no-salt-added diet

Pruitt-Inahara
P.-I. carotid shunt
P.-I. vascular shunt

prune
p. belly anomaly
p. belly syndrome

pruned tree appearance

prurigo
melanotic prurigo of Hebra
melanotic prurigo of Pierini

pruritic
eosinophilic, polymorphic, and pruritic eruption associated with radiotherapy
p. lesion
p. papular eruption
p. rash
p. urticarial papules and plaques

pruritic *(continued)*
p. urticarial papules and plaques of pregnancy
pruritus
anal p.
p. ani
aquagenic p.
jaundice p.
perineal p.
symptomatic p.
p. vulvae
vulvar p.
psammomatous meningioma
pseudarthrosis
Anderson tibial pseudarthrosis classification
failed back syndrome with documented p.
pseudoachievement syndrome
pseudoamniotic fluid
pseudoanemia
athlete's p.
pseudoaneurysm
anastomotic p.
aortic p.
arterial p.
peripancreatic p.
radial artery p.
ventricular p.
pseudoangiosarcoma
Masson p.
pseudoanodontia
growth retardation, alopecia, pseudoanodontia, and optic atrophy syndrome
pseudoarthrosis
long bone p.
pseudobulbar
p. palsy
p. paralysis
pseudocholinesterase
atypical p.
pseudocoloboma
macular p.
pseudocyesis
monosymptomatic delusional p.
pseudocyst
p. abscessed
auricular endochondral p.
p. formation
myxoid p.
necrotic bone p.
p. of pancreas
pancreatic p.
pseudoepithelioma
macrocephaly, pseudoepithelioma, multiple hemangiomas syndrome
pseudoepitheliomatous hyperplasia
pseudoexfoliation
p. of lens capsule
p. syndrome
pseudoexfoliative glaucoma
pseudofollicular growth center
pseudofracture
Looser p.
pseudoheart disease
pseudohemophilia hepatica
pseudohermaphrodites
male p.
pseudohermaphroditism
dysgenetic male p.
incomplete male p.
male p.
pseudohydrocephalic
neonatal pseudohydrocephalic progeroid syndrome
pseudohypoaldosteronism
p. type I, II
pseudohypoparathyroidism
Auerbach p.
pseudoidiopathic thrombocytopenic purpura
pseudoinflammatory
Sorsby pseudoinflammatory macular degeneration
pseudointimal hyperplasia
pseudoisochromatic
pseudoleukemica
anemia infantum p.
anemia pseudoleukemica infantum
pseudolupus erythematosus syndrome
pseudolymphocytic choriomeningitis
pseudomallei
melioidosis *Pseudomonas pseudomallei* vaccine
pseudomembranous
antibiotic-associated pseudomembranous colitis
p. bronchitis
p. candidiasis
p. cheilitis
p. colitis
p. conjunctivitis
p. enteritis
p. gastritis
p. gingivitis
p. lesion
p. necrotizing enterocolitis
necrotizing pseudomembranous colitis
p. rhinitis
pseudomonad
non-*Aeruginosa* p.
Pseudomonas
P. aeruginosa
Pseudomonas aeruginosa bacteremia
Pseudomonas aeruginosa pneumonia
anti-*Pseudomonas* human plasma
Pseudomonas cellulitis
Pseudomonas cepacia bacteremia
Pseudomonas exotoxin
P. infection
melioidosis *Pseudomonas pseudomallei* vaccine
Pseudomonas septicemia
pseudomucinous cyst
pseudomuscular hypertrophy
pseudomyxoma
peritoneal p.
p. peritonei
pseudonephritis
athlete's p.
pseudo-obstruction
chronic idiopathic intestinal pseudo-obstruction syndrome
idiopathic intestinal p.-o.
intestinal p.-o.
polyneuropathy, ophthalmoplegia, leukoencephalopathy, and intestinal p.-o.
pseudoparalysis
arthritic general p.
congenital atonic p.
pseudoparalytica
myasthenia gravis p.
pseudoparesis
alcoholic p.
pseudoperiodic lateralized paroxysmal discharge
pseudophakic
p. bullous keratopathy
p. corneal edema
p. eye
pseudopresumed ocular histoplasmosis syndrome

pseudoprogeria/Hallermann-Streiff

pseudorabies virus

pseudo-renal artery syndrome

pseudosarcomatous
p. fasciitis
p. fibromyxoid tumor
p. myofibroblastic tumor
nodular pseudosarcomatous fasciitis

pseudotabes
diphtheric p.

pseudotsugata
Orgyia pseudotsugata MNPV

pseudotumor
atelectatic asbestos p.
p. cerebri
p. cerebri syndrome
p. effect
fibroosseous p.
inflammatory p.
lymphoid inflammatory p.
nuchal fibrocartilaginous p.
ocular adnexal inflammatory p.

pseudovaginal perineoscrotal hypospadias

pseudovascular adenoid squamous cell carcinoma

pseudovitamin D deficiency rickets

pseudoxanthoma
p. elasticum
localized acquired cutaneous pseudoxanthoma elasticum

pseudo-Zollinger-Ellison syndrome

psi-interactive biomolecule

psittacosis
p. infection
p., lymphogranuloma venereum, trachoma
p. virus

psoas
p. abscess
greater psoas muscle
p. major
p. major muscle
p. shadow
p. sign

psoralen
p. plus ultraviolet light of A wavelength
trimethyl p.

psoriasiform
p. dermatitis
p. eruption
p. rash

psoriasis
anti-CD11a humanized monoclonal antibody for p.
p. area sensitivity index
p. area and severity index
arthritis-associated p.
erythrodermic p.
p. guttata
P. Life Stress Inventory
localized pustular p.
microabscess of p.
napkin p.
p. nummularis
p. orbicularis
pustular p.
p. severity scale

psoriatic
p. arthritis
p. arthropathy
axial psoriatic arthritis
p. dermatitis
p. diaper rash
noninvolved psoriatic skin
p. onychopachydermoperiostitis

psoriatica
arthropathia p.

psychasthenia
mixed compulsive states p.

psychedelic
distressing psychedelic experience
p. drug ingestion

psychiatric
accredited psychiatric hospital
p. admission
adult psychiatric hospital
p. aide
alcohol, epilepsy, insulin, overdose, uremia, trauma, infection, psychiatric, stroke
alcohol-related psychiatric problem
American P. Association
anger and violence psychiatric syndrome
anxiety-related psychiatric syndrome
p. assessment
Brief P. Rating Scale for Children
p. care
Child and Adolescent P. Assessment
childhood severity of psychiatric illness
Children's Interview for P. Disorders
Children's P. Rating Scale
p. clinician
coexisting psychiatric disorders
community-based psychiatric program
p. comorbidity
Computer-Assisted P. Evaluation and Review System
p. condition
p. conflict
p. consequence
p. deviate, subtle
p. diagnosis
p. diagnostic interview
p. disability
p. disease
p. disorder
distinct psychiatric disorder
p. disturbance
p. drug
p. education
p. effect
p. emergency service
p. emergency team
p. evaluation
P. Evaluation Form
P. Evaluation Profile
exacerbation of preexisting psychiatric illness
p. examination
p. family history
family psychiatric history
General Audit Inpatient P. Assessment Scale
General Purpose P. Questionnaire
genetic predisposition to psychiatric illness
Hamburg Rating Scale for P. Disorders
p. hospital
p. hospitalization
p. illness
initial psychiatric development
initial psychiatric treatment plan
innovative psychiatric nursing intervention
Inpatient Multidimensional P. Scale
inpatient psychiatric care
inpatient psychiatric consultation
inpatient psychiatric treatment
p. instability
p. intensive care unit

psychiatric *(continued)*
interruption of pregnancy for psychiatric indication
p. intervention
Iowa Structured P. Interview
P. Knowledge and Skills Self-Assessment Program
maximum-security forensic psychiatric hospital
National Association of P. Health Systems
paranoia and delusions psychiatric syndrome
post-Vietnam psychiatric syndrome
preschool-age psychiatric assessment
previous psychiatric history
private psychiatric hospital
P. Questionnaire Obsessive-Compulsive Neurosis
semistructured psychiatric interview
p. services section
p. social worker
p. specialist
P. Status Rating scale
P. Status Schedule
Wittenborn P. Rating Scale
Wittenborn P. Symptoms Inventory
young adult psychiatric assessment

psychiatrically impaired

psychiatrist
board certified p.
child p.
court-appointed p.
independent p.

psychiatry
administrative p.
adolescent p.
child p.
hospital and community p.
intermediate p.
military forensic p.
minority group p.
multidisciplinary group p.
p. and neurology
open p.
organized care p.
Pascal-Suttle Test psychiatry
Standard System of P.
Tell a Tale psychiatry
Trail-Making Test psychiatry

psychiatry-neurology

psychic
p. ability
p. aftershock
p. disorder
p. distress
p. energy
p. equivalent
p. experience
p. impotence
p. insomnia
Inventory of P. and Somatic Complaints in the Elderly

psychoacoustic
p. test
p. testing

psychoactive
p. doses of hallucinogen
p. drug
p. drug abuse
p. effect
intense psychoactive drug effect
other or unspecified psychoactive substance intoxication
p. properties of hallucinogen
self-administration of psychoactive drug
p. substance abuse and dependence
p. substance use disorder

psychoaffective disorder

psychoanalysis
child and adolescent p.

psychoanalytical
American P. Association

Psychodevelopment Checklist

psychodynamic
individual psychodynamic psychotherapy
p. and therapeutic education

psychoeducational
p. group therapy
P. Profile
Woodcock-Johnson P. Battery

Psycho-Epistemological Profile

psychogalvanic
p. reflex
p. response
p. skin resistance
p. skin response audiometry

psychogenic
allergic psychogenic disorder
p. alopecia
p. amnesia
p. anxiety
anxiety psychogenic disorder
p. aphasia
p. aphonia
appetite psychogenic disorder
p. arthralgia
p. aspermia
p. ataxia
p. chest pain
p. constipation
p. deafness
p. depression
p. dermatitis
p. diarrhea
p. disorder
p. dizziness
p. drug
p. dysmenorrhea
p. dyspareunia
p. dyspepsia
p. eczema
p. enuresis
p. erectile dysfunction
p. excitation
p. factor
p. fugue
p. gastric ulcer
p. headache
p. hearing impairment
p. hearing loss
p. illness
p. impotence
p. limp
low back pain psychogenic disorder
mass psychogenic illness
p. nocturnal polydipsia
p. paralysis
p. pelvic pain
p. rumination
p. vomiting

psychogeriatric
London P. Scale

psychokinesis
recurrent spontaneous p.

psychologic
p. adjustment
p. dysfunction
House-Tree-Person Projective Technique psychologic test
Myers-Briggs Type Indicator psychologic test
Object Sorting Scales psychologic test

psychological
p. abnormality
p. abuse

acute adverse psychological reaction
adverse psychological response
American P. Association
p. approach
Assessment in Infancy Ordinal Scales of P. Development
automatic psychological process
Bipolar Psychological Inventory
California P. Inventory
delirium, infection, atrophic urethritis and vaginitis, pharmaceuticals, psychological disorders, excessive urine output, restricted mobility, stool impaction
p. dependency
p. disorder
p. dysfunction
p. effects of hallucinogen
p. evaluation
p. examination
factitious illness with psychological symptoms
p. factor
p. first aid
P. General Well-Being Scale
p. growth
p. health
p. history as screening device
p. illness
p. impact
improved psychological adjustment
p. information, acquisition, processing, and control system
internal psychological conflict
presurgical psychological screening
P. Screening Inventory
p., social, and vocational
p. stress of hospitalization
p. warfare

psychologically impaired

psychologist
adolescent p.

psychology
child p.
nonturning against self psychology
Photo Articulation Test psychology
Picture Arrangement p.
Quick Test psychology, pregnancy, prothrombin
Yerkes-Bridges Test psychology

psychomotor
p. abnormality
p. activity
p. agitation
p. behavior
p. change
p. convulsion
p. delay
p. development
P. Development Index
p. disturbance
p. function
p. impairment
increased psychomotor activity
microcephaly, infantile spasm, psychomotor retardation, nephrotic syndrome
p. retardation
skeletal abnormalities, cutis laxa, craniostenosis, psychomotor retardation, facial abnormalities

psychoneurosis
anxiety p.
compulsion p.
depersonalization p.

psychoneurotic
anxiety psychoneurotic reaction

psychoorganic syndrome

psychopathic
amoral psychopathic personality
antisocial psychopathic Q factor
antisocial trends p.
antisocial trends psychopathic personality
asocial trends psychopathic personality
constitutional psychopathic state
p. deviate
inferiority

psychopathological
Comprehensive P. Rating Scale
Manchester and Oxford Universities Scale for the P. Assessment of Dementia

psychopathology
adult p.
comorbid p.
Current and Past P. Scales
deep-seated p.
human p.
Systematic Nursing Observation of P.

psychopathy
autistic p.
dull p.

psychopharmacology
adolescent p.

psychophysiologic
p. gastrointestinal reaction
p. musculoskeletal reaction

psychophysiological
complex psychophysiological process

psychosexual
adult-life psychosexual identity disorder
anal stage psychosexual development
atypical psychosexual dysfunction
p. development
disorders of psychosexual identity
p. dysfunction
p. history
p. identity

psychosis, pl. **psychoses**
active p.
affective alcoholic p.
affective paranoid organic p.
affective schizophreniform p.
akinetic p.
alcoholic Korsakoff p.
alcoholic liver disease-type organic p.
alcoholic paranoid p.
alcoholic polyneuritic p.
alcoholism organic p.
alternating p.
alternative p.
Alzheimer p.
amphetamine p.
anergastic organic p.
anxiety-blissfulness p.
arteriosclerotic brain disease-type organic p.
arteriosclerotic psychosis confusional state
atropine p.
atypical childhood p.
autistic p.
autoscopic p.
bipolar p.
cannabis p.
p. in childbirth
childbirth organic p.
p. of childhood
delusional transient organic p.
depressive p.
depressive-type p.
p. during pregnancy
p. in the elderly
electroshock-induced p.

psychosis *(continued)*
embarrassment p.
emotional stress depressive p.
endocrine disease organic p.
excitative-type p.
febrile p.
full-blown p.
hereditary psychoses
hysteria p.
intensive care unit p.
p., intermittent hyponatremia, polydipsia syndrome
Korsakoff p.
liver disease organic p.
major depressive affective p.
manic-depressive p.
melancholia affective p.
metabolic disease organic p.
mixed bipolar affective p.
monosymptomatic hypochondriacal p.
organic p.
paranoid p.
paranoid-type alcoholic p.
paranoid-type arteriosclerotic p.
pathologic drug intoxication drug p.
postictal p.
postpartum p.
scale of p.
self-induced water intoxication and p.
unipolar p.

psychosocial
P. Adjustment to Illness Scale
adverse psychosocial environment
p. assessment
P. Assessment of Childhood Experiences
p. care
clinical appraisal of psychosocial problem
complete psychosocial history
p. deprivation
p. development
p. evaluation
p. function
p. functioning
Giannetti Online P. History
p. history
P. History Screening Questionnaire
P. History Screening Test
Inventory of P. Development
Measures of P. Development
p. stressors
p. therapy

psychosocial-labile

psychosomatic
p. aches and pains
p. complaint
p. disease
p. disorder
Freeman Anxiety Neurosis and P. Test
p. illness
p. inventory
p. medicine

psychostimulant
p. dependence
p. drug

psychosyndrome
algogenic p.

psychotherapeutic
p. agent
p. drug
p. intervention

psychotherapy
activity-interview group p.
analytic group p.
P. Competence Assessment Schedule
exploratory insight-oriented p.
harm reduction p.
individual psychodynamic p.
intensive insight-oriented p.
interpersonal p.
marathon group p.
p. responder
short-term anxiety-provoking p.
time-limited p.

psychotic
acute psychotic episode
aggressive psychotic behavior
aggressive psychotic inpatient
alcohol-induced psychotic disorder
alcohol-induced psychotic disorder with delusions
alcohol-induced psychotic disorder with hallucinations
amphetamine-induced psychotic disorder with delusions
amphetamine-induced psychotic disorder with hallucinations
anxiolytic-induced psychotic disorder with delusions
anxiolytic-induced psychotic disorder with hallucinations
p. attack
p. behavior
p. brain syndrome
cannabis-induced psychotic disorder with delusions
cannabis-induced psychotic disorder with hallucinations
p. dementia
p. depression
p. disturbance
electroshock-induced psychotic syndrome
explosive psychotic state
p. factor
p. illness
p. individual
P. Inpatient Profile
mood-congruent psychotic feature
nonaffective psychotic disorder
other than p.
P. Reaction Profile
p. symptom
p. thought disorder
p. trigger reaction

psychotropic
p. agent
p. drug
p. medication
p. medication plan
self-administration of psychotropic drug
p. therapy

psyllium hydrophilic mucilloid

pteroyltriglutamic acid

pterygium
Arlt p.
Arlt pterygium excision
head of p.
McReynolds pterygium scissors
McReynolds pterygium transplant
multiple pterygium syndrome

pterygoalar bar

pterygoarthromyodysplasia, congenital

pterygoid
artery of pterygoid canal
p. branch
p. branch of maxillary artery
p. branch of posterior deep temporal artery
p. canal
p. chest
p. depression
p. fissure
p. fossa
lateral pterygoid muscle
lateral pterygoid plate
medial pterygoid muscle
medial pterygoid plate
p. muscle

pharyngeal branch of artery of pterygoid canal
p. plate
p. process

pterygoidei
arteria canalis p.
nervus canalis p.

pterygomaxillary
p. area
p. buttress
p. dysjunction
p. fissure
p. fossa

pterygomeningealis
arteria p.

pterygopalatine
p. canal
p. fossa
p. fossa syndrome
p. ganglion
p. groove
orbital branch of pterygopalatine ganglion

PTH-related protein

ptosis, pl. **ptoses**
age-related p.
aponeurogenic p.
aponeurotic p.
blepharophimosis, ptosis, epicanthus inversus syndrome
p. of chin
p. of eyelid
p. of kidney
Machek ptosis operation
Marcus Gunn jaw-winking p.
mechanical acquired p.
midbrain p.
morning p.
myogenic acquired p.
myopathic p.
neurogenic acquired p.
neuromuscular p.

ptotic
p. brow
p. ear
p. eyebrow
p. kidney

pubarche
precocious p.

pubertal
hypothalamic pubertal syndrome
Marshall and Tanner pubertal stage

puberty
central precocious p.
idiopathic isosexual p.
male-limited familial precocious p.
male precocious p.
neurogenic precocious p.
Williams syndrome, early p.
Williams syndrome, late p.

pubic
absence of facial and pubic hair
p. angle
p. arch
arcuate pubic ligament
p. bone
p. crest
p. hair
p. hair line
inferior point of pubic bone
p. lice
masculine pubic hair
narrow pubic arch
obturator branch of pubic branch of inferior epigastric vein
parallel development of pubic hair
p. ramus
sacrococcygeal to inferior pubic point
p. symphysis
p. tubercle

pubis
arcuate ligament of p.
arcus p.
hair of p.
mons p.
os p.
osteitis symphysis p.
pectineal line of p.
pediculosis p.
sacrum to p.
xiphoid to p.

public
p. access defibrillation
p. access defibrillator
p. health
p. health education program
p. health hazard
p. health nurse
p. health official
p. relations
p. service announcement

publication
not for p.

publish
do not p.

published
not yet p.

pubocervical
p. fascia
p. ligament

pubococcygeal
p. line
p. muscle

puboprostatic ligament

puborectal muscle

pubourethral ligament

pubovaginal
minimal-incision pubovaginal suspension
p. muscle

pubovesicale

pubovesicalis
plica p.

pubovesical ligament

Puchong virus

pucker
macular p.

puckering
macular p.

pudding-thick liquid diet consistency

pudenda, pl. **pudendae**

pudendal
p. anesthesia
anterior labial branch of deep external pudendal artery
anterior scrotal branch of deep external pudendal artery
p. area
p. artery
p. block
p. branch
p. canal
p. cleavage
p. cleft
disposable pudendal nerve electrode
p. evoked response
p. hernia
internal pudendal vein
p. nerve
superficial external pudendal artery
p. ulcer
p. vein

pudendal-nerve terminal motor latency

pudendi
noma p.

puerperal
- p. convulsion
- p. eclampsia
- p. endometritis
- p. fever
- p. hematoma
- p. hemiplegia
- p. infection
- p. insanity
- p. mastitis
- p. ovarian vein thrombophlebitis
- p. ovarian vein thrombosis
- p. sepsis

puffer
- pink puffer sign of emphysema

puffiness
- p. of face
- p. of feet
- p. of hands
- molimina of p.
- periorbital p.

puffy
- p. ankles
- p. face
- p. gums
- gums red and p.
- Pott puffy tumor

pugilistic
- median cleft upper lip, mental retardation, pugilistic facies syndrome

pullback
- aortic p.
- aortic pullback pressure

pulled catheter out

pulley
- annular p.
- anular p.
- bone p.
- p. tendon

pulling
- compulsive hair p.
- ear p.
- fidgeting, aching, pulling, or itching feeling
- pathological hair p.

pulling-boat hands

pulls
- patient pulls hair

pullthrough
- slow p.

pull-through
- endorectal ileal p.-t.
- endorectal ileoanal p.-t.
- station p.-t.

pulmocutaneous exchange

pulmonales
- lymphonodus juxta-esophageales p.

pulmonalis
- arteria p.
- pars basalis arteriae p.

pulmonary
- abnormal pulmonary function
- p. abscess
- absence of branch pulmonary artery
- accessory pulmonary blood flow
- active pulmonary disease
- acute bovine pulmonary edema
- acute cardiogenic pulmonary edema
- acute pulmonary edema
- acute pulmonary hemorrhage
- p. adenopathy
- adventitial pulmonary sound
- p. agenesis
- allergic pulmonary edema
- p. alveolar hemorrhage
- p. alveolar hypoxic vasoconstriction
- p. alveolar macrophage
- p. alveolar microlithiasis
- p. alveolar proteinosis
- alveolar pulmonary edema
- p. alveoli
- p. angiogram
- p. angiography
- p. angioma
- p. angiotensin I converting enzyme
- anomalous left coronary artery from pulmonary artery
- anomalous left coronary artery from pulmonary artery syndrome
- anomalous left pulmonary artery
- anomalous origin of left coronary artery from pulmonary artery
- anomalous pulmonary vein
- anomalous pulmonary venous connection, total or partial
- anomalous pulmonary venous drainage
- anomalous pulmonary venous return
- anomalous right pulmonary vein dextroposition
- p. anomalous superior venous return
- anomaly of drainage of pulmonary vein
- anterior pulmonary branch of vagus nerve
- anterior pulmonary plexus
- aortic p.
- aortic second sound, pulmonary second sound
- p. apex
- apical branch of inferior lobar branch of right pulmonary artery
- apical branch of right superior pulmonary vein
- apicoposterior branch of left superior pulmonary vein
- p. area
- p. arterial diastolic pressure
- p. arterial pressure-pulmonary venous pressure
- p. arterial stenosis
- p. arteriolar resistance
- p. arteriovenous aneurysm
- p. arteriovenous fistula
- p. arteriovenous malformation
- arteriovenous pulmonary aneurysm
- p. artery
- p. artery anastomosis
- p. artery aneurysm
- p. artery atresia
- p. artery balloon pump
- p. artery banding
- p. artery bifurcation
- p. artery blockage
- p. artery catheter
- p. artery catheterization
- p. artery counterpulsation
- p. artery diastolic
- p. artery diastolic and wedge pressure
- p. artery embolization
- p. artery end-diastolic pressure
- p. artery filling defect
- p. artery hemorrhage
- p. artery hypertension
- p. artery hypotension
- p. artery line
- p. artery obstruction
- p. artery occlusion pressure
- p. artery pressure monitoring
- p. artery rupture
- p. artery steal
- p. artery stenosis
- p. artery stenting
- p. artery systolic
- p. artery systolic/diastolic
- p. artery systolic pressure
- p. artery thromboembolism
- p. artery thromboendarterectomy
- p. artery trunk
- p. artery wedge
- p. asbestosis

p. aspergillosis
asymmetric pulmonary congestion
p. atelectasis
atherosclerotic pulmonary vascular disease
p. atresia/pulmonary stenosis
p. atresia with intact ventricular septum
p. atresia with ventricular septal defect
p. autograft
balloon pulmonary valvuloplasty
p. balloon valvuloplasty
basilar pulmonary infiltrate
bilateral alveolar pulmonary infiltrate
p. bleb
p. blood clot
p. blood flow
p. blood mixing volume
p. blood volume index
p. branch stenosis
p. bypass
p. capillary
p. capillary blood flow perfusion
p. capillary blood volume
p. capillary gas volume
p. capillary hemangiomatosis
p. capillary protein leakage
p. capillary wedge
p. capillary wedge pressure
p. carcinoma
cardiac and pulmonary rehabilitation
p. care team
p. cavitation
central pulmonary vasculature
chronic obstructive pulmonary disease
chronic obstructive pulmonary emphysema
chronic pulmonary insufficiency of prematurity
chronic pulmonary interstitial fibrosis
chronic restrictive pulmonary disease
chronic thromboembolic pulmonary hypertension
chronic thrombotic pulmonary vascular obstruction
p. circulation
p. clearance delay
clinical pulmonary infection score
coarctation of pulmonary arteries
p. collagen vascular disease
p. collapse
p. complication
congenital pulmonary cystic lymphangiectasia
congenital pulmonary lymphangiectasia
p. congestion
p. consolidation
p. contusion
p. cyst
delayed pulmonary toxicity syndrome
diaphragmatic pulmonary infarct
diastolic pulmonary artery pressure
diffuse interstitial pulmonary calcification
diffuse interstitial pulmonary disease
diffuse interstitial pulmonary fibrosis
diffuse obstructive pulmonary syndrome
diffuse pulmonary alveolar hemorrhage
diffuse pulmonary hemorrhage
diffuse pulmonary infiltrate
p. diffusing capacity
p. diffusing study
p. diffusion capacity
p. disease
p. disease anemia
p. disorder
dynamic pulmonary imaging
p. dysfunction
p. dysplasia
p. edema
p. edema fluid
effective pulmonary blood flow
p. effusion
p. ejection click
p. embolectomy
p. embolism
p. embolus
p. embolus with small infarct
p. emphysema
p. endodermal tumor
p. endothelial membrane
epibronchial right pulmonary artery syndrome
essential pulmonary hemosiderosis
p. extravascular fluid volume
p. extravascular water volume
p. factor
p. failure
familial primary pulmonary hypertension
fatal pulmonary hemorrhage
fluffy pulmonary infiltrate
p. flushing
fulminant pulmonary edema
p. function
P. Functional Status and Dyspnea Questionnaire
p. function score
p. function study
p. function test
p. gas exchange
p. granuloma
p. granulomatosis
p. groove
p. hamartoma
hantavirus pulmonary syndrome
p. heart disease
p. heart valve disorder
p. hemorrhagic necrosis
p. hemosiderosis
high-altitude pulmonary edema
p. hilum
p. histiocytosis
p. hyaline membrane
p. hyalinizing granuloma
hydrostatic pulmonary edema
hypercarbia pulmonary hypertension
p. hypertension pressure
hypertensive pulmonary vascular disease
p. hypertrophic osteoarthropathy
hypertrophic pulmonary osteoarthritis
hypertrophic pulmonary osteoarthropathy
p. hypoplasia
p. hypoplasia membrane disease
p. hypothalamic stimulation
hypoxia-induced pulmonary hypertension
hypoxic pulmonary vasoconstriction
idiopathic interstitial pulmonary fibrosis
idiopathic pulmonary arteriosclerosis
idiopathic pulmonary hemorrhage
p. immaturity
p. immaturity and atelectasis
p. immaturity of prematurity
p. incompetence
increased pulmonary artery pressure
index of pulmonary vascular disease
p. infarct
p. infarction

pulmonary *(continued)*
p. infection
p. infiltrate
p. infiltrate fever
p. infiltrate with eosinophilia
p. infiltration
p. infiltration with eosinophilia
infundibular pulmonary stenosis
p. injury
injury pulmonary edema
p. insufficiency
p. insufficiency of the premature
p. insufficiency of prematurity
p. intensive care unit
p. interstitial disorder
p. interstitial edema
p. interstitial emphysema
p. interstitial fibrosis
interstitial pulmonary edema
interstitial pulmonary emphysema
p. intimal sarcoma
intratracheal pulmonary ventilation
invasive pulmonary aspergillosis
p. Kaposi sarcoma
p. lavage
left inferior pulmonary vein
left pulmonary artery oxygen saturation
lentigines, electrocardiographic abnormalities, ocular hypertelorism, pulmonary stenosis, abnormalities of genitalia, retardation of growth, deafness syndrome
p. lesion
p. ligament
p. lymphoid hyperplasia
p. lymphoma
malposition of the branch pulmonary artery
malposition of branch pulmonary artery
p. markings
massive pulmonary embolus
massive pulmonary hemorrhage
p. maturation
p. maturity
mean pulmonary artery wedge pressure
mean pulmonary capillary wedge pressure
mean pulmonary transit time
p. mean transit time
medial basal branch of pulmonary artery
p. metastasis
p. microvascular permeability to protein
middle lobe branch of right superior pulmonary vein
miliary pulmonary aspergillosis
multiple interstitial pulmonary hemorrhage
multiple pulmonary infarct
p. mycosis
narrow pulmonary outflow tract
p. necrosis
neonatal cystic pulmonary emphysema
Neonatal P. Insufficiency Index
p. neuroendocrine cell
p. neuroepithelial endocrine
no active pulmonary disease
nodular pulmonary amyloidosis
p. nodule
no evidence of pulmonary disease
noncardiac pulmonary edema
noncavitating pulmonary nodule
nonhydrostatic pulmonary edema
normal pulmonary function
obliterative pulmonary hypotension
p. obstruction
obstructive pulmonary emphysema
occult pulmonary embolus
oxygen concentration in pulmonary capillary blood
p. parenchyma
p. parenchymal disease
p. parenchymal tissue volume
p. parenchymal window
partial anomalous pulmonary veins
partial anomalous pulmonary venous connection
partial anomalous pulmonary venous drainage
partial anomalous pulmonary venous return
passive pulmonary hypertension
p. perfusion scanning
peripheral pulmonary artery stenosis
permeability pulmonary edema
persistent fetal circulation with pulmonary hypertension
persistent interstitial pulmonary emphysema
persistent pulmonary hypertension
persistent pulmonary hypertension of newborn
p. platelet trapping
p. pleura
p. pleurisy
postoperative pulmonary function
postoperative pulmonary problem
posttraumatic pulmonary insufficiency
primary pulmonary hypertension murmur
primary pulmonary hypertension risk factor
primary pulmonary non-Hodgkin lymphoma
progressive interstitial pulmonary fibrosis
prominence of pulmonary markings
prominence of pulmonary vasculature
prominence of pulmonary vessel
pure pulmonary atresia
ratio of pulmonary to systemic circulation
recurrent pulmonary emboli
regional pediatric pulmonary center
regional pulmonary blood flow
p. regurgitation
p. rehabilitation
p. reimplantation response
right descending pulmonary artery
right pulmonary artery withdrawal
right pulmonary vein
p. scintigraphy
p. scleroderma
secondary pulmonary hypertension
secondary pulmonary hypoplasia
septic pulmonary edema
p. sequestration
sheep pulmonary adenomatosis
p. siderosis
solitary pulmonary nodule
p. stretch receptor
submassive pulmonary embolism
superior pulmonary vein isolated
surgical pulmonary intensive care unit
p. talcosis
p. thromboembolectomy
p. thromboembolic disease
thromboembolic pulmonary hypertension
p. thrombosis
thrombotic pulmonary artery
p. tissue concentration
p. toilet
total anomalous pulmonary circulation

total anomalous pulmonary venous connection
total anomalous pulmonary venous drainage
total anomalous pulmonary venous return
total pulmonary blood flow
total pulmonary vascular resistance
p. tuberculosis
upper lobe pulmonary edema
p. valve anomaly
p. valve area
p. valve disease
p. valve dysplasia
p. valve gradient
p. valve opening
p. valve stenosis
p. valvotomy
p. valvuloplasty
p. valvulotomy
p. vascular disorder
p. vascular hyperplasia
p. vascular hypertension
p. vascularity
p. vascular obstruction
p. vascular obstructive disease
p. vascular resistance
p. vascular resistance index
p. vasculature
p. vein
p. vein atrial reversal
p. vein stenosis
p. venoocclusive disease
p. venous capillary
p. venous congestion
p. venous flow
p. venous obstruction
p. venous occlusion
p. venous pressure
p. venous redistribution
p. venous return
p. ventilation
p. ventilation impairment
vigorous pulmonary toilet
Wegener pulmonary granulomatosis

pulmonary-to-systemic flow ratio

pulmonic

p. area
p. closure
p. closure sound
p. endocarditis
p. heart sound less than aortic second heart sound
p. incompetence
p. insufficiency
mild pulmonic stenosis
p. murmur
percutaneous balloon pulmonic valvuloplasty
p. regurgitation
second aortic sound equals second pulmonic sound
second aortic sound greater than second pulmonic sound
second aortic sound less than second pulmonic sound
p. second heart sound equal to aortic second heart sound
p. second heart sound greater than aortic second heart sound
p. second sound split
p. valve
p. valve stenosis
valvular pulmonic stenosis

pulp

p. abscess
p. amputation
artery of p.
atrophic p.
axial wall of pulp chamber
p. canal
p. canal sealer
p. chamber
chronic perforating hyperplasia of p.
devitalized p.
finger p.
gangrenous pulp necrosis
p. hernia
p. horn
p. hyperemia
microsurgical free pulp flap
white p.
wood pulp worker lung

pulposus

herniated nucleus p.
herniation of nucleus p.
nucleus pulposus herniation

pulpotomy

formocresol p.

pulsatile

p. assist device
p. discharge
p. epigastric mass
p. fontanelle
p. hematoma
p. tinnitus

pulsatility

anterior cerebral artery pulsatility index
arterial p.
femoral pulsatility index
hepatic arterial pulsatility index
p. index

pulsating

p. aneurysm
p. aorta
p. current
p. electromagnetic field
p. empyema
p. exophthalmos
p. headache
p. hematoma
p. mass
p. neck vein

pulsation

arterial pulsation artifact
ascending aorta synchronized p.
intraaortic balloon p.
jugular venous p.
spontaneous venous p.

pulse

p. amplitude
p. amplitude ratio
apical p.
p. apical
apical-radial p.
asynchronous pulse generator
atrial liver p.
atrial synchronous pulse generator
atrial triggered pulse generator
average pulse magnitude
bilateral pedal pulses present
blood pressure and p.
blood pressure, pulse, respiration, and temperature
blood volume p.
carotid pulse tracing
cine pulse system
p. code modulation
p. cytophotometry
deep p.
p. deficit
differential pulse polarography
dorsalis pedis p.
p. duration
electromagnetic p.
p. frequency
p. generated runoff
p. generator
half amplitude pulse duration
implantable pulse generator
increased pulse rate
p. interval
irregularity of p.
irregularly irregular p.
jugular venous p.

pulse *(continued)*
jugular venous pulse tracing
key pulse rate
MARS pulse oximetry
Masimo SET signal extraction pulse oximetry
maximal pulse rate measurement
p. mode
motion compensation gradient p.
motion-resistant pulse oximetry
nerve net p.
normal resting p.
normal resting pulse rate
Ohmeda Minx pulse oximeter
p. oximeter
p. oximeter/end tidal CO_2
p. oximetry
p. oximetry monitoring
p. oximetry on 2 liters of oxygen
p. oximetry waveform systolic blood pressure
oxygen saturation as measured using pulse oximetry
pacemaker pulse generator
pain, pallor, pulse loss, paresthesia, and paralysis
palpable carotid p.
palpable femoral p.
palpable radial p.
paradoxical p.
pedal p.
pedal p.'s equal and strong
pedal pulse not palpable
pedal pulse palpable
pedal pulse present
pedal pulse weak
penile-brachial pulse index
periodic short p.
peripheral p.
peripheral p.'s full and equal bilaterally
peripheral p.'s intact
peripheral p.'s palpable both legs
peripheral pulse palpable
p.'s per minute
posterior tibial p.
p., motor, and sensory
Quincke capillary p.
radial p.
p. rate
reflectance pulse oximetry
p. regular
p. repetition
p. repetition frequency
p. and respiration
p. sequence
sequential p.
spontaneous venous p.
standard temperature and p.
temperature and p.
temperature, pulse, and respiration
p. transmission time
p. value recording
vertical synchronization p.
p. volume recorder
p. volume recording
p. wave velocity
p. weak
p. weak and rapid
p. width
xylol pulse indicator

pulsed
p. ablation
p. diathermy
p. Doppler cross-sectional echocardiography
p. Doppler echo
p. Doppler echocardiogram
p. Doppler echocardiography
p. Doppler flowmetry
p. Doppler ultrasonic flowmeter
p. Doppler ultrasonography
p. dose rate
p. electromagnetic field
p. electromagnetic stimulator
endoscopic pulsed dye laser
endoscopic pulsed dye laser lithotripsy
flashlamp pulsed dye laser
flashlamp-pumped pulsed dye laser
p. gradient
high-energy pulsed ruby laser
high-pH anion exchange chromatography coupled with pulsed amperometric detection
high-voltage pulsed current
high-voltage pulsed galvanic stimulation
p. idioventricular rhythm
p. inotrope therapy
intense pulsed light source
p. irrigation for enhanced evacuation
p. laser ablation
p. light therapy
p. ultrasonic blood velocity detector
p. ultraviolet actinotherapy
p. wave

pulsed-field gradient gel electrophoresis

pulsed-gradient spin echo

pulsed-wave
p.-w. Doppler echocardiogram
p.-w. Doppler echocardiography
p.-w. Doppler mapping
p.-w. tissue Doppler

pulse-height analyzer

pulse-inversion
p.-i. contrast harmonic imaging
p.-i. mode ultrasound

pulseless
p. electrical activity
p. idioventricular rhythm

pulse-synchronized contractions

pulse-wave speed

pulsus paradoxus

Pulvertaft fishmouth incision

pump
artificial left heart p.
bile salt export p.
cardiac balloon p.
continuous subcutaneous insulin infusion p.
external insulin p.
implantable drug infusion p.
implantable insulin infusion p.
infusion p.
insulin pen p.
internal insulin p.
intraaortic balloon p.
left ventricle bypass p.
low-pressure breast p.
manual breast p.
mechanical heart p.
mechanical insulin p.
Na^+-K^+ ATPase p.
open-loop pump therapy
p. oxygenation
pain control infusion p.
portable insulin infusion p.
proton pump blocker
pulmonary artery balloon p.
rapid infusion p.
subcutaneous morphine p.

pumping
p. ability of failing heart
p. ability of weakened heart
p. function of heart
heart p.
heart pumping action
heart pumping chamber
impaired pumping ability
inefficient pumping of blood
intraaortic balloon pumping assistance

Rasor blood pumping system
single-action pumping system
venoarterial bypass p.

pump-operated penile implant

punch
antrum punch forceps
arthroscopic p.
Australian p.
backward-biting ostrum p.
p. biopsy
bone-biting p.
bone graft p.
disc p.
dural p.
kidney punch
kidney punch test
lunate facet dye punch injury
Luntz-Dodick p.
Murphy punch maneuver test
negative punch biopsy
Orentreich p.
sclerotomy p.
sclerotomy with p.

punched-out area

puncta (*pl. of* punctum)

punctal
p. occlusion
p. plug

punctata
chondrodysplasia p.
keratitis p.
rhizomelic chondrodysplasia p.

punctate
p. area of increased signal
p. calcification
p. epithelial erosion
p. epithelial keratopathy
p. hemorrhage
orange punctate pigmentation
p. rash
p. subepithelial infiltrate
superficial punctate erosion
superficial punctate keratitis

punctuate
p. hemorrhage
multiple punctuate hemorrhage

punctum, pl. **puncta**
p. lacrimale
lower p.
Micro punctum plug
one-snip p.
one-snip punctum operation
p. proximum
p. remotum

puncture
apical left ventricular p.
arterial puncture site closure device
p., aspiration, injection, reaspiration
cecal ligation and p.
direct cardiac p.
fluoroscopic-assisted lumbar p.
follicle puncture for oocyte retrieval
p. headache
hemostatic puncture closure device
p. laceration
lumbar p.
lumbar puncture headache
lumbar puncture manometry
Marfan epigastric p.
multiple puncture tuberculin test
p. needle
percutaneous cord cyst p.
percutaneous needle p.
postdural puncture headache
postlumbar puncture headache
prostate puncture biopsy
p. site
skin puncture test
suprapubic p.
tracheoesophageal p.
tracheojejunal p.
transesophageal p.
transvaginal amniotic p.
p. wound
p. wound of foot

punctured lung

punishing behavior of bulimic

punishment
corporal p.
cruel p.

Punta
P. Salinas virus
P. Toro virus

pupil
Adie tonic p.
Argyll-Robertson pupil sign
asymmetric p.
attention reflex of p.
change in color of p.
contraction of p.
dark-adapted pupil size
dilated p.'s and hypothermia
p. dilation
p.'s equal and reactive to light and accommodation
p.'s equal, round, reactive to light and accommodation
p.'s equal, round, reactive to light and accommodation directly and consensually
p.'s equal in size and reaction
fixed and dilated p.
iris and p.
light response of p.
local tonic p.
Marcus Gunn p.
p.'s mid-position, fixed
p. miosis
moderately constricted and equally reactive p.
moderately constricted and slightly reactive p.
moderately dilated and equally reactive p.
moderately dilated and slightly reactive p.
neuropathic tonic p.
p. nonreactive
occlusion of p.
p. pinpoint
p. rating scale
p. reaction and size
p. reactive
reactive to light p.
p.'s react to light and accommodation
p.'s react sluggishly
P. Record of Education Behavior
Rhode Island P. Identification Scale
round pupil intracapsular cataract extraction
p. round and regular
round, regular, and equal p.
p. stretching
p.'s, tension, media, disc, and fundus
p.'s unreactive

pupilla, pl. **pupillae**
ectopia pupillae congenita
musculus dilator pupillae
musculus dilator p.
musculus sphincter p.

pupillaris
membrana p.

pupillary
p. abnormality
afferent pupillary defect
aphakic pupillary block
p. center
p. change
consensual pupillary response

pupillary *(continued)*
p. constriction
p. defect
p. dilatation
p. distance
p. entrapment
Gunn pupillary reflex
hyperplastic persistent pupillary membrane
increase in pupillary diameter
p. light reflex
Marcus Gunn pupillary sign
p. membrane
normal pupillary reaction to light
orbicularis pupillary reflex
paradoxical pupillary phenomenon
paradoxical pupillary reflex
p. paralysis
persistent pupillary membrane
persistent pupillary membrane remnant
pigmented pupillary membrane
p. reaction
p. reflex
relative afferent pupillary defect
p. sphincter muscle
Westphal pupillary reflex
p. zone

pupillography
electronic p.

Purdue
P. Perceptual-Motor Survey
P. Student-Teacher Opinionnaire
P. Teacher Questionnaire

pure
p. agraphia
p. aphasia
p. blowout fracture
chemically p.
chronic, acquired, pure red cell aplasia
commercially p.
depression pure disease
p. dysarthria
familial pure depressive disease
p. free acid
p. gonadal dysgenesis
marbled pure tone
minimal pure radium equivalent
p. motor hemiparesis
p. pancreatic juice
partially pure human leukocyte interferon
p. pulmonary atresia
p. red blood cell agenesis
p. red blood cell aplasia
p. red cell aplasia
p. sensory stroke
p. sensory syndrome
p. tone acuity
p. tone audiometry
p. tone average
p. tone threshold
p. ultrafiltration
p. vegetarian

pureed, mechanical, soft diet

purge
binge and p.
binge and purge syndrome
bulimic p.

purging
p. behavior
p. behavior of bulimic
bingeing and p.

purified
p. alternate pathway
p. *Brucella* protein
p. cell walls
p. chick embryo cell culture
p. diphtheria toxoid precipitated by aluminum phosphate
p. fibrillar collagen
p. fusion protein
highly p.
micronized purified flavonoid fracture
monocomponent highly purified pork insulin
p. placental protein
p. placental protein, human
p. porcine insulin
p. pork insulin
p. protein derivative
p. protein derivative–Battey
p. protein derivative of tuberculin
p. protein derivative–standard
p. protein derivative test
rabies vaccine, purified chick embryo cell culture
Siebert purified protein derivative of tuberculin
p. spleen extract

purine
p. base
p. body
p. metabolism
p. nucleotide cycle

purine-free diet

purinergic agonist

Puritan heated nebulizer

purity
radionuclide p.
ultrahigh p.

Purkinje
P. cell
cerebellar Purkinje cell
P. corpuscle
P. fiber
P. layer
P. phenomenon
P. tumor

puromycin
p. aminonucleoside nephropathy

purple
p. agarbase medium
bromcresol p.
p. urine bag syndrome

purplish hemorrhagic spot on skin

purpose
cosmetic and functional p.
general all p.
General P. Psychiatric Questionnaire
p. in life

purposeful
autism, dementia, ataxia, loss of purposeful hand use syndrome
inability to perform purposeful movements
p. movements
patient has no purposeful movement

purpura
acute idiopathic thrombocytopenic p.
allergic nonthrombocytopenic p.
alloimmune neonatal thrombocytopenic p.
autoimmune thrombocytopenic p.
Bauhinia purpura agglutinin
chronic pigmental p.
p. fulminans
hemolytic uremic syndrome/thrombotic thrombocytopenia p.
p. hemorrhagica
Henoch-Schönlein p.
Henoch-Schönlein purpura nephritis
hyperglobulinemia p.
idiopathic thrombocytopenia p.
idiopathic thrombocytopenic p.
immune thrombocytopenic p.
Moschcowitz thrombotic thrombocytopenic purpura disease

neonatal alloimmune thrombocytopenic p.
posttransfusion p.
pseudoidiopathic thrombocytopenic p.
Schönlein-Henoch p.
Schönlein -Henoch p.
thrombocytopenic p.
thrombotic thrombocytopenic p.
thrombotic thrombocytopenic purpura and hemolytic uremic syndrome

purpuric
Brazilian purpuric fever
p. hemorrhage
p. lesion
patchy purpuric hemorrhage

pursed-lip breathing

purse-string suture

pursuit
p. abnormality
p. eye movement
p. goal
smooth pursuit eye movement
p. testing
p. tracking

purulent
p. appendicitis
p. arthritis
p. ascites
p. conjunctivitis
p. discharge
drainage of purulent material
p. encephalitis
p. enterocolitis
p. exudate
p. fluid
p. and foul smelling
p. gastritis
Gram stain of purulent discharge
p. iritis
p. keratitis
p. material
p. meningitis
p. nasal drainage
necrotic purulent material
oozing of purulent material
p. otitis media
otitis media, purulent, acute
p. pericarditis
p. pharyngitis
p. pneumonia
p. retinitis
p. rhinitis
p. secretion
p. sputum
p. synovitis
p. wound

purulenta
myositis p.
myositis purulenta tropica

Purus virus

pus
p. accumulation
p. at incision site
cheesy p.
p. coating stool
p. collection
curdy p.
p. in ear
frank p.
p. from conjunctivitis
heat, absence of use, redness, pain, pus, swelling
loculated p.
pocket of p.
p. pocket
p. in urine

push
p. fluids
intravenous push dose
slow intravenous p.

pusher
band p.
endoscopic knot p.
femoral component p.

pushup
neck p.

pustular
contagious pustular dermatitis
contagious pustular stomatitis
eosinophilic pustular folliculitis
p. eruption
infectious pustular vaginitis
p. lesion
localized pustular psoriasis
neonatal pustular melanosis
p. pharyngitis
p. psoriasis
subcorneal pustular dermatosis
p. tonsillitis
transient neonatal pustular melanosis
p. varicella

pustule
anthrax malignant p.
malignant p.
rash p.

pustulosa
miliaria p.

pustulosis
acute generalized exanthematous p.
p. palmaris et plantaris
palmoplantar p.
synovitis, acne, pustulosis, hyperostosis, osteomyelitis syndrome

putamen
caudate p.
dorsal caudate p.

putty

Puumala
P. hantavirus
P. virus

Puusepp reflex

P-wave
diphasic P.-w.

pyelitis
calculous p.
encrusted p.
p. glandularis
p. granulosa
p. gravidarum
hematogenous p.
hemorrhagic p.

pyelocalyceal system

pyelogram
drip-infusion p.
intravenous p.
limited intravenous p.
retrograde p.

pyelographic
infusion pyelographic study
p. study

pyelography
antegrade pyelography imaging
cystoscopy and p.
intravenous p.
percutaneous antegrade p.
rapid-sequence intravenous p.

pyelolithotomy
percutaneous ultrasonic p.

pyelonephritis
acute p.
chronic p.
emphysematous p.
xanthogranulomatous p.

pyeloplasty
Anderson-Hynes dismembered p.

pyelotomy incision

pyeloureterography
antegrade p.

pyemia
arterial p.

***Pygeum africanum* extract**

pylori
anti-*Helicobacter pylori* IgM
anti-*Helicobacter pylori* treatment
Helicobacter p.
Helicobacter pylori eradication therapy
Helicobacter pylori-like organism
Helicobacter pylori stool antigen
Helicobacter pylori vaccine
metronidazole, amoxicillin, clarithromycin, *H. pylori*, one-week therapy
musculus dilator pylori gastroduodenalis

pyloric
p. antrum
p. atresia
attenuated pyloric canal
p. canal
p. channel
p. channel ulcer
p. constriction
p. diameter
p. dilator
hypertrophic pyloric stenosis
p. incompetence
infantile hypertrophic pyloric stenosis
p. insufficiency
p. lymph node
p. mass
metaplastic pyloric gland
p. obstruction
p. region
p. sphincter
p. stenosis
p. vein

pylorici
nodi lymphoidei p.

pyloricum
antrum p.

pyloroduodenal perforation

pyloroplasty
Finney p.
Heineke-Mikulicz p.
selective vagotomy with p.
truncal vagotomy plus p.
p. and vagotomy
vagotomy and p.

pylorus
gastric p.
gastroduodenal p.
lateral p.
p. of stomach

pylorus-preserving
p.-p. gastrectomy
p.-p. pancreatoduodenectomy
p.-p. Whipple modification

pyoderma
p. gangrenosum
malignant p.
pyogenic sterile arthritis, pyoderma gangrenosum, and acne

pyogenic
p. abscess
p. abscess of liver
p. arthritis
p. culture
p. exudate
p. granuloma
p. infection
recurrent pyogenic cholangiogram
recurrent pyogenic cholangiohepatitis
p. sterile arthritis, pyoderma gangrenosum, and acne

pyomyositis
tropical p.

pyorrhea
p. alveolaris
p. around lower and upper teeth
Schmutz p.

pyosis
Manson p.

pyramid
anterior p.
Malacarne p.
malpighian p.
nasal p.
p. surface

pyramidal
anterior pyramidal cataract
anterior pyramidal fasciculus
anterior pyramidal tract
p. bone
p. cataract
p. cell
p. cell layer
p. disease
p. eminence
p. eye implant
p. fiber
p. fracture
hippocampal pyramidal cell
p. lesion
p. lobe
p. lobe of thyroid gland
p. response
small pyramidal cell
p. tract

pyretic tick-borne encephalitis

pyrexia
maternal p.
Pel-Ebstein p.
p. of undetermined origin
p. of unknown etiology
p. of unknown origin

pyrexial headache

pyridine
p. acetic acid
p. aldoxime methiodide
alum-precipitated p.
p. nucleotide

pyridoxalated
stroma-free hemoglobin p.
p. stroma-free hemoglobin

pyridoxine-deficient diet

pyridoxylated
p. hemoglobin
p. hemoglobin-polyoxyethylene

pyriform
p. apparatus
congenital nasal pyriform aperture stenosis
nasal pyriform aperture stenosis
p. sinus

pyrimethamine
chloroquine, pyrimethamine, and sulfisoxazole

pyrindinol carbamate

pyrithione
zinc p.

pyrogen
endogenous p.
leukocytic p.

pyrogenic
p. exotoxin
p. exotoxin C
streptococcal pyrogenic exotoxin B, C
streptococcal pyrogenic exotoxin

pyrogen-releasing factor

pyromania
erotic p.

pyronin
methyl green pyronin dye

pyrophosphate
alkaline phosphatase and p.
p. arthropathy

calcium pyrophosphate crystal deposition disease
calcium pyrophosphate dehydrate deposition disease
calcium pyrophosphate deposition
calcium pyrophosphate deposition disease
calcium pyrophosphate dihydrate
calcium pyrophosphate dihydrate crystal deposition
calcium pyrophosphate dihydrate deposition disease
chronic pyrophosphate arthropathy
crystalline calcium pyrophosphate dihydrate
free p.
inorganic p.

pyrophosphohydrolase
ATP p.

pyropoikilocytosis
hereditary p.

pyrrolizidine alkaloid

pyruvate
p. dehydrogenase
p. dehydrogenase complex deficiency
p., inosine, glucose phosphate, and adenine
inosine, pyruvate, and inorganic phosphate
liver pyruvate kinase
p. oxidation factor
serum pyruvate kinase

pyruvic acid

6-pyruvoyltetrahydropterin synthase

pyuria and hematuria

Q
Q angle
Q compound

Q10
coenzyme Q.

Qalyub virus

Q-H interval

qigong
q. deviation syndrome
q. meridian massage
self-healing style of q.

Qi and Yin deficiency

QKD interval

Q-M interval

Q-R interval

Q-stress
Q.-s. treadmill

Q-switched
Q.-s. neodymium:YAG laser
Q.-s. ruby laser

QT
QT corrected for heart rate
QT dispersion
QT interval
prolonged QT interval
prolonged QT syndrome

QT/QTc dispersion

quad
active quad strengthening exercise
ambulates with a quad cane
q. cane
q. ex
isometric quad strengthening exercise
large-base quad cane
narrow-base quad cane
patient independent with small based quad cane
small-based quad cane
wide-base quad cane

quadrangular cartilage

quadrangularis
pars anterior lobuli quadrangularis anterioris

quadrant
all 4 q.'s
four quadrant biopsy
q. hemianopia
inferior nasal q.
inferior temporal q.
left lower quadrant of abdomen
left upper outer q.
left upper quadrant of abdomen
lower left q.
lower outer q.
lower right q.
lowest q.
low inner q.
outer upper left q.
outer upper right q.
q. pain
right anterior q.
right lower q.
right lower quadrant of abdomen
right lower quadrant defect
right upper outer q.
right upper quadrant of abdomen
superior nasal q.
superior temporal q.
upper inner q.
upper left q.
upper outer q.
upper right q.

quadrantectomy,
q. axillary dissection, radiation therapy
q. axillary dissection and radiotherapy

quadrate
q. ligament
q. lobe
q. lobule
lumbar quadrate muscle

quadratic hemianopia

quadrature phase detector

quadriceps
q. angle
anterior quadriceps musculocutaneous flap technique
q. aponeurosis
q. atrophy
q. contracture
q. contusion
q. extension exercise
q. fatigue
q. femoris muscle
q. jerk
q. neutral angle
q. set
short-arc quadriceps test
q. tendon
q. tendon bearing

quadricusp mitral valve

quadrigeminal
anterior quadrigeminal body
q. cistern lipoma
q. plate cistern
q. pulse
q. rhythm

quadrigeminalis
arteria q.

quadrilateral socket

quadriplegia
partial q.
ventilator dependent q.

quadriplegic
cervical vent-dependent q.

quadruple
nuclear quadruple resonance

Quaglino operation

Quain
Q. degeneration
Q. fatty heart

qualified Medicare beneficiary

qualifying
additional qualifying symptoms

qualitative
q. alteration
q. analysis
q. assessment
q. coronary ultrasound
fibrinogen qualitative test
q. radiocardiography

quality
Arthritis Q. of Life Scale
q. assessment
q. assurance
q. assurance monitor
q. assurance program
q. assurance reagent
q. assurance/risk management
q. assurance standards
q. assurance and utilization review
Asthma Q. of Life Questionnaire
beam quality comparison
q. buffy coat
q. of caring
concurrent quality assurance
Q. of Contact
q. control
q. control nurse
diabetes quality of life
external quality assessment
Q. Extinction Test
Gastrointestinal Q. of Life Index
q. healthcare
health-related quality of life
human immunodeficiency virus quality audit marker
q. improvement
improve quality of life
indoor air q.
q. information monitoring system

quality *(continued)*
q. of life
q. of life in epilepsy
Q. of Life Index
Q. of Life Interview
Q. of Life Inventory
Q. of Life Questionnaire-C30
Q. of Life Scale
microbiologic quality control
q. of motion
q. of movement
Multidimensional Q. of Life Questionnaire for Persons with Human Immunodeficiency Virus
nursing quality assurance
palliation, quality, radiation, severity, time
Parkinson Disease Q. of Life Scale
q. of patient care
Pediatric Asthma Q. of Life Questionnaire
perceived quality of life
Q. Point of Service
position, quality, radiation, severity, time
preservation of quality of life
Respiratory Q. of Life Questionnaire
rhinoconjunctivitis-specific quality of life questionnaire
Sleep Apnea Q. of Life Index
statistical analysis and quality control
stroke-specific quality of life
therapeutic q.'s of ice
total quality management
Q. of Upper Extremities Test
Vital Signs Q. of Life
voice q.
Q. of Well Being Index
Q. of Well-Being Scale Self-Administered
q. of working life
World Health Organization Quality of Life 100-Item

quality-adjusted
q.-a. life expectancy
q.-a. life-year
q.-a. life-year saved
q.-a. survival
q.-a. time without symptoms or toxicity

quality-of-life issue

quality-related event

quantification
acoustic q.
digital echo q.

quantified
axial quantified computed tomography
q. computed tomography

quanti-Pirquet reaction

quantitation
amniotic fluid q.
immunoglobulin q.
q. standard

quantitative
q. analysis
q. approach
q. autonomic functioning testing
q. autoradiographic
q. bone ultrasound
q. buffy coat
q. buffy-coat analysis
q. competitive PCR
q. competitive polymerase chain reaction
q. computed tomography
q. coronary angiography
q. coronary arteriography
q. digital radiography
q. Doppler
q. electroencephalogram
q. electroencephalography
q. evaluation
q. gated SPECT
q. hepatobiliary scintigraphy
q. hyperplasia
q. immunoelectrophoresis
q. immunoglobulin
q. inhalation challenge apparatus
q. insulin sensitivity check index
Q. Inventory of Alcohol Disorders
q. light induced fluorescence
q. muscle testing
peripheral quantitative computed tomography
q. pharmacoelectroencephalography
q. sacroiliac scintigraphy
Q. Sensory Testing
q. structure-activity relationship
Q. Sudomotor Axon Reflex Test
q. test
q. tip culture
q. trait locus
q. wall motion score

quantity
any q.
limited quantity test performed on small specimen
minimal detectable q.
not sufficient q.
patient vomited large q.'s of blood
protein, quantity not sufficient
summation of all q.'s following the symbol
unknown q.

quantization
q. matrix
sequential scalar q.
wavelet scalar q.

Quant sign

quantum
atomic orbital with angular momentum quantum number zero
q. chromodynamics
q. detection efficiency
detective quantum efficiency
q. electrodynamics
Q. inflation device
magnetic quantum number
principal quantum number
spin quantum number
superconducting quantum interference device susceptometer
q. yield

quarantine period

quart
liquid q.

quarta
macula cribrosa q.

quartan fever

quarter
left caudal quarter ganglion
left rostral quarter ganglion
right caudal quarter ganglion
right rostral quarter ganglion
sick in q.'s military

quarti
apertura lateralis ventriculi q.
apertura mediana ventriculi q.

quartus
musculus gluteus q.

quartz
cold quartz mercury vapor lamp

quasi-continuous wave

quasielastic laser light-scattering spectroscope

quasimorphine withdrawal syndrome

quasiresonant nucleus

quasistatic
q. compliance
q. pressure volume

quaternary ammonium compounds

queasiness
intestinal q.

Queckenstedt
Q. maneuver
Q. sign
Q. test

Queckenstedt-Stookey test

Queensland
Q. fever
North Queensland tick fever
North Queensland tick typhus

Quénu-Muret sign

querulous paranoia

Quervain
de Quervain disease
de Quervain fracture
de Quervain injury
de Quervain syndrome
de Quervain tendinitis
de Quervain tenolysis
de Quervain tenosynovitis

query
Physician Data Q.
protocol data q.

quest
Fear Avoidance Beliefs Q.

question
answers q.'s appropriately
frequently asked q.'s
multiple choice q.
survey, question, read, review, recite

questionable Babinski sign

questioning
dull on q.
on direct q.

questionnaire
Abbreviated Parent Symptom Q.
Acquired Immunodeficiency Syndrome Beliefs and Behavior Q.
acquired immunodeficiency syndrome health assessment q.
Acute Low Back Pain Screening Q.
Adolescent Life Change Event Q.
Adult Neuropsychological Q.
Adult Suicidal Ideation Q.
Ages and Stages Q.
Alcohol Usage Q.
anxiety scale q.
Asthma Quality of Life Q.
Attitude to School Q.
Attributional Style Q.
autism spectrum screening q.
Behavioral Assessment of Pain Q.
Behavior Style Q.
Berne pain q.
Big Five Q.
Change Agent Q.
child health q.
Childhood Asthma Q.
Childhood Health Assessment Q.
childhood trauma q.
Child Neuropsychological Q.
Children's Comprehensive Pain Q.
Children's Personality Q.
Chronic Respiratory Q.
Clinical Analysis Q.
Clinical Health Assessment Q.
clinical-symptom/self-evaluation q.
Cognitive Failures Q.
College Student Satisfaction Q.
Community College Student Experiences Q.
Community Integration Q.
Conners Parent Q.
Conners Teacher Q.
Coping Strategies Q.
Depressive Experiences Q.
Diagnostic Assessment Q.
Dimensional Assessment of Personality Pathology-Basic Q.
Early School Personality Q.
Eysenck Personality Q.
Fagerstrom tolerance q.
Family Attitudes Q.
Fibromyalgia Impact Q.
Functional Outcomes of Sleep Q.
Functional Status Q.
General Health Perception Q.
General High Altitude Q.
General Purpose Psychiatric Q.
Headache Assessment Q.
Health Assessment Q. Disability Index
health-related quality-of-life q.
High School Personality Q.
Hilton Drinking Behavior Q.
Hostility and Direction of Hostility Q.
human health and behavior q.
Q. for Identifying Children with Chronic Conditions
Illness Behavior Q.
Inflammatory Bowel Disease Q.
Inquiry Mode Q.: A Measure of How You Think and Make Decisions
Insight and Treatment Attitudes Q.
Leader Behavior Description Q.
Life Situation Q.
Living with Asthma Q.
Low Back Pain Q.
Managerial Style Q.
Mauldsley Medical Q.
McGill Pain Assessment Q.
Menstrual Distress Management Q.
mental status q.
Michigan Hand Outcomes Q.
Minnesota Importance Q.
Modified Autonomic Perception Q.
Modified Health Assessment Q.
Modified Somatic Perception Q.
Multidimensional Personality Q.
Multidimensional Quality of Life Q. for Persons with Human Immunodeficiency Virus
National Eye Institute Visual Function Q.
Neuroticism Scale Q.
OARS Multidimensional Functional Assessment Q.
Occupational Roles Q.
Offer Self-Image Q. for Adolescents
Organizational Value Dimensions Q.
Osteoporosis Knowledge Q.
Owestry Disability Q.
Pain Coping Q.
parental development q.
Parent Symptom Q.
Parent-Teacher Q.
Parkinson Disease Q.
PARS III q.
patient satisfaction q.
Pediatric Asthma Quality of Life Q.
Personal Experience and Attitude Q.
Personal Experience Screening Q.
16 Personality Factor Q.
personality factor q.
Personal Strain Q.
Philadelphia Head Injury Q.

questionnaire *(continued)*
Physical Activity Readiness Q.
Postoperative Pain Q.
Postpartum Self-Evaluation Q.
Premenstrual Distress Q.
Preschool Behavior Q.
Prescreening Development Q.
Psychiatric Q. Obsessive-Compulsive Neurosis
Psychosocial History Screening Q.
Pulmonary Functional Status and Dyspnea Q.
Purdue Teacher Q.
Readiness to Change q.
respiratory disease q.
Respiratory Quality of Life Q.
Revised Denver Prescreening Development Q.
rhinoconjunctivitis-specific quality of life q.
Roland-Morris Q.
Sales Personality Q.
School Atmosphere Q.
Seasonal Pattern Assessment Q.
Seattle angina q.
Self-Administered Dependency Q.
Self-Description Questionnaire II
Sexual Adjustment Q.
Sexual Function Inventory Q.
Short Inflammatory Bowel Disease Q.
Short Portable Mental Status Q.
side-effects q.
Smoking Behavior Q.
Speech and Language Screening Q.
Stanford Health Assessment Q.
St. Georges Respiratory Q.
Student Adaptation to College Q.
Substance Abuse Q.
Suicide Opinion Q.
Toronto Functional Capacity Q.
verbalizer-visualization q.
Vocational Interest Q.
Waring Intimacy Q.
Work Attitudes Q.

Questionnaire-C30
Quality of Life Q.-C.

Questionnaire-Revised
Incontinence Impact Q.-R.
Personality Diagnostic Q.-R.

Queyrat erythroplasia

quick
q. catheter
child quick to anger
q. and early diagnosis
q. early warning
q. fraction
q. freeze
Otis Q. Scoring Mental Abilities Test
Q. Picture Vocabulary Test
q. prothrombin time
repeated quick stretch
repeated quick stretch from elongation
repeated quick stretch superimposed upon an existing contraction
Q. test
Q. Test psychology, pregnancy, prothrombin
Voc-Tech Quick Screener

quickening
fetal q.

quiescent
q. hepatitis
q. phase of cells leaving the mitotic cycle

quiet
q. breath sound
deep q.
q. heart sound
Paget quiet necrosis

quiet-alert state

quieting
q. reflex
q. response

quilt suture

Quimby dose distribution system

quinacrine
q. mustard

quinaldine red

Quincke
Q. capillary pulse
Q. disease
Q. edema
Q. puncture
Q. sign

quinidine effect

quinine
q. and colchicine
q. fever

quinolone-resistant ***Neisseria gonorrhoeae***

quinone
NADPH dehydrogenase q.

quinti
abductor digiti q.
abductor digiti quinti muscle
abductor digiti quinti tendon
adductor digiti q.
extensor digiti q.
extensor digiti quinti muscle
extensor digiti quinti proprius
extensor digiti quinti tendon
extensor quinti proprius
flexor digiti quinti brevis
flexor digiti quinti muscle
flexor digitorum quinti brevis
Littler-Cooley abductor digiti quinti transfer
musculus abductor digiti q.
musculus extensor digiti quinti proprius
opponens digiti q.
opponens digiti quinti muscle

quisqualic acid

quo
status q.

quotient
accomplishment q.
achievement q.
adolescent language q.
aphasia q.
average perturbation q.
brain-age q.
cerebral glucose oxygen q.
circadian q.
cognitive laterality q.
conceptual q.
corrected development q.
developmental q.
developmental motor q.
discomfort relief q.
education q.
encephalization q.
energy q.
eudismic affinity q.
Freedom from Distractibility Deviation Q.
Full-Scale Intelligence Q.
glucose oxidation q.
Hilson Personnel Profile/Success Q.
intelligence quotient test
longevity q.
lordosis q.
mean developmental q.
memory deviation q.
metabolic respiratory q.
oxygen q.
Perceptual Organization Deviation Q.

Performance Intelligence Q.
permeability q.
positive-negative ambivalent q.
reading q.
recovery q.
respiratory q.
social q.
total living q.
verbal comprehension deviation q.
Verbal Intelligence Q.

Q-wave myocardial infarction

rabbit
r. antibladder antibody
r. antibladder cancer
r. antibody to human ovary
r. antibody to pig ovary
r. antidog-thymus serum
r. antimouse-thymocyte antiserum, r.
r. antithymocyte globulin
r. antithymocyte serum
citrated normal rabbit serum
cottontail rabbit herpesvirus
r. erythrocyte
r. ileal loop test
isolated perfused rabbit lung
r. kidney vacuolating virus
malignant rabbit fibroma virus
nonimmunized rabbit serum
normal inactivated rabbit serum
r. ovarian antitumor serum
primary rabbit kidney
r. serum albumin
r. thymus extract
r. trachea
tumor-bearing r.
venereal spirochetosis of r.'s
zymosan-activated plasma rabbit

rabies
fluorescent rabies antibody
human rabies immune globulin
human rabies immunoglobulin
r. immunoglobulin
indirect fluorescent rabies antibody test
r. postexposure prophylaxis
rapid rabies enzyme immunodiagnosis
Rhesus diploid cell strain rabies vaccine
r. vaccine adsorbed
r. vaccine, duck embryo culture
r. vaccine, human diploid cell culture
r. vaccine, purified chick embryo cell culture
r. viral culture
r. virus

Rabok
Tanjong Rabok virus

Rabson-Mendenhall syndrome

racemosa
livedo r.

racemose aneurysm

racemosum

rachitic
r. diet
r. dwarf
r. rosary
r. scoliosis

Racial Perceptions Inventory

racing
disconnected and racing thoughts
r. heart
r. heartbeat
r. heart rhythm
r. thoughts

racism
aversive r.

racquet incision

radar absorbent material

radial
annular radial rupture
anterior radial collateral artery
r. arterial line
r. artery
r. artery bypass surgery
r. artery catheter
r. artery graft
r. artery pseudoaneurysm
r. artery systolic pressure
articular facet of radial head
r. aspect
r. and astigmatic keratotomy
atraumatic, multidirectional, bilateral radial instability
r. bone
brachial, radial, femoral
r. collateral ligament
collateral radial ligament
r. condyle
controlled radial expansion
r. deviation
double radial immunodiffusion
r. drift
r. dysplasia
r. eminence of wrist
r. extensor muscle
r. fiber of cochlea
r. flow chromatography
r. forearm free flap
r. fossa
r. groove
r. head
r. head dislocation
r. head epiphysis
r. head fracture
r. head subluxation
r. hemolysis
r. hemolysis in gel
r. immunity
r. immunodiffusion cerebrospinal fluid
r. incision
inverted radial reflex
r. keratectomy
keratoneuritis
left radial artery
long radial extensor muscle of wrist
malformed radial head
midcarpal r.
Nadler superior radial scissors
r. nerve
Newman classification of radial neck and head fracture
nonarticular distal radial fracture
O'Brien classification of radial fracture
palmar carpal branch of radial artery
palpable radial pulse
pathognomonic radial keratoneuritis
r. photon absorptiometry
prospective evaluation of radial keratotomy
r. pulse
r. rate
right radial artery
sensory branch of radial nerve
single radial diffusion test
single radial hemolysis
single radial immunodiffusion
superficial radial nerve
Swanson radial head implant
ventricular radial dysplasia
vertebral abnormality, anal imperforation, tracheoesophageal fistula, and radial, ray, or renal anomalies

radialis
arteria collateralis r.
brachial radialis jerk
extensor carpi r.
extensor carpi radialis brevis
extensor carpi radialis brevis muscle
extensor carpi radialis brevis tendon
extensor carpi radialis longus
extensor carpi radialis longus flap
extensor carpi radialis longus muscle
extensor carpi radialis longus tendon
flexor carpi r.

R

radialis *(continued)*
flexor carpi radialis brevis
musculus extensor carpi radialis brevis
musculus extensor carpi radialis longus
musculus flexor carpi r.

radiant
r. energy
r. flux
r. heat
r. heat device
r. heat warmer
r. intensity
out of radiant warmer
r. power

radiate
r. carpal ligament
r. ligament of head of rib

radiated
effective isotropic radiated power

radiating
r. chest pain
chest pain radiating to jaw and shoulder
pain radiating to back
pain radiating down legs
pain radiating into back
pain radiating to jaw
pain radiating to jaw and shoulder

radiation
r. absorbed dose
acute radiation disease
acute radiation pneumonitis
adjuvant whole-brain radiation therapy
airline flight r.
r. alopecia
anatomical considerations in radiation therapy
anterior thalamic r.
artificial UV r.
as low as reasonably achievable radiation exposure
r. assault on tumor
average radiation dose
r. beam
biologic effects of ionizing r.
r. bowel reaction
r. burn
cell sensitivity to r.
cerebral radiation necrosis
r. and chemotherapy
r. colitis
combined drug and radiation modality
combined hyperthermia and radiation treatment
conformal radiation therapy
coronary radiation therapy
cranial radiation therapy
cumulative radiation effect
r. cystitis
r. damage
r. dermatitis
r. dermatosis
r. dose
r. dose limit
effective direct r.
r. effect unit
electromagnetic r.
electron-beam intraoperative radiation therapy
r. emergency area
endoluminal radiation therapy
r. enteritis
r. equivalent in man
r. equivalent therapy
r. experience data
r. exposure
r. exposure guide
r. exposure in pregnancy
extended abdominal radiation therapy
extended field r.
extended field radiation therapy
external beam radiation therapy
field of r.
focal cranial radiation therapy
full course of r.
full course radiation therapy
full radiation of brain
r. gastritis
r. hazard
hazards from microwave r.
health effects of ionizing r.
heat loss by r.
high-dose fractional radiation therapy
high-dose fractionation radiation therapy
high-dose radiation therapy
high-dose radiation to tumor mass
high-energy ionizing r.
high linear energy transfer r.
humeral block in radiation therapy
hyperfractionated accelerated radiation therapy
hysterectomy and r.
r. implant
r. induced emesis
infrared r.
r. injury
r. intensity
intensity-modulated radiation therapy
internal radiation therapy
interstitial radiation pneumonitis
interstitial radiation therapy
r. intoxication
intracavitary radiation sources
intracavitary radiation therapy
intracoronary radiation therapy
intraluminal radiation therapy
intraoperative radiation surgery
ionizing radiation unit
r. laboratory
lead shielding in r.
lens-sparing external beam radiation therapy
r. leukemia protection
r. leukemia virus
light activation by stimulated emission of r.
light amplification by stimulated emission of r.
r. linked antibodies
r. linked disease
local recurrence after radiation therapy
low-dose of ionizing r.
low-dose mediastinal radiation therapy
low-linear energy transfer r.
lumpectomy and r.
medical internal radiation dose
microwave amplification by stimulated emission of r.
microwave radiation injury
r. myeloid leukemia
natural UV r.
r. necrosis
neutron beam r.
noninvasive evaluation of radiation output
nonionizing electromagnetic r.
occipitofrontal r.
ocular radiation therapy
r. oncology
optic r.
r. optic neuropathy
optic radiation lesion
oral radiation death
palliation, quality, radiation, severity, time
palliative radiation therapy

palliative radiation treatment
particle beam radiation therapy
patient tolerated full course of r.
peroral cone radiation therapy
photon irradiation technique in radiation therapy
photosynthetically active r.
r. pneumonitis
position, quality, radiation, severity, time
preoperative radiation therapy
prophylactic whole brain radiation therapy
r. protection guide
proton beam r.
quadrantectomy, axillary dissection, radiation therapy
r. rash
r. reaction
r. response
staging system in radiation therapy
stereotactic-assisted radiation therapy
tenth value layer radiation
therapeutic external r.
r. therapy for intact breast
r. therapy oncology group
r. therapy on prophylactic basis
r. therapy planning
r. therapy planning system
thoracic radiation therapy
three-dimensional conformal radiation therapy
thymic radiation therapy
total body r.
total lymphoid r.
r. treatment
r. treatment of glandular tissue
r. treatment planning
true radiation emission
ultraviolet r.
vertical radiation topography
whole-body r.
whole brain r.
whole brain versus local brain radiation therapy
wide-field radiation therapy

radiation-absorbed dose

radiation-equivalent-man

radiation-equivalent-manikin

r.-e.-m. absorption
r.-e.-m. calibration

radiation-induced

r.-i. atrophy
r.-i. carcinogenesis
r.-i. change
r.-i. colitis
r.-i. fibrosis
r.-i. heart disease
r.-i. leukemia
r.-i. liver disease
r.-i. nausea and vomiting
r.-i. neoplasm
r.-i. sarcoma of the head and neck
r.-i. thyroiditis
r.-i. xerostomia

radiation-related eosinophilia

radiative

mass radiative stopping power

radical

r. abdominal hysterectomy
ascorbic free r.
Auchincloss modified radical mastectomy
r. behavior change
r. cystectomy
r. en bloc removal
r. excision
r. exenteration
extended radical mastectomy
free r.
free radical assay technique
Halsted radical mastectomy
hand-assisted laparoscopic radical nephrectomy
r. hemorrhoidectomy
hydroxyl r.
r. hysterectomy
r. hysterectomy and bilateral salpingo-oophorectomy
inhibitor of radical processes
laparoscopic radical nephrectomy
laparoscopic radical prostatectomy
left modified radical mastectomy
left radical neck dissection
r. mastectomy
mitochondrial free radical generation
modified radical hysterectomy
r. neck dissection
nitron radical trap
organic r.
oxygen free r.
r. pair mechanism
Patey radical mastectomy
r. perineal prostatectomy
r. posteromedial and plantar release
r. prostate surgery
r. retropubic prostatectomy
right modified radical mastectomy
right radical neck dissection
Schauta radical vaginal hysterectomy
r. vulvectomy
Wertheim radical hysterectomy
Willy Meyer radical mastectomy

radices (*pl. of* radix)

radicis

apex radicis dentis

radicular

r. abscess
anterior and posterior radicular artery
anterior radicular artery
apical radicular cyst
r. cyst
inferior radicular vein
lower radicular obstetrical paralysis
superior radicular vein
transient radicular irritation

radiculares

radicularis

arteria radicularis anterior magna
arteria radicularis magna
arteria radicularis magna of Adamkiewicz

radiculomyelitis

ascending r.

radiculoneuritis

Lyme r.

radiculopathy

motor r.
spondylotic caudal r.

radii (*pl. of* radius)

radioactive

r. antigen microprecipitin
r. bead
r. cesium
r. constant
r. decay
r. drug
r. drug research committee
effective half-life of radioactive substance
r. fibrinogen uptake
r. gallium
r. gold
r. Hippuran test
r. hydrogen isotope
r. implant
r. injection
insert radioactive implant
interstitial implantation of radioactive isotope

radioactive *(continued)*
r. iodinated human serum albumin
r. iodinated serum albumin
r. iodine
r. iodine uptake
r. iron
r. isotopic venogram, bilateral
low-level radioactive tracer
r. material
^{13}N ammonia radioactive tracer
r. seed implant
r. seeding of prostate
r. tag
r. technetium
thyroidal radioactive iodine uptake test
r. tracer
r. waste

radioactivity
extrathyroidal neck r.
r. of vegetative cells

radioallergosorbent assay test

radioantigen-binding assay

radioassayable neurotensin

radiobiologic equivalent

radiocardiography
qualitative r.

radiocarpal
r. angle
r. arthrodesis
r. articulation
r. dislocation
dorsal radiocarpal ligament
r. implant
r. joint

radiocarpalis
articulatio r.

radiocarpea
articulatio r.

radiochemical neutron activation analysis

radiocontrast
r. dye
r. material

radiocurable tumor

radiodermatitis emulsion

radioenzymatic assay

radiofluorescent antibody

radiofrequency
r. ablation
capacitive r.
r. catheter ablation
r. coil
computed tomography-guided percutaneous radiofrequency denervation of the sacroiliac joint
conductive radiofrequency electric field
r. current
r. interference
interstitial r.
r. magnetic field in nuclear magnetic resonance
percutaneous r.
percutaneous radiofrequency facet nerve block
r. percutaneous myocardial revascularization
percutaneous radiofrequency denervation
percutaneous radiofrequency rhizolysis
percutaneous stereotactic radiofrequency rhizotomy
r. thermal ablation
r. thermocoagulation
r. tissue volume reduction

radio-gas chromatography

radiograph
anterior drawer stress r.
bite-wing r.
chest r.
digitally reconstructed r.
dual-energy r.
lateral decubitus r.
mandibular cuspid-first bicuspid r.
mandibular cuspid r.
maxillary bicuspid r.
maxillary cuspid r.
occlusal cross-section r.
plain abdominal r.
plain spine r.
portable chest r.

radiographic
r. absorptiometry
r. baseline
r. bone strength index
r. contrast
r. contrast agent
r. contrast media
r. contrast medium
r. coronary calcification
r. criterion
r. evaluation
r. and fluoroscopic
r. healing
r. imaging system
intensified radiographic imaging system
r. lung area
r. planimetry
spinal cord injury without radiographic abnormality
r. study

radiographically
no radiographically visible recurrence

radiography
advanced multiple-beam equalization r.
anterior-posterior dual energy r.
computed digital r.
digital r.
direct digital r.
electron r.
film screen r.
flat plate r.
invasion depth r.
lateral-view dual-energy r.
mass miniature r.
mass radiography unit
mental extraoral r.
nonionic contrast r.
occlusal film r.
panoral r.
panoramic extraoral r.
photostimulable phosphor dental r.
plain abdominal r.
quantitative digital r.
scanned projection r.
scanning equalization r.
scan projection r.

radioimmune antiglobulin test

radioimmunoassay
Australia antigen r.
automated r.
r. double antibody test
r. of hair
human myoglobulin r.
indirect r.
insulin r.
Packard radioimmunoassay system
polystyrene-tube r.
solid phase r.
tetraiodothyronine thyroxine r.
thyroid r.
triiodothyronine r.
tritium r.

radioimmunoblot assay

radioimmunoelectrophoresis
crossed r.

radioimmunoglobulin
r. scintigraphy
r. therapy

radioimmunoguided surgery

radioimmunologic assay antithyroid antibody

radioimmunoprecipitation
- r. assay
- r. test

radioimmunosorbent
- r. assay
- paper radioimmunosorbent technique
- paper radioimmunosorbent test
- r. test

radioiodinated
- r. fatty acid
- macroaggregated radioiodinated albumin
- r. rose bengal dye
- r. serum albumin
- r. triolein

radioiodine
- r. test
- r. uptake

radioisotope
- double radioisotope derivative
- r. imaging
- r. implant
- life of r.
- local-acting r.
- r. medicine
- r. of phosphorus
- thyroxine radioisotope assay
- r. uptake study

radiolabeled
- r. antibody imaging
- r. antigen
- r. fibrinogen
- r. iodine
- r. microsphere
- Oncolym radiolabeled monoclonal antibody

radiolabeling
- area of increased r.

radiolocalization
- gamma probe r.

radiologic
- antiestrogen radiologic therapy
- chemical, bacteriologic, and radiologic warfare
- r. contrast-induced renal failure
- r. control center
- r. emergency assistance team
- r. evaluation
- r. half-life
- r. health
- r. health data
- r. osteoarthritis
- right posterior oblique radiologic view
- r. warfare

radiological
- chemical, biological, radiological or nuclear weapons
- chemical, radiological, and biological
- interventional radiological technique

radiology
- barium contrast r.
- computed r.
- diagnostic r.
- pediatric r.
- r. telephone access system
- therapeutic r.
- vascular r.

radiolucency
- apical r.
- linear band of maximal r.
- periventricular r.

radiolucent crescent sign

radiolunate
- long r.
- short r.

radiometer
- scanning r.

radiometric
- automated radiometric technique
- rapid r.

radio nonopaque stone

radionuclear bone scan

radionucleotide
- antibody r.
- antibody radionucleotide conjugate

radionuclide
- adenosine radionuclide perfusion imaging
- r. angiocardiography
- r. angiography
- r. bone scan
- r. cardiography
- r. cerebral angiogram
- cerebral radionuclide angiography
- r. cholescintigraphy
- r. cineangiography
- r. cisternography
- r. cystography
- equilibrium-gated radionuclide angiography
- esophageal radionuclide transit
- r. esophageal scintigraphy
- first-pass radionuclide angiogram
- r. functional lymphoscintigraphy
- r. gastric emptying study
- gated radionuclide angiography
- r. imaging
- r. imaging of inferior vena cava
- indirect radionuclide cystography
- intravenous radionuclide venography
- r. joint imaging
- low-dose dobutamine stress radionuclide ventriculography
- maximal permissible concentration of unidentified r.'s
- r. purity
- resting radionuclide ejection fraction
- r. scanning
- r. scintigraphy
- subcutaneous radionuclide venography
- r. superior cavography
- three-phase radionuclide bone scanning
- r. thyroid imaging
- r. venography
- r. ventriculogram
- r. ventriculography

radiopaque
- r. bone cement
- r. calculus
- r. contrast medium
- r. density
- r. dye
- injection of radiopaque material
- open end flow-through radiopaque tip
- r. tantalum stent

radiopharmaceutical drug product

radiopharmaceuticals
- accelerator-produced r.

radioreceptor
- r. activity
- r. assay
- r. assay pregnancy blood

radioscope
- Lombart r.

radiosensitivity test

radiosurgery
- advanced design LINAC r.
- arteriovenous malformation r.
- fractionated stereotactic r.
- gamma knife stereotactic r.
- linear accelerator-based r.
- linear accelerator r.

radiosurgery *(continued)*
megavoltage computed tomography-assisted stereotactic r.
megavoltage CT-assisted stereotactic r.
particle beam r.
photon beam r.
proton beam r.
stereotactic r.

radiotherapy
chemotherapy and r.
computer-controlled r.
continuous hyperfractionated accelerated r.
electron-beam intraoperative r.
eosinophilic, polymorphic, and pruritic eruption associated with r.
external beam r.
fractionated stereotactic r.
hypofractionated stereotactic r.
r. implant
intraoperative electron beam r.
locoregional r.
locoregional field r.
mathematical optimization and logical dimensioning for r.
megavoltage external r.
mixed neutron and photon r.
palladium 103 ophthalmic plaque r.
pelvic boost r.
postoperative r.
preoperative r.
quadrantectomy, axillary dissection and r.
tumorectomy, axillary dissection, r.
whole-brain r.

radioulnar
articular disc of distal radioulnar joint
congenital radioulnar synostosis
r. dislocation
distal radioulnar joint
proximal radioulnar joint
r. synostosis

radioulnaris
articulatio radioulnaris proximalis

radium
adenoidectomy with r.
cervical insertion of r.
r. emanation
Ernst radium applicator
Ernst radium capsule
Ernst radium tandem
r. implant
implantation of r.
r. insertion
intracavitary r.
Manchester system for radium therapy
minimal pure radium equivalent
Paris method for radium therapy
Plummer-Vinson radium applicator
resting r.
r. seed
r. therapy

radius, pl. **radii**
anterior border of r.
antcrior oblique line of r.
anular ligament of r.
anular ligament of r.
arc radius system
articular circumference of head of r.
articular pit of head of r.
axial length/corneal radius ratio
back optic zone r.
r. cap prosthesis
dislocation head of r.
front optic zone r.
full radius cutter
Galeazzi fracture of r.
head of r.
inside r.
interosseous border of r.
neck of r.
notch of r.
nutrient artery of r.
open reduction of radius and ulna
orbicular ligament of r.
posterior apical r.
progressive curvature of r.
resection head of r.
thrombocytopenia and absent r.
ulnar notch of r.
r. of view

Radi virus

radix, pl. **radices**
morselized cartilage onlay radix graft

radon seed implantation

Raeder syndrome

rage
hidden r.
r. impotence
narcissistic r.
r. reduction therapy
unprovoked rage attack

ragged red fiber

ragpicker's disease

ragsorter's disease

ragweed
r. antigen
r. antigen E
giant ragweed test
r. pollen
polymerized r.
r. sensitivity
short ragweed test
whole ragweed extract

railroad
r. track appearance
r. track sign

rainbow vision

Rainey tubes

Rainville test

raise
arm r.'s maneuver
double seated straight leg r.
r. head of bed
negative straight leg r.
reverse straight leg r.
straight leg r.

raising
crossed straight leg r.
straight leg raising test

Raji
R. cell assay
R. cell-binding material
R. cell-binding unit

raking
endoscopic r.

rales
r. audible at bases
basilar r.
bronchial r.
coarse r.
crackling r.
de retour r.
few fine r.
fine crepitant r.
medium r.
moderate number of medium r.
musical r.
numerous coarse r.
r. and rhonchi
r., rhonchi, or wheezes
Skoda r.
snoring r.

raloxifene
multiple outcomes of raloxifene evaluation trial

rami (*pl. of* ramus)

ramification
apical r.

Ramirez
ashy dermatosis of R.

Ramsay Hunt syndrome

ramus, pl. **rami**
angular position of r.
anterior ramus of cervical nerve
anterior ramus of lateral sulcus of cerebrum
anterior ramus of lumbar nerve
anterior ramus of sacral nerve
anterior ramus of spinal nerve
anterior ramus of thoracic nerve
ascending r.
ascending ramus of ischium
ascending ramus of lateral sulcus of cerebrum
ascending ramus of mandible
bilateral sagittal split ramus osteotomies
bilateral vertical ramus osteotomy
r., body, symphysis, palate
bone r.
coronoid process of r.
r. fracture
intraoral vertical ramus osteotomy
ischial r.
r. of mandible
mandible r.
mandibular r.
medial branch of posterior rami of spinal nerve
pubic r.
sagittal split ramus osteotomy

Randall-Baker Soucek

random
r. access
r. activity
r. amplified polymorphic DNA
r. blood glucose
r. blood sugar
r. chemistry profile
dynamic random access memory
longitudinal random coefficient model
r. migration
mixed discrete-continuous random variable
r. sample
r. single donor platelet
static random access memory
r. transfusion
r. urine
r. variable

random-access memory

random-donor platelet

randomized
completely randomized design
r. controlled clinical trial
double-blind placebo-controlled randomized clinical trial
r. double-blind trial
prospective randomized trial
r. prospective trial
r. response technique
r. trial

range
r. of ability
r. of accommodation
active ankle joint complex range of motion
active-assisted range of motion
active integral range of motion
active and passive range of motion
active resistive range of motion
affect within normal r.
alpha frequency r.
alternating range of motion
ankle dorsiflexion range of motion
ankle inversion-eversion range of motion
asymmetry, range of motion abnormality, tissue texture abnormality
back range of motion
boiling r.
brain wave frequency r.
cervical range of motion
r. of comfortable loudness
complete and pain-free range of motion
r. of convergence
critical bandwidth range of frequencies
dynamic range control
end range of motion
r. of frequency
full r.
full, free range of motion
full joint range of motion
full joint range of movement
full range of affect
heart rate r.
intersegmental range of motion palpation
r. of joint motion
joint range of motion
maximum frequency r.
median range score
medium r.
most comfortable loudness r.
r. of motion complete and pain-free
r. of motion within normal limits
r. of movement
neck full range of motion
normal r.
normal range of motion
pain-free range of motion
pain sensitivity r.
passive assistance range of motion
resistive range of motion
restricted range of motion
spinal range of motion
total range of motion
visual auditory r.
voluntary range of motion
wide r.
Wide R. Achievement Test-Revised
Wide R. Assessment of Memory and Learning
wide dynamic range compression
within normal r.

range-gated Doppler

ranina
arteria r.

raninus
arcus r.

ranitidine
r. bismuth citrate
r. bismuth citrate, amoxicillin, clarithromycin
r. bismuth citrate, metronidazole, tetracycline

rank
r. correlation coefficient
first rank symptom
Mann-Whitney rank sum statistic
matched pairs signed rank test
percentile r.
Wilcoxon rank sum statistic
Wilcoxon rank sum test

Ranke
R. angle
R. complex
R. stage

Rankine
absolute temperature on the Rankine scale
degree R.
R. scale

rank-order stability analysis

Ranvier
R. cross
R. disk
R. membrane
node of R.

rapamycin
mammalian target of r.
target of rapamycin inhibitor

rape
anal r.
anal rape fantasy
r. crisis center
r. crisis intervention program
r. intervention

rapeseed
adulterated rapeseed oil-associated toxic oil syndrome

raphe
attenuated media r.
dorsal r.
dorsal raphe nucleus
median r.
median longitudinal raphe of tongue
median raphe cyst of the penis
mesencephalic r.
midbrain raphe nucleus
nucleus centralis superior r.
nucleus raphe magnus
r. transection

raphespinal
anterior raphespinal tract

rapid
abbreviated rapid processing
abnormally rapid heart rate
r. acquisition computed axial tomography
r. acquisition with relaxation enhancement
r. acquisition with resolution enhancement
r. alternating movements
r. amplification of polymorphic DNA
r. antigen-detection test
r. assay delivery systems
r. atrial fibrillation
AuraTek rapid cancer test
r. beating of heart
r. body shaper
r. bone loss
burst of rapid atrial pacing
r. cooling
r. detox
r. dissolution formula
dizziness from rapid and deep breathing
r. dyssynchronous depolarization
r. electrophoresis
r. electrophoresis creatine kinase
r. erythrocyte degeneration
R. Estimation of Adult Literacy in Medicine
excessively rapid heart rate
r. exchange
r. extinction effect
r. eye movement
r. eye movement sleep
r. filling
r. filling period
r. filling rate
r. filling wave
fine rapid nystagmus
r. fluorescent focus inhibition test
r. frozen section
r. gait
gold-labeled optical rapid immunoassay
r. head movement
r. heart action
r. heartbeat
r. heart rhythm
heparin assay rapid easy method
r. high
hybrid rapid acquisition with relaxation enhancement
r. identification method
r. identification method-*Neisseria*
r. immunofluorescence staining
increased rapid eye movement sleep
r. infusion pump
r. ingestion
r. ingestion of large amounts of food
locally made rapid urease test
r. loss of bone
magnetization-prepared rapid gradient echo-water excitation
r. manual processing
r. maxillary expansion
method of rapid determination
r. micromedia method
modified rapid fermentation test
mood disorder with rapid cycling
r. movement disorder
r. muscle growth
nonrapid eye movement-rapid eye movement cycle
r. onset of jaundice
r. opiate detoxification under anesthesia
r. opioid detoxification
Parkland R. Exam
r. plasma reagent
r. plasma reagin
r. plasma reagin circle card test
r. plasma reagin complement fixation
r. processing mode
r. pull-through technique
pulse weak and r.
r. rabies enzyme immunodiagnosis
r. radiometric
R. Rare Event Detection
r. recompression-high pressure oxygen
r. reintegration unit
r. rhythmic alternating movements
r. sequence induction orotracheal intubation
r. sequence intubation
r. shallow breathing
R. Shallow Breathing Index
r. simple tests
sleep-onset rapid eye movement period
r. smoking
r. straight pacing
r. surfactant test
surgically assisted rapid maxillary expansion
surgically assisted rapid palatal expansion
Ultegra rapid platelet function assay
r. urease test
r. ventricular response
r. weight gain
r. whole blood test

rapid-acquisition spin echo

rapidly
r. accumulating ascites
R. Alternating Speech Perception Test
r. growing lesion
r. growing tumor
idiopathic rapidly progressive glomerulonephritis
r. miscible pool
patient rapidly intubated

r. progressing bilateral hearing loss
r. progressive crescenting glomerulonephritis
r. progressive necrotizing glomerulonephritis

rapid-sequence
r.-s. induction
r.-s. intravenous pyelography

rapist
adolescent r.

Rappaport
R. classification
R. classification of lymphoma

rapport
patient has good rapport with others

rare
r. detail response
r. earth element
Rapid R. Event Detection
unusual rare detail response

rarefaction
mottled r.

rarer
frequency of rarer allele of a gene pair

Ras
mutant Ras peptide-pulsed dendritic cell therapy

Rasch sign

rash
allergic diaper r.
angiectatic skin r.
arthropod-borne viral arthritis and r.
atopic dermatitis r.
atopic diaper r.
eczematoid skin r.
erythematous maculopapular r.
exanthematous drug r.
funny-looking r.
generalized r.
glue sniffer's r.
intractable skin r.
itchy skin r.
juvenile rheumatoid arthritis r.
lupus erythematous-like r.
malar r.
malar butterfly r.
monilial diaper r.
morbilliform skin r.
Murray Valley r.
polymorphous macular r.
prickly heat r.
psoriatic diaper r.
r. pustule
road r.
seborrheic diaper r.
warm weather r.

Rashkind procedure

Rasmussen
R. aneurysm
bundle of R.
R. encephalitis
olivocochlear bundle of R.

Rasor blood pumping system

rasp
angled r.
bone r.
carbon-tungsten r.
custom r.
Miltner rotary bone r.
Wiener-Pierce r.

raspberry mark

rat
r. aortic tissue
r. basophilic leukemia
r. embryo tissue culture
r. growth hormone
r. insulinoma
r. insulin receptor
r. intrinsic factor concentrate
iodinated rat serum albumin
isolated perfused rat liver
lactating rat serum factor
r. lung strip
r. mast cell protease
r. mast cell technique
r. nephroma tissue culture
normal rat kidney
normotensive Wistar r.
northern rat flea
northern rat flea bite
r. ovarian weight
pink-eyed, tan-hooded rat
r. serum albumin
r. serum protein
spontaneously diabetic r.
r. stomach strip
r. synaptic ending
r. thymus antiserum
r. urine protein
r. virus

rate
abnormality in heart r.
abnormally rapid heart r.
abnormally slow heart r.
absolute catabolic r.
accelerating heart r.
accelerating rate calorimetry
activity metabolic r.
age-specific cumulative incidence r.
age-specific fertility r.
albumin excretion r.
aldosterone excretion r.
aldosterone secretion r.
aldosterone secretory r.
allograft survival r.
alteration in rate of speech
alternate motion r.
alternating motion r.
amebic prevalence r.
amphotericin B-induced reduction glomerular filtration r.
r. analysis
angina threshold heart r.
angiotensin generation r.
anticipatory bogus heart rate feedback
apneic infant with decreased heart r.
apparent net transfer r.
apparent norepinephrine secretion r.
arousal heart r.
atrial overdrive stimulation r.
atrial tachycardia detection r.
attack r.
attrition rate scale
average daily metabolic r.
average flow r.
axillary count r.
basal heart r.
basal metabolic r.
basal secretory flow r.
baseline variability of fetal heart r.
basic incidence r.
blood filtration r.
blood flow r.
blood oxygen release r.
blood production r.
blood sedimentation r.
body acceleration synchronous with heart r.
bone formation r.
breathing r.
calcification r.
cerebral cortex perfusion r.
cerebral metabolic r.
cerebral metabolic rate of glucose
cerebral metabolic rate of lactate
cerebral metabolic rate of oxygen
cerebral rate of glucose metabolism

rate *(continued)*
change in heart r.
r. change induced
compliance, rate, oxygenation, and pressure
compliance, rate, oxygenation, and pressure index
r. constant
constant dose r.
constant exposure r.
r. constants
contraceptive failure r.
r. control
control of heart rate during oxygen deprivation
conversion r.
cooling r.
corrected sedimentation r.
corrected survival r.
cortisol production r.
cortisol secretion r.
crevicular fluid flow r.
crude birth r.
crying, requirement for oxygen supplementation, increases in heart rate and blood pressure
crypt cell production r.
cumulative conception r.
cumulative potency r.
cumulative survival r.
daily fractionation rate of rad
r. of decay
decreased heart r.
deoxycorticosterone secretion r.
dialysate filtration r.
diastolic descent r.
r. difference
differential reinforcement of low response rates
disease-free survival r.
disordered breathing r.
drip rate of infusion
effective filtration r.
ejection r.
elevated heart r.
elimination rate constant
r. of energy loss
entomological inoculation r.
eradication r.'s
erythrocyte sedimentation r.
estradiol production r.
ethanol metabolic r.
excessively rapid heart r.
exercise heart r.
external fetal heart rate monitoring
false-negative r.
fast growth r.
fast heart r.
fasting intestinal flow r.
fetal heart r.
fetal heart rate acceleration
fetal heart rate baseline
fetal heart rate deceleration
fetal heart rate monitoring
fetal heart rate nonstress test
fetal heart rate reactivity
fetal heart rate reading
fetal heart rate variability
filled voiding flow r.
filtered atrial rate interval
five-year cure r.
five-year survival r.
fixed rate pacemaker
flocculation rate in antigen-antibody reaction
r. of flow
flow r.
r. of fluid filtration
fractional albuminuria r.
fractional catabolic r.
fractional disappearance r.
fractional esterification r.
fractional turnover r.
fractionated high dose r.
full outpatient r.
gallbladder ejection r.
glomerular filtration r.
glucose disposal r.
glucose production r.
graft survival r.
granulocyte turnover r.
growth r.
r. of healing
heart rate audiometry
heart rate condition ability
heart rate control
heart rate control learning and awareness
heart rate disorder
heart rate feedback
heart rate monitor
heart rate monitored
heart rate peak
heart rate perception
heart rate power spectral analysis
heart rate range
heart rate responses
high cure r.
high death r.
high dose r.
high dose rate brachytherapy
higher r.
highest equivalent heart r.
hourly fetal urine production r.
human operant heart rate conditioning
immunization r.
increased flow r.
increased heart and breathing r.
increased pulse r.
increased respiratory r.
increasing heart r.
infant mortality r.
information outflow r.
inspiratory flow r.
instrumental heart rate responses
insulin production r.
insulin secretion r.
internal fetal heart rate monitoring
interval patency r.
intrauterine growth r.
intrinsic heart r.
ionization exposure r.
irregular rate and rhythm
irreversible loss r.
keep open r.
key pulse r.
large magnitude voluntary heart rate changes
left ventricular peak filling r.
low absolute glomerular filtration r.
low-dose r.
low-dose rate intracavity therapy
low-dose rate irradiation
low flow r.
lymphatic return r.
marrow production r.
marrow release r.
maternal death r.
maternal mortality r.
maximal expiratory flow r.
maximal inspiratory flow r.
maximal midexpiratory flow r.
maximal midflow r.
maximal predicted heart r.
maximal pulse r.
maximal rate of urea synthesis
maximal relation r.
maximal relaxation r.
maximal tubular reabsorption rate for glucose
maximal urinary flow r.
maximal ventilation r.
maximum determined heart r.
maximum expiratory flow r.
maximum free flow r.
maximum midexpiratory flow r.
maximum predicted heart r.

mean atrial r.
mean axillary count r.
mean midexpiratory flow r.
mean normalized systolic ejection r.
mean systolic ejection r.
metabolic clearance r.
midinspiratory flow r.
mineral apposition r.
minimum flow r.
R. Modulated Pacing
modulation r.
moisture vapor transmission r.
molar esterification r.
mortality r.
mortality rate doubling time
movement-associated fetal heart rate accelerations
mucociliary clearance r.
mucus flow r.
multiplication r.
mutation r.
myocardial metabolic r.
myocardial ventilation, oxygen r.
neonatal death r.
neonatal mortality r.
net reproduction r.
nipple flow r.
normalized protein catabolic r.
normal resting pulse r.
normal sinus rate and rhythm
one-year survival r.
operant acceleration of heart r.
operant deceleration of heart r.
operative mortality r.
outflow r.
oxygen extraction r.
oxygen transport r.
pacemaker adaptive r.
pancreatic secretory flow r.
parathyroid hormone secretion r.
parotid flow r.
peak diastolic filling r.
peak ejection r.
peak emptying r.
peak expiratory flow r.
peak heart r.
peak inspiratory flow r.
peak jet flow r.
peak secretory flow r.
peak work r.
r. of perceived exertion
perfusion flow r.
perinatal morbidity r.
perinatal mortality r.
periodontal disease r.
physiologic aging r.
plasma appearance r.
plasma clearance r.
plasma glucose disappearance r.
plasma glucose tolerance r.
plasma iron turnover r.
precordial heart r.
predicted maximal heart r.
pregnancy r.
pressure increment r.
pressure rate product
production r.
protein catabolic r.
proton relaxation r.
pulse r.
pulsed dose r.
QT corrected for heart r.
radial r.
rapid filling r.
r. ratio
r. of reaction catalyzed by an enzyme
reaction rate constant
red blood cell iron turnover r.
red blood cell precursor production r.
reduced heart r.
regional cerebral metabolic rate for oxygen
regular heart r.
regular rate, clear tones, no murmurs
regular rate and rhythm
relative consumption r.
relative corrected death r.
relative growth r.
relatively slow sinus r.
relative survival r.
renal excretion r.
renin-release r.
respiratory r.
respiratory rate per minute
respiratory rate:pulse rate index
response r.
resting heart r.
resting metabolic r.
r. and rhythm
right ventricular peak filling r.
rising heart r.
sebum excretion r.
secretion r.
sedimentation rate test
single-nephron glomerular filtration r.
sinusoidal heart r.
sister chromatid exchange r.
slew r.
slow growth r.
slow heart r.
somnolent metabolic r.
specific absorption r.
standardized metabolic r.
standardized rate ratio
standing heart r.
steady-state heart r.
steroid metabolic clearance r.
stillbirth r.
sustained response r.
systolic ejection r.
target heart r.
target heart rate zone
testosterone production r.
time of peak emptying rate of mouth
time of peak emptying rate of pharynx
time to peak filling r.
time of peak filling rate of esophagus
total abortion r.
total fertility r.
total matrix formation r.
training heart r.
transcapillary escape r.
true negative r.
true positive r.
turnover r.
ultrafiltration r.
ultralow dose r.
urinary calcium volume excretion r.
urinary potassium volume excretion r.
urinary production r.
urine filtration r.
variable r.
vasoconstriction r.
r. of velocity constant
ventilation r.
ventricular rate variability
ventricular response r.
very low birth r.
voiding flow r.
volume clearance r.
voluntary heart rate control
Westergren erythrocyte sedimentation r.
Wintrobe erythrocyte sedimentation r.
work r.
work metabolic r.
5-year survival r.
zeta erythrocyte sedimentation r.

rate-adaptive pacemaker

rated
Clinician R. Anxiety Scale
Patient R. Anxiety Scale
r. perceived exertion
Sheehan Patient R. Anxiety Scale

rate-dependent
r.-d. angina
r.-d. left bundle-branch block

rate-drop response

rate-pressure product

rate/pulse
respiratory rate:pulse rate index

rate-responsive
dual-chamber r.-r.
r.-r. pacing

Rathke
R. bundle
R. cleft cyst
R. diverticulum
R. duct
R. fold
R. pocket
R. pouch
R. pouch homeobox transcription factor
R. tumor

rating
Abbreviated Conners Teacher R. Scale
Adjective R. Form
Alzheimer Disease R. Scale
Amphetamine Interview R. Scale
anxiety rating for children
anxiety rating scale
Atkinson Life Happiness R.
Attention Deficit Disorder Behavior R. Scale
average impairment r.
Behavioral and Emotional R. Scale
Behavior R. Profile, Second Edition
Behavior R. Scale
Blessed Dementia R. Scale
r. board
Brief Cognitive R. Scale
Brief Psychiatric Rating Scale for Children
Burks Behavior R. Scale
child behavior rating form
Childhood Autism R. Scale
Children's Affective R. Scale
Children's Depression R. Scale-Revised
Children's Psychiatric R. Scale
Clinical Dementia R.
Clinical R. Scale
Clinician's Global R. Scale
Comprehensive Psychopathological R. Scale
Conners Teacher R. Scale
Cooper-Farran Behavioral R. Scale
Devereux Elementary School Behavior Rating Scale II
Disability R. Scale
Dyskinesia R. Scale
extrapyramidal symptom rating scale
flight aptitude r.
R. Form of IBD Patient Concerns
Gait Abnormality R. Scale Modified
Gastrointestinal Symptom R. Scale
Global Improvement R.
Graphic R. Scale
Group Conformity R.
Hamburg R. Scale for Psychiatric Disorders
Hamilton Anxiety R. Scale
Hamilton Depression R. Scale
Hamilton R. Scale for Depression
Health-Sickness R. Scale
Hemiballism/Hemichorea Outcome R. Score
Himmelsbach R. Scale
Infant/Toddler Environment R. Scale
Inpatient Behavior R. Scale
Karnofsky rating scale
Lengyeh-Kerman-Vargar rating
Life Satisfaction R.
Living Conditions R. Scale
mania rating scale
Mattis Dementia R. Scale
Mazur ankle r.
Merle d'Aubigné and Postel hip rating scale
modified Gait Abnormality R. Scale
Neurobehavioral R. Scale
neuropsychiatric acquired immunodeficiency syndrome rating scale
newborn maturity r.
Noise Reduction R.
numeric rating scale
Pain R. Index
parent anxiety rating scale
parent's rating scale
patient evaluation rating scale
r. of perceived breathing difficulty
r. of perceived exertion
Permanent Disability Rating Board
Personality R. Scale
Process Skills R. Scale
Psychiatric Status Rating scale
pupil rating scale
Rehabilitation Client R. Scale
risk rescue r.
R. Scale of Communication in Cognitive Decline
sexual maturity r.
Short Clinical R. Scale
Social Readjustment R. Scale
Social Skills R. System
Symptom R. Scale
Symptom R. Test
Teacher R. Form
Timed Behavioral R. Sheet
Toronto Western Spasmodic Torticollis R. Scale
Treatment R. Assessment Matrix
Unified Parkinson Disease R. Scale
Verdun Depression R. Scale
Verdun Target Symptom R. Scale
Ward Behavior R. Scale
Wender Utah R. Scale
Wittenborn Psychiatric R. Scale
Young Mania R. Scale

ratio
accommodative convergence/accommodation r.
achievement r.
acid-base r.
adherence r.
adrenal-to-spleen r.
adrenal vein aldosterone r.
age-standardized mortality r.
amplitude r.
amylase to creatinine r.
amylase-creatinine clearance r.
ankle-brachial blood pressure r.
aortic root r.
aortic valve opening to aortic valve closing r.
apolipoprotein CII-CIII r.
arterial to alveolar oxygen tension r.
artery:aortic velocity r.
artery bronchus r.
artery-to-vein r.
association sensation r.

automated ventricular brain r.
axial length/corneal radius r.
r. of basal acid output to maximal acid output
benefit/cost r.
bile duct-to-portal space r.
bilirubin to albumin r.
blood urea nitrogen/creatinine r.
body hematocrit-venous hematocrit r.
bone age r.
bone-contacting surface r.
bound/free antigen r.
calcium to phosphorus r.
carbon-to-nitrogen r.
cardiothoracic r.
case-fatality r.
category ratio 0–10
cerebral blood volume/cerebral blood flow r.
cholesterol to phospholipid r.
compression to traction r.
contrast-to-noise r.
coronary observation r.
cremaster r.
critical r.
crossmatch to transfusion r.
crude mortality r.
cup-to-disc ratio horizontal
cup-to-disc ratio vertical
dead-space gas volume to tidal gas volume r.
r. of decayed and filled surfaces
r. of decayed and filled teeth
deuterium/hydrogen ratio
distribution r.
doctor/population r.
dose nonuniformity r.
effective thyroxine r.
effector to target r.
efficacy r.
r. of electron charge to mass
embolus-to-blood r.
endocardial viability r.
enhancement r.
essential metabolism r.
estimated thyroid r.
r. of expiration time and total time of breathing cycle
expiratory to inspiratory r.
extracellular mass to body cell mass r.
extraction r.
fixed r.
fixed ratio combination drugs
flow r.
fluorescein to protein r.
forced expiratory volume in one second to forced vital capacity r.
forced expiratory volume timed to forced vital capacity r.
functional terminal innervation r.
galvanic tetanus r.
gas isotope ratio mass spectrometry
glucose/nitrogen ratio in urine
glucose/nitrogen ratio in water
graft-to-recipient weight r.
hazard r.
head-to-abdomen ratio
heart-to-lung r.
immunoreactive insulin to serum or plasma glucose r.
r. of inspiration time and total time of breathing cycle
inspiratory to expiratory r.
inspiratory expiratory r.
r. of inspiratory time to total cycle time
intelligence r.
international calibrated r.
international normalized r.
intrapulmonary shunt r.
isotope ratio mass spectrometry
ketogenic/antiketogenic ratio
ketone body r.
left-to-right r.
left-to-right shunt r.
length-to-diameter r.
light/dark amplitude r.
limb bone length r.
lithocholic acid-deoxycholic acid r.
log magnitude r.
lung-body weight r.
r. of magnetic moment of a particle to Bohr magneton
magnetization transfer r.
Mantel-Haenszel weighted odds r.
mass-to-charge r.
maximal aggregation r.
maximum diameter to minimum diameter r.
mean diameter-thickness r.
message competition r.
metaphysial to diaphysial width r.
r. of midsagittal diameter
modified gain r.
molecular weight r.
monocyte-lymphocyte r.
mortality rate r.
myeloid to erythroid r.
N-acetylaspartate/creatine r.
neck-to-thigh r.
neopterin to biopterin r.
net histocompatibility r.
net protein r.
nitrous oxide to oxygen r.
noise-to-harmonic r.
nonglucogenic/glucogenic r.
nuclear-cytoplasmic r.
nutrition r.
odds r.
off-axis r.
off-center r.
oil-water ratio
optic cup-to-disk r.
oral-nasal acoustic r.
oronasal acoustic r.
oxidative phosphorylation r.
oxygen enhancement r.
oxygen extraction r.
PAC lateralization r.
parent-metabolite ratio
peak respiratory r.
peak-to-resting-velocity r.
pepsinogen A-C r.
platelet aggregate r.
polyunsaturated-to-saturated fatty acids r.
positive to negative r.
potency r.
pressure-controlled inverse ratio ventilation
pressure transmission r.
presumed circle area r.
productivity to respiration r.
proportional morbidity r.
proportional mortality r.
proportionate morbidity r.
protein efficiency r.
protein kinase activation r.
prothrombin time r.
r. of pulmonary to systemic circulation
pulmonary-to-systemic flow r.
pulse amplitude r.
rate r.
red blood cell to plasma r.
relative standardized mortality r.
renal vein/renal activity r.
renin-release r.
respiratory control r.
respiratory exchange r.
response-stimulus r.
retention time r.
right lung-to-head circumference r.
right-to-left shunt r.

ratio *(continued)*
scatter-air r.
scatter-maximum r.
segmented venous capacitance r.
sentinel node-to-background r.
sequential probability ratio test
r. of serum alanine aminotransferase to serum aspartate aminotransferase
sex r.
signal-difference to noise r.
signal enhancement r.
signal-to-noise r.
speech-to-noise r.
spleen-to-body weight r.
standardized incidence r.
standardized mortality r.
standardized rate r.
standard morbidity r.
standard mortality r.
stimulation r.
surface area to volume r.
terminal innervation r.
testosterone to epitestosterone r.
thermal enhancement r.
thyroid hormone-binding r.
thyroid-serum r.
tissue-air r.
tissue-maximum r.
tissue-phantom r.
triiodothyronine uptake r.
trough-to-peak r.
type-to-token r.
upper body segment to lower body segment r.
urea reduction r.
urine-plasma r.
variable r.
variance r.
velocity r.
venous diameter r.
ventilation r.
ventilation/perfusion r.
ventricle-to-brain r.
ventricular-brain r.
visceral abdominal fat to total abdominal fat r.
r. of waist to hip circumference
waist-to-hip r.

rational
r. behavior therapy
r. hypertensive therapy
systematic rational restructuring
r. thinking

rational-emotive therapy

rationality
irrational r.

rationing
healthcare rationing plan

rat-tail configuration

rattle
death r.
tobacco rattle virus

Rau
apophysis of R.

Rauchfuss
R. sling
R. triangle

Raulerson
Arrow Raulerson syringe

Rauscher
R. murine leukemia virus

Raven
R. Colored Progressive Matrices Test
R. Standard Progressive Matrices

raw
r. area under curve
certified raw milk

ray
r. amputation
axial ray of light
r. axis
capture gamma r.
cathode r.
cathode ray oscilloscope
central r.
detection of gamma r.
gamma ray spectrometer
gamma ray surgery
gamma ray therapy
hard r.'s
indirect r.'s
intensity of roentgen r.
Leonard cathode ray unit
long axis r.
marginal ray of light
oblique ray of light
optical ray tracing
paraxial ray of light
peripheral ray of light
photon gamma r.
r. resection
specific gamma ray constant
r. tracing
vertebral abnormality, anal imperforation, tracheoesophageal fistula, and radial, ray, or renal anomalies

Rayleigh
R. number
R. test

Raymond apoplexy

Raynaud
calcification, Raynaud phenomenon, scleroderma, telangiectasis syndrome
R. disease
R. gangrene
idiopathic Raynaud disease
R. phenomenon
R. sign
R. syndrome

Rayner-Choyce implant

Razdan virus

razor

reabsorption
absolute proximal r.
fractional r.
maximal tubular reabsorption rate for glucose
phosphate reabsorption index
tubular r.
tubular reabsorption of phosphate

reach
R. in Four Directions Test
functional r.

reached
r. maximum hospital benefit
not r.
patient reached maximum hospital benefit

reacher
long-handled dressing r.

react
febrile nonhemolytic transfusion r.
hemolytic transfusion r.
pupils react to light and accommodation
pupils react sluggishly
round, regular, react normally

reactant
acute phase r.
acute-phase reactant protein

reacting
melanoma antigen reacting to T cell
minimum reacting dose
not r.

reaction
absence of heat in a r.
absolute reaction of degeneration
acetic acid r.
active avoidance r.
acute adverse psychological r.
acute anxiety r.
acute dystonic r.

acute paranoid schizophrenic r.
acute phase r.
acute stress r.
acute undifferentiated schizophrenic r.
adjustment reaction of adolescence
adjustment reaction of childhood
adjustment reaction conduct disorder
adjustment reaction disturbance
adjustment reaction of infancy
adjustment reaction of later life
adjustment reaction of menopause
adjustment reaction of middle age
adjustment reaction physical symptom
adjustment situational r.
r. of adolescence
adolescent turmoil r.
adult situation stress r.
adverse drug r.
adverse drug-induced r.
affective depressive r.
affective reaction type
agglutinative r.'s
aggressive undersocialized r.
alarm r.
alarm reaction stage
allele-specific polymerase chain r.
allergic drug r.
allergic transfusion r.
amplification refractory mutation system-polymerase chain r.
anaphylactic transfusion r.
anesthetic conversion r.
angry back r.
angry reaction to minor stimuli
anterior chamber r.
antibody reaction site
antigen-antibody r.
antigen-antiglobulin r.
anxiety panic r.
anxiety psychoneurotic r.
anxiety reaction, intense
anxious mood adjustment r.
arbitrarily-primed polymerase chain r.
arbitrary-primed polymerase chain r.
argentaffin reaction test
aseptic meningeal r.
Asian alcohol flush r.
association reaction time
autoimmune type of r.
autologous mixed leukocyte r.
autologous mixed lymphocyte r.
automatic movement r.
autonomic conversion r.
BCR-ABL multiplex reverse transcriptase polymerase chain reaction assay
r. center
central reaction time
cerebrospinal fluid–Wassermann r.
characteristic inflammatory r.
r. of childhood
choice r.
choice reaction time
chronic paranoid schizophrenic r.
clinical manifestation of drug r.
clinical manifestation of panic r.
competitive polymerase chain r.
competitive reverse transcription-polymerase chain r.
complement-fixation r.
complete reaction of degeneration
complex reaction time
conduct disturbance adjustment r.
consensual light r.
countertransference r.'s
cutaneous graft-versus-host r.
r. to death
r. of degeneration
degeneration r.
delayed asthmatic r.
delayed cutaneous r.
delayed hemolytic r.
delayed skin hypersensitivity r.
r. of denervation
dextran-induced anaphylactoid r.
direct transverse r.
drug-induced skin r.'s
dual asthmatic r.
early-phase r.
emotional disturbance adjustment r.
emotional disturbance stress r.
r. energy
erythema-edema reaction
family reaction to illness
fatal hypersensitivity r.
Felix-Weil r.
fight or flight r.
first-dose r.
flashback reaction with hallucinogen
flocculation rate in antigen-antibody r.
Folin-Wu r.
generalized Sanarelli-Shwartzman r.
generalized Shwartzman r.
gonococcal antibody r.
graft-versus-host disease r.
granulomatous hypersensitivity r.
r. half-time
heightened startle r.'s
hot plate reaction time
hyperimmune r.
hyperkinetic reaction of childhood
hypersensitivity r.
hysterical conversion r.
r. of identity
idiosyncratic drug r.
immediate asthmatic r.
immediate generalized r.
immediate phase r.
immediate transfusion r.
immune complex r.
r. immunity
immunologic hypersensitivity r.
individual r.
injection site r.
interpersonal reaction test
intradermal r.
ipsilateral instinctive grasp r.
irritant r.
Jarisch-Herxheimer r.
Jolly r.
large local r.
late cutaneous anaphylactic r.
latency r.
late-phase cutaneous r.
latex direct agglutination r.
leukocyte migration inhibition r.
leukoerythroblastic r.
R. Level Scale
lid closure r.
ligase-chain reaction assay
ligase-chain reaction testing
light r.
limit of r.
limiting dilution polymerase chain r.
linear Koebner r.
local anesthetic r.
localized immune r.
lymphocyte transfer r.
lymphocytic leukemoid r.
marked localized r.
massive vitreous r.
median reaction time
Meinicke turbidity r.
mild anxiety r.
mixed antiglobulin r.
mixed cell agglutination r.
mixed disturbance stress r.
mixed lymphocyte culture r.

reaction *(continued)*
mixed lymphocyte reaction blocking factor
mixed skin cell leukocyte r.
modified Gomori trichrome r.
monocytic leukemoid r.
mucus escape r.
multiple marker reverse transcriptase-polymerase chain reaction assay
multiplex polymerase chain r.
myelocytic leukemoid r.
myeloproliferative r.
near reaction to light
negative therapeutic r.
Neill-Mooser r.
neonatal leukemoid r.
neurotic depressive r.
neutrophil antibody and transfusion r.
no adverse r.
nonanaphylactic r.
nonhemolytic febrile transfusion r.
nonimmediate-type immunologic drug r.
nonimmunologic drug r.
nonspecific r.
nonsystemic r.
normal r.
normal pupillary reaction to light
ocular tilt r.
painful withdrawal r.
panic reactions with hallucinogen
paradoxical darkness r.
partial reaction of degeneration
passive Arthus r.
passive avoidance r.
passive cutaneous anaphylactic r.
pathologic grief r.
peracetic acid-Schiff r.
performic acid-Schiff r.
periodic acid-Schiff r.
peritumor glial r.
persistent light r.
photoallergic drug r.
phototoxic r.
physiological musculoskeletal r.
polymerase chain r.
polymerase chain reaction analysis of prostate-specific antigen
polymerase chain reaction in situ hybridization
possible allergic r.
Price precipitation r.
r. product
proprioceptive neuromuscular fasciculation reaction
psychophysiologic gastrointestinal reaction
psychophysiologic musculoskeletal reaction
psychotic trigger r.
pupil reaction and size
pupils equal in size and r.
quanti-Pirquet r.
quantitative competitive polymerase chain r.
radiation r.
radiation bowel r.
r. rate constant
rate of reaction catalyzed by an enzyme
red blood cell-linked antigen-antiglobulin r.
repetitive extragenic palindromic polymerase chain r.
reversed passive hemagglutination r.
reverse transcriptase polymerase chain r.
ribonucleic acid-polymerase chain r.
Sachs-Georgi r.
schizophrenic r.
schizophrenic reaction, acute, paranoid
schizophrenic reaction, acute undifferentiated
schizophrenic reaction, chronic, paranoid
schizophrenic reaction, chronic, undifferentiated
serum Wassermann r.
severe withdrawal r.
Shwartzman generalized r.
Shwartzman local r.
sigma r.
simple reaction time
in situ polymerase chain r.
slowed reaction time
suspected adverse drug r.
systemic r.
therapeutic r.
r. time
transfusion r.
transient situational r.
treatment of acute drug reaction to hallucinogen
tryptophan-acid r.
Wassermann r.
wheal-and-flare r.
wiping r.
xanthine oxidase r.

reaction–single

reactiva
meningitis necrotoxica r.

reactivated tuberculosis

reactivation
enhanced r.
host-cell r.
multiplicity r.
ultraviolet-enhanced r.

reactive
r. airway
r. arthritis
atypical favor r.
autologous reactive T cell
r. bowel
r. confusion
r. cutaneous angioendotheliomatosis
r. dermatitis
r. eosinophilic pleuritis
equal and r.
exertional reactive airway disease
r. extensor postural synergy
highly reactive oxygen molecules
r. hyperemia
r. hyperemia blood flow
r. hyperplasia
r. to light pupil
r. lymphoid hyperplasia
r. lymphoid tissue
moderately constricted and equally reactive pupil
moderately constricted and slightly reactive pupil
moderately dilated and equally reactive pupil
moderately dilated and slightly reactive pupil
r. neurotic depression
r. nitrogen intermediate
r. nonstress test
r. oxygen intermediate
r. oxygen species
panel of reactive antibodies
peak reactive hyperemia blood flow
percent reactive antibody
percent reactive antibody/panel reactive antibody
r. perforating collagenosis
postocclusive reactive hyperemia
postoperative reactive hyperemia
poststreptococcal reactive arthritis
r. power

r. protein
pupils equal, reactive, and contracting
pupils equal and reactive to light and accommodation
pupils equal, round, reactive to light and accommodation
pupils equal, round, reactive to light and accommodation directly and consensually
sexually acquired reactive arthritis
r. site
r. spindle cell nodule
r. subdural effusion
r. upper airways dysfunction syndrome
weakly r.

reactivity
airway reactivity index
B-cell r.
cellular immunologic r.
cerebrovascular r.
digital vascular r.
fetal cardiac reactivity test
fetal heart rate r.
lymphocyte reactivity index
persistent reactivity to light
skin test r.
T-cell r.

reactor
biologic false-positive r.
hot reactor syndrome

read
survey, question, read, review, recite
unable to read lab result

readily
as low as readily practicable

readiness
Academic R. Scale
California Marriage R. Evaluation
Caregiver's School R. Inventory
R. to Change questionnaire
Discharge R. Inventory
Hess School R. Scale
Kindergarten R. Test
Metropolitan R. Test
Pediatric Examination of Educational R.
Phelps Kindergarten R. Scale
Physical Activity R. Questionnaire
r. potential
Printing Performance School R. Test
self-directed learning readiness scale
Simultaneous Technique for Acuity and R. Testing
Slosson Test of Reading R.
Teacher School R. Inventory
Thackray Reading R. Profile

reading
r. age
albumin r.
Basic R. Inventory
r. card
r. chart
Diagnostic Assessments of R.
fetal heart rate r.
general reading backwardness
Gilmore Oral R. Test
r. glasses
Gray Oral R. Test-Revised
Gray Oral R. Test, Third Edition
Group R. Test
Individualized Criterion Reference Testing R.
keratometric r.'s
R. Miscue Inventory
National Adult R. Test
Neale Reading Analysis
Pepper Visual Skills for R. Test
Prescriptive R. Inventory
r. quotient
r. retarded
Slosson Oral Reading Test-Revised
Slosson Test of R. Readiness
specific reading disability
specific reading retarded
r. of standard
Stanford Diagnostic R. Test
r. task
r. test
Test of Early R. Comprehension
Thackray R. Readiness Profile
r. time
tonometer r.
total reading time
unidentified reading frame
r. of unknown
visual, association, kinesthetic, tactile r.
Woodcock R. Mastery Test

Reading-Free Vocational Interest Inventory

readjustment
Social R. Rating Scale

read-only memory

reagent
analyte-specific r.
analytical r.
blood glucose reagent strip
Bolton-Hunter r.
heated serum r.
microanalytical r.
quality assurance r.
rapid plasma r.
r. strip
Woodward reagent K

reagin
atopic r.
automated r.
automated reagin test
rapid plasma r.
rapid plasma reagin circle card test
rapid plasma reagin complement fixation
Reiter protein r.
r. screen test
unheated serum r.

real
r. anxiety
Estero Real virus
r. oxygen transport
simulated real ear measurement

reality
R. Check Survey
contact with r.
r. denial
flight from r.
hallucinations and loss of r.
impaired reality testing
r. of injury
interpretation of r.
r. orientation
r. oriented
severe impairment in interpretation of r.

reality-adaptive supportive

real-time
r.-t. Doppler
r.-t. dose area product
r.-t. fine-needle aspiration
r.-t., low-intensity x-ray
r.-t. position management
r.-t. scan
r.-t. ultrasonography

reamer
A-type r.
Aufranc r.
Austin Moore r.
ball r.
blunt tapered T-handled r.

reamer *(continued)*
congruous cup-shaped r.
conical r.
cup r.
fenestrated r.
flexible medullary r.
fluted r.
humeral r.

reaming
cannulated reaming technique

reanastomosis
limb r.

reaper's keratitis

rearend collision

rearfoot stability system

rearranged during transfection

rearrangement
Amadori-type r.
lymphocyte gene r.

reason
R.'s for Living Inventory
not guilty by reason of insanity
other administrative r.'s
r. for visit

reasonable
r. compensation equivalent
r. and customary
customary, prevailing, and r.
usual, customary, and reasonable fees

reasonably
as low as reasonably achievable radiation exposure
r. expected as safe

reasoning
abstract r.
age of r.
arithmetical r.
Critical R. Test
functioning, reasoning, orientation, memory, arithmetic, judgment, and emotion
Picture R. Test
Toronto Biculture Test of Nonverbal R.
verbal, numerical, and r.

reaspiration
puncture, aspiration, injection, r.

reassessment
attitude r.
sexual attitude r.

reassignment
sex reassignment surgery

reattachment
Amstutz r.
r. of retina

Réaumur scale

rebellion
adolescent r.
r. in home

rebleed
aneurysmal r.

rebleeding
decreased rebleeding risk

rebound
r. and/or guarding
r. angina
guarding and/or r.
r. guarding or rigidity
r. headache
medication rebound syndrome
postinhibition r.
REM r.
r. tenderness
tenderness and r.

rebreathing
aerosol rebreathing method
controlled partial rebreathing anesthesia method
r. mask
multiple gas r.
partial rebreathing mask
r. ventilation

Rebuck skin window technique

recalcification
whole-blood recalcification time

recalcified whole-blood activated clotting time

recalcitrant
r. benign paroxysmal positional vertigo
r. hypertension

recall
delayed r.
delayed work recall test
diminished r.
evaluate orientation, attention, and recent r.
failure of immediate r.
immediate auditory r.
immediate and delayed r.
immediate sensory trace r.
inability to r.
inability to recall events
intentional r.
multiplanar gradient r.
short-term r.
r. urticaria

recalled
spoiled gradient r.

recanalization
angiographic r.
endoscopic laser r.
excimer vascular r.
intraoperative r.
percutaneous endoscopic r.
percutaneous transluminal coronary r.

recanalizing thrombosis

receded gums

receding
r. hairline
r. lower jaw

received
positive attention r.

receiver
bone-conduction r.
r. operating characteristic
r. operating characteristic curve

receiving
medical receiving station
patient receiving respiratory assistance

recent
area of recent hemorrhage
evaluate orientation, attention, and recent recall
r. event memory
impaired memory for recent events
r. infarct
r. life event
loss of recent memory, confusion and poor judgment
r. memory impairment and confabulation
most recent episode
no recent illnesses
r. and remote
Schedule of R. Experiences
signs of recent hemorrhage
small, deep, recent infarct
r. soft tissue hemorrhage
stigmata of recent hemorrhage

receptacle
fecal collection receptacle assembly
solid phase r.

reception
speech reception test
speech reception threshold

receptive
r. aphasia

r. deficit
developmental receptive language disorder
r. dysphagia
r. field of visual cortex
r. language
R. One-Word Picture Vocabulary Test

Receptive-Expressive
R.-E. Observation Scale

receptor
acetylcholine r.
acetylcholine receptor antibody
activated estrogen r.
r. activator of NF-κB
r. activator of nuclear factor kappa B ligand
activin r.
activin receptor IB, II, IIB
activin receptor IB, II, IIB
adrenergic r.
adrenergic receptor binder
adrenergic receptor kinase
adrenergic receptor material
alpha-adrenergic r.'s
alpha-2 adrenergic r.
alpha-adrenergic receptor agonist
alpha-adrenergic receptor antagonist
alpha-2-adrenergic receptor antagonist
alpha receptor blocking agent
androgen r.
androgen receptor antagonist
androgen receptor element
androgen receptor gene
androgen receptor gene mutation
angiotensin II r.
angiotensin II receptor blocker
ANP clearance r.
antiacetylcholine receptor antibody
antiacetylcholine receptor antibody assay
anti-ACh receptor antibody
antiandrogen receptor blocker
antiasialoglycoprotein r.
antidiuretic arginine vasopressin V2 r.
anti-EGF receptor antibody for cancer
antiepidermal growth factor r.
antiepidermal growth factor receptor antibody for cancer
antiepidermal growth factor receptor monoclonal antibody
antigenic binding r.
antigen receptor gene
antiinsulin receptor antibody
anti-interleukin-2 receptor alpha monoclonal antibody
antimuscarinic acetylcholine r.
aryl hydrocarbon r.
aryl hydrocarbon receptor nuclear translocator
atrial natriuretic factor r.
autocrine motility factor r.
B-cell antigen r.
benzodiazepine r.
beta-adrenergic r.
beta-adrenergic receptor kinase
r. blockade
calcium-sensing r.
cAMP receptor protein
r. cells of hearing
chemokine receptor 2, 3, 5
chemokine-related r.
ciliary-derived neurotrophic factor r.
9-*cis* retinoic acid r.
complement receptor 1–4
complement receptor location
complement receptor lymphocyte
corticotropin-releasing hormone receptor type 1, 2
decreased estrogen r.
dihydrotestosterone receptor deficiency
dopamine receptor agonist property
drug r.
early receptor potential
early receptor potential mottling
epidermal growth factor r.
erythrocyte r.
estradiol r.
estradiol receptor assay
estrogen r.
estrogen receptor alpha
estrogen receptor assay
estrogen receptor beta
estrogen receptor immunocytochemistry assay
estrogen receptor/progesterone r.
estrogen receptor protein
fibroblast growth factor r.
fibroblast growth factor receptor 2
glucocorticoid r.
glutamide receptor subunit
gonadotropin-releasing hormone r.
G protein-coupled r.
granulocyte colony-stimulating factor r.
growth hormone receptor deficiency
growth hormone-releasing hormone r.
growth hormone secretagogue r.
high-density lipoprotein-cell surface r.
histamine-2 r.
histamine-2 receptor antagonist
histamine$_2$ receptor antagonist
histamine receptor type 1
hormone receptor site
hormone receptor test
human androgen receptor assay
human androgen receptor gene
human epidermal growth receptor 2
humanized antihuman IL-2 receptor antibody
human thyroid hormone r.
r. for hyaluronan-mediated motility
imidazoline r.
increased estrogen r.
infectious mononucleosis r.
inhibitory r.
insulinlike growth factor-II r.
insulin receptor binding test
insulin receptor knockout
insulin receptor-related r.
insulin receptor species
r. interacting protein
interleukin-2 r.
interleukin-1 receptor antagonist protein
intravenous H2 receptor antagonist
keratinocyte growth factor r.
killer cell inhibitory r.
leukotriene receptor antagonist
ligand r.
ligand-dependent action of thyroid hormone r.
ligand-independent action of thyroid hormone r.
limbic dopamine r.
lipopolysaccharide r.
low affinity antigen r.
low-density lipoprotein receptor disorder
luteinizing hormone r.
lymphocyte homing r.
macula densa r.
malfunctioning insulin receptor cells
mamillary nuclei r.

receptor *(continued)*
maternal thyrotropin receptor blocking antibody-induced congenital hypothyroidism
Mel1a melatonin r.
melanocortin-2, -3, -4 r.
melanocortin receptor isoform
Mel1b melatonin r.
membrane-associated estrogen r.
membrane-bound receptor molecule
metabotropic glutamate r.
metenkephalin receptor binding
MHC receptor expression
mineralocorticoid r.
MIS II r.
motilin receptor agonist
müllerian-inhibiting substance r.
muscarinic acetylcholine r.
muscarinic cholinergic r.
muscarinic receptor autoantibody
muscle r.
muscle receptor organ
myocardial beta-adrenergic r.
myometrial oxytocin r.
natriuretic peptide r.
natural cytotoxicity r.
nerve growth factor r.
neural growth factor r.
neurokinin-1 receptor antagonist
neurotensin receptor type 1, 2
neurotrophic tyrosine kinase receptor, type 1
nicotinic acetylcholine r.
nicotinic cholinergic r.
nicotinic receptor blockade therapy
nonselective adenosine receptor antagonist
nuclear hormone r.
nuclear receptor corepressor
opiate receptor agonist
opioid cell membrane r.
opioid receptor agonist
opioid receptor antagonist
r. organ of hearing
parathyroid extracellular calcium-sensing r.
peptic cell r.
peptide growth factor receptor signal
peripheral benzodiazepine r.
peripheral catecholamine r.
peripheral-type benzodiazepine r.
peroxisomal proliferator r.
peroxisome proliferator-activated r.
peroxisome proliferator-activated receptor gamma
polyimmunoglobulin r.
premenopausal hormone receptor positive
progesterone r.
progesterone receptor assay
progestin r.
prostaglandin F r.
protease-activated r.
r. protein tyrosine kinase
pulmonary stretch r.
rat insulin r.
r. activator of nuclear factor-kappa B
retinoic acid r.
retinoic acid-related orphan r.
retinoid X, Z r.
selective estrogen receptor modulator
silencing mediator of retinoic acid and thyroid hormone r.
soluble complement r.
soluble transferrin r.
soluble tumor necrosis factor-a receptor type I
somatostatin r.
somatostatin receptor scintigraphy
source-to-image receptor distance
stimulatory r.
sulfonylurea r.
T_3 r.
T-cell antigen r.
T cell antigen receptor Vb
thrombin r.
thyroid hormone r.
thyroid hormone receptor-retinoid X r.
thyroid-stimulating hormone r.
thyroid-stimulating hormone receptor antibody
thyroid-stimulating hormone receptor autoantibody
thyrotropin r.
thyrotropin receptor autoantibody
thyrotropin-releasing hormone r.
total cellular receptor pool
transferrin r.
r. transforming
TSH receptor antibody
tumor necrosis factor r.
r. tyrosine kinase
urokinase plasminogen activator r.
vasopressin r.
virus entry mediator, a receptor expressed by T lymphocyte
vitamin D r.
X-linked human androgen r.

receptor-activating
thrombin receptor-activating peptide
thrombin receptor-activating peptide 6

receptor-associated
r.-a. coactivator 3
r.-a. protein

receptor-binding abnormality

receptor-chemoeffector complex

receptor-destroying enzyme

receptor-negative
estrogen r.-n.

receptor-positive
estrogen r.-p.

receptor/progesterone
estrogen receptor/progesterone receptor

recess
anterior recess of interpeduncular fossa
anterior recess of ischiorectal fossa
anterior recess of tympanic membrane
anular periradial r.
costodiaphragmatic recess of pleura
costomediastinal recess of pleura
epitympanic r.
lateral recess stenosis
lateral recess syndrome
superior duodenal r.

recession
r. index
inferior oblique r.
optic muscle r.
r. and resection

recessive
r. allele
autosomal r.
autosomal recessive disorder
autosomal recessive hereditary optic neuropathy
autosomal recessive hypophosphatemic rickets
autosomal recessive ichthyosis
autosomal recessive inheritance
autosomal recessive juvenile parkinsonism
autosomal recessive kidney disease
autosomal recessive mode

autosomal recessive mutation
autosomal recessive nonsyndromic hearing loss
autosomal recessive ocular albinism
autosomal recessive ocular Ehlers-Danlos syndrome
autosomal recessive renal proximal tubulopathy and hypercalciuria
autosomal recessive severe combined immunodeficiency disorder
autosomal recessive spastic ataxia of Charlevoix-Saguenay
autosomal recessive syndrome of encephalopathy
autosomal recessive trait
cerebral autosomal recessive arteriopathy with subcortical infarcts and leukoencephalopathy
r. disorder
r. dystrophic epidermolysis bullosa
r. epidermolysis bullosa dystrophica–Hallopeau-Siemens syndrome
r. gene
inheritance
mild X-linked recessive muscular dystrophy
nonsyndromic autosomal recessive disorder
severe childhood autosomal recessive muscular dystrophy
type 1 autosomal recessive vitamin D dependency
r. X-linked ichthyosis
X-linked recessive lymphoproliferative syndrome
X-linked recessive nephrolithiasis

recessively
autosomally recessively inherited disease

recheck
bladder tumor r.

recidivans
leishmaniasis r.

recipient
artificial heart r.
heart transplant r.
high-risk r.
r. hospital
organ recipient candidate
organ and recipient match
organ transplant r.
renal allograft r.
renal transplant r.
transplant r.

reciprocal
r. asymmetrical
r. beat
r. geometric mean titer
r. hindlimb-scratching syndrome
r. innervation
lack of reciprocal interest
r. ohm
r. ohm centimeter
r. ohm meter
paroxysmal atrioventricular nodal reciprocal tachycardia
r. ST depression
r. tension membrane
r. translocation

reciprocating
Adjustable Advanced R. Gait Orthosis
atrioventricular reciprocating tachycardia
end-cutting reciprocating saw
r. gait orthosis
junctional reciprocating tachycardia
permanent junctional reciprocating tachycardia

recirculating
molecular adsorbent recirculating system
r. single pass

recirculation
instrument recirculation center
lymphocyte r.
oxygenation before r.

recite
survey, question, read, review, r.

reckless
r. behavior
r. and impulsive activity
involvement in reckless activity

Recklinghausen
canal of R.
R. disease
R. disease of bone
von Recklinghausen disease

reclining
r. chair
left arm, r.
right arm r.

recognition
antigen r.
antisignal recognition particle antibody
Continuing Education Approval and R. Program
Depression: Awareness, R., and Treatment
r. factor
immediate and delayed r.
leukocyte automatic recognition computer
median recognition threshold
molecular recognition unit
optical character r.
oral form r.
Pantomime R. Test
patient burned beyond r.
pattern r.
perception, thought and recognition of information
serial probe r.
signal recognition particle
signal recognition protein
speech recognition threshold
Tactile Finger R. Test
Tactile Form R. Test
tissue-stone recognition system
within-list r.
Y chromosome RNA recognition motif

recognizable
minimal recognizable odor
r. viral syndrome

recognizance
own r.

recognize
inability to recognize objects
r., empathize, think, hear, integrate, notice, keep

recognized
Generally R. As Safe
Generally R. as Safe and Effective
melanoma antigen recognized by T cell

recognizer
precision encoder and pattern r.

recoil
arm r.
elastic recoil pressure of lung
increased r.
lung elastic recoil pressure
maximal expiratory flow-static recoil curve
maximum expiratory airflow-static lung elastic recoil pressure

recoil *(continued)*
partial expiratory flow-static recoil curve

recollection
conscious r.
distressing recollection of incident

recombinant
r. alpha-1 antitrypsin
r. chromosome
r. deoxyribonucleic acid
r. desmoglein
r. DNA
r. factor VIIA
r. follicle-stimulating hormone
r. HBcAg
r. hirudin
r. human activated protein C
r. human albumin
r. human bone morphogenetic protein
r. human erythropoietin
r. human granulocyte-macrophage colony-stimulating factor
r. human growth hormone
r. human IL-10
r. human insulinlike growth factor
r. human insulin-like growth factor-1
r. human interleukin
r. human interleukin-2, -3, -11
r. human leukocyte interferon A
r. human MIP-1 alpha
r. human platelet-derived growth factor
r. human superoxide dismutase
r. human thyroid-stimulating hormone
r. human tissue factor pathway inhibitor
r. human TSH
r. human vascular endothelial growth factor
r. immunoblot assay
r. immunosorbent assay
r. inbred strain
r. interferon alpha
r. interferon gamma
live-attenuated recombinant *Salmonella typhi*
r. methioninase
r. Norwalk virus
r. outer surface protein A
r. plasminogen activator
r. platelet factor-4
r. polyethylene glycol
r., single-chain, urokinase-type plasminogen activator
r. soluble CD4
soluble recombinant human CD4
r. tissue-type plasminogen activator
r. tumor necrosis factor alpha
r. urokinase
r. virus assay

recombinase
lymphocyte r.

recombination
high-frequency r.
smallest unit of DNA capable of r.

recommendation
evidence-based r.'s
physician's nutritional r.

recommended
r. daily dietary allowance
r. daily intake
r. dietary intake
r. dose
r. exposure level
r. international nonproprietary name
maximal recommended human dose
maximum recommended daily dose
maximum recommended human dose
r. nutrient intake

reconditioned heart

reconditioning
physical reconditioning exercise

reconstituted
immunopotentiating reconstituted influenza virosomes

reconstitution
artery r.
multilineage r.

reconstruct
r. heart muscle
r. knee

reconstructed
digitally reconstructed radiograph

reconstruction
algebraic reconstruction technique
Allman modification of Evans ankle r.
allograft reconstruction of fibular collateral ligament
anterior capsulolabral r.
anterior cruciate ligament r.
aortic root r.
arthroscopically assisted anterior cruciate ligament r.
arthroscopic anterior cruciate ligament r.
arthroscopic transhumeral r.
autogenous patellar tendon r.
breast mound reduction and nipple reconstruction with wraparound flap
breast reconstruction after mastectomy
Brent eyebrow r.
Cabral coronary r.
ceramic r.
composite mandibular r.
computed tomography with multiplanar r.'s
computer-assisted reconstruction by tracing of serial sections
cruciate ligament r.
double-looped semitendinous and gracilis hamstring graft knee reconstruction technique
end-to-end reconstruction technique
gated 3D r.
immediate breast r.
inferior vena cava r.
Integrated Auricular R. Protocol
laryngotracheal r.
lateral compartment r.
ligament reconstruction with tendon interposition
lower extremity r.
lymphatic r.
mandibular functional r.
mandibular reconstruction plate
Millard advancement rotation flap r.
Mladick ear r.
modified Chrisman-Snook ankle r.
modified double-opposing tab flap nipple r.
nasal alar rim r.
nasoseptal r.
Nicholas five-in-one r.
Nicholas five-in-one reconstruction technique
r. occlusal surface
O'Donoghue ACL r.
one-stage reconstruction of eye socket and eyelids
ossicular chain r.
segmental correction using spine r.
Sheen airway r.

simultaneous multiple-angle reconstruction technique
Tanzer auricle r.
titanium hollow-screw osseointegrating reconstruction plate
total anorectal r.
total ossicular reconstruction prosthesis
Wookey pharyngoesophageal r.

reconstructive
aortic reconstructive surgery
arterial reconstructive procedure
arterial reconstructive surgery
r. dentistry
r. hip surgery
plastic and reconstructive surgery

reconstructor
dynamic planar r.
dynamic spatial r.

record
abnormal r.
American Pediatric Gross Assessment R.
automated anesthesia r.
automated clinical r.
chronologic drinking r.
clinical r.
computer-based patient r.
Computerized Healthcare And R. Transfer System
computerized patient r.
computer-stored ambulatory r.
confidentiality of r.
contact r.
r. of contact
current medical evidence of r.
daily fetal movement r.
echo record access
r. of electrocerebral inactivity
electronic patient medical r.
empty, measure, and r.
fetal movement r.
Functional Performance R.
Graduate R. Examination
individual medical r.
Infant Behavior R.
measure and r.
medication administration r.
Mental Status Examination R.
Minimal R. of Disability
normal r.
note, record, report
occluding centric relation r.
patient contact r.
patient progress r.
patient termination r.
periodic evaluation r.
physician of r.
preference r.
prior medical r.
problem-oriented medical r.
Pupil R. of Education Behavior
self-medication administration r.
service r.
treatment administration r.
virtual patient r.
vital r.

recorded electrical brain activity

recorder
blood pressure r.
cardiac output r.
circadian event r.
graphic level r.
intraocular tension r.
pulse volume r.
video cassette r.

recording
all night sleep r.
bipolar needle recording electrode
cardiopneumographic r.
cine loop r.
double simultaneous r.
r. of electrical activity
r. electrode
eye movement r.
high frequency of r.
His bundle r.
intracardiac catheter r.
night sleep r.
paired electrode r.
pulse value r.
pulse volume r.

Record—Vocational
Kuder Preference R.

recoverable
heat-activated recoverable temporary stent

recovered
r. avian sarcoma virus
r. memory

recovery
adult recovery services
anesthetic immediate r.
arrhythmia-insensitive flow-sensitive alternating inversion r.
at-home recovery period
automaticity recovery phase
automaticity recovery time
baseline r.
bereavement recovery group
cardiac catheterization r.
cardiovascular recovery room
corrected adjusted sinus node recovery time
corrected sinus nodal recovery time
corrected time of sinoatrial node function r.
critical care recovery unit
digital temperature recovery time test
fluid attenuated inversion r.
fluid attenuation inversion r.
fluorescence photobleaching r.
fluorescence recovery after photobleaching
full recovery time
good r.
r. group
r. incision
inversion recovery spin-echo sequence
liquid holding r.
myocardial infarction recovery index
organ recovery coordinator
organ recovery team
organ and tissue r.
patient recovery plan
photostress recovery test
photostress recovery time
postanesthesia recovery area
postanesthesia recovery score
postanesthetic recovery unit
r. quotient
saturation r.
short inversion imaging r.
short tau inversion r.
short T1 inversion r.
sinoatrial recovery time
sinus node recovery time
skin temperature recovery time
stroke with full r.
r. time
transient ischemic attack, incomplete r.

recreation
social r.
therapeutic r.
therapeutic recreation associate

recreational
r. drinking
r. drug
r. drug use
r. injury
r. therapy

recrudescent
r. typhus
r. typhus fever

recruitment
lung r.
lymphocyte r.
mononuclear cell r.

recta (*pl. of* rectum)

rectae

rectal
r. abscess
acute rectal hemorrhage
advancement of rectal flap
r. ampulla
autoerotic rectal trauma
r. biopsy
r. bleeding
r. bleeding secondary to hemorrhoid
r. canal
r. cancer
r. carcinoid tumor
descending rectal septum
digital rectal examination
digital rectal test
distal rectal adenocarcinoma
endoluminal rectal ultrasonography
r. endoscopic ultrasonography
r. evacuation
r. evacuatory disorder
r. examination
r. fissure
r. floor
r. hernia
hyperplastic rectal polyp
r. incontinence
r. injury
low rectal resection
r. morphine sulfate suppository
r. mucosa
Nova R.
pelvic and rectal examination
per anum intersphincteric rectal dissection
r. prolapse
r. sinus
solitary rectal ulcer
solitary rectal ulcer syndrome
r. swab
r. temperature
r. ulcer
r. vault

rectales
nodi lymphoidei rectales superiores
venae rectales inferiores

rectal-expander-assisted transanal endoscopic microsurgery

rectangular
r. amputation
axis of three-dimensional rectangular coordinate system
horizontal axis of rectangular coordinate system
vertical axis of rectangular coordinate system

rectification
anomalous r.

rectified average

rectifier
silicon-controlled r.

recto
hernia in r.

rectoanal inhibitory reflex

rectocolic hemorrhage

rectoperineal
anterior rectoperineal fistula

rectopexy
anterior resection r.

rectosigmoid
r. anastomosis
r. cancer
r. carcinoma
r. colon
r. function
r. junction

rectosphincteric reflex

rectouterina
plica r.

rectouterine fold

rectovaginal
r. examination
r. fascia
r. fistula
r. fold
r. hernia

rectovesical
r. fascia
r. fistula
r. fold

rectum, pl. **recta**
adenomatosis of colon and r.
ampulla of r.
augmented valved r.
blood per r.
bright red blood per r.
colonoscopy per r.
flexure of r.
gastric mucosal ectopia in r.
hereditary adenomatosis of colon and r.
horizontal fold of r.
implantation of ureter into r.
internal hemorrhoid of r.
inverted polypoid hamartoma of r.
muscular coat of r.
muscular layer of r.
nothing per r.
pars recta
per r.
perineal flexure of r.
solitary ulcer of rectum syndrome
transverse fold of r.

rectus
r. abdominis
r. abdominis free flap
r. abdominis muscle
r. abdominis muscle flap
r. abdominis muscle transfer
r. abdominis musculocutaneous flap
r. abdominis myocutaneous flap
anterior layer of rectus abdominis sheath
anterior rectus capitis
anterior rectus fascia
anterior rectus muscle
anterior rectus muscle of head
arcuate line of rectus sheath
autologous rectus fascia sling
de-epithelialized rectus abdominis muscle graft
r. diastasis
r. fascia
r. femoris
r. femoris muscle
r. femoris muscle flap
r. femoris tendon
free transverse rectus abdominis myocutaneous flap
free transverse rectus abdominis musculocutaneous flap
r. inferior
inferior rectus muscle
lateral rectus, both eyes
lateral rectus eye muscle
lateral rectus incision
left inferior r.
left lateral rectus eye muscle
left medial rectus eye muscle
left rectus femoris
left superior r.
r. and longus capitis muscle
medial rectus, both eyes

medial rectus extraocular muscle
medial rectus function
medial rectus muscle
medial rectus palsy
medial rectus transposition
r. muscle splitting incision
musculus rectus lateralis bulbi
musculus rectus lateralis oculi
musculus rectus medialis bulbi
musculus rectus medialis oculi
overactive superior r.
right inferior r.
right lateral rectus muscle
right medial rectus muscle
right rectus femoris
right superior rectus muscle
r. sheath
r. sheath hematoma
superior rectus muscle
superior rectus traction suture
transverse rectus abdominis musculocutaneous flap
transverse rectus abdominis musculoperitoneal flap
transverse rectus abdominis muscle

recumbency cramp

recumbent

dorsal recumbent position
left arm, r.
measurement
right arm r.

recuperation

rest and r.

recurrence

Composite Laryngeal R. Staging System
early ischemic r.
ipsilateral breast tumor r.
local r.
local recurrence after radiation therapy
no evidence of r.
no radiographically visible r.
regional recurrence of tumor

recurrence-free interval

recurrent

r. abdominal pain
r. abdominal pain syndrome
r. abortion
acute recurrent pancreatitis
anterior recurrent tibial artery
anterior tibial recurrent artery
anterior ulnar recurrent artery
r. aphthous stomatitis
r. aphthous ulcer
r. appendicitis
r. arthralgia
articular recurrent nerve
r. ascites
r. aspiration
ataxia, myoclonic encephalopathy, macular degeneration, recurrent infections syndrome
r. attack
benign recurrent hematuria
benign recurrent intrahepatic cholestasis
r. calcium urolithiasis
r. caries
r. cholangitis
r. choroiditis
r. chronic depression
r. chronic dissecting aneurysm
chronic recurrent multifocal osteomyelitis
r. colitis
r. colorectal cancer
r. congestive heart failure
r. corneal lesion
r. cystitis
r. deep vein thrombosis
r. depression
r. dysphagia
r. early pregnancy loss
r. empyema
r. epistaxis
r. erosion syndrome
r. excruciating headache
r. fetal loss
r. fever
r. genital herpes
r. gingivitis
r. glioblastoma multiforme
r. gross hematuria
r. heart attack
r. hemorrhage from aneurysm
r. hernia
r. herpes labialis
Hodgkin disease, r.
idiopathic recurrent pancreatitis
r. illness
r. induced malaria
r. infection
r. insanity
r. intrahepatic obstructive jaundice
intrastent recurrent disease
r. laryngeal nerve
r. lobar hemorrhage
r. lower respiratory tract disease
r. mesenteric ischemia
r. miscarriage
multifocal and recurrent choroidopathy
r. myocardial infarction
no evidence of recurrent disease
r. nonulcer dyspepsia
ophthalmic recurrent nerve
r. oral ulcer
pharyngeal branch of recurrent laryngeal nerve
r. pleomorphic adenoma
posterior branch of recurrent ulnar artery
r. pulmonary emboli
r. pyogenic cholangiogram
r. pyogenic cholangiohepatitis
r. respiratory papilloma
r. respiratory papillomatosis
r. seizures
r. spontaneous abortion
r. spontaneous psychokinesis
r. ulcerative scarifying stomatitis
r. upper respiratory tract infection
r. variceal hemorrhage
r. vomiting

recurring

r. blackouts
chronic recurring depression
r. digital fibroma of childhood
r. dream
r. hallucination
r. headache
r. hemorrhage
idiopathic recurring stupor
r. infection
r. venous thromboembolism

recurvatum

r. deformity
genu r.
pectus r.

recycled human blood substitute

recycling

maximal recycling capacity
medullary r.

red

absolute nucleated red blood cell
accelerated destruction of red blood cells
acquired red-cell aplasia
AS red cell
autologous red blood cell
autologous red cell salvage
blanchable red lesion
blister red, scaly, and itchy
r. blood cell

red *(continued)*
r. blood cell adenosine deaminase
r. blood cell adherence
r. blood cell agglutination
r. blood cell cast
r. blood cell concentrate
r. blood cell count
r. blood cell diameter width
r. blood cell distribution width index
r. blood cell fallout
r. blood cell filter ability
r. blood cell folate
r. blood cell fragility
r. blood cell immune adherence
r. blood cell iron turnover rate
r. blood cell-linked antigen-antiglobulin reaction
r. blood cell mass
r. blood cell to plasma ratio
r. blood cell precursor production rate
r. blood cells per high-power field
r. blood cell spun filtration
r. blood cell suspension
r. blood cell transfusion
r. blood cell volume
r. blood corpuscle
bovine red blood cell
bright red blood per rectum
r. cell
r. cell cast
r. cell index
r. cell morphology index
r. cell peroxide hemolysis
r. cells too numerous to count
r. cell volume
cerebral red blood cell volume
cherry red spot
chicken red blood cell
chlorophenyl r.
chronic, acquired, pure red cell aplasia
r. colloidal test
r. color sign
concentrated red blood cell
Congo red stain
contact lens-induced acute red eye
copious bright red blood
r. corpuscle
crenated red blood cell
cresyl r.
deglycerolized frozen red cell
denatured red blood cell
dog red blood cell
donkey red blood cell
fast red B salt
frozen section red blood cell
Gerbich red cell antigen
r. glass test
guinea pig red blood cell
r. gums from dentures
gums red and puffy
r. hemorrhagic fluid
r. herring
horse red blood cell
r. hypertension
immature red blood cell
indole, methyl red, Voges-Proskauer, and citrate test
r. induration
r. infarct
infected red blood cell
intraoperative endoscopic Congo red test
intravascular red cell aggregation
intravascular red light therapy
irradiated red blood cell
r. laser illumination
leukocyte-poor red blood cell
r. light therapy
liver, iron, red bone marrow
r. marrow
methyl r.
methyl red test
methyl red, Voges-Proskauer medium
microcytic red cell
monkey red blood cell
mouse red blood cell
neutral r.
normal sheep red blood cell
nuclear fast red stain
nucleated red blood cell mass
nucleated red cell
r. nucleus
oil red O
ox red blood cell
packed red blood cell
packed red blood cell transfusion
parvovirus B19 red cell aplasia
r. patch or blister on arm
phenol r.
plasma-free red cell
production of red blood cells
pure red blood cell agenesis
pure red blood cell aplasia
pure red cell aplasia
quinaldine r.
ragged red fiber
r. reflex
ruthenium r.
sedimented red cell
sheep red cell rosette-forming cell
sheep red blood cell
sickle red blood cell
specific red cell adherence
r. spider vein
r. spot on breast
r. strawberry tongue
r., swollen, and itchy
r. swollen joint
r., swollen, tender gums
tanned red blood cell agglutination
tanned red blood cell hemagglutination
tanned red blood cell hemagglutination inhibition
tanned red cell
r. tetrazolium
thick, red itchy patch of skin
toluidine red unheated serum test
total red blood cells
total red cell volume
trypsinized sheep red blood cell
unit of packed red blood cells
r. venous blood
r. veterinary petrolatum
volume of packed red blood cells
r. and warm breast
washed red blood cell

reddening
heat, reddening, swelling, or tenderness

red-green color perception deficiency

redistribution
cell cycle r.
cell cycle redistribution and dose fractionation
cell redistribution and dose hyperfractionation
cycle redistribution and dose
r. imaging
pulmonary venous r.

Redlich-Fisher miliary plaque

red-man syndrome

redness
r. along incision site
r. at incision site
diffuse r.
r., dryness and itching
heat, absence of use, redness, pain, pus, swelling

r. and inflammation
without redness or swelling

redraped skin

redressing
sterile r.

reduce
restore mobility and reduce pain
r. risk of hospital-associated infection
r. salt intake
r. sodium intake
r. swelling in brain
r. tension headache frequency

reduced
r. agitation
r. anxiety
r. blood flow to brain
r. blood supply to heart
cardiac output markedly r.
flavin phosphate, r.
r. folate carrier
r. form of flavin mononucleotide
r. glutathione
r. glutathione peroxidase
r. haloperidol
r. hearing at high frequency
r. heart rate
heart reduced to normal size
r. hemoglobin
r. joint survey
lactose reduced diet
Listing reduced eye
r. liver transplant
methylene blue, r.
r. nasal fracture
r. profile
r. coenzyme A
r. renal mass
r. space symbologies
r. tolerance for physical activity
r. vascular response
r. vestibular response
r. yellow enzyme

reduced-acquisition matrix

reduced-size liver transplant

reducer
Honan pressure r.
McCannel ocular pressure r.
nitrate r.
ocular pressure r.

reducible hernia

reducing
fracture reducing elevator
r. substances
total reducing sugars
turbidity r.

reductase
aldose r.
aldose reductase inhibitor
biliverdin r.
dihydrofolate r.
dihydropteridine r.
erythrocyte glutathione r.
glutathione r.
gluthathione r.
17-ketosteroid r.
methemoglobin r.
methylene tetrahydrofolate r.
methylenetetrahydrofolate reductase gene
methylene tetrahydrofolate reductase thermolability
nitrate r.
nitrite r.
ribonucleotide r.
thioredoxin r.

reduction
absolute risk r.
acetylene reduction activity
air pressure enema r.
AmB-induced reduction GFR
amphotericin B-induced reduction glomerular filtration rate
r. in amplitude
anterior disc displacement without r.
anterior displacement no r.
anterior displacement with r.
Aries-Pitanguy breast r.
arousal reduction mechanism
arousal reduction technique
assisted reduction and internal fixation
axillary endoscopic r.
breast mound reduction and nipple reconstruction with wraparound flap
bulbous tip r.
cardiac risk r.
closed r.
closed reduction and cast
closed reduction of fracture
closed reduction and internal fixation
closed reduction and percutaneous pin fixation
closed reduction and percutaneous pin ring
copper reduction test
Crutchfield reduction technique
cyclic flow r.
decimal reduction time
r. deformity
digoxin reduction product
dose reduction effectiveness factor
Essex-Lopresti reduction technique
r. of examination anxiety
external r.
feedback reduction circuit
fog reduction elimination device
gastric reduction surgery
gradient moment r.
gravity lumbar r.
harm reduction psychotherapy
r. headache
health care cost r.
heart reduction surgery
internal r.
left ventricular r.
r. level
limb reduction defects
log reduction value
Lorenz hip r.
Lottes reduction technique
lung volume r.
lung volume reduction surgery
Magnuson reduction technique
manual fracture r.
Martin reduction technique
McBride hallux abductovalgus r.
McBride hallux valgus r.
methemoglobin reduction test
methylene blue reduction time
Molulsky dye reduction test
multifetal pregnancy r.
nitrate reduction test
nitrite reduction test
noise r.
Noise R. Rating
noise reduction coefficient
nonsurgical septal reduction therapy
open r.
open reduction and external fixation
open reduction of humerus
open reduction and internal fixation
open reduction metallic fixation
open reduction of radius and ulna
open reduction of skull fracture
PDI-mediated disulfide bond r.
percent reduction in urea
posterior reduction device
radiofrequency tissue volume r.
rage reduction therapy
relative risk r.

reduction *(continued)*
resazurin reduction time
risk factor r.
risk reduction component
rotation and reduction of fracture
r. of salt intake
single lung reduction surgery
skin exposure reduction paste against chemical warfare agent
Speed and Boyd reduction technique
stress reduction technique
tetrazolium r.
tetrazolium reduction inhibition
Thomson reduction technique
r. time
unilateral lung reduction surgery
urea reduction ratio
volume reduction surgery
Wagner reduction technique

redundant cusp syndrome

reduplication
r. cataract
r. murmur

reduplicative paramnesia

Reed-Sternberg cell

reeducation
neuromuscular reeducation technique

Reef
Saumarez Reef virus

reeling
gait reeling, staggering

reemergent symptom

reemerging infection

reentrant
r. arrhythmia
r. atrial tachycardia
atrioventricular junctional r.
atrioventricular nodal reentrant tachycardia
atrioventricular reentrant paroxysmal tachycardia
atypical atrioventricular nodal reentrant tachycardia
AV nodal reentrant tachycardia
intraatrial reentrant tachycardia
nodal reentrant paroxysmal tachycardia
paroxysmal reentrant supraventricular tachycardia
r. pathway
sustained reentrant ventricular tachyarrhythmia
r. ventricular arrhythmia

reentry
atrioventricular nodal r.
atrioventricular reentry tachycardia
AV nodal reentry tachycardia
bundle-branch r.
intraatrial reentry tachycardia
Schmitt-Erlanger model of r.
sinoatrial nodal r.

Reese
R. Ellsworth classification
R. syndrome

Rees and Ecker diluting fluid

Reeves treadmill protocol

reexcision
tumor r.

refeeding syndrome

reference
angiographic reference system
anterior commissure-posterior commissure reference point
articulatory specified neutral r.
assay reference plasma
delusional or ideas of r.
delusion of r.
distal reference axis
distorted ideas of r.
ideas of r.
Individualized Criterion R. Testing Mathematics
Individualized Criterion R. Testing Reading
integrated reference air-kerma
interferon reference unit
internal visual r.
International R. Preparation
r. interval
laboratory r.
r. material
McMaster-Toronto Arthritis Patient R.
mean reference diameter
normal reference serum
r. normal serum
olfactory reference syndrome
r. point following QRS complex, at beginning of ST segment
Primary R. Material
proximal reference axis
single reference electrode
single reference point
Standard R. Material
Systematized Nomenclature of Medicine R. Terminology
total reference air-kerma
transient ideas of r.
unaided equalization r.
Universal Control R. Plasma
r. value
r. vessel diameter

referential
r. montage
r. thinking

referral
Alzheimer Disease Education and R.
r., diagnosis, treatment, and discharge
discharged during r.
physician referral service
School Health Additional R. Program

referred
r. care
r. pain

referring
r. doctor
r. physician

refill
brisk capillary r.
capillary r.
capillary refill, sensation, motor function, temperature
capillary refill time
no r.
prolonged capillary r.
transcapillary r.
venous refill time

refine
selective tubal assessment to refine reproductive therapy

refinement
nasal r.

reflectance
affinity attenuated total reflectance spectroscopy
diffuse reflectance spectroscopy
r. oximetry
r. pulse oximetry
tissue reflectance oximeter

reflected
r. light
muscle reflected from insertion
ophthalmoscopy with reflected light

reflecting
ligament reflecting edge

reflection
angle of r.
attenuated total r.
r. coefficient
r. high-energy electron diffraction

r. interference microscopy
light reflection rheography
line of pleural r.
total internal reflection microscopy

reflection-absorption infrared spectroscopy

reflectometry
spectral gradient acoustic r.

reflector
parabolic r.

reflex
abnormal jugular r.
Abrams heart r.
r. absent
Achilles tendon r.
Achilles tendon reflex time
acoustic muscle r.
acoustic reflex test
acoustic reflex threshold
acquired gustolacrimal r.
r. action
r. activity
airway dilation r.
ankle jerk r.
ankle reflex time
Arnold nerve reflex cough syndrome
asymmetric incurvatum r.
asymmetric tonic neck r.
attention reflex of pupil
auditory oculogyric r.
auropalpebral r.
automatic neonatal walking r.
autonomic walking r.
Babinski reflex, sign
balloon reflex manometry
baroreceptor reflex response
baroreceptor reflex sensitivity
basal joint r.
Bezold-type r.
biceps tendon r.
bladder cooling r.
blink r.
bulbocavernosus r.
cardiac depressor r.
cardiovascular reflex conditioning
cardiovascular reflex conditioning system
cervicoocular r.
chiropractic manipulative reflex technique
cochleopalpebral r.
conditioned r.
conditioned orientation reflex audiometry
conditioned reflex skill
conditioned reflex therapy
condition orientation reflex audiometry
consensual light r.
corneal blink r.
r. cough
r. decay
deep abdominal r.
deep tendon r.
deep tendon r.'s active and equal bilaterally
deep tendon r.'s bilaterally
delayed r.
diminished gag r.
r. disorder
dorsal root r.
electrically induced spinal r.
eyelid closure r.
flexion reflex testing
fontanelle r.
galvanic skin r.
gastric component of reflex barrier
gastrosalivary r.
generalized time r.
r. grasp
great toe r.
Gunn pupillary r.
hair-trigger gag r.
r. hallucination
hand grasp r.
r. headache
hepatojugular reflex test
Hering-Breuer inflation r.
hyperactive carotid sinus r.
hyperactive tendon r.
hypoactive deep tendon r.
r. ileus
incomplete Moro r.
r. incontinence
increased action of r.
increased deep tendon r.
increased reflex activity
r. inhibition
inhibitory anal r.
inverted radial r.
iris contraction r.
r. irritability
jaw jerk r.
jaw-opening r.
knee jerk r.
labyrinthine righting r.
laryngeal adductor r.
laryngeal cough reflex test
lid closure r.
light optometer r.
light reflex ring
linguomandibular r.
Lockwood light r.
loss of righting reflex
lower abdominal periosteal r.
macular light r.
Magnus and de Kleijn tonic neck r.
mandibular r.
margin reflex distance
markedly decreased r.
Mendel dorsal foot r.
middle ear muscle r.
milk ejection r.
milk let-down r.
monosynaptic r.
Morley peritoneocutaneous r.
motor, pain, touch, reflex deficit
muscle stretch r.
myotactic r.
near gaze r.
near light r.
r. nephropathy
nonoptic reflex eye movement
normal detrusor r.
norm physiological r.
ocular countertorsion r.
oculocardiac r.
oculogyric auricular r.
oculosensory cell r.
opticofacial winking r.
orbicularis pupillary r.
orienting r.
oval window r.
palmar grasp r.
palmar reflex grasp
palmomental reflex of Marinesco-Radovici
palpebral oculogyric r.
paradoxical ankle r.
paradoxical extensor r.
paradoxical flexor r.
paradoxical pupillary r.
paradoxic gustolacrimal r.
patellar tendon r.
perimeter corneal reflex test
perineobulbar detrusor facilitative r.
perineobulbar detrusor inhibitory r.
photopalpebral r.
plantar flexor r.
postural r.
present and active r.'s
Preyer r.
psychogalvanic r.
pupillary light r.

reflex *(continued)*
Quantitative Sudomotor Axon R. Test
quieting r.
rectoanal inhibitory r.
rectosphincteric r.
red r.
r. relaxation index
retinal r.
Riddoch mass r.
sacral r.'s
sensitivity prediction by acoustic r.
single lens r.
skin potential r.
stretch r.
suppress reflex contraction
symmetrical tendon r.
symmetric tonic neck r.
r. sympathetic dystrophy
r. symptom
tendo Achillis r.
r. therapy
tonic labyrinthine r.
tonic neck r.
tonic vibration r.
total vibration r.
triceps tendon r.
unconditioned r.
r. vasculopathic activity
ventral root r.
vestibuloocular r.
visually enhanced vestibuloocular r.
visual vestibuloocular r.
von Mering r.
Westphal pupillary r.
wrist flexion r.

reflexa
placenta r.

reflex-activating stimulus

reflex-inhibiting pattern

reflexive ileus

reflexively
patient gags r.

reflex-type ileus

reflux
acid reflux test
r. activity
r. of air
alkaline reflux esophagitis
alkaline reflux gastritis
r. of barium
r. of bile
r. bile gastritis
delayed reflex
duodenal-gastric reflux gastropathy
duodenogastric r.
duodenogastroesophageal r.
r. dyspepsia
r. esophagitis
r. gastritis
gastroesophageal r.
gastroesophageal reflux disease
gynecological chylous reflux syndrome
r. into terminal ileum normal
intrarenal r.
mitral r.
nasopharyngeal r.
nocturnal acid r.
nocturnal gastric r.
nonerosive gastroesophageal reflux disease
normal gastroesophageal reflux of infancy
pharyngeal acid r.
physiologic reflux test
standard acid reflux test
valves, unilateral reflux, dysplasia
venous r.
vesicoureteral reflux grade I–V

refocused
multiplanar gradient r.

reform
conventional reform eye implant
mental health r.
Snellen conventional reform implant
Snellen reform eye

reformation
anterior chamber r.
axial multiplanar reformation technique

reformatted
curved, reformatted mandibular image

reformatting
multiplanar reformatting view

reformulated
newly r.

refract
cell refract ability

refracted ray

refractile body

refracting angle of prism

refraction
angle of r.
cycloplegic r.
index of r.
manifest r.
parallax and r.
r. test

refractive
r. amblyopia
r. ametropia
astigmatic refractive error
asymmetric refractive error
r. disease
r. error
r. index
r. keratoplasty
photoastigmatic refractive keratectomy
r. power

refractometer
meridional r.

refractometry
infrared r.

refractor
automatic r.
objective r.

refractory
absolute refractory period
amplification refractory mutation system
amplification refractory mutation system-polymerase chain reaction
r. anemia
r. anemia, erythroblastic
r. anemia with excess blasts
r. anemia with excess of blasts in transformation
r. anemia with excess blasts in transition
r. anemia with excess myeloblasts
r. anemia with partial myeloblastosis
r. anemia with ring sideroblasts
antegrade refractory period
r. ascites
atrial effective refractory period
atrioventricular refractory period
cardiac refractory period
r. convergence nystagmus
r. Crohn disease
r. depression
r. duodenal ulcer
effective refractory length
effective refractory period
effective refractory period of the left ventricle
r. emesis
r. epistaxis
r. esophagitis
functional refractory period

r. heart failure
r. hypertension
r. hypoglycemia
idiopathic acquired refractory sideroblastic anemia
idiopathic refractory sideroblastic anemia
r. illness
r. period
r. period of transmission
postventricular atrial refractory period
r. rickets
right ventricular refractory period
r. sprue
r. status epilepticus
total atrial refractory period
ventricular effective refractory period

Refsum
R. disease
infantile Refsum syndrome
R. syndrome

refusal
blood transfusion refusal form
r. to eat
r. of medical aid

refuse
right to refuse intervention

refused admission

regained
patient regained active status

regard
area of conscious r.
object of r.
plane of r.
point of r.

regarded
generally regarded as effective

regenerated cellulose

regenerating
liver regenerating serum factor
r. bone marrow extract

regeneration
guided bone r.
guided tissue r.
impaired regeneration syndrome
r. of nerve
osteoblastic bone r.

regenerative
atypical regenerative hyperplasia
r. index
nodular regenerative hyperplasia
nodular regenerative hyperplasia of liver

Regen flexion exercise

regia

regimen
anticoagulation regimen of aspirin
anticonstipation r.
antimicrobial dosing r.
Atzpodien regimen for renal cell carcinoma
birth control r.
bowel emptying r.
drug regimen review
Einhorn regimen of chemotherapy
low-intensity preparative r.
multiple injection r.
nonmyeloablative conditioning r.
postoperative regimen for oral early feeding
premedication r.

region
abnormally contracting r.'s
r. of activation
argyrophilic nucleolar organizer r.
argyrophilic nucleolar organizer region staining
argyrophil organizer region protein
artery of chiasmal r.
r. of back
beta-chain variable r.
r. of body
breakpoint cluster r.
breakpoint cluster region negative
breakpoint cluster region positive
r. of chest
complementarity-determining r.
deltoid r.
diseased r.
epigastric r.
Epstein-Barr early region protein
external abdominal r.
r. of face
germ cell tumor with synchronous lesions in pineal and suprasellar r.
r. of head
homogeneous staining region of chromosome
hypogastric region of abdomen
immune region-associated antigen
r. of interest
intertrochanteric region fracture
lateral abdominal r.
major breakpoint r.
major histocompatibility r.
mid lumbar r.
minor cluster r.
mutation cluster r.
negatively correlated r.
negatively staining region of chromosome
nucleolar organizing r.
nucleolus-organizing r.
occipital regions of head
operative r.
proximal alveolar r.
r. of sarcomere containing only myosin filaments
scaffold-associated r.'s
sex-determining r.
silver-staining nucleolar organizer r.
superior labial r.
temporomesial r.
third framework r.
untranslated r.
5′-untranslated r.
upstream regulatory r.

regional
r. adenitis
r. alveolar damage
r. analgesia
r. anesthetic
r. block
r. block anesthesia
r. bone mass
r. cerebral blood flow
r. cerebral blood volume
r. cerebral metabolic rate for oxygen
r. cerebral perfusion pressure
r. chemotherapy
r. colitis
complex regional pain syndrome
continuous intravenous regional anesthesia
continuous regional arterial infusion
r. deep heating
r. differentiation
r. disease
r. distribution
r. distribution of hepatic blood flow
r. ejection fraction image
elective regional lymph node dissection
r. enteritis
r. enterocolitis
r. gas exchange
r. heparinization
high regional wall motion velocity
r. ileitis
r. ileocolitis

regional *(continued)*
intravenous regional anesthesia
intravenous regional sympathetic block
r. involvement
r. irradiation
local regional metastases
r. lymphadenitis
r. lymphadenopathy
r. lymph involvement
r. lymph node
r. lymph node cell
r. lymph node dissection
r. lymph nodes cannot be addressed
r. myocardial blood flow
r. neonatal intensive care unit
r. organ procurement
r. oxygen saturation
r. pediatric pulmonary center
r. perfusion
r. perinatal intensive care center
primary tumor, regional lymph node, remote metastases classification, staging
r. pulmonary blood flow
r. recurrence of tumor
r. wall motion
r. wall motion abnormality

register
high-risk r.

registered
r. nurse
visiting registered nurse

registration
Broadbent registration point
photoelectric registration device

registry
antiretroviral pregnancy r.
balloon valvuloplasty r.
cord blood r.
ovarian tumor r.
r. and tissue bank
tumor r.

Regitine test

regloving and regowning carried out

regressing atypical histiocytosis

regression
age r.
r. analysis
atavistic r.
caudal regression syndrome
Classification and R. Tree analysis
r. coefficient
linear regression analysis
Mevacor Atherosclerosis Regression Study
multinomial polytomous logistic regression method
multiple linear regression analysis
multiple logistic r.
multivariate logistic r.
multivariate logistic regression analysis
myopic r.
nonlinear least squares regression analysis
trophoblast in r.
tumor regression antigen
tumor regression grade

regression-associated protein

regressive
r. electric shock therapy
r. electroshock treatment
r. resistive exercise

regrowth
goiter r.
nerve tissue r.

regular
advance to regular diet
bowel sounds r.
deep and regular respiration
r. education
r. foot hygiene
r. heart rate
r. heart rhythm
r. heart tones
r. hemodialysis treatment
human insulin regular
r. insulin
r. insulin infusion
neutral regular insulin
no regular medicines
r. nursing floor
pulse r.
pupil round and r.
r. rate, clear tones, no murmurs
r. rate and rhythm
r. respiration
round, regular, react normally
round, regular, and equal
round, regular, and equal pupil
r. sinus rhythm
r. spiking activity
r., wide QRS tachycardia

regularity
surface regularity index

regularly irregular rhythm

regulated
cocaine and amphetamine regulated transcript
extracellular regulated kinase
r. upon activation, normal T-cell expressed and secreted

regulation
arginine vasopressin r.
r. of body temperature
feedback r.
interleukin regulation of immune system
menstrual cycle r.
negative feedback r.

regulator
antiviral r.
autocrine-paracrine growth r.
autoimmune r.
autoimmune regulator gene
calcium-dependent r.
cystic fibrosis transmembrane conductance r.
r. gene
lysosomal trafficking regulator protein
lysosome trafficking r.
master regulator gene
retinitis pigmentosa GTPase regulator gene
tyrosine aminotransferase r.

regulatory
r. albuminuria
assimilation regulatory protein
autoimmune r.
autoimmune regulatory gene
downstream regulatory element antagonistic modulator gene
follicle regulatory protein
guanine nucleotide regulatory protein
r. hormone
integrating regulatory transcription unit
interferon regulatory factor
interferon regulatory factor-1
interferon regulatory factor-2
peptide regulatory factor
r. protein
steroid acute regulatory protein
steroidogenic acute regulatory protein
sterol regulatory element binding protein
type I, II regulatory dimer
upstream regulatory region

regurgitant
effective regurgitant orifice
r. fraction
r. jet area
mitral regurgitant murmur
r. orifice area
r. stroke volume

regurgitation
acute mitral r.
aortic r.
aortic regurgitation murmur
aortic valve r.
atrial r.
r. of bile
cardiac valvular r.
combined mitral stenosis and r.
congenital mitral r.
ischemic mitral r.
massive aortic r.
mitral valve r.
r. murmur
prosthetic valve r.
pulmonary r.
pulmonic r.
tricuspid r.
valvular r.

rehabilitation
accredited rehabilitation worker
alcohol rehabilitation center
alcohol rehabilitation program
atraumatic, multidirectional, bilateral rehabilitation inferior capsular shift
aural r.
cardiac and pulmonary r.
cardiac rehabilitation mental stress
cardiac rehabilitation program
cardiac rehabilitation team
cardiac rehabilitation unit
r. center
r. center for physically handicapped
R. Client Rating Scale
comprehensive outpatient rehabilitation facility
convalescence and r.
coronary rehabilitation program
Edinburgh R. Status Scale
halfway house for penal r.
heart attack r.
r. of heart disease
heart rehabilitation program
r. hospital
industrial rehabilitation unit
Level of R. Scale 1
medical r.
r. medicine
musculoskeletal evaluation, rehabilitation and conditioning
myocardial infarction rehabilitation program
open-heart rehabilitation program
outpatient rehabilitation center
phased knee r.
physical medicine and r.
r. program
pulmonary r.
r. team goal
testing, orientation, work, evaluation, r.
r. therapist
ventilator rehabilitation unit
vocational r.
vocational rehabilitation counselor
vocational rehabilitation and education
vocational rehabilitation program
vocational rehabilitation therapy

Rehabilitative Addicted Family Treatment

rehydrated
patient r.

rehydrating solution

rehydration
r. and detoxification
growth monitoring, oral rehydration, breast feeding, and immunization
oral r.
oral rehydration salt
oral rehydration solution

Reichel chondromatosis

Reichert
R. cartilage
R. scar

Reichmann
R. disease
R. rod

Reid baseline

Reider cell leukemia

Reifenstein syndrome

Reil
R. ansa
R. band
circular sulcus of R.
island of R.
limiting sulcus of R.

reimbursement
insufficient government r.'s
maximal reimbursement point
medical reimbursement plan

reimplantation
aortorenal r.
pulmonary reimplantation response

reimplanted tooth

reinfection
graft r.

reinforced
metal frame reinforced plastic bracket
r. clostridial medium

reinforcement
brain stimulation r.
continuous r.
differential reinforcement of other behavior
differential reinforcement of low response rates
giant prosthetic reinforcement of the visceral sac
intracranial r.
partial r.
partial reinforcement extinction effect
tangible reinforcement of operant conditioned audiometry
r. value
visual reinforcement audiometry

reinforcing stimulus

reinfusion
autologous bone marrow r.

Reinke crystalloid

reinoculate
remove, replace, reinoculate, repair

reinsertion
aponeurosis r.

reintegration
rapid reintegration unit

reintervention
target lesion r.

Reisberg scale

Reis-Bücklers superficial corneal dystrophy

Reissner
R. canal
R. membrane

Reis-Wertheim hysterectomy

Reitan-Indiana
R.-I. aphasic screening test
R.-I. Neuropsychological Battery

Reiter
R. disease

Reiter *(continued)*
R. protein complement-fixation test
R. protein reagin
R. syndrome

rejected
heart r.
total graft area r.

rejection
acute allograft r.
acute cellular r.
acute humoral r.
acute lung r.
acute organ r.
acute vascular xenograft r.
allograft corneal r.
autologous tumor rejection antigen
bone marrow transplant r.
bout of r.
cardiomyopathy transplant r.
chronic organ r.
classical signs of r.
combat rejection of transplanted organ
common mode r.
daily observation for r.
delayed xenograft r.
hyperacute xenograft r.
immediate good function followed by accelerated r.
immediate graft r.
immune to r.
immune rejection of transplanted heart
late graft r.
liver transplant r.
lung transplant r.
marrow graft r.
mean rejection grading
motion artifact rejection system
multiple acute rejection episode
organ rejection of transplantation
renal allograft r.
steroid-resistant r.
tumor-associated rejection antigen

rejuvenation
multiplanar endoscopic facial rejuvenation technique
r. with sparing of vascular perforators

relapse
fluctuating periods of remission and r.
freedom from r.
r. hazard
Hodgkin disease in r.
r. incidence
median relapse time
r. and remission
remission, relapse, and life expectancy

relapse-free survival

relapsing
African endemic relapsing fever
r. appendicitis
chronic relapsing demyelinating inflammatory polyneuropathy
chronic relapsing disorder
chronic relapsing pancreatitis
r. fever
frequently relapsing nephrotic syndrome
hereditary multifocal relapsing inflammation
louse-borne relapsing fever
r. malaria
r. pancreatitis
r. polychondritis
r. hepatitis B

relapsing-remitting
r.-r. course
r.-r. multiple sclerosis

relate
inability to relate to people

related
abuse related depression
adult-to-adult living related donor living transplant
alcohol r.
Alzheimer Disease and R. Disorders Association
anemia related to chemotherapy
Assessment of Aphasia and R. Disorders, Second Edition
Austin-Kartush group C patient related to ossiculoplasty
cardiovascular problems related to drug abuse
centrally active phenethylamine derivative related to amphetamine and methamphetamine
compliance related acute complication
condition related to stress
fibrinogen r.
Functional R. Groups
r. hemorrhage
hepatic problems related to drug abuse
hypersomnia related to another mental disorder
hypersomnia related to a known organic factor
implant related complications
insomnia related to a known organic factor
insomnia related to mental disorder
International Classification of Diseases and R. Health Problems, 10th Edition
lower extremity equipment r.
mismatched related donor
pain related to exertion
Screening Children for R. Early Educational Needs
skeletal related event
treatment and education of autistic and related communications handicapped children

relation
Allport group relations theory
centric r.
centric relation occlusion
concentration effect r.
Family R.'s Test
Fundamental Interpersonal R.'s Orientation-Behavior
Fundamental Interpersonal R.'s Orientation-Feelings
heterosexual relations scale
human r.'s
impaired interpersonal r.'s
interpersonal r.'s
mandibular centric r.
maximal relation rate
Minnesota Spatial R.'s Test
occluding centric relation record
patient r.'s
potential r.
professional r.'s
public r.'s
Social R. Test

relational
ethnic relational behavior
Global Assessment of R. Functioning
mean relational utterance

relationship
r. addiction
Caring R. Inventory
centric jaw r.
conscious-subconscious r.'s
decline in social r.'s
diastolic pressure-flow r.

disturbed interpersonal r.'s
end-systolic pressure-length r.
intense interpersonal r.
linear free-energy r.
log dose-response r.
mother-child r.
Mother-Child R. Evaluation
mutually monogamous r.
Partner R. Inventory
patient-physician r.
Perception of R.'s Test
Personal Assessment of Intimacy in R.'s
Personal R. Inventory
probable causal r.
protrusive r.
quantitative structure-activity r.
structure-activity r.
unstable and intense r.'s
unstable interpersonal r.

relative

r. accommodation
r. afferent pupillary defect
r. area of cardiac dullness
r. average perturbation
r. binding affinity
r. biologic effectiveness
r. body weight
California R. Value Studies
r. centrifugal field
r. centrifugal force
r. chemotactic activity
r. consumption rate
r. coronary flow reserve
r. corrected death rate
r. divergence
r. dose intensity
r. flow
r. fluorescence
r. fluorescence efficiency
r. gas expansion
r. growth rate
haplotype relative risk
r. hemianopia
r. hemoglobin
r. hepatic dullness
r. humidity
r. hyperemia
r. hypoxia
r. immunity
r. incompetence
r. inspiratory effort
r. light units
Marcus Gunn relative afferent defect
r. medullary area of kidney
r. medullary thickness
r. mobility
r. molecular mass
nonmatching donor r.
r. odds
r. operating characteristic
patient released in care of r.
r. polycythemia
r. potency
r. proliferative capacity
resource-based relative value scale
r. response
r. response attributable to the maneuver
r. response index
r. retention time
r. risk
r. risk cohort
r. risk reduction
r. to rotation of a beam of polarized light
r. sagittal depth
r. shunt flow
r. size
r. specific activity
stabilized relative response
r. standard accuracy
r. standard deviation
r. standardized mortality ratio
r. storage capacity
r. supersaturation
r. survival rate
survival relative to nodal involvement in breast carcinoma
r. time unit
r. tumor size
r. value guide
r. value index
r. value scale
r. value schedule
r. value study
r. value unit
r. vascular resistance
r. vertebral density
r. volume decrease
r. wall thickness

relative-intensity measure

relatively slow sinus rate

relativistic mass

relax

contract relax agonist contract
inability to r.

relaxant

muscle r.
skeletal muscle r.

relaxation

r. and biofeedback
breathing and relaxation technique
contraction and relaxation of heart
desensitization and relaxation group
r., distraction and imagery
early diastolic r.
electrochemical relaxation method
epithelium-derived relaxation factor
half relaxation time
r. of heart muscle
hybrid rapid acquisition with relaxation enhancement
hypnotic relaxation for insomnia
r. internal sphincter
isometric relaxation period
isometric relaxation time
isovolumetric r.
isovolumetric relaxation period
isovolumic relaxation time
r. of joint
latency r.
longitudinal relaxation time
lower esophageal sphincter r.
maximal relaxation rate
pelvic floor r.
pelvic girdle r.
progressive muscle r.
progressive relaxation for insomnia
progressive relaxation training
progressive relaxation under hyperactivity
proton relaxation enhancement
proton relaxation rate
rapid acquisition with relaxation enhancement
reflex relaxation index
r. response in headache therapy
spin-lattice or longitudinal relaxation time
spin-spin or transverse relaxation time MRI scan
stress r.
surgical relaxation of contracture
r. technique
r. therapy
r. therapy for hyperactivity
r. time
total apexcardiographic relaxation time index
r. training
transient lower esophageal r.
transverse r.
upper esophageal sphincter r.
volume of r.

relaxation-induced anxiety

relaxed
heart relaxed phase
r. introitus
r. pelvic floor
repair relaxed vaginal outlet
r. skin tension line
squarely face person, open posture, lean toward person, eye contact, r.
r. vaginal outlet

relaxin
synthetic human r.

relaxing
endothelium-derived relaxing factor

relaxing incision

relaxivity
longitudinal r.
transverse r.

relay
thalamocortical r.

release
airway pressure release ventilation
anterior hip r.
anterior release posterior fusion
anterior shoulder r.
blood oxygen release rate
carpal tunnel r.
carpal tunnel release system
chromium release test
complete subtalar r.
controlled r.
controlled release infusion syndrome
date of r.
distal soft tissue r.
egg-laying release hormone
endoscopic carpal tunnel r.
extended release tablet
facilitated positional r.
formation and release of hormones
growth hormone r.
r. of hormones
r. of information
r. inhibition
labeled release experiment
leukocyte histamine release test
long-acting r.
lysozymal enzyme r.
marrow release rate
medication release consent
Mital elbow r.
Mital elbow release operation
Mital elbow release technique
morphine sulfate immediate r.
myofascial r.
nocturnal vasopressin r.
octreotide long-acting r.
open carpal tunnel r.
ostomotic release oral system
patient release form
physiologic pattern r.
pituitary hormone r.
plantar fascial r.
posteromedial r.
potassium chloride sustained release tablet
radical posteromedial and plantar r.
renin r.
sign own r.
slow r.
slow release of hormones
somatotropin release factor
specific immune r.
sustained ethanol release tube
sustained release medication
sustained release theophylline
tarsal tunnel r.
tendo Achillis lengthening and toe flexor r.
tethered cord r.
theophylline-sustained r.
thyrotropin release factor
timed r.
trigger finger r.
vastus lateralis r.

released
advised and r.
r. from active duty
kinetic energy released in the medium
patient released in care of relative
patient released against medical advice
patient released on overnight pass

release-inhibiting
growth hormone release-inhibiting factor
growth hormone release-inhibiting hormone

releasing
antenatal thyrotropin releasing hormone
r. factor
growth hormone releasing factor
histamine inhibitory releasing factor
histamine releasing factor
r. hormone
inherited releasing mechanism
innate releasing mechanism

relevant
past relevant history
past relevant work
syndrome of approximate relevant answers

reliability
alternate forms reliability coefficient
r. coefficient
Employee R. Inventory
Weidel Yes/No R. Test

relief
allergy relief medicine
anxiety relief response
discomfort relief quotient
general r.
improved symptom r.
r. incision
r. of intracranial pressure
r. medication unit index
temporary relief of headache pain
tinnitus relief device
total pain r.

reliever
nonprescription pain r.
pain r.

relieving
nonbreathing pressure r.
pain relieving injection

religious
r. affiliation
r. approach
r. attitude
r. background
r. behavior
r. commitment
r. ecstasy
r. experience
r. faith

reloading
anode tube r.

REM
rapid eye movement
REM behavior disorder
REM density
REM rebound
REM sleep
REM spindle

remaining
average remaining lifetime

Remak
fiber of R.

R. fiber
R. ganglion
R. reflex

remarkable
family history not r.
mental retardation, pre-and postnatal overgrowth, remarkable face, acanthosis nigricans syndrome
not r.
past history not r.

remedial occupational therapy

remediation
cognitive remediation therapy
orientation/alertness r.

remedy
acceptable dental r.'s
herbal r.
homeopathic r.
magnetically influenced homeopathic r.
traditional Chinese herbal r.

remember
inability to remember spoken words

remission
cancer in r.
character, onset, location, duration, exacerbation, r.
complete clinical r.
complete continuous r.
continuous complete r.
cumulative duration of the first r.
disease in complete r.
exacerbation and r.
fluctuating periods of remission and relapse
r. induced
r. induction
partial r.
pathologically confirmed complete r.
prolonged r.
r., relapse, and life expectancy
relapse and r.
unconfirmed/uncertain complete r.

remission-inducing drug

remittance advice

remittent
r. malaria
r. malarial fever

remitting
r. fever
r. seronegative symmetric synovitis with pitting edema

remnant
aneurysm remnant neck
gastric r.
r. gastric cancer
gastric remnant cancer
lipoprotein r.
r. lipoprotein
omphalomesenteric duct r.
ovarian r.
persistent pupillary membrane r.
r. stomach

remnant-like lipoprotein particle

remodeling
adrenal r.
bony r.
coronary r.
cortical bone r.
fracture r.
heart r.
neural foramen r.
paraarticular bone r.

remote
r. access perfusion
r. afterload brachytherapy
R. Associates Test
contralateral remote masking
r. data entry
r. data entry system
r. hospital
r. point of convergence
primary tumor, regional lymph node, remote metastases classification, staging
recent and r.
r. study monitoring

remottling fracture site

remotum
punctum r.

removable
r. implant
r. partial denture
r. silicone plug

removal
angled nucleus removal loupe
antibiotic removal device
antimicrobial removal device
Arana-Iniquez intracranial cyst removal technique
authorization form for removal of tissue for grafting
consent form for removal of tissue for grafting
digital removal of stool
en bloc r.
endoscopic stone r.
r. of excess cement
extracorporeal carbon dioxide r.
r. of foreign body
foreign body r.
hair removal efficiency
hair removal treatment
insertion and r.
r. of life support
nail fold r.
nucleus removal loupe
r. of
pack r.
percutaneous endoscopic r.
percutaneous stone r.
peritoneal dialysis urea r.
piecemeal removal of kidney stone
radical en bloc r.
smoke removal tube
suture r.
r. of vermiform appendix

remove
r. intoxicated driver
r. and replace intraocular lens
r., replace, reinoculate, repair

removed
bone marrow removed and stored
cast removed, take x-ray
placenta removed manually
r. in toto

remover
anterior band r.
dental stain r.

renal
r. abnormality
r. abscess
acquired renal cystic disease
acute on chronic renal failure
acute postoperative renal failure
acute renal failure and chronic renal failure
acute renal insufficiency
acute renal necrosis
r. adenoma
adipose renal capsule
r. agenesis
r. allograft
r. allograft recipient
r. allograft rejection
r. amyloidosis
r. anastomosis
anemia associated with chronic renal failure
anemia of chronic renal failure

renal *(continued)*
anemia of end-stage renal disease
anterior branch of the renal artery
anterior renal fascia
anterior superior renal segment
r. anuria
arterial renal plasma flow
r. arteriole
arteriosclerotic cardiovascular renal disease
arteriosclerotic renal artery disease
r. artery
r. artery aneurysm
r. artery bypass graft
r. artery pressure
r. artery response
r. artery stenosis
r. artery thrombosis
Ask-Upmark renal segment
asphyxial renal trauma
asphyxia-related renal necrosis
atheroembolic renal disease
atherosclerotic renal artery
atherosclerotic renal artery stenosis
atypical renal cyst
Atzpodien regimen for renal cell carcinoma
autolymphocyte-based treatment for renal cell carcinoma
autosomal recessive renal proximal tubulopathy and hypercalciuria
avascular renal mass
AVF-induced renal ischemia
r. axis
azoospermia, renal anomaly, cervicothoracic spine dysplasia
bilateral renal agenesis
bilateral renal tumor
bilateral renal vein thrombosis
r. biopsy
r. blood flow
cadaver renal transplant
calcium oxalate renal stone
r. calculus
r. calix
r. capsule
r. carcinoma
cardiovascular renal disease
r. cast
r. cell cancer
r. cell carcinoma
r. cholesterol embolization
chromophobe renal cell carcinoma
chronic renal disease
chronic renal failure
chronic renal insufficiency
r. clearance
clear cell renal cell carcinoma
r. colic
r. collar
comprehensive renal scintillation procedure
compromised renal function
computed renal tomography
r. congestion
continuous renal replacement therapy
contralateral renal plasma flow
r. corpuscle
r. cortex
r. cortical blood flow
r. cortical vascular resistance
r. crisis
crush injury renal problem
r. cyst
cystic renal cell carcinoma
r. diabetes
r. disease
dissecting renal artery aneurysm
distal renal tubular acidosis
r. dose dopamine
drug-induced renal disease
r. duplex scan
r. duplication
dynamic renal scintigraphy
r. dysfunction
r. dysgenesis
r. dysplasia
r. ectopia
effective renal blood flow
effective renal plasma flow
efferent renal sympathetic nerve activity
r. and electrolyte
end-stage renal disease
end-stage renal failure
r. epistaxis
r. epithelioid oxyphilic neoplasm
equivalent residual renal urea clearance
r. erythropoietic factor
r. excretion
r. excretion rate
r. exploration
r. failure
r. failure index
r. fascia
r. fibroma
r. fistula
r. fossa
r. function
functional renal failure of cirrhosis
r. function panel
r. function study
r. function test
r. ganglion
r. glomerular basement membrane thickness
r. glycosuria
r. helical computed tomography
r. hematoma
r. hematuria
r. hemorrhage
hemorrhagic fever with renal symptoms
hemorrhagic fever with renal syndrome
hereditary clear cell renal carcinoma
hereditary papillary renal cell carcinoma
hereditary papillary renal cancer
high-output renal failure
r. hilum
r. hilus
Hipputope renal function
r. homotransplantation
hyperchloremic renal acidosis
r. hyperplasia
r. hypertension
hypertension secondary to renal disease
r. hypertensive disease
hypertensive renal failure
idiopathic calcium renal stone formation
immune renal disease
r. impaired patient
impaired renal function
r. impairment
impending renal failure
incised renal parenchyma
r. infarct
r. injury
r. insufficiency
r. involvement
ischemic acute renal failure
r. kalium wasting
r. kidney stone
r. laboratory profile
r. labyrinth
left renal artery
left renal vein
living renal donor
living renal transplant
r. lobe

local bulge renal contour
main renal artery
main renal artery stenosis
main renal vein
malignant renal neoplasm
r. mass
mean renal blood flow
medullary renal carcinoma
metastatic renal cell carcinoma
microcystic disease of renal medulla
minimal renal disease
moderate renal failure
moderate renal insufficiency
müllerian duct, unilateral renal agenesis, and anomalies of the cervicothoracic somites
müllerian, renal, cervicothoracic, somite abnormalities
müllerian, renal, cervicothoracic, somite abnormalities syndrome
multicystic renal dysplasia
muscular layer of renal pelvis
myoglobinuric rhabdomyolytic acute renal failure
nephrotoxic acute renal failure
nodular renal blastoma
nonimmune renal disease
normal renal function
obstruction of renal artery
r. osteodystrophy
outpatient renal dialysis unit
r. papilla
r. papillary necrosis
papillary renal cell carcinoma
parenchymatous acute renal failure
patchy atrophy of renal cortex
patent renal agenesis
pediatric renal osteodystrophy
r. pelvic hemorrhage
r. pelvis
penetrating renal injury
r. percutaneous transluminal angioplasty
percutaneous transluminal renal angioplasty
r. plasma flow
posterior branch of renal artery
postischemic acute renal failure
posttransplant acute renal failure
posttraumatic acute renal failure
potential renal solute load
prerenal acute renal failure
r. pressor substance
progressive renal failure
radiologic contrast-induced renal failure
reduced renal mass
r. reserve filtration capacity
residual renal function
r. resistive index
r. retention
r. rickets
right renal artery
right renal vein
sarcomatoid renal cell carcinoma
scleroderma renal crisis
segmental bronchus renal artery waveform
segmented renal artery
severely impaired renal function
severe renal failure
severe renal insufficiency
r. solute load
split renal function
superficial renal cortical perfusion
theoretical renal phosphorus threshold
r. threshold
total renal blood flow
r. toxicity
r. transplant
r. transplantation
r. transplant patient
r. transplant recipient
transplant renal artery stenosis
r. tubular acidosis
r. tubular antigen
r. tubular cell
r. tubular dysgenesis
r. tubular epithelial
r. tubular necrosis
r. tubule hypokalemia
ultrasonic renal scanning
r. ultrasound
unilateral renal agenesis
unilateral renal artery stenosis
ureteric branch of renal artery
r. vascular failure
r. vascular resistance index
r. vasculature
r. vein plasma renin activity
r. vein/renal activity ratio
r. vein renin
r. vein renin activity
r. vein renin assay
r. vein renin concentration
r. vein thrombosis
r. venous
venous renal plasma flow
vertebral abnormality, anal imperforation, tracheoesophageal fistula, and radial, ray, or renal anomalies
wedged renal vein pressure

renal-anal-lung-polydactyly-hamartoblastoma syndrome

Renaut body

Rendu-Osler-Weber
R.-O.-W. disease
R.-O.-W. syndrome

renewed tumor activity

reniformis
placenta r.

renin
active renin concentration
r. activity
r. angiotensin blocker
r. essential hypertension
inactive renin activity
low renin, normal aldosterone
normal renin essential hypertension
peripheral vein renin activity
plasma renin concentration
plasma renin substrate activity
plasmin renin activity
r. release
renal vein r.
renal vein plasma renin activity
renal vein renin activity
renal vein renin assay
renal vein renin concentration
submandibular gland r.
total renin activity
total renin concentration
upright peripheral plasma renin activity
venous renin concentration

renin-angiotensin-aldosterone
r.-a.-a. system

renin-release
r.-r. rate
r.-r. ratio

reniportal anastomosis

ren mai channel

rennin
high level of kidney protein r.

renogram

renointestinal reflex

renomedullary
antihypertensive neural renomedullary lipids
r. interstitial cell

Rénon-Delille syndrome

renoprival hypertension

renovascular
atherosclerotic renovascular disease
r. hypertension
r. pressure
unilateral renovascular disease

rent of intestine

reoperative coronary artery bypass graft

reorientation
community leave for r.

reovirus
channel catfish r.
Coho salmon r.

reovirus-like
human r.-l.

repair
Abraham-Pankovich tendo calcaneus r.
Achilles tendon r.
Allison hiatal hernia r.
alpha-BSM bone repair material
Anson-McVay hernia r.
anterior cruciate ligament r.
anterior and posterior r.
aortic valve r.
Arlt epicanthus r.
Arlt eyelid r.
arthroscopic Bankart r.
Asopa hypospadias r.
Atasoy-type flap for nail injury r.
Bassini inguinal hernia r.
Bassini-type hernia r.
carpal tunnel r.
central episiotomy and r.
customized joint r.
DeBakey-Creech aneurysm r.
delayed primary r.
dentition in poor r.
Effler hiatal hernia r.
endovascular r.
end-to-end tendon r.
flexor tendon r.
hiatal hernia r.
inadequate tissue r.
inguinal hernia r.
intraperitoneal onlay mesh hernia repair
r. of joint
laparoscopic paraesophageal hernia r.
laparoscopic repair of paraesophageal hernia
Lichtenstein hernial r.
ligamentous and capsular r.
Lotheissen hernia r.
Lynn Achilles tendon repair technique
Magpi hypospadias r.
Marcy hernia r.
Marlex hernial r.
McVay repair of hernia
medial canthal r.
Millard bilateral cleft lip r.
minimally invasive valve r.
mismatch r.
mitral valve r.
modified Bardach r.
modified Becker r.
Moloney hernia r.
Mustard atrial baffle r.
mutation mismatch r.
nasoseptal r.
neonatal exstrophic bladder r.
Nicoll fracture repair procedure
Noble-Mengert perineal r.
nuclear excision repair instability
pants-over-vest hernial r.
paravaginal cystocele r.
paravaginal defect r.
paravaginal fascial r.
percutaneous Achilles tendon r.
poor dental r.
postreplication r.
r. of potentially lethal damage
r. relaxed vaginal outlet
remove, replace, reinoculate, r.
retinal detachment r.
rotator cuff r.
Sever-L'Episcopo repair of shoulder
skeletal repair system
staged abdominal r.
r. of sublethal damage
teeth in good dental r.
total r.
total extraperitoneal laparoscopic hernia r.
transabdominal preperitoneal laparoscopic hernia r.
ultrasound-guided compression r.
vaginal vault r.
vascularized double-sided preputial island flap and W flap glanuloplasty hypospadias r.
vesicovaginal fistula r.
VL stow r.

reparative
peripheral giant cell reparative granuloma

repeat
r. action tablet
r. heart attack
r. hip replacement surgery
inverted r.'s
leucine rich r.
long terminal repeat sequence
r. low transverse cesarean section
may r.
may repeat one time
r. open-application testing
short tandem repeat polymorphism
simple tandem repeat polymorphism
telomere repeat amplification protocol
telomeric repeat amplification protocol
terminal r.
time to r.
variable numbers of tandem r.'s

repeated
r. abuse
r. ear infection
r. exposure
r. oral doses of activated charcoal
r. partial asphyxia
r. quick stretch
r. quick stretch from elongation
r. quick stretch superimposed upon an existing contraction
r. skin grafting
r. spontaneous abortion
R. Test of Sustained Wakefulness

repeating
structural repeating unit

repellent
extended-duration topical arthropod r.

repens

reperfusion
r. arrhythmia
atherolytic reperfusion wire device
hepatic ischemia and r.
r. injury
ischemia and r.
ischemic reperfusion injury
ischemic tissue r.
postischemic reperfusion injury

reperfusion-induced hemorrhage

repetition
r. maximum
peak repetition frequency
pulse r.

pulse repetition frequency
Spreen-Benton Sentence R. Test
r. time

repetitious
r. activity
r. behavior

repetitive
r. action
acute repetitive seizure
adjust repetitive behavior
r. bending and stooping
r. bursts of action potential
complex repetitive discharge
r. excess mixed anhydride method
r. extragenic palindromic polymerase chain reaction
fast-frequency repetitive transcranial magnetic stimulation
r. fibrillation potential
r. hand motion
involuntary repetitive movement
r. motion disorder
r. motion injury
r. motion in the joint
r. motion syndrome
r. nerve stimulation
r. strain injury
r. stress injury
r. stress syndrome
r. task
timed repetitive ankle jerk
r. trauma disorder
r. ventricular response

rephasing
field-echo sequence with even-echo r.
gradient moment r.
gradient motion r.

replace
remove and replace intraocular lens
remove, replace, reinoculate, repair

replaced
liver volume replaced by tumor
r. with new bone

replacement
adequate fluid r.
aggression replacement training
allograft joint r.
allograft ligament r.
alumina-alumina total hip replacement prosthesis
alumina bioceramic joint r.
anatomic porous r.
anatomic porous replacement hemispheric acetabular component
androgen replacement therapy
antibody replacement therapy
aortic root r.
aortic valve r.
bipolar hip r.
bipolar hip replacement prosthesis
r. bone
cementless surface replacement arthroplasty
cementless total hip r.
colloid replacement solution
continuous-combined hormone replacement therapy
continuous hormone replacement therapy
continuous renal replacement therapy
r. culture medium
daily replacement factor of lymphocytes
double isomorphous r.
double valve r.
dual lock total hip r.
elastic-type disc r.
elective replacement indicator
electrolyte replacement with glucose
endoprosthetic femoral head r.
extended aortic root r.
failed joint r.
filtration replacement fluid
frozen embryo r.
gamma globulin r.
glandular replacement therapy
growth hormone r.
hair replacement surgery
hand/wrist joint r.
hard tissue r.
head-neck r.
heart valve r.
hip replacement surgery
hormonal replacement therapy
hormone replacement medication
hormone replacement therapy
incus replacement prosthesis
joint replacement center
low-dose estrogen r.
menopausal estrogen replacement therapy
metal-on-metal hip r.
metal-on-plastic hip r.
mineralocorticoid replacement therapy
minimally invasive valve replacement surgery
mitral and aortic valve r.
multiple isomorphous r.
nasogastric r.
oral hormone replacement therapy
pancreatic enzyme replacement therapy
partial ossicular replacement prosthesis
P.C.A. E-Series hip r.
postmenopausal estrogen r.
primary high-risk replacement surgery
repeat hip replacement surgery
revision hip replacement surgery
Scandinavian total ankle r.
self-articulating femoral hip r.
single isomorphous r.
stapes replacement prosthesis
supraannular mitral valve r.
surfactant replacement therapy
r. therapy
thyroid hormone r.
total ankle r.
total articular replacement arthroplasty
total elbow r.
total hip r.
total hip articular replacement by internal eccentric shells
total hip replacement operation
total hip replacement procedure
total joint r.
total knee r.
total knee replacement, left
total knee replacement, right
total ossicular chain replacement prosthesis
total shoulder r.
total wrist r.
tricuspid valve r.
valve r.

replacing
T-cell replacing factor

replantation
autogenous meniscal cartilage r.
r. of finger
intentional r.

repletion
nutrition r.
volume r.

replica of donor tissue

replicate
r. organism detection and counting
r. organism direct agar contact

replication
autonomous replication sequence
baboon virus r.
cell replication potential
r. error negative
r. error positive
low-level viral r.
lytic viral r.
morphine-potentiated HIV r.
morphine-potentiated human immunodeficiency virus r.
r. and transfer

replication-competent retrovirus assay

replicative
r. form
r. intermediate

repolarization
benign early r.
early r.
early repolarization pattern
early ventricular repolarization syndrome
electrocardiographic wave corresponding to repolarization of ventricles

repopulating
spleen repopulating activity

repopulation
marrow repopulation activity

report
attached r.
case r.
case report form
cumulative r.
data case report form
r. of event
examination and r.
failed to r.
hospital r.
Individual Case Safety R.'s
Juvenile Arthritis Functional Assessment R.
laboratory r.
mental status examination r.
no r.
note has been dictated/look for r.
note, record, r.
r. of
patient care r.
patient report form
problem-analysis r.
problem status r.
Proficiency Assessment R.
Teacher R. Form

reported
incurred but not r.
Structured Interview of R. Symptoms
r. visual sensation

reporter
catalyzed reporter deposition
luciferase reporter gene

reporting
drug abuse reporting program
periodic safety update r.
problem reporting program

repositioned
apically repositioned flap in mucogingival surgery

repositioning
adjustable leg and ankle repositioning mechanism
auricular r.
canalith r.
canalith repositioning maneuver
canalith repositioning procedure
craniomandibular orthopedic repositioning device
mandibular orthopedic repositioning appliance
maneuver

repositor

repository
cell repository line
Clinical Data R.
human genetic mutant cell r.
soluble r.

representational difference analysis

representative sample sectioned

representing
part of the electrocardio-graphic cycle representing atrial depolarization

repressed
r. feeling
testosterone repressed prostate message-2

repression
apoT3R-mediated r.
dissociation and r.
negative control r.

Repression-Sensitization Scale

repressor
heme-controlled r.
human-controlled r.
inducible cAMP early r.
r. molecule

reprimand
verbal r.

reprocessing
eye movement desensitization r.

reprocessor
automatic endoscopic r.

reproduction
asexual r.
assisted r.
net reproduction rate
Tactile R. Pegboard
visual r.

reproductive
assisted reproductive technique
r. cycle
r. disorder
r. endocrinology
r. failure
female reproductive tract
r. function
r. history
male reproductive organ
male reproductive tract
r. medicine
minimal reproductive unit
pituitary reproductive hormone
r. potential
selective tubal assessment to refine reproductive therapy
r. success
surgical myomectomy as reproductive therapy

reptilase time

request
life-terminating acts without the explicit r.
r. for payment
r. for proposal
treatment authorization r.

requesting
patient requesting admission

required
r. consent
14-hour fast r.
no further action r.
time required to complete G_1 phase of cell cycle
time required to complete G_2 phase of cell cycle
time required to complete M phase of cell cycle
time required to complete S phase of cell cycle
time required to double number of cells in given population

requirement
anticoagulation monitoring r.
caloric r.'s for burn patients
crying, requirement for oxygen supplementation, increases in heart rate and blood pressure
estimated protein r.
insulin r.
minimal daily r.
minimum daily r.
Parkland fluid requirement formula for burn patients
total energy r.

requisite
health deviation self-care r.

reroute
r. blood
r. digestive system

resazurin reduction time

rescripting nightmare

rescue
autologous bone marrow r.
autologous stem cell r.
r. breathing apparatus
citrovorum-factor r.
emergency medical care and r.
high-dose chemotherapy and stem cell r.
methotrexate, calcium leucovorin rescue, Adriamycin, cisplatin, bleomycin, cyclophosphamide, dactinomycin
peripheral blood stem cell r.
risk rescue rating
stem cell r.

research
ambulatory care research facility
arrhythmia research technology
r. assistant
r. aviation medicine
r. clinic
clinical r.
clinical research center
clinical research trial
clinical research unit
colony-stimulating factor developed by Venereal Disease R. Laboratory
computer-assisted r.
cooperative institutional research program
r. and development
r. and development board
r. diagnostic criteria
r. and education
eye r.
family history research diagnostic criteria
general r.
history of r.
motivation r.
myocardial infarction research unit
operations r.
orthopedic r.
Patient Outcomes R. Team
Personality R. Form
pharmaceutical research and testing
r. protocol
radioactive drug research committee
systems r.
r. and training center

resectable
r. carcinoma
r. lesion

resected
advanced resected head and neck cancer
carotid bodies r.
r. end-to-end ileal colostomy
intercostal nerve r.

resecting fracture

resection
abdominoperineal r.
activation map-guided surgical r.
anterior craniofacial r.
anterior mesial temporal r.
anterior pituitary r.
anterior resection rectopexy
anterior tarsal r.
anteromedial temporal lobe r.
atretic extrahepatic bile duct r.
atrial septal r.
Balfour gastric r.
bilateral carotid body r.
bladder neck r.
coagulation and hemostatic resection of prostate
colon r.
cricotracheal r.
cutting endoscopic mucosal r.
dilated bowel loop r.
duodenum-preserving pancreatic head r.
en bloc r.
endocardial resection procedure
endocervical r.
endometrial resection and ablation
endomyometrial r.
endoscopic mucosal r.
endoscopic mucosal resection, cap method
endoscopic mucosal resection, tube method
endoscopic mucosal resection with ligation
extended endocardial r.
extended endocardial resection procedure
gastric r.
gross total r.
r. head of pancreas
r. head of radius
holmium laser resection of the prostate
ileal r.
infundibular wedge r.
r. of intestine
laparoscopic resection of the ureterosacral ligament
laser r.
lift-and-cut endoscopic mucosal r.
low anterior r.
low anterior resection in combination with coloanal anastomosis
low rectal r.
major liver r.
margin of r.
massive bowel r.
massive bowel resection syndrome
medial eminence r.
metaphysial head resection with prosthesis
metastasis, age, completeness of resection, local invasion, and tumor size
metatarsal head r.
Milch cuff resection of ulna technique
Miles abdominoperineal r.
minimal transurethral resection of prostate
Mohs microsurgical r.
r. of muscle
neural arch resection technique
ovarian wedge r.
pancreatic head r.
panmetatarsal head r.
partial cricotracheal r.
partial dural r.
partial gastric r.
partial resection of stomach
proximal gastric r.
recession and r.
segmental colonic r.

resection *(continued)*
segment-oriented hepatic r.
status post transurethral resection of prostate
submucous resection and rhinoplasty
subtotal r.
total bladder r.
total transurethral resection of prostate
transcervical resection of the endometrium
transperineal urethral r.
transsphenoidal pituitary r.
transurethral prostatic r.
transurethral resection of bladder
transurethral resection of prostate
transurethral resection syndrome
transurethral resection of valves
transurethral resection of vesical neck
wedge matrix r.

resection/ablation
outpatient endometrial resection/ablation procedure

resector
full-radius r.
full-radius resector knife

resectoscope
specialized tissue aspirating r.

resembling
uterine tumor resembling an ovarian sex-cord tumor

resentment
covert r.

reserve
bone marrow neutrophil r.
breathing r.
cerebrovascular reserve capacity
coronary flow velocity r.
coronary reserve flow
expiratory r.
fractional flow r.
fractional velocity r.
heart rate r.
impaired coronary vascular r.
inspiratory reserve capacity
marrow neutrophil r.
myocardial fractional flow r.
myocardial perfusion r.
ovary r.
peripheral blood stem cell r.
relative coronary flow r.
renal reserve filtration capacity
respiratory r.
serum reserve cholesterol binding capacity
stenotic flow r.
r. volume
r. zone

reservoir
double-bubble flushing r.
double-stapled ileoanal r.
Neville upper reservoir buffer
on-off flushing r.
orthotopic colonic r.
orthotopic continent r.

reshaping
heart r.

residence
gastric residence time
mean residence time
University R. Environment Scale
usual place of r.

residency
hospital residency program
r. review committee

resident
r. admission notes
r. assessment protocol
r. progress note
variance of resident time

residential
acquired immune deficiency syndrome residential treatment facility
r. care
r. care facility for the elderly
r. care home
r. center
juvenile residential care
r. treatment center

residua (*pl. of* residuum)

residual
abnormal residual tissue
r. air
r. albuminuria
r. appendix
attention deficit disorder, residual type
r. disability
r. dye
equivalent residual renal urea clearance
r. fat
r. functional capacity
functional residual volume
gastric residual volume
r. gradient
r. handicap
r. hematoma
r. immunity
r. infiltrate
r. lung capacity
r. lymphocyte output
r. lymphoid tissue
macroscopic residual disease
mean residual gap
r. necrotic tissue
r. organic carbon
placental residual blood volume
postvoiding residual volume
postvoid residual volume
predicted functional residual capacity
r. renal function
retroperitoneal residual tumor mass
schizophrenia, residual type, subchronic
schizophrenic residual state
r. thermal damage
r. tuberculin
tumor r.
r. type schizophrenia
r. urine
r. urine volume
ventricular residual volume
well-healed, no r.'s

residue
cartilage r.
chemically bound r.
insoluble r.
liver residue factor
maximum residue limits of veterinary drugs
methanol extraction r.
nucleotide r.
root mean square r.
tuberculin r.

residue-free diet

residuum, pl. **residua**
microscopic r.
stroke with minimal r.

resilience
orbital r.

resin
anion exchange r.
autopolymerizing acrylic r.
cast resin lens
Harleco synthetic r.
r. hemoperfusion column
melamine-formaldehyde resin
microfilled composite r.
serum resin triiodothyronine uptake

strong exchange capacity r.
r. thyroxin
T_3 resin uptake
r. triiodothyronine
triiodothyronine resin uptake

resin-uptake ratio

resistance

acquired resistance to antibiotic
activated protein C r.
active r.
airway r.
r. airway
androgen resistance syndrome
antibiotic resistance gene
aortic valve r.
arterial arteriolar r.
axial resistance exerciser
basal skin r.
r. and capacitance
cardiovascular r.
cardiovascular resistance index
cerebrovascular r.
chromosomal mediated r.
circuit resistance training
coronary vascular r.
coronary vascular resistance index
decreasing peripheral vascular r.
r. determinant
diffusion r.
early progressive r.
efferent arteriolar r.
electric skin r.
environmental r.
estimated cerebrovascular r.
extended r.
external r.
extraparenchymal r.
extreme drug r.
factor essential for resistance to methicillin
fasting insulin resistance index
fold increase in r.
forearm vascular r.
frequency dependence of r.
galvanic skin r.
generalized resistance to thyroid hormone
generalized thyroid hormone r.
genotypic antiretroviral resistance testing
heavy resistance strength training
heterogeneous resistance to vancomycin
high-level gentamicin r.
hirsutism, androgen excess, insulin resistance, acanthosis nigricans syndrome
hyperandrogenism, insulin resistance, and acanthosis nigricans syndrome
increasing airway r.
r. index
r. to infection
inspiratory r.
inspiratory resistance and positive expiratory pressure
insulin resistance index
internal r.
intrahepatic r.
intraparenchymal r.
intrinsic flow r.
intrinsic resistance to antibiotic
limb vascular r.
loss of r.
lowered resistance to infection
malignant hyperthermia r.
manual resistance exercise
mean airway r.
mean resistance time
mechanical bladder outlet r.
minimal coronary vascular resistance index
minimal forearm vascular r.
moderate r.
r. to movement of lung tissue
multidrug resistance associated protein
multidrug resistance detoxification
multidrug resistance gene
multidrug resistance modulator
multiple-drug resistance gene
nasal airway r.
natural resistance macrophage-associated protein
overt compliance masking covert r.
parathyroid hormone resistance syndrome
partial insulin r.
passive resistance exercise
peripheral resistance unit
peripheral tissue resistance to thyroid hormone
peripheral total r.
peripheral vascular r.
peripheral vascular resistance index
pituitary resistance to thyroid hormone
pituitary thyroid hormone r.
r. plasmid
pleiotropic drug r.
primary drug r.
progressive r.
progressive resistance exercise
psychogalvanic skin r.
pulmonary arteriolar r.
pulmonary vascular r.
pulmonary vascular resistance index
relative vascular r.
renal cortical vascular r.
renal vascular resistance index
r. activated protein C
respiratory r.
respiratory resistance unit
respiratory system r.
screen-filtration r.
selective pituitary resistance to thyroid hormone
skin r.
specific r.
specific airway r.
stage of r.
stimulating insulin r.
syndrome of generalized thyroid hormone r.
systemic peripheral vascular r.
systemic vascular resistance index
r. to thyroid hormone
thyroid hormone r.
tissue r.
total airway r.
total flow r.
total peripheral resistance index
total peripheral vascular r.
total pulmonary vascular r.
total respiratory r.
total systemic arterial r.
r. training
r. transfer
r. transfer factor
transhepatic r.
transthoracic r.
r. unit
upper airway r.
upper airway resistance syndrome
urethral resistance factor
vascular r.
velocity-enhanced resistance training
venous r.
r. to venous return

resistance-inducing factor

resistant

caries r.
chromosomally mediated resistant *Neisseria gonorrhoeae*
cortisone resistant thymocyte
r. Friend leukemia cell
r. hypertension

resistant *(continued)*
r. individual
multiple resistant cell lines
periodic acid-Schiff r.
r. pneumococcus
seizure r.
steroid resistant asthma
steroid resistant graft-versus-host disease
r. strains of bacteria

resisted
shortened, held, resisted, contracted

Resistencia virus

resistive
active resistive range of motion
Doppler R. Index
r. exercise
r. exercise product
r. exercises to upper extremities
graded resistive exercise
r. index
r. load
r. load detection
r. movement
r. range of motion
regressive resistive exercise
renal resistive index

resistivity
electrical r.

resistor
input r.

resolution
angle variation r.
atomic resolution microscopy
crisis resolution center
high r.
incomplete resolution, scan to follow
logarithmic Minimum Angle of R.
minimal angle r.
Ophthimus High-Pass Resolution perimeter
rapid acquisition with resolution enhancement

resolved
angular resolved photoelectron spectroscopy
not r.
r. sarcoidosis
spatially resolved spectroscopy

resolving
r. ischemic neurologic deficit
spontaneously resolving thyrotoxicosis

resonance
axial breath-hold gradient-echo cine magnetic resonance imaging
axial magnetic resonance image
canal resonance response
cervical magnetic resonance phlebography
cine magnetic resonance imaging
constant magnetic field in nuclear magnetic r.
continuous arterial spin-labeled perfusion magnetic resonance imaging
contrast-enhanced magnetic resonance angiography
contrast medium-enhanced magnetic resonance imaging
conventional magnetic resonance imaging
diffusion-weighted imaging/magnetic resonance imaging
diffusion-weighted magnetic resonance imaging
dynamic contrast-enhanced magnetic resonance imaging
dynamic enhanced magnetic resonance imaging
electromagnetic molecular electronic r.
electron nuclear double r.
electron paramagnetic r.
electron spin r.
endoesophageal magnetic resonance imaging
endoesophageal magnetic resonance imaging coil
endorectal magnetic resonance imaging
endoscopic magnetic r.
enhancement of magnetic resonance imaging
fast imaging steady precession sequence three-dimensional magnetic resonance imaging
field focused nuclear magnetic r.
fluorescence resonance energy transfer
functional magnetic resonance angiography
functional magnetic resonance imaging
gadolinium-enhanced magnetic resonance imaging
instantaneous resonance curve
r. ionization mass spectrometry
r. ionization spectroscopy
localized magnetic r.
low-field magnetic resonance imaging
magnetic r.
magnetic resonance arteriography
magnetic resonance cholangiogram
magnetic resonance colonography
magnetic resonance coronary angiography
magnetic resonance elastography
magnetic resonance flowmetry
magnetic resonance imaging
magnetic resonance imaging thermometry
magnetic resonance pancreatography
magnetic resonance spectroscopic imaging-guided brachytherapy
magnetic resonance tomographic angiography
magnetic resonance tomography
magnetization transfer magnetic resonance imaging
minimum basis set magnetic resonance angiography
multisection diffuse-weighted magnetic resonance imaging
nuclear magnetic r.
nuclear magnetic resonance imaging
nuclear magnetic resonance spectroscopy
nuclear quadruple r.
perfusion-weighted magnetic resonance imaging
phase-contrast cine magnetic resonance imaging
phosphorus magnetic resonance imaging
phosphorus magnetic resonance spectroscopy
phosphorus-31 magnetic resonance spectroscopy
phosphorus nuclear magnetic resonance spectroscopy
proton magnetic r.
proton magnetic resonance spectroscopy
radiofrequency magnetic field in nuclear magnetic r.
rotating delivery of excitation off r.
surface plasmon r.

three-dimensional contrast-enhanced magnetic resonance angiography
topical magnetic r.
tritium nuclear magnetic r.
velocity-encoded cine-magnetic resonance imaging
vocal r.

resonant
fully resonant nucleus
thorax resonant on percussion

resorbable blast media

resorcinol
r. formaldehyde
gelatin, resorcinol, formaldehyde
latex and resorcinol formaldehyde

resorcinol-sulfur

resorcylic acid lactone

resorption
apical root r.
compensatory bone r.
cortical bone r.
external apical root r.
fractional proximal r.
osteoclast-activated bone r.
osteoclast-driven bone r.
osteoclastic bone r.
osteoclastic resorption lacuna
osteoclast-mediated bone r.
paracellular calcium r.
periprosthetic bone r.
progressive condylar r.

resource
Coping R.'s Inventory
Family Inventory of R.'s for Management
measure of resource use
medical resource utilization
mental health r.
r. utilization group

resource-based relative value scale

respiration
absence of r.
accessory muscles of r.
artificial r.
assisted r.
Austin Flint r.
blood pressure, pulse, respiration, and temperature
r. cease
Cheyne-Stokes r.
circulation, respiration, abdomen, motor, and speech
controlled r.
deep and regular r.
electrophrenic r.
frequency of r.
r. has ceased
intermittent positive pressure r.
irregular r.'s
percutaneous aspiration, instillation of hypertonic saline, r.
phonation, respiration, articulation-resonance
positive-negative pressure r.
productivity to respiration ratio
pulse and r.
regular r.
Schafer method of artificial r.
temperature, pulse, and r.

respirator
breathing supported by mechanical r.
drinker r.
mechanical r.
Monaghan r.
Morch r.
Morsch-Retec r.
Moynihan r.
negative-pressure r.
negative pressure r.
patient weaned from r.
volumetric diffusive r.

respiratorius
apparatus r.

respiratory
r. acidosis
acoustic respiratory motion sensor
acute febrile respiratory disease
acute febrile respiratory illness
acute hypoxemic respiratory failure
acute respiratory distress syndrome
acute respiratory insufficiency
acute respiratory tract illness
acute viral respiratory infection
adult respiratory distress syndrome
r. alkalosis
allergic respiratory disease
alopecia, nail dystrophy, ophthalmic complication, thyroid dysfunction, hypohidrosis, ephelides and enteropathy, and respiratory tract infection
alteration in respiratory function
amphoric respiratory sound
anaerobic respiratory infection
r. arrest
r. arrhythmia
aspirin-sensitive respiratory disease
atopic respiratory disease
r. battery, acute
r. bronchiole
r. bronchiolitis
r. bronchiolitis-associated interstitial lung disease
r. burst
Canadian Acute R. Illness and Flu Scale
cardiac and r.
r. care
r. care plan
r. center
central respiratory depression
chronic aspecific respiratory ailment
chronic obstructive respiratory disease
Chronic R. Questionnaire
chronic respiratory failure
chronic respiratory insufficiency
cocaine-induced respiratory failure
r. collapse
community-acquired respiratory infection
compliance of the respiratory system
r. complication
concurrent upper respiratory tract infection
r. control index
r. control ratio
cranial-sacral respiratory mechanism
declining respiratory status
decrease in respiratory effort
r. depression
r. depression inhalation anesthesia
r. disease
r. disease questionnaire
r. disorder
r. distress
r. distress index
r. distress syndrome
r. disturbance index
dorsal respiratory group
drug-induced postanesthetic respiratory depression
r. enteric orphan virus
r. exchange ratio
exercise-induced respiratory distress syndrome
r. failure
r. feedback
r. flora
r. frequency

respiratory *(continued)*
r. gas equation
r. glycoconjugate
r. heat exchange
hereditary respiratory disease
hospital-acquired lower respiratory infection
hospital-associated respiratory tract infection
human respiratory syncytial virus
idiopathic respiratory distress of newborn
idiopathic respiratory distress syndrome
r. illness
r. impairment
incipient respiratory infection
increased respiratory rate
increasing respiratory acidosis
r. index score
r. inductance plethysmography
r. inductive plethysmography
infant in acute respiratory distress
infant respiratory distress syndrome
r. inflammation
r. injury
r. insufficiency
r. intensive care unit
r. inversion point
r. irritation
r. isolation implementation efficiency
r. isolation implementation sensitivity
late respiratory systemic syndrome
lower respiratory tract illness
lower respiratory tract infection
lower respiratory tract inflammation
measurable undesirable respiratory contaminants
metabolic respiratory quotient
r. metabolism
minute respiratory volume
r. minute volume
mitochondrial respiratory chain defect
mitochondrial respiratory chain enzyme
mitochondrial respiratory chain enzyme complex
mixed r.
mixed respiratory failure
mixed respiratory vaccine
mixed vaccine, respiratory infection
mixed virus respiratory infection
r. movement
r. muscle strength
narcotic-induced respiratory depression
navigator echo-based real-time respiratory gating and triggering
necrotizing respiratory granulomatosis
neonatal respiratory distress syndrome
neutrophil respiratory burst activity
newborn respiratory distress syndrome
nosocomial respiratory tract infection
obstructive respiratory disease
r. ordered phase encoding
r. papillomatosis
r. paralysis
patient in cardiac or respiratory distress
patient receiving respiratory assistance
patient suffered respiratory arrest
peak respiratory ratio
perioperative respiratory therapy
poor respiratory effort
portable monitor of respiratory parameters
postanesthetic respiratory depression
postoperative respiratory therapy
postoperative respiratory treatment
primarily respiratory alkalosis
prolonged respiratory support
R. Quality of Life Questionnaire
r. quotient
r. rale
r. rate
r. rate per minute
r. rate:pulse rate index
recurrent lower respiratory tract disease
recurrent respiratory papilloma
recurrent respiratory papillomatosis
recurrent upper respiratory tract infection
r. reserve
r. resistance
r. resistance unit
routine respiratory care
severe respiratory insufficiency
r. sinus arrhythmia
R. Special Care Unit
steroid acute respiratory protein
St. Georges R. Questionnaire
r. stridor
surgical respiratory intensive care unit
r. symptom
r. syncytial virus
r. syncytial virus bronchiolitis
r. syncytial virus immune globulin
r. syncytial virus intravenous immunoglobulin
r. system
system for anesthetic and respiratory administration
r. system compliance score
r. system elastance
r. system resistance
terminal respiratory acidosis
terminal respiratory unit
r. therapy
r. toilet
total respiratory conductance
total respiratory resistance
total respiratory time
r. tract
r. tract fluid
r. tract infection
r. tract inflammation
r. tract lining fluid
transient respiratory distress of the newborn
transient respiratory distress syndrome
undifferentiated respiratory disease
upper r.
upper airway respiratory syndrome
upper respiratory disease
upper respiratory obstruction
upper respiratory tract infection
ventilator-dependent respiratory failure
wheezing-associated respiratory infection

respiratory-surgical intensive care unit

respirogram
transthoracic electric impedance r.

respirometer
speech-controlled respirometer for ambulatory measurement

respite and in-home care

respond
did not r.

failed to r.
patient failed to r.
r. to verbal command

responded

patient responded to treatment
patient responded verbally

responder

complete r.'s
first r.
hypoxic r.
isolated volume r.
medication r.
psychotherapy r.

responding

r. to internal stimuli
spontaneously responding hyperthyroidism

response

abnormal muscle r.
acoustic evoked r.
acoustic response technology
acquiescent response scale
acute insulin r.
acute phase r.
acute phase response element
adverse autonomic r.
adverse psychological r.
age-related pharmacodynamic r.
aided equalization r.
alertness, response to voice, response to pain, unresponsive
alert, verbal stimulus response, painful stimulus response, unresponsive
alternate response test
alternating failure of response mechanical to electrical depolarization
amplitude of successive r.'s
anatomy r.
antibody directed cytotoxic r.
antibody immune r.
anticipatory goal r.
antigen-specific immune r.
antiidiotype immune r.
antiidiotypic immunoglobulin r.
antistreptolysin O r.
anxiety relief r.
appropriateness of emotional r.
aqueous flare r.
assessing severity: age of patient, systems involved, stage of disease, complications, response to therapy
associative detail response to white space
associative response to a white space on a card
atrial flutter r.
atrial tachy r.
attenuated fever r.
audiometric brainstem r.
auditory brainstem-evoked r.
auditory brainstem response audiometry
auditory brainstem response test
auditory middle latency r.
auditory oculogyric r.
auditory response to bell
auditory response cradle
auditory visual evoked r.
automated auditory brainstem r.
automated auditory brainstem response hearing screening
average electroencephalic r.
average evoked r.
average evoked response audiometry
average evoked response technique
average response computer
baroreceptor reflex r.
best motor r.
biologic r.
Biological R. Modification Program
biologic response modifier
brainstem auditory evoked r.
brainstem electrical response audiometry
brainstem electric response audiometry
brainstem evoked r.
brain wave r.
cAMP response element-binding
canal resonance r.
cardiac-evoked response audiometry
cell-mediated immune r.
cell response to estrogen
cellular mediated immune r.
cephalic vasomotor r.
clinical partial r.
compensatory antiinflammatory response syndrome
complete r.
conditioned avoidance r.
conditioned behavior r.
conditioned emotional r.
conditioned fear r.
confabulated detail r.
confabulated whole r.
consensual pupillary r.
controlled ventricular r.
correct r.
cortical auditory evoked r.
cortical somatosensory evoked r.
r. criteria
Cushing pressure r.
cytotoxic T-cell lymphocyte r.
data, action, r.
data, action, response, and evaluation
defective immune r.
defibrillation response interval
detail r.
detail response elaborating the whole
detail response to small white space
differential reinforcement of low response rates
direct cortical r.
double ventricular r.
early asthmatic r.
edge response function
electrical response activity
electric response audiometry
electrocardiographic r.
electrodermal response biofeedback
electrodermal response audiometry
electroencephalic response audiometry
electroencephalographic r.
electronically provoked r.
electron paramagnetic r.
Environmental R. Inventory
Equal Listener R. scale
evoked cortical r.
evoked potential r.
evoked response audiometer
evoked response audiometry
evoked response test
evoked somatosensory r.
evoked visual r.
fastigial pressor r.
first-phase insulin r.
fixed frequency r.
flexor plantar r.
form r.
frequency-following r.
galvanic skin response audiometry
gamma band r.
gastrocolonic r.
glucocorticoid response element
glucose r.
good form r.
good partial r.
graft-versus-host r.

response *(continued)*
r. grasp
growth hormone r.
Hazardous Materials R. Unit
heart rate r.'s
heart response to stress
heparin dose r.
heparin response test
high irradiance r.
histoculture drug response assay
hormonal r.
hormone response element
hormone response unit
host-versus-graft r.
human figure parts r.
hypercapnic ventilatory r.
hypoxic ventilatory r.
Immediate R. Mobile Analysis
immune r.
immune response and combined modality treatment
immunologic r.
index of r.
indices predicting r.
inhibitory response element
initial immune r.
instrumental heart rate r.'s
insulin secretory r.
integrated gastrin r.
integrated pancreatic polypeptide r.
integrated secretory r.
r. interruption
item response theory
late asthmatic r.
late auditory evoked r.
late cortical r.
late-phase r.
Lewis triple r.
light response of pupil
Likert-type response pattern
local inflammatory r.
local twitch r.
long-duration r.
lymphocyte adenylate cyclase r.
mammalian diving r.
maternal humoral immune r.
maternal inflammatory r.
maternal vascular r.
maximal static response assay
mean length of r.
median duration of r.
menstrual cycle hemodynamic r.
methacholine inhalation challenge r.
middle latency r.
minimal response level
mixed leukocyte r.
mixed lymphocyte r.
motor-evoked r.
motor-evoked response to transcranial stimulation
mucosal immune r.
multimodality evoked r.
muscle response test
muscular response to electrical stimulation of motor nerve
negative T_3 response element
negative triiodothyronine response element
neonatal auditory response cradle
nephropathic immune r.
neurological evoked r.
neurologically evoked r.
neutrophil chemotactic r.
nictitating membrane r.
no r.
nodular complete r.
nonadrenergic inhibitory r.
normal plantar r.
orienting r.
paced ventricular evoked r.
paradoxical cold r.
partial r.
patient's immune r.
pattern evoked retinal r.
pattern-shift visual-evoked r.
pattern visual-evoked r.
peak thyroid-stimulating hormone r.
peak TSH r.
peroxisome proliferator response element
personal emergency response system
phase response curve
plantar response downgoing
plantar response upgoing
polymorphonuclear leukocyte r.
poor form r.
poor partial r.
popular r.
position r.
postocclusive oscillatory r.
primary immune r.
protamine response test
psychogalvanic r.
psychogalvanic skin response audiometry
pudendal evoked r.
pulmonary reimplantation r.
pyramidal r.
quieting r.
radiation r.
randomized response technique
rapid ventricular r.
rare detail r.
r. rate
rate-drop r.
reduced vascular r.
reduced vestibular r.
relative r.
relative response attributable to the maneuver
relative response index
relaxation response in headache therapy
renal artery r.
repetitive ventricular r.
reversal speed of bronchoconstriction in response to methacholine
screening auditory brainstem r.
secondary immune r.
selective estrogen response modifier
sensitivity r.
sensitization response cell
sensory evoked r.
sequential vascular r.
Sexual Assault R. Team
shade response to light gray area
shading response to black areas
shading response to gray areas
short-duration r.
simple response paradigm
skin conductance orienting r.
slow immune r.
soluble immune response suppressor
somatosensory evoked r.
specific r.
speed of bronchoconstriction in response to methacholine
stabilized relative r.
standardized response mean
steady-state auditory evoked r.
stimulus r.
stimulus-organism r.
suppressed immune r.
sustained response rate
sympathetic skin r.
systemic inflammatory response syndrome
thyroid hormone response element
thyroid response element
tonic vibration r.
total r.
total response index
trabecular meshwork-inducible glucocorticoid r.

transient auditory evoked r.
Treatment R. Assessment Method
unconditioned r.
unusual rare detail r.
vasomotor r.
ventricular r.
ventricular response rate
vestibuloocular r.
visual auditory evoked r.
visually evoked flow r.
visual response audiometry
volume-pressure r.
r. to white space
whole r.
whole response to detail

response-stimulus ratio

response-to-injury theory

responsibility

ascriptive r.
assigned r.
R. and Independence Scale for Adolescents
obsessive feelings of r.

responsible

diagnosis responsible for length of stay

responsive

attentive and r.
r. and attentive
magnetically responsive microsphere
patient responsive to noxious stimuli
patient responsive to painful stimuli
patient responsive to verbal command
T_3 responsive element

responsiveness

bronchial r.
mutual affective r.

rest

adrenal cell rest tumor
adrenal rest tissue
auxiliary implant r.
auxiliary occlusal r.
auxiliary rest implant substructure
bowel r.
Chan wrist r.
congenital cartilaginous rest of neck
r. cure
ejection fraction at r.
electron rest mass
evaluation of denervated heart at r.
r. and exercise
r. home
hot packs and bed r.
r., ice, compression, elevation
intralobar nephrogenic r.
ischemic rest angina
Malassez epithelial r.'s
maximal force at rest length
metabolism at r.
multigated blood pool image at r.
nephrogenic r.
r. pain
pain at r.
patient at complete bed r.
perilobar nephrogenic r.
physiologic rest position
postural rest position
protection, rest, ice, compression, elevation, support
r. and recuperation
steady-state r.
total bed r.
r. tremor
Veley head r.
Walthard cell r.

Restan virus

restaurant

Chinese restaurant asthma
Chinese restaurant syndrome

rested state contraction

restenosis

aortic valve r.
in-stent r.
intrastent r.
r. postangioplasty
post balloon angioplasty r.

rest-exercise program

restful awareness

resting

r. ankle-arm pressure index
r. ankle index
r. blood pressure
r. calcaneal stance position
r. cardiac output
r. electroencephalogram
r. energy
r. energy expenditure
evaluation of resting activity
r. expiratory level
functional resting position splint
r. hair
r. head pressure
heart r.
r. heart rate
maximal resting anal pressure
mean resting diastolic blood pressure
mean resting potential
r. membrane potential
r. metabolic expenditure
r. metabolic rate
r. muscle activity
normal resting pulse
normal resting pulse rate
r. phase of facial hair
r. radionuclide ejection fraction
r. radium
teboroxime resting washout
r. tremor
uterine resting tone
r. value
r. venous pressure

restless

r. leg syndrome
vegetative and r.

restlessness

irritability, agitation and r.
irritability, restlessness, and intense craving
motor r.

Reston virus

restoration

alloy r.
electrolyte balance r.
full cast r.
hair restoration surgery
Marzola hair restoration surgery
r. of normal anatomic alignment
r. of spontaneous circulation

restorative

r. care
full-mouth restorative dentistry
intermediate restorative material
r. nursing program
r. proctocolectomy
r. sleep
temporary endodontic restorative material
totally stapled restorative proctocolectomy

restore

r. lost or thinning hair
r. mobility and reduce pain
r. tissue to affected area

restored mobility

restrain

supportive device to restrain hernia

restrained

patient restrained with vest

restraining tape

restraint
Charcot restraint orthotic walker
emergency chemical r.
emergency mechanical r.
emergency physical r.
nonambulatory r.
patient in complete r.
patient in partial r.
r. and seclusion
r. and water immersion stress

restricted
r. activity
r. behavior
calorie r.
delirium, infection, atrophic urethritis and vaginitis, pharmaceuticals, psychological disorders, excessive urine output, restricted mobility, stool impaction
R. Environment Stimulation Therapy
r. eye movement
r. fluids
medically restricted diet
painful and restricted movement
phosphate restricted diet
protection, restricted activity, ice, compression, elevation
r. range of motion
r. ROM
tenderness, asymmetry, restricted motion, and tissue texture changes

restricting
lysis of restricting strand
r. food intake

restriction
asymmetric fetal growth r.
r. endonuclease analysis
r. endonucleases from *Haemophilus influenzae*
r. of environmental stimulation therapy
r. enzyme analysis
fetal growth r.
fluid r.
r. fragment length polymorphism
human leukocyte antigen restriction element
intrauterine growth r.
r. landmark genomic scanning
major histocompatibility complex r.
mutation-enriched restriction fragment length polymorphism assay
normotensive intrauterine growth r.
sleep restriction therapy
tissue texture changes, asymmetry, restriction of motion, tenderness

restrictive
r. abnormality
r. cardiomyopathy
chronic restrictive pulmonary disease
r. functional impairment
r. heart disease
idiopathic restrictive cardiomyopathy
interstitial restrictive lung disease
least restrictive environment
maximal restrictive exercise

restrictor
beam r.

restructuring
attitude r.
confrontational cognitive r.
sexual attitude r.
systematic rational r.

resubmission turnaround document

result
r.'s of clinical controlled trial
false-negative r.'s
false-positive r.'s
r.'s to follow
good cosmetic r.
knowledge of r.
unable to read lab result

resultant
r. current
r. physiologic acceleration

resulting
overstimulation and resulting confusion

resumption
menstrual cycle r.
r. of normal sinus rhythm

resurface skin

resurfacing
Achilles tendon r.
carbon dioxide laser skin r.
cosmetic skin r.
face laser skin r.
laser skin r.
total articular resurfacing arthroplasty
transconjunctival blepharoplasty laser r.

resuscitate
do not r.
orders not to r.

resuscitated
heart r.
not to be r.

resuscitation
attempted cardiopulmonary r.
baby expired following resuscitation attempt
cardiac resuscitation team
cardiopulmonary r.
cardiopulmonary-cerebral r.
closed chest cardiac r.
dead despite resuscitation attempt
r. of depressed newborn
despite resuscitation attempts
expired following resuscitation attempt
external cardiopulmonary r.
heart-lung r.
interposed abdominal compressions-cardiopulmonary r.
no cardiopulmonary r.
open chest cardiac r.
open-chest cardiopulmonary r.
Parkland burn resuscitation formula
Parkland formula for fluid resuscitation for burn trauma
simultaneous compression ventilation-cardiopulmonary r.
standard external cardiopulmonary r.

resuscitative
cardiac automatic resuscitative device
dead on arrival despite resuscitative attempts

resuscitator
heart-lung r.
infant Ambu r.

retained
r. alpha activity
r. cortical activity
evacuation of retained products of conception
r. fetal lung fluid
r. foreign body
foreign body r.
r. gastric antrum
r. gastric antrum syndrome

r. lung fluid
r. placenta
r. placental tissue
r. products of conception
r. urine

retainer
band and spur r.
bonded r.
flexible spiral wire r.
lingual canine-to-canine r.

retaining
r. new information

retard
r. bone activity
r. fetal growth

retardates
Sheridan Tests for Young Children and R.

retardation
agonadism, mental retardation, short stature, retarded bone age syndrome
alopecia, contracture, dwarfism, mental retardation syndrome
alopecia, mental retardation, epilepsy, microcephaly syndrome
alpha-thalassemia mental r.
aniridia, ambiguous genitalia, mental r.
aniridia, ambiguous genitalia, mental retardation triad syndrome
anophthalmia, hand-foot defects-mental retardation syndrome
aortic arch anomaly-peculiar facies mental retardation syndrome
aortic stenosis, corneal clouding, growth and mental retardation syndrome
arithmetical skills learning r.
asymmetric intrauterine growth r.
basal ganglion disorder-mental r.
brachydactyly, mesomelia, mental retardation, aortic dilation, mitral valve prolapse, characteristic facies syndrome
cataract, hypertrichosis, mental r.
caudal appendage, short terminal phalanges, deafness, cryptorchidism, mental retardation syndrome
Charcot-Marie-Tooth syndrome, X-linked type II with deafness and mental r.
coloboma, heart anomaly, ichthyosis, mental retardation, and ear abnormality syndrome
congenital cataracts, sensorineural deafness, Down syndrome facial appearance, short stature, mental retardation syndrome
congenital emphysema, cryptorchidism, penoscrotal web, deafness, mental retardation syndrome
deafness, onychoosteodystrophy, and mental retardation syndrome
dislocated elbow, bowed tibiae, scoliosis, deafness, cataract, microcephaly, mental retardation syndrome
distal arthrogryposis, hypopituitarism, mental retardation, facial anomalies syndrome
early onset Parkinsonism-mental retardation syndrome
ectodermal dysplasia, cleft lip and palate, mental retardation, syndactyly syndrome I, II
facial dysplasia, hyperextensibility of joints, clinodactyly, growth retardation, mental retardation syndrome
r. factor
fetal alcohol r.
fetal growth r.
fragile site mental retardation 1, 2
fragile X mental retardation protein
gingival fibromatosis, hypertrichosis, cherubism, mental retardation, epilepsy syndrome
gonadal failure, short stature, mitral valve prolapse, mental retardation syndrome
goniodysgenesis, mental retardation, short stature
growth retardation, alopecia, pseudoanodontia, and optic atrophy syndrome
growth retardation in children
growth retardation, ocular abnormalities, microcephaly, brachydactyly, oligophrenia
hereditary motor sensory neuropathy II-deafness-mental r.
insulin-resistant diabetes, acanthosis nigricans, hypogonadism pigmentary retinopathy, deafness, mental retardation syndrome
intrauterine fetal growth r.
lentigines, electrocardiographic abnormalities, ocular hypertelorism, pulmonary stenosis, abnormalities of genitalia, retardation of growth, deafness syndrome
linear growth r.
macrocephaly, facial abnormalities, disproportionate tall stature mental retardation syndrome
macrosomia-mental retardation syndrome
marfanoid habitus-mental retardation syndrome
median cleft upper lip, mental retardation, pugilistic facies syndrome
megalocornea, developmental retardation, dysmorphic syndrome
mental r.
Mental R. and Development Disabilities
mental health and mental r.
mental and physical retardation, speech disorders, peculiar facies syndrome
mental retardation, ataxia, hypotonia, hypogonadism, retinal dystrophy syndrome
mental retardation, blepharonasofacial abnormalities, hand malformations syndrome
mental retardation, cerebral palsy
mental retardation, coarse face, microcephaly, epilepsy, skeletal abnormalities syndrome
mental retardation, coarse facies, epilepsy, joint contracture syndrome
mental retardation, congenital contracture, low fingertip arches syndrome
mental retardation, congenital heart disease, blepharophimosis, blepharoptosis, hypoplastic teeth
mental retardation, dysmorphism, cerebral atrophy syndrome
mental retardation, dystonic movements, ataxia, seizures syndrome
mental retardation, epilepsy, short stature, skeletal dysplasia syndrome

retardation *(continued)*
mental retardation, facial anomalies, hypopituitarism, distal arthrogryposis syndrome
mental retardation, gynecomastia, obesity syndrome
mental retardation, hearing impairment, distinct facies, skeletal anomalies syndrome
mental retardation, macroorchidism syndrome
mental retardation, microcephaly, blepharochalasis syndrome
mental retardation, mitral valve prolapse, characteristic face syndrome
mental retardation, optic atrophy, deafness, seizures syndrome
mental retardation, overgrowth, craniosynostosis, distal arthrogryposis, sacral dimple, joint laxity
mental retardation, polydactyly, phalangeal hypoplasia, syndactyly, unusual face, uncombable hair
mental retardation, pre-and postnatal overgrowth, remarkable face, acanthosis nigricans syndrome
mental retardation, retinopathy, microcephaly syndrome
mental retardation, scapuloperoneal muscular dystrophy, lethal cardiomyopathy syndrome
mental retardation, short stature, hypertelorism syndrome
mental retardation, short stature, obesity, hypogonadism syndrome
mental retardation, skeletal dysplasia, abducens palsy syndrome
mental retardation, spasticity, distal transverse limb defects syndrome
mental retardation, spastic paraplegia, palmoplantar hyperkeratosis syndrome
mental retardation, typical facies, aortic stenosis syndrome
microcephaly, infantile spasm, psychomotor retardation, nephrotic syndrome
microcephaly, mental retardation, cataract, hypogonadism syndrome
microcephaly, mental retardation, retinopathy syndrome
microcephaly, mild mental retardation, short stature, skeletal anomalies syndrome
microcephaly, sparse hair, mental retardation, seizures syndrome
mild mental r.
mixed sclerosing bone dysplasia, small stature, seizures, mental retardation syndrome
moderate mental r.
motor-sensory neuropathy, X-linked Type II, with deafness and mental r.
multiple congenital anomalies/mental retardation syndrome
multiple exostoses-mental retardation syndrome
multiple exostosis mental retardation syndrome
nasal hypoplasia, peripheral dysostosis, mental retardation syndrome
nonprogressive cerebellar disorder with mental r.
nonspecific mental r.
Northern epilepsy with mental r.
pandevelopmental r.
parietal foramina, brachymicrocephaly, mental retardation syndrome
peripheral dysostosis, nail hypoplasia, mental retardation syndrome
profound mental r.
psychomotor r.
severe mental r.
skeletal abnormalities, cutis laxa, craniostenosis, psychomotor retardation, facial abnormalities
undifferentiated mental r.
Wilms tumor, aniridia, genitourinary abnormalities, and mental r.
X-linked alpha-thalassemia/mental retardation syndrome
X-linked mental r.
X-linked mental retardation, microphthalmia, microcornea, cataract, hypogenitalism-mental retardation-spasticity syndrome
X-linked mental retardation, seizures, acquired microcephaly, agenesis of corpus callosum
X-linked mental retardation syndrome 1–6

retardation-absent
mental retardation-absent nails of hallux and pollex syndrome

retarded
agonadism, mental retardation, short stature, retarded bone age syndrome
coloboma, heart disease, atresia choanae, retarded growth and retarded development and/or CNS anomalies, genital hypoplasia, and ear anomalies and/or deafness syndrome
educable mentally r.
mentally r.
mentally retarded and developmentally disabled
profoundly mentally r.
reading r.
specific reading r.
trainable mentally r.

rete
malpighian r.
r. peg
r. ridge
r. testis aspiration

retention
absolute retention time
acute urinary r.
apocrine retention cyst
r. band
Benton Visual R. Test, Revised
r. catheter
chronic urinary r.
coefficient of fat r.
r. of contrast material
corrected retention time
r. cyst
debridement and prosthesis r.
fluid r.
fluid retention syndrome
heavy retention suture
mucous retention cyst
nylon retention suture
oil retention enema
partial denture r.
relative retention time
r. suture
r. time
r. time ratio
urinary r.
Visual R. Test
water r.
whole-body r.

reticula (*pl. of* reticulum)

reticular
r. activating system
ascending reticular activation
ascending reticular arousal system
r. cartilage
r. cell
r. degeneration
r. degeneration of pigment epithelium
dorsal medullary reticular formation
r. dysgenesis
r. erythematous mucinosis
r. fiber
r. formation
r. keratitis
r. lamina
lateral reticular nucleus
mesencephalic reticular formation
midbrain reticular formation
r. nucleus
paramedian pontine reticular formation
paramedian reticular nucleus
pontine paramedian reticular formation
pontine reticular formation

reticular-activating
ascending reticular-activating system

reticulare
magma r.

reticulate
r. body
confluent, reticulate papillomatosis

reticulated
r. bone
r. corpuscle
r. siderocyte
subpleural reticulated carbon deposition
r. tissue

reticulocyte
automated reticulocyte counting
r. cell-free system
r. count
early r.
hemoglobin content of r.
r. hemoglobin distribution width
large r.
r. mean corpuscular volume
r. production index
r. standard buffer

reticulocytic production index

reticuloendothelial
r. cell
r. depressing substance
hepatic reticuloendothelial cell
r. phagocytic capacity
r. system

reticuloendotheliosis
avian r.
leukemic r.
r. virus

reticuloid
actinic reticuloid dermatitis

reticulopathy
malignant r.

reticulosis
histiocytic medullary r.
localized pagetoid r.
lymphoid follicular r.
mast cell r.
midline malignant r.
polymorphic r.

reticulospinal tract

reticulum, pl. **reticula**
agranular endoplasmic r.
r. cell
r. cell carcinoma
dendritic reticulum cell
fragmented sarcoplasmic r.
Golgi endoplasmic reticulum lysosome
granular endoplasmic r.
rough endoplasmic r.
sarcoplasmic r.
smooth endoplasmic r.
total endoplasmic r.

retina
active hyperemia of r.
angiomatosis of r.
arteriosclerosis of r.
r. asthenopia
avascular peripheral r.
cyanosis of r.
Heidelberg retina tomograph
hemangioma of r.
hemorrhage in r.
lattice degeneration of r.
limiting membrane of r.
lipemic r.
lower r.
macula of r.
medial arteriole of r.
medial venulae of r.
molecular layer of r.
mottled r.
murine r.
nasal arteriole of r.
nasal venule of r.
neovascularization of r.
neovascularization elsewhere on r.
nerve layer of r.
neural layer of optic part of r.
neuroepithelial element of r.
neuroepithelial layer of r.
neurosensory r.
nuclear layers of r.
outer r.
passive hyperemia of r.
peripheral r.
periphery of r.
physiologic r.
pigmented retina epithelial cell
pigmented layer of r.
r. pigment epithelium detachment
plexiform layers of r.
reattachment of r.
shot-silk r.
tear of r.
tigroid r.
vascularization elsewhere in the r.
watered-silk r.

retinacular
oblique retinacular ligament

retinaculotome
Paine carpal tunnel r.

retinal
r. abiotrophy
r. abnormality
abnormal retinal correspondence
aneurysm of retinal arteriole
angioid retinal streak
anomalous retinal correspondence
anterior retinal orbital canal
aphakic retinal detachment
r. aplasia
arcuate retinal fold
r. arterial narrowing and straightening
r. arteritis
r. artery
bilateral acute retinal necrosis
branch retinal artery occlusion
branch retinal vein occlusion
r. camera
r. capillary microaneurysm
central retinal artery
central retinal artery occlusion
central retinal vein
central retinal vein occlusion
complex retinal detachment
r. cone
congenital hypertrophy of retinal pigment epithelium
r. damage threshold
r. degeneration

retinal *(continued)*
r. detachment
r. detachment, oculus dexter
r. detachment, oculus sinister
r. detachment repair
endophlebitis of retinal vein
r. examination
r. flap
r. fold
r. fundus photography
r. ganglion cell
giant retinal tear
r. hemorrhage
high-altitude retinal hemorrhage
r. hole
hydrocephalus, agyria, retinal dysplasia with or without encephalocele syndrome
Iwanoff retinal edema
macula-off rhegmatogenous retinal detachment
macular branch retinal vein occlusion
mental retardation, ataxia, hypotonia, hypogonadism, retinal dystrophy syndrome
morning glory retinal detachment
myelinated retinal nerve fiber
myelination of retinal nerve
myopic retinal degeneration
narrowing of retinal arteriole
r. necrosis
r. nerve fiber layer
neurosensory retinal detachment
nicking of retinal vein
nonmydriatic retinal photography
nonrhegmatogenous retinal detachment
normal retinal correspondence
normal retinal movement
obstructive retinal vasculitis
occlusion of retinal arteriole
occlusion of retinal vein
occlusive retinal arteritis
pattern evoked retinal response
pellucid marginal retinal degeneration
peripapillary retinal height
peripapillary retinal nerve
peripapillary retinal nerve fiber
peripheral branch retinal vein occlusion
peripheral retinal ablation
peripheral retinal operculum
peripheral retinal vascular sheathing
r. pigment epithelial cell
r. pigment epithelium
preferred retinal locus
progressive outer retinal necrosis
r. reflex
r. rod
senile retinal neovascular membrane
tractional retinal detachment
traction retinal detachment
r. vasculature
r. vasculitis
r. vein occlusion
r. venous dilation and tortuosity
r. vessel

retinalis
lipemia r.

retinitis
actinic r.
AIDS-related r.
apoplectic r.
central angiospastic r.
congenital retinitis blindness
diabetic r.
r. gravidarum
herpes simplex r.
hypertensive r.
metastatic r.
necrotizing r.
neurogenic muscle weakness, ataxia, and retinitis pigmentosa
peripheral necrotizing r.
Pick r.
r. pigmentosa
r. pigmentosa GTPase regulator gene
r. proliferans
purulent r.
serous r.
simple r.
suppurative r.
uremic r.
Wagener r.
X-linked retinitis pigmentosa

retinoblastoma
r. gene
intraocular r.
r. protein
trilateral r.

retinocerebellar angiomatosis

retinochoroiditis
nosocomial r.
toxoplasmic r.

retinoic
r. acid
r. acid-binding protein
r. acid metabolism blocking agent
r. acid receptor
r. acid-related orphan receptor
cellular retinoic acid-binding protein
9-*cis* retinoic acid receptor
9-*cis* retinoic acid
silencing mediator of retinoic acid and thyroid hormone receptor

retinoid
combination retinoid and PUVA therapy
r. X, Z receptor

retinol-binding
r.-b. globulin
r.-b. protein

retinol equivalent

Retinopan

retinopathy
acute zonal occult outer r.
background diabetic r.
carotid occlusive disease r.
central disk-shaped r.
central serous r.
diabetic r.
early diabetic r.
full florid diabetic r.
hemorrhagic r.
high-altitude r.
high oxygen percentage in retinopathy of prematurity
hypertensive r.
insulin-resistant diabetes, acanthosis nigricans, hypogonadism pigmentary retinopathy, deafness, mental retardation syndrome
mental retardation, retinopathy, microcephaly syndrome
microcephaly, mental retardation, retinopathy syndrome
nonproliferative diabetic r.
optic disc drusen r.
osteogenesis imperfecta, optic atrophy, retinopathy, developmental delay syndrome
peripheral diabetic r.
peripheral exudative choroidal hemorrhagic r.
r. of prematurity
preproliferative diabetic r.
proliferative diabetic r.
proliferative diabetic retinopathy with vitreous hemorrhage

proliferative sickle r.
sickle cell r.
surface wrinkling r.
threshold stage III of retinopathy of prematurity
venous stasis r.

retinoschisis
congenital hereditary r.
X-linked juvenile r.

retinoscope
luminous r.

retinoscopy
monocular-estimate-method dynamic r.
noncycloplegic distance static r.

retirement
R. Descriptive Index
Employee R. Income Security Act

retour
de retour rales

retracted
Ashford retracted nipple operation
periosteum incised and r.

retracting
grunting, flaring, and retracting breathing
infant retracting and grunting

retraction
anterior retraction archwire
axonal retraction ball
clot r.
clot retraction test
clot retraction time
distortion or retraction of nipple
Duane syndrome r.
r. or grunting
grunting and r.
grunting or r.
intercostal space r.
massive preretinal r.
massive vitreous r.
mechanical lid r.
mesencephalic lid r.
myopathic eyelid r.
neuromuscular eyelid r.
neuropathic eyelid r.
sternal intercostal r.
substernal r.
r. syndrome

retraining
bladder retraining drill
computerized diaphragmatic breathing r.

retrieval
egg retrieval procedure
follicle puncture for oocyte r.
heat-induced epitope r.
immature oocyte r.
information storage and r.
instrument retrieval container
intravascular foreign body r.
low-temperature, heat-mediated antigen r.
microwave epitope retrieval technique
organ retrieval and preservation
pancreas antigen r.
Short-Term Auditory R. and Storage Test
sonication-induced epitope r.
sperm microaspiration retrieval technique
transvaginal ultrasound-directed oocyte r.

retrieved
donor heart r.

retroactive
r. amnesia
r. inhibition
r. interference

retroambigualis
nucleus r.

retroauricular
postauricular and retroauricular scalping

retrobulbar
r. abscess
r. lid block
r. neuritis
r. optic neuritis
r. space

retrocalcaneal bursa

retrocaval catheter

retrocecal
r. abscess
r. appendix
r. hernia
r. lymph node
perforated retrocecal appendix

retrocecales
nodi lymphoidei r.

retrocedent gout

retrocentral sulcus

retrocerebellar
arachnoid retrocerebellar pouch

retrochiasmatica
area r.

retrococcygeal air study

retrocochlear hearing loss

retrocolic anastomosis

retrocorneal pigmentation

retroduodenal
r. artery
r. fossa

retroduodenalis
arteria r.

retroflexed uterus

retroflexus
fasciculus r.

retrogasserian
percutaneous retrogasserian glycerol injection

retrograde
r. amnesia
r. approach
balloon-occluded retrograde transvenous obliteration
r. blood flow
r. cerebral perfusion
r. cholangiogram
r. cholangiography
computed tomography under endoscopic retrograde pancreatography
r. conduction time
cystocopy and r.
r. cystogram
r. cystourethrogram
r. direction
r. duodenogastroscopy
r. ejaculation
endoscopic retrograde balloon dilatation
endoscopic retrograde biliary drainage
endoscopic retrograde biliary stenting
endoscopic retrograde cholangiogram
endoscopic retrograde cholangiography
endoscopic retrograde cholangiopancreatogram
endoscopic retrograde cholangiopancreatography
endoscopic retrograde cholecystoendoprosthesis
endoscopic retrograde pancreatogram
endoscopic retrograde pancreatography

retrograde *(continued)*
endoscopic retrograde parenchymography of pancreas
endoscopic retrograde sphincterotomy
r. fashion
r. femoral catheter
r. filling
r. flow of barium
r. hernia
r. infection
intravenous r.
intravenous retrograde access port
r. kidney study
mother endoscopic retrograde cholangiopancreatoscopy system
r. percutaneous gastrostomy
r. pyelogram
r. pyelography
r. ureterogram
r. urethrogram
r. urethrography
r. urogram

retrolabyrinthine vestibular neurectomy

retrolental fibroplasia

retromanubrial dullness

retromolar
r. triangle
r. trigone

retroorbicularis oculi fat

retropatellar
r. fat pad
r. pain syndrome

retroperitoneal
anterior retroperitoneal decompression
anterior retroperitoneal flank approach
balloon-assisted, endoscopic, retroperitoneal, gasless
r. fibromatosis
r. gas insufflation
r. hemorrhage
r. hernia
idiopathic retroperitoneal fibrosis
r. lymphadenectomy
r. pelvic lymph node dissection
r. residual tumor mass

retroperitoneum irrigated

retropharyngeal
r. abscess
anteromedial retropharyngeal approach
r. lymph node
r. soft tissue space

retropharyngeales
nodi lymphoidei r.

retroplacental gamma globulin

retropubic
r. cytourethropexy
r. hernia
r. prostatectomy
radical retropubic prostatectomy
r. urethropexy

retropylorici
nodi lymphoidei r.

retrorectal space

retrosigmoid approach

retrosternal
r. abnormality
anterior retrosternal hernia of Morgagni
r. area
r. chest pain
r. hematoma
r. hernia

retrouterine hematoma

retrovaginal space

retroversion
angle of r.

retroverted/retroflexed

retroverted uterus

retroviral
acute retroviral syndrome
human retroviral disease
r. infection
r. vaccine

retrovirus
AIDS-associated r.
avian type C retrovirus group
porcine endogenous r.
replication-competent retrovirus assay

retruded contact position

return
anomalous pulmonary venous r.
r. to baseline
r. to clinic
decreased venous return to heart
r. electrode monitor
r. to flow
r. flow enema
r. flow hemostatic catheter
good blood r.
Harris return flow
lymphatic return rate
no blood r.
partial anomalous pulmonary venous r.
patient to r.
pulmonary anomalous superior venous r.
pulmonary venous r.
resistance to venous r.
sluggish blood r.
r. of spontaneous circulation
to r.
total anomalous pulmonary venous r.
venous r.
venous return to heart
venous return time

returned
cecum returned to abdomen

Retzius
R. cavity
R. fiber
foramen of Key and R.
R. gyrus
R. ligament
lines of R.
R. space

reuptake
dopamine reuptake inhibitor
noradrenaline reuptake inhibitor
norepinephrine reuptake inhibitor
selective serotonin reuptake inhibitor
serotonin noradrenergic reuptake inhibitor
serotonin-norepinephrine reuptake inhibitor
serotonin reuptake transporter

Reusner sign

Reuss
R. color chart
R. table

Reuter button

revascularization
arrested-heart revascularization technique
arterial revascularization therapy study
r. of blood vessels of heart
cardiac revascularization procedure
coronary artery revascularization procedure
direct myocardial r.
heart laser r.
laser transmyocardial r.
lower extremity r.
myocardial laser r.
percutaneous coronary r.

percutaneous transluminal coronary r.
percutaneous transluminal endomyocardial r.
percutaneous transluminal myocardial r.
percutaneous transmyocardial laser r.
radiofrequency percutaneous myocardial r.
target lesion r.
target vessel r.
transmyocardial laser r.

revealed
lungs revealed hyperresonance to percussion

revealing
lymph node revealing solution

reveals
bone scan reveals increased activity

revenge
Montezuma's r.

reverberation artifact

Reverdin
R. graft
R. operation

Reverdin-Green bunionectomy

reversal
r. of antagonist
dosage-sensitive sex reversal
habit reversal training
isotonic r.
pattern reversal visual evoked potential
r. phase
pulmonary vein atrial r.
r. speed of bronchoconstriction in response to methacholine
stabilizing r.

reverse
r. analgesia
autologous reverse graft
autologous reverse graft to ankle
avian myeloblastosis leukemia virus reverse transcriptase
avian myeloblastosis virus reverse transcriptase
BCR-ABL multiplex reverse transcriptase polymerase chain reaction assay
competitive reverse transcription-polymerase chain reaction
r. curve
r. fast imaging with steady-state free precession
r. filling
r. filling procedure
r. flow island flap
r. forearm island flap
r. heart disease
r. heart failure
r. hemolytic plaque assay
human milk reverse transcriptase enzyme
human telomerase reverse transcriptase
r. immune cytoadhesion
r. isolation
McIntyre reverse cystitome
mixed reverse passive antiglobulin hemagglutination
multiple marker reverse transcriptase-polymerase chain reaction assay
nonnucleoside reverse transcriptase inhibitor
nucleoside analog reverse transcriptase inhibitor
nucleoside reverse transcriptase inhibitor
nucleotide reverse transcriptase inhibitor
r. osmosis
r. passive anaphylaxis
r. phase
r. pivot shift
product-enhanced reverse transcriptase
r. straight leg raise
r. sutured eye
r. T_3
r. transcriptase inhibitor
r. transcriptase polymerase chain reaction
r. transcriptase primer extension
r. transcriptase-producing agent
r. triiodothyronine

reversed
r. anaphylaxis
r. coarctation
r. digital artery flap
r. dorsal digital flap
r. ductus arteriosus
electrodialysis with reversed polarity
r. gastric tube
r. ophthalmic artery flow
r. passive hemagglutination
r. passive hemagglutination by miniature centrifugal fast analysis
r. passive hemagglutination reaction
r. passive latex particle agglutination
r. phase high-performance liquid chromatography
r. phase ion-pair partition
r. saphenous vein graft
twin reversed arterial perfusion
r. vertebral blood flow

reversed-phase liquid chromatography

reverse-shape implant

reversible
r. blockade
r. colloid
r. inhibitor of monoamine oxidase-type A
r. ischemia
r. ischemic attack
r. ischemic neurologic deficit
r. ischemic neurologic disability
r. obstructive airways disease
poorly reversible asthma
r. posterior leukoencephalopathy
r. posterior leukoencephalopathy syndrome
prolonged reversible ischemic neurologic deficit
r. sickle cell

reverting scope

review
antibiotic utilization r.
capital expenditure r.
cardiovascular r.
Computer-Assisted Psychiatric Evaluation and R. System
continued-stay r.
continuing disability r.
critical incident r.
drug regimen r.
drug use r.
focused medical r.
health care r.
hospital peer r.
independent professional r.
institutional review board
local medical review policy
medical history r.
online prospective drug utilization r.
peer review committee
periodic medical r.
program evaluation and review technique
prospective drug r.

review *(continued)*
quality assurance and utilization r.
residency review committee
r. of outside film
r. of signs and symptoms
r. of subjective symptoms
survey, question, read, review, recite

reviewing physician

revised
Benton Visual Retention Test, R.
R. Children's Depression Scale
R. Children's Manifest Anxiety Scale
R. Denver Prescreening Development Questionnaire
R. Memory and Behavior Problems Checklist
Michigan Picture Test, R.
Optimism-Pessimism Scale, r.
Revised European-American Classification of Lymphoid Neoplasms
Symptoms Checklist 90 R.
R. Trauma Score

revising sleep habits

revision
r. of amputation stump
r. arthroplasty
r. and debridement
debridement and r.
exploration and r.
fusiform skin r.
r. hip arthroplasty
r. hip replacement surgery
lip scar r.
Modular Acetabular R. System

revitalize hair growth

rewarming
extracorporeal r.
passive external r.

Rey Auditory Verbal Learning Test

Reye
adult Reye syndrome
meningitis or encephalitis, metabolic, Reye syndrome
R. syndrome

Rey-Estreich Complex Figure Test

Reynell Development Language Scales

Reynier
Nager-de Reynier syndrome

Reynolds
R. Adolescent Depression Scale
R. Child Depression Scale
R. number

Rey-Osterrieth complex figure

RFX-associated protein

Rh
R. agglutinin
antepartum Rh isoimmunization
R. antibody titer
R. antigen
R. blood factor
R. blood group
R. immune globulin
R. incompatibility
R. negative
negative Rh blood
parental Rh incompatibility
R. positive
R. sensitization

rhabdoid
composite extrarenal rhabdoid tumor
extrarenal rhabdoid tumor
malignant extrarenal rhabdoid tumor
malignant rhabdoid tumor of kidney
malignant rhabdoid tumor of soft tissue
r. suture
r. tumor of the kidney

rhabdomyolysis
acute exertional r.
malignant hyperthermic r.

rhabdomyolytic
myoglobinuric rhabdomyolytic acute renal failure
r. syndrome

rhabdomyomatous
fetal rhabdomyomatous nephroblastoma

rhabdomyosarcoma
alveolar r.
embryonal r.
r. of head and neck
paratesticular r.
r. of soft tissue

rhamnosus
Lactobacillus rhamnosus strain GG

rhegmatogenous
r. detachment
macula-off rhegmatogenous retinal detachment
r. retinal detachment

rheography
light reflection r.

rhesus
r. antigen C
r. D antigen
R. diploid cell strain rabies vaccine
R. diploid cell strain rabies vaccine
r. E antigen
R. factor
r. gene CE, D
R. hemolytic disease
R. immune globulin
R. monkey kidney
R. negative
R. positive
Rhesus hemolytic disease
R. rotavirus
r. rotavirus-tetravalent vaccine

rheumatic
acute rheumatic arthritis
acute rheumatic fever
r. aortic valve disease
r. arteritis
r. arthralgia
r. arthritis
arthritis and rheumatic diseases
arthritis of rheumatic fever
r. carditis
childhood rheumatic disease
r. chorea
r. disease
r. disorder
environmentally associated rheumatic disorder
r. exanthema
r. fever
r. fever vaccine
r. gout
r. granuloma
healed rheumatic valvulitis
r. mitral stenosis
r. nodule
r. pain modulation disorder
r. valvular heart disease

rheumatica
peliosis r.
polymyalgia r.
polymyalgia rheumatica syndrome

rheumatism
acute articular r.
chronic articular r.

r. of heart
Macleod capsular r.
nodules, eosinophilia, rheumatism, dermatitis, and swelling syndrome
palindromic r.
soft-tissue r.

rheumatoid
r. agglutinator
ankle rheumatoid arthritis
r. arthritis
r. arthritis agglutinin
r. arthritis, diffuse idiopathic skeletal hyperostosis
r. arthritis factor test
r. arthritis nuclear antigen
r. arthritis precipitin
r. arthritis serum factor
r. arthritis and Sjögren syndrome
assignment criteria for rheumatoid arthritis
r. biologically active factor
r. cervical myelopathy
chronic rheumatoid arthritis
chronic rheumatoid nodular fibrositis
debilitating rheumatoid arthritis
r. deformity
differential rheumatoid agglutination test
r. disease
elderly-onset rheumatoid arthritis
r. factor
r. factor binding
r. factorlike activity
r. factorlike substance
r. factor test
r. foot
immunoglobulin G rheumatoid factor
juvenile-onset rheumatoid arthritis
juvenile rheumatoid arthritis rash
Mayo classification of rheumatoid elbow
mixed rheumatoid and degenerative arthritis
monoclonal rheumatoid factor
r. nodule
oligoarticular seronegative rheumatoid arthritis
pauciarticular juvenile rheumatoid arthritis
r. pocket
r. polyarthritis
polyarticular juvenile rheumatoid arthritis
polyclonal rheumatoid factor
r. rosette
systemic juvenile rheumatoid arthritis
test for rheumatoid factor
r. vasculitis
younger-onset rheumatoid arthritis

rhinitis
allergic r.
allergic rhinitis perennial
atrophic r.
atrophic rhinitis of swine
blood eosinophilic nonallergic r.
congestive seasonal allergic r.
eosinophilic nonallergic r.
nonallergic noninfectious perennial r.
nonallergic rhinitis with eosinophilia syndrome
noneosinophilic nonallergic r.
perennial allergic r.
postnasal drip due to r.
probable allergic r.
seasonal allergic r.
r. sicca
total vasomotor rhinitis symptom score
vasomotor r.

rhinobronchitis
allergic r.

rhinocerebral
r. aspergillosis
r. infection

rhinoconjunctivitis
allergic r.
perennial allergic r.
seasonal allergic r.

rhinoconjunctivitis-specific quality of life questionnaire

rhinology
ophthalmology, otology, laryngology, and r.
otology, laryngology, and r.

rhinomanometry
anterior active mask r.

rhinometry
acoustic r.

rhinoplasty
Carpue r.
conservative subtraction-addition r.
submucous resection and r.

rhinopneumonia
equine r.

rhinopneumonitis
equine r.
equine rhinopneumonitis virus

rhinorrhea
ipsilateral r.

rhinoscopy
anterior r.
fiberoptic r.

rhinoseptoplasty procedure

rhinosinusitis
acute bacterial r.
viral r.

rhinotracheitis
feline viral r.
infectious bovine r.
infectious bovine rhinotracheitis virus

rhinoviral cold

rhinovirus inhibitor

rhizolysis
percutaneous glycerol r.
percutaneous radiofrequency r.

rhizomelic chondrodysplasia punctata

rhizotomy
anterior r.
facet r.
percutaneous stereotactic radiofrequency rhizotomy
selective dorsal r.
selective posterior r.
trigeminal r.

Rh-negative
immune globulin to an Rh-negative woman

RhO
R. D immune globulin

rhodamine
r. isothiocyanate
r. isothiocyanate conjugated

Rhode Island Pupil Identification Scale

RhO D immune globulin

rhodopsin-lipid complex

rhombencephalic gustatory nucleus

rhombic groove

rhomboid
r. fossa
greater rhomboid muscle
r. impression
r. ligament
limiting sulcus of rhomboid fossa
r. major muscle
medial eminence of r.
median rhomboid glossitis

rhomboideus major

rhonchi
coarse r.
expiratory r.
inspiratory r.
rales and r.
rales, rhonchi or, wheezes
sibilant r.

rhyme
modified rhyme hearing test
phonetically balanced rhyme test

rhythm
abnormal cardiac r.
abnormal heart r.
abnormally slow r.
accelerated idioventricular r.
accelerated intraventricular r.
accelerated junctional r.
accelerated ventricular r.
r. of alpha frequency
alpha rhythm frequency
alternate with alpha r.
arteriovenous junctional r.
artificial pacemaker-induced ventricular r.
atrial bigeminal r.
atrioventricular junctional r.
atrioventricular junction escape r.
atrioventricular nodal r.
AV junctional r.
basic electrical r.
cardiac r.
change in heart r.
chaotic heart r.
circadian biological r.
circadian rhythm dyssomnia
control electrical r.
coronary nodal r.
daily affective r.
decelerate breathing r.
disturbance in cardiac r.
diurnal r.
endogenous circadian r.
endogenous circadian rhythm phase
erratic heart r.
erratic speech r.
fast alpha variant r.
fatal heart rhythm disturbance
fetal heart r.
frontocentral beta r.
r. of heartbeat disorder
heart electrical r.
heart rhythm abnormality
heart rhythm disorder
heart rhythm disturbance
heart rhythm drug
heart rhythm problem
idiojunctional r.
idioventricular r.
increased rhythm disturbances
r. instability of head and trunk
irregular heartbeat r.
irregular heart r.
irregularly irregular r.
irregular rate and r.
junctional escape r.
junctional rhythm after cardiac surgery
life-threatening heart r.
maternal estradiol r.
r. method
nodal escape r.
nonparoxysmal nodal r.
normal alpha r.
normal heart r.
normal rhythm of heart
normal sinus heart r.
normal sinus rate and r.
pacemaker r.
paroxysmal nodal r.
pulsed idioventricular r.
pulseless idioventricular r.
racing heart r.
rapid heart r.
rate and r.
regular heart r.
regularly irregular r.
regular rate and r.
regular sinus r.
resumption of normal sinus r.
scapulohumeral r.
Seashore R. Test
sensorimotor r.
shock heart into normal r.
sinus r.
sinus rhythm, no ectopy
slow alpha variant r.
slow heart r.
steady alpha r.
r. strip
supraventricular r.
systolic gallop r.
underlying heart r.
ventricular r.
ventricular escape r.
ventricular paced r.

rhythmic
r. chorea
r. contraction
cranial rhythmic impulse
r. discharge
frontal intermittent rhythmic delta activity
frontal irregular rhythmic delta activity
r. horizontal oscillation of eyeball
hyperventilation-induced high-amplitude rhythmic slowing
r. inhibitory pattern
r. initiation
r. instability of head and trunk
intermittent rhythmic delta activity
involuntary rhythmic oscillation
r. jerking movements
occipital dominant intermittent rhythmic delta activity
rapid rhythmic alternating movements
r. sensory bombardment therapy
subclinical rhythmic epileptiform discharge of adult
wave lengths of rhythmic activity

rhythmical
continuous high-amplitude electroencephalogram rhythmical synchronous slowing
r. midtemporal discharge

rhytidectomy
facial r.

rib
angle of anterior r.
angle of posterior r.
anterior angle of r.
anterior rib impingement syndrome
articular facet of head of r.
articular facet of tubercle of r.
articular surface of head of r.
articular surface of tubercle of r.
autologous r.
autologous rib bone graft
r. belt
r. cage
caliper rib movement
r. cartilage
r. contusion
cough fracture of r.
floating r.
r. fracture
intact rib cage
lumbar r.
Majewski short rib polydactyly
multiple nevoid, basal cell epithelioma, jaw cysts, bifid rib syndrome
nevoid basal cell epithelioma, jaw cysts, bifid rib syndrome
proximal end of r.

radiate ligament of head of r.
slipping rib syndrome
smaller rib incision
r. spreader inserted
supernumerary r.
upper rib cage
Zahn r.

ribbon gut

ribcage intact

Ribes ganglion

riboflavin
r. carrier protein
r. deficiency
r. tetrabutyrate

riboflavin-binding protein

ribonuclear
soluble ribonuclear protein

ribonuclease protection assay

ribonucleic
r. acid
r. acid-binding motif
r. acid-dependent deoxyribonucleic acid polymerase
r. acid-polymerase chain reaction
alanyl-transfer ribonucleic acid synthetase
chromosomal ribonucleic acid
cold-inducible ribonucleic acid-binding protein
heterogeneous nuclear ribonucleic acid
heterogeneous ribonucleic acid
immune ribonucleic acid
informational ribonucleic acid
messenger ribonucleic acid
mini-exon-derived ribonucleic acid gene
nuclear ribonucleic acid
oncogene ribonucleic acid
ribosomal ribonucleic acid
ribosomal ribonucleic acid transcription unit
small nuclear ribonucleic acid
soluble ribonucleic acid
transfer ribonucleic acid
translational control ribonucleic acid
viral ribonucleic acid

ribonucleoprotein
heterogeneous nuclear r.
messenger r.
messenger ribonucleoprotein acid
nuclear r.
small nuclear r.

ribonucleotide
aminoimidazole carboxamide r.
imidazoleacetic acid r.
r. reductase
total adenine r.

riboprobe
antisense r.

ribose
adenosine diphosphate r.

riboside
hypoxanthine r.
methylmercaptopurine r.
6-methylmercaptopurine r.

ribosomal
r. deoxyribonucleic acid
r. DNA
r. ribonucleic acid
r. ribonucleic acid transcription unit
r. RNA

ribosome
internal ribosome entry site
total cytoplasmic r.

ribosome-like particle

ribothymidylic acid

ribotide
aminoimidazole carboxamide r.
N-formylglycinamide r.
succinyl aminoimidazole carboxamide r.

Ricard amputation

rice
bananas, rice, applesauce, tea, toast diet
bananas, rice, applesauce, toast diet
bananas, rice cereal, applesauce, toast diet

rich
leucine rich repeat

Richardson
Modified Richardson technique

Richards-Rundle syndrome

Richart Pap smear

Richet
R. aneurysm
R. operation

Richner-Hanhart syndrome

Richter hernia

ricin
anti-B4 blocked r.

rickets
autosomal recessive hypophosphatemic r.
familial hypophosphatemic r.
hereditary hypophosphatemic rickets with hypercalciuria syndrome
pseudovitamin D deficiency r.
sex-linked hypophosphatemic r.
vitamin D-dependent rickets type II
vitamin D-resistant r.
X-linked hypophosphatemic r.

Rickett organism

Rickettsiae
typhus *Rickettsiae* species vaccine

rickettsial disorder

rickettsiosis
Eastern tick-borne r.

Riddoch
R. mass reflex
R. syndrome

Rideal-Walker coefficient

rider
intravenous r.

rider's
r. bone
r. bursa

ridge
apical ectodermal r.
buccal triangular r.
Cowbone Ridge virus
distal cusp r.
distal marginal r.
distobuccal cusp r.
distolingual cusp r.
incisal r.
lingual alveolar r.
lower alveolar r.
mandibular anteroposterior ridge slope
maxillary alveolar r.
medial epicondylar r.
mesial cusp r.
mesial marginal r.
mesiobuccal cusp r.
mesiolingual cusp r.
oblique r.
Palmer classification of trapezial ridge fracture
total ridge count
transverse groove of oblique r.
trapezius ridge sign

ridging
metopic r.

Riedel
R. disease
R. lobe
R. thyroiditis
Rieder cell
Riegel
R. pulse
R. test meal
Rieger
R. anomaly
short stature, hyperextensibility of joints or hernia or both, ocular depression, Rieger anomaly, teething, delayed
R. syndrome
Riehl melanosis
Rietti
microelliptopoikilocytic anemia of Rietti, Greppi, and Micheli
Rieux hernia
rifampin-isoniazid-streptomycin-ethambutol
rifamycin
newer r.
Rifkind sign
rifle
air r.
assault r.
Rift Valley fever virus
right
r. abdominal pain
aberrant right subclavian artery
abnormal right axis deviation
r. acromiodorsoanterior fetal position
r. acromiodorsoposterior fetal position
acute right heart syndrome
acute right ventricular heart failure
r. angle
r. angle clamp
anomalous nonrecurrent right inferior laryngeal nerve
anomalous right pulmonary vein dextroposition
anomalous right subclavian artery
r. antecubital
r. anterior
r. anterior caudocranial oblique
anterior cusp of right atrioventricular valve
r. anterior descending
r. anterior descending coronary artery
r. anterior hemiblock
r. anterior measurement
r. anterior oblique
r. anterior oblique position
r. anterior oblique projection
r. anterior oblique view
r. anterior occipital
r. anterior quadrant
r. anterior thigh
anterior right ventricular wall
r. aortic arch
aortic sinus to right ventricle fistula
apical branch of inferior lobar branch of right pulmonary artery
apical branch of right superior pulmonary vein
apical segmental artery of superior lobar artery of right lung
r. arm
r. arm electrode for electrocardiogram
r. arm hemiparesis
r. arm reclining
r. arm recumbent
r. arm, sitting
arrhythmogenic right ventricular cardiomyopathy
arrhythmogenic right ventricular dysplasia
r. atrial abnormality
r. atrial appendage
r. atrial contraction
r. atrial diameter
r. atrial enlargement
r. atrial function
r. atrial hypertrophy
r. atrial involvement
r. atrial mean pressure
r. atrial pressure elevation
r. atrium
r. atrium body
r. atrium of heart
augmented filling of right ventricle
augmented voltage unipolar right arm lead
r. auricle
auricle of right atrium
r. axis deviation
r. basilar artery
r. to be assisted to die
r. and below
below right costal margin
blood pressure, right arm
r. border cardiac dullness
r. border of heart
r. brachial artery
r. brachial vein
r. brachial vein occlusion
r. brain
r. brain damage
r. brain stroke
r. branch
r. breast
r. breast biopsy
r. breast biopsy examination
r. bundle
r. bundle-branch
r. bundle-branch block
r. bundle-branch system block
r. bundle ventricular
r. buttock
r. carotid artery
r. carotid endarterectomy
catheter stimulation of right atrium
r. caudal quarter ganglion
r. caudate nucleus
r. cerebral hemisphere
r. cerebrovascular accident
chest and right arm
r. colic artery
r. colic vein
r. colon
r. common carotid
r. common carotid artery
r. common femoral angioplasty
r. common femoral artery
complete right bundle branch block
congestive right ventricular failure
contraction of right atrium
r. coronary
r. coronary angiography
r. coronary artery
r. coronary cusp
r. coronary sinus
r. costal margin
r. crus
r. crus of diaphragm
r. deltoid
r. deltoid muscle
r. descending pulmonary artery
r. deviation of electrical axis
deviation to the r.
dextroduction of right eye
diaphragmatic surface of right lung
r. direct inguinal hernia
disregard rights of others
distal right coronary artery
r. dorsoanterior

r. dorsogluteal
r. dorsoposterior
r. ductus arteriosus
dullness over right lung
duplication of right collecting system
duplication of right kidney
r. ear
r. ear advantage
r. ear, cold stimulus
r. ear, warm stimulus
easy normal r.
emptying of right atrium
r. end-expiratory pressure
epibronchial right pulmonary artery syndrome
r. esotropia
r. exotropia
r. external carotid
r. external carotid artery
r. eye
r. eye patched
r. femoral artery
r. femoral vein
r. fibrous trigone
filling of right atrium
fingerbreadth below right costal margin
fixing right eye
r. foot
r. foot switch
r. forearm
r. frontal craniotomy
r. frontal hematoma
r. frontal lobe
r. frontal sinus
r. frontoanterior fetal position
r. frontolateral fetal position
r. frontoposterior fetal position
r. frontotransverse fetal position
r. gastric lymph node
r. gastric vein
r. gaze
r. giant cell
r. gluteal
r. gluteus maximus
r. gutter
r. hand
r. hand grip
head rotation to r.
r. heart
r. heart blood volume
r. heart border
r. heart bypass
r. heart catheterization
r. heart failure
r. heart mixing volume
r. heart strain
r. heeloff
r. heel strike
r. hemicolectomy
r. hemiplegia
r. hemisphere
r. hemisphere of brain
r. hemisphere brain damage
r. hemisphere deficit
R. Hemisphere Language Battery
r. hemisphere lesion
r. hemothorax
r. hepatic artery
r. hepatic duct
r. hepatic lobe
r. hepatic vein
high right parasternal view
high right atrium
high right atrium electrocardiogram
r. hilar lymph node
r. homonymous hemianopia
human rights committee
hypermetropia, r.
r. hyperphoria
r. hypertropia
hypesthesia of right leg
r. hypochondrium
hypoplastic right heart syndrome
r. iliac artery
r. iliac crest
r. iliac fossa
impaired right discrimination
incomplete right bundle-branch block
r. index finger
r. inferior oblique muscle
r. inferior rectus
r. inferior vena cava
r. inguinal hernia
r. innominate artery
r. innominate vein
r. intercostal margin
r. intercostal space
r. internal capsule
r. internal jugular vein
r. internal mammary anastomosis
r. internal mammary artery
r. internal thoracic artery
r. kidney
r. lateral
r. lateral bending
r. lateral decubital position
r. lateral femoral
r. lateral gaze
r. lateral position
r. lateral rectus muscle
r. lateral thigh
r. leg
r. liver lobe
r. lower
r. lower arm
r. lower border of cardiac dullness
r. lower extremity
r. lower lid
r. lower limb
r. lower lobe
r. lower lobe infiltrate
r. lower quadrant
r. lower quadrant of abdomen
r. lower quadrant defect
lower right quadrant
r. lower scapular border
r. lower sternal border
low right atrium
low septal right atrium
r. lung
r. lung-to-head circumference ratio
r. main bronchus
r. main coronary artery
r. main-stem bronchus
r. manubrial dullness
marginal atrial branch of right coronary artery
marginal branch of right coronary artery
r. margin of heart
r. mastoid
maximal r.
mean right atrial pressure
mean right ventricular pressure
r. medial rectus muscle
r. median
r. mediolateral
r. mediolateral episiotomy
r. mentoanterior fetal position
r. mentolateral fetal position
r. mentoposterior fetal position
r. mentotransverse position
r. midclavicular line
r. middle cerebral artery thrombosis
r. middle ear exploration
r. middle finger
middle lobar artery of right lung
r. middle lobe
middle lobe branch of right superior pulmonary vein
r. middle lobe bronchus
r. middle lobe of lung
middle lobe of right lung
r. middle lobe syndrome

right *(continued)*
r. middle sternal border
Mini Inventory of R. Brain Injury
r. modified radical mastectomy
neutral, sidebent right, rotated left
nonweightbearing, r.
r. nostril naris
r. oblique inguinal hernia
r. occipitoanterior position
r. occipitolateral fetal position
r. occipitoposterior position
r. occipitoposterior presentation
r. occipitotransverse fetal position
occiput right anterior
occiput right posterior
occlusion of right carotid artery
r. otitis externa
r. otitis media
r. otitis media, suppurative, acute
r. otitis media, suppurative, chronic
outer upper right quadrant
pain down right arm
r. parasternal impulse
patient's bill of r.'s
phacoemulsification of the right eye
pole of right kidney
r. portal vein
r. posterior internal carotid artery
r. posterior oblique radiologic view
r. posterior ventricular preexcitation
r. preejection period
prominence of right hilum
r. pulmonary artery withdrawal
r. pulmonary vein
r. radial artery
r. radical neck dissection
r. rectus femoris
r. to refuse intervention
r. renal artery
r. renal vein
r. rostral quarter ganglion
r. sacroanterior fetal position
r. sacrolateral fetal position
r. sacroposterior fetal position
r. sacrotransverse
r. sacrum
r. sacrum anterior
r. salpingo-oophorectomy
r. scapuloanterior
r. scapuloposterior
scleral buckle, right eye
r. septum
r. short leg brace
r. single lung transplant
r. somatosensory evoked potential
spontaneous right hemothorax
r. stellate ganglion
r. sternal border
r. sternal edge
r. subclavian
r. subclavian artery
r. subclavian central venous
r. subclavian vein
r. substantia nigra
r. superior intercostal vein
r. superior oblique muscle
r. superior oblique palsy
r. superior rectus muscle
r. superior vena cava
r. toe off
r. toe strike
total knee replacement, r.
r. triceps
r. uninjured
r. uninvolved
unpatched right eye
r. upper
upper r.
r. upper extremity
r. upper eyelid
r. upper lateral
upper lid right eye
r. upper limb
r. upper lobe
r. upper lung
r. upper medial
r. upper outer quadrant
r. upper pole
r. upper quadrant of abdomen
upper right quadrant
upper right sternal border
r. upper sternal border
r. ureteral orifice
r. vastus lateralis
vector cardiography electrode right midaxillary line
r. ventricle
r. ventricle anterior wall
r. ventricle of heart
r. ventricle infarction
r. ventricle internal dimension diastole
r. ventricle stroke output
r. ventricular
r. ventricular activation
r. ventricular apex
r. ventricular apical
r. ventricular assist device
ventricular atrial height right atrium
r. ventricular cardiomyopathy
r. ventricular copulsation balloon
r. ventricular diastolic overload
r. ventricular diastolic pressure
r. ventricular diastolic volume
r. ventricular dimension
r. ventricular ejection fraction
r. ventricular ejection time
r. ventricular end-diastolic diameter
r. ventricular end-diastolic pressure
r. ventricular end-diastolic volume
r. ventricular end-diastolic volume index
r. ventricular end-flow
r. ventricular endocardial potential
r. ventricular end-systolic volume
r. ventricular end-systolic volume index
r. ventricular enlargement
r. ventricular failure
r. ventricular filling pressure
r. ventricular function
r. ventricular heart failure
r. ventricular heave
r. ventricular hypertrophy
r. ventricular hypoplasia
r. ventricular inflow tract
r. ventricular initial diastolic pressure
r. ventricular internal dimension
r. ventricular mass
r. ventricular outflow
r. ventricular outflow tract
r. ventricular overactivity
r. ventricular peak filling rate
r. ventricular refractory period
r. ventricular stroke work index
r. ventricular systolic pressure
r. ventricular wall device
r. ventrogluteal
r. ventrolateral gluteal
r. vertebral artery
r. vertebral density
r. visceral ganglion
vision right eye
visual acuity, right eye
r. visual field
r. X chromosome

right-angle forceps

right-beating nystagmus

right-hand dominant

right-handed
r.-h. individual
r.-h. orthogonal coordinate system
patient r.-h.

righting
labyrinthine righting reflex
loss of righting reflex
optic labyrinthine r.
r. reflex

right-left
r.-l. discrimination
r.-l. disorientation

right/left discrimination

Right-Left Orientation Test

right-sided
r.-s. clonus
r.-s. congestive heart failure
r.-s. endocarditis
r.-s. heart failure
r.-s. lesion
r.-s. weakness

right-to-left shunt ratio

rigid
r. abdomen
r. bronchoscopy
r. cervical immobilization
chevron osteotomy with rigid screw fixation
r. clubfoot
r. collar
r. contact lens
r. flatfoot deformity
r. gait
r. gas-permeable contact lens
r. hymen
r. internal fixation
peptidoglycan rigid cell wall
r. rockerbottom

rigidity
r. and/or guarding
board-like rigidity of abdomen
coefficient of scleral r.
guarding and/or r.
multiple articular r.
progressive encephalomyelitis with rigidity and myoclonus
rebound guarding or r.

rigid-man syndrome

rigidus
hallux r.
hallux rigidus arthrodesis

rigor
calcium r.
frank r.'s
r. mortis

Riley
R. Articulation and Language Test
R. Inventory of Basic Learning Skills
R. Preschool Developmental Screening Inventory

Riley-Day syndrome

Riley-Shwachman syndrome

rim
acetabular r.
acetabular rim fracture
alar r.
alar rim excision
anterior helical rim free flap
Antia-Buch helical rim advancement flap
anular rim of cartilage
r. of cartilage
r. of fascia
helical r.
inferior orbital r.
intact outer r.
narrow rim of cytoplasm
nasal alar r.
nasal alar rim reconstruction
neural r.
neuroretinal r.
orbital inferior r.
orbital rim fracture

rimming
anal r.

Rincoe human action bionic

Rindfleisch cell

ring
r. abscess
adjustable ring gastroplasty
anterior limiting r.
apex of external r.
A ring of esophagus
r. block
r. of bone
Cabot ring body
carbon fiber half r.
cartilaginous ring incised
Caspar ring opacity
r. chromosome 1–22
closed reduction and percutaneous pin r.
r. constriction
contractile ring dysphagia
deep inguinal r.
r. enhancement
enhancing ring lesion
esophageal mucosal r.
esophageal muscular r.
external inguinal r.
fibrocartilaginous ring of tympanic membrane
r. finger
r. fracture
r. graft
greater ring of iris
implantable rings in eyes
internal abdominal r.
internal inguinal r.
intrastromal corneal ring segments
intravaginal r.
Japanese erection r.
left ring finger
light reflex r.
lower esophageal B r.
lower esophageal contraction r.
lower esophageal mucosal r.
lower esophageal r.
lymphatic ring of cardia
lymphatic ring of cardiac part of stomach
marginal ring ulcer of cornea
medial crus of the superficial inguinal r.
milk r.
milk ring test
Mose concentric r.'s
mucosal esophageal r.
multiple concentric GI r.'s
multiple concentric ring sign
multistate drug distribution r.
muscular esophageal r.
napkin ring calcar allograft
napkin ring compression
napkin ring defect
Ophthimus ring perimeter
orthosis drop-lock r.
paracentral ring scotoma
peripheral ring of hemoglobin
peripheral ring infiltrate
r. pessary
prosthetic ring anuloplasty
refractory anemia with ring sideroblasts
r. scotoma
segmented ring tripolar
sewing ring area
r. sideroblast
Silastic ring vertical-banded gastric bypass
silicone elastomer ring vertical gastroplasty
St. Jude annuloplasty r.
vertical ring gastroplasty
Waldeyer r.

Ringer
buffered Ringer solution
lactated Ringer solution
R. lactate solution

ringspot
tobacco ringspot virus

ringworm
nail r.
Oriental r.

Rinman sign

Rinne
R. hearing test
R. sign
R. test negative
R. test positive

Rio
R. Bravo virus
Del Rio Language Screening Test
R. Grande virus
mal de Rio Cuarto virus

Riolan
R. anastomosis
R. arc
R. arcade
R. arch
arch of R.
R. artery
R. bone
R. bouquet
R. muscle

ripe
r. cataract
r. cervix
r. ovum

ripening
cervical r.

rippling muscle disease

Risdon
R. approach
R. wire

rising
r. health care costs
r. heart rate

risk
absolute risk reduction
adolescent at r.
adolescents risk for violence
age, metastases, extent and size risk criteria
age-specific risk factor
alcohol-related risk for accident
alcohol-related risk for suicide
alcohol-related risk for violence
alloantigen-independent risk factor
r. of anesthesia
r. assessment
attitudinal risk factor
averse to r.
r.'s, benefits, and alternatives
Cardiac R. Index
cardiac risk factor
cardiac risk factor modification
cardiac risk reduction
cardiovascular risk factor
cardiovascular risk status
Clinical R. Index for Babies
clinical risk assessment
Composite R. Index
computerized risk assessment
controllable risk factor
coronary risk factor
damage risk criteria
decreased rebleeding r.
decreased risk of heart disease
direct suicide r.
Distress R. Assessment Method
Driver R. Inventory
ergonomic assessment of risk and liability
r. evaluation
r. of exposure
r. factor
r. factor for mortality
r. factor reduction
fairly good risk for anesthesia
fall risk assessment
family risk assessment program
r. of first heart attack
r. group for infection
haplotype relative r.
health risks from smoking
health risk appraisal
health risk assessment
health risk factor
heart attack r.
heart attack risk factor
r. of heart disease
heart disease, low r.
heart disease risk factor
heart risk assessment
high risk for breast cancer
high clotting r.
high degree of r.
highest risk for disease
high fracture r.
high genetic r.
high medical-social r.
high risk for breast cancer
high risk of HIV
high risk of HIV infection
high risk of suicide
Hospital Admission R. Profile
hypermobility as a risk factor
increased medical r.
increased risk of breast cancer
increased risk for illness
r. indicator
r. of infection
r. of infectious disease
lower risk of heart disease
r. management
maternal age-related r.
maternal health risk factor
maximal risk estimate
r. model
mortality risk factor
Multiple R. Factor Intervention Trial
neonatal/high risk
neonatal/medium risk
neonatal mortality r.
not at r.
Nursery Neurobiological R. Score
obstetric risk factor
occupational health r.
organs at r.
parents at r.
patient is a poor surgical r.
Pediatric Risk of Mortality Score
percutaneous exposure r.
platelet aggregation as a risk of diabetes
poor risk for anesthesia
positive cardiac disease risk factors
positive risk factors for cardiac disease
Pregnancy R. Monitoring System
Prematurity R. Evaluation Measure
pressure sore risk assessment
primary pulmonary hypertension risk factor
reduce risk of hospital-associated infection
r. reduction component
relative r.
relative risk cohort
relative risk reduction
r. rescue rating
Screening Instrument for Targeting Educational R.
serious health r.
Simple Calculated Osteoporosis R. Estimation
specified risk materials
r. stratification
suicide risk classification

suicide risk screen
youth risk behavioral survey

Risk-Adjusted Mortality Index

risk-benefit threshold

risk-screening model

risk-taking
r.-t., Attitude, Values Inventory
r.-t. behavior

Risley prism

ristocetin cofactor

ristocetin-induced platelet agglutination

Ritchie sedimentation

Rite
Atlanta-Scottish Rite abduction orthosis
Atlanta-Scottish Rite brace

Ritgen
R. maneuver
modified Ritgen maneuver

Ritter-Oleson technique

ritual
r. abuse
ADHD r.'s
detailed r.'s and routine
idiosyncratic obsessions and r.'s

ritualistic behavior

Riva-Rocci sphygmomanometer

river
Adelaide R. virus
r.'s cocktail
Haw R. syndrome
Ross R. fever
Shark R. virus
Virgin R. virus
Yangtze R. disease

Rivermead
R. Behavioral Memory Test
R. Mobility Index
R. motor assessment
R. Perceptual Assessment Battery

Riviere sign

Rivinus
R. canal
R. duct
R. gland
R. incisure

rna
antisense r.

RNA-binding motif

RNase
R. D, H
nonisotopic RNase cleavage assay
R. P

road
r. rash
r. traffic accident

roaming optical access multiscope

Robert Apperception Test for Children

Robertson
R. pupil

Robin
congenital thrombocytopenia, Robin sequence, agenesis of corpus callosum, distinctive facies, developmental delay syndrome

Robinow
R. dwarfism
R. syndrome

robustus
arthritis r.

Rocha-Lima inclusion

Rochambeau virus

Rochester Epidemiology Project

Roche, Wainer, and Thissen method of height prediction

Rocio virus

rock
pelvic r.

rockerbottom
r. flatfoot
r. flatfoot deformity
r. foot
rigid r.

rocket immunoelectrophoresis

rocking
head rolling, rocking and crying
mirror rocking test
paradoxical rocking impulse

Rockwell hardness number

Rocky-Davis incision

Rocky Mountain spotted fever vaccine

rod
aerobic gram-negative r.
aluminum master r.
anaerobic gram-negative r.
auto-reinforced polyglycolide r.
cluster of short gram-negative r.'s
compression rod treatment
r.'s and cones
darkly-staining gram-positive r.'s
r. disc membrane
r. fiber
flared spinal r.
fluted medullary r.
Gram-negative r.
Gram-negative rod and coccus
Gram-positive r.
Gram-positive rod and coccus
r. granule
Harrington r.
intramedullary rod fixation
Küntscher r.
lactose fermenting Gram-negative r.
long alignment r.
Maddox rod hyperphoria
Maddox rod method
Maddox rod occluder
Maddox rod test
microglial rod cell
modified Harrington r.
r. myopathy
nonlactose fermenting gram-negative r.
r. outer segment
peripheral rod function
Rush rod insertion
silicone rod implant
thermoluminescent dosimeter rod
r. vision

rod-and-frame test

rodent
enterocytopathogenic rodent orphan virus
r. thyroid-stimulating antibody

Rodgers antibody

Rodman
modified Rodman skin thickness score

Rodney Smith tubes

Rodrigues aneurysm

rod-shaped bacteria

Roeder
modified Roeder knot

roentgen
r. absorbed dose
r. administered dose
r. equivalent-physical
equivalent roentgen unit
gamma r.
intensity of roentgen ray
r. kymography
r. meter
r. per hour

roentgen *(continued)*
r. per hour at one meter
r. ray
roentgen-equivalent biologic
roentgen-equivalent-man
r.-e.-m. period
roentgenogram
chest r.
roentgenographically occult lung cancer
roentgenographic pelvimetry
roentgenography
chest r.
mass miniature r.
roentgenology
diagnostic r.
Roesler-Dressler infarction
roger
R. bruit
R. disease
maladie de r.
Rohrer index
Rohr stria
Rokeach Value Survey
Rokitansky
R. disease
R. hernia
Rokitansky-Aschoff sinus
Rokitansky-Kuster-Hauser syndrome
rolandic
r. artery
benign rolandic epilepsy
r. epilepsy
positive rolandic spike
r. region
Roland-Morris Questionnaire
Rolando
R. angle
R. area
R. cell
R. column
fissure of R.
R. gelatinous substance
role
alternating r.
altruistic r.
anticipation of r.
attacker r.
Bem Sex R. Inventory
contributing r.
r. exchange/education-practice
gender role definition
identity and role counseling
major role therapy
morality of conventional role conformity
Occupational R.'s Questionnaire
r. perception picture inventory
Personal Adjustment and R. Skills Scale
Personal and R. Skills
r. playing
Professional Sexual R. Inventory
sick role tendency
Rolf lance
roll
cotton r.
hip r.
log roll maneuver
narrow gauze r.
peripheral iris r.
Rolland-Desbuquois syndrome
Rollet
R. secondary substance
R. stroma
rolling
head r.
head rolling, rocking and crying
r. hernia
patient independent in boosting and r.
Romaña sign
Romano-Ward syndrome
Romberg
R. disease
R. sign
R. syndrome
R. test
Rommel cautery
rongeur
angled jaw r.
angled pituitary r.
angular bone r.
basket r.
bayonet r.
bone r.
curved bone r.
end-biting blunt nosed r.
ethmoidal r.
McIndoe bone r.
micropituitary r.
pediatric bone r.
R-on-T phenomenon
roof
orbital r.
room
r. air blood gas
blood gas at room temperature
capillary blood gas at room air
cardiovascular operating r.
cardiovascular recovery r.
emergency room computerized tomography
emergency room physician
emergency room triage documentation
exclusive operating r.
isocapnic hyperventilation with room air
laminar air flow r.
negative-pressure isolation r.
on-call to operating r.
r. temperature vulcanization
void on-call to operating r.
Roos test
root
r. abscess
ansa cervicalis r.
anterior r.
anterior nerve r.
anterior root of spinal nerve
r. of aorta
aortic root angiogram
aortic root cineangiography
aortic root diameter
aortic root dilatation
aortic root dimension
aortic root echocardiography
aortic root homograft
aortic root pressure
aortic root ratio
aortic root reconstruction
aortic root replacement
aortic root velocity waveform
apical portion of r.
apical root perforation
apical root resorption
arachnoidal root sleeve
arachnoid nerve root sheath dilation
r. avulsion injury
basal optic r.
bifurcation of r.
buccal r.
calciobiotic root canal sealer
r. canal filling
r. canal therapy
r. canal of tooth
r. caries
r. cause analysis
r. compression
conjoined nerve root anomaly

r. curettage
dilatation of aortic r.
distal r.
distobuccal r.
dorsal nerve r.
dorsal root, cervical
dorsal root dilator
dorsal root entry zone
dorsal root, lumbar
dorsal root potential
dorsal root reflex
dorsal root, sacral
dorsal root, thoracic
r. exit zone
extended aortic root replacement
external apical root resorption
first lumbar ventral nerve r.
r. fracture
r. of helix
r. hernia
incomplete vertical root fracture
r. injection
lingual r.
long root of ciliary ganglion
lower sacral nerve root compression
lumbar root disease
lumbosacral root lesion
r. of lung
May apple r.
r. mean square residue
mesiobuccal r.
motor root of ciliary ganglion
multiple cone root canal filling method
nerve root anomaly
nerve root compression
nerve root involvement
nerve root stimulation
nerve root syndrome
normalized mean square r.
oculomotor root of ciliary ganglion
peripheral nerve root syndrome
peripheral root compression
r. plane
r. planing and curettage
posterior r.
posterior root entry zone
scaling and root planing
second lumbar ventral nerve r.
selective nerve root block
ventral nerve r.
ventral root, lumbar
ventral root reflex
ventral root, thoracic

rooting reflex

root-mean-square
r.-m.-s. deviation
r.-m.-s. error

rope graft

ropy
breasts ropy or granular

roqueforti
Penicillium roqueforti toxin

Rorschach Inkblot Test

rosa
mal de la r.
Santa Rosa virus

rosacea
acne r.
facial r.
r. keratitis
ocular r.

rosae
Diplocarpon rosae virus

Rosai-Dorfman disease

rosary
rachitic r.

rose
attar of r.
r. bengal antigen
r. bengal dye
r. bengal scan
r. bengal staining
radioiodinated rose bengal dye
R. tamponade

rosea
atypical pityriasis r.
pityriasis r.

Rose-Bradford kidney

Rosenbach
R. sign
R. syndrome

Rosenberg Self-Esteem Scale

Rosenmüller
R. fossa
R. gland
R. node

Rosenthal
R. ascending vein
basal vein of R.
R. canal
R. fiber

Rosenthal-Melkersson syndrome

Rosenzweig Picture-Frustration Study

roseola
r. infantilis
r. infantum
syphilitic r.
r. typhosa

Roser-Braun sign

Rose-Thompson repair

rosette
erythrocyte rosette inhibitor
r. formation
r. of hemorrhoids
r. inhibition
r. inhibition titer
r. inhibitory factor
malarial r.
mucosal r.
rheumatoid r.
T-cell r.
vesicular r.

rosette-forming
r.-f. cell
direct antiglobulin r.-f.

Rose-Waaler test

Ross
R. carbohydrate free
R. cycle
R. River fever
R. River virus

Rossetti modification of Nissen fundoplication

Rossolimo reflex

Rostan shunt

rostellum
armed r.

rostral
r. basilar artery syndrome
r. direction
r. end
r. lamina
r. layer
left rostral quarter ganglion
right rostral quarter ganglion
r. sulcus
r. ventrolateral medulla

rostralis
nucleus cuneatus pars, r.

rostrum of corpus callosum

rotary
r. ankle instability
anterior rotary drawer test
anterolateral-anteromedial rotary instability
anterolateral rotary knee instability
anteromedial-posteromedial rotary instability
AO rotary prism

rotary *(continued)*
atlantoaxial rotary displacement
atlantoaxial rotary fixation
diamond rotary instrument
r. displacement
r. door flap
r. joint
Miltner rotary bone rasp
r. vertigo

rotated
abducted and externally r.
extended, rotated, sidebent
flexed, rotated, sidebent
neutral, sidebent right, rotated left

rotate fetal head

rotating
r. aspiration thromboembolectomy
automatic rotating tourniquet
counter rotating saw
r. delivery of excitation off resonance
r. hemostatic valve
molybdenum rotating anode x-ray tube
total rotating knee

rotation
abduction-external r.
active wrist rotation unit
adduction-internal rotation deformity
anterior innominate r.
arc of r.
arc of rotation of fasciocutaneous flap
axial rotation joint
r. axis
backward internal r.
center of r.
extended external r.
external rotation in extension
external rotation in flexion
external rotation/internal r.
fabere external rotation test
r. flap
flexion, abduction, external r.
flexion, abduction, external rotation contracture
flexion, abduction, external rotation, extension
flexion, extension, and r.
forced passive internal r.
glabellar rotation flap
head rotation to right
hip rotation test
internal r.
internal rotation contracture of hip
internal rotation in extension
internal rotation in flexion
lateral r.
left r.
r. left
lower trunk r.
medial hip r.
medial hip rotation in extension
medial rotation clubfoot
midforceps r.
Millard advancement rotation flap reconstruction
optical r.
pronation-eversion-external r.
pronation-external r.
pronation-lateral rotation fracture
r. and reduction of fracture
relative to rotation of a beam of polarized light
sagittal, frontal, transverse, r.
specific optical r.
supination external rotation
thoracolumbosacral orthosis—flexion, extension, lateral bending, and transverse r.

rotational
r. ablation
anisotropically rotational diffusion
anisotropically rotational diffusion imaging
anterolateral rotational instability
r. atherectomy system
r. axis
complex rotational movement
r. contracture
r. coronary atherectomy
coronary rotational atherectomy
r. deformity
r. deformity of finger
digital rotational angiography
r. dislocation
excimer laser, rotational atherectomy, and balloon angioplasty
r. flap
r. frequency
low-frequency head-only rotational testing
Mustardé rotational cheek flap
nonuniform rotational defect
r. nystagmus
percutaneous coronary rotational atherectomy
percutaneous rotational thrombectomy
percutaneous rotational transluminal coronary angioplasty
percutaneous transluminal coronary rotational ablation
percutaneous transluminal coronary rotational atherectomy
varus rotational osteotomy

rotation/internal
external rotation/internal rotation

rotator
r. cuff
r. cuff buttress
r. cuff calcific tendinitis
r. cuff impingement syndrome
r. cuff injury
r. cuff repair
r. cuff of shoulder
r. cuff tear
r. cuff tendon
r. cuff tendonitis
long external r.
long rotator muscle
lumbar rotator muscle
Neer acromioplasty for rotator cuff tear
Western Ontario R. Cuff

rotatory
anteromedial rotatory instability
atlantoaxial rotatory fixation
atlantoaxial rotatory subluxation
computer-driven rotatory chair
magnetic optical rotatory dispersion
r. nystagmus
optical rotatory dispersion
r. subluxation of scaphoid
r. vertigo

rotavirus
adult diarrhea r.
attenuated human r.
r. diarrhea
r. enteritis
r. gastroenteritis
human r.
nosocomial rotavirus infection
oral tetravalent rotavirus vaccine
Rhesus r.
r. vaccine

Rothera test

Rothmann-Makai syndrome

Rothmund syndrome

Rothmund-Thomson syndrome

Roth spot

Rotor syndrome

Rotter
R. Incomplete Sentences Blank
R. Sentence Completion Test

Rotterdam
Amsterdam R.
R. Symptom Check List

rotund abdomen

rouge
L'Homme r.
mal r.

rough
r. bacterial colony
r. endoplasmic reticulum
grade, rough, breathy, asthenic, strained
r. hard sphere
r., noncapsulated, avirulent bacterial culture

round
artery of round ligament of uterus
r. body
r. bur
r. eminence
r. and equal
r. facies
full-jacketed military r.
r. heart
r. heart disease
intact round window
r. ligament
malignant small round cell tumor
r. pupil intracapsular cataract extraction
pupil round and regular
pupils equal, round, reactive to light and accommodation
pupils equal, round, reactive to light and accommodation directly and consensually
r., regular, and equal
r., regular, and equal pupil
r., regular, react normally
small round structured virus
r. spermatid nuclear injection
r. window electrocochleography

round-cell
desmoplastic small round-cell tumor

rounded border of lung

Rous
Prague strain Rous sarcoma virus
R. sarcoma virus immunoglobulin intravenous
Schmidt-Ruppin strain Rous sarcoma virus

Rous-associated virus

Roussel
Hoechst Marion Roussel stain

Roussy-Lévy disease

route
r. of infection
nonpulmonary route of elimination
oral r.

Routier operation

routine
r. admission laboratory test
r. antenatal diagnostic imaging with ultrasound
appendectomy performed in routine fashion
cardiac ambulation r.
r. cholecystectomy
decline in ability to perform routine tasks
detailed rituals and r.
diabetic floor r.
r. dialysis therapy
r. fever therapy
r. followup
r. gynecological examination
head injury r.
r. health care
r. health management
r. home care
intermittent catheter r.
r. laboratory work done
r. medical care
r. and microscopic
not routine care
r. order
r. prophylaxis
r. respiratory care
r. test dilution
r. urinalysis
urinalysis, routine and microscopic
r. urine analysis

routing
bilateral contralateral routing of signals
contralateral routing of signals
focal contralateral routing of signals
front routing of signal
high-frequency contralateral routing of offside signals
ipsilateral frontal routing of signals

Rouviere
nodes of R.

Roux conditioned medium

Roux-en-Y
R.-e.-Y. anastomosis
R.-e.-Y. bypass
R.-e.-Y. gastrectomy

Roux-Goldthwait operation

roving
disconjugate roving eye movement

Rovsing sign

Rowden uterine manipulator-injector

rowing ergometer

Rowinski operation

Royal Farm virus

rub
alcohol r.
audible r.
bilateral pleural r.
centripetal r.
friction r.
murmurs, gallops, or r.'s
murmurs, r.'s, and gallops
pericardial friction r.
peritoneal friction r.
pleural friction r.
pleuritic r.

Rubarth disease virus

rubber
r. band hemorrhoidectomy
r. band ligation of hemorrhoid
r. band ligator
r. base impression
r. bolster
r. dam
natural rubber latex allergy
occupational rubber dermatitis
silicone r.
styrene-butadiene r.

rubber-reinforced bandage

rubbing
constant skin irritation and r.
habitual eye r.
r. heart sound

Rubbrecht operation

rubella
r. cataract
congenital r.
congenital rubella deafness
congenital rubella infection
congenital rubella syndrome
r. immunization

rubella *(continued)*
r. infection
measles, mumps, rubella immunization
measles, mumps, and rubella vaccine
measles and r.
measles and rubella vaccine
measles, rubella and zoster
progressive rubella panencephalitis
r. syndrome
syphilis, toxoplasmosis, other agents, rubella, cytomegalovirus, herpes simplex virus
r. titer
toxoplasmosis, other infections, rubella, cytomegalovirus infection, herpes simplex syndrome
r. vaccine
r. vaccine-like virus

rubeola scarlatinosa

ruber
lichen r.
lichen ruber acuminatus
lichen ruber moniliformis
lichen ruber planus
lichen ruber verrucosus

rubidium dihydrogenarsenate

Rubinstein-Taybi syndrome

Rubin test

rubor
dependent r.

rubra
lochia r.
miliaria r.
moderate rubra lochia
r. pityriasis
pityriasis rubra pilaris
polycythemia r.
polycythemia rubra vera
r. trichomycosis

rubrospinal tract

ruby
high-energy pulsed ruby laser
Q-switched ruby laser

Rucker-Gable Educational Programming Scale

Ruckland
tuberculin Ruckland new tuberculin

rudimentary disc space

Rud syndrome

ruff
papillary r.

Ruffini corpuscle

ruffling
membrane r.

rugal fold

rugby knee

Ruggeri reflex

Ruiz-Morgan procedure

rule
10% r.
analytic r.
Anstie r.
Arey r.
assimilation r.
astigmatism against the r.
astigmatism with the r.
r. bending
r. of evidence
Gibson r.
Hasse r.
His r.
r. in
Jackson r.
Liebermeister r.
Lossen r.
Luedde transparent r.
mental treatment r.'s
Mittendorf-Williams r.
modified Simpson r.
Nägele r.
New Hampshire r.
nines r.
r. of nines
Ogino-Knaus r.
only handle it once r.
Out r.
r. out
r. out appendicitis
r. out myocardial infarct
r. out myocardial infarction
Simpson r.
r. of thumb
Trauma Triage R.

ruled
carcinoma to be ruled out

rulemaking
notice of proposed r.

ruler
calibration r.

rumble
mid-diastolic r.

rumbling in abdomen

Rumel
R. technique
R. tourniquet

rumination
anxious r.
endless r.
guilty r.
manie de r.
obsessive r.
pessimistic r.
psychogenic r.
r. syndrome

rump
crown r.
head to rump length
r. heel length

Rumpel-Leede
R.-L. capillary fragility
R.-L. phenomenon

Rumpf sign

Rumple-Leede phenomenon

runaway
adolescent r.
halfway house for r.'s

Runeberg type

Runger test

runner's high

running
continuous running lock suture
continuous running monofilament suture
en bloc running locking suture
fracture running length of bone
Free R. Asthma Test
r. frequency and intensity
r. injury
r. total

runny
r. itchy nose
r. nose and eyes itchy

runoff
aortofemoral r.
aortogram with distal r.
arterial r.
digital r.
nuclear runoff assay
poor distal r.
pulse generated r.
venous r.

runs of slow activity

Runström projection

Runyon classification

rupture
aortic aneurysm r.

rupture
Achilles tendon r.
acute hepatic r.
adventitial r.
alveolar r.
annular radial r.
anterior talofibular ligament r.
aortic aneurysm r.
aortic arch r.
arterial dilatation and r.
arthrographic capsular distension and rupture technique
artificial membrane r.
artificial rupture of bag of waters
artificial rupture of membranes
atherosclerotic plaque r.
attrition rupture of tendon
r. of bag of waters
balloon r.
breast prosthesis r.
cardiac r.
chamber r.
collateral ligament r.
cruciate ligament r.
esophageal r.
flexor tendon r.
r. follicle
follicle aspiration, sperm injection, and assisted r.
r. of heart
r. of implant
interventricular septal r.
r. of intervertebral disc
intervertebral disc r.
liver r.
lumbar disc r.
marginal sinus r.
medial head of the gastrocnemius r.
r. of membranes
papillary muscle r.
prelabor rupture of the membranes
premature rupture of fetal membranes
premature spontaneous rupture of bag of waters
preterm premature rupture of membranes
preterm spontaneous rupture of membranes
prolonged premature rupture of membranes
prolonged rupture of fetal membranes
pulmonary artery r.
spleen r.
r. spontaneous
spontaneous premature rupture of membranes
spontaneous rupture of bag of waters
traumatic r.
traumatic rupture of the diaphragm
traumatic rupture of thoracic aorta
urinary bladder r.
uterine r.

ruptured
r. abdominal aortic aneurysm
r. Achilles tendon
r. aneurysm
r. appendix
artificially r.
bag of waters r.
r. Baker cyst
r. bladder
r. blood vessels
r. brain aneurysm
r. cuff
r. disc
r. eardrum
r. ectopic pregnancy
r. iliac aneurysm
r. interventricular septum
r. intervertebral disc
r. lumbar disc
r. membranes
prematurely ruptured membrane
r. sinus of Valsalva aneurysm
r. spleen
r. tympanic membrane
r. uterus

rupture-delivery interval

rural
health in underserved rural areas
r. general practitioner

rush
R. intramedullary nail
peristaltic r.
peristaltic r.
R. rod
R. rod insertion

Russe bone graft

Russell
R. body
R. brain disease
R. dwarf
Halstead Russell Neuropsychological Evaluation System
R. syndrome
R. viper

Russian
R. autumn encephalitis
R. autumn encephalitis virus
Eastern subtype Russian spring-summer encephalitis
R. influenza
R. spring-summer encephalitis
R. spring-summer encephalitis virus

rust
concentrated rust inhibitor

rusty sputum

ruthenium red

rutherford
r. ion backscattering
R. syndrome

Ruvalcaba-Myhre-Smith syndrome

ruyschiana
membrana r.

Ruysch membrane

R-wave
R-w. progression
R-w. threshold electrocardiography

rye
R. classification
r. whole-grain

Ryle tube

S-A
S.-A. arrest
S.-A. node
saber
s. shin
s. tibia
saber-shin deformity
Sabia virus
Sabin dye test
Sabin-Feldman dye test
sabot
coeur en s.
s. heart
Sabouraud agar
Saboya virus
sac
abnormal sac containing gas
alveolar s.
amniotic s.
aneurysmal s.
aortic s.
caudal s.
colostomy s.
double decidual s.
dural s.
empty gestational s.
endolymphatic s.
fluid-filled s.
fluid in heart s.
s. formation
gestational s.
gestational sac and maternal date
gestational sac size
giant prosthetic reinforcement of the visceral s.
high ligation of hernia s.
indirect hernial s.
intrauterine gestational s.
large inguinal hernia s.
lesser s.
mean gestational sac diameter
mean sac size
mean sac size and crown-rump length
mediastinal yolk sac tumor
pleural s.
polyp in lacrimal s.
scrotal s.
yolk s.
yolk sac carcinoma
saccade
corrective s.
gaze s.
memory guidance saccade test
ocular s.
scanning s.
saccadic
s. eye movement
s. pulse
saccharide
O-linked s.
sacciform kidney
saccular
s. aneurysm
s. duct
s. gland
sacculated
s. aneurysm
s. bladder
sacculation of colon
saccule
air s.
laryngeal s.
s. of larynx
maculae of utricle and s.
vestibular s.
sacculus, pl. **sacculi**
macula sacculi
Sachs-Georgi
S.-G. reaction
S.-G. test
Sacks Sentence Completion Test
sac-like gallbladder
sacra (*pl. of* sacrum)
sacral
s. ala
s. anesthesia
s. aneurysm
anterior ramus of sacral nerve
anterior sacral foramen
anterior sacral meningocele
s. approach
s. block
s. bone
s. bursa
s. canal
central sacral line
s. cornu
s. crest
s. cyst
s. decubitus ulcer
dorsal root, s.
s. dysgenesis
s. edema
first to fifth sacral nerves
first to fifth sacral vertebrae
s. flexure
s. foramen
s. fracture
s. ganglia
s. ganglion
s. hiatus
s. horizontal plane line
s. horn
s. index
s. insufficiency fracture
s. kyphosis
lower sacral nerve root compression
lumbar fifth vertebra to sacral first vertebra
s. lymph node
mental retardation, overgrowth, craniosynostosis, distal arthrogryposis, sacral dimple, joint laxity
middle sacral artery
s. nerve
s. nerve stimulation
s. plexus
s. prominence
s. promontory
s. reflexes
s. segment
s. tuberosity
s. vein
sacrales
nodi lymphoidei s.
sacralis
ansa s.
arteria sacralis lateralis
sacrifice
endovascular carotid s.
sacroanterior
left sacroanterior position
right sacroanterior fetal position
sacrococcygea
articulatio s.
sacrococcygeal
s. abscess
s. agenesis
anterior sacrococcygeal ligament
s. defect
s. disk
s. to inferior pubic point
s. joint
s. junction
sacrogenital fold
sacroiliac
anterior sacroiliac joint plate
anterior sacroiliac ligament
s. approach

sacroiliac *(continued)*
s. articulation
s. block
computed tomography-guided percutaneous radiofrequency denervation of the sacroiliac joint
s. disarticulation
s. dislocation
s. joint
s. orthosis
posterior sacroiliac spine
quantitative sacroiliac scintigraphy

sacroiliaca
articulatio s.

sacrolateral
right sacrolateral fetal position

sacrooccipital technique

sacroposterior
left sacroposterior fetal position
right sacroposterior fetal position

sacrosciatic
anterior sacrosciatic ligament
greater sacrosciatic notch

sacrospinous

sacrospinous ligament

sacrotransverse
left s.
right s.

sacrum, pl. **sacra**
ala of s.
apex of s.
assimilation s.
auricular surface of s.
left s.
s. posterior
s. to pubis
right s.
right sacrum anterior
spontaneous osteoporotic fracture of s.
s. transverse

saddle
s. block
s. block anesthesia
s. defect
s. deformity
s. embolus
s. nose
s. nose deformity
s. sensation

sadism
anal s.

sadism/masochism

sadistic behavior

sadness
increased s.

Saemisch
S. operation
S. section
S. ulcer

Saenger
S. macular
S. operation
S. reflex
S. sign

Saethre-Chotzen syndrome

safe
s. blood
s. and effective dosage
estimated safe and adequate daily dietary intake
Generally Recognized As S.
Generally Recognized as S. and Effective
S. Medical Device Act
permitting safe expression of anger
reasonably expected as s.
virtually safe dose

safety
bathroom safety device
s. belt
contract for s.
Diameter Index S. system
s. and efficiency
evaluate safety and stability at home
health and safety executive
Individual Case S. Reports
Integrated Summary of S.
s. lens
margin of s.
material safety data sheet
s., monitoring, intervention, length of stay, and evaluation
National Institute for Occupational S. and Health
occupational health and s.
periodic safety update reporting
s. technique goal

Safran Student's Interest Inventory

Sage rod

sagging
cracked mouth corners from sagging cheek

sagittal
anterior sagittal anorectoplasty
anterior sagittal diameter
anterior sagittal pelvic inlet
anterior-to-posterior sagittal canal diameter
s. area
s. axis
bilateral sagittal split ramus osteotomies
s. crest
s. depth of cornea
s. diameter
s., frontal, transverse, rotation
s. groove
inferior sagittal sinus
posterior sagittal diameter
posterior sagittal index
relative sagittal depth
s. sinus
s. sinus thrombosis
s. split advancement
s. split ramus osteotomy
s. split setback
superior sagittal sinus thrombosis
superior sagittal sinus velocity
vertical sagittal split osteotomy
s. view

Sagiyama virus

Sagnac ray

sago-grain stool

saimiri
herpesvirus s.

Saint
S. Anthony dance
S. Anthony fire
S. Ignatius itch

Saint-Floris virus

Sakhalin virus

salaam
s. activity
s. convulsion

Sala cell

Salamon-Conte Life Satisfaction in the Elderly Scale

Salanga virus

Salehabad virus

Sales
S. Attitude Check List
S. Personality Questionnaire

salicylamide, phenacetin, caffeine

salicylanilide

salicylate
lithium s.

physostigmine salicylate ophthalmic
s. poisoning
s. toxicity

salicylic
s. acid
s. and lactic acid paint

salicylsalicylic acid

Salience Inventory

salient symptom

Salinas
Punta Salinas virus

saline
adjustable saline breast implant
anterior chamber irrigated with s.
antibiotic and saline solution
area lavaged with sterile s.
balanced saline solution
buffered s.
buffered saline solution
catheter aspirated and flushed with s.
citrate-buffered s.
s. diuresis
s. and dopamine infusion
Dulbecco phosphate-buffered s.
s. enema
extraamniotic saline infusion
s. filled breast implant
s. flush
glucose in normal s.
glucose and s.
glycerine-buffered s.
Grey balanced saline solution
half-normal s.
half-strength s.
heparinized s.
hypertonic s.
imidazole-buffered s.
s. implant
s. infusion
s. infusion sonography
s. infusion sonohysterography
s. injection
intraamniotic saline infusion
invert sugar 10% in s.
10% invert sugar in 0.9% sodium chloride saline injection
irrigated with s.
s. lavage
leaky saline implant
normal s.
normal saline bolus
operative area irrigated with normal s.
operative site irrigated with normal s.
Page ameba s.
percutaneous aspiration, instillation of hypertonic saline, respiration
phosphate-buffered s.
phosphate, saline, glucose
physiologic saline solution
replacement normal s.
s. slush
s. soak
s. sodium citrate
s. solution
s. solution enema
standard saline citrate
sterile normal s.
sterile saline soak
tetradecyl sulfate, ethanol, and s.
triethanolamine-buffered s.
tris-buffered s.
tube-fed s.
Tween-TRIS-buffered saline solution
Veronal-buffered oxalated s.
wound irrigated with normal s.

saline-assisted polypectomy

saline-filled breast implant

Salinem
S. fever
S. infection

salinity
temperature, depth, and s.

saliva
artificial s.
ganglionic s.
oral transmission of s.
overproduction of s.
s. sample
s. substitute

salivary
acute salivary adenitis
s. calculus
s. colic
s. corpuscle
cribriform salivary carcinoma of excretory duct
s. duct
s. duct carcinoma
s. duct cyst
s. duct obstruction
s. epidermal growth factor
s. fistula
s. gland
s. gland anlage tumor
s. gland carcinoma
s. gland disease
s. gland enlargement
s. gland lymphocyte
s. gland pleomorphic adenoma
s. gland swelling
s. gland virus
s. gland virus disease
human immunodeficiency virus-associated salivary gland disease
labial salivary gland
s. and lacrimal secretion
major salivary gland
mixed tumor of salivary gland
mouse salivary gland virus
s. progesterone
s. scintiscan
sublabial salivary gland

salivation, lacrimation, urination, defecation, gastrointestinal distress and emesis

sallow skin

salmon
s. calcitonin
Coho salmon reovirus
S. sign

Salmonella
antimicrobial-resistant *Salmonella*
Salmonella illness
Salmonella infection
live-attenuated recombinant *Salmonella typhi*
non-typhi *Salmonella*
nontyphoidal *Salmonella* species
nontyphoid *Salmonella* bacteremia
oral attenuated *Salmonella typhi* vaccine
S. typhi

salmonella
nontyphoid s.
nontyphoidal salmonella infection

salmonellae

Salmonella-Shigella
Salmonella-Shigella agar

salmonellosis
nontyphoidal s.
nosocomial s.

salmon-poisoning disease

Salomon test

salpingectomy
bilateral partial s.
laparoscopic bilateral partial s.

salpingitis
s. after previous tubal occlusion
chronic interstitial s.
granulomatous s.
hemorrhagic s.

salpingitis *(continued)*
hypertrophic s.
nongranulomatous s.
s. in previously occluded tubes

salpingolysis
salpingo-ovarian s.

salpingo-oophorectomy
bilateral s.-o.
left s.-o.
radical hysterectomy and bilateral s.-o.
right s.-o.
total abdominal hysterectomy and bilateral s.-o.
unilateral s.-o.

salpingo-ovarian salpingolysis

salpingopharyngea
plica s.

salpingostomy
linear s.

Salpix contrast medium

salt
s. added
artificial vichy s.
balanced salt solution
bile s.
bile salt concentrate
bile salt concentration
bile salt export pump
bile salt metabolism
bile salt output
s. cedar
cerebral salt wasting
conjugated bile s.'s
s. craving
s. depletion
s. depletion syndrome
diminished salt intake
Earle balanced salt solution
fast red B s.
s. free
gelatin Hanks buffered salt solution
gold salt therapy
Hanks balanced salt solution
Hanks balanced salt solution plus glucose
s. intake
limit salt intake
s. loser
low s.
mannitol salt agar
mineral s.'s medium
modified Hanks balanced salt solution
no added s.
oral rehydration s.
physiologic salt solution
reduce salt intake
reduction of salt intake
s. resistant
Seligmann buffered salt solution
universal salt iodization
s. wasting
s. and water imbalance
s. water implant

saltatory tic

salt-dependent agglutinin

Salter
S. fracture
S. osteotomy

Salter-Harris
S.-H. classification
S.-H. classification of fracture

salt-losing adrenogenital syndrome

salt-poor albumin

salt-wasting
s.-w. congenital adrenal hyperplasia
s.-w. crisis

Salus arch

salute
allergic s.

salvage
s. angioplasty
autologous red cell s.
cell s.
s. chemotherapy
s. cystectomy
s. highly active antiretroviral therapy
intraoperative s.
limb s.
Predictive S. Index
severed limb salvage technique
s. technique
s. therapy

salvarsan throat irrigation tube

Sal Vieja virus

Salzmann nodular corneal dystrophy

Samaritan
Good Samaritan Act

same
cold to the opposite, warm to the s.
continue same treatment
s. day admission

same-day microsurgical arthroscopic lateral-approach laser-assisted

sample
arterial blood s.
cord blood s.
s. correlation coefficient
discrete time s.
drawing of blood s.
fingerstick blood s.
s. and hold
Life Study S.
Linguistic Analysis of Speech S.'s
s. mean
midstream urine s.
multiple automated sample harvester
no s.
peritoneal cytology s.
population s.
random s.
representative sample sectioned
saliva s.
s. size
sound production s.
s. standard deviation
s. variance
venous blood s.
verbal sample evaluation method

sampler
Anderson s.
sequential impaction cascade sieve volumetric air s.

sampling
adrenal venous s.
arterial gas s.
asymmetric data s.
cavernous sinus s.
chorionic villus s.
continuous interleaved s.
fetal scalp s.
inferior petrosal sinus s.
Language S. Analysis
limited sampling model
lymph node s.
optimal sampling theory
paraaortic node s.
pelvic node s.
percutaneous fetal tissue s.
percutaneous umbilical blood s.
periaortic node s.
portal venous s.
primary sampling unit

Sampson cyst

San
S. Angelo virus
S. Joaquin Valley disease
S. Juan virus
Maestre de San Juan-Kallmann-de Morsier syndrome
mal de San Lazaro
S. Miguel sea lion virus
S. Perlita virus

Sanarelli-Shwartzman phenomenon

Sanchez-Cascos cardioauditory syndrome

sandbag placed for support

Sanders bed

Sanders-Retzlaff-Kraff formula

sandfly
s. fever
s. fever Naples virus
s. fever Sicilian virus

Sandhoff disease

Sandjimba virus

sandwich
alloplastic sandwich augmentation
anterior sandwich patch technique
s. counterelectrophoresis

Sanfilippo
mucopolysaccharidosis type III Sanfilippo A, B, C
S. syndrome

Sanger-Brown syndrome

Sango virus

sanguinareus
mycetism s.

sanguineous
s. cyst
s. exudate

sanguineus
nevus s.

sanguis
Streptococcus s.

sanitary
s. engineering
s. napkin

Sansom sign

Santarem virus

Santa Rosa virus

Santavuori
muscle-eye-brain disease of S.

Santorini
S. canal
S. cartilage
cartilage of S.
circular Santorini muscles
S. concha
S. duct
S. fissure
fissure of S.
S. incisure
S. labyrinth
S. major caruncle
plexus of S.
S. plexus

São
S. Paulo fever
S. Paulo typhus

saphenofemoral bypass

saphenous
s. artery
s. flap
greater saphenous phlebectomy
greater saphenous vein
greater saphenous vein cutdown
high saphenous vein ligation
long saphenous nerve
long saphenous vein
medial crural cutaneous branch of saphenous nerve
s. nerve
reversed saphenous vein graft
temperature in saphenous vein
s. vein
s. vein bypass
s. vein bypass graft
s. vein graft
s. vein graft de novo
s. vein graft stenosis

saponification
index of s.

sapophore group

Sappey
S. fiber
S. vein

Saraca virus

Sarbo sign

sarcasm
displays extreme s.

sarcofetal pregnancy

sarcoid
granuloma s.
s. granuloma
miliary s.
morpheaform s.
Spiegler-Fendt s.

sarcoidosis
alveolar s.
cardiac sarcoidosis myocarditis
noncured s.
ocular s.
pediatric ocular s.
resolved s.
stable s.
thyroiditis, Addison disease, Sjögren syndrome, sarcoidosis syndrome

sarcolemma lipid

sarcoma
acquired immunodeficiency syndrome with Kaposi s.
African cutaneous Kaposi s.
African lymphadenopathic Kaposi s.
AIDS-related Kaposi s.
alveolar soft part s.
appendiceal Kaposi s.
avian sarcoma and leukosis virus
biphasic synovial s.
s., breast and brain tumors, leukemia, laryngeal and lung cancer adenoma
clear cell sarcoma of the kidney
clear cell sarcoma of the liver
embryonal s.
endometrial stromal s.
epithelioid s.
Ewing sarcoma family of tumors
extraosseous Ewing s.
Gross sarcoma virus antigen
s. growth factor
Harvey murine sarcoma virus
human herpesvirus 8/Kaposi sarcoma herpesvirus
human osteogenic s.
interdigitating dendritic cell s.
Kaposi s.
Kaposi sarcoma herpesvirus
Kaposi sarcoma human growth factor
Kaposi sarcoma and opportunistic infection
low-grade central osteogenic s.
low-grade fibromyxoid s.
lymphosarcoma-reticulum cell s.
Maloney murine s.
mast cell s.
McDonough feline sarcoma virus
Mediterranean Kaposi s.
meningeal s.
metastatic s.
methylcholanthrene-induced s.
mixed cell s.
mixed müllerian s.
mixed ovarian mesodermal s.
Moloney murine sarcoma virus

sarcoma *(continued)*
monophasic synovial s.
multifocal hemorrhagic s.
multiple idiopathic hemorrhagic s.
myeloid s.
myeloproliferative sarcoma virus
nonrhabdomyosarcoma soft tissue s.
obesity in endometrial s.
orbital granulocytic s.
osteogenic s.
periosteal s.
Prague strain Rous sarcoma virus
primary bone s.
prostate gland s.
pulmonary intimal s.
pulmonary Kaposi s.
radiation-induced sarcoma of the head and neck
recovered avian sarcoma virus
Rous sarcoma virus immunoglobulin intravenous
Schmidt-Ruppin strain Rous sarcoma virus
simian sarcoma virus
small cell s.
soft tissue s.
spindle cell s.
undifferentiated embryonal s.
vasoablative endothelial s.
s. virus
Yoshida s.

sarcoma-like mural nodule

sarcoma/peripheral
Ewing sarcoma/peripheral neuroectodermal tumor

sarcoma-primitive

sarcomatoid
s. renal cell carcinoma
s. thymic carcinoma

sarcomatosum
glioma s.
lipoma s.
myxoma s.

sarcomatous
adenocarcinoma of the uterus with sarcomatous overgrowth

sarcomere
region of sarcomere containing only myosin filaments

sarcoplasmic
fragmented sarcoplasmic reticulum
s. reticulum

sarcosporidian cyst

sarcotubular system

sarcous substance

Sarns membrane oxygenator

sartorius
s. bursa
s. flap

SAT1
Aphthovirus S.

SAT2
Aphthovirus S.

SAT3
Aphthovirus S.

satellite
s. abscess
s. cell
chromosomal s.
s. chromosome
s. clinic
erythematous satellite lesion
s. lesion
s. tobacco necrosis virus

Sathuperi virus

satisfaction
College Student S. Questionnaire
Global Sexual S. Index
Index of Work S.
life s.
Life Satisfaction Index A, B
Marital S. Scale
Minnesota S. Scale
Multidimensional Student Life S. Scale
patient satisfaction questionnaire
Salamon-Conte Life S. in the Elderly Scale

satisfactorily
bowel fills and evacuates s.

satisfactory
s. condition
following satisfactory general anesthesia
s. postanesthesia course
under satisfactory general anesthesia
s. wound healing

sativa
cannabis s.

sativum
Pisum sativum agglutinin

Sattler veil

saturated
s. base excess
s. calomel electrode
cholesterol saturated fat index
end of saturated bombardment
s. fat
s. fat intake
s. fatty acid
s. for intake
low saturated fat
s. phosphatidylcholine
potassium iodide, saturated solution
s. potassium iodide solution
s. solution of potassium iodide

saturating
single saturating dose

saturation
s. analysis
aortic oxygen s.
arterial oxygen s.
arterial oxyhemoglobin s.
cholesterol saturation index
fetal arterial oxygen s.
frequency-selective s.
s. of hemoglobin
s. index
s. inversion projection
iron saturation level
iron saturation of serum transferrin
jugular venous oxygen s.
left pulmonary artery oxygen s.
low oxyhemoglobin s.
mixed venous oxygen s.
O2 saturation level
O2 saturation on three liters nasal cannula
O2 saturation on two liters nasal cannula
s. of oxygen in arterial blood
oxygen saturation on 2 liters nasal cannula
oxygen saturation on 3 liters nasal cannula
oxygen saturation as measured using pulse oximetry
oxygen saturation index
oxygen saturation level
oxygen saturation meter
partial saturation spin echo
s. recovery
regional oxygen s.
s. sound pressure level

saturnina
arthralgia s.

saturnine
arthralgia s.
s. colic
s. encephalopathy
s. gout

satyri
apex s.

sauce
apple sauce appearance

Sauerbruch prosthesis

Saumarez Reef virus

sausage
s. digit
s. finger

Sauvineau ophthalmoplegia

Savage syndrome

Savary bougie

saved
marginal cost per year of life s.
quality-adjusted life-year s.

Saver disease

saw
air-driven oscillating s.
bayonet s.
counter rotating s.
crosscut s.
electric cast s.
end-cutting reciprocating s.
fine-tooth electric s.
Oto-Flex crura s.
s. palmetto berry extract

sawgrass virus

sawtooth
s. appearance
s. configuration

Saxtorph maneuver

Sayre head sling

scabbard trachea

scabetic infection

scabies
animal s.
canine s.
s. mite
nodular s.
Norwegian s.

scaffold-associated regions

scala
Löwenberg s.
s. tympani

scalar
sequential scalar quantization
wavelet scalar quantization

scalded
s. mouth syndrome
s. skin syndrome
staphylococcal scalded skin syndrome

Scale-2
Behavior Evaluation S.

scale
Abbreviated Conners Teacher Rating S.
Abbreviated Injury S.
absolute temperature on the Rankine s.
absorbance units, full s.
Academic Readiness S.
Ackerman-Schoendorf S.'s for Parent Evaluation of Custody
acquiescent response s.
activities of daily living s.
Activities-Specific Balance Confidence S.
Adaptive Behavior Evaluation S.
Adolescent and Pediatric Pain Tool S.
Adult Self-Expression S.
Affect Balance S.
Alberta Infant Motor S.
Albert Einstein Neonatal Developmental S.
alcohol abuse s.
Alcohol Dependence S.
Alzheimer Disease Assessment S.
Alzheimer Disease Assessment Scale, cognitive subscale
Alzheimer Disease Rating S.
Amphetamine Interview Rating S.
Anger Expression S.
Anxiety S.'s for Children and Adults
S. of Anxiety and Depression
anxiety rating s.
anxiety scale questionnaire
Aphasia Language Performance S.
Arizona Articulation Proficiency S.
Arthritis Impact Measurement S.
Arthritis Quality of Life S.
Arthur Adaptation of the Leiter International Performance S.
ASIA impairment scale for classification of spinal cord injury
Assessment in Infancy Ordinal S.'s of Psychological Development
S. for the Assessment of Negative Symptoms
S. for the Assessment of Positive Symptoms
S. for the Assessment of Unawareness of Mental Disorder
Attention Deficit Disorder Behavior Rating S.
Attitudes Toward Mainstreaming S.
attrition rate s.
Balthazar S.'s of Adaptive Behavior
Barnes Akathisia S.
Barron-Welsh Art S.
Baumé s.
Bayley Scales of Infant Development-II
Beck Hopelessness S.
bedside s.
Behavioral Assessment S. for Children
Behavioral Dyscontrol S.
Behavioral and Emotional Rating S.
Behavior Disorders Identification S.
Behavior Rating S.
bench scale calorimeter
Benoist s.
Blessed Dementia Rating S.
Blessed-Roth Dementia S.
Body Dysmorphic Disorder Modification of Yale-Brown Obsessive-Compulsive S., McLean version
Brazelton Neonatal Behavioral Assessment S.
Brief Cognitive Rating S.
Brief Psychiatric Rating Scale for Children
Brief Social Phobia S.
Bristol Language Development S.
British Ability S.
Burks Behavior Rating S.
California Infant S. for Motor Development
California Preschool Social Competency S.
Canadian Acute Respiratory Illness and Flu S.
cardiac adjustment s.
Cattell Infant Intelligence S.
Cattell Infant S. Inventory
Celsius temperature s.
Centers for Epidemiologic Studies Depression s.
centigrade temperature s.
Child and Adolescent Functional Assessment S.
Childhood Autism Rating S.
Childhood Myositis Assessment S.

scale *(continued)*
Child Personality S.
Children's Affective Rating S.
Children's Depression S.
Children's Global Assessment S.
Children's Manifest Anxiety S.
Children's Psychiatric Rating S.
Children's Self-Concept S.
Children's Yale-Brown Obsessive Compulsive S.
Classroom Environmental S.
Claude Mood S.
Clinical Adaptive Test/Clinical Linguistic and Auditory Milestone S.
Clinical Global Impression-Severity of Illness S.
Clinical Linguistic and Auditory Milestone S.
Clinical Rating S.
Clinician Rated Anxiety S.
Clinician's Global Rating S.
Clyde Mood S.
S.'s of Cognitive Ability for Traumatic Brain Injury
College and University Environment S.'s
Colored Visual Analogue S.
Columbia Mental Maturity S.
Community-Oriented Programs Environment S.
Comprehensive Career Assessment S.
Comprehensive Level of Consciousness S.
Comprehensive Psychopathological Rating S.
Comrey Personality S.
Concept-Specific Anxiety S.
Conflict in Marriage S.
Conners Teacher Rating S.
Cooper-Farran Behavioral Rating S.
Cornell S. for Depression, Dementia
Correctional Institutions Environment S.
S.'s of Creativity and Learning Environment
Cultural Attitude S.
Current and Past Psychopathology S.'s
death anxiety s.
decimal scale of potency or dilution
Defensive Functioning S.
Dementia Mood Assessment S.
Derogatis Affects Balance S.
Devereux Elementary School Behavior Rating Scale II
Disability Rating S.
Disability Status S.
disease disability s.
Distress S. for Ventilated Newborn Infants
Dyskinesia Rating S.
Early Language Milestone S.
Early Neonatal Neurobehavior S.
Early Social Communication S.
Edinburgh 2 Coma S.
Edinburgh Postnatal Depression S.
Edinburgh Rehabilitation Status S.
Edmonton Symptom Assessment S.
Ego Development S.
Einstein Neonatal Neurobehavioral Assessment S.
Emotional and Behavior Problem S.
S. for Emotional Blunting
Emotionality Activity Sociability S.
Endler Multidimensional Anxiety S.
Epworth Sleepiness S.
Equal Listener Response scale
European Stroke S.
Expanded Disability Status Scale
extrapyramidal symptom rating s.
Facial Impairment S.'s for Children
Fahrenheit temperature s.
Fairview Language Evaluation S.
Falls Efficacy S.
Family Adaptability and Cohesion Evaluation S.
Family Drawing Depression S.
Family Environment S.
Family Therapist Behavioral S.
Flint Colon Injury S.
Flint Infant Security S.
foot and ankle severity s.
French s.
frequency of contact s.
Functional Impairment S. for Children and Adolescents
Functional Life S.
Gait Abnormality Rating S. Modified
Gastrointestinal Symptom Rating S.
General Audit Inpatient Psychiatric Assessment S.
Generalized Contentment S.
Geriatric Depression S.
Gesell Child Development Age S.
Gifted Evaluation S.
Glasgow Coma S.
Glasgow Outcome S.
Global Deterioration S.
Global Obsessive-Compulsive S.
global ward behavior s.
Goal Attainment S.
Goldberg Anorectic Attitude S.
Graphic Rating S.
Griffiths Mental Developmental S.
Group Encounter S.
Group Environment S.
hallux metatarsophalangeal interphalangeal s.
Hamburg Rating S. for Psychiatric Disorders
Hamilton Anxiety Rating S.
Hamilton Depression Rating S.
Hamilton Rating S. for Depression
Haptic Intelligence S.
Harvard Group Scale of Hypnotic Susceptibility, Form A
Health Behavior S.
Health Intention S.
Health-Sickness Rating S.
Hearing Handicap S.
Hess School Readiness S.
Heterosexual Attitudes Toward Homosexuality s.
heterosexual relations scale
Himmelsbach Rating S.
HIV Dementia S.
Home Incapacity S.
homeopathic symbol for decimal scale of potencies
Homes-Rahe S.
Hopelessness S.
Hospital Anxiety and Depression S.
House-Brackmann Grading S.
How I See Myself Scale
hypochondriasis s.
illness attitude s.
Impact of Events S.
Individual Self-Rating S.
Infant/Toddler Environment Rating S.
Infant/Toddler Environment Rating S.
Injury Severity S.
Inpatient Behavior Rating S.

Inpatient Multidimensional Psychiatric S.
Interpersonal Perception S.
It Scale for Children
Job Attitude S.
Karnofsky rating s.
Kaufman Development S.
Kent Infant Development S.
Kurtzke Disability Status S.
Learning Disability Evaluation S.
Leiter International Performance S.
Level of Rehabilitation S. 1
Likert s.
linear analog pain s.
linear visual analog s.
Liverpool Seizure Severity S.
Living Conditions Rating S.
Livingston insomnia s.
Locus of Control S.
London Psychogeriatric S.
Lovett clinical scale of strength
Lower Extremity Functional S.
Lund-Browder burn s.
Lung Cancer Symptom S.
MacAndrew Addiction S.
Management Philosophies Scale I-V
Manchester and Oxford Universities S. for the Psychopathological Assessment of Dementia
Mandel Social Adjustment S.
mania rating s.
Manifest Anxiety S.
Mankin histologic/histochemical s.
Marcus grading scale for avascular necrosis
Marital Satisfaction S.
Marlowe-Crown Social Desirability S.
Maryland coma s.
Maternal Attitude S.
Mattis Dementia Rating S.
McAndrews Alcoholism S.
McCarthy Memory S.
mean scale value
Mecham Verbal Language S.
Memorial Delirium Assessment S.
Memorial University of Newfoundland S. of Happiness
Memory Assessment S.
Mental Adjustment to Cancer s.
Merle d'Aubigné and Postel hip rating s.
Merrill-Palmer S. of Mental Tests
Migraine Disability Assessment S.
Miller Behavioral Style S.
Minnesota Cocaine Craving S.
Minnesota Multiphasic Personality Inventory Depression Scale
Minnesota Satisfaction S.
modified Gait Abnormality Rating S.
Mohs hardness s.
Montgomery-Asberg Depression Rating S.
Mood and Physical Symptoms S.
Morphine-Benzedrine Group S.
Motor Assessment S.
Mullen S.'s of Early Learning
Multidimensional S. of Perceived Social Support
Multidimensional Self Concept S.
Multidimensional Student Life Satisfaction S.
narcotic withdrawal s.
National Institute of Mental Health-Global Obsessive Compulsive S.
Naylor-Harwood Adult Intelligence S.
Neonatal Behavioral Assessment S.
Neonatal Behavioral Assessment S. with Kansas Supplements
Neonatal Infant Pain S.
Neurobehavioral Rating S.
neuropsychiatric acquired immunodeficiency syndrome rating s.
Neurosurgical Cervical Spine S.
Neuroticism S. Questionnaire
Newborn Behavior Assessment S.
NIMH global s.
Numeric Pain Intensity S.
numeric rating s.
Nurses' Observation S. for Inpatient Evaluation
Nursing-Care Dependency scale
Object Sorting S.'s psychologic test
Obsessive-Compulsive Drinking S.
Obsessive-Compulsive Neurosis S.
Odorant Confusion Matrix s.
Optimism-Pessimism Scale, revised
Oral Analogue S.
Orpington prognostic s.
overcontrolled hostility s.
Overt Aggression S.
Overt Agitation Severity S.
Pain Anxiety Symptoms S.
pain catastrophizing s.
Pain Observation S. for Young Children
pain on a scale from 1 to 10
Parental Stressor S.: Neonatal Intensive Care Unit
parent anxiety rating s.
Parent Attitude S.
parent's rating s.
Parkinson Disease Quality of Life S.
patient evaluation rating s.
Patient Rated Anxiety S.
Patterns of Individual Change S.
Peabody Developmental Motor S.
Pediatric Behavior S.
Pediatric Liver Transplant-Specific S.
Pediatric Overall Performance Category s.
Pediatric Trauma S.
Perception of Ability S. for Students
performance status scale for head and neck cancer
performing scale
Personal Adjustment and Role Skills S.
Personality Rating S.
Personal Preference S.
Phelps Kindergarten Readiness S.
Philadelphia Geriatric Center Morale S.
Physical Self Maintenance S.
58-point Scandinavian Stroke S.
Positive and Negative Stroke S.
Positive and Negative Syndrome S.
Positive Well-being scale
Postural Assessment S. for Stroke Patients
Pre-Reading Expectancy Screening S.
Preschool Language S.
Pressure Ulcer S. for Healing
Process Skills Rating S.
Progressive Deterioration S.
psoriasis severity s.
Psychiatric Status Rating s.
Psychological General Well-Being S.
s. of psychosis
Psychosocial Adjustment to Illness S.
pupil rating s.
Quality of Life S.

scale *(continued)*
Quality of Well-Being S. Self-Administered
Rankine scale
Rating S. of Communication in Cognitive Decline
Reaction Level S.
Receptive-Expressive Observation Scale
Rehabilitation Client Rating S.
relative value s.
Repression-Sensitization Scale
resource-based relative value s.
Responsibility and Independence S. for Adolescents
Revised Children's Depression S.
Revised Children's Manifest Anxiety S.
Reynell Development Language S.'s
Reynolds Adolescent Depression S.
Reynolds Child Depression S.
Rhode Island Pupil Identification S.
Rosenberg Self-Esteem S.
Rucker-Gable Educational Programming S.
Salamon-Conte Life Satisfaction in the Elderly S.
School Handicap Condition S.
Self-Assessment Depression S.
Self-Control S.
self-directed learning readiness s.
Self-Evaluation of Life Function s.
Self-Rating Depression S.
sensation-seeking s.
sexual differentiation s.
Sexual Myths S.
Sheehan Patient Rated Anxiety S.
Shipley-Hartford S.
Shipley Institute of Living S.
Shipman Anxiety Depression S.
Short Clinical Rating S.
simple descriptive s.
Situational Attitude S.
Sklar Aphasia S.
sliding fee s.
sliding scale insulin
sliding scale insulin therapy
Social Adaptation Self-Evaluation S.
Social Adjustment Self-Report S.
Social Climate S.
Social Readjustment Rating S.
Specific Activity S.
Spiritual Well-Being S.
staff burnout s.
Stanford-Binet Intelligence S.
Stanford Hypnotic Susceptibility S.
Stanford Sleepiness S.
State-Trait Anger S.
Stress Impact S.
Stroke Impact S.
Subjective Units of Distress S.
Suinn Test Anxiety Behavior S.
Symptom Distress S.
Symptom Rating S.
Tale-Brown Obsessive-Compulsive S.
Tanner Developmental S.
Taylor Manifest Anxiety S.
Teacher Evaluation S.
Tennessee Self-Concept S.
The Instructional Environment S.
Toddler-Preschooler Postoperative Pain S.
Toronto Alexithymia S.
Toronto Western Spasmodic Torticollis Rating S.
Transition Behavior S.
Treatment Emergent Symptom S.
Treatment Outcome PTSD s.
trial assessment procedure s.
tridimensional evaluation s.
Unified Parkinson Disease Rating S.
University Residence Environment S.
Vane Evaluation of Language S.
Verbal Language Development S.
Verdun Depression Rating S.
Verdun Target Symptom Rating S.
very large scale integration
Veteran's Adjustment S.
Vineland Social Maturity S.
viral analog s.
Visual Analogue Mood S.
Visual Analogue Self Assessment S.'s For Pain Intensity
Vocabulary Comprehension S.
Ward Atmosphere S.
Ward Behavior Rating S.
Ward Incapacity S.
Ward Initiation S.
Wechsler-Bellevue S.
Wechsler Intelligence S.
Wechsler Memory S.
Wechsler Preschool and Primary S. of Intelligence
Wender Utah Rating S.
Wittenborn Psychiatric Rating S.
Yale-Brown Obsessive-Compulsive S.
Yale Global Tic Severity S.
Young Mania Rating S.
Zimmerman Preschool Language S.
Zung Self-Rating Depression S.

Scaled
S. Curriculum Achievement Levels Test
Structured and Scaled Interview to Assess Maladjustment

scalene
s. adenopathy
anterior scalene muscle
s. fat pad biopsy
s. hiatus
s. lymph node biopsy
s. muscle
s. muscle, anterior, posterior, middle
s. node
s. node biopsy

scalenus
s. anterior muscle
anterior scalenus muscle
s. anticus syndrome

Scale-Physical
Memorial Symptom Assessment S.-P.

Scale-Psychological
Memorial Symptom Assessment S.-P.

scaler
anterior s.

Scale-Revised
Children's Depression Rating S.-R.

scaling
age-grade s.
s. device
electrosurgical s.
goal attainment s.
heavy scaling of skin
keratotic s.
multidimensional s.
Organ Injury S.
s. and root planing

scall
milk s.

scalloped
s. appearance
s. appearance of white matter
s. border
s. pupil

scalloping
anterior s.
anterior scalloping of vertebra
peripheral s.

Scalogram
Multidimensional Scalogram Analysis

scalp
s. abrasion
anterior port scalp excision
axial pattern scalp flap
s. closure
coarse scalp hair
s. contusion
dermatophyte infection of s.
s. electrocardiogram
s. electroencephalogram
electron beam scalp irradiation
expanded free scalp flap
fetal scalp blood
fetal scalp electrode
fetal scalp sampling
s. flap
s. folliculitis
hematoma of s.
s. hematoma
s. infection
internal fetal scalp electrode
s. laceration
s. louse

scalpel
#11 bayonet-handled s.
s. biopsy
harmonic s.

scalping
postauricular and retroauricular s.

scalp-sphenoidal electroencephalography

scaly
blister red, scaly, and itchy

scan
abdominal CT s.
adenosine thallium s.
aerosol ventilation s.
amniotic fluid s.
ATL real-time Neurosector scan imaging
attenuation coefficient on MRI s.
attenuation value on MRI s.
axial unenhanced CT s.
bone scan reveals increased activity
bone scan showed increased activity
cardiac nuclear probe s.
carotid duplex s.
color Doppler s.
color-flow duplex s.
computed tomographic s.
computed tomography brain s.
computed topographic s.
computerized axial tomography s.
coronary artery s.
cranial sector s.
dual-energy x-ray absorptiometry scan
duplex Doppler s.
enhanced CT s.
esophageal transit s.
fluorescence-activated cell sorter s.
full scan with interpolation projection
gallbladder and liver s.
gallium citrate s.
gastric emptying s.
heel bone density s.
high-resolution computed tomography s.
high-resolution CT s.
incomplete resolution, scan to follow
indium-labeled leukocyte s.
injection scan interval
s. interpretation
iodine-131 total body s.
isotope bone s.
limited gallium s.
linear profile s.
liver s.
low-dose CT s.
mechanical compound s.
methydiphosphonate bone s.
monoclonal antibody scintigraphic s.
multiplanar computed tomography s.
multiplanar CT s.
multiple gated acquisition s.
multiple line s.
multiple scan average dose
myocardial isotopic perfusion s.
negative bone s.
negative brain s.
noncontrast CT s.
nonenhanced CT s.
nuclear bleeding s.
nuclear cardiac s.
nuclear medicine s.
Opthascan Mini-A s.
orbital CT s.
panoramic CT s.
paraisopropyliminodiacetic acid s.
perfusion lung s.
positron emission tomography s.
s. projection radiography
radionuclear bone s.
radionuclide bone s.
real-time s.
renal duplex s.
rose bengal s.
segmenting dual-echo MR head s.
serial duplex s.
spin-spin or transverse relaxation time MRI scan
spiral CT s.
technetium diisopropyliminodiacetic acid s.
technetium hepatoiminodiacetic acid s.
thallium exercise heart s.
thyroid uptake s.
total body s.
transvaginal sector s.
tumor localization s.
unenhanced CAT s.
ventilation/perfusion lung s.
V/Q lung s.
white blood cell s.
whole-body s.
whole-body bone s.

Scandinavian
58-point Scandinavian Stroke Scale
S. total ankle replacement

scanned projection radiography

scanner
ATL real-time Neurosector s.
biplane sector s.
CardioData MK-3 Holter s.
computed tomographic s.
gated CT s.
infrared liver s.
laser tomography s.
megavoltage computed tomography s.
megavoltage CT s.
MR catheter imaging and spectroscopy system s.
multidetector CT s.
supercam scintillation s.
whole-body digital s.

scanning
automatic computed transverse axial s.
computerized scanning equipment
confocal laser scanning microscopy
differential scanning colorimeter
diffusion-weighted s.
Doppler s.
electrical impedance breast s.
s. electron micrograph
s. electron microscopy
electrophoresis s.
s. equalization radiography
field emission scanning electron microscopy
s. force microscopy
gallium s.
gated blood pool s.
isotope scanning study
s. laser acoustic microscope
s. laser ophthalmoscope
s. laser tomography
low-dose helical scanning technique
low-voltage high-resolution scanning electron microscopy
multigated cardiac blood pool s.
near field scanning optical microscope
optical s.
s. photoacoustic microscopy
s. probe microscopy
pulmonary perfusion s.
s. radiometer
radionuclide s.
restriction landmark genomic s.
s. saccade
speech s.
stress thallium s.
three-phase radionuclide bone s.
Topographic S. System
total body s.
s. transmission electron microscope
transmission scanning electron microscopy
s. tunneling microscope
ultrasonic renal s.
ultrasound s.
venous duplex s.

scanning-beam digital x-ray

scant infiltration

scanty menstrual flow

Scanzoni maneuver

scaphocapitolunate arthrodesis

scaphocephalic idiocy

scaphoconchal angle

scaphoid
s. abdomen
avascular scaphoid necrosis
avascular tarsal scaphoid necrosis
s. bone
s. fossa
s. fossa of sphenoid bone
s. nonunion advanced collapse
rotatory subluxation of s.
s. scapula
s. shift maneuver
s., trapezium, trapezoid

scaphoiditis
tarsal s.

scaphoid-lunate advanced collapse

scapholunate
s. advanced collapse
s. arthritic collapse
s. articulation
s. ligament

scaphotrapezoid-trapezial

scapula, pl. **scapulae**
angle of inferior s.
angle of superior s.
angulus inferior scapulae
angulus lateralis scapulae
angulus superior scapulae
arteria circumflexa scapulae
Graves s.
medial border of s.
neck of s.
scaphoid s.
wing of s.
winged s.

scapular
s. border
left lower scapular border
left upper scapular border
s. line
right lower scapular border

scapuloanterior
left s.
right s.

scapuloclavicular joint

scapulohumeral
s. atrophy
s. reflex
s. rhythm

scapuloperoneal
mental retardation, scapuloperoneal muscular dystrophy, lethal cardiomyopathy syndrome

scapuloposterior
left s.
right s.

scapulothoracic joint

scar
abdominal s.'s
abnormal development of scar tissue
acne s.
appendectomy s.
argon laser-induced s.
atrophic facial acne s.
atrophic white s.
s. band
bilateral mastectomy s.
broad based s.
burn scar contracture
chickenpox s.
s. contracture
corneal s.
s. dehiscence
dehiscence of cesarean section s.
s. formation
formation s.
hypertrophic burn s.
hypertrophied s.
internal scar tissue
lip scar revision
lower midline scar with hernia
Marchac and Chiari short scar technique
medial epicanthal scar band
operative s.
sternal splitting s.
vaccination s.
vaccination scar upper left arm
well-healed midline s.
well-healed previous excisional s.'s

Scardino ureteropelvioplasty

scarf sign

scarifying
recurrent ulcerative scarifying stomatitis

scarlatina
stomatitis s.

scarlatinal nephritis

scarlatinosa
angina s.
rubeola s.

scarlet
s. fever
s. fever antitoxin
Martius scarlet blue
miniature scarlet fever

Scarpa
canal of S.
S. fascia
S. fluid
S. foramen
S. ganglion
S. hiatus
S. ligament
S. staphyloma

scarred heart

scarring
s. alopecia
apical s.
central centrifugal scarring alopecia
corneal s.
cortical scarring of kidney
duodenal bulb s.
focal interstitial s.
s. and furrowing
s. of heart muscle
s. of heart valve
hilar s.
interstitial s.
linear s.
mild focal interstitial s.
s. and narrowing of esophagus
parenchymal s.
perihilar s.
pleural s.

Scatchard plot

scatter
s. activity
Compton scatter tomography
s. dose
light s.
light scatter technique
multiangle polarized scatter separation
s. pattern
peak scatter factor
peripheral light s.
s. photocoagulation
photocoagulation s.
s. and veiling glare

scatter-air ratio

scattered
s. chronic inflammatory infiltrate
s. ray

scattering
dynamic light s.
high-energy ion s.
ion surface s.
light scattering index
low-angle laser light s.
low-energy ion s.
tissue attenuation and s.

scatter-maximum ratio

scavenger
s. cell
s. receptor

scene
dead at s.

Schacher ganglion

Schafer
S. method of artificial respiration
S. syndrome

Schamberg fever

Schanz
S. disease
S. syndrome

Schapiro sign

Schatzki ring

Schatz maneuver

Schaumann
S. benign lymphogranuloma
S. body

Schauta radical vaginal hysterectomy

Schauta-Wertheim operation

Scheck

Schede thoracoplasty

schedule
S. for Affective Disorders and Schizophrenia-Change
S. for Affective Disorders and Schizophrenia-Lifetime
S. for Affective Disorders and Schizophrenia for School-Age Children
S. for Affective Disorders and Schizophrenia for School-Age Children-Epidemiologic Version
S. for Affective Disorders and Schizophrenia for School-Age Children-Present Episode
altered sleep s.
S. for Assessment of Insight
Autism Diagnostic Observation S.
s. change
chronic sleep schedule disturbance
Diagnostic Interview S.
Edwards Personal Preference S.
Fear Survey S.
Gesell Developmental S.'s
Glasgow Assessment S.
gradual dosage s.
Interview S. for Children and Adolescents
Interview S. for Events and Difficulties
Life Events and Difficulty S. Interview
s. of maximal allowance
maximal surgical blood order s.
medical fee s.
mental status s.
National Institute of Mental Health Diagnostic Interview S.
s. for negative symptoms
parent-child communication s.
Pleasant Events S.
Psychiatric Status S.
Psychotherapy Competence Assessment S.
S. of Recent Experiences
relative value s.
Self Care Assessment S.
strict voiding s.
Support Team Assessment S.
symptom schedule for the diagnosis of borderline schizophrenia
Unpleasant Events S.
Wolpe Fear Survey S.

Schedule-Controlled Operant Behavior

scheduled nursing activities program

Scheibe hearing impairment

Scheie
mucopolysaccharidosis type I S.
S. syndrome

Schema Assessment instrument

schematic
affective schematic mental model
affect-related schematic mental model
Listing schematic eye

scheme
Integrated Child Development S.
Multi-Environment S.

Schepelmann sign

Schepens-Okamura-Brockhurst technique

Scheuermann
S. disease
S. juvenile kyphosis

Scheuthauer-Marie-Sainton syndrome

Schick
negative Schick test
S. sign

Schiff
S. base
lead tetraacetate S.
S. stain

Schiller
S. method
S. stain

Schilling
S. leukemia
S. test

Schinzel-Giedion syndrome

Schiotz
S. scale
tension by Schiotz tonometer

Schirmer test

schistosomal
s. dermatitis
s. dysentery

schistosome granuloma

schistosomiasis
Asiatic s.
hepatic s.
Manson s.
Oriental s.

schizoaffective disorder

schizoaffective-type schizophrenia

schizoid
anesthetic variant of schizoid behavior
s. personality disorder

schizoid-schizotypal personality disorder

schizophrenia
agitation catatonic s.
alternative dimensional descriptors for s.
arrest of s.
borderline s.
catatonic s.
s., catatonic type, subchronic
childhood-onset s.
chronic undifferentiated s.
s., chronic undifferentiated type
comorbidity of schizophrenia and substance abuse
disorganized type s.
s., disorganized type, subchronic
distorted communication in s.
early-onset s.
s. family history
s. index
s. non-family history
paranoid s.
s., paranoid type, subchronic
prepubescent s.
residual type s.
s., residual type, subchronic
slow-progressive s.
symptom schedule for the diagnosis of borderline s.
undifferentiated s.
very early onset s.
s. with premorbid association

Schizophrenia-Change
Schedule for Affective Disorders and S.-C.

schizophrenic
acute paranoid schizophrenic reaction
acute undifferentiated schizophrenic reaction
s. affect
anergic s.
s. brain abnormality
catatonic schizophrenic disorder
chronic paranoid schizophrenic reaction
s. delusion
disorganized schizophrenic disorder
Grid Test of S. Thought Disorder
s. hallucination
s. hallucinations and delusions
s. reaction
s. reaction, acute, paranoid
s. reaction, acute undifferentiated
s. reaction, chronic, paranoid
s. reaction, chronic, undifferentiated
s. residual state
s. spectrum
s. spectrum disorder
S. Subscale of Present State Examination
Whitaker Index of S. Thinking

schizophreniform
affective schizophreniform psychosis
s. disorder

schizotypal personality disorder

Schlatter disease

Schlein-type elbow arthroplasty

Schlemm
canal of S.
S. canal
canal of S.

Schlesinger sign

Schmidt
S. diet
S. keratitis
S. syndrome

Schmidt-Lanterman
S.-L. cleft
S.-L. incisure

Schmidt-Ruppin strain Rous sarcoma virus

Schmincke tumor

Schmitt-Erlanger model of reentry

Schmorl
S. body
S. jaundice
S. nodule

Schmutz pyorrhea

Schnabel atrophy

schneiderian
s. carcinoma
s. membrane
oncocytic schneiderian papilloma

Schneider rod

Schnyder crystalline corneal dystrophy

Scholastic
S. Aptitude Test
Minnesota Scholastic Aptitude Test

Scholz disease

Schönlein-Henoch
S.-H. purpura
S.-H. syndrome
S.-H. vasculitis

school
s. achievement
s. age
S. Assessment Survey
S. Atmosphere Questionnaire
Attitude to S. Questionnaire
S. Attitude Survey
S. Attitude Test
s. avoidance
Basic S. Skills Inventory
Caregiver's S. Readiness Inventory
S. and College Ability Test
Devereux Elementary School Behavior Rating Scale II
Early S. Assessment
Early S. Personality Questionnaire
Effective S. Battery
S. Handicap Condition Scale

S. Health Additional Referral Program
Hess S. Readiness Scale
High S. Personality Questionnaire
Meeting Street S. Screening Test
S. Motivation Analysis Test
Ottawa S. Behavior Checklist
Printing Performance S. Readiness Test
S. Problem Screening Inventory
S. Situation Survey
Teacher S. Readiness Inventory
Test of Attitude Toward S.

school-age child

school-based health center

Schott treatment

Schreger line

Schroeder operation

Schroetter
Paget-von Schroetter syndrome

Schrötter chorea

Schuchardt operation

Schüffner
S. dot
S. granule

Schüller
S. disease
S. duct

Schüller-Christian disease

Schultz
S. angina
S. syndrome

Schultze
S. bundle
S. cell
S. fold
S. mechanism
S. sign

Schumann ray

Schütz bundle

Schwabach test

Schwalbe
S. corpuscle
S. line
S. space

Schwann
S. cell membrane
S. sheath
white substance of S.

schwannoma
acoustic s.
ancient s.
Antoni classification of schwannoma morphology
granular cell s.
intracerebral s.
malignant glandular s.
melanotic s.
vestibular s.

Schwartz
S. sign
S. syndrome

Schwartz-Jampel disease

Schweninger-Buzzi
anetoderma of S.-B.

Sciana blood group

sciatic
artery to sciatic nerve
s. function index
greater sciatic foramen
greater sciatic notch
s. hernia
s. nerve
s. nerve compression
s. nerve entrapment
s. nerve syndrome
s. neuritis
s. notch
pinched sciatic nerve
s. radiation
s. scoliosis

science
Medical S.'s Knowledge Profile
National Institute of General Medical S.'s

scientific
intensive scientific investigation

scientifically treated petroleum

scientist
Association of Clinical S.'s
Tests of Perception of S.'s and Self

scimitar
s. sign
s. syndrome

scintigraphic
s. angiography
monoclonal antibody scintigraphic scan

scintigraphy
dipyridamole myocardial s.
direct vesicoureteral s.
dynamic renal s.
esophageal s.
exercise thallium 201 s.
gated blood pool s.
hepatic arterial perfusion s.
infarct avid hot spot s.
infarct avid myocardial s.
marrow agent bone s.
multiple gated equilibrium s.
myocardial stress perfusion s.
planar thallium s.
quantitative hepatobiliary s.
quantitative sacroiliac s.
radioimmunoglobulin s.
radionuclide esophageal s.
single-photon gamma s.
single-photon planar s.
somatostatin receptor s.
SPECT brain perfusion s.
thallium myocardial s.
three-phase bone s.
whole-gut transit s.

scintillating
s. scotoma
s. speckled pattern

scintillation
comprehensive renal scintillation procedure
gamma scintillation camera
liquid scintillation counting
supercam scintillation scanner
time-resolved liquid scintillation counting

scintiscan
salivary s.

scintography
gallium s.

scirrhous
s. cancer
s. carcinoma

scissor gait

scissors
adventitial s.
alligator s.
angled cartilage s.
arthroscopic s.
bipolar electrosurgical s.
blepharoplasty s.
blunt Metzenbaum s.
blunt-tip iris s.
bulldog nasal s.
collar and crown s.
ethmoidal s.
s. gait
iridotomy s.
iris s.
Lister s.
Manson-Aebli corneal section s.
Mattis corneal s.
Mayo s.
McReynolds pterygium s.

scissors *(continued)*
mechanized s.
Metzenbaum s.
micro Westcott s.
mini-keratoplasty stitch s.
Moore-Troutman corneal s.
Nadler superior radial s.
Northbent s.
Noyes iridectomy s.
Nugent-Gradle s.
O'Brien stitch s.
Olivecrona dura s.

sclera, pl. **sclerae**
sclerae anicteric
s. and conjunctiva
conjunctivae and sclerae
cornea, sclera, and conjunctiva
corneas, conjunctivae, and sclerae
s. cryotherapy
ectasia of s.
limbus of s.
sclerae markedly icteric
s. marker
massive granuloma of s.
perforated layer of s.
superficial s.

scleral
s. band
s. bed
s. buckle
s. buckle, left eye
s. buckle, right eye
s. buckling
s. buckling procedure
coefficient of scleral rigidity
s. crescent
s. depression
encircling of scleral buckle operation
s. flap
s. hemorrhage
s. hook
s. icterus
s. implant
s. insertion
Lopez-Enriquez scleral trephine
s. pigmentation
s. show
s. spur
s. tissue
s. tunnel incision

sclerectasia
partial s.

scleredema of Buschke

sclerema neonatorum

scleritis
annular s.
anterior s.
anular s.
malignant s.
necrotizing nodular s.
necrotizing scleritis with adjacent inflammation
necrotizing scleritis without adjacent inflammation
nodular s.
nonrheumatoid s.

scleroatrophy
anetoderma s.
atrophoderma s.
lichen sclerosus s.

sclerochoroiditis
anterior s.

sclerocornea
microphthalmia, dermal aplasia, sclerocornea syndrome

sclerocorneal
s. junction
necrotizing sclerocorneal ulceration

sclerocystic disease of the ovary

sclerodactyly

scleroderma
calcification, Raynaud phenomenon, scleroderma, telangiectasis syndrome
diffuse cutaneous s.
limited systemic s.
linear scleroderma variant
progressive systemic s.
s. renal crisis
systemic sclerosis sine s.

scleroderma-like syndrome

sclerosed leiomyoma

sclerose en plaques

sclerosing
acute sclerosing hyaline necrosis
s. adenosis
s. agent
diffuse sclerosing osteomyelitis
s. encapsulating peritonitis
focal sclerosing glomerulonephritis
s. hemangioma
s. hepatic carcinoma
hereditary sclerosing poikiloderma
intravascular sclerosing bronchioloalveolar tumor
s. keratitis
s. leukoencephalopathy
mixed sclerosing bone dysplasia, small stature, seizures, mental retardation syndrome
mixed sclerosing bone dystrophy
s. mucoepidermoid carcinoma with eosinophilia
nodular sclerosing Hodgkin disease
nonencapsulated sclerosing tumor
onchocercal sclerosing keratitis
s. pancreatocholangitis
primary sclerosing cholangitis
s. stromal tumor
subacute sclerosing panencephalitis

sclerosis
acute lateral s.
adrenocortical atrophy-cerebral sclerosis syndrome
amyotrophic lateral s.
anterolateral s.
arterial fibrosing s.
ash-leaf spot in tuberous s.
chronic progressive multiple s.
coronary s.
diffuse cortical s.
diffuse mesangial s.
disseminated s.
endoscopic injection s.
endoscopic variceal s.
esophageal variceal s.
exacerbating-remitting multiple s.
familial amyotrophic lateral s.
focal segmental glomerular hyalinosis and s.
focal segmental glomerular sclerosis and hyalinosis
global focal s.
glomerular s.
hippocampal s.
Hodgkin disease, nodular s.
infantile diffuse brain s.
isolated diffuse mesangial s.
lateral amyotrophic s.
limited progressive systemic s.
linear progressive systemic s.
localized progressive systemic s.
medial calcific s.
mediastinal B-cell lymphoma with s.
mesial temporal s.
multiple combined s.
multiple sclerosis susceptibility gene
myelinoclastic diffuse cerebral s.
nodular cortical s.
nuclear s.
nuclear sclerosis of lens

Prausnitz-Küstner s.
primary lateral s.
primary mediastinal large cell lymphoma with s.
primary-progressive multiple s.
progressive systemic s.
relapsing-remitting multiple s.
systemic progressive s.
systemic sclerosis sine scleroderma
transverse spinal s.
tuberous s.
tuberous sclerosis complex

sclerostomy
March laser sclerostomy needle

sclerosus
genital lichen s.
lichen s.
lichen sclerosus et atrophicans
lichen sclerosus scleroatrophy

sclerotherapy
antegrade scrotal s.
endoscopic injection s.
endoscopic variceal s.
esophageal variceal s.
fiberoptic injection s.
injection s.
long-term injection s.

sclerotic
s. aorta
atonic sclerotic muscle dystrophy
s. body
s. bone
s. cemental mass
s. coat
congenital atonic sclerotic muscular dystrophy
s. leiomyoma

sclerotome

sclerotomy
anterior s.
Lindner s.
s. punch
s. with punch
s. with trephine

sclerouvectomy
partial lamellar s.

scoliosis
adolescent idiopathic s.
Aussies-Isseis unstable s.
s. correction
dislocated elbow, bowed tibiae, scoliosis, deafness, cataract, microcephaly, mental retardation syndrome
s. film
juvenile idiopathic s.

scoliotic
s. curve
s. curve fixation

scombroid poisoning

scoop
Arlt s.
Moore gallstone s.
Moynihan gallstone s.
Mules s.

scope passed per ora

scopic
thor scopic talc pleurodesis

scopolamine-Eukodal-Ephetonin

scorbutic
s. anemia
s. dysentery

score
Abbreviated Injury S.
Abbreviated Injury Score/Injury Severity S.
acute change clinical s.
acute physiology and chronic health evaluation s.
amputation index s.
Ashworth score of muscle spasticity
Asthma Severity S.
Ballard Assessment S.
Baylor bleeding s.
biophysical profile s.
Birmingham Vasculitis Activity S.
Boix-Ochoa s.
Champion Trauma S.
Children's Coma S.
clinical performance s.
clinical pulmonary infection s.
composite treatment s.
cumulative pain s.
Danish Prostate Symptom S.
discrimination s.
Dubowitz s.
Duke treadmill prognostic s.
Expectation S.
extent of pleural carcinomatosis s.
five-factor s.
Friesinger s.
full-scale s.
Glasgow Coma S.
Glasgow Dyspepsia Severity S.
Glasgow Meningococcal Septicemia Prognostic S.
Glasgow Outcome S.
Gleason s.
Hanover Intensive S.
Harris hip s.
Hemiballism/Hemichorea Outcome Rating S.
Hopkins Symptom Checklist-90 Total S.
Idiopathic Headache S.
initial Apgar s.
initial prognostic s.
Injury Severity S.
International Classification of Diseases 9th Ed. Injury Severity S.
International Prostate Symptom S.
ischemic s.
Karnofsky performance s.
liberal cutoff s.
linear analog pain s.
Logistic Organ Dysfunction S.
Lung Cancer Symptom S.
lung injury s.
maladjustment s.
Mangled Extremity Severity S.
Manning score of fetal activity
Maryland Foot S.
Maternal Trait Anxiety S.
maximum likelihood s.
Mayo Clinic forefoot s.
Mayo elbow performance s.
McGill-Melzack Pain S.
M.D. Anderson tumor score system
median range s.
Merchant and Dietz ankle s.
Merle d'Aubigné hip s.
Methods for the Epidemiology of Child and Adolescent Disorders T s.
Michigan Diabetic Neuropathy S.
modified Harris hip s.
Modified Injury Severity S.
modified Rodman skin thickness s.
mood cluster s.
nasal congestion s.
nasal symptom s.
S. for Neonatal Acute Physiology-Perinatal Extension
Nerve Disability S.
Nerve Symptom S.
Neurologic and Adaptive Capacity S.
Neurologic Disability S.
neuropsychological test Z s.
neurotic s.
New Ballard S.

score *(continued)*
newborn Apgar s.
New Injury Severity S.
normalized alignment s.
Objective Pain S.'s
Odorant Confusion Matrix s.
Oswestry Disability S.
pain and distress s.
pain intensity difference score
peak pain intensity difference s.
Pediatric Risk of Mortality Score
Pediatric Trauma S.
periodontal disease s.
Peritonitis Severity S.
personality disorder s.
postanesthesia recovery s.
pressure s.
prognostic s.
pulmonary function s.
quantitative wall motion s.
respiratory index s.
respiratory system compliance s.
Revised Trauma S.
sexual function s.
Simplified Acute Physiology S.
Skin Intensity S.
speech discrimination s.
standard deviation s.
surgical Gleason s.
total cellular s.
total coronary s.
total corrected incremental s.
total nuclear s.
total vasomotor rhinitis symptom s.
Trauma and Injury Severity S.'s
treadmill s.
tumor score system
visual analog pain s.
Visual Memory S.
visual observation shivering s.
wall motion score index
War Head-Injury S.
word discrimination s.

scored tablet

scoring
Adhesion S. Group
AFS adhesion scoring system
ankle scoring system of Baird and Jackson
anterior scoring technique
Atkinson scoring system for dysphagia
Developmental Sentence S.
dysfunctional voiding scoring system
Mayo Clinic hip scoring system
modified anterior scoring technique
Neonatal Abstinence Scoring System
Otis Quick S. Mental Abilities Test
Post Anesthesia Discharge S. System
Severity S. of Atopic Dermatitis
Therapeutic Intervention S. System

scotoma, pl. **scotomata**
absolute s.
annular s.
arcuate Bjerrum s.
aural s.
central s.
filtering s.
flashing lights and/or s.
paracentral ring s.
scintillating s.

scotopic
s. adaptation
s. eye
s. perimetry
s. vision

scours
Nebraska calf scours virus

scout film

Scoville

scraped
iris scraped free

scraper
cervical s.

scrapie
prion protein scrapie isoform-reactive plaque

scraping
nasal s.
skin s.

scratch
Apley scratch test
Means-Lerman s.
Means-Lerman scratch murmur
s. reflex
s. test

screen
antibody s.
S. for Child Anxiety-Related Emotional Disorders
children of alcoholic screen testing
coagulation s.
computer screen chart
crystal examination s.
drug screen blood
Early Years Easy S.
film screen radiography
s. filtration pressure
future order s.
heavy metal s.
medical data s.
molecular target-based s.
multicopy suppressor s.
multiphasic health screen test
newborn screen serum thyroxine and phenylketonuria
nonreflective glass s.
organic acid s.
reagin screen test
sickle hemoglobin screen
substance abuse evaluation screen unit
suicide risk s.
The Primary Language S.
type and s.
urine drug s.
urine toxicology s.
Verbal Auditory S. for Children
video display terminal glare s.
Visual Auditory S. for Children

screen-containing cassette

screener
Bayley Infant Neurodevelopmental S.
Oregon Adolescent Depression Project-Conduct Disorder S.
Voc-Tech Quick S.

screen-filtration resistance

screening
s. and acute care
Acute Low Back Pain S. Questionnaire
Adolescent Language S. Test
antibody screening test
antinuclear antibody screening by enzyme immunoassay
antinuclear antibody screening test
Aphasia S. Test
S. Assessment for Gifted Elementary Students, Primary
s. audiometry
s. auditory brainstem response
autism spectrum screening questionnaire
automated auditory brainstem response hearing s.
automated multiphasic s.
s. bacteriuria
Bankson Language Screening Test
Beery Picture Vocabulary S.

breast cancer screening indicator
Brief Aphasia S. Examination
Canterbury Alcoholism S. Test
chemistry screening batteries I and II
chemistry screening profile
Chick Embryotoxicity S. Test
Children of Alcoholics S. Test
S. Children for Related Early Educational Needs
color allergy screening test
S. and Crisis Intervention Program
s. cystometry
Del Rio Language S. Test
Denver Articulation S. Exam
Denver Developmental S. Test
Denver Eye S. Test
Developmental Activities S. Inventory
s. and diagnostic technique
s. dipstick
Draw-A-Person S. Procedure for Emotional Disturbance
Drug Abuse S. Test
Early and Periodic Screening, Diagnosis, and Treatment program
s. endoscopy
s. examination
Fein Articulation S. Test
Flowers Auditory S. Test
Fluharty Preschool Speech and Language S. Test
Frenchay Aphasia S. Test
health screening center
health screening test
hearing acuity s.
heart disease s.
hemostatic screening profile
high-throughput s.
hypertension screening program
Individual Learning Disabilities Classroom S. Instrument
initial drug screening test
initial screening examination
S. Instrument for Targeting Educational Risk
Kindergarten Auditory S. Test
Kindergarten Language S. Test
S. Kit of Language Development
s. laboratory test
limited toxicology s.
s. mammography
medical history as screening device for drug abuse
Meeting Street School S. Test
metabolic disorder s.
metabolic screening disorder
Michigan Abuse S. Test
Michigan Alcoholism S. Test
Michigan Neuropathy S. Test
microsatellite instability s.
Mother/Infant Communication S.
multiphasic s.
multiple health s.
multiple marker s.
neurodevelopmental screening test
newborn screening kit
newborn screening program
Northwestern Syntax S. Test
nuchal translucency s.
oral cancer s.
Oral Language Sentence Imitation S. Test
Patterned Elicitation Syntax S. Test
pediatric infectious disease developmental screening test
Personal Experience S. Questionnaire
Picture Articulation and Language S. Test
preadmission s.
preadmission screening and assessment team
preadmission screening summary
prenatal screening test
Pre-Reading Expectancy S. Scale
presurgical psychological s.
Problem-Oriented S. Instrument for Teenagers
prostate cancer s.
psychological history as screening device
Psychological S. Inventory
Psychosocial History S. Questionnaire
Psychosocial History S. Test
Reitan-Indiana aphasic screening test
Riley Preschool Developmental S. Inventory
School Problem S. Inventory
Self-Administered Alcoholism S. test
Sheffield S. Test for Acquired Language Disorders
Short Michigan Alcoholism S. Test
sickle cell s.
Slingerland S. Tests
social history as screening device for drug abuse
Speech and Language S. Questionnaire
Stephens Oral Language Screening Test
Substance Abuse Subtle S. Inventory
S. Test for Auditory Comprehension of Language
S. Test for Educational Prerequisite Skills
thromboplastin screening test
Universal Neonatal Hearing S.
universal newborn hearing screening program
s. urinalysis
visual acuity s.

screen-intensifying factor

screw

adjunctive screw fixation
s. angulation
anterior C1-C2 screw fixation
anterior screw fixation
arthroscopic screw fixation
arthroscopic screw installation
axial anchor s.
axial compression s.
s. breakage
buttress thread s.
cannulated hip s.
chevron osteotomy with rigid screw fixation
compression hip s.
compression lag s.
compression plate and s.
condylar screw fixation
coracoclavicular screw fixation
cortical bone s.
cortical cancellous s.
countersink screw head
dynamic hip s.
European compression technique bone screw and internal fixation
s. fixation
s. fusion
s. head
installation
mini lag screw system
plate and screw fixation of fracture
transfixion s.'s
variable screw placement
variable screw plate

screwdriver

cannulated s.
s. teeth

screw-plate fixation

screwworm
s. fly
New World s.

Scribner arteriovenous shunt

scrofular conjunctivitis

scrofulosis
lichen s.

scrofulosorum
lichen s.

scrofulous
s. keratitis
lichen s.
s. rhinitis

scrotal
s. abscess
s. anatomy
antegrade scrotal sclerotherapy
anterior scrotal branch of deep external pudendal artery
anterior scrotal nerve
anterior scrotal vein
s. artery
s. calcification
s. compartment
s. edema
s. encroachment
s. fat necrosis
s. hernia
s. hydrocele
s. mass
s. sac

scrotum, pl. **scrota**
angiokeratoma of s.
arterial scrotum supply
dartos muscle of s.
malignant neoplasm of s.
necrotizing fasciitis of the s.
shawl s.
watering-can s.

scrub
Betadine scrub solution
s. nurse
Ocusoft s.
surgical hand s.
warm compresses and lid s.'s

scrubbed
abdomen scrubbed, prepped, and draped

Scully tumor

scurf
lid s.

scurvy
chronic subclinical s.
s. rickets

sea
modified sea water yeast extract agar
San Miguel sea lion virus
s. scurvy
s. sickness

sea-blue histiocyte

seal
Bennett s.
closed water seal drainage system
long s.
water seal chest tube
water seal drainage

sealant
autologous fibrin sealant glue

seal-bark cough

sealed
intrapleural sealed drainage unit

sealer
calciobiotic root canal s.
pulp canal s.

sealing
collagen vascular s.

seam
osteoid seam thickness
stocking seam incision

search
MEDLINE s.
Self-Directed S.
Visual S. and Attention Test
visual search task

Seashore Rhythm Test

seasonal
s. affective disorder
s. affective disorder syndrome
s. allergic conjunctivitis
s. allergic rhinitis
s. allergic rhinoconjunctivitis
s. allergy
s. asthma
congestive seasonal allergic rhinitis
mood disorder with seasonal pattern
S. Pattern Assessment Questionnaire

seated
double seated straight leg raise
s. diastolic blood pressure

seater
band s.

Seattle angina questionnaire

seawater
artificial s.

sebaceous
anogenital sebaceous cyst
s. cyst
s. duct
s. epithelioma
s. gland
s. gland hyperplasia
s. horn
linear sebaceous nevus sequence
linear sebaceous nevus syndrome
lupus s.
nevus s.
nevus sebaceous of Feuerstein and Mims

sebaceum
adenoma s.
molluscum s.

sebaceus
lupus s.
nevus s.
nevus sebaceus of Jadassohn

seborrhea
s. capitis
eczematoid s.
s. sicca

seborrheic
s. dermatitis
s. dermatosis
s. diaper rash
s. eczema
s. external otitis
s. keratitis
s. keratosis

sebum excretion rate

secant integral

Seckel
S. dwarfism
S. syndrome

seclusion
locked door s.
restraint and s.

second
ampere per s.
aortic second sound, pulmonary second sound
s. aortic sound equals second pulmonic sound
s. aortic sound greater than second pulmonic sound
s. aortic sound less than second pulmonic sound
Assessment of Aphasia and Related Disorders, S. Edition

s. auditory area
Behavior Rating Profile, S. Edition
Culture-Free Self-Esteem Inventories, S. Edition
Detroit Tests of Learning Aptitude - Primary, S. Edition
Diagnostic Achievement Battery, S. Edition
English as a second language
s. filial generation
forced expiratory time in s.'s
forced expiratory volume at one s.
forced expiratory volume in one second as percent of FVC
forced expiratory volume in one second to forced vital capacity ratio
forced inspiratory volume in one s.
s. generation sulfonylurea
s. harmonic imaging
healing by first, second, or third intention
S. International Standard
kilogram-meter per second squared
s. left interspace
liposomally entrapped second antibody
lithium action on second messenger
s. lumbar ventral nerve root
s. malignant neoplasm
medial deviation of the second toe
Mendel second law
s. midstream bladder specimen
Minnesota Multiphasic Personality Inventory, S. Edition
s. obtuse marginal artery
s. obtuse marginal branch
s. opinion
oral airflow in liters per s.
pulmonic heart sound less than aortic second heart sound
pulmonic second heart sound equal to aortic second heart sound
pulmonic second heart sound greater than aortic second heart sound
pulmonic second sound split
s. set of followup data
s. stage of decreased intraocular tension
Test of Early Language Development, S. Edition
tricuspid second heart sound
s. trimester abortion
wound healed by first, second or third intention
X-linked second site of fragility

secondarily generalized tonic-clonic seizure

secondary

acute lymphoblastic leukemia secondary to Burkitt lymphoma
s. alopecia
s. amenorrhea
s. anemia
anemia secondary to blood loss
s. anticoagulation system
s. arrest
s. articulation
autosympathectomy secondary to neuropathy
s. axillary adenopathy
s. carcinoma of the upper mediastinum
s. cleavage
s. closure
coma secondary to head trauma
congenital paucity of secondary synaptic clefts syndrome
s. cutaneous large B-cell lymphoma
delayed secondary closure
s. dementia
s. dysmenorrhea
s. effect of treatment
emphysema secondary to heavy smoking
s. encephalitis
s. enrichment medium
s. enuresis
s. focal point of lens
s. generalized epilepsy
s. glaucoma
headache secondary to cervical spinal disease
healing by secondary intention
s. hemorrhage
hemorrhagic diathesis secondary to hepatic failure
s. high blood pressure
s. hydrocephalus
s. hyperparathyroidism
s. hypertension
hypertension secondary to renal disease
s. hyperthyroidism
s. hypertrophic arthropathy
s. hypertrophic osteoarthropathy
s. hypogammaglobulinemia
s. hypogonadism
s. hypoparathyroidism
s. hypothyroidism
s. immune response
s. immunodeficiency
s. infection
s. infertility
s. integration
s. interpretation
s. intervention
s. ion mass spectroscopy
s. leukemia
lipid-soluble secondary antioxidant
s. lymphatic tissue
s. malignancy
s. myelodysplastic syndrome
neutrophil-specific secondary granule deficiency
nutritional secondary hyperparathyroidism
pancreatitis secondary to gallstones
pathologic secondary erythrocytosis
s. plating efficiency
s. pulmonary hemosiderosis
s. pulmonary hypertension
s. pulmonary hypoplasia
rectal bleeding secondary to hemorrhoid
Rollet secondary substance
s. sex characteristic
s. Sjögren syndrome
s. spermatocyte
s. syphilis
wound healed by secondary intention

second-degree

s.-d. AV block
s.-d. burn
s.-d. heart block

second-generation

s.-g. antipsychotic
s.-g. cephalosporin
s.-g. enzyme immunoassay

secondhand smoke

second-line

s.-l. chemotherapy
s.-l. drug

second-look

s.-l. biopsy
s.-l. laparotomy
s.-l. operation
s.-l. sonography

secreta and excrement

secretagogue
growth hormone s.
growth hormone secretagogue receptor

secreted
aminooxypentane regulated-on-activation normal T-expressed and s.
s. insulin
regulated upon activation, normal T-cell expressed and s.

secretes gastric juice

secretin
s., cholecystokinin, pancreozymin
duodenal secretin test
immunoreactive s.
intraarterial s.
intraductal secretin test
pancreozymin s.
s. pancreozymin
pancreozymin secretin test
s. test

secreting
prolactin secreting pituitary tumor

secretin-like immunoreactivity

secretion
aldosterone secretion defect
aldosterone secretion rate
anti-*Toxoplasma gondii* antibody secretion assay
apparent norepinephrine secretion rate
basal gastric s.
blood and s.
conjunctival s.
continuous aspiration of subglottic s.'s
control gastric s.
cortisol secretion rate
deoxycorticosterone secretion rate
distal effective potassium s.
s. droplet
enzymatic pancreatic s.
excessive acid s.
excessive insulin s.
s. and excretion
expressed prostatic s.'s
gastric acid s.
glucagon s.
glucose-stimulated insulin s.
growth hormone s.
s. of hormones
inappropriate gonadotropin s.
inappropriate secretion of antidiuretic hormone
inappropriate vasopressin s.
insulin secretion rate
Leydig cell s.
luteinizing hormone s.
ovarian androgen s.
pancreatic enzyme s.
parathyroid hormone s.
parathyroid hormone secretion rate
persistent estrogen s.
pituitary gonadotropin s.
plasma immunoreactive s.
prostate gland s.
prostatic s.
s. rate
salivary and lacrimal s.
s. and spill from acquired immune deficiency syndrome
s. spills from hepatitis patients
syndrome of inappropriate antidiuretic hormone s.
syndrome of inappropriate secretion of antidiuretic hormone
thick bronchial s.'s
total parathyroid hormone s.

secretory
aldosterone secretory rate
basal secretory flow rate
s. carcinoma of the endometrium
s. coil
s. component
s. cyst
s. duct
s. endometrial
endometrial secretory adenocarcinoma
free secretory component
free secretory piece
gastric secretory testing
s. granule
hypothalamic secretory factor
s. IgA
insulin secretory response
integrated secretory response
s. leukocyte protease inhibitor
s. leukoprotease inhibitor
s. leukoproteinase inhibitor
Leydig cell secretory function
s. otitis media
pancreatic secretory flow rate
pancreatic secretory trypsin inhibitor
parathyroid secretory protein
peak secretory flow rate
pentagastrin gastric secretory test
s. piece
s. sphingomyelinase

section
attached cranial s.
axial celloidin s.
biopsy submitted for frozen s.
cardiac section of stomach
central material s.
cesarean s.
classic cesarean s.
computer-assisted reconstruction by tracing of serial s.'s
decalcified section of vertebral body
dehiscence of cesarean section scar
frozen section red blood cell
frozen section assay
histologic section of ganglion
intrauterine pregnancy, term birth, cesarean s.
low cervical transverse cesarean s.
lower cervical cesarean s.
lower uterine segment transverse cesarean s.
low flap cesarean s.
low vertical cesarean s.
Manson-Aebli corneal section scissors
median longitudinal s.
middle fossa vestibular nerve s.
s. modulus
nerve cross s.
paraffin-embedded semithin s.
primary cesarean s.
psychiatric services s.
rapid frozen s.
repeat low transverse cesarean s.
serial transverse s.
transverse s.
transverse section of heart
vaginal birth after cesarean s.

sectional impression

sectionally processed antibody coated

sectioned
doubly ligated and s.
representative sample s.

sectioning
Albert-Linder bone s.
fixation and sectioning of the brain
s. technique

sector
biplane sector scanner
cranial sector scan
s. scan

superior sector iridectomy
transvaginal sector scan

secundum
s. atrial septal defect
per secundum healing

secure
patient-centered access to secure systems online

secured
bleeding points s.
hemostasis s.
hemostasis secured with ties

security
Employee Retirement Income S. Act
Flint Infant S. Scale
Personnel S. Preview

sedation
conscious s.
heavy s.
intravenous s.
level of s.
meperidine conscious s.
midazolam conscious s.
Observer Assessment of Alertness and S.
patient-controlled s.
pediatric sedation unit
procedural sedation and analgesia
terminal s.

sedative cabinet bath

Seddon nerve graft

sedentary
cyclic s.
s. habit
s. individual

sediment
barium sediment in urine
strained urinary s.

sedimentation
blood sedimentation rate
s. coefficient
s. constant
corrected sedimentation rate
erythrocyte sedimentation rate
s. field flow fractionation
negative sedimentation Svedberg unit
s. rate test
Ritchie s.
s. time
Westergren erythrocyte sedimentation rate
Wintrobe erythrocyte sedimentation rate
zeta erythrocyte sedimentation rate

sedimented red cell

see
How I See Myself Scale

seed
s. graft
horse chestnut seed extract
Mick seed applicator
millet seed nodule
radioactive seed implant
radium s.
radon seed implantation

seeding
s. of joint
microscopic s.
perichondral cell s.
radioactive seeding of prostate

seeing
S. Essential English
S. Eye

seeker
bone s.
care s.

seeking
coronary seeking catheter
lymph node seeking equivalent

seen
no apparent disease seen in chest

seepage
fecal s.

segment
A1-A5 s.'s of anterior cerebral artery
aganglionic segment of colon
anterior basal bronchopulmonary s.
anterior basal s.
anterior bronchopulmonary s.
anterior ocular s.
anterior portion of left medial segment IV of liver
anterior segment angiography
anterior segment examination
anterior segment of eye
anterior segment inflammation
anterior segment necrosis
anterior segment sleeve
anterior superior renal s.
aperistaltic distal ureteral s.
apical bronchopulmonary s.
apical segment of lung
apicoposterior bronchopulmonary s.
arterial segment of kidney
artery of anterior inferior segment of kidney
artery of anterior superior segment of kidney
artery of posterior segment of kidney
A1 segment of anterior cerebral artery
A2 segment of anterior cerebral artery
Ask-Upmark renal s.
atretic aortic s.
body segment parameter
s. of bowel
clinoidal s.
demucosalized augmentation with gastric s.
depressed ST s.
diseased segment of bowel
dorsal intercalated segment instability
dorsiflexed intercalated segment instability
electrocardiographic junction between QRS complex and ST s.
electrocardiographic wave s.
end-diastolic segment length
end-systolic segment length
fixed segment of bowel
flow-limiting s.
hypervariable segment II
ileal segment
ilial s.
s. inertial properties
s. inferior
initial s.
instability
intrastromal corneal ring s.'s
jejunal s.
s.'s of liver
s. long-spacing collagen
lower s.
lower esophageal s.
lower uterine s.
lower uterine segment transverse cesarean section
low segment transverse incision
M2 artery s.
medial basal bronchopulmonary segment S VII
medial basal s.
mesodermal dysgenesis of anterior s.
middle ear s.

segment *(continued)*
M2 segment of middle cerebral artery
nonspecific abnormality of ST segment and T wave
nonspecific ST wave segment changes on electroencephalogram
ophthalmic s.
reference point following QRS complex, at beginning of ST s.
rod outer s.
sacral s.
ST segment depression
superior segment of lung
trypsin-insoluble s.
upper s.
upper body segment to lower body segment ratio
volar flexed intercalated segment instability

segmental
akinetic segmental wall motion abnormality
s. alveolar osteotomy
s. alveolar pattern
anterior basal segmental artery
anterior-posterior fusion with segmental spinal instrumentation
anterior segmental artery
anterior segmental dentoalveolar osteotomy
anterior superior segmental artery of kidney
s. antigen challenge
apical segmental artery
apical segmental artery of superior lobar artery of right lung
s. arterial disorganization
s. artery of kidney
s. artery of liver
s. atelectasis
s. bile duct fibrosis
s. biliary obstruction
s. bone defect
s. bone loss
s. bowel infarct
s. branch
s. branch of artery
bronchopulmonary segmental artery
bronchopulmonary segmental drainage
s. bronchus consolidation
s. bronchus defect
s. bronchus fracture
s. bronchus ischemia
s. bronchus lesion
s. bronchus lower extremity Doppler pressure
s. bronchus narrowing
s. bronchus orifice
s. bronchus perfusion abnormality
s. bronchus plethysmography
s. bronchus renal artery waveform
s. bronchus sign
s. bronchus symptom
s. cement extraction system
s. colonic adenomatous polyposis syndrome
s. colonic resection
s. colonic tuberculosis
s. continuity defect
s. correction using spine reconstruction
s. correction using x-ray measurement
s. demyelinating polyneuropathy
s. epidural analgesia
s. epidural anesthesia
s. fixation
focal segmental glomerular hyalinosis and sclerosis
focal segmental glomerular sclerosis and hyalinosis
focal segmental glomerulosclerosis
focal and segmental hyalinosis
s. fracture
s. hyalinizing vasculitis
interspinous segmental spinal instrumentation technique
intraoral vertical segmental osteotomy
s. iris atrophy
s. limb systolic pressure
living segmental donor pancreas transplantation
medial basal segmental artery
medial basal segmental bronchus
s. mesangial hypercellularity
s. multileaf collimator
s. pancreas donation
s. sequential irradiation
s. spinal correction system
s. spinal instrumentation
s. stenosis
s. venous capacitance
s. wall motion
s. wall motion abnormality

segmentales
arteriae medullares s.

segmentary syndrome

segmentation
s. anomaly
automated airway tree segmentation method
automatic lumen edge s.
s. cavity
costovertebral segmentation defect with mesomelia syndrome
s. defect
phonemic segmentation test
time-resolved imaging by automatic data s.

segmented
s. cell
focused segmented ultrasound machine
s. neutrophils
s. renal artery
s. ring tripolar
s. venous capacitance ratio

segmenting
s. body
s. dual-echo MR head scan
s. dual-echo MR imaging

segment-oriented hepatic resection

Segond fracture

segregation
administrative s.
chromosomal s.

Seidelin body

Seidel scotoma

Seitz sign

seizure
absence s.
s. activity
acute repetitive s.
affective symptom of s.
alcohol as cause of s.
alcohol withdrawal s.
atonic absence s.
atypical absence s.
atypical petit mal s.
breastfeeding and s.
characteristic of seizure abnormality
clinically observed s.
complex febrile s.
complex motor s.
complex partial nocturnal s.
continuous seizure activity
s. control
conversion disorder, seizure type
s. diathesis
electrographic seizure activity

electroshock seizure threshold
epilepsy with grand mal seizures on awakening
s. exacerbation
first-trimester maternal s.
fluent aphasic s.
s. frequency
frontal lobe s.
generalized tonic-clonic s.
grand mal s.
s. history
idiopathic seizure disorder
s. impulse
s. induction
infantile myoclonic s.
infant with s.'s
intractable s.'s
isolated grand mal s.
Liverpool S. Severity Scale
localization-related epilepsy s.
localized electroencephalographic seizure pattern
major motor s.
maximal electroshock s.
maximal electroshock-induced s.
mental retardation, dystonic movements, ataxia, seizures syndrome
mental retardation, optic atrophy, deafness, seizures syndrome
Metrazol-electroshock s.
microcephaly, sparse hair, mental retardation, seizures syndrome
minor motor s.
mixed sclerosing bone dysplasia, small stature, seizures, mental retardation syndrome
multifocal clonic s.
neonatal drug addiction s.
neonatal hypoglycemic s.
new-onset s.'s
nonepileptic s.
nonfluent aphasic s.
painful tonic s.
partial complex s.
partial epileptic s.
partial motor s.
partial seizures with or without generalized tonic-clonic s.'s
petit mal s.
posttraumatic s.
previous seizure disorder
recurrent s.'s
s. resistant
secondarily generalized tonic-clonic s.
s. sensitive
serial focus s.'s
simple partial s.
sleep-related epileptic s.
temporal lobe s.
s. threshold
tonic-clonic s.
typical absence s.
uncontrolled generalized grand mal s.
X-linked mental retardation, s.'s, acquired microcephaly, agenesis of corpus callosum

seizure-brain damage

seizure-producing areas of brain

Seldinger technique

selected

above selected threshold
s. ion flow tube
s. ion monitoring
s. mucosal biopsy

selection

adverse s.
antibiotic s.
artificial s.
s. coefficient
equal probability of selection method
gametic s.
natural s.
natural selection theory
negative s.
negative selection procedure
optimal dose s.
Pacemaker S. in the Elderly
product selection allowed

selective

s. ablation
s. amnesia
s. androgen-receptor modulator
s. angiography
s. antipolysaccharide antibody deficiency
s. apoptotic antineoplastic drugs
auditory selective listening
s. broth medium
s. catheterization
chemical shift s.
s. chemotherapy
s. complete lymph node dissection
s. deafness
s. decontamination of the digestive tract
s. digestive decontamination
s. digestive tract decontamination
s. dorsal rhizotomy
s. estrogen receptor modulator
s. estrogen response modifier
Flowers Auditory Test of S. Attention
s. gastric vagotomy
s. grinding
s. hearing loss
highly selective vagotomy
horizontally selective visual cell
s. imaging and graphics for stereotactic surgery
s. intestinal decontamination
s. intracoronary thrombolysis
s. intrapartum chemoprophylaxis
s. laser trabeculoplasty
s. lymphoid irradiation
s. neck dissection
s. nerve root block
s. pituitary resistance to thyroid hormone
s. posterior rhizotomy
s. protein index
s. proximal vagotomy
s. serotonin reuptake inhibitor
transtracheal selective bronchial brushing
s. tubal assessment to refine reproductive therapy
s. tubal occlusion procedure
s. vagotomy with antrectomy
s. vagotomy with pyloroplasty
s. vascular clamping
s. visceral angiography

selectivity

thermokinetic s.

selector

patient-operated selector mechanism

selenite brilliant green

selenium-labeled homocholic acid conjugated with taurine

Seletar virus

self

s. blood-glucose monitoring
S. Care Assessment Schedule
caring for s.
dangerous to one's s.
s. harm
missing self hypothesis
Multidimensional S. Concept Scale
multiple domains of s.
nonturning against self psychology

self *(continued)*
patient incapacitated of caring for s.
Physical S. Maintenance Scale
Tests of Perception of Scientists and S.
threat to self or others
totally incapacitated of caring for s.
turning against s.
Visual Analogue S. Assessment Scales For Pain Intensity

self-administered
S.-a. Alcoholism Screening test
S.-a. Dependency Questionnaire
s.-a. injection
s.-a. medication
Quality of Well-Being Scale S.-a.
s.-a. therapy

self-administration
s.-a. of psychoactive drug
s.-a. of psychotropic drug

Self-Analysis
S.-A. Form
S.-A. Inventory

self-applied health enhancement method

self-articulating
s.-a. femoral
s.-a. femoral hip replacement

self-assertion
healthy s.-a.

self-assessment
computer-assisted s.-a.
S.-a. Depression Scale

self-awareness in illness

self-blood sugar monitoring

self-breast examination

self-care
s.-c. activity
s.-c. deficit
independent s.-c.

self-catheterization
intermittent s.-c.

self-centeredness
destructive s.-c.

self-concept
S.-c. as a Learner
disturbance in s.-c.
improved s.-c.
S.-c. and Motivation Inventory

self-contained
s.-c. enzymatic membrane immunoassay
s.-c. underwater breathing apparatus

self-controlled intravenous system

Self-Control Scale

self-damaging behavior

self-defense
fighting, injuries, sex, threats, s.-d.

Self-Description
S.-D. Inventory
S.-D. Questionnaire II

self-destructive behavior

self-directed
s.-d. learning
s.-d. learning readiness scale
S.-d. Search

self-emptying blind loop

self-esteem
Children's Inventory of S.-e.
chronic low s.-e.
improve health s.-e.
S.-e. Index
inflated s.-e.
S.-e. Inventory

Self-Evaluation of Life Function scale

self-examination
breast s.-e.
genital s.-e.
skin s.-e.
testicular s.-e.

self-expanding
s.-e. metallic stent
s.-e. microporous stent

self-expectation
high s.-e.

self-filling blind loop

self-harm
adult self-harm behavior
deliberate s.-h.
self-reported s.-h.

self-healing
s.-h. personality
self-massage acupressure for s.-h.
s.-h. style of qigong

self-help
s.-h. abortion
medical s.-h.
s.-h. support group
s.-h. technique

self-hypnosis
patient under s.-h.

self-image
disturbance in s.-i.
good s.-i.
improve s.-i.
negative s.-i.

Offer Self-Image Questionnaire for Adolescents

self-importance
grandiose sense of s.-i.

self-induced
s.-i. alopecia
s.-i. illness
s.-i. injury
s.-i. water intoxication and psychosis

self-inflating bulb

self-inflicted
s.-i. bodily injury
s.-i. wound

self-inhibiting behavioral injury device

self-injection
penile s.-i.

self-injuring behavior

self-injurious
s.-i. behavior
s.-i. habit

self-injurious-behavior inhibiting system

self-injury
adult s.-i.

self-intermittent catheterization

self-limited disease

self-limiting illness

self-managing arthritis

self-massage acupressure for self-healing

self-medication administration record

self-monitored blood glucose

self-monitoring
drugs, exercise, education, diet, and s.-m.

Self-Motivation Inventory

self-mutilation
compulsive s.-m.

self-object transference

self-obtained smear

Self-Perception Inventory

self-phase modulation

Self-Rating
Anorexia Nervosa Inventory for S.-R.
S.-R. Depression Scale
S.-R. Obsessive-Compulsive Personality Inventory

self-regulation
cardiac s.-r.

self-reinforced poly-L-lactide

self-reinforcing polylevolactic acid

self-report
youth s.-r.

self-reported
s.-r. history
s.-r. self-harm

self-retaining catheter

self-sealing breast implant

self-stimulation
apnea/bradycardia s.-s.
intracranial s.-s.

self-terminating tachycardia

self-worth
augment individual sense of s.-w.

Seligmann buffered salt solution

Selivanoff reaction

Seliwanow test

sella
atrophy of dorsum s.
empty sella turcica syndrome
gourd-shaped s.
midpoint of sella turcica
most anterior point of anterior contour of the sella turcica
most posterior point on posterior contour of sella turcica
s. to nasion cephalometrics
primary empty sella syndrome
s. turcica

sellaris
articulatio s.

Sellick maneuver

selvagem

semantic
s. aphasia
s. argument
s. cueing
s. dementia
s. memory

semen
s. analysis
computer-assisted semen analysis
s., hair and blood
hyaluronidase unit for s.

semiadjustable
arcon semiadjustable articulator

semialdehyde
succinate semialdehyde dehydrogenase

semicircular
anterior semicircular canal
anterior semicircular duct
s. canal
s. duct
horizontal semicircular canal
membranous ampullae of the semicircular duct
membranous limb of semicircular duct
posterior semicircular canal
superior semicircular canal
superior semicircular canal deficiency

semiconductor
complementary metal-oxide semiconductor logic
metal oxide semiconductor field effect transistor
N-type metal oxide s.

semicontinuous activated sludge

semielemental diet

semihorizontal heart position

semi-invasive aspergillosis

semilunar
anterior semilunar valve
s. bone
s. cartilage
s. conjunctival fold
s. cusp
s. fascia
s. fasciculus
s. flap
s. ganglion
s. hiatus
s. incision
s. line
s. valve
s. valve closure

semilunaris

semimembranous bursa

seminal
s. capsule
s. colliculus
s. duct
s. fluid
s. fluid analysis
s. fluid assay
s. gland
s. granule
s. hillock
human seminal plasma inhibitor
s. lake
muscular layer of seminal gland
sheep seminal vesicle
s. vesicle
s. vesicle invasion
s. vesicle microsome
s. vesiculography

seminiferous
s. epithelium
s. tubule

seminis
musculus ejaculator s.

seminoma
extragonadal s.

semipermeable
s. film
s. membrane

semiprone position

semiquantitative culture

semirigid fiberglass cast

semishell implant

semispinalis
s. capitis
s. capitis muscle
s. cervicis muscle

semispinal muscle of head

semistructured psychiatric interview

semisynthetic
human semisynthetic insulin
s. penicillin

semitendinosus
biceps s.

semitendinous
double-looped semitendinous and gracilis hamstring graft knee reconstruction technique

semithin
paraffin-embedded semithin section

semiupright film

Semliki Forest virus

Semm
classic abdominal Semm hysterectomy

Semmes-Weinstein monofilament

Semon sign

Sena Madureira virus

Sendai virus

Senear-Usher
- S.-U. disease
- S.-U. syndrome

senescent heart

Sengstaken-Blakemore tube

senile
- s. alopecia
- Alzheimer-like senile dementia
- s. amyloidosis
- atrophic senile gingivitis
- s. atrophoderma
- s. atrophy
- s. cataract
- s. chorea
- s. choroidal macular degeneration
- s. delirium
- s. dementia
- s. dementia of the Alzheimer type
- s. dwarfism
- s. gait disorder
- s. gangrene
- s. insanity
- s. keratoderma
- s. keratoma
- s. keratosis
- s. lenticular myopia
- s. lentigo
- s. macular chorioretinal degeneration
- s. macular degeneration
- neuritis senile plaque
- s. onset
- s. paraplegia
- s. parkinsonism
- s. plaque
- s. retinal neovascular membrane
- s. tremor

senility
- s. and disorientation
- onset of s.

senior
- S. Apperception Technique
- S. Apperception Test
- medication information leaflet for s.'s

Senning procedure

Senoussi Multiphasic Marital Inventory

sensation
- association sensation ratio
- auditory and kinesthetic s.
- burning sensation in stomach
- burning sensation in upper chest
- capillary refill, sensation, motor function, temperature
- circulation and s.
- s., circulation, motion
- circulation, motor ability, sensation, and swelling
- circulation, sensation, mobility
- color, warmth, movement s.
- creeping sensation in extremity
- crushing sensation in chest
- decibels sensation level
- diminished sensation to pinprick
- disorder of s.
- s. disturbance
- disturbance of s.
- fine tactile s.
- flushing sensation of heaviness
- foreign body s.
- grating sensation under kneecap
- s. of heaviness
- hot and cold s.
- impaired discriminatory, vibratory and position s.
- s. impairment
- s. of intense dread
- itching or burning s.
- joint position s.
- s. level of hearing
- liminal s.
- loaded breathing s.
- loss of protective s.
- s. and motor function
- painful burning sensation in chest
- pressure sensation in chest
- propagated sensation along the channel
- propagated sensation along the meridian
- reported visual s.
- skin crawling s.
- terminal s.
- tingling and burning s.
- tingling sensation in hand
- s. unit

sensation-seeking scale

sense
- augment individual sense of self-worth
- blanked ventricular s.
- color s.
- common sense judgment
- s. of detachment
- deteriorating sense of balance
- distorted sense of time and perception
- disturbed sense of time
- s. of equilibrium
- s. of failure
- grandiose sense of self-importance
- s. of guilt
- s. of hearing
- heightened sense of awareness
- s. of helplessness
- s. of hopelessness
- s. of identity
- s. of increasing helplessness
- intensive stimulation of s.'s
- joint position s.
- light s.
- overwhelming sense of panic
- special sense organs
- stimulation of s.'s
- ventricular s.

sensibility
- articular s.
- epicritic s.
- somesthetic s.

sensing
- integrated bipolar s.
- pacing and sensing threshold
- ventricular pacing, atrial sensing, triggered mode, pacemaker

sensitive
- arrhythmia-insensitive flow-sensitive alternating IR
- corticoid s.
- corticosteroid sensitive asthma
- hormone sensitive lipase
- s. index
- light s.
- ouabain s.
- seizure s.
- suppressor s.
- very s.

sensitivity
- anaphylactoid food s.
- angiotensin sensitivity test
- animal dander s.
- antibiotic sensitivity test
- antibiotic sensitivity testing
- anxiety sensitivity index
- anxiety sensitivity theory
- baroreceptor reflex s.
- baroreflex s.
- cell sensitivity to radiation
- chemical sensitivity syndrome
- circulatory problem with cold s.
- confusion with light s.
- contact s.
- culture and s.
- culture and sensitivity and colony count

delayed s.
diphtheria toxin s.
heightened sensitivity to odors
heightened sensitivity to sounds
herpesvirus s.
high-anxiety s.
high methacholine s.
human corona virus s.
s. to hyperthermia
idiopathic leucine s.
immediate s.
International S. Index
leukocyte-antigen sensitivity testing
s. to light and glare
liminal s.
s. of method
microculture and s.
modal s.
multiple chemical s.
multiple chemical sensitivity syndrome
mumps sensitivity test
pain sensitivity range
partial androgen s.
peak flow s.
Pelli-Robson contrast sensitivity chart
periocular drug s.
peripheral insulin s.
poliovirus s.
s. prediction by acoustic reflex
Profile of Nonverbal S.
psoriasis area sensitivity index
quantitative insulin sensitivity check index
ragweed s.
s. reaction
respiratory isolation implementation s.
s. response
short increment sensitivity index
slice sensitivity profile
small increment sensitivity index
steroid s.
T-cell-mediating contact s.
temperature s.
urine culture and s.

sensitization
aerosol s.
autoerythrocyte s.
autoerythrocyte sensitization syndrome
s. response cell
Rh s.
s. test

sensitized
s. antigen
s. cell
s. culture
s. sheep cell agglutination

sensitize heart muscle to digitalis toxicity

sensitizing
s. antibody
s. dose
s. injection
s. substance

sensitometer
electroluminescent s.

sensitometric
cineangiography and sensitometric ejection fraction

sensor
acoustic respiratory motion s.
anterior oesophageal s.
differential temperature s.
electromyogram s.'s
implantable glucose s.
multiparameter intraarterial s.
ocular vergance and accommodation s.
s. position indicator

sensorimotor
anorectal sensorimotor dysfunction
s. area
chronic sensorimotor neuropathy
s. cortex
mitochondrial encephalomyopathy with sensorimotor polyneuropathy
mitochondrial encephalomyopathy with sensorimotor polyneuropathy, ophthalmoplegia, and paralysis
mixed sensorimotor polyneuropathy
s. polyneuropathy
primary sensorimotor cortex
s. rhythm

sensorineural
s. acuity level
autoimmune sensorineural hearing loss
congenital cataracts, sensorineural deafness, Down syndrome facial appearance, short stature, mental retardation syndrome
s. deafness
diabetes insipidus, diabetes mellitus, progressive bilateral optic atrophy, and sensorineural deafness
fluctuating sensorineural hearing loss
s. hearing impairment
s. hearing loss
high-frequency sensorineural hearing loss
idiopathic sudden sensorineural hearing loss
low-frequency sensorineural hearing loss
ocular albinism with late-onset sensorineural deafness
severe sensorineural hearing loss

sensorium
appearance, mood, sensorium, intelligence, and thought process
clear s.
clearing of s.
clouded s.

sensory
s. abnormality
s. acuity level
altered sensory perception
s. anesthesia
s. aphasia
s. apraxia
s. ataxia
s. ataxic neuropathy with dysarthria and ophthalmoplegia
atypical sensory modality
s. aura
s. awareness
s. binocular cooperation
blurred sensory perceptions
s. branch of radial nerve
Clinical Test of S. Interaction & Balance
computer-assisted sensory examination
s. conduction velocity
s. cortex
cortical sensory loss
s. decision theory
decreased sensory perception
s. defect
s. deficit
s. deprivation
s. deprivation syndrome
s. detection method
distal sensory latency
distal sensory polyneuropathy
distal symmetric sensory neuropathy
distal symmetric sensory polyneuropathy
distortion of sensory perception
s. distribution

sensory *(continued)*
s. disturbance
effective sensory projection
elbow sensory potential
enhanced sensory awareness
evoked sensory nerve action potential
s. evoked potential
s. evoked response
Familiar S. Stimulation
s. feedback therapy
fiberoptic endoscopic evaluation of swallowing with sensory testing
s. finding
flexible endoscopic evaluation of swallowing with sensory testing
s. function
s. functioning
s. ganglion
gross sensory deficit
s. hair
s. hair cells
hereditary sensory and autonomic neuropathy types I-IV
hereditary sensory motor neuropathy type I–III
hereditary motor sensory neuropathy II-deafness-mental retardation
hereditary sensory neuropathy
idiopathic sudden sensory hearing loss
immediate sensory trace recall
s. impaired support
s. impairment
s. impression
individual sensory modality
s. integration
S. Integration and Praxis Tests
s. integration training
s. isolation
laryngopharyngeal sensory stimulation
s. latency
s. loss
low sensory threshold
main sensory nucleus
mixed sensory polyneuritis
s. motor integration
motor, vascular, and s.
multiple sensory defect dizziness
multiple sensory deficit
s. nerve
s. nerve action potential
s. nerve conduction velocity
s. neural hearing loss
s. neuron
nondermatomal sensory abnormality
S. Organization Test
S. Perceptual Examination
pulse, motor, and s.
pure sensory stroke
pure sensory syndrome
Quantitative S. Testing
rhythmic sensory bombardment therapy
s. seizure
Southern California S. Integration Tests
s. stimuli
structured sensory stimulation
subacute sensory neuropathy
supplementary sensory feedback
terminal sensory latency
s. tract intact
s. urgency
Weinstein enhanced sensory test

sent
slip s.

sentence
Auditory Comprehension Test for S.'s
Auditory Comprehension Test for S.'s
Completing S. Test
Developmental S. Scoring
Fokes sentence builder
Forer S. Completion Test
Oral Language S. Imitation Diagnostic Inventory
Oral Language S. Imitation Screening Test
Rotter S. Completion Test
Rotter Incomplete S.'s Blank
Sacks S. Completion Test
Spreen-Benton S. Repetition Test
Stein Sentence Completion Test
synthetic sentence identification
synthetic sentence list

sentinel
s. cell
s. lymphadenectomy
s. lymph node
s. lymph node biopsy
s. lymph node detection
s. lymph node mapping
s. node-to-background ratio

Seoul virus

separable
minimum separable acuity
minimum separable angle

separated
carbon separated from the carboxyl group by 2 other carbon atoms
legally s.

separation
s. anxiety disorder
S. Anxiety Symptom Inventory
aortic valve cusp s.
articular mass s.
articular mass separation fracture
s. of circle-diamond
dermal-epidermal s.
E-point to septal s.
s. of ghosts
s. or loss abandonment
lymphocyte separation medium
multiangle polarized scatter s.
premature separation of placenta
trabecular s.

separator
blood cell s.

Sepik virus

sepsis
alcoholism, leukopenia, pneumococcal s.
catheter-related s.
Escherichia coli sepsis peritonitis
Gram-negative s.
group B streptococcal s.
infant with s.
intraabdominal s.
jaundice associated with s.
Listeria monocytogenes s.
suspected catheter s.
uremia and s.

sepsis-related organ failure assessment

septa (*pl. of* septum)

septal
acquired ventricular septal defect
anterior septal branch of anterior ethmoidal artery
aorticopulmonary septal defect
aortic septal defect
aortopulmonary septal defect
s. apical
apical interventricular septal amplitude
s. area
s. artery
s. asymmetry
atrial septal aneurysm
atrial septal defect
atrial septal defect occlusion
atrial septal heart disease

atrial septal resection
atrioventricular canal septal defect
atrioventricular nodal septal defect
atrioventricular septal defect
s. band
s. basal
basal septal hypertrophy
s. bone
s. branch
calibrated triangle of septal cartilage
s. cartilage
cartilaginous autologous thin septal graft
clamshell closure of atrial septal defect
closure interatrial septal defect
s. defect
s. deformity
s. deviation
disproportionate septal thickening
s. edema
Eisenmenger ventricular septal defect
endocardial cushion-type ventricular septal defect
E-point to septal distance
E-point to septal separation
s. fracture
s. hematoma
hydrogen-detected ventricular septal defect
s. hypertrophy
iatrogenic atrial septal defect
s. impaction
s. infarction
infundibular septal defect
interatrial septal aneurysm
interatrial septal defect
interatrial septal defect closure
interventricular septal defect
interventricular septal excursion
interventricular septal motion
interventricular septal rupture
interventricular septal thickness
isolated asymmetric septal hypertrophy
lateral s.
left transatrial s.
left ventricular septal wall
s. line
low septal right atrium
medial septal nucleus
muscular ventricular septal defect
s. myectomy
s. myotomy
nasal septal perforation button
nonsurgical septal reduction therapy
percutaneous transluminal septal myocardial ablation
s. pore
pulmonary atresia with ventricular septal defect
secundum atrial septal defect
s. spur
s. thickness
transcoronary ablation of septal hypertrophy
vascular septal defect
ventral septal defect
ventricular septal heart defect

septate
s. appearance
s. hymen

septation
aorticopulmonary s.
deficient atrioventricular s.
s. of heart

septectomy
atrial s.

septi
arteria nasalis posterior s.

septic
s. abortion
s. arthritis
s. bursitis
s. complication
s. disease
s. encephalitis
s. fever
s. finger joint
s. granuloma
s. inflammation
s. meningitis
nongonococcal septic arthritis
s. pelvic thrombophlebitis
s. phlebitis
s. pulmonary edema
s. shock
s. shock syndrome
Simon septic factor
s. thrombosis
s. workup
s. wound

septicemia
acute s.
anthrax s.
catheter-related s.
Glasgow Meningococcal S. Prognostic Score
Gram-negative s.
meningococcal s.
metastasizing s.
morphine injector's s.
neonatal s.
nosocomial s.
Pseudomonas s.
s. sputum
s. treatment
viral hemorrhagic septicemia virus

septicemic
s. abscess
s. cutaneous ulcerative disease
s. meningitis

septooptic dysplasia

septoplasty
atrial septoplasty procedure
graft s.
nasal s.

septorhinoplasty
corrective s.

septostomy
atrial balloon s.
atrial septostomy procedure
atrial septostomy via balloon
balloon atrial s.
echo-guided balloon atrial s.

septum, pl. **septa**
anal intermuscular s.
aneurysm of atrial s.
aneurysm of membranous ventricular s.
anterior crural s.
anterior intermuscular s.
anterior nasal s.
anterior vein of septum pellucidum
anteroapical trabecular s.
anteromedial intermuscular s.
ascending bladder s.
atrial septum excision
atrioventricular nodal s.
congenital defect interventricular septum of heart
deflection of nasal s.
depressor muscle of septum of nose
descending rectal s.
deviated nasal s.
s. of glans penis
s. of heart
high membranous interventricular s.
s. intact
intact ventricular s.
interatrial s.
interventricular s.
interventricular septum aneurysm

septum *(continued)*
left s.
medial intermuscular s.
midvaginal transverse s.
muscular atrioventricular s.
muscular ventricular s.
s. pellucidum
s. pellucidum absent with porencephalia syndrome
pulmonary atresia with intact ventricular s.
right s.
ruptured interventricular s.
supravaginal s.
Swiss cheese interventricular s.
syndrome of absence of septum pellucidum with poerencephaly
ventricular s.

sequela, pl. **sequelae**
delayed neuropsychological s.
long-term sequelae
no sequelae
s. of therapy
well-healed, no sequelae

sequence
adenomatous polyp-cancer s.
amino acid s.
amniotic band s.
autonomous replication s.
Carr-Purcell s.
Carr-Purcell-Meiboom-Gill s.
congenital thrombocytopenia, Robin sequence, agenesis of corpus callosum, distinctive facies, developmental delay syndrome
contrast-enhanced fast s.
developmental sequence posture
esophageal manometric s.
s. of events
expressed sequence tag
expression sequence tagged
fast imaging steady precession sequence three-dimensional magnetic resonance imaging
fast-repeating high s.
fetal akinesia deformation s.
field-echo sequence with even-echo rephasing
gene-activating s.
immunostimulatory DNA s.
ingressive-egressive s.
insertion s.
intervening s.
inversion recovery spin-echo s.
linear sebaceous nevus s.
long terminal repeat s.
magnetization-prepared 3D gradient-echo s.
melanocyte-stimulating hormone s.
mental retardation-overgrowth s.
missed ostium s.
mitochondrial targeting s.
nucleotide sequence analysis
operon promoter s.
out of s.
pancreatic islet cell-specific enhancer s.
pulse s.
rapid sequence induction orotracheal intubation
rapid sequence intubation
upstream activating s.

sequenced
Adapted S. Inventory of Communication Development
S. Inventory of Language Development

sequenced-based typing

sequence-independent single primer amplification

sequence-specific
s.-s. DNA primer
s.-s. oligonucleotide probe hybridization

sequence-tagged sites

sequencing
auditory vocal s.
Denver Auditory Phoneme S. Test
s. by hybridization
massively parallel signature s.
molecular cloning and s.
nucleic acid s.
Visual-Motor S. Test

sequential
s. access
s. analysis
s. analysis of twelve chemistry constituents
s. atrioventricular pacing
atrioventricular sequential pacing
s. combination chemotherapy
s. compression device
s. developmental exercises
s. free flap
s. hemibody irradiation
s. impaction cascade sieve volumetric air sampler
s. multichannel autoanalyzer
s. multiple analysis
s. multiple analyzer
s. oral contraceptive
s. organ failure assessment
s. paired opposed plaque
point estimation by sequential testing
s. postremission chemotherapy
s. probability ratio test
s. pulse
s. scalar quantization
segmental sequential irradiation
S. Tests of Educational Progress, Series III
s. treatment employing pharmacologic support
s. ultrafiltration
s. vascular response
s. ventriculoatrial pacing
s. volitional oral movement

sequestered
s. antigen
s. lung

sequestration
acute splenic sequestration crisis
bronchopulmonary s.
s. cyst
extralobar s.
pulmonary s.

sequestrum
associated s.
avascular s.

sera (*pl. of* serum)

Serafini hernia

serenity, tranquility, peace user's term for dimethoxymethylamphetamine

Sergent white line

serial
s. analysis of gene expression
s. autocorrelation
s. blood sugar
computer-assisted reconstruction by tracing of serial sections
s. CT
s. duplex scan
s. focus seizures
incision closed in serial fashion
s. multiple analysis
S.'s on Line
Paced Auditory S. Addition Test
s. probe recognition
s. 7's
s. sevens test
s. thrombin time
s. transverse section

serial-agitated dilution

series
acute abdominal s.
acute infectious disease s.
anion of the Hofmeister s.
s. elastic component of muscles
s. elastic element
first in alpha series or group
Fourier s.
fourth in a series or group
full-mouth s.
gallbladder s.
gastrointestinal s.
liver function s.
metabolic bone s.
Missouri Children's Picture Series
Sequential Tests of Educational Progress, S. III
small bowel s.
upper gastrointestinal series with small bowel follow-through
upper GI s.

serine
s. dehydrase
s. glycerophosphatide
lymphocyte serine esterase
s. protease inhibitor
s. proteinase
s. threonine kinase gene 11

serious
s. adverse event
s. emotional disturbance
s. gum disease
s. health risk
s. illness
s. impulsive dyscontrol
no serious abnormality
warning signs of serious illness

seriously ill list

seroconversion
HIV s.
human immunodeficiency virus s.

serodiagnosis
hepatitis s.

seroenzyme reaction

seroepidemiological study

serogroup
s. C meningococcal vaccine
meningococcal *Neisseria meningitidis* s.'s unspecified vaccine

serologic
s. assay
biological false-positive serologic test for syphilis
blood serologic test
major serologic antigen
nontreponemal serologic test
s. test for syphilis
s. typing
Youman-Parlett serologic test

serological
ascariasis serological test
s. marker of disease

serologically
s. defined
s. detectable
s. determined

serologic-blocking factor

serology
AIDS s.
Aspergillus s.
hepatitis C s.
HIV s.
Lyme arthritis s.
Lyme disease s.
mumps s.
Mycoplasma s.
s. nonreactive
nonreactive s.
nontreponemal s.
parainfluenza virus s.
parvovirus B19 s.
pertussis s.
RSV s.

seroma
auricular s.

seromucous cell

seromuscular
s. enterocystoplasty lined with urothelium
s. layer
s. stitch
s. suture

seromyotomy
anterior s.

seronegative
s. arthritis
s. arthropathy
oligoarticular seronegative rheumatoid arthritis
s. polyarthritis
remitting seronegative symmetric synovitis with pitting edema
s. spondyloarthropathy

seronegativity, enthesopathy, arthropathy

seropositive
ANA s.
anti-HCV s.
antihepatitis C virus s.
s. disease
s. reaction

seropositivity
HIV s.

seropurulent discharge

serosa
s. of colon
s. of esophagus
s. of gallbladder
intestinal s.
s. of large intestine
s. of liver
lochia s.

serosal
s. adhesion
s. fluid
s. fold
s. hemorrhage
metastatic adenocarcinoma serosal surfaces
s. surface

serosanguineous
s. discharge
s. drainage
s. fluid

seroserous suture

serositis
multiple s.

serotherapy
percutaneous alcohol s.

serotonergic
noradrenergic and specific serotonergic antidepressant

serotonin
s. antagonist
s. deficiency
5-hydroxytryptamine serotonin
monoamine s.
s. noradrenergic reuptake inhibitor
s. reuptake transporter
selective serotonin reuptake inhibitor
s. syndrome

serotonin-binding protein

serotonin/dopamine antagonist

serotonin-norepinephrine reuptake inhibitor

serotype
s. A, B, C virus
homologous s.
human astrovirus serotype 1–7
nonvaccine s.
vaccine s.

serous
s. adenocarcinoma
bilateral serous otitis media
s. borderline tumor
s. cell
central serous chorioretinopathy
central serous choroidopathy
central serous retinopathy
s. cyst
s. cystadenoma
s. diarrhea
s. effusion
s. epithelial ovarian carcinoma
s. fluid
s. gland
s. granule
s. hemorrhage
idiopathic central serous chorioretinopathy
s. iritis
s. ligament
s. membrane
micropapillary serous ovarian carcinoma
s. otitis
s. otitis media
ovarian papillary serous adenocarcinoma
ovarian serous borderline tumor
papillary serous carcinoma of the peritoneum
papillary serous cystadenocarcinoma
parietal layer of serous pericardium
s. pericardium
peripapillary central serous choroidopathy
s. retinitis
uterine papillary serous carcinoma
visceral layer of serous pericardium
yellow-brown serous ascites

serpentine
s. aneurysm
s. incision

serpiginosa

serpiginosum
angioma s.

serpiginosus
lupus s.

serpiginous
s. border
s. chancroid
s. choroidopathy
s. corneal ulcer

Serra do Navio virus

serrata
nasal ora s.

serrated appearance

serratus
s. anterior
s. anterior muscle flap
anterior serratus muscle
aponeurosis of posterior superior s.

Serres
S. angle
S. gland

Sertoli
S. cell
S. cell culture medium
S. cell index
S. cell mesenchyme tumor
S. cell-only tumor
S. column
large cell calcifying Sertoli cell tumor

sertoliform endometrioid carcinoma

Sertoli-Leydig cell tumor

serum, pl. **sera**
s. accelerator factor
acetone-extracted s.
acidified serum, acidified complement
s. acid phosphatase
acute serum sickness
adult bovine s.
s. albumin
s. alcohol level
s. aldolase
s. aldosterone
s. alkaline phosphatase
s. aminoglycoside concentration
amoxicilloyl-human serum albumin
ampicillin-human serum albumin
s. amylase
s. amyloid P component
s. amyloid type A
s. angiotensin-converting enzyme
anomalous serum chemistry
anti-B s.
antibiotic concentration in serum and tissue
antibovine serum albumin antibody
s. antichymotrypsin
antifibroblast s.
antigas gangrene s.
anti-HIV immune serum globulin
antihuman immunodeficiency virus immune serum globulin
antihuman lymphocyte s.
antihuman thymus s.
antiinsulin s.
antikidney serum nephritis
antilymphocyte s.
antimacrophage s.
antimouse lymphocyte s.
antineutrophilic s.
antirabies s.
antireticular cytotoxic s.
antitetanus s.
antithymocyte s.
s. antitrypsin
antiviral lymphocyte s.
anti-Yo serum antibody
s. ascites-albumin gradient
Australia serum hepatitis antigen
autologous serum application
s. bactericidal activity
s. bactericidal concentration
s. bactericidal level
s. bactericidal test
s. bactericidal titer
s. bacteriologic titer
beef serum albumin
beekeeper s.
s. bicarbonate
s. bile acid
s. bilirubin
s. blocking factor
s. blood sugar
bound serum iron
bovine serum albumin
s. calcium
calculated serum osmolality
calf s.
cancer serum index
s. carboxypeptidase N
s., casein, glucose, yeast extract medium
s. chemistry graft
s. chemistry graph
s. chemogram
s. chloride
s. cholesterol
s. cholinesterase
citrated normal rabbit s.
s. complement C1–C9
control s.
s. copper level
s. creatine kinase
s. creatine phosphokinase
s. creatinine
s. creatinine test

s. cryptococcal antigen
s. defect
delipidized serum protein
despeciated bovine s.
s. digoxin concentration
s. digoxin level
s. disease
disease control s.
s. drug concentration
s. drug level
Dubois oleic serum complex
electrolytes, blood urea nitrogen, and serum creatinine
s. electrophoresis
s. enzyme study
equine antihuman lymphoblast s.
equine serum hepatitis
s. factor
fasting serum glucose
fasting serum level
s. ferritin
fetal bovine s.
fetal calf s.
s. fibrinogen
fluorescein-labeled serum protein
s. folic acid
s. fungicidal
s. fungistatic
gamma globulin-free calf s.
s. gamma-glutamyltransferase
s. gentamicin concentration
s. globulin
s. glucose
glucose, lactalbumin, serum, and hemoglobin
s. glucose monitoring
s. glutamic-oxaloacetic transaminase
s. glutamic-oxaloacetic transferase
s. glutamic-pyruvic transaminase
glycosylated serum protein
goat s.
guinea pig antiinsulin s.
s. half-life
heated serum reagent
heat-inactivated fetal bovine s.
heat-inactivated fetal calf s.
hemopexin serum protein
s. hepatitis
s. hepatitis antigen
s. hepatitis-associated antigen antibody
hereditary erythroblastic multinuclearity with positive acidified s.
homologous s.
homologous serum jaundice
horse s.
human cord s.
human hypopituitary s.
human immune serum globulin
human serum albumin
human serum esterase
human serum prealbumin
human serum protein
human serum thymus factor
s. hydroxybutyrate dehydrogenase
s. hydroxybutyric dehydrogenase
hyperimmune s.
hyperimmune serum globulin
immune s.
s. immunoelectrophoresis
s. immunofixation electrophoresis
s. immunoglobulin
immunoreactive bovine serum albumin
immunoreactive insulin to serum or plasma glucose ratio
s. immunoreactive parathyroid hormone
inactivated fetal calf s.
inactivated horse s.
s. index
s. inhibitor of streptolysin S
s. inhibitory activity
s. inhibitory concentration
s. inhibitory factor
s. inhibitory titer
s. insulin
s. insulin concentration
s. intoxication
intravenous immune serum globulin
iodinated bovine serum albumin
iodinated human serum albumin
iodinated rat serum albumin
s. iron
s. iron-binding capacity
iron saturation of serum transferrin
s. isocitrate dehydrogenase
s. lactate dehydrogenase
lactating rat serum factor
s. leucine aminopeptidase
s. lidocaine level
s. lipophosphoprotein
liquid human s.
liver enzyme serum level
liver regenerating serum factor
Locke egg serum medium
Löffler coagulated serum medium
s. lysozyme
MacFarlane serum method
maleated bovine serum albumin
maternal serum alpha fetoprotein
maternal serum level
measles convalescent s.
s. methyl alcohol level
methylated bovine serum albumin
s. methylguanidine
microaggregated human serum albumin
microdilution serum bactericidal test
modified immune serum globulin
s. monoamine oxidase
mouse antirat s.
mouse serum albumin
muscle enzyme serum level
s. myelin basic protein
nephrotoxic s.
s. neutralization
newborn calf s.
newborn screen serum thyroxine and phenylketonuria
noncurrent s.
nonimmune sheep serum
nonimmunized rabbit s.
normal s.
s. normal agglutinator
normal blood s.
normal burro s.
normal dog s.
normal goat s.
normal horse s.
normal human s.
normal inactivated rabbit s.
normal mouse s.
normal reference s.
normal serum albumin
normal serum thyroxine
North American antisnakebite s.
s. ornithine carbamoyltransferase
osmolality s.
s. osmolality
Osteomark NTx serum test
s. parvo virus-like virus
patient-heated s.
patient's s.
peak maximum serum concentration
peak serum level
s. phenylalanine concentration
phosphatase acid s.
pigeon s.
pooled human s.
s. precipitable iodine
predialyzed human s.
pregnancy s.
pregnant mare s.

serum *(continued)*
pregnant mare serum gonadotropin
s. protein-bound iodine
s. protein electrolytes
s. protein electrophoresis
s. protein electrophoretogram
s. protein and immunofixation electrophoresis system
s. protein level
s. prothrombin activity
s. prothrombin conversion accelerator
s. pyruvate kinase
rabbit antidog-thymus s.
rabbit antithymocyte s.
rabbit ovarian antitumor s.
rabbit serum albumin
radioactive iodinated human serum albumin
radioactive iodinated serum albumin
radioiodinated serum albumin
ratio of serum alanine aminotransferase to serum aspartate aminotransferase
rat serum albumin
rat serum protein
reference normal s.
s. reserve cholesterol binding capacity
s. resin triiodothyronine uptake
rheumatoid arthritis serum factor
s. inhibitor of streptolysin S
s. shock
s. sickness
s. sodium
s. soluble antigen
sulfation factor of blood s.
technetium-99m galactosyl-human serum albumin
tetanus antitoxic s.
s. theophylline concentration
s. theophylline level
theophylline serum concentration
s. thiocyanate
s. thrombotic accelerator
s. thymus factor
s. thyroxine measured by column chromatography
s. thyroxine measured by displacement analysis
s. tissue polypeptide antigen
s. tobramycin assay
toluidine red unheated serum test
total serum hemolytic complement
total immunoreactive serum pepsinogen
total serum bile acid
total serum bilirubin
total serum prostatic acid phosphatase
total serum protein
total serum solids
s. transferrin
s. triglyceride level
trough minimum serum concentration
s. trypsin inhibition capacity
s. trypsin inhibitor
tumor necrosis s.
unheated serum reagin
s. urea nitrogen
s. uric acid
Veronal-buffered saline-fetal bovine s.
s. viscosity
s. Wassermann reaction
s. xanthine oxidase
zoster serum immunoglobulin
zymosan-activated autologous s.
zymosan-treated s.

serum-bound
iron low s.-b.

serum-free
s.-f. fatty acid
s.-f. hemoglobin
s.-f. thyroxin

serum-inhibiting titer

serum-killing level

serum-neutralizing

serum-platelet bindable immunoglobulin G

service
adult recovery s.'s
S. Assessment for Children and Adolescents
Child Protective S.'s
clinical pharmacokinetics consulting s.
s. connected
consultation s.
disability determination s.
existed prior to s.
home, no services needed
s. hours
Individualized Family S. Plan
inpatient geriatric consultation s.'s
integrated medical s.'s
maternal and child health s.
nutritional support s.
palliative care s.
personal care s.
pharmacokinetic drug-monitoring s.
physical therapy s.'s
physician referral s.
point of s.
pregnancy advisory s.
pregnancy interruption s.
protective s.'s
psychiatric emergency s.
psychiatric services section
public service announcement
Quality Point of S.
s. record
specialty inpatient s.
training and placement s.
transfusion therapy s.
Utilization Information S.
Visual Impairment S.
volunteer transport s.

service-connected
s.-c. disability
outpatient treatment, s.-c.

service-related disability

Servo
Isolette Servo control

sesamoid
axial sesamoid projection
axial sesamoid view
s. bone
s. cartilage
fibular s.
s. fracture
tibial sesamoid position

sesamoidectomy
fibular s.

sesquioleate
sorbitan s.

sessile
gastric antral sessile polyp
s. hydatid
s. lesion
s. polyp

session
adjunctive individual s.
alpha conditioning s.
auditory training s.'s
group support s.
group therapy s.
individual counseling s.'s

sestamibi
s. imaging
s. scan
s. stress test
thallium s.

set
altered set point
aluminum contouring template s.
articular set angle
automatic zero s.
distal articular set angle
first set of followup data
gluteal s.'s
hamstring s.'s
intermittent infusion s.
minimum basis set magnetic resonance angiography
minimum data s.
Outcomes and Assessment Information S.
pediatric vitrectomy lens s.
proximal articular set angle
quadriceps s.
second set of followup data

setback
sagittal split s.

seton
s. operation
s. wound

Settegast position

setter
bone plug s.
fire s.
non-fire s.

setting
aperture current s.
assisted living s.
partial hospital s.

settling
gravity settling culture plate

set-up
new patient s.-u.

seven
health level s.
serial s.'s test

seventh
Metropolitan Achievement Test, S. Edition
s. cranial nerve

Sever disease

severe
s. acidosis
acquired severe aplastic anemia
s. acute pancreatitis
acute severe hypotension
s. agitation
s. allergies
s. anoxic encephalopathy
s. anxiety
s. aplastic anemia
s. ataxia
Athabascan type of severe combined immunodeficiency disease
s. atheromatous change of aorta
s. autoimmune disease
s. autonomic insufficiency
autosomal recessive severe combined immunodeficiency disorder
s. bone loss
Boston Assessment of S. Aphasia
s. childhood autosomal recessive muscular dystrophy
s. chronic neutropenia
s. combined immune deficiency
s. combined immune deficiency syndrome
s. combined immunodeficiency disease
s. combined immunodeficient mice
s. congenital anomaly
s. congenital neutropenia
s. coronary arteriosclerosis
s. debilitating symptom
s. deficit
s. dehydration
s. dementia
s. depression
s. depressive illness
s. disability
s. disabling handicap
s. dissociative symptom
s. emotional handicap
s. functional insufficiency
s. gastritis
s. gastrointestinal bleeding
s. headache
s. head trauma
s. hearing loss
s. heartburn
s. heart valve narrowing
s. hemophilia
s. hemorrhagic pancreatitis
s. hypertension
s. impairment
s. impairment of hearing
s. impairment in interpretation of reality
s. impairment in thinking
s. impairment of ventricle
s. infection
s. insomnia
intermittent attacks of severe vertigo
s. intestinal infection
s. intracranial lesion
s. invasion streptococcal syndrome
s., jabbing facial pain
s. joint pain and fatigue
s. ketoacidosis
s. latex allergy
s. mental illness
s. mental retardation
s. myoclonic epilepsy
s. myoclonic epilepsy in infancy
s. myopia
s. nail-biting habit
s. neurological impairment
s. obstruction
s. ovarian hyperstimulation syndrome
s. pancreatic insufficiency
s. paralytic illness
patient with severe systemic disease limiting activity but not incapacitating
s. and persistent mental illness
s. renal failure
s. renal insufficiency
s. respiratory insufficiency
s. sensorineural hearing loss
sudden, severe headache
s. throbbing headache
s. visual loss
s. withdrawal reaction
X-linked severe combined immunodeficiency

severed
s. jugular vein
s. limb salvage technique
s. surface of bone

severely
s. affected individual
Assessment for Persons Profoundly or S. Impaired
s. disabled
s. impaired renal function
s. low birth weight
s. mentally impaired
s. and profoundly handicapped
s. subnormal
s. swollen ankle
s. traumatized brain
s. weakened heart

Severin
anatomical classification system of S.

severity
Abbreviated Injury Score/Injury S. Score

severity *(continued)*
Addiction S. Index
Adolescent Problem S. Index
APACHE II measure of disease s.
assessing severity: age of patient, systems involved, stage of disease, complications, response to therapy
Asthma S. Score
Atopic Dermatitis Area and S. Index
childhood severity of psychiatric illness
computed tomography severity index
Crohn Disease Endoscopic Index of S.
Dermatology Index of Disease S.
Eczema Area and S. Index
foot and ankle severity scale
Functional Bowel Disorder S. Index
Glasgow Dyspepsia S. Score
Global S. Index of Brief Symptom Inventory
s. index
s. of injury
Injury S. Scale
Injury S. Score
injury severity index
insufficient severity of duration
International Classification of Diseases 9th Ed. Injury S. Score
Liverpool Seizure S. Scale
Mangled Extremity S. Score
Modified Injury S. Score
Multiple S. of Illness System
New Injury S. Score
Overt Agitation S. Scale
pain increasing in s.
palliation, quality, radiation, severity, time
Pediatric Acute Admission S. classification
Peritonitis S. Score
Pneumonia S. Index
position, quality, radiation, severity, time
psoriasis area and severity index
psoriasis severity scale
S. Scoring of Atopic Dermatitis
stuttering severity instrument
symptom severity index
symptoms increased in s.
Teen Addiction S. Index
Total S. Assessment
Trauma and Injury S. Scores
Yale Global Tic S. Scale

Sever-L'Episcopo repair of shoulder

Sewall-Boyden flap

sewing ring area

sex
absence of sex chromosome
adolescent sex offender
adult-child s.
anal s.
s. arousal mechanism
assigned s.
Bem S. Role Inventory
casual s.
s. cell
s. change
s. chromatin
s. chromatin test
s. chromosome
s. cord
s. cord tumors with annular tubules
s. counseling
decline in interest of opposite s.
s. determination
s. deviant
s. difference in life expectancy
dosage-sensitive sex reversal
s. drive
s. education
environmental sex determination
female sex chromosome
female sex hormone
fighting, injuries, sex, threats, self-defense
s. headache
s. hormone
s. hormone-binding globulin
illicit s.
indeterminate s.
s. inventory
s. karyotypes
S. Knowledge and Attitude Test
s. and love addictions
male sex chromosome
male sex differentiation
male sex hormone
mentally disordered sex offender
men who have sex with men
mesenchymal sex cord stromal tumor
mixed sex cord-stromal tumor
morphological s.
normal female sex chromosome type
normal male sex chromosome type
nuclear s.
s. offender
opposite biological s.
parental attitudes toward s.
presence of only one sex chromosome
production of sex hormone
s. ratio
s. reassignment surgery
secondary sex characteristic
s. steroid-binding globulin

sex-cord
uterine tumor resembling an ovarian sex-cord tumor

sex-determining region

sex-limited protein

sex-linked
s.-l. disease
s.-l. disorder
s.-l. heredity
s.-l. hypophosphatemic rickets
s.-l. trait

sextant
transrectal ultrasound-guided sextant biopsy

sexual
aberrant sexual behavior
s. aberration
s. abstinence
s. abuse
s. abuse of child
s. abuse group
s. abuse history
s. activity
S. Adjustment Questionnaire
adolescent sexual activity
adolescent sexual change
adolescent sexual ideation
adolescent sexual identity
age-inappropriate knowledge of sexual behavior
alcohol-induced sexual dysfunction
amphetamine-induced sexual dysfunction
anomalous sexual behavior
anomalous sexual urge
antipsychotic-associated sexual dysfunction
anxiolytic-induced sexual dysfunction
S. Arousability Inventory
s. arousal

s. assault forensic evidence
s. assault nurse examiner
S. Assault Response Team
s. attitude reassessment
s. attitude restructuring
s. battering
Brief Index of S. Functioning for Women
change in sexual habit
Child S. Behavior Inventory
childhood sexual abuse
S. Compatibility Test
s. complications of drug abuse
compulsive sexual behavior
consensual sexual behavior
criminal sexual psychopath
decline in sexual function
decreased sexual interest
delayed sexual development
s. desire
destructive sexual behavior
s. deviant
s. differentiation scale
dissociation and sexual abuse
s. dysfunction
s. dysfunction after heart attack
s. encounter
s. excitement
s. experience
female sexual arousal disorder
female sexual dysfunction
forced sexual encounter
s. functioning
S. Functioning Index
S. Function Inventory Questionnaire
s. function score
s. function of women
Global S. Satisfaction Index
s. harassment
heightened sexual drive
high-risk sexual activity
high-risk sexual behavior
s. history
hypoactive sexual desire disorder
s. identity
impaired sexual development
s. impairment
s. impotence
s. impulsiveness
s. inadequacy
inadequate sexual function
inappropriate sexual behavior
increased sexual appetite
increased sexual desire
inhibited sexual desire
inhibited sexual excitement
s. intercourse
s. interest
s. inversion
involuntary deviate sexual intercourse
s. issue
last sexual contact
loss of sexual interest
male hypoactive sexual desire disorder
s. maturity rating
s. molestation
S. Myths Scale
painful sexual intercourse
postponing sexual involvement
Professional S. Role Inventory
s. transmission of viral hepatitis
s. tubal sterilization

sexuality
index of s.
s. issue
S. Preference Profile

sexually
s. acquired reactive arthritis
s. active homosexual men
s. dimorphic nucleus
inappropriate sexually provocative behavior
s. oriented hallucination
s. transmitted condition
s. transmitted disease
s. transmitted infection

sexual/reproductive system impairment

Sézary
S. cell
S. erythroderma
S. syndrome

Sgambati reaction

shaded-surface display

shade response to light gray area

shading
s. response to black areas
s. response to gray areas

shadow
s. cell
s. corpuscle
gallbladder s.
heart s.
hilar s.
liver s.
mitral configuration of cardiac s.
nipple s.
nodular s.
opaque s.
overlying bowel s.'s
overlying gas s.
psoas s.
snowstorm s.
soft tissue s.
superimposition of bowel s.
s. test
wall-echo s.

shaft
s. of bone
s. of clavicle
endoscope s.
femoral shaft axis
femoral shaft malunion
s. of femur
s. of fibula
s. fracture
hair s.
head, neck, and s.
humeral s.
humeral shaft fracture
s. of humerus
medulla of hair s.
penile s.
proximal s.
tibial s.
ulnar s.

shag
aortic s.

shaggy pericardium

shagreen
anterior capsule s.
anterior mosaic crocodile s.
s. of the lens

shake
nonalcoholic white shake lotion
wet dog s.'s syndrome
withdrawal body s.'s

shaken baby syndrome

shaking
s. chills and night sweats
disabling shaking and trembling
hyperventilating, sweating and s.

shaky
handwriting progressively s.

shallow
s. affected
s. breathing
s. compartment
s. distance
focal shallow subpleural hemorrhage
Rapid S. Breathing Index

shallow *(continued)*
rapid shallow breathing
s. respiration
shallowing
anterior chamber s.
sham
s. feeding
modified sham feeding
s. operation
s. transcutaneous nerve stimulation
Shambaugh endaural incision
shambling gait
shame
guilt and s.
s. and guilt
Shamonda virus
shampoo
bath, laxative, enema, shampoo, and shower
shape
S.'s Analysis Test
anatomical position of duodenum
aneurysm with simple s.
fundus anterior, normal size and shape, and mobile
heart size and s.
s. of incisions in V-Y plasty
s. memory alloy
normal size and s.
normal size, shape, and position, anteverted and anteflexed uterus
normal size, shape, and consistency
normal size, shape, and location
normal size, shape, and position
s. of surgical incisions W-plasty
s. of surgical incision Z-plasty
vertebral body s.
shaped
irregularly shaped bone
shaper
automated corneal s.
rapid body s.
shaping
s. of breast
shaping of breast
Shapiro sign
shared haplotypes
sharing
history of needle s.
s. infected intravenous drug needle
needle s.
organ s.
shark
s. liver oil
S. River virus
sharp
s. and blunt dissection
blunt and sharp dissection
s. Bragg peak
carina midline sharp and mobile
central sharp wave transient
centrotemporal sharp wave
contaminated s.'s
s. curettage
s. dissection
s. dissection technique
s., jabbing or electrical pain
periodic sharp wave complex
s. and pink
positive occipital sharp transients of sleep
positive sharp wave fibrillations
significant sharp spike or delta wave
small sharp spike
vertex sharp transient electroencephalography
sharper hearing
Sharpey
S. fiber
perforating fibers of S.
sharply demarcated circumferential lesion
Sharrard-type kyphectomy
shave
s. excision
s. excisional biopsy
lip s.
shaved
s. biopsy
s. plaque
shaver
arthroscopic s.
automated s.
cartilage shaver blade
cutting s.
S. disease
shaving
arthroscopic s.
femoral condylar s.
shawl scrotum
shear
anterior s.
s. force
s. fracture
s. stress
vertical s.
shearing force
Shea stapedectomy
sheath
anterior layer of rectus abdominis s.
anterior tarsal tendinous s.
anular part of fibrous digital sheath of digits of hand and foot
anulus of fibrous s.
arachnoid nerve root sheath dilation
arcuate line of rectus s.
carotid s.
connective tissue s.
s. and dilator system
extensor carpi ulnaris s.
flexor tendon s.
giant cell tumor of tendon s.
s. ligament
malignant nerve sheath tumor
malignant peripheral nerve sheath tumor
Mullins long transseptal s.
nerve s.
nerve sheath malignant tumor
nerve sheath meningioma
optic nerve s.
optic nerve sheath decompression
optic nerve sheath fenestration
optic nerve sheath meningioma
palmar carpal tendinous s.
periarterial lymphatic s.
periarteriolar lymphocyte s.
perioptic sheath meningioma
peripheral nerve sheath tumor
rectus sheath hematoma
Spectranetics laser s.
sport s.
sheathed artery
sheathing
arteriolar s.
peripheral retinal vascular s.
perivascular s.
shed
mediastinal shed blood
shedding
asymptomatic viral s.
chronic fecal s.
excessive hair s.
herpes simplex viral s.
nail s.
s. of nails

Sheehan
S. disease
S. Patient Rated Anxiety Scale
S. syndrome
Sheehy syndrome
sheen
S. airway reconstruction
skin s.
sheep
s. cell agglutination test
s. cell agglutination titer
s. erythrocyte
s. erythrocyte agglutination test
s. erythrocyte antibody
s. erythrocyte antigen
s. factor delta
s. hemolysate supernatant
nonimmune sheep serum
normal sheep lung fibroblast
normal sheep red blood cell
s. pulmonary adenomatosis
s. red blood cell
s. red cell rosette-forming cell
s. seminal vesicle
sensitized sheep cell agglutination
trypsinized sheep red blood cell
sheet
investigational drug data s.
material safety data s.
Timed Behavioral Rating S.
sheeting
architectural s.
micromesh s.
occlusive s.
silicone gel s.
Sheffield
S. Screening Test for Acquired Language Disorders
S. treadmill protocol
shelf
crescentic shelf osteotomy
shelf-type implant
shell
acetabular s.
s. fragment
s. fragment wound
s. implant
total hip articular replacement by internal eccentric s.'s
shelled
gallbladder shelled out from the gallbladder bed
shellfish
diarrheic shellfish poisoning
shelving
s. border of inguinal ligament
s. incision
ligament shelving edge
Shenstone tourniquet
Shenton arch
Sheridan Tests for Young Children and Retardates
Sherman
Fort Sherman virus
Sherrington law
shiatsu massage
Shibley sign
shield
eye pad and shield applied
Fox eye s.
gastric s.
high-humidity tracheostomy s.
lead apron s.
Mueller eye s.
protective eye s.
splatter control s.
shielding
critical organ shielding blocks
lead shielding in radiation
lung s.
shift
anterior ankle shift operation
anterior capsular s.
anterior talus s.
aromatic solvent-induced s.
atraumatic, multidirectional, bilateral rehabilitation inferior capsular s.
s. in attention
attention shift ability
change of s.
chemical shift imaging
chemical shift misregistration artifact
chemical shift selective
contralateral threshold s.
s. in direction and pattern of brain electrical activity
electrophoretic mobility shift analysis
electrophoretic mobility shift assay
extradimensional s.
inferior capsular s.
microbial antigenic phase s.
mobility shift assay
Neer capsular shift procedure
noise-induced permanent threshold s.
noise-induced temporary threshold s.
O'Brien capsular shift procedure
paramagnetic enhancement accentuation by chemical shift imaging
paroxysmal depolarization s.
paroxysmal depolarizing s.
permanent threshold s.
phase shift artifact
pivot shift test
proximal brain s.
reverse pivot s.
scaphoid shift maneuver
sustained depolarizing s.
temporary threshold s.
shifting
associative s.
s. goal
Shiga
S. bacillus
Shiga-like toxin
Shigella
Shigella diarrhea
Shigella dysentery
Shigella infection
Shigella mutant
Shigella-like toxin-producing *Escherichia coli*
shin
anterior shin splint
s. bone
s. bone fever
saber s.
shiner
allergic s.
golden shiner virus
shingles
chills from s.
Shinowara-Jones-Reinhart unit
ship
hospital s.
Shipley
S. Institute of Living Scale
S. Personal Inventory
Shipley-Hartford Scale
Shirley drain
Shirodkar
S. needle
S. operation
shivering
visual observation shivering score
shock
anaphylactic shock prophylaxis

shock *(continued)*
s. antigen
cardiac shock wave therapy
cardiogenic s.
confusion from insulin s.
convulsive shock therapy
deep shock insulin
delayed s.
dengue hemorrhagic fever shock syndrome
diarrhea from toxic shock syndrome
electric shock therapy
electric shock treatment
electroconvulsive shock therapy
electroconvulsive shock treatment
electrohydraulic shock wave lithotripsy
extracorporeal shock wave therapy
extracorporeal shock wave lithotripsy
Gram-negative endotoxic s.
Gram-negative endotoxin-induced s.
gut-derived infectious toxic s.
heart defibrillated with single s.
s. heart into normal rhythm
heat shock protein
hemorrhage and s.
hemorrhagic shock and encephalopathy
hemorrhagic shock syndrome
high-energy transthoracic s.
hypoosmotic shock treatment
s. index
insulin shock therapy
insulin shock treatment
intraperitoneal s.
laser-induced intracorporeal shock wave lithotripsy
levels of shock intensity
s. lung
Mengert shock syndrome
menstrual toxic shock syndrome
nonmenstrual toxic shock syndrome
patient in cardiogenic s.
s.'s per minute
peroral shock wave lithotripsy
postcardiotomy s.
regressive electric shock therapy
septic s.
septic shock syndrome
staphylococcal toxic shock syndrome
streptococcal toxic shock syndrome
s. therapy
toxic shock antigen
toxic shock syndrome exoprotein
toxic shock syndrome exotoxin
toxic shock syndrome toxin
s. trauma unit
uncontrolled hemorrhagic s.
s. wave lithotripsy

shocked
heart shocked during cardiac arrest

shock-elicited aggression

shock-induced suppression of drinking

shock-wave therapy

shocky
pallid and s.

shoe
arthritic s.
athletic shoe carbon fiber plate
bone graft shoe horn
corrective s.
custom-made s.
custom-molded s.
ill-fitting s.'s
long-handled shoe horn
metatarsal bar shoe modification
navicular cookie in s.
orthotic s.
swing-out s.

Shokwe virus

Shone
S. anomaly
S. complex

Shope papillomavirus

Shorr stain

short
s. above-elbow cast
agonadism, mental retardation, short stature, retarded bone age syndrome
anatomic short leg
s. arc motion
s. arm brace
s. arm cast
s. arm of chromosome X
s. arm cylinder cast
s. arm fiberglass cast
s. arm navicular cast
s. arm plaster splint
s. arm posterior-molded splint
s. arm sugar-tong splint
s. arm thumb spica cast
asymmetric short stature syndrome
s. attention span
autosomal dominant mild short limb dwarfism
s. axis
s. axis image
s. axis plane
Beck Depression Index S. Form
s. below-elbow cast
bilateral short leg cane
s. bowel syndrome
brittle hair, intellectual impairment, decreased fertility, short stature syndrome
s. calcaneocuboid
cataract, motor system disorder, short stature, learning difficulty, skeletal abnormalities syndrome
caudal appendage, short terminal phalanges, deafness, cryptorchidism, mental retardation syndrome
s. circuit current
S. Clinical Rating Scale
cluster of short gram-negative rods
congenital cataracts, sensorineural deafness, Down syndrome facial appearance, short stature, mental retardation syndrome
s. course chemotherapy
s. crus of incus
deafness, femoral epiphysial dysplasia, short stature, developmental delay syndrome
deep sleep of short duration
deletion of short arm of chromosome X
diathermy short wave
digital anomalies, short palpebral fissures, atresia of esophagus or duodenum syndrome
directly observed treatment, short course
s. distance group
s. double upright
s. duration, unilateral, neuralgic, conjunctival injection and tearing
ear, patella, short stature syndrome
end of short arm of chromosome
Factor Analyzed S. Form
s. foot drape
S. Form Test of Academic Aptitude
s. gastric vein

gonadal failure, short stature, mitral valve prolapse, mental retardation syndrome
goniodysgenesis, mental retardation, short stature
s. gut syndrome
s. half-life
s. hydrophobic
ichthyosis, brittle hair, impaired intelligence, decreased fertility, short stature syndrome
idiopathic short stature
s. increment sensitivity index
S. Inflammatory Bowel Disease Questionnaire
s. intense course
s. interspersed elements
s. inversion imaging recovery
36-item short form health survey
s. latent-evoked potential
left short leg
s. leg brace
s. leg cylinder cast
s. leg nonwalking cast
s. leg nonweightbearing cast
s. leg posterior-molded splint
s. leg walking cast
s. limb dwarfism
low-dose short synacthen test
s. luteal phase
macrocephaly, hypertelorism, short limbs, hearing loss, developmental delay syndrome
Majewski short rib polydactyly
Marchac and Chiari short scar technique
medical short procedure unit
mental retardation, epilepsy, short stature, skeletal dysplasia syndrome
mental retardation, short stature, hypertelorism syndrome
mental retardation, short stature, obesity, hypogonadism syndrome
S. Michigan Alcoholism Screening Test
microcephaly, hypergonadotropic hypogonadism, short stature syndrome
microcephaly, mild developmental delay, short stature, distinctive face syndrome
microcephaly, mild mental retardation, short stature, skeletal anomalies syndrome
S. Musculoskeletal Function Assessment
nongrowth hormone deficient short stature
normal variant short stature
obesity, short stature, mental deficiency, hypogonadism, micropenis, finger contracture, cleft lip-palate syndrome
s. orientation-memory-concentration test
parasternal short axis
periodic short pulse
s. plantar ligament
S. Portable Mental Status Questionnaire
s. radiolunate
s. ragweed test
s. rib-polydactyly syndrome
right short leg brace
s. small bowel
s. spike burst
s. stature homeobox gene
s. stature, hyperextensibility of joints or hernia or both, ocular depression, Rieger anomaly, teething, delayed
subcostal short axis
surgical short procedure unit
s. tandem repeat polymorphism
s. tau inversion recovery
Temple University S. Syntax Inventory
s. T1 inversion recovery
S. Transitional Edge Protection
upper fossa active, medial knee pain, and short leg on the side ipsilateral to the weak fossa
very short below-elbow cast
s. wavelength automated perimetry

short-acting
s.-a. benzodiazepine
s.-a. block
s.-a. hallucinogen
s.-a. insulin

short-arc quadriceps test

short-bowel syndrome

short-chain
s.-c. acyl-CoA dehydrogenase deficiency
s.-c. fatty acid
s.-c. gram-positive cocci
s.-c. hydroxyacyl-coenzyme A dehydrogenase
s.-c. polyunsaturated fatty acid

short-contact treatment

short-duration response

shortened
s. attention span from anxiety
attention span shortened from anxiety
s. electrochemical systole
s., held, resisted, contracted

shortening
Achilles tendon s.
circumferential shortening fraction
fiber shortening velocity
fractional s.
s. fraction percentage
functional s.
left ventricular functional s.
long-axis fractional s.
minor axis shortening of left ventricle
muscle s.
percent fractional s.
velocity of circumferential fiber s.
wall shortening index

short-gut syndrome

short-latency somatosensory-evoked potential

short-lived high

shortness
acute shortness of breath
s. of air
s. of breath
s. of breath on exertion
head of bed up for shortness of breath
increased shortness of breath
palpitation and shortness of breath
sudden shortness of breath

short-segment Barrett esophagus

short-stay ward

short-term
s.-t. anxiety intense
s.-t. anxiety-provoking psychotherapy
S.-t. Auditory Retrieval and Storage Test
s.-t. detoxification
s.-t. dialysis
s.-t. exposure limit
flow-assisted s.-t.
s.-t. goal
s.-t. immunotherapy
s.-t. insomnia
s.-t. irritability intense
s.-t. memory

short-term *(continued)*
s.-t. moodiness intense
s.-t. recall
s.-t. variability
s.-t. visual storage

shortwave diathermy

Shoshin disease

shot
axial single shot fast spin-echo
fast low-angle s.
single shot fast spin echo
sinus s.

shot-silk
s.-s. reflex
s.-s. retina

shotted suture

shotty lymph node

shoulder
airplane splint shoulder brace
all-fours maneuver for shoulder dystocia
s. ankylosis
anterior labrum periosteum shoulder arthroscopic lesion
anterior shoulder dislocation
anterior shoulder instability
anterior shoulder release
AO group shoulder arthrodesis
arm and s.
s. arm system
s. arthritis
s. arthrodesis
arthrotomography of s.
atrophy in shoulder area
autogenous interpositional shoulder arthroplasty
axilla, shoulder, elbow bandage
s. bone
cervical, skull, and shoulder block
chest pain radiating to jaw and s.
chronic intractable shoulder pain
s. contracture
curvilinear threshold s.
disabilities of the arm, shoulder, and hand
s. disarticulation
s. dislocation
double-contrast shoulder arthrography
dynamic ultrasound of s.
s. dystocia
s., elbow, wrist, hand orthosis
s. flap
s. girdle
s. groove
s. horizontal flexion
s. joint
Little League s.
luxatio erecta shoulder dislocation
Milwaukee shoulder syndrome
neck and shoulder pain
Neer classification of shoulder fracture
Neviaser frozen shoulder classification
s. pain
pain between s.'s
painful shoulder syndrome
pain radiating to jaw and s.
pain spreading to s.
s. pain and stiffness
partial s.
pillow inserted under s.
s. press
prominent shoulder blade
rotator cuff of s.
Sever-L'Episcopo repair of s.
s. shrug exercise
simple shoulder test
single shoulder contrast arthrography
s. subluxation inhibitor
s. subluxed
total shoulder replacement

shoulder-hand syndrome

shoulder-strap incision

show
do not s.

showed
abdomen showed evidence of weight loss
bone scan showed increased activity

shower
bath, laxative, enema, shampoo, and s.
embolic s.
needle s.

showing
carcinoma showing thymus-like differentiation

shrapnel fragment wound

Shrapnell membrane

shredding embolectomy thrombectomy

shrinkage
gum s.
s. of hemorrhoid

shrinking
s. field technique
gums s.
s. lungs syndrome
stump s.

shrink inoperable tumor

shrug
shoulder shrug exercise

shrunken atrophied neurons

shuckers'
oyster shuckers' keratitis

shuffling gait

Shuni virus

shunt
adjustable pressure s.
aorticopulmonary window s.
arterioportal venous s.
arteriovenous s.
arteriovenous shunt imaging
arteriovenous shunt infection
bidirectional shunt calculation
Blalock-Taussig s.
cardiac atrial s.
cardiac shunt detection
cerebral fluid s.
Denver peritoneal venous s.
Denver pleuroperitoneal s.
distal splenorenal s.
drainage about shunt site
end-to-side portacaval s.
end-to-side splenorenal s.
s. flow
hexose monophosphate s.
s. index via the inferior mesenteric vein
s. index via superior mesenteric vein
s. infection
initial venous s.
intrapulmonary shunt fraction
intrapulmonary shunt ratio
left-right s.
left-to-right shunt ratio
LeVeen dialysis s.
lumbar arachnoid peritoneal s.
lumboperitoneal s.
s. malfunction
mesoatrial s.
mesocaval H-graft s.
modified Blalock-Taussig s.
Molteno shunt tube
oozing about shunt site
opticociliary shunt vein
opticociliary shunt vessel
Orbis-Sigma cerebrospinal fluid shunt valve

palliative cerebrospinal shunt procedure
peritoneojugular s.
peritoneovenous s.
physiologic shunt flow
portal shunt index
s. pressure
s. procedure
Pruitt-Inahara carotid s.
Pruitt-Inahara vascular s.
relative shunt flow
right-to-left shunt ratio
Scribner arteriovenous s.
side-to-side portacaval s.
Spetzler lumboperitoneal s.
spontaneous portal-systemic s.
total cavopulmonary s.
transjugular intrahepatic portosystemic stent s.
ventricles to peritoneal cavity s.
ventriculojugular s.
ventriculoperitoneal s.
ventriculovenous s.

shunted blood

shunting
arterioportal vein s.
arterioportal venous s.
interatrial s.
portosystemic s.
syringosubarachnoid s.

shut-in personality

shuttlemaker disease

Shwachman syndrome

Shwartzman
S. generalized reaction
generalized Shwartzman reaction
S. local reaction

Shy-Drager syndrome

Shy-Magee syndrome

shyness
childhood shyness disorder

sialadenitis
allergic s.
autoimmune s.
granulomatous s.
myoepithelial s.

sialic
infantile sialic acid storage disorder

sialoglycoprotein
human s.

sialography
parotid s.

sialometaplasia
necrotizing s.

sialoprotein
bone s.

sib
multiple sib case

sibilant
expiratory s.
s. rhonchi

Sibley-Lehninger unit

sibling
subsequent s.
S. Training Program

Sibson
S. aponeurosis
S. fascia
S. groove

Sicar sign

sicca
s. complex
keratoconjunctivitis s.
non-Sjögren keratoconjunctivitis s.
s. syndrome
systemic sicca syndrome

siccus
pannus s.

Sicilian
sandfly fever Sicilian virus

sick
s. bay
s. boy
s. building syndrome
s. call
euthyroid sick syndrome
s. in quarters military
s. role tendency
s. sinus syndrome

sickle
acute sickle chest syndrome
s. cell
s. cell anemia
s. cell anemia test
s. cell beta
s. cell chronic lung disease
s. cell crisis
s. cell disease
s. cell hemoglobin
s. cell hemoglobin C disease
s. cell hemoglobin D disease
s. cell hemoglobin F
s. cell lung disease
s. cell retinopathy
s. cell screening
s. cell thalassemia
s. cell-thalassemia disease
s. cell trait
s. hemoglobin screen
homozygous for sickle cell hemoglobin
irreversible sickle cell
mild sickle cell disease
proliferative sickle retinopathy
s. red blood cell
reversible sickle cell

sickle-shaped particle cell

sickling hemoglobin

sickness
acute mountain s.
acute serum s.
African horse s.
African horse sickness virus 1–9
African sleeping s.
decompression s.
high altitude-related s.
S. Impact Profile
motion sickness susceptibility
serum s.
West African sleeping s.

side
anticholinergic side effect
antimesocolic side of cecum
antipsychotic side effect
autonomic side effect
s. of bed
s. bend
s. bending
s. branch
s. chain in amino acid formula
contralateral side of cerebellum
s. effect
extrapyramidal side effect
s. glide
left-hand s.
local side effect
lower fossa active, lateral knee pain, and long leg on the side ipsilateral to the weak fossa
muscarinic cholinergic side effect
peripheral antimuscarinic side effect
s. platelet aggregation test
s. port
progressive weakness on one side of the body
side to back to s.
upper fossa active, medial knee pain, and short leg on the side ipsilateral to the weak fossa

side-arm nebulizer

sidebent
extended, rotated, s.

sidebent *(continued)*
flexed, rotated, s.
neutral, sidebent right, rotated left

side-chain cleavage

side-effects
adverse s.-e.
s.-e. questionnaire

side-entry access

sideline assessment of concussion

sideplate
barreled s.
compression s.

sideroblast
refractory anemia with ring s.'s
ring s.

sideroblastic
acquired idiopathic sideroblastic anemia
idiopathic acquired refractory sideroblastic anemia
idiopathic acquired sideroblastic anemia
idiopathic refractory sideroblastic anemia
primary acquired sideroblastic anemia

siderochestica

siderocyte
reticulated s.

sideropenic
s. anemia
s. dysphagia

siderosis
hematogenous s.
hepatic s.
myocardial s.
ocular s.
pulmonary s.

siderotic
s. nodule
s. splenomegaly

siderotica
granulomatosis s.

sidestream
low-flow sidestream capnography

sideswipe fracture

side-to-end anastomosis

side-to-side
s.-t.-s. anastomosis
s.-t.-s. gastroenterostomy
s.-t.-s. hepatojejunostomy
s.-t.-s. isoperistaltic strictureplasty
s.-t.-s. portacaval shunt

side-view
s.-v. MRI
s.-v. scan

Sidler-Huguenin endothelioma

Siebert purified protein derivative of tuberculin

Siegel
method of Bernie S.

Siegert sign

Siegrist-Hutchinson syndrome

Siemens
ichthyosis bullosa of S.

sieve
s. bone
s. graft
sequential impaction cascade sieve volumetric air sampler

sievert
s. integral
s. unit

sieving coefficient for sodium

sighing
s. dyspnea
s. respiration

sighs per hour

sight
loss of s.
night s.

sighted
partially s.

sigma reaction

sigmoid
alpha sigmoid loop
s. colon carcinoma
s. colostomy
s. disease
s. diverticulitis
s. diverticulum
s. flexure
s. flexure of colon
s. fossa
s. loop
s. loop colostomy
s. mesocolon
s. septum
s. sinus
s. sulcus
s. volvulus

sigmoideae
arteriae s.

sigmoidei
nodi lymphoidei s.

sigmoidoscope
fiberoptic s.

sigmoidoscopy
fiberoptic s.
flexible fiberoptic s.

sign
abducens nerve s.
afebrile, vital signs stable
air bronchogram s.
Albright dimpling s.
alien hand s.
alien limb s.
American Indian S. Language
anchor signs of withdrawal
anterior drawer s.
anterior hiatal s.
anterior tibialis s.
anterior tibial s.
antral nipple s.
aortic calcification s.
aortic nipple s.
apical cap s.
Argyll-Robertson pupil s.
arterial occlusion s.
auditory and visual s.'s
autonomic hyperactivity s.
Babinski s.
barber pole s.
Battle s.
Braxton-Hicks s.
Brudzinski s.
cardinal sign of alcoholism
chandelier s.
classical signs of rejection
Claude hyperkinesis s.
clenched fist s.
clinical s.'s and symptoms
coiled spring s.
communication in sign language
cranial nerve s.
crescent sign of hydronephrosis
current vital s.'s
cutaneous signs of drug abuse
decreased signs and symptoms of anxiety
decreased signs and symptoms of depression
doll's eye s.
epicardial fat pad s.
failing lung s.
glossopharyngeal nerve s.
Grey Turner s.
hyperdense middle cerebral artery s.
hypoglossal nerve s.

intravascular fetal air s.
s. language
liver flap s.
localized abdominal s.
localizing s.
long tract s.
Lotze local s.
Lovibond profile s.
1-2-3 lung s.
Marcus Gunn pupillary s.
melanoma warning s.
Mexican hat s.
Möbius-von Graefe-Stellway s.
motor neuron s.
mouse bed s.
mucous bronchogram s.
Muehrcke s.
multiple concentric ring s.
negative delta s.
neonatal abstinence s.
neurological signs stable
neurologic vital s.'s
no signs of acute disease
no inflammatory s.'s
normal vital s.'s
no sign of infection
no sign of inflammation
notch chest s.
objective neurologic s.'s
oculodigital sign of Franchesseti
oil drop s.
open bronchus s.
orbital coke-bottle s.
s. own release
painful arc s.
parallel channel s.
patellar apprehension s.
patent bronchus s.
physical and neurologic examination for soft s.'s
Pidgin Sign English
pink puffer sign of emphysema
posttraumatic s.'s or symptoms
prognostically bad signs during pregnancy
Quant s.
Quénu-Muret s.
questionable Babinski s.
radiolucent crescent s.
railroad track s.
s.'s of recent hemorrhage
red color s.
review of s.'s and symptoms
segmental bronchus s.
stable vital s.'s
Steinberg thumb s.
s. symptom complex
s.'s and symptoms
Tinel sign distal tingling on percussion
toe s.
trapezius ridge s.
vital s.
vital signs normal
Vital S.'s Quality of Life
vital signs stable
vital signs stable, afebrile
von Graefe s.
warning signs of hearing loss
warning signs of heart attack
warning signs of serious illness
warning sign of drug abuse
warning sign identification

signal

s. acquisition
amplitude of s.
asymmetrical signal change
s. attenuation
automatic signal processing
autoregressive model for signal analysis
s. averaging
bilateral contralateral routing of s.'s
color Doppler s.
contralateral routing of s.'s
contralateral routing of s.'s
digital signal processing
s. enhancement ratio
evoked potential signal averaging
extra ABL signal fluorescent in situ hybridization
s. extraction technology
feedback s.
focal contralateral routing of s.'s
front routing of s.
high-frequency contralateral routing of offside s.'s
high-frequency contralateral routing of offside s.'s
high-intensity transient s.
input signal processor
insufficient s.
s. intensity
ipsilateral frontal routing of s.'s
linear degenerative signal intensity
long-loop feedback s.
low-amplitude s.
low–pass-filtered s.
Masimo SET signal extraction pulse oximetry
microembolic s.
myoelectric s.
nuclear localization s.
nuclear localization signal motif
optical intrinsic signal imaging
output signal processor
ovarian Doppler s.
peptide growth factor receptor s.
percentage signal intensity loss
punctate area of increased s.
s. recognition particle
s. recognition protein
therapeutic error s.
time domain signal processor
s. transducer and activator of transcription-4
s. transducer and activator of transcription-5
tyramide signal amplification
variable-angle uniform signal excitation
white matter signal abnormality

signal-averaged

s.-a. echocardiogram
s.-a. electrocardiogram
s.-a. electrocardiography
s.-a. P-wave duration

signal-difference to noise ratio

signaling

antiapoptotic signaling pathway
death-inducing signaling complex
Notch signaling pathway
peptide growth factor signaling mechanism
s. lymphocytic activation molecule
suppressor of cytokine signaling 3

signal-to-noise

s.-t.-n. calculation
s.-t.-n. ratio

signature

massively parallel signature sequencing
phase-invariant signature algorithm
s. prescription

signed

autopsy permit s.
S. English
matched pairs signed rank test
multichannel signed averager
operative permit s.
s. out against medical advice

signet-ring cell carcinoma

significance

atypical endocervical cells of undetermined s.

significance *(continued)*
atypical glandular cells of uncertain s.
atypical glandular cells of unknown s.
atypical glandular cell of undetermined s.
atypical squamous cell of undetermined s.
granulomatous lesions of unknown s.
honest significance difference
McNemar test of s.
monoclonal gammopathy of undetermined s.
monoclonal gammopathy of unknown s.
plasma cell dyscrasia of unknown s.
s. probability mapping
s. probability value
squamous intraepithelial lesion/atypical squamous cell of undetermined s.

significant
s. abnormality
s. asymptomatic bacteriuria
clinically significant arrhythmia
finding of no significant impact
s. gain in weight
s. glandular enlargement
hemodynamically significant stenosis
least significant change
least significant difference
s. medial event
most significant bit
most significant digit
most significant other
no significant anomaly
no significant change from previous tracing
no significant defect
no significant deficiency
no significant deviation
no significant difference
no significant findings
s. sharp spike or delta wave
statistically s.
s. weight gain

Signing Exact English

Signorelli sign

Silapap
Children's S.

Silastic
S. mushroom catheter
S. ring vertical-banded gastric bypass

silence
s. of apneic episode
code of s.
electrocerebral s.

silencer of death domain

silencing mediator of retinoic acid and thyroid hormone receptor

silent
s. abdomen
s. allele
s. angina
s. area
s. belch
s. brain infarction
s. carcinoma
s. cerebral infarct
s. cerebral infarction
documented silent ischemia
exercise-induced silent myocardial ischemia
s. gallstone
s. gap
s. heart attack
s. heart damage
s. heart muscle distress
s. ischemia
s. ischemic brain damage
s. ischemic heart disease
s. mitral stenosis
s. myocardial infarction
s. myocardial ischemia
s. period
s. treatment

silhouette
cardiac silhouette enlargement
cardiomediastinal s.
enlarged cardiac s.
s. of heart
s. sign

silica gel filtered

silicate
magnesium aluminum s.
zirconium s.

silicon
amorphous hydrogenated silicon carbide
arsenic nickel s.
s. carbide
s. photodiode

silicon-controlled
s.-c. rectifier
s.-c. switch

silicone
adhesive silicone implant
adjustable silicone gastric banding
s. band
breast silicone implant
s. coated
conventional silicone elastomer
detachable silicone balloon
direct injection of silicone into breast
s. elastomer ring vertical gastroplasty
flexible silicone implant
fluted silicone drain
s. gel-filled breast implant
s. gel-filled mammary implant
s. gel sheeting
s. immersion
s. implant material
s. injection
laser adjustable silicone gastric banding
occlusion balloon catheter with silicone balloon
one-piece plate haptic silicone intraocular lens
open adjustable silicone gastric banding
Packer tunnel silicone sponge
removable silicone plug
s. rod implant
s. rubber
s. shunt
s. sponge implant
s. thermoplastic splinting

silicone-based artificial joint

silicone-filled breast implant

silicone-only suspension

silicon-intensified target

silicotic
s. granuloma
s. pneumonoconiosis

siliculose cataract

siliquose cataract

silk
artificial silk keratitis
black silk suture
s. braided suture
continuous silk suture
s. implantation
interrupted black silk suture
interrupted fine silk suture
s. interrupted mattress suture
skin closed with interrupted s.

silkworm gut suture

silo-filler's
s.-f. disease
s.-f. lung

Silon test

Silva-Costa operation

silver
S. bunionectomy
S. dwarf
Grocott-Gomori methenamine silver nitrate
Grocott methenamine silver stain
Masson-Fontana ammoniac silver stain
methenamine silver stain
s. nitrate
s. nitrate immunoperoxidase
s. nitrate solution
polyacrylamide gel electrophoresis with silver stain
sulfadiazine s.
s. sulfadiazine
S. syndrome
Wilder silver stain

silver-fork
s.-f. deformity
s.-f. fracture

Silverman
S. needle biopsy
S. score

silver-staining nucleolar organizer region

Silverwater virus

Silvestroni-Bianco syndrome

Simbu virus

simethicone
magaldrate and s.

simian
s. acquired immunodeficiency syndrome
s. adenovirus
s. crease
s. crease of palm
s. fissure
s. foamy viruses
s. hand
s. hemorrhagic fever
s. herpes virus
s. immunodeficiency virus
s. malaria
s. sarcoma-associated virus
s. sarcoma virus
s. sign
s. T-cell lymphotropic virus
s. vacuolating virus 40

Similac with iron

similar
number of similar negatives
number of similar positives

similarity
assumed s.
vocabulary, information, block design, and s.'s

similarly
amphetamine or similarly acting sympathomimetic intoxication
s. tested

Simmond disease

Simmons
occult temporal arteritis of S.

Simonart
S. bands
S. ligament

Simon septic factor

simple
s. absence
aneurysm with simple shape
s. aphasia
s. atrophy
S. Calculated Osteoporosis Risk Estimation
chronic simple glaucoma
complete simple mastectomy
complex simple fracture
s. cyst
s. decompression
s. descriptive scale
s. diplopia
s. dislocation
s. fracture
fracture simple and complete
fracture simple complete and comminuted
fracture simple and depressed
s. ganglion
s. glaucoma
s. goiter
s. harmonic motion
s. hyperplasia
s. hypocalcemic tetany
s. interrupted fashion
s. joint
s. knee test
s. mastectomy
s. myopia
s. necrosis
s. neonatal procedure
s. obesity
s. partial seizure
s. phobia
rapid simple tests
s. reaction time
s. response paradigm
s. retinitis
s. shoulder test
s. tandem repeat polymorphism
s. virilizing congenital adrenal hyperplasia

simplex
dominant epidermolysis bullosa s.
epidermolysis bullosa s.
herpes s.
herpes simplex antibody titer
herpes simplex genitalis
herpes simplex gingivostomatitis
herpes simplex infection
herpes simplex keratitis
herpes simplex labialis
herpes simplex neonatorum
herpes simplex pneumonitis
herpes simplex retinitis
herpes simplex viral shedding
herpes simplex virus encephalitis
herpes simplex virus thymidine kinase
herpes simplex type 1, 2
herpes simplex virus 1, 2
herpes simplex virus type 1, 2, 6, 7
lichen chronicus s.
localized epidermolysis bullosa s.
McKrae herpes simplex virus
mucocutaneous herpes s.
neonatal herpes s.
neonatal herpes simplex virus
neonatal herpes simplex virus infection
ocular herpes s.
orofacial herpes s.
syphilis, toxoplasmosis, other agents, rubella, cytomegalovirus, herpes simplex virus
toxoplasmosis, other infections, rubella, cytomegalovirus infection, herpes simplex syndrome
visceral herpes s.

simplified
S. Acute Physiology Score
S. Acute Physiology Score version II
S. Calculus Index
s. nocturnal home hemodialysis
S. Oral Hygiene Index

Simpson
S. dysmorphia syndrome
modified Simpson rule
S. rule

Simpson-Golabi-Behmel syndrome

Sims-Huhner test

simulated

s. activities of daily living
s. aircraft fire and emergency
s. echo artifact
s. fluorescence process
s. gastric fluid
s. intestinal fluid
s. moving bed chromatography
professional simulated patient
s. real ear measurement
topographic simulated keratometric power

simulation

computer graphic s.
high-altitude simulation test
s. kinetics analysis
Monte Carlo photon transport s.
osteotomy analysis simulation software
work s.

simulator

video display terminal s.

simultaneous

s. activity
s. analog stimulation
s. areolar mastopexy and breast augmentation
s. auditory feedback
s. bilateral percutaneous nephrolithotomy
s. bilateral spontaneous pneumothorax
s. binaural bithermal
s. binaural midplace localization
s. communication
s. compression ventilation-cardiopulmonary resuscitation
s. contrast
s. double kidney transplantation
double simultaneous recording
double simultaneous stimulation
dual-isotope simultaneous acquisition single-photon emission computed tomography
s. equation
s. foveal perception
s. independent lung ventilation
s. insanity
S. Interview Technique
s. kidney-pancreas transplantation
s. macular perception
s. multichannel autoanalyzer
s. multiple analyzer
s. multiple-angle reconstruction technique
s. peripheral operation on-line
s. prism and cover test
S. Technique for Acuity and Readiness Testing
s. thermoradiotherapy

simultaneously stapled pneumonectomy

sin

capital s.
S. Nombre virus

since

s. last visit
slightly more marked s.
zero stool since birth

Sindbis virus

Sinding-Larsen-Johansson disease

sine

depression sine depression
migraine sine hemicrania
pellagra sine pellagra
systemic sclerosis sine scleroderma
s. wave
s. wave pattern
s. wave threshold

Singapore

S. ear
S. epidemic conjunctivitis

singe

main en s.

singer's

s. node
s. nodule

Singer-Loomis Inventory of Personality

Singh Index

single

anaplastic infiltrating single cell
s. antibody millipore filtration
axial single shot fast spin-echo
s. axis
s. base cane
binocular single vision
s. binocular vision
s. blind
s. breath
buffered single substrate
s. central maxillary incisor
s. chemical
s. coronary artery bypass graft
s. coronary artery graft
s. crystal gamma camera
deoxyribonucleic acid single stranded
disabled infectious single cycle virus
s., divorced, married
s. dose suppression
s. enhancing CT lesion
s. episode
s. fiber electromyography
Fowler single breath test
gastric augment and single pedicle tube
s. gene disorder
greatest single allergen present
s. harelip
heart defibrillated with single shock
high single dose alternate day
s. injection
s. internal mammary artery
s. isomorphous replacement
s. knee to chest
s. lens reflex
s. limb support
s. lumen
s. lung reduction surgery
s. major locus
s. needle device
s. nephron
nitrogen washout, single breath
nominal single dose
normal single dose
s. nucleopolyhedrovirus
s. nucleotide polymorphism
s. nucleotide polymorphisms - linkage disequilibrium
number equal to one; single patient trial
s. palmar crease
s. parent keeping baby
s. parent not keeping baby
s. patient system
s. photoelectron counting
s. potential analysis cavernous electrical activity
s. presentation phenotype
s. proton counting
s. radial diffusion test
s. radial hemolysis
s. radial immunodiffusion
random single donor platelet
recirculating single pass
s. reference electrode
s. reference point
right single lung transplant
s. saturating dose

sequence-independent single primer amplification
s. shot fast spin echo
s. shoulder contrast arthrography
s. stranded
s. umbilical artery
s. unit activity
upper single tooth
s. ventricle
s. vibration
s. vision glasses

single-action pumping system

single-agent chemotherapy

single-axis
s.-a. friction knee prosthesis
s.-a. locking knee prosthesis

single-breath
s.-b. carbon monoxide diffusing capacity of lung
s.-b. diffusing capacity
s.-b. nitrogen test
s.-b. nitrogen washout

single-celled protein

single-cell liquid cytotoxic assay

single-chain
s.-c. antigen-binding protein
s.-c. variable fragment

single-channel analyzer

single-contrast
s.-c. barium enema
s.-c. study

single-donor
s.-d. apheresis platelet
s.-d. frozen plasma
s.-d. transfusion

single-electrode current perception threshold

single-energy x-ray absorptiometer

single-frequency bioimpedance

single-limb progression

single-lumen catheter

single-lung transplant

single-nephron
s.-n. glomerular blood flow
s.-n. glomerular filtration rate
s.-n. glomerular plasma flow

single-photon
s.-p. absorptiometry
s.-p. counting system
s.-p. emission computed tomography
s.-p. emission imaging tomography
s.-p. gamma scintigraphy
s.-p. planar imaging
s.-p. planar scintigraphy

single-stage exercise stress test

single-stranded
s.-s. conformational polymorphism
s.-s. deoxyribonucleic acid
s.-s. DNA

single-stripe colitis

singleton
s. breech presentation
s. fetus
s. infant

singlet oxygen

single-unit delivery system

single-use
s.-u. catheter
s.-u. electrode

single-vessel disease

singly and consensually

singular
s. value decomposition

sinister
lower lid, oculus s.
retinal detachment, oculus s.
tension oculus sinister

sink-side bathing

sinoaortic denervation

sinoatrial
s. arrest
artery to the sinoatrial node
s. block
s. bundle
s. conduction time
corrected time of sinoatrial node function recovery
direct sinoatrial conduction time
s. entrance block
s. ganglion
s. heart block
s. nodal reentry
s. node
s. node artery
s. recovery time

sinoauricular heart block

sinobronchial syndrome

Sinografin contrast medium

sinonasal
s. adenocarcinoma
S. Outcome Test-16
s. undifferentiated carcinoma

sinopulmonary disease

sinotubular
aortic sinotubular junction

sinovenous occlusive disease

sinoventricular tachyarrhythmia

sinuatrialis
nodus s.

sinuatrial node

sinus
angular aqueous sinus plexus
anterior cavernous sinus space
anterior cavernous sinus syndrome
anterior chamber s.
anterior ethmoid s.
anterior intercavernous s.
aortic sinus aneurysm
aortic sinus fistula
aortic sinus to right ventricle fistula
aortic valve s.
apertura sinus frontalis
aperture of sphenoid s.
s. arrest
s. arrhythmia
artery of inferior cavernous s.
s. block
s. bradycardia
s. breakthrough beat
s. cancer
carotid s.
carotid-cavernous sinus fistula
carotid sinus compression
carotid sinus denervation
carotid sinus nerve
carotid sinus nerve stimulation
carotid sinus pressure
carotid sinus syncope
carotid sinus test
cavernous s.
cavernous sinus infiltration
cavernous sinus sampling
cavernous sinus thrombosis
s. cavity
cerebral venous sinus thrombosis
clouding of s.'s
complex unroofed coronary s.
computer-guided endoscopic sinus surgery
s. congestion
coronary s.
coronary sinus blood flow
coronary sinus flow
coronary sinus occlusion pressure
coronary sinus stimulation

sinus *(continued)*
corrected adjusted sinus node recovery time
corrected sinus nodal recovery time
s. cycle length
s. cyst
distal coronary s.
endodermal sinus tumor
endoscopic sinus surgery
s. endoscopy
ethmoid sinus
ethmoid sinus adenocarcinoma
functional endoscopic s.
functional endoscopic sinus surgery
s. ganglion
granuloma of s.
s. groove
s. headache
s. headache from cold
s. histiocytosis
s. histiocytosis with massive lymphadenopathy
hyperactive carotid sinus reflex
hypersensitive carotid sinus syndrome
image-guided functional endoscopic sinus surgery
s. infection
inferior petrosal sinus sampling
inferior sagittal s.
intermittent coronary sinus occlusion
intracranial sinus thrombosis
s. irregularity
lateral sinus thrombophlebitis
lateral venous s.
left coronary s.
longitudinal vertebral venous s.
lumbosacral dermal s.
marginal sinus of placenta
marginal sinus rupture
massage of the carotid s.
maxillary sinus aspiration
maxillary sinus carcinoma
middle coronary s.
mini-functional endoscopic sinus surgery
nasal sinus disease
nerve to carotid s.
s. node
s. node cycle length
s. node dysfunction
s. node electrogram
s. node formation
s. node impulse
s. node potential
s. node recovery time
noncoronary s.
normal sinus heart rhythm
normal sinus rate and rhythm
s.'s, nose, throat
open dermal s.
opening of coronary s.
opening of frontal s.
osteoplastic frontal sinus procedure
paranasal sinus lymphoma
paranasal sinus tumor
paroxysmal sinus tachycardia
pilonidal sinus disease
powered endoscopic sinus surgery
pressure-controlled intermittent coronary sinus occlusion
proximal coronary s.
pyriform s.
rectal s.
relatively slow sinus rate
respiratory sinus arrhythmia
resumption of normal sinus rhythm
s. rhythm
s. rhythm, no ectopy
right coronary s.
right frontal s.
Rokitansky-Aschoff s.
ruptured sinus of Valsalva aneurysm
sagittal sinus thrombosis
s. shot
space of the cavernous s.
sphenoid s.
superior sagittal s.
superior sagittal sinus thrombosis
superior sagittal sinus velocity
s. tachycardia
s. tract
transverse s.
transverse/sigmoid s.
s. tympani
urogenital s.
s. venosus
venous s.
ventricular atrial distal coronary s.
ventricular atrial proximal coronary s.
s. x-ray

sinusitis
acute maxillary s.
allergic fungal s.
chronic hyperplastic sinusitis with nasal polyposis
postnasal drip due to s.

sinusography
cerebral s.

sinusoidal
s. capillary
s. circulation
s. endothelial cell
s. heart rate
s. wave

sinusotomy
transseptal frontal s.

sinus-vein thrombosis

sinuvertebral nerve

sip-and-puff mouthpiece

siphon
carotid s.

sireniform fetus

sister
s. chromatid exchange
s. chromatid exchange rate

site
active oozing from s.
angulation at fracture s.
antibody combining s.
antibody reaction s.
antigen binding s.
arterial bleeding s.
arterial entry s.
arterial puncture site closure device
ATP binding s.
bleeding at site of injection
bleeding from multiple s.'s
bleeding site cauterized
bone graft s.
cancer of unknown primary s.
cannula insertion s.
carcinoma of uncertain primary s.
carcinoma of unknown primary s.
catheter insertion s.
chromosome modification s.
crepitus at fracture s.
s. of disease
donor site of bone graft
donor site dressing
donor site of skin graft
drainage about shunt s.
drainage at incision s.
estrogen binding s.
extralymphatic organ s.
extramedullary s.

fracture s.
fragile chromosome s.
fragile site mental retardation 1
fragile site mental retardation 2
healed cutdown s.
healed incision s.
healing incision s.
hormone receptor s.
s. of illness
incisional site draining
incision carried down to the fracture s.
infected incision s.
injection site reaction
insertion site infection
internal ribosome entry s.
intravenous infection s.
intravenous needle site care
intravenous site of infection
irritation of incision s.
lesion on erythrocyte cell membrane at the site of complement fixation
lump at site of injection
Morrison donor site design
multiple noninguinal s.'s
nerve entrapment s.
N-linked glycosylated s.
nonunion of fracture s.
Norwood donor site design
oozing about shunt s.
oozing from s.
operative site complication
operative site infection
operative site irrigated
operative site irrigated with antibiotic solution
operative site irrigated with normal saline
s. of origin
original injection s.
original tumor s.
pain at incision s.
patellar tendon graft donor s.
pedicled enteric donor s.
placental bleeding s.
placental site trophoblastic tumor
primary cancer s.
primary tumor s.
primary tumor site unknown
pus at incision s.
reactive s.
redness along incision s.
redness at incision s.
remottling fracture s.
sequence-tagged s.'s
swelling at incision s.
tenderness at site of incision
vesicle attachment s.
warmth at incision s.
X-linked first site of fragility
X-linked mental retardation-fragile site 1, 2
X-linked second site of fragility

sitting
s. balance
s. height
left arm, s.
long leg s.
mean sitting diastolic blood pressure
right arm, s.
s. tolerance
transfer from supine to s.

sit-to-stand transfer

situ
adenocarcinoma in s.
apocrine ductal carcinoma in s.
argyrophilic ductal carcinoma in s.
bladder carcinoma in s.
cancer in s.
carcinoma in s.
double-fusion fluorescent in situ hybridization
ductal carcinoma in s.
endocrine ductal carcinoma in s.
endometrial carcinoma in s.
Epstein-Barr virus-encoded RNA in situ hybridization
extra ABL signal fluorescent in situ hybridization
fluorescent in situ hybridization
glansplasty in situ tubularization of urethral plate
glanuloplasty in situ tubularization of urethral plate
isolated gland carcinoma in s.
laser-assisted in situ keratomileusis
lobular carcinoma in s.
malignant melanoma in s.
melanoma in s.
multiple in situ hybridization
multispectral fluorescent in situ hybridization
nasopharyngeal carcinoma in s.
neuroendocrine ductal carcinoma in s.
nonisotopic in situ hybridization
nonradioactive in situ hybridization
polymerase chain reaction in situ hybridization
primed in situ labeling
in situ end labeling
in situ hybridization
in situ hybridization histochemistry
in situ polymerase chain reaction
squamous cell carcinoma in s.
surface carcinoma in s.
transitional carcinoma in s.
tumor in s.
ultrasensitive fluorescence in situ hybridization

situation
adult situation stress reaction
s. anxiety
anxiety-provoking s.
Asch s.
Life S. Questionnaire
School S. Survey
social or interpersonal s.

situational
adjustment situational reaction
s. anger disorder with aggression
s. anger disorder without aggression
S. Attitude Scale
s. crisis
s. depression
s. disturbance
s. ethics
s. syncope
transient situational reaction

situs
s. ambiguus with polysplenia
atrial s.
atrial situs solitus
complete situs inversus
dextrocardia with situs inversus
incomplete situs inversus
inversus
s. inversus viscerum

sitz bath

six-area, six-sign atopic dermatitis

Sixgun City virus

six-meal bland diet

Sixteen Personality Factors Test

sixth
band form in sixth stage of myelocyte maturation
s. disease

size
age, distant metastases, extent and s.

size *(continued)*
age, metastases, extent and size risk criteria
appropriate blood pressure cuff s.
cardiac size and function
configuration and s.
dark-adapted pupil s.
doubling time of tumor s.
s. exclusion chromatography
field size in half body irradiation
finger joint s.
focal spot s.
fundus anterior, normal size and shape, and mobile
gestational sac s.
heart reduced to normal s.
heart size and outline
heart size and shape
increased dose size per fraction
increased heart s.
s. of infarct
infarct size index
mean particle s.
mean sac s.
mean sac size and crown-rump length
metastasis, age, completeness of resection, local invasion, and tumor s.
normal heart s.
normal size, shape, and position, anteverted and anteflexed uterus
normal size and configuration
normal size heart
normal size and shape
normal size, shape, and consistency
normal size, shape, and location
normal size, shape, and position
optimal group s.
optimum information s.
particle size distribution
population s.
pupil reaction and s.
pupils equal in size and reaction
relative tumor s.
sample s.
total burn s.
tumor increased in s.
vertebral body s.

size/date
s. consistency
s. inconsistency

Sjögren
S. disease
primary Sjögren syndrome
rheumatoid arthritis and Sjögren syndrome
S. syndrome
S. syndrome antigen A
thyroiditis, Addison disease, Sjögren syndrome, sarcoidosis syndrome

Sjögren-Larsson syndrome

skate
arm s.
s. flap
s. graft

skein
s. cell

skeletal
s. abnormalities, cutis laxa, craniostenosis, psychomotor retardation, facial abnormalities
s. abnormality
s. age
s. anomaly
s. antibody
appendicular skeletal muscle
balanced skeletal traction
s. biopsy
bovine embryo skeletal muscle
calcinosis cutis, osteoma cutis, poikiloderma, and skeletal abnormalities syndrome
cataract, motor system disorder, short stature, learning difficulty, skeletal abnormalities syndrome
cerebral, ocular, dental, auricular, skeletal syndrome
congenital hyperphosphatasemic skeletal dysplasia
s. correction
s. defect
s. deformity
diffuse idiopathic skeletal hyperostosis
s. disruption
s. distraction
s. dysplasia
s. dysplasia in fetus
external skeletal fixation
external spinal skeletal fixator
s. growth factor
human skeletal growth factor
idiopathic skeletal hyperostosis
intramedullary skeletal kinetic distractor
ischemic skeletal muscle
s. mass
s. maturation
mental retardation, coarse face, microcephaly, epilepsy, skeletal abnormalities syndrome
mental retardation, epilepsy, short stature, skeletal dysplasia syndrome
mental retardation, hearing impairment, distinct facies, skeletal anomalies syndrome
mental retardation, skeletal dysplasia, abducens palsy syndrome
s. metastasis
microcephaly, mild mental retardation, short stature, skeletal anomalies syndrome
mitral valve prolapse, aortic anomalies, skeletal changes, and skin changes syndrome
s. muscle
s. muscle ischemia
s. muscle protein
s. muscle relaxant
s. myxoid chondrosarcoma
s. neoplasm
s. related event
s. repair system
s. resistance
rheumatoid arthritis, diffuse idiopathic skeletal hyperostosis
s. scintigraphy
s. survey
s. traction

skeletogenous cell

skeleton
cell wall s.
computer tomographic methods of axial s.
computer tomographic methods of peripheral s.
s. hand
mitral valve, aorta, skeleton, skin
osseocartilaginous craniofacial s.

Skene
Bartholin, Skene, and urethral glands
Bartholin, urethral, and Skene glands, and external genitalia
S. gland

skepticism
adolescent s.

Skevas-Zerfus disease

skew
s. deviation
s. distribution

skiagram study

skier's thumb

ski graft

skill

adaptive hand s.'s
ambulation s.'s
anger management s.
arithmetical skills learning retardation
articulatory s.
assertiveness s.
attending s.
attentional s.'s
auditory s.
Basic School S.'s Inventory
bed mobility s.
Boston Diagnostic Inventory of Basic S.'s
California Critical Thinking S.'s Test
California Test of Basic S.'s
Campbell Interest and S. Survey
Canadian Test of Basic S.'s
Checklist of Adaptive Living S.'s
Cognitive S.'s Assessment
cognitive coping s.
cognitive perceptual motor s.'s
cognitive skills training approach
communication skills assessment
conditioned reflex s.
control motor s.'s
coping s.
Cornell Learning and Study S.'s Inventory
daily living s.'s
s.'s of daily living
decision-making s.'s
Developing S.'s Checklist
Differentiation of Auditory Perception S.
donning-doffing s.
Evaluating Acquired S.'s in Communication
fine motor s.
Frostig Movement S.'s Test Battery
Goldman-Fristoe-Woodcock Auditory S.'s Test Battery
gross motor s.
higher level s.
impulse control s.'s
inadequate literacy s.'s
independent living s.'s
S. Indicators
intact motor s.'s
intellectual and motor s.'s
interpersonal s.'s
Interpersonal Language S.'s and Assessment
Inventory of Perceptual S.'s
Iowa Tests of Basic S.'s
Kaufman Survey of Early Academic and Language S.'s
knowledge, s.'s, and abilities
limited interpersonal s.'s
Marriage S.'s Analysis
meal-time s.
Modern Occupational S.'s Test
motor s.
negotiating goals s.'s
nonconfrontational communication s.'s
nonverbal communication s.
Parent Awareness S.'s Survey
Pepper Visual S.'s for Reading Test
perceptual motor s.'s
Personal Adjustment and Role S.'s Scale
Personal and Role S.'s
physical daily living s.'s
Primary Test of Cognitive S.'s
problem-solving s.
Process S.'s Rating Scale
Psychiatric Knowledge and S.'s Self-Assessment Program
Riley Inventory of Basic Learning S.'s
Screening Test for Educational Prerequisite S.'s
social interpersonal s.'s
Social S.'s Rating System
social skills training
spatial skills and attention
special skills training
vocational skills assessment and development program
Vocational Interest, Experience, and S. Assessment

skilled

certified skilled nursing facility
geriatric skilled care unit
intermittent skilled nursing care
s. nursing care
s. nursing extended care facility
s. nursing facility
s. nursing visit
patient discharged to skilled nursing facility
patient transferred to skilled nursing facility

Skillern fracture

skim

dried skim milk
s. milk

skimming

plasma s.
platelet s.

skin

adnexal skin tumor
anal skin tag
anergy skin test battery
anesthetic skin lesion
angiectatic skin rash
anterior skin flap
Apligraf tissue-engineered s.
appendage of s.
approximate skin edges
apron skin incision
asymmetric skin fold
atrophic brown s.
s. atrophy
autologous cultured skin grafting
autologous cultured skin transplantation
autologous skin transplant
axial pattern vascularized skin flap
s. barrier
basal skin resistance
s. biopsy
s. bleeding time
blue skin from blood clot
bovine lumpy skin disease
s. breakdown
break in the s.
s. bridge
s. caliper
s. cancer
carbon dioxide laser skin resurfacing
s. carcinoma
cavernous hemangioma of s.
s. change
clamminess of s.
s. closed with interrupted silk
s. closure
closure of skin wound
collagen skin treatment
color change of s.
composite cultured s.
s. conductance level
s. conductance orienting response
s. conduction
congenital localized absence of s.
constant skin irritation and rubbing
continual skin peeling syndrome
cosmetic skin resurfacing

skin *(continued)*
s. coverage
s. crawling sensation
s. crease
curvilinear skin incision
cyanotic discoloration of s.
s. cyst
debridement infected s.
defatted skin graft
s. defect
delayed skin hypersensitivity reaction
s. depth
dermatophyte infection of s.
s. destruction
dimpling of breast s.
s. discoloration
donor site of skin graft
s. dose
drug-induced skin reactions
drying and wrinkling of s.
dry itching s.
dry skin and hair
eczematoid skin rash
eczematous skin lesion
electric skin resistance
electrodispersive skin potential
s. endpoint titration
s. eruption
s. erythema dose
excited skin syndrome
exophytic skin lesion
s. exposure reduction paste against chemical warfare agent
extent of skin involvement
face laser skin resurfacing
s. and fascia stapler
s. fibroblast
s. flap
s. flora
s. fluorescence
s. fold
s. fold caliper
s. fold incision
s. fold measurement
s. fold thickness
s. fold thickness test
s. fragility
fusiform skin revision
galvanic skin potential
galvanic skin reflex
galvanic skin resistance
galvanic skin response audiometry
genital skin fibroblast
s. glue
good contact with s.
s. goose bumps
s. graft
s. graft defatted
s. graft donor
s. grafting
s. graft slough
Gram stain of skin lesion
s. growth
growth and maturation of new s.
s. hardening from dermatitis
heavy scaling of s.
hemihypertrophy, intestinal web, preauricular skin tag, and congenital corneal opacity syndrome
hemorrhoidal skin tag
histoplasmin skin test
s. homograft
horseshoe-shaped skin flap
human embryonic s.
human skin collagenase
human skin equivalent
human skin nurse cell
s. hydration
immunoreactive human skin collagenase
impaired skin integrity
impairment of skin integrity
s. impedance
s. incision
s. incision closed
increased skin temperature
induration along skin incision
infant skin control
s. infection
s. inflammation
s. integrity
S. Intensity Score
intermediate split-thickness skin graft
intractable skin rash
s. involvement
s. irritation
itchy or chapped s.
itchy skin rash
s. jaundiced
laser skin resurfacing
s. lesion
s. line incision
lumbosacral skin pigment change
lumpy skin disease
lymphocytic infiltration of the s.
lymphoepithelioma-like carcinoma of s.
lymphoproliferative skin lesion
maculopapular skin lesion
Mantoux tuberculin skin test
McFarlane skin flap
mechanical creep of s.
Mecholyl skin test
s. melanoma
metallic skin staple
methacholine chloride skin test
microphthalmia with linear skin defects
midline skin incision
midpoint skin test
mild skin irritation
Milian citrine s.
mitral valve, aorta, skeleton, s.
mitral valve prolapse, aortic anomalies, skeletal changes, and skin changes syndrome
mixed skin cell leukocyte reaction
mixed tumor of s.
modified Rodman skin thickness score
monoclonal protein, s.
Montenegro skin test
morbilliform skin rash
mottling of s.
multiple benign circumferential skin creases on limb
mumps skin test antigen
s. necrosis
neonatal skin allograft
new skin growth
nicotine skin patch
noncancerous skin growth
nongenital skin fibroblast
noninvolved psoriatic s.
pacemaker implanted under s.
pale and clammy s.
s. pale and diaphoretic
s. pallor
pallor of s.
papillomatous skin lesion
papulosquamous skin lesion
patch skin test
penicillin allergy skin testing
penicilloyl polylysine skin test
s. perfusion pressure
perineal skin tag
petechial hemorrhage of s.
polyneuropathy, organomegaly, endocrinopathy, monoclonal gammopathy, and skin changes syndrome
polyneuropathy, organomegaly, endocrinopathy, M protein, and skin changes syndrome
s. potential level
s. potential reflex
precancerous skin spot

preoperative skin preparation
prick skin test
s. prick test
primary neuroendocrine carcinoma of s.
s. protection factor
psychogalvanic skin resistance
psychogalvanic skin response audiometry
s. puncture test
purplish hemorrhagic spot on s.
Rebuck skin window technique
relaxed skin tension line
repeated skin grafting
s. resistance
s. scraping
s. self-examination
s. sheen
s., eye, mucocutaneous
s., head, eyes, ears, nose, and throat
source to skin distance
split-thickness skin excision
staphylococcal scalded skin syndrome
subscapular skin fold thickness
s. surface lipid
s. surface microscopy
s. suture intact
s. sympathetic activity
sympathetic skin response
s. tag
TB skin test
s. temperature recovery time
s. temperature test
s. tension line
tenting of s.
s. test for delayed-type hypersensitivity
s. test done
s. test dose
s. test reactivity
s. test unit
tetanus antitoxin skin test
s. thickness
thickness of skin fold
thick, red itchy patch of s.
through the s.
topical skin protection
total skin electron beam
total skin examination
toxoplasmin skin test antigen
triceps skin fold thickness
tuberculin skin test
tuberculosis skin test
tumor skin test
s. turgor
s. ulcer
s. ulceration
s. undermined
unique facies, anorexia, cachexia, and eye and skin syndrome
s. unit dose
wide skin incision
wound and s.
s. and wound isolation
wrinkly skin syndrome

skin-adipose superficial musculoaponeurotic system

skin-associated lymphoid tissue

skin-film distance

skin-muscle free flap

skinny needle aspiration

skin-reactive factor

skin-sensitizing antibody

skin-soft tissue envelope

skin-sparing
s.-s. effect
s.-s. mastectomy

skin-to-tumor distance

skive
medial heel skive technique

Sklar Aphasia Scale

Skoda
S. rales
S. sign
S. tympany

skodaic resonance

Skoog procedure

skull
anterior cerebral artery crawling under the s.
anterior fossa skull base glabellar
anterior skull base
anterior skull base malignancy
AP-PA skull block
AP-PA skull immobilizer
apposition of skull suture
basal skull fracture
base of s.
s. base tumor
bleeding inside s.
bur holes drilled in s.
s. cap
cervical skull pillow
cervical, skull, and shoulder block
closed skull fracture
comminuted skull fracture
conformation of the s.
crushing procedure skull of fetus
debridement of compound skull fracture
depressed fracture s.
depressed skull fracture
s. fracture
Frankfort horizontal plane of s.
intracranial pressure monitor in s.
linear skull fracture
longitudinal arc of s.
open reduction of skull fracture
s. survey
s. suture line
trauma s.
whole skull irradiation
s. x-ray

skullcap
autumn skullcap mushroom

slant
antimongoloid eye s.
antimongoloid eyelid s.
modified whole-egg slant medium
mongoloid s.
palpebral s.

slant-hole tomography

slanting
antimongoloid s.

slap
foot s.

slapping gait

sleep
s. abnormality
active sleep state
s. activity
alcohol-dependent sleep disorder
alcohol-induced nighttime s.
alcohol sleep disorder
all night sleep recording
alpha, delta sleep anomaly
alpha-nonrapid eye movement s.
altered sleep schedule
amnesia for sleep and dreaming
amnesia for sleep terror event
s. anomaly
s. apnea
s. apnea-hypersomnolence syndrome associated with upper airway obstruction
s. apnea monitor
S. Apnea Quality of Life Index
s. apnea syndrome
s. architecture
s. arousal
arousal from s.
before s.
benign epileptiform transients of s.

sleep *(continued)*
s. bruxism
caffeine-induced sleep disorder
cardiopulmonary sleep study
central sleep apnea
central sleep apnea syndrome
chronic sleep schedule disturbance
circadian rhythm-based sleep disorder
combined central and obstructive sleep apnea
cumulative sleep deficit
daytime multiple sleep latency test
daytime sleep episodes
decreased need for s.
deep s.
deep sleep of short duration
s. deficit
delayed sleep phase
delayed sleep phase syndrome
delta sleep stage
deprivation of s.
desynchronized s.
s. disorder
s. disorders center
disorders of initiating and maintaining s.
s. disruption
s. disturbance
disturbed sleep pattern
drowsiness from sleep apnea
duration of sleep interruption
s. dysfunction
early stages of s.
electroencephalographic sleep study
s. enuresis
s. epilepsy
epilepsy with continuous spikes and waves during s.
epileptic postictal s.
Functional Outcomes of S. Questionnaire
s. hallucination
s. hygiene
s. hygiene abnormality
s. hypoxia
inability to s.
increased rapid eye movement s.
induction of s.
infantile sleep apnea
initial sleep disturbance
s. interruption
s. latency
s. maintenance insomnia
mixed sleep apnea
Multiple S. Latency Test
negative conditioning for s.
night sleep deprivation
night sleep recording
nonrapid eye movement s.
obstructive sleep apnea-hypopnea syndrome
obstructive sleep apnea-hypoventilation
Obstructive S. Disorders-6 test
obstructive sleep apnea syndrome
obstructive sleep disorder
s. onset
s. onset insomnia
overnight sleep evaluation
paradoxical s.
s. paralysis
s. patterns of insomniac
periodic limb movements during s.
periodic limb movement in s.
positive occipital sharp transients of s.
primary sleep disorder
prolonged sleep apnea
rapid eye movement s.
restorative s.
s. restriction therapy
revising sleep habits
slow wave s.
s. spindle
s. stage change frequency
symmetrical sleep pattern
synchronized s.
s. terror disorder
total sleep time
transitional s.
upper airway sleep apnea
wake after sleep onset
wake after sleep onset time
wakefulness after sleep onset

sleep-deprivation therapy

sleep-disordered breathing

sleep-dream study

sleeper
stomach s.

sleepiness
disorders of excessive s.
Epworth S. Scale
excessive daytime s.
Stanford S. Scale

sleeping
African sleeping sickness
West African sleeping sickness

sleep-onset rapid eye movement period

sleep-related
s.-r. asthma
s.-r. cluster headache
s.-r. epileptic seizure
s.-r. hallucination
s.-r. head banging
s.-r. tumescence

sleep-wake
s.-w. abnormality
s.-w. cycle
s.-w. shift

sleepwalker
current s.
past s.

sleeve
advancement sleeve flap
anterior labroligamentous periosteal s.
anterior labroligamentous periosteal sleeve avulsion lesion
anterior labrum periosteal sleeve avulsion
anterior segment s.
arachnoid s.
arachnoidal root s.
arthroscopic monopolar thermal stabilization forefoot compression s.
drill s.
elastic knee sleeve brace
s. graft
malleolar gel s.
pneumatic compression s.

slew rate

slice
angled s.
apical short-axis s.
axial s.
s. excitation wave
s. graft
s. sensitivity profile
transaxial s.
whole tomography s.

slick-gut syndrome

slide
s. agglutination test
automated slide staining
s. board
Hemoccult slide test
s. latex agglutination
microscope s.
tube slide agglutination test

sliding
anterior sliding tibial graft
s. esophageal hiatal hernia

s. fee scale
s. hernia
s. inlay bone graft
massive sliding graft
s. scale insulin
s. scale insulin therapy

slight
s. hearing impairment
s. hearing loss
s. intention tremor
s. trace

slightly
s. active
moderately constricted and slightly reactive pupil
moderately dilated and slightly reactive pupil
s. more marked since

slim disease

sling
autogenous fascia lata sling procedure
autologous rectus fascia s.
continuous sling suture
head s.
knee sling exercises
lower lid sling procedure
Martius flap and fascial s.
Mersilene mesh s.
s. procedure
Sayre head s.
s. suspension
s. and swathe
vaginal wall s.

Slingerland Screening Tests

slip
s. made out
s. sent

slipped
s. capital femoral epiphysis
s. disk
s. elbow
s. hernia
s. meniscus
s. on ice
s. upper femoral epiphysis

slipping
s. dentures
s. rib syndrome

slit
s. diaphragm
fixed slit lamp
s. graft
peripheral capillary filtration slit length
s. ventricle syndrome

slit-lamp examination

Slocum operation

slope
electromechanical slope computer
initial slope index
International S. Index
mandibular anteroposterior ridge s.
mitral deceleration s.
oxygen uptake efficiency s.

Slosson
S. Articulation Language Test with Phonology
S. Intelligence Test
S. Oral Reading Test-Revised
S. Test of Reading Readiness

slot
anterior slot graft arthrodesis

slot-blot hybridization analysis

slotted
AO slotted medullary nail

slouch
arch and slouch position

slough
skin graft s.

sloughed-off skin

sloughing
endometrial s.
mucosal s.
tissue s.

slow
abnormally slow heart rate
abnormally slow rhythm
s. activity
s. alpha variant rhythm
background of slow activity
s. blood clotting
central slow wave focus
s. channel blocker
s. cognitive processing
s. component
continuous slow ultrafiltration
coronary slow flow syndrome
s. death factor
disoriented or slow thought process
s. down cancer growth
s. expressive language development
s. eye movement
s. fetal growth
s. filling wave
focus of slow activity
generalized slow activity
s. growth rate
s. heartbeat
s. heart rate
s. heart rhythm
s. hemoglobin
high-voltage arrhythmic slow wave
high-voltage diphasic slow wave
high-voltage slow activity
s. high-voltage wave
s. immune response
independent slow wave
s. infusion
s. inhibitory potential
s. initial function
s. intravenous drip
s. intravenous infusion
s. intravenous push
large amplitude, slow wave activity
s. lateral eye movement
left ventricular slow filling time
s. low-efficiency dialysis
s. mitten pattern
s. oxidative
s. paroxysmal atrial tachycardia
paroxysmal high-voltage slow wave
pressure at slow component intercept
s. pullthrough
relatively slow sinus rate
s. release
s. release of hormones
runs of slow activity
s. spinal cord compression syndrome
s. transit constipation
s. twitch
s. twitch fiber
s. vital capacity
s. volume encephalography
s. waking activity
s. wave activity
s. wave sleep
zone of slow conduction

slow-acting antirheumatic drug

slow-binding target-attaching globulin

slow-channel congenital myasthenic syndrome

slow-component velocity

slowed
s. intellectual function
s. reaction time

slower
conduction velocity of slower fibers

slowest moving protease

slow-fast tachycardia

slow-growing
s.-g. acoustic neuroma
s.-g. cortical neoplasm
s.-g. invasive adenocarcinoma

slowing
continuous high-amplitude electroencephalogram rhythmical synchronous s.
hyperventilation-induced high-amplitude rhythmic s.
junctional s.
macrophage slowing factor

slowly
s. developing atelectasis
s. developing lesion
disease progressed s.
s. growing invasive adenocarcinoma
s. growing tumor
moves all extremities s.
s. progressive hereditary disorder

slow-moving
s.-m. protease
s.-m. vehicle

slowness of mental action

slow-phase velocity

slow-progressive schizophrenia

slow-reacting
s.-r. factor
s.-r. factor of anaphylaxis
s.-r. substance
s.-r. substance of anaphylaxis

slow-twitch fiber

slow-wave
s.-w. abnormality
s.-w. encephalography

Sluder
lower half headache of S.
S. neuralgia

sludge
s. ball
gallbladder s.
semicontinuous activated s.

sludged blood

sluggish
s. blood return
s. gallbladder

sluggishly
pupils react s.

slumber
affective s.

slumping
spinal s.

slurred
chronic slurred speech
s. indistinct speech
s. speech

slurring
s. of ST
s. of QRS

slurry
autogenous bone s.
bone s.
talc s.

slush
saline s.

Sly
mucopolysaccharidosis type VII S.
S. syndrome

small
s. airway disease
s. airway dysfunction
s. airway obstruction
s. aorta syndrome
s. artery
asymmetric small foramen magnum
atypical small acinar proliferation of prostate
s. blood pressure cuff
s. bone structure
s. bowel
s. bowel adenocarcinoma
s. bowel adenoma
s. bowel anastomosis
s. bowel atresia
s. bowel bacterial overgrowth
s. bowel biopsy
s. bowel carcinoma
s. bowel disease
s. bowel dysmotility
s. bowel enteroscopy
s. bowel followthrough
s. bowel ischemia
s. bowel loop
s. bowel motility
s. bowel mucosa
s. bowel obstruction
s. bowel peristalsis
s. bowel phytobezoar
s. bowel series
s. bowel thickening
s. bowel transit time
s. bowel transplantation
s. bowel tumor
s. bowel volvulus
s. brain hemorrhage
brief, small, abundant motor-unit action potential
brief, small, abundant, polyphasic potential
s. caliber vessel
s. cell bronchogenic carcinoma
s. cell cancer of bladder
s. cell carcinoma
s. cell carcinoma of bronchus
s. cell carcinoma of lung
s. cell malignant lymphoma
s. cell osteosarcoma
s. cell sarcoma
s. cell tumor
s. cell undifferentiated carcinoma of the prostate
s. cell undifferentiated neuroendocrine carcinoma
s. cleaved cell
complete small bowel obstruction
contaminated small bowel syndrome
s. cystic infarct
s., deep, recent infarct
desmoplastic small round-cell tumor
detail response to small white space
distal portion of small intestine
s. end-expiratory pressure
extrapulmonary small cell carcinoma
fluid-filled small bowel
s. focus hemorrhage
s. focus of hepatic necrosis
full-term, small for gestational age
gangrenous small bowel
s. for gestational age
s. gram-negative coccobacilli
s. granular vesicle
s. group therapy
immunoproliferative small intestine disease
s. incision cataract surgery
s. increment sensitivity index
s., intensely fluorescent ganglion

intermittent small bowel obstruction
s. intestinal atresia
s. intestinal submucosa
s. intestinal wall
s. intestine absorption
s. intestine as a defense barrier
s. intestine bacterial overgrowth
s. intestine cancer
s. intestine channel acupuncture
s. intestine mesentery
s. intestine transplant
left anterior small thoracotomy
s. leukocyte
limited anterior small thoracotomy
limited quantity test performed on small specimen
limited-stage small cell lung cancer
longitudinal layer of muscle coat of small intestine
s. lymphocyte
s. lymphocytic lymphoma
malignant small round cell tumor
mixed sclerosing bone dysplasia, small stature, seizures, mental retardation syndrome
mixed small cleaved and large cell lymphoma
mucosal surface of small intestine
multiple loops of small bowel
s. muscle atrophy
muscular coat of small intestine
muscular layer of small intestine
neonatal small left colon syndrome
neuroendocrine small cell carcinoma
s. noncleaved cell lymphoma
s. noncleaved cell, non-Burkitt lymphoma
s. nuclear ribonucleic acid
s. nuclear ribonucleoprotein
s. nuclear ribonucleoprotein-associated polypeptide
painless, small intact blister
partial small bowel obstruction
patient independent with small based quad cane
s. pedunculated adenomatous polyps
s. protein
proximal small bowel
pulmonary embolus with small infarct
s. pyramidal cell
s. round-cell tumor
s. round structured virus
s. sharp spike
short small bowel
s. spherical particle
stenting in small arteries
strangulated small bowel
s. third-trimester fetus
total small intestinal allotransplantation
upper gastrointestinal series with small bowel follow-through
s. vein of heart
s. vessel disease
s. vessel inadequate blood flow
s. volume
s. volume parenteral infusion
s. whirlpool
s., yellow, constipated stool

small-angle double-incidence angiogram

small-based quad cane

Small-Carrion penile prosthesis

smaller rib incision

smallest unit of DNA capable of recombination

small-intestine transplantation

small-particle aerosol generator

smallpox
malignant s.
modified s.
s. vaccination

small-scale integration

small-vessel infarction

small-volume nebulizer

Sma- and Mad-related protein

smart anesthesia multigas

smear
abnormal Pap s.
acid-fast bacilli s.
acid-fast sputum s.
anal Pap s.
bacteria in blood s.
s. and culture
fungus s.
fungus, smear, and culture
last Pap s.
low-grade positive s.
LSIL Pap s.
peripheral blood s.
Richart Pap s.
self-obtained s.
special Pap s.
sputum s.
stained smear and culture
vaginal cervical endocervical s.
vaginal irrigation s.
wet s.

smell
University of Pennsylvania S. Identification Test

smelling
foul-smelling urine
purulent and foul s.

Smeloff-Cutter

Smeloff heart valve

smile incision

Smillie nail

Smith
Eustace Smith murmur
S. fracture
S. physical capacities evaluation
Rodney Smith tubes
S. subtalar joint arthroereisis peg

Smith-Fineman-Myers syndrome

Smith-Lemli-Opitz syndrome

Smith-Magenis syndrome

smoke
cigarette s.
cigarette smoke asthma
cigarette smoke condensate
cigarette smoke solution
environmental tobacco s.
s. exposure
s. exposure machine
s. extract
filtered smoke exposure
s. inhalation
passive smoke exposure
passive tobacco s.
patient treated for smoke inhalation
s. removal tube

smoke-induced lung injury

smokeless tobacco

smoker
s. bronchitis
cigarette s.
continuing s.
habitual cocaine s.
s. hack
s. heart

smoking
S. Behavior Questionnaire
s. cessation
emphysema secondary to heavy s.
s. habit

smoking *(continued)*
hazard of s.
health risks from s.
s. history
involuntary s.
kicking smoking habit
long smoking history
maternal s.
Office on S. and Health
opium s.
rapid s.

Smoky
Great Smoky Mountains Study of Youth

smoldering myeloma

smooth
airway smooth muscle
alpha smooth muscle actin
arterial smooth muscle cell
s. bacterial colony
s. border
capsular surface smooth and glistening
s., capsulated, virulent bacteria
s. cell
s. colony
s. contour
s. cortical surface
s. endoplasmic reticulum
s. excimer laser coronary angioplasty
gastrointestinal smooth muscle tumor
guinea pig tracheal smooth muscle
human aortic smooth muscle cell
hypertrophic smooth muscle layer
s. muscle
s. muscle actin
s. muscle activating factor
s. muscle antibody
s. muscle autoantibody
s. muscle cell
s. muscle contracting agent
s. muscle contraction
s. muscle tumors
myometrial smooth muscle
peritoneum smooth and glistening
s. pursuit eye movement
soft and smooth prostate
vascular smooth muscle cell

smooth-rough bacterial colony

smudge cell

snake
Arizona coral s.
moccasin snake bite
s. venom

snap
chemical snap pack
mitral opening s.
opening mitral valve s.
opening snap ejection systolic click
opening tricuspid valve s.

snapping
s. finger
hip s.
medial snapping hip syndrome

snare
angiographic 2-wire s.
s. cautery
dissection and s.
dissection and snare tonsillectomy
electrosurgical s.
electrosurgical snare polypectomy
endoscopic s.

sneeze syncope

sneezing
control itching and s.

Snellen
S. conventional reform implant
S. eye chart
S. reform eye
S. sign

Snider Match Test

sniff
alcohol sniff test

sniffer's
glue sniffer's rash

sniffing
sudden sniffing death

snooze-induced excitation of sympathetic triggered activity

snoring
apneic spell associated with loud s.
habitual s.
s. rales

snow
anesthetizing effect of ice and s.
s. glasses

snowball
mycotic snowball opacity

snowman
s. abnormality
s. heart

snowshoe hare virus

snowstorm shadow

snuff
moist s.

snuffbox
anatomical s.

Snyder-Robinson syndrome

soak
astringent s.
saline s.
sterile saline s.

soap
animal s.
cola tar s.
strong soap solution
tincture of green s.
s. and water

soapsuds
high soapsuds enema

soapy kidney

Sociability
Emotionality Activity Sociability Scale

social
s. ability
s. acquiescence
S. Adaptation Self-Evaluation Scale
S. Adaptation Status
S. Adequacy Index
S. Adjustment Self-Report Scale
adult social dysfunction
s. age
s. anxiety disorder
anxiety-induced impaired social functioning
Automated Child/Adolescent S. History
s. avoidance and distress
S. Behavior Assessment Inventory
s. breakdown syndrome
Brief Social Phobia Scale
Bristol S. Adjustment Guides
California Preschool S. Competency Scale
certified social worker
S. Climate Scale
conforms to social normal
s. consciousness
decline in social relationships
s. desirability
diagnostic, social and addiction history form
s. drinker
Early S. Communication Scale
emotional, spiritual, and s.
s. environmental therapy

ethical, legal, and social implications
Facial Disability Index S.
feelings of social inadequacy
S. Function Index
generalized social phobia
s. growth
s. handicap
heavy social drinkers
hepatitis virus social history
s. history
s. history as screening device for drug abuse
impaired social interaction
impairment of social function
inappropriate social behavior
s. information system
s. inhibition
s. interaction
s. or interpersonal situation
s. interpersonal skills
s. intervention
s. introversion
s. isolation
s. issue
key integrative social system
loss of interest in peer social activity
Mandel S. Adjustment Scale
Marlowe-Crown S. Desirability Scale
Multidimensional Scale of Perceived S. Support
S. and Occupational Functioning Assessment
occupational and social impairment
past social history
personal and social history
S. and Prevocational Information Battery
Progress Assessment Chart of S. and Personal Development
psychiatric social worker
psychological, social, and vocational
s. quotient
S. Readjustment Rating Scale
s. recreation
S. Relations Test
S. Skills Rating System
s. skills training
s. stigma
s. stress and functionality inventory
s. stressor
supportive social structure
Teacher Assessment of S. Behavior
Test of S. Inferences
Vineland S. Maturity Scale
Vineland Measurement of S. Competence

social/family well-being

socialization
adult s.

socialized
s. delinquency
s. dementia
s. medicine

socially
s. acceptable monitoring instrument
s. and emotionally disturbed
s. inappropriate behavior
s. incompetent
s. isolated

societal
age-appropriate societal norm

socioeconomic
s. factor
s. status

sociogenic
mass sociogenic illness

sociopathic personality disorder

Sociopolitical Locus of Control

sock
ankle-foot orthosis brace s.
arthritis s.
cast s.
gloves and s.'s syndrome
knee-high s.'s
long-handled sock donner
papular-purpuric gloves and socks syndrome
thigh-high s.'s

socket
adjustable postoperative protective prosthetic s.
s. joint
one-stage reconstruction of eye socket and eyelids
patella tendon s.
quadrilateral s.
suction s.
universal frame outer s.
variable circumference suprapatellar s.

soda
s. headache
s. lime

sodium
s. amylosulfate
s. amytal interview
anhydrous sodium sulfite
s. antimony gluconate
s. aurothiomalate
s. balance
s. bicarbonate
s. bicarbonate in invert sugar
caffeine sodium benzoate
carbazochrome sodium sulfonate
s. carboxymethylcellulose
s. chloride
s. chloride, adenine, glucose, mannitol
s. chloride-sodium citrate solution
s. citrate
s. clearance
congenital sodium diarrhea
s. cromoglycate
s. current
s. deficiency
s. deoxycholate
s. depletion
dextran sodium sulfate
s. dialysate
s. diphenylhydantoin
docusate s.
s. dodecyl sulfate
s. dodecyl sulfate-polyacrylamide gel electrophoresis
epithelial sodium channel
filtered s.
s. fluorescein
fractional excretion of s.
s. glucose cotransporter
gold sodium thioglucose
gold sodium thiomalate
s. hypochlorite
10% invert sugar in 0.9% sodium chloride saline injection
s. iodide
s. lactate
low sodium intake
menadiol sodium diphosphate
2-mercaptoethane sulphonate s.
s. monofluoroacetate
s. nitroprusside
normal sodium diet
s. perborate
phenobarbital s.
phosphate-buffered s.
plasma s.
potassium, sodium chloride, and sodium lactate solution
s. and potassium spot urine test
s. pregnanediol glucuronide

sodium *(continued)*
reduce sodium intake
saline sodium citrate
s. sensitivity
sieving coefficient for s.
s. sulfite titration
supplemental minimal s.
sustained-release sodium fluoride
s. tetradecylsulfate
thallium-activated sodium iodide crystal
s. thiocyanate
s. thiopental
s. thiosulfate
total body s.
total exchangeable s.
s. tripolyphosphate
s. urate crystal
urinary concentration of s.
urinary sodium excretion
s. wasting

sodium/hydrogen exchanger

sodium-iodide symporter

sodium-lithium
s.-l. countertransport
s.-l. countertransporter

sodium-potassium

sodium-potassium-2 chloride cotransporter

sodium- and potassium-activated adenosine triphosphatase

sodium-restricted diet

Soemmerring
S. crystalline swelling
S. ganglion
S. gray substance

soft
s. abdomen
abdominal soft tissue density
acute soft tissue injury
alveolar soft part sarcoma
s. ankle, cushioned heel orthopaedic appliance
anterior soft tissue impingement
ASTM augmented soft tissue mobilization
augmented soft tissue mobilization
baby soft diet
breasts soft and nontender
California soft spinal system
s. callus stage
s. cartilage
s. cataract
closed soft tissue injury
daily-wear soft contact lens
devitalized soft tissue
distal soft tissue release
s. drusen
s. drusen maculopathy
s. elastic capsule
s. elastic gelatin capsule
elastic soft tissue
extended-wear soft contact lens
s. exudate
s. feces
fibrosarcoma of soft tissue
s. and flat
s. fleshy lesion
s. fleshy nodule
s. fluctuant nodular lesion
foreign body soft tissue
full and soft diet
hard and soft palates
histiocytoma of soft tissue
large green soft stool
large yellow soft stools
s. lesion
malignant fibrous histiocytoma of soft tissue
malignant rhabdoid tumor of soft tissue
medium yellow soft stools
Modane S.
multiple soft tissue injuries
myxomatous soft connective tissue
s. nevus
nonrhabdomyosarcoma soft tissue sarcoma
orbital, mandibular, ear, neural, soft tissue
orbit, mandible, ear, cranial nerves, soft tissue syndrome
s. organs not palpable
s. palate
s. parts giant cell tumor
periarticular soft tissue
periorbital soft tissue
physical and neurologic examination for soft signs
s. and pliable
posterior nasal spine to soft palate
prevertebral soft tissue
pureed, mechanical, soft diet
recent soft tissue hemorrhage
retropharyngeal soft tissue space
rhabdomyosarcoma of soft tissue
s. and smooth prostate
s. tissue abscess
s. tissue calcification
s. tissue carcinoma
s. tissue compression injury
s. tissue density
s. tissue hematoma
s. tissue hemorrhage
s. tissue hemorrhage into mesentery
s. tissue infection
s. tissue invasion
s. tissue involvement
s. tissue laceration
s. tissue loss
s. tissue mass
s. tissue metastasis
s. tissue nodule
s. tissue sarcoma
s. tissue shadow
s. tissue swelling
s. tissue treatment
s. tissue tumor
s. tissue view

softener
stool s.

softening
s. of the brain
s. of cartilage
diffuse hepatic s.
gray s.
hemorrhagic s.

softness
variable s.

soft-tissue rheumatism

software
linear combination model s.
osteotomy analysis simulation s.

soil
night s.

soiling
fecal s.

Sokuluk virus

solar
s. cheilitis
s. comedo
s. dermatitis
s. elastosis
s. fever
s. ganglion
s. keratosis
s. lentigo
nasal solar dermatitis
s. retinopathy
s. therapy
s. urticaria

solaris
macula s.
Soldado virus
soldering flux
sole
s. community hospital
hyperkeratosis of s.
soleus
gastrocnemius s.
gastrocnemius and soleus muscles
line for soleus muscle
s. muscle
tendinous arch of soleus muscle
solid
s. ankle flexible endoskeletal
s. bone mass
s. cystic tumor
s. and cystic tumor of the pancreas
dissolved s.'s
double antibody solid phase
s. extract
fat-free s.
s. food
gastric emptying of s.'s
glycogen- and fat-free s.
Knoop hardness number of s.'s
mixed echogenic solid mass
s. organs not palpable
s. organ transplant
s. phase
s. phase fluorescence immunoassay
s. phase peptide synthesis
s. phase radioimmunoassay
s. phase receptacle
total body s.'s
total serum s.'s
total s.'s in urine
s. tumor
solidified liquid
solid-phase
s.-p. enzyme-linked immunospot
s.-p. extraction
s.-p. immunoabsorbent assay
s.-p. immunoassay
s.-p. immunoassay fluorescence
s.-p. microextraction
solid-state transducer intracompartment
solitarii
lymphatici s.
noduli lymphoidei s.
solitary
s. autonomous nodule
s. bone cyst
s. bone lesion
s. bundle
extramedullary solitary plasmacytoma
s. fasciculus
s. fibrous tumor
s. follicle
s. gland
s. kidney
s. lesion
s. lymphatic nodule
s. lymph node
s. plasmacytoma of bone
s. pulmonary nodule
s. rectal ulcer
s. rectal ulcer syndrome
s. ulcer of rectum syndrome
solitus
atrial situs s.
solubility
Bunsen solubility coefficient
Ostwald solubility coefficient
potassium solubility product
soluble
s. in alkaline medium
s. antigen fluorescent antibody test
s. c-kit
cold water s.
collagenase soluble glomerular basement membrane
s. complement receptor
s. complex
s. cytoplasmic protein
s. cytotoxic medium
s. egg antigen
epidermal soluble protein
s. fibrin-fibrinogen complex
s. fibrin monomer
s. fibrin monomer complex
fumarate hydratase, s.
s. gelatin
glutamic-oxaloacetic transaminase, s.
s. glycoprotein
s. HLA antigen
hot water s.
s. human leukocyte antigen
s. immune response suppressor
s. insulin
s. intracellular adhesion molecule
s. liver antigen
nonionic detergent s.
partly s.
s. recombinant human CD4
recombinant soluble CD4
s. repository
s. ribonuclear protein
s. ribonucleic acid
serum soluble antigen
sparingly s.
s. specific substance
s. suppressor factor
thymidine kinase, s.
s. transferrin receptor
s. tumor necrosis factor-a receptor type I
s. viral extract
water s.
Soluset
intravenous S.
solute
potential renal solute load
renal solute load
total body s.
total solute absorption
weight of solute per volume of solution
weight of solute per weight of solvent
solution
acid test s.
alcohol, ether, and acetone s.
aluminum chloride s.
amino acid-enriched cardioplegic s.
antibiotic and saline s.
anticoagulant heparin s.
apparatus for maintaining pH of s.
arterial line flush s.
balanced electrolyte s.
balanced saline s.
balanced salt s.
Betadine scrub s.
boric acid s.
buffered Ringer s.
buffered saline s.
cardioplegic perfusion s.
cervical mucous s.
cigarette smoke s.
Collins s.
colloid replacement s.
commercial dialysis s.
contamination from irrigating s.'s
crystalline amino acid s.
crystalloid cardioplegic s.
dilute volume of s.
double-normal solution
Earle balanced salt s.
enteral nutrition s.
erythromycin topical s.
extracellular-like, calcium-free s.

solution *(continued)*
extravasation irrigation s.
s. focused group therapy
formaldehyde, acetic acid, and alcohol s.
formalin, acetic, and alcohol s.
fortified aqueous s.
gelatin Hanks buffered salt s.
glucose-electrolyte s.
glucose-free Hanks solution
glucose-insulin-potassium solution
glucose-Ringer-phosphate s.
Grey balanced saline s.
half-normal solution
Hanks balanced salt s.
Hanks balanced salt solution plus glucose
Hartmann s.
heparinized solution infusion
hundredth molar s.
hydroxyethyl starch solution
hyperalimentation s.
inside bathing s.
Krebs-Henseleit s.
Krebs-Ringer bicarbonate s.
Krebs-Ringer phosphate s.
lactated Ringer s.
Los Angeles preservation solution 1
low ionic strength solution
Lugol iodine s.
lymph node revealing s.
maintenance electrolyte s.
merthiolate formaldehyde s.
merthiolate, iodine, formalin solution
metered solution inhaler
minimal essential s.
modified Hanks balanced salt s.
modified University of Wisconsin s.
molar s.
molecular dispersed s.
neonatal morphine s.
neonatal opium s.
nonstandard electrolyte s.
normal Krebs-Henseleit s.
normal saline s.
operative area irrigated with antibiotic s.
operative site irrigated with antibiotic s.
ophthalmic s.
oral rehydration s.
original University of Wisconsin s.
oxidation of s.
peripheral protein sparing s.
physiologic saline s.
physiologic salt s.
pilocarpine 1% ophthalmic s.
polyethylene glycol electrolyte lavage s.
potassium iodide, saturated s.
potassium, sodium chloride, and sodium lactate s.
preservative-free solution system
rehydrating s.
Ringer lactate s.
saline s.
saline solution enema
saturated potassium iodide s.
saturated solution of potassium iodide
Seligmann buffered salt s.
silver nitrate s.
sodium chloride-sodium citrate s.
stable plasma protein s.
standard electrolyte s.
sterile s.
sterile aqueous s.
sterile injectable s.
strong soap s.
tenth molar s.
tenth-normal s.
tobramycin solution for inhalation
tris-buffered Grey solution
tropicamide 1% ophthalmic solution Mydriacyl
Tween-TRIS-buffered saline s.
University of Wisconsin s.
volumetric s.
weight of solute per volume of s.

solvent
automatic computerized solvent litholysis
brain protein s.
nearly ideal binary s.
organic solvent poisoning
weight of solute per weight of s.

solving
Interpersonal Cognitive Problem S.
means-end problem s.
problem s.
problem solving information

Somagyi reflex

somata
neuronal s.

somatic
s. agglutinin
anxious somatic depression
s. artery
s. cell-derived growth factor
s. cell human gene therapy
s. complaint
s. crossing-over
s. delusion
s. depression
s. dysfunction
s. dysfunction lower extremity
s. dysfunction upper extremity
general somatic afferent nerve
general somatic efferent nerve
s. induction
Inventory of Psychic and S. Complaints in the Elderly
Modified S. Perception Questionnaire
s. pain
s. reaction
special somatic afferent
s. symptom

somatically evoked field

somatoform
atypical somatoform disorder

somatomammotropin
chorionic s.
human chorionic s.
immunoradioassayable human chorionic s.
immunoreactive human chorionic s.

somatomedin
s. A, C

somatosensory
s. aura
s. brainstem evoked potential
central somatosensory conduction time
cervical somatosensory evoked potential
s. cortex
s. cortical evoked potential
cortical somatosensory evoked potential
cortical somatosensory evoked response
s. deficit
s. dysfunction
s. evoked response
evoked somatosensory response
extreme somatosensory evoked potential
s. impairment
left somatosensory evoked potential

lower extremity somatosensory evoked potential
median nerve somatosensory evoked potential
right somatosensory evoked potential
s. thalamus
upper extremity somatosensory evoked potential

somatostatin
intraluminal s.
s. receptor
s. receptor scintigraphy

somatostatin-like immunoreactivity

somatotroph hormone

somatotropic hormone

somatotropin
human chorionic s.
s. release factor
s. release-inhibiting factor
s. release-inhibiting hormone

somatotropin-releasing
s.-r. factor
s.-r. hormone

somatotyping ponderal index

somatropin deficiency syndrome

some appreciable change

somesthetic sensibility

somite
s. embryo
müllerian duct, unilateral renal agenesis, and anomalies of the cervicothoracic s.'s
müllerian, renal, cervicothoracic, somite abnormalities
müllerian, renal, cervicothoracic, somite abnormalities syndrome

sommeil

somnambulism
cataleptic s.
s. disorder

somnolence
disorders of excessive s.
excessive daytime s.

somnolent
s. metabolic rate
s. and obtunded

Somogyi
S. effect
S. phenomenon
S. unit

Sondermann canal

Songo fever

sonic
prefrontal sonic treatment
s. imaging technique

sonic-accelerated fracture-healing system

sonication-induced epitope retrieval

Sonne-Duval bacillus

sonogram
fatty meal s.
s. of heart
ophthalmic Doppler s.

sonographic
growth-adjusted sonographic age
s. planning of oncology treatment

sonography
Aspen sonography unit
colonic transabdominal s.
color-coded duplex s.
color Doppler s.
color-flow Doppler s.
contrast-enhanced transcranial color-coded real-time s.
diagnostic medical s.
directional Doppler s.
Doppler s.
extracranial Doppler s.
focused abdominal s.
focused abdominal sonography for trauma
focused assessment by sonography for trauma
functional transcranial Doppler s.
high-frequency ultrasound probe s.
high-resolution endoluminal s.
intraoperative s.
saline infusion s.
second-look s.
s. of subfascial hematoma
transcranial color-coded duplex s.
transcranial color-coded real-time s.
transcranial Doppler s.
transvaginal color Doppler s.
two-dimensional transcranial color-coded s.
ultra–Doppler s.

sonohysterography
saline infusion s.

sonolucent area

sonometer
ultrasound bone imaging s.

sonorous rale

soot cancer

sophistication
Vocational Interest and S. Assessment

soporific drug

sorbent unit

sorbitan sesquioleate

sorbitol
s. dehydrogenase
s. MacConkey agar

sore
burning mouth from cold s.
canker sore from anxiety
fungating s.
gaping, draining s.
mixed s.
Naga s.
natal s.
nonhealing s.
open s.
oriental s.
pressure s.
pressure sore risk assessment

soreness
delayed muscle s.
delayed-onset muscle s.
pain and s.

Soret band

Soria operation

Sororoca virus

Sorsby
S. pseudoinflammatory macular degeneration
S. syndrome

sorted
mean sorted difference

sorter
fluorescence-activated cell s.
fluorescence-activated cell sorter scan
magnetically activated cell s.

sorting
density-adjusted cell s.
S. of Figures Test
fluorescence-activated cell s.
fluorescent-activated cell s.
Object S. Scales psychologic test
Object S. Test
Wisconsin Card S. Test

Soto-Hall sign

Soucek
Randall-Baker S.

souffle
fetal s.
mammary s.

sound
s. abatement
absent bowel s.'s
absent breath s.'s
active bowel s.'s
adventitial pulmonary s.
adventitious breath s.
amphoric respiratory s.
anodal closure s.
anodal opening s.
aortic ejection s.
aortic first s.
aortic second sound, pulmonary second s.
artificial sound generator
association of s.'s and symbols
attention to s.
auditory perception of speech s.'s
auscultation of bowel s.'s
bilateral breath s.'s
bilateral equal breath s.'s
bowel s.'s
bowel sounds normal
bowel sounds normal and active
bowel sounds present and active
bowel sounds regular
breath s.'s
breath sounds equal bilaterally
cardiac sounds normal
coarse breath s.'s
crackling s.'s in lungs
crowing breath s.'s
decibels sound pressure level
dichotic environmental sounds test
digital sound processing
diminished bowel s.'s
diminished breath s.'s
distant breath s.
distant heart s.'s
Doppler sound device
dry crackling s.
ejection s.
equal bilateral breath s.'s
equal breath sounds bilaterally
extra heart s.
fetal heart s.
s. field
first to fourth heart s.'s
first heart s.
first through fourth heart s.'s
fourth heart s.
French steel s.
good breath s.
gradual distortion of s.
s. guided into bladder
gurgling bowel s.'s
heart sounds normal
heightened sensitivity to s.'s
high-frequency sound wave
high-pitched bowel s.
hyperactive bowel s.
hypoactive bowel s.'s
s. intensity
s. level
s. level meter
lung s.'s
muffled heart s.
normal bowel s.'s
normal cardiac s.
normoactive bowel s.'s
Ohio Tests of Articulation and Perception of S.'s
output sound pressure level
palpable aortic ejection s.
passage of s.
peak equivalent sound pressure level
perceptually adequate s.
pericardial friction s.
physiologic third heart s.
positive bowel s.'s
s. power
s. pressure
s. pressure level
s. production sample
s. production tasks
pulmonic closure s.
pulmonic heart sound less than aortic second heart s.
pulmonic second heart sound equal to aortic second heart s.
pulmonic second heart sound greater than aortic second heart s.
pulmonic second sound split
quiet breath s.
quiet heart s.
rubbing heart s.
saturation sound pressure level
second aortic sound equals second pulmonic s.
second aortic sound greater than second pulmonic s.
second aortic sound less than second pulmonic s.
splitting of heart s.
s. stimulus
thinking creatively with s.'s and words
third heart s.
tracheal breath s.
tricuspid first heart s.
tricuspid second heart s.
tubular breath s.'s
van Buren s.
velocity of sound of blood
vesicular breath s.'s
xiphisternal crunching s.

sounded
endometrial cavity s.

sound-sensing cell

soup
malt soup extract

soupy
cell soupy cytoplasm

source
common source outbreak
confront source of anxiety
s. of contamination
contamination of exogenous s.'s
discrete bleeding s.
s. of embolism
endoscopic light s.
s. film distance
high-intensity light s.
s. image distance
s. of infection
intense pulsed light s.
intracavitary radiation s.'s
s. of intraperitoneal bleeding
monochromatic light s.
possible source of bleeding
potential source of infection
s. to skin distance

source-skin distance

source-surface distance

source-to-axis distance

source-to-image receptor distance

source-to-skin distance

source-tray distance

South
S. African tick-bite fever
S. African tick fever
S. African type porphyria
S. American blastomycosis
S. American hemorrhagic fever
S. American trypanosomiasis

Southeast
S. Asia mosquito-borne hemorrhagic fever
S. Asian ovalocytosis

Southern
S. blot
S. blot analysis

S. California Figure Ground Test
S. California Postrotary Nystagmus Test
S. California Sensory Integration Tests
S. California Space Visualization Test
S. transfer analysis

soy
s. phytoestrogen extract
trypticase soy plate
trypticase soy broth
trypticase soy yeast
tryptone soy broth
wheat soy blend

soybean
s. agglutinin
cornmeal, soybean, milk
heated soybean flower
s. lecithin
s. oil meal
s. trypsin inhibitor

soybean-casein digest medium

soy-free diet

spa
holistic health s.

space
air space disease
algebraic unknown or space coordinate
anatomic dead s.
anterior cavernous sinus s.
anterior clear s.
anterior incisural s.
anterior pararenal s.
apical air s.
associative detail response to white s.
associative response to a white space on a card
auditory space perception
s. available for the cord
band and bar space maintainer
band and crib space maintainer
bile duct-to-portal space ratio
bonded space maintainer
cantilever space maintainer
s. of the cavernous sinus
change in space and time
color and space perceptual disturbance
dead air s.
deep space neck infection
detail response to small white s.
diffuse air space disease
dilated perivascular s.'s
disc space height
disc space narrowing
distortion of time and s.
s. of Donders
drainage of cerebral epidural s.
epidural space infection
extracellular s.
fifth intercostal s.
s. of His
His perivascular s.
hyaline membranes lining alveolar s.
intercellular tissue s.
intercostal space retraction
interstitial fluid s.
intervertebral disc space infection
lateral intercellular s.
lateral pharyngeal s.
left intercostal s.
mechanical dead s.
medial clear s.
medial hemijoint articular s.
medial joint s.
s. medicine
middle ear s.
narrowed disc s.
narrowing of intervertebral disc s.
narrowing of joint s.
nerve, artery, vein, empty space, lymphatics
obliteration of apophyseal s.
occupying space lesion
oropharyngeal airway s.
parafoveal cystic s.
paralaryngeal s.
parapharyngeal s.
pararectal s.
paravesical s.
patient alert to space, time, and person
perianal anorectal s.
peribronchial alveolar s.
perioptic subarachnoid s.
peripheral air space disease
perivascular lymph s.
physiologic dead s.
point of maximum impulse fifth intercostal s.
Poiseuille s.
posterior airway s.
post space preparation
preepiglottic s.
prevesicle s.
reduced space symbologies
response to white s.
retropharyngeal soft tissue s.
retrorectal s.
retrovaginal s.
right intercostal s.
rudimentary disc s.
Southern California S. Visualization Test
subarachnoid s.
subendothelial s.
subtrapezial s.
tissue s.
ventilation of alveolar dead s.
ventilation of anatomic dead s.
ventilation per minute of dead s.
vesicocervical s.
vesicovaginal s.
visual pleural s.
volume of alveolar dead s.
volume of anatomic dead s.
volume of mechanical dead s.
wide intervertebral s.

space-adaptation syndrome

space-occupying lesion

spacer
internal transcribed s.
temporary articulating methylmethacrylate antibiotic s.

spacing
parallel line equal s.

spagyric medicine

Spalding sign

span
Arithmetic, Coding, Information, and Digit S.
attention span shortened from anxiety
auditory memory s.
digit s.
increased attention s.
increase in life s.
life s.
Life S. Study
limited attention s.
mean life s.
median life s.
perceptual span time
short attention s.
shortened attention span from anxiety
Visual Aural Digit S. Test
visual memory s.

Spanish
S. American
S. American black
S. American female

Spanish *(continued)*
S. American male
Austin Spanish Articulation Test

Spanish-speaking only

spanner
multimembrane s.

spanning
glycosylated protein spanning viral envelope

sparganosis
nodules in s.
ocular s.

sparing
arytenoid s.
limb sparing surgery
macular s.
peripheral protein sparing solution
rejuvenation with sparing of vascular perforators

sparingly soluble

sparse
microcephaly, sparse hair, mental retardation, seizures syndrome

spasm
carpal pedal s.
catheter-induced s.
compulsive s.'s and tics
constriction or spasm of blood vessel
coronary artery s.
coronary spasm induction
coronary spasm and prolapse
diffuse esophageal s.
hemifacial s.
intermittent or continuous s.'s
s. of intestinal wall
involuntary spasm of diaphragm
lightning attacks in infantile s.
microcephaly, infantile spasm, psychomotor retardation, nephrotic syndrome
mixed infantile s.
muscle s.
nocturnal painful tonic s.
oculomotor paresis with cyclic s.
painful muscle s.
pain and spasm of muscles
paraspinal muscle s.
paravertebral muscle s.
piriformis muscle s.
primary symptomatic diffuse esophageal s.
sphincter of Oddi s.
sudden torsion s.
symptomatic diffuse esophageal s.
winking s.'s

spasmodic
abductor spasmodic dysphonia
adductor spasmodic dysphonia
s. asthma
s. dysmenorrhea
s. dysphonia
s. strabismus
s. tabes
Toronto Western S. Torticollis Rating Scale

spasmolytic
pancreatic spasmolytic peptide

spastic
s. aphonia
ataxic and spastic dysarthria
autosomal recessive spastic ataxia of Charlevoix-Saguenay
s. bladder
s. bowel syndrome
s. colon
s. dysarthria
s. dysphonia
s. entropion
familial spastic paraplegia
s. flatfoot
s. gait
s. hemiplegia
hereditary spastic paraparesis
hereditary spastic paraplegia
s. ileus
mental retardation, spastic paraplegia, palmoplantar hyperkeratosis syndrome
mild spastic diplegic cerebral palsy
s. muscle activity
s. mydriasis
neuromuscular firing in spastic subject
s. paraplegia
s. stricture
tropical spastic paraparesis
tropical spastic paraparesis/HTLV-I associated myelopathy

spasticity
adductor spasticity of hip
s. of arm
Ashworth score of muscle s.
counteract s.
mental deficiency, spasticity, congenital ichthyosis syndrome
mental retardation, spasticity, distal transverse limb defects syndrome

spatial
s. acuity
altered spatial perception
s. aptitude
s. average
s. average-pulse average
s. average-temporal average
s. average temporal peak
s. deficit
dynamic spatial reconstructor
s. emotional stimuli
s. intensity
left maximal spatial voltage
maximal spatial vector to left
Minnesota S. Relations Test
s. modulation of magnetization
s. nonemotional stimuli
S. Orientation Memory Test
s. peak temporal average
s. sense
s. skills and attention
unilateral spatial neglect
s. vectorcardiogram
Weber Advanced S. Perception test

spatially resolved spectroscopy

spatula
metal handle mixing s.
microvitreoretinal s.
needle s.
nucleus s.
Obstbaum synechia s.

spatulated
ASSI breast dissector s.

spatulation
graft s.

Spatz-Lindenberg disease

Spaulding-Richardson hysterectomy

speak
difficulty or inability to s.
inability to s.

speaking
avoidance s.
s. fundamental frequency
s. phonation

spear
Merocel surgical s.

special
S. Aptitude Test Battery
s. baby Travesol
s. care
s. care baby unit
s. care formula
s. care nursery

Children with S. Health Care Needs
s. education
s. handicap
infant-toddler special care unit
intensive special care nursery
intensive special care unit
s. interest group
s. intervention
medical special care unit
s. monthly compensation
s. monthly pension
s. mouth care
newborn special care unit
no special preparation necessary for test
s. observation
orthopedic examination, s.
s. Pap smear
pediatric special care unit
Respiratory S. Care Unit
s. sense organs
s. skills training
s. somatic afferent
s. teaching issue
s. tube feeding
s. visceral afferent
s. visceral efferent

specialist
work capacity s.

specialized
s. columnar epithelium
s. intestinal metaplasia
s. tissue aspirating resectoscope
s. treatment facility
ventricular specialized conduction system

specialty
cardiovascular specialty unit
clinical specialty unit
s. inpatient service

species
bacillus species enzyme
s. immunity
insulin receptor s.
methicillin-resistant *Staphylococcus* s.
nontyphoidal *Salmonella* s.
paramagnetic iron s.
Pasteurella species taxon 16
reactive oxygen s.
typhus *Rickettsiae* species vaccine

specific
s. absorption coefficient
s. absorption rate
s. absorptivity
s. action exercise
active specific immunotherapy
s. activity
S. Activity Scale
s. airway conductance
s. airway resistance
allergen specific nasal challenge
s. anergy
s. antibody deficiency
s. antigen
s. antithymocytic
atypical specific developmental disorder
s. blocking factor
s. capsular substance
s. characteristic
s. clotting factor and inhibitor
s. conductance
s. COX-2 inhibitor
decreased specific gravity
s. developmental disorder
s. disease
disturbance of emotions specific to adolescence
disturbance of emotions specific to childhood
donor transfusion, s.
s. dynamic action
s. dynamic effect
s. enthalpy
s. expressive language impairment
s. gamma ray constant
s. gravity
s. gravity test
group s.
s. heat at constant volume
s. heat capacity
s. immune release
s. immune-response-enhancing factor
s. immunity
s. immunotherapy allergy
s. injection immunotherapy
intolerance to specific drugs
intolerance to specific foods
s. isolation precautions
s. language disorder
s. latent heat
s. macrophage-arming factor
male specific antigen
maximal specific binding capacity
melanoma specific antigen
nonantigenic specific mediator
noradrenergic and specific serotonergic antidepressant
s. optical rotation
s. paroxysmal discharge
s. pathogen free
permission, limited information, specific suggestions, and intensive therapy
prostatic specific antigen
s. reading disability
s. reading retarded
s. red cell adherence
relative specific activity
s. resistance
s. response
soluble specific substance
s. soluble substance
s. strain of bacteria
s. thalamic projection system
tumor s.
type s.
X inactive, specific transcript

specification
out of specification deviation from standard

specificity
anti-P blood group s.
assay s.

specified
alcohol-related use disorder, not otherwise s.
s. antilymphocytic
articulatory specified neutral reference
s. bovine offals
cannabis-related disorder, not otherwise s.
dissociative disorder not otherwise s.
nicotine-related disorder, not otherwise s.
not elsewhere s.
not otherwise s.
pervasive developmental disorder not otherwise s.
s. risk materials
typhoid vaccine, not otherwise s.

specifier
longitudinal course s.

specimen
catheterized urine s.
clean-voided s.
culture midvoid s.
early morning specimen of urine
first voided bladder s.
initial urine s.
limited quantity test performed on small s.
lost surgical s.
mammary aspiration s.

specimen *(continued)*
mammary aspiration specimen cytology test
s. mass measurement device
midstream specimen of urine
midstream urine s.
midvoid urine s.
nature of s.
needle biopsy s.
open-wedge biopsy s.
potentially infectious blood s.
protected catheter brushing s.
protected specimen brushing
second midstream bladder s.
s. submitted for biopsy
third midstream bladder s.
urine specimen after prostate massage
urine specimen before prostate massage
urine specimen volume measuring device
urine specimen volume measuring system

speckle
electronic speckle pattern interferometry

speckled
scintillating speckled pattern

spectacle
aphakic s.'s
aspheric spectacle lens
bioptic telescopic s.
lid crutch s.'s
Masselon s.'s
minus spectacle lens
multifocal spectacle lens
optical center of spectacle lens
orthoscopic s.'s
pantoscopic s.'s
periscopic s.'s
telescopic s.'s
without s.'s

spectometry
time-of-flight mass s.

spectra (*pl. of* spectrum)

spectral
s. analysis
compressed spectral array
compressed spectral assay
density-modulated spectral array
density spectral array
s. edge frequency
s. envelope
s. frequency distribution
s. gradient acoustic reflectometry
heart rate power spectral analysis
s. karyotype
s. karyotyping
orthogonal polarization s.
s. peak
s. power distribution
power spectral analysis
power spectral density
s. sensitivity
s. transmittance

Spectranetics laser sheath

spectrometer
atomic absorption s.
energy-dispersive s.
gamma ray s.
hard x-ray imaging s.
inductively-coupled plasma-mass s.
laser desorption/ionization time-of-flight-mass s.
nondispersive infrared s.

spectrometric
emission spectrometric detector
mass spectrometric analysis

spectrometry
accelerator mass s.
chemical ionization mass s.
electrohydrodynamic ionization mass s.
electron ionization mass s.
electrospray ionization mass s.
emission s.
fast atom bombardment mass s.
gas chromatographic-mass s.
gas isotope ratio mass s.
gas-liquid chromatography/mass s.
inductively-coupled plasma-optical emission s.
isotope dilution-mass s.
isotope ratio mass s.
liquid chromatography coupled to tandem mass s.
mass s.
matrix-assisted laser desorption and ionization mass s.
matrix-assisted laser desorption ionization-time-of-flight mass s.
proportional counter s.
resonance ionization mass s.
x-ray energy s.

spectrophotometer
atomic absorption s.
digital imaging s.
mass s.
narrow band s.

spectrophotometric
mass spectrophotometric detector

spectrophotometry
colorimetry, including spectrophotometry and photometry
electrothermal atomic absorption s.
infrared s.

spectroscope
quasielastic laser light-scattering s.

spectroscopic
magnetic resonance spectroscopic imaging-guided brachytherapy

spectroscopy
affinity attenuated total reflectance s.
affinity evanescent wave s.
affinity fluorescence s.
angular resolved photoelectron s.
atomic absorption s.
depth-resolved surface coil s.
difference s.
diffuse reflectance s.
electron energy loss s.
electron spectroscopy for chemical analysis
extended x-ray absorption fine structure s.
flame emission s.
fluorescence correlation s.
Fourier transform infrared s.
laser correlational s.
laser-induced fluorescence s.
longitudinal proton MR s.
low-energy electron diffraction s.
magnetic resonance s.
medical optical s.
MR catheter imaging and spectroscopy system scanner
near-infrared s.
nuclear magnetic resonance s.
optical emission s.
phosphorus magnetic resonance s.
phosphorus-31 magnetic resonance s.
phosphorus nuclear magnetic resonance s.
photoacoustic s.
photoelectron s.
point-resolved s.
proton magnetic resonance s.
reflection-absorption infrared s.
resonance ionization s.
secondary ion mass s.
spatially resolved s.
spin-echo correlated s.
ultraviolet photoelectron s.

in vivo optical s.
x-ray photoemission s.

spectroscopy-directed laser

spectrum, pl. **spectra**
adult/adolescent spectrum of HIV disease
affective spectrum disorder
s. analysis
autism spectrum screening questionnaire
autistic spectrum disorder
clinical spectrum of cancer
depressed spectrum disease
electroencephalogram interval spectrum analysis
midrange spectrum ultraviolet light
oculoauriculovertebral s.
pediatric spectrum of disease
schizophrenic s.
schizophrenic spectrum disorder

specula (*pl. of* speculum)

specular
endothelial specular microscope
s. glare
s. image

speculoscopy
Pap plus s.

speculum, pl. **specula**
bivalved s.
s. examination
flat-bladed nasal s.
s. inserted
lid s.
long weighted s.
Murdoon eye s.
nasal s.
pediatric lid s.
vaginal s.

speech
alteration in rate of s.
anterior speech zone
aprosody of s.
arrest of s.
articulation of s.
Assessment of Intelligibility of Dysarthric S.
audible blocking in s.
audible speech blockade
s. audiometry
auditory perception of speech sounds
avoidance of speech dysfluency
s. awareness threshold
s. center
child speech impaired
chronic slurred s.
circulation, respiration, abdomen, motor, and s.
computerized speech lab
confused or impoverished thought and s.
s. defect
delayed development of s.
delayed or impaired s.
s. detectability threshold
s. detection threshold
deterioration of coordination, gait, and s.
s. development
developmental apraxia of s.
s. discrimination
s. discrimination loss
s. discrimination score
s. discrimination test
s. discrimination testing
s. disorder
s. disturbance
s. dysfunction
Early S. Perception Test
erratic speech rhythm
Filtered Audiometer S. Test
fluent aphasic s.
fluent paraphasic s.
Fluharty Preschool S. and Language Screening Test
garbled s.
s. and hearing
s. and hearing impairment
impaired difficult s.
s. impaired individual
s. interference level
Kent State University S. Discrimination Test
s. and language impaired
s. and language pathologist
s. and language pathology
S. and Language Screening Questionnaire
Linguistic Analysis of Speech Samples
mental and physical retardation, speech disorders, peculiar facies syndrome
neuromuscular development of s.
nonfluent aphasic s.
Northwestern University Children's Perception of S. Test
outpatient speech therapy
s. pathology and audiology
Pediatric S. Intelligibility Test
perseveration of s.
poverty of content of s.
preferred frequency speech interference level
s. processor interface
Rapidly Alternating S. Perception Test
s. reception test
s. reception threshold
s. recognition threshold
s. scanning
slurred s.
slurred indistinct s.
tangential speech pattern
s. therapist
s. therapy
wearable speech processor
S. Weber Test
S. with Alternating Masking Index

speech-controlled respirometer for ambulatory measurement

speech-language pathologist

speech-sound
s.-s. discrimination
S.-s. Perception Test

speech-to-noise ratio

speed
S. and Boyd reduction technique
s. of bronchoconstriction in response to methacholine
comfortable walking s.
naming speed deficit
perceptual s.
pulse-wave s.
reversal speed of bronchoconstriction in response to methacholine
super high s.
walking s.

spell
apneic spell associated with loud snoring
breath-holding s.
falling spells of Tumarkin
neonatal breath-holding s.
pallid breath-holding s.
paroxysmal hypoxic s.

Spemann induction

Spence
axillary tail of S.

Spencer-Watson operation

spender
binge s.

sperm
s. abnormality
s. agglutinin

sperm *(continued)*
altered sperm motility
anonymous donor s.
artificial insemination with donor s.
s. bank
s. count
s. cytotoxic
direct oocyte sperm transfer
s. donor
s. entry point
epididymal sperm aspiration
fallopian tube sperm perfusion
follicle aspiration, sperm injection, and assisted rupture
head-to-head sperm agglutination
head-to-tail sperm agglutination
healthy mobile s.
s. immobilization test
S. Immobilization Test-Fjabrant
S. Immobilization Test-Isojima
maternal sperm antibody
s. microaspiration retrieval technique
microepididymal sperm aspiration
microscopic epididymal sperm aspiration
microsurgical epididymal sperm aspiration
microsurgical epididymal sperm aspiration procedure
microsurgical extraction of ductal s.
microsurgical extraction of sperm from epididymis
motile s.
s. motility
s. penetration assay
percutaneous epididymal sperm aspiration
peritoneal oocyte and sperm transfer
testicular sperm aspiration
testicular sperm extraction
transvaginal intrafallopian sperm transfer

spermatic
s. cord
s. cord torsion
s. filament
s. fistula
inferior spermatic plexus
internal spermatic fascia
internal spermatic vessel
microsurgical denervation of the spermatic cord
s. plexus

spermatid
round spermatid nuclear injection

spermatocele
alloplastic s.
artificial s.
autogenous s.

spermatocyte
secondary s.

spermatogenic activity test

spermatozoon, pl. **spermatozoa**
nonmigrating fraction of spermatozoa
outer dense fibers of s.

sperm-cervical mucus contact

sperm-coating antigen

spermicide-germicide compound

sperm-specific
s.-s. antigen
s.-s. antiserum

sperm-ubiquitin tag immunoassay

sperm-washing insemination method

Spetzler lumboperitoneal shunt

sphenoccipital fissure

sphenoethmoidal suture

sphenofrontal suture

sphenoid
aperture of sphenoid sinus
s. bone fracture
s. dysplasia
limbus of sphenoid bone
malar crest of great wing of sphenoid bone
orbital border of sphenoid bone
orbital wing of sphenoid bone
parietal angle of s.
parietal border of sphenoid bone
parietal margin of greater wing of s.
scaphoid fossa of sphenoid bone
s. septum
s. sinus
s. sinusitis
s. turbinate

sphenoidal
s. border
s. fissure
s. fontanelle
s. herniation

sphenoidale
os s.

sphenoidectomy
antral ethmoidal s.

sphenomaxillary
s. fissure
s. fossa
s. ganglion

sphenooccipital
s. joint
s. synchondrosis

sphenoorbital suture

sphenopalatine
s. artery
s. foramen
s. ganglion

sphenopetrosal fissure

sphere
diopter s.
double minute s.
hollow sphere prosthesis
s. implant
method of the s.
Mules vitreous s.
oriented in all s.'s
plastic sphere implant
rough hard s.

spherical
s. aberration
s. candle power
s. equivalent
floating spherical gaussian orbital
s. implant
s. lens
mean spherical candle power
small spherical particle

sphericity index

spherocytic
s. anemia
s. jaundice

spherocytosis
hereditary s.

spheroid
hereditary diffuse leukoencephalopathy with s.'s
s. joint
multicellular tumor s.

spheroidal oral drug absorption system

spherule wall

sphincter
s. of ampulla
anal ileostomy with preservation of s.
anal sphincter dysplasia
anal sphincter laceration

anal sphincter squeeze pressure
artificial genitourinary sphincter implantation
artificial urethral s.
artificial urinary s.
artificial urinary sphincter implantation
s. of bile duct
s. of common bile duct
s. deficiency
detrusor external sphincter dyssynergia
detrusor sphincter dyssynergia
endoscopic balloon sphincter dilation
external anal s.
external urethral s.
s. of eye
s. of gastric antrum
genitourinary s.
s. of hepatic flexure of colon
ileocecal s.
incompetent esophageal s.
inferior esophageal s.
internal anal s.
internal sphincter muscle of anus
intrinsic sphincter deficiency
intrinsic sphincter dysfunction
lesser esophageal s.
long anal s.
lower esophageal s.
lower esophageal sphincter circular muscle
lower esophageal sphincter locator
lower esophageal sphincter pressure
lower esophageal sphincter relaxation
lower esophageal sphincter tone
s. muscle
musculus sphincter pupilla
normal sphincter tone
s. of Oddi
s. of Oddi dysfunction
s. of Oddi manometry
s. of Oddi pressure
s. of Oddi spasm
pancreatic duct s.
pupillary sphincter muscle
relaxation internal s.
s. stenosis
s. tear
s. tone
upper esophageal s.
upper esophageal sphincter pressure
upper esophageal sphincter relaxation
vesical external sphincter dyssynergia

sphincterotomy
biliary sphincterotomy and stent placement
endoscopic pancreatic s.
endoscopic retrograde s.
multiple anal s.'s
needle-knife endoscopic pancreatic s.
pancreatic duct s.

sphincter-preserving operation

sphingolipid activator protein-1

sphingomyelin
lipid s.

sphingomyelinase
secretory s.

sphygmomanometer
aneroid s.
cuff s.
mercury s.
Riva-Rocci s.

spica
s. case
hip s.
hip spica cast
short arm thumb spica cast
thumb spica bandage
thumb spica splint

spicy
caffeine, alcohol, pepper, spicy foods

spider
s. angioma
arterial s.
black widow spider toxin
black widow spider venom
s. hemangioma
s. nevi
s. nevus
red spider vein
s. telangiectasia
s. vein

Spiegler-Fendt sarcoid

Spielberger State-Trait Anxiety Inventory

spigelian hernia

Spigelius
S. line
S. lobe

spike
anterior temporal focal s.
benign partial epilepsy with centrotemporal s.
central spike focus
data spike detection error artifact
epilepsy with continuous spikes and waves during sleep
epilepsy with multiple independent spike focus
hemisphere s.'s
isolated spike transients
long spike burst
noise spike artifact
s. occurrence density
peak absorption s.
pontogeniculooccipital s.
positive rolandic s.
positive spike pattern
s. potential
short spike burst
significant sharp spike or delta wave
small sharp s.
spontaneous interictal s.
s. wave

spiked
fenestrated spiked open-span jumbo biopsy forceps
patient spiked a fever

spike-processed contraction

spike-wave stupor

spiking
s. activity
irregular spiking activity in electroencephalography
regular spiking activity

spill
hazardous s.'s of fluid
prompt spill into duodenum
secretion s.'s from hepatitis patients
secretion and spill from acquired immune deficiency syndrome

spillage
fecal s.

spilled
patient spilled protein
patient spilled sugar
sugar s.

spilling
fluid spilling into upper abdomen

spillway
axial s.

spilus
nevus s.
nevus spilus lentigo

spin
axial spin density
s. density
s. diffusion
s. echo
s. echo imaging
electron spin resonance
fast asymmetric spin echo
partial saturation spin echo
pulsed-gradient spin echo
s. quantum number
rapid-acquisition spin echo
single shot fast spin echo
turbo spin echo

spina
adolescent spina bifida
s. bifida
s. bifida aperta
s. bifida cystica
s. bifida cystica
s. bifida occulta

spinal
abnormal spinal posture
s. abscess
s. accessory-hypoglossal neuroanastomosis
s. accessory nerve
s. accessory nerve palsy
acute atrophic spinal paralysis
acute central cervical spinal cord injury
acute spinal cord injury
acute spinal stenosis
Adkins spinal fusion
Adkins technique spinal arthrodesis
adult-onset spinal muscular atrophy
agonal spinal cord hemorrhage
Albee lumbar spinal fusion
Albee spinal fusion
s. analgesia
s. analysis machine
s. anesthesia
ankylosing spinal hyperostosis
ankylosing spinal stenosis
s. anomaly
anterior column of spinal cord
anterior horn of spinal cord
anterior median fissure of spinal cord
anterior-posterior fusion with segmental spinal instrumentation
anterior ramus of spinal nerve
anterior root of spinal nerve
anterior spinal artery syndrome
anterior spinal cord syndrome
anterior spinal fixation
anterior spinal fusion
anterior spinal instrumentation
anterior spinal line
anterior spinal plating
anterolateral column of spinal cord
AO spinal internal fixation
apex of dorsal horn of spinal cord
apex of posterior horn of spinal cord
s. apoplexy
arachnoid of spinal cord
s. arthritis
artificial spinal disk
ASIA impairment scale for classification of spinal cord injury
s. attunement technique
autonomic column of spinal cord
axial spinal system
s. block
s. blockade
bovine spinal cord protein
California soft spinal system
s. canal
s. canal stenosis
s. canal tumor
central cervical spinal cord syndrome
chronic spinal muscular atrophy
s. column
s. compression fracture
compression of spinal nerve
s. computed tomography
s. concussion
continuous spinal anesthesia
contoured anterior spinal plate
s. cord
s. cord abscess
s. cord blood flow
s. cord compression
s. cord concussion
s. cord decompression
s. cord demyelinization
s. cord disease
s. cord disorder
s. cord dysfunction
s. cord infarction
s. cord injury
s. cord injury unit
s. cord injury without radiographic abnormality
s. cord laceration
s. cord pain
s. cord perfusion pressure
s. cord stimulation
s. cord tract
cruciform anterior spinal hyperextension
s. curvature
s. decompression
s. defect
s. degeneration
degenerative spinal disease
s. detrusor hyperreflexia
diagnostic spinal tap
s. disorder
s. dorsal horn
dorsal horns of spinal cord
dowel spinal fusion
s. dural arteriovenous fistula
s. dysraphism
electrically induced spinal reflex
electrical spinal cord stimulation
s. epidural abscess
s. epidural hematoma
s. epidural hemorrhage
epidural spinal cord compression
s. evoked potential
external spinal skeletal fixator
s. fixation
flared spinal rod
s. fluid
s. fluid count
s. fluid Gram stain
s. fluid leak
s. fluid pressure
functional spinal unit
s. fusion
s. fusion surgery
s. ganglion
s. gliosis
graduated spinal block
gray matter of spinal cord
gray substance of spinal cord
s. headache
headache after spinal tap
headache secondary to cervical spinal disease
head and spinal cord injury
s. hemianesthesia
s. hemiplegia
hemisection of spinal cord
s. herniation
high spinal anesthesia
s. immobilization
immobilization of spinal injury
impingement on spinal nerve
s. induction
infantile spinal muscular atrophy
intact spinal cord
s. intensive care unit

interspinous segmental spinal instrumentation technique
intramedullary spinal cord metastasis
invasive spinal surgery
s. irritation
laser-assisted spinal endoscopy
left anterior spinal artery
s. length
s. lesion
lumbar enlargement of spinal cord
lumbar spinal block
lumbar spinal stenosis
lumbosacral enlargement of spinal cord
malignant spinal disease
s. manipulative therapy
s. marrow
medial branch of posterior branch of spinal nerve
medial branch of posterior rami of spinal nerve
meningeal branch of spinal nerve
metastatic cancer of spinal fluid
metastatic epidural spinal cord compression
minimal access spinal technology
s. muscular atrophy
narrowing of spinal canal
narrow spinal channel
neoplastic destruction of spinal element
neuron in spinal cord
nontraumatic spinal tap
normal spinal fluid
s. opioid analgesia
s. orthosis
percutaneously inserted spinal cord electrical stimulation
posterior branch of spinal nerve
posterior spinal fusion
posterolateral spinal artery
pressure on spinal cord
s. progressive amyotrophy
s. progressive muscular atrophy
progressive spinal ataxia
progressive spinal muscular atrophy
proximal spinal muscular atrophy
s. range of motion
s. scoliosis
segmental spinal correction system
segmental spinal instrumentation
slow spinal cord compression syndrome
s. slumping
split spinal cord malformation
spontaneous spinal epidural hematoma
s. stenosis
s. stroke
subacute combined degeneration of spinal cord
s. subdural hemorrhage
s. tap
thoracolumbar spinal orthosis
thoracolumbosacral spinal orthosis
transected spinal cord
transverse spinal sclerosis
variable spinal plating
ventral derotating spinal implant
Vermont spinal fixator

spindle

anulospiral ending of muscle s.
aortic s.
Axenfeld-Krukenberg s.
s. cataract
s. cell
s. cell carcinoma
s. cell epithelial tumor with thymus-like differentiation
s. cell lipoma
s. cell nevus
s. cell sarcoma
His s.
s. microtubule
mitotic spindle apparatus
mitotic spindle inhibitor
neuromuscular s.
pigmented spindle cell
plexiform spindle cell nevus
potato spindle tuber viroid
reactive spindle cell nodule
REM s.
sleep s.

spindliform activity

spine

airway, breathing, circulation, cervical spine, and consciousness level
alertness, airway, breathing, circulation, and cervical s.
angulation of s.
anterior column of s.
anterior lower cervical spine surgery
anterior lumbar spine interbody fusion
anterior maxillary s.
anterior nasal s.
anterior nasal spine of maxilla
anterior occipitocervical s.
anterior spine fusion
anterior-superior s.
anterior tibial s.
anterior upper s.
anteroposterior iliac s.
anterosuperior iliac spine graft
arachnoid loculation of the s.
arachnoid spine cyst
axial loading of s.
azoospermia, renal anomaly, cervicothoracic spine dysplasia
cervical s.
cervical spine injury
cervical spine screw-plate fixation
collapsed vertebra of s.
compression fracture of s.
concavity of s.
dendritic s.
distance between iliac s.'s
dorsal s.
flexion-compression spine injury stabilization
full cervical s.
full spine board
Gait, Arms, Legs, and S.
greater tympanic s.
s. of helix
hyperextension of s.
lateral electrical spine stimulation
lower cervical spine fusion
lower cervical spine posterior stabilization
lumbar s.
lumbar spine bone density
lumbar spine bone mineral density
lumbar spine index
lumbosacral s.
microcephaly-cervical spine fusion anomalies
minimally invasive spine surgery
Neurosurgical Cervical S. Scale
osseous cervical spine injury
osteoarthritis of the s.
palpation of anterior superior iliac s.
plain spine radiograph
portable cervical s.
posterior inferior iliac s.
posterior nasal s.
posterior nasal spine to soft palate
posterior sacroiliac s.
posterior superior iliac s.
segmental correction using spine reconstruction
s. spot film

spine *(continued)*
spurring of lumbar s.
spurring of thoracic s.
stable cervical spine injury
superior iliac s.
thoracic s.
Universal S. System

spin-echo
s.-e. correlated spectroscopy
fat-suppressed s.-e.
half-Fourier acquisition single-shot turbo s.-e.
s.-e. imaging

spin-lattice or longitudinal relaxation time

spinnbarkeit testing

spinning
magic angle spinning NMR

spinocerebellar
adult-onset spinocerebellar ataxia
anterior spinocerebellar tract
s. ataxia
s. degeneration
dorsal spinocerebellar tract

spinopelvic transiliac fixation

spinothalamic
anterior spinothalamic tract
s. cordotomy
lateral spinothalamic tract
s. tract

spinous process

spin-spin or transverse relaxation time MRI scan

spinulosa
trichostasis s.

spinulosus
lichen s.

spiradenoma
angiolipoma, posttraumatic neuroma, glomus tumor, eccrine spiradenoma, and leiomyoma cutis
malignant eccrine s.

Spira disease

spiral
Archimedes s.
s. artery
s. bandage
s. canal of cochlea
childhood accidental spiral tibial fracture
s. computed tomography arteriography
s. crest
s. CT angiography
s. CT scan
s. dissection
flexible spiral wire retainer
s. fold
s. fracture
s. ganglion
s. ganglion of cochlea
s. groove
s. incision
limbus of osseous spiral lamina
outer spiral fibers of cochlea
s. tip catheter
tracheal s.
s. vein of modiolus
s. wound
s. x-ray computed tomography

spiral-shaped bacteria

spirillum
Obermeier s.

spirit
aromatic ammonia s.
controlling external s.
industrial methylated s.

spiritual
s. approach
s. assessment
emotional, spiritual, and social
human spiritual concerns
S. Well-Being Scale

spirituality
awareness of s.

spirochetal
s. disease
s. icterus
s. jaundice
nonpathogenic s.

spirochete
syphilitic s.

spirochetosis
venereal spirochetosis of rabbits

spirogram
forced expiratory s.
forced inspiratory s.

spirometer
incentive s.

spirometric screening

spirometry
incentive s.
incentive spirometry breathing

spit
swish and s.

Spitz
angiomatoid Spitz nevus
S. nevus

splanchnic
s. aneurysm
s. artery occlusion
s. blood flow
s. cavity
central splanchnic venous thrombosis
s. ganglion
greater splanchnic nerve
s. layer
lowest splanchnic nerve
lumbar splanchnic nerve
s. nerve
s. occluded portal pressure

splatter control shield

splayed artery

spleen
adenosine-coupled spleen cell
anterior extremity of s.
bovine embryonic spleen cell
s. cell
s. cell conditioned medium
s. colony assay
ellipsoid of s.
Friend spleen focus virus
guanosine-coupled spleen cell
guinea pig s.
hilum of s.
human embryonic s.
inverted Y and spleen pedicle
kidneys, ureters, and spleen x-ray
liver, kidneys, and s.
liver, kidneys, spleen, and bladder
liver, kidneys, and spleen not palpable
liver, spleen masses
long axis of s.
malpighian body of s.
multiple accessory s.'s
s. necrosis virus
palpable liver, spleen and kidneys
pokeweed activated spleen conditioned medium
purified spleen extract
s. repopulating activity
s. rupture
ruptured s.
s. scan
syngeneic spleen cell

spleen-to-body weight ratio

splenic
s. abscess
acute splenic sequestration crisis
s. adherent cell
s. agenesis syndrome
s. artery
s. artery aneurysm
autotransplantation of splenic fragment
s. blood flow
s. cell
s. cord
s. corpuscle
s. dullness
s. flexure
s. flexure syndrome
s. fossa
s. hilum
s. infarct
s. localization index
low-dose splenic irradiation
s. lymph node
s. lymphoma with villous lymphocyte
s. macrophage
s. marginal zone lymphoma
partial splenic embolization
transcatheter splenic arterial embolization
s. vascular supply
s. vein
s. vein obstruction

splenomegaly
hyperactive malarial splenomegaly syndrome
persistent gross s.
tropical splenomegaly syndrome

splenoportal hypertension

splenorenal
distal s.
distal splenorenal shunt
end-to-side splenorenal shunt
s. ligament
s. shunt

splice junction

splint
airplane splint orthosis
airplane splint shoulder brace
air pressure s.
aluminum foam s.
aluminum hand s.
aluminum wire s.
alveolar arch acrylic s.
ankle stirrup s.
anterior acute flexion elbow s.
anterior shin s.
cast bar s.
cock-up hand s.
cock-up splint orthosis
cock-up wrist s.
constant tension s.
continuous clasp s.
cubital tunnel s.
Denis Browne s.
dorsal wrist s.
felt collar s.
flexor hinge s.
folded aluminum ear s.
functional resting position s.
gait lock s.
hip-knee orthosis s.
inflatable limb s.
knuckle-bender splint
long arm posterior-molded s.
long leg posterior molded s.
Lorenz night s.
out of s.
palmar cock-up s.
Pearson attachment to Thomas s.
short arm plaster s.
short arm posterior-molded s.
short arm sugar-tong s.
short leg posterior-molded s.
sugar-tong s.
tension night s.
thumb spica s.

splinted
hand splinted in flexion

splintered fraction

splinter hemorrhage

splinting
manual splinting of thoracic cage
silicone thermoplastic s.

splint/stent
kidney internal s.

split
anterior cricoid s.
anterior cricoid split procedure
s. anterior tibial tendon transfer
bilateral sagittal split ramus osteotomies
cantilevered split cranial bone graft
s. course technique
s. course treatment
fibrinogen split product
fibrinolytic split product
fibrin split product
s. function study
s. graft
s. hand
s. hand-cleft lip/palate and ectodermal dysplasia
s. image artifact
influenza virion vaccine, split virion
influenza virus inactivated vaccine, split virion, types A, B, trivalent
peroneus brevis s.
s. products of fibrin
pulmonic second sound s.
s. renal function
sagittal split advancement
sagittal split ramus osteotomy
sagittal split setback
s. spinal cord malformation
s. thickness
vertical sagittal split osteotomy

split-brain
s.-b. patient
s.-b. syndrome

split-cord malformation

split-course regimen

split-liver transplantation

split-skin graft

split-thickness
s.-t. autogenous graft
s.-t. skin excision
s.-t. skin graft

splitting
s. of heart sound
macular s.
Minsky intramarginal s.
muscle s.
muscle splitting incision
paradoxic s.
physiologic s.
rectus muscle splitting incision
sternal splitting incision
sternal splitting scar

Spofford-Christopher oxygen optimizing program

spoiled
fast multiplanar spoiled gradient-recalled imaging
s. gradient recalled

spoiler
lucite beam s.

spoken
inability to remember spoken words

spoking
cortical s.

Spondaic
Staggered Spondaic Word Test

Spondee
S. Error Index
S. Picture Test

Spondweni virus

spondylar changes, nasal anomaly, striated metaphyses

spondylitis
ankylosing s.
ankylosing spondylitis, lung
s., enthesitis, arthritis
idiopathic ankylosing s.
juvenile ankylosing s.
lung ankylosis s.

spondyloarthropathy
ankylosing s.
seronegative s.

spondylodesis
ventral derotation s.

spondyloepimetaphyseal dysplasia with joint laxity

spondyloepiphyseal
s. dysplasia
s. dysplasia congnita

spondylolisthesis
anteroinferior s.

spondylosis
ankylosis s.
Nurick classification of s.
ochronotic s.

spondylotic
s. caudal myelopathy
s. caudal radiculopathy
cervical spondylotic myelopathy

sponge
absorbable gelatin s.
s. blood loss
collagen sponge contraceptive
correct sponge and needle count
s. count correct
s. graft
s. implant
s. and lap count
long-handled s.
s. and needle count
needle and sponge count correct times two
needle, sponge, and instrument count correct times three
needle, sponge, and instrument count correct times two
needle and sponge count
needle and sponge count correct times three
Packer tunnel silicone s.
polyvinyl sponge implant
silicone sponge implant

sponge-like holes in brain

spongiform
amyotrophic type of spongiform encephalopathy
bovine spongiform encephalopathy
s. encephalopathy
transmissible spongiform encephalopathy

spongioblastoma multiforme

spongiosa
intramedullary and spongiosa graft

spongiosus
nevus spongiosus albus mucosa

spongy
s. bone
s. degeneration
s. degeneration of infancy
s. iritis
s. layer of female urethra
s. layer of vagina
s. mass
muscular coat of spongy part of male urethra
s. part of bone
porous and spongy bone

spontaneous
s. abortion
s. activity test
s. acute bacterial peritonitis
s. agglutination
s. amputation
s. assisted vaginal delivery
s. autoimmune thyroiditis
s. biliary perforation
s. blastogenesis
s. breech extraction
s. cell-mediated cytotoxicity
s. cervical artery dissection
s. coronary artery dissection
s. delivery
s. descent of testis
s. echo contrast
s. electrical activity
s. fibrillation
s. fluctuation
s. fracture
full-term, normal, spontaneous delivery
s. generation
s. hemorrhage
s. hemorrhagic necrosis
s. hypoglycemia
s. interictal spike
s. intermittent mandatory ventilation
s. intracerebral hemorrhage
s. intracranial hypotension
s. intramural hematoma of the esophagus
s. ischemia
s. killer cell
s. labor
left atrial spontaneous echo contrast
s. left hemothorax
s. lesion
s. lymphocyte-mediated cytotoxicity
s. mammary tumor
s. miscarriage
s. motor activity
s. neonatal chylothorax
normal spontaneous full-term delivery
normal spontaneous vaginal birth
no spontaneous movement of limbs
s. nystagmus
s. onset of labor
onset of spontaneous labor
s. osteonecrosis of knee
s. osteoporotic fracture of sacrum
s. otoacoustic emission
pathologic spontaneous activity
s. peak inspiratory force
Performance Assessment of Syntax Elicited and S.
s. platelet aggregation
s. pneumothorax
s. portal-systemic shunt
s. positive end expiratory pressure
s. premature rupture of membranes
premature spontaneous rupture of bag of waters
s. preterm birth
preterm spontaneous rupture of membranes
s. primary hypothyroidism
primary spontaneous pneumothorax
recurrent spontaneous abortion
recurrent spontaneous psychokinesis
repeated spontaneous abortion
s. respiration
restoration of spontaneous circulation

return of spontaneous circulation
s. right hemothorax
rupture s.
s. rupture of bag of waters
s. seizure
simultaneous bilateral spontaneous pneumothorax
s. spinal epidural hematoma
sterile spontaneous controlled vaginal delivery
sterile, spontaneous vaginal delivery
stimulate adequate spontaneous breathing
stroke-prone spontaneous hypertensive
s. suppressor cell activity
s. venous pulsation
s. venous pulse
s. vertex vaginal delivery
s. voiding

spontaneously
s. aborted human fetus
s. breathing
s. diabetic rat
s. resolving thyrotoxicosis
s. responding hyperthyroidism

spoon
brain s.
needle s.

sporadic
s. adenomatous polyps
s. cerebral amyloid angiopathy
s. depression
s. depressive disease
nontoxic sporadic goiter
s. olivopontocerebellar ataxia

spore
airborne s.
anthrax s.
mold s.

sporotrichosis
extracutaneous s.
lymphocutaneous s.
mucocutaneous s.
osteoarticular s.

sporozoan parasite

sport
s. cord
s. physical
preparticipation sports examination
s. sheath

Sportono
cementless S.

sports-related
s.-r. injury
s.-r. osteoarthritis

sporulation
nutrient sporulation medium

spot
amylase urine spot test
ash leaf s.
ash-leaf spot in tuberous sclerosis
café au lait s.
calcium-urine spot test
cherry red s.
cherry-red spot myoclonus
cold spots and hot spots with electron beam dosimetry
cotton-wool s.'s
creatinine urine spot test
focal s.
focal spot size
Grafenberg s.
hematocystic s.
hot spot imaging
infarct avid hot spot scintigraphy
macular cherry-red s.
Mariotte blind s.
mental blind s.
mongolian s.
opacification cherry-red s.
osmolality urine spot test
pathognomonic Koplik s.
peripheral chorioretinal atrophic s.
physiologic blind s.
precancerous skin s.
purplish hemorrhagic spot on skin
s. radiation
red spot on breast
sodium and potassium spot urine test
spine spot film
Tay cherry-red s.
uric acid urine spot test
urine glucose spot test
yellow s.

spotted
s. fever
s. fever group
Japanese spotted fever
Mexican spotted fever
Rocky Mountain spotted fever vaccine

spotting
s. and cramping
intermenstrual s.
intermittent spotting and cramping

midcycle s.
postcoital s.

spousal abuse

spouse's perception of disease

sprain
acute cervical traumatic sprain or syndrome
ankle s.
anterior cruciate s.
anterior talofibular s.
s. fracture
inversion s.
knee s.
medial collateral s.
posterior cruciate s.

sprained ankle

spray
aerosol spray abuse
aerosol spray dependence
air plasma s.
budesonide aqueous nasal s.
low-pressure plasma s.
nasal nicotine s.
nasal spray insulin
nasal steroid s.
nicotine nasal s.
Nitrolingual Translingual S.
steam spray inhaler

sprayed
titanium plasma s.

spread
extracapsular s.
s. of infection
line spread function
lymphangitic spread of prostatic adenocarcinoma
pattern of cancer s.
prevent spread of infection

spreader
bone s.
conjunctiva s.
rib spreader inserted

spreading
cortically spreading depression
s. depression
macrophage spreading factor
pain spreading to arm
pain spreading to neck
pain spreading to shoulder
superficial spreading melanoma

Spreen-Benton Sentence Repetition Test

Sprengel deformity

spring
coiled spring sign

spring *(continued)*
constant s.
s. finger
hemoglobin Constant S.
Malpais Spring virus
Muir Springs virus
pronation spring control

spring-summer
Russian spring-summer encephalitis virus

sprouting
collateral nerve s.
mossy fiber s.
nerve s.

sprue
celiac s.
celiac sprue disease
tropical s.

spud
gouge s.
needle s.
O'Brien s.

spun
Gram stain of UN spun urine
red blood cell spun filtration

spur
anterior impingement s.
band and spur retainer
detection of bone s.
heel s.
heel spur excision
heel spur syndrome
osteoarthritic hypertrophic spur formation
painful heel s.
plantar calcaneal s.
scleral s.

spuria
melena s.
placenta s.

spurious
s. cast
hydrops s.
s. parasite

Spurling sign

spurring
anterior s.
degenerative anterior s.
hypertrophic s.
s. of lumbar spine
s. of thoracic spine

spurt
growth s.

sputum, pl. **sputa**
abnormal s.
acid-fast sputum smear
acid-fast stain of s.
blood-tinged s.
coughing conductive of s.
cough productive of bloody s.
cough and s.
s. culture
currant jelly s.
s. cytology
s. examination
s. Gram stain
induced s.
induced sputum analysis
s. induction
mucopurulent s.
Papanicolaou stain of s.
purulent s.
s. smear
tenacious s.
wet s.
yellow s.

squamocolumnar
original squamocolumnar junction
physiologic s.

squamosal
s. border
s. margin

squamous
adenocarcinoma with squamous differentiation
advanced squamous cell cervical carcinoma
anal squamous intraepithelial lesion
anogenital squamous intraepithelial neoplasia
atypical squamous cell of undetermined significance
basaloid squamous cell carcinoma
s. border
s. carcinoma of cervix
s. cell
s. cell cancer
s. cell carcinoma
s. cell carcinoma antigen
s. cell carcinoma dorsum of hand
s. cell carcinoma of the esophagus
s. cell carcinoma of head and neck
s. cell carcinoma inhibitory factor
s. cell carcinoma in situ
s. cell carcinoma of the thyroid
s. cell carcinoma of tongue
s. cell carcinoma of vocal cord
s. cell carcinoma of vulva
s. cell head and neck cancer
s. cell hyperplasia
s. cell lung tumor
s. cell papilloma
s. dysplasia
s. epithelial cell
s. epithelium
esophageal squamous cell carcinoma
head and neck squamous cell carcinoma
high-grade squamous intraepithelial lesion
infiltrating squamous cell carcinoma
s. intraepithelial cell
s. intraepithelial lesion
s. intraepithelial lesion/atypical squamous cell of undetermined significance
laryngeal squamous cell carcinoma
low-grade squamous intraepithelial lesion
s. margin
s. metaplasia
metastatic squamous carcinoma of head and neck
multiple self-healing squamous carcinoma
native squamous epithelium
s. odontogenic tumor
oral squamous cell carcinoma
parietal border of squamous part of temporal bone
perianal squamous cell carcinoma
poorly differentiated squamous cell carcinoma
pseudovascular adenoid squamous cell carcinoma

square
integrated square error
least s.
linear-nonlinear least s.'s
liter per minute per square meter
lumen per square foot
lumen per square meter
mean square deviation
mean square error
meganewton per square meter
newton per square centimeter
newton per square meter
newton-second per square meter
nonlinear least s.'s method
nonlinear least s.'s regression analysis

normalized mean square root
ordinary least s.'s
root mean square residue
sum of square deviations
s. waves of high frequency
weighted nonlinear least s.'s

squarely face person, open posture, lean toward person, eye contact, relaxed

squat
heel squat exercise

squeeze
anal sphincter squeeze pressure
maximum squeeze pressure
pause and squeeze technique

squint
angle of s.
noncomitant s.

squinting eye

squirrel plague conjunctivitis

Sripur virus

S-shaped
S.-s. scar
S.-s. scoliosis

St.
S. Anthony fire
S. Georges Respiratory Questionnaire
S. Jude annuloplasty ring
S. Jude valve
S. Louis encephalitis virus
S. Vitus dance

stabbing
intense stabbing pain
s. joint pain

stability
collateral ligament s.
evaluate safety and stability at home
foam stability index
immediate postoperative s.
physiologic stability index
rank-order stability analysis
rearfoot stability system
Test of Work Competency and S.

stabilization
anterior internal s.
anterior short-segment s.
anterior stabilization procedure
aquatic stabilization program
arthroscopic monopolar thermal stabilization forefoot compression sleeve
arthroscopic transglenoid suture stabilization procedure
clot stabilization test
crystal field stabilization energy
dynamic integrated stabilization chair
femoral access s.
flexion-compression spine injury s.
isometric trunk s.
lower cervical spine posterior s.
odontoid fracture s.
patellar tendon s.
pelvic stabilization orthosis
percutaneous bladder neck s.
vertical stabilization program

stabilized
joint s.
patient's condition s.
s. relative response

stabilize heart function

stabilizer
mast cell s.

stabilizing
ankle stabilizing orthosis
ankle stabilizing orthosis support
dynamic stabilizing innersole system
membrane stabilizing action
patellar stabilizing brace
s. reversal

stabkernige band neutrophil

stable
s. access cannula
afebrile, vital signs s.
s. angina pectoris
s. burst fracture
s. cervical spine injury
chronic stable angina
s. disease
s. eating habit
elastic stable intramedullary nailing
s. factor
s. fetal heart tones
s. gait
s. health status
heat s.
s. hypertension
mentally stable and oriented
microsatellite s.
neurological signs s.
patient in stable condition
s. plasma protein solution
s. sarcoidosis
s. vision
s. vital signs
vital signs s.
vital signs stable, afebrile

staccato
s. speech
s. syndrome

staff
s. burnout scale
dysfunctional staff behavior
s. escort
intake assessment s.

stage
adolescence developmental s.
adulthood developmental s.
advanced stage of congestive heart failure
advanced stage group
Ages and S.'s Questionnaire
alarm reaction s.
anal stage psychosexual development
anhepatic stage of liver transplantation
Ann Arbor Hodgkin lymphoma stage I, IE, II, IIE, IIIE, IIIS, IIISE, IV
assessing severity: age of patient, systems involved, stage of disease, complications, response to therapy
attending to language s.
band form in sixth stage of myelocyte maturation
carcinoma stage irresectable
clinical s.
clinically active s.
delta sleep s.
early stage breast cancer
early stages of sleep
first stage of anesthesia
first stage of labor
grammar development s.
grammar formation s.
s.'s of labor
Marshall and Tanner pubertal s.
myelocyte at fourth stage of maturation
myelocyte at third stage of maturation
PAHO stage 0, 1a, 1b, 2, 3
pronuclear stage transfer
pronucleate stage embryo transfer
pronucleate stage tubal transfer
s. of resistance
second stage of decreased intraocular tension
sleep stage change frequency

stage *(continued)*
soft callus s.
stress injury s.
Tanner genital s.
terminal stage of illness
third stage of labor
threshold stage III of retinopathy of prematurity
tubal embryo stage transfer
WHO classification for transitional cell carcinoma of the urinary bladder: stages Ta through T4

staged
s. abdominal repair
s. ulcer diet

stage-specific embryonic antigen

Staggered Spondaic Word Test

staggering
s. gait
gait reeling, s.

staghorn calculus

staging
Ann Arbor cancer s.
Ann Arbor classification of Hodgkin disease s.
Ann Arbor staging classification
Arizona Cancer Center multiple myeloma staging system
Astwood-Coller staging system for carcinoma
s. of cancer
casualty staging unit
clinical diagnostic s.
clinical staging of tumors, nodes, and metastases as determined by noninvasive examination
Composite Laryngeal Recurrence S. System
diagnostic workup and s.
Functional Assessment S.
Hodgkin disease s.
International Federation of Gynecology and Obstetrics classification of tumor s.
invasive surgical s.
lymph node s.
Masaoka staging system for thymoma
M.D. Anderson cancer s.
Memorial Sloan-Kettering staging of childhood lymphoma
Mitsuyasu staging system
multiple myeloma s.
Murphy staging system
nodal staging procedure
Outerbridge degenerative arthritis s.
pathological tumor, nodes, metastases staging of cancer
pathology and s.
preoperative staging of cancer
s. process and imaging
s. system in radiation therapy
s. workup

stagnant hypoxia

stagnate loop syndrome

Stahl ear

stain
acid-fast stain of sputum
Alcian blue s.
aldehyde-fuchsin s.
aniline blue modified trichrome s.
auramine fluorochrome s.
auramine O fluorescent s.
auramine-rhodamine acid-fast s.
aurintricarboxylic acid s.
avidin-biotin stain technique
brilliant cresyl blue s.
calcofluor white s.
Congo red s.
Coomassie brilliant blue R-250 s.
dental stain remover
dried blood s.
fluorescence plus Giemsa s.
fluorescent antibody s.
Giemsa banding s.
Gram stain of body fluid
Gram stain of cervix
Gram stain of exudates
Gram stain of facial abscess
Gram stain negative bacteremias
Gram stain of pelvic abscess
Gram stain of peritoneal fluid
Gram stain procedure
Gram stain of purulent discharge
Gram stain of skin lesion
Gram stain of stool test
Gram stain of throat
Gram stain of UN spun urine
Gram stain of urethra
Grocott methenamine silver s.
heavy metal s.
hematoxylin-eosin s.
hematoxylin and eosin s.
hematoxylin-phloxine-saffron s.
hematoxylin and van Gieson s.
Hoechst Marion Roussel stain
India ink s.
indigo carmine s.
leukocyte alkaline phosphatase s.
Lillie allochrome connective tissue s.
Lillie azure-eosin s.
Lillie ferrous iron s.
Loeffler caustic s.
Loeffler methylene blue s.
Lugol iodine s.
Luna-Parker acid fuscin s.
Luxol fast blue s.
lymphocyte enzyme s.
Mallory aniline blue s.
Mallory collagen s.
Maloney stain for aluminum
Masson argentaffin s.
Masson-Fontana ammoniac silver s.
Masson trichrome s.
Mayer acid alum hematoxylin s.
Mayer mucicarmine s.
methenamine silver s.
methylene blue s.
modified acid-fast s.
modified Dieterle s.
modified Kinyoun acid-fast s.
modified trichrome s.
MPO bone marrow s.
myeloperoxidase bone marrow s.
Nair buffered methylene blue s.
neuron-specific enolase s.
new methylene blue N s.
Nile blue fat s.
nonspecific esterase s.
nuclear fast red s.
orange green stain
overnight Giemsa s.
oxalic acid s.
oxytalan fiber s.
Papanicolaou stain of sputum
periodic acid-Schiff-Alcian blue combination s.
periodic acid-Schiff-hematoxylin s.
periodic acid-Schiff s.
periodic acid-silver methenamine s.
periodic acid-thiocarbohydrazide-silver proteinate stain
phosphotungstic acid-hematoxylin s.
polyacrylamide gel electrophoresis with silver s.
polychrome methylene blue s.
port-wine stain birthmark
potassium hydroxide stain
spinal fluid Gram s.
sputum Gram s.
thiosemicarbazide s.

toluidine blue s.
Unna-Pappenheim s.
Warthin-Starry s.
Weigert hematoxylin s.
Wilder silver s.
Wright-Giemsa s.
Ziehl-Neelsen s.

stainable iron

stained
dark blood stained fluid
healthy tissue s.
meconium s.
s. smear and culture

staining
acid-fast staining method
argyrophilic nucleolar organizer region s.
Attwood staining method
automated slide s.
fluorescent actin s.
fluorescent antibody staining technique
Gram staining technique
homogeneous staining region of chromosome
immunogold-silver s.
lightly staining coiled bacteria
mast cell s.
May-Grünwald-Giemsa staining
meconium staining of liquor
MicroTrak direct fluorescent antibody s.
monoclonal antibody s.
negatively staining region of chromosome
periodic acid s.
rapid immunofluorescence s.
rose bengal s.
tannic acid, polyphosphomolybdic acid, and amido acid staining technique

stainless
austenitic stainless steel
s. steel crown
s. steel implant
s. steel and molybdenum
s. steel suture

stalemate
analytic s.

stalk
allantoic s.
infundibular s.
mesenteric s.
narrow mesenteric s.
neural s.
neurohypophysial s.
optic s.
pituitary s.
pituitary stalk distortion

stalked hydatid

Stallard operation

stall the healing process

stammering of the bladder

Stamm gastrostomy

stance
approach-avoidance s.
disturbance of gait and s.
gait and s.
resting calcaneal stance position

stand
Mayo s.
s. and pivot

standard
s. above-elbow cast
s. accuracy
s. acid reflux test
s. bicarbonate
British S. Unit
Consolidated S.'s Manual
density optical s.
s. dentures
s. deviation interval
s. deviation of mean
s. deviation of normal-to-normal beat
s. deviation score
S. Deviation Unit
s. dose administration
s. electrode potential
s. electrolyte solution
s. error of difference
s. error of estimate
s. error of the mean
s. external cardiopulmonary resuscitation
s. fixation preference test
s. free energy
s. gait
s. glucose tolerance test
s. heparin infusion
s. hospital treatment
s. hyperalimentation
S. Industrial Classification
s. infertility treatment algorithm
s. inpatient care
insulin s.
internal s.
internal telomerase s.
s. isolation technique
s. language test for aphasia
s. laparoscopy
s. method agar
s. metropolitan statistical area
s. mineral base
s. morbidity ratio
s. mortality ratio
s. mycological identification technique
S. Nomenclature of Athletic Injuries
S. Nomenclature of Diseases and Operations
s. normal deviation
s. observed minus expected
s. operating procedure
OSHA blood-borne pathogen s.
out of specification deviation from standard
s. peak dilution
S.'s for Pediatric Immunization
s. perfusion fluid
s. platelet count
population standard deviation
s. practice
Provisional International S.
quality assurance s.'s
quantitation s.
Raven Standard Progressive Matrices
reading of s.
S. Reference Material
relative standard accuracy
relative standard deviation
reticulocyte standard buffer
s. saline citrate
sample standard deviation
Second International S.
S. System of Psychiatry
s. temperature and pressure, dry
s. temperature and pulse
s. test dose
s. thickness
s. tone-decay test
s. triple therapy
s. tube agglutination test
s. tube feeding
S. Units and Nomenclature
s. uptake value
s. wire gauge
s. Y incision

standardization
Medicare Bone Mass Measurement S. Act

standardized
S. Assessment of Depressive Disorders
s. care plan
s. deviate

standardized *(continued)*
s. device
s. incidence ratio
s. metabolic rate
s. mortality ratio
S. Nomenclature of Medicine
s. proportionate mortality
s. rate ratio
relative standardized mortality ratio
s. response mean
s. test
s. uptake value

standby
anesthesia s.
s. angioplasty
s. assistance in transfers and ambulation
s. assist with ambulation
patient transfers with standby assistance
s. transfer and ambulation

standing
s. ambulation
s. balance
copied standing order
s. diastolic blood pressure
s. heart rate
s. order
s. pivotal transfer
s. tolerance
s. venous pressure

standstill
atrial s.
auricular s.
inspiratory s.
persistent atrial s.

Stanford
S. Achievement Test
S. biopsy method
S. Diagnostic Reading Test
S. Health Assessment Questionnaire
S. Hypnotic Susceptibility Scale
S. Sleepiness Scale

Stanford-Binet
S.-B. Fourth Edition
S.-B. Intelligence Scale
S.-B. Intelligence Test-Form LM

Stanford-type aortic dissection

stannous fluoride

stapedectomy
Shea s.

stapedial
s. artery
s. fold

stapedis
caput s.
plica s.

stapedius muscle

stapes
anterior crest of s.
anterior crus of s.
anterior limb of s.
anular ligament of s.
anular ligament of s.
capitulum of s.
fold of s.
footplate of the s.
head of s.
posterior crus of s.
s. replacement prosthesis

staphylococcal
s. abscess
s. bacteremia
s. blepharitis
s. clumping test
s. conjunctivitis
s. enterotoxin A, B, D, F
s. enterotoxin B antiserum
s. hemagglutinating antibody
s. infection
s. infection of heart valve
neonatal staphylococcal disease
s. phage lysate
platelet ^{125}I-labeled staphylococcal protein A
s. pneumonia
s. protease
s. scalded skin syndrome
s. protein A
s. toxic shock syndrome

Staphylococcus
Staphylococcus aureus hyperimmunoglobulinemia E syndrome
Staphylococcus aureus pneumonia
Staphylococcus aureus prosthetic joint infection
Staphylococcus aureus protease
borderline-resistant *Staphylococcus aureus*
epidemic methicillin-resistant *Staphylococcus aureus*
glycopeptide-insensitive *Staphylococcus aureus*
glycopeptide-intermediate *Staphylococcus aureus*
glycopeptide-resistant *Staphylococcus aureus*
hemolytic Staphylococcus aureus
methicillin-aminoglycoside-resistant *Staphylococcus aureus*
methicillin-resistant coagulase-negative *Staphylococcus*
methicillin-resistant *Staphylococcus epidermidis*
methicillin-resistant *Staphylococcus* species
methicillin-susceptible coagulase-negative *Staphylococcus*
mupirocin-resistant, methicillin-resistant *Staphylococcus aureus*
mupirocin-resistant *Staphylococcus aureus*
mutiresistant *Staphylococcus aureus*
oxacillin aminoglycoside-resistant *Staphylococcus aureus*
vancomycin-insensitive *Staphylococcus aureus*
vancomycin-intermediate-resistant *Staphylococcus aureus*
vancomycin-resistant *Staphylococcus aureus*

staphylococcus
coagulase-negative s.
coagulase-negative staphylococcus bacteremia
coagulase-positive s.
s. medium

***Staphylococcus aureus* hyperimmunoglobulinemia E syndrome**

***Staphylococcus aureus* pneumonia**

Staphylococcus epidermidis
methicillin-resistant e.

staphylogenes
impetigo s.

staphylolysin
epsilon s.
gamma s.

staphyloma
anterior corneal s.
congenital anterior s.

staphylomata
peripapillary s.

staple
automatic s.
barbed s.
metallic skin s.
s. suture

stapled
simultaneously stapled pneumonectomy
s. intestinal anastomosis

totally stapled restorative proctocolectomy

stapler
circular stapler donut
intraluminal s.
skin and fascia s.
thoracoabdominal s.

stapling
double stapling technique
gastric stapling procedure
gastric vertical s.
stomach stapling technique

star
S. Cancellation Test
Lindstrom S.
Lindstrom Star nucleus manipulator
Lone S. fever
Lone S. tick
macular s.
macular star formation
optic disc edema with a macular s.
Winslow s.

star-cancellation test

starch
amylase-resistant s.
Argo corn starch test
degradable starch microsphere
s. equivalent
hydroxyethyl starch solution
magnetic starch microspheres
s. methylenedianiline

Stargardt
S. disease
S. syndrome

Starling
S. curve
S. hypothesis
S. law

start
s. of anesthesia
s. of anesthetic
s. of care
hypnagogic s.'s

started
intravenous fluids s.

starting
difficulty in starting urinary stream
s. and stopping of urinary stream

startle
s. epilepsy
heightened startle reactions
hypnagogic s.
s. reflex
s. test

starvation
s. acidosis
s. diabetes

starving behavior of bulimic

stasis
antral s.
atrial stasis index
chronic stasis leg ulcer
s. cirrhosis
s. dermatitis
s. eczema
gallbladder s.
ileal s.
intestinal s.
malleolus stasis ulcer
papillary s.
s. ulcer
venous stasis changes
venous stasis retinopathy
venous stasis ulcer

state
active sleep s.
acute confusional s.
adult ego s.
affective and paranoid s.
alcoholic confusional s.
alcoholic paranoid s.
alcoholic twilight s.
alcohol-induced paranoid s.
alert awake s.
s. of alertness
alert state of consciousness
altered mental s.
altered state of conscious awareness
altered state of consciousness
anxiety state neurotic disorder
anxiety tension s.
aroused state of disturbed behavior
arteriosclerotic dementia confusional s.
arteriosclerotic paranoid s.
arteriosclerotic psychosis confusional s.
atypical neurotic anxiety s.
awake and active s.
calm-wakefulness s.
cardiovascular steady s.
central excitatory s.
central inhibitory s.
chronic anxiety s.
s. of consciousness
constitutional psychopathic s.
contrast-enhanced Fourier-acquired steady s.
deficiency state immunity
Ego S. Inventory
epileptic confusional s.
explosive psychotic s.
fast adiabatic trajectory in steady s.
Fatigue-Inertia Subscale of the Profile of Mood S.'s
Golombok-Rust Inventory of Marital S.
gradient-recalled acquisition in steady s.
gradient-refocused acquisition in a steady s.
hallucinatory state induced by drug
heightened attention s.
heightened awareness s.
hyperosmolar nonketotic diabetic s.
immunity deficiency s.
Kent S. University Speech Discrimination Test
litigious delusional s.
local excitatory s.
low excitatory s.
s. medical facilities plan
meningococcal carrier s.
s. mental hospital
Mini-Mental State Examination of Folstein
mixed bipolar s.
mixed compulsive states psychasthenia
Modified Mini-Mental S. Examination
multiple ego s.
muscle in elongated s.
myocardial contractile s.
neurohumoral excitation s.
neuromuscular tension s.
neurotic anxiety s.
neurotic depressive s.
nonketotic hyperosmolar s.
opposite affect s.
panic attack neurotic anxiety s.
parasomniac conscious s.
parent ego s.
paroxysmal emotional s.
patient in catatonic s.
persistent vegetative s.
Present S. Examination
Profile of Mood S.'s
rested state contraction

state *(continued)*
schizophrenic residual s.
Schizophrenic Subscale of Present S. Examination
subacute confusional s.
tolerate immune s.
S. Trait Anxiety Index-I
transition state theory
United S.'s Pharmacopeia Drug Information

state-and-trait anxiety

statement
anatomic gift s.
attending physician's s.
Environmental Impact S.
Twenty S.'s Test
Vaccine Information S.

State-Trait
S.-T. Anger Expression Inventory
S.-T. Anger Scale
S.-T. Anxiety Inventory
S.-T. Personality Inventory

static
s. arthropathy
s. ataxia
automated static threshold perimetry
s. cervical traction
s. compliance
s. elastance
s. gangrene
s. lung compliance
maximal static response assay
noncycloplegic distance static retinoscopy
s. pelvic traction
s. random access memory
s. shock
total static compliance
s. two-point discrimination
s. volume pressure

station
abnormal gait and s.
adequate gait and s.
balance, gait, and s.
casualty clearing s.
central patient s.
gait and s.
Lawrence Experimental Station agar
lymph node s.
mediastinal nodal s.
medical receiving s.
nursing s.
s. pull-through

stationary
s. ankle flexible endoskeleton
s. attachment flexible endoskeletal
s. cataract
congenital stationary night blindness
s. phase

statistic
cooperative health statistics system
Mann-Whitney rank sum s.
Wilcoxon rank sum s.

statistical
s. analysis and quality control
s. control
s. deviation
metropolitan statistical area
Neyman-Pearson statistical hypothesis
standard metropolitan statistical area

statistically significant

stature
agonadism, mental retardation, short stature, retarded bone age syndrome
asymmetric short stature syndrome
brittle hair, intellectual impairment, decreased fertility, short stature syndrome
cataract, motor system disorder, short stature, learning difficulty, skeletal abnormalities syndrome
congenital cataracts, sensorineural deafness, Down syndrome facial appearance, short stature, mental retardation syndrome
deafness, femoral epiphysial dysplasia, short stature, developmental delay syndrome
ear, patella, short stature syndrome
gonadal failure, short stature, mitral valve prolapse, mental retardation syndrome
goniodysgenesis, mental retardation, short s.
ichthyosis, brittle hair, impaired intelligence, decreased fertility, short stature syndrome
idiopathic short s.
macrocephaly, facial abnormalities, disproportionate tall stature mental retardation syndrome
mental retardation, epilepsy, short stature, skeletal dysplasia syndrome
mental retardation, short stature, hypertelorism syndrome
mental retardation, short stature, obesity, hypogonadism syndrome
microcephaly, hypergonadotropic hypogonadism, short stature syndrome
microcephaly, mild developmental delay, short stature, distinctive face syndrome
microcephaly, mild mental retardation, short stature, skeletal anomalies syndrome
microdontia-microcephaly-short stature syndrome
mixed sclerosing bone dysplasia, small stature, seizures, mental retardation syndrome
nongrowth hormone deficient short s.
normal variant short s.
obesity, short stature, mental deficiency, hypogonadism, micropenis, finger contracture, cleft lip-palate syndrome
short stature homeobox gene
short stature, hyperextensibility of joints or hernia or both, ocular depression, Rieger anomaly, teething, delayed

status
acute change in mental s.
altered mental s.
Anxiety S. Index
Anxiety S. Inventory
apical biopsy s.
ASA physical s.
assessment of health s.
Behavior S. Inventory
Brief Neuropsychological Mental Status Examination
cardiovascular risk s.
clinical status of node
compensated cardiac s.
complex partial status epilepticus
convulsive status epilepticus
Current, Global, Psychiatric-Social S.
declining respiratory s.
Depression S. Inventory
Disability S. Scale
Duke Activity S. Index
Edinburgh Rehabilitation S. Scale
elopement s.

s. epilepticus
Expanded Disability Status Scale
febrile status epilepticus
fluctuating mental s.
functional s.
Functional S. Index
Functional S. Questionnaire
functional status measures
grand mal s.
human immune status survey
human immunodeficiency virus-patient-reported status and experience
individualized functional status assessment
Inventory of Functional S. After Childbirth
Karnofsky performance s.
knowledge, attitude, behavior, and improvement in nutritional s.
Kurtzke Disability S. Scale
limbic status epilepticus
male biological s.
Mental S. Examination Record
mental health s.
mental status change
mental status evaluation
mental status examination report
mental status, oriented
mental status questionnaire
mental status schedule
modified version of the mini mental status examination
mutation carrier s.
Neurobehavioral Cognitive S. examination
neurovascular s.
nonconvulsive status epilepticus
nonreassuring fetal s.
nutritional status assessment
nutritional status type
oral health s.
patient regained active s.
performance status scale for head and neck cancer
physical status patient classifications
s. post
postmenopausal hormonal s.
s. post myocardial infarction
s. postoperative
s. post surgery
s. post transurethral resection of prostate
problem status report
Psychiatric S. Schedule
Psychiatric Status Rating scale
Pulmonary Functional S. and Dyspnea Questionnaire
s. quo
refractory status epilepticus
Short Portable Mental S. Questionnaire
Social Adaptation S.
socioeconomic s.
stable health s.
suicidal observation s.
s. thymicolymphaticus

Staunig position

stave
barrel stave osteotomy procedure

staved
barrel staved graft

stay
diagnosis responsible for length of s.
safety, monitoring, intervention, length of stay, and evaluation

steady
s. alpha rhythm
cardiovascular steady state
central, steady and maintained fixation
contrast-enhanced Fourier-acquired steady state
fast adiabatic trajectory in steady state
fast imaging steady precession sequence three-dimensional magnetic resonance imaging
fast imaging with steady precession
s. gait
gradient-recalled acquisition in steady state
gradient-refocused acquisition in a steady state

steady-state
s.-s. auditory evoked response
s.-s. carbon monoxide diffusing capacity of lung
s.-s. exercise
Fourier-acquired steady-state technique
s.-s. free precession
s.-s. free progression
s.-s. heart rate
s.-s. plasma glucose
s.-s. plasma insulin
s.-s. rest

steal
carotid steal syndrome
cerebral ischemia s.
coronary artery s.
coronary steal mechanism
coronary steal phenomenon
coronary steal syndrome
coronary-subclavian steal syndrome
s. effect
lateral crural s.
myocardial steal syndrome
pulmonary artery s.

stealth liposomal doxorubicin

steam
heat, steam, gum, yawn, and Valsalva maneuver
s. inhalation
s. inhalation therapy
s. spray inhaler

steam-fitter's asthma

steatocystoma
multiplex s.
s. multiplex

steatohepatitis
alcoholic s.
nonalcoholic s.

steatorrhea
idiopathic s.
pancreatic s.

steatosis
s. cordis
macrovesicular s.
microvesicular hepatic s.

steel
austenitic stainless s.
carbon steel drill point
French steel sound
stainless steel crown
stainless steel implant
stainless steel and molybdenum
stainless steel suture

steeple sign

steering wheel injury

Stefan-Boltzmann constant

Steinberg thumb sign

Stein-Leventhal syndrome

Stein Sentence Completion Test

stellate
s. abnormality
s. abscess
s. block anesthesia
s. cell of cerebral cortex
s. cell of liver
s. configuration
s. fracture
s. ganglion nerve block

stellate *(continued)*
s. hair
hepatic stellate cell
s. incision
s. laceration
left stellate ganglionic blockade
s. ligament
right stellate ganglion

Stellwag
S. brawny edema
S. sign

stem
allogeneic stem cell
allogeneic stem cell transplant
allogenic hematopoietic stem cell transplantation
allographic stem cell transplant
APR hip s.
autologous hematopoietic stem cell transplantation
autologous peripheral blood stem cell bone marrow transplantation
autologous peripheral hematopoietic stem cell support
autologous stem cell
autologous stem cell rescue
autologous stem cell transplantation
bone marrow stem cell
brain stem glioma
brain stem hemorrhage
s. bronchus
s. cell
s. cell apheresis
s. cell factor
s. cell indicated by transplantation assay
s. cell leukemia
s. cell proliferation factor
s. cell rescue
s. cell support
contoured femoral s.
cryopreserved stem cell
debonded femoral stem prosthesis
dorsal brain stem lipoma
embryonic stem cell
erythropoietin-sensitive stem cell
harvested stem cell
hematopoietic stem cell transplantation
hemopoietic blood stem cell
high-dose chemotherapy and stem cell rescue
human mesenchymal stem cell
human tumor stem cell assay
impairment of functions of brain s.
left main stem bronchus
left main stem coronary artery disease
limbal stem cell transplantation
long s.
lymphoid stem cell
MacArthur Story S. Battery
main stem bronchus
marrow hematopoietic stem cell
massive infarct of brain s.
matched unrelated donor stem cell transplant
monoblock femoral stem prosthesis
mouse stem cell-like cell
myeloid stem cell
nonmyeloablative allogeneic stem cell transplant
normal brain s.
pediatric brain stem glioma
peripheral blood stem cell
peripheral blood stem cell autografting
peripheral blood stem cell infusion
peripheral blood stem cell rescue
peripheral blood stem cell reserve
peripheral blood stem cell support
peripheral blood stem cell transplantation
peripheral stem cell harvest
peripheral stem cell transplant
pluripotent hemopoietic stem cell
pluripotent myeloid stem cell
primary s.
temporal s.
totipotent hematopoietic stem cell
transient brain stem ischemia

Stenger hearing test

stenoregurgitation
mitral s.

stenosing
s. peripheral arterial disease
s. tenosynovitis

stenosis, pl. **stenoses**
acute spinal s.
ankylosing spinal s.
aortic ostial s.
aortic stenosis and aortic insufficiency murmurs
aortic stenosis, corneal clouding, growth and mental retardation syndrome
aortic valve s.
aortic valvular s.
asymptomatic carotid artery s.
atherosclerotic renal artery s.
atypical aortic valve s.
calcific aortic valve s.
calcific mitral s.
calcific nodular aortic s.
carotid artery s.
Carotid Artery S. with Asymptomatic Narrowing: Operation Versus Aspirin Study
cervical canal s.
combined mitral stenosis and regurgitation
congenital nasal pyriform aperture s.
coronary stenosis index
craniofacial s.
critical coronary s.
discrete subaortic s.
distal urethral s.
dynamic subaortic s.
hemodynamically significant s.
hydrocephalus due to congenital stenosis of aqueduct of Sylvius
hypertrophic muscular subaortic s.
hypertrophic pyloric s.
idiopathic hypertrophic aortic s.
idiopathic hypertrophic subaortic s.
infantile hypercalcemia s.
infantile hypertrophic pyloric s.
infundibular pulmonary s.
internal carotid s.
laryngotracheal s.
lateral recess s.
lentigines, electrocardiographic abnormalities, ocular hypertelorism, pulmonary stenosis, abnormalities of genitalia, retardation of growth, deafness syndrome
long-segment congenital tracheal s.
lumbar canal s.
lumbar spinal s.
main renal artery s.
mental retardation, typical facies, aortic stenosis syndrome
mild pulmonic s.
mitral stenosis in pregnancy
mitral valve s.
muscular subaortic s.
myocardial infundibular s.
napkin ring anular s.
nasal pyriform aperture s.
nasal vestibular s.

nasopharyngeal s.
neural foraminal s.
nodular calcific aortic s.
noncalcified coronary s.
noncircumferential s.
papillary bile duct s.
peripheral pulmonary artery s.
piriform aperture s.
posterior glottic s.
prosthetic valve s.
pulmonary arterial s.
pulmonary artery s.
pulmonary atresia/pulmonary s.
pulmonary branch s.
pulmonary valve s.
pulmonary vein s.
pulmonic valve s.
pyloric s.
renal artery s.
rheumatic mitral s.
saphenous vein graft s.
silent mitral s.
spinal canal s.
subaortic s.
subglottic s.
supravalvular hypertrophic aortic s.
tetracycline-induced s.
transplant renal artery s.
tricuspid s.
unilateral renal artery s.
urethral meatal s.
valvular aortic s.
valvular pulmonic s.
X-linked aqueductal s.

stenotic
s. disease
s. flow reserve
s. hymen

Stensen
S. duct
S. foramen

stent
antireflux double-J s.
s. apposition
autologous vein graft s.
autologous vein graft-coated s.
balloon expandable intravascular s.
balloon-expandable tantalum s.
biliary sphincterotomy and stent placement
s. coil
common bile duct s.
s. delivery system
s. deployment
endoscopic biliary s.
endovascular stent graft
expandable esophageal s.
s. expansion
s. graft
heat-activated recoverable temporary s.
s. implantation
insertion of s.
internal biliary s.
metallic biliary s.
metallic biliary stent migration
percutaneous transluminal angioplasty with stent placement
percutaneous ureteral s.
peripheral anterior stent keratopathy
pigtail curl of stent tube
radiopaque tantalum s.
self-expanding metallic s.
self-expanding microporous s.
s. thrombosis
transjugular intrahepatic portosystemic stent shunt

stented coronary artery

stenting
antegrade ureteral s.
carotid angioplasty and s.
endoscopic pancreatic s.
endoscopic retrograde biliary s.
innominate artery s.
pulmonary artery s.
s. in small arteries

stentless porcine valve

stent-mounted heterograft valve

Stenver x-ray view

steochondritis
syphilitic s.

step
American Heart Association S. One Diet
s. deformity
nasal step defect
s. out, turn out

stepdown
cardiac stepdown unit and telemetry
neonatal stepdown unit

Stephens Oral Language Screening Test

stepladder
s. appearance
s. stage

steppage gait

stercoraceous abscess

stercoral
s. appendicitis
s. colic
s. ulcer

stereoacuity
Titmus stereoacuity test

stereocampimeter
Lloyd s.

stereochemical structure

stereopsis
macular s.

stereoscope
binocular s.

stereoscopic
s. acuity
s. parallax
s. vision

stereospecific binding

stereotactic
s. ablation
s. aspiration
s. brachytherapy
s. brain biopsy
s. breast biopsy
computer assisted stereotactic laser microsurgery
computer-assisted stereotactic surgery
s. cordotomy
s. core biopsy
s. core-needle biopsy
s. depth electroencephalogram
s. electroencephalogram
s. external-beam irradiation
fractionated stereotactic radiosurgery
fractionated stereotactic radiotherapy
s. frame
frameless stereotactic device
frameless stereotactic guidance
frameless stereotactic microsurgery
gamma knife stereotactic radiosurgery
s. guidance
s. guide
s. guided core-needle biopsy
hypofractionated stereotactic radiotherapy
Mayfield/ACCISS stereotactic workstation
megavoltage computed tomography-assisted stereotactic radiosurgery

stereotactic *(continued)*
megavoltage CT-assisted stereotactic radiosurgery
s. mesencephalic tractotomy
MRI-based stereotactic biopsy
s. needle biopsy
percutaneous stereotactic radiofrequency rhizotomy
s. radiosurgery
selective imaging and graphics for stereotactic surgery
s. surface projection

stereotactically guided core needle biopsy

stereotactic-assisted radiation therapy

stereotaxy
frameless s.
frameless stereotaxy system

stereotyped
atypical stereotyped movement disorder
s. behavior

stereotype habits disorder

stereotypical behavior

stereotypic movement disorder

steric exclusion chromatography

sterile
absorbent sterile towel
s. aqueous solution
s. aqueous suspension
area lavaged with sterile saline
central sterile supply department
s. drapes applied
s. dressing
s. dressing applied
s. dry dressing
dry sterile dressing applied
dry sterile fluff
dry sterile gauze
s. elective low forceps vaginal delivery
s. female
fenestrated sterile field barrier
s. field
s. immunity
s. indicated low forceps vaginal delivery
s. injectable solution
s. injectable suspension
s. irrigation
s. low midforceps vaginal delivery
s. normal saline
operating theatre sterile supply unit
patient is prepped and draped in usual sterile fashion
pyogenic sterile arthritis, pyoderma gangrenosum, and acne
s. redressing
s. saline soak
s. solution
s. spontaneous controlled vaginal delivery
s., spontaneous vaginal delivery
s. urine culture
urine sterile on culture
s. vaginal examination
s. water gastric drip
s. water for injection

sterilely prepped and draped

sterility
aspermatogenic s.
s. assurance level
male s.
normospermatogenic s.
one-child s.

sterilization
cold gas s.
hysterectomy and s.
laparoscopic tubal s.
liquid chemical s.
postpartum s.
sexual tubal s.
voluntary s.

sterilized
autoclave s.
gas sterilized instrument
s. gown and mask
prereduced anaerobically sterilized medium

sterilizer
bead s.

sternal
s. abscess
s. angle
s. bar
s. border
s. cartilage
deep sternal wound infection
heard best at left lower sternal border
heard best at left upper sternal border
s. intercostal retraction
s. joint
left lower sternal border
left sternal border
left sternal edge
left upper sternal border
lower sternal border
s. notch to nipple
s. occipital mandibular immobilization
right lower sternal border
right middle sternal border
right sternal border
right sternal edge
right upper sternal border
s. splitting incision
s. splitting scar
s. synchondrosis
upper left sternal border
upper right sternal border

Sternberg
S. cell
S. sarcoma
S. sign

Sternberg-Reed cell

sternochondral junction

sternoclavicular
s. angle
anterior sternoclavicular joint
anterior sternoclavicular ligament
articular disc of sternoclavicular joint
s. disk
s. joint
s. junction
s. ligament

sternoclavicularis
articulatio s.

sternocleidomastoid
s. diameter
s. hemorrhage
s. muscle

sternocostales

sternocostal joint

sternocostoclavicular hyperostosis

sternohyoid muscle

sternomastoid
anterior sternomastoid approach
s. artery

sternooccipital-mandibular
s.-m. immobilization brace
s.-m. immobilization orthosis
s.-m. immobilizer

sternothyroid muscle

sternotomy
s. dehiscence
horizontal s.

median sternotomy incision
vertical s.

sternum
anterior bowing of s.
clavicular notch of s.
costal notches of s.
manubrium of s.
notch of s.

steroid
s. acute regulatory protein
s. acute respiratory protein
adrenal steroid hormone
adrenal steroid precursor
alkylated androgenic s.
anabolic steroid abuse
androgenic-anabolic s.
cancer and steroid hormone
carbohydrate-active s.
s. cell tumor
cervical epidural steroid injection
s. dependence
electrolyte steroid cardiopathy by calcification
electrolyte and steroid cardiopathy with necrosis
epidural steroid injection
glucocorticoid steroid-induced osteoporosis
gonadal steroid suppression
s. hormone
s. hormone-binding globulin
s. implantation
s. inhaler
s. injection
ketogenic s.
17-ketogenic s.
long-acting contraceptive s.
low steroid content combined oral contraceptive
lumbar epidural s.
lumbar epidural steroid injection
maternal steroid concentration
s. metabolic clearance rate
nasal s.
nasal steroid spray
normal gonadal steroid level
oral contraceptive s.
oral steroid drug
s. protein activity index
s. resistant asthma
s. resistant graft-versus-host disease
s. sensitivity
s. sulfatase
s. sulfate
s. sulfurylation
tapered steroid dosing package
s. therapy
thoracic epidural steroid injection

steroidal-cell antibody

steroid-binding plasma protein

steroid-dependent
s.-d. asthma
s.-d. asthmatic
s.-d. Crohn disease
s.-d. tumor

steroidogenesis
adrenal s.
gonadal s.
ovarian s.

steroidogenic
s. acute regulatory protein
adrenal steroidogenic cascade
s. diabetes
s. factor-1
ovarian steroidogenic dysfunction

steroid-resistant rejection

steroid-responsive nephrotic syndrome

steroid-sensitive idiopathic nephrotic syndrome

sterol
s. carrier protein-2
s. ester
s. regulatory element binding protein

stertorous respiration

stethoscope
Doppler ultrasound s.
oral esophageal s.
pacing esophageal s.
precordial s.

Stetson Auditory Discrimination Test

Stevens-Johnson syndrome

Stewart-Morel syndrome

Stewart-Treves syndrome

S-thalassemia
hemoglobin S.-t.

stick
blood gas s.
heel stick pain
hockey stick incision
needle stick injury
s. swab

Stickler syndrome

Stierlin sign

stiff
s. joint
s. man syndrome
swollen, stiff, inflamed joint

stiffening
arterial s.
cautery-assisted palatal stiffening operation
joint s.

stiff-heart syndrome

stiffness
early morning s.
end-diastolic chamber s.
glands, goiter, or stiffness of neck
goiter or stiffness of glands
s. or heaviness of limbs
joint pain and s.
morning s.
shoulder pain and s.
s., tremors and immobility

stigma, pl. **stigmata**
hysteric s.
malpighian s.
stigmata of recent hemorrhage
social s.

still
adult-onset systemic Still disease
S. disease
S. murmur

stillbirth
intrapartum s.
s., mummification, embryonic death, infertility syndrome
s. rate

stillborn
infant s.

Still-Chauffard syndrome

Stilling
canal of S.
S. canal
S. column

stimulant
appetite s.
s. effect
heart s.
hepatic s.
intestinal s.
s. laxative
local s.
luteinization s.
nerve s.
nervous s.
overdosed with s.'s
vasomotor s.

stimulate
s. adequate spontaneous breathing

stimulate *(continued)*
s. bone formation
s. to cry
s. heart muscle
s. the immune system
s. nerve impulse
s. new vessel growth

stimulated
anti-CD3 stimulated peripheral blood lymphocytes transduced with a gene encoding a chimeric
autologous T lymphocytes stimulated with the patient's tumor-specific mutated RAS peptides
s. echo acquisition mode
s. echo artifact
s. fibrinolytic activity
intellectually s.
light activation by stimulated emission of radiation
light amplification by stimulated emission of radiation
microwave amplification by stimulated emission of radiation
s. protein synthesis

stimulating
adrenal androgen corticotropic stimulating hormone
alpha-adrenergic stimulating drug
bipolar stimulating electrode
corpus luteum stimulating hormone
s. factor
growth stimulating hormone
s. insulin resistance
intrinsic stimulating activity
isolated follicle-stimulating hormone deficiency syndrome
labile aggregation stimulating substance
nerve growth stimulating activity

stimulation
acoustic stimulation test
acupuncture and transcutaneous electrical nerve s.
alpha-adrenergic s.
apnea/bradycardia mild s.
arginine-insulin stimulation test
arginine stimulation test
atrial overdrive stimulation rate
brain stimulation reinforcement
breast stimulation contraction test
calibrated electrical s.
caloric stimulation test for vestibular function
carotid chemoreceptor s.
carotid sinus nerve s.
catheter stimulation of right atrium
cervical s.
chest wall s.
cognitive environmental s.
contralateral acoustic s.
coronary sinus s.
cosyntropin stimulation test
cranial electrical s.
deep brain s.
diaphragm s.
diaphragmatic nerve s.
direct brain s.
direct electrical nerve s.
dorsal column s.
dorsal cord s.
double simultaneous s.
drug-induced lymphocyte stimulation test
electrical bone-growth s.
electrical bone s.
electrical brain s.
electrical intracranial s.
electrical muscle s.
electrical nerve s.
electrical spinal cord s.
electrical stimulation of hand
electrical stimulation of heart
electrical stimulation mapping
electrical transcranial s.
electric field s.
electric stimulation of brain
electrogalvanic s.
electrotherapeutic point s.
environmental s.
eosinophil stimulation promoter
Familiar Sensory S.
fast-frequency repetitive transcranial magnetic s.
fetal acoustic stimulation testing
field s.
field-electrical neural s.
fluids, aeration, nutrition, communication, activity, and s.
functional electrical s.
functional neuromuscular s.
functional transcutaneous nerve s.
galvanic muscle s.
galvanic vestibular s.
gonadotropin agonist stimulation test
growth hormone stimulation test
Hallpike caloric stimulation test
high-voltage pulsed galvanic s.
histamine stimulation test
intensive stimulation of senses
interferential s.
intermittent photic stimulation
intracranial s.
intraduodenal s.
intraoperative electrical cortical s.
laryngopharyngeal sensory s.
lateral electrical spine s.
lateral electrical surface s.
Leydig cell s.
s. of lower bowel
low-frequency tetanic s.
mammary parenchymal s.
manual organ stimulation technique
maximum stimulation test
mechanical s.
microamperage electrical nerve s.
microamperage neural s.
motor-evoked response to transcranial s.
multiple antigen stimulation test
muscular response to electrical stimulation of motor nerve
nerve root s.
neuromuscular electrical stimulation therapy
nipple s.
nipple stimulation contraction stress test
noninvasive carotid baroceptor s.
noninvasive programmed s.
paired electrical s.
peak acid output after pentagastrin s.
pelvic floor electrical s.
percutaneous electrical nerve s.
percutaneously inserted spinal cord electrical s.
percutaneous on-surface s.
photic stimulation procedure
phrenic nerve s.
positional feedback stimulation trainer
postganglionic vagal s.
postural stimulation test
programmed electrical s.
programmed ventricular s.
promontory stimulation test
pulmonary hypothalamic s.
s. ratio
repetitive nerve s.
Restricted Environment S. Therapy
restriction of environmental stimulation therapy
sacral nerve s.

s. of senses
sham transcutaneous nerve s.
simultaneous analog s.
spinal cord s.
Stoller afferent nerve s.
structured sensory s.
subcutaneous nerve s.
support and s.
therapeutic electrical s.
thyrotropin-releasing hormone stimulation test
transcranial cortical magnetic s.
transcutaneous acupoint electrical s.
transcutaneous cranial electrical s.
transcutaneous electrical nerve s.
transesophageal atrial s.
transmural electrical field s.
transurethral electrical bladder s.
s. of trigger area
TSH stimulation blocking antibody
vagal s.
vagus nerve s.
vibratory acoustic s.
vibroacoustic s.
visual or auditory s.

stimulation-bound behavior

stimulation-induced
s.-i. analgesia
s.-i. hypalgesia

stimulation-produced analgesia

stimulator
direct-current bone growth s.
dorsal column s.
electrical bone-growth s.
human-specific thyroid s.
human thyroid adenylcyclase s.
implantable bone growth s.
long-acting thyroid stimulator protector
long-acting transmural s.
lumbar anterior-root stimulator implant
metabolic heat load s.
monopolar cathodal s.
neuromuscular electrical s.
Ortho DX electromedical s.
percutaneous epidural nerve s.
peripheral nervous s.
personal portable s.
point locator s.
pulsed electromagnetic s.
transcutaneous electrical nerve s.

stimulatory
B-lymphocyte stimulatory factor
hepatic stimulatory substance
s. receptor

stimulus, pl. **stimuli**
abnormal electrical s.
afferent stimulus interaction
alerting stimulus on electroencephalogram
alert, verbal stimulus response, painful stimulus response, unresponsive
alert, vocal stimulus, painful stimulus, unresponsive
ambiguous external stimuli
angry reaction to minor stimuli
anxiolytic stimuli
s. artifact
brief stimulus therapy
s., conditioned
conditioned s.
s. control
critical stimulus duration
discriminative s.
s. drive
s. generalization
s. hunger
hyperreactivity to stimuli
s. intensity
s. isolation
s. isolation unit
method of constant stimuli
moderate tactile s.
movement-produced s.
neonatal amblyogenic s.
patient responsive to noxious stimuli
patient responsive to painful stimuli
perceptual emotive s.
premature atrial s.
proprioceptive stimuli
reflex-activating s.
reinforcing s.
responding to internal stimuli
s. response
right ear, cold s.
right ear, warm s.
sensory stimuli
spatial emotional stimuli
spatial nonemotional stimuli
unconditional s.
unconditioned s.
verbal nonemotional stimuli

stimulus-action hunger

stimulus-organism response

sting
Africanized honeybee s.
s. allergy
ant s.
Apis mellifera s.
arthropod s.
ashgray blister beetle s.
bee sting hypersensitivity
dizziness from insect s.
insect s.
Lytta vesicata s.
marine animal s.
Megabombus s.
Megalopyge opercularis s.
millipede s.

stinger
barbed s.

stippled
s. appearance
s. epiphysis

stippling
basophilic s.

stirrer
magnetic s.

stirrup
ankle stirrup brace
ankle stirrup splint
Finochietto s.

stitch
s. abscess
apical s.
baseball s.
bow-tie s.
corner s.
episiotomy s.
figure-of-eight s.
horizontal mattress s.
McCall s.
mini-keratoplasty stitch scissors
O'Brien stitch scissors
s.'s out in afternoon
s.'s out in morning
perineal support s.
seromuscular s.

stock
osteopenic bone s.
out of s.
poor bone s.

Stocker line

stockinette
s. bandage
basket s.
s. dressing
dressing and stockinette applied

stocking
adjustable thigh antiembolism s.'s
antiembolic s.'s

stocking *(continued)*
antiembolism s.
elastic s.
elastic compression s.
s. glove distribution
s. and glove type hypesthesia
graduated compression s.'s
nylon stocking dermatitis
pneumatic antiembolic s.
pneumatic compression s.
s. seam incision
support s.
thigh-high antiembolic s.
thromboembolic disease s.
venous pressure gradient support s.'s

stocking-and-glove
s.-a.-g. anesthesia
s.-a.-g. distribution

stoichiometric number

stokes
S. amputation
S. basket
collar of S.

Stokes-Adams
S.-A. attack
S.-A. disease
S.-A. syndrome

Stoller afferent nerve stimulation

stoloniferum
Penicillium stoloniferum F virus
Penicillium stoloniferum S virus

stoma, pl. **stomas, stomata**
abdominal s.
anastomotic s.
appendicoumbilical s.
Assura stoma cap
colonoscopy per s.
diverting stoma creation
end s.
end-loop s.
gastric s.
ileal loop s.
s. irrigated
Malone antegrade colonic enema stoma procedure
Mitrofanoff continent urinary s.
tracheostomy s.

stomach
s. acid
air contrast view of the s.
angular notch of s.
angulus of s.
anterior wall of s.
antral stomach narrowing
antrum of s.
aphthous stomach ulcer
barium passed through esophagus into s.
s. bed
s. bubble
burning sensation in s.
s. carcinoma
cardiac notch of s.
cardiac section of s.
diffuse histiocytic lymphoma of s.
s. and duodenum
s., duodenum, and pancreas
early gastric cancer of the upper s.
esophagus, stomach, and duodenum
gas in s.
hourglass contraction of s.
human stomach cancer-transforming factor-1
human stomach cancer-transforming factor-2
irritable stomach syndrome
s. irritation
s. lining
lymphatic ring of cardiac part of s.
muscular coat of s.
muscular layer of s.
neutralize stomach acidity
neutralizing acid in s.
oblique fibers of muscular layer of s.
partial emptying of s.
partial resection of s.
passed through esophagus into s.
pineapple test for butyric acid in s.
polyp of antrum of s.
polyp of body of s.
polyp of fundus of s.
pylorus of s.
rat stomach strip
remnant s.
s. sleeper
s. stapling technique
total stomach volume
watermelon s.

stomal bag

stomas (*pl. of* stoma)

stomata (*pl. of* stoma)

stomatitis
acute herpetic gingival s.
allergic contact s.
atypical lichenoid s.
bovine papular s.
contagious pustular s.
s. herpetica
necrotizing ulcerative s.
periodic fever, aphthous stomatitis, pharyngitis, cervical adenitis
recurrent aphthous s.
recurrent ulcerative scarifying s.
s. scarlatina
vesicular s.
vesicular stomatitis Alagoas virus
vesicular stomatitis Indiana virus

stone
s. basketing
biliary tract s.
s. burden
calcium apatite s.
calcium oxalate renal s.
calcium oxalate stone former
calcium phosphate s.
carbonate apatite s.
cholesterol s.
chronically inflamed gallbladder with s.'s
common bile duct s.
common duct pigment s.
s. disintegration
endoscopic stone disintegration
endoscopic stone manipulation
endoscopic stone removal
s. extraction
gallbladder pigment s.'s
hepatic duct s.
idiopathic calcium renal stone formation
s. imaging and localization
kidney s.
magnesium ammonium phosphate s.
manipulation
metabolic stone workup
occluded common bile duct s.
pancreatic duct s.
pancreatic stone protein
passage of s.
passing of kidney s.
percutaneous stone removal
piecemeal removal of kidney s.
radio nonopaque s.
renal kidney s.

stone-tissue detection system

Stookey reflex

stool
antigen stool detection test
APC stool test
change in color and consistency of s.
s. culture
dark bloody s.
delirium, infection, atrophic urethritis and vaginitis, pharmaceuticals, psychological disorders, excessive urine output, restricted mobility, stool impaction
digital removal of s.
electron microscopy of s.
s. elimination
s. evacuation
s. examination
frank blood in s.
Gram stain of stool specimen
Gram stain of stool test
grossly bloody s.
guaiac stool test
Helicobacter pylori stool antigen
Hematest s.'s
Hemoccult negative s.'s
Hemoccult positive s.'s
inability to control s.
incontinence of s.
large green soft s.
large yellow soft s.'s
medium brown loose s.
medium yellow soft s.'s
occult blood in s.
patient incontinent of s.
s. positive for occult blood
s. preservative
pus coating s.
small, yellow, constipated s.
s. softener
tarry black s.
test of stool guaiac
zero stool since birth

stooping
repetitive bending and s.

stop
automatic stop order
venous stop flow pressure

stopped flow pressure

stopping
mass collision stopping power
mass radiative stopping power
starting and stopping of urinary stream
voluntarily stopping eating and drinking

stopwatch
Astrand 30-beat stopwatch method

storage
autologous leukapheresis, processing, and s.
cholesterol ester storage disease
cold s.
cryogenic storage container
s. disease
glycogen storage disease, types 1–10
glycogen storage disorder
glycogen storage test
ichthyosis and neutral lipid storage disease
infantile sialic acid storage disorder
information storage and retrieval
iron storage disease
lipid content of storage fat
lipid storage disease
lysis, storage, and transportation
lysosomal storage disease
lysosomal storage disorder
mucopolysaccharide storage disease I–VIII
neutral lipid storage disease
polysaccharide storage disease
relative storage capacity
Short-Term Auditory Retrieval and S. Test
short-term visual s.
visual information s.

stored
bone marrow removed and s.

stories
Michigan Picture S.

storiform pattern

storm
affective s.
thyroid s.
thyrotoxic s.

stormy
postoperatively stormy course

story
MacArthur S. Stem Battery
Make A Picture S. test
Picture S. Language Test

stow
VL stow repair

strabismus
arteriovenous strabismus syndrome
AV strabismus syndrome
convergent s.
correction of s.

Strachan-Scott syndrome

straddling
limbus parallel orientation straddling tattoo mark

straight
s. back syndrome
s. bag drainage
s. conjugate
crossed straight leg raising
dentate straight fissure bur
double seated straight leg raise
s. drainage
s. gravity drainage
s. gyrus
intermittent straight catheterization
s. leg raise
s. leg raising tenderness
s. leg raising test
s. line velocity
negative straight leg raise
neutral axis of straight beam
Oaks straight cannula
proximal straight tubule
rapid straight pacing
reverse straight leg raise

straighten
arm straighten maneuver
inability to straighten back

straightening
retinal arterial narrowing and s.

strain
alpha wave s.
beta hemolytic s.
Caregiver S. Index
challenge virus s.
chronic low back s.
s. energy density
human diploid cell s.
hypothetical mean s.
ingrown positive s.
inversion strain x-ray
Lactobacillus rhamnosus strain GG
left heart s.
left ventricular s.
LGV strain of *Chlamydia*
live vaccine s.
macrophage-tropic HIV s.
macrophage-tropic human immunodeficiency virus s.
Moloney s.
mumps virus vaccine Jeryl Lynn s.
overuse strain injury

strain *(continued)*
Personal S. Questionnaire
Prague strain Rous sarcoma virus
recombinant inbred s.
resistant strains of bacteria
Rhesus diploid cell strain rabies vaccine
right heart s.
Schmidt-Ruppin strain Rous sarcoma virus
specific strain of bacteria
swine influenza s.
thoracolumbosacral s.
wild type s.

strained
grade, rough, breathy, asthenic, s.
s. urinary sediment

straining
coughing and s.
s. on bowel movement

strait
dire s.'s
entrance of fetal head into superior pelvic s.

straitjacket
chemical s.

strand
anticoding s.
antiparallel s.
antisense s.
s. displacement amplification
lysis of restricting s.
mucin s.
mucus s.
negative strand virus
nests and s.'s of cells
nonrejoining DNA strand break

stranded
deoxyribonucleic acid double s.
deoxyribonucleic acid single s.
single s.

strandy infiltrate

strange

strangulated
s. bowel obstruction
s. hemorrhoid
s. hernia
s. small bowel

strangulation of bladder

strap
chest s.
control adjustment s.
distal over-shoulder s.
elastic back s.
forearm flexion control s.
front support s.
infrahyoid s.
s. muscle
over-shoulder s.
proximal over-shoulder s.

strapping
figure-of-eight s.
loop and hook s.

strata (*pl. of* stratum)

strategy, pl. **strategies**
age-appropriate s.
alternative s.
ankle s.
antisense s.
augmentation s.
Children's Coping Strategies Checklist
coping s.
coping strategy enhancement
expected intervention s.
hard-nose s.
healthy coping s.
intervention strategies
Learning and Study Strategies Inventory
maladaptive coping s.
mutational s.
neurorehabilitation s.

Stratford virus

stratification
risk s.

stratified epithelium

stratum, pl. **strata**
atrophia strata et maculosa
autoantibody to stratum corneum
s. corneum
s. corneum basic protein
s. granulosum
lateral nuclear s.
malpighian s.
medial nuclear s.
paraventricular nuclear s.

strawberry
s. birthmark
s. cervix
s. gallbladder
s. hemangioma
s. nevus
red strawberry tongue

straw-colored urine

Strayer procedure

streak
angioid retinal s.
s. artifact
atherosclerotic fatty s.
s. culture
s. gonad
gonadal s.
lightning s.
linear streak lesion
marbled hypopigmented s.
meningitic s.
Moore lightning s.
nonfunctional s.

streaking
linear s.

streaky infiltrate

stream
s. of consciousness
difficulty initiating urinary s.
difficulty in starting urinary s.
s. dilution factor
extended data s.
starting and stopping of urinary s.
s. of thought
weak of interrupted urine s.

street
Meeting S. School Screening Test

Streeter horizon

strength
abdominal muscle s.
antagonistic muscle s.
area of strength and weakness
artery weld s.
axial gripping s.
bilateral leg s.
breaking s.
current s.
density and strength of bone mass
dilute s.
dioptric s.
double s.
Ego S. test
extra s.
full s.
s. grasp
grip s.
guaranteed yield s.
half s.
hand grip s.
hand strength test
heavy resistance strength training
increased muscle s.
inherent strength of myocardial contraction
ionic s.
leg s.
Lovett clinical scale of s.

low ionic s.
low ionic strength solution
magnetic field s.
measure of acid s.
muscle s.
peripheral muscle s.
s. of pole
radiographic bone strength index
respiratory muscle s.
symmetrical s.
s. training exercise
ultimate tensile s.
wound-breaking s.

strength-duration curve

strengthened
gas atomized dispersion s.

strengthening
active quad strengthening exercise
isometric quad strengthening exercise

streptavidin
labeled streptavidin biotin

streptavidin-biotin peroxidase complex

streptobacillary fever

streptocerca
Mansonella streptocerca infection

streptococcal
antecedent streptococcal infection
s. antibody
s. cell membrane
s. empyema
s. exotoxin-A
group B streptococcal infection
group B streptococcal meningitis
group B streptococcal pneumonia
group B streptococcal sepsis
pediatric autoimmune neuropsychiatric diseases associated with streptococcal infection
pediatric autoimmune neuropsychiatric disorders associated with streptococcal infection
perianal streptococcal cellulitis
s. pneumonia
s. proliferative factor
s. pyrogenic exotoxin
s. pyrogenic exotoxin B, C
severe invasion streptococcal syndrome
s. superantigen
s. tonsillitis
s. toxic shock syndrome

streptococcus, pl. **streptococci**
alpha hemolytic s.
beta-hemolytic s.
beta-hemolytic streptococcus group A
drug-resistant *Streptococcus pneumoniae*
group A beta hemolytic s.
group A s.
group A streptococcus direct test
group A streptococcus infection
group B s.
group C s.
group D s.
group G s.
multidrug-resistant *Streptococcus pneumoniae*
multidrug-resistant *Streptococcus pneumoniae*
mutans streptococci
nutritionally variant s.
Optochin-resistant *Streptococcus pneumoniae*
penicillin-nonsusceptible *Streptococcus pneumoniae*
penicillin-resistant *Streptococcus pneumoniae*
penicillin-sensitive *Streptococcus pneumoniae*
pneumococcal conjugate vaccine
pneumococcal *Streptococcus pneumoniae* polysaccharide
Streptococcus pneumoniae
Streptococcus sanguis
Streptococcus viridans endocarditis

streptogenes
impetigo s.

streptogramins
macrolides, lincosamides, and s.

streptokinase
anisoylated plasminogen streptokinase activator complex

streptolysin
s. O test
serum inhibitor of streptolysin S

streptomycin
conditionally streptomycin dependent
penicillin, bacitracin, streptomycin, caprylate
penicillin, streptomycin, tetracycline

streptothrix organism

streptozotocin
MeCCNU, Oncovin, 5-fluorouracil plus s.

stress
ability to cope with s.
acute posttraumatic stress syndrome
acute stress disorder
acute stress erosion
acute stress reaction
adolescent stress hematuria
adult situation stress reaction
affected by s.
anatomic stress incontinence
s., anger and hopelessness
anterior drawer stress radiograph
anteroposterior stress test
AP inversion stress vagina view
avulsion stress fracture
brief exposure to heat s.
Bruce maximal stress test
cardiac rehabilitation mental s.
cardiac stress test
Cardiolite stress test
cardiopulmonary stress test
s. caused health problem
circumferential end-systolic s.
circumferential wall s.
combat stress exposure
condition related to s.
contraction stress test
cope with daily s.
critical incident stress management
dipyridamole thallium stress imaging
s. disorder
s. distribution factor
dobutamine-atropine stress echocardiography
dobutamine stress echocardiography
dobutamine stress test
s. electrocardiography
electrophilic s.
elevated-arm stress test
Ellestad exercise stress test
emotional disturbance stress reaction
emotional stress depressive psychosis
emotional stress precipitating tremor
end-diastolic circumferential s.
end-systolic wall s.
exercise stress echocardiography
exercise stress electrocardiography

stress *(continued)*
exercise stress test
external rotation-abduction stress test
finite element stress analysis
s. formula
s. fracture
S. From Life Experience
s. gastritis
genuine stress urinary incontinence
graphic stress telethermometry
graphic stress thermography
gravity stress test
s. headache
s. of heart disease
heart response to s.
heat stress index
s. hematuria
s. hormone
hospital-based stress management
s. in hypertensive patient
S. Impact Scale
s. incontinence
increased stress incontinence
s. injury
s. injury stage
s. inoculation
s. inoculation training
inversion stress test
low-contact s.
low-dose dobutamine stress radionuclide ventriculography
low-load prolonged s.
s. management and imagery
maximal treadmill stress test
medial tibial stress syndrome
mental stress test
meridional end-systolic s.
metabolic stress episode
metatarsal stress fracture
mixed disturbance stress reaction
Miyazaki-Bonney test for stress incontinence
MUGA exercise stress test
s. myocardial image
myocardial stress perfusion scintigraphy
nipple stimulation contraction stress test
nuclear stress test
Occupational S. Indicator
occupational stress syndrome
oxidative s.
pacing stress test
Parental S. Index
parent-infant traumatic s.
Parenting S. Index
perinatal stress test
physiologic low stress angioplasty
porcine stress syndrome
postmenstrual s.
postural stress test
progressive accumulated s.
progressively lowered stress threshold
Psoriasis Life S. Inventory
psychological stress of hospitalization
s. reduction technique
s. relaxation
repetitive stress syndrome
restraint and water immersion s.
sestamibi stress test
shear s.
single-stage exercise stress test
social stress and functionality inventory
supine bicycle stress echocardiography
supine empty stress test
technetium Cardiolite stress test
tethered median nerve stress test
s. thallium scanning
thallium stress test
transesophageal dobutamine stress echocardiograph
transesophageal echocardiography-dobutamine stress echocardiography
treadmill exercise stress test
true positive stress test
s. ulcer prophylaxis
s. urinary incontinence
urinary stress incontinence
valgus stress test
valgus-varus stress test
varus stress test

stress-activated protein 1

stressful
s. encounter
s. imagery
modify stressful living habits

stress-generated potential

stress-induced
s.-i. alopecia
s.-i. analgesia
s.-i. anesthesia
s.-i. angina
s.-i. hyperthermia

stressor
Parental S. Scale: Neonatal Intensive Care Unit
psychosocial s.'s
social s.
traumatic s.

stress-related
s.-r. arrhythmia
s.-r. disorder
s.-r. disturbance
s.-r. headache
s.-r. heart condition
s.-r. hormone
s.-r. hypertension
s.-r. mucosal damage

stress-released hormone

stretch
calf-heel stretch exercise
carbon-hydrogen s.
chest stretch exercise
hamstring stretch exercise
heel-cord s.'s
hip adductor stretch exercise
low-load prolonged s.
s. mark
muscle stretch reflex
pulmonary stretch receptor
s. reflex
repeated quick s.
repeated quick stretch from elongation
repeated quick stretch superimposed upon an existing contraction

stretching
s. and breathing exercise
s. calf, thigh and hamstring
iris stretching operation
s. and neck isometric
pupil s.
s. syncope

stretching-yawning syndrome

stria, pl. **striae**
abdominal s.
anterior acoustic s.
atrophic s.
auditory striae
striae keratopathy
malleolar s.
medial longitudinal s.
Rohr s.
Vogt s.

striatal
infantile bilateral striatal necrosis syndrome

striate
anterolateral striate artery
s. area

s. body
s. cortex
s. keratopathy

striated
anisotropic band in striated muscle
s. border
isotropic band striated muscle fiber
isotropic disc striated muscle fiber
s. muscle
s. reticulum
spondylar changes, nasal anomaly, striated metaphyses

striation
longitudinal dense s.

striatonigral degeneration

striatum
atrophoderma striatum et maculatum
corpus s.
xanthoma striatum palmare

striatus
lichen s.
lichen striatus epidermal nevus
limbus s.

strict
s. bed confinement
s. bedrest
s. isolation
s. no information in paper
s. voiding schedule

striction
group s.

strictly confined to bed

stricture
anastomotic stricture formation
anular esophageal s.
anular esophageal s.
area of s.
benign bile duct s.
biliary tract s.
caustic strictures of cervical esophagus
caustic strictures of hypopharynx
common bile duct s.
granular stricture of urethra
longitudinal esophageal s.
lower esophageal s.
nonsteroidal antiinflammatory drug-induced intestinal s.
pancreatic duct s.
peptic esophageal s.
percutaneous stricture dilatation
Wickwitz esophageal s.

strictureplasty
Heineke-Mikulicz s.
side-to-side isoperistaltic s.

stridor
audible s.
expiratory s.
inspiratory s.
respiratory s.

strike
left heel s.
right heel s.
right toe s.

striker
forefoot-to-rearfoot s.

string
auditory s.
duodenal string test

string-of-beads appearance

string-of-pearls appearance

String-Oriented Symbolic Language

stringy mucus

striopallidodentate calcinosis

strip
s. biopsy
blood glucose reagent s.
capsule strip easily
s. gauze
s. graft
guinea pig lung s.
LiPA strip assay
lung s.
marginal tear s.
Mersilene fascial s.
Micral urine test s.
rat lung s.
rat stomach s.
rhythm s.

stripe
aortopulmonary mediastinal s.
endometrial s.
mallear s.
Mees s.

striped tag myocardial tagging system

stripper
intraluminal s.
maple bark stripper disease
Oesch perforation invagination s.
vein s.

stripping
anodic stripping voltametry
apical pleural s.
continuous s.
dissection and s.
high ligation and s.
ligation and s.
varicose vein stripping and ligation
vocal cord s.

striving
emancipatory s.

stroke
acute ischemic s.
acute stroke unit
adequate stroke volume
alcohol, epilepsy, insulin, overdose, uremia, trauma, infection, psychiatric, s.
American Heart Association S. Outcome Classification
anterior circulation s.
antiphospholipid antibodies in stroke study
aortic valve stroke volume
aqueductal CSF stroke volume
augmented stroke volume
Burke Stroke Time-Oriented profile
cardioembolic s.
completed s.
conductance stroke volume
s. count
dizziness from heat s.
s. due to cerebral hemorrhage
early progressing s.
S. Education Program
European S. Scale
s. in evolution
exertional heat s.
footdrop after s.
forward stroke volume
s. guidance system
heat stroke in aging
hemorrhage and s.
history of s.
S. Impact Scale
s. index
late progressing s.
left hemisphere s.
left ventricular stroke volume index
left ventricular stroke work
left ventricular stroke work index
life-threatening heat s.
partial nonprogressive s.
percent stroke length
58-point Scandinavian S. Scale
Positive and Negative S. Scale

stroke *(continued)*
Postural Assessment Scale for S. Patients
s. in progression
pure sensory s.
regurgitant stroke volume
right brain s.
right ventricle stroke output
right ventricular stroke work index
s. screening
s. survivor
total stroke volume
s. treatment center
s. unit
ventricular stroke work
s. volume
s. volume of heart
s. volume index
s. with full recovery
s. with minimal residuum
s. work

strokelike
mitochondrial myopathy, encephalopathy, lactic acidosis, strokelike episodes
myopathy, encephalopathy, lactic acidosis, strokelike episodes

stroke-prone spontaneous hypertensive

stroke-specific quality of life

stroke-work index

stroking
cast stroking maneuver during massage
fan stroking maneuver during massage

stroma, pl. **stromata**
avascular corneal s.
endometrial s.
gonadal s.
s. of iris
limbal s.
lymphatic s.
myxoid s.
ovarian s.
perilimbal s.
Rollet s.

stroma-free
s.-f. hemoglobin
s.-f. hemoglobin pyridoxalated

stromal
anterior stromal micropuncture
s. cell-derived factor-1
s. cell tumor
cortical stromal hyperplasia
s. disease
s. edema
endolymphatic stromal myosis
endometrial stromal sarcoma
gastrointestinal stromal tumor
s. herpetic keratitis
herpetic stromal keratitis
s. hyperplasia
s. hypertrophy
immune stromal keratitis
mesenchymal sex cord stromal tumor
mesenchymal stromal cell
mixed germ cell-sex cord stromal tumor
nebular stromal opacity
necrotizing stromal keratitis
s. osteoclast-forming activity
ovarian stromal hyperplasia
patchy anterior stromal infiltrate
prostatic stromal proliferation of uncertain malignant potential
pseudoangiomatous stromal hyperplasia
sclerosing stromal tumor
s. thickness
s. thinning
s. tumor of unknown malignant potential

stromata (*pl. of* stroma)

stromelysin
human stromelysin aggregated proteoglycan

stromuhr
Ludwig s.

strong
s. exchange capacity resin
grips strong and equal
handgrasp equal and s.
s. partial maternal behavior
pedal pulses equal and s.
s. soap solution
S. Vocational Interest Blank

Strong-Campbell Interest Inventory

strongyloidiasis with massive hyperinfection

strophulosus
lichen s.

structural
s. abnormality
s. alignment
s. alteration
s. aluminum malleable
antigenic structural grouping
s. atrophy
s. atypia
basic structural unit
s. change in heart
s. changes in joint
S. Classification of Proteins
epileptogenic structural lesion
s. heart defect
s. heart disease
objective structural clinical examination
s. repeating unit
s. valve deterioration

structure
alteration of memory s.
coiled bony s.
congested vascular s.
s. of the cytoplasmic matrix
demineralized bony s.
differentiated internal s.
ductlike s.
extended electron-loss line fine s.
extended x-ray absorption fine structure spectroscopy
fine s.
hyperfine s.
intact bone s.
s. of intellect
limbic forebrain s.
mediobasal brain s.
mesial cerebral s.
midline cystic s.
mosaic genome s.
müllerian duct derived s.
multilaminated s.
narcissistic character s.
natural killer target s.
opaque branching s.
ossification of cartilaginous s.
S. Photographic Expressive Language Test-II
small bone s.
stereochemical s.
supportive social s.
surface extended x-ray absorption fine s.
tubuloreticular s.

structure-activity
quantitative structure-activity relationship
s.-a. relationship

structured
assertion structured therapy
s. clinical interview
S. Clinical Interview for DSM

S. Clinical Interview for DSM-IV Axis I Disorders: Clinician Version
S. Clinical Interview for DSM-IV Dissociative Disorders
S. Clinical Interview for DSM-IV Dissociative Disorders
S. Clinical Interview for DSM-IV Patient Version
S. Clinical Interview for DSM-IV Psychotic Disorders
intensive structured hospitalization
s. interview for diagnosis of Alzheimer dementia
S. Interview of Reported Symptoms
Iowa S. Psychiatric Interview
s. pain interview
S. and Scaled Interview to Assess Maladjustment
s. sensory stimulation
small round structured virus

struggle
anticipatory and struggle behavior theories

strumipriva
cachexia s.

Strümpell disease

Strunsky sign

strut
allograft s.
cartilage s.
cartilage strut placement
columellar s.
corticocancellous s.
medial crural strut graft
nonvascularized fibular strut graft
optic s.
outlet strut fracture
polyethylene s.

Struthers
arcade of S.
ligament of S.

struvite calculus

strychnine
aloin, belladonna, strychnine laxative
lysergic acid diethylamide and s.

Stryker
S. frame
S. walking heel

Stryker-Halbeisen syndrome

ST-segment
S.-s. abnormality
S.-s. depression
S.-s. elevation

ST-T
S.-T. abnormality
S.-T. wave change

Stuart
prothrombin, proconvertin, Stuart factor, antihemophilic B factor

Stuart-Prower factor

studded
peritoneum studded with tumor nodules
s. with numerous tumor nodules

student
S. Adaptation to College Questionnaire
S. Adjustment Inventory
College S. Satisfaction Questionnaire
Community College S. Experiences Questionnaire
S. Disability Survey
Multidimensional S. Life Satisfaction Scale
S. Opinion Inventory
S. Orientations Survey
Perception of Ability Scale for S.'s
Screening Assessment for Gifted Elementary S.'s, Primary

Student's
Safran Student's Interest Inventory

study
aerosol ventilation s.
air contrast s.
Allport-Vernon-Linzey S. of Values
anisotropic volume s.
antegrade contrast s.
antegrade pressure s.
anti-DNA immunological s.
antihepatitis A-IgM immunological s.
antinuclear antibody immunological s.
antiphospholipid antibodies in stroke s.
anti-SSA immunological s.
anti-SSB immunological s.
arterial revascularization therapy s.
asymptomatic carotid atherosclerosis s.
S. Attitudes and Methods Survey
Austrian Breast Cancer S. Group
autopsy-based neurochemical s.
barium swallow s.
blood gas s.
brain imaging s.
brain perfusion s.
California Relative Value S.'s
cancer biotherapy study group
cardiac gated s.
cardiopulmonary sleep s.
cardiovascular diagnostic s.
carotid Doppler s.
carotid duplex s.
Centers for Epidemiologic Studies Depression scale
cerebral blood flow s.'s
cerebral vascular profile s.
child behavioral s.
Children's Health S.
chronic electrophysiologic s.
cine phonation s.
coagulation s.
Collaborative Transplant S.
compared with previous s.
Cornell Learning and S. Skills Inventory
detrusor muscle pressure-flow micturition s.
Diagnostic Interview for Genetic S.
Doppler flow s.
double-blind s.
drug efficacy study implementation
dynamic flow s.
electroencephalographic sleep s.
electrophysiologic s.
equilibrium-gated blood pool s.
evoked potential s.
fat absorption s.
fluorourodynamic s.
function s.
gated blood pool s.
Great Smoky Mountains S. of Youth
hearing loss s.'s
hemodynamic angiographic s.
hepatic enzyme s.
hepatitis surface antigen s.'s
horizontal beam s.
hormone binding s.
hypertension optical treatment s.
infertility s.'s
infusion pyelographic s.
isotope scanning s.
laboratory admission baseline s.'s
Learning and S. Strategies Inventory

study *(continued)*
Life S. Sample
Life Span S.
longitudinal experimental study design
luminal contrast s.
Medical Outcomes S.
medical studies unit
meglumine diatrizoate enema s.
metrizamide contrast s.
mineral balance s.
mini-invasive vascular s.
molecular genetic s.
molecular hybridization s.
National Comorbidity S.
National Cooperative Dialysis S.
National Cooperative Growth S.
National Health and Nutrition Examination Follow-Up S.
National Wilms Tumor S.
naturalistic followup s.
nerve conduction velocity s.
neural crest tumor localization s.
New Haven s.
noninvasive brain imaging s.
noninvasive carotid s.
noninvasive flow s.
noninvasive neurovascular s.'s
noninvasive vascular laboratory s.'s
normal exercise s.
nuclear ventricular function s.
paramagnetic contrast-enhanced MR s.
patterns of care s.
penile blood flow s.
peripheral blood s.'s
perirenal air s.
Physicians Health Study II
picture frustration s.
picture-frustration study, test
placebo-controlled drug s.
platelet function s.
preliminary s.'s
pressure-flow s.
primary dependence s.
pulmonary diffusing s.
pulmonary function s.
radioisotope uptake s.
radionuclide gastric emptying s.
relative value s.
remote study monitoring
renal function s.
retrococcygeal air s.
retrograde kidney s.
Rosenzweig Picture-Frustration S.
seroepidemiological s.
serum enzyme s.
split function s.
S. Attitudes and Methods Survey
Survey of S. Habits and Attitudes
technetium albumin s.
thyroid function s.
urodynamic flow s.
venous Doppler s.
videoendoscopic swallowing s.
videofluoroscopic swallowing s.
wall-motion s.

stuffiness
nasal s.
nose s.

stump
amputated s.
amputation s.
amputation stump neuroma
anastomotic stump leak
aortic stump blowout
appendiceal s.
s. of bone
bury stump of appendix
cardiac stump inverted
cone-shaped amputation s.
doubly clamped, transected and stump ligated
s. edema
s. hallucination
revision of amputation s.
s. shrinking

stun
cardiac s.

stunned atrium

stunning
myocardial s.

stunt
Pangola stunt virus

stunted growth

stunting
growth s.

stupor
idiopathic recurring s.
spike-wave s.

Sturge disease

Sturge-Weber
S.-W. disease
S.-W. syndrome

Sturmdorf suture

stuttering
s. gait
medication-induced s.
s. severity instrument

Stüve-Wiedemann syndrome

sty
meibomian s.
zeisian s.

style
Affective S. Index
analysis of coping s.
arrogant s.
attachment s.
Attributional S. Questionnaire
avoidance s.
Behavior S. Questionnaire
coping s.
dysfunctional parenting s.
Group S.'s Inventory
Learning S. Profile
Managerial S. Questionnaire
Miller Behavioral S. Scale
S. of Mind Inventory
Personal S. Inventory
self-healing style of qigong
Test of Cognitive S. in Mathematics
Vocational Learning S.'s

stylet
blunt s.
endotracheal s.
heart catheterization s.

stylohyoid ligament

styloid
s. cornu
s. process
ulnar styloid bone

stylomastoid
s. artery
s. foramen

stylomastoidea
arteria s.

styptic bitter

styrene-butadiene rubber

Suarez-Villafranca operation

subacromial
s. bursa
s. bursitis
s. decompression

subacute
s. bacterial endocarditis
s. combined degeneration of spinal cord
s. confusional state
s. cortical cerebellar degeneration
s. cutaneous lupus erythematosus
s. dialysis

diffuse unilateral subacute neuroretinitis "wipe-out" syndrome
s. hepatic necrosis
s. hepatitis with bridging
s. inclusion body encephalitis
s. infectious arthritis
s. inflammation
s. liver failure
myelomonocytic leukemia, s.
s. necrotizing encephalomyelopathy
painful subacute thyroiditis
s. sclerosing panencephalitis
s. sensory neuropathy
s. tamponade
s. thrombosis
s. thyroiditis
s. thyroiditis-like syndrome
s. treatment of acute drug intoxication
s. yellow atrophy

subannular mattress suture

subaortic
discrete subaortic stenosis
dynamic subaortic stenosis
hypertrophic muscular subaortic stenosis
idiopathic hypertrophic subaortic stenosis
muscular subaortic stenosis
s. stenosis

subarachnoid
acute subarachnoid hemorrhage
aneurysmal subarachnoid hemorrhage
s. bleed
s. block
s. cavity
cerebral subarachnoid venous pressure
s. cerebrospinal fluid
s. cistern
s. fluid collection
s. hemorrhage
s. hemorrhage in cranium
interhemispheric subarachnoid hemorrhage
intracerebral and subarachnoid hemorrhage
perimesencephalic nonaneurysmal subarachnoid hemorrhage
perioptic subarachnoid space
s. septum
s. space
surgical procedure for subarachnoid hemorrhage
traumatic subarachnoid hemorrhage

subarachnoidal sinus

subareolar duct papillomatosis

subastragalar amputation

subaxial subluxation

subbasement membrane

subcallosa
area s.

subcallosal
s. area
s. fasciculus
s. gyrus

subcapital fracture

subcapsular
anterior s.
anterior subcapsular cataract
s. cataract
s. hematoma
s. hematoma of liver
posterior subcapsular cataract
posterior subcapsular cataractous plaque
posterior subcapsular precipitates

subchondral bone

subchronic
schizophrenia, catatonic type, s.
schizophrenia, disorganized type, s.
schizophrenia, paranoid type, s.
schizophrenia, residual type, s.

subcitrate
colloidal bismuth s.
omeprazole, bismuth subcitrate, tetracycline, and metronidazole

subclass
immunoglobulin A subclass 1, 2
immunoglobulin D subclass 1, 2
s. of immunoglobulin E, M

subclavian
aberrant right subclavian artery
anomalous right subclavian artery
arteriovenous subclavian fistula
s. artery
carotid subclavian bypass
double lumen subclavian catheter
s. duct
s. flap aortoplasty
s. groove
s. hemodialysis catheter
indwelling subclavian catheter
s. intravenous line
left subclavian artery
left subclavian central venous pressure
left subclavian vein
s. loop
right s.
right subclavian artery
right subclavian central venous pressure
right subclavian vein
s. steal syndrome
s. vein
s. vein catheterization
s. vein compression
s. vein thrombosis
Waldhausen subclavian flap technique

subclinical
chronic subclinical scurvy
s. diabetes
s. hepatic encephalopathy
s. papillomavirus infection
s. rhythmic epileptiform discharge of adult

subcoma insulin treatment

subcommissural organ

subcondylar
s. deformity
s. fracture
vertical subcondylar oblique

subconjunctival
s. hemorrhage of eye
s. injection

subcontact
proximal subcontact area

subcoracoid
s. bursa
s. bursitis
s. type displacement

subcorneal pustular dermatosis

subcortical
s. arteriosclerotic encephalopathy
s. atherosclerotic encephalopathy
cerebral autosomal recessive arteriopathy with subcortical infarcts and leukoencephalopathy
multiple subcortical infarction
s. vascular encephalopathy

subcostal
apical and subcostal four-chambered view
s. flank incision
s. incision
s. long axis
s. short axis
transperitoneal anterior subcostal incision

subcutanea

subcutaneous
s. abdominal
s. acromial bursa
s. adipose tissue
arm-implanted subcutaneous reservoir-catheter system
s. augmentation material
s. bursa of lateral malleolus
s. bursa of medial malleolus
s. bursa of teres major
s. bursitis
s. continuous infusion
continuous subcutaneous infusion
continuous subcutaneous insulin infusion
continuous subcutaneous insulin infusion pump
continuous subcutaneous insulin injection
dermal subcutaneous junction
s. electrode implantation
s. emphysema
s. fascia
s. fat atrophy
s. fat necrosis
s. felon
s. flap
hard subcutaneous nodule
s. hematoma
s. histamine test
s. immunoglobulin
s. injection
s. intraocular node
s. intravenous
linear subcutaneous atrophy
s. lupus erythematosis
medial malleolar subcutaneous bursa
membranous layer of subcutaneous tissue of abdomen
s. morphine pump
multiple synchronous subcutaneous metastases
muscle layer in fatty layer of subcutaneous tissue
s. nerve stimulation
s. panniculitis-like T-cell lymphoma
s. peritoneal administration device
s. radionuclide venography
s. swelling
s. tissue
s. tissues approximated
s. vaginal

subcuticular fat

subdeltoid
s. bursa
s. bursitis

subdermal
s. graft
s. implant material
s. levonorgestrel implant
levonorgestrel subdermal implant

subdiaphragmatic
s. hernia
s. sympathectomy

subdural
s. abscess
acute subdural hematoma
s. cavity
chronic subdural hematoma
s. effusion with hydrocephalus
s. electrode array
s. empyema
s. hematoma
s. hemorrhage in cranium
s. hygroma
interhemispheric subdural hematoma
liquefaction of subdural hematoma
s. peritoneal
s. puncture
reactive subdural effusion
spinal subdural hemorrhage

subendocardial
acute subendocardial myocardial infarction
atrial subendocardial hemorrhage
s. fibrosis
focal subendocardial hemorrhage
impairment of subendocardial blood flow
s. infarct
s. ischemia
left ventricular subendocardial myocardial ischemia
s. myocardial infarction
s. myocardial injury
s. petechial hemorrhage
superficial subendocardial focal hemorrhage

subendothelial space

subependymal
s. giant cell astrocytoma
s. hemorrhage

subepithelial
s. basement membrane
s. corneal infiltrate
s. hemorrhage
s. plaque
punctate subepithelial infiltrate

suberythemal dose

subfascial
sonography of subfascial hematoma
s. endoscopic perforator surgery

subfornical organ

subgaleal
s. abscess
s. hematoma

subgallate
bismuth s.

subgingival curettage

subglenoid dislocation

subglottic
s. area
continuous aspiration of subglottic secretions
s. stenosis

subgroup
myxoma virus s.
orf virus s.

subhepatic
s. abscess
s. area

subhuman primate model

subhyoid laryngotomy

subiculum
ventral s.

subischial leg length

subisthmic
atypical subisthmic coarctation

subitum
exanthema s.

subjacent dorsal horn

subject
escape and avoidance conditioning in human s.'s
lethal dose in all exposed s.'s
neuromuscular firing in normal s.
neuromuscular firing in spastic s.

subjective
s. finding
s. fremitus
s. global assessment
s., objective, management, and analytic
s. paranormal experience
point of subjective equality
s. posttraumatic syndrome
review of subjective symptoms
s. symptom

S. Units of Distress Scale
s. vertigo

subjunctional heart block

sublabial salivary gland

sublentiform nucleus

sublethal
s. dose
repair of sublethal damage

subleukemic leukemia

subligamentous
partial subligamentous calcification

subliminal
s. perception
s. seizure

sublingual
s. artery
s. bursa
s. caruncle
s. crescent
s. cyst
s. duct
s. fold
s. fossa
s. ganglion
s. gland
s. hematoma
s. immunotherapy
major sublingual duct
s. nitroglycerin
s. tablet

sublingualis
arteria s.

subluxation
anterior tibial s.
atlantoaxial rotatory s.
atlas vertebral subluxation complex
congenital hip s.
metacarpophalangeal joint s.
s. of patella
radial head s.
rotatory subluxation of scaphoid
shoulder subluxation inhibitor
subaxial s.
unilateral interfacetal dislocation or s.
vertebral subluxation complex

subluxed
shoulder s.

submammary
s. crease
s. mastitis

submandibular
s. duct calculus
s. fossa
s. ganglion
s. gland
s. gland renin
sympathetic branch to submandibular ganglion

submanubrial dullness

submassive pulmonary embolism

submaxillary
s. duct
s. fossa
s. ganglion
s. gland
ovine submaxillary mucin

submaximal
s. neuromuscular block
s. treadmill exercise test
s. working capacity

submental
s. artery
s. fat pad
s. hematoma
s. lymph node
s. region
s. vertex view

submentalis
arteria s.

subminiature end-plate potential

submission
electronic claims s.

submitochondrial

submitted
s. for biopsy
biopsy submitted for frozen section
s. for microsection
specimen submitted for biopsy

submucosa
hemorrhage into s.
small intestinal s.
tracheobronchial s.

submucosal
s. aponeurotic system flap
s. dissection
s. fat
s. gland hypertrophy
s. hemorrhage
s. implant
lobulated submucosal mass

submucous
s. cleft palate
oral submucous fibrosis
s. resection and rhinoplasty

subnormal
educationally s.
mildly s.
severely s.

subnormality
mental s.

subnormal-moderate
educationally s.-m.

subnormal-severe
educationally s.-s.

suboccipital
s. approach
s. craniectomy
s. craniotomy
s. decompression
far lateral inferior suboccipital approach
s. incision

suboptimal
zinc s.

suborbicularis oculi fat

subordinance
double s.

subpectoral
axillary subpectoral approach
s. implantation of cardioverter-defibrillator

subperiosteal
s. abscess
s. amputation
anterior subperiosteal implant
s. fracture
s. implant material
s. minimally invasive laser endoscopic facelift
s. orbital abscess
s. tissue expander

subperitoneal
s. appendicitis
s. fascia

subphrenic abscess

subpleural
s. bleb
s. bulla
focal shallow subpleural hemorrhage
focal subpleural interstitial fibrosis
s. hemorrhage
s. reticulated carbon deposition

subpopulation
lymphocyte s.

subpubic hernia

subpubicus
angulus s.

subpylorici
nodi lymphoidei s.

subretinal
choroidal or subretinal neovascularization
disciform macular degeneration with subretinal neovascular membrane
drainage subretinal fluid
s. fluid
s. hemorrhage
s. neovascularization
s. neovascular membrane
peripapillary subretinal neovascularization
surrounding subretinal fluid cuff

subsalicylate
bismuth s.
bismuth subsalicylate, metronidazole, and amoxicillin

subsartorial
s. canal
s. fascia

subscale
Alzheimer Disease Assessment Scale, cognitive s.
cognitive anxiety s.
Fatigue-Inertia S. of the Profile of Mood States
Schizophrenic S. of Present State Examination
Western Ontario and McMaster Universities Osteoarthritis Index Physical Functioning subscale and chair-performance
Western Ontario and McMaster Universities Osteoarthritis Index Physical Functioning subscale and chair-stand performance

subscapular
s. angle
s. artery
s. branch
s. bursa
s. cataract
s. fossa
long subscapular nerve
s. nerve
s. skin fold thickness

subsegmental
s. airway
s. atelectasis
s. bronchus
s. transcatheter arterial embolization

subseptus hymen

subsequent
s. hospital care
s. sibling
s. weight gain

subserosal fibroid

subserous
s. fascia
s. fibroid

subset
lymphocyte s.
lymphocyte subset count
lymphocyte subset panel

subshock insulin treatment

subspecialist
medical s.

substance
s. abuse counselor
s. abuse disorder
s. abuse evaluation screen unit
S. Abuse Questionnaire
s. abuser
S. Abuse Subtle Screening Inventory
s. abuse treatment
s. abuse treatment clinic
s. abuse treatment program
s. abuse treatment unit
angiotensin-like s.
anterior perforated s.
anterior pituitary-like s.
antidiuretic s.
anxiety due to a s.
anxious substance abuser
arborescent white substance of cerebellum
blood group s.
body substance isolation
child of substance abuser
chronic substance abuse
comorbidity of schizophrenia and substance abuse
compact substance of bone
controlled substance analog
cortical substance of bone
digitalis-like s.'s
digoxin-like immunoreactive s.
effective half-life of radioactive s.
endogenous digitalis-like s.
excitor s.
exophthalmos-producing s.
exposure to industrial s.'s
fat-mobilizing s.
ferredoxin-reducing s.
gamete-shedding s.
gelatinous substance of gray substance
granulocyte s.
gray substance of spinal cord
Hazardous S.'s Act
hepatic stimulatory s.
hilar substance of lung
illegal controlled s.'s
illicit substance use
immunoreactive substance P
immunosuppressive acidic s.
ingestion of poisonous s.
ingestion of potentially poisonous s.
inhalation of foreign s.
inhibitor s.
interstitial fluids and ground s.
labile aggregation stimulating s.
maternal substance abuse
meiosis-inducing s.
methylene blue active s.
mucus-stimulating s.
müllerian-inhibiting s.
müllerian inhibiting s.
müllerian-inhibiting substance receptor
myocardial depressant s.
nonirritating test s.
osmotically active s.
other or unspecified psychoactive substance intoxication
ouabain-like s.
s. P
periaqueductal gray s.
perinatal substance abuse
periventricular gray s.
polysaccharide substance tumor
prostaglandin-like s.
psychoactive substance abuse and dependence
psychoactive substance use disorder
reducing s.'s
renal pressor s.
reticuloendothelial depressing s.
rheumatoid factorlike s.
Rolando gelatinous s.
Rollet secondary s.
slow-reacting s.
slow-reacting substance of anaphylaxis
Soemmerring gray s.
soluble specific s.
specific capsular s.

specific soluble s.
surface-active s.
toxic s.
Toxic S. Control Act
tumor polysaccharide s.
s. use disorder
vasoconstrictor s.
vasodilator s.
white substance of Schwann

substance-abusing
infant of substance-abusing mother

substantia
left substantia nigra
s. nigra
right substantia nigra

substantivity
antibacterial s.
antimicrobial s.

substation
outpatient clinic s.

substernal
s. angle
s. burning
s. chest pain
s. gastric bypass
s. goiter
s. retraction

substitute
alpha bone substitute material
alpha-BSM bone substitute material
s. for morphine
protein plasma s.
recycled human blood s.
saliva s.

substituted metabolite

substitution
arthroscopy-assisted patellar tendon s.
creeping substitution of bone
digit substitution test
orthotopic bladder s.

substitutional
digit symbol substitutional test

substrate
aged substrate plasma
artificial blood s.
buffered single s.
defined s.
enzyme s.
enzyme substrate inhibitor
myocardial substrate uptake
plasma renin substrate activity

substrate-1

substrate-2

substrate-labeled fluorescent immunoassay

substrate-linked fluorescent immunoassay

substructure
auxiliary rest implant s.
peripheral frame implant s.

subsynaptic
s. membrane
s. plate perforation

subtalar
arthroscopic subtalar arthrodesis
s. arthrosis
asymmetric subtalar joint development
complete subtalar release
s. joint axis
s. joint function
s. joint neutral position
Smith subtalar joint arthroereisis peg

subtemporal decompression

subtest
arithmetic s.
Paired Associate Learning S.

subthalamic
s. nucleus
s. nucleus implant

subtle
s. and nonspecific symptom
psychiatric deviate, s.
Substance Abuse S. Screening Inventory

subtotal
s. amputation
s. colectomy
s. gastrectomy
s. hysterectomy
s. lymphoid irradiation
s. nodal irradiation
s. resection
s. supraglottic laryngectomy
s. thyroidectomy
s. villous atrophy

subtraction
s. angiography
computer-assisted blood background s.
contrast subtraction mammography
digital subtraction angiogram
digital subtraction arteriography
digital subtraction echocardiogram
digital subtraction echocardiography
digital subtraction imaging
digital subtraction indocyanine green angiography
digital subtraction phlebography
digital subtraction ventriculography
digital venous subtraction angiography
intraarterial digital subtraction angiogram
intraarterial digital subtraction angiography
intraoperative digital subtraction angiography
intravenous digital subtraction angiography

subtrapezial space

subtype
Eastern subtype Russian spring-summer encephalitis
human immunodeficiency virus-1 subtype C
male alcoholism s.
myxoid histopathologic s.
non-Burkitt s.

subungual
s. abscess
distal subungual onychomycosis
s. hematoma
s. keratoacanthoma
s. melanoma
proximal subungual onychomycosis

subunit
functional s.
glutamide receptor s.
nicked free beta subunit of human chorionic gonadotropin
proteoglycan s.

subureteric Teflon injection

subzonal
s. injection
s. insemination
s. insertion

succedaneous teeth

succenturiatus
lien s.

success
cumulative probability of s.
reproductive s.

successive
amplitude of successive responses

succinate
s. dehydrogenase
ethylene glycol s.

succinate *(continued)*
methylprednisolone sodium s.
neopentyl glycol s.
s. semialdehyde dehydrogenase
vitamin E s.

succinic dehydrogenase activity

succinyl aminoimidazole carboxamide ribotide

succinylcholine chloride

succulent
Marinesco succulent hand

suck
infant suck is poor
s. reflex

sucking
s. blister
s. chest wound
chewing, sucking, swallowing
high-amplitude sucking technique
nonnutritive s.
nonnutritive sucking opportunity
nutritive s.

suckle
inability to s.

suckling
s. mouse
s. mouse brain
s. reflex

Sucquet
S. anastomosis
S. canal

Sucquet-Hoyer
S.-H. anastomosis
S.-H. canal

sucrase-isomaltase deficiency

sucrose
s. density gradient
s. density gradient centrifugation
s. density gradient ultracentrifugation
s. intolerance
s. medium
s. polyester

sucrose-phosphate-glutamic acid

suction
angled suction tube
aortic vent suction line
s. aspiration
s. aspiration abortion
s. banding
s. biopsy instrument
continuous suction drainage
dilation and s.
s., dilation, and curettage
s. dissection
endotracheal s.
foot pedal suction control
high intermittent s.
intubation and s.
Jackson-Pratt to bulb s.
low constant s.
low continuous wall s.
low Gomco s.
low intermittent wall s.
s. method
moderate constant s.
moderate intermittent s.
nasal Fraser suction technique
nasotracheal s.
open endotracheal s.
orotracheal s.
paracentesis and s.
percussion, vibration, and s.
perilimbal suction cup
s. socket
s. tubes inserted
vitreous infusion suction cutter

suction-assisted
s.-a. lipectomy
s.-a. lipoplasty

suctioning
airway s.
DeLee s.
malar bag s.
nasogastric tube s.
nasopharyngeal s.
nasotracheal s.
open endotracheal s.
ultrasonic fat s.

suction-irrigator
Nezhat-Dorsey s.-i.

sudamina
miliary s.

Sudan
S. Black B
S. stain

sudden
s. body jerk
s. cardiac arrest
s. cardiac death
s. cardiopulmonary arrest
s. congestive heart failure
s. coronary death
s. deafness
s. death due to cocaine ingestion
s. death in infancy
s. death ischemic heart disease
exercise-induced sudden death
s. fatal heart attack
s. headache
s. hearing loss
s. heart attack death
s. heart failure
idiopathic sudden sensorineural hearing loss
idiopathic sudden sensory hearing loss
s. illness
s. impulse
s. inexplicable death
s. infant crib death
s. infant death syndrome
ischemic sudden death
near-miss sudden infant death syndrome
out-of-hospital sudden cardiac death
partially unexplained sudden infant death syndrome
s., severe headache
s. shortness of breath
s. sniffing death
s. torsion spasm
totally unexplained sudden infant death syndrome
s. transient freezing
s. unexpected infant death
s. unexpected, unexplained death
s. unexplained death syndrome
s. unexplained infant death
s. weight gain

sudden-dosage onset

Sudeck
S. atrophy
S. critical point
S. disease

Sudeck-LeRiche syndrome

sudomotor
s. fiber
Quantitative S. Axon Reflex Test

sudoriferous
s. abscess
s. cyst
s. duct
s. gland
nevus s.

suffered
patient suffered respiratory arrest

suffering
anticipated emotional s.
chronic emotional s.
pain and s.

sufficient
s. impairment
not sufficient quantity

pancreas s.
protein, quantity not s.

suffocation
mechanical s.

suffocative goiter

sugar
s. and acetone determination
s., acetone, diacetic acid test
admitting blood s.
blood fasting s.
blood sugar level
capillary blood s.
capillary whole blood true s.
evening blood s.
fasting blood s.
fingerstick blood s.
high-dose urea in invert s.
home blood sugar monitoring
2-hour postprandial blood s.
increased level of blood s.
s. intake
10% invert sugar injection in water
10% invert sugar in 0.9% sodium chloride saline injection
invert sugar 10% in saline
invert sugar 5% in water
low blood s.
low-dose urea in invert s.
nucleoside diphosphate s.
patient spilled s.
postprandial blood s.
random blood s.
self-blood sugar monitoring
serial blood s.
serum blood s.
sodium bicarbonate in invert s.
s. spilled
total reducing s.'s
triple sugar iron agar

sugar-coated tablet

sugar-tong
s.-t. cast
s.-t. splint

suggested
s. brain dysfunction
s. indication of diagnosis
s. minimum increment

suggestion
affective s.
permission, limited information, specific suggestions, and intensive therapy
posthypnotic s.
undisciplined interpretation and s.

suggestive of good

Sugiura operation

suicidal
actively s.
Adult S. Ideation Questionnaire
s. behavior
s. and eloper
s. gesture
s. or homicidal feeling
s. ideation
s. intent
s. observation status
s. overture
s. tendency
s. thought train of thought

suicidal/homicidal ideation

suicide
actual suicide attempt
alcohol-related risk for s.
s. alert
s. attempt
cluster s.'s
completed s.
contagious suicide syndrome
contract against s.
direct suicide risk
ethical validity of assisted s.
failed suicide attempt
high risk of s.
history of suicide attempt
hospitalized attempted s.
s. ideation
Inventory of S. Orientation-30
Martin S. Depression Inventory
new age suicide prevention
nonfatal attempt at s.
S. Opinion Questionnaire
s. precautions number 1, 2
s. risk classification
s. risk screen

Suicide-Depression Proneness Checklist

suit
circumferential pneumatic compression s.

suite
endoscopy s.
minor surgery s.
operating s.
operative s.
surgical s.

sulcated tongue

sulci (*pl. of* sulcus)

sulcoplasty
mandibular vestibulolingual s.

sulcular
s. epithelium
s. fluid

sulcus, pl. **sulci**
anterior intermediate s.
anterior interventricular s.
anterior parolfactory s.
anterior ramus of lateral sulcus of cerebrum
artery of central s.
artery of postcentral s.
artery of precentral s.
ascending ramus of lateral sulcus of cerebrum
calcarine s.
cingulate s.
circular sulcus of Reil
interventricular sulcus of heart
intraparietal s.
limiting sulcus of Reil
limiting sulcus of rhomboid fossa
longitudinal sulcus of heart
mapping of cerebral s.
marginal branch of cingulate s.
marginal branch of parietooccipital s.
medial bicipital s.
medial orbital s.
median frontal s.
middle frontal s.
occipital temporal s.
Pancoast superior sulcus syndrome
principal s.
rostral s.
superior frontal s.
superior sulcus tumor syndrome
transverse sulcus of heart

sulfadiazine
silver s.
s. silver

sulfamethoxazole and trimethoprim

sulfatase
iduronate sulfatase deficiency
multiple sulfatase deficiency syndrome
steroid s.
sulfoiduronate sulfatase deficiency

sulfate
anhydrous magnesium s.
bacitracin, polymyxin B, neomycin s.
barium s.
chondroitin s.
chondroitin sulfate A

sulfate *(continued)*
dermatan s.
dextran sodium s.
dihydrostreptomycin s.
dimethyl s.
dimethylamine s.
ferrous s.
fluorometholone and neomycin s.
glucosamine s.
heparin s.
hypodermic morphine s.
magnesium s.
magnesium sulfate, glycerin, and water enema
morphine s.
morphine sulfate controlled-release suppository
morphine sulfate immediate release
Mycifradin S.
nebulized preservative-free morphine s.
oral morphine s.
orthotoluidine manganese s.
polymyxin B sulfate, bacitracin, and neomycin
protamine s.
rectal morphine sulfate suppository
sodium dodecyl s.
steroid s.
sustained-release morphine s.
testosterone s.
tetradecyl sulfate, ethanol, and saline
triglycine s.
yeast, peptone, and adenine s.

sulfated
s. acid mucopolysaccharide
s. glycoprotein-2
s. hydrogenated caster oil
s. insulin
s. lithocholic conjugate

sulfation factor of blood serum

sulfhydryl
boron s.
s. variant

sulfide
dimethyl s.
s., indole, motility medium

sulfinic
cysteine sulfinic acid decarboxylase

sulfisoxazole
chloroquine, pyrimethamine, and s.

sulfite
s. allergy
anhydrous sodium s.
s. sensitivity
sodium sulfite titration

sulfobenzyl penicillin

sulfocyanate

sulfoglycoprotein
fetal sulfoglycoprotein antigen

sulfoiduronate sulfatase deficiency

sulfonamide
long-acting s.

sulfonamide-resistant

sulfonate
alkylbenzene s.
carbazochrome sodium s.
cyanide s.
linear alkyl s.
2-mercaptoethane s.
methylene dimethane s.
tricaine methane s.

sulfonated polymer

sulfonic
s. group
para-chloromercuribenzine sulfonic acid
toluene sulfonic acid

sulfonylurea
s. receptor
second generation s.
suppertime mixed insulin and daytime s.'s

sulfosalicylic acid

sulfosuccinate

sulfoximine
buthionine s.

sulfphonate
2-mercaptoethane sulphonate sodium

sulfur
aniline, sulfur, formaldehyde
s. colloid
s. containing
s. dioxide
s. hexafluoride
s. sugar
technetium-99m sulfur colloid
technetium sulfur colloid
volatile sulfur compound

sulfur-carbon drug

sulfurylation
steroid s.

Sulkowitch test

sum
Mann-Whitney rank sum statistic
s. of square deviations
Wilcoxon rank sum statistic
Wilcoxon rank sum test

summarized
behavior summarized evaluation

summary
discharge summary dictated
Integrated S. of Safety
Mental Component S.
Physical Component S.
preadmission screening s.
S. of Product Characteristics
transfer summary dictated

summating potential

summation
s. of all quantities following the symbol
computer summation technique
electronic summation device
s. gallop
impulse s.
s. potential

summed pain intensity difference

summer
s. asthma
s. diarrhea
s. itch

summer-type hypersensitivity pneumonitis

sump
Argyle-Salem sump tube
arterial sump effect
s. catheter

sun
cumulative effects of unprotected s.
overexposed to s.
s. protection factor

sunburn cell

sunburst
s. appearance
s. effect

Sunday Canyon virus

sundowner effect

sundowning behavior

sundown syndrome

sunflower cataract

sunken acetabulum

sunlight
overexposure to s.
suntan photoprotection factor
super
s. high frequency
s. high speed
s. packed platelet
superantigen
streptococcal s.
supercam scintillation scanner
superciliaris
arcus s.
superciliary arch
supercilii
superconducting quantum interference device susceptometer
supercritical
s. fluid
s. fluid extraction
superego
autonomous s.
superficial
s. abrasion
anterior auricular branch of superficial temporal artery
anterior superficial cervical lymph node
ascending branch of superficial cervical artery
s. bladder cancer
s. branch of lateral plantar nerve
s. branch of medial circumflex femoral artery
s. branch of medial plantar artery
s. branch of superior gluteal artery
s. branch of transverse cervical artery
s. branch of ulnar nerve
chronic superficial gastritis
s. circumflex iliac artery
s. circumflex iliac vein
s. cortical hemorrhage
disseminated superficial actinic porokeratosis
s. distal axillary node
s. distal esophagus hemorrhage
s. esophageal carcinoma
s. external pudendal artery
s. fascia
s. fascial system
s. fat
s. femoral angioplasty
s. femoral artery
s. femoral vein
s. frostbite
s. gastric ulcer
s. gastritis
greater superficial petrosal neurectomy
greater superficial temporal artery biopsy
healed superficial laceration
s. hemangioma
s. implant
s. implantation
s. incision
s. infection
s. inferior epigastric artery
s. inguinal lymph node
s. irritation
s. layer
s. linear array
medial crus of the superficial inguinal ring
membranous layer of superficial fascia
membranous layer of superficial fascia of perineum
s. musculoaponeurotic system
necrotizing superficial tracheobronchitis
s. occipital artery to middle cerebral artery
s. ocular trauma
parietal branch of superficial temporal artery
s. punctate erosion
s. punctate keratitis
s. radial nerve
Reis-Bücklers superficial corneal dystrophy
s. renal cortical perfusion
s. sclera
skin-adipose superficial musculoaponeurotic system
s. spreading melanoma
s. subendocardial focal hemorrhage
s. temporal artery-middle cerebral artery
s. temporal artery-posterior cerebral artery
s. temporal artery-superior cerebellar artery
s. temporal fascia
three-dimensional superficial liposculpture
s. thrombophlebitis
s. tibiotalar
s. transitional cell carcinoma
s. ulceration
s. varicosity
s. vascular plexus
s. vastus lateralis
s. white onychomycosis
superfluous hair
super-heated aerosol
superimposed
s. acute inflammatory episode
s. bowel gas
s. dorsiflexion of foot
s. pregnancy-induced hypertension
repeated quick stretch superimposed upon an existing contraction
superimposition of bowel shadow
superior
s. angle
angle of superior scapula
angulus superior scapulae
ankyloglossia superior syndrome
anterior glandular branch of superior thyroid artery
anterior/lateral/posterior glandular branch of superior thyroid artery
anterior middle superior alveolar
anterior and posterior superior pancreaticoduodenal artery
anterior superior alveolar artery
anterior superior alveolar branch of infraorbital nerve
anterior superior dental artery
anterior superior pancreaticoduodenal artery
anterior superior renal segment
anterior superior segmental artery of kidney
anteromedial superior humeral head impaction
apertura pelvis s.
apertura thoracis s.
apical branch of right superior pulmonary vein
apical segmental artery of superior lobar artery of right lung
apicoposterior branch of left superior pulmonary vein
aponeurosis of posterior superior serratus
aponeurosis of superior levator palpebra
arcus dentalis s.
arcus palpebralis s.

superior *(continued)*
area vestibularis s.
arteria cerebelli s.
arteria collateralis ulnaris s.
arteria epigastrica s.
arteria glutea s.
arteria lingularis s.
arteria mesenterica s.
arteria pancreaticoduodenalis s.
arteria pancreaticoduodenalis superior anterior
arteria pancreaticoduodenalis superior posterior
arteria phrenica s.
arteria superior cerebelli
arteria thoracica s.
arteria thyroidea s.
arteria tympanica s.
arteria vesicalis s.
artery of anterior superior segment of kidney
s. articular process
s. aspect
auricularis superior muscle
s. axis deviation
bidirectional superior cavopulmonary anastomosis
s. border
s. border of body of pancreas
s. branch
s. carotid artery
s. carotid ganglion
s. cerebellar artery
s. cerebellar peduncle
s. cervical ganglion
s. colliculus
s. constrictor muscles of pharynx
s. cornu
s. cul-de-sac
decussation of superior cerebellar peduncles
deep superior epigastric artery
s. dental arch
s. duodenal flexure
s. duodenal fold
s. duodenal fossa
s. duodenal recess
s. edge
s. endplate
entrance of fetal head into superior pelvic strait
s. epigastric artery
s. epigastric vein
external branch of superior laryngeal
s. facet
s. fascia
s. flap
s. frontal convolution
s. frontal gyrus
s. frontal sulcus
s. ganglion of vagus nerve
s. gaze
s. gemellus muscle
s. gluteal artery
s. gluteal artery perforator
s. gluteal nerve
s. gluteal vein
gyrus frontalis s.
gyrus temporalis s.
s. hemiazygos vein
s. hemorrhagic polioencephalitis
s. hemorrhoidal plexus
s. hemorrhoidal vein
s. horn
s. hypophysial artery
s. iliac crest
s. iliac spine
inferior parietal and superior temporal lobe
internal branch of superior laryngeal nerve
s. internal laryngeal nerve
s. labial region
s. labrum anterior and posterior
s. lacrimal duct
lateral superior olive
left anterior s.
left superior intercostal vein
left superior oblique
left superior rectus
left superior vena cava
s. ligament of epididymis
ligament of epididymis inferior and s.
s. ligament of incus
ligament of left superior vena cava
s. ligament of malleus
s. limb
s. limbic keratoconjunctivitis
s. lobe of heart
macula cribrosa s.
s. margin
s. margin of cerebral hemisphere
medial superior olive
medial superior temporal visual area
s. mesenteric
s. mesenteric artery
s. mesenteric artery blood flow
s. mesenteric artery blood velocity
s. mesenteric artery embolus
s. mesenteric artery occlusion
s. mesenteric artery syndrome
s. mesenteric ganglion
s. mesenteric-portal vein confluence
s. mesenteric vein
middle gray layer of superior colliculus
middle lobe branch of right superior pulmonary vein
musculus auricularis s.
musculus gemellus s.
musculus longitudinalis s.
musculus obliquus superior bulbi
musculus obliquus superior oculi
Nadler superior radial scissors
s. nasal
s. nasal artery
s. nasal quadrant
s. nasal vein
nervus gluteus s.
nucleus centralis superior raphe
nucleus centralis tegmenti s.
s. oblique
obliquity superior muscle
obliquus capitis s.
obliquus capitis superior muscle
s. orbital fissure
s. orbital fissure syndrome
orbital superior fissure
overactive superior oblique
overactive superior rectus
palpation of anterior superior iliac spine
Pancoast superior sulcus syndrome
paries superior orbitae
s. parietal lobule
posterior superior iliac spine
posterior superior pancreaticoduodenal vein
pulmonary anomalous superior venous return
s. pulmonary vein isolated
s. QRS axis
s. radicular vein
radionuclide superior cavography
s. rectus muscle
s. rectus traction suture
right superior oblique muscle
right superior rectus muscle
right superior intercostal vein
right superior oblique palsy
right superior vena cava
s. sagittal sinus
s. sagittal sinus thrombosis
s. sagittal sinus velocity

s. sector iridectomy
s. segment of lung
s. semicircular canal
s. semicircular canal deficiency
shunt index via superior mesenteric vein
s. sulcus tumor syndrome
superficial branch of superior gluteal artery
s. tarsal muscle
s. temporal artery
s. temporal gyrus
s. temporal quadrant
s. temporal vein
s. thyroid notch
s. turbinate
s. vagal ganglion
s. vena cava
s. vena cava compression syndrome
s. vena cava obstruction
vena cava s.

superioris
musculi levatoris palpebrae s.
palpebrae superioris muscle

superiority complex

supernatant
high-speed s.
normal lymphocyte s.
postmitochondrial s.
protein-free s.
sheep hemolysate s.
T-cell s.
thymic epithelial s.

supernormal
s. artery
s. excitability

supernumerary
s. bone
s. breast
s. kidney
s. marker chromosome
s. nipple
s. rib

superoinferior heart

superolateral aspect

superoxide
human superoxide dismutase
manganese superoxide dismutase gene
polyethylene glycol-conjugated superoxide dismutase pegorgotein
recombinant human superoxide dismutase

superparamagnetic
ultrasmall-particle superparamagnetic iron oxide

supersaturated potassium iodide

supersaturation
relative s.

supersensitivity perception

superstitious false ideas

superstructure
attaching material implant s.
attachment to implant s.

supervised intermittent ambulatory treatment

supervision
close s.
noncontact s.
patient does ADL with s.
person in need of s.

supervisory
S. Behavior Description
S. Practices Test

supination
s. contracture
s. deformity
s. external rotation
s. of foot
forearm s.
s. of forearm
pronation and s.

supine
AP supine portable view
s. bicycle stress echocardiography
s. diastolic blood pressure
s. empty stress test
s. hypotensive syndrome
mean daily supine blood pressure
transfer from supine to sitting
s. and upright

supine-to-sit transfer

Suppan nail technique

supper
fat-free s.

suppertime mixed insulin and daytime sulfonylureas

supple
neck s.

supplement
daily high fiber s.
endothelial cell growth s.
enteral nutritional s.
high-protein s.
S. to HIV/AIDS Surveillance
mycobacteria antibiotic s.
Neonatal Behavioral Assessment Scale with Kansas S.'s
Pediatrician infant dietary s.

supplemental
Children's Apperception Test, S.
s. groove
s. growth hormone therapy
s. insurance
s. minimal sodium
s. motor area
s. oxygen
s. oxygen system
phosphate supplemental diet
physician supplemental order
s. thyroid hormone

supplementary
s. canal
s. medical insurance
s. menstruation
s. motor area
s. parenteral nutrition
s. sensory feedback

supplementation
appropriate nutritional s.
crying, requirement for oxygen supplementation, increases in heart rate and blood pressure
macronutrient s.
micronutrient s.
mineral s.
nutritional s.

supplemented
s. Eagle minimal essential medium
high cholesterol and tocopherol s.
improved minimal essential medium, hormone s.
tocopherol s.

supply
adequate blood s.
arterial blood s.
arterial scrotum s.
battery-charging power s.
blood supply of brain
blood supply to heart
central material s.
central sterile supply department
collateral blood s.
compensatory blood s.
inadequate blood s.
insufficient blood s.
interruption of blood s.
longitudinal blood s.
operating theatre sterile supply unit

supply *(continued)*
oxygenated blood s.
s., processing, and distribution department
reduced blood supply to heart
splenic vascular s.
uninterruptible power s.

support
adaptive support ventilation
adolescent support group
adolescent support system
advanced cardiac life s.
advanced pediatric life s.
advanced trauma life s.
aeromedical evacuation support team
ankle stabilizing orthosis s.
anorexia support group
arterial cannulation s.
artificial hepatic s.
autologous bone marrow s.
autologous hematopoietic stem cell s.
autologous peripheral hematopoietic stem cell s.
basic trauma life s.
bioartificial extracorporeal liver support system
biventricular s.
cardiopulmonary s.
Children's Perception of S. Inventory
combat support hospital
comprehensive health enhancement support system
comprehensive support care team
divorce support group
donut support brace
s., empathy, and truth
enteral nutritional s.
esophageal-directed pressure s.
extracorporeal life s.
front support strap
good pelvic s.
grief support group
s. group for epilepsy
group support session
hypotensive and ventilatory s.
ice, compression, elevation, and s.
introitus with good s.
life support unit
longitudinal arch s.
long-term support group
luteal phase s.
medical support equipment
minimal s.
mobile arm s.
Multidimensional Scale of Perceived Social S.
multiple abutment s.
neonatal adjuvant life s.
noninvasive ventilatory s.
nutritional support service
nutritional support team
pain support group
s. parenteral nutrition
pediatric advanced life s.
pelvic support index
percutaneous cardiopulmonary bypass s.
perineal support stitch
perineal support suture
peripheral blood stem cell s.
plantar arch support orthosis
positive support ventilator
pressure support ventilation
prolonged respiratory s.
prone cranial support device
protection, rest, ice, compression, elevation, support
removal of life s.
sandbag placed for s.
self-help support group
sensory impaired s.
sequential treatment employing pharmacologic s.
single limb s.
stem cell s.
s. and stimulation
s. stocking
s. suture
S. Team Assessment Schedule
tibial fracture brace proximal s.
uterus has good s.
venous pressure gradient support stockings
volume-assured pressure s.
wide base of s.
wrist hand extension compression s.
youth/parent support group

supported
s. arm exercise
breathing supported by mechanical respirator
externally s.
extrinsically s.
pressure supported ventilation

supporting tissue of brain

supportive
s. care
s. device to restrain hernia
s. halo cast
intensive supportive care
intensive supportive programs
patient treated with supportive care
reality-adaptive s.
s. social structure

suppository
contraceptive suppository capsule
Monistat-3 vaginal s.
morphine sulfate controlled-release s.
rectal morphine sulfate s.

suppressant
appetite s.
cough s.

suppressed
hyperimmunized s.
s. immune response

suppression
s. amblyopia
androgen suppression therapy
antibody-mediated immune s.
atropine suppression test
bone marrow s.
cardiac arrhythmia suppression trial
electroencephalogram burst suppression pattern
failure of fixation s.
gonadal steroid s.
gonadal suppression treatment
intermittent androgen s.
Liddle dexamethasone suppression test
light chain isotype s.
low-dose dexamethasone suppression test
motion artifact suppression technique
s. and mutation
orbital fat s.
overnight high-dose dexamethasone suppression test
overnight 1-mg dexamethasone suppression test
pancreatic suppression test
pituitary gonadotropin s.
shock-induced suppression of drinking
single dose s.
s. for tumor growth

suppressive medication

suppressor
antigen-specific suppressor T cell
APC tumor suppressor gene
s. cell

s. cell activity
s. of cytokine signaling 3
histamine-induced suppressor factor
immune s.
s. lymphocyte
multicopy suppressor screen
nonspecific suppressor cell
ochre suppressor genetic mutation
s. sensitive
soluble immune response s.
soluble suppressor factor
spontaneous suppressor cell activity
T s.
T-helper suppressor cell

suppressor-activating determinant

suppress reflex contraction

suppurating
s. gastritis
otitis media, acute, s.
otitis media, chronic, s.

suppurativa
axillary hidradenitis s.
hidradenitis s.

suppurative
acute obstructive suppurative cholangitis
acute suppurative appendicitis
acute suppurative cholangitis
acute suppurative parotitis
s. appendicitis
s. arthritis
s. cerebritis
chronic suppurative lung disease
chronic suppurative otitis media
cystic suppurative necrosis
s. encephalitis
s. exudate
s. gastritis
s. gingivitis
s. hepatitis
s. infection
s. keratitis
s. mastitis
s. mediastinitis
s. pneumonia
s. retinitis
right otitis media, suppurative, acute
right otitis media, suppurative, chronic
s. thrombophlebitis
s. tonsillitis

supraannular
s. mitral valve replacement
s. valve

supracapsular nerve entrapment syndrome

supracervical
s. hysterectomy
s. incision
laparoscopic supracervical hysterectomy

suprachiasmatica
arteria s.

suprachiasmatic nucleus

suprachoroidal hemorrhage

supraclavicular
s. adenopathy
anterior supraclavicular nerve
s. approach
s. compression
s. fascia
s. fat pad
s. fossa
greater supraclavicular fossa
s. lymph node
s. muscle
s. nerve block
s. node biopsy

supraclinoid carotid aneurysm

supracondylar
femoral supracondylar fracture
intramedullary s.
s. knee-ankle orthosis
s. line
Mueller femoral supracondylar fracture classification

supracondylar-suprapatellar

supracricoid
s. hemilaryngopharyngectomy

supracristal plane

supraduodenalis
arteria s.

supragenicular popliteal artery

supraglottic
s. horizontal laryngectomy
s. structure
subtotal supraglottic laryngectomy

suprahepatic
s. abscess
s. inferior vena cava

supra-Hisian block

suprahyoid
s. gland
s. muscle

supralevator abscess

supramalleolar orthosis

supramamillary nucleus

supramarginal gyrus

supramentale craniometric point

supranormal excitation

supranuclear
progressive supranuclear palsy
s. gaze palsy

supraoptica
arteria s.

supraoptical hypophysial diabetes insipidus

supraoptic hypothalamic nucleus

supraopticus
nucleus s.

supraorbital
s. akinesia
s. arch
s. artery
s. foramen
s. fracture
s. groove
s. margin
s. nerve
s. reflex
s. ridge
s. vein

suprapatellar
s. amputation
s. bursa
s. cuff
s. pouch
variable circumference suprapatellar socket

supraplatysmal
extended supraplatysmal plane

suprapubic
s. aspiration
s. bladder tap
s. catheter
s. cystotomy
s. discomfort
s. drainage
epiurethral suprapubic vaginal suspension
s. incision
s. mass
5-mm suprapubic trocar
percussion of suprapubic area
percutaneous suprapubic cystostomy
s. prostatectomy

suprapubic *(continued)*
s. puncture
s. tenderness
s. tube

suprapubically
opened s.

suprapyloricus
nodus lymphoideus s.

suprarenal
s. body
s. capsule
s. cortex
s. ganglion
s. gland
medial border of suprarenal gland
ureteric branch of inferior suprarenal artery

suprarenale
melasma s.

suprascapular
s. artery
s. ligament
s. nerve compression

suprasellar
s. cistern
s. cyst
germ cell tumor with synchronous lesions in pineal and suprasellar region
s. lesion
s. region
s. tumor

supraspinatus
s. fossa

supraspinous ligament

suprasternal
s. examination
s. fossa
s. notch
s. region

Suprathreshold Adaptation Test

supratonsillaris
plica s.

supratrochlear
s. artery
s. nerve
s. nucleus

supratrochlearis
arteria s.

supravaginal
s. hysterectomy
s. septum

supravalvular
s. aortic hypercalcemia syndrome
s. hypertrophic aortic stenosis

supraventricular
s. arrhythmia
s. crest
s. ectopy
narrow complex supraventricular tachycardia
paroxysmal reentrant supraventricular tachycardia
paroxysmal supraventricular arrhythmia
s. premature beat
s. premature contraction
s. rhythm
sustained supraventricular tachyarrhythmia
s. tachyarrhythmia
s. tachycardia ablation

surae
s. reflex

sural
adipofascial sural flap

suralis
arteria s.

surdocardiac syndrome

Suretee Events Index

surface
active trabecular calcification s.
s. adherent monocyte
anatomic surface prosthesis
anterior articular surface of dens
anterior part of diaphragmatic surface of liver
anterior talar articular surface of calcaneus
antibody to hepatitis B surface antigen
s. antigen
apical surface of heart
apposing articular s.
approximal surface of tooth
s. area
s. area to volume ratio
articular surface of acromion
articular surface of arytenoid cartilage
articular surface of head of fibula
articular surface of head of rib
articular surface of knee
articular surface of mandibular fossa
articular surface of mandibular fossa of temporal bone
articular surface on calcaneus for cuboid bone
articular surface of patella
articular surface of talus
articular surface of temporal bone
articular surface of tubercle of rib
arytenoidal articular s.
arytenoidal articular surface of cricoid
s. asymmetry index
attenuated cortical s.
auricular surface of ilium
auricular surface of sacrum
axial surface cavity
s. binding protein
biometal s.
s. biopsy
body surface area
body surface burned
body surface Laplacian mapping
body surface potential mapping
bone-contacting surface ratio
buccal surface of tooth
Calculus S. Index
capsular surface smooth and glistening
s. carcinoma in situ
cell surface antigen
cell surface protein
cementless surface replacement arthroplasty
s. coil MR
s. colony
concave anterior s.
concave posterior s.
débrided bone s.'s
depth-resolved surface coil spectroscopy
diaphragmatic surface of left lung
diaphragmatic surface of right lung
dorsolateral surface of knee
eburnated bone s.
electrodes placed on the surface of head
s. electromyography
enamel surface index
endorectal surface coil MRI
s. enhanced laser desorption/ionization
epidermal cell surface protein
s. epithelium
erosion of articular s.
erosion surface per bone s.

s. extended x-ray absorption fine structure
exterior s.
fibular articular surface of tibia
fractional osteoid s.
Gross cell surface antigen
s. of head
hepatitis B s.
hepatitis B surface antibody
hepatitis B surface antigen
hepatitis B surface associated
hepatitis surface antigen studies
high-density lipoprotein-cell surface receptor
s. immunoglobulin A
s. implant
s. inductive plethysmography
s. infiltration by hemorrhage
internal surface area
ion surface scattering
islet cell surface antibody
lateral electrical surface stimulation
lingual surface of tooth
lunate surface of acetabulum
macular surface wrinkling
malleolar articular surface of fibula
malleolar articular surface of tibia
medial cerebral s.
medial malleolar surface of talus
medial surface of cerebral hemisphere
s. membrane immunoglobulin
mesial incisal lingual s.
metastatic adenocarcinoma serosal s.'s
Moloney cell surface antigen
mucosal surface of large intestine
mucosal surface of small intestine
navicular articular surface of talus
normal ovarian surface epithelium
occlusal surface of tooth
opposing articular s.'s
optical surface imaging
osteoid s.
outer surface protein
ovarian surface epithelium
palmar surface desensitization
parallelism of articular s.
partial bursal surface tear
permeability s.
s. plasmon resonance
proximal isovelocity surface area
pyramid s.
rad surface dose
ratio of decayed and filled s.'s
recombinant outer surface protein A
reconstruction occlusal s.
s. regularity index
severed surface of bone
skin surface lipid
skin surface microscopy
smooth cortical s.
stereotactic surface projection
s. tension
total blood volume predicted from body s.
total body s.
total body surface area
total burn surface area
tumor-associated surface antigen
tumor-specific cell surface antigen
variable antigen, s.
variant-specific surface antigen
variant surface glycoprotein
viral cell surface antigen
s. wrinkling retinopathy
xenograph surface area

surface-active
s.-a. material
s.-a. substance

surface-connecting membrane

surfaced
hyperkeratotic verrucoid surfaced lesion

surfactant
bovine lavage extract s.
calf lung surfactant extract
exogenous natural s.
human lung s.
nonionic surfactant vesicle
s. protein-A
s. protein-B
s. protein-C
rapid surfactant test
s. replacement therapy

surfactant-like activity

surge
estrogen s.
gonadotropin surge attenuating factor
LH s.
midcycle s.
nocturnal thyroid-stimulating hormone s.
nocturnal TSH s.

surgeon
curved-needle s. knot
partial throw s. knot

surgery
abdominal s.
ambulatory surgery center
anterior cervical surgery vocal cord damage
anterior cervicothoracic junction s.
anterior cranial fossa s.
anterior lower cervical spine s.
aortic reconstructive s.
apically repositioned flap in mucogingival s.
arterial reconstructive s.
arthroscopic knee s.
arthroscopic laser s.
artificial divergency s.
asymptomatic carotid surgery trial
beating-heart bypass s.
brain graft s.
brain implant s.
breast enhancement s.
cardiac s.
cardiac surgery intensive care unit
cardiopulmonary bypass s.
cardiothoracic s.
cardiovascular s.
cardiovascular surgery unit
cardiovascular-thoracic s.
cataract surgery with implant
closed heart s.
colorectal s.
s. complication
computer-aided s.
computer-assisted orthopedic s.
computer-assisted stereotactic s.
computer-guided endoscopic sinus s.
consent for s.
coronary artery bypass graft s.
coronary artery bypass grafting s.
cosmetic implant s.
cosmetic nasal s.
cosmetic surgery authorization form
cosmetic surgery consent form
day surgery unit
detoxification before s.
elective cosmetic s.
endoscopic sinus s.
endoscopic video-assisted s.
exenterative surgery for pelvic cancer
failed back surgery syndrome

surgery *(continued)*
functional endoscopic sinus s.
gamma ray s.
gastric bypass s.
gastric reduction s.
general medicine and s.
glaucoma filtering s.
s., gynecology, and obstetrics
hair replacement s.
hair restoration s.
hand s.
hand-assisted laparoscopic s.
heart bypass s.
heart reduction s.
heart valve s.
hip replacement s.
hypothermic cardiac arrest s.
ileus following abdominal s.
image-guided functional endoscopic sinus s.
intestinal bypass s.
intraoperative radiation s.
invasive brain s.
invasive spinal s.
irradiation and s.
junctional rhythm after cardiac s.
laparoscopically assisted s.
laparoscopic antireflux s.
laparoscopic gallbladder s.
laser glaucoma s.
laser heart s.
limb sparing s.
lower abdominal s.
lower extremity s.
lung volume reduction s.
macular hole s.
major abdominal s.
major GI s.
Marzola hair restoration s.
McCash hand s.
medicine and s.
microscopically controlled s.
microscopic endoscopy s.
middle ear s.
mini-functional endoscopic sinus s.
minimal access general s.
minimally invasive brain s.
minimally invasive cardiac s.
minimally invasive laparoscopic s.
minimally invasive spine s.
minimally invasive valve replacement s.
minimum-access s.
minimum incision s.
minor surgery suite
mitral valve s.
Mohs micrographic s.
nasal endoscopic s.
navigated brain tumor s.
nonvascular abdominal s.
no-stitch phacoemulsification s.
open anti-reflux s.
open disc s.
ophthalmology, otorhinolaryngology, and head and neck s.
oral and maxillofacial s.
oral surgery handpiece
osteopathic medicine and s.
patient is prepped and draped for s.
pediatric cardiovascular s.
pediatric lung s.
pelvic colonic s.
peripheral ablative s.
peripheral vascular s.
permission for s.
plastic and reconstructive s.
postcardiac s.
postoperative open heart s.
powered endoscopic sinus s.
preoperative contraindication to s.
primary high-risk replacement s.
prosthetic heart valve s.
radial artery bypass s.
radical prostate s.
radioimmunoguided s.
reconstructive hip s.
repeat hip replacement s.
revision hip replacement s.
selective imaging and graphics for stereotactic s.
sex reassignment s.
single lung reduction s.
small incision cataract s.
spinal fusion s.
status post s.
subfascial endoscopic perforator s.
sutureless cataract s.
thoracic s.
traumatic unidirectional Bankart lesion s.
triple bypass heart s.
triple cardiac bypass s.
unilateral lung reduction s.
upper abdominal s.
video-assisted thoracic s.
video-assisted thoracoscopic s.
video-assisted transthoracic s.
videoendoscopic s.
videoscopic hernia s.
volume reduction s.

surgical
s. abdomen
s. ablation
s. abortion
s. absence of breast
absorbable surgical suture
s. access
s. Achilles tendon lengthening
activation map-guided surgical resection
acute surgical abdomen
s. adjuvant therapy
aggressive surgical approach
ambulatory surgical unit
s. anatomy
s. anesthesia
anterior surgical exposure
AO surgical technique
appendix brought into surgical incision
arachnophlebectomy surgical device
s. artifact
s. blood order equation
s. care
clear surgical diet
complete surgical exploration
s. complication of drug abuse
s. cone
day care surgical unit
s. debridement
s. debulking
s. decompression
diagnostic and s.
s. diagnostic oncology
s. drain
s. emergency
s. excision
s. followup
s. foreign body
free-standing ambulatory surgical center
s. Gleason score
Gram-positive surgical pathogen
s. hand scrub
healing surgical incision
s. history
s. hypoparathyroidism
image-guided surgical technique
s. immobilization of joint
s. implant
s. incision
incisional surgical wound infection
s. inpatient care
intensive care, s.
s. intensive therapy

s. intermediate care unit
intermediate surgical unit
s. intervention
invasive surgical staging
invasive surgical technique
irradiated surgical defects
lost surgical specimen
s. lung biopsy
maximal surgical blood order schedule
Medpor surgical implant
s. menopause
Merocel surgical spear
s. microscope navigation
mobile surgical unit
s. myomectomy as reproductive therapy
s. neck of humerus
nonabsorbable surgical suture
nonphysician surgical assistant
open surgical biopsy
ophthalmic vitreous surgical technique
s. orthotopic implantation
outpatient surgical unit
s. overhead canopy
past surgical history
patient is a poor surgical risk
pediatric surgical intensive care
s. peripheral iridectomy
primary surgical ward
s. procedure for subarachnoid hemorrhage
s. pulmonary intensive care unit
s. relaxation of contracture
s. respiratory intensive care unit
shape of surgical incisions W-plasty
shape of surgical incision Z-plasty
s. short procedure unit
s. suite
s. termination of pregnancy
s. treatment for brain tumor
s. treatment for epidural hemorrhage
s. treatment objective
video-assisted thoracic surgical non-rib-spreading lobectomy
voluntary surgical contraception
s. wound infection

surgically

s. assisted rapid maxillary expansion
s. assisted rapid palatal expansion
s. implanted hemodialysis catheter

surrogate

s. end-point biomarker
s. father
s. mother
s. tolerogenesis

surrounded

pelvic viscera surrounded by hematoma

surrounding subretinal fluid cuff

sursumduction of eye

Surtees Difficulties Index

surveillance

antepartum fetal s.
s. artifact
Cancer S. Program
Cancer S. System
cardiac surveillance unit
s. colonoscopy
S. and Control of Pathogens of Epidemiologic Importance
endoscopic s.
s. endoscopy
graft s.
infection surveillance and control program
maternal s.
nutritional s.
postmarketing s.
Supplement to HIV/AIDS S.

survey

Access Management S.
Adult Performance Level S.
California Occupational Preference S.
Campbell Interest and Skill S.
Cancer Attitude S.
Children's Attention and Adjustment S.
Conflict Management S.
Creativity Attitude S.
current population s.
S. of Employee Access
Fear S. Schedule
Gardner Analysis of Personality S.
Group Encounter S.
Guilford-Zimmerman Aptitude S.
Guilford-Zimmerman Temperament S.
Health and Activity Limitation S.
health and nutrition examination s.
Hereford Parental Attitude S.
hospital discharge s.
human immune status s.
Interpersonal Behavior S.
S. of Interpersonal Values
36-item short form health s.
Jackson Vocational Interest S.
Juvenile Wellness and Health S.
Kaufman S. of Early Academic and Language Skills
Keystone Telebinocular Visual S.
Kuder Occupational Interest S.
Life Experience S.
long bone s.
Management Appraisal S.
medical s.
metabolic bone s.
metastatic bone s.
Meyer-Kendall Assessment S.
National Ambulatory Medical Care S.
Ohio Vocational Interest S.
S. of Pain Attitudes
Parent Awareness Skills S.
Picture Interest Exploration S.
point-prevalent s.
Priority Counseling S.
Purdue Perceptual-Motor S.
s., question, read, review, recite
Reality Check S.
reduced joint s.
Rokeach Value S.
School Assessment S.
School Attitude S.
School Situation S.
skeletal s.
Student Disability S.
Student Orientations S.
Study Attitudes and Methods S.
S. of Study Habits and Attitudes
Team Effectiveness S.
Transactional Analysis Life Position S.
voice outcome s.
Wolpe Fear S. Schedule
youth risk behavioral s.

surveyor

Occupational Interests S.

survival

allograft survival rate
s. analysis
breast cancer-specific s.
cause-specific s.
clinical estimation of s.
corrected survival rate
cumulative duration of s.
cumulative survival rate
disease-free s.
disease-free survival rate
disease-specific s.

survival *(continued)*
distant-disease-free s.
distant recurrence-free s.
event-free s.
failure-free s.
s. of the fittest
five-year survival rate
s. fraction
graft s.
graft survival rate
high probability of s.
leukemia-free s.
life table s.
local recurrence-free s.
locoregional recurrence-free s.
mean allograft s.
mean survival time
s. motor neuron telomeric gene
nerve cell s.
one-year survival rate
overall s.
platelet survival time
progression-free s.
quality-adjusted s.
relapse-free s.
s. relative to nodal involvement in breast carcinoma
relative survival rate
surviving and survival guilt
s. time
total lymphoid irradiation for allograft s.
5-year survival rate

surviving
long-term s.
s. and survival guilt

survivor
s. of abuse
adult survivor of neglect
Alzheimer s.
depressed heart attack s.
s. guilt
heart attack s.
long-term s.
long-term survivor of heart transplant
stroke s.

Susan
Wistar Institute Susan Hayflick cell

susceptibility
antibacterial agent susceptibility testing
antimicrobial susceptibility test
antimicrobial susceptibility testing
antimicrobiology susceptibility testing
antimycobacterial susceptibility testing
culture and s.
dynamic susceptibility contrast
electric s.
Harvard Group Scale of Hypnotic Susceptibility, Form A
hereditary neuropathy with susceptibility to pressure palsy
increased susceptibility to infection
lysostaphin susceptibility test
magnetic s.
malignant hypothermia s.
microbial susceptibility test
microdilution broth susceptibility test
microdilution susceptibility testing
minimum inhibitory concentration susceptibility test
motion sickness s.
multiple sclerosis susceptibility gene
Neisseria gonorrhoeae susceptibility testing
novobiocin susceptibility test
Optochin susceptibility test
penicillinase-producing organisms susceptibility testing
Stanford Hypnotic S. Scale
s. testing

susceptible
caries s.
s. host
moderately s.

susceptometer
superconducting quantum interference device s.

suspect
s. glaucoma
ocular hypertensive glaucoma suspect

suspected
s. adverse drug reaction
s. catheter sepsis
s. child abuse or neglect
s. heart attack
s. nonaccidental trauma

suspended
fine suspended particulate
s. heart
s. particulate matter
total suspended particulate

suspension
anterior suspension of hyoid bone
bladder neck s.
budesonide inhalation s.
cable suspension system
endoscopic bladder neck s.
epiurethral suprapubic vaginal s.
extraperitoneal laparoscopic bladder neck s.
human platelet s.
insulin zinc s.
laparoscopic bladder neck s.
liquid barium s.
magnesia and alumina oral s.
magnesium hydroxide s.
minimal-incision pubovaginal s.
modified Peyronie bladder neck s.
needle bladder neck s.
oral barium s.
patellar tendon s.
patellar tendon-bearing s.
percutaneous bladder neck s.
Pereyra bladder neck s.
Pereyra needle s.
platelet suspension immunofluorescence test
red blood cell s.
silicone-only s.
sterile aqueous s.
sterile injectable s.
transvaginal bladder neck s.

suspensor
elastic s.
lateral loop s.
lateral suspensor ligament

suspensorii

suspensory
anterior suspensory ligament
s. bandage
s. ligament
s. ligament of axilla
s. ligament of breast
s. ligament of clitoris
s. ligament of Cooper
s. ligament of duodenum
s. ligament of esophagus
s. ligament of eye
s. ligament of gonad
s. ligament of lens
s. ligament of ovary
s. ligament of penis
s. ligament of testis
s. ligament of thyroid gland

suspicion
high index of s.
inappropriate s.

suspicious behavior

sustain
inability to sustain consistent work behavior

sustainable
maximal sustainable ventilatory capacity

sustained
s. action
s. activity
s. apical impulse
s. cardiac arrest
s. depolarizing shift
s. engraftment
s. ethanol release tube
s. horizontal nystagmus
s. hypertension
s. low-efficiency dialysis
s. maximal inspiration
s. maximal inspiratory lung exercise
maximal sustained level of ventilation
maximal sustained ventilatory capacity
maximum duration of sustained blowing
s. monomorphic ventricular tachycardia
s. natural apophysial glide
s. periods of grandiosity
potassium chloride sustained release tablet
s. reentrant ventricular tachyarrhythmia
s. release medication
s. release theophylline
Repeated Test of S. Wakefulness
s. response rate
s. supraventricular tachyarrhythmia
s. ventricular tachycardia
ventricular tachycardia s.

sustained-release
s.-r. morphine sulfate
s.-r. nitroglycerin
s.-r. oral
s.-r. sodium fluoride

sustentacular
s. cell
s. fiber
s. tissue

Sutherland-Haan syndrome

sutural
s. bone
s. cataract
s. ligament

suture
absorbable surgical s.
adjustable external s.
Albert suture technique
anchor with suture ligature
angle suture technique
anterior palatine s.
Appolito suture technique
apposition of skull s.
apposition suture technique
approximation suture technique
arcuate suture technique
Argyll-Robertson suture technique
Arlt suture technique
Arroyo encircling s.
Arruga encircling s.
arthroscopic transglenoid suture stabilization procedure
atraumatic suture technique
Axenfeld suture technique
bastard suture technique
black silk s.
bolster suture technique
cable wire suture technique
catgut s.
chromic catgut mattress s.
chromic gut s.
circumferential suture tie
continuous circular inverting s.
continuous hemostatic s.
continuous inverting s.
continuous mattress s.
continuous over-and-over s.
continuous running lock s.
continuous running monofilament s.
continuous silk s.
continuous sling s.
continuous suture technique
coracoclavicular suture fixation
coronal suture synostosis
cutaneous suture of palate
cutaneous suture technique
double-armed mattress s.
doubly ligated with transfixion s.
early postoperative suture adjustment
en bloc running locking s.
evening interrupted s.
s. failure
figure-of-eight suture technique
frontomaxillonasal s.
s. harelip
heavy retention s.
horizontal mattress s.
interrupted black silk s.
interrupted chromic s.
interrupted cotton s.
interrupted fine silk s.
interrupted mattress s.
interrupted pledgeted s.
intraoperative suture adjustment
s. of iris
late postoperative suture adjustment
Lee double-loop locking s.
s. ligated
s. line
locking horizontal mattress s.
Maxon delayed-absorbable s.
McCannel suture technique
medial crural s.
median palatine s.
metal suture material
mild chromic s.
modified Frost s.
monofilament nylon s.
nonabsorbable surgical s.
nylon retention s.
nylon suture material
occipitomastoid suture lines
perineal support s.
persistent frontal s.
plain catgut s.
plain 2-0 catgut s.
plain 3-0 catgut s.
plain 4-0 catgut s.
plain gut s.
plication s.'s
polydioxanone s.
s. removal
silk braided s.
silk interrupted mattress s.
silkworm gut s.
skin suture intact
skull suture line
stainless steel s.
subannular mattress s.
superior rectus traction s.
synthetic absorbable s.
transverse palatine s.
zygomaticofrontal suture line

sutured
cleaned, sutured, and dressed
reverse sutured eye
transsclerally sutured posterior chamber lens

sutureless
s. anastomosis
s. cataract surgery

suturing
bone suturing wire chisel-tip wire
freehand suturing technique
magnetic control s.
transvaginal s.

Svedberg
S. equation
S. flotation unit
negative sedimentation Svedberg unit

SvO2
continuous cardiac output with SvO_2

swab
antibiotic-soaked s.
cotton s.
cotton-tipped s.
nasal s.
nasal swab culture
nasopharyngeal s.
rectal s.
stick s.
throat s.
urethral s.
wound s.

swallow
barium s.
barium swallow study
dry s.
impaired ability to s.
inability to chew or s.
modified barium s.
modified barium swallow with videofluoroscopy
swish and s.
videofluoroscopic barium s.
water s.
wet s.

swallowed blood syndrome

swallowing
chewing, sucking, s.
s. difficulty
s. disorder
s. dysfunction
fiberoptic endoscopic evaluation of s.
fiberoptic endoscopic evaluation of swallowing with sensory testing
fiberoptic endoscopic examination of s.
flexible endoscopic evaluation of s.
flexible endoscopic evaluation of swallowing with sensory testing
flexible endoscopic swallowing examination
impaired breaking and s.
s. mechanism
pain on s.
patient has difficulty s.
s. therapy
videoendoscopic swallowing study
videofluorographic evaluation of s.
videofluoroscopic swallowing study

Swan-Ganz catheter

swan-neck finger deformity

Swanson
S. carpal lunate implant
S. radial head implant
S. wrist joint implant

Swan syndrome

swathe
arm s.
sling and s.

sway
anteroposterior lateral s.
aphysiologic s.
s. back

swayback deformity

swaying gait

sweat
apocrine sweat gland
chills, fever, and night s.'s
drenching night s.'s
s. duct
fever and night s.'s
Gibson-Cooke sweat test
s. gland
s. gland carcinoma
malodorous s.
shaking chills and night s.'s

sweating
fever, chills, and s.
fever, chills, sweating, nausea, vomiting, and diarrhea
hyperventilating, sweating and shaking
s. sickness

sweep
adductor sweep of thumb
audiometry sweep test
duodenal bulb and s.

sweet
s. clover disease
S. disease
gated sweet magnetic imaging
increased craving for s.'s
no concentrated s.'s

swell
mean swell time botulism test

swelling
s. of abdomen
abdominal swelling and pain
s. of ankles
s. at incision site
circulation, motor ability, sensation, and s.
s. deformity of affected bone
diarrhea with abdominal pain and s.
diffuse brain s.
s. of disc
ecchymosis and s.
focal axonal s.
footpad s.
s. of gums
s. of hands or feet
heat, absence of use, redness, pain, pus, s.
heat, reddening, swelling, or tenderness
hypoosmotic s.
induration and s.
inflammation and/or s.
joint contracture and s.
joint pain and s.
joint swelling in hemodialysis
loss of appetite with joint s.
Neufeld capsular s.
nodules, eosinophilia, rheumatism, dermatitis, and swelling syndrome
optical disc s.
optic disc s.
painful swelling of breast
pain and s.
reduce swelling in brain
salivary gland s.
Soemmerring crystalline s.
soft tissue s.
s., tenderness, limitation of motion
without redness or s.

swimmer's
s. dermatitis
s. ear

swimming
s. injury
s. pool granuloma

swimming-related illness

swine
African swine fever virus

African swine pox
atrophic rhinitis of s.
s. dysentery
edema disease of s.
enterocytopathogenic swine orphan virus
s. flu vaccine
s. influenza
s. influenza strain
s. influenza virus
s. kidney
s. vesicular disease
s. vesicular disease virus
vesicular exanthema of swine virus

swine-associated mucoprotein

swinepox virus

swing light test

swing-out shoe

swings
irritability and mood s.

swing-through gait

swish
s. and spit
s. and swallow

Swiss
S. cheese defect
S. cheese hyperplasia
S. cheese interventricular septum
S. Webster mouse

Swiss-type agammaglobulinemia

switch
arterial switch operation
arterial switch procedure
atrial switch operation
atrial switch procedure
gain control s.
left foot s.
lineage switch leukemia
Mustard atrial switch procedure
right foot s.
silicon-controlled s.

switching
automatic mode s.

swollen
s. belly disease
s. belly syndrome
hot, swollen, and tender
inflamed swollen joint
s. joint count
joint swollen and inflamed
s. and painful joint
painful swollen gland
red, swollen, and itchy
red swollen joint
red, swollen, tender gums
severely swollen ankle
s., stiff, inflamed joint
s. and tender gums

Swyer syndrome

sycosis
lupoid s.
nonparasitic s.

Sydenham
S. chorea
S. disease

Sydney line

syllable
weak syllable deletion

sylvian
s. angle
s. approach
s. aqueduct
s. area
s. cistern
s. dissection
s. fissure
ischemic sylvian wave
s. line

sylvii
aqueductus s.

Sylvius
angle of S.
aqueduct of S.
cistern fossa of S.
fissure of S.
hydrocephalus due to congenital stenosis of aqueduct of S.

symblepharon
anterior s.
total s.

symbol
association of sounds and s.'s
digit s.
S. Digit Modalities Test
digit symbol substitutional test
homeopathic symbol for decimal scale of potencies
Kahn Test of S. Arrangement
picture s.'s
programmed s.'s
summation of all quantities following the s.

symbolic
memory for symbolic unit
S. Play Test
String-Oriented S. Language

symbolism
anagogic s.

symbologies
reduced space s.

Syme amputation

Symmers clay pipestem fibrosis

symmetric
acute symmetric polyarthritis
benign symmetric lipomatosis
bilateral s.
s. chest
s. consolidation
distal symmetric sensory neuropathy
distal symmetric sensory polyneuropathy
s. distribution
lipomatosis
progressive symmetric erythrokeratodermia
remitting seronegative symmetric synovitis with pitting edema
s. tonic neck reflex

symmetrical
bilateral, symmetrical, equal
s. brain
s. calcification of basal cerebral ganglion
diffuse symmetrical uterine enlargement
distal acquired demyelinating symmetrical neuropathy
distal symmetrical polyneuropathy
s. peripheral gangrene
s. sleep pattern
s. strength
s. tendon reflex
uterus symmetrical in contour

symmetry
detailed evaluation of facial s.
point of s.

sympathectomy
bilateral upper dorsal s.
chemical s.
peripheral chemical s.

sympathetic
s. activity
s. agent
alpha sympathetic blockade
s. autonomic nervous system
autonomic sympathetic ganglion
s. block
s. blockade
s. blockade anesthetic technique
s. block anesthesia
s. branch
s. branch to submandibular ganglion

sympathetic *(continued)*
cardiac sympathetic nerve
s. component
s. efferent nerve activity
efferent renal sympathetic nerve activity
efferent sympathetic activity
s. ganglion
s. ganglion block anesthetic technique
ganglion of sympathetic plexus
ganglion of sympathetic trunk
s. heterochromia
s. hypertonia
s. imbalance
s. inhibitor
intravenous regional sympathetic block
s. iritis
left cardiac sympathetic ganglionectomy
left sympathetic nerve
lumbar sympathetic block
lumbar sympathetic blockade
s. maintained plan
muscle sympathetic nerve activity
s. nerve
s. nerve block
s. nervous system
s. ophthalmia
s. orthostatic hypotension
s. plexus
s. preganglionic neuron
reflex sympathetic dystrophy
s. skin response
skin sympathetic activity
snooze-induced excitation of sympathetic triggered activity
s. uveitis

sympathetically
s. independent pain syndrome
s. mediated pain syndrome

sympathoadrenal system

sympathomimetic
s. agent
s. amine
amphetamine or similarly acting sympathomimetic intoxication
autonomic sympathomimetic drug
s. drug
intrinsic sympathomimetic activity
s. syndrome

sympathovagal imbalance

symphathectomy
endoscopic transthoracic s.

symphyseal bar

symphysis, pl. **symphyses**
s., buttocks, and xiphoid
s. mandibulae
mandibular s.
manubriosternal s.
osteitis symphysis pubis
pubic s.
ramus, body, symphysis, palate

symporter
sodium-iodide s.

symptom
Abbreviated Parent S. Questionnaire
s.'s of acute drug intoxication
additional qualifying s.'s
adjustment reaction physical s.
adolescent depression s.
affective symptom of seizure
alcohol-induced gastrointestinal s.
s. of apnea
array of s.'s
s. assessment
asthma symptom checklist
attention deficit s.
atypical factitious disorder with physical s.'s
AUA S. Index
Brief S. Inventory
S.'s Checklist 90 Revised
chronic factitious illness with physical s.'s
clearing of mental s.'s
clinical signs and s.'s
cluster of s.
comprehensive assessment of symptoms and history
Danish Prostate S. Score
dearth of s.'s
decreased signs and symptoms of anxiety
decreased signs and symptoms of depression
disease-related s.'s
disease-related symptom improvement
s. distress check list
S. Distress Scale
s. of drug abuse
dry eye s.
early identification of s.
Edmonton S. Assessment Scale
s. evaluation
extrapyramidal s.
extrapyramidal symptom rating scale
factitious disorder with physical s.'s
factitious illness with psychological s.'s
Fatigue S. Checklist
first rank s.
s. free
gastrointestinal s.
Gastrointestinal S. Rating Scale
Global Severity Index of Brief S. Inventory
s. grouping
hay fever s.'s
heart attack s.'s
s. of heartbeat
s.'s of heart failure
hemorrhagic fever with renal s.'s
history and symptoms of emergency cardiac care
Hopkins S. Checklist-90 Total Score
improved symptom relief
s.'s increased in severity
International Prostate S. Score
Low Back Pain S. Checklist
lower urinary tract s.
Lung Cancer S. Scale
s. magnification
major symptom complex
Memorial Symptom Assessment Scale-Physical
Memorial Symptom Assessment Scale-Psychological
Mood and Physical S.'s Scale
motor conversion s.
Multidimensional Fatigue S. Inventory
multiple occurrence of unexplained s.'s
National Institutes of Health Chronic Prostatitis S. Index
Nerve S. Score
neurovegetative functioning or s.
obstructive voiding s.
onset of s.'s
opiate withdrawal s.
overall depressive s.
overt symptom of heart disease
Pain Anxiety S.'s Scale
Parent S. Questionnaire
Pediatric S. Checklist
physical withdrawal s.'s
Positive S. Distress Index
positive symptom total
posttraumatic signs or s.'s
premenstrual s.'s
prevent withdrawal s.

s. problem index
progression of s.'s
quality-adjusted time without symptoms or toxicity
S. Rating Scale
S. Rating Test
respiratory s.
review of signs and s.'s
review of subjective s.'s
Rotterdam S. Check List
Scale for the Assessment of Negative S.'s
Scale for the Assessment of Positive S.'s
s. schedule for the diagnosis of borderline schizophrenia
schedule for negative s.'s
segmental bronchus s.
Separation Anxiety S. Inventory
severe debilitating s.
severe dissociative s.
s. severity index
signs and s.'s
sign symptom complex
Structured Interview of Reported s.'s
subtle and nonspecific s.
time without symptoms of progression or toxicity
total symptom complex
total vasomotor rhinitis symptom score
transient neurologic s.'s
Trauma S. Checklist for Children
treatment of emergent s.
Treatment Emergent S. Scale
Verdun Target S. Rating Scale
Wittenborn Psychiatric S.'s Inventory

symptomatic
s. alcohol heart muscle disease
s. asthma
s. coarctation of aorta
s. diffuse esophageal spasm
s. erythema
s. fever
s. fibroid
s. fistula
s. gallbladder disease
s. gallstone
s. headache
s. hearing loss
s. hemorrhage
s. HIV infection
s. hypertension
s. hypoglycemia
s. impotence
s. improvement
s. infection
not s.
patient s.
s. porphyria
primary symptomatic diffuse esophageal spasm
s. progression of disease
prolonged symptomatic illness
s. pruritus
s. purpura
s. treatment
s. urinary tract infection
s. uterine prolapse
Warfarin-Aspirin S. Intracranial Disease

symptomatically
patient symptomatically improved

symptomatology
increasing s.
neurologic s.

symptom-free
patient s.-f.
s.-f. walking distance

symptomless autoimmune thyroiditis

symptom-limited graded exercise test

symptomologic factor

synacthen
low-dose short synacthen test

synalbumin-insulin antagonism

synapse
autonomic ganglionic s.

synaptic
s. bouton
s. cleft
s. conduction
congenital paucity of secondary synaptic clefts syndrome
s. electronic activation
s. ending
evoked synaptic potential
hippocampal synaptic plasma membrane
s. level
s. membrane
s. plasma membrane
rat synaptic ending
s. transmission
s. vesicle

synaptosome

synchondrosis, pl. **synchondroses**
anterior intraoccipital s.
anterior synchondrosis intraoccipital
sphenooccipital s.

synchronization
vertical synchronization pulse

synchronized
ascending aorta synchronized pulsation
s. cardioversion
s. intermittent mandatory ventilation
s. nasal intermittent positive-pressure ventilation
s. sleep

synchronous
s. activity
s. adenoma
atrial synchronous pulse generator
atrial synchronous ventricular inhibited pacing
body acceleration synchronous with heart rate
s. colonic adenocarcinoma
continuous high-amplitude electroencephalogram rhythmical synchronous slowing
germ cell tumor with synchronous lesions in pineal and suprasellar region
s. ipsilateral breast cancer
multiple synchronous subcutaneous metastases
s. pacemaker
periodic synchronous discharge
ventricular synchronous pacing
s. with heartbeat

synchrony
arm heel-strike s.

synclonic spasm

syncopal
s. episode
s. migraine headache

syncope
cardiac obstruction in s.
cardioinhibitory s.
carotid sinus s.
cough s.
defecation s.
heat s.
hypoglycemic s.
hysterical s.
micturition s.
near s.
neurally mediated vasovagal s.
neurocardiogenic s.
neuromediated s.

syncope *(continued)*
noncardiac s.
orthostatic s.
situational s.
sneeze s.
stretching s.
s. of unknown origin
vasodepressor s.
vasomotor s.
vasovagal s.
vertigo, syncope and hypotension

syncytia (*pl. of* syncytium)

syncytial
antirespiratory syncytial virus
s. bud
s. cell
chick syncytial virus
human respiratory syncytial virus
s. knot
s. knot formation
respiratory syncytial virus
respiratory syncytial virus bronchiolitis
respiratory syncytial virus immune globulin
respiratory syncytial virus intravenous immunoglobulin
s. trophoblast

syncytiotrophoblast
malignant s.
s. microvillar plasma membrane

syncytiotrophoblastic giant cell

syncytiovascular membrane

syncytium, pl. **syncytia**
syncytia induction assay

syndactylism release

syndactyly
ectodermal dysplasia, cleft lip and palate, mental retardation, syndactyly syndrome I, II
mental retardation, polydactyly, phalangeal hypoplasia, syndactyly, unusual face, uncombable hair
microcephalus, imperforate anus, syndactyly, hamartoblastoma, abnormal lung lobulation, polydactyly
microphallus, imperforate anus, syndactyly, hamartoblastoma, abnormal lung

syndesmosis, pl. **syndesmoses**
tibiofibular s.

syndrome
Aarskog-Scott s.
abdominal compartment s.
ablepharon macrostomia s.
s. of absence of septum pellucidum with poerencephaly
acid aspiration s.
acquired cellular immunodeficiency s.
acquired hyperostosis s.
acquired immune deficiency s.
acquired immune deficiency syndrome-related complex
acquired immune deficiency syndrome-related dementia
acquired immune deficiency syndrome-related macular degeneration
acquired immune deficiency syndrome antibody
acquired immune deficiency syndrome antibody test
acquired immune deficiency syndrome carrier
acquired immune deficiency syndrome crisis
acquired immune deficiency syndrome dementia complex
acquired immune deficiency syndrome epidemic
acquired immune deficiency syndrome infected child
acquired immune deficiency syndrome mandatory testing
acquired immune deficiency syndrome prevention
acquired immune deficiency syndrome primary pathogen
acquired immune deficiency syndrome residential treatment facility
acquired immune deficiency syndrome tainted transfusion
acquired immune deficiency syndrome transmission
acquired immune deficiency syndrome treatment
acquired immune deficiency syndrome virus infection
acquired immunodeficiency s.
Acquired Immunodeficiency S. Beliefs and Behavior Questionnaire
acquired immunodeficiency syndrome health assessment questionnaire
acquired immunodeficiency syndrome with Kaposi sarcoma
acquired prothrombin complex deficiency s.
acquired violence immune deficiency s.
acrocallosal s.
acromegaloid facial s.
actinic reticuloid s.
acute aseptic meningitis s.
acute brain s.
acute cervical traumatic sprain or s.
acute chest s.
acute compartment s.
acute coronary s.
acute death s.
acute diarrheal s.
acute exertional compartment s.
acute hemolytic uremic s.
acute ischemic coronary s.
acute joint s.
acute low back s.
acute lumbar trauma s.
acute organic brain s.
acute posttraumatic stress s.
acute respiratory distress s.
acute retinal necrosis s.
acute retroviral s.
acute right heart s.
acute sickle chest s.
acute tumor lysis s.
acute urethral s.
acute viral s.
adrenal feminization s.
adrenal virilizing s.
adrenocortical atrophy-cerebral sclerosis s.
adrenocorticotropic hormone-dependent Cushing s.
adrenogenital s.
adult adrenogenital s.
adulterated rapeseed oil-associated toxic oil s.
adult-onset polyglandular s.
adult respiratory distress s.
adult Reye s.
advanced sleep-phase s.
affective disorder s.
afferent loop s.
age-dependent epilepsy s.
agenesis of corpus callosum-mental retardation-osseous lesions s.
aging brain s.
agonadism, mental retardation, short stature, retarded bone age s.
AIDS-related s.

AIDS wasting s.
air pollution s.
Alagille-Watson s.
alcohol abstinence s.
alcohol amnestic s.
alcohol dependence s.
alcoholic abstinence s.
alcoholic brain s.
alcoholic Korsakoff s.
alcoholic malabsorption s.
alcohol-induced organic mental s.
alcohol withdrawal s.
Alice in Wonderland s.
alien hand s.
Allen-Herndon-Dudley s.
allopurinol hypersensitivity s.
alopecia, contracture, dwarfism, mental retardation s.
alopecia, epilepsy, oligophrenia s.
alopecia, mental retardation, epilepsy, microcephaly s.
alveolar hypoventilation s.
Amish brittle hair s.
amniotic fluid infection s.
androgen insensitivity s.
androgen resistance s.
anencephaly-spina bifida s.
anger and violence psychiatric s.
angiotensin-converting enzyme dysfunction s.
angry back s.
angry woman s.
angular gyrus s.
aniridia, ambiguous genitalia, mental retardation triad s.
aniridia, cerebellar ataxia-oligophrenia s.
aniridia, Wilms tumor, gonadoblastoma s.
ankyloblepharon, ectodermal dysplasia, clefting s.
ankyloglossia superior s.
anomalous innominate artery compression s.
anomalous left coronary artery from pulmonary artery s.
anophthalmia, hand-foot defects-mental retardation s.
anophthalmic orbit s.
anophthalmos-limb anomalies s.
anosmia and hypogonadotropic hypogonadism s.
antenatal Bartter s.
anterior abdominal wall s.
anterior bulb s.
anterior cavernous sinus s.
anterior cervical cord s.
anterior chamber cleavage s.
anterior chamber dysgenesis s.
anterior chest wall s.
anterior cingulate prefrontal s.
anterior cleavage s.
anterior compartment s.
anterior cord s.
anterior cornual s.
anterior impingement s.
anterior interosseous nerve s.
anterior optic chiasmal s.
anterior rib impingement s.
anterior spinal artery s.
anterior spinal cord s.
anterior tarsal tunnel s.
anterior tibial compartment s.
anterior vermis s.
anterolateral impingement s.
anti-acquired immune deficiency syndrome vaccine
antiandrogen withdrawal s.
antibody deficiency s.
anticardiolipin antibody s.
anticonvulsant hypersensitivity s.
antiepileptic drug hypersensitivity s.
antimüllerian derivative s.
antiphospholipid antibody s.
anti-Sjögren syndrome A, B antibody
anular constricting band s.
anxiety-related psychiatric s.
aortic arch anomaly-peculiar facies mental retardation s.
aortic stenosis, corneal clouding, growth and mental retardation s.
aplastic abdominal muscle s.
aplastic anemia s.
apparent mineral corticoid excess s.
apparent mineralocorticoid excess s.
apple-peel bowel s.
approximate answers s.
s. of approximate relevant answers
apraxia-ataxia-mental deficiency s.
apraxia-oculomotor contracture-muscle atrophy s.
Argonz-Del Castillo s.
Arnold nerve reflex cough s.
arrhinia, choanal atresia, microphthalmia s.
arterial-ecchymotic type Ehlers-Danlos s.
arterial thoracic outlet s.
arteriomesenteric duodenal compression s.
arteriosclerotic brain s.
arteriovenous strabismus s.
arthritis-hives-angioedema s.
arthrochalasis multiplex congenita Ehlers-Danlos s.
arthrogryposis congenita, distal, type I, II s.
arthrogryposis, ectodermal dysplasia, cleft lip/palate developmental delay s.
arylsulfatase B s.
aseptic meningitis s.
asphyxiating thoracic dysplasia s.
aspirin-sensitive asthma s.
asplenia s.
association with hydrocephalus s.
asymmetric short stature s.
ataxia, myoclonic encephalopathy, macular degeneration, recurrent infections s.
atherosclerotic occlusive s.
athletic heart s.
atypical hemolytic uremia s.
atypical measles s.
atypical or mixed organic brain s.
atypical mole s.
auriculotemporal nerve s.
autism, dementia, ataxia, loss of purposeful hand use s.
autism-fragile X s.
autoerythrocyte sensitization s.
autoimmune deficiency s.
autoimmune lymphoproliferative s.
autoimmune paraneoplastic s.
autoimmune polyendocrine-candidiasis s.
autoimmune polyendocrine s.
autoimmune polyglandular s.
autonomic imbalance s.
autosomal dominant compelling helioophthalmic outburst s.
autosomal dominant macrocephaly s.
autosomal dominant Opitz s.
autosomal-dominant periodic fever s.
autosomal-recessive Alport s.
autosomal recessive ocular Ehlers-Danlos s.
autosomal recessive syndrome of encephalopathy
aviator's effort s.
AV strabismus s.

syndrome *(continued)*
axonopathic neurogenic thoracic outlet s.
Baller-Gerold s.
Bannayan-Riley-Ruvalcaba s.
Bannayan-Zonna s.
Bartter s.
basal cell nevus s.
bashful bladder s.
battered child s.
battered husband s.
battered woman s.
Behçet s.
benign breast s.
Bernard-Soulier s.
billowing mitral leaflet s.
binge eating s.
binge and purge s.
bioenergy imbalance s.
Birt-Hogg-Dubé s.
blepharophimosis, ptosis, epicanthus inversus s.
bloating and irritable bowel s.
blood product contaminated by acquired immune deficiency s.
Bloom s.
blue diaper s.
blue toe s.
bone cement implantation s.
borderline syndrome index
brachioskeletogenital s.
Brachmann-Cornelia de Lange s.
brachydactyly, mesomelia, mental retardation, aortic dilation, mitral valve prolapse, characteristic facies s.
bradycardia-tachycardia s.
branchiooculofacial s.
branchiootorenal s.
brittle hair, intellectual impairment, decreased fertility, short stature s.
bronchiolitis obliterans s.
brown bowel s.
Budd-Chiari s.
building illness s.
burning feet s.
burning mouth s.
calcification, Raynaud phenomenon, scleroderma, telangiectasis s.
calcinosis cutis, osteoma cutis, poikiloderma, and skeletal abnormalities s.
camptodactyly-arthropathy-pericarditis s.
camptomelic s.
cancer, anorexia, cachexia s.
cancer family s.
capillary leak s.
capsular thrombosis s.
carbohydrate-deficient glycoprotein syndrome
carbonless paper s.
carcinoid s.
cardiofaciocutaneous s.
cardiomyopathy and woolly haircoat s.
cardiorespiratory syndrome of obesity in child
cardiovascular dysmetabolic s.
carotid sinus s.
carotid steal s.
carpal tunnel s.
carrier of acquired immune deficiency s.
cataract, motor system disorder, short stature, learning difficulty, skeletal abnormalities s.
cat's eye s.
cauda equina s.
caudal appendage, short terminal phalanges, deafness, cryptorchidism, mental retardation s.
caudal dysplasia s.
caudal regression s.
celiac artery compression s.
cellular immunity deficiency s.
central alveolar hypoventilation s.
central anticholinergic s.
central cervical spinal cord s.
central sleep apnea s.
cerebral, ocular, dental, auricular, skeletal s.
cerebrocostomandibular s.
cerebrofacioarticular s.
cerebrohepatorenal s.
cerebrooculofacial-skeletal s.
cerebrooculomuscular s.
cervical disc s.
cervicobrachial s.
cervicooculoacusticus s.
Charcot-Marie-Tooth syndrome, X-linked type II with deafness and mental retardation
Charles Bonnet s.
cheirooral s.
chemical sensitivity s.
Chiari-Frommel s.
Chinese restaurant s.
Christ-Siemens-Touraine s.
chronic alcoholic brain s.
chronic anovulation s.
chronic anterior exertional compartment s.
chronic compartment s.
chronic fatigue immune deficiency s.
chronic fatigue and immune dysfunction s.
chronic heel pain s.
chronic hyperventilation s.
chronic idiopathic intestinal pseudo-obstruction s.
chronic infantile hypotonic s.
chronic itch-and-scratch s.
chronic itching s.'s
chronic muscle pain s.
chronic musculoskeletal pain s.
chronic myelodysplastic s.
chronic nervous exhaustion s.
chronic organic brain s.
chronic organic mental s.
chronic pelvic pain s.
chronic prostatitis/pelvic pain s.
cleft lip, cleft palate, lobster-claw deformity s.
cleft palate-lateral synechia s.
Clerc-Levy-Cristeco s.
click-murmur s.
climacteric s.
clinically isolated s.
clitoris tourniquet s.
clofibrate-induced muscular s.
closed head s.
cloudy-cornea s.
Cockayne s.
cold agglutinin s.
Collet-Sicard s.
coloboma, heart anomaly, ichthyosis, mental retardation, and ear abnormality s.
coloboma, heart disease, atresia choanae, retarded growth and retarded development and/or CNS anomalies, genital hypoplasia, and ear anomalies and/or deafness s.
combined immunodeficiency s.
community-acquired immunodeficiency s.
compensatory antiinflammatory response s.
complete androgen insensitivity s.
complex regional pain s.
compression s.
computer vision s.
concentration-camp s.
confused language s.
congenital alcoholic s.

congenital asplenia s.
congenital cataracts, sensorineural deafness, Down syndrome facial appearance, short stature, mental retardation syndrome
congenital central hypoventilation s.
congenital emphysema, cryptorchidism, penoscrotal web, deafness, mental retardation s.
congenital hemidysplasia with ichthyosiform erythroderma and limb defects s.
congenital high airway obstruction s.
congenital nephrotic s.
congenital paucity of secondary synaptic clefts s.
congenital rubella s.
congenital thrombocytopenia, Robin sequence, agenesis of corpus callosum, distinctive facies, developmental delay s.
congenital vascular-bone s.
congenital versus acquired s.
congenital vs. acquired s.
conotruncal anomaly face s.
contact urticaria s.
contagious suicide s.
contaminated small bowel s.
continual skin peeling s.
controlled release infusion s.
Cornelia de Lange s.
coronary insufficiency s.
coronary slow flow s.
coronary steal s.
coronary-subclavian steal s.
corpus luteum deficiency s.
costoclavicular s.
costovertebral segmentation defect with mesomelia s.
crack baby s.
craniofacial dysmorphism, absent corpus callosum, iris colobomas, connective tissue dysplasia s.
craniofrontonasal s.
craniosynostosis, ataxia, trigeminal anesthesia, parietal anesthesia and pons, vermis fusion s.
creepy-crawly syndrome of legs
cricopharyngeal achalasia s.
cri du chat s.
Crigler-Najjar s.
crush s.
crush fracture s.
crush injury s.
Cruveilhier-Baumgarten s.
crying cat s.
cubital tunnel s.
culture-bound s.
curly hair-ankyloblepharon-nail dysplasia s.
Cushing virilizing s.
cyclic vomiting s.
damaged disc s.
Dandy-Walker s.
dead-in-bed s.
deafness, femoral epiphysial dysplasia, short stature, developmental delay s.
deafness, onychoosteodystrophy, and mental retardation s.
delayed anovulatory s.
delayed microembolism s.
delayed pulmonary toxicity s.
delayed sleep phase s.
dementia syndrome of depression
dengue hemorrhagic fever shock s.
dental distress s.
dental enamel dysplasia s.
Denys-Drash s.
deprivation s.
de Quervain s.
developmental Gerstmann s.
diabetic foot s.
dialysis disequilibrium s.
dialysis encephalopathy s.
diarrhea from toxic shock s.
diencephalic s.
diffuse infiltrative lymphocytosis s.
diffuse obstructive pulmonary s.
diffuse unilateral subacute neuroretinitis "wipe-out" s.
DiGeorge s.
digital anomalies, short palpebral fissures, atresia of esophagus or duodenum s.
digitorenocerebral s.
disequilibrium s.
dislocated elbow, bowed tibiae, scoliosis, deafness, cataract, microcephaly, mental retardation s.
disseminated intravascular coagulation s.
distal arthrogryposis, hypopituitarism, mental retardation, facial anomalies s.
distal ileal obstruction s.
distal intestinal obstruction s.
disturbance of function occlusion s.
dorsal wrist s.
Down syndrome child
drowned newborn s.
drug-induced delayed multiorgan hypersensitivity s.
drug-induced lupus s.
Duane syndrome retraction
dumping s.
Dyke Davidoff-Masson s.
dysarthria-clumsy hand s.
dysequilibrium s.
dysesthetic pain s.
dyskinetic cilia s.
dysmyelopoietic s.
dysplastic nevus s.
early onset Parkinsonism-mental retardation s.
early ventricular repolarization s.
ear, patella, short stature s.
ectodermal dysplasia, cleft lip and palate, mental retardation, syndactyly syndrome I, II
ectodermal dysplasia, ectrodactyly, macular dystrophy s.
ectopic ACTH s.
ectopic Cushing s.
ectrodactyly-cleft palate s.
ectrodactyly, ectodermal dysplasia, clefting s.
efferent loop s.
egg drop s.
Ehlers-Danlos s.
Eisenmenger s.
electroshock-induced psychotic s.
Elejalde s.
elfin facies hypercalcemia s.
Ellis-van Creveld s.
embryofetal alcohol s.
emotional effects of acquired immune deficiency s.
empty sella turcica s.
endovascular hemolytic-uremic s.
enlarged vestibular aqueduct s.
eosinophilia-myalgia s.
epibronchial right pulmonary artery s.
epigastric distress s.
epileptic s.
Erb-Charcot s.
Erb-Goldflam s.
euthyroid sick s.
excessive lateral pressure s.
excited skin s.
exercise-induced respiratory distress s.
exertional anterior compartment s.

syndrome *(continued)*
exertional deep posterior compartment s.
exfoliation s.
exfoliation syndrome glaucoma
exhaustion s.
exophthalmos, myxedema circumscriptum praetibiale, and osteoarthropathia hypertrophicans s.
extended lymphadenopathy s.
extrapyramidal s.
facial dysplasia, hyperextensibility of joints, clinodactyly, growth retardation, mental retardation s.
failed back surgery s.
failed back syndrome with documented pseudarthrosis
failing ovary s.
familial advanced sleep-phase s.
familial atypical multiple-mole melanoma s.
familial dysplastic nevus s.
fat embolism s.
fatty liver and kidney s.
feline urologic s.
female pseudo-Turner s.
feminizing testis s.
femoral hypoplasia unusual facies s.
femur-fibula-ulna s.
fetal alcohol s.
fetal gigantism-renal hamartoma-nephroblastomatosis s.
fetal hydantoin s.
fetal tobacco s.
fetal valproate s.
fetal varicella s.
fetal warfarin s.
fibromyalgia s.
fidgety leg s.
first-use s.
fissured tongue s.
flat back s.
floating harbor s.
floppy infant s.
fluid retention s.
focal dermal hypoplasia s.
foot compartment s.
fragile X s.
frequently relapsing nephrotic s.
functional bowel s.
galactorrhea-amenorrhea hyperprolactinemia s.
Galloway-Mowat s.
general adaptation s.
generalized lymphadenopathy s.
s. of generalized thyroid hormone resistance
genital neoplasm-papilloma s.
genitoanorectal s.
Gerstmann-Straüssler-Scheinker s.
Gilles de la Tourette s.
gingival fibromatosis, hypertrichosis, cherubism, mental retardation, epilepsy s.
gloves and socks s.
Golabi-Rosen s.
Goldberg-Maxwell-Morris s.
gonadal agenesis s.
gonadal dysgenesis s.
gonadal failure, short stature, mitral valve prolapse, mental retardation s.
gonadotrophin-resistant ovary s.
gonococcal arthritis/dermatitis s.
gray baby s.
gray platelet s.
Greig cephalopolysyndactyly s.
Griscelli s.
growth retardation, alopecia, pseudoanodontia, and optic atrophy s.
Guérin-Stern s.
Guillain-Barré s.
Gulf War s.
gynecological chylous reflux s.
Hamman-Rich s.
hammertoe s.
hand-foot s.
hand-foot-genital s.
hantavirus cardiopulmonary s.
hantavirus pulmonary s.
Haw River s.
headache, insomnia, and depression s.
head trauma s.
heat illness s.
heel spur s.
hemangioma-thrombocytopenia s.
hematuria-dysuria s.
hemiconvulsion-hemiplegia-epilepsy s.
hemihypertrophy, intestinal web, preauricular skin tag, and congenital corneal opacity s.
hemolytic uremic s.
hemophagocytic s.
hemorrhagic fever with renal s.
hemorrhagic shock-encephalopathy s.
hemorrhagic shock s.
heparin-induced thrombosis-thrombocytopenia s.
hepatopulmonary s.
hepatorenal s.
hereditary flat adenoma s.
hereditary hemolytic s.
hereditary hypophosphatemic rickets with hypercalciuria s.
hereditary onychoosteodysplasia s.
herniated disc s.
herniated disc s.
high-altitude hypertrophic cardiomyopathy s.
high-pressure neurologic s.
hirsutism, androgen excess, insulin resistance, acanthosis nigricans s.
holiday heart s.
hot reactor s.
Hoyeraal-Hreidarsson s.
hydrocephalus, agyria, retinal dysplasia with or without encephalocele s.
hyperactive malarial splenomegaly s.
hyperandrogenism, insulin resistance, and acanthosis nigricans s.
hypercalcemia-osteolysis-T-cell s.
hypereosinophilic s.
hyperglycemic hyperosmolar nonketotic s.
hyper-IgM s.
hyperimmunoglobulin E s.
hyperimmunoglobulinemia s.
hyperimmunoglobulinemia D s.
hyperkinesis s.
hyperkinetic behavior s.
hyperkinetic heart s.
hyperkinetic syndrome of childhood
hyperlucent lung s.
hypermobility s.
hyperosmolar hyperglycemic nonketotic s.
hypersensitive carotid sinus s.
hyperstimulation s.
hypertelorism-microtia-clefting s.
hyperventilation s.
hyperviscosity s.
hypocomplementemic urticarial vasculitis s.
hypocomplementemic vasculitis urticaria s.
hypogonadotropic hypogonadism-anosmia s.
hypoparathyroidism, Addison disease, and mucocutaneous candidiasis s.

hypoparathyroidism, adrenal insufficiency, mucocutaneous candidiasis s.
hypoplastic left heart s.
hypoplastic left ventricular s.
hypoplastic lung s.
hypoplastic right heart s.
s. of hyporeninemic hypoaldosteronism
hypothalamic pubertal s.
hypothenar hammer s.
hypotonia, hypomentia, hypogonadism, and obesity s.
ichthyosis, brittle hair, impaired intelligence, decreased fertility, short stature s.
ichthyosis-cheek-eyebrow syndrome
ichthyosis, follicularis, atrichia or alopecia, photophobia s.
idiopathic carpal tunnel s.
idiopathic hypereosinophilic s.
idiopathic hyperkinetic heart s.
idiopathic long Q-T interval s.
idiopathic lymphadenopathy s.
idiopathic minimal lesion nephrotic s.
idiopathic nephrotic s.
idiopathic orbital inflammatory s.
idiopathic postprandial s.
idiopathic respiratory distress s.
iliotibial band friction s.
iliotibial tract friction s.
immotile cilia s.
immunodeficiency, centromeric instability, facial anomalies s.
impaired regeneration s.
s. of inappropriate antidiuresis
s. of inappropriate antidiuretic hormone
inappropriate antidiuretic hormone s.
s. of inappropriate antidiuretic hormone secretion
s. of inappropriate secretion of antidiuretic hormone
incomplete testicular feminization s.
indirect optic nerve injury s.
infant apnea s.
infantile bilateral striatal necrosis s.
infantile nephrotic s.
infantile Refsum s.
infant respiratory distress s.
infection-associated hemophagocytic s.
inflammatory bowel s.
infrapatellar contracture s.
inspissated bile s.
insulin-resistance s.
insulin-resistant diabetes, acanthosis nigricans, hypogonadism pigmentary retinopathy, deafness, mental retardation s.
intermediate coronary artery s.
intraamniotic infection s.
intraepithelial dyskeratosis syndrome, hereditary benign
intravascular coagulation and fibrinolysis s.
iridocorneal endothelial syndrome
irritable bowel syndrome with constipation
irritable colon s.
irritable stomach s.
irritable voiding s.
Irvine s.
s. of isolated diastolic dysfunction
isolated follicle-stimulating hormone deficiency s.
Jackson-Weiss s.
jugular foramen s.
juvenile polyposis s.
juvenile tropical pancreatitis s.
Kabuki makeup s.
kinky hair s.
kwashiorkor-marasmus s.
lacunar s.
Lambert-Eaton myasthenic s.
Landry-Guillain-Barré s.
late dumping s.
lateral facet s.
lateral hypothalamic s.
lateral medullary s.
lateral recess s.
late respiratory systemic s.
later onset nephrotic s.
Laurence-Moon-Biedl s.
Laurence-Moon-Biedl-Bardet s.
laxative abuse s.
lazy leukocyte s.
lentigines, electrocardiographic abnormalities, ocular hypertelorism, pulmonary stenosis, abnormalities of genitalia, retardation of growth, deafness s.
lexical-syntactic s.
lichen planus overlap s.
lid imbrication s.
Li-Fraumeni familial cancer s.
limb abnormality s.
limb-girdle s.
s. of limited joint mobility
limp infant s.
linear sebaceous nevus s.
lipodystrophy-acromegaloid gigantism s.
lip pseudocleft-hemangiomatous branchial cyst s.
local adaptation s.
locked-in s.
loin pain hematuria s.
long face s.
loose anagen hair s.
low back s.
low cardiac output s.
Lowe oculocerebrorenal s.
low natural killer s.
Lown-Ganong-Levine s.
Lowry-Wood s.
low T3 s.
lumbar disc s.
lumbar flat back s.
lumboradicular s.
lumpy jaw s.
lupus anticoagulant s.
lupus obstetric s.
lupus-scleroderma overlap s.
luteinized unruptured follicle s.
Luys body s.
lymphadenopathy s.
lymphoma syndrome leukemia
Lynch cancer family syndrome I, II
lysine malabsorption s.
macrocephaly, facial abnormalities, disproportionate tall stature mental retardation s.
macrocephaly, hypertelorism, short limbs, hearing loss, developmental delay s.
macrocephaly, multiple lipomas, hemangiomata s.
macrocephaly, pseudoepithelioma, multiple hemangiomas s.
macronutrient deficiency s.
macroorchidism marker X s.
macrophage activation s.
macrosomia-mental retardation s.
macrosomia, obesity, macrocephaly, ocular abnormality s.
macular ocular histoplasmosis s.
Mad Hatter s.
Maestre de San Juan-Kallmann-de Morsier s.
Maestre-Kallmann-de Morsier s.

syndrome *(continued)*
magnesium deficiency infantile tremor s.
male climacteric s.
male Turner s.
malignant B-cell s.
malignant carcinoid s.
malignant external otitis s.
malignant hyperthermia s.
malignant mole s.
malignant neuroleptic s.
Mallory-Weiss s.
mandatory acquired immune deficiency syndrome testing
mandibular pain dysfunction s.
mandibulofacial dysostosis with epibulbar dermoids s.
mandibulofacial dysostosis with limb malformations s.
mandibulofacial dysotosis s.
mangled extremity syndrome index
Marcus Gunn jaw-winking s.
Marden-Walker s.
marfanoid craniosynostosis s.
marfanoid habitus-mental retardation s.
marfanoid habitus-microcephaly-glomerulonephritis s.
marfanoid hypermobility s.
marfanoid hypermobility s.
Marin Amat s.
marker X s.
Maroteaux-Lamy s.
marrow failure s.
Martin-Albright s.
Martin-Bell s.
Martorell aortic arch s.
massive bowel resection s.
mastitis, metritis, agalactia s.
maternal Bernard-Soulier s.
maternal deprivation s.
maternal hydrops s.
Meckel s.
meconium aspiration s.
meconium blockage s.
meconium plug s.
medial frontal lobe s.
medial snapping hip s.
medial tibial stress s.
median cleft face s.
median cleft upper lip, mental retardation, pugilistic facies s.
median face s.
median facial cleft s.
medication-induced depressive s.
medication rebound s.
megacystic microcolon s.
megacystis-microcolon-intestinal hypoperistalsis s.
megalocornea, developmental retardation, dysmorphic s.
megalocornea-mental retardation s.
megalocystis microcolon intestinal hypoperistalsis s.
Mengert shock s.
meningitis or encephalitis, metabolic, Reye s.
Menkes kinky hair s.
menopausal s.
menstrual toxic shock s.
mental deficiency, spasticity, congenital ichthyosis s.
mental and growth retardation-amblyopia s.
mental and physical retardation, speech disorders, peculiar facies s.
mental retardation-absent nails of hallux and pollex s.
mental retardation-adducted thumbs s.
mental retardation, ataxia, hypotonia, hypogonadism, retinal dystrophy s.
mental retardation, blepharonasofacial abnormalities, hand malformations s.
mental retardation-clasped thumb s.
mental retardation, coarse face, microcephaly, epilepsy, skeletal abnormalities s.
mental retardation, coarse facies, epilepsy, joint contracture s.
mental retardation, congenital contracture, low fingertip arches s.
mental retardation-distal arthrogryposis s.
mental retardation, dysmorphism, cerebral atrophy s.
mental retardation, dystonic movements, ataxia, seizures s.
mental retardation, epilepsy, short stature, skeletal dysplasia s.
mental retardation, facial anomalies, hypopituitarism, distal arthrogryposis s.
mental retardation, gynecomastia, obesity s.
mental retardation, hearing impairment, distinct facies, skeletal anomalies s.
mental retardation, macroorchidism s.
mental retardation, microcephaly, blepharochalasis s.
mental retardation, mitral valve prolapse, characteristic face s.
mental retardation, optic atrophy, deafness, seizures s.
mental retardation-overgrowth s.
mental retardation, pre-and postnatal overgrowth, remarkable face, acanthosis nigricans s.
mental retardation-psoriasis s.
mental retardation, retinopathy, microcephaly s.
mental retardation, scapuloperoneal muscular dystrophy, lethal cardiomyopathy s.
mental retardation, short stature, hypertelorism s.
mental retardation, short stature, obesity, hypogonadism s.
mental retardation, skeletal dysplasia, abducens palsy s.
mental retardation-sparse hair s.
mental retardation, spasticity, distal transverse limb defects s.
mental retardation, spastic paraplegia, palmoplantar hyperkeratosis s.
mental retardation-spastic paraplegia s.
mental retardation, typical facies, aortic stenosis s.
mesenteric artery s.
mesomelic dwarfism-small genitalia s.
metabolic acidosis s.
metabolic syndrome cataract
metabolic syndrome X
metastatic carcinoid s.
methionine malabsorption s.
Meyer-Schwickerath and Weyers s.
Michelin tire baby s.
Mickety-Wilson s.
microangiopathic hemolytic uremic s.
microcephalic primordial dwarfism-cataracts s.
microcephaly-calcification of cerebral white matter s.
microcephaly-digital anomalies s.
microcephaly, hiatus hernia, nephrotic s.
microcephaly, hypergonadotropic hypogonadism, short stature s.

microcephaly, infantile spasm, psychomotor retardation, nephrotic s.
microcephaly, mental retardation, cataract, hypogonadism s.
microcephaly, mental retardation, retinopathy s.
microcephaly, mesobrachyphalangy, tracheoesophageal fistula s.
microcephaly, microphthalmia, ectrodactyly, prognathism s.
microcephaly, mild developmental delay, short stature, distinctive face s.
microcephaly, mild mental retardation, short stature, skeletal anomalies s.
microcephaly, muscular build, rhizomelia-cataracts s.
microcephaly, oculodigital, esophageal, duodenal s.
microcephaly, sparse hair, mental retardation, seizures s.
microcephaly-spastic diplegia s.
microdontia-microcephaly-short stature s.
microphthalmia, dermal aplasia, sclerocornea s.
microphthalmia-mental deficiency s.
micropolycystic ovary s.
microscopic colitis s.
microtia-absent patellae-micrognathia s.
microvascular compression s.
middle aortic s.
middle cerebral artery s.
middle fossa s.
middle lobe s.
midface hypoplasia s.
midline cleft s.
Milch fracture classification s.
Miles-Carpenter s.
milk alkali s.
milk drinker's s.
Miller-Dieker lissencephaly s.
Miller Fisher s.
Milwaukee knee s.
Milwaukee shoulder s.
minimal brain dysfunction s.
minimal change idiopathic nephrotic s.
minimal change nephrotic s.
minimal lesion nephrotic s.
Minot-von Willebrand s.
misery perfusion s.
Mitis-type Ehlers-Danlos s.
mitochondrial DNA s.
mitral leaflet s.
mitral valve prolapse, aortic anomalies, skeletal changes, and skin changes s.
mixed antiinflammatory s.
mixed cord s.
mixed cryoglobulin s.
mixed sclerosing bone dysplasia, small stature, seizures, mental retardation s.
modified varicella-like s.
Moersch-Woltman s.
Mohr-Tranebjaerg s.
monoclonal lymphoproliferative s.
monofixation s.
monosomy G s.
monosomy 7 s.
Montreal platelet s.
morning glory s.
mosaic tetrasomy 8p s.
mosaic Turner s.
mother infected with acquired immune deficiency s.
moving toes, painful leg s.
Moynahan alopecia s.
mucocutaneous lymph node s.
mucocutaneous ocular s.
mucosal neuroma s.
Muir-Torre syndrome of hereditary nonpolyposis colon cancer
müllerian duct derivation s.
müllerian duct s.
müllerian, renal, cervicothoracic, somite abnormalities s.
multiorgan dysfunction s.
multiple basal cell carcinoma syndrome multiple basal cell nevus syndrome
multiple basal cell neuroma s.
multiple basal cell nevoid s.
multiple chemical sensitivity s.
multiple cholesterol emboli s.
multiple congenital anomalies/mental retardation s.
multiple endocrine deficiency, Addison disease, and candidiasis s.
multiple endocrine neoplasia syndrome, type 1, 2A, 2B, 3
multiple epiphysial dysplasia-early onset diabetes mellitus s.
multiple epiphysial dysplasia tarda s.
multiple evanescent white dot s.
multiple exostoses-mental retardation s.
multiple exostosis mental retardation s.
multiple glandular deficiency s.
multiple hamartoma s.
multiple lentigines s.
multiple mucosal neuroma s.
multiple nevoid-basal cell carcinoma s.
multiple nevoid, basal cell epithelioma, jaw cysts, bifid rib s.
multiple organ dysfunction s.
multiple organ failure s.
multiple organ malrotation s.
multiple pterygium s.
multiple sulfatase deficiency s.
multiple synostoses s.
multiple X s.
Münchausen by proxy s.
Münchausen syndrome by proxy
murine-acquired immunodeficiency s.
muscle atrophy-contracture-oculomuscle apraxia s.
muscle-eye-brain s.
muscle pain, allergy, tachycardia and tiredness, headache s.
muscular hypertrophy s.
muscular pain-fasciculation s.
musculoskeletal pain s.
musician's overuse s.
myasthenia gravis s.
myasthenic syndrome of Eaton-Lambert
mycosis fungoides/Sézary s.
myelodysplastic s.
myocardial ischemic s.
myocardial steal s.
myoclonic alien hand s.
myoclonic encephalopathy s.
myofascial pain-dysfunction s.
myonephropathic metabolic s.
myopathic limb-girdle s.
myopathy-lactic acidosis-sideroblastic anemia s.
myxedema-myotonic dystrophy s.
Nager-de Reynier s.
nail patella s.
Nance-Horan s.
nanism-constrictive pericarditis s.
narcolepsy cataplexy s.
narcotic bowel s.
narcotic withdrawal s.
nasal hypoplasia, peripheral dysostosis, mental retardation s.

syndrome *(continued)*
Navajo brainstem s.
naviculocapitate fracture s.
near-miss sudden infant death s.
neonatal air leak s.
neonatal Bartter s.
neonatal Guillain-Barré s.
neonatal hepatitis s.
neonatal lupus s.
neonatal Marfan s.
neonatal myasthenic s.
neonatal narcotic abstinence s.
neonatal pseudohydrocephalic progeroid s.
neonatal respiratory distress s.
neonatal small left colon s.
nephrosis, microcephaly, hiatus hernia s.
nephrosis-neuronal dysmigration s.
nephrotic s.
Neri-Barré s.
nerve compression-degeneration s.
nerve compression s.
nerve entrapment s.
nerve root s.
Netherton s.
Neu-Laxova s.
neural crest s.
neuroallergic s.
neurocutaneous melanosis s.
neurofacial-digitorenal s.
neurofibromatosis-Noonan s.
neurofibromatosis, type 1 s.
neuroleptic malignant s.
neurological disease s.
neurologic paraneoplastic s.
neuropsychiatric acquired immunodeficiency syndrome rating scale
neuropsychiatric syndrome of systemic lupus erythematosus
neurovascular compression s.
nevi, atrial myxoma, myxoid neurofibroma, and ephelides s.
nevoid basal cell carcinoma s.
nevoid basal cell epithelioma, jaw cysts, bifid rib s.
newborn respiratory distress s.
night eating s.
Nijmegen breakage s.
nocturnal drinking s.
nocturnal eating s.
nodules, eosinophilia, rheumatism, dermatitis, and swelling s.
nonallergic rhinitis with eosinophilia s.
nonketotic hyperosmolar s.
nonmenstrual toxic shock s.
nonneoplastic s.
nonprogressive hypoplastic s.
nonprogressive motor impairment s.
nonsalt-losing adrenogenital s.
nonthyroidal illness s.
Noonan s.
Noonan-like giant cell lesion s.
Norman-Roberts lissencephaly s.
numb cheek s.
numb chin s.
nutritional deprivation s.
Nyhan-Lesch s.
nystagmus blockage s.
obesity hypoventilation s.
obesity, short stature, mental deficiency, hypogonadism, micropenis, finger contracture, cleft lip-palate s.
obesity/type 2 diabetes s.
obstruction of s.
obstructive sleep apnea s.
obstructive sleep apnea-hypopnea s.
occipital condyle s.
occipital horn s.
occupational maladjustment s.
occupational stress s.
ocular coloboma-imperforate anus s.
ocular histoplasmosis s.
ocular hypoperfusion s.
ocular ischemic s.
ocular motor s.
ocular-mucous membrane s.
ocular-scoliotic type Ehlers-Danlos s.
oculocerebral hypopigmentation s.
oculocerebral syndrome of Cross and McKusick
oculocerebrorenal s.
oculomucous membrane s.
oculopalatal myoclonus s.
oculopalatocerebral s.
odontogenic keratocytosis-skeletal anomalies s.
Oestreicher-Turner s.
OFD syndrome, type I–IV, VI–IX
Ohdo blepharophimosis s.
oil-associated pneumoparalytic eosinophilic s.
olfactory reference s.
oligoasthenoteratozoospermia s.
oligomenorrheic polycystic ovary s.
Omenn s.
omphalocele-cleft palate s.
Ondine curse s.
one hand-two foot s.
onychodystrophy-congenital deafness s.
ophthalmoplegia-hypotonia-ataxia-hypacusis-athetosis s.
opiate abstinence s.
opiate withdrawal s.
Opitz BBB s.
opsoclonus-myoclonus s.
optic atrophy-ataxia s.
optic chiasmal s.
optic tract s.
oral allergy s.
oral-facial-digital s.
orbital apex s.
orbital compartment s.
orbital floor s.
orbit, mandible, ear, cranial nerves, soft tissue s.
organic affective s.
organic amnestic s.
organic anxiety s.
organic brain syndrome with hallucinogen
organic delusional s.
organic dust toxic s.
organic hallucinosis s.
organic hyperkinetic s.
organic mental s.
organic mood s.
organic personality s.
Oriental nocturnal death s.
orofacial dysfunction s.
orofaciodigital s.
Osler syndrome II
Osler-Weber-Rendu s.
osmotic demyelination s.
osteogenesis imperfecta congenita s.
osteogenesis imperfecta, optic atrophy, retinopathy, developmental delay s.
osteogenesis imperfecta s.
osteoporosis-pseudoglioma s.
Ostrum-Furst s.
Ota nevus s.
otomandibular s.
otopalatodigital s.
ovarian dysgenesis-sensorineural deafness s.
ovarian hyperstimulation s.
overuse s.
overwear s.
pacemaker s.

pachyonychia congenita syndrome of nail
Paget abscess s.
Paget-von Schroetter s.
pain dysfunction s.
painful arc s.
painful articular s.
painful bruising s.
painful heel s.
painful shoulder s.
Pallister mosaic s.
palmar fasciitis and polyarthritis s.
palmar-plantar erythrodysesthesia s.
palmoplantar erythrodysesthesia s.
Pancoast superior sulcus s.
pancreatic cholera s.
pancreatic insufficiency s.
papular-purpuric gloves and socks s.
papulovesicular acrolocated s.
paramedian clefting s.
paraneoplastic antiphospholipid s.
paraneoplastic neurologic s.
paranoia and delusions psychiatric s.
parathyroid hormone resistance s.
parietal foramina, brachymicrocephaly, mental retardation s.
Parinaud oculoglandular s.
partial androgen insensitivity s.
partial anterior circulation s.
partial form of DiGeorge s.
partially unexplained sudden infant death s.
Partington s.
patellar clunk s.
patellar femoral s.
patellofemoral joint s.
patellofemoral pain s.
patient unknown acquired immune deficiency syndrome carrier
4p deletion s.
Pearson marrow-pancreas s.
pediatric acquired immunodeficiency s.
pelvic congestion s.
pelvic floor s.
Pendred s.
Pendred syndrome gene
penis at twelve s.
pentalogy of Cantrell s.
pericardial constriction-growth failure s.
pericolic membrane s.
perilymphatic fistula s.
perimenstrual s.
periodic fever s.
periodontitis Ehlers-Danlos s.
peripheral dysostosis, nail hypoplasia, mental retardation s.
peripheral nerve root s.
pernicious anemia-like syndrome and immunoglobulin deficiency
peroneal compartment s.
Persian Gulf s.
persistent müllerian duct s.
persistent viral s.
persisting galactorrhea-amenorrhea s.
Pettigrew s.
Peutz-Jeghers s.
phantom limb s.
pharmacogenic confusional s.
pheochromocytoma, thyroid carcinoma s.
phonologic programming deficit s.
pigment dispersion s.
pineal gonadal s.
Pitt-Rogers-Danks s.
plantar fascia s.
plantar fasciitis s.
polycystic ovarian s.
polydactyly, imperforate anus, vertebral anomalies s.
polyglandular autoimmune syndrome type I, II
polymyalgia rheumatica s.
polyneuropathy, organomegaly, endocrinopathy, monoclonal gammopathy, and skin changes s.
polyneuropathy, organomegaly, endocrinopathy, M protein, and skin changes s.
Porak-Durante s.
porcine stress s.
Positive and Negative S. Scale
postaxial acrofacial dysostosis s.
postcardiac injury s.
postcardiotomy s.
postcholecystectomy s.
postconcussion s.
posterior circulation s.
post-head injury s.
postmalarial neurological s.
postmastectomy pain s.
postmaturity s.
postmenopausal s.
postmyocardial infarction s.
postnasal drainage s.
postnasal drip s.
postneonatal mortality s.
postperfusion s.
postpericardiotomy s.
postphlebitic s.
postpolio atrophy s.
postpoliomyelitis s.
postpump s.
postsurgical gastroparesis s.
postthrombophlebitis s.
postthrombotic s.
posttraumatic brain s.
posttraumatic fibromyalgia s.
posttraumatic hyperirritability s.
postural orthostatic tachycardia s.
post-Vietnam psychiatric s.
postviral fatigue s.
pre-acquired immune deficiency s.
preexcitation s.
preleukemic s.
premenstrual dysphoric s.
premenstrual tension s.
presumed ocular histoplasmosis s.
Prieto s.
primary acquired preleukemic s.
s. of primary aldosteronism
primary antiphospholipid antibody s.
primary empty sella syndrome
primary fibromyalgia s.
primary immunodeficiency s.
primary myelodysplastic s.
primary Sjögren s.
prison-acquired lymphoproliferative s.
prolapsed mitral valve s.
prolapse gastropathy s.
prolonged QT s.
Proteus s.
prune belly s.
pseudoachievement s.
pseudoexfoliation s.
pseudolupus erythematosus s.
pseudopresumed ocular histoplasmosis s.
pseudo-renal artery s.
pseudotumor cerebri s.
pseudo-Zollinger-Ellison s.
psychoorganic s.
psychosis, intermittent hyponatremia, polydipsia s.
psychotic brain s.
pterygopalatine fossa s.
pure sensory s.
purple urine bag s.
qigong deviation s.
quasimorphine withdrawal s.
Ramsay Hunt s.

syndrome *(continued)*
Raynaud s.
reactive upper airways dysfunction s.
recessive epidermolysis bullosa dystrophica–Hallopeau-Siemens s.
reciprocal hindlimb-scratching syndrome
recognizable viral s.
recurrent abdominal pain s.
recurrent erosion s.
red-man s.
redundant cusp s.
refeeding s.
renal-anal-lung-polydactyly-hamartoblastoma s.
Rénon-Delille s.
repetitive motion s.
repetitive stress s.
respiratory distress s.
restless leg s.
retained gastric antrum s.
retropatellar pain s.
reversible posterior leukoencephalopathy s.
Reye s.
rheumatoid arthritis and Sjögren s.
Richner-Hanhart s.
right middle lobe s.
rigid-man s.
Roberts s.
Rokitansky-Kuster-Hauser s.
Rolland-Desbuquois s.
Rosenthal-Melkersson s.
rostral basilar artery s.
rotator cuff impingement s.
Rothmann-Makai s.
rumination s.
Ruvalcaba-Myhre-Smith s.
salt depletion s.
salt-losing adrenogenital s.
Sanchez-Cascos cardioauditory s.
scalded mouth s.
scalded skin s.
scalenus anticus s.
Schinzel-Giedion s.
sciatic nerve s.
scleroderma-like s.
seasonal affective disorder s.
secondary myelodysplastic s.
secondary Sjögren s.
secretion and spill from acquired immune deficiency s.
segmental colonic adenomatous polyposis s.
sensory deprivation s.
septic shock s.
septum pellucidum absent with porencephalia s.
serotonin s.
severe combined immune deficiency s.
severe invasion streptococcal s.
severe ovarian hyperstimulation s.
Sézary s.
shaken baby s.
short bowel s.
short gut s.
short rib-polydactyly s.
shoulder-hand s.
shrinking lungs s.
sick building s.
sick sinus s.
Silvestroni-Bianco s.
simian acquired immunodeficiency s.
Simpson dysmorphia s.
Simpson-Golabi-Behmel s.
sinobronchial s.
Sjögren syndrome antigen A
sleep apnea s.
sleep apnea-hypersomnolence syndrome associated with upper airway obstruction
slipping rib s.
slit ventricle s.
slow-channel congenital myasthenic s.
slow spinal cord compression s.
small aorta s.
Smith-Fineman-Myers s.
Smith-Lemli-Opitz s.
Smith-Magenis s.
Snyder-Robinson s.
social breakdown s.
solitary rectal ulcer s.
solitary ulcer of rectum s.
somatropin deficiency s.
space-adaptation s.
spastic bowel s.
splenic agenesis s.
splenic flexure s.
staccato s.
stagnate loop s.
staphylococcal scalded skin s.
staphylococcal toxic shock s.
Staphylococcus aureus hyperimmunoglobulinemia E s.
steroid-responsive nephrotic s.
steroid-sensitive idiopathic nephrotic s.
Stickler s.
stiff man s.
stillbirth, mummification, embryonic death, infertility s.
straight back s.
streptococcal toxic shock s.
stretching-yawning s.
Sturge-Weber s.
Stüve-Wiedemann s.
subacute thyroiditis-like s.
subclavian steal s.
subjective posttraumatic s.
sudden infant death s.
sudden unexplained death s.
superior mesenteric artery s.
superior orbital fissure s.
superior sulcus tumor s.
superior vena cava compression s.
supine hypotensive s.
supracapsular nerve entrapment s.
supravalvular aortic hypercalcemia s.
Sutherland-Haan s.
swallowed blood s.
swollen belly s.
sympathetically independent pain s.
sympathetically mediated pain s.
synovitis, acne, pustulosis, hyperostosis, osteomyelitis s.
systemic capillary leak s.
systemic inflammatory response s.
systemic sicca s.
systolic click murmur s.
tarsal tunnel s.
temporomandibular joint-pain dysfunction s.
testicular feminization s.
tethered cord s.
therapy-related myelodysplastic s.
thoracic endometriosis s.
thoracic outlet s.
thoracoabdominal s.
thrombotic thrombocytopenic purpura and hemolytic uremic s.
thyroiditis, Addison disease, Sjögren syndrome, sarcoidosis s.
tight lens s.
total allergy s.
total anterior circulation s.
totally unexplained sudden infant death s.
toxic epidemic s.
toxic oil epidemic s.
toxic shock s.
toxic shock-like s.
toxic shock syndrome exoprotein
toxic shock syndrome exotoxin

toxic shock syndrome toxin
toxoplasmosis, other infections, rubella, cytomegalovirus infection, herpes simplex s.
tracheoesophageal fistula, esophageal atresia, multiple congenital anomaly s.
transfusion-associated acquired immune deficiency s.
transfusion-transmitted acquired immune deficiency s.
transient respiratory distress s.
transurethral resection s.
Treacher Collins s.
trichodentoosseous s.
trichorhinophalangeal s.
trigeminal trophic s.
trisomy 18, 21 s.
tropical diarrhea-malabsorption s.
tropical splenomegaly s.
Troyer s.
tubulointerstitial nephritis and uveitis s.
tumor lysis s.
tumor necrosis factor receptor-associated periodic s.
Turner s.
twin-twin transfusion s.
ulnar tunnel s.
undifferentiated autoimmune s.
undifferentiated connective tissue s.
unique facies, anorexia, cachexia, and eye and skin s.
universal joint s.
upper airway resistance s.
upper airway respiratory s.
urethral manipulation s.
Usher s.
uterine compression s.
uveitis, glaucoma, hyphema s.
Van der Hoeve s.
vanishing lung s.
vascular fragility s.
vascular headache s.
vascular leak s.
velocardiofacial s.
venous insufficiency s.
vertebral irritation s.
vestibular aqueduct s.
virus-associated hemophagocytic s.
vitreal corneal touch s.
vitreoretinal choroidopathy s.
vitreoretinal traction s.
Vogt-Koyanagi-Harada s.
von Hippel-Landau s.
vulvar vestibulitis s.
Wardenburg s.
watery diarrhea, hypokalemia, and achlorhydria s.
Weaver-Smith s.
Werner s.
Wernicke-Korsakoff s.
West s.
wet dog shakes s.
wet lung s.
whistling face s.
white coat s.
Wiedemann-Rautenstrauch s.
Williams s.
Williams syndrome, early puberty
Williams syndrome, late puberty
Wilson-Mikity s.
Wilson-Turner s.
Wiskott-Aldrich syndrome protein
Wolf-Hirschhorn s.
wrinkly skin s.
X-linked alpha-thalassemia/mental retardation s.
X-linked Alport s.
X-linked dysplasia-gigantism s.
X-linked mental retardation syndrome 1–6
X-linked mental retardation-aphasia s.
X-linked mental retardation-blindness-deafness-multiple congenital anomalies s.
X-linked mental retardation, microphthalmia, microcornea, cataract, hypogenitalism-mental retardation-spasticity s.
X-linked Opitz s.
X-linked recessive lymphoproliferative s.
yellow nail s.
yellow vernix s.
yin deficiency-yang excess s.
zinc depletion s.
Zollinger-Ellison s.

syndrome-related
acquired immunodeficiency syndrome-related virus

syndromethrombotic
hemolytic uremic syndrome/thrombotic thrombocytopenia purpura

synechia, pl. **synechiae**
annular s.
anterior s.
anterior synechia formation
anular s.
asymptomatic s.
cleft palate-lateral synechia syndrome
Obstbaum synechia spatula
peripheral anterior s.
posterior synechiae

synechiotomy
Paufique s.
posterior s.

synergistic
s. affect
s. effect
Meleney synergistic gangrene

synergy
reactive extensor postural s.

synesthesia
auditory s.

Syngamus trachea

syngeneic
s. graft
s. spleen cell

synkinesis
mouth-and-hand s.
oculocephalic s.
oculomotor nerve s.

synkinetic movement

synostosis, pl. **synostoses**
congenital radioulnar s.
coronal suture s.
humeroradial s.
multiple synostoses syndrome
nonsyndromic bicoronal s.
radioulnar s.
unicoronal s.

synostotic frontal plagiocephaly

synovectomy
Albright s.
arthroscopic s.
arthroscopically assisted s.

synovia (*pl. of* synovium)

synovial
biphasic synovial sarcoma
s. bursa
s. capsule
s. cavity
s. cell
s. chondromatosis
s. chondrosarcoma
s. crypt
s. cyst
s. fistula
s. fluid
s. fluid lymphocyte
s. fold of hip
s. fringe

synovial *(continued)*
s. ganglion
s. hernia
s. inflammation
s. joint
s. ligament
s. lining cell
s. membrane
s. membrane of joint
monophasic synovial sarcoma
patellar synovial fold
s. sheath
temporomandibular joint synovial fluid

synovialis
articulatio s.

synoviocyte
fibroblast-like s.

synovitis
s., acne, pustulosis, hyperostosis, osteomyelitis syndrome
asymptomatic cricoarytenoid s.
diffuse pigmented villonodular s.
localized nodular s.
pigmented villonodular s.
remitting seronegative symmetric synovitis with pitting edema
villonodular s.

synovium, pl. **synovia**
fibrous s.
hyperplastic s.

syntactical aphasia

syntax
Bilingual S. Measure II Test
Northwestern S. Screening Test
Patterned Elicitation S. Screening Test
Performance Assessment of S. Elicited and Spontaneous
Temple University Short S. Inventory

synthase
antithymidylate synthase polyclonal antibody
argininosuccinic acid synthase deficiency
citrate s.
constitutive nitric oxide s.
dihydopteroate s.
endogenous inhibitor of prostaglandin s.
endothelial constitutive nitric oxide s.
endothelial nitric oxide s.
glycogen synthase kinase-3
heme s.
induced nitric oxide s.
inducible nitric oxide s.
methionine synthase deficiency
nitric oxide synthase gene
nitric oxide synthase inhibitor
s. phosphatase
porphobilinogen s.
prostaglandin H s.
6-pyruvoyltetrahydropterin s.
thymidylate s.
uroporphyrinogen s.

synthesis, pl. **syntheses**
de novo thymidylate synthesis
depressed DNA s.
inhibitor of DNA s.
lipid s.
maximal rate of urea s.
ovarian estrogen s.
protein s.
solid phase peptide s.
stimulated protein s.
unscheduled deoxynucleic acid s.

synthesize gamma globulin

synthesizing
Oliphant Auditory S. Test
s. protein complex

synthetase
alanyl-transfer ribonucleic acid s.
aminolevulinic acid s.
argininosuccinate s.
argininosuccinate synthetase deficiency
argininosuccinic acid synthetase deficiency
dihydrobiopterin s.
endothelial constitutive nitric oxide s.
glutamine s.
glutamylcysteine s.
glutathione synthetase deficiency
glycogen synthetase kinase
glycogen synthetase phosphatase
heme s.
holocarboxylase s.
inducible nitric oxide s.
prostaglandin s.
prostaglandin synthetase inhibitor
tryptophan s.
uroporphyrinogen s.

synthetic
s. absorbable suture
s., adhesive, moisture vapor permeable
s. amino acid
s. androgen
aqueous synthetic dual phenolic disinfectant
cardiolipin synthetic lecithin
s. chemistry
s. detergent
s. DNA
s. graft
s. graft material
Harleco synthetic resin
s. heart valve
s. hemoglobin
s. human gastrin
s. human growth hormone
s. human relaxin
s. insulin
s. male hormone
s. medium old tuberculin trichloroacetic acid precipitated
natural or synthetic hormone
penicillinase-resistant synthetic penicillin
s. RNA polymer
s. sentence identification
s. sentence list
s. thyroid hormone

syntonic type

syphilid
annular s.
macular s.
miliary papular s.
nodular s.
nummular s.

syphilis
biological false-positive serologic test for s.
s. of bone
congenital s.
hemagglutination treponemal test for s.
Hinton flocculation test for s.
noduloulcerative tertiary s.
nontreponemal syphilis test
parenchymatous congenital s.
primary s.
secondary s.
serologic test for s.
tertiary s.
s., toxoplasmosis, other agents, rubella, cytomegalovirus, herpes simplex virus

syphilitic
s. alopecia
amyotrophic syphilitic myelitis
s. aortitis
s. cataract
chronic syphilitic infection

congenital syphilitic conjunctivitis
congenital syphilitic infection
congenital syphilitic paralytic dementia
s. fever
initial syphilitic lesion
s. meningitis
ocular syphilitic disease
s. roseola
s. spirochete
s. steochondritis

syphiliticus
lichen s.
pemphigus s.

syphilology
dermatology and s.

Syrian hamster embryo

syringe
Arrow Raulerson s.
aspiration s.
s. exchange program
hypodermic s.

syringe-driven system

syringoma
malignant chondroid s.

syringomyelia
ape hand of s.
s. disorder
lumbar s.

syringomyelic
s. clawhand
s. dissociation
s. hemorrhage

syringosubarachnoid shunting

syrup
Apathy gum syrup medium
ipecac s.
maple syrup urine disease

system
abusive family s.
active immune s.
adnexal adhesion classification s.
adolescent support s.
Advanced Catheter S.
Advanced Interventional S.'s
AFS adhesion scoring s.
AIDS-related primary central nervous system lymphoma
air abrasion s.
air filtration s.
allergy immune s.
alternative delivery s.
amplification refractory mutation s.
anatomical classification system of Severin
anatomic medullary locking hip s.
s. for anesthetic and respiratory administration
angiographic reference s.
angled-vision lens s.
ankle scoring system of Baird and Jackson
annular phased array s.
anomalous arrangement of pancreaticobiliary ductal s.
anterior cervical plate fixation s.
anterior locking plate s.
antibody-based detection s.
antimigration s.
arc-centered guidance s.
arc radius s.
Arizona Cancer Center multiple myeloma staging s.
arm-implanted subcutaneous reservoir-catheter s.
Arndorfer capillary perfusion s.
arrhythmia mapping system catheter
arterial port catheter s.
artificial heart energy s.
Artisan cement s.
ascending neurotransmitter s.
ascending reticular-activating s.
ascending reticular arousal s.
Ashhurst fracture classification s.
assessing severity: age of patient, systems involved, stage of disease, complications, response to therapy
Astwood-Coller staging system for carcinoma
Atkinson scoring system for dysphagia
atrial septal defect occlusion s.
atrioventricular conduction s.
augmentative communication s.
autofluorescent endoscopic s.
autologous melanoma s.
automated cytochemical s.
automated eligibility verification s.
automated endoscopic system for optimal positioning
automated hospital information s.
automatic endoscopic system for optimal positioning
automatic karyotype system database
automatic positioning s.
automatic titration s.
autonomic division of nervous s.
autonomic nervous system disorder
autonomic nervous system dysfunction
autonomic part of peripheral nervous s.
avidin-biotin-based detection s.
avidin-biotin complex immunodetection s.
avidin-biotin detection s.
axial spinal s.
axis of three-dimensional rectangular coordinate s.
behavioral family systems therapy
behavioral inhibition s.
bioartificial extracorporeal liver support s.
biologic detection s.
biomedical monitoring s.
blood factor in the MNS blood group s.
blood and lymphatic s.
blood plasma measuring s.
cable suspension s.
California soft spinal s.
Cancer Surveillance S.
Cardiovascular Measurement s.
cardiovascular reflex conditioning s.
carotid artery s.
carpal tunnel release s.
cataract, motor system disorder, short stature, learning difficulty, skeletal abnormalities syndrome
central auditory nervous s.
centralized cancer patient data s.
central nervous s.
central nervous system depression
central nervous system leukemia
cine pulse s.
closed-loop system passing electrode
closed water seal drainage s.
combined system disease
community health management information s.
compliance of the respiratory s.
compliant prestress s.
Composite Laryngeal Recurrence Staging S.
comprehensive health enhancement support s.
Computer-Assisted Psychiatric Evaluation and Review S.
computer imaging s.

system *(continued)*
Computerized Healthcare And Record Transfer S.
computerized notation s.
Conceptual S.'s Test
condom catheter collecting s.
conduction system disease
continuous distention-irrigation s.
continuous glucose monitoring s.
continuous insulin delivery s.
cooperative health statistics s.
cruciate condylar knee s.
cytochrome s.
deep muscular aponeurotic s.
demarcation membrane s.
dense canalicular s.
dense tubular s.
development and/or central nervous system anomalies, genital hypoplasia, ear anomalies
Diameter Index Safety s.
diffuse neuroendocrine s.
digital cardiac imaging s.
digital vascular imaging s.
direct bonding s.
Disaster Warning S.
distal perfusion s.
drug reaction-monitoring s.
duplication of left collecting s.
duplication of right collecting s.
dynamic optical breast imaging s.
dynamic stabilizing innersole s.
dysfunctional immune s.
dysfunctional voiding scoring s.
Education and Career Exploration S.
enteric nervous s.
ethmoidal infundibular s.
Facial Action Coding S.
Facial Grading S.
Family Tracking S.
fecal containment s.
fiducial alignment s.
flavin-containing mono-oxygenase metabolic s.
foot-pound-second system, unit
four-in-one positioning block s.
frameless stereotaxy s.
French-American-British leukemia classification s.
gastrointestinal therapeutic s.
glucose transport s.
Gordon diagnostic s.
granulomatous angiitis of the central nervous s.
gravity extension locking s.
hereditary disease of nervous s.
His-Purkinje s.
horizontal axis of rectangular coordinate s.
human diploid cell s.
human immunodeficiency virus overview of problems evaluation s.
human leukocyte antigen s.
hyperactive immune s.
hypothalamic-hypophysial-adrenal s.
hypothalamic-pituitary-adrenocortical system
hypothalamohypophysial portal s.
idiopathic central nervous system hypersomnolence
implantable left ventricular assist s.
impulse-conducting s.
incomplete development of autonomic nervous s.
indirect blood pressure measuring s.
information processing in central nervous s.
inhibit immune s.
Integrated Assessment S.
intensified radiographic imaging s.
interleukin regulation of immune s.
intrauterine progesterone contraceptive s.
inventory of s.'s
Irvine viable organ-tissue transport s.
isolated angiitis of central nervous s.
Kell blood s.
key integrative social s.
late central nervous system toxicity
left bundle-branch system block
Lens Opacification Classification S.
Lens Opacities Classification S. II
limbic GABAergic s.
lower collecting s.
luciferase enzyme-based luminescence s.
lumbosacral cartilaginous s.
Lutheran blood group s.
Magerl hook-plate s.
magnocellular neurosecretory s.
major histocompatibility s.
malfunctioning immune s.
management information s.
Manchester system for brachytherapy
Manchester system for radium therapy
Masaoka staging system for thymoma
Mason fracture classification s.
Massachusetts General Hospital Utility Multi-Programming S.
massive parallel processing s.
matrix transdermal s.
Mayo Clinic hip scoring s.
Mayo Clinic system test for primary biliary cirrhosis
McAllister grading s.
McGuire I/A s.
McIntyre I/A s.
M.D. Anderson grading s.
M.D. Anderson tumor score s.
mechanical assist s.
medical data s.
Medical Examination and Diagnostic Coding S.
Medical Inventory Management S.
medicated urethral s.
medication monitoring event s.
mental health s.
mesenteric arterial s.
mesocortical dopaminergic s.
mesolimbic dopamine s.
microdilution s.
Micro Drop yeast identification s.
microendoscopic discectomy s.
micromultileaf collimator s.
microscopic angiogenesis grading s.
microsomal enzyme s.
microsomal ethanol oxidizing s.
microsurgical drill s.
microtiter blood typing s.
microwave cardiac ablation s.
middle ear implantable s.
Millennium LX microsurgical s.
Minaar classification s.
mini lag screw s.
mini Vidas automated immunoassay s.
Minnesota Occupational Classification S.
minocycline periodontal therapeutic s.
mitochondrial ethanol oxidase s.
mitochondrial glycine cleavage s.
Mitsuyasu staging s.

mixed function oxidase s.
mobile artery and vein imaging s.
Modular Acetabular Revision S.
Modulus CD anesthesia s.
molecular adsorbent recirculating s.
monocular heads-up display imaging s.
mononuclear phagocyte s.
Moore hip endoprosthesis s.
morphology system CAS-200
mother endoscopic retrograde cholangiopancreatoscopy s.
motion analysis s.
motion artifact rejection s.
Mot-R-Pak vitrectomy s.
MR catheter imaging and spectroscopy system scanner
mucosal oral therapeutic s.
multiaxial classification s.
Multi Balance S.
S. of Multicultural Assessment
S. of Multicultural Pluralistic Assessment
multihormonal system disorder
multihospital s.
multiorgan system failure
multiple organ system dysfunction
multiple organ system failure
Multiple Severity of Illness S.
MultiPulse laser s.
multistate information s.
Multitest CMI s.
Murphy staging s.
mycobacteria growth indicator tube s.
myeloperoxidase s.
myocardial protection s.
NADPH oxidase s.
nasolacrimal drainage s.
near-UV excited autofluorescence diagnosis s.
needle-free injection s.
needle management s.
Nelson grading s.
Neonatal Abstinence Scoring S.
Neonatal Facial Coding S.
nervous s.
nervous system effect
nervous system involvement
s.'s network architecture
network operating s.
Neurotrend continuous multiparameter s.
Newport hip s.
Niamtu video imaging s.
nicotine transdermal s.
nigrostriatal dopaminergic s.
nigrostriatal dopamine s.
NIH Classification S. for Prostatitis
nonisotopic detection s.
nonoral estradiol delivery s.
nonrebreathing s.
normal immune system function
Norwood classification s.
nuclear medicine information s.
Nuvolase 660 laser s.
object coordinate s.
ocular motor s.
Ocutome II fragmentation s.
Ogden fracture classification s.
Olympus endoscopy s.
open anesthesia s.
open canalicular system of platelets
open double-decked hook cervical s.
open-loop insulin delivery s.
organic central nervous system deterioration
organized delivery s.
organ system failure index
osteochondral autograft transfer s.
osteocytic membrane s.
ostomotic release oral s.
Outpatient Prospective Payment S.
overactive immune s.
oxidation-reduction s.
pacing system analyzer
Packard radioimmunoassay s.
pancreaticobiliary ductal s.
Panoview arthroscopic s.
paranoid belief s.
parasympathetic division of antonomic nervous s.
parasympathetic nerve s.
Passport disposable injection s.
Patient Care Information S.
patient-centered access to secure systems online
patient data s.
Patient Data Management S.'s
P blood group s.
pediatric anesthesia s.
PE-400 ERG/VEP s.
percutaneous excimer laser coronary angioplasty s.
performance measurement s.
peripapillary choroidal arterial s.
Peripheral Access S.
peripheral nervous s.
peripheral nervous system disorder
peripheral vascular s.
peritoneal dialysis s.
personal emergency response s.
personality assessment s.
phosphotransferase s.
photon-activated drug delivery s.
picture archival communication s.
portal insulin infusion s.
possible vertebrobasilar s.
Post Anesthesia Discharge Scoring S.
Pregnancy Risk Monitoring S.
preservative-free solution s.
primary angiitis of the central nervous s.
primary central nervous s.
primary central nervous system lymphoma
problem-oriented system of charting
programmable implantable medication s.
prospective outcomes monitoring evaluation s.
psychological information, acquisition, processing, and control s.
quality information monitoring s.
Quimby dose distribution s.
radiation therapy planning s.
radiographic imaging s.
radiology telephone access s.
rapid assay delivery s.'s
Rasor blood pumping s.
rearfoot stability s.
remote data entry s.
renin-angiotensin s.
renin-angiotensin-aldosterone s.
reroute digestive s.
s.'s research
respiratory s.
respiratory system compliance score
respiratory system elastance
respiratory system resistance
reticular activating s.
reticulocyte cell-free s.
reticuloendothelial s.
right bundle-branch system block
right-handed orthogonal coordinate s.
rotational atherectomy s.
secondary anticoagulation s.
segmental cement extraction s.
segmental spinal correction s.

system *(continued)*
self-controlled intravenous s.
self-injurious-behavior inhibiting s.
serum protein and immunofixation electrophoresis s.
sexual/reproductive system impairment
sheath and dilator s.
shoulder arm s.
single-action pumping s.
single patient s.
single-photon counting s.
single-unit delivery s.
skeletal repair s.
skin-adipose superficial musculoaponeurotic s.
social information s.
Social Skills Rating S.
sonic-accelerated fracture-healing s.
specific thalamic projection s.
spheroidal oral drug absorption s.
staging system in radiation therapy
Standard S. of Psychiatry
stent delivery s.
stimulate the immune s.
stone-tissue detection s.
striped tag myocardial tagging s.
stroke guidance s.
submucosal aponeurotic system flap
superficial fascial s.
superficial musculoaponeurotic s.
supplemental oxygen s.
sympathetic autonomic nervous s.
sympathetic nervous s.
syringe-driven s.
tear drainage s.
testosterone transdermal s.
Therapeutic Intervention Scoring S.
thread mate s.
tissue-stone recognition s.
Topographic Scanning S.
transdermal delivery s.
transdermal infusion s.
transdermal therapeutic s.
transtelephonic ambulatory monitoring s.
transurethral ultrasound-guided laser-induced prostatectomy s.
transvenous s.
Trex digital mammography s.
trigeminovascular s.
Tri-Service Medical Information S.
tuberoinfundibular dopamine s.
tumor score s.
underactive immune s.
Unified Medical Language S.
Universal Spine S.
s. universal verbotonol audition Guberina
urine specimen volume measuring s.
uterine progesterone s.
valve s.
ventricular specialized conduction s.
vertebrobasilar artery s.
vertical axis of rectangular coordinate s.
vesicular transport s.
video imaging s.
von Herrick grading s.
weakened immune s.
Wisconsin Compression S.
work evaluation systems technology

systematic
s. anatomy
S. Assessment for Treatment of Emergent Events
s. bacteriology
s. comparison
s., complete, objective, practical, empirical
s. desensitization
s. followup
S. Inquiry
S. Nursing Observation of Psychopathology
s. nutritional muscle testing
s. rational restructuring

systematized
s. assertive therapy
S. Nomenclature of Medicine Clinical Terms
S. Nomenclature of Medicine Reference Terminology
S. Nomenclature of Pathology

systemic
s. active immunotherapy
active systemic anaphylaxis
acute systemic lupus erythematosus
adult-onset systemic Still disease
s. anaphylaxis
ANCA-associated systemic vasculitis
s. anterior motion
s. arterial hypertension
s. arterial pressure
s. artery
s. aspergillosis
s. assertive therapy
s. bacterial infection
s. blastomycosis
s. blood flow
s. blood pressure
bullous systemic lupus erythematosus
s. candidiasis
s. capillary leak syndrome
s. carnitine deficiency
s. chemotherapy
control of local and systemic disease
s. cutaneous basophil hypersensitivity
s. death
s. disorder
s. drug
s. hemodynamic parameters
s. hemodynamics
s. hyperbaric oxygen therapy
s. hypertension
s. hyperthermia
s. illness
s. impact
inadequacy of systemic circulation
s. infection
s. inflammatory disease
s. inflammatory response syndrome
s. infusion
s. injection
s. juvenile rheumatoid arthritis
late respiratory systemic syndrome
limited progressive systemic sclerosis
limited systemic scleroderma
linear progressive systemic sclerosis
localized progressive systemic sclerosis
S. Lupus Activity Measure
lupus erythematosus, s.
S. Lupus Erythematosus Disease Activity Index
malignant systemic mastocytosis
s. mast cell disease
s. mean arterial pressure
mean systemic arterial pressure
mild systemic atherosclerosis
modified systemic Berlin-Frankfurt-Munster therapy
necrotizing granulomatous systemic arteritis

s. necrotizing vasculitis
neonatal systemic candidiasis
neurologic complication of systemic cancer
neuropsychiatric syndrome of systemic lupus erythematosus
nonneuropathic systemic amyloidosis
opportunistic systemic fungal infection
opportunistic systemic mycosis
s. oxygen transport
patient with incapacitating systemic disease
patient with mild to moderate systemic disease
patient with severe systemic disease limiting activity but not incapacitating
s. peripheral vascular resistance
primary systemic vasculitis
s. progressive sclerosis
progressive systemic scleroderma
progressive systemic sclerosis
ratio of pulmonary to systemic circulation
s. reaction
s. sclerosis sine scleroderma
s. sepsis
s. sicca syndrome
targeted systemic exposure
total systemic arterial resistance
total systemic flow
s. vascular hypertension
s. vascular resistance index
s. venous collateral
s. venous hypertension

Systemized Nomenclature of Medicine

systole

duration of s.
end of atrial s.
left ventricular internal dimension s.
left ventricular internal dimension at end s.
premature auricular s.
premature junctional s.
premature ventricular s.
shortened electrochemical s.
total electromechanical s.

systolic

ankle systolic pressure
s. anterior motion of mitral valve
aortic systolic ejection murmur
aortic systolic pressure
s. apical impulse
apical systolic heart murmur
area systolic pressure
arterial peak systolic pressure
s. arterial pressure
s. blood pressure
blowing systolic murmur
borderline systolic hypertension
s. bruit
s. click
s. click murmur syndrome
s. coronary artery narrowing
s., diastolic, mean blood pressure
s. discharge
Doppler systolic velocity index
s. dysfunction
early systolic acceleration
early systolic paradox
effective systolic pressure
ejection fraction s.
s. ejection murmur
s. ejection period
s. ejection rate
s. ejection time
finger systolic blood pressure
s. gallop
s. gallop rhythm
s. gradient
harsh systolic murmur
s. heart failure
s. heart murmur
heart rate-systolic blood pressure product
s. heave
s. honk
s. hypertension
s. hypertension in the elderly
s. hypotension
impaired systolic function
impairment of systolic and diastolic performance
s. index
isometric systolic tension
late systolic click
late systolic murmur
left ventricular peak systolic pressure
left ventricular systolic diameter
left ventricular systolic dimension
left ventricular systolic dysfunction
left ventricular systolic index
left ventricular systolic output
maximal exercise systolic pressure
s. mean
mean ankle-brachial systolic pressure index
mean left ventricular systolic pressure
mean normalized systolic ejection rate
mean systolic ejection rate
s. motion
opening snap ejection systolic click
paradoxical systolic expansion
peak systolic aortic pressure
peak systolic gradient pressure
s. pressure time index
pulmonary artery s.
pulmonary artery systolic pressure
pulse oximetry waveform systolic blood pressure
radial artery systolic pressure
right ventricular systolic pressure
segmental limb systolic pressure
s. thrill
s. time interval
tumor peak systolic velocity
unassisted systolic pressure
s. velocity integral
s. wall motion velocity

systolic/diastolic

pulmonary artery s.

systolic-diastolic hypertension

Szabo test

Szondi Experimental Diagnostics of Drives

Szymanowski operation

T45′
T_45'-deiodinase type 2

Ta
WHO classification for transitional cell carcinoma of the urinary bladder: stages Ta through T4

tab
modified double-opposing tab flap nipple reconstruction

tabes
cerebral t.
cervical t.
Diabetic t.
Friedreich t.
hereditary t.
t. infantum
interstitial t.
t. mesenterica
nerve t.
spasmodic t.

tabetic
t. arthropathy
t. crisis
t. dissociation

table
Everyman Contingency T. Analysis
harmonic attenuation t.
inner table thickness
International T. calorie
life table method
life table survival
long axis traction chiropractic t.

tablet
chocolate-coated t.
coated compressed t.
compressed tablet triturate
cyanide t.
delayed-action t.
dispensing t.
emergency drinking water germicidal t.
extended release t.
hypodermic t.
immediate-release t.
modified double-opposing t.
multiple compressed t.
orally disintegrating t.
oral triphasic tablets
placebo capsule or t.
potassium chloride sustained release t.
repeat action t.
sublingual t.
sugar-coated t.
t. triturate

Tacaiuma virus

Tacaribe virus

tache
t. blanche

tachography study

tachy
atrial tachy response

tachyarrhythmia
atrial t.
external tachyarrhythmia control device
t. pacing
paroxysmal t.
sinoventricular t.
supraventricular t.
sustained reentrant ventricular t.
sustained supraventricular t.
ventricular t.

tachy-brady
t.-b. arrhythmia
t.-b. syndrome

tachycardia
accelerated idioventricular t.
alternating bidirectional t.
arteriovenous junctional t.
artificial circus-movement t.
atrial chaotic t.
atrial ectopic automatic t.
atrial paroxysmal t.
atrial tachycardia detection rate
atrial tachycardia with block
atrioventricular functional t.
atrioventricular junctional t.
atrioventricular nodal reentrant t.
atrioventricular reciprocating t.
atrioventricular reentrant paroxysmal t.
atrioventricular reentry t.
atypical atrioventricular nodal reentrant t.
atypical ventricular t.
automatic atrial t.
automatic ectopic t.
AV junctional t.
AV nodal reentrant t.
AV nodal reentry t.
chaotic atrial t.
double t.
ectopic atrial t.
endless loop t.
exercise-induced ventricular t.
extrasystolic atrial t.
hypertension and t.
hypotension and t.
idiojunctional t.
idiopathic ventricular t.
implantable cardioverter-defibrillator/atrial tachycardia pacing
intraatrial reentrant t.
intraatrial reentry t.
intractable junctional t.
junctional ectopic t.
junctional reciprocating t.
long R-P t.
malignant ventricular t.
monomorphic ventricular t.
multifocal atrial t.
multiform ventricular t.
muscle pain, allergy, tachycardia and tiredness, headache syndrome
narrow complex supraventricular t.
narrow complex t.
nodal paroxysmal t.
nodal reentrant paroxysmal t.
nonparoxysmal atrial t.
nonparoxysmal atrioventricular junctional t.
nonparoxysmal nodal t.
nonsustained monomorphic ventricular t.
nonsustained polymorphic ventricular t.
orthodromic reciprocating t.
pacemaker circus-movement t.
pacemaker-mediated t.
parasystolic ventricular t.
paroxysmal atrial t.
paroxysmal atrioventricular nodal reciprocal t.
paroxysmal auricular t.
paroxysmal junctional ventricular t.
paroxysmal nodal t.
paroxysmal reentrant supraventricular t.
paroxysmal sinus t.
permanent junctional reciprocating t.
postural orthostatic tachycardia syndrome
primary ventricular t.
reentrant atrial t.
regular, wide QRS t.
sinus t.
slow paroxysmal atrial t.
supraventricular tachycardia ablation

tachycardia *(continued)*
sustained monomorphic ventricular t.
sustained ventricular t.
torsade de pointes ventricular t.
unsustained ventricular t.
ventricular tachycardia cycle length
ventricular tachycardia event
ventricular tachycardia nonsustained
ventricular tachycardia sustained
wide-complex t.

tachycardia-induced cardiomyopathy

tachykinin-like immunoreactivity

tachypnea
nervous t.
t. of newborn
transient t.
transient tachypnea of newborn

tachyzoite
extracellular t.
intracellular t.

tack
carpet tack follicular keratotic plug

tacking suture

tactic
confrontational t.
diversionary t.

tactile
t. afferent
t. amnesia
t. anesthesia
t. aphasia
t. cell
t. corpuscle
t. delusion
t. disk
t. extinction
t. feedback
t. fever
fine tactile sensation
T. Finger Recognition Test
T. Form Recognition Test
t. fremitus
t. hair
t. hallucination
t. hyperesthesia
t. image
moderate tactile stimulus
occasional tactile hallucination
T. Performance Test
t. pressure
T. Reproduction Pegboard
t. sensation
t. stimulation
t. tension
visual, association, kinesthetic, tactile reading
t. vocal fremitus

taeniasis
Asian t.

tag
anal skin t.
epicardial fat t.
expressed sequence t.
hemihypertrophy, intestinal web, preauricular skin tag, and congenital corneal opacity syndrome
hemorrhoidal skin t.
perineal skin t.
sperm-ubiquitin tag immunoassay
striped tag myocardial tagging system

tagged
expression sequence t.
muscles isolated and t.

Taggert virus

tagging
barium-based fecal t.
fecal t.
striped tag myocardial tagging system

Tahyna virus

tail
artery of the pancreatic t.
artery to tail of pancreas
axillary tail of Spence
t. of breast
t. of helix
lipid t.
long dural t.
mare's tail line
t. pinch
wet tail disease

tailgut cyst

tailoring
custom t.
t. of flap

tainted
acquired immune deficiency syndrome tainted transfusion
t. blood transfusion

Tai virus

Takayasu
T. arteriopathy
T. arteritis
T. disease

take
cast removed, take x-ray
t. home pack
to take out

takedown
t. of adhesion
bilateral ureterostomy t.
t. of colostomy
colostomy t.

taken
biopsy of area t.
multiple biopsies t.

takeoff of artery

taking down of adhesion

Talairach
atlas of Talairach and Tournoux

talar
anterior talar articular surface of calcaneus
anterior talar dome
anterior talar translation
t. axis–first metatarsal base angle
t. dislocation
t. dome
t. dome cyst
t. dome fracture
t. head
tibial talar tilt/tibiotalar tilt
t. tilt

talcosis
pulmonary t.

Tale
Tell a Tale psychiatry

Tale-Brown Obsessive-Compulsive Scale

talipes
t. cavus
t. equinovalgus
t. equinovarus
t. valgus
t. varus

talk
inability to t.

talking
compulsive t.
increased t.
t. task

tall
macrocephaly, facial abnormalities, disproportionate tall stature mental retardation syndrome
t. cell variant

talocalcanea
articulatio t.

talocalcaneal
t. angle
anterior talocalcaneal angle
anterior talocalcaneal ligament
anteroposterior talocalcaneal angle
anteroposterior talocalcaneal divergence
t. fusion
interosseous talocalcaneal ligament
t. joint
lateral talocalcaneal angle
lateral talocalcaneal ligament
t. ligament
medial talocalcaneal facet

talocalcaneonavicular
t. articulation
t. joint

talocrural
t. articulation
t. joint
medial ligament of talocrural joint

talofibular
anterior talofibular ligament rupture
anterior talofibular sprain
t. ligament
posterior t.
posterior talofibular ligament

talonavicular
arthritic talonavicular change
t. arthrodesis
t. articulation
t. dislocation
t. joint
t. ligament

talotibial
anterior talotibial ligament

talus
anterior talus shift
articular surface of t.
congenital vertical t.
congenital vertical talus foot deformity
head of t.
medial malleolar facet of t.
medial malleolar surface of t.
navicular articular surface of t.
oblique t.
osteochondral fracture of the dome of the t.
osteochondral lesion of the t.

Tamdy virus

Tamiami virus

Tamm-Horsfall
T.-H. mucoprotein
T.-H. protein

tampon
nasal t.
tracheal t.
Trendelenburg t.

tamponade
cardiac t.
esophagogastric balloon t.
ferromagnetic t.
low-pressure cardiac t.
nontraumatic cardiac t.
pericardial chyle with t.

tandem
afterloading tandem and ovoids
t. autotransplants
t. colonoscopy
Ernst radium t.
Fletcher afterloading t.
Fletcher-Suit afterloading t.
forward tandem gait
t. gait test
t. insertion
liquid chromatography coupled to tandem mass spectrometry
t. and ovoids
short tandem repeat polymorphism
simple tandem repeat polymorphism
t. translocation
t. transplant
variable numbers of tandem repeats

Tanga virus

tangential
alignment of tangential beam
t. beam
t. field
t. flow filtration
t. speech pattern
t. thinking
t. view

tangent screen

tangible reinforcement of operant conditioned audiometry

tangle
neurofibrillary t.

Tanjong Rabok virus

tank
Hubbard t.
nitrous oxide t.
portable oxygen t.
walking t.

tanned
t. erythrocyte electrophoretic mobility
t. red blood cell agglutination
t. red blood cell hemagglutination
t. red blood cell hemagglutination inhibition
t. red cell

Tanner
T. Developmental Scale
T. genital stage
Marshall and Tanner pubertal stage
T. stage
T. staging

Tanner-Whitehouse Mark 2 bone-age assessment

tannic acid, polyphosphomolybdic acid, and amido acid staining technique

tantalum
balloon-expandable tantalum stent
t. mesh graft
t. mesh implant material
radiopaque tantalum stent
t. wire fixation

tanycyte ependymal cell

Tanzer auricle reconstruction

tap
anterior chamber t.
AO t.
ascites fluid t.
bloody t.
bone marrow t.
diagnostic spinal t.
headache after spinal t.
heel t.
lung t.
nontraumatic spinal t.
percutaneous lung t.
pericardial t.
peritoneal t.
pleural t.
spinal t.
suprapubic bladder t.
t. water enema
t. water enema til clear
t. water wet dressing

tapasin
novel glycoprotein t.

tape
anthropometric measuring t.
appendectomy t.
cast t.
circular t.
collagen tape prosthesis
fiberglass casting t.
foam t.
optokinetic t.
restraining t.
tension-free vaginal t.

tapered
blunt tapered T-handled reamer
collarless, polished, t.
t. crown
dentate tapered fissure bur
t. steroid dosing package

tapering
t. dose
t. schedule

tapetochoroidal
peripheral tapetochoroidal degeneration

taping
Achilles tendon taping technique
buddy t.
figure-of-eight t.

tapped
ascitic fluid tapped daily

tar
t. acne
t. camphor
coal tar bath
coal tar pitch volatiles
cola tar soap
crude coal t.
crude coal tar in petroleum
t. keratosis
t. and nicotine
ointment of t.
pine t.

tarda
lues t.
lymphedema t.
multiple epiphysial dysplasia tarda syndrome
osteogenesis imperfecta t.

Tardieu ecchymosis

tardive
antipsychotic-induced tardive dyskinesia
t. cyanosis
t. dyskinesia
t. dystonia
t. muscular dystrophy
neuroleptic-induced tardive dyskinesia

target
angiographic t.
antigenic t.
t. area
t. area under the curve
aspartate t.
assay t.
asymmetric target appearance
automated test target calibration
average target absorbed dose
t. cell
t. cell anemia
clinical target volume
Dameshek oval target cell
t. dry weight
effector to target ratio
t. gland
t. heart rate
t. heart rate zone
initial target volume
t. lesion
t. lesion reintervention
t. lesion revascularization
liver-kidney-microsomal type 1 antibody target assay
macular t.
mammalian target of rapamycin
maximum target absorbed dose
minimal deformation t.
minimum target absorbed dose
mixed lymphocyte target interaction
molybdenum t.
natural killer target structure
t. organ
t. organ disease
oval target cell
peritoneal dialysis creatinine clearance t.
planning target volume
t. plasma concentration
policy target adjustment factor
t. of rapamycin inhibitor
silicon-intensified t.
Verdun T. Symptom Rating Scale
t. vessel revascularization
t. volume

target-attaching
t.-a. globulin
t.-a. globulin precursor

target-controlled infusion

targeted
doxorubicin adsorbed to magnetic targeted carrier
t. systemic exposure

target-film distance

targeting
t. agent
angiographic t.
magnetite in tumor t.
Screening Instrument for T. Educational Risk

targetoid hemosiderotic hemangioma

targetry
angiographic t.

target-skin distance

tarry
t. black bowel movement
t. black stool

tarsal
t. amputation
anterior tarsal resection
anterior tarsal tendinitis
anterior tarsal tendinous sheath
anterior tarsal tunnel syndrome
t. arch
avascular tarsal scaphoid necrosis
t. bone
t. bone fracture
t. canal
t. cartilage
t. cyst
t. fold
inferior tarsal muscle
t. joint
t. laceration
t. plate
t. scaphoiditis
t. sinus
superior tarsal muscle
t. synostosis
t. tunnel decompression
t. tunnel release
t. tunnel syndrome

tarsometatarsal
t. amputation
t. angle
t. dislocation
t. fracture-dislocation
t. joint
t. ligament

tarsometatarsales

tarsometatarseae

tarsophalangeal reflex

tarsorrhaphy
internal t.

tarsus inferior

tartaric dimalonate

tartrate
metoprolol t.
nicotine t.
noradrenaline acid t.
pentolinium t.

tartrate-resistant acid phosphatase

task
auditory continuous performance t.
auditory 3-stimuli oddball t.
continuous performance t.
decline in ability to perform routine t.'s
T.'s of Emotional Development
goal oriented t.
job task analysis
linguistic content of t.
metabolic equivalent of t.
modal adaptive t.
Paired Associate Learning T.
reading t.
sound production t.'s
talking t.
visual search t.

task-oriented
t.-o. approach
t.-o. assessment
t.-o. group

taste
t. abnormality
t. aversion
t. bud
t. cell
t. corpuscle
t. deficiency
t. hair
heightened awareness of touch or t.
metallic t.

Tataguine virus

tattoo
amalgam t.
t. of cornea
limbus parallel orientation straddling tattoo mark
oral t.

tattooing
medical t.

tau
altered tau processing
short tau inversion recovery

taught
patient taught deep breathing

taurine
t. cotransporter
selenium-labeled homocholic acid conjugated with t.

taurodeoxycholic acid

tauroursodeoxycholic acid

Taussig-Bing disease

taut and distended abdomen

Tawara
node of Aschoff and T.

taxon
Pasteurella species taxon 16

taxonomic
operational taxonomic unit

taxonomy
numerical t.

Tay cherry-red spot

Taylor
T. apparatus
T. back brace
T. Manifest Anxiety Scale
occipital cortical dysplasia of T.

Taylor-Johnson Temperament Analysis

Tay-Sachs disease

99mtc diphosphonate

T-cell
T.-c. acute lymphoblastic leukemia
adult T-cell leukemia virus
T.-c. antigen receptor
cardiac abnormality, T-cell deficit, clefting, hypocalcemia
CD4 T.-c.
T.-c. chronic lymphatic leukemia
T.-c. crossmatch
T.-c. defect
T.-c. dependent
T.-c. depletion
T.-c. dysfunction
T.-c. enriched
T.-c. function
T.-c. growth factor-1
T.-c. growth factor-2
human T-cell leukemia virus type 1, 2, 3
human T-cell leukemia-lymphoma virus
human T-cell leukemia virus
human T-cell lymphoma virus
human T-cell lymphotropic virus
lymphoid precursor T.-c.
T.-c. lymphoma
T.-c. prolymphocytic leukemia
T.-c. reactivity
T.-c. receptor-rearrangement excision circle
T.-c. replacing factor
T.-c. rosette
simian T-cell lymphotropic virus
T.-c. supernatant
T.-c. trophic

T cell cytotoxic

T-cell-mediating contact sensitivity

T-cell-restricted intracellular antigen

T-cell-rich B-cell lymphoma

^{99m}Tc-hexamethylpropyleneamine oxime

99mTc-labeled antigranulocyte antibody

^{99m}Tc MDP uptake

$T_4$5′-deiodinase type 2

tea
bananas, rice, applesauce, tea, toast diet
decaffeinated green t.
green tea extract
green tea polyphenol
t. tree oil

teacher
Abbreviated Conners T. Rating Scale
T. Assessment of Social Behavior
Conners T. Questionnaire
Conners T. Rating Scale
dental auxiliary teacher education
T. Evaluation Scale
Minnesota T. Attitude Inventory
Parent as a T. Inventory
Purdue T. Questionnaire
T. Rating Form
T. Report Form
T. School Readiness Inventory

teaching
discharge t.
t. hospital
special teaching issue

team
aeromedical evacuation support t.
aged care assessment t.
Bimodality Lung Oncology T.

team *(continued)*
cardiac rehabilitation t.
cardiac resuscitation t.
child protection t.
clinical pharmacokinetics t.
comprehensive support care t.
coronary care t.
diagnostic and therapeutic t.
disaster medical assistance t.
T. Effectiveness Survey
emergency medical t.
geriatric assessment t.
medication administration t.
mobile crisis outreach t.
multidisciplinary team approach
nutritional support t.
organ recovery t.
Patient Outcomes Research T.
perinatal mortality counseling t.
preadmission screening and assessment t.
psychiatric emergency t.
pulmonary care t.
radiologic emergency assistance t.
rehabilitation team goal
Sexual Assault Response T.
Support T. Assessment Schedule

tear
anterior cruciate ligament t.
anterior horn meniscal t.
anterior oblique meniscal t.
anular tear classification
anular tear extent
anular tear pattern
anulus fibrosus t.
aqueous layer of tear film
aqueous tear deficiency
aqueous tear layer
artificial t.'s
t. away
t. break-up test
t. breakup time
bucket-handle meniscus t.
bucket-handle tear of meniscus
circular tear capsulotomy
cruciate ligament t.
cuff tear arthropathy
cuff tear arthroplasty
t. down
t. drainage system
t. duct
t. flow
t. gas
giant retinal t.
horseshoe t.
t. lake
lipid tear layer
longitudinal displaced complete t.
Mallory-Weiss t.
marginal tear strip
meniscus
mop-end Achilles tendon t.
mucin of t.
t. in mucosa at cardioesophageal junction
mucous tear layer
Neer acromioplasty for rotator cuff t.
noninvasive tear film break-up time
nonpreserved artificial t.'s
partial bursal surface t.
t. pool
posterior cruciate ligament t.
preocular tear film
t. of retina
rotator cuff t.
t. sac
t. secretion
triangular fibrocartilage complex t.

teardrop
t. appearance
axial load teardrop fracture
t. burst fracture
extension teardrop fracture
t. fracture
t. heart
t. pupil

tearing
excessive t.
medial collateral ligament t.
meniscal t.
short duration, unilateral, neuralgic, conjunctival injection and t.

teboroxime resting washout

technetium
t. albumin study
t. bond
t. Cardiolite stress test
t. diisopropyliminodiacetic acid scan
t. hepatoiminodiacetic acid scan
radioactive t.
t. sulfur colloid

technetium-99m
t. galactosyl-human serum albumin
t. hexamethylpropylene amine oxime single-photon emission computed tomography
t. imaging
t. macroaggregated albumin
t. MDP uptake
t. methoxyisobutylisonitrile
t. MIBI imaging
t. mini-microaggregated albumin
t. sulfur colloid

technique
Achilles tendon taping t.
active-release t.
Adkins technique spinal arthrodesis
advance cochlear echo t.
Albert suture t.
algebraic reconstruction t.
angiographic road-mapping t.
angle bisection t.
angle suture t.
antegrade double balloon-double wire t.
antegrade/retrograde cardioplegia t.
antegrade transseptal t.
anterior iliofemoral t.
anterior quadriceps musculocutaneous flap t.
anterior sandwich patch t.
anterior scoring t.
anterograde transseptal t.
anthrone colorimetric t.
antireflux ureteral implantation t.
anxiety control t.
AO-ASIF compression t.
AO surgical t.
Appolito suture t.
apposition suture t.
approximation suture t.
Arana-Iniquez intracranial cyst removal t.
arc therapy t.
arcuate suture t.
Argyll-Robertson suture t.
Arlt suture t.
arousal reduction t.
arrested-heart revascularization t.
arterial cannulation anesthetic t.
arthrographic capsular distension and rupture t.
ascending technique audiometry
aseptic catheterization t.
Asher physical build assessment t.
assisted reproductive t.
Atasoy V-Y t.
atraumatic suture t.
automated radiometric t.
avascular cuff t.
average evoked response t.
avidin-biotin immunoperoxidase t.

avidin-biotin stain t.
Axenfeld suture t.
axial multiplanar reformation t.
axial pin t.
axillary block anesthetic t.
axillary perivascular t.
bacterial automated identification t.
balloon catheter and basket-retrieval t.
bastard suture t.
behavioral management t.
behavior modification t.
bolster suture t.
brain imaging t.
Braun pinch graft t.
breathing and relaxation t.
cable wire suture t.
cannulated reaming t.
cardiac catheterization t.
cardiac imaging t.
Carr-Purcell-Meiboom-Gill spin-echo t.
cerclage wire t.
chevron marking t.
chiropractic manipulative reflex t.
classic t.
clean needle t.
cognitive behavioral t.
computer averaging t.
computerized display t.
computerized imaging t.
computer summation t.
conjugated-immunoglobulin t.
continuous pull-through t.
continuous suture t.
coronal arc t.
Crawford graft inclusion t.
Crutchfield reduction t.
Cumulative T.'s and Procedures in Clinical Microbiology
cutaneous suture t.
dental implant t.
develop isolation t.
Dimon-Hughston intertrochanteric osteotomy t.
direct insertion t.
dosimetry and t.
double immunodiffusion t.
double-looped semitendinous and gracilis hamstring graft knee reconstruction t.
double-sampling dye dilution t.
double stapling t.
drip infusion t.
en bloc no touch t.
endobronchial intubation anesthetic t.
endoforehead-biplanar face t.
endoforehead fixation t.
end-to-end reconstruction t.
enzyme-linked immunocytochemical t.
enzyme-multiplied immunoassay t.
epidural blood patch anesthetic t.
esophageal banding t.
Essex-Lopresti reduction t.
European compression technique bone screw and internal fixation
excisional biopsy t.
ex vivo t.
Ficoll-Hypaque t.
figure-of-eight suture t.
flap transplant t.
fluorescent antibody staining t.
forced oscillation t.
four field t.
Fourier-acquired steady-state t.
freehand suturing t.
free radical assay t.
gold-labeled antigen detection t.
gradient-recalled echo t.
Gram staining t.
great toe arthroplasty implant t.
guidewire exchange t.
hand washing t.
high-amplitude sucking t.
Holtzman Inkblot T.
hot biopsy t.
House-Tree-Person Projective Technique psychologic test
image-guided surgical t.
immunofluorescence t.
immunoperoxidase t.
implantation t.
interspinous segmental spinal instrumentation t.
interventional radiological t.
invasive surgical t.
irrigation t.
kissing atherectomy t.
leukocyte migration t.
Lich extravesical t.
light around wire t.
light scatter t.
Lightspeed canal preparation t.
Lloyd-Roberts fracture t.
long axis t.
long cone t.
loop gastric bypass t.
Lottes reduction t.
Louisiana ankle wrap t.
low-dose helical scanning t.
low-flow anesthetic t.
lumbar accessory movement t.
lumbar anesthetic t.
Lynn Achilles tendon repair t.
lysis centrifugation t.
Magnuson reduction t.
Malawer excision t.
manual organ stimulation t.
Marchac and Chiari short scar t.
Marcus-Balourdas-Heiple ankle fusion t.
Markov chain Monte Carlo t.
Martin reduction t.
mathematical modeling t.
Maurice corneal depot t.
McCannel suture t.
McKeever-Buck elbow t.
McSpadden endodontic t.
medial cortical overlap t.
medial graft t.
medial heel skive t.
membrane catheter t.
membrane filter t.
Menghini biopsy t.
merthiolate, iodine, formaldehyde t.
M-FISH cytogenetic t.
microwave epitope retrieval t.
midface degloving t.
Mikulicz drain t.
Milch cuff resection of ulna t.
Milch elbow t.
Millard forked flap t.
Mital elbow release t.
mixed photon-electron t.
modified anterior scoring t.
modified Belsey fundoplication t.
modified Bernard-Burow t.
modified brachial t.
modified Cantwell t.
modified Child t.
modified Crawford Campbell inlaid bone-grafting t.
modified Gilsbach t.
modified Hassan open t.
modified Pomeroy t.
Modified Richardson t.
modulus blipped echo-planar single-pulse t.
Mohs fresh tissue chemosurgery t.
Mohs fresh-tissue t.
molecular diagnostic t.
molecular genetic t.
monitored anesthesia care anesthetic t.
Monte Carlo t.

technique *(continued)*
Monticelli-Spinelli distraction t.
motion artifact suppression t.
Mowlem-Jackson t.
Mubarak-Hargens decompression t.
mucoperiosteal flap t.
Mullins blade t.
multicoil array t.
multicolor FISH cytogenetic t.
multiplanar endoscopic facial rejuvenation t.
multiple inert gas elimination t.
multiple-site perineal applicator t.
muscle energy t.
Myers bunching t.
nasal Fraser suction t.
nasovesicular catheter t.
natural holistic t.
navigator echo motion correction t.
neural arch resection t.
neurodevelopmental t.
neuroleptanalgesia anesthetic t.
neuromuscular reeducation t.
neutralization t.
Neviaser acromioclavicular t.
Nicholas five-in-one reconstruction t.
Nissen fundoplication t.
Nissen-Rosseti fundoplication t.
nitrous oxide-oxygen-opioid anesthetic t.
nonaxial beam t.
noncoplanar arch t.
noncoplanar arc t.
noncoplanar beam t.
nonoperative biopsy t.
nonsterile irrigation t.
Northern blot t.
nucleic acid amplification t.
O'Brien akinesia t.
open drop t.
open flap t.
open harvesting t.
open Hasson t.
ophthalmic vitreous surgical t.
oral anesthetic t.
orbital exenteration gastroscopic access t.
Osborne-Cotterill elbow t.
osteopathic manipulative t.
Ostrup harvesting t.
Ouchterlony double diffusion t.
Ouchterlony gel diffusion t.
paper radioimmunosorbent t.
Parkland Hospital t.
Parvin gravity t.
passive gliding t.
patch clamp t.
patient-controlled analgesia anesthetic t.
pause and squeeze t.
pelviscopic clip ligation t.
percutaneous conchotome biopsy t.
percutaneous multipuncture t.
peribulbar anesthetic t.
perichondrial double cartilage block t.
periodic acid-Schiff t.
peroxidase-antiperoxidase t.
photon irradiation technique in radiation therapy
portal venous and enteric drainage t.
positron emission tomography t.
pressure half-time t.
problem elicitation t.
program evaluation and review t.
protein A-gold t.
randomized response t.
rapid pull-through t.
rat mast cell t.
Rebuck skin window t.
sacrooccipital t.
safety technique goal
screening and diagnostic t.
Senior Apperception T.
severed limb salvage t.
sharp dissection t.
shrinking field t.
Simultaneous T. for Acuity and Readiness Testing
Simultaneous Interview T.
simultaneous multiple-angle reconstruction t.
sonic imaging t.
Speed and Boyd reduction t.
sperm microaspiration retrieval t.
spinal attunement t.
split course t.
standard isolation t.
standard mycological identification t.
stomach stapling t.
stress reduction t.
Suppan nail t.
sympathetic blockade anesthetic t.
sympathetic ganglion block anesthetic t.
tannic acid, polyphosphomolybdic acid, and amido acid staining t.
Thomson reduction t.
tumor-infiltrating lymphocyte t.
update isolation t.
V-Y advancement t.
Wagner reduction t.
Waldhausen subclavian flap t.
whole-body antibody t.

technologist
electroneurodiagnostic t.
histologic t.

technology
acoustic response t.
arrhythmia research t.
assistive technology device
automated cell-counter t.
minimal access spinal t.
signal extraction t.
video graphic tool t.
in vivo expression t.
work evaluation systems t.

tectorial membrane

tectum, pl. **tecta**
contralateral optic t.
ipsilateral optic t.

teen
T. Addiction Severity Index

teenage mother

teenager
antisocial t.
Problem-Oriented Screening Instrument for T.'s

teeth (*pl. of* tooth)

teething

Teflon
angiographic Teflon dilator
subureteric Teflon injection
T. tube insertion

Teflon tube insertion

tegmental
anterior tegmental decussation
central tegmental tract
medial central tegmental field
ventral tegmental area

tegmenti
nucleus centralis tegmenti superior

tegmentum
ventromedial t.

Tehran virus

teichoic acid crude extract

telangiectasis
calcification, Raynaud phenomenon, scleroderma, telangiectasis syndrome
conjunctival t.

hemorrhagic t.
linear t.
multiple hereditary hemorrhagic t.

telangiectatic
t. angioma
t. cancer
t. change
t. fibroma
t. glioma

Telebinocular
Keystone Telebinocular Visual Survey

telecommunication
t. device for the deaf

telemetric
t. monitoring

telemetry
cardiac stepdown unit and t.
home-based t.
t. monitor

telencephalic
perinatal telencephalic leukoencephalopathy

telephone
radiology telephone access system

telescope
angled t.
forward-viewing t.
monocular t.

telescopic
bidirectional telescopic distractor
bioptic telescopic spectacle
t. denture
t. glasses
t. spectacles

telescoping
t. crossbite
t. plugged catheter

telethermometry
graphic stress t.

Tellina virus

Tell a Tale psychiatry

Telok Forest virus

telomerase
human telomerase reverse transcriptase
internal telomerase standard

telomere repeat amplification protocol

telomeric
SMN telomeric gene
survival motor neuron telomeric gene
t. repeat amplification protocol

telopeptide
N-terminal telopeptide of type I collagen

telopeptide-poor collagen

Tembe virus

Tembusu virus

temperament
Guilford-Zimmerman T. Survey
Taylor-Johnson T. Analysis
T. and Values Inventory

temperate
mibuna temperate virus

temperature
absolute temperature
absolute temperature on the Rankine scale
altered body t.
ambient temperature and pressure
ambient temperature and pressure, dry
t., axillary
axillary t.
basal body t.
basal temperature chart
blood gas at room t.
blood pressure, pulse, respiration, and t.
blood temperature chart
t., body
body t.
body temperature, pressure, dry
capillary refill, sensation, motor function, t.
Celsius temperature scale
centigrade temperature scale
central venous t.
cervical mucous basal body t.
chilly ambient t.
t. coefficient
color and t.
color and temperature normal, both lower extremities
t. compensation
controlled t.
core body t.
customary t.
t., depth, and salinity
t. difference integrator
t. differential
differential temperature sensor
digital temperature recovery time test
dry bulb t.
t. effect
effective t.
t. factor
Fahrenheit temperature scale
t. fluctuation
t., freezing
glass transition t.
t. gradient
heat temperature vulcanized
increased skin t.
internal body t.
t. interval
t. inversion
low temperature isotropic
maximum t.
mean perfusate t.
melting t.
t. midpoint Celsius
t. by mouth
t., muscle
normal body t.
normal pressure and t.
normal temperature and pressure
optimal cutting t.
t., oral
oral t.
oral temperature device
t. and pressure
pressure, volume, t.
t. and pulse
t., pulse, and respiration
rectal t.
regulation of body t.
room temperature vulcanization
t. in saphenous vein
t. sensitivity
skin temperature recovery time
skin temperature test
standard temperature and pressure, dry
standard temperature and pulse
temporalis muscle t.
temporal temperature gradient gel electrophoresis
thermodynamic t.
time and t.
tympanic t.
ultrahigh t.
ultralow t.
water t.
wet bulb t.

temperature-gradient gel electrophoresis

template
aluminum contouring template set
bleeding time t.

template *(continued)*
Martinez Universal Perineal Interstitial T.

temple
library t.
loafer t.
paddle t.
T. University Short Syntax Inventory

temporal
alternative temporal forced choice
anterior auricular branch of superficial temporal artery
anterior mesial temporal resection
anterior temporal atrophy
anterior temporal branch
anterior temporal branch of posterior cerebral artery
anterior temporal diploic vein
anterior temporal focal spike
anterior temporal lobectomy
anterior tip of temporal lobe
anterior transverse temporal gyrus
anteromedial temporal lobe resection
anteromesial temporal lobectomy
apex of petrous part of temporal bone
apex of petrous portion of temporal bone
t. aponeurosis
t. arcade
t. arteritis
t. artery
t. artery biopsy
t. arthritis
articular eminence of temporal bone
articular fossa of temporal bone
articular surface of mandibular fossa of temporal bone
articular surface of temporal bone
articular tubercle of temporal bone
attic temporal bone
autosomal dominant temporal lobe epilepsy
t. average
t. bone
t. bone fracture
t. branch
t. canal
t. complex
t. cortex
deep temporal fascia
t. difference limen
epileptogenic temporal lesion
t. external artery
t. field of vision
t. fossa
granulomatous temporal arteritis
greater superficial temporal artery biopsy
t. headache
t. hemianopia
t. horn
inferior t.
inferior parietal and superior temporal lobe
inferior temporal artery
inferior temporal cortex
inferior temporal quadrant
inferior temporal vein
t. instability artifact
t. integration
interclavicular notch of temporal bone
jugular notch of temporal bone
t. line
t. lobe
t. lobe epilepsy
t. lobe seizure
medial t.
medial superior temporal visual area
medial temporal visual area
mesial aspect of temporal lobe
mesial temporal lobe
middle temporal visual area
monocular temporal arcuate defect
monocular temporal crescent
t. muscle wasting
occipital border of temporal bone
occipital margin of temporal bone
t., occipital, parietal
occipital temporal sulcus
occult temporal arteritis of Simmons
parietal border of squamous part of temporal bone
parietal branch of superficial temporal artery
t. peak
t. plane
pterygoid branch of posterior deep temporal artery
spatial average temporal peak
spatial peak temporal average
t. stem
superficial temporal artery-middle cerebral artery
superficial temporal artery-posterior cerebral artery
superficial temporal artery-superior cerebellar artery
superficial temporal fascia
superior temporal artery
superior temporal gyrus
superior temporal quadrant
superior temporal vein
t. temperature gradient gel electrophoresis
t. wedge

temporary
t. articulating methylmethacrylate antibiotic spacer
t. base
t. blindness
t. breast implant
t. callus
t. cartilage
t. conservatorship
t. deafness
t. dentition
t. denture
t. disability
t. endodontic restorative material
t. filling
t. global amnesia
t. hair loss
t. hearing loss
t. heart transplant
heat-activated recoverable temporary stent
t. impairment
t. impotence
t. ischemia
t. leave of absence
t. master apical file
noise-induced temporary threshold shift
t. pacemaker
t. pacemaker implant
t. partial disability
t. portacaval anastomosis
t. relief of headache pain
t. threshold shift
t. total disability
total temporary disability
t. transvenous pacemaker
t. visit

temporobasal
anterior temporobasal vein

temporofacial graft

temporomandibular
alloplastic temporomandibular joint prosthesis

t. arthralgia
articular disc of temporomandibular joint
t. articulation
t. disorder
t. joint
t. joint dislocation
t. joint disorder
t. joint dysfunction
t. joint osteoarthritis
t. joint-pain dysfunction syndrome
t. joint synovial fluid
t. ligament
medial ligament of temporomandibular joint

temporomesial region

temporoparietal
axial temporoparietal fascial flap
deep temporoparietal fascia
t. fascial flap
t. white matter

temporopolar artery

temporozygomatic suture

tenacious sputum

tenaculum
cleft palate t.

tenax
Eristalis t.

tendency
antisocial t.
exhibitionistic t.
hereditary t.
homicidal t.
invasive t.
measure of central t.
sick role t.
suicidal t.

tender
abdomen distended, tender, tympanitic
abdomen tender to palpation
hot, swollen, and t.
t. joint
t. joint count
markedly t.
t. to palpation
t. point
t. to pressure
red, swollen, tender gums
swollen and tender gums

tenderness
t. of abdomen
t. in abdomen due to hepatitis
t. in abdomen from appendicitis
t. in abdomen from gastritis
abdominal distention and t.
abdominal tenderness from appendicitis
t., asymmetry, restricted motion, and tissue texture changes
t. at site of incision
cervical motion t.
costovertebral angle t.
costovertebral angle tenderness to percussion
deep abdominal t.
diffuse abdominal t.
t. to digital palpation
heat, reddening, swelling, or t.
low back t.
lower abdominal t.
masses or t.
mass, induration, or t.
t. on palpation
pain and t.
t. to palpation or percussion
parasternal intercostal t.
patellar t.
point of maximum t.
point of t.
t. and rebound
straight leg raising t.
suprapubic t.
swelling, tenderness, limitation of motion
t. to touch
tssue texture changes, asymmetry, restriction of motion, t.
vertebral body t.

tendinitis
anterior tarsal t.
de Quervain t.
hypertrophic infiltrative t.
posterior tibial t.
rotator cuff calcific t.

tendinopathy
Achilles t.
peroneus longus t.

tendinosis
angiofibroblastic hyperplasia t.

tendinosum
xanthoma t.

tendinous
anterior tarsal tendinous sheath
t. arch
t. arch of levator ani
t. arch of pelvic fascia
t. arch of soleus muscle
t. band
t. cord
t. fiber
t. galea
palmar carpal tendinous sheath

tendo
Abraham-Pankovich tendo calcaneus repair
t. Achillis
t. Achillis lengthening
t. Achillis lengthening and toe flexor release
t. Achillis reflex

tendon
abductor digiti quinti t.
abductor hallucis t.
abductor pollicis brevis t.
accessory communicating t.
Achilles t.
Achilles tendon advancement
Achilles tendon bursa
Achilles tendon bursitis
Achilles tendon enthesis
Achilles tendon enthesis calcification
Achilles tendon insertion
Achilles tendon lengthening
Achilles tendon pain
Achilles tendon reflex
Achilles tendon reflex time
Achilles tendon repair
Achilles tendon resurfacing
Achilles tendon rupture
Achilles tendon shortening
Achilles tendon taping technique
Achilles tendon test
Achilles tendon xanthoma
Achilles tendon Z-lengthening
adductor hallucis t.
adductor pollicis brevis t.
t. advancement
anterior tibialis t.
anterior tibial t.
aponeurosis of t.
arthroscopy-assisted patellar tendon substitution
aspiration and injection of t.'s
attenuation of t.
attrition rupture of t.
attrition of t.
autogenous patellar tendon reconstruction
biceps femoris t.
biceps tendon reflex
t. bundle
calcaneonavicular ligament-tibialis posterior tendon advancement
deep tendon reflexes active and equal bilaterally
deep tendon reflexes bilaterally

tendon *(continued)*
t. dislocation
end-to-end tendon repair
t. entrapment
extensor carpi radialis brevis t.
extensor carpi radialis longus t.
extensor carpi ulnaris t.
extensor digiti minimi t.
extensor digiti quinti t.
extensor digitorum communis t.
extensor pollicis brevis t.
extensor tendon lengthening
extensor tendon tenolysis
extensor tendon transfer
flexor t.
flexor digitorum profundus t.
flexor profundus t.
flexor tendon adhesion
flexor tendon anastomosis
flexor tendon graft
flexor tendon grafting
flexor tendon laceration
flexor tendon repair
flexor tendon rupture
flexor tendon sheath
Ganley tendon transfer
giant cell tumor of tendon sheath
Golgi tendon organ
t. graft
hyperactive tendon reflex
hypoactive deep tendon reflex
identified proximal ends of t.
t. implant
increased deep tendon reflex
t. insertion
t.'s intact
t. jerk
t. lengthening
ligament reconstruction with tendon interposition
long abductor t.
Lynn Achilles tendon repair technique
mechanoreceptor Golgi tendon organ
medial canthal t.
medial transplantation of patellar tendon insertion
minimal active muscle tendon tension
Moberg free tendon graft
mop-end Achilles tendon tear
Murphy Achilles tendon advancement
muscle and t.
neck flexor t.
palmaris brevis t.
patellar tendon advancement
patellar tendon autograft
patellar tendon bearing
patellar tendon graft donor site
patellar tendon insertion
patellar tendon reflex
patellar tendon stabilization
patellar tendon suspension
patellar tendon transplant
patellar tendon transposition
patella tendon socket
percutaneous Achilles tendon repair
peroneus brevis t.
pollicis brevis extensor t.
posterior tibial t.
posterior tibial tendon dysfunction
postoperative flexor t.
profundus flexor digitorum t.
quadriceps tendon bearing
rectus femoris t.
rotator cuff t.
t. rupture
ruptured Achilles t.
t. sheath
t. shortening
split anterior tibial tendon transfer
surgical Achilles tendon lengthening
symmetrical tendon reflex
t. transfer
t. transposition
triceps tendon reflex
vascularized patellar t.
wrist extensor t.

tendon-bone
bone-patellar t.-b.

tendonitis
iliotibial band t.
infiltrative t.
pes t.
rotator cuff t.

tenens

tenia, pl. **teniae**
teniae coli
colic t.

Tennessee Self-Concept Scale

tennis elbow

tenodesis
anterolateral femorotibial ligament t.
extensor t.
MacIntosh extraarticular t.
Mueller anterolateral femorotibial ligament t.

tenolysis
de Quervain t.
extensor tendon t.

Tenon
capsule of T.
T. space

tenosynovectomy
extensor t.
flexor t.

tenosynovitis
de Quervain t.
flexor t.
granulomatous t.
stenosing t.

tenotomy
adductor t.
adductor tenotomy and obturator neurectomy
Arroyo t.
Arruga t.
extensor t.
flexor t.
graduated t.
percutaneous adductor t.

tenovagosynovitis
pigmented villonodular t.

tensa
pars t.

Tensaw virus

tense ascites

tensile
ultimate tensile strength

tensin
phosphatase and tensin homologue deleted on chromosome

tension
alveolar-arterial oxygen tension difference
alveolar-arterial oxygen tension gradient
anxiety, tension, and headache
anxiety tension state
AO tension band
applanation t.
t. by applanation
t., arterial
arterial to alveolar oxygen tension ratio
arterial blood hydrogen t.
arterial oxygen t.
articulated tension device

balanced ligamentous tension treatment
t. band
t. band fixation
carbon monoxide pressure or t.
cervical tension myositis
chronic tension and anxiety
chronic tension headache
constant tension splint
t. curve
decreased tension pressure
difference in nitrogen tension between mixed alveolar gas and mixed arterial blood
extrapolated end-tidal carbon dioxide t.
finger t.
t. fracture
group t.
t. headache
headache and t.
high lateral t.
increased eye t.
increased intraocular t.
increased mental t.
increased tension line
induced muscular t.
inspired oxygen t.
integrated isometric t.
intraalveolar oxygen t.
intraocular tension, normal
intraocular tension recorder
t. irritability
isometric systolic t.
left ventricular t.
t. line
low t.
McKay-Marg t.
minimal active muscle tendon t.
mixed expired carbon dioxide t.
muscle tension headache
t. and nervousness
nervous tension headache
neuromuscular t.
neuromuscular tension state
t. night splint
normal intraocular t.
ocular t.
t. oculus sinister
partial arterial gas tension of carbon dioxide
partial pressure tension of carbon dioxide, vein
partial pressure tension of oxygen, vein
partial venous gas tension of oxygen
postmenstrual t.
premenstrual t.
premenstrual tension syndrome
pupils, tension, media, disc, and fundus
reciprocal tension membrane
reduce tension headache frequency
relaxed skin tension line
t. by Schiotz tonometer
second stage of decreased intraocular t.
skin tension line
surface t.
tactile t.
time to peak t.
transcutaneous carbon dioxide t.
twitch t.
upper limb tension test
volume and t.
voluntary control of tension headache

tension-free

t.-f. anastomosis
t.-f. closure
t.-f. hernioplasty
transvaginal t.-f.
t.-f. vaginal tape

tension-reducing hypothesis

tension-time

t.-t. index
t.-t. index per beat

tensor

t. fasciae latae muscle
t. veli palatini

tent

aerosol t.
Ohio pediatric tent with compressed air
Ohio pediatric tent with oxygen

tentative

t. diagnosis
t. discharge tomorrow
t. finding

tenth

t. cranial nerve
t. molar solution
t. value layer radiation

tenth-normal solution

tenting

t. of diaphragm
t. of skin

tentorial

t. angle
t. herniation
marginal tentorial branch of internal carotid artery
t. nerve
t. notch
t. region

tentorium

t. cerebelli attachment
t. of hypophysis

tepid water enema

teratogenic effect

teratoma

adult cystic t.
atypical brain t.
benign cystic t.
t. differentiated
immature ovarian t.
malignant ovarian t.
malignant teratoma, anaplastic
malignant teratoma, trophoblastic
malignant teratoma, undifferentiated
malignant trophoblastic t.
mature cystic ovarian t.
mature mediastinal t.
mature ovarian t.
ovarian cystic t.
ovarian embryonal t.
ovarian immature t.
t. with malignant transformation

teratosis

atresic t.

teres

anterior pronator t.
t. major muscle
t. muscle
notch for ligamentum t.
pronator t.
pronator teres muscle
subcutaneous bursa of teres major

term

amniotic fluid at t.
t. birth appropriate for gestational age
t. birth, living child
t. birth, living female
t. birth, living infant
t. birth, living male
chronic long term illness
t. delivery
t. delivery intrapartum death
full term, born dead
t. gestation
t. infant
t. intrauterine pregnancy
intrauterine pregnancy at t.

term *(continued)*
intrauterine pregnancy, term birth, cesarean section
intrauterine pregnancy, term birth, living infant
t. living newborn
lowest level t.
t. milk
t. newborn
newborn, term, normal, female
newborn, term, normal, male
t. normal delivery
pregnancy at t.
pregnancy, term, complicated delivered, living female
pregnancy, term, complicated delivered, living male
pregnancy, term, uncomplicated
pregnancy, term, uncomplicated delivered, living female
pregnancy, term, uncomplicated delivered, living male
serenity, tranquility, peace user's term for dimethoxymethylamphetamine
Systematized Nomenclature of Medicine Clinical T.'s

Termeil virus

terminal
amino t.
anterior terminal vein
t. antrum
t. antrum contraction
t. arteriole
t. artery
t. aspiration of gastric contents
autonomic postganglionic nerve t.
axonal t.
t. banding
t. banding of chromosome
t. bar
t. blush
t. bouton
t. bronchiole
t. cancer
t. capillary network
carboxyl t.
carboxyl terminal peptide
t. carcinoma
t. care
caudal appendage, short terminal phalanges, deafness, cryptorchidism, mental retardation syndrome
central terminal of Wilson
certification of terminal illness
t. crest
t. deletion
t. dementia
t. deoxynucleotide transferase
t. deoxynucleotidyl transferase
t. device
t. dribbling
t. ductal lobular unit
t. or end
t. extension
t. extensor mechanism
functional terminal innervation ratio
t. ganglion
t. hair
t. half-life of isotopes
t. hepatic vein obliteration
t. ileal loop
t. ileitis
t. ileum
t. ileum intubation
t. ileus
t. illness
t. infection
t. innervation ratio
t. internal carotid artery
t. interphalangeal
t. knee extension
t. latency
t. limen
t. line
long terminal repeat sequence
maximal terminal flow
t. motor latency
t. nerve ending
neurohypophysial nerve t.
t. phalanx
posterior terminal vein
pudendal-nerve terminal motor latency
reflux into terminal ileum normal
t. repeat
t. respiratory acidosis
t. respiratory unit
t. sedation
t. sensation
t. sensory latency
t. stage of illness
t. transferase
t. vein
video display t.
video display terminal glare screen
video display terminal simulator
visual display t.
t. web
Wilson central t.

terminale
tight filum t.

terminally
t. ill
patient terminally ill

terminated
pregnancy t.
t. pregnancy

termination
early-phase t.
elective termination of pregnancy
intentional termination of pregnancy
medical termination of pregnancy
patient termination record
t. of pregnancy
surgical termination of pregnancy
voice termination time
voluntary termination of pregnancy

terminology
current medical information and t.
Current Procedural T.
Systematized Nomenclature of Medicine Reference T.

Terpeniya
Zaliv Terpeniya virus

terpin
elixir terpin hydrate
elixir terpin hydrate with codeine

terrain
biological terrain assessment

terramycin
triamcinolone t.

territory
vertebrobasilar territory ischemia

terror
amnesia for sleep terror event
attack of intense t.
current night t.'s
t. dream
night t.'s
sleep terror disorder

Terry
T. nail
T. syndrome

Terson syndrome

tert
methyl-*tert*-butyl ether therapy
triamcinolone acetomide *tert*-butyl acetate

tertian
benign tertian malaria

t. fever
t. malaria
malignant tertian fever
malignant tertian malaria
malignant tertian malarial parasite
t. parasite

tertiary
t. amputation
t. butyl acetate
t. care
t. care facility
t. cleavage
t. closure
t. contraction
t. hyperparathyroidism
methyl tertiary butyl ether
noduloulcerative tertiary syphilis
t. syphilis

tesla
joule per t.

Tessier classification

Test-16
Sinonasal Outcome T.

test
Aachen aphasia t.
abdominal jugular t.
abnormal glucose tolerance t.
abnormal liver function t.
abortus-Bang-ring t.
absorbed test plasma
academic aptitude t.
acetic acid t.
achievement t.
Achilles tendon reflex t.
Achilles tendon t.
acid challenge t.
acid clearance t.
acid reflux t.
acid test solution
acoustic noise t.
acoustic reflex t.
acoustic stimulation t.
acquired immune deficiency syndrome antibody t.
adenosine thallium t.
T. of Adolescent/Adult Word Finding
T. of Adolescent Language
Adolescent Language Screening T.
adonitol fermentation t.
agar diffusion t.
agar dilution t.
agar gel diffusion t.
agar gel precipitation t.
Age Projection T.
agglutination-flocculation t.
agglutination test for brucellosis
air caloric t.
airway function t.
alcohol sniff t.
Alcohol Use Disorders Identification T.
aldehyde-thionine-periodic acid-Schiff t.
alkaline phosphatase t.
alkali patch t.
Allen vision t.
allergen inhalation challenge t.
alpha fetoprotein t.
alpha verbal t.
alternate cover t.
alternate monaural loudness balance t.
alternate response t.
alternate uses t.
ambulatory uterine contraction t.
aminopyrine breath t.
amplified *Mycobacterium tuberculosis* direct t.
Amsler grid t.
amylase urine spot t.
analyst anchor t.
Anderson and Goldberger t.
Andrews anterior instability t.
anergy skin test battery
angiotensin I, II infusion t.
angiotensinogen t.
angiotensin sensitivity t.
anion gap t.
ankle clonus t.
ankle dorsiflexion t.
anorectal function t.
anterior apprehension t.
anterior rotary drawer t.
anteroposterior drawer t.
anteroposterior stress t.
anthropomorphic test dummy
anti-B19 antibody t.
antibiotic-associated colitis toxin t.
antibiotic sensitivity t.
anti-blood group A antiglobulin t.
antibody-dependent cytotoxicity t.
antibody screening t.
anti-*Chlamydia* antibody t.
anticytoplasmic antibody t.
antideoxyribonuclease B titer t.
antiendomysial antibody t.
antigen detection t.
antigen stool detection t.
antigliadin IgA ELISA autoimmune t.
antigliadin IgG ELISA autoimmune t.
antigliadin IgG, IgA t.
anti-GM_1 antibody t.
antihuman globulin t.
antimalignant antibody t.
antimicrobial susceptibility t.
antineuronal enteric antibody t.
antinuclear antibody screening t.
anti-Rho-D titer t.
antistreptococcal polysaccharide A t.
antistreptolysin t.
antistreptozyme t.
antithrombin III t.
antitreponemal antibody t.
Antivirogram test procedure
T. Anxiety Inventory
aortic jugular t.
APC stool t.
Aphasia Screening T.
API Staph-IDENT t.
Apley compression t.
Apley distraction t.
Apley grinding t.
Apley knee t.
Apley scratch t.
Apt-Downey alkali denaturation t.
APTT coagulation t.
Arabic eye t.
arabinose fermentation t.
D-arabitol fermentation t.
argentaffin reaction t.
arginine infusion t.
arginine-insulin stimulation t.
arginine-insulin tolerance t.
arginine stimulation t.
Argo corn starch t.
arm fossa t.
arm-tongue time t.
Army Alpha t.
Army Beta t.
Army General Classification T.
arterial blood gas point-of-care t.
T. of Articulation Performance-Diagnostic
T. of Articulation Performance-Screen
artificial erection t.
arylsulfatase activity t.
ascariasis serological t.
Aschheim-Zondek t.
ascitic fluid t.
ascorbic acid t.
Aspergillus antibody t.

test *(continued)*
aspirin tolerance t.
ASTRA profile t.
atopy patch t.
atropine suppression t.
attached proton t.
attention alertness t.
T. of Attitude Toward School
audiometry sweep t.
Auditory Analysis T.
auditory apperception t.
auditory brainstem response t.
T.'s for Auditory Comprehension of Language
T.'s for Auditory Comprehension of Language-Revised
Auditory Comprehension T. for Sentences
T. of Auditory Discrimination
Auditory Discrimination T.
auditory discrimination t.
Auditory Pointing T.
augmented histamine t.
AuraTek rapid cancer t.
Austin Spanish Articulation T.
automated dithionite t.
automated factor V Leiden mutation t.
automated reagin t.
automated test target calibration
autonomic function t.
Autopath QC t.
axial compression t.
axial load t.
axial manual traction t.
balloon test occlusion
Bankson-Bernthal Test of Phonology
Barlow and Ortolani t.
basic assurance t.
t.'s of basic experience
Basic Occupational Literacy T.
basophil granulation t.
battery of t.'s
Beery Developmental T. of Visual-Motor Integration
Békésy Functionality Detection T.
Bender-Gestalt t.
Bender Visual-Motor Gestalt T.
bentonite flocculation t.
Benton Visual Retention T., Revised
bicolor guaiac t.
bile esculin t.
Bilingual Syntax Measure II T.
Binet-Simon t.
Bingham Button T.
Binocular Visual Acuity T.
biological false-positive serologic test for syphilis
Blind Learning Aptitude T.
block design t.
blood serologic t.
Boehm T. of Basic Concepts
t. bolus
borderline glucose tolerance t.
Boston T. for Examining Aphasia
Boston Naming T.
breast stimulation contraction t.
breath hydrogen t.
Brief T. of Head Injury
Brief Vestibular Disorientation T.
Brightness Acuity T.
Bruce maximal stress t.
Bryant-Schwan Design T.
bulimia t.
Buschke Memory T.
caffeine and halothane contracture t.
calcium tolerance t.
calcium-urine spot t.
California Achievement T.
California T. of Basic Skills
California Critical Thinking Skills T.
California mastitis t.
California T. of Mental Maturity-Short Form
California Test of Personality
California Verbal Learning T.
caloric stimulation test for vestibular function
CAMP t.
Canadian T. of Basic Skills
Canadian Cognitive Abilities T.
Canterbury Alcoholism Screening T.
capillary agglutination t.
capillary fragility t.
carbon-13 urea breath t.
carbon-14 urea breath t.
card agglutination trypanosomiasis t.
cardiac stress t.
cardiolipin flocculation t.
cardiolipin Wassermann t.
Cardiolite stress t.
cardiopulmonary exercise t.
cardiopulmonary stress t.
carotid sinus t.
Carrow T. for Auditory Comprehension
Casoni intradermal t.
catch and clunk t.
Category T.
cephalin flocculation t.
cervical mucus penetration t.
Chick Embryotoxicity Screening T.
Children of Alcoholics Screening T.
Children's Apperception T., Supplemental
Children's Apperceptive Story-Telling T.
Children's Articulation T.
Children's Embedded Figures T.
Children's Orientation and Amnesia T.
chi-squared t.
chlormerodrin accumulation t.
cholesteric analysis profile t.
chorionic gonadotropin t.
Christie-Atkins-Munch-Petersen t.
chromium release t.
Clinical Adaptive T.
Clinical T. of Sensory Interaction & Balance
clomiphene citrate challenge t.
clot retraction t.
clot stabilization t.
coagglutination t.
cognitive function t.'s
T. of Cognitive Style in Mathematics
coil t.
cold pressor t.
cold-stimulation time t.
College Ability T.
colloidal gold t.
colony overlay t.
colony-stimulating factor fluorescent treponemal antibody-absorption t.
colony-stimulating factor microhemagglutination-*Treponema pallidum* t.
color allergy screening t.
combining power t.
Communication Abilities Diagnostic T.
complement fixation antibody t.
Completing Sentence T.
Complex Figure T.
Comprehensive T. of Visual Functioning
Concept Mastery T.
Conceptual Systems T.
T. of Concept Utilization

conglutinating complement absorption t.
conjunctival provocation t.
contact, control, test, evaluate, treatment
continuous performance t.
Continuous Visual Memory T.
contraction stress t.
Controlled Oral Word Association T.
Coombs t.
copper reduction t.
copy intersecting pentagons t.
corneal impression t.
cortisone-glucose tolerance t.
cortisone-primed oral glucose tolerance t.
cosyntropin stimulation t.
countercurrent immunoelectrophoresis t.
cover t.
cover-uncover eye t.
creatinine clearance t.
creatinine urine spot t.
Creativity T.'s for Children
critical flicker fusion t.
Critical Reasoning T.
t. and crossmatch
Culture-Free Intelligence T.
t. of cure
C-urea breath t.
cutaneous tuberculin t.
dark adaptation t.
Davidson protocol exercise t.
daytime multiple sleep latency t.
decibel hearing t.
delayed double diffusion t.
delayed hypersensitivity t.
delayed work recall t.
Del Rio Language Screening T.
Dennis T. of Child Development
dental aptitude t.
Denver Auditory Phoneme Sequencing T.
Denver Developmental Screening T.
Denver Eye Screening T.
dermatophyte test media
desensitization t.
Detroit T.'s of Learning Aptitude - Primary, Second Edition
Detroit T.'s of Learning Aptitude, Third Edition
Developmental Articulation T.
developmental hand function t.
Developmental T. of Visual Perception
Diabetes: Basic Knowledge T.
Diabetes: Basic Knowledge T.
diagnostic test and procedure
dichotic environmental sounds t.
dichotic pitch discrimination t.
Dichotic Word T.
did not t.
differential agglutination t.
Differential Aptitude T.
differential rheumatoid agglutination t.
Digital Finger Tapping T.
digital rectal t.
digital temperature recovery time t.
digit substitution t.
digit symbol substitutional t.
dihydroepiandrosterone loading t.
dipyridamole echocardiography t.
direct agglutination t.
direct amplification t.
direct antiglobulin Coombs t.
direct fluorescent antibody t.
direct fluorescent antigen t.
direct immunofluorescence t.
direct latex agglutination pregnancy t.
diurnal cortisol t.
dobutamine stress t.
Doerfler-Stewart t.
Doppler flow t.
Doppler ophthalmic t.
t. dose
dot ELISA t.
Draw-A-Family t.
Draw-A-Person t.
Drug Abuse Screening T.
drug-induced lymphocyte stimulation t.
dumping provocation t.
duodenal secretin t.
duodenal string t.
duration of voluntary apnea t.
dye disappearance t.
t. ear
T. of Early Language Development, Second Edition
early pregnancy t.
T. of Early Reading Comprehension
Early Speech Perception T.
Eating Attitudes T.
Ebbinghaus t.
T. of Economic Literacy
Eddy hot plate t.
Edinburgh Articulation T.
Educational Goal Attainment T.
Education Apperception T.
effective thyroxine t.
egg yolk-cobalamin absorption t.
Ego-Ideal and Conscience Development T.
Ego Strength t.
Eidetic Parents T.
elevated-arm stress t.
ELISA-I, -II, -III t.
Ellestad exercise stress t.
Embedded Figures T.
empty can t.
enzyme allergosorbent t.
enzyme-linked antiglobulin t.
enzyme-multiplied immunoassay t.
epsilometer t.
t. equivocal possible low titer
ergonovine provocation t.
erythrocyte fragility t.
erythromycin breath t.
ethanol gelation t.
etiocholanolone t.
euglobulin clot t.
euglobulin lysis t.
evoked response t.
Ewald test meat
T. for Examining Expressive Morphology
exercise stress t.
exercise tolerance t.
exercise treadmill t.
exercise treadmill test with thallium
Expressive One-Word Picture Vocabulary T.
external rotation-abduction stress t.
fabere abduction t.
fabere extension t.
fabere external rotation t.
fabere fixation t.
factor V Leiden mutation t.
Fagerstrom T. for Nicotine Dependence
Fairview Language Evaluation T.
Family Apperception T.
family attitudes t.
Family Relations T.
Farnsworth panel D-15 color vision t.
fasting t.
fat tolerance t.
fecal leukocyte count t.
fecal occult blood t.
Fein Articulation Screening T.
Fetal Activity T.
fetal cardiac reactivity t.

test *(continued)*
fetal heart rate nonstress t.
fetal hemoglobin t.
fetal movement acceleration t.
fibrinogen qualitative t.
fibrinogen uptake t.
Figurative Language Interpretation T.
Filtered Audiometer Speech T.
filter paper microscopic t.
finger-counting vision t.
finger extension t.
finger-nose-finger coordination t.
Finger Oscillation T.
finger-to-finger-to-nose t.
finger-to-nose coordination t.
Fisher exact t.
Fisher-Logemann T. of Articulation Competence
Flanagan Aptitude Classification T.
Flanagan Industrial T.
flexion-rotation-drawer knee instability t.
flicker fusion frequency t.
Flowers Auditory Screening T.
Flowers Auditory T. of Selective Attention
Fluharty Preschool Speech and Language Screening T.
fluorescein clearance t.
fluorescein treponemal antibody t.
fluorescent allergosorbent t.
fluorescent antibody to membrane antigen t.
fluorescent antimembrane antibody t.
fluorescent focus inhibition t.
fluorescent gonorrhea t.
fluoroallergosorbent t.
focus-reduction neutralization t.
Forer Sentence Completion T.
formiminoglutamic acid t.
Fowler single breath t.
fractional test meal
Franck Drawing Completion T.
Free-Floating Anxiety T.
Freeman Anxiety Neurosis and Psychosomatic T.
Free Running Asthma T.
Frenchay Aphasia Screening T.
Friedman test for pregnancy
Frostig Developmental T. of Visual Motor Perception
Frostig Movement Skills T. Battery
fructose tolerance t.
Fullerton Language T. for Adolescents
function t.
Functional Acuity Contrast T.
functional hearing t.
Functional Integration t.
functional muscle t.
fusion-inferred threshold t.
galactose tolerance t.
gallbladder function t.
Galveston Orientation and Amnesia T.
Galveston Orientation and Awareness T.
gelatin agglutination t.
General Aptitude T. Battery
General Clerical T.
giant ragweed t.
Gibson-Cooke sweat t.
Gilmore Oral Reading T.
glucagon t.
glucose absorption t.
glucose-insulin tolerance t.
glucose-lactate tolerance t.
glucose oxidase t.
glucose tolerance test
glycogen storage t.
glycosylated hemoglobin t.
Goldman-Fristoe T. of Articulation
Goldman-Fristoe-Woodcock Auditory Skills T. Battery
golfer's elbow t.
gonadotropin agonist stimulation t.
gonococcal complement-fixation t.
gonorrhea complement-fixation t.
Goodenough-Harris Drawing T.
graded exercise t.
graded treadmill exercise t.
Graham-Kendall Memory for Designs T.
Gram stain of stool t.
granulocyte immunofluorescence t.
gravity stress t.
Gray Oral Reading T., Third Edition
Grid T. of Schizophrenic Thought Disorder
group A streptococcus direct t.
Group Embedded Figures T.
Group Reading T.
growth hormone-releasing factor t.
growth hormone stimulation t.
guaiac stool t.
Guilford-Zimmerman Personality T.
guinea pig kidney absorption t.
guinea pig maximization t.
Haemophilus test medium
hair analysis t.
Hallpike caloric stimulation t.
Halstead Aphasia T.
Halstead-Reitan Neuropsychological T. Battery
Hamburg-Wechsler Intelligence T. for Children
hamster oocyte penetration t.
hamster zona-free ovum t.
Hand Dynamometer T.
handgrip apexcardiographic t.
hand motion at 3 feet vision t.
hand strength t.
hand thrust t.
Hardy-Rand-Ritter color vision test kit
harmonic attenuation t.
Harris Infant Neuromotor T.
head distraction t.
head-down tilt t.
head thrust t.
head tilt t.
head-up tilt-table t.
Health Check T.
health screening t.
hearing distraction t.
hearing-for-speech t.
heart t.
heat detection t.
heel-knee-shin t.
heel-to-knee t.
heel-to-shin t.
hemadsorption t.
hemagglutination inhibition morphine t.
hemagglutination treponemal test for syphilis
Hemoccult slide t.
Hendler T. for Chronic Pain
heparin response t.
hepatojugular reflex t.
hereditary hemolytic anemia t.
Heston Personality Inventory Test
high-altitude simulation t.
Hinton flocculation test for syphilis
hip rotation t.
Hiskey-Nebraska T. of Learning Aptitude
histamine challenge t.
histamine inhalation t.
histamine provocation t.

histamine stimulation t.
histoplasmin skin t.
Hodkinson Mental T.
home medical test kit
home pregnancy t.
Hooper Visual Organization T.
hormone receptor t.
hot plate t.
5-hour glucose tolerance t.
2-hour pregnancy t.
House-Tree T.
House-Tree-Person Projective Technique psychologic t.
Huhner t.
human basophil degranulation t.
human chorionic gonadotropin t.
human erythrocyte agglutination t.
Hundred Pictures Naming T.
hydrocortisone t.
hydrogen breath t.
hyperventilation provocation t.
ice water t.
icterus index t.
immune diffusion t.
immunity t.
immunobead t.
immunodiffusion t.
immunodouble diffusion t.
immunofluorescence t.
immunoglobulin consumption t.
immunologic t.
immunological fecal occult blood t.
implantation t.
indigo carmine t.
indirect antiglobulin t.
indirect bilirubin t.
indirect Coombs t.
indirect fluorescent rabies antibody t.
indirect hemagglutination antibody t.
indirect microhemagglutination t.
indole, methyl red, Voges-Proskauer, and citrate t.
T. of Infant Motor Performance
infertility t.'s
inhalation t.
initial drug screening t.
insulin clearance t.
insulin hypoglycemia t.
insulin receptor binding t.
insulin sensitivity t.
insulin tolerance t.
intelligence quotient t.
interpersonal reaction t.
Inter-Person Perception T.
intracellular magnesium t.
intracutaneous t.
intradermal cancer t.
intraductal secretin t.
intraoperative endoscopic Congo red t.
intraoral cariogenicity t.
intraperitoneal glucose tolerance t.
intravenous glucose tolerance t.
intravenous histamine t.
intravenous tolbutamide tolerance t.
invasive activity t.
inversion stress t.
iodine azide t.
Iowa Achievement T.
Iowa Algebra Aptitude T.
Iowa T.'s of Basic Skills
Iowa Pressure Articulation T.
iron tolerance t.
irresistible impulse t.
isometric hand grip t.
isotonic endurance t.
jugular compression t.
Kahn intelligence t.
Kahn T. of Symbol Arrangement
Kaufman T. of Educational Achievement
Kent State University Speech Discrimination T.
kidney punch test
Kindergarten Auditory Screening T.
Kindergarten Language Screening T.
Kindergarten Readiness T.
Kleihauer-Betke t.
Knowledge of Occupations T.
Kuder Performance T.
lactose tolerance t.
T. of Language Competence
T. of Language Development - Intermediate, Second Edition
Language Modalities T. for Aphasia
Language Proficiency T.
laryngeal cough reflex t.
lateral position t.
latex agglutination-inhibition t.
latex fixation t.
latex flocculation t.
T. of Learning Accuracy in Children
Lee and Desus D t.
left atrial transesophageal pacing t.
leucine aminopeptidase t.
leucine tolerance t.
leukocyte esterase t.
leukocyte histamine release t.
leukocyte migration inhibition t.
LH Color t.
Liddle dexamethasone suppression t.
Lighthouse Distance Visual Acuity T.
light projection t.
limited quantity test performed on small specimen
limited treadmill t.
linear visual acuity t.
lipoprotein electrophoresis t.
T. of Listening Accuracy in Children
Listening Comprehension T.
liver enzyme t.
liver flocculation t.
liver function t.'s
liver injury t.
loaded breathing t.
locally made rapid urease t.
Locke-Wallace Marital Adjustment t.
low-calcium test diet
low-dose dexamethasone suppression t.
low-dose short synacthen t.
low-level graded exercise t.
lues t.
lumbar extension t.
lung connectivity t.
lupus band t.
lupus erythematosus cell t.
Luria-Delbruck fluctuation t.
Luscher Color T.
Lyme disease antibody t.
lymphoblastic transformation t.
lymphocyte immunofluorescence t.
lymphocyte transformation t.
lymphocytotoxicity t.
lymphogranuloma venereum complement fixation t.
lysine decarboxylase t.
lysostaphin susceptibility t.
Macherey-Nagel strep t.
Machover Draw-A-Person T.
macrophage migration inhibition t.
macroscopic agglutination t.
macroscopic broth dilution t.
Macro-Vue RPR Card T.
Maddox rod t.
Maddox wing t.
magnetic field-search coil t.

test *(continued)*
maintenance of wakefulness t.
Make A Picture Story t.
making change t.
malaria film t.
male frog t.
male impotence t.
malonate utilization t.
maltose fermentation t.
mammary aspiration specimen cytology t.
Manipulative Aptitude T.
mannitol fermentation t.
mannose fermentation t.
D-mannose fermentation t.
Mann-Whitney U t.
Mantel-Haenszel test for linearity
Mantoux tuberculin skin t.
manual muscle t.
Marcus Gunn t.
MAS cytology t.
MASS cytology t.
MAST blood t.
mast cell degranulation t.
matched pairs signed rank t.
Matching Familiar Figures T.
Maudsley Mentation T.
Maurer optimization t.
maximal exercise tolerance t.
maximal treadmill stress t.
maximum stimulation t.
Mayo Clinic system test for primary biliary cirrhosis
McDonald Deep T. of Articulation
McNemar test of significance
meal tolerance t.
mean swell time botulism t.
Mecholyl skin t.
Medical College Admission T.
medical test cabinet
Meeting Street School Screening T.
Melastatin test kit
melezitose fermentation t.
melibiose fermentation t.
Memory for Designs t.
memory guidance saccade t.
Mental Alternation T.
mental arithmetic t.
mental stress t.
Merrill-Palmer Scale of Mental T.'s
Mertens Visual Perception T.
metabolic products t.
metabolism inhibition t.
methacholine challenge t.
methacholine chloride skin t.
methasone-suppressed corticotropin-releasing hormone t.
methemoglobin reduction t.
methylene blue t.
methylphenidate challenge t.
methyl red t.
Metropolitan Achievement T., Seventh Edition
Metropolitan Readiness T.
Michigan Abuse Screening T.
Michigan Alcoholism Screening T.
Michigan Neuropathy Screening T.
Michigan Picture T., Revised
Micral urine dipstick t.
Micral urine test strip
microagglutination t.
microbial susceptibility t.
microdilution broth dilution t.
microdilution broth susceptibility t.
microdilution serum bactericidal t.
microendoscopic test card
microhemagglutination test for *Treponema pallidum*
microscopic agglutination t.
MicroTrak direct fluorescent antibody t.
microtube dilution t.
Middlebrook-Dubos hemagglutination t.
midpoint skin t.
migration inhibition t.
milk proteolysis t.
milk ring t.
Miller Analogies T.
Miller-Yoder T. of Grammatical Comprehension
Millon Clinical Multiaxial Inventory t.
Minimum Auditory Capabilities T.
minimum bactericidal concentration t.
Minimum Essentials T.
minimum inhibitory concentration susceptibility t.
mini object t.
Minnesota Clerical Aptitude T.
Minnesota T. for Differential Diagnosis of Aphasia
Minnesota Engineering Analogies T.
Minnesota Mechanical Assembly T.
Minnesota Paper Form Board T.
Minnesota Percepto-Diagnostic T.
Minnesota Scholastic Aptitude T.
Minnesota Spatial Relations T.
Minor iodine-starch t.
6-minute walking t.
miracidial immobilization t.
mirror rocking t.
mixed agglutination t.
mixed lymphocyte culture t.
Miyazaki-Bonney test for stress incontinence
Modern Occupational Skills T.
Modified Clinical Technique t.
modified Draize t.
modified oxidase t.
modified rapid fermentation t.
modified rhyme hearing t.
modified tone decay t.
Modified Word Learning T.
Moeller decarboxylation t.
Mohs hardness t.
Molulsky dye reduction t.
molybdenum-99 breakthrough t.
monaural loudness balance t.
monoclonal antibody coagglutination t.
monocular confrontation visual field t.
monocyte function t.
Monospot t.
Monosticon Dri-Dot t.
Monotic Word Memory T.
Montenegro skin t.
morning corticotropin-releasing hormone t.
motility test medium
motivation analysis t.
motor control t.
motor coordination t.
Motor-Free Visual Perception T.
Motor Impersistence T.
mouse antibody production t.
mouse neutralization t.
Mr. Color t.
mucate fermentation t.
mucin clot prevention t.
mucin clot t.
MUGA exercise stress t.
multiphasic health screen t.
multiple antigen stimulation t.
multiple choice discrimination t.
multiple puncture tuberculin t.
Multiple Sleep Latency T.
multipuncture t.
multistage graded exercise t.
multithread allergosorbent t.
mumps sensitivity t.

mumps skin test antigen
Murex *Candida albicans* t.
Murphy punch maneuver t.
muscle enzyme t.
muscle function t.
muscle response t.
Music Achievement T. 1-4
mydriatic provocative t.
mydriatic test for angle-closure glaucoma
Myers-Briggs Type Indicator psychologic test
myoglobin clearance t.
N-acetylglucosamine fermentation t.
nalidixic acid t.
Names Learning T.
NAP differentiation t.
nasal antigen challenge t.
nasal provocation t.
National Adult Reading T.
National Attention T.
navicular drop t.
NBT dye t.
near patient t.
near vision t.
negative control t.
negative patch t.
negative Schick t.
Neisseria gonorrhoeae DNA detection t.
neoprecipitin t.
nerve compression t.
nerve conduction velocity t.
nerve excitability t.
Neufeld capsular t.
neurodevelopmental screening t.
neurometric test battery
neuropsychological t.
neuropsychological test battery
neuropsychological test profile
neuropsychological test Z score
Neurotic Personality Factor T.
neutral density filter t.
neutralization t.
New Mexico Attitude Toward Work T.
New Mexico Career Planning T.
New Mexico Knowledge of Occupations T.
niacin accumulation t.
ninety hue discrimination t.
nipple stimulation contraction stress t.
nitrate disc t.
nitrate reduction t.
Nitrazine fern t.
nitric acid t.
nitrite reduction t.
nitroblue tetrazolium dye t.
nitrogen washout t.
no t.
no new laboratory test orders
noninvasive diagnostic t.
nonirritating test substance
Nonne globulin t.
Non-Reading Aptitude T. Battery
Non-Reading Intelligence Test, Levels 1-3
nonstress test fetal monitoring
nontreponemal flocculation t.
nontreponemal serologic t.
nontreponemal syphilis t.
Nonverbal Ability T.
T. of Nonverbal Auditory Discrimination
T. of Nonverbal Intelligence
normal lymphocyte transfer t.
Norris Educational Achievement T.
Northern blot t.
Northwestern Syntax Screening T.
Northwestern University Children's Perception of Speech T.
no special preparation necessary for t.
novobiocin susceptibility t.
N-telopeptide urine t.
nuclear stress t.
nucleic acid amplification t.
nucleic acid hybridization t.
number connection t.
Numerical Attention T.
t. object
object t.
object assembly t.
Object Classification T.
objective prism-neutralized cover t.
Object Sorting T.
Object Sorting Scales psychologic test
Obstructive Sleep Disorders-6 t.
obtained under test conditions
occlusive patch t.
occult blood t.
O'Connor finger dexterity t.
Octopus 201 perimeter t.
ocular dysmetria t.
ocular motility t.
oculodynamic t.
Ohio T.'s of Articulation and Perception of Sounds
oleic acid uptake t.
Oliphant Auditory Discrimination Memory T.
Oliphant Auditory Synthesizing T.
one-hour glucose tolerance t.
one-leg hop for distance t.
open application t.
open epicutaneous t.
open patch t.
Optochin susceptibility t.
oral glucose challenge t.
oral glucose tolerance t.
Oral Language Sentence Imitation Screening T.
Oral Verbal Intelligence T.
Organic Integrity T.
orientation t.
t. orientation procedure
ornithine tolerance t.
orthogonal-hole test pattern
osmolality dehydration t.
osmolality urine spot t.
osmotic fragility t.
Osteomark NTx serum t.
Otis-Lennon Mental Ability T.
Otis Quick Scoring Mental Abilities T.
otoacoustic emission t.
ovarian ascorbic acid depletion t.
ovarian cholesterol depletion t.
overhead exercise t.
overnight high-dose dexamethasone suppression t.
overnight metyrapone t.
overnight 1-mg dexamethasone suppression t.
oxacillin disc diffusion t.
oxaloacetic acid t.
oxytocin challenge t.
Paced Auditory Serial Addition T.
pacing stress t.
Pain Apperception T.
Palmer acid test for peptic ulcer
pancreatic exocrine function t.
pancreatic suppression t.
pancreozymin secretin t.
Pantomime Recognition T.
paper radioimmunosorbent t.
paracetamol absorption t.
parainfluenza antibody t.
particle agglutination t.
Pascal-Suttle Test psychiatry
passive accessory motion t.
passive cutaneous anaphylaxis t.
passive forced duction t.
passive head-up tilt t.

test *(continued)*
passive hemagglutination t.
patch skin t.
patch test for allergy
patch test for tuberculosis
patellar apprehension t.
patellar glide t.
patellar inhibition t.
Patterned Elicitation Syntax Screening T.
Paul-Bunnell antibody t.
PCR amplification t.
Peabody Individual Achievement T.
Pease-Allen Color t.
pediatric infectious disease developmental screening t.
Pediatric Speech Intelligibility T.
pendular eye-tracking t.
penicillin disc t.
penicilloyl polylysine skin t.
pentagastrin gastric secretory t.
pentagastrin provocation t.
Pepper Visual Skills for Reading T.
Perception of Relationships T.
T.'s of Perception of Scientists and Self
perchlorate discharge t.
performance-intensity function t.
perimeter corneal reflex t.
perinatal nonstress t.
perinatal stress t.
periodic acid-Schiff t.
peripheral cue t.
peripheral detection t.
peritoneal equilibration t.
peroxidase-labeled antibodies t.
peroxide hemolysis t.
Personnel T.'s for Industry
pertussis agglutination t.
phenacetin breath t.
phonemic segmentation t.
phonetically balanced rhyme t.
Photo Articulation T. psychology
photostress recovery t.
Physical Ability T.
Physical Performance T.
physical volume t.
Physiognomic Cue Test
physiologic reflux t.
Pictorial T. of Intelligence
Picture Articulation and Language Screening T.
picture-frustration study, t.
Picture Identification T.
Picture Reasoning T.
Picture Story Language T.
pineapple test for butyric acid in stomach
pituitary function t.
pivot shift t.
placental function t.
planar thallium t.
plantar ischemia t.
plant protease t.
platelet aggregation t.
platelet complement fixation t.
platelet function t.
platelet suspension immunofluorescence t.
Porter-Silber chromogen t.
Porteus maze t.
postcoital t.
posterior drawer t.
postural stimulation t.
postural stress t.
T. of Pragmatic Language
Prausnitz-Küstner t.
Predictive Ability T.
predictive value of a negative t.
predictive value of a positive t.
predischarge graded exercise t.
prednisolone glucose tolerance t.
prenatal screening t.
prick skin t.
Primary T. of Cognitive Skills
Primary Mental Abilities T.
Primary Visual Motor T.
primed lymphocyte t.
Printing Performance School Readiness T.
prism adaptation t.
prism and alternate cover t.
Professional Employment T.
progesterone challenge t.
progestin challenge t.
Progressive Achievement T.'s of Listening Comprehension
progressive exercise t.
promontory stimulation t.
protamine response t.
prothrombin and proconvertin t.
provocative use t.
psychoacoustic t.
Psychosocial History Screening T.
pulmonary function t.
purified protein derivative test
Quality Extinction T.
Quality of Upper Extremities T.
quantitative t.
Quantitative Sudomotor Axon Reflex T.
Queckenstedt-Stookey t.
Quick Picture Vocabulary T.
Quick T. psychology, pregnancy, prothrombin
RA t.
rabbit ileal loop t.
radioactive Hippuran t.
radioallergosorbent assay t.
radioimmune antiglobulin t.
radioimmunoassay double antibody t.
radioimmunoprecipitation test
radioimmunosorbent t.
radiosensitivity t.
rapid antigen-detection t.
rapid fluorescent focus inhibition t.
Rapidly Alternating Speech Perception T.
rapid plasma reagin circle card t.
rapid simple t.'s
rapid surfactant t.
rapid urease t.
rapid whole blood t.
Raven Colored Progressive Matrices T.
Reach in Four Directions T.
reactive nonstress t.
reading t.
reagin screen t.
Receptive One-Word Picture Vocabulary T.
red colloidal t.
red glass t.
Reitan-Indiana aphasic screening t.
Reiter protein complement-fixation t.
Remote Associates T.
renal function t.
Repeated T. of Sustained Wakefulness
Rey Auditory Verbal Learning T.
Rey-Estreich Complex Figure T.
rheumatoid arthritis factor t.
t. for rheumatoid factor
rheumatoid factor t.
Riegel test meal
Right-Left Orientation T.
Riley Articulation and Language T.
Rinne hearing t.
Rinne test negative
Rinne test positive
Rivermead Behavioral Memory T.
Robert Apperception T. for Children
rod-and-frame t.

Rorschach Inkblot T.
Rotter Sentence Completion T.
routine admission laboratory t.
routine test dilution
Sabin dye t.
Sabin-Feldman dye t.
Sachs-Georgi t.
Sacks Sentence Completion T.
Scaled Curriculum Achievement Levels T.
Scholastic Aptitude T.
School Attitude T.
School and College Ability T.
School Motivation Analysis T.
Screening T. for Auditory Comprehension of Language
Screening T. for Educational Prerequisite Skills
screening laboratory t.
Seashore Rhythm T.
sedimentation rate t.
Self-Administered Alcoholism Screening t.
Senior Apperception T.
sensitization t.
Sensory Integration and Praxis T.'s
Sensory Organization T.
Sequential T.'s of Educational Progress, Series III
sequential probability ratio t.
serial sevens t.
serologic test for syphilis
serum bactericidal t.
serum creatinine t.
sestamibi stress t.
sex chromatin t.
Sex Knowledge and Attitude T.
Sexual Compatibility T.
Shapes Analysis T.
sheep cell agglutination t.
sheep erythrocyte agglutination t.
Sheffield Screening T. for Acquired Language Disorders
Sheridan Tests for Young Children and Retardates
short-arc quadriceps t.
Short Form T. of Academic Aptitude
Short Michigan Alcoholism Screening T.
short orientation-memory-concentration t.
short ragweed t.
Short-Term Auditory Retrieval and Storage T.
sickle cell anemia t.
side platelet aggregation t.
simple knee t.
simple shoulder t.
simultaneous prism and cover t.
single-breath nitrogen t.
single radial diffusion t.
single-stage exercise stress t.
Sixteen Personality Factors T.
skin fold thickness t.
skin prick t.
skin puncture t.
skin temperature t.
skin test for delayed-type hypersensitivity
skin test done
skin test reactivity
slide agglutination t.
Slingerland Screening T.'s
Slosson Articulation Language Test with Phonology
Slosson Intelligence T.
Slosson T. of Reading Readiness
Snider Match T.
T. of Social Inferences
Social Relations T.
sodium and potassium spot urine t.
soluble antigen fluorescent antibody t.
Sorting of Figures T.
Southern California Figure Ground T.
Southern California Postrotary Nystagmus T.
Southern California Sensory Integration T.'s
Southern California Space Visualization T.
Spatial Orientation Memory T.
Special Aptitude T. Battery
specific gravity t.
speech discrimination t.
speech reception t.
Speech-Sound Perception T.
Speech Weber T.
spermatogenic activity t.
sperm immobilization t.
Spondee Picture T.
spontaneous activity t.
Spreen-Benton Sentence Repetition T.
Staggered Spondaic Word T.
standard acid reflux t.
standard fixation preference t.
standard glucose tolerance t.
standardized t.
standard language test for aphasia
standard test dose
standard tone-decay t.
standard tube agglutination t.
Stanford Achievement T.
Stanford Diagnostic Reading T.
staphylococcal clumping t.
Star Cancellation T.
star-cancellation t.
Stein Sentence Completion T.
Stenger hearing t.
Stephens Oral Language Screening T.
Stetson Auditory Discrimination T.
t. of stool guaiac
straight leg raising t.
streptolysin O t.
STYCAR Hearing T.
STYCAR Language T.
STYCAR Vision T.
subcutaneous histamine t.
t. subject
submaximal treadmill exercise t.
sugar, acetone, diacetic acid t.
Suinn T. Anxiety Behavior Scale
Supervisory Practices T.
supine empty stress t.
Suprathreshold Adaptation T.
swing light t.
Symbol Digit Modalities T.
Symbolic Play T.
Symonds Picture-Story T.
symptom-limited graded exercise t.
Symptom Rating T.
Tactile Finger Recognition T.
Tactile Form Recognition T.
Tactile Performance T.
tandem gait t.
TB patch t.
TB skin t.
tear break-up t.
technetium Cardiolite stress t.
test tube turbidity t.
tetanus antitoxin skin t.
tethered median nerve stress t.
thallium-graded exercise t.
thallium stress t.
thematic apperception t.
thematic aptitude t.
This I Believe t.
Thomas-Binetti t.
Three-Dimensional Block Construction T.
thromboplastin activation t.

test *(continued)*
thromboplastin generation t.
thromboplastin screening t.
thumb-finding t.
thymol turbidity t.
thyroidal radioactive iodine uptake t.
thyroid function t.
thyrotropin-releasing hormone stimulation t.
tilt-table t.
tine t.
tissue thromboplastin inhibition t.
Titmus stereoacuity t.
Toglia Category Assessment T.
token t.
tolbutamide-glucagon t.
tolbutamide tolerance t.
toluidine red unheated serum t.
tone decay t.
Tone in Noise t.
Toronto Biculture T. of Nonverbal Reasoning
Torrance Tests of Creative thinking
toxoplasmin skin test antigen
Trail-Making Test psychiatry
training and test lung
transfer factor t.
Translating and Congruent Mobile-Bearing Knee t.
transmission disequilibrium t.
tray agglutination t.
treadmill exercise stress t.
treadmill performance t.
treponemal antibody t.
Treponema pallidum hemagglutination t.
Trieger Dot T.
true positive stress t.
Trunk Control T.
tryptophan load t.
tuberculin skin t.
tuberculin tine t.
tuberculosis patch t.
tuberculosis skin t.
tube slide agglutination t.
tumor activity t.
tumor skin t.
tuning fork t.
Twenty Statements T.
University of Pennsylvania Smell Identification T.
upper limb tension t.
urea breath t.
uric acid urine spot t.
urinary coproporphyrin t.
urine glucose spot t.
urine pregnancy t.
Utah T. of Language Development
valgus stress t.
valgus-varus stress t.
van den Bergh t.
T. of Variables of Attention
varus stress t.
Verbal Fluency T.
vertebral artery t.
vestibular autorotation t.
visual acuity t.
visual apperception t.
Visual Aural Digit Span T.
visual distortion t.
visual field t.
Visual Form Discrimination T.
Visual-Motor Gestalt T.
visual-motor integration t.
Visual-Motor Sequencing T.
Visual Organization T.
Visual Retention T.
Visual Search and Attention T.
Vocational Apperception T.
Voges-Proskauer medium, t.
Walter bromide t.
Wassermann t.
waterload t.
Weber Advanced Spatial Perception t.
Wechsler Intelligence for Children T.
Weidel Auditory Processing T.
Weidel Yes/No Reliability T.
t. weight
Weinstein enhanced sensory t.
Western Aphasia Battery T.
Western blot t.
Wilcoxon rank sum t.
Wisconsin Card Sorting T.
Wolf Motor Function T.
Woodcock Reading Mastery T.
Word Association T.
T. of Word Finding
T. of Word Finding in Discourse
T. of Work Competency and Stability
Worth four-dot test for fusion
wrist flexion t.
T. of Written Language
wrong test requested-floor error
xylose breath t.
xylose concentration t.
Yerkes-Bridges Test psychology
Youman-Parlett serologic t.
Yvon coefficient t.
Ziehen t.
zinc flocculation t.
zinc turbidity t.

Test/Clinical
Clinical Adaptive Test/Clinical Linguistic and Auditory Milestone Scale

tested
differently t.
not t.
similarly t.

tester
alcohol breath t.

testes (*pl. of* testis)

test-estrin timed action

Test-Fjabrant
Sperm Immobilization T.-F.

Test-Human
Children's Apperception T.-H.

testicle
undescended t.

testicular
t. abscess
t. adrenal-like tissue
t. agenesis
t. atrophy
t. cancer
t. carcinoma
combined testicular weight
t. cord
t. dysfunction
t. feminization
t. feminization mutation
t. feminization syndrome
t. growth
t. implant
incomplete testicular feminization syndrome
t. interstitial fluid
Lugano classification for testicular tumor
metachronous testicular germ cell tumor
Mostofi classification of testicular tumor
nonseminomatous germ cell testicular tumor
prepubertal testicular tumor
t. self-examination
t. sperm aspiration
t. sperm extraction
t. torsion
t. tubular adenoma
T. Tumor Panel

testicularis
arteria t.

testing
acquired immune deficiency syndrome mandatory t.
active motion t.
air conduction t.
angle isometric t.
anorectal physiology t.
antibacterial agent susceptibility t.
antibiotic sensitivity t.
antimicrobial susceptibility t.
antimicrobiology susceptibility t.
antimycobacterial susceptibility t.
antiphosphatidylserine-prothrombin complex antibody t.
aquatic cardiac evaluation and t.
autoantibody assay t.
automated multiphasic health t.
axial closed-loop hydraulic mechanical t.
bedside t.
caloric testing of vestibular function
Cattell's Institute for Personality and Ability Testing Anxiety Scale
children of alcoholic screen t.
confrontation visual field t.
cortical function t.
counseling and t.
early exercise t.
t. and evaluation
fetal acoustic stimulation t.
fiberoptic endoscopic evaluation of swallowing with sensory t.
flexible endoscopic evaluation of swallowing with sensory t.
flexion reflex t.
forensic urine drug t.
gastric secretory t.
genotypic antiretroviral resistance t.
impaired reality t.
Individualized Criterion Reference T. Mathematics
Individualized Criterion Reference T. Reading
information overload testing aid
lactose hydrogen breath t.
leukocyte-antigen sensitivity t.
ligase-chain reaction t.
light touch t.
low-frequency head-only rotational t.
lung function t.
mandatory acquired immune deficiency syndrome t.
manual muscle t.
Materials T. System
maximal treadmill t.
methacholine provocative t.
microdilution susceptibility t.
microsatellite instability t.
modified treadmill exercise t.
molecular probe t.
motivation analysis t.
multiphasic health t.
muscle t.
National Collegiate Athletic Association drug testing policy
near acuity t.
near vision t.
Neisseria gonorrhoeae susceptibility t.
nocturnal penile tumescence t.
nondestructive t.
noninvasive cardiac t.
nonreassuring fetal t.
nucleic acid amplification t.
occult blood t.
oral glucose tolerance t.
t., orientation, work, evaluation, rehabilitation
otoacoustic emission t.
panel-reactive antibody t.
p24 antigen t.
PAR Admissions Testing program
penicillin allergy skin t.
penicillinase-producing organisms susceptibility t.
percutaneous allergy t.
pharmaceutical research and t.
placebo-controlled oral challenge t.
point estimation by sequential t.
point-of-care t.
preadmission t.
preadmission testing program
protein truncation t.
psychoacoustic t.
quantitative autonomic functioning t.
quantitative muscle t.
Quantitative Sensory T.
repeat open-application t.
Simultaneous Technique for Acuity and Readiness T.
speech discrimination t.
systematic nutritional muscle t.
vestibular autorotational t.
vibration perception t.
viral lode t.
visual field t.
voluntary counseling and t.

Testing-Teaching Module of Auditory Discrimination

testis, pl. **testes**
anterior border of t.
appendix testis torsion
calf t.
t. cord
testes down
t. ectopia
feminizing testis syndrome
Leydig cells of the t.
lobule of t.
lower pole of t.
parietal layer of tunica vaginalis of t.
rete testis aspiration
spontaneous descent of t.
suspensory ligament of t.
tunica vaginalis t.
vestigial t.

testis-determining
t.-d. antigen
t.-d. factor

Test-Isojima
Sperm Immobilization T.-I.

testis-specific binding protein

testolactone
aromatase inhibitor t.

testosterone
apparent free testosterone concentration
circadian testosterone pattern
t. deficiency
t. to epitestosterone ratio
free t.
free testosterone level
t. glucuronide
t. level
long-acting testosterone ester
male hormone t.
nonsex hormone-binding globulin bound t.
t. production rate
t. propionate
t. repressed prostate message-2
t. sulfate
t. transdermal system
transscrotal t.
unbound t.

testosterone-binding
t.-b. affinity
t.-b. globulin
t.-b. protein

testosterone-estradiol-binding globulin

Test-Revised
Gray Oral Reading T.-R.
Peabody Picture Vocabulary T.-R.
Slosson Oral Reading T.-R.

tetanic
t. contraction
t. convulsion
low-frequency tetanic stimulation

tetanus
acellular pertussis vaccine with diphtheria and tetanus toxoid
anodal closure t.
anodal duration t.
anodal opening t.
t. antitoxic serum
t. antitoxin
t. antitoxin skin test
cathodal closure t.
cathodal-duration t.
cathodal-opening t.
cathode-duration t.
combined diphtheria t.
t. and diphtheria
diphtheria, pertussis, tetanus, poliomyelitis, and measles vaccine
diphtheria, pertussis, and t.
diphtheria, pertussis, and tetanus immunization
diphtheria, pertussis, and tetanus vaccine
diphtheria, tetanus, pertussis, *Haemophilus influenzae* type b vaccine
diphtheria, tetanus toxoids, whole-cell pertussis, and *Haemophilus influenzae* type b conjugate
diphtheria, tetanus toxoid, and acellular pertussis vaccine
t. and diphtheria toxoid immunization
diphtheria, tetanus toxoids, whole-cell pertussis vaccine
galvanic tetanus ratio
homologous tetanus immune globulin
human tetanus antitoxin
human tetanus immune globulin
human tetanus immunoglobulin
t. immune globulin
t. immunization
t. immunoglobulin
low-frequency t.
t. neonatorum
polysaccharide tetanus conjugate vaccine
t. toxin
t. toxoid antibody
t. toxoid immunization
t. toxoid outdated
t. toxoid toxoplasmic choroiditis
t. toxoid up-to-date
typhoid, paratyphoid A, B, tetanus toxoid, and diphtheria toxoid vaccine

tetanus-diphtheria
t.-d. toxoid, adult type

tetanus-pertussis
t.-p. vaccine

tetany
contraction of hand in t.
duration of t.
simple hypocalcemic t.

Tete virus

tethered
t. cord
t. cord release
t. cord syndrome
t. median nerve stress test

tethering effect

tetraacetate
lead tetraacetate Schiff

tetrabutyrate
riboflavin t.

tetracaine
t., Adrenalin, and cocaine
lidocaine, adrenaline, t.
liposome-encapsulated t.

tetrachloride
carbon tetrachloride poisoning

tetrachlorodiphenyl ethane

tetracyclic antidepressant

tetracycline
bismuth, metronidazole, t.
omeprazole, bismuth subcitrate, tetracycline, and metronidazole
penicillin, streptomycin, t.
ranitidine bismuth citrate, metronidazole, t.

tetracycline-induced stenosis

tetracycline-resistant *Neisseria gonorrhoeae*

tetrad
congenital eyelid t.

tetradecadiene acetate

tetradecylsulfate
sodium t.

tetradecyl sulfate, ethanol, and saline

tetraethyl
t. lead

tetraethylammonium bromide

tetraethylene glycol dimethacrylate

tetrafluor
ethylene tetrafluor ethylene

tetrahydrocannabinol cross-reacting cannabinoid

tetrahydro-compound S

tetrahydrofolate
methylene tetrahydrofolate reductase thermolability

tetrahydrofolic
methyl tetrahydrofolic acid

tetrahydrofurfuryl

tetraiodothyronine
t. thyroxine
t. thyroxine radioimmunoassay

tetralogy
Eisenmenger t.
Fallot t.
t. of Fallot

tetramethyl
t. benzidine
t. lead

tetramethylammonium hydroxide

tetramethylrhodamine
t. isothiocyanate
t. isothionate

tetrapeptide
cholecystokinin t.

tetraphosphate
adenosine t.

tetrasodium-meso-tetra
manganese t.-m.-t.

tetrasomy
mosaic tetrasomy 8p syndrome

tetravalent
oral tetravalent rotavirus vaccine

tetrazolium
blue t.
microculture tetrazolium dye assay
nitroblue tetrazolium dye
nitroblue tetrazolium dye test
red t.
t. reduction
t. reduction inhibition
t. violet

tetter
milk t.
moist t.

texture
asymmetry, range of motion abnormality, tissue texture abnormality
color and texture normal
hair normal t.
tenderness, asymmetry, restricted motion, and tissue texture changes
tissue texture changes, asymmetry, restriction of motion, tenderness
tissue texture abnormality

textured vegetable protein

T-file
Mity engine T.-f.

Thackray Reading Readiness Profile

thalami
nuclei anteriores t.
nuclei dorsales t.
nucleus anteroinferior t.
nucleus anterosuperior t.
nucleus anteroventralis t.
nucleus arcuatus t.
nucleus centralis lateralis t.
nucleus centralis medialis t.
nucleus dorsales t.

thalamic
anterior thalamic radiation
anterior thalamic tubercle
anterodorsal thalamic nucleus
anteromedial thalamic nucleus
anteroventral thalamic nucleus
t. gustatory nucleus
t. projection neuron
specific thalamic projection system

thalamocortical
t. fiber
t. relay

thalamostriatae

thalamostriate
anterolateral thalamostriate artery
anteromedial thalamostriate artery

thalamotomy
anterior t.
parafascicular t.

thalamus
anterior nucleus of t.
anterior peduncle of t.
anterior tubercle of t.
anterodorsal nucleus of t.
anteromedial nucleus of t.
anteroventral nucleus of t.
arcuate nucleus of t.
medial central nucleus of t.
medial dorsal nucleus of t.
medullary layers of t.
nucleus ventralis anterior of t.
optic t.
somatosensory t.

thalassemia
alpha-thalassemia
t. intermedia
t. major
t. minor
sickle cell t.
t. trait

thalassemia/mental
X-linked alpha-thalassemia/mental retardation syndrome

Thal fundoplication procedure

thallium
adenosine thallium scan
adenosine thallium test
t. chloride
dipyridamole thallium stress imaging
dobutamine thallium angiography
t. exercise heart scan
exercise thallium 201 scintigraphy
exercise treadmill test with t.
t. imaging
t. myocardial perfusion
t. myocardial scintigraphy
t. perfusion imaging
planar thallium scintigraphy
planar thallium test
t. poisoning
t. scan
t. sestamibi
t. stress test
stress thallium scanning

thallium-activated sodium iodide crystal

thallium-graded exercise test

thallous
polymyxin, lysozyme, EDTA, and thallous acetate in heart infusion agar

than
air greater than bone conduction
bone conduction greater than air conduction
bone conduction less than air conduction
head higher than heart
higher t.
legs elevated higher than heart
less than effective
mycobacteria other than *Mycobacterium tuberculosis*
Mycobacteria other than tuberculosis
other than psychotic
particulate matter less than 10 micrometers diameter
pulmonic heart sound less than aortic second heart sound
pulmonic second heart sound greater than aortic second heart sound
second aortic sound greater than second pulmonic sound
second aortic sound less than second pulmonic sound

that
amino acid that gives aspartic acid after hydrolysis
concentration that inhibits 50%

Thayer-Martin
T.-M. medium
T.-M., modified agar

the
T. Injury Prevention Program
T. Instructional Environment Scale
T. Primary Language Screen

theatre
operating theatre sterile supply unit

theca
t. cell
t. cell tumor
t. cordis
lumbar t.
luteinized theca cell
multiple luteinized theca cyst

thecocellulare
xanthofibroma t.

thecoma
luteinized t.
luteinized thecoma of ovary

Theiler
T. murine encephalomyelitis virus

T-helper
T.-h. cell type 1, 2, 3
T.-h. suppressor cell

thematic
t. apperception test
t. aptitude test
t. content modification program

thenar
t. eminence
t. fascia
t. muscle atrophy
t. muscle contraction
t. palmar crease
t. space

theophylline
t. serum concentration
serum theophylline concentration
serum theophylline level
sustained release t.

theophylline-guaifenesin

theophylline-sustained release

theoretical
t. growth evaluation
t. renal phosphorus threshold

theory
affective arousal t.
aggressive behavior t.
Allport group relations t.
Allport personality trait t.
anticipatory and struggle behavior t.'s
anxiety sensitivity t.
Bloembergen, Purcell, and Pound t.
crystal field t.
endorphin, dopamine, and prostaglandin t.
item response theory
life cycle t.
lipoid theory of narcosis
local circuit t.
lymphatic dissemination theory of endometriosis
mass action t.
membrane expansion t.
Metchnikoff cellular immunity t.
Miller chemicoparasitic t.
molecular dissociation t.
natural selection t.
operant behavior t.
opponent colors t.
optimal sampling t.
oxygen deprivation theory of narcosis
peripheral arterial vasodilation t.
sensory decision t.
transition state t.
Young-Helmholtz t.

therapeutic
t. abortion
t. abortion, dilation, aspiration, and curettage
accepted dental t.'s
t. agent
aggressive therapeutic trial
t. alternative
t. amniocentesis
t. anesthesia
t. approach
t. benefits of humor
t. class profile
t. community
t. concentrate
t. continuous penicillin
diagnostic and therapeutic team
t. dietitian
t. dissection
t. donor insemination
t. dose
t. drug assay
t. drug monitoring
t. effect
t. electrical stimulation
t. electromembrane
t. endpoint
t. error signal
t. exercise
t. external radiation
t. failure
t. gain factor
gastrointestinal therapeutic system
general therapeutic exercise
t. hemapheresis
t. home pass
t. home trial visit
human therapeutic dose
t. humor
t. humor movement
t. husband-insemination
t. impact
t. incompatibility
t. index
insufficient therapeutic effect
t. intervention
T. Intervention Scoring System
t. iridectomy
t. lifestyle change
t. lymph node dissection
minocycline periodontal therapeutic system
mucosal oral therapeutic system
narrow band UVB therapeutic light exposure
narrow therapeutic index
negative therapeutic reaction
nonsurgical therapeutic abortion
t. nutritional intake
optimal therapeutic dose
t. outcomes monitoring
overall therapeutic goal
t. paracentesis
t. pass
pharmacy and t.'s
t. plasma exchange
t. play group
psychodynamic and therapeutic education
t. qualities of ice
rad equivalent t.
t. radiology
t. reaction
t. recreation
t. recreation associate
timed therapeutic absence
t. touch
transdermal therapeutic system

therapist
enterostomal t.
Family T. Behavioral Scale
guided imagery t.
industrial physical t.
inhalation t.
manual arts t.
physical t.
speech t.

therapist-driven protocol

therapy
ablative hormonal t.
activity group t.
additive hormonal t.
adjunctive t.
adjunctive glucocorticoid t.
adjuvant chemoradiation t.
adjuvant drug t.
adjuvant medical t.
adjuvant post-radiation t.
adjuvant therapy for breast cancer
adjuvant whole-brain radiation t.
adolescent group t.
adoptive cellular t.
Adriamycin therapy toxicity
adult group t.
alcoholism therapy class
alkylating agent t.
allogeneic cellular immune t.
alpha interferon t.
alpha-receptor blockade t.
alternating triple t.
alternative cancer t.
5-aminolevulinic acid photodynamic t.
amplitude-summation interferential current t.
analytical play t.
anatomical considerations in radiation t.

androgen ablation t.
androgen deprivation t.
androgen replacement t.
androgen suppression t.
androgen withdrawal endocrine t.
animal-assisted t.
antenatal corticosteroid t.
antiangiogenesis gene t.
antibiotic combination t.
antibiotic infusion t.
antibody-dependent enzyme-prodrug t.
antibody-directed enzyme prodrug t.
antibody-directed, enzyme-producing t.
antibody-directed enzyme t.
antibody induction t.
antibody replacement t.
anticholinergic medicine t.
anticoagulant t.
antiestrogen radiologic t.
antifungal drug t.
antigen-specific preventive t.
anti-IIb-IIIA mAB t.
antimonial drug therapy for leishmaniasis
antiparasitic drug t.
antipsychotic drug t.
antiretroviral triple combination t.
antisense oligonucleotide viral t.
antithyroid drug t.
antitumor necrosis factor-based t.
aquatic therapy pool
arc therapy technique
argon laser t.
around-the-clock oral maintenance bronchodilator t.
art t.
arterial revascularization therapy study
aspirin tolerance t.
assertion structured t.
assessing severity: age of patient, systems involved, stage of disease, complications, response to t.
atropine coma t.
attractor field t.
autologous cellular t.
axillary irradiation t.
behavioral family systems t.
behavioral marital t.
beta blocker t.
blood component t.
blood transfusion t.
boron neutron capture t.
breast conservation t.
breast-conserving t.
brief stimulus t.
British anti-Lewisite t.
cancer multistep t.
cancer therapy facility
carbon dioxide t.
cardiac shock wave t.
T. Carrot finger contracture orthosis
cell t.
cellular breast cancer t.
central axis depth dose of electron beam t.
cerebral protective t.
chemoradiation t.
chest physical t.
chronic antidepressant t.
chronic opioid analgesic t.
Clinitron air-fluidized t.
clitoral therapy device
cognitive behavior t.
cognitive behavioral t.
Cognitive Behavior T. Package
cognitive remediation t.
cognitive therapy group
combination high- and low-energy x-ray t.
combination hormone t.
combination retinoid and PUVA t.
combined antiretroviral t.
combined chemotherapy/radiation therapy
combined hormone t.
combined intermittent t.
combined modality t.
complex oncologic therapy protocol
composite cyclic t.
computer therapy program
conditioned reflex t.
conformal radiation t.
continuous-combined hormone replacement t.
continuous hormone replacement t.
continuous nebulization t.
continuous oxygen t.
continuous renal replacement t.
conventional asthma t.
conventional immunosuppressive t.
conventional insulin t.
conventional therapy group
convulsive shock t.
cord blood cell t.
coronary radiation t.
corrective t.
corrective therapy department
corticosteroid t.
couples group t.
cranial radiation t.
craniosacral t.
cryosurgery and laser t.
cytotoxic immunosuppressive t.
daily group t.
deep chest t.
deep x-ray t.
diagnostic t.
dialectical behavior t.
directive group play t.
directive play therapy group
directly observed t.
t. discontinued
disease-controlling antirheumatic t.
diversional t.
drainage, irrigation, fibrinolytic t.
educational t.
ego-oriented individual t.
electrical aversion t.
electric differential t.
electric shock t.
electroaerosol t.
electroconvulsive shock t.
electron-beam intraoperative radiation t.
electron and photon t.
electroshock t.
electrosleep t.
electrostimulation t.
endoluminal radiation t.
endometrial laser intrauterine thermal t.
endoscopic injection t.
endoscopic laser t.
enteral nutritional t.
enterostomal t.
estrogen add back t.
estrogen replacement t.
extended abdominal radiation t.
extended family t.
extended field radiation t.
external beam photon t.
external beam radiation t.
external irradiation t.
extracorporeal shock wave t.
family group t.
fever unresponsive to antibiotic t.
focal cranial radiation t.
frequency-difference interferential current t.
full course radiation t.
Functional Assessment of Cancer T.

therapy *(continued)*
gamma globulin t.
gamma ray t.
gene therapy for heart
genetic t.
glandular replacement t.
gold salt t.
group adjustment t.
group therapy session
growth hormone t.
heart disease t.
heater probe t.
heat and massage t.
Helicobacter pylori eradication t.
hemofiltration t.
high-dose aspirin t.
high-dose fractional radiation t.
high-dose fractionation radiation t.
high-dose immunosuppressive t.
high-dose radiation t.
highly active antiretroviral t.
high-velocity lead t.
home infusion t.
home intravenous antibiotic t.
home nutrition t.
home oxygen t.
home parenteral antibiotic t.
hormonal replacement t.
hormonal therapy in endometrial carcinoma
hormone replacement t.
human gene t.
humeral block in radiation t.
hyperbaric oxygen t.
hyperfractionated accelerated radiation t.
hypertensive hypervolemic t.
iatrogenic effects of behavior t.
immune augmentative t.
immune-based t.
immunoaugmentative t.
immunosuppressive drug t.
immunotoxin t.
incentive t.
independent toxicity in combined modality t.
individual solution-based t.
inhalation t.
insulin coma t.
insulin convulsive t.
insulin shock t.
integrative couple t.
intensified conventional insulin t.
intensity-modulated proton t.
intensity-modulated radiation t.
intensive antimicrobial t.
intensive conventional t.
intensive dietary t.
intensive group t.
intensive insulin t.
intensive therapy observation unit
intensive topical antibiotic t.
intermittent diuretic t.
intermittent needle t.
internal radiation t.
interpersonal group t.
interstitial radiation t.
intraarterial thrombolytic t.
intracavitary cesium t.
intracavitary radiation t.
intracoronary radiation t.
intradiscal electrothermal t.
intraluminal radiation t.
intraoperative electron beam t.
intraoperative intraarterial fibrinolytic t.
intraoperative radiation t.
intraoral cone for electron beam t.
intraperitoneal photodynamic t.
intravascular red light t.
intravenous antioxidant t.
intravenous nutritional t.
ischemia-guided medical t.
language enrichment t.
laser therapy of hemorrhoid
lens-sparing external beam radiation t.
LH-releasing hormone agonist t.
local recurrence after radiation t.
long-term aspirin t.
long-term oxygen t.
long-term RBC transfusion t.
low air loss therapy mattress
low-dose aspirin t.
low-dose intravenous insulin t.
low-dose mediastinal radiation t.
low-dose rate intracavity t.
low-dose VV t.
low insulin t.
low-level laser t.
luteal phase t.
maggot debridement t.
maintenance drug t.
major role t.
malaria t.
Manchester system for radium t.
marital couples group t.
maternal blood clot patch t.
maximum tolerated medical t.
medical therapy unit
melodic intonation t.
menopausal estrogen replacement t.
methylprednisolone pulse t.
methyl-*tert*-butyl ether t.
metronidazole, amoxicillin, clarithromycin, *H. pylori*, one-week t.
microwave coagulation t.
migraine abortive t.
mineralocorticoid replacement t.
mobile electroconvulsive therapy apparatus
modified directly observed t.
modified systemic Berlin-Frankfurt-Munster t.
moist heat t.
molecular-based conceptual t.
monoclonal antibody t.
morning bright light t.
motivational enhancement t.
multidimensional family t.
multidrug t.
multimodal adjuvant t.
multimodal behavior t.
multimodal physical t.
multiple agent t.
multiple family t.
multiple injection therapy of insulin
multiple monitored electroconvulsive t.
multiport collimated cobalt-60 t.
multisystemic t.
music t.
mutant Ras peptide-pulsed dendritic cell t.
myoblast transfer t.
nasopharyngoscopy biofeedback t.
neoadjuvant androgen derivation t.
neoadjuvant hormonal t.
neurodevelopmental treatment physical therapy
neuromuscular electrical stimulation t.
neutron beam t.
neutron capture t.
neutron therapy machine
new approaches to brain tumor t.
Newcastle disease virus t.
new drug t.
nicotine patch t.
nicotine replacement t.
nicotinic receptor blockade t.
nitrogen mustard t.
nocturnal oxygen t.
nocturnal oxygen therapy trial
nonsurgical septal reduction t.

NordiCare Back Therapy System
occlusal appliance t.
occupational therapy/recreational t.
ocular radiation t.
oestrogen estrogen-replacement t.
oncologic therapy protocol
open-loop pump t.
oral antiarrhythmic t.
oral anticoagulant t.
oral appliance t.
oral contraceptive t.
oral drug t.
oral estrogen t.
oral hormone replacement t.
oral iron t.
oral rehydration t.
osteomanipulative t.
osteopathic manipulative t.
outpatient occupational t.
outpatient parenteral antibiotic t.
outpatient physical t.
outpatient speech t.
palliative radiation t.
pancreatic enzyme replacement t.
paraffin heat t.
parent-child group t.
Paris method for radium t.
particle beam radiation t.
passive immunization t.
patient intolerant to aspirin t.
percutaneous embolization t.
percutaneous microwave coagulation t.
percutaneous neuromodulatory t.
perioperative antibiotic t.
perioperative respiratory t.
permanent implant t.
permission, limited information, specific suggestions, and intensive t.
peroral cone radiation t.
photodynamic t.
photon irradiation technique in radiation t.
photon-radiosurgical t.
photoradiation t.
physical t.
physical therapy assistant
physical therapy services
platelet transfusion t.
play group t.
pneumatic compression t.
postmenopausal estrogen t.
postmenopausal hormonal t.
postmenopausal hormone t.
postoperative radiation t.
postoperative respiratory t.
preoperative radiation t.
preventive aspirin t.
preventive aspirin t.
profile-based t.
prolonged antibiotic t.
prophylactic whole brain radiation t.
prostate hormone t.
protein-sparing t.
proton beam t.
psychoeducational group t.
pulsed inotrope t.
pulsed light t.
quadrantectomy, axillary dissection, radiation t.
radiation equivalent t.
radiation therapy for intact breast
radiation therapy oncology group
radiation therapy on prophylactic basis
radiation therapy planning
radiation therapy planning system
radioimmunoglobulin t.
radium t.
rage reduction t.
rational behavior t.
rational-emotive t.
rational hypertensive t.
recreational t.
red light t.
regressive electric shock t.
relaxation response in headache t.
relaxation therapy for hyperactivity
remedial occupational t.
respiratory t.
Restricted Environment Stimulation T.
restriction of environmental stimulation t.
rhythmic sensory bombardment t.
root canal t.
routine dialysis t.
routine fever t.
salvage highly active antiretroviral t.
selective tubal assessment to refine reproductive t.
self-administered t.
sensory feedback t.
sequela of t.
shock t.
shock-wave t.
sleep restriction t.
sliding scale insulin t.
small group t.
social environmental t.
solution focused group t.
somatic cell human gene t.
spinal manipulative t.
staging system in radiation t.
standard triple t.
steam inhalation t.
stereotactic-assisted radiation t.
supplemental growth hormone t.
surfactant replacement t.
surgical adjuvant t.
surgical intensive t.
surgical myomectomy as reproductive t.
systematized assertive t.
systemic assertive t.
systemic hyperbaric oxygen t.
thoracic radiation t.
Thought Field T.
three-dimensional conformal radiation t.
thrombolytic t.
thymic radiation t.
traditional behavior t.
traditional Chinese herbal t.
transcatheter t.
transcranial electrostimulation t.
transfusion therapy service
transpupillary thermal t.
transtracheal oxygen t.
triple intrathecal t.
tumor amplified protein expression t.
ultrasound-guided injection t.
uterine balloon t.
validation t.
vertical float aquatic t.
vertical float progression aquatic t.
visual communication t.
vitamin B t.
vocational rehabilitation t.
whole brain versus local brain radiation t.
wide-field radiation t.
work t.

therapy/audiokinetics
music t.

Therapy-Breast
Functional Assessment of Cancer T.-B.

Therapy-Fatigue
Functional Assessment of Cancer T.-F.

Therapy-General
Functional Assessment of Cancer T.-G.
Therapy–Head
Functional Assessment of Cancer Therapy–Head and Neck
Therapy-Lung
Functional Assessment of Cancer T.-L.
Therapy-Prostate
Functional Assessment of Cancer T.-P.
therapy/recreational
occupational therapy/recreational therapy
therapy-related
t.-r. acute myelogenous leukemia
t.-r. acute myeloid leukemia
t.-r. myelodysplasia
t.-r. myelodysplastic syndrome
there is no evidence of malignancy
thermal
t. ablation
arthroscopic monopolar thermal stabilization forefoot compression sleeve
British thermal unit
t. burn
centigrade thermal unit
t. conductivity
t. conductivity detector
t. death point
t. death time
t. destruction
t. dilution
t. dilution catheter
t. effect of exercise
t. effect of food
endometrial laser intrauterine thermal therapy
t. energy analyzer
t. enhancement ratio
extravascular thermal volume
t. flushing
t. green dye
t. inactivation point
t. injury
t. keratoplasty
t. laser keratoplasty
lung thermal volume
neutral thermal environment
noncontact holmium:yttrium-argon-garnet laser thermal keratoplasty
t. perception
radiofrequency thermal ablation
residual thermal damage
transpupillary thermal therapy
thermal/perfusion balloon angioplasty
thermic
t. anesthesia
t. effect of exercise
t. effect of feeding
t. effect of food
t. effect of physical activity
t. fever
thermica
myalgia t.
thermistor
nasal tip t.
thermoacidurans agar modified
thermoanalysis
differential t.
thermochemiluminescence
thermocoagulation
radiofrequency t.
thermodilution
bolus t.
cardiac output by t.
t. cardiac output
thermodynamic
t. activity
t. temperature
thermoeffector
antagonistic t.
thermogenesis
adaptive t.
dietary t.
diet-induced t.
nonexercise activity t.
nonshivering t.
thermogenic action
thermogram
liquid crystal t.
thermographic
infrared thermographic calorimetry
thermography
graphic stress t.
laser-induced t.
liquid crystal t.
liquid crystal contact t.
thermokinetic selectivity
thermolability
methylene tetrahydrofolate reductase t.
thermoluminescent dosimeter rod
thermolysin-like metalloendopeptidase
thermometer
axilla t.
axillary t.
glass t.
t. monitoring in hyperthermia
oral t.
tympanic membrane t.
thermometry
magnetic resonance imaging t.
MRI t.
thermoplastic
t. elastomer
silicone thermoplastic splinting
thermoradiotherapy
simultaneous t.
thermoregulatory
t. mechanism
t. system
thermostable direct hemolysin
thermotherapy
adjuvant microwave t.
high-energy transurethral microwave t.
laser-induced t.
low-energy transurethral microwave t.
microwave plaque t.
periurethral transurethral microwave t.
transpupillary t.
transurethral microwave t.
water-induced t.
theta
t. activity
t. antigen
Thiafora virus
thiamine
t. deficiency encephalopathy
t. diphosphate
t. propyldisulfide
thiazole
thick
t. ascending limb
t. ascending limb of Henle loop
t. bronchial secretions
cervix long, thick and closed
cortical thick ascending limb
t. cutaneous melanoma
t. filament
medullary thick ascending limb
medullary thick ascending limb of Henle

t., red itchy patch of skin
t. walled

thickened
t. aortic valve
t. bladder
bladder wall t.
t. bladder wall
t. bone
t. bowel loop
t. duodenal fold
t. gallbladder wall
t. heart muscle
t. mitral valve
t. pericardium

thickening
anterior joint capsule t.
antral mucosal t.
aortic valve t.
aortic wall t.
apical pleural t.
apical thickening of left ventricle
asbestos-related pleural t.
cardiac wall t.
diffuse intimal t.
disproportionate septal t.
fibrous intimal t.
heart wall t.
indistinct semi-circumferential fibrous t.
intimal t.
medial t.
mesangial t.
muscle capillary basement membrane t.
small bowel t.
urinary bladder wall t.

thickly padded

thickness
absorption-equivalent t.
antropyloric muscle t.
arterial wall t.
basement membrane t.
capillary basement membrane t.
central corneal t.
combined cortical t.
common carotid artery intima-media t.
corneal t.
cortical t.
diploë t.
edge t.
end-diastolic cardiac wall t.
endometrial t.
end-systolic wall t.
esophageal wall t.
half-value t.
inner table t.
interventricular septal t.
intimal medial t.
left ventricular posterior wall t.
mean cell t.
mean corpuscular t.
membrane t.
modified Rodman skin thickness score
mucous gel t.
myocardial wall t.
nuchal translucency t.
osteoid seam t.
parietal bone t.
patellar cartilage t.
posterior wall t.
posterior wall thickness at end-diastole
relative medullary t.
relative wall t.
renal glomerular basement membrane t.
septal t.
skin t.
skin fold t.
t. of skin fold
skin fold thickness test
split t.
split-thickness autogenous graft
subscapular skin fold t.
trabecular t.
triceps skin fold t.
volume thickness index
wall t.

thick-split graft

thigh
adductor compartment of t.
adjustable thigh antiembolism stockings
anterior compartment of t.
anterolateral thigh free flap
t. atrophy
t. bone
t. circumference
extensor compartment of t.
t. flap
t. hair
lateral cutaneous nerve of t.
left anterior t.
left lateral t.
medial circumflex artery of t.
medial compartment of t.
medial cutaneous thigh flap
perineal branch of posterior cutaneous nerve of t.
posterior compartment of t.
posterior cutaneous nerve of t.
right anterior t.
right lateral t.
stretching calf, thigh and hamstring

thigh-foot angle

thigh-high
t.-h. antiembolic stocking
t.-h. socks

thigh-leg angle

Thimiri virus

thin
t. adhesion
t. basement membrane
t. basement membrane disease
cartilaginous autologous thin septal graft
t. film dressing
long thin extremity

think
ability to think or concentrate
diminished ability to think or concentration
Inquiry Mode Questionnaire: A Measure of How You T. and Make Decisions
recognize, empathize, think, hear, integrate, notice, keep

thinking
t. ability
abstract t.
adolescent t.
allusive t.
animistic t.
archaic-paralogical t.
associative t.
asyndetic t.
autistic t.
bizarre incoherent t.
bizarre way of t.
California Critical T. Dispositions Inventory
California Critical T. Skills Test
circular t.
clear t.
concrete t.
creative-associate t.
t. creatively with sounds and words
deficient cognitive t.
delusional t.
disordered t.
disorganized t.
distorted t.
distorted negative t.
T. Disturbance Factor
erratic t.

thinking *(continued)*
illogical t.
impaired abstract t.
impaired thinking or concentration
incoherent t.
inconsistent and inappropriate t.
irrational t.
rational t.
referential t.
severe impairment in t.
tangential t.
Torrance Tests of Creative t.
Whitaker Index of Schizophrenic T.
woolly t.

thin-layer
t.-l. chromatography
t.-l. electrophoresis

thinning
apical t.
blood thinning agent
t. hair
t. infarct
parietal bone t.
t. process of bone
restore lost or thinning hair
stromal t.
white matter t.

thin-section
t.-s. axial image
t.-s. CT

thin-walled
t.-w. blood vessel
t.-w. catheter
t.-w. cyst

thiobarbituric acid

thiocarbohydrazide

thiocyanate
serum t.
sodium t.

thioglucose
gold t.
gold sodium t.

thioglycolate
t. broth
fluid thioglycolate medium

6-thioguanine
ara-C plus -t.

thiomalate
gold sodium t.

thiopental
sodium t.

thiophosphate

thiophosphoramide
t. Thiotepa
triethylene t.

thiopurine methyltransferase

thioredoxin reductase

thiosemicarbazide stain

thiosemicarbazone

thiosulfate
sodium t.

thiosulfate-citrate-bile salts-sucrose agar

thiotepa
thiophosphoramide Thiotepa
triethylenethiophosphoramide t.

thiourea
fluorescence t.

third
t. cranial nerve
t. cuneiform bone
t. degree heart block
Detroit Tests of Learning Aptitude, T. Edition
t. disease
distal t.
t. framework region
Gray Oral Reading Test, T. Edition
healing by first, second, or third intention
t. heart sound
intention
junction of distal t.
lower third of leg bone
middle third of long bone
t. midstream bladder specimen
Mycobacterium fortuitum third biovar complex
myelocyte at third stage of maturation
t. nerve palsy
physiologic third heart sound
t. pregnancy
proximal third of bone
t. stage of labor
t. trimester
upper third of long bone
t. ventricle cyst
wound healed by first, second or third intention

third-degree
t.-d. atrioventricular block
t.-d. AV block
t.-d. burn
t.-d. frostbite
t.-d. heart block
t.-d. hemorrhoid
t.-d. hypospadias
t.-d. uterine prolapse

third-generation antidepressant

third-party administrator

thirst
excessive t.
t. fever
increased t.
morbid t.

Thiry-Vella fistula

this
not found this examination

Thissen
Roche, Wainer, and Thissen method of height prediction

thistle
milk t.

Thogoto virus

Thoma ampulla

Thomas
Pearson attachment to Thomas splint

Thomas-Binetti test

Thomsen disease

Thomson reduction technique

thoracentesis
blind t.
diagnostic t.
emergency t.
t. fluid

thoraces (*pl. of* thorax)

thoracic
t. angiography
angle of thoracic inclination
anterior branch of thoracic nerve
anterior intercostal branch of internal thoracic artery
anterior ramus of thoracic nerve
anterior thoracic meningocele
anterior thoracic nerve
anterior thoracic wall
t. aorta
t. aortic aneurysm
t. aortic coarctation
t. aortic cross-clamping
t. aortic disease
t. aortic dissection
t. approach
t. arch aortography
arch of thoracic duct
arterial thoracic outlet syndrome
t. asphyxiant dystrophy

asphyxiating thoracic chondrodystrophy
asphyxiating thoracic dysplasia
asphyxiating thoracic dysplasia syndrome
asphyxiating thoracic dystrophy
axonopathic neurogenic thoracic outlet syndrome
t. cage
t. cage volume
t. cavity
cervical, thoracic, and lumbar
cervical and thoracic vertebrae
t. circumference
t. computed tomography
descending thoracic aortofemoral-femoral bypass
dorsal root, t.
t. duct
t. duct drainage
t. duct fistula
t. duct flow
t. duct lymphocyte
t. duct pressure
ectasia of thoracic aorta
t. electrical bioimpedance
t. endometriosis syndrome
t. epidural steroid injection
t. fascia
first to twelfth thoracic nerves
first to twelfth thoracic vertebrae
t. fluid content
t. ganglion
t. gas volume
t. girdle
t. goiter
high thoracic cord lesion
t. index
t. inferior vena cava
t. inlet
t. intensive care unit
intensive thoracic cardiovascular unit
internal thoracic artery graft
internal thoracic vein
t. laminectomy
lateral thoracic arteries
left internal thoracic artery
long thoracic artery
long thoracic nerve entrapment
long thoracic nerve palsy
long thoracic vein
t. lymphatic duct
manual splinting of thoracic cage
medial anterior thoracic nerve
mediastinal branch of internal thoracic artery
mediastinal branch of thoracic aorta
meningocele
t. nerve
t. orthosis
t. outlet decompression
t. outlet syndrome
t. pain
perforating artery of internal thoracic artery
perforating branch of internal thoracic artery
pericardial branch of thoracic aorta
t. radiation therapy
right internal thoracic artery
t. spine
spurring of thoracic spine
t. surgery
total thoracic esophagectomy
transverse thoracic diameter
traumatic rupture of thoracic aorta
upper t.
ventral root, t.
t. vertebra
video-assisted thoracic surgical non-rib-spreading lobectomy
volume thoracic gas

thoracica
aorta t.
arteria thoracica lateralis
arteria thoracica superior

thoracic-pelvic-phalangeal dystrophy

thoracoabdominal
t. aortic aneurysm
t. approach
arteriosclerotic thoracoabdominal aortic aneurysm
t. irradiation
t. stapler
t. syndrome

thoracoacromial
t. artery
pectoral branch of thoracoacromial artery

thoracoacromialis
arteria t.

thoracodorsal artery

thoracodorsalis
arteria t.

thoracolumbar
anterior layer of thoracolumbar fascia
t. fascia
t. spinal orthosis
t. spine

thoracolumbosacral
t. orthosis—flexion, extension, lateral bending, and transverse rotation
t. spinal orthosis
t. strain

thoracoplasty
Schede t.

thoracopulmonary
Askin thoracopulmonary neuroepithelial tumor

thoracoscopic
video-assisted thoracoscopic surgery

thoracoscopy
video-assisted t.

thoracostomy
closed chest t.
tube t.
t. tube

thoracotomy
anterolateral thoracotomy incision
closed t.
emergency department t.
t. incision
left anterior small t.
limited anterior small t.
t. tube
t. tube in place
t. with exploration

thorax, pl. **thoraces**
asymmetric t.
barrel-shaped t.
bony t.
milk lines of t.
t. resonant on percussion

Thorndike-Lorge written frequency

thorny-headed worm

thor scopic talc pleurodesis

Thottapalayam virus

thought
adaptive control of t.
altered thought process
appearance, mood, sensorium, intelligence, and thought process
t. blocking
blocking of thought process
t. broadcasting
concrete thought process

thought *(continued)*
confused or impoverished thought and speech
constraint of t.
t. content
content of t.
decreased capacity for abstract t.
delusional thought pattern
t. deprivation
destructive thought pattern
diminution of t.
disconnected and racing t.'s
t. disorder
disoriented or slow thought process
egocentric thought process
endorsement of deviant t.'s and beliefs
T. Field Therapy
form of t.
Grid Test of Schizophrenic T. Disorder
improved thought process
incoherent t.'s
t. insertion
irrational t.'s
logical analysis of automatic t.
perception, thought and recognition of information
poverty of content of t.
t. process
psychotic thought disorder
racing t.'s
stream of t.
suicidal thought train of thought
train of t.
vague obsessional t.'s
t. withdrawal

thoughtless hostility

thread
buttress thread screw
t. mate system
mucous t.
mucus t.
neural thread protein

threaded
t. fusion cage
t. titanium acetabular prosthesis

thready pulse

threat
fighting, injuries, sex, threats, self-defense
high-risk model of threat perception
t. to life
perceived illness t.
t. to self or others

threatened
t. abortion
t. miscarriage
t. myocardial infarction

threatening behavior

three
t. concept view
t. dimensional
needle and sponge count correct times t.
needle, sponge, and instrument count correct times t.
O2 saturation on three liters nasal cannula
Pediatric Extended Examination at T.
plasma exchange number t.
t. times daily with meal
t. times a week
t. times weekly

three-chambered heart

three-dimensional
T.-d. Block Construction Test
t.-d. computed tomographic angiography
t.-d. computed tomography pancreatography
t.-d. conformal radiation therapy
t.-d. contouring
t.-d. contrast-enhanced magnetic resonance angiography
t.-d. echocardiography
t.-d. Fourier transform
t.-d. superficial liposculpture
t.-d. ultrasound
t.-d. view

three-phase
t.-p. bone scintigraphy
t.-p. radionuclide bone scanning

three-point
t.-p. fixation
t.-p. gait

three-vessel disease

threonine
t. dehydrogenase
serine threonine kinase gene 11

threshold
above selected t.
acoustic reflex t.
anaerobic t.
angina threshold heart rate
atrial defibrillation t.
automated static threshold perimetry
capital expenditure t.
contralateral threshold shift
contrast threshold for motion perception
cough t.
current perception t.
curvilinear threshold shoulder
defibrillation t.
t. of detectability
difference limen t.
t. of discomfort
t. dose
electroshock seizure t.
t. energy
t. erythema dose
expiratory threshold load
exposure duration t.
flicker fusion t.
frequency threshold curve
fusion-inferred threshold test
hearing t.
hearing threshold level
impedance threshold valve
increased pain t.
inspiratory threshold load
t. of intelligibility
lactate t.
lactic acidosis t.
light differential t.
t. limit value
low anger t.
low sensory t.
mean cell t.
mechanical pain t.
median detection t.
median recognition t.
minimal t.
minimum elicitation t.
minimum light t.
motion detection t.
noise detection t.
noise-induced permanent threshold shift
noise-induced temporary threshold shift
olfactory t.
outlier t.
pacing and sensing t.
peak-to-peak t.
permanent threshold shift
t. potential
pressure pain t.
progressively lowered stress t.
pure tone t.
retinal damage t.

R-wave threshold electrocardiography
sine wave t.
single-electrode current perception t.
speech awareness t.
speech detectability t.
speech detection t.
speech reception t.
speech recognition t.
t. stage III of retinopathy of prematurity
temporary threshold shift
theoretical renal phosphorus t.
ventilatory anaerobic t.
ventricular fibrillation t.
ventricular premature contraction t.
vibration perception t.

thresholding
Swedish interactive thresholding algorithm

thrill
aortic t.
coarse t.
diastolic t.
no palpable t.
palpable t.
precordial t.
presystolic t.
systolic t.

thrive
cataract, microcephaly, failure to thrive, kyphoscoliosis
failure to t.
nonorganic failure to t.
organic failure to t.

throat
t. abscess
acute throat infection
acute throat irritation
t. clearing from anxiety
collapsed tissue in t.
t. culture
ears, nose, and t.
eyes, ears, nose and t.
Gram stain of t.
head, eyes, ears, nose, and t.
head, eyes, ears, nose, and throat unremarkable
t. injected
normal throat flora
salvarsan throat irrigation tube
sinuses, nose, t.
skin, head, eyes, ears, nose, and t.
t. smear
stab wound of t.
t. swab
usual throat flora

throbbing
t. headache
intense throbbing pain
t. pain in head
severe throbbing headache
unilateral throbbing headache

thrombasthenia
Glanzmann t.

thrombectomy
Arrow-Trerotola percutaneous thrombectomy device
intracoronary aspiration t.
percutaneous mechanical t.
percutaneous rotational t.
shredding embolectomy t.

thrombi (*pl. of* thrombus)

thrombin
t. activation device
t. clotting time
t. control
heparin neutralized thrombin time
high-dose thrombin time
human t.
t. receptor
t. receptor-activating peptide
t. receptor-activating peptide 6
serial thrombin time

thrombin-antithrombin III

thrombin-increasing fibrinopeptide B

thromblastic activity of amniotic fluid

thromboangiitis

thromboangiitis obliterans

thrombocythemia
essential t.
primary t.

thrombocytopenia
t. and absent radius
amegakaryocytic t.
atypical immune-mediated t.
autoimmune neonatal t.
congenital thrombocytopenia, Robin sequence, agenesis of corpus callosum, distinctive facies, developmental delay syndrome
drug-induced t.
drug-related t.
fetomaternal alloimmune t.
hemolytic uremic syndrome/thrombotic thrombocytopenia purpura
heparin-associated t.
heparin-associated thrombocytopenia and thrombosis
heparin-induced t.
idiopathic thrombocytopenia purpura
neonatal alloimmune t.
neonatal autoimmune t.
neonatal isoimmune t.
passive alloimmune t.
transplant-associated t.
X-linked t.

thrombocytopenia-thrombosis
heparin-induced t.-t.

thrombocytopenic
acute idiopathic thrombocytopenic purpura
alloimmune neonatal thrombocytopenic purpura
autoimmune thrombocytopenic purpura
idiopathic thrombocytopenic purpura
immune thrombocytopenic purpura
Moschcowitz thrombotic thrombocytopenic purpura disease
neonatal alloimmune thrombocytopenic purpura
pseudoidiopathic thrombocytopenic purpura
t. purpura
thrombotic thrombocytopenic purpura
thrombotic thrombocytopenic purpura and hemolytic uremic syndrome

thrombocytosis
essential t.

thromboembolectomy
percutaneous aspiration t.
pulmonary t.
rotating aspiration t.

thromboembolic
t. cerebral vascular accident
chronic thromboembolic pulmonary hypertension
t. complication
t. disease
t. disease stocking
t. event
t. pulmonary hypertension

thromboembolic *(continued)*
- pulmonary thromboembolic disease
- venous thromboembolic disease

thromboembolism
- aortic t.
- pulmonary artery t.
- recurring venous t.
- venous t.

thromboembolization
- deep venous t.

thromboendarterectomy
- pulmonary artery t.

thrombolysis
- high-frequency t.
- intracoronary thrombolysis balloon valvuloplasty
- selective intracoronary t.

thrombolysis-related intracranial hemorrhage

thrombolytic
- clot dissolving thrombolytic drug
- t. drug
- intraarterial thrombolytic therapy
- percutaneous thrombolytic device
- t. therapy

thrombomodulin glycoprotein

thrombonecrosis
- arteriolar t.

thrombopenia
- essential t.

thrombopenic purpura

thrombophilia
- factor V Leiden t.
- lupus t.

thrombophlebitis
- lateral sinus t.
- t. migrans
- migratory deep vein t.
- pelvic t.
- puerperal ovarian vein t.
- septic pelvic t.
- superficial t.
- suppurative t.

thromboplastic
- t. cell component
- t. plasma component

thromboplastin
- activated partial thromboplastin time
- t. activation test
- automated activated partial t.
- t. generation test
- t. generation time
- human brain t.
- leukocyte t.
- partial thromboplastin time control
- plasma t.
- plasma thromboplastin antecedent
- plasma thromboplastin component
- plasma thromboplastin factor
- platelet thromboplastin antecedent
- prothrombin time and partial thromboplastin time
- t. screening test
- tissue thromboplastin inhibition test
- whole-blood partial thromboplastin time

thrombopoiesis-stimulating factor

thromboscintigram
- deep venous t.

thrombosed
- arteriosclerotic thrombosed aneurysm
- t. graft
- t. hemorrhoid
- t. oral varix
- t. vein

thrombosis, pl. **thromboses**
- acute t.
- ascending medullary vein t.
- bilateral renal vein t.
- capsular thrombosis syndrome
- cavernous sinus t.
- central splanchnic venous t.
- cerebral artery t.
- cerebral vein t.
- cerebral venous sinus t.
- coronary t.
- deep vein t.
- deep venous t.
- deep venous thrombosis prophylaxis
- femoral artery t.
- hemoglobinuria and glomerular t.
- heparin-associated thrombocytopenia and t.
- hepatic artery t.
- iliac vein t.
- iliofemoral deep vein t.
- inferior vena cava t.
- infrarenal aortic t.
- intracranial sinus t.
- left middle cerebral artery t.
- maternal cortical vein t.
- mesenteric arterial t.
- mesenteric vein t.
- mesenteric venous t.
- middle cerebral artery t.
- orbital vein t.
- ovarian vein t.
- pelvic ovarian vein t.
- portal vein t.
- postoperative deep venous t.
- prosthetic valve t.
- proximal vein t.
- puerperal ovarian vein t.
- pulmonary t.
- recurrent deep vein t.
- renal artery t.
- renal vein t.
- right middle cerebral artery t.
- sagittal sinus t.
- sinus-vein t.
- stent t.
- subacute t.
- subclavian vein t.
- superior sagittal sinus t.
- venous t.

thrombospondin
- Asserachrom t.

thrombotic
- t. brain infarction
- chronic thrombotic pulmonary vascular obstruction
- t. complication
- t. disease
- t. endocarditis
- t. episode
- fetal thrombotic vasculopathy
- t. gangrene
- hemisphere thrombotic infarction
- t. hydrocephalus
- ischemic thrombotic cerebrovascular disease
- t. microangiopathy
- Moschcowitz thrombotic thrombocytopenic purpura disease
- nonbacterial thrombotic endocardial lesion
- nonbacterial thrombotic vegetation
- t. occlusion
- t. pulmonary artery
- serum thrombotic accelerator
- t. thrombocytopenic purpura
- t. thrombocytopenic purpura and hemolytic uremic syndrome

thrombus, pl. **thrombi**
- echogenic intraluminal t.
- t. formation time
- free-floating t.
- t. grade
- intracardiac t.
- left atrial ball-valve t.

occlusive arterial t.
percutaneous dissolution of t.
portal vein tumor t.
t. precursor protein
tumor t.
tumor thrombus in the portal vein

through
achievement through counseling and treatment
Awareness T. Movement
barium passed through esophagus into stomach
bronchoscope inserted through vocal cords with ease
drain brought out through stab wound
factor I through XIII
first through fifth digits of hand
first through fifth lumbar vertebrae or lumbar nerve
first through fourth heart sounds
first through twelfth dorsal vertebrae
forceps passed up through incision
t. illumination
incision through wall of cavity
jejunal tube through percutaneous endoscopic gastrostomy
t. the knee
opening through lens
passed through esophagus into stomach
t. the skin
WHO classification for transitional cell carcinoma of the urinary bladder: stages Ta through T4

through-and-through
t.-a.-t. avulsion injury
t.-a.-t. defect

throughout hospitalization

through-the-scope balloon dilation

throw
partial throw surgeon's knot

thrower's
grenade thrower's arm
grenade thrower's fracture

thrush
lid t.
oral t.

thrust
hand thrust test
head thrust test
jaw thrust maneuver
manual t.
t. plate prosthesis
tongue t.

thulium-holmium-chromium:YAG laser

thumb
t. abduction
adductor sweep of t.
t. deformity
t. fusion
gamekeeper's t.
gamekeeper's thumb dislocation
hitchhiker's t.
long abductor muscle of t.
long extensor muscle of t.
long flexor muscle of t.
mental retardation-adducted thumbs syndrome
mental retardation-clasped thumb syndrome
opposing muscle of t.
rule of t.
short arm thumb spica cast
skier's t.
t. spica bandage
t. spica splint
Steinberg thumb sign
trigger t.

thumb-finding test

thunderclap headache

Thygeson keratitis

thymectomy
neonatal t.

thymi (*pl. of* thymus)

thymic
t. alymphoplasia
t. carcinoid
t. carcinoid tumor
cardiac abnormality, abnormal facies, thymic hypoplasia, cleft palate, hypocalcemia
congenital thymic dysplasia
conotruncal cardiac defect, abnormal face, thymic hypoplasia, cleft palate
t. corpuscle
cultured thymic epithelium
t. depletion
t. dysplasia
t. epithelial supernatant
human thymic leukemia
t. humoral factor
humoral thymic factor
t. hypoplasia
t. irradiation
t. lymphocyte antigen
lymphoepithelioma-like thymic carcinoma
lymphopenic thymic dysplasia
mouse thymic virus
Nezelof type of thymic alymphoplasia
t. polypeptide
primary thymic carcinoma
t. radiation therapy
sarcomatoid thymic carcinoma
t. weight

thymica
mors t.

thymicae
arteriae t.

thymicolymphaticus
status t.

thymidine
cytosolic thymidine kinase
t. diphosphate
t. 5′-diphosphate
herpes simplex virus thymidine kinase
hypoxanthine, azaserine, and t.
t. kinase
t. kinase deficiency
t. kinase, mitochondrial
t. kinase, soluble
t. labeling index
t. monophosphate
t. 5′-monophosphate
t. triphosphate
t. 5′-triphosphate
tritiated t.
tritiated thymidine labeling index

thymidylate
de novo thymidylate synthesis
t. synthase

thymine, adenine, and guanine

thymitis
experimental autoimmune t.

thymocyte
antihuman thymocyte globulin
antihuman thymocyte plasma
cortisone resistant t.
horse antihuman thymocyte globulin
human thymocyte antigen

thymocytotoxic
t. autoantibody
natural thymocytotoxic autoantibody

thymol
t. flocculation
Maclagan thymol turbidity test
t. turbidity
t. turbidity test

thymoma
atypical t.
invasive t.
lymphocyte-predominant t.
Masaoka staging system for t.
medullary t.
mixed t.
murine t.
noninvasive t.
predominantly epithelial t.

thymopoietin pentapeptide

thymosin
t. $alpha_1$
t. $beta_4$
t. fraction 5

thymus, pl. **thymi**
activated thymus cell
t. and activation-regulated chemokine
antihuman thymus serum
bovine thymus extract
calf thymus extract
t. cell
t. cell growth factor
t. epithelium
fetal thymus organ culture
t. gland excision
t. gland function
homeostatic thymus hormone
horse antihuman thymus globulin
human serum thymus factor
human thymus antiserum
t. independent
t. leukemia antigen
lobule of t.
t. lymphoma
t. permeability factor
t. protein
rabbit thymus extract
rat thymus antiserum
serum thymus factor
t. tolerance factor
t. transfer factor

thymus-dependent
t.-d. lymphocyte
t.-d. zone of lymph node

thymus-derived lymphocyte

thyreopriva
cachexia t.

thyrocervical trunk

thyroepiglottic ligament

thyrogenic
nonpapillary thyrogenic carcinoma

thyroglobulin
t. antibody
autoantibodies to human t.
t. autoprecipitin
human t.
mouse t.

thyroglossal
t. diverticulum
t. duct
t. duct carcinoma
t. duct cyst

thyrohyoid
t. arch
t. branch of ansa cervicalis
t. laryngotomy
t. ligament
t. membrane
t. muscle

thyroid
t. abscess
t. adenoma
aggressive thyroid carcinoma
alopecia, nail dystrophy, ophthalmic complication, thyroid dysfunction, hypohidrosis, ephelides and enteropathy, and respiratory tract infection
anaplastic thyroid carcinoma
anterior glandular branch of superior thyroid artery
anterior/lateral/posterior glandular branch of superior thyroid artery
t. antibody
t. artery
t. autoantibody
autoimmune thyroid disease
autoimmune thyroid disorder
autoimmune thyroid hyperfunction
autonomously functioning thyroid nodule
autonomous thyroid adenoma
autonomous thyroid nodule
autosomal dominant toxic thyroid hyperplasia
benign granuloma of t.
t. biopsy
t. body
calcified thyroid adenoma
t. capsule
t. carcinoma
t. cartilage
colloid nodule of t.
t. crisis
t. deficiency
desiccated thyroid extract
differentiated thyroid carcinoma
diffusely enlarged t.
t. disease
t. disorder
t. diverticulum
t. dysfunction
t. dysgenesis
t. eye disease
familial medullary thyroid cancer
familial medullary thyroid carcinoma
familial nonmedullary thyroid carcinoma
fluorescent thyroid imaging
follicular variant of papillary thyroid carcinoma
t. foramen
t. function profile
t. function study
t. function test
t. ganglion
generalized resistance to thyroid hormone
generalized thyroid hormone resistance
t. gland
t. gland carcinoma
t. gland dysfunction
t. growth-blocking immunoglobulin
t. growth immunoglobulin
high-lying thyroid gland
t. hormone
t. hormone autoantibodies
t. hormone-binding index
t. hormone-binding ratio
t. hormone production
t. hormone receptor
t. hormone receptor-retinoid X receptor
t. hormone replacement
t. hormone resistance
t. hormone response element
t. hormone treatment
human-specific thyroid stimulator
human thyroid adenylcyclase stimulator
human thyroid hormone receptor
hypothalamic, pituitary, t.
increased thyroid activity
inferior thyroid gland
inferior thyroid notch
t. insufficiency
t. intoxication
t. isthmus

isthmus of thyroid gland
ligand-dependent action of thyroid hormone receptor
ligand-independent action of thyroid hormone receptor
light cells of t.
lingual thyroid gland
t. lobe
lobe of thyroid gland
lobule of thyroid gland
long-acting thyroid stimulator protector
lowest thyroid artery
low thyroid function
macrofollicular thyroid papillary carcinoma
malignant thyroid nodule
masked thyroid autonomy
maternal postpartum thyroid dysfunction
medullary carcinoma of t.
medullary carcinoma of the t.
t. microsomal antibody
mild thyroid failure
multinodular thyroid gland
multinodular thyroid nodule
t. necrosis
neonatal thyroid dysfunction
t. neoplasia
t. nodule
t. nodule ablation
nontoxic thyroid adenoma
oblique line of thyroid cartilage
overactive thyroid disorder
overactive thyroid gland
t. overactivity
papillary carcinoma of t.
papillary thyroid cancer
peripheral thyroid hormone metabolism
peripheral tissue resistance to thyroid hormone
t. peroxidase
pharyngeal branch of inferior thyroid artery
pheochromocytoma, thyroid carcinoma syndrome
pituitary resistance to thyroid hormone
pituitary thyroid hormone resistance
postpartum thyroid dysfunction
t. profile
pyramidal lobe of thyroid gland
t. radioimmunoassay
radionuclide thyroid imaging
resistance to thyroid hormone
t. response element
selective pituitary resistance to thyroid hormone
silencing mediator of retinoic acid and thyroid hormone receptor
squamous cell carcinoma of the t.
t. stimulation-blocking antibody
t. storm
superior thyroid notch
supplemental thyroid hormone
suspensory ligament of thyroid gland
syndrome of generalized thyroid hormone resistance
synthetic thyroid hormone
t. T-cell line
t. transcription factor
t. transcription factor-1
t. transcription factor 2
t. ultrasound
underactive thyroid gland
t. uptake gradient
t. uptake scan

thyroidal
t. ablation
t. hernia
t. radioactive iodine uptake test

thyroid-associated ophthalmopathy

thyroid-binding
t.-b. globulin
t.-b. globulin index
t.-b. inhibitory immunoglobulin
t.-b. prealbumin

thyroid-blocking antibody

thyroidectomy
medical t.
nearly total t.
near-total t.
partial t.
subtotal t.
total t.

thyroidei
nodi lymphoidei t.

thyroiditis
t., Addison disease, Sjögren syndrome, sarcoidosis syndrome
atrophic chronic autoimmune t.
atrophic Hashimoto t.
chronic lymphocytic t.
experimental autoimmune t.
giant cell t.
Hashimoto t.
lymphocytic t.
lymphocytic thyroiditis neoplasia
nonspecific chronic lymphocytic t.
painful subacute t.
painless postpartum t.
postpartum t.
postpartum painless thyroiditis with transient thyrotoxicosis
spontaneous autoimmune t.
subacute t.
symptomless autoimmune t.

thyroid-parathyroidectomy

thyroid-related ophthalmopathy

thyroid-releasing hormone

thyroid-serum ratio

thyroid-specific enhancer binding protein-1

thyroid-stimulating
t.-s. hormone-binding inhibitor antibody
t.-s. hormone receptor
t.-s. hormone receptor antibody
t.-s. hormone receptor autoantibody
t.-s. hormone-releasing factor
t.-s. hormone-releasing hormone
t.-s. hormone-secreting tumor
human thyroid-stimulating hormone
t.-s. immunoglobulin

thyromegaly
palpable t.

thyronine-binding prealbumin

thyroparathyroidectomy
acute t.

thyroperoxidase antibody

thyroplasty
anterior and posterior medialization t.

thyrotoxic
t. coma
t. crisis
t. exophthalmos
t. goiter
t. heart disease
t. myopathy
t. phase
t. storm

thyrotoxicosis
amiodarone-induced destructive t.
gestational transient t.
mild overt t.
postpartum painless thyroiditis with transient t.
spontaneously resolving t.

thyrotroph embryonic factor

thyrotropic
- t. hormone
- t. hormone-releasing factor

thyrotropin
- antenatal thyrotropin releasing hormone
- human chorionic t.
- human molar t.
- human placental t.
- Junkman-Schoeller unit of t.
- maternal thyrotropin receptor blocking antibody-induced congenital hypothyroidism
- t. receptor
- t. receptor autoantibody
- t. receptor-stimulating antibody
- t. release factor

thyrotropin-binding inhibitory immunoglobulin

thyrotropin-displacing activity

thyrotropin-producing adenoma

thyrotropin-receptor antibody

thyrotropin-releasing
- t.-r. factor
- t.-r. hormone
- t.-r. hormone receptor
- t.-r. hormone stimulation test

thyrotropin-stimulating hormone

thyroxin
- resin t.
- serum-free t.

thyroxine
- absolute free t.
- t. binding globulin
- dialyzable free t.
- effective thyroxine test
- effective thyroxine ratio
- extrathyroidal t.
- free thyroxine factor
- free thyroxine fraction
- free unbound t.
- t. iodine
- newborn screen serum thyroxine and phenylketonuria
- normal serum t.
- proportion free t.
- protein-bound t.
- t. radioisotope assay
- serum thyroxine measured by column chromatography
- serum thyroxine measured by displacement analysis
- tetraiodothyronine t.
- tetraiodothyronine thyroxine radioimmunoassay
- total exchangeable t.
- triiodothyronine to thyroxine index

thyroxine-binding
- t.-b. albumin
- t.-b. coagulin
- t.-b. globulin
- t.-b. globulin, estimated
- t.-b. globulin index
- t.-b. index
- t.-b. meningitis
- t.-b. prealbumin
- t.-b. protein

thyroxine-specific activity

tibia
- adolescent tibia vara
- anterior t.
- anterior border of t.
- anterior bowing t.
- anterior intercondylar area of t.
- t. bone
- t. and fibula
- fibular articular facet of t.
- fibular articular surface of t.
- infantile tibia vara
- interosseous border of t.
- lateral condyle of t.
- malleolar articular surface of t.
- medial border of t.
- medial condyle of t.
- medial malleolus of t.
- medullary nailing of t.
- nutrient artery of the t.
- nutrient artery of t.

tibiae
- arteria nutricia t.
- arteria nutriens t.
- dislocated elbow, bowed tibiae, scoliosis, deafness, cataract, microcephaly, mental retardation syndrome

tibial
- Anderson tibial pseudarthrosis classification
- anterior recurrent tibial artery
- anterior sliding tibial graft
- anterior tibial artery
- anterior tibial bowing
- anterior tibial bursa
- anterior tibial compartment
- anterior tibial compartment syndrome
- anterior tibial fasciocutaneous flap
- anterior tibial lymph node
- anterior tibial margin
- anterior tibial muscle
- anterior tibial nerve
- anterior tibial nerve dermatome
- anterior tibial recurrent artery
- anterior tibial sign
- anterior tibial spine
- anterior tibial subluxation
- anterior tibial tendon
- anterior tibial tubercle
- anterior tibial vein
- anterolateral tibial bowing
- t. base plate
- t. border of foot
- t. bowing
- childhood accidental spiral tibial fracture
- t. collateral ligament
- collateral tibial ligament
- comminuted tibial fracture
- t. condyle
- t. crest
- t. defect
- t. eminence
- femoral tibial bypass
- t. fracture brace proximal support
- t. graft
- high tibial osteotomy
- internal tibial torsion
- lateral tibial plateau
- lateral tibial torsion
- t. malleolus
- medial calcaneal branch of tibial nerve
- medial malleolar branch of posterior tibial artery
- medial tibial plateau
- medial tibial stress syndrome
- modified Boyd amputation of ankle and distal tibial physis
- Ovadia-Beals classification of tibial plafond fracture
- t. plateau
- t. plateau fracture
- popliteal tibial bypass vein graft
- posterial t.
- posterior t.
- posterior tibial artery
- posterior tibial muscle
- posterior tibial nerve
- posterior tibial tendinitis
- posterior tibial tendon
- posterior tibial tendon dysfunction
- posterior tibial transfer
- Potts tibial osteotomy
- proximal tibial epiphysis
- t. sesamoid position

t. shaft
split anterior tibial tendon transfer
t. talar tilt/tibiotalar tilt
t. tuberosity
upper tibial osteotomy

tibialis
t. anterior muscle
anterior tibialis sign
anterior tibialis tendon
anterior tibialis transfer
arteria nutriens t.
arteria tibialis anterior
arteria tibialis posterior
dorsalis t.
nodus lymphoideus tibialis posterior

tibiarum

tibiofemoral
t. alignment
t. angle
t. index

tibiofibular
anterior-inferior tibiofibular ligament
anterior tibiofibular ligament
t. articulation
t. fracture
t. joint
t. ligament
t. mortise
t. syndesmosis

tibiofibularis
articulatio t.

tibiotalar
anterior tibiotalar fascicle
anterior tibiotalar part
anterior tibiotalar part of deltoid ligament
anterior tibiotalar part of medial ligament of ankle joint
deep anterior t.
deep posterior t.
superficial t.

Tibrogargan virus

tic
atypical tic disorder
autoimmune obsessive-compulsive tic disorder
chronic motor t.
chronic motor or vocal tic disorder
chronic tic disorder
complex motor t.
compulsive spasms and t.'s
dizziness from tic douloureux
t. douloureux
generalized degenerative t.
involuntary motor t.
involuntary verbal t.
multiple t.'s
multiple tic disorder
transient tic disorder
verbal involuntary t.
Yale Global T. Severity Scale

ticarcillin
tobramycin and t.

ticarcillin-clavulanate

tick
African tick bite fever
African tick typhus
African tick virus
Australian tick typhus
Colorado tick fever
Colorado tick fever virus
hard t.
Lone Star t.
North Asian tick typhus
North Queensland tick fever
North Queensland tick typhus
pajaroello t.
t. paralysis
South African tick fever
t. typhus

tick-borne
central European tick-borne encephalitis
Eastern tick-borne rickettsiosis
t.-b. encephalitis
t.-b. encephalitis virus
Far Eastern tick-borne encephalitis
focal tick-borne encephalitis
t.-b. illness
meningeal tick-borne encephalitis
progressive form of tick-borne encephalitis
pyretic tick-borne encephalitis

ticking

tickler
brain t.

ticlopidine plus aspirin

tidal
t. air
alveolar tidal volume
t. breathing flow-volume
t. breathing flow-volume loop
dead-space gas volume to tidal gas volume ratio
t. drainage
exercise tidal flow-volume loop
exhaled tidal volume
t. expiratory flow at 25% of tidal volume
t. expiratory flow at 50% of tidal volume
t. expiratory flow at 75% of tidal volume
t. expiratory volume
t. flow-volume loop
frequency to tidal volume
t. inspiratory flow
t. inspiratory flow at 50% of tidal volume
t. inspiratory volume
t. liquid ventilation
mechanical tidal volume
nocturnal tidal peritoneal dialysis
peak tidal expiratory flow
peak tidal inspiratory flow
pulse oximeter/end tidal CO_2
time to peak tidal expiratory flow

tie
breast tissue approximated with t.'s
catgut plain t.
circumferential suture t.
hemostasis secured with t.'s

tied
bleeder clamped and t.
clamped, divided and t.

tie-over-stent

tight
air t.
t. feeling in head
t. filum terminale
t. junction
t. lens syndrome
t. nuchal cord around infant's neck

tightness
capsular t.
chest pain and t.
hamstring t.

tight-to-shaft

tigroid
t. body
t. fundus
t. retina

til
tap water enema til clear

Tilligerry virus

tilt
anterior pelvic t.

tilt *(continued)*
head-down tilt test
head tilt and chin lift maneuver
head tilt method
head tilt test
head tilt with chin tilt
head tilt with neck lift
head-up t.
passive head-up tilt test
pelvic tilt exercise
posterior pelvic t.
talar t.
tibial talar tilt/tibiotalar t.

tilted
t. disk
t. optimized nonsaturating excitation

tilting
head t.

tilt-table
head-up tilt-table test
t.-t. test

tilt/tibiotalar
tibial talar tilt/tibiotalar tilt

Timboteua virus

Timbo virus

time
t. above minimum inhibitory concentration
absolute retention t.
Achilles tendon reflex t.
activated clotting t.
activated coagulation t.
activated partial thromboplastin t.
alert and oriented to person, place, and t.
alert and oriented to person, place, time, and date
alteration in time perception
altered time perception
t. and amount
ankle reflex t.
arm-tongue time test
t. of arrival
arteriovenous passage t.
ascites euglobulin lysis t.
aspirin tolerance t.
association reaction t.
asymmetric appearance t.
atrial activation t.
automaticity recovery t.
average extubation t.
before time of operation
t. between P wave and beginning of QRS complex in electrocardiography
bleeding t.
bleeding time template
blood-clot lysis t.
blood coagulation t.
buildup t.
capillary filling t.
capillary refill t.
carcinoembryonic antigen doubling t.
carotid ejection t.
central motor conduction t.
central reaction t.
central somatosensory conduction t.
cerebral transit t.
change in space and t.
choice reaction t.
cine densitometric assessment of transit t.
circulation t.
clot lysis t.
clot retraction t.
clotting t.
coagulation t.
cold ischemia t.
cold ischemic t.
cold-stimulation time test
t. compensation gain
complex reaction t.
concentration multiplied by t.
confusion about time and place
t. constant
contraction t.
corrected adjusted sinus node recovery t.
corrected ejection t.
corrected retention t.
corrected sinus nodal recovery t.
corrected time of sinoatrial node function recovery
crest t.
cross clamp t.
t.'s daily
Dale-Laidlaw clotting t.
t. of death
deceleration t.
decimal reduction t.
dedicated time block
delayed transit t.
t. of departure
diastolic amplitude time index
differential time to positivity
diffusion t.
digital temperature recovery time test
direct sinoatrial conduction t.
direct vision times one
discrete time sample
disordered breathing t.
disorientation to time and place
t. to distant failure
distorted sense of time and perception
distortion of time and space
disturbed sense of t.
t. domain signal processor
t. domain ultrasound
donor organ ischemic t.
doubling time of tumor size
dream t.
echo delay t.
ejection t.
ejective time index
endurance t.
esophageal transit t.
estimated time of arrival
estimated time of conception
estimated time of ovulation
t. estimation
euglobulin clot lysis t.
expiration t.
expiratory t.
external isovolumic contraction t.
filling t.
five times a day
five times a week
t. to following commands
forced expiratory t.
forced expiratory time in seconds
full recovery t.
function, appearance, t.
gastric bleeding t.
gastric emptying t.
gastric residence t.
gastrointestinal transit t.
gel development t.
generalized time reflex
generation t.
generation time of cell cycle
granulation t.
ground-glass clotting t.
half relaxation t.
helium equilibration t.
heparin neutralized thrombin t.
high-dose thrombin t.
high temperature-short time pasteurization
home prothrombin time monitoring
hospital arrival t.
hot plate reaction t.
t. information
inspiration t.
inspiratory t.

instillation abortion t.
instillation delivery t.
t. interval
t. interval between cessation of contraception and conception
t. interval between doses
t. interval difference
t. interval histogram
inversion t.
isometric endurance t.
isometric relaxation t.
isovolumic contraction t.
isovolumic relaxation t.
t. lapse
Lee-White tritium clotting t.
left ventricular activation t.
left ventricular ejection t.
left ventricular ejection time index
left ventricular fast filling t.
left ventricular slow filling t.
lethal t.
t. limited
t. to local failure
long time dialysis
longitudinal relaxation t.
lung capillary t.
lung-to-finger circulation t.
t. marker
marking time pattern
mass doubling t.
t. of maximal concentration
maximal extrapolated clotting t.
maximal flow per unit of t.
maximal predicted phonation t.
maximal ventilation t.
maximum walking t.
may repeat one t.
mean absorption t.
mean time between or before failures
mean circulating t.
mean circulation t.
mean disintegration t.
mean dissolution t.
mean generation t.
mean input t.
mean latency t.
mean pulmonary transit t.
mean residence t.
mean resistance t.
mean survival t.
mean swell time botulism test
mean transit t.
median lethal t.
median reaction t.
median relapse t.
median survival t.
membrane closure t.
methylene blue reduction t.
midexpiratory t.
mineralization lag t.
minimal time interval
t. and modifying
mortality rate doubling t.
t. motion
mucociliary clearance t.
myocardial contrast appearance t.
needle and sponge count correct times three
needle and sponge count correct times two
needle, sponge, and instrument count correct times three
needle, sponge, and instrument count correct times two
next t.
t. to nondetectable
noninvasive tear film break-up t.
not available at the present t.
no time limit
not invasive break-up t.
nucleation t.
occlusion t.
t. off
one day at a t.
oriented to t.
oriented times one
oriented to person, place, and t.
oriented to time and place
oriented to time, place, and person
oriented to time, place, person, and objects watch, pen, book
oriented times two
orocecal transit t.
t. out
overall treatment t.
PA conduction t.
pain-free walking t.
palliation, quality, radiation, severity, t.
partial prothrombin t.
partial thromboplastin t.
partial thromboplastin time control
particle transport t.
patient alert to space, time, and person
patient oriented to person, place and t.
patient's t.
t. to peak
t. to peak contrast
peak ejection t.
t. of peak emptying rate of mouth
t. of peak emptying rate of pharynx
peak expiratory flow t.
t. to peak expiratory flow
t. to peak filling rate
t. of peak filling rate of esophagus
t. to peak inspiratory flow
peak occupancy t.
t. to peak tension
t. to peak tidal expiratory flow
percentage of acceleration t.
perceptual span t.
peristimulus t.
personal time off
person, place, and t.
phonation t.
photostress recovery t.
place, person, and t.
place, time, and person
place and t.
plasma clotting t.
plasma iron disappearance t.
platelet survival t.
population doubling t.
position, quality, radiation, severity, t.
poststimulus t.
poststimulus time histogram
poststimulus time histograph
predetermined interval of t.
preejection period/left ventricular ejection t.
t. to pregnancy
pressure one-half t.
pressure time index
pressure time per minute
pressure time product
t. to progression
prolonged bleeding t.
prostate-specific antigen doubling t.
prothrombin consumption t.
prothrombin time control
prothrombin time control
prothrombin time fixing agent
prothrombin time and partial thromboplastin t.
prothrombin time ratio
pulmonary mean transit t.
pulse transmission t.
quality-adjusted time without symptoms or toxicity
quick prothrombin t.

time *(continued)*
ratio of expiration time and total time of breathing cycle
ratio of inspiration time and total time of breathing cycle
ratio of inspiratory time to total cycle t.
reaction t.
reading t.
recalcified whole-blood activated clotting t.
recovery t.
reduction t.
relative retention t.
relative time unit
relaxation t.
t. to repeat
repetition t.
reptilase t.
t. required to complete G_1 phase of cell cycle
t. required to complete G_2 phase of cell cycle
t. required to complete M phase of cell cycle
t. required to complete S phase of cell cycle
t. required to double number of cells in given population
resazurin reduction t.
retention t.
retention time ratio
retrograde conduction t.
right ventricular ejection t.
sedimentation t.
serial thrombin t.
simple reaction t.
sinoatrial conduction t.
sinoatrial recovery t.
sinus node recovery t.
skin bleeding t.
skin temperature recovery t.
slowed reaction t.
small bowel transit t.
spin-lattice or longitudinal relaxation time
spin-spin or transverse relaxation time MRI scan
survival t.
systolic ejection t.
systolic pressure time index
systolic time interval
tear breakup t.
t. and temperature
thermal death t.
three times daily with meal
three times a week
three times weekly
thrombin clotting t.
thromboplastin generation t.
thrombus formation t.
time to peak expiratory flow and total expiration t.
tincture of t.
total apexcardiographic relaxation time index
total end-range t.
total expiratory t.
total operating t.
total reading t.
total respiratory t.
total sleep t.
total time to intubation
total tourniquet t.
total twitch t.
t. trade-off
transient time of barium
transit t.
tumor doubling t.
t. to tumor progression
turnaround t.
turnover t.
unit of medical t.
t.'s upper limit of normal
t.'s upper limit of normal
variance of resident t.
t. velocity integral
venous clotting t.
venous filling t.
venous refill t.
venous return t.
ventricular activation t.
visual action t.
voice onset t.
voice termination t.
volume airflow per unit of t.
volume of oxygen consumption per unit of t.
Wagner-Nelson time 50 hours
wake after sleep onset t.
whole-blood activated clotting t.
whole-blood partial thromboplastin t.
whole-blood recalcification t.
whole time equivalent
t. without symptoms of progression or toxicity

time-activity curve

time-averaged urea concentration

timed
T. Behavioral Rating Sheet
t. contractions
t. disintegration
forced expiratory volume t.
t. forced expiratory volume
forced expiratory volume timed to forced vital capacity ratio
t. release
t. repetitive ankle jerk
test-estrin timed action
t. therapeutic absence
t. up and go
t. ventilatory capacity
t. vital capacity

time-delayed exponential

time-dose fractionation factor

timed-temperature gradient electrophoresis

time-gain
t.-g. compensation
t.-g. compensator
t.-g. control

time-limited psychotherapy

time-motion mode

time-of-flight
t.-o.-f. and absorbance
t.-o.-f. angiography
electron t.-o.-f.
laser desorption/ionization time-of-flight mass spectrometer
t.-o.-f. mass spectometry
two-dimensional t.-o.-f.

Time-oriented Data Bank

time-resolved
t.-r. imaging by automatic data segmentation
t.-r. imaging contrast kinetics
t.-r. liquid scintillation counting

Time-Sample Behavioral Checklist

time-tension index

time-to-disease progression

time-to-pulse-height converter

time-to-treatment failure

time-varied
t.-v. gain
t.-v. gain control

time-weighted average

TIMI
corrected TIMI frame count

timing
main timing event
meal t.

tin
t. ethyl

t. oxide
t. protoporphyrin

Tinaroo virus

tincture
Arning t.
deodorized tincture of opium
t. of green soap
t. of opium
t. of time

Tindholmur virus

tine
tuberculin tine test

tinea
t. capitis
t. corporis
t. cruris
moccasin-type tinea pedis
t. pedis
t. versicolor

Tinel
T. sign distal tingling on percussion

tine test

tingling
t. and burning sensation
distal tingling on percussion
numbness or t.
numbness and t.
numbness, tingling, and burning
t. and numbness in feet
numbness, tingling, and pain
numbness and tingling around mouth
numbness and tingling in finger
prickly, burning, and tingling feeling
t. sensation
t. sensation in hand
Tinel sign distal tingling on percussion

tinnitus
t. aurium
bilateral t.
t. cerebri
deafness with t.
Medical Audiologic T. Patient Protocol
nervous t.
objective t.
pulsatile t.
t. relief device
tonal t.
unilateral t.

tinted contact lens

tip
anterior tip of temporal lobe
t. of auricle
ball tip electrode
t. bossing
bulbous nasal t.
bulbous tip reduction
cannula t.
diamond tip wire
t. of ear
t. of elbow
endolaser probe t.
glomerular tip lesion
t. graft
hot tip laser probe
mastoid t.
nasal tip cautery
nasal tip thermistor
needle t.
nonaspirating ultrasonic phaco chopper t.
nonfrosted t.
open end flow-through radiopaque t.
pedicle tip amputation
petrous t.
quantitative tip culture
spiral tip catheter

tip-of-the-tongue

tipped
transbronchoscopic balloon t.
t. uterus

tire
Michelin tire baby syndrome

tiredness
muscle pain, allergy, tachycardia and tiredness, headache syndrome

tire implant

tirilazad mesylate

tissue
abdominal soft tissue density
t. ablation
t. ablation, incision and excision
abnormal development of scar t.
abnormal mass of tissue growth
abnormal residual t.
abnormal tissue mass
active brain t.
acute soft tissue injury
adipose t.
adipose tissue extract
adrenal rest t.
allograft tissue transplantation
t. angiogenesis factor
angiomatous neoplastic t.
annular atrophic connective tissue panniculitis of the ankle
t. antagonist of interferon
anterior soft tissue impingement
antibiotic concentration in serum and t.
Antoni A, B t.
aortic aneurysm t.
areolar connective t.
arrhythmogenic myocardial tissue ablation
articular joint tissue catabolism
ASTM augmented soft tissue mobilization
asymmetry, range of motion abnormality, tissue texture abnormality
atrioventricular conduction t.
atrophy of glandular t.
t. attenuation and scattering
augmented soft tissue mobilization
authorization form for removal of tissue for grafting
autodigestion of connective t.
autogenous composite t.
autoimmune connective tissue disorder
autologous adrenal medullary t.
autologous tissue flap
automatic tissue processing
axillary breast t.
t. band
t. biopsy
blood forming t.'s
blood-starved heart muscle t.
brain tissue implant
brain tissue partial pressure of oxygen
breast tissue approximated with ties
breast tissue expander
bronchus-associated lymphoid t.
brown adipose t.
burn healthy t.
cerebral tissue perfusion pressure
closed soft tissue injury
coagulation of t.
collapsed tissue in throat
collar of t.
composite free tissue transfer
t. concentrations of antibiotics
condensation of connective t.
connective t.
connective tissue disease
connective tissue growth factor
connective tissue massage

tissue *(continued)*
connective tissue sheath
consent form for removal of tissue for grafting
continuously cultured carcinoma cell line used for tissue cultures
Cooperative Human T. Network
craniofacial dysmorphism, absent corpus callosum, iris colobomas, connective tissue dysplasia syndrome
crescent-shaped flap of t.
cryopreserved tissue banking
t. culture
t. culture assay
t. culture infectious dose
t. culture infective dose
t. culture inoculated dose
t. culture medium
damage to healthy t.
death of heart muscle t.
débrided necrotic t.
debridement of bruised t.
debridement of necrotic t.
t. debris
deep bites of t.
degenerated tissue disease
dense collagenous t.
dense fibroelastic connective t.
dense fibrous t.
denuded connective t.
dermal fat free tissue transfer
destroy healthy t.
devitalized soft t.
diffuse connective tissue disease
t. displacement
t. dissection
distal soft tissue release
dog kidney tissue culture
t. Doppler imaging
elastic connective t.
elastic soft t.
endoscopic tissue culture
engrafted allogenic t.
t. equivalent
eroding gum t.
excess hemorrhoidal t.
t. expansion
extracellular t.
extranodular t.
exuberant granulation t.
t. factor pathway inhibitor
fetal mesencephalic t.
fetal tissue transplant
fibrin tissue adhesive
fibroelastic connective t.
fibrosarcoma of soft t.
fibrous connective t.
fibrovascular tissue on disc
fibrovascular tissue elsewhere
flap of abdominal t.
foreign body soft t.
fragment of endometrial t.
free tissue transfer
friable necrotic t.
gastrointestinal-associated lymphoid t.
glass factor tissue culture
t. glue
good tissue turgor
gradual loss of bone t.
t. graft
granulation t.
gross examination of t.
guided tissue regeneration
gum tissue breakdown
gut-associated lymphoid t.
hardening of breast t.
hard tissue replacement
hard tissue replacement-malleable facial implant
healthy tissue stained
heart muscle t.
hepatoma tissue culture
histiocytoma of soft t.
histoplasma tissue inhibitory factor
hyalinized fibrous t.
t. hydrostatic pressure
t. immunity
impaired tissue integrity
inadequate tissue maintenance
inadequate tissue repair
induration of t.
infected tissue culture
inflamed airway t.
inflammation of biopsy t.
inflammation of connective t.
t. inhibitor of metalloproteinase
intercellular tissue space
internal scar t.
interstitial t.
intracranial calcification benign glandular t.
intravesical prostatic t.
investing t.'s
ischemic tissue reperfusion
joint t.'s
t. lactase activity
laser tissue interaction
late effects of normal t.
lidocaine tissue concentration
Lillie allochrome connective tissue stain
liver tissue abnormality
localized tissue irritation
local tissue advancement flap
loose fibroelastic connective t.
lung biopsy t.
lymphoid tissue lymphoma
lyophilized anterior pituitary t.
malignant fibrous histiocytoma of soft t.
malignant rhabdoid tumor of soft t.
marginal zone/mucosa-associated lymphoid t.
median tissue culture infective dose
mediator chemical released in the t.'s
membranous layer of subcutaneous tissue of abdomen
metachronous tissue lesion
Miami STAR tissue expander
micronized AlloDerm t.
microscopically normal t.
microvascular free tissue transfer
mixed connective tissue disease
mixed connective tissue disorder
mixed tissue tumor
Mohs fresh tissue chemosurgery technique
monkey kidney tissue culture
monocyte tissue factor
mononuclear cell tissue factor
mucosa-associated lymphoid t.
mucosa-associated lymphoid tissue function
mucosa-associated lymphoid tissue lymphoma
mucosa-associated lymph t.
mucous connective t.
multilocular adipose t.
multiple soft tissue injuries
muscle layer in fatty layer of subcutaneous t.
mutation in hematopoietic t.
myxomatous soft connective t.
nasopharyngeal-associated lymphoid t.
native tissue harmonic imaging
t. necrosis
t. necrosis factor
necrotic gangrene t.
necrotic gangrenous t.
necrotic kidney t.
necrotic placental t.
nerve tissue regrowth
nervous tissue vaccine
neural crest t.

Nexacryl tissue adhesive
nodular connective tissue disease nevus
nodular growth of t.
non–mucosa-associated lymphoid tissue lymphoma
nonrhabdomyosarcoma soft tissue sarcoma
normal breast t.
normal immature brain t.
occipital cortex t.
t. oncotic pressure
orbital adipose t.
orbital, mandibular, ear, neural, soft t.
orbit, mandible, ear, cranial nerves, soft tissue syndrome
organ-cultured corneal t.
organ and tissue distribution
organ and tissue recovery
Pacific Coast T. Bank
paraffin-embedded t.
parietal pleural t.
passage of t.
passively congested lung t.
pathological endocrine t.
pathological tissue examination
percutaneous fetal tissue sampling
t. perfusion
periarticular soft t.
peribronchial connective t.
pericanalicular connective t.
pericardial bioprosthetic t.
perilobular connective t.
periorbital soft t.
peripheral tissue resistance to thyroid hormone
t. plasminogen activator
t. polypeptide antigen
prevertebral soft t.
procurement of donor organs and t.
prolonged acute tissue expansion
pulmonary parenchymal tissue volume
pulmonary tissue concentration
pulsed-wave tissue Doppler
radiation treatment of glandular t.
radiofrequency tissue volume reduction
rat aortic t.
rat embryo tissue culture
rat nephroma tissue culture
reactive lymphoid t.
recent soft tissue hemorrhage
recombinant human tissue factor pathway inhibitor
t. reflectance oximeter
t. regeneration
registry and tissue bank
t. repair
replica of donor t.
residual lymphoid t.
residual necrotic t.
t. resistance
resistance to movement of lung t.
restore tissue to affected area
retained placental t.
retropharyngeal soft tissue space
rhabdomyosarcoma of soft t.
secondary lymphatic t.
serum tissue polypeptide antigen
skin-associated lymphoid t.
skin-soft tissue envelope
t. sloughing
soft tissue abscess
soft tissue carcinoma
soft tissue compression injury
soft tissue density
soft tissue hematoma
soft tissue hemorrhage into mesentery
soft tissue infection
soft tissue invasion
soft tissue involvement
soft tissue laceration
soft tissue loss
soft tissue mass
soft tissue metastasis
soft tissue nodule
soft tissue sarcoma
soft tissue shadow
soft tissue treatment
soft tissue tumor
soft tissue view
t. space
specialized tissue aspirating resectoscope
subcutaneous adipose t.
subcutaneous tissues approximated
subperiosteal tissue expander
supporting tissue of brain
tenderness, asymmetry, restricted motion, and tissue texture changes
testicular adrenal-like t.
t. texture abnormality
t. texture changes, asymmetry, restriction of motion, tenderness
t. thromboplastin inhibition test
t. tolerance dose
total adipose t.
t. transglutaminase
t. transglutaminase ELISA
transplanting human fetal t.
tumor-associated tissue eosinophilia
tumor-specific tissue antigen
t. typing
unclassifiable connective tissue disease
underlying connective t.
undifferentiated connective tissue disease
undifferentiated connective tissue syndrome
vaporized hemorrhoidal t.
visceral adipose t.
white adipose t.

tissue-activating
connective tissue-activating peptide

tissue-air ratio

tissue-coding factor

tissue-damaging factor

tissue-infiltrating macrophage

tissue-invasive cytomegalovirus

tissue-maximum ratio

tissue-phantom ratio

tissue-protective, end-cutting

tissue-specific antigen

tissue-stone recognition system

titanium
t. cage
t. elastic nailing
fluted titanium nail
t. hollow-screw osseointegrating reconstruction plate
t. implant
t. linear cutter
t. mesh
t. plasma sprayed
threaded titanium acetabular prosthesis

titanyl
potassium titanyl phosphate laser

titer
antideoxyribonuclease B titer test
anti-DNase B t.
anti-HHV8 antibody t.
anti-HSV IgM Ab t.
antihuman herpesvirus 8 antibody t.
antihyaluronidase t.
antineutrophil cytoplasmic antibody t.
antinuclear antibody t.

titer *(continued)*
anti-Rho-D titer test
antirotavirus IgA t.
antistreptococcal DNase-B t.
antistreptolysin O t.
antithyroid antibody t.
Aspergillus IgG t.
atypical antibody t.
Bryan high t.
cold agglutinin t.
differential agglutination t.
fluorescent titer antibody
geometric mean t.
hemagglutination inhibition t.
herpes simplex antibody t.
heterophil antibody t.
high titer, low acidity
indirect Coombs t.
log infectious virus t.
microsomal antibody t.
mumps antibody t.
mycoplasma IgM t.
reciprocal geometric mean t.
Rh antibody t.
rosette inhibition t.
serum bactericidal t.
serum bacteriologic t.
serum-inhibiting t.
serum inhibitory t.
sheep cell agglutination t.

title peritoneal dialysis

Titmus stereoacuity test

titrable
urinary titrable acidity

titratable acid

titrated
t. extract of *Centella asiatica*
t. initial dose
t. norepinephrine excretion
t. water

titrating

titration
automatic titration system
heparin protamine t.
intragastric t.
skin endpoint t.
sodium sulfite t.

Tlacotalpan virus

T-lymphocyte-associated antigen

T/natural killer cell

TNF-related apoptosis inducing ligand

TNF-weak homologue

to
abdomen tender to palpation
ability to cope with stress
ability to function independently
ability to hold head up
ability to perform
ability to think or concentrate
abnormal intolerance to light
acclimation to heat and work
acetabular depth to femoral head diameter
acquired resistance to antibiotic
acute injury to brain
acute lymphoblastic leukemia secondary to Burkitt lymphoma
advance to regular diet
t. affected areas
aggression to people and animals
aid to the blind
Aid to Dependent Children
Aid to Permanently and Totally Disabled
aids to ambulation
alertness, response to voice, response to pain, unresponsive
alert and oriented to person, place, and time
alert and oriented to person, place, time, and date
allergy to insulin
alternating failure of response mechanical to electrical depolarization
alternative to violent behavior
amylase to creatinine ratio
analog to digital
anastomosed to loop of bowel
anemia related to chemotherapy
anemia secondary to blood loss
angry reaction to minor stimuli
anterior cervical approach to cervicothoracic junction
antibodies to the Epstein-Barr virus transactivator protein
antibodies to HIV
antibody to bromodeoxyuridine
antibody to C22-3
antibody to c100 protein
antibody to hepatitis A–E virus
antibody to hepatitis-associated antigen
antibody to hepatitis B core antigen
antibody to hepatitis Be antigen
antibody to hepatitis B surface antigen
antibody to HTLV-I
antibody to keratin
antibody to murine cardiac myosin
anxiety due to physical disorder
anxiety due to a substance
aortic sinus to right ventricle fistula
aortic valve opening to aortic valve closing ratio
apply to affected area
arterial to alveolar
arterial to alveolar gradient
arterial to alveolar oxygen tension ratio
arterial branch to dura mater
artery to atrioventricular node
artery to ductus deferens
artery to sciatic nerve
artery to the sinoatrial node
artery to tail of pancreas
artery to vas deferens
ascites due to bile leak
assessing severity: age of patient, systems involved, stage of disease, complications, response to therapy
associative detail response to white space
associative response to a white space on a card
asymbolia to pain
attachment to implant superstructure
attending to language stage
attention to sound
attitude to death
attitude to medication
Attitude to School Questionnaire
auditory response to bell
Austin-Kartush group C patient related to ossiculoplasty
autoantibodies to human thyroglobulin
autoantibody to stratum corneum
autologous reverse graft to ankle
autopsy limited to abdomen
autopsy limited to brain
autopsy limited to heart and lungs
autosympathectomy secondary to neuropathy
averse to risk
barium adherent to esophageal walls
t. be absorbed
t. be administered
t. be admitted

t. be announced
t. be arranged
t. be assessed
bed to chair transfer
t. be determined
t. be evaluated
belly button to medial malleolus
bilirubin to albumin ratio
blood flow to brain
blood from flow heart to lungs
blood supply to heart
blow to head
blunt injury to heart
bone to femur graft
bowel adherent to omentum
brief exposure to heat stress
calcium to phosphorus ratio
t. call back
capacity to function
carcinoma to be ruled out
cardiovascular problems related to drug abuse
cast off, to x-ray
cataract, microcephaly, failure to thrive, kyphoscoliosis
ceased to breathe
ceased to function
cecum returned to abdomen
cell response to estrogen
cell sensitivity to radiation
centrally active phenethylamine derivative related to amphetamine and methamphetamine
chest clear to auscultation and percussion
chest clear to percussion and auscultation
chest pain radiating to jaw and shoulder
child quick to anger
cholesterol to phospholipid ratio
clear to auscultation
clear to auscultation and percussion
clot to hold
cold to the opposite, warm to the same
collateral arterial flow to brain
coma secondary to head trauma
compression to traction ratio
condition related to stress
conforms to social normal
consent form to delivery by alternative physician
consent to intervention
controlled access to fluid
Coping Orientations to Problems Experienced
coronary mastoid-to-mastoid incision
costovertebral angle tenderness to percussion
crossmatch to transfusion ratio
cruelty to animals
damage to healthy tissue
danger to others
dangerous to one's self
dangerous to others
death due to drug abuse
decline in ability to perform routine tasks
decreased ability to concentrate
decreased ability to function
decreased venous return to heart
dementia due to Creutzfeldt-Jakob disease
dementia due to head trauma
dementia due to hepatic condition
dementia due to multiple etiologies
dementia due to traumatic brain injury
dementia due to vitamin deficiency
detail response to small white space
deviation to the left
deviation to the right
did not exist prior to enlistment
differential time to positivity
difficulty or inability to speak
diminished ability to think or concentration
diminished sensation to pinprick
discharge to duty
disorientation to time and place
disturbance of emotions specific to adolescence
disturbance of emotions specific to childhood
double knee to chest
doxorubicin adsorbed to magnetic targeted carrier
dry to wet
due to void
dullness to percussion
eclampsia due to uremia
effector to target ratio
electrical impulse to heart
electrocardiographic interval from the beginning of QRS complex to end of the T wave
electrocardiographic wave corresponding to repolarization of ventricles
emergency assistance to families
emphysema secondary to heavy smoking
encourage to cough and deep breathe
E-point to septal distance
E-point to septal separation
equal t.
etiology to be determined
existed prior to enlistment
existed prior to service
expiratory to inspiratory ratio
exposure to allergen
exposure to blood or body fluid
exposure to industrial substances
extracellular mass to body cell mass ratio
face to face
factor essential for resistance to methicillin
failed to report
failed to respond
failure to descend
failure to engraft
failure to progress in labor
failure to thrive
failure to wean
family reaction to illness
fever unresponsive to antibiotic therapy
first to fifth sacral nerves
first to fifth sacral vertebrae
first to fourth heart sounds
first to twelfth thoracic nerves
first to twelfth thoracic vertebrae
fit to be detained
flow of blood and oxygen to heart
fluorescein to protein ratio
fluorescent antibody to membrane antigen test
t. follow
forced expiratory volume in one second to forced vital capacity ratio
forced expiratory volume timed to forced vital capacity ratio
forceps to aftercoming head
free to total prostate-specific antigen
frequency to tidal volume
full to confrontation
gallbladder anastomosed to duodenum

to *(continued)*
generalized resistance to thyroid hormone
genetic predisposition to psychiatric illness
grams of nitrogen to nonprotein kilocalories
gunshot wound to abdomen
gunshot wound to head
headache secondary to cervical spinal disease
head rotation to right
head to rump length
heart reduced to normal size
heart response to stress
heel to buttock
heightened sensitivity to odors
heightened sensitivity to sounds
hemorrhagic diathesis secondary to hepatic failure
hepatic problems related to drug abuse
hepatitis C antiviral long-term treatment to prevent cirrhosis
hereditary neuropathy with susceptibility to pressure palsy
heterogeneous resistance to vancomycin
high-dose radiation to tumor mass
highly prone to fantasy
home evaluation prior to discharge
hydrated to hydration
hydrocephalus due to congenital stenosis of aqueduct of Sylvius
hyperreactivity to stimuli
hyperresonance to percussion
hypersensitivity to aspirin
hypersomnia related to a known organic factor
hypertension secondary to renal disease
immediate intense need to void
immune globulin to an Rh-negative woman
immune to rejection
immunoreactive insulin to serum or plasma glucose ratio
impaired ability to swallow
impulsivity to plan ahead
inability to arrange words
inability to arrange words properly
inability to chew or swallow
inability to close eye
inability to communicate
inability to concentrate
inability to control appetite
inability to control blood pressure
inability to control drinking
inability to control stool
inability to control urine
inability to control weight
inability to cope
inability to defecate
inability to exercise
inability to feel pleasure
inability to focus
inability to focus attention
inability to function
inability to interpret written word
inability to maintain attention
inability to make decisions
inability to move a joint
inability to move tongue
inability to pass urine
inability to perform purposeful movements
inability to recall
inability to recall events
inability to recognize objects
inability to relate to people
inability to relax
inability to remember spoken words
inability to sleep
inability to speak
inability to straighten back
inability to suckle
inability to sustain consistent work behavior
inability to talk
inability to tolerate boredom
inability to walk
incipient cataract grade 11 to 41
incision carried down to the fracture site
incomplete resolution, scan to follow
increased blood flow to ear
increased blood flow to heart muscle
increased susceptibility to infection
Index to Dental Literature
inpatient to outpatient transfer
insomnia related to a known organic factor
insomnia related to mental disorder
inspiratory to expiratory ratio
insufficient blood flow to heart
intense need to void immediate
intent to control
intolerance to certain foods
intolerance to cold
intolerance to specific drugs
intolerance to specific foods
intracranial to intracranial anastomosis
intrinsic resistance to antibiotic
irreversible damage to brain cell
ischemic damage to heart
Jackson-Pratt to bulb suction
job hazardous to health
t. keep needle open
t. keep vein open
lateral to the incision
lateral ventricular width to hemispheric width
lecithin to sphingomyelin
left border dullness of heart to percussion
left to count
left ventricle to aorta pressure gradient
liability to pressure palsy
licensed to practice
linked to dipalmitoyl phosphatidylethanolamine
liquid chromatography coupled to tandem mass spectrometry
long-term variability-average to moderate
loss of ability to hold head up
lowered resistance to infection
lower fossa active, lateral knee pain, and long leg on the side ipsilateral to the weak fossa
lumbar fifth vertebra to sacral first vertebra
lungs clear to auscultation
lungs clear to auscultation and percussion
lungs revealed hyperresonance to percussion
manipulates to gain power
manipulates to gain profit
maximal spatial vector to left
maximum diameter to minimum diameter ratio
melanoma antigen reacting to T cell
mental disorder due to alcoholism
mental disorder due to a general medical condition
metaphysial to diaphysial width ratio

9- to 5-MHz convex array
microhemagglutination assay for antibodies to *Treponema pallidum*
midclavicular line to nipple
mild down-slant to palpebral fissure
mild to moderately impaired
minus two hours two hours prior to treatment
Moberg deltoid-to-triceps transfer
mood disorder due to a general medical condition
moribund patient not expected to live
motor-evoked response to transcranial stimulation
muscular response to electrical stimulation of motor nerve
myeloid to erythroid ratio
navicular to first metatarsal angle
near reaction to light
need to control
negative to date
nerve to carotid sinus
neutralizing antibody to vascular endothelial growth factor
new approaches to brain tumor therapy
new approaches to coronary intervention
nitrate to gas
nitrous oxide to oxygen ratio
noncontributory to present illness
nonorganic failure to thrive
nonresponsive to antibiotic
normal pupillary reaction to light
nose to ear to xiphoid
not to be resuscitated
not to exceed
number equal to one; single patient trial
number needed to treat
occupational exposure to chemicals
on-call to operating room
open to air
O-plasty to Z-plasty
orders not to resuscitate
organic damage to brain
organic failure to thrive
orientation to hospital
oriented to person, place, and time
oriented to time
oriented to time and place
oriented to time, place, and person
oriented to time, place, person, and objects watch, pen, book
overexposed to sun
overexposure to heat
overexposure to sunlight
painful inability to urinate
pain on a scale from 1 to 10
pain radiating to back
pain radiating to jaw
pain radiating to jaw and shoulder
pain related to exertion
pain spreading to arm
pain spreading to neck
pain spreading to shoulder
pancreatitis secondary to gallstones
parental failure to guide
parent to child
patient alert to space, time, and person
patient to call
patient-centered access to secure systems online
patient difficult to arouse
patient discharged to home care
patient discharged to nursing home
patient discharged to office followup
patient discharged to skilled nursing facility
patient discharged to SNF
patient failed to respond
patient guide to medication
patient has natural immunity to hepatitis B virus
patient hypersensitive to aspirin
patient immune to hepatitis B infection
patient intolerant to aspirin therapy
patient oriented to person, place and time
patient responded to treatment
patient responsive to noxious stimuli
patient responsive to painful stimuli
patient responsive to verbal command
patient to return
patient's ability to perform
patient transferred to nursing home
patient transferred to skilled nursing facility
patient transferred to SNF
patient with mild to moderate systemic disease
Pearson attachment to Thomas splint
period to discharge
peripheral tissue resistance to thyroid hormone
peroxidase antibody to peroxidase
persistent reactivity to light
pharmacy to dose
pituitary resistance to thyroid hormone
point to point
positive to negative ratio
posterior nasal spine to soft palate
postnasal drip due to rhinitis
postnasal drip due to sinusitis
potential tolerance to hallucinogen
P to P
pre-aid to the disabled
preoperative contraindication to surgery
prepatient periods to oocyst
pressure to control bleeding
prior to birth
prior to conception
prior to delivery
prior to exposure
prior to hospitalization
productivity to respiration ratio
Profile of Adaptation to Life
progressive inability to walk
prone to developing pigment gallstones
in proportion to age
prostate-specific antigen bound to alpha-1 antichymotrypsin
Psychosocial Adjustment to Illness Scale
pulmonary microvascular permeability to protein
pulmonic second heart sound equal to aortic second heart sound
pupils equal and reactive to light and accommodation
pupils equal, round, reactive to light and accommodation
pupils equal, round, reactive to light and accommodation directly and consensually
pupils react to light and accommodation
rabbit antibody to human ovary
rabbit antibody to pig ovary

to *(continued)*
ratio of basal acid output to maximal acid output
ratio of electron charge to mass
ratio of inspiratory time to total cycle time
ratio of magnetic moment of a particle to Bohr magneton
ratio of pulmonary to systemic circulation
ratio of serum alanine aminotransferase to serum aspartate aminotransferase
reaction to death
reactive to light pupil
Readiness to Change questionnaire
rectal bleeding secondary to hemorrhoid
red blood cell to plasma ratio
red cells too numerous to count
reduced blood flow to brain
reduced blood supply to heart
refusal to eat
relative response attributable to the maneuver
relative to rotation of a beam of polarized light
resistance to infection
resistance to movement of lung tissue
resistance to thyroid hormone
resistance to venous return
resistive exercises to upper extremities
responding to internal stimuli
respond to verbal command
response to white space
restore tissue to affected area
results to follow
t. return
return to baseline
return to clinic
return to flow
reversal speed of bronchoconstriction in response to methacholine
right to be assisted to die
right to refuse intervention
sacrococcygeal to inferior pubic point
sacrum to pubis
selective pituitary resistance to thyroid hormone
selective tubal assessment to refine reproductive therapy
sensitivity to hyperthermia
sensitivity to light and glare
sensitize heart muscle to digitalis toxicity
shade response to light gray area
shading response to black areas
shading response to gray areas
side to back to side
signal-difference to noise ratio
single knee to chest
source to skin distance
speed of bronchoconstriction in response to methacholine
sternal notch to nipple
stimulate to cry
strictly confined to bed
stroke due to cerebral hemorrhage
Structured and Scaled Interview to Assess Maladjustment
Student Adaptation to College Questionnaire
sudden death due to cocaine ingestion
superficial occipital artery to middle cerebral artery
Supplement to HIV/AIDS Surveillance
supportive device to restrain hernia
surface area to volume ratio
survival relative to nodal involvement in breast carcinoma
sympathetic branch to submandibular ganglion
t. take out
tenderness in abdomen due to hepatitis
tenderness to digital palpation
tenderness to palpation or percussion
tenderness to touch
tender to palpation
tender to pressure
testosterone to epitestosterone ratio
threat to life
threat to self or others
time to distant failure
time to following commands
time to local failure
time to nondetectable
time to peak
time to peak contrast
time to peak expiratory flow
time to peak expiratory flow and total expiration time
time to peak filling rate
time to peak inspiratory flow
time to peak tension
time to peak tidal expiratory flow
time to pregnancy
time to progression
time to repeat
time required to complete G_1 phase of cell cycle
time required to complete G_2 phase of cell cycle
time required to complete M phase of cell cycle
time required to complete S phase of cell cycle
time required to double number of cells in given population
time to tumor progression
tolerance to hallucinogen
too early to evaluate
too many to count
too numerous to count
total inability to urinate
total time to intubation
tracking blood flow to the brain
traction applied to extremity
transfer from supine to sitting
transfer to intermediate
transfer to nursing home
transfer to open
transferred t.
transmission of infected mother to infant
transmission of microbe to host
transmitting electrochemical messages to the brain
treatment of acute drug reaction to hallucinogen
triiodothyronine to thyroxine index
twisting injury to joint
umbilical vein to maternal vein
unable to determine
unable to locate
unable to obtain
unable to read lab result
up to date
upper body segment to lower body segment ratio
upper fossa active, medial knee pain, and short leg on the side ipsilateral to the weak fossa
venous return to heart
visceral abdominal fat to total abdominal fat ratio
visual fields full to confrontation
void on-call to operating room

volume to be infused
volume to peak expiratory flow and total expiratory volume
weightbearing to tolerance
whole response to detail
willful exposure to unwanted pregnancy
xiphoid to pubis
year to date

to-and-fro
t.-a.-f. flow
t.-a.-f. murmur

toast
bananas, rice, applesauce, toast diet
bananas, rice, applesauce, tea, toast diet
bananas, rice cereal, applesauce, toast diet

tobacco
t. addiction
alcohol, tobacco, and other drugs
t. dependence
environmental tobacco smoke
fetal tobacco syndrome
t. glycoprotein
history of tobacco use
loose-leaf t.
t. mosaic virus
t. necrosis virus
t. nonuser
passive tobacco smoke
t. rattle virus
t. ringspot virus
satellite tobacco necrosis virus
smokeless t.

tobacco-specific nitrosamine

tobramycin
serum tobramycin assay
t. solution for inhalation
t. and ticarcillin

tocolytic agent

tocopherol
alpha tocopherol beta carotene
t. deficient
high cholesterol and tocopherol deficient
high cholesterol and tocopherol supplemented
t. supplemented

Todd
T. paralysis
T. unit

toddler and infant motor evaluation

Toddler-Preschooler Postoperative Pain Scale

toe
adducted great t.
t. amputation
anterior long toe flexor
t. blood pressure
blue toe syndrome
cast with dorsal toe plate extension
cast with volar toe plate extension
t. clawing
claw toe position
clubbing of t.
cramping of t.
t.'s downgoing
t. extensor muscle
fanning of t.'s
t. flexion
t. gait
t. grasp
great t.
great toe amputation
great toe arthroplasty implant technique
great toe bone
great toe implant
great toe implant prosthesis
great toe reflex
great toe transplant
great toe wraparound flap
heel and toe walking
long extensor muscle of great t.
long flexor muscle of great t.
medial crossover t.
medial deviation of the second t.
microvascular free toe transfer
modified Cocklin toe operation
moving toes, painful leg syndrome
normal flexion of great t.
numbness in t.
pressure on toe joint
right toe off
right toe strike
t. sign
tendo Achillis lengthening and toe flexor release
total toe arthroplasty
t. touch as tolerated
t. touch exercise
t.'s upgoing
t. walking and heel walking

toeing in

toenail
ingrown t.

toe-to-thumb transplant

toe-walker
idiopathic t.-w.

toe-walking
idiopathic t.-w.

together
bring t.

Toglia Category Assessment Test

toilet
bronchial t.
joint t.
pulmonary t.
respiratory t.
tracheal bronchial t.
tracheobronchial t.
vigorous pulmonary t.

toileting self-care deficit

token
t. economy unit
t. test

tolbutamide
intravenous tolbutamide tolerance test
t. tolerance test

tolbutamide-glucagon test

Toldt
T. fascia
ligament of T.
line of T.
white line of T.

tolerable
maximal tolerable daily intake
maximum tolerable volume
t. daily intake

tolerance
abnormal glucose t.
alcohol dependence with t.
arginine-insulin tolerance test
arginine/insulin tolerance test
aspirin tolerance test
aspirin tolerance therapy
aspirin tolerance time
borderline glucose tolerance test
calcium tolerance test
cortisone-primed oral glucose tolerance test
t. dose
t. and endurance
exercise tolerance test
Fagerstrom tolerance questionnaire

tolerance *(continued)*
fat tolerance test
fructose tolerance test
glucose t.
glucose-insulin tolerance test
glucose-lactate tolerance test
glucose tolerance factor
glucose tolerance test
t. to hallucinogen
5-hour glucose tolerance test
impaired glucose t.
improved performance and t.
increased pain t.
increased tolerance of pain
intraperitoneal glucose tolerance test
intravenous glucose tolerance test
intravenous tolbutamide tolerance test
iron tolerance test
lactose t.
leucine tolerance test
t. level
low frustration t.
maximal exercise tolerance test
meal tolerance test
minimum tolerance dose
normal glucose t.
one-hour glucose tolerance test
oral glucose t.
oral glucose tolerance test
oral glucose tolerance testing
ornithine tolerance test
Physical T. Profile
plasma glucose tolerance rate
polyvalent t.
poor exercise t.
potential abnormality of glucose t.
potential tolerance to hallucinogen
prednisolone glucose tolerance test
pressure pain tolerance level
previous abnormality of glucose t.
reduced tolerance for physical activity
sitting t.
standard glucose tolerance test
standing t.
t. threshold
thymus tolerance factor
tissue tolerance dose
tolbutamide tolerance test
weightbearing to t.
zero work t.

tolerant
neonatally t.
persistent tolerant infection

tolerate
t. immune state
inability to tolerate boredom

tolerated
activity as t.
diet as t.
maximal tolerated concentration
maximal tolerated dose
maximal tolerated pressure
maximum tolerated medical therapy
patient tolerated full course of radiation
patient tolerated the procedure well
patient tolerated traction well
toe touch as t.
up out of bed as t.
weightbearing as t.

toleration
maximal t.
maximal toleration volume

tolerogenesis
surrogate t.

tolonium chloride

toluene
t. diisocyanate
t. sulfonic acid

toluidine
t. blue
t. blue stain
t. red unheated serum test

tomogram
computed electroencephalogram t.
transaxial t.
t. with oscillating Bucky

tomograph
Heidelberg retina t.

tomographic
computed t.
computed tomographic angiography
computed tomographic cisternography
computed tomographic colonography
computed tomographic metrizamide myelography
computed tomographic myelography
computed tomographic pelvimetry
computed tomographic scan
computed tomographic scanner
computerized tomographic hepatic angiography
computerized tomographic holography
computer tomographic methods of axial skeleton
computer tomographic methods of peripheral skeleton
coronal computed tomographic arthrography
t. cut
delay computer tomographic myelography
helical computed tomographic angiography
hepatic computed tomographic density
t. image of the head
magnetic resonance tomographic angiography
metrizamide computed tomographic cisternography
three-dimensional computed tomographic angiography
x-ray tomographic microscope

tomography
adenosine triphosphate single-photon emission computed t.
adrenal computerized t.
atrial bolus dynamic computed t.
automated computed axial t.
automated computerized axial t.
axial quantified computed t.
axial transverse t.
cardiovascular computed t.
carotid compression t.
cine computed t.
Compton scatter t.
computed abdominal t.
computed body t.
computed renal t.
computed tomography angiography
computed tomography arterial portography
computed tomography brain scan
computed tomography dose index
computed tomography laser mammography
computed tomography number
computed tomography severity index
computed tomography under endoscopic retrograde pancreatography
computed tomography with multiplanar reconstructions

computed transaxial t.
computer-assisted axial t.
computerized axial t.
computerized axial tomography scan
computerized transaxial t.
contrast-enhanced computed t.
cranial computed t.
double-dose–delay computed t.
dual-isotope simultaneous acquisition single-photon emission computed t.
dynamic computed t.
electrical impedance t.
electron-beam computed t.
electron-beam computerized t.
electron beam computerized t.
emergency room computerized t.
emission computed t.
emission computer-assisted t.
emission computerized axial t.
expiratory computed t.
fluoride ion positron emission t.
focused appendix computed t.
gated single-photon emission computed t.
gradient-echo single-photon emission computed t.
head computed t.
head computerized axial t.
high-resolution computed t.
high-resolution computed tomography scan
high-spatial-resolution cine computed t.
laminar t.
laser tomography scanner
magnetic resonance t.
megavoltage computed t.
megavoltage computed tomography scanner
methoxyisobutyl isonitrile single-photon emission computed t.
metrizamide-assisted computed t.
metrizamide computed tomography cisternography
multidetector computed t.
multiplanar computed tomography scan
multislice computed t.
noncontrast helical computed t.
nonenhanced computed t.
ocular coherence t.
optical coherence t.
optical coherence tomography in uveitis
optical coherent t.
parathyroid computed t.
perfusion computed t.
peripheral quantitative computed t.
pluridirectional t.
positron emission computed t.
positron emission tomography balloon
positron emission tomography scan
positron emission tomography technique
positron emission transaxial t.
positron emission transverse t.
quantified computed t.
quantitative computed t.
rapid acquisition computed axial t.
renal helical computed t.
scanning laser t.
single-photon emission computed t.
single-photon emission imaging t.
spinal computed t.
spiral computed tomography arteriography
spiral x-ray computed t.
technetium-99m hexamethylpropylene amine oxime single-photon emission computed t.
thoracic computed t.
three-dimensional computed tomography pancreatography
transmission computer-assisted t.
transverse axial t.
triple-phase helical computer t.
ultrafast computed t.
ultrasound computed t.
unenhanced helical computed t.
volumetric computed t.
whole-lung t.
whole tomography slice
xenon-enhanced computed t.
x-ray computed t.

tomorrow
anticipate discharge t.
discharge t.
tentative discharge t.

tonal tinnitus

tone
abdominal muscle t.
abnormal muscle t.
brief tone audiometry
continuous tone masking
t. deafness
t. decay
t. decay test
fetal heart t.'s
heart t.'s
hyperactive bowel t.'s
hypoactive bowel t.'s
improved muscle t.
increased flexor t.
increased muscle t.
lower esophageal sphincter t.
low muscle t.
marbled pure t.
modified tone decay test
muscle t.
T. in Noise test
noise tone difference
normal sphincter t.
normoactive bowel t.
peripheral arterial t.
poor muscle t.
t. and positioning
pure tone audiometry
pure tone acuity
pure tone average
pure tone threshold
regular heart t.'s
regular rate, clear t.'s, no murmurs
sphincter t.
stable fetal heart t.'s
touch and t.
uterine muscle t.
uterine resting t.
vasomotor t.
Williams tracheal t.

tone-reducing ankle-foot orthosis

tongs
cranial t.

tongue
anomalous tongue position
anterior part of t.
apex of t.
base of t.
base of tongue carcinoma
black hairy t.
blue t.
t. bone
t. of cerebellum
t. clucking
t. deviation
fissured tongue syndrome
inability to move t.
t. inflammation from pernicious anemia
t., jaw, neck dissection
lingual tongue flap
lymphatic follicle of t.

tongue *(continued)*
margin of t.
median groove of t.
median longitudinal raphe of t.
t. midline
mucoepidermoid carcinoma of t.
numbness of t.
osseous choristoma of the t.
outstretched hand or t.
petechiae of t.
t. protrudes in midline
t. protrusion
protrusion of t.
red strawberry t.
squamous cell carcinoma of t.
t. thrust

tongue-retaining device

tonic
Adie tonic pupil
asymmetric tonic neck reflex
t. contraction
t. control
t. convulsion
t. epilepsy
generalized tonic clonic
t. heart level
t. hind limb extension
t. immobility
intermittent tonic muscle contractions
t. labyrinthine inverted
t. labyrinthine reflex
local tonic pupil
Magnus and de Kleijn tonic neck reflex
t. neck reflex
neuropathic tonic pupil
nocturnal painful tonic spasm
painful tonic seizure
t. postural epilepsy
t. pupil
t. seizure
t. spasm
symmetric tonic neck reflex
t. vibration reflex
t. vibration response

tonic-clonic
t.-c. activity
t.-c. convulsion
t.-c. movement
secondarily generalized tonic-clonic seizure
t.-c. seizure

tonicity
muscle t.

tonofilament
desmosome with bundle of t.

tonography
carotid compression t.

tonometer
air-puff contact t.
air-puff noncontact t.
impression t.
Lombart t.
Maklakoff t.
McLean t.
noncontact t.
t. reading
tension by Schiotz t.

tonometry
applanation t.
t. by applanation
carotid applanation t.
noncontact t.

Tono-Pen
Oculab T.-P.

tonsil
t.'s and adenoids
t. of cerebellum
crypts of pharyngeal t.
fetal t.
t. grasped
hypertrophy of t.'s and adenoids
t.'s inflamed
t.'s intact

tonsillar
anterior tonsillar pillar
t. biopsy
t. calculus
t. coblation
t. concretion
t. crypt
t. debris
t. exudate
t. fold
t. fossa
t. fossa carcinoma
t. hernia
t. herniation
mucosal intact laser tonsillar ablation
t. pillar
t. tissue

tonsillectomy
t. and adenoidectomy
adenoidectomy and t.
dissection and snare t.
t. with operating microscope

tonsillitis
diphtherial t.
exudative t.
herpetic t.
necrotizing t.
pustular t.
streptococcal t.
suppurative t.

tonus
arterial t.
neurogenic t.

too
t. early to evaluate
t. many to count
t. numerous to count
red cells too numerous to count

tool
Adolescent and Pediatric Pain T. Scale
Apraxia Profile: A Descriptive Assessment T. for Children
Nursing Care Intervention T.
video graphic tool technology

tooth, pl. **teeth**
t. abscess
anchor t.
ankylosed t.
ankylosis of t.
anterior flared t.
apex of cusp of t.
apical foramen of t.
approximal surface of t.
artificial t.
auditory t.
autogenous tooth transplantation
avulsed t.
t. avulsion
t. banding
buccal surface of t.
t. bud
canine t.
t. contour
t. decay
embedded t.
erupted wisdom teeth
t. eruption
t. etching
t. extracted
t. extraction
t. fracture
t. germ
teeth in good dental condition
teeth in good dental repair
t. grinding
impacted t.
lingual surface of t.
t. loss
malpositioned wisdom teeth

mandibular t.
marginal crest of t.
maxillary anterior t.
medial incisor t.
molar permanent tooth
occlusal surface of t.
partially impacted wisdom teeth
t. pocket
ratio of decayed and filled teeth
reimplanted t.
t. restoration
root canal of t.
t. treatment
upper single t.
wisdom teeth

tooth-brushing instruction

top
child-resistant bottle t.
premature top codon

Topamax
topiramate Topamax

tophaceous
t. deposit
t. gout

tophus, pl. **tophi**
gouty t.

topical
t. anesthesia
t. anesthetic
t. antibiotic
t. corticosteroid
t. decongestant
t. eczema
erythromycin topical solution
t. estrogen
extended-duration topical arthropod repellent
t. fluoride
t. fluoride application
gentamicin, clindamycin, and polymyxin topical preparation
t. hypothermia
intensive topical antibiotic therapy
t. magnetic resonance
t. moisturizer
Monistat-Derm T.
Mycelex-G t.
Mycogen II T.
Mycolog-II T.
Myconel t.
Mytrex F T.
t. oropharyngeal anesthesia
t. skin protection
t. steroid

topic-oriented process group

topiramate Topamax

topographic
t. anatomy
computed topographic scan
T. Scanning System
t. simulated keratometric power

topography
arterial t.
corneal t.
vertical radiation t.

topoisomerase
DNA topoisomerase I
t. II
t. II-alpha
lipophilic topoisomerase I inhibitor
liposomal topoisomerase I inhibitor

toppling gait

toric contact lens

torn
t. lateral meniscus
t. medial meniscus

Tornwaldt
T. abscess
T. cyst
T. disease

Toro
Punta Toro virus

toroidal coil chromatography

Toronto
T. Alexithymia Scale
T. Biculture Test of Nonverbal Reasoning
T. Functional Capacity Questionnaire
T. Western Spasmodic Torticollis Rating Scale

torpedo
axon torpedo appearance

torque
peak isometric t.

Torrance Tests of Creative thinking

torsade
t. de pointes
t. de pointes ventricular tachycardia

torsion
angle of femoral t.
angle of t.
appendix testis t.
t. dystonia
t. fracture
internal tibial t.
lateral femoral t.
lateral tibial t.
medial femoral t.
medial tibial t.
ovarian cyst t.
spermatic cord t.
sudden torsion spasm
t. test

torsional
t. deformity
t. diplopia
upbeat torsional nystagmus

torso phased-array coil

torticollis
benign paroxysmal t.
Toronto Western Spasmodic T. Rating Scale

tortuosity
retinal venous dilation and t.
venous t.

tortuous
t. aorta
t. aortic arch
t. blood vessel
t. varicosity
t. vein
t. vessel

torus
mandibular t.

Toscana virus

tosylarginine methyl ester

tosylate
bretylium t.

total
t. abdominal colectomy
t. abdominal evisceration
t. abdominal fat
t. abdominal hysterectomy
t. abdominal hysterectomy and bilateral salpingo-oophorectomy
t. ablation
t. abortion rate
t. abstinence
t. acid
t. acidity
t. active motion
t. adenine deoxyribonucleotide
t. adenine nucleotide
t. adenine ribonucleotide
t. adipose tissue
t. administered dose
affinity attenuated total reflectance spectroscopy
t. aganglionosis coli

total *(continued)*
t. agenesis
t. air
t. air volume
t. airway resistance
t. alkaline phosphatase
t. alkaloid
t. allergen content
t. allergy syndrome
alumina-alumina total hip replacement prosthesis
alumina cemented total hip prosthesis
t. ammonia nitrogen
t. amnesia
t. ankle arthroplasty
t. ankle replacement
t. anomalous pulmonary circulation
t. anomalous pulmonary venous connection
anomalous pulmonary venous connection, total or partial
t. anomalous pulmonary venous drainage
t. anomalous pulmonary venous return
t. anorectal reconstruction
t. anterior circulation infarct
t. anterior circulation syndrome
anthropometric total hip
t. antitryptic activity
t. apexcardiographic relaxation time index
t. aphasia
t. arm length
t. articular replacement arthroplasty
t. articular resurfacing arthroplasty
t. artificial heart
ascitic fluid total protein
t. atrial blanking
t. atrial refractory period
attenuated total reflection
t. autogenous latissimus
t. axial node irradiation
t. base
t. bed capacity
t. bed rest
t. bile acid
t. biopsy
t. bladder capacity
t. bladder resection
t. blood granulocyte pool
t. blood volume
t. blood volume predicted from body surface
t. body
t. body bone mineral
t. body bone mineral density
t. body calcium
t. body clearance
t. body counting
t. body density
t. body electrical conductivity
t. body fat
t. body hematocrit
t. body hyperthermia
t. body irritation
t. body mass
t. body neutron activation
t. body neutron activation analysis
t. body nitrogen
t. body phosphorus
t. body photograph
t. body potassium
t. body protein
t. body protein turnover
t. body radiation
t. body scan
t. body scanning
t. body sodium
t. body solids
t. body solute
t. body surface
t. body surface area
t. body washout
t. body water
t. body weight
t. bound
t. burn size
t. burn surface area
t. bypass
t. calcium
t. capacity
t. capacity of lung
t. carbon dioxide content
t. cardiopulmonary bypass
CardioWest total artificial heart
t. cavopulmonary connection
t. cavopulmonary shunt
t. cellular receptor pool
t. cellular score
cementless total hip arthroplasty
cementless total hip replacement
ceramic total hip
t. cerebral blood flow
t. cerebral ischemia
t. cholesterol
t. cholic acid
t. cholinesterase
chronic total occlusion
t. circulating albumin
t. circulating hemoglobin
t. circulating protein
t. circulatory arrest
t. colectomy
t. colon examination
t. colonic aganglionosis
t. colonoscopy
concentration of total carbon dioxide
concentration of total oxygen
t. condylar prosthesis III
t. conjunctival flap
t. contact casting
t. contact orthosis
t. continence
t. cordectomy
t. coronary flow
t. coronary score
t. corrected incremental score
t. correction
t. counts bound
cyclic total parenteral nutrition
t. cystectomy
t. cytoplasmic ribosome
t. daily dose
t. daily energy expenditure
t. decreased histamine
t. dehiscence
delivered total dose
t. dietary calorie
t. digestible energy
t. digestible nutrients
t. digitalizing dose
t. disability
t. dose
t. dose infusion
dual lock total hip replacement
t. elbow arthroplasty
t. elbow replacement
t. electromechanical systole
t. end-diastolic diameter
t. endoplasmic reticulum
t. endoprosthesis
t. end-range time
t. end-systolic diameter
t. energy expended
t. energy expenditure
t. energy requirement
t. enteral nutrition
T. Environment Control
t. eosinophil count
t. epidermal necrolysis
t. episode of illness
t. esophagectomy
t. estrogen excretion
t. ethmoidectomy
t. exchangeable potassium

t. exchangeable sodium
t. exchangeable thyroxine
t. exchange capacity
t. excretory nitrogen
t. expiratory time
t. extraperitoneal laparoscopic hernia repair
t. fat intake
t. fat mass
t. fatty acid
t. fecal nitrogen
femoral total density
t. fertility rate
t. flow
t. flow resistance
t. fluid movement
fractionated total body irradiation
free to total prostate-specific antigen
Full-Scale Score T.
t. fundoplication
t. fundoplication procedure
t. gastrectomy
gastric analysis, free and t.
t. glossectomy
t. glottic transverse laryngectomy
t. glycoalkaloids
t. graft area rejected
grand t.
gross total resection
t. healthcare
t. heme mass
t. hemoglobin
t. hemolytic complement
t. hip arthroplasty
t. hip articular replacement by internal eccentric shells
t. hip prosthesis
t. hip replacement
t. hip replacement operation
t. hip replacement procedure
home total parenteral nutrition
t. homocysteine level
Hopkins Symptom Checklist-90 T. Score
t. hydroperoxide
t. hydroxyapatite
t. hypermetropia
hypermetropia, t.
t. hyperopia
hyperopia, t.
t. hysterectomy
t. immobility
t. immunoreactive
t. immunoreactive serum pepsinogen
t. implantation of artificial heart
t. inability to urinate
t. incontinence
t. infections versus total admission
t. infusion
t. infusion period
t. internal reflection microscopy
t. intrauterine volume
t. intravenous anesthesia
iodine-131 total body scan
t. iron
t. iron-binding capacity
t. joint arthroplasty
t. joint replacement
t. keratoplasty
t. knee arthroplasty
t. knee arthroscopy
t. knee prosthesis
t. knee replacement
t. knee replacement, left
t. knee replacement, right
lactic dehydrogenase t.
laparoscopic total occlusion
t. laryngectomy
t. laryngopharyngectomy
t. L-chain concentration
t. life expectancy
t. lipid extract
t. lipids
t. liquid ventilation
t. living quotient
t. lung capacity
t. lung compliance
t. lung volume
t. lung water
t. lymphocyte
t. lymphocyte count
t. lymphoid irradiation
t. lymphoid irradiation for allograft survival
t. lymphoid radiation
t. mastectomy
t. matrix formation rate
Mayo modified total elbow arthroplasty
mean total dose
t. meniscectomy
t. mesorectal excision
t. metabolizable energy
t. monocular blindness
t. muscle mass
nearly total thyroidectomy
t. negatives
t. nerve deafness
t. net positive
t. nodal irradiation
nonacute total occlusion
t. nuclear score
t. nutrient admixture
t. obstruction
t. occlusion of basilar artery
t. operating time
t. organic carbon
t. ossicular chain replacement prosthesis
t. ossicular reconstruction prosthesis
t. oxyhemoglobin
t. packed cell volume
t. pain relief
t. parathyroid hormone secretion
t. parenteral alimentation
t. particulate matter
t. passive motion
t. patient care
t. pelvic exenteration
t. peripheral parenteral nutrition
t. peripheral resistance index
peripheral total resistance
t. peripheral vascular resistance
peripheral vein total parenteral nutrition
permanent and t.
permanent total disability
t. peroxyl radical-trapping antioxidant potential
t. phobic anxiety
t. placental estrogen
t. placenta previa
t. plasma catecholamines
t. plasma cholesterol
t. population
t. positives
positive symptom t.
t. pressure
t. protective environment
t. protein tuberculin
t. pulmonary blood flow
t. pulmonary vascular resistance
t. quality management
t. radical-trapping antioxidant parameter
t. range of motion
ratio of expiration time and total time of breathing cycle
ratio of inspiration time and total time of breathing cycle
ratio of inspiratory time to total cycle time
t. reading time
t. red blood cells
t. red cell volume
t. reducing sugars
t. reference air-kerma

total *(continued)*
t. renal blood flow
t. renin activity
t. renin concentration
t. repair
t. respiratory conductance
t. respiratory resistance
t. respiratory time
t. response
t. response index
t. ridge count
t. rosette-forming cell
t. rotating knee
running t.
Scandinavian total ankle replacement
t. serum bile acid
t. serum bilirubin
t. serum hemolytic complement
t. serum prostatic acid phosphatase
t. serum protein
t. serum solids
T. Severity Assessment
t. shoulder arthroplasty
t. shoulder replacement
t. skin electron beam
t. skin examination
t. sleep time
t. small intestinal allotransplantation
t. solids in urine
t. solute absorption
t. static compliance
t. stomach volume
t. stroke volume
t. suspended particulate
t. symblepharon
t. symptom complex
t. systemic arterial resistance
t. systemic flow
t. T_3
t. T_4
t. temporary disability
temporary total disability
t. thoracic esophagectomy
t. thyroidectomy
t. time to intubation
time to peak expiratory flow and total expiration time
t. toe arthroplasty
t. tourniquet time
t. trabecular bone volume
t. transfer
t. transurethral resection of prostate
true total lung capacity
t. tumor dose
t. tumor mass
t. twitch time
t. ultrafiltration
t. urethral discharge
t. urinary gonadotropin
t. urinary nitrogen
t. vaginal hysterectomy
t. vascular isolation
t. vasomotor rhinitis symptom score
t. ventilatory assistance
t. viable cells
t. vibration reflex
visceral abdominal fat to total abdominal fat ratio
t. vital capacity
t. vitamin B_{12} binding capacity
t. volume capacity
volume to peak expiratory flow and total expiratory volume
t. volume of urine
t. weight gain
t. white blood cells
t. white and differential cell count
t. wrist arthroplasty
t. wrist replacement

total-blood cholesterol

total-body magnesium

total-dietary fiber

total-dose infusion

total-head excursion

totalis
hyperostosis t.
ophthalmoplegia t.

totally
Aid to Permanently and T. Disabled
t. dependent individual
t. disabled
t. endoscopic coronary artery bypass
t. extraperitoneal
t. functional neutrophil
t. incapacitated of caring for self
patient totally inoperable
t. stapled restorative proctocolectomy
t. unexplained sudden infant death syndrome

total-retinal detachment

total-serum bilirubin

totipotent hematopoietic stem cell

Totman
T. Change Index
T. Loss Index

toto
in t.
removed in t.

touch
bleeding on t.
en bloc no touch technique
healing t.
heightened awareness of touch or taste
light t.
light moving t.
light touch testing
motor, pain, touch, reflex deficit
One T. glucometer
One T. Profile
One T. Ultra meter
tenderness to t.
therapeutic t.
toe touch as tolerated
toe touch exercise
t. and tone
vitreal corneal touch syndrome

touchdown
t. nonweightbearing
t. partial weightbearing

touch-toe weightbearing

Toupet hemifundoplication fundoplication

Tourette
T. disease
T. disorder
Gilles de la Tourette syndrome
T. syndrome

Tournay
T. phenomenon
T. sign

tourniquet
applied t.
t. applied
arthroscopic t.
automatic rotating t.
clitoris tourniquet syndrome
t. control
t. ischemia
pneumatic t.
pneumatic tourniquet control
Rumel t.
Shenstone t.
total tourniquet time
upper arm t.

Tournoux
atlas of Talairach and T.

toward
Attitudes T. Disabled Persons
Attitudes T. Mainstreaming Scale
Heterosexual Attitudes T. Homosexuality scale
New Mexico Attitude T. Work Test
Opinions toward Adolescents
parental attitudes toward sex
predisposition t.'s illness
squarely face person, open posture, lean toward person, eye contact, relaxed
Test of Attitude T. School

towel
absorbent sterile t.
Ann Arbor double towel clamp
gowns and t.'s

tower
T. of Hanoi
T. of London

town
out of t.

toxemia
eclamptic t.
metabolic toxemia of late pregnancy
preeclamptic t.

toxic
acute toxic encephalopathy
acute toxic hepatitis
t. adenoma
adulterated rapeseed oil-associated toxic oil syndrome
alimentary toxic aleukia
t. amaurosis
t. amblyopia
t. appearance
autonomous toxic nodule
autosomal dominant toxic thyroid hyperplasia
t. cardiomyopathy
t. cirrhosis
t. deafness
t. dementia
diarrhea from toxic shock syndrome
diffuse toxic non-nodular goiter
t. dilatation of bowel
t. dose
t. dose, low
t. encephalopathy
t. epidemic syndrome
t. epidermal necrolysis
t. epidermal necrosis
t. equivalent
t. *Escherichia coli*
t. gas
t. gastritis
t. granulation differential
gut-derived infectious toxic shock
t. headache
t. hepatitis
ingestion of toxic agent
ingestion of toxic drug
t. insanity
lowest effective toxic dose
marrow toxic drug
maternal toxic effect
median toxic concentration
median toxic dose
medical toxic environment
t. megacolon
menstrual toxic shock syndrome
t. metabolic encephalopathy
t. metabolic etiology
minimum toxic dose
multiheteronodular toxic goiter
t. multinodular goiter
t. myocarditis
t. neuropathy
t. nodular goiter
nonmenstrual toxic shock syndrome
t. oil epidemic syndrome
t. optic nerve atrophy
organic dust toxic syndrome
t. overdose
t. retinopathy
t. shock
t. shock antigen
t. shock-associated protein
t. shock-like syndrome
t. shock syndrome
t. shock syndrome exoprotein
t. shock syndrome exotoxin
t. shock syndrome toxin
staphylococcal toxic shock syndrome
streptococcal toxic shock syndrome
t. substance
T. Substance Control Act
t. thyroid nodule
t. unit
t. vertigo

toxica
periostitis ossificans t.

toxicity
Adriamycin therapy t.
bone marrow t.
delayed pulmonary toxicity syndrome
digitalis t.
dose-limiting t.
t. or drug interaction
ethylene glycol t.
t. of hallucinogen
independent toxicity in combined modality therapy
t. information
intolerance and t.
late central nervous system t.
late neurological t.
lowest effect level of t.
mesalamine-related lung t.
methyl alcohol t.
newborn drug t.
nucleoside-associated mitochondrial t.
oxygen toxicity in immature lung
quality-adjusted time without symptoms or t.
sensitize heart muscle to digitalis t.
time without symptoms of progression or t.
treatment-related t.
vitamin A t.

toxicology
T. Data Base
T. Information Center
T. Information Conversational On-Line Network
limited toxicology screening
t. screen
urine toxicology screen

toxicosis
triiodothyronine t.

toxin
adenylate cyclase t.
ampicillin-resistant *Escherichia coli*
antibiotic-associated colitis toxin test
anticholera toxin antibody
black widow spider t.
botulinum t.
botulinum toxin A
cholera t.
cobra t.
dermonecrotic t.
diphtheria t.
diphtheria toxin normal
diphtheria toxin sensitivity
Escherichia coli heat-labile toxin vaccine
t. exposure
heat-labile t.
methyl alcohol t.

toxin *(continued)*
mixed bacterial t.
t. neutralization
Penicillium roqueforti t.
pentavalent botulism t.
pertussis t.
Shiga-like t.
tetanus t.
toxic shock syndrome t.
t. unit
vacuolating toxin gene A
zonula occludens t.

toxin-antitoxin
t.-a. immunity

toxin-induced
t.-i. diarrhea
t.-i. myopathy

toxin-mediated disease

toxin-negative
culture-positive t.-n.

toxin-positive
culture-positive t.-p.

toxipathic hepatitis

toxocariasis
ocular t.

toxoid
acellular pertussis vaccine with diphtheria and tetanus t.
alum-precipitated diphtheria t.
diphtheria-tetanus t.
diphtheria, tetanus toxoid, and acellular pertussis vaccine
diphtheria, tetanus t.'s, whole-cell pertussis, and *Haemophilus influenzae* type b conjugate
formol t.
horse antitetanus toxoid globulin
pertussis t.
polyribosylribitol phosphate-diphtheria toxoid conjugate
purified diphtheria toxoid precipitated by aluminum phosphate
tetanus-diphtheria toxoid, adult type
tetanus and diphtheria toxoid immunization
tetanus toxoid antibody
tetanus toxoid immunization
tetanus toxoid outdated
tetanus toxoid toxoplasmic choroiditis
tetanus toxoid up-to-date
typhoid, paratyphoid A, B, tetanus toxoid, and diphtheria toxoid vaccine

toxoid-antitoxin floccule

toxoid-antitoxoid
t.-a. floccule
t.-a. mixture
t.-a. mixture esterase

Toxoplasma
anti-*Toxoplasma gondii* antibody
anti-*Toxoplasma gondii* antibody secretion assay
Toxoplasma encephalitis
T. gondii

toxoplasmic
t. encephalitis
t. retinochoroiditis
tetanus toxoid toxoplasmic choroiditis

toxoplasmin skin test antigen

toxoplasmosis
AIDS-related t.
t. chorioretinitis
congenital t.
t. infection
neonatal t.
ocular t.
t., other infections, rubella, cytomegalovirus infection, herpes simplex syndrome
syphilis, toxoplasmosis, other agents, rubella, cytomegalovirus, herpes simplex virus
t. titer

T-plate
ASIF T.-p.

trabecula, pl. **trabeculae**
anterior chamber t.
arachnoid t.

trabecular
absolute volume of trabecular bone
active trabecular calcification surface
anteroapical trabecular septum
t. bone
t. bone volume
t. carcinoma
t. degeneration
t. hypertrophy
t. meshwork
t. meshwork-inducible glucocorticoid response
t. network
t. pattern
posterior trabecular meshwork
t. separation
t. thickness
total trabecular bone volume

trabeculated
bladder wall t.
t. bone
t. bone lesion

trabeculation
arachnoid t.
coarse t.
mild t.
vesical t.

trabeculectomy
argon laser t.
Pearce t.

trabeculopexy
argon laser t.

trabeculoplasty
argon laser t.
diode laser t.
laser t.
selective laser t.

trabeculotome
McPherson t.

trace
t. ankle edema
t. element
immediate sensory trace recall
t. metal elements injection
multiple trace elements
t. occult blood
slight t.

tracer
t. abnormality
arrow-point t.
low-level radioactive t.
National Biomedical T. Facility
nuclear t.
patchy distribution of t.
radioactive t.
t. study
t. uptake

trachea
anular ligaments of t.
anular ligament of t.
bifurcation of t.
carina of t.
deviation of t.
extrinsic compression of t.
guinea pig t.
t. incised
t. markedly inflamed
meconium in t.
t. midline
muscular coat of t.

muscular layer of t.
rabbit t.
scope inserted into trachea with ease

tracheal
anterior tracheal displacement
t. aspirate
t. atresia
t. bifurcation
t. biopsy
t. blood flow
t. branch
t. breath sound
t. bronchial toilet
t. bronchitis
t. bronchus
t. button
t. cartilage
t. catheterization
closure of tracheal fistula
t. collar
t. compression
t. deviation
t. diameter
t. displacement
t. fenestration
t. fistula
t. gas insufflation
t. gland
guinea pig tracheal smooth muscle
t. incision
t. intubation
t. intubation fiberscope
laryngeal tracheal anesthesia
t. lavage
local tracheal anesthesia
long-segment congenital tracheal stenosis
t. mucous velocity
t. occlusion
t. ring
t. spiral
t. tampon
t. transport velocity
Williams tracheal tone

tracheitis
erosive t.
t. sicca

tracheloplasty
ex utero intrapartum t.

tracheobronchial
t. amyloidosis
t. aspirate fluid
t. diverticulum
t. dyskinesia
t. foreign body
t. groove
t. injury
t. lavage
t. submucosa
t. toilet
t. tree

tracheobronchiales
nodi lymphoidei tracheobronchiales inferiores
nodi lymphoidei tracheobronchiales superiores

tracheobronchitis
acute t.
necrotizing superficial t.

tracheoesophageal
t. atresia
t. cleft
t. dysraphism
t. fistula
t. fistula, esophageal atresia, multiple congenital anomaly syndrome
t. junction
microcephaly, mesobrachyphalangy, tracheoesophageal fistula syndrome
t. prosthesis
t. puncture
vertebral abnormality, anal imperforation, tracheoesophageal fistula, and radial, ray, or renal anomalies

tracheojejunal puncture

tracheoscopy
t. with biopsy
t. with irrigation

tracheostomy
t. button
cricothyroidotomy and t.
t. cuff
cuffed tracheostomy tube
fenestrated tracheostomy tube
heated tracheostomy collar
high-humidity tracheostomy collar
high-humidity tracheostomy mask
high-humidity tracheostomy shield
t. mask anesthesia
percutaneous dilational t.
t. stoma
t. tube
t. tube inserted

tracheotomy
t. bar
emergency t.
high t.
percutaneous dilatational t.
percutaneous dilational t.
permanent t.

trachoma
Arlt t.
Arlt-Jaesche t.
t. and inclusion conjunctivitis
ocular t.
psittacosis, lymphogranuloma venereum, t.

trachomatis
Chlamydia t.

trachomatous
t. conjunctivitis
t. dacryocystitis
t. keratitis
t. pannus

tracing
carotid pulse t.
computer-assisted reconstruction by tracing of serial sections
computer-based case t.
computerized edge t.
definitely abnormal t.
dipole t.
t.'s of electrocerebral inactivity
fetal heart monitor t.
interrupted t.
jugular venous pulse t.
no prior t.'s
no significant change from previous t.
optical ray t.
precordial acceleration t.

track
fast track program
infant t.'s movement
needle t.
Nordic T.
nuclear track emulsion
railroad track appearance
railroad track sign

tracker-assisted
t.-a. photorefractive keratectomy
t.-a. PRK

tracking
atrial tracking pacemaker
automatic peak t.
t. blood flow to the brain
double tracking of barium
t. dye
Family T. System
magnetic bolus t.

tract
accessory optic t.
acute respiratory tract illness

tract *(continued)*
alimentary tract calcification
alimentary tract duplication
alopecia, nail dystrophy, ophthalmic complication, thyroid dysfunction, hypohidrosis, ephelides and enteropathy, and respiratory tract infection
angular tract of cervical fascia
anterior corticospinal t.
anterior internodal tract of Bachmann
anterior pyramidal t.
anterior raphespinal t.
anterior spinocerebellar t.
anterior spinothalamic t.
anterior trigeminothalamic t.
anterolateral t.
aortic tract complex hypoplasia
apple-peel appearance of the GI t.
asymptomatic urinary tract infection
atretic outflow t.
atrio-His bypass t.
atrio-hisian bypass t.
atrionodal bypass t.
atrioventricular nodal bypass t.
biliary tract infection
biliary tract obstruction
biliary tract pain
biliary tract stone
biliary tract stricture
Candida urinary tract infection
catheter-related urinary tract infection
central tegmental t.
chronic gastrointestinal tract bleeding
chronic obstruction of biliary t.
chronic urinary tract infection
concealed bypass t.
concurrent upper respiratory tract infection
congenital urinary tract deformities
corticobulbar t.
corticospinal t.
device-related urinary tract infection
dorsal spinocerebellar t.
dorsolateral t.
double-contrast barium examination of the upper gastrointestinal t.
female genital t.
female genital tract carcinosarcoma
female genital tract mutilation
female reproductive t.
frontal outflow t.
gastric tract disorder
gastrointestinal t.
gastrointestinal tract lymphoma
gastrointestinal tract bleeding
geniculohypothalamic t.
t. of Goll
hepatobiliary tract disease
hospital-acquired urinary tract infection
hospital-associated respiratory tract infection
iliotibial t.
iliotibial tract friction syndrome
incision and drainage of fistulous t.
intact motor t.
intestinal tract carcinoid
intestinal tract gas
lateral olfactory t.
lateral spinothalamic t.
lateral vestibulospinal t.
left ventricular outflow tract obstruction
long tract sign
lower genital tract infection
lower GI tract foreign body
lower respiratory t.
lower respiratory tract illness
lower respiratory tract infection
lower respiratory tract inflammation
lower urinary t.
lower urinary tract cancer
lower urinary tract dysfunction
lower urinary tract infection
lower urinary tract obstruction
lower urinary tract symptom
lower urinary tract tumor
male reproductive t.
mammillothalamic t.
mesolimbic dopamine t.
milk of calcium urinary tract cyst
Moore classification for vascular anomalies of the gastrointestinal t.
multicentric lower genital tract neoplasia
multisite lower genital tract involvement
narrow pulmonary outflow t.
neospinothalamic t.
nosocomial respiratory tract infection
nosocomial urinary tract infection
nucleus of optic t.
optic t.
optic tract compression
optic tract damage
optic tract lesion
optic tract pituitary tumor
optic tract syndrome
outflow biliary t.
outflow tract obstruction
percutaneous transhepatic liver biopsy with tract embolization
pyramidal t.
recurrent lower respiratory tract disease
recurrent upper respiratory tract infection
respiratory tract inflammation
respiratory tract lining fluid
reticulospinal t.
right ventricular inflow t.
right ventricular outflow t.
rubrospinal t.
selective decontamination of the digestive t.
selective digestive tract decontamination
sensory tract intact
spinal cord t.
spinothalamic t.
symptomatic urinary tract infection
upper aerodigestive t.
upper gastrointestinal tract hemorrhage
upper respiratory t.
upper respiratory tract illness
upper respiratory tract infection
urinary tract anomaly
urinary tract candidiasis
urinary tract infection cleared
urinary tract malformation
ventricular outflow t.

traction
t. alopecia
ankle traction bandage
anterior loop t.
application of traction device
t. applied to extremity
t. atrophy
axial manual traction test
axis traction forceps
balanced skeletal t.
t. band
bipolar vertebral t.

brachial plexus traction injury
cervical t.
compression to traction ratio
controlled cord t.
device for transverse t.
diathermy, traction, and ultrasound
t. diverticulum
t. epiphysis
finger trap t.
t. fracture
t. headache
head halter t.
home cervical traction unit
intermittent cervical t.
intermittent pelvic t.
long axis traction chiropractic table
low-profile halo t.
lumbar t.
manual cervical t.
obstetric traction injury
patient tolerated traction well
peripheral vitreoretinal t.
placed in t.
point of entry, traction and twist
t. retinal detachment
skeletal t.
static cervical t.
static pelvic t.
superior rectus traction suture
treated with ultrasound, diathermy, and t.
vitreoretinal traction syndrome

tractional retinal detachment

tractor
variable-width forms t.

tractotomy
anterolateral t.
stereotactic mesencephalic t.

trade-off
time t.-o.

traditional
t. behavior therapy
t. belief
t. birth attendant
t. Chinese herbal remedy
t. Chinese herbal therapy
t. Chinese medicine
t. counseling
t. home care
integral traditional Chinese medicine
t. psychotherapy

traffic
t. accident
illegal drug t.
road traffic accident

trafficking
lysosomal trafficking regulator protein

tragal cartilage

trailing pole

Trail-Making Test psychiatry

train
apin-echo t.
suicidal thought train of thought
t. of thought

trainable
t. mentally handicapped
t. mentally retarded

trained
t. participating father birth
t. participating husband birth

trainer
computer-aided fluency establishment t.
kinesthetic ability t.
positional feedback stimulation t.

Trainer's Assessment of Proficiency

training
activity t.
aggression replacement t.
alpha wave t.
ambulation training orthosis
ankle disc t.
anxiety control t.
anxiety management t.
asthma care t.
auditory integration t.
auditory training sessions
auditory training units
autogenic training for headache
autogenic training for hypertension
autogenic training for insomnia
awareness training model
Basic Aid T.
biofeedback t.
bowel training program
circuit resistance t.
cognitive skills training approach
crutch t.
t. and experience
field training exercise
food awareness t.
gait t.
t. group
habit reversal t.
heart-circulation t.
t. heart rate
heavy resistance strength t.
hospital inservice t.
inspiratory muscle t.
medical training center
neurofeedback t.
neuromuscular feedback t.
Nurse T. Act
parent effectiveness t.
physical t.
t. and placement service
progressive relaxation t.
research and training center
resistance t.
sensory integration t.
Sibling T. Program
social skills t.
special skills t.
strength training exercise
stress inoculation t.
t. and test lung
velocity-enhanced resistance t.
ventilatory muscle t.
walking t.
weight training exercise
Youth Effectiveness T.

trait
Allport personality trait theory
alpha-thalassemia-1, -2 t.
antisocial personality t.
anxious-neurotic personality t.
autosomal dominant t.
autosomal recessive t.
chromosomal t.
cognitive personality t.
gait t.
health enhancing t.
histrionic personality t.
Maternal T. Anxiety Score
mendelian t.
multifactorial t.
narcissistic t.
personality t.
personality trait disorder
quantitative trait locus
sex-linked t.
sickle cell t.
State T. Anxiety Index-I
thalassemia t.

trajectory
dying t.
emotional t.
fast adiabatic trajectory in steady state

trance
amnesia after t.
t. coma

tranquility
serenity, tranquility, peace user's term for dimethoxymethylamphetamine

tranquilizer
major t.
minor t.

trans
t. fatty acid
t. pars plana vitrectomy

transabdominal
anterior transabdominal approach
t. approach
axial transabdominal image
axial transabdominal imaging
colonic transabdominal sonography
t. preperitoneal laparoscopic hernia repair
t. sonography
t. thin-gauge embryofetoscopy

transabdominal/transvaginal ultrasound

transaction
Management T.'s Audit
online transaction processing

transactional
t. analysis
t. Analysis Life Position Survey

transactivation factor

transactivator
antibodies to the Epstein-Barr virus transactivator protein

transairway laryngeal control

transaminase
alanine t.
alanine amino t.
aspartate t.
erythrocyte glutamic oxaloacetic t.
gamma-aminobutyric acid t.
glutamic-oxaloacetic transaminase, mitochondrial
glutamic-oxaloacetic transaminase, soluble
glutamic-pyruvic t.
ornithine-ketoacid t.
serum glutamic-oxaloacetic t.
serum glutamic-pyruvic t.
tyrosine t.

transanal
rectal-expander-assisted transanal endoscopic microsurgery
t. endoscopic microsurgery

transaortic
peak transaortic valve gradient
t. valve gradient

transarterial
t. catheter embolization
t. chemoembolization

transatrial
left transatrial septal
percutaneous transatrial mitral commissurotomy

transaxial
computed transaxial tomography
computerized transaxial tomography
t. plane
positron emission transaxial tomography
t. slice
t. tomogram

transbrachial arch aortogram

transbronchial
t. brush biopsy
t. lung biopsy
t. needle aspiration
protected transbronchial needle aspirate

transbronchoscopic balloon tipped

transcapillary
t. escape rate
t. refill

transcarbamoylase

transcarbamylase
heterozygous ornithine t.
ornithine transcarbamylase deficiency

transcatheter
t. ablation
t. arterial chemoembolization
t. arterial embolization
t. arterial infusion
t. biopsy
t. closure
t. embolotherapy
t. oily chemoembolization
t. splenic arterial embolization
subsegmental transcatheter arterial embolization
t. therapy
t. umbrella

transcerebellar diameter

transcerebral electrotherapy

transcervical
t. approach
t. balloon tuboplasty
t. femoral fracture
t. intrafallopian tube transfer
t. resection of the endometrium
t. tubal access catheter

transcobalamin I, II

transcondylar
t. amputation
t. axis
t. fracture

transconjunctival
t. blepharoplasty
t. blepharoplasty laser resurfacing

transcoronary
t. ablation of septal hypertrophy
t. alcohol ablation

transcortical
t. apraxia
motor aphasia t.
t. motor aphasia

transcranial
t. color-coded duplex sonography
t. color-coded real-time sonography
contrast-enhanced transcranial color-coded real-time sonography
t. cortical magnetic stimulation
t. Doppler sonography
t. Doppler ultrasound
electrical transcranial stimulation
t. electrostimulation therapy
fast-frequency repetitive transcranial magnetic stimulation
functional transcranial Doppler sonography
motor-evoked response to transcranial stimulation
two-dimensional transcranial color-coded sonography

transcribed
internal transcribed spacer

transcript
cocaine and amphetamine regulated t.
latency-associated t.
X inactive, specific t.

transcriptase
avian myeloblastosis leukemia virus reverse t.
avian myeloblastosis virus reverse t.
BCR-ABL multiplex reverse transcriptase polymerase chain reaction assay
human milk reverse transcriptase enzyme
human telomerase reverse t.

nonnucleoside reverse transcriptase inhibitor
nucleoside analog reverse transcriptase inhibitor
nucleoside reverse transcriptase inhibitor
nucleotide reverse transcriptase inhibitor
product-enhanced reverse t.
reverse transcriptase inhibitor
reverse transcriptase polymerase chain reaction
reverse transcriptase primer extension

transcription
activating transcription factor
computer-assisted real-time t.
constitutive transcription unit
date of t.
integrating regulatory transcription unit
Janus kinase/signal transducer and activator of t.
NF-1 transcription factor
nuclear factor kappa B transcription factor protein
nuclear transcription factor
octamer-binding transcription factor
parathyroid hormone gene t.
pituitary-specific transcription factor-1
Rathke pouch homeobox transcription factor
ribosomal ribonucleic acid transcription unit
thyroid transcription factor
thyroid transcription factor-1
thyroid transcription factor 2

transcription-4
signal transducer and activator of t.

transcription-5
signal transducer and activator of t.

transcriptional intermediary factor 2

transcriptionist
medical t.

transcription-mediated amplification

transcutaneous
t. acupoint electrical stimulation
acupuncture and transcutaneous electrical nerve stimulation
t. aortovelography
t. bilirubin
t. carbon dioxide monitor
t. carbon dioxide pressure
t. carbon dioxide tension
t. cranial electrical stimulation
t. electrical nerve stimulation
t. electrical nerve stimulator
functional transcutaneous nerve stimulation
indwelling transcutaneous vascular access device
t. oxygen monitor
t. oxygen pressure measurement
t. pacing
t. partial pressure of oxygen
sham transcutaneous nerve stimulation

transcystic
t. duct
laparoscopic transcystic common bile duct exploration
laparoscopic transcystic lithotripsy

transdermal
t. absorption
t. administration
t. analgesic
t. anesthesia
t. delivery system
t. estrogen
t. fentanyl device
t. glyceryl trinitrate
t. infusion system
matrix transdermal system
t. nicotine patch
nicotine transdermal patch
t. nitroglycerin
t. testosterone
testosterone transdermal system
t. therapeutic system

transdiaphragmatic
maximal sniff-induced transdiaphragmatic pressure
t. pressure

transduced
anti-CD3 stimulated peripheral blood lymphocytes transduced with a gene encoding a chimeric

transducer
antral pressure t.
anular array t.
t. cell
floating mass t.
intracompartment
Janus kinase/signal transducer and activator of transcription
linear array B-mode ultrasound t.
neuro convex t.
Ocuscan 400 t.
signal transducer and activator of transcription-4
signal transducer and activator of transcription-5
solid-state transducer intracompartment

transduction
high-frequency t.
low-frequency t.

transduodenal approach

transected
doubly clamped, transected and stump ligated
t. spinal cord

transection
cranial nerve t.
esophagogastric devascularization and t.
lower esophageal t.
multiple subpial t.
raphe t.

transepidermal water loss

transepithelial
t. elimination
no-touch transepithelial photorefractive keratectomy

transesophageal
t. atrial pacing
t. atrial stimulation
t. dobutamine stress echocardiograph
t. Doppler color flow imaging
t. echocardiogram
t. echocardiography-dobutamine stress echocardiography
t. echocardiography with pacing
t. fistula
intraoperative transesophageal echocardiography
left atrial transesophageal pacing test
t. probe
t. puncture
two-dimensional transesophageal echocardiography
t. ventricular pacing

transfection
adenoviral gene t.
locoregional t.
rearranged during t.

transfemoral amputation

transfer
adenovirus-mediated gene t.
admission, discharge, t.
anterior tibialis t.
anteromedial tubercle t.
antibody transplacental t.
apparent net transfer rate
asynchronous transfer mode
auditory transfer deficit
autogenous osteocartilage t.
autologous fat t.
bed to chair t.
carbon monoxide transfer factor
cholesteryl ester transfer protein
chromosome-mediated gene t.
coefficient of heat t.
composite free tissue t.
Computerized Healthcare And Record T. System
t. coping
correctional t.
date of t.
delayed transfer flap
t. deoxyribonucleic acid
dermal fat free tissue t.
detector transfer function
direct oocyte sperm t.
egg t.
electric field mediated t.
electron transfer flavoprotein
electron transfer flavoprotein dehydrogenase
embryo intrafallopian t.
extensor tendon t.
t. factor
t. factor, dialyzable
t. factor test
fluorescence energy transfer immunoassay
fluorescence excitation transfer immunoassay
fluorescence resonance energy t.
free tissue t.
t. from supine to sitting
gamete intrafallopian tube t.
Ganley tendon t.
t. gene
heat transfer agent
heat transfer factor
high-frequency t.
high linear energy transfer radiation
high-risk t.
histamine ion t.
hospital transfer order
immediate transfer flap
inpatient to outpatient t.
t. to intermediate
intraocular t.
leg transfer device
ligand-to-metal charge t.
linear energy t.
Littler-Cooley abductor digiti quinti t.
low energy t.
low-frequency t.
low-linear energy transfer radiation
lymphocyte transfer reaction
magnetization transfer magnetic resonance imaging
magnetization transfer ratio
mass transfer area coefficient
mass transfer coefficient
maximum assisted t.
metal-to-ligand charge t.
microsomal triglyceride transfer protein
microvascular bone t.
microvascular free flap t.
microvascular free tissue t.
microvascular free toe t.
minimal assistance for transfers
minimal assisted t.
Moberg deltoid muscle t.
Moberg deltoid-to-triceps t.
modulation transfer factor
myoblast transfer therapy
normal lymphocyte transfer test
t. to nursing home
nursing home t.
Ober anterior t.
t. to open
oral transfer factor
osteochondral autograft transfer system
osteomyocutaneous free-tissue t.
t. out
patellar tendon t.
patient completes independent t.'s
patient transfer form
patient t.'s with standby assistance
pedicled colon t.
pedicled fibular t.
peritoneal oocyte and sperm t.
peroneus brevis t.
pes anserine t.
phase transfer catalyst
pivot transfer from wheelchair
posterior tibial t.
pronuclear stage t.
pronucleate stage embryo t.
pronucleate stage tubal t.
rectus abdominis muscle t.
replication and t.
resistance t.
resistance transfer factor
t. ribonucleic acid
Southern transfer analysis
split anterior tibial tendon t.
standby assistance in t.'s and ambulation
standby transfer and ambulation
standing pivotal t.
t. summary dictated
thymus transfer factor
total t.
transcervical intrafallopian tube t.
transvaginal intrafallopian sperm t.
tubal embryo stage t.
t. vesicle
in vitro fertilization-embryo t.
zygote intrafallopian t.

transfer

transferase
6-alkyl guanine alkyl t.
galactosyl t.
gamma-glutamyl t.
glucuronyl t.
oligosaccharide transferase enzyme
ornithine carbamoyl transferase deficiency
serum glutamic-oxaloacetic t.
terminal t.
terminal deoxynucleotide t.
terminal deoxynucleotidyl t.
uridine diphosphoglucuronyl t.

transference
affectionate t.
aim t.
alter ego t.
erotic t.
t. neurosis
self-object t.

transferral
weight transferral frequency

transferred
patient transferred to nursing home
patient transferred to skilled nursing facility
patient transferred to SNF
t. sensation
t. to

transferrin
carbohydrate-deficient t.
iron saturation of serum t.
t. receptor

serum t.
soluble transferrin receptor

transferrin-bound iron

transferring
t. immature muscle cell

transferring immature muscle cell

transfixation
t. of iris

transfixation of iris

transfixion
beaded transfixion wire
doubly ligated with transfixion suture
t. screws

transform
automated Hough t.
discrete Fourier t.
driven equilibrium Fourier t.
Fourier transform infrared spectroscopy
gradient field t.
Hough t.
inverse Fourier t.
multidimensional Fourier t.
three-dimensional Fourier t.
two-dimensional Fourier t.

transformation
atypical transformation zone
cavernous transformation of the portal vein
t. frequency
giant cell t.
growth and t.
hemorrhagic t.
human lymphocyte t.
large loop excision of transformation zone/loop electrosurgical excision procedure
loop excision of the transformation zone
lymphoblastic transformation test
lymphocyte transformation test
murine fibroblast t.
needle diathermy excision of the transformation zone
normal transformation zone colposcopy
partial nodular t.
peripheral blood lymphocyte t.
progressive transformation of germinal center
refractory anemia with excess of blasts in t.
teratoma with malignant t.
t. zone

transformational
endoscopic transformational diskectomy

transformed
large transformed cell
t. mink fibroblast

transformer
high-voltage t.
linear variable differential t.

transforming
t. growth factor
t. growth factor-1
t. growth factor alpha
t. growth factor beta-1, -2, -3
pituitary tumor transforming gene
t. principle
receptor t.

transfused
patient admitted and transfused with whole blood

transfusion
acquired immune deficiency syndrome-associated t.
acquired immune deficiency syndrome tainted t.
allergic transfusion reaction
allogeneic blood t.
allogenic blood t.
anaphylactic transfusion reaction
antenatal fetofetal t.
autologous blood t.
blood transfusion refusal form
blood transfusion therapy
crossmatch to transfusion ratio
directed donor t.
donor-specific blood t.
donor transfusion, specific
exchange blood t.
febrile nonhemolytic transfusion react
fresh frozen plasma t.
hemolytic blood transfusion disease
hemolytic transfusion react
t. hepatitis
immediate transfusion reaction
incompatible blood t.
incompatible hemolytic blood t.
intraoperative autologous t.
intrauterine fetal t.
intravenous fetal t.
long-term RBC transfusion therapy
matched lymphocyte t.
neonatal exchange t.
neutrophil antibody and transfusion reaction
nonhemolytic febrile transfusion reaction
packed red blood cell t.
partial exchange t.
percutaneous fetal t.
periodic blood t.
permission for blood t.
placentofetal t.
platelet transfusion therapy
random t.
t. reaction
red blood cell t.
single-donor t.
tainted blood t.
t. therapy service
t. transmission of viral hepatitis
t. transmitted
turn-to-turn t.
twin-twin transfusion syndrome
white blood cell t.
whole blood t.

transfusional hemosiderosis

transfusion-associated
t.-a. acquired immune deficiency syndrome
t.-a. AIDS
t.-a. graft-versus-host disease
t.-a. lung injury

transfusion-related
t.-r. acute lung injury
t.-r. AIDS

transfusion-transmitted
t.-t. acquired immune deficiency syndrome
t.-t. virus

transgastrostomic enteroscopy

transgenesis
mammalian t.

transglenoid
arthroscopic transglenoid suture stabilization procedure

transglutaminase
immunoglobulin A transglutaminase antibody
tissue t.
tissue transglutaminase ELISA

transhepatic
anterior transhepatic approach
t. cholangiogram
t. cholangiography
t. embolization

transhepatic *(continued)*
fine-needle transhepatic cholangiogram
fine-needle transhepatic cholangiography
percutaneous transhepatic biliary drainage
percutaneous transhepatic biliary drainage-enteric feeding
percutaneous transhepatic catheterization
percutaneous transhepatic cholangio-drainage
percutaneous transhepatic cholangioscopic lithotomy
percutaneous transhepatic cholangioscopy
percutaneous transhepatic cholecystolithotomy
percutaneous transhepatic cholecystoscopy
percutaneous transhepatic gallbladder drainage
percutaneous transhepatic liver biopsy with tract embolization
percutaneous transhepatic obliteration
percutaneous transhepatic portography
t. portal vein
t. portography
t. resistance

transhepatitic
direct percutaneous transhepatitic cholangiography

transhiatal esophagectomy

transhumeral
arthroscopic transhumeral reconstruction

transhydrogenase
glutathione-insulin t.

transient
t. abnormal myelopoiesis
t. abnormal Q wave
t. acantholytic dermatosis
t. aplastic crisis
t. asystole
t. ataxia
t. auditory evoked response
benign epileptiform t.'s of sleep
t. brain stem ischemia
t. cardiac arrest
central sharp wave t.
t. cerebral ischemia
t. cerebral ischemic episode
t. clinical hepatitis
computer of average t.'s
t. cortical blindness
crescendo transient ischemic attack
delusional transient organic psychosis
t. disorder
t. dizziness
t. dystonia
t. edema
t. emboligenic aortoarteritis
t. episodes of myocardial ischemia
t. erythroblastopenia of childhood
t. evoked otoacoustic emission
t. focal neurologic event
t. gastroparesis
gestational transient thyrotoxicosis
t. global amnesia
t. heart block
t. hemispheric attack
high-intensity transient signal
t. hyperammonemia of newborn
t. hypertension
t. hypogammaglobulinemia of infancy
t. ideas of reference
t. impairment
t. incontinence
t. infection
t. insomnia
t. ischemia
t. ischemic attack
t. ischemic attack and aging
t. ischemic attack, incomplete recovery
t. ischemic dilation
t. ischemic episode
t. ischemic event
isolated spike t.'s
t. joint pain
t. loss of consciousness
t. lower esophageal relaxation
t. mesenteric ischemia
t. monocular blindness
t. neonatal diabetes
t. neonatal diabetes mellitus
t. neonatal hyperammonemia
t. neonatal pustular melanosis
t. neurologic symptoms
t. osteoporosis of hip
t. paralysis
t. paranoid ideation
positive occipital sharp t.'s of sleep
postpartum painless thyroiditis with transient thyrotoxicosis
t. radicular irritation
t. respiratory distress of the newborn
t. respiratory distress syndrome
t. response imaging
t. situational reaction
sudden transient freezing
t. tachypnea
t. tachypnea of newborn
t. tic disorder
t. time
t. time of barium
vertex sharp transient electroencephalography
t. visual loss

transiently amplifying cell

transiliac
spinopelvic transiliac fixation

transillumination procedure

transistor
insulated gate field effect t.
junction field-effect t.
metal oxide semiconductor field effect t.
unijunction t.

transit
cerebral transit time
cine densitometric assessment of transit time
delayed transit time
esophageal radionuclide t.
esophageal transit scan
esophageal transit time
gastrointestinal transit time
mean colonic t.
mean pulmonary transit time
mean transit time
orocecal transit time
pulmonary mean transit time
slow transit constipation
small bowel transit time
t. time
whole-gut transit scintigraphy

transition
age t.
augmented transition network
T. Behavior Scale
t. breathing
glass transition temperature
isometric t.
large loop excision of transition zone
t. point
prostate-specific antigen transition zone

refractory anemia with excess blasts in t.
t. state theory
t. zone

transitional
anal transitional zone
t. bladder cell carcinoma
t. carcinoma in situ
t. care unit
t. cell
t. cell cancer
t. cell cancer-associated virus
t. cell carcinoma
t. cell carcinoma of bladder
t. cell papilloma
t. cell tumor
t. cell zone
t. denture
t. feeding
t. living program
lymphocyte t.
t. mucosa
Short T. Edge Protection
t. sleep
superficial transitional cell carcinoma
WHO classification for transitional cell carcinoma of the urinary bladder: stages Ta through T4

transitory
t. hallucination
t. hypertension

transjugular
t. cholangiography
t. fibrocartilage complex
t. intrahepatic portosystemic stent shunt

transketolase
t. activity
erythrocyte t.

translabyrinthine
middle fossa transtentorial translabyrinthine approach

translaryngeal
t. aspiration
t. intubation

translating
T. and Congruent Mobile-Bearing Knee test

translation
anterior talar t.
anterior translation of knee
force t.
formula t.

translational
t. control
t. control ribonucleic acid
t. displacement
t. inhibition

translation-inhibiting protein

translatory
AP translatory motion

translingual
Nitrolingual T. Spray

translocase
fatty acid t.

translocation
autosome t.
t. between 2 X chromosome
macular t.
medial extended facial t.
mosaic t.
nuclear t.
reciprocal t.
tandem t.
variegated translocation mosaicism

translocator
adenosine nucleotide t.
aryl hydrocarbon receptor nuclear t.

translucency
nuchal t.
nuchal translucency in a fetus
nuchal translucency measurement
nuchal translucency screening

translumbar
t. aortogram
t. aortography

transluminal
antegrade transluminal balloon dilatation
t. balloon valvuloplasty
t. coronary angioplasty
t. endarterectomy catheter
t. extraction atherectomy
t. extraction catheter
t. extraction-endarterectomy catheter
percutaneous coronary transluminal angioplasty
percutaneous transluminal myocardial revascularization
percutaneous rotational transluminal coronary angioplasty
percutaneous transluminal angioplasty with stent placement
percutaneous transluminal angioscopy
percutaneous transluminal balloon angioplasty
percutaneous transluminal balloon dilatation
percutaneous transluminal balloon valvuloplasty
percutaneous transluminal coronary angioplasty
percutaneous transluminal coronary arteriography
percutaneous transluminal coronary recanalization
percutaneous transluminal coronary revascularization
percutaneous transluminal coronary rotational ablation
percutaneous transluminal coronary rotational atherectomy
percutaneous transluminal dilatation
percutaneous transluminal endomyocardial revascularization
percutaneous transluminal renal angioplasty
percutaneous transluminal septal myocardial ablation
percutaneous transluminal ultrasonic coronary angioplasty
primary percutaneous transluminal coronary angioplasty
renal percutaneous transluminal angioplasty

transluminescent dosimeter

transmalleolar axis

transmandibular
t. approach
t. implant

transmaxillary approach

transmembrane
cystic fibrosis transmembrane conductance regulator
diastolic transmembrane voltage, maximum
t. hydrostatic pressure
t. potential
t. potential gradient

transmesenteric hernia

transmetatarsal amputation

transmissible
t. gastroenteritis
t. gastroenteritis virus
t. infection
t. mink encephalopathy
t. spongiform encephalopathy

transmissible *(continued)*
t. venereal tumor
t. virus dementia

transmission
acquired immune deficiency syndrome t.
analytic transmission electron microscope
asynchronous data t.
autosomal dominant t.
t. of bacteria
t. coefficient
t. computer-assisted tomography
confirmed transmission of viral hepatitis
t. by contact
conventional transmission electron microscope
conventional transmission electron microscopy
deficient transmission chemoreceptor
depression of t.
t. disequilibrium test
t. electron microscope
t. electron microscopy
food-borne transmission of viral hepatitis
hemodialysis transmission of viral hepatitis
t. hepatitis
high-resolution transmission electron microscopy
high-voltage transmission electron microscopy
index of vertical t.
t. of infected mother to infant
t. of infection
inoculation transmission of viral hepatitis
irregular dopamine t.
maternal-fetal transmission of antibody
maternal-neonatal transmission of viral hepatitis
t. of microbe to host
moisture vapor transmission rate
mother-to-child t.
neuromuscular t.
neuromuscular transmission blockade
oral transmission of saliva
oral transmission of viral hepatitis
pain transmission neuron
perinatal HIV t.
pressure transmission ratio
prevent transmission of disease
pulse transmission time
refractory period of t.
t. scanning electron microscopy
scanning transmission electron microscope
sexual transmission of viral hepatitis
transfusion transmission of viral hepatitis
t. unit
volumetric multiple exposure transmission holography
waterborne transmission of viral hepatitis

transmittance
spectral t.

transmitted
enterically transmitted non-A, non-B hepatitis
impulse transmitted pain
nonsexually transmitted disease
parenterally transmitted non-A non-B hepatitis
sexually transmitted condition
sexually transmitted infection
transfusion t.

transmitter
false t.
false neurochemical t.

transmitting electrochemical messages to the brain

transmucosal
oral t.
oral transmucosal fentanyl citrate
t. potential difference

transmural
t. colitis
t. drainage
t. electrical field stimulation
t. enteritis
t. hemorrhage
left atrial transmural pressure
long-acting transmural stimulator
t. myocardial infarction
t. pressure
t. pressure airway
t. steal

transmyocardial
t. laser revascularization
laser transmyocardial revascularization
percutaneous transmyocardial laser revascularization

transnasal
t. approach
t. butorphanol
t. endoscopic ethmoidectomy
t. esophagoscopy
t. fiberoptic laryngoplasty

transorbital leukotomy

transpalatal bar

transpapillary
endoscopic transpapillary catheterization of gallbladder
endoscopic transpapillary cyst drainage
t. endoscopic cholecystotomy

transparency
illusion of t.

transparent
highly permeable transparent dressing
Luedde transparent rule
optically transparent electrode

transpedicular
percutaneous transpedicular diskectomy

transpeptidase
gamma-glutamyl t.
glutamyl t.

transperineal
t. interstitial permanent prostate brachytherapy
t. urethral resection

transperitoneal
t. anterior subcostal incision
t. laparoscopic adrenalectomy
t. laparoscopic nephrectomy

transplacental
antibody transplacental transfer
t. gradient
t. hemorrhage
t. infection
t. transfer

transplant
adult-to-adult living related donor living t.
allogeneic bone marrow t.
allogeneic peripheral cell t.
allogeneic stem cell t.
allogenic kidney t.
allographic stem cell t.
antigen-modulated mini-stem cell t.
arteriovenous fistula t.
autologous bone marrow t.
autologous skin t.
bilateral lung t.

bone marrow t.
bone marrow transplant neutropenia
bone marrow transplant rejection
bone marrow transplant unit
cadaveric whole organ t.
cadaver renal t.
cardiomyopathy transplant rejection
t. center
chronic transplant nephropathy
clinical transplant coordinator
Collaborative T. Study
combined kidney and pancreas t.
corneal t.
t. coronary artery disease
double lung t.
en bloc bilateral lung t.
endocrine organ transplant complication
fetal tissue t.
flap transplant technique
great toe t.
heart-lung t.
heart transplant patient
heart transplant recipient
heterotopic cardiac t.
heterotopic heart t.
heterotopic kidney t.
human fetal pancreas t.
identical twin t.'s
t. intensive care unit
islet cell t.
kidney t.
kidney transplant unit
liver transplant rejection
living donor bilobar t.
living relative transplant donor
living renal t.
long-term survivor of heart t.
lung t.
lung transplant rejection
matched unrelated donor stem cell t.
McReynolds pterygium t.
metabolic organ transplant complication
National Lung T. Patient Association
nonmyeloablative allogeneic stem cell t.
nonmyeloablative allogenic t.
ocular muscle t.
organ transplant center
organ transplant infection
organ transplant recipient
orthotopic heart t.
orthotopic hepatic t.
orthotopic liver t.
pancreas after kidney t.
patellar tendon t.
Paton transplant speculum
penetrating corneal t.
peripheral blood progenitor cell t.
peripheral stem cell t.
peroneus brevis t.
t. recipient
reduced liver t.
reduced-size liver t.
t. rejection
renal t.
t. renal artery stenosis
renal transplant patient
renal transplant recipient
right single lung t.
single-lung t.
small intestine t.
solid organ t.
tandem t.
temporary heart t.
unrelated cord-blood t.
unrelated donor t.
whole bone transplant graft

transplantable

t. hepatocellular carcinoma

transplant-associated thrombocytopenia

transplantation

allogeneic bone marrow t.
allogeneic marrow t.
allogeneic stem cell t.
allogenic bone marrow t.
allogenic hematopoietic stem cell t.
allograft tissue t.
anhepatic stage of liver t.
t. antigen
antral t.
autogenous cartilage t.
autogenous tooth t.
autograft hair t.
autologous and allogeneic marrow t.
autologous blood and marrow t.
autologous chondrocyte t.
autologous cultured skin t.
autologous hematopoietic progenitor cell t.
autologous hematopoietic stem cell t.
autologous ovarian t.
autologous peripheral blood stem cell bone marrow t.
autologous stem cell t.
auxiliary heterotopic liver t.
auxiliary liver t.
auxiliary orthotopic liver t.
auxiliary partial orthotopic living donor t.
cadaveric donor t.
cardiac t.
cord blood t.
cryopreserved venous t.
displacement bone marrow t.
domino heart t.
heart-lung t.
hematopoietic stem cell t.
heterophil transplantation antigen
intrasplenic t.
isolated pancreatic islet t.
kidney t.
limbal autograft t.
limbal stem cell t.
liver and intestinal t.
liver and kidney t.
living donor liver t.
living-related donor t.
living-related liver t.
living segmental donor pancreas t.
lung t.
medial transplantation of patellar tendon insertion
meniscal autograft t.
non-heart-beating donor liver t.
nude bone graft t.
organ rejection of t.
organ for t.
orthotopic heart t.
orthotopic liver t.
osteoarticular allograft t.
pancreas transplantation alone
pancreatic islet cell t.
pancreatic transplantation alone
partial auxiliary orthotopic liver t.
peripheral blood stem cell t.
porcine bone marrow t.
procurement of cadaver organs for t.
simultaneous double kidney t.
simultaneous kidney-pancreas t.
small bowel t.
small-intestine t.
split-liver t.
stem cell indicated by transplantation assay
tumor-associated transplantation antigen
tumor-specific transplantation antigen

transplantation *(continued)*
tumor-specific transplantation immunity
vascularized bone marrow t.

transplanted
combat rejection of transplanted organ
t. hand
immune rejection of transplanted heart
t. immunity
t. marrow

transplanting
hair t.
t. human fetal tissue

transplant-related mortality

transport
air critical-care t.
anion transport inhibitor
anterograde axonal t.
atrial transport function
charcoal viral transport medium
Chlamydia transport media
ciliary particle t.
critical care air t.
effective oxygen t.
electron transport particle
fast axoplasmic t.
fatty acid transport protein
glucose t.
glucose transport system
high-affinity choline t.
Irvine viable organ-tissue transport system
t. maximum
McCarey-Kaufman transport medium
t. mechanism
t. medium
membrane transport defect
Monte Carlo photon t.
Monte Carlo photon transport simulation
mucociliary t.
oxygen transport rate
particle transport time
real oxygen t.
systemic oxygen t.
tracheal transport velocity
t. tube
tubular transport maximum
vesicular transport system
t. vial
virus transport medium
volunteer transport service

transportable
medical unit, self-contained and t.

transport-associated protein

transportation
air medical t.
lysis, storage, and t.
portacaval t.

transporter
ATP-binding cassette t.
canicular multispecific organic anion t.
glucose t.
monocarboxylate t.
norepinephrine t.
organic anion transporter polypeptide
serotonin reuptake t.
urea t.
vesicular monoamine t.

transposition
antrocolic t.
t. of aorta
bilateral advancement t.
complete transposition of great arteries
complete transposition of great vessels
t. complex
congenitally corrected transposition of the great arteries
corrected congenital transposition of the great vessels
t. flap
t. of the great arteries
t. of great vessel
left transposition of great artery
medial rectus t.
mesiolabial bilobed transposition flap
parotid duct t.
patellar tendon t.
portacaval t.
triple advancement t.

transpulmonary
t. pressure
t. thermal-dye dilution

transpupillary
t. thermal therapy
t. thermotherapy

transpyloric tube

transrectal
linear array transrectal ultrasound probe
t. needle biopsy
t. needle biopsy of prostate
t. probe
t. prostatic hyperthermia
t. ultrasonography
t. ultrasound
t. ultrasound-guided sextant biopsy
t. ultrasound of prostate

transscleral
contact transscleral laser cytophotocoagulation

transsclerally sutured posterior chamber lens

transscrotal testosterone

transsection
aortic t.

transseptal
t. angiocardiography
antegrade transseptal technique
anterograde transseptal technique
t. approach
t. frontal sinusotomy
t. left heart catheterization
Mullins long transseptal sheath

transsphenoidal
t. approach
t. pituitary resection

transtelephonic
t. ambulatory monitoring system
t. arrhythmia monitoring
t. electrocardiographic monitoring
t. exercise monitor
t. monitoring
pacemaker monitoring t.

transtentorial
t. herniation
middle fossa transtentorial translabyrinthine approach
traumatic transtentorial herniation

transthoracic
anterior transthoracic approach
t. approach
t. biopsy
t. color Doppler echocardiography
t. echocardiogram
t. electric impedance respirogram
endoscopic transthoracic symphathectomy
high-energy transthoracic shock
t. intracardiac monitoring
t. needle aspiration
t. needle aspiration biopsy
percutaneous transthoracic needle biopsy
t. projection

t. resistance
two-dimensional transthoracic echocardiography
video-assisted transthoracic surgery

transtrabecular plane

transtracheal
t. aspiration
t. catheter
t. insufflation
t. jet ventilation
t. oxygen
t. oxygen therapy
percutaneous transtracheal jet ventilation
t. selective bronchial brushing

transtrochanteric valgus osteotomy

transtubular potassium concentration gradient

transudate
oral mucosal t.
periarteriolar t.

transudative
t. ascites
t. pleural effusion

transumbilical
t. breast augmentation
t. plane

transureteroureteral anastomosis

transurethral
t. ablation
t. electrical bladder stimulation
t. electroresection
t. electrovaporization of prostate
t. evaporation of prostate
t. extraction
high-energy transurethral microwave thermotherapy
t. incision
t. incision of bladder neck
t. incision of prostate
low-energy transurethral microwave thermotherapy
t. microwave
t. microwave thermotherapy
minimal transurethral resection of prostate
t. needle ablation
t. needle biopsy of the prostate
periurethral transurethral microwave thermotherapy
t. prostate procedure
t. prostatic resection
t. resection of bladder
t. resection of prostate
t. resection syndrome
t. resection of valves
t. resection of vesical neck
status post transurethral resection of prostate
total transurethral resection of prostate
t. ultrasound
t. ultrasound-guided laser-induced prostatectomy
t. ultrasound-guided laser-induced prostatectomy system
t. ureterolithotripsy
t. ureterorenoscopy
t. vaporization of prostate
t. vaporization-resection of prostate

transvaginal
t. amniotic puncture
t. approach
t. bladder neck suspension
t. Burch procedure
t. color Doppler sonography
t. cone
t. fine-needle biopsy
t. hydrolaparoscopy
t. hysterosonography
t. intrafallopian sperm transfer
t. sector scan
t. suturing
t. tension-free
t. ultrasonography
t. ultrasound-directed oocyte retrieval

transvalvular
t. aortic gradient
t. pressure gradient

transvenous
t. angiography
t. aortovelography
balloon-occluded retrograde transvenous obliteration
t. catheter pacemaker
t. defibrillation lead
t. electrode
t. implantation of cardioverter-defibrillator
t. pacemaker
percutaneous transvenous mitral commissurotomy
permanent transvenous demand pacemaker
t. system

transversalis
arcus pedis t.

transverse
t. abdominal diameter
acute transverse myelitis
acute transverse myelopathy
t. amputation
ankle inferior transverse ligament
anterior transverse temporal gyrus
t. aortic arch
apical t.
aponeurosis of plantar transverse fasciculi
aponeurosis of transverse abdominal
t. approach
arcuate transverse keratotomy
t. arrest
t. arytenoid muscle
atlantal transverse ligament
automatic computed transverse axial scanning
t. axial tomography
axial transverse tomography
t. cardiac diameter
t. carpal ligament
t. colon
t. colostomy
t. commissure
deep transverse friction
device for transverse traction
t. diameter
t. diameter between ischia
t. diameter of heart
direct transverse reaction
t. electromagnetic
t. electromagnetic mode
t. fascia
t. fascicular area
five-chamber t.
t. fold of rectum
four-chamber t.
t. fracture
free transverse rectus abdominis myocutaneous flap
free transverse rectus abdominis musculocutaneous flap
t. friction massage
great transverse commissure
great transverse fissure of cerebrum
t. groove of oblique ridge
t. heart diameter
t. hermaphroditism
t. incision
t. inlet
t. lie
t. lie presentation
t. ligament of elbow

transverse *(continued)*
t. ligament of leg
t. line
t. linear incision
low cervical t.
low cervical transverse cesarean section
lower abdominal transverse incision
lower transverse abdominal incision
lower uterine segment transverse cesarean section
low flap t.
low segment transverse incision
low transverse hysterotomy
low transverse uterine incision
t. magnetization
mental retardation, spasticity, distal transverse limb defects syndrome
mentum transverse position
midpapillary t.
midvaginal transverse septum
t. muscle of abdomen
t. myelitis
normal functioning ileal transverse colostomy
occiput t.
t. palatine suture
t. polarization
positron emission transverse tomography
t. process
t. rectus abdominis muscle
t. rectus abdominis musculocutaneous flap
t. rectus abdominis musculoperitoneal flap
t. relaxation
t. relaxivity
repeat low transverse cesarean section
sacrum t.
sagittal, frontal, transverse, rotation
t. section
t. section of heart
serial transverse section
t. sinus
t. spinal sclerosis
spin-spin or transverse relaxation time MRI scan
t. sulcus of heart
superficial branch of transverse cervical artery
t. thoracic diameter
thoracolumbosacral orthosis—flexion, extension, lateral bending, and transverse rotation
total glottic transverse laryngectomy

transversely
t. excited atmospheric pressure
fascia incised t.
opened t.

transverse/sigmoid sinus

transversus
t. abdominis muscle
aponeurosis of musculus transversus abdominis
musculus arytenoideus t.

transvesical prostatectomy

transvestic fetishism

trap
finger trap traction
Luekens t.
nitron radical t.
osseous coagulum t.

trapeze
overhead frame t.

trapezial
Palmer classification of trapezial ridge fracture

trapezium
scaphoid, trapezium, trapezoid

trapezium-metacarpal eburnation

trapezius
ascending part of trapezius muscle
t. flap
t. ridge sign

trapezoid
anterior nucleus of trapezoid body
t. body
t. bone
t. implant
t. ligament
t. line
medial nucleus of trapezoid body
scaphoid, trapezium, t.

trapezoidal
Nordin-Ruiz trapezoidal marker
t. paddle pectoralis major myocutaneous flap

trapezoidei

trapped
t. air
t. air volume
t. gas volume

trapping
air t.
t. of air
expiratory trapping of air
pulmonary platelet t.

trash
isolation t.

Traube
T. bruit
T. corpuscle
T. dyspnea

trauma
abdominal trauma index
acute head t.
acute lumbar trauma syndrome
advanced trauma life support
affect trauma model
aftermath of t.
alcohol, epilepsy, insulin, overdose, uremia, trauma, infection, psychiatric, stroke
amnesia for t.
asphyxial renal t.
autoerotic rectal t.
basic trauma life support
cardiac arrest following t.
t. care
t. center
Champion T. Score
childhood trauma questionnaire
closed cerebral t.
closed craniocerebral t.
closed head t.
coma secondary to head t.
cumulative effects of t.
cumulative trauma disorder
dehydration, poisoning, t.
dementia due to head t.
destabilizing impact of t.
t. and emergency center
emergency medical trauma center
emergency and trauma center
emergency and trauma unit
focused abdominal sonography for t.
focused assessment by sonography for t.
forceps birth t.
head trauma syndrome
T. and Injury Severity Scores
t. intensive care unit
long-term effects of t.
multiple blunt t.
no acute t.

nonaccidental t.
nonpenetrating head t.
nonunion fracture t.
occult head t.
occult trauma, postanoxia, ventriculoperitoneal
pain and t.
Parkland formula for fluid resuscitation for burn t.
Pediatric T. Scale
Pediatric T. Score
penetrating abdominal t.
penetrating abdominal trauma index
perinatal craniocerebral t.
postdisaster t.
repetitive trauma disorder
Revised T. Score
severe head t.
shock trauma unit
t. skull
superficial ocular t.
suspected nonaccidental t.
T. Symptom Checklist for Children
T. Triage Rule

traumatic

t. abnormality
t. abscess
acute cervical traumatic sprain or syndrome
acute traumatic aortic injury
t. amaurosis
t. amnesia
t. amputation
t. aneurysm
t. aphasia
t. arthritis
t. avulsion
t. birth injury
t. bone cyst
t. brain death
t. brain injury
t. burn injury
t. cardiopulmonary arrest
chronic traumatic encephalopathy
communal traumatic experiences inventory
delayed traumatic intracerebral hematoma
dementia due to traumatic brain injury
t. dermatitis
t. dislocation
t. displacement
early traumatic epilepsy
t. epiphysial coxa vara
t. fat necrosis
t. fracture
t. glaucoma
t. headache
t. hemorrhage
t. hemorrhagic bursitis
t. hemothorax
t. intracranial aneurysm
t. lesion
mild traumatic brain injury
t. multiple hemorrhages
parent-infant traumatic stress
t. rupture
t. rupture of the diaphragm
t. rupture of thoracic aorta
Scales of Cognitive Ability for T. Brain Injury
t. stressor
t. subarachnoid hemorrhage
t. tamponade
t. thrombus
t. transtentorial herniation
t. unidirectional Bankart lesion surgery
t. vaginal delivery

traumatized

severely traumatized brain

traveler's diarrhea

Travesol

special baby T.

tray

t. agglutination test
automated tray assembly
infant cardiac arrest t.

Treacher Collins syndrome

treadmill

Bruce treadmill protocol
Duke treadmill prognostic score
t. exercise
exercise t.
t. exercise stress test
exercise treadmill test
exercise treadmill test with thallium
graded treadmill exercise test
limited treadmill test
maximal treadmill stress test
maximal treadmill testing
modified treadmill exercise testing
t. performance test
Reeves treadmill protocol
t. score
Sheffield treadmill protocol
submaximal treadmill exercise test

treat

t. empirically
number needed to t.

treatable illness

treated

t. but not admitted
diagnosed and t.
t. group
ineffectively t.
t. on an outpatient basis
patient empirically t.
patient treated conservatively
patient treated empirically
patient treated in hospital
patient treated initially
patient treated initially with intravenous fluids
patient treated medically
patient treated for smoke inhalation
patient treated with comfort care only
patient treated with supportive care
scientifically treated petroleum
volume treated in external irradiation
t. with ultrasound, diathermy, and traction

treating physician

treatment

achievement through counseling and t.
acquired immune deficiency syndrome residential treatment facility
acquired immune deficiency syndrome t.
active treatment period
t. of acute drug reaction to hallucinogen
acute intensive t.
t. of acute intoxication
acute treatment for acute drug intoxication
addiction treatment program
adequacy of t.
adjuvant hormonal or chemotherapy t.
adjuvant treatment option
t. administration record
adolescent day treatment program
adult diagnostic and treatment center
advanced coronary t.
aerosol treatment chamber

treatment *(continued)*
aggressive laser t.
AIDS/HIV Treatment Directory
alcohol dependence treatment program
alcohol treatment unit
allergy t.
allocation of t.
alternative method of t.
ambulatory antibiotic t.
antenatal corticosteroid t.
antenatal phenobarbital t.
anterior capsulotomy for treatment of OCD
anterior cingulotomy for treatment of OCD
anti-D globulin t.
anti-*Helicobacter pylori* t.
Antihypertensive and Lipid-Lowering T. to Prevent Heart Attack Trial
antioxidant eye t.
antipsychotic drug t.
antiretroviral t.
arrest-and-reversal t.
articulation t.
assertive-community treatment approach
t. assignment
T. Authorization Number
t. authorization request
autolymphocyte-based treatment for renal cell carcinoma
balanced ligamentous tension t.
behavioral health t.
care and treatment during pregnancy
catheter administered t.
cognitive behavior t.
cold or ice whirlpool t.
cold water t.
collagen skin t.
combined hyperthermia and radiation t.
community-based mental health t.
community periodontal index of treatment needs
t. completed
composite treatment score
comprehensive inpatient t.
comprehensive outpatient t.
comprehensive treatment plan
compression rod t.
confidential evaluation and t.
contact, control, test, evaluate, t.
continue same t.
controlled environment t.
cornerstones of t.
course of t.
court-ordered involuntary outpatient t.
court-ordered medical t.
date of t.
day treatment center
denial of lifesaving medical t.
Depression: Awareness, Recognition, and T.
Depression: Awareness, Recognition, and T.
detoxification and brief t.
diagnosis and t.
diagnostic procedure and t.
direct t.
directly observed treatment, short course
t. discontinued
drug dependence treatment program
drug treatment group
Early and Periodic Screening, Diagnosis, and Treatment program
t. and education of autistic and related communications handicapped children
electric shock t.
electroconvulsive shock t.
electroshock t.
emergency diagnostic and treatment unit
emergency medical t.
t. of emergent symptom
T. Emergent Symptom Scale
endovascular graft t.
entire treatment period
episodic treatment group
evaluation and t.
experimental breast cancer t.
ex utero intrapartum t.
Fletcher-Suit afterloading tandem
general care and t.
gingiva t.
Gliadel wafer treatment protocol
t. goal
goals of t.
gonadal suppression t.
graphite t.
group treatment for children
group treatment for insomnia
habilitative day t.
t. for hair loss
hair removal t.
t. of heart disease
heart failure t.
hepatitis C antiviral long-term treatment to prevent cirrhosis
highly active antiretroviral t.
high-quality and effective t.
HIV/AIDS Treatment Information Service
home t.
hormonal cancer t.
hospital t.
hospitalization and t.
hyperbaric oxygen t.
hypertension optical treatment study
hypertension optimal t.
hypoosmotic shock t.
immune response and combined modality t.
impaired employee alcohol and drug treatment issue
incontinence treatment center
increased overall treatment of duration
indirect t.
individual treatment assessment
individual treatment plan
inhalation chemotherapy t.
initial diagnosis and t.
initial evaluation and t.
initial psychiatric treatment plan
inpatient drug t.
inpatient psychiatric t.
inpatient treatment facility
inpatient treatment protocol
Insight and T. Attitudes Questionnaire
insulin shock t.
intensive chemotherapy t.
intensive diabetes t.
intensive outpatient treatment program
intensive treatment unit
interim treatment plan
t. intervention
inverse treatment planning
joint treatment planning
kidney t.
left without completing t.
life-sustaining medical t.
long-term aftercare t.
low-friction ion t.
manual lymphedema t.
master treatment plan
medical emergency t.
medically managed intensive addiction treatment unit
medical treatment facility

Mental Health Early Intervention, Treatment, and Prevention Act of 2000
mental health t.
mental health treatment facility
t. of mental illness
mental treatment rules
mercury bougienage t.
methadone maintenance t.
methadone maintenance and aftercare treatment program
microwave diathermy t.
minus two hours two hours prior to treatment
moist heat t.
Multicenter Myocarditis T. Trial
multicomponent behavioral t.
multidisciplinary pain t.
multidisciplinary treatment plan
multidose insulin t.
multimodality treatment program
multimodal treatment plan
multimonitored electroconvulsive t.
MultiPulse cosmetic treatment laser
narcotics treatment center
narcotic treatment facility
narcotic treatment program
nebulized mist t.
neoadjuvant antiandrogenic t.
neurodevelopmental treatment physical therapy
no further t.
noncompliance with medical t.
no treatment indicated
no treatment necessary
t. and observation
observation and t.
office t.
Optic Neuritis T. Trial
orthopedic t.
osteopathic manipulation t.
T. Outcome PTSD scale
outpatient drug t.
outpatient treatment, nonservice-connected
outpatient treatment, service-connected
overall treatment time
pain treatment unit
palliative radiation t.
partial hospital treatment program
patient admitted for observation and t.
patient responded to t.
patient treatment file
percutaneous endovascular t.
t. plan
t. planning conference
plans of t.
postexposure t.
postoperative respiratory t.
post treatment abstinence
preferred treatment in cancer
prefrontal sonic t.
t. prescribed
t. prescription
prevention and treatment of depression
preventive allergy t.
T. Priority Index
prophylactic antibiotic t.
prostate cancer t.
t. protocol
radiation treatment of glandular tissue
radiation treatment planning
T. Rating Assessment Matrix
referral, diagnosis, treatment, and discharge
t. regimen
regressive electroshock t.
regular hemodialysis t.
Rehabilitative Addicted Family T.
residential treatment center
T. Response Assessment Method
secondary effect of t.
sequential treatment employing pharmacologic support
short-contact t.
silent t.
t. simulation
soft tissue t.
sonographic planning of oncology t.
specialized treatment facility
split course t.
standard hospital t.
standard infertility treatment algorithm
stroke treatment center
subacute treatment of acute drug intoxication
subcoma insulin t.
subshock insulin t.
substance abuse t.
substance abuse treatment clinic
substance abuse treatment program
substance abuse treatment unit
supervised intermittent ambulatory t.
surgical treatment for brain tumor
surgical treatment for epidural hemorrhage
surgical treatment objective
Systematic Assessment for T. of Emergent Events
thyroid hormone t.
tooth t.
unchanged conventional t.
Vietnam Veterans Evaluation and T. Program
visceral manipulative t.
visualized treatment objective
wastewater treatment plant
Weir Mitchell t.

treatment-related

t.-r. death
t.-r. mortality
t.-r. toxicity

treatment-resistant depression

tree

alder t.
alder tree pollen
arbor vitae t.
Arizona ash t.
Arizona cypress t.
Arizona/Fremont cottonwood t.
arterial t.
ash t.
ash tree pollen
Australian pine t.
automated airway tree segmentation method
biliary t.
Classification and Regression T. analysis
endobronchial t.
live oak t.
lodgepole pine t.
Lombardy poplar t.
maple t.
maple tree pollen
melaleuca t.
mesquite t.
Monterey cypress t.
mountain cedar t.
oak t.
oak tree pollen
olive t.
olive tree pollen
paper mulberry t.
plugging of bronchial t.
pruned tree appearance
tea tree oil
tracheobronchial t.

trefoil factor family

Treitz
T. arch
T. fascia
T. fossa
T. ligament
ligament of T.

trembling
disabling shaking and t.
t. from atherosclerosis
t. of hand
involuntary trembling of body
involuntary trembling of limb

tremens
delirium t.

tremor
alcoholic withdrawal t.
anticonvulsant medication-induced postural t.
ataxia and intention t.
benign essential t.
clubbing or t.
coarse hand t.'s
counting money t.
disabling essential t.
emotional stress precipitating t.
essential t.
fine postural t.
head and neck t.
hereditary essential t.
intentional t.
intention tremor of extremity
irritability and t.
t.'s and jerky movements
magnesium deficiency infantile tremor syndrome
optic atrophy t.
Parkinson tremor disorder
rest t.
slight intention t.
stiffness, t.'s and immobility

tremulousness
alcohol withdrawal t.

tremulous patient

trench
t. fever
t. foot
t. hand
t. mouth
t. mouth from anxiety

trend
age-related t.
amoral t.

Trendelenburg
T. gait
Lloyd Davies Trendelenburg position
T. position
T. tampon

trends
antisocial trends psychopathic
antisocial trends psychopathic personality
asocial trends psychopathic personality

trephination
elliptical t.
nail t.
nonmechanical t.
open-sky t.
partial-thickness t.

trephine
automatic t.
bone-biting t.
lid t.
Londermann corneal t.
Lopez-Enriquez scleral t.
Moria t.
Paton corneal t.
Paufique t.
sclerotomy with t.

Treponema
colony-stimulating factor microhemagglutination-*Treponema pallidum* test
direct fluorescent antibody examination for *Treponema pallidum*
intrathecal *Treponema pallidum* antibody
microhemagglutination assay for antibodies to *Treponema pallidum*
microhemagglutination test for *Treponema pallidum*
Treponema pallidum agglutination
Treponema pallidum complement fixation
Treponema pallidum cryolysis complement
Treponema pallidum hemagglutination test
Treponema pallidum immobilization immune adherence
Treponema pallidum immobilization test

treponemal
t. antibody test
colony-stimulating factor fluorescent treponemal antibody-absorption test
t. false positive
fluorescein treponemal antibody test
fluorescence treponemal antibody absorption
hemagglutination treponemal test for syphilis

treponematosis
nonsyphilitic t.
nonvenereal t.

Trex digital mammography system

TRH-degrading ectoenzyme

triacrylate

triad
aniridia, ambiguous genitalia, mental retardation triad syndrome
female athlete t.
fragile histidine t.

triage
emergency room triage documentation
myocardial infarction triage and intervention
nursing t.
Trauma T. Rule

trial
aggressive therapeutic t.
Antihypertensive and Lipid-Lowering Treatment to Prevent Heart Attack T.
Antioxidant Polyp Prevention T.
antiplatelet t.
t. assessment procedure scale
asymptomatic carotid surgery t.
cardiac arrhythmia suppression t.
clinical research t.
controlled clinical t.
double-blind placebo-controlled randomized clinical t.
t. and error
Fracture Intervention T.
functional trial visit
high-frequency ventilation t.
historic control t.
t. of labor
t. leave
lower hook t.
Multicenter Myocarditis Treatment T.
multiple outcomes of raloxifene evaluation t.
nocturnal oxygen therapy t.
number equal to one; single patient t.
ongoing clinical t.
t. prescription order

prospective randomized t.
randomized controlled clinical t.
randomized double-blind t.
randomized prospective t.
results of clinical controlled t.
therapeutic home trial visit
Veteran's Administration Cooperative Study on Glycemic Control and Complications in Type 2 Diabetes t.
t. visit
t. of void
t. without catheter

triamcinolone
t. acetomide *tert*-butyl acetate
t. acetonide cream
t. lotion
t. and nystatin
t. ointment
t. terramycin

triamide
hexamethylphosphoric t.

triangle
Alsberg t.
anterior t.
anterior triangle approach
anterior triangle of neck
apex of Koch t.
aponeurotic t.
Arlt t.
Assézat t.
auricular t.
ausculatory t.
axillary t.
calibrated triangle of septal cartilage
Calot t.
Einthoven t.
Hesselbach t.
Kiesselbach t.
Langenbeck t.
Lieutaud t.
lumbar t.
lumbocostal triangle of diaphragm
lumbocostoabdominal t.
Macewen t.
Malgaigne t.
Marcille t.
muscle of anal t.
paravertebral t.
Rauchfuss t.
retromolar t.

triangular
anteroinferior triangular fragment
Atasoy triangular advancement flap
t. bone
buccal triangular ridge
t. crest
t. defect
t. disk
distal triangular fossa
t. fascia
t. fibrocartilage
t. fibrocartilage complex
t. fibrocartilage complex tear
t. fibrocartilaginous complex
t. fossa
t. infarct
t. ligament
t. ligament of liver
mesial triangular fossa

triangularis
plica t.

Tribec virus

tributaries
perforators and t.

tricaine methane sulfonate

triceps
t. bursa
t. flap
t. jerk
left t.
right t.
t. skin fold thickness
t. tendon reflex

trichilemma
malignant trichilemma tumor

trichilemmal cyst

trichloride
antimony t.

trichloroacetic
synthetic medium old tuberculin trichloroacetic acid precipitated

trichloroethylene-extracted soybean-oil meal

trichodentoosseous syndrome

trichoepithelioma
multiple t.

trichomonas
T. vaginalis
t. and yeast

trichomycosis
rubra t.

trichophyticus
lichen t.

***Trichoplusia ni* SNPV**

tricho-rhino-auriculo-phalangeal multiple exostoses

trichorhinophalangeal
t. multiple exostoses
t. syndrome

trichosporosis nodosa

trichostasis spinulosa

trichromatism
anomalous t.

trichromatopsia
anomalous t.

trichrome
aniline blue modified trichrome stain
Masson t.
Masson trichrome stain
modified Gomori trichrome reaction
modified trichrome stain
t. stain

tricuspid
t. annular motion
anterior cusp of tricuspid valve
anterior tricuspid leaflet
anterior tricuspid valve leaflet
t. anuloplasty
t. aortic valve
t. atresia
balloon tricuspid valvotomy
t. first heart sound
t. heart valve
t. incompetence
t. insufficiency
t. murmur
opening tricuspid valve snap
posterior tricuspid valve leaflet
premature tricuspid closure
t. regurgitation
t. second heart sound
t. stenosis
t. valve closure
t. valve gradient
t. valve prolapse
t. valve replacement
t. valve vegetation
t. valvular leaflet
t. valvuloplasty
t. valvulotomy

tricyclic
t. amine
anticholinergic t.
t. antidepressant drug
t. antipsychotic
t. drug

trident hand

tridimensional evaluation scale

Trieger Dot Test

triethanolamine
epichlorohydrin and t.
triethanolamine-buffered saline
triethyl citrate
triethylene
t. thiophosphoramide
triethylenethiophosphoramide thiotepa
triethylphosphine gold
trifascicular heart block
trifocal glasses
trifunctional protein deficiency
trigeminal
aneurysm of persistent trigeminal artery
atypical trigeminal neuralgia
t. cave
t. cavity
congenital trigeminal anesthesia
craniosynostosis, ataxia, trigeminal anesthesia, parietal anesthesia and pons, vermis fusion syndrome
t. crest
t. decompression
t. evoked potential
t. ganglion
idiopathic trigeminal neuralgia
t. impression
t. nerve
t. nerve irritation
t. nerve, mandibular division
t. nerve, maxillary division
t. nerve, ophthalmic division
t. neuralgia
t. nucleus
t. pain
persistent trigeminal artery
primitive trigeminal artery
t. rhizotomy
t. rhythm
t. trophic syndrome
t. zoster
trigemini
nuclei nervi t.
trigeminothalamic
anterior trigeminothalamic tract
trigeminovascular system
trigeminus
nervus t.
trigeminy
ventricular t.
trigger
t. action
anticipation of t.
associated myofascial trigger point
t. of asthma
chemoreceptor trigger zone
t. finger
t. finger release
headache t.'s
heart attack t.
hot flash t.
pituitary hormone trigger ovulation
t. point
t. point injection
psychotic trigger reaction
stimulation of trigger area
t. thumb
triggered
atrial triggered pulse generator
depression triggered by physical illness
snooze-induced excitation of sympathetic triggered activity
ventricular pacing, atrial sensing, triggered mode, pacemaker
triggering
navigator echo-based real-time respiratory gating and t.
triglyceride
elevated t.'s
hepatic triglyceride lipase
t.'s incalculable
t. lipase
long-chain t.
medium-chain t.
medium-chain triglyceride oil
microsomal triglyceride transfer protein
normal t.'s
normal triglyceride levels
plasma t.
serum triglyceride level
triglyceridemia
normal t.
triglyceride-rich
t.-r. lipoprotein
t.-r. protein
triglycine sulfate
trigone
angles of t.
t. of bladder
hypertrophy of t.
hypoglossal t.
Lieutaud t.
Mueller t.
retromolar t.
right fibrous t.
trigonum
os t.
trihexoside
ceramide t.
triiodothyronine
absolute free t.
erythrocyte t.
free t.
free triiodothyronine index
negative triiodothyronine response element
t. radioimmunoassay
resin t.
t. resin uptake
reverse t.
serum resin triiodothyronine uptake
t. to thyroxine index
t. toxicosis
t., amino acids, glucagon, and heparin
t. uptake ratio
trilateral retinoblastoma
trileaflet aortic prosthesis
trillion
parts per t.
triloba
placenta t.
trilobar hyperplasia
trilocular heart
trilogy of Fallot
trimalleolar fracture
trimandibular plate
trimester
third t.
trimethoprim
sulfamethoxazole and t.
t. and sulfamethoxazole
trimethoprim-sulfamethoxazole
trimethylacetate
deoxycorticosterone t.
trimethylamine oxide
trimethyl psoralen
trimethylxanthine amphetamine
trimmer
gingival margin t.
trimming
heart trimming procedure
improper nail t.
mucoperiosteal flap t.

trinitrate
glyceryl trinitrate
transdermal glyceryl t.

trinitroglycerol nitroglycerin

triolate

triolein
radioiodinated t.

triose isomerase

triose-kinase

triosephosphate
t. isomerase
trioxide arsenic t.

trioxide
arsenic t.
t. arsenic triosephosphate
mineral trioxide aggregate

tripartita
placenta t.

tripartite
t. fracture of patella
t. placenta

tripeptide
muramyl t.

trip-hammer pulse

triphasic
oral triphasic tablets
t. action potential

triphenylacetate
desoxycorticosterone t.

triphosphatase
adenosine t.
adenosine triphosphatase activity
F_1 adenosine t.
guanosine t.
hydrogen adenosine t.
inosine t.
sodium- and potassium-activated adenosine t.

triphosphate
adenosine t.
adenosine triphosphate disodium
adenosine triphosphate single-photon emission computed tomography
azidothymidine t.
cytosine t.
deoxycytidine t.
deoxyguanosine t.
deoxynucleotide t.
deoxythymidine t.
deoxyuridine t.
fluorouridine t.
guanosine t.
guanosine 5′ t.
inosine t.
inositol t.
t. of lime
nucleoside t.
thymidine t.
uridine t.
xanthosine t.

1,4,5-triphosphate

5′-triphosphate
adenosine -t.
guanosine -t.
inosine -t.
thymidine -t.
uridine -t.

triphosphopyridine nucleotide

triple
t. advancement transposition
alternating triple therapy
t. antibiotic
antiretroviral triple combination therapy
t. balloon valvuloplasty
t. bypass heart surgery
t. cardiac bypass surgery
t. coronary artery bypass graft
t. helix
Hoke triple arthrodesis
t. intrathecal therapy
Lewis triple response
t. lumen catheter
Nichamin triple chopper
primary glaucoma triple procedure
t. staining
standard triple therapy
t. sugar iron agar
t. vessel disease
t. vessel disease with abnormal left ventricle
t. voiding cystogram

triple-lumen Arrow catheter

triple-phase helical computer tomography

triplet
neurofilament t.'s antibody
neurofilament triplet polypeptide
nonsense t.

triplex
placenta t.

triplex-forming oligonucleotide

triploid chromosome number

tripod
t. cane
t. fracture

tripolar
t. lead
segmented ring t.

tripolyphosphate
sodium t.

triquetral bone

triquetrolunate dislocation

triquetropisiform articulation

triquetrum
os t.

tris-buffered
t.-b. Grey solution
t.-b. saline

Tri-Service Medical Information System

tris-maleate buffer

trismus neonatorum

trisodium edetate

trisomy
autosomal t.
mosaic trisomy 14
noninvasive detection of trisomy 18
t. 18, 21 syndrome

tritiated
t. thymidine
t. thymidine labeling index

tritium
Lee-White tritium clotting time
t. nuclear magnetic resonance
t. radioimmunoassay

triton
malignant triton tumor

triturate
compressed tablet t.
tablet t.

trivalent
botulism equine trivalent antitoxin
cold-adapted influenza virus vaccine, t.
influenza virus inactivated vaccine, split virion, types A, B, t.
t. oral poliovirus vaccine
poliovirus vaccine trivalent oral

trivittatus virus

trocar
Argyll trocar catheter
conical t.
disposable t.
gallbladder t.
laparoscopic t.

trocar *(continued)*
10-mm t.
5-mm suprapubic t.

trochanter
greater t.
greater trochanter muscle

trochanteric
ball-and-socket trochanteric osteotomy
t. bursa
t. bursitis
t. crest
t. fossa
greater trochanteric apophysial arrest
greater trochanteric bursa
greater trochanteric femoral fracture
t. tendinitis

trochanteric/controlled

trochanter-knee-ankle

Troche
Mycelex T.

trochlea femoris

trochlear
t. defect
t. fossa
t. fovea
t. groove
t. nerve
t. notch
nuclear-fascicular trochlear nerve palsy
t. nucleus

trochlearis
nervus t.

trochoidea
articulatio t.

troika
aponeurotic t.

tromethamine
lodoxamide t.

trophectoderm
mural t.

Trophermyma whippleii

trophic
t. change
t. fracture
t. gangrene
t. hormone
t. keratitis
t. nucleus
T-cell t.
trigeminal trophic syndrome
t. ulcer

trophoblast
t. antigen
t. in regression
syncytial t.

trophoblastic
gestational trophoblastic disease
gestational trophoblastic neoplasm
gestational trophoblastic tumor
t. lacuna
malignant teratoma, t.
malignant trophoblastic teratoma
t. malignant tumor
metastatic trophoblastic disease
neoplastic trophoblastic disease
nonmetastatic gestational trophoblastic disease
nonmetastatic trophoblastic disease
persistent trophoblastic disease
placental site trophoblastic tumor

trophoblast-lymphocyte
t.-l. cross-reactive
t.-l. cross-reactivity

trophopathic hepatitis

tropic
chronic calcific pancreatitis of the t.'s
t. immersion foot
macrophage t.
monocyte tropic virus

tropica
myositis purulenta t.

tropical
t. abscess
t. acne
t. anemia
t. ataxic neuropathy
t. calcific pancreatitis
t. diarrhea
t. diarrhea-malabsorption syndrome
t. disease
t. eczema
t. hypereosinophilia
juvenile tropical pancreatitis syndrome
macrocytic anemia t.
t. mask
t. medicine
t. myositis
t. pancreatic diabetes
t. phagedenic ulcer
t. pyomyositis
t. spastic paraparesis
t. spastic paraparesis/HTLV-I associated myelopathy
t. splenomegaly syndrome
t. sprue

tropicamide
t. 1% ophthalmic solution Mydriacyl

tropicum
angiofibroma contagiosum t.

tropicus
lichen t.

tropism
macrophage t.

troponin
cardiac troponin I
cardiac troponin T
t. I level

trouble
low back t.
previous t.

troubled
t. adolescent
t. child

trough
bone t.
gentamicin trough level
t. minimum serum concentration
peak and t.
peak and trough levels

trough-to-peak ratio

trousers
antishock t.
medical antishock t.
military antishock t.

Trousseau sign

troy
ounce t.

Troyer syndrome

Trubanaman virus

Tru-Cut needle biopsy

true
t. aneurysm
t. ankylosis
t. anomaly
capillary whole blood true sugar
t. conjugate
t. dwarfism
t. epilepsy
t. hemianopia
t. hernia
t. histiocytic lymphoma
t. hyperplasia
t. hypertrophy
t. incontinence
t. knot in cord
t. labor

t. metatarsus adductus
t. negative
t. negative fraction
t. negative rate
t. positive
t. positive fraction
t. positive rate
t. positive stress test
t. radiation emission
t. total lung capacity
t. vertebra
t. visual acuity
t. vocal cords
t. vocal fold

trumpet
angel's t.

truncal
t. abrasion
t. asymmetry
t. ataxia
t. instability
t. obesity
t. vagotomy
t. vagotomy plus antrectomy
t. vagotomy plus pyloroplasty

truncated
McIntyre truncated cone

truncation
protein truncation testing
uterine positioning via ligament investment fixation t.

truncus
t. arteriosus
persistent truncus arteriosus

trunk
anterior division of brachial plexus
anterior gastric branch of anterior vagal t.
anterior vagal t.
anterior vaginal t.
arterial brachiocephalic t.
t.'s of brachial plexus
brachiocephalic arterial t.
T. Control Test
t. of corpus callosum
t. extension-flexion unit
ganglion of sympathetic t.
head, arms, and t.
t. and hip flexibility
t. index
isometric trunk stabilization
left main t.
lower trunk rotation
lumbar t.'s
lumbosacral nerve t.
meningohypophyseal t.
pulmonary artery t.
rhythmic instability of head and t.
rhythm instability of head and t.

trunk-hip-knee-ankle-foot orthosis

trust
atmosphere of t.

truth
t. disclosure
support, empathy, and t.

trypanosome growth factor

trypanosomiasis
African t.
American t.
card agglutination trypanosomiasis test
human African trypanosomiasis
South American t.

trypsin
t. activation peptide
bovine t.
bovine pancreatic trypsin inhibitor
human pancreatic trypsin inhibitor
immunoreactive t.
immunoreactive trypsin output
Kunitz pancreatic trypsin inhibitor
lima bean trypsin inhibitor
ovomucoid trypsin inhibitor
pancreatic secretory trypsin inhibitor
pancreatic trypsin inhibitor
porcine t.
serum trypsin inhibition capacity
serum trypsin inhibitor
soybean trypsin inhibitor
urinary trypsin inhibitor

trypsin-aldehyde-fuchsin

trypsin-binding activity

trypsin-inhibiting unit

trypsin-inhibitory
t.-i. capability
t.-i. capacity

trypsin-insoluble segment

trypsinized sheep red blood cell

trypsin-like
t.-l. amidase
t.-l. immunoactivity

trypsinogen
anionic t.
bovine t.
cationic t.
immunoreactive t.

trypsinogen-activating peptide

tryptase
mast cell t.
mast cell containing both tryptase and chymase
mast cell containing tryptase but not chymase

trypticase
cystine trypticase agar
t. soy broth
t. soy plate
t. soy yeast

trypticase-peptone-glucose-yeast extract-trypsin medium

trypticase-soy agar

tryptone
t. glucose extract
t. glucose yeast agar
t. phosphate broth
t. soy broth

tryptophan
t. deaminase agar
t. hydroxylase
t. load test
t. peptone glucose broth
t. peroxidase
t. synthetase

L-tryptophan

tryptophan-acid reaction

tryptophan-rich prealbumin

tryptose agar

tryptose/blood/agar base

Tsai
area ventralis of T.

T-shaped
T.-s. capsulotomy
T.-s. fracture
T.-s. graft
T.-s. incision

TSH-binding inhibitory immunoglobulin

TSH-displacing antibody

TSH-secreting
T.-s. pituitary adenoma
T.-s. pituitary tumor

T-strain
Mycoplasma T.-s.

T-suppressor factor

Tsuruse virus

T-tube
T.-t. cholangiogram
T.-t. cholangiography
T.-t. drainage

tub
t. bath
continuous-flow t.
hot tub bath

tubal
t. abortion
t. air cell
t. banding
bilateral tubal coagulation
bilateral tubal ligation
bilateral tubal occlusion
t. diverticulum
t. ectopic pregnancy
t. embryo stage transfer
t. endometriosis
t. fulguration
t. gestation
t. infertility
t. inflammatory damage
t. insufflation
laparoscopic tubal banding
laparoscopic tubal cautery
laparoscopic tubal coagulation
laparoscopic tubal sterilization
t. ligation
t. mass
modified Irving-type tubal ligation
t. obstruction
t. occlusion device
t. perfusion pressure
Pomeroy tubal ligation
postpartum tubal ligation
pronucleate stage tubal transfer
proximal tubal obstruction
salpingitis after previous tubal occlusion
selective tubal assessment to refine reproductive therapy
selective tubal occlusion procedure
sexual tubal sterilization
transcervical tubal access catheter
tuboovarian abscess after previous tubal occlusion

tubam
per t.

tubariae
plicae tubariae tubae uterinae

tube
t. agglutination
ampulla of uterine t.
angled pleural t.
angled suction t.
angulated buccal t.
anode tube reloading
anterior chamber t.
anterior neural tube closure
anterior neural tube defect
aortic tube graft
apically directed chest t.
Argyle chest t.
Argyle-Salem sump t.
Armstrong tube line
ascites drainage t.
aspiration and dissection t.
attenuation-based on-line modulation of the tube current
auditory tube nerve
bilateral myringotomy and t.'s
bilateral ventilation t.'s
bladder flap t.
blenderized tube feeding
t. cast
catheterization of eustachian t.
cathode-ray t.
chest t.
chest tube drainage
chest tube output
chest tube placement
chest tube present in abdomen
collar button t.
continuous tube feeding
cuffed endotracheal t.
cuffed tracheostomy t.
damaged or blocked fallopian t.'s
double-lumen endobronchial t.
endoscopic mucosal resection, tube method
endotracheal tube placement
enteral feeding t.
esophageal gastric tube airway
esophagogastric tube airway
esophagotracheal combination t.
eustachian t.
eustachian tube dysfunction
eustachian tube function
eustachian tube obstruction
eustachian tube pressure
fallopian tube sperm perfusion
t. feeding
feeding gastrostomy t.
feeding tube placement
fenestrated tracheostomy t.
fimbriae of ovarian t.
fimbriae of uterine t.
fimbriated end of fallopian t.
gamete intrafallopian tube transfer
gastric augment and single pedicle t.
gastric lavage t.
gastrojejunostomy t.
gastrostomy tube feeding
gastrostomy tube migration
t. graft
t. holder
home enteral tube feeding
house tube feeding
hydrosalpinx, both t.'s
hyperreactive bronchial t.
immunodiffusion tube precipitin
infant feeding t.
t. inserted
intratracheal t.
isthmus of auditory t.
jejunal extension t.
jejunal feeding t.
jejunal tube through percutaneous endoscopic gastrostomy
jejunostomy tube feeding
knuckle of t.
laser office ventilation of ears with insertion of t.'s
limiting membrane of neural t.
lines and t.'s
medial lamina of cartilage of pharyngotympanic auditory t.
mediastinal t.
metallic distal end of t.
microfocal direct magnification in vitro x-ray t.
microhematocrit capillary t.
Miller-Abbott t.
Molteno shunt t.
molybdenum rotating anode x-ray t.
mucous gland of auditory t.
muscular coat of uterine t.
muscular layer of uterine t.
mycobacteria growth indicator t.
mycobacteria growth indicator tube system
nasal duodenostomy t.
nasal endotracheal t.
nasoendotracheal t.
nasogastric feeding t.
nasogastric tube suctioning
nasogastrojejunal t.
nasointestinal t.
nasojejunal feeding t.
nasotracheal t.
NJ feeding t.
obstruction of fallopian t.
open gastrostomy tube placement
oral endotracheal t.
oral esophageal t.
oral gastric t.

orogastric t.
orotracheal t.
t.'s and ovaries
t.'s and ovaries
pars plana Baerveldt tube insertion with vitrectomy
patent fallopian t.
pear-shaped extension t.
pediatric feeding t.
percutaneous endoluminal gastrostomy t.
percutaneous endoscopic gastrostomy and jejunal extension t.
percutaneous endoscopic gastrostomy t.
percutaneous endoscopic placement of jejunal t.
percutaneous nephrostomy t.
photoelectric multiplier t.
photomultiplier t.
pigtail curl of stent t.
pigtail nephrostomy t.
polyethylene t.
posterior chest t.
t. precipitin
pressure equalization t.
pressure equalizing t.
primary fallopian tube carcinoma
reversed gastric t.
Rodney Smith t.'s
salpingitis in previously occluded t.'s
salvarsan throat irrigation t.
selected ion flow t.
Sengstaken-Blakemore t.
t. slide agglutination test
smoke removal t.
special tube feeding
standard tube agglutination test
standard tube feeding
suction t.'s inserted
suprapubic t.
sustained ethanol release t.
Teflon tube insertion
test tube turbidity test
t. thoracostomy
thoracotomy tube in place
tracheostomy tube inserted
transcervical intrafallopian tube transfer
transpyloric t.
tympanostomy tube insertion
tympanotomy and tube insertion
vacuum t.
vacuum tube voltmeter
water seal chest t.

tubed pedicle flap

tube-fed
t.-f. food
t.-f. saline

tuber
artery of tuber cinereum
ashen t.
medial branch of artery of tuber cinereum
potato spindle tuber viroid

tuberalis
pars t.

tubercle
anterior thalamic t.
anterior tibial t.
anterior tubercle of atlas
anterior tubercle of cervi
anterior tubercle of cervical vertebrae
anterior tubercle of thalamus
anteromedial tubercle transfer
areolar t.'s
articular bone t.
articular facet of tubercle of rib
articular surface of tubercle of rib
articular tubercle of temporal bone
ashen t.
auditory t.
auricular t.
auricular tubercle of Darwin
avian tubercle bacillus
t. bacillus
cluster of t.'s
greater t.
lesser t.
Lisfranc t.
Lister t.
Lower t.
mamillary t.
mamillary tubercle of hypothalamus
marginal t.
marginal tubercle of zygomatic bone
middle greater tubercle of facet of humerus
Montgomery t.
Morgagni t.
Müller t.
naked t.
necrogenic t.
nucleus cuneatus t.
nucleus gracilis t.
olfactory t.
optic disc t.
pubic t.
Whitnall t.

tuberculid
micronodular t.
micropapular t.
nodular t.
papulonecrotic t.

tuberculin
albumose-free t.
alkaline t.
t. bacillary emulsion
cutaneous tuberculin test
derivative of contagious t.
t. filtrate
human old t.
Mantoux tuberculin skin test
multiple puncture tuberculin test
old tuberculin [Tuberkulin]
original t.
t. precipitate
t. precipitation
purified protein derivative of t.
t. reaction
residual t.
t. residue
Siebert purified protein derivative of tuberculin
t. skin test
synthetic medium old tuberculin trichloroacetic acid precipitated
t. tine test
total protein t.
tuberculin R new tuberculin
tuberculin Ruckland new tuberculin
t. unit
1 tuberculin unit
5 tuberculin unit
250 tuberculin unit
vacuum t.
t. volutin

tuberculin-delayed hypersensitivity

tuberculoid
borderline t.

tuberculoma
optochiasmatic t.

tuberculosis
acute generalized t.
acute miliary t.
amplified *Mycobacterium tuberculosis* direct test
atypical t.
t., contagious
late generalized t.

tuberculosis *(continued)*
multidrug-resistant t.
multiple-drug resistant t.
mycobacteria other than *Mycobacterium tuberculosis*
Mycobacteria other than t.
Mycobacterium t.
Mycobacterium tuberculosis detection
Mycobacterium tuberculosis direct test
oral cavity t.
parotid gland t.
t. patch test
patch test for t.
peripheral osteoarticular t.
pulmonary t.
segmental colonic t.
t. skin test

tuberculosis-respiratory disease

tuberculosus
lupus t.

tuberculous
ancient tuberculous arthritis
Assmann tuberculous infiltrate
t. bronchopneumonia
t. enteritis
t. iritis
localized tuberculous meningitis
t. lymphadenitis
t. mediastinal adenopathy
t. meningitis
metastatic tuberculous abscess
t. nephritis
t. pericarditis
t. peritonitis
t. pleurisy
t. pneumonia
t. spondylitis

tuberis
nucleus lateralis t.

Tuberkulin
old tuberculin [Tuberkulin]

tuberohypophyseal dopaminergic neuron

tuberoinfundibular
t. dopaminergic
t. dopaminergic neuron
t. dopamine system

tuberosity, pl. **tuberosities**
between ischial tuberosities
t. of carpal bone
t. of cuboid bone
t. of fifth metatarsal
t. of fifth metatarsal bone
greater tuberosity fracture
greater tuberosity osteotomy
ischial t.
medial femoral t.
omental tuberosity of liver
omental tuberosity of pancreas
tibial t.

tuberosum
lymphangioma tuberosum multiplex
xanthoma t.
xanthoma tuberosum multiplex

tuberous
ash-leaf spot in tuberous sclerosis
t. sclerosis
t. sclerosis complex

tubing
elastic t.
hyperalimentation t.
Mini-Med t.
paracentesis and tubing of ears

tubocornual
microsurgical tubocornual anastomosis

tuboovarian
t. abscess
t. abscess after previous tubal occlusion
t. complex

tuboplasty
transcervical balloon t.

tuboreticular
intracytoplasmic tuboreticular inclusion

tubular
abnormal tubular myelin
acute interstitial tubular nephritis
acute tubular necrosis
t. adenocarcinoma
t. adenoma
t. aneurysm
autosomal congenital tubular dysgenesis
t. basement membrane
t. breath sounds
t. carcinoma
cytoplasmic tubular aggregate
dense tubular system
distal renal tubular acidosis
t. ectasia
t. fluid
t. graft
t. hypoplasia aortic arch
t. hypoplasia left aortic arch
maximal tubular reabsorption rate for glucose
mean tubular diameter
t. myelin
t. necrosis
Pick tubular adenoma
postischemic acute tubular necrosis
proximal tubular pressure
t. reabsorption
t. reabsorption of phosphate
renal tubular antigen
renal tubular cell
renal tubular dysgenesis
renal tubular epithelial
testicular tubular adenoma
t. transport maximum
wall coated open t.

tubular-fertility index

tubularization
glansplasty in situ tubularization of urethral plate
glanuloplasty in situ tubularization of urethral plate

tubularized incised plate

tubule
apical membrane of proximal convoluted tubule cell
collecting t.
distal convoluted t.
early distal proximal t.
human proximal t.
isolated cortical t.
late distal cortical t.
late proximal cortical t.
medullary collecting t.
proximal convoluted t.
proximal straight t.
renal tubule hypokalemia
sex cord tumors with annular t.'s

tubuloglomerular feedback

tubulointerstitial
t. nephritis
t. nephritis and uveitis syndrome
t. nephropathy

tubulopapillary adenoma

tubulopathy
autosomal recessive renal proximal tubulopathy and hypercalciuria

tubuloreticular
t. inclusion
t. structure

tuck
chin t.

tuft
distal t.
finger t.
t. fracture
t. of hair
lumbosacral tuft of hair
malpighian t.
neovascular t.
phalangeal t.

tufted
acquired tufted angioma

tularemia
oculoglandular t.
oropharyngeal t.

Tumarkin
falling spells of T.

tumescence
nocturnal penile t.
nocturnal penile tumescence testing
nocturnal tumescence monitor
sleep-related t.

tumescent
t. absorbent bandage
t. liposuction

tumidus
lupus erythematosus t.

tumor
t. ablation
acral arteriovenous t.
t. activity
t. activity test
acute tumor lysis
acute tumor lysis syndrome
adenomatoid odontogenic t.
adnexal skin t.
adrenal cell rest t.
adrenal cortex estrogen-secreting t.
adrenal cortex testosterone-secreting t.
adrenocorticotrophic hormone-secreting pituitary t.
adult granulosa cell t.
aggressive papillary middle ear t.
AJCC TNM tumor classification
alcohol injection of t.
alkaline phosphatase isoenzyme tumor marker
allogeneic tumor cell immunization
allogeneic tumor cell vaccine
ameloblastic adenomatoid t.
t. amplified protein expression therapy
anaplastic Wilms t.
anemone cell t.
t. angiogenesis factor
t. angiogenic factor
angiolipoma, posttraumatic neuroma, glomus tumor, eccrine spiradenoma, and leiomyoma cutis
angiosarcoma bone t.
aniridia, Wilms tumor association
aniridia, Wilms tumor, gonadoblastoma syndrome
Ann Arbor tumor classification
anterior cingulate gyrus t.
anterior pillar t.
t. antigen
t. antigen 4
t. antigenicity
aortic body t.
APC tumor suppressor gene
argentaffin carcinoid t.
t. ascites
ascites tumor fluid
ascitic tumor fluid
Askin thoracopulmonary neuroepithelial t.
t. associated
at autopsy tumor, nodes, and metastases
atypical carcinoid t.
atypical giant cell t.
autologous tumor cell immunization
autologous tumor extract
autologous tumor rejection antigen
autologous tumor vaccine
autonomic nerve t.
avian tumor virus
t. bearing
t. bed
benign epithelial t.
benign glandular cell t.
benign mesenchymal t.
bilateral renal t.
bladder t.
bladder tumor antigen
bladder tumor check
bladder tumor recheck
t. blush
brain adjacent t.
breast t.
bronchogenic Pancoast-type t.
t. bulk
t. burden
t. burden index
calcifying epithelial odontogenic t.
t. capsule
carcinoid tumor of intestine
carotid body t.
t. cell
t. cell burden
t. cell hypoxia
cell kinetics of t.'s
t. cell migration-inhibition factor
central granular cell odontogenic t.
central primitive neuroectodermal t.
cerebral t.
t. chemosensitivity assay
classification of malignant t.'s
classification of malignant t.'s
clear cell odontogenic t.
clinical staging of tumors, nodes, and metastases as determined by noninvasive examination
clinical tumor volume
t. clonogenic assay
cluster of tumor cells
t. colony-forming unit
combined germ cell t.
composite extrarenal rhabdoid t.
contaminating tumor cell
cutaneous neural t.
t. debulking
debulking of t.
deep-seated benign t.
t. defect
desmoplastic small round-cell t.
t. destruction
t. dose fractionation
t. doubling time
doubling time of tumor size
ductus deferens t.
dysembryoplastic neuroepithelial t.
ectomesenchymal chondromyxoid t.
Ehrlich ascites t.
Ehrlich ascites tumor cell
t. embolism
embryonal cell t.
endocervical mucinous borderline t.
endocrine inactive pituitary t.
endodermal sinus t.
enzootic nasal t.
epithelial t.
estrogen receptor-positive t.
ethanol-induced tumor necrosis
Ewing sarcoma family of t.'s
Ewing sarcoma/peripheral neuroectodermal t.
excisional biopsy of tumor mass

tumor *(continued)*
extrarenal rhabdoid t.
female adnexal tumor of probable wolffian origin
t. of the follicular infundibulum
gadolinium-enhancing tumor volume
gastrointestinal autonomic nerve t.
gastrointestinal pacemaker cell t.
gastrointestinal smooth muscle t.
gastrointestinal stromal t.
germ cell t.
germ cell tumor with synchronous lesions in pineal and suprasellar region
gestational trophoblastic t.
giant cell tumor of low malignant potential
giant cell tumor of tendon sheath
giant cell t.
t. glycoprotein assay
glycoprotein-secreting pituitary t.
t. grade
t. grading
granular cell t.
granulosa cell t.
granulosa-stromal cell t.
granulosa-theca cell t.
gross tumor volume
t. growth
t. growth delay
t. growth factor
growth hormone-releasing factor t.
hair follicle t.
hair-like t.
hamster tumor line
hemorrhagic tumor metastasis
hepatic tumor index
6-HIAA tumor marker
high-dose radiation to tumor mass
t. histology
hormone-secreting adrenal t.
hormone-secreting pituitary t.
hot vs. cold breast t.
human breast t.
human laryngeal tumor cell
human mammary tumor virus
human tumor bank
human tumor colony assay
human tumor stem cell assay
Hürthle cell t.
t. identified
t. immunology bank
t. implant
t. increased in size
t. inducing
t. induction
infiltrating irregular tumor mass
inflammatory myofibroblastic t.
t. inoperable
inoperable brain t.
International Federation of Gynecology and Obstetrics classification of tumor staging
interstitial cell t.
intestinal mucinous borderline t.
intracranial t.
intraductal papillary mucinous t.
intravascular sclerosing bronchioloalveolar t.
t. invasion
ipsilateral breast tumor recurrence
juvenile granulosa cell t.
juxtaglomerular cell t.
large cell calcifying Sertoli cell t.
largest tumor dimension
t. lethal dose
Leydig cell t.
lipid cell ovarian t.
lipoid cell t.
lipoid ovarian t.
liposclerosing myxofibrous t.
liver cell t.
liver volume replaced by t.
lobuloalveolar t.
t. localization scan
localized fibrous t.
local tumor excision
local tumor excision with irradiation
local tumor hyperthermia
lowered tumor antigenicity
lower urinary tract t.
low malignant potential epithelial ovarian t.
low-risk t.
Lucké tumor virus
Lugano classification for testicular t.
luteinizing hormone-secreting t.
lysed tumor cell
t. lysis
t. lysis syndrome
macrophage-derived tumor necrosis factor
magnetite in tumor targeting
male germ line t.
malignant brain t.
malignant breast t.
malignant duodenal t.
malignant epithelial t.
malignant extrarenal rhabdoid t.
malignant giant cell t.
malignant glandular cell t.
malignant glomus t.
malignant islet cell t.
malignant mesenchymal t.
malignant mixed mesodermal t.
malignant mixed müllerian t.
malignant nerve sheath t.
malignant ovarian germ cell t.
malignant peripheral nerve sheath t.
malignant rhabdoid tumor of kidney
malignant rhabdoid tumor of soft tissue
malignant small round cell t.
malignant trichilemma t.
malignant triton t.
malignant tumor of cervix
mammary t.
mammary tumor agent
mammary tumor virus
mammary tumor virus of mice
t. margin
t. marker
mast cell t.
MCA tumor marker
M.D. Anderson tumor score system
mediastinal germ cell t.
mediastinal mesenchymal t.
mediastinal yolk sac t.
melanocytic iris t.
melanotic neuroectodermal t.
melanotic neuroectodermal tumor of infancy
meningeal cell t.
Merkel cell t.
mesenchymal bone t.
mesenchymal sex cord stromal t.
metachronous testicular germ cell t.
t. metastasis
metastasis, age, completeness of resection, local invasion, and tumor size
metastasis of t.
metastatic brain t.
metastatic cardiac t.
metastatic choroidal t.
metastatic lymph node t.
metastatic mixed müllerian t.
metastatic tumor of unknown origin
microscopic granular cell t.

midline craniofacial t.
mixed epithelial-mesenchymal t.
mixed germ cell t.
mixed germ cell-sex cord stromal t.
mixed histology t.
mixed mesodermal t.
mixed müllerian t.
mixed phenotype t.
mixed sex cord-stromal t.
mixed tissue t.
mixed tumor of salivary gland
mixed tumor of skin
mixed uterine t.
Mostofi classification of testicular t.
mouse mammary t.
mouse mammary tumor virus
mouse ovarian t.
mouse parotid tumor virus
MSA tumor marker
mucinous adenocarcinoma t.
mucinous borderline ovarian t.'s
mucinous cystic t.
mucinous ductectatic tumor of pancreas
mucin-producing tumor of the pancreas
mucosa-associated lymphoid t.
müllerian mixed t.
multicellular tumor spheroid
multicentric carcinoid t.
multifocal bladder t.
multifocal brain t.
murine mammary tumor virus
murine tumor cell
myasthenia gravis and mediastinal t.'s
napkin ring anular t.
National Wilms T. Study
navigated brain tumor surgery
t. necrosis factor
t. necrosis factor-alpha
t. necrosis factor-beta
t. necrosis factor-binding protein
t. necrosis factor receptor
t. necrosis factor receptor-associated factor
t. necrosis factor receptor-associated periodic syndrome
t. necrosis factor-related activation-induced cytokine
t. necrosis factor-related apoptosis-inducing ligand
t. necrosis serum
necrosis of t.
nerve cell t.
nerve sheath malignant t.
neural crest t.
neural crest tumor localization study
neuraxial desmoplastic neuroepithelial t.
neuroectodermal t.
neuroendocrine t.
neuronal cell origin t.
neuron-specific enolase tumor marker
new approaches to brain tumor therapy
4-nitroquinolin-1-oxide-induced t.
node-negative primary t.
t., nodes, metastasis
no evidence of primary t.
non-beta cell t.
nonencapsulated sclerosing t.
nonfunctional pituitary t.
nonfunctioning pituitary t.
nongerminoma germ cell t.
nonimmunogenic murine tumor cell
non-islet cell tumor hypoglycemia
nonsecreting pituitary t.
nonseminomatous germ cell testicular t.
North American Brain Tumor Consortium
NSE lung cancer tumor marker
null cell t.
oat cell t.
ocular adnexal t.
odontogenic adenomatoid t.
olfactory groove t.
oncocytic hepatocellular t.
ophthalmic t.
optic chiasm t.
optic complex t.
optic nerve t.
optic tract pituitary t.
oral cavity t.'s
orbital childhood t.
original tumor site
ovarian borderline t.
ovarian carcinoid t.
ovarian epithelial t.
ovarian germ cell t.
ovarian granulosa-stromal cell t.
ovarian granulosa-theca cell t.
ovarian hilar cell t.
ovarian malignant germ cell t.
ovarian serous borderline t.
ovarian tumor registry
Page grade for breast t.
pancreatic alpha-cell t.
pancreatic endocrine t.
pancreatic islet cell t.
pancreatic polypeptide-secreting t.
papillary tumor projection
paranasal sinus t.
parasellar dermoid t.
paraumbilical vein t.
pathological tumor, nodes, metastases staging of cancer
t. peak systolic velocity
pearly CNS t.
percutaneous ethanol ablation of t.
percutaneous tumor ablation
periampullary duodenal t.
peripheral giant cell t.
peripheral nerve sheath t.
peripheral neuroectodermal t.
peripheral primitive neuroectodermal t.
peritoneal borderline t.
peritoneum desmoid t.
peritoneum studded with tumor nodules
petrous apex t.
pineal cell t.
pineal gland t.
pituitary gland t.
pituitary tumor transforming gene
placental site trophoblastic t.
pleomorphic hyalinizing angiectatic t.
t. polypeptide antigen
t. polysaccharide substance
polysaccharide substance t.
poorly differentiated embryonal cell t.
popliteal fossa t.
portal vein tumor thrombus
posterior fossa t.
Pott puffy t.
prepubertal testicular t.
primary brain t.
primary malignant t.
primary mediastinal germ-cell t.
primary neuroectodermal t.
primary tumor, regional lymph node, remote metastases classification, staging
primary tumor site
primary tumor site unknown
primitive neuroectodermal t.
primitive tumor cell
prolactin secreting pituitary t.
pseudosarcomatous fibromyxoid t.
pseudosarcomatous myofibroblastic t.

tumor *(continued)*
pulmonary endodermal t.
radiation assault on t.
rapidly growing t.
t. receptor-associated factor
recombinant tumor necrosis factor alpha
rectal carcinoid t.
t. reexcision
regional recurrence of t.
t. registry
t. regression antigen
t. regression grade
relative tumor size
t. removal
renewed tumor activity
t. residual
retroperitoneal residual tumor mass
rhabdoid tumor of the kidney
salivary gland anlage t.
sarcoma, breast and brain tumors, leukemia, laryngeal and lung cancer adenoma
sclerosing stromal t.
t. score system
serous borderline t.
Sertoli cell mesenchyme t.
Sertoli cell-only t.
Sertoli-Leydig cell t.
sex cord t.'s with annular tubules
shrink inoperable t.
t. in situ
t. skin test
skull base t.
slowly growing t.
small bowel t.
small cell t.
small round-cell t.
smooth muscle t.'s
soft parts giant cell t.
soft tissue t.
solid cystic t.
solid and cystic tumor of the pancreas
solitary fibrous t.
soluble tumor necrosis factor-a receptor type I
t. specific
spinal canal t.
spindle cell epithelial tumor with thymus-like differentiation
spontaneous mammary t.
squamous cell lung t.
squamous odontogenic t.
steroid cell t.
stromal cell t.
stromal tumor of unknown malignant potential
studded with numerous tumor nodules
superior sulcus tumor syndrome
t. suppression
suppression for tumor growth
surgical treatment for brain t.
Testicular T. Panel
theca cell t.
t. thrombus
t. thrombus in the portal vein
thymic carcinoid t.
thyroid-stimulating hormone-secreting t.
time to tumor progression
total tumor dose
total tumor mass
transitional cell t.
transmissible venereal t.
trophoblastic malignant t.
TSH-secreting pituitary t.
unknown primary t.
urinary bladder t.
uterine tumor resembling an ovarian sex-cord t.
vasoactive intestinal peptide-secreting t.
vasoactive intestinal polypeptide t.
Wilms t.
Wilms tumor 1
t. with lymph node metastases
wound tumor virus

tumor-activated prodrug

tumor-associated
t.-a. glycoprotein
t.-a. glycoprotein-72
t.-a. lymphocyte
t.-a. macrophage
t.-a. rejection antigen
t.-a. surface antigen
t.-a. tissue eosinophilia
t.-a. transplantation antigen

tumor-bearing
t.-b. animal
t.-b. mice
t.-b. rabbit

tumor-cased headache

tumor-cell-induced platelet aggregation

tumor-derived
t.-d. activated cell
t.-d. antigen

tumor-direct cell-mediated hypersensitivity

tumor-draining
t.-d. lymph node
t.-d. lymph node cell

tumorectomy, axillary dissection, radiotherapy

tumoricidal
macrophage tumoricidal activity

tumorigenesis
mammary t.

tumor-induced
t.-i. angiogenesis
t.-i. marrow cytotoxicity

tumor-inducing
t.-i. complex
t.-i. factor
t.-i. hypercalcemia

tumor-infiltrating
t.-i. lymphocyte
t.-i. lymphocyte technique

tumor-inhibiting
t.-i. factor
t.-i. principle

tumor-medulloblastoma
primitive neuroectodermal t.-m.

tumor-producing dose

tumor-resistant antigen

tumor-specific
t.-s. cell surface antigen
t.-s. glycoprotein
t.-s. tissue antigen
t.-s. transplantation antigen
t.-s. transplantation immunity

tumor-suppressor gene

tumor-susceptible antigen

tuneable
argon tuneable dye laser

tungsten-188

tungsten carbide

tunic
longitudinal layers of muscular t.

tunica
t. albuginea oculi
aortic tunica adventitia
aortic tunica intima
aortic tunica media
autogenous tunica vaginalis graft intima
malignant mesothelioma of the tunica vaginalis
media t.
parietal layer of tunica vaginalis of testis
t. vaginalis testis

tunicary hernia

tuning
- t. fork
- t. fork examination
- t. fork test

tunnel
- anterior tarsal tunnel syndrome
- aortic and left ventricular t.
- aortic-left ventricular t.
- carpal t.
- carpal tunnel decompression
- carpal tunnel endoscopy
- carpal tunnel release
- carpal tunnel release system
- carpal tunnel repair
- carpal tunnel syndrome
- t. cell
- cubital tunnel splint
- cubital tunnel syndrome
- t. disease
- driver tunnel locator apparatus
- endoscopic carpal tunnel release
- t. flap
- t. graft
- idiopathic carpal tunnel syndrome
- lateral atrial t.
- open carpal tunnel release
- Packer tunnel silicone sponge
- Paine carpal tunnel retinaculotome
- scleral tunnel incision
- tarsal tunnel decompression
- tarsal tunnel release
- tarsal tunnel syndrome
- ulnar tunnel syndrome
- t. vision

tunneled implant

tunneling
- scanning tunneling microscope

turbid
- t. fluid
- t., no creamy layer

turbidimetric
- particle-enhanced turbidimetric inhibition immunoassay

turbidity
- Maclagan thymol turbidity test
- Meinicke turbidity reaction
- nephelometric turbidity units
- picric acid t.
- t. reducing
- test tube turbidity test
- thymol t.
- thymol turbidity test
- zinc turbidity test

turbidity-reducing unit

turbinate
- t. bone
- bovine t.
- hypertrophied inferior t.
- inferior t.
- middle t.

turbine
- air-bearing turbine handpiece

turbo
- half-Fourier acquisition single-shot turbo spin-echo
- t. spin echo

turbulent
- patient's hospital course t.

turcica
- empty sella turcica syndrome
- midpoint of sella t.
- most anterior point of anterior contour of the sella t.
- most posterior point on posterior contour of sella t.
- sella t.

Türck
- T. bundle
- T. column
- T. degeneration

TUR-Cue photometer

turgor
- good tissue t.
- hydration and t.
- skin t.

turkey
- t. gamma globulin
- herpesvirus of t.'s
- t. virus hepatitis

Turlock virus

turmoil
- adolescent t.
- adolescent turmoil reaction

turn
- ampere t.
- apical turn of the cochlea
- t. and cough
- t., cough, deep breath
- t., cough, and hyperventilate
- please turn the patient over
- t. and position
- step out, turn out

turnaround
- resubmission turnaround document
- t. time

Turner
- gonadal dysgenesis of Turner type
- Grey Turner sign
- male Turner syndrome
- mosaic Turner syndrome
- T. sign
- T. syndrome

turning
- t. against object
- t. against self
- conjunctivitis with eyelashes turning in
- contralateral head t.
- ipsilateral head t.

turnover
- adipofascial turnover flap
- erythroid iron t.
- fixed erythrocyte t.
- fixed parenchymal t.
- fractional turnover rate
- granulocyte turnover rate
- ineffective iron t.
- low bone turnover disease
- marrow iron t.
- t. number
- plasma iron turnover rate
- t. rate
- red blood cell iron turnover rate
- t. time
- total body protein t.

turn-to-turn transfusion

Turuna virus

T-wave
- T.-w. abnormality
- T.-w. alternans
- asymmetric negative T.-w.
- diphasic T.-w.
- T.-w. flattening
- flipped T.-w.
- T.-w. inversion
- inverted T.-w.

Tween
- human blood bilayer T.

Tween-TRIS-buffered saline solution

T1-weighted
- T.-w. axial image
- T.-w. coronal image

T2-weighted image

twelfth
- t. cranial nerve
- first through twelfth dorsal vertebrae
- first to twelfth thoracic nerves

twelfth *(continued)*
first to twelfth thoracic vertebrae
t. nerve palsy
twelve
penis at twelve syndrome
sequential analysis of twelve chemistry constituents
Twenty Statements Test
twice
t. a day
t. weekly
twilight
alcoholic twilight state
t. anesthesia
t. state
twin
asymmetrical conjoined t.'s
t. birth
t. birth weight discordance
curved base twin bracket
t. delivery
dizygotic t.'s
equal conjoined t.'s
t. gestation
identical t.
identical twin transplants
impacted t.
t. jet nebulizer
MacArthur Longitudinal Twin Study
monochorionic diamniotic placenta t.'s
monochorionic diamniotic twin pregnancy
monochorionic, monoamniotic twins
t. reversed arterial perfusion
unequal conjoined t.
twin-twin transfusion syndrome
twist
point of entry, traction and t.
twisted hair
twister
elastic twister orthosis
twisting injury to joint
twitch
fast t.
first twitch height
t.'s and involuntary movements
local twitch response
myoclonic twitch activity
slow t.
slow twitch fiber
t. tension
total twitch time
twitching
arrhythmic t.
involuntary t.
myoclonic t.
pain and t.
two
t. cerebral hemisphere vegetal hemisphere
t. dimensional
limb lead t.
minus two hours two hours prior to treatment
needle and sponge count correct times t.
needle, sponge, and instrument count correct times t.
oriented times t.
O2 saturation on two liters nasal cannula
two-chamber
two-dimensional
t.-d. echo-derived ejection fraction
t.-d. Fourier transform
t.-d. time-of-flight
t.-d. transcranial color-coded sonography
t.-d. transesophageal echocardiography
t.-d. transthoracic echocardiography
two-phase CT imaging
two-photon laser-scanning microscope
two-point
t.-p. discrimination
t.-p. gait
two-stage
ultrathin-walled t.-s.
two-step nested PCR
Tylenol with codeine
tympanae
tympanic
t. air cell
anterior recess of tympanic membrane
anterior tympanic artery
anterior wall of tympanic cavity
t. antrum
t. attic
bilateral tympanic membranes
t. body
t. bone
bulging tympanic membrane
t. canal
t. cavity
t. cell
fibrocartilaginous ring of tympanic membrane
t. ganglion
t. gland
greater tympanic spine
t. groove
limbus of tympanic membrane
mastoid branch of posterior tympanic artery
t. membrane
t. membrane gray
t. membrane inflammation
t. membrane injected
t. membrane perforation
t. membrane thermometer
otitis media with perforated tympanic membrane
perforated tympanic membrane
perforation of tympanic membrane
ruptured tympanic membrane
t. temperature
tympanicity auscultation of chest
tympanicus
annulus t.
anulus t.
tympanitic
abdomen distended, tender, t.
t. resonance
t. sound
tympanomastoidectomy
canal wall down t.
tympanomeatal flap
tympanometry test
tympanoplasty
canal wall down t.
canal wall up t.
t. with mastoidectomy
t. without mastoidectomy
Wullstein type t.
tympanostapedial junction
tympanostomy tube insertion
tympanotomy
t. tube
t. and tube insertion
tympany
abdominal t.
acute abdominal t.
chronic abdominal t.
Tyndall
T. effect
T. phenomenon

type

t. A behavior
AB negative blood t.
ABO blood t.
t. A, B personality
affective reaction t.
aggressive predatory t.
aggressive type undersocialized conduct disorder
5-alpha-reductase type I, II
Alzheimer type I, II astrocyte
American T. Culture Collection
amyotrophic type of spongiform encephalopathy
Antoni type A, B neurilemoma
apolipoprotein type 3
arterial-ecchymotic type Ehlers-Danlos syndrome
arthrogryposis congenita, distal, type I, II syndrome
asthenic constitutional t.
AT3 deficiency type II
Athabascan type of severe combined immunodeficiency disease
athletic constitutional t.
attention deficit disorder, residual t.
attention deficit hyperactivity disorder, combined t.
attention deficit hyperactivity disorder, predominantly hyperactive-impulsive t.
autoimmune type of reaction
t. 1 autosomal recessive vitamin D dependency
avian type C retrovirus group
t. B behavior
behavioral, anxiety, mood, and other t.'s of disorders
bipolar disorder type 1, 2
blood t.
blood type in ABO blood group
blood type A negative
blood type A positive
blood type O negative
B negative blood t.
bone morphogenetic protein type 2
carboxyterminal propeptide of type 1 procollagen
chairback type brace
Charcot-Marie-Tooth syndrome, X-linked type II with deafness and mental retardation
chronic active viral hepatitis, type B
conduct disorder type group
congenital dyserythropoietic anemia t.'s I–III
conversion disorder, mixed t.
conversion disorder, motor t.
conversion disorder, seizure t.
corticotropin-releasing hormone receptor type 1, 2
C propeptide of type II collagen
t. and crossmatch
t. and crossmatch blood
degenerative dementia of Alzheimer t.
t. 1, 2, 3 deiodinase
delusional type of activity
dementia of Alzheimer t.
t. 1, 2 diabetes mellitus
diabetes mellitus type 1
diabetes mellitus type 2
diphtheria, tetanus, pertussis, *Haemophilus influenzae* type b vaccine
diphtheria, tetanus toxoids, whole-cell pertussis, and *Haemophilus influenzae* type b conjugate
disorganized type schizophrenia
enterochromaffin-like t.
epidermolysis bullosa, macular t.
fragile X type A
gender identity disorder of adolescence or adulthood, nontranssexual t.
gestational diabetes mellitus, diet controlled, type 2
gestational diabetes mellitus, insulin controlled, type 1
glycogen storage disease, t.'s 1–10
gonadal dysgenesis of Turner t.
Haemophilus influenzae type b
Haemophilus influenzae type b conjugate vaccine
Haemophilus influenzae type b polysaccharide vaccine
Haemophilus influenzae type b vaccine
Haemophilus influenzae type b vaccine, PRP-D conjugate vaccine
Haemophilus influenzae type b vaccine, PRP-OMP conjugate vaccine
Haemophilus influenzae type b vaccine, PRP-T conjugate vaccine
Haemophilus influenzae type vaccine oligosaccharide-CRM197 vaccine conjugate
hereditary motor-sensory neuropathy type IA, II, III–VII
hereditary sensory and autonomic neuropathy t.'s I-IV
hereditary sensory motor neuropathy type I–III
herpes simplex type 1
herpes simplex virus type 1, 2, 6, 7
histamine receptor type 1
Hodgkin disease of diffuse histiocytic lymphocyte depleted t.
Hodgkin disease, mixed nodular t.
t. and hold
human immunodeficiency virus type 1, 2
human papillomavirus type 16
human T-cell leukemia virus type 1, 2, 3
human T-cell lymphotrophic virus type I–III
human T-cell lymphotropic virus type I associated myelopathy
human T-lymphotrophic virus type I
t. I, II regulatory dimer
t. II procollagen gene
influenza virus inactivated vaccine, split virion, t.'s A, B, trivalent
intratubular germ cell neoplasia, unclassified t.
isolated gastric varices type 1, 2
isolated growth hormone deficiency type IB, II, III
leukocyte adhesion deficiency type 1–4
liver-kidney-microsomal type 1 antibody target assay
low-grade B-cell lymphoma of MALT t.
Lutheran blood antibody t.
Lynch and Crues type 2 lesion
major histocompatibility t.
maleylacetoacetate hydrolase, type Ib
malignant lymphoma, lymphoblastic t.
mammalian type B, C, D oncovirus group
Margarita Island type ectodermal dysplasia
maternal blood t.

type *(continued)*
melancholic constitutional t.
membrane type 1–6
membranoproliferative glomerulonephritis type I, II
mesangiocapillary glomerulonephritis type I, II
mixed hyperlipoproteinemia familial type 5 hyperlipidemia
mixed type of incontinence
MMPI Code T.
Mobitz type I, II block
t. of molecular bond
monoamine oxidase type A, B
motor-sensory neuropathy, X-linked Type II, with deafness and mental retardation
mucolipidosis type II, III
mucopolysaccharidosis t.'s I, II, III, IIIB, III, IIID, IVA, IVB, VI, VII
mucopolysaccharidosis type III Sanfilippo A, B, C
mucopolysaccharidosis type I Hurler
mucopolysaccharidosis type I Hurler-Scheie
mucopolysaccharidosis type I Scheie
mucopolysaccharidosis type IV Morquio
mucopolysaccharidosis type VII Sly
mucopolysaccharidosis type VI Maroteaux-Lamy
multiple endocrine adenomatosis type I, II
multiple endocrine neoplasia type 1, 2, 2a, 2b, 3
multiple endocrine neoplasia syndrome, type 1, 2A, 2B, 3
Murphy-Meisgeier T. Indicator for Children
muscle fiber type disproportion
Myers-Briggs Type Indicator psychologic test
Naegeli type of monocytic leukemia
National T. Culture Collection
native type anti-DNA antibody
nephronophthisis type 1
neurofibromatosis type 1, 2
neurofibromatosis, type I
neurofibromatosis, type II
neurofibromatosis, type 1 syndrome
neurogenic fiber type group
neurotensin receptor type 1, 2
neurotrophic tyrosine kinase receptor, type 1
Nezelof type of thymic alymphoplasia
Niemann-Pick disease, type A, B, C, D
Niemann-Pick disease type I, II
nonhistiocytic type lymphoma
non-insulin-dependent diabetes mellitus type 1, 2
nonobese type 2 NIDDM
normal female sex chromosome t.
normal male sex chromosome t.
nosotropic drug dementia of Alzheimer t.
N-terminal telopeptide of type I collagen
nutritional status t.
obese type 2 noninsulin-dependent diabetes mellitus
obsessive-compulsive disorder with poor insight t.
ocular-scoliotic type Ehlers-Danlos syndrome
oculocutaneous albinism type I
OFD syndrome, type I–IV, VI–IX
osteogenesis imperfecta type I–IV
paraesophageal hernia type I, II
parainfluenza type 1, 2, 3, 4A, 4B
paratyphoid fever, t.'s A, B, C
persistent viral hepatitis, type B
phosphodiesterase type 5 inhibitor
plasminogen activator inhibitor type 1, 2
polyglandular autoimmune syndrome type I, II
posterior urethral valve type I–IV
primary degenerative dementia of Alzheimer t.
probability of type I, II error
procollagen type III aminoterminal peptide
pseudohypoaldosteronism type I, II
residual type schizophrenia
schizophrenia, catatonic type, subchronic
schizophrenia, chronic undifferentiated t.
schizophrenia, disorganized type, subchronic
schizophrenia, paranoid type, subchronic
schizophrenia, residual type, subchronic
t. and screen
senile dementia of the Alzheimer t.
serum amyloid type A
soluble tumor necrosis factor-a receptor type I
South African type porphyria
t. specific
stocking and glove type hypesthesia
subcoracoid type displacement
$T_4$5′-deiodinase type 2
tetanus-diphtheria toxoid, adult t.
T-helper cell type 1, 2, 3
usual type papillary carcinoma
variable antigen t.
vitamin D-dependent rickets type II
wild type strain
Wullstein type tympanoplasty

typed
dictated and t.

type-specific
t.-s. antibody
t.-s. M protein

type-to-token ratio

typhi
live-attenuated recombinant *Salmonella typhi*
oral attenuated *Salmonella typhi* vaccine

typhoid
apyretic t.
t. cholera
t. dysentery
t. fever
intradermal typhoid and paratyphoid vaccine
Malaysian t.
t., paratyphoid A, B, C vaccine
t., paratyphoid A, B, tetanus toxoid, and diphtheria toxoid vaccine
t. pneumonia
t. vaccine, acetone-killed and dried
t. vaccine, attenuated live
t. vaccine, heat and phenol inactivated, dried
t. vaccine, not otherwise specified
t. vaccine, Vi capsular polysaccharide

typhoid-paratyphoid vaccine

typhosa
roseola t.

typhus
African tick t.
Australian tick t.
louse-borne t.
Manchurian t.
Mexican t.
mite t.
mite-borne t.
Moscow t.
murine t.
North Asian tick t.
North Queensland tick t.
prison fever t.
recrudescent t.
recrudescent typhus fever
t. *Rickettsiae* species vaccine
São Paulo t.
tick t.

typical
t. absence seizure
t. carcinoid
intraluminal typical bronchial carcinoid
t. measles
mental retardation, typical facies, aortic stenosis syndrome

typing
blood t.
homozygous typing cell
microtiter blood typing system
Mostofi histologic t.
multilocus sequence t.
primed lymphocyte t.
sequenced-based t.
serologic t.

typology
anxiety t.

tyramide signal amplification

tyrosinase-negative oculocutaneous albinism

tyrosine
t. aminotransferase
t. aminotransferase deficiency
t. aminotransferase regulator
Bruton tyrosine kinase
diiodinated t.
t. ethyl ester
t. hydroxylase
Janus family tyrosine kinase
t. kinase-2
t. kinase activity
monoiodinated t.
neurotrophic tyrosine kinase receptor, type 1
t. phenol-lyase
protein tyrosine kinase
receptor protein tyrosine kinase
receptor tyrosine kinase
t. transaminase

tyrosinemia
neonatal t.
oculocutaneous tyrosinemia or tyrosinosis

tyrosinosis
oculocutaneous tyrosinemia or t.

Tyuleniy virus

ubiquinone-50

ubiquitous
conserved helix-loop-helix ubiquitous kinase

Uganda S virus

ugliness
irrational obsession with imagined u.

ulatrophy
afunctional u.
atrophic u.

ulcer
acute decubitus u.
acute duodenal u.
anterior duodenal u.
anterior wall antral u.
aortic penetrating u.
aphthous genital u.
aphthous ileal u.
aphthous oral u.
aphthous stomach u.
apical duodenal u.
arteriolar ischemic u.
atherosclerotic aortic u.
u. base
u. bed
benign gastric u.
chronic gastric u.
chronic stasis leg u.
u. crater
decubitus u.
dendritic corneal u.
dermal u.
diabetic foot u.
u. disease
duodenal peptic ulcer disease
duodenal ulcer perforation
u. dyspepsia
genital ulcer disease
giant gastric u.
gravitational u.
healing duodenal u.
idiopathic esophageal u.
U. Index
infected decubitus u.
malleolus stasis u.
marginal catarrhal u.
marginal corneal u.
marginal ring ulcer of cornea
Meleney chronic undermining u.
minute bleeding u.
Mooren corneal u.
mucosal gastric u.
mycotic corneal ulcer disease
necrotic palatal u.
neurotrophic food u.
in noma u.
nontreponemal genital ulcer disease
oral aphthous u.
oval-shaped vernal u.
Palmer acid test for peptic u.
patchy colonic u.
penetrating aortic u.
penetrating atherosclerotic u.
perforated acid peptic u.
perforated corneal u.
perforated duodenal u.
perforated gastric u.
perforated peptic u.
peripheral corneal u.
pressure u.
Pressure U. Scale for Healing
psychogenic gastric u.
pyloric channel u.
recurrent aphthous u.
recurrent oral u.
refractory duodenal u.
sacral decubitus u.
serpiginous corneal u.
solitary rectal u.
solitary rectal ulcer syndrome
solitary ulcer of rectum syndrome
staged ulcer diet
stress ulcer prophylaxis
superficial gastric u.
tropical phagedenic u.
varicose u.
venous stasis u.

ulcer-associated cell lineage

ulcerated
u. lesion
u. nodule
u. plaque

ulcerating
u. carcinoma
u. form
u. lesion

ulceration
anal u.
anastomotic u.
aphthoid u.
aphthous u.
ASA-induced gastric u.
u. of cornea
corneal u.
erosive gastritis with u.
gastrointestinal irritation and u.
u. of the globe
herpetic u.
metaherpetic ulceration of the cornea
mucous membrane u.
nasal mucosal u.
necrosis and u.
necrotic u.
necrotizing sclerocorneal u.
neuropathic forefoot u.
nonhealing u.
oral u.
patchy colonic u.
peptic u.
perilimbal u.
skin u.
superficial u.
vulvovaginal u.

ulcerative
acute necrotizing ulcerative gingivitis
acute ulcerative colitis
acute ulcerative gingivitis
u. blepharitis
u. bowel disease
chronic ulcerative colitis
u. colitis
u. dermatosis
diarrhea from ulcerative colitis
u. esophagitis
idiopathic ulcerative colitis
u. keratitis
u. lesion
mild ulcerative colitis
moderate ulcerative colitis
mucosal ulcerative colitis
necrotizing ulcerative keratitis
necrotizing ulcerative periodontitis
necrotizing ulcerative stomatitis
u. proctitis
recurrent ulcerative scarifying stomatitis
septicemic cutaneous ulcerative disease
u. stomatitis

Uldall catheter

ulerythematosa
atrophoderma u.

***Ulex europaeus* agglutinin I**

ulitis
aphthous u.

ulna
anterior border of u.
articular circumference of head of u.
interosseous border of u.
Milch cuff resection of ulna technique

ulna *(continued)*
Monteggia fracture-dislocation of u.
nutrient artery of u.
open reduction of radius and u.
proximal end of u.

ulnae
arteria nutricia u.
arteria nutriens u.

ulnar
anterior ulnar recurrent artery
Armistead ulnar lengthening operation
u. artery
u. artery injury
u. bone
u. border of forearm
u. branch
u. branch of medial antebrachial cutaneous nerve
u. collateral ligament
u. collateral ligament of elbow joint
u. collateral ligament of wrist joint
collateral ulnar ligament
common palmar digital nerve of ulnar nerve
u. compression neuropathy
u. cutaneous vein
u. deviation
u. deviation deformity
u. drift
u. fracture
u. groove
lateral ulnar collateral ligament
u. ligament
medial ulnar collateral ligament
midcarpal u.
negative ulnar variance
u. nerve compression
u. nerve conduction velocity
u. nerve distribution
u. nerve entrapment
u. nerve palsy
u. notch
u. notch of radius
palmar carpal branch of ulnar artery
palmar cutaneous branch of the ulnar nerve
u. palsy
positive ulnar variance
posterior branch of recurrent ulnar artery
u. resection
u. shaft
u. styloid bone
superficial branch of ulnar nerve
u. tunnel syndrome
u. vein

ulnocarpal ligament

Ultegra rapid platelet function assay

ultimate
u. goal
u. tensile strength

ultimobranchial
u. body
u. gland

Ultra
One Touch Ultra meter

ultracentrifugation
sucrose density gradient u.

ultra–Doppler sonography

ultrafast
u. computed tomography
u. contrast-enhanced MRA
u. CT imaging

ultrafiltration
u. coefficient
continuous arteriovenous u.
continuous slow u.
dialytic u.
extracorporeal u.
u. hemodialyzer
isolated u.
pure u.
u. rate
sequential u.
total u.
u. volume

ultrafine
u. fiber
u. fraction

ultrahigh
u. carbon
u. frequency
u. magnification mammography
u. molecular weight
u. molecular weight polyethylene
u. purity
u. temperature
u. vacuum
u. voltage

ultrahigh-frequency ventilation

ultralow
u. birth weight
u. dose rate
u. particulate air
u. profile
u. temperaturc
u. volume

Ultramark
ATL Ultramark 4,8,9 ultrasound

Ultramatic Project-O-Chart projector

ultrasensitive fluorescence in situ hybridization

ultrashort wave

ultrasmall-particle superparamagnetic iron oxide

ultrasonic
u. arteriogram
u. assessment
u. attenuation
u. cardiogram
u. cardiography
u. cephalometry
u. cleaning
Doppler ultrasonic flowmeter
u. echography
u. encephalography
u. fat suctioning
u. flow detector
u. frequency
u. handpiece
u. heat
u. humidifier
u. liposuction
u. mist
u. nebulizer
nonaspirating ultrasonic phaco chopper tip
percutaneous transluminal ultrasonic coronary angioplasty
percutaneous ultrasonic lithotripsy
percutaneous ultrasonic nephrolithotripsy
percutaneous ultrasonic pyelolithotomy
pulsed ultrasonic blood velocity detector
pulsed Doppler ultrasonic flowmeter
u. renal scanning
u. therapy

ultrasonically guided needle biopsy

ultrasonic-assisted
u.-a. lipoplasty
u.-a. liposuction

ultrasonogram
B-scan u.

ultrasonography
advanced u.

carotid duplex u.
catheter probe-assisted endoluminal u.
color Doppler u.
color duplex u.
contrast-enhanced endoscopic u.
duplex color u.
endoluminal rectal u.
endorectal u.
high-intensity focused u.
intraductal u.
intraoperative u.
laparoscopic contact u.
laparoscopic intracorporeal u.
microvascular Doppler u.
penile duplex u.
periorbital directional Doppler u.
pulsed Doppler u.
real-time u.
rectal endoscopic u.
transrectal u.
transvaginal u.

ultrasound

u. assessment
ATL HDI4000 u.
ATL Ultramark 4,8,9 u.
automated cardiac flow measurement u.
u. backscatter microscopy
u. biomicroscopy
u. bone imaging sonometer
bone ultrasound attenuation
carotid artery u.
carotid ultrasound examination
u. catheter probe
colonoscopic endoluminal u.
color duplex u.
color flow Doppler u.
compression u.
u. computed tomography
condom catheter endoscopic u.
continuous-wave Doppler u.
u. contrast agent
u. diagnosis
diathermy, traction, and u.
digital u.
Doppler ultrasound imaging
Doppler ultrasound stethoscope
duplex B-mode u.
duplex carotid u.
duplex Doppler u.
dynamic ultrasound of shoulder
u. echocardiography
echo guided u.
endoanal u.
endorectal u.
endoscopic u.
endovaginal u.
esophageal u.
u. examination
focused segmented ultrasound machine
front-loading ultrasound probe
u. gallstone detection
u. guidance
heat, ultrasound, and massage
high-frequency ultrasound probe sonography
high-intensity focused u.
hydrogen peroxide u.
u. hyperthermia
hypoechoic area of u.
u. imaging
intracoronary vascular u.
intraductal u.
intraluminal u.
intraocular u.
intraoperative u.
intravascular ultrasound catheter
intravenous ultrasound catheter
kidney ultrasound biopsy
laparoscopic intraoperative u.
linear array B-mode ultrasound transducer
linear array transrectal ultrasound probe
MAGGI disposable biopsy needle guide for u.
u. mammography
medical ultrasound 3D portable, with advanced communication
neonatal adrenal u.
obstetric u.
obstetrical u.
ophthalmic biometry by ultrasound echography
preoperative u.
pulse-inversion mode u.
qualitative coronary u.
quantitative bone u.
routine antenatal diagnostic imaging with u.
u. scanning
three-dimensional u.
time domain u.
transabdominal/transvaginal u.
transcranial Doppler u.
u. transducer
transrectal u.
transrectal ultrasound of prostate
transurethral u.
treated with ultrasound, diathermy, and traction
weeks by u.

ultrasound-assisted lipectomy

ultrasound-guided

u.-g. bronchoscopy
u.-g. compression repair
u.-g. core breast biopsy
u.-g. core-needle biopsy
u.-g. fine-needle aspiration
u.-g. fine-needle aspiration biopsy
u.-g. injection therapy
u.-g. vascular access

ultrastructure

osteoclast u.

ultrathin-walled two-stage

ultraviolet

u. A, B, C
u. blood irradiation
damaging u.
u. exposure
extreme u.
extreme ultraviolet laser
u. germicidal irradiation
u. light
u. light, long wavelength
u. light, midrange-wavelength
midrange spectrum ultraviolet light
midrange-wavelength ultraviolet light
u. photoelectron spectroscopy
u. photometry
psoralen plus ultraviolet light of A wavelength
pulsed ultraviolet actinotherapy
u. radiation
u. ray
vacuum u.

ultraviolet-enhanced reactivation

Umatilla virus

umbilical

u. arterial
u. arterial line
u. artery
u. artery catheter
u. artery catheterization
u. artery line
u. cholesterol
u. coiling index
u. cord
u. cord blood
u. cord blood culture
u. cord blood leukocyte
u. cord compression
u. cord prolapse
u. cyst
u. fascia
u. fissure

umbilical *(continued)*
u. fistula
u. fold
u. fossa
u. graft
u. granuloma
u. hernia
human umbilical cord blood
human umbilical vein
human umbilical vein endothelial cell
infant with umbilical catheter
late clamped umbilical cord
milking of umbilical cord
mixed umbilical arterial acidemia
10-mm umbilical port
mucoid degeneration of umbilical cord
percutaneous umbilical blood sampling
single umbilical artery
u. vein
u. vein catheter
u. vein catheterization
u. vein to maternal vein
u. venous catheter
u. venous line

umbilicalis
anulus u.
arteria u.
arteritis u.

umbilicus
below the u.
fingers above u.
fingers below u.
fundus firm at u.
fundus firm 1, 2 cm above u.
fundus firm 1, 2 cm below u.
one fingerbreadth above u.
one fingerbreadth below u.

umbrella
u. closure
double u.
double umbrella closure
double umbrella device
u. iris
transcatheter u.

Umbre virus

unable
u. to determine
u. to locate
u. to obtain
u. to read lab result

unaided equalization reference

unassisted
u. diastolic pressure
u. systolic pressure

unauthorized
u. absence
u. leave

unavailable
emotionally u.

Una virus

unavoidable hemorrhage

unawareness
Scale for the Assessment of U. of Mental Disorder

unbound
fraction u.
free unbound thyroxine
u. iron-binding capacity
u. testosterone
u. thyroxine-binding globulin

uncal
bilateral uncal herniation
u. herniation

uncalis
arteria u.

uncaring
caregiver withholding and u.

uncertain
atypical glandular cells of uncertain significance
carcinoma of uncertain primary site
u. etiology
prostatic stromal proliferation of uncertain malignant potential

uncertainty
fear, uncertainty, and doubt

unchanged conventional treatment

uncinate
u. gyrus
u. process

unclassifiable connective tissue disease

unclassified
arbovirus group u.
u. fecal virus
intratubular germ cell neoplasia, unclassified type

uncle
maternal u.

uncombable
mental retardation, polydactyly, phalangeal hypoplasia, syndactyly, unusual face, uncombable hair

uncombined coenzyme A

uncomfortable
u. listening level
u. loudness level

uncompensated
u. acidosis
u. alkalosis

uncomplicated
u. arteriosclerotic dementia
u. delivery
full-term uncomplicated pregnancy, labor, and delivery
multiinfarct dementia, u.
u. postoperative course
postoperative course u.
pregnancy, term, u.
pregnancy, term, uncomplicated delivered, living female
pregnancy, term, uncomplicated delivered, living male

unconditional stimulus

unconditioned
u. reflex
u. response
u. stimulus

unconfirmed/uncertain complete remission

unconjugated
u. bilirubin
u. estriol

unconscious
airway obstruction in unconscious patient
immobilized and u.

unconsciousness
onset of u.

unconstrained
cruciate condylar unconstrained prosthesis

uncontrollable
u. crying
u. hemorrhaging

uncontrolled
u. cell division growth
u. generalized grand mal seizure
u. hemorrhagic shock
u. high blood pressure
u. hypertension
u. unsterile delivery
unsterile uncontrolled vaginal delivery
u. variable

uncorrected visual acuity

uncoupling
u. protein
u. protein 1, 2, 3

uncus
arachnoid of u.

undedicated logic array

undegraded insulin factor

undelivered
pregnancy uterine, u.

undenatured bacterial antigen

under
u. care of
u. direct vision
u. elbow
u. observation
u. satisfactory general anesthesia

underactive
u. immune system
u. thyroid
u. thyroid gland

underdeveloped
u. chin
u. mandible

underdevelopment
middle one-third of face u.

underfilling
arterial u.

underlay fascial graft

underlying
u. cause
u. condition
u. connective tissue
u. disorder
u. emotional issue
u. fascia
u. heart rhythm
u. physical illness

undermined
edges u.
skin u.
wound margin u.

undermining
Meleney chronic undermining ulcer

undernutrition
protein-calorie u.

underperfused myocardium

undersensing
pacemaker u.

underserved
health in underserved rural areas

undersocialized
aggressive type undersocialized conduct disorder
aggressive undersocialized reaction

understanding
memorandum of u.
verbalize u.

underwater
self-contained underwater breathing apparatus

undescended
u. testicle
u. testis

undesirable
u. discharge
measurable undesirable respiratory contaminants

undetected infarct

undetermined
atypical endocervical cells of undetermined significance
atypical glandular cell of undetermined significance
atypical squamous cell of undetermined significance
bilirubin of undetermined origin
bleeding of undetermined origin
bruising of undetermined origin
cause u.
u. cause
diagnosis u.
u. etiology
fever of undetermined origin
u. malignant potential
monoclonal gammopathy of undetermined significance
u. origin
pyrexia of undetermined origin
squamous intraepithelial lesion/atypical squamous cell of undetermined significance

undiagnosed
u. hepatitis
u. hydrocephalus

undifferentiated
acute undifferentiated leukemia
acute undifferentiated schizophrenic reaction
u. adenocarcinoma
u. autoimmune syndrome
u. B-cell lymphoma
u. carcinoma
u. cell
u. cell adenoma
u. connective tissue disease
u. connective tissue syndrome
diffuse and u.
diffuse undifferentiated lymphoma
u. embryonal sarcoma
u. large cell carcinoma
malignant teratoma, u.
u. mental retardation
u. neoplasm
u. osteosarcoma
u. pattern
u. respiratory disease
u. schizophrenia
schizophrenia, chronic undifferentiated type
schizophrenic reaction, acute u.
schizophrenic reaction, chronic, u.
sinonasal undifferentiated carcinoma
small cell undifferentiated carcinoma of the prostate
small cell undifferentiated neuroendocrine carcinoma

undisciplined interpretation and suggestion

undulating membrane

undulatory nystagmus

Unemployment Insurance Benefits

unenhanced
axial unenhanced CT scan
u. CAT scan
u. helical computed tomography
u. study

unequal conjoined twin

unesterified free fatty acid

uneventful
postoperative course u.
u. postoperative course

unexpected
sudden unexpected infant death
sudden unexpected, unexplained death

unexplained
u. apparent life-threatening event
u. fever
u. infertility
multiple occurrence of unexplained symptoms
partially unexplained sudden infant death syndrome
sudden unexpected, unexplained death
sudden unexplained death syndrome
sudden unexplained infant death

unexplained *(continued)*
totally unexplained sudden infant death syndrome
unfavorable history
unfixed cryostat
unflagged order
unfractionated
u. heparin
low-dose unfractionated heparin
unguis
matrix u.
os u.
unguium
arcus u.
unheated
toluidine red unheated serum test
u. serum reagin
uniaxial balance evaluation
unicompartmental knee arthroplasty
unicondylar fracture
unicornis
uterus u.
unicoronal synostosis
unicryptal adenoma
unicystic ameloblastoma
unidentified
u. bright object
u. endosteal marrow cell
u. foreign object
u. growth factor
maximal permissible concentration of unidentified radionuclides
u. reading frame
unidirectional
traumatic unidirectional Bankart lesion surgery
unified
u. atomic mass unit
U. Medical Language System
U. Parkinson Disease Rating Scale
unifocal
u. eosinophilic granuloma
u. premature ventricular contractions
u. ventricular ectopic beat
uniform
u. food encoding
variable-angle uniform signal excitation
uniformly positive
unijunction transistor
unilamellar
large unilamellar vesicle
unilateral
u. absence of excretion
u. amputee
u. anesthesia
u. approach
u. calcaneal brace
u. cleft
u. cleft of lip and palate
diffuse unilateral subacute neuroretinitis "wipe-out" syndrome
u. epileptiform discharges
u. gliosis
u. head pain
u. hearing loss
u. hemianopia
u. hydrocephalus
u. hyperplasia
u. hypertrophy
u. interfacetal dislocation or subluxation
u. laterothoracic exanthem
u. lung reduction surgery
müllerian duct, unilateral renal agenesis, and anomalies of the cervicothoracic somites
occipital lobe unilateral cerebral hemisphere lesion
parietal lobe unilateral cerebral hemisphere lesion
u. posterior lumbar interbody fusion
progressive unilateral hearing loss
u. renal agenesis
u. renal artery stenosis
u. renovascular disease
u. salpingo-oophorectomy
short duration, unilateral, neuralgic, conjunctival injection and tearing
u. spatial neglect
u. strabismus
u. throbbing headache
u. tinnitus
u. ureteral obstruction
u. ureteral occlusion
valves, unilateral reflux, dysplasia
u. vocal cord paralysis
u. weakness
unilateralis
nevus acneiformis u.
unilobar
u. emphysema
idiopathic unilobar emphysema
unilobular cirrhosis
unilocular
u. cyst
u. fat
u. joint
unimpaired motor function
uninhibited
u. detrusor muscle capacity
u. neurogenic bladder
u. overactive bladder
uninjured
left u.
right u.
uninterruptible power supply
uninvolved
u. epidermis
left u.
right u.
uniocular hemianopia
union
anomalous pancreaticobiliary ductal u.
delayed union of fracture
fracture with delayed u.
osteonal bone u.
unipara
uniparental
u. disomy
maternal uniparental heterodisomy
unipolar
augmented voltage unipolar left arm lead
augmented voltage unipolar left foot lead
augmented voltage unipolar right arm lead
u. cell
u. chest lead
u. depression
implantable unipolar endocardial electrode
u. limb lead
u. pacemaker
u. pacing
u. precordial lead
u. psychosis
unique
u. facies, anorexia, cachexia, and eye and skin syndrome
u. patient number

unit

absorbance units, full scale
active wrist rotation u.
acute care u.
acute stroke u.
addictive disease u.
admission, entrance, and evaluation u.
adolescent drug abuse u.
adolescent inpatient u.
afferent motor u.
alcohol and drug dependence u.
alcohol treatment u.
allercoat enzyme allergosorbent u.
allergy u.
ambulatory care u.
ambulatory surgical u.
u. of analysis
antigen-inducing u.
antitoxin u.
arbitrary valve u.
arithmetic and logic u.
Aspen sonography u.
asymmetric unit membrane
atomic mass u.
atomic weight u.
auditory training u.'s
Autoflex II, III CPM u.
autologous blood u.
autologous RBC u.
barrier isolation u.
basic health u.
basic multicellular u.
basic structural u.
Behnken unit of roentgen-ray exposure
Bessey-Lowry u.
Bessey-Lowry-Brock method or u.
Bethesda u.
biological allergic u.
bipolar cautery u.
Bod u.
Bodansky u.
bone marrow transplant u.
British Standard U.
British thermal u.
burn care u.
burst-forming u.
cardiac ambulatory monitoring u.
cardiac observation u.
cardiac rehabilitation u.
cardiac stepdown unit and telemetry
cardiac surgery intensive care u.
cardiac surveillance u.
cardiology intensive care u.
cardiothoracic intensive care u.
cardiovascular inpatient care u.
cardiovascular specialty u.
cardiovascular surgery u.
cardiovascular-thoracic intensive care u.
C-arm fluoroscopy u.
casein u.
casualty staging u.
centigrade thermal u.
central processing u.
chemical dependency u.
Cherry-Crandall u.
chick-cell agglutination u.
chymotrypsin u.
u. clerk
clinical research u.
clinical specialty u.
closed head u.
colony-forming u.
color u.
community care u.
complex motor u.
comprehensive cardiac care u.
conscious control of motor u.'s
constitutive transcription u.
continuing education u.
continuous motor unit activity control u.
convalescent u.
u. of convergence
coronary arrhythmia monitoring u.
coronary intensive care u.
critical care medicine u.
critical care recovery u.
cumulative dose u.
custom fit in ear u.
day care surgical u.
day surgery u.
developmental u.
dial u.
diffusion per unit of alveolar volume
direct observation u.
dog u.
dolorimetric unit of pain intensity
u. dose
dose u.
early clinical drug evaluation u.
eating disorder u.
Ehrlich u.
electrocautery u.
electromagnetic u.
electrostatic u.
electrosurgical u.
ELISA u.
emergency diagnostic and treatment u.
emergency and trauma u.
endotoxin u.
energy u.
entropy u.
environmental control u.
environmental exposure u.
enzyme u.
epidemic observation u.
epilepsy monitoring u.
epithelial focus-forming u.
equivalent roentgen u.
esterase u.
extended care u.
family-centered care u.
family participation u.
fetal intensive care u.
fetoplacental u.
fibrinogen equivalent u.
fingertip u.
Finsen u.
focus-forming u.
foot-pound-second system, u.
u. of force
u. of force of acceleration
functional spinal u.
gastrointestinal procedure u.
geriatric assessment u.
geriatric evaluation and management u.
geriatric skilled care u.
germ-free isolation u.
glycogenic u.
gracilis myocutaneous u.
granulocyte-macrophage colony-forming u.
gravitational u.
gravity u.
group of units of analysis
guinea pig u.
Hazardous Materials Response U.
headache unit index
head-drop u.
head injury u.
u. of heat
heater probe u.
hemagglutinating u.
hemagglutinin u.
hemodialysis u.
hemolytic u.
Holzknecht u.
home cervical traction u.
hormone response u.
Hounsfield u.
hyaluronidase unit for semen
hyperemia u.

unit *(continued)*
u. hyperemia
immunizing u.
individual motor unit action potential
industrial rehabilitation u.
infant intensive care u.
infant-toddler special care u.
infectious disease u.
infectious units per million
infusoria killing u.
inpatient dialysis u.
inpatient hospice u.
integrating regulatory transcription u.
intensive care unit psychosis
intensive coronary care u.
intensive special care u.
intensive therapy observation u.
intensive thoracic cardiovascular u.
intensive treatment u.
interferon reference u.
intermediate coronary care u.
intermediate medical care u.
intermediate medicine u.
intermediate surgical u.
International U.
international benzoate u.
international opacity u.
International U. per liter
International U. per minute
intrapleural sealed drainage u.
ionizing radiation u.
Junkman-Schoeller unit of thyrotropin
kallikrein inactivating u.
kallikrein inactivation u.
kallikrein inhibiting u.
Karmen u.
kidney transplant u.
Kienböck unit of x-ray exposure
Kimbrel u.
King-Armstrong u.
laminar air flow u.
Leonard cathode ray u.
leukocyte colony-forming u.
leukocyte equivalent u.
life change u.
life support u.
limit flocculation u.
lipid fluidity u.
liver dialysis u.
living u.
locked hospital u.
loudness u.
lytic u.
Mache u.
macro motor unit action potential
maintenance dialysis u.
malaria control u.
mass radiography u.
maternal pediatric u.
mature burst-forming unit erythroid
maximal care u.
maximal flow per unit of time
McIntyre irrigating/aspirating u.
mean dose per unit cumulated activity
medical intensive care u.
medically managed intensive addiction treatment u.
medical maintenance u.
medical oncology u.
medical progressive care u.
medical short procedure u.
medical special care u.
medical studies u.
medical therapy u.
u. of medical time
medical unit, self-contained and transportable
megakaryocyte colony-forming u.
memory for symbolic u.
mental health care u.
mescaline u.
milli-International unit one-thousandth of an International U.
millimass u.
million u.'s
million international u.'s
minimal reproductive u.
Mira diathermy u.
mobile coronary care u.
mobile intensive care u.
mobile surgical u.
molecular recognition u.
monitor u.
Montevideo u.
motor cortex u.
motor unit action potential
mouse uterine weight u.
multiple unit activity
Multistar angiographic u.
murine colony-forming u.
Murphy u.
myocardial infarction research u.
nectary of floral u.
negative sedimentation Svedberg u.
neonatal intensive care u.
neonatal stepdown u.
nephelometric turbidity u.'s
neurointermediate nursing u.
neurologic intensive care u.
neuromuscular u.
neurosurgery intensive care u.
neurosurgical continuous care u.
neurosurgical intensive care u.
u. of neutron dosage
newborn convalescent care u.
newborn intensive care u.
newborn special care u.
N_2O cryosurgical u.
Noon pollen u.
not on u.
nursing home care u.
observation care u.
Ocutome vitrectomy u.
one-millionth International U.
operating theatre sterile supply u.
operational taxonomic u.
optical density u.
ostiomeatal u.
outpatient renal dialysis u.
outpatient surgical u.
u. of packed red blood cells
pain control u.
pain treatment u.
palliative care u.
pantothenic acid u.
Parental Stressor Scale: Neonatal Intensive Care U.
partial denture u.
patient care u.
Pebax counter u.
Peczon I/A u.
pediatric intensive care u.
pediatric sedation u.
pediatric special care u.
pepsin u.
peripheral resistance u.
u. per liter
100 units per milliliter
photosynthetic u.
plaque-forming u.
plasma equivalent u.
pock-forming u.
polymerase-inducing u.
portable dialysis u.
postanesthesia care u.
postanesthetic recovery u.
postcoronary care u.
postsurgical u.
prenatal intensive care u.
primary care u.
primary sampling u.
progressive care u.

protected environment units and prophylactic antibiotic
protective care u.
protein nitrogen u.
psychiatric intensive care u.
pulmonary intensive care u.
radiation effect u.
Raji cell-binding u.
rapid reintegration u.
regional neonatal intensive care u.
relative light u.'s
relative time u.
relative value u.
relief medication unit index
resistance u.
respiratory intensive care u.
respiratory resistance u.
Respiratory Special Care U.
respiratory-surgical intensive care u.
ribosomal ribonucleic acid transcription u.
sensation u.
Shinowara-Jones-Reinhart u.
shock trauma u.
Sibley-Lehninger u.
sievert u.
single unit activity
skin test u.
skin unit dose
smallest unit of DNA capable of recombination
Somogyi u.
sorbent u.
special care baby u.
spinal cord injury u.
spinal intensive care u.
Standard Deviation U.
Standard U.'s and Nomenclature
stimulus isolation u.
stroke u.
structural repeating u.
Subjective U.'s of Distress Scale
substance abuse evaluation screen u.
substance abuse treatment u.
surgical intermediate care u.
surgical pulmonary intensive care u.
surgical respiratory intensive care u.
surgical short procedure u.
Svedberg flotation u.
terminal ductal lobular u.
terminal respiratory u.
thoracic intensive care u.
Todd u.
token economy u.
toxic u.
toxin u.
transitional care u.
transmission u.
transplant intensive care u.
trauma intensive care u.
trunk extension-flexion u.
trypsin-inhibiting u.
tuberculin u.
1 tuberculin u.
5 tuberculin u.
250 tuberculin u.
tumor colony-forming u.
turbidity-reducing u.
unified atomic mass u.
urinary care u.
uterine activity u.
u. of variance
ventilator rehabilitation u.
vertebral motion u.
video display u.
visual display u.
volume airflow per unit of time
volume unit meter
volume of oxygen consumption per unit of time
weighted patient care u.
u. of whole blood
workload u.
X u.

unitas
oculi u.
oculus u.

unit-culture
colony-forming u.-c.

united
U. States Pharmacopeia Drug Information

unit-eosinophil
colony-forming u.-e.

unit-erythrocyte
colony-forming u.-e.

unit-erythroid
burst-forming u.-e.
colony-forming u.-e.

unit-fibroblast
colony-forming u.-f.

unit-fibroblastoid
colony-forming u.-f.

unit-granulocyte-macrophage
colony-forming u.-g.-m.

unit-lymphoid
colony-forming u.-l.

unit-megakaryocyte
colony-forming u.-m.

unit-neutrophil-monocyte
colony-forming u.-n.-m.

units/mL
colony-forming u.

unit-spleen
colony-forming u.-s.

unius
nevus unius lateralis

univentricular
u. atrioventricular connection
u. heart
orthotopic univentricular artificial heart

universal
u. blood donor
U. bone plate
U. Control Reference Plasma
u. donor
u. electron microscope
u. feeder
u. frame outer socket
u. joint syndrome
Martinez U. Perineal Interstitial Template
U. Neonatal Hearing Screening
u. newborn hearing screening program
U. plantar fasciitis orthotic
u. precautions
u. proximal femur prosthesis
u. salt iodization
U. Spine System
system universal verbotonol audition Guberina

universale
melasma u.

universalis
calcinosis u.
neurinomatosis u.

University
College and University Environment Scales
Kent State University Speech Discrimination Test
Manchester and Oxford U.'s Scale for the Psychopathological Assessment of Dementia
Memorial University of Newfoundland Scale of Happiness
modified University of Wisconsin solution

University *(continued)*
Northwestern University Children's Perception of Speech Test
original University of Wisconsin solution
U. of Pennsylvania Smell Identification Test
U. Residence Environment Scale
Temple University Short Syntax Inventory
Western Ontario and McMaster U.'s Osteoarthritis Index Physical Functioning subscale and chair-performance
Western Ontario and McMaster U.'s Osteoarthritis Index Physical Functioning subscale and chair-stand performance
U. of Wisconsin solution

unknown
algebraic unknown or space coordinate
u. amino acid
amyloid of unknown origin
arthritis of unknown diagnosis
atypical glandular cells of unknown significance
u. black female
u. black male
cancer of unknown primary
cancer of unknown primary site
carcinoma of unknown primary
carcinoma of unknown primary site
cause u.
chest pain of unknown etiology
density optical u.
etiology u.
u. etiology
u. factor
fever of unknown etiology
fever of unknown origin
granulomatous lesions of unknown significance
impaired memory of unknown cause
metastatic carcinoma of unknown primary origin
metastatic tumor of unknown origin
monoarticular arthritis of unknown etiology
monoclonal gammopathy of unknown significance
myocardial disease of unknown origin
myocardiopathy of unknown origin
name u.
u. origin
patient unknown acquired immune deficiency syndrome carrier
plasma cell dyscrasia of unknown significance
u. primary carcinoma
primary carcinoma u.
u. primary tumor
primary tumor site u.
prolonged fever of unknown origin
pyrexia of unknown etiology
pyrexia of unknown origin
u. quantity
reading of u.
stromal tumor of unknown malignant potential
syncope of unknown origin
villitis of unknown etiology
u. white female
u. white male

unlicensed assistive personnel

unlocked
closed unlocked nail

unmasking
antigen u.

unmet dependency need

Unna boot

Unna-Pappenheim stain

unoccupied
lowest unoccupied molecular orbital

unopposed estrogen

unpaired

unpatched
u. left eye
u. right eye

unpersuasive false ideas

Unpleasant Events Schedule

unprotected
cumulative effects of unprotected sun
u. left main

unproven health claim

unprovoked
u. anger
u. rage attack

unreactive
pupils u.

unreasonable fear

unrecognized
previously unrecognized mental illness

unrelated
u. cord-blood transplant
u. donor
u. donor transplant
living unrelated donor
matched unrelated donor stem cell transplant

unremarkable
head u.
head, eyes, ears, nose, and throat u.
past medical history u.

unresectable tumor

unresolved
u. bereavement
u. grief

unresponsive
alertness, response to voice, response to pain, u.
alert, verbal stimulus response, painful stimulus response, u.
alert, vocal stimulus, painful stimulus, u.
fever unresponsive to antibiotic therapy
patient weak, hypotensive and u.

unresponsiveness
ACTH u.

unripe
cervix u.

unroofed
complex unroofed coronary sinus

unroofing
endoscopic u.

unruptured
u. brain aneurysm
u. ectopic pregnancy
luteinized unruptured follicle
luteinized unruptured follicle syndrome

unsatisfactory condition

unsaturated
u. binding capacity
u. fatty acid
u. iron-binding capacity
u. vitamin B_{12}-binding capacity

unscheduled
u. deoxynucleic acid synthesis

unspecified
meningococcal *Neisseria meningitidis* serogroups unspecified vaccine
other or unspecified psychoactive substance intoxication

unstable
u. angina
u. angina/non-Q-wave myocardial infarction
u. angina pectoris
Aussies-Isseis unstable scoliosis
u. bladder
u. coronary artery disease
emotionally u.
emotionally unstable character disorder
u. fracture
heart electrically u.
u. hemoglobin disease
u. and intense relationships
u. interpersonal relationship

unstained
large unstained cell

unsteady
u. gait
patient unsteady in gait

unsterile
uncontrolled unsterile delivery
u. controlled vaginal delivery
u. uncontrolled vaginal delivery
warm moist pack unsterile

unsterile
u. controlled vaginal delivery
u. uncontrolled vaginal delivery

unstirred water layer

unsupported arm exercise

unsuspected hydrocephalus

unsustained ventricular tachycardia

until
u. finished
u. further notice
u. gone
plug the lung until it grows

untoward reaction

5′-untranslated region

untranslated region

untreatable
chronic untreatable condition
u. injury

untreated cell

unusual
u. facial features
femoral hypoplasia unusual facies syndrome
u. interstitial pneumonitis
mental retardation, polydactyly, phalangeal hypoplasia, syndactyly, unusual face, uncombable hair
u. position of limbs
u. rare detail response

unusually hostile or aggressive behavior

unverifiable memories of incest

unwanted
willful exposure to unwanted pregnancy

unwed mother

unwinding
fluorometric analysis of DNA u.

up
ability to hold head u.
appendix freed u.
baby up for adoption
canal wall up mastoidectomy
canal wall up tympanoplasty
coughing up blood
coughing up blood with chest pain
u. to date
follow u.
follow up intervention for normal development
forceps passed up through incision
freeing up of adhesion
head of bed up for shortness of breath
loss of ability to hold head u.
u. out of bed as tolerated
patient up ad lib
patient up in chair
timed up and go

upbeat torsional nystagmus

update
periodic safety update reporting
u. isolation technique

update isolation technique

updraft nebulizer

upgoing
plantar response u.
toes u.

upheaval
emotional u.

Upolu virus

upon
catheter coiled upon itself
regulated upon activation, normal T-cell expressed and secreted
repeated quick stretch superimposed upon an existing contraction
u. arrival patient found

upper
u. abdomen
u. abdominal area
u. abdominal flap
u. abdominal pain
u. abdominal surgery
acute upper gastrointestinal bleeding
acute upper gastrointestinal hemorrhage
u. aerodigestive
u. aerodigestive tract
u. airway
u. airway closing pressure
u. airway congestion
u. airway disease
u. airway disorder
u. airway obstruction
u. airway opening pressure
u. airway resistance
u. airway resistance syndrome
u. airway respiratory syndrome
u. airway sleep apnea
anterior upper spine
u. arm
u. arm flap
u. arm tourniquet
arterial arch of upper eyelid
artery of upper limb
bilateral upper dorsal sympathectomy
u. body ergometer
u. body segment to lower body segment ratio
both upper extremities
buccal of upper and lingual of lower
burning sensation in upper chest
u. chamber of heart
clubbing and cyanosis upper extremity
u. completely edentulous
complete upper and lower dentures
concurrent upper respiratory tract infection
u. confidence limit
Cupid's bow upper lip
diagonal 1, 2 upper extremity

upper *(continued)*
double-contrast barium examination of the upper gastrointestinal tract
early gastric cancer of the upper stomach
u. esophageal constriction
u. esophageal sphincter
u. esophageal sphincter pressure
u. esophageal sphincter relaxation
u. esophagus
expected upper limit
u. extremity
u. extremity arterial
u. extremity nerve block
u. extremity somatosensory evoked potential
u. eyelid
fluid spilling into upper abdomen
u. fossa active, medial knee pain, and short leg on the side ipsilateral to the weak fossa
full upper denture
full upper denture, partial lower denture
u. ganglion
u. gastrointestinal biopsy
u. gastrointestinal bleeding
u. gastrointestinal endoscopy
u. gastrointestinal series with small bowel follow-through
u. gastrointestinal tract hemorrhage
u. GI
u. GI lesion
u. GI series
u. gut
u. half
u. hand
heard best at left upper sternal border
u. hemianopia
u. hemibody irradiation
hump in upper back
u. impression
u. inner quadrant
intramuscular artery of upper extremity
u. jaw
u. jawbone
u. left
left upper eyelid
u. left quadrant
u. left sternal border
left upper arm
left upper extremity
left upper limb
left upper lobe
left upper lung
left upper outer buttock
left upper outer quadrant
left upper quadrant of abdomen
left upper scapular border
left upper sternal border
u. lid right eye
u. limb
u. limb orthosis
u. limb prosthesis
u. limb tension test
u. limits of normal
u. lip
u. lobe
u. lobe pulmonary edema
u. and lower
lower and upper extremities
u. and lower extremities within normal limits
lymph node of upper limb
maximum assistance for upper body dressing
median cleft upper lip, mental retardation, pugilistic facies syndrome
microcomputer upper limb exerciser
u. midclavicular line
middle upper arm circumference
minimal assistance for upper body dressing
u. motor neurogenic bladder
u. motor neuron
u. motor neuron lesion
muscle of upper extremity atrophic
Neville upper reservoir buffer
nonlingular branch of upper lobe bronchus
u. outer quadrant
outer upper left quadrant
outer upper right quadrant
u. partially edentulous
partial upper and lower dentures
patient independent in upper body dressing
u. pole of kidney
u. pole of uterine incision
pyorrhea around lower and upper teeth
Quality of U. Extremities Test
reactive upper airways dysfunction syndrome
recurrent upper respiratory tract infection
resistive exercises to upper extremities
u. respiratory
u. respiratory disease
u. respiratory obstruction
u. respiratory tract
u. respiratory tract illness
u. respiratory tract infection
u. rib cage
right u.
u. right
right upper eyelid
u. right quadrant
u. right sternal border
right upper extremity
right upper lateral
right upper limb
right upper lung
right upper medial
right upper outer quadrant
right upper pole
right upper quadrant of abdomen
right upper sternal border
secondary carcinoma of the upper mediastinum
u. segment
u. single tooth
sleep apnea-hypersomnolence syndrome associated with upper airway obstruction
slipped upper femoral epiphysis
somatic dysfunction upper extremity
u. third of long bone
u. thoracic
u. tibial osteotomy
times upper limit of normal
vaccination scar upper left arm
u. yield point

upright
u. chest film
u. film of abdomen
long double upright brace
u. peripheral plasma renin activity
u. posture
short double u.
supine and u.

upset
intestinal u.

upstream
u. activating sequence
chicken ovalbumin upstream promoter
u. regulatory region

upstroke
carotid u.
delayed u.
u. pattern on apex cardiogram
u. velocity

uptake
absolute iodine u.
amine precursor uptake and decarboxylation cell
amine uptake and decarboxylation cell
area of increased u.
asymmetric limb u.
brain uptake index
diffused lung u.
duroxide u.
fibrinogen uptake test
functional uptake of carbon monoxide
glucose u.
increased uptake of isotope
insulin-mediated glucose u.
maximum oxygen u.
minute oxygen u.
myocardial substrate u.
^{13}N ammonia u.
net hepatic glucose u.
oleic acid uptake test
oxygen uptake efficiency slope
peak oxygen u.
peripheral glucose u.
precursor u.
radioactive fibrinogen u.
radioactive iodine u.
radioiodine u.
radioisotope uptake study
serum resin triiodothyronine u.
standardized uptake value
standard uptake value
^{99m}Tc MDP u.
technetium-99m MDP u.
thyroidal radioactive iodine uptake test
thyroid uptake gradient
thyroid uptake scan
T_3 resin u.
triiodothyronine resin u.
triiodothyronine uptake ratio

up-to-date
immunizations u.-t.-d.
tetanus toxoid u.-t.-d.

upward
blunt dissection carried u.
conjugate upward gaze
u. gaze
u. gaze weakness
nystagmus on upward gaze
paralysis of conjugate upward gaze

urachal
u. cyst
u. fistula
u. fold
u. ligament

urachus
patent u.

uracil
arginine, hypoxanthine, and u.
u. deoxyriboside
u. mustard

uranium

urate
monosodium u.
monosodium urate monohydrate
monosodium urate monohydrate crystal
sodium urate crystal

uratic iritis

urban
National U. League

urea
blood u.
blood urea nitrogen/creatinine ratio
u. breath test
carbon-13 urea breath test
carbon-14 urea breath test
u. clearance
u. cycle enzymopathy
u. dialysance
dialysate urea kinetic modeling
dialysate urea nitrogen
dialysis/plasma urea ratio
dichloral u.
electrolytes, blood urea nitrogen, and serum creatinine
equivalent residual renal urea clearance
u. formaldehyde
u. formaldehyde foam insulation
high-dose urea in invert sugar
u. kinetic modeling
low-dose urea in invert sugar
maximal rate of urea synthesis
u. nitrogen
percent reduction in u.
peritoneal dialysis urea removal
plasma urea nitrogen
u. reduction ratio
time-averaged urea concentration
u. transporter
urinary concentration of u.
urinary urea nitrogen excretion
urine urea nitrogen

urease
locally made rapid urease test
rapid urease test

uremia
alcohol, epilepsy, insulin, overdose, uremia, trauma, infection, psychiatric, stroke
atypical hemolytic uremia syndrome
eclampsia due to u.
extrarenal u.
perforating disorder of u.
prerenal u.
u. and sepsis

uremic
u. acidosis
acute hemolytic uremic syndrome
aplastic uremic osteodystrophy
aseptic uremic meningitis
u. colitis
u. coma
hemolytic uremic syndrome/thrombotic thrombocytopenia purpura
u. medullary cystic disease
microangiopathic hemolytic uremic syndrome
mixed uremic osteodystrophy
u. retinitis
thrombotic thrombocytopenic purpura and hemolytic uremic syndrome

ureter
atonic u.
atretic u.
congenital absence of u.
corkscrew u.
dilatation of u.
implantation of ureter into rectum
moderately dilated u.
muscular coat of u.
muscular layer of u.
obstruction of u.
partially duplicated u.
patent u.
pelvis, calix and u.
proximal u.

ureteral
antegrade ureteral drainage
antegrade ureteral stenting
antireflux ureteral implantation technique
aperistaltic distal ureteral segment

ureteral *(continued)*
u. atresia
u. back pressure
bilateral ureteral obstruction
u. branch
u. calculus
u. colic
u. dilatation
u. ectopia
iatrogenic ureteral injury
u. implant
u. implantation
u. implant material
LeDuc ureteral anastomosis
left u.
left ureteral orifice
u. orifice
percutaneous ureteral dilatation
percutaneous ureteral stent
u. ridge
right ureteral orifice
u. stent
u. stone
unilateral ureteral obstruction
unilateral ureteral occlusion

ureteric
u. branch of inferior suprarenal artery
u. branch of ovarian artery
u. branch of renal artery

ureterocystoplasty
augmentation u.

ureterogram
retrograde u.

ureteroileocutaneous anastomosis

ureterolithiasis
proximal u.

ureterolithotomy
proximal u.

ureterolithotripsy
transurethral u.

ureteroneocystostomy
Lich-Gregoire u.

ureteropelvic junction

ureteropelvioplasty
Scardino u.

ureterorenoscopy
transurethral u.

ureterosacral
laparoscopic resection of the ureterosacral ligament

ureteroscope
flexible u.

ureterostomy
bilateral ureterostomy takedown
cutaneous u.

ureterovesical
u. angle
u. junction
u. obstruction

ureters
kidneys, ureters, bladder x-ray
kidneys, ureters, and spleen x-ray

urethane dimethacrylate

urethra
angle of inclination of u.
anterior u.
Gram stain of u.
granular stricture of u.
low-pressure u.
membranous u.
mucosa of female u.
mucosa of male u.
muscular coat of female u.
muscular coat of intermediate part of male u.
muscular coat of prostatic u.
muscular coat of spongy part of male u.
muscular layer of female u.
muscular layer of intermediate part of male u.
muscular layer of prostatic u.
narrowed u.
navicular fossa of male u.
obstruction of u.
penile u.
posterior u.
prolapse of urethra and bladder
prostatic u.
spongy layer of female u.

urethral
acute urethral syndrome
u. angle
anterior urethral injury
anterior urethral valve
u. artery
artificial urethral sphincter
Bartholin, Skene, and urethral glands
Bartholin, urethral, and Skene glands, and external genitalia
u. calculus
u. caruncle
u. catheter in
u. catheterization
u. catheter out
u. and cervical cultures
u. closure pressure
u. closure pressure profile
u. crest
u. cyst
u. dilatation
u. dilation
u. discharge
distal urethral stenosis
u. duplication
external urethral meatus
external urethral orifice
external urethral sphincter
u. function
functional urethral length
u. gland
glansplasty in situ tubularization of urethral plate
glanuloplasty in situ tubularization of urethral plate
u. hematuria
u. incompetence
indwelling urethral catheter
internal urethral meatus
internal urethral orifice
low urethral pressure
u. manipulation syndrome
maximal urethral pressure
maximum urethral closure pressure
u. meatal stenosis
u. meatus
medicated urethral system
u. opening
patulous urethral wall
posterior urethral injury
posterior urethral valve type I–IV
u. pressure profilometry
u. resistance factor
u. stenosis
u. stricture
u. swab
total urethral discharge
transperineal urethral resection
voiding urethral pressure measurement

urethralis
annulus u.
anulus u.
arteria u.

urethritica
arthritis u.

urethritis
delirium, infection, atrophic urethritis and vaginitis, pharmaceuticals, psychological disorders, excessive urine output, restricted mobility, stool impaction

gonococcal u.
Neisseria gonorrhoeae u.
nongonococcal u.
nonspecific u.
postgonococcal u.

urethrocystometry
direct electronic u.

urethrogram
cystoscopy and voiding u.
retrograde u.

urethrography
retrograde u.

urethropexy
retropubic u.

urethroplasty
mesh graft u.
patch graft u.
pedicle flap u.

urethrotomy
direct vision internal u.
optical internal u.
visual internal u.

urge
anomalous sexual u.
cravings and u.'s
u. incontinence

urgency
frequency and urgency of urination
hypertensive u.
sensory u.
urinary urgency and frequency

urgent
u. care center
u. care clinic
very u.
u. visit center

uric
u. acid
u. acid calculus
u. acid infarct
u. acid nitrogen
u. acid urine spot test
blood uric acid
serum uric acid

uridine
cyclic uridine 3,′5′-monophosphate
u. diphosphate
u. 5′-diphosphate
u. diphosphate-galactose-4-epimerase deficiency
u. diphosphate glucuronosyltransferase
u. diphosphogalactose
u. diphosphoglucose
u. diphosphoglucuronic acid
u. diphosphoglucuronyl transferase
u. 5′-monophosphate
u. monophosphate kinase
u. triphosphate
u. 5′-triphosphate

uridylic acid

uridyltransferase

urinal
assist with u.

urinalysis, pl. **urinalyses**
clean-catch midstream u.
elements on u.
fractional u.
u. and microscopy
midstream u.
routine u.
u., routine and microscopic

urinary
u. abnormality
u. abscess
acute urinary retention
u. albumin excretion
u. aldosterone
u. ammonium
u. amylase
apex of urinary bladder
artificial urinary sphincter
artificial urinary sphincter implantation
u. ascites
asymptomatic urinary lithiasis
asymptomatic urinary tract infection
atonic urinary bladder
u. basic fetoprotein
u. beta-core fragment
u. bladder
u. bladder adenocarcinoma
u. bladder atony
u. bladder calculus
u. bladder capacity
u. bladder fistula
u. bladder hernia
u. bladder rupture
u. bladder tumor
u. bladder wall mass
u. bladder wall thickening
u. burning
calcium phosphate urinary lithiasis
u. calcium volume excretion rate
u. calculus
Candida urinary tract infection
u. care unit
u. cast
u. catheter
u. catheter in
u. catheter out
catheter-related urinary tract infection
u. chorionic gonadotropin
chronic urinary retention
chronic urinary tract infection
closed urinary drainage bag with drip chamber
u. concentration of sodium
u. concentration of urea
congenital urinary tract deformities
u. coproporphyrin
u. coproporphyrin test
u. C-peptide
cumulative urinary excretion
device-related urinary tract infection
u. diagnostic index
difficulty initiating urinary stream
difficulty in starting urinary stream
distended urinary bladder
dynamic urinary graciloplasty
u. excretion of protein
external urinary device
u. fistula
u. flow
u. follicle-stimulating hormone
u. free cortisol
free monoclonal urinary light chain
u. frequency
frequent urinary incontinence
u. FSH
genuine stress urinary incontinence
u. glucose
u. gonadotropin fragment
u. gonadotropin peptide
gravity urinary incontinence
u. hemorrhage
u. hesitancy
hospital-acquired urinary tract infection
human u.
human urinary CSF
human urinary follicle-stimulating hormone
human urinary kallikrein
u. incontinence
increased urinary flow
increasing urinary excretion
indwelling urinary catheter
u. kallikrein

urinary *(continued)*
kidneys and urinary bladder
lower urinary tract
lower urinary tract cancer
lower urinary tract dysfunction
lower urinary tract infection
lower urinary tract obstruction
lower urinary tract symptom
lower urinary tract tumor
u. luteinizing hormone
magnesium ammonium phosphate urinary lithiasis
u. magnesium volume
major urinary protein
maximal urinary concentration
maximal urinary flow rate
maximal urinary osmolality
menopausal urinary gonadotropin
micturition urinary incontinence
milk of calcium urinary tract cyst
minimize or delay urinary incontinence
Mitrofanoff continent urinary stoma
u. muramidase activity
muscular coat of urinary bladder
muscular layer of urinary bladder
u. nitrogen
u. nitrogen appearance
nocturnal urinary frequency
nocturnal urinary incontinence
noninvasive assessment of urinary flow
u. norepinephrine
normal urinary function
nosocomial urinary tract infection
u. osmolality
u. output
u. potassium volume excretion rate
u. production rate
u. reflux
u. retention
u. sodium excretion
starting and stopping of urinary stream
strained urinary sediment
u. stress incontinence
stress urinary incontinence
symptomatic urinary tract infection
u. titrable acidity
total urinary gonadotropin
total urinary nitrogen
u. tract anomaly
u. tract candidiasis
u. tract infection
u. tract infection cleared
u. tract malformation
u. trypsin inhibitor
u. urea nitrogen excretion
u. urgency and frequency
u. volume
u. washings
WHO classification for transitional cell carcinoma of the urinary bladder: stages Ta through T4

urinary-derived human follicle-stimulating hormone

urinate
painful inability to u.
total inability to u.

urination
burning on u.
dribbling at end of u.
dribbling on u.
frequency and urgency of u.
increased frequency of u.
interruption of flow of u.
pain during u.
pain on u.
salivation, lacrimation, urination, defecation, gastrointestinal distress and emesis

urine
abnormally high concentration of u.
u. acid output
adequate urine output
u. aliquot
amylase urine spot test
u. analysis
bacteria in u.
barium sediment in u.
calcium-urine spot test
u. cast
catheterized urine specimen
change in urine flow from constipation
clean-catch midstream u.
clean, midstream u.
u. collection
u. collection device
u. collection pads
u. concentrate
u. concentration
concentration of insulin in u.
u. creatinine
creatinine urine spot test
u. culture
u. culture and sensitivity
u. cytology
delirium, infection, atrophic urethritis and vaginitis, pharmaceuticals, psychological disorders, excessive urine output, restricted mobility, stool impaction
diabetic u.
u. dipstick
u. diribose phosphate
drug abuse u.
u. drug panel
u. drug screen
early morning specimen of u.
effluxed clear u.
u. electrolytes
u. filtration rate
first morning u.
first-void u.
forensic urine drug testing
foul-smelling u.
fractional u.'s
u. free cortisol
u. glucose
u. glucose ketone
u. glucose spot test
Gram stain of UN spun u.
green urine from antidepressant
u. hazy
24-hour urine collection
hourly fetal urine production rate
human u.
u. immunoelectrophoresis
u. immunofixation electrophoresis
inability to control u.
inability to pass u.
incontinence of u.
increased urine osmolality
initial urine specimen
interrupted urine flow
involuntary discharge of u.
involuntary dribbling of u.
iron in u.
low urine pH
maple syrup urine disease
Micral urine dipstick test
Micral urine test strip
midstream clean-catch u.
midstream clean-catch urine culture
midstream specimen of u.
midstream urine sample
midstream urine specimen
midvoid urine specimen
u. net charge
normal urine flow
normal urine output

N-telopeptide urine test
oasthouse urine disease
osmolality u.
u. osmolality
osmolality urine spot test
osmolarity of blood and u.
u. output
passage of dark brown u.
patient incontinent of u.
pediatric urine collector
u. pH
porphyrin in u.
postvoid dribbling of u.
u. potassium
potassium in 24-hour u.
u. pregnancy test
pregnancy urine hormone
u. protein
u. protein electrophoresis
purple urine bag syndrome
pus in u.
random u.
rat urine protein
residual u.
residual urine volume
routine urine analysis
sodium and potassium spot urine test
u. specimen after prostate massage
u. specimen before prostate massage
u. specimen volume measuring device
u. specimen volume measuring system
u. sterile on culture
sterile urine culture
total solids in u.
total volume of u.
u. toxicology screen
u. urea nitrogen
uric acid urine spot test
u. urobilinogen
u. uroporphyrin
voiding urine cytology
u. volume
weak of interrupted urine stream

urine-plasma ratio

urobilin icterus

urobilinogen
fecal u.
urine u.

urobilinogen—2 hours

urocanic acid

urodynamic
ambulatory u.'s
u. assessment
u. evaluation
u. flow study
u. testing

urogenital
u. atrophy
u. cleft
u. diaphragm
u. disorder
U. Distress Inventory
u. fistula
u. sinus
u. tract
u. vestibule

urogenitalis
apparatus u.

urogram
constant infusion excretory u.
excretory u.
infusion u.
intravenous u.
micturating u.
retrograde u.

urography
excretory u.
intravenous u.
magnetic resonance u.
percutaneous antegrade u.

urokinase
2-chain urokinase plasminogen activator
u. intracoronary
u. plasminogen activator
u. plasminogen activator receptor
recombinant u.

urokinase-type plasminogen activator

urolithiasis
asymptomatic u.
recurrent calcium u.

urologic
feline urologic syndrome

Urological
National Kidney and Urological Diseases Information Clearinghouse

urologic disease

urology
gynecologic u.

uronate
macromolecular u.

uropathy
lower obstructive u.
obstructive u.

uroporphyrin
u. isomerase
urine u.

uroporphyrinogen
u. decarboxylase
u. synthase
u. synthetase

urostomy
Assura convex urostomy pouch

urothelial
u. basement membrane
u. carcinoma

urothelium
neoplastic u.
seromuscular enterocystoplasty lined with u.

ursodeoxycholic acid

urticaria
acquired cold u.
acute allergic u.
chronic idiopathic u.
contact u.
contact urticaria syndrome
delayed pressure u.
dermodistortive u.
u. hemorrhagica
hypocomplementemic vasculitis urticaria syndrome
immunological contact u.
nonallergic contact u.
nonimmunologic contact u.
u. pigmentosa
recall u.
solar u.

urticarial
hypocomplementemic urticarial vasculitis syndrome
minimal urticarial dose
pruritic urticarial papules and plaques
pruritic urticarial papules and plaques of pregnancy
u. rash
u. reaction

urticatus
lichen u.

Urucuri virus

usage
Alcohol U. Questionnaire
hard drug u.
heavy alcohol u.

usage *(continued)*
intravenous u.
women years of u.
Working Formulation for Clinical U.

use
adolescent drug u.
age at onset of u.
Alcohol U. Disorders Identification Test
alcohol-related use disorder, not otherwise specified
alcohol use disorder
alcohol use inventory
alternate u.'s test
amount of u.
antibiotic use and abuse
anxiolytic use disorder
autism, dementia, ataxia, loss of purposeful hand use syndrome
cannabis use disorder
curb intravenous use of drugs
drug use evaluation
drug use monitoring
drug use review
excessive drug u.
for external use only
fatal complications of illicit drug u.
heat, absence of use, redness, pain, pus, swelling
history of pathological u.
history of tobacco u.
illegal intravenous drug u.
illicit drug u.
illicit substance u.
improper use of prescription
for internal use only
intravenous drug u.
long-term catheter u.
long-term heavy u.
maternal cocaine u.
measure of resource u.
medication use evaluation
oral contraceptive u.
polysubstance use and abuse
provocative use test
psychoactive substance use disorder
recreational drug u.
substance use disorder

useful field of view

user
casual drug u.
hard alcoholic u.
heavy alcohol u.
injecting drug u.
injection drug u.
number user identification
serenity, tranquility, peace u. term for dimethoxymethylamphetamine

U-shaped incision

Usher syndrome

using
contrast chromoscopy using indigo carmine
longitudinal expert evaluation using all available data
MRCP using HASTE with a phased array coil
oxygen saturation as measured using pulse oximetry
segmental correction using spine reconstruction
segmental correction using x-ray measurement

usual
u. anatomic position
u. body weight
u. care
u. childhood diseases
u. childhood illnesses
u. and customary
u., customary, and reasonable fees
u. diseases of childhood
u. interstitial pneumonia
u. interstitial pneumonia of Liebow
u. interstitial pneumonitis
loss of interest in usual activity
patient is prepped and draped in usual sterile fashion
u. place of residence
u. provider continuity
u. throat flora
u. type papillary carcinoma

Usutu virus

Utah
U. Test of Language Development
Wender Utah Rating Scale

uterina
arteria u.
pars uterina placentae

uterine
abnormal uterine bleeding
u. activity
u. activity integral
u. activity unit
u. adenocarcinoma
ambulatory uterine contraction test
ampulla of uterine tube
u. anomaly
anterior lip of uterine os
u. appendage
u. artery
u. artery embolization
u. aspiration
u. atony
u. balloon therapy
balloon uterine elevator cannula
u. bleeding
u. blood flow
u. body
u. calculus
u. canal
u. cavity
u. colic
u. compression syndrome
u. contraction
u. cornual access catheter
u. cramping
u. cry
u. curetting
diffuse symmetrical uterine enlargement
u. distention
dorsal uterine artery
u. dysfunction
dysfunctional uterine bleeding
u. dysmenorrhea
u. endometrial carcinoma
u. enlargement
essential uterine hemorrhage
estrogen-agonist uterine effect
u. evacuation
evacuation of uterine contents
u. evaluation
extra uterine life
u. fibroid
fimbriae of uterine tube
functional uterine bleeding
u. fundus
u. hemorrhage
u. hernia
home uterine activity monitor
home uterine activity monitoring
home uterine monitoring
horizontal uterine incision
u. horn
u. hyperplasia
hypertonic uterine dysfunction
u. hypotonia

u. incision
u. infection
u. insufficiency
irregular uterine bleeding
u. irritability
left uterine displacement device
u. leiomyosarcoma
u. lining
lower uterine segment transverse cesarean section
low transverse uterine incision
low vertical uterine incision
u. malposition
manipulator-injector
u. manipulator-injector
u. mass
middle uterine artery
midline vertical uterine extension
mixed uterine tumor
mouse uterine weight unit
u. muscle tone
muscular coat of uterine tube
muscular layer of uterine tube
u. myoma
u. myomectomy
u. necrosis
u. neoplasm
noncommunicating uterine horn
u. ostial access catheter
ovarian branch of uterine artery
u. papillary serous carcinoma
u. positioning via ligament investment fixation truncation
precancerous overgrowth of uterine lining
pregnancy uterine, undelivered
u. progesterone system
u. prolapse
u. resting tone
Rowden uterine manipulator-injector
u. rupture
u. sarcoma
u. suspension
symptomatic uterine prolapse
third-degree uterine prolapse
u. tumor resembling an ovarian sex-cord tumor
upper pole of uterine incision
u. vacuum aspirating curette
vacuum uterine cannula
vertical uterine incision
Zinnanti uterine manipulator-injector

uterine-relaxing factor

uterine-stimulating potency

utero
dead fetus in u.
death in u.
ex utero intrapartum tracheloplasty
ex utero intrapartum treatment
fetal death in u.
in u.
in utero drug exposure

uteroplacental
u. insufficiency
u. ischemia

uterosacral
laser uterosacral nerve ablation
u. ligament

uterotropic
human placental uterotropic hormone

uterotubal junction

uterovaginal fistula

uterovesical
u. fold
u. ligament

uterque
auris u.
oculi u.
visio oculus uterque

uterus
adenocarcinoma of the uterus with sarcomatous overgrowth
anatomical internal os of u.
anomalous u.
anteflexed u.
u. anteflexed
anterior lip of external os of u.
anteversion of u.
anteverted u.
aplastic u.
arbor vitae u.
arcuate u.
arcuatus u.
artery of round ligament of u.
asymmetric u.
AV/AF u.
bicornuate u.
boggy u.
calcified leiomyoma of u.
cauterize lining of u.
cervical ganglion of u.
configuration of u.
cornual position of u.
dehiscence of u.
u. delivery
dextrorotation of u.
u. didelphys
external os of u.
extirpation of uterus and cervix
firm and midline u.
fundal portion of u.
gravid u.
u. has good support
horn of u.
leiomyoma of u.
liposarcoma of u.
masculine u.
membrane of cervix u.
muscular coat of u.
normal size, shape, and position, anteverted and anteflexed u.
one-horned u.
outer border of the u.
perforated u.
placenta, ovaries, u.
pregnant u.
procidentia of u.
prolapse of u.
retroflexed u.
retroverted u.
ruptured u.
u. symmetrical in contour
tipped u.
u. unicornis

utility
Health U.'s Index
Massachusetts General Hospital U. Multi-Programming System

utilization
antibiotic utilization review
apparent oxygen u.
Dental Auxiliary U.
u. healthcare
Hospital U. Project
U. Information Service
local cerebral glucose u.
malonate utilization test
U. Management
medical resource u.
net nitrogen u.
net protein u.
online prospective drug utilization review
oxygen u.
quality assurance and utilization review
resource utilization group
Test of Concept U.

Utinga virus

utricle
macula of u.
maculae of utricle and saccule

utriculi
macula u.

utriculosaccularis
maculae u.

utterance
extended length of u.
gradual increase in length and complexity of u.
u. length
mean length of u.
mean relational u.
voluntary control of involuntary utterances

Uukuniemi virus

uveae
congenital ectropion u.
ectropion u.

uveal
u. atrophy
u. staphyloma

uvealis
pars u.

uveitis
acute anterior u.
chronic anterior u.
experimental autoimmune u.
u., glaucoma, hyphema syndrome
nongranulomatous anterior u.
optical coherence tomography in u.
tubulointerstitial nephritis and uveitis syndrome

uvula, pl. **uvulae**
Lieutaud u.
musculus uvulae
musculus azygos uvulae
palatine u.

uvulopalatoplasty
Bovie-assisted u.
laser u.
laser-assisted u.

vaccinated
not v.

vaccination
anticytokine v.
influenza v.
nucleic acid v.
pneumonia v.
v. scar
v. scar upper left arm
smallpox v.

vaccine
acellular pertussis vaccine with diphtheria and tetanus toxoid
allogeneic tumor cell v.
alum-precipitated v.
anti-acquired immune deficiency syndrome v.
antipertussis acellular v.
autologous tumor v.
bacille Calmette-Guérin v.
v. body
Children's V. Initiative
cold-adapted influenza virus vaccine, trivalent
cold-attenuated intranasal influenza v.
dengue fever v.
diphtheria, pertussis, and tetanus v.
diphtheria, pertussis, tetanus, poliomyelitis, and measles v.
diphtheria, tetanus, pertussis, *Haemophilus influenzae* type b v.
diphtheria, tetanus toxoid, and acellular pertussis v.
diphtheria, tetanus toxoids, whole-cell pertussis v.
duck embryo origin v.
Eastern and Western encephalomyelitis v.
Edmonston-Zagreb high-titer v.
enhanced inactivated polio v.
Escherichia coli heat-labile toxin v.
Haemophilus b conjugate v.
Haemophilus influenzae type b conjugate v.
Haemophilus influenzae type b polysaccharide v.
Haemophilus influenzae type b vaccine, PRP-D conjugate v.
Haemophilus influenzae type b vaccine, PRP-OMP conjugate v.
Haemophilus influenzae type b vaccine, PRP-T conjugate v.
Haemophilus influenzae type vaccine oligosaccharide-CRM197 vaccine conjugate
Haemophilus pertussis v.
Helicobacter pylori v.
hepatitis A, B, C, E, G v.
hepatitis B oligosaccharide-CRM197 v.
human diploid cell v.
inactivated polio v.
inactivated poliovirus v.
infectious bronchitis v.
influenza virion vaccine, split virion
influenza virion vaccine, whole virion
influenza virus, attenuated live v.
influenza virus inactivated v.
influenza virus inactivated vaccine, split virion, types A, B, trivalent
V. Information Statement
intradermal typhoid and paratyphoid v.
Japanese encephalitis virus v.
killed measles virus v.
killed polio v.
Klebsiella v.
Lactobacillus acidophilus v.
la Peste v.
leishmaniasis v.
live v.
live-attenuated lentiviral v.
live-attenuated virus v.
live oral poliovirus v.
live varicella v.
live vector v.
low virulence v.
lungworm v.
Lyme disease v.
v. lymph
malaria v.
measles, mumps, and rubella v.
measles and rubella v.
melanoma whole-cell v.
melioidosis *Pseudomonas pseudomallei* v.
meningococcal *Neisseria meningitidis* serogroups unspecified v.
meningococcal polysaccharide v.
mixed respiratory v.
mixed vaccine, respiratory infection
modified vaccine virus Ankara
monoclonal antibody anticancer v.
monovalent oral polio virus v.
Moraxella catarrhalis v.
mumps virus v.
mumps virus vaccine Jeryl Lynn strain
naked DNA vector v.
nervous tissue v.
nonvalent pneumococcal conjugate v.
oral attenuated poliomyelitis virus v.
oral attenuated poliovirus v.
oral attenuated *Salmonella typhi* v.
oral polio v.
oral poliovirus v.
oral tetravalent rotavirus v.
parainfluenza paramyxovirus v.
Pasteur Institute bacillus Calmette-Guérin v.
pertussis, acellular antigens, v.
pertussis, whole-cell antigens, v.
pneumococcal conjugate v.
pneumococcal polysaccharide v.
pneumococcal 7-valent conjugate v.
pneumococcus v.
polio v.
poliomyelitis live v.
poliomyelitis vaccine inactivated
poliomyelitis vaccine killed
poliovirus vaccine monovalent oral
poliovirus vaccine trivalent oral
polysaccharide tetanus conjugate v.
rabies vaccine adsorbed
rabies vaccine, duck embryo culture
rabies vaccine, human diploid cell culture
rabies vaccine, purified chick embryo cell culture
Rhesus diploid cell strain rabies v.
rhesus rotavirus-tetravalent v.
rheumatic fever v.
Rocky Mountain spotted fever v.
rubella v.
serogroup C meningococcal v.
v. serotype
swine flu v.
tetanus-pertussis v.
trivalent oral poliovirus v.
typhoid vaccine, acetone-killed and dried
typhoid vaccine, attenuated live
typhoid-paratyphoid v.

V

vaccine *(continued)*
typhoid, paratyphoid A, B, C v.
typhoid, paratyphoid A, B, tetanus toxoid, and diphtheria toxoid v.
typhoid vaccine, heat and phenol inactivated, dried
typhoid vaccine, not otherwise specified
typhoid vaccine, Vi capsular polysaccharide
typhus *Rickettsiae* species v.
varicella chickenpox varicella zoster virus v.
varicella-zoster virus v.
Venezuelan equine encephalitis vaccine, attenuated live
Venezuelan equine encephalitis vaccine, inactivated
whooping cough v.
yellow fever v.

vaccine-associated
v.-a. paralytic polio
v.-a. paralytic poliomyelitis

vaccine-induced immunity

vaccinia
v. immunoglobulin
New York vaccinia virus
v. virus

vaccinia-immune globulin

vaccinial
ocular vaccinial conjunctivitis

vacuo
ex vacuo dilatation
hydrocephalus ex v.
hydrocephalus ex vacuo change

vacuolar
AIDS-associated vacuolar myelopathy

vacuolated cell

vacuolating
rabbit kidney vacuolating virus
simian vacuolating virus 40
v. toxin gene A

vacuolation
neuronal v.

vacuolative
papilloma virus, polyoma virus, vacuolative virus

vacuole
autophagic v.
parasitophorous v.

vacuolization
cytoplasmic v.
fatty v.
marrow cell v.

vacuum
v. aspiration
v. constriction device
v. curettage
v. erection device
v. extraction
v. extraction delivery
v. extractor
v. headache
high v.
manual vacuum aspiration
Marshall-Taylor vacuum extraction
permeability of v.
polyethylene vacuum cup
v. tube
v. tuberculin
v. tube voltmeter
ultrahigh v.
v. ultraviolet
v. uterine cannula
uterine vacuum aspirating curette
v. vaginal delivery

vacuum-assisted
v.-a. closure dressing
v.-a. core biopsy

vagabonds' disease

vagal
v. accessory nerve
v. action
adrenergic vagal function
anterior gastric branch of anterior vagal trunk
anterior vagal trunk
v. attack
v. bradycardia
dorsal vagal nucleus
inferior vagal ganglion
postganglionic vagal stimulation
v. reaction
v. response
v. stimulation
superior vagal ganglion
v. tone

vagi

vagina
anterior fornix of v.
anterior wall of v.
apex of v.
AP inversion stress vagina view
v. bulbi
congenital absence of v.
v., ectocervix, and endocervix
muscular coat of v.
muscular layer of v.
nothing per v.
passage of flatus per v.
posterior cul-de-sac of v.
spongy layer of v.
vulva and v.

vaginal
laparoscopic-assisted vaginal hysteroscopy

vaginal
abnormal vaginal bleeding
v. acidity
allantoin vaginal cream
v. anomaly
anterior vaginal fornix
anterior vaginal trunk
v. apex
artificial vaginal epithelium
v. atresia
atrophic vaginal mucosa
v. atrophy
v. birth after cesarean section
v. birth after cesarean—trial of labor
v. bleeding
bloody vaginal discharge
v. breech delivery
v. canal
v. cancer
v. cervical endocervical smear
v. cone biopsy
v. contraceptive film
v. cuff
v. culture
v. delivery
v. delivery after cesarean
dysfunctional vaginal bleeding
epiurethral suprapubic vaginal suspension
v. examination
v. flora
v. fluid ferning
v. fold
frank vaginal breech delivery
heavy vaginal discharge
v. hemorrhage
v. hernia
v. hysterectomy
v. inclusion cyst
v. infection
v. intercourse
v. interruption of pregnancy with dilatation and curettage
v. intraepithelial dysplasia
v. intraepithelial neoplasia
v. intraepithelial neoplasm
v. introitus
irregular vaginal bleeding

v. irrigation
v. irrigation smear
v. irritation
v. itch
v. itching
itchy, whitish vaginal discharge
v. laceration
laparoscopic-assisted vaginal hysterectomy
lateral vaginal wall
v. lesion
v. ligament
low-dose vaginal estrogen
v. lubricant
v. lumen
midforceps vaginal delivery
Monistat-3 vaginal suppository
v. mucosa
normal spontaneous vaginal birth
normal vaginal delivery
v. opening
operative vaginal delivery
persistent vaginal cornification
posterior vaginal hernia
posterior vaginal wall
v. prolapse
prolapsed vaginal wall
relaxed vaginal outlet
repair relaxed vaginal outlet
Schauta radical vaginal hysterectomy
v. smear
v. speculum
spontaneous assisted vaginal delivery
spontaneous vertex vaginal delivery
sterile elective low forceps vaginal delivery
sterile indicated low forceps vaginal delivery
sterile low midforceps vaginal delivery
sterile spontaneous controlled vaginal delivery
sterile, spontaneous vaginal delivery
sterile vaginal examination
subcutaneous v.
v. suppository
tension-free vaginal tape
total vaginal hysterectomy
traumatic vaginal delivery
unsterile controlled vaginal delivery
unsterile uncontrolled vaginal delivery
vacuum vaginal delivery
v. varicose vein
v. vault
v. vault repair
v. vertex delivery
v. wall sling
v. yeast infection

vaginalis
arteria v.
autogenous tunica vaginalis graft
malignant mesothelioma of the tunica v.
parietal layer of tunica vaginalis of testis
patent processus v.
Trichomonas v.
tunica vaginalis testis

vaginitis
bacterial v.
delirium, infection, atrophic urethritis and vaginitis, pharmaceuticals, psychological disorders, excessive urine output, restricted mobility, stool impaction
infectious pustular v.
nonspecific v.

vaginolabial hernia

vaginoperineal fistula

vaginopexy
Norman Miller v.

vaginosis
bacterial v.

vaginotomy
anterior v.

vagotomy
v. and antrectomy
v. and Billroth gastroenterostomy
v. and gastroenterotomy
hemigastrectomy and v.
highly selective v.
parietal cell v.
proximal gastric v.
v. and pyloroplasty
pyloroplasty and v.
selective gastric v.
selective proximal v.
selective vagotomy with antrectomy
selective vagotomy with pyloroplasty
truncal v.
truncal vagotomy plus pyloroplasty
truncal vagotomy plus antrectomy

vagovagal spasm

vague
v. abdominal complaints
v. abdominal pain
delusions with vague conspiracy
v. obsessional thoughts

vagus
anterior pulmonary branch of vagus nerve
v. area
auricular branch of vagus nerve
communicating branch of glossopharyngeal nerve with auricular branch of vagus nerve
dorsal motor nucleus of v.
inferior ganglion of vagus nerve
jugular ganglion of vagus nerve
lower ganglion of vagus nerve
meningeal branch of vagus nerve
v. nerve
v. nerve palsy
v. nerve paralysis
v. nerve stimulation
pharyngeal branch of vagus nerve
superior ganglion of vagus nerve

valence bond

7-valent pneumococcal conjugate

valerate
estradiol v.

valeric acid

valgum
idiopathic genu v.

valgus
adolescent hallux v.
anatomic genu v.
v. deformity
hallux v.
hallux valgus angle
hallux valgus deformity
hallux valgus orthosis
Mayo hallux valgus modified operation
McBride bunion hallux valgus operation
McBride hallux valgus reduction
Mitchell hallux valgus procedure
obligatory heel v.
v. strain
v. stress test
transtrochanteric valgus osteotomy

valgus-varus stress test

validation
consensual validation consent
v. therapy

validity
ethical validity of assisted suicide
V. Indicator Profile

valise handle graft

vallecula
epiglottic v.

valley
Murray Valley encephalitis virus
Murray V. rash
Pahvant V. fever
Pahvant V. plague
peak and v.
Rift V. fever virus
San Joaquin V. disease

valproate
fetal valproate syndrome

valproic acid

Valsalva
heat, steam, gum, yawn, and Valsalva maneuver
V. leak point pressure
V. maneuver
V. procedure
ruptured sinus of Valsalva aneurysm

value
Allport-Vernon-Linzey Study of V.'s
alpha beta v.
Astrup blood gas v.
attenuation value on MRI scan
biologic v.
California Relative V. Studies
core v.'s
critical v.
crossover v.
derived value on apex cardiogram
expected v.
expected value of clinical information
high biological value protein
V.'s Inventory for Children
iodine v.
law of initial v.
log reduction v.
low biological v.
Maferr Inventory of Masculine V.'s
mean clinical v.
mean scale v.
negative predictive v.
normal v.
ocular hemodynamic v.
Ohio Work V.'s Inventory
Organizational V. Dimensions Questionnaire
Personal V.'s Abstract
Personal V.'s Inventory
physiologic full v.
positive predictive v.
predictive value of a negative test
predictive value of a positive test
pulse value recording
reference v.
reinforcement v.
relative value guide
relative value scale
relative value schedule
relative value study
relative value unit
resource-based relative value scale
Risk-Taking, Attitude, V.'s Inventory
Rokeach V. Survey
significance probability v.
singular value decomposition
standardized uptake v.
standard uptake v.
Survey of Interpersonal V.'s
Temperament and V.'s Inventory
tenth value layer radiation
threshold limit v.

valve
v. ablation
anterior cusp of left atrioventricular v.
anterior cusp of mitral v.
anterior cusp of right atrioventricular v.
anterior cusp of tricuspid v.
anterior leaflet of the mitral v.
anterior mitral valve leaflet
anterior motion of posterior mitral valve leaflet
anterior nasal v.
anterior semilunar v.
anterior tricuspid valve leaflet
anterior urethral v.
antibiotic-sterilized aortic valve homograft
antisiphon v.
v. anulus
aortic valve anulus
aortic valve area
aortic valve atresia
aortic valve calcification
aortic valve cusp separation
aortic valve deformity
aortic valve disease
aortic valve echocardiogram
aortic valve echocardiography
aortic valve endocarditis
aortic valve insufficiency
aortic valve leaflet
aortic valve leaflet prolapse
aortic valve lesion
aortic valve nodule
aortic valve obstruction
aortic valve opening
aortic valve opening to aortic valve closing ratio
aortic valve peak instantaneous gradient
aortic valve pressure gradient
aortic valve prosthesis
aortic valve regurgitation
aortic valve repair
aortic valve replacement
aortic valve resistance
aortic valve restenosis
aortic valve sinus
aortic valve stenosis
aortic valve stroke volume
aortic valve thickening
aortic valve vegetation
aortic valve velocity profile
arbitrary valve unit
arching of mitral valve leaflet
Argyle anti-reflux v.
artificial cardiac v.
artificial heart v.
artificial valve endocarditis
atrioventricular nodal v.
atrioventricular valve insufficiency
atrioventricular valve opening
atypical aortic valve stenosis
auriculoventricular valve opening
bag, valve, mask
bicommissural aortic v.
bicuspid aortic v.
biological heart v.
bioprosthetic heart v.
bovine heart v.
bowing of mitral valve leaflet
brachydactyly, mesomelia, mental retardation, aortic dilation, mitral valve prolapse, characteristic facies syndrome
breast implant v.
caged-ball prosthetic v.
calcific aortic valve stenosis
calcified aortic v.
calcium deposit on heart v.'s

cardiac valve procedure
cardiac valve prosthesis
clicking of malfunctioning v.
composite valve graft
congenital anomaly of mitral v.
crisscross atrioventricular v.
cryopreserved heart valve allograft
cryopreserved heart valve graft
cryopreserved homograft v.
v. cusp
defective artificial heart v.
degeneration of myxomatous heart v.
v. diameter
disc cage v.
double valve replacement
drip infusion v.
early mitral valve closure
early opening of v.
ectatic aortic v.
esophageal v.
faulty valve action
fishmouth configuration of mitral v.
floppy aortic v.
floppy mitral v.
gonadal failure, short stature, mitral valve prolapse, mental retardation syndrome
heart valve abnormality
heart valve damage
heart valve defect
heart valve disease
heart valve disorder
heart valve function
heart valve infection
heart valve prosthesis
heart valve replacement
heart valve surgery
heart valve vegetation
Heimlich heart v.
idiopathic mitral valve prolapse
impedance threshold v.
incompetence of cardiac v.
incompetent atrioventricular v.
v. of Kerckring
leaking heart v.
leaky heart v.
LeVeen v.
malformed heart or heart v.
mechanical heart v.
mental retardation, mitral valve prolapse, characteristic face syndrome
metal heart v.
midsystolic buckling of mitral v.
minimally invasive valve repair
minimally invasive valve replacement surgery
mitral and aortic valve replacement
mitral valve leaflet excursion
mitral valve aneurysm
mitral valve anterior leaflet
mitral valve, aorta, skeleton, skin
mitral valve atresia
mitral valve closure
mitral valve echo
mitral valve endocarditis
mitral valve gradient
mitral valve hypoplasia
mitral valve insufficiency
mitral valve opening
mitral valve orifice
mitral valve orifice area
mitral valve prolapse, aortic anomalies, skeletal changes, and skin changes syndrome
mitral valve prosthesis
mitral valve repair
mitral valve surgery
mixed aortic valve disease
narrowed atrial ventricular v.
narrowing of aortic v.
narrowing of heart v.
native aortic v.
native aortic valve closure
opening of aortic v.
opening mitral valve snap
opening tricuspid valve snap
open mitral valve commissurotomy
Orbis-Sigma cerebrospinal fluid shunt v.
parachute deformity of mitral v.
peak transaortic valve gradient
plastic heart v.
porcine aortic valve prosthesis
porcine heart v.
porcine prosthetic v.
porcine valve bioprosthesis
posterior leaf mitral v.
posterior mitral valve leaflet
posterior tricuspid valve leaflet
posterior urethral valve type I–IV
premature closure of v.
v. prolapse
prolapse of aortic v.
prolapsed mitral v.
prolapsed mitral valve syndrome
prolapse of mitral v.
prosthetic aortic v.
prosthetic ball v.
prosthetic cardiac v.
prosthetic heart v.
prosthetic heart valve surgery
prosthetic valve dysfunction
prosthetic valve regurgitation
prosthetic valve stenosis
prosthetic valve thrombosis
prosthetic valve vegetation
pulmonary heart valve disorder
pulmonary valve anomaly
pulmonary valve area
pulmonary valve disease
pulmonary valve dysplasia
pulmonary valve gradient
pulmonary valve opening
pulmonary valve stenosis
pulmonic v.
pulmonic valve stenosis
quadricusp mitral v.
v. replacement
rheumatic aortic valve disease
rotating hemostatic v.
scarring of heart v.
semilunar v.
semilunar valve closure
severe heart valve narrowing
Smeloff heart v.
staphylococcal infection of heart v.
stentless porcine v.
stent-mounted heterograft v.
St. Jude v.
structural valve deterioration
supraannular v.
supraannular mitral valve replacement
synthetic heart v.
v. system
systolic anterior motion of mitral v.
thickened aortic v.
thickened mitral v.
transaortic valve gradient
transurethral resection of v.'s
tricuspid aortic v.
tricuspid heart v.
tricuspid valve closure
tricuspid valve gradient
tricuspid valve replacement
tricuspid valve vegetation
v.'s, unilateral reflux, dysplasia

valved

augmented valved rectum
v. holding chamber

valve-transverse

mitral v.-t.

valvoplasty
percutaneous mitral v.

valvotomy
balloon aortic v.
balloon mitral v.
balloon tricuspid v.
mitral balloon v.
percutaneous mitral balloon v.

valvulae

valvular
acquired valvular heart disease
v. aortic disease
v. aortic insufficiency
v. aortic stenosis
aortic valvular disease
aortic valvular incompetence
aortic valvular insufficiency
aortic valvular stenosis
cardiac valvular regurgitation
chronic valvular heart disease
v. disease
v. disease of heart
v. dysfunction
v. endocarditis
v. heart disease
v. incompetence
v. insufficiency
mitral valvular disease
v. pulmonic stenosis
v. regurgitation
rheumatic valvular heart disease
tricuspid valvular leaflet
venous valvular insufficiency

valvule
lymphatic v.

valvulitis
healed rheumatic v.
murmur of v.

valvuloplasty
v. and angioplasty of congenital anomalies
balloon aortic v.
balloon dilation v.
balloon mitral v.
balloon pulmonary v.
balloon valvuloplasty registry
catheter balloon v.
intracoronary thrombolysis balloon v.
percutaneous balloon aortic v.
percutaneous balloon pulmonic v.
percutaneous mitral balloon v.
percutaneous transluminal balloon v.
pulmonary balloon v.
transluminal balloon v.
triple balloon v.

valvulotomy
bicuspid v.
mitral v.
percutaneous mitral balloon v.
pulmonary v.
tricuspid v.

van
V. Buren catheter
v. Buren disease
v. Buren sound
v. den Bergh test
V. der Hoeve syndrome
v. der Waals force
hematoxylin and van Gieson stain
modified V. Lint anesthesia
modified V. Lint block

VanB *Enterococcus faecium*

vancomycin
gentamicin, vancomycin, and nystatin
heterogeneous resistance to v.

vancomycin-insensitive *Staphylococcus aureus*

vancomycin-intermediate-resistant *Staphylococcus aureus*

vancomycin-resistant
v.-r. *Enterococcus*
v.-r. *Enterococcus faecium*
v.-r. *Staphylococcus aureus*

Vane Evaluation of Language Scale

vanillacetic acid

vanilla milkshake

vanillylmandelic acid

vanishing
v. lung
v. lung syndrome

Vantage Performance monitor

vapor
anesthetic v.
cold quartz mercury vapor lamp
v. density
formaldehyde v.'s
mercury vapor poisoning
moisture vapor transmission rate
partial pressure of water v.
v. pressure
synthetic, adhesive, moisture vapor permeable

vaporization
carbon dioxide laser v.
contact laser vaporization of the prostate
v. laser ablation of prostate
laser coagulation vaporization procedure
laser vaporization and excisional conization
transurethral vaporization of prostate

vaporized
v. hemorrhoidal tissue
v. hydrogen peroxide

vaporizer
cool mist v.

vaporize water in herniated disc

vapor-phase chromatography

vara
adolescent tibia v.
infantile tibia v.
traumatic epiphysial coxa v.

variabilis
erythrokeratodermia v.

variability
baseline variability of fetal heart rate
beat-to-beat v.
fetal heart rate v.
heart rate v.
long-term v.
short-term v.
ventricular rate v.
within-person v.

variability-absent
long-term v.-a.

variable
angular coordinate v.
v. antigen, surface
v. antigen type
beta-chain variable region
v. circumference suprapatellar socket
common variable hypogammaglobulinemia
common variable immunodeficiency
v. coupling
dependent v.
v. diversity joining
v. domain of heavy chain immunoglobulin
v. domain of light chain immunoglobulin
v. flexion overhinge
v. immunodeficiency

insulin v.
v. interval
v. life-adjusted display
linear variable differential transformer
mixed discrete-continuous random v.
v. numbers of tandem repeats
v. positive airway pressure
v. projection method
random v.
v. rate
v. ratio
v. screw placement
v. screw plate
single-chain variable fragment
v. softness
v. spinal plating
v. strabismus
Test of V.'s of Attention
uncontrolled v.

variable-angle uniform signal excitation

variable-dose patient-controlled anesthesia

variable-width forms tractor

variably positive

variance
analysis of v.
environmental v.
genetic v.
multiple abstract variance analysis
multiple analysis of v.
multivariate analysis of v.
negative ulnar v.
positive ulnar v.
v. ratio
v. of resident time
sample v.
unit of v.

varians
metamorphopsia v.

variant
anatomic bile duct v.
anesthetic variant of schizoid behavior
v. angina
v. angina pectoris
blastoid variant of mantel cell lymphoma
chronic and dilute v.
chronic lymphocytic leukemia v.
columnar cell v.
corticosteroid-binding globulin v.
v. Creutzfeldt-Jakob disease
fast alpha variant rhythm
fibrosarcomatous variant of dermatofibrosarcoma protuberans
floral variant of follicular lymphoma
follicular variant of papillary thyroid carcinoma
v. frequency
growth hormone v.
hairy cell leukemia v.
linear scleroderma v.
Los Angeles variant galactosemia
mediastinal arterial v.
new variant Creutzfeldt-Jakob disease
non-syncytium-inducing variant of AIDS virus
normal variant short stature
petit mal v.
slow alpha variant rhythm
sulfhydryl v.
v. surface glycoprotein
tall cell v.

variant-specific surface antigen

variation
angle variation resolution
coefficient of v.
conative negative v.
contingent negative v.
diurnal and matutinal v.
v.'s in electrical activity
negative v.
normal anatomic v.
postimperative negative v.

variceal
angiographic variceal embolization
anorectal variceal bleeding
endoscopic variceal band ligation
endoscopic variceal sclerosis
endoscopic variceal sclerotherapy
esophageal variceal bleeding
esophageal variceal hemorrhage
esophageal variceal sclerosis
esophageal variceal sclerotherapy
esophagogastric variceal bleeding
intraesophageal variceal pressure
massive variceal hemorrhage
recurrent variceal hemorrhage

varicella
v. chickenpox varicella zoster virus vaccine
fetal varicella syndrome
live varicella vaccine
pustular v.
v. virus infection

varicella-zoster
v.-z. immune globulin
v.-z. virus
v.-z. virus vaccine

varicelliform
Kaposi varicelliform eruption

varices (*pl. of* varix)

varicocele
ovarian v.

varicose
v. eczema
persistent varicose veins
v. ulcer
vaginal varicose vein
v. vein
v. vein stripping and ligation

varicosity
autonomic v.
neurophysin-positive v.
superficial v.
tortuous v.

varicosus
nevus varicosus osteohypertrophicus

variegated translocation mosaicism

variegate porphyria

variety
v.'s of human leukocyte antigen
v. of abuse patterns

variolosa
orchitis v.

varix, pl. **varices**
bleeding esophageal v.
bleeding gastric v.
isolated gastric varices type 1, 2
thrombosed oral v.

varum
genu v.

varus
Axer varus derotational osteotomy
v. deformity
v. derotational osteotomy
derotational varus osteotomy
forefoot v.
fracture complete and varus deformity
genu v.
hallux v.
v. hindfoot
v. hindfoot deformity
metatarsus primus v.
pes v.
v. rotational osteotomy
v. strain

varus *(continued)*
v. stress test
talipes v.

varus-valgus
v.-v. angulation

varying amplitude

vasa
aortic vasa vasorum

vasal
laser-assisted vasal anastomosis
maximum vasal pressure

vascular
v. abnormality
v. access device
v. access dressing
v. access graft
v. access in hemodialysis
v. accident
acute mesenteric vascular insufficiency
acute vascular compromise
acute vascular xenograft rejection
v. anastomosis
angiographically occult intracranial vascular malformation
angiographically occult vascular malformation
angiographically visualized vascular malformation
anomalous vascular distribution
antral vascular ectasia
v. arcade
arterial noninvasive vascular assessment
arterial vascular bed
arterial vascular disease
arteriosclerotic mesenteric vascular occlusive disease
arteriosclerotic peripheral vascular disease
articular vascular circle
articular vascular network
articular vascular network of elbow
articular vascular network of knee
articular vascular plexus
atherosclerotic pulmonary vascular disease
autoimmune collagen vascular disease
v. bed
benign vascular neoplasm
BI cranial vascular headache
v. bruit
cardiac allograft vascular disease
v. cell adhesion molecule
v. cell adhesion molecule-1
cerebral vascular profile study
v. change
chronic graft vascular disease
chronic thrombotic pulmonary vascular obstruction
clinical vascular laboratory
cocaine-related vascular headache
collagen vascular disease
collagen vascular sealing
complex-combined vascular malformation
v. compression
v. compromise
congenital vascular malformation
congested vascular structure
v. congestion of interstitial vessel
conjunctival vascular injection
coronary vascular resistance
coronary vascular resistance index
cryptic vascular malformation
v. decompensation
decreasing peripheral vascular resistance
v. defect
v. dementia
v. depression
digital vascular imaging system
digital vascular reactivity
v. disease
v. disease in diabetic heart
v. disease of heart
v. dysfunction
v. endothelial cell growth inhibitor
v. endothelial growth factor 2, 3
v. endothelial growth factor/vascular permeability factor
excimer vascular recanalization
v. flow headache
focal vascular headache
v. fold
forearm vascular resistance
v. fragility syndrome
gastric antral vascular ectasia
gastric vascular ectasia
v. goiter
v. graft infection
v. grafting
v. headache
v. headache syndrome
v. heart disease
hemicranial vascular headache
v. hemostatic device
hepatic vascular exclusion
hepatic vascular isolation
v. hypertension
hypertensive pulmonary vascular disease
hypertensive vascular crisis
v. hypotension
v. imaging
impaired coronary vascular reserve
implantable vascular access device
index of pulmonary vascular disease
indwelling transcutaneous vascular access device
indwelling vascular access catheter
v. inflammation
v. injury
v. insufficiency
v. insult
intracoronary vascular ultrasound
intracranial vascular abnormality
intracranial vascular evaluation
intracranial vascular malformation
v. invasion
v. involvement
v. irregularity
ischemic vascular disease
v. keratitis
laser-assisted vascular anastomosis
v. layer
v. leak syndrome
v. lesion
limb vascular resistance
v. malformation
maternal vascular response
mesenteric vascular occlusive disease
mini-invasive vascular study
minimal coronary vascular resistance index
minimal forearm vascular resistance
Moore classification for vascular anomalies of the gastrointestinal tract
motor, vascular, and sensory
myocardial vascular capacity
neural axis vascular malformation
neutralizing antibody to vascular endothelial growth factor
noninvasive vascular laboratory studies
obliterative vascular disease
v. occlusion
v. occlusive episode
occlusive vascular disease

occult cerebral vascular malformation
oculocephalic vascular anomaly
partial hepatic vascular exclusion
peripheral v.
peripheral retinal vascular sheathing
peripheral vascular insufficiency
peripheral vascular laboratory
peripheral vascular occlusion
peripheral vascular occlusive disease
peripheral vascular resistance index
peripheral vascular surgery
peripheral vascular system
v. permeability
v. plasminogen activator
v. plexus
premature vascular disease
Pruitt-Inahara vascular shunt
pulmonary collagen vascular disease
pulmonary vascular disorder
pulmonary vascular hyperplasia
pulmonary vascular hypertension
pulmonary vascular obstruction
pulmonary vascular obstructive disease
pulmonary vascular resistance index
v. radiology
recombinant human vascular endothelial growth factor
reduced vascular response
rejuvenation with sparing of vascular perforators
relative vascular resistance
renal cortical vascular resistance
renal vascular failure
renal vascular resistance index
v. resistance
selective vascular clamping
v. septal defect
sequential vascular response
v. smooth muscle cell
splenic vascular supply
subcortical vascular encephalopathy
superficial vascular plexus
systemic peripheral vascular resistance
systemic vascular hypertension
systemic vascular resistance index
thromboembolic cerebral vascular accident
v. thrombosis
total peripheral vascular resistance
total pulmonary vascular resistance
total vascular isolation
ultrasound-guided vascular access
v. volume of distribution
v. wall

vasculare
poikiloderma atrophicans v.

vascularis
nevus v.

vascularity
pulmonary v.

vascularization elsewhere in the retina

vascularized
allogenically vascularized prefabricated flap
axial pattern vascularized skin flap
v. bone graft
v. bone marrow transplantation
v. double-sided preputial island flap and W flap glanuloplasty hypospadias repair
metatarsal free vascularized graft
v. patellar tendon

vasculature
atypical v.
central pulmonary v.
choroidal v.
hilar v.
perimacular v.
prominence of pulmonary v.
pulmonary v.
renal v.
retinal v.

vasculi
nodular v.

vasculitides

vasculitis
allergic v.
ANCA-associated v.
ANCA-associated systemic v.
ANCA-positive v.
antineutrophilic cytoplasmic autoantibody-small vessel v.
asthma with v.
Birmingham V. Activity Score
cutaneous necrotizing v.
hypocomplementemic urticarial vasculitis syndrome
hypocomplementemic vasculitis urticaria syndrome
leukocytoclastic v.
necrotizing bowel v.
necrotizing granulomatous v.
nodular granulomatous v.
obstructive retinal v.
primary systemic v.
retinal v.
rheumatoid v.
segmental hyalinizing v.
systemic necrotizing v.

vasculogenic impotence

vasculopathic
reflex vasculopathic activity

vasculopathy
cardiac allograft v.
fetal thrombotic v.
idiopathic polypoidal choroidal v.
portal hypertensive intestinal v.

vasculosus
nevus v.
nevus vasculosus osteohypertrophicus

vasectomy
no-scalpel v.
open-ended v.

vasoablative endothelial sarcoma

vasoactive
v. intestinal peptide
v. intestinal peptide-secreting tumor
v. intestinal polypeptide immunoreactivity
v. intestinal polypeptide tumor
v. intracorporeal pharmacotherapy

vasoconstriction
delayed cerebral v.
hypoxic pulmonary v.
peripheral circulatory v.
peripheral cutaneous v.
pulmonary alveolar hypoxic v.
v. rate

vasoconstrictor
v. assay
v. center
v. substance

vasodepressor
v. lipid
v. material
v. syncope

vasodilating agent

vasodilation
flow-mediated v.
increased peripheral vasodilation and hypotension
myocardial v.

vasodilation *(continued)*
peripheral arterial vasodilation theory
vasodilator
v. agent
arterial-selective intravenous v.
v. center
oral v.
parenteral v.
v. substance
vasoexcitor material
vasogenic shock
vasoinhibitory
v. center
v. peptide
vasomotor
v. activity
acute vasomotor nephropathy
v. angina
v. ataxia
v. center
cephalic vasomotor response
v. fiber
v. flushing
v. headache
v. imbalance
v. instability
v. response
v. rhinitis
v. stimulant
v. syncope
v. tone
total vasomotor rhinitis symptom score
vasoocclusive
v. angiotherapy
v. crisis
vasopeptidase inhibitor
vasopressin
antidiuretic arginine vasopressin V2 receptor
aqueous v.
arginine v.
arginine vasopressin regulation
inappropriate vasopressin secretion
intraarterial v.
intravenous v.
neonatal arginine v.
neurophysin associated with v.
nocturnal vasopressin release
v. receptor
vasopressor
arginine vasopressor precursor
vasorum
aortic vasa v.
vasospasm
cerebral v.
painless cold-sensitive digital v.
vasospastic angina
vasotocin
arginine v.
vasotonin
lysine v.
vasovagal
v. attack
v. epilepsy
v. episode
v. hypotension
neurally mediated vasovagal syncope
v. reaction
v. syncope
v. syndrome
vastus
aponeurosis of vastus muscle
deep vastus lateralis
v. intermedius
v. lateralis
v. lateralis muscle
v. lateralis release
left vastus lateralis muscle
v. medialis
v. medialis advancement
v. medialis muscle
v. medialis oblique muscle
v. medialis obliquus musculus
obliquus v.
right vastus lateralis
superficial vastus lateralis
Vater
ampulla of V.
ampulla of Vater anatomy
ampulla of Vater cyst
V. corpuscle
V. fold
papilla of V.
Vater-Pacini corpuscle
vault
anterior apical vault defect
craniosacral v.
craniosacral vault 4
rectal v.
vaginal vault repair
Vb
T cell antigen receptor V.
V-dimercaptosuccinic acid
vectis
aspirating/irrigating v.
Peczon I/A v.
vector
v. analysis
astigmatic vector analysis
attenuated bacterial v.
attenuated poxvirus v.
augmented v.
v. cardiography electrode right midaxillary line
electric field v.
v. electrocardiogram
electrocardiographic angle between QRS and T v.'s
integrated vector control
live vector vaccine
live viral v.
magnetic field v.
magnetic heart v.
v. magnitude
major injury v.
maximal spatial vector to left
mean cardiac v.
movement arm v.
naked DNA vector vaccine
nucleic acid v.
vectorcardiogram
spatial v.
vectorcardiography electrode
vegetable
brominated vegetable oil
v. protein diet plus fiber
textured vegetable protein
vegetal
two cerebral hemisphere vegetal hemisphere
vegetans
pemphigus v.
vegetarian
pure v.
vegetation
aortic valve v.
bacterial v.'s
cardiac v.
endocardial v.
heart valve v.
nonbacterial thrombotic v.
prosthetic v.
prosthetic valve v.
tricuspid valve v.
verrucous v.
vegetative
v. disturbance
v. endocarditis
v. lesion
v. process

radioactivity of vegetative cells
v. and restless

vehicle

emergency v.
v. for initial crawling
motor vehicle collision
operating motor vehicle while intoxicated
pedestrian hit by motor v.
slow-moving v.

vehicular accident

veil

aqueduct v.
Sattler v.

veiling

scatter and veiling glare

vein

accompanying vein of hypoglossal nerve
adrenal vein aldosterone ratio
v. allograft
aneurysm of Galen v.
aneurysm of vein of Galen
angular facial v.
anomalous pulmonary v.
anomalous right pulmonary vein dextroposition
anomaly of drainage of pulmonary v.
anterior auricular v.
anterior basal v.
anterior cardiac v.
anterior cardinal v.
anterior cerebral v.
anterior ciliary v.
anterior circumflex humeral v.
anterior condylar v.
anterior conjunctival v.
anterior facial v.
anterior horizontal jugular v.
anterior intercostal v.
anterior internal vertebral v.
anterior interosseous v.
anterior labial v.
anterior pontomesencephalic v.
anterior and posterior vestibular v.'s
anterior scrotal v.
anterior temporal diploic v.
anterior temporobasal v.
anterior terminal v.
anterior tibial v.
anterior vein of the leg
anterior vein of septum pellucidum
anterior vertebral v.
aortocoronary-saphenous vein bypass graft
apical branch of right superior pulmonary v.
apicoposterior branch of left superior pulmonary v.
aplasia of deep v.
arciform vein of kidney
arcuate vein of kidney
arterialization of portal v.
arterialized leptomeningeal v.
arterioportal vein shunting
v., artery, nerve
ascending lumbar v.
ascending medullary vein thrombosis
autogenous vein bypass graft
autogenous vein graft conduit
autologous internal jugular v.
autologous vein graft
basal vein of Rosenthal
bilateral renal vein thrombosis
branch retinal vein occlusion
branch vein occlusion
v. bypass graft
bypass vein graft
cavernous transformation of the portal v.
central retinal v.
central retinal vein occlusion
central vein of hepatic lobule
cerebral vein thrombosis
collapsed jugular v.
collecting v.
common iliac v.
communicating vein incompetence
conducting v.
v. cutdown
deep circumflex iliac v.
deep vein thrombosis
dorsal interosseous metacarpal v.
dorsal interosseous vein of foot
dorsal vein complex
double vein graft
endophlebitis of retinal v.
esophageal collateral v.
external iliac v.
external jugular v.
extrahepatic portal vein obstruction
femoral v.
femoral-popliteal vein bypass
femoral vein ligation
first jejunal v.
flat jugular v.
v. of Galen
v. of Galen aneurysmal dilatation
v. of Galen aneurysmal malformation
v. graft
great cardiac v.
great cardiac vein flow
greater saphenous v.
greater saphenous vein cutdown
great vein of Galen
hepatic portal v.
hepatic vein catheterization
hepatic vein free pressure
hepatic vein injury
hepatic vein occlusion
highest intercostal v.
high saphenous vein ligation
human umbilical v.
human umbilical vein endothelial cell
iliac vein thrombosis
iliofemoral deep vein thrombosis
incompetent perforating v.
incompetent perforator v.
inferior gluteal v.
inferior hemorrhoidal v.
inferior mesenteric v.
inferior nasal v.
inferior radicular v.
inferior temporal v.
intercostal vein of hand
interlobar vein of kidney
interlobular vein of kidney
interlobular vein of liver
internal auricular v.
internal cerebral v.
internal iliac v.
internal jugular vein cannulation
internal pudendal v.
internal thoracic v.
interventricular v.'s
intrapulmonary v.
jugular v.
jugular neck vein distention
keep vein open
to keep vein open
lateral sacral v.
left brachial vein occlusion
left coronary v.
left gastric v.
left hepatic v.
left inferior pulmonary v.
left innominate v.
left internal jugular v.
left renal v.
left subclavian v.
left superior intercostal v.
lobe of azygos v.
long saphenous v.

vein *(continued)*
long thoracic v.
lumen of v.
macular branch retinal vein occlusion
main portal vein peak velocity
main renal v.
Marshall oblique v.
mastoid emissary v.
maternal cortical v.
maternal cortical vein thrombosis
medial atrial v.
medial circumflex femoral v.
medial genicular v.
median antebrachial v.
median basilic v.
median cephalic v.
median cubital v.
mesenteric vein thrombosis
middle cardiac v.
middle colic v.
middle genicular v.
middle hemorrhoidal v.
middle hepatic v.
middle lobe branch of right superior pulmonary v.
middle lobe v.
migratory deep vein thrombophlebitis
mobile artery and vein imaging system
neck vein distended
neck vein distention
nerve, artery, vein, empty space, lymphatics
nicking of retinal v.
obturator branch of pubic branch of inferior epigastric v.
occipital cerebral v.
occipital diploic v.
occipital emissary v.
occlusion of branch v.
occlusion of retinal v.
opticociliary shunt v.
orbital vein thrombosis
palmar cutaneous v.
palmar digital v.
pancreatic v.
paraesophageal collateral v.
paraumbilical vein tumor
parietal emissary v.
partial anomalous pulmonary v.'s
partial pressure tension of carbon dioxide, v.
partial pressure tension of oxygen, v.
patency of v.
pelvic ovarian vein thrombosis
percutaneous femoral v.
percutaneous femoral vein catheter
peripheral acinar v.
peripheral branch retinal vein occlusion
peripheral vein total parenteral nutrition
peripheral vein plasma
peripheral vein renin activity
persistent varicose v.'s
popliteal v.
popliteal tibial bypass vein graft
portal v.
portal vein aneurysm
portal vein congestive index
portal vein dilation
portal vein infusion
portal vein obstruction
portal vein occlusion
portal vein tumor thrombus
posterior arch v.
posterior auricular v.
posterior intercostal v.
posterior interosseous v.
posterior superior pancreaticoduodenal v.
posterior terminal v.
posterior tibial v.
precentral cerebellar v.
primary head v.
profunda femoris v.
proximal vein thrombosis
puerperal ovarian vein thrombophlebitis
puerperal ovarian vein thrombosis
pulmonary v.
pulmonary vein atrial reversal
pulmonary vein stenosis
pulsating neck v.
recurrent deep vein thrombosis
red spider v.
renal vein plasma renin activity
renal vein renin
renal vein renin activity
renal vein renin assay
renal vein renin concentration
reversed saphenous vein graft
right brachial v.
right brachial vein occlusion
right colic v.
right femoral v.
right gastric v.
right hepatic v.
right innominate v.
right internal jugular v.
right portal v.
right pulmonary v.
right renal v.
right subclavian v.
right superior intercostal v.
Rosenthal ascending v.
sacral v.
saphenous v.
saphenous vein bypass
saphenous vein bypass graft
saphenous vein graft
saphenous vein graft de novo
saphenous vein graft stenosis
severed jugular v.
short gastric v.
shunt index via the inferior mesenteric v.
shunt index via superior mesenteric v.
small vein of heart
spiral vein of modiolus
splenic v.
splenic vein obstruction
v. stripper
subclavian v.
subclavian vein catheterization
subclavian vein compression
subclavian vein thrombosis
superficial circumflex iliac v.
superficial femoral v.
superior epigastric v.
superior gluteal v.
superior hemiazygos v.
superior hemorrhoidal v.
superior mesenteric v.
superior mesenteric-portal vein confluence
superior nasal v.
superior pulmonary vein isolated
superior radicular v.
superior temporal v.
temperature in saphenous v.
terminal hepatic vein obliteration
transhepatic portal v.
tumor thrombus in the portal v.
ulnar cutaneous v.
umbilical v.
umbilical vein catheter
umbilical vein catheterization
umbilical vein to maternal v.
vaginal varicose v.
varicose v.
varicose vein stripping and ligation
wedged renal vein pressure

3-vein graft

vein/renal
renal vein/renal activity ratio

vela (*pl. of* velum)

Veley head rest

veli
levator veli palatini muscle
tensor veli palatini

Vellore virus

velocardiofacial syndrome

velocimetry
laser Doppler v.

velocity
air velocity index
angular eye v.
angular head v.
aortic blood flow velocity waveform
aortic root velocity waveform
aortic valve velocity profile
artery:aortic velocity ratio
average path v.
average peak v.
baseline average peak v.
blood flow v.
blood flow velocity waveform
capillary blood flow v.
cerebral blood flow v.
v. of circumferential fiber shortening
v. coefficient
v., common carotid artery
conduction v.
conduction velocity of slower fibers
constant angular v.
constant linear v.
v. constants
v. of contractile element
coronary blood flow v.
coronary flow velocity reserve
curvilinear v.
v. distribution function
Doppler systolic velocity index
Doppler velocity probe
end-diastolic v.
end-diastolic velocity measurement
end-systolic force velocity index
fiber shortening v.
flow v.
force, velocity, length
fractional velocity reserve
growth v.
height v.
high regional wall motion v.
v. index
v. internal carotid artery
v. of light
linear growth v.
main portal vein peak v.
maximal v.
maximum conduction v.
maximum eversion v.
mean aortic flow v.
mean pulmonary-blood-flow v.
midshunt peak v.
minimal height v.
motor nerve conduction v.
muscle fiber conduction v.
myocardial Doppler v.
nerve conduction v.
nerve conduction velocity study
nerve conduction velocity test
peak aortic flow v.
peak diastolic v.
peak early diastolic filling v.
peak ejection v.
peak growth v.
peak height v.
peak hyperemic average v.
peak systolic v.
peak weight v.
portal vein blood flow v.
portal venous v.
posterior wall v.
prostate-specific antigen v.
PSA v.
pulsed ultrasonic blood velocity detector
pulse wave v.
rate of velocity constant
v. ratio
sensory conduction v.
sensory nerve conduction v.
slow-component v.
slow-phase v.
v. of sound of blood
straight line v.
superior mesenteric artery blood v.
superior sagittal sinus v.
systolic velocity integral
systolic wall motion v.
time velocity integral
tracheal mucous v.
tracheal transport v.
tumor peak systolic v.
ulnar nerve conduction v.
ventricular conduction v.
vocal velocity index
v. waveform

velocity-encoded
v.-e. cine
v.-e. cine-magnetic resonance imaging

velocity-enhanced resistance training

velopharyngeal
v. closure
v. competence
v. dysfunction
v. gap
v. incompetence
v. insufficiency
v. opening

Velpeau
V. canal
V. deformity
V. fossa
V. hernia

velum, pl. **vela**
anterior medullary v.
aponeurosis of v.
artificial v.
palatine v.

vena
apertura mediana v.
v. cava
v. cava inferior
v. caval filter
v. cava superior
v. comitans
Greenfield vena cava filter
inferior vena cava
inferior vena cava filter
inferior vena cava pressure
inferior vena cava reconstruction
inferior vena cava thrombosis
infrahepatic interruption of inferior vena cava
left inferior vena cava
left superior vena cava
ligament of left superior vena cava
ligament of left vena cava
lymphonodus arcus vena azygos
membranous obstruction of the inferior vena cava
opening of inferior vena cava
orifice of inferior vena cava
radionuclide imaging of inferior vena cava
right inferior vena cava
right superior vena cava
superior vena cava compression syndrome
superior vena cava obstruction

vena *(continued)*
suprahepatic inferior vena cava
thoracic inferior vena cava

venacavogram
inferior v.

venacavography
inferior v.

venae rectales inferiores

veneer
acrylic veneer crown
etched porcelain v.
full veneer crown
partial veneer crown
porcelain v.
porcelain veneer bridge
porcelain veneer crown

venerea
lues v.

venereal
colony-stimulating factor developed by V. Disease Research Laboratory
v. condyloma
v. disease
v. disease, gonorrhea
v. disease-syphilis
v. granuloma
v. infection
not v.
no venereal disease
v. spirochetosis of rabbits
transmissible venereal tumor
v. wart

venereum
lymphogranuloma v.
lymphogranuloma venereum antigen
lymphogranuloma venereum complement fixation test
lymphogranuloma venereum conjunctivitis
lymphogranuloma venereum infection
lymphogranuloma venereum keratitis
lymphogranuloma venereum virus
lymphopathia v.
psittacosis, lymphogranuloma venereum, trachoma

Venezuelan
V. equine encephalitis vaccine, attenuated live
V. equine encephalitis vaccine, inactivated
V. equine encephalitis virus
V. equine encephalomyelitis virus

venoarterial
v. bypass pumping

venogram
nuclear v.
radioactive isotopic venogram, bilateral

venography
ascending contrast v.
intravenous radionuclide v.
magnetic resonance v.
pedal control v.
radionuclide v.
subcutaneous radionuclide v.

venom
antisnake v.
axillary venom gland
black widow spider v.
cobra venom factor
v. hemolysis
honeybee v.
v. immunotherapy
mixed vespid v.
Polistes wasp v.
snake v.
yellow jacket v.

venoocclusive
v. disease
hepatic venoocclusive disease
mesenteric inflammatory venoocclusive disease
pulmonary venoocclusive disease

venosum

venous
v. access
v. access device
v. access port
v. admixture
adrenal venous sampling
v. air embolism
ambulatory venous pressure
v. anastomosis
v. anatomy
v. angiocardiography
v. angioplasty
anomalous pulmonary venous connection, total or partial
anomalous pulmonary venous drainage
anomalous pulmonary venous return
v. anomaly
antiseptic-impregnated central venous catheter
aortocoronary venous bypass
areolar venous plexus
arterial/deep v.
arterial/deep venous difference
arterialization of venous blood
arterioportal venous shunt
arterioportal venous shunting
arteriosuperficial venous difference
v. artery
v. backflow
v. bifurcation
bioimpedance venous analysis
v. blood
v. blood circulation
v. blood gas
v. blood pressure
v. blood sample
v. bypass graft
v. cannulation
v. capacitance
v. capillary
v. carbon dioxide production
central v.
central splanchnic venous thrombosis
central venous access
central venous access device
central venous catheter infection
central venous line
central venous nutrition
central venous oxygen
central venous pressure
central venous temperature
cerebral subarachnoid venous pressure
cerebral venous malformation
cerebral venous sinus thrombosis
cervical venous hum
v. circulation
v. clotting time
v. collateral circulation
continuous venous infusion
cryopreserved venous transplantation
v. cutdown
decreased venous return to heart
deep venous insufficiency
deep venous occlusion
deep venous thromboembolization
deep venous thromboscintigram
deep venous thrombosis
deep venous thrombosis prophylaxis
v. defect
Denver peritoneal venous shunt
developmental venous anomaly
v. dialysis pressure
v. diameter ratio

v. digital angiogram
digital venous subtraction angiography
v. distensibility index
v. distention
v. distention or mass
v. Doppler study
Doppler venous examination
Doppler venous imaging
downstream venous pressure
v. duplex scanning
v. ectasia
v. emptying
end-to-end venous anastomosis
end-to-side venous anastomosis
episcleral venous pressure
v. extension
v. filling time
v. flow
v. flow controller
v. foramen
free hepatic venous pressure
v. graft
v. groove
v. heart
v. hematocrit
v. hemorrhage
hepatic portal venous gas
hepatic venous effluence
hepatic venous isolation by direct hemoperfusion
hepatic venous outflow obstruction
hepatic venous pressure gradient
v. hyperemia
v. hypertension
v. impedance plethysmography
implantable venous access device
v. incompetence
increased central venous pressure
increased venous pressure
indwelling venous catheter
indwelling venous line
initial venous shunt
v. insufficiency
v. insufficiency syndrome
intracranial venous malformation
jugular venous arch
jugular venous catheter
jugular venous oxygen saturation
jugular venous pressure
jugular venous pulsation
jugular venous pulse
jugular venous pulse tracing
lateral venous sinus
left subclavian central venous pressure
longitudinal vertebral venous sinus
long-term central venous access catheter placement
long-term venous catheter
low central venous pressure anesthesia
lower extremity v.
v. malformation
maternal v.
maximal venous oxygen consumption
maximal venous outflow
maximum venous outflow
mean venous outflow
mean venous pressure
medullary venous malformation
mesenteric venous thrombosis
minimal venous oxygen consumption
mixed v.
mixed venous blood
mixed venous hypoxia
mixed venous oxygen
mixed venous oxygen content
mixed venous oxygen saturation
multilumen central venous pressure
no venous distention
v. occlusion plethysmography
v. oozing
ovarian venous plasma oxytocin
oxygen content of mixed venous blood
partial anomalous pulmonary venous connection
partial anomalous pulmonary venous drainage
partial anomalous pulmonary venous return
partial oxygen pressure in mixed venous blood
partial pressure of carbon dioxide in mixed venous blood
partial pressure of mesenteric venous carbon dioxide
partial venous gas tension of oxygen
passive venous congestion
pelvic venous incompetence
percutaneous central venous catheter
percutaneous femoral venous catheter
peripherally inserted central venous catheter
peripheral venous disease
peripheral venous nutrition
peripheral venous pressure
portal venous and enteric drainage technique
portal venous access
portal venous phase
portal venous sampling
portal venous velocity
postoperative deep venous thrombosis
v. pressure gradient support stockings
v. pressure module
prolonged venous access devices
protracted venous infusion
pulmonary anomalous superior venous return
pulmonary arterial pressure-pulmonary venous pressure
pulmonary venous capillary
pulmonary venous flow
pulmonary venous obstruction
pulmonary venous occlusion
pulmonary venous redistribution
pulmonary venous return
recurring venous thromboembolism
red venous blood
v. refill time
v. reflux
renal v.
v. renal plasma flow
v. renin concentration
v. resistance
resistance to venous return
resting venous pressure
retinal venous dilation and tortuosity
v. return
v. return to heart
v. return time
right subclavian central v.
v. runoff
segmental venous capacitance
segmented venous capacitance ratio
v. sinus
spontaneous venous pulsation
spontaneous venous pulse
standing venous pressure
v. stasis changes
v. stasis retinopathy
v. stasis ulcer
v. stop flow pressure
systemic venous collateral
systemic venous hypertension
v. thromboembolic disease

venous *(continued)*
v. thromboembolism
v. thrombosis
v. tortuosity
total anomalous pulmonary venous connection
total anomalous pulmonary venous drainage
total anomalous pulmonary venous return
umbilical venous catheter
umbilical venous line
v. valvular insufficiency
ventral venous line
v. volume plethysmograph
wedge hepatic venous pressure

venous/arterial management protection

venous-to-venous anastomosis

venovenous
v. bypass
continuous venovenous hemodiafiltration
continuous venovenous hemodialysis
continuous venovenous hemofiltration

ventilated
Distress Scale for V. Newborn Infants
v. group
v. mask
paralyzed and mechanically v.

ventilating
heating, ventilating, and air conditioning

ventilation
adaptive support v.
aerosol ventilation scan
aerosol ventilation study
airway pressure release v.
alveolar v.
v. of alveolar dead space
alveolar minute v.
alveolar ventilation per minute
v. of anatomic dead space
artificial v.
assist-controlled mechanical v.
assist-control mode v.
assisted mechanical v.
backup v.
bilateral ventilation tubes
combined high-frequency v.
compression and v.
computer-assisted v.
continuous flow v.
continuous mandatory v.
continuous mechanical v.
continuous negative-pressure v.
continuous positive-pressure v.
controlled mechanical v.
control mode v.
conventional mechanical v.
v. defect
distribution of v.
effective alveolar v.
endotracheal intubation and mechanical v.
excessive v.
expiration-synchronized intermittent mandatory v.
extended mandatory minute v.
forced mandatory intermittent v.
high-frequency oscillation v.
high-frequency oscillatory v.
high-frequency percussive v.
high-frequency positive-pressure v.
high-frequency ventilation trial
v. index
inspired v.
intermittent assisted v.
intermittent demand v.
intermittent mechanical v.
intermittent negative pressure-assisted v.
intermittent percussive v.
intermittent positive pressure v.
intrapulmonary percussive v.
intratracheal pulmonary v.
laser office ventilation of ears with insertion of tubes
liquid v.
liquid-assisted high-frequency oscillatory v.
local exhaust v.
low-frequency positive pressure v.
lung-protective pressure-targeted v.
mandatory minute v.
v. by mask
mask and bag v.
maximal exercise v.
maximal sustained level of v.
maximal ventilation time
maximal voluntary v.
maximum voluntary v.
mechanical v.
minute v.
myocardial ventilation, oxygen rate
nasal nocturnal v.
nasal positive pressure v.
negative-pressure v.
noninvasive motion v.
noninvasive positive pressure v.
one-lung v.
oxygen ventilation equivalent
partial liquid v.
peak exercise v.
percutaneous transtracheal jet v.
v. and perfusion
v. perfusion defect
v. per minute of dead space
positive airway pressure v.
positive-pressure v.
pressure control v.
pressure-controlled inverse ratio v.
pressure support v.
pressure supported v.
proportional assist v.
pulmonary ventilation impairment
v. rate
v. ratio
rebreathing v.
simultaneous independent lung v.
spontaneous intermittent mandatory v.
synchronized intermittent mandatory v.
synchronized nasal intermittent positive-pressure v.
tidal liquid v.
total liquid v.
transtracheal jet v.
ultrahigh-frequency v.
volume-controlled v.
volume-cycled decelerating-flow v.
walking v.
xenon lung ventilation imaging

ventilation/carbon dioxide production

ventilation/perfusion
v. imaging
v. lung scan
v. ratio

ventilator-associated
v.-a. lung injury
v.-a. pneumonia

ventilator-dependent respiratory failure

ventilator-induced lung injury

ventilatory
accumulated alveolar ventilatory volume
v. anaerobic threshold
v. assistance
v. capacity
continuous mechanical ventilatory assistance

v. dysfunction
v. failure
hypercapnic ventilatory response
hypotensive and ventilatory support
hypoxic ventilatory drive
hypoxic ventilatory response
maximal sustainable ventilatory capacity
maximal sustained ventilatory capacity
maximal ventilatory volume
minute ventilatory volume
v. muscle training
noninvasive ventilatory support
timed ventilatory capacity
total ventilatory assistance

venting percutaneous gastrostomy

ventral

v. border
v. branch
v. cell column
v. column
v. decubitus
v. derotating spinal implant
v. derotation spondylodesis
first lumbar ventral nerve root
v. fold
v. gland
v. hernia
v. mesentery
v. nerve root
v. posterior inferior
v. posterolateral nucleus
v. root, lumbar
v. root reflex
v. root, thoracic
second lumbar ventral nerve root
v. septal defect
v. subiculum
v. tegmental area
v. venous line
v. wall defect

ventrale

ventralis

area ventralis of Tsai
v. intermedius
v. lateralis
nucleus ventralis anterior of thalamus
v. oralis anterior
v. oralis posterior
v. posteromedialis

ventricle

akinetic left v.
anteroventral 3rd v.
aortic sinus to right ventricle fistula
aortic ventricle of heart
aortic vestibule of v.
apex of left v.
apical thickening of left v.
appendix of laryngeal v.
appendix of ventricle of larynx
atrium of lateral v.
atrium of v.
augmented filling of right v.
v. of cerebral hemisphere
dilatation of v.
v.'s dilated and hypertrophied
double-inlet v.
double-outlet left v.
double-outlet right v.
effective refractory period of the left v.
electrocardiographic wave corresponding to repolarization of v.'s
hypoplastic left v.
ischemic left v.
lateral v.
left v.
left ventricle to aorta pressure gradient
left ventricle bypass pump
left ventricle of heart
mechanical auxiliary v.
median aperture of fourth v.
minor axis shortening of left v.
one ventricle heart
v.'s to peritoneal cavity shunt
poorly contractile globular left v.
posterior wall of left v.
right v.
right ventricle anterior wall
right ventricle of heart
right ventricle infarction
right ventricle internal dimension diastole
right ventricle stroke output
severe impairment of v.
single v.
slit ventricle syndrome
third ventricle cyst
triple vessel disease with abnormal left v.

ventricle-to-brain ratio

ventricular

abdominal left ventricular assist device
v. access
acquired ventricular septal defect
v. activation time
acute left ventricular heart failure
acute right ventricular heart failure
acute ventricular assist device
v. aneurysm
v. aneurysmectomy
aneurysm of membranous ventricular septum
v. angiography
anterior right ventricular wall
aorta-left ventricular fistula
aorta-right ventricular fistula
aortic-left ventricular tunnel
aortic and left ventricular tunnel
apical left ventricular puncture
v. arrhythmia
v. arrhythmia ablation
v. arrhythmia monitor
arrhythmogenic right ventricular cardiomyopathy
arrhythmogenic right ventricular dysplasia
artificial left ventricular assist device
artificial pacemaker-induced ventricular rhythm
Arvidsson dimension-length method for ventricular volume
v. assist device
v. asynchronous pacemaker
v. asystole
v. atresia
v. atrial distal coronary sinus
v. atrial height right atrium
v. atrial His bundle electrocardiogram
v. atrial proximal coronary sinus
atrial synchronous ventricular inhibited pacing
atrial ventricular canal defect
atrial and ventricular implantable cardioverter-defibrillator
atypical ventricular tachycardia
automated ventricular brain ratio
v. bigeminy
bilateral ventricular assist device
blanked ventricular sense
v. block
v. bradycardia
burst of ventricular pacing
v. capture
v. capture beat
v. cavity
v. cerebrospinal fluid
chaotic activity of ventricular fibrillation

ventricular *(continued)*
combined ventricular hypertrophy
concentric left ventricular hypertrophy
v. conduction
v. conduction velocity
congestive right ventricular failure
continuous ventricular asynchronous pacing
v. contractility function
controlled ventricular response
v. defibrillation
v. demand pacing
v. diastolic fragmentation
v. diastolic gallop
diastolic left ventricular index
v. diastolic pressure
v. dilator
direct mechanical ventricular actuation
double ventricular response
v. dysfunction
v. dysrhythmia
early ventricular repolarization syndrome
v. ectopic activity
v. ectopic arrhythmia
v. ectopic beat
v. ectopic depolarization
ectopic ventricular beat
v. ectopy
v. effective refractory period
Eisenmenger ventricular septal defect
v. ejection fraction
v. elasticity
end-diastolic aortic-left ventricular pressure gradient
end-diastolic left ventricular pressure
v. end-diastolic pressure
v. end-diastolic volume
endocardial cushion-type ventricular septal defect
end-systolic left ventricular pressure
end-systolic ventricular volume
v. escape
escaped ventricular contraction
v. escape rhythm
exercise-induced ventricular tachycardia
external ventricular drainage
v. extra beat
v. extrasystole
v. fibrillation threshold
v. filling pressure
v. fluid
v. fluid pressure
v. flutter
frequency ectopic ventricular beat
v. function curve
v. fusion
v. ganglion
global left ventricular ejection fraction
v. gradient
v. heart disease
v. heave
hydrogen-detected ventricular septal defect
v. hypertrophy
hypoplastic left ventricular syndrome
idiopathic ventricular fibrillation
idiopathic ventricular tachycardia
impaired left ventricular function
v. implantable cardioverter-defibrillator
implantable left ventricular assist system
intact ventricular septum
interstitial left ventricular myocardial fibrosis
v. inversion
isolated noncompaction of the ventricular myocardium
isolated ventricular noncompaction
v. late potential
lateral ventricular nerve
lateral ventricular width to hemispheric width
left v.
left ventricular dimension in end-diastole
left ventricular end-diastole
left lateral ventricular preexcitation
left posterior ventricular preexcitation
left ventricular activation time
left ventricular aneurysm
left ventricular aneurysmectomy
left ventricular angiogram
left ventricular assist device
left ventricular bundle-branch block
left ventricular diastolic dimension
left ventricular diastolic volume
left ventricular dysfunction
left ventricular ejection
left ventricular ejection fraction
left ventricular ejection time
left ventricular ejection time index
left ventricular end-diastolic area
left ventricular end-diastolic circumference
left ventricular end-diastolic diameter
left ventricular end-diastolic dimension
left ventricular end-diastolic pressure
left ventricular end-diastolic volume
left ventricular end-diastolic volume index
left ventricular end-systolic area
left ventricular end-systolic dimension
left ventricular end-systolic volume
left ventricular end-systolic volume index
left ventricular enlargement
left ventricular failure
left ventricular fast filling time
left ventricular filling pressure
left ventricular free wall
left ventricular function
left ventricular functional shortening
left ventricular heart failure
left ventricular hemodynamic abnormalities
left ventricular hypertrophy
left ventricular infarct volume
left ventricular inflow volume
left ventricular initial diastolic pressure
left ventricular injection
left ventricular insufficiency
left ventricular internal diameter
left ventricular internal diastolic diameter
left ventricular internal diastolic dimension
left ventricular internal dimension at end systole
left ventricular internal dimension diastole
left ventricular internal dimension systole
left ventricular mass
left ventricular mass index
left ventricular minute flow
left ventricular muscle mass
left ventricular outflow

left ventricular outflow tract obstruction
left ventricular outflow volume
left ventricular overactivity
left ventricular peak filling rate
left ventricular peak systolic pressure
left ventricular posterior wall
left ventricular posterior wall thickness
left ventricular preejection period
left ventricular reduction
left ventricular septal wall
left ventricular slow filling time
left ventricular strain
left ventricular stroke volume index
left ventricular stroke work
left ventricular stroke work index
left ventricular subendocardial myocardial ischemia
left ventricular systolic diameter
left ventricular systolic dimension
left ventricular systolic dysfunction
left ventricular systolic index
left ventricular systolic output
left ventricular tension
left ventricular wall motion
left ventricular wall motion abnormality
left ventricular wall motion index
malignant ventricular arrhythmia
malignant ventricular tachycardia
marked left ventricular hypertrophy
v. mass
maximal left ventricular developed pressure
maximum ventricular elastance
mean diastolic left ventricular pressure
mean left ventricular systolic pressure
mean right ventricular pressure
mechanical ventricular assistance
multifocal premature ventricular contraction
multiform ventricular tachycardia
muscular ventricular septal defect
muscular ventricular septum
narrowed atrial ventricular valve
nonsustained monomorphic ventricular tachycardia
nonsustained polymorphic ventricular tachycardia
nuclear ventricular function study
onset of ventricular depolarization
v. outflow tract
v. paced rhythm
paced ventricular evoked response
v. pacing, atrial sensing, triggered mode, pacemaker
parasystolic ventricular tachycardia
paroxysmal junctional ventricular tachycardia
v. peritoneal
permanent demand ventricular pacemaker
permanently implanted ventricular assist device
v. pleural pressure gradient
posterior left v.
posthemorrhagic ventricular dilatation
posthemorrhagic ventricular dilation
preejection period/left ventricular ejection time
v. preexcitation
v. premature activation
v. premature beat
v. premature complex
v. premature contraction
v. premature contraction threshold
v. premature depolarization
v. premature depolarization contraction
premature ventricular complex
premature ventricular contraction with coupling
premature ventricular depolarization
premature ventricular extrasystole
primary ventricular fibrillation
programmed ventricular stimulation
v. pseudoaneurysm
pulmonary atresia with intact ventricular septum
pulmonary atresia with ventricular septal defect
v. radial dysplasia
rapid ventricular response
v. rate variability
reentrant ventricular arrhythmia
v. region
repetitive ventricular response
v. residual volume
v. response
v. response rate
v. rhythm
right v.
right bundle v.
right ventricular inflow tract
right posterior ventricular preexcitation
right ventricular activation
right ventricular apex
right ventricular apical
right ventricular assist device
right ventricular cardiomyopathy
right ventricular copulsation balloon
right ventricular diastolic overload
right ventricular diastolic pressure
right ventricular diastolic volume
right ventricular dimension
right ventricular ejection fraction
right ventricular ejection time
right ventricular end-diastolic diameter
right ventricular end-diastolic pressure
right ventricular end-diastolic volume
right ventricular end-diastolic volume index
right ventricular end-flow
right ventricular endocardial potential
right ventricular end-systolic volume
right ventricular end-systolic volume index
right ventricular filling pressure
right ventricular function
right ventricular heart failure
right ventricular heave
right ventricular hypertrophy
right ventricular hypoplasia
right ventricular initial diastolic pressure
right ventricular internal dimension
right ventricular mass
right ventricular outflow
right ventricular outflow tract
right ventricular overactivity
right ventricular peak filling rate
right ventricular refractory period
right ventricular stroke work index
right ventricular systolic pressure
right ventricular wall device
v. sense
v. septal heart defect
v. septum
v. shunt
v. specialized conduction system
v. stroke work

ventricular *(continued)*
sustained monomorphic ventricular tachycardia
sustained reentrant ventricular tachyarrhythmia
sustained ventricular tachycardia
v. synchronous pacing
v. tachyarrhythmia
v. tachycardia cycle length
v. tachycardia event
v. tachycardia nonsustained
v. tachycardia sustained
torsade de pointes ventricular tachycardia
transesophageal ventricular pacing
v. trigeminy
unifocal premature ventricular contractions
unifocal ventricular ectopic beat
unsustained ventricular tachycardia
v. wall motion
v. wall motion abnormality
v. wave

ventricular-brain ratio

ventriculares
arteriae v.

ventriculi
apertura lateralis ventriculi quarti
apertura mediana ventriculi quarti
atrium ventriculi lateralis
Merkel filtrum v.
paries anterior v.
pars centralis ventriculi lateralis

ventriculitis

ventriculoarterial connection

ventriculoatrial
v. condition
v. conduction
sequential ventriculoatrial pacing

ventriculogram
axial left anterior oblique v.
gated blood pool v.
left v.
radionuclide v.

ventriculography
contrast v.
digital subtraction v.
echocardiography-radionuclide v.
low-dose dobutamine stress radionuclide v.
pacing digital v.
radionuclide v.

ventriculojugular shunt

ventriculolumbar perfusion

ventriculomegaly
posthemorrhagic v.

ventriculoperitoneal
occult trauma, postanoxia, v.
v. shunt

ventriculoseptal defect

ventriculotomy
encircling endocardial v.
partial encircling endocardial v.

ventriculovenous shunt

ventrocaudal nucleus

ventrogluteal
left v.
right v.

ventrolateral
v. medulla
v. nucleus of hypothalamus
right ventrolateral gluteal
rostral ventrolateral medulla

ventrolateralis

ventromedial
hypothalamic ventromedial nucleus
lateral ventromedial nucleus
medial ventromedial nucleus
v. nucleus
v. nucleus of the hypothalamus
v. tegmentum
v. hypothalamic neuron, nucleus

ventromedialis

Venturi mask

venulae
medial venulae of retina

venule
high-endothelial v.
main v.
nasal venule of retina
postcapillary v.

Venus
necklace of V.

vera
anodontia v.
melena v.
neuralgia facialis v.
polycythemia rubra v.
polycythemia vera with myeloid metaplasia

verb
auxiliary v.

verbal
v. aggression
v. agraphia
alert, verbal stimulus response, painful stimulus response, unresponsive
alpha verbal test
v. aphasia
v. apraxia
V. Auditory Screen for Children
auditory verbal agnosia
auditory verbal memory
California V. Learning Test
Children's Auditory V. Learning Test-2
v. communication
v. comprehension
v. comprehension deviation quotient
v. comprehension factor
constant verbal cueing
v. cue
v. deficit
eyes, motor, v.
V. Fluency Test
impaired verbal communication
V. Intelligence Quotient
v. involuntary tic
involuntary verbal tic
V. Language Development Scale
Mecham V. Language Scale
v. nonemotional stimuli
v., numerical, and reasoning
Oral V. Intelligence Test
v. order
patient responsive to verbal command
v. reprimand
respond to verbal command
Rey Auditory V. Learning Test
v. sample evaluation method

verbal-auditory agnosia

verbalization
inappropriate v.

verbalizer-visualization questionnaire

verbalize understanding

verbally
patient responded v.

verbotonol
system universal verbotonol audition Guberina

Verdun
V. Depression Rating Scale
V. Target Symptom Rating Scale

vergance
ocular vergance and accommodation sensor

verge
anal v.
nasal v.

vergence
v. eye movements
negative vertical v.

verification
automated eligibility verification system

vermicularis
atrophoderma v.

vermiculatum
atrophoderma v.

vermiform
v. appendage
v. appendix
appendix v.
v. body
removal of vermiform appendix

vermilion
v. border
lip v.

vermis
anterior v.
anterior vermis syndrome
cerebellar vermis hypoplasia, oligophrenia, congenital ataxia, coloboma, hepatic fibrosis
craniosynostosis, ataxia, trigeminal anesthesia, parietal anesthesia and pons, vermis fusion syndrome
v. incision
medullary body of v.
partial agenesis of v.

Vermont spinal fixator

vernal
v. keratoconjunctivitis
limbic vernal keratoconjunctivitis
oval-shaped vernal ulcer

vernix
yellow vernix syndrome

verocytotoxin-producing ***Escherichia coli***

Veronal
V. buffer
gelatin, glucose, and Veronal buffer
glucose-gelatin Veronal buffer

Veronal-buffered
V.-b. diluent
V.-b. oxalated saline
V.-b. saline-fetal bovine serum

verotoxin-producing ***Escherichia coli***

verruca, pl. **verrucae**
mosaic v.
v. plana juvenilis
v. plantaris
v. vulgaris
v. vulgaris of the larynx

verruciformis
epidermal dysplastic v.
epidermodysplasia v.

verrucoid
hyperkeratotic verrucoid surfaced lesion

verrucosa hyperplasia

verrucosis
lymphostatic v.
nevus v.

verrucosum
molluscum v.

verrucosus
lichen planus v.
lichen ruber v.
lupus v.

verrucous
atypical verrucous endocarditis
v. carcinoma
v. endocarditis
v. hemangioma
inflamed linear verrucous epidermal nevus
inflammatory linear verrucous epidermal nevus
v. lesion
leukoplakia
linear inflammatory verrucous epidermal nevus
nonbacterial verrucous endocarditis
proliferative verrucous leukoplakia
v. vegetation

versatility
attachment v.

versicolor
pityriasis v.
tinea v.

version
Body Dysmorphic Disorder Modification of Yale-Brown Obsessive-Compulsive Scale, McLean v.
Diagnostic Interview for Children and Adolescents-Child V.
Diagnostic Interview for Children and Adolescents-Parent V.
ductions and v.'s
external cephalic v.
femoral neck v.
modified version of the mini mental status examination
Schedule for Affective Disorders and Schizophrenia for School-Age Children-Epidemiologic V.
Simplified Acute Physiology Score version II
Structured Clinical Interview for DSM-IV Axis I Disorders: Clinician V.
Structured Clinical Interview for DSM-IV Patient V.

versus
cancellous versus cortical bone
Carotid Artery Stenosis with Asymptomatic Narrowing: Operation V. Aspirin Study
congenital versus acquired syndrome
eloquent versus noneloquent area
internal versus external
performance versus intensity function for phonetically balanced words
total infections versus total admission
whole brain versus local brain radiation therapy

vertebra, pl. **vertebrae**
anterior scalloping of v.
anterior tubercle of cervical vertebrae
arch of v.
articular process of v.
cervical v.
cervical and thoracic vertebrae
collapsed vertebra of spine
first to fifth sacral vertebrae
first through fifth lumbar vertebrae or lumbar nerve
first through twelfth dorsal vertebrae
first to twelfth thoracic vertebrae
last normal v.
lumbar fifth vertebra to sacral first v.
mammillary process of lumbar v.
neural arch of v.
pedicle of arch of v.
thoracic v.
true v.

vertebral
v. abnormality, anal imperforation, tracheoesophageal

vertebral *(continued)*
fistula, and radial, ray, or renal anomalies
alignment of vertebral bodies
v. ankylosing hyperostosis
anomalous vertebral artery
anterior internal vertebral vein
anterior lumbar vertebral interbody fusion
anterior vertebral body margin
anterior vertebral vein
v. arch
v. arch defect
v. arteries of intracerebral vessels
v. artery
v. artery bypass graft
v. artery dissection
v. artery injury
v. artery occlusion
v. artery test
v. arthritis
artificial vertebral body
atlantic part of vertebral artery
atlas vertebral subluxation complex
avascular vertebral body necrosis
v. axial decompression
v. basilar insufficiency
bipolar vertebral traction
v. block
v. body decompression
v. body endplate
v. body fracture
v. body shape
v. body size
v. body tenderness
v. bone loss
v. bone mass
v. canal
v. collapse
v. column
v. column defect
v. compression
decalcified section of vertebral body
v. disk
v. dissection
v. endplate
v. exposure
v. fracture
v. fusion
v. ganglion
v. groove
v. hemangioma
v. interspace
v. irritation syndrome
left vertebral artery
longitudinal vertebral venous sinus
meningeal branch of intracranial part of vertebral artery
v. motion unit
v. osteomyelitis
pain from herniated vertebral disc
v. plexus
polydactyly, imperforate anus, vertebral anomalies syndrome
relative vertebral density
reversed vertebral blood flow
right vertebral artery
right vertebral density
v. subluxation complex

vertebrobasilar
v. artery insufficiency
v. artery system
v. insufficiency
v. occlusive disease
possible vertebrobasilar system
v. territory ischemia

vertebroplasty
percutaneous v.

vertex, pl. **vertices**
back vertex power
v. delivery
v. headache
v. potential
v. presentation
v. sharp transient electroencephalography
spontaneous vertex vaginal delivery
submental vertex view

vertical
v. angulation
anterior vertical canal
v. axis
v. axis of rectangular coordinate system
v. banded gastroplasty
bilateral vertical ramus osteotomy
v. and centric bite
v. compression
congenital vertical talus
congenital vertical talus foot deformity
cup-to-disc ratio v.
v. deviation
dissociated vertical deviation
v. float aquatic therapy
v. float progression aquatic therapy
v. flow clean bench
v. fracture
gastric vertical stapling
v. gaze palsy
v. groove
v. heart
v. hemianopia
v. hymen
v. incision
incomplete vertical root fracture
v. index
index of vertical transmission
intraoral vertical ramus osteotomy
intraoral vertical segmental osteotomy
low v.
low cervical vertical incision
low vertical cesarean section
low vertical uterine incision
v. maxillary deficiency
v. maxillary excess
midline vertical uterine extension
v. movement
negative vertical divergence
negative vertical vergence
Nichamin vertical chopper
v. nystagmus
occlusal vertical dimension
v. plane
positive vertical divergence
postural vertical dimension
v. radiation topography
v. ring gastroplasty
v. sagittal split osteotomy
v. shear
silicone elastomer ring vertical gastroplasty
v. stabilization program
v. sternotomy
v. strabismus
v. subcondylar oblique
v. synchronization pulse
v. uterine incision
v. vesicomyotomy

vertically
opened v.

vertices (*pl. of* vertex)

verticis

vertiginous episode

vertigo
benign paroxysmal positional v.
chronic posttraumatic v.
disabling positional v.
v. and imbalance
initial attack of v.
intermittent attacks of severe v.
paroxysmal positional v.

recalcitrant benign paroxysmal positional v.
v., syncope and hypotension
toxic v.

very
v. early onset schizophrenia
v. fast death factor
v. good
v. good health
v. high density lipoprotein
v. high dose phenobarbital
v. high frequency
v. important patient
v. large scale integration
v. late activation
v. late antigen-4
v. long chain acyl-CoA dehydrogenase
v. long chain fatty acid
long-chain very long-chain acyl-CoA dehydrogenase deficiency
v. low birth rate
v. low birth weight
v. low birth weight infant
v. low birth weight preterm neonate
v. low calorie diet
v. low density
v. low density lipoprotein
v. low density lipoprotein C
v. low density lipoprotein-triglyceride
v. low frequency
v. narrow anterior chamber angle
patient very disturbed
v. sensitive
v. short below-elbow cast
v. urgent

very-late antigen

Vesalius
canal of V.
foramen of V.

vesicae
apex v.
ectopia v.

vesical
v. calculus
v. external sphincter dyssynergia
v. fistula
v. hematuria
v. hernia
v. neck
v. neck contracture
v. trabeculation
transurethral resection of vesical neck

vesicalis
anus v.
arteria vesicalis superior
plica vesicalis transversa

vesicata
Lytta vesicata sting

vesicle
v. attachment site
carotenoid v.
germinal v.
germinal vesicle breakdown
v. hernia
herpes virus v.'s
inside-out v.
intraepithelial v.'s
large dense-cored v.
large granular v.
large opaque v.
large unilamellar v.
multilaminar v.
nonionic surfactant v.
pinocytotic v.
seminal v.
seminal vesicle invasion
seminal vesicle microsome
sheep seminal v.
small granular v.
transfer v.

vesicocervical space

vesicomyotomy
circular v.
vertical v.

vesicoureteral
direct vesicoureteral scintigraphy
v. junction
v. reflux grade I–V

vesicourethral
v. anastomosis
v. angle
v. canal

vesicouterine
v. fistula
v. ligament

vesicovaginal
v. fistula
v. fistula repair
v. space

vesicular
v. appendage
v. breathing
v. breath sounds
v. exanthema
v. exanthema of swine virus
v. monoamine transporter
v. rale
v. rosette
v. stomatitis
v. stomatitis Alagoas virus
v. stomatitis Indiana virus
swine vesicular disease
swine vesicular disease virus
v. transport system

vesiculography
seminal v.

vesiculosa
appendix v.
miliaria v.

vesiculosae

vespid
mixed vespid antigen
mixed vespid venom

vessel
advanced vessel analysis
afferent lymphatic v.
angiographically occult v.
angioplasty-related vessel occlusion
antegrade filling of v.
anterior great v.
antineutrophilic cytoplasmic autoantibody-small vessel vasculitis
arteriosclerosis of eye v.
atherosclerosis of intracerebral v.'s
atypical vessel colposcopic pattern
ballooning-out of blood v.
blood v.
blood vessel endothelium
blood vessel graft
blood vessel inflammation
blood vessel invasion
blood vessel prosthesis
caliber of v.
collateralizing v.
complete transposition of great v.'s
conceptional v.
constriction or spasm of blood v.
coronary vessel anatomy
corrected congenital transposition of the great vessels
dextratransposition of great v.'s
disc, macula, v.'s, periphery
discs and v.'s
elevated new v.'s elsewhere
elevated new v.'s on the disc
extraalveolar v.
frond of v.
governing v.

vessel *(continued)*
graft vessel disease
heart and great v.'s
hemangioma of meningeal v.'s
hilar v.'s exposed
impaired blood vessel elasticity
intercostal vessel ligated
internal spermatic v.
invasive growth of blood v.
large vessel hematocrit
laser photocoagulation of the communicating v.
lymph vessel invasion
mechanical vessel blockage
mucosal blood v.
narrowed blood v.
narrowing of blood v.
neovascularization of new v.'s elsewhere
new v.
new vessel disc
new v.'s elsewhere
nonbleeding visible v.
occluded carotid v.
occluded coronary v.
opticociliary shunt v.
palliation of great v.'s
pancreaticoduodenal arcade v.
pelvic collateral v.
periesophageal blood v.
peripelvic collateral v.
peripheral v.
plaque in blood v.
prominence of pulmonary v.
proximal and distal portion of v.
reference vessel diameter
revascularization of blood v.'s of heart
ruptured blood v.'s
small caliber v.
small vessel disease
small vessel inadequate blood flow
stimulate new vessel growth
target vessel revascularization
thin-walled blood v.
tortuous blood v.
transposition of great v.
triple vessel disease with abnormal left ventricle
vascular congestion of interstitial v.
vertebral arteries of intracerebral v.'s
v. wall

vest
halo v.
patient restrained with v.

vestibular
angular vestibular nucleus
anogenital vestibular cyst
anogenital vestibular papilla
anterior and posterior vestibular veins
anterior vestibular artery
v. aqueduct
v. aqueduct syndrome
v. autorotational testing
v. autorotation test
Brief V. Disorientation Test
caloric stimulation test for vestibular function
caloric testing of vestibular function
v. canal
central audio vestibular dysfunction
v. compensation
v. damage
v. deficit
v. disease
v. disorder
v. dizziness
v. dysfunction
enlarged vestibular aqueduct syndrome
v. fold
v. fossa
galvanic vestibular stimulation
v. ganglion
v. gland
greater vestibular gland
great vestibular gland
v. hair cell
v. hyperreactivity
lateral vestibular nucleus
v. ligament
little fossa of oval vestibular window
v. membrane
middle fossa vestibular nerve section
middle fossa vestibular neurectomy
nasal vestibular stenosis
v. nerve
v. neurectomy
nonsyndromic familial enlarged vestibular aqueduct
v. nucleus
v. nystagmus
peripheral vestibular deficit
peripheral vestibular nystagmus
reduced vestibular response
retrolabyrinthine vestibular neurectomy
v. saccule
v. schwannoma
v. vertigo

vestibularis
anus v.
area v.
area vestibularis superior
arteria vestibularis anterior
pars caudalis nervi v.

vestibule
aortic v.
aortic vestibule of ventricle
aqueduct of v.
artery of bulb of v.
laryngeal v.
v. of larynx
nasal v.
nasal vestibule cancer
urogenital v.

vestibulitis
vulvar vestibulitis syndrome

vestibulocerebellar ataxia

vestibulocochlearis
arteria v.

vestibulocochlear nerve

vestibulolingual
mandibular vestibulolingual sulcoplasty

vestibuloocular
v. reflex
v. response
visually enhanced vestibuloocular reflex
visual vestibuloocular reflex

vestibulospinal
lateral vestibulospinal tract

vestigial
Marshall vestigial fold
v. testis

vestimenti
pediculosis v.

vestimentorum

vest-over-pants
v.-o.-p. herniorrhaphy

veteran
combat v.
Vietnam V.'s Evaluation and Treatment Program

Veteran's
V. Adjustment Scale

V. Administration Cooperative Study on Glycemic Control and Complications in Type 2 Diabetes Trial
V. Administration hospital

veterinarian

veterinary
maximum residue limits of veterinary drugs
red veterinary petrolatum

Vi
typhoid vaccine, Vi capsular polysaccharide

via
atrial septostomy via balloon
shunt index via superior mesenteric vein
shunt index via the inferior mesenteric vein
uterine positioning via ligament investment fixation truncation

viability
endocardial viability ratio
fetal v.
organ v.

viable
v. alternative
v. birth
v. female infant
v. fetus
v. heart
individually viable cell
Irvine viable organ-tissue transport system
v. male infant
number of pregnancies producing viable offspring
total viable cells

vial
glass v.
multiple dose v.
transport v.

vibrate
percuss and v.

vibrating ossicular prosthesis

vibration
chest percussion and v.
double v.
v. perception testing
v. perception threshold
percussion and v.
percussion, vibration, and drainage
percussion, vibration, and suction
v. per minute
postural drainage, percussion and v.
v. sense
single v.
v. threshold
tonic vibration reflex
tonic vibration response
total vibration reflex

vibrational circular dichroism

vibration-induced white finger

vibrator
automatic v.
bone-conduction v.

vibratory
impaired discriminatory, vibratory and position sensation
v. acoustic stimulation

vibrio
V. cholerae neuraminidase
marine v.'s
Nasik *Vibrio*
noncholera *Vibrio*

vibroacoustic stimulation

vicarious
v. hemoptysis
v. hemorrhage
v. hyperplasia
v. hypertrophy

vichy
artificial vichy salt

vicinal isomer

Vickers
V. hardness number

victim
accident v.
cocaine-related heart attack v.
heart attack v.
high-risk potential v.'s
ice v.
irradiated v.
National Organization of V. Assistance

Vidas
mini Vidas automated immunoassay system

video
v. arthroscopy
v. cassette recorder
v. densitometry
v. dimensional analysis
v. disc
v. display terminal
v. display terminal glare screen
v. display terminal simulator
v. display unit
v. endoscopy
v. esophagoscopy
flexible video laparoscope
v. fluoroscopy
forward-viewing video colonoscope
v. frequency
v. gambling
v. graphic tool technology
high-definition video display
v. imaging
v. imaging system
v. monitoring
Niamtu video imaging system

video-assisted
v.-a. excisional biopsy
v.-a. gastrectomy
v.-a. thoracic surgery
v.-a. thoracic surgical non-rib-spreading lobectomy
v.-a. thoracoscopic surgery
v.-a. thoracoscopy
v.-a. transthoracic surgery

videoendoscopic
v. surgery
v. swallowing study

videofluorographic evaluation of swallowing

videofluoroscopic
v. barium swallow
v. swallowing study

videofluoroscopy
modified barium swallow with v.

video-intensification microscopy

videokeratography
computerized v.

videoscope
Olympus v.

videoscopic
v. evaluation
v. hernia surgery

vidian
v. artery
v. canal
v. nerve
v. neuralgia

Vieja
Sal Vieja virus

Vietnam
V. era
V. Veterans Evaluation and Treatment Program

Vieussens
annulus of V.
ansa of V.
V. anulus
anulus of V.
circle of V.
V. ganglion
V. isthmus
loop of V.

view
air contrast view of the stomach
angled craniocaudal v.
anterior feet v.
anterior-posterior, posterior-anterior v.
anteroposterior and lateral v.'s
apical 2-chamber v.
apical 2-chamber view echocardiography
apical 4-chamber v.
apical 2-chamber view echocardiogram
apical 4-chamber view echocardiogram
apical 5-chamber view echocardiogram
apical 5-chamber view echocardiography
apical lordotic v.
apical and subcostal four-chambered v.
AP inversion stress vagina v.
AP and lateral v.
AP supine portable v.
axial calcaneus v.
axial sesamoid v.
beam's eye v.
Caldwell x-ray v.
caudocranial hemiaxial v.
color enhanced v.
cross-table lateral v.
exaggerated craniocaudal lateral v.
field of v.
high right parasternal v.
large field of v.
lateral distant v.
lateral oblique x-ray v.
left portal v.
long axial oblique v.
long axis parasternal v.
medial oblique v.
medial oblique x-ray v.
multiplanar reformatting v.
normal anteroposterior v.
normal AP v.
owl's eyes view of hydrocele
radius of v.
right anterior oblique v.
right posterior oblique radiologic v.
soft tissue v.
Stenver x-ray v.
submental vertex v.
three concept v.
useful field of v.

viewing
exophoria, near v.

viewpoint
alternative v.

vigilance-controlled electroencephalogram

vigorous pulmonary toilet

VII
factor VII
factor VII antigen
factor VII deficiency
factor VII inhibitor
factor VII, VIII inhibitor
medial basal bronchopulmonary segment S VII
mucopolysaccharidosis types I, II, III, IIIB, III, IIID, IVA, IVB, VI, VII
mucopolysaccharidosis type VII Sly

VII
nervus facialis [CN V.]

VIIA
recombinant factor V.

VII:Ag10000
Asserachrom V.

VIII
factor VIII
factor VIII antigen
factor VIII coagulation function
factor VIII deficiency
factor VIII gene
factor VIII hemophilia
factor VIII inhibitor
factor VIII inhibitor bypassing activity
factor VIII, IX deficiency
factor VII, VIII inhibitor

VIII:C
factor VIII:C heat-treated antihemophilic factor
factor VIII:C inhibitor

VI–IX
OFD syndrome, type I–IV, V.

villi (*pl. of* villous)

villitis of unknown etiology

villoglandular adenocarcinoma

villonodular
diffuse pigmented villonodular synovitis
pigmented villonodular bundle
pigmented villonodular synovitis
pigmented villonodular tenovagosynovitis
v. synovitis

villotubular adenoma

villous, pl. **villi**
v. adenoma
arachnoid villi
arachnoid granulation villi
arachnoid villi obstruction
atrophic villi
v. atrophy
v. carcinoma
chorionic villi
chronic villous arthritis
jejunal villi
multiple villous infarcts
partial villous atrophy
pectinate villi
pleural villi
splenic lymphoma with villous lymphocyte
v. structure
subtotal villous atrophy

villus
arachnoid v.
chorionic villus biopsy
chorionic villus infarction
chorionic villus ischemia
chorionic villus sampling
intestinal v.
mature abnormal chorionic v.

vinblastine
Adriamycin, vinblastine, methotrexate
chlorambucil, vinblastine, procarbazine, prednisone, etoposide, vincristine, Adriamycin
doxorubicin, vinblastine, mechlorethamine, vincristine, bleomycin, etoposide, prednisone
L-phenylalanine mustard, v.
methotrexate, vinblastine, Adriamycin, cisplatin
mitomycin, vinblastine, Platinol
nitrogen mustard, vincristine, procarbazine, prednisone/doxorubicin, bleomycin, v.

Vincent
V. bacillus
V. disease
Vinces virus
vinculum, pl. **vincula**
long v.
vinegar
Vineland
V. Measurement of Social Competence
V. Social Maturity Scale
Vinethine and ether anesthesia
vinosus
nevus v.
vinyl
v. chloride
v. chloride monomer
ethylene vinyl acetate
violaceous hue
violation
articular cartilage v.
violence
acquired violence immune deficiency syndrome
acts of v.
adolescents risk for v.
alcohol-related risk for v.
alleviating violence in aggressive behavior
anger and violence psychiatric syndrome
antecedents of v.
domestic v.
v. and eloper
physical harm or v.
violence-induced handicap
violent
aggressive or violent behavior
alternative to violent behavior
hyperactive and v.
v. and irregular jerking motion
violet
aniline gentian v.
cresyl v.
cresyl violet acetate
crystal v.
ethyl violet azide broth
gentian v.
tetrazolium v.
viper
Russell v.
viral
acute viral hepatitis
acute viral infection
acute viral respiratory infection
acute viral syndrome
v. agent
v. analog scale
anicteric viral hepatitis
v. antigen
antisense oligonucleotide viral therapy
arthropod-borne viral arthritis and rash
arthropod-borne viral disease
arthropod-borne viral encephalitis
arthropod-borne viral hemorrhagic fever
asymptomatic viral shedding
avian viral arthritis virus
bovine viral diarrhea virus 1, 2
bovine viral diarrhea
bovine viral diarrhea mucosal disease
v. capsid antigen
v. capsid antigen, Epstein-Barr
v. cell surface antigen
charcoal viral transport medium
cholestatic viral hepatitis
chronic active viral hepatitis
chronic active viral hepatitis, non-A, non-B
chronic active viral hepatitis, type B
confirmed transmission of viral hepatitis
Coxsackie viral infection
v. cystitis
v. diarrhea
v. disease
documented viral infection
v. dysentery
v. encephalitis
v. enteritis
v. envelope antigen
Epstein-Barr viral capsid antigen
feline viral rhinotracheitis
food-borne transmission of viral hepatitis
fulminant viral hepatitis
v. gastritis
v. gastroenteritis
v. glycoprotein
glycosylated protein spanning viral envelope
v. hematodepressive disease
hemodialysis transmission of viral hepatitis
v. hemorrhagic fever
v. hemorrhagic septicemia virus
v. hepatitis
v. hepatitis panel
herpes simplex viral shedding
hibernal epidemic viral infection
hospital-acquired viral hepatitis
v. illness
v. infection
v. inflammation
inoculation transmission of viral hepatitis
intrauterine viral infection
v. isolation
live viral vector
v. load
v. lode testing
low-level viral replication
lytic viral replication
maternal-neonatal transmission of viral hepatitis
v. myocarditis
nosocomial viral conjunctivitis
oral transmission of viral hepatitis
parainfluenza viral disease
persistent viral hepatitis
persistent viral hepatitis, non-A, non-B
persistent viral hepatitis, type B
persistent viral syndrome
plasma viral load
v. pneumonia
v. porcine pneumonia
v. protein
v. protein R
rabies viral culture
recognizable viral syndrome
v. respiratory infection
v. rhinosinusitis
v. ribonucleic acid
sexual transmission of viral hepatitis
soluble viral extract
v. titer
transfusion transmission of viral hepatitis
v. protein R
waterborne transmission of viral hepatitis
viral-associated arthritis
viral-like infection
Virchow
V. angle
V. cell
V. corpuscle
V. disease
V. node
Virchow-Robin space

viremia
asymptomatic v.
hepatitis v.
low-titer v.
maternal v.
virginal introitus
Virgin River virus
viridans
icterus v.
Streptococcus viridans endocarditis
viridescens
Lactobacillus v.
virile
virilis
mamma v.
virilism
congenital adrenal v.
virilizing
adrenal virilizing syndrome
congenital virilizing adrenal hyperplasia
Cushing virilizing syndrome
simple virilizing congenital adrenal hyperplasia
v. adrenal hyperplasia
virion
influenza virion vaccine, split v.
influenza virion vaccine, whole v.
influenza virus inactivated vaccine, split virion, types A, B, trivalent
viroid
potato spindle tuber v.
virosomes
immunopotentiating reconstituted influenza v.
virtual
ARTMA virtual patient
v. bronchoscopy
v. colonoscopy
v. endoscopy
v. labor monitor
parallel virtual machine
v. patient record
virtually safe dose
virulence
low virulence vaccine
virulent
smooth, capsulated, virulent bacteria
virus
Abelson leukemia v.
Abelson murine leukemia v.
Abras v.
Acado v.
acquired immune deficiency syndrome virus infection
acquired immunodeficiency syndrome-related v.
Adelaide River v.
adenoassociated virus 1–5
adenoassociated virus for cystic fibrosis
adult T-cell leukemia v.
African horse sickness virus 1–9
African swine fever v.
African tick v.
Aguacate v.
v. A hepatitis
AIDS-related v.
Akabane v.
Alenquer v.
Aleutian mink disease v.
Almeirim v.
Almpiwar v.
Altamira v.
Amapari v.
American eel v.
amphotropic murine leukemia v.
anal human papilloma virus infection
Ananindeua v.
Andasibe v.
Anhanga v.
Anhembi v.
anicteric virus hepatitis
animal v.'s
Anopheles A, B v.
Antequera v.
antibodies to the Epstein-Barr virus transactivator protein
antibody to hepatitis A–E v.
anti-Epstein-Barr v.
anti-Epstein-Barr virus antibody
antihepatitis A, E v.
antihepatitis C virus seropositive
antihepatitis delta virus immunoglobulin
antihepatitis E virus immunoglobulin
antihuman immunodeficiency virus immune serum globulin
antihuman immunodeficiency virus protease inhibitor
antirespiratory syncytial v.
Apeu v.
aphid lethal paralysis v.
Aphthovirus A virus
Apoi v.
Aransas Bay v.
Arbia v.
Arboledas v.
arboviral virus disease
Argentine hemorrhagic fever v.
Arkonam v.
Aroa v.
Arracacha virus A, B, Y
Arracacha latent v.
arthropod-borne v.
arthropod-borne virus encephalitis
Aruac v.
Arumowot v.
attenuated mumps v.
Aujeszky disease v.
Aura v.
Australian X disease v.
Australian X encephalitis v.
Auzduk disease v.
Avalon v.
avian encephalomyelitis v.
avian erythroblastosis v.
avian infectious bronchitis v.
avian infectious laryngotracheitis v.
avian influenza v.
avian leukosis v.
avian leukosis-sarcoma v.
avian lymphomatosis v.
avian myeloblastosis leukemia virus reverse transcriptase
avian myeloblastosis virus reverse transcriptase
avian myelocytomatosis v.
avian neurolymphomatosis v.
avian paramyxovirus virus 1–9
avian pneumoencephalitis v.
avian sarcoma and leukosis virus
avian tumor v.
avian viral arthritis v.
A virus hepatitis
Babahoya v.
baboon virus replication
Bagaza v.
Bahig v.
Bakau v.
Baku v.
Bandia v.
Bangoran v.
Bangui v.
Banna v.
Barmah Forest v.
Barranqueras v.
Barur v.
Batai v.
Batama v.
Bauline v.
Bayou v.

bean golden mosaic v.
Bebaru v.
Belem v.
Belmont v.
Belterra v.
Benevides v.
Benfica v.
Berne v.
Berrimah v.
v. B hepatitis
Bimbo v.
Bimiti v.
Birao v.
black beetle v.
Black Creek Canal v.
v. blockade
bluetongue virus 1–24
Bobaya v.
Bobia v.
Boletus virus X
Boraceia v.
border disease v.
Borna disease v.
Botambi v.
Boteke v.
Bouboui v.
bovine leukemia v.
bovine viral diarrhea virus 1, 2
Buenaventura v.
Bunyamwera v.
Bunyip Creek v.
Bushbush v.
Bussuquara v.
Buttonwillow v.
Bwamba v.
Cache Valley v.
Cacipacore v.
Caimito v.
Calchaqui v.
California encephalitis v.
Cananeia v.
Caninde v.
canine distemper v.
Cape Wrath v.
Capim v.
caprine arthritis encephalitis v.
Caraparu v.
Carey Island v.
carrier of human immunodeficiency v.
Catu v.
cauliflower mosaic v.
central European encephalitis v.
Chaco v.
Chagres v.
challenge virus strain
Chandipura v.
Changuinola v.
Charleville v.
Chenuda v.
chick syncytial v.
Chikungunya v.
Chilibre v.
Chim v.
chimpanzee coryza agent v.
Chobar Gorge v.
chronic Epstein-Barr v.
Clo Mor v.
coastal plains v.
cold-adapted influenza virus vaccine, trivalent
Colorado tick fever v.
Connecticut v.
Corfou v.
Corriparta v.
Cotia v.
Cowbone Ridge v.
Coxsackie virus myocarditis
Crimean-Congo hemorrhagic fever v.
croup-associated v.
cucumber mosaic v.
cytomegalic inclusion disease v.
cytoplasmic polyhedrosis v.
Dakar bat v.
D'Aoust Fineman v.
deer kidney v.
defective leukemia v.
dengue virus 1–4
Dera Ghazi Khan v.
Diplocarpon rosae v.
disabled infectious single cycle v.
distemper v.
Douglas v.
Drosophila A, C, P, X v.
duck embryo v.
duck hepatitis B v.
duck virus enteritis
Dugbe v.
Eastern equine encephalitis v.
Eastern equine encephalomyelitis v.
Ebola v.
Ebola virus outbreak
Edge Hill v.
encephalomyocarditis v.
Enseada v.
Entebbe bat v.
enterocytopathogenic avian orphan v.
enterocytopathogenic bovine orphan v.
enterocytopathogenic cat orphan v.
enterocytopathogenic dog orphan v.
enterocytopathogenic equine orphan v.
enterocytopathogenic human orphan v.
enterocytopathogenic human orphan-rhinocoryza v.
enterocytopathogenic monkey orphan v.
enterocytopathogenic porcine orphan v.
enterocytopathogenic rodent orphan v.
enterocytopathogenic swine orphan v.
v. entry mediator, a receptor expressed by T lymphocyte
epizootic hemorrhagic disease virus 1–8
Epstein-Barr v.
Epstein-Barr virus early antigen
Epstein-Barr virus nuclear antigen
equine abortion v.
equine morbilli v.
equine rhinopneumonitis v.
erythroid leukemia v.
Estero Real v.
Eubenangee v.
Everglades v.
Eyach v.
Farallon v.
feline ataxia v.
feline fibrosarcoma v.
feline immunodeficiency v.
feline infectious peritonitis v.
feline leukemia v.
feline panleukopenia v.
fer-de-lance v.
Fiji disease v.
Flanders v.
Flexal v.
Fomede v.
foot-and-mouth disease v.
Forecariah v.
Fort Morgan v.
Fort Sherman v.
fowl plague v.
Friend disease v.
Friend leukemia v.
Friend spleen focus v.
Friend virus anemia
Friend virus polycythemia
Frijoles v.
Gabek Forest v.

virus *(continued)*
Gadget's Gully v.
Gamboa v.
Gan Gan v.
gastrointestinal v.
genital herpes v.
Germiston v.
Getah v.
gibbon ape leukemia v.
gibbon ape lymphosarcoma v.
golden shiner v.
Gomoka v.
goose hepatitis v.
Gordil v.
Gossas v.
Grand Arbaud v.
granulosis v.
Gray Lodge v.
Great Island v.
Gross leukemia v.
Gross sarcoma virus antigen
Guajara v.
Guama v.
Guaroa v.
Gumbo Limbo v.
Gurupi v.
hamster leukemia v.
Hantaan v.
Hart Park v.
Harvey murine sarcoma v.
Hazara v.
hemadsorption v.
hemagglutinating virus of Japan
hemagglutination encephalomyelitis v.
hepatitis virus A, B, IH
hepatitis A–G v.
hepatitis-associated virus
hepatitis A virus antibody
hepatitis B virus immunoglobulin
hepatitis C virus enzyme immunoassay
hepatitis C virus RNA
hepatitis delta v.
hepatitis G virus RNA
hepatitis virus social history
hepatoencephalomyelitis v.
herpes family of v.'s
herpes simplex virus 1, 2
herpes simplex virus type 1, 2, 6, 7
herpes simplex virus encephalitis
herpes simplex virus thymidine kinase
herpes-type v.
herpes virus of the eye
herpes virus vesicles
herpes zoster v.
herpes zoster virus infection
Highlands J v.
Huacho v.
Hughes v.
human B lymphotropic v.
human coronary v.
human corona virus sensitivity
human enteric v.
human hepatitis A v.
human immunodeficiency v.
human immunodeficiency virus type 1, 2
human immunodeficiency virus antibody
human immunodeficiency virus associated dementia
human immunodeficiency virus associated motor cognitive disorder
human immunodeficiency virus dementia
human immunodeficiency virus encephalopathy
human immunodeficiency virus gingivitis
human immunodeficiency virus immunoglobulin
human immunodeficiency virus infected blood
human immunodeficiency virus overview of problems evaluation system
human immunodeficiency virus quality audit marker
human immunodeficiency virus seroconversion
human mammary tumor v.
human papilloma v.
human respiratory syncytial v.
human T-cell leukemia v.
human T-cell leukemia-lymphoma v.
human T-cell leukemia virus type 1, 2, 3
human T-cell lymphoma v.
human T-cell lymphotrophic virus type I–III
human T-cell lymphotropic v.
human T-cell lymphotropic virus II
human T-cell lymphotropic virus III
human T-cell lymphotropic virus type I associated myelopathy
human T-lymphotrophic virus/lymphadenopathy associated v.
human T-lymphotropic virus 1, 2
Humpty Doo v.
Iaco v.
Ibaraki v.
Icoaraci v.
Ieri v.
Ife v.
Ilesha v.
Ilheus v.
immunodeficiency-associated v.
v. inclusion conjunctivitis
v. infection-associated antigen
infectious bovine rhinotracheitis v.
infectious bronchitis v.
infectious bursal disease v.
infectious hematopoietic necrosis v.
infectious pancreatic necrosis v.
infectious papilloma v.
influenza virus inactivated vaccine, split virion, types A, B, trivalent
influenza virus, attenuated live vaccine
influenza virus inactivated vaccine
influenza virus pneumonia
Ingwavuma v.
Inini v.
Inkoo v.
Ippy v.
v.'s isolated from patients
Japanaut v.
Japanese encephalitis virus vaccine
Kaeng Khoi v.
Kamese v.
Kammavanpettai v.
Ketapang v.
Keystone v.
killed measles virus vaccine
Klamath v.
Kolongo v.
Kowanyama v.
lactate dehydrogenase elevating v.
lactic dehydrogenase v.
Landjia v.
Langat v.
Lassa fever v.
Latino v.
Lebombo v.
Le Dantec v.
leukemia v.
Lipovnik v.

live v.
live-attenuated human immunodeficiency v.
live-attenuated virus vaccine
Llano Seco v.
log infectious virus titer
Lokern v.
Lone Star v.
louping ill v.
Lucké tumor v.
Lukuni v.
lymphadenopathy-associated v.
lymphatic leukemia v.
lymphocyte-associated v.
lymphocytic choriomeningitis v.
lymphocytic choriomeningitis virus encephalitis
lymphocytic choriomeningitis virus group
lymphogranuloma venereum v.
lymphoid leukosis v.
lymphoproliferative virus group
lytic Epstein-Barr v.
Macaua v.
Machupo v.
macrophage-tropic human immunodeficiency virus strain
Madrid v.
Maguari v.
Main Drain v.
Malakal v.
mal de Rio Cuarto v.
malignant catarrhal fever v.
malignant rabbit fibroma v.
Maloney leukemia v.
Malpais Spring v.
mammary cancer virus of mice
mammary tumor v.
mammary tumor virus of mice
Manawa v.
Mapputta v.
Maprik v.
Mapuera v.
Marburg v.
Marburg-like v.'s
Marburg virus group
Marco v.
Marek disease v.
Marek disease-like viruses
Marituba v.
Marrakai v.
Mason-Pfizer monkey v.
Matruh v.
Matucare v.
Mayaro virus disease
McDonough feline sarcoma v.
McKrae herpes simplex v.
Meaban v.
measles v.
measles-rinderpest-distemper virus group
measles virus enzyme-linked immunosorbent assay
Melao v.
Mermet v.
mibuna temperate v.
milkers' nodule v.
Minatitlan v.
mink enteritis v.
Minnal v.
minute virus of canines
minute virus of mice
Mirim v.
Mitchell River v.
mixed virus respiratory infection
Mobala v.
modified vaccine virus Ankara
Moju v.
molluscum contagiosum v.
Moloney leukemogenic v.
Moloney murine leukemia v.
Moloney murine sarcoma v.
monkey B v.
monkey polyoma v.
monocyte tropic v.
Mono Lake v.
monovalent oral polio virus vaccine
Montana myotis leukoencephalitis v.
Monte Dourado v.
Moriche v.
morphine-potentiated human immunodeficiency virus replication
Mosqueiro v.
Mossuril v.
Mount Elgon bat v.
mouse encephalomyelitis v.
mouse hepatitis v.
mouse leukemia v.
mouse mammary tumor v.
mouse parotid tumor v.
mouse poliomyelitis v.
mouse salivary gland v.
mouse thymic v.
Mucambo v.
mucosal disease v.
mucosal disease virus group
Muerto Canyon v.
Muir Springs v.
Multidimensional Quality of Life Questionnaire for Persons with Human Immunodeficiency V.
multimammate papilloma v.
multiple hepatitis virus infection
multiple nucleocapsid v.
mumps virus culture
mumps virus vaccine
mumps virus vaccine Jeryl Lynn strain
Munguba v.
murine erythroblastosis v.
murine leukemia v.
murine lymphocytic choriomeningitis v.
murine mammary tumor v.
murine sarcoma v.
Murray Valley encephalitis v.
Murutucu v.
myeloblastosis-associated v.
myeloproliferative leukemia v.
myeloproliferative sarcoma v.
Mykines v.
myxoma virus subgroup
Naranjal v.
Nasoule v.
Navarro v.
Ndelle v.
Ndumu v.
Nebraska calf diarrhea v.
Nebraska calf scours v.
Neckar river v.
nef gene-deleted v.
negative strand v.
neonatal calf diarrhea v.
neonatal herpes simplex v.
neonatal herpes simplex virus infection
Nepuyo v.
v. neutralization
Newcastle disease v.
Newcastle disease virus therapy
Newcastle virus disease
New Minto v.
New York vaccinia v.
Ngaingan v.
Ngari v.
Nique v.
Nkolbisson v.
nodule-inducing v.
non-A hepatitis v.
non-A, non-B hepatitis v.
nonbacterial gastroenteritis v.
non-B hepatitis v.
nonsyncytia-forming human immunodeficiency v.
non-syncytium-inducing variant of AIDS v.
Northway v.
Norwalk-like agent v.

virus *(continued)*
Ntaya v.
nt-1, -2 v.
nuclear polyhidrosis v.
Nugget v.
Nyando v.
Odrenisrou v.
Okhotskiy v.
Okola v.
Olifantsvlei v.
Omo v.
Omsk hemorrhagic fever v.
O'nyong-nyong v.
oral attenuated poliomyelitis virus vaccine
orf virus subgroup
Oriboca v.
Oriximina v.
Oropouche v.
Orungo v.
Ossa v.
Ouango v.
Oubi v.
ovine AAV v.
oyster v.
Pacora v.
Pacui v.
Pahayokee v.
Palestina v.
Palyam v.
Pangola stunt v.
panleukopenia v.
papilloma-polyoma-vacuolating agent v.
papilloma virus, polyoma virus, vacuolative v.
pappataci fever v.
parainfluenza virus type 1–4, 4B
parainfluenza virus antigen
parainfluenza virus culture
parainfluenza virus serology
Paramushir v.
Paraná v.
paravaccinia virus infection
Paroo River v.
Parry Creek v.
Pata v.
Pathum Thani v.
patient has natural immunity to hepatitis B v.
Patois v.
Penicillium brevicompactum v.
Penicillium chrysogenum v.
Penicillium cyaneo-fulvum v.
Penicillium stoloniferum F, S v.
Perinet v.
peripheral blood mononuclear cell hepatitis B virus measurement
pharyngoconjunctival fever v.
Phnom Penh bat v.
Pichinde v.
Picola v.
Piry v.
Pixuna v.
Playas v.
pneumonia virus of mice
polyoma v.
Pongola v.
Ponteves v.
Powassan v.
Prague strain Rous sarcoma v.
Precarious Point v.
Pretoria v.
progressive pneumonia v.
Prospect Hill v.
v. protein
pseudorabies v.
Puchong v.
Punta Salinas v.
Punta Toro v.
Purus v.
Puumala v.
Qalyub v.
rabbit kidney vacuolating v.
Radi v.
radiation leukemia v.
rat v.
Rauscher murine leukemia v.
Razdan v.
recombinant Norwalk v.
recombinant virus assay
recovered avian sarcoma v.
Resistencia v.
respiratory enteric orphan v.
respiratory syncytial v.
respiratory syncytial virus bronchiolitis
respiratory syncytial virus immune globulin
respiratory syncytial virus intravenous immunoglobulin
Restan v.
reticuloendotheliosis v.
Rift Valley fever v.
Rio Bravo v.
Rio Grande v.
Rochambeau v.
Rocio v.
Ross River v.
Rous-associated v.
Rous sarcoma virus immunoglobulin intravenous
Royal Farm v.
Rubarth disease v.
rubella vaccine-like v.
Russian autumn encephalitis v.
Russian spring-summer encephalitis v.
Saboya v.
Sagiyama v.
Saint-Floris v.
Sakhalin v.
Salanga v.
Salehabad v.
salivary gland v.
salivary gland virus disease
Sal Vieja v.
San Angelo v.
sandfly fever Naples v.
sandfly fever Sicilian v.
Sandjimba v.
Sango v.
San Juan v.
San Miguel sea lion v.
San Perlita v.
Santarem v.
Santa Rosa v.
Saraca v.
sarcoma v.
satellite tobacco necrosis v.
Sathuperi v.
Saumarez Reef v.
sawgrass v.
Schmidt-Ruppin strain Rous sarcoma v.
Seletar v.
Semliki Forest v.
Sena Madureira v.
Sendai v.
Seoul v.
Sepik v.
serotype A, B, C v.
Serra do Navio v.
serum parvo virus-like v.
Shamonda v.
Shark River v.
Shokwe v.
Shuni v.
Silverwater v.
Simbu v.
simian foamy v.'s
simian herpes v.
simian immunodeficiency v.
simian sarcoma v.
simian sarcoma-associated v.
simian T-cell lymphotropic v.
simian vacuolating virus 40
Sindbis v.
Sin Nombre v.
Sixgun City v.

small round structured v.
snowshoe hare v.
Sokuluk v.
Soldado v.
Sororoca v.
spleen necrosis v.
Spondweni v.
Sripur v.
St. Louis encephalitis v.
Stratford v.
Sunday Canyon v.
swine influenza v.
swine vesicular disease v.
syphilis, toxoplasmosis, other agents, rubella, cytomegalovirus, herpes simplex v.
Tacaiuma v.
Tacaribe v.
Taggert v.
Tahyna v.
Tai v.
Tamdy v.
Tamiami v.
Tanga v.
Tanjong Rabok v.
Tataguine v.
Tehran v.
Tellina v.
Telok Forest v.
Tembe v.
Tembusu v.
Tensaw v.
Termeil v.
Tete v.
Theiler murine encephalomyelitis v.
Thiafora v.
Thimiri v.
Thogoto v.
Thottapalayam v.
Tibrogargan v.
tick-borne encephalitis v.
Tilligerry v.
Timbo v.
Timboteua v.
Tinaroo v.
Tindholmur v.
v. titer
Tlacotalpan v.
tobacco mosaic v.
tobacco necrosis v.
tobacco rattle v.
tobacco ringspot v.
Toscana v.
transfusion-transmitted v.
transitional cell cancer-associated v.
transmissible gastroenteritis v.
transmissible virus dementia
v. transport medium
Tribec v.
trivittatus v.
Trubanaman v.
Tsuruse v.
TT v.
turkey virus hepatitis
Turuna v.
Tyuleniy v.
Uganda S v.
Umatilla v.
Umbre v.
Una v.
unclassified fecal v.
Upolu v.
Urucuri v.
Usutu v.
Utinga v.
Uukuniemi v.
vaccinia v.
varicella chickenpox vaccine
varicella virus infection
varicella-zoster v.
varicella-zoster virus vaccine
Vellore v.
Venezuelan equine encephalitis v.
Venezuelan equine encephalomyelitis v.
vesicular exanthema of swine v.
vesicular stomatitis Alagoas v.
vesicular stomatitis Indiana v.
Vinces v.
viral hemorrhagic septicemia v.
Virgin River v.
Wad Medani v.
Wallal v.
Wanowrie v.
Warrego v.
Wesselsbron disease v.
western equine encephalomyelitis v.
West Nile encephalitis v.
Whataroa v.
Witwatersrand v.
Wongal v.
Wongorr v.
woodchuck hepatic v.
wound tumor v.
Xiburema v.
Yaba monkey v.
Yacaaba v.
yam mosaic v.
Yaquina Head v.
Yata v.
yellow fever v.
Yogue v.
Yug Bogdanovac v.
Zaliv Terpeniya v.
Zegla v.
Zika v.
Zirqa v.

virus-adjusting diluent

virus-associated

v.-a. hemophagocytic syndrome
human immunodeficiency virus-associated nephropathy

virus-inactivating agent

virus-induced interferon

virus-like

v.-l. action
v.-l. infectious agent
v.-l. particle
serum parvo virus-like virus

virus/lymphadenopathy

human T-lymphotrophic virus/lymphadenopathy associated virus

virus-neutralizing antibody

viscera (*pl. of* viscus)

visceral

v. abdominal fat
v. abdominal fat to total abdominal fat ratio
v. abscess
v. adipose tissue
v. anesthesia
v. arch
autonomic visceral motor nucleus
v. brain
v. cavity
childhood visceral myopathy
v. cleft
v. distension
v. dysfunction
v. edema
familial visceral myopathy
familial visceral neuropathy
general visceral afferent nerve
general visceral efferent nerve
generalized visceral hypersensitivity
giant prosthetic reinforcement of the visceral sac
v. herpes simplex
v. larva migrans
v. layer
v. layer of serous pericardium
v. leishmaniasis
v. manipulative treatment
v. nucleus

visceral *(continued)*
v. pain
v. pleura incised
right visceral ganglion
selective visceral angiography
special visceral afferent
special visceral efferent

viscerales
lymphonodus abdominis v.
nodi lymphoidei abdominis v.

visceralium

viscerotropic leishmaniasis

viscerum
situs inversus v.

viscoelastic agent

viscosity
absolute v.
blood v.
dynamic v.
v. index
kinematic v.
limiting viscosity number
minimal apparent v.
plasma v.
serum v.

viscous
dark green viscous bile

viscus, pl. **viscera**
abdominal viscera
herniated v.
hollow viscus injury
hollow viscus organ
intraabdominal viscera
intraperitoneal v.
pelvic viscera
pelvic viscera surrounded by hematoma
perforated v.

vise
hemodynamic v.

visible
autokinetic visible light phenomenon
horizontal visible iris diameter
minimum visible angle
nonbleeding visible vessel
no radiographically visible recurrence
v. iris diameter

vision
abrupt change in v.
binocular single v.
blurred or fuzzy v.
blurred vision from anemia
blurred vision from diabetes
blurred vision in one eye
blurring or dimming of v.
blurring of v.
center of field of v.
central vision loss
v., color
color v.
colored v.
color vision deviant
computer vision syndrome
degeneration of v.
diminished hearing and v.
dimness or loss of v.
direct vision internal urethrotomy
direct vision times one
distance and near vision
double v.
double vision from myasthenia gravis
double vision with headache
episode of blurred v.
Erhardt Developmental V. Assessment
Farnsworth panel D-15 color vision test
field of v.
field of vision intact
finger-counting vision test
gradual blurring of v.
hand motion at 3 feet vision test
Hardy-Rand-Ritter color vision test kit
v. impairment
intermittent double v.
laser vision correction
v. left eye
Lighthouse National Center for V. and Aging
line of v.
loss of v.
low vision aid
low vision clinic
macular binocular v.
Massachusetts V. Kit
migrainous vision loss
naked v.
near v.
near vision test
near vision testing
normal color v.
organ of v.
painless progressive loss of v.
progressive impairment of v.
v. right eye
single binocular v.
single vision glasses
STYCAR V. Test
temporal field of v.
under direct v.
v. with correction

visio oculus uterque

visit
ambulatory visit groups
date of v.
discharged on v.
domiciliary v.
emergency center v.'s
follow-up office v.
functional trial v.
home health v.
hospital v.
initial office v.
next v.
office v.
outpatient v.
postoperative office v.
reason for v.
since last v.
skilled nursing v.
temporary v.
therapeutic home trial v.
trial v.
urgent visit center

visiting registered nurse

VISU
OPMI VISU 200 microscope

visual
v. action time
v. activity
v. acuity
v. acuity, left eye
v. acuity, left eye, left perception with projection
v. acuity loss
v. acuity, right eye
v. acuity screening
v. acuity test
afferent visual pathway
age-related visual impairment
v. agnosia
v. aid
v. analog pain score
V. Analogue Mood Scale
V. Analogue Self Assessment Scales For Pain Intensity
v. angle
anterior visual pathway
anterior visual pathway dysfunction
v. apperception test
apperceptive visual agnosia
arcuate visual field defect

v., association, kinesthetic, tactile reading
associative visual agnosia
associative visual cortex
asymptomatic visual field defect
auditory visual evoked response
v. auditory evoked response
v. auditory range
V. Auditory Screen for Children
v. or auditory stimulation
auditory and visual signs
v. aura
V. Aural Digit Span Test
automated visual field
v. axis
Benton V. Retention Test, Revised
best-corrected visual acuity
Binocular V. Acuity Test
binocular visual efficiency
v. blurring
v. capacity
v. center
central visual acuity
central visual field
v. change
Colored V. Analogue Scale
v. communication therapy
Comprehensive Test of V. Functioning
computerized visual field machine
confrontation of visual field
confrontation visual field testing
Continuous V. Memory Test
v. cortex
cortical visual impairment
v. cue
v. cut
v. deficit
v. detection level
Developmental Test of V. Perception
v. discriminatory acuity
v. display terminal
v. display unit
distance visual acuity
distance visual acuity with correction
distance visual acuity without correction
distorted visual images and hallucinations
v. distortion
v. distortion test
v. disturbance
disturbance of visual function
dynamic visual acuity
v. efficiency
evoked visual potential
evoked visual response
v. examination
v. feedback display
v. field
v. field cut
v. field defect
v. field deficit
v. field disturbance
v. field floater
v. field intact
v. field loss
v. fields full to confrontation
v. fields by Goldmann-type perimeter
v. field test
v. field testing
v. floater
V. Form Discrimination Test
Frostig Developmental Test of V. Motor Perception
Frostig Program for the Development of V. Perception
v. function
V. Functioning index
gaze-evoked visual loss
glaucomatous visual field loss
good visual fields
v. habit
v. half-field
v. hallucinations
v. hearing
v. hearing loss
Hooper V. Organization Test
horizontally selective visual cell
Humphrey visual field
v. illusion
v. imagery
v. imagery exercise
immediate visual memory
v. impairment
V. Impairment Service
v. impulse
v. information
v. information storage
v. inspection
integrated visual and auditory
v. internal urethrotomy
internal visual reference
v. interpretation
Keystone Telebinocular V. Survey
v. laser ablation of prostate
v. laser-assisted prostatectomy
left visual field
Lighthouse Distance V. Acuity Test
linear visual acuity test
linear visual analog scale
v. loss
loss of visual acuity
magnocellular visual pathway
medial superior temporal visual area
medial temporal visual area
V. Memory Score
v. memory span
Mertens V. Perception Test
middle temporal visual area
minimum visual angle
monocular confrontation visual field test
Motor-Free V. Perception Test
MST visual area
MT visual area
myoid visual cell
v. naming
narrowing of visual field
National Eye Institute V. Function Questionnaire
negative visual phenomenon
nonorganic visual loss
nonphysiologic visual field loss
normal visual acuity
V. Numerical Discrimination Pretest
numerical visual acuity
v. observation shivering score
V. Organization Test
paracentral visual field
v. pathway
pattern reversal visual evoked potential
Pepper V. Skills for Reading Test
v. perception
peripheral visual field loss
peristriate visual cortex
permanent visual impairment
v. plane
v. pleural space
potential visual acuity meter
Primary V. Motor Test
primary visual cortex
receptive field of visual cortex
v. reinforcement audiometry
reported visual sensation
v. reproduction
v. response audiometry
V. Retention Test
right visual field
V. Search and Attention Test
v. search task
severe visual loss

visual *(continued)*
short-term visual storage
transient visual loss
true visual acuity
uncorrected visual acuity
v. vestibuloocular reflex
vivid visual, auditory and olfactory hallucinations
vivid visual imagery

visual-evoked cortical potential

visualization
direct visualization of vocal cords
endoscopic v.
fluoroscopic v.
imagery and v.
panoramic v.
Southern California Space V. Test

visualized
angiographically visualized vascular malformation
gallbladder v.
poorly visualized gallbladder
v. treatment objective

visualizing
poorly visualizing gallbladder

visually
v. enhanced vestibuloocular reflex
v. evoked cortical potential
v. evoked field
v. evoked flow response
v. handicapped
v. impaired

visual-motor
V.-m. Gestalt Test
v.-m. integration
v.-m. integration test
V.-m. Sequencing Test
v.-m. task

vitae
arbor vitae cerebelli
arbor vitae tree
arbor vitae uterus
curriculum v.

vital
afebrile, vital signs stable
v. capacity
current vital signs
v. exhaustion and depression
failure of all vital forces
forced expiratory volume in one second to forced vital capacity ratio
forced expiratory volume timed to forced vital capacity ratio
forced inspiratory vital capacity
forced vital capacity analysis
functional vital capacity
v. health information
inspiratory vital capacity
inspired vital capacity
maximum expiratory flow at 50% vital capacity
midinspiratory flow at 50% of vital capacity
neurologic vital signs
normal vital signs
normal vital capacity
predicted vital capacity
v. record
v. sign
v. signs normal
V. Signs Quality of Life
v. signs stable
v. signs stable, afebrile
slow vital capacity
stable vital signs
timed vital capacity
total vital capacity

vitality index

vitamin
v.'s A and D
v. A deficiency
ataxia with isolated vitamin E deficiency
v. A toxicity
v. B complex
v. B deficiency
v. B_{12} deficiency
v. B_6 deficiency
v. B_1 deficiency
v. B_{12} level
v. B therapy
v. capsule
v. D-binding protein
v. D-dependent rickets type II
v. deficiency
dementia due to vitamin deficiency
v. D receptor
v. D-resistant rickets
v. D-response element
v. E, K, K_2
v. E succinate
fat-soluble vitamin deficiency
high v.
v. K deficiency bleeding
menaquinone vitamin K_2
multiple oral v.
multiple vitamin injection
prenatal v.'s
proteins, v.'s, and minerals
prothrombin induced by vitamin K absence or antagonist-II
total vitamin B_{12} binding capacity
type 1 autosomal recessive vitamin D dependency
unsaturated vitamin B_{12}-binding capacity

viteae
Acanthocheilonema viteae excretory-secretory antigen

vitelliform macular degeneration

vitellina
arteria v.

vitelline
patent vitelline duct

vitellointestinal duct

vitiligo
v. disease activity
localized v.
occupational v.
perilimbal v.

vitrea
membrana v.

vitreal
v. bleed
v. corneal touch syndrome
v. membrane
posterior vitreal detachment

vitrectomy
closed v.
Lightning high-speed vitrectomy handpiece
Mot-R-Pak vitrectomy system
Ocutome vitrectomy unit
pars plana v.
pars plana Baerveldt tube insertion with v.
pediatric vitrectomy lens set
v. procedure
trans pars plana v.

vitrector
mechanical v.
Microvit v.

vitreoglial
perifoveolar vitreoglial membrane

vitreoretinal
v. choroidopathy syndrome
peripheral vitreoretinal traction
v. traction syndrome

vitreoretinochoroidopathy
autosomal-dominant v.

vitreoretinopathy
dominant exudative v.
familial exudative v.
proliferative v.

vitreous
v. aspiration
v. body
v. cell
v. chamber
v. clouding
coloboma of v.
v. detachment
v. exudate
v. floater
v. fluid
v. fluorophotometry
hemorrhage in v.
v. hemorrhage
v. hernia
v. herniation
v. humor
v. infusion suction cutter
liquefaction of v.
liquified v.
v. loss
loss of v.
man-made vitreous fiber
massive vitreous hemorrhage
massive vitreous reaction
massive vitreous retraction
v. membrane
micelles in v.
Mules vitreous sphere
v. opacity
ophthalmic vitreous surgical technique
organized v.
patellar fossa of v.
persistent hyperplasia of primary v.
persistent hyperplastic primary v.
persistent hypertrophic v.
persistent primary hyperplastic v.
posterior v.
primary persistent hyperplastic v.
proliferative diabetic retinopathy with vitreous hemorrhage

vitreous-block glaucoma

vitro
in vitro antibody production assay
microfocal direct magnification in vitro x-ray tube
in vitro fertilization
in vitro fertilization-embryo transfer
in vitro protein digestibility

vitrum

Vitus
St. Vitus dance

vivid
v. hallucination
v. visual, auditory and olfactory hallucinations
v. visual imagery

VI–VIII
mucopolysaccharidosis MPS V.

vivo
ex vivo cannulation
ex vivo count
ex vivo fertilization
ex vivo perfusion
ex vivo technique
in vivo adhesive platelet
in vivo fertilization
in vivo optical spectroscopy

vocabulary
auditory v.
Beery Picture V. Screening
completion, arithmetic problems, vocabulary, following directions
V. Comprehension Scale
Expressive One-Word Picture V. Test
v., information, block design, and similarities
Peabody Picture Vocabulary Test-Revised
Quick Picture V. Test
Receptive One-Word Picture V. Test

vocal
alert, vocal stimulus, painful stimulus, unresponsive
anomalous parental vocal pattern
anterior cervical surgery vocal cord damage
auditory vocal sequencing
bilateral abductor vocal cord paralysis
bilateral vocal fold immobility
bilateral vocal fold paralysis
bronchoscope inserted through vocal cords with ease
chronic motor or vocal tic disorder
v. cord
v. cord activity
v. cord atrophy
v. cord carcinoma
v. cord dysfunction
v. cord movement
v. cord nodule
v. cord palsy
v. cord paralysis
v. cord stripping
direct visualization of vocal cords
v. dysfunction
false vocal cord
false vocal fold
v. fold
v. fold dysfunction
v. fold injection
v. fremitus
paradoxical vocal cord motion
paradoxical vocal fold dysfunction
v. paralysis
paralysis of vocal cord
paralyzed vocal cord
V. Profiles Analysis
v. resonance
squamous cell carcinoma of vocal cord
tactile vocal fremitus
true vocal cords
true vocal fold
unilateral vocal cord paralysis
v. velocity index

vocalis
plica v.

vocational
V. Apperception Test
v. counseling
v. evaluation
V. Evaluation and Work Adjustment
v. guidance
V. Interest Blank
V. Interest, Experience, and Skill Assessment
V. Interest Questionnaire
V. Interest and Sophistication Assessment
Jackson V. Interest Survey
V. Learning Styles
licensed vocational nurse
Minnesota V. Interest Inventory
Ohio V. Interest Survey
V. Opinion Index
V. Planning Inventory
V. Preference Inventory
psychological, social, and vocational
Reading-Free V. Interest Inventory
v. rehabilitation
v. rehabilitation counselor
v. rehabilitation and education
v. rehabilitation program

vocational *(continued)*
v. rehabilitation therapy
v. skills assessment and development program
Strong V. Interest Blank

Voc-Tech Quick Screener

Vogel-Johnson agar

Voges-Proskauer medium, test

Vogt
V. angle
V. cornea
V. degeneration
limbal girdle of V.
limbal palisades of V.
palisades of V.
V. stria
V. syndrome

Vogt-Koyanagi-Harada syndrome

Vohwinkel
mutilating keratoderma of V.

voice
alertness, response to voice, response to pain, unresponsive
automatic voice analysis
v. change from antihistamine
conversational v.
duckbill voice prosthesis
v. handicap index
hearing v.'s
v. intensity controller
monitored live v.
Multi-Dimensional V. Program 4305
v. onset time
ordinary conversational v.
v. outcome survey
v. quality
v. termination time
whispered v.

voice-activated
v.-a. computer
v.-a. unit

voicelessness
degree of v.

void
due to v.
immediate intense need to v.
intense need to void immediate
v. metal composite
v. on-call to operating room
trial of v.

voided
v. bladder
first voided bladder specimen
has v.
has not v.
v. specimen
v. urine

voiding
alarm clock v.
bladder emptied on v.
v. cystogram
v. cystography
cystoscopy and voiding urethrogram
v. cystourethrogram
v. cystourethrograph
v. cystourethrography
v. diary
v. difficulty
v. dysfunction
dysfunctional voiding scoring system
filled voiding flow rate
v. flow rate
irritable voiding syndrome
isotope voiding cystourethrography
night frequency of v.
nighttime v.
obstructive voiding symptom
v. pressure
spontaneous v.
strict voiding schedule
v. urethral pressure measurement
v. urine cytology

volar
Atasoy-Kleinert volar V-Y advancement flap
Atasoy volar V-Y flap
v. carpal ligament
cast with volar toe plate extension
v. flexed intercalated segment instability
v. interosseous artery
v. interosseous muscle
v. interosseous nerve

volaris
arcus volaris profundus

volatile
v. anesthetic
coal tar pitch v.'s
v. corrosion inhibitor
v. fatty acid
free volatile fatty acid
not v.
v. organic compound
v. organic compounds
v. sulfur compound

volatiles
coal tar pitch v.

volcanic ash

volitantes
muscae v.

volitional
v. intent
sequential volitional oral movement

Volkmann
V. canal
V. cheilitis
V. contracture

volley
antidromic v.

volt
billion electron v.'s
coulomb per v.
electrical potential in v.'s
electron v.
gigaelectron v.
kiloelectron v.
megaelectron v.
million electron v.'s
peak electron v.
v. per meter
potential difference in v.'s

voltage
v. activity
augmented voltage unipolar left arm lead
augmented voltage unipolar left foot lead
augmented voltage unipolar right arm lead
diastolic transmembrane voltage, maximum
v. drop
v. gradient
high-voltage can
left maximal spatial v.
medium voltage activity
v. peak
periodic bursts of high v.
ultrahigh v.

voltage-dependent
v.-d. anion channel
v.-d. calcium channel

voltage-gated calcium channel

voltage-sensitive calcium channel

voltametry
anodic stripping v.

voltmeter
digital v.

electronic v.
vacuum tube v.

volubility
excessive v.

volume
absolute volume of trabecular bone
v. acquisition
adequacy of intravascular v.
adequate stroke v.
v. airflow per unit of time
alcohol-induced extracellular volume contraction
v. of alveolar dead space
alveolar tidal v.
amniotic fluid v.
v. of anatomic dead space
anisotropic volume study
aortic flow v.
aortic valve stroke v.
apparent volume of distribution
aqueductal CSF stroke v.
arterial gas v.
articular cartilage v.
Arvidsson dimension-length method for ventricular v.
atomic v.
atrial emptying v.
augmented stroke v.
automatic volume control
average volume of air
v. averaging
v. to be infused
blood v.
v. of blood flow
blood volume expander
blood volume expansion
blood volume pulse
v., capillary
cardiac v.
cardiopulmonary blood v.
cell v.
cell volume profile
central circulating blood v.
cerebral red blood cell v.
cerebrospinal fluid v.
choroidal blood v.
circulating blood v.
v. clearance rate
clinical target v.
clinical tumor v.
closing v.
collective v.
concentrated v.
conductance stroke v.
conductivity cell v.
v. control
corpuscular v.
corrected blood v.
cortical blood v.
dead-space gas volume to tidal gas volume ratio
v. depletion
diastolic atrial v.
diffusion per unit of alveolar v.
dilute volume of solution
diminished lung v.
v. of distribution
v. of distribution of bilirubin
effective arterial blood v.
effective circulating blood v.
v. ejection
elastic equilibrium v.
v. element
end-diastolic v.
end-diastolic volume index
end-expiratory lung v.
end-inspiratory lung v.
end-systolic ventricular v.
end-systolic volume index
ethanol volume fraction
exhaled tidal v.
v. expander
expiratory flow v.
expiratory reserve v.
expired v.
v. of expired gas
extracellular fluid v.
extracellular fluid volume depletion
extracellular fluid volume excess
extracellular volume of distribution
extracellular volume expansion
extracorporeal v.
extravascular thermal v.
fiber bundle v.
flow v.
v. flow
fluid v.
fluid volume overload
forced expiratory flow v.
forced expiratory volume at one second
forced expiratory volume in one second as percent of FVC
forced expiratory volume in one second to forced vital capacity ratio
forced expiratory volume timed
forced expiratory volume timed to forced vital capacity ratio
forced inspiratory v.
forced inspiratory volume in one second
forced volume, expiratory
forward stroke v.
frequency to tidal v.
functional extracellular fluid v.
functional residual v.
gadolinium-enhancing tumor v.
gas v.
gastric residual v.
gram-molecular v.
gross tumor v.
heart v.
hepatic distribution v.
hepatocycle volume fraction
high lung v.
hippocampal volume loss
v. index
initial target v.
inspiratory reserve v.
v. of inspired gas per minute
interstitial fluid v.
intracellular fluid v.
intrathoracic blood v.
intrathoracic gas v.
intravascular volume expansion
v. of Isoflow
isolated volume responder
left atrial end-diastolic v.
left atrial end-systolic v.
left heart blood v.
left ventricular diastolic v.
left ventricular end-diastolic v.
left ventricular end-diastolic volume index
left ventricular end-systolic v.
left ventricular end-systolic volume index
left ventricular infarct v.
left ventricular inflow v.
left ventricular outflow v.
left ventricular stroke volume index
liver volume replaced by tumor
v. load hypertrophy
low v.
low volume disease
lung blood v.
lung thermal v.
lung volume reduction surgery
mamillary body v.
mandatory minute v.
maximal expiratory flow v.
maximal expiratory flow volume curve
maximal midexpiratory flow v.
maximal toleration v.

volume *(continued)*
maximal ventilatory v.
maximum expiratory flow v.
maximum tolerable v.
mean cell v.
mean corpuscular v.
mean plasma v.
mean platelet v.
v. of mechanical dead space
mechanical expiratory flow volume curve
mechanical tidal v.
median biopsy v.
minimum obstructive v.
minute alveolar v.
minute respiratory v.
minute ventilatory v.
minute volume of air or blood
neonatal blood v.
normal extracellular fluid v.
osteoid v.
outflow v.
v. overload
v. oxygen consumption
v. of oxygen consumption per unit of time
packed cell v.
v. of packed red blood cells
partial expiratory flow v.
v. percent
v. percentage
periorbital volume augmentation
v. per weight
phonation v.
physical volume test
placental residual blood v.
planning target v.
plasma v.
postvoiding residual v.
postvoid residual v.
predicted blood v.
pressure-regulated volume control
pressure, volume, temperature
pulmonary blood mixing v.
pulmonary blood volume index
pulmonary capillary blood v.
pulmonary capillary gas v.
pulmonary extravascular fluid v.
pulmonary extravascular water v.
pulmonary parenchymal tissue v.
pulse volume recorder
pulse volume recording
quasistatic pressure v.
radiofrequency tissue volume reduction
red blood cell v.
red cell v.
v. reduction surgery
regional cerebral blood v.
regurgitant stroke v.
relative volume decrease
v. of relaxation
v. repletion
reserve v.
residual urine v.
respiratory minute v.
reticulocyte mean corpuscular v.
right heart blood v.
right heart mixing v.
right ventricular diastolic v.
right ventricular end-diastolic v.
right ventricular end-diastolic volume index
right ventricular end-systolic v.
right ventricular end-systolic volume index
slow volume encephalography
small v.
small volume parenteral infusion
specific heat at constant v.
static volume pressure
stroke v.
stroke volume of heart
surface area to volume ratio
target v.
v. and tension
v. thickness index
thoracic cage v.
v. thoracic gas
thoracic gas v.
tidal expiratory v.
tidal expiratory flow at 25% of tidal v.
tidal expiratory flow at 50% of tidal v.
tidal expiratory flow at 75% of tidal v.
tidal inspiratory v.
tidal inspiratory flow at 50% of tidal v.
timed forced expiratory v.
total air v.
total blood v.
total blood volume predicted from body surface
total intrauterine v.
total lung v.
total packed cell v.
total red cell v.
total stomach v.
total stroke v.
total trabecular bone v.
total volume capacity
total volume of urine
trabecular bone v.
trapped air v.
trapped gas v.
v. treated in external irradiation
ultrafiltration v.
ultralow v.
v. unit meter
urinary v.
urinary calcium volume excretion rate
urinary magnesium v.
urinary potassium volume excretion rate
urine v.
urine specimen volume measuring device
urine specimen volume measuring system
vascular volume of distribution
venous volume plethysmograph
ventricular end-diastolic v.
ventricular residual v.
volume to peak expiratory flow and total expiratory v.
weight of solute per volume of solution
whole blood v.

volume-assured pressure support

volume/cerebral
cerebral blood volume/cerebral blood flow ratio

volume-controlled ventilation

volume-cycled decelerating-flow ventilation

volume-guaranteed pressure option

volume-packed cells

volume-pressure response

volume/total
residual volume/total lung capacity ratio

volumetric
v. analysis
atrial-phase volumetric function
v. bone mineral density
v. computed tomography
v. diffusive respirator
v. flask
high-speed volumetric imaging
v. lung depth
v. multiple exposure transmission holography

sequential impaction cascade sieve volumetric air sampler
v. solution

voluminous hernia

voluntarily stopping eating and drinking

voluntary
absence of voluntary muscle movement
v. admission
central voluntary control
v. closing
v. control
v. control of bleeding
v. control of involuntary utterances
v. control of tension headache
v. counseling and testing
duration of voluntary apnea test
v. effort
v. guarding
v. heart rate control
impairment of power of voluntary movement
individual voluntary control
v. interruption of pregnancy
large magnitude voluntary heart rate changes
maximal voluntary contraction
maximum voluntary contraction
v. muscle action
no voluntary activity
v. opening
v. range of motion
v. sterilization
v. subluxation
v. surgical contraception
v. termination of pregnancy

volunteer
hospice v.
normal v.
v. transport service

volutin
tuberculin v.

volvulus
cecal v.
gastric v.
malrotation with midgut v.
mesenteroaxial v.
midgut v.
sigmoid v.
small bowel v.

vomer
ala of v.
v. bone

vomerine
v. canal
v. cartilage
v. crest of choana

vomeronasal
v. cartilage
v. organ

vomited
patient vomited large quantities of blood

vomiting
anticipatory v.
v. center
cyclic vomiting syndrome
v. and diarrhea
diarrhea with fever and v.
fever, chills, sweating, nausea, vomiting, and diarrhea
fever, cough, nausea, and v.
v. from appendicitis
v. and headache
nausea and v.
nausea, vomiting, and diarrhea
nausea, vomiting, diarrhea, and constipation
nausea and vomiting of pregnancy
no nausea, vomiting, or diarrhea
no nausea or v.
no nausea, vomiting, diarrhea or constipation
pain in abdomen with v.
pain with v.
patient vomiting blood
persistent vomiting or confusion headache
postchemotherapy nausea and v.
postoperative nausea and v.
projectile v.
radiation-induced nausea and v.
winter vomiting disease

vomitus coffee-ground

von
acquired von Willebrand disease
v. Economo encephalitis
v. Graefe sign
v. Herrick grading system
v. Hippel-Landau syndrome
v. Mering reflex
v. Meyenburg complex
nest of von Brunn
v. Recklinghausen disease
v. Willebrand disease
v. Willebrand factor

voracious appetite

vorax
lupus v.

vortex of heart

voyeurism
adolescent v.

V-pattern exotropia

vs.
congenital vs. acquired syndrome
hot vs. cold breast tumor

V-shaped
V.-s. fracture
V.-s. incision

vulcanization
room temperature v.

vulcanized
heat temperature v.

vulgaris
apple jelly papule of lupus v.
ichthyosis v.
pemphigus v.
verruca vulgaris of the larynx

vulnerability
individual v.

vulnerable period

vulva, pl. **vulvae**
elephantiasis of v.
focal herpes of v.
multinucleated atypia of the v.
nevus of v.
noma vulvae
Paget disease of v.
pruritus vulvae
squamous cell carcinoma of v.
v. and vagina

vulvar
v. adenocystic adenocarcinoma
v. atrophy
v. atypia
v. biopsy
v. carcinoma
v. condylomata
v. dystrophy
v. infection
v. intraepithelial neoplasia
invasive vulvar carcinoma
v. irritation
v. itch
v. itching
v. lesion
localized vulvar pemphigoid of childhood
v. malignancy
v. melanoma
v. nevus

vulvar *(continued)*
v. pruritus
v. vestibulitis syndrome

vulvectomy
en bloc v.
radical v.

vulvitis
herpes v.

vulvovaginal
v. anus
v. candidiasis
v. gland
v. ulceration

vulvovaginitis
candidal v.
herpetic v.

Waals
van der Waals force
Waardenburg syndrome
waddling gait
Wade-Fite-Faraco stain
Wad Medani virus
Wadsworth-Todd cautery
wafer
aluminum w.
chemo w.'s implanted
Gliadel wafer treatment protocol
Wagener retinitis
Wagner
W. disease
W. operation
W. reduction technique
W. syndrome
Wagner-Nelson time 50 hours
wagon wheel fracture
Wagstaffe fracture
wailing
weeping, whining, and w.
Wainer
Roche, Wainer, and Thissen method of height prediction
waist
above w.
below w.
w. belt
narrow mediastinal w.
waist-hip ratio
waist-to-hip
w.-t.-h. ratio
waiting
w. list
patient w.
watchful w.
waiver
informed waiver and consent
wake
w. after sleep onset
w. after sleep onset time
w. response
Wakefield Inventory
wakefulness
w. after sleep onset
maintenance of wakefulness test
Repeated Test of Sustained W.
wakeful state
waking
normal waking activity
normal waking electroencephalogram
normal waking electroencephalogram pattern
slow waking activity
Waldenström macroglobulinemia
Waldeyer
W. fluid
W. fossa
W. gland
pelvic colon of W.
W. ring
W. sulcus
Waldhauer operation
Waldhausen subclavian flap technique
walk
dynamic wall w.
inability to w.
lift-off of heel in w.
nonweightbearing crutch w.
progressive inability to w.
w. with aid of cane
walker
ambulation with w.
Charcot restraint orthotic w.
front wheel w.
jump w.
patient ambulates with w.
pick-up w.
wheeled w.
walk-in
w.-i. emergency department
w.-i. high-pressure chamber
w.-i. patient
walking
w. aid
assistance with w.
automatic neonatal walking reflex
autonomic walking reflex
below-knee walking cast
below-knee walking plaster
w. boot cast
comfortable walking speed
crutch w.
health benefits of w.
w. heel
w. heel cast
heel and toe w.
long leg walking cast
maximum walking distance
maximum walking time
6-minute walking test
nonweightbearing crutch w.
pain-free walking time
pain on w.
w. pneumonia
short leg walking cast
w. speed
Stryker walking heel
symptom-free walking distance
w. tank
toe walking and heel w.
w. training
w. ventilation
wall
abdominal w.
akinetic segmental wall motion abnormality
alveolar w.
alveolar wall basement membrane
w. of aneurysm
aneurysmal wall calcification
aneurysmal wall gas
anterior abdominal w.
anterior abdominal wall syndrome
anterior aortic w.
anterior chest wall flap
anterior chest wall syndrome
anterior right ventricular w.
anterior thoracic w.
anterior wall antral ulcer
anterior wall infarction
anterior wall ischemia
anterior wall of middle ear
anterior wall motion
anterior wall myocardial infarct
anterior wall myocardial infarction
anterior wall of stomach
anterior wall of tympanic cavity
anterior wall of vagina
anterolateral abdominal w.
aortic posterior w.
aortic wall deterioration
aortic wall necrosis
aortic wall thickening
apical-lateral wall myocardial infarct
apical wall motion
arterial wall dissection
arterial wall integrity
arterial wall thickness
axial wall of pulp chamber
ballooning-out of artery w.
barium adherent to esophageal walls
bladder wall thickened
bladder wall trabeculated
bladder wall weakened
bowel wall hemorrhage
bowel wall induration

W

wall *(continued)*
brisk wall motion
calcified wall of gallbladder
canal wall down mastoidectomy
canal wall down tympanomastoidectomy
canal wall down tympanoplasty
canal wall up mastoidectomy
canal wall up tympanoplasty
cardiac wall hypokinesis
cardiac wall motion
cardiac wall thickening
cell w.
cell wall defective
cell wall skeleton
chest w.
chest wall compliance
chest wall stimulation
circumferential wall stress
w. coated open tubular
degeneration of wall of artery
dynamic wall walk
end-diastolic cardiac wall thickness
end-systolic wall index
end-systolic wall stress
end-systolic wall thickness
esophageal wall thickness
fracturing w.
glomerular capillary w.
hardening of w.'s of artery
heart wall thickening
hematoma of chest w.
hemorrhage into wall of bladder
high-frequency chest wall compression
high-frequency chest wall oscillation
high regional wall motion velocity
incision through wall of cavity
inferior wall ischemia
inferior wall myocardial infarction
inherent weakness in arterial w.
inner w.
intact canal w.
intestinal wall perforation
ischemic heart w.
lateral pharyngeal w.
lateral vaginal w.
lateral wall ischemia
lateral wall pressure
left atrial posterior w.
left ventricular free w.
left ventricular posterior w.
left ventricular posterior wall thickness
left ventricular septal w.
left ventricular wall motion
left ventricular wall motion abnormality
left ventricular wall motion index
limb-body wall complex
low continuous wall suction
low intermittent wall suction
w. motion
w. motion abnormality
w. motion index
w. motion score index
multiple bull's eye lesions bowel w.
musculoskeletal chest wall pain
Mycobacterium cell wall complex
myocardial wall thickness
nasal cavity w.
old inferior wall myocardial infarction
orbital wall fracture
outer w.
paradoxical chest wall motion
paraumbilical anterior abdominal w.
patulous urethral w.
peptidoglycan rigid cell w.
peripheral cavity w.
perpendicular antcrior w.
posterior w.
posterior aspect of pharyngeal w.
posterior vaginal w.
posterior wall of heart
posterior wall of left ventricle
posterior wall myocardial infarction
posterior wall thickness
posterior wall thickness at end-diastole
posterior wall velocity
prolapsed vaginal w.
purified cell w.'s
quantitative wall motion score
regional wall motion
regional wall motion abnormality
relative wall thickness
right ventricle anterior w.
right ventricular wall device
segmental wall motion
segmental wall motion abnormality
w. shortening index
small intestinal w.
spasm of intestinal w.
spherule w.
systolic wall motion velocity
thickened bladder w.
thickened gallbladder w.
w. thickness
urinary bladder wall mass
urinary bladder wall thickening
vaginal wall sling
vascular w.
ventral wall defect
ventricular wall motion
ventricular wall motion abnormality
vessel w.

Wallal virus

Walldius prosthesis

wall-echo shadow

walled
thick w.

Wallenberg syndrome

wallerian
w. degeneration
w. law

wall-eyed
w.-e. bilateral internuclear ophthalmoplegia
w.-e. monocular internuclear ophthalmoplegia

wall-motion study

Walsh
neurovascular bundle of W.

Walter bromide test

Walthard
W. cell
W. cell rest
W. inclusion

Walther
W. canal
W. duct
W. ganglion

Wampole test

wandering
aimless w.
w. atrial pacemaker
episodic nocturnal w.
w. gallbladder
w. goiter
w. heart
increased w.
Marchand wandering cell
night w.

Wangensteen
W. awl
W. carrier
W. colostomy
W. drainage

W. suction
W. tube

Wanowrie virus

Wanscher mask

war
Gulf War syndrome
W. Head-Injury Score
w. nephritis
not prisoner of w.
prisoner of w.

warble
ox w.

Warburg apparatus

ward
W. Atmosphere Scale
W. Behavior Rating Scale
children's w.
w. confinement
emergency w.
general w.
global ward behavior scale
W. Incapacity Scale
W. Initiation Scale
intensive care w.
w. manager
w. pack
primary surgical w.
short-stay w.

Wardenburg syndrome

warfare
atomic, biological, chemical w.
bacteriologic w.
biologic and chemical w.
chemical, bacteriologic, and radiologic w.
chemical and biological w.
germ w.
ordinary w.
psychological w.
radiologic w.
skin exposure reduction paste against chemical warfare agent

warfarin
w. dose index
fetal warfarin syndrome
w. sodium
w. therapy

Warfarin-Aspirin Symptomatic Intracranial Disease

Waring Intimacy Questionnaire

warm
w. autoimmune hemolytic anemia
cold to the opposite, warm to the same
combined cold and warm antibody autoimmune hemolytic anemia
w. compress
w. compresses and lid scrubs
donor-related warm ischemia
w. and dry
healing power of warm baths
w. joint
w. mist humidifier
w. moist heat
w. moist pack unsterile
pink, moist, and warm mucous membranes
red and warm breast
right ear, warm stimulus
w. water immersion foot
w. weather rash

warmer
hypothermia oxygen w.
infant placed in w.
open bed w.
out of radiant w.
placed in w.
radiant heat w.

warmth
color, warmth, movement sensation
w. at incision site

warning
Disaster W. System
Drug Abuse W. Network
melanoma warning sign
quick early w.
w. sign of drug abuse
w. sign identification
w. signs of hearing loss
w. signs of heart attack
w. signs of serious illness

warrant
detention w.
mental inquest w.

Warrego virus

Warren
W. incision
W. operation
W. shunt

wart
anal w.
anogenital w.
asbestos w.
juvenile w.
moist w.
mosaic w.
mucous membrane w.
myrmecia w.
nail w.
necrogenic w.
perianal w.
periungual w.
plantar w.
venereal w.

Wartenberg sign

Warthin
W. sign
W. tumor

Warthin-Starry stain

wart-like growth

wash
alveolar w.
nasal w.
pHisoHex face w.

washable base

washed
w. bladder
w. packed cells
w. red blood cell

washer
anchor w.

washing
bronchoalveolar w.
w. and brushing
culture of nasal w.
gastric w.
hand washing compulsion
hand washing in critical care area
hand washing in nursery
hand washing technique
nasal w.
nasopharyngeal w.
pelvic w.'s
urinary w.'s

washout
anterior chamber w.
bladder w.
multiple-breath nitrogen w.
nitrogen washout, multiple breath
nitrogen washout, single breath
nitrogen washout test
single-breath nitrogen w.
teboroxime resting w.
total body w.

wasp
Polistes wasp venom

Wassermann
W. antibody
blood W.
cardiolipin Wassermann test
W. reaction

Wassermann *(continued)*
serum Wassermann reaction
W. test
wastage
air w.
early pregnancy w.
fetal w.
waste
hazardous w.
low-level w.
radioactive w.
wastewater treatment plant
wasting
AIDS wasting syndrome
cerebral salt w.
peripheral fat w.
renal kalium w.
temporal muscle w.
watch
careful w.
hearing distance with w.
oriented to time, place, person, and objects watch, pen, book
watchful waiting
water
acetone in w.
aquaporin-2 water channel
aqua PT water massage
artificial rupture of bag of w.'s
autoprotolysis constant of w.
bacteriostatic water for injection
bag of w.'s
bag of waters ruptured
bladder distended with w.
w. blister
body w.
w. bottle
w. bowel movement
w. brash
buffered distilled w.
bulging bag of w.'s
w. canker
carbonaceous activated w.
catalyst altered w.
centimeters of water cuff pressure
centimeters of w.
chronic disordered water balance
w. clearance
closed water seal drainage system
cold water immersion foot
cold water soluble
cold water treatment
cutaneous water loss
deionized w.
w. deprivation
dissociation constant of w.
distilled w.
double distilled w.
doubly labeled w.
emergency drinking water germicidal tablet
evaporation water loss
extracellular w.
extravascular lung w.
free water clearance
free water deficit
fresh w.
w. gauge
glass-distilled w.
glucose in w.
glucose water feeding
glycerin in w.
glycerin and w.
glycerin and water enema
hot water bottle
hot water extract
hot water soluble
ice water test
w. immersion
w. ingestion
w. for injection
insensible water loss
intact bag of w.'s
w. intake
intercellular w.
interstitial w.
w. intoxication
intracellular w.
invert sugar 5% in w.
10% invert sugar injection in w.
liters per centimeter of w.
w. loss
magnesium sulfate, glycerin, and water enema
millimeters of w.
modified sea water yeast extract agar
nonrenal water loss
w. in oil
oil in water emulsion
w. packed
partial pressure of water vapor
premature spontaneous rupture of bag of w.'s
pulmonary extravascular water volume
restraint and water immersion stress
w. retention
rupture of bag of w.'s
salt and water imbalance
salt water implant
w. seal chest tube
w. seal drainage
self-induced water intoxication and psychosis
soap and w.
w. soluble
spontaneous rupture of bag of w.'s
sterile water gastric drip
sterile water for injection
w. swallow
tap water enema
tap water enema til clear
tap water wet dressing
w. temperature
tepid water enema
titrated w.
total body w.
total lung w.
transepidermal water loss
unstirred water layer
vaporize water in herniated disc
warm water immersion foot
waterborne
w. illness outbreak
w. transmission of viral hepatitis
watercraft
personal watercraft accident
watered-silk retina
water-ethyleneglycol
waterfall
w. appearance
w. stomach
water-hammer pulse
Waterhouse-Friderichsen syndrome
water-induced thermotherapy
watering-can scrotum
waterload test
watermelon stomach
water-retaining laxative
water-retention coefficient
watershed
w. infarct
w. infarction
w. region
water-silk reflex
water-soluble antibiotic
Waterson
Cooley modification of Waterson anastomosis
waterwheel sound

watery
w. and bloody diarrhea
w. diarrhea
w. diarrhea, hypokalemia, and achlorhydria syndrome
w. diarrhea with hypokalemic alkalosis
w. discharge
explosive watery diarrhea
w., itchy eyes
itchy, watery eye

Watkins operation

Watkins-Wertheim operation

Watson
W. method
W. reagent

Watson-Crick helix

watt
w. hour
lumen per w.
w. per kilogram
w. second

Watzke band

wave
abnormal w.
abnormal brain wave discharge
abnormal brain wave function
abnormal wave form
affinity evanescent wave spectroscopy
alpha brain w.
w.'s of alpha frequency
alpha wave intrusion
alpha wave strain
alpha wave training
w. amplitude
w. analyzer
brain wave activity
brain wave cycle
brain wave frequency range
brain wave pattern
brain wave response
cardiac shock wave therapy
central sharp wave transient
central slow wave focus
centrotemporal sharp w.
clustered w.'s
complex wave form
continuous w.
continuous wave ablation
continuous wave laser ablation
decreased brain wave activity
delta w.
diathermy short w.
distal mean wave pressure
early diastolic w.
electrocardiographic w.
electrocardiographic interval from the beginning of QRS complex to end of the T w.
electrocardiographic wave corresponding to repolarization of ventricles
electrocardiographic wave in QRS complex
electrocardiographic wave segment
electrohydraulic shock wave lithotripsy
electromagnetic w.'s
epilepsy with continuous spikes and w.'s during sleep
excessive diffuse low and medium wave beta activity
excessive fast brain wave activity
expectancy w.
extracorporeal shock wave therapy
flipped T w.
flutter w.
w. form
w. function
high-frequency sound w.
high-voltage arrhythmic slow w.
high-voltage brain w.
high-voltage diphasic slow w.
w.'s of increasing amplitude
independent slow w.
w. interval
inverted T w.
ischemic sylvian w.
large amplitude, slow wave activity
laser-induced intracorporeal shock wave lithotripsy
w. lengths of rhythmic activity
longitudinal acoustic w.
long wave irradiation
low-voltage brain w.
monophasic R w.
nonspecific abnormality of ST segment and T w.
nonspecific ST wave segment changes on electroencephalogram
nonspecific ST and T w.
nonspecific ST-T wave abnormality
nonspecific ST-T wave change
normal P w.
w. number
w. on electrocardiogram
w. on phlebogram
paroxysmal high-voltage slow w.
periodic sharp wave complex
peristaltic w.
peroral shock wave lithotripsy
point of maximum amplitude of w.
poor progression of R wave in precordial leads
positive sharp wave fibrillations
precordial A w.
pressures and w.'s
pulsed w.
pulse wave velocity
P wave in electrocardiography
quasi-continuous w.
rapid filling w.
significant sharp spike or delta w.
sine wave threshold
sine wave pattern
slice excitation w.
slow filling w.
slow high-voltage w.
slow wave activity
slow wave sleep
spike w.
square w.'s of high frequency
ST-T wave change
time between P wave and beginning of QRS complex in electrocardiography
transient abnormal Q w.
ultrashort w.
ventricular w.

waveform
w. amplitude
aortic blood flow velocity w.
aortic root velocity w.
blood flow velocity w.
w. distortion
Doppler waveform analysis
Doppler waveform dampening
epidural pressure w.
flow-velocity w.'s
pulse oximetry waveform systolic blood pressure
segmental bronchus renal artery w.
velocity w.

wavelength
w. accuracy
psoralen plus ultraviolet light of A w.
short wavelength automated perimetry
ultraviolet light, long w.

wavelength-dispersive x-ray fluorescence

wavelet scalar quantization

waviness index

wax
animal w.
w. bean agglutinin
w. bite
candle wax appearance of bone
w. ester
model denture w.
mouth denture w.
w. pattern

waxy
w. cast
w. deposit on brain
w. exudate hard
w. finger

way
bizarre way of thinking
by way of

weak
w. and dizzy all over
infant had weak cry
w. of interrupted urine stream
lower fossa active, lateral knee pain, and long leg on the side ipsilateral to the weak fossa
mixed lymphocyte culture, w.
patient weak, hypotensive and unresponsive
pedal pulse w.
pulse w.
pulse weak and rapid
w. syllable deletion
upper fossa active, medial knee pain, and short leg on the side ipsilateral to the weak fossa

weakened
bladder wall w.
w. heart
w. heart muscle
w. host
w. immune system
w. immunity
pumping ability of weakened heart
severely weakened heart

weakening
muscle weakening myasthenia gravis

weakly
w. interacting massive particle
w. reactive

weakness
area of strength and w.
w. or atrophy
back pain and w.
cataplexy muscle w.
decreased energy, fatigue and w.
w. and fatigue
generalized body w.
w. in hand
heart muscle w.
increasing debility and w.
increasing weakness, debility, and dyspnea
inherent weakness in arterial wall
left-sided w.
limb-girdle muscular weakness and atrophy
motor neuron w.
neurogenic muscle weakness, ataxia, and retinitis pigmentosa
numbness or w.
numbness, weakness and paralysis of arm
onset of facial w.
pelvic floor w.
progressive fatigue and w.
progressive weakness of extremity
progressive weakness on one side of the body
proximal muscle w.
right-sided w.
unilateral w.
upward gaze w.
w., atrophy, and fasciculation
w., dizziness and joint pain

wean
failure to w.

weaned
patient weaned from respirator

weaning
w. brash
w. index

weapon
aerosolized plague w.
anthrax as a biological w.
assault with deadly w.
assault with a deadly w.
availability of w.'s
biologic w.
chemical, biological, radiological or nuclear w.'s
w.'s of mass destruction

wear
asymmetric w.
patient w.'s dentures

wearable
w. artificial kidney
w. cardioverter-defibrillator
w. speech processor

wearing
w. glasses
glove w.
w. patch on arrival

weather
hot weather ear
warm weather rash

weaver bottom

Weaver-Smith syndrome

weaving
head w.

web
antral w.
congenital emphysema, cryptorchidism, penoscrotal web, deafness, mental retardation syndrome
esophageal w.
w. of finger
hemihypertrophy, intestinal web, preauricular skin tag, and congenital corneal opacity syndrome
metabolic w.
terminal w.
World Wide W.

webbed toe

weber
W. Advanced Spatial Perception test
circle of W.
W. gland
W. implant
W. law
w. per ampere
W. sign
Speech W. Test
W. syndrome

Weber-Christian disease

Weber-Cockayne disease

Webster
W. operation
Swiss Webster mouse

Wechsler
W. Intelligence for Adult
W. Intelligence for Children Test
W. Intelligence Scale
W. Memory Scale
W. Preschool and Primary Scale of Intelligence

Wechsler-Bellevue Scale

wedge
w. adjustable cushioned heel
alar wedge excision

Amspacher-Messenbaugh closing wedge osteotomy
Axer lateral opening wedge osteotomy
w. biopsy
w. bone
capillary wedge pressure
closed base wedge osteotomy
closed wedge osteotomy/bunionectomy
closing abductory wedge osteotomy
coronary wedge pressure
dorsiflexory wedge osteotomy
w. excision
w. excisional biopsy
excision and wedge biopsy
excision and wedge biopsy of breast
w. heel
w. hepatic venous pressure
hepatic wedge pressure
infundibular wedge resection
inner heel w.
Livingston peribulbar w.
w. matrix resection
mean pulmonary artery wedge pressure
mean pulmonary capillary wedge pressure
medial closing wedge phalangeal osteotomy
medial heel w.
medial heel-and-sole w.
medial heel wedge orthosis
oblique closing wedge osteotomy
open w.
open base wedge osteotomy
open base wedge osteotomy/bunionectomy
opening abductory wedge osteotomy
open wedge osteotomy
ovarian wedge resection
w. pressure
pulmonary artery w.
pulmonary artery diastolic and wedge pressure
pulmonary capillary w.
pulmonary capillary wedge pressure
w. resection

wedged
w. fetal head
w. renal vein pressure

wedge-shaped
w.-s. appearance
w.-s. cut into bone
w.-s. defect

wedging
anterior w.
w. deformity

wedlock
out of w.
out of wedlock and not keeping child

weed
alfalfa weed pollen
mugwort weed pollen

week
W.'s bacillus
every w.
every four w.'s
five times a w.
w.'s old
once a w.
person gametocyte w.
three times a w.
w.'s by ultrasound

weekend
w. drinker
every w.
w. pass

Weeker operation

weekly
w. interval
once w.
three times w.
twice w.

weeks
every four w.
w. by ultrasound

weeping
w. eczema
w. lesion
w., whining, and wailing

Wegener
W. disease
limited Wegener granulomatosis
W. pulmonary granulomatosis

Wegner disease

Weidel
W. Auditory Processing Test
W. Yes/No Reliability Test

Weigert hematoxylin stain

weighed
not w.

weight
abdomen showed evidence of weight loss
abnormal diurnal weight gain
actual body w.
adrenal weight factor
antipsychotic-induced weight gain
atomic w.
atomic weight unit
axial weight loading
birth w.
birth weight for gestational age
body w.
body weight gain
by w.
combined testicular w.
daily w.
desirable body w.
diurnal weight fluctuation
dry body w.
episodic weight gain
erratic weight gain
estimated dry w.
estimated fetal body w.
estimated weight loss
excessive weight gain
excessive weight loss
expected weight gain
extremely low birth w.
fat-free dry w.
fat-free wet w.
fetal w.
w. gain
gradual weight gain
graft-to-recipient weight ratio
gram-molecular w.
gross w.
hand-held w.
heart w.
high birth w.
high molecular w.
high molecular weight component
high molecular weight dextran
high molecular weight glycoprotein
high molecular weight hemoglobin
high molecular weight kininogen
high molecular weight melanoma-associated antigen
high molecular weight polyethylene
ideal body w.
inability to control w.
infant weight gain
infant weight loss
ischial weight bearing leg brace
kidney w.
lean body w.
light molecular weight meromyosin

weight *(continued)*
w. loss
w. loss from anxiety
w. loss from pernicious anemia
low birth w.
low birth weight infant
low molecular w.
low molecular weight dextran
low molecular weight heparin
low molecular weight oxidizing agent
low molecular weight proteinuria
lung w.
lung-body weight ratio
w. management program
maternal weight gain
maximal increment in growth and w.
mean birth w.
mean percentage of desirable w.
minimal weight bearing
moderately low birth w.
molecular w.
molecular weight distribution
molecular weight ratio
mouse uterine weight unit
naked w.
normal birth w.
nutrition and weight control
ova w.
patient's weight in kilograms
peak weight velocity
postmenopausal weight gain
rapid weight gain
rat ovarian w.
relative body w.
severely low birth w.
significant gain in w.
significant weight gain
w. of solute per volume of solution
w. of solute per weight of solvent
spleen-to-body weight ratio
subsequent weight gain
sudden weight gain
target dry w.
test w.
thymic w.
total body w.
total weight gain
w. training exercise
w. transferral frequency
twin birth weight discordance
ultrahigh molecular w.
ultrahigh molecular weight polyethylene
ultralow birth w.
usual body w.
very low birth w.
very low birth weight infant
very low birth weight preterm neonate
volume per w.
wet w.

weight-activated locking knee prosthesis

weight-based heparin dosing

weightbearing
w. activity
w. as tolerated
full w.
ischial weightbearing prosthesis
w. joint
long leg weightbearing cast
no w.
partial w.
w. to tolerance
touchdown partial w.
touch-toe w.
w. with crutches

weighted
axial echo planar diffusion weighted imaging
long weighted speculum
Mantel-Haenszel weighted odds ratio
w. mean index
w. nonlinear least squares
w. patient care unit
T2 weighted image

weight-length index

weight-matched control

weight-related health problem

Weil
W. disease
W. syndrome

Weil-Felix
W.-F. reaction
W.-F. test

Weill-Marchesani syndrome

Weill sign

Weinberger Adjustment Inventory

Weinberg test

Weinstein enhanced sensory test

Weir Mitchell treatment

Weiss
W. procedure
W. reflex

Weissmann bundle

Weitbrecht
W. cartilage
W. fiber
W. foramen
W. ligament

weld
artery weld strength

Welder keratoconjunctivitis

welder's
arc welder's lung

welding
arc w.

welfare
Pension and W. Benefits Administration

Welin technique

well
alive and w.
as well as
w. baby
w. differentiated
diffuse lymphocytic, well differentiated
doing w.
fairly well developed
w. flexed
gamma well counter
w. groomed
w. healed
healing w.
heparin w.
living and w.
moves all extremities equally w.
normal well developed
nursed fairly w.
pain well controlled
patient tolerated the procedure w.
patient tolerated traction w.
patient well developed
patient well developed, well nourished
patient well hydrated
patient well nourished
Quality of W. Being Index
wound healing w.

well-baby
w.-b. clinic
w.-b. nursery

well-being
cognitive aspect of w.-b.
emotional w.-b.
functional w.-b.
Index of W.-b.
social/family w.-b.

well-born nursery

well-child care

well-circumscribed
- w.-c. carcinoma
- w.-c. lesion

well-developed
- w.-d. agar
- w.-d. collateral circulation

well-differentiated
- w.-d. adenoma
- w.-d. fetal adenocarcinoma
- w.-d. hepatocellular carcinoma
- w.-d. lymphocytic

well-healed
- w.-h. midline scar
- w.-h., nonsymptomatic
- w.-h., no residuals
- w.-h., no sequelae
- w.-h. previous excisional scars

well-known fact

wellness
- health w.
- Juvenile W. and Health Survey

well-nourished
- w.-n. female
- w.-n. male
- w.-n. man

Wenckebach
- W. atrioventricular block
- atrioventricular Wenckebach block
- AV Wenckebach heart block
- W. cycle
- W. heart block
- W. period
- W. phenomena

wen cyst

Wender Utah Rating Scale

Werdnig-Hoffman
- W.-H. disease
- W.-H.n muscular atrophy
- W.-H. syndrome

Wermer syndrome

Wernekinck
- W. commissure
- W. decussation

Werner
- W. disease
- W. syndrome

Wernicke
- W. aphasia
- W. area
- W. disease
- W. encephalopathy
- W. reaction
- W. sign

Wernicke-Korsakoff
- W.-K. encephalitis
- W.-K. syndrome

Wernicke-Mann hemiplegia

Wertheim
- W. operation
- W. radical hysterectomy

Wesselsbron
- W. disease
- W. disease virus

West
- W. African fever
- W. African sleeping sickness
- W. Nile encephalitis
- W. Nile encephalitis virus
- W. Nile fever
- W. Nile-like fever
- W. operation
- W. syndrome

Westberg space

Westcott
- micro Westcott scissors
- W. test

Westergren
- W. erythrocyte sedimentation rate
- W. method

Westermark sign

western
- W. Aphasia Battery
- W. Aphasia Battery Test
- W. blot
- W. blot analysis
- W. blot test
- W. blotting
- Eastern and W. encephalomyelitis vaccine
- w. equine encephalitis
- w. equine encephalomyelitis
- w. equine encephalomyelitis virus
- W. ligand blot
- W. Ontario Instability Index
- W. Ontario and McMaster Universities Osteoarthritis Index Physical Functioning subscale and chair-performance
- W. Ontario and McMaster Universities Osteoarthritis Index Physical Functioning subscale and chair-stand performance
- W. Ontario Rotator Cuff
- Toronto W. Spasmodic Torticollis Rating Scale

Westhaven Yale Multidimensional Pain Inventory

Westphal
- W. pupillary reflex
- W. sign

wet
- w. bulb
- w. bulb temperature
- w. compress
- w. dog shakes syndrome
- w. dressing
- dry to w.
- fat-free wet weight
- w. film
- w. gangrene
- hot wet pack
- w. lung
- w. lung syndrome
- w. mount
- w. nurse
- open wet dressing
- w. pack
- w. prep
- w. smear
- w. sputum
- w. swallow
- w. tail disease
- tap water wet dressing
- w. weight

wettable powder

wetting
- w. agent
- bed w.

Wetzel grid

Weve
- W. electrode
- W. operation

Weyers
- Meyer-Schwickerath and Weyers syndrome

Wharton
- W. duct
- W. jelly
- W. operation

Whataroa virus

wheal
- erythematous w.
- w. and flare
- w. and plaque

wheal-and-flare reaction

wheal-flare reaction

wheat
- w. amylase inhibitor

wheat *(continued)*
w. germ agglutinin
w. soy blend

wheel
diamond w.
front wheel walker
Meals on W.'s
Meals on W.'s Association of America
mill wheel murmur
steering wheel injury
wagon wheel fracture

wheelchair
w. access
w. artifact
w. confinement
patient needs minimal assistance for wheelchair mobility
pivot transfer from w.

wheeled walker

Wheeler
W. implant
W. method
W. operation

wheeze
bilateral w.'s
expiratory w.
forced end-expiratory w.
inspiratory w.
rales, rhonchi, or w.'s

wheezing
coughing and/or w.
expiratory w.
high-pitched w.
inspiratory w.
monophonic w.
nocturnal w.
w. on inspiration
patient w.
w. while breathing

wheezing-associated respiratory infection

whiff test

while
w. awake
driving while impaired
driving while intoxicated
operating motor vehicle while intoxicated
wheezing while breathing
whistling in nose while breathing

whining
weeping, whining, and wailing

whiplash
acute w.
w. injury
patient has whiplash injury

whiplash-associated disorder

Whipple
antrum-sparing modified Whipple procedure
W. disease
W. operation
W. procedure
pylorus-preserving Whipple modification

whippleii
Tropheryma w.

whirlpool
w. bath
cold or ice whirlpool treatment
large w.
w., massage, exercise
small w.
w. therapy
w. treatment

whiskey equivalent

whisper
forced w.

whispered
w. bronchophony
w. voice

whispering
w. pectoriloquy
w. resistance
w. resonance

whistle
peak flow w.

whistling
w. deformity
w. face syndrome
w. in nose while breathing

Whitacre operation

Whitaker Index of Schizophrenic Thinking

white
w. adipose tissue
w. American
w. Anglo-Saxon Protestant
anisotropy of white matter
anterior white commissure
anterolateral white matter of cord
arborescent white substance of cerebellum
associative detail response to white space
associative response to a white space on a card
atrophic white scar
autologous white cell localization
automated white blood cell differential
bacillary white diarrhea
w. blood cell
w. blood cell count
w. blood cell depletion
w. blood cell scan
w. blood cells per high-power field
w. blood cell transfusion
w. blood corpuscle
calcofluor white stain
w. cell
w. cell cast
w. cell count
w. cell count
w. child
w. coat effect
w. coat hypertension
w. coat syndrome
deep white matter hyperintensity
deep white matter infarct
deep white matter lesion
detail response to small white space
w. divorced female
echogenicity of periventricular white matter
w. female living child
generalized white matter atrophy
idiopathic white matter lesion
infection-fighting white cell
large white kidney
w. line of Toldt
long-term low-level white noise
w. male living child
w. matter
w. matter damage
w. matter edema
w. matter hyperintensity
w. matter lesion cerebral
w. matter signal abnormality
w. matter thinning
microcephaly-calcification of cerebral white matter syndrome
multifocal white matter inflammatory lesion
multiple evanescent white dot syndrome
New Zealand white mouse
Nicolle white mycetoma
nonalcoholic white shake lotion
normal-appearing white matter

normal human white matter
w. or pale nails from anemia
w. patches from anemia
pearl white mounds
peripheral white blood cell
w. pulp
response to white space
scalloped appearance of white matter
Sergent white line
w. substance of Schwann
superficial white onychomycosis
temporoparietal white matter
total white and differential cell count
total white blood cells
unknown white female
unknown white male
vibration-induced white finger
zinc oxide-eugenol white zinc

white-faced hornet

Whitehead deformity

whitish
itchy, whitish vaginal discharge

whitlow
w. herpetic
melanotic w.

Whitman
W. frame
W. operation

Whitmore
W. bacillus
W. disease

Whitnall tubercle

who
men who have sex with men
woman who has given birth

whole
w. abdominopelvic irradiation
w. blood
w. blood transfusion
w. blood volume
w. body
w. boiled milk
w. bone transplant graft
w. brain irradiation
w. brain radiation
w. brain versus local brain radiation therapy
cadaveric whole organ transplant
capillary whole blood true sugar
w. chromosome paint
w. complement
confabulated whole response
w. cow's milk
detail response elaborating the w.
extracorporeal whole body hyperthermia
w. homogenate
influenza virion vaccine, whole virion
w. lymphocyte fraction
w. milk
w. mount microscopy
Pall-filtered whole blood
patient admitted and transfused with whole blood
prophylactic whole brain radiation therapy
w. ragweed extract
rapid whole blood test
w. response
w. response to detail
w. skull irradiation
w. time equivalent
w. tomography slice
unit of whole blood

whole-blood
w.-b. activated clotting time
w.-b. folate
w.-b. hematocrit
w.-b. partial thromboplastin time
w.-b. recalcification time

whole-body
w.-b. activity
w.-b. antibody technique
w.-b. bone scan
w.-b. counting
w.-b. CT
w.-b. digital scanner
w.-b. extract
w.-b. hyperthermia
w.-b. protein
w.-b. radiation
w.-b. retention
w.-b. scan
w.-b. scintigraphy

whole-bowel irrigation

whole-brain
w.-b. radiotherapy

whole-cell lysate

whole-grain
rye w.-g.

whole-gut transit scintigraphy

whole-lung tomography

whooping
w. cough
w. cough vaccine

whorled
w. cells
w. enamel
linear and whorled nevoid hypermelanosis
w. pattern

whorl motion

Wiberg
angle of W.
capital epiphysis angle of W.
CE angle of W.
W. classification

Wicherkiewicz operation

wick
gauze w.

Wickersheimer
W. fluid
W. medium

wicket rhythm

Wickwitz esophageal stricture

Widal reaction

wide
w. awake
w. band noise
w. base of support
w. dynamic range compression
w. excision
w. field
w. intervertebral space
w. local excision
moderately wide open anterior chamber angle
w. open
w. open anterior chamber angle
w. range
W. Range Achievement Test-Revised
W. Range Assessment of Memory and Learning
regular, wide QRS tachycardia
w. skin incision
World W. Web

wide-angle glaucoma

wide-based gait

wide-base quad cane

wide-complex tachycardia

wide-field
w.-f. eyepiece
w.-f. radiation therapy

widely
w. invasive follicular carcinoma
w. patent

widened
incision w.

widening
aneurysmal widening of aorta
ankle mortise w.
w. of interspace
mediastinal w.
palpebral fissure w.

widespread
w. anoxic change
chronic widespread pain
w. ecchymosis and hematoma

Widmark conjunctivitis

widow
black widow spider toxin
black widow spider venom

widow's hump

Widowitz sign

width
anterior arch w.
arch width analysis
arm girth, chest depth, and hip w.
aryepiglottic fold w.
capillary basement membrane w.
distal phalangeal w.
full width at half maximum
full width of photopeak measured at half maximal count
hemisphere w.
interphalangeal w.
lateral ventricular width to hemispheric w.
lung w.
maximal cardiac w.
maximal chest w.
metaphysial to diaphysial width ratio
notch width index
orbital fissure w.
platelet distribution w.
pulse w.
red blood cell diameter w.
red blood cell distribution width index
reticulocyte hemoglobin distribution w.

Wiedemann-Rautenstrauch syndrome

Wiedemann syndrome

Wiener operation

Wiener-Pierce rasp

Wies
modified Wies procedure

wife
bereaved w.

Wigand
W. maneuver
W. version

Wigby-Taylor position

Wiktor stent

Wilcoxon
W. rank sum statistic
W. rank sum test

wild
w. limb jerk
w. type strain

Wilde incision

Wilder
W. diet
W. sign
W. silver stain

Wildermuth ear

Wilke boot brace

will
w. be in
w. call
w. call back
w. follow in office
living w.

Willebrand
acquired von Willebrand disease
anti-von Willebrand factor
anti-von Willebrand factor antibody
Minot-von Willebrand syndrome
von Willebrand disease
von Willebrand factor

willful exposure to unwanted pregnancy

Williams
W. exercise
W. operation
W. position
W. sign
W. syndrome
W. syndrome, early puberty
W. syndrome, late puberty
W. tracheal tone

Williamson sign

Williams-Richardson operation

Willis
antrum of W.
arterial circle of W.
artery of W.
circle of W.
W. cord
nerve of W.
W. pancreas

Willowbrook virus

willow fracture

Wills test

Willy Meyer radical mastectomy

Wilmer operation

Wilms
anaplastic Wilms tumor
aniridia, Wilms tumor association
aniridia, Wilms tumor, gonadoblastoma syndrome
National Wilms Tumor Study
W. operation
W. tumor
W. tumor 1
W. tumor, aniridia, genitourinary abnormalities, and mental retardation

Wilson
W. block
central terminal of W.
W. central terminal
W. cloud chamber
W. disease
W. method
W. muscle
W. operation
W. syndrome
W. test

Wilson-Kimmelstiel disease

Wilson-McKeever operation

Wilson-Mikity syndrome

Wilson-Turner syndrome

winder dysentery

windmill
periodic alternating windmill nystagmus

window
aorticopulmonary window defect
aorticopulmonary window shunt
aortic window node
aortopulmonary w.
aortopulmonary window mass
fenestration of oval w.
intact round w.
lateral frontal bone w.
little fossa of cochlear w.
little fossa of oval vestibular w.
middle meatus nasal antral w.
nasal antral w.
oval w.
oval window defect
oval window reflex
paramedian frontal bone w.
patchy window defect
pulmonary parenchymal w.
Rebuck skin window technique

round window electrocochleography

windsock
w. aneurysm
w. sign

wine
port wine hemangioma
port wine mark

wineglass appearance

wing
angel w.
ashen w.
W. Autistic Disorder Interview Checklist
w. cell
Maddox wing test
malar crest of great wing of sphenoid bone
modified gull wing incision
orbital wing of sphenoid bone
parietal margin of greater wing of sphenoid
posterior bite w.
w. of scapula
w. suture

winged
w. incisor
w. scapula
w. shunt

wink
anal w.

Winkelman disease

winking
jaw w.
opticofacial winking reflex
w. spasms

Winslow
epiploic foramen of W.
foramen of W.
W. ligament
W. pancreas
W. star

winter
W. arch bar
w. blues
w. bronchitis
w. cough
w. depression
w. exercise
W. technique
w. vomiting disease

Wintrich sign

Wintrobe
W. erythrocyte sedimentation rate
W. index
W. test

wiping reaction

wire
aluminum wire splint
antegrade double balloon-double wire technique
atherolytic reperfusion wire device
beaded transfixion w.
bone suturing wire chisel-tip wire
cable wire suture technique
cerclage wire fixation
cerclage wire inserter
cerclage wire technique
circular wire fixator
continuous loop w.
diamond-point wire double-strand wire
diamond tip w.
figure-of-eight wire loop
w. fixation
flexible spiral wire retainer
ideal arch w.
Kirschner w.
light around wire technique
loop circumferential w.
w. mesh implant
w. mesh implant material
over the w.
pacemaker w.
pacing electrode w.
standard wire gauge
tantalum wire fixation

wired
jaw w.

wireless endoscopy capsule

wiring
circumferential w.
circumzygomatic w.
continuous loop w.
jaw w.
oblique facet w.

Wirsung
canal of W.
W. canal
duct of W.
W. duct
main duct of W.

wiry pulse

Wisconsin
W. Card Sorting Test
W. Compression System
modified University of Wisconsin solution
original University of Wisconsin solution
University of Wisconsin solution

wisdom
erupted wisdom teeth
impacted wisdom teeth
malpositioned wisdom teeth
partially impacted wisdom teeth
w. teeth

Wise areola mastopexy breast augmentation

wish
asymptotic wish fulfillment

Wiskott-Aldrich
W.-A. syndrome
W.-A. syndrome protein

Wistar
W. Institute Susan Hayflick cell
normotensive Wistar rat

wit
allusion in w.

with
w. assistance
compare w.
compatible w.
in connection w.
consistent w.
crossed w.
w. disease
w. feedings
followed w.
w. meal

withdrawal
abrupt w.
alcoholic withdrawal tremor
alcohol intake w.
alcohol withdrawal delirium
alcohol withdrawal hallucinosis
alcohol withdrawal seizure
alcohol withdrawal syndrome
alcohol withdrawal tremulousness
anchor signs of w.
androgen withdrawal endocrine therapy
antiandrogen withdrawal syndrome
w. body shakes
clinical manifestation of w.
drug withdrawal insomnia
w. dyskinesia
w. dystonia
w. effect
estrogen-progesterone withdrawal bleeding
estrogen withdrawal bleeding
w. from hallucinogen

withdrawal *(continued)*
gradual w.
w. headache
isolation and w.
narcotic withdrawal scale
narcotic withdrawal syndrome
negotiable order of w.
Neonatal W. Inventory
Neonatal Narcotic W. Index
neuroleptic w.
newborn drug w.
opiate w.
opiate withdrawal symptom
opiate withdrawal syndrome
painful withdrawal reaction
persistent withdrawal occlusion
physical withdrawal symptoms
precipitated withdrawal diarrhea
prevent withdrawal symptom
progesterone w.
quasimorphine withdrawal syndrome
right pulmonary artery w.
w. seizure
severe withdrawal reaction
thought w.

withdrawal-emergent dyskinesia

withering cancer

withholding
caregiver withholding and uncaring

within
accumulation of blood within joint
affect within normal range
w. defined limits
w. full limits
w. functional limits
inflammation within affected area
w. normal limits
w. normal range
range of motion within normal limits
upper and lower extremities within normal limits

within-list recognition

within-person variability

without
absent without leave
aggression without provocation
agoraphobia without history of panic disorder
alexia without agraphia
anterior disc displacement without reduction
arthritis without deformity
attention deficit disorder without hyperactivity
away without authorization
blister without infection
w. correction/without glasses
distance visual acuity without correction
Doctors W. Borders
w. dyskinesia
hydrocephalus, agyria, retinal dysplasia with or without encephalocele syndrome
jaundice without inflammation
leave without consent
left without completing treatment
life-terminating acts without the explicit request
light perception without projection
migraine without aura
necrotizing scleritis without adjacent inflammation
otitis media without effusion
panic disorder without agoraphobia
partial seizures with or without generalized tonic-clonic seizures
passed without difficulty
quality-adjusted time without symptoms or toxicity
w. redness or swelling
situational anger disorder without aggression
w. spectacles
spinal cord injury without radiographic abnormality
time without symptoms of progression or toxicity
trial without catheter
tympanoplasty without mastoidectomy

with-the-rule astigmatism

witness
autopsy w.

Wittenborn
W. Psychiatric Rating Scale
W. Psychiatric Symptoms Inventory

Witwatersrand virus

Wladimiroff-Mikulicz amputation

Wladimiroff operation

Wohlgemuth unit

Woillez disease

Wolf
W. method
W. Motor Function Test
W. syndrome

Wolfe
W. graft
W. operation

Wolfe-Krause graft

Wolff-Chaikoff
W.-C. block
W.-C. effect

wolffian
w. body
w. cyst
w. duct
w. duct carcinoma
female adnexal tumor of probable wolffian origin

Wolf-Hirschhorn syndrome

Wölfler gland

Wolfring gland

Wolman xanthomatosis

Wolpe Fear Survey Schedule

woman, pl. **women**
alcohol abuse among women
amenorrheic w.
androgenized w.
angry woman syndrome
antibody-positive w.
Brief Index of Sexual Functioning for Women
healthy pregnant women
heterosexual development of women
hundred woman years of exposure
immune globulin to an Rh-negative w.
W., Infants, and Children Program
infertility in women
men and women
w. milk
normoprolactinemic w.
sexual function of women
w. who has given birth
w. years
women years of usage

womb
falling of the w.

Women's
W. Health Initiative
National Women's Health Information Center
National Women's Health Network
Older Women's League

Wonderland
Alice in Wonderland syndrome
Wongal virus
Wongorr virus
wood
W. light examination of eye
w. pulp worker lung
W. unit
woodchuck hepatic virus
Woodcock-Johnson Psychoeducational Battery
Woodcock Reading Mastery Test
Wood-Downes-Lecks
wooden
w. belly
w. resistance
w. resonance
wooden-shoe heart
Woodward reagent K
woody
w. edema
w. thyroiditis
Wookey
W. neck flap
W. pharyngoesophageal reconstruction
woolly
cardiomyopathy and woolly hair-coat syndrome
w. hair
w. thinking
woolsorter's
w. disease
w. pneumonia
word
angry word exchange
w. association
W. Association Test
auditory word center
clipped w.
Controlled Oral W. Association Test
Cornell W. Form
Dichotic W. Test
w. discrimination score
echoing words of others
w. fluency
inability to arrange w.'s
inability to arrange words properly
inability to interpret written w.
inability to remember spoken w.'s
W. Intelligibility by Picture Identification
Modified W. Learning Test
Monotic W. Memory Test
number of words chosen
number of different w.'s
performance versus intensity function for phonetically balanced w.'s
phonetically balanced w.
phonetically balanced percentage of word lists
w. processor
Staggered Spondaic W. Test
Test of Adolescent/Adult W. Finding
Test of W. Finding
Test of W. Finding in Discourse
thinking creatively with sounds and w.'s
word-finding
w.-f. ability
w.-f. difficulty
work
acclimation to heat and w.
admission blood w.
W. Attitudes Questionnaire
w. of breathing
w. capacity
w. capacity assessment
w. capacity evaluation
w. capacity specialist
cardiac w.
cardiac work index
cardiovascular work capacity
case w.
w. conditioning
delayed work recall test
w. evaluation systems technology
fasting blood w.
fasting laboratory w.
functional work capacity assessment
group w.
w. hardening
w. hardening exercise
w. hardening program
hold breakfast for blood w.
hostile work environment
w. hypertrophy
inability to sustain consistent work behavior
Index of W. Satisfaction
w. and interest
left ventricular stroke w.
left ventricular stroke work index
w. metabolic rate
New Mexico Attitude Toward W. Test
off w.
Ohio W. Values Inventory
parent guidance w.
past relevant w.
peak work capacity
peak work rate
physical work capacity
w. rate
right ventricular stroke work index
routine laboratory work done
w. simulation
stroke w.
Test of W. Competency and Stability
testing, orientation, work, evaluation, rehabilitation
w. therapy
ventricular stroke w.
Vocational Evaluation and W. Adjustment
zero work tolerance
worker
accredited rehabilitation w.
case w.
certified social w.
childcare w.
coal w. lung
coal w. pneumoconiosis
direct care w.
health care w.
laboratory w.
machine worker dermatitis
malt w. lung
mental health w.
mushroom w. lung
paper mill w. disease
psychiatric social w.
wood pulp worker lung
workers'
bauxite workers' disease
w. compensation
Workgroup
National Arthritis Data W.
working
w. distance
W. Formulation for Clinical Usage
metal working fluid
new working formulation
w. point
quality of working life
submaximal working capacity
work-level month

workload unit

workout
high-stress w.

work-related injury

workshop
International W. and Conference on Human Leukocyte Differentiation Antigens

workup
diagnostic workup and staging
gastrointestinal w.
metabolic stone w.
neonatal cholestasis w.
patient admitted for evaluation and w.
patient hospitalized for w.
preoperative laboratory w.
presurgical laboratory w.
septic w.

world
Experiential W. Inventory
W. Health Organization classification of lupus nephritis I, IIA, IIB, III, IV, V
W. Health Organization Quality of Life 100-Item
W. Medical Association
New W. hemorrhagic fever
New W. leishmaniasis
New W. screwworm
Old W. leishmaniasis
W. Wide Web

worm
bag of w.'s appearance
Guinea worm disease
heart w.
Manson eye w.
meal w.
parasitic w.
thorny-headed w.

wormseed
oil of American w.

worn
body worn hearing aid
w. facet joint
has not worn glasses
has worn prescription glasses

worship
ancestral w.

Worth four-dot test for fusion

worthlessness
feeling of guilt, worthlessness and helplessness

wound
w. abscess
active oozing from w.
alginate wound cover
approximate wound edges
w. bed
w. biopsy
w. botulism
w. breakdown
w. care
chronic granulating w.
w. clean and healed
closed over w.
w. closure
closure of skin w.
clot expressed from w.
contaminated operative wound classification
w. contraction
counter stab wound incision
w. culture
débrided wound edge
w. debridement
deep sternal wound infection
dehydration of w.
delayed closure of accidental w.
delayed closure of operative w.
died from w.'s
dirty operative wound classification
w. drainage
drain brought out through stab w.
drain placed into w.
w. dressing emulsion
w. examined for hemostasis
w. excision
w. of exit
fasciotomy wound biopsy
fragment w.
full-jacketed bullet w.
gaping wound edges
gas gangrene w.
w. granulating in
gunshot w.
gunshot wound to abdomen
gunshot wound to head
w. healed by first, second or third intention
w. healed per primam
w. healed by secondary intention
w. healing
w. healing capability
w. healing well
w. hematoma
incisional surgical wound infection
w. infection
intraocular leaking w.
w. irrigated with normal saline
w. isolation
knife stab w.
w. loosely approximated
margins of wound brought into apposition
w. margin undermined
multiple fragment w.'s
multiple gunshot w.
multiple stab w.'s
nonhealing w.
nosocomial wound infection
oozing from w.
open w.
open fracture wound drain
open-sky cataract w.
operative wound clean and healed
penetrating abdominal w.
penetrating cardiac w.
penetrating neck w.
penetrating wound of the abdomen
penetrating wound of heart
plantar puncture w.
platelet-derived wound healing factor
poor wound healing
postoperative wound infection
probing of w.
puncture w.
puncture wound of foot
satisfactory wound healing
self-inflicted w.
shell fragment w.
shrapnel fragment w.
w. and skin
skin and wound isolation
spiral w.
stab w.
stab wound incision
stab wound of throat
sucking chest w.
w. swab
w. tumor virus

wound-breaking strength

wounded in action

wound-induced

W-plasty
shape of surgical incisions -p.

wrap
cardiac muscle w.
double w.
gastric w.
Louisiana ankle wrap technique
Nissen 360-degree wrap fundoplication
Nissen fundoplication w.

wraparound
breast mound reduction and nipple reconstruction with wraparound flap
great toe wraparound flap

wrapping aneurysm

wrath
Cape W. virus

Wreden sign

wrench
beaded-pin w.
box-end w.
cannulated w.
hex w.

Wright
W. antigen
W. peak flowmeter
W. plate
W. stain
W. version

Wright-Giemsa stain

wringing
hand w.

wrinkle artifact

wrinkling
drying and wrinkling of skin
macular surface w.
surface wrinkling retinopathy

wrinkly skin syndrome

Wrisberg
W. cartilage
W. ganglion
ligament of W.
W. ligament
W. nerve

wrist
active wrist rotation unit
w. arthroscopy
articular wrist disorder
w. block
w. bone
carcinomatous arthritis in w.
Chan wrist rest
cock-up wrist splint
w. contracture
w. deformity
w. disarticulation
w. dislocation
dorsal wrist splint
dorsal wrist syndrome
w. drop
w. extensor tendon
w. flexion
w. flexion reflex
w. flexion test
w. ganglion
golfer's w.
w. hand extension compression support
hand flexed at w.
w. joint
long radial extensor muscle of w.
lunate acrylic cement wrist prosthesis
medial ligament of w.
radial eminence of w.
shoulder, elbow, wrist, hand orthosis
Swanson wrist joint implant
total wrist arthroplasty
total wrist replacement
ulnar collateral ligament of wrist joint

wrist-hand orthosis

wristlet
elastic w.

writer's cramp

writing
ataxic w.
automatic w.
developmental expressive writing disorder
w. hand

written
dispense as w.
w. home exercise program
inability to interpret written word
w. order
Test of W. Language
Thorndike-Lorge written frequency

wrong test requested-floor error

Wucherer conjunctivitis

Wullstein type tympanoplasty

WW/1 virus

Wyeomyia virus

Wyeth operation

Wylie
W. operation
W. pessary

X:Ag
Asserachrom X:Ag

xanthelasma palpebrarum

xanthelasmoideum
lymphangioma x.

xanthine
x. dehydrogenase
x. diphosphate
x. monophosphate
x. oxidase
x. oxidase reaction
serum xanthine oxidase

Xanthium pensylvanicum

xanthoastrocytoma
pleomorphic x.

xanthochromic fluid

xanthoerythrodermia perstans

xanthofibroma thecocellulare

xanthogranuloma
adult-type x.
juvenile x.

xanthogranulomatous pyelonephritis

xanthoma
Achilles tendon x.
x. disseminatum
x. eruptivum
malignant fibrous x.
x. multiplex
x. palpebrarum
x. planum
x. striatum palmare
x. tendinosum
x. tuberosum
x. tuberosum multiplex

xanthomatosis
x. bulbi
cerebrotendinous x.
chronic idiopathic x.
x. iridis
normal cholesteremic x.

xanthomatous granuloma

xanthosine
x. 5′-monophosphate
x. triphosphate

xanthurenic acid

X-chromosome
adhesion molecule-like from the X.-c.

X-E
fragile X.-E.

xenobiotic-response element

xenogeneic
x. antigen
x. graft

xenograft
acute vascular xenograft rejection
delayed xenograft rejection
x. dressing
hyperacute xenograft rejection
x. transplantation

xenograph surface area

xenon
x. arch photocoagulator
x. arc laser
x. arc light
x. chloride
x. lung ventilation imaging

xenon-enhanced computed tomography

xenopi
Mycobacterium xenopi infection

xenoreactive natural antibody

xenotransplantation procedure

xeroderma
x. of Kaposi
x. pigmentosum
x. pigmentosum group A, C

xerodermic idiocy

xeromammogram study

xerophthalmic fundus

xerosis
x. conjunctivae
x. cutis
x. parenchymatosus
x. superficialis

xerostomia
radiation-induced x.

xerotica
balanitis xerotica obliterans
x. obliterans

xerotic keratitis

XI
Factor XI
factor XI deficiency

Xiburema virus

XII
factor XII deficiency
factor XII inhibitor

XIII
factor I through X.
factor XIII deficiency

XIIIa
factor XIIIa

xiphoid
x. angle
x. bone
x. cartilage
nose to ear to x.
x. process
x. to pubis
symphysis, buttocks, and x.

X-linked
X.-l. abnormality
X.-l. agammaglobulinemia
X.-l. alpha-thalassemia/mental retardation syndrome
X.-l. Alport syndrome
X.-l. aqueductal stenosis
X.-l. cardiomyopathy
X.-l. cerebral ataxia
X.-l. dilated cardiomyopathy
X.-l. disease
X.-l. disorder
X.-l. dominant
X.-l. dysplasia-gigantism syndrome
X.-l. first site of fragility
X.-l. genetic defect
X.-l. heredity
X.-l. human androgen receptor
X.-l. hydrocephalus
X.-l. hypercalciuric nephrolithiasis
X.-l. hypogammaglobulinemia
X.-l. hypophosphatemia
X.-l. hypophosphatemic rickets
X.-l. ichthyosis
X.-l. inheritance
X.-l. juvenile retinoschisis
X.-l. lymphoproliferative disease
X.-l. mental retardation
X.-l. mental retardation-aphasia syndrome
X.-l. mental retardation-blindness-deafness-multiple congenital anomalies syndrome
X.-l. mental retardation, microphthalmia, microcornea, cataract, hypogenitalism-mental retardation-spasticity syndrome
X.-l. mental retardation, seizures, acquired microcephaly, agenesis of corpus callosum
X.-l. mental retardation syndrome 1–6
X.-l. myotubular myopathy
X.-l. ocular albinism
X.-l. olivopontocerebellar ataxia
X.-l. Opitz syndrome
X.-l. progressive mixed deafness with perilymphatic gusher

X-linked *(continued)*
X.-l. recessive lymphoproliferative syndrome
X.-l. recessive nephrolithiasis
X.-l. retinitis pigmentosa
X.-l. second site of fragility
X.-l. severe combined immunodeficiency
X.-l. thrombocytopenia

Xonics electron mammography

XP21
partial monosomy XP21, XP22

XP22
partial monosomy XP21, X.

x-ray
abdominal x.-r.
admission chest x.-r.
x.-r. analysis
x.-r. arteriography
cast-off x.-r.
cast off, to x.-r.
cast removed, take x.-r.
check-up x.-r.
x.-r. computed tomography
deep x.-r.
x.-r. dermatitis
x.-r. diffraction
x.-r. dosimetry
x.-r. energy spectrometry
x.-r. film
x.-r. finding
x.-r. fluorescence
full-mouth x.-r.
hard x-ray imaging spectrometer
high-dose beam of x.-r.'s
x.-r. imaging
x.-r. immunosuppressive measure
kidneys, ureters, bladder x.-r.
kidneys, ureters, and spleen x.-r.
x.-r. mammogram
mobile mass x.-r.
x.-r. out of plaster
periapical x.-r.
x.-r. photoemission spectroscopy
x.-r. in plaster
portable chest x.-r.
real-time, low-intensity x.-r.
scanning-beam digital x.-r.
skull x.-r.
x.-r. tomographic microscope

XXX
mosaicism for XXX

XXY syndrome

xylene-alcohol mixture

xylol
formalin, ethanol, xylol, and ethanol
x. pulse indicator

xylose
x. breath test
x. concentration test

xylose-lysine-deoxycholate agar

Xytron pacemaker

X,Y,Z
cardinal axes X,Y,Z

Yaba monkey virus

Yacaaba virus

YAG posterior capsulotomy

Yale
- Westhaven Yale Multidimensional Pain Inventory
- Y. Global Tic Severity Scale

Yale-Brown Obsessive-Compulsive Scale

yam mosaic virus

yang meridian

Yangtze River disease

Yaquina Head virus

yard
- cubic y.

Yasargil
- Y. neurological instrument
- Y. technique

Yata virus

Yates correction

yaw
- foot y.
- mother y.

yawn
- heat, steam, gum, yawn, and Valsalva maneuver

year
- y. of birth
- y. to date
- y. of death
- disability-adjusted life y.'s
- Early Y.'s Easy Screen
- epidemiology y.
- fiscal y.
- full y.
- healthy y.'s of life
- y.'s of healthy life
- healthy y.'s of life lost
- hundred woman y.'s of exposure
- y.'s of life lost
- y.'s of life with disability
- lost y.'s of expected life
- marginal cost per year of life saved
- month, date, y.
- y.'s old
- packs per year cigarettes
- packs per year history
- per member per y.
- postoperative chronologic y.
- potential y.'s of life lost
- y.'s of potential life lost before age 65
- women y.'s
- women y.'s of usage

yearbook
- Mental Measurements Y.

5-year survival rate

yeast
- acid bismuth yeast medium
- y. alcohol dehydrogenase
- y. artificial chromosome
- autolyzed yeast protein
- brewers' y.
- buffered charcoal yeast extract
- y. carbon base
- casein yeast lactate medium
- y. cell
- charcoal yeast extract medium
- y. extract
- facultative yeast carrier
- y. fungus
- y. infection
- lipophilic y.
- live yeast cell derivative
- y. and mannitol
- Micro Drop yeast identification system
- modified sea water yeast extract agar
- y. morphology agar
- multitest yeast plate
- y. nitrogen base
- oral yeast infection
- y., peptone, and adenine sulfate
- peptone, glucose, and yeast extract medium
- y. phase
- serum, casein, glucose, yeast extract medium
- trichomonas and y.
- trypticase soy y.
- tryptone glucose yeast agar
- vaginal yeast infection

yellow
- y. body
- y. bone marrow
- y. enzyme
- y. fat
- y. fever
- y. fever immunization
- y. fever vaccine
- y. fever virus
- fuchsin, amido black, and naphthol y.
- healed yellow atrophy
- y. hyaline membrane disease
- y. jacket venom
- jungle yellow fever
- large yellow soft stools
- y. ligament
- lustrous central yellow point
- medium yellow soft stools
- y. nail
- y. nail syndrome
- old yellow enzyme
- reduced yellow enzyme
- y. skin
- small, yellow, constipated stool
- y. spot
- y. sputum
- subacute yellow atrophy
- y. vernix syndrome
- y. vision

yellow-brown serous ascites

yellow-faced hornet

Yeo treatment

Yerkes-Bridges Test psychology

Yersinia
- *Yersinia* arthritis
- *Yersinia* enterocolitica colitis

yersiniosis
- nonplague y.

Yes/No
- Weidel Yes/No Reliability Test

yet
- not yet discovered
- not yet published

yield
- ectocervical cell y.
- guaranteed yield strength
- lower yield point
- y. point
- y. pressure
- quantum y.
- upper yield point

Yin
- Qi and Yin deficiency

yin deficiency-yang excess syndrome

yoga
- Hatha y.

Yogue virus

yokes
- cerebral yokes of bone of cranium

yolk
- y. cell
- y. cleavage
- egg y.
- egg yolk agar
- mediastinal yolk sac tumor
- neomycin egg yolk agar

yolk *(continued)*
- y. sac
- y. sac carcinoma

York
- Y. antibody
- New York City medium
- New York erysiphake
- New York Heart Association
- New York Heart Association classification of heart disease
- New York vaccinia virus

Yorke-Mason incision

Yoshida sarcoma

You
- Inquiry Mode Questionnaire: A Measure of How You Think and Make Decisions

Youman-Parlett serologic test

young
- y. adult chronic patient
- y. adult psychiatric assessment
- y. male Caucasian
- Y. Mania Rating Scale
- mature-onset diabetes of the y.
- maturity-onset diabetes of the y.
- Y. operation
- Pain Observation Scale for Y. Children
- Y. procedure
- Sheridan Tests for Young Children and Retardates

younger-onset rheumatoid arthritis

youngest living child

Young-Helmholtz theory

Yount operation

youth
- y. counselor
- Y. Effectiveness Training
- Great Smoky Mountains Study of Y.
- mature-onset diabetes of y.
- presexual y.
- y. risk behavioral survey
- y. self-report

youth/parent support group

Y-shaped
- Y.-s. cartilage
- Y.-s. ligament

Y-suspensor
- inverted Y.-s.

yttrium
- y., aluminum, garnet
- y., argon, garnet
- y. lithium fluoride

yttrium-aluminum-garnet laser

Y-type incision

Yug Bogdanovac virus

yuppie
- y. flu
- y. influenza

Yvon
- Y. coefficient
- Y. coefficient test

YY
- peptide YY

Zahn
anomaly of Z.
line of Z.
Z. line
pocket of Z.
Z. rib
Zaliv Terpeniya virus
Zancolli operation
Zanelli position
Zang space
Zappert chamber
Zaufal sign
Z-cut osteotomy
Zealand
New Zealand obese mouse
New Zealand white mouse
New Zealand green-lipped mussel
New Zealand mice
zebra body
Zeeman effect
Zegla virus
Zeis gland
zeisian
z. gland
z. sty
Zeiss
Z. instruments
Z. microscope
Zellweger syndrome
Zenker
Z. crystal
Z. degeneration
Z. diverticulum
Z. fluid
Z. necrosis
Z. solution
Zephiran
Z. irrigation
Z. solution
zero
z. amplitude
atomic orbital with angular momentum quantum number z.
audiometric z.
automatic zero set
z. defect
z. differential overlap
z. discharge
z. end-expiratory pressure
z. frequency
parietal midline zero electrode placement in electroencephalography
z. point of charge
z. population growth
z. stool since birth
z. work tolerance
zero-flow pressure
zeta
z. erythrocyte sedimentation rate
hemoglobin z.
Z-flap incision
Ziegler
Z. cautery
Z. operation
Z. scale
Ziehen-Oppenheim disease
Ziehen test
Ziehl-Neelsen
Z.-N. method
Z.-N. stain
Zielke
Ziemann dot
Zieve
Z. method
Z. syndrome
Zika
Z. fever
Z. virus
Zimaloy femoral head prosthesis
Zimany
Z. bilobed flap
Z. flap
Zimmerman
Z. arch
Z. Preschool Language Scale
Zimmermann
Z. corpuscle
Z. granule
Zimmer method
zinc
z. adequate pair-fed
z. chloride poisoning
crystalline zinc insulin
z. deficient
z. depletion syndrome
z. finger protein
z. flocculation test
z. gluconate glycine
z. glycinate marker
insulin-protamine z.
insulin zinc suspension
z. meta-arsenite
z. oxide
z. peroxide
promyelocytic leukemia zinc finger
protamine zinc insulin
z. protoporphyrin
z. protoporphyrin/heme
z. pyrithione
z. suboptimal
z. turbidity test
zinc oxide-eugenol white zinc
Zinn
annulus of Z.
aponeurosis of Z.
Z. aponeurosis
Z. artery
Z. cap
Z. circle
Z. circlet
Z. corona
Z. ligament
Z. membrane
Z. tendon
Z. zone
Z. zonule
Zinnanti uterine manipulator-injector
zinnii
annulus z.
Zinsser inconsistency
zip
apical z.
zipper
z. artifact
z. scar
zirconium
z. granuloma
z. silicate
Zirqa virus
Z-lengthening
Achilles tendon Z.-l.
Zollinger-Ellison syndrome
Zöllner line
zona, pl. **zonae**
z. aberration
z. drilling
z. fasciculata
z. glomerulosa
z. glomerulosa protein
partial zona dissection
partial zona drilling
z. pellucida
z. pellucida 1, 2, 3
zonal
acute zonal occult outer retinopathy

Z

zonal *(continued)*
z. anatomy
assisted zonal hatching
continuous-flow zonal centrifugation
partial zonal dissection

zonary placenta

zone
adrenal cortex z.
anal transitional z.
anterior optical z.
anterior speech z.
antibasement membrane zone autoantibody
antibody excess z.
apical zone of cornea
arrhythmogenic border z.
arterial border z.
atypical transformation z.
avascular z.
back optic zone radius
basement membrane z.
capillary-free z.
capillary zone electrophoresis
chemoreceptor trigger z.
dorsal root entry z.
epidermal basement z.
fetal danger z.
focal z.
foveal avascular z.
front optic zone radius
high-intensity z.
high-pressure z.
hypertrophic z.
infarction z.
iron z.
landing z.
large loop excision of transition z.
Lissauer marginal z.
loop excision of the transformation z.
lower esophageal high-pressure z.
MALT/marginal zone lymphoma
mantle z.
mantle zone hyperplasia
mantle zone nodule
mantle zone pattern
marginal z.
marginal zone cell lymphoma
marginal zone B-cell lymphoma
marginal zone cell
marginal zone lymphocyte
marginal zone lymphoma
marginal zone macrophage
marginal zone pattern
markers for z.
McDonald optic zone marker
needle diathermy excision of the transformation z.
neutral z.
nodal marginal zone B-cell lymphoma
noninfarct z.
normal transformation zone colposcopy
optical z.
optical zone centration
optical zone of contact lens
optical zone diameter
optical zone marker
orbicular zone of hip
peripheral z.
z. of polarizing activity
posterior necrotic z.
posterior optical z.
posterior root entry z.
pregnancy z.
pregnancy zone protein
z. of preparatory calcification
pressure zone microphone
proliferative z.
prostate-specific antigen transition z.
reserve z.
root exit z.
z. of slow conduction
splenic marginal zone lymphoma
target heart rate z.
thymus-dependent zone of lymph node
transformation z.
transition z.
transitional cell z.

zone/loop
large loop excision of transformation zone/loop electrosurgical excision procedure

zone/mucosa
marginal zone/mucosa-associated lymphoid tissue

zonula, pl. **zonulae**
z. ciliaris
z. occludens
z. occludens toxin

zonular
z. band
z. cataract
z. fiber
z. layer
z. placenta
z. space

zonule
Zinn z.

zoom
acquisition z.

Zoon erythroplasia

zoonotic disease

zoster
disseminated herpes zoster infection
z. encephalomyelitis
herpes z.
herpes zoster of cornea
herpes zoster dermatitis
herpes zoster infection
herpes zoster of iris
herpes zoster ophthalmicus
herpes zoster pain
herpes zoster virus
herpes zoster virus infection
z. immune globulin
z. immune plasma
z. immune platelet
measles, rubella and z.
multidermatomal herpes z.
z. serum immunoglobulin
varicella chickenpox vaccine

zoster-associated pain

Zosyn

Z-shaped
Z.-s. anastomosis
Z.-s. incision
Z.-s. scar

Zuckerkandl
Z. body
Z. convolution
Z. fascia
organ of Z.

Zung Self-Rating Depression Scale

Zürich
hemoglobin Z.

Z-wave tube

zygapophyseales

zygapophysiales

zygapophysial joint

zygomatic
z. arch
z. bone
z. branch
z. fossa
greater zygomatic muscle
z. malar complex
marginal tubercle of zygomatic bone

z. maxillary complex
z. muscle
z. nerve
orbital eminence of zygomatic bone
z. process
z. reflex
z. region
z. suture

zygomaticofacial
z. foramen
z. nerve

zygomaticofrontal suture line

zygomaticomaxillary
z. complex
z. fracture
z. suture

zygomaticoorbitalis
arteria z.

zygomaticotemporal
z. nerve
z. suture

zygomaticum
os z.

zygomaticus
arcus z.
nervus z.

zygomaxillary complex

zygote intrafallopian transfer

zymogen
z. cell
z. granule
pancreatic digestive z.

zymoplastic substance

zymosan-activated
z.-a. autologous serum
z.-a. plasma rabbit

zymosan-treated serum

Common Medical Abbreviations and Acronyms

α alpha: Bunsen's solubility coefficient; first in a series; specific rotation term; heavy chain class corresponding to IgA
a (specific) absorption (coefficient) (USUALLY ITALIC); (total) acidity; area; (systemic) arterial (blood) (SUBSCRIPT); asymmetric; atto-
A absorbance
A adenosine (or adenylic acid); alveolar gas (SUBSCRIPT); ampere
Å angstrom; Ångström unit
AA amino acid; aminoacyl
AB abortion
Ab antibody
ABG arterial blood gas
abl Abelson murine leukemia virus
ABLB alternate binaural loudness balance (test)
ABO blood group system
ABR abortus-Bang-ring (test); auditory brainstem response (audiometry)
γ-Abu γ-aminobutyric acid
ABVD adriamycin (doxorubicin), bleomycin, vinblastine, and dacarbazine
a.c. [L.] *ante cibum,* before a meal
aC arabinosylcytosine
Ac acetyl; actinium
AC acetate; acromioclavicular; atriocarotid
AC/A accommodation convergence-accommodation (ratio)
ACE angiotensin-converting enzyme
ACEI angiotensin-converting enzyme inhibitor
ac-g accelerator globulin
AcG accelerator globulin
Ach acetylcholine
aCL anticardiolipin (antibody)
ACP acyl carrier protein
ACTH adrenocorticotropic hormone (corticotropin)
AD [L.] *auris dextra,* right ear; Alzheimer disease
ADA Americans with Disabilities Act
Ade adenine
ADH antidiuretic hormone
ADLs activities of daily living
ad lib [L.] *ad libitum,* freely, as desired
Ado adenosine
ADP adenosine 5′-diphosphate
A-E above-the-elbow (amputation)
AFB acid-fast bacillus
AFORMED alternating failure of response, mechanical, to electrical depolarization
AFP α-fetoprotein
Ag antigen; [L.] *argentum,* silver
A/G R albumin-globulin ratio
AHF antihemophilic factor
AHG antihemophilic globulin
AID artificial insemination donor
AIDS acquired immunodeficiency syndrome
AIH artificial insemination by husband; artificial insemination, homologous
A-K above-the-knee (amputation)
Al aluminum
Ala alanine (or its mono- or diradical)
ALA δ-aminolevulinic acid
ALD adrenoleukodystrophy
ALL acute lymphocytic leukemia
ALS antilymphocyte serum; advanced life support
ALT alanine aminotransferase
Am americium
AML acute myelogenous leukemia
AMP adenosine monophosphate (adenylic acid)
amu atomic mass unit
ANA antinuclear antibody
ANF antinuclear factor
ANOVA analysis of variance
ANS autonomic nervous system
ANUG acute necrotizing ulcerative gingivitis
APA antipernicious anemia (factor)
APC antigen-presenting cells
A-P-C adenoidal-pharyngeal-conjunctival (virus); antigen-presenting cell
aPS antiphospholipid antibody syndrome
APTT activated partial thromboplastin time
Ar argon
araC arabinosylcytosine (cytarabine)
ARDS adult respiratory distress syndrome
ARF acute renal failure; acute rheumatic fever
Arg arginine (or its mono- or diradical)
As arsenic
AS [L.] *auris sinistra,* left ear
ASA acetylsalicylic acid (aspirin)
ASCUS abnormal squamous cells of undetermined significance
ASHD arteriosclerotic heart disease
Asn asparagine (or its mono- or diradical)
ASO antistreptolysin O
Asp aspartic acid (or its radical forms)
AST aspartate aminotransferase
At astatine
ATFL anterior talofibular ligament
ATL adult T-cell leukemia; adult T-cell lymphoma
atm (standard) atmosphere
ATP adenosine 5′-triphosphate
ATPase adenosine triphosphatase
ATPD ambient temperature and pressure, dry
ATPS ambient temperature and pressure, saturated (with water vapor)
at. wt. atomic weight
Au [L.] *aurum,* gold
AU [L.] *auris utraque,* each ear, both ears
AV arteriovenous
A-V arteriovenous; atrioventricular
AVN atrioventricular node
AVP antiviral protein
AW atomic weight
ax. axis
AZT azidothymidine (zidovudine)
b second in a series; blood (SUBSCRIPT)
B barometric (pressure) (SUBSCRIPT); boron
Ba barium
BADL basic activities of daily living
BAER brainstem auditory evoked response
BAL British anti-Lewisite (dimercaprol); bronchoalveolar lavage
BALB binaural alternate loudness balance (test)
BBB blood-brain barrier
BCG bacille bilié de Calmette-Guérin (vaccine)
BE barium enema
Be beryllium
B-E below-the-elbow (amputation)
Bi bismuth
b.i.d. [L.] *bis in die,* twice a day
BIDS brittle hair, impaired intelligence, decreased fertility, and short stature (syndrome)
BIPAP bilevel positive airway pressure
Bk berkelium

APP

BM bowel movement
BMI body mass index
bp base pair
BP blood pressure; boiling point; *British Pharmacopoeia*
BPF bronchopleural fistula
BPH benign prostatic hyperplasia
Bq becquerel (SI unit of radionuclide activity)
Br bromine
BRAT (diet) banana, rice cereal, applesauce, toast
BSA body surface area
BSER brainstem evoked response (audiometry)
BT bleeding time
BTPS body temperature, ambient pressure, saturated (with water vapor)
BTU British thermal unit
BUN blood urea nitrogen
BUS Bartholin glands, urethra, Skene glands
C calorie (large); carbon; Celsius; centigrade; clearance (rate, renal) (FOLLOWED BY A SUBSCRIPT); compliance; concentration; cylindrical (lens); cytidine
c calorie (small); capillary (blood) (SUBSCRIPT); centi-
ca. [L.] *circa,* about, approximately
c-a cardioarterial
Ca calcium; cathodal; cathode
CA cancer; carcinoma; cardiac arrest; chronologic age; croup-associated (virus); cytosine arabinoside
CABG coronary artery bypass graft
cal calorie (small)
Cal calorie (large)
cAMP cyclic AMP (adenosine monophosphate)
CAP catabolite (gene) activator protein
CAPD continuous ambulatory peritoneal dialysis
CAT computerized axial tomography
CBC complete blood (cell) count
CBG corticosteroid-binding globulin
Cbz carbobenzoxy (chloride)
cc, c.c. cubic centimeter
C.C. chief complaint
CCK cholecystokinin
CCNU chloroethylcyclohexylnitrosourea (lomustine)
CCU coronary care unit; critical care unit
cd candela
Cd cadmium
CDC Centers for Disease Control and Prevention
cDNA complementary DNA
CDP cytidine 5′-diphosphate
Ce cerium
CEA carcinoembryonic antigen
CELO chicken embryo lethal orphan (virus)
CEP congenital erythropoietic porphyria
Cf californium
CF complement fixation; cystic fibrosis; coupling factor
CG chorionic gonadotropin
CGA catabolite gene activator
cGMP cyclic GMP (guanosine monophosphate)
cgs, CGS centimeter-gram-second (system, unit)
Ch^1 Christchurch (chromosome)
CHF congestive heart failure
CHO carbohydrate
Ci curie
μCi microcurie
CI color index; *Colour Index*
CIB [L.] *cibus,* food
CJD Creutzfeldt-Jakob disease
CK creatine kinase
Cl chlorine
CL cardiolipin
CLIA Clinical Laboratory Improvement Amendments
CLL chronic lymphocytic leukemia
CLQ cognitive laterality quotient
cm centimeter
cM centimorgan
Cm curium
CMC carpometacarpal
CMI cell-mediated immunity
CML chronic myelogenous leukemia
CMP cytidine 5′-phosphate (or any cytidine monophosphate)
CMV controlled mechanical ventilation; ctomegalovirus
CNS central nervous system
Co cobalt
c/o complains of
CoA coenzyme A
COG center of gravity
conA concanavalin A
COPD chronic obstructive pulmonary disease
CP cerebral palsy; costophrenic
CPAP continuous (or constant) positive airway pressure
CPD cephalopelvic disproportion
CPM continuous passive motility
CPPB continuous (or constant) positive-pressure breathing
CPPV continuous positive-pressure ventilation
CPR cardiopulmonary resuscitation
cps cycles per second
Cr chromium; creatinine
CR conditioned reflex; crown-rump (length)
CRD chronic respiratory disease
CRH corticotropin-releasing hormone
CRL crown-rump length
CRP cross-reacting protein
CRST calcinosis cutis, Raynaud phenomenon, sclerodactyly, and telangiectasia (syndrome)
Cs cesium
C&S culture and sensitivity
CSD catscratch disease
CSF cerebrospinal fluid
CT computed tomography
CTP cytidine 5′-triphosphate
CTR cardiothoracic ratio
Cu [L.] *cuprum,* copper
CV cardiovascular
CVA cerebrovascular accident
CVP central venous pressure
CXR chest x-ray
Cyd cytidine
cyl cylinder; cylindrical (lens)
CYP cytochrome P-450 (enzyme)
Cys cysteine
Cyt cytosine
δ delta; heavy chain class corresponding to IgD
Δ delta; change; heat
d deci-
d deuterium
d- dextrorotatory
D dead (space gas) (SUBSCRIPT); deciduous; deuterium; diffusing (capacity); dihydrouridine (in nucleic acids); diopter; [L.] *dexter,* right (opposite of left); vitamin D potency of cod liver oil
D- prefix indicating that a molecule is sterically analogous to D-glyceraldehyde
da deca-
dA deoxyadenosine
Da diabetes
DA developmental age
dAdo deoxyadenosine
dAMP deoxyadenylic acid
DANS 1-dimethylaminonaphthalene-5-sulfonic acid
db diabetes
dB decibel
DC Dental Corps
D&C dilation and curettage
DCG dacryocystography
DCI dichloroisoproterenol
dCMP deoxycytidylic acid
DDT dichlorodiphenyl-trichloroethane (chlorophenothane)

D&E dilation and evacuation
def decayed, extracted, or filled (deciduous teeth)
DEF decayed, extracted, or filled (permanent teeth)
DES diethylstilbestrol
DET diethyltryptamine
DEV duck embryo vaccine; duck embryo virus
DEXA dual-energy x-ray absorptiometry
df decayed and filled (deciduous teeth)
Df deficiency (absence or inactivation of a gene)
DF decayed and filled (permanent teeth)
dGMP deoxyguanosine monophosphate (deoxyguanylic acid)
DHEA dehydro-3-epiandrosterone
DIC disseminated intravascular coagulation
DIP desquamative interstitial pneumonia; distal inter-phalangeal (joint)
DJD degenerative joint disease
dk deca-, deka-
dM decimorgan
DMD Duchenne muscular dystrophy
dmf decayed, missing, or filled (deciduous teeth)
DMF decayed, missing, or filled (permanent teeth)
DMSO dimethyl sulfoxide
DMT *N,N*-dimethyltryptamine
DN dibucaine number
DNA deoxyribonucleic acid
DNAase deoxyribonucleic acid nuclease
DNase deoxyribonuclease
DNAse deoxyribonuclease
DNP deoxyribonucleoprotein; 2,4-dinitrophenol
DNR do not resuscitate
DNS director of nursing service(s)
DOA dead on arrival
DOC deoxycholic acid; deoxycorticosterone
DOM 2,5-dimethoxy-4-methylamphetamine
Dp duplication of a gene or chromosomal segment
2,3-DPG 2,3-diphosphoglycerate
DPI dry powder inhaler
DPN diphosphopyridine nucleotide
DPT dipropyltryptamine; diphtheria, pertussis, and tetanus (vaccines)
dr dram
DR degeneration reaction, reaction of degeneration
DRG diagnosis-related group
DRVVT dilute Russell's viper venom test
D-S Doerfler-Stewart (test)
DSA digital subtraction angiography
dsDNA double-stranded DNA
dT deoxythymidine
DT delirium tremens; duration of tetany
dTDP deoxythymidine 5-diphosphate
dThd thymidine
DTIC dimethyltrizenoimidazole carboxamide (dacarbazine)
dTMP deoxythymidylic acid
DTP diphtheria and tetanus toxoids and pertussis vaccine; distal tingling on percussion (Tinel sign)
DTPA diethylenetriamine pentaacetic acid
DTR deep tendon reflex
dTTP deoxythymidine 5′-triphosphate
Dx diagnosis
Dy dysprosium
ϵ epsilon; molar absorption coefficient; heavy chain class corresponding to IgE
E exa-; extraction (ratio)
EB Epstein-Barr (virus)
EBV Epstein-Barr virus
ECF extracellular fluid
ECF-A eosinophilic chemotactic factor of anaphylaxis
ECG electrocardiogram
ECHO enterocytopathogenic human orphan (virus)
ECM erythema chronicum migrans
ECMO extracorporeal membrane oxygenation
ECS electrocerebral silence
ECT electroconvulsive therapy
ED effective dose
EDTA ethylenediamine-tetraacetic acid (edathamil, edetic acid)
EEG electroencephalogram
EENT eye, ear, nose, and throat
EIA enzyme immunoassay
EKG [German] *Elektrokardiogramme,* electrocardiogram
EKY electrokymogram
ELISA enzyme-linked immunosorbent assay
EMC encephalomyocarditis (virus)
EMF electromotive force
EMG electromyogram; exomphalos, macroglossia, and gigantism (syndrome)
EMS emergency medical services
ENG electronystagmography
ENT ear, nose, and throat
EOG electrooculography
EPAP expiratory positive airway pressure
Er erbium
ER endoplasmic reticulum; emergency room
ERBF effective renal blood flow
ERCP endoscopic retrograde cholangiopancreatography
ERG electroretinogram
ERPF effective renal plasma flow
ERV expiratory reserve volume
Es einsteinium
ESEP extreme somatosensory evoked potential
ESP extrasensory perception
ESR electron spin resonance; erythrocyte sedimentation rate
ESRD end-stage renal disease
EtOH ethyl alcohol
Eu europium
ev electron-volt
eV electron-volt
f femto-; (respiratory) frequency
F Fahrenheit; faraday (constant); fertility (factor); field (of vision); fluorine; force; fractional (concentration); free (energy)
F1.2 (prothrombin) fragment 1.2
F_1 first filial generation
Fab fragment of antibody molecule involved in antigen binding
FAD flavin(e) adenine dinucleotide; familial Alzheimer disease
FANA fluorescent antinuclear antibody (test)
FB foreign body
FBS fasting blood sugar
Fc constant fragment of an antibody molecule
FDA Food and Drug Administration
Fe [L.] *ferrum,* iron
FEF forced expiratory flow
FET forced expiratory time
FEV forced expiratory volume
FF filtration fraction
FFD focus-film distance
FHR fetal heart rate
FHT fetal heart tones
FIA fluorescent immunoassay
FIGLU formiminoglutamic (acid)
FISH fluorescent in situ hybridization
Fm fermium
FMN flavin(e) mononucleotide
fps foot-pound-second (system, unit)
FPS foot-pound-second (system, unit)
Fr francium; French (gauge, scale)
FRC functional residual capacity (of lungs)
FRF follicle-stimulating hormone-releasing factor
FRS first-rank symptom
Fru fructose
FSH follicle-stimulating hormone

FSH-RF follicle-stimulating hormone-releasing factor
FSH-RH follicle-stimulating hormone-releasing hormone
FTA-ABS fluorescent treponemal antibody-absorption (test)
FU fluorouracil
FUO fever of unknown origin
FVC forced vital capacity
Fw F wave (fibrillary wave, flutter wave)
Fx fracture
γ gamma; Ostwald solubility coefficient; the third in a series; heavy chain class corresponding to IgG
μg microgram
g gram
G giga-; glucose; gravitation (newtonian constant of); guanosine (or guanylic acid) residues in polynucleotides; gravida (obstetric history)
G 1 gap 1
G 2 gap 2
G6P glucose 6-phosphate
Ga gallium
GABA γ-aminobutyric acid
GABHS group-A β-hemolytic streptococcus
Gal galactose
GC gonococcus, gonorrhea
Gd gadolinium
GDP mannose-1-phosphate guanylyltransferase
Ge germanium
GERD gastroesophageal reflux disease
GFR glomerular filtration rate
GGT γ-glutamyl transferase
GH glenohumeral; growth hormone
GHB γ-hydroxybutyrate
GHRF growth hormone-releasing factor
GH-RF growth hormone-releasing factor
GHRH growth hormone-releasing hormone
GH-RH growth hormone-releasing hormone
GI gastrointestinal; Gingival Index
GIP gastric inhibitory polypeptide
GLC gas-liquid chromatography
Gln glutamine; glutaminyl
Glu glutamic acid; glutamyl
Gly glycine; glycyl
GMP guanosine monophosphate (guanylic acid)
GMS Gomori (or Grocott) methenamine silver (stain)
GnRH gonadotropin-releasing hormone
GOT glutamic-oxaloacetic transaminase (aspartate aminotransferase)
GPI Gingival-Periodontal Index
GPT glutamic-pyruvic transaminase (alanine aminotransferase)
gr grain
GSH reduced glutathione
GSR galvanic skin response
GSSG oxidized glutathione
gt. [L.] *gutta,* a drop
GTP guanosine 5′-triphosphate
gtt. [L.] *guttae,* drops
GTT glucose tolerance test
GU genitourinary
Guo guanosine
GVHD graft-versus-host disease
Gy gray (unit of absorbed dose of ionizing radiation)
GYN gynecology
h hecto-
h Planck constant
α-h the right-handed helical form assumed by many proteins
H henry; hydrogen; hyperopia; hyperopic
^{1}H hydrogen-1 (protium, light hydrogen)
^{2}H hydrogen-2 (deuterium, heavy hydrogen)
^{3}H hydrogen-3 (tritium, radioactive hydrogen)
H^+ hydrogen ion
Ha hahnium
HA hyaluronic acid; hemagglutinin
HAV hepatitis A virus
Hb hemoglobin
HbA adult hemoglobin
HbA_1 major component of adult hemoglobin
HbA_2 minor fraction of adult hemoglobin
HbAS heterozygosity for hemoglobin A and hemoglobin S (sickle cell trait)
HB_cAg hepatitis B core antigen
HbCO carboxyhemoglobin
HB_e hepatitis B early antigen
HB_eAb hepatitis B early antibody
Hb_eAg hepatitis B early antigen
HBIG hepatitis B immune globulin
HbF fetal hemoglobin
HbO_2 oxyhemoglobin, oxygenated hemoglobin
HbS sickle cell hemoglobin
HB_sAb hepatitis B surface antibody
HB_sAg hepatitis B surface antigen
HBV hepatitis B virus
HCFA Health Care Financing Administration
HCG human chorionic gonadotropin
HCS human chorionic somatomammotropin (human placental lactogen)
Hct hematocrit
HDL high-density lipoprotein
HDRV human diploid (cell strain) rabies vaccine
He helium
H&E hematoxylin and eosin
HEMPAS hereditary erythroblastic multinuclearity associated with positive acidified serum
Hf hafnium
HFJV high-frequency jet ventilation
HFOV high-frequency oscillatory ventilation
HFPPV high-frequency positive pressure ventilation
HFV high-frequency ventilation
Hg [L.] *hydrargyrum,* mercury
HGE human granulocytic ehrlichiosis
HGH human (pituitary) growth hormone
HGSIL high-grade squamous intraepithelial lesion
HI hemagglutination inhibition (test, titer)
His histidine
His- histidyl
-His histidino
HIV human immunodeficiency virus
Hl hyperopia, latent
HLA human lymphocyte antigen
Hm hyperopia, manifest (hypermetropia)
HME human monocytic ehrlichiosis
HMG human menopausal gonadotropin
HMG CoA 3-hydroxy-3-methylglutaryl coenzyme A
HMO health maintenance organization
HMWK high molecular weight kininogen (Fletcher factor)
Ho holmium
HPF high-power field
HPI history of present illness
HPL human placental lactogen
HPLC high-performance liquid chromatography
HPV human papilloma virus
h. s. [L.] *hora somni,* at bedtime
HS [L.] *hora somni,* at bedtime
HSV herpes simplex virus
Ht hyperopia, total
5-HT 5-hydroxytryptamine (serotonin)
HTLV human T-cell lymphocytotrophic virus; human T-cell lymphoma/leukemia virus
HVL half-value layer
Hx (medical) history
Hyp hydroxyproline
Hz hertz
I inspired (gas) (SUBSCRIPT); iodine
^{123}I iodine-123 (radioisotope)
^{125}I iodine-125
^{131}I iodine-131

IADL instrumental activities of daily living
IAP intermittent acute porphyria
ICD *International Classification of Diseases of the World Health Organization*
ICDA *International Classification of Diseases, Adapted for Use in the United States*
ICF intracellular fluid
ICP intracranial pressure
ICSH interstitial cell-stimulating hormone
ICU intensive care unit
ID infective dose
I&D incision and drainage
IDU idoxuridine
IF initiation factor; intrinsic factor
IFN interferon
Ig immunoglobulin
IGF insulin-like growth factor
IH infectious hepatitis
IL interleukin
ILA insulin-like activity
Ile isoleucine
IM internal medicine; intramuscular(ly); infectious mononucleosis
IMP inosine monophosphate (inosinic acid)
IMV intermittent mandatory ventilation
In indium
Ino inosine
INR international normalized ratio
I&O (fluid) intake and output
IOML infraorbitomeatal line
IP interphalangeal; intraperitoneal(ly)
IPAP inspiratory positive airway pressure
IPPB intermittent positive-pressure breathing
IPPV intermittent positive-pressure ventilation
IPV inactivated poliovirus vaccine
IQ intelligence quotient
Ir iridium
IRV inspiratory reserve volume
ISI International Sensitivity Index
ITP idiopathic thrombocytopenic purpura; inosine 5′-triphosphate
IU International Unit
IUCD intrauterine contraceptive device
IUD intrauterine device
I.V. intravenous, intravenously; intraventricular
J joule
J flux (density)
k kilo-
K [Modern L.] *kalium,* potassium; kelvin
K_M Michaelis constant
kat katal
kb kilobase
kc kilocycle
kcal kilocalorie
KCT kaolin clotting time
kDa kilodalton
kg kilogram
KJ knee jerk
Kr krypton
KS Kaposi sarcoma
17-KS 17-ketosteroid
kv kilovolt
kVp kilovolt peak
KW Kimmelstiel-Wilson (disease); Keith-Wagener (retinal changes)
μl, μL microliter
l liter
L inductance; left; [L.] *limes,* boundary, limit; liter
L- prefix indicating that a molecule is sterically analogous to L-glyceraldehyde
La lanthanum
LA lupus anticoagulant
LAP leucine aminopeptidase
LATS long-acting thyroid stimulator
LBT lupus band test
LC lethal concentration
LCAT lecithin-cholesterol acyltransferase
LCM lymphocytic choriomeningitis (virus)
LD lethal dose
LDH lactate dehydrogenase
LDL low-density lipoprotein
LE left eye; lupus erythematosus
LEEP loop electrosurgical excision procedure
LES lower esophageal sphincter
LETS large external transformation-sensitive (fibronectin)
Leu leucine
LFA left frontoanterior (fetal position)
LFP left frontoposterior (fetal position)
LFT left frontotransverse (fetal position)
LGSIL low-grade squamous intraepithelial lesion
LGV lymphogranuloma venereum
LH luteinizing hormone
LH/FSH-RF luteinizing hormone/follicle-stimulating hormone-releasing factor
LH-RF luteinizing hormone-releasing factor
LH-RH luteinizing hormone-releasing hormone
Li lithium
LLQ left lower quadrant
LMA left mentoanterior (fetal position)
LMP left mentoposterior (fetal position)
LMT left mentotransverse (fetal position)
LNPF lymph node permeability factor
LOA left occipitoanterior (fetal position)
LOP left occipitoposterior (fetal position)
LOT left occipitotransverse (fetal position)
LPF low-power field
LPH lipotropic pituitary hormone (lipotropin)
Lr lawrencium
LRH luteinizing hormone-releasing hormone
LSA left sacroanterior (fetal position)
LSD lysergic acid diethylamide
LSP left sacroposterior (fetal position)
L/S R lecithin/sphingomyelin ratio
LST left sacrotransverse (fetal position)
LTH luteotropic hormone
LTM long-term memory
LTR long terminal repeat
Lu lutetium
LUQ left upper quadrant
LVET left ventricular ejection time
LVH left ventricular hypertrophy
Lw (FORMER SYMBOL FOR) lawrencium (now Lr)
Lys lysine (or its radicals in peptides)
μ mu; micro-; heavy chain class corresponding to IgM
m mass; meter; milliminim; molar
m- meta-
M mega-, meg-; molar; moles (per liter); morgan; myopic; myopia
M molar; moles (per liter)
m moles (per liter)
μμ micromicro-
μm micrometer
mμ millimicron
mA milliampere
MA mental age
MAA macroaggregated albumin
M-Am compound myopic astigmatism
MAC *Mycobacterium avium* complex
MAI *Mycobacterium avium intracellulare*
MAO monoamine oxidase
MAOI monoamine oxidase inhibitor
MAP morning-after pill
mA-S milliampere-second
Mb myoglobin
MBC maximum breathing capacity
MbCO carbon monoxided myoglobin
MbO_2 oxymyoglobin
MC Medical Corps
MCH mean corpuscular hemoglobin
MCHC mean corpuscular hemoglobin concentration
mCi millicurie

MCP metacarpophalangeal
MCV mean corpuscular volume
Md mendelevium
MDF myocardial depressant factor
MDI metered-dose inhaler
Me methyl
MEDLARS Medical Literature Analysis and Retrieval System
MEP maximal expiratory pressure
meq, mEq milliequivalent
Met methionine
MET metabolic equivalent of task
met-Hb methemoglobin
met-Mb metmyoglobin
MEV million electron-volts (10^6 ev)
mg milligram
Mg magnesium
MHC major histocompatibility complex
mho siemens unit
MHz megahertz
MI myocardial infarction
MID minimal infecting dose
MIP maximum inspiratory pressure
MK menaquinone (vitamin K_2)
mks, MKS meter-kilogram-second (system, unit)
ml, mL milliliter
MLC mixed lymphocyte culture (test)
MLD minimal lethal dose
mm millimeter
mmol millimole
MMPI Minnesota Multiphasic Personality Inventory
MMR measles-mumps-rubella (vaccine)
Mn manganese
Mo molybdenum
MO medical officer; mineral oil
mol mole
mol wt molecular weight
MOM milk of magnesia
MOPP Mustargen (mechlorethamine hydrochloride), Oncovin (vincristine sulfate), procarbazine hydrochloride, and prednisone
mor. sol. [L.] *more solito,* as usual, as customary
MPD maximal permissible dose
MPS mononuclear phagocyte system
MR milk-ring (test)
M_r molecular (weight) ratio
mrd, MRD minimal reacting dose
MRI magnetic resonance imaging
mRNA messenger RNA
ms millisecond
MS multiple sclerosis; morphine sulfate
msec millisecond
MSG monosodium glutamate
MSH melanocyte-stimulating hormone
mtDNA mitochondrial DNA
MTP metatarsophalangeal (joint)
Mu Mache unit
MUGA multiple-gated acquisition (imaging)
mV millivolt
Mv mendelevium
MVE Murray Valley encephalitis (virus)
MVV maximal voluntary ventilation
MW molecular weight
My myopia
ν nu; kinematic viscosity
n index of refraction; nano-
N newton; nitrogen; normal (concentration)
N normal (SMALL CAPS)
Na [Modern L.] *natrium,* sodium
NA *Nomina Anatomica*
NAD nicotinamide adenine dinucleotide; no acute distress
NAD⁺ nicotinamide adenine dinucleotide (oxidized form)
NADH nicotinamide adenine dinucleotide (reduced form)
NADP nicotinamide adenine dinucleotide phosphate
NADP⁺ nicotinamide adenine dinucleotide phosphate (oxidized form)
NADPH nicotinamide adenine dinucleotide phosphate (reduced form)
NAME nevi, atrial myxoma, myxoid neurofibromas, and ephelides (syndrome)
Nb niobium
NCV nerve conduction velocity
Nd neodymium
Ne neon
NE norepinephrine; not examined
NEEP negative end-expiratory pressure
NF National Formulary
ng nanogram
NGF nerve growth factor (antigen)
Ni nickel
NIH National Institutes of Health
NK natural killer (cell)
NKA no known allergies
NLM National Library of Medicine
nm nanometer
NMN nicotinamide mononucleotide
No nobelium
Np neptunium
NREM non-rapid eye movement (sleep)
nRNA nuclear RNA
NS normal saline
NSAID nonsteroidal anti-inflammatory drug
NSR normal sinus rhythm
NUG necrotizing ulcerative gingivitis
Ω omega; ohm
o- ortho-
O [L.] *oculus,* eye; opening (in formulas for electrical reactions); oxygen
OAV oculoauriculovertebral (dysplasia, syndrome)
OB obstetrics
OB/GYN obstetrics (and) gynecology
OBS organic brain syndrome
OC oral contraceptive
OCD obsessive-compulsive disorder
OD [L.] *oculus dexter,* right eye; overdose
ODD oculodentodigital (dysplasia, syndrome)
Oe oersted (centimeter-gram-second unit of magnetic field strength)
OFD orofaciodigital (dysostosis, syndrome)
OKT Ortho-Kung T (cell)
OML orbitomeatal line
OMM ophthalmomandibulomelic (dysplasia, syndrome)
OMS organic mental syndrome
OP osmotic pressure; outpatient
O&P ova and parasites
OPV oral poliovirus vaccine
OR operating room
ORD optical rotatory dispersion
Orn ornithine (or its radical)
Oro orotate; orotic acid
Os osmium
OS [L.] *oculus sinister,* left eye
OSHA Occupational Safety and Health Administration
OT occupational therapy; Koch old tuberculin
OTC over the counter (nonprescription drug)
OU [L.] *oculus uterque,* each eye (both eyes)
OXT oxytocin
oz ounce
p pico-; pupil
p- para-
P partial (pressure); peta-; phosphorus, phosphoric (residue); plasma (concentration); pressure; para (obstetric history)
^{32}**P** phosphorus-32
P_1 first parental generation
Pa pascal; protactinium
PABA paraaminobenzoic acid
PAF platelet-aggregating (or -activating) factor
PAH paraaminohippuric (acid)
PAO_2 partial pressure of arterial oxygen
PAS paraaminosalicylic (acid), periodic acid-Schiff (reagent)

PASA paraaminosalicylic acid
PAT paroxysmal atrial tachycardia
Pb [L.] *plumbum,* lead
PBG porphobilinogen
p.c. [L.] *post cibum,* after a meal
PCB polychlorinated biphenyl
Pco_2 partial pressure of carbon dioxide
PCP phencyclidine
Pd palladium
PD prism diopter
PDGF platelet-derived growth factor
PDLL poorly differentiated lymphocytic lymphoma
PEEP positive end-expiratory pressure
PEG polyethylene glycol
PET positron emission tomography
PF_4 platelet factor 4
PFT pulmonary function test
pg picogram
PG prostaglandin
PGA prostaglandin A
PGB prostaglandin B
PGE prostaglandin E
PGF prostaglandin F
pH hydrogen ion concentration; p (power) of $[H^+]_{10}$
Ph phenyl
Ph^1 Philadelphia (chromosome)
PHA phytohemagglutinin (antigen)
Phe phenylalanine (or its radical)
PhG [L.] *Pharmacopoeia Germanica,* German Pharmacopeia
PICC peripherally inserted central catheter
PID pelvic inflammatory disease
PIF prolactin-inhibiting factor
PIP proximal interphalangeal (joint)
pK negative logarithm of the ionization constant (K_a) of an acid
PK pyruvate kinase
PKU phenylketonuria
pm picometer
Pm promethium
PM post mortem
PMN polymorphonuclear (leukocyte)
PMS premenstrual syndrome
PND paroxysmal nocturnal dyspnea; postnasal drip
PNP platelet neutralization procedure
PNPB positive-negative pressure breathing
Po polonium
PO [L.] *per os,* by mouth
PO_2, Po_2 partial pressure of oxygen
POEMS polyneuropathy, organomegaly, endocrinopathy, monoclonal protein, and skin changes (syndrome)
POMP prednisone, Oncovin (vincristine sulfate), methotrexate, and Purinethol (6-mercaptopurine)
POR problem-oriented (medical) record
PP pyrophosphate
PPCA proserum prothrombin conversion accelerator
PPD purified protein derivative (of tuberculin)
PPLO pleuropneumonia-like organism
ppm parts per million
PPO 2,5-diphenyloxazole
PPPPP pain, pallor, pulselessness, paresthesia, paralysis
PPPPPP pain, pallor, pulselessness, paresthesia, paralysis, prostration
PPV positive pressure ventilation
Pr praseodymium; presbyopia
PRA plasma renin activity
PRF prolactin-releasing factor
PRL prolactin
p.r.n. [L.] *pro re nata,* as needed
PRN [L.] *pro re nata,* as needed
Pro proline (or its radicals)
psi pounds per square inch
PSV pressure-supported ventilation
Pt platinum
PT physical therapy; prothrombin time
PTA plasma thromboplastin antecedent; phosphotungstic acid; prior to admission
PTAH phosphotungstic acid hematoxylin
PTCA percutaneous transluminal coronary angioplasty
PTH parathyroid hormone
PTU prophylthiouracil
Pu plutonium
PUO pyrexia of unknown origin
PUPPP pruritic urticarial papules and plaques of pregnancy
PUVA (oral administration of) psoralen (and subsequent exposure to) ultraviolet light of A wavelength (UV-A)
PVC polyvinyl chloride; premature ventricular contraction
PVP polyvinylpyrrolidone (povidone)
$\dot{Q}$ volume of blood flow
Q coulomb
Qco_2 microliters CO_2 given off per milligram of dry weight of tissue per hour
q.d. [L.] *quaque die,* every day
q.i.d. [L.] *quater in die,* four times a day
QNS quantity not sufficient
Qo oxygen consumption
Qo_2 oxygen consumption
q.s. [L.] *quantum satis,* as much as is enough; [L.] *quantum sufficiat,* as much as may suffice; quantity sufficient
r racemic; roentgen
R gas constant (8.315 joules); (organic) radical; Réaumur (scale) ; [L.] *recipe,* take; resistance determinant (plasmid); resistance (electrical); resistance (unit) (in the cardiovascular system); resolution; respiration; respiratory (exchange ratio); roentgen
Ra radium
RA rheumatoid arthritis
rad radian
RAS reticular activating system
RAST radioallergosorbent test
RAV Rous-associated virus
RAW resistance, airway
Rb rubidium
rbc red blood cell; red blood (cell) count
RBC red blood cell; red blood (cell) count
RBF renal blood flow
RD reaction of degeneration; reaction of denervation
RDA recommended daily allowance
rDNA ribosomal DNA
RDS respiratory distress syndrome
RDW red (cell) diameter (or distribution) width
Re rhenium
RE right ear; right eye
rem roentgen equivalent, man
REM rapid eye movement (sleep); reticular erythematous mucinosis
rep roentgen equivalent, physical
RF release factor; rheumatoid factor
RFA right frontoanterior (fetal position)
RFLP restriction fragment length polymorphism
RFP right frontoposterior (fetal position)
RFT right frontotransverse (fetal position)
Rh Rhesus (Rh blood group); rhodium
RH releasing hormone
RIA radioimmunoassay
Rib ribose
RLL right lower lobe
RLQ right lower quadrant
RMA right mentoanterior (fetal position)
RML right middle lobe
RMP right mentoposterior (fetal position)
RMT right mentotransverse (fetal position)
Rn radon
RNA ribonucleic acid
RNase ribonuclease
RNP ribonucleoprotein
ROA right occipitoanterior (fetal position)
ROM range of motion
ROP right occipitoposterior (fetal position)

ROT right occipitotransverse (fetal position)
RP retinitis pigmentosa
RPF renal plasma flow
rpm revolutions per minute
RPR rapid plasma reagin (test)
RQ respiratory quotient
rRNA ribosomal RNA
Rs response
RS respiratory syncytial (virus)
RSA right sacroanterior (fetal position)
RSP right sacroposterior (fetal position)
RST right sacrotransverse (fetal position)
RSV Rous-sarcoma virus; respiratory syncytial virus
rTMP ribothymidylic acid
Ru ruthenium
RUL right upper lobe
RUQ right upper quadrant
RV residual volume
RVH right ventricular hypertrophy
℞ [L.] *recipe,* (the first word on a prescription), take; prescription; treatment
σ sigma; reflection coefficient; standard deviation; 1 millisecond (0.001 sec)
s [L.] *semis,* half; steady state (SUBSCRIPT); [L.] *sinister,* left
S [L.] *sinister,* left; saturation of hemoglobin (percentage of) (FOLLOWED BY SUBSCRIPT O_2 or CO_2); siemens; spherical; spherical (lens); sulfur; Svedberg (unit)
S_1 first selfing generation
S-A sinoatrial
SaO_2 oxygen saturation (of) arterial (oxyhemoglobin)
sat. saturated
sat. sol. saturated solution
Sb [L.] *stibium,* antimony
SBE subacute bacterial endocarditis
sc subcutaneous(ly)
Sc scandium
SC sternoclavicular; subcutaneous(ly)
SCID severe combined immunodeficiency
SD standard deviation; streptodornase
SDA specific dynamic action
Se selenium
Ser serine
Sf Svedberg flotation (constant, unit)
SGOT serum glutamic-oxaloacetic transaminase (aspartate aminotransferase)
SGPT serum glutamic-pyruvic transaminase (alanine aminotransferase)
SH serum hepatitis
Si silicon
SI [French] Système International d'Unités; International System of Units
SID source-to-image (-receptor) distance
SIDS sudden infant death syndrome
sig. [L.] *signa,* affix a label, inscribe
SIMV spontaneous intermittent mandatory ventilation; synchronized intermittent mandatory ventilation
SIRD source-to-image-receptor distance
SISI small-increment (or short-increment) sensitivity index (test)
SK streptokinase
SLE systemic lupus erythematosus
SLR straight leg raising
Sm samarium
Sn [L.] *stannum,* tin
SOAP subjective data, objective data, assessment, and plan (problem-oriented medical record)
SOB short(ness) of breath
sol. solution
soln. solution
sp. species
SPCA serum prothrombin conversion accelerator (factor VII)
SPECT single photon emission computed tomography
SPF sun protection (or protective) factor
sp. gr. specific gravity
sph spherical (lens)
spm suppression and mutation
spp. species (plural)
SQ subcutaneous
Sr strontium
SRF somatotropin-releasing factor
SRF-A slow-reacting factor of anaphylaxis
SRIF somatotropin-release-inhibiting factor
sRNA soluble RNA
SRS slow-reacting substance
SRS-A slow-reacting substance of anaphylaxis
ssDNA single-stranded DNA
ssp. subspecies
SSRI selective serotonin reuptake inhibitor
ST scapulothoracic
stat [L.] *statim,* immediately, at once
STD sexually transmitted disease
STEL short-term exposure limit
STH somatotropic hormone
STM short-term memory
STPD standard temperature (0° C) and pressure (760 mm Hg absolute), dry
Sv, SV sievert (unit)
SVT supraventricular tachycardia
t metric ton
t temperature (Celsius); tritium
α-T α-tocopherol
T temperature, absolute (Kelvin); tension (intraocular); tera-; tesla; tetanus (toxoid); tidal (volume) (SUBSCRIPT); tocopherol; transverse (tubule); tritium; tumor (antigen)
T absolute temperature (Kelvin)
T_3 3,5,5′-triiodothyronine
T_4 tetraiodothyronine (thyroxine)
T− (FOLLOWED BY NUMBER) decreased tension (intraocular)
T+ (FOLLOWED BY NUMBER) increased tension (intraocular)
Ta tantalum
TA *Terminologia Anatomica*
TAD transient acantholytic dermatosis
TAF tumor angiogenesis factor
TAR thrombocytopenia with absent radius (syndrome)
TAT thematic apperception test
Tb terbium
TB tuberculosis
TBP thyroxine-binding protein
TBV total blood volume
Tc technetium
^{99m}Tc technetium-99m
T&C type and crossmatch
TCA tricarboxylic acid; trichloracetic acid
TCN talocalcaneonavicular (joint)
Td tetanus-diphtheria (toxoids, adult type)
TDP ribothymidine 5′-diphosphate
Te tellurium
TEDD total end-diastolic diameter
TEN toxic epidermal necrolysis
TESD total end-systolic diameter
Th thorium
THC tetrahydrocannabinol
Thr threonine (or its radicals)
t_i/t_{tot} duty cycle
Ti titanium
TIA transient ischemic attack
t.i.d. [L.] *ter in die,* three times a day
tinct. tincture
TITh 3,5,3′-triiodothyronine
TKO to keep (venous infusion line) open
Tl thallium
TLC thin-layer chromatography; total lung capacity; tender, loving care
TLV threshold-limit value
t_m temperature midpoint (Celsius)
Tm thulium; tubular maximal (excretory capacity of kidneys)
T_m temperature midpoint (Kelvin)
TM transport maximum
TMJ temporomandibular joint
TMP ribothymidine 5′-monophosphate
TMT tarsometatarsal

TMV tobacco mosaic virus
Tn normal intraocular tension
TNF tumor necrosis factor
TNM tumor, node, metastasis (tumor staging)
TORCH toxoplasmosis, other, rubella, cytomegalovirus, and herpes simplex (maternal infections)
t-PA, TPA tissue plasminogen activator
TPHA *Treponema pallidum* hemagglutination (test)
TPI *Treponema pallidum* immobilization (test)
TPN total parenteral nutrition
TPR temperature, pulse, and respirations
tr. tincture
TRH thyrotropin-releasing hormone (stimulation test)
TRIC trachoma inclusion conjunctivitis (organism)
tRNA transfer RNA
Trp tryptophan (and its radicals)
TSH thyroid-stimulating hormone
TSS toxic shock syndrome
TSTA tumor-specific transplantation antigen
TTP thrombotic thrombocytopenic purpura
TU toxic unit, toxin unit
Tyr tyrosine (and its radicals)
U unit; uranium; uridine (in polymers); urinary (concentration)
UA urinalysis
UDP uridine diphosphate
UDPG UDP-glucose
UGIS upper gastrointestinal series
UMP uridine monophosphate (uridylic acid)
ung. [L.] *unguentum,* ointment
u-PA urokinase
Urd uridine
URI upper respiratory infection
USAN United States Adopted Names (Council)
USP *United States Pharmacopeia*
USPHS United States Public Health Service
UTI urinary tract infection
UTP uridine triphosphate
UV ultraviolet
v venous (blood); volt
V vanadium; vision; visual (acuity); volt; volume (frequently with subscripts denoting location, chemical species, and conditions)
$\dot{V}$ ventilation; gas flow (frequently with subscripts indicating location and chemical species); ventilation
V_1-V_6 unipolar precordial electrocardiogram chest leads
VA viral antigen
$\dot{V}_A$ alveolar ventilation
V-A ventriculoatrial
Val valine (and its radicals)
V/Q ventilation/perfusion ratio
VATER vertebral defects, imperforate anus, tracheoesophageal fistula with esophageal atresia, and radial and renal dysplasia (complex)
VC vision, color; vital capacity
VCE vagina, (ecto)cervix, endocervical canal
V_D (physiologic) dead space
VDRL Venereal Disease Research Laboratory (test)
VHDL very-high-density lipoprotein
VIP vasoactive intestinal polypeptide
VLDL very-low-density lipoprotein
VMA vanillylmandelic acid (test)
V_{max} maximal velocity
VP vasopressin
VR vocal resonance
VS volumetric solution
V_T tidal volume
W watt; [German] *Wolfram,* tungsten
Wb weber
WBC white blood cell; white blood (cell) count
WD well-developed
WDLL well-differentiated lymphocytic (or lymphatic) lymphoma
WHO World Health Organization
WN well-nourished
X xanthosine
Xao xanthosine
Xe xenon
^{133}Xe xenon-133
XU excretory urogram
Y yttrium
YAG yttrium-aluminum-garnet (laser)
Yb ytterbium
Z carbobenzoxy (chloride)
ZEEP zero end-expiratory pressure
ZES Zollinger-Ellison syndrome
Zn zinc
^{65}Zn zinc-65
Zr zirconium
ZSR zeta sedimentation ratio

Medical Prefixes, Suffixes, and Combining Forms: The Building Blocks of Medical Language

a- not, without, -less
ab-, abs- from, away from, off
acanth(o)- thorn
acou- hearing
acr(o)- extremity
acu- hearing; needle
ad- increase, adherence, motion toward; very
-ad toward, in the direction of; -ward
aden(o)- gland
adip(o)- fat
-agog, -agogue promoter, stimulator
aidoio- genitals
-al pertaining to
alb(o)- white
alge(si)-, algio-, algo- pain
allo- other, different
ambi- around, on (both) sides, on all sides, both
ambly(o)- dull
amyl(o)- starch, polysaccharide
an- not, without, -less
ana- up, toward, apart
andr(o)- male
angi(o)- vessel
ankylo- crooked
ante- before
anthraco- coal, carbon
anti- against, opposing; curative; antibody
apo- separated from, derived from
aque(o)- water
-ar pertaining to
-arche beginning
arteri(o)- artery
arthr(o)- joint, articulation
-ary pertaining to
-ase an enzyme
-ate a salt or ester of an "-ic" acid
athero- pasty, fatty
atto- one-quintillionth (10^{-18})
audi(o)- hearing
aur(i)-, auro- ear
aut(o)- self, same
bacteri(o)- bacteria
balan(o)- glans penis
bi- twice, double
bio- life
blasto- budding by cells or tissue
blephar(o)- eyelid
brachi(o)- arm
brachy- short
bronch- bronchus
bronch(i)-, bronch(i)o- bronchus
carcin(o)- cancer
cardi(o)- heart; esophageal opening of stomach
carpo- wrist
cata- down
caud(o)- tail, lower part of body
-cele hernia, swelling
celio- abdomen
-centesis surgical puncture
centi- one-hundredth (10^{-2})
cephal(o)- the head
cervic(o)- neck; uterine cervix
cheil(o)- lip
cheir(o)- hand
chem(o)- chemistry; drug
chir(o)- hand
chlor(o)- green; chlorine
chol(e)- bile
chondrio-, chondr(o)- cartilage; granular; gritty
chrom-, chromat-, chromo- color
chron(o)- time
-cidal, -cide killing, destroying
cis- on this side, on the near side
-clast breaker
-clysis washing
co- with, together, in association, very, complete
col- with, together, in association, very, complete
colp(o)- vagina
com-, con- with, together, in association, very, complete
conio- dust
cor- with, together, in association, very, complete
coreo- pupil
cost(o)- rib
crani(o)- cranium
-crine secretion
cry(o)- cold
crypt(o)- hidden
culdo- cul-de-sac
cyan(o)- blue; cyanide
cycl- circle, cycle; ciliary body
cyst(i)-, cysto- bladder; cyst; cystic duct
cyt-, -cyte, cyto- cell
dacry(o)- tears
dactyl(o)- finger, toe
de- away from; cessation
deca- ten
deci- one-tenth (10^{-1})
deka- ten
dent(i)- tooth
derm-, derma-, dermat(o)-, dermo- skin
-desis binding
dextr(o)- right, toward or on the right side
di- separation, taking apart, reversal, not, un-
dif- separation, taking apart, reversal, not, un-
dipso- thirst
dir-, dis- separation, taking apart, reversal, not, un-
duo- two
duodeno- duodenum
-dynia pain
dynamo- force, energy
dys- bad, difficult
ect- outer, on the outside
-ectasia, -ectasis dilation, stretching
ecto- outer, on the outside
-ectomy excision
-emphraxis obstruction
encephal(o)- brain
end(o)- within, inner
enter(o)- intestine
ent(o)- inner, within
ep-, epi- upon, following, subsequent to
ergo- work
erythr(o)- red, redness
eso- inward
esthesio- sensation, perception
eu- good, well
ex- out of, from, away from
exo- exterior, external, outward
extra- without, outside of
ferri- ferric ion (Fe^{3+})
ferro- metallic iron; ferrous ion (Fe^{2+})
fibr(o)- fiber
-form in the form or shape of

galact(o)- milk
gastr(o)- stomach; belly
gen-, -gen producing, coming to be; precursor
giga- one billion (10^9)
gingiv(o)- gums
gloss(o)- tongue
gluco- glucose
glyco- sugars
gnath(o)- jaw
gon- seed, semen
gonio- angle
gono- seed, semen
-gram writing, recording
granul(o)- granular, granule
-graph recording instrument
gyn(e)-, gyneco-, gyno- woman
hecto- one hundred (10^2)
hem(a)-, hemat(o)- blood
hemi- one-half
hemo- blood
hepat-, hepatico-, hepato- liver
hept(a)- seven
hidr(o)- sweat
hist-, histio-, histo- tissue
homeo- same, constant
hydr(o)- water; hydrogen
hyper- above, excessive
hypo- below, deficient
hyster(o)- uterus; hysteria; late, following
-ia condition
-iasis condition, infestation, infection
-ic pertaining to
-ics organized knowledge, practice, treatment
ileo- ileum
ilio- ilium
in- in; not
-in chemical suffix
-ine chemical suffix
infra- below
inguino- groin
inter- between, among
intra-, intro- within
irid(o)- iris
ischi(o)- ischium
-ism condition, disease; practice, doctrine
-ismus spasm; contraction
iso- equal, like; isomer; sameness
-ite of the nature of, resembling
-ites -y, -like
-itides plural of -itis
-itis inflammation
kal(i)- potassium
kary(o)- nucleus
kerat(o)- cornea, cornified epithelium
kilo- one thousand (10^3)
kin(e)-, kinesi(o)-, kineso-, kino- movement
labio- lip
lacrim(o)- tears
lact(i)-, lacto- milk
laparo- abdomen, abdominal wall
laryng(o)- larynx
lateri-, latero- lateral, to one side, side
-lepsis, -lepsy seizure
lepto- light, slender, thin, frail
leuk(o)- white
lien(o)- spleen
linguo- tongue
lip(o)- fat, lipid
lith(o)- stone, calculus, calcification
-log speech, words
log(o)- speech, words
-logy study of; collecting
lymph(o)- lymph; lymphocyte
lys(o)-, -lysis, -lytic dissolution, disintegration; release
macr(o)- large; long
mal- bad, deficient
-malacia softening
mamm-, mamm(a)-, mammo- breast
mast(o)- breast
meg- large, oversize
mega- large, oversize; one million (10^6)
megal(o)- large
-megaly enlargement
melan(o)- black
men- menstruation
mening(o)- meninges
meno- menstruation
ment(o)- chin
-mer member of a series
mes(o)- middle, mean, intermediate; attaching membrane
meta- after, behind; joint action, sharing
-meter measurement, measuring device
metr(o)- uterus
micr- small, microscopic
micro- small, microscopic; one-millionth (10^{-6})
milli- one-thousandth (10^{-3})
mon(o)- single
morph(o)- form, shape, structure
my(o)- muscle
myel(o)- bone marrow; spinal cord
myring(o)- tympanic membrane
myx(o)- mucus
nano- dwarf; one-billionth (10^{-9})
nas(o)- nose
natr(i)- sodium
necr(o)- death, necrosis
neo- new
nephr(o)- kidney
neur(i)-, neuro- nerve, nervous system
norm(o)- normal
octo- eight
oculo- eye
odont(o)- tooth
odyn(o)-, -odynia pain
-oid resemblance to
olig(o)- few, little
-oma tumor, neoplasm
-omata plural of -oma
oncho-, onco- tumor, bulk, volume
-one ketone (-CO- group)
onych(o)-, -onychia fingernail, toenail
oo- egg, ovary
oophor(o)- ovary
ophthalm(o)- eye
-opia, -opsia, -opsis vision
or- mouth
orchi-, orchid(o)-, orchio- testis
ori-, oro- mouth
-ose sugar
-oses plural of -osis
-osis process, condition, state
osseo- bony
ossi- bone
ost(e)-, osteo- bone
ovari(o)- ovary
ov(i)-, ovo- egg
ox(a)-, oxo- oxygen
oxy- sharp, acid; acute, shrill, quick; oxygen
pachy- thick
pan-, pant(o)- all, entire
para- beside, near; similar; subordinate; abnormal
pari- equal
path(o)- disease, abnormality
-pathy disease, abnormality
ped(i)-, pedo- child; foot
-penia deficiency
penta- five
per- through, thoroughly, intensely
peri- around, about
-pexy fixation, usually surgical
phaco- lens
-phage, -phagia, phago-, -phagy eating, devouring
phako- lens
phanero- visible, evident
pharmaco- drug, medicine

pharyng(o)- pharynx
phil- attraction; chemical affinity
-philia attraction; chemical affinity
philo- attraction; chemical affinity
phleb(o)- vein
-phobe, -phobia fear; chemical repulsion
phon(o)- sound, speech
phor(o)- carrying, bearing
phos-, phot(o)- light
phren(i)- diaphragm; mind; phrenic
-phrenia mind
phrenico-, phreno- diaphragm; mind; phrenic
-phylaxis protection
phyll(o)- leaf
physi(o)- physical; natural
physo- swelling, inflation; air, gas
phyt(o)- plants
pico- one-trillionth (10^{-12})
plan(i)-, plano- flat
-plasia formation
plasm(a)-, plasmat(o)-, plasmo- plasma
platy- wide, flat
-plegia paralysis
pleo- more
plesio- near, similar
pleur(a)-, pleuro- rib, side, pleura
pluri- several, more
-pnea breath, respiration
pneo- breath, respiration
pneum(a)-, pneumat(o)- air, gas; lung; breathing
pod(o)- foot, foot-shaped
-poiesis, -poietic production
poikilo- irregular, variable
polio- gray
poly- many, multiple; polymer
post- after, behind, posterior
pre- anterior, before
presby- old
pro- before, forward; precursor
proct(o)- anus, rectum
prot(o)- first
pseud(o)- false
psych(e)-, psycho- mind
-ptosis sagging, falling
pyel(o)- (renal) pelvis
pykn(o)- dense, compact
pyo- suppuration, pus
pyreto- fever
pyro- fire, heat, fever
quadr(i)- four
rachi(o)- spinal column
radio- radiation, x-ray; radius
re- again, back, backward
rect(i)- straight
rect(o)- rectum
ren(o)- kidney
retro- backward, behind
rhin(o)- nose
-rrhagia discharge, bleeding
-rrhaphy surgical suturing
-rrhea flow
-rrhexis rupture
salping(o)- tube
sarco- flesh, muscle
schisto-, schiz(o)- split, cleft, division
scler(o)- hardness, sclerosis; ocular sclera
scolio- crooked
-scope instrument for viewing
-scopy viewing
scot(o)- shadow, darkness
semi- one-half; partly
sept- seven; septum; sepsis, infection
septi- seven
septo- seven; septum; sepsis, infection
sial(o)- saliva, salivary gland
sider(o)- iron
sigmoid(o)- S-shaped; sigmoid colon
sin-, sin(o)-, sinu- sinus
sito- food, grain
somat-, somato-, somatico- body, bodily
somno- sleep
son(o)- sound; ultrasound
spasmo- spasm
sperm(a), spermat(o), spermo- semen, spermatozoa
sphygmo- pulse
spir(o)- breathing
splanchn(i)-, splanchno- viscera
splen(o)- spleen
staphyl(o)- grape, bunch of grapes; staphylococci
-stasis stopping
-stat arresting change or movement
steno- narrowness, constriction
stereo- solid
stheno- strength, force, power
stom(a)-, stomat(o)- mouth
sub- beneath, less than normal, inferior
super- above, in excess, superior
supra- above
sy-, syl-, sym-, syn-, sys- together
tachy- rapid
tel(e)- distant
ten-, tendin-, teno-, tenont(o)- tendon
tera- one quadrillion (10^{15})
tetra- four
thel(o)- nipple
therm(o)- heat
thora-, thorac(i)-, thoracico, thoraco- chest, thorax
thromb(o)- blood clot
thyre(o)-, thyr(o)- thyroid gland
toco-, toko- childbirth
-tome cutting instrument; segment, section
-tomy cutting operation
tono- tone, tension, pressure
top(o)- place, topical
tox(i)-, toxico-, toxo- toxin, poison
trache(o)- trachea
trans- across, through, beyond
tri- three
trich(i)- hair
-trichia hair **tricho-** hair
tris- three
-trophic, tropho-, -trophy food, nutrition
-tropia, -tropic, -tropy turning, tendency, affinity
ultra- beyond
uni- one, single
uri- uric acid
-uria urine, urination
uric(o)- uric acid
uro- urine; urinary tract
vas- duct; blood vessel
vasculo- blood vessel
vaso- duct, blood vessel
vesic(o)- urinary bladder, vesicle
xanth(o)- yellow
xero- dry
zo(o)- animal; life
zym(o)- fermentation, enzyme